369 0235408

DIAGNOSTIC PATHOLOGY

Kidney Diseases

SECOND EDITION

COLVIN | CHANG

FARRIS • KAMBHAM • CORNELL • MEEHAN • LIAPIS
GAUT • BONSIB • SESHAN • JAIN • LARSEN

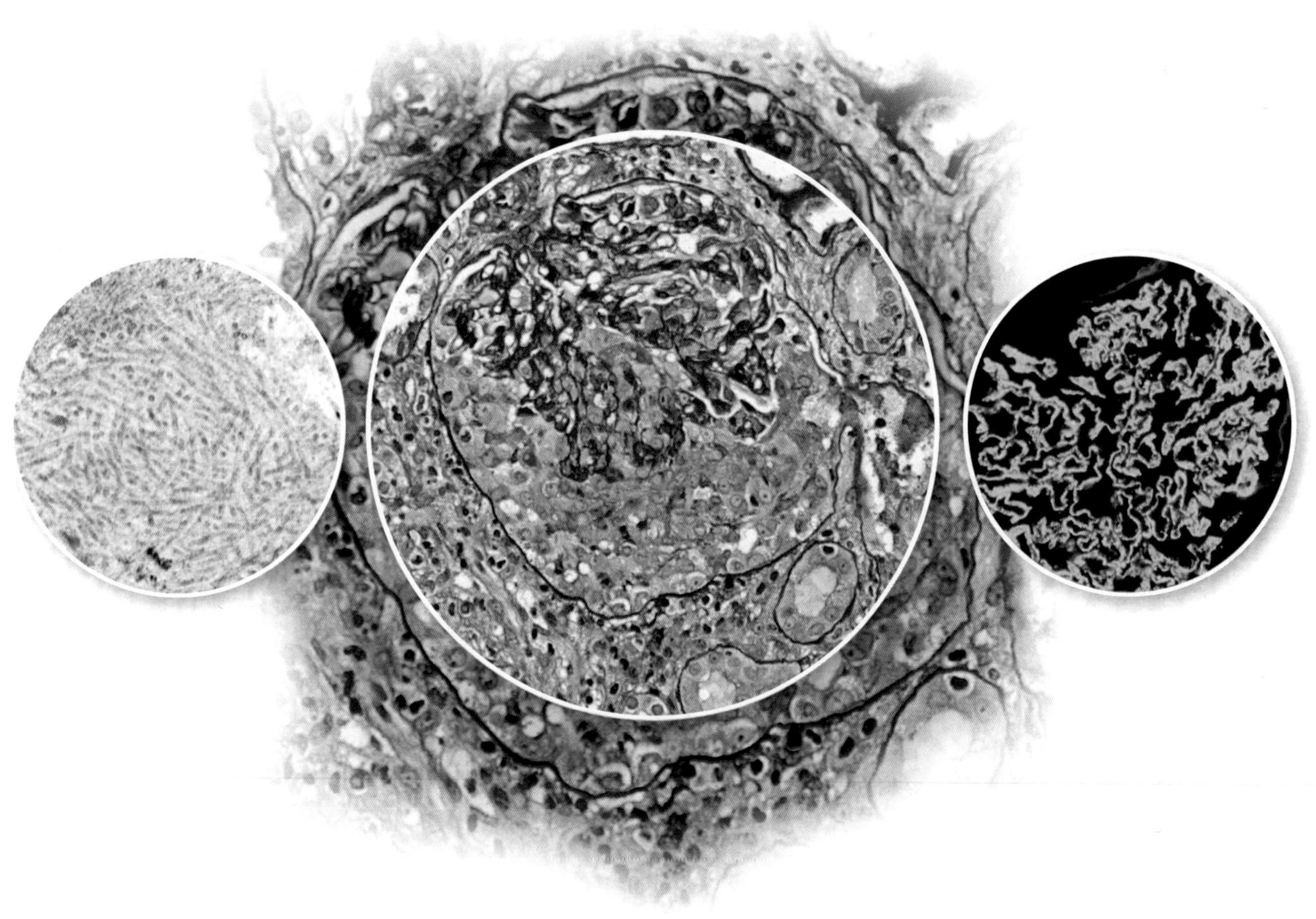

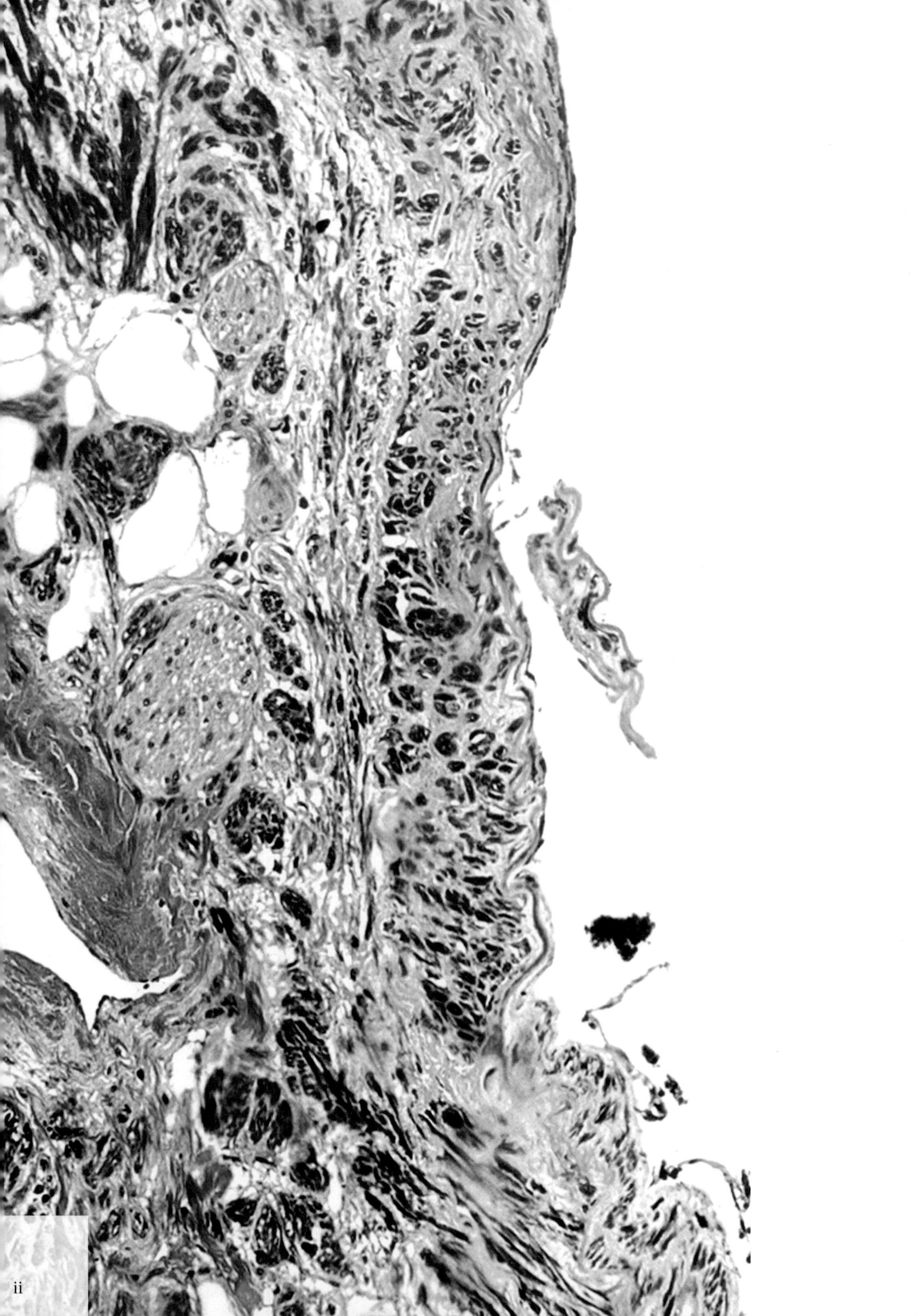
ii

DIAGNOSTIC PATHOLOGY

Kidney Diseases

SECOND EDITION

Robert B. Colvin, MD
Benjamin Castleman Distinguished Professor of Pathology
Department of Pathology
Harvard Medical School
Massachusetts General Hospital
Boston, Massachusetts

Anthony Chang, MD
Associate Professor of Pathology
Associate Director, Pathology Residency Program Director
Medical Director, UC MedLabs Outreach Program
Renal Pathology and Renal Pathology Fellowship
The University of Chicago Medicine
Chicago, Illinois

A. Brad Farris III, MD
Director, Laboratory of Nephropathology and
Electron Microscopy
Assistant Professor of Pathology
Department of Pathology
Emory University School of Medicine
Atlanta, Georgia

Neeraja Kambham, MD
Professor of Pathology
Department of Pathology
Stanford University
Stanford, California

Lynn D. Cornell, MD
Associate Professor of Laboratory
Medicine and Pathology
Consultant, Division of Anatomic Pathology
Mayo Clinic College of Medicine
Rochester, Minnesota

Shane M. Meehan, MBBCh
Renal Pathology Service
Sharp Memorial Hospital
San Diego, California

Helen Liapis, MD
Nephropath
Little Rock, Arkansas

Joseph P. Gaut, MD, PhD
Assistant Professor
Department of Pathology and Immunology
Washington University School of Medicine
St. Louis, Missouri

Stephen M. Bonsib, MD
Nephropathologist
Nephropath
Little Rock, Arkansas

Surya V. Seshan, MD
Professor of Clinical Pathology
Weill Cornell Medical College
Cornell University
New York, New York

Sanjay Jain, MD, PhD
Associate Professor
Departments of Internal Medicine & Pathology
Washington University School of Medicine
St. Louis, Missouri

Christopher P. Larsen, MD
Nephropath
Little Rock, Arkansas

ELSEVIER

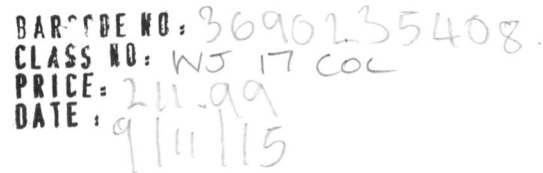

1600 John F. Kennedy Blvd.
Ste 1800
Philadelphia, PA 19103-2899

DIAGNOSTIC PATHOLOGY: KIDNEY DISEASES, SECOND EDITION

ISBN: 978-0-323-37707-2

Notices

Knowledge and best practice in this field are constantly changing. As new research and experience broaden our understanding, changes in research methods, professional practices, or medical treatment may become necessary.

Practitioners and researchers must always rely on their own experience and knowledge in evaluating and using any information, methods, compounds, or experiments described herein. In using such information or methods they should be mindful of their own safety and the safety of others, including parties for whom they have a professional responsibility.

With respect to any drug or pharmaceutical products identified, readers are advised to check the most current information provided (i) on procedures featured or (ii) by the manufacturer of each product to be administered, to verify the recommended dose or formula, the method and duration of administration, and contraindications. It is the responsibility of practitioners, relying on their own experience and knowledge of their patients, to make diagnoses, to determine dosages and the best treatment for each individual patient, and to take all appropriate safety precautions.

To the fullest extent of the law, neither the Publisher nor the authors, contributors, or editors, assume any liability for any injury and/or damage to persons or property as a matter of products liability, negligence or otherwise, or from any use or operation of any methods, products, instructions, or ideas contained in the material herein.

Publisher Cataloging-in-Publication Data

Diagnostic pathology. Kidney diseases / [edited by] Robert B. Colvin and Anthony Chang.
pages ; cm
Kidney diseases
Includes bibliographical references and index.
ISBN 978-0-323-37707-2 (hardback)
1. Kidneys--Diseases--Diagnosis--Atlases. I. Colvin, Robert B.
II. Chang, Anthony. III. Title: Kidney diseases.
[DNLM: 1. Kidney Diseases--diagnosis--Atlases. 2. Kidney Diseases--pathology--Atlases. WJ 17]
RC904.D519 2015
616.6/1075--dc23

International Standard Book Number: 978-0-323-37707-2

Cover Designer: Tom M. Olson, BA

Printed in Canada by Friesens, Altona, Manitoba, Canada

Last digit is the print number: 9 8 7 6 5 4 3 2 1

Dedications

The authors thank our teachers, students, and families who gave us guidance, inspiration, and love. We owe you everything. You know who you are!

We also thank the many investigators, pathologists, and clinicians who created the knowledge we have summarized, and the patients whose renal biopsies revealed so many of the insights.

Bob and Tony

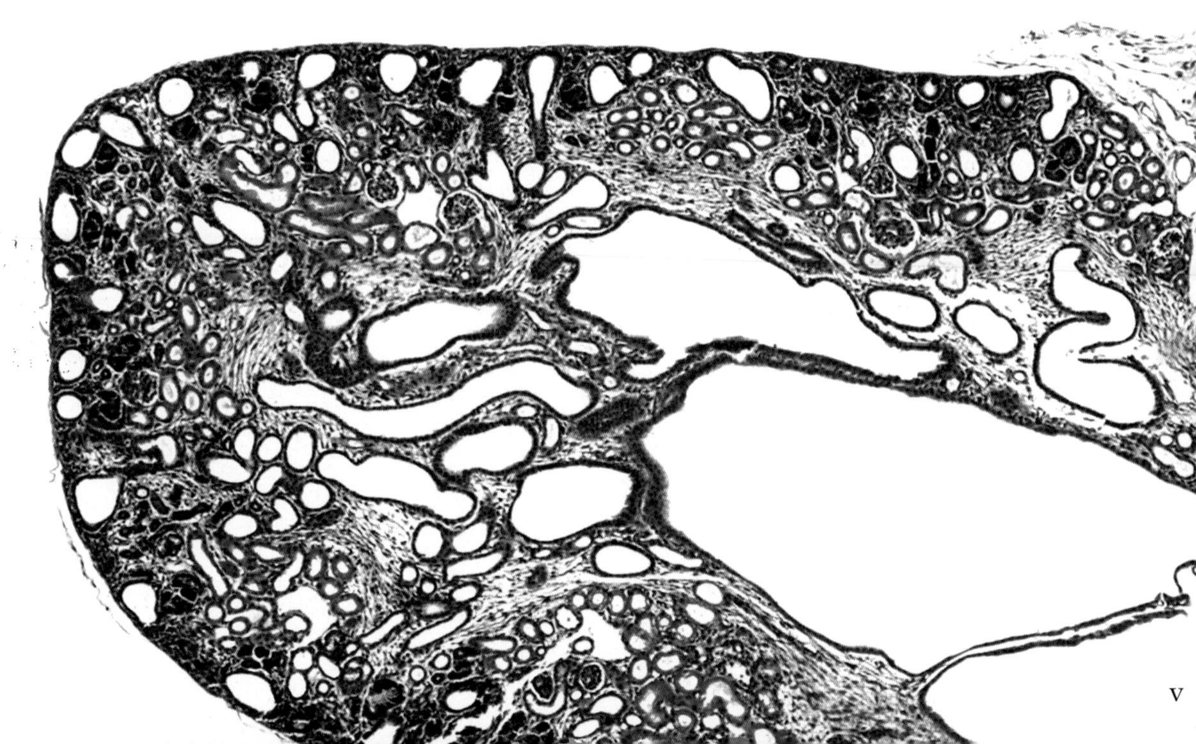

Contributing Authors

L. Nicholas Cossey, MD, FCAP
Nephropathologist
Nephropath
Little Rock, Arkansas

Christie L. Boils, MD
Nephropathologist
Nephropath
Little Rock, Arkansas

Marie Claire Gubler, MD
Director of Research Emeritus
INSERM U1163
Hôpital Necker Enfants Malades
Paris, France

Josephine Ambruzs, MD, MPH
Nephropathologist
Nephropath
Little Rock, Arkansas

Nidia Messias, MD
Nephropathologist
Nephropath
Little Rock, Arkansas

A. Bernard Collins, BS
Technical Director Immunopathology Unit
Department of Pathology
Massachusetts General Hospital
Associate in Pathology Harvard Medical School
Boston, Massachusetts

Aleksandr Vasilyev, MD, PhD
Assistant Professor
Department of Biomedical Sciences
New York Institute of Technology
College of Osteopathic Medicine
Old Westbury, New York

Xin Gu, MD
Department of Pathology
Louisiana State University Health Sciences
Center in Shreveport
Shreveport, Louisiana

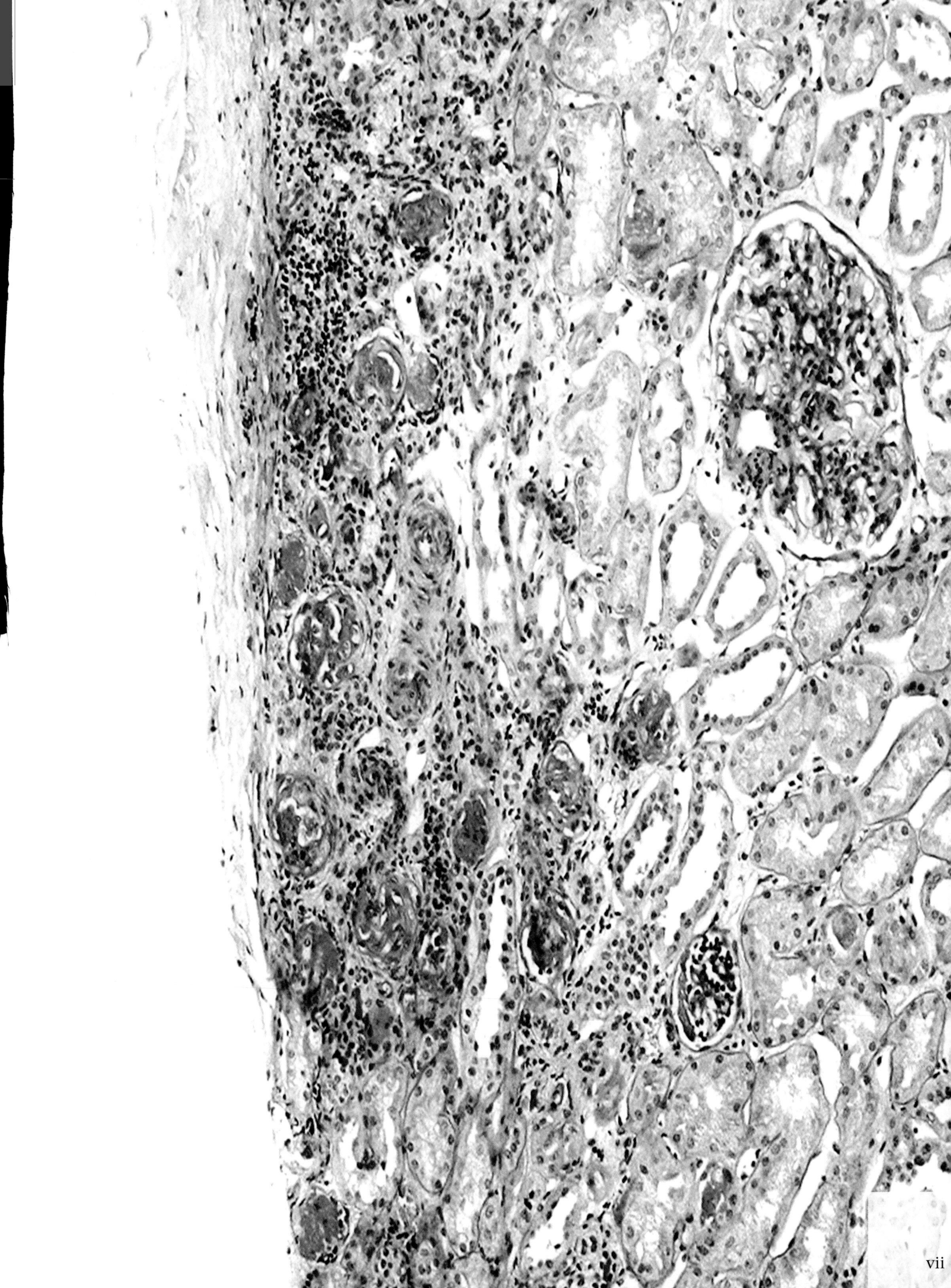

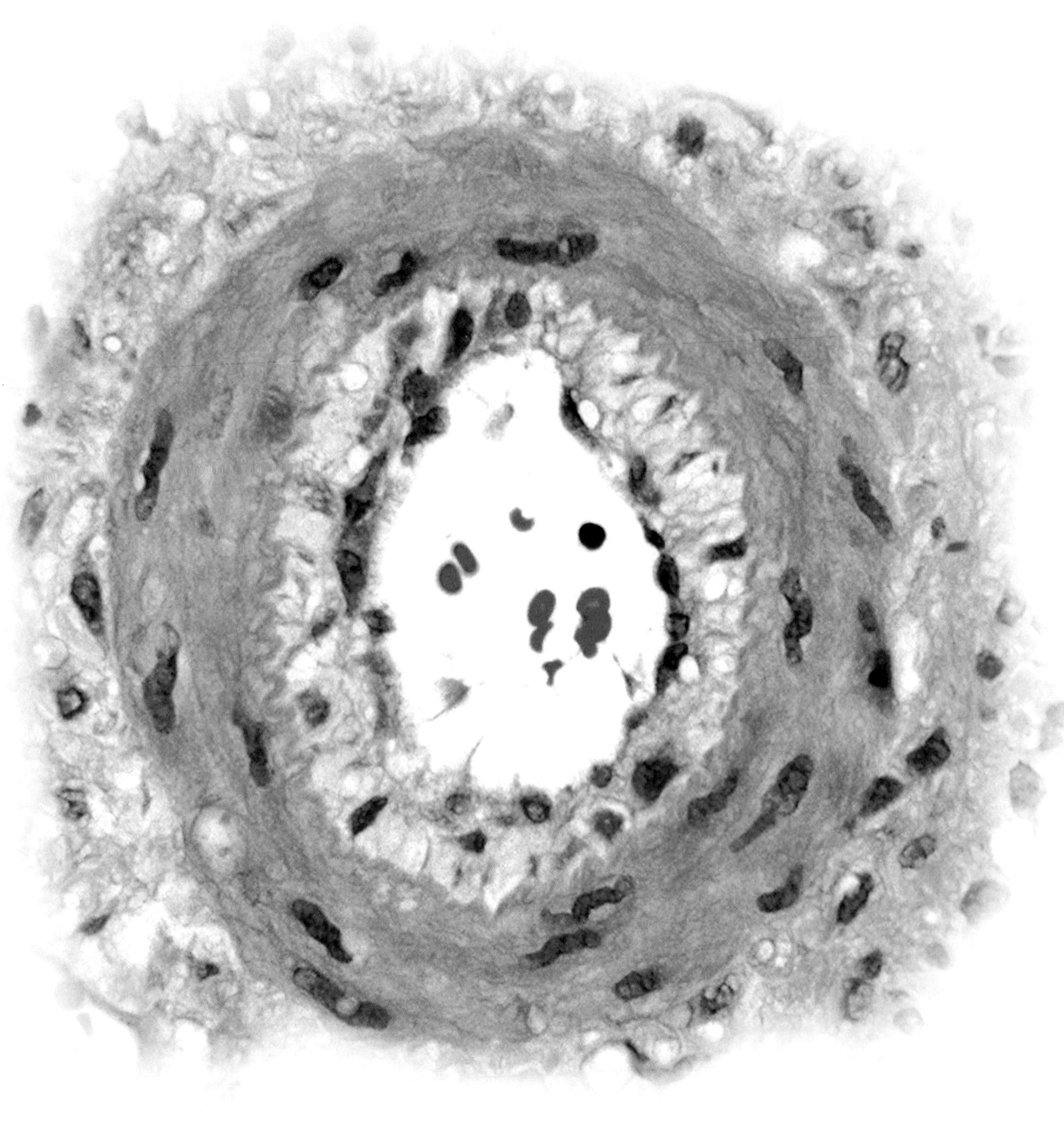

Image Contributors

We are grateful to the collaborators listed below, who kindly and without hesitation shared their digital images of unusual or unique cases, published and unpublished. They are cited individually in the figure legends, but we also wish to acknowledge them as a group. Their help was essential in our endeavor to create a comprehensive text. We are also indebted to our patients who contributed their specimens for research to find better treatment, diagnosis, and understanding of our renal diseases.

Anila Abraham, MD
Cyril Abrahams, MD
Shreeram Akilesh, MD
Kerstin Amann, MD
Thomas Atwell, MD
Niaz Banaei, MD
Laura Barisoni-Thomas, MD
Jay Bernstein, MD
William D. Bates, MBChB, MMed, PhD
Gerald Berry, MD
Athanase Billis, MD
Erika Bracamonte, MD
Helen Catthro, MD
Maggie (Ying) Chen, MD, PhD
Jacob Churg, MD
Arthur Cohen, MD
Terence Cook, MD
Vivette D'Agati, MD
Cinthia Drachenberg, MD
Andrew Evan, MD
Luis Fajardo, MD
John Fallon, MD, PhD
Evan Farkash, MD, PhD
Dusan Ferluga, MD
Judith Ferry, MD
Mary Fidler, MD
Sandrin Florquin, MD, PhD
Andreas Friedl, MD
Billie Fyfe, MD
Neriman Gokden, MD
Paul Grimm, MD
Marie-Claire Gubler, MD
Nancy Harris, MD
Joel Henderson, MD, PhD
Randolph Hennigar, MD
Colin Hébert, MD
Leal Herlitz, MD
Guillermo Herrara, MD
Aliya Husain, MD
Bela Ivanyi, MD
George Jarad, MD
J. Charles Jennette, MD
Jason Karamchadani, MD
Jolanta Kowalewska, MD
Shaila Khubchandani, MD
Lisa Kim, MD
Christopher Larsen, MD
Reinhold Linke, MD
Alexander Magil, MD
Cynthia Magro, MD
Christine Menias, MD
Michael Mihatsch, MD
Jeffery Miner, PhD
Guido Monga, MD
Jose Montoya, MD
Jocelyn Moore, MD
Tibor Nadasdy, MD
Samih Nasr, MD
Cynthia Nast, MD
Volker Nickeleit, MD
Louis Novoa-Takara, MD
Ryuji Ohashi, MD
Juan Olano, MD
Victor Pardo, MD
Kwan-Kyu Park, MD, PhD
Vesna Petronic-Rosic, MD
Maria Picken, MD, PhD
Alkis Pieridis, MD
James Pullman, MD
Lorraine Racusen, MD
Emilio Ramos, MD
Parmjeet Randhawa, MD
Ian Roberts, MD
Ivy Rosales, MD
Seymour Rosen, MD
Robert Rouse, MD
Virginie Royal, MD
Luis Salinas-Madrigal, MD
Paula Santos do Carmo, MD
J.A. Schroeder, MD, PhD
Athena Shih, MD
Akira Shimizu, MD, PhD
R. Neal Smith, MD, PhD
Keyoumars Soltani, MD
Jie Song, MD
Christine Swett, AB
Gerald Spear, MD
J. Steinmetz, MD
Osamu Takasu, MD
Robert Tanenberg, MD
Jerome Taxy, MD
Nguyen Trang, MD
William Travis, MD
Megan Troxell, MD
Alenka Vizjak, PhD
Rosemary Wieczorek, MD
Ioanna Zouvani, MD

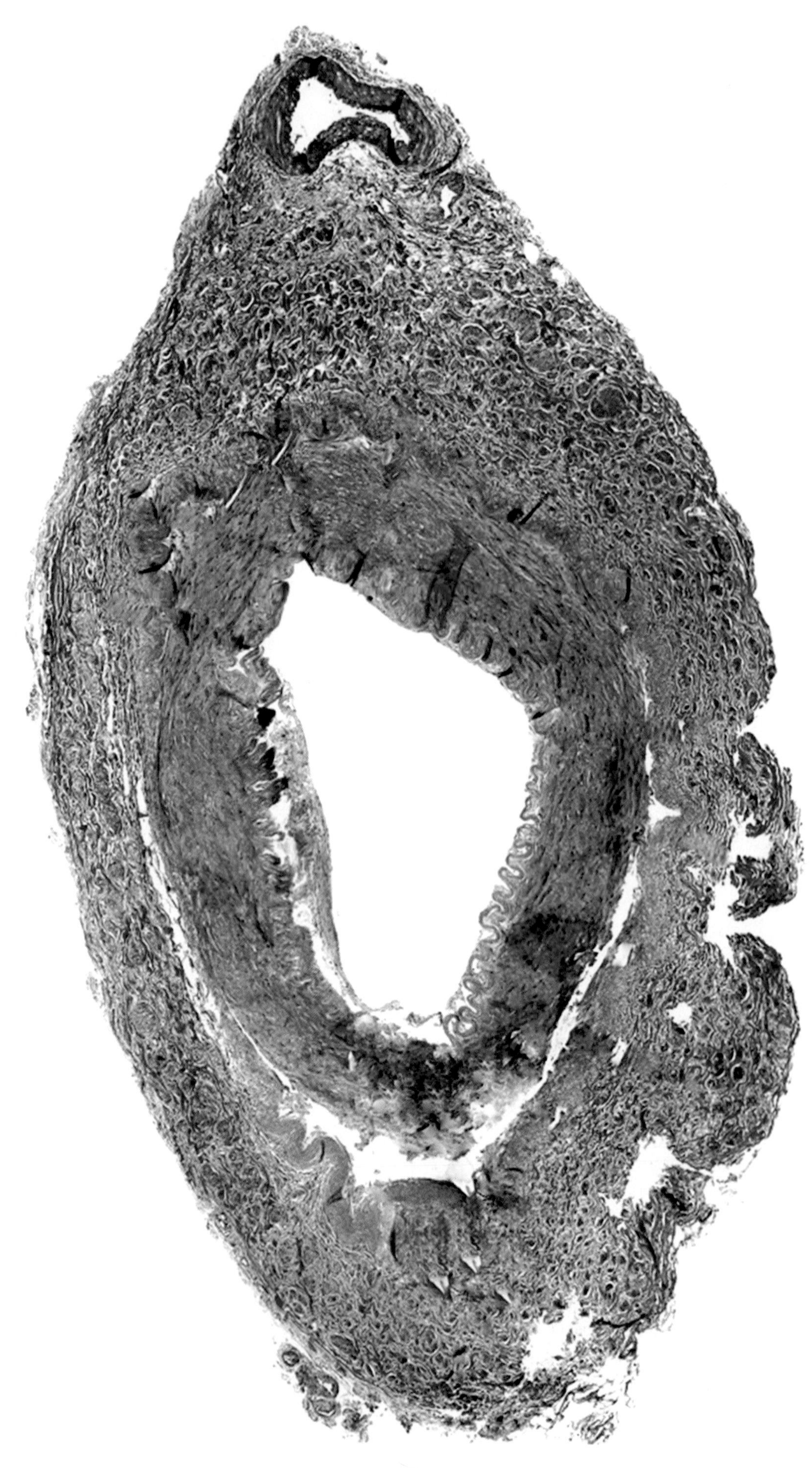

Preface

Welcome to the world of renal pathology! The team who developed this book has over 250 years of combined experience in renal pathology. We were motivated by the desire to create a comprehensive, succinct, and diagnostically useful resource for practicing pathologists, nephrologists, and all students of kidney diseases. Here, you will find the most complete survey available of nonneoplastic diseases of native and transplant kidneys, amply illustrated by over 3,500 pathology images of classic and variant features. The information and images are web accessible to all owners of the book through Expert Consult and to subscribers of ExpertPath© by Elsevier.

Renal pathologists typically consider pathogenesis and etiology in addition to the diagnosis. This approach requires knowledge of the clinical presentation, relevant laboratory and molecular data, and evidence from mechanistic research studies. We provide all of these elements in a highly structured format for each disease entity.

The authors are particularly delighted to present the second edition of this text. The excellent reception to the first edition has encouraged us to update and expand the content. We have added 40 chapters and 5 new authors, reorganized some of the sections, updated and polished text in all of the chapters, and added current references and innumerable new images. Overall, we are pleased that the book reflects significant progress in our quest to provide a useful, accurate, and accessible compendium of all nonneoplastic renal diseases for clinicians, pathologists, and investigators.

One may ask, "Why so many chapters?" The answer is that medical research has led to an increasing number of distinct diseases, once categorized by clinical and pathologic characteristics and now increasingly further defined and separated by etiologic and genetic criteria. The structured format of the book is conducive to presenting this expanding list that will continue to grow in the era of personalized medicine.

We hope this text will help improve the diagnosis of renal disease and stimulate advances in the field.

Robert B. Colvin, MD
Benjamin Castleman Distinguished Professor of Pathology
Department of Pathology
Harvard Medical School
Massachusetts General Hospital
Boston, Massachusetts

Anthony Chang, MD
Associate Professor of Pathology
Associate Director, Pathology Residency Program Director
Medical Director, UC MedLabs Outreach Program
Renal Pathology and Renal Pathology Fellowship
The University of Chicago Medicine
Chicago, Illinois

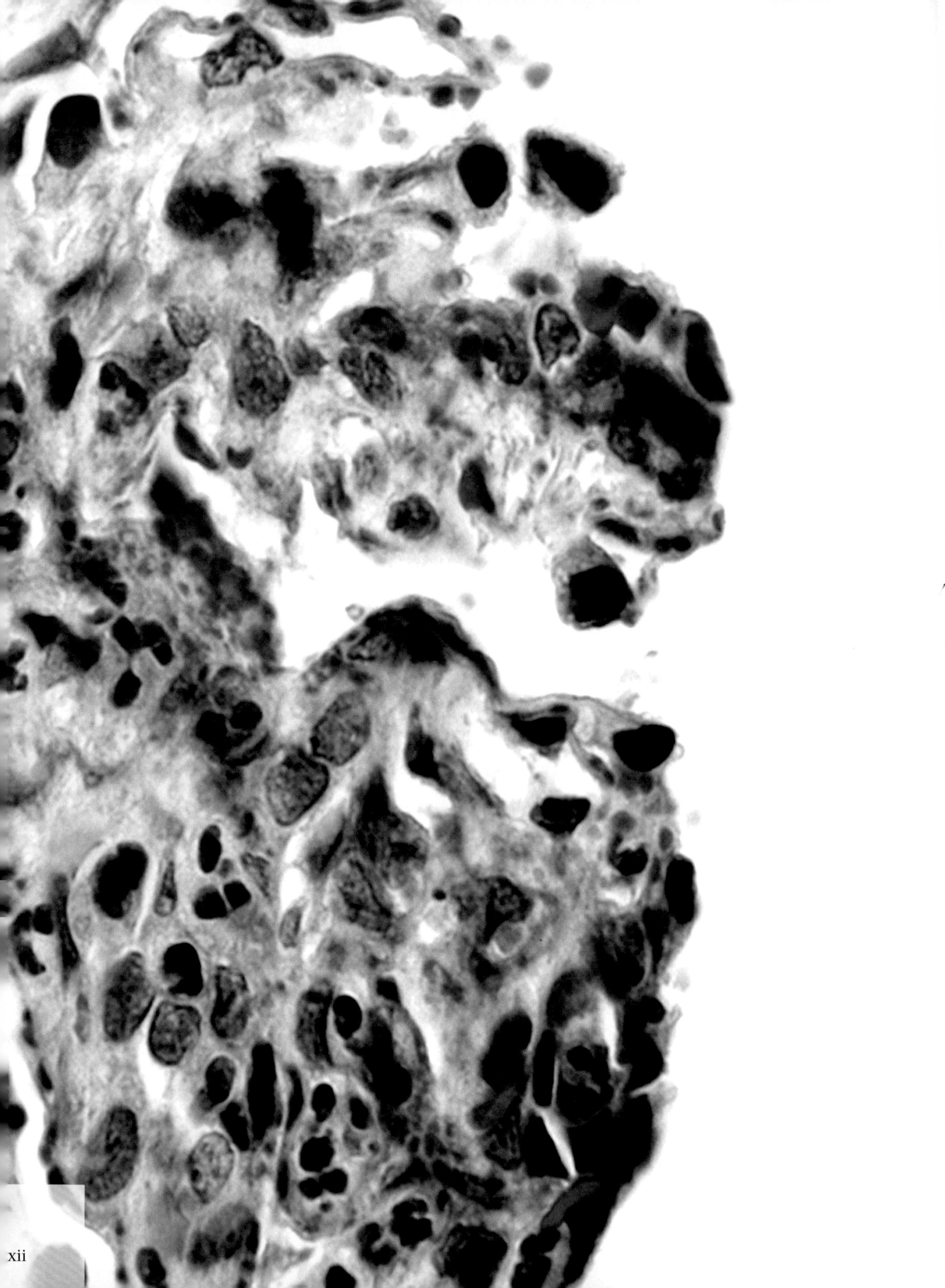

Acknowledgments

Text Editors

Dave L. Chance, MA, ELS
Nina I. Bennett, BA
Sarah J. Connor, BA
Tricia L. Cannon, BA
Terry W. Ferrell, MS
Lisa A. Gervais, BS
Karen E. Concannon, MA, PhD

Image Editors

Jeffrey J. Marmorstone, BS
Lisa A. M. Steadman, BS

Medical Editors

Ivy A. Rosales, MD
Kammi J. Henriksen, MD

Illustrations

Laura C. Sesto, MA
Lane R. Bennion, MS
Richard Coombs, MS

Art Direction and Design

Tom M. Olson, BA
Laura C. Sesto, MA

Lead Editor

Arthur G. Gelsinger, MA

Production Coordinators

Angela M. Terry, BA
Rebecca L. Hutchinson, BA

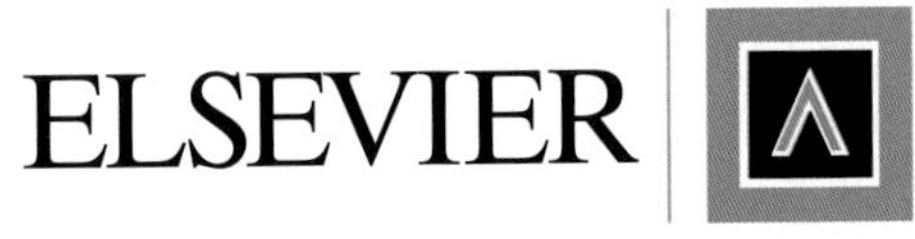

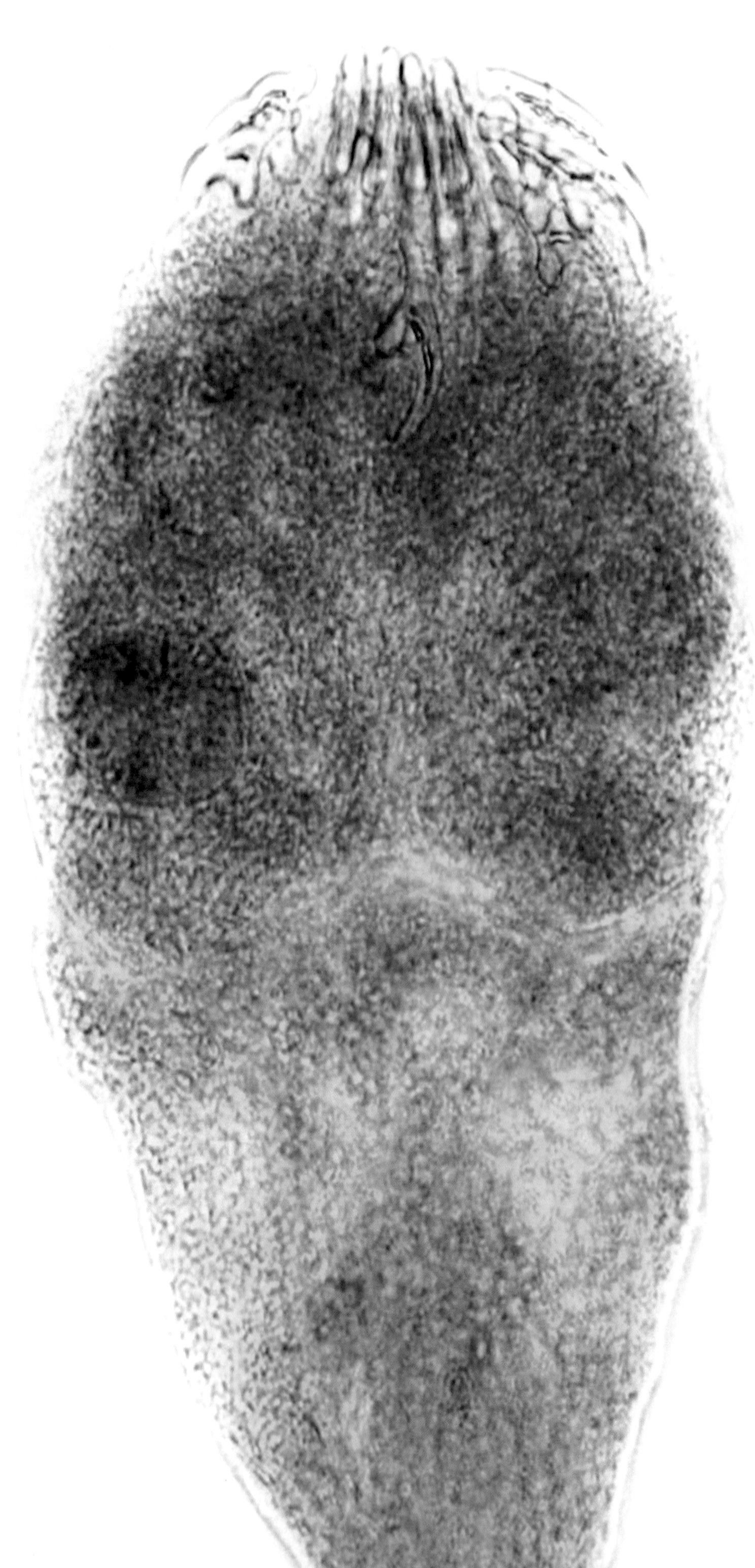

Sections

TABLE OF CONTENTS

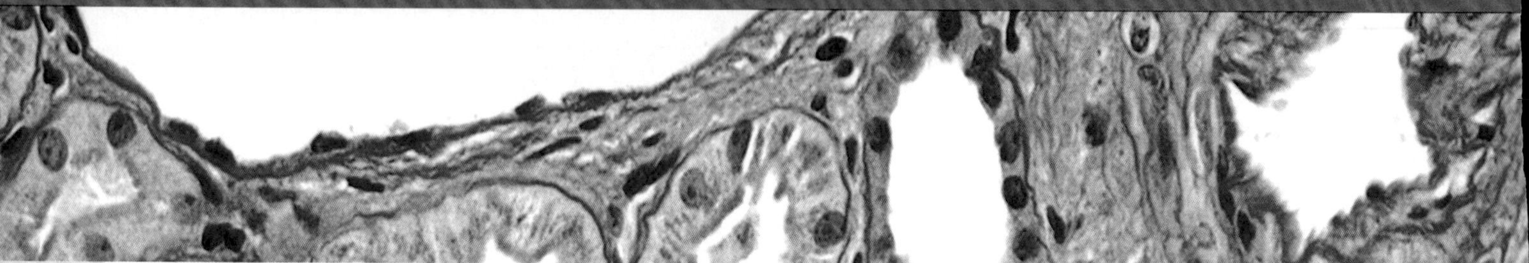

SECTION 1: INTRODUCTION

INTRODUCTION AND OVERVIEW

SECTION 2: GLOMERULAR DISEASES

MINIMAL CHANGE DISEASE

FOCAL SEGMENTAL GLOMERULOSCLEROSIS

MEMBRANOUS GLOMERULONEPHRITIS

C3-RELATED GLOMERULONEPHRITIS AND MEMBRANOPROLIFERATIVE GLOMERULONEPHRITIS

IgA-RELATED GLOMERULONEPHRITIS

SLE AND RELATED AUTOANTIBODY-MEDIATED GN

ANTI-GBM NEPHRITIS

MONOCLONAL IMMUNOGLOBULIN DISEASES

TABLE OF CONTENTS

TABLE OF CONTENTS

TABLE OF CONTENTS

TABLE OF CONTENTS

TABLE OF CONTENTS

TABLE OF CONTENTS

DIAGNOSTIC PATHOLOGY

Kidney Diseases

SECOND EDITION

COLVIN | CHANG

FARRIS • KAMBHAM • CORNELL • MEEHAN • LIAPIS
GAUT • BONSIB • SESHAN • JAIN • LARSEN

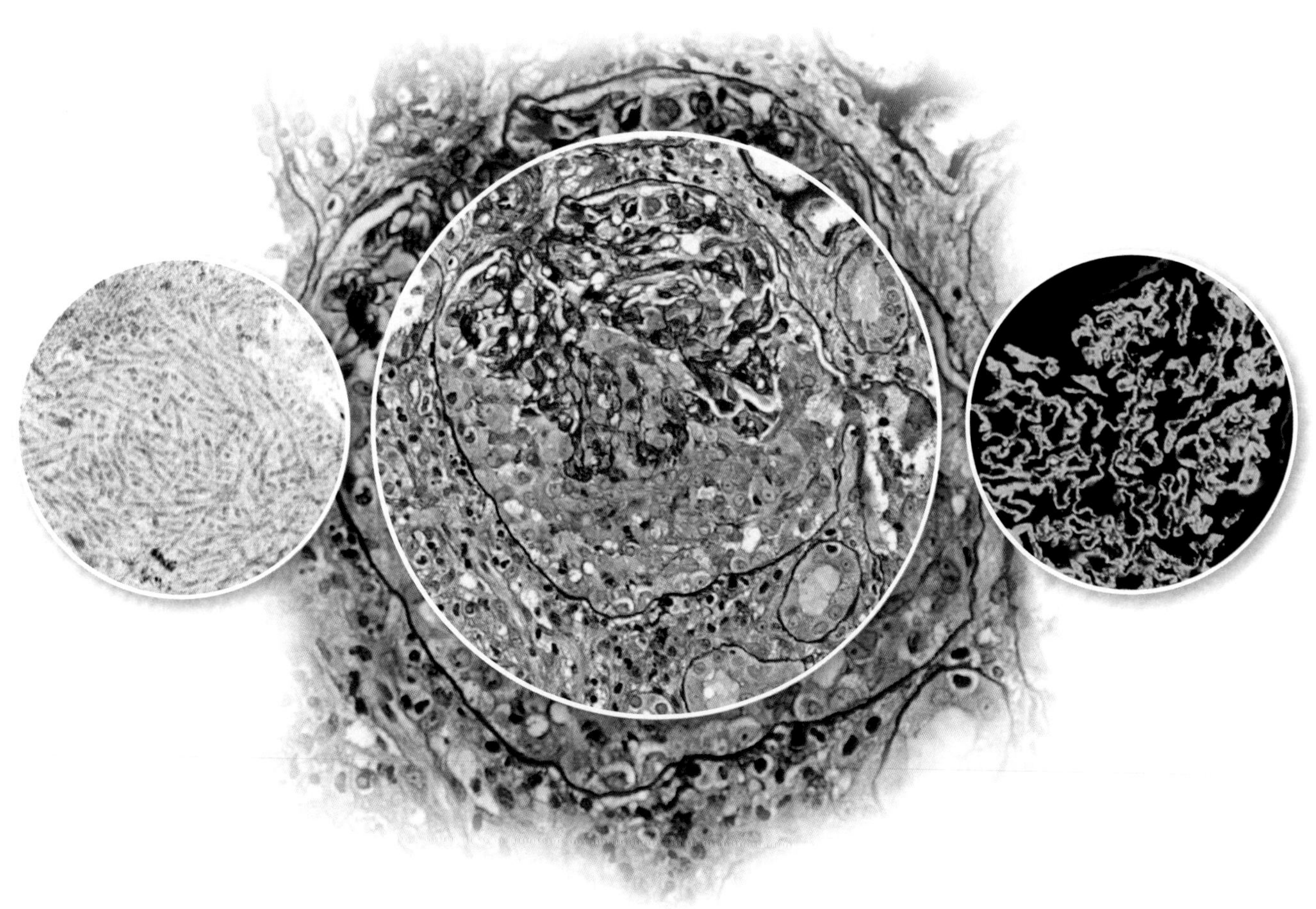

SECTION 1

Introduction

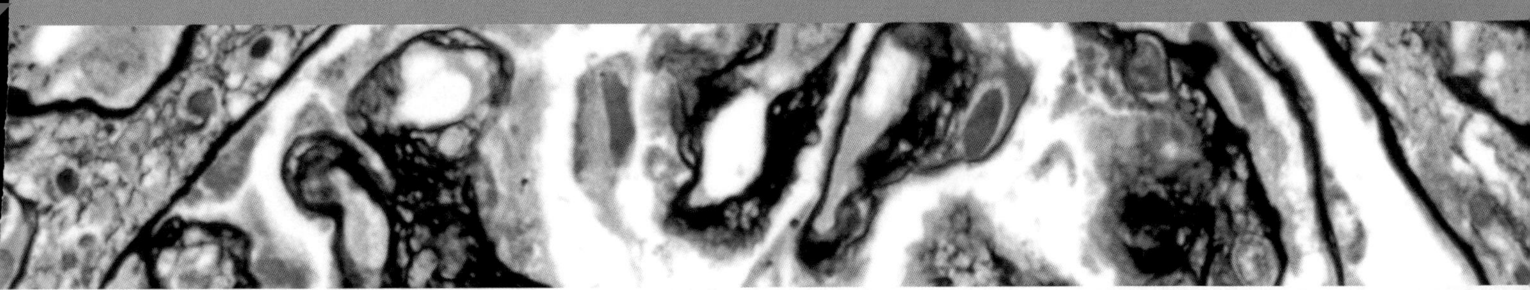

Introduction and Overview

VALUE OF RENAL BIOPSY

Provides Diagnosis

- Alters clinical diagnosis 24-47%

Guides Treatment

- Changes therapy 31-42%
- Determines reversibility and activity

Predicts Prognosis

- Specific pathologic features and extent of changes
- Changes prognosis 31-57%

Reveals Pathogenesis

- Molecular and cellular mechanisms

Validates Outcome

- Used as endpoint in clinical trials

INDICATIONS FOR RENAL BIOPSY

Elevated Cr or BUN (Acute or Chronic)

- Elevated with decreased renal filtration
- Measure creatinine clearance or estimated glomerular filtration rate (eGFR) based on gender, body weight, race, age

Proteinuria

- May be asymptomatic or symptomatic
- Usually a sign of increased permeability of glomerulus
  - Failure of reabsorption by tubules can lead to low-level proteinuria
- 1-3 g/d usually asymptomatic
- Higher levels lead to edema and nephrotic syndrome

Nephrotic Syndrome

- Proteinuria > 3.5 g/d, hypoalbuminemia, edema, hyperlipidemia, lipiduria
- Increased glomerular permeability to albumin and other plasma proteins

Hematuria (Microscopic or Gross)

- May be asymptomatic or symptomatic (gross hematuria)
- Usually a sign of glomerular inflammation and ruptured glomerular basement membrane (GBM), especially with red blood cell (RBC) casts
- When combined with acute renal failure and RBC casts, termed nephritic syndrome

Nephritic Syndrome

- Hematuria, proteinuria, elevated Cr, hypertension, edema
- Loss of function due to decreased glomerular blood flow, salt retention

BIOPSY TECHNIQUE AND SAFETY

Percutaneous (Needle) Biopsy

- Ultrasound guided, automated gun
  - Generally regarded as safe outpatient procedure
  - 14-16 gauge needle recommended for adults; 16-18 gauge for children < 8 years old
  - At least 2 cores if possible
- Complications varies with technique
  - Microscopic (~ 35%) or gross hematuria (4.5%)
  - Complications requiring intervention 6.6% (Korbet 2014)
    - Hematoma 3.5%
    - Transfusion 5.3%
    - Embolization 0.8%
    - Obstruction 0.2%
    - Mortality 0.09%
- Adequacy
  - Excellent diagnostic yield with two 14-g cores (99%; mean: 32 glomeruli)
  - 94% adequacy with 18-g needle (mean 9 glomeruli)

Open (Wedge) Biopsy

- Primarily samples outer cortex

Transjugular Vein Biopsy

- High-risk patients

PROCESSING OF TISSUE

Gross Examination

- Determine whether glomeruli in sample

Gross Appearance of Renal Biopsy Cores

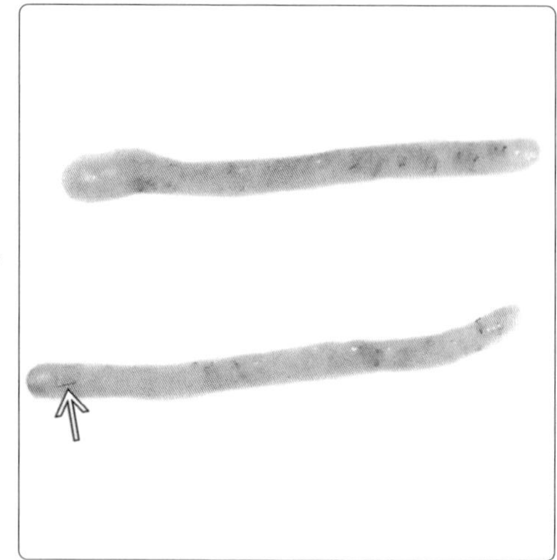

Division of Renal Biopsy Cores

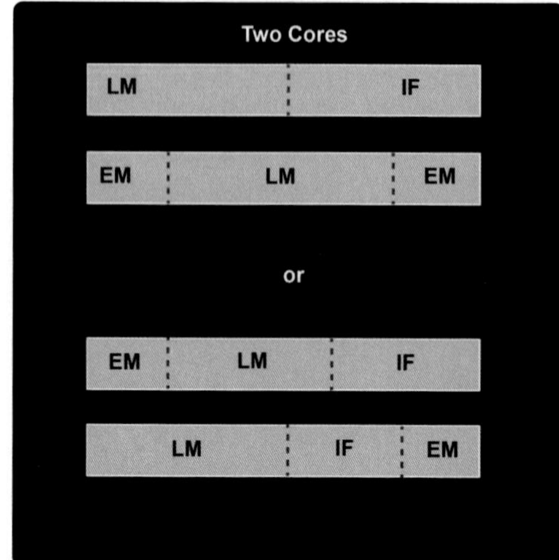

(Left) *Renal biopsy cores from 16-g needle show glomeruli appearing as pale or congested bulges and red cell casts as brown streaks ➡ or dots.* **(Right)** *Renal biopsy cores are divided into 3 portions for light microscopy (LM), immunofluorescence (IF), and electron microscopy (EM). Two cores are generally taken and divided transversely with effort to ensure that each of the 3 portions include cortex. Longitudinal division is not recommended.*

- Dissecting microscope, loupe

Division of Sample

- Divide into 3 parts for light (LM), immunofluorescence (IF), and electron microscopy (EM)
  - Take LM portions from both cores, EM from ends

Light Microscopy

- Formalin-fixed, paraffin-embedded, 2-3 μm sections
  - Multiple levels
- H&E, PAS, silver and trichrome stains usual
  - Other stains as indicated

Immunofluorescence

- Quick freeze on cryostat chuck or liquid N_2
- Frozen sections cut at 3-4 μm
- Stain for IgG, IgA, IgM, kappa, lambda, C1q, C3, fibrinogen, albumin
  - C4d on transplant biopsies

Electron Microscopy

- 2% paraformaldehyde/2.5% glutaraldehyde in cacodylate or phosphate buffered fixative (Karnovsky half strength, "K2") and osmium post fix
- 1 μm toluidine blue-stained sections to screen for glomeruli
- Choose 1-2 blocks with glomeruli and trim for EM sectioning and staining (Pb/Ur)

Recording Results

- Digital cameras commonly used for IF and EM
- Whole slide scans for LM for clinical trials/teaching
- EM morphometry to measure GBM thickness

SYSTEMATIC APPROACH

Light Microscopy

- Examine each of 4 components
  - Glomeruli, tubules, interstitium, and vessels
  - Try to decide which component is primarily affected
- Describe and quantitate changes in each compartment
  - Distinguish acute and chronic changes
  - Examine each section
- Examine frozen and plastic section by light microscopy

Immunofluorescence

- Assess pattern, extent, and intensity of glomerular staining
- Assess presence and pattern of deposits in other sites (tubular basement membrane [TBM], vessels, interstitium)

Electron Microscopy

- GBM thickness and appearance
- Presence and location of electron dense deposits
  - Substructure and periodicity, if any
- Podocyte changes (effacement)
- Endothelial changes
- Mesangial features
- TBM, interstitium, peritubular capillaries

ISSUES IN INTERPRETATION

Sampling

- Adequacy of sample is dependent on nature of disease
  - Small samples are adequate for diffuse diseases
  - Large samples are needed for focal diseases
- The rarer the lesion, the greater the sample needed
  - S = 1 - (1 - p) ^ n, where S = probability of obtaining at least 1 affected glomerulus, p = fraction of affected glomeruli in kidney, and n = number of glomeruli in sample (binomial distribution)
  - For example, if 10% of glomeruli are affected, need 30 glomeruli to have > 95% chance of sampling at least 1 affected glomerulus
- Estimation of % affected glomeruli in kidney is similarly subject to sampling error (e.g., distinction between > 50% and < 50%)
- Distribution of lesions is not random in some diseases (e.g., focal segmental glomerular sclerosis FSGS)
- Options when inadequate
  - Reprocess paraffin or frozen block for EM or frozen for paraffin
  - Immunohistochemistry for Ig in paraffin block

Scoring Systems and Definitions

- Described by several classification systems
  - Lupus (ISN/RPS), IgA (Oxford), transplants (Banff)
- Do not always agree on definitions or method of scoring for same features

Complex Biopsies

- > 1 disease may be present
  - Common in allografts
  - Residue from past disease persists

Functional Interrelationships

- Disease of 1 component affects others
  - Loss of glomeruli affects blood supply of tubules
  - Vascular disease affects tubules and glomeruli

REPORTING RECOMMENDATIONS

Diagnosis

- Use current classification system for particular disease (e.g., lupus, IgA, diabetes, vasculitis, transplant)
- Include severity and activity whenever possible

Description

- Indicate sample (number of cores, cortex, medulla, corticomedullary junction)
- Glomeruli
  - Count number in sample (can count section with greatest number)
  - Give % of globally and segmentally sclerotic glomeruli
  - Mesangial cellularity
  - Thickening of capillary wall/GBM
  - Presence or absence of inflammation, necrosis, crescents, thrombi, adhesions, hyaline, periglomerular fibrosis
    - Indicate fraction of glomeruli involved
  - Useful to give % of normal glomeruli
- Tubules
  - Acute injury, necrosis
  - Atrophy (give %)
  - Casts (RBC, protein, pigment, neutrophils)
  - Tubular reabsorption droplets
  - Vacuolization, nuclear inclusions, giant mitochondria

- Interstitium
  - Inflammation, type of cells, granuloma
  - Fibrosis, pattern, extent (%)
- Vessels
  - Count arteries
  - Intimal fibrosis, arteries (% luminal occlusion)
  - Arteriolar hyalinization (extent)
  - Vasculitis
  - Peritubular capillaritis
- Immunofluorescence
  - Indicate number of glomeruli in sample
  - Give pattern and intensity of glomerular staining for each positive reactant and score 0-4(+)
  - Note other relevant staining: TBM, interstitium, vessels, reabsorption droplets
  - List all stains used, including negative
- Electron microscopy
  - Indicate number of glomeruli
  - Status of podocytes (effacement, hypertrophy, separation from GBM)
  - GBM (thickness, lamination, deposits)
  - Extent and position of deposits
    - Give substructure, if any, and dimensions
  - Mesangial features (fibrils, cells, deposits)

Summary

- Link to clinical information
- Compare with previous biopsy
- Discuss differential and basis of conclusion

DEFINITIONS FOR GLOMERULI

Adhesion

- Abnormal attachment of glomerular tuft to Bowman capsule; area of continuity between glomerular tuft and Bowman capsule separate from extracapillary lesion or from area of segmental sclerosis

Bowman Capsule

- Layer of basement membrane surrounding Bowman space on which parietal epithelial cells rest; continuous with GBM at base of glomerulus

Bowman Space

- Space between glomerular tuft and surrounding Bowman capsule, in continuity with lumen of proximal tubule

Capillary Wall Thickening

- Used for H&E sections in which GBM, deposits, and cellular elements all contribute to thickness

Collapsing Lesion

- Collapse of glomerular capillaries with overlying podocyte hypercellularity

Crescent

- Extracapillary proliferation of > 2 cell layers occupying 25% or more of glomerular capsular circumference or > 10%
  - Sometimes graded: < 10% (tiny focus), 10-25%, 25-50%, > 50% of glomerular capsular circumference

Crescent, Cellular

- Crescent with cells and no fibrosis; usually have fibrin and inflammatory cells

Crescent, Fibrocellular

- Crescent with mixture of cellular and fibrous components

Crescent, Fibrous

- Predominantly fibrous tissue in Bowman space; no fibrin or inflammatory cells

Diffuse

- Majority of glomeruli (≥ 50%)

Disappearing Glomerulosclerosis

- Global glomerulosclerosis with some dissolution of Bowman capsule

Duplication of GBM

- Double layer of GBM separated by clear zone on silver or PAS stains; sometimes likened to tram tracks; sometimes redundantly called "reduplication"

Endocapillary Hypercellularity (Proliferation)

- Increased numbers of intracapillary cells causing narrowing of glomerular capillary lumina

Extracapillary Hypercellularity (Proliferation)

- Synonym for crescent

Fenestrations (Fenestrae)

- Openings through endothelial cells (~ 50 nm in diameter) that allow fluid passage but retain formed elements

Fibrinoid Necrosis

- Area of necrosis that stains brick red with eosin due to denatured proteins and fibrin

Filtration Slit Diaphragm

- Connection between podocyte foot processes consisting of nephrin and other components
- Thought to be responsible for macromolecular filtration
- a.k.a. "zipper" for its en face appearance

Focal

- Minority of glomeruli (< 50%)

Global Glomerulosclerosis

- Sclerotic remnant of glomerulus largely consisting of extracellular material; sometimes subdivided into obsolescent, solified, and disappearing types

Glomerular Basement Membrane

- Continuous layer of collagen type IV and matrix components on which podocytes and endothelial cells rest; does not include Bowman capsule

GBM Thickening

- Used for PAS and silver stains that distinguish GBM elements

Hyaline Deposits

- Homogeneous, dense eosinophilic deposits, often with clear fine lipid droplets; composition not well defined

Hyaline Thrombi

- Synonym for pseudothrombi

Hypertrophy

- Increase in size (diameter) of glomerulus (normally < radius of a 40x field ≈ 440μm); typically accompanied by increased mesangium and thickened GBM

Inflammation

- Increased numbers of leukocytes (granulocytes, monocytes, lymphocytes) in capillaries (normally < 2 per glomerulus)

Global

- Entire glomerulus involved (> 50% in lupus)

Ischemic Collapse (Sclerosis)

- Glomerulus showing collapse of capillary tuft ± thickening of Bowman capsule and fibrosis in Bowman space

Karyorrhexis

- Pyknotic and fragmented nuclei

Mesangial Cell

- Normal resident of mesangium in glomerulus; has contractile and phagocytic properties

Mesangial Hypercellularity

- 3 or more mesangial nuclei in 1 mesangial area in a 3 μm section (lupus classification); 4 or more in IgA classification, subdivided into mild (4-5), moderate (6-7), and severe (8 or more)

Mesangial Matrix

- Extracellular component of normal mesangium, includes collagen IV alpha 1, 2 chains, fibronectin, and variety of glycosaminoglycans

Mesangial Matrix Expansion

- Width of mesangial interspace exceeds 2 mesangial cell nuclei in at least 2 glomerular lobules (IgA)

Mesangiolysis

- Loss of integrity of mesangium so that glomerular capillary forms aneurysmal dilation

Necrosis

- Loss of integrity of glomerulus; typically manifested by fragmented nuclei (karyorrhexis), disruption of GBM, and deposition of fibrin; minimum requirement is extravascular fibrin (IgA)

Nodules

- Rounded expansion of mesangial matrix &/or cells with peripheral necklace of capillaries

Nuclear Dust

- Fragments of neutrophil nuclei (karyorrhexis) in site of inflammation

Obsolescent Glomeruli

- Retracted, globally sclerotic glomeruli with Bowman space filled with matrix

Parietal Epithelium

- Cells that line Bowman capsule

Pseudothrombi

- Eosinophilic, rounded aggregates in glomerular capillaries due to immune complex precipitates rather than fibrin (typically due to cryoglobulins with IgG, IgM, and C3); a.k.a. hyaline thrombi

Podocyte

- Cell on outside of GBM with extensive foot processes connected with filtration slit diaphragms; terminally differentiated

Sclerosis

- Obliteration of capillary lumen by increased extracellular matrix ± hyalinosis or foam cells

Segmental

- Part of glomerulus involved; definitions varies from any amount to < 50%

Solidified Glomerulosclerosis

- Globally sclerotic glomeruli filling Bowman space

Spikes

- "Hair on end" pattern of subepithelial GBM on silver or PAS stain; need 40-100x to appreciate

Visceral Epithelium

- Normally synonymous with podocyte. Preferred term when nature of cell on the GBM is uncertain, as in collapsing glomerulopathy

DEFINITIONS FOR TUBULES

Acute Tubular Injury

- Loss of brush border on PAS stain, thin cytoplasm, loss of nuclei; simplification of epithelium without TBM thickening

Acute Tubular Necrosis

- Epithelial cell death, as manifested by loss of or pale-staining nuclei and eosinophilic cytoplasm; usually not conspicuous unless toxin or vessel occlusion; sometimes used as synonym for acute tubular injury

Apoptosis

- Programmed cell death, as manifested by pyknosis and fragmentation of nuclei

Casts

- Presence of protein or cells in tubular lumen taking shape of tubule

Casts, Red Cell

- Presence of compacted red cells in tubular lumen; may be hemolyzed or fragmented; need to distinguish loose red cells from biopsy artifact

Casts, Tamm-Horsfall Protein (Uromodulin)

- Cast of protein normally produced in distal tubule; pale on H&E, strongly PAS positive

Dystrophic Calcification

- Calcification of necrotic cells or debris; typically in casts as variably sized basophilic granules

Fatty Change

- Tubules with clear cytoplasm containing lipid (demonstrable in Oil red O-stained frozen sections), a feature of nephrotic syndrome

Intranuclear Inclusions

- Homogeneous dense or pale transformation of nucleus
  - Indicative of active viral replication

Isometric Vacuolization

- Abundant clear cytoplasmic vacuoles of about same size

Nephrocalcinosis

- Accumulation of calcium salts, typically in TBM as basophilic, linear deposit; also present in casts

Osmotic Nephrosis

- Fine, clear vacuolization in tubules

Thyroidization

- Dilated tubular segments with eosinophilic proteinaceous casts and thin epithelial lining

Tubular Atrophy

- Loss of cytoplasmic organelles (pale cytoplasm) accompanied by shrinkage of tubular diameter and often thickened TBM

Tubular Hypertrophy

- Increased diameter of tubules with increased size of epithelial cells

Tubular Reabsorption Droplets (Hyaline Droplets)

- PAS(+) small round granules in tubular cells; contain albumin and often other plasma proteins and indicate glomerular proteinuria

Tubular Rupture

- Disruption of TBM with localized inflammatory response; may have granulomatous reaction and spilling of Tamm-Horsfall protein into interstitium (piss granuloma)

Tubulitis

- Mononuclear leukocytes within epithelial layer of tubules

DEFINITIONS FOR INTERSTITIUM

Abscess

- Localized collection of neutrophils in area of destruction of normal tissue components

Interstitial Fibrosis

- Expansion of normal interstitial connective tissue by increased collagen (I and III, typically); may or may not be accompanied by tubular atrophy; may be diffuse or focal
  - Scored by % of cortex involved or area of fibrosis

Interstitial Inflammation

- Increased numbers of leukocytes between tubules; may be focal or diffuse, nodular, perivascular, subcapsular
- Should be noted whether or not inflammation is confined to areas of interstitial fibrosis

Granuloma

- Nodular collection of epithelioid macrophages, sometimes with multinucleated macrophages (a.k.a histocytes), usually with lymphocytes

DEFINITIONS FOR VESSELS

Arteriolar Hyalinosis

- Accumulation of eosinophilic, amorphous material (usually containing plasma proteins) in arteriolar wall; may be subendothelial, peripheral nodular, or transmural; focal or circumferential

Capillaritis

- Accumulation of leukocytes in peritubular capillaries

Endarteritis

- Mononuclear inflammatory cells under endothelium of arteries and arterioles

Fibrinoid Necrosis

- Brick red staining of vessel wall on H&E with loss of smooth muscle nuclei; may have inflammatory component

Intimal Fibroelastosis

- Thickening of arterial intima with multiple layers of elastic fibers and collagen; usually not very cellular

Intimal Fibrosis

- Accumulation of fibrous tissue in intima, usually concentric, causing stenosis of lumen

Mucoid Intimal Thickening

- Accumulation of edematous extracellular matrix in intima resembling mucus; pale blue on H&E, Alcian blue positive

Onion Skinning

- Multilayered cells and matrix in intima of small arteries and arterioles

Vasculitis

- Inflammation in wall of vessel, as manifested by neutrophil karyorrhexis, fibrinoid necrosis of media; may occur in any sized vessel, artery, capillary, or vein

SELECTED REFERENCES

1. Korbet SM et al: Percutaneous renal biopsy of native kidneys: a single-center experience of 1,055 biopsies. Am J Nephrol. 39(2):153-62, 2014
2. Sis B et al: Banff '09 meeting report: antibody mediated graft deterioration and implementation of Banff working groups. Am J Transplant. 10(3):464-71, 2010
3. Walker PD: The renal biopsy. Arch Pathol Lab Med. 133(2):181-8, 2009
4. Working Group of the International IgA Nephropathy Network and the Renal Pathology Society et al: The Oxford classification of IgA nephropathy: pathology definitions, correlations, and reproducibility. Kidney Int. 76(5):546-56, 2009
5. Weening JJ et al: The classification of glomerulonephritis in systemic lupus erythematosus revisited. J Am Soc Nephrol. 15(2):241-50, 2004
6. Nicholson ML et al: A prospective randomized trial of three different sizes of core-cutting needle for renal transplant biopsy. Kidney Int. 58(1):390-5, 2000
7. Khajehdehi P et al: Percutaneous renal biopsy in the 1990s: safety, value, and implications for early hospital discharge. Am J Kidney Dis. 34(1):92-7, 1999
8. Huang FY et al: The role of percutaneous renal biopsy in the diagnosis and management of renal diseases in children. Zhonghua Min Guo Xiao Er Ke Yi Xue Hui Za Zhi. 39(1):43-7, 1998
9. Al-Rasheed SA: The impact of renal biopsy in the clinical management of childhood renal disease. Saudi J Kidney Dis Transpl. 8(1):11-5, 1997
10. Corwin HL et al: The importance of sample size in the interpretation of the renal biopsy. Am J Nephrol. 8(2):85-9, 1988

Normal Glomerulus

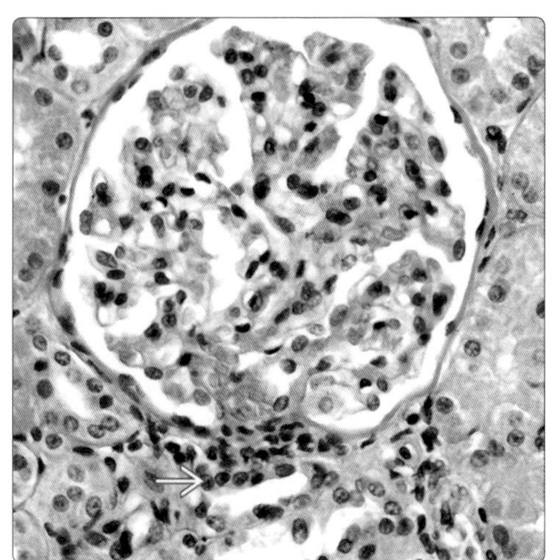

Normal Glomerulus

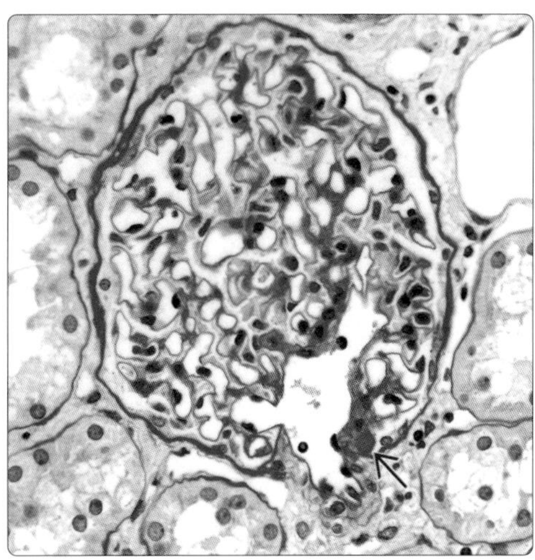

(Left) *H&E shows a normal glomerulus from a biopsy for asymptomatic microhematuria. The juxtaglomerular apparatus is at the base ➡. The capillaries are open, and the cellularity is normal although it is difficult to define the mesangium.* **(Right)** *Glomerulus in a donor biopsy stained with PAS reveals a thin GBM, open capillaries, an inconspicuous mesangium, and normal podocytes. A small hyaline deposit is present at the hilum ➡, but it is otherwise normal.*

Normal Glomerulus

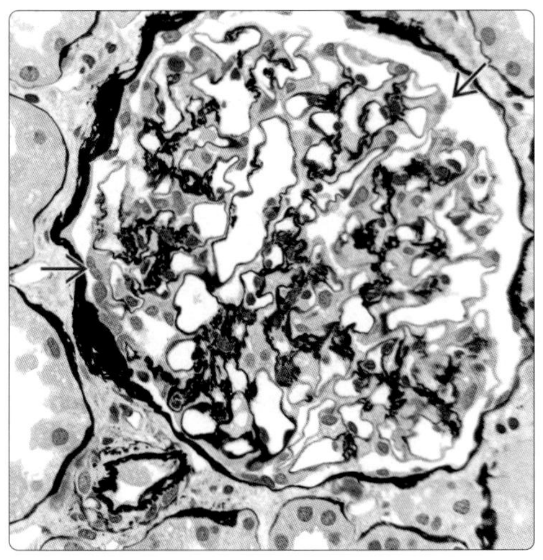

Minimal Mesangial Hypercellularity

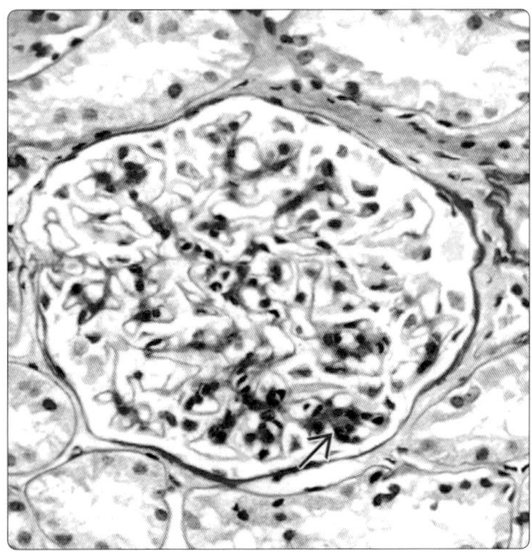

(Left) *Donor biopsy stained with Jones silver stain highlights the normal GBM. The podocytes ➡ are well seen, but the mesangial cells are lost in the densely stained mesangial matrix. This and the PAS stain are most valuable for appreciating the LM glomerular anatomy.* **(Right)** *PAS stain shows minimal mesangial hypercellularity ➡ in a patient with lupus nephritis. The threshold for mesangial hypercellularity is 3-4 mesangial cells per mesangial area in a 2-3 µm section.*

Moderate Mesangial Hypercellularity

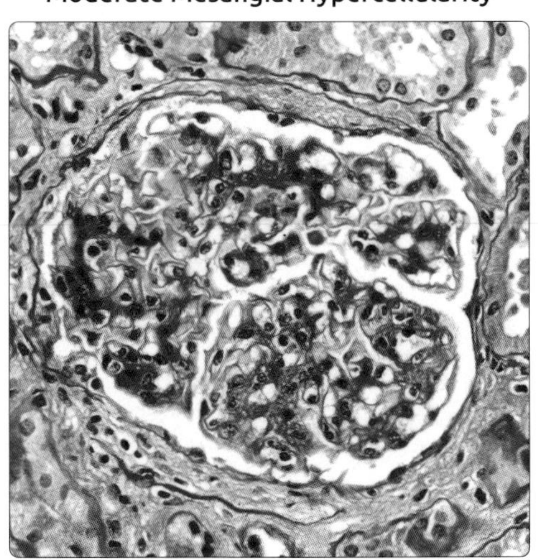

Mesangial Hypercellularity and Nodules

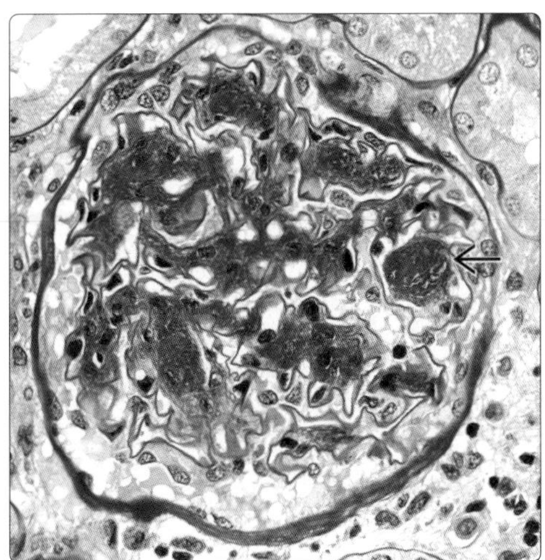

(Left) *PAS stain shows moderate global mesangial hypercellularity in a patient with IgA nephropathy. All segments of the glomerulus have increased mesangial cells and matrix.* **(Right)** *Marked global expansion of the mesangial matrix and cellularity with a segmental nodular pattern ➡ is evident in this PAS-stained glomerulus with diabetic glomerulosclerosis.*

(**Left**) *Neutrophils can be seen in glomerular capillaries with swollen endothelial cells that occlude the capillary lumina in a lupus nephritis case. Fragments of nuclei (nuclear dust) or karyorrhexis are present.* (**Right**) *Necrosis of a glomerulus is shown with loss of nuclei and obliteration of the normal architecture of the glomerulus. Thrombi are evident in arterioles in this case of thrombotic microangiopathy.*

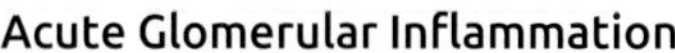

Acute Glomerular Inflammation

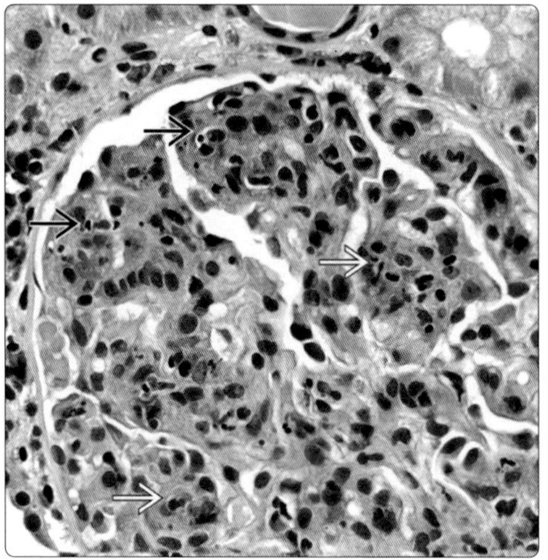

Segmental Glomerular Necrosis

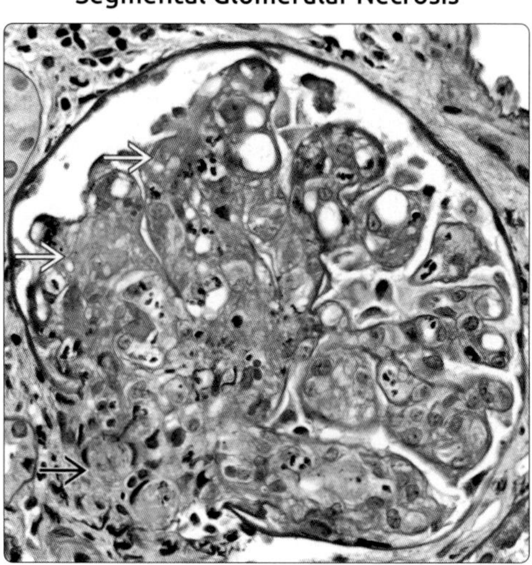

(**Left**) *Fibrinoid necrosis is best seen on H&E-stained sections in which the fibrin and denatured protein stain brick red with nearby nuclear dust. An area of old necrosis with loss of the normal architecture but without fibrin is also present. Patient has ANCA-related glomerulonephritis.* (**Right**) *Thrombi in capillaries and fibrinoid necrosis are shown in a glomerular tuft from a patient with endocarditis.*

Fibrinoid Necrosis in Glomerulus

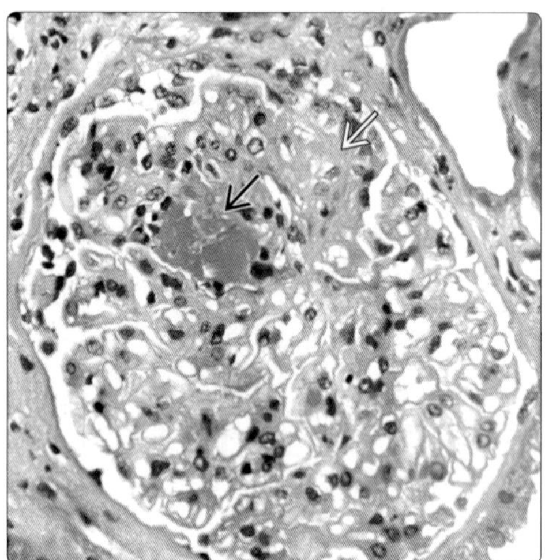

Thrombi in Glomerulus

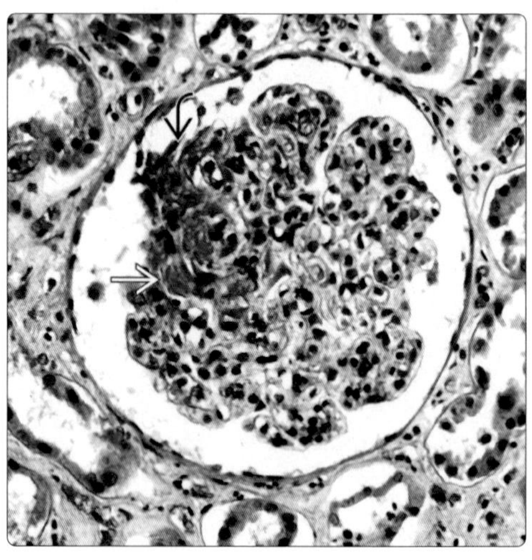

(**Left**) *Endocapillary hypercellularity illustrated in this glomerulus from a patient with lupus nephritis is defined as leukocytes or other cells filling the capillary loops. Here there are both mononuclear and polymorphonuclear cells. The capillary walls are also thickened, but this is better appreciated in PAS or silver stains.* (**Right**) *This glomerulus has an infiltrate of monocytes in the capillaries, occluding the lumina. Patient has mixed cryoglobulinemia.*

Endocapillary Hypercellularity

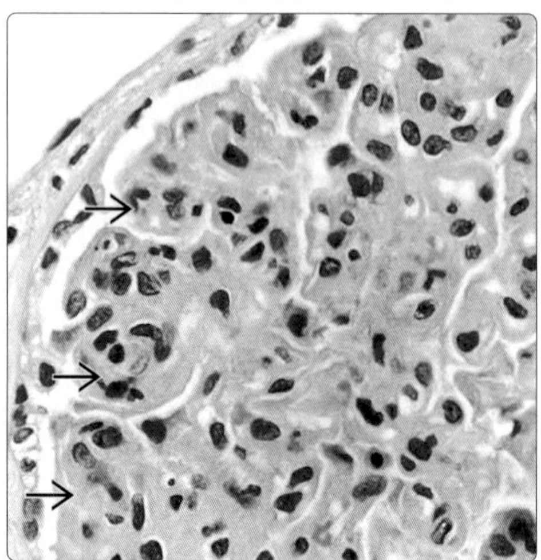

Mononuclear Endocapillary Hypercellularity

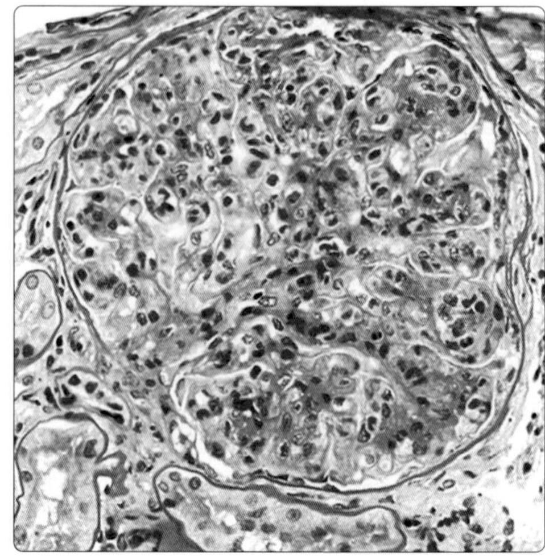

Cellular Crescent

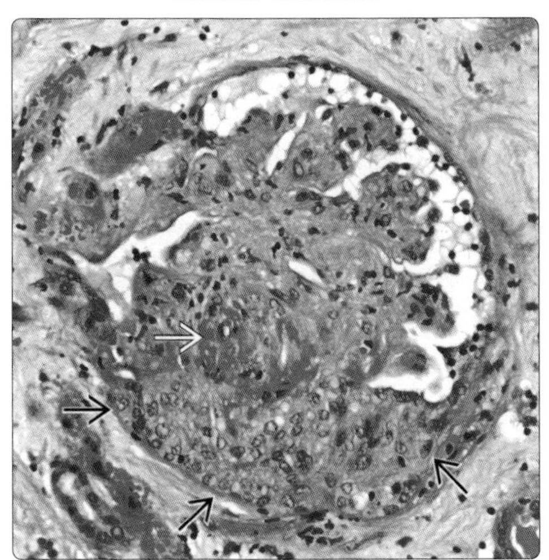

Cellular Crescent Blocking Tubule

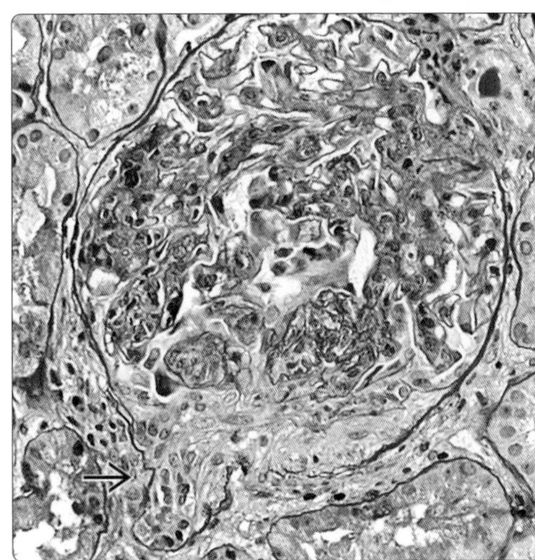

(Left) *H&E shows a cellular crescent ⇨ occupying 1/3 of the circumference of Bowman capsule with associated fibrinoid necrosis ➡. A crescent is defined as a layer of > 2 cells in Bowman space occupying ≥ 25% of the circumference of Bowman capsule. Crescents are also known as extracapillary proliferation.* **(Right)** *Crescents interfere with glomerular function by compressing the tuft and blocking the outlet of Bowman space into the proximal tubule ⇨.*

Fibrocellular Crescent

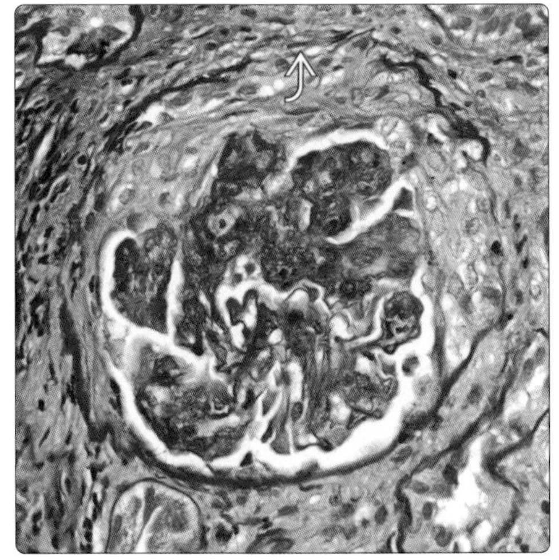

Fibrous Crescent

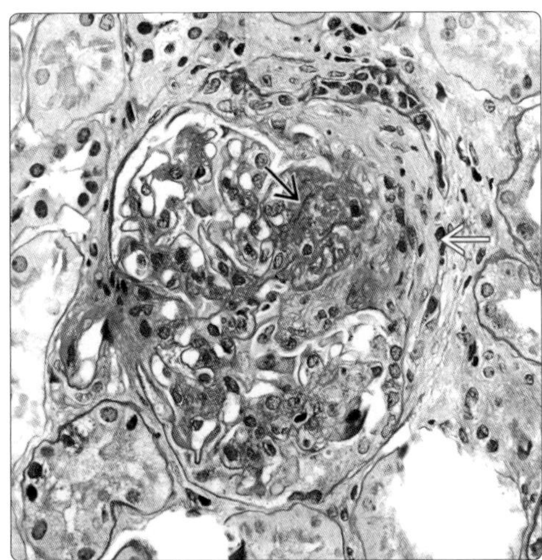

(Left) *Crescents start as a cellular proliferation of parietal epithelial cells and evolve into fibrocellular crescents (shown here), which have less cellularity and more collagen deposition. Disruption ➡ of Bowman capsule is present, a typical feature of crescents.* **(Right)** *A fibrous crescent remains in this glomerulus with associated adherent segmental sclerosis ⇨ of the tuft due to prior necrosis. Bowman capsule is disrupted ➡.*

Evolution of Crescents

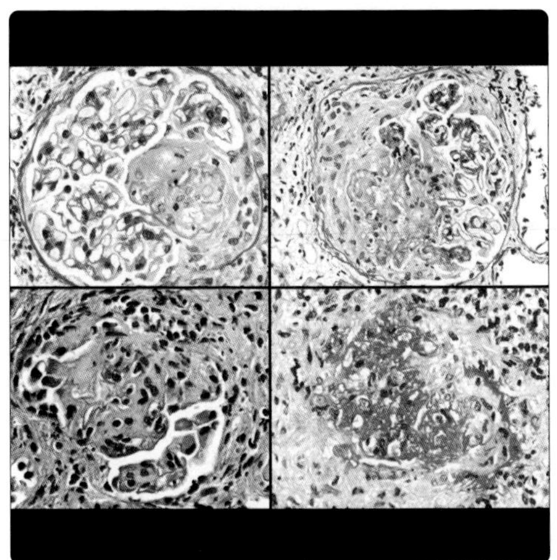

Global Glomerulosclerosis

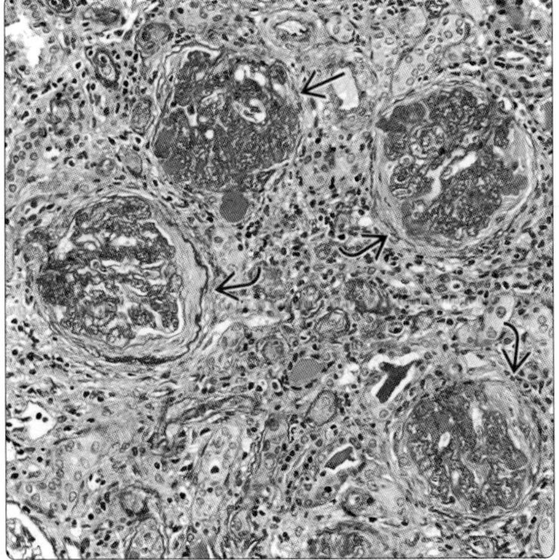

(Left) *Evolution of crescents is shown from cellular (upper left) to partial destruction of tuft (upper right), to global destruction of architecture (lower left), to "dissolving" global glomerulosclerosis with remnants of GBM and disrupted Bowman capsule (lower right).* **(Right)** *Global glomerulosclerosis is best appreciated in PAS stains because of the definition of the GBM and Bowman capsule. Three are "obsolescent" with matrix filling Bowman space ⇨ and one is "solidified" filling Bowman capsule ⇨.*

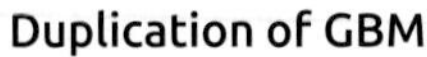

Duplication of GBM

Spikes in GBM

(Left) *Silver stain is useful to demonstrate abnormalities of the GBM in this patient with an allograft with transplant glomerulopathy, as shown here in a glomerulus with prominent duplication of the GBM (tram tracks)* . **(Right)** *GBM "spikes" can be appreciated in membranous glomerulonephritis on a thin (2 μm) silver-stained section. These protrusions of the GBM surround the silver-negative immune complex deposits.*

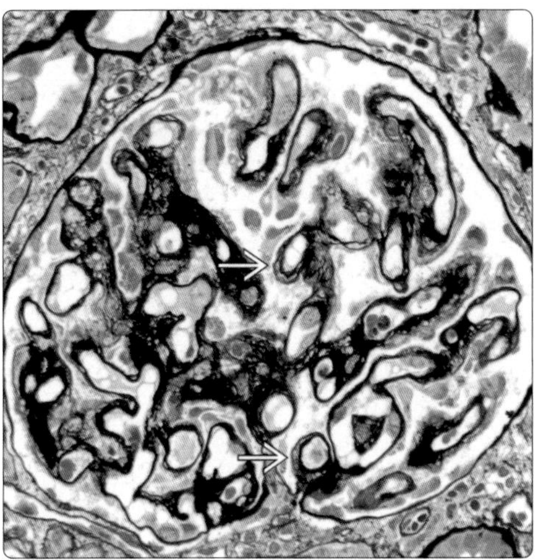

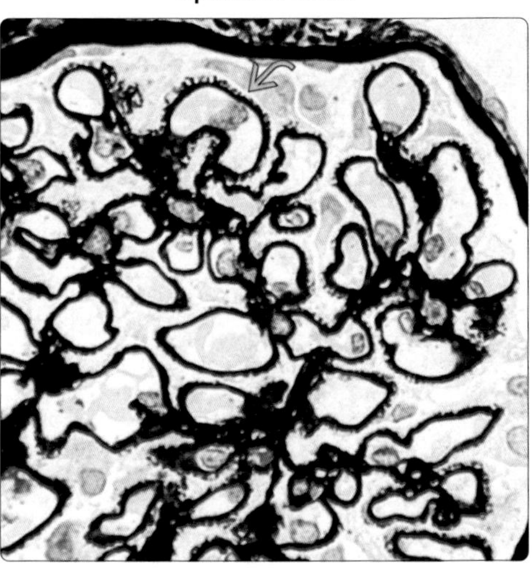

Wire Loops

Segmental Adhesion

(Left) *Wire loops are eosinophilic thickening of the glomerular capillary wall due to subendothelial deposits, shown here in a case of active lupus nephritis, class IV.* **(Right)** *Adhesion of a sclerotic glomerular segment to Bowman capsule is shown in a patient with idiopathic focal segmental glomerulosclerosis (FSGS). A useful feature to distinguish an adhesion from artifactual compression of the tuft against the Bowman capsule is the tenting of Bowman capsule toward the glomerulus.*

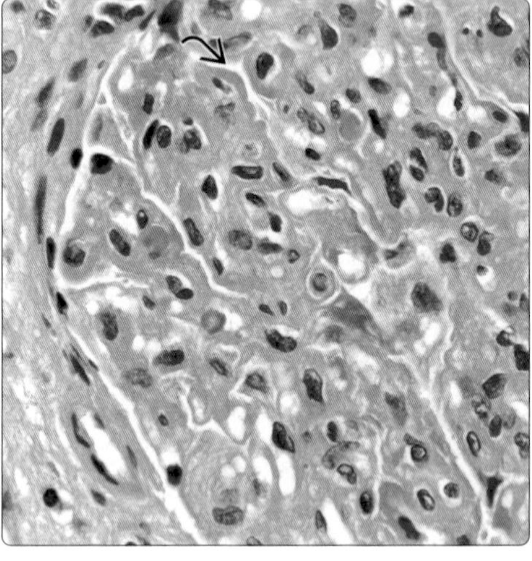

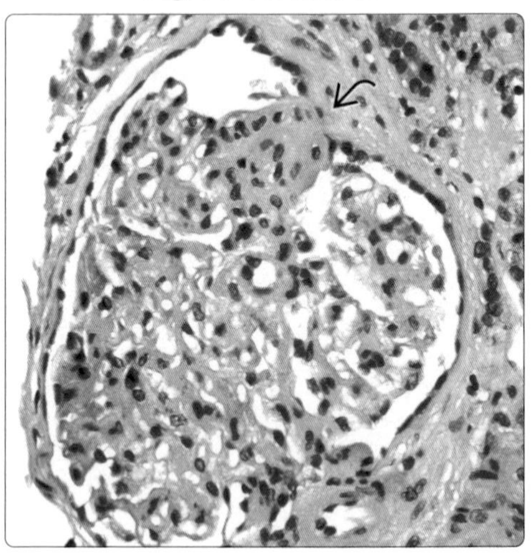

Adhesion With Hyaline Deposits

Collapsing Glomerulopathy With Pseudocrescent

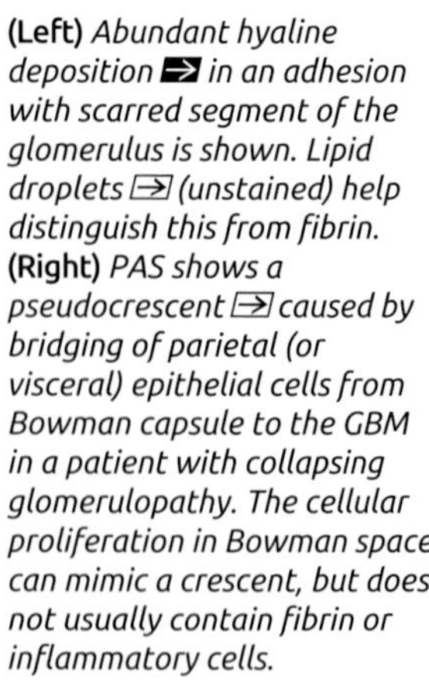

(Left) *Abundant hyaline deposition in an adhesion with scarred segment of the glomerulus is shown. Lipid droplets (unstained) help distinguish this from fibrin.* **(Right)** *PAS shows a pseudocrescent caused by bridging of parietal (or visceral) epithelial cells from Bowman capsule to the GBM in a patient with collapsing glomerulopathy. The cellular proliferation in Bowman space can mimic a crescent, but does not usually contain fibrin or inflammatory cells.*

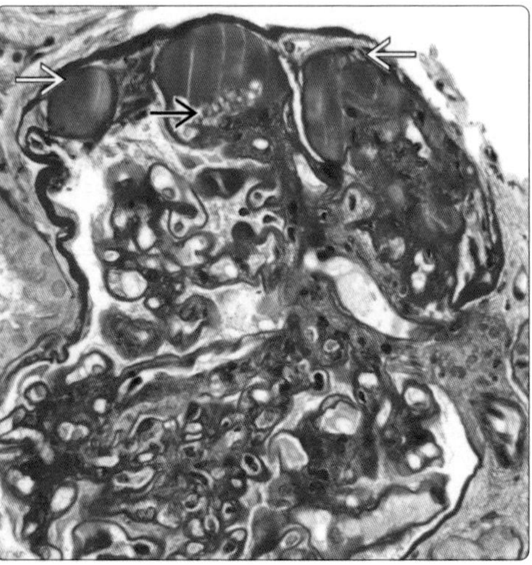

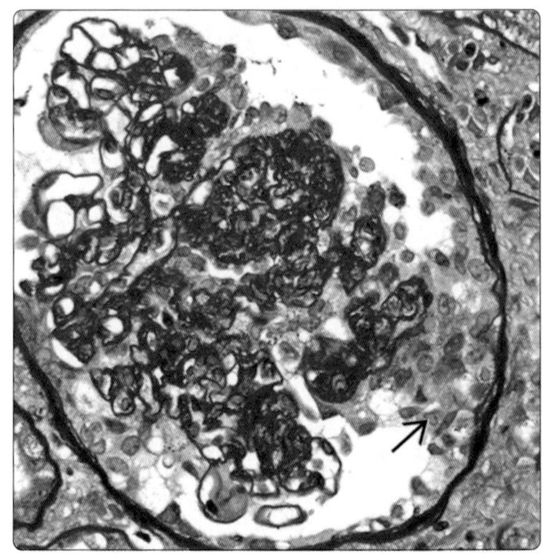

Red Cell Cast

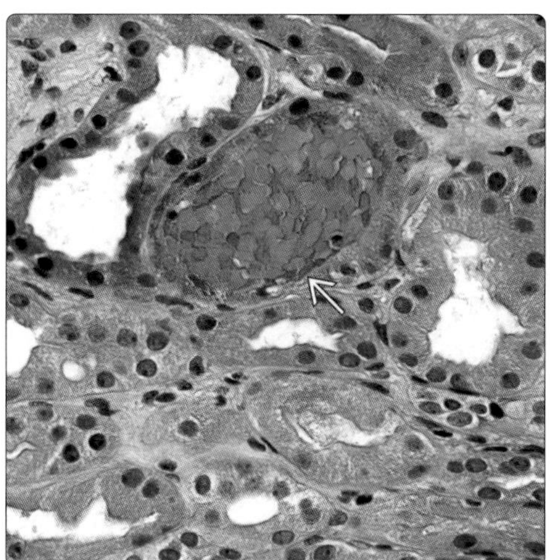

Hemolyzed Red Cell Cast

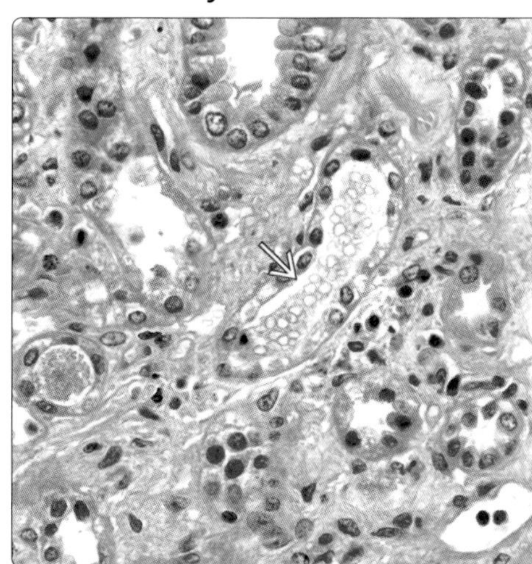

(Left) *Red cell cast in a tubule ➡ is shown. The compaction of the erythrocytes and complete filling of the tubule indicate that this is not an artifact of the biopsy procedure.* **(Right)** *Hemolyzed red cell cast in a tubule is shown ➡. The ghost cells can still be recognized on H&E. Hemolysis indicates that these are not artifacts of the biopsy. Patient has Henoch-Schönlein purpura.*

Pigmented Cast

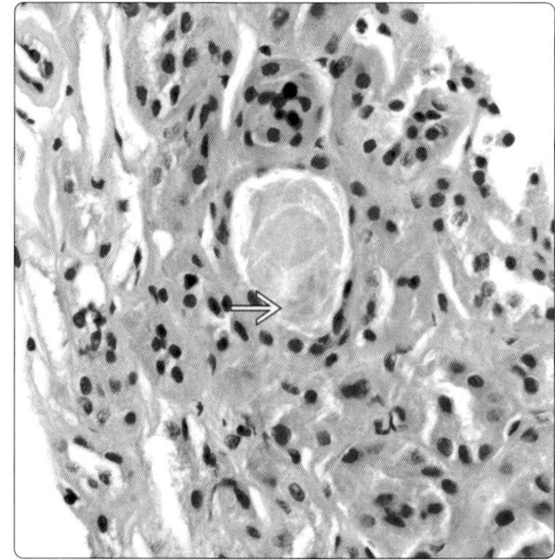

Cellular Cast

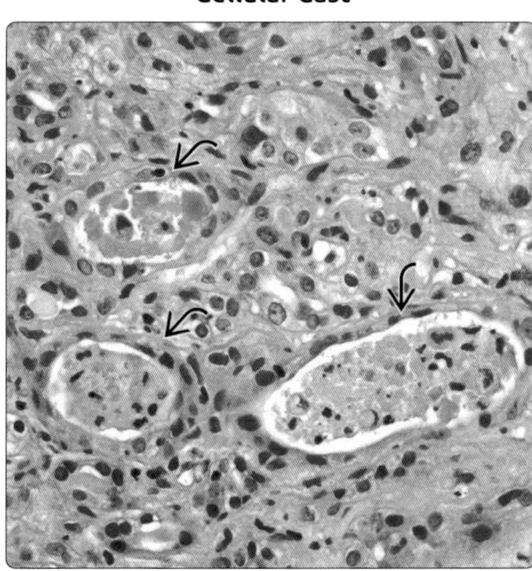

(Left) *A pigmented cast ➡ was all that remained as evidence of prior glomerular bleeding in a patient with IgA nephropathy.* **(Right)** *Casts ➡ in acute tubular necrosis typically contain nuclear fragments and eosinophilic cytoplasmic debris derived from necrotic tubular epithelial cells.*

Neutrophil Cast

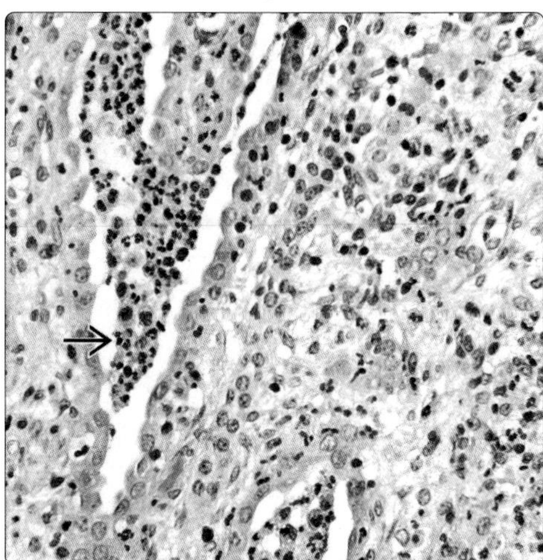

Myeloma Casts

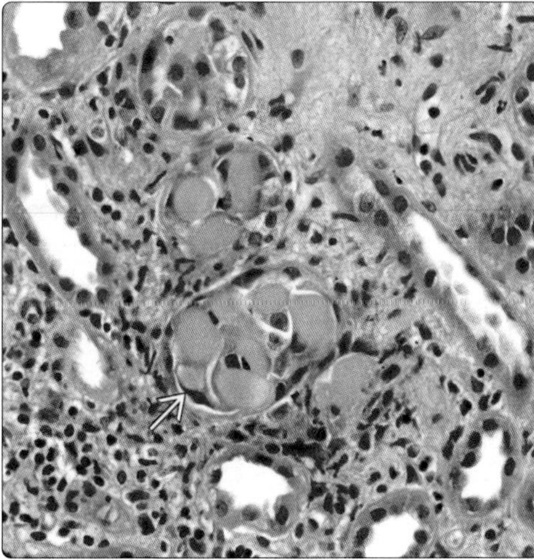

(Left) *In acute pyelonephritis (not often diagnosed in biopsy), prominent neutrophil casts ➡ can be seen in a collecting duct identifiable by its branching.* **(Right)** *Eosinophilic casts with attached mononuclear cells ➡ should raise suspicion of myeloma cast nephropathy, as illustrated in this case.*

(Left) *Normal tubules and interstitium in a donor biopsy stained with PAS are shown. Tubules are separated by peritubular capillaries, and there is minimal fibrous tissue.* **(Right)** *Tubular reabsorption droplets in the cytoplasm of proximal tubular cells are round granules that are positive ➢ with PAS stain. The distal tubules are negative →. Patient had minimal change disease.*

Normal Cortical Tubules and Capillaries

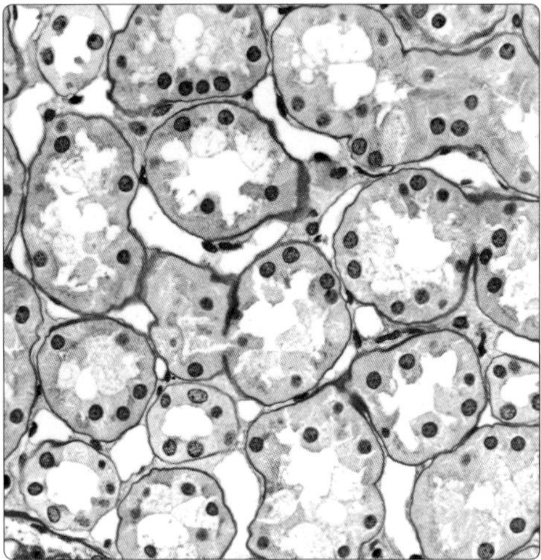

Tubular Reabsorption Droplets

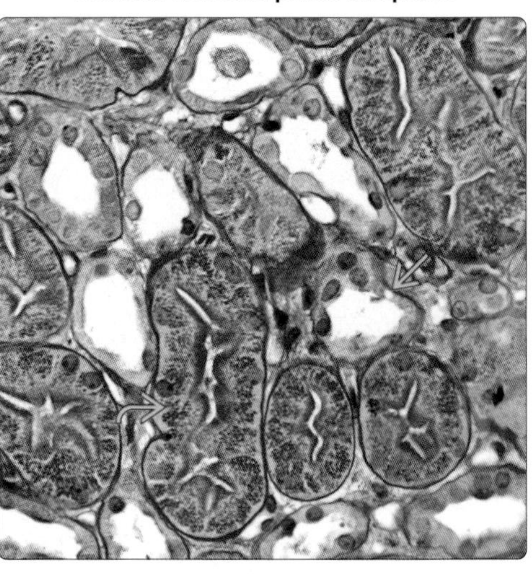

(Left) *PAS shows acute tubular injury with thinned cytoplasm ➢ with loss of brush border, decreased numbers of nuclei ➢, and granular casts →.* **(Right)** *Myoglobin casts are typically strongly eosinophilic and granular. They can be identified with antimyoglobin immunohistochemistry.*

Acute Tubular Injury

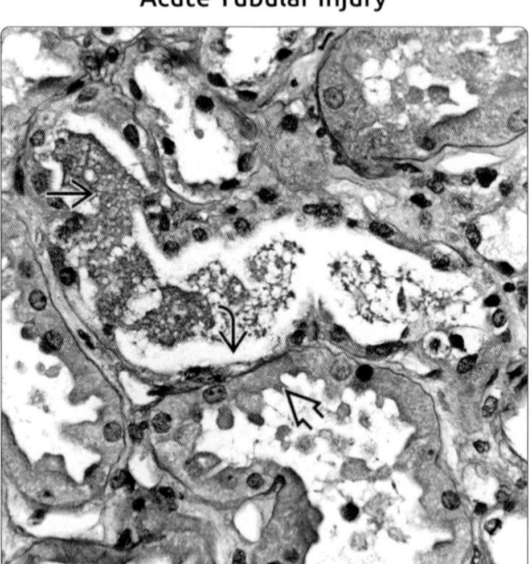

Myoglobin Casts

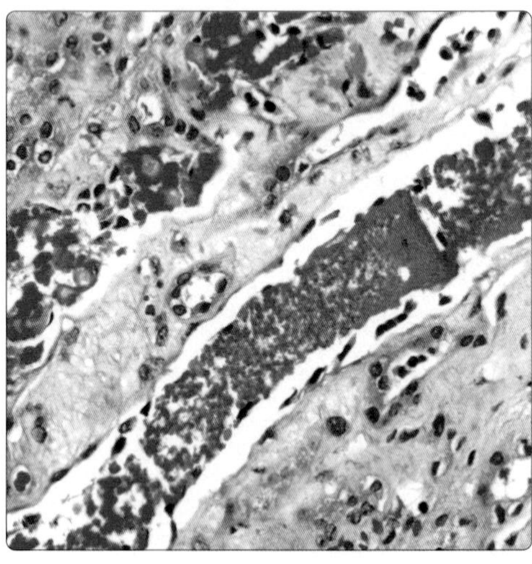

(Left) *Thyroidization is a term applied to the eosinophilic casts in atrophic, microcystic tubules. These are generally associated with chronic pyelonephritis but are not specific. They are caused by disruption of the tubules by scar and retention of Tamm-Horsfall protein.* **(Right)** *Nephrocalcinosis is manifested by TBM deposits of basophilic calcium salts ➢. Nephrocalcinosis can be seen in a variety of conditions with hypercalcemia and in nephrogenic systemic sclerosis related to gadolinium scans.*

Atrophic Tubules in Thyroidization Pattern

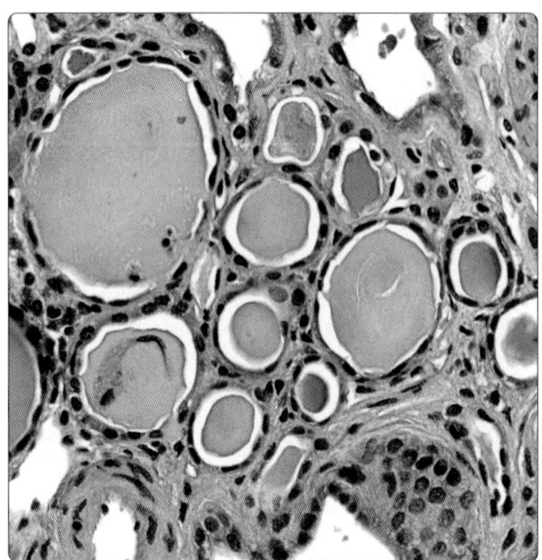

Nephrocalcinosis

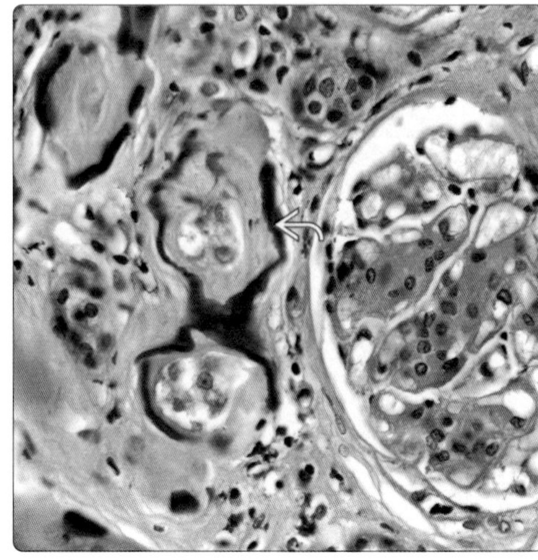

Urate Deposition With Giant Cells

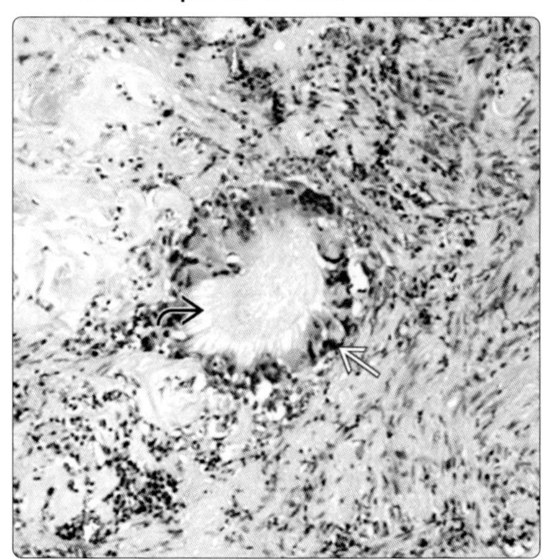

Acute Interstitial Inflammation

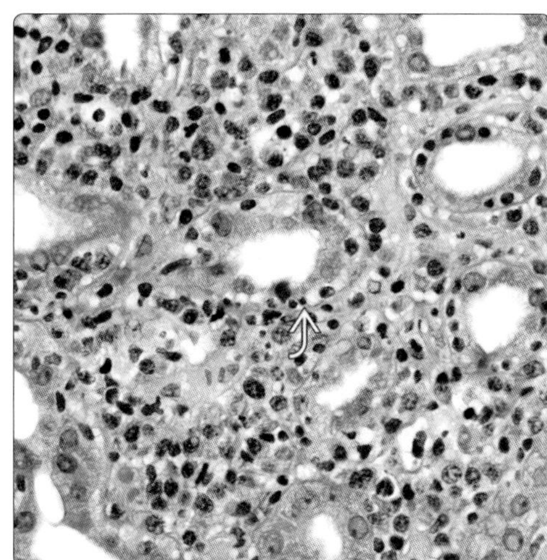

(Left) *H&E shows a urate deposit ➩ with a giant cell reaction ➡ in the medulla of kidney from a patient with gout. The crystals dissolve, in contrast to oxalates, but can be seen in frozen tissue.* **(Right)** *Acute interstitial inflammation with mononuclear cells separates and invades the tubules (tubulitis) ➡. This pattern can be seen in acute rejection (as in this case) or in drug allergy and other conditions.*

Granuloma Interstitium

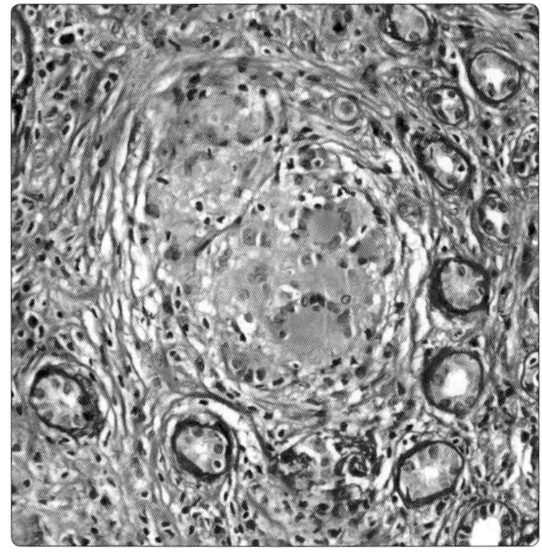

Neutrophils in Peritubular Capillaries

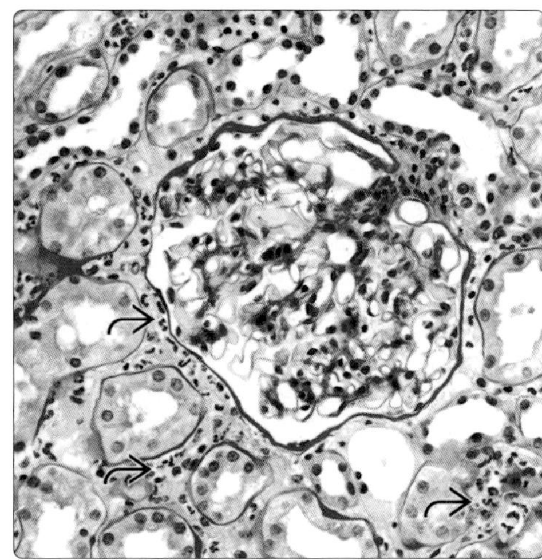

(Left) *Interstitial granuloma with multinucleated giant cells is shown. Granulomatous interstitial nephritis has a broad differential, including infection (mycobacteria, adenovirus), sarcoidosis, Crohn disease, and drug allergy.* **(Right)** *Neutrophils in peritubular capillaries (capillaritis) ➩ are a sign of acute antibody-mediated rejection. Neutrophils can be relatively inconspicuous.*

Mononuclear Cells and C4d in Peritubular Capillaries

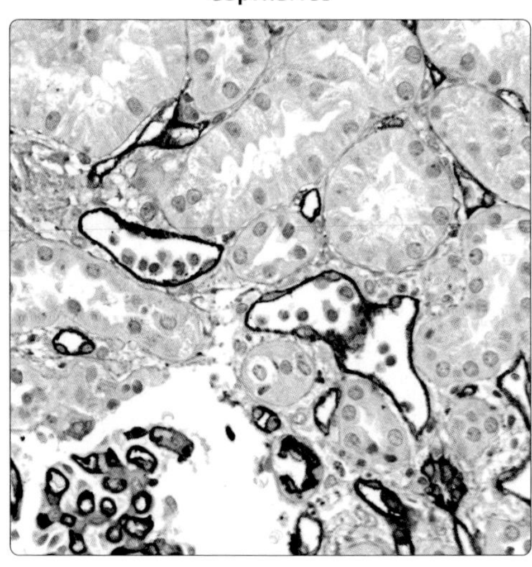

Focal Cortical Fibrosis

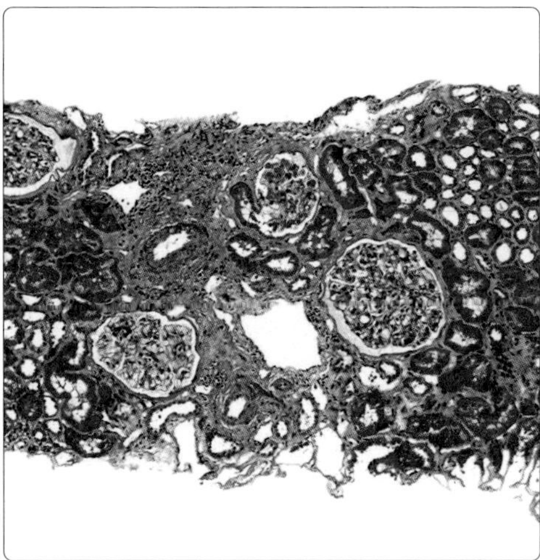

(Left) *Intracapillary mononuclear cells and positive staining for C4d in peritubular capillaries are defining characteristics of chronic humoral rejection.* **(Right)** *Trichrome stain allows more accurate assessment of interstitial fibrosis; illustrated here is focal fibrosis that is typical of vascular disease, with loss of tubules and relative preservation of glomeruli.*

(**Left**) *Arteriolar hyalinosis is PAS positive and may be focal, circumferential, or nodular . This case is a donor biopsy. Arteriolar hyalinosis is caused by hypertension, diabetes, aging, and calcineurin inhibitors.* (**Right**) *Leukocytoclastic vasculitis with nuclear dust and fibrinoid necrosis is evident in a small artery . Microscopic polyangiitis in a renal biopsy is associated with ANCA(+), cryoglobulinemia, and Henoch-Schönlein purpura.*

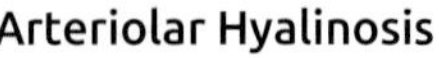

Arteriolar Hyalinosis

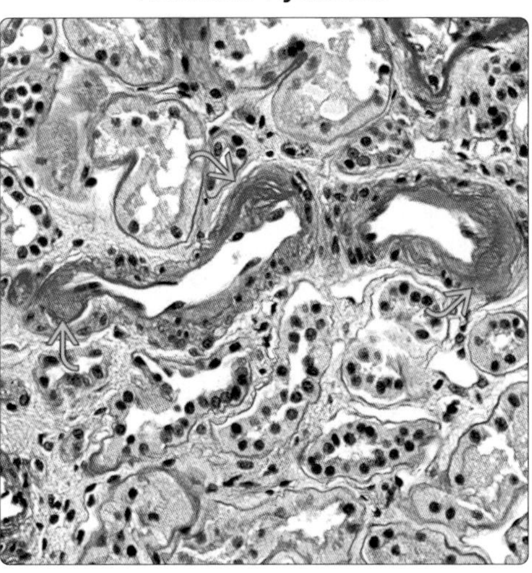

Leukocytoclastic Vasculitis

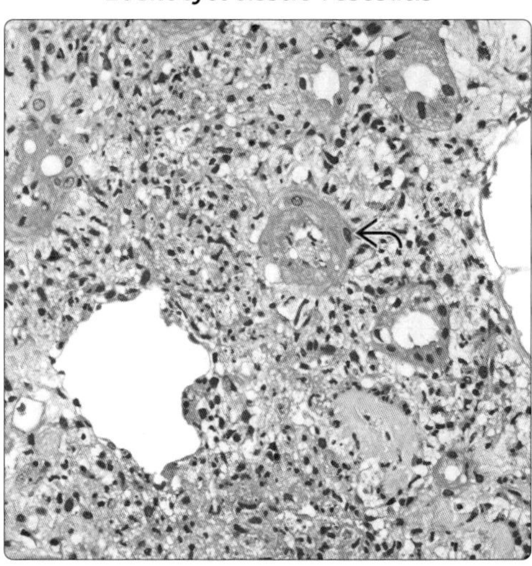

(**Left**) *Mucoid intimal thickening appears as a loose, slightly basophilic accumulation of matrix in the intima, a sign of thrombotic microangiopathy (TMA). In this case, it was related to a factor H mutation.* (**Right**) *Organized thrombus in an arcuate-sized artery in a patient with TMA is shown.*

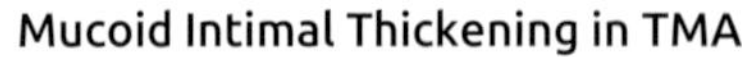

Mucoid Intimal Thickening in TMA

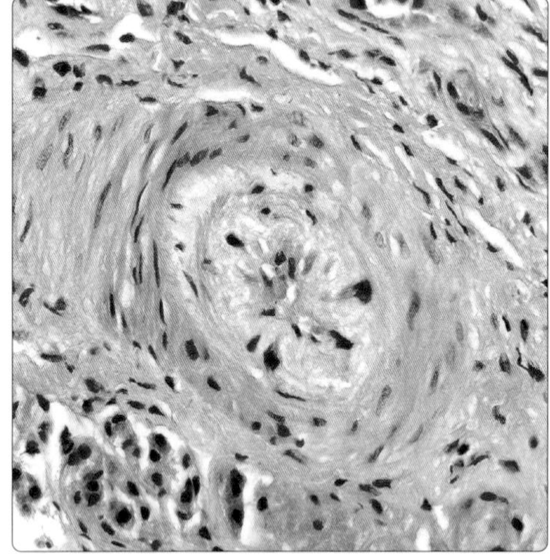

Organized Arterial Thrombus in TMA

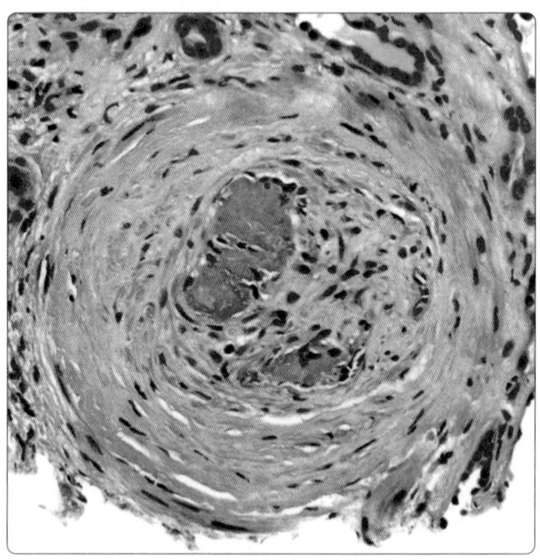

(**Left**) *Onion skin pattern of intimal thickening in a small artery in a patient with severe hypertension is shown.* (**Right**) *Elastic fiber stain highlights the fibroelastosis of the intima that occurs in longstanding hypertension.*

Onion Skin Thickening of Arteriole

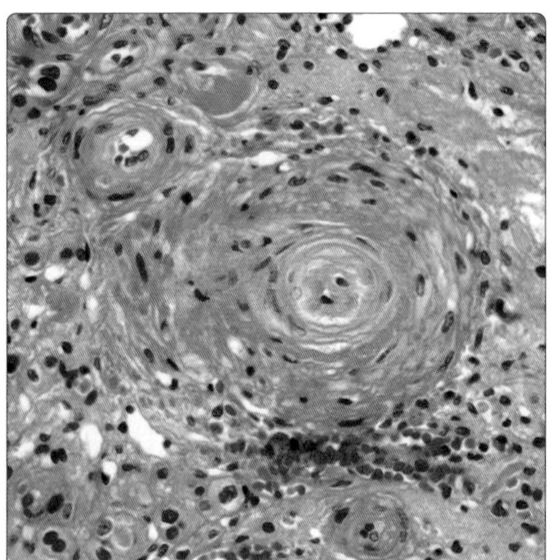

Fibroelastosis of Arterial Intima

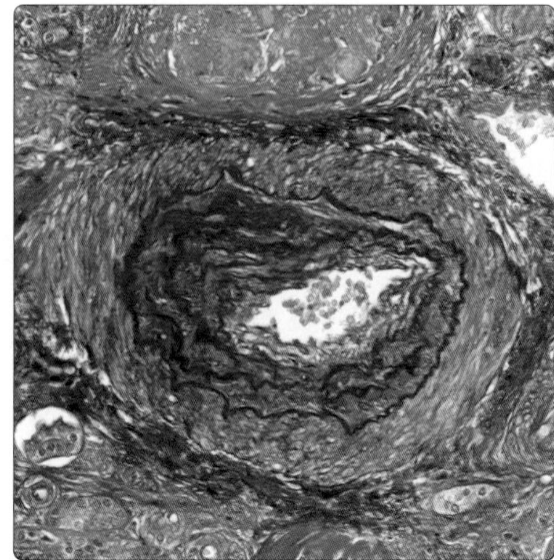

Finely Granular GBM Deposits (IgG)

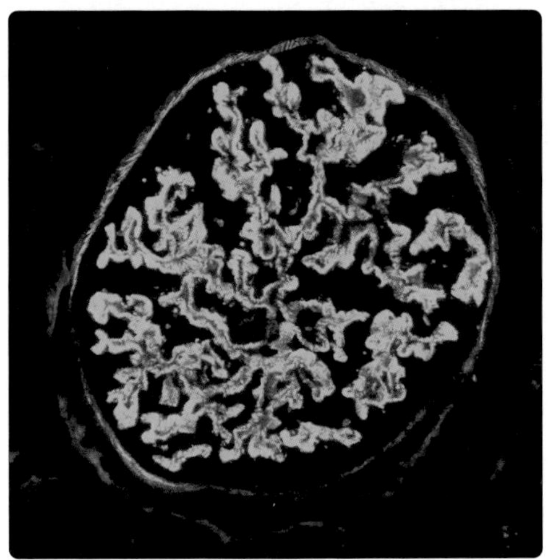

Coarse Granular GBM Deposits ("Humps") (IgG)

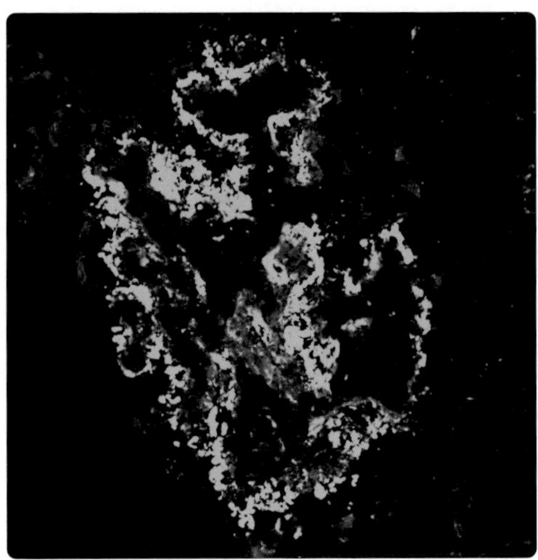

(Left) *Fine, uniform, granular deposits all along the GBM are typical of subepithelial deposits in membranous glomerulonephritis, here stained for IgG. Some appear to be in the mesangium, but these may be tangential cuts of the GBM.* **(Right)** *Rounded granular deposits of IgG along the GBM are typical of the "humps" of post-infectious glomerulonephritis (GN), as in this case of post-streptococcal GN.*

Broad Segmental GBM Deposits (IgG)

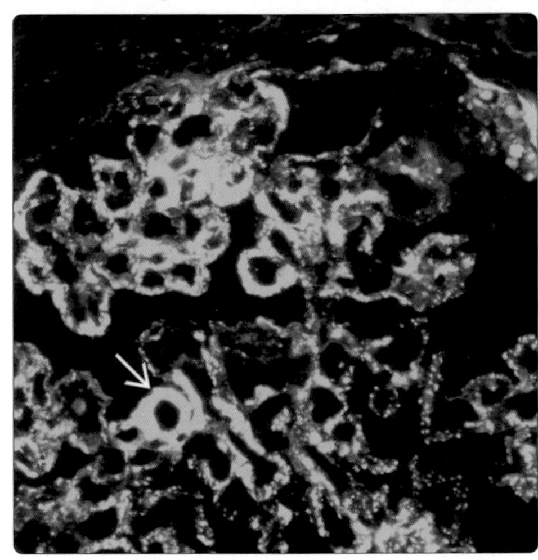

Mesangial Deposits

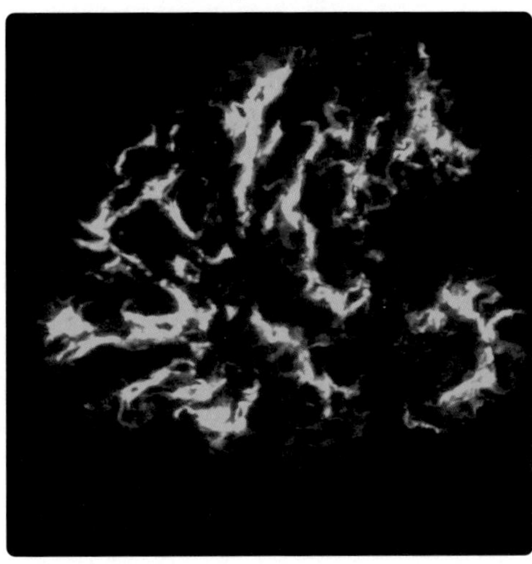

(Left) *Broad, granular, and elongated deposits ➡ along the GBM (sometimes referred to as "wire loop" lesions) are typical of subendothelial deposits, as in this case of lupus nephritis.* **(Right)** *Classical mesangial deposition pattern in glomerulus resembles the branches of a tree, as in this IgA stain in IgA nephropathy.*

Linear GBM Deposits

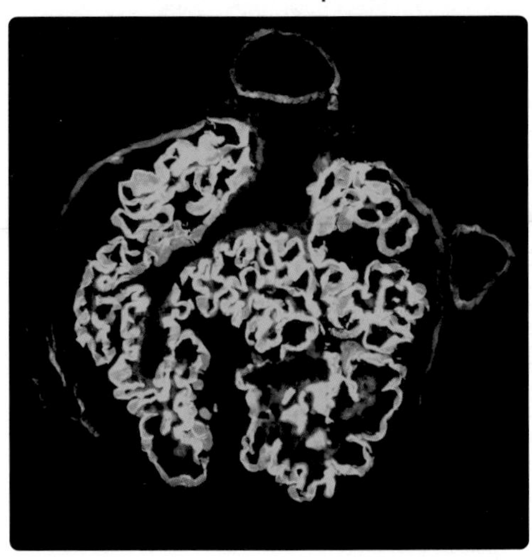

Coarse Granular Mesangial Deposits

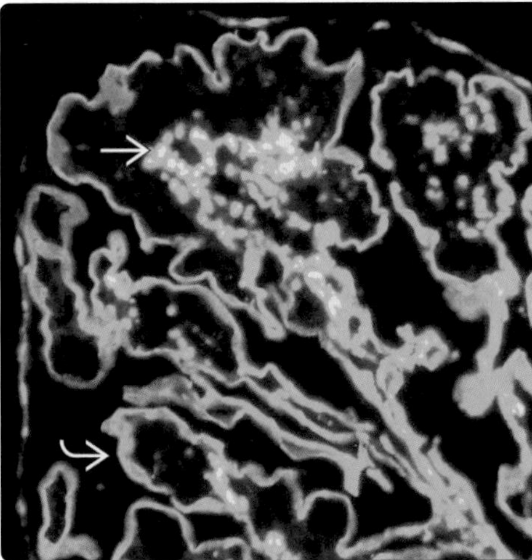

(Left) *Linear IgG in the GBM is characteristic of anti-GBM disease, as shown in this case. Diabetes can also have prominent linear IgG, but in that case, albumin is similarly present.* **(Right)** *Dense deposit disease has a unique IF pattern. C3 is deposited in coarse, brightly staining granules ➡ in the mesangium, sometimes with a dark center. Linear GBM staining ➡ is also present.*

(Left) *Glomerular pseudothrombi (hyaline thrombi)* ➡ *of mixed cryoglobulinemia appear as rounded, brightly stained deposits in glomerular capillaries when stained for IgM. These are not fibrin thrombi but rather are precipitates of immune complexes.* **(Right)** *IgM and C3 commonly are present in segments of glomeruli that are sclerotic, as shown here in a case of FSGS stained for IgM.*

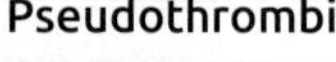

Pseudothrombi

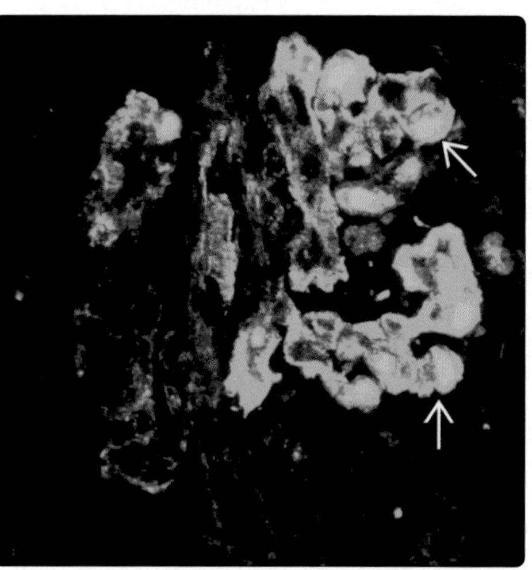

Segmental Glomerulosclerosis

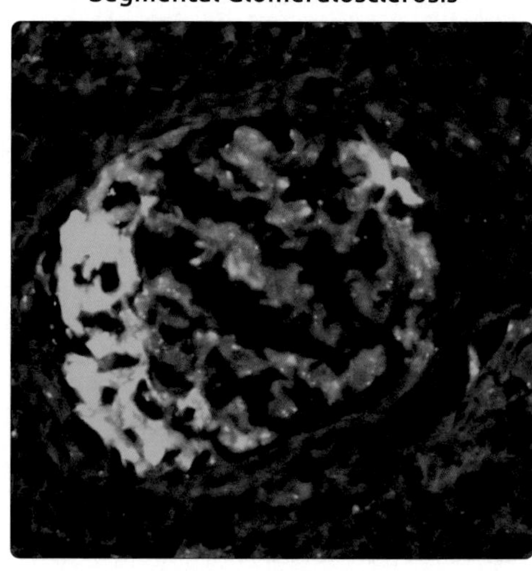

(Left) *Coarse granular C3 deposits in the mesangium and along the GBM* ➡ *are seen in diseases with mesangial and subendothelial deposits, as in this case of C3 glomerulopathy (or membranoproliferative glomerulonephritis, type I).* **(Right)** *Fibrillary GN has a distinctive pattern with deposits of IgG in the mesangium and segmentally along the GBM in a broad linear distribution.*

Coarse Granular GBM and Mesangial Deposits

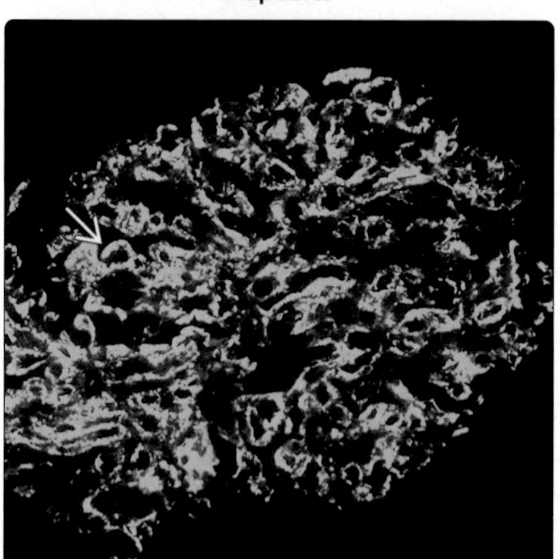

Broad Linear GBM Deposits

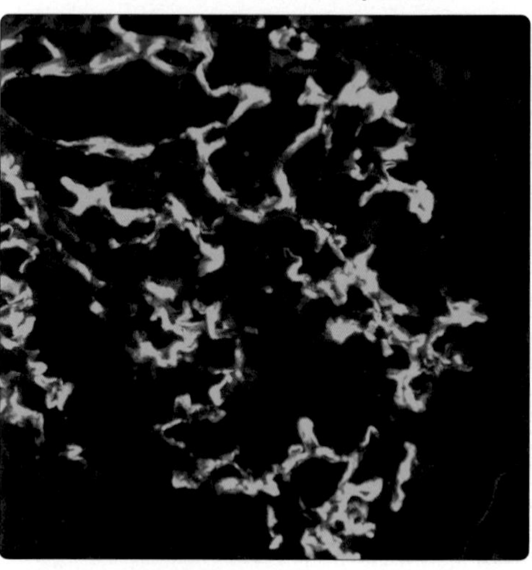

(Left) *Amyloid deposits in the glomeruli have broad, fairly homogeneous staining in the mesangium and GBM for the components of the amyloid (light chains, amyloid A protein, fibrinogen, etc.). This case is stained for amyloid A protein.* **(Right)** *Crescents typically have deposition of fibrin among the proliferating parietal epithelial cells. Activation of the clotting system in Bowman space is a general mechanism of formation of crescents, whatever the underlying glomerular disease.*

Broad Global Deposits (AA Protein)

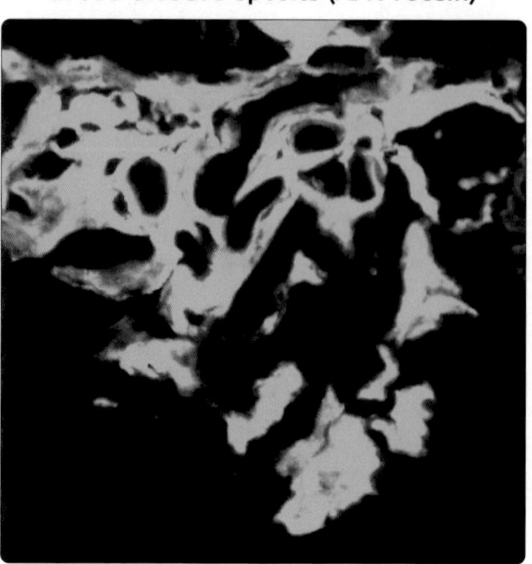

Fibrin in Crescent

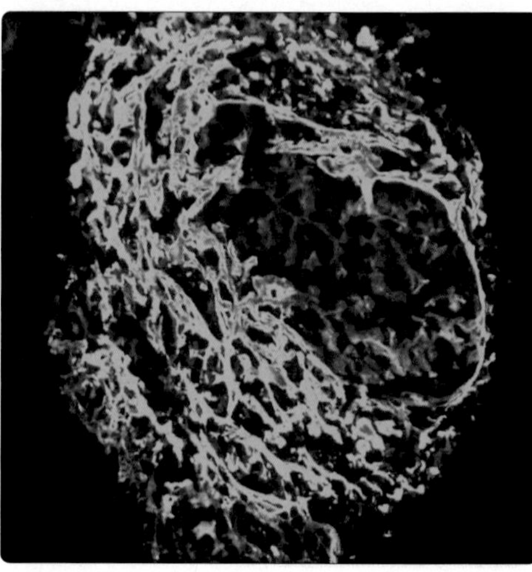

Tubular Reabsorption Droplets

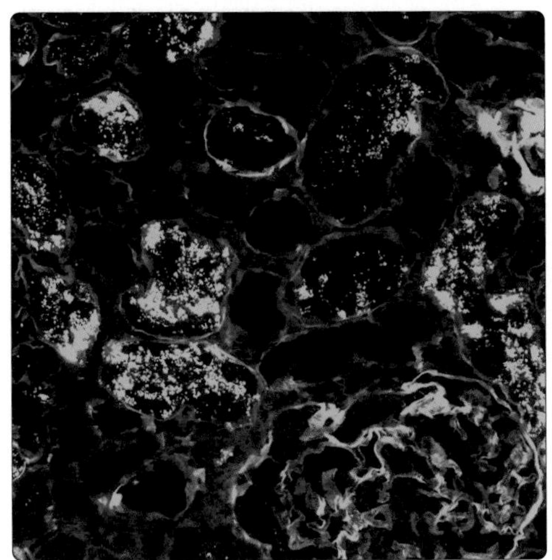

Granular TBM Deposits

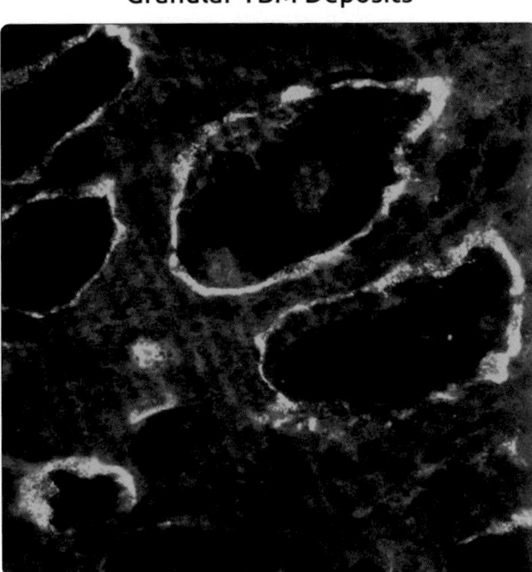

(Left) *Tubular reabsorption droplets stain for albumin (as in this image) and other plasma proteins (IgG, C3, fibrinogen, etc.). This is an indication of glomerular proteinuria in this case of minimal change disease.* **(Right)** *Granular deposits of IgG along the TBM can be seen in lupus nephritis and occasionally in other diseases, such as polyoma infections. In contrast, C3 deposits segmentally in the TBM are common and should not be taken as evidence of immune complex deposition.*

Myeloma Casts

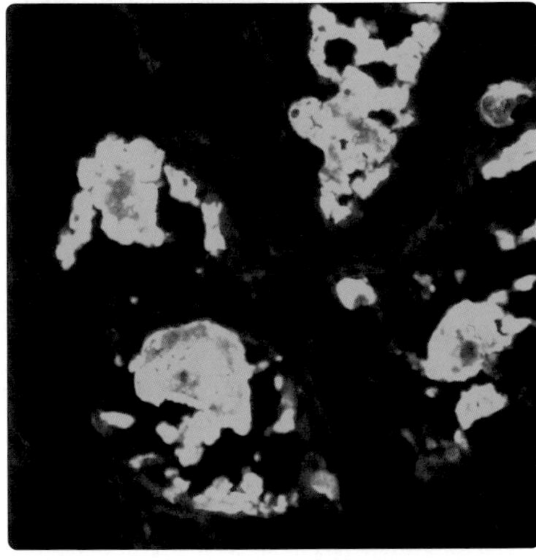

Fibrin in Arteriole in TMA

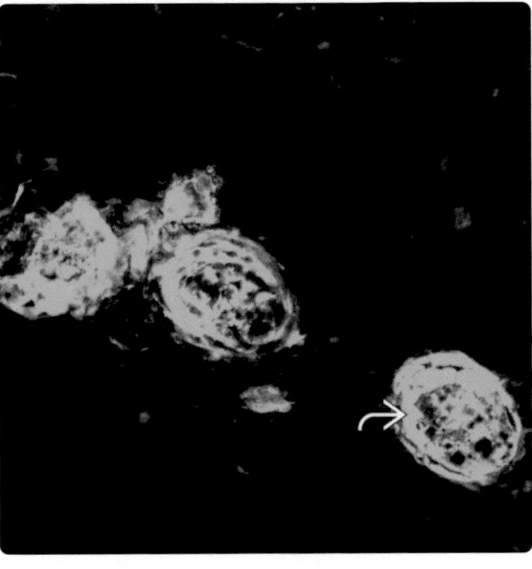

(Left) *Light chain staining is essential for the diagnosis of monoclonal gammopathies. In this patient with myeloma cast nephropathy, kappa, but not lambda, was detected in the casts in the tubules.* **(Right)** *Fibrin* ➦ *is detected in the arterioles in this case of thrombotic microangiopathy due to Avastin therapy. Fibrin also permeates the wall, a reflection of fibrinoid necrosis of the vessels.*

Broad Deposits in TBM

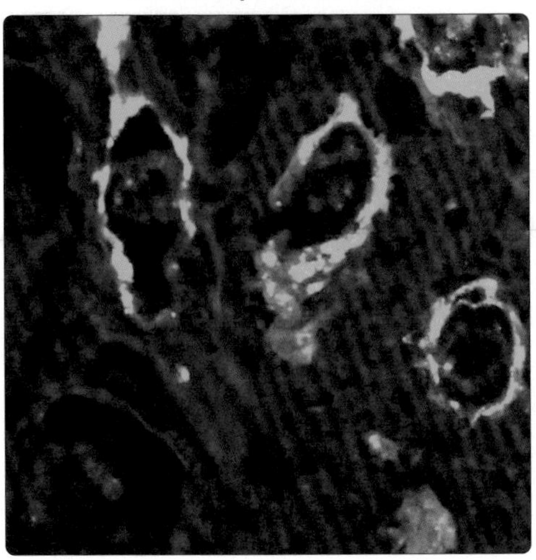

Tissue ANA

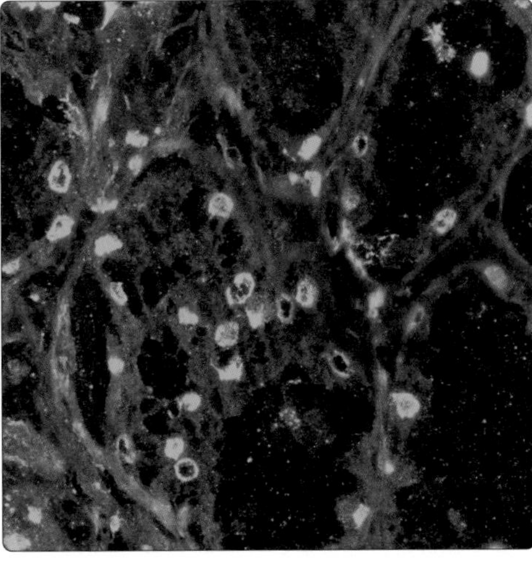

(Left) *C3 is not uncommonly detected in the tubular basement membrane, as in this case of calcineurin inhibitor toxicity in an allograft. Tubular cells activate the alternative complement pathway, and this is probably a manifestation of tubular injury.* **(Right)** *Lupus biopsies sometimes show antinuclear antibody (ANA) in tubular cells, here stained with anti-IgM. These are probably due to plasma ANA artifactually depositing during the IF staining procedure in permeabilized cells.*

(Left) *EM shows normal glomerulus with podocyte foot processes and a normal GBM. The normal GBM is thicker than a typical foot process.* (Right) *Widespread effacement of foot processes is a feature of minimal change disease and, to some degree, of other diseases with glomerular proteinuria.*

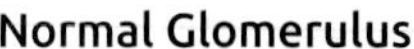

Normal Glomerulus

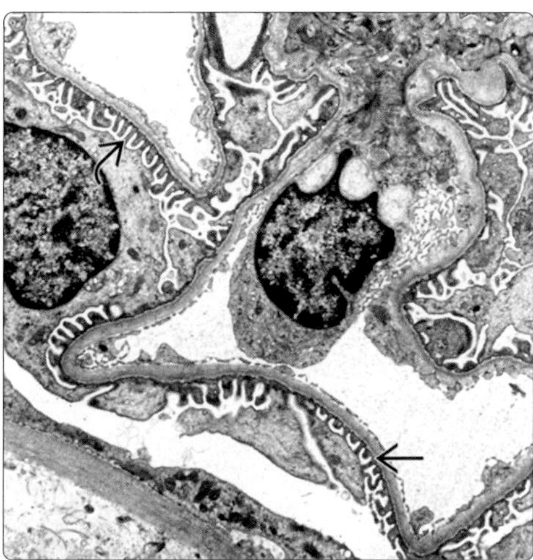

Foot Process Effacement

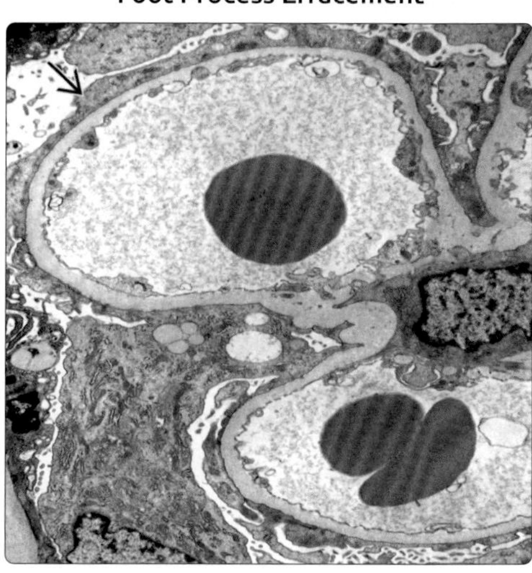

(Left) *Thin basement membrane disease has thin but otherwise normal GBM. The measurements are taken using a grid overlay. The distance is measured where the grid crosses the GBM, and the harmonic mean is calculated. Normal mean ± 2 s.d. is 373 ± 84 nm for men, 326 ± 90 nm for women.* (Right) *Diabetes has a uniformly thickened but otherwise normal GBM. The thickness has been measured using a grid overlay. Normal mean ± 2 s.d. is 373 ± 84 nm for men, 326 ± 90 nm for women.*

Thin GBM

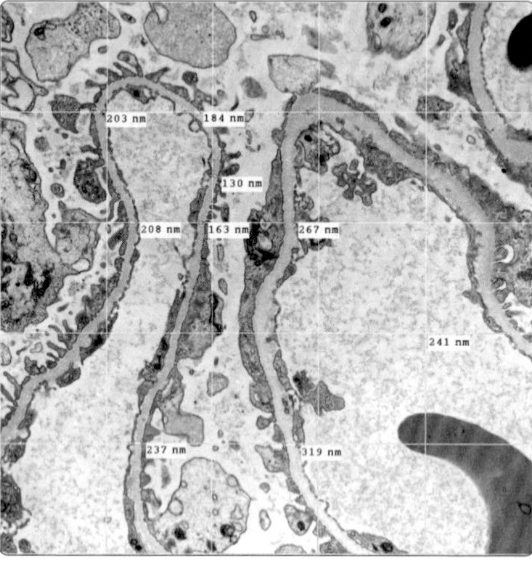

Thick GBM (Diabetes)

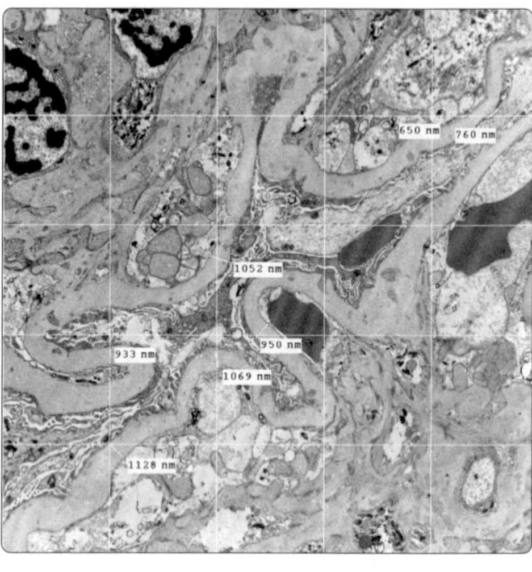

(Left) *Podocyte injury is sometimes reflected by new subepithelial layers of basement membrane matrix between the podocyte and original GBM. This is a characteristic feature of collapsing glomerulopathy. Intracapillary endothelial cells or macrophages contain lipid (foam cells).* (Right) *Fine reticulated lamination of a thickened GBM with scalloping of the subepithelial surface is a characteristic feature of Alport syndrome.*

Subepithelial New GBM

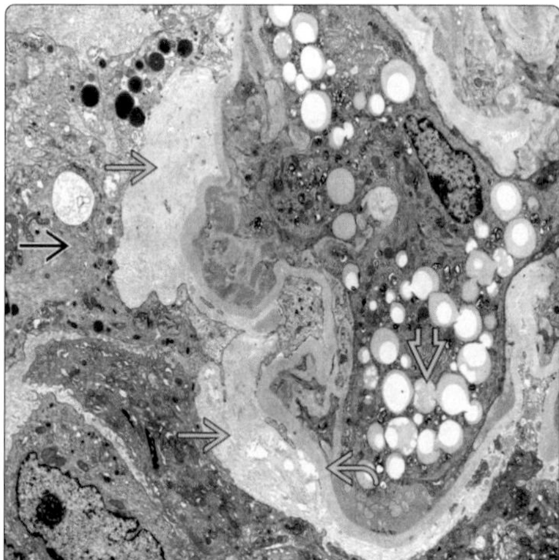

Lamination of GBM (Alport)

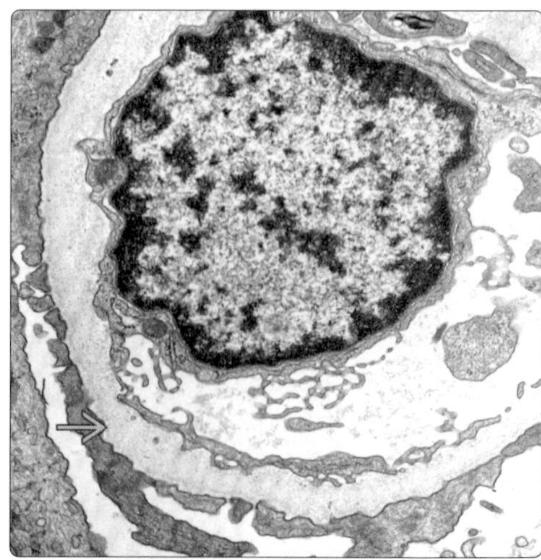

Microtubular Deposits (Cryoglobulinemia)

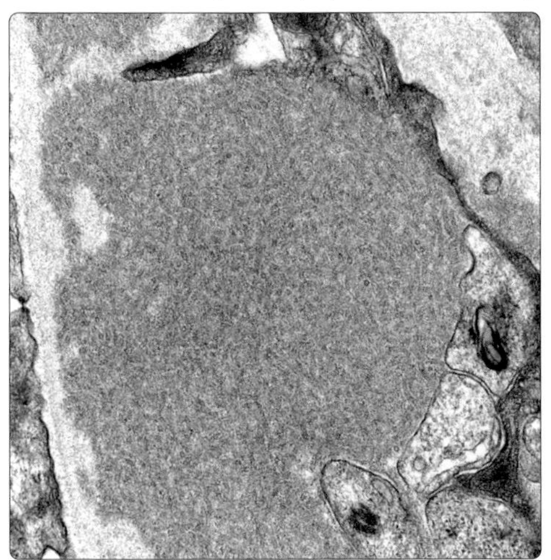

Microtubular Deposits (Immunotactoid Glomerulopathy)

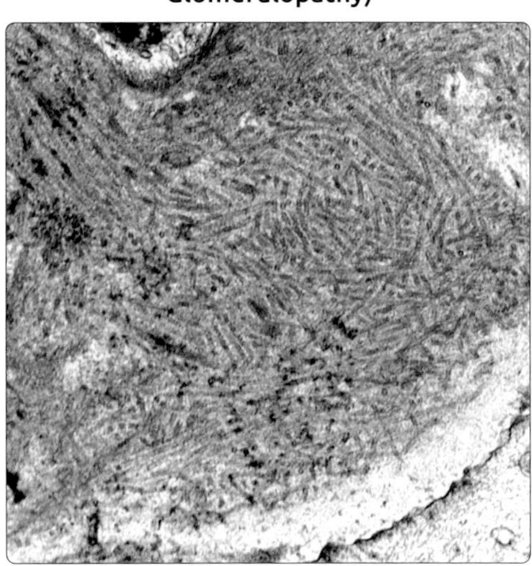

(Left) *EM shows an organized mesangial deposit in a patient with mixed cryoglobulinemia.* **(Right)** *Immunotactoid glomerulopathy has tubular deposits typically > 25 nm in diameter; in this case they measured ~ 35 nm.*

Fibrillar Deposits (Fibrillary GN)

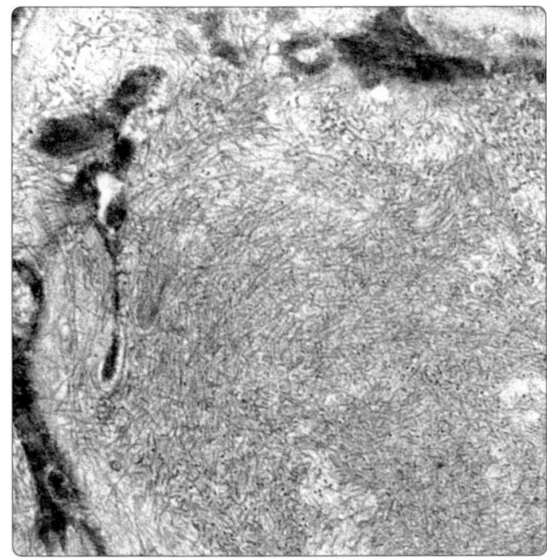

Amyloid Fibrils

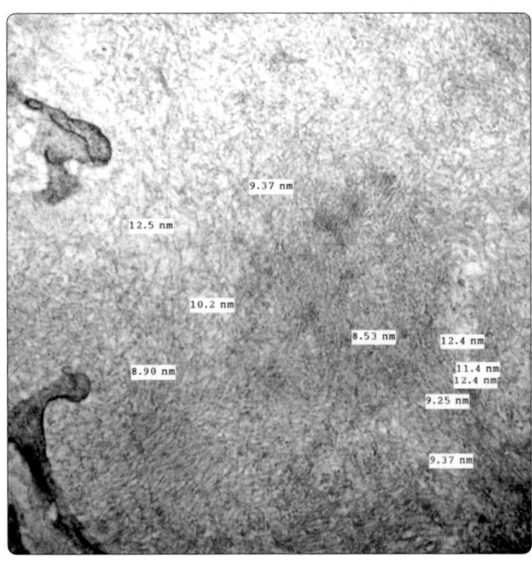

(Left) *Fibrillary glomerulonephritis has nonperiodic fibrils that are typically 10-20 nm in diameter; in this case they were ~ 13 nm in diameter.* **(Right)** *Amyloid fibrils are typically 8-12 nm in diameter without periodicity. These averaged ~ 10 nm. The appearance is similar to fibrillary glomerulonephritis, and a Congo red stain is necessary to confirm their identity.*

Type III Collagen Deposits

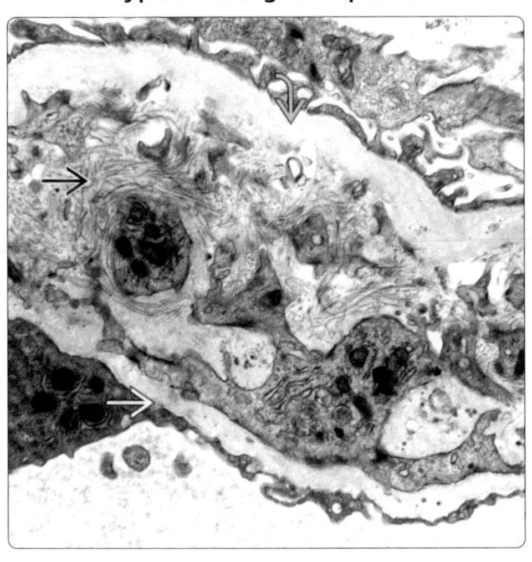

Fibrillar Collagen in Mesangium

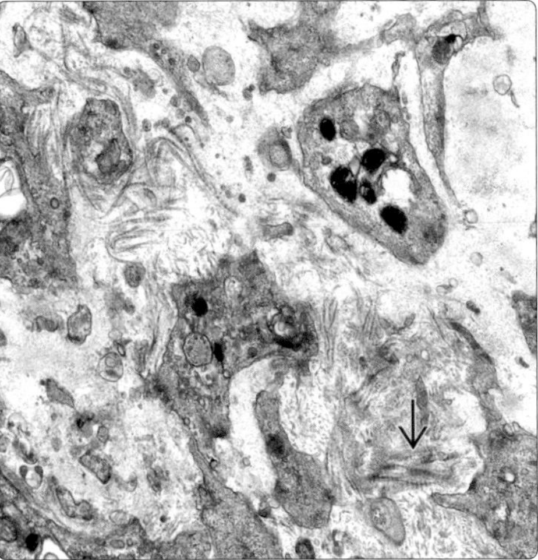

(Left) *Type III collagen glomerulopathy (collagenofibrotic glomerulopathy) has deposits of fibrillar collagen with a periodicity of 62 nm →. The GBM is duplicated; original ⇗ and new ➡ subendothelial layers are indicated.* **(Right)** *Fibrillar collagen → is sometimes detected in the mesangium as part of a pathologic process of sclerosis. Here the fibrils are seen in a case of IgA nephropathy. This should not be confused with type III collagen glomerulopathy.*

(Left) *EM of a glomerulus from a patient with poststreptococcal GN shows the characteristic humps located along the GBM in the subepithelial space ➡. These do not elicit a GBM response of spikes in contrast to membranous GN.* (Right) *A glomerular capillary has subepithelial deposits with spikes of GBM between them ➡. This is a typical feature of membranous GN in contrast to postinfectious GN. The neutrophil ➡ in the capillary may be a sign of renal vein thrombosis.*

Subepithelial "Humps"

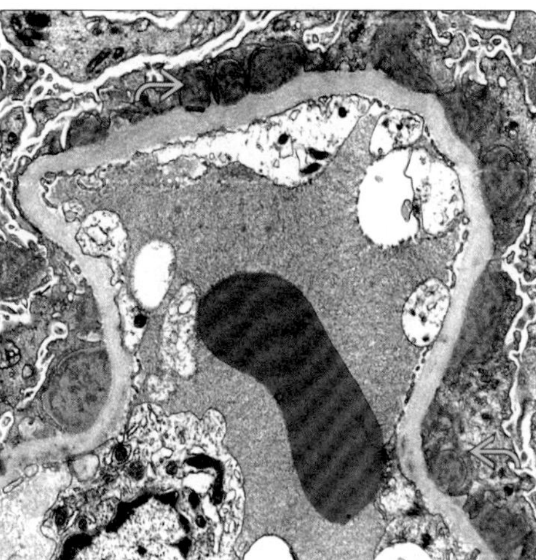

Subepithelial Deposits and GBM Spikes

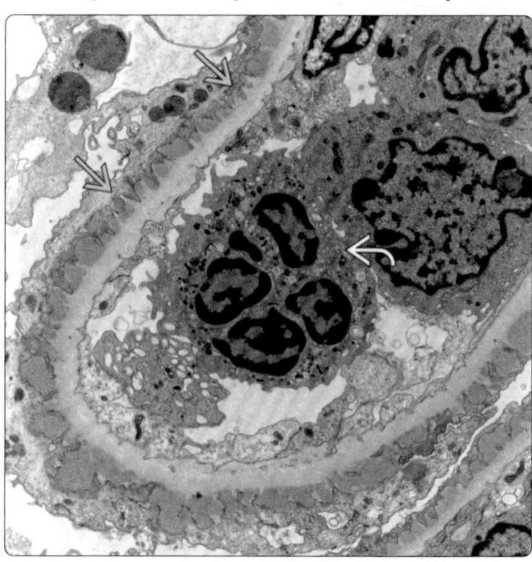

(Left) *Mesangial deposits ➡ in IgA nephropathy typically hug the mesangial cells ➡ and are amorphous.* (Right) *Subendothelial deposits ➡ are present in many glomerular diseases and usually elicit a new layer of GBM over their surface, as in this case from a patient with lupus nephritis. Subepithelial deposits are also present and penetrate the GBM ➡.*

Mesangial Deposits

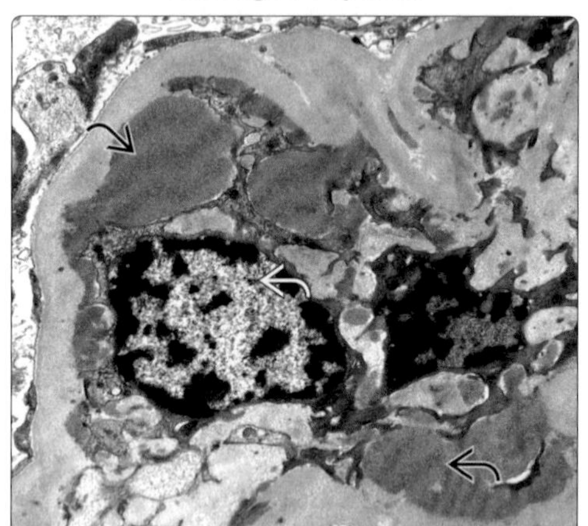

Subendothelial and Subepithelial Deposits

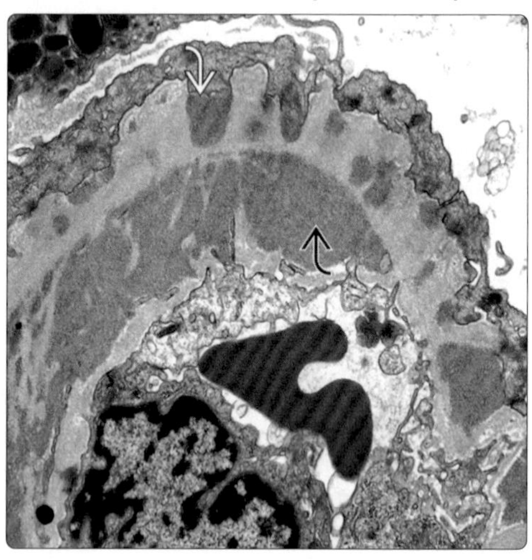

(Left) *Immune complex deposits can be reabsorbed or dissolved with time, in which case they begin to lose their electron density ➡, as in this case of membranous GN.* (Right) *The reabsorption of deposits occurs with time in most diseases; here, a subepithelial deposit in membranous GN is almost completely removed ➡ and resurfaced with a new layer of subepithelial GBM ➡.*

Partial Reabsorption of Deposits

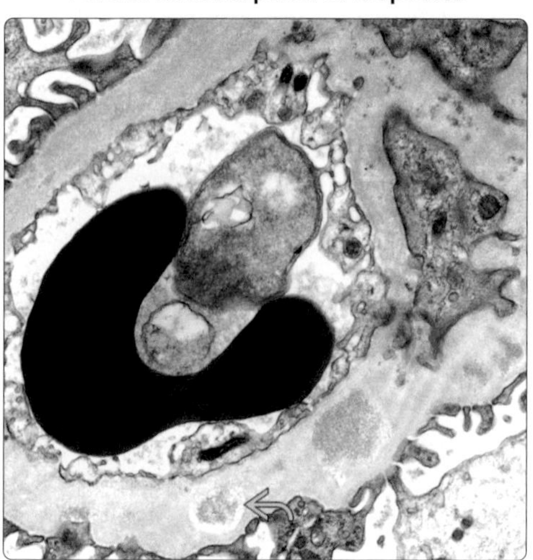

Reabsorbed Deposit

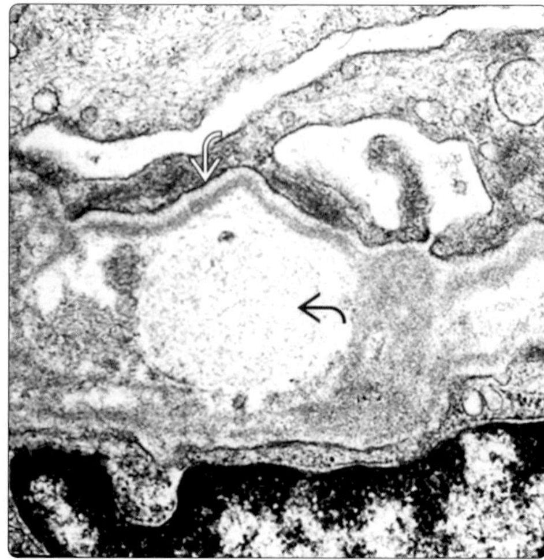

Granular GBM Dense Deposits

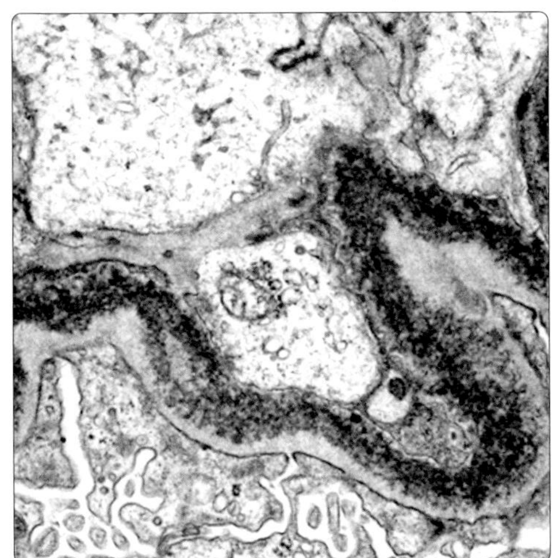

Dense Deposit Disease

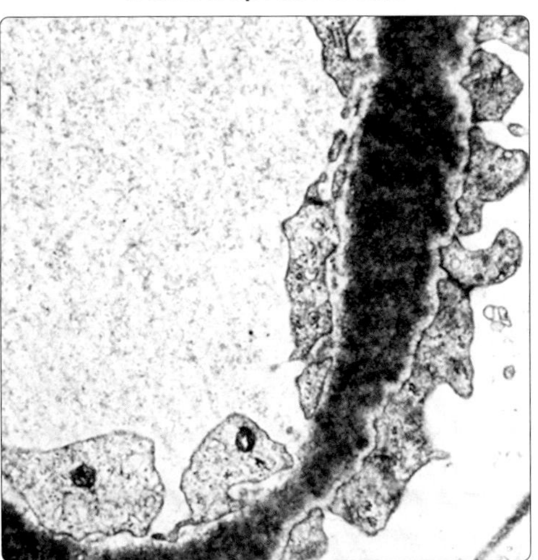

(Left) *Granular dense deposits in the GBM, mesangium, TBM, and vascular basement membrane characterize systemic light chain deposition, here shown in a glomerular capillary in a patient with κ light chain deposition by IF.* **(Right)** *The densest deposit in renal pathology by EM is that in dense deposit disease (DDD), here shown replacing the GBM in a glomerular capillary in a child with DDD. The deposits contain C3 and factor H.*

Fingerprint Deposits

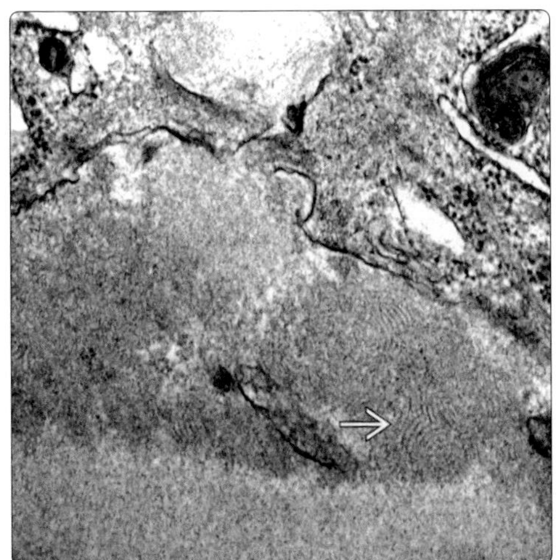

Fibrin in Bowman Space

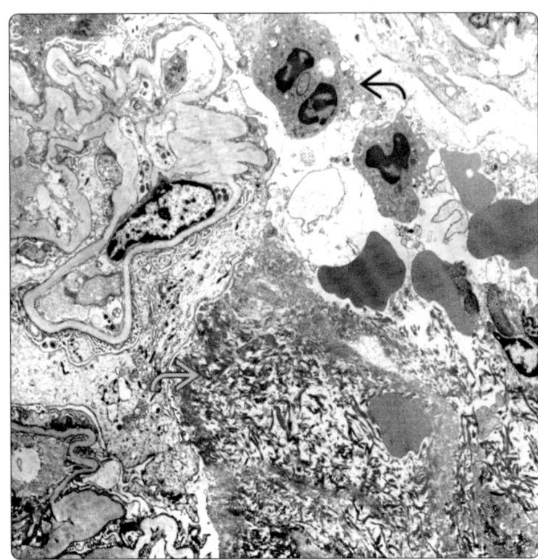

(Left) *Deposits with periodicity are sometimes evident in lupus nephritis, where they have been called "Churg's thumbprints" for the renal pathologist who 1st described them.* **(Right)** *Fibrin by EM appears denser than the usual immune complex deposit and has a fibrillar tactoid pattern; sometimes the 22 nm periodicity is evident. Shown here are fibrin and neutrophils in Bowman space in a patient with ANCA-related GN and crescents.*

Tubuloreticular Structure

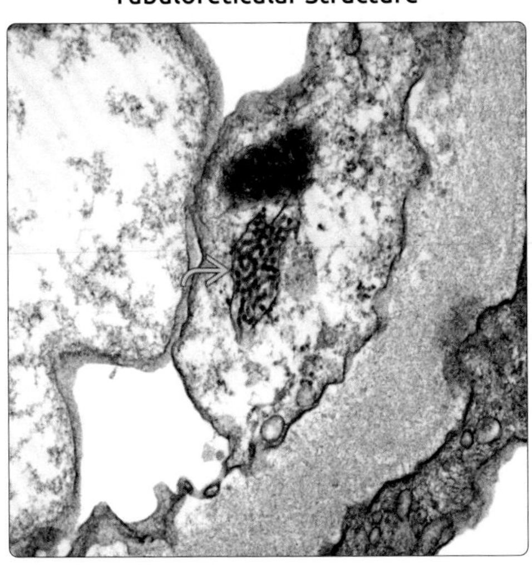

Particulate Subepithelial Deposit

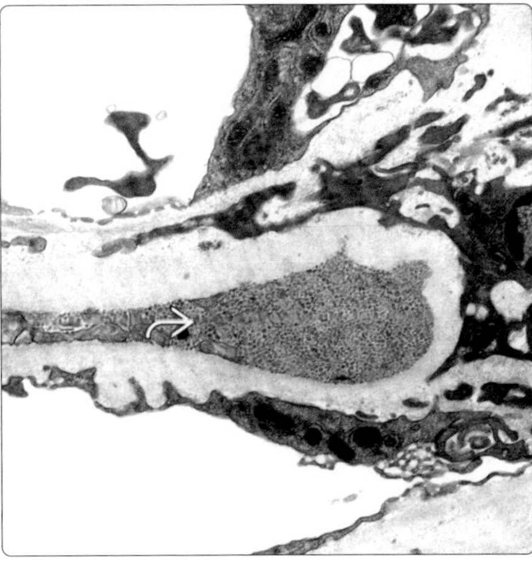

(Left) *Once thought to be a virus, this intracellular tubular aggregate in a glomerular endothelial cell is known as a "tubuloreticular structure" . This is a cellular response to interferons and is most often found in lupus and in patients treated with interferons.* **(Right)** *A particulate subepithelial deposit of unknown nature is sometimes found without clear explanation. This is almost certainly not a virus; theories include lipoproteins or components of the podocyte.*

TERMINOLOGY

Abbreviations

- Glomerular basement membrane (GBM)
- Peritubular capillaries (PTC)

MACROSCOPIC

Anatomic Features

- Kidneys
  - Paired, bean-shaped organs
    - Each weighs 150 g, measures 11 cm in length, 5-7 cm wide, and 3 cm thick
      - Smaller in women, but size best correlates with body surface area and weight
      - After 3rd decade, progressive decline in renal mass due to glomerulosclerosis
  - Located in retroperitoneal space, extending from 12th thoracic to 3rd lumbar vertebrae
    - Hilum oriented slightly anteriorly
    - Renal sinus refers to concave space at hilum composed of adipose tissue, renal pelvis, and neurovascular structures
    - Calyces converge into renal pelvis, which narrows inferiorly as ureter
  - Smooth outer surface covered by translucent, fibrous capsule surrounded by perinephric fat
  - Fetal lobulations demarcated by surface grooves seen mostly in infants

Longitudinal Cross Section of Kidney

- Dark brown outer cortex and paler inner medullary "pyramids"
- Cortex ~ 1 cm in thickness
  - Extends between medullary pyramids
    - Referred to as "columns of Bertin"
- Pyramid and surrounding cortex constitute renal lobe
  - Normal kidney has 11-14 lobes
- Each kidney has 7-10 medullary pyramids
  - Papillae are tips of medullary pyramids

Podocyte Foot Process and Slit Diaphragm Complex

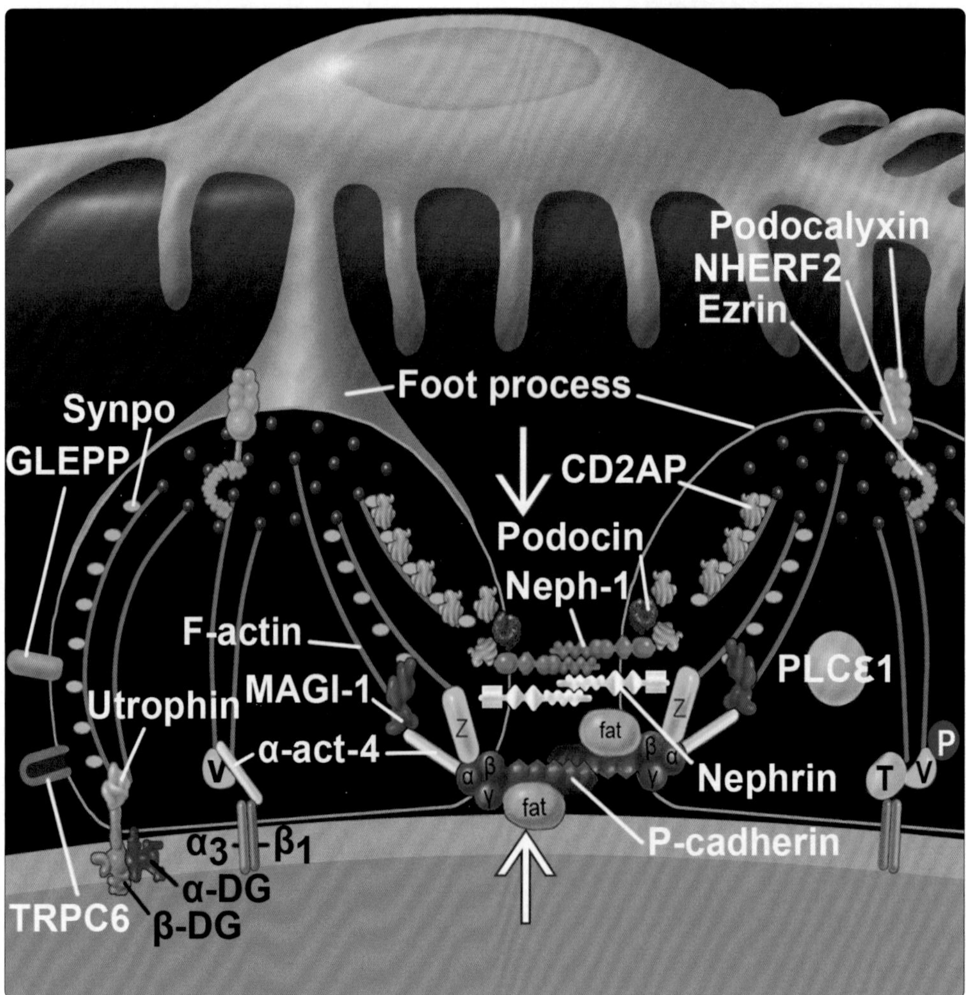

The slit diaphragm complex ➡ is a highly specialized cell junction connecting the foot processes of adjacent podocytes. It is composed of proteins (e.g., nephrin, podocin, CD2AP) expressed by the podocytes.

- Most central papillae drain single lobe termed "simple papillae"
  - Have slit-like openings of ducts of Bellini
  - Convex tips aid prevention of urinary reflux from pelvis into kidney
- Papillae in superior and inferior poles drain 2-3 lobes termed "compound papillae"
  - Orifices of ducts of Bellini rounded and gaping open
    - Susceptible to intrarenal reflux

Vascular Supply and Nerve Innervation

- Arterial supply
  - Kidney receives 25% of cardiac output
  - End arteries have no collateral blood flow
  - Renal artery from aorta enters hilum and divides into anterior and posterior segmental branches
    - Segmental arteries divide into 6-8 interlobar arteries
      - Traverse between renal lobes and penetrate renal parenchyma at corticomedullary junction
    - Interlobar arteries continue as arcuate arteries at right angles along corticomedullary junction
      - Branch as afferent arterioles that terminate as glomerular capillary tufts
    - Arcuate arteries give rise to interlobular arteries that extend into outer cortex at right angles
- Venous drainage
  - Blood from PTCs and vasa recta drains sequentially into interlobular, arcuate, and interlobar veins
  - Larger veins traverse parallel to arteries, merge into renal veins, and drain into inferior vena cava
  - Due to high perfusion rates, renal arteriovenous oxygen gradient much lower than other organs
- Lymphatic supply
  - Lymphatic drainage follows vasculature
    - Begin in adventitia of interlobular arteries, merge with other lymphatics, and exit from renal hilus
      - Drain into hilar and paraaortic lymph nodes
    - No periglomerular or peritubular lymphatic vessels
    - Superficial outer cortex drained by transcapsular lymphatics that join hilar lymphatics
- Nerve supply
  - Sympathetic fibers from celiac plexus traverse via splanchnic nerves to ganglia in renal plexus
  - Nerve fibers traverse along arterial system and innervate vessels, cortical tubules, and juxtaglomerular apparatus
  - Sensory fibers from kidney also travel along sympathetic pathways to T10-T11 nerves

MICROSCOPIC

Architectural Organization

- Cortex organized into 2 architectural components
  - Cortical labyrinth
    - Consist of glomeruli, proximal and distal convoluted tubules, and initial portions of collecting ducts
    - Vasculature includes interlobular arteries and veins, arterioles, venules, and capillaries
    - Scant interstitium has PTCs and interstitial cells
  - Medullary rays
    - Elongated medullary projections extend into cortex
    - Composed of tubular segments arranged at right angles to corticomedullary junction
    - Tubular segments include collecting ducts and straight segments of proximal and distal tubules
- Medulla composed of inner and outer segments
  - Outer medulla has outer and inner stripes
    - Outer stripe composed of straight portions of proximal tubule, collecting ducts, and thick ascending loops of Henle
    - Inner stripe has thin descending and thick ascending loops of Henle and collecting ducts
  - Inner medulla has thin descending and ascending loops of Henle and collecting ducts of Bellini

Nephron

- Functional unit derived from metanephric blastema
- ~ 1,000,000 nephrons per kidney
- Each nephron contains glomerulus and tubule
  - Glomeruli confined to cortex
  - Tubule consist of proximal tubule, loop of Henle, and distal tubule
  - Outer and midcortical glomeruli extend short loops of Henle into inner stripe of outer medulla
  - Glomeruli at corticomedullary junction (juxtamedullary glomeruli) have long loops of Henle that dip deep into inner medulla
- Distal nephron tubule drains into collecting ducts and eventually into renal pelvis
  - Both embryologically derived from ureteric bud
- Renal progenitor/stem cells are in 3 intrarenal "niches"
  - Identified in renal papillae, proximal tubules and in parietal layer of glomerulus
  - Progenitor cells are identified by various markers including CD24 and CD133

Glomerulus

- Consists of capillary tuft anchored at vascular pole and floats in Bowman space surrounded by Bowman capsule
- Mean adult diameter of glomerulus is 200 μm
  - Juxtamedullary glomeruli slightly larger
- Cellular components include endothelial cell, mesangial cell, podocyte, and parietal epithelial cell
  - Evidence for cross talk via signaling pathways between glomerular cells
  - Cytokines synthesized by 1 cell type may influence receptors on other cells
    - For example, vascular endothelial growth factor (VEGF) produced by podocytes affects endothelial cells
- Extracellular matrix includes mesangial matrix, GBM, and Bowman capsule
- Glomerular filtration barrier composed of endothelial cell surface layer, endothelial cells, GBM, slit diaphragm, and subpodocyte space
  - Components restrict filtrate flow based on charge, shape, and size of molecules
- Endothelial cells
  - Cytoplasm covers inner aspect of capillary loop
    - Has microtubules and filaments that provide cytoskeletal support
  - Nucleus and nonfenestrated cytoplasm usually reside over mesangial interface

- Thin, attenuated layer of fenestrated cytoplasm extends along GBM
  - Fenestrations 70-100 nm in diameter
- Surface polyanionic glycoproteins, such as podocalyxin, impart negative charge
  - Restrict filtration of plasma molecules
- Endothelial surface layer is carbohydrate-rich meshwork coating luminal aspect of endothelial cells
  - Important component of glomerular filtration barrier
- Secrete molecules involved in immune response and coagulation system
- Express MHC class II molecules

- Mesangial cells
  - Restricted to 1-2 nuclei per matrix area (for 2 μm thick tissue section)
  - Numerous cytoplasmic processes extend to endothelial cells, mesangial GBM, and other mesangial cells
    - Make direct contact and form gap junctions with endothelial cells through fenestrations at interface
  - Smooth muscle properties of mesangial cells mediated by vimentin intermediate filaments, actin-based cytoskeleton, and contractile proteins
  - Phagocytic properties for degradation of immune complexes
  - Secrete molecules that participate in matrix production and degradation in response to injury
- Podocytes or visceral epithelial cells
  - Specialized cell with large cell body and multiple elongated arborizing cell processes that end in terminal structures called foot processes
  - Terminally differentiated with tight control of cell cycle
  - Participate in GBM synthesis, contribute to glomerular filtration barrier, and help maintain hydraulic regulation of capillary loop diameter
  - Express unique set of molecules including Wt1, C3b receptors, and vimentin, but not cytokeratin intermediate filaments
  - Reside in urinary space and attached to GBMs via foot processes
  - Cell body resides near GBM reflection of adjacent capillary loops and consists of major organelles
    - Separated from GBM by subpodocyte space and layer of foot processes
    - Subpodocyte space is dynamic and restrictive compartment that covers 60% of glomerular filtration barrier and helps modulate glomerular permeability
  - Cell processes rich in microtubules and intermediate filaments
  - Foot processes are cytoplasmic extensions arranged at right angles to long axis of GBM
    - Extensively interdigitate with foot processes of adjacent podocytes
    - Anchor to GBM by α3β1-integrins and dystroglycans
    - Space between foot processes bridged by zipper-like slit diaphragms
    - Foot process structure maintained by actin-based cytoskeleton
    - Several molecules described in podocyte foot processes and slit diaphragms contribute to structural integrity and permselectivity of filtration barrier
- Parietal epithelial cells (PEC)
  - Flattened cells that line inner surface of Bowman capsule
  - Express pax-2, claudin-1, and other PEC proteins
  - In continuity with podocytes at vascular pole and with tubular epithelial cells at urinary pole
  - Recent evidence suggests an important role in glomerular repair and injury
    - Parietal epithelial layer has stem cells that are highlighted by CD24 and CD133
      - PEC stem cells may be involved in regeneration of podocytes and tubular epithelial cells
      - Subset at vascular pole, referred to as transitional cell/peripolar cell/parietal podocyte, also expresses podocyte markers and forms foot processes
      - Subset resides near tubular pole
      - Podocyte-committed progenitor cells reside between tubular and vascular poles and show graded expression of both stem cell and podocyte markers
    - Activated PEC are formed in response to injury
      - These cells are cuboidal with larger cytoplasm
      - Coexpress PEC proteins and CD44
      - Form cellular crescents and migrate to sclerotic segments of FSGS
      - Per some authors, the pseudocrescents of collapsing FSGS are derived from PEC
      - Secrete extracellular matrix in response to TGF-b secretion by podocytes
- Mesangial matrix
  - Mesangial matrix and cells support glomerular infrastructure
  - Composed of microfibrils, type IV (α-1 and α-2) and V collagen, laminin, and fibronectin
  - More porous to macromolecules than GBM
- Glomerular basement membrane
  - Composed of fused basal lamina of endothelial cells and podocytes
  - 3 layers
    - Lamina rara interna (inner)
    - Lamina densa (central)
    - Lamina rara externa (outer)
  - Measures ~ 300-350 nm in thickness with slightly thicker GBM in males
  - Children have thinner basement membranes but achieve adult thickness by age 10-12 years
  - Composed predominantly of type IV collagen, noncollagenous glycoproteins (laminin, entactin), and sulfated proteoglycans
    - Collagen type IV is triple helix substructure has heterodimers of 3 α chain combinations (from α1-α6)
    - GBM composed of collagen type IV with α3.α4.α5 chain network
    - Collagen type IV structure has attachment sites for other basement membrane molecules
    - Noncollagenous glycoproteins and collagen type IV are crosslinked for structural integrity
    - Sulfated proteoglycans impart anionic charge
  - GBM restricts flow of molecules in filtrate, provides structural support, and has attachment sites for various molecules that affect cell signaling and polarity
- Bowman capsule

- Connective tissue barrier between interstitium and urinary space
- Continuous with proximal tubular basement membrane at urinary pole and with GBM at vascular pole
- Components include collagen type IV (α-1, α-2, α-5, α-6), laminin, and entactin

Juxtaglomerular Apparatus

- Located at glomerular vascular pole that comes in contact with distal tubule as it ascends toward glomerulus
- Glomerular component includes terminal afferent arteriole and initial portion of efferent arteriole
- Tubular component includes "macula densa," which refers to specialized distal tubular epithelial cells
  - Macula densa cells are elongated with reverse polarity of apical nuclei
  - Responsible for "tubuloglomerular feedback," which regulates glomerular blood flow based on NaCl concentration in distal tubular lumen
- Extraglomerular mesangial cells in continuity with arteriolar smooth muscle cells
- Renin-secreting juxtaglomerular granular cells are mostly within muscularis of afferent arterioles
  - Receive rich sympathetic innervation, which regulates renin secretion
  - Renin secretion also regulated by NaCl within tubular lumens near macula densa

Tubules

- Tubular segments of nephron include proximal tubule, loop of Henle, and distal convoluted tubule
- Collecting duct derived from ureteric bud and not embryologically part of nephron
- Connecting segment between distal tubule and collecting duct not well delineated in humans
- Proximal tubule
  - Begins at tubular pole of glomerulus and composed of proximal convoluted segment in cortex and straight segment residing in medulla
  - Lining cells are eosinophilic with abundant mitochondria
  - Have prominent brush border
- Loop of Henle
  - Proximal tubule descends as thin descending limb, thin ascending limb, and thick ascending limb
  - Thick ascending limb merges with distal tubule at junction of macula densa
  - Glomeruli from outer and middle cortex have short descending thin loops extending only to outer medulla
  - Juxtamedullary glomeruli have long descending thin loops that extend deep into papillary tips
  - Epithelium of thin limbs flattened and mimic capillaries
- Distal tubule
  - Distal tubules drain into collecting ducts
  - Composed of small paler epithelial cells without brush borders
- Collecting duct
  - Cuboidal epithelium; cells increase in height as ducts descend into medulla
  - Lining cells include principal and intercalated cells
  - Intercalated cells mainly in cortex and outer medulla with progressively fewer in deep medulla
  - Coalesce into larger ducts of Bellini

Interstitium

- Renal cortex has minimal interstitium
- Interstitium prominent in inner medulla and papillary tips

Capillary Network

- Renal circulation has dual capillary beds in series: Glomerular network and PTC network
- Glomerular capillary network
  - Afferent arteriole breaks into glomerular capillaries
  - Glomerular capillaries coalesce into efferent arteriole, which immediately bifurcates into PTC network
  - Higher pressures (40-50 mm Hg) compared with other capillary beds, including PTCs (5-10 mm Hg)
  - Efferent arterioles usually smaller than afferent arterioles, but converse for juxtamedullary arterioles
- Peritubular capillaries
  - Form extensive vascular network in cortex
  - Return reabsorbed fluid from tubules into circulation
  - Receive postglomerular blood with high oncotic pressure due to increased concentration of proteins and red blood cells
  - Specialized PTC in medulla called vasa recta
    - Arise from postglomerular efferent arterioles of juxtamedullary glomeruli
    - Form hairpin loops that descend into outer renal medulla forming rich vascular bundles
    - Countercurrent mechanism in vasa recta responsible for high osmotic concentration of medullary interstitium relative to collecting duct lumens and plasma
    - Seen throughout medulla except in papillae
  - PTC coalesce to form venules and, eventually, renal vein

SELECTED REFERENCES

1. Shankland SJ et al: The emergence of the glomerular parietal epithelial cell. Nat Rev Nephrol. 10(3):158-73, 2014
2. Winyard PJ et al: Experimental renal progenitor cells: repairing and recreating kidneys? Pediatr Nephrol. 29(4):665-72, 2014
3. Lasagni L et al: Glomerular epithelial stem cells: the good, the bad, and the ugly. J Am Soc Nephrol. 21(10):1612-9, 2010
4. Mathieson PW: Update on the podocyte. Curr Opin Nephrol Hypertens. 18(3):206-11, 2009
5. Salmon AH et al: New aspects of glomerular filtration barrier structure and function: five layers (at least) not three. Curr Opin Nephrol Hypertens. 18(3):197-205, 2009
6. Satchell SC et al: Glomerular endothelial cell fenestrations: an integral component of the glomerular filtration barrier. Am J Physiol Renal Physiol. 296(5):F947-56, 2009
7. Schlöndorff D et al: The mesangial cell revisited: no cell is an island. J Am Soc Nephrol. 20(6):1179-87, 2009
8. Barisoni L et al: Update in podocyte biology: putting one's best foot forward. Curr Opin Nephrol Hypertens. 12(3):251-8, 2003
9. Kurokawa K: Tubuloglomerular feedback: its physiological and pathophysiological significance. Kidney Int Suppl. 67:S71-4, 1998
10. Pesce C: Glomerular number and size: facts and artefacts. Anat Rec. 251(1):66-71, 1998
11. Epstein M: Aging and the kidney. J Am Soc Nephrol. 7(8):1106-22, 1996
12. Hudson BG et al: Structure and organization of type IV collagen of renal glomerular basement membrane. Contrib Nephrol. 107:163-7, 1994
13. Lingrel JB et al: Structure-function studies of the Na,K-ATPase. Kidney Int Suppl. 44:S32-9, 1994
14. Latta H: An approach to the structure and function of the glomerular mesangium. J Am Soc Nephrol. 2(10 Suppl):S65-73, 1992

Podocyte and Slit Diaphragm Molecules

Molecule	Gene	Functional Properties
Podocyte-Slit Diaphragm Complex		
Nephrin	*NPHS1*	Major structural protein of slit diaphragm; member of immunoglobulin superfamily; associates with signaling domains of foot process cell membranes (lipid rafts) & interacts with CD2AP and podocin
Podocin	*NPHS2*	Transmembrane molecule that maintains structural integrity of slit diaphragm; interacts with nephrin, CD2AP, & NEPH-1 & thus signaling
CD2AP	*CD2AP*	Intracellular adapter podocyte protein binds to cytoplasmic domain of nephrin & links it to actin-based cytoskeleton
NEPH-1	*KIRREL*	Transmembrane protein of immunoglobulin superfamily; NEPH-1 interacts with podocin, ZO-1, & nephrin
ZO-1	*TJP1*	Membrane protein located at attachment between slit diaphragm & foot process; interacts with NEPH-1 & actin-based cytoskeleton; may participate in signaling events through tyrosine phosphorylation
mFAT1	*FAT*	Protocadherin in slit diaphragm; functions may include cell adhesion & role to maintain extracellular space
P-cadherin	*CDH3*	Slit diaphragm molecule involved in cell adhesion
Podocyte-Glomerular Basement Membrane (GBM) Complex		
α3β1-integrin		Anchor podocyte foot processes to GBM; bridge structural proteins of GBM (collagen IV, laminin) to cytoskeleton
Dystroglycan		Podocyte transmembrane molecule with α & β subunits; α subunit binds to cationic components of GBM, & intracellular β subunit binds to actin cytoskeleton
Podocyte		
Podocalyxin	*PODXL*	Major determinant of podocyte anionic glycocalyx located along luminal (facing urinary space) aspect of podocyte; maintains glomerular architecture & foot process integrity via its connections to actin-based cytoskeleton
GLEPP-1		Transmembrane protein along luminal aspect & a receptor tyrosine phosphatase; may help regulate glomerular filtration rate through effects on podocyte structure and function
WT-1	*WT-1*	Transcription factor restricted to podocytes in adult kidney
Cytoskeletal and others		Cytoskeletal proteins (actin, myosin, α-actinin, & synaptopodin) for integrity of foot processes; C3b receptor, vimentin, TRPC6 ion channel, cell cycling molecules such as p27, p57, cyclin D3; transcription factors such as PAX2, Pod1, LMX1B

Characteristics of Tubular Segments of Nephron

Structural Characteristics	Functional Considerations	Other Comments
Proximal Tubule		
Eosinophilic cytoplasm & prominent apical brush border; abundant mitochondria & basolateral infoldings that interdigitate	Absorb bulk of solutes in glomerular filtrate: 60% of Na^+, Cl^-, K^+, $Ca2^+$, & water, & 90% of $HCO3^-$, glucose, & amino acids	Na^+/K^+ ATPase in basolateral membrane derives energy from abundant mitochondria; water channel aquaporin I in microvilli
Have tight intercellular junctions with zona occludens	Secretion of solutes, such as organic anions and cations, into lumina	Also has Na^+/H^+ exchanger (sensitive to angiotensin II), Cl^- anion exchanger
Loop of Henle		
Includes thin descending/ascending limb; thick ascending limb terminates with macula densa; flattened epithelium of thin limbs	Maintains high concentrations of medullary interstitium & countercurrent mechanisms	Thick ascending limb: Na^+ K^+ $2Cl^-$ (NKCC2) membrane cotransporter, target of furosemide
Basolateral infolding & mitochondria are fewer, especially thin descending and ascending loops	Thick ascending limb is water impermeable (diluting segment), site of $Mg2^+$ reabsorption, & secretes uromodulin	Thin descending limb: Na^+/K^+ ATPase, carbonic anhydrase, and aquaporin I
Distal Convoluted Tubule		
Lining cells are smaller, less eosinophilic than proximal tubular cells, & lack brush border	Determines final urine tonicity, volume, & concentrations of Na^+, K^+, and Cl^-	Site of Na^+/Cl^- cotransporter (NCCT), a thiazide diuretic-sensitive carrier protein
Basolateral infoldings are well developed, and mitochondria are abundant	Site of action of regulatory hormones such as aldosterone and vasopressin	
Collecting Duct		
Have principal (paler cytoplasm) & intercalated cells (darker with more organelles)	Principal cells are mainly involved in Na^+ & water transport	Principal cells have vasopressin receptors & water channel aquaporins 2, 3, and 4
Cuboidal epithelial cells with mild basal infolding	Intercalated cells are site of acid base regulation	Intercalated cells have H^+ ATPase, $HCO3^-/Cl^-$ exchanger & carbonic anhydrase; colloidal Fe^+
Papillary tips lined by urothelium		Distal tubule has epithelial Na^+ channel (ENaC), amiloride diuretic-sensitive channel

Schematic of Kidney

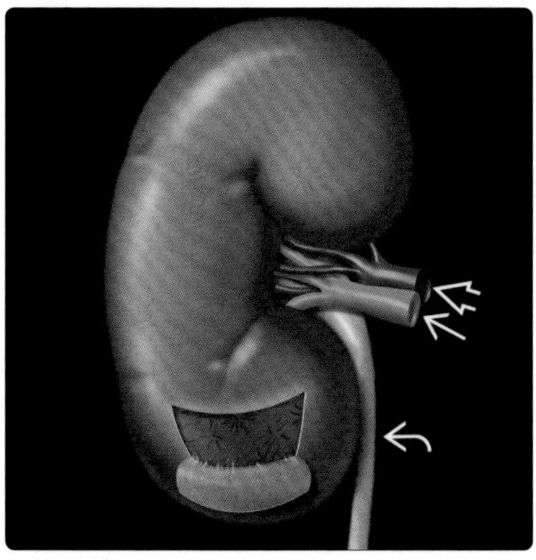

Schematic Cross Section of Kidney

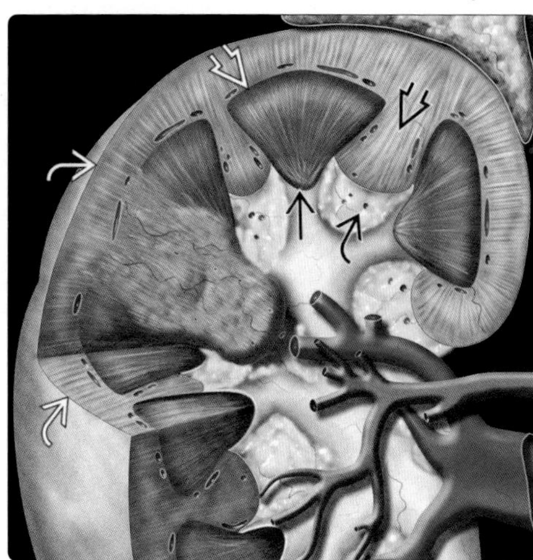

(Left) *Every day 1,800 L of blood (roughly 25% of the cardiac output) flow into the kidneys through the renal artery ➡ and exit the renal vein ➡. Up to 1 L of urine is produced, which exits through the ureter ➡ into the bladder.* **(Right)** *The cortex runs along the outer rim ➡ and extends as columns ➡ between the medullary pyramids ➡. Urine drains into the minor calyces through the papillae ➡. A capsule is not present to contain tumors from gaining access to lymphatics in the sinus fat region ➡.*

Schematic of 2 Nephrons With Blood Supply

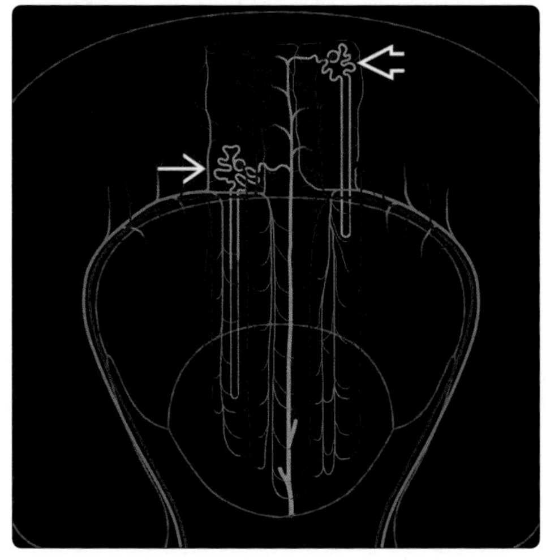

Normal Cortex

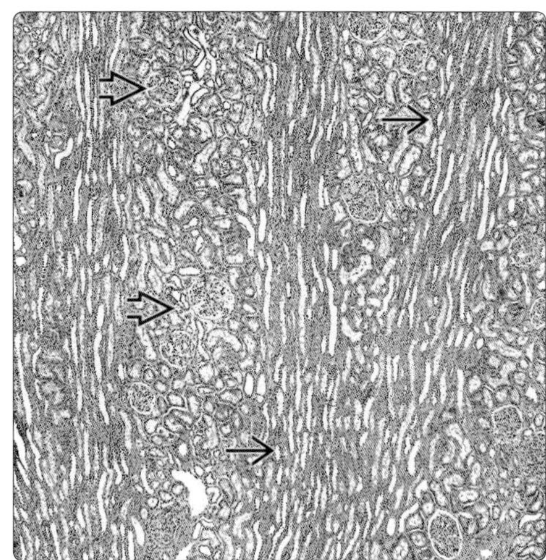

(Left) *Juxtamedullary glomeruli/nephrons ➡ have a longer loop of Henle compared with cortical glomeruli/nephrons ➡. The efferent arterioles of cortical nephrons supply the peritubular capillary network, while the efferent arterioles of juxtamedullary nephrons may supply the vasa recta.* **(Right)** *Glomeruli ➡ are present only in the cortex. Medullary rays ➡ are part of the cortex and run up toward the capsule and down toward the medulla in this photomicrograph. The tubules are closely packed in the cortex.*

Schematic View of Nephron

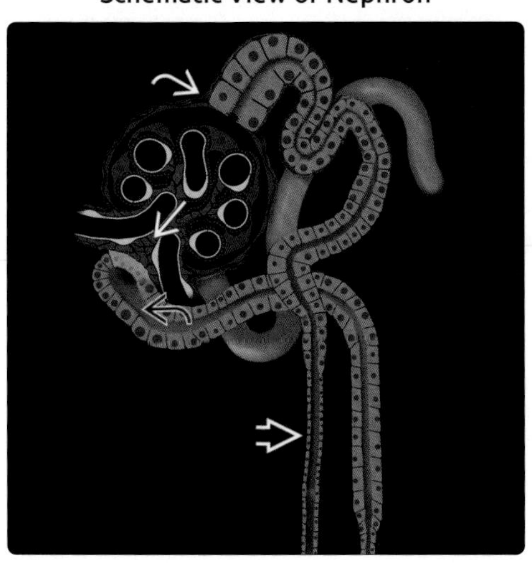

Normal Medulla

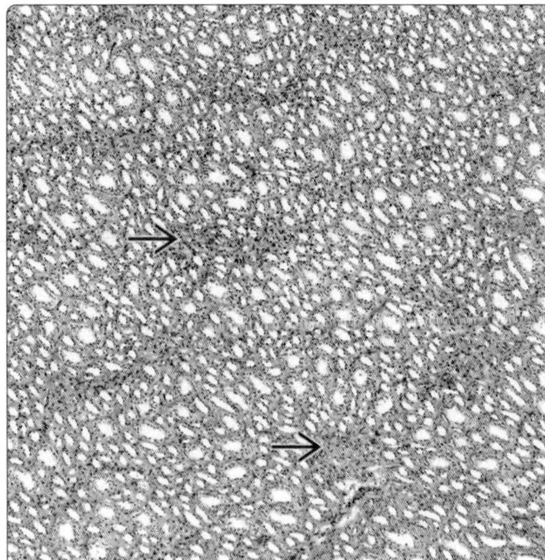

(Left) *The renal corpuscle consists of a Bowman capsule and its included glomerulus. The proximal tubule joins the renal corpuscle at the urinary pole ➡. The diagram also shows the descending portion of the loop of Henle ➡, the distal tubule ➡, and the macula densa (light brown), which is in continuity with the juxtaglomerular apparatus ➡.* **(Right)** *Efferent arterioles of juxtamedullary glomeruli become the vasa recta and form bundles ➡.*

Normal Glomerulus Schematic

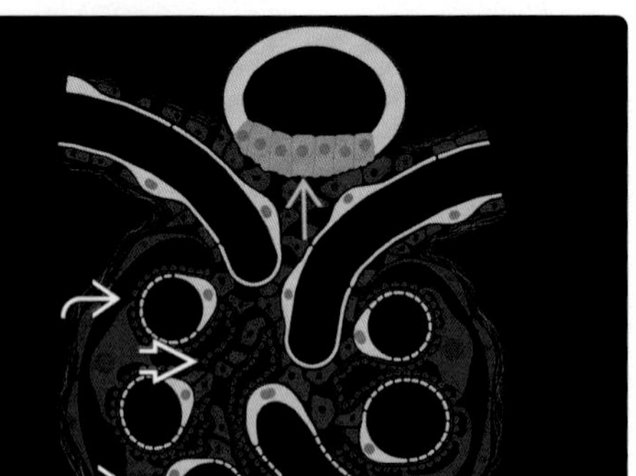

Normal Pediatric Glomerulus

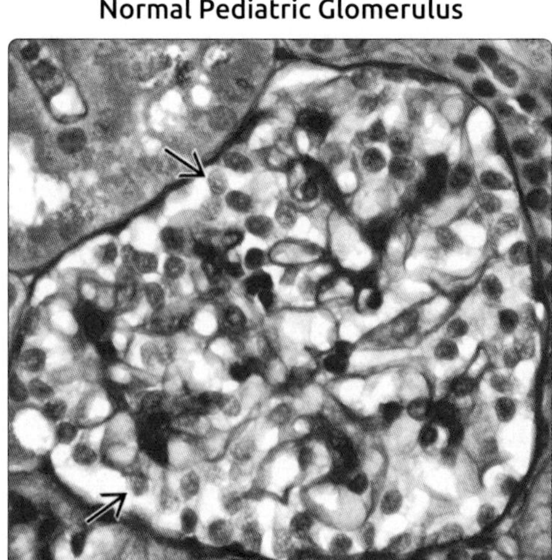

(Left) *The glomerulus consists of mesangial cells ➡, fenestrated endothelial cells ➡, and podocytes ➡ overlying the glomerular basement membrane. The macula densa ➡ is adjacent to the juxtaglomerular apparatus. It is a group of densely staining cells in the distal tubule that may function as receptors that feed information to the juxtaglomerular cells.* **(Right)** *Pediatric glomeruli are smaller than adult glomeruli and have prominent podocytes ➡ (visceral epithelial cells).*

Normal Glomerulus: PAS

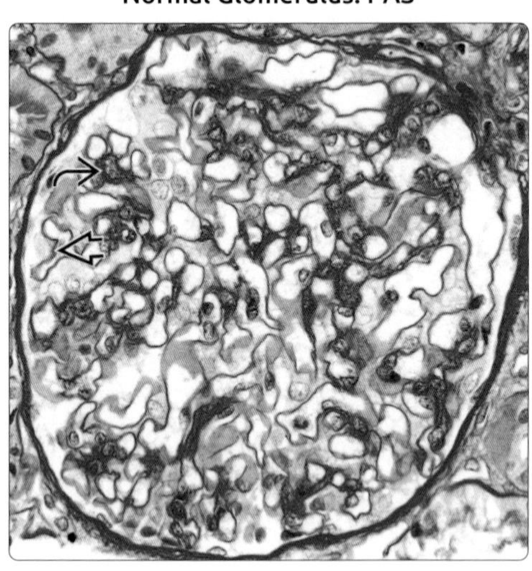

Normal Glomerulus on JMS

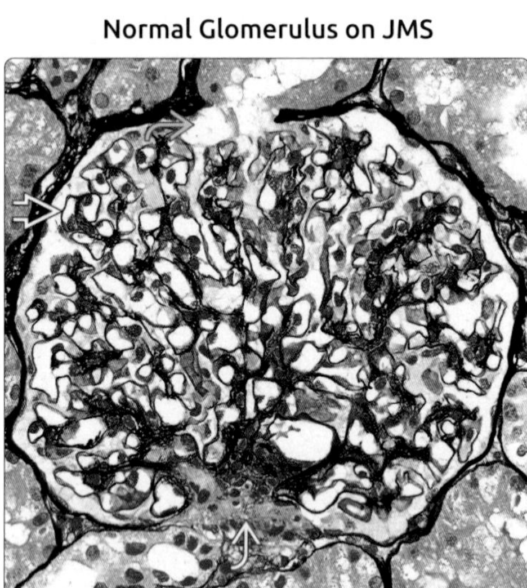

(Left) *PAS outlines the glomerular basement membrane ➡, facilitating assessment of the glomerulus. Mesangial areas ➡ normally have < 3 nuclei per region in a 2 µm thick section.* **(Right)** *JMS allows optimal visualization of the normal glomerular basement membranes ➡ and mesangial cellularity. The juxtaglomerular apparatus ➡ is next to the hilar arteriole at the vascular pole. The tip of the glomerulus empties into the urinary pole ➡ (or proximal portion of the proximal tubule).*

Schematic of Glomerular Capillaries

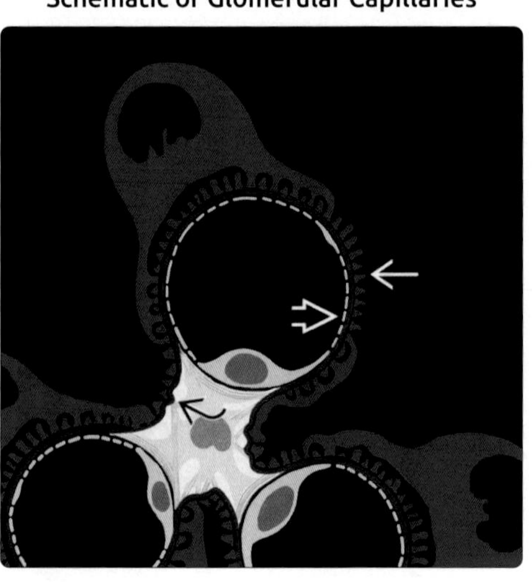

Normal Glomerular Capillaries

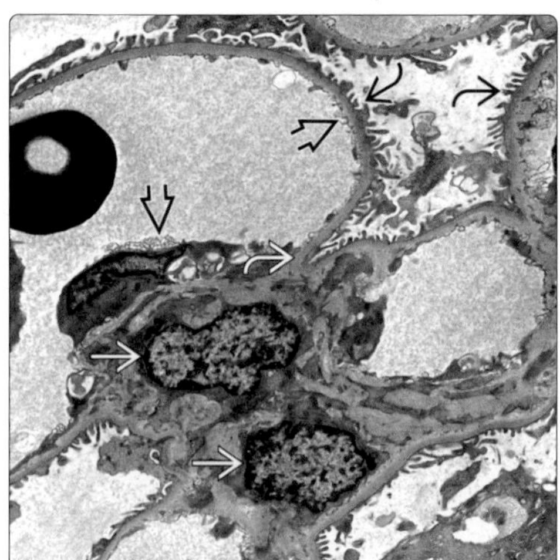

(Left) *The podocytes and their foot processes ➡ cover the glomerular basement membranes. The fenestrated endothelial cells ➡ also contribute to the glomerular filtration barrier. The glomerular basement membranes are anchored to the mesangium ➡.* **(Right)** *The glomerular capillary basement membrane anchors in the mesangium ➡. It is lined by fenestrated endothelial cells ➡ and covered by podocytes ➡. Normally, 2 mesangial cells ➡ are present per mesangial region.*

Renal Cortex: Proximal Tubules

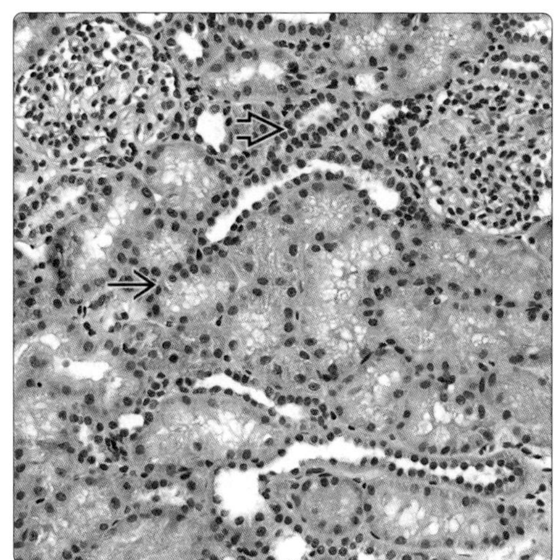

Renal Cortex: Proximal Tubules

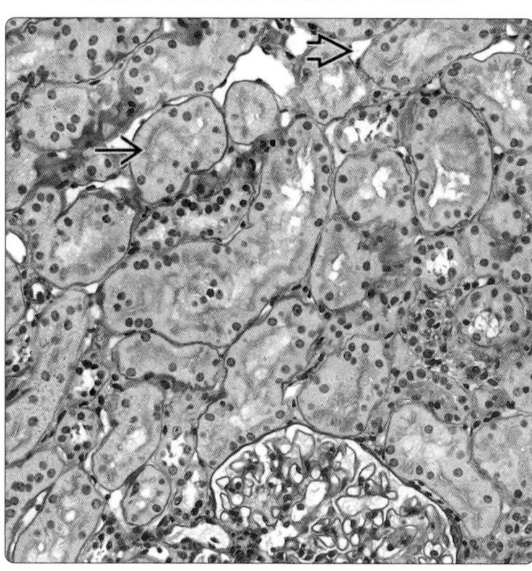

(Left) *The convoluted proximal tubules ➡ comprise the majority of tubules seen in the renal cortex. They are characterized by abundant eosinophilic cytoplasm, in contrast with the distal nephron segments ➡ that have much smaller cells and thus more nuclei per tubule length.* **(Right)** *PAS shows the abundant cytoplasm of the proximal tubular epithelial cells ➡. No significant space is present between tubules except for the network of peritubular capillaries ➡.*

Proximal Tubules on H&E

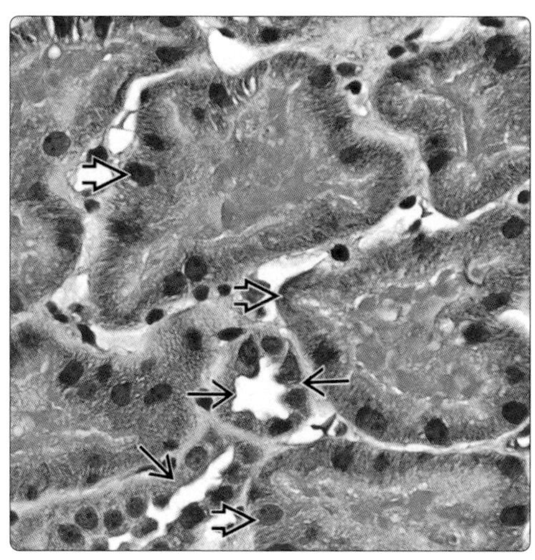

Proximal Tubules on PAS

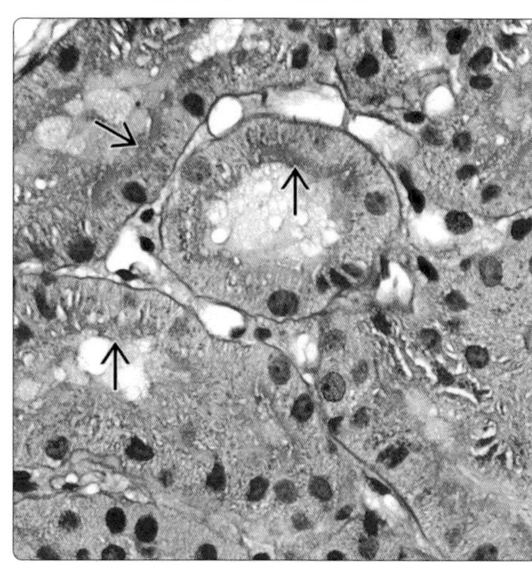

(Left) *Proximal tubular cells ➡ have abundant eosinophilic cytoplasm (due to high mitochondrial content) compared with distal tubules ➡. 60% (~ 110 L) of the total glomerular filtrate (180 L) is reabsorbed by the proximal tubules daily. The ratio of proximal tubular profiles to distal nephron segments is roughly 3:1 in the cortex.* **(Right)** *The brush border ➡ at the apical aspect of the proximal tubules is best visualized with PAS stain and may be attenuated in acute tubular injury/necrosis.*

Proximal Tubules on CD10

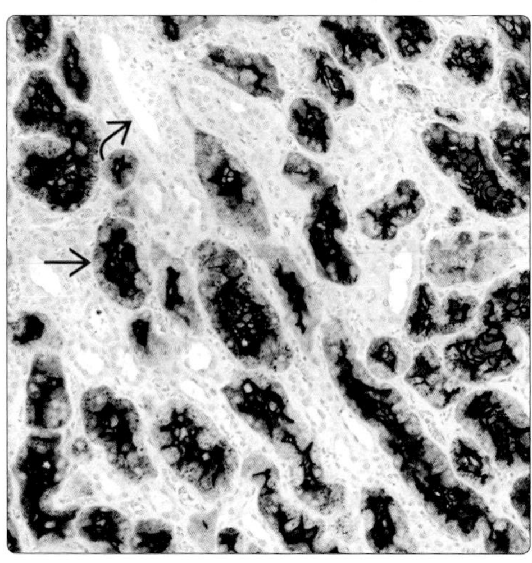

Proximal Tubular Epithelial Cell

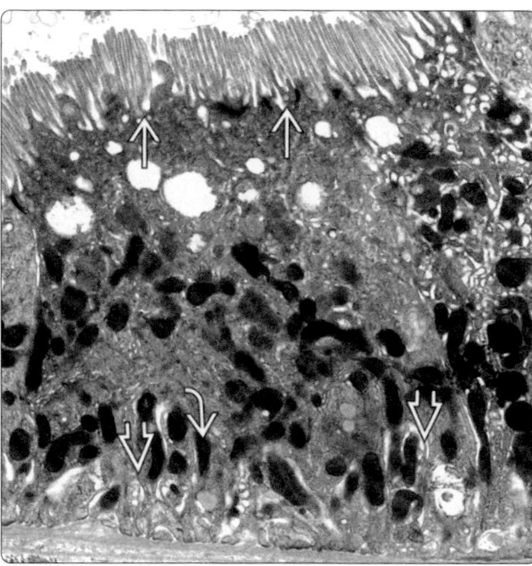

(Left) *CD10 strongly stains the brush borders ➡ on the apical aspect of the proximal tubular epithelial cells. The distal nephron segments ➡ are negative.* **(Right)** *This electron micrograph shows the brush border ➡ along the apical surface that is characteristic of proximal tubular epithelial cells. Many mitochondria ➡ are associated with the basolateral interdigitations ➡ along the tubular basement membrane.*

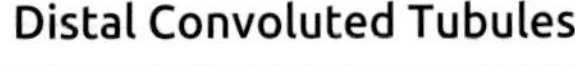

Distal Convoluted Tubules

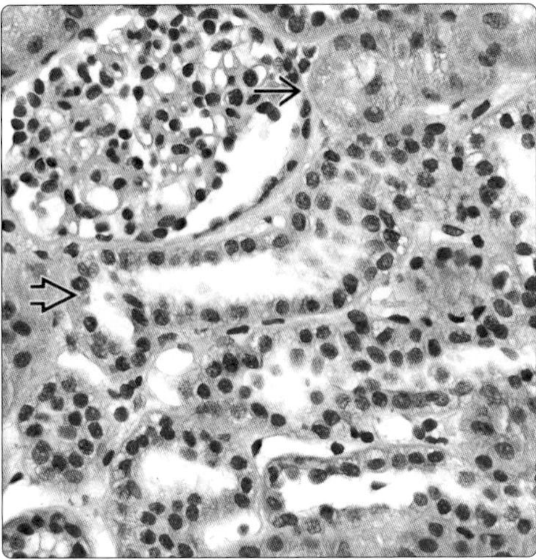

Loops of Henle

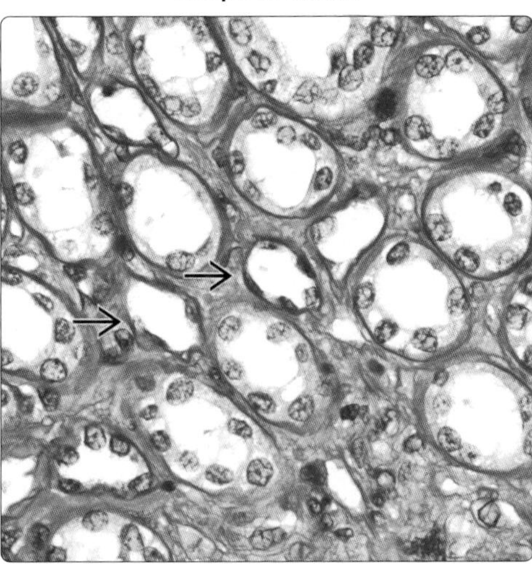

(Left) *The distal tubules → are easily distinguished from the larger proximal tubular epithelial cells → as they have many more cells and nuclei per tubule length and each cell has much less cytoplasm (and thus a less eosinophilic appearance).* **(Right)** *Cross sections of the loops of Henle → show their nuclei protruding into the tubular lumina with attenuated cell cytoplasm. Adjacent peritubular capillaries have a smaller caliber.*

Macula Densa

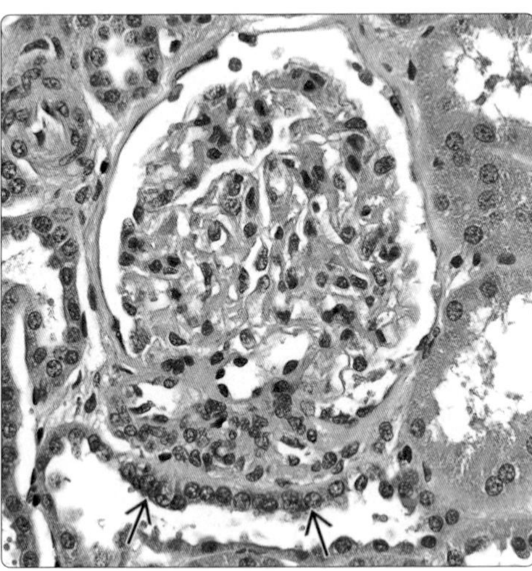

Tubules and Collecting Ducts on EMA

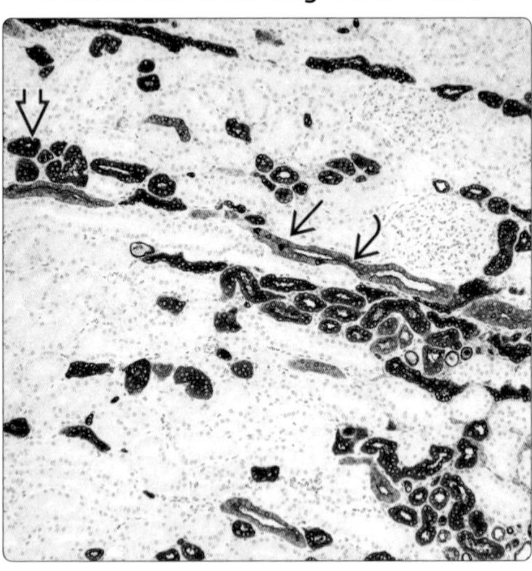

(Left) *The cells of the macula densa → are columnar; they represent a specialized portion of the distal tubule that is adjacent to the juxtaglomerular apparatus and should not be mistaken for a cellular crescent.* **(Right)** *Epithelial membrane antigen (EMA) is expressed in the distal tubules → but not in glomeruli or proximal tubules. The principal cells of the collecting ducts → demonstrate less intense cytoplasmic staining, whereas the scattered intercalated cells → have strong staining.*

Collecting Duct on H&E Stain

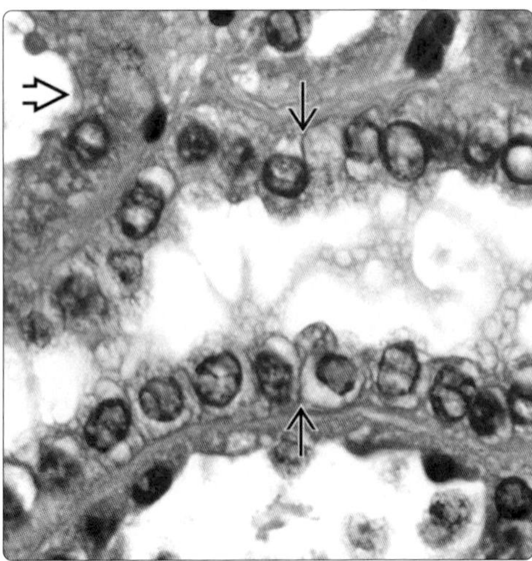

Cytokeratin 7

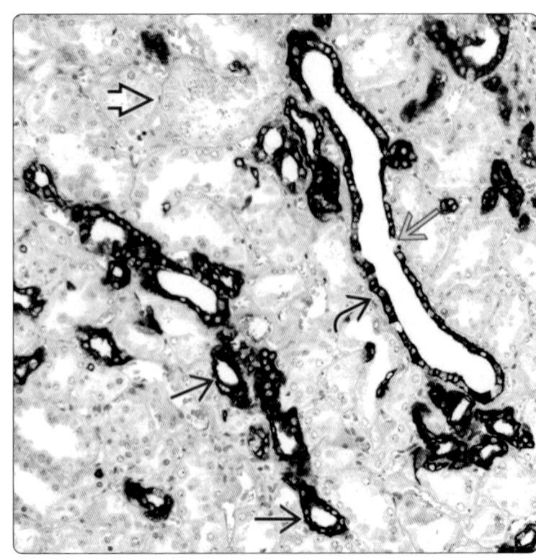

(Left) *The lateral cell borders → of the collecting ducts are often distinct in contrast to the adjacent proximal tubular epithelial cells → that lack this feature.* **(Right)** *Cytokeratin 7 highlights the distal tubules → and collecting ducts →, but there is no expression in the proximal tubules →. The principal cells within the collecting ducts express cytokeratin 7, while the intercalated cells → show no expression.*

Collecting Duct on AE1/AE3

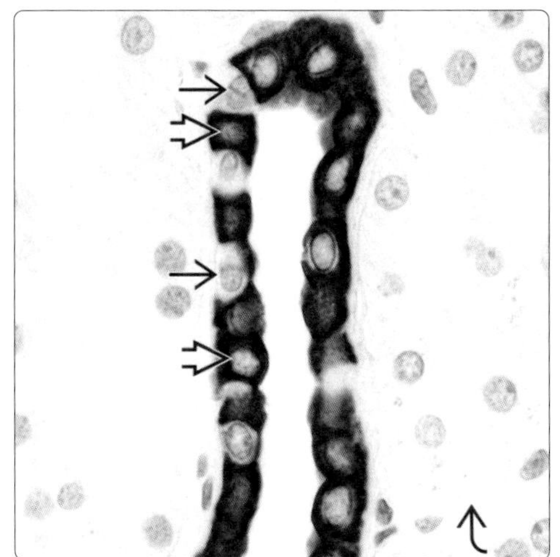

Renal Medulla on Masson Trichrome

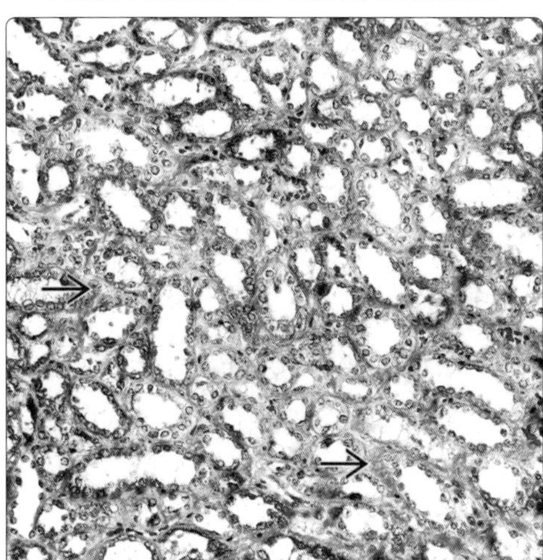

(Left) *AE1/AE3 immunohistochemistry strongly stains the cytoplasm of principal cells ⇨ of the collecting duct, while intercalated cells → are negative. The adjacent proximal tubules ↪ demonstrate no staining.* **(Right)** *Masson trichrome stains tubular basement membranes and interstitial fibrosis blue →. The tubules have more space between them in the medulla, where assessing the extent of interstitial fibrosis and tubular atrophy is much more difficult than in the cortex.*

Principal Cell

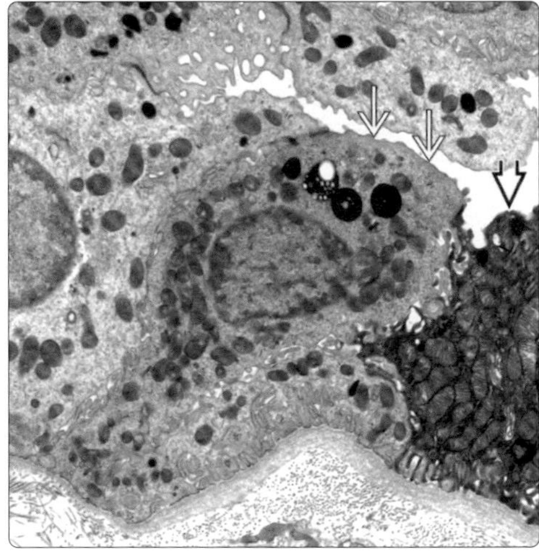

Intercalated Cell

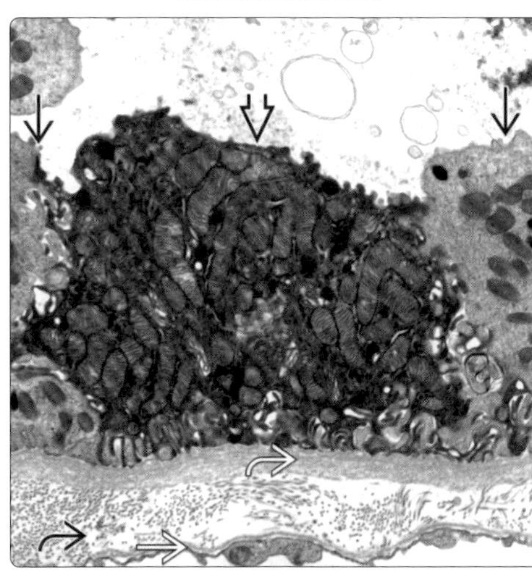

(Left) *The principal cell ➡ contains fewer mitochondria and other organelles and has a distinctly lighter cytoplasmic color compared with the adjacent intercalated cell ⇨.* **(Right)** *Abundant mitochondria are present in the cytoplasm of this intercalated cell ⇨ and give the darker cytoplasmic hue. Two principal cells → are adjacent in this collecting duct. Collagen fibrils ↪ are present between the tubular basement membrane ↪ and the peritubular capillary basement membrane ➡.*

Nerves

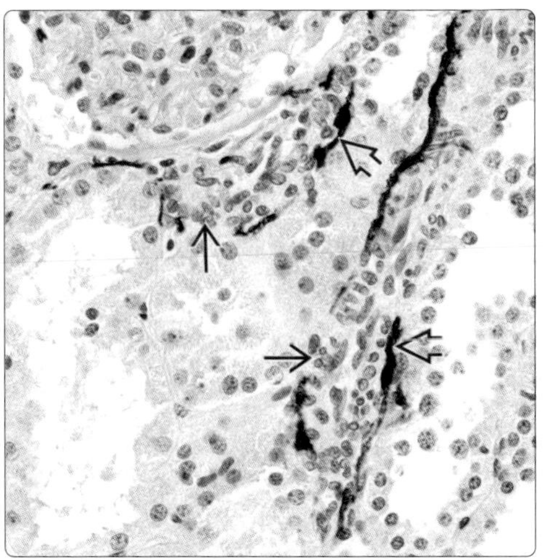

Nerves

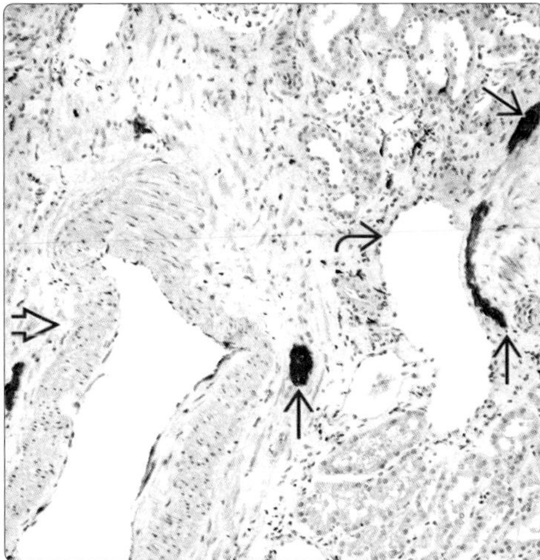

(Left) *Nerves are not generally abundant in the renal cortex, but S100 highlights small nerves ⇨ that course along the arterioles →. Renal denervation is currently gaining attention as a potential safe and effective treatment for refractory hypertension.* **(Right)** *S100 immunohistochemistry reveals the larger nerves → that accompany large-caliber arteries ⇨ and venules ↪ in the medulla and hilum of the kidney.*

(Left) *The internal elastic lamina → has a refractile quality that is best appreciated when viewed under the microscope while focusing the slide up and down. This structure is not present in the veins.* **(Right)** *This interlobular artery → extends from the arcuate artery (not shown) into the cortex adjacent to a medullary ray as afferent arterioles branch off into glomeruli.*

Renal Artery

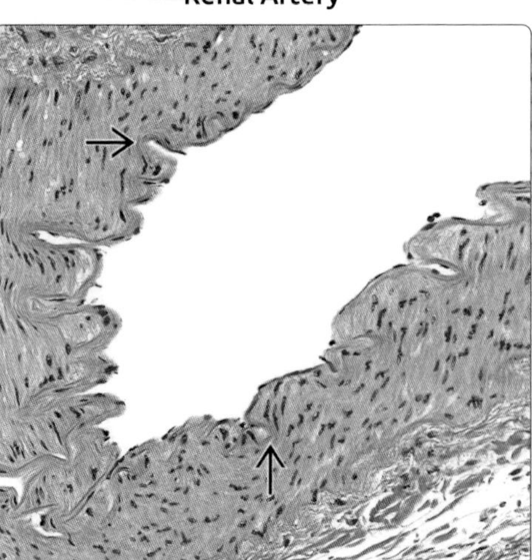

Interlobular Artery

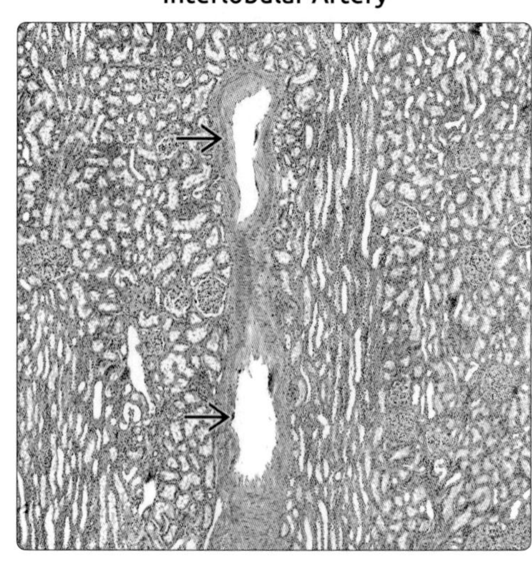

(Left) *This interlobular artery → branches into an afferent arteriole → before entering a glomerulus (not shown). The arteriole wall thickness normally consists of ≤ 2 layers of smooth muscle cells.* **(Right)** *Jones methenamine silver shows an afferent arteriole →, which often has a thicker vessel wall and larger caliber than the efferent arteriole →. A fortuitous section to visualize both arterioles simultaneously may be necessary to distinguish one from the other.*

Artery and Arteriole

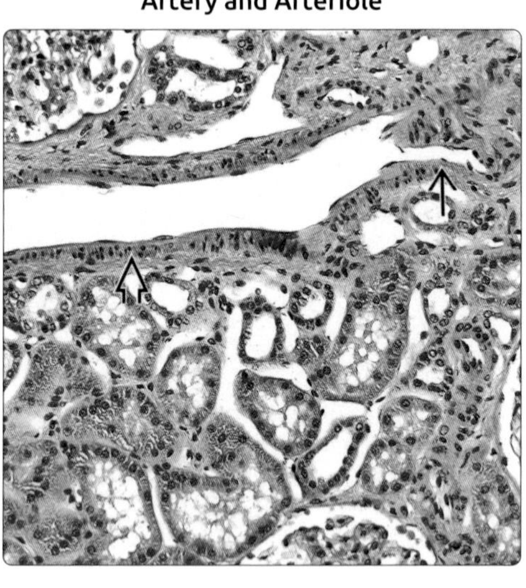

Afferent and Efferent Arterioles

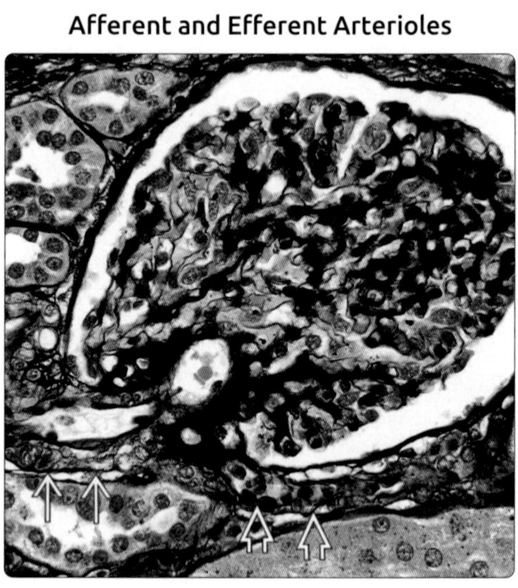

(Left) *CD31 highlights the intricate peritubular capillary network → as well as the glomerular capillaries → and 1 artery →. Pathologic glomerular injury can decrease blood flow to the peritubular capillaries, which results in tubular atrophy and interstitial fibrosis.* **(Right)** *This peritubular capillary → contains a red blood cell →. The endothelial cell → sits atop a single basement membrane layer →, which may be multilayered in chronic antibody-mediated rejection in renal allografts.*

Peritubular Capillary Network

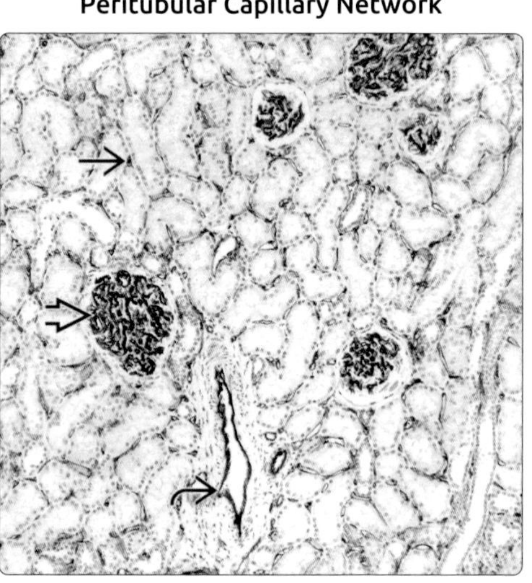

Peritubular Capillary

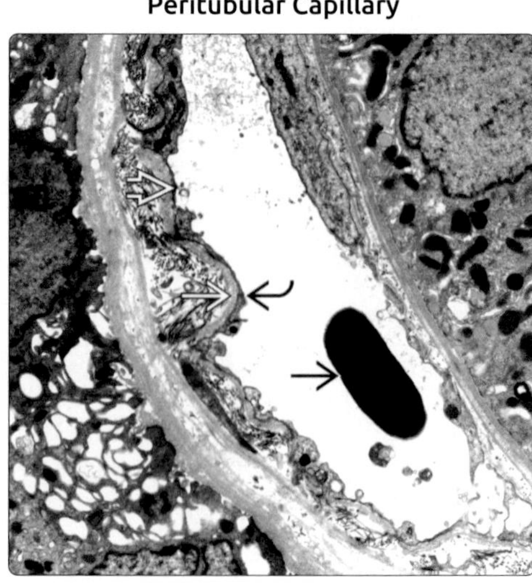

CD31

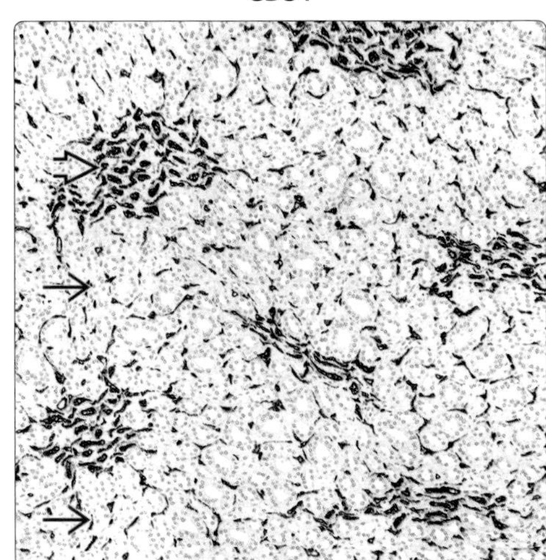

Vascular Bundle on α-Smooth Muscle Actin

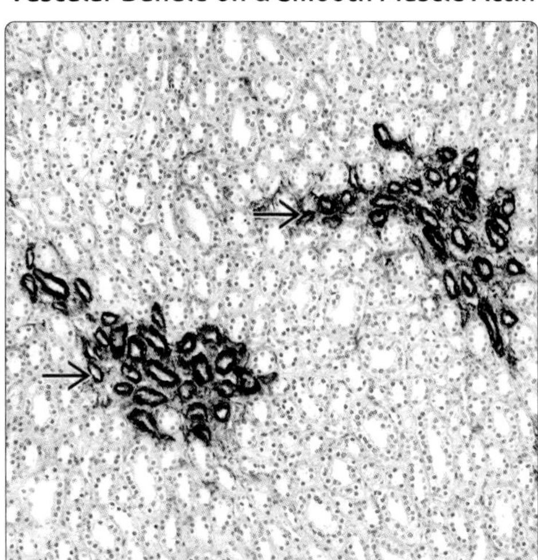

(Left) *CD31 immunohistochemistry highlights the vascular bundles ⇨ and individual peritubular capillaries → that course through the renal medulla.* **(Right)** *α-smooth muscle actin highlights the vasa recta →, which travel in bundles through the renal medulla. Note that the peritubular capillary network that is present between the tubules is not highlighted by this immunostain.*

Lymphatics

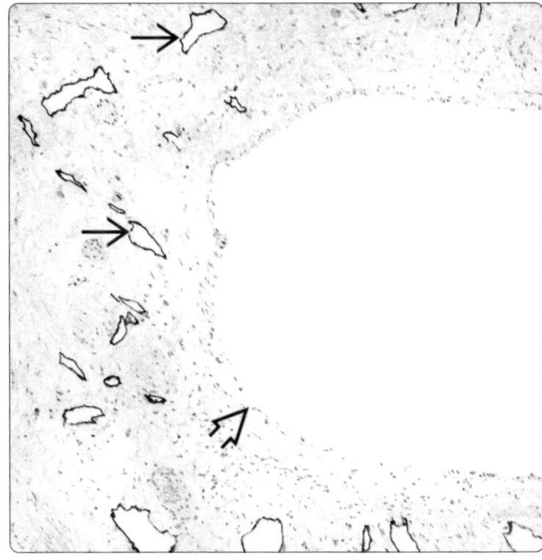

Lymphatics in Renal Sinus

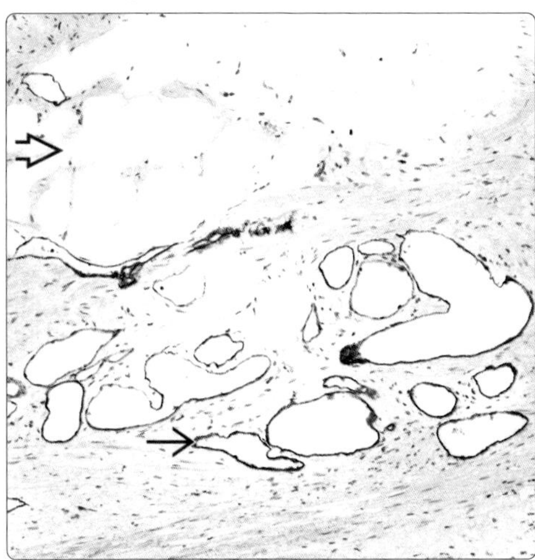

(Left) *D2-40 immunohistochemistry outlines the numerous lymphatic channels → that are present in the wall of this renal vein ⇨.* **(Right)** *D2-40 immunohistochemistry highlights the many lymphatic vessels → that are present in close proximity to the renal sinus fat ⇨. In contrast to the outer aspect of the kidney, a capsule does not exist between the medulla and renal sinus. Therefore, large malignant renal neoplasms can extend into this region and easily gain access to these lymphatic vessels.*

Resident Dendritic Cells

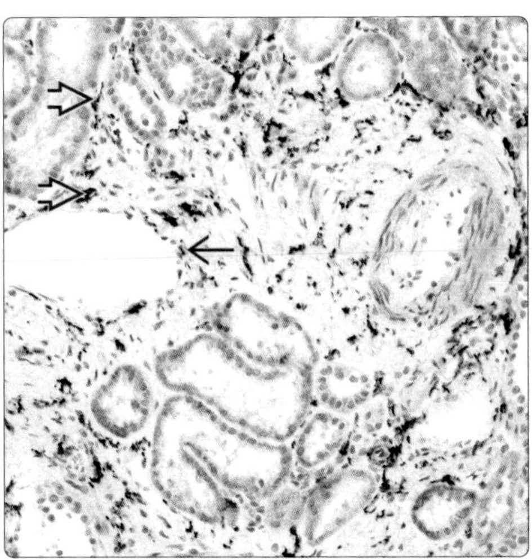

Resident Dendritic Cells

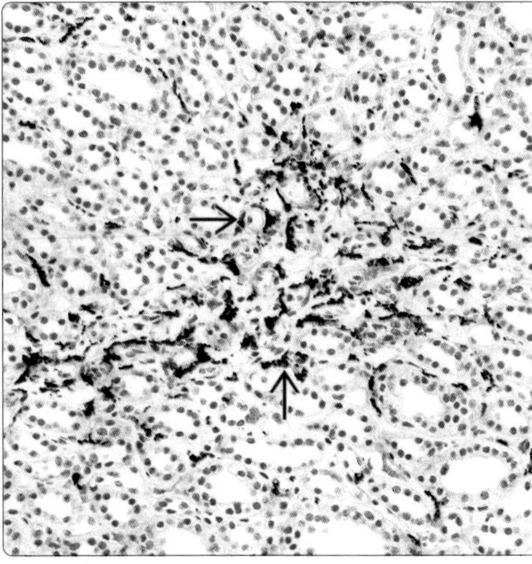

(Left) *CD163 immunohistochemistry reveals numerous dendritic cells ⇨ in the normal renal cortex, which are closely approximated with venules →, peritubular capillaries, and lymphatics. They may have a role in immune surveillance.* **(Right)** *CD163 highlights the resident dendritic cells that are present in greater density along the vascular bundles → that course through the medulla.*

TERMINOLOGY

Abbreviations

- Wolffian duct (WD) (a.k.a. nephric duct)
- Ureteric bud (UB)
- Collecting duct (CD)
- Metanephric mesenchyme (MM)
- Intermediate mesoderm (IM)
- Mesenchymal to epithelial transition (MET)

STAGES OF KIDNEY DEVELOPMENT

Overview

- Embryonic kidney development begins from collection of cells in intermediate mesoderm, a layer of tissue between paraxial mesoderm and lateral plate mesoderm
- 3 sets of embryonic kidneys (pronephros, mesonephros, and metanephros) develop in anterior (rostral) to posterior (caudal) direction
- Pronephros and mesonephros precede definitive kidney (metanephros)

Pronephros

- Transient collection of cells in intermediate mesoderm at ~ 3 weeks of gestation that undergo mesenchymal to epithelial transition
- Epithelialized tube may induce formation of rudimentary tubules in intermediate mesoderm that degenerate by 4 weeks of gestation
- Involution of pronephros coincides with beginning of mesonephros

Mesonephros

- Epithelialized intermediate mesoderm cells form a tube called the nephric duct (wolffian duct) that grows in rostrocaudal direction towards cloaca; continued wolffian duct growth progressively induces adjacent mesenchyme to form mesonephros, starting at ~ 3.5 weeks of gestation
- Transient **linear organization** of functional nephrons connected to nephric duct (about 34)
- Regresses at ~ 16 weeks of gestation in humans except most of anterior/cranial mesonephric tubules, which in males, become part of epididymis
- Wolffian duct becomes vas deferens in males
- Many genes/processes that regulate mesonephros and metanephros development are thought to be similar
- Without wolffian duct, kidneys, ureters, and male genital tract do not develop

Metanephros

- Definitive kidney
- Begins at ~ 4th-5th week of gestation, giving rise to ~ 1 million nephrons/kidney
- Starts from distal end of wolffian duct as diverticulum
- **Branched organization** of urinary collecting system and proximal nephrons (tubules and glomeruli)
- Fetal and embryonic kidneys have **lobulated** appearance
- As nephrons are added, grooves distend and kidney surface becomes smooth
- Lateral fusion of cortex of lobules produces columns of Bertin

MAJOR COMPONENTS OF DEVELOPING METANEPHROS, ORIGIN, AND DERIVATIVES

Overview

- > 40 different cell types in mammalian kidney
- Fate mapping and lineage tracing studies help determine origin and destiny of various cell types

Ureteric Bud

- Derived from wolffian duct
- Produces cortical and medullary collecting ducts (principal and intercalated cells), calyces, pelvis, and ureter

Metanephric Mesenchyme

- Derived from intermediate mesoderm; produces glomeruli (podocytes, parietal epithelium of Bowman capsule), proximal tubules, loop of Henle, distal tubules, connecting tubules

Early Morphogenesis

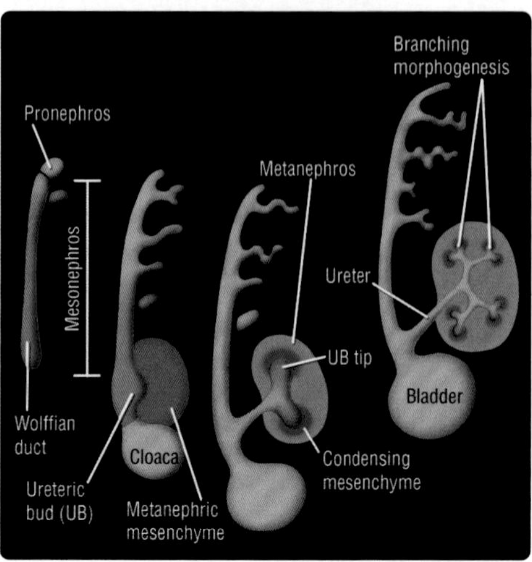

Metanephric Nephrogenesis

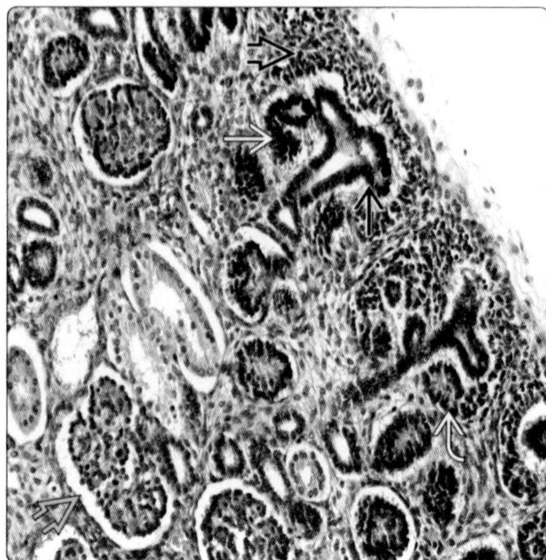

(Left) *The pronephros is formed at ~ 3rd gestational week from intermediate mesoderm. The mesonephros begins at 3.5 weeks forming the wolffian ducts and a linear arrangement of nephrons. The metanephros, forming the definitive kidney begins at 4 weeks with UB that invades metanephric mesenchyme and undergoes branching morphogenesis.* **(Right)** *Branching UB shows tips ➡, mesenchymal condensation ➡, pretubular aggregates ➡, and renal vesicles ➡. Earlier glomeruli are toward the medulla ➡.*

Stroma

- Likely originates from paraxial mesoderm
- Source for interstitial cells, pericytes, smooth muscle cells, mesangium, capsule, angioblasts, and nerves

Vasculature

- Blood vessels derived from sacral branches of descending aorta
- Lymphatics follow vessels and drain into lumbar lymph nodes

Innervation

- Sympathetic innervation from renal ganglia regulates blood flow (activation reduces flow)
- Afferent or sensory nerve fibers follow along sympathetic tracts to lower thoracic levels
- Parasympathetic innervation to ureter and lower urinary tract by pelvic ganglia located adjacent to bladder neck

STEPS IN METANEPHRIC KIDNEY DEVELOPMENT

Ureteral Bud Induction

- Signals from metanephric mesenchyme induce ureteric bud outgrowth from caudal end of each wolffian duct; ureteric bud grows in dorsal direction toward metanephric mesenchyme

Ureteral Bud Invasion Into Metanephric Mesenchyme

- Inductive signals induce branching as T-shaped structure
  - Trunk of this structure is ureteric bud stalk, which will become ureter
  - Tips are called ureteric bud tips or ampulla
  - Rapid proliferation and subsequent branching occur in ureteral bud tips
  - Ureteral bud tips regulate subsequent nephrogenesis

Mesenchymal Condensation

- Mesenchymal cells aggregate around ureteric bud tips, reciprocal interactions follow
  - Metanephric mesenchyme signals ureteral bud to branch
  - Ureteric bud signals metanephric mesenchyme to undergo condensation
  - Stromal cells instruct condensing cells and ureteric bud to continue to grow and differentiate

Branching Morphogenesis

- Stroma and condensed mesenchyme stimulate repetitive branching of ureteric bud tip, giving rise to new stalks and ureteral bud tips in each cycle (branching morphogenesis), resulting in centripetal growth of developing kidney
  - 1st few generations of branching produce pelvis and major and minor calyces; later generations of branching produce collecting duct system in kidney
  - Lateral branching may also occur from stalks but definitive proof in vivo is lacking
- 3 main stages
  - Initial rapid branching
  - Slower rate of branching to promote lengthening of stalks
  - Rapid branching, many nephrons are induced from each ureteral bud tip, forming arcades

Pretubular Aggregates

- Form next to junction of ureteral bud stalk and node from subset of cap mesenchyme cells that have undergone mesenchymal to epithelial transition

Comma-Shaped Body

- Formed from pretubular aggregates
- Cleft in comma-shaped body is infiltrated by capillaries, mainly from extrarenal sites, although stromal endothelial progenitors may participate

S-Shaped Body (Tubulogenesis and Glomerulogenesis)

- Formed from proliferation of comma-shaped body; indicates that patterning of nephron has occurred
  - Outer portion of proximal end of this structure (farther from ureteric bud stalk) becomes parietal epithelium of Bowman capsule and inner layer becomes visceral epithelium (podocytes)
    - Cleft invaded by capillaries (glomerular tuft)
  - Proximal end gives rise to podocytes
  - Distal ends produce proximal and distal tubules
    - Distal end fuses with collecting ducts
- Glomerulogenesis completed ~ 2 weeks before birth in humans
- Fetal glomeruli appear compact with closely aligned podocytes, known as immature glomeruli
- Tubulogenesis continues for a few weeks after birth
- After birth, kidney growth occurs by adding length and diameter to tubules and diameter to glomeruli
  - No more glomeruli added after birth, with total numbers of 227,000-1,825,000/kidney
  - Varies by birth weight

Glomerulogenesis

- Begins at ~ 8 weeks of gestation
- Developing glomeruli grow in rows (generations) from tips of ureteric bud
- More mature (older) glomeruli located toward corticomedullary area and newer ones toward capsule due to centripetal branching of ureteric bud
- Gestational age fairly accurately determined by number of glomerular rows in cortex between 23-33 weeks of gestation
  - Gestational age (weeks) = 4.7 x number of glomerular layers + 0.1
  - Total of 9-14 glomerular generations by end of gestation (variation due to methodology)

Collecting Ducts

- Ureteral bud stalk and tip differentiate into collecting ducts
  - Principal cells (ion pumps, Na, K)
  - Intercalated cells (acid-base balance)

FINAL POSITION OF KIDNEYS

Kidney Ascent: Pelvis to Abdomen

- Not true migration
  - Apparent ascent due to disparate caudal growth of fetus relative to trunk, leaving kidneys behind
- Begins at ~ 6 weeks of gestation

- Initially, kidneys posteriorly located and hila pointing anteriorly
- By 7-8 weeks, kidneys start medial rotation and apparent ascent
- By 9 weeks, hila anteromedially positioned and kidneys in retroperitoneal cavity in abdomen
  - ~ located at T12-L1
  - Positioned underneath adrenal glands, result in flattening of adrenal inferior surface

Blood Supply of Ascending Kidneys

- Blood vessels change with ascent, thus are transient until final location in abdomen
  - While located in pelvis, kidneys derive blood supply from lower segments of aorta
  - Abdominally positioned kidneys derive from higher segments of aorta and caudal branches degenerate
- Accessory blood supply and variations due to persistence of early vessels
- Failure of lower vessels to degenerate can lead to ureteral obstruction as they may cross over ureter

GENES IMPORTANT IN KIDNEY DEVELOPMENT

Major Genes by Stage Identified From Model Organisms

- Genes in upper-case shown to be important in humans
  - Wolffian duct growth or development
    - *LIM1, PAX2, GATA3, Emx2, EYA1, FOXC1, Odd1, RET*
  - Ensuring single ureteral bud outgrowth
    - *RET, GDNF, Spry1, ROBO2, Slit2, LIM1, Bmp4, GATA3*
  - Ureteral bud induction
    - *RET, Gfra1, GDNF*
  - Ureteral bud branching
    - *RET, Ralph2, FoxB2, WT1, PAX2, GDNF, Wnt11, BMP7, Wnt4, Foxd1, SALL1, Bcl2, Fgf7, Fgf10, Fgfrl1, Fgfr2IIIb, Fgfr1, Fgfr2, FRAS1*
  - Metanephric mesenchyme condensation, tubulogenesis, glomerulogenesis
    - *AGT, AGTR1, Notch1, Notch2, Fgf2, Fgf8, Fgfr1, Six2, BMP7, PdgfB, CD2AP, Vegf, Wnt4, A3b1, At2, LAMB2, WT1, PAX2, Wnt9*

CELLULAR PROCESSES IN KIDNEY DEVELOPMENT

Stages and Different Compartments

- Wolffian duct growth: Proliferation, migration, and cell structure changes, particularly at distal tip
- Ureteric bud outgrowth and branching
  - Proliferation occurs mainly in ureteral bud tip and differentiation toward more distal region
  - Low cell death
- Metanephric mesenchyme and nephrogenesis
  - in absence of mesenchymal induction or proper branching
  - Initially proliferates to synchronize with ureteral bud branching
  - Cell death occurs in both metanephric mesenchyme and stroma
  - Balance maintained between cell death and proliferation as growth continues
  - Migration involved in generation of pretubular aggregates and various cell types of tubules and glomerulus

SELECTED REFERENCES

1. Davis TK et al: To bud or not to bud: the RET perspective in CAKUT. Pediatr Nephrol. 29(4):597-608, 2014
2. Hoshi M et al: Novel mechanisms of early upper and lower urinary tract patterning regulated by RetY1015 docking tyrosine in mice. Development. 139(13):2405-15, 2012
3. Chi X et al: Ret-dependent cell rearrangements in the Wolffian duct epithelium initiate ureteric bud morphogenesis. Dev Cell. 17(2):199-209, 2009
4. Dressler GR: Advances in early kidney specification, development and patterning. Development. 136(23):3863-74, 2009
5. Guillaume R et al: Paraxial mesoderm contributes stromal cells to the developing kidney. Dev Biol. 329(2):169-75, 2009
6. Grote D et al: Gata3 acts downstream of beta-catenin signaling to prevent ectopic metanephric kidney induction. PLoS Genet. 4(12):e1000316, 2008
7. Jennette JC et al: Heptinstall's Pathology of the Kidney. 6th ed. Philadelphia: Lippincott Williams & Wilkins, 2007
8. Kopan R et al: Molecular insights into segmentation along the proximal-distal axis of the nephron. J Am Soc Nephrol. 18(7):2014-20, 2007
9. Basson MA et al: Branching morphogenesis of the ureteric epithelium during kidney development is coordinated by the opposing functions of GDNF and Sprouty1. Dev Biol. 299(2):466-77, 2006
10. Costantini F: Renal branching morphogenesis: concepts, questions, and recent advances. Differentiation. 74(7):402-21, 2006
11. dos Santos AM et al: Assessment of renal maturity by assisted morphometry in autopsied fetuses. Early Hum Dev. 82(11):709-13, 2006
12. Dressler GR: The cellular basis of kidney development. Annu Rev Cell Dev Biol. 22:509-29, 2006
13. Jain S et al: Critical and distinct roles for key RET tyrosine docking sites in renal development. Genes Dev. 20(3):321-33, 2006
14. Basson MA et al: Sprouty1 is a critical regulator of GDNF/RET-mediated kidney induction. Dev Cell. 8(2):229-39, 2005
15. Grieshammer U et al: SLIT2-mediated ROBO2 signaling restricts kidney induction to a single site. Dev Cell. 6(5):709-17, 2004
16. Hughson M et al: Glomerular number and size in autopsy kidneys: the relationship to birth weight. Kidney Int. 63(6):2113-22, 2003
17. Vize PD et al: The Kidney: From Normal Development to Congenital Disease. London: Academic Press, 2003
18. Lechner MS et al: The molecular basis of embryonic kidney development. Mech Dev. 62(2):105-20, 1997
19. Kriz W et al: Structural organization of the mammalian kidney. In Seldin DW et al: The Kidney: Physiology and Pathophysiology. New York: Raven Press. 2nd ed. 661-698,1992
20. Saxen L: Organogenesis of the Kidney. Cambridge: Cambridge University Press. 1987
21. Dorovini-Zis K et al: Gestational development of brain. Arch Pathol Lab Med. 101(4):192-5, 1977

Expression of Selected Proteins in Developing Murine Kidney

Mesonephros and Wolffian Duct	Ureteric Bud Stalk	Ureteric Bud Tip	Metanephric Mesenchyme	Stroma	C-, S-Shaped Bodies, Tubules	Glomerulus
Pax2	Met	Ret	Gfra1	Foxd1	Pax2	Wt1
Lhx1	Wnt9b	Gfra1	Gdnf	Pod1	Wnt4	Pax2
Odd1	Wnt7	Wnt11	Robo2	Bmp5	Lhx1	Pod1
Ret		Spry1	Wt1	Fgf7	Bm1	Glepp1
Gfra1		Slit2	Pax2	Fgf10	Dll1	Neph
Spry1		Pax2	Foxc1	Rarα1	Notch1	Vegf
Bmp4		Lhx1	Eya1	Rarβ2	Notch2	Pdgf
Pax8		Hspg	Sal1	Raraldh2	Jag1	Lmx1b
Robo2		Emx2	Six2		Hes	Cd2AP
Slit2		Agt	Pax3		Hey	Nck
FoxC1		Fgfr2 (IIIb)	Bmp7		Cdh6, 11	ColIV
Gata3		Gpc3	Hox11		Jnk	
α3β1		Erm	Pleiotrophin			
Emx2		Pea3	Bmp4			
Lama1		Wnt9b	Agtr2			
Wnt4		Spry2	Midkine			
		Grip1	Pbx1			

For a more detailed list, see www.gudmap.org.

Human Fetal Gestational Age and Glomerular Development

Gestational Age in Weeks	Rows of Glomeruli in Cortex from Medulla to Capsule*	Number of Mature Glomerular Layers (NGL)**
16-23	3	-
24	3-5	4.3 ± 0.8
25	4-6	4.6 ± 0.7
26	5-7	-
27	6-8	6.1 ± 1.1
28	7-9	6.0 ± 1.2
29	8-10	6.3 ± 1.3
30	9-11	-
31	10-12	7.1 ± 0.9
32	11-13	-
33	12-13	7.7 ± 0.8
34	12-14	-
35-42	12-14	7.6 ± 0.4 - 8.6 ± 1.3
Newborn-adult	12-14	-
	Cortex between columns of Bertin	Radial counts; excludes columns of Bertin

*Adapted from Dorovini-Zis K et al: Gestational development of brain. Arch Pathol Lab Med. 101(4):192-5, 1977. **Adapted from dos Santos AM et al: Assessment of renal maturity by assisted morphometry in autopsied fetuses. Early Hum Dev. 82(11):709-13, 2006.

(Left) *Graphic shows cloaca ➙ and kidney ➙.* **(Right)** *Initial ureteric bud (UB) invasion into mesenchyme results in mesenchymal condensation around the UB tip.*

Fetal Kidney Drains Into Cloaca

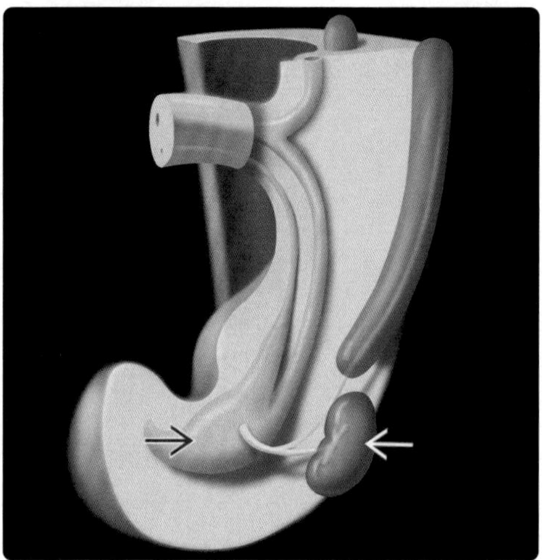

Ureteric Bud

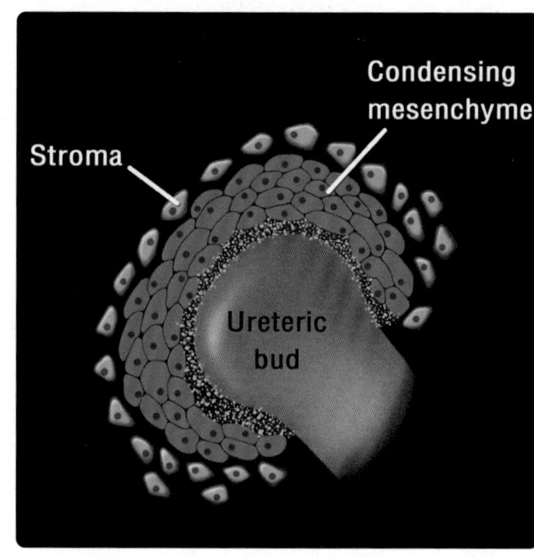

(Left) *Reciprocal interactions between the condensing mesenchyme, stroma, and UB lead to branching and renal vesicle formation through epithelial to mesenchymal transformation. The initial UB stalk that grows from the wolffian duct becomes the ureter. Selected genes in the process are indicated.* **(Right)** *Pretubular aggregates lead to comma-shaped bodies that give rise to S-shaped bodies. The proximal part of these become tubules and the distal part glomerular epithelial cells.*

1st Branching of Ureteric Bud

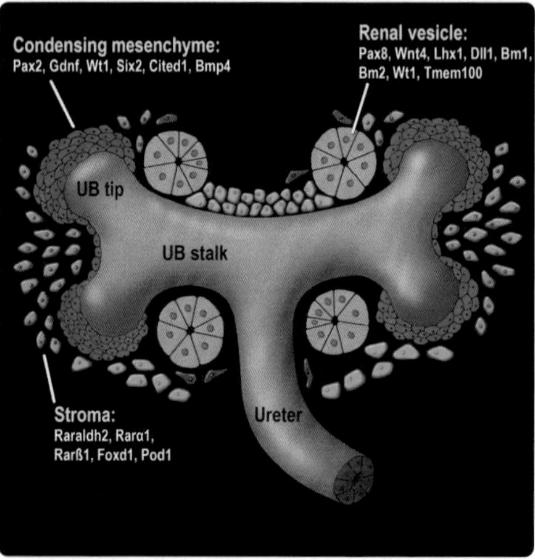

Stages of Glomerulogenesis

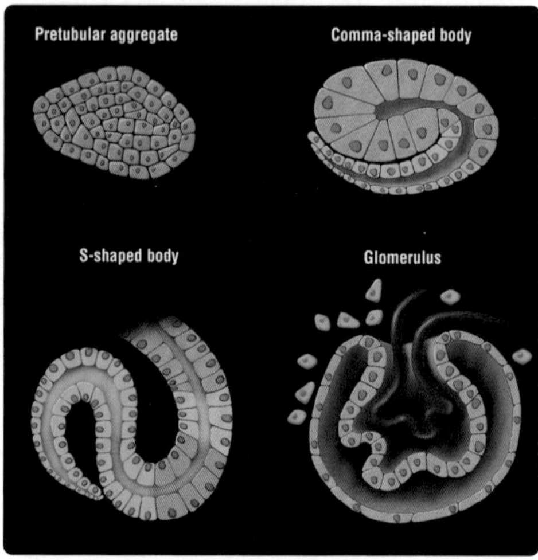

(Left) *A renal vesicle undergoes further patterning and differentiation to form a comma-shaped body and then an S-shaped structure. Endothelial cells invade the proximal cleft of the S-shaped body, the proximal end becomes the glomerulus, and the distal end becomes the connecting tubule, which joins to the collecting ducts. (Modified from Dressler, 2009.)* **(Right)** *Relationship between blood vessels and nephron, and major cell types in the glomerulus are shown. (Modified from Dressler, 2009.)*

S-Shaped Body and Collecting Duct

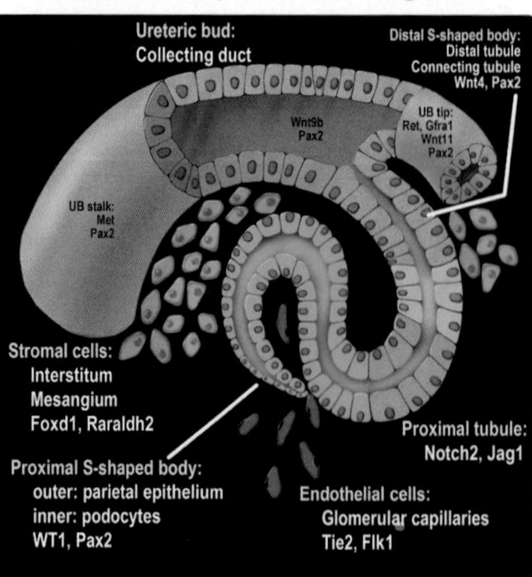

Nephron and Blood Vessels

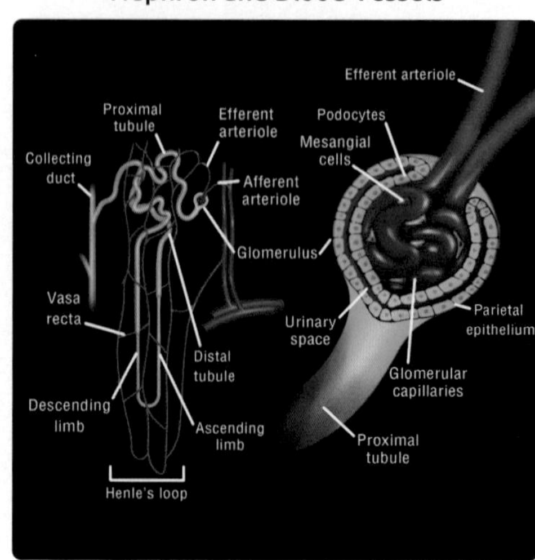

Kidneys Begin in Pelvic Cavity

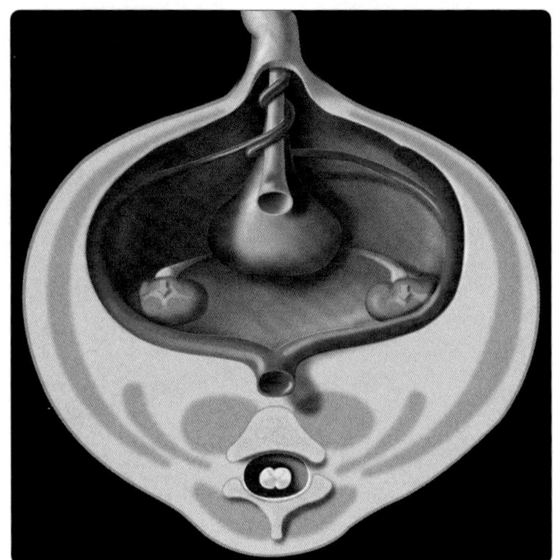

Anterior Hilum During Early Development

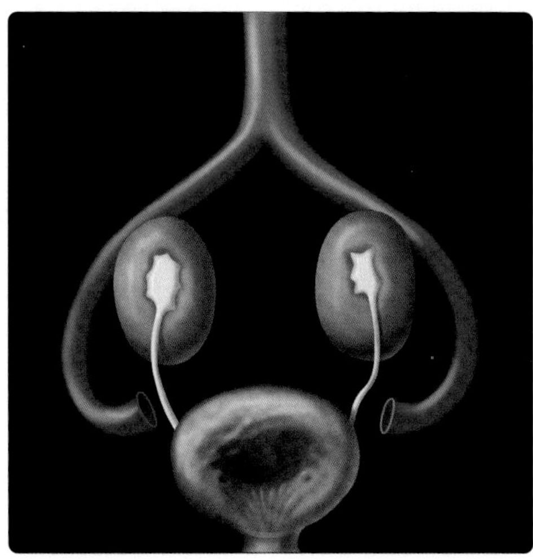

(Left) *Axial view shows posteriorly facing kidneys in the pelvic cavity during early development (~ 6 weeks).* **(Right)** *Coronal view at 6 weeks shows posteriorly facing kidneys in the pelvis with the hila point anteriorly. The blood supply is from the lower transient branches of the aorta.*

Pelvic Kidneys During Early Development

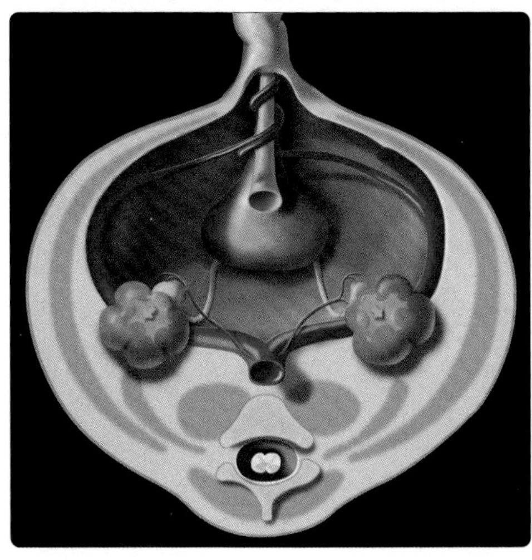

Medial Rotation of Kidneys

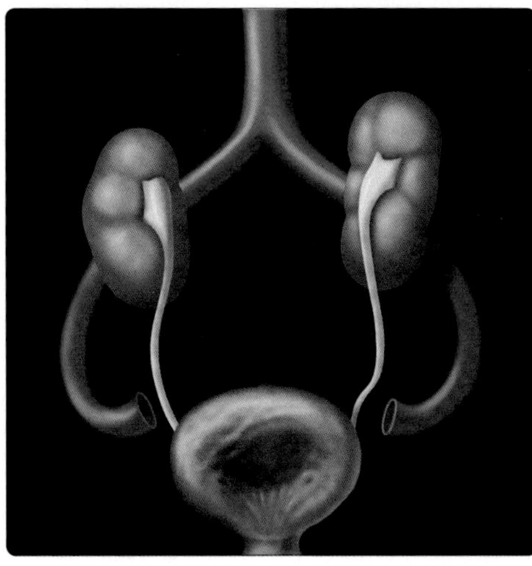

(Left) *Axial view shows kidneys beginning ascent and medial rotation. Note the blood supply is from the lower levels of the aorta.* **(Right)** *Illustration depicts middle stages of kidney ascent as they begin medial rotation (7 weeks), with the blood supply from more superiorly located transient vessels from the aorta than in previous stages. There is actually no true migration but apparent ascent due to disparate caudal growth of the fetus, leaving the kidney behind.*

Final Retroperitoneal Position of Kidneys

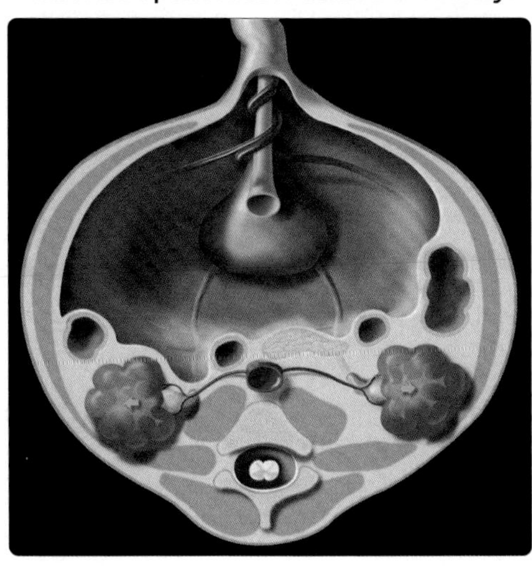

Final Position of Fetal Urinary System

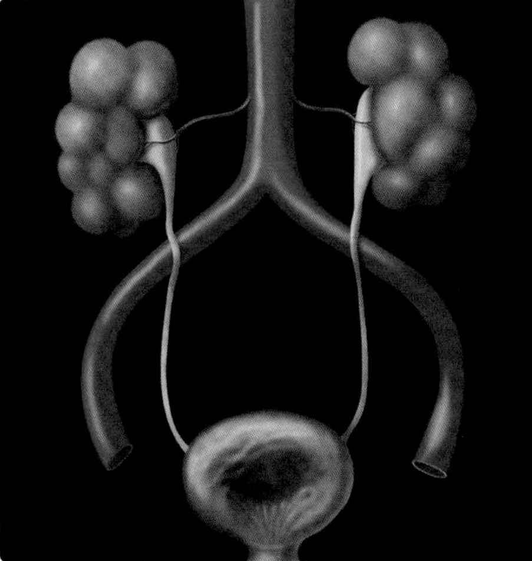

(Left) *Axial view shows that the kidneys have completed their ascent and are located retroperitoneally. Note the hila are pointing medially and blood supply is from the aorta.* **(Right)** *The final retroperitoneal location of the kidneys in the abdomen is shown. The hila face anteromedially. The blood supply is from renal arteries emanating from the aorta before aortic bifurcation.*

Mesonephros

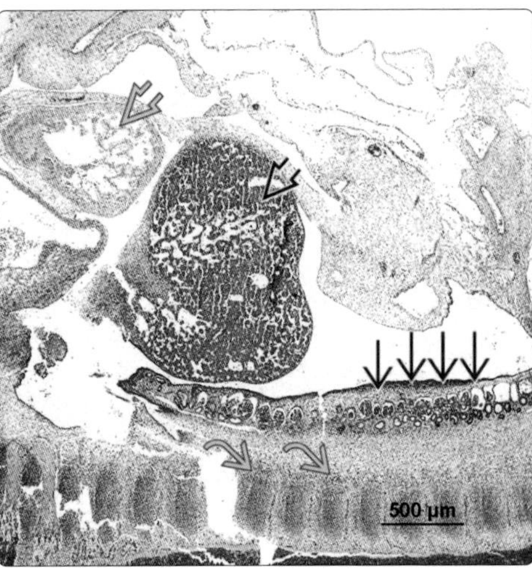

Immature Mesonephritic Nephron

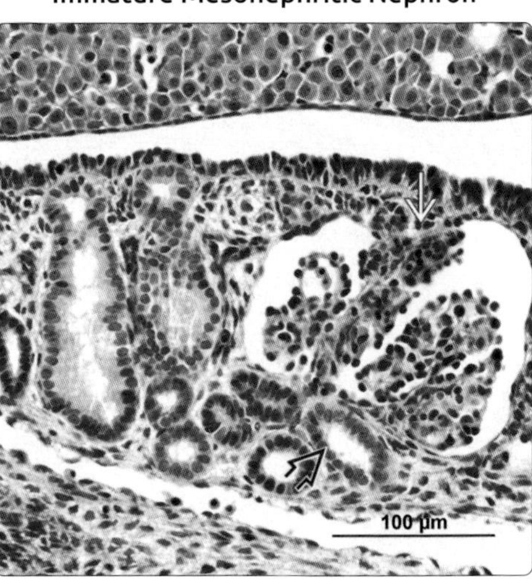

(Left) *Low-power image from a sagittal section of 1st trimester human products of conception shows the location of the developing mesonephros and its organization in a linear fashion ➡. The rostral side is on the left and the caudal end is on the right. Note the relationship of the mesonephros with respect to other organs such as the liver ➡, heart ➡, and somites ➡.* **(Right)** *High-power view of human fetal mesonephros shows a primitive glomerulus ➡ and tubules ➡.*

Ureteral Branching in Mouse

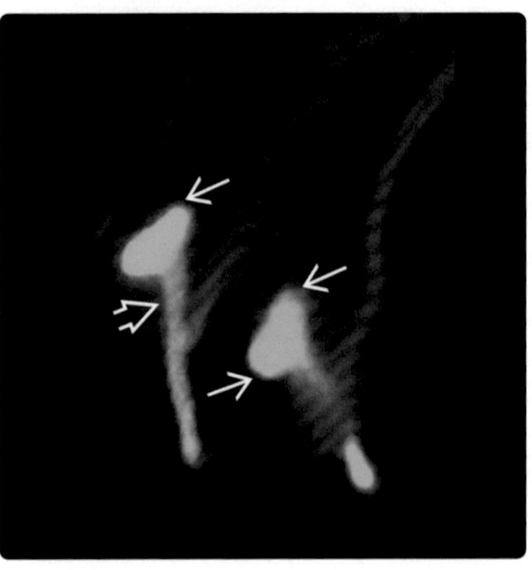

Branching Morphogenesis In Vitro

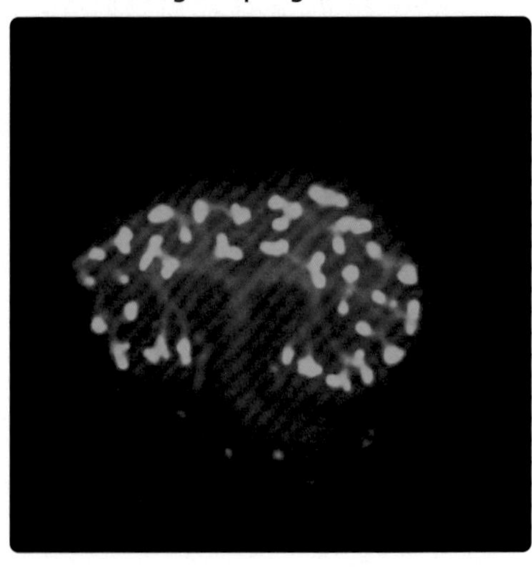

(Left) *Live detection shows 1st UB branching to produce T-shaped structure, visualized by green fluorescent protein (GFP) from the Ret locus in mice. This image is from E11.5d mouse urinary tract. The intense green signal in the UB tip ➡ represents sites of Ret expression that regulate UB branching. The initial UB stalk ➡ will become the ureter.* **(Right)** *Shown here is branching morphogenesis depicted by GFP expression in UB tips in a mouse metanephric kidney organ culture.*

Early Metanephric Condensation

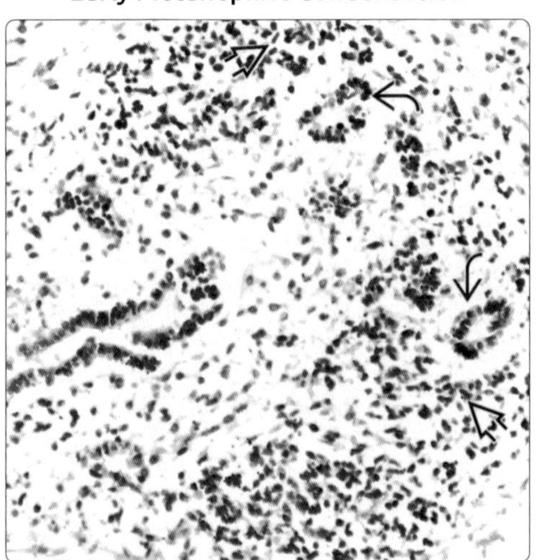

Mesonephros

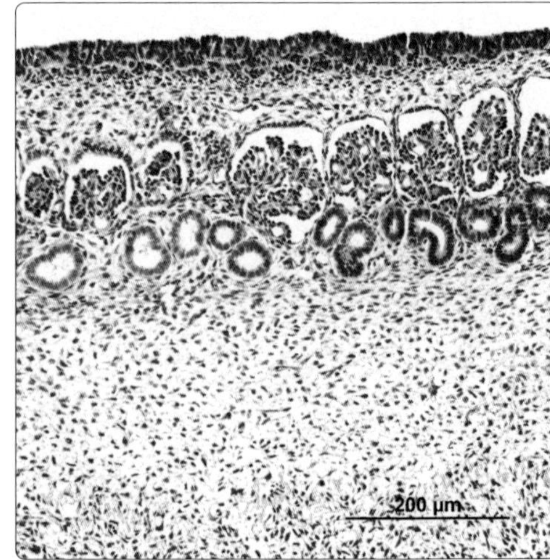

(Left) *Early stage of metanephric development shows ureteric bud (UB) invasion into the metanephric mesenchyme. The cells surrounding UB tips ➡ are the condensing mesenchyme ➡ that undergo mesenchymal to epithelial transformation to produce tubules and glomeruli.* **(Right)** *H&E-stained section shows linear organization of mesonephros in a human fetus with glomeruli and tubules.*

Sequential Glomerular Generations

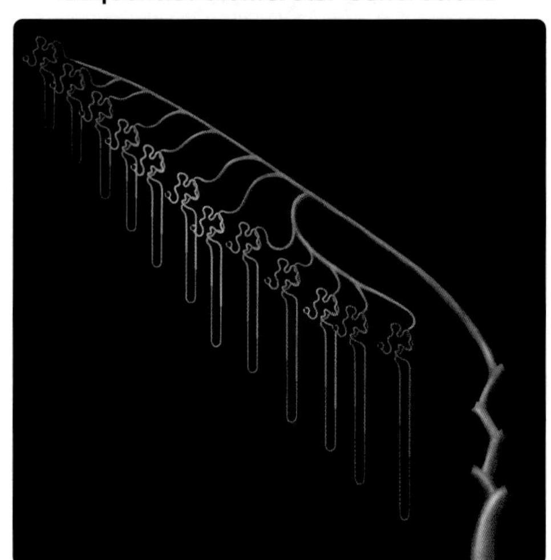

S-Shaped Body

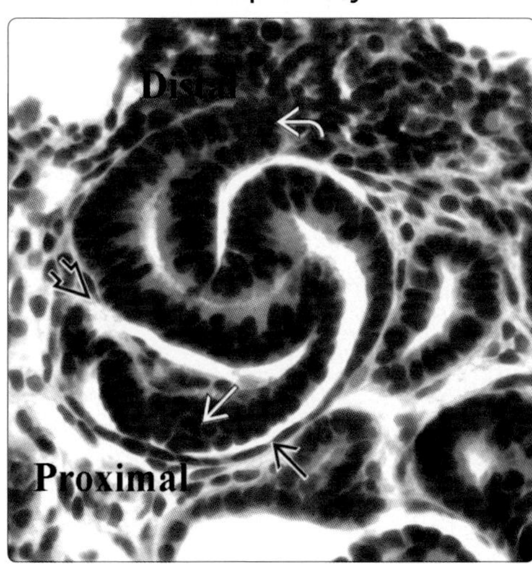

(Left) *12-14 glomerular generations develop centripetally, with the oldest glomeruli nearest the medulla. Glomerulogenesis is complete by birth; no new glomeruli form postnatally in humans.* **(Right)** *Human S-shaped body has a proximal end, glomerulus, distal end, and connecting tubule ➡. Endothelial cells migrate to the cleft ➡ to form the glomerular tuft. The outer cells ➡ become parietal epithelium of Bowman capsule, and the inner cells ➡ become podocytes.*

Metanephric Nephrogenesis

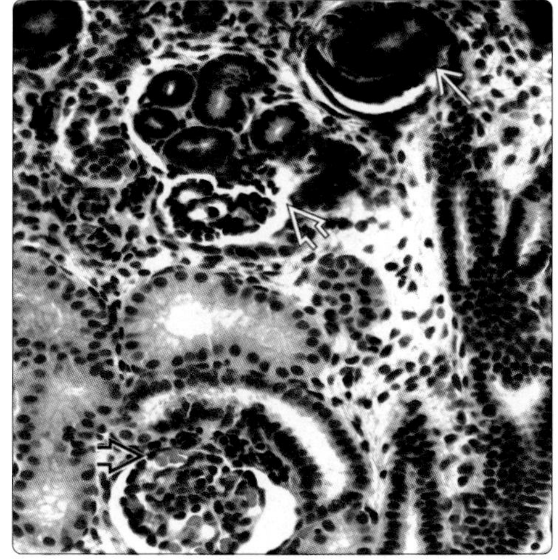

Fetal Glomeruli

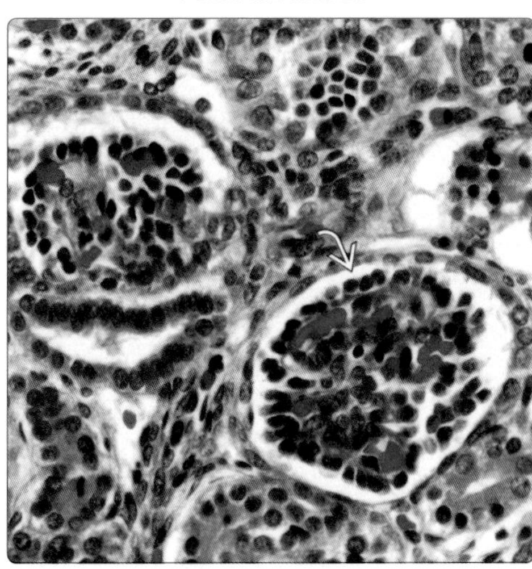

(Left) *Image of human metanephros shows different stages of nephrogenesis: Early comma-shaped body ➡, intermediate ➡, and more advanced ➡ stage.* **(Right)** *Early human fetal glomeruli are not fully vascularized. Eventually, 10-12 capillary loops will fill each glomerulus. Podocytes ➡ are densely arranged, forming a corona at the periphery of the capillary loops. As the loops develop, the podocytes flatten.*

S-Shaped Body

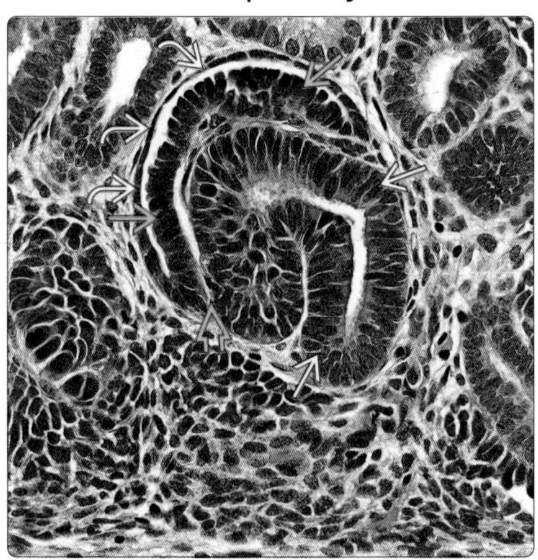

Developing Glomerulus

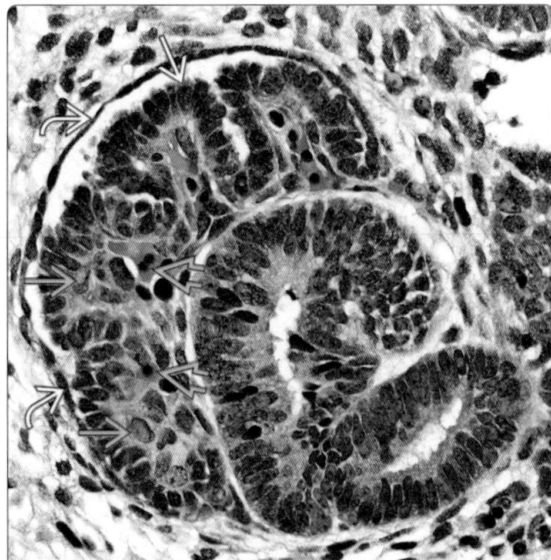

(Left) *S-shaped body is a precursor to different parts of the proximal nephron. Illustrated are the parietal layer ➡, podocytes arranged like a "picket-fence" ➡, the cleft through which endothelial and capillary progenitors enter ➡, and the proximal tubules ➡.* **(Right)** *Image from a fetal kidney demonstrates parietal cells ➡, fetal podocytes ➡ arranged perpendicular to the Bowman capsule, and mesangial cells ➡ & immature nucleated red blood cells in the developing vascular network in the glomerulus ➡.*

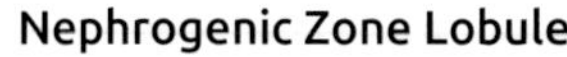

Nephrogenic Zone Lobule

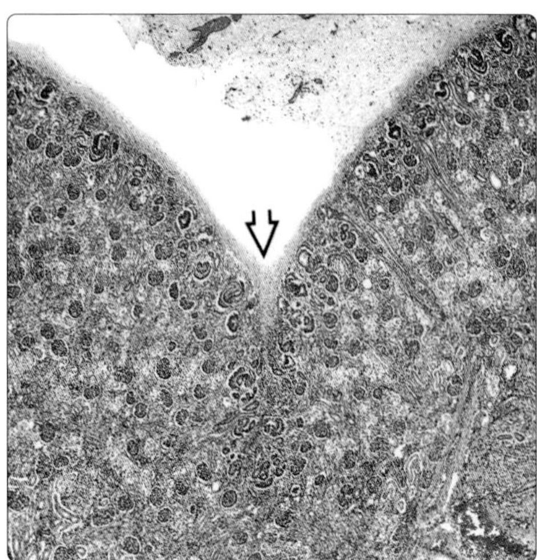

Nephrogenic Zone

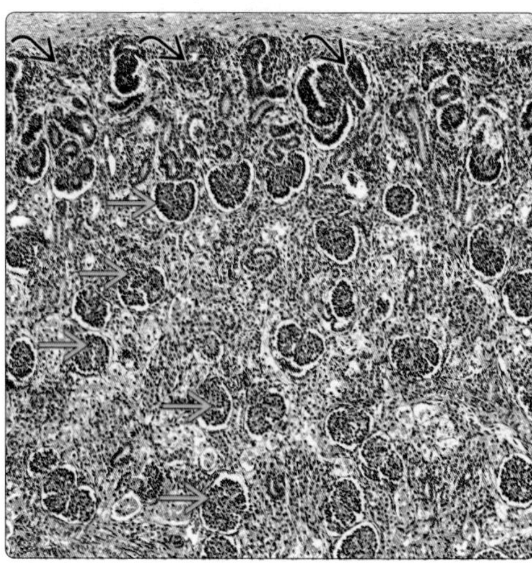

(Left) *Human fetal kidney is lobulated. This section shows junction of the nephrogenic zone between adjacent lobules.* **(Right)** *Image shows the nephrogenic zone at the top and newly formed glomeruli underneath. This shows that kidneys grow in a centripetal fashion with older glomeruli toward the center.*

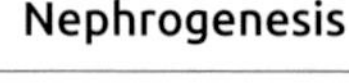

Nephrogenesis

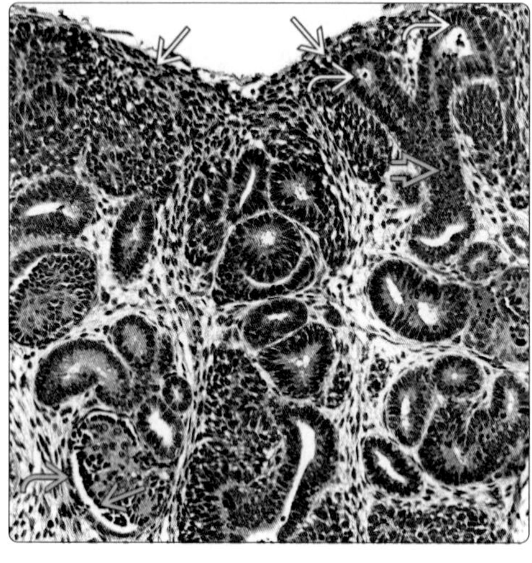

Branching Ureteric Bud

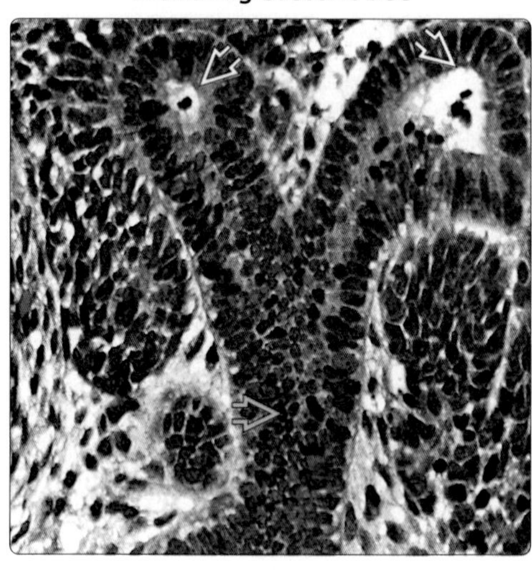

(Left) *The nephrogenic zone is toward the periphery of the developing kidney. Note the branching UB tip and stalk surrounded by cap mesenchyme cells and the outermost parietal and inner visceral fetal podocytes in a developing glomerulus.* **(Right)** *Image shows branching UB including the UB tips and the UB stalk. The tip cells are collecting duct progenitors that will renew to give more UB tips, and some will differentiate and incorporate into the stalk to form collecting ducts.*

Nephrogenic Zone

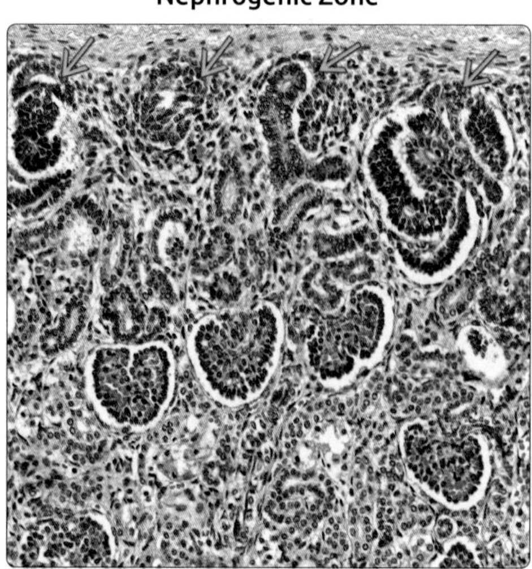

Collecting Duct

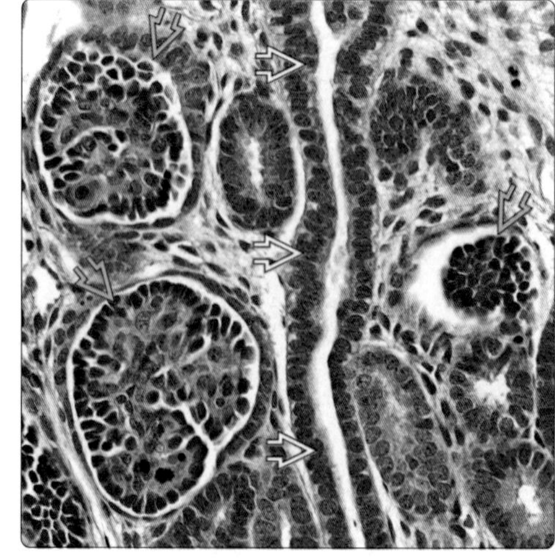

(Left) *High magnification of the nephrogenic zone shows 4 different nephrons at different stages of nephrogenesis.* **(Right)** *Longitudinal section through the collecting duct is shown. Notice a single layer of cuboidal appearing epithelium. Few immature fetal glomeruli are also in the field.*

pax-2

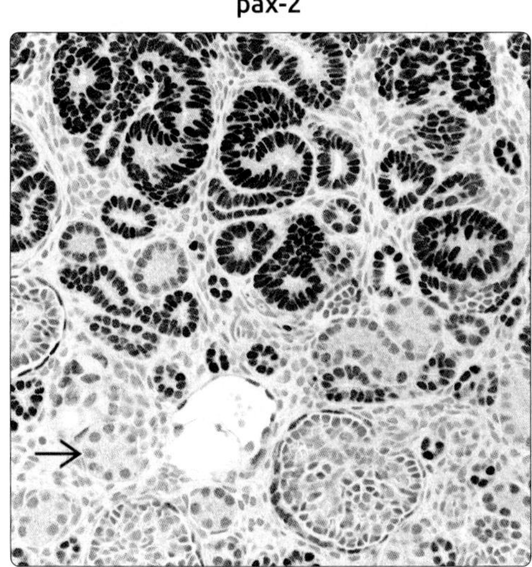

CD34

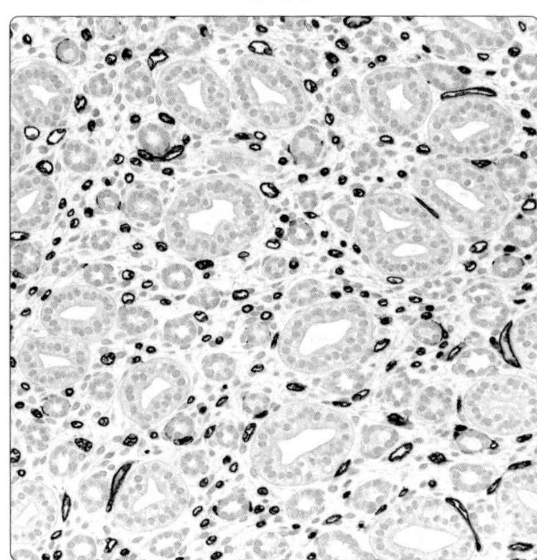

(Left) *pax-2 strongly highlights tubular epithelial cell nuclei in the nephrogenic zone in this fetal kidney at 12 weeks gestation. The cells closest to the capsule are the most strongly stained while deeper tubules* → *demonstrate weak to no nuclear staining.* **(Right)** *CD34 immunohistochemistry highlights the peritubular capillary network within the renal medulla of this fetal kidney at 12 weeks gestation.*

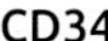

CD34

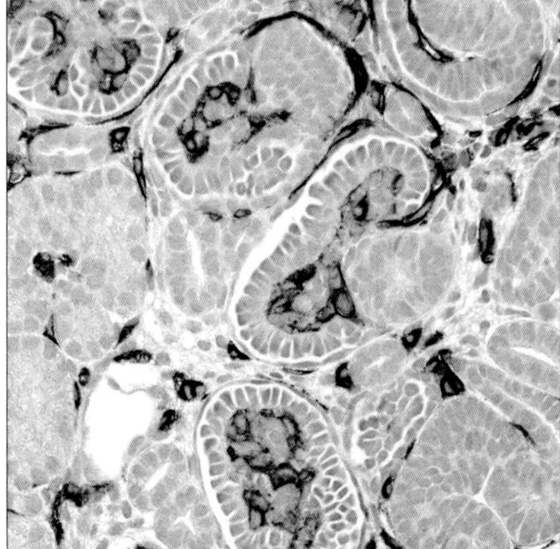

CD34

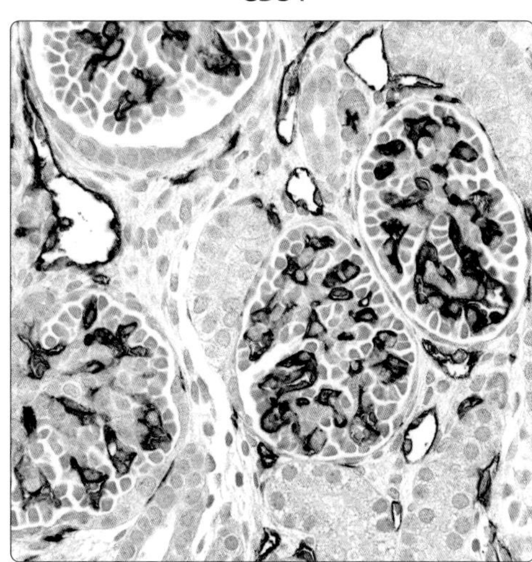

(Left) *CD34 IHC highlights glomerular capillaries in a fetal kidney at 12 weeks gestation.* **(Right)** *The glomerular capillaries are difficult to identify in fetal glomeruli. CD34 immunohistochemistry reveals the glomerular capillaries at 12 weeks gestation as the podocytes remain prominent and mesangial cells are inconspicuous.*

Newborn Kidney

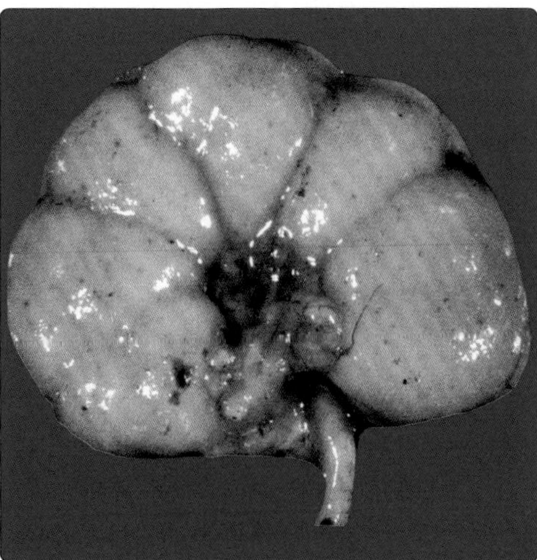

Newborn Kidney

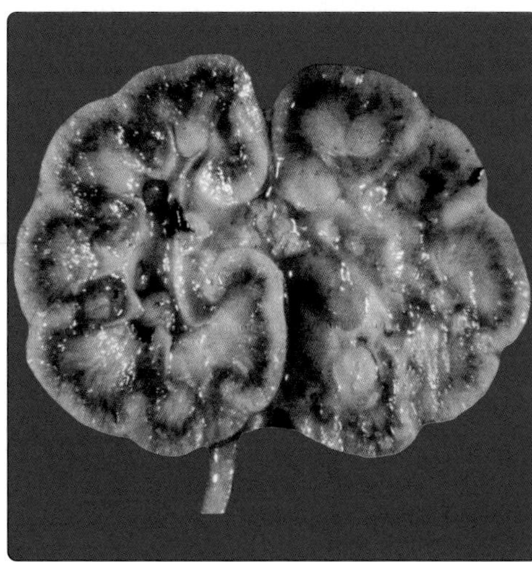

(Left) *Gross photograph of a normal neonatal kidney shows prominent fetal lobulations. These lobulations disappear with continued growth postnatally to give rise to a smooth-surfaced adult kidney.* **(Right)** *Coronal section of a newborn kidney is shown. Note that the cut surface shows lobulations and a well-organized cortex and medulla.*

SECTION 2

Glomerular Diseases

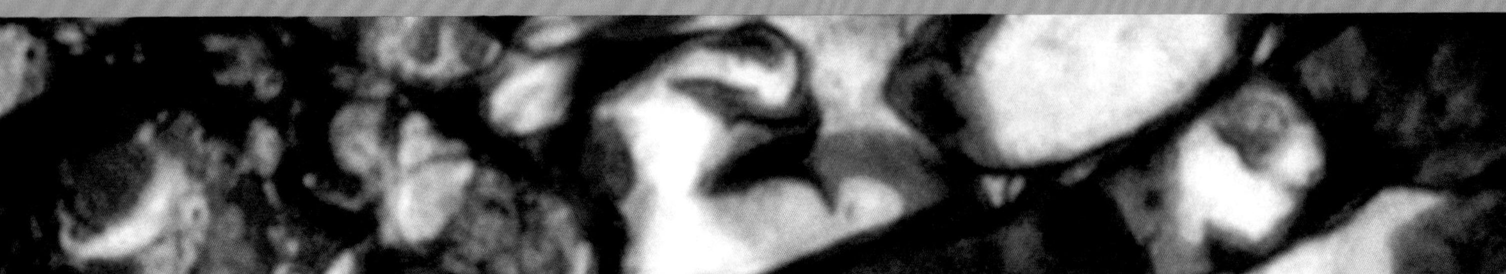

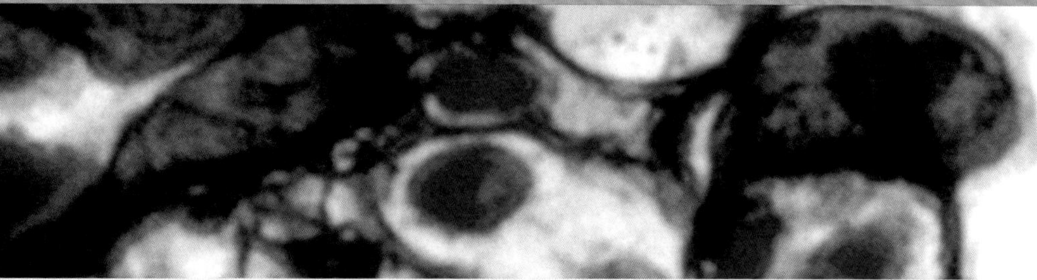

Diabetic Renal Disease

Infection-Related Glomerular Disease

Genetic Diseases of the Glomerulus

Genetic Diseases of the Glomerular Basement Membrane

Genetic Diseases of the Podocyte

Genetic Storage and Lipid Diseases

Other Genetic Diseases Affecting the Glomerulus

Miscellaneous Glomerular Diseases

Minimal Change Disease

KEY FACTS

TERMINOLOGY

- Idiopathic glomerular disease that causes nephrotic syndrome, with little or no light or immunofluorescent microscopic abnormalities and podocyte foot process effacement on electron microscopy

ETIOLOGY/PATHOGENESIS

- Usually idiopathic
- Involves loss of glomerular negative charge
- Circulating permeability factor
- Secondary forms due to virus, drugs, lymphoma

CLINICAL ISSUES

- Nephrotic syndrome
- Most common in young children, boys > girls
- 90-95% respond to corticosteroids
- Can present as acute renal insufficiency in adults

MICROSCOPIC

- Glomerulus normal by light microscopy except for variable podocyte hypertrophy
- Protein reabsorption droplets in tubules

ANCILLARY TESTS

- Immunofluorescence negative except for variable focal IgM ± C3
- Electron microscopy has characteristic findings
  - Podocyte foot process effacement, swelling, and microvillous transformation
  - Slit diaphragms lost
  - Normal glomerular basement membrane and no deposits

TOP DIFFERENTIAL DIAGNOSES

- Focal segmental glomerulosclerosis (FSGS)
- Diffuse mesangial hypercellularity (DMH)
- IgA, IgM, or C1q nephropathy

(Left) *The glomerulus appears normal by light microscopy PAS stain in a 5-year-old boy with nephrotic syndrome due to minimal change disease (MCD) with multiple relapses off steroids. Immunofluorescence studies were negative.* **(Right)** *IgG stain in a case of MCD shows little or no IgG present in the form of immune complexes. IgG and other plasma proteins may be found in podocytes as reabsorption droplets, which may be confused with deposits.*

Normal Glomerulus

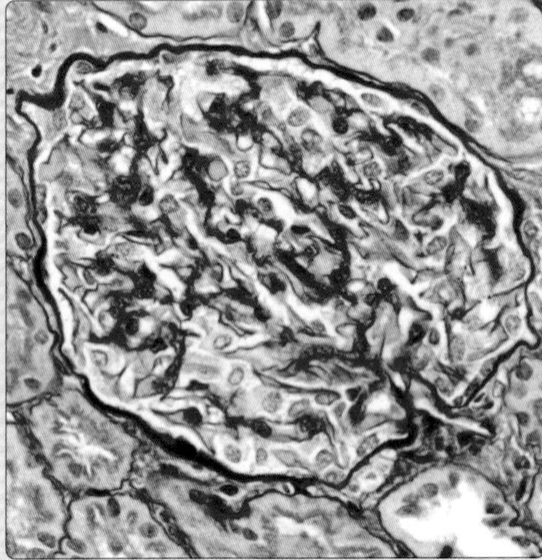

Negative Immunofluorescence

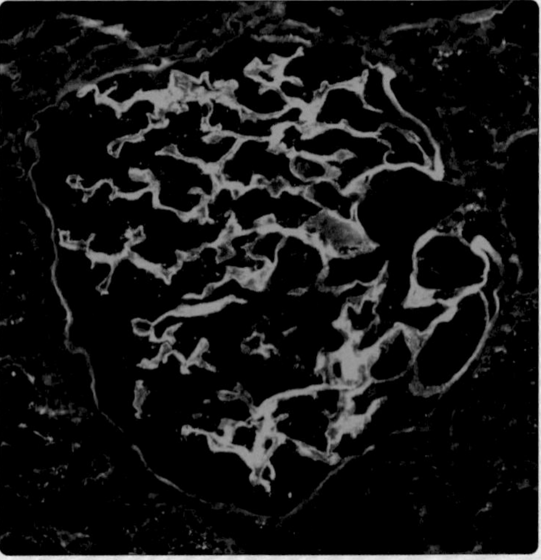

(Left) *Extensive effacement of foot processes ➡ is present in these glomerular capillaries from a 37-year-old woman with sudden onset of edema and 15 lb weight gain. Microvillous change in podocytes ➡ can also be seen. She responded completely to steroids.* **(Right)** *Prominent foot process effacement ➡ is present in this case of MCD. The glomerular basement membrane (GBM) has a normal thickness, and no electron-dense deposits are present.*

Foot Process Effacement

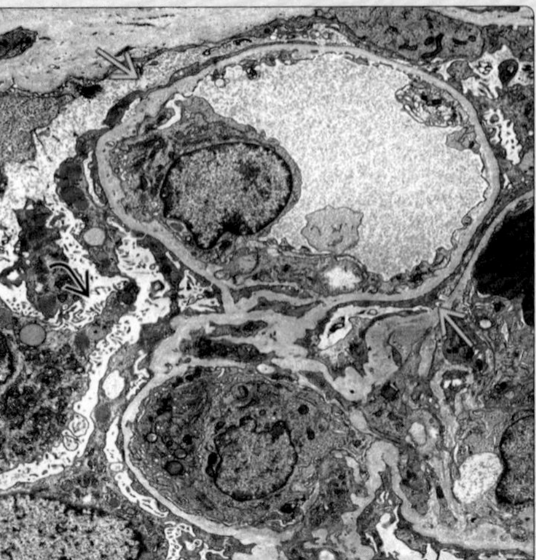

Foot Process Effacement

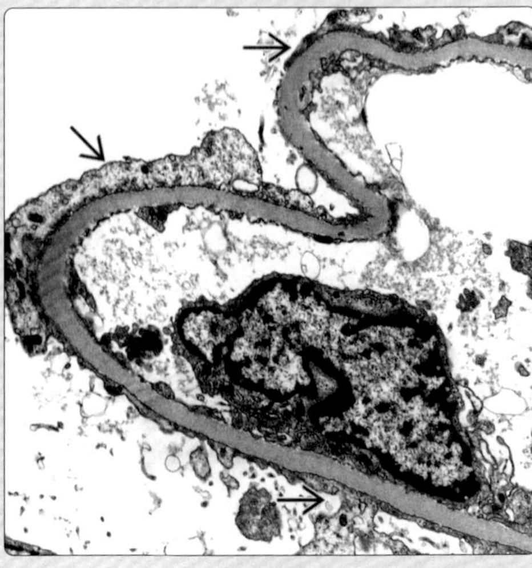

TERMINOLOGY

Abbreviations

- Minimal change disease (MCD)

Synonyms

- Idiopathic nephrotic syndrome, minimal change nephrotic syndrome, lipoid nephrosis, nil disease

Definitions

- Idiopathic glomerular disease that causes nephrotic syndrome, with little or no light or immunofluorescent microscopic abnormalities and podocyte foot process effacement (FPE) on electron microscopy
- Occurs as primary (idiopathic) disease, especially in children, and secondary to drugs, allergic reactions, immunologic diseases, and neoplasia at all ages

ETIOLOGY/PATHOGENESIS

Idiopathic (Primary)

- Classified as disease of podocytes, a "podocytopathy"
- Loss of podocyte negatively charged glycocalyx a central feature
  - Cause unknown; possibilities include
    - Enzymatic cleavage (e.g., neuraminidase)
    - Neutralizing positively charged molecule
    - Decreased synthesis
  - Loss of negative (anionic) charge leads to
    - Selective leakage of albumin (most negatively charged of major plasma proteins)
    - Foot process effacement
- Circulating permeability factor or cytokine abnormality postulated
  - Various substances have been suggested, ranging in molecular weight from 12-160 kDa
  - T-cell IL-13 content increases during relapse
    - Anti-inflammatory Th2 cytokine for B cells and monocytes
  - Podocyte CD80 (B7.1) may be involved
  - Increased serum IgE, IgG4 in some patients
- Rarely familial, no strong genetic associations

Secondary Forms of MCD

- Infection
  - Human immunodeficiency virus (HIV)
  - Upper respiratory tract infection
  - Mononucleosis
- Lymphoma (Hodgkin, mantle cell)
  - Possibly related to abnormal T-cell function
  - MCD may precede lymphoma by a year or more
- Allergy
  - Drugs, especially nonsteroidal anti-inflammatory drugs
  - Bee venom
  - Immunization
- Systemic lupus erythematosus
- Graft-vs.-host disease
- Acute renal allograft rejection (rare)

Experimental Studies

- Key features of MCD (e.g., FPE, proteinuria) reproduced in rats or mice by
  - Overexpression of IL-13
  - Administration of puromycin aminonucleoside or Adriamycin
  - Supernatants from hybridomas made from T cells from patients with MCD
  - Administration of neuraminidase or protamine sulfate (removes sialic acid or neutralizes anionic charge, respectively)

Relationship to Idiopathic Focal Segmental Glomerulosclerosis (FSGS)

- FSGS differs in podocyte loss and scarring, with evidence for replacement by parietal epithelial cells
- Some believe they form spectrum of same disease

CLINICAL ISSUES

Epidemiology

- Age
  - Most common cause of nephrotic syndrome in children younger than 10 years (70-90% of cases)
    - Median age of onset is 2.5 years; peak incidence at 2-3 years
  - ~ 50% of nephrotic syndrome in adolescents
  - ~ 10-15% of nephrotic syndrome in adults, with late peak incidence
    - 46% are 80-91 years
- Sex
  - In children, M:F = 2:1
  - In adults, M = F
- Ethnicity
  - More common in whites and Asians than in blacks

Presentation

- Sudden (days) onset of nephrotic syndrome
- Nephrotic syndrome
  - Proteinuria defined as ≥ 3.5 g/d in adults and ≥ 40 mg/m^2 body surface area (BSA)/hr in timed overnight collection in children
    - Selective proteinuria (chiefly albumin)
  - Edema
  - Hypoalbuminemia defined as serum albumin < 2.5 g/dL in children and < 3.5 g/dL in adults
  - Hypercholesterolemia
  - Lipiduria
    - Lipid-laden enucleated tubular cells may be seen as "oval fat bodies" in urinary sediment, with polarizable lipid
    - Gave rise to the term "lipoid nephrosis," original term for MCD
- Hematuria
  - Microscopic hematuria (10-30% of cases)
- Renal dysfunction
  - Acute renal failure occurs in 25% of adults with MCD
    - Associated with proteinuria > 10 g/d, serum albumin < 2 g/dL, hypertension, male gender, older age
    - Most recover in 4-8 weeks
      - Elevated serum Cr often persists (mean 2.11 ± 0.44)
  - Serum Cr > 98th percentile in < 1/3 of children with MCD
    - Reduced glomerular hydraulic conductivity for small molecules from loss of filtration slit pores

Laboratory Tests

- CD80 in urine may be marker for MCD vs. FSGS

Treatment

- Drugs
  - Corticosteroids primary treatment
    - 90-95% of children respond within 8 weeks, and 85-90% of adults respond within 20 weeks
    - 8-week course of daily or alternate day steroids often used as 1st treatment in children
      - If no response, renal biopsy performed to identify causes of nephrotic syndrome
    - Relapse within 1st year in up to 50% of children and 60-75% of adults
      - Usually treated with another course of steroids
  - Treatment for steroid failures
    - Cyclophosphamide, levamisole, cyclosporine
    - Rituximab (off label)
    - Abatacept (CTLA4-Ig) (off label)
      - Thought to bind to podocyte CD80
    - Repeat biopsy to detect FSGS

Prognosis

- Primary (idiopathic)
  - Rarely, if ever, leads to end-stage renal disease (ESRD) without development of FSGS
  - Adults with MCD and acute renal failure also usually fully recover
  - Relapses common and often lead to steroid dependence
- Secondary
  - Remits if underlying condition can be cured
- MCD may be initial manifestation of FSGS (~ 5%), in which case prognosis is that of FSGS

MACROSCOPIC

General Features

- Enlarged, waxy, yellow cortex due to lipid accumulation in proximal tubules

MICROSCOPIC

Histologic Features

- Glomeruli
  - Normal by light microscopy
    - Slight increases in mesangial cellularity and matrix in minority
    - Normal GBM
    - Normal glomerular size
  - Podocytes may be swollen and prominent with basophilic cytoplasm, resembling plasma cells
    - Resorption droplets in visceral epithelial cells
  - Loss of negative charge revealed by ↓ colloidal iron stain along GBM
  - Globally sclerotic glomeruli may be seen in MCD in adults
    - 10% of glomeruli may be sclerotic by age 40 and 30% by age 80
  - In children, involuted glomeruli are sometimes present
    - Lack of atrophic tubules indicates developmental rather than acquired glomerular sclerosis
- Tubules
  - Protein resorption droplets ("hyaline droplets")
    - PAS(+) and red on trichrome stain
  - Lipid droplets
    - Origin of term "lipoid nephrosis"
    - Clear vacuoles on H&E, PAS, and trichrome
    - Red droplets on oil red O-stained frozen sections
  - Usually little to no tubular atrophy
    - Older patients with concurrent arteriosclerosis may have underlying glomerular obsolescence and tubular atrophy
  - Tubular regenerative changes and injury in adults with acute renal failure
- Interstitial inflammation and fibrosis are usually absent
  - Interstitial foam cells may be seen but are rare

ANCILLARY TESTS

Immunofluorescence

- Typically no deposits of immunoglobulin or complement
- Minority have faint (≤ 1+) staining in glomeruli for IgM ± C3
  - < 5% of MCD cases have mesangial staining for IgG, IgM, IgA, C1q, &/or C3, particularly in children
    - May predict higher rate of steroid resistance
- Renal tubular resorption droplets stain for albumin
  - Usually, there is little immunoglobulin or C3 droplets in tubules (variable)

Electron Microscopy

- Podocyte FPE
  - Foot processes retract and cell body spreads on GBM (not "fusion")
  - Diffuse, usually involving > 75% of capillary surface
    - Extent (% of surface) correlates with severity of proteinuria in some but not all reports
  - Morphometry
    - Mean foot process width (1,566 ± 429 nm vs. 472 ± 52 nm normal); median 1,725 nm vs. 562 nm
    - Number of feet/10 µm of GBM (0.84 ± 0.24 vs. 3.84 ± 1.8 normal)
  - After remission, foot processes return toward normal, although some persistent change observed
  - FPE occurs in any renal disease with severe glomerular proteinuria
- Other usual podocyte abnormalities
  - Vacuolization and microvillous transformation
  - Resorption droplets and increased cellular organelles
  - Decreased numbers of filtration slit diaphragms
- Mild mesangial expansion in minority of cases
  - Vague mesangial and paramesangial electron densities, probably due to nonspecific protein insudation
- Tubules
  - Proximal tubules contain electron-dense resorption droplets (secondary lysosomes) and electron-lucent lipid droplets

Immunohistochemistry

- Decreased nephrin along GBM, corresponding with loss of slit diaphragms
  - Nephrin loss is seen in other diseases with FPE
- Markers that favor FSGS over MCD
  - CD44 in parietal epithelial cells (PEC), a marker of activation
  - Ectopic PEC markers in glomerular tuft

- Claudin-1, A-kinase anchor protein, annexin-A3
  - Preservation of α- and β-dystroglycan in some but not all studies
- Markers that favor MCD over FSGS
  - Podocyte CD80 (B7.1)

DIFFERENTIAL DIAGNOSIS

Focal Segmental Glomerulosclerosis (FSGS)

- Segmental hyalinosis or synechiae to Bowman capsule
- Minority of cases with MCD on initial biopsy show FSGS later due to sampling or progression
- FSGS cases with unsampled glomerulosclerosis may be misdiagnosed as MCD
  - Serial sectioning required to detect segmental glomerulosclerosis, most common at corticomedullary junction
    - Sections of segmentally sclerotic glomeruli may appear normal if plane of section does not include segmental sclerosis
  - Probability of detecting focal glomerular lesion (P) is a function of % of glomeruli affected in kidney (p) and number of glomeruli in biopsy (n)
    - $P = (1-p)^n$
    - e.g., to detect lesions with > 95% probability, if 5% affected in kidney, 60 glomeruli needed; if 10% affected, 30 glomeruli needed
  - Clues to underlying FSGS
    - Glomerular hypertrophy or tubular atrophy
      - Glomerular area of 1.75x age-matched controls
    - Expression of PEC proteins in glomerular tuft
    - Endocapillary foam cells
- Recurrent FSGS in transplants begins as MCD-like lesions in 1st month after transplant, followed by FSGS lesions later

Diffuse Mesangial Hypercellularity (DMH)

- Possibly a variant of MCD
  - > 4 mesangial cells per mesangial region in ≥ 80% of glomeruli in 2-3 µm tissue sections
- ~ 3% of pediatric cases of idiopathic nephrotic syndrome
- IF may show IgM or C3; EM shows electron-dense deposits in 50%
- More likely to have hematuria and hypertension
- Higher rate of steroid resistance

IgM Nephropathy

- Possibly a variant of MCD/FSGS
- Diffuse, global mesangial IgM (≥ 2+); C3 in 30+%
- EM shows FPE and occasional scanty paramesangial deposits
- Hematuria and hypertension more common than in MCD
- 6x increased rate of progression to FSGS in children compared with MCD

IgA Nephropathy

- MCD superimposed on IgA nephropathy should be entertained if nephrotic syndrome is of rapid onset and complete FPE is present
- Most respond to steroids (80%)

C1q Nephropathy

- C1q in mesangium (≥ 2+) ± immunoglobulins on IF
- Occasional electron-dense deposits on EM

Chyluria

- Normal podocytes (no FPE) with heavy proteinuria

Amyloidosis

- Has been missed in early cases without EM or Congo red

Congenital Nephrotic Syndrome (Finnish Type)

- Onset in in utero/infancy
- Absence of podocyte slit diaphragm by EM

DIAGNOSTIC CHECKLIST

Pathologic Interpretation Pearls

- Podocyte hypertrophy (cytoplasmic basophilia) and tubular reabsorption droplets are LM clues to diagnosis
- Multiple levels important to detect FSGS
  - Note whether biopsy includes corticomedullary junction (site initially affected by FSGS)
  - Prudent to always state "FSGS cannot be excluded"
- Acute tubular necrosis may be present and account for acute renal failure

SELECTED REFERENCES

1. Ling C et al: Urinary CD80 levels as a diagnostic biomarker of minimal change disease. Pediatr Nephrol. 30(2):309-16, 2015
2. Garin EH et al: Case series: CTLA4-IgG1 therapy in minimal change disease and focal segmental glomerulosclerosis. Pediatr Nephrol. ePub, 2014
3. Iwabuchi Y et al: Long-term prognosis of adult patients with steroid-dependent minimal change nephrotic syndrome following rituximab treatment. Medicine (Baltimore). 93(29):e300, 2014
4. Kofman T et al: Minimal change nephrotic syndrome associated with non-Hodgkin lymphoid disorders: a retrospective study of 18 cases. Medicine (Baltimore). 93(24):350-8, 2014
5. Liu XJ et al: Ultrastructural changes of podocyte foot processes during the remission phase of minimal change disease of human kidney. Nephrology (Carlton). 19(7):392-7, 2014
6. Smeets B et al: Detection of Activated Parietal Epithelial Cells on the Glomerular Tuft Distinguishes Early Focal Segmental Glomerulosclerosis from Minimal Change Disease. Am J Pathol. ePub, 2014
7. Munyentwali H et al: Rituximab is an efficient and safe treatment in adults with steroid-dependent minimal change disease. Kidney Int. 83(3):511-6, 2013
8. Chugh SS et al: New insights into human minimal change disease: lessons from animal models. Am J Kidney Dis. 59(2):284-92, 2012
9. Wei C et al: Minimal change disease as a modifiable podocyte paracrine disorder. Nephrol Dial Transplant. 26(6):1776-7, 2011
10. Garin EH et al: Urinary CD80 excretion increases in idiopathic minimal-change disease. J Am Soc Nephrol. 20(2):260-6, 2009
11. Deegens JK et al: Podocyte foot process effacement as a diagnostic tool in focal segmental glomerulosclerosis. Kidney Int. 74(12):1568-76, 2008
12. Waldman M et al: Adult minimal-change disease: clinical characteristics, treatment, and outcomes. Clin J Am Soc Nephrol. 2(3):445-53, 2007
13. Stokes MB et al: Glomerular tip lesion: a distinct entity within the minimal change disease/focal segmental glomerulosclerosis spectrum. Kidney Int. 65(5):1690-702, 2004
14. Fogo A et al: Glomerular hypertrophy in minimal change disease predicts subsequent progression to focal glomerular sclerosis. Kidney Int. 38(1):115-23, 1990
15. Jennette JC et al: Adult minimal change glomerulopathy with acute renal failure. Am J Kidney Dis. 16(5):432-7, 1990
16. Childhood nephrotic syndrome associated with diffuse mesangial hypercellularity. A report of the Southwest Pediatric Nephrology Study Group. Kidney Int. 24(1):87-94, 1983

(Left) *Jones methenamine silver stain shows that the GBMs have a normal thickness* → *in minimal change disease with no duplication or glomerular hypercellularity.* **(Right)** *Glomerulus from a patient with MCD appears normal by light microscopy. The only clue that there is proteinuria is the presence of hypertrophied podocytes* →*, which have increased, basophilic cytoplasm* →*.*

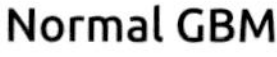

Normal GBM

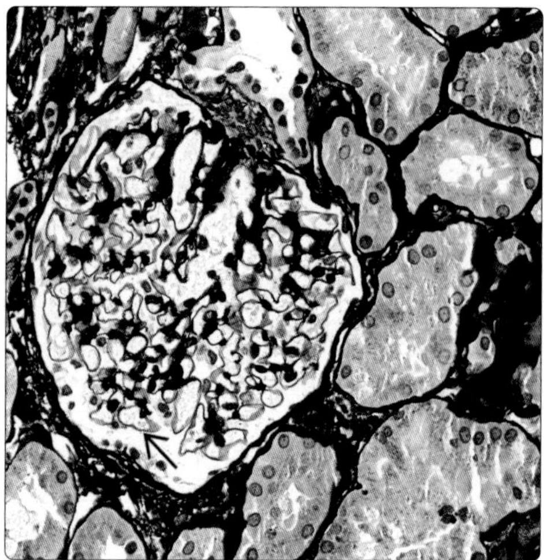

Hypertrophied Podocytes

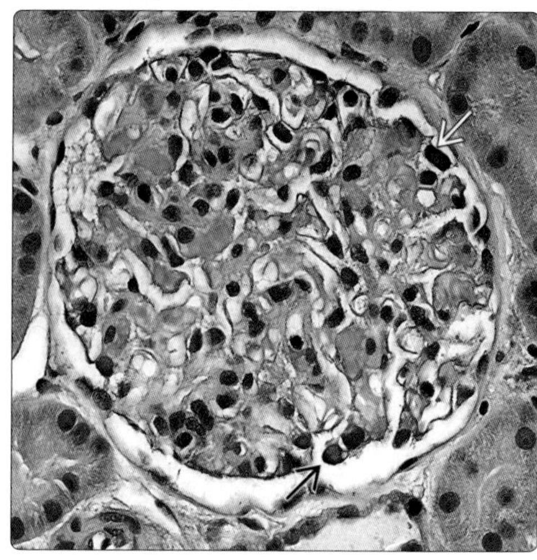

(Left) *This specimen is from a 5-year-old boy who presented with MCD. Glomeruli with an immature appearance are present, with crowded podocytes* →*. This should not be confused with collapsing glomerulopathy.* **(Right)** *This "pseudo-adhesion"* → *is due to a tangential section through the GBM in a patient with MCD. In presumed MCD, it is essential to search for evidence of FSGS in multiple levels, as adhesions and artifacts such as this can confound interpretation.*

Crowded Podocytes

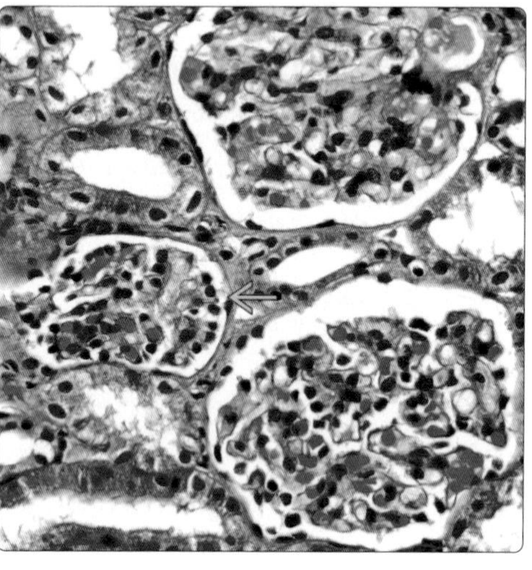

"Pseudo-Adhesion"

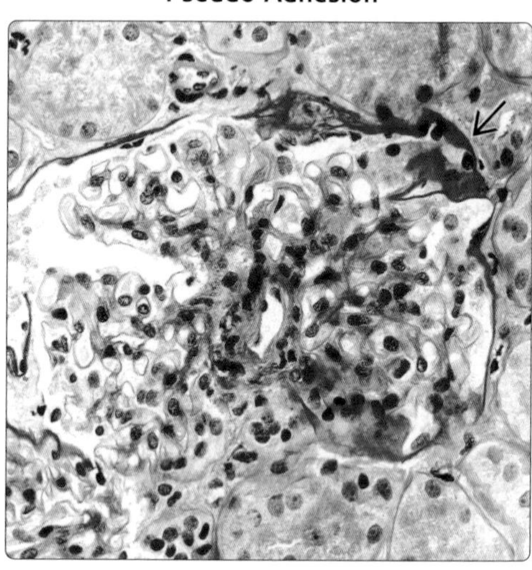

(Left) *PAS-positive tubular resorption droplets* → *in MCD are predominantly in the proximal renal tubules. These are found in any disease with glomerular proteinuria.* **(Right)** *Oil red O stain of a frozen section from a patient with MCD shows the characteristic lipid* → *in proximal tubules. These accumulate in tubules in all diseases with nephrotic-range proteinuria, but since the lipid was the only feature noted originally in MCD it lead to the term "lipoid nephrosis."*

Tubular Resorption Droplets

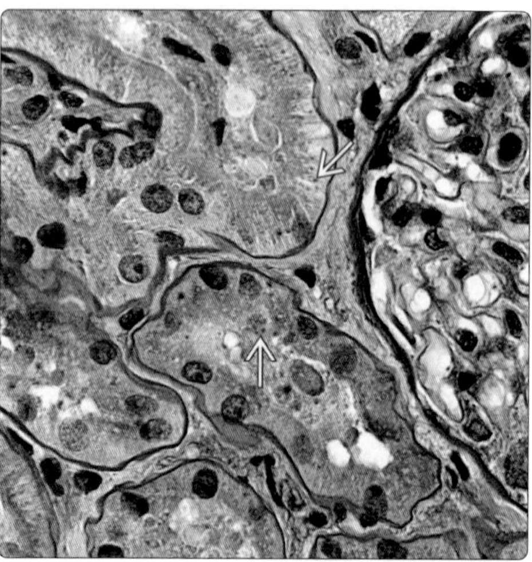

Lipid in Tubules

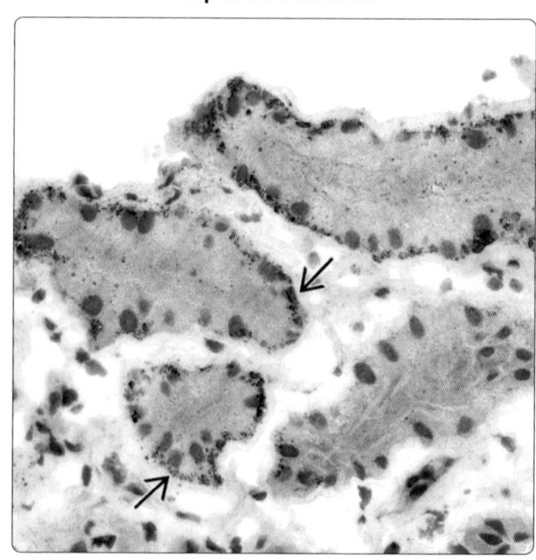

Minimal IgM Deposits

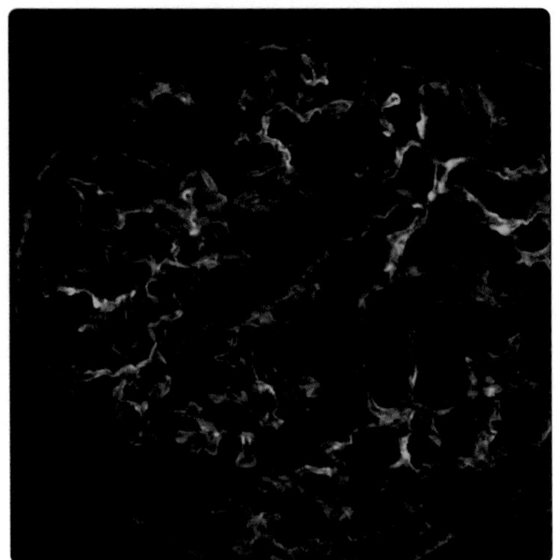

IgM Deposits

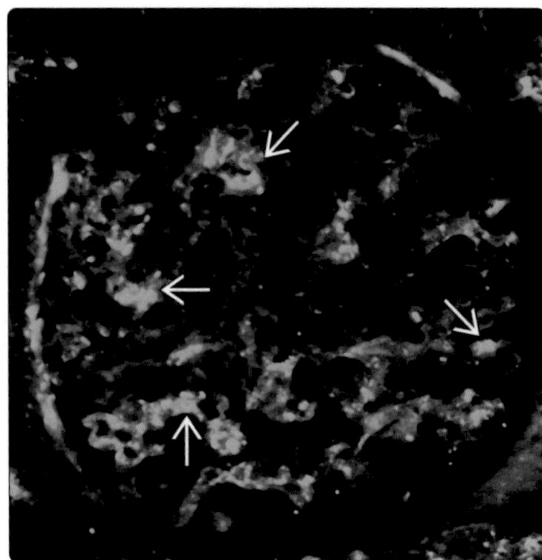

(Left) *Trace mesangial IgM can sometimes be seen in MCD. When 2+ IgM is present along with electron-dense deposits by EM, some categorize the lesion as IgM nephropathy.* **(Right)** *In MCD, there can be mesangial staining for IgM as in this case, which some might categorize as IgM nephropathy ➡. This may be associated with decreased responsiveness to steroids.*

Negative IgA

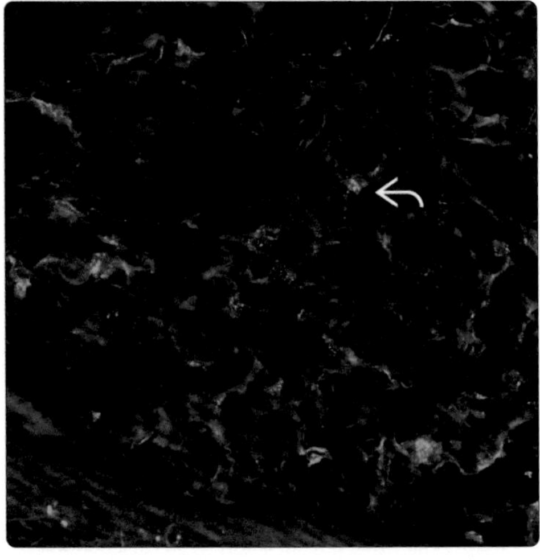

Glomerular C3

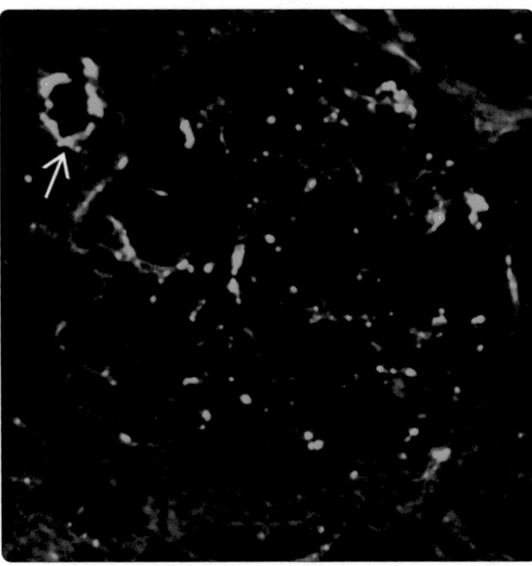

(Left) *In MCD, little or no immunoglobulin is typically present. In this case of MCD, no IgA is detected in the glomerulus aside from a few faint granules that are probably protein reabsorption droplets in the podocyte ➦.* **(Right)** *This patient with MCD has more prominent C3 in the glomerulus. Most is probably in podocyte reabsorption droplets, and some is in the mesangium. The arterial wall also has C3 ➡, a common, nonspecific finding.*

Tubular Reabsorption Droplets

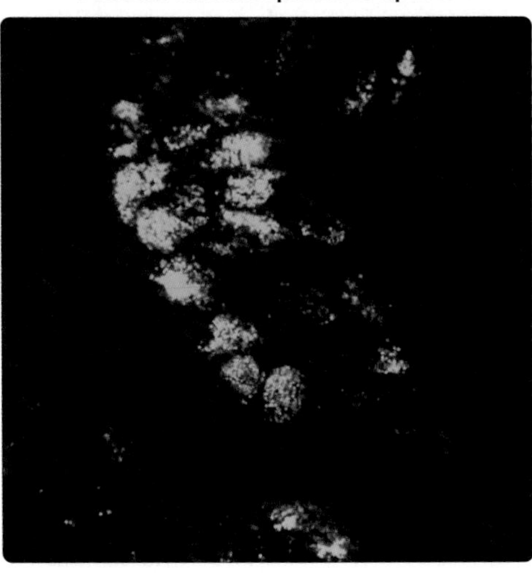

Reabsorption Droplets

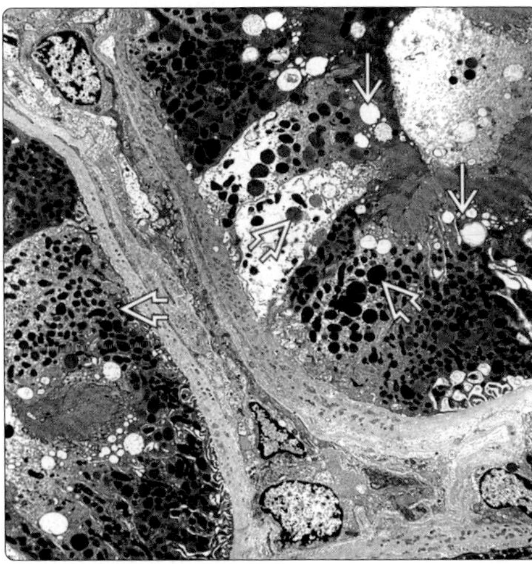

(Left) *Proximal tubules show abundant reabsorption droplets that stain for albumin in this patient with MCD. Other plasma proteins are commonly found as well. This may be the only abnormality by immunofluorescence.* **(Right)** *The tubules in MCD may have frequent resorption droplets, some of which are clear ➡ on EM, representing lipid vacuoles, and some of which are electron dense ⇨, representing proteinaceous droplets.*

(Left) *This patient with MCD shows expansion of the cell body surface area, a classic feature of the podocyte reaction to heavy proteinuria that produces villous hypertrophy* ⇨*. Foot processes are effaced, and the GBM is normal.* (Right) *Patient with MCD has swollen podocytes* ⇨ *but only patchy foot process effacement in this capillary.*

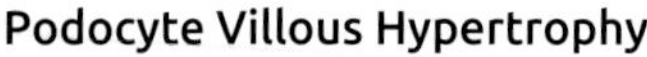

Podocyte Villous Hypertrophy

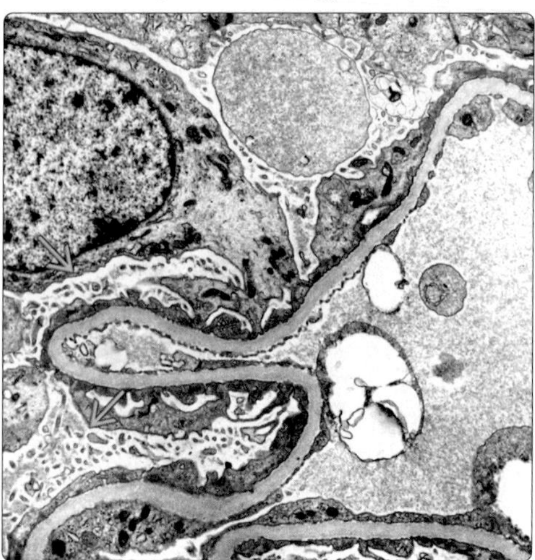

Swollen Podocytes

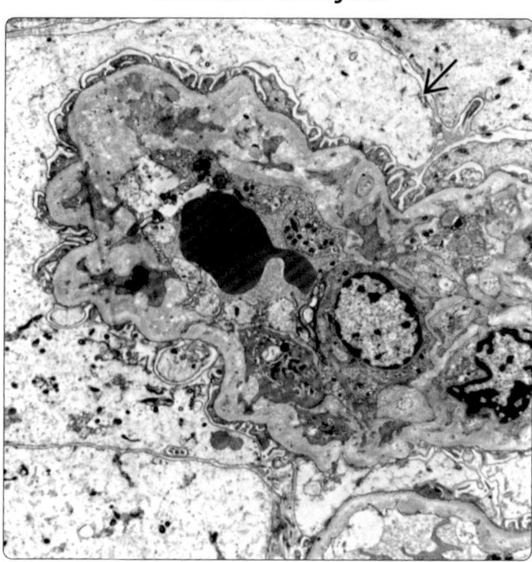

(Left) *In MCD, the mesangium can be mildly expanded with cellular debris* ⇨*. Vague densities* ➡ *may be present although these are not considered evidence of an immune complex-mediated disorder but rather of nonspecific entrapment.* (Right) *This specimen is from an 18-year-old man who presented with nephrotic syndrome due to MCD associated with retroperitoneal masses, later shown to be Hodgkin disease. Lymphoma is a cause of MCD but usually remits with remission of the lymphoma.*

Mildly Expanded Mesangium

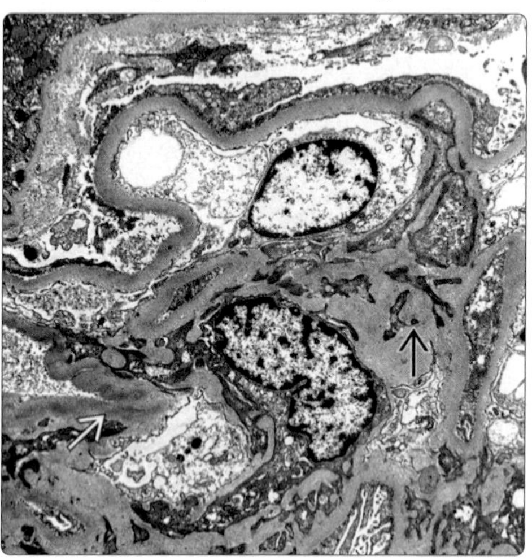

MCD Due to Lymphoma

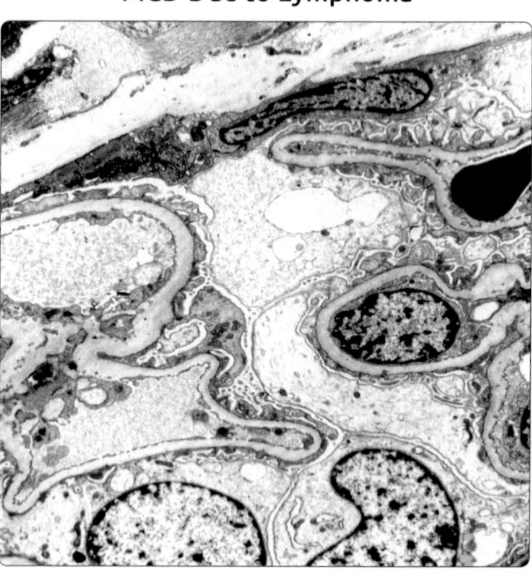

(Left) *A 68-year-old woman presented with 3.4 g protein/day and edema associated with NSAIDs. Acute interstitial nephritis was also present. Drugs, especially NSAIDs, are associated with MCD.* (Right) *A 9-year-old girl with nephrotic syndrome was treated successfully with corticosteroids and biopsied when the proteinuria was in remission. EM shows complete recovery of foot processes* ⇨*.*

MCD Due to NSAIDs

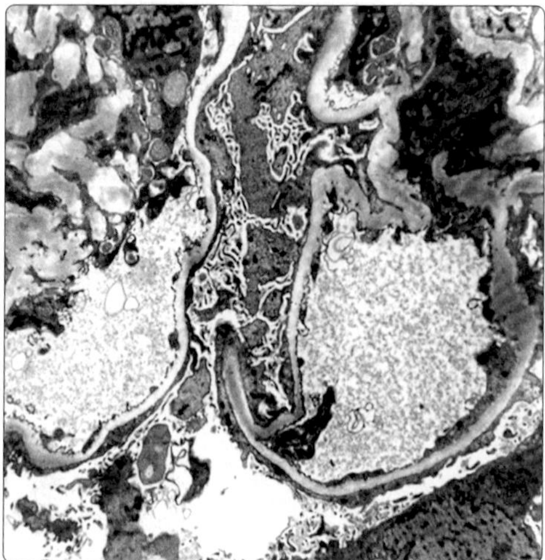

Recovery of Podocyte Foot Processes

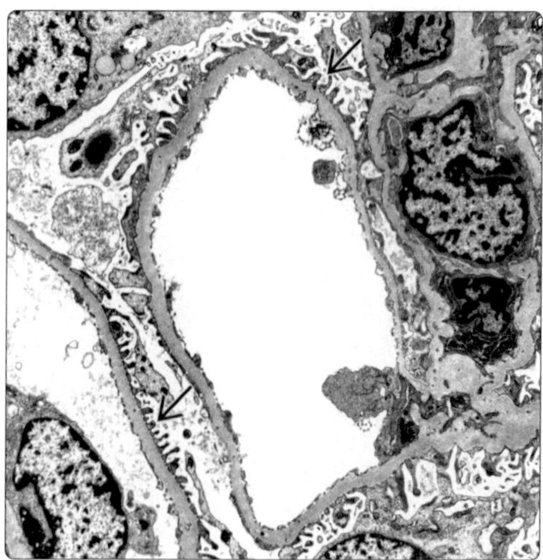

MCD and IgA Nephropathy

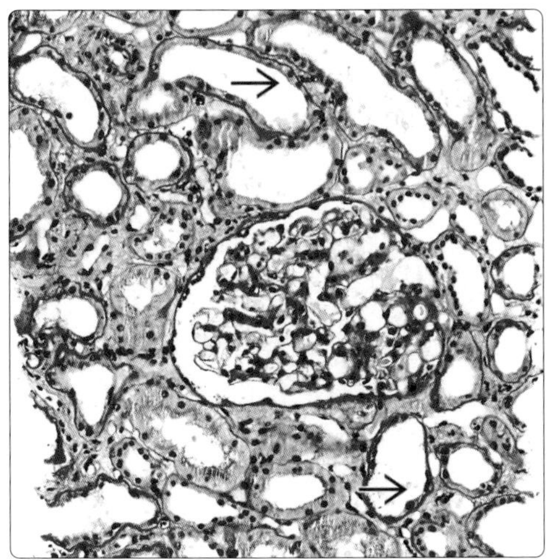

MCD and IgA Nephropathy

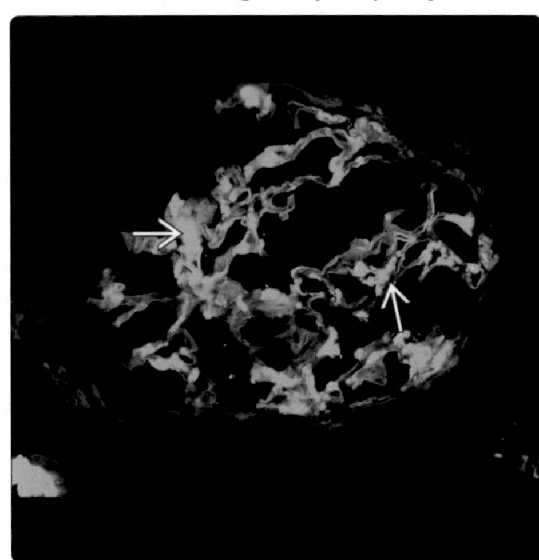

(Left) *Glomeruli in a 48-year-old man with acute onset of nephrotic syndrome and renal failure (albumin 1 g/dl, 15 g/d proteinuria, Cr 1.5 mg/dL) show mild mesangial hypercellularity. Dilated tubules show flattened epithelium ⇒. IgA was prominent by IF.* **(Right)** *IF in a patient with an acute nephrotic syndrome clinically suspicious for MCD reveals bright granular mesangial staining for IgA ➡. The glomeruli showed similar staining for C3 and both light chains. There was widespread FPE by EM.*

MCD and IgA Nephropathy

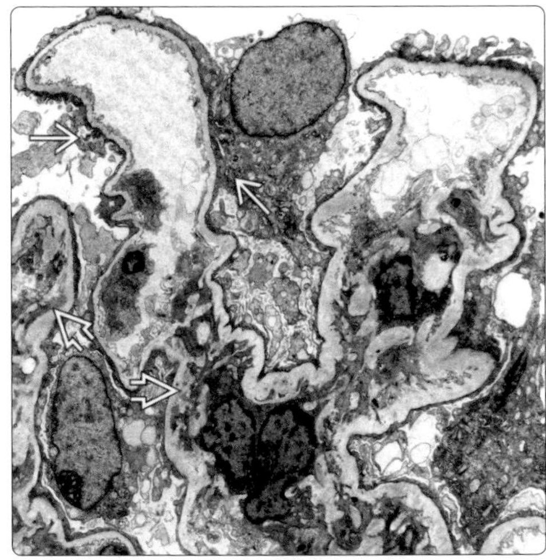

MCD With C1q Nephropathy

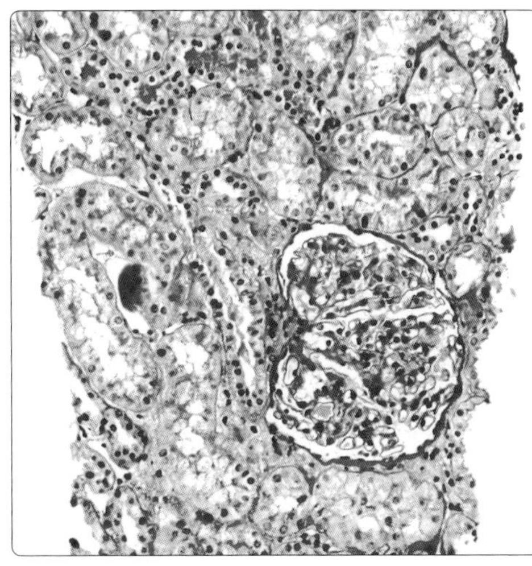

(Left) *Ultrastructural study reveals diffuse podocyte FPE, typical of MCD ➡. Mesangial and paramesangial electron-dense deposits are present as well ➡, part of IgA nephropathy.* **(Right)** *Biopsy from a 20-year-old man with sudden onset of nephrotic syndrome with anasarca and 10 g/d proteinuria shows glomeruli appearing normal. C1q was 2+ in the mesangium associated with electron-dense deposits.*

MCD With C1q Nephropathy

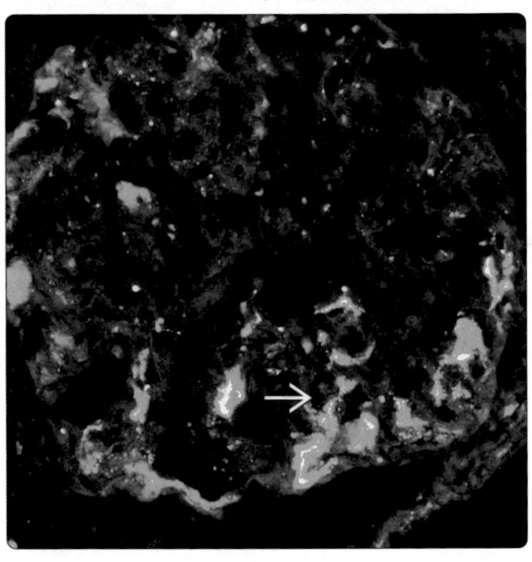

MCD With C1q Nephropathy

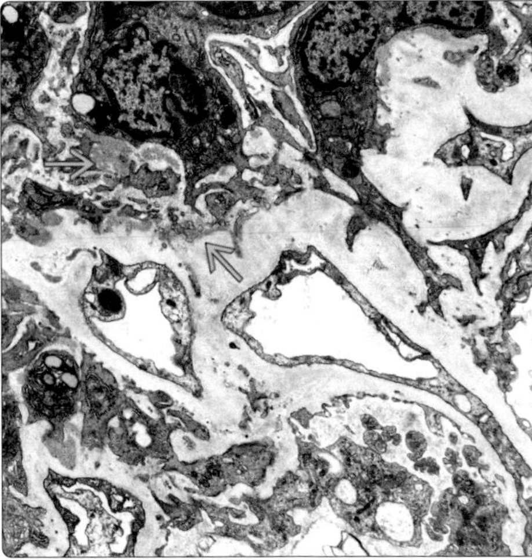

(Left) *Staining for C1q reveals 2+ granular mesangial staining ➡. C1q was the dominant immunoreactant in this case; there was lesser staining of glomeruli for IgG, kappa, and lambda, and stains for IgA were negative. The patient did not have clinical or laboratory evidence of systemic lupus erythematosus and otherwise had MCD.* **(Right)** *There are scattered amorphous mesangial electron-dense deposits within the glomeruli in this patient with MCD and C1q nephropathy ⇒.*

KEY FACTS

ETIOLOGY/PATHOGENESIS

- Nonsteroidal anti-inflammatory drugs (NSAIDs)
  - Diclofenac
  - 5-aminosalicylic acid (ASA)
- Cyclooxygenase 2 inhibitors
  - Celecoxib
- Mercury skin cream
- Interferon-α and interferon-β
- Pamidronate
- Gold
- Lithium
- Amoxicillin
- Rifampin
- Penicillamine
- Gongjin-dan (Chinese folk medicine)

CLINICAL ISSUES

- Nephrotic syndrome
- Treatment
  - Discontinue offending pharmacologic agent
- Prognosis
  - Excellent with generally rapid remission after drug withdrawal

MICROSCOPIC

- Normal glomeruli by light microscopy
- Diffuse podocyte foot process effacement

ANCILLARY TESTS

- No immune deposits by IF or electron dense deposits by EM

TOP DIFFERENTIAL DIAGNOSES

- Minimal change disease, primary
- Focal segmental glomerulosclerosis (unsampled)
- Acute interstitial nephritis
  - May occur concurrently with drug-induced MCD
- IgM nephropathy
- Lithium nephrotoxicity

(Left) *PAS shows a normal glomerulus by light microscopy. Diagnostic findings can only be observed by electron microscopy. Interstitial inflammation is also present adjacent to Bowman capsule, but some patients may only manifest with proteinuria.* **(Right)** *Jones methenamine silver reveals a normal glomerulus with delicate basement membranes and normal cellularity. Prominent podocyte protein droplets ⇒ correlate with the clinical history of severe proteinuria (13 g/d).*

Normal Glomerulus (PAS)

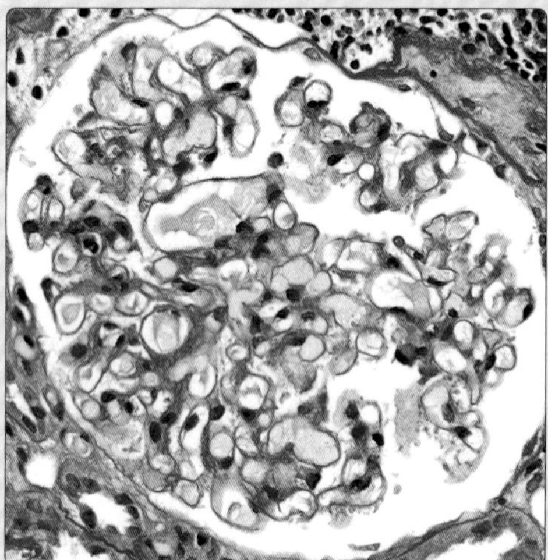

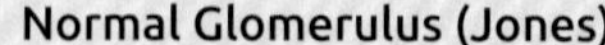

Normal Glomerulus (Jones)

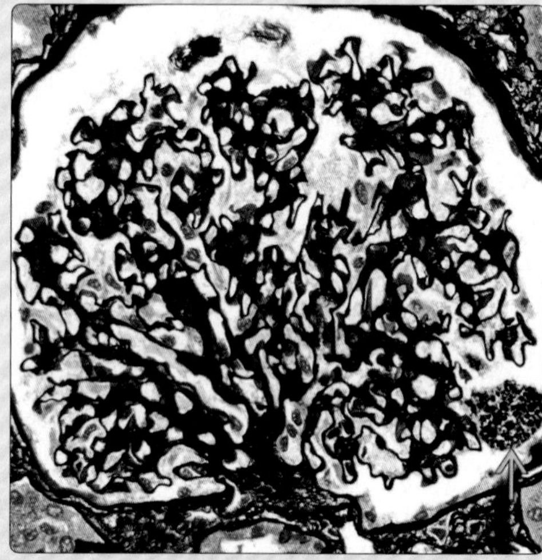

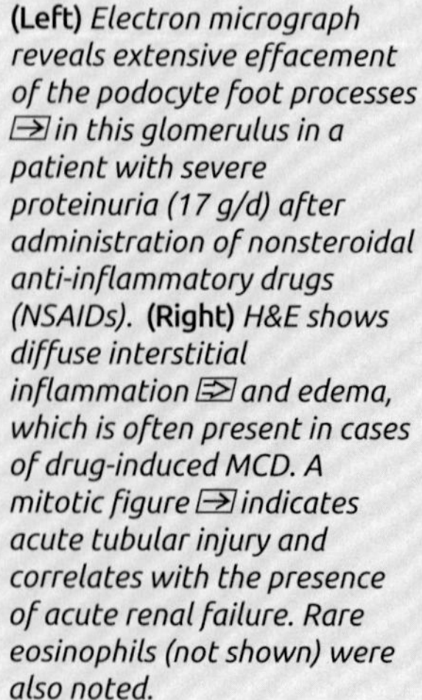

(Left) *Electron micrograph reveals extensive effacement of the podocyte foot processes ⇒ in this glomerulus in a patient with severe proteinuria (17 g/d) after administration of nonsteroidal anti-inflammatory drugs (NSAIDs).* **(Right)** *H&E shows diffuse interstitial inflammation ⇒ and edema, which is often present in cases of drug-induced MCD. A mitotic figure ⇒ indicates acute tubular injury and correlates with the presence of acute renal failure. Rare eosinophils (not shown) were also noted.*

Podocyte Foot Process Effacement (EM)

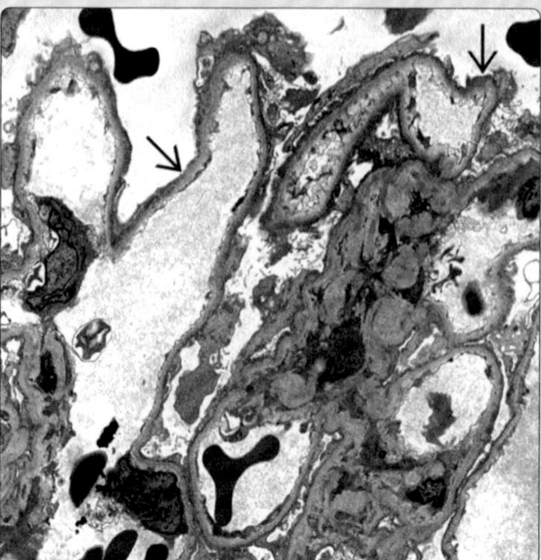

Interstitial Inflammation (H&E)

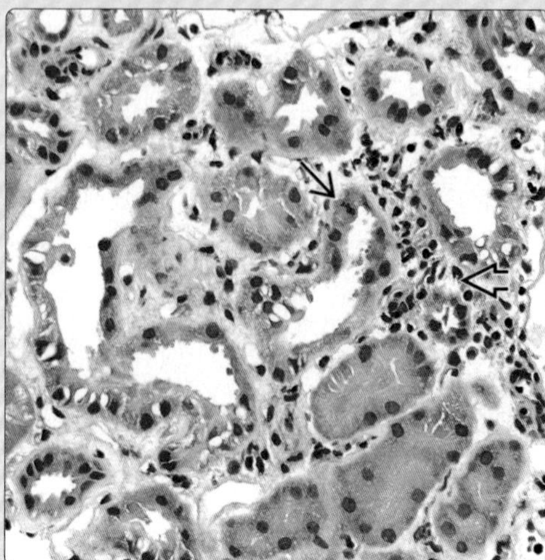

TERMINOLOGY

Abbreviations

- Minimal change disease (MCD)

ETIOLOGY/PATHOGENESIS

Implicated Drugs

- Nonsteroidal anti-inflammatory drugs (NSAIDs)
  - Diclofenac
  - 5-aminosalicylic acid (ASA)
- Cyclooxygenase 2 inhibitor
  - Celecoxib
- Pamidronate
  - Can also result in focal segmental glomerulosclerosis or collapsing glomerulopathy
- Amoxicillin
- Rifampin
- Penicillamine
- Interferon-α or -β
- Mercury skin cream
- Lithium
- Gold
- Gongjin-dan (Chinese folk medicine)

Mechanism Unknown

- T lymphocytes and chemokines have been implicated in pathogenesis of MCD
  - Not clear if these play a role in drug-induced MCD

CLINICAL ISSUES

Epidemiology

- Ethnicity
  - No ethnic predilection

Presentation

- Nephrotic syndrome
- Acute renal failure
  - Occasionally present

Laboratory Tests

- Urine dipstick
- 24-hour urine collection

Treatment

- Drugs
  - Steroids
    - Rarely needed
- Discontinuation of offending pharmacologic agent

Prognosis

- Excellent
  - Generally rapid remission after drug withdrawal

MICROSCOPIC

Histologic Features

- Normal glomeruli by light microscopy
- Interstitial inflammation
  - Often present
  - Acute tubular injury may be present

ANCILLARY TESTS

Immunofluorescence

- No immune deposits

Electron Microscopy

- Extensive effacement of podocyte foot processes
- No electron-dense deposits present

DIFFERENTIAL DIAGNOSIS

Minimal Change Disease

- Absence of administration of new pharmacologic agent would distinguish idiopathic form from drug-induced MCD

Focal Segmental Glomerulosclerosis

- Diffuse effacement of podocyte foot processes should always raise this diagnostic consideration
- Sampling issue if < 20 glomeruli are present for evaluation or if corticomedullary junction is absent
- Interstitial fibrosis and tubular atrophy may be related to aging but also raise this consideration

Acute Interstitial Nephritis

- Prominent interstitial inflammation with tubulitis
- May occur concurrently with drug-induced MCD

IgM Nephropathy

- Normal glomeruli by light microscopy
- Mesangial IgM immune complexes detected by immunofluorescence and electron microscopy

Lithium Nephrotoxicity

- Severe proteinuria may be present
- Cystic dilatation of distal nephron segments
- Clinical history of bipolar or other psychiatric disorder

DIAGNOSTIC CHECKLIST

Pathologic Interpretation Pearls

- Knowledge of clinical history of medications is critical
- Electron microscopy is essential to establish diagnosis

SELECTED REFERENCES

1. Kikuchi H et al: Nephrotic-range proteinuria and interstitial nephritis associated with the use of a topical loxoprofen patch. Intern Med. 53(11):1131-5, 2014
2. Tang HL et al: Minimal change disease caused by exposure to mercury-containing skin lightening cream: a report of 4 cases. Clin Nephrol. 79(4):326-9, 2013
3. Galesic K et al: Minimal change disease and acute tubular necrosis caused by diclofenac. Nephrology (Carlton). 13(1):87-8, 2008
4. Almansori M et al: Cyclooxygenase-2 inhibitor-associated minimal-change disease. Clin Nephrol. 63(5):381-4, 2005
5. Kohno K et al: Minimal change nephrotic syndrome associated with rifampicin treatment. Nephrol Dial Transplant. 15(7):1056-9, 2000
6. Tam VK et al: Nephrotic syndrome and renal insufficiency associated with lithium therapy. Am J Kidney Dis. 27(5):715-20, 1996
7. Savill JS et al: Minimal change nephropathy and pemphigus vulgaris associated with penicillamine treatment of rheumatoid arthritis. Clin Nephrol. 29(5):267-70, 1988
8. Wolters J et al: Minimal change nephropathy during gold treatment. A case with unusual histopathological and immunopathological features. Neth J Med. 31(5-6):234-40, 1987
9. Bander SJ: Reversible renal failure and nephrotic syndrome without interstitial nephritis from zomepirac. Am J Kidney Dis. 6(4):233-6, 1985

Etiology of Focal Segmental Glomerulosclerosis (FSGS)

Disease	Distinctive Pathology Features	Comments	PMID
Primary			
Idiopathic FSGS	75-90% NOS, 8-10% CG, 1-10% TIP, 1-5% perihilar, ~ 1% cellular variant; extensive FPE	Circulating factor, various candidates, none confirmed; recurs in transplants; worst prognosis CG, best TIP; *APOL1* risk alleles in ~ 70% of recent African ancestry	25416821 25561578
Genetic: Nonsyndromic			
Congenital nephrotic syndrome (Finnish) *NPHS1*	May have only DMS	7% of famialial SRNS; usually congenital nephrotic syndrome, milder cases detected in adulthood (AR)	19812541
Podocin deficiency *NPHS2*	May have diffuse mesangial hypercellularity without FSGS	10% of familial SRNS; childhood or congenital; ~ 7% of sporadic FSGS in children; ± *NPHS1* mutations (AR)	24856380 11805168
Phospholipase C ε 1 *PLCE1*	DMS 18-40%	2% of familial SRNS (AR); not found in sporadic FSGS	25349199
Autosomal dominant FSGS *INF2*	NOS, CG; segmental FPE, jagged foot processes	0.5% of familial SRNS; 12% have Charcot-Marie-Tooth disease (AD)	21258034 20023659
Familial collapsing FSGS *TRPC6*	CG	0.5% of familial SRNS (AR); ESRD 21 years or older (AD)	23689571
CD2AP deficiency *CD2AP*	CG; diffuse mesangial IgM	Heterozygote in ~ 3% sporadic SRNS (AR)	17713465
α-actinin-4 *ACTN4*	Podocyte cytoplasmic aggregates	Adult onset, may have hematuria (AD)	19357256
Apolipoprotein L1 *APOL1*	CG	Also FSGS superimposed on other renal diseases (AR)	25530085
Dent disease *CLCN5*	FPE usually < 50%; CaPhos; metachromatic casts	Hypercalciuria, tubular proteinuria, nephrotic range (X); ESRD	22735364 24810952
Genetic: Syndromic			
Frasier and Denys-Drash syndromes *WT1*	PH, NOS; DMS common (23%) (especially Denys-Drash)	4.8% of familial SRNS; Wilms tumor (Denys-Drash); male pseudohermaphroditism (Frasier); (AD)	20419325
Alport syndrome *COL4A3, COL4A4*	NOS or PH; GBM irregularities but not diagnostic of Alport	Familial FSGS with proteinuria, hematuria (AR); may be no eye or hearing signs	25229338 21908087
Pierson syndrome *LAMB2*	DMS 14%	1% of familial SRNS; microcoria (AR)	20591883
Schimke immuno-osseous dysplasia *SMARCAL1*	CG, TIP; TUNEL+ podocytes, parietal and tubular epithelium	T-cell deficiency, spondyloepiphyseal dysplasia; 0.9% of familial SRNS (AR)	25319549
Nail-patella syndrome *LMX1B*	Banded collagen in GBM	FSGS can occur without extrarenal signs (AD)	23687361
Galloway-Mowat *WDR73*	CG, CG	Microcephaly (AR)	25873735
Fabry disease *GLA*	CG, NOS; EM lipid inclusions	Late change (X)	19833663
CoQ10 deficiency *COQ2*	CG; dysmorphic mitochondria	0.2% of familial SRNS (AR); treated with oral CoQ10	17855635
MELAS syndrome (*MTTL1*)	NOS; dysmorphic mitochondria	Encephalomyopathy, lactic acidosis, stroke-like episodes	22909780
Other genes: *ADCK4, DGKE, ARHGAP24, ARHGDIA, CFH, COQ6, CUBN, ITGA3, ITGB4, MYO1E, PDSS2*	Scant pathology information	Each < 0.5% of familial SRNS	25349199
Infection			
HIV	CG histologic variant, TRS common, tubular dilation, infiltrate	*APOL1* risk variants (recent African descent)	25848879
Parvovirus B19	CG, TRS, tubular dilation, infiltrate	Anemia; weak association	23372939
CMV	CG, TIP, abundant TRS	Strong but not conclusive association	25852866
HCV	CG		16142571
Tuberculosis	CG, NOS		23594801
Filariasis (*Loa loa*)	CG; microfilariae in vessels		9398129
Schistosomiasis	CG	Black race a risk factor; persist after schistosomal therapy	22124564
Drugs			
Interferon (alpha, beta or gamma)	Abundant endothelial tubuloreticular structures	Treatment for multiple sclerosis, HCV and other diseases; *APOL1* risk alleles found in 7/7; improved after discontinuation of drug	20203164 25100047
Lithium		Progression even with drug withdrawal if Cr > 2.5	10906157
Bisphosphonates	CG	Occasionally with a single dose	25473406
Calcineurin inhibitors	CG, severe hyaline arteriolopathy	Allografts and native kidneys in recipients of other organs	9603167
Sirolimus	NOS, ↓ VEGF expression	Improved after discontinuation of drug	17699432

Etiology of Focal Segmental Glomerulosclerosis (FSGS) (Continued)

Disease	Distinctive Pathology Features	Comments	PMID
Anthracyclines	CG, NOS	Improved after discontinuation of drug (doxorubicin, daunorubicin)	23219112
Immunological Diseases			
SLE	CG	Superimposed on class II or other	21279391
MCTD	CG		21269591
Adult Stills disease	CG		15112192
Behçet syndrome	CG	Remission on cyclosporine	21833522
Guillain-Barré syndrome		Remission of nephropathy with neuropathy	24726719
C1q nephropathy	CG, NOS	*APOL1* association	20116156
Membranous GN	NOS, PH; ↓ glomerular CD34(+) cells		25875837
Lymphoma/Leukemia			
Mantle cell lymphoma	NOS	Remission with chemotherapy	17497453
Multiple myeloma	CG	Partial remision with myeloma treatment	14750118
Acute monoblastic leukemia	CG	May be related to chemotherapy or GVHD	10594796
Chronic neutrophilic leukemia	Interstitial neutrophil infiltrate	Remission with hydroxyurea/interferon	25366011
Natural killer cell leukemia	CG		21908087
Hemophagocytic syndrome	CG; MCD	Rare survival	16557222
Vascular Diseases			
Diabetes (hyalinosis)	CG	APOL1 risk alleles	21074826
Atheroembolism	CG; emboli		9041208
Thrombotic microangiopathy	CG	Anti-VEGF therapy, transplants	25500702
Sickle cell disease	CG, NOS, sickled cells in capillaries		21338490
Adaptive (Maladaptive or Post-Adaptive)			
All causes	PH, glomerular hypertrophy, thickened GBM, patchy or little FPE	Usually slow progression	28583334, 25447132
Congenital Deficiency of Nephrons			
Dysplasia/hypoplasia	Cartilage, decreased lobes		2302871
Unilateral renal agenesis	NOS, PH	May be familial	8503422
Oligomeganephronia (*PAX2, EYA1, SIX5, SIX1, TCF1*)	Small kidneys, < 50% normal	Presents in infancy, ESRD later	6490319
Prematurity/low birth weight	PH	Birth weight < 1,500 g; FSGS in adolescence or later	19019999
Acquired Loss of Nephrons			
Reflux nephropathy	Dilated ureter, hydronephrosis	Associated with hypertension	8008693
Any disease that severely reduces nephrons	Pathologic features of underlying disease (e.g., IgA, pyelonephritis)		21178978
Increased Metabolic Demand			
Anabolic steroid abuse	PH, CG	Stablized off drugs; relapse when resumed	19917783
Morbid obesity	PH	BMI ≥ 30; remission after bariatric surgery or treatment of obstructive sleep apnea	21657818 22185970
Acromegaly	Glomerulomegaly	Remission reported after pituitary surgery	11499662
Cyanotic congenital heart disease	PH, NOS	Remission with ACE inhibitor	11773480
Diabetes mellitus	GBM thickening	Obesity and *APOL1* also contribute	24795211
Preeclampsia	Endothelial swelling	FSGS, if present, may come first	7924017
Glycogen storage disease	NOS	Onset 13-47 years	21620087

Isolated case reports: HTLV-1, HHV-8, Prader-Willi, familial dysautonomia, Turner syndrome, renal tubular acidosis. Abbreviations: AD = autosomal dominant, AR = autosomal recessive, CG = collapsing glomerulopathy, DMS = diffuse mesangial sclerosis, FPE = foot process effacement, NOS = not otherwise specified variant, PH = perihilar variant, PMID = PubMed identifier, SRNS = steroid resistant nephrotic syndrome, TIP = tip variant, X = X-linked

General references: Fogo, AB. Causes and pathogenesis of focal segmental glomerulosclerosis. Nat Revi Nephrol 11: 76-87. 2015; Sadowski et al. A single-gene cause in 29.5% of cases of steroid-resistant nephrotic syndrome. J Am Soc Nephrol (ePub). 2014

TERMINOLOGY

Abbreviations

- Focal segmental glomerulosclerosis (FSGS)

Definitions

- Group of podocytopathies (of varied etiology) sharing feature of focal segmental glomerulosclerosis, typically with moderate to heavy proteinuria

CLASSIFICATION SYSTEMS

Morphologic Classification

- Based on glomerular morphology categories defined by Columbia classification
  - Collapsing variant
  - Glomerular tip lesion
  - Cellular variant
  - Perihilar variant
  - FSGS not otherwise specified (NOS)

Etiologic Classification

- Based on identified causes of FSGS: Some correspondence with morphologic variants
- Idiopathic (primary)
  - Usual form, either NOS or collapsing variant
  - Plasma factor responsible, identity elusive
- Genetic
  - Nonsyndromic
    - *NPHS1* (nephrin)
    - *NPHS2* (podocin)
    - *PLCE1* (phospholipase C ε1)
    - *INF2* (familial FSGS)
    - *ACTN4* (α-actinin-4)
    - *TRPC6* (familial CG)
    - *CD2AP* (CD2 associated protein)
  - Syndromic
    - *WT1* (Frasier, Denys-Drash syndromes)
    - *COL4A3, COL4A4* (Alport syndrome)
    - *LAMB2* (Pierson syndrome)
    - *LMB1X* (nail-patella syndrome)
    - *WDR73* (Galloway-Mowat syndrome)
    - *COQ2* (CoQ10 deficiency)
    - *MTTL1* (MELAS syndrome)
  - Other genetic causes, newly described and rare
    - *ADCK4, GLA, DGKE, ARHGAP24, ARHGDIA, CFH, COQ6, CUBN, ITGA3, ITGB4, MYO1E, PDSS2, SMARCAL1*
- Infections
  - HIV, parvovirus B19, Cytomegalovirus (CMV), hepatitis C virus (HCV), tuberculosis, filariasis, schistosomiasis
- Drug-induced
  - Interferon-α and -β, lithium, bisphosphonates, heroin, calcineurin inhibitors, sirolimus, anthracyclines
- Immunologic diseases
  - Systemic lupus erythematosus (SLE), mixed connective tissue disease (MCTD), Stills disease, Behçet syndome, Guillain-Barré syndrome, C1q nephropathy
- Lymphoma/leukemia
  - Mantle cell lymphoma, multiple myeloma, acute monoblastic leukemia, chronic neutrophilic leukemia, NK cell leukemia, hemophagocytic syndrome
- Vascular
  - Hypertension, atheromatous emboli, sickle cell disease, thrombotic microangiopathy
- Adaptive, structural-functional responses
  - Congenital deficiency of nephrons
    - Unilateral renal agenesis, dysplasia/hypoplasia, oligomeganephronia, prematurity/low birth weight
  - Acquired loss of nephrons
    - Reflux nephropathy
    - Any scarring disease that severely reduces nephrons (glomerular, tubular, interstitial, vascular)
  - Increased metabolic demand
    - Morbid obesity, anabolic steroid abuse, acromegaly, cyanotic congenital heart disease, diabetes mellitus, preeclampsia, glycogen storage disease

EPIDEMIOLOGY

Incidence

- Most common cause of nephrotic syndrome in adults

Collapsing Variant of FSGS

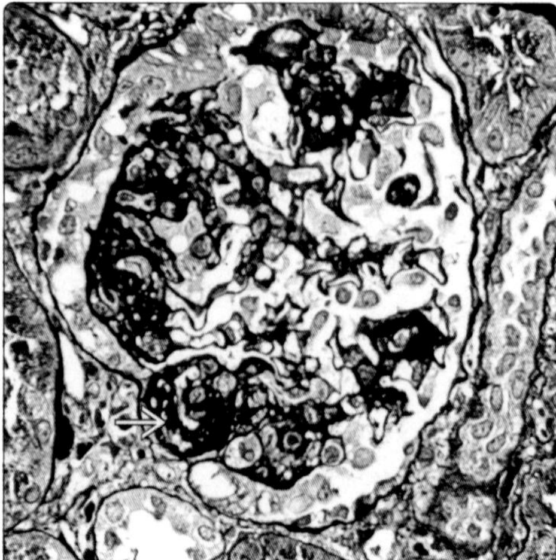

Segmental C3 Deposition

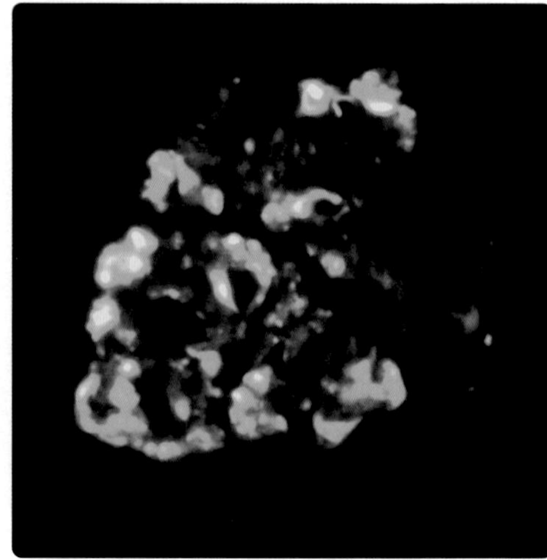

(Left) *Light microscopy of a case of collapsing focal segmental glomerulosclerosis (FSGS) shows a glomerulus with areas of sclerosis ➡ (silver stain).* **(Right)** *Immunofluorescence for C3 shows a predominantly segmental pattern of staining in the mesangium and in areas of glomerular capillary loop collapse in a case of FSGS.*

- Apparent increased incidence over past 2 decades
  - ~ 25% of adult nephropathies, compared with < 10% 20 years ago

History

- Focal and segmental glomerular hyalinization and capillary loop degradation described by Fahr in 1925
- Arnold Rich described juxtamedullary glomerulosclerosis in children dying with nephrotic syndrome in 1957
- FSGS was recognized as a distinct entity by International Study of Kidney Diseases in Children in 1970s
- Collapsing variant was recognized by Mark Weiss in 1980s and later as usual pattern of HIV-associated nephropathy (HIVAN)

ETIOLOGY/PATHOGENESIS

Pathogenesis

- Now classified as podocytopathies
  - Familial podocyte protein defects
    - Mutations in *TRPC6*, a calcium-permeable cation channel, lead to abnormal podocyte function and hereditary FSGS
    - FSGS with defects in α-actinin-4 (*ACTN4*), podocin (*NPHS2*, defective in corticosteroid-resistant nephrotic syndrome), and nephrin (*NPHS1*, defective in congenital nephrotic syndrome of Finnish type) are relatively rare familial forms of FSGS
    - Nephrin interacts with CD2-associated protein (CD2AP), and podocin interacts with nephrin-CD2AP complex
    - Mutations in WT1 transcription factor, which regulates several podocyte genes, lead to FSGS syndromes (Denys-Drash and Frasier syndromes)
  - Abnormal cytokines thought to play major role in idiopathic FSGS development
    - Circulating factor identified in patients who have recurrent FSGS after transplant, typically occurring within months after transplantation
  - Podocyte dysregulation/dysfunction
    - Differentiation markers of podocytes (e.g., Wilms tumor WT1 protein, podocalyxin, and synaptopodin) disappear in collapsing FSGS and HIVAN
  - Loss of podocytes leads to adhesions
  - Risk factor in African descent is *APOL1* gene
- Relationship with minimal change disease (MCD) unclear
  - Dystroglycan, an integral component of GBM, is decreased in MCD but maintained in nonsclerotic segments in FSGS

CLINICAL IMPLICATIONS

Prognosis

- Generally poor with substantial fraction progressing to end-stage renal disease

Clinical Presentation

- Proteinuria
- Nephrotic syndrome
- Azotemia

Treatment

- Plasmapheresis has been used to induce remission in some patients with recurrent FSGS

MACROSCOPIC

General Features

- Pale yellow kidneys due to lipid in tubules

MICROSCOPIC

General Features

- Glomeruli
  - Sclerosis involves some glomeruli (focal) and only a portion of glomerular tuft (segmental)
    - Diagnosed even when only 1 glomerulus involved
    - Global sclerosis may be incidental finding and is not particularly useful in making diagnosis of FSGS
  - Adhesions (synechiae) of glomerular tuft to Bowman space often accompany segmental sclerosis and are often seen early in sclerosis process
  - Hyalinosis
    - Portion of glomerular involvement has smooth, glassy (hyaline) appearance
    - Typically thought to occur from insudation of plasma proteins
  - Increased matrix with obliteration of glomerular capillary lumen
  - FSGS has zonal distribution, beginning in corticomedullary (juxtamedullary) junction (CMJ)
    - Important to note whether sampling of CMJ is included
  - Glomerular hypertrophy often accompanies FSGS
    - Potential surrogate marker in cases without sampled segmental sclerosis
- Tubules
  - Tubular epithelial cells contain PAS(+) reabsorption droplets due to glomerular proteinuria
  - Tubular atrophy is typically only focal early in course of FSGS
    - TBM thickened in areas of atrophy
    - Tubular atrophy may be more prominent late in course of disease
  - Tubulointerstitial changes pronounced in collapsing variants of FSGS and in HIVAN
    - Cystic dilatation and more prominent lymphoid infiltrate
- Interstitium
  - Interstitial fibrosis (IF) may be present and is typically focal
    - Some cases have extensive IF ± tubular atrophy (TA), and IF/TA in young patients may indicate unsampled FSGS in patients without identified glomerulosclerosis
  - Interstitial inflammation is absent or minimal
- Vessels
  - Arteriolar hyalinosis and arterial intimal fibrosis may be prominent late in course of FSGS

FSGS Morphologic Classification Algorithm

Variant	Diagnostic Criteria	Exclude	Prognosis	% of 1° FSGS
Collapsing	≥ 1 glomerulus with collapse with segmental or global collapse and podocyte hyperplasia and hypertrophy	None	Poor	8-12%
Tip	≥ 1 segmental lesion in tip domain (outer 25% of tuft next to proximal tubule origin), adhesion is required at tubular lumen or neck	Collapsing variant, perihilar sclerosis	Possibly better prognosis	1-10%
Cellular	≥ 1 glomerulus with segmental or global endocapillary hypercellularity occluding lumina, ± karyorrhexis and foam cells	Collapsing and tip variants	Possibly early-stage lesion	1-3%
Perihilar	≥ 1 glomerulus with perihilar hyalinosis, ± sclerosis	Collapsing, tip, and cellular variants	Might often be a secondary type of FSGS	1-7%
FSGS (NOS)	≥ 1 glomerulus with segmental increase in matrix obliterating capillary lumina	Collapsing, tip, cellular, and perihilar variants	Usual course	68-90%

FSGS Morphologic Features

Variant	Location	Distribution	Hyaline	Adhesion	PCH	MHC	GM	AH
Collapsing	Anywhere	Segmental or global	-/+	-/+	+++	-/+	-/+	-/+
Tip	Tip domain	Segmental	+/-	+++/-	-	-/+	-/+	-/+
Cellular	Anywhere	Segmental	-/+	-/+	-	-/+	-/+	-/+
Perihilar	Perihilar	Segmental	++/-	+++/-	-	-/+	+++/-	++/-
FSGS (NOS)	Anywhere	Segmental	+/-	++/-	-/+	-/+	+/-	+/-

AH = arteriolar hyalinosis, FSGS) focal segmental glomerulosclerosis, GM = glomerulomegaly, MHC = mesangial hypercellularity, PCH = podocyte hyperplasia. Features are expressed as "most common/least common presentation." Each (+) denotes the approximate frequency at which the features occur; (-) denotes that this feature may be absent. Adapted from D'Agati et al: Pathologic classification of focal segmental glomerulosclerosis: a working proposal. Am J Kidney Dis. 43(2):368-82, 2004.

ANCILLARY TESTS

Immunofluorescence

- IgM and C3 often positive in sclerotic areas or areas of mesangial matrix increase
  - Thought to be nonspecific entrapment
  - IgM staining without EM deposits does not appear to have etiologic, prognostic, or diagnostic significance

Electron Microscopy

- Foot process effacement (FPE) typically not complete
- Secondary FSGS usually shows less FPE than idiopathic forms of FSGS
- In HIVAN, tubuloreticular inclusions can sometimes be identified
- Subepithelial multilamination of GBM in collapsing variant

DIFFERENTIAL DIAGNOSIS

Focal Glomerulonephritis (GN)

- IgA nephropathy, lupus, and other inflammatory GNs can result in segmental scars in glomeruli
- Breaks in GBM sometimes evident in PAS/silver stains (not seen in FSGS)

Minimal Change Disease (MCD)

- No segmental sclerosis
- FPE is usually complete in MCD but is typically less in most cases of FSGS
- Numerous globally sclerotic glomeruli, interstitial fibrosis, and vascular changes in patient with nephrotic syndrome are suggestive of FSGS even if no segmental lesions are seen

DIAGNOSTIC CHECKLIST

Pathologic Interpretation Pearls

- Multiple levels (step sections) may be needed to identify focal segmental lesions
- Note whether corticomedullary junction is sampled
- Adequate sample of glomeruli is crucial to make diagnosis of FSGS since focal lesions may be missed with small samples
  - For example, biopsy with 10 glomeruli has 35% probability of missing a focal lesion present in 10% of glomeruli in kidney, whereas probability decreases to 12% if 20 glomeruli are sampled

SELECTED REFERENCES

1. Fogo AB: Causes and pathogenesis of focal segmental glomerulosclerosis. Nat Rev Nephrol. ePub, 2014
2. Sadowski CE et al: A Single-Gene Cause in 29.5% of Cases of Steroid-Resistant Nephrotic Syndrome. J Am Soc Nephrol. ePub, 2014
3. Stokes MB et al: Morphologic variants of focal segmental glomerulosclerosis and their significance. Adv Chronic Kidney Dis. 21(5):400-7, 2014

Normal Glomerulus

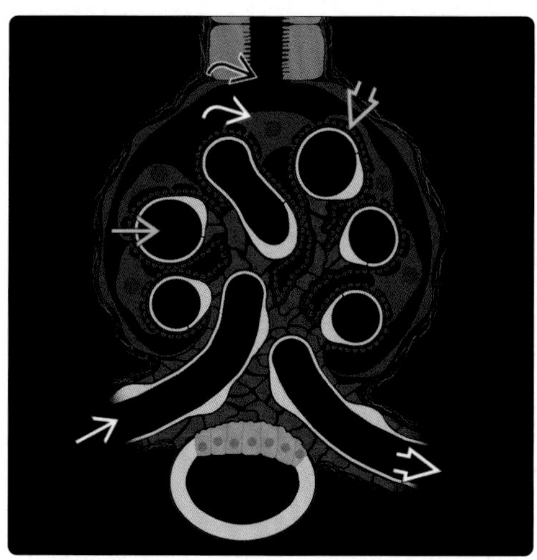

Collapsing Variant

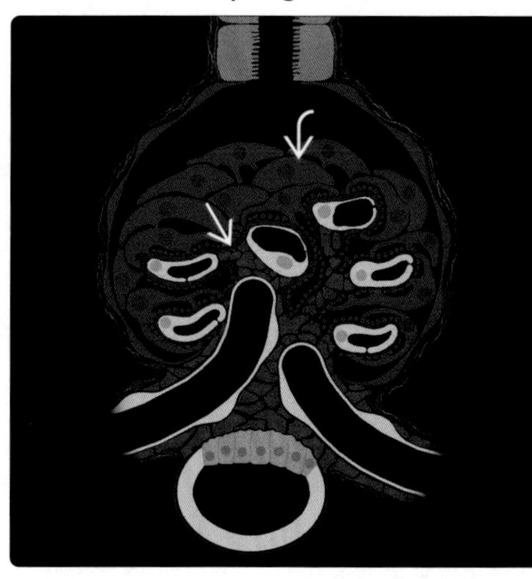

(Left) *Features that are important to consider in FSGS include the podocytes ➡, the hilar region with the afferent ➡ and efferent ➡ arterioles, the endocapillary cells ➡, sclerosis along glomerular basement membranes ➡, and the "tip" of the glomerulus at the tubular pole ➡.* **(Right)** *In FSGS collapsing variant, at least 1 glomerulus has collapse and an overlying podocyte hypertrophy/hyperplasia ➡, together with glomerulosclerosis ➡.*

Tip Variant

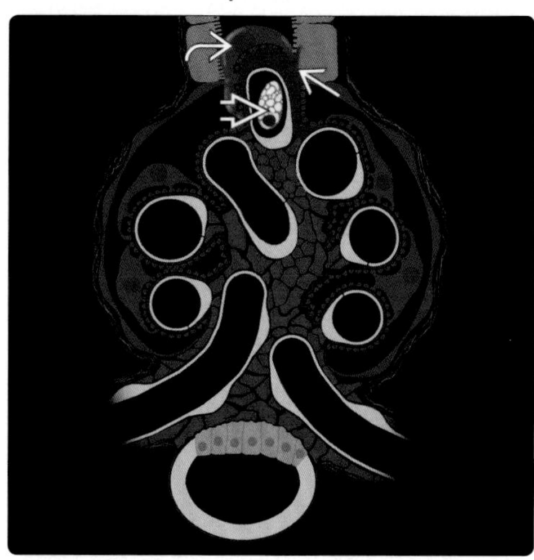

Cellular Variant

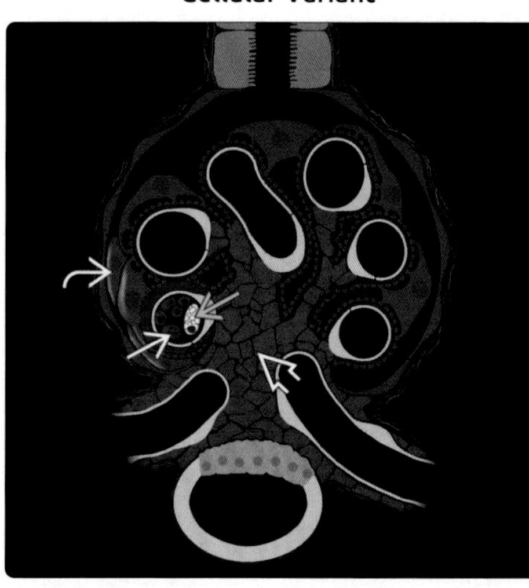

(Left) *In FSGS "tip" variant, there is at least 1 segmental lesion involving the tip domain, often coupled with an adhesion ➡, podocyte hypertrophy ➡, and intraluminal foam cells ➡.* **(Right)** *In FSGS cellular variant (rarest type), there is at least 1 glomerulus with segmental endocapillary hypercellularity occluding lumina, often with inflammatory cells, foam cells ➡, karyorrhexis ➡, overlying podocyte hyperplasia ➡, and mesangial hypercellularity ➡. Some consider this within the collapsing group.*

Perihilar Variant

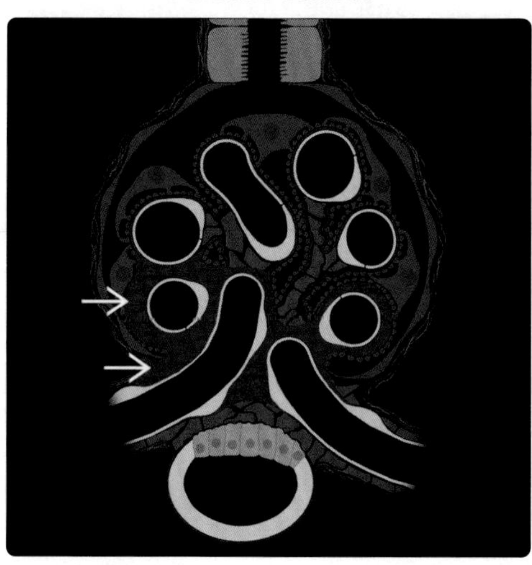

FSGS, Not Otherwise Specified Variant

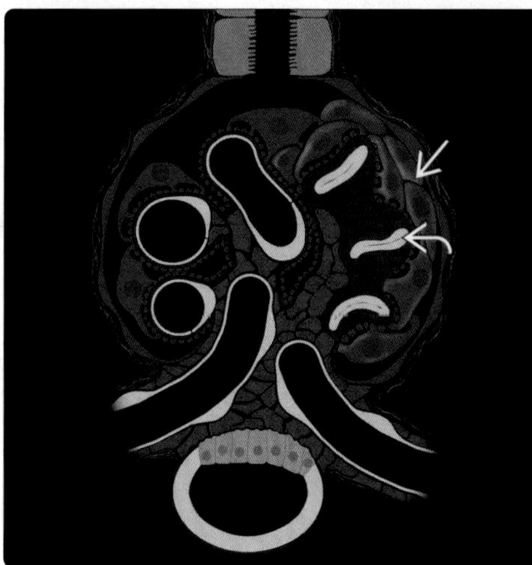

(Left) *In FSGS perihilar variant, at least 1 glomerulus has perihilar hyalinosis/sclerosis ➡, which must be present in over 50% of glomeruli with segmental lesions. This is typical of adaptive FSGS.* **(Right)** *In FSGS (NOS), at least 1 glomerulus must have segmental increase in the matrix that obliterates the capillary lumina. This is often in a peripheral, nonspecific pattern of sclerosis ➡ ± overlying podocyte hypertrophy ➡. This random distribution of scarring is the most common pattern in idiopathic (primary) FSGS.*

Focal Segmental Glomerulosclerosis, Primary

KEY FACTS

ETIOLOGY/PATHOGENESIS

- Idiopathic disease with podocytopenia
- Plasma factor & genetic predisposition

CLINICAL ISSUES

- Common cause of nephrotic syndrome in children and adults
- 15-20% of biopsies
- More common in blacks
- Therapy
  - Minority respond to steroids (~ 33%)
  - Cyclophosphamide, cyclosporine, plasmapheresis
  - Under study: Rituximab, abatacept
- Recurs in transplants

MICROSCOPIC

- 5 pathologic variants (Columbia classification)
  - Not otherwise specified (NOS): Random distribution of adhesions (commonest)
  - Tip: Adhesion at inlet of proximal tubule
  - Perihilar: Adhesion around hilum
  - Cellular: Luminal occlusion by endocapillary hypercellularity
  - Collapsing: Collapse and hypercellularity of podocytes
- Juxtamedullary glomeruli affected early
- Hyaline can accumulate at adhesion
- Foot process effacement and loss by electron microscopy
- IgM & C3 in segmental scars by immunofluorescence

TOP DIFFERENTIAL DIAGNOSES

- Forms of FSGS with known cause (genetic, drug, infection)
- Minimal change disease if no segmental scar sampled
- FSGS superimposed on other glomerular diseases

DIAGNOSTIC CHECKLIST

- Multiple levels may be needed to see segmental lesion
- FSGS, NOS is diagnosis of exclusion since other diseases can cause segmental glomerular scars

(Left) *Focal segmental glomerulosclerosis (FSGS) has segmental scars in some glomeruli, typically with hyaline ➡ and adhesion ➡ to Bowman capsule. Most of the glomerulus appears normal.* **(Right)** *Defining features of FSGS are sparing of some glomeruli ("focal") & partial involvement of affected tufts ("segmental"). Affected glomerulus has broad adhesion & hyalinosis ➡.*

Segmental Glomerulosclerosis

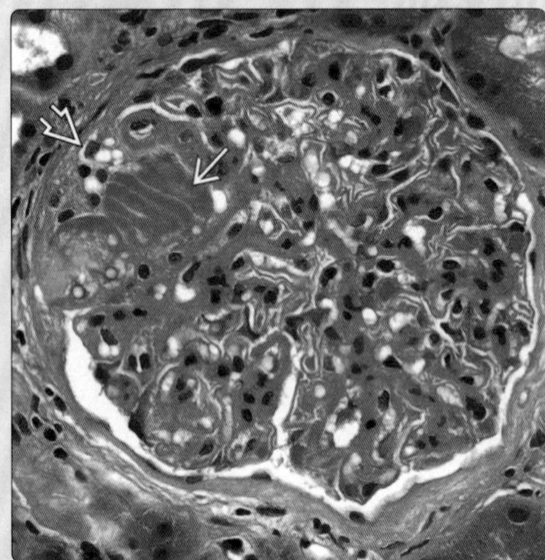

Adhesion and Hyalinosis

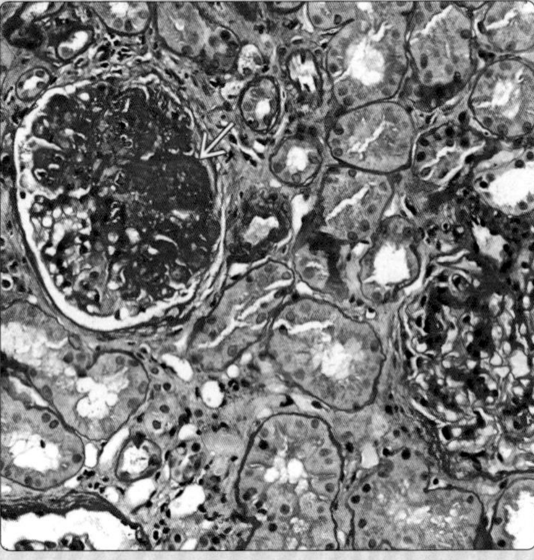

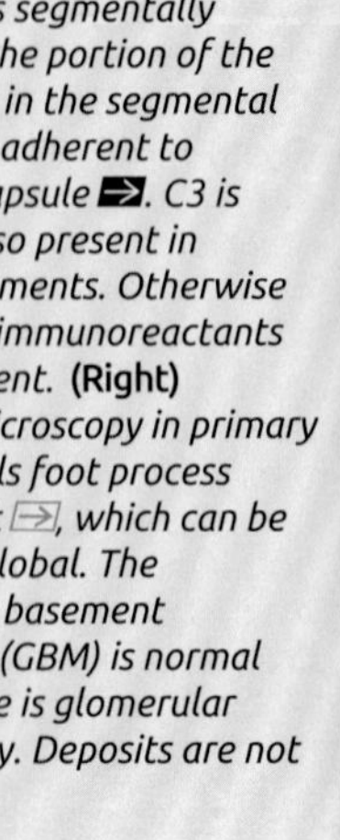

(Left) *IgM is segmentally present in the portion of the glomerulus in the segmental scar that is adherent to Bowman capsule ➡. C3 is typically also present in scarred segments. Otherwise little or no immunoreactants are prominent.* **(Right)** *Electron microscopy in primary FSGS reveals foot process effacement ➡, which can be patchy or global. The glomerular basement membrane (GBM) is normal unless there is glomerular hypertrophy. Deposits are not prominent.*

IgM in Segmental Scar

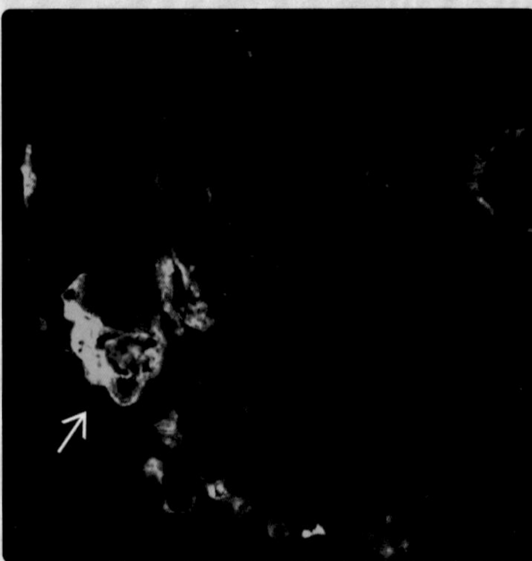

Foot Process Effacement

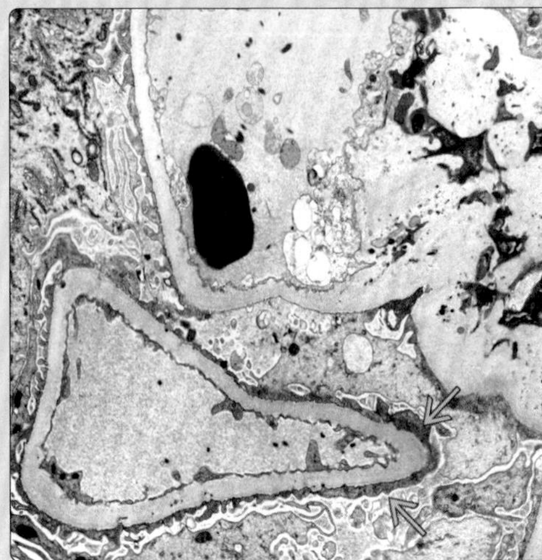

TERMINOLOGY

Abbreviations

- Focal segmental glomerulosclerosis (FSGS)

Synonyms

- Idiopathic FSGS

Definitions

- Idiopathic glomerular disease manifested by marked proteinuria, often nephrotic syndrome, with segmental scars in some glomeruli, adhesion of tuft to Bowman capsule (BC), & foot process effacement (FPE)
  - Classified separately from FSGS secondary to known causes, including genetic disorders, infection, drugs, and adaptive responses
  - As more specific genetic, metabolic, & microbial causes are identified, this category will diminish & be replaced by FSGS of known etiologies
- Pathologic classification (Columbia): Adhesions are randomly distributed (not otherwise specified [NOS]) at origin of proximal tubule (tip variant) or at hilum (perihilar variant); glomeruli may show endocapillary hypercellularity (cellular variant) or collapse (collapsing variant)

ETIOLOGY/PATHOGENESIS

Podocyte Disease/Podocytopathy

- Podocyte depletion believed to be central mechanism (podocytopenia)
  - Podocytes have limited replicative ability
  - Podocyte loss leads to bare GBM, promoting adhesion & repopulation by parietal epithelial cells (PEC)
  - Cause of podocytopenia not established
    - TGF-β is mediator in animal models

Plasma Factor

- Proteinuria often recurs after renal transplant, sometimes within minutes of reperfusion
- Protein fractions of patient serum cause proteinuria in rats, & glomeruli isolated from these rats have ↑ glomerular albumin permeability
- Identification of plasma factor remains elusive and controversial
  - Cardiotrophin-like cytokine-1
  - Soluble urokinase plasminogen activator receptor (suPAR)

Genetic Factors

- Genetic factors can predispose and even cause FSGS
- Several forms of FSGS with similar morphology have genetic defect (*NPHS2*, *ACTN4*)
- ↑ FSGS risk in African Americans with *APOL-1* gene variants

Tubulointerstitial Injury

- Proteinuria thought to cause tubulointerstitial damage by ↑ tubular chemokine expression & endoplasmic stress

CLINICAL ISSUES

Epidemiology

- Incidence
  - 2.2% of end-stage renal disease (ESRD) in USA (2004-2008)
    - 11.6% of ESRD in children (2008-2014)
  - Increasing incidence in children and adults
    - FSGS-related ESRD increased 49x from 1980 to 2000
  - ~ 20% of adult renal biopsies for nephrotic syndrome
  - 30-70% NOS, 20-40% tip, 3-5% cellular (more common in children)
- Age
  - Mean age at onset: ~ 37-50 years in adults, ~ 6-7 years in children
- Sex
  - Male preponderance (1.5-3x)
- Ethnicity
  - ESRD from FSGS 4-5x more common in those of African descent than Caucasians or Asians
    - African descent: 23.6/million per year in 2000; lifetime risk: 1:556
    - Caucasians: 5.4/million per year in 2000; lifetime risk: 1:2,500

Presentation

- Nephrotic-range proteinuria (> 3.5 g/d)
  - ~ 60% with NOS variant
  - ~ 97% with tip variant
    - Often sudden onset
- Hypertension (~ 65%)

Treatment

- Drugs
  - Steroids
    - Limited response rate (~ 33%) and frequent relapse of therapy
    - Tip variant often responds to steroids (80%) with complete remission in 60%, similar MCD
  - 2nd-line therapies: Cyclosporine, cyclophosphamide, mycophenolate mofetil, rituximab, plasmapheresis
  - Angiotensin-converting enzyme (ACE) inhibitors to ↓ proteinuria & tubular injury
  - Abatacept under study: Targets B7-1 (CD80) and led to complete remission of proteinuria in small series

Prognosis

- Wide range due to diverse patient selection and therapies
- ESRD in 3-5 years according to pathologic classification
  - NOS variant: 20-37%
  - Tip variant: 6-24%
  - Cellular variant: 0-33%
  - Perihilar: 0-37%
  - Collapsing: 18-70%
- Risk factors for ESRD: Heavy proteinuria, elevated Cr, hypertension at time of biopsy; failure to respond to therapy; nontip lesions in tip variant

MICROSCOPIC

Histologic Features

- Glomeruli (NOS variant)
  - Adhesion of glomerular capillaries to BC
    - Randomly distributed (by definition, not at tip or perihilar)
    - Sometimes observe cells from BC bridging between BC & GBM
  - Accumulation of hyaline at site of adhesion

- Segmental sclerosis of glomerular capillaries
- Zonal cortical distribution (worst at corticomedullary junction)
- Mild, variable mesangial hypercellularity
- Normal GBM by light microscopy
- By definition, no glomerular collapse with podocyte proliferation (a feature of collapsing variant)
- Tubules: Tubular resorption droplets & focal atrophy, associated with glomerulosclerosis areas
- Interstitium: Fibrosis, correlated with FSGS lesions
- Vessels: Intimal fibrosis and arteriolar hyalinosis

Other Variants

- Tip variant (Howie and Brewer)
    - Adhesion in tip region: Outer 25% of glomerulus next to proximal tubule origin
        - Affected segment may "herniate" into tubular lumen
    - Segmental lesions contain endocapillary hypercellularity or sclerosis (often intracapillary foam cells)
    - May have adhesions in other sites (except perihilar)
    - Tip lesion can be seen in glomerular diseases other than primary FSGS (e.g., thrombotic microangiopathy [TMA], glomerulonephritis [GN])
- Cellular variant
    - Expansile endocapillary hypercellularity occluding lumina
        - Intracapillary endothelial cells and macrophage-type foam cells ± neutrophils & lymphocytes
        - ± apoptosis with pyknotic or karyorrhectic debris
        - ± fibrin within glomerular capillaries
        - May not have segmental scar
- Perihilar variant
    - Sclerosis restricted to vascular pole in > 50% of glomeruli
    - Not often found in primary FSGS (< 10%), common in adaptive (secondary) FSGS
- Collapsing variant
    - ≥ 1 glomerulus with segmental collapse and hypercellularity of visceral epithelium (podocytes)

ANCILLARY TESTS

Immunohistochemistry

- Parietal epithelial cells (PEC) on GBM stain for claudin-1
    - Activated PEC express CD44
- Ki-67(+) visceral epithelial cells in collapsing variant

Immunofluorescence

- IgM and C3 in scarred segments
    - IgM and C3 deposition long regarded as nonspecific trapping
        - Evidence that IgM contributes to glomerular injury based on inhibition of FSGS in mice by deficiency of immunoglobulin or depletion of B cells
- Kappa & lambda stain equivalent and similar to IgM
- Other stains typically negative or minimal scattered deposits (IgG, IgA, C1q, fibrin)

Electron Microscopy

- Podocyte foot process effacement (FPE) typically > 50% of capillary surface area
    - Average foot process width > 1,500 μm distinguishes primary FSGS from secondary FSGS due to adaptive response with ~ 100% sensitivity and ~ 70% specificity
- Normal GBM without rupture
- No or minor deposits
- Loss of podocytes with bridging of parietal epithelium to GBM in areas of adhesion
- Cellular variant: Intracapillary foam cells
    - Segmental glomerular capillary occlusion
- Collapsing variant: Subepithelial laminations of new GBM

DIFFERENTIAL DIAGNOSIS

FSGS Secondary to Adaptive Response

- Glomerular hypertrophy
- Perihilar distribution of adhesions & hyaline
- Less extensive FPE (by measure of foot process width)

Minimal Change Disease

- Cannot distinguish without presence of segmental glomerulosclerosis
- Sampling an issue without corticomedullary junction or small number of glomeruli

FSGS Due to Genetic Causes

- NOS variant usual pattern; genetic testing required

FSGS Superimposed on Other Glomerular Diseases

- Segmental scars, collapse, and tip lesions may complicate other glomerular diseases, suggested by
    - Immune complexes by IF
    - Deposits or GBM abnormalities by EM
    - Disrupted GBM in GN scars by LM

DIAGNOSTIC CHECKLIST

Pathologic Interpretation Pearls

- In setting of nephrotic syndrome and lesions of minimal change disease, FSGS cannot be ruled out
    - Presence of tubular atrophy even without glomerular scar is suspicious
    - Multiple levels may be necessary to demonstrate segmental lesion
- FSGS NOS is diagnosis of exclusion since other diseases can cause segmental glomerular scars

SELECTED REFERENCES

1. Fogo AB: Causes and pathogenesis of focal segmental glomerulosclerosis. Nat Rev Nephrol. ePub, 2014
2. Hakroush S et al: Extensive podocyte loss triggers a rapid parietal epithelial cell response. J Am Soc Nephrol. 25(5):927-38, 2014
3. Smeets B et al: Detection of activated parietal epithelial cells on the glomerular tuft distinguishes early focal segmental glomerulosclerosis from minimal change disease. Am J Pathol. ePub, 2014
4. Stokes MB et al: Morphologic variants of focal segmental glomerulosclerosis and their significance. Adv Chronic Kidney Dis. 21(5):400-7, 2014
5. D'Agati VD et al: Association of histologic variants in FSGS clinical trial with presenting features and outcomes. Clin J Am Soc Nephrol. 8(3):399-406, 2013
6. Strassheim D et al: IgM contributes to glomerular injury in FSGS. J Am Soc Nephrol. 24(3):393-406, 2013
7. Yu CC et al: Abatacept in B7-1-positive proteinuric kidney disease. N Engl J Med. 369(25):2416-23, 2013
8. Deegens JK et al: Podocyte foot process effacement as a diagnostic tool in focal segmental glomerulosclerosis. Kidney Int. 74(12):1568-76, 2008
9. Thomas DB et al: Clinical and pathologic characteristics of focal segmental glomerulosclerosis pathologic variants. Kidney Int. 69(5):920-6, 2006
10. D'Agati VD et al: Pathologic classification of focal segmental glomerulosclerosis: a working proposal. Am J Kidney Dis. 43(2):368-82, 2004

Corticomedullary Junction Predisposition

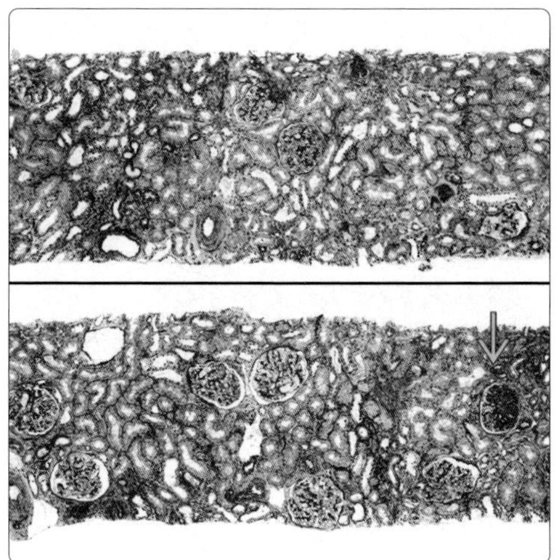

Adhesion

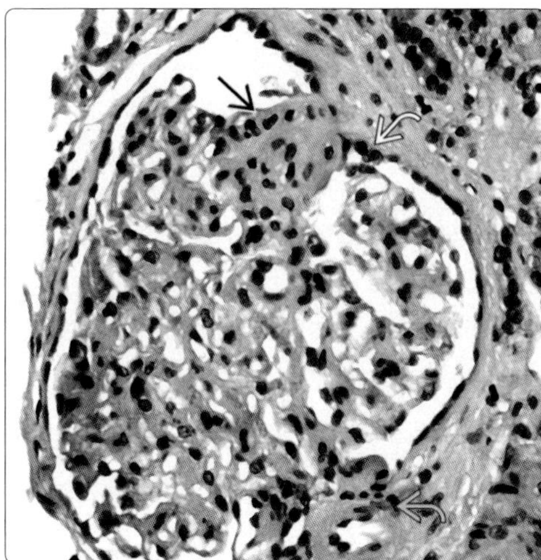

(Left) *Low-power view biopsy of FSGS reveals 1 glomerulus ➡ with segmental GS in an African American man. These glomeruli are preferentially located at the corticomedullary junction, which should be included to consider the sample adequate.* **(Right)** *Glomerular tuft adhesion ➡ to Bowman capsule (BC) is shown. Note BC tenting ➡, a useful feature indicating that the adhesion is not an artifact. Identification of the glomerular base ➡ helps exclude that structure, which sometimes resembles an adhesion.*

Adhesion to Bowman Capsule

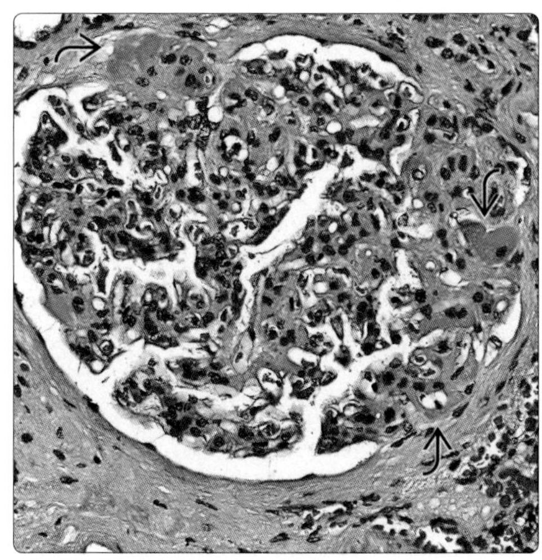

Adhesion in FSGS

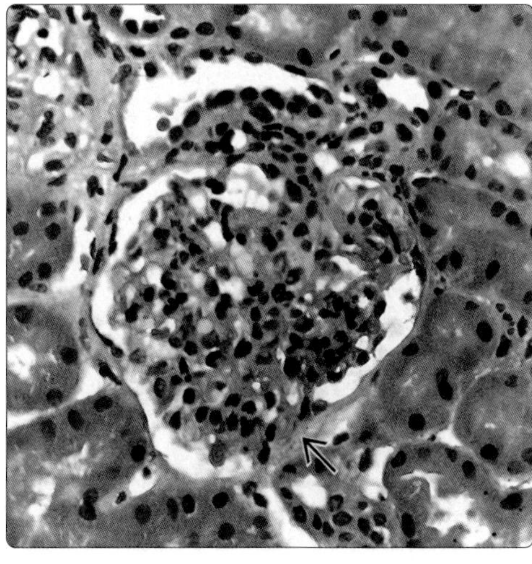

(Left) *This glomerulus has 3 sites of adhesion to BC with accompanying deposition of hyaline ➡. The rest of the glomerulus has mild mesangial hypercellularity but is otherwise unremarkable.* **(Right)** *Subtle adhesion ➡ in a 6 year old with nephrotic syndrome is shown. The tenting of Bowman capsule is useful to distinguish real from artifactual adhesions.*

Adhesion With Bridging by Parietal Epithelium

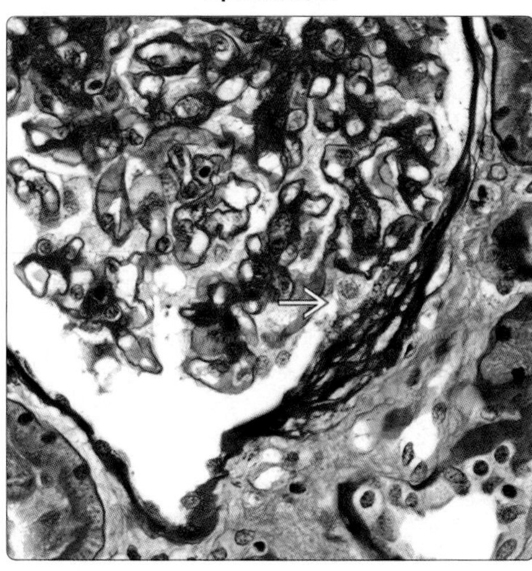

Perihilar Adhesion and Hyaline

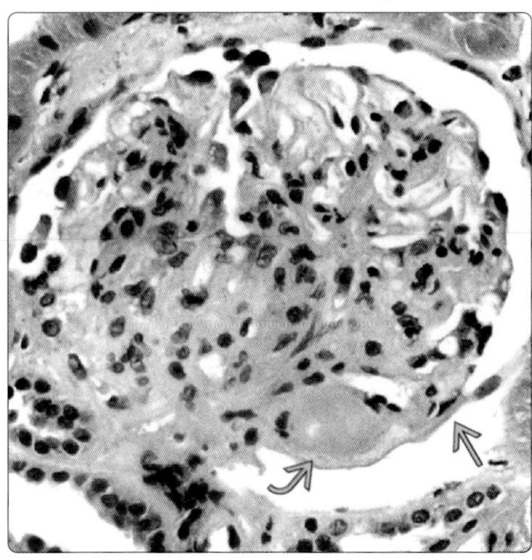

(Left) *An adhesion has a cell ➡ bridging between the laminated Bowman capsule and the GBM. The presence of a Bowman capsule reaction helps distinguish a real adhesion from one created as a biopsy artifact, with compression of the tuft against the capsule.* **(Right)** *Perihilar adhesion ➡ and hyaline ➡ deposition are present in > 50% of glomeruli in the perihilar variant. This pattern is most common in secondary, maladaptive FSGS (nephron overload).*

(Left) *Segmental IgM deposits ➡ in the sclerotic segments of the involved glomeruli in FSGS are shown. Mesangial IgM is also not uncommon. IgM in scarred areas is thought to be due to nonspecific trapping, although there is no proof of that interpretation.* **(Right)** *C3 deposits in sclerotic segments of glomeruli ➡ in FSGS are seen here. C3 is also present in the rest of the glomerulus in the mesangium ⇨. Glomeruli with segmental sclerosis, whatever the cause, may have IgM and C3 deposits.*

Segmental IgM Deposit in FSGS

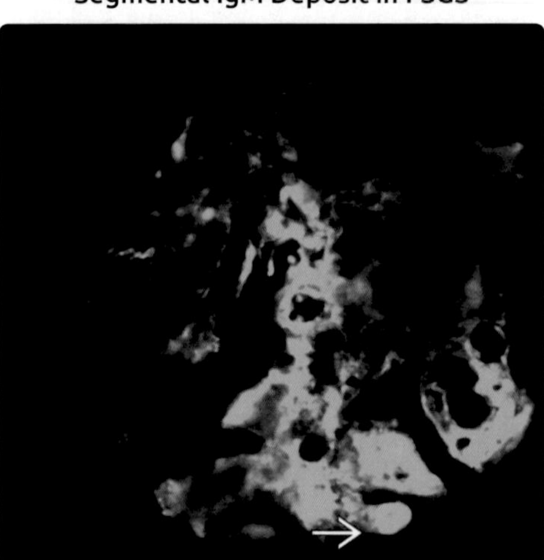

C3 Deposit in FSGS

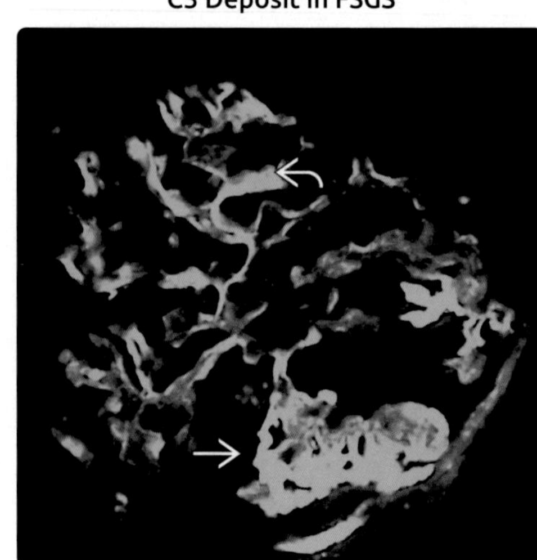

(Left) *Segmental IgM ➡ in a case of FSGS is shown. Typical of FSGS, this case also had C3 but no IgG or IgA staining.* **(Right)** *C3 is present in a capsular adhesion. Whether this has a role in the pathogenesis is unknown, but it is almost invariably present, along with IgM.*

Segmental IgM in FSGS

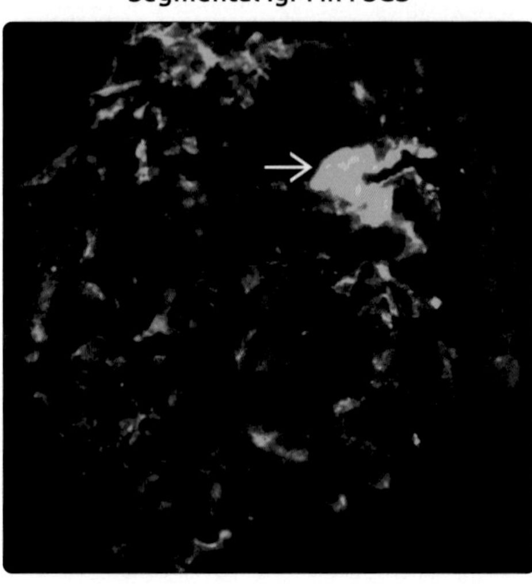

C3 at Capsular Adhesion in FSGS

(Left) *FSGS can be superimposed on almost any glomerular disease, including membranous glomerulonephritis (GN) (shown) as well as IgA, diabetic glomerulopathy, and Alport syndrome. The presence of FSGS lesions can be an adverse prognostic feature, as in IgA nephropathy.* **(Right)** *Segmental scars can be the result of focal glomerular inflammation, as in this case of IgA nephropathy. One clue that the scar is due to inflammatory injury rather than podocyte loss is a fragmented GBM ⇨.*

FSGS Superimposed on Membranous GN

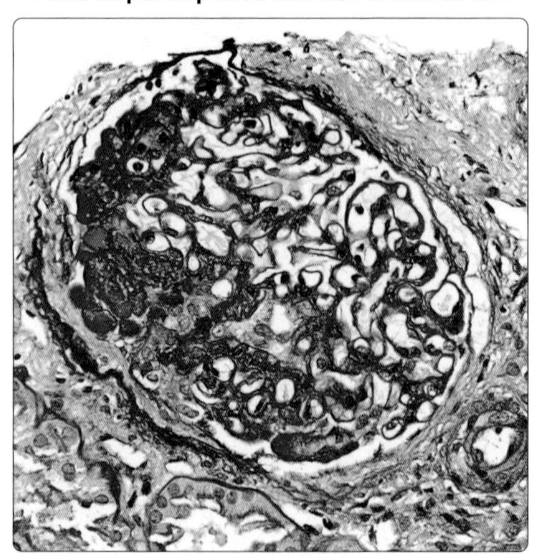

Broken GBM in Segmental Scar in IgA Nephropathy

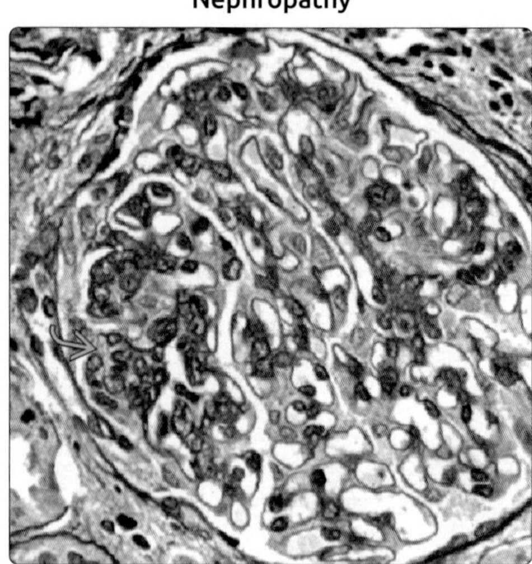

Foot Process Effacement

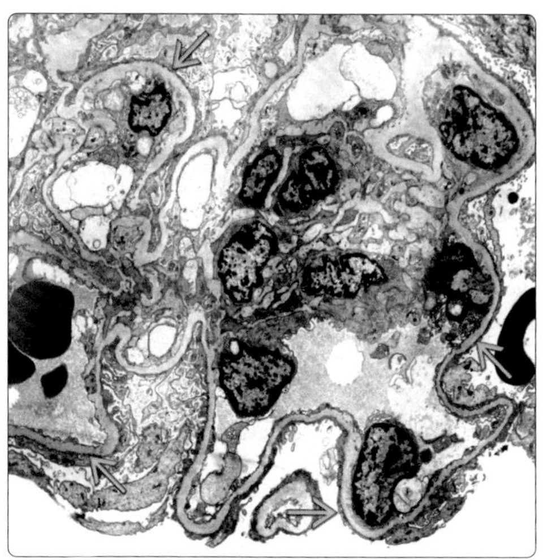

GBM Wrinkling and Foot Process Effacement

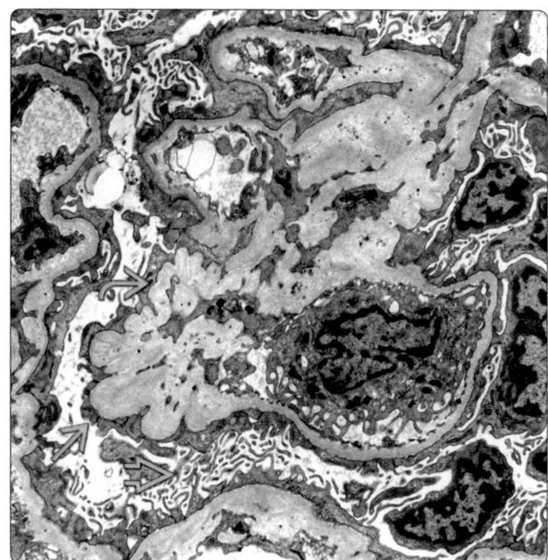

(Left) *Electron microscopy at low power in FSGS reveals extensive foot process effacement* ➙ *and a normal GBM in a 25 year old with nephrotic-range proteinuria and FSGS seen in the light microscopic portion of the biopsy.* **(Right)** *In FSGS, there is often extensive foot process effacement* ➙, *which may be accompanied by podocyte microvillous transformation* ➙ *and glomerular basement membrane (GBM) wrinkling* ➙.

Podocyte Hypertrophy

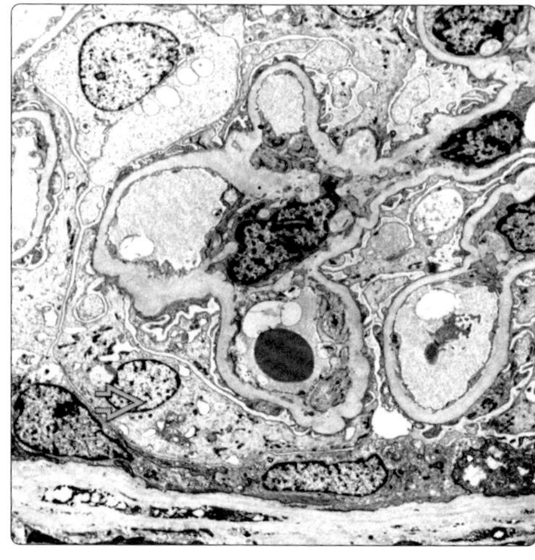

Foot Process Effacement and Adhesion

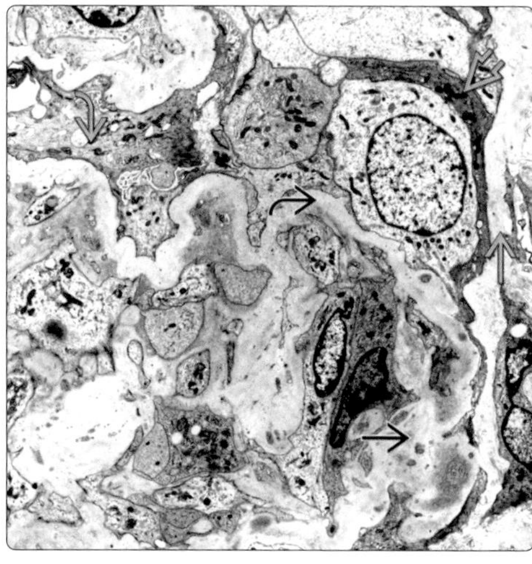

(Left) *In this 22-year-old African-American with 1.8 g/d proteinuria and FSGS, patchy foot process effacement affects ~ 20% of glomerular capillaries. A podocyte* ➙ *is stretched & is in close contact with parietal epithelium but not the Bowman capsule (BC).* **(Right)** *Segmental glomerulosclerosis* ➙ *with adhesion to BC* ➙ *in a 25-year-old African-American with nephrotic syndrome is shown. A cell* ➙ *bridges the GBM* ➙ *& BC. Podocyte foot process effacement is widespread* ➙.

Segmental Scar and Podocyte Loss

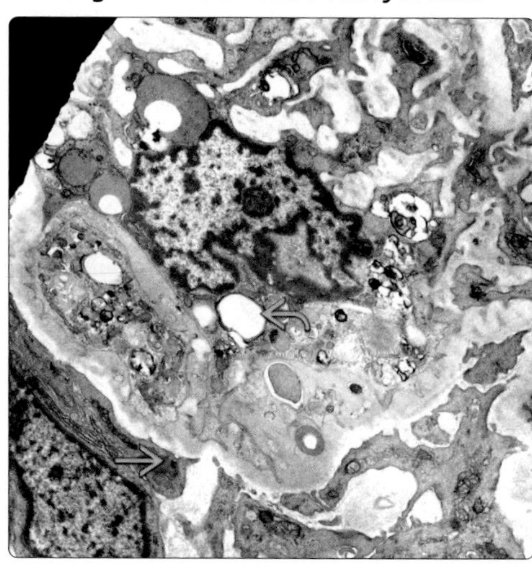

Cellular Bridging of Bowman Capsule in FSGS

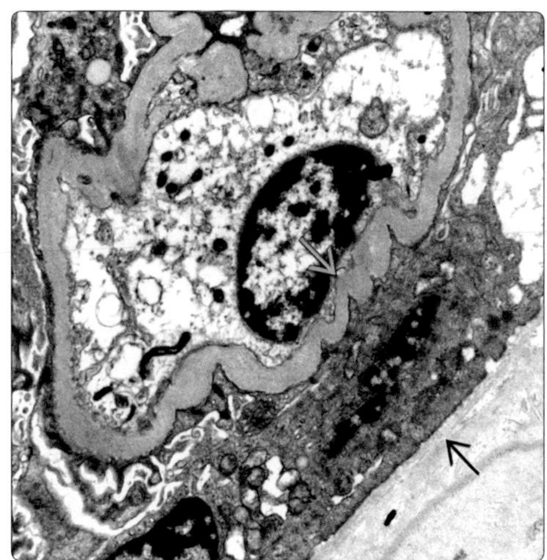

(Left) *Segmental scar shows lipid in mesangial cells* ➙ *and loss of the podocytes* ➙. **(Right)** *A single cell bridges the Bowman capsule* ➙ *and the GBM* ➙, *probably the earliest phase of an adhesion in FSGS. The nature of the cell is not certain, but based on experimental evidence, it is probably a parietal epithelial cell that attached to a bare GBM.*

(Left) *In this case of FSGS, tip variant, there is herniation of the glomerular tuft ➔ into the proximal tubule where it exits the Bowman space.* **(Right)** *In this case of FSGS, tip variant, a glomerular capillary contains foam cells and is adherent to Bowman capsule ➔ at the inlet of the proximal tubule ➔. Enlarged, reactive podocytes are also at the site ➔.*

Tip Variant

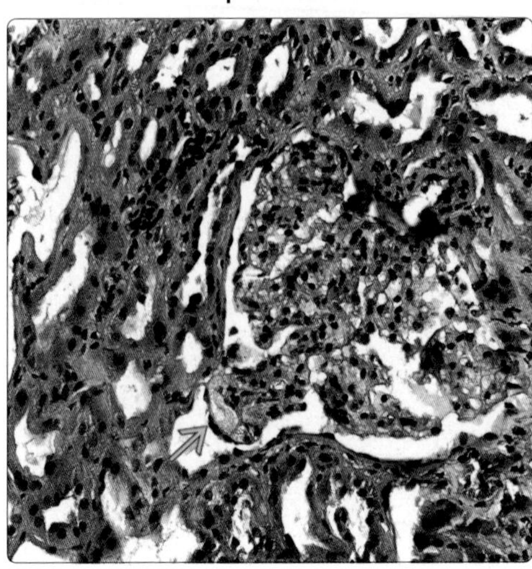

Tip Variant With Adhesion

(Left) *Even though the proximal tubule is not seen in this section, the characteristic intracapillary foam cells ➔ are seen in the tip quadrant opposite the glomerular hilum at the bottom.* **(Right)** *In this tip variant, the glomerular capillary loops are adherent to BC ➔. Hypertrophic podocytes ➔ are "herniating" through the site at which the tubular pole exits ➔, and adjacent foam cells are in capillaries.*

Tip Lesion With Foam Cells

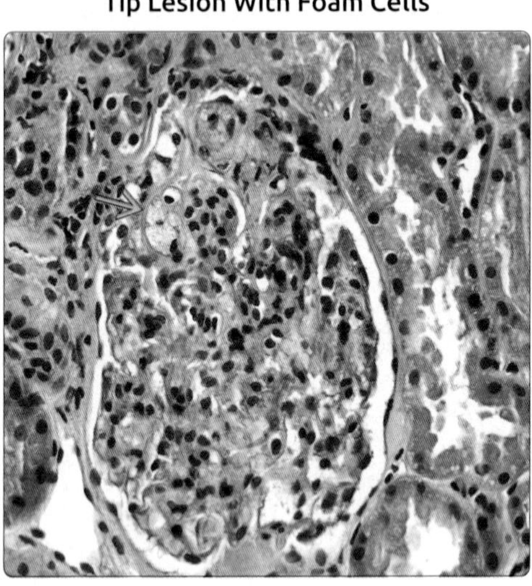

Podocyte Hypertrophy and Endocapillary Foam Cells

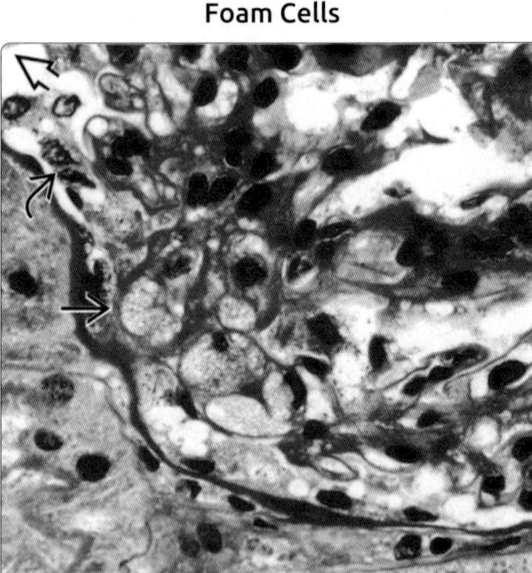

(Left) *In this case of FSGS, tip variant, EM shows wrinkled glomerular basement membranes ➔ and endocapillary hypercellularity ➔ at the portion adjacent to the tubular pole.* **(Right)** *In this case of FSGS, tip variant, there is widespread podocyte foot process effacement ➔ by electron microscopy.*

GBM Wrinkling in Tip Variant

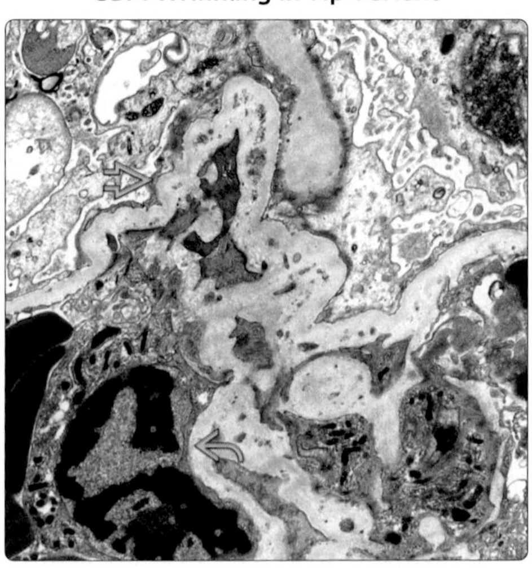

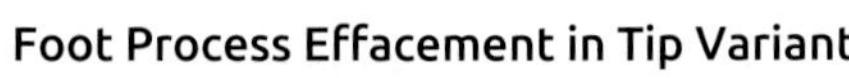

Foot Process Effacement in Tip Variant

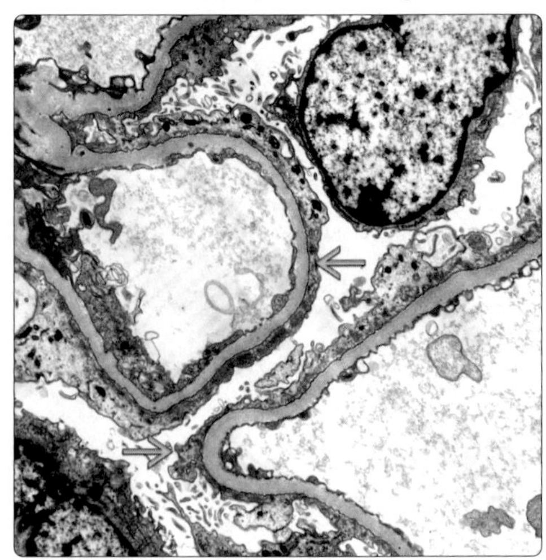

Cellular Variant With Mononuclear Cells Filling Capillaries

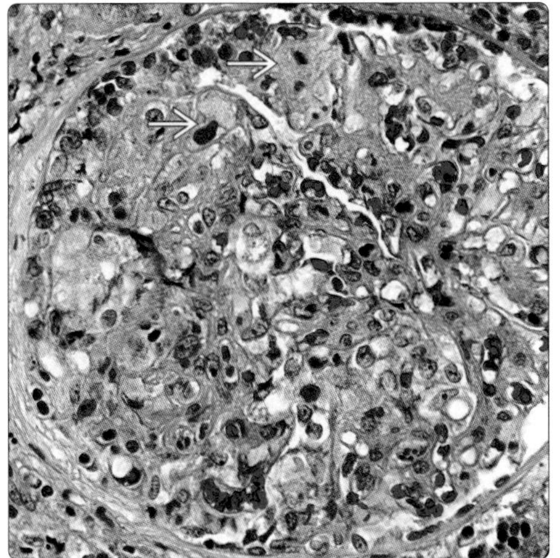

Cellular Variant With Intracapillary Cells

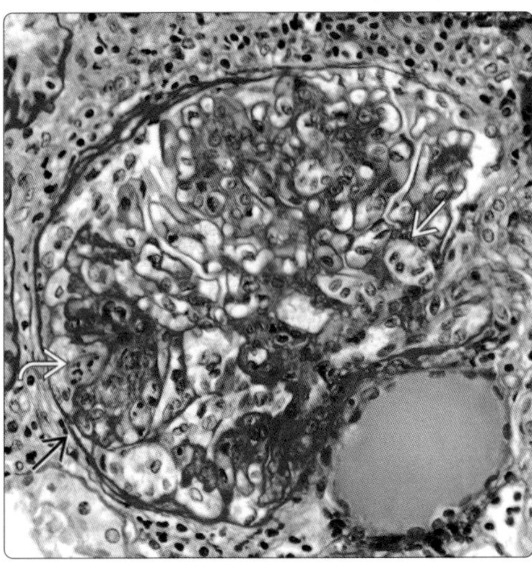

(Left) *Trichrome stain of a biopsy with the cellular variant of FSGS shows most glomerular capillaries filled with mononuclear cells with abundant, sometimes foamy cytoplasm* ➡. **(Right)** *In this case of FSGS, cellular variant, the glomerulus shows intracapillary cells* ➡ *and adhesions to Bowman capsule* ➡. *Karyorrhexis is also present* ➡.

Segmental IgM in Cellular Variant

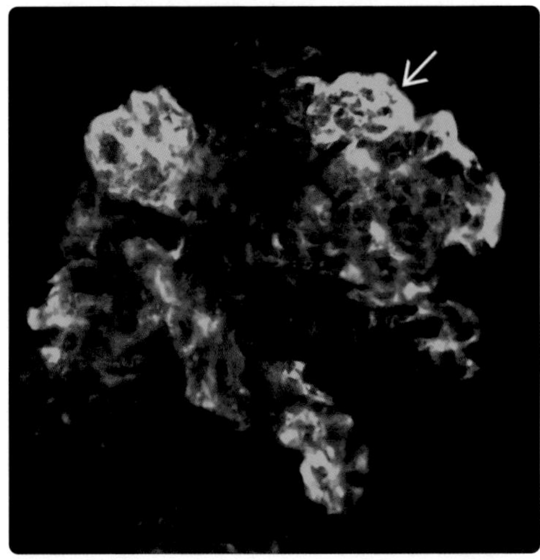

Segmental C3 in Cellular Variant

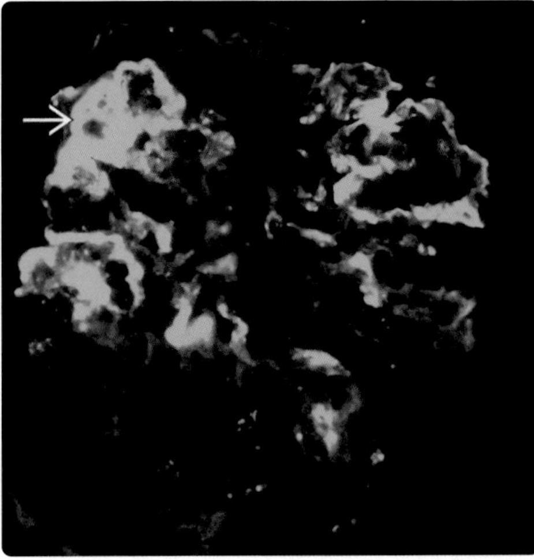

(Left) *IgM by immunofluorescence shows segmental positivity* ➡ *in the cellular variant of FSGS.* **(Right)** *In this case of FSGS, cellular variant, there is segmental deposition of C3* ➡ *by immunofluorescence.*

Cellular Variant With Intracapillary Cells

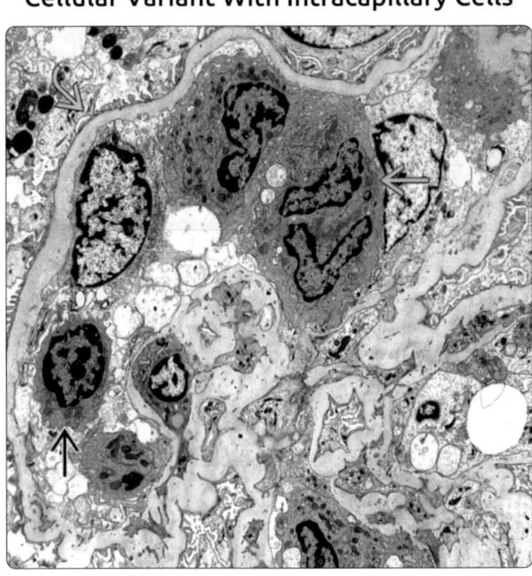

Podocyte Foot Process Effacement in Cellular Variant of FSGS

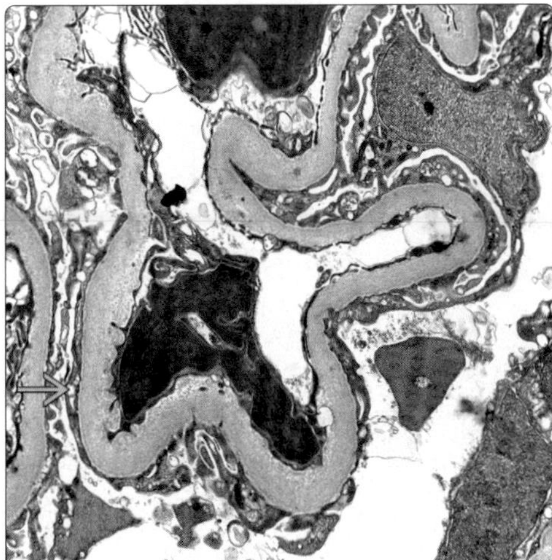

(Left) *The cellular variant of FSGS is defined by intracapillary cells, here shown to be monocytes* ➡ *and lymphocytes* ➡. *Foam cells, either macrophages or endothelial cells, can also be conspicuous. Foot process effacement is present but patchy* ➡. **(Right)** *In the cellular variant of FSGS, there is podocyte foot process effacement* ➡ *&/or blunting around many of the glomerular capillary loops.*

KEY FACTS

TERMINOLOGY

- FSGS due to adaptive response to excess demand on glomerular function

ETIOLOGY/PATHOGENESIS

- Adaptive structural-functional response
  - Reduced nephron mass: Oligomeganephronia, reflux nephropathy, renal agenesis/dysplasia, ablation, cortical necrosis, advanced renal disease of any cause
  - Normal nephron mass: HTN, obesity-related glomerulopathy (ORG), atheroemboli/vasoocclusion, sickle cell anemia, congenital heart disease, drugs (anabolic steroids, calcineurin inhibitors)
- Glomerular HTN, podocytopenia

CLINICAL ISSUES

- Proteinuria & systemic HTN
- Treatment
  - Angiotensin II receptor antagonists &/or ACE inhibitors
  - Low-protein diet, bariatric surgery (obesity)
  - Steroids not usually effective

MICROSCOPIC

- Glomerulomegaly
- Perihilar glomerular adhesion and hyaline
- Compensatory tubular hypertrophy
- Often arteriolar hyalinosis, arteriosclerosis
- IF: Most notable for segmental IgM & C3
- EM: Segmental podocyte foot process effacement (FPE)
  - Increased thickness of otherwise normal GBM

TOP DIFFERENTIAL DIAGNOSES

- Primary FSGS
- Underlying renal disease that caused nephron loss

DIAGNOSTIC CHECKLIST

- Assess glomerular size in biopsies
- Rough guide: Normal glomeruli are < 50% of diameter of 40x field of 440 μm

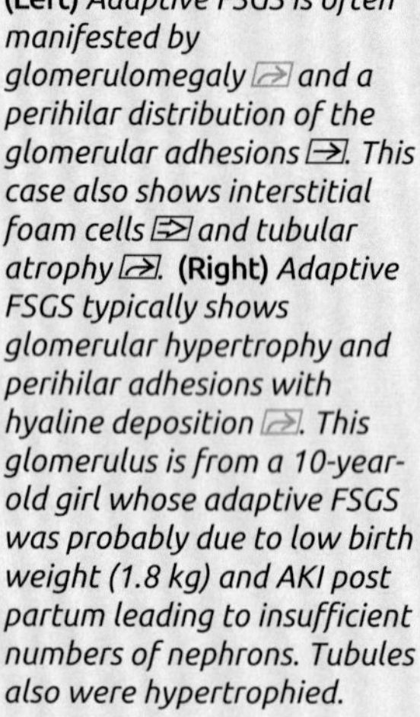

Perihilar Adhesion and Sclerosis

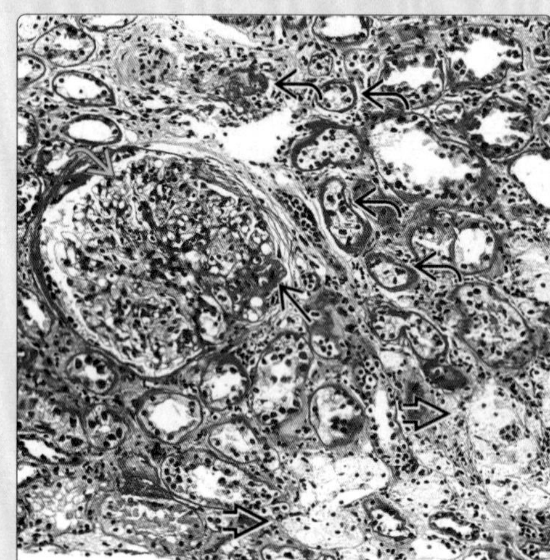

Glomerular Hypertrophy and Perihilar Hyaline

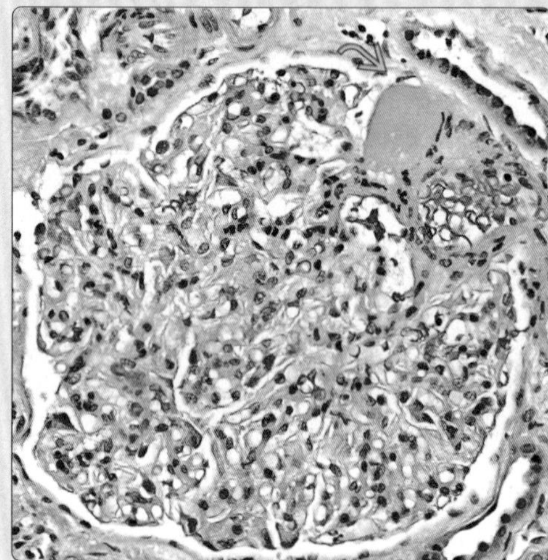

(Left) *Adaptive FSGS is often manifested by glomerulomegaly* ➢ *and a perihilar distribution of the glomerular adhesions* ➔. *This case also shows interstitial foam cells* ➡ *and tubular atrophy* ➢. **(Right)** *Adaptive FSGS typically shows glomerular hypertrophy and perihilar adhesions with hyaline deposition* ➢. *This glomerulus is from a 10-year-old girl whose adaptive FSGS was probably due to low birth weight (1.8 kg) and AKI post partum leading to insufficient numbers of nephrons. Tubules also were hypertrophied.*

Segmental C3 Deposition

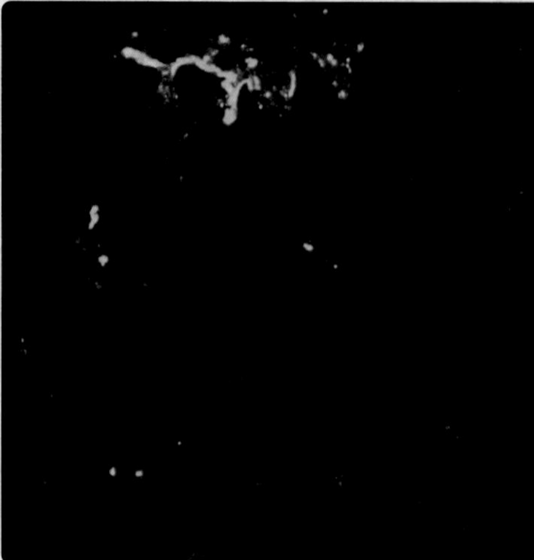

Thickened GBM and Preservation of Foot Processes

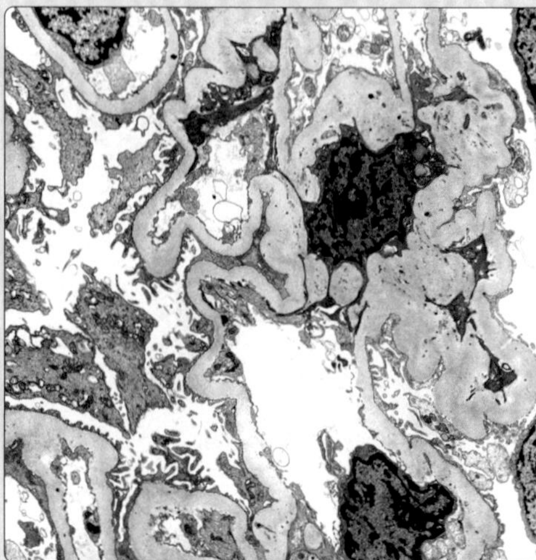

(Left) *Segmental C3 deposition occurs in areas of glomerular scarring and adhesion in FSGS due to any cause, including, as illustrated in this case, with adaptive FSGS. IgM shows a similar pattern. This has been assumed to be nonspecific trapping.* **(Right)** *The manifestation of glomerular hypertrophy by EM is a diffusely thickened GBM. Secondary FSGS often has relatively little foot process effacement despite moderately heavy proteinuria (in this case due to hypertension, ~ 3 g/d).*

TERMINOLOGY

Abbreviations

- Focal segmental glomerulosclerosis (FSGS)

Synonyms

- Secondary FSGS
  - Less specific term
- Perihilar variant of FSGS
  - Common histologic pattern of adaptive FSGS but also occurs in minority (< 10%) of primary FSGS

Definitions

- Adaptive FSGS arises as response to loss of nephrons or increased demand, probably due to increased filtration/perfusion of glomeruli, insufficient numbers of podocytes for filtration area, and podocyte stress

ETIOLOGY/PATHOGENESIS

Adaptive Structural-Functional Response

- Imbalance between glomerular capacity & metabolic demands
  - Thought to act through glomerular hypertension (HTN), ↑ filtration, relative podocytopenia, and podocyte stress
  - ↑ glomerular capillary pressures & flow rates
- Arises from several pathways
  - Failure to develop normal number of glomeruli
    - Unilateral renal agenesis, dysplasia, oligomeganephronia, low birth weight, & other congenital renal developmental diseases
  - Acquired disease that causes ↓ of functional nephrons
    - Sequelae of chronic renal disease of any etiology that destroys nephrons: Final common pathway
    - Reflux nephropathy, Alport syndrome, HTN, cortical necrosis, & virtually any other chronic renal disease
  - Normal number of glomeruli but increased "demand"
    - Obesity, body builders, anabolic steroids, possibly HTN

Specific Mechanisms

- Obesity-related glomerulopathy (ORG)
  - Receptor for advanced glycation end products (RAGE) may mediate obesity-associated renal injury
  - RAGE may also be important to diabetes, doxorubicin-induced nephropathy, HTN, lupus nephritis, ischemic renal injury, & renal amyloidosis
- Calcineurin inhibitors (CNIs)
  - Arteriolar constriction leads to variable glomerular perfusion
  - Particularly important in renal transplant recipients since FSGS can sometimes be ascribed to CNIs
- Anabolic steroids used in bodybuilding
  - Possibly due to direct nephrotoxic effect of anabolic steroids and increase in lean body mass
- Sleep apnea
  - Hypoxia leads to sympathetic nervous system activation & stimulates renin-angiotensin system
- Unilateral renal agenesis
  - Higher risk of FSGS than general population
- Unilateral nephrectomy in adults does not increase risk for FSGS

Pathologic Consequences

- Glomerular hypertrophy
  - Increase in diameter & number of mesangial cells
  - Thickened glomerular basement membrane (GBM)
  - Relative deficiency of podocytes, which have limited replicative ability
- Segmental glomerular capillary scars and adhesions to Bowman capsule
  - Classically, adhesion & hyaline in perihilar region
  - Known as the "hilar" variant of FSGS

Murine Model

- Removal/infarction of upper & lower pole of kidney followed by contralateral nephrectomy (5/6 nephrectomy)
- Results in HTN, glomerulomegaly, and later, FSGS over 8-12 weeks with proteinuria & loss of renal function
- Ameliorated by inhibitors of renin-angiotensin system (angiotensin II receptor inhibitors)

CLINICAL ISSUES

Epidemiology

- Incidence
  - Coincident with increase in obesity incidence: Apparent increased incidence of ORG

Presentation

- Proteinuria is often > 3.5 g/d but usually without hypoalbuminemia, hypercholesterolemia, & edema
  - Specifically, ORG shows decreased incidence of nephrotic syndrome than idiopathic FSGS
- Renal dysfunction
  - Most have ↑ serum creatinine and ↓ glomerular filtration rate (GFR) preceding development of nephrotic proteinuria
    - ORG is notable exception since it may have ↑ GFR (supernormal, > 120 mL/min) 2° to hyperfiltration/overwork state caused by ↑ ratio of body mass to renal mass
- Hypertension
- ORG patients typically have a BMI > 30
  - BMI 30-34.9, grade 1 obesity; BMI 35.0-39.9, grade 2 obesity; & BMI ≥ 40, grade 3 obesity (morbid obesity)

Treatment

- Drugs
  - Steroids are not typically effective
    - Often contraindicated in many patients (e.g., in obesity) due to stimulation of weight gain & diabetes
  - Angiotensin II receptor antagonists &/or ACE inhibitors
  - Stop anabolic steroid use
- Other treatment
  - Bariatric surgery may normalize proteinuria in ORG
  - Low-protein diet

Prognosis

- Adaptive FSGS more indolent than primary FSGS
- Studies regarding prognosis of perihilar variant of FSGS are mixed
  - Probably relates to underlying causes

MICROSCOPIC

Histologic Features

- Glomeruli
  - Glomerulomegaly
    - Glomeruli enlarged with expanded hypercellular mesangium
    - Universal definition of glomerulomegaly not established, even by "gold standard" morphometric methods due to significant population variability
    - Rule of thumb: Glomerular diameter > 220 μm (~ 1/2 diameter of typical 40x objective field)
    - Variable degrees, heterogeneity
  - Segmental glomerulosclerosis (GS)
    - Loss of intrinsic cells & structure of glomerulus
    - Global GS may also be present
  - Adhesion to Bowman capsule
    - Typically in perihilar region
    - Contains hyaline deposits in capillary loops
    - Hyalinosis composed of protein insudation between GBM & endothelial cells
    - To qualify for hilar variant, > 50% of glomeruli with segmental lesions must have perihilar GS &/or hyalinosis
    - Foam cells may be entrapped in sclerotic lesions
  - Podocyte hypertrophy & hyperplasia may be present
- Vessels
  - Arteriolar hyalinosis may be in continuity with perihilar segment of arteriole
- Tubules and interstitium
  - Tubular hypertrophy (↑ tubular diameter & cell size)
  - Atrophy and interstitial fibrosis related to decreased nephron number

Specific Features by Cause

- Obesity
  - Mesangial expansion, GBM thickening, & glomerulomegaly
  - Segmental lesions often perihilar with hyalinosis
  - Tubulointerstitial disease often mild in comparison with glomerular changes
- Hypertension
  - Glomerulosclerosis often occurs in outer cortex, forming subcapsular scars
  - Arteriosclerosis and arteriolar hyalinosis present
  - Glomerular hypertrophy
  - Segmental sclerosis often perihilar
  - Atubular glomeruli often form, leading to cystic dilatation of Bowman space
  - Interstitial fibrosis and tubular atrophy prominent
- Reflux nephropathy
  - Reflux nephropathy shows prominent periglomerular fibrosis and thickening of Bowman capsule
  - Interstitial fibrosis in "geographic" pattern
- Sickle cell disease
  - Glomerular hypertrophy & capillary loop congestion by sickled erythrocytes
  - Glomerular capillaries may have double contours due to thrombotic microangiopathy

ANCILLARY TESTS

Immunofluorescence

- Segmental IgM & C3 in glomerulosclerotic lesions
- Little or no immunoglobulin otherwise

Electron Microscopy

- Podocyte foot process effacement (FPE) is cardinal feature
  - Typically segmental FPE (often < 50%)
    - Average foot process width of < 1,500 μm distinguishes adaptive FSGS from primary FSGS (100% sensitive and 70% specific)
  - Podocyte hypertrophy & hyperplasia typically < in primary FSGS
  - Podocytes may detach from GBM and may contain protein resorption droplets
  - Podocytes may detach, leaving bare GBM segments
- Features of particular etiologies
  - Obesity-associated FSGS: Subtotal FPE & marked glomerulomegaly
  - HTN: Ischemic wrinkling & thickening of GBM

DIFFERENTIAL DIAGNOSIS

Primary FSGS

- Less glomerulomegaly, more diffuse foot process effacement
- Majority NOS variant rather than perihilar

Identification of Underlying Renal Disease

- Look for features of underlying immune complex, proliferative, or nonimmune diseases
- Immune complexes may be difficult to find in end-stage kidneys, making diligent search necessary

Focal Glomerulonephritis (GN)

- Segmental scars may be residue of past inflammatory GN

DIAGNOSTIC CHECKLIST

Pathologic Interpretation Pearls

- Perihilar glomerulosclerosis and hypertrophy are clues to diagnosis
- Routinely assess glomerular size in biopsies
  - Normal is < 50% of diameter of 40x field (440 μm)

SELECTED REFERENCES

1. Fogo AB: Causes and pathogenesis of focal segmental glomerulosclerosis. Nat Rev Nephrol. ePub, 2014
2. Ikezumi Y et al: Low birthweight and premature birth are risk factors for podocytopenia and focal segmental glomerulosclerosis. Am J Nephrol. 38(2):149-57, 2013
3. D'Agati VD et al: Focal segmental glomerulosclerosis. N Engl J Med. 365(25):2398-411, 2011
4. D'Agati V et al: RAGE and the pathogenesis of chronic kidney disease. Nat Rev Nephrol. 6(6):352-60, 2010
5. Herlitz LC et al: Development of focal segmental glomerulosclerosis after anabolic steroid abuse. J Am Soc Nephrol. 21(1):163-72, 2010
6. D'Agati VD et al: Pathologic classification of focal segmental glomerulosclerosis: a working proposal. Am J Kidney Dis. 43(2):368-82, 2004
7. Rennke HG et al: Pathogenesis and significance of nonprimary focal and segmental glomerulosclerosis. Am J Kidney Dis. 13(6):443-56, 1989

Global and Segmental Glomerulosclerosis

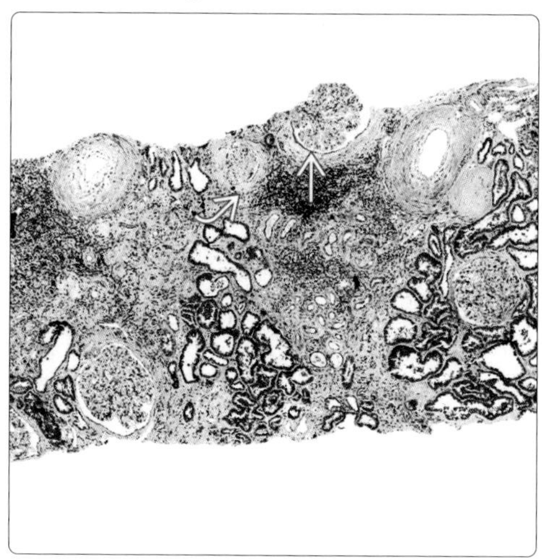

Perihilar Adhesion and Scar in Hypertensive Renal Disease

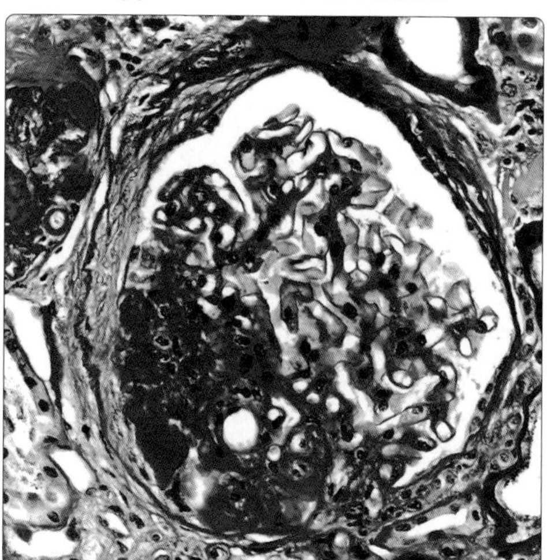

(Left) *One of the more common causes of adaptive FSGS is HTN, which causes progressive loss of functional nephrons and produces global ➭ & segmental ➡ glomerulosclerosis, as shown here in a 63-year-old woman with poorly controlled HTN for 30 years.* **(Right)** *Adaptive FSGS can arise from many causes; in this case, hilar sclerosis & adhesions were due to chronic renal disease presumed to be hypertensive nephropathy. Cr was 2.2, and the urine protein/Cr ratio was 2.8.*

Sclerosis at Glomerular Hilum With Lipid Droplets

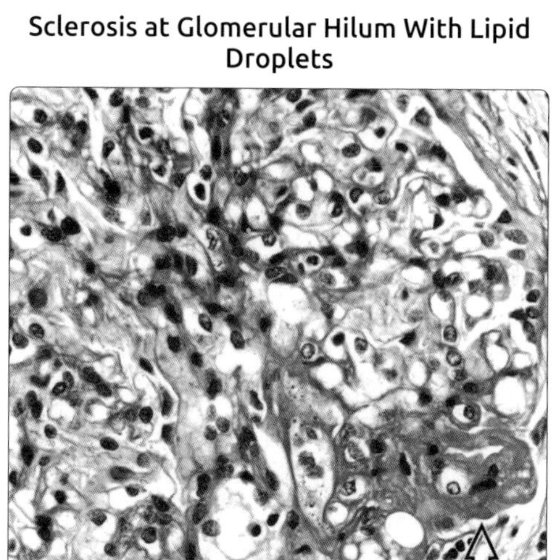

Perihilar Segmental Glomerulosclerosis

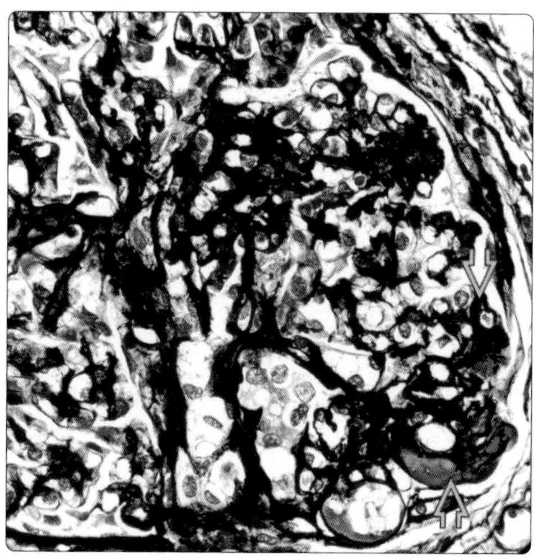

(Left) *High power of a PAS stain shows sclerosis at the glomerular hilum ⇨ containing lipid droplets ➩.* **(Right)** *High-power view of a silver stain in a 21-year-old man with nephrotic syndrome and perihilar segmental GS shows that intracapillary hyaline ⇨ is present in the segmental sclerosis lesion.*

Adaptive FSGS in Reflux Nephropathy

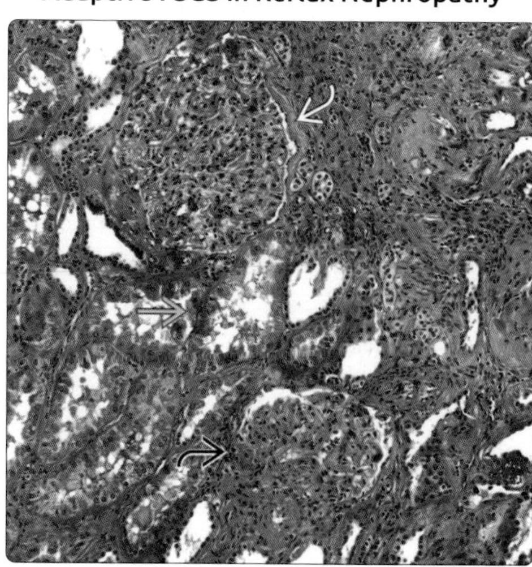

IgM Deposits Segmentally in FSGS

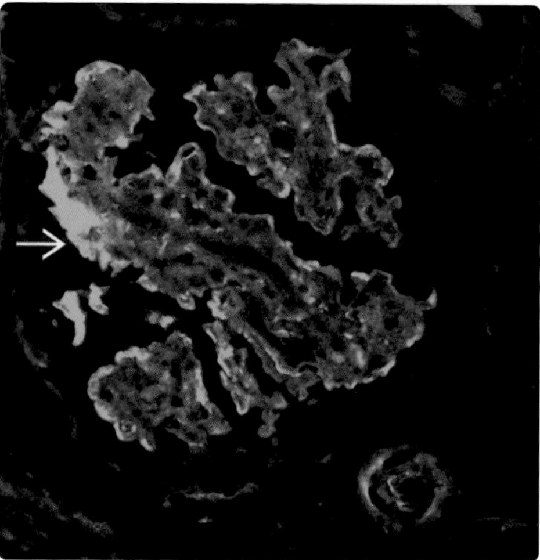

(Left) *Late-stage bilateral reflux nephropathy is one of the classic causes of adaptive FSGS. The remaining glomeruli are hypertrophied ➭; the spared tubules are also hypertrophied ⇨. Perihilar adhesions are present ➩.* **(Right)** *The main value of IF in cases with FSGS is to rule out underlying glomerular disease. In FSGS of all types, segmental deposits of IgM ➡ & C3 are in the segmental lesions, sometimes with segmental granular deposits along the GBM.*

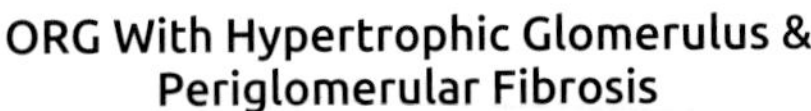

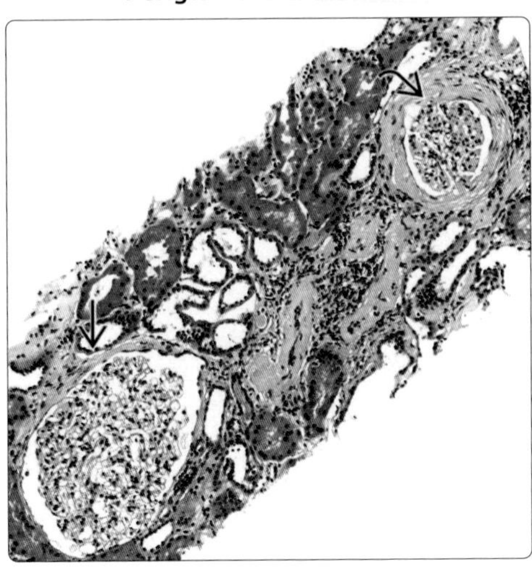

ORG With Glomerular Capillary Loop Condensation

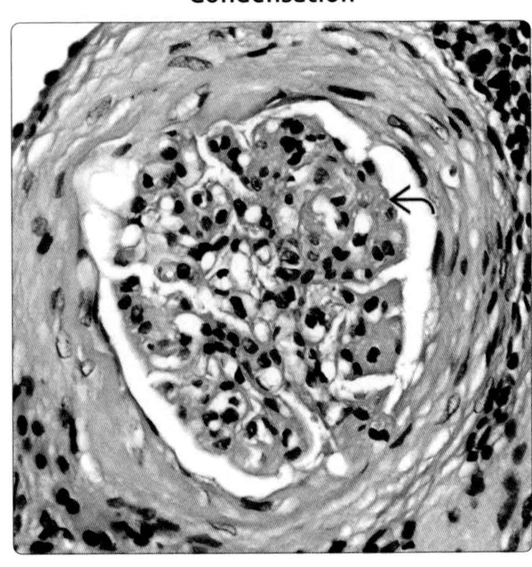

(Left) *H&E from a 37-year-old African-American woman with morbid obesity (> 350 lb), HTN, and proteinuria shows a hypertrophic glomerulus* ➡ *and a relatively normal-sized glomerulus with periglomerular fibrosis* ➡. *Overall, this is clinicopathologically compatible with obesity-related glomerulopathy (ORG).* **(Right)** *In an ORG case, there is peripheral condensation of the glomerular capillary loops* ➡, *suggestive of evolving FSGS.*

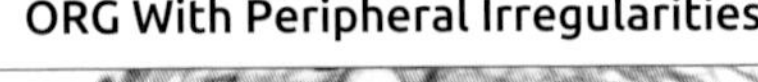

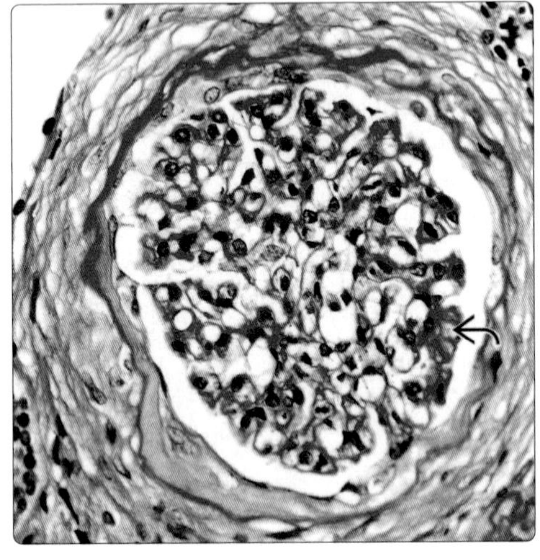

ORG With Peripheral Irregularities

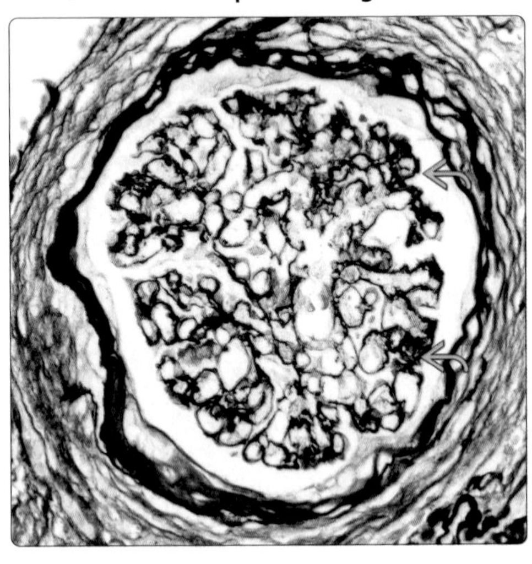

(Left) *A PAS stain shows the peripheral irregularities in glomerular capillary loops* ➡ *in a case most compatible with obesity-related glomerulopathy in a 37 year old with morbid obesity.* **(Right)** *A periodic acid-methenamine-silver (PAMS) stain shows peripheral irregularities* ➡ *in the glomerular capillary loops in the same patient.*

ORG With Glomerular Hypertrophy

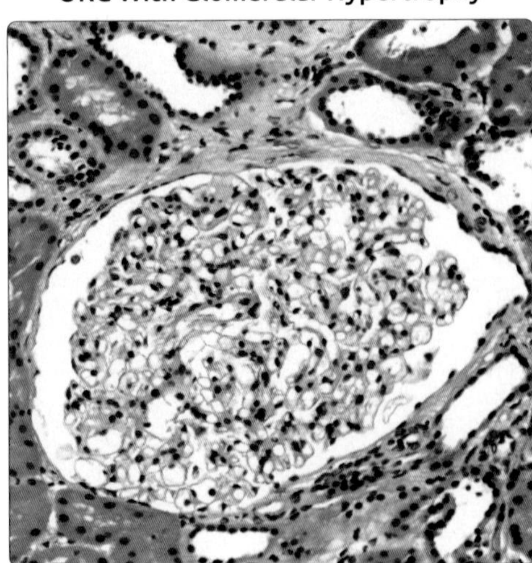

ORG With Glomerular Hypertrophy

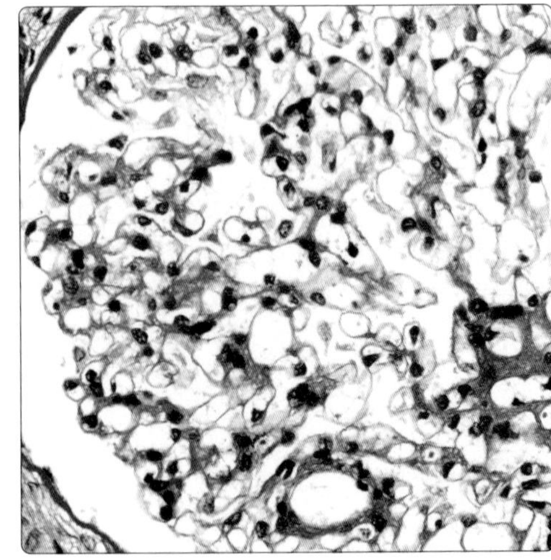

(Left) *Glomerulus shows marked hypertrophy in the same patient.* **(Right)** *Glomerulus shows marked hypertrophy in the same patient. Normally, a glomerulus should fit into a 40x field, but in this case, less than 2/3 of the glomerulus fits.*

ORG

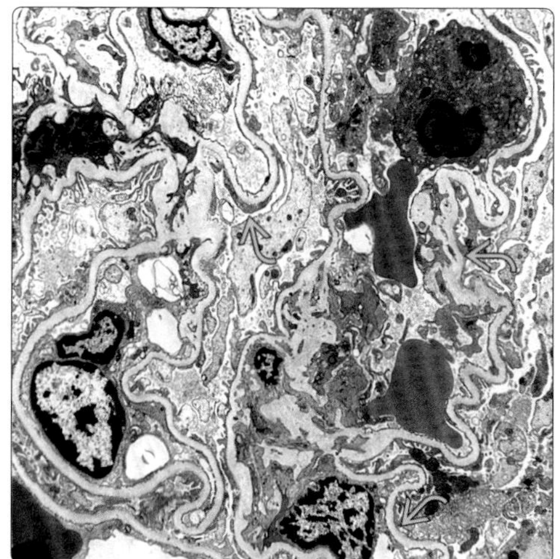

ORG With Segmental Podocyte FPE

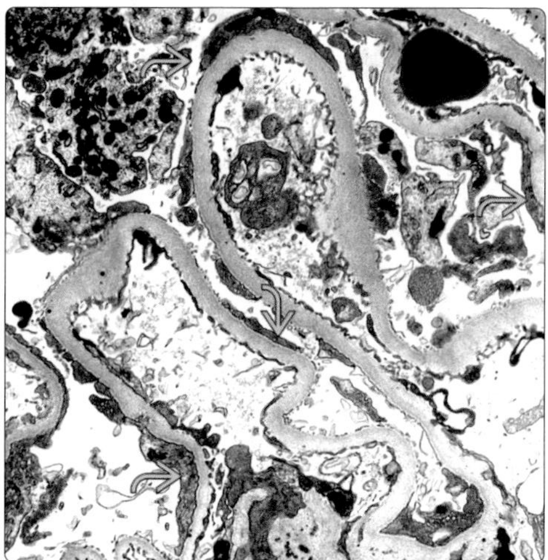

(Left) *In a 53-year-old man with morbid obesity (BMI 41.9), creatinine 10 mg/dL, and a urine protein/creatinine ratio of 12.96, there is only patchy effacement of foot processes (FPE)* ➢. **(Right)** *In the same patient, there was segmental FPE* ➢, *compatible with adaptive FSGS.*

ORG With Segmental Podocyte FPE

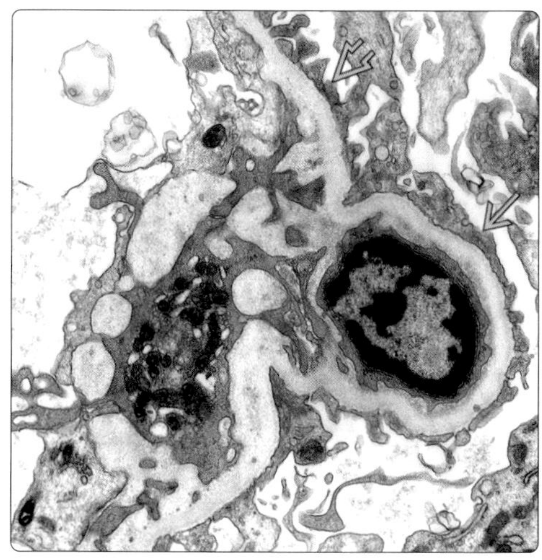

Segmental Podocyte FPE in FSGS From Anabolic Steroids

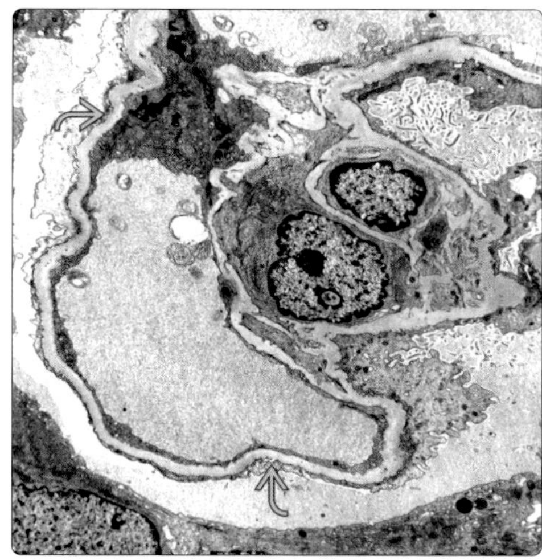

(Left) *In the same patient, there was prominent segmental podocyte foot process effacement* ➢, *together with more preserved foot processes* ➢, *compatible with obesity-related FSGS in this case to ORG.* **(Right)** *In a 40-year-old male bodybuilder with years of anabolic steroid use, there is segmental podocyte foot process effacement* ➢. *This adaptive FSGA is attributed to increased glomerular demand due to anabolic steroid use.*

Segmental Podocyte FPE in FSGS From Anabolic Steroids

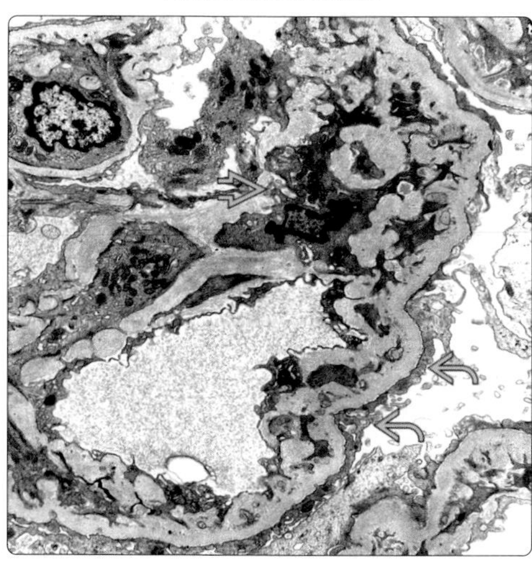

Vague Densities in FSGS from Anabolic Steroids

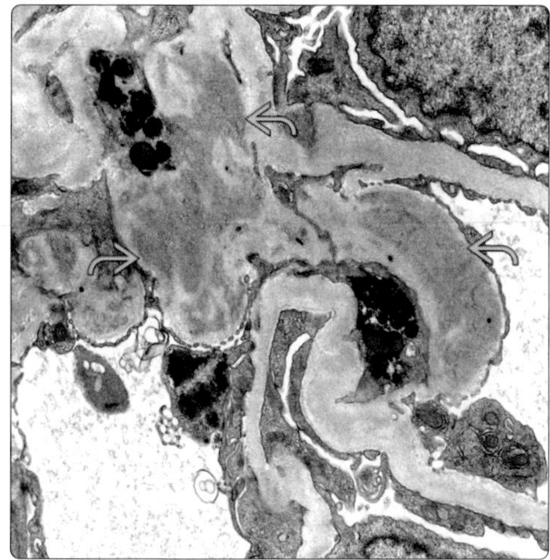

(Left) *In the same patient with a history of years of anabolic steroid use for bodybuilding, there is segmental podocyte foot process effacement* ➢ *and mesangial expansion* ➢. **(Right)** *In FSGS attributed to anabolic steroids, there were occasional vague densities* ➢, *some having a hyaline quality. IF did not impart specificity to the densities, suggesting that their presence is secondary to entrapment.*

Collapsing Glomerulopathy

KEY FACTS

TERMINOLOGY

- Glomerular diseases defined by prominent capillary loop collapse, glomerular visceral epithelial cell hypercellularity, and proliferation

ETIOLOGY/PATHOGENESIS

- Loss of podocytes and replacement with parietal epithelial cells
- Causes
  - Idiopathic believed to be due to circulating factor
  - Infection: HIV, parvovirus B19, and many others
  - Drugs: Interferons, bisphosphonates, calcineurin inhibitors
  - Genetic: Most commonly *APOL1* in blacks

CLINICAL ISSUES

- Blacks disproportionately affected in most forms
- Nephrotic syndrome and nephrotic-range proteinuria
- Renal dysfunction
- Often refractory to steroid therapy
- Rapid progression to renal failure

MICROSCOPIC

- At least 1 glomerulus with
  - Global or segmental collapse
  - Overlying podocyte hyperplasia and hypertrophy
- Tubulointerstitial fibrosis, cysts, and inflammation
- Ki-67-positive visceral epithelial cells (proliferation)
- Immunofluorescence: Segmental IgM and C3
- Electron microscopy
  - Segmental foot process effacement and separation from GBM
  - Wrinkled GBM with capillary loop collapse

TOP DIFFERENTIAL DIAGNOSES

- Crescentic glomerulonephritis
- Other variants of FSGS
- Secondary to underlying glomerular disease

(Left) *In collapsing glomerulopathy, glomerular capillary loops are not well defined ⇨, and a rim of crowded, reactive podocytes is present →.* **(Right)** *Podocyte proliferation in collapsing glomerulopathy can resemble a cellular crescent ↷. However, the cells are more rounded than the more spindle-shaped parietal epithelial cells typically seen in a crescent.*

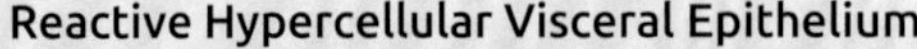

Reactive Hypercellular Visceral Epithelium

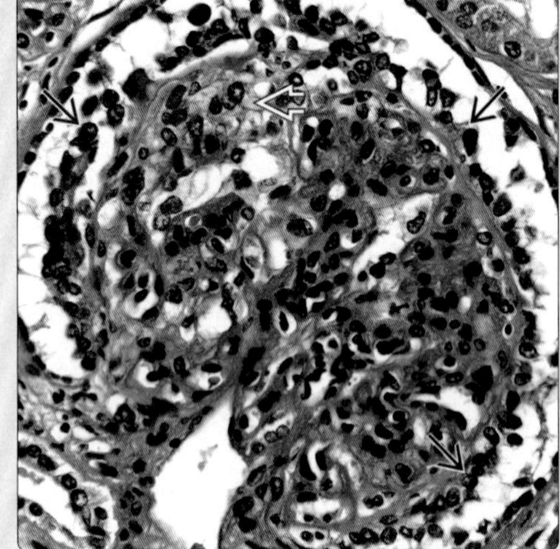

Pseudocrescent

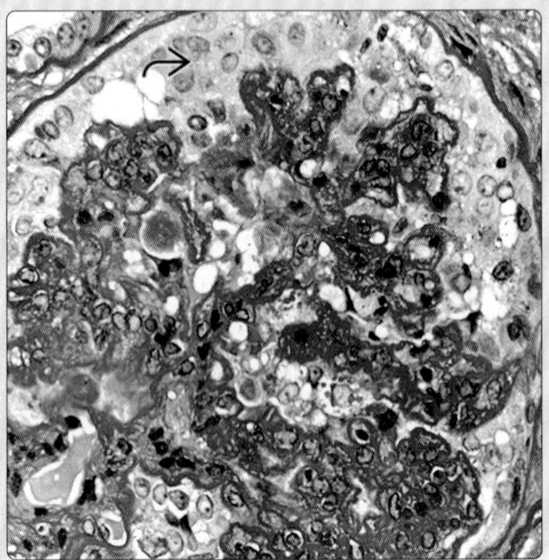

(Left) *Proliferating podocytes → are highlighted by Ki-67 immunohistochemistry in this case of collapsing glomerulopathy.* **(Right)** *EM shows prominent glomerular basement membrane wrinkling with collapse of glomerular capillary loops →.*

Visceral Epithelium is Ki-67(+)

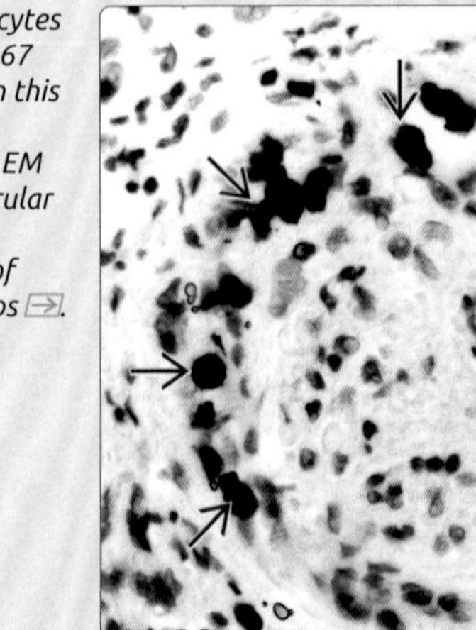

Glomerular Capillary Loop Collapse

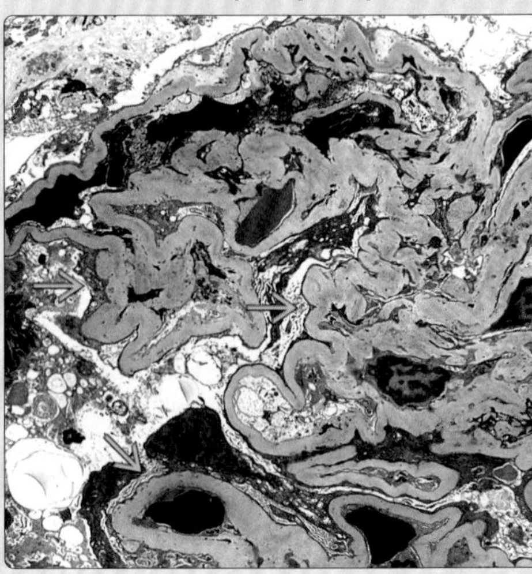

TERMINOLOGY

Abbreviations

- Collapsing glomerulopathy (CG)

Synonyms

- Focal segmental glomerulosclerosis (FSGS), collapsing variant
- Idiopathic collapsing FSGS

Definitions

- "Podocytopathy" defined pathologically by prominent capillary loop collapse, glomerular visceral epithelial cell hypercellularity, and proliferation

ETIOLOGY/PATHOGENESIS

Diverse Etiologies

- Primary (idiopathic)
- Secondary
  - Infection
  - Drugs
  - Vascular disease
  - Malignancy
  - Genetic disorders
  - Superimposed on other glomerular diseases

Common Features

- Prominent proliferation of epithelial cells on urinary side of glomerular basement membrane (GBM) that lack normal podocyte markers
  - These cells characteristically lack expression of WT1 of normal podocyte and increase expression of proteins involved in cell division (e.g., Ki-67)
  - Originally attributed to dedifferentiation or dysregulation of podocyte
  - Now considered to be repopulation with parietal epithelial cells from Bowman capsule
    - Cells on GBM have markers of parietal epithelial cells
      - pax-2, cytokeratin (CK) 8/18 and 19, claudin-1
      - CD44 (activation marker)
  - Podocyte bridging between Bowman capsule and glomerulus can be seen
    - Forms pseudocrescent
- Primary event probably podocyte loss (podocytopenia), as demonstrated in other types of FSGS
  - CG differs in its much greater degree of proliferation and repopulation with parietal epithelial cells
- Normal podocytes have low rate of turnover
  - WT1 transcription factor inhibits proliferation
- Proximal tubular cells also affected and show increased cell turnover

Specific Mechanisms in Idiopathic (Primary) CG

- Circulating permeability factor shown by recurrence in allografts, but molecular identification remains elusive

Genetic Factors

- 2 *APOL1* risk alleles in patients of recent African descent
  - Affects risk of CG due to drugs and other glomerular diseases
- Mitochondrial genes
  - Coenzyme Q2

Experimental Models

- Adriamycin podocyte toxicity in mouse

CLINICAL ISSUES

Epidemiology

- Incidence
  - Second most common FSGS pattern in biopsies (~ 12%) in adults
  - Rare in children < 10 years old
    - Except for genetic forms
  - Geographic/racial differences
    - Blacks are disproportionately affected (20-50x rate of nonblacks)
    - More common in FSGS series in Brazil (37%) than Korea (1%) or India (2%)

Presentation

- Nephrotic syndrome or nephrotic-range proteinuria
  - Hypoalbuminemia
  - Hypercholesterolemia
- Renal dysfunction
  - Elevated serum Cr at presentation, higher than FSGS of other types

Treatment

- Drugs
  - None effective
  - Typically refractory to steroids
  - Treatment of underlying condition such as infection or tumor can lead to remission

Prognosis

- Poor prognosis of idiopathic CG in all series
  - 47% progress to end-stage renal disease (ESRD) in 3 years
  - 50% ESRD in 6 months
  - More rapid progression than other types of FSGS
    - "Malignant" FSGS
- Improvement can occur in cases with recovery from or removal of etiologic agent

MICROSCOPIC

Histologic Features

- Glomeruli
  - At least 1 glomerulus with global or segmental collapse and overlying epithelial hyperplasia and hypertrophy, according to Columbia Working Proposal
    - This is lowest possible threshold and has led to marked increase in diagnosis of CG
  - Visceral epithelial cells with hypertrophy and hyperplasia
    - Urinary space may be filled with podocytes, forming pseudocrescents
    - Enlarged nuclei with open, vesicular chromatin and frequent nucleoli
    - Binucleate forms may be seen
    - Mitotic figures and apoptosis occasionally sampled
    - Protein resorption droplets may be seen in pseudocrescent podocytes
  - GBMs wrinkled in areas of collapse

- PAS and Jones methenamine silver stains are useful in highlighting basement membrane collapse
  - Mesangial and intracapillary matrix are not appreciably increased, except in cases superimposed upon diabetes
- Tubules
  - Tubular microcysts in 40% of cases
    - Proximal tubules dilated with proteinaceous casts, sometimes with "peripheral scalloping"
    - Enlarged hyperchromatic nuclei, mitotic figures, nucleoli, and focal apoptosis
  - Tubular atrophy/injury
    - Tubular epithelial simplification and flattening
  - Tubulitis can be present, often composed of neutrophilic tubulitis
- Interstitium
  - Inflammation
    - Interstitial mononuclear inflammation can be prominent
  - Edema
- Arteries/arterioles
  - Renal vessels may have changes of thrombotic microangiopathy if etiology involves TMA

ANCILLARY TESTS

Immunofluorescence

- IgM and C3 with segmental or global deposits in collapsed segments with less common deposits of C1q
- IgG, IgA, and albumin in visceral epithelial protein resorption droplets
- Tubules have epithelial protein resorption droplets containing plasma proteins (IgG, IgA, C3, albumin, and others)

Electron Microscopy

- Podocyte hypertrophy overlying areas of collapse
  - Foot processes are extensively effaced
  - Contain electron-dense protein resorption droplets, electron-lucent transport vesicles, and increased numbers of organelles, including prominent rough endoplasmic reticulum
  - Podocytes detached from GBM with interposition of newly formed extracellular matrix
  - Multiple layers of newly formed GBM between podocyte and original GBM
  - Actin cytoskeleton is disrupted, making cytoplasm appear open and pale
  - Podocytes become cuboidal
- GBM
  - Wrinkled GBM in areas of collapse
  - GBM not appreciably thickened
  - Absent electron-dense deposits except for small, rare paramesangial deposits
- Glomerular endothelium
  - Absent tubuloreticular inclusions in all forms except for HIV-associated CG, interferon-mediated forms, and lupus-associated forms

Immunohistochemistry

- Ki-67 (MIB1), a proliferation marker, is positive in visceral epithelial cells
  - Normal podocytes rarely express Ki-67 (< 1/glomerulus)
  - Proximal tubular cells also have increased Ki-67 staining
- Loss of normal podocyte differentiation markers
  - WT1, synaptopodin, podocin, podocalyxin, glomerular epithelial protein 1 [GLEPP1], α-actinin, C3b receptor, and CD10
- Gain of markers of parietal epithelial cells
  - pax-2, Claudin-1, CK8/18
- These alternations in visceral epithelial phenotype are most marked and most common in CG, but present in lesser degrees in other forms of FSGS

DIFFERENTIAL DIAGNOSIS

FSGS, Not Otherwise Specified (NOS)

- If glomerulus has collapsing lesion, forces classification to CG
- Podocyte proliferation and hypercellularity absent or minimal
- More hyalinosis, sclerosis, and adhesions to Bowman capsule

FSGS, Cellular Variant

- Endocapillary hypercellularity is more evident in cellular variant
- Some consider cellular variant to be in CG spectrum because of overlapping features
  - Cellular variant has increased Ki-67 and cytokeratin expression in visceral epithelial cells, with loss of normal podocyte markers (WT1, CD10, α-actinin)

Glomerulonephritis With Crescents

- True crescents usually contain fibrin and spindle-shaped cells that lack reabsorption droplets
- Necrotizing lesions in capillary tuft and GBM breaks absent in CG

Superimposed on Other Glomerular Diseases

- Characteristic features of underlying glomerular disease also present
  - IgA nephropathy, lupus nephritis, diabetes
- Associated with marked proteinuria and progression to ESRD

Superimposed on Arterial Disease

- Characteristic vascular lesions
  - Thrombotic microangiopathy
  - Severe arteriolar hyalinosis

HIV-Associated Nephropathy

- Prominent tubuloreticular structures in endothelial cells
- May have mitochondrial abnormalities in tubules due to highly active antiretroviral therapy (HAART)

SELECTED REFERENCES

1. Hakroush S et al: Extensive podocyte loss triggers a rapid parietal epithelial cell response. J Am Soc Nephrol. 25(5):927-38, 2014
2. Nichols B et al: Innate immunity pathways regulate the nephropathy gene Apolipoprotein L1. Kidney Int. ePub, 2014
3. Larsen CP et al: Apolipoprotein L1 risk variants associate with systemic lupus erythematosus-associated collapsing glomerulopathy. J Am Soc Nephrol. 24(5):722-5, 2013
4. Testagrossa L et al: Immunohistochemical expression of podocyte markers in the variants of focal segmental glomerulosclerosis. Nephrol Dial Transplant. 28(1):91-8, 2013

Pathogenetic Classification of Collapsing Glomerulopathy

Category	Cause	Comments
Idiopathic		
	Putative circulating factor	Most common form
Infection		
	HIV	Most common form of HIV glomerular disease in blacks; tubuloreticular inclusions prominent
	Cytomegalovirus	Immunocompromised patients; improved with steroids and ganciclovir
	Parvovirus B19	Post kidney transplant; in situ demonstration of virus in parietal epithelial cells
	Tuberculosis	Recovery reported
	Leishmaniasis	Visceral form; recovery reported
	Malaria	*Plasmodium falciparum* or *vivax* with hemolytic uremic syndrome; recovery reported
Drugs		
	Calcineurin inhibitors	Renal and non-renal transplant recipients; probably related to vascular disease (TMA, hyalinosis); poor prognosis
	IV drug abuse (e.g., heroin)	Often associated with HIV
	Bisphosphonates	High-dose pamidronate, especially IV; recovery reported
	Interferons (IFNα, β, γ)	IFNα for HCV; IFNβ for multiple sclerosis; IFNγ for pulmonary fibrosis; tubuloreticular inclusions usually prominent; *APOL1* alleles increase risk
	Griseofulvin	Recovered on drug withdrawal
Vascular		
	Thrombotic microangiopathy	Transplant, also in hemolytic uremic syndrome
	Periinfarct	Shows that acute glomerular ischemia can lead to CG pattern of injury
Autoimmune Disease		
	Still disease	Remission reported with steroids
Malignancy		
	Leukemia/lymphoma	Associated with hemophagocytic syndrome, anthracycline therapy, myeloma
Superimposed on Other Glomerular Diseases		
	IgA nephropathy	Poor prognosis; 90% ESRD
	Diabetes	Associated with severe hyalinosis; 75% ESRD in 7 months
	SLE and SLE-like	With class IV; partial remission reported with steroids, cyclophosphamide; 2 *APOL1* risk alleles increase odds 5.4x
Genetic		
	APOL1	Apolioprotein-1 variant alleles in blacks protect from trypanosomiasis but increase risk of CG, including idiopathic SLE- and IFN-related forms; expressed in podocytes
	COQ2	CoQ10 pathway; dysmorphic mitochondria in podocytes; onset < 2 years; ± CNS signs
	ZMPSTE24	Metalloproteinase cleaves prelamin A to mature lamin A; manifested systemically as mandibuloacral dysplasia
	SCARB2	Lysosomal protein; manifested as myoclonic epilepsy and renal failure
	TRPC6	Early onset CG in infants (6 months)
	SMARCAL1	Helicase; Schimke immuno-osseous dysplasia

Single case reports: Campylobacter, Loa loa, Epstein-Barr virus, HTLV-1, mixed connective tissue disorder, Guillain-Barré syndrome, giant cell arteritis, sickle cell anemia, valproic acid, and sirolimus. Abbreviations: CG = collapsing glomerulopathy; ESRD = end-stage renal disease; HCV = hepatitis C virus; IFN = interferon; SLE = systemic lupus erythematosus; TMA = thrombotic microangiopathy.

5. Kopp JB et al: APOL1 genetic variants in focal segmental glomerulosclerosis and HIV-associated nephropathy. J Am Soc Nephrol. 22(11):2129-37, 2011

(Left) *Minimal collapsing lesion is seen in 2 segments of this glomerulus, 1 with podocyte hypercellularity and 1 with adhesion or bridging to Bowman capsule.* **(Right)** *This Jones methenamine silver (JMS) stain illustrates areas of glomerular capillary loop collapse. The podocytes in the Bowman space resemble a crescent.*

Adhesion With Bridging Epithelial Cells

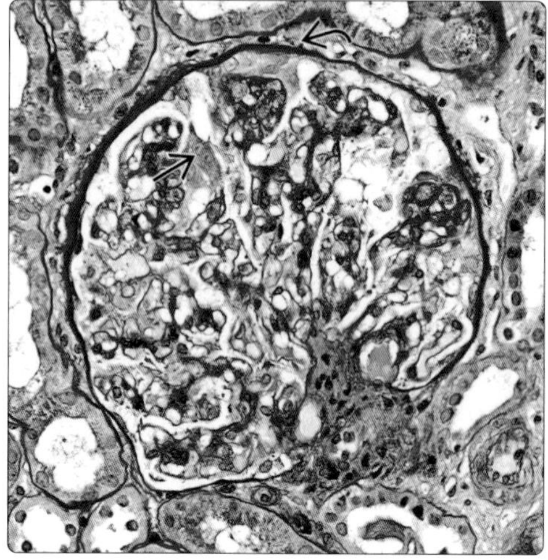

Pseudocrescent

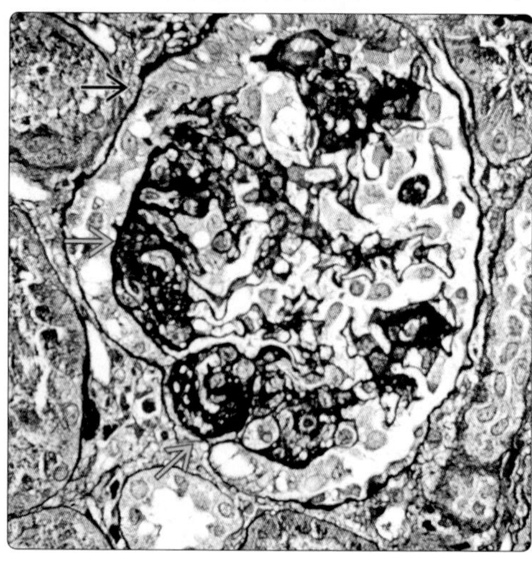

(Left) *Apoptosis in podocytes in a 29-year-old woman with new onset of nephrotic syndrome over 1 month due to idiopathic CG provides evidence of podocyte injury in the pathogenesis of collapsing glomerulopathy. (Courtesy I. Rosales, MD.)* **(Right)** *A glomerulus has undergone prominent collapse with overlying podocyte hypertrophy and marked dilatation of Bowman space.*

Apoptosis in Podocytes

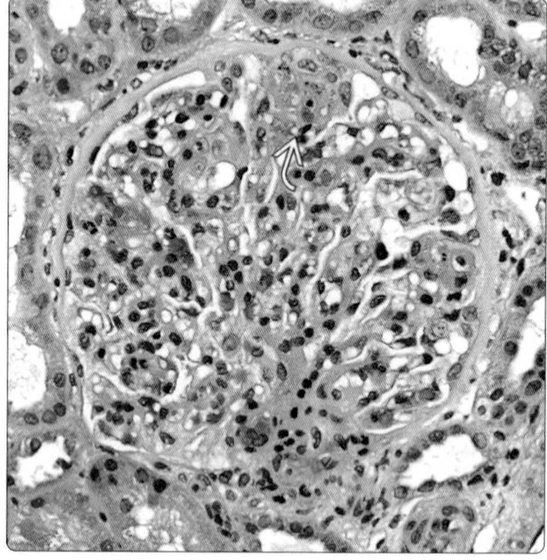

Bowman Space Dilatation and Glomerular Collapse

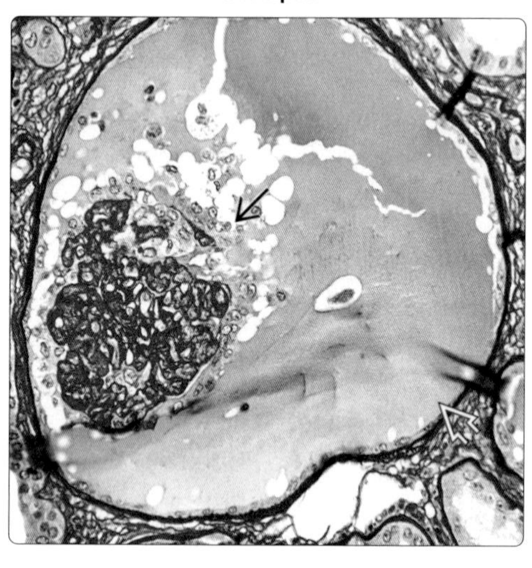

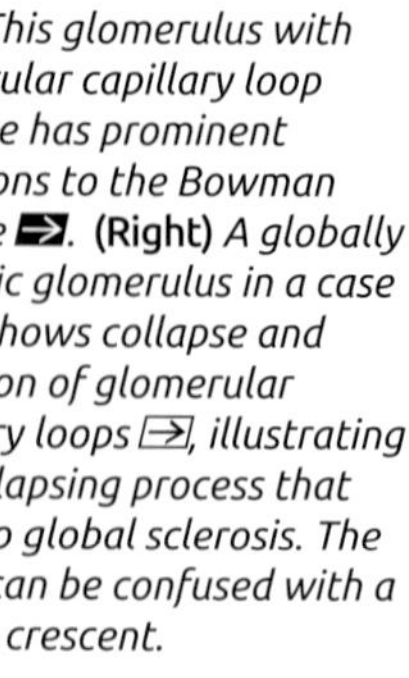

(Left) *This glomerulus with glomerular capillary loop collapse has prominent adhesions to the Bowman capsule.* **(Right)** *A globally sclerotic glomerulus in a case of CG shows collapse and occlusion of glomerular capillary loops, illustrating the collapsing process that leads to global sclerosis. The lesion can be confused with a fibrous crescent.*

Adhesion to Bowman Capsule

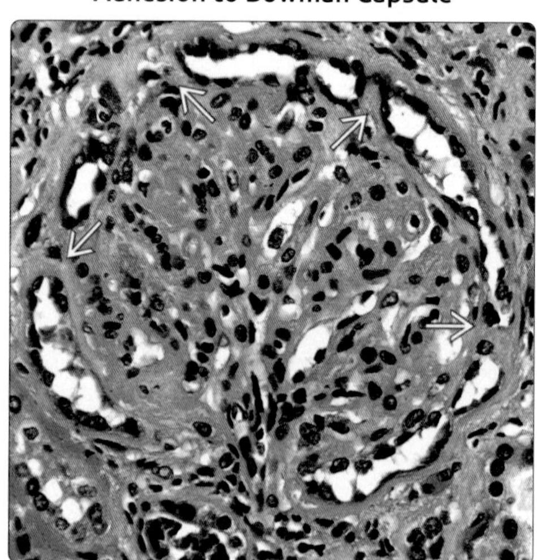

Global Glomerulosclerosis

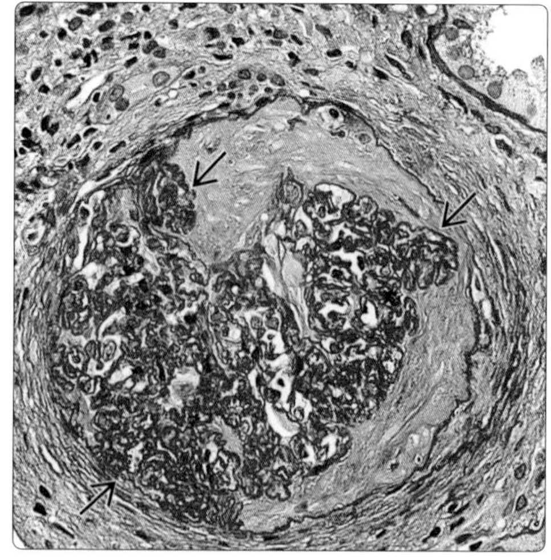

Bridging Epithelial Cells from Tuft to Capsule

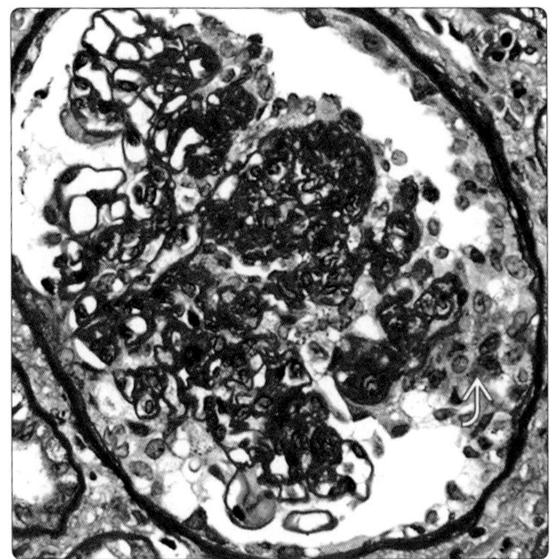

Mitosis

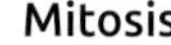

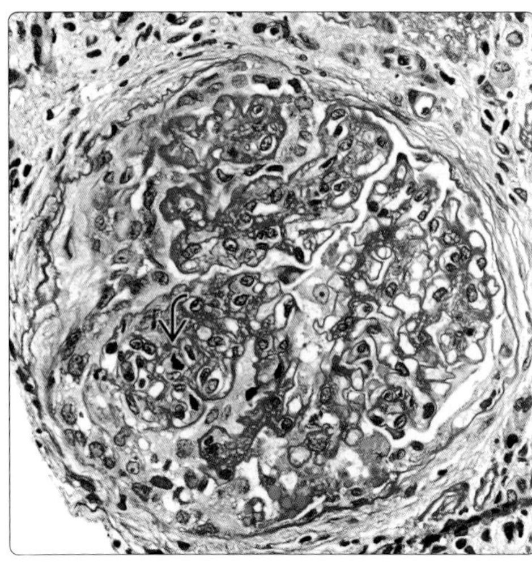

(Left) *Collapsing glomerulopathy with a pseudocrescent is shown. This glomerulus has podocytes that bridge → between the glomerular tuft and BC. These cells may actually arise from the podocyte progenitor cells that normally reside in the BC, which are repopulating the glomerular tuft.* **(Right)** *CG is present in a 74-year-old Caucasian man with nephrotic syndrome. Severe vascular disease was present and may have contributed. An unidentified cell (perhaps a podocyte) is in mitosis →.*

Segmental IgM

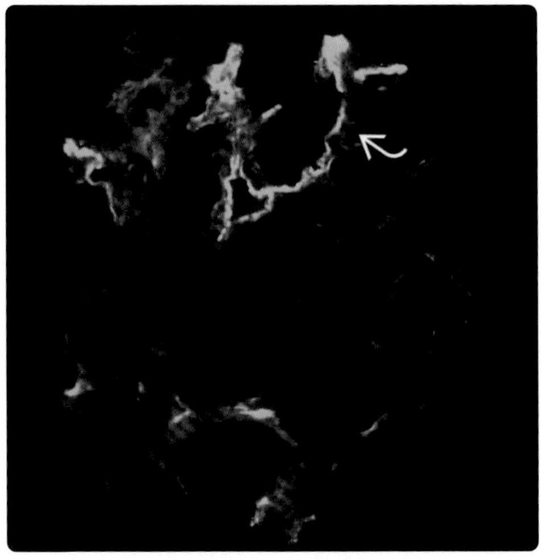

Segmental C3

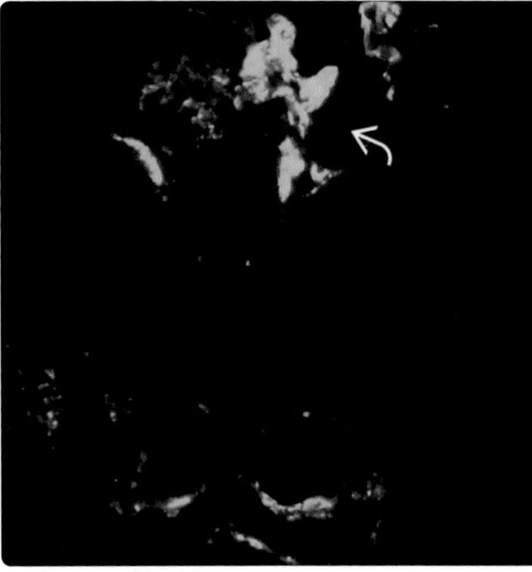

(Left) *Segmental IgM is commonly present in all forms of FSGS, including CG, as illustrated here →. While this is generally regarded as "nonspecific" trapping, there is some recent experimental evidence that IgM is necessary for development of FSGS.* **(Right)** *Segmental C3 → is commonly present in all variants of FSGS including the collapsing variant. Other immunoreactants are generally absent or minimally detected.*

Reabsorption Droplets in Visceral Epithelial Cells

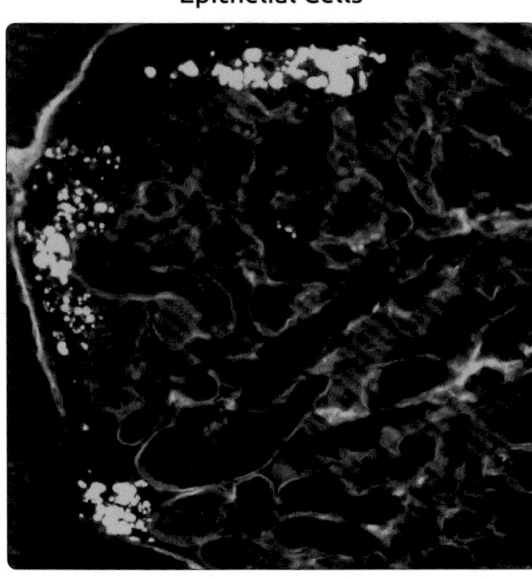

Large Reabsorption Droplets in Visceral Epithelium

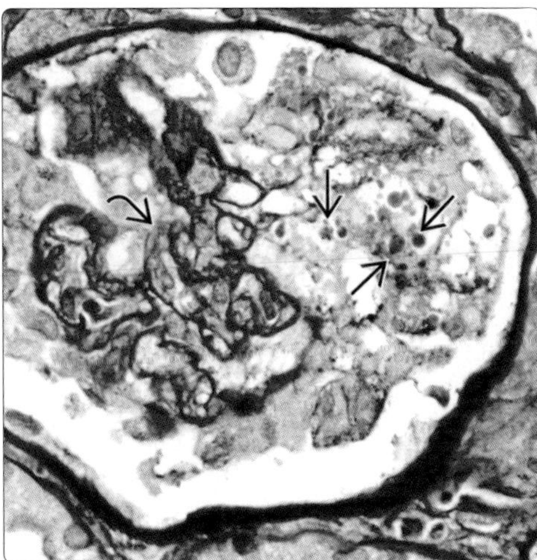

(Left) *Prominent, large protein reabsorption droplets are commonly present in CG. Immunoglobulin and complement components can also be present in these droplets and should not be mistaken for immune complexes.* **(Right)** *This collapsed glomerulus → has prominent podocyte proliferation with tubular reabsorption droplets evident in the podocytes →.*

(Left) *Wrinkled GBM leads to collapse of glomerular capillary loops. Podocytes are segmentally separated from the original GBM with multiple layers of newly formed GBM. Swollen reactive endothelial cells are also present.* (Right) *Podocytes are separated from the original GBM by multiple layers of newly formed matrix, indicating past podocyte injury and repair. The segmental process was first described in FSGS associated with heroin addiction.*

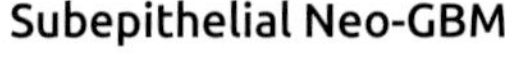

Subepithelial Neo-GBM

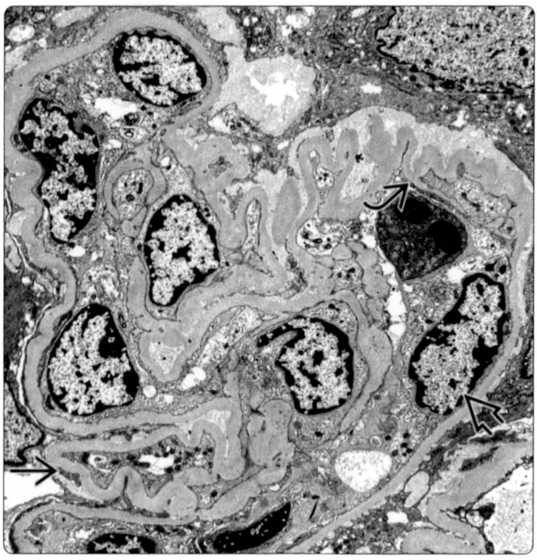

Newly Formed GBM Matrix

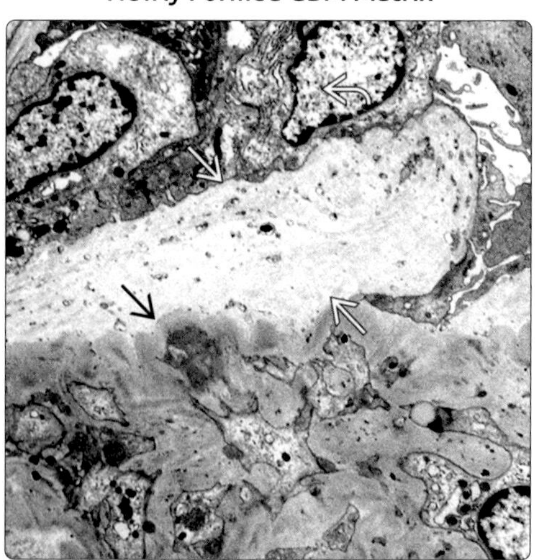

(Left) *Capillary loops are occluded in this CG, and podocytes are diffusely effaced. Endocapillary cells are swollen and reactive; however, this case did not have enough endocapillary cellularity to suggest the "cellular lesion."* (Right) *Prominent laminations on the outer aspect of the collapsed GBM are evident in this case of CG. Intracapillary foam cells were present, a feature more commonly associated with the cellular variant of FSGS.*

Occluded Capillary Loops

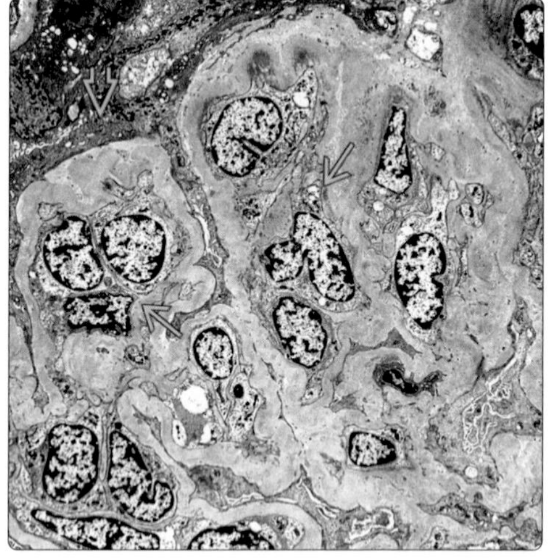

Intracapillary Foam Cells

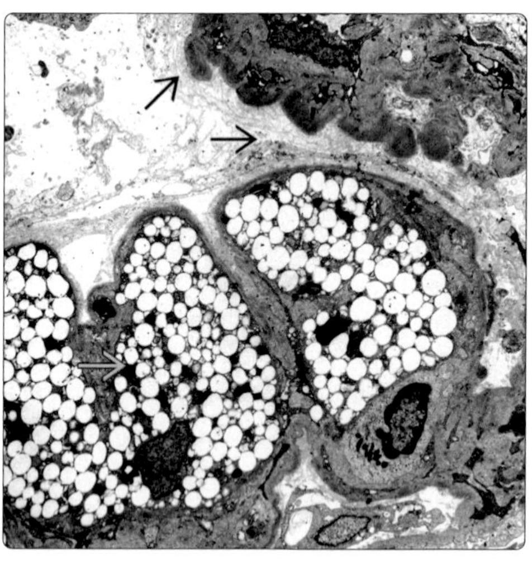

(Left) *This biopsy was taken from a 7-year-old boy with recurrent CG 2 days post transplant and shows widespread effacement of foot processes but no collapse, resembling minimal change disease.* (Right) *In a nephrectomy performed for intractable protein loss in a 9-year-old boy with recurrent CG 2 years after transplant, collapse of glomerular capillaries and prominent podocyte hypertrophy are shown with villous transformation. Recurrence began 2 days after transplant.*

Foot Process Effacement

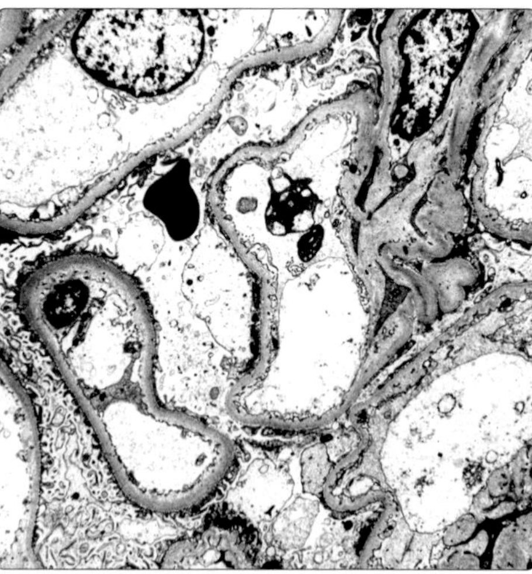

Recurrent CG With Glomerular Capillary Loop Collapse

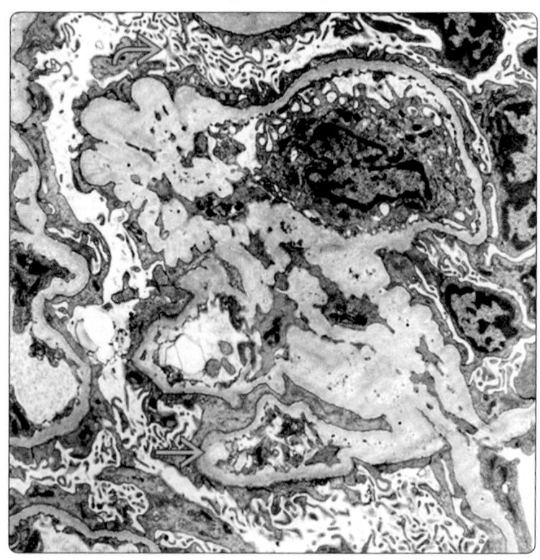

Tubular Dilatation

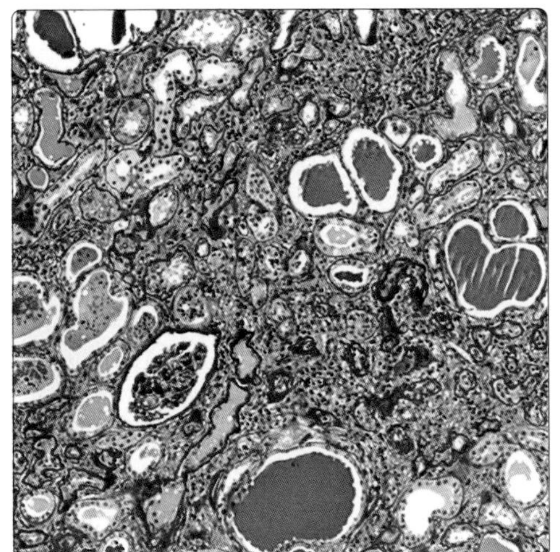

Ectatic Tubules With PAS(+) Casts

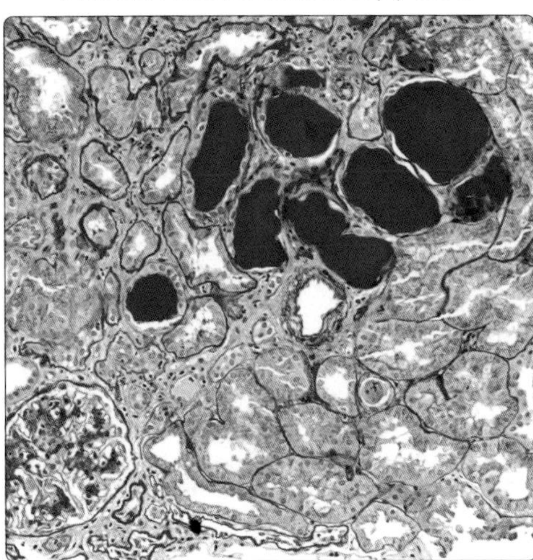

(Left) *CG is typically accompanied by tubulointerstitial disease, here shown at low power. Marked dilation of proximal tubules filled with PAS-positive protein is evident, as well as tubular atrophy and interstitial inflammation.* **(Right)** *Markedly dilated tubules distended with PAS(+) material are characteristic of CG of all causes. Tubular epithelial cells proliferate as well as glomerular epithelial cells.*

Interstitial Inflammation

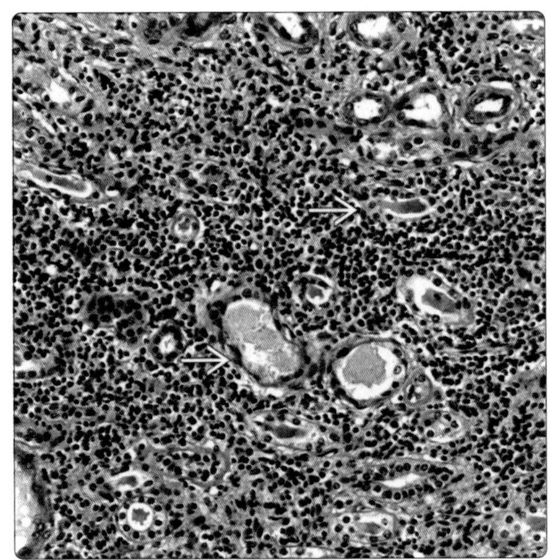

Interstitial Inflammation

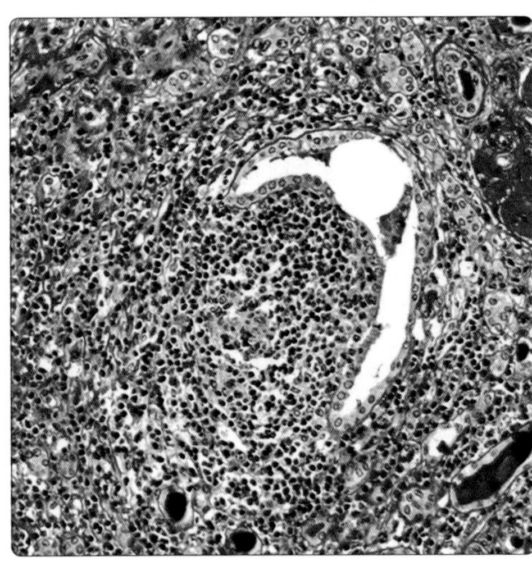

(Left) *There is prominent interstitial inflammation amidst these atrophic tubules, many of which have proteinaceous casts ➡.* **(Right)** *Lymphoid interstitial infiltrates are often prominent in CG and sometimes form lymphoepithelial structures with tubules, as shown here. The presence of tubulointerstitial disease indicates that CG is not exclusively a "podocytopathy."*

Sloughed Cells in Tubules

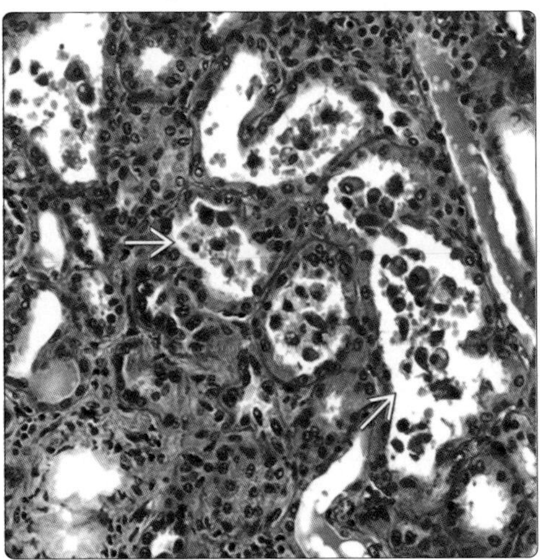

Lipid Accumulation

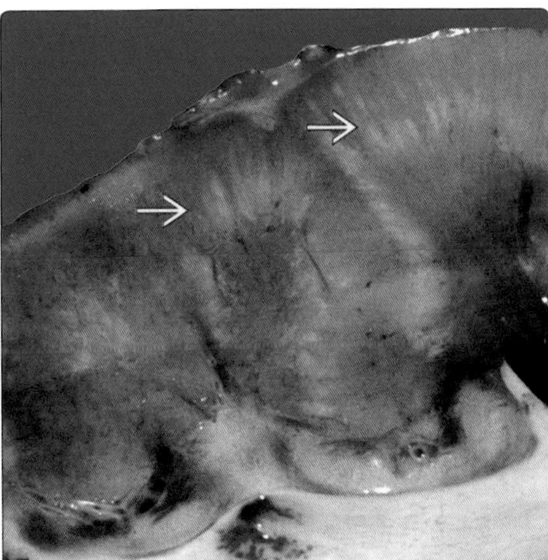

(Left) *The reactive tubular cells in CG are shed in the tubule, as shown here ➡. The sloughed cells may also include podocytes, which have been detected in the urine.* **(Right)** *This nephrectomy specimen from a 7-year-old boy with idiopathic CG was done in preparation for renal transplantation. Yellow areas at the corticomedullary junction ➡ are due to lipid in tubules.*

(Left) *De novo CG developed in the native kidneys of this patient 10 years post heart and lung transplant. Severe arteriolar hyalinosis was also present, related to cyclosporin therapy.* **(Right)** *IgA nephropathy can present with superimposed CG as in this case, which had mesangial IgA (3+) and electron dense deposits. The course is typically rapidly downhill with ESRD in 90%.*

De Novo CG Due to Calcineurin Inhibitor Therapy

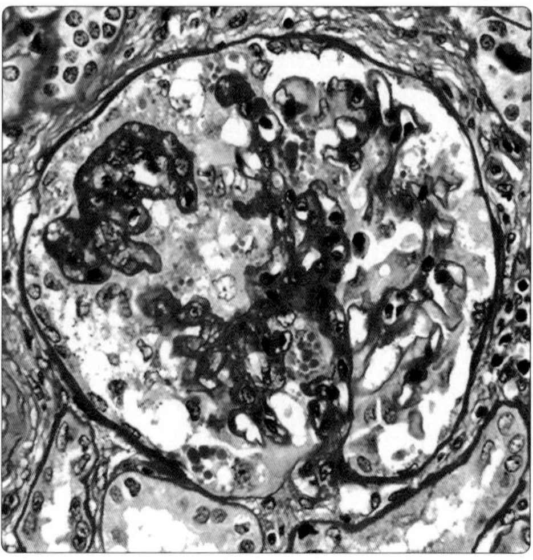

Collapsing Glomerulopathy Complicating IgA Nephropathy

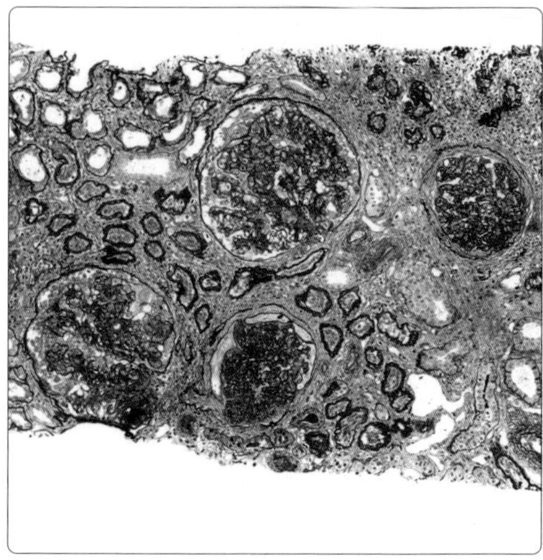

(Left) *A biopsy is depicted from a 28-year-old black woman who returned from South Africa with Plasmodium falciparum malaria and new onset of nephrotic syndrome. Blacks with certain APOL1 variants have a much greater risk of developing CG from other causes.* **(Right)** *Tubuloreticular inclusions ⇨ are present in endothelial cells in CG secondary to HIV infection; these are not often present in other causes of CG except those related to interferon therapy.*

CG Related to *P. falciparum* Malaria

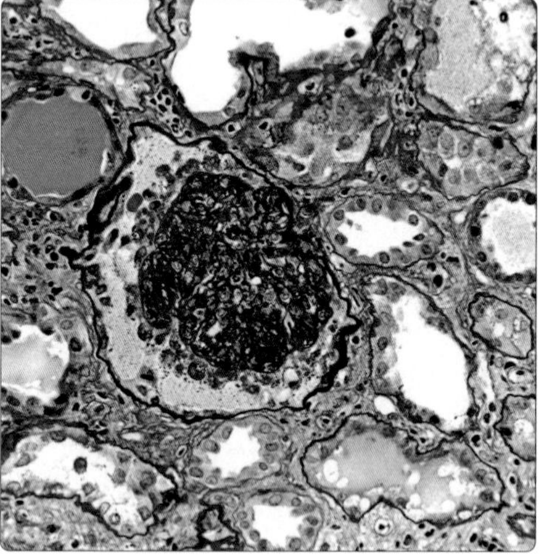

Tubuloreticular Inclusion in HIV

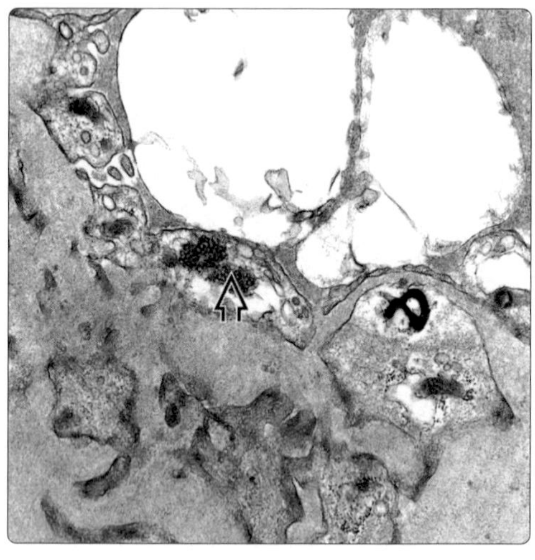

(Left) *CG is shown in a woman who developed nephrotic syndrome while on interferon-β for treatment of multiple sclerosis. Collapse and prominent podocyte hyperplasia are present. Intracapillary leukocytes are also present, a feature of the cellular variant of FSGS.* **(Right)** *In CG present in a woman on interferon-β for treatment of multiple sclerosis, numerous tubuloreticular structures → were present in the glomerular endothelium, an effect of interferon-α, -β, or -γ.*

CG Due to Interferon Therapy

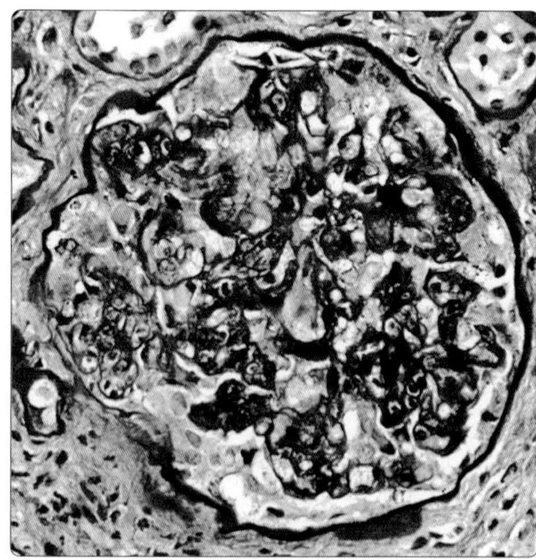

Tubuloreticular Structures Due to Interferon Therapy

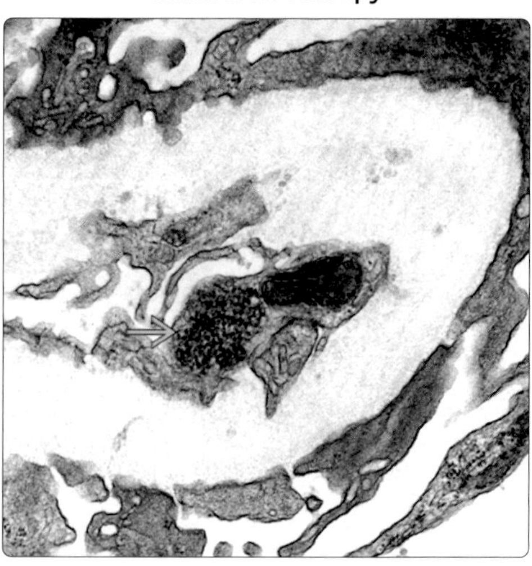

Ki-67 Highlights Proliferating Visceral and Parietal Epithelium

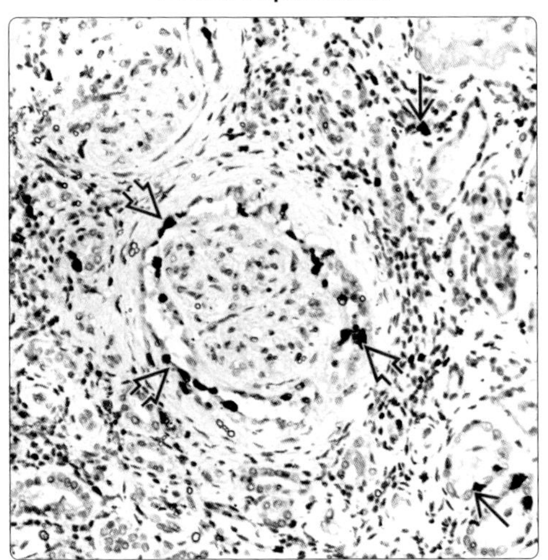

Ki-67(+) Tubular Epithelium

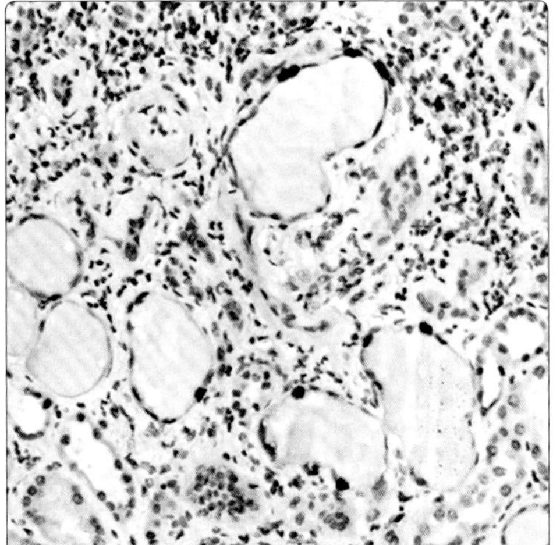

(Left) *Ki-67 immunohistochemistry highlights proliferating podocytes →. Occasional Ki-67(+) proliferating tubular epithelial cells → are also present, compatible with the tubular injury that can be seen in CG.* **(Right)** *Just as proliferation of podocytes occurs in CG, proliferation of proximal tubular cells also occurs, as shown here with a Ki-67 stain. This indicates that proliferation is a more generalized phenomenon in CG.*

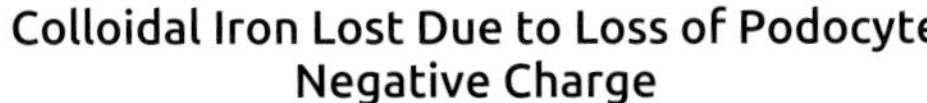

Colloidal Iron Lost Due to Loss of Podocyte Negative Charge

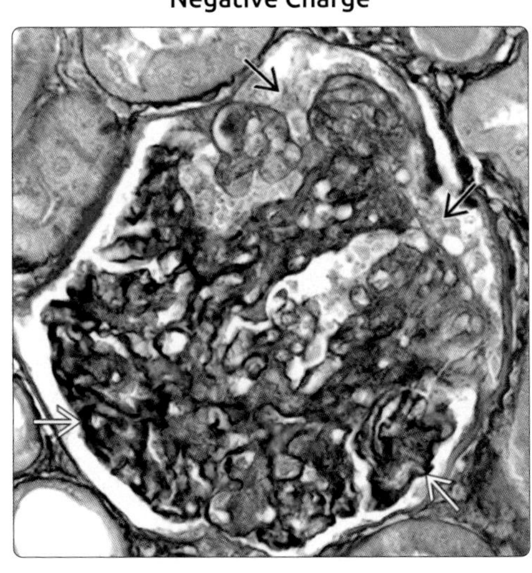

Visceral Epithelium Loses WT1 Expression

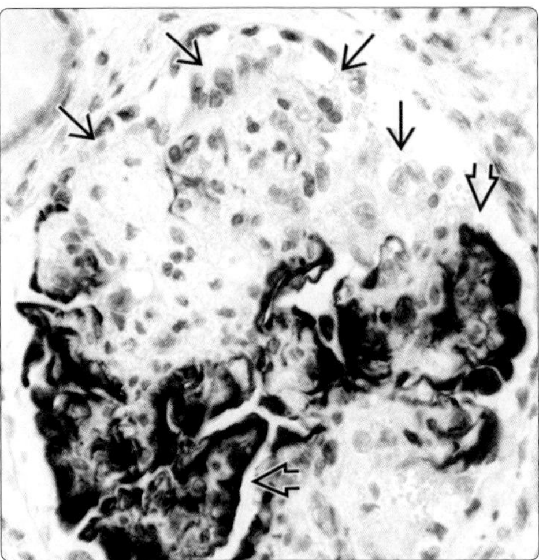

(Left) *Loss of the negative charge of the podocytes can be detected by loss of colloidal iron staining → as shown segmentally in this glomerulus. Normal staining is seen in 1/2 of the glomerulus →.* **(Right)** *WT1 stain of glomerulus in CG shows segmental loss of expression in podocytes, a sign of dedifferentiation →. The other 1/2 of the glomerulus stains normally for WT1 →. WT1 inhibits cell proliferation and is characteristically lost in CG.*

Ectopic Expression of CK8/18 in Visceral Epithelial Cells

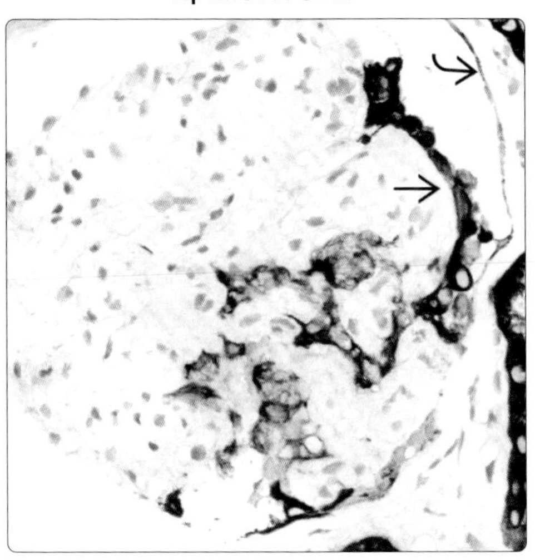

Ectopic Expression of CK19 in Visceral Epithelial Cells

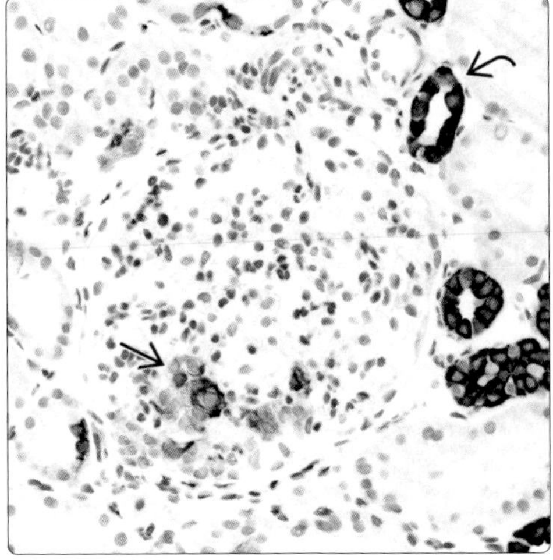

(Left) *CK8/18 shows ectoptic expression in visceral epithelial cells → in a patient with CG. This cytokeratin is normally expressed by parietal epithelial cells → but not podocytes. This is taken as evidence of podocyte dysregulation or more likely replacement of podocytes by the parietal epithelium.* **(Right)** *Ectopic expression of CK19 in visceral epithelial cells → is characteristic of CG. Podocytes do not normally express CK19, although distal tubules do →.*

Bisphosphonate-Induced Collapsing Glomerulopathy

KEY FACTS

TERMINOLOGY

- Collapsing focal segmental glomerulosclerosis (FSGS) secondary to use of pamidronate, bisphosphonate inhibitor of bone resorption
  - Can also occur from other bisphosphonates (e.g., alendronate and zoledronate)

ETIOLOGY/PATHOGENESIS

- Bisphosphonate binds calcium phosphate crystals within bone matrix, thus inhibiting osteoclast activity
- Pamidronate is thought to interfere with podocyte function and metabolism, similar to its metabolic effects on osteoclasts
- Renal excretion appears to be only by glomerular ultrafiltration
  - Tubular injury suggests that tubules can take up bisphosphonates, although, no tubular transport for bisphosphonates identified

CLINICAL ISSUES

- HIV-negative patients with nephrotic syndrome and severe renal insufficiency, typically older and white
- Treatment: Cessation of pamidronate
- Monitor serum creatinine and adjust dosage if renal insufficiency occurs

MICROSCOPIC

- Collapsing FSGS
- Hyperplastic and hypertrophic glomerular epithelial cells
- Tubular injury and simplification
- Increased Ki-67 positive cells in Bowman space
- IF: IgM and C3 segmentally stain glomerular tuft
- Electron microscopy
  - GBM wrinkling and collapse
  - Podocyte foot processes totally effaced

TOP DIFFERENTIAL DIAGNOSES

- Collapsing glomerulopathy of other causes

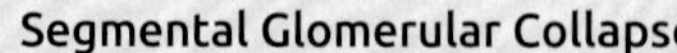

Segmental Glomerular Collapse

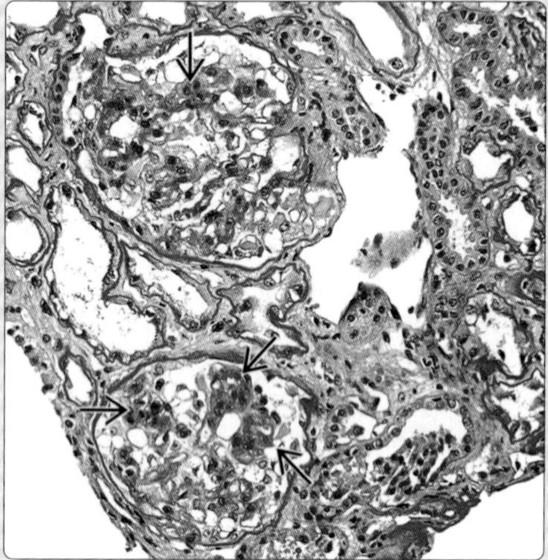

Segmental Podocyte Hypercellularity

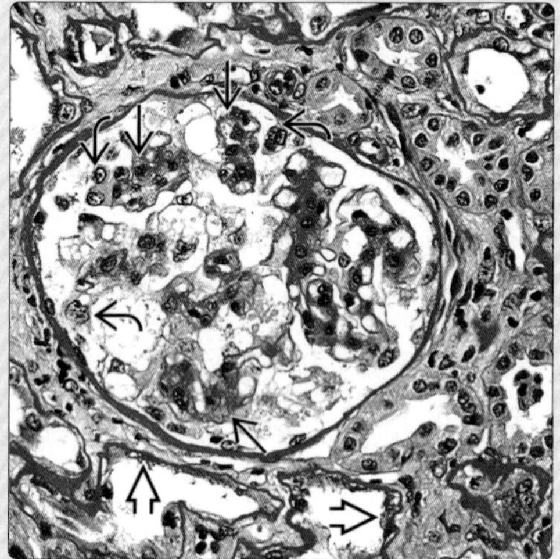

(Left) *Glomerular capillary loops show segmental occlusion and clustering of podocytes. Biopsy is from a 67-year-old woman with multiple myeloma who received pamidronate and developed 50 g/d proteinuria requiring hemodialysis.* **(Right)** *Glomerular capillary loops show segmental collapse with overlying podocyte hypercellularity. Tubular injury can be observed with flattening of the tubular epithelium.*

Podocyte Foot Process Effacement

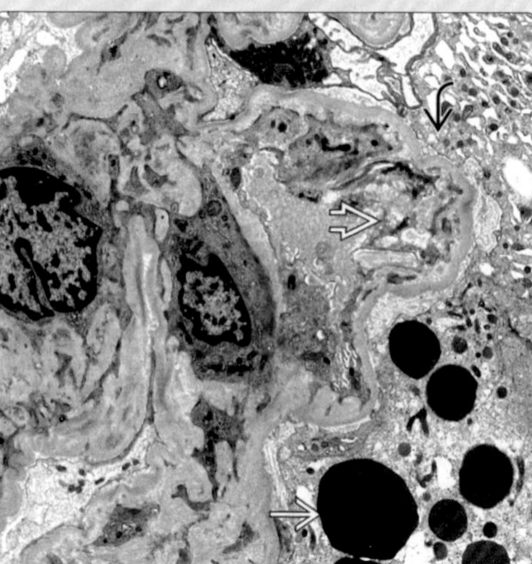

Subepithelial Duplication of the GBM

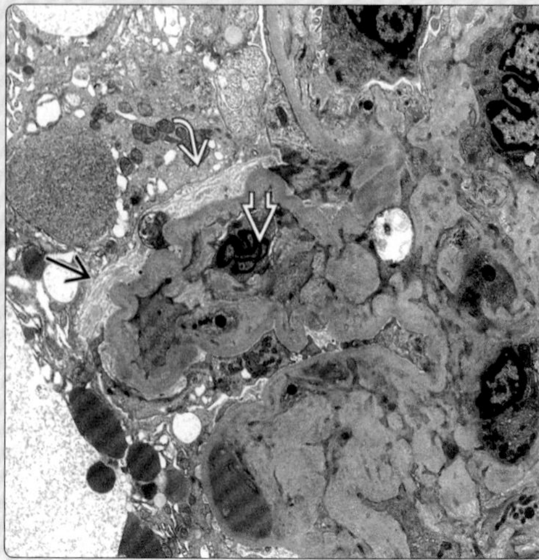

(Left) *EM shows extensive foot process effacement, glomerular capillary loop collapse, and resorption droplets within podocytes.* **(Right)** *EM shows subepithelial layers of glomerular basement membrane (GBM) probably due to repeated podocyte injury and repair. There is extensive foot process effacement, and glomerular capillary loops show nearly complete collapse.*

TERMINOLOGY

Abbreviations

- Focal segmental glomerulosclerosis (FSGS)

Definitions

- Collapsing FSGS secondary to bisphosphonates, such as pamidronate (Aredia), used in treatment of osteolytic metastases, Paget disease, hypercalcemia of malignancy, and postmenopausal osteoporosis (PMO)

ETIOLOGY/PATHOGENESIS

Pamidronate Exposure

- Renal glomerular toxicity depends on dose and route
  - Patients typically used higher than recommended doses
  - Intravenous route of administration implicated
    - Oral bisphosphonates do not produce significant nephrotoxicity
  - Rare case with single dose in patient of African descent
    - *APOL1* alleles may be risk factor (not yet reported)
- Zoledronate appears to mainly be associated with tubular injury, in contrast to pamidronate
- Ibandronate not reported to produce renal toxicity
- Protein excretion may increase when drug is restarted

Mechanism of Podocyte Toxicity Unknown

- Bisphosphonates binds calcium phosphate crystals within bone matrix, thus inhibiting osteoclast activity
- Podocyte and tubular mitochondrial injury may contribute
- Injured podocytes fall off glomerular basement membrane (GBM) and are replaced by parietal epithelium
  - Evidenced by loss of podocyte synaptopodin and increased Ki-67 expression

CLINICAL ISSUES

Presentation

- Initial description by Markowitz et al was in older, white, HIV-negative patients
  - Cohort consisted of 5 women and 2 men, 6 with multiple myeloma and 1 with breast cancer with mean serum creatinine of 3.6 mg/dL and mean urine protein of 12.4 g/d
  - Collapsing FSGS otherwise more common in blacks
- Nephrotic syndrome
- Renal dysfunction/severe renal insufficiency
- Fanconi syndrome

Treatment

- Cessation of pamidronate use
- Prevented by monitoring serum creatinine and adjusting dosage if renal insufficiency is present

Prognosis

- Renal function improves with drug discontinuance in ~ 50%
- End-stage renal disease (ESRD) reported in ~ 35%

MICROSCOPIC

Histologic Features

- Glomeruli
  - Collapsing or noncollapsing FSGS
    - Hyperplastic and hypertrophic visceral epithelial cells (podocytes)
    - Global wrinkling and retraction of GBM
    - Swollen and contain protein resorption droplets
    - Increased Ki-67(+) cells in Bowman space
  - Minimal change disease has also been described
- Tubules
  - Tubular injury and simplification, attributable to toxic acute tubular necrosis
    - Regenerative nuclear atypia
    - No tubulitis
  - Tubular microcyst formation
- Interstitium
  - Edema
  - Inflammation is only sparse, without eosinophils
  - Fibrosis eventually occurs
- Vessels
  - No specific changes

ANCILLARY TESTS

Immunofluorescence

- Segmental IgM and C3 in glomeruli

Electron Microscopy

- Global GBM wrinkling and collapse of glomerular capillaries
- Podocyte foot processes totally effaced
- Podocyte hypertrophy

DIFFERENTIAL DIAGNOSIS

Collapsing Glomerulopathy of Other Causes

- Careful history is needed since there is no distinguishing feature

DIAGNOSTIC CHECKLIST

Pathologic Interpretation Pearls

- Collapsing FSGS has many specific causes, and etiologic diagnosis should be sought

SELECTED REFERENCES

1. Neyra JA et al: Collapsing focal segmental glomerulosclerosis resulting from a single dose of zoledronate. Nephron Extra. 4(3):168-74, 2014
2. Hirschberg R: Renal complications from bisphosphonate treatment. Curr Opin Support Palliat Care. 6(3):342-7, 2012
3. ten Dam MA et al: Nephrotic syndrome induced by pamidronate. Med Oncol. 28(4):1196-200, 2011
4. Perazella MA et al: Bisphosphonate nephrotoxicity. Kidney Int. 74(11):1385-93, 2008
5. Dijkman HB et al: Proliferating cells in HIV and pamidronate-associated collapsing focal segmental glomerulosclerosis are parietal epithelial cells. Kidney Int. 70(2):338-44, 2006
6. Markowitz GS et al: Collapsing focal segmental glomerulosclerosis following treatment with high-dose pamidronate. J Am Soc Nephrol. 12(6):1164-72, 2001

Causes of Membranous Glomerulonephritis

Cause	Distinctive Pathologic Features	Comments	Outcome	PLA2R*
Autoimmune Disease				
Autoantibodies to phospholipase A2 receptor (PLA2R)	PLA2R in deposits; IgG4 usually present	Most common form of primary MGN (~ 80%); PLA2R antibodies correlate with activity and outcome	30-40% develop ESRD; recurs in transplants	> 90% circulating antibody, some have only PLA2R in deposits
Autoantibodies to thrombospondin type-1 domain-containing 7A (THSD7A)	THSD7A and IgG4 in deposits	2nd most common antigen in primary MGN (~10%)		0% (0/15)
Systemic lupus erythematosus	96% mesangial deposits, 32% TBM deposits; 67% intense C1q; IgG3	May be 1st manifestation of SLE	Variable response to immunosuppression	1.4% (1/68)
Rheumatoid arthritis		~ 25% occur without drug therapy	Remission with steroids or with infliximab	
Mixed connective tissue disease	all IgG3- (vs. SLE)	Anti-U1-RNP		0% (0/2)
IgG4-related systemic disease	56% had tubulointerstitial nephritis	Extrarenal disease ~ 80%; antigen unknown	6/6 improved with immunosuppression	0% (0/8)
Sjögren syndrome		rare; 1 had EBV+ lymphoma		16% (1/6)
ANCA Disease	Crescents, MPO in deposits; IgG4- (60%)	1-3% of ANCA cases	25% ESRD; 50% Cr <2.0	16% (1/6)
Anti-GBM Disease	100% crescents; 75% stage I; 100% IgG4-; linear IgG sometimes discernible		~ 50% 2-year renal survival; vs. anti-GBM alone (10%)	0% (0/8)
Sarcoidosis	Granulomatous interstitial nephritis ~ 20%	42% of patients with sarcoidosis and glomerular disease; precedes sarcoid diagnosis in ~ 45%; PLA2R antibodies correlate with sarcoid activity	Remission reported with steroids	64% (6/6) with active disease
Alloimmune Response				
Kidney allograft	Associated with chronic antibody mediated rejection	Late complication; antigen unknown		0% (0/17)
Hematopoietic cell transplantation	Associated with graft-vs.-host disease	Antigen unknown		0%
Neutral endopeptidase	Neutral endopeptidase in deposits; annular deposits by EM	Infants born to mothers with genetic absence of neutral endopeptidase	IgG1 antibodies more severe disease than IgG4	0%
α-glucosidase	α-glucosidase in deposits; mesangial deposits	Recombinant α-glucosidase for Pompe disease	Resolved with decreased drug	
Aryl sulfatase	Aryl sulfatase B in deposits	Recombinant aryl sulfatase B for mucopolysaccharidosis type VI	Remission while continuing drug after immunosuppressive therapy	0% (0/1)
Exogenous Antigen				
Bovine milk	IgG1, IgG4, bovine serum albumin (BSA) in deposits	Young children with cationic BSA in blood and anti-BSA antibodies; no other evidence of milk allergy	Complete remission in 75% with prednisone and or cyclosporine	0% (0/4)
Infection				
Hepatitis B virus	HBeAg, HBcAg, or HBsAg in deposits; C1q+ in 55%; subendothelial &/or mesangial deposits	Common cause of MGN in children prior to vaccination era (40-90%)	Prevented by HBV vaccination; remission with antiviral therapy (lamiduvir, entecavir)	11% (4/37)
Hepatitis C virus	individual cases with IgG1λ or IgA1λ; virus-like particles		Remission reported with interferon-alpha or	65% (7/11)

Causes of Membranous Glomerulonephritis (Continued)

Cause	Distinctive Pathologic Features	Comments	Outcome	PLA2R*
	within deposits		rituximab	
Syphilis	Treponemal antigen reported in deposits; stage I often	Congenital or adult	Histologic remission in 6 months with penicillin	0% (0/2)
HIV		May be HBV or syphilis coinfection	Remission with HAART reported	0% (0/1)
Epstein-Barr virus			Remission with clearance of viremia	
Drugs (Antigen Unknown)				
Nonsteroidal anti-inflammatory drugs	Often stage I	~ 10% of early MGN; ampiroxicam, celecoxib,diclofenac, etodolac, fenoprofen, ibuprofen, nabumetone, naproxen, oxaprozin, piroxicam, tolmetin	Remission on drug withdrawal; recurrence with rechallenge	Unknown (1/1+)
Penicillamine	± mesangial deposits, can have crescents	Rheumatoid arthritis, scleroderma; Wilson disease thiol group; (60% with crescents ANCA+)	Remission with drug withdrawal ± immunosuppression	
Bucillamine	Can have crescents (ANCA-)	Rheumatoid arthritis, thiol group similar to penicillamine	Stabilized off drug	
Gold	± mesangial deposits	thiol group		
Etanercept and adalimumab		Anti-TNF agents in rheumatoid arthritis and ankylosing spondylitis	Remission with drug withdrawal ± rituximab	
Lithium	With tubulointerstitial disease	Children and adults	Remission off lithium	
Mercury	IgG1 dominant; 50% mesangial deposits; ~ 30% tubulointerstitial nephritis	Skin creams, hair dye, vapor, i.v., Chinese "pills"	90% remission after drug withdrawal	
Captopril		0.5-1% of patients on drug; thiol group; causal role debated	Proteinuria remits on drug withdrawal	
Mercaptopropionyl glycine		Therapy for cystinuria and rheumatoid arthritis (Tiopronin); thiol group	Remission with drug withdrawal	
Malignant Neoplasm				
Carcinoma, lymphoma, leukemia, melanoma	Carcinoembryonic antigen reported in deposits in a few cases	~ 10% of MGN patients have cancer, 26% lung; 15% prostate; 14% hematopoietic (lymphoma, CLL), colorectal, breast, stomach, esophagus, kidney, cervix/uterus et al	Remission of nephrotic syndrome after tumor excision reported in many cases	22% (6/22)

Individual case reports with other viruses (e.g., cytomegalovirus, hepatitis E virus), other autoimmune diseases (Hashimoto thyroiditis, Churg-Strauss syndrome, Kimura disease, C3Nef), other neoplasms, various drugs (fluconazole, bevacizumab, pegylated interferon alpha-2a, anti-seizure drugs), iron overload, sickle cell trait, neurofibromatosis; causal association with MGN not proved. blank field indicates no relevant information available.

* Serum antibody or PLA2R localization in deposits. General review: Debiec H et al: Immunopathogenesis of membranous nephropathy: an update. Semin Immunopathol. 36:381-97, 2014; complete references in Secondary Membranous Glomerulonephritis chapter.

Membranous Glomerulonephritis, Primary

KEY FACTS

TERMINOLOGY

- Autoimmune glomerular disease characterized by diffuse subepithelial immune complex deposition with nephrotic-range proteinuria, without known systemic cause

ETIOLOGY/PATHOGENESIS

- Autoantibodies to PLA2R1 on podocyte (70-80%)
- Autoantibodies to thrombospondin type-1 domain-containing 7A (~ 5%)
- Rare congenital MGN due to MME antibodies

CLINICAL ISSUES

- Nephrotic syndrome
- Insidious onset, ~ 33% progress to end-stage renal disease
- Peak age: 30-50 years

MICROSCOPIC

- Diffuse thickening of glomerular capillary wall
- Subepithelial "spikes" in PAS and Jones methenamine silver stains
- Immunofluorescence
  - Diffuse granular deposits along GBM that stain for IgG, usually C3
  - IgG4 usually dominant subclass
- Electron microscopy
  - Subepithelial amorphous deposits
  - Intervening "spikes" of GBM
  - Deposits resurfaced by GBM and resorbed
  - Staging based on status of deposits

TOP DIFFERENTIAL DIAGNOSES

- Lupus glomerulonephritis, class 5
- Secondary MGN due to drugs, infection, and other causes
- Postinfectious glomerulonephritis

DIAGNOSTIC CHECKLIST

- Adverse pathologic prognostic features include interstitial fibrosis and tubular atrophy, FSGS, arteriosclerosis, and mixed-stage deposits

GBM Alterations

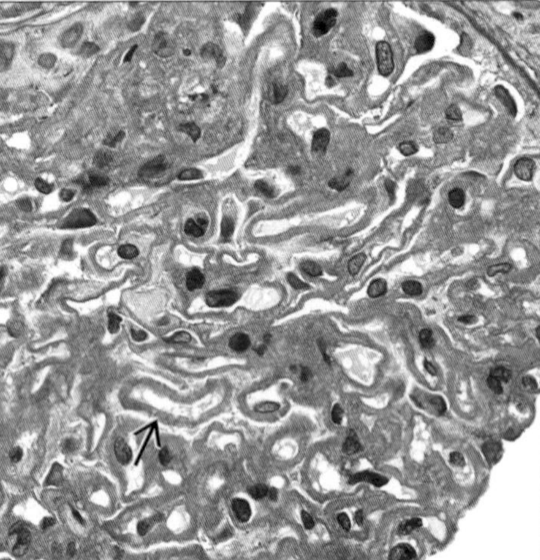

Subepithelial "Spikes"

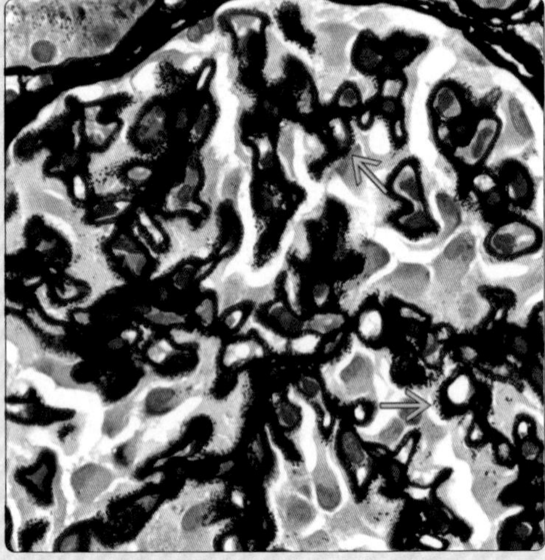

(Left) *Periodic acid-Schiff shows prominent thickening of the GBM with a hint of a vacuolated appearance → that is not as distinct when compared with the Jones methenamine silver stain.* **(Right)** *Jones methenamine silver reveals a "hair on end" pattern of subepithelial "spikes" of GBM in most capillaries →, best appreciated on well-stained 2-3 μm silver or PAS stains under 100x oil.*

IgG

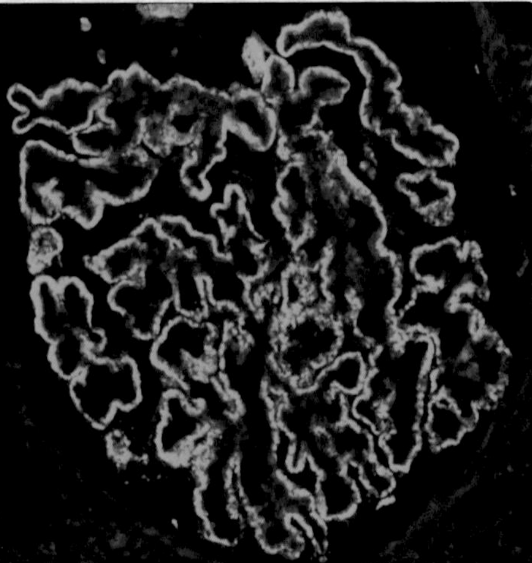

Subepithelial Deposits and GBM "Spikes"

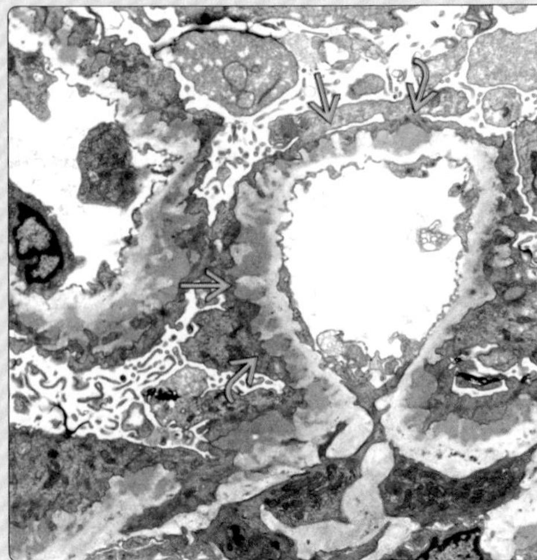

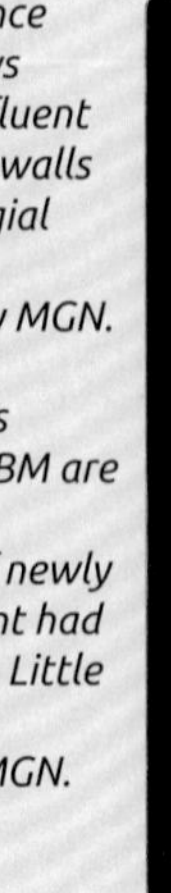

(Left) *Immunofluorescence microscopy for IgG shows intense granular to confluent staining of the capillary walls without definite mesangial staining, which is characteristic of primary MGN.* **(Right)** *Widespread subepithelial amorphous deposits → along the GBM are typical of MGN, with intervening spikes → of newly formed GBM. This patient had anti-PLA2R1 antibodies. Little or no deposits are in the mesangium in primary MGN.*

TERMINOLOGY

Abbreviations

- Membranous glomerulonephritis (MGN)

Synonyms

- Membranous nephropathy
- Membranous glomerulopathy

Definitions

- Autoimmune glomerular disease characterized by diffuse subepithelial immune complex deposition with nephrotic-range proteinuria, without known systemic cause

ETIOLOGY/PATHOGENESIS

Autoimmune Disease With In Situ Glomerular Immune Complex Formation

- 5 autoantigens identified
  - Phospholipase A2 receptor 1 (PLA2R1)
    - Expressed on podocytes and proximal tubules
      - Dominant epitope in N-terminal cysteine-rich ricin domain
    - IgG4 anti-PLA2R1 detected in ~ 70% of primary MGN
      - Colocalized with IgG4 in glomeruli
    - Proteinuria can persist for months after autoantibodies undetectable
  - Thrombospondin type 1 domain-containing 7A
    - Detected in 2.5-5% of primary MGN
    - Similar biochemical properties to PLA2R1
  - Membrane metalloendopeptidase (MME), a.k.a. neutral endopeptidase or CD10
    - Expressed on human podocytes and proximal tubular brush borders
    - Rare neonatal form of MGN in mothers with absent MME
      - Negligible role in adult MGN
    - Maternal anti-MME antibodies cross placenta and deposit on fetal podocytes
    - 1st human antigenic target of MGN identified
      - Subsequently, other families reported
  - Aldose reductase (AR) and manganese superoxide dismutase 2 (SOD2)
    - Expressed in tubular epithelial cells, **not** glomeruli
    - May be upregulated on podocytes in primary MGN
      - IgG4 recognizes these antigens & colocalizes to subepithelial deposits of MGN
- Antigenic target(s) in secondary forms different from PLA2R1 but not yet identified

Genetic Factors

- 2 strongly linked loci in genome-wide association studies
  - HLA-DQA1 allele
  - PLA2R allele
- May facilitate presentation of autoantigen

CLINICAL ISSUES

Epidemiology

- Incidence
  - 6-10% of native adult biopsies
  - ~ 3% in children (< 18 years old)
- Age
  - Peak: 30-50 years
- Sex
  - M:F ratio = 2:1
- Ethnicity
  - Caucasian predilection

Presentation

- Nephrotic syndrome
- Proteinuria, asymptomatic
- Hematuria
  - Usually microscopic, rarely gross hematuria
- Renal vein thrombosis

Laboratory Tests

- Anti-PLA2R1 autoantibodies
  - Used for diagnosis, monitoring therapeutic response, and predicting recurrence

Treatment

- Drugs
  - Variety used with limited success
    - Prednisone, mycophenolate mofetil, rituximab, cyclophosphamide, chlorambucil

Prognosis

- 50% 10-year renal survival (90% in Japan)
- 33% spontaneously remit
- 33% stable with proteinuria with little progression
- 33% progress to end-stage renal disease (ESRD)
  - 10-30% recur after kidney transplantation
    - 1 week to many years
    - Graft loss in 10-50% of recurrent MGN
  - Adverse clinical prognostic features: Nephrotic syndrome, azotemia, hypertension

MICROSCOPIC

Histologic Features

- Glomerulus
  - Appear normal when only stage 1 deposits seen by EM
  - Glomerular basement membrane (GBM) thickened on H&E
    - Subepithelial "spike" formation or vacuolated appearance (when sectioned en face) on PAS or Jones silver stain
  - Little or no increase in mesangial hypercellularity
  - Glomerulosclerosis
    - Segmental
    - Global
  - No inflammatory infiltrate in glomerulus
    - Presence of leukocytes suggests renal vein thrombosis or other mechanisms superimposed (anti-GBM, antineutrophil cytoplasmic antibody [ANCA])
      - > 8 neutrophils per glomerulus reported in MGN associated with cancer
  - Crescents (rare in absence of positive ANCA or anti-GBM titer)
- Tubules
  - Protein resorption droplets
- Interstitium
  - Foam cells variably present

- Interstitial fibrosis and tubular atrophy in later stages
- Vessels
  - Arteriosclerosis common

Variants

- MGN and anti-GBM disease (rare)
  - Crescentic glomerular injury often diffuse
    - Linear IgG staining of GBM along with granular staining of capillary walls
    - Positive anti-GBM antibody titer
- MGN and antineutrophil cytoplasmic antibody (ANCA) disease (rare)
  - Necrotizing glomerular lesions with crescents
  - Positive ANCA titer
- MGN and anti-tubular basement membrane (TBM) disease (rare)
  - Linear IgG staining of tubular basement membranes and prominent interstitial inflammation
  - Typically < 5 years of age

ANCILLARY TESTS

Immunohistochemistry

- PLA2R1
  - Positive in 70% of primary MGN

Immunofluorescence

- Diffuse, granular deposits along GBM
  - Stain for IgG, kappa and lambda light chains ± complement components
    - IgA and IgM usually not prominent
  - IgG4 dominant subclass
  - Global (> 50% of single glomerulus) involvement of capillary walls typical
    - Segmental involvement suggestive of secondary MGN
  - Extent of complement deposition may correlate with renal function deterioration
- Little or no mesangial deposits
  - Tangential sections of GBM may be hard to distinguish from mesangial deposits
- No TBM immunoglobulin deposits

Electron Microscopy

- 4 stages described by Ehrenreich and Churg
  - 1: Subepithelial deposits without significant basement membrane reaction between deposits
  - 2: Subepithelial deposits with basement membrane material ("spikes") between deposits
  - 3: Subepithelial (or intramembranous) deposits with basement membrane material between and surrounding deposits
  - 4: Electron-lucent areas represent probable resorption of prior subepithelial immune complexes
- Location
  - Strictly subepithelial (and later, intramembranous)
  - Bowman capsular deposits, rare
  - Mesangial deposits suggest secondary forms (e.g., hepatitis C-associated MGN)
    - Few deposits can be observed in PLA2R-positive MGN
  - Subendothelial or TBM deposits generally suggest secondary MGN (e.g., lupus nephritis)
- Substructure
  - Usually amorphous
  - Microspherular substructural organization reported in primary MGN
    - Neonatal MGN due to *MME* mutation shows microspherular substructure in subepithelial deposits

DIFFERENTIAL DIAGNOSIS

Membranous Glomerulonephritis, Secondary

- Requires clinical correlation
- Mesangial deposits often present
- PLA2R(+) deposits in < 10% (depends on cause)

Postinfectious Glomerulonephritis

- Lack of "spikes" around "humps"
- Segmental distribution of subepithelial deposits
- Deposits in mesangium and subendothelial space
- Intraglomerular inflammation and hypercellularity
  - Neutrophils may be present in MGN associated with malignancy or renal vein thrombosis

Membranous Lupus Nephritis

- Favored by mesangial deposits, full-house IF (IgG, IgA, IgM, C3, C1q), tubuloreticular structures, and TBM deposits
- Deposits sometimes penetrate GBM and associate with subendothelial deposits

DIAGNOSTIC CHECKLIST

Clinically Relevant Pathologic Features

- Adverse prognostic features
  - Interstitial fibrosis and tubular atrophy
  - Focal segmental glomerulosclerosis (FSGS)
  - Arteriosclerosis
  - Heterogeneous (multistage) deposits
- Extent and stage of deposits not consistently correlated with outcome

Pathologic Interpretation Pearls

- MGN can occur concurrently with many renal diseases, such as diabetic nephropathy or crescentic GN

SELECTED REFERENCES

1. Fresquet M et al: Identification of a major epitope recognized by PLA2R autoantibodies in primary membranous nephropathy. J Am Soc Nephrol. 26(2):302-13, 2015
2. Kao L et al: Identification of the immunodominant epitope region in phospholipase A2 receptor-mediating autoantibody binding in idiopathic membranous nephropathy. J Am Soc Nephrol. 26(2):291-301, 2015
3. Kattah A et al: Anti-Phospholipase A_2 Receptor Antibodies in Recurrent Membranous Nephropathy. Am J Transplant. ePub, 2015
4. Quintana LF et al: Antiphospholipase A2 Receptor Antibody Levels Predict the Risk of Posttransplantation Recurrence of Membranous Nephropathy. Transplantation. ePub, 2015
5. Rodriguez EF et al: Membranous nephropathy with crescents: a series of 19 cases. Am J Kidney Dis. 64(1):66-73, 2014
6. Tomas NM et al: Thrombospondin type-1 domain-containing 7A in idiopathic membranous nephropathy. N Engl J Med. ePub, 2014
7. Huang CC et al: IgG subclass staining in renal biopsies with membranous glomerulonephritis indicates subclass switch during disease progression. Mod Pathol. 26(6):799-805, 2013
8. Larsen CP et al: Determination of primary versus secondary membranous glomerulopathy utilizing phospholipase A2 receptor staining in renal biopsies. Mod Pathol. 26(5):709-15, 2013
9. Beck LH Jr et al: M-type phospholipase A2 receptor as target antigen in idiopathic membranous nephropathy. N Engl J Med. 361(1):11-21, 2009
10. Debiec H et al: Antenatal membranous glomerulonephritis due to anti-neutral endopeptidase antibodies. N Engl J Med. 346(26):2053-60, 2002

Mild Mesangial Hypercellularity

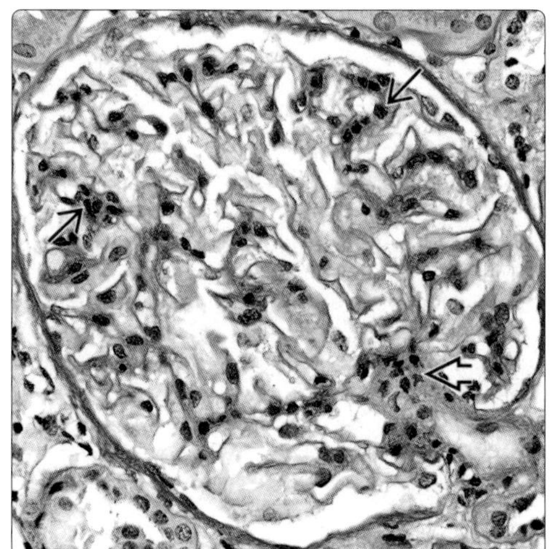

Fine GBM Vacuolization

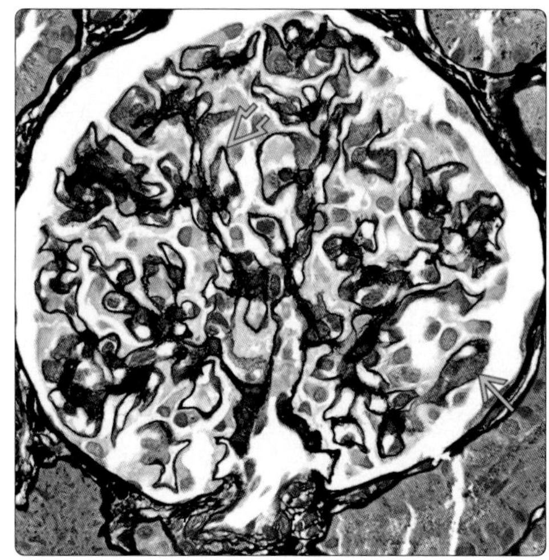

(Left) *Periodic acid-Schiff may not demonstrate apparent GBM abnormalities when changes associated with MGN occur early. There is mild mesangial hypercellularity ➡, which should be assessed in areas removed from the vascular pole ⇨.* **(Right)** *Jones methenamine silver reveals a finely vacuolated appearance of the GBM, which is accentuated when sectioned en face ➡. A hint of subepithelial "spike" formation ⇨ is also noted along some segments.*

Subepithelial "Spikes" and "Domes"

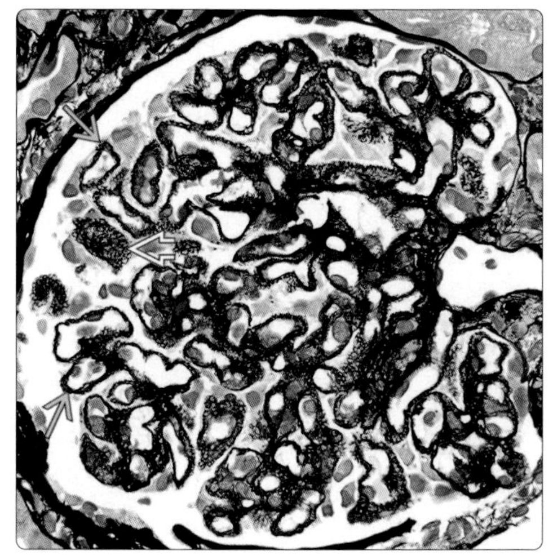

Segmental Sclerosis

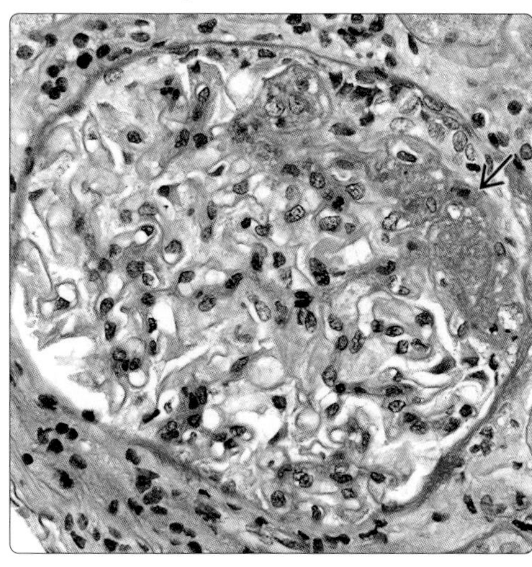

(Left) *Jones methenamine silver stain shows focal subepithelial "spike" formation ➡ and a prominent vacuolated appearance ⇨, which correlates with Ehrenreich-Churg stages 3-4.* **(Right)** *Periodic acid-Schiff demonstrates segmental sclerosis ➡ in a case of MGN. By light microscopy, the GBM abnormalities are not obvious, and the pathologic findings could be mistaken for focal segmental glomerulosclerosis in the absence of immunofluorescence or electron microscopy.*

Pauci-Immune GN & MGN

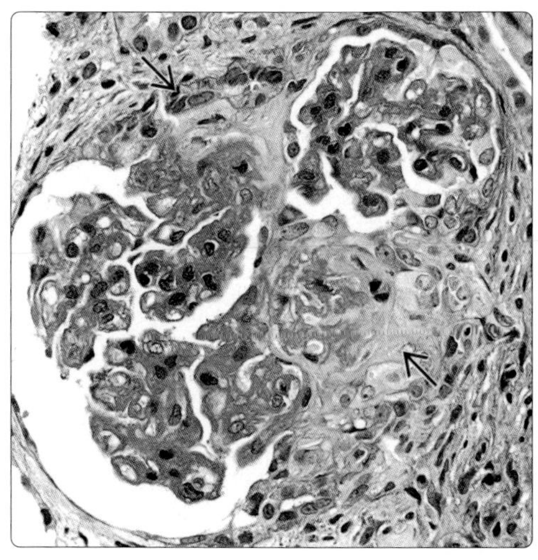

Anti-GBM Nephritis & MGN

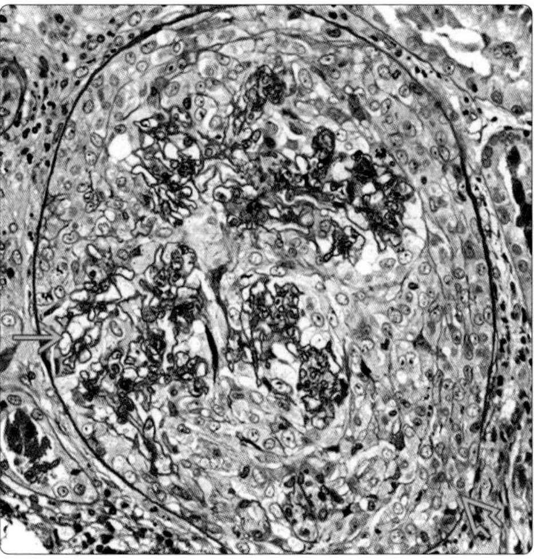

(Left) *Periodic acid-Schiff reveals a fibrocellular crescent ➡ with prominent thickening of the GBM in a patient with positive ANCA titers. The constellation of findings is consistent with pauci-immune, ANCA-associated crescentic GN superimposed upon MGN.* **(Right)** *Periodic acid-Schiff shows a cellular crescent ➡ filling up Bowman space in a glomerulus with anti-GBM disease superimposed upon MGN. The residual glomerular tufts show no evidence of endocapillary hypercellularity ⇨. (Courtesy M. Troxell, MD, PhD.)*

(Left) *Immunofluorescence microscopy for IgG reveals strong and diffuse granular staining along the glomerular capillaries ➡ without mesangial staining in a case of MGN. This pattern of staining is characteristic of MGN.* **(Right)** *The granular deposits along the GBM stain moderately well with antibody to the IgG1 subclass in MGN, which may be more dominant with stage 1 deposits. However, the most prominent subclass is usually IgG4.*

IgG

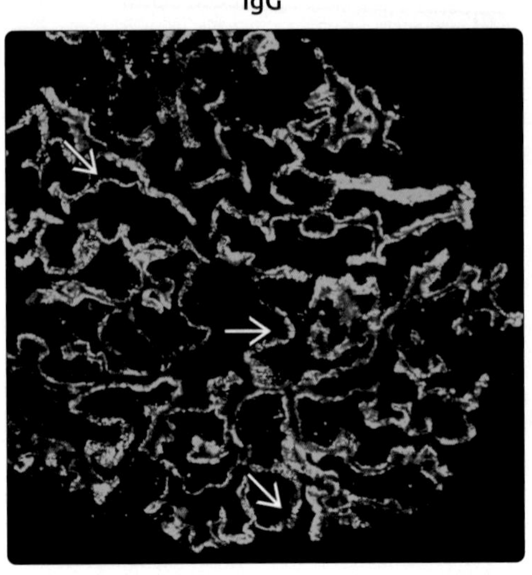

IgG1

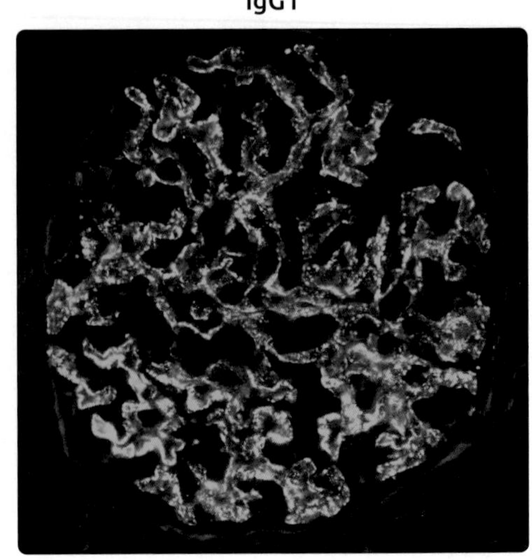

(Left) *Double stain with anti-IgG4-FITC (green) and anti-PLA2R-Cy3 (red) shows the granular deposits of PLA2R colocalize with IgG4 in the merged image, giving a yellow color. This is diagnostic of anti-PLA2R-related MGN.* **(Right)** *Double stain with anti-IgG4-FITC (green) and anti-PLA2R-Cy3 (red) shows the granular deposits of PLA2R do not co-localize with IgG4 in the merged image. This patient was suspected of having SLE, although the serology for ANA and dsDNA were negative.*

Colocalization of IgG4 and PLA2R

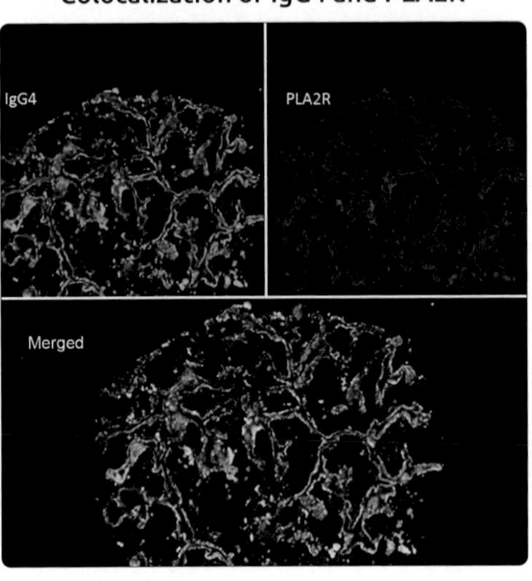

Non-PLA2R MGN

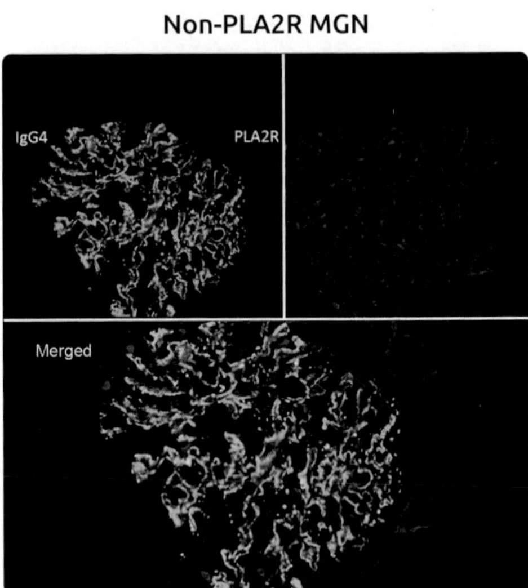

(Left) *Immunofluorescence microscopy for kappa light chain demonstrates a granular staining pattern of the glomerular capillary walls similar to lambda, but the intensity is typically less than IgG.* **(Right)** *Immunofluorescence microscopy for IgG shows both strong linear ➡ and granular ➡ staining of the glomerular basement membranes consistent with anti-GBM disease and concurrent MGN. (Courtesy M. Troxell, MD, PhD.)*

Kappa Light Chain

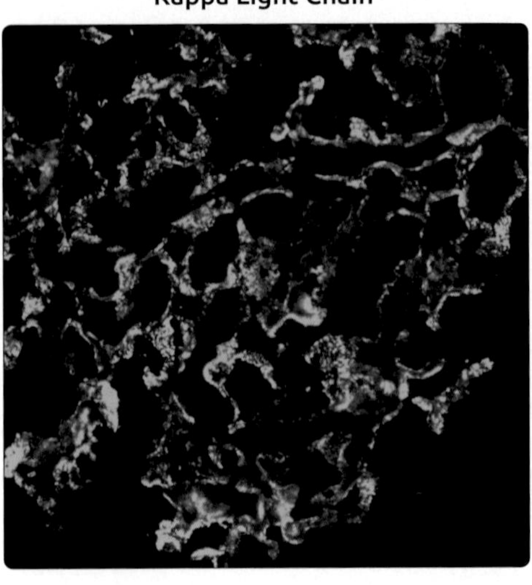

Anti-GBM Nephritis With MGN

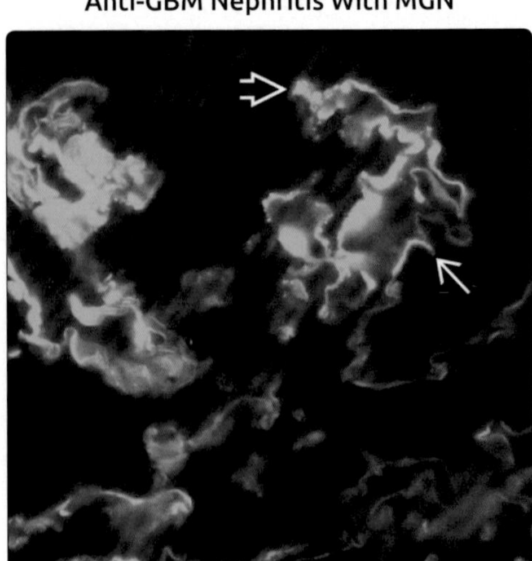

Stage 1 MGN

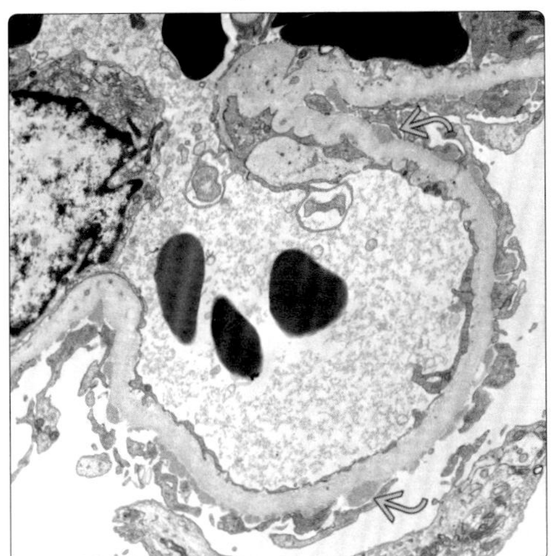

Stage 2 MGN

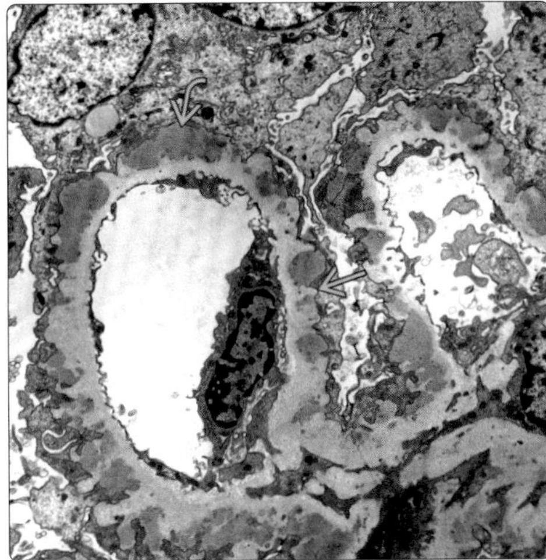

(Left) *Ehrenreich-Churg stage 1 is defined by the presence of sparse subepithelial deposits ⇨ with few GBM "spikes." This stage can resemble postinfectious GN.* **(Right)** *Ehrenreich-Churg stage 2 is defined by the presence of abundant subepithelial deposits ⇨ with intervening GBM "spikes" ⇨. The overlying podocyte foot processes are diffusely effaced. It is not uncommon to see deposits of varied stages of evolution in the same glomerulus.*

Stage 3 MGN

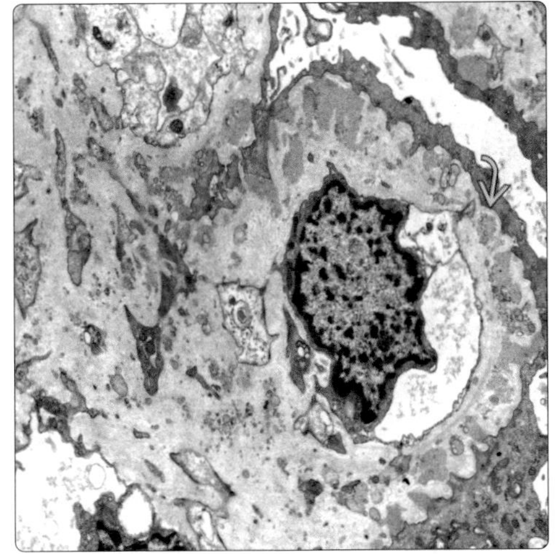

Stage 4 MGN

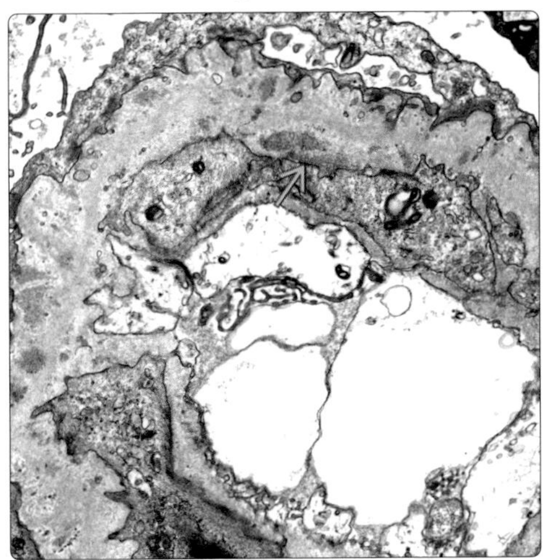

(Left) *Ehrenreich-Churg stage 3 is defined by the presence of abundant subepithelial deposits with intervening GBM "spikes" that enclose the deposits and form a layer ⇨ between the deposits and the podocyte.* **(Right)** *Ehrenreich-Churg stage 4 is defined by the dissolution of the subepithelial deposits, which become incorporated into the irregularly thickened GBM. Occasional deposits ⇨ are seen on the endothelial side of the GBM, presumably because of new GBM laid down by the podocyte or a secondary form of membranous nephropathy.*

Microspherular Substructure

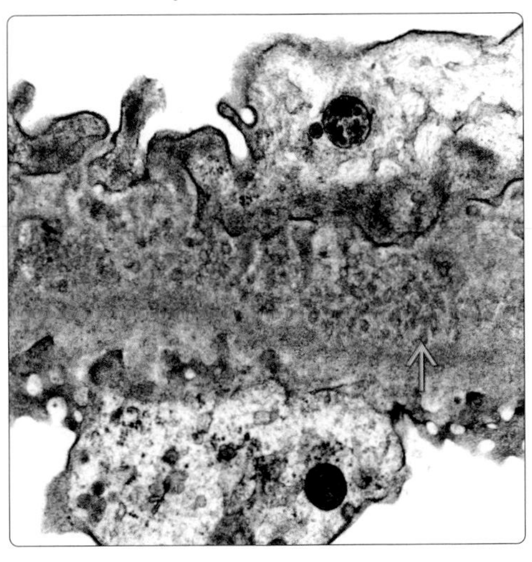

MGN With Renal Vein Thrombosis

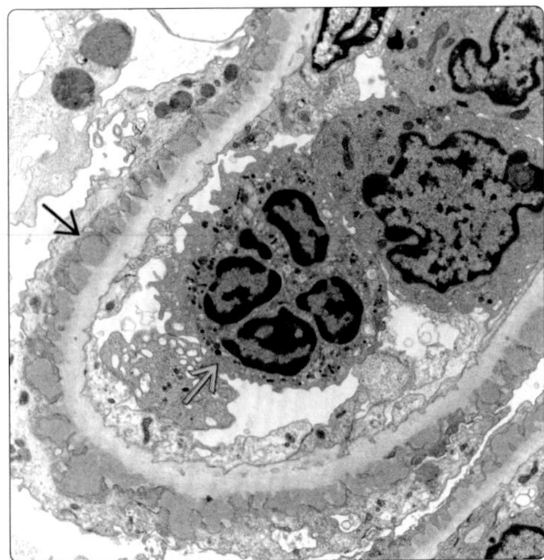

(Left) *Electron microscopy reveals a microspherular substructure ⇨ in the subepithelial deposits of this MGN case. (Courtesy J. Kowalewska, MD.)* **(Right)** *Electron micrograph shows a glomerular capillary loop with numerous subepithelial deposits ⇨, typical of stage 2 MGN. Luminal neutrophils ⇨ and monocytes have been associated with renal vein thrombosis, although this is not highly specific or sensitive.*

Membranous Glomerulonephritis, Secondary

KEY FACTS

TERMINOLOGY

- MGN in association with underlying disorder, infection, or administration of therapeutic agent

ETIOLOGY/PATHOGENESIS

- Common disease associations in secondary MGN include
  - Hepatitis B and C
  - Carcinoma, lymphoma/leukemia
  - Systemic lupus erythematosus, rheumatoid arthritis
  - Drugs (especially NSAIDs)
  - Sarcoidosis

CLINICAL ISSUES

- Nephrotic syndrome

MICROSCOPIC

- GBM thickening or subepithelial "spike" formation
- Mesangial hypercellularity
- Glomerulitis, or increased circulating leukocytes within glomerular capillaries, reported in association with underlying malignancy
- Immunofluorescence
  - Granular GBM deposits of IgG, C3 and variable other components
- Electron microscopy
  - Subepithelial electron-dense deposits, often stage I
  - ± mesangial electron-dense deposits

TOP DIFFERENTIAL DIAGNOSES

- Primary (idiopathic) MGN
- Membranous (class V) lupus nephritis

DIAGNOSTIC CHECKLIST

- Mesangial immune complex deposition suggests secondary MGN
  - Primary MGN 2° to PLA2R antibodies rarely has mesangial immune complexes

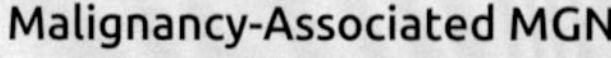

Malignancy-Associated MGN

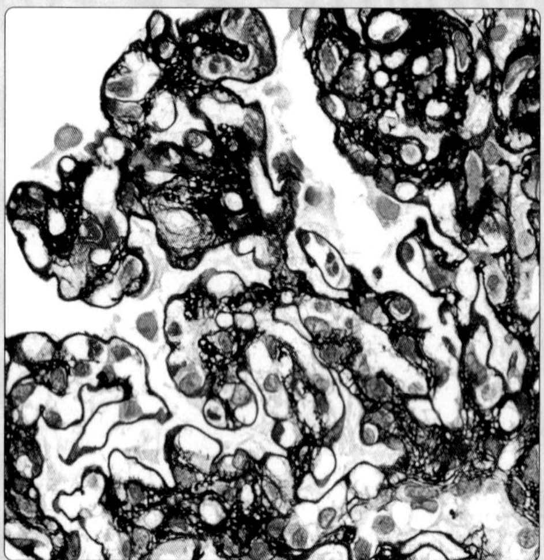

Sjögren Syndrome-Associated MGN

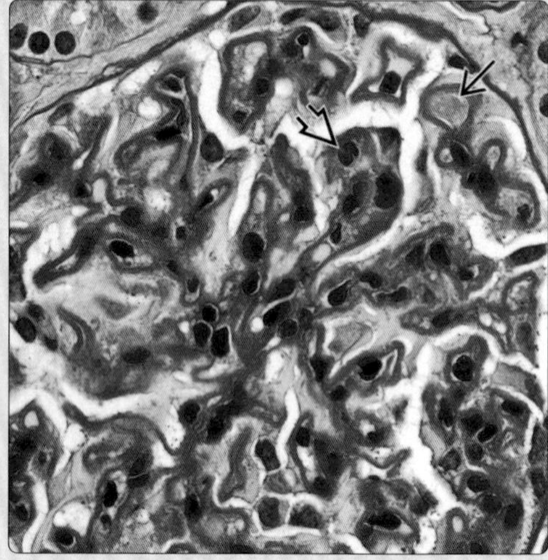

(Left) *Jones methenamine silver of MGN shows occasional circulating neutrophils within a few glomerular capillaries in this patient with an underlying malignancy. No apparent glomerular basement membrane abnormalities are noted.* **(Right)** *Periodic acid-Schiff shows a glomerular thrombus ⇒ in this Sjögren syndrome patient with deep venous and renal vein thrombosis. Congestion by neutrophils ⇒ in glomerular capillaries may be seen but was not a prominent feature in this biopsy.*

IgG

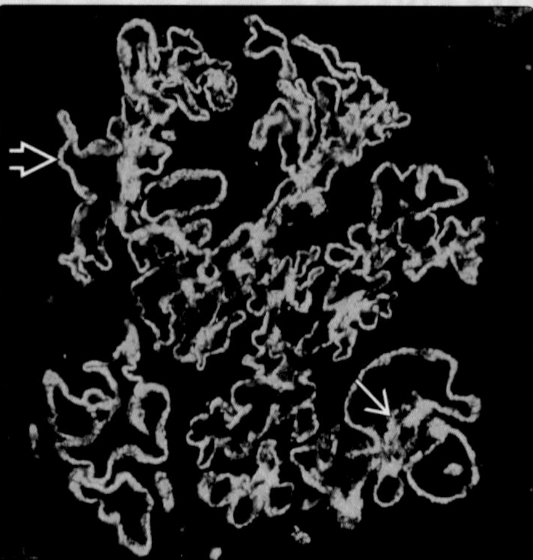

Mesangial Deposits and Stage I MGN

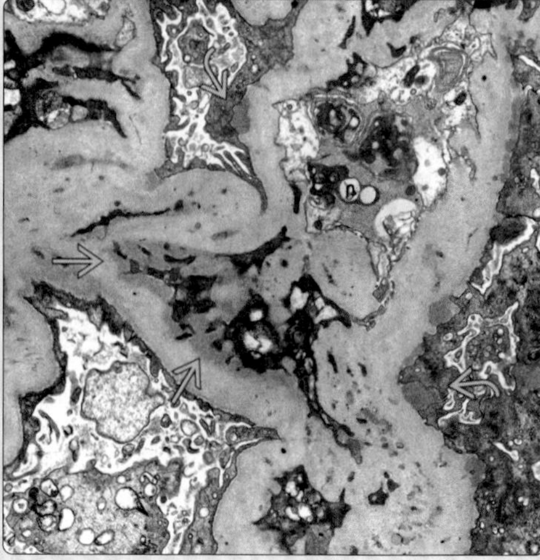

(Left) *Immunofluorescence microscopy for IgG shows characteristic granular staining of the capillary walls ⇒ in MGN. Additional granular mesangial staining ⇒ is suggestive of secondary MGN.* **(Right)** *If mesangial deposits ⇒ are present in MGN, secondary causes should be considered as in this case due to mercury ingestion. Stage I deposits (sparse and with little spike formation) are also common in the secondary forms ⇒.*

TERMINOLOGY

Abbreviations

- Membranous glomerulonephritis (MGN)

Definitions

- MGN in association with underlying disorder, infection, or administration of therapeutic agents.

ETIOLOGY/PATHOGENESIS

Antibody Response

- Chronic response to organisms, self-antigens, alloantigens or exogenous antigens that persist for months to years
  - Subepithelial deposits probably result from in situ immune complex formation (glomerular antigen)
  - Mesangial immune complexes probably caused by circulating immune complexes
  - Mesangial and subepithelial deposits may also be result of "planted" circulating antigens

Conditions Associated With Secondary MGN

- Chronic infections
- Autoimmune diseases
- Malignant neoplasms
- Transplantation (organ or hematopoietic)
- Drugs
- Sarcoidosis

CLINICAL ISSUES

Presentation

- Proteinuria, nephrotic syndrome, edema
- Microscopic hematuria, rarely gross hematuria
- Renal vein thrombosis < 10%

Treatment

- Withdrawal of suspected drug
- Antibiotics for infection
- Immunosuppression for autoimmune disease
- Excision/chemotherapy for neoplasm

Prognosis

- Generally good if cause can be eliminated

MICROSCOPIC

Histologic Features

- Subepithelial "spikes" in PAS and silver stains; subepithelial deposits on trichrome
- Mesangial hypercellularity variable
- Increased circulating leukocytes in glomerular capillaries
  - Reported in association with underlying malignancy or renal vein thrombosis
- Glomerular thrombi associated with malignancies
- Tubules, interstitium, and vessels have no specific lesions

ANCILLARY TESTS

Immunofluorescence

- Granular capillary wall staining for IgG and kappa and lambda light chains ± complement components
  - IgG1 and IgG2 described in subepithelial deposits of MGN associated with carcinoma
  - IgG3 is dominant subclass in membranous lupus nephritis
- Many examples of putative antigen localization in deposits (e.g., carcinoembryonic antigen, bovine serum albumin, enzyme replacement, hepatitis B)
  - Caveat that proteins can be trapped nonspecifically in deposits
- Tubular basement membrane Ig deposits common in lupus

Electron Microscopy

- Subepithelial electron-dense deposits, often stage I
- Mesangial electron-dense deposits
  - Non-PLA2R associated MGN has mesangial deposits in ~ 70% (Cossey)
  - MGN 2° with PLA2R deposition has mesangial deposits in ~ 30% (Cossey)
- Endothelial tubuloreticular inclusions
  - In systemic lupus erythematosus or viral infections, such as hepatitis or HIV
- Bowman capsular electron-dense deposits in lupus
  - Also reported in a few primary MGN cases with substantial clinical follow-up

DIFFERENTIAL DIAGNOSIS

Primary (Idiopathic) MGN

- Minority have mesangial deposits and TBM deposits very rare

Membranous (Class V) Lupus Nephritis

- Mesangial electron-dense deposits almost universal
- C1q deposits in 67%; TBM deposits in >30%
- Endothelial tubuloreticular inclusions &/or subendothelial deposits

Other Causes of Secondary MGN

- History of drug, infection, autoimmune disease, neoplasm, allograft
- Demonstration of putative antigen in deposits

DIAGNOSTIC CHECKLIST

Clinically Relevant Pathologic Features

- Remission of nephrotic syndrome in 93% with mesangial deposits vs. 60% of those without

SELECTED REFERENCES

1. Stehlé T et al: Phospholipase A2 receptor and sarcoidosis-associated membranous nephropathy. Nephrol Dial Transplant. ePub, 2015
2. Vivarelli M et al: Genetic homogeneity but IgG subclass-dependent clinical variability of alloimmune membranous nephropathy with anti-neutral endopeptidase antibodies. Kidney Int. 87(3):602-9, 2015
3. Debiec H et al: Immunopathogenesis of membranous nephropathy: an update. Semin Immunopathol. 36(4):381-97, 2014
4. Tomas NM et al: Thrombospondin Type-1 Domain-Containing 7A in Idiopathic Membranous Nephropathy. N Engl J Med. ePub, 2014
5. Larsen CP et al: Determination of primary versus secondary membranous glomerulopathy utilizing phospholipase A2 receptor staining in renal biopsies. Mod Pathol. 26(5):709-15, 2013
6. Li P et al: Clinical and pathological analysis of hepatitis B virus-related membranous nephropathy and idiopathic membranous nephropathy. Clin Nephrol. 78(6):456-64, 2012
7. Debiec H et al: Early-childhood membranous nephropathy due to cationic bovine serum albumin. N Engl J Med. 364(22):2101-10, 2011

(Left) *Jones methenamine silver reveals discrete subepithelial "spike" formation along all of the glomerular capillaries in this patient with both Sjögren syndrome and MGN.* **(Right)** *Immunofluorescence shows widespread granular deposits of IgG typical of membranous glomerulonephritis in a patient with nephrotic syndrome 3 years after a bone marrow transplant. Bowman capsule granular staining is noted.*

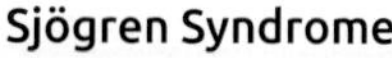

Sjögren Syndrome

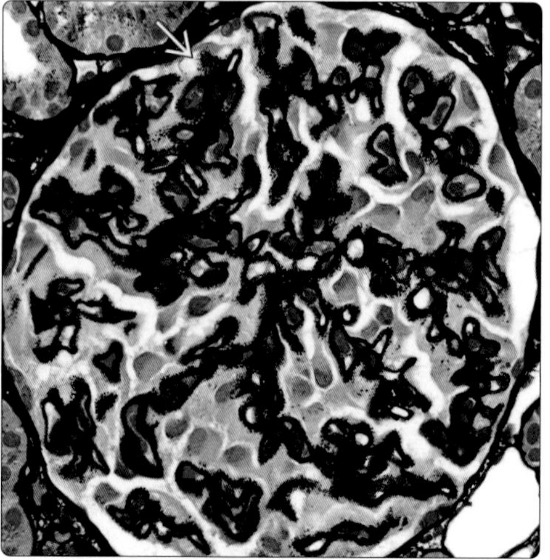

IgG in Bone Marrow Transplantation

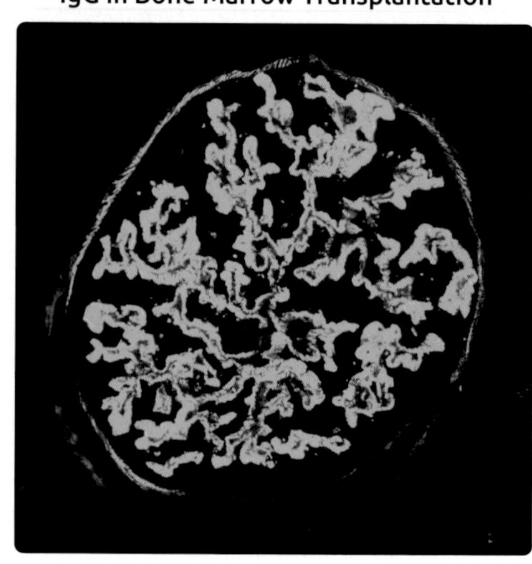

(Left) *H&E shows prominent thickening of the glomerular basement membranes in this case of MGN. A glomerular thrombus is noted in a capillary of this patient with renal vein thrombosis.* **(Right)** *H&E shows several neutrophils and small thrombi within glomerular capillaries in MGN associated with colon carcinoma and renal vein thrombosis. Both features (neutrophils and thrombi) have been observed in both clinical settings of renal vein thrombosis and malignancy.*

Glomerular Capillary Thrombus

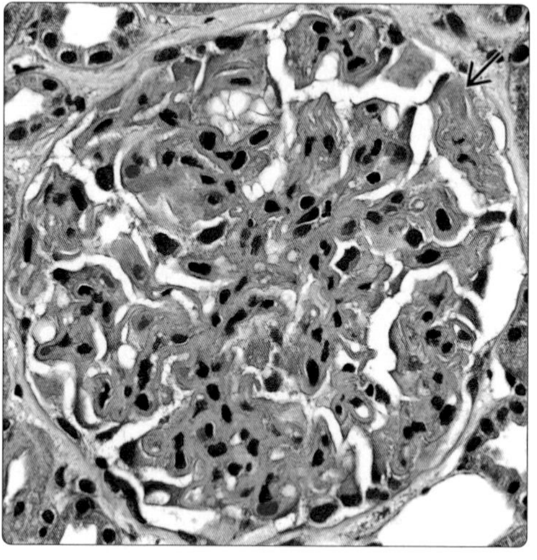

Intracapillary Neutrophils

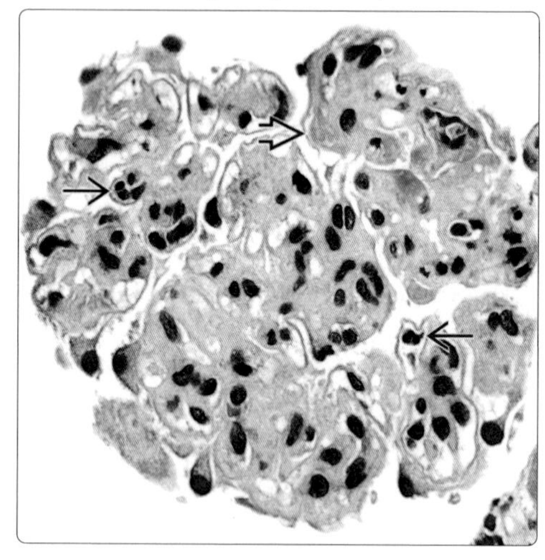

(Left) *Granular GBM deposits are present segmentally as well as in the mesangium in this glomerulus from a patient with drug-induced MGN. Mesangial deposits are more common in patients with secondary MGN.* **(Right)** *MGN in a patient with a renal cell carcinoma is shown. The deposits appear to be restricted to the GBM (without mesangial deposits) and contained IgG4, which co-localized with PLA2R, indicating this is a primary MGN and not related to the neoplasm.*

GBM and Mesangial IgG

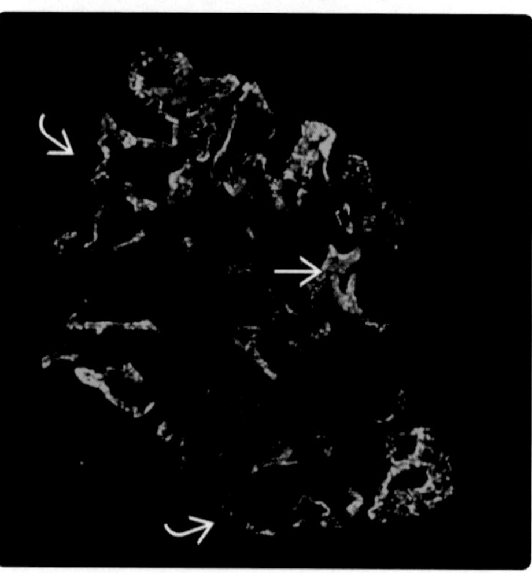

Granular IgG GBM Deposits

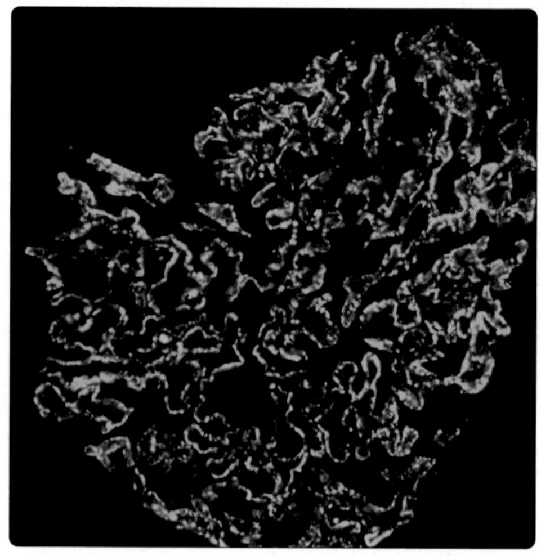

Stage I MGN

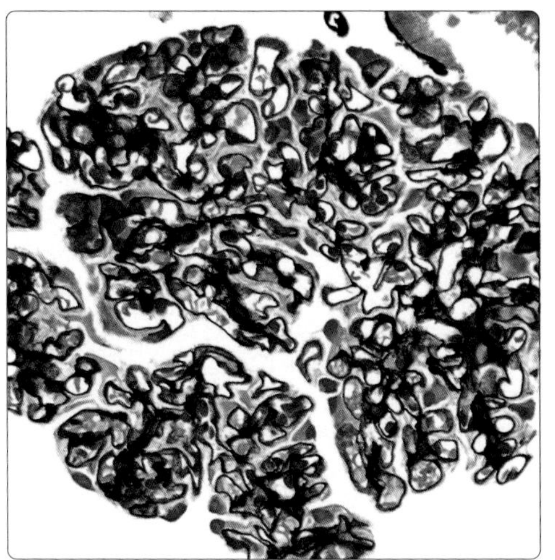

Sparse Subepithelial Deposits

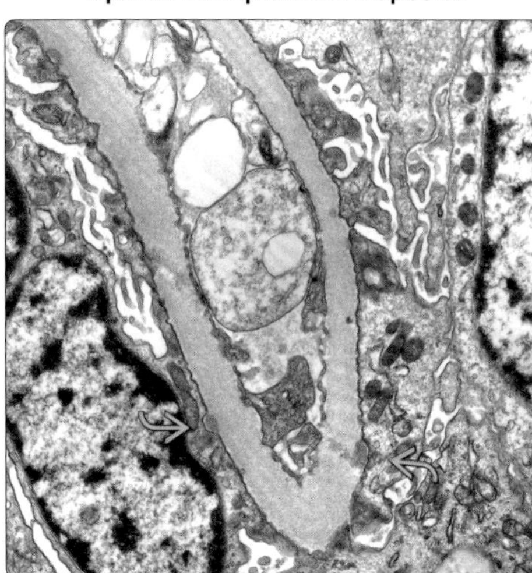

(Left) *Jones methenamine silver stain shows a glomerulus without significant pathologic abnormalities. There is no significant mesangial or endocapillary hypercellularity. Early stages of MGN may resemble minimal change disease by light microscopy.* **(Right)** *Drug-induced MGN is often stage I, with sparse deposits ➡ and little or no GBM spike formation, as in this adolescent who developed nephrotic-range proteinuria due to thiola (tiopronin) therapy for cystinuria.*

Endothelial Tubuloreticular Inclusion

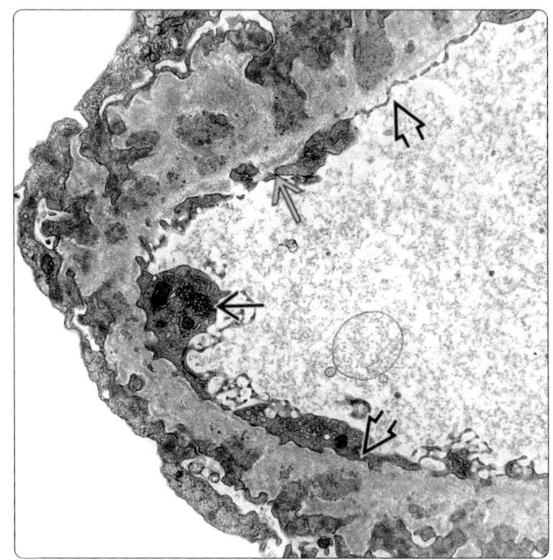

C1q

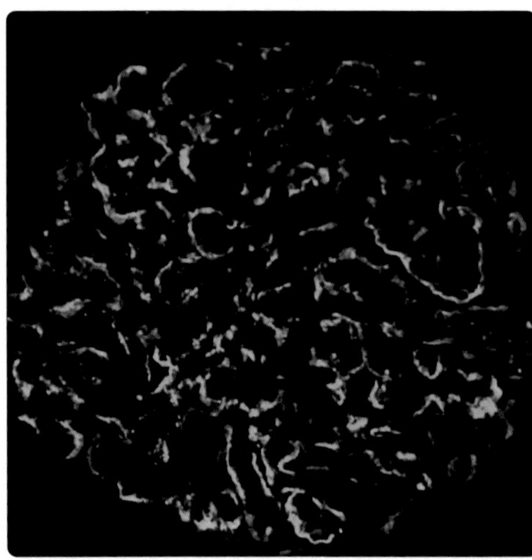

(Left) *A tubuloreticular inclusion ➡ in an endothelial cell, subepithelial deposits ➡ which sometimes penetrate into the GBM, and occasional subendothelial deposits ➡ are clues for the diagnosis of lupus MGN.* **(Right)** *Immunofluorescence Microscopy for C1q shows granular staining of the glomerular capillary walls in a patient with a clinical diagnosis of lupus.*

Lack of PLA2R in Deposits

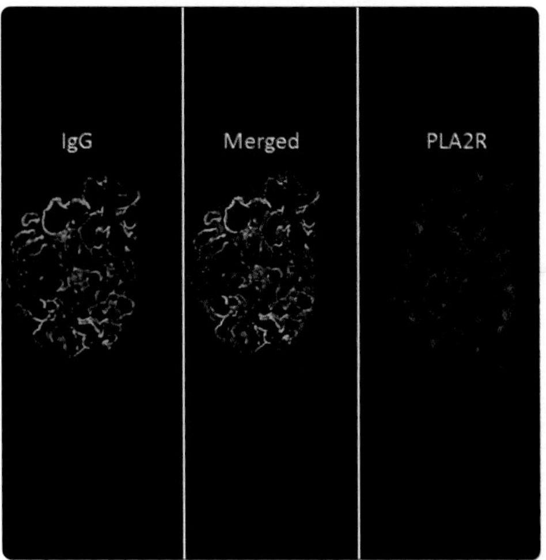

PLA2R Colocalization

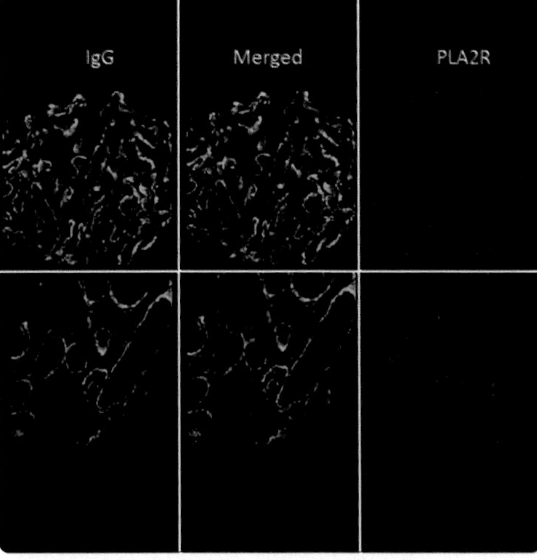

(Left) *PLA2R in IgG4 deposits is assessed by double IF stains. In this case the merged image shows no yellow areas, which would indicate co-localization. The cause of the MGN was not determined, the patient had a spontaneous remission 3 months later.* **(Right)** *Double stain for IgG (green) & PLA2R (red) in a patient with class V lupus GN Is shown. Merged images in top row show yellow areas of colocalization, indicating PLA2R in the deposits. TBM deposits in lower row show no yellow areas. Rare patients with SLE have PLA2R antibodies.*

Membranous Glomerulonephritis With Anti-TBM Antibodies

KEY FACTS

TERMINOLOGY

- Autoimmune disease characterized by membranous glomerulonephritis (MGN) and autoantibodies to tubular basement membrane (TBM)

ETIOLOGY/PATHOGENESIS

- Noncollagenous 48-58 kd proximal TBM autoantigen
- Does not cross-react with glomerular basement membrane (GBM)

CLINICAL ISSUES

- Age: < 5 years old
- Fanconi syndrome
- Nephrotic syndrome

MICROSCOPIC

- Typical features of MGN plus interstitial nephritis
  - Thickened TBM
- Linear IgG staining of proximal TBM
- Finely granular deposits of IgG along GBM

ANCILLARY TESTS

- Subepithelial amorphous deposits in GBM ± intervening membrane "spikes"

TOP DIFFERENTIAL DIAGNOSES

- MGN with TBM immune complex deposits
- Idiopathic MGN

DIAGNOSTIC CHECKLIST

- Anti-TBM antibodies may appear after MGN
- IgG TBM deposits are linear
- Segmental C3 deposition along TBM is a common incidental finding and nondiagnostic

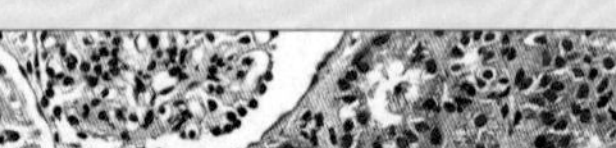

Interstitial Inflammation

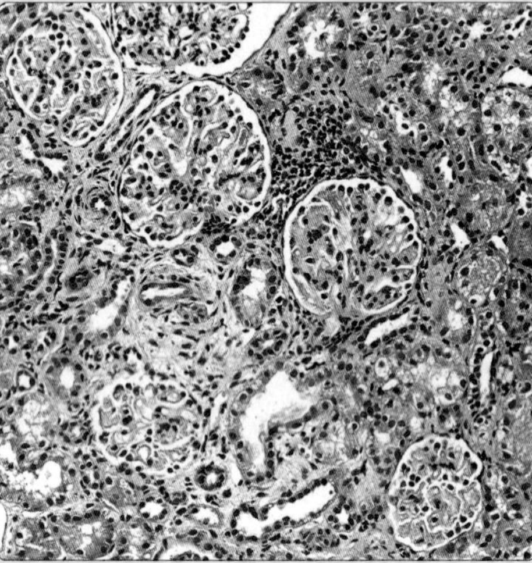

Glomerular Subepithelial Deposits

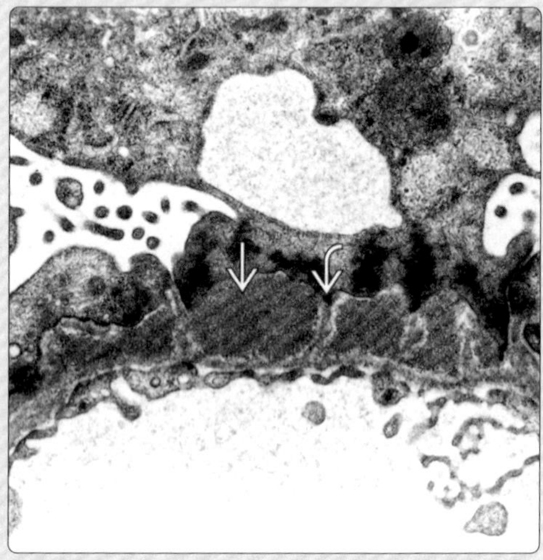

(Left) *Glomeruli have focal, segmental proliferation and increased matrix in a child who has membranous glomerulonephritis (MGN) with anti-tubular basement membrane (TBM) antibodies. The interstitium has foci of periglomerular lymphocytic infiltrate. (Courtesy B. Ivanyi, MD.)* **(Right)** *Subepithelial deposits with intervening spikes are conspicuous in this sample from a 1-year-old child with MGN with anti-TBM antibodies. (Courtesy B. Ivanyi, MD.)*

Linear IgG Along TBM

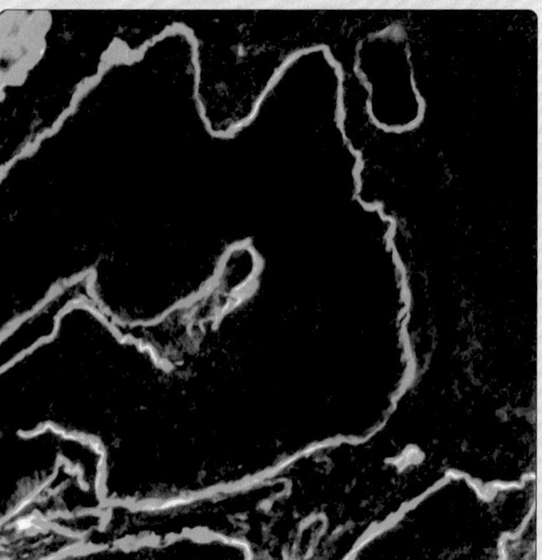

Linear IgG Along TBM in Recurrence

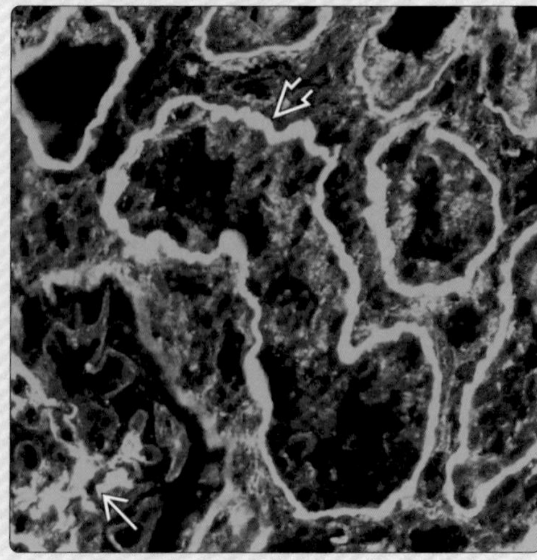

(Left) *Linear staining of the proximal TBM for IgG is shown in a child who has MGN with anti-TBM antibodies. C3 may also be present. (Courtesy B. Ivanyi, MD.)* **(Right)** *Recurrent anti-TBM disease in a transplant shows linear immunostaining along the TBM. Glomeruli have granular staining in the mesangium. (Courtesy B. Ivanyi, MD.)*

TERMINOLOGY

Abbreviations

- Membranous glomerulonephritis (MGN)

Definitions

- Autoimmune disease characterized by MGN and autoantibodies to tubular basement membrane (TBM)

ETIOLOGY/PATHOGENESIS

Autoantibodies to TBM

- Noncollagenous 48-58 kd TBM autoantigen in TBM of proximal tubules
- Does not cross-react with glomerular basement membrane (GBM) by indirect immunofluorescence
- Anti-TBM may be a later complication since a younger sibling of an affected boy had MGN without anti-TBM

Autoantibodies Form Immune Complexes in Glomerulus

- Antigen in GBM deposits unknown
- MGN occurs without anti-TBM

Animal Models

- Anti-TBM disease in guinea pigs
  - No MGN component
  - Marked giant cell response around TBM
  - Response linked to MHC
    - Strain XIII susceptible, strain II not
    - Restricted idiotypes of autoantibodies
- Anti-TBM disease in rats
  - Pathology same as in guinea pig
  - Antigen and disease restricted to Brown-Norway (BN) rats
    - Lewis rats lack antigen, develop disease in BN renal allografts
- Anti-TBM disease in mice
  - T-cell reactivity in addition to anti-TBM antibodies necessary

CLINICAL ISSUES

Epidemiology

- Incidence
  - Rare; 11 cases reported (1998)
  - HLA-B7 (4/5) and HLA-DR8 (2/5) may be risk factors
- Age
  - < 5 years old

Presentation

- Nephrotic syndrome in childhood
- Microhematuria
- Hypertension
- Fanconi syndrome (glycosuria, aminoaciduria)
- Diarrhea
- Neurological and ocular symptoms

Treatment

- None effective
- Recurrence reported in 1 transplant followed 2 years

MICROSCOPIC

Histologic Features

- Typical features of MGN plus interstitial nephritis
- Glomeruli
  - Diffusely thickened GBM with "spikes" on PAS and silver stains
  - Mesangial hypercellularity
- Tubules
  - Thickened TBM
  - Atrophic tubules
  - Tubular resorption droplets
- Interstitium
  - Mononuclear inflammation

ANCILLARY TESTS

Immunofluorescence

- Finely granular deposits of IgG along GBM
  - IgA, C3, C1q, and IgM variably present
- Linear staining of TBM of proximal tubules for IgG ± other components
- Segmental C3 deposition along TBM is a common incidental finding and nondiagnostic

Electron Microscopy

- Subepithelial amorphous deposits in GBM ± intervening membrane "spikes"
- Thickening of TBM without electron-dense deposits

DIFFERENTIAL DIAGNOSIS

MGN With TBM Immune Complex Deposits

- Granular vs. linear IgG along TBM

Idiopathic MGN

- No linear deposits

DIAGNOSTIC CHECKLIST

Pathologic Interpretation Pearls

- Anti-TBM antibodies may appear after MGN

SELECTED REFERENCES

1. Markowitz GS: Membranous glomerulopathy: emphasis on secondary forms and disease variants. Adv Anat Pathol. 8(3):119-25, 2001
2. Iványi B et al: Childhood membranous nephropathy, circulating antibodies to the 58-kD TIN antigen, and anti-tubular basement membrane nephritis: an 11-year follow-up. Am J Kidney Dis. 32(6):1068-74, 1998
3. Katz A et al: Role of antibodies to tubulointerstitial nephritis antigen in human anti-tubular basement membrane nephritis associated with membranous nephropathy. Am J Med. 93(6):691-8, 1992
4. Butkowski RJ et al: Characterization of a tubular basement membrane component reactive with autoantibodies associated with tubulointerstitial nephritis. J Biol Chem. 265(34):21091-8, 1990
5. Ueda S et al: Autoimmune interstitial nephritis induced in inbred mice. Analysis of mouse tubular basement membrane antigen and genetic control of immune response to it. Am J Pathol. 132(2):304-18, 1988
6. Clayman MD et al: Isolation and characterization of the nephritogenic antigen producing anti-tubular basement membrane disease. J Exp Med. 161(2):290-305, 1985
7. Dumas R et al: [Membranous glomerulonephritis in two brothers associated in one with tubulo-interstitial disease, Fanconi syndrome and anti-TBM antibodies (author's transl).] Arch Fr Pediatr. 39(2):75-8, 1982

TERMINOLOGY

Abbreviations

- Membranoproliferative glomerulonephritis (MPGN)

Background

- MPGN historically divided into 3 **morphologic** categories, all with glomerular C3 deposition, chronic hypocomplementemia, and sometimes C3 nephritic factor
  - MPGN I defined by mesangial hypercellularity, subendothelial deposits, and duplication of GBM
  - MPGN II or dense deposit disease defined originally by EM feature of hyperdense deposits
  - MPGN III defined by prominent subepithelial deposits or diffuse intramembranous GBM deposits
- Problems recognized in classification
  - Same complement abnormality can lead to different glomerular pathologies
  - Same pathologic pattern can be caused by different complement abnormalities
- Those with prominent C3 and little or no immunoglobulin deposition were recently separated into the category "C3 glomerulopathy" in which the demonstrable abnormality is dysregulation of alternative pathway of complement
  - Dense deposit disease is prototype; but a spectrum of morphologic patterns are associated with alternative pathway dysregulation
- Idiopathic MPGN with prominent immunoglobulin deposits are probably a type of chronic immune complex disease, as in chronic infections
  - Includes ~ 70% of MPGN type I and 60% type III cases
  - However, ~ 50% have identified abnormality in alternative pathway
  - Classification system is evolving
- These 2 categories are not sharply separated
- Dysregulation of complement system, if present, may magnify pathologic consequences of otherwise banal immune complex disease
  - Can also manifest as atypical HUS and age-related macular degeneration

Complement Dysregulation in C3 Glomerulopathies

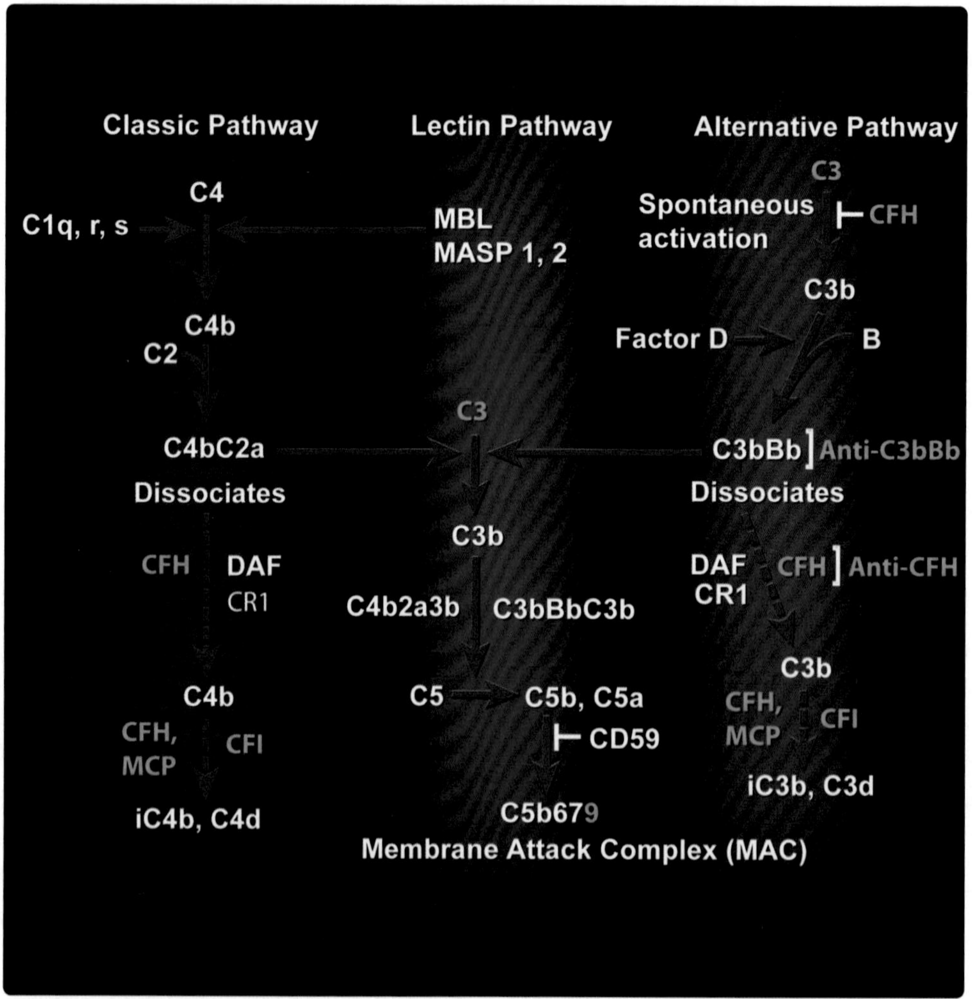

Schematic of the complement system is illustrated. Components known to be abnormal in C3-related glomerular diseases are indicated in green. Mutations involve loss of function of the complement inhibitors (CFH, CFI, MCP), lack of binding to inhibitors (C3), and autoantibodies that protect C3 convertase (C3bBb) from dissociation (C3NeF). CFH-related proteins have also been implicated. The alternate pathway "ticks over" spontaneously in the plasma by reaction with water and is activated by microbial surfaces. The classical pathway is activated by IgG or IgM complexes with antigen. The lectin pathway is triggered by carbohydrate structures on microbes.

Classification of C3-Related Glomerular Diseases

Category	Defining Features	Complement Abnormalities
C3 Glomerulopathies		
Dense deposit disease (DDD)	Extremely dense GBM and mesangial deposits by EM; variable histologic patterns: MPGN, AGN, mesangial proliferative and crescentic GN; C3 dominant	Autoantibody to C3bBb (> 80%) or C3 (rare); mutation in CFH (minority), C3 (rare), CFHR1 (rare)
C3 glomerulonephritis (primary GN with isolated C3 deposits)	C3 in mesangium/GBM with Ig and C1q at least 2 IF levels less; deposits not as dense as DDD; "humps" occasionally; 3 patterns: MPGN type I or III and epimembranous deposits without MPGN	Autoantibody to C3bBb (~ 30%); mutation in CFH (minority), CFI (rare), MCP (rare)
Familial C3 glomerulopathy	MPGN type III (one family)	Hybrid CFHR3-1
CFHR5 nephropathy	MPGN I or III pattern, autosomal dominant	Mutation in CFHR5
Atypical acute glomerulonephritis	Persistent hematuria/proteinuria with or without history of infection; endocapillary and mesangial proliferation + subepithelial "humps"; C3 > Ig	Autoantibody to C3bBb (C3NeF) ~ 70%; mutations in CFH5 or CFH5R ~ 30%
Idiopathic MPGN With Immune Complex Deposition		
MPGN, type I	Mesangial proliferation + subendothelial and mesangial deposits, duplication of GBM; C3 in mesangium/GBM with Ig &/or C1q greater than or within 1 IF level of C3	Autoantibody to C3bBb (20-50%); CFH mutation (minority); CFI mutation (minority); C9 (rare); often evidence of classic pathway activation (low C4)
MPGN, type III	Mesangial proliferation + subepithelial or intramembranous deposits; C3 in mesangium/GBM with Ig &/or C1q greater than or within 1 IF level of C3	Sparse genetic and autoimmune data in type III with Ig/C1q

CFH = complement factor H; CFI = complement factor I; MPGN = membranoproliferative glomerulonephritis; AGN = acute glomerulonephritis; CFHR = complement factor H-related proteins.

C3 GLOMERULOPATHIES

Definition

- Disease process due to abnormal control of complement activation, deposition, or degradation and characterized by predominant glomerular C3 fragment deposition with electron-dense deposits on EM
- Proposed definition of "predominant C3"
  - C3 IF intensity ≥ 2 levels above immunoglobulins or C1q on a scale of 0, trace, 1+, 2+, -3+

Causes

- Genetic abnormalities in complement regulatory proteins or complement components
  - Complement factor H (CFH) and related (CFHR) proteins
    - CFH, CFHR5, CFHR1, CFHR3-1 hybrid
  - Membrane cofactor protein (MCP)
    - Cell-bound protein that inactivates C3b & C4b
  - CFI
    - Inhibits active C3b by cleaving to iC3b & C3f
  - C3
- Autoantibodies
  - C3bBb (C3 nephritic factor)
    - Stabilizes and prolongs activity of C3bBb
  - CFH, C3, factor B
    - Some anti-CFH are monoclonal Ig
- Either genetic abnormalities or autoantibodies lead to dysregulation of alternative pathway of complement activation, low serum levels of C3, and glomerular deposition of C3 and related components

Identified Subtypes

- Dense deposit disease
- C3 glomerulonephritis
- CFHR5 nephropathy
- Familial C3 glomerulopathy
- Atypical acute GN

IDIOPATHIC MPGN WITH IMMUNE COMPLEX DEPOSITION

Definition

- MPGN I or III morphologic pattern with C3 in mesangium/GBM and Ig &/or C1q greater than or within 1 IF level of C3
- Those with identifiable cause are not included and classified by cause (e.g., infection, lupus etc)

Relationship to C3 Glomerulopathy

- ~ 50% also have dysregulation of alternative pathway
- Dysregulation is thought to predispose or prolong injury initiated by immune complexes

SELECTED REFERENCES

1. Cook HT et al: Histopathology of MPGN and C3 glomerulopathies. Nat Rev Nephrol. 11(1):14-22, 2015
2. De Vriese AS et al: Kidney Disease Caused by Dysregulation of the Complement Alternative Pathway: An Etiologic Approach. J Am Soc Nephrol. ePub, 2015
3. Hou J et al: Toward a working definition of C3 glomerulopathy by immunofluorescence. Kidney Int. 85(2):450-56, 2014
4. Xiao X et al: C3 glomerulopathy: the genetic and clinical findings in dense deposit disease and C3 glomerulonephritis. Semin Thromb Hemost. 40(4):465-71, 2014
5. Pickering MC et al: C3 glomerulopathy: consensus report. Kidney Int. 84(6):1079-89, 2013
6. Tortajada A et al: C3 glomerulopathy-associated CFHR1 mutation alters FHR oligomerization and complement regulation. J Clin Invest. 123(6):2434-46, 2013

(Left) *The characteristic hyperdense deposits in the GBM seen by EM are pathognomonic of dense deposit disease, and even persist in globally sclerotic glomeruli as shown. These deposits are also seen in the mesangium, Bowman capsule, and TBM.* (Right) *At high power, the hyperdense deposits have no substructure and permeate the GBM. The podocyte foot processes at the top are normal.*

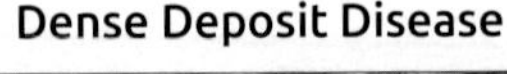

Dense Deposit Disease

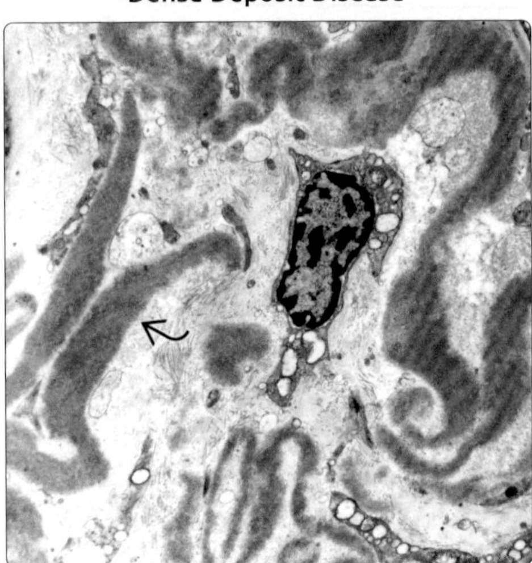

Dense Deposit Disease

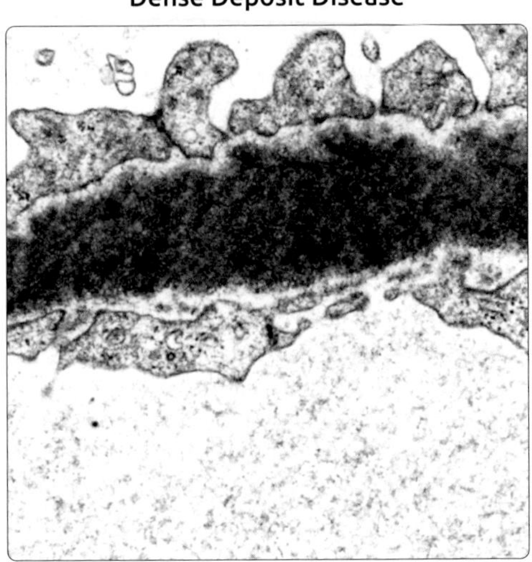

(Left) *Type I MPGN pattern begins as subendothelial and mesangial deposits. These are amorphous and less electron dense than in DDD. Subepithelial deposits may also be present, but if prominent, classified as type III.* (Right) *As type I MPGN evolves, duplication of the GBM develops on the endothelial side. Mesangial cells are interposed between the layers and the electron-dense deposits become less conspicuous. This case is C3 glomerulonephritis of 5 years duration in a 14-year-old boy with persistent low C3.*

Type I MPGN

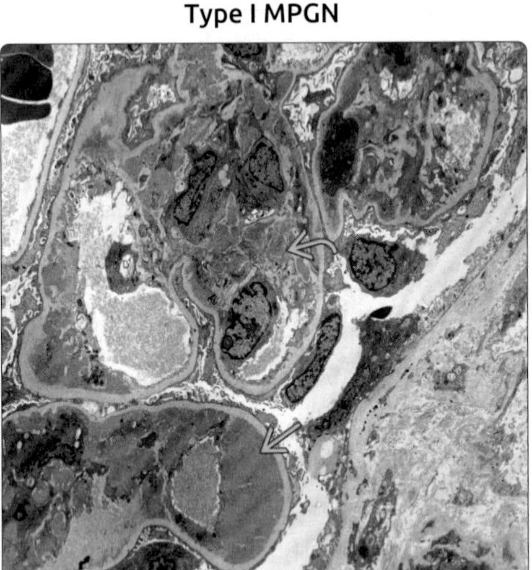

Type I MPGN

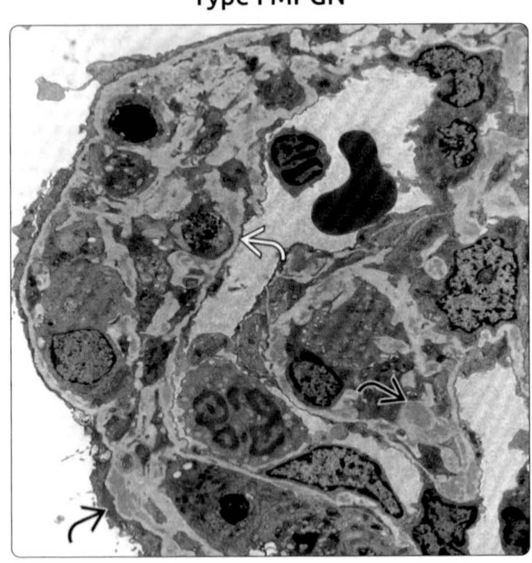

(Left) *In type III MPGN of the Anders and Strife pattern, the deposits permeate the GBM but are not as dense as in DDD. This pattern is common in C3 glomerulopathies, which this patient had. Permeating deposits of type III can occur together with subendothelial deposits, even in the same glomerulus.* (Right) *In type III MPGN of the Burkholder type, subepithelial deposits are prominent, resembling membranous glomerulonephritis, along with subendothelial deposits of MPGN type I.*

Type III MPGN

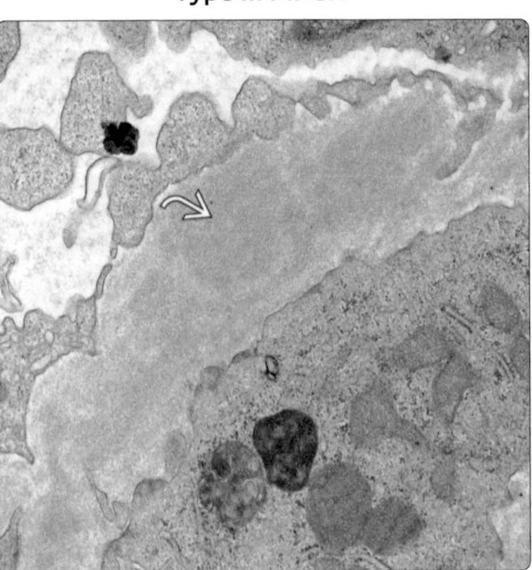

Type III MPGN

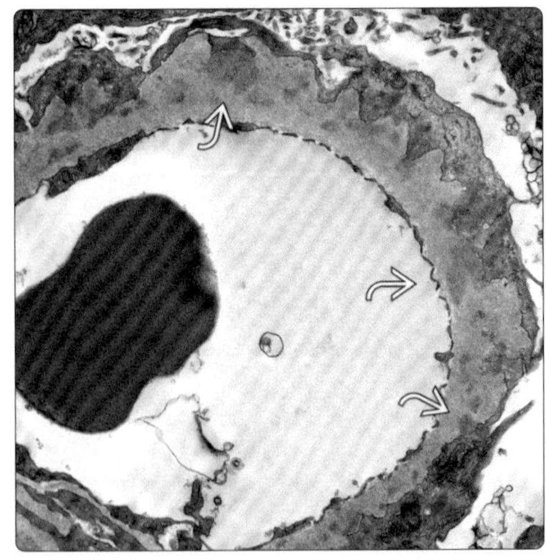

Strong C3 Staining With Negative IgG

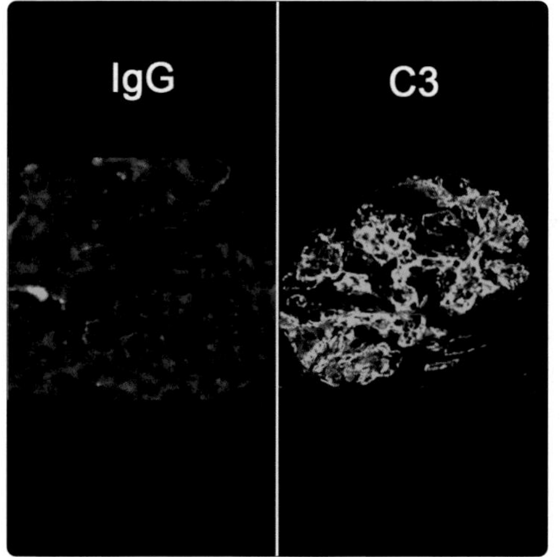

Strong C3 Staining With Focal IgM

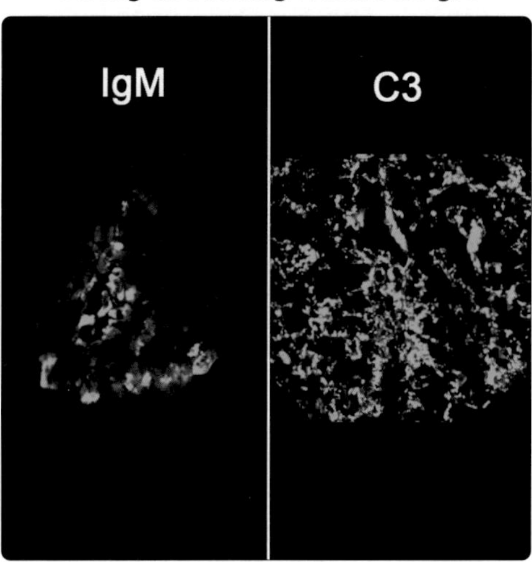

(Left) *The relative staining of C3 compared with IgG, IgA, IgM &/or C1q is proposed as a diagnostic criterion for C3 glomerulopathies. In this case of DDD, C3 is 4+ and IgG is negative, meeting the criteria of an IF score of 2 or more higher for C3 than IgG.* **(Right)** *In this case of DDD, C3 is 3+ and IgM is focally and segmentally positive (1+), meeting the criteria for C3 glomerulopathy with an IF score of 2 or more higher for C3 than Ig or C1q.*

Strong C3 (3+) and Weak IgG (Trace-1+)

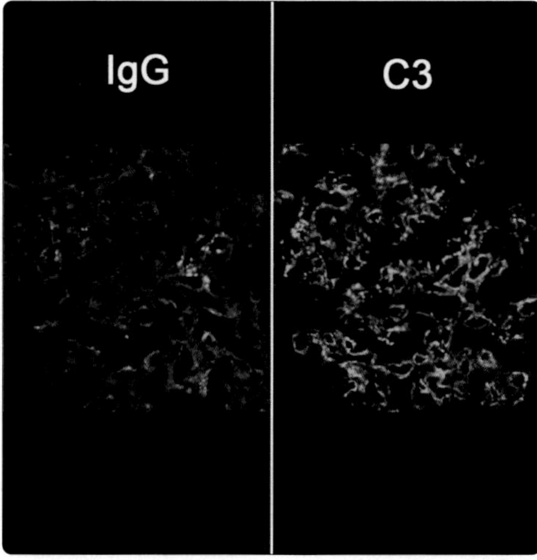

Strong C3 (3+) and Weak IgG (Trace)

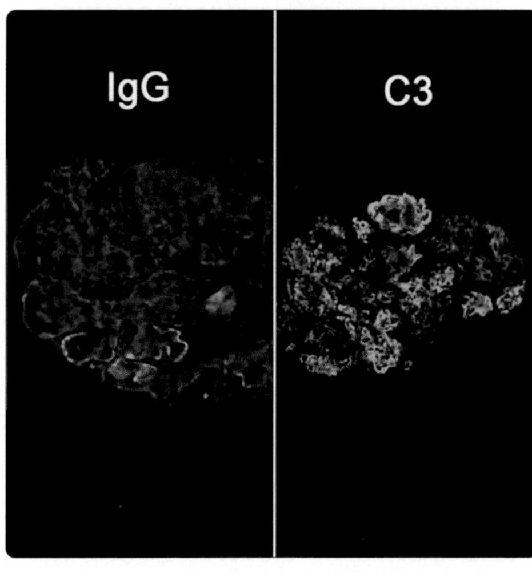

(Left) *In this case, C3 (3+) was stronger than IgG (trace-1+), and therefore the case meets the proposed criterion for C3 glomerulopathy. The patient had persistent low C3 and recurrence in a transplant at 4 months.* **(Right)** *C3 (3+) is stronger than IgG (trace), and therefore this biopsy of MPGN meets the proposed criterion for C3 glomerulopathy. The patient had persistent low C3 and normal C4. However, biopsy a year before had strong IgG staining (2+), showing C3GN can start with immune complexes.*

Strong C3 (3+) and IgG (2+)

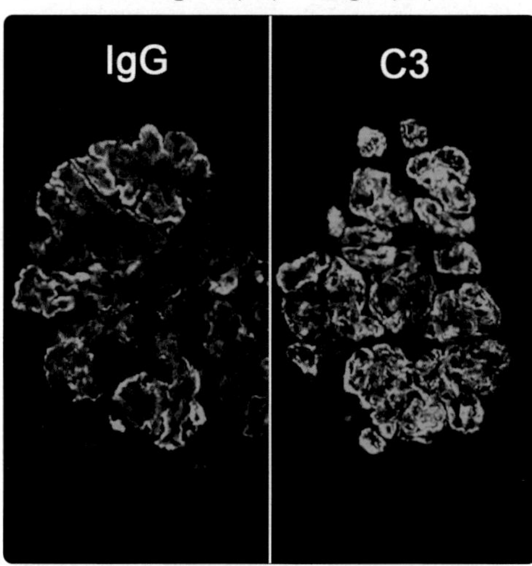

Strong C3 (3+) and IgG (2+)

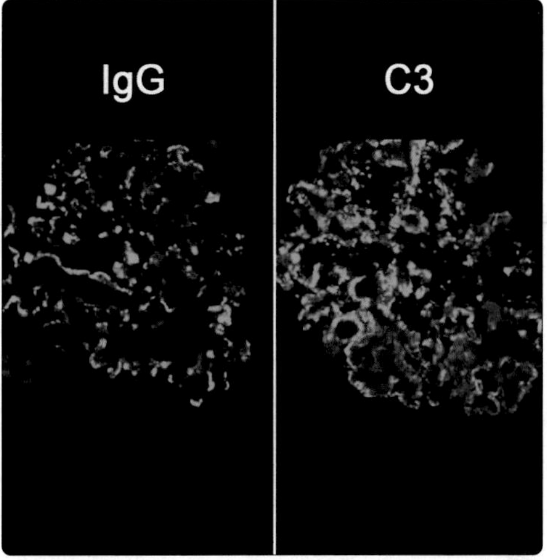

(Left) *In this case, C3 (3+) was only 1 level stronger than IgG (2+), and therefore does not meet the proposed criterion for C3 glomerulopathy. However, the patient had persistently low C3. Biopsy a year later had trace IgG and 3+ C3, meeting the criteria for C3GN, showing these categories can evolve with time.* **(Right)** *In this case, C3 is 3+ and IgG is 2+. C1q was also strong (3+). This case does not meet the proposed IF criteria for C3 glomerulopathy and is classified as MPGN with immune complexes (type I or III depending on EM).*

Dense Deposit Disease

KEY FACTS

TERMINOLOGY

- C3-related glomerulopathy manifested by broad, linear, extremely electron-dense deposits with C3 within GBM, mesangium, Bowman capsule, and TBM

CLINICAL ISSUES

- Rare (1-3 cases/million); affects both children and adults
- Etiology: (1) autoantibodies (e.g., C3 nephritic factor [C3NeF] in > 80%), (2) complement component gene mutations (e.g., complement factor H), (3) infections
- Proteinuria/hematuria, nephritic or nephrotic syndrome
- Ocular drusen (↓ visual acuity)
- Acquired partial lipodystrophy (APL) (~ 5%)
- No effective treatment, ~ 50% develop ESRD in 10-15 years
- Complement inhibitors under evaluation
- Usually recurs in renal allografts

MICROSCOPIC

- Varied glomerular pathology
  - Mesangial proliferation, acute exudative GN, membranoproliferative glomerulonephritis (MPGN), crescentic GN
- GBMs are thickened, eosinophilic, and refractile and stain strongly with PAS
- IF: Garland and granular mesangial pattern of C3 in 100%
  - Minimal immunoglobulin and C1q, almost always 2 fluorescence levels less than C3
- EM: Highly osmiophilic, dense deposits within GBM, mesangium, Bowman capsule, and TBM
- Deposits in Bruch membrane and spleen

TOP DIFFERENTIAL DIAGNOSES

- C3 glomerulonephritis; acute GN, MIDD; C4-dense deposit disease

DIAGNOSTIC CHECKLIST

- Hyperdense GBM deposits are pathognomic

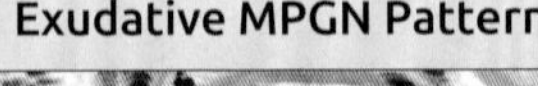

Exudative MPGN Pattern

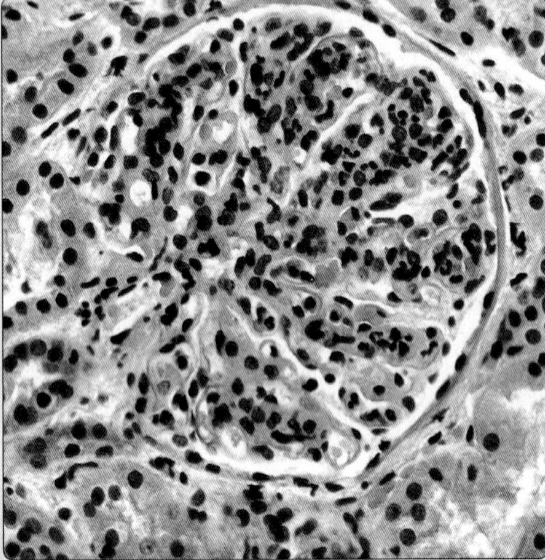

Dense Deposits in GBM

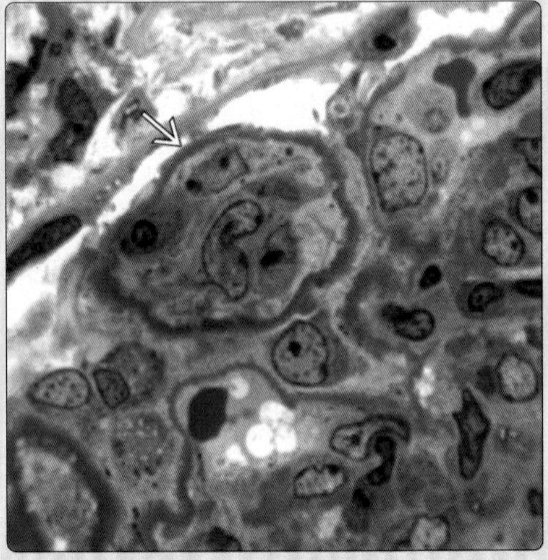

(Left) *Dense deposit disease (DDD) often presents with an membranoproliferative glomerulonephritis (MPGN) pattern, shown here in a biopsy from a 13-year-old boy with gross hematuria and proteinuria 3 days after a meningococcal septicemia. Serum C3 was undetectable and remained so on follow-up.* **(Right)** *On a toluidine blue "scout" section for EM, ribbon-like dense deposits* ➡ *can be seen within the thickened GBM.*

C3 Deposition in Glomerulus

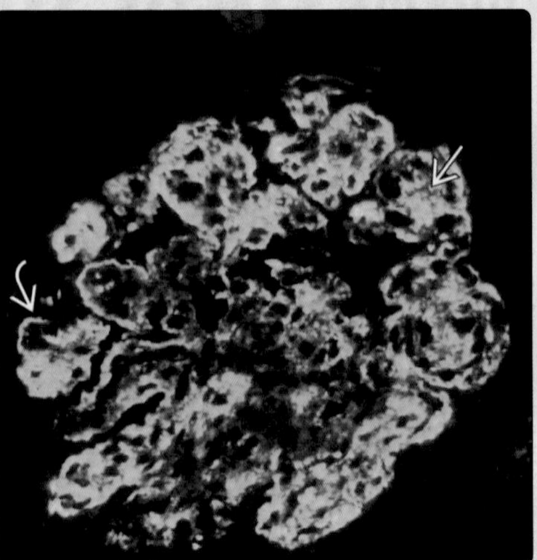

Hyperdense Deposits

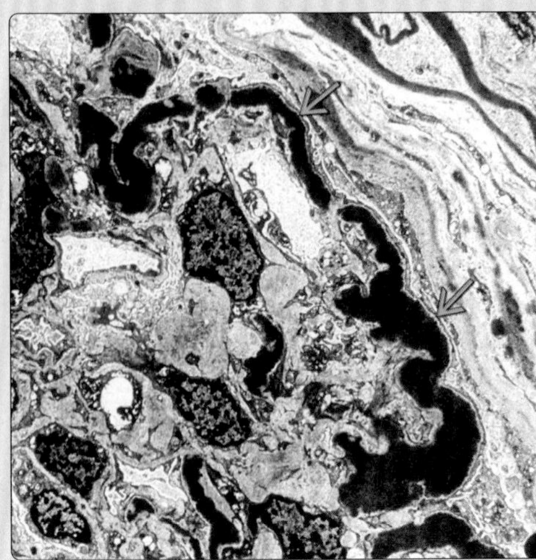

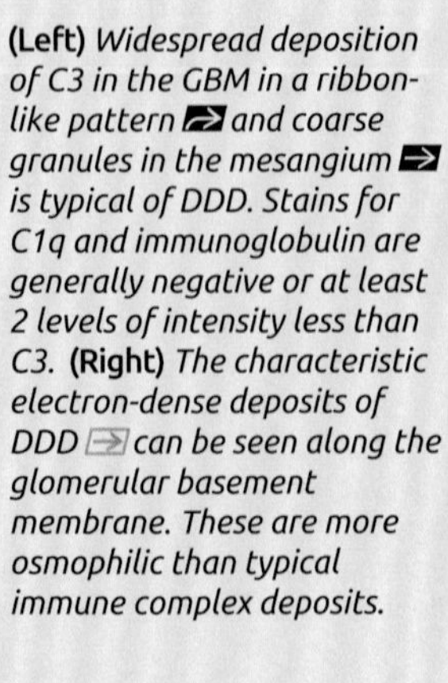

(Left) *Widespread deposition of C3 in the GBM in a ribbon-like pattern* ➡ *and coarse granules in the mesangium* ➡ *is typical of DDD. Stains for C1q and immunoglobulin are generally negative or at least 2 levels of intensity less than C3.* **(Right)** *The characteristic electron-dense deposits of DDD* ➡ *can be seen along the glomerular basement membrane. These are more osmophilic than typical immune complex deposits.*

TERMINOLOGY

Abbreviations

- Dense deposit disease (DDD)

Synonyms

- Membranoproliferative glomerulonephritis (MPGN), type II

Definitions

- C3-related glomerulopathy manifested by broad, linear, extremely electron-dense deposits with C3 within GBM, mesangium, Bowman capsule, and tubular basement membrane (TBM)
  - Once classified as variant of MPGN, but MPGN pattern present in < 50%
  - Hyperdense deposits by EM pathognomonic; therefore, DDD is preferred name
  - Initially reported by Galle and Berger in 1962

ETIOLOGY/PATHOGENESIS

Chronic Activation of Alternative Complement Pathway

- Autoantibodies (AutoAbs) to complement components
  - C3 nephritic factor (C3NeF): AutoAb to C3 convertase of alternative pathway (C3bBb) prevents inactivation, resulting in complement alternative pathway continuous activation
    - C3NeF present in > 80% (~ 100% children, ~ 40% adults)
    - C3NeF may also be present in healthy individuals
  - AutoAbs to complement factor H (CFH), factor B, or C3
- Genetic predisposition in complement component genes
  - 17% have factor H mutation, leads to ↓ plasma levels or affect its C3bBb decay function
  - *CFH*, *CFI*, *C3*, and *CFHR5* are rare allele variants associated with DDD
    - *CFH* Y402H is risk variant associated with DDD, not other forms of C3GN
  - *C3* mutation resistant to factor H in fluid phase described

Accumulation of Complement Components in Tissue

- Recruitment of leukocytes and inflammatory damage of glomerulus

Precipitating Factors

- Infection, various (pneumonia, upper respiratory)
  - Group A streptococcal or meningococcal infections
- Post chemotherapy for breast cancer
- ~ 20% of adults with DDD have monoclonal gammopathy, including myeloma
- ~ 70% of patients have monoclonal gammopathy of undetermined significance
- Some patients have multiple susceptibility factors

Animal Models

- *CFH* mutation in Norwegian Yorkshire pigs
- Mouse strain with *CFH* knockout
  - Prevented by combined factor B or factor I knockout
    - Proves necessity of alternative pathway convertase (C3bBb) and factor I-generated degradation products (iC3b, C3c, C3dg)

CLINICAL ISSUES

Epidemiology

- Incidence
  - Rare; estimated at 1-3 cases/million
    - Familial cases even rarer (~ 6 patients reported)
  - ~1% of renal biopsies
- Age
  - Mean age at diagnosis 19 years; 45-60% in children 5-15 years old; 40% > 60 years old
- Sex
  - F:M = 1.5:2

Presentation

- Hematuria (~ 90%); macrohematuria (~ 15%)
- Proteinuria (~ 95%), may rapidly fluctuate and sometimes, nephrotic range (~ 60%)
- Renal insufficiency (~ 50%)
- Acquired partial lipodystrophy (APL) (3-5%)
  - Loss of subcutaneous fat in upper 1/2 of body
  - ~ 83% have ↓ C3 levels & polyclonal C3NeF
  - ~ 20% develop MPGN after median of 8 years after onset of lipodystrophy
- Ocular drusen common (~ 10% develop ↓ visual acuity)

Laboratory Tests

- ↓ serum C3 in ~ 80% of patients (↓ C3dg & C3d)
  - More common in children (100%) than adults (40%)
- C3NeF (Ab to C3bBb) present in > 80%
  - Persists in > 50%
- *CFH* mutations 17%

Treatment

- Drugs
  - Steroids, immunosuppression not yet proven effective
  - Complement inhibitors such as Eculizumab (anti-CD5 Ab) under evaluation
  - In patients with *CFH* mutations, plasma exchange and recombinant CFH

Prognosis

- Spontaneous remission rare
- ~ 50% develop end-stage renal disease (ESRD) within 10-15 years
  - Mean time to ESRD = 5 years in adults, 20 years in children
- Recurs in almost all renal allografts
  - ~ 50% of allografts ultimately fail, typically in first 3 years

MICROSCOPIC

Histologic Features

- Glomeruli
  - Membranoproliferative GN pattern (25-45%)
    - Mesangial proliferation, GBM thickened ± duplication
    - Eosinophilic and refractile and brightly PAS(+); fuchsinophilic on trichrome
    - DDD deposits stain poorly with Jones stain
  - Mild mesangial hypercellularity (30-50%)
    - Normal GBM by light microscopy
  - Crescentic GN (10-20%); primarily children
    - Focal crescents in > 50% of cases

- Acute GN (10-20%)
  - Poly- or mononuclear cells, mesangial hypercellularity, normal GBM thickness
- Necrosis uncommon (~ 15%)
- Focal, segmental, and global glomerulosclerosis, late
- Transitions
  - Progression of mesangial proliferative GN → MPGN pattern
  - Resolution of crescentic GN → mesangial proliferative GN
- Tubules and interstitium
  - Usually not affected early in disease
  - ± thickened TBM due to deposits
  - Tubular atrophy and interstitial fibrosis develop late in disease
- Vessels: No specific changes
- Follow-up biopsies: ↓ acute glomerular inflammation and ↑ glomerulosclerosis, tubular atrophy, fibrosis

ANCILLARY TESTS

Immunofluorescence

- Prominent C3 deposits (100%)
  - Ribbon-like (garland) pattern in GBM
    - ± railroad track or double contour pattern along GBM
  - Coarse mesangial spherules or ring-like deposits
  - C3c appears to be main constituent of dense deposits
    - Some C3d(+) (absent from C3c): Detects C3b, iC3b, and C3d
  - Broad linear TBM deposits (~ 60%) & Bowman capsule deposits (~ 30%)
  - C3 present before dense deposits detected in transplants
- Focal Ig deposits in minority
  - IgM (35%), IgG (25%), IgA (15%), C1q (10%)
  - Almost always 2 levels of fluorescence intensity less than C3 (88%)
  - Paucity of Ig indicates that dense deposits are not immune complexes
- DDD variant with C4d and no C3 associated with lectin activation

Electron Microscopy

- Highly osmiophilic dense deposits in lamina densa of GBM, resulting in very electron-dense appearance
  - Lack organized substructure and have dark, homogeneous, smudgy, hazy appearance
  - Segmental, discontinuous, or diffuse pattern of dense deposits along GBM
    - Sausage string pattern
  - ± subendothelial deposits ± same deposits in mesangium and small vessels
  - Similar deposits in Bowman capsule (~ 45%) and TBM (~ 50%)
  - Reason for osmophilia unknown; may be due to unsaturated lipids associated with apolipoprotein E (ApoE) accumulation
- ± subepithelial "humps" (~ 30%) less dense than intramembranous deposits
- Podocyte injury eventually occurs with actin cytoskeleton and slit diaphragm disruption, resulting in podocyte hypertrophy, detachment, and death

Special Stains

- Deposits stain with fluorescent dye thioflavin T

Laser Capture-Mass Spectroscopy

- Deposits contain C3, C5, C8α, C9, CFH-related protein 1 (FHR1), clusterin, vitronectin, and ApoE
- In contrast, immune complex GN rarely had C9 or vitronectin; none had ApoE

Other Organs

- Deposits in choroidal blood vessels and splenic sinusoidal basement membrane
- Deposits along choriocapillaris-Bruch membrane-retinal pigment epithelial interface
  - Responsible for ocular drusen detectable in 2nd decade of life
  - Similar to age-related macular degeneration

DIFFERENTIAL DIAGNOSIS

C3 Glomerulonephritis

- Lack hyperdense deposits, duplication more prominent

Acute Glomerulonephritis (AGN)

- IgG present and lacks hyperdense deposits
- DDD can follow typical AGN

Monoclonal Ig Deposition Disease (MIDD)

- By definition, has Ig deposition (single light chain &/or heavy chain)
- May have DDD and monoclonal gammopathy

C4 Dense Deposit Disease

- C4d present in deposits, but little or no C3
- Lectin pathway activated rather than alternative pathway

DIAGNOSTIC CHECKLIST

Clinically Relevant Pathologic Features

- ESRD associated with older age & higher creatinine at presentation, "humps" possibly crescents

Pathologic Interpretation Pearls

- Most important findings are very dense, osmiophilic deposits on EM

SELECTED REFERENCES

1. Figuères ML et al: Heterogeneous histologic and clinical evolution in 3 cases of dense deposit disease with long-term follow-up. Hum Pathol. ePub, 2014
2. Prasto J et al: Streptococcal infection as possible trigger for dense deposit disease (C3 glomerulopathy). Eur J Pediatr. 173(6):767-72, 2014
3. Sethi S et al: C4 dense-deposit disease. N Engl J Med. 370(8):784-6, 2014
4. Xiao X et al: C3 glomerulopathy: the genetic and clinical findings in dense deposit disease and C3 glomerulonephritis. Semin Thromb Hemost. 40(4):465-71, 2014
5. Barbour TD et al: Dense deposit disease and C3 glomerulopathy. Semin Nephrol. 33(6):493-507, 2013
6. Herlitz LC et al: Pathology after eculizumab in dense deposit disease and C3 GN. J Am Soc Nephrol. 23(7):1229-37, 2012
7. Servais A et al: Acquired and genetic complement abnormalities play a critical role in dense deposit disease and other C3 glomerulopathies. Kidney Int. 82(4):454-64, 2012

Intracapillary Neutrophils

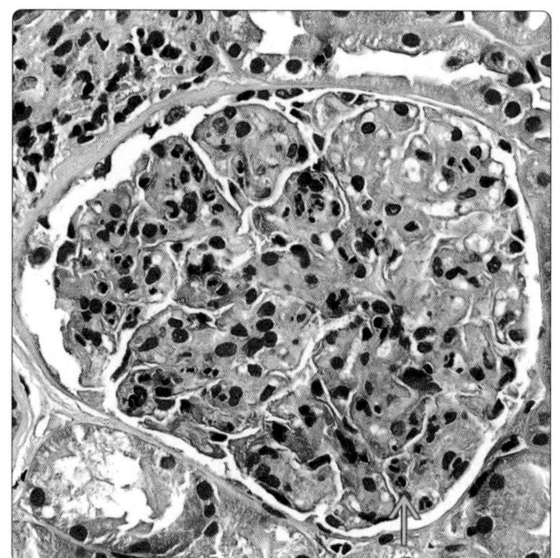

Mesangial Hypercellularity

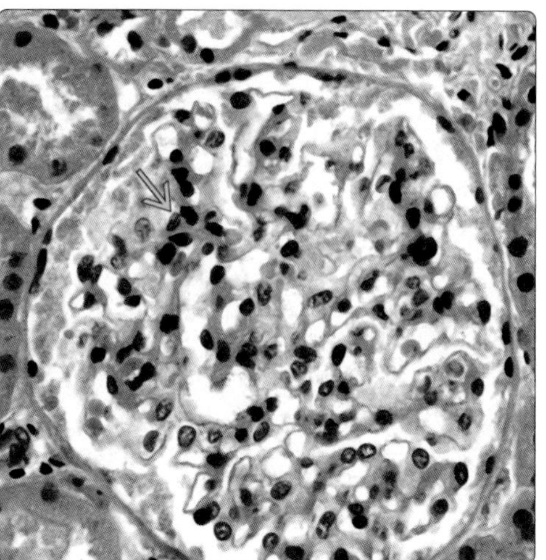

(Left) *Approximately 15% of DDD cases show an acute glomerulonephritis-type morphology with a vaguely lobular configuration of the glomerular tuft and numerous intracapillary neutrophils* ➩. **(Right)** *About 40% of DDD biopsies present with a mild mesangial hypercellularity* ➩ *and a normal GBM by light microscopy. This 8-year-old boy had repeated microhematuria with Strep infections. The diagnosis requires EM, which showed the characteristic dense deposits.*

Crescent

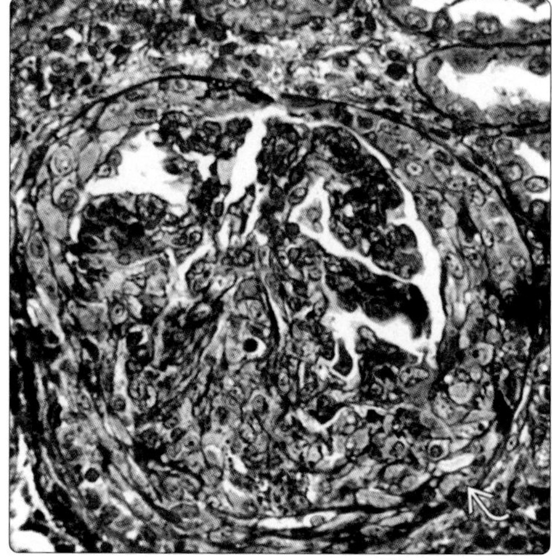

Decreased Jones Staining

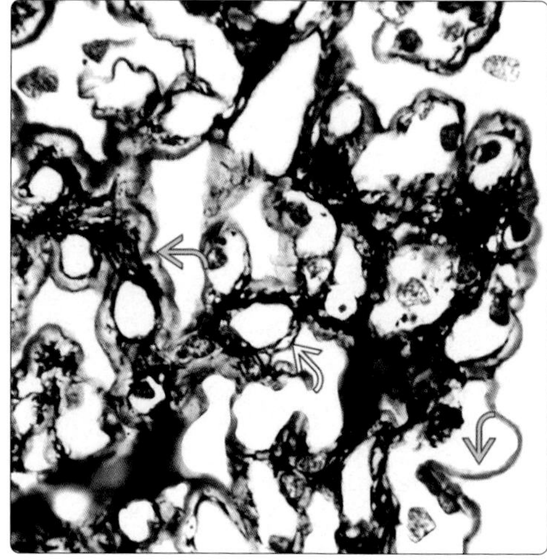

(Left) *Crescents* ➩, *as seen in this biopsy from a 13-year-old girl, are common in DDD and extensive in ~ 15% of cases. Characteristic hyperdense deposits and subepithelial "humps" were evident by EM.* **(Right)** *The Jones stain in DDD shows decreased staining of the GBM* ➩, *which is normally argyrophilic. The loss is due to the dense deposits in the GBM. Double contours are segmentally present* ➩ *but uncommon, in contrast to MPGN, type I.*

GBM Thickening and Intracapillary Inflammation

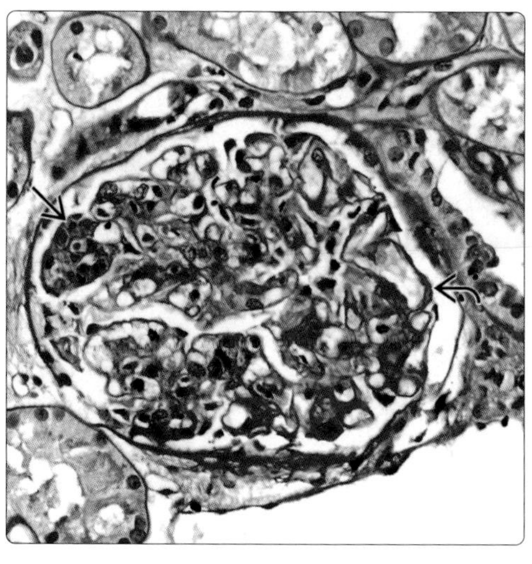

GBM Thickening and Glomerular Inflammation

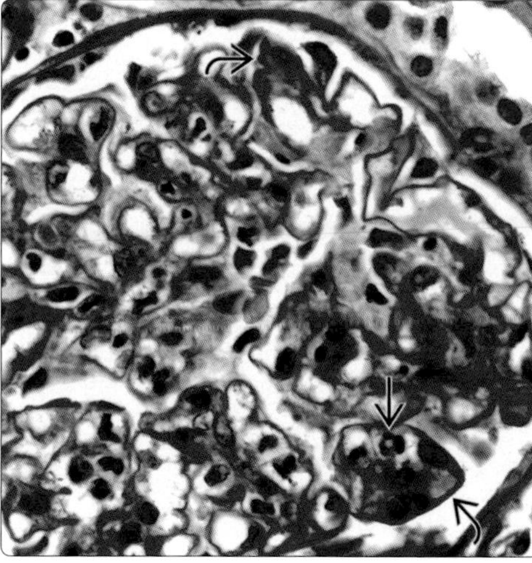

(Left) *This case of DDD has PAS(+) thickening of the GBM* ➩ *and a mild acute glomerulonephritis-type morphology with increased numbers of inflammatory cells in glomerular capillaries* ➩. **(Right)** *DDD is characterized by segmental PAS(+) thickening of the glomerular basement membrane (GBM)* ➩, *visible by light microscopy and variable degrees of inflammation, seen here with neutrophils* ➩.

(Left) *DDD classically has prominent bright granular deposits of C3 in the mesangium → and segmentally linear → deposits along the GBM. Immunoglobulins and C1q are typically absent or minimally present.* (Right) *The garland pattern → of GBM staining for C3 in DDD is illustrated in a biopsy from a 9-year-old girl who developed end-stage renal disease 25 years later. Bowman capsule → also stains, and the distinctive dark cores of mesangial deposits → can be appreciated.*

Mesangial C3 Deposits

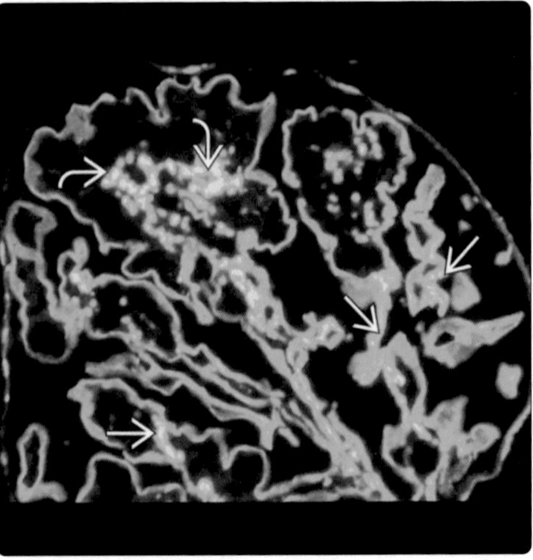

Mesangial and Garland GBM C3

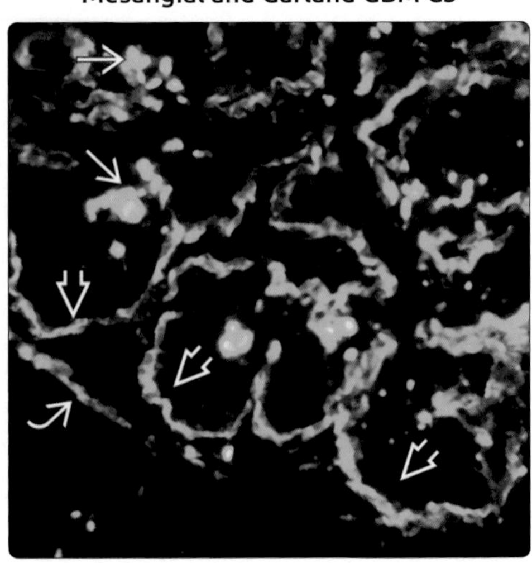

(Left) *This case of DDD has prominent bright deposits of C3 in the mesangium → and only segmental deposits in the GBM →.* (Right) *Scattered granular deposits of IgM are sometimes found in DDD, as illustrated in this case. IgG is almost always negative or minimally present.*

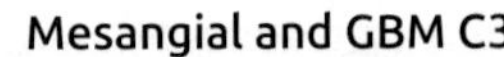

Mesangial and GBM C3

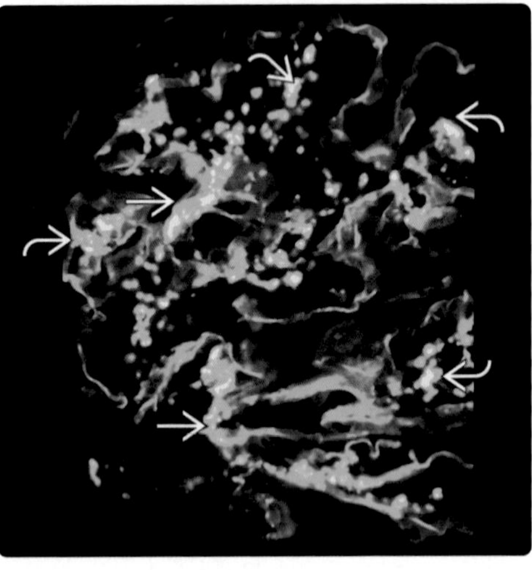

Granular IgM

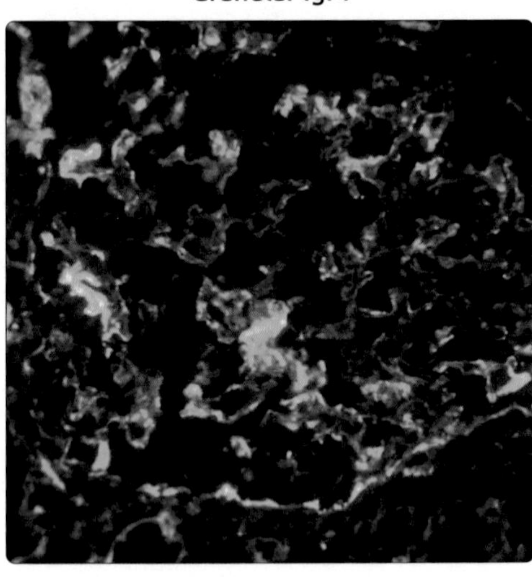

(Left) *The tubular basement membranes (TBM) in DDD focally contain dense deposits and stain for C3 in a broad segmental pattern →, as illustrated in this case of familial DDD in a 35-year-old man who received a renal transplant. His daughter also had DDD in a biopsy at age 6 years.* (Right) *Thioflavin T stain of a case of DDD viewed under fluorescence illumination (UV) is shown. The dense deposits → characteristically have a blue autofluorescence, which is not seen in MPGN, type I.*

TBM C3

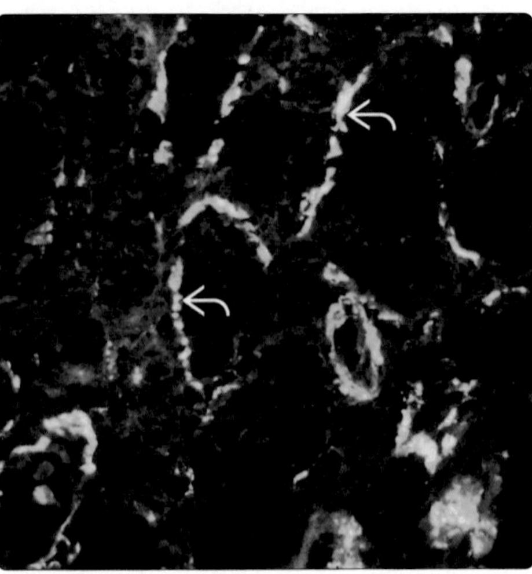

Thioflavin T in DDD

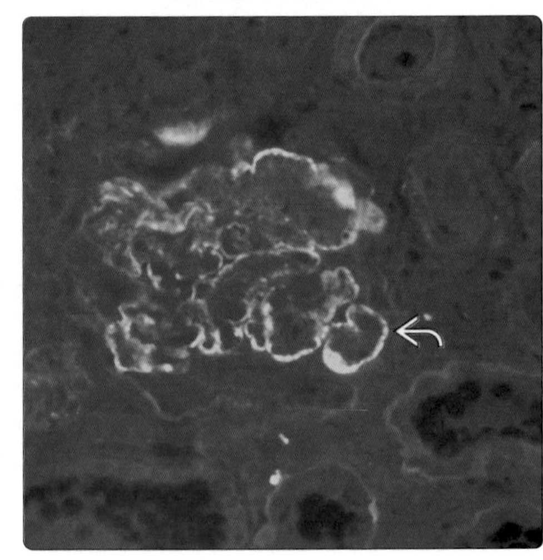

Dense GBM Deposits

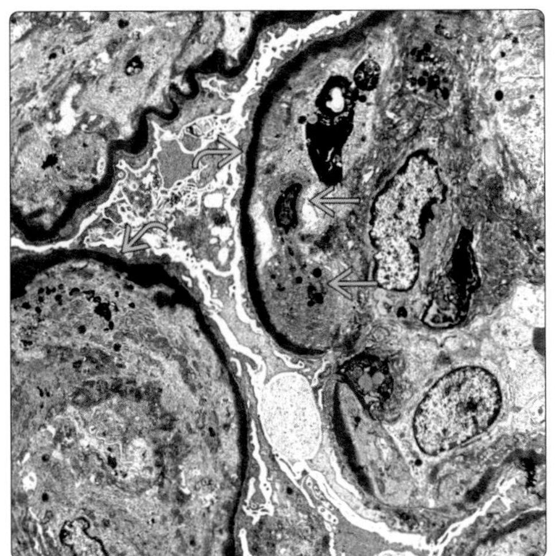

"Hump" and GBM Deposits

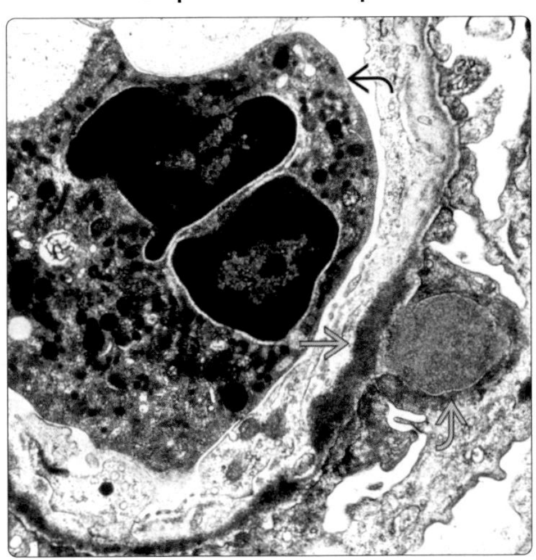

(Left) *The classic lesions in DDD are extremely electron-dense deposits in the GBM ➚ and mesangium. This biopsy from a 9-year-old girl also has prominent intracapillary inflammatory cells ➙. She developed renal failure over the next 25 years and received a transplant.* **(Right)** *This case shows DDD in a 13-year-old girl who presented with acute glomerulonephritis, clinically. In addition to the distinctive hyperdense deposits ➙ in the GBM, there is a subepithelial "hump" ➚, which has lower density. A neutrophil is in the capillary loop ➚.*

Segmental GBM Deposits

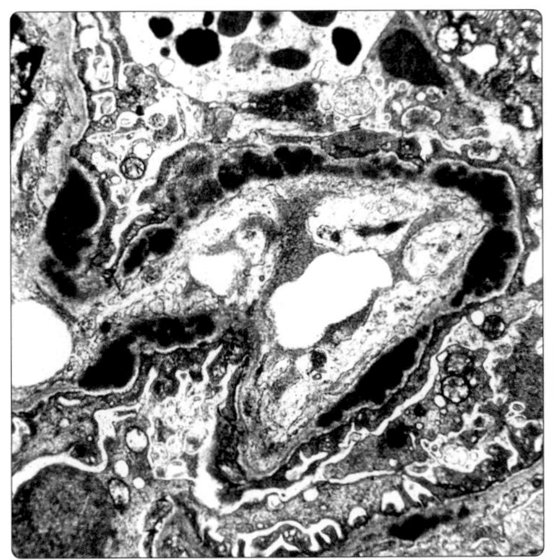

Dense Deposits

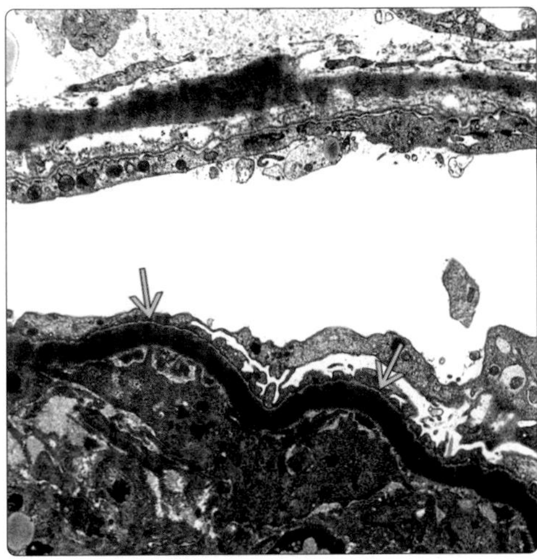

(Left) *This case of DDD in an 8-year-old boy who had repeated episodes of gross hematuria associated with streptococcal infections shows a variant pattern with interrupted, segmental deposition in the GBM.* **(Right)** *Electron-dense deposits ➙ can be seen along the glomerular basement membrane in a case of dense deposit disease.*

Subendothelial Deposits

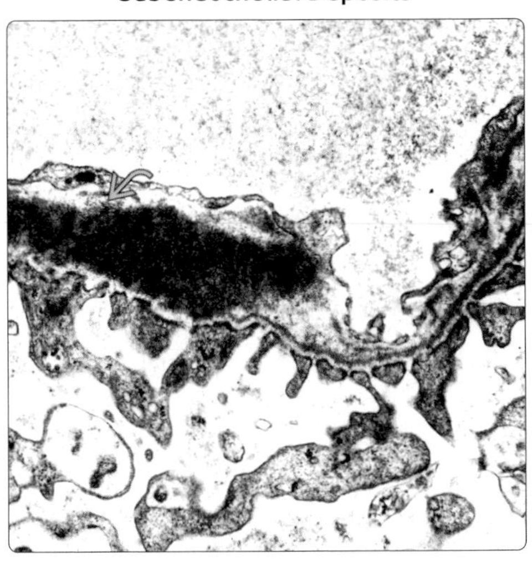

TBM Deposits

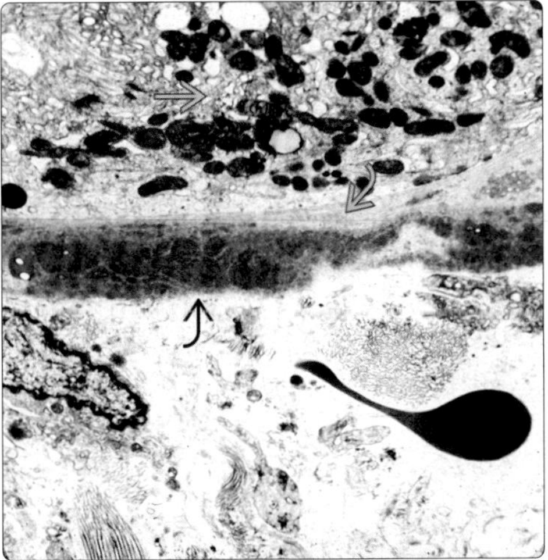

(Left) *Sometimes the dense deposits in DDD are predominantly subendothelial, as in this case ➚. This may be an early stage of the disease.* **(Right)** *The dense deposits of DDD are found in the tubular basement membrane (TBM), as illustrated here ➚. A layer of uninvolved TBM can be seen ➚ between the tubular epithelial cells ➙ and the dense deposits. Other sites with deposits are the splenic sinusoids, the choroidal vessels, and the retina (ocular drusen).*

C3 Glomerulonephritis

KEY FACTS

TERMINOLOGY

- Glomerulonephritis secondary to dysfunction of alternative complement pathway
- Dominant C3 deposits by immunofluorescence with intermediately electron-dense deposits in glomeruli
- Member of C3 glomerulopathy group, which includes dense deposit disease (DDD)

ETIOLOGY/PATHOGENESIS

- Genetic and acquired defects in alternative complement pathway
  - Mutations: *CFH, CFH5R, CFHR3-1, CFI, CD46*
  - Autoantibodies to C3 convertase (C3NeF)

CLINICAL ISSUES

- Heterogeneous presenting features
  - Proteinuria
  - Hematuria
  - Hypertension
- Low C3 in ~ 40%; normal C4
- Need to evaluate for complement system abnormalities

MICROSCOPIC

- Various glomerular patterns by light microscopy
  - MPGN
  - Mesangial and subepithelial to intramembranous deposits without MPGN
- C3 deposits in mesangium and GBM
- Significantly less immunoglobulin deposits
- Amorphous mesangial and subendothelial deposits by EM

TOP DIFFERENTIAL DIAGNOSES

- Dense deposit disease
- MPGN with immune complex deposits
- Postinfectious glomerulonephritis

DIAGNOSTIC CHECKLIST

- Key feature is C3 with little or no immunoglobulin and deposits less dense than those seen in DDD

Mesangial Proliferation

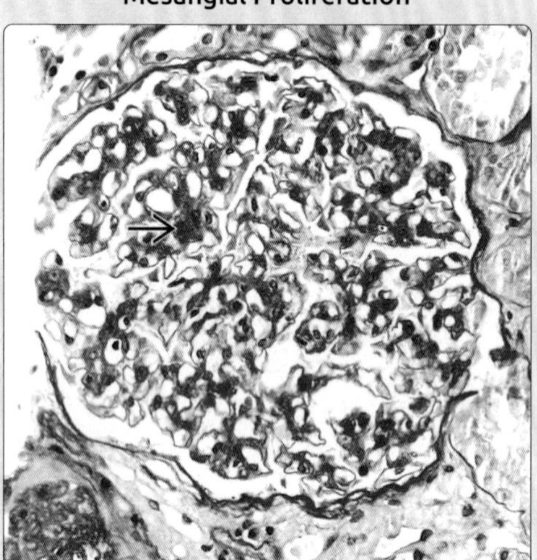

MPGN Pattern

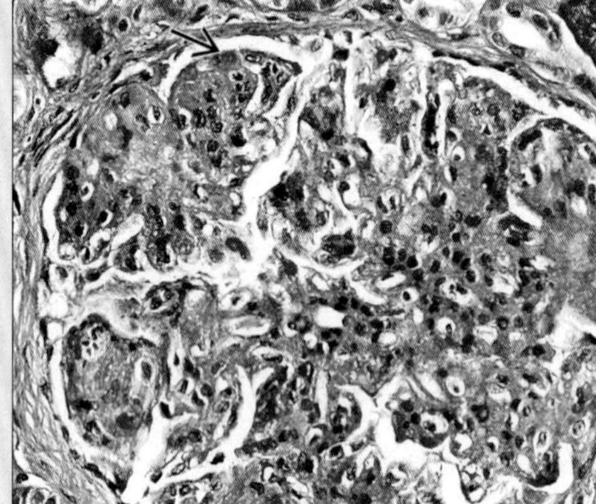

(Left) *Mesangioproliferative ⇨ pattern of C3 glomerulonephritis is shown. Expansion and hypercellularity of the mesangium is present without duplication or thickening of the glomerular basement membrane (GBM) that define the MPGN pattern.* **(Right)** *C3GN with a membranoproliferative glomerulonephritis (MPGN) pattern shows lobular accentuation of the glomerulus. Subendothelial deposits ⇨, which appear red on this trichrome stain, can be seen.*

Strong Staining for C3 in Glomerulus

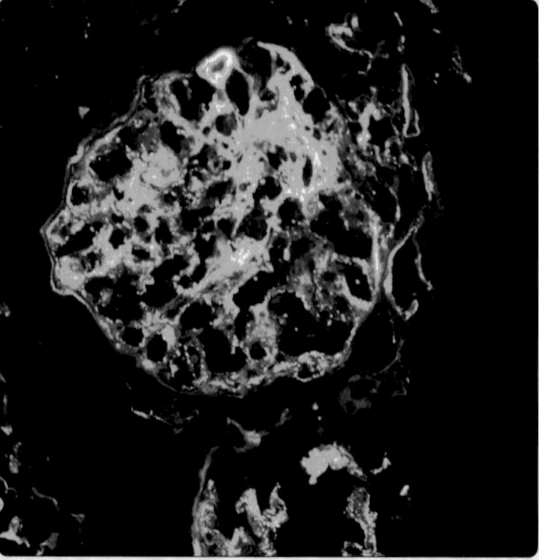

Intramembranous and Mesangial Deposits

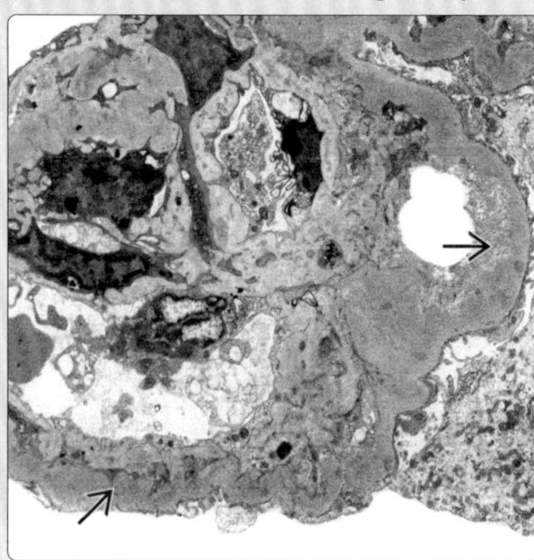

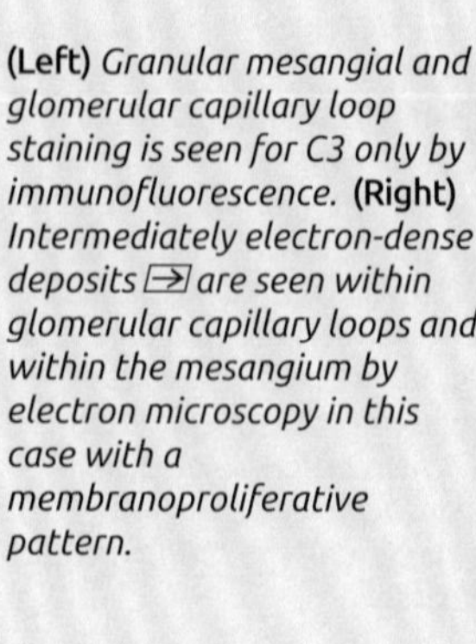

(Left) *Granular mesangial and glomerular capillary loop staining is seen for C3 only by immunofluorescence.* **(Right)** *Intermediately electron-dense deposits ⇨ are seen within glomerular capillary loops and within the mesangium by electron microscopy in this case with a membranoproliferative pattern.*

TERMINOLOGY

Abbreviations

- C3 glomerulonephritis (C3GN)

Synonyms

- Primary glomerulonephritis with isolated C3 deposits
- Glomerulonephritis with dominant C3

Definitions

- Glomerulonephritis with isolated C3 deposits secondary to dysfunction of alternative complement pathway and electron-dense deposits in glomeruli not as electron dense as dense deposit disease (DDD)
  - Some entities previously classified as type I or III membranoproliferative glomerulonephritis (MPGN) belong in this category
  - Some cases have minimal immunoglobulin deposition (threshold not yet defined)
- C3 glomerulonephritis is a member of C3 glomerulopathy spectrum of glomerular diseases, which also includes DDD and CFH5R nephropathy, diseases that share dependence on alternative pathway dysregulation and C3 dominant deposition

ETIOLOGY/PATHOGENESIS

Dysregulation of Alternative Complement Pathway

- Initial activation of complement and complement amplification via alternative pathway amplification loop
- Defect in complement regulatory proteins or complement activators
- Both acquired and inherited abnormalities in alternative complement pathway may be present in single patient with C3GN

CLINICAL ISSUES

Epidemiology

- Age
  - Mean presentation: 30 years; range: 7 to > 70 years

Presentation

- Heterogeneous presenting features
- Proteinuria, mild to nephrotic range (average 3.6 g/d)
- Microhematuria (~ 64%)
- Hypertension
- Chronic renal failure (Cr >1.5 mg/dl ~ 46%)

Laboratory Tests

- Complement levels
  - Serum C3 levels decreased in ~ 40% of patients
  - Serum C4 level normal
- Specialized complement tests
  - Factor H, factor I, factor B
  - Serum soluble membrane attack complex
    - Increased levels in some patients
  - Alternative complement pathway functional and hemolytic assays
- Autoantibodies
  - C3 nephritic factor (C3NeF) detectable in 45%
  - Anti-C3 convertase and anti-factor H autoantibodies
- Genetic tests
  - Factor H, factor I, membrane co-factor protein (MCP; CD46)
    - H402 allele in cases with factor H mutation
  - Complement factor H-related protein family: CFHR1-5
    - *CFHR5* mutation causing C3GN identified in families of Cypriot origin
  - Complement factor B, C3
- Circulating monoclonal immunoglobulin in ~ 30%
  - Older patients (mean: 54 years)
  - Underlying monoclonal gammopathy of undetermined significance (MGUS) or hematologic malignancy
  - Causal link suspected but not yet proved

Treatment

- Surgical approaches
  - Renal transplantation
    - C3GN recurs in ~ 67% of allografts
    - Graft failure in 50% with recurrent C3GN
    - Median time to graft loss is 77 months post transplant
- Drugs
  - Treatment approach depends on cause
    - Plasma infusions for complement factor deficiencies
    - Plasmapheresis or rituximab for autoantibodies
    - Chemotherapy if underlying hematologic malignancy
  - Steroid responsive in some patients
  - Inhibition of complement pathway
    - C5 inhibition with eculizumab (experimental)
      - May be effective in a subset of patients
    - New drugs under development

Prognosis

- Variable; some progress to end-stage renal disease while others retain normal renal function

MICROSCOPIC

Histologic Features

- Glomeruli
  - Mesangial and subepithelial to intramembranous deposits without MPGN pattern
    - No mesangial proliferation
    - No or minimal glomerular basement membrane (GBM) duplication
  - Membranoproliferative glomerulonephritis (MPGN), type I pattern
    - Mesangial hypercellularity
    - Mainly subendothelial and mesangial deposits; may have some subepithelial deposits
    - Diffuse GBM duplication
    - Renal disease more severe in patients with MPGN pattern than non-MPGN pattern
  - Endocapillary proliferation
    - May show neutrophils (mimicking postinfectious glomerulonephritis) &/or mononuclear cells
  - Crescents occasionally prominent
- Tubules and interstitium
  - Interstitial fibrosis and tubular atrophy, usually mild to moderate
- Vessels
  - No specific changes

Complement Pathway Abnormalities Associated With C3GN

Autoantibodies Against Complement Pathway Components (Acquired Factors)	Mutations in Complement Regulatory Factors	Allele Variants or Mutations in Complement Factors
C3 convertase (C3bBb)	Factor H	Factor H
Factor H	Factor I	C3
Factor I	Membrane cofactor protein/CD46	Membrane cofactor protein
Factor B	CFHR5	
	CFHR3-1	
One or more acquired or inherited abnormalities may be present in a single patient.		

Sethi S and Fervenza FC: Membranoproliferative glomerulonephritis--a new look at an old entity. N Engl J Med. 366(12):1119-31, 2012

ANCILLARY TESTS

Immunofluorescence

- Prominent granular C3 deposits in mesangium and GBMs
- Little or no immunoglobulin
  - IgG, IgM, IgA and C1q, at least 2 levels of intensity less than C3
- C4d typically shows little or no staining
- Follow-up biopsies show same pattern in 57%, others gain or lose immunoglobulin intensity

Electron Microscopy

- Amorphous deposits in mesangium
- Subendothelial electron-dense deposits (MPGN pattern) &/or scattered subepithelial deposits, intramembranous deposits
  - Often permeates GBM (MPGN 3 pattern of Strife and Anders)
  - Subepithelial hump-shaped deposits may be present
- Deposits may be electron dense or intermediately dense
  - Not as dense as dense deposit disease (DDD)
  - "Fluffy" or indistinct borders of deposits
  - Rarely, a few deposits may show fibrillary substructure that merges with electron-dense deposits
- Some cases may show overlapping features with DDD with intramembranous deposits

Mass Spectrometry

- Deposits composed of alternative and terminal complement pathway components, similar to DDD

DIFFERENTIAL DIAGNOSIS

MPGN With Immune Complex Deposits

- Prominent immunoglobulin deposition by IF along with C3
- Associated with infection, autoimmune disease, paraproteins

Dense Deposit Disease

- Deposits more electron dense

C4 Dense Deposit Disease

- C4 and C4d deposits rather than C3

Postinfectious Glomerulonephritis

- Usually shows immunoglobulin deposits by IF
  - C3 can persist longer than immunoglobulin
- Acute exudative pattern with numerous neutrophils
- Resolving postinfectious GN may not show neutrophils
- History of infection not decisive because C3GN may first manifest at time of infection
- Hypocomplementemia transient

Atypical Postinfectious Glomerulonephritis

- Associated with abnormalities in alternative complement pathway
- Probably predisposes to acute GN response in infection

Infection-Related Glomerulonephritis/Endocarditis-Associated Glomerulonephritis

- May have C3 dominant pattern (e.g., *Bartonella*)

Membranous-Like Glomerulonephritis With Masked IgG-Kappa Deposits

- IF on pronase-digested paraffin sections reveals monotypic IgG kappa staining
- Large subepithelial deposits by EM; may be hump-shaped

Focal Segmental Glomerulosclerosis

- Nonspecific "trapping" of C3 in scarred glomeruli usually with IgM
- No deposits by electron microscopy

DIAGNOSTIC CHECKLIST

Pathologic Interpretation Pearls

- Key features are C3 with little or no immunoglobulin and deposits less dense by EM than DDD

SELECTED REFERENCES

1. Le Quintrec M et al: Eculizumab for treatment of rapidly progressive C3 glomerulopathy. Am J Kidney Dis. 65(3):484-9, 2015
2. Sethi S et al: C4d as a Diagnostic Tool in Proliferative GN. J Am Soc Nephrol. ePub, 2015 May 19
3. Hou J et al: Toward a working definition of C3 glomerulopathy by immunofluorescence. Kidney Int. 85(2):450-56, 2014
4. Zand L et al: Clinical findings, pathology, and outcomes of C3GN after kidney transplantation. J Am Soc Nephrol. 25(5):1110-7, 2014
5. Zhang Y et al: Defining the Complement Biomarker Profile of C3 Glomerulopathy. Clin J Am Soc Nephrol. ePub, 2014
6. Pickering MC et al: C3 glomerulopathy: consensus report. Kidney Int. 84(6):1079-89, 2013
7. Sethi S et al: Atypical postinfectious glomerulonephritis is associated with abnormalities in the alternative pathway of complement. Kidney Int. 83(2):293-9, 2013
8. Gale DP et al: Identification of a mutation in complement factor H-related protein 5 in patients of Cypriot origin with glomerulonephritis. Lancet. 376(9743):794-801, 2010

MPGN Pattern

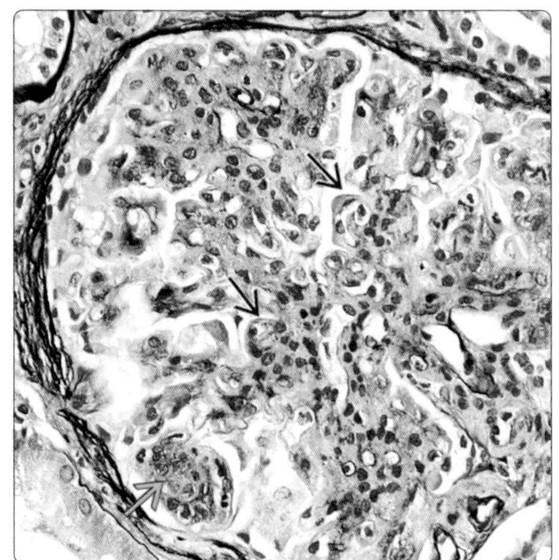

Mesangial and Endocapillary Proliferation

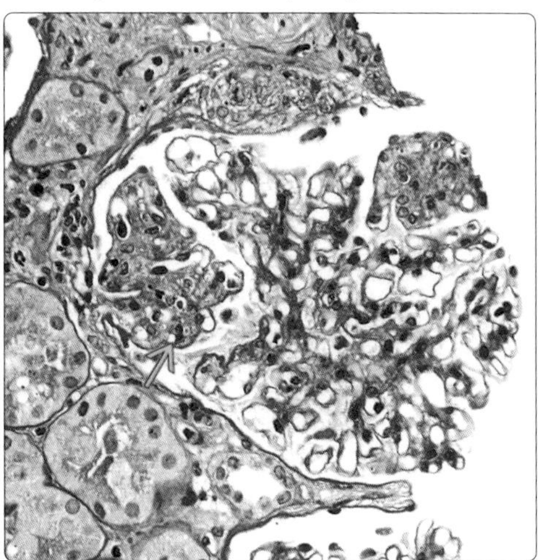

(Left) *This example of C3GN shows a membranoproliferative pattern of injury, with mesangial hypercellularity* ⇨ *and glomerular basement membrane duplication* ➡. **(Right)** *A biopsy from a patient with chronic kidney disease and hematuria showed C3GN with segmental endocapillary proliferation* ⇨. *The patient had a monoclonal IgG lambda protein in the serum. C3GN is sometimes associated with monoclonal proteins, although glomeruli only stain for C3 by immunofluorescence.*

MPGN Pattern

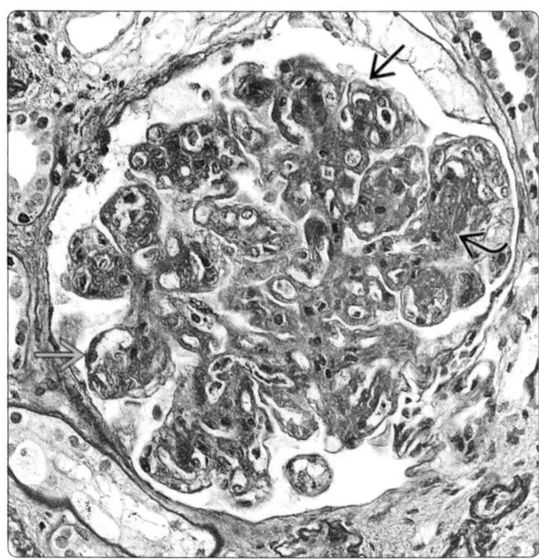

Mesangial Proliferation and Segmental Scars

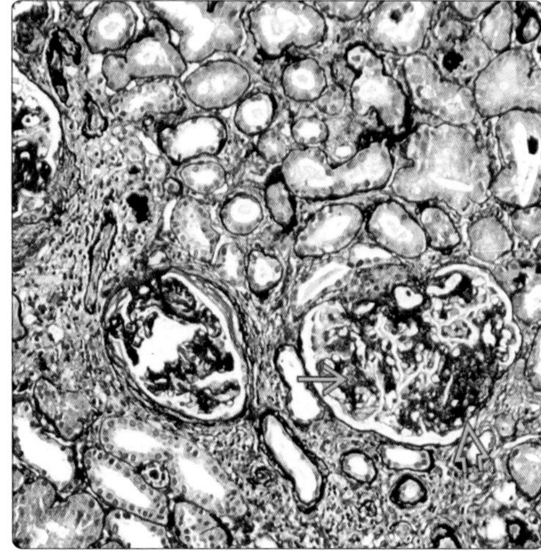

(Left) *This glomerulus with C3GN shows an MPGN pattern, with lobular accentuation of the glomerulus, mesangial expansion* ➬ *and hypercellularity, and glomerular basement membrane duplication* ➡ *and thickening* ⇨. **(Right)** *C3GN with a mesangioproliferative* ⇨ *and segmental sclerosing* ⇨ *pattern is shown. The patient was a young man with nephrotic-range proteinuria and normal renal function.*

C3

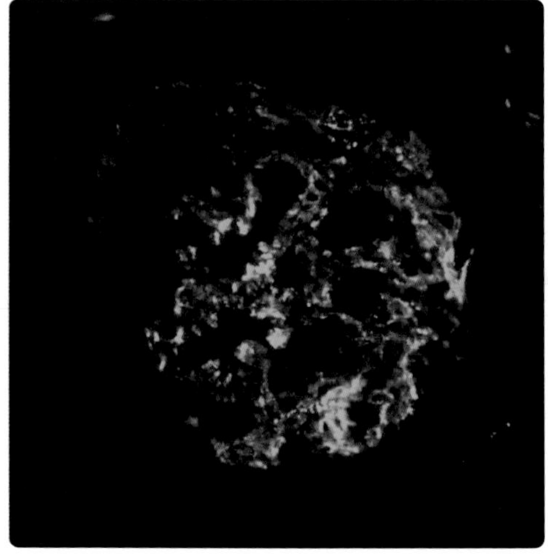

Negative IgG

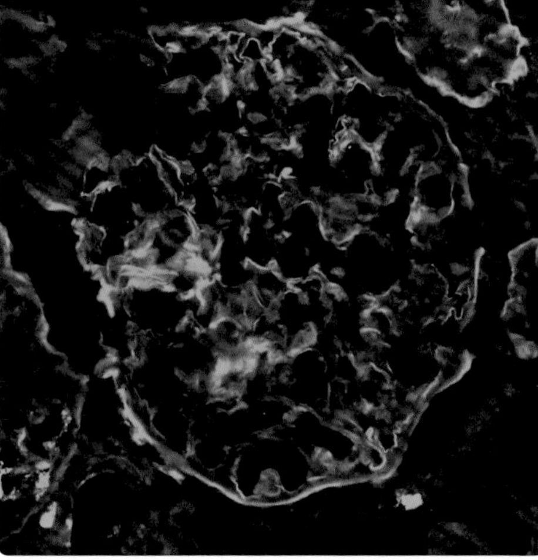

(Left) *Immunofluorescence for C3 (2-3+) stains a glomerulus with C3GN. By light microscopy, the glomeruli in this case showed mild mesangial expansion and segmental and global glomerulosclerosis.* **(Right)** *IF is negative for IgG and for other immunoglobulins. Negativity for immunoglobulins, with only staining for C3, raises the possibility of C3GN, and evaluation for complement system abnormalities is warranted.*

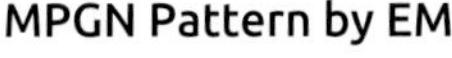

MPGN Pattern by EM

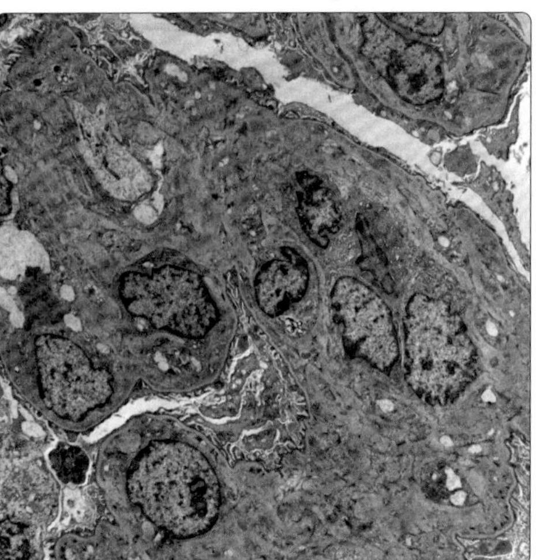
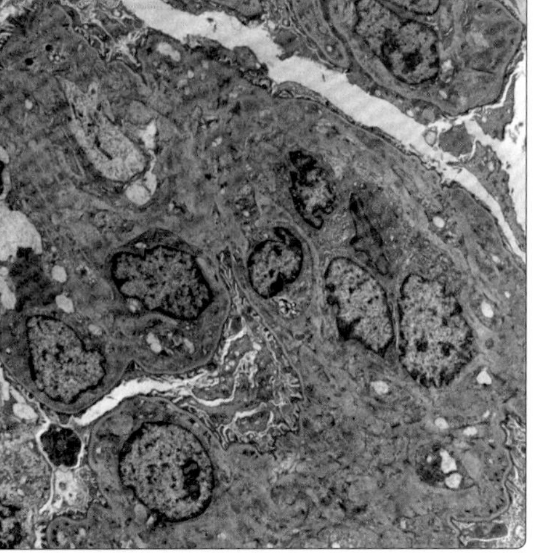

Subepithelial Hump

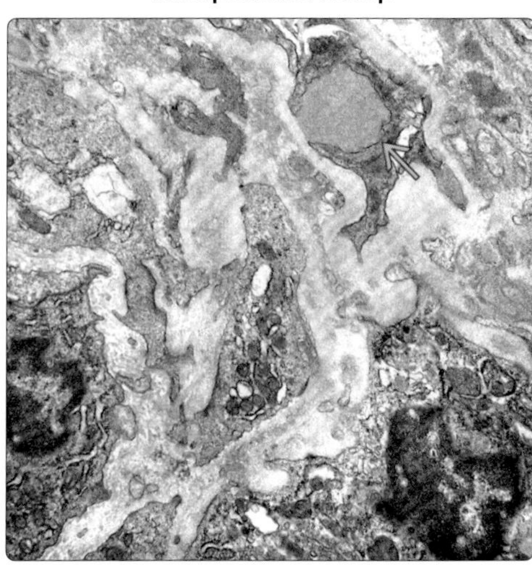

(Left) *Membranoproliferative pattern is shown in an older woman with C3GN and a family history of glomerulonephritis. C3GN may be familial or acquired, and is associated with a defect in the alternative pathway of complement.* **(Right)** *C3GN in the same patient shows a hump-shaped subepithelial deposit (nonspecific) along with subendothelial deposits.*

Subepithelial Hump and Subendothelial Deposits

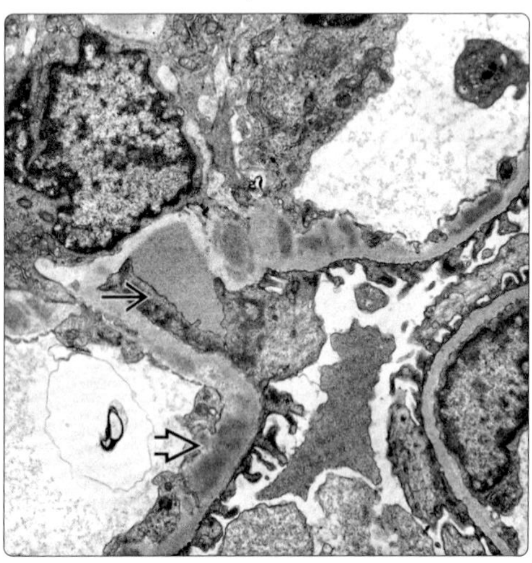

Mesangial Deposits

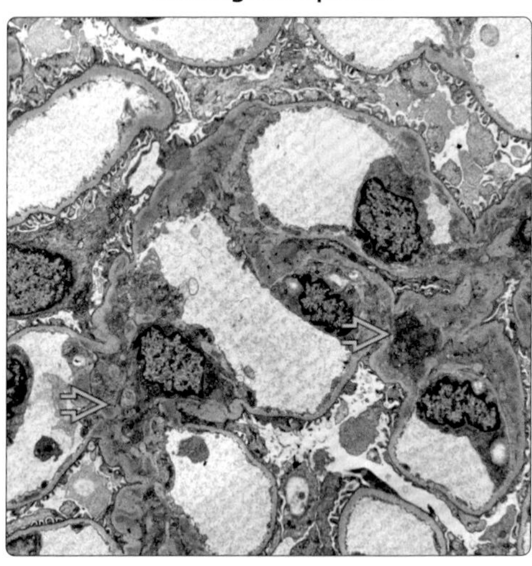

(Left) *Paramesangial to subendothelial and subepithelial amorphous electron-dense deposits are shown. Hump-shaped subepithelial deposits are reminiscent of postinfectious glomerulonephritis but are not specific. Findings are compatible with early recurrent C3GN or early MPGN.* **(Right)** *Amorphous electron-dense deposits, mostly within mesangium, are seen by electron microscopy. Podocytes show largely preserved foot processes.*

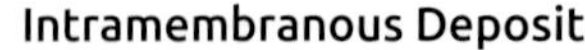

Intramembranous Deposits

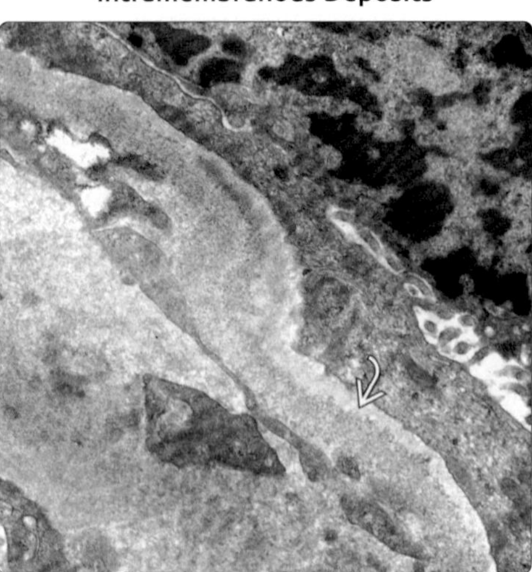

Intramembranous Deposits and "Humps"

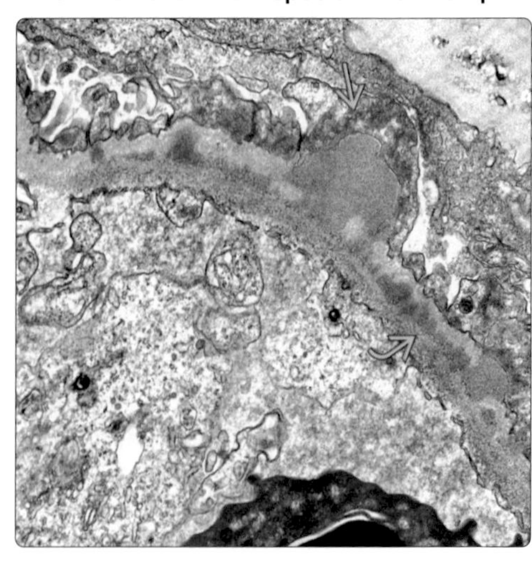

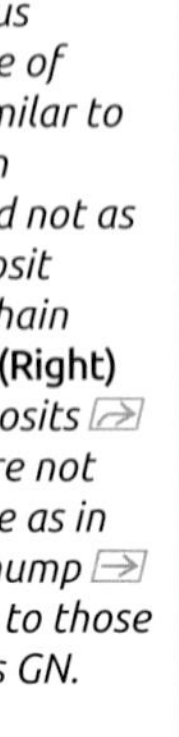

(Left) *Intramembranous deposits in this case of C3GN are granular, similar to monoclonal light chain deposition disease, and not as dense as in dense deposit disease (DDD). Light chain stains were negative.* **(Right)** *Intramembranous deposits in this case of C3GN are not quite as electron-dense as in DDD. A subepithelial hump is also present, similar to those in acute postinfectious GN.*

Monoclonal Gammopathy and C3GN

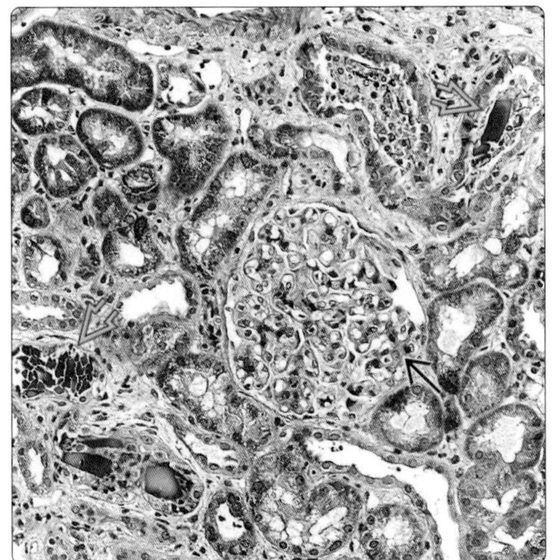

C3GN With Monoclonal Gammopathy

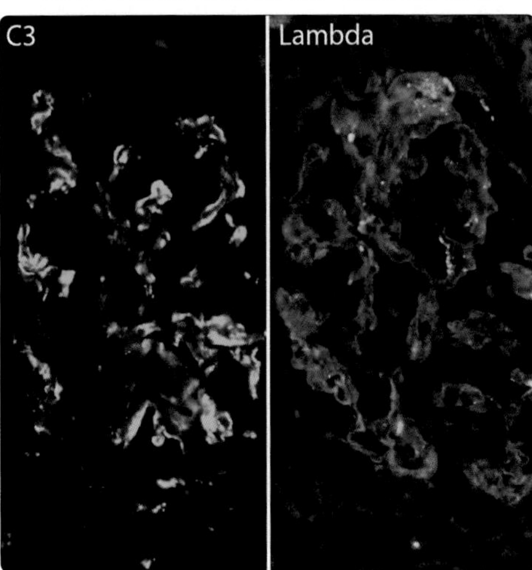

(Left) *This case of C3GN shows mild mesangial expansion ⇒. There is a concurrent light chain cast nephropathy, with atypical casts ⇨ that stained for lambda by immunofluorescence.* **(Right)** *In a case of C3GN associated with lambda light chain cast nephropathy, glomeruli show bright mesangial and capillary loop staining for C3 and absence of significant granular staining by IF for lambda light chain. The C3GN is likely causally related to the monoclonal protein.*

C4d

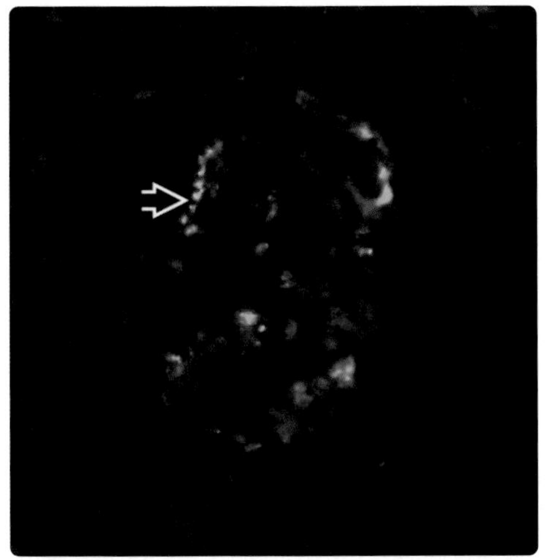

Recurrent C3GN in Transplant

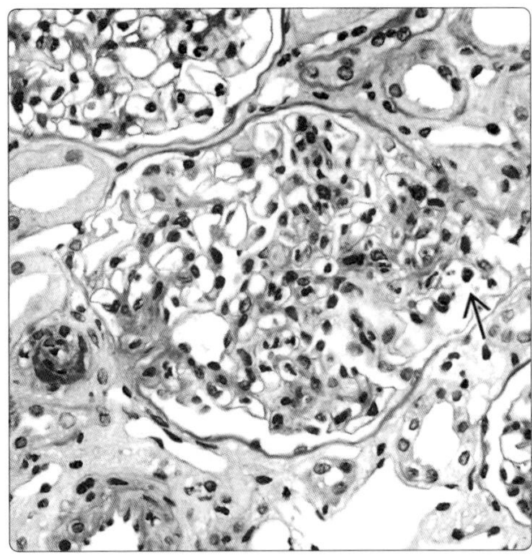

(Left) *C4d shows trace mesangial and segmental capillary loop staining ➡ in a glomerulus with C3GN. IF staining for C4d can help distinguish between immune complex GN, which shows bright staining for C4d, and C3GN.* **(Right)** *A glomerulus in a kidney transplant patient with recurrent C3GN shows mild mesangial hypercellularity and mesangial matrix expansion. Neutrophils ⇒ are present within segmental glomerular capillary loops.*

Recurrent C3GN in Transplant

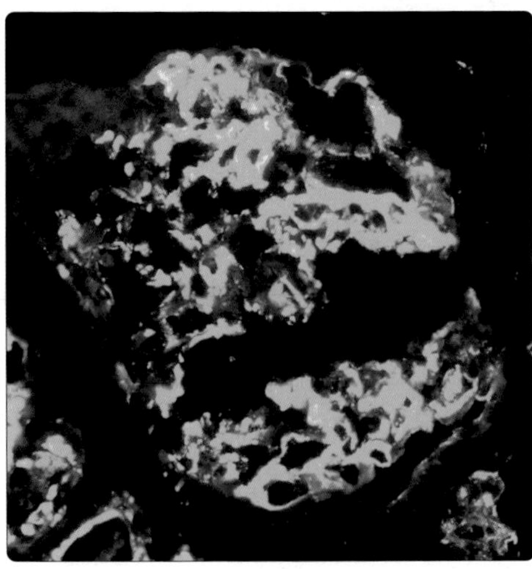

Eculizumab-Treated C3GN

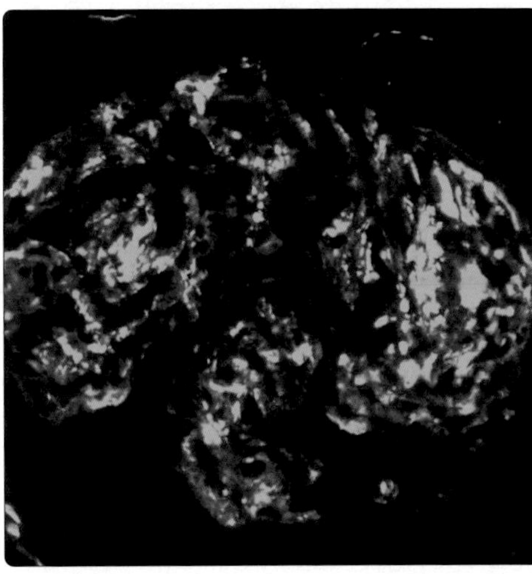

(Left) *By IF, a glomerulus in a transplant biopsy shows bright granular staining for C3 in the mesangium and segmental glomerular capillary loops. Recurrence in allograft of C3GN may resemble postinfectious GN.* **(Right)** *Kappa light chain in glomerulus in recurrent C3GN treated with eculizumab. Lambda staining was negative. IgG2 and IgG4 were also detected, indicative of deposition of the eculizumab (IgG2/4 kappa) in the glomerulus.*

Membranoproliferative Glomerulonephritis With Immune Complexes

KEY FACTS

TERMINOLOGY

- Glomerular disease characterized by mesangial hypercellularity and duplication of GBM with subendothelial and mesangial immune complex deposits without known cause (infections, autoimmune disease)

CLINICAL ISSUES

- Older children, adolescents, & young adults
- Nephrotic syndrome: > 50% of patients
- Hematuria: 10-20% with acute nephritic syndrome
- Hypocomplementemia
- ~ 50% have detectable abnormalities in alternative complement pathway

MICROSCOPIC

- Lobular, hypercellular glomerulus with thickened capillary walls & increased mesangial substance
- "Tram tracks" or duplication of GBM on PAS & silver stains
- Crescents in ~ 20% of cases
- Endocapillary hypercellularity ± neutrophils and monocytes
- IF: Classic feature is C3 in capillary walls & mesangium, "railroad track," "lumpy bumpy" granular C3
  - Distinguished from C3 glomerulopathy by prominent Ig &/or C1q & C4
- EM: Amorphous, dense subendothelial and mesangial deposits ± intramembranous or subepithelial deposits
  - 3 types based on predominant location of deposits: Type I, subendothelial; type III (Burkholder), subepithelial deposits; type III (Anders and Strife) complex intramembranous deposits

TOP DIFFERENTIAL DIAGNOSES

- C3 glomerulopathies
  - Overlap with C3 glomerulonephritis with MPGN pattern
  - Dense deposit disease (formerly type II MPGN)
- Cryoglobulinemic GN
- Chronic Infections
- Lupus erythematosus

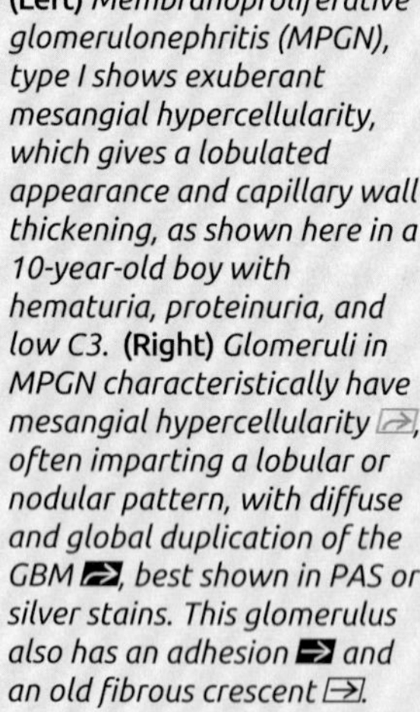

(Left) *Membranoproliferative glomerulonephritis (MPGN), type I shows exuberant mesangial hypercellularity, which gives a lobulated appearance and capillary wall thickening, as shown here in a 10-year-old boy with hematuria, proteinuria, and low C3.* **(Right)** *Glomeruli in MPGN characteristically have mesangial hypercellularity →, often imparting a lobular or nodular pattern, with diffuse and global duplication of the GBM →, best shown in PAS or silver stains. This glomerulus also has an adhesion → and an old fibrous crescent →.*

Lobulated Proliferative Appearance

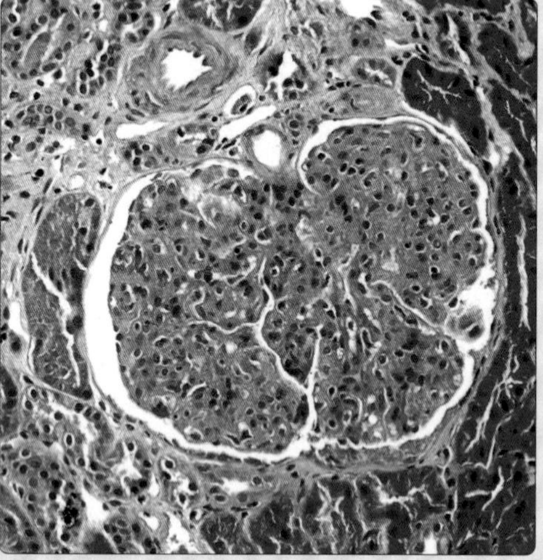

Mesangial Expansion and Duplication of GBM

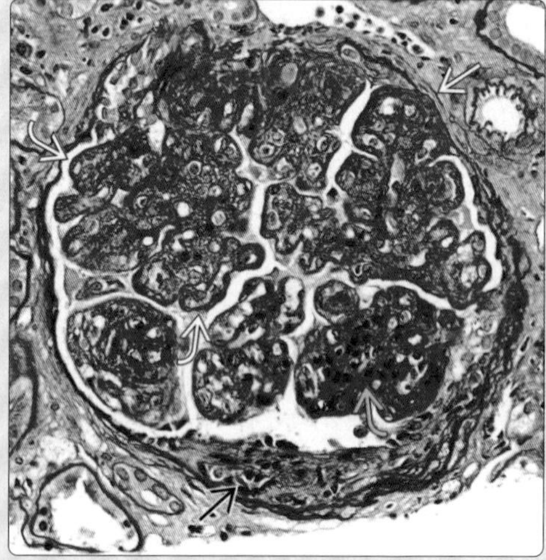

(Left) *Prominent immunoglobulins &/or C1q in addition to C3 distinguishes MPGN with immune complexes from C3 glomerulopathies.* **(Right)** *By EM, MPGN, type I shows numerous amorphous subendothelial electron-dense deposits → along the GBM and new GBM layers →, giving a "tram-track" appearance in PAS or silver stains.*

Prominent IgG and C3

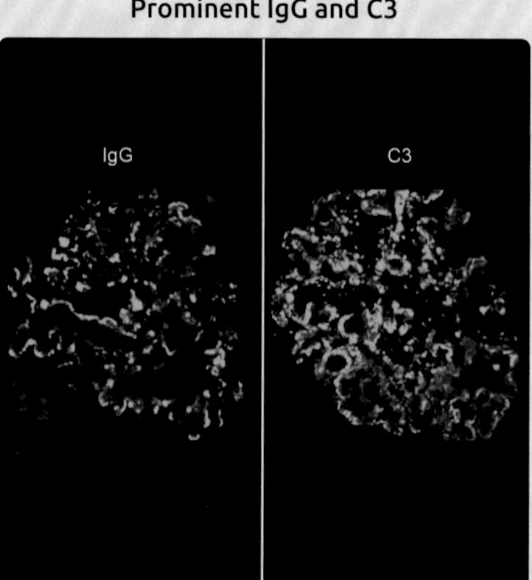

Subendothelial Deposits

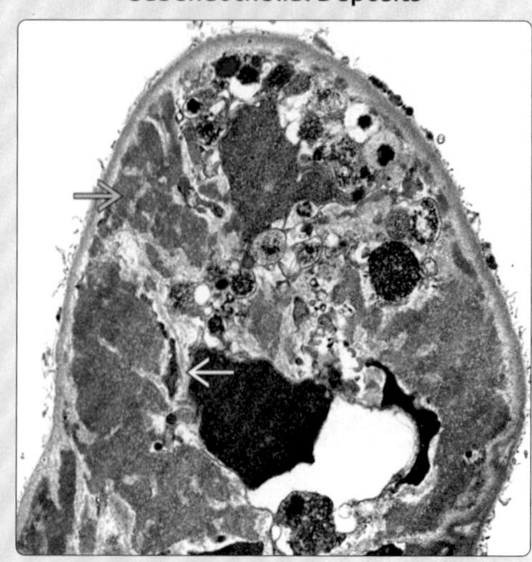

TERMINOLOGY

Abbreviations

- Membranoproliferative glomerulonephritis with immune complexes (MPGN-IC)

Synonyms

- Mesangiocapillary GN
- Lobular GN

Definitions

- Glomerular disease characterized by mesangial hypercellularity and duplication of GBM with subendothelial and mesangial immune complex deposits without known cause (infections, autoimmune disease)
- Ultrastructural variants include type I: Predominately subendothelial deposits and type III permeation of GBM with deposits (Strife and Anders) or prominent subepithelial deposits (Burkholder)
- Dense deposit disease (DDD) now classified as C3 glomerulopathy
  - Previously known as MPGN, type II

Relationship With C3 Glomerulopathies

- Prominent immunoglobulin or C1q distinguishes from new category of C3 glomerulopathies
  - 60-65% of biopsies with MPGN I or III have sufficient immunoglobulin or C1q deposition that they would not be classified as C3 glomerulopathies by definition proposed by Columbia University group
  - Overlaps C3 glomerulopathy, as ~ 50% have abnormalities in alternative pathway

ETIOLOGY/PATHOGENESIS

Infectious Agents

- Pattern of glomerular disease common in chronic infections
  - When known infection present (e.g., hepatitis C virus [HCV]), termed secondary MPGN

Immune Complex Deposition

- Circulating immune complexes detected in many MPGN patients
  - Activate classical and alternative complement pathways
- Chronic serum sickness in animals caused by repeated injection of antigen leads to MPGN pattern

Complement System

- Some have dysfunction or persistent activity of alternative complement pathway, including C3 nephritic factor (C3NeF)

CLINICAL ISSUES

Epidemiology

- Incidence
  - ~ 3% of GN in biopsies of children and adults
  - ~ 60% of primary MPGN type I or III cases (others meet criteria for C3 glomerulopathy)
- Age
  - Primarily older children, adolescents, and young adults (~ 7-30 years old)
    - Rare in children < 2 years old or adults > 50 years old
- Sex
  - No gender predilection
- Ethnicity
  - Higher incidence in whites
  - Navajo Indians in USA may have high rates of nondiabetic end-stage renal disease (ESRD) due to GN of this type

Presentation

- Proteinuria
  - Nephrotic syndrome in > 50% of patients
  - May be subnephrotic
  - Syndrome often initially nephritic and eventually nephrotic
- Hematuria
  - ± recurrent episodes of gross or microscopic hematuria
  - Acute nephritic syndrome in 10-20%
- Hypertension
  - Usually mild but may be malignant
  - ~ 1/3 of patients
- Renal vein thrombosis may be present

Laboratory Tests

- Hypocomplementemia similar to C3 nephropathies
  - Low C3: 46%
  - Low C4: 2%
  - Low factor B: 34%
  - C3NeF 54%: (Type I)
- Mutations in *CFH* (10%) or *CFI* (6%) (type I)

Treatment

- Drugs
  - Steroids
    - Long-term, low dose used in children with 1° MPGN
    - Rebiopsy often after 5 years of therapy initiation to ascertain if continuation needed
  - Other agents (antiplatelet agents, eculizumab, rituximab); none dramatically effective
  - Recurrence rate: 27-65%
  - ~ 30% of children with MPGN, type I recur in 6 months to 1 year after transplant
    - ~ 40% of recurrences lead to graft failure
- Treat underlying disorder, if known
  - Infection, autoimmune disease, hematologic dyscrasia
- Transplantation

Prognosis

- Renal survival ~ 50% at ~ 10 years
  - Therapy improves to 60-85% at 10 years
  - Median renal survival time for MPGN, type I or III: 9-12 years
- 5-20% have clinical remission
- Risk factors for poor outcome
  - Sclerotic glomeruli, crescents, interstitial fibrosis, and tubular atrophy
  - Severe nephrotic syndrome, ↑ creatinine, hypertension
- Predictors of good outcome
  - Focal/mild MPGN features on biopsy, asymptomatic hematuria, subnephrotic proteinuria

MACROSCOPIC

General Features

- Pale kidneys

- ○ ± cortical yellow flecks, representing tubular lipid & interstitial foam cells
- Advanced disease: Small granular kidneys ± prominent vessels

MICROSCOPIC

Histologic Features

- Glomeruli
  - Lobular, hypercellular with thickened capillary walls and increased mesangial substance
  - Mesangial interposition: Mesangial cells migrate into peripheral capillary walls between GBM and endothelium
    - Partial if only capillary wall segment involved
    - Circumferential if involving entire circumference of individual capillary
    - Produces "tram tracks," "double contours," or GBM duplication secondary to GBM synthesis
      - Best seen on PAS and silver stains
    - ± subendothelial immune deposits (between duplicated GBMs) seen as PAS[+], nonargyrophilic on Jones methenamine silver (JMS), & fuchsinophilic on trichrome
  - ± sclerosis; ± sclerotic mesangial nodules
  - Crescents in ~ 20% of cases
  - ± neutrophils & monocytes
  - Sometimes hyaline aggregates of immune complexes in capillary lumina
  - Silver stains in type III show frayed GBM with disrupted, moth-eaten appearance (Anders and Strife) or "spikes" (Burkholder)
- Tubules and interstitium
  - Variable interstitial fibrosis and tubular atrophy, inflammation, & edema
  - Tubular resorption droplets
  - Interstitial foam cells
  - Red cell casts
- Vascular changes nonspecific

ANCILLARY TESTS

Immunofluorescence

- MPGN, type I
  - C3 in capillary walls & mesangium is classic feature
    - IgG or IgM present and prominent (C3 not 2 levels greater according to criteria proposed by Columbia University group)
  - Also "lumpy bumpy" granular C3, IgG, & early complement (C1q & C4)
  - Railroad track pattern may be seen on IF at high power
- MPGN, type III subtypes have similar findings
  - ~ 50% of cases have IgG & C3 (& less intense IgM, IgA, & C1q)
  - ~ 50% stain only for C3 and are thus classified as "C3 GN/glomerulopathy"

Electron Microscopy

- **Type I: Common variant**
  - Large, dense deposits throughout glomerulus; primarily subendothelial and mesangial
  - Produces GBM duplication with mesangial interposition
  - "Mesangialization" of capillary loops
  - Increased mesangial matrix
- Podocyte foot process effacement
- **Type III: Strife and Anders variant (IIIS/A)**
  - Intramembranous deposits in addition to subendothelial & mesangial deposits
  - Deposits extend from GBM subendothelial to subepithelial portion, disrupting GBM lamina densa, giving a laminated, woven appearance (referred to as a "complex intramembranous" pattern)
    - GBM can have a "sausage string" or fusiform appearance
    - Less dense than DDD
    - Silver stains show frayed GBM with disrupted, moth-eaten appearance
  - TBM deposits present in ~ 1/3 of cases, which prompts consideration of DDD
- **Type III: Burkholder variant (IIIB)**
  - Subepithelial deposits similar to membranous GN in addition to subendothelial and mesangial deposits

Laser Microdissection and Mass Spectrometry

- Can be useful in MPGN cases, particularly in suspected monoclonal gammopathy-related GN

DIFFERENTIAL DIAGNOSIS

Complement Deficiencies/C3 Glomerulonephritis

- MPGN-type pattern seen in a number of genetic complement deficiencies (e.g., inherited C2, C3, C6, C7, & C8 deficiencies, etc.)
- Autoimmunity can also contribute to an MPGN pattern (e.g., anticomplement factor H)
- Subset with C3 and no immunoglobulin now classified as "C3 glomerulonephritis"
- Patients may also show signs of meningococcal infections & MPGN

Dense Deposit Disease (DDD)

- EM: Highly electron-dense deposits
- IF: Tubular basement membrane (TBM) deposits, rarely prominent immunoglobulin (~ 10%)

Mixed Cryoglobulinemia

- Characteristic PAS(+) "pseudothrombi" can be seen in glomerular capillary loops in cryoglobulinemic GN
- Cryoglobulin present

Infectious Diseases

- History, physical, & clinical laboratory data help favor diagnosis of infectious disease
- Bacterial
  - Endocarditis & infected vascular shunts
  - Poststreptococcal acute glomerulonephritis: Elevated antistreptolysin-O (ASLO) titers
- Viral: Hepatitis B & C, HIV
- Protozoal: Malarial & schistosomiasis
- Other: Mycoplasma, mycobacteria

Systemic Lupus Erythematosus (SLE)

- ANA(+), anti-ds DNA(+)
- IF shows full-house staining pattern
  - Granular TBM deposits

Membranoproliferative Glomerulonephritis Variants

Type	LM	IF	EM	Other Characteristic Features
I	GBM duplication & mesangial expansion	IgG & C3 ± IgM, C1q	Subendothelial & mesangial deposits	(1) infection, (2) autoimmunity, (3) neoplasia; some are C3 GP variant of MPGN type I
III: Burkholder variant (IIIB)	Mesangial proliferation, double contours, "spikes"	IgG & C3 ± IgM, C1q	Subendothelial, subepithelial, intramembranous, & mesangial deposits	Combination of type I MPGN & membranous GN; some are C3 GP variant of MPGN type IIIB
III: Strife/Anders variant (IIIS/A)	Subendothelial, subepithelial, intramembranous, & mesangial deposits	IgG & C3 ± IgM, C1q	Subendothelial, subepithelial, & complex intramembranous deposits, may be electron lucent without silver impregnation	Combination of type I and type II (DDD) MPGN; some are C3 GP variant of MPGN type IIIS/A

EM: Electron microscopy; IF: Immunofluorescence microscopy; GBM: Glomerular basement membrane; GP: Glomerulopathy; LM: Light microscopy; MPGN: Membranoproliferative glomerulonephritis. The proposed IF distinction between C3 GP and MPGN with immune complexes is based on the presence of immune complexes in the latter, as judged by Ig &/or C1q within 2 IF levels of C3 staining.

Table reference: Zhou XJ and Silva FG: Membranoproliferative glomerulonephritis. In Jennette JC et al: Heptinstall's Pathology of the Kidney. 7th ed. Philadelphia: Wolters Kluwer. 301-339, 2015.

- EM: Tubuloreticular structures, organized deposits (thumbprint)

Sjögren Syndrome

- ANA(+)
- SSB/La(+) (more specific)
- SSA/Ro(+) (less specific than SSB, also seen in other autoimmune conditions)

Thrombotic Microangiopathy (TMA)

- GBM duplication lacking immunoglobulin deposits except for IgM
- Subendothelial accumulation of electron-lucent, flocculent material rather than electron-dense deposits

α-1 Antitrypsin (A1AT) Deficiency

- Severe liver disease or cirrhosis necessary prior to developing MPGN
- A1AT deposits and PiZ protein detected in subendothelial space
- Glomerular injury possibly reversible with liver transplantation

Chronic, Active Antibody-Mediated Rejection

- GBM duplication prominent (transplant glomerulopathy)
- Minimal Ig and C3 deposits and electron-dense deposits
- Usually C4d in peritubular capillaries and donor-specific antibody

DIAGNOSTIC CHECKLIST

Pathologic Interpretation Pearls

- MPGN may initially mimic poststreptococcal GN
  - Upper respiratory infection often precedes both
  - Biopsy kidney if hematuria, proteinuria, & hypocomplementemia last ≥ 6 weeks to exclude MPGN
- Nosology of MPGN in transition
  - MPGN cases with little or no immunoglobulin now classified as "C3 glomerulonephritis"
    - Due to genetic or acquired abnormalities in alternative complement pathway
  - MPGN with prominent IF evidence of classical pathway activation (immunoglobulin &/or C1q) are considered MPGN I/III with immune complexes
  - However, overlap between 2 categories suggests either or both mechanisms may be operative in an individual patient
  - "Idiopathic" MPGN is diagnosis of exclusion and becoming less common as causes of MPGN are better understood

SELECTED REFERENCES

1. Jain D et al: Membranoproliferative glomerulonephritis: the role for laser microdissection and mass spectrometry. Am J Kidney Dis. 63(2):324-8, 2014
2. Appel GB: Membranoproliferative glomerulonephritis - mechanisms and treatment. Contrib Nephrol. 181:163-74, 2013
3. D'Agati VD et al: C3 glomerulopathy: what's in a name? Kidney Int. 82(4):379-81, 2012
4. Dillon JJ et al: Rituximab therapy for Type I membranoproliferative glomerulonephritis. Clin Nephrol. 77(4):290-5, 2012
5. Fervenza FC et al: Idiopathic membranoproliferative glomerulonephritis: does it exist? Nephrol Dial Transplant. 27(12):4288-94, 2012
6. Radhakrishnan S et al: Eculizumab and refractory membranoproliferative glomerulonephritis. N Engl J Med. 366(12):1165-6, 2012
7. Sethi S et al: Membranoproliferative glomerulonephritis–a new look at an old entity. N Engl J Med. 366(12):1119-31, 2012
8. Vernon KA et al: Experimental models of membranoproliferative glomerulonephritis, including dense deposit disease. Contrib Nephrol. 169:198-210, 2011
9. Lorenz EC et al: Recurrent membranoproliferative glomerulonephritis after kidney transplantation. Kidney Int. 77(8):721-8, 2010
10. Strife CF et al: Type III membranoproliferative glomerulonephritis: long-term clinical and morphologic evaluation. Clin Nephrol. 21(6):323-34, 1984
11. Anders D et al: Basement membrane changes in membranoproliferative glomerulonephritis. II. Characterization of a third type by silver impregnation of ultra thin sections. Virchows Arch A Pathol Anat Histol. 376(1):1-19, 1977
12. Burkholder PM et al: Mixed membranous and proliferative glomerulonephritis. A correlative light, immunofluorescence, and electron microscopic study. Lab Invest. 23(5):459-79, 1970
13. Zhou XJ and Silva FG: Membranoproliferative glomerulonephritis. In Jennette JC et al: Heptinstall's Pathology of the Kidney. 7th ed. Philadelphia: Wolters Kluwer. 301-339, 2015

(Left) *Characteristically in MPGN I and III, all glomeruli show similar features (diffuse) and all of the tuft is involved (global). The glomeruli are enlarged, with prominent mesangial hypercellularity that gives a lobular pattern. Secondary focal changes occur, such as crescents, adhesions, and glomerulosclerosis.* (Right) *This glomerulus with MPGN I has marked mesangial hypercellularity and increased matrix with a lobular pattern. Capillary loops are not open, due to endocapillary leukocytes.*

Diffuse and Global Mesangial Hypercellularity

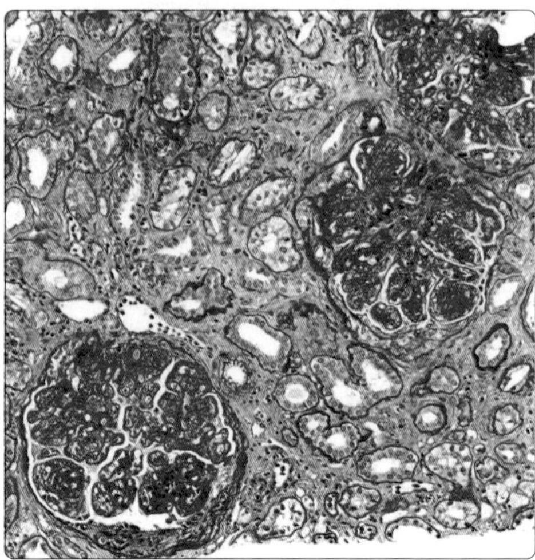

Marked Mesangial Hypercellularity

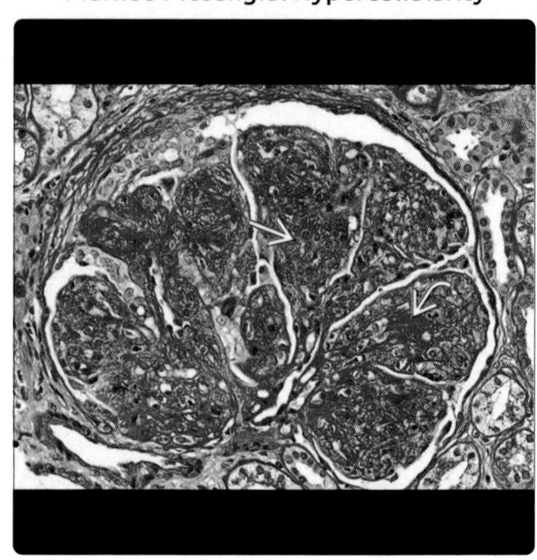

(Left) *The "membrano" component of MPGN is due to widespread duplication of the GBM, which can be seen in a PAS stain. This is a case of recurrent MPGN I in an allograft 7 years after transplantation.* (Right) *The duplicated GBM is well shown in silver stains. Mesangial cells extend between the layers of GBM and can be appreciated by light microscopy.*

Duplicated GBM

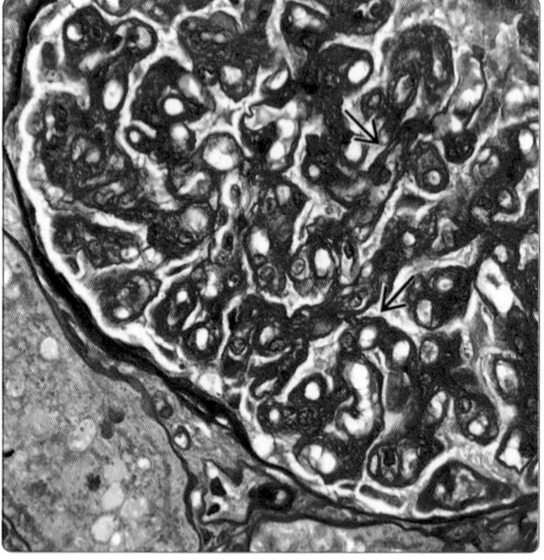

GBM Duplication

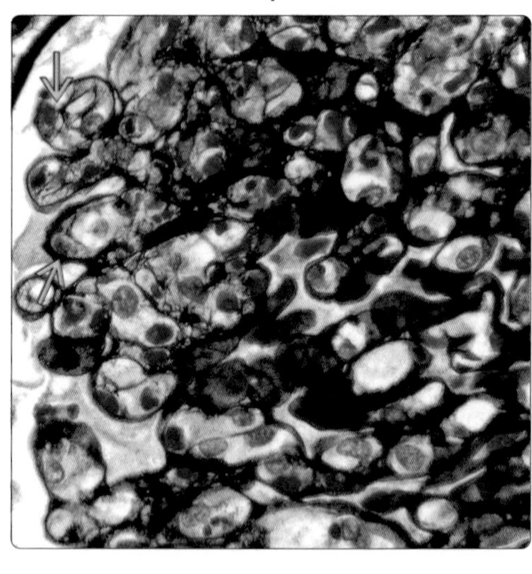

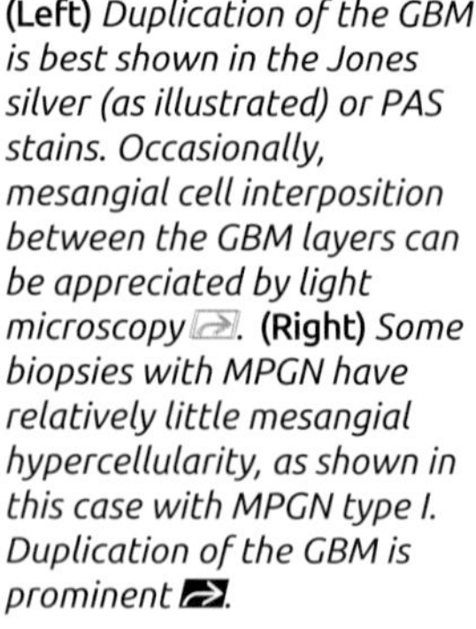

(Left) *Duplication of the GBM is best shown in the Jones silver (as illustrated) or PAS stains. Occasionally, mesangial cell interposition between the GBM layers can be appreciated by light microscopy.* (Right) *Some biopsies with MPGN have relatively little mesangial hypercellularity, as shown in this case with MPGN type I. Duplication of the GBM is prominent.*

GBM Duplication

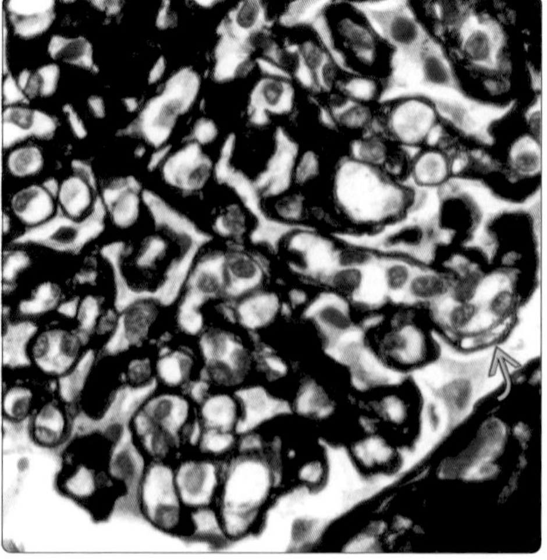

MPGN With Relatively Little Mesangial Hypercellularity

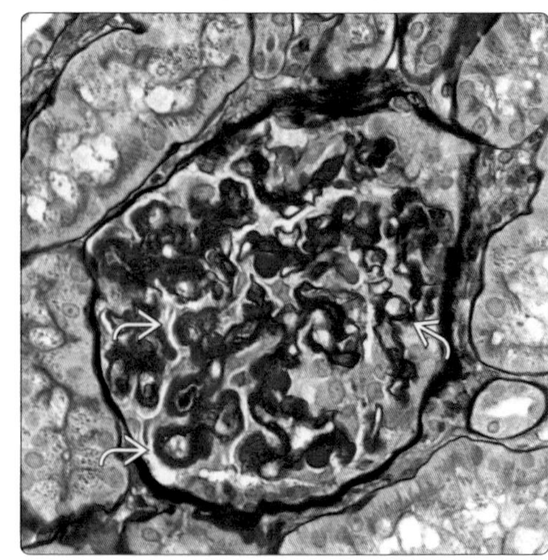

Intracapillary Inflammatory Cells

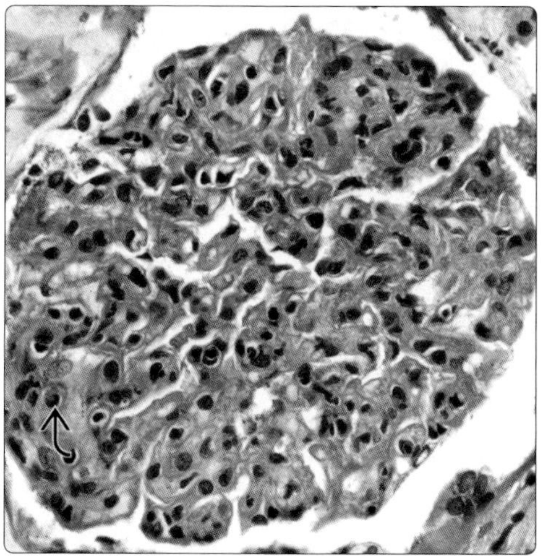

Endocapillary Hypercellularity

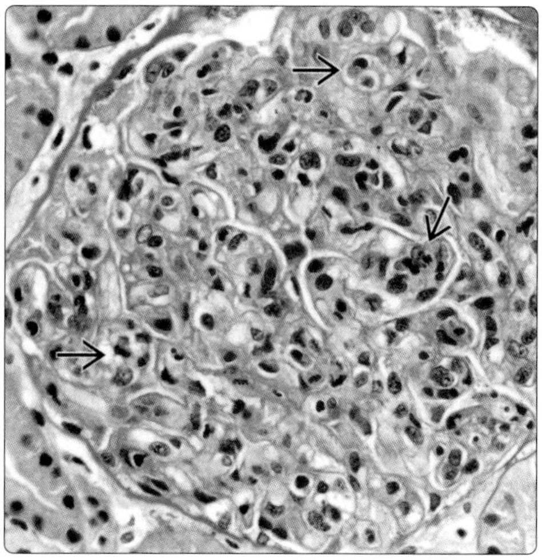

(Left) *In this 41-year-old patient with MPGN, type I, the glomerulus is hypercellular with increased numbers of intracapillary cells ↪, some of which appear to be infiltrating inflammatory cells in an exudative/acute GN-type process.* **(Right)** *In MPGN, type I, glomeruli are hypercellular with increased numbers of intracapillary cells →. The increased lobularity of the glomerular tuft is not prominent in this sample.*

GBM and Mesangial Hypercellularity

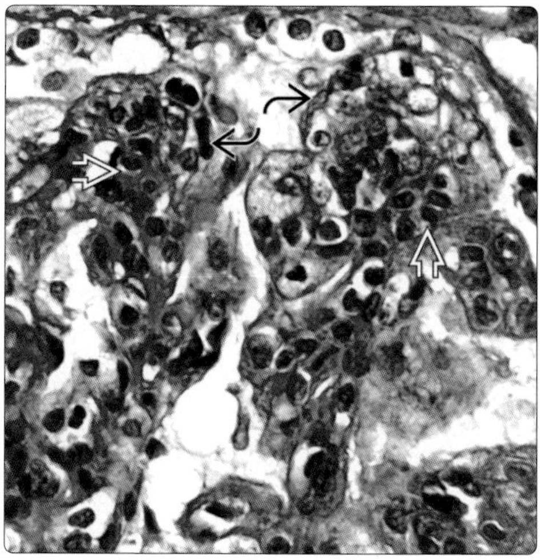

Subendothelial and Subepithelial Deposits

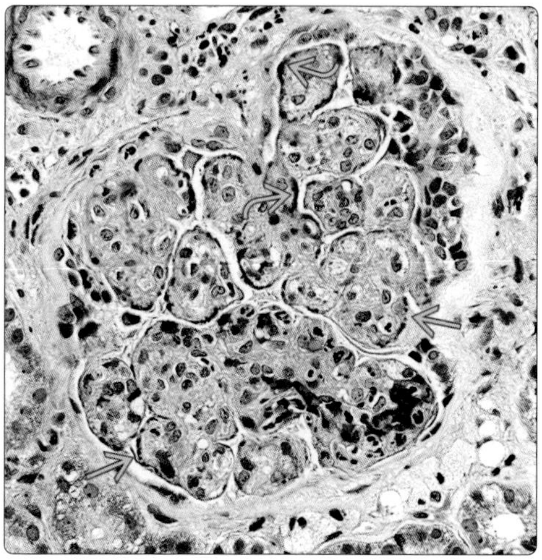

(Left) *In a 9-year-old boy with MPGN, type III-Burkholder variant, peripheral capillary loops showed GBM duplication ↪ with cellular interposition and increased mesangial cellularity ⇨.* **(Right)** *The broad, elongated subendothelial deposits ↪ and the smaller, rounded subepithelial immune complex deposits → can be appreciated in trichrome stains in which they typically are red-purple and darker than the GBM.*

Loss of GBM Argyrophilia in MPGN Type IIIS/A

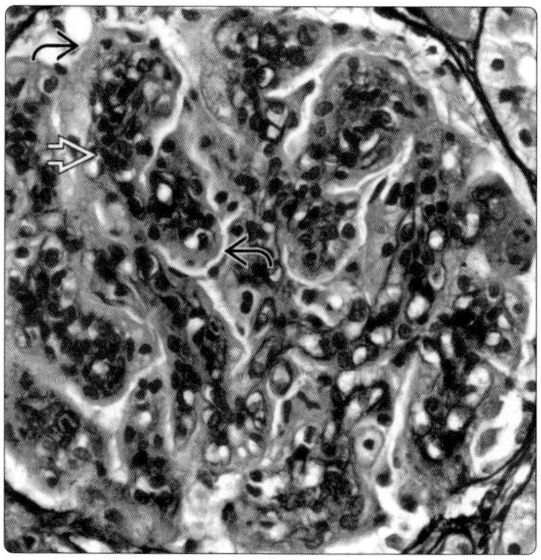

Crescent

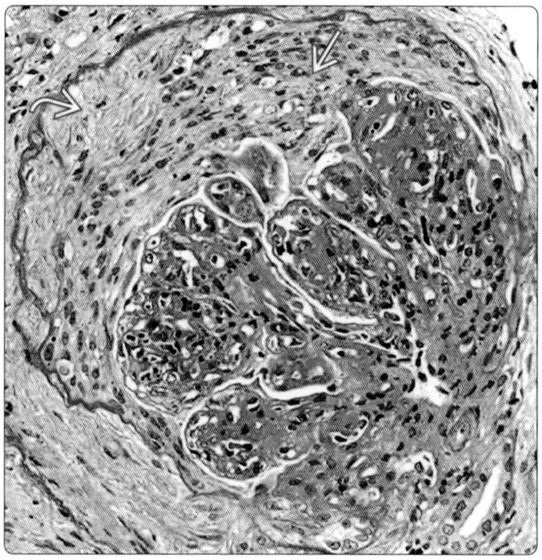

(Left) *Peripheral capillary loops show less argyrophilia ↪ than the mesangium ⇨, a feature of MPGN, type III of the Strife-Anders variant (IIIS/A). This results from a disorganized GBM permeated with deposits.* **(Right)** *Fibrocellular crescent in MPGN appears to have an outer, older fibrous component ↪ next to Bowman capsule and an inner, more recent component → in contact with the glomerular tuft. The glomerulus has prominent mesangial and endocapillary hypercellularity.*

Granular IgG

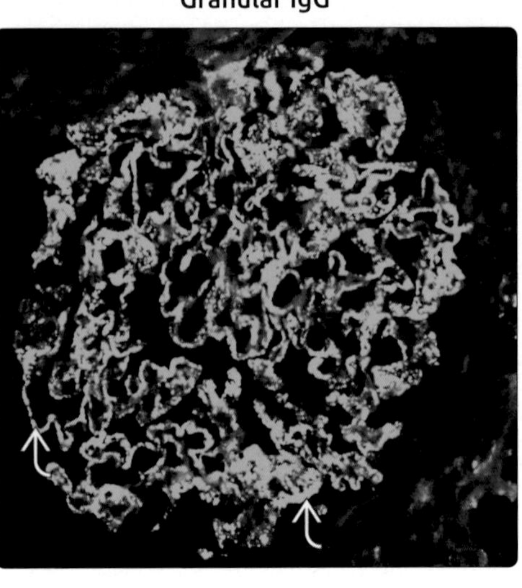

C3 Along GBM and Mesangium

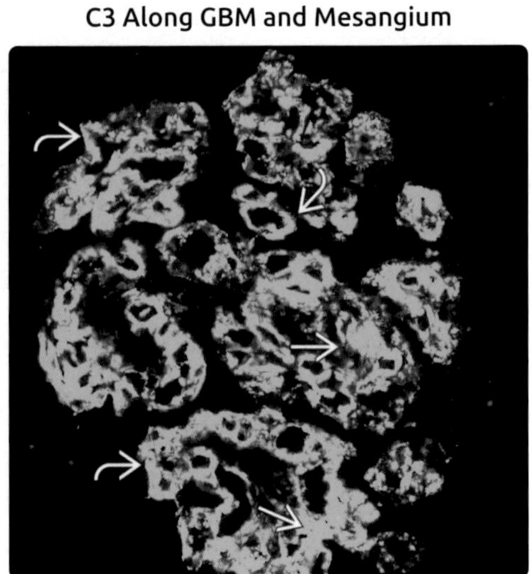

(Left) *In this case of MPGN I, IgG has a confluent distribution along the GBM in some foci, compatible with subendothelial deposits. Similar staining intensity was seen for C3.* **(Right)** *In MPGN, deposits stain brightly for C3 along the capillary walls and in the mesangium. This 14-year-old girl had hypocomplementemia, hematuria, proteinuria (protein:creatinine ratio = 4), creatinine 0.4 mg/dL, and a negative serologic work-up.*

C1q Along GBM

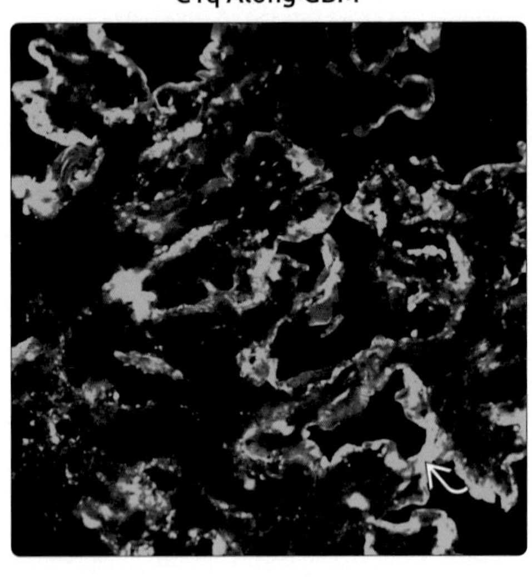

IgM in GBM

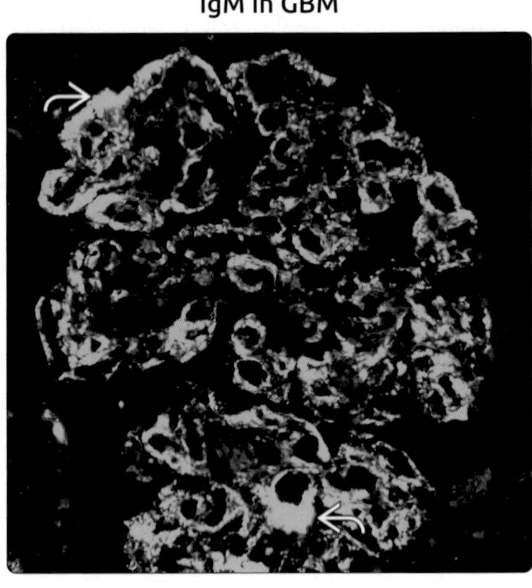

(Left) *Immunofluorescence staining for C1q can be appreciated in a confluent pattern along the GBM, compatible with subendothelial deposits in MPGN, type I with immune complex deposits.* **(Right)** *In a 14-year-old girl with MPGN, type III, there is bright IgM by IF, appreciable as broad deposits along the GBM.*

MPGN Type I With Immune Complexes

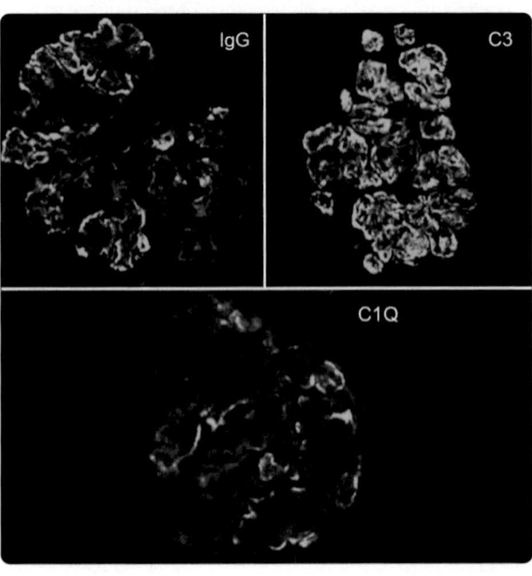

C3 Glomerulonephritis

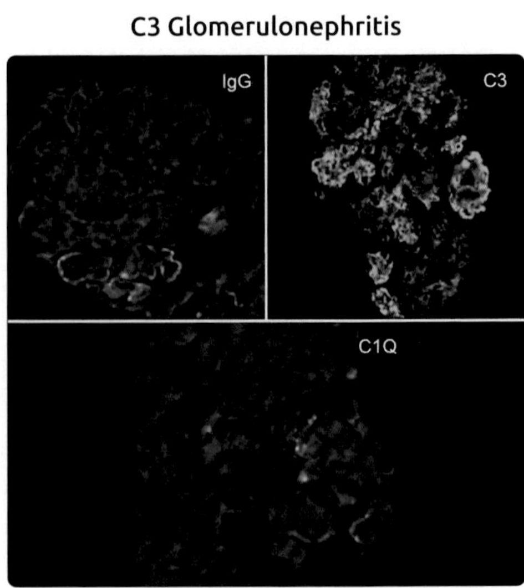

(Left) *This biopsy meets criteria for MPGN-IC: The IF level of IgG (2+) and C1q (1-2+) are within 2 levels of the C3 (3+). However, a repeat biopsy 1 year later showed scant IgG and C1q with persistence of bright C3, meeting the criteria for C3 GN.* **(Right)** *This biopsy meets the criteria for C3GN because of the weak IgG (trace) and C1q (trace) with bright C3 (3+). A biopsy 1 year previously met the criteria for MPGN-IC, with prominent IgG (2+) and C1q (1-2+), showing that these can be phases in the same disease process.*

MPGN Type I, Early Stage

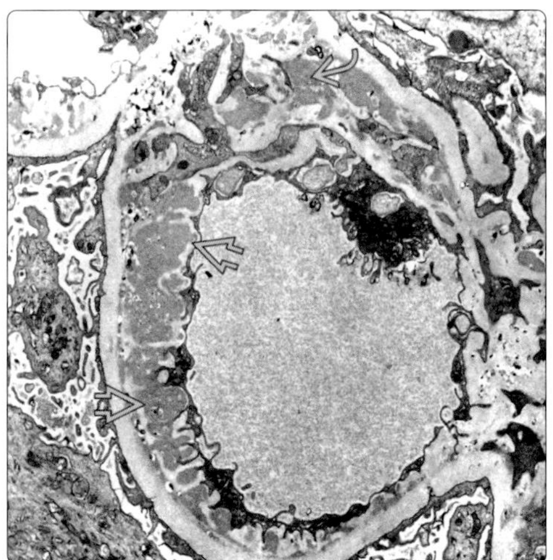

MPGN Type I, Late Stage

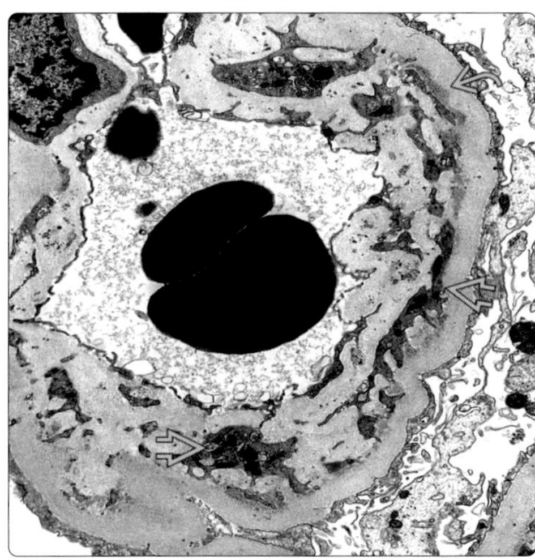

(Left) *MPGN is classified by EM. Most common is type I, defined by the presence of predominantly subendothelial deposits in addition to mesangial deposits. These become resurfaced by new GBM on the endothelial side, leading to GBM duplication evident in PAS stained slides.* **(Right)** *Late in the evolution of MPGN type I, the deposits can diminish, but the GBM duplication persists. Mesangial cell interposition is characteristically present between the layers of GBM.*

MPGN Type III B

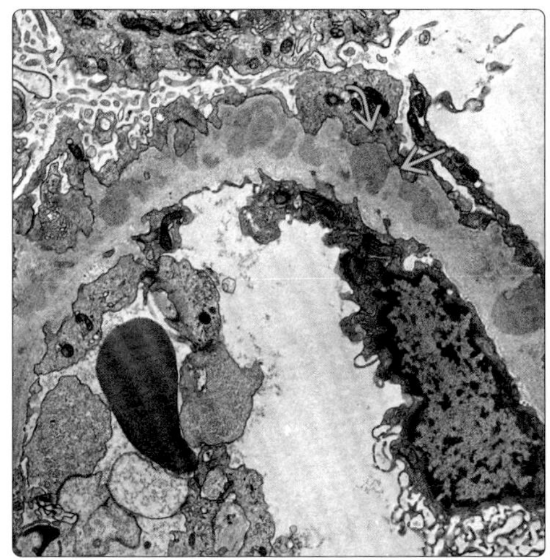

MPGN Type III B

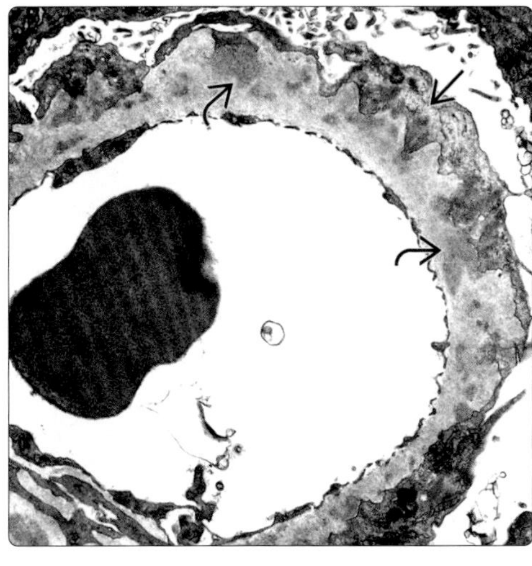

(Left) *One variant of MPGN, type III of Burkholder (IIIB), has prominent subepithelial deposits with "spikes" of GBM resembling membranous GN. Mesangial and subendothelial deposits are present in addition.* **(Right)** *In MPGN, type III of Burkholder (IIIB), subepithelial electron-dense deposits can be seen, some of which extend into the GBM. In addition, there is overlying podocyte foot process effacement.*

MPGN Type III S/A

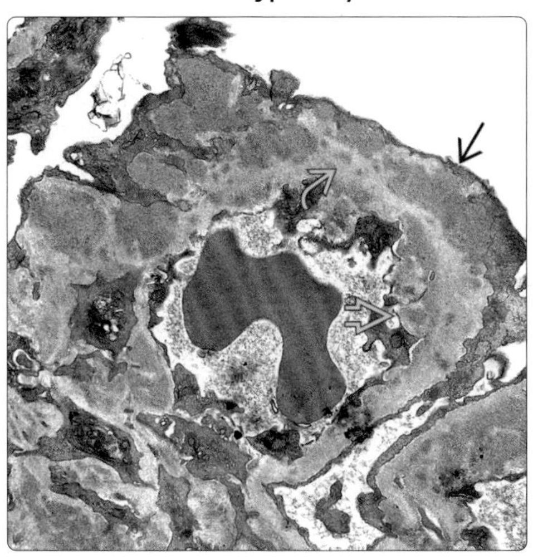

Lucent/Pale Deposits in MPGN, Type III S/A

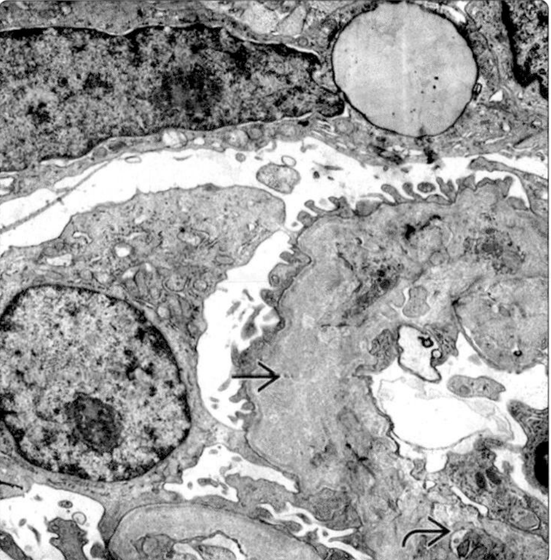

(Left) *In type III MPGN of the Strife-Anders variety, the electron-dense deposits permeate the GBM. Here they are seen in subendothelial, intramembranous, and subepithelial locations.* **(Right)** *In MPGN, type III Strife-Anders variant, the GBM can appear disorganized with GBMs thickened by deposits that are less electron dense than typical deposits and disrupted by cellular interposition.*

IgA Nephropathy

KEY FACTS

TERMINOLOGY

- Glomerulonephritis with dominant or codominant IgA deposits in mesangium in absence of systemic disease

ETIOLOGY/PATHOGENESIS

- Genetic factors (> 7 loci by GWAS)
- Abnormal glycosylation of IgA1
- Autoantibodies to galactose deficient IgA1
- Abnormally active IgA response

CLINICAL ISSUES

- Most common cause of glomerulonephritis worldwide
- Asia > USA/Europe > Africa
- Often asymptomatic hematuria ± proteinuria
- ↑ circulating serum IgA
- Recurs in transplants (30%)

MICROSCOPIC

- Usual: Mesangial hypercellularity and ↑ matrix
- Common: Focal, segmental inflammation of glomeruli
- Less common: Crescents ± necrosis
- Interstitial inflammation with eosinophils
- Histologically normal (10%)

ANCILLARY TESTS

- IF: IgA mesangial deposits (100%)
  - C3 (90%), IgG, IgM (50%), C1q (10%)
- EM: Amorphous electron-dense deposits in mesangium
  - Subepithelial or subendothelial deposits occasionally

TOP DIFFERENTIAL DIAGNOSES

- Henoch-Schönlein purpura
- Postinfectious glomerulonephritis (IgA-dominant)
- IgA nephropathy in cirrhosis of liver

GRADING

- Oxford classification: Mesangial hypercellularity (M), tubular atrophy/interstitial fibrosis (T), and segmental glomerulosclerosis (S) correlate with outcome

Mesangial Hypercellularity

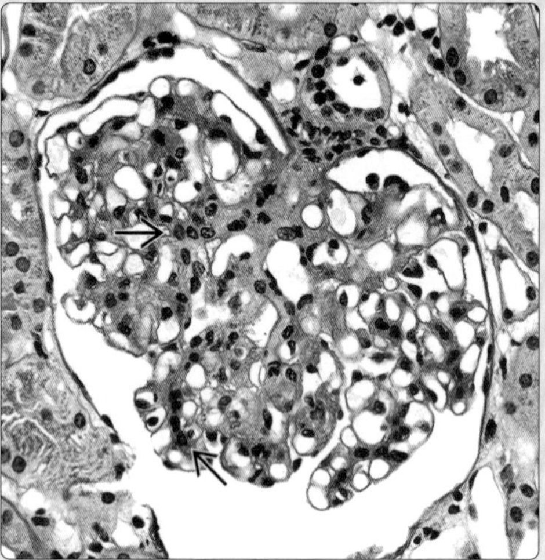

Segmental Glomerulosclerosis

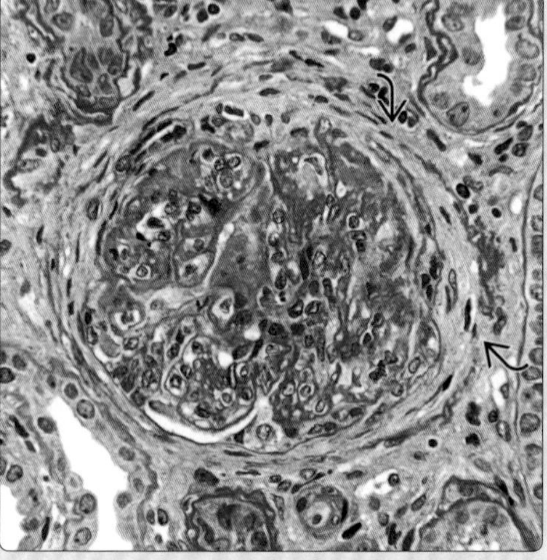

(Left) *This glomerulus in IgA nephropathy (IgAN) shows mesangial hypercellularity → and expanded mesangial matrix. Most cases show this feature, but the additional pathology is quite variable.* **(Right)** *PAS shows subtotal segmental glomerulosclerosis with adhesions to Bowman capsule over most of the surface in this 27-year-old man with elevated serum creatinine (5.6 mg/dL), hematuria, and urine protein to creatinine ratio of 7. Fragmentation of Bowman capsule ↷ is suggestive of past crescent formation.*

Typical IgA Mesangial Deposition

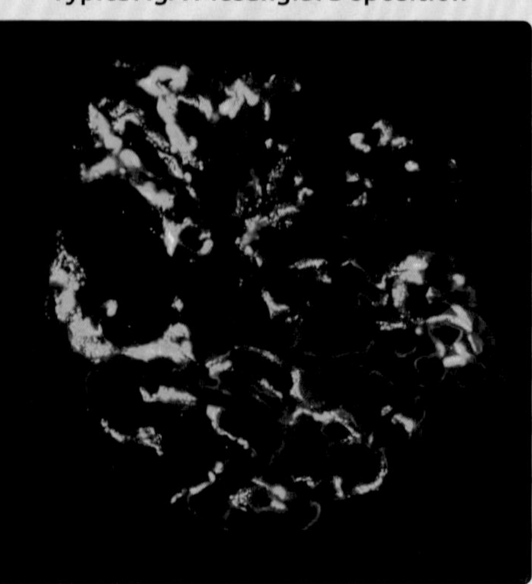

Amorphous Mesangial Deposits

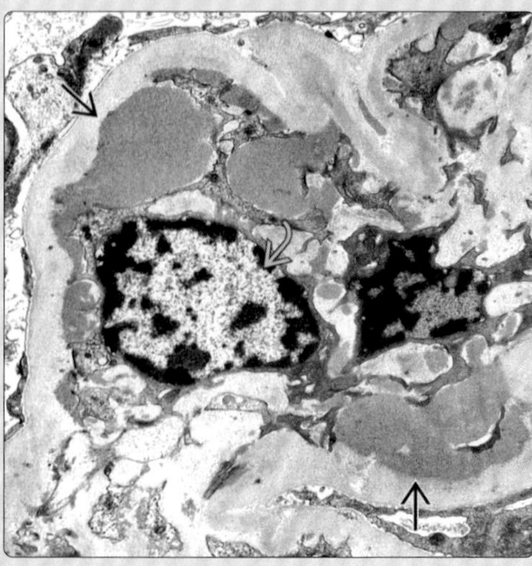

(Left) *Immunofluorescence shows prominent IgA deposits, typical of IgAN. Indeed, IgAN was initially defined by immunofluorescence, due to characteristic deposition in the mesangium with a tree trunk and branches pattern.* **(Right)** *Electron-dense mesangial deposits → are uniformly present in IgA nephropathy and do not show substructure. The deposits are typically in close association with a mesangial cell ↷.*

TERMINOLOGY

Abbreviations

- IgA nephropathy (IgAN)

Definitions

- Glomerulonephritis with dominant or codominant IgA deposits in absence of systemic disease
  - Initially described by Berger and Hinglais (1968)

ETIOLOGY/PATHOGENESIS

Genetic Factors

- Family history of nephritis in ~ 10%
- Several susceptibility loci revealed in genome wide associated studies (GWAS) using single nucleotide polymorphisms (SNP)
  - Strongest signal in MHC locus: *6p21* (*HLA-DQB1/DRB1, PSMB9/TAP1, DPA1/DPB2*); also *CFHR1/CFHR3* (1q32) and *HORMAD2-MTMR3* (22q12)
    - Loci explain ~ 4-7% of disease variance and correlate with geographic distribution
    - CFHR3-1 risk allele is deletion and protective
      - ↑ serum CFH and C3
      - ↓ C3 in glomeruli
    - Additional risk loci: 17p13 (α-defensin gene cluster) and 8q23 (*TNFSF13* encodes APRIL), 16p11 (*ITGAM-ITGAX*), 1p13 (*VAV3*), and 9q34 (*CARD9*)
- Abnormal glycosylation of IgA
  - Autosomal dominant pattern of inheritance
    - ~ 25-33% of 1st-degree family members (without IgAN) have ↑ GD-IgA
    - Henoch-Schönlein purpura have ↑ GD-IgA
  - IgAN patients have IgA1 that is deficient in galactose (GD-IgA) in serum and in glomeruli
    - ↓ galactose attached to GalNAc in IgA1 hinge region
    - GD-IgA level independent risk factor for progression
  - Intrinsic property of IgAN B cells in vitro
- Autosomal dominant IgA nephropathy
  - *SPRY2* mutation in Sicilian family
    - Mutation causes inhibition of MAPK/ERK1/2

Abnormal IgA Response

- Increased IgA response to intranasal antigens
- Elevated serum IgA levels in ~ 50%

Autoantibodies to GD-IgA

- GD-IgA serves as autoantigen
- IgG or IgA1 autoantibodies bind to GalNAc neoepitopes on GD-IgA
  - GD-IgA immune complexes detected in blood
  - GD-IgA may also be planted in mesangium
    - GD-IgA binds to transferrin receptor
- Progression involves interaction between IgA and mesangial cells and ↑ cytokines
  - IgA/anti-IgA complexes stimulate mesangial cell proliferation
  - Activate mesangial cell MAPK/ERK pathway via CD71 (IgA1 Fc receptor)

Complement System

- C3 almost universally present with IgA (~ 90%)
- Accompanied by classic, alternative, or lectin pathway components

Progression/Precipitating Factors

- Asymptomatic individuals can have mesangial IgA
- 2nd hit thought necessary to precipitate disease
  - Often exacerbated by upper respiratory infections
- Complement fixation by lectin pathway may contribute

CLINICAL ISSUES

Epidemiology

- Incidence
  - Most common glomerulonephritis worldwide
    - 10 cases per 1 million person-years in USA
    - 1-3% of end-stage renal disease in USA and Europe
    - Biopsy prevalence: USA (5%), Europe (15%), Japan (30%)
  - Lanthanic IgA
    - 6-16% of donor biopsies have IgA (usually no C3 or IgG)
    - Unclear whether this is precursor or incidental
- Age
  - Wide spectrum (1 to > 65 years)
  - Peak age: 20-30 years
- Sex
  - M:F = 2:1
- Ethnicity
  - Asians > whites > blacks
  - Asian descent risk factor for ESRD (HR = 1.56)

Presentation

- Microhematuria (88%)
- Macrohematuria (43%)
- Hypertension (25%)
- Proteinuria
  - Nephrotic-range proteinuria (10%)
  - > 1 g/d proteinuria (47%)
- Asymptomatic urinary abnormalities (40%)
- Loin or abdominal pain (30%)
- Acute renal failure (7%)
- Chronic renal failure
- Thrombotic microangiopathy

Laboratory Tests

- Elevated circulating IgA (50%)
- Elevated GD-IgA
- IgG and IgA autoantibodies to GD-IgA
- Normal complement levels

Treatment

- Recommendations vary with clinical setting
  - Minor urinary abnormalities: Follow-up for hypertension and progression
  - Microhematuria, proteinuria: Optimized support, corticosteroids if proteinuria > 1g/d
  - Nephrotic syndrome or rapidly progressive kidney injury: Corticosteroids, immunosuppression if vasculitis or crescents
  - Recurrent IgA nephropathy: Supportive care
- Corticosteroids reduce risk of progression in direct proportion to proteinuria (VALIGA)

- Fish oil has debated benefit on renal function
- Tonsillectomy benefit long debated
  - Meta-analysis of 1794 patients shows 3.4x remission with tonsillectomy
- Transplantation
  - Recurrence rate: 32% in protocol biopsies
    - Decreased by cyclosporine (21% vs. 45%)
  - Graft loss from recurrent disease rare (3-4%)

Prognosis

- ~ 80% 10-year renal survival
- Varies with pathological and clinical features
  - 92% of patients with normal Cr and ≤ 0.5 g/d proteinuria
    - Have renal function preservation over 20 years (↑ Cr < 50%) without steroids or immunosuppressants
  - Better survival in children
    - 68% with minor glomerular abnormalities had recurrence free remission at 10 years
  - Paradoxically, recurrent macrohematuria has better 20-year renal survival (91%) than isolated (64%) or no macrohematuria (57%)
- Spontaneous remissions reported
  - 20% who present with nephrotic syndrome (may be minimal change disease)
- Independent clinical predictors of progression to ESRD
  - Reduced eGFR, severe proteinuria, hypertension
- Recurs in transplants in 30%
  - 4-5% graft loss due to recurrence at 10 years
  - Steroid maintenance reduces risk of recurrence 50%

MICROSCOPIC

Histologic Features

- Glomeruli
  - Highly variable glomerular pathology
  - Mesangial hypercellularity and increased matrix usual
    - > 3 mesangial cell nuclei per mesangial area not adjacent to vascular pole, in 3 µm thick section
    - PAS(+) mesangial deposits in adults
  - Focal, segmental inflammation of glomeruli common
  - Endocapillary hypercellularity
  - Necrotizing glomerulonephritis (10%)
  - Crescentic glomerulonephritis (5% have > 50% glomeruli involved)
  - Focal segmental glomerulosclerosis common
    - Broken glomerular basement membrane (GBM) sometimes in scarred areas
    - Collapsing glomerulopathy (~ 10%), associated with more rapid progression
  - Global glomerulosclerosis
  - Glomerulomegaly
  - Minor GBM thickening or duplication
  - Histologically normal in 10%
- Interstitium and tubules
  - Interstitial inflammation with eosinophils, mononuclear cells, plasma cells, and mast cells
  - Red blood cell (RBC) casts
    - Sometimes tubules packed with RBCs, suggesting brisk bleeding from glomerulus
    - Pigmented casts indicate prior red cell leakage
- Vessels
  - Thrombotic microangiopathy (acute or chronic) present (53% in El Karoui series)
  - Associated with more severe glomerular and interstitial scarring and more rapid progression of renal failure
- Repeat biopsies after immunosuppression show reduced endocapillary hypercellularity, crescents, and necrosis

ANCILLARY TESTS

Immunofluorescence

- IgA-dominant or codominant staining of mesangium (100%)
  - Segmental granular GBM deposits in ~ 15%
  - Lambda > kappa (64%)
    - Occasionally only lambda (3%)
- IgA deposits accompanied by IgG (~ 50%), IgM (~ 50%), C3 (~ 90%)
  - C1q uncommon (< 10%)
- Fibrinogen/fibrin in mesangium (~ 30-70%)
- Capillary wall deposits of IgA or presence of IgG correlates with mesangial and endocapillary cellularity, but not with outcome
- Repeat biopsies
  - After clinical response to immunosuppression, persistence but reduced intensity of IgA and C3
  - In 2-year protocol biopsies, IgA deposits disappeared in 20% of children treated with prednisone ± azathioprine

Electron Microscopy

- Electron-dense mesangial deposits
  - Mesangium and paramesangium (100%)
  - Subendothelial deposits (11%)
  - Subepithelial deposits (6%)
  - Intramembranous deposits (2%)
  - Hump-like subepithelial deposits rare
  - Immune deposits do not show substructure
- GBM abnormalities often present
  - Thinning of GBM in 40%
  - May be coincidental (or synergistic) thin basement membrane disease
- Podocytes
  - Extensive foot process effacement with severe proteinuria
  - May be due to minimal change disease
- Mesangium
  - Hypercellularity
  - Increased matrix

Immunohistochemistry

- Mesangial C4d present in 30-38%
  - Independent risk factor for ↓ 20-year renal survival (28% vs. 85%)

DIFFERENTIAL DIAGNOSIS

Henoch-Schönlein Purpura (HSP) Nephritis

- Cannot be distinguished by renal biopsy
  - ~ 1% have vasculitis in kidney
- Clinical evidence crucial in diagnosis: Skin rash, arthritis, abdominal pain, or GI bleeding

Familial IgA Nephropathy

- Indistinguishable by biopsy
- Has poorer prognosis (36% 15-year renal survival)

Lupus Nephritis

- IgA accompanied by "full house" staining pattern by immunofluorescence (IgG, IgM, C3, C1q)
- Nearly all cases of lupus nephritis will show brighter IgG staining than IgA and C1q

Postinfectious Glomerulonephritis (IgA Dominant)

- Subepithelial hump-shaped deposits prominent
- Deposits do not persist

IgA Deposits in HIV Infection

- Prominent tubuloreticular structures in endothelial cells
- Mesangial proliferation ± collapsing glomerulopathy

Hepatic Glomerulosclerosis

- > 60% of cirrhotics have mesangial IgA at autopsy
- Rarely causes severe glomerular pathology

Incidental Mesangial IgA Deposits

- Commonly present (~ 10%) without symptoms
- Typically, little mesangial proliferation, no IgA or C3
- Incidental finding in minimal change disease, membranous GN, thin basement membrane disease, or ANCA-related GN

Minimal Change Disease With IgA Deposits

- Diffuse effacement of foot processes and mild histologic changes with IgA deposits by immunofluorescence likely represents dual glomerulopathy, as nearly all respond to steroids

Focal Segmental Glomerulosclerosis (FSGS)

- IgAN may have histologic pattern of FSGS
- FSGS lacks IgA dominant deposits

DIAGNOSTIC CHECKLIST

Clinically Relevant Pathologic Features

- Independent predictors of progression to ESRD
    - Extent of tubular atrophy/interstitial fibrosis (T)
    - Segmental glomerulosclerosis (S)
    - Mesangial hypercellularity (E)
- Other proposed predictive indicators
    - Crescents (some studies); may not be independent of Cr
    - C4d, C1q

Pathologic Interpretation Pearls

- Acute renal failure may be caused by severe hematuria due to red cell casts
- Broken GBM fragments in scarred areas distinguish from focal, segmental glomerulosclerosis
- PAS(+) mesangial deposits are histologic clue
- IgAN may be entirely normal by light microscopy
- Histologic lesions focal but IgA deposition diffuse
- C1q stain usually negative in IgA nephropathy vs. lupus nephritis
- IgA deposits persistent in IgA nephropathy vs. HSP

GRADING

Historical Classifications

- Lee (1982)
    - Based on proliferation and extent of crescents
- Haas (1997)
    - Modeled on lupus classification
    - Predicts outcome

Oxford Classification System (2009)

- Evidence-based system developed with international group of pathologists and nephrologists led by Ian Roberts and Daniel Cattran
- Scores individual features, does not further classify
- Several individual features correlate with outcome
    - Mesangial hypercellularity (M), segmental glomerulosclerosis (S), endocapillary hypercellularity (E), tubular atrophy/interstitial fibrosis (T)
- Widely used, many studies confirm and extend prognostic significance

SELECTED REFERENCES

1. Milillo A et al: A SPRY2 mutation leading to MAPK/ERK pathway inhibition is associated with an autosomal dominant form of IgA nephropathy. Eur J Hum Genet. ePub, 2015
2. Tesar V et al: Corticosteroids in IgA nephropathy: a retrospective analysis from the VALIGA study. J Am Soc Nephrol. ePub, 2015
3. Zhu L et al: Variants in complement factor H and complement factor H-related protein genes, CFHR3 and CFHR1, affect complement activation in IgA nephropathy. J Am Soc Nephrol. 26(5):1195-204, 2015
4. Coppo R et al: Validation of the Oxford classification of IgA nephropathy in cohorts with different presentations and treatments. Kidney Int. 86(4):828-36, 2014
5. Espinosa M et al: Association of C4d deposition with clinical outcomes in IgA nephropathy. Clin J Am Soc Nephrol. 9(5):897-904, 2014
6. Herlitz LC et al: IgA nephropathy with minimal change disease. Clin J Am Soc Nephrol. 9(6):1033-9, 2014
7. Kiryluk K et al: The genetics and immunobiology of IgA nephropathy. J Clin Invest. 124(6):2325-32, 2014
8. Roberts IS: Pathology of IgA nephropathy. Nat Rev Nephrol. 10(8):445-54, 2014
9. Lee HJ et al: Association of C1q deposition with renal outcomes in IgA nephropathy. Clin Nephrol. 80(2):98-104, 2013
10. Berthoux F et al: Autoantibodies targeting galactose-deficient IgA1 associate with progression of IgA nephropathy. J Am Soc Nephrol. 23(9):1579-87, 2012
11. El Karoui K et al: A clinicopathologic study of thrombotic microangiopathy in IgA nephropathy. J Am Soc Nephrol. 23(1):137-48, 2012
12. Gutiérrez E et al: Long-term outcomes of IgA nephropathy presenting with minimal or no proteinuria. J Am Soc Nephrol. 23(10):1753-60, 2012
13. Zhao N et al: The level of galactose-deficient IgA1 in the sera of patients with IgA nephropathy is associated with disease progression. Kidney Int. 82(7):790-6, 2012
14. Bellur SS et al: Immunostaining findings in IgA nephropathy: correlation with histology and clinical outcome in the Oxford classification patient cohort. Nephrol Dial Transplant. 26(8):2533-6, 2011
15. El Karoui K et al: Focal segmental glomerulosclerosis plays a major role in the progression of IgA nephropathy. II. Light microscopic and clinical studies. Kidney Int. 79(6):643-54, 2011
16. Floege J et al: Current therapy for IgA nephropathy. J Am Soc Nephrol. 22(10):1785-94, 2011
17. Gharavi AG et al: Genome-wide association study identifies susceptibility loci for IgA nephropathy. Nat Genet. 43(4):321-7, 2011
18. Hill GS et al: Focal segmental glomerulosclerosis plays a major role in the progression of IgA nephropathy. I. Immunohistochemical studies. Kidney Int. 79(6):635-42, 2011
19. Shima Y et al: Disappearance of glomerular IgA deposits in childhood IgA nephropathy showing diffuse mesangial proliferation after 2 years of combination/prednisolone therapy. Nephrol Dial Transplant. 26(1):163-9, 2011

Haas IgA Nephropathy Classification

Class	Definition	5-Year Renal Survival, Adults	10-Year Renal Survival, Adults	5-Year Renal Survival, Children	10-Year Renal Survival, Children
Class 1: Minimal histologic lesions	No more than minimal mesangial hypercellularity without FSGS or crescents	100%	> 90%	100%	100%
Class 2: Focal segmental glomerulosclerosis-like	FSGS lesions with at most minimal mesangial hypercellularity and no crescents	100%	> 90%	100%	100%
Class 3: Focal proliferative glomerulonephritis	< 50% glomeruli are hypercellular (segmental or global), including mesangial and endocapillary hypercellularity and crescents	90%	60%	100%	90%
Class 4: Diffuse proliferative	> 50% glomeruli are hypercellular (segmental or global), including mesangial and endocapillary hypercellularity and crescents	60%	20%	85%	60%
Class 5: Advanced chronic glomerulonephritis	> 40% global glomerulosclerosis or > 40% tubular atrophy/loss in PAS-stained sections (trumps other classes if present)	20%	15%	-	-

125 adults ≥ 18 years old; 99 children < 18 years old.

Renal survival data from Haas M et al: IgA nephropathy in children and adults: comparison of histologic features and clinical outcomes. Nephrol Dial Transplant 23: 2537, 2008.

Oxford IgA Nephropathy Classification

Score	Definition	Comments	Hazard Ratio for 50% ↓ eGFR or ESRD (Coppo)	Hazard Ratio for 50% ↓ eGFR Doubling Cr or ESRD (Lv)
Mesangial Hypercellularity				
M0	Mean of < 4 cells per mesangial area			0.6 ($p < 0.001$)
M1	Mean of ≥ 4 cells per mesangial area	If > 50% of glomeruli have > 3, no need to do formal count	2.3 ($p < 0.001$)	
Segmental Glomerulosclerosis				
S0	Absent			
S1	Present		4.1 ($p < 0.001$)*	1.8 ($p < 0.001$)
Endocapillary Hypercellularity				
E0	Absent			1.4 ($p = 0.1$)
E1			Not significant	
Interstitial Fibrosis/Tubular Atrophy				
T0	≤ 25%	% cortical area involved by tubular atrophy or interstitial fibrosis, whichever is greater	5.6 ($p < 0.001$)* (T1 + T2)	3.2 ($p < 0.001$) (T1+T2)
T1	26-50%			
T2	> 50%			
Crescents				
	Present/absent		Not significant	2.3 ($p < 0.001$)

**Significant in multivariate ($p < 0.02$) adjusted for eGFR, follow-up blood pressure, and proteinuria.*

Roberts IS et al: The Oxford classification of IgA nephropathy: pathology definitions, correlations, and reproducibility. Kidney Int 76: 546, 2009. Cattran DC et al: The Oxford classification of IgA nephropathy: rationale, clinicopathological correlations, and classification. Kidney Int 76: 534, 2009. Coppo et al: Validation of the Oxford classification of IgA nephropathy in cohorts with different presentations and treatments. Kidney Int 86: 828, 2014 (n =1147). Lv et al: Evaluation of the Oxford Classification of IgA nephropathy: a systematic review and meta-analysis. Am J Kidney Dis 62: 891, 2013 (n = 3893).

Minimal Mesangial Hypercellularity (M0)

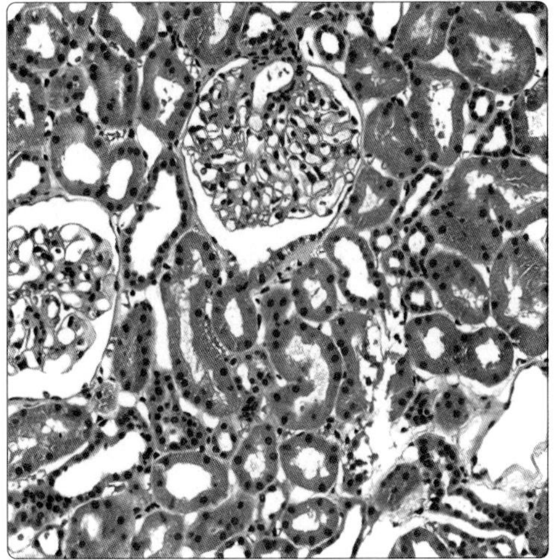

Mesangial Hypercellularity (M0)

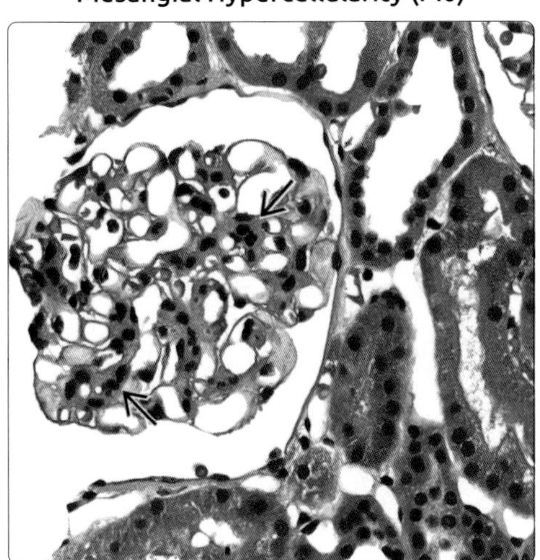

(Left) *H&E of the cortex shows focal minimal mesangial hypercellularity and normal tubules and interstitium. In the Oxford classification, mesangial hypercellularity is scored as a mean of < 4 cells (M0) and ≥ 4 cells/mesangial area (M1).* **(Right)** *This glomerulus shows mild mesangial hypercellularity. Although some mesangial areas have > 10 cells ⇒, this was a focal finding, involving a minority of the glomeruli. Mesangial hypercellularity is scored as a mean of < 4 (M0) and ≥ 4 cells/mesangial area (M1).*

Mesangial Hypercellularity (M1)

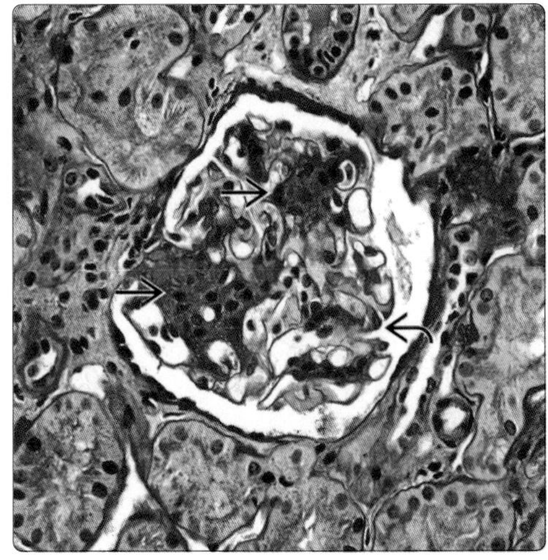

Segmental Glomerulosclerosis (S1)

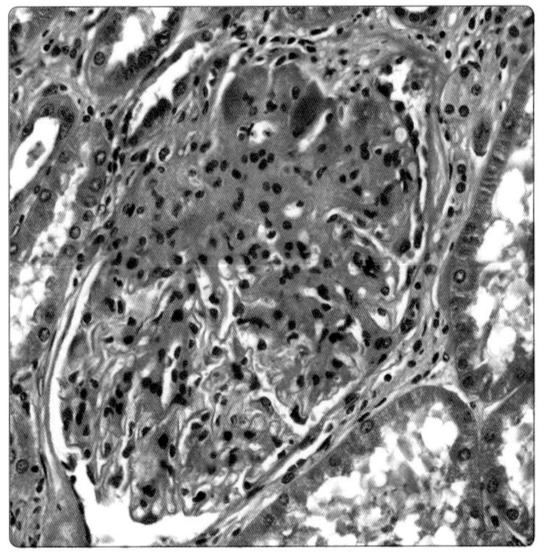

(Left) *This section shows irregular, marked mesangial hypercellularity ⇒ and a normal GBM. Podocytes are basophilic and enlarged ⇒ in this 19-year-old man with a 3-year history of proteinuria and episodes of gross hematuria. Serum IgA was 397 mg/dL (normal: 68-309).* **(Right)** *This glomerulus shows segmental glomerulosclerosis, adhesion to Bowman capsule, and hyaline deposits in this case of advanced IgAN nephropathy. In the Oxford classification, segmental glomerulosclerosis is scored present (S1) or absent (S0).*

Cellular Crescent

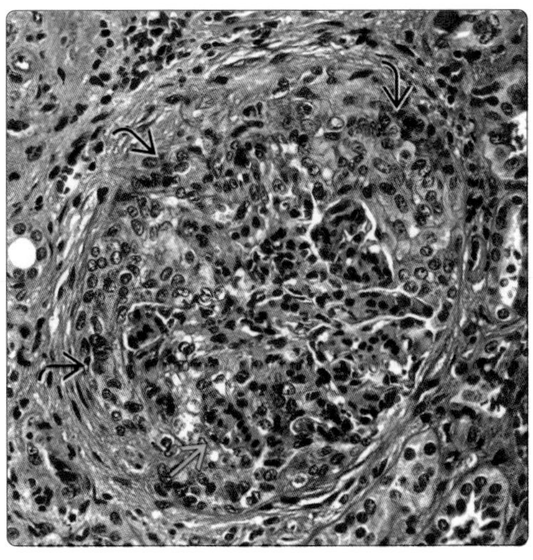

Marked Mesangial Hypercellularity

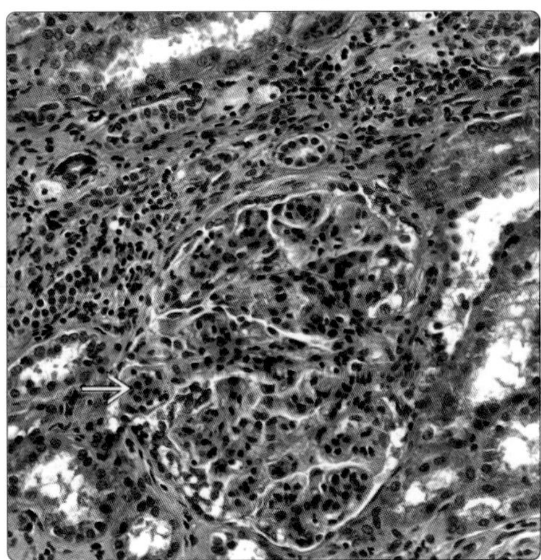

(Left) *Cellular crescent ⇒ is present in a glomerulus that also shows mesangial hypercellularity and glomerulitis ⇒. The distinction between IgAN and Henoch-Schönlein purpura is best made by clinical features.* **(Right)** *This end-stage kidney removed during transplantation shows persistence of mesangial hypercellularity ⇒ even at this late stage. IgA deposits also persist in end-stage kidneys.*

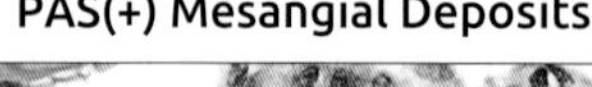

(Left) *A 68-year-old man with microhematuria, proteinuria, Cr 1.2, and elevated serum IgA shows increased mesangial matrix with PAS(+) deposits, a diagnostically helpful feature sometimes found in IgAN. The GBM is segmentally duplicated.* **(Right)** *This PAS(+) "pseudothrombus" was in a glomerular capillary of a 33-year-old man with proteinuria (1.2 g/d), normal Cr (1.1 mg/dL), and recurrent episodes of macrohematuria associated with exercise. A minority of cases of IgAN have cryoglobulins.*

PAS(+) Mesangial Deposits

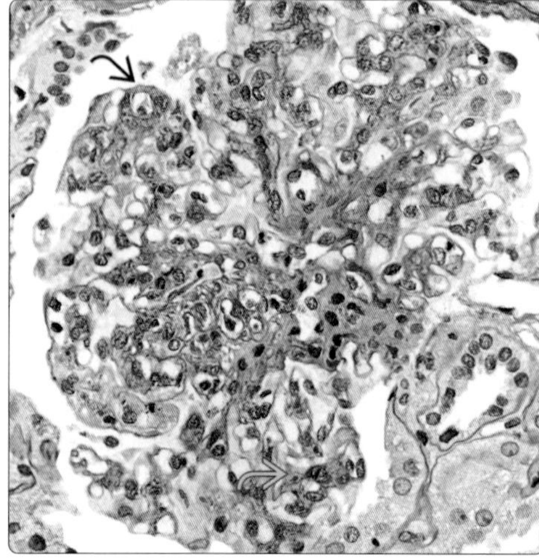

IgAN: Pseudothrombus

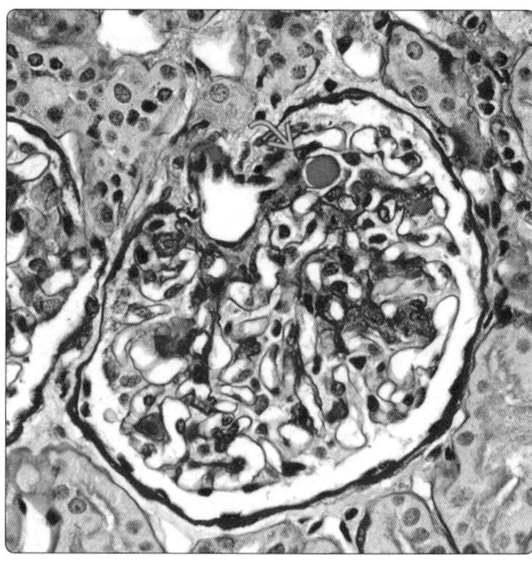

(Left) *Mild mesangial hypercellularity is seen in this biopsy from a patient with sudden onset nephrotic syndrome. IF showed IgA-dominant mesangial deposits. Electron microscopy showed diffuse podocyte foot process effacement, typical of minimal change disease.* **(Right)** *This case shows a mononuclear infiltrate with eosinophils, typical of IgA nephropathy. Prominent interstitial infiltrates in IgAN may be confused with acute interstitial nephritis.*

IgAN With Minimal Change Disease

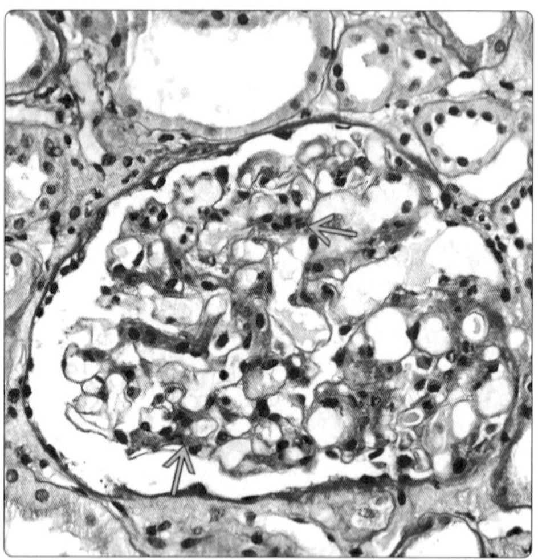

Eosinophils in IgAN

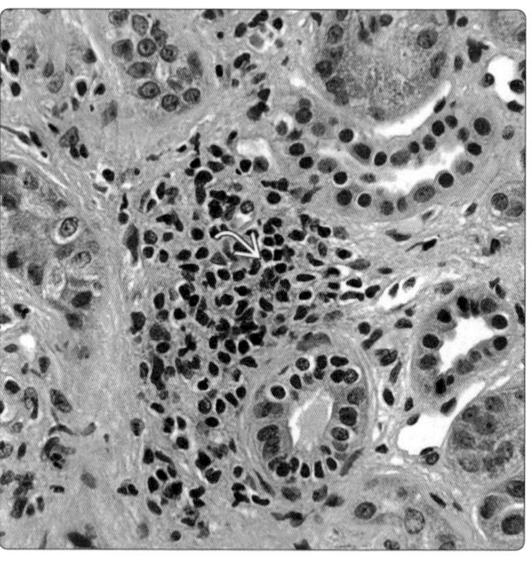

(Left) *Various types of casts are seen, including pigmented with red cell ghosts, red cells mixed with proteinaceous material, and compacted red cells.* **(Right)** *Immunoperoxidase staining for hemoglobin shows staining of red cells and red cell fragments in tubules.*

IgAN: Red Cell Casts

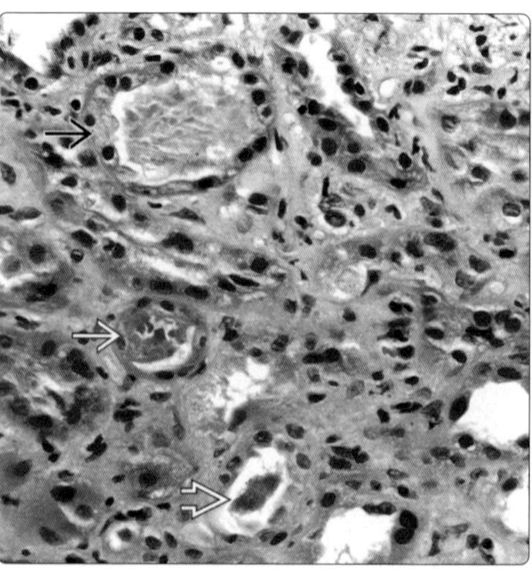

RBC Casts Stained for Hemoglobin

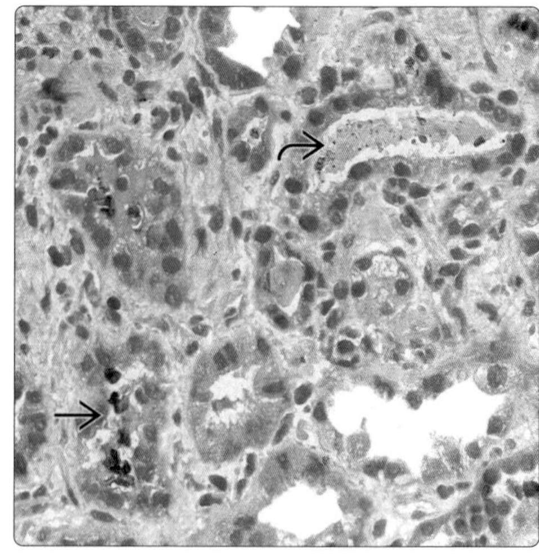

Minimal IgAN: RBC Casts

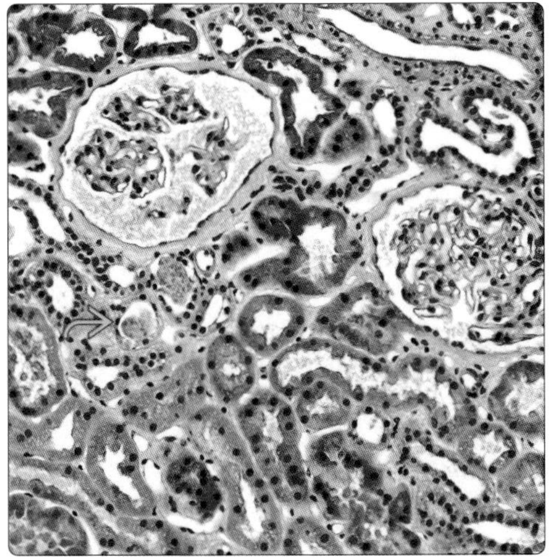

Minimal IgAN: Normal Glomerulus

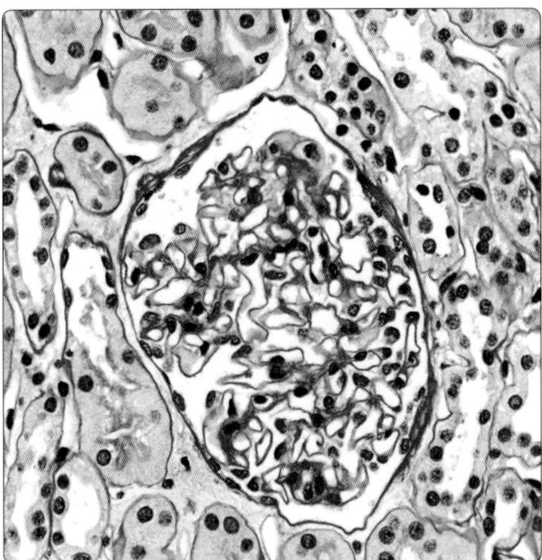

(Left) *Red blood cell casts within tubules* ⮳ *are shown. In this case, the red blood cell casts were the only light microscopic evidence of glomerular disease.* **(Right)** *PAS-stained section shows a normal glomerulus without mesangial expansion or glomerular basement membrane abnormalities.*

Minimal IgAN: Mesangial IgA

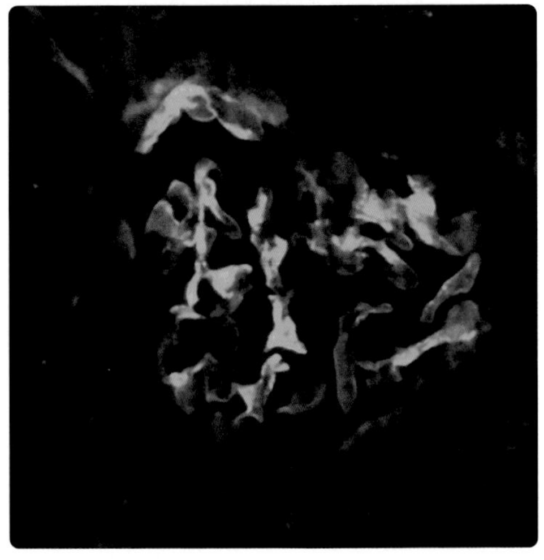

Minimal IgAN: Rare Mesangial Deposits

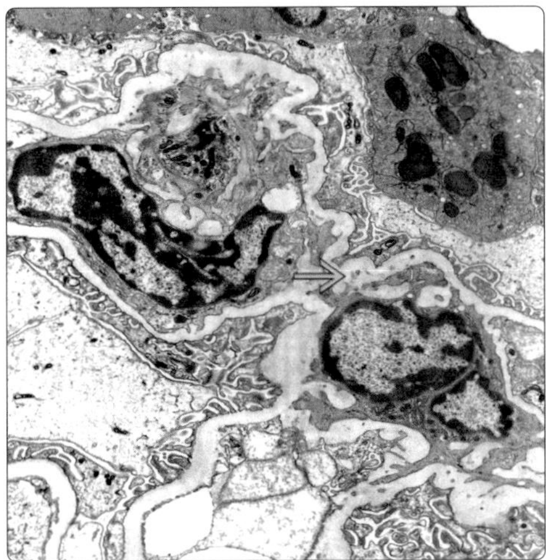

(Left) *Immunofluorescence for IgA shows distinct granular mesangial deposits, 1-2+ in intensity, that affected all of the glomeruli despite their normal appearance by light microscopy. C3 was also present but less intense (1+). The IgA deposits by IF and the presence of electron-dense deposits on electron microscopy made the diagnosis.* **(Right)** *Electron microscopy of a glomerulus shows rare scattered electron-dense deposits in the mesangium* ⇒ *in this example.*

IgAN With Acute Renal Failure

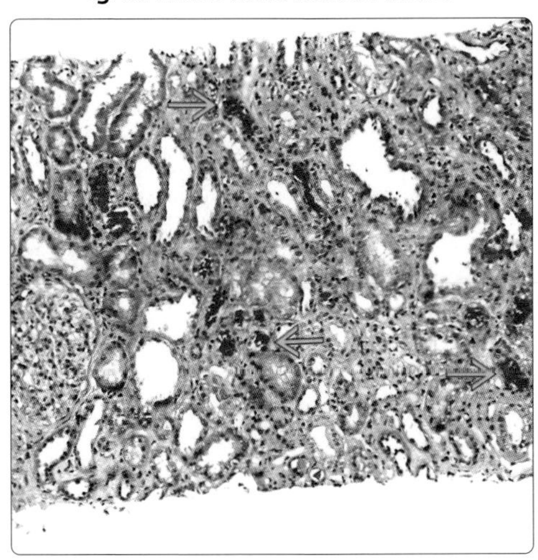

IgAN With Acute Renal Failure

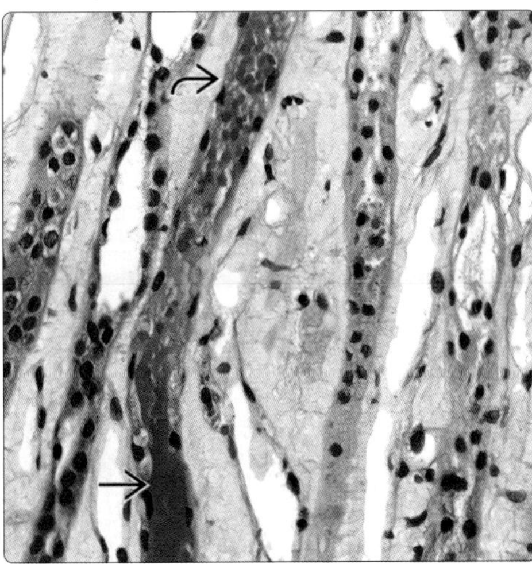

(Left) *Numerous red blood cell casts* ⇒ *are seen in this case of IgAN in a patient on warfarin with acute kidney injury & creatinine of 4.5 mg/dL, increased from 0.8 mg/dL. Red cell casts likely contribute to acute kidney injury; in the setting of a predisposing factor for hematuria, anticoagulant likely contributes to hematuria.* **(Right)** *At high magnification, medulla shows loose red cells in a tubule at the top* ⮳*, embedded in a proteinaceous matrix, with red cells becoming more compacted distally* ➔*.*

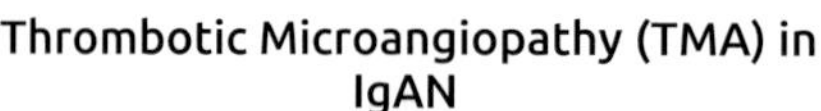

Thrombotic Microangiopathy (TMA) in IgAN

Mucoid Intimal Thickening

(Left) *Thrombotic microangiopathy is a risk factor for progression of IgAN and is associated with severe hypertension. This arteriole shows a thrombus ➙. In addition to IgAN, this patient was pregnant at the time of biopsy and was later found to have a thrombomodulin gene mutation.* **(Right)** *Mucoid intimal thickening is characteristic of thrombotic microangiopathy and a risk factor for progression of IgAN. This patient presented with malignant hypertension and acute renal failure, associated with IgAN.*

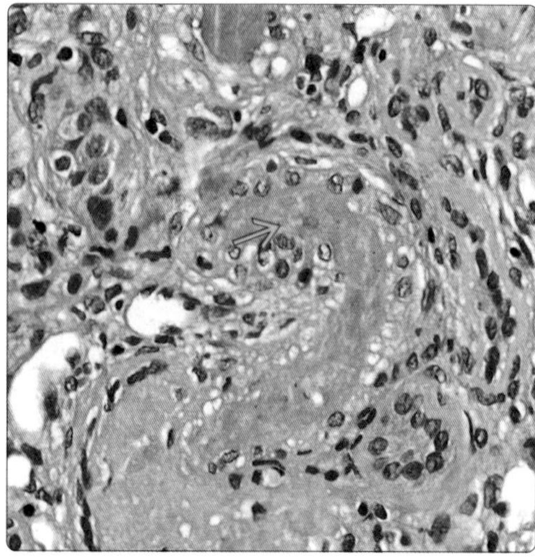

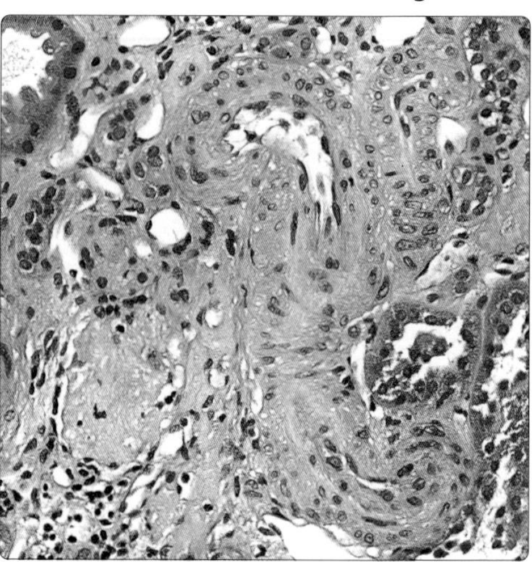

Early Adhesion

Collapsing Lesion in IgAN

(Left) *The initial stage of FSGS is bridging of the glomerular tuft to Bowman capsule by epithelial cells ➙, probably derived from the capsule. A clue that this is not a squeeze artifact is the lamination of Bowman capsule in the same region ➙.* **(Right)** *Collapsing glomerulopathy can be a feature of IgAN and, when present, is a risk factor for progression to ESRD. The epithelial nuclei ➙ are crowded in the area of collapse and bridge to Bowman capsule. Reabsorption droplets ➙ are prominent.*

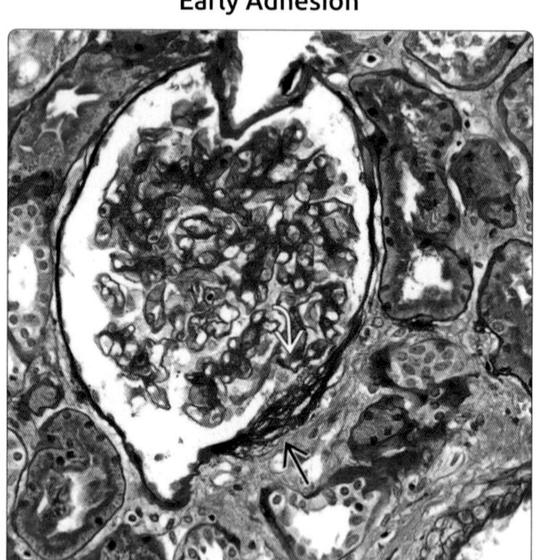

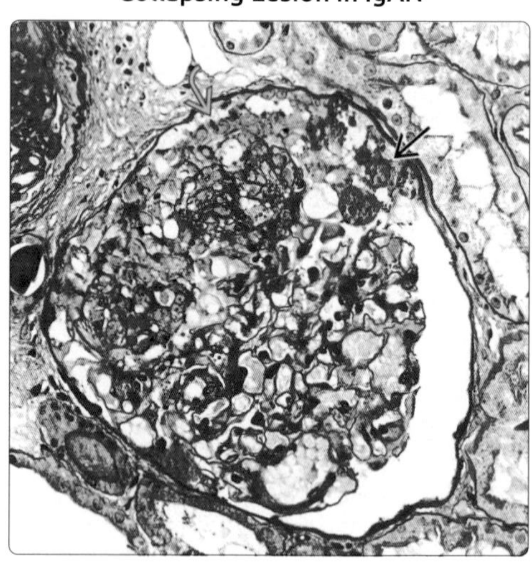

Collapsing Lesion in IgAN

Interstitial Fibrosis and Tubular Atrophy (T2)

(Left) *The collapsing lesions in IgAN have the same phenotype as in primary collapsing glomerulopathy, with loss of normal podocyte differential markers (e.g., WT1) and acquisition of those of Bowman capsule ➙, such as cytokeratin 18 ➙.* **(Right)** *Interstitial fibrosis and tubular atrophy are strong independent predictors of progression of IgAN (and most other forms of renal disease). The Oxford classification scores it as T0 ≤ 25%, T1 = 26-50%, and T2 > 50%. In this case, > 50% of the cortex is fibrotic.*

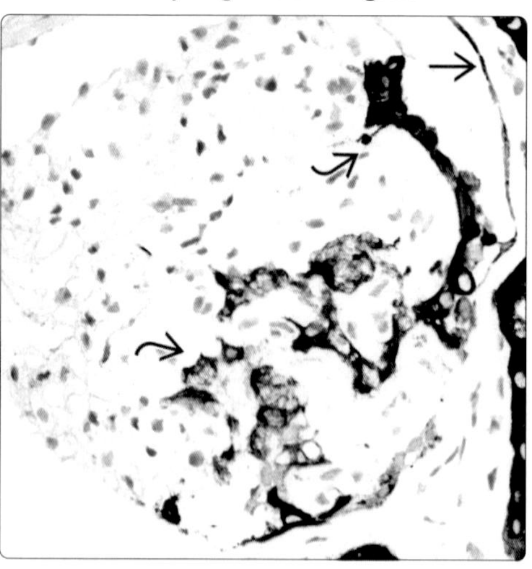

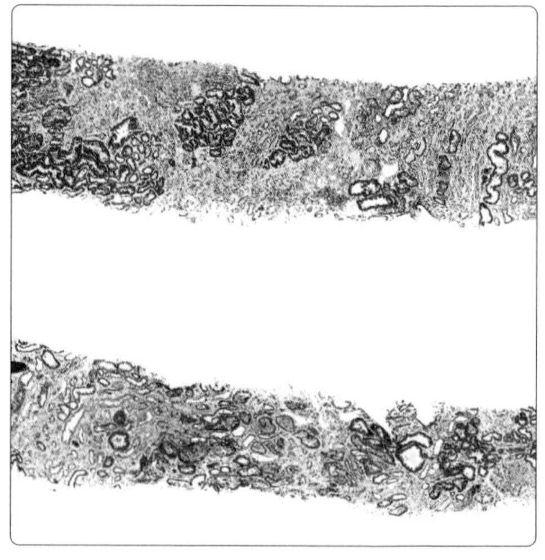

Typical Mesangial IgA Pattern

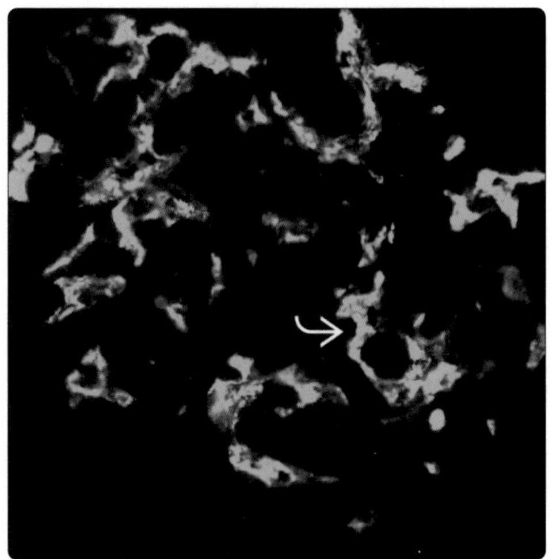

Paramesangial IgA

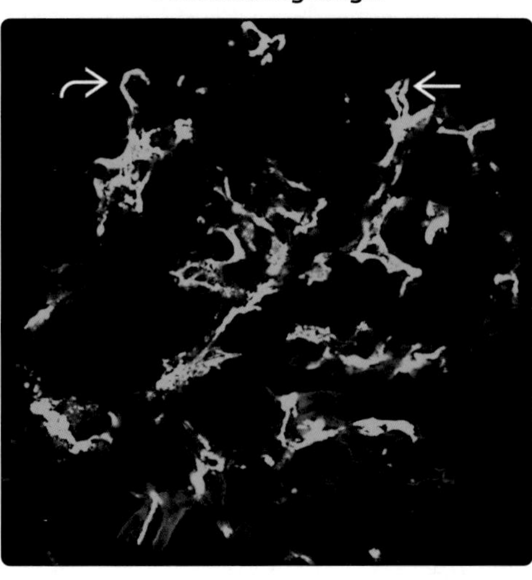

(Left) *The typical tree trunk and branch pattern of IgAN is illustrated here. In areas, the granular pattern of the deposits can be seen ➢. In this glomerulus, little or no IgA is evident along the GBM.* **(Right)** *A stain for IgA shows mostly mesangial deposits; a few capillaries have peripheral loop deposits ➢. It is often difficult to be certain that the deposits are in the capillary wall, as the mesangial deposits typically line up along the GBM bordering the mesangium ➡. A parallel pattern helps distinguish the latter site.*

Mesangial and GBM IgA

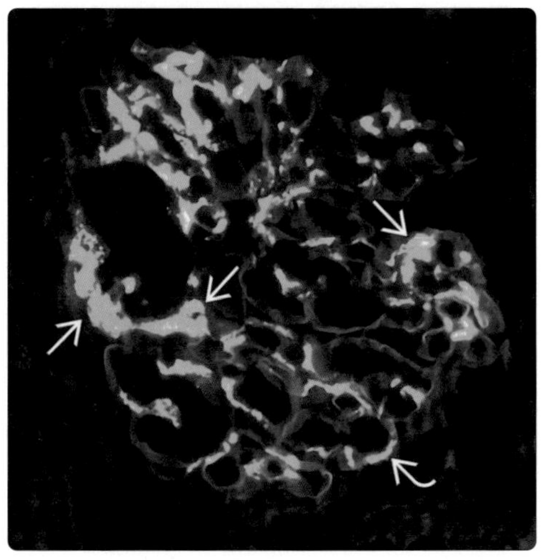

IgAN: Typical IgG Staining

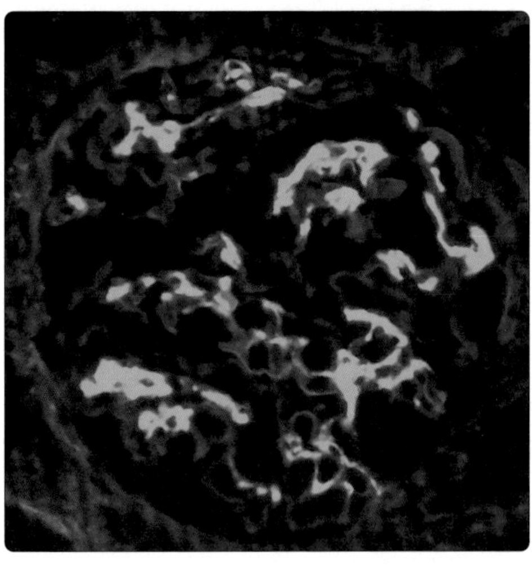

(Left) *Immunofluorescence stain for IgA shows bright granular staining, predominantly mesangial ➡. IgA is the dominant immunoglobulin. Segmental deposits are present along the glomerular basement membrane ➢.* **(Right)** *Immunofluorescence for IgG shows strictly mesangial deposition, somewhat less intense than IgA. About 50% of IgAN cases have IgG, but not more intense than IgA.*

IgAN: Typical C3 Staining

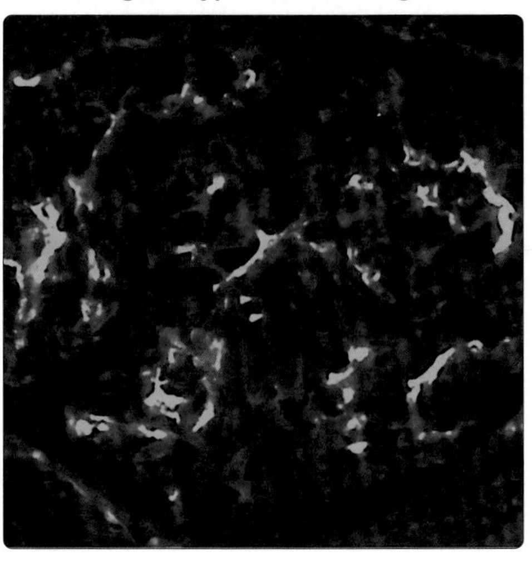

IgAN: Typical Fibrinogen/Fibrin

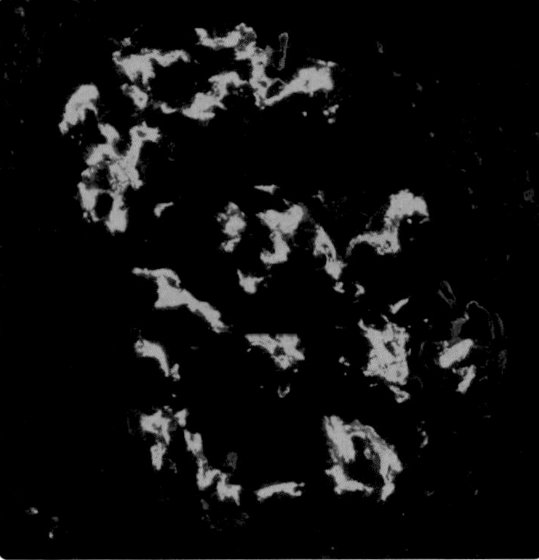

(Left) *Immunofluorescence for C3 shows a sparse, more discrete deposition in the mesangium in this 23-year-old man with IgAN and a 3-year history of episodic gross hematuria, minimal proteinuria (0.7 g/d), and a normal Cr (0.9 mg/dL). C3 is present in > 90% of IgAN cases.* **(Right)** *Immunofluorescence for fibrin or fibrinogen shows 3+ granular deposition that is strictly mesangial in location. Fibrin is commonly present in IgAN; whether it has pathogenetic significance is unknown.*

(Left) *In IgA nephropathy, lambda is often somewhat stronger than kappa, as shown in this panel.* **(Right)** *Immunofluorescence of a glomerulus stained for C1q is trace positive. The paucity of C1q commonly observed in ~ 90% of IgAN helps distinguish the disease from SLE, which usually has prominent C1q in glomeruli.*

Lambda Greater than Kappa

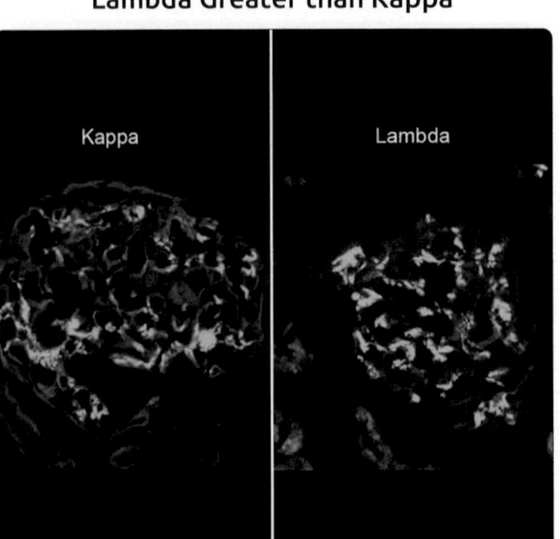

C1q Trace Positive

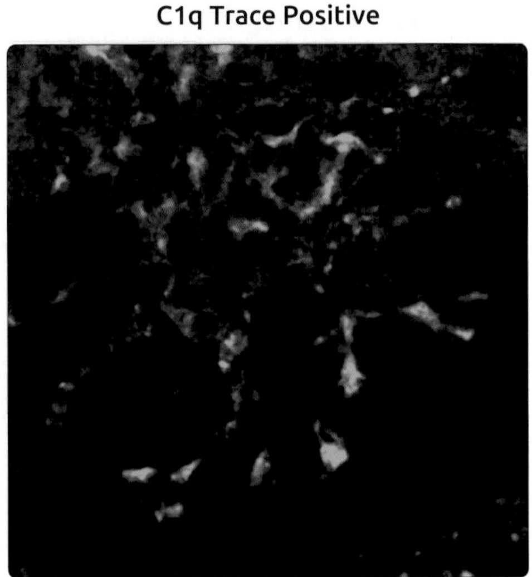

(Left) *Immunofluorescence microscopy shows deposition of fibrin in a crescent ➔, which should be contrasted to the mesangial pattern. Fibrin is present in active (cellular or fibrocellular) crescents in all types of glomerulonephritis.* **(Right)** *Immunofluorescence of an end-stage case of IgAN shows persistence of the IgA deposits in the mesangium. This finding is typical of IgAN, in contrast to Henoch-Schönlein purpura, in which the IgA deposits are usually transient.*

Crescent With Fibrin

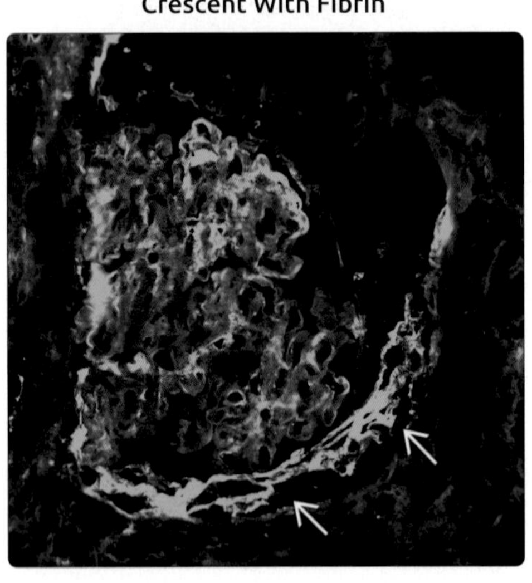

End-Stage IgAN

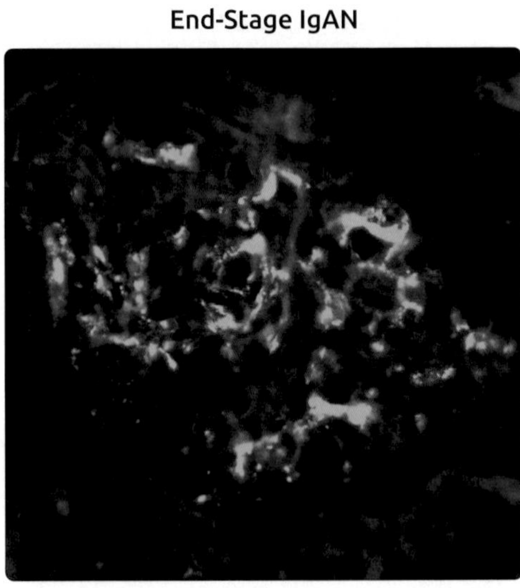

(Left) *Incidental IgA deposition is detected in ~ 10% of donor biopsies. It disappears with time after transplant, and it is not clear whether this is an early stage of IgAN or a "normal" finding. In this case, no C3 was present, and no mesangial deposits were seen on EM.* **(Right)** *IgA in a donor biopsy at the time of transplantation shows 1-2+ mesangial deposition. The donor was asymptomatic. A protocol biopsy 3 months after transplantation shows complete resolution of the IgA deposits.*

Incidental IgA Deposition in Donor Biopsy

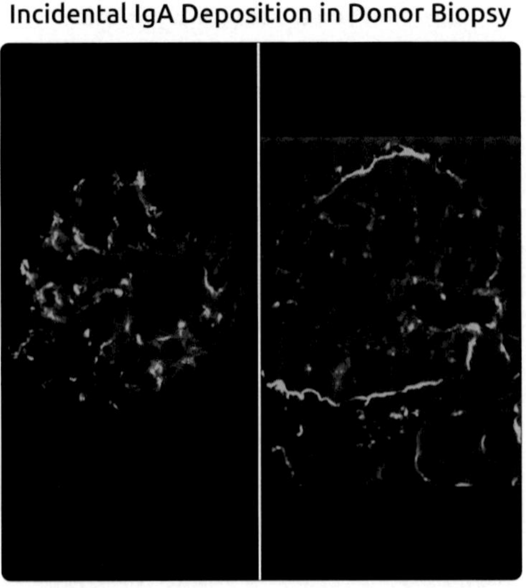

Loss of IgA From Donor Kidney

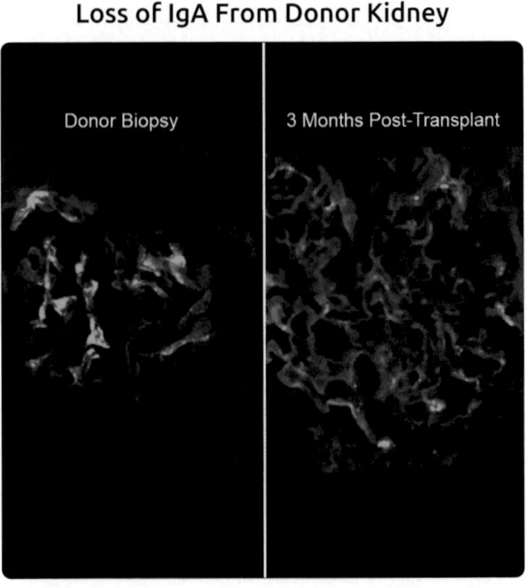

Typical Mesangial Deposits

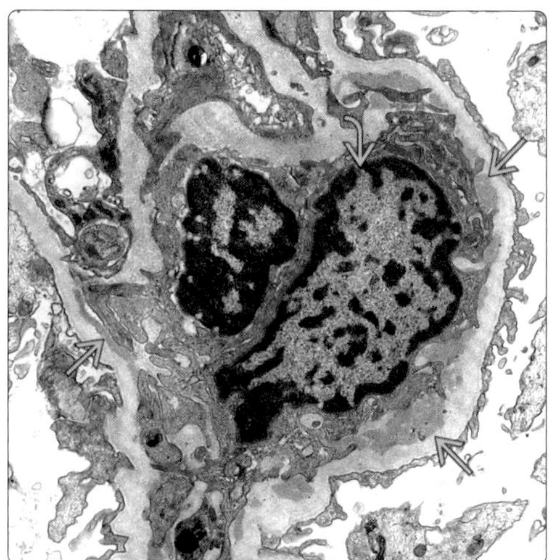

Amorphous Mesangial Deposits

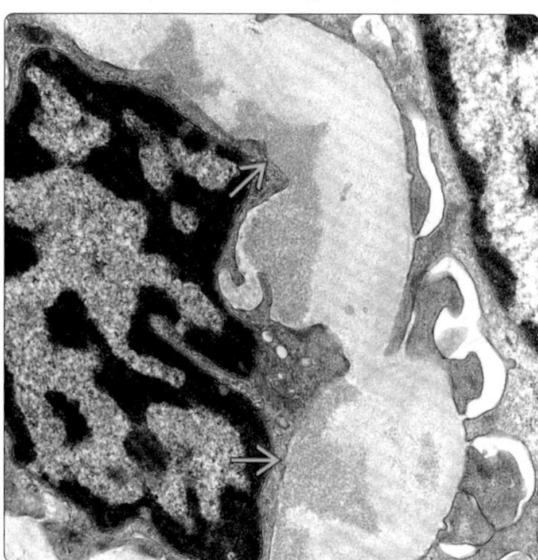

(Left) *EM of a typical case of IgAN shows amorphous electron-dense mesangial deposits ➡ in close contact with a mesangial cell ➡.* **(Right)** *High magnification shows the finely granular texture and lack of substructure in the mesangial deposits and the close contact with the mesangial cell membrane ➡. Interaction of the deposits with the mesangial cell is thought to be important in the pathogenesis of IgAN.*

Subendothelial and Subepithelial Deposits

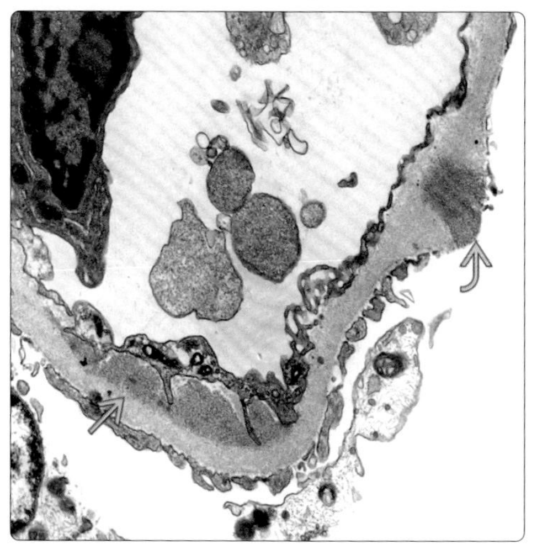

Subendothelial Deposits

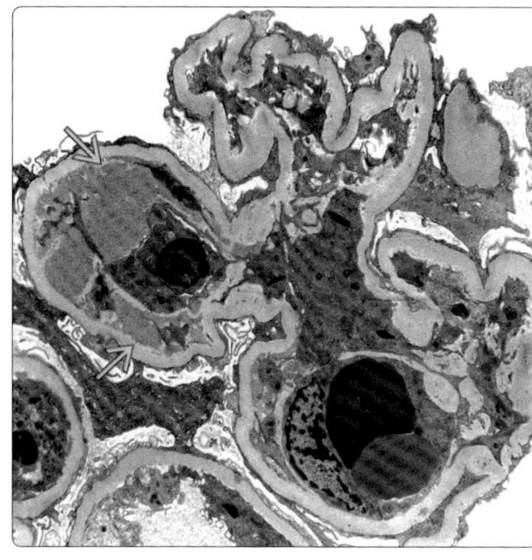

(Left) *EM of a glomerular capillary loop shows subendothelial ➡ and subepithelial ➡ deposits. Deposits along the GBM, although less commonly seen, may be important in causing GBM injury and consequent hematuria and proteinuria.* **(Right)** *EM of a glomerulus shows prominent subendothelial deposits ➡ segmentally, a pattern less commonly seen in IgAN and raises the possibility of other immune complex diseases, such as SLE.*

Expanding Mesangial Deposits

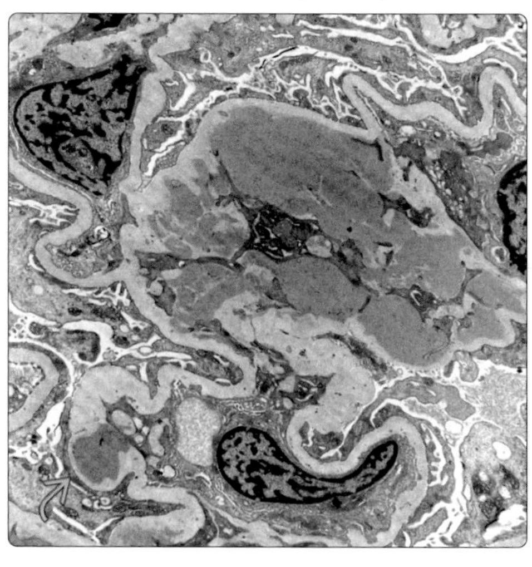

Mesangial Deposits Disrupt GBM

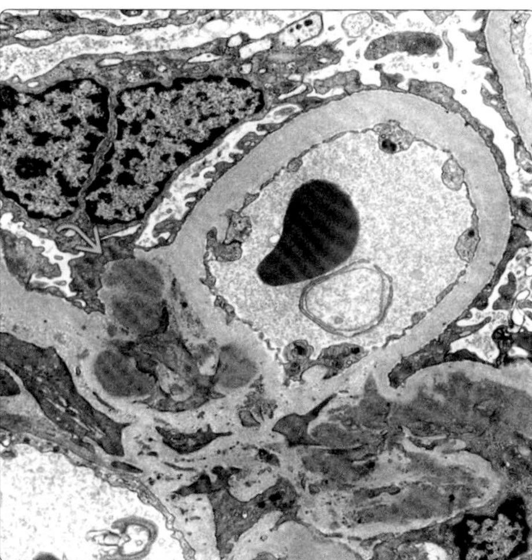

(Left) *EM of a mesangial region shows large mesangial deposits, one of which appears to push through the GBM ➡. This may be a mechanism of GBM disruption in IgAN.* **(Right)** *EM of a mesangial region shows large mesangial deposits, several of which are in a region of GBM disruption and in contact with a podocyte ➡. This may be a mechanism of GBM disruption in IgAN.*

Fragmented GBM

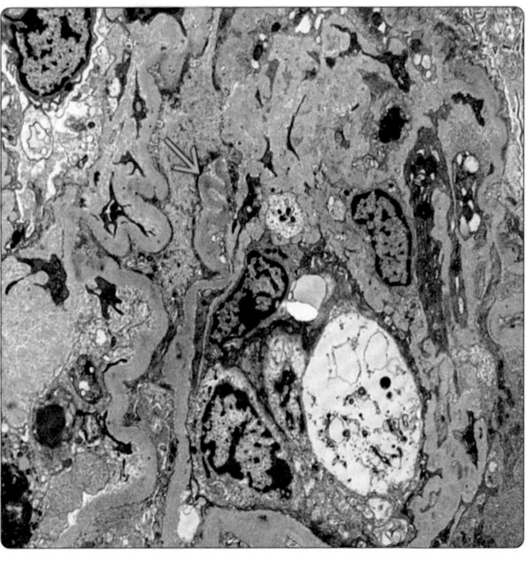

Extreme Thinning of GBM

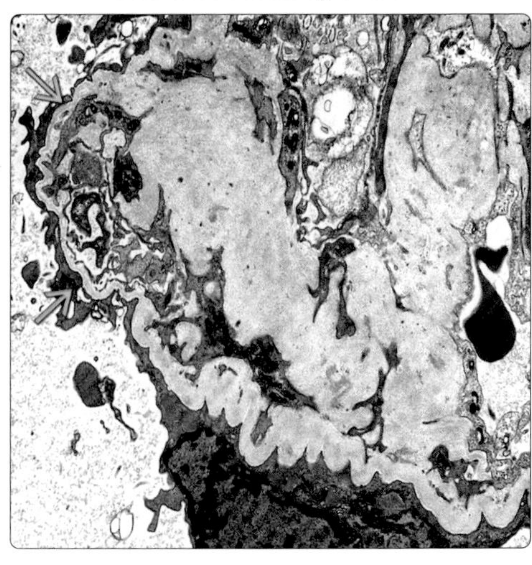

(Left) *EM shows a fragmented portion of GBM → that has been partially repaired with new matrix formation. For hematuria to arise from an injured glomerulus, the GBM has to be disrupted; however, it is uncommon to observe the disruption in histologic or EM preparations.* **(Right)** *EM shows a segment of GBM with extreme thinning →. Overlying this segment is a podocyte with effaced foot processes. This is believed to be a site of previous disruption/injury and the beginning of a repair.*

Diffuse Foot Process Effacement

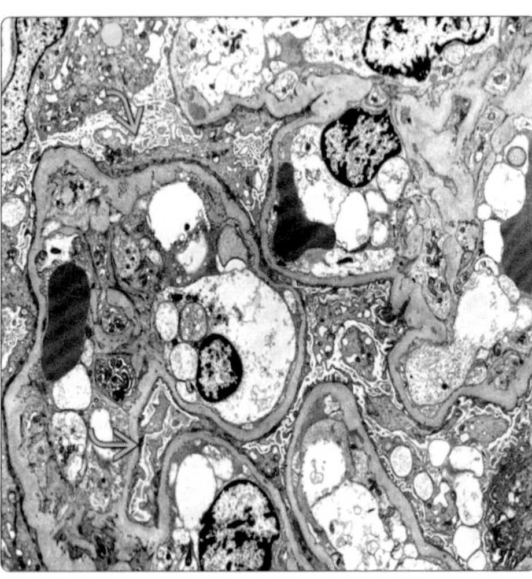

Coincidental Thin Basement Membrane Disease

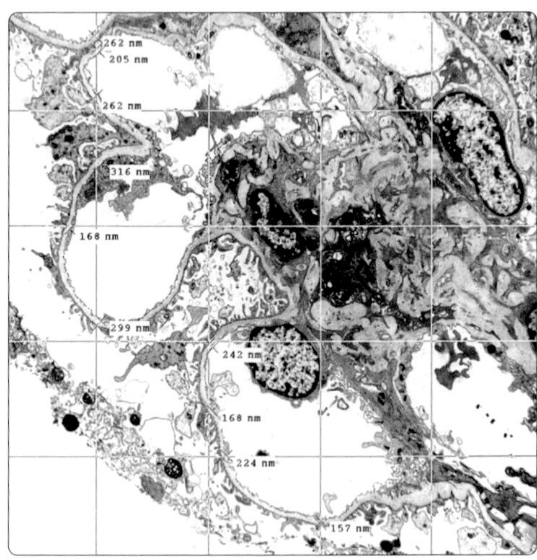

(Left) *Widespread foot process effacement →, as shown, can sometimes be seen in patients with IgA mesangial deposits, nephrotic syndrome, and mild histologic lesions. The nephrotic syndrome often responds to corticosteroids and is thought to be due to superimposed minimal change disease.* **(Right)** *EM shows a thin but normal-appearing GBM in a patient with IgAN. This provides evidence of a 2nd disease, thin basement membrane disease, which may be synergistic with IgAN in causing hematuria.*

GBM Laminations

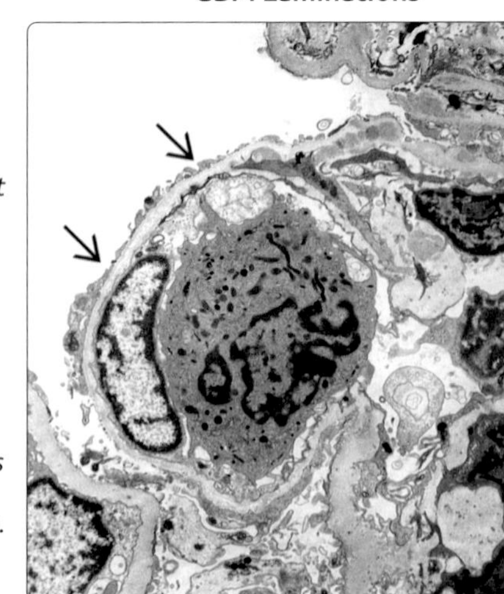

Pseudo-Alport GBM Lesions in IgAN

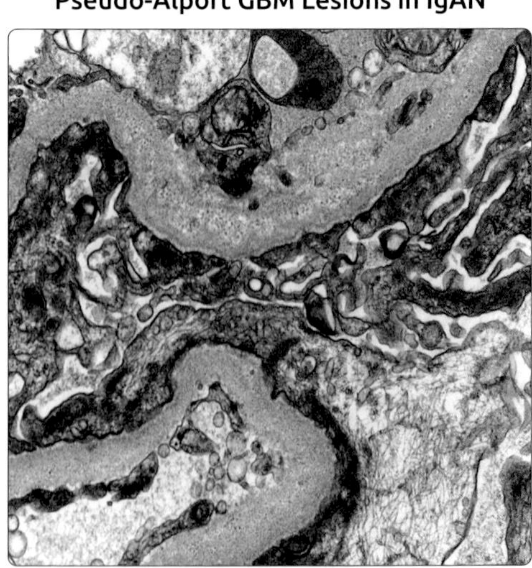

(Left) *EM shows a multilaminated segment of GBM → with irregular layers of matrix. This repair process resembles the GBM lesions of Alport syndrome from which it is distinguished, primarily by the segmental nature and preservation of a3(IV) and a5 (IV) collagen staining.* **(Right)** *A segment of laminated GBM has intervening particles that closely resembles Alport syndrome. IgAN typically has only a few capillaries with this pattern and stains normally for a3(IV) and a5 (IV) collagen.*

Recurrent IgAN 8 Years Post Transplant

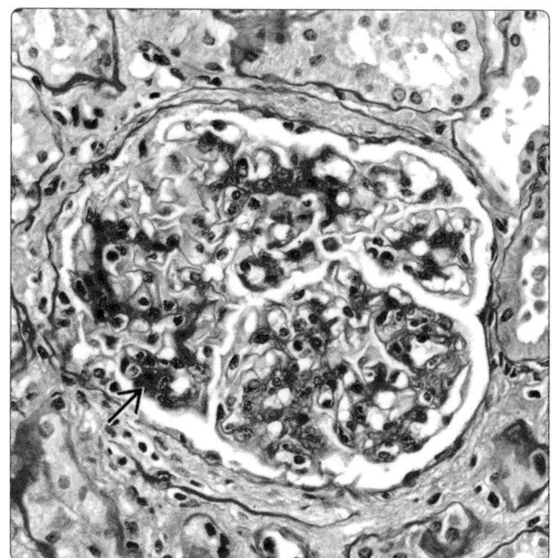

Recurrent IgAN 8 Years Post Transplant

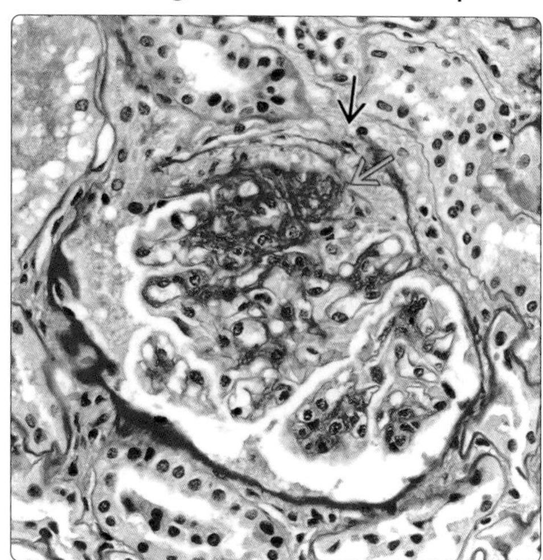

(Left) *PAS shows mesangial hypercellularity ⇨ and a generally normal GBM in a 43-year-old woman with recurrent IgAN 8 years after living unrelated renal transplantation.* **(Right)** *This glomerulus with recurrent IgAN has a segmental scar and adhesion to Bowman capsule, which is disrupted ⇨. The broken GBM ⇨ is indicative of inflammatory injury (vs. the usual FSGS), and the disrupted Bowman capsule suggests a past crescent.*

IgA Deposition in Recurrent IgAN

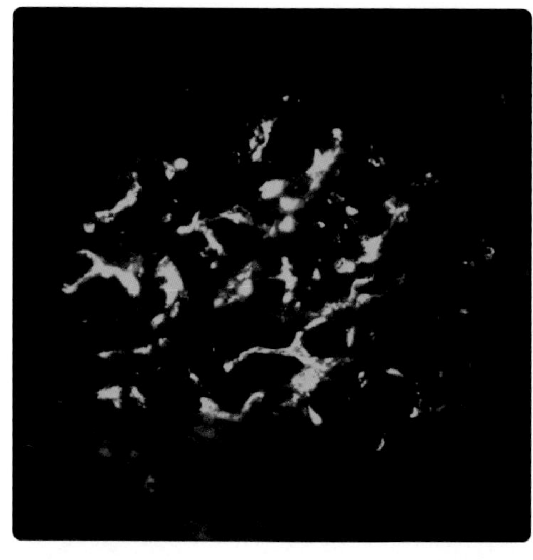

Recurrent IgAN

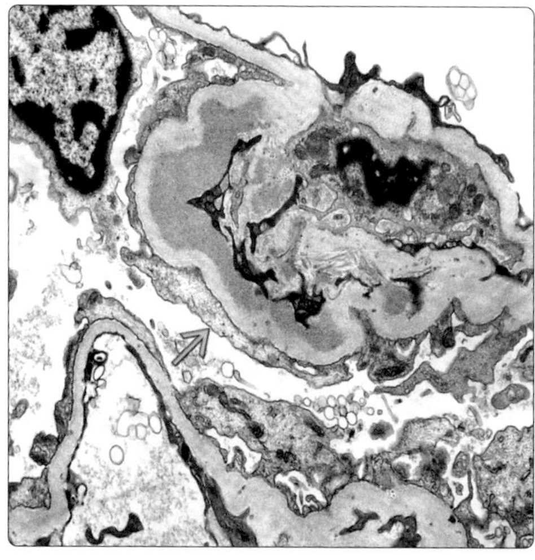

(Left) *This biopsy from a 43-year-old woman with a living unrelated renal transplant and elevated serum creatinine has prominent IgA deposition in the mesangium 8 years post transplant.* **(Right)** *EM shows amorphous electron-dense deposits closely applied to the mesangial cell. Segmental podocyte foot process effacement ⇨ is also present in this case of recurrent IgAN 8 years after living unrelated renal transplantation.*

Recurrent IgAN 4 Months Post Transplant

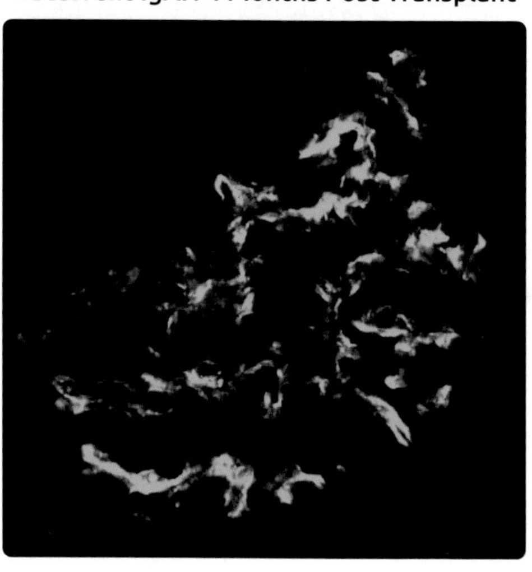

Early Recurrence With Mesangial Deposits

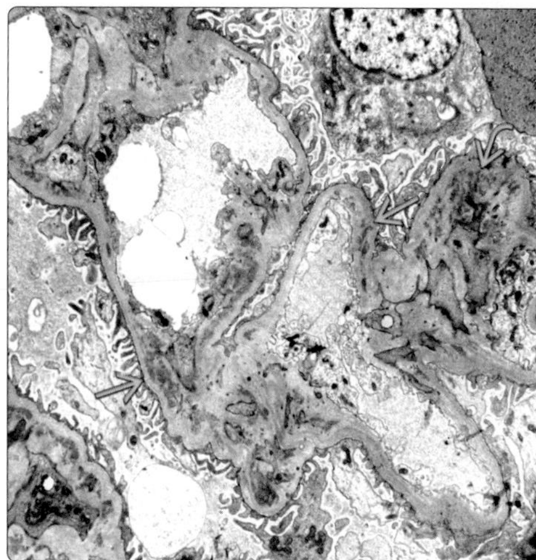

(Left) *Immunofluorescence shows prominent IgA mesangial deposits in recurrent IgA nephropathy 4 months after transplantation. A biopsy at 15 days post transplant previously had only a trace IgA in this 22-year-old man.* **(Right)** *EM shows paramesangial ⇨ and mesangial ⇨ amorphous electron-dense deposits 4 months after transplantation in this 22-year-old man with recurrent IgAN.*

Henoch-Schönlein Purpura

KEY FACTS

TERMINOLOGY

- Glomerular IgA immune complex deposition with extrarenal manifestations, such as purpura

ETIOLOGY/PATHOGENESIS

- Unknown, abnormal glycosylation of IgA1

CLINICAL ISSUES

- Most common childhood vasculitis
- 90% of cases occur before age of 10 years
- Purpura
  - Often involves lower extremities and buttocks
  - Skin biopsy demonstrates leukocytoclastic vasculitis with IgA deposition in acute lesions
- Abdominal pain
- Arthritis
- Hematuria
  - More renal involvement in adults (50-80%) than in children (20-50%)
- Prognosis depends on extent of renal involvement
  - Often worse in adults vs. children

MICROSCOPIC

- Variable mesangial hypercellularity
- Cellular crescents variable extent
- IF: Prominent IgA deposits, primarily in mesangium
- EM: Amorphous deposits in mesangium
  - Also subendothelial and sometimes subepithelial deposits

TOP DIFFERENTIAL DIAGNOSES

- IgA nephropathy
- IgA-dominant postinfectious GN
- Mesangial proliferative lupus nephritis

DIAGNOSTIC CHECKLIST

- Use International Study of Kidney Disease in Children (ISKDC) Histologic Classification (1977)

(Left) *In this Henoch-Schönlein purpura (HSP) patient, purpura is diffusely present on the lower extremities, which is a common site for skin manifestations. (Courtesy V. Petronic-Rosic, MD.)* **(Right)** *Segmental fibrinoid necrosis ⇒ with the prominence of adjacent epithelial cells is a common finding in HSP patients. Marked accumulation of red blood cells within the adjacent tubular lumina ⇨ correlates with the presence of gross hematuria.*

Purpura

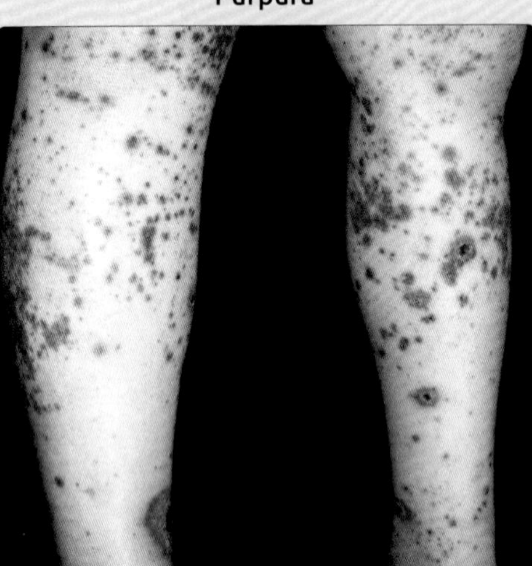

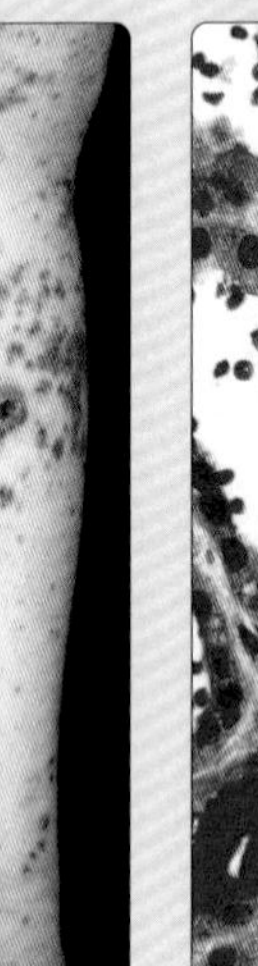

Fibrinoid Necrosis Glomerulus

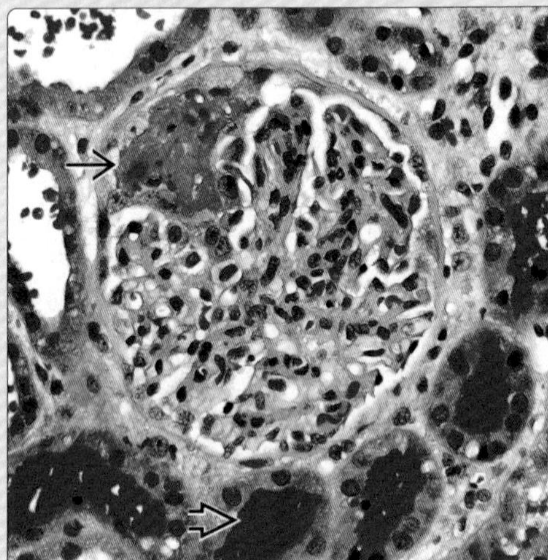

(Left) *Glomerular IgA deposition in primarily mesangial areas ➡ is the characteristic pathologic finding for the diagnosis of HSP along with the presence of extrarenal manifestations.* **(Right)** *Electron-dense deposits consistent with immune complexes are present in the mesangial region ⇨ of this glomerulus from a patient with HSP, which appears identical to IgA nephropathy.*

Mesangial IgA

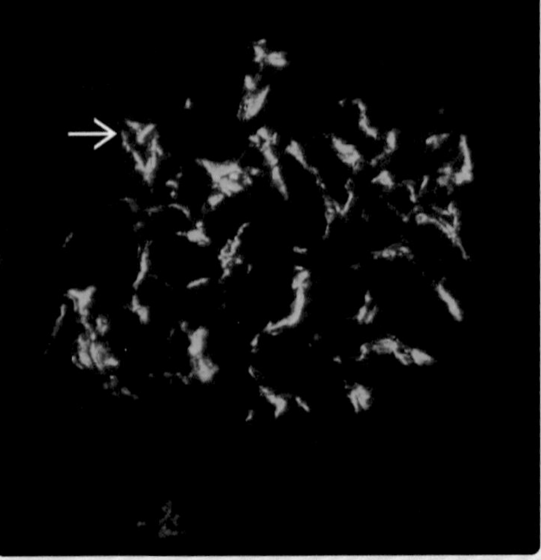

Mesangial Amorphous Electron Dense Deposits

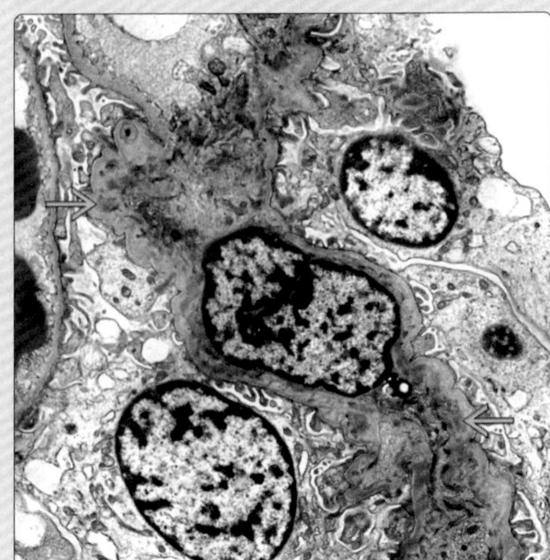

TERMINOLOGY

Abbreviations

- Henoch-Schönlein purpura (HSP)
  - Johann Schönlein (1793-1864)
    - Described entity in 1837
  - Eduard Henoch (1820-1910)

Synonyms

- HSP nephritis
- Anaphylactoid purpura
- Purpura rheumatica
- Heberden-Willan disease
  - William Heberden (1710-1801) and Robert Willan (1757-1812) described 1st cases in 1802 and 1808, respectively

Definitions

- Glomerular IgA immune complex deposition with extrarenal manifestations, such as purpura

ETIOLOGY/PATHOGENESIS

Infectious Agents

- Upper respiratory infection often precedes onset of HSP
  - HSP more common in winter months
- No definitive infectious agent identified as cause of HSP
  - IgA binding streptococcal M binding proteins identified in glomerular immune complexes of subset of HSP patients
  - Nephritis-associated plasmin receptor, group A streptococcal antigen, detected in mesangium of 30% of HSP patients

Abnormal Glycosylation of IgA1

- Galactose deficient or decreased galactosylation at hinge region of IgA molecule
  - HSP patients without renal involvement lack abnormal glycosylation of IgA1
- Increased binding of abnormal IgA1 to mesangial cells in vitro
- IgA1 bound with IgG specific for galactose-deficient IgA1 stimulates cultured mesangial cell proliferation
- Hepatic clearance of abnormal IgA1 is decreased in IgA nephropathy and possibly in HSP patients

Genetic Factors

- Complement deficiency
  - C2 deficiency or complete C4 deficiency increases likelihood of HSP development
  - C4B deficiency increases likelihood of nephritis in HSP patients
  - C4A deficiency worsens HSP nephritis severity

Possible Relationship With IgA Nephropathy

- IgA nephropathy precedes development of HSP in some patients
- Many similarities with clinical and pathologic features of HSP and IgA nephropathy
  - HSP may represent systemic form of IgA nephropathy
  - Systemic immune complexes also consist of IgA1 subclass

CLINICAL ISSUES

Epidemiology

- Incidence
  - 6-20 cases per 100,000 children
    - Most common childhood vasculitis
- Age
  - 90% of cases occur before age of 10 years
  - Can occur at any age
- Sex
  - Male > female
- Ethnicity
  - Caucasian > African descent

Presentation

- European League Against Rheumatism and Paediatric Rheumatology European Society (2006) HSP criteria
  - Palpable purpura (mandatory criterion)
    - Usual initial sign
    - Often involves lower extremities and buttocks
    - May also involve face, trunk, and arms
  - And at least 1 of following criterion
    - Hematuria &/or proteinuria
      - 40% of pediatric patients develop nephritis within 4-6 weeks after purpura
      - Renal involvement in adults (50-80%) > children (20-50%)
    - Diffuse abdominal pain
      - Gastrointestinal tract bleeding &/or obstruction
    - Arthritis or acute arthralgia in any joint
    - Any biopsy with dominant IgA deposition

Laboratory Tests

- Serum IgA level elevated in ~ 50%
- Plasma IgE level increased in > 70%
- Low C3 in ~ 10%

Natural History

- Spontaneous regression common when no renal involvement is present

Treatment

- Surgical approaches
  - Tonsillectomy
    - Combination with steroid therapy may be useful
    - Clinical studies of tonsillectomy alone show mixed outcomes
- Drugs
  - High-dose corticosteroids
  - No treatment necessary in mild cases
- Kidney transplantation
  - Recurrence rate of 15-20%
    - Recurrence in related > unrelated donors
    - Necrotizing and crescentic HSP glomerulonephritis (GN) recurred compared to 12% with mesangial proliferation
    - 10% graft loss due to recurrence
  - 10-year graft survival ~ 90% in children and 75% in adults

Prognosis

- Dependent on extent of renal involvement

International Study of Kidney Disease in Children Classification

Class	Progression to Chronic Kidney Disease
I (minimal alterations)	< 15% (often grouped with class II)
II (pure mesangial proliferation)	15%
III (focal [IIIa] or diffuse [IIIb] mesangial proliferation with < 50% crescents)	15%
IV (focal [IVa] or diffuse [IVb] mesangial proliferation with 50-75% crescents)	37%
V (focal [Va] or diffuse [Vb] mesangial proliferation with > 75% crescents)	70%
VI (membranoproliferative-like GN)	Paucity of data

- End-stage renal disease in ~ 30% of adults and 2% of children
- Severe proteinuria correlates with worse outcome

MICROSCOPIC

Histologic Features

- Glomerular alterations
  - May be normal
  - Variable mesangial hypercellularity
    - Mesangial hypercellularity defined as > 2 mesangial cell nuclei (per 2 μm thick section) or > 3 mesangial cell nuclei (per 3 μm thick section)
    - Mesangial PAS(+) granules representing IgA immune complexes may be present
  - Cellular crescent formation
    - Focal to diffuse
- Necrotizing vasculitis (rare)
  - Rare necrotizing capillaritis of peritubular capillaries of renal medulla
- Acute tubular injury
- Interstitial inflammation
  - May be prominent with significant crescentic glomerular injury
- Interstitial fibrosis and tubular atrophy

Other Sites

- Skin
  - Leukocytoclastic vasculitis
    - IgA deposition in vessels may be patchy and present primarily in acute lesions
- GI tract
  - Leukocytoclastic vasculitis with IgA deposits

ANCILLARY TESTS

Immunofluorescence

- IgA dominant, primarily mesangial, and focally along GBM
  - Other reactants usually present: C3, IgG
  - Variable IgM, fibrin; little C1q
- Late in disease course, IgA disappears vs. persistence of IgA in IgA nephropathy

Electron Microscopy

- Amorphous deposits in mesangium
  - May be absent in some cases despite strong IgA staining
- Often subendothelial deposits
  - May correlate with crescent formation and necrosis
- Segmental subepithelial "humps" sometimes present
  - Must exclude IgA-dominant postinfectious GN

DIFFERENTIAL DIAGNOSIS

IgA Nephropathy

- Identical pathologic features as HSP
- Absence of extrarenal manifestations
- IgA deposits persist in contrast to HSP

Mesangial Proliferative Lupus Nephritis

- Requires clinical diagnosis of systemic lupus erythematosus
- IgA not dominant or codominant immunoglobulin

IgA-Dominant Postinfectious GN

- May be associated with staphylococcal infection
- Large subepithelial electron-dense deposits ("humps")

Pauci-Immune Crescentic GN

- 85% positive for antineutrophil cytoplasmic antibodies (antimyeloperoxidase or antiproteinase 3)
- Mesangial IgA deposits may be present, typically 1+ staining or less
- No significant mesangial or endocapillary hypercellularity

DIAGNOSTIC CHECKLIST

Pathologic Interpretation Pearls

- Endocapillary hypercellularity and interstitial fibrosis/tubular atrophy but not crescents are independent risk factors for progression (Oxford IgA classification)
- Renal biopsy findings cannot distinguish between HSP and IgA nephropathy

Grading

- Meadow Histologic Classification System (1972)
- International Study of Kidney Disease in Children (ISKDC) Histologic Classification (1977)

SELECTED REFERENCES

1. Davin JC et al: Henoch-Schönlein purpura nephritis in children. Nat Rev Nephrol. 10(10):563-73, 2014
2. Kim CH et al: Using the Oxford classification of IgA nephropathy to predict long-term outcomes of Henoch-Schönlein purpura nephritis in adults. Mod Pathol. 27(7):972-82, 2014
3. Edström Halling S et al: Predictors of outcome in Henoch-Schönlein nephritis. Pediatr Nephrol. 25(6):1101-8, 2010
4. Lau KK et al: Pathogenesis of Henoch-Schönlein purpura nephritis. Pediatr Nephrol. 25(1):19-26, 2010
5. Hung SP et al: Clinical manifestations and outcomes of Henoch-Schönlein purpura: comparison between adults and children. Pediatr Neonatol. 50(4):162-8, 2009
6. Counahan R et al: Prognosis of Henoch-Schönlein nephritis in children. Br Med J. 2(6078):11-4, 1977

Normal Glomerulus by LM

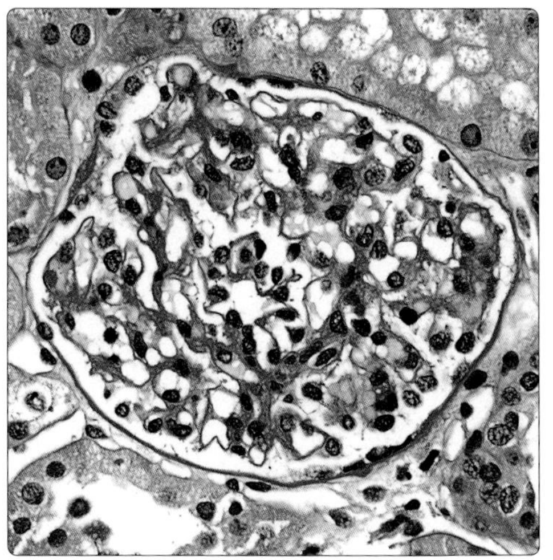

Segmental Mesangial Hypercellularity

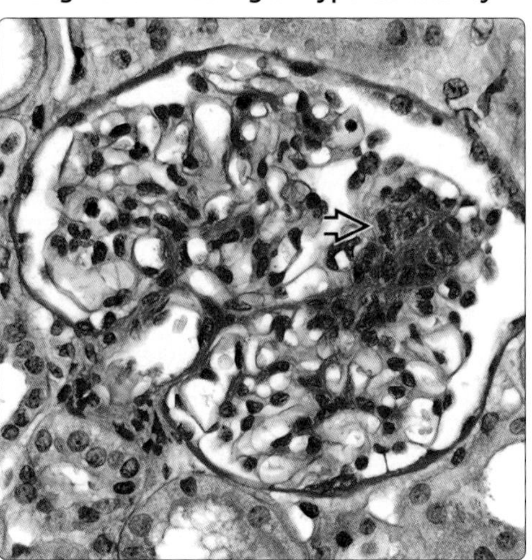

(Left) *This glomerulus from a 4-year-old girl with HSP appears normal, but a necrotizing and crescentic injury (not shown) involved 20% of her glomeruli. Antineutrophil cytoplasmic antibodies were also present and may have contributed to the crescentic injury.* **(Right)** *Marked segmental mesangial hypercellularity ⇨ is present in this glomerulus from an 8-year-old girl with HSP.*

Focal Crescent Formation and Interstitial Nephritis

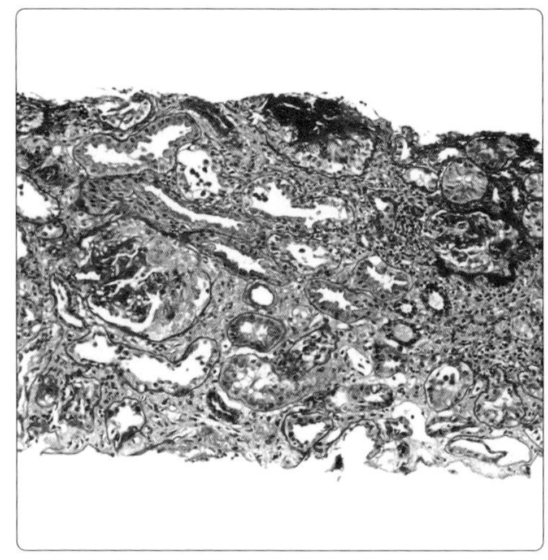

Cellular Crescent

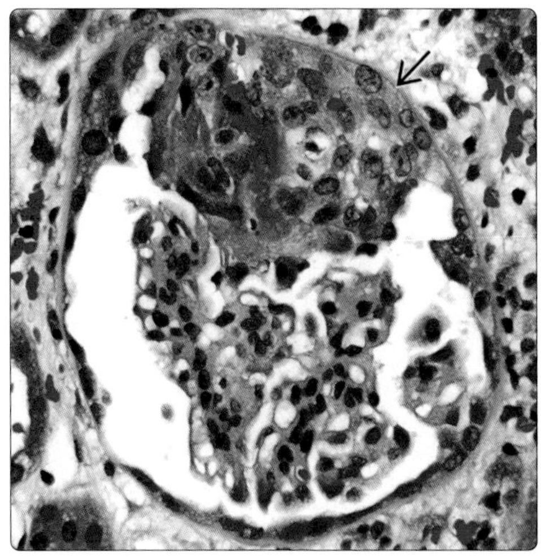

(Left) *Crescents are evident in this low-power view of a case of HSP. If crescents are > 50% of glomeruli, the prognosis is worse. However, HSP with crescents still has a good prognosis. Interstitial nephritis is also commonly present.* **(Right)** *A small cellular crescent ➙ with fibrinoid necrosis occupies the upper portion of the urinary space and compresses the remaining glomerular tufts, which reveal mild mesangial hypercellularity in an HSP patient.*

Endocapillary Hypercellularity

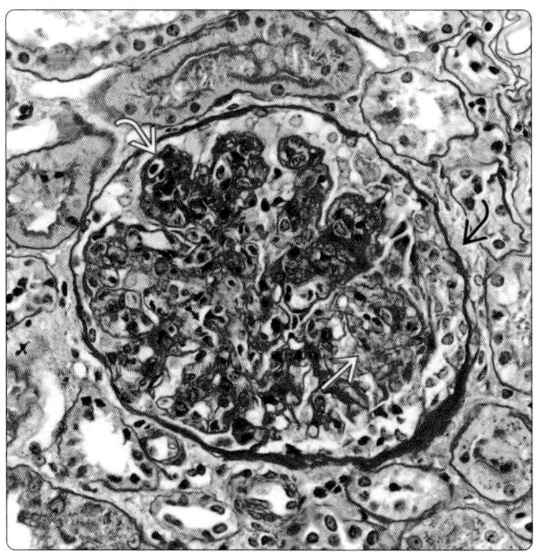

PAS Positive Deposits in the Mesangium

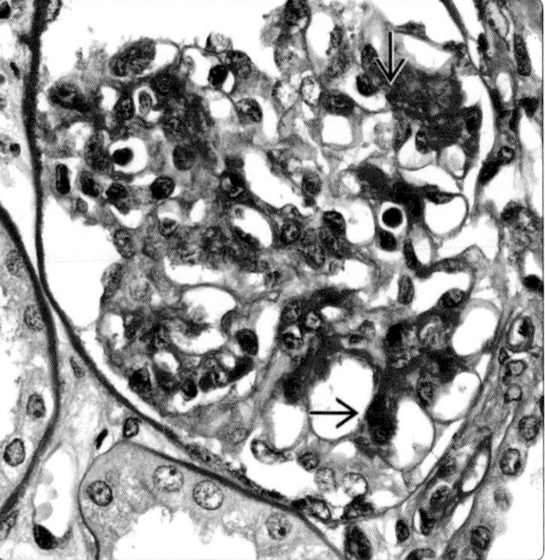

(Left) *Endocapillary leukocytes are present in most glomerular capillary loops ➙. In addition, there is segmental disruption of the GBM ➙ and early cellular crescent reaction ➙. In HSP, histologic changes are typically focal and normal glomeruli are present.* **(Right)** *Many PAS(+) granules are present in the mesangium ➙ in an 84-year-old man with HSP. Similar PAS(+) mesangial deposits are sometimes found in IgA nephropathy.*

Lambda Light Chain Deposition

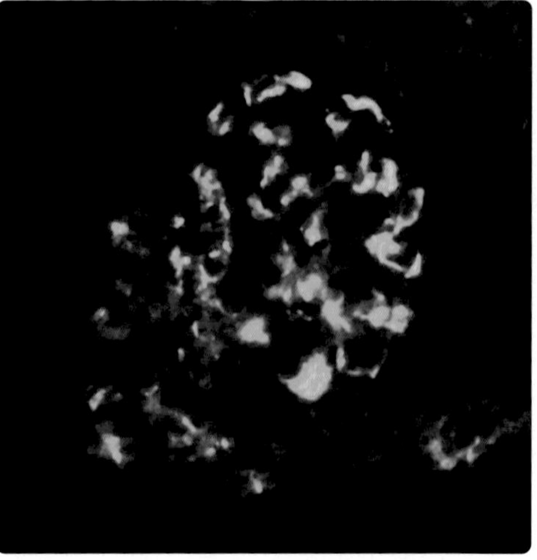

C3 Deposition

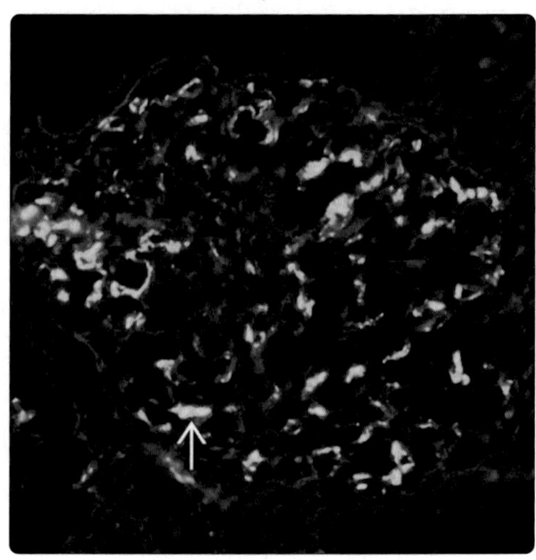

(Left) *Lambda light chain shows strong staining intensity of the glomerular immune complexes, often more intense than kappa, which can be a useful finding to help support the diagnosis of HSP, although similar lambda predominance is typical of IgA nephropathy.* **(Right)** *Granular C3 immunofluorescence staining can be observed in some of the mesangial areas ➔ in a glomerulus from a patient with HSP. This is a variable finding and may be negative in a significant subset of cases.*

Fibrinogen in Mesangium

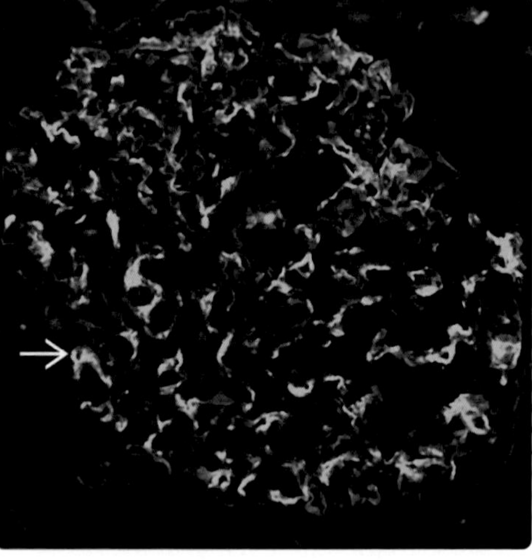

Mesangial Deposits

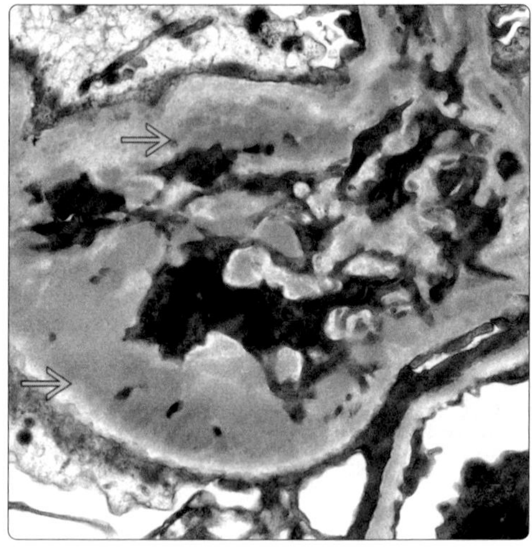

(Left) *Immunofluorescence microscopy for fibrinogen can highlight the mesangial ➔ immune complexes of HSP in a subset of cases, which is due to the glomerular deposition of cross-linked fibrin degradation products. This can also be observed in IgA nephropathy.* **(Right)** *Large aggregates of electron-dense deposits ➔ may accumulate in mesangial regions, which are characteristic of HSP and appear identical to IgA nephropathy or mesangial proliferative lupus nephritis.*

Subendothelial Deposits

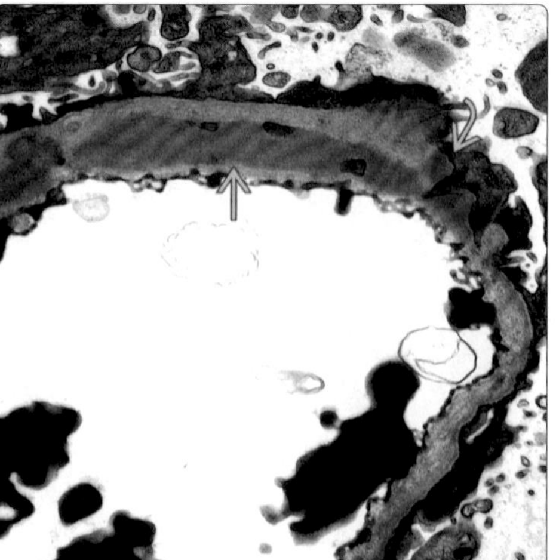

Subepithelial Deposits

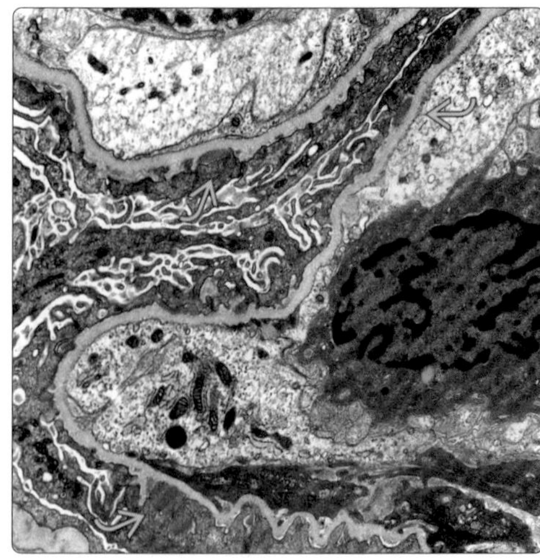

(Left) *Prominent subendothelial electron-dense deposits ➔ may be present, and this finding often correlates with the presence of cellular crescent formation. A subepithelial deposit is also present ➔.* **(Right)** *HSP can sometimes have subepithelial deposits ➔, although these are much less common than mesangial or subendothelial deposits.*

Purpura

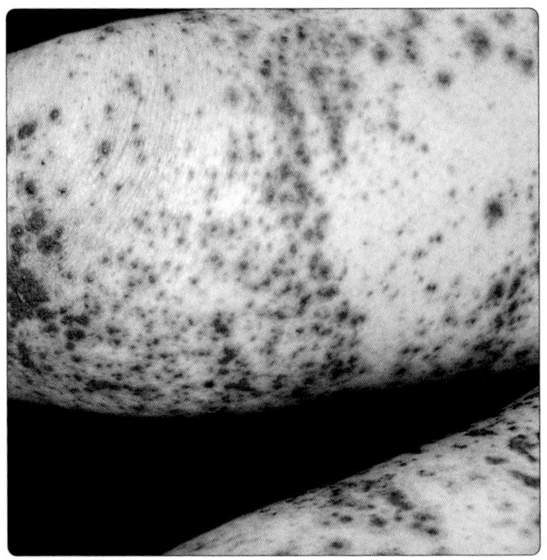

Leukocytoclastic Vasculitis in Purpuric Lesion

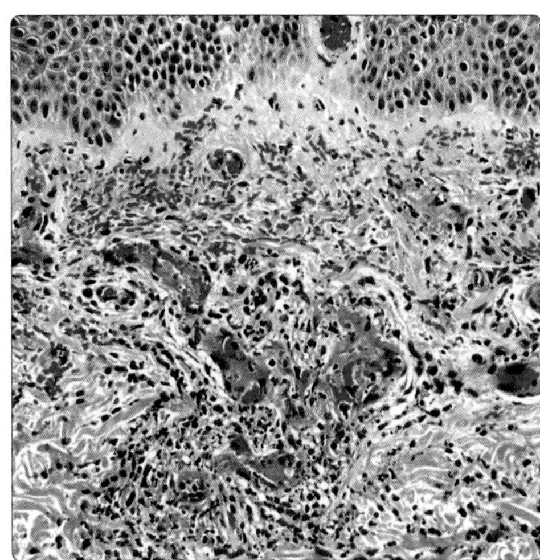

(Left) *Purpuric macules, papules, patches, and plaques are diffusely present on the lower extremities of this patient with HSP. (Courtesy V. Petronic-Rosic, MD.)* **(Right)** *Leukocytoclastic vasculitis is the typical skin biopsy finding for HSP. Prominent inflammation is present in the dermal capillaries, and there are marked, extravasated red blood cells in the dermis. (Courtesy J. Song, MD.)*

IgA Deposition in Dermal Microvasculature

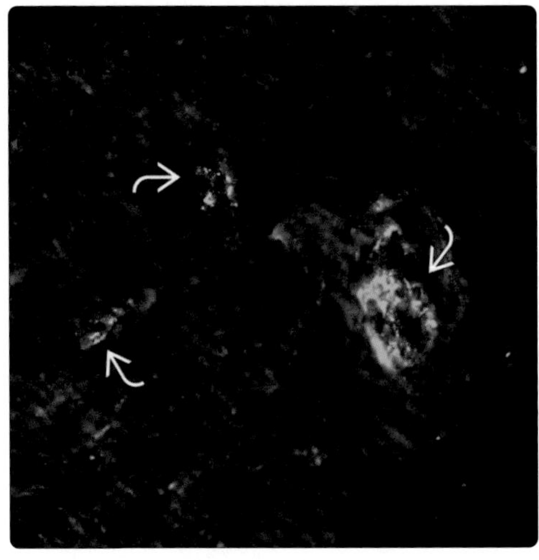

Small Bowel With Petechiae

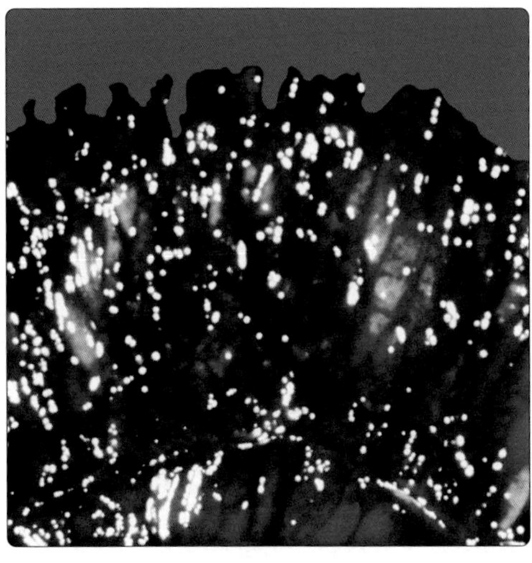

(Left) *Granular IgA deposition in dermal microvasculature ➡ is characteristic of HSP. The staining can be quite focal and mild and is easily overlooked. C3 and fibrin are also commonly present. Early lesions are more likely to contain IgA.* **(Right)** *Small bowel in a patient with HSP shows submucosal petechial hemorrhages due to vasculitis. Intussusception can result from the intramural hemorrhage.*

Focal Hemorrhage in Small Bowel Mucosa

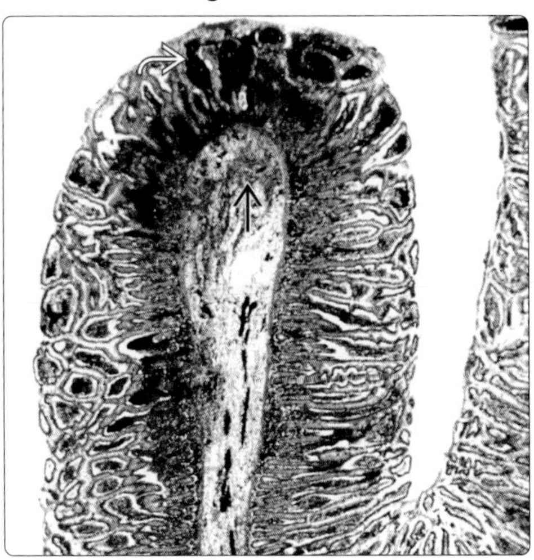

Vasculitis With Fibrinoid Necrosis in Bowel

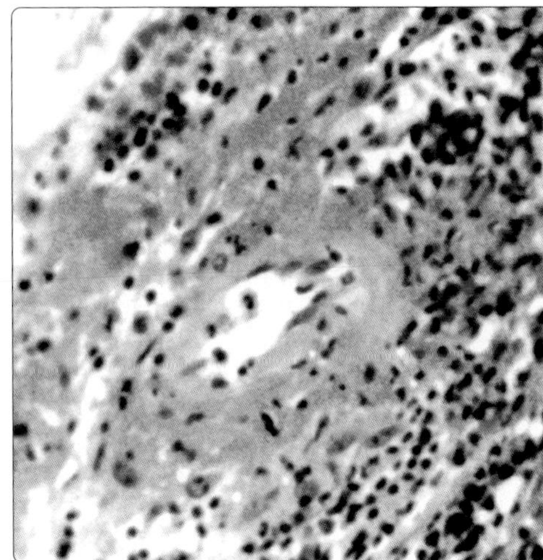

(Left) *Small bowel in HSP shows focal hemorrhage ➡ in a fold of mucosa, the cause of which is vasculitis in the lamina propria ➡.* **(Right)** *H&E shows vasculitis in the small bowel lamina propria in HSP. The wall of this small artery has fibrinoid necrosis with neutrophils, nuclear dust, and local hemorrhage.*

KEY FACTS

TERMINOLOGY

- Systemic autoimmune disease manifested by inflammation of skin, joints, kidneys and central nervous system
  - IgG autoantibodies to DNA, RNA, proteins, phospholipids

ETIOLOGY/PATHOGENESIS

- Autoantibodies cause immune complex deposition, vasculitis, thrombotic microangiopathy
- Multiple genetic risk factors

MICROSCOPIC

- Glomerular pathology is quite varied and is basis of ISN/RPS classification
  - Mesangial proliferation
  - Thickened GBM (extreme is wire loop)
  - Endocapillary hypercellularity
  - Necrosis, crescents
  - Thrombotic microangiopathy may dominate
- Tubulointerstitial inflammation common
- IF: IgG deposits in glomeruli are essential for diagnosis
  - Usually accompanied by IgM, IgA, C1q, and C3 (full house)
  - TBM deposits in ~ 60%
- EM: Amorphous and structured deposits
  - Mesangial, subendothelial, and subepithelial deposits

TOP DIFFERENTIAL DIAGNOSES

- MPGN with immune complexes
- Cryoglobulinemia
- Drug-induced lupus nephritis
- Postinfectious GN

DIAGNOSTIC CHECKLIST

- Important diagnostic clues include heterogeneity of glomerular lesions; "full house" pattern (IgG, IgA, IgM, C3, C1q) and TBM deposits of IgG; and endothelial tubuloreticular inclusions and thumbprint pattern in deposits

Endocapillary and Mesangial Hypercellularity

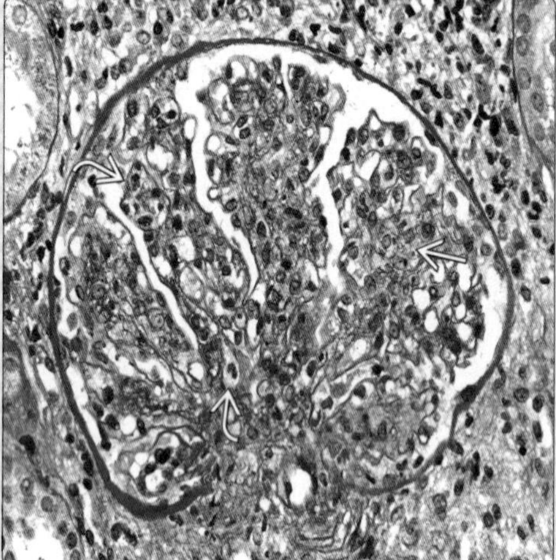

Wire Loop Lesions

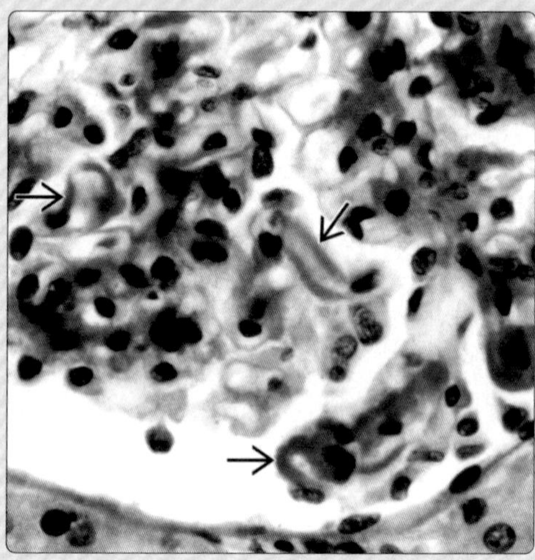

(Left) *Endocapillary hypercellularity ➡ with a mixture of neutrophils and mononuclear cells is present segmentally. Mesangial hypercellularity ➡ affects all lobules of the glomerulus. These are two common histologic manifestations of active lupus glomerulonephritis.* **(Right)** *"Wire loop" thickening of the glomerular capillary wall ➡ in a patient with lupus GN is shown. "Wire loops" are due to subendothelial deposits and were initially described in lupus by Baehr, Klemperer, and Shifrin in 1935.*

Prominent Granular GBM Deposits

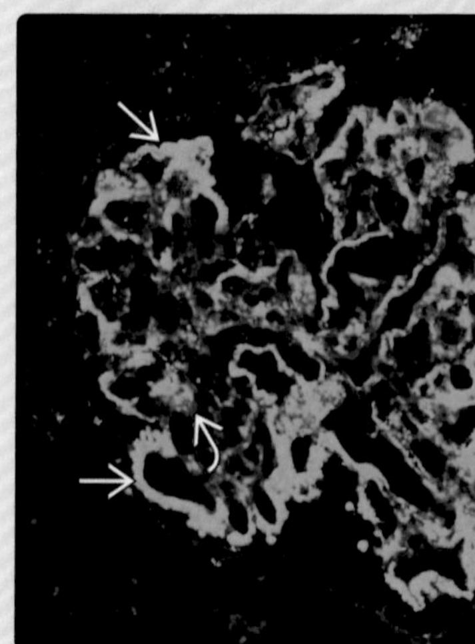

Glomerular Electron-Dense Deposits

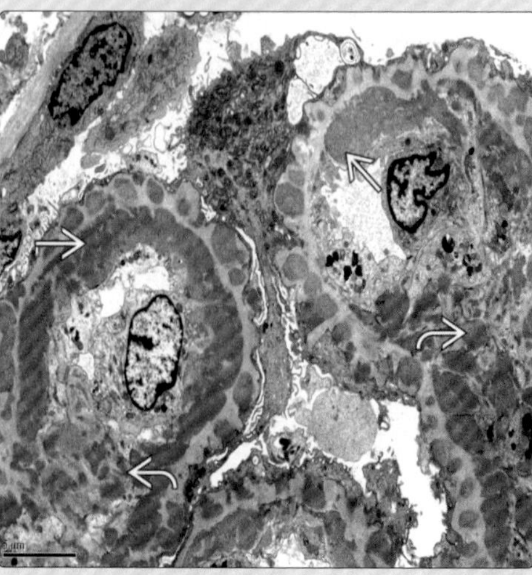

(Left) *Granular capillary wall staining for IgG ➡ is a feature of lupus nephritis and a pattern frequently seen in ISN/RPS classes III and IV-S. Mesangial deposits are also present ➡.* **(Right)** *Deposits can be found in 4 locations in the glomerulus in LN in different relative amounts. Here, subepithelial, intramembranous, subendothelial ➡, and mesangial ➡ dense deposits are evident in a biopsy with diffuse proliferative and membranous LN.*

TERMINOLOGY

Abbreviations

- Systemic lupus erythematosus (SLE)

Definitions

- Systemic autoimmune disease manifested by inflammation of skin, joints, kidneys, and central nervous system, with pathogenic IgG autoantibodies targeting nuclear, cell surface, and plasma protein self-antigens
- Diagnostic criteria (Systemic Lupus Collaborating Clinics, SLICC): Biopsy-confirmed nephritis (ISN/RPS classification) and anti-nuclear or anti-dsDNA antibodies; if not, must meet 4/17 clinical and immunologic criteria
  - Clinical: Acute or chronic cutaneous lesions, oral ulcers, nonscarring alopecia, synovitis, serositis, renal, neurologic, hemolytic anemia, leukopenia, thrombocytopenia
  - Immunologic: Antinuclear antibodies (ANA), anti-dsDNA, anti-Sm, antiphospholipid antibody, low complement, direct Coombs test

ETIOLOGY/PATHOGENESIS

Autoimmune Disease

- Autoantibodies
  - ANA in 95%
    - Double-stranded (ds) DNA (nucleosomes), Ro/SSA (ribonucleoprotein), La (RNA binding protein), Sm (ribonucleoprotein)
    - Occasional LN with negative ANA, especially class V
  - Cardiolipin (false-positive test for syphilis)
  - Phospholipids, ADAMTS13, lupus anticoagulant
  - C1q, laminin, heparan sulfate proteoglycans, podocyte antigens, and others
- Autoantibodies may be detectable years before disease
- Breakdown of tolerance to self-antigens, trigger unknown
  - "Waste disposal" hypothesis
    - Defective phagocytosis of apoptotic cells exposures immune system to intracellular sequestered antigens
    - Activation of self-reactive T and B cells and development of autoantibodies

Environmental Triggers and Aggravating Factors

- Sunlight (UV)
- Estrogens
- Drugs: Hydralazine, procainamide, quinidine

Genetic Factors

- 10% have relatives with SLE
- Higher concordance in monozygotic twins (25-69%) than dizygotic twins (1-2%)
- Deficiencies in complement or nuclease enzymes
  - C1q, C2, or C4; rarely other complement components
  - Nuclease genes *TREX1*, *DNASE1*
- Polymorphisms (SNPs) of > 25 genes increase risk in genome-wide association studies
  - Fcγ receptor IIB (inhibitory receptor on B cells)
  - Toll-like receptors (TLR 7 and 9)
  - Interferon and tumor necrosis factor signaling
  - HLA-DR2 and 3

Pathogenesis of Renal Disease

- Immune complex (IC) formation and deposition in kidney
  - Circulating IC trapped in capillaries and mesangium
  - In situ formation of IC due to planted or intrinsic antigen
    - Histone-rich nucleosomal antigens trapped in glomeruli, may initiate IC formation
  - Complement fixation: C3a and C5a attract neutrophils and macrophages
  - Inflammatory cells bind IC via Fc and complement receptors and are activated
  - Persistent or recurrent inflammation leads to changes in intrinsic glomerular cell numbers and function, and matrix homeostasis
- Thrombotic microangiopathy
  - Due to lupus anticoagulant, antiphospholipid antibodies, or antibodies to ADAMTS13
  - May arise independently of immune complex LN
- Vasculitic GN: Necrosis with little or no IC deposition and endothelial damage by uncertain mechanism
- Podocytopathy: Minimal change lesion, FSGS, or collapsing glomerulopathy
- T-cell-mediated autoimmune reactivity particularly in tubulointerstitial disease

Insights From Animal Studies

- NZB/NZW F1, MRL/lpr, and BSXB mice develop lupus-like GN
  - Multigenic risk factors
  - Promoted by deficiency of C4, C3, FcγRIIB, CD19, fas, Ro

CLINICAL ISSUES

Epidemiology

- Age
  - Peak incidence of LN: ~ 34 years (range: < 5 to > 75)
- Sex
  - F:M ~ 9:1
- Prevalence
  - 7-159/100,000 worldwide; varied methodologies
    - Asians 30-50/100000; blacks 9-30/100000; whites 5-10/100000
  - ~ 80% have LN during course of disease
    - 20% have nephritis at onset, > 90% at autopsy

Presentation

- Gradual or sudden onset
- Presentation correlates partially with ISN/RPS classification
  - Acute renal failure: Class IV (~ 85%)
  - Nephrotic syndrome: Class V (~ 45%); IV (~ 35%); non-LN (~ 10%)
  - Isolated proteinuria: Class V (~ 45%); IV (~ 35%); II (~ 15%); III (~ 15%)
  - Isolated hematuria: Class II (~ 40%), V (~ 30%); non-LN (~ 30%)
- Can have subclinical ("silent") LN, even with class IV
- Nonrenal manifestations: Serositis, synovitis, skin rash (malar, butterfly), oral ulcers, non-scarring alopecia, hemolytic anemia, leukopenia/lymphopenia, thrombocytopenia, lymphadenopathy, thrombosis, neuropathy, seizures, psychosis

Laboratory Tests

- Autoantibodies
  - 95% have antinuclear antibodies (ANA)
    - > 95% ANA (speckled pattern)
      - ~ 5% in general population have positive ANA
    - 30-80% anti-dsDNA; 20-30% anti-Sm (99% have SLE); 30-50% anti-Ro (SSA); 30-40% anti-U1RNP; ~ 60% anti-histone
  - 40-50% anticardiolipin; 15% antiphospholipid; 30-50% anti-C1q
  - Nephritis associated with anti-dsDNA and anti-C1q
- Complement levels
  - 30-50% ↓ C3, 67-80% ↓ C4, association with active disease

Treatment

- Drugs
  - Immunosuppressive therapy to decrease or arrest IC deposits, inflammation, and necrosis
    - Glucocorticoids, mycophenolate mofetil, cyclophosphamide, chlorambucil and azathioprine
  - Antibodies targeting CD20 (rituximab) and BLys (Belimumab) under evaluation
- Transplantation
  - Clinical recurrence ~ 2%; subclinical recurrence ~ 40%

Prognosis

- Typically remitting and recurring course
- 20-25% develop end-stage renal disease (ESRD)
  - ESRD or doubling of Cr at 10 years by ISN/RPS class
    - Class I, II: 0%
    - Class III: 0-8%
    - Class IV: 8-50%
    - Class V: 0-10%
  - Risk factors for ESRD: Class III or IV biopsy: Male gender, hypertension, proteinuria

MICROSCOPIC

Histologic Features

- Lupus nephritis affects glomeruli, peritubular capillaries, muscular blood vessels, tubules, and interstitium with a spectrum of lesions
- Glomeruli
  - Glomerular lesions determine ISN/RPS classification (classes I-VI)
    - Lesions can be active (acute) or chronic (sclerosing)
    - Focal (< 50% of glomeruli affected; III) or diffuse (≥ 50% of glomeruli affected; IV)
    - Segmental (part of a glomerulus) or global (> 50% of a glomerulus)
    - Distinction between III and IV is by extent of glomerular lesions (< or ≥ 50%, respectively)
  - Normal (class I)
    - Requires mesangial IgG to diagnose lupus class I
    - Class I is seen in < 1% of biopsies for cause
  - Mesangial hypercellularity (class II)
    - By itself is not considered an active lesion
    - Class II is seen in 8-17% of biopsies
  - Endocapillary hypercellularity (class III, IV)
    - Proliferation of intrinsic glomerular cells and accumulation of leukocytes with capillary luminal reduction
    - Class III is seen in 9-24% of biopsies
    - Class IV is seen in 37-66% of biopsies
      - Segmental glomerulonephritis designated IV-S (10-20%); global glomerulonephritis as IV-G (21-46%)
  - Extracapillary hypercellularity (crescents) (class III, IV)
    - Proliferation of parietal epithelium and accumulation of leukocytes, especially macrophages
    - Defined as ≥ 2 cells thick, > 25% of circumference of capsule
  - Karyorrhexis, fibrinoid necrosis ± GBM rupture (class III, IV)
  - Prominent subendothelial deposits ("wire loops") (class III, IV)
    - Trichrome stain highlights bright red wire loops
  - Hyaline "pseudothrombi" (class III, IV)
  - Hematoxylin bodies specific but rare (class III, IV): In vivo LE cell
  - Membranous lesions (class V)
    - Diffuse thickening of GBM with granular subepithelial deposits (trichrome) with silver-positive "spikes"
    - Class V is seen in 8-29% of biopsies; often mixed with other classes (II, III, IV)
  - Chronic glomerular lesions
    - Included in count of involved glomeruli for III vs. IV, if believed to be due to LN
    - Glomerular sclerosis, segmental or global and fibrous adhesions
    - Fibrous crescents
    - GBM duplication
    - End stage (class VI); ≥ 90% global glomerulosclerosis; 1-3% of biopsies
  - Variants
    - Some patients with minimal lupus (I-II) have podocytopathy (minimal change disease and focal segmental glomerulosclerosis)
    - Focal segmental glomerular sclerosis can also be late scarring phase of lupus nephritis or maladaptive/hemodynamic secondary to loss of nephrons
    - Rarely thrombotic microangiopathy with little immune complex disease
- Tubules and interstitium
  - Tubulointerstitial lesions most commonly seen in association with class III and IV GN
    - May be active or chronic; ± IgG and C3 positive tubulointerstitial immune deposits
    - Tubulointerstitial immune deposits strongly correlated with interstitial lymphoid follicles
    - Anti-vimentin autoantibody titers commonly found and correlate with degree of interstitial inflammation
  - Active lesions have T cells, macrophages, B cells, plasma cells, neutrophils, edema and tubulitis
  - Chronic lesions are characterized by interstitial fibrosis and tubular atrophy
  - Tubulointerstitial disease with little or no glomerular disease (e.g., class I and II) occurs rarely (15 cases reported); beware of unsampled class III.
- Vessels: 6 patterns observed

- Normal (negative IF)
- Uncomplicated vascular immune deposits: Normal-looking vessels with Ig and C by IF
- Noninflammatory lupus vasculopathy: Hyaline deposits with Ig and C by IF
- Necrotizing lupus vasculitis: Fibrinoid necrosis and leukocytoclasis ± immune deposits
- Thrombotic microangiopathy: ± class III or IV glomerular lesions
- Arterial and arteriolar sclerosis: Nonlupus vasculopathy without immune deposits

ANCILLARY TESTS

Immunofluorescence

- Detection of IgG deposits in glomeruli essential for diagnosis
  - Usually accompanied by IgA, IgM, C3, and C1q ("full house")
  - Kappa and lambda equal
  - IgG1 and IgG3 are predominate subclasses
  - Fibrin in necrotizing lesions, thrombi and crescents
- Glomerular patterns
  - Mesangial only (class I, II)
  - Capillary wall, focal or diffuse, coarse granular, elongated (class III, IV)
  - Capillary wall, diffuse, finely granular (class V)
- Tubules focal granular IgG in ~ 60% of cases, ± other components (Ig, C3, C1q)
  - IgG subclass distribution different from those in glomerulus in 70%
  - No strong correlation with interstitial inflammation
- Vessels: Granular IgG in small arteries &/or arterioles (~ 48%) &/or peritubular capillaries (6%) along with various other components

Electron Microscopy

- Amorphous electron-dense deposits present in glomeruli in varied locations and extent
  - Mesangium, subendothelium, subepithelium
  - Subepithelial deposits sometimes penetrate GBM
  - Substructure may be focally manifested as "fingerprint" pattern
- Extraglomerular deposits of similar nature
  - Tubular basement membrane, Bowman capsule, peritubular capillaries, interstitium, small arteries
- Endothelial cells have tubuloreticular inclusions
  - Clusters of vesicles and tubules of diameter 20-25 nm in endoplasmic reticulum
  - Consequence of elevated levels of interferon: So-called "interferon footprints"

DIFFERENTIAL DIAGNOSIS

Type II Mixed Cryoglobulinemia

- Cryoglobulins in serum
- Microtubular substructure of deposits
- Usually no subepithelial deposits
- Deposits can be sparse, macrophages prominent, IgM dominant

Membranoproliferative GN With Immune Deposits

- Little or no C1q
- Negative lupus serologies

Idiopathic Membranous GN

- Absence of subendothelial, mesangial, and TBM deposits or tubuloreticular inclusions
- Deposits typically do not penetrate the GBM
- Antibodies to phospholipase A2 receptors in~70%

Lupus-Like GN in HIV

- Negative or low titer ANA and negative dsDNA antibodies by definition
- ~ 20% of renal biopsies in HIV-infected patients

C1q Nephropathy

- No clinical or serologic evidence of lupus (by definition)
- Abundant mesangial immune deposits, with predominance of C1q

Drug-Induced LN

- Propylthiouracil, isoniazid, hydralazine, procainamide, chlorpromazine
- Usually no dsDNA antibodies or renal disease (5%)
  - High frequency of antihistone antibodies
- Proof requires improvement after drug withdrawal and absence of SLE prior to drug exposure

Postinfectious GN

- IgG and C3 in a characteristic coarse granular ("lumpy-bumpy") pattern, with hump-like deposits along subepithelium; usually little C1q
- Deposits in subepithelium ("humps") do not have "spikes"

ANCA-Related GN

- Little or no endocapillary hypercellularity or Ig or complement deposition

DIAGNOSTIC CHECKLIST

Clinically Relevant Pathologic Features

- Kidneys are biopsied in SLE to determine type of renal disease, acute inflammatory activity, and extent of glomerular and tubulointerstitial scarring
- Histologic predictors of poor renal outcome
  - ISN/RPS class of LN broadly correlates with outcome but tendency for class changes in follow-up biopsies reduces predictive value
    - Mesangial and membranous lesions have better prognosis than focal or diffuse GN
  - Amount of subendothelial deposits
  - Crescents (cellular and fibrous)
  - Glomerulosclerosis, tubular atrophy
  - Activity and chronicity index

Pathologic Interpretation Pearls

- Lupus nephritis is in differential diagnosis of almost every renal biopsy
- Heterogeneity of glomerular lesions, extraglomerular IgG, and endothelial tubuloreticular inclusions are most important diagnostic clues to LN
- Hematoxylin bodies are pathognomonic but rare

ISN/RPS Classification of Lupus Glomerulonephritis (2004)

Class	Name	Definition	Comments
I	Minimal mesangial LN	Normal by LM with mesangial deposits by IF or EM	May have other features such as podocytopathy or tubulointerstitial disease (beware of unsampled class III)
II	Mesangial proliferative LN	Purely mesangial hypercellularity by LM with mesangial deposits by IF; may be rare subepithelial or subendothelial deposits by IF or EM (not by LM)	May have other features such as podocytopathy, tubulointerstitial disease (beware of unsampled class III), or TMA
III	Focal LN	Active or inactive segmental or global endocapillary &/or extracapillary GN by LM in < 50% of glomeruli; usually with subendothelial deposits; designate whether lesions are active (A) &/or chronic (C)	Active lesions include endocapillary hypercellularity, cellular crescents, neutrophils/karyorrhexis, necrosis, and "wire loops"; chronic lesions include segmental or global glomerulosclerosis considered to be due to LN, and fibrous crescents
IV	Diffuse segmental or global LN	Active or inactive endocapillary &/or extracapillary GN by LM in ≥ 50% of glomeruli; designate whether lesions are active (A) &/or chronic (C) and whether lesions are either segmental (S) or global (G)	e.g., class IV-S (A), segmental lesions with active features; class IV-G (A/C), global lesions with both active and chronic features
V	Membranous LN	Global or segmental granular subepithelial deposits along the GBM by LM and IF or EM; if class III or IV present, these need to be in > 50% of capillaries of > 50% of glomeruli; ± mesangial alterations	May occur with class III or IV, which are designated class III/V or class IV/V, respectively
VI	Advanced sclerosing LN	≥ 90% of glomerular sclerosis without residual activity	Need to attribute sclerosis to LN rather than ischemia

Weening JJ et al: The classification of glomerulonephritis in systemic lupus erythematosus revisited. J Am Soc Nephrol. 15(2):241-50, 2004

GRADING

ISN/RPS Classification of Lupus Glomerulonephritis (2004)

- Based on light and immunofluorescence microscopy; electron microscopy not required
  - ≥ 20 glomeruli should be sampled for accurate classification
  - Classification requires distinction of active and chronic lesions and determination of extent of glomerular involvement by these injury processes
    - One glomerulus may have both acute/active lesions and chronic/sclerosing lesions
    - Heterogeneity of interglomerular and intraglomerular changes makes classification difficult
  - Majority of reported cases have no change of class in follow-up biopsies
    - Class III and IV lesions rarely downgrade to class II
  - Classification upgrades reported in repeat biopsies over months to years
    - Class II upgrades to class III, IV, and V lesions in ~ 33%
    - Class III upgrades to class IV and V in ~ 50%
    - Class IV upgrades to class V and VI lesions in ~ 15%
    - Class V develop proliferative (class III or IV) lesions in ~ 45% of cases
- Classes broadly correlate with outcome
  - Class I and II: Best survival
  - Class IV: Worse survival than III in many studies
    - Little or no difference in outcome of (G) vs. (S)
  - Class V: Good long-term survival
  - Class VI: End-stage disease

Activity and Chronicity Indices

- Histologic lesions scored 0 (none), 1 (mild), 2 (moderate), 3 (severe), and summed
- Activity index (AI) (range 0-24)
  - Components: Endocapillary hypercellularity, neutrophils, fibrinoid necrosis/karyorrhexis, cellular crescents, "pseudothrombi"/"wire loops"
    - Scores for necrosis/karyorrhexis and cellular crescents are doubled
- Chronicity index (CI) (range 0-12)
  - Components: Glomerular sclerosis, fibrous crescents, interstitial fibrosis, and tubular atrophy
- Limited reproducibility and correlation with outcome, however widely used by nephrologists as a guide and particularly for comparing repeat biopsies

SELECTED REFERENCES

1. Dhingra S et al: Tubulointerstitial nephritis in systemic lupus erythematosus: innocent bystander or ominous presage. Histol Histopathol. 29(5):553-65, 2014
2. Haring CM et al: Segmental and global subclasses of class IV lupus nephritis have similar renal outcomes. J Am Soc Nephrol. 23(1):149-54, 2012
3. Vozmediano C et al: Risk factors for renal failure in patients with lupus nephritis: data from the spanish registry of glomerulonephritis. Nephron Extra. 2(1):269-77, 2012
4. Chang A et al: In situ B cell-mediated immune responses and tubulointerstitial inflammation in human lupus nephritis. J Immunol. 186(3):1849-60, 2011
5. Hiramatsu N et al: Revised classification of lupus nephritis is valuable in predicting renal outcome with an indication of the proportion of glomeruli affected by chronic lesions. Rheumatology (Oxford). 47(5):702-7, 2008
6. Weening JJ et al: The classification of glomerulonephritis in systemic lupus erythematosus revisited. J Am Soc Nephrol. 15(2):241-50, 2004
7. Austin HA 3rd et al: Diffuse proliferative lupus nephritis: identification of specific pathologic features affecting renal outcome. Kidney Int. 25(4):689-95, 1984

Minimal Mesangial (Class I) LN

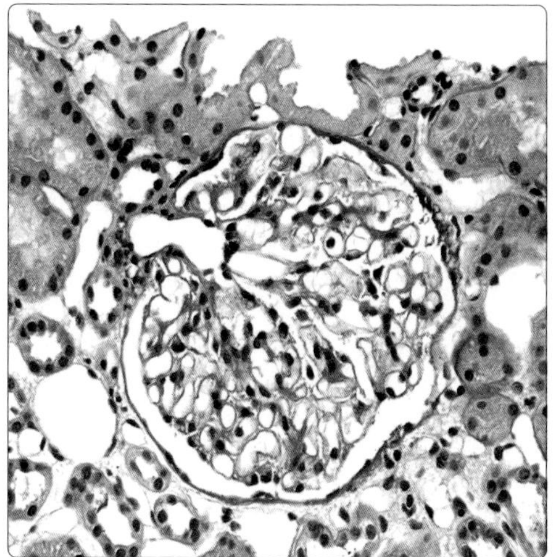

Mesangial Proliferative (Class II) LN

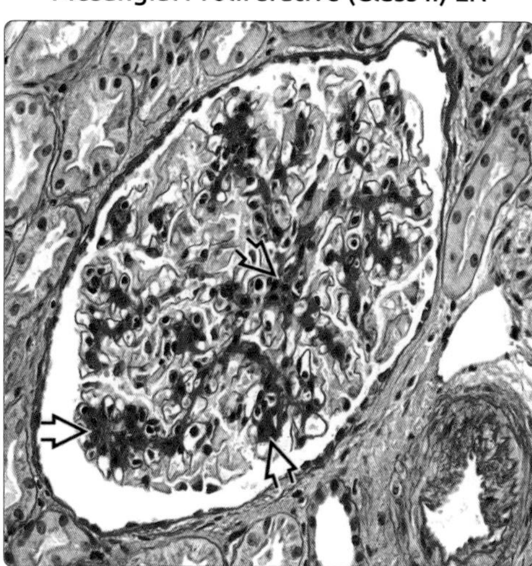

(Left) *Normal-appearing glomerulus with IgG deposits is identified in the mesangium by immunofluorescence, characteristic of minimal mesangial LN. This is rarely seen in biopsies.* **(Right)** *Class II lupus GN may have moderate mesangial hypercellularity and matrix expansion ➡. Class II lesions do not have capillary deposits or active inflammation. Mesangial hypercellularity is defined as ≥ 4 nuclei in 1 mesangial area in sections cut at 3 μm.*

Segmental Lupus GN (Class III or IV)

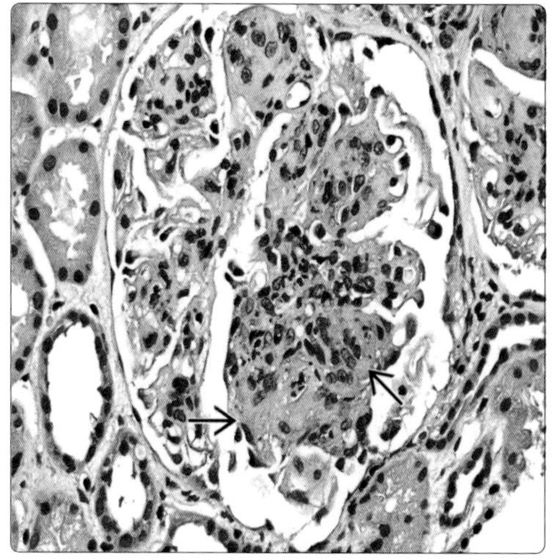

Endocapillary Hypercellularity

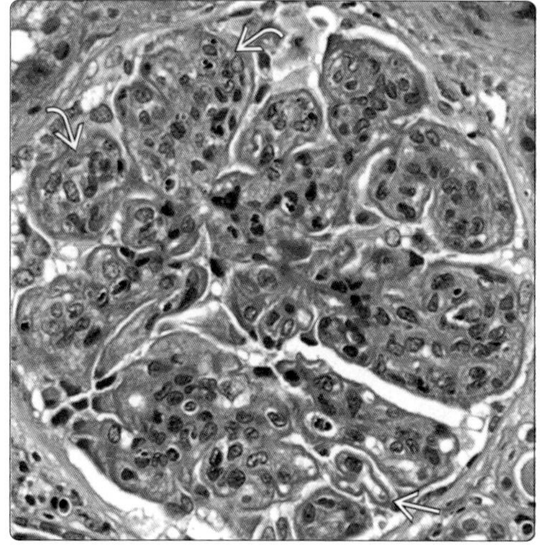

(Left) *A typical pattern of segmental GN is segmental capillary necrosis, with fibrinous and neutrophilic exudation, and karyorrhexis →. These are common in class III (A) and IV-S (A) lupus GN. If < 50% of glomeruli are affected, this is termed class III, and if ≥ 50% affected, it is termed class IV.* **(Right)** *This glomerulus has global endocapillary hypercellularity ↪. The endocapillary cells are a combination of macrophages, neutrophils, and endothelial cells. One capillary loop is has no hypercellularity ➡.*

Membranous (Class V) LN

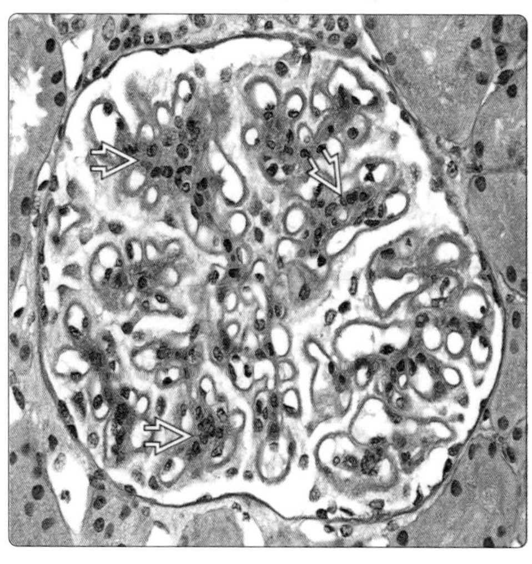

Global Glomerulosclerosis (Class VI)

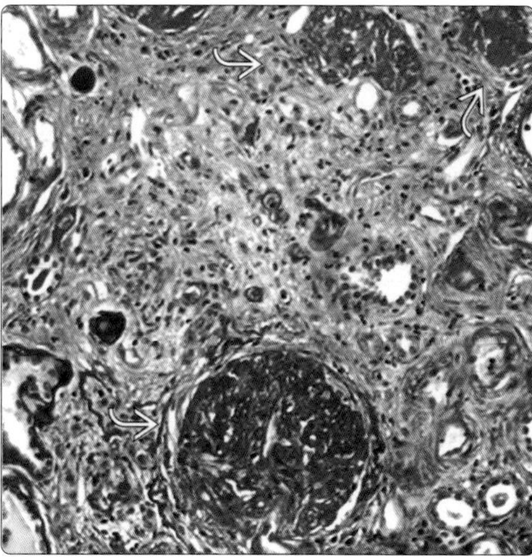

(Left) *Class V lupus GN has diffuse and global thickening of the GBM, "spikes" and prominent podocytes, often with mesangial expansion and hypercellularity ➡.* **(Right)** *When global glomerulosclerosis exceeds 90% due to LN and there is no evidence of activity, this is termed class VI. PAS stain shows 3 glomeruli with global glomerulosclerosis ↪, and there is extensive interstitial fibrosis and tubular atrophy.*

(Left) *Segmental endocapillary and extracapillary hypercellularity* ➲ *is evident in a glomerulus with largely open capillaries and mesangial hypercellularity. These lesions are seen in focal (class III [A]) and diffuse segmental (IV-S [A]) lupus GN.* **(Right)** *Segmental endocapillary hypercellularity and capillary basement membrane rupture* ➲ *may be subtle. In this case, 1 of 30 glomeruli had such a lesion. The diagnosis is focal LN (class III [A]).*

Segmental Lupus GN

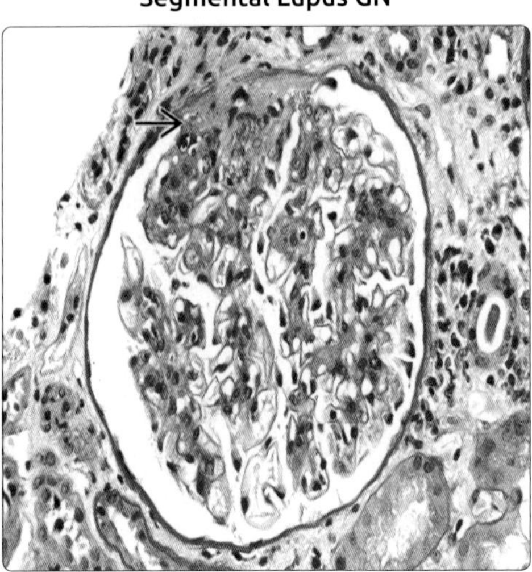

Focal (Class III [A]) LN

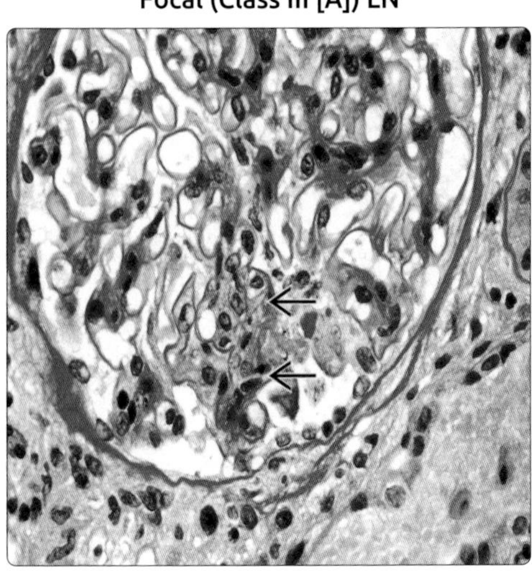

(Left) *A little over 50% of the glomerular cross-sectional area has endocapillary hypercellularity, and some capillaries have "wire loop" thickening* ➲*. Lesions like these are typical in ISN/RPS class IV-G lesions.* **(Right)** *Global endocapillary hypercellularity with neutrophils, mononuclear cells, and numerous karyorrhectic fragments are seen typically in diffuse lupus nephritis, class IV-G (A). Exudative lesions like this resemble postinfectious GN.*

Global Lupus GN (Class III or IV)

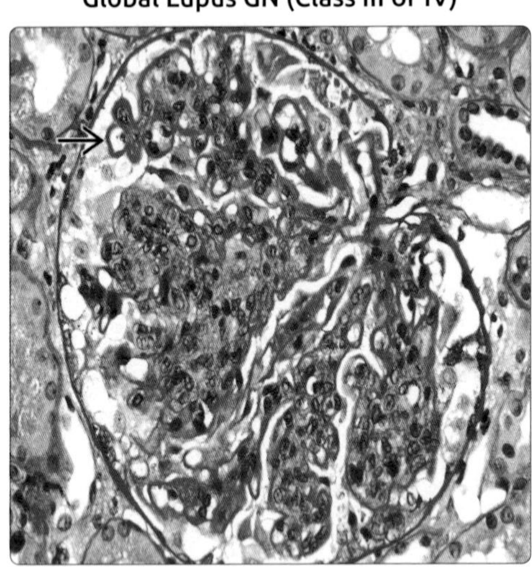

Global Lupus GN (Class IV)

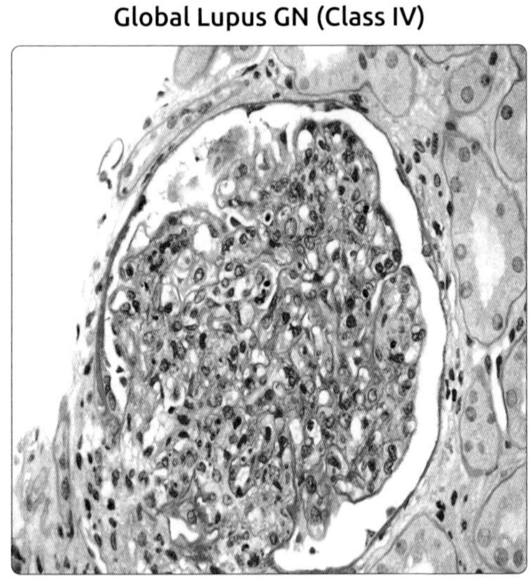

(Left) *The glomerular capillary wall is markedly and uniformly thickened* ➲ *in this H&E stained section. The thickening is due to subendothelial immune deposits and is a sign of activity.* **(Right)** *Duplication of the GBM can be marked* ➲*, shown here in a silver stain. There is lobular expansion and increased mesangial matrix, imparting a membranoproliferative glomerulonephritis-like appearance. Lesions like this are seen in ISN/RPS class IV-G LN.*

Extensive Wire Loops (Class IV)

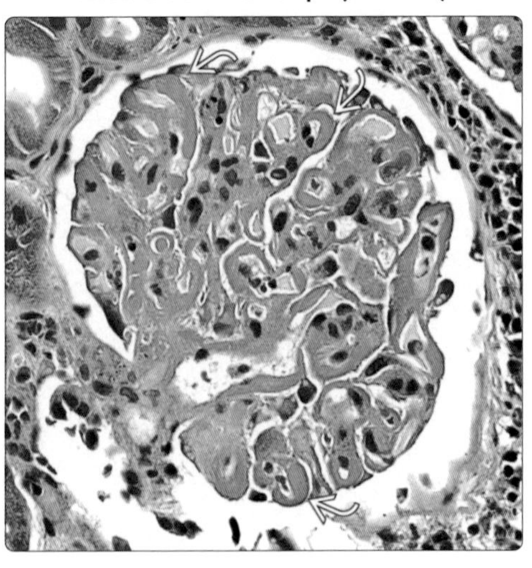

GBM Duplication

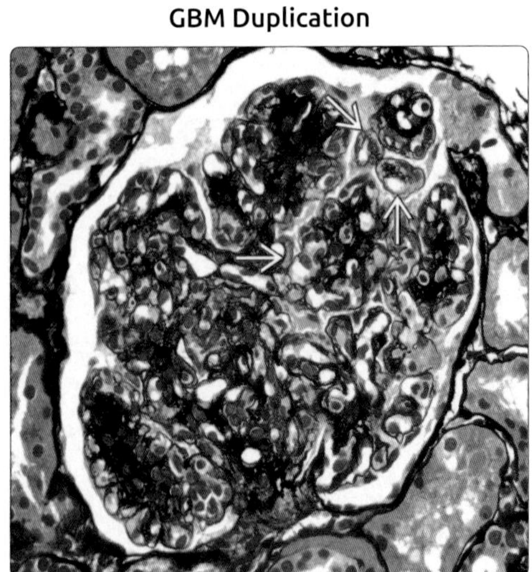

Mesangial Proliferative (Class II) LN

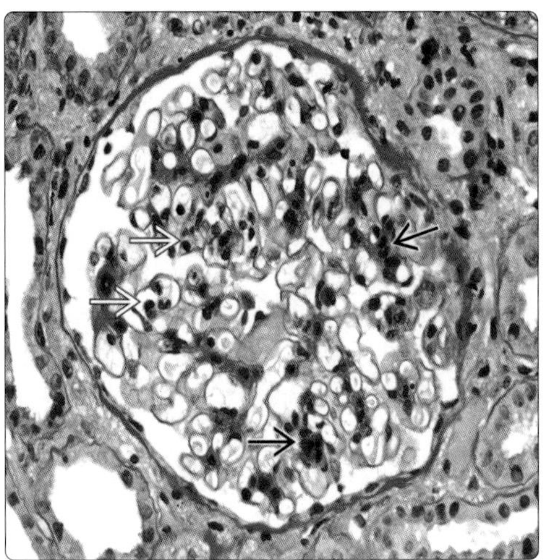

Focal Necrotizing (Class III [A]) LN

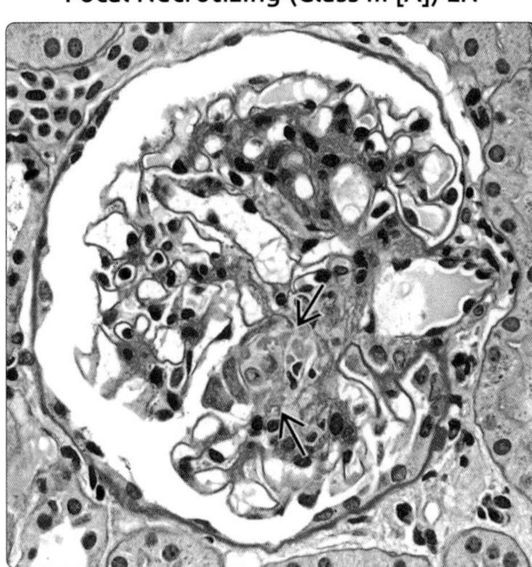

(Left) *A glomerulus with minimal mesangial thickening and hypercellularity ⇨, and detectable immune complex deposits containing immunoglobulins and complement by IF, is characteristic of mild class II lupus GN. A few intracapillary leukocytes are present ➡.* **(Right)** *Segmental capillary basement membrane rupture ⇨ with fibrinous and cellular exudation may be focal and is easy to miss. This was the only lesion in a sample of 38 glomeruli, and the diagnosis is focal (class III [A]) LN.*

Global Lupus GN

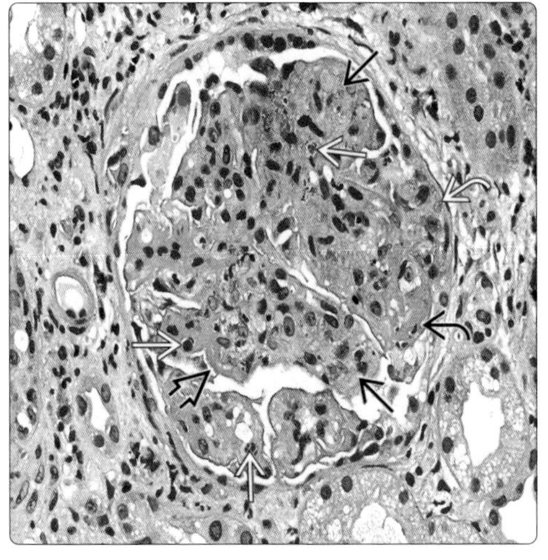

Crescentic and Membranous GN

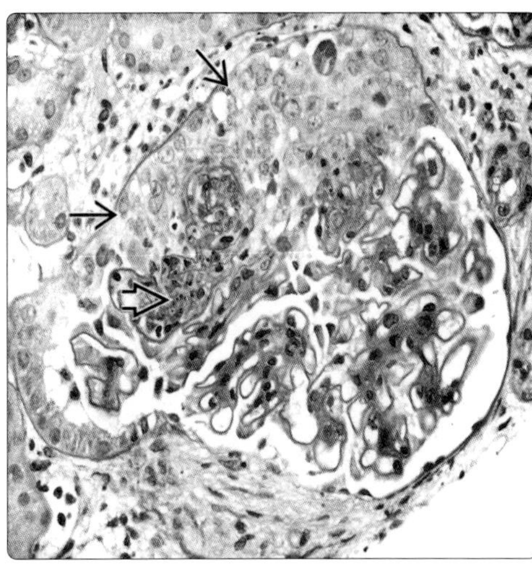

(Left) *Endocapillary hypercellularity ⇨, "wire loop" thickened capillary walls ⇨, fibrinoid exudate with karyorrhexis ⇨, a small cellular crescent ➡, and the rarely seen hematoxylin bodies ➡ indicate active lupus glomerulonephritis.* **(Right)** *Cellular crescents ⇨ can be seen in glomeruli with karyorrhexis ⇨ but without overt fibrinoid necrosis. Segmental endocapillary hypercellularity is present in the upper part of this glomerulus. The lower portion has mesangial hypercellularity and GBM thickening (class V).*

Active and Sclerosing Lupus GN

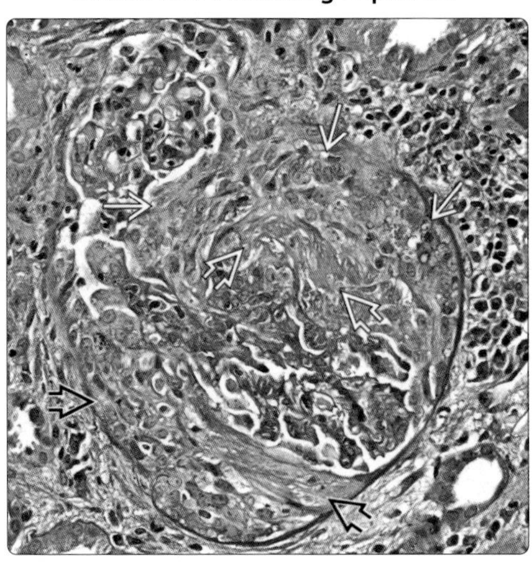

Segmental Glomerulosclerosis

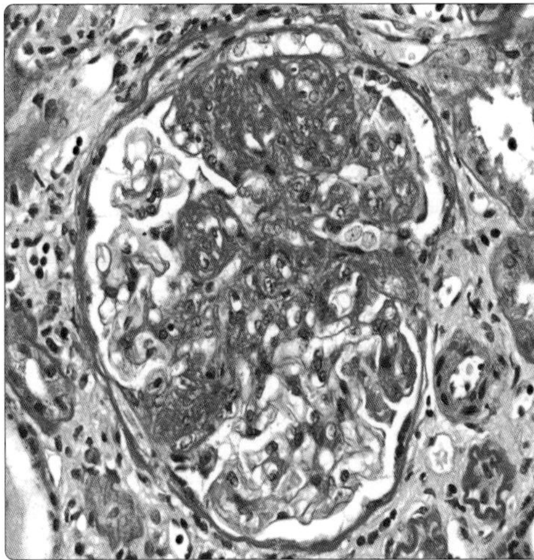

(Left) *Individual glomeruli may have active fibrinoid necrosis ➡ and cellular crescents ➡ adjacent to fibrocellular crescents ⇨. These dyssynchronous lesions indicate separate episodes of glomerular injury.* **(Right)** *Broad segmental irregular scars with adhesions to Bowman capsule and endocapillary hypercellularity are features indicative of sclerosing GN. Such lesions can be seen in class III (C) or IV-S (C) lupus nephritis.*

(Left) *Global subepithelial "spike" formation is barely evident → at this power in a glomerulus from a patient with SLE. There is little hypercellularity. Pure membranous glomerulopathy, ISN/RPS class V, is rare in lupus nephritis biopsies.* **(Right)** *Global subepithelial basement membrane projections or "spike" formation → is evident on Jones silver methenamine stain in this example of membranous lupus nephritis.*

Membranous Lupus GN (Class V)

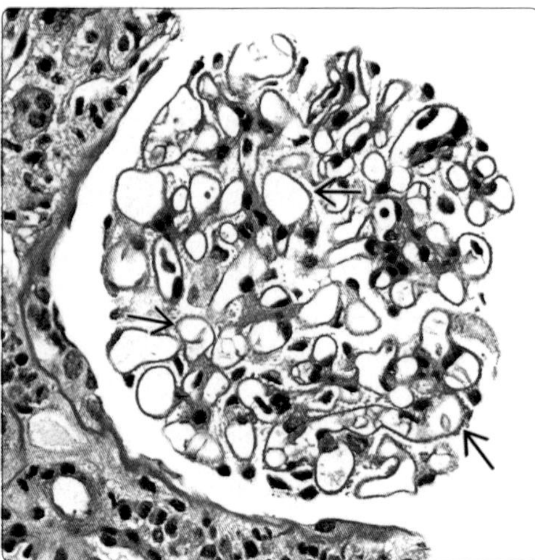

Membranous (Class V) LN

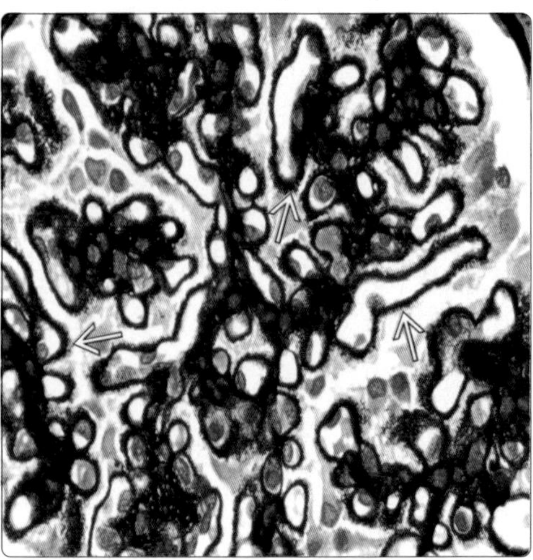

(Left) *Hyaline "pseudothrombi" → and "wire loop" thickening → are often evident together in capillaries in lupus nephritis. Such lesions may be associated with cryoglobulinemia in SLE.* **(Right)** *Class IV LN with prominent pseudothrombi in capillary loops → is shown in this PAS stained slide. In addition there is global endocapillary hypercellularity →. Karyorrhexis is abundant →.*

Pseudothrombi

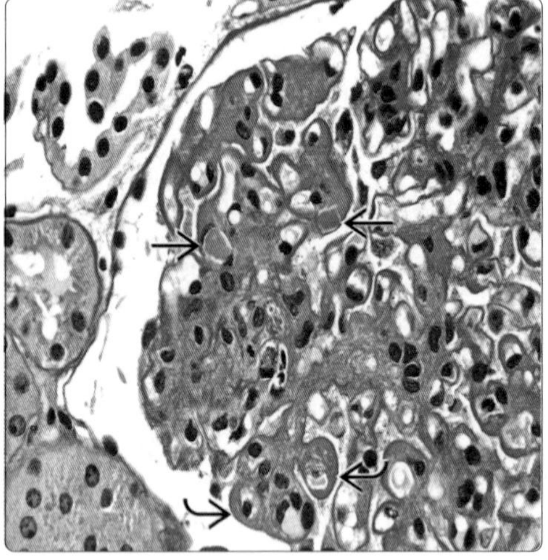

Pseudothrombi

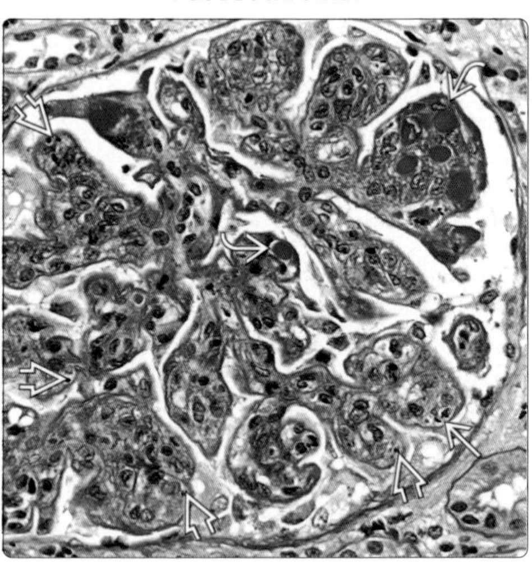

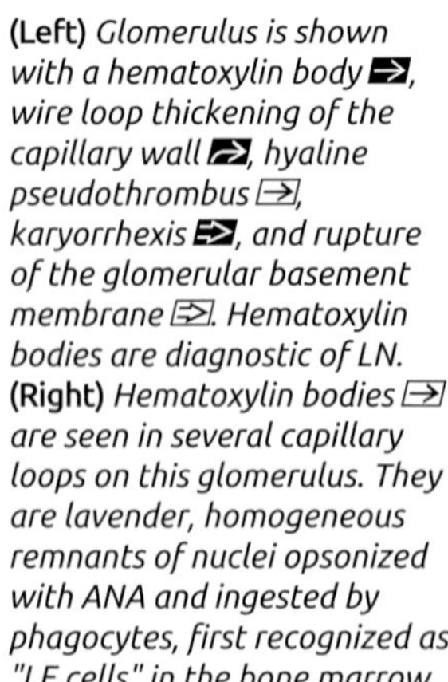

(Left) *Glomerulus is shown with a hematoxylin body →, wire loop thickening of the capillary wall →, hyaline pseudothrombus →, karyorrhexis →, and rupture of the glomerular basement membrane →. Hematoxylin bodies are diagnostic of LN.* **(Right)** *Hematoxylin bodies → are seen in several capillary loops on this glomerulus. They are lavender, homogeneous remnants of nuclei opsonized with ANA and ingested by phagocytes, first recognized as "LE cells" in the bone marrow.*

Hematoxylin Body

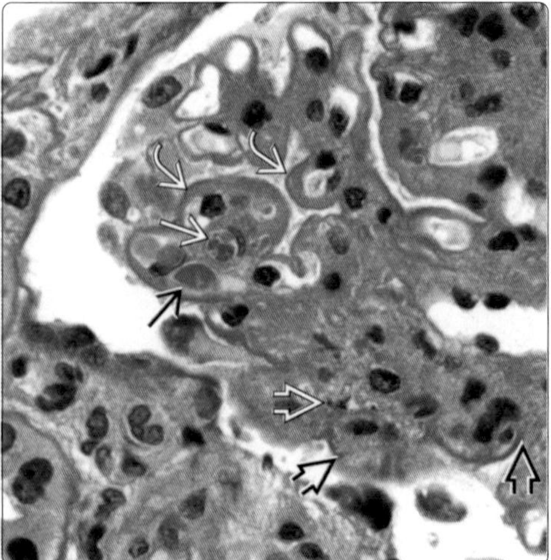

Hematoxylin Bodies

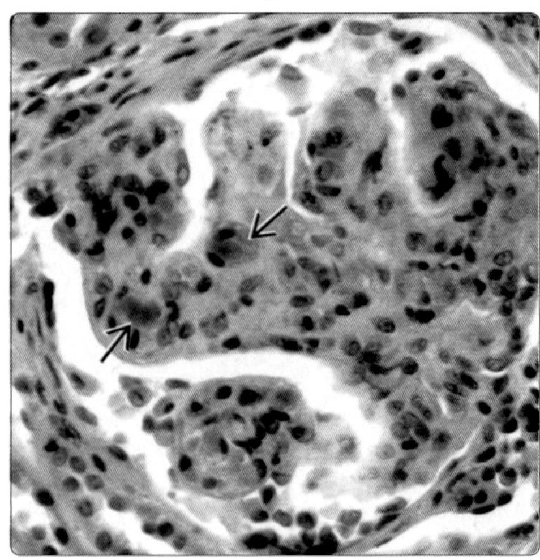

Mesangial Immune Deposits

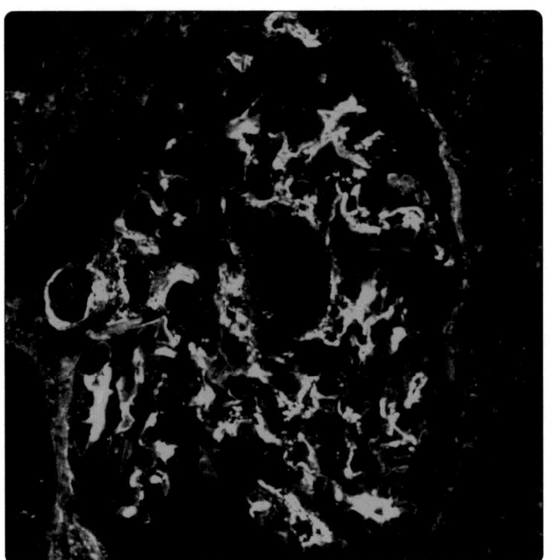

Broad GBM Deposits (Class III, IV)

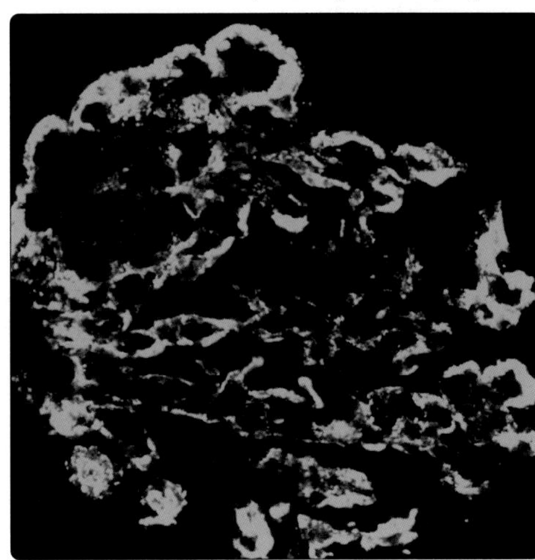

(Left) *In minimal mesangial (class I) and mesangial proliferative GN (class II), there is typically global and diffuse mesangial granular staining for IgG. Mesangial deposits are usually found in the higher classes as well (III, IV, V).* **(Right)** *The "wire loop" lesions of lupus are due to subendothelial deposits, which, like the mesangial deposits, typically stain for all of the usual reactants (IgG, IgM, IgA, C3, C1q), a "full house." Here, C1q is illustrated.*

Mesangial and GBM Deposits (Class III, IV)

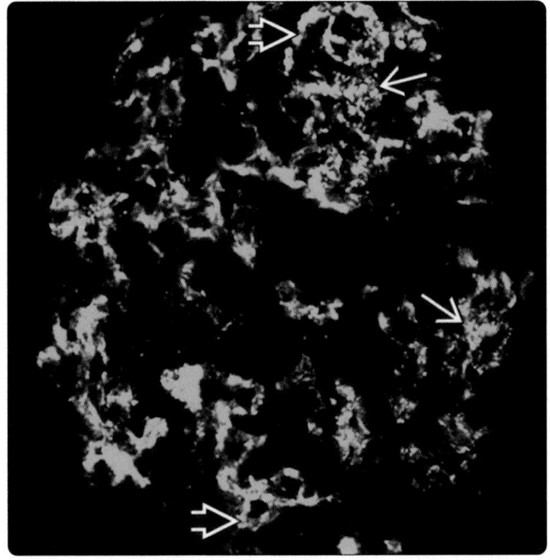

Membranous Pattern (Class V)

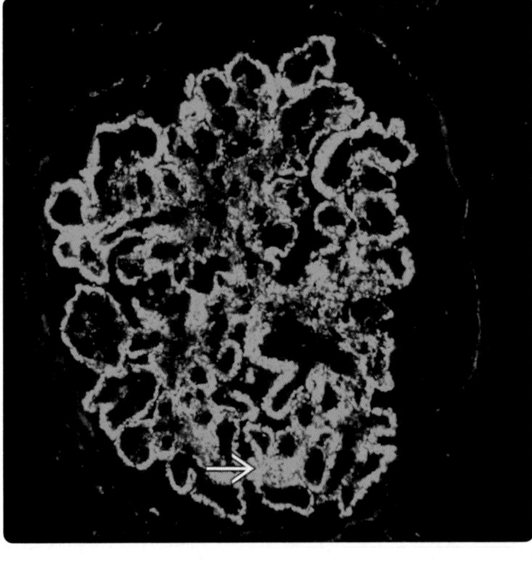

(Left) *In focal and diffuse lupus GN granular immune deposits containing IgG are seen in the mesangium ➡ and in capillary walls ➡.* **(Right)** *Finely granular and confluent staining of the glomerular capillary walls and segmental staining of the mesangium ➡ are seen in membranous lupus nephritis, class V.*

Finely Granular GBM Deposits (Class V) and Pseudothrombi

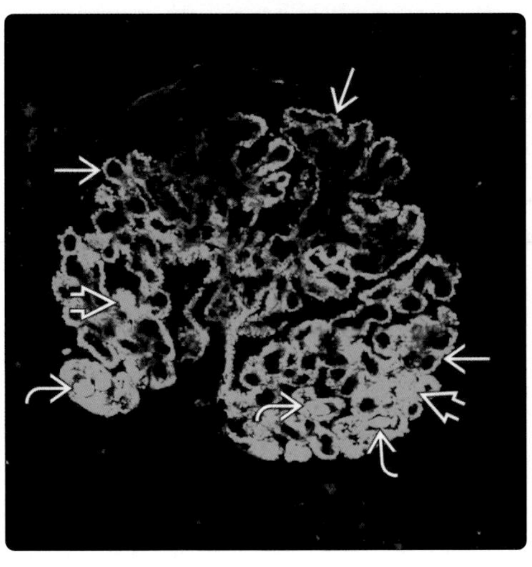

GBM and Mesangial Deposits With Reabsorption Droplets

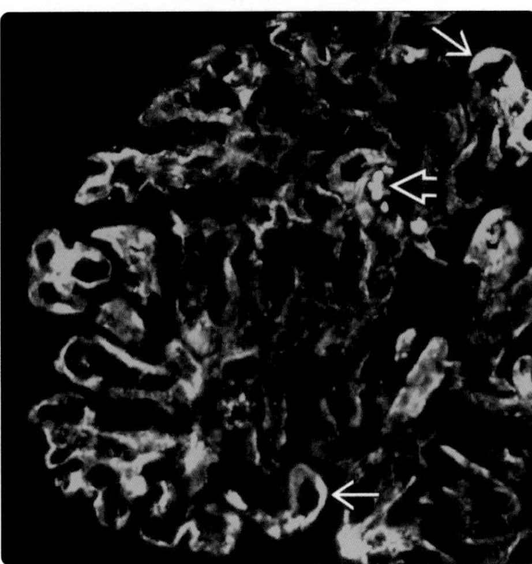

(Left) *Finely granular capillary wall staining ➡ in a membranous pattern with segmental mesangial staining ➡ is shown for IgG. Hyaline "pseudothrombi" ➡, are intracapillary globulin-antiglobulin complexes with a globular staining pattern.* **(Right)** *Band-like staining of capillary walls corresponds to "wire-loop" type immune deposits ➡. Globular staining of podocyte protein droplets ➡ should not be confused with hyaline pseudothrombi.*

(Left) *Immunofluorescence staining for IgA shows widespread granular deposits predominately along the GBM. In contrast, IgA nephropathy shows predominantly mesangial IgA deposits and minor GBM deposits.* **(Right)** *Segmental staining for fibrin/fibrinogen is evident at sites of glomerular fibrinoid necrosis. Such lesions are typical of class III (A) and IV-S (A) lupus GN.*

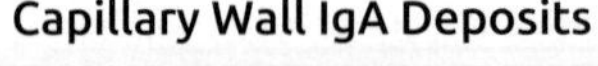

Capillary Wall IgA Deposits

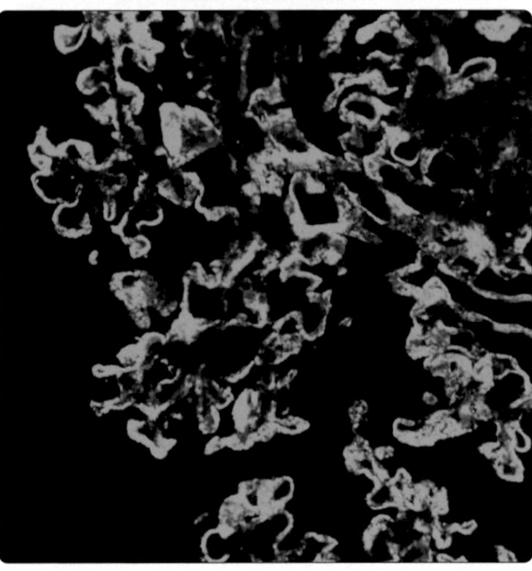

Glomerular Fibrinogen Deposition

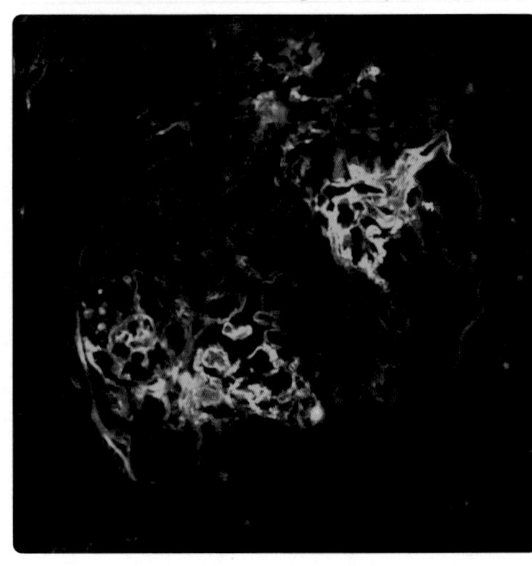

(Left) *Immunofluorescence for fibrin/ogen shows strong staining of a crescent in Bowman space ➞. Fibrin deposition is characteristically present in active crescents of all types of glomerulonephritis, including class III and IV lupus GN.* **(Right)** *Globally sclerosed glomeruli may retain staining for IgG even in advanced stages. This is helpful in making the diagnosis of diffuse sclerosing lupus GN (class VI) when light microscopy presents diffuse global glomerular sclerosis.*

Crescentic Lupus GN With Fibrinogen

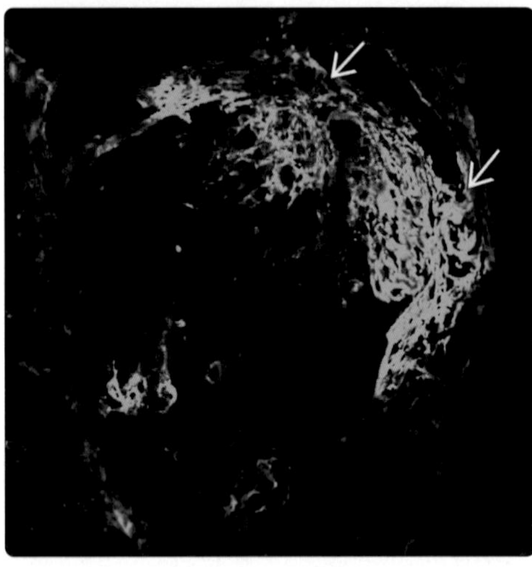

Global Glomerulosclerosis With IgG

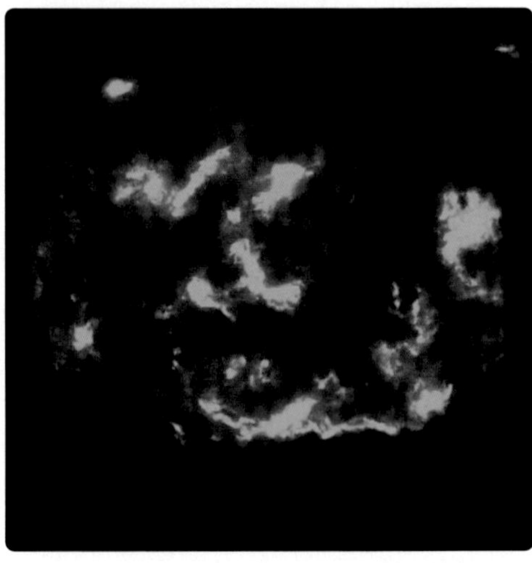

(Left) *Class IV/V lupus nephritis with numerous pseudothrombi, which appear as rounded structures in glomerular capillaries, are stained for IgG ↪. These also stained strongly for IgA, IgM C1q and C3, but not for fibrin.* **(Right)** *Fibrin is present in an arteriole in the vascular pole ↪ and segmentally in the glomerular tuft ➞ in a lupus patient with a high titer of IgG anticardiolipin antibodies. The dominant feature was thrombotic microangiopathy.*

Pseudothrombi

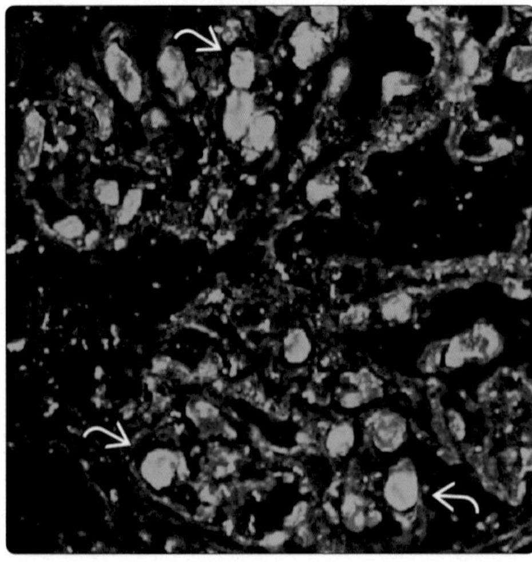

Fibrin in Thrombotic Microangiopathy

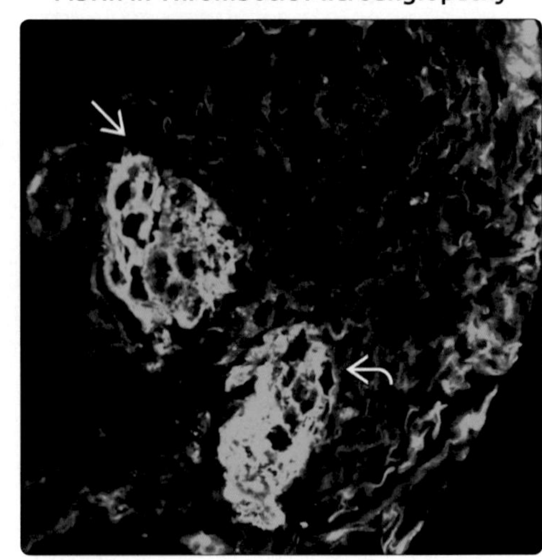

Mesangial Deposits

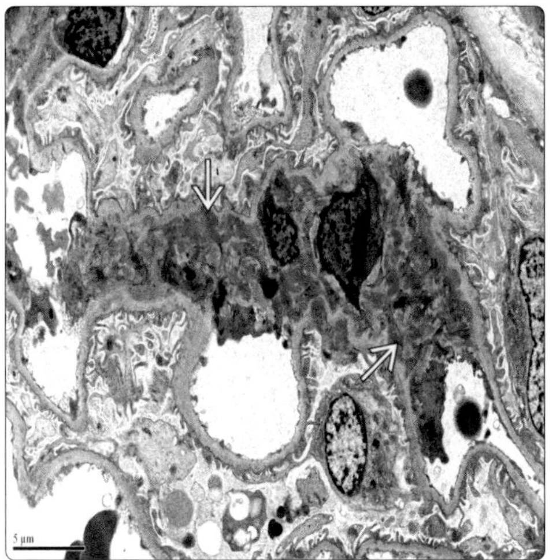

Subendothelial Deposits

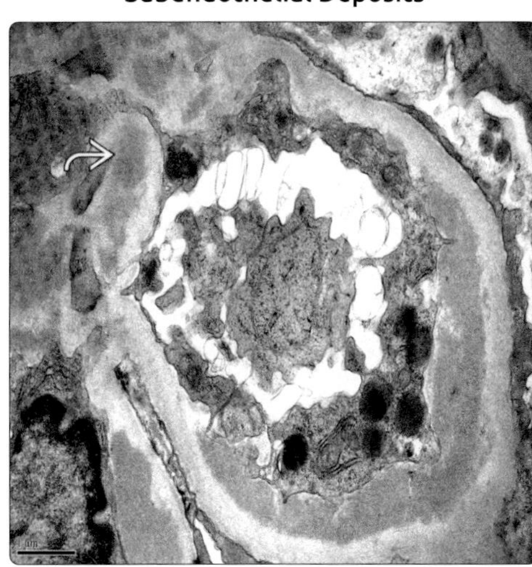

(Left) *Mesangial proliferative lupus nephritis has abundant amorphous granular electron-dense deposits ➡. These are absent from the capillary walls. Podocyte foot processes are preserved.* **(Right)** *Large, confluent, subendothelial electron-dense deposits, the ultrastructural correlate of "wire loop" thickening, are evident in this capillary from a biopsy with diffuse LN. The endothelium is swollen. There are numerous mesangial deposits ➡.*

Membranous LN

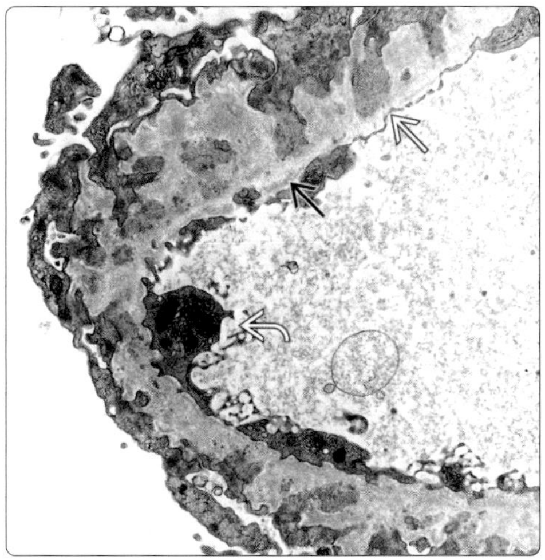

Subepithelial and Mesangial Deposits

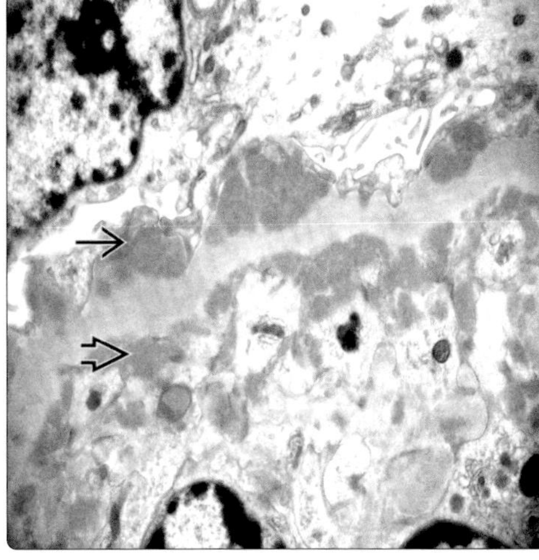

(Left) *Deposits in class V lupus nephritis may penetrate the GBM ➡, in contrast to idiopathic membranous glomerulonephritis (MGN). Mesangial deposits, subendothelial deposits ➡, and tubuloreticular structures ➡ also favor lupus over idiopathic MGN.* **(Right)** *Epimembranous ➡ and mesangial ➡ electron-dense deposits are shown in an example of membranous lupus nephritis (class V) with mesangial immune complex deposits.*

Mesangial and Capillary Wall Deposits

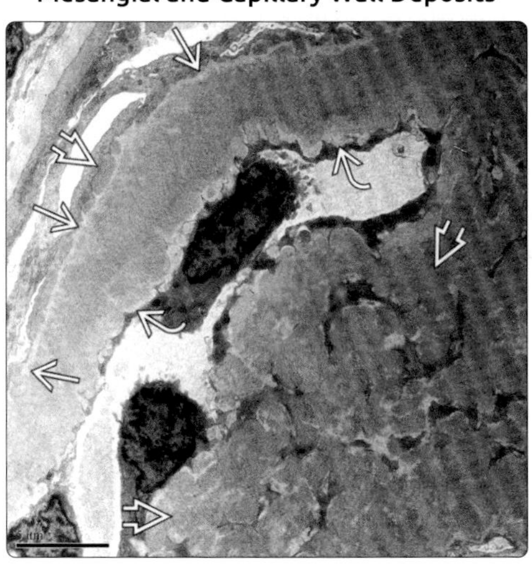

Subepithelial Deposits and Tubuloreticular Inclusions

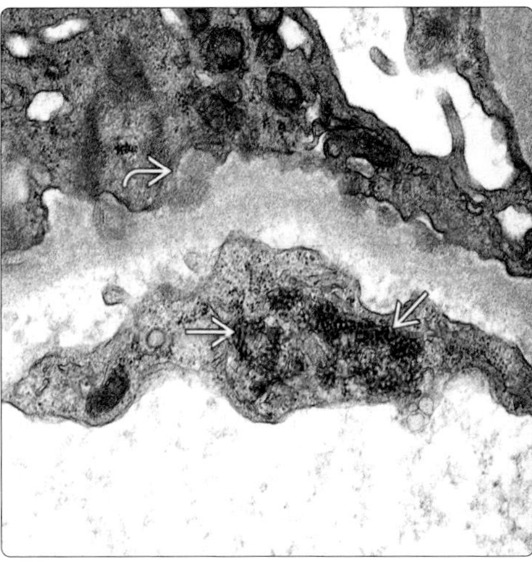

(Left) *Abundant "wire loop" electron-dense deposits fill the subendothelium and encroach on the GBM ➡, and are associated with new subendothelial basement membrane formation ➡. Abundant mesangial and subepithelial deposits ➡ are also present.* **(Right)** *A swollen glomerular capillary endothelial cell has a tubuloreticular inclusion ➡. There is subendothelial widening without electron-dense deposits at this site. Small subepithelial deposits are evident ➡.*

Mesangial Immune Deposits (Class I or II)

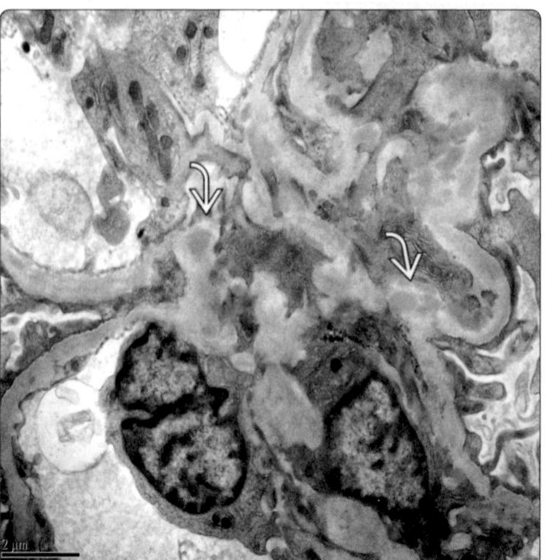

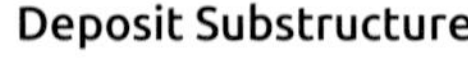

Abundant Mesangial Deposits

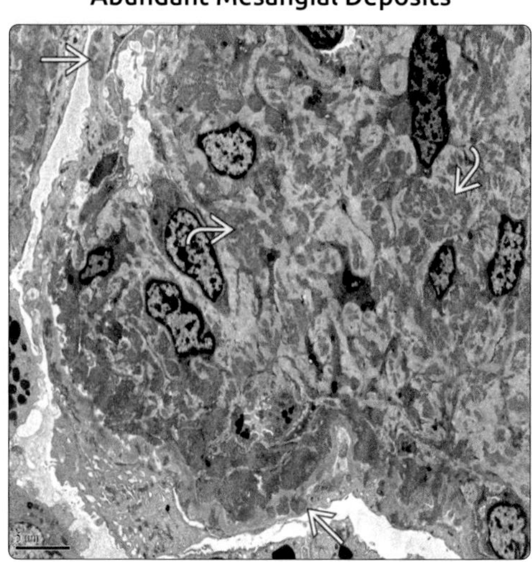

(Left) *Electron dense deposits are present in the mesangium with few in other locations. This pattern can resemble IgA nephropathy, although the prominence of C1q and IgG typically is greater in LN than IgA nephropathy.* **(Right)** *The glomerulus has advanced mesangial sclerosis with increased cellularity and an abundance of electron-dense deposits within the mesangium. Subepithelial deposits are also seen.*

Deposit Substructure

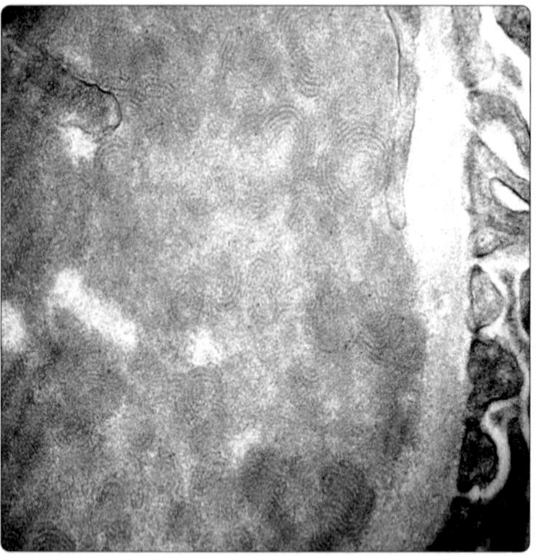

Deposit Substructure

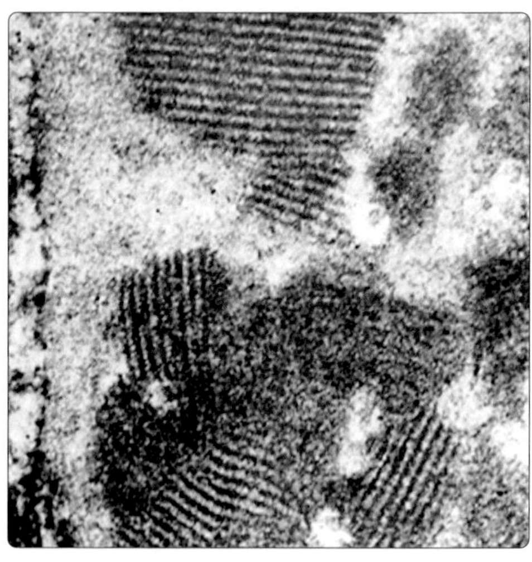

(Left) *This large accumulation of mesangial electron-dense deposit has a distinctive concentric tubular substructure, giving rise to the term "fingerprint deposits."* **(Right)** *High-power electron micrograph of the glomerular mesangium shows the parallel arrays of deposits with regular spacing, resembling fingerprints in lupus nephritis. These distinctive deposits are unrelated to cryoglobulins and are found in about 6-20% of lupus biopsies.*

Penetrating Deposits

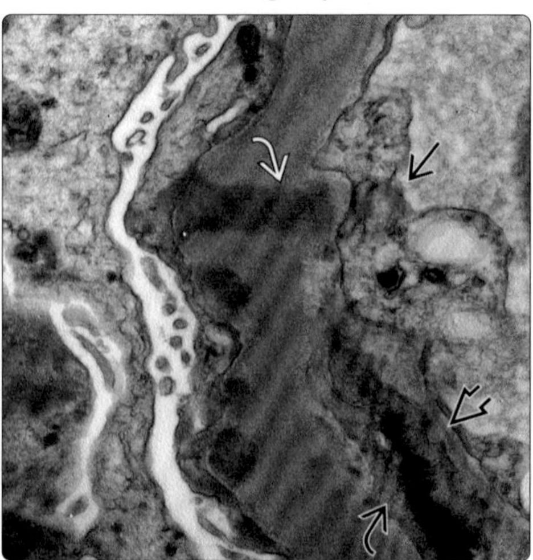

Hematoxylin Body

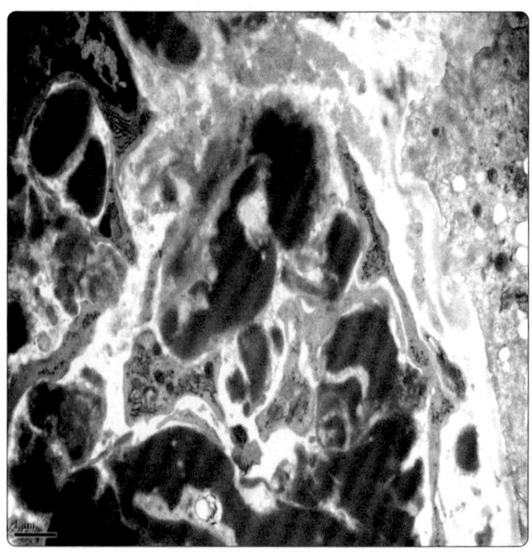

(Left) *Subepithelial deposits sometimes penetrate through the GBM to the subendothelium and may be in continuity with subendothelial deposits. This is not typical of primary membranous glomerulonephritis. Subendothelial neomembrane and interposition are also evident.* **(Right)** *Electron-dense nuclear fragments comprise the bulk of these hematoxylin bodies seen by electron microscopy. These are composed of nuclear histone proteins, nucleic acids, and bound antinuclear antibodies.*

Thrombotic Microangiopathy

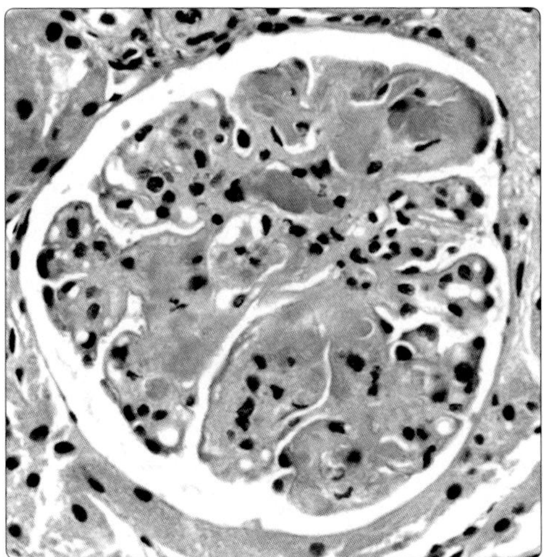

Thrombotic Microangiopathy

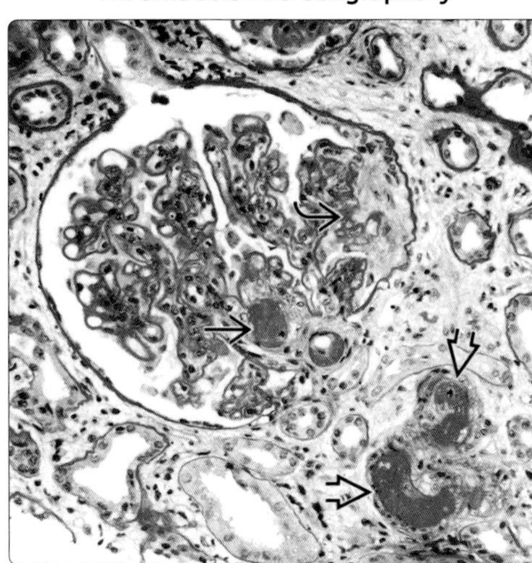

(Left) *Thrombotic microangiopathy in a 13-year-old girl with lupus anticoagulant is shown. Antiphospholipid syndrome occurs in about 1/3 of lupus patients with renal biopsies. TMA may be present in the absence of immune complex-mediated lesions of lupus.* **(Right)** *PAS shows thrombotic microangiopathy (TMA) ➔ involving the perihilar glomerular vessels and an adjacent arteriole ➔. This biopsy has mixed membranous and segmental sclerosing GN (ISN/RPS class III [C] and V) ➔, in addition.*

Segmental Glomerular Sclerosis in LN

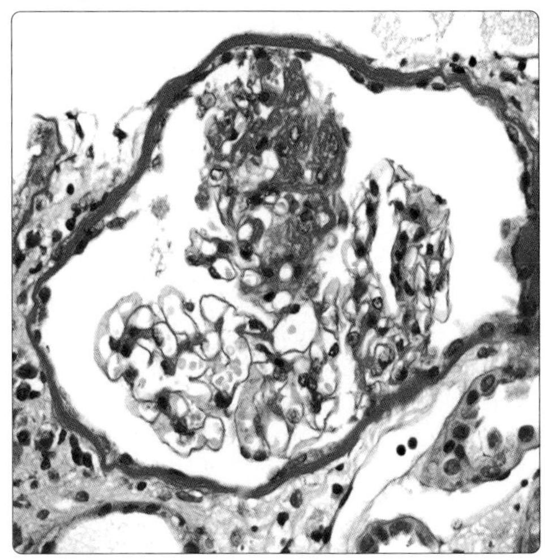

Lupus Podocytopathy

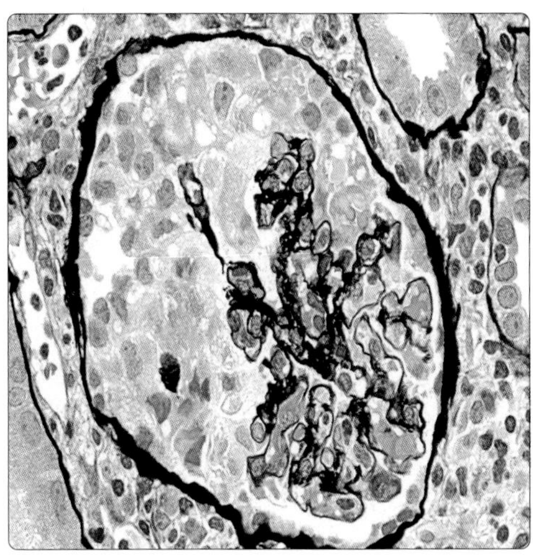

(Left) *PAS shows segmental glomerular sclerosis in a biopsy with lupus nephritis. The distinction of segmental glomerular sclerosis due to prior inflammation from a lupus podocytopathy can be difficult. Diffuse foot process effacement and nephrotic-range proteinuria favor a lupus podocytopathy.* **(Right)** *Lupus podocytopathy with capillary collapse and visceral epithelial cell hyperplasia are features of collapsing glomerulopathy, arising in this case in a patient with SLE.*

Lupus Podocytopathy

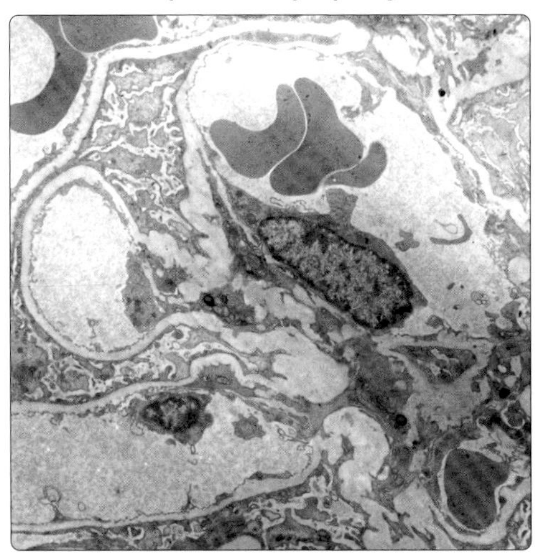

Lupus Podocytopathy

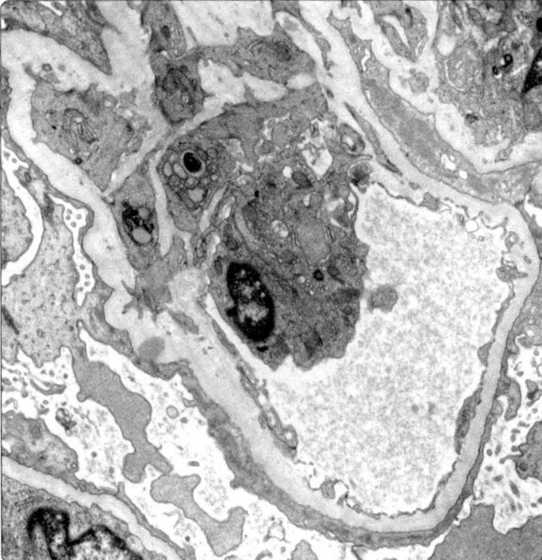

(Left) *Widespread effacement of podocyte foot processes is present in this patient with SLE (ANA[+], dsDNA[+]) and ↑ proteinuria. Rare mesangial deposits were present and IF had minimal IgM, C3 and C1q (trace -1+). Minimal-change-like lesions have been reported occasionally in SLE patients.* **(Right)** *Diffuse effacement of foot processes is present in this patient with class II lupus nephritis. Electron-dense deposits were mainly mesangial with rare subepithelial deposits, insufficient for a diagnosis of class V LN.*

(Left) *Tubulointerstitial nephritis in SLE has an infiltrate composed of lymphocytes and numerous plasma cells. This can occur in SLE with little or no glomerular disease and is not associated with TBM deposits, suggesting cell-mediated mechanisms.* (Right) *Granular staining of the TBM and the interstitium for IgG is detected in 60% of LN. These deposits are often, but not always, accompanied by tubulointerstitial inflammation or fibrosis. C3, C1q, and both light chains are commonly present with IgG.*

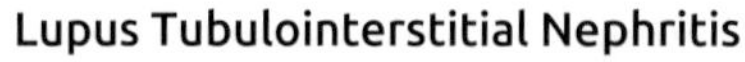

Lupus Tubulointerstitial Nephritis

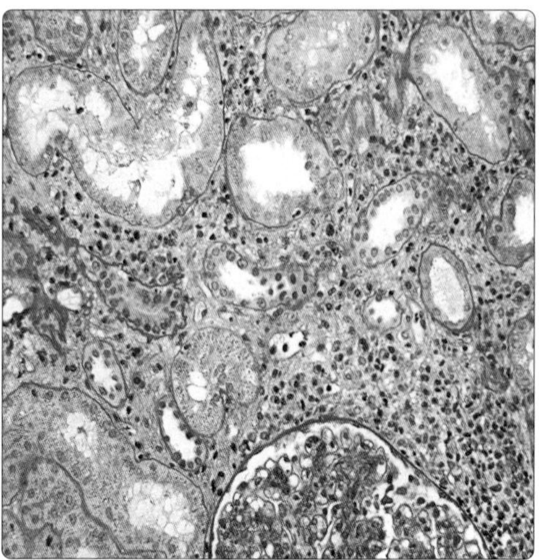

Tubulointerstitial Immune Deposits

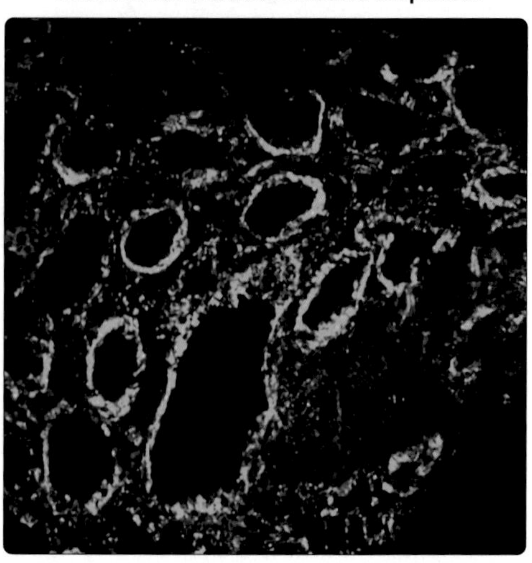

(Left) *Immunoglobulin deposits are present along the TBM and in the interstitium, typical of lupus nephritis. Mixed cryoglobulinemia and occasionally Sjögren syndrome can have similar deposits.* (Right) *Deposits are found in occasional lupus cases in the peritubular capillaries, here detected with an antibody to C4d. The coarse granular pattern contrasts with the linear stain found in humoral rejection of allografts. The TBM also contains C4d.*

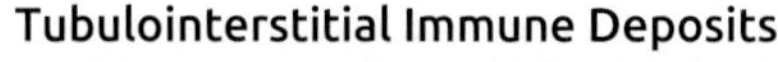

Tubulointerstitial Immune Deposits

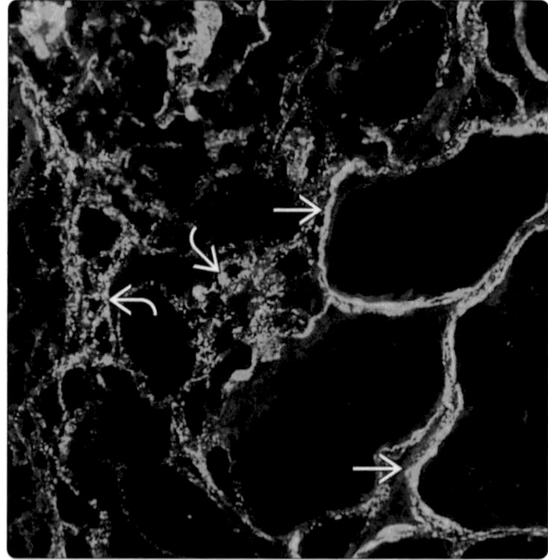

Peritubular Capillary Immune Deposits

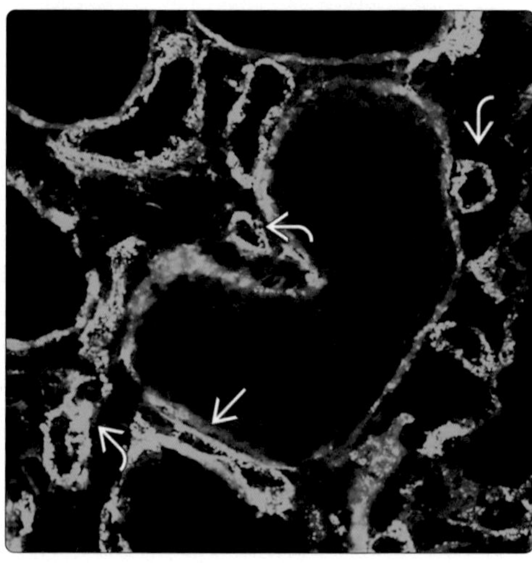

(Left) *Electron-dense deposits beneath the tubular epithelium, within the tubular basement, and on the outer aspect of the tubular basement membrane of an adjacent tubule are shown. Such deposits are not always associated with tubulointerstitial inflammation.* (Right) *Electron-dense immune deposits are present within and on the outside of the tubular basement membrane. Interstitial deposits are also seen.*

Tubular Basement Membrane Deposits

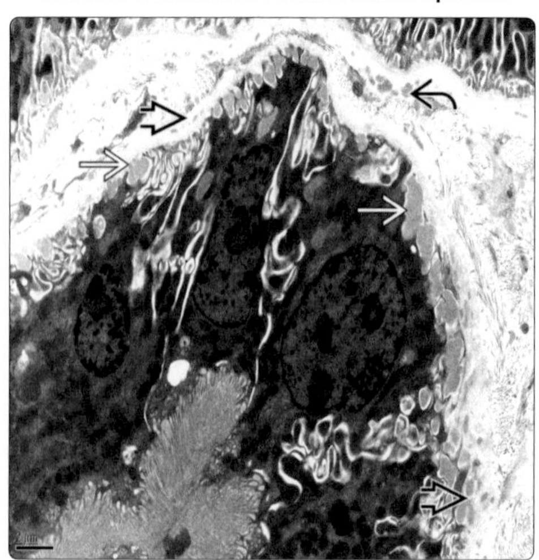

TBM Electron-Dense Deposits

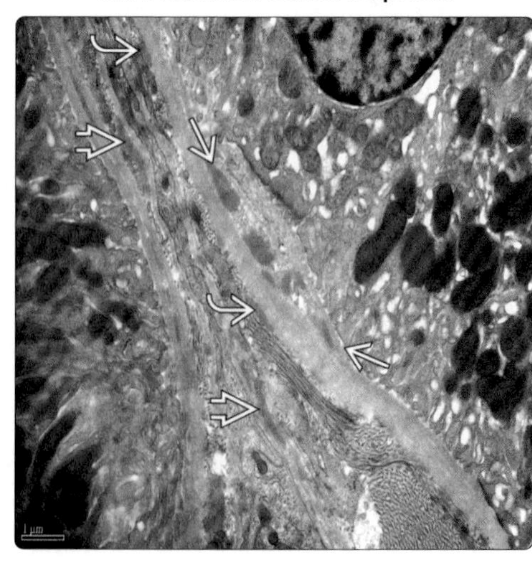

Tubulointerstitial Nephritis With Minimal Glomerular Disease

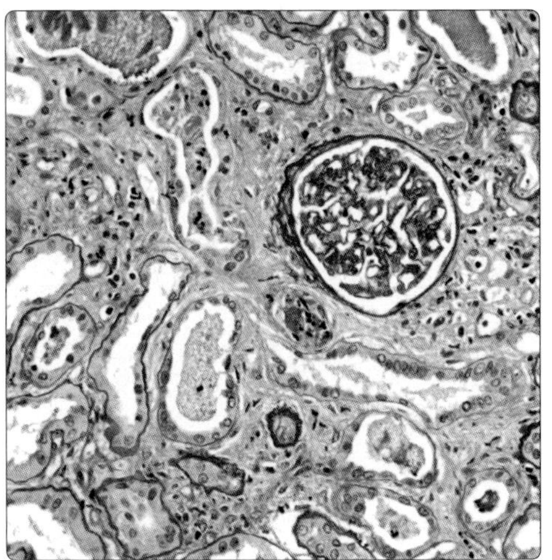

Acute Tubulointerstitial Nephritis in SLE

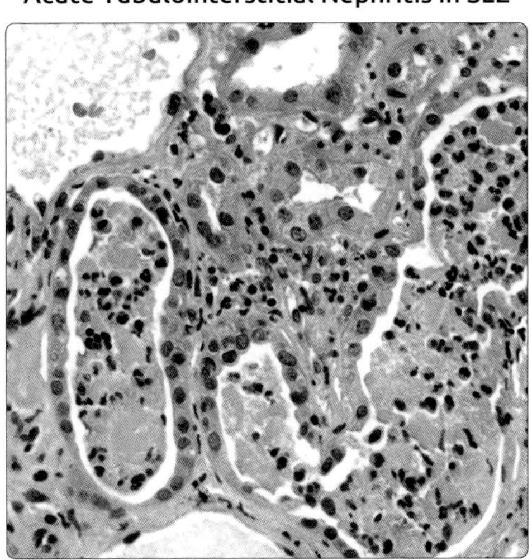

(Left) *LN biopsies may rarely have tubulointerstitial disease with minimal glomerular involvement (≤ class II). This case had IgG, IgM, and C3 deposits in the TBM, with only faint staining for C3 in glomeruli.* **(Right)** *Biopsy from a 52-year-old woman with SLE (positive ANA, pancytopenia, polyarthritis low C3, Cr 2.4, proteinuria ++) shows acute tubulointerstitial nephritis with tubular injury and prominent cellular casts. There was no active glomerular disease.*

Lymphoid Follicles

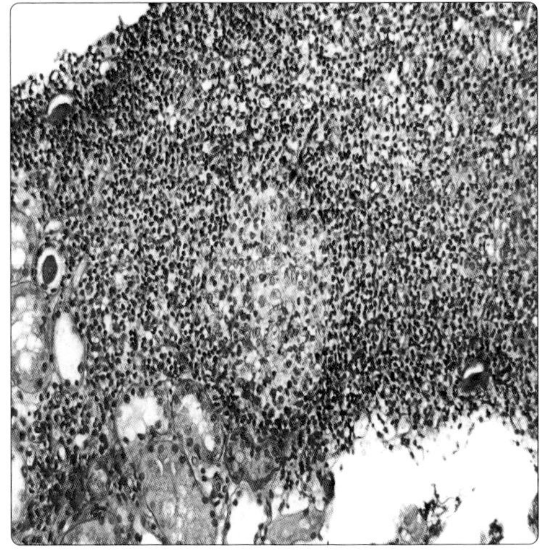

Lymphoid Follicles

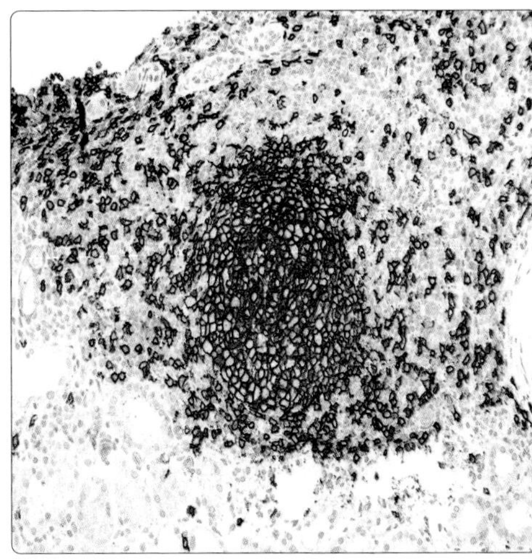

(Left) *Lymphoid aggregates with germinal centers may sometimes be evident in tubulointerstitial nephritis of SLE. Immunohistochemical staining for T and B cells may be helpful in the exclusion of lymphoma in these instances.* **(Right)** *This tubulointerstitial lymphoid follicle, stained for B cells (anti-CD20), demonstrates prominent B-cell populations in the reactive germinal center with scattered B cells in the surrounding interstitium.*

Lymphoid Follicles

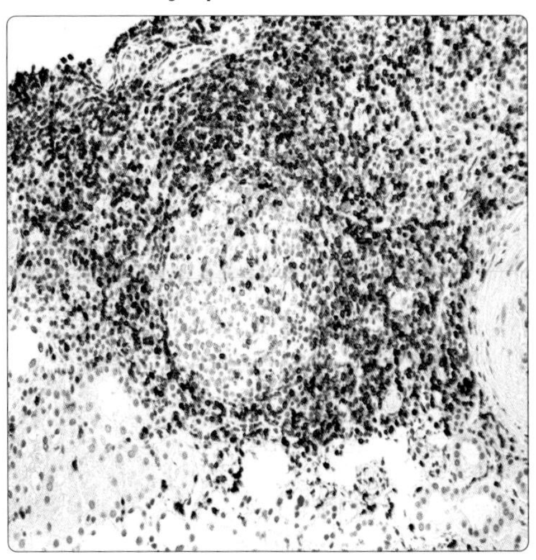

Lymphoid Follicles

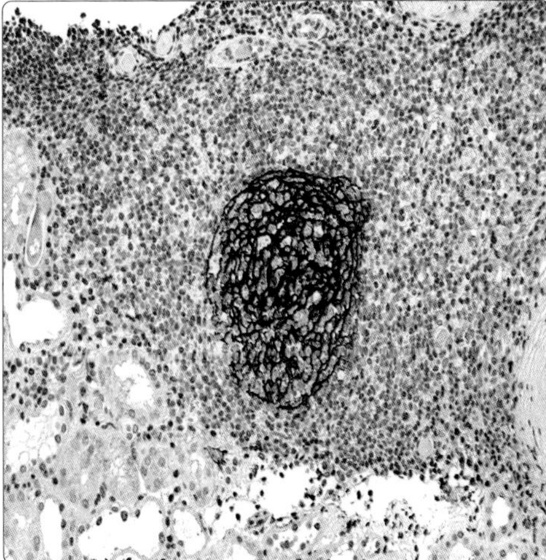

(Left) *This tubulointerstitial lymphoid follicle, stained for T cells by anti-CD3, highlights scattered T cells in the germinal center and numerous cells in the marginal zone and surrounding interstitium.* **(Right)** *This tubulointerstitial lymphoid follicle has a prominent network of follicular dendritic cells that stain for CD21. This staining pattern confirms the reactive nature of these follicles. Lymphoid follicles are strongly correlated with the presence of tubulointerstitial immune deposits.*

(Left) *This artery profile has normal endothelium, minimal intimal thickening, and an unremarkable tunica media and adventitia.* **(Right)** *Identification of uncomplicated vascular immune deposits requires detection of IgG ± complement deposits by IF, and normal-appearing arteries. Deposits may be seen on EM. This lesion is unique to lupus nephritis and is helpful in confirming the diagnosis.*

Uncomplicated Vascular Immune Deposits

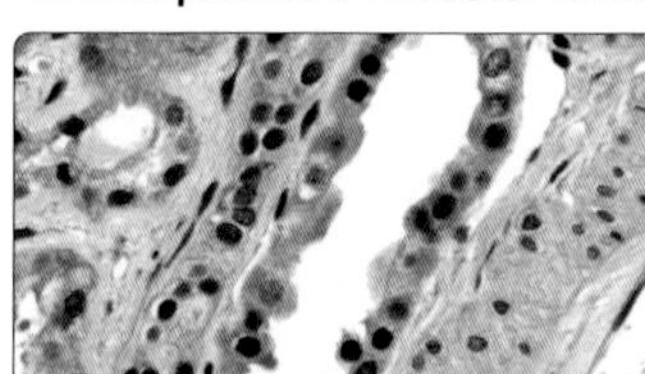

Arterial Immune Deposits

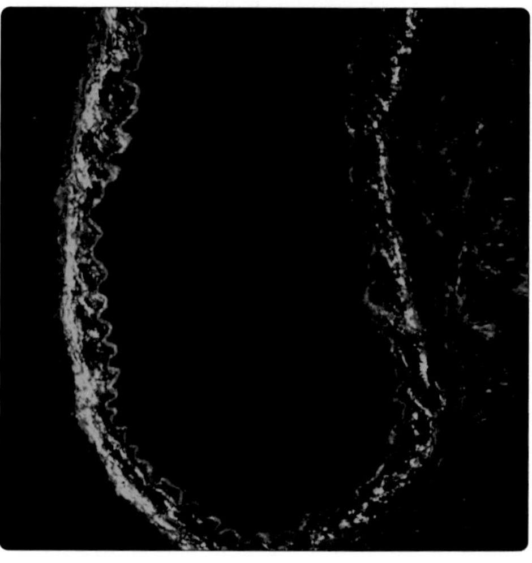

(Left) *High-intensity granular staining for IgG may be detectable by IF in the intima and media of arteries, frequently without morphologic abnormalities. This is characteristic of uncomplicated vascular immune deposits in LN.* **(Right)** *Arterial medial immune deposits → may frequently be seen in lupus nephritis. The deposits are located between the smooth muscle cells. The endothelium (below) and adventitia (above) appear normal. The vessels were unremarkable by light microscopy.*

Arterial Immune Deposits

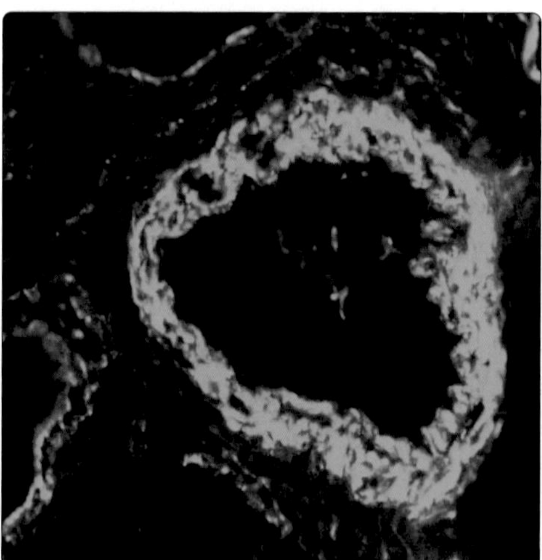

Tunica Media Vasorum Deposits

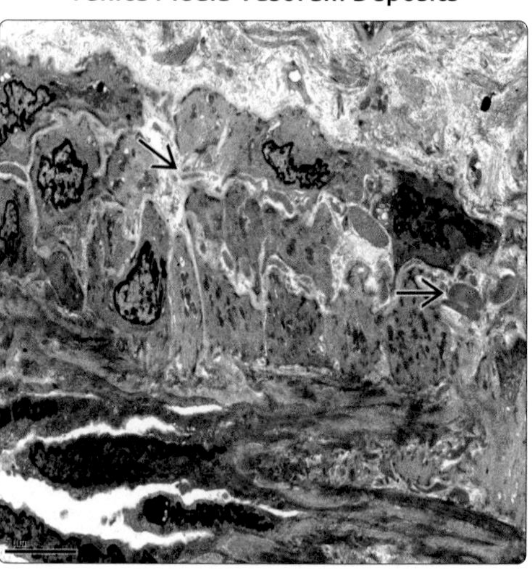

(Left) *Noninflammatory "necrotizing" lupus vasculopathy affects primarily afferent arterioles and has intimal and medial deposits of hyaline material replacing myocytes. These can be distinguished from severe hyalinization or TMA by their content of immunoglobulins and complement.* **(Right)** *Noninflammatory lupus vasculopathy has abundant staining of the affected vessels for IgG, IgM, IgA, kappa and lambda light chains, C3, C1q, and fibrin/ogen.*

Noninflammatory Lupus Vasculopathy

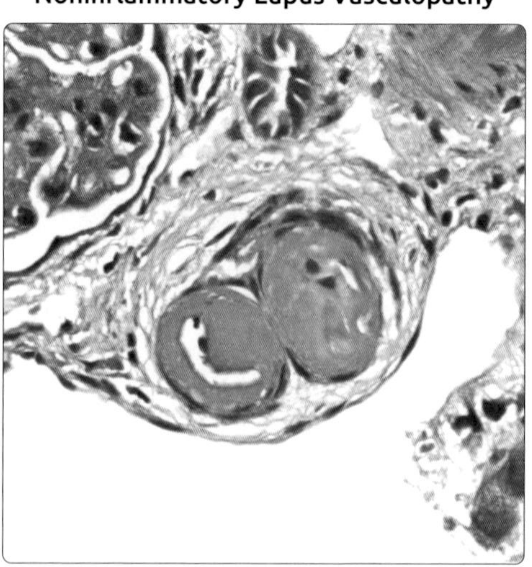

Noninflammatory Lupus Vasculopathy

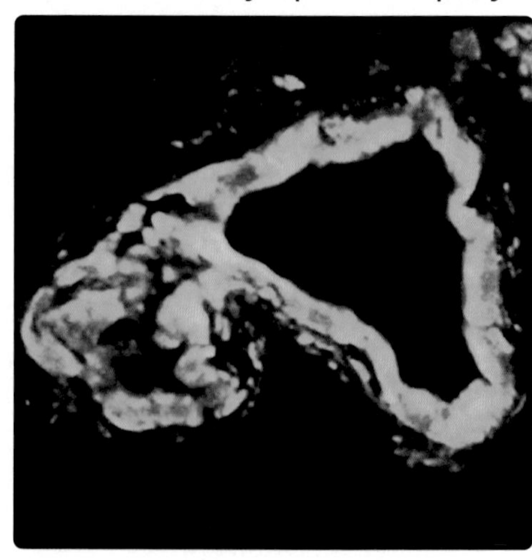

Noninflammatory Lupus Vasculopathy

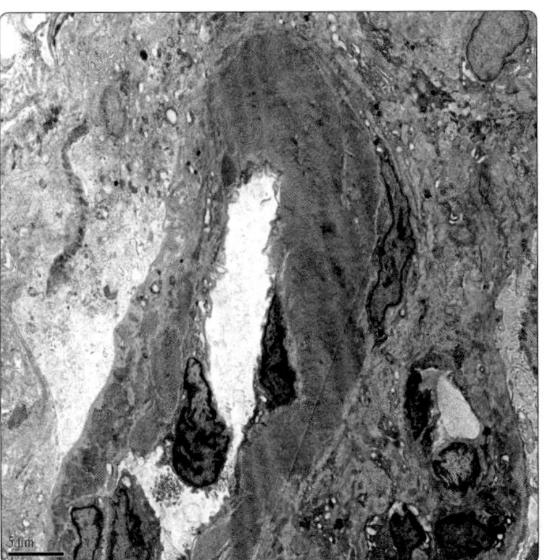

Necrotizing Lupus Vasculitis

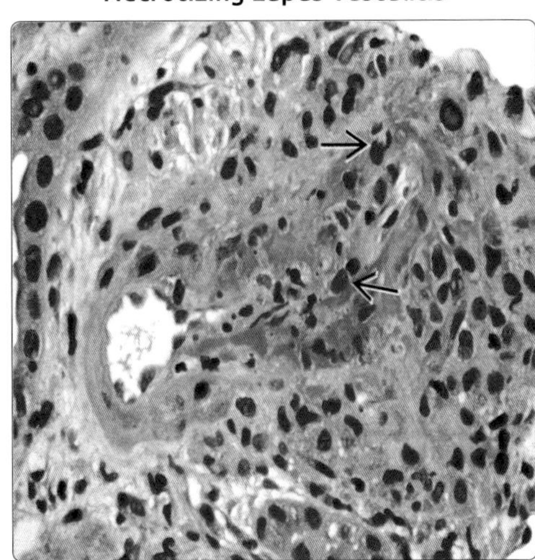

(Left) *This uncommon lesion is characterized by replacement of myocytes by homogeneous electron-dense material. This stains for Ig, complement and fibrin/ogen by IF, and may arise by a combination of immune deposition and coagulation.* **(Right)** *Necrotizing lupus arteritis has transmural fibrinoid necrosis and exceptionally numerous hematoxylin bodies ⇨. Perivascular macrophages are also evident.*

Necrotizing Lupus Arteritis and TMA

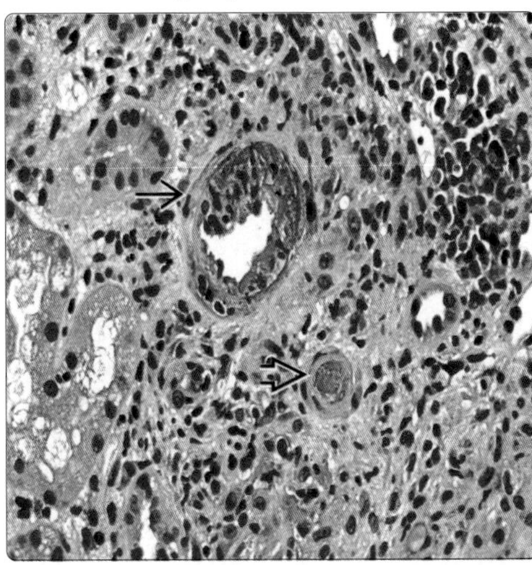

Necrotizing Lupus Vasculitis

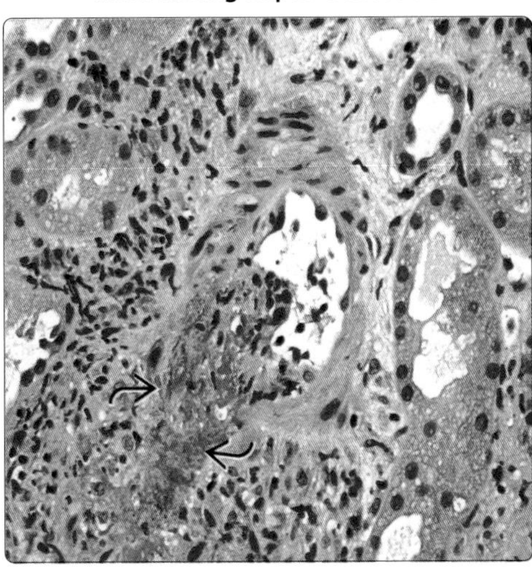

(Left) *Necrotizing lupus arteritis ⇨ has intimal and medial inflammation, leukocytoclasis, and fibrinoid necrosis. Thrombotic occlusion of a noninflamed arteriole is also evident ⇨ in this biopsy with active lupus nephritis.* **(Right)** *Necrotizing lupus arteritis with intimal inflammation, fibrin exudation, and medial necrosis with hematoxyphilic material is shown ⇨ (Azzopardi effect).*

IgG in Necrotizing Lupus Vasculitis

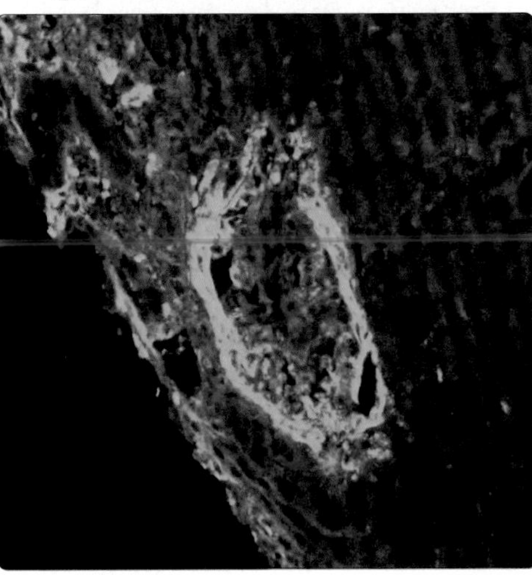

Fibrinogen in Necrotizing Lupus Vasculitis

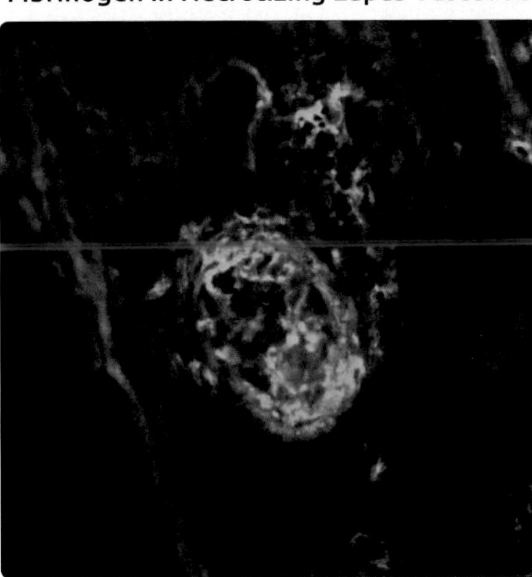

(Left) *Mural IgG deposits are present in the wall of an interlobular artery. This vessel had fibrinoid necrosis by light microscopy.* **(Right)** *Necrotizing lupus arteritis has fibrin/fibrinogen deposits at sites of fibrinoid necrosis. These lesions may or may not have Ig and complement deposits.*

Mixed Connective Tissue Disease

KEY FACTS

TERMINOLOGY

- Autoimmune disease with features of systemic lupus erythematosus (SLE), polymyositis, and scleroderma and high titers of anti-U1 ribonucleoprotein (RNP)
- Debated whether a distinct disease or overlap syndrome

CLINICAL ISSUES

- F:M ~ 16:1
- 2nd to 3rd decades of life
- Proteinuria up to nephrotic range ± hematuria
- Systemic and pulmonary hypertension
- Cutaneous lesions: Ulcers, hand swelling, acrosclerosis, Raynaud, and vasculitis-like lesions
- Arthritis/arthralgias
- Myositis, synovitis, esophageal/other GI dysmotility, mitral valve prolapse
- ANA often > 1:1,000 to 1:10,000
- Various anti-ribonucleoproteins (RNPs)
- Steroid (i.e., corticosteroids) treatment used

MICROSCOPIC

- 35-40% membranous glomerulonephritis
- Focal proliferative GN equivalent to SLE class III
- Also mesangial and membranoproliferative patterns
- If crescents and fibrinoid necrosis may be ANCA associated
- Sometimes thrombotic microangiopathy equivalent to scleroderma renal crisis
- Rarely amyloidosis, minimal change disease, collapsing glomerulopathy

ANCILLARY TESTS

- Deposits on IF, IgG, and C3 most commonly ± others
- Deposits and tubuloreticular inclusions on EM

TOP DIFFERENTIAL DIAGNOSES

- Systemic lupus erythematosus
- Membranous glomerulonephritis
- Scleroderma
- ANCA-related disease

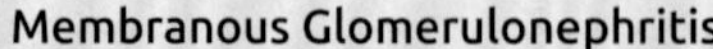
Membranous Glomerulonephritis

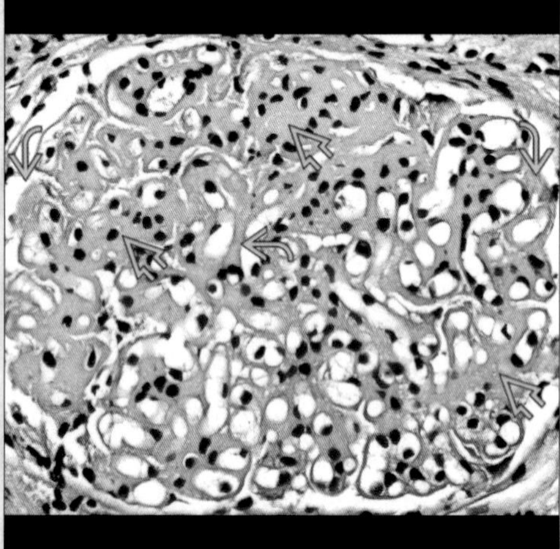

Granular GBM Deposits

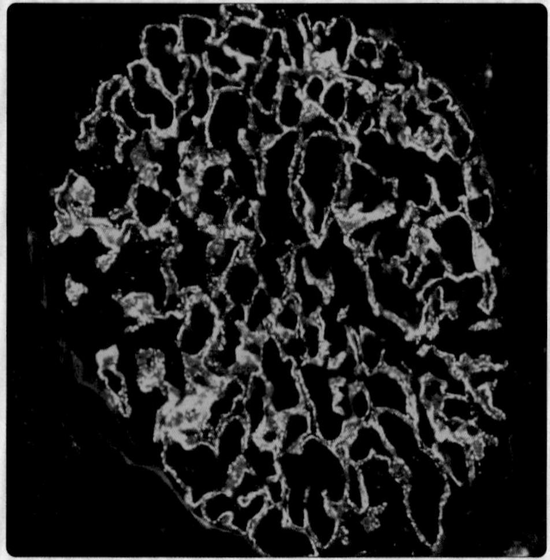

(Left) *In this case of mixed connective tissue disease (MCTD) with membranous glomerulopathy, there are areas of basement membrane thickening* → *as well as mesangial expansion* →, *culminating in segmental sclerosis. This is the most common glomerular disease in MCTD.* **(Right)** *Widespread granular deposits along the GBM stain for IgG (and C3) in this patient with MCTD. Mesangial and small subendothelial deposits were evident by EM and no PLA2R containing deposits were seen, similar to lupus class V.*

Subepithelial Deposits and GBM "Spikes"

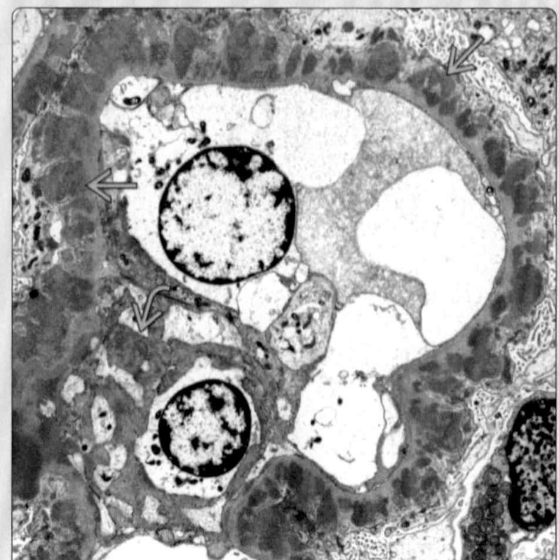

Tubuloreticular Structure

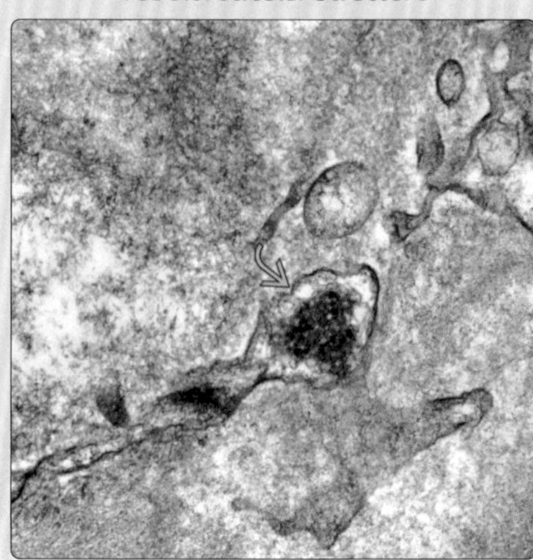

(Left) *By electron microscopy, multiple immune deposits are seen along the basement membrane* → *in a case of membranous glomerulopathy due to MCTD. Mesangial deposits are also typically present* →, *similar to systemic lupus erythematosus (SLE).* **(Right)** *Glomerular endothelial cells commonly contain tubuloreticular structures* → *in MCTD just as in lupus nephritis. This is a cellular response to increased exposure to interferons.*

TERMINOLOGY

Abbreviations

- Mixed connective tissue disease (MCTD)

Definitions

- Autoimmune disease with features of systemic lupus erythematosus (SLE), polymyositis, and scleroderma and high titers of anti-U1 ribonucleoprotein (RNP)
- Debated whether a distinct disease or overlap syndrome

ETIOLOGY/PATHOGENESIS

Autoimmune Disease of Unknown Etiology

- Pathogenesis involves mechanisms related to SLE (e.g., immune complex glomerulonephritis) and scleroderma (e.g., vasculopathy/thrombotic microangiopathy)
- IL-10 gene polymorphism associated with anti-U1RNP
- DRB1*04:01 (HLA-DR4) major risk allele (different from SLE)

CLINICAL ISSUES

Epidemiology

- Age
  - Usually 2nd to 3rd decades of life
- Sex
  - F:M ~ 16:1

Presentation

- Kidney involved in 10-26% of adults, 33-50% of children
- Proteinuria
  - ~ 20% at least mild (~ 500 mg/d)
  - ~ 30% nephrotic-range proteinuria
- Microhematuria
- Hypocomplementemia (± renal disease)
- Hypertension (HTN)
- Acute renal failure (rare, scleroderma renal crisis)
- Scleroderma symptoms
  - Esophageal dysmotility, digital gangrene, Raynaud phenomenon, swelling or sclerodermatous hand changes, restrictive lung disease, pulmonary HTN
- SLE symptoms
  - Alopecia, malar erythema, photosensitivity, pericarditis, arthritis/arthralgias, discoid, lupus-like disease, lymphadenopathy, serositis, mitral valve prolapse, hepatosplenomegaly
- Polymyositis symptoms
  - Myalgia

Laboratory Tests

- Antinuclear antibody (ANA) often > 1:1,000 to 1:10,000
- Anti-U1RNP most characteristic of MCTD
  - Small and heterogeneous nuclear RNP (U1-snRNP and U1-hnRNP-A2)
- Absence of anti-DNA, anti-Sm, and histone antibodies

Treatment

- Drugs
  - Corticosteroids

Prognosis

- Chronic renal failure in ~ 14%

MICROSCOPIC

Histologic Features

- Glomeruli
  - 35-40% membranous glomerulonephritis (MGN)
  - 7% membranoproliferative glomerulonephritis
  - 7% mesangial proliferative glomerulonephritis
  - Focal proliferative GN equivalent to SLE class III
  - Rarely amyloidosis, minimal change disease, collapsing glomerulopathy
  - Glomerular fibrinoid necrosis and crescents (associated with ANCA[+])
- Interstitial disease in 15%
- Vascular disease in 22%
  - Arterial intimal fibrosis, medial hyperplasia
  - Medial hyperplasia
  - Rarely scleroderma-like renal crisis with mucoid intimal change, fibrinoid necrosis

ANCILLARY TESTS

Immunofluorescence

- GBM granular IgG and C3 (~ 30% of patients) ± IgA
  - May accompany diffuse mesangial and focal proliferative changes
  - ± subendothelial IgG, IgA, IgM, and C3
- Mesangial deposits alone
- Tubular basement membrane deposits noted rarely

Electron Microscopy

- Amorphous deposits and tubuloreticular inclusions as in SLE
- "Fingerprint" lesions (± cryoglobulin)

DIFFERENTIAL DIAGNOSIS

Lupus Erythematosus

- Kidney pathology completely overlaps with SLE
- Distinction between SLE and MCTD based on clinical features and autoantibodies

Membranous Glomerulonephritis

- Mesangial and TBM deposits argue against idiopathic MGN
- Anti-PLA2R negative in MCTD (limited experience)

DIAGNOSTIC CHECKLIST

Diagnostic Criteria

- Anti-RNP > 1:600 and 3 of the following: Hand edema, synovitis, myositis, Raynaud phenomenon, and acrosclerosis (100% sensitive, 99.6% specific)

SELECTED REFERENCES

1. Flåm ST et al: The HLA profiles of mixed connective tissue disease differ distinctly from the profiles of clinically related connective tissue diseases. Rheumatology (Oxford). 54(3):528-35, 2015
2. Paradowska-Gorycka A et al: IL-10, IL-12B and IL-17 gene polymorphisms in patients with mixed connective tissue disease. Mod Rheumatol. 25(3):487-9, 2015
3. Ortega-Hernandez OD et al: Mixed connective tissue disease: an overview of clinical manifestations, diagnosis and treatment. Best Pract Res Clin Rheumatol. 26(1):61-72, 2012
4. Sawai T et al: Morphometric analysis of the kidney lesions in mixed connective tissue disease (MCTD). Tohoku J Exp Med. 174(2):141-54, 1994

Rheumatoid Arthritis

KEY FACTS

TERMINOLOGY

- Kidney disease in RA patients, due to therapy or RA inflammatory processes

ETIOLOGY/PATHOGENESIS

- Therapy related most common
  - Tubulointerstitial nephritis caused by NSAIDs
  - Membranous glomerulonephritis (MGN) caused by gold salts, penicillamine, and TNF-α antagonists
  - ANCA-related disease precipitated by penicillamine and TNF-α antagonists
  - Arteriolar hyalinosis and interstitial fibrosis caused by calcineurin inhibitors
  - Papillary necrosis in analgesic nephropathy
- Disease related
  - AA amyloidosis with long duration RA (> 15 years)
  - Mesangial proliferative glomerulonephritis (GN), some cases of MGN, ANCA-related disease

CLINICAL ISSUES

- Clinical presentation varies based on type and extent of renal involvement
- Withdrawal of offending drug resolves most renal manifestations

MICROSCOPIC

- Tubulointerstitial nephritis with acute tubular injury
- MGN with IgG, C3 deposits
- Cyclosporine toxicity with arteriolar hyalinosis or TMA
- Pauci-immune GN with glomerular necrosis and crescents
- Amyloidosis, AA subtype
- Mesangioproliferative immune complex-mediated GN
- Minimal change disease

TOP DIFFERENTIAL DIAGNOSES

- Primary MGN
- ANCA-related diseases
- Amyloidosis AL and other types

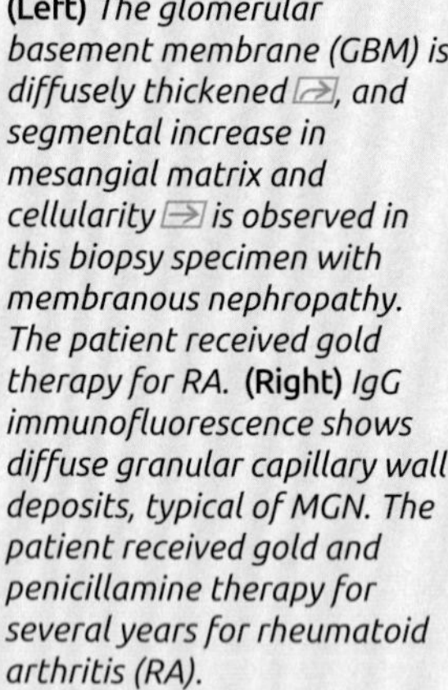

(Left) *The glomerular basement membrane (GBM) is diffusely thickened →, and segmental increase in mesangial matrix and cellularity → is observed in this biopsy specimen with membranous nephropathy. The patient received gold therapy for RA.* **(Right)** *IgG immunofluorescence shows diffuse granular capillary wall deposits, typical of MGN. The patient received gold and penicillamine therapy for several years for rheumatoid arthritis (RA).*

Therapy-Related Membranous Nephropathy

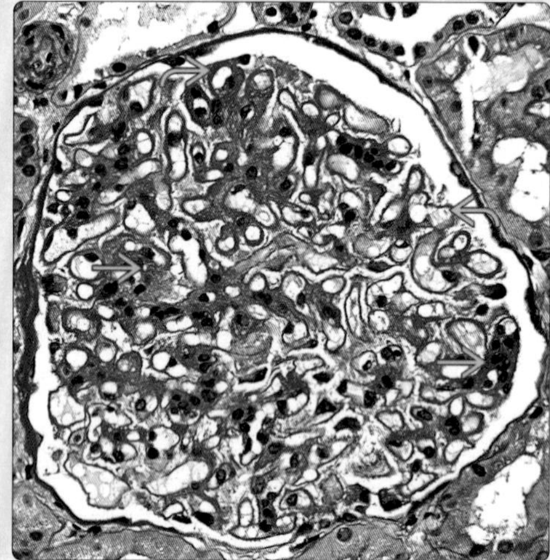

Glomerular Capillary Wall IgG Deposits

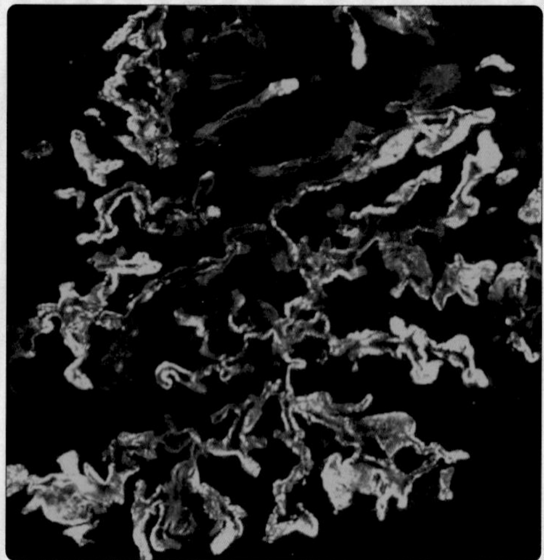

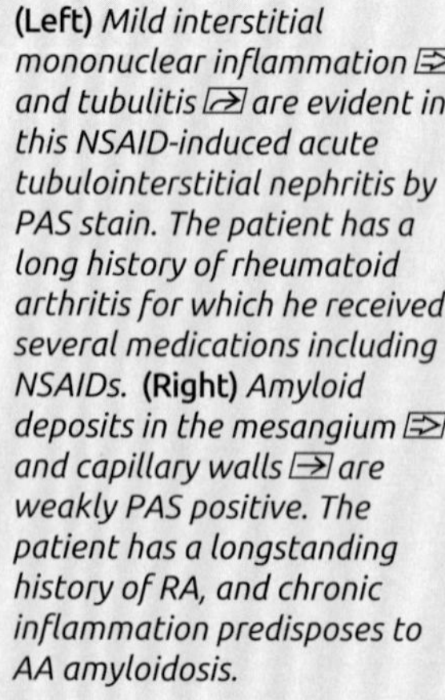

(Left) *Mild interstitial mononuclear inflammation → and tubulitis → are evident in this NSAID-induced acute tubulointerstitial nephritis by PAS stain. The patient has a long history of rheumatoid arthritis for which he received several medications including NSAIDs.* **(Right)** *Amyloid deposits in the mesangium → and capillary walls → are weakly PAS positive. The patient has a longstanding history of RA, and chronic inflammation predisposes to AA amyloidosis.*

NSAID-Related Tubulointerstitial Nephritis

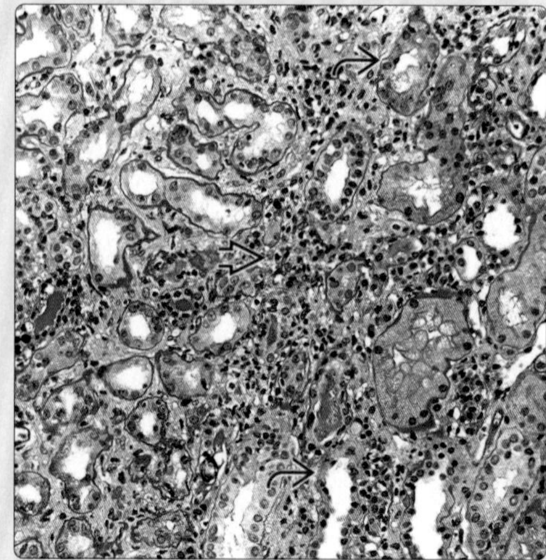

Weakly PAS-Positive Amyloid Deposits

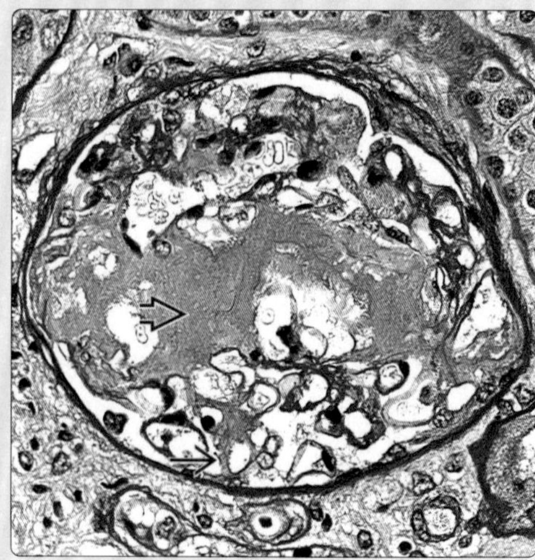

TERMINOLOGY

Abbreviations

- Rheumatoid arthritis (RA)

Definitions

- Kidney disease in RA patients, due to drug therapy or RA inflammatory processes

ETIOLOGY/PATHOGENESIS

Complications of Treatment

- Nonsteroidal anti-inflammatory drugs (NSAIDs) cause tubulointerstitial nephritis and acute renal failure
  - Often occurs after months of NSAID use
  - Inhibition of cyclooxygenase and reduced synthesis of vasodilatory prostaglandins cause acute renal failure
  - NSAID-related minimal change disease less common
- Gold salts and penicillamine therapy results in membranous glomerulonephritis (MGN)
  - No correlation between cumulative dose and disease development
- Penicillamine therapy linked to pauci-immune GN and Goodpasture-like pulmonary renal syndrome
- Cyclosporine nephrotoxicity
  - Related to vasoconstrictor or endothelial injury effects
- Analgesic nephropathy due to phenacetin
  - Much less common in modern era, after withdrawal of phenacetin from market
  - Chronic interstitial nephritis and papillary necrosis
- Tumor necrosis factor (TNF)-α inhibitors can precipitate autoimmune disease
  - Causes proliferative or membranous lupus nephritis, pauci-immune glomerulonephritis (GN), or vasculitis

AA Amyloidosis

- Duration of RA disease often > 15 years
- Chronic inflammation can result in AA amyloidosis

Renal Disease Directly Related to RA

- Rare but documented in absence of drug therapy
- Includes glomerular involvement by mesangial proliferative GN, MGN, and pauci-immune GN
- Reports of vasculitis involving renal artery and its branches
- Thrombotic microangiopathy due to concomitant antiphospholipid antibody syndrome

CLINICAL ISSUES

Epidemiology

- Incidence
  - Renal involvement mainly therapy related
    - MGN secondary to gold and penicillamine therapy occurs in 1-10% of RA patients
  - Based on autopsy series, prevalence of AA amyloidosis ~ 15%
  - Rare direct kidney involvement as part of systemic RA

Presentation

- Kidney involvement
  - Presentation varies based on type and extent of renal involvement
  - Nephrotic syndrome common in MGN and amyloidosis
  - Rapidly progressive renal failure in ANCA-related GN and vasculitis
  - Acute renal failure with NSAID-related interstitial nephritis and acute tubular injury
  - Isolated hematuria &/or proteinuria in mesangioproliferative GN related directly to RA
  - Variable decline in renal function and mild proteinuria in most other instances
- Systemic manifestations of RA
  - Arthritis due to autoimmune inflammation of joints
  - Various extraarticular manifestations include pericarditis, pulmonary nodules, pulmonary interstitial fibrosis, mononeuritis multiplex, and systemic vasculitis
  - Diagnosis of RA is based on criteria established by collaborative efforts of American College of Rheumatology and European League Against Rheumatism

Laboratory Tests

- p-ANCA test positive in pauci-immune GN secondary to RA or treatment complication
- ANA, anti-DNA antibodies, and low serum complement levels in anti-TNF-α therapy-induced autoimmune disease

Treatment

- Drugs
  - Withdrawal of offending drug (NSAIDs; gold, penicillamine) causes resolution of tubulointerstitial nephritis and MGN, respectively, in most cases
    - Resolution of disease after drug withdrawal takes up to 1 year
    - If renal dysfunction persists, steroids accelerate recovery in NSAID interstitial nephritis
  - Corticosteroids, colchicine, and cyclophosphamide may be useful in treatment of AA amyloidosis
    - Strict control of RA inflammation and hypertension may lead to remission of proteinuria and preservation of renal function
  - Immunosuppressive therapy for pauci-immune GN and mesangioproliferative GN

MICROSCOPIC

Histologic Features

- Tubulointerstitial nephritis
  - Interstitial inflammation due to NSAIDs usually sparse
  - Interstitial edema and inflammation is present in nonatrophic parenchyma
  - Acute tubular injury may be evident with loss of proximal tubular brush borders and sloughed epithelial cells
- Membranous glomerulonephritis (MGN)
  - Glomerular basement membrane (GBM) may be thickened or show basement membrane "spikes," depending on MGN stage
    - Subepithelial deposits may be seen on PAS and trichrome stains
  - Mild mesangial proliferation can be present, especially in therapy-induced membranous lupus nephritis
- Cyclosporine toxicity
  - Normal histology in vasoconstriction-induced acute nephrotoxicity
  - Tubular isometric cytoplasmic vacuoles in acute toxicity

- Arteriolar hyaline insudation, particularly with medial or peripheral beaded appearance
- Interstitial fibrosis with striped pattern due to non-uniform involvement of arterioles
- Acute thrombotic microangiopathy with endothelial swelling, mesangiolysis, and fragmented RBCs

- Pauci-immune GN
  - Variable degree of glomerular fibrinoid necrosis and crescents
  - Small vessel vasculitis may be present
- Amyloidosis
  - Amyloid AA deposits in glomeruli, tubular basement membranes, interstitium, and blood vessels
    - Distribution of amorphous deposits typical of AA amyloidosis
      - Deposits weakly PAS and trichrome positive
    - Congo red stain also positive with apple-green birefringence under polarized light
- Mesangioproliferative GN
  - Mild to moderate mesangial proliferation
  - No endocapillary proliferation, necrosis, or crescents
- Analgesic nephropathy
  - Predominant tubular atrophy and interstitial fibrosis with relatively mild chronic interstitial inflammation
  - Tubulointerstitial compartment disproportionately affected compared to extent of glomerulosclerosis
  - Papillary necrosis may be identified on biopsy
- Minimal change disease
  - Normal glomerular histology
  - Acute tubular injury may be evident in setting of acute renal failure
- Other
  - Rare cases of fibrillary glomerulonephritis reported
  - Variable extent of tubular atrophy and interstitial fibrosis
  - Arterio- and arteriolosclerosis present in setting of hypertensive nephrosclerosis
  - Vasculitis of renal artery and its branches rare and may not be sampled

ANCILLARY TESTS

Immunofluorescence

- Diffuse or segmental capillary wall deposits identified in MGN with IgG and C3
  - Therapy-induced membranous lupus nephritis may have mesangial and capillary wall deposits with "full house" staining
- Mesangial IgM immune deposits often dominant with weaker staining for other Ig and complement components in mesangioproliferative GN related to RA
- Amyloid can be typed by immunofluorescence or immunohistochemistry
  - Subtyping of amyloid demonstrates AA protein with no evidence of immunoglobulin light or heavy chains
- No immune complexes in NSAID interstitial nephritis, cyclosporine toxicity, analgesic nephropathy, pauci-immune GN, and minimal change disease

Electron Microscopy

- Subepithelial electron-dense deposits in MGN
  - Proximal tubular lysosomal gold inclusions characterized by electron-dense filaments in gold-induced MGN
- Mesangial deposits in mesangioproliferative GN and membranous lupus nephritis
- Amyloid deposits composed of nonbranching randomly oriented fibrils, 8-12 nm thick
- No deposits in interstitial nephritis, cyclosporine toxicity, analgesic nephropathy, and pauci-immune GN
- Extensive foot process effacement in NSAID-induced minimal change disease

DIFFERENTIAL DIAGNOSIS

Primary MGN

- PLA2R antibodies and IF staining in 70-80% of idiopathic MGN

ANCA-Related Diseases

- Drug history helpful

Amyloidosis AL and Other Types

- Typing of deposits by IF or IHC

SELECTED REFERENCES

1. Kuroda T et al: Significant association between renal function and area of amyloid deposition in kidney biopsy specimens in reactive amyloidosis associated with rheumatoid arthritis. Rheumatol Int. 32(10):3155-62, 2012
2. Ueno T et al: Remission of proteinuria and preservation of renal function in patients with renal AA amyloidosis secondary to rheumatoid arthritis. Nephrol Dial Transplant. 27(2):633-9, 2012
3. Aletaha D et al: 2010 Rheumatoid arthritis classification criteria: an American College of Rheumatology/European League Against Rheumatism collaborative initiative. Arthritis Rheum. 62(9):2569-81, 2010
4. Kurita N et al: Myeloperoxidase-antineutrophil cytoplasmic antibody-associated crescentic glomerulonephritis with rheumatoid arthritis: a comparison of patients without rheumatoid arthritis. Clin Exp Nephrol. 14(4):325-32, 2010
5. Yun YS et al: Fibrillary glomerulonephritis in rheumatoid arthritis. Nephrology (Carlton). 15(2):266-7, 2010
6. Pruzanski W: Renal amyloidosis in rheumatoid arthritis. J Rheumatol. 34(4):889; author reply 889, 2007
7. Stokes MB et al: Development of glomerulonephritis during anti-TNF-alpha therapy for rheumatoid arthritis. Nephrol Dial Transplant. 20(7):1400-6, 2005
8. Bruyn GA et al: Anti-glomerular basement membrane antibody-associated renal failure in a patient with leflunomide-treated rheumatoid arthritis. Arthritis Rheum. 48(4):1164-5, 2003
9. Chevrel G et al: Renal type AA amyloidosis associated with rheumatoid arthritis: a cohort study showing improved survival on treatment with pulse cyclophosphamide. Rheumatology (Oxford). 40(7):821-5, 2001
10. Murakami H et al: Rheumatoid arthritis associated with renal amyloidosis and crescentic glomerulonephritis. Intern Med. 37(1):94-7, 1998
11. Almirall J et al: Penicillamine-induced rapidly progressive glomerulonephritis in a patient with rheumatoid arthritis. Am J Nephrol. 13(4):286-8, 1993
12. Ludwin D et al: Cyclosporin A nephropathy in patients with rheumatoid arthritis. Br J Rheumatol. 32 Suppl 1:60-4, 1993
13. Boers M: Renal disorders in rheumatoid arthritis. Semin Arthritis Rheum. 20(1):57-68, 1990
14. Hall CL: The natural course of gold and penicillamine nephropathy: a longterm study of 54 patients. Adv Exp Med Biol. 252:247-56, 1989
15. Boers M et al: Renal findings in rheumatoid arthritis: clinical aspects of 132 necropsies. Ann Rheum Dis. 46(9):658-63, 1987
16. Honkanen E et al: Membranous glomerulonephritis in rheumatoid arthritis not related to gold or D-penicillamine therapy: a report of four cases and review of the literature. Clin Nephrol. 27(2):87-93, 1987
17. Antonovych TT: Gold nephropathy. Ann Clin Lab Sci. 11(5):386-91, 1981

Therapy-Related Interstitial Nephritis

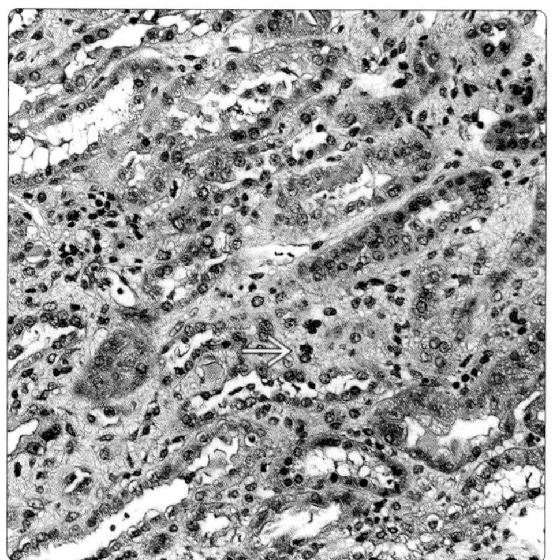

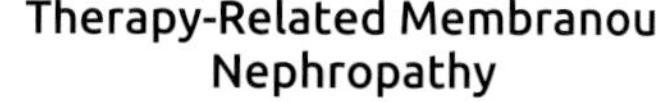

Therapy-Related Membranous Nephropathy

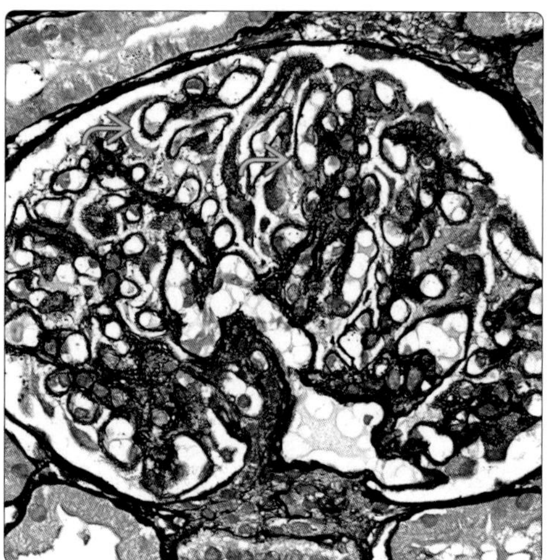

(Left) *Mild interstitial edema is evident in this H&E-stained kidney biopsy in RA with acute renal failure. Sparse interstitial infiltrate of lymphocytes and eosinophils is seen →. The drug history is significant for NSAID use.* **(Right)** *This 65-year-old woman with a 20-year history of RA has been treated with gold, penicillamine, steroids, and methotrexate over the years. The glomerulus shows MGN with thickened GBM with basement membrane "spikes" →, probably related to gold &/or penicillamine therapy (silver stain).*

GBM "Spikes" in Membranous Nephropathy

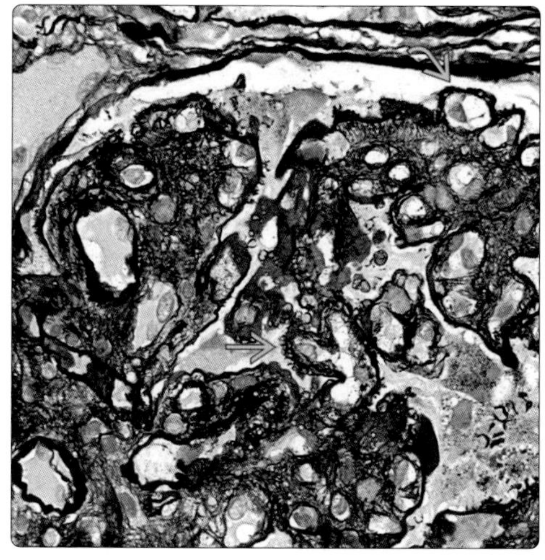

Interstitial Foam Cells

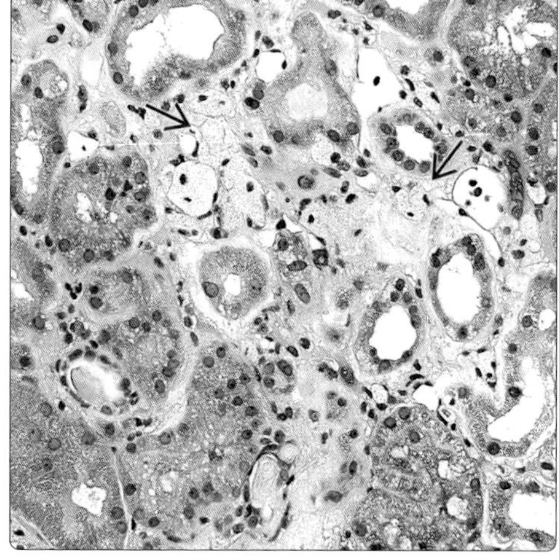

(Left) *The thickened GBMs have "spikes" → and narrow reduplication →. The biopsy is from a patient with membranous nephropathy likely related to gold therapy in the setting of RA.* **(Right)** *Small collections of interstitial foam cells → are seen in the setting of chronic membranous nephropathy. The biopsy is from a patient treated with gold for RA.*

Therapy-Related Membranoproliferative GN

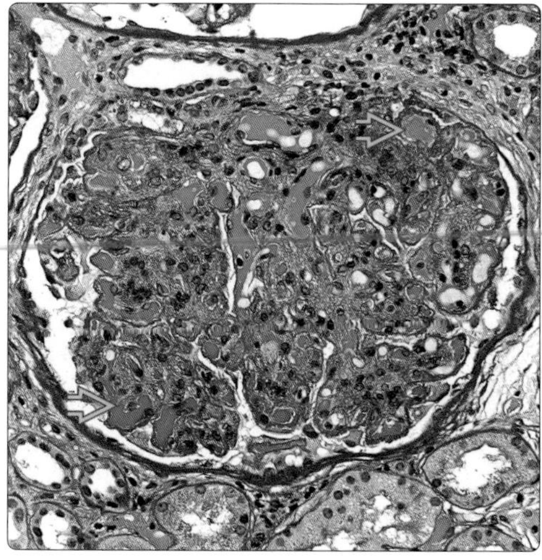

Electron Dense Deposits in Membranoproliferative GN

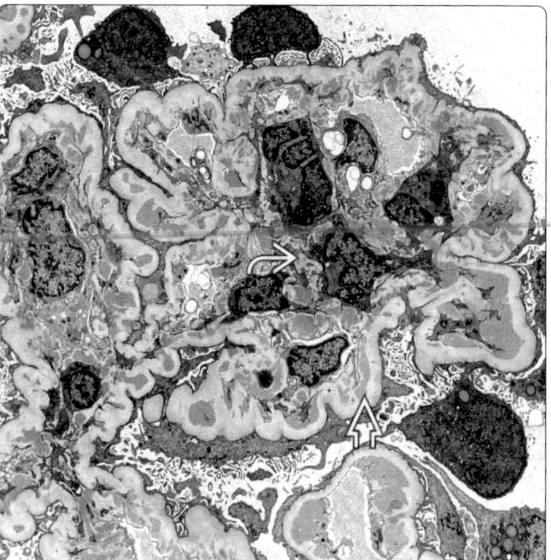

(Left) *Membranoproliferative GN is seen in this RA patient treated with anti-TNF-α. The patient presented with nephrotic syndrome, positive ANA, and anti-ds DNA. Abundant deposits → are seen in capillary lumens, and "full house" staining was evident on IF.* **(Right)** *Mesangial → and subendothelial → electron-dense deposits are seen in a patient with a several-year history of RA and recent treatment with anti-TNF-α. Patient developed lupus-like syndrome, including positive serologies.*

(Left) *Amyloid deposits* ➦ *in the mesangium stain grayish blue on trichrome stain. The patient is a 71-year-old man with a several-year history of RA treated with steroids and methotrexate. The amyloid material is of AA subtype.* (Right) *The Congo red stain highlights the mesangial* ⇨ *and capillary wall* → *amyloid, which was further characterized as AA subtype. The patient presented with nephrotic syndrome, and prior history was significant for RA for many years.*

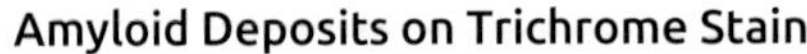

Amyloid Deposits on Trichrome Stain

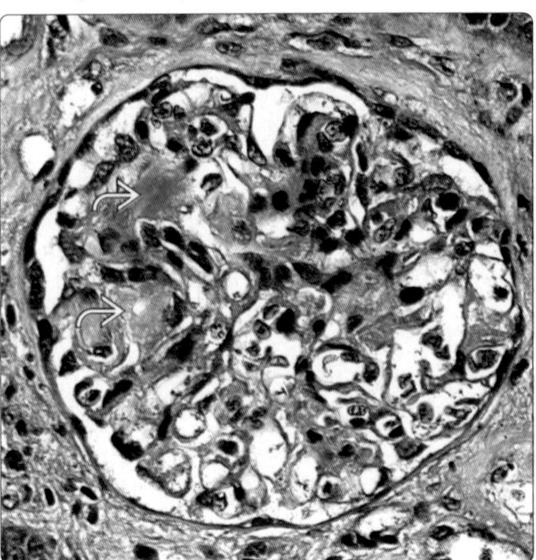

Congo Red(+) Amyloid Deposits

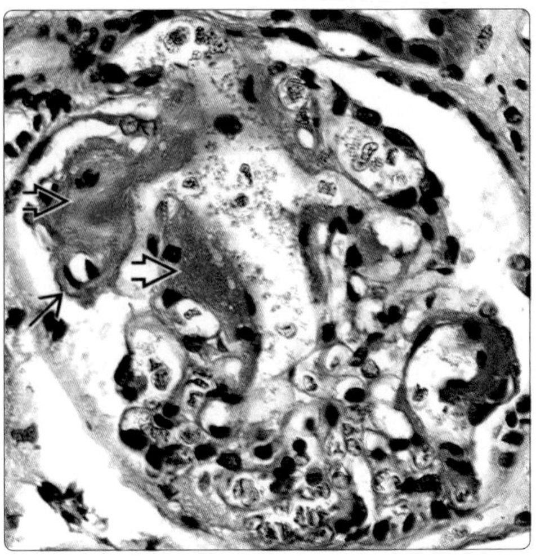

(Left) *Apple-green birefringence* ➦ *is observed on Congo red stain when examined under polarized light. The findings are characteristic of amyloid deposits, which were characterized as AA type in this patient with RA.* (Right) *Antibodies to amyloid A show positive staining* ⇨ *in glomeruli. The biopsy is from a patient with RA who presented with nephrotic syndrome. The prolonged chronic inflammation in RA predisposes to amyloid deposition.*

Amyloid Deposits Under Polarized Light

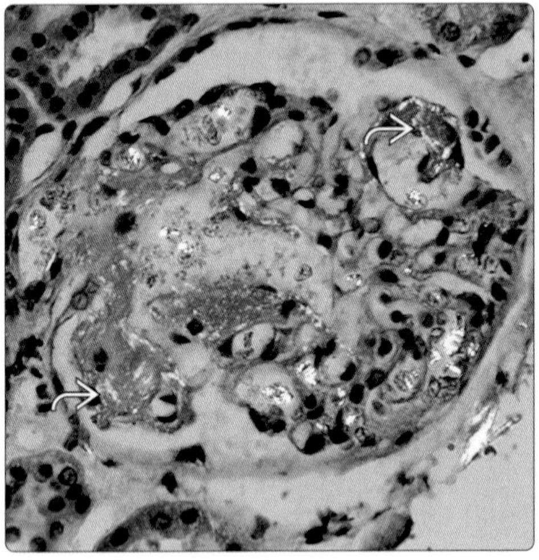

AA Amyloidosis: Immunohistochemistry

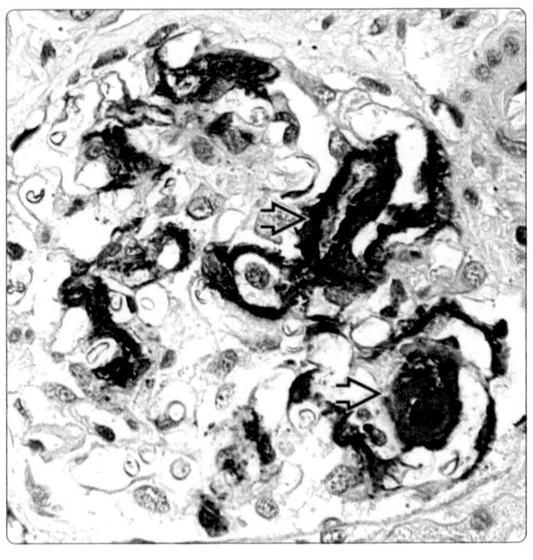

(Left) *On ultrastructural examination, the amyloid deposits in this RA patient are composed of ill-defined electron-dense material in the mesangium* ➦ *and lamina densa of the GBM* ➡. (Right) *On high magnification, the amyloid deposits are composed of randomly oriented fibrils* → *that measure 8-12 nm in thickness. The AA amyloid in this patient with RA is indistinguishable from other forms of amyloid.*

Electron Dense Amyloid Deposits

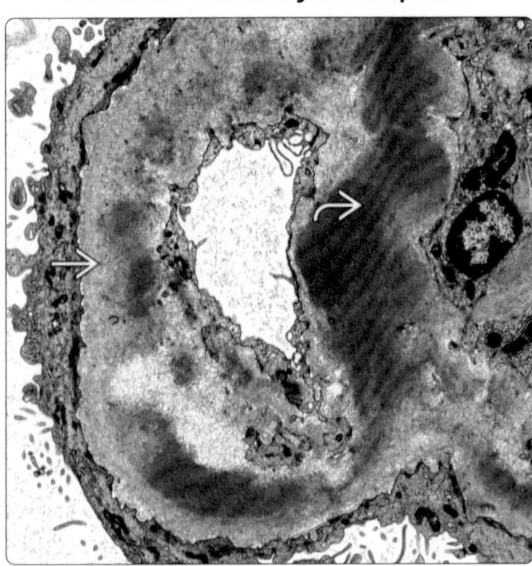

Fibrillar Ultrastructure of Amyloid

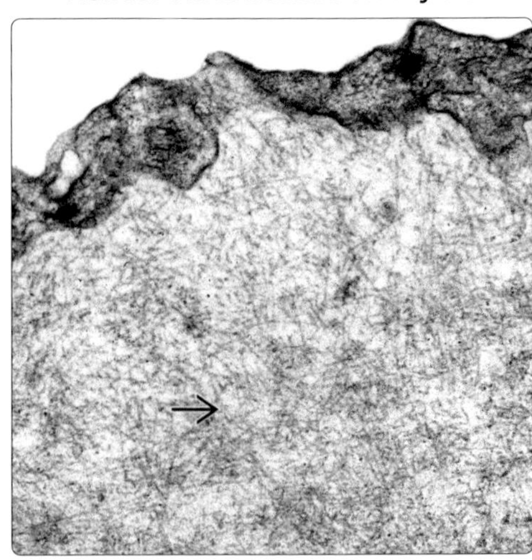

Segmental Mesangial Proliferation in RA

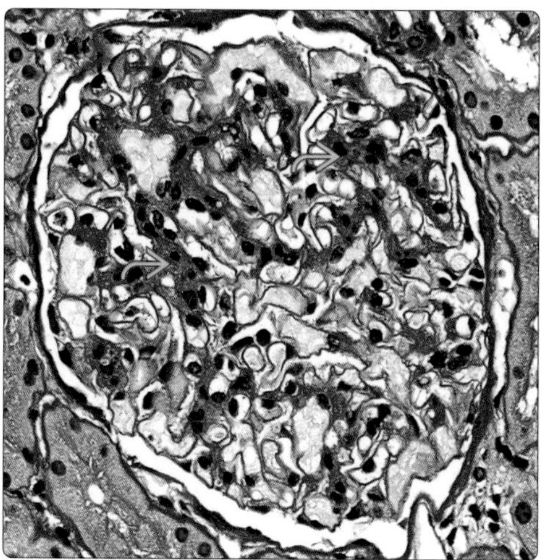

Mesangial Immune Deposits With IgG

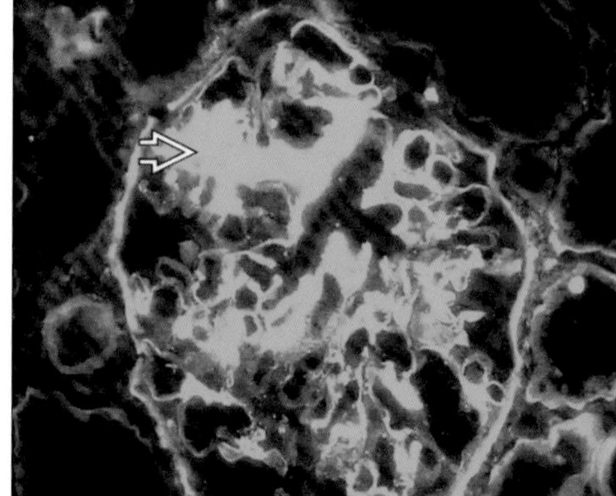

(Left) *The PAS-stained renal biopsy is from a 29-year-old woman with RA, treated with steroids alone. She presented with mild proteinuria and hematuria, normal serum creatinine, ANA positive in low titers, but anti-ds DNA negative. Mild segmental mesangial proliferation is seen* ⇨. **(Right)** *IgG immunofluorescence staining demonstrates mesangial immune complexes* ➡. *The patient has RA treated with steroids alone, and biopsy showed mild segmental mesangial proliferation.*

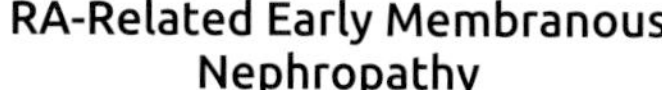

RA-Related Early Membranous Nephropathy

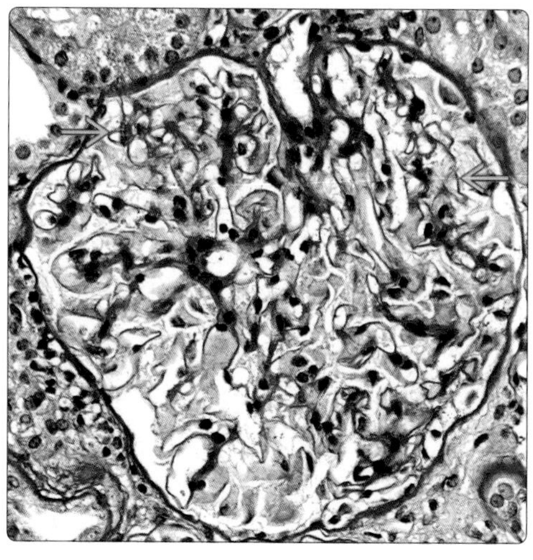

Subepithelial Electron Dense Deposits

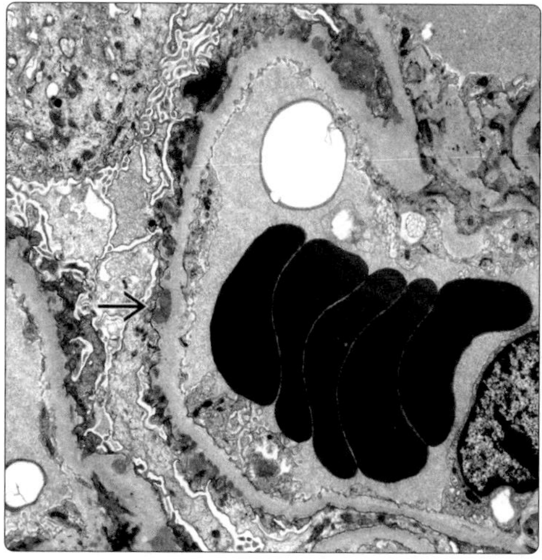

(Left) *A 64-year-old man with RA, treated with methotrexate for several years until 9 months before the biopsy and no treatment with gold or penicillamine, presented with nephrotic syndrome. Biopsy shows minimally thickened GBM* ⇨*, and IF showed diffuse granular capillary wall deposits with IgG and C3, typical of MGN.* **(Right)** *Subepithelial deposits* → *are compatible with MGN in an RA patient. In absence of gold or penicillamine treatment, MGN is probably directly related to RA.*

Glomerular Crescents in RA

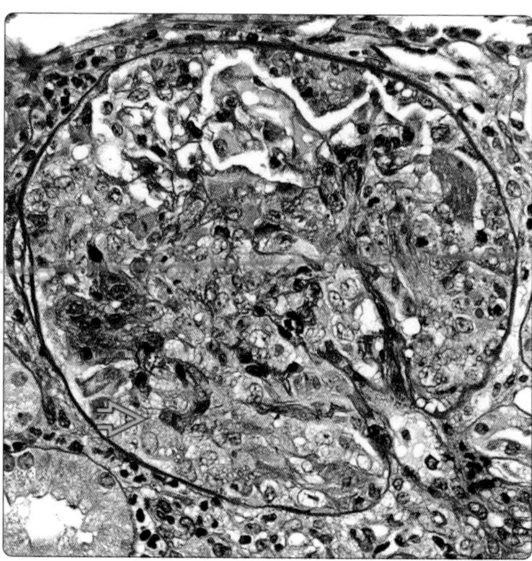

Normal Glomerulus in Pauci-Immune GN

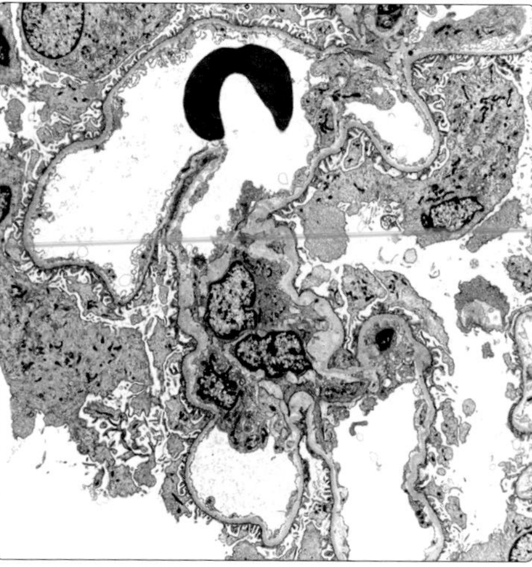

(Left) *ANCA-related glomerular disease is seen in a 51-year-old RA patient with nephrotic proteinuria, hematuria, acute renal failure, and hemoptysis who was p-ANCA positive. Prior therapy was only steroids. The glomerulus shows capillary wall necrosis and a cellular crescent* ⇨*. No immune complexes were identified on IF.* **(Right)** *Normal glomerulus with no deposits in an RA patient with pauci-immune GN is shown. Cellular crescents were seen elsewhere in this patient, who was treated with steroids alone.*

Mixed Cryoglobulinemic Glomerulonephritis

KEY FACTS

TERMINOLOGY

- Immune complex chronic GN and vasculitis due to type II cryoglobulins, typically containing monoclonal IgMκ rheumatoid factor and polyclonal IgG, and most often related to hepatitis C virus (HCV) infection

ETIOLOGY/PATHOGENESIS

- HCV causes ≥ 90% of cases
- Other causes autoimmune diseases, other infections

CLINICAL ISSUES

- Cutaneous purpura, urticaria, weakness, & arthralgias
- Proteinuria &/or hematuria
- Cryoglobulin serum precipitate, typically IgG and IgMκ

MICROSCOPIC

- ~ 85% have diffuse membranoproliferative pattern of glomerular disease
  - Glomerular basement membrane duplication, mesangial proliferation
  - Diffuse intracapillary hypercellularity largely due to monocytes (CD68[+])
  - PAS(+) pseudothrombi in glomerular capillaries in > 50%
  - Crescents in ~15%
- Vasculitis in ~ 20%
- Immunofluorescence
  - Granular GBM and mesangial deposits of IgG, IgM, C3, C1q
  - Pseudothrombi have similar staining (fibrin negative)
  - Kappa > lambda occasionally
- Electron microscopy
  - Microtubular structures 10-25 nm wide, rings 30 nm wide, curved cylinders, and annular structures with spokes ~ 3 nm in diameter

TOP DIFFERENTIAL DIAGNOSES

- Lupus nephritis, idiopathic MPGN, other GNs
- Immunotactoid glomerulopathy
- Thrombotic microangiopathy (TMA)

Glomerular Cryoglobulin Pseudothrombi

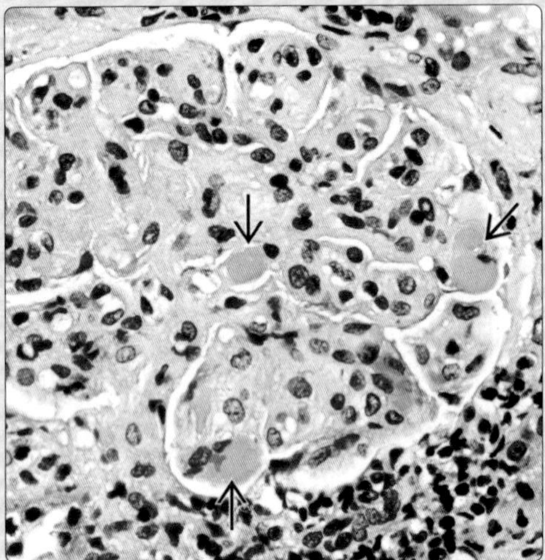

Pseudothrombi and GBM Duplication

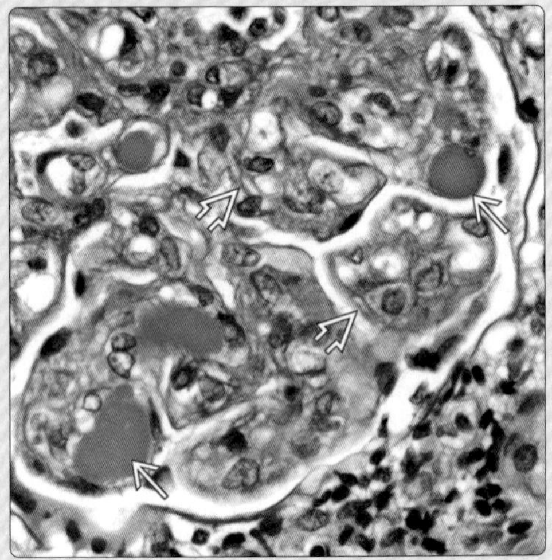

(Left) *H&E stain shows an enlarged glomerulus with pseudothrombi → that are eosinophilic. Fibrin is typically brighter red and less PAS positive.* **(Right)** *High-power view of a PAS stain shows hyaline, refractile pseudothrombi ➡ (also known as PAS-positive "coagulum"), and glomerular basement membrane duplication ➡ in a case of cryoglobulinemic GN.*

Pseudothrombi

Microtubular Ultrastructure

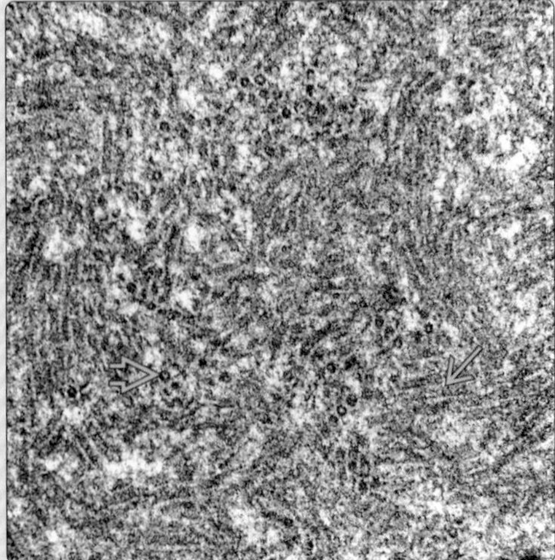

(Left) *This glomerulus from a patient with HCV infection shows prominent rounded structures in capillary loops that stain brightly for IgM ➡. They also stained for IgG, C3, and kappa and lambda. Scattered granular deposits are also along the GBM ➡.* **(Right)** *High-power EM of cryoglobulinemic GN shows curved microtubular structures → and rings →. Without a history of cryoglobulinemia, this might be interpreted as immunotactoid glomerulopathy.*

TERMINOLOGY

Abbreviations

- Cryoglobulinemic glomerulonephritis (CryoGN)

Synonyms

- Originally termed "essential mixed cryoglobulinemia" by Meltzer, McCluskey and colleagues, before HCV was identified

Definitions

- Immune complex chronic GN and vasculitis due to type II cryoglobulins, typically containing monoclonal IgMκ rheumatoid factor and polyclonal IgG, and most often related to hepatitis C virus infection
- Cryoglobulins precipitate at 4° C and redissolve at 37° C
- Type II cryoglobulins consist of a monoclonal Ig and a polyclonal Ig

ETIOLOGY/PATHOGENESIS

Infectious Agents

- ~ 90% due to active hepatitis C virus (HCV) infection (Saadoun 2006 series, 1301/1434)
- ~ 3% hepatitis B virus, HIV, leishmaniasis

Autoimmune Diseases

- ~ 2% SLE, Sjögren syndrome, rheumatoid arthritis

B-Cell Neoplasia

- ~ 2% related to B-cell non-Hodgkin lymphoma

Idiopathic (Essential)

- ~ 2% have no identified cause

B-Cell Proliferation

- Clonal expansion and functional exhaustion of monoclonal marginal zone B cells

CLINICAL ISSUES

Presentation

- Purpura, urticaria, weakness, arthralgias, splenomegaly
- Renal disease in 10-60%
  - ~ 20% have nephrotic-range proteinuria or nephrotic syndrome
  - ~ 25% of patients have acute nephritic syndrome with hypertension, increased serum creatinine, proteinuria, and macroscopic hematuria
  - < 5% of patients develop oliguric or anuric renal failure

Laboratory Tests

- Cryoglobulins reported as a "cryocrit" (% of serum composed of precipitate) or g/L
  - > 0.05 g/L on 2 occasions considered potentially clinically significant
  - Caveats
    - Blood sample must be maintained at 37° C until serum is retrieved
    - Cryoglobulin may take 7 days or more to precipitate
- C4 low in > 90%; C3 decreased in ~ 50%

Treatment

- Drugs
  - Drugs for HCV
    - New oral agents, such as simeprevir and sofosbuvir, are curative
    - Ribavirin, interferon-α used extensively in past
  - Immunosuppression
    - Steroids and cyclophosphamide used with caution because of potential HCV reactivation
    - Rituximab
- Plasmapheresis
  - For relief of acute exacerbation of renal disease
- Transplantation
  - Renal transplantation uncommonly performed because of usual indolent nature
  - May recur in transplant

Prognosis

- 5-year survival ~ 80% for HCV and non-HCV related mixed cryoglobulinemia
  - Deaths primarily from infections, cirrhosis, lymphoma, hepatocellular carcinoma
  - Renal disease is adverse risk factor
- ~ 10% of cases of cryoGN progress to ESRD in 5-10 years
- Early evidence suggests that curing HCV ameliorates cryoGN

MICROSCOPIC

Histologic Features

- Glomeruli
  - ~ 85% have diffuse membranoproliferative pattern (MPGN)
    - Duplication or "tram tracking" of GBM appreciated most readily on PAS or Jones stain
    - Mesangial hypercellularity and increased matrix
    - Diffuse intracapillary hypercellularity with glomerular capillary loop occlusion
      - Leukocytes, particularly monocytes, compose the hypercellularity
      - May be exudative (neutrophils prominent)
    - > 50% have pseudothrombi
      - Eosinophilic, rounded refractile PAS(+) deposits in capillary lumina
      - Known as pseudothrombi since they are not actually composed of fibrin
    - ~ 15% have crescents
  - ~ 8% have mesangial proliferative pattern
    - Global and diffuse slight mesangial matrix expansion; 30% pseudothrombi
  - ~ 8% have focal membranoproliferative pattern
    - Mild and irregular proliferation, exudation, and thickening of capillary wall; 10% pseudothrombi
  - Diffuse MPGN pattern associated with cases having heavy proteinuria and renal failure
- Tubulointerstitium
  - Interstitial fibrosis and tubular atrophy is usually mild/localized
  - Erythrocyte casts in tubular lumina, particularly during acute episodes
- Vessels
  - Vasculitis of small- and medium-sized arteries and arterioles (20-25% of cases)

- Intimal and medial fibrinoid necrosis
- Intraluminal and vessel wall glassy or refractile deposits in arterioles
  - PAS positive as they are in glomerular capillary loops
- Intimal fibrosis eventually replaces areas of fibrinoid necrosis

ANCILLARY TESTS

Immunohistochemistry

- CD68 (KP-1) used to reveal glomerular intracapillary macrophages
  - Express CXCL9, a classical macrophage activation marker
- HCV antigen has been difficult to demonstrate
  - 3 cases reported glomerular deposits that reacted with mouse monoclonal antibody to HCV-NS3 protein (Millipore, Temecula CA)

Immunofluorescence

- Glomeruli
  - Granular IgM and IgG staining in glomerular capillaries in subendothelial location & often in mesangium
  - IgA occasionally (< 5%)
  - Glomerular capillary lumina often with intense IgG and IgM in intraluminal thrombi
  - Kappa sometimes more prominent than lambda, but rarely conspicuous light chain restriction
  - C3 in > 90%, C4d in ~ 33% of cases; C1q common
  - Deposits can be sparse, probably due to macrophage clearance
- Vessels
  - IgG, IgM, C3 in arteriolar walls and intraluminal deposits in arterioles
  - Fibrin may be present

Electron Microscopy

- Organized deposits
  - Microtubular structures 10-25 nm wide, rings 30 nm wide, curved cylinders, and annular structures with spokes ~ 3 nm in diameter
  - Tubular and annular pattern may be present in same case
  - Deposits may also be fibrillar, may show "fingerprinting," or may show crystalloid substructure
  - Usually in subendothelial and intramembranous location and within intraluminal thrombi in glomerular capillaries
    - Subepithelial deposits uncommon
  - Rhomboid, membrane-bound osmiophilic cytoplasmic structures in mesangial and glomerular epithelial cells may be seen, resembling crystalloid structures seen in Fanconi lesion associated with plasma cell dyscrasias
  - Some cases have amorphous electron-dense deposits (i.e., without clear organization)
- Monocyte/macrophages are often associated with deposits, often in subendothelial location interposed between GBM and endothelial lining
  - Monocyte-type cells lead to GBM "reduplication" that is caused by mesangial cells in idiopathic MPGN
  - Neutrophils may be present

DIFFERENTIAL DIAGNOSIS

Idiopathic MPGN

- Cryoglobulinemic GN favored by
  - Large number of monocytes in glomerular capillary tuft
  - Glomerular capillary intraluminal thrombi
  - Vasculitis in small and medium-sized arterioles
  - EM with substructure characteristic of cryoglobulin
  - Positive cryoglobulin assay

Immunotactoid Glomerulopathy

- Microtubular structures in cryoglobulinemic GN are typically shorter and are against amorphous or granular, electron-dense background
- Cases otherwise classified as immunotactoid glomerulopathy are diagnosed as cryoglobulinemic GN if they fulfill clinical or laboratory criteria for cryoglobulinemia

Immune Glomerulonephritis of Other Etiologies

- Cryoglobulins may be present in glomerulonephritis of various forms including
  - Systemic lupus erythematosus, postinfectious GN, Henoch-Schönlein purpura, and others
- Distinguishing clinical and pathologic features of those diseases are usually present, such as characteristic serologic findings

Thrombotic Microangiopathy (TMA)

- Presence of glomerular capillary pseudothrombi raises possibility of TMA
- Ultrastructural demonstration of immune-type deposits helps favor cryoglobulinemic GN

DIAGNOSTIC CHECKLIST

Pathologic Interpretation Pearls

- Though important in diagnosing cryoglobulinemic GN, intraluminal thrombi or pseudothrombi can be very focal and may be missed
- EM shows microtubular &/or annular deposits

SELECTED REFERENCES

1. Cacoub P et al: Cryoglobulinemia Vasculitis. Am J Med. ePub, 2015
2. Cornella SL et al: Persistence of mixed cryoglobulinemia despite cure of hepatitis C with new oral antiviral therapy including direct-acting antiviral sofosbuvir: A case series. Postgrad Med. 1-5, 2015
3. Fabrizi F et al: Hepatitis C virus infection, mixed cryoglobulinemia, and kidney disease. Am J Kidney Dis. 61(4):623-37, 2013
4. Kowalewska J et al: Expression of macrophage markers in cryoglobulinemic glomerulonephritis - a possible role of CXCL9. Adv Med Sci. 58(2):394-400, 2013
5. Visentini M et al: Clonal expansion and functional exhaustion of monoclonal marginal zone B cells in mixed cryoglobulinemia: the yin and yang of HCV-driven lymphoproliferation and autoimmunity. Autoimmun Rev. 12(3):430-5, 2013
6. Bataille S et al: Membranoproliferative glomerulonephritis and mixed cryoglobulinemia after hepatitis C virus infection secondary to glomerular NS3 viral antigen deposits. Am J Nephrol. 35(2):134-40, 2012
7. Tsuboi N et al: Rapidly progressive cryoglobulinemic glomerulonephritis. Clin Exp Nephrol. 14(5):492-5, 2010
8. Roccatello D et al: Multicenter study on hepatitis C virus-related cryoglobulinemic glomerulonephritis. Am J Kidney Dis. 49(1):69-82, 2007
9. Saadoun D et al: Increased risks of lymphoma and death among patients with non-hepatitis C virus-related mixed cryoglobulinemia. Arch Intern Med. 166(19):2101-8, 2006
10. Meltzer M et al: Cryoglobulinemia–a clinical and laboratory study. II. Cryoglobulins with rheumatoid factor activity. Am J Med. 40(6):837-56, 1966

Membranoproliferative Pattern

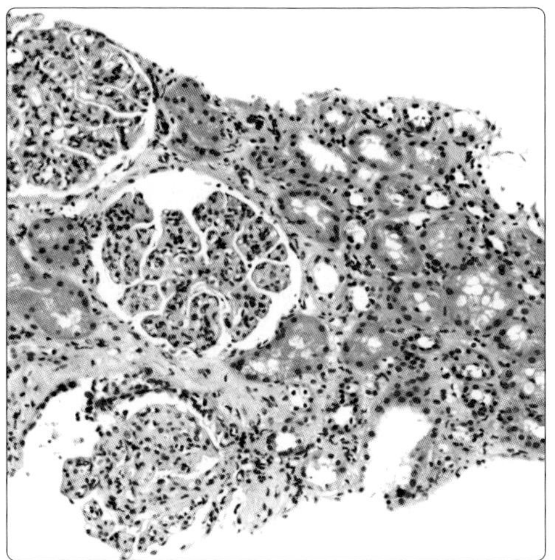

PAS(+) Pseudothrombi

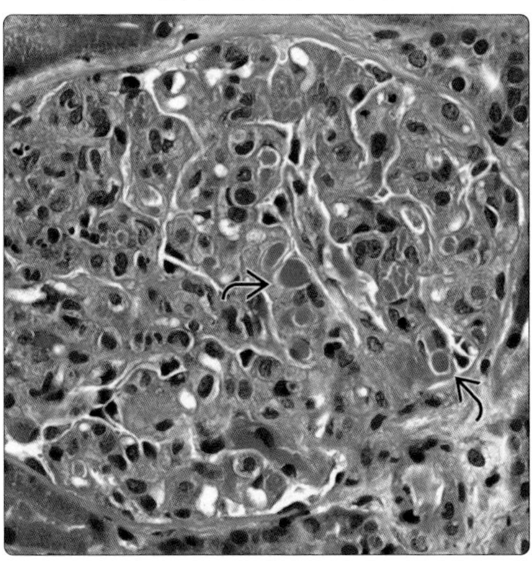

(Left) *Low-power view of an H&E shows lobular hypercellular glomeruli in a case of cryoglobulinemic GN. This pattern can be seen in many diseases, including lupus and membranoproliferative glomerulonephritis.* **(Right)** *Abundant "pseudothrombi" are present in this patient who presented with acute renal failure, low C3, and no skin lesions. Macrophages and neutrophils occlude the capillaries. Her cryocrit was 5%. This case was idiopathic with negative HCV studies, even in the cryoprecipitate.*

Membranoproliferative Pattern

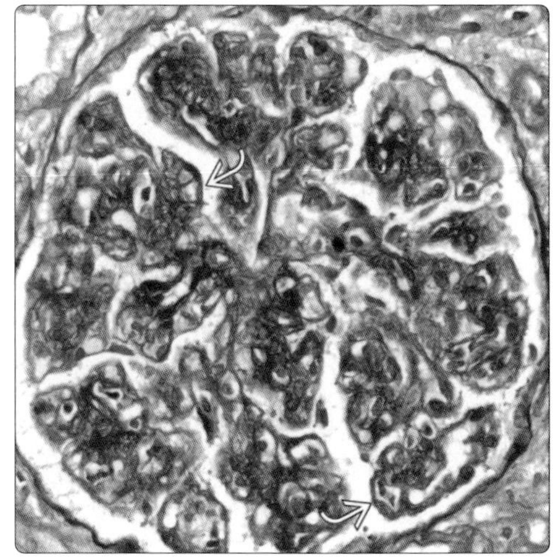

Crescent

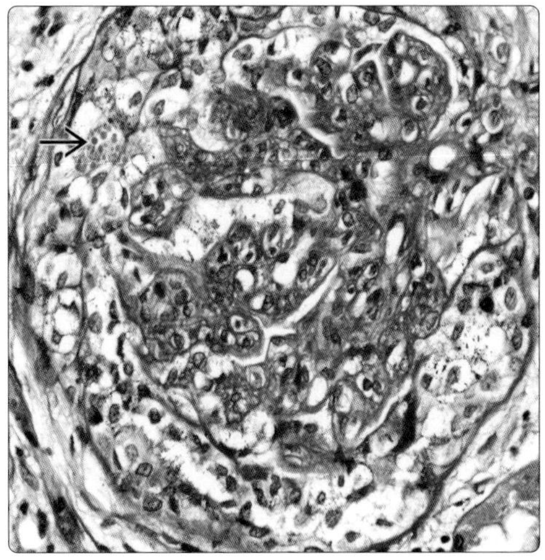

(Left) *Diffuse duplication of the GBM and lobular mesangial hypercellularity are seen in this glomerulus, the most common pattern in mixed cryoglobulinemia.* **(Right)** *A glomerulus is surrounded by a crescent in a case of cryoglobulinemic GN. The differential includes "tubularization"; however, the cells in this case were negative for CD10, which would be expected for a tubularization of Bowman space. Prominent resorption droplets are seen.*

Acute GN Pattern

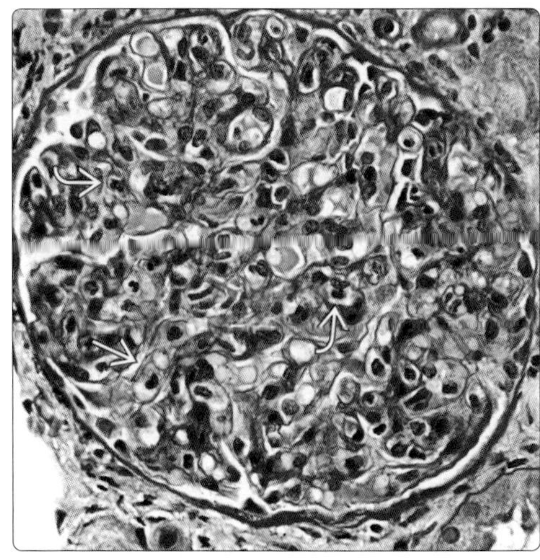

CD68(+) Intracapillary Macrophages

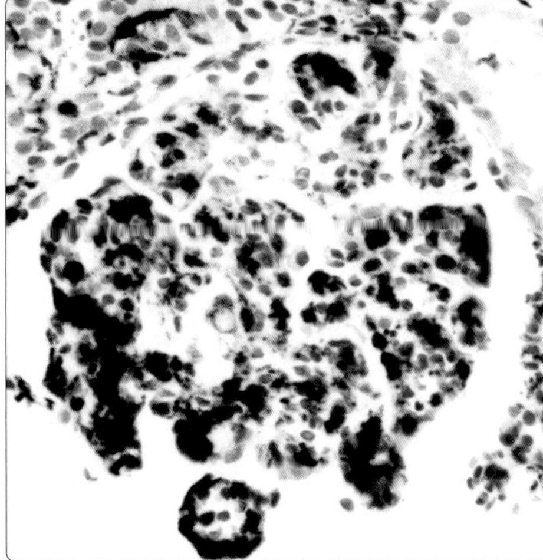

(Left) *This glomerulus from a patient with cryoglobulinemia has an exudative pattern, with neutrophils as well as mononuclear cells in capillary loops and segmental GBM duplication.* **(Right)** *CD68 immunohistochemical stain is positive in many glomerular monocytes/macrophages in this case of cryoglobulinemic GN. This positivity is commonly a prominent and characteristic feature.*

IgG in Pseudothrombi

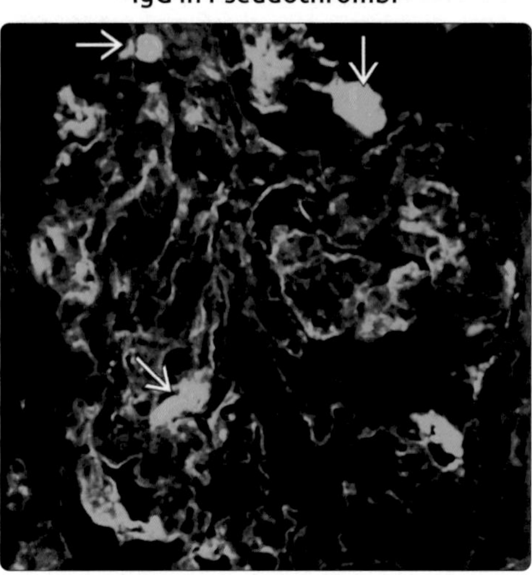

Kappa/Lambda Deposits

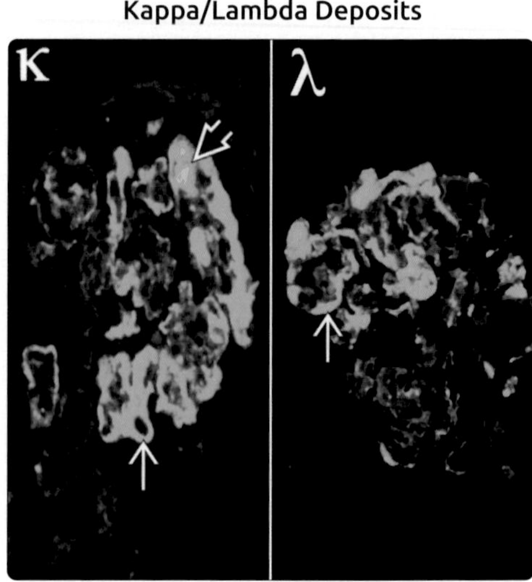

(Left) *IgG immunofluorescence shows patchy staining ➡, particularly within glomerular capillary loops. In mixed cryoglobulinemia, the deposits can be quite sparse, presumably because of degradation by the mononuclear cells.* **(Right)** *Kappa and lambda immunofluorescence show glomerular staining along capillary loops ➡ and in capillary lumens ➡. The deposits are not usually light chain restricted because the IgG is polyclonal.*

C3 Deposits

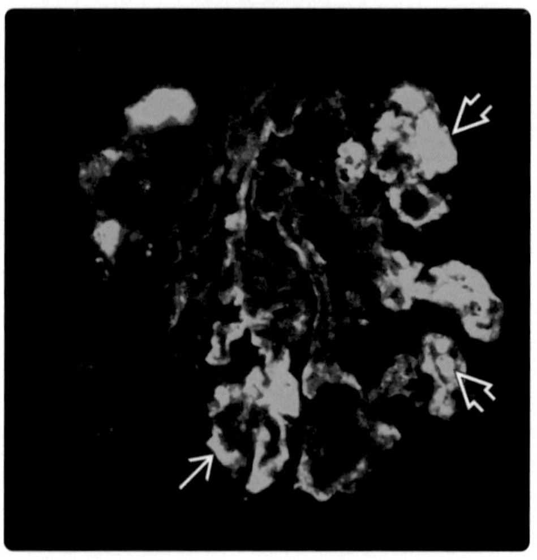

C1q Deposits

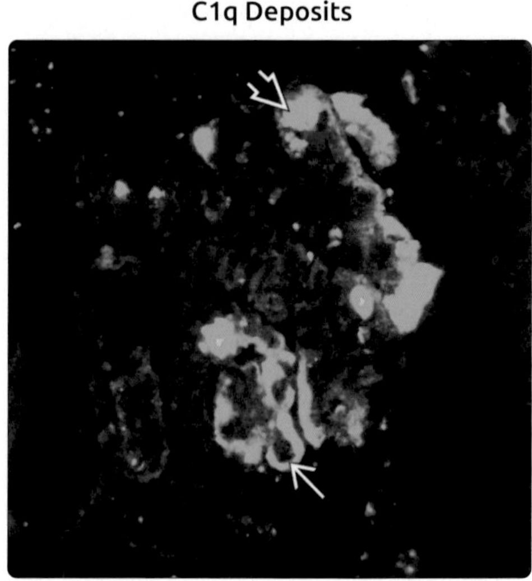

(Left) *C3 immunofluorescence shows staining within glomerular capillary lumina ➡ and along glomerular capillary loops ➡.* **(Right)** *C1q immunofluorescence shows staining along glomerular capillary loops ➡ and within glomerular capillary lumina ➡.*

Cryoglobulinemic Vasculitis

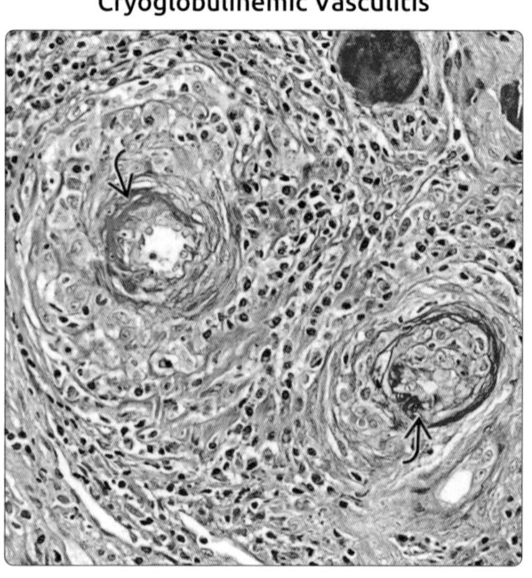

Immune Complexes in Vasculitis

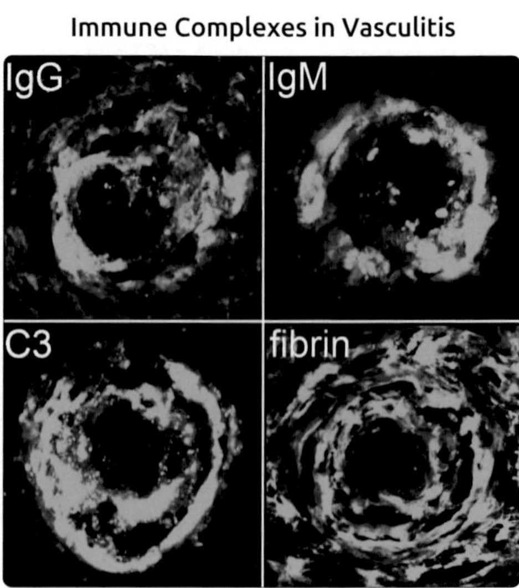

(Left) *Two renal arterioles show vasculitis in this patient with type II cryoglobulinemia associated with Sjögren syndrome. In contrast to other forms of vasculitis, the deposits ➡ in cryoglobulinemia are PAS positive because they are immune complexes rather than fibrin.* **(Right)** *An arteriole stains for the labeled immunoreactant, illustrating that this arteriole contains cryoglobulin. The arteriole is likely involved by vasculitis since it also contains fibrin, making this a "true" thrombus.*

Capillary With Phagocytosed Material in Endothelium

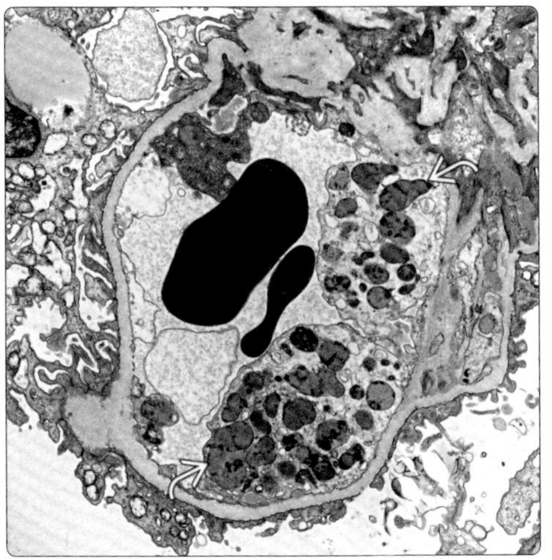

Macrophage With Ingested Cryoproteins

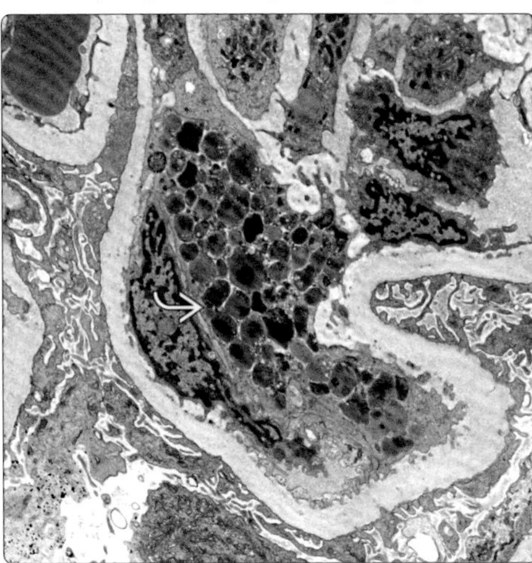

(Left) *This capillary loop has 2 endothelial cells distended with ingested material ➡, probably derived from pseudothrombi. There are no immune complex deposits, which can be sparse in mixed cryoglobulinemia.* **(Right)** *This glomerular capillary is occluded by a macrophage filled with phagocytosed material ➡. This was presumably derived from ingesting complexes.*

GBM Duplication and Pseudothrombus

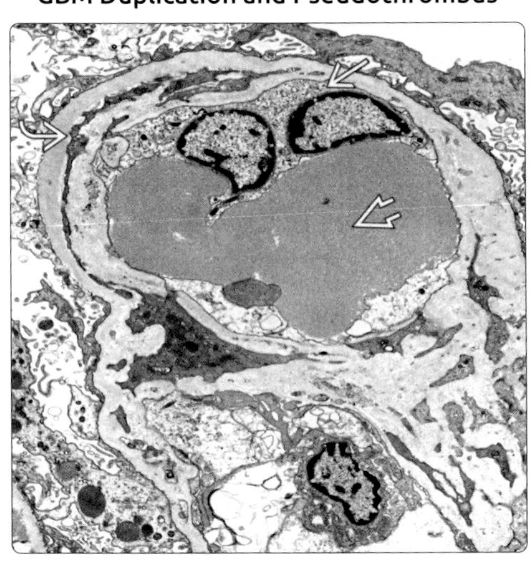

Substructure in Pseudothrombus and Subendothelial Deposits

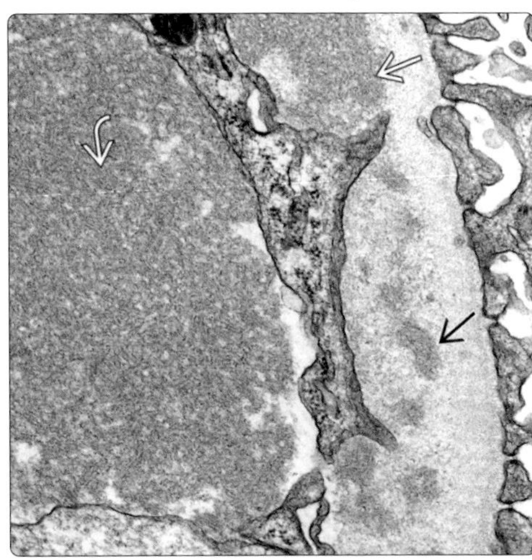

(Left) *The glomerular capillary is occluded by a pseudothrombus ➡ and the GBM is duplicated and has cellular interposition ➡, features that indicate chronicity. The endothelium ➡ is markedly reactive with almost complete loss of fenestrations.* **(Right)** *The pseudothrombus ➡ in the glomerular capillary and a subendothelial deposit ➡ have a tubular substructure typical of cryoglobulins. Intramembranous amorphous deposits are also present ➡.*

GBM Duplication

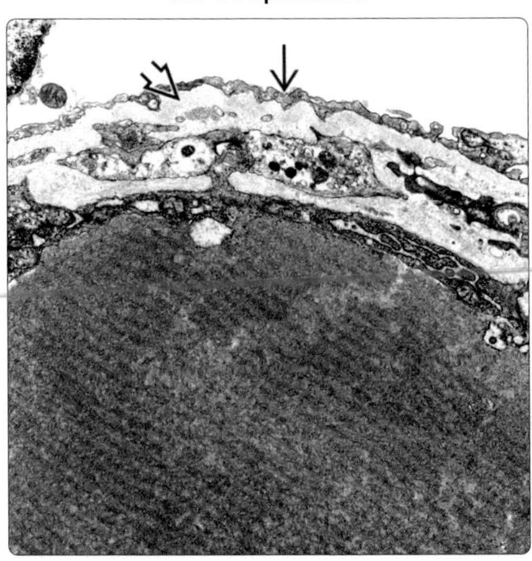

Substructure of Deposits

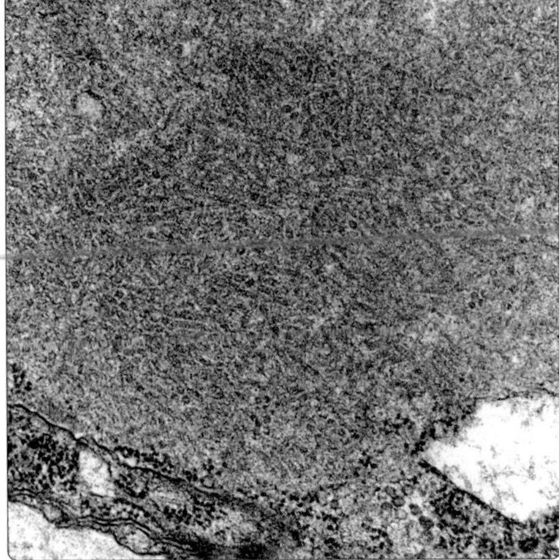

(Left) *The glomerular basement membrane (GBM) is duplicated ➡ in this case of cryoglobulinemic GN, leading to "tram-tracking" or "double contours." There is cellular interposition leading to GBM duplication, typically due to monocytes/macrophages. In addition, podocytes are extensively effaced ➡.* **(Right)** *Higher power of the material in this case of cryoglobulinemic GN shows only a vague fibrillar/microtubular substructure. The appearance and prominence of the fibrils is highly variable.*

Anti-GBM Glomerulonephritis

KEY FACTS

TERMINOLOGY

- Disease caused by autoantibody to glomerular basement membrane collagen, typically manifested by necrotizing, crescentic GN, and sometimes lung hemorrhage

ETIOLOGY/PATHOGENESIS

- Autoantibody targets neoepitope in noncollagenous-1 (NC1) domain of α-3 chain of collagen IV (Goodpasture antigen)
- Risk factors
  - Hydrocarbon exposure &/or cigarette smoking
  - Certain HLA-DR and DQ antigens

CLINICAL ISSUES

- Rare: 1 case per 1 million per year in United States
- Peak incidence in 2nd and 6th decades of age
- Presents with acute kidney injury (> 90%)
- 25-50% pulmonary hemorrhage
- Treatment: Plasmapheresis, immunosuppression
- Rare renal function recovery if ≥ 75% crescents
- Poor prognostic factors include Cr > 5 mg/dL at time of diagnosis and anuria

MICROSCOPIC

- Cellular crescent formation ± segmental fibrinoid necrosis
  - Often involves > 75% of glomeruli
- Linear IgG and C3 staining of GBM
  - IgG4 staining reported in cases with mild or no renal involvement
  - Rare monoclonal IgG, IgA, or IgM staining reported
- EM: Breaks in GBM, but otherwise normal (no deposits)

TOP DIFFERENTIAL DIAGNOSES

- Pauci-immune crescentic glomerulonephritis
- Atypical forms of anti-GBM disease
- Membranous GN and anti-GBM disease

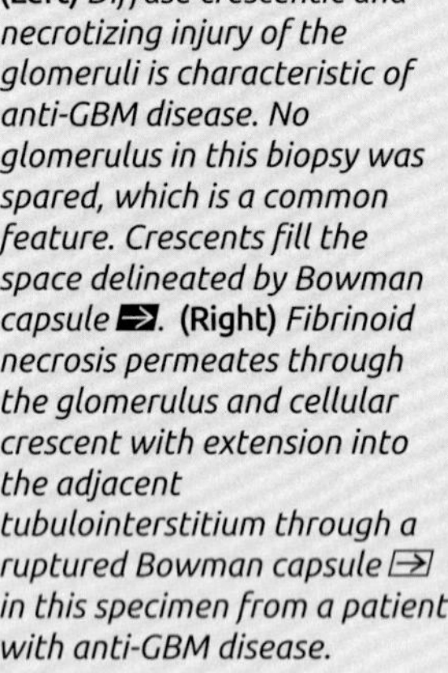

(Left) *Diffuse crescentic and necrotizing injury of the glomeruli is characteristic of anti-GBM disease. No glomerulus in this biopsy was spared, which is a common feature. Crescents fill the space delineated by Bowman capsule.* **(Right)** *Fibrinoid necrosis permeates through the glomerulus and cellular crescent with extension into the adjacent tubulointerstitium through a ruptured Bowman capsule in this specimen from a patient with anti-GBM disease.*

Cellular Crescents

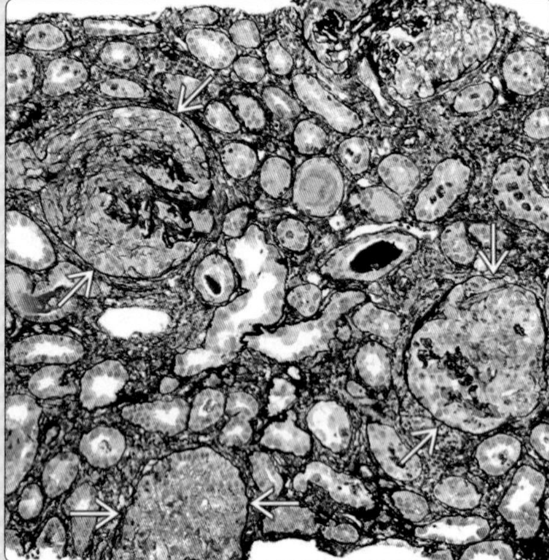

Fibrinoid Necrosis and Crescent Formation

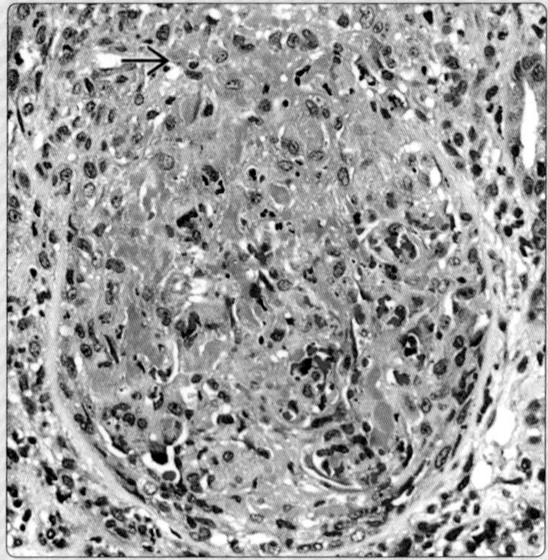

(Left) *Strong linear IgG staining of the GBM is characteristic of anti-GBM disease. The glomerulus has a break in the GBM and is compressed by a crescent, which does not stain. The α-3 chain of type IV collagen is the target antigen in the GBM and is not normally expressed in Bowman capsule.* **(Right)** *Rupture of the GBM is typically found in areas of fibrin extravasation and crescent formation. Deposits are usually inconspicuous or absent, and the GBM is otherwise unremarkable.*

Linear IgG in GBM

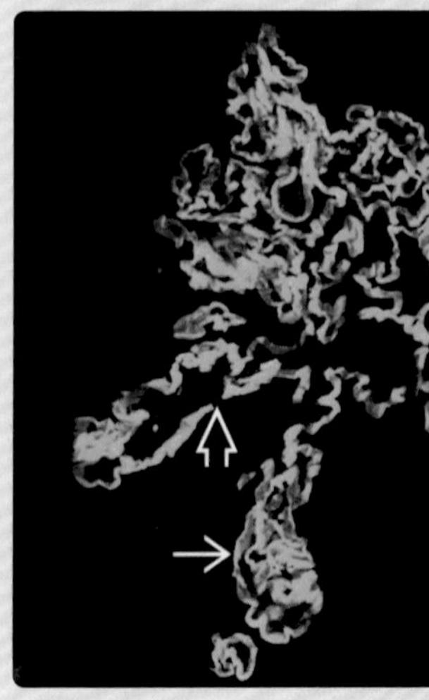

GBM Rupture and Crescent

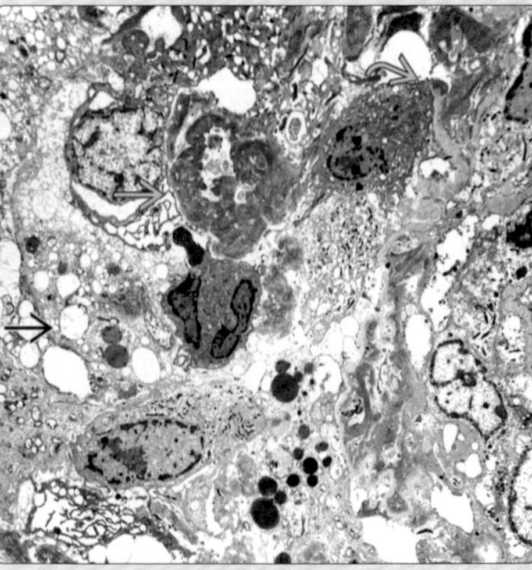

TERMINOLOGY

Abbreviations

- Anti-glomerular basement membrane glomerulonephritis (anti-GBM GN)

Synonyms

- Anti-GBM disease
- Goodpasture syndrome

Definitions

- Disease caused by autoantibody to glomerular basement membrane collagen, typically manifested by necrotizing, crescentic GN, and sometimes lung hemorrhage

ETIOLOGY/PATHOGENESIS

Autoantibody Deposition

- Autoantibody targets noncollagenous-1 (NC1) domain of α-3 chain of collagen IV (Goodpasture antigen)
- Autoantibody targeting noncollagenous-1 (NC1) domain of α-5 chain of collagen IV may also be present
    - Autoantibodies reactive to α-3 NC1 and α-5 NC1 are nonreactive to normal collagen
    - Conformational changes allow formation of neoepitopes for autoantibodies
    - Dissociation of α-3 chain of collagen IV in both kidney and lung increases binding affinity of autoantibodies
- Anti-GBM antibody response is typically transient (2-3 months)

Genetic Predisposition

- Strong association with certain HLA class II antigens: DRB1-1501 and DQB1-0602

Precipitating Events

- Pulmonary injury
    - Hydrocarbon exposure
        - Inhibition of putative enzyme that catalyzes formation of sulfilimine bonds between collagen hexamers
        - May trigger neoepitope formation for Goodpasture autoantibody development
    - Cigarette smoking
        - Increases risk of pulmonary hemorrhage
- Infectious agent postulated
    - Flu-like symptoms prior to onset in some patients
    - Mini-epidemics documented (4-7 cases over a few months)
        - 2005 (April-June): 7 cases in Chicago, IL, USA
        - 2013 (March-April): 4 cases in Seattle, WA, USA
        - Causative agent not identified
- Sequelae of glomerular injury, including ANCA disease, membranous glomerulonephritis
- Exposure to allogeneic GBM antigens
    - 3-5% of Alport syndrome patients develop de novo anti-GBM GN after transplantation
    - Associated with large *COL4A3* deletions

Inflammatory Mediators

- FcγRIII, classic and alternative complement pathway

CLINICAL ISSUES

Epidemiology

- Incidence
    - Rare: 1 case per 1 million per year in United States
- Age
    - Bimodal distribution with peaks in 2nd and 6th decades of age; rare in children < 11 years old
- Sex
    - Male predilection in 2nd decade
        - Pulmonary and renal involvement common
    - Female predilection in 6th decade
        - Crescentic GN without pulmonary involvement common
- Ethnicity
    - Rare in African Americans

Presentation

- Acute kidney injury in > 90%
    - Rare cases with renal sparing
- Hematuria
- Proteinuria
    - Rarely nephrotic range
- Pulmonary hemorrhage (25-50%)
    - Hemoptysis, dyspnea, rales, rhonchi
    - 5-10% lung only involved

Laboratory Tests

- Anti-GBM titer
    - Western blot and ELISA
        - Titers do not correlate with severity
    - IgG1 and IgG3
    - Some female patients have high IgG4 titers associated with pulmonary hemorrhage
        - False-negative immunoassay
- Antineutrophil cytoplasmic antibodies (ANCA)
    - Present in 1/3 of anti-GBM disease patients

Treatment

- Drugs
    - Cyclophosphamide and high-dose corticosteroids
- Plasmapheresis/plasma exchange
- Renal transplantation
    - Recurrence uncommon if negative anti-GBM antibodies

Prognosis

- Poor prognostic factors
    - Dialysis requirement at presentation or Cr > 5 mg/dL
    - Oligoanuria
    - Extensive crescents on biopsy
        - If ≥ 75% crescents, all dialysis dependent by 3 months (15/15) vs. 38% with < 75% crescents (7/12)
- Rarely recurs if anti-GBM alone (no ANCA)

MACROSCOPIC

General Features

- Petechiae on cortical surface ("flea-bitten")
    - Due to blood within tubular lumina or Bowman space
- Normal to slightly enlarged kidneys
- Lung: Airless alveoli filled with red/brown blood diffusely

MICROSCOPIC

Histologic Features

- Glomeruli
  - Cellular crescents ± segmental fibrinoid necrosis
    - Often involves > 75% of glomeruli
    - Rupture or GBM breaks in PAS or silver stains
    - Disruption of Bowman capsule
    - Periglomerular granulomatous inflammation with multinucleated giant cells
      - Not specific for anti-GBM GN
  - Uninvolved glomerular tufts without significant endocapillary or mesangial hypercellularity
    - Neutrophils may be present adjacent to crescents or fibrinoid necrosis
    - Contrasts with immune complex-mediated GN with crescents
  - Thrombotic microangiopathy involving glomerular capillaries
    - Present in subset of anti-GBM GN
  - Atypical, mild forms with lobular mesangial expansion or minimal glomerular lesions and few crescents
- Tubules
  - Red blood cell casts
    - Aggregates of red blood cells in tubular lumina
  - Tubulitis
- Interstitium
  - Interstitial inflammation
    - Consists of lymphocytes, plasma cells, neutrophils, and macrophages
    - More prominent with TBM IgG
    - Prominent eosinophilic infiltrate may suggest Churg-Strauss syndrome
- Vessels
  - Necrotizing vasculitis rare (8%)
    - May be due to presence of ANCA

ANCILLARY TESTS

Immunofluorescence

- Bright linear IgG in GBM (99%)
  - Predominately IgG3 by IHC (Qu); IgG1 and IgG4 by IF (Noël)
- Linear staining with IgM (~ 50%), IgA (~ 10%), C3 (~ 90%) or C1q (~ 20%)
  - Rare strong linear IgA without IgG
- Both light chains, kappa > lambda in ~ 95%
  - Rare light chain restriction with IgG, IgA, or IgM reported
- Linear TBM IgG staining in 10-67%
  - Distal tubules express α-3 chain
  - IgG3 by IHC correlated with increased interstitial inflammation
- Rare IgG4 predominance with mild or no renal involvement
  - May be due to inability of IgG4 to fix complement

Electron Microscopy

- Break or disruption of GBM
- Neutrophils and monocytes in capillary loops
- Fibrin tactoids present where fibrinoid necrosis occurs
- Absence of immune complex deposition
- Crescents contain leukocytes, fibrin, parietal epithelium
- Ultrastructural findings not specific for anti-GBM GN

DIFFERENTIAL DIAGNOSIS

Pauci-Immune Crescentic GN

- Lacks strong linear immunoglobulin deposition in GBM
- Presence of fibrocellular to fibrous crescents favors pauci-immune GN

Membranous GN and Anti-GBM GN

- Anti-GBM disease superimposed upon very small subset of membranous GN patients
- Careful evaluation of immunofluorescence and serologic test for anti-GBM necessary to establish diagnosis

Atypical Forms of Anti-GBM Disease

- Mild forms with lobular glomerular pattern or minimal glomerular lesions
  - Few cases associated with nodular glomerulosclerosis and cigarette smoking
- Some associated with IgG4 anti-GBM antibodies

Monoclonal Immunoglobulin Deposition Disease

- Light chain restricted linear deposits along GBM and TBM
- Cellular crescents rare

Diabetic Nephropathy

- Linear immunofluorescence of GBM for albumin and IgG
  - Segmental sclerosis or collapsed tufts with prominent overlying podocytes **not** to be mistaken as crescents
  - Superimposed pauci-immune crescentic GN observed in small subset of diabetic patients

DIAGNOSTIC CHECKLIST

Pathologic Interpretation Pearls

- Cellular crescents typically involve most glomeruli
  - Extent correlates with serum Cr
  - Rarely recover if ≥ 75% crescents
- Uninvolved glomerular tufts lack endocapillary hypercellularity, in contrast to other forms of GN, except pauci-immune GN
- Anti-GBM autoantibodies may complicate other renal diseases, such as membranous GN, ANCA-related GN

SELECTED REFERENCES

1. Alchi B et al: Predictors of renal and patient outcomes in anti-GBM disease: clinicopathologic analysis of a two-centre cohort. Nephrol Dial Transplant. ePub, 2015
2. Batal I et al: Nodular glomerulosclerosis with anti-glomerular basement membrane-like glomerulonephritis; a distinct pattern of kidney injury observed in smokers. Clin Kidney J. 7(4):361-366, 2014
3. Coley SM et al: Monoclonal IgG1κ anti-glomerular basement membrane disease: a case report. Am J Kidney Dis. ePub, 2014
4. Cui Z et al: Advances in human antiglomerular basement membrane disease. Nat Rev Nephrol. 7(12):697-705, 2011
5. Williamson SR et al: A 25-year experience with pediatric anti-glomerular basement membrane disease. Pediatr Nephrol. 26(1):85-91, 2011
6. Pedchenko V et al: Molecular architecture of the Goodpasture autoantigen in anti-GBM nephritis. N Engl J Med. 363(4):343-54, 2010
7. Yang R et al: The role of HLA-DRB1 alleles on susceptibility of Chinese patients with anti-GBM disease. Clin Immunol. 133(2):245-50, 2009
8. Sethi S et al: Linear anti-glomerular basement membrane IgG but no glomerular disease: Goodpasture's syndrome restricted to the lung. Nephrol Dial Transplant. 22(4):1233-5, 2007
9. Fischer EG et al: Anti-glomerular basement membrane glomerulonephritis: a morphologic study of 80 cases. Am J Clin Pathol. 125(3):445-50, 2006

Petechiae on Surface of Kidney

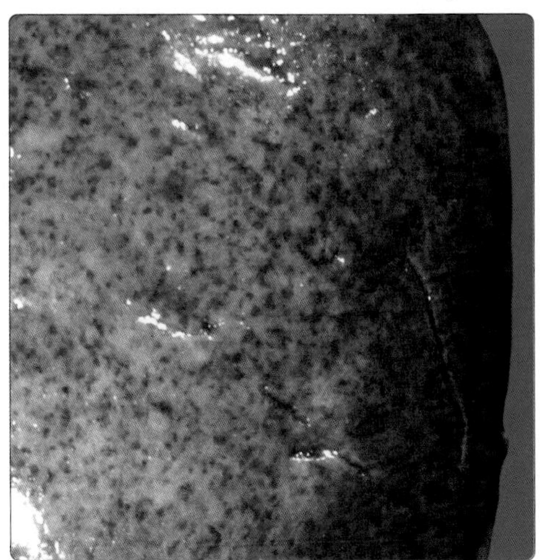

Extensive Cellular Crescents

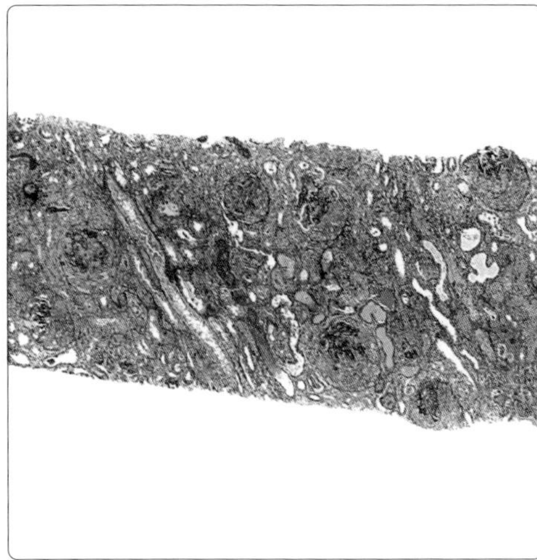

(Left) *In anti-GBM disease, the surface of the kidney has innumerable petechiae, which are the result of extensive foci of blood in tubules and Bowman space.* **(Right)** *Anti-GBM disease typically has extensive crescents. In this patient, 75% of the glomeruli had cellular crescents, all of the same appearance (no fibrocellular or fibrous crescents). This low-power field has 7/7 glomeruli with crescents.*

Cellular Crescents

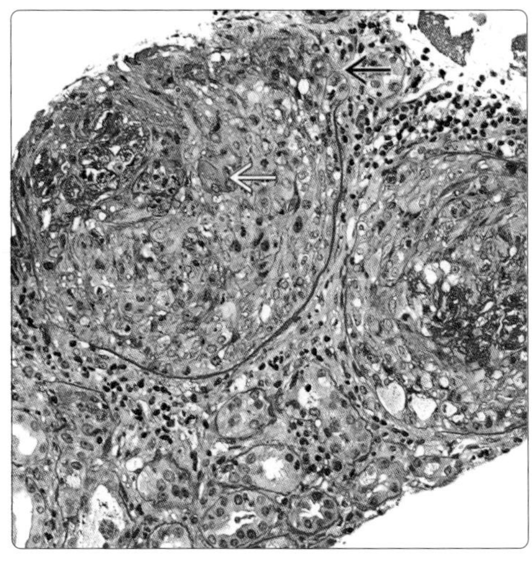

Fragmented GBM and Crescent

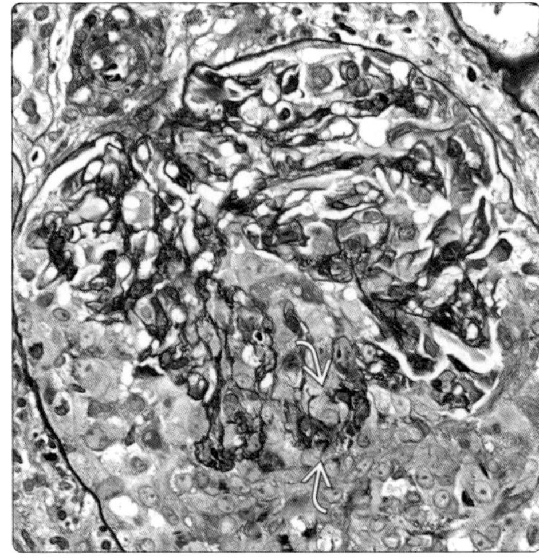

(Left) *Large cellular crescents occupy nearly every glomerulus in a biopsy with anti-GBM disease. Focal fibrinoid necrosis ➔ and disruption of Bowman capsule ➔ are associated with interstitial inflammation.* **(Right)** *The GBM is commonly fragmented ➔ in glomeruli with crescents. This can be seen in PAS or silver-stained sections.*

Cellular Crescent

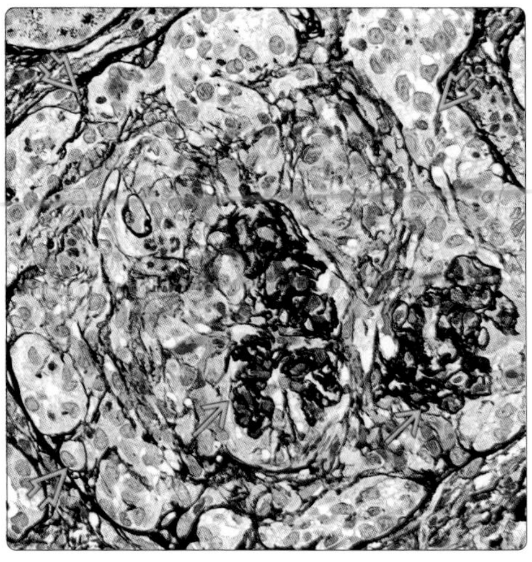

Focal Epithelial Cell Prominence

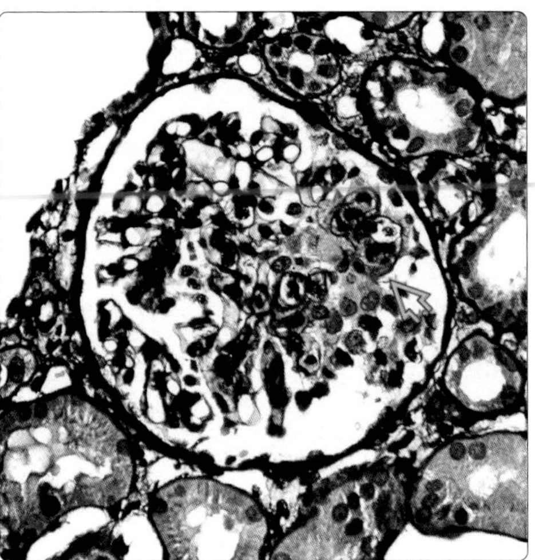

(Left) *Jones silver stain from a patient with anti-GBM glomerulonephritis reveals a few remnants of GBM ➔ surrounded by a cellular crescent ➔ occupying all of Bowman space.* **(Right)** *One of 25 glomeruli in this case of mild anti-GBM GN shows segmental necrosis with prominence of adjacent epithelial cells and rupture of the GBM ➔ (silver stain). A biopsy 2 months previously showed 1 cellular crescent of 18 glomeruli sampled.*

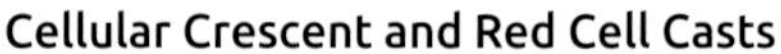

Cellular Crescent and Red Cell Casts

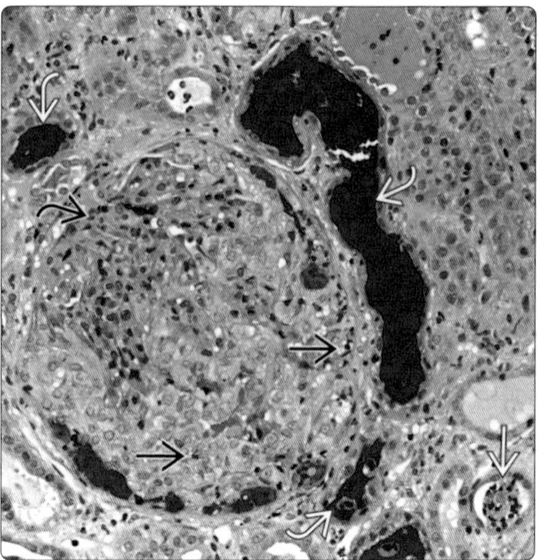

Tubulointerstitial Nephritis

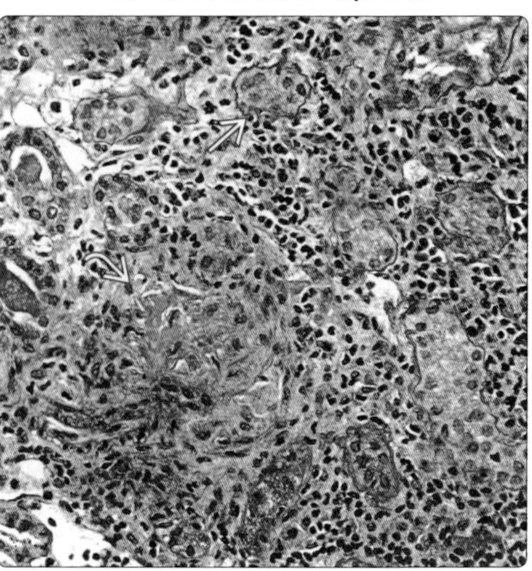

(Left) *Red cell casts* ↪ *are present as well as loose red cells embedded in proteinaceous casts* ➡. *Red cells* ⇨ *can also be seen trapped in the cellular crescent. The glomerulus* ↪ *is compressed and largely bloodless.* **(Right)** *Tubulointerstitial nephritis can be prominent in anti-GBM disease, associated with deposition of IgG along the distal tubular TBM. Tubulitis is present* ➡. *A glomerulus shows loss of Bowman capsule and dissolution of GBM* ↪, *characteristic of severe anti-GBM disease.*

Multinucleated Giant Cell in Urinary Space

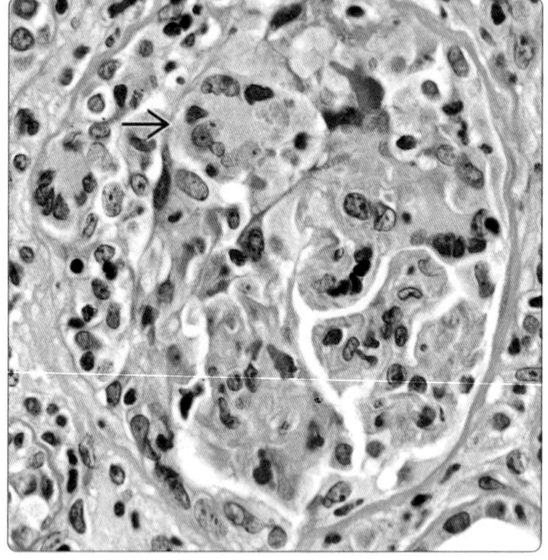

Periglomerular Granulomata

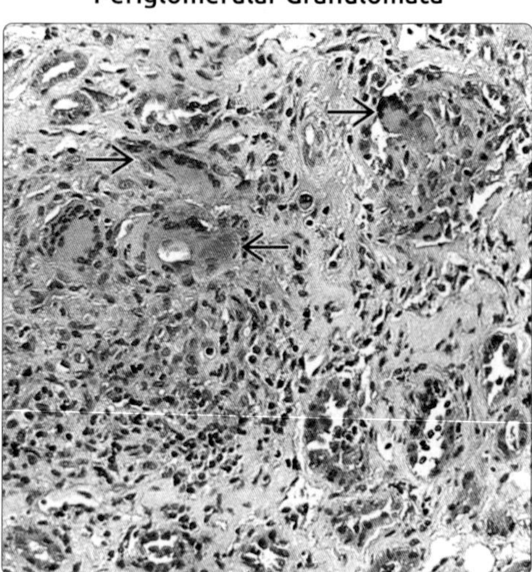

(Left) *Giant cell reaction* ⇨ *within Bowman space is not pathognomic for anti-GBM disease, but it is rarely observed in other causes of crescentic GN.* **(Right)** *Isolated interstitial granulomata that are not associated with crescentic or necrotizing GN are a suggestive feature of Wegener granulomatosis, but these multinucleated giant cells* ⇨ *are within and adjacent to glomeruli from anti-GBM GN.*

CD68

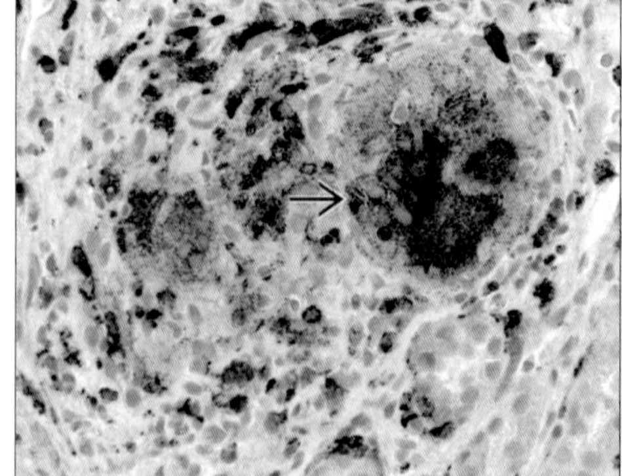

Normal Glomerulus

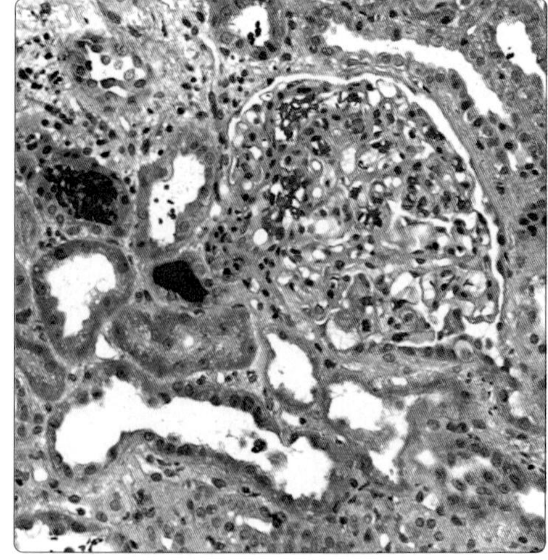

(Left) *CD68 immunohistochemistry confirms that the multinucleated giant cells* ⇨ *consist of macrophages, and many scattered macrophages are also present throughout the glomerular crescent as well as the adjacent tubules and interstitium.* **(Right)** *Occasional histologically normal glomeruli are present in anti-GBM disease, despite deposition of anti-GBM antibodies in all glomeruli, which argues that an additional component is needed to trigger the glomerular damage.*

Linear IgG Deposition and GBM Fragmentation

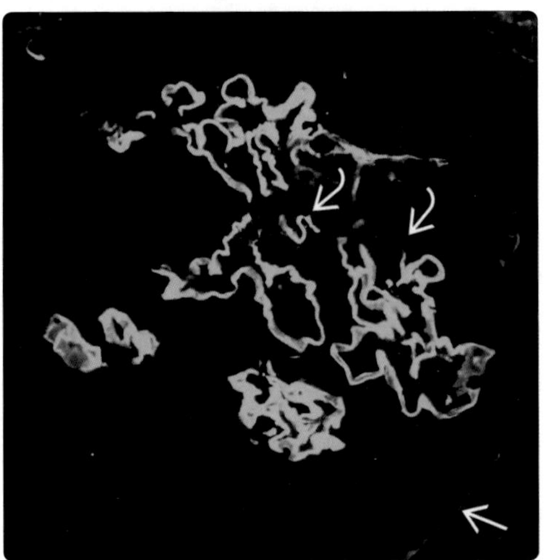

Linear Staining for IgG Greater Than Albumin

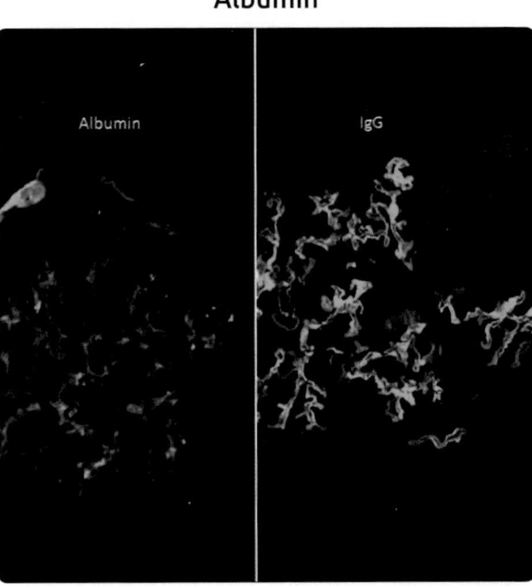

(Left) *Diffuse, bright, linear staining of the GBM for IgG is characteristic of anti-GBM disease. The fragmentation of the GBM is evident ➡ in this glomerulus surrounded by a cellular crescent, which fills the space between the glomerulus and Bowman capsule ➡ (both negative).* **(Right)** *Linear staining for IgG is the principal defining IF feature of anti-GBM disease. In contrast to diabetic glomerulopathy, IgG staining of the GBM is of greater intensity than albumin.*

Linear TBM Staining

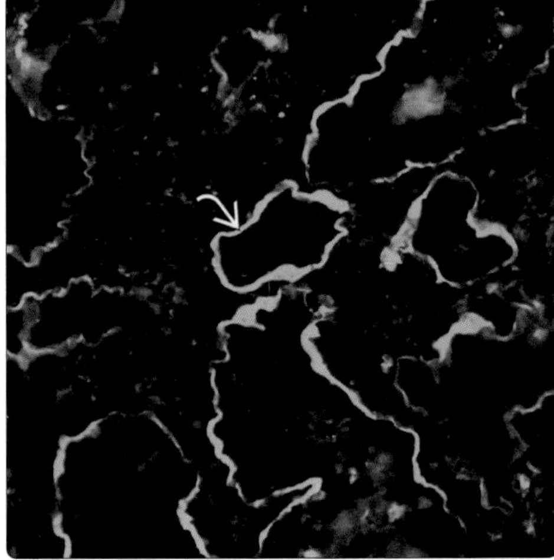

C3 Deposition

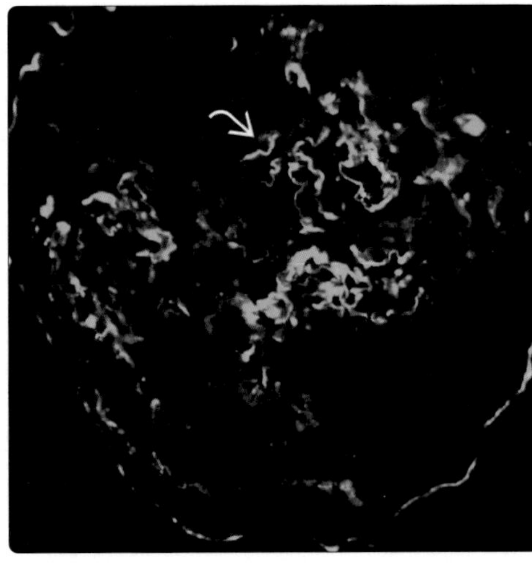

(Left) *Linear IgG staining of distal tubule basement membranes ➡ is present in 10-67% of anti-GBM GN cases. The a-3 chain is normally present in distal tubule TBM but is probably less accessible than the GBM to circulating autoantibodies. Tubulointerstitial nephritis may be the consequence of this deposition.* **(Right)** *C3 deposits are typically not as extensive as IgG in anti-GBM disease, although segmental linear staining of the GBM ➡ can be seen, here probably due to disruption and destruction of the GBM.*

Fibrinogen

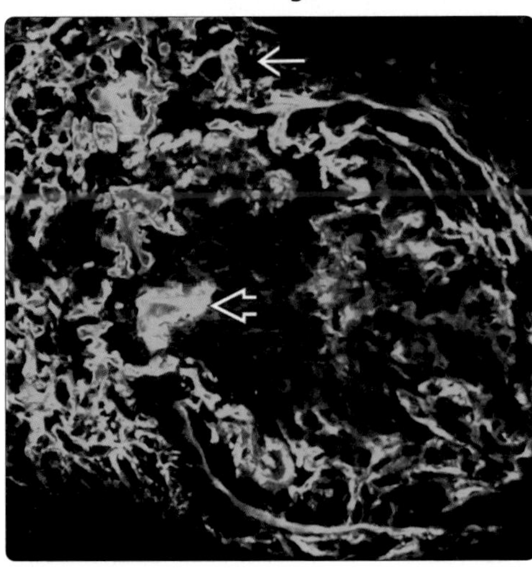

IgG4

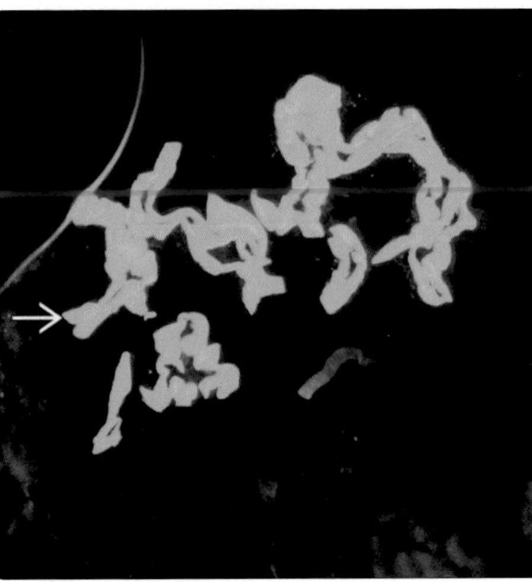

(Left) *Fibrinoid necrosis is highlighted by strong fibrinogen staining ➡ in the crescent that has extended beyond Bowman capsule ➡ in this glomerulus. Fibrin is usually conspicuous in cellular crescents regardless of etiology.* **(Right)** *Occasional anti-GBM cases show bright linear GBM ➡ staining for IgG4 and have a milder course. IgG4, in contrast to IgG1 and IgG3, does not fix complement or bind to Fc receptors and may account for the milder disease phenotype.*

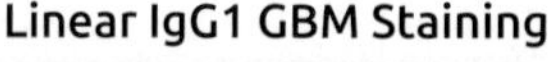

Linear IgG1 GBM Staining

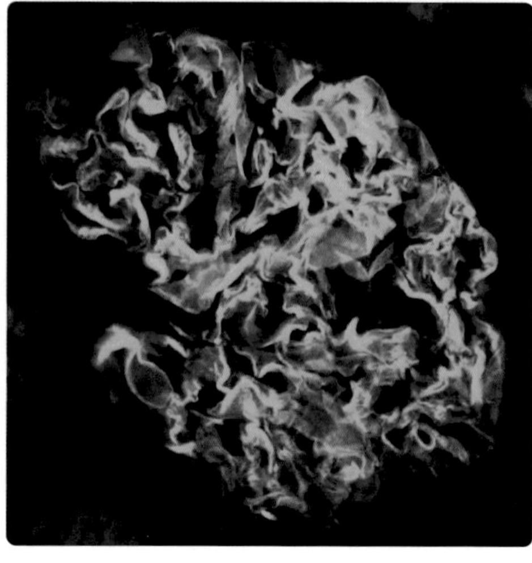

Granular and Linear IgG Deposition

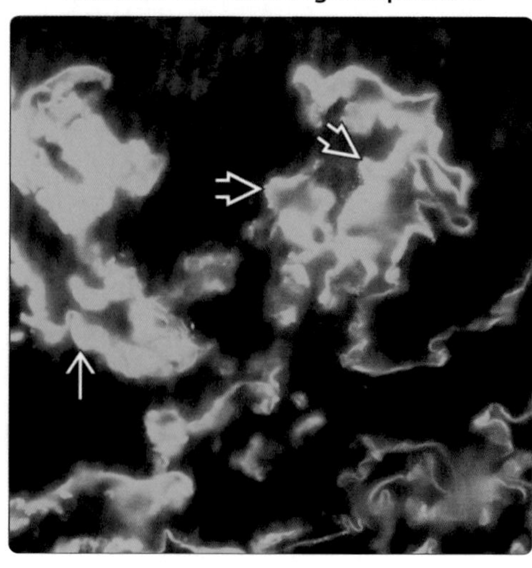

(Left) *IgG1 typically shows strong linear staining of the GBM in a young male patient with anti-GBM disease and no significant renal injury, but extensive pulmonary hemorrhage resulted in the death of this adolescent male.* **(Right)** *IgG immunofluorescence staining demonstrates both granular ➡ capillary wall staining, which indicates membranous GN, and linear staining of the GBM ➡ in this rare patient with concurrent anti-GBM GN. (Courtesy M. Troxell, MD, PhD.)*

Neutrophils and Fibrin Tactoids

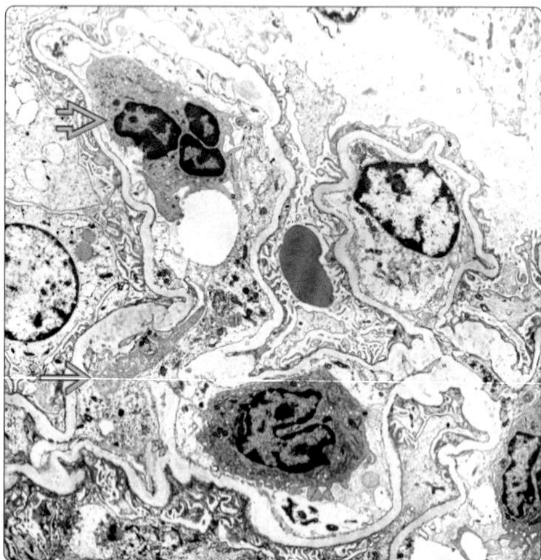

Intracapillary Neutrophil

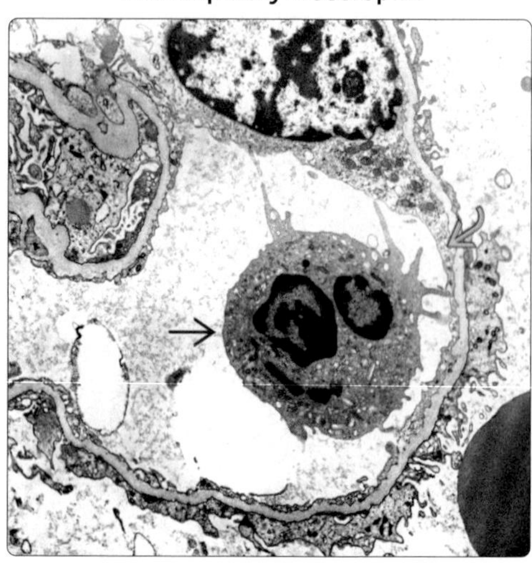

(Left) *Fibrin tactoids ➡ and neutrophils ➡ are present in glomerular capillaries in anti-GBM disease. No immune complexes are present, and some glomeruli may lack any pathologic abnormalities. EM corroborates light microscopic features, but there are no unique findings in anti-GBM disease.* **(Right)** *A neutrophil ➡ in a glomerular capillary in a case of anti-GBM disease is associated with endothelium that shows signs of an injury response in the form of expanded cytoplasm and loss of fenestrations ➡. The GBM appears normal.*

Fragmentation of GBM

Fibrin Deposition in Bowman Space

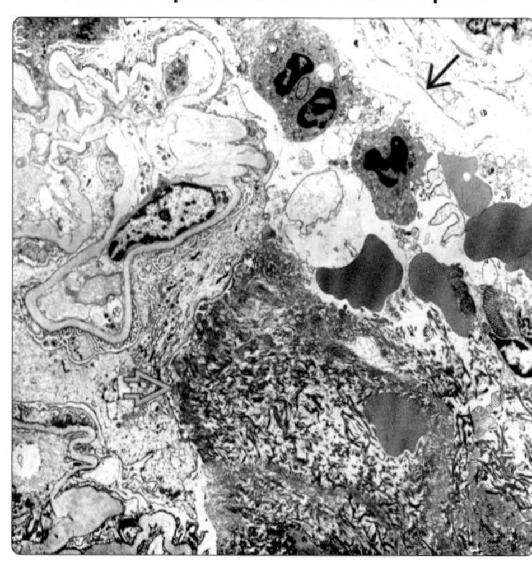

(Left) *The GBM should be 1 continuous structure, but focal rupture of the GBM is present ➡, a feature associated with crescent formation regardless of diagnosis.* **(Right)** *Fibrin ➡ has spilled into the urinary space with neutrophils in this glomerulus from a patient with anti-GBM GN. A segment of Bowman capsule ➡ is present. Crescents are formed in response to coagulation activation and fibrin deposition in the urinary space.*

Glomerular Destruction

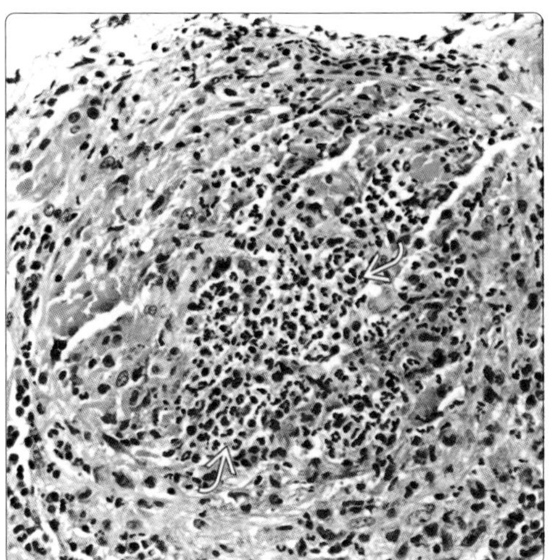

Pulmonary Hemorrhage

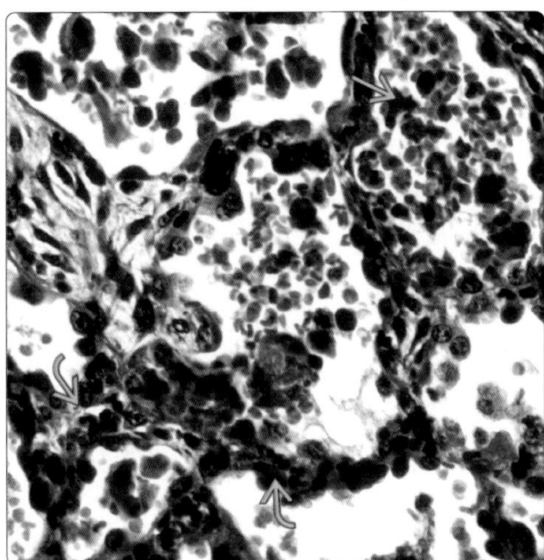

(Left) *Extreme and rapid destruction of the glomerular tuft can occur in anti-GBM disease as shown here in a biopsy from a 63-year-old woman whose Cr was 0.9 13 days previously. Bowman space is filled with neutrophils and no glomerular tuft is recognizable.* **(Right)** *Pulmonary hemorrhage is detected in about 25-50% of patients with anti-GBM disease, associated with a smoking history. Histologic changes are blood-filling alveolar spaces and focal capillaritis .*

Differential Diagnosis: Pauci-Immune GN

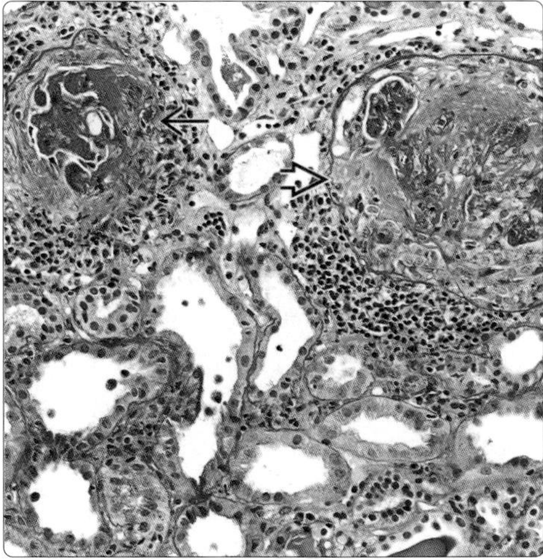

Differential Diagnosis: Vasculitis

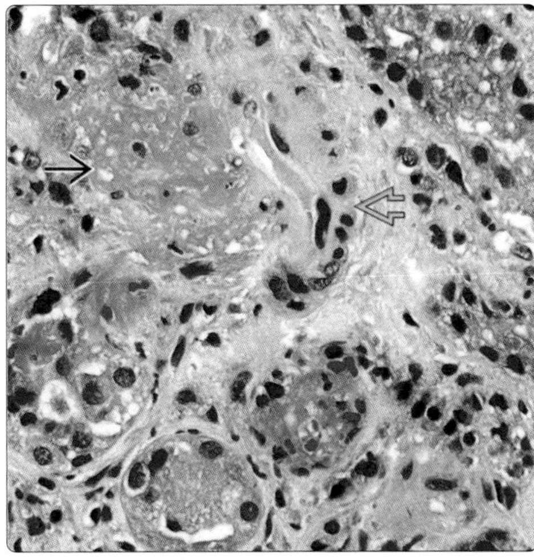

(Left) *Crescents in various temporal stages are characteristic of pauci-immune crescentic GN, such as this fibrous and fibrocellular crescent, but immunofluorescence is the definitive way to distinguish it from anti-GBM GN.* **(Right)** *Fibrinoid necrosis is present in an arteriole . This patient had anti-GBM and anti-myeloperoxidase antibodies (ANCA). ANCA is probably the cause of the necrotizing vasculitis, since pure anti-GBM disease does not typically have vasculitis.*

Differential Diagnosis: Diabetic Glomerulopathy

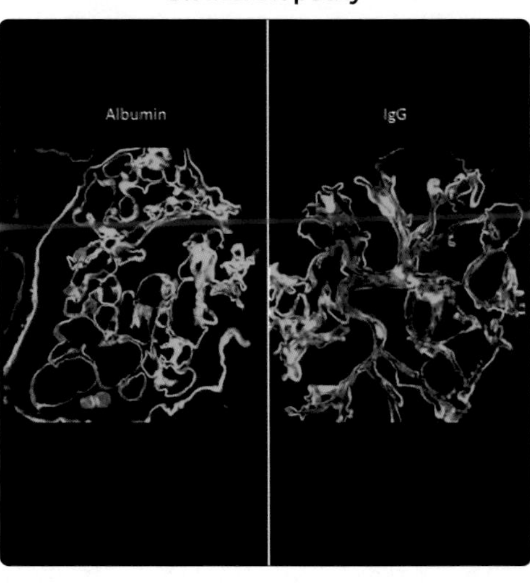

Differential Diagnosis: Monoclonal Immunoglobulin Deposition Disease

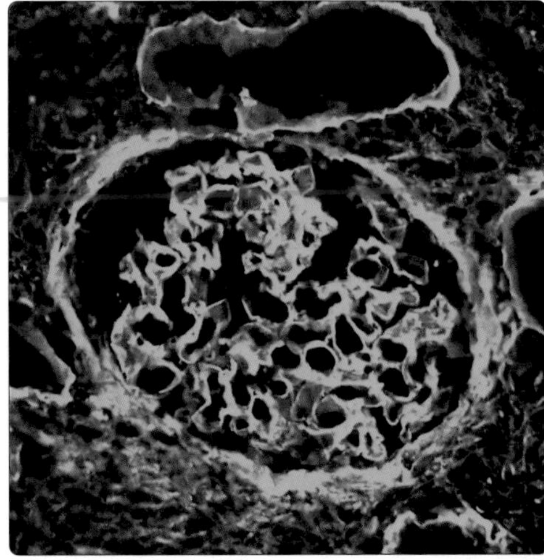

(Left) *In diabetic glomerulopathy, linear staining of the GBM and TBM for IgG is usually prominent. In contrast to anti-GBM disease, however, the GBM and TBM stain equally brightly for albumin. Thickened basement membranes and abnormal glycosylation are probably responsible.* **(Right)** *Confluent IgG staining of the glomerular and tubular basement membranes in this case of monoclonal immunoglobulin deposition disease mimics anti-GBM disease, but monoclonal lambda light chain staining was present.*

Atypical Anti-GBM Nephritis

KEY FACTS

TERMINOLOGY

- Linear glomerular basement membrane (GBM) staining for immunoglobulins and different histologic appearance from typical anti-GBM disease

ETIOLOGY/PATHOGENESIS

- Presumably disease caused by circulating pathogenic immunoglobulin that recognizes different GBM epitope than anti-GBM disease

CLINICAL ISSUES

- Hematuria (gross or microscopic)
- Proteinuria
- Nephrotic syndrome
- Renal insufficiency (generally mild)
- Absence of pulmonary hemorrhage
- Better outcome compared to classic anti-GBM disease

MICROSCOPIC

- Proliferative glomerulonephritis
- Nodular glomerulosclerosis
- Glomerular microangiopathy
- Features may overlap

ANCILLARY TESTS

- Linear GBM staining for immunoglobulin heavy chain (usually IgG) and light chain(s)
  - Approximately 50% of cases show light chain restriction by immunofluorescence (IF)
- Undetectable anti-GBM antibodies by commercially available ELISA

TOP DIFFERENTIAL DIAGNOSES

- Classic anti-GBM disease
- Light and heavy chain deposition disease
- Nodular diabetic glomerulosclerosis
- Idiopathic nodular glomerulopathy

(Left) *This biopsy shows a pattern of diffuse mesangial and endocapillary proliferative glomerulonephritis. By immunofluorescence, there was bright linear GBM staining for monotypic IgG lambda; electron microscopy did not show deposits.* **(Right)** *Endocapillary hypercellularity ⇒ is noted in this example of atypical anti-GBM nephritis. Glomerular basement membrane duplication ⇒ is also present.*

Proliferative Glomerulonephritis Pattern

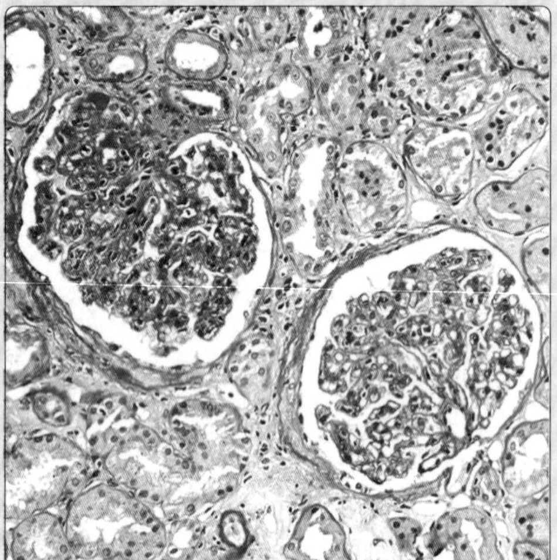

Proliferative Glomerulonephritis Pattern

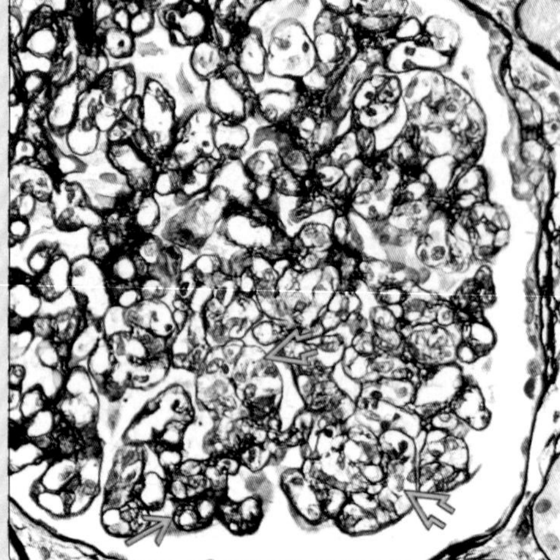

(Left) *By EM, this example of atypical anti-GBM nephritis shows subendothelial lucency ⇒ and early GBM duplication.* **(Right)** *In this example of atypical anti-GBM nephritis, there was focal and segmental necrosis of the glomerular tuft with GBM disruption ⇒.*

Microangiopathy in Atypical Anti-GBM Nephritis

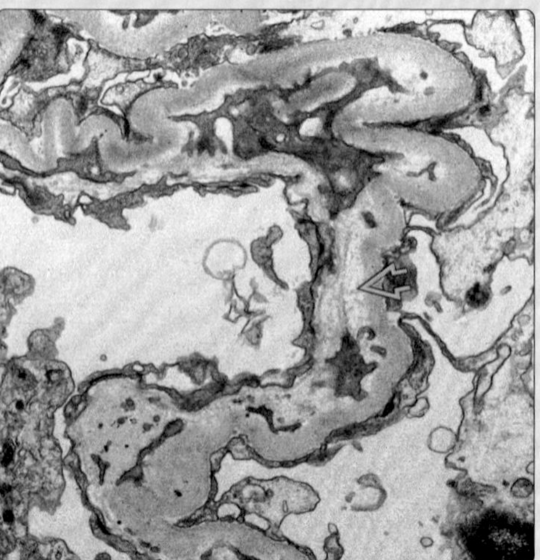

Segmental Necrosis

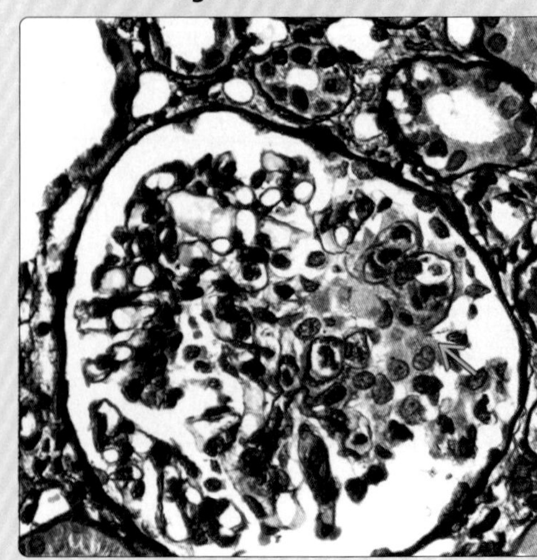

TERMINOLOGY

Abbreviations

- Anti-glomerular basement membrane (anti-GBM)

Definitions

- Linear glomerular basement membrane (GBM) staining for immunoglobulins
  - Different histologic appearance than typical anti-GBM disease

ETIOLOGY/PATHOGENESIS

Unknown Etiology

- Linear GBM staining for heavy and light chain(s) but negative anti-GBM assay by ELISA
- Presumably caused by circulating immunoglobulins that recognize different GBM epitopes than classic anti-GBM disease
  - Causative immunoglobulin may be polyclonal or monoclonal
  - Different antigen target may result in different histologic patterns and different disease course

CLINICAL ISSUES

Presentation

- Hematuria (gross or microscopic)
- Proteinuria
- Nephrotic syndrome
- Renal insufficiency (generally mild)
- Absence of pulmonary hemorrhage

Prognosis

- Better outcome than classic anti-GBM disease
  - 1-year renal survival: 85%
  - 1-year patient survival: 93%

MICROSCOPIC

Histologic Features

- Range of glomerular features
  - Proliferative glomerulonephritis
    - Endocapillary proliferative
    - Mesangial proliferative
    - Membranoproliferative
  - Nodular glomerulosclerosis
  - Glomerular microangiopathy
    - Mesangiolysis
    - GBM duplication
    - Thrombi
  - Focal crescents (cellular or fibrous)
  - Focal segmental glomerular scarring
  - Features may overlap

ANCILLARY TESTS

Immunofluorescence

- Linear GBM staining for immunoglobulin heavy chain (usually IgG) and light chain(s)
  - Approximately 50% of cases show light chain restriction by immunofluorescence (IF)
- Focal linear tubular basement membrane staining
- Absence of granular staining in glomeruli or tubular basement membranes

Serologic Testing

- Undetectable anti-GBM antibodies by commercially available ELISA
- Most with undetectable anti-GBM antibodies by western blot technique
  - Single report with negative anti-GBM ELISA and positive western blot

Electron Microscopy

- Features of glomerular microangiopathy
  - Subendothelial lucency
  - Swollen endothelial cells
- Absence of electron-dense immune complex-type deposits
- Absence of finely granular "powdery" deposits in basement membranes

DIFFERENTIAL DIAGNOSIS

Classic Anti-GBM Glomerulonephritis

- Usually diffuse (> 50%) crescentic glomerulonephritis
- IF stains for IgG, kappa, and lambda
  - Not light chain restricted
- Focal linear tubular basement membrane staining
- Clinical presentation and course different from atypical anti-GBM nephritis
  - Rapidly progressive glomerulonephritis ± pulmonary hemorrhage

Light and Heavy Chain Deposition Disease

- Diffuse linear GBM and TBM staining for monotypic heavy and light chain
- Finely granular "powdery" deposits by EM

Nodular Diabetic Glomerulosclerosis

- Absence of GBM-restricted linear staining for immunoglobulin by IF

Idiopathic Nodular Glomerulopathy

- Absence of GBM-restricted linear staining for immunoglobulin by IF
- Association with smoking and hypertension

SELECTED REFERENCES

1. Batal I et al: Nodular glomerulosclerosis with anti-glomerular basement membrane-like glomerulonephritis; a distinct pattern of kidney injury observed in smokers. Clin Kidney J. 7(4):361-366, 2014
2. Coley SM et al: Monoclonal IgG1κ anti-glomerular basement membrane disease: a case report. Am J Kidney Dis. ePub, 2014
3. Bazari H et al: Case records of the Massachusetts General Hospital. Case 20-2012. A 77-year-old man with leg edema, hematuria, and acute renal failure. N Engl J Med. 366(26):2503-15, 2012
4. Pedchenko V et al: Molecular architecture of the Goodpasture autoantigen in anti-GBM nephritis. N Engl J Med. 363(4):343-54, 2010
5. Fischer EG et al: Anti-glomerular basement membrane glomerulonephritis: a morphologic study of 80 cases. Am J Clin Pathol. 125(3):445-50, 2006
6. Kalluri R et al: Identification of the alpha 3 chain of type IV collagen as the common autoantigen in antibasement membrane disease and Goodpasture syndrome. J Am Soc Nephrol. 6(4):1178-85, 1995
7. Hellmark T et al: Characterization of anti-GBM antibodies involved in Goodpasture's syndrome. Kidney Int. 46(3):823-9, 1994
8. Nasr SH et al: Atypical anti-glomerular basement membrane nephritis: clinicopathologic characteristics and outcome (submitted 2015)

(Left) *This glomerulus shows a fibrous crescent ⇨ with segmental scarring. The biopsy also showed features of microangiopathy in glomeruli.* **(Right)** *A focal glomerulus shows segmental karyorrhexis ⇨ in an example of atypical anti-GBM nephritis.*

Fibrous Crescent

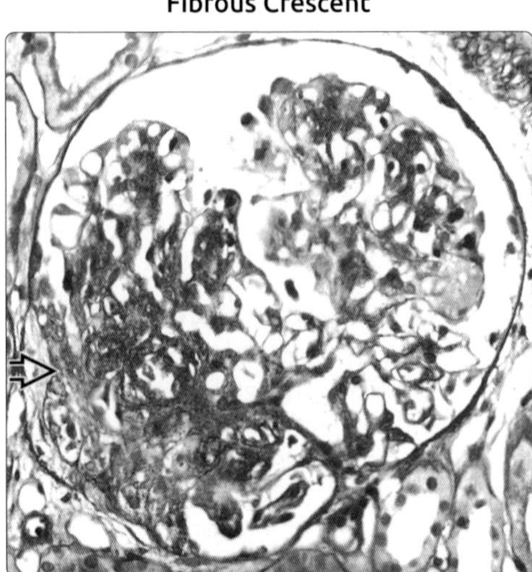

Segmental Karyorrhexis

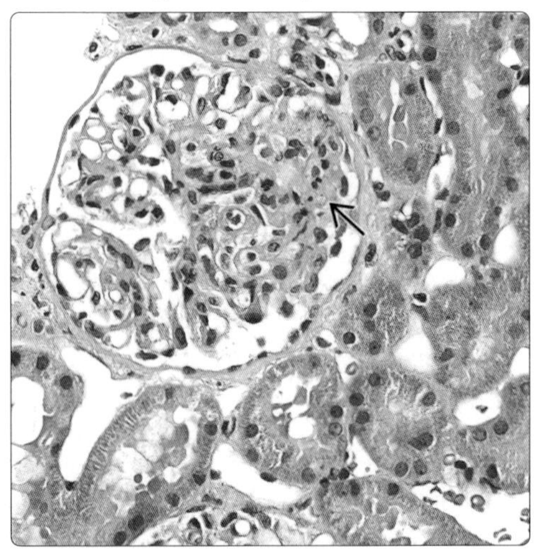

(Left) *In this example of atypical anti-GBM nephritis with polytypic staining, there was bright linear GBM staining for IgG, IgG4 (shown), kappa, and lambda.* **(Right)** *This example of atypical anti-GBM nephritis shows bright linear GBM staining for kappa light chain (left) and for lambda light chain (right). There was linear GBM staining for IgG as well.*

Linear GBM for IgG4

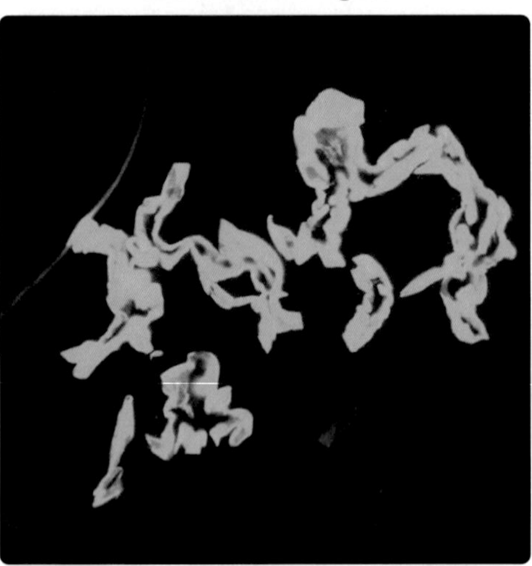

Linear GBM Staining for Kappa and Lambda

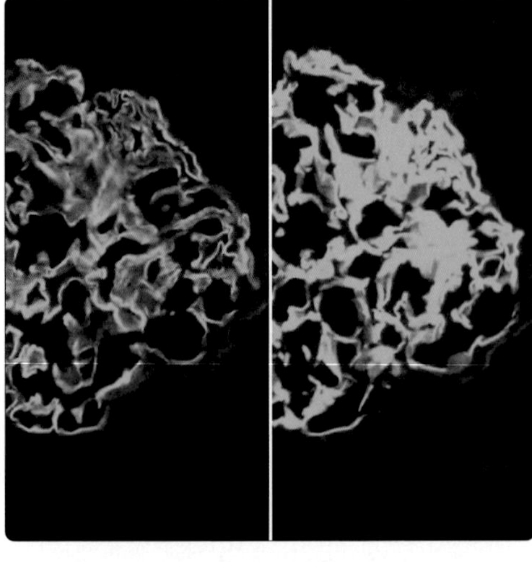

(Left) *This case of atypical anti-GBM nephritis showed bright linear GBM staining for IgG with monotypic staining for IgG2 (shown here) and lambda light chain.* **(Right)** *This example of atypical anti-GBM nephritis shows negative glomerular staining for kappa light chain (left) and bright linear GBM staining for lambda light chain (right). There was linear GBM staining for IgG as well. Approximately half of atypical anti-GBM cases show monotypic staining by IF.*

Atypical Anti-GBM Nephritis With Monotypic IgG2 Lambda Staining

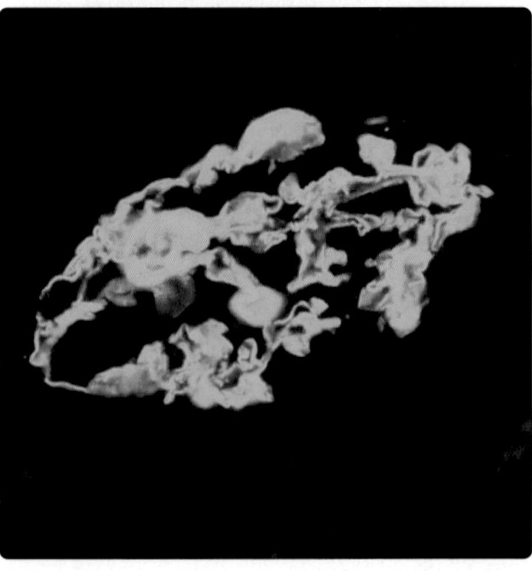

Atypical Anti-GBM Nephritis With Monotypic IgG Lambda Staining

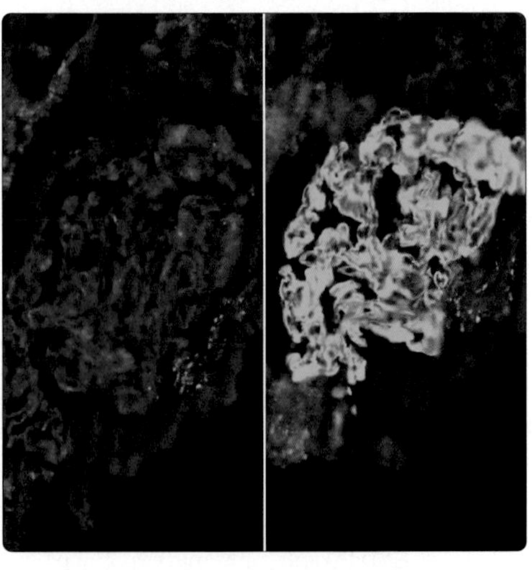

Glomerular Microangiopathy

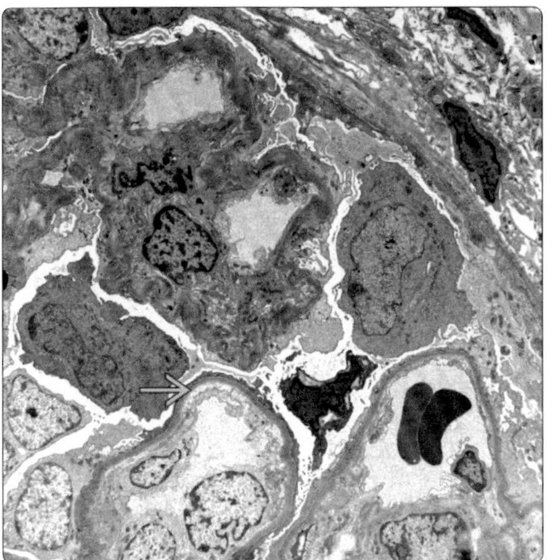

Glomerular Microangiopathy

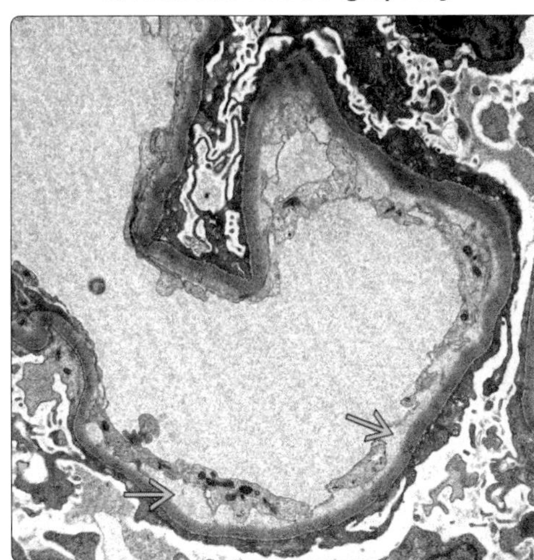

(Left) *By EM, subendothelial lucency ⇒ is seen, a feature of thrombotic microangiopathy. There is diffuse podocyte foot process effacement as well.* **(Right)** *By EM, there is subendothelial lucency ⇒, a feature of glomerular microangiopathy (thrombotic microangiopathy).*

Podocyte Foot Process Effacement

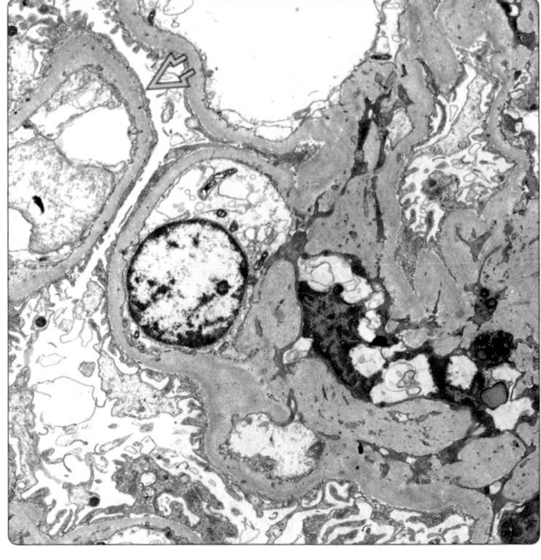

Diffuse Podocyte Foot Process Effacement

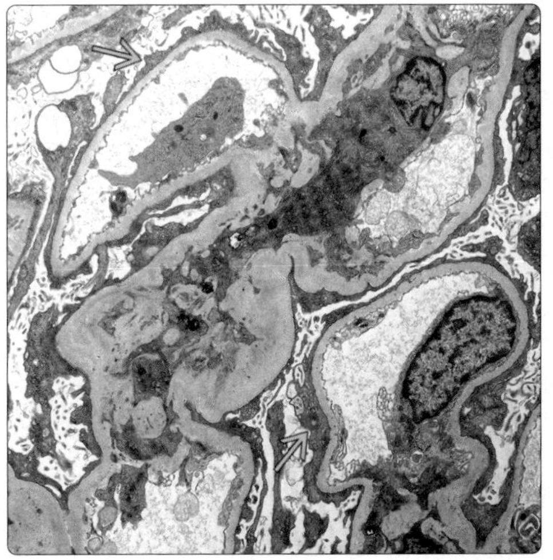

(Left) *This example of atypical anti-GBM nephritis shows moderate segmental podocyte foot process effacement ⇒. Note absence of "powdery" deposits along the glomerular basement membranes.* **(Right)** *In this biopsy, light microscopy slides showed a pattern of FSGS. EM shows diffuse podocyte foot process effacement ⇒. By IF, there was linear GBM staining for IgG, kappa, and lambda, of unclear significance. This may represent primary FSGS with superimposed "nonpathogenic" anti-GBM antibodies.*

Focal Segmental Glomerulosclerosis

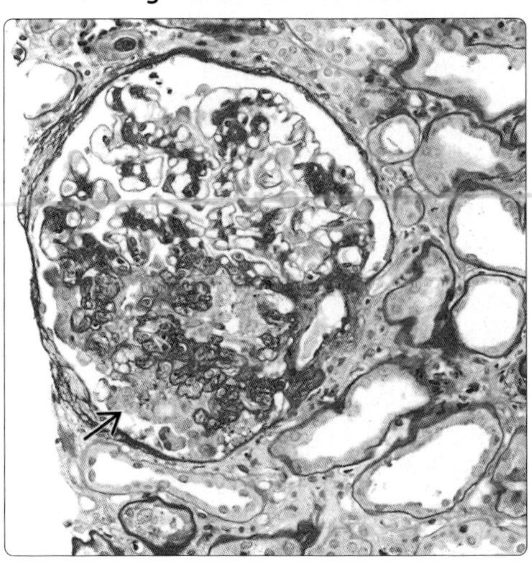

Nodular Glomerulosclerosis With Anti-GBM Antibodies

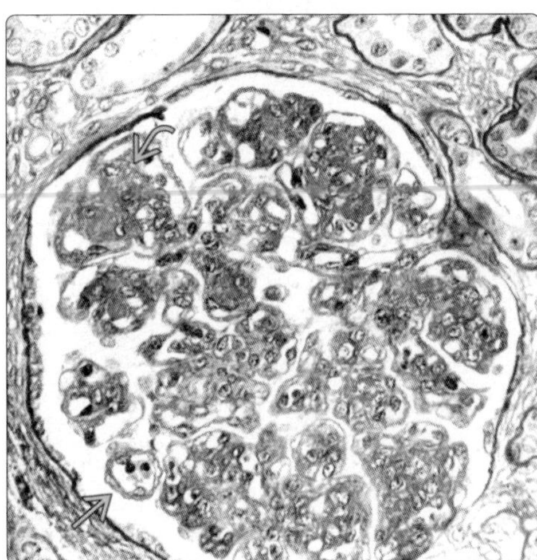

(Left) *This biopsy showed a pattern of FSGS with collapsing features ⇒. EM showed diffuse podocyte foot process effacement. IF showed bright linear GBM staining for IgG, kappa, and lambda.* **(Right)** *This 50-year-old nondiabetic woman presented with advanced renal failure for transplant. Glomeruli showed nodular mesangial expansion ⇒ and hypercellularity with duplication of the GBM ⇒. The glomeruli had bright linear IgG and eluates from nephrectomy contained anti-GBM antibodies by indirect IF.*

ETIOLOGY/PATHOGENESIS

Monoclonal Immunoglobulin

- May be produced by malignant lymphoid or plasma cell neoplasm

Reactive (Benign Monoclonal Proliferation)

- Some represent "monoclonal gammopathy of undetermined significance" (MGUS) without identifiable underlying neoplasm at time of renal biopsy
- Some cases never manifest an identified neoplastic proliferation
  - Appear to be clonal, but not malignant
- MGUS associated with renal disease termed "monoclonal gammopathy of renal significance"

APPROACH

Light Microscopy

- Quite variable appearances
  - Mimic membranoproliferative GN, acute GN, membranous GN (MIDD, type I cryo, PGNMID)
  - Mimic diabetes with nodular mesangial glomerulopathy (MIDD)
  - Tubulointerstitial disease may predominate (MIDD, cast nephropathy, light chain proximal tubulopathy ± crystals)

Special Stains

- Congo red stain with polarization essential to distinguish amyloidosis
  - Amyloidosis can be due to monoclonal immunoglobulin or other proteins
  - Thicker tissue sections more sensitive
  - High-quality polarizing microscope more sensitive

Immunofluorescence

- Stains for light chains essential to distinguish this group of diseases
- Light chain restriction may be seen in glomerular deposits, TBM deposits or in tubules
- Some monotypic light chains truncated and stain poorly

Algorithm for Diseases With Monoclonal Immunoglobulin Deposits

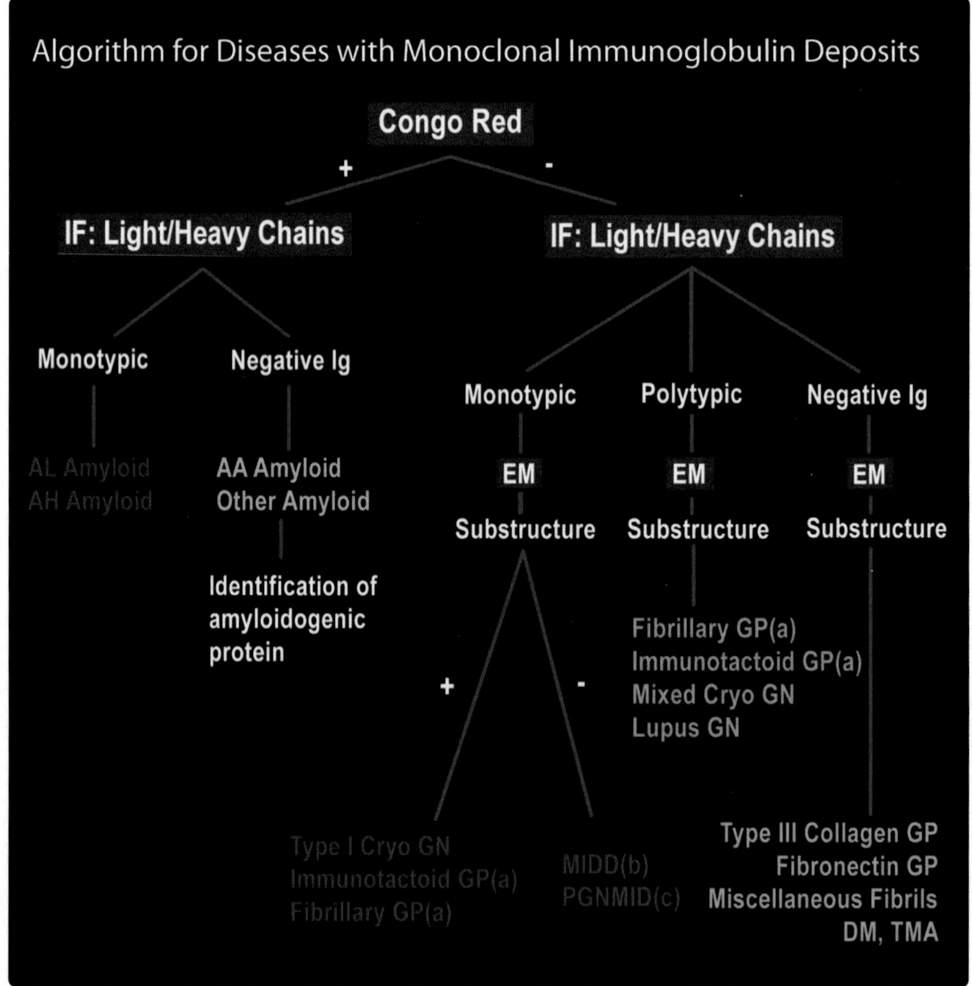

This algorithm begins with whether deposits are Congo red positive, followed by immunofluorescence (IF) for monotypic immunoglobulin chains (single light &/or heavy chain), equal staining of light chains (polyclonal) or no immunoglobulin staining. EM assesses the substructure of deposits. Immunotactoid and fibrillary GP sometimes have monotypic light chain (a). MIDD has either light chain, heavy chain, or both (b) and has no organized substructure. PGNMID usually, but not always, has amorphous deposits (c).

Diseases With Monoclonal Immunoglobulin Deposits

Disease	Light Microscopy	Congo Red	IF	EM	Underlying Diseases
AL or AH amyloid	Amorphous eosinophilic material in GBM, mesangium; sometimes interstitium, vessels	+	Monotypic light (AL) or heavy (AH) chains	Fibrils, abundant, 8-12 nm, nonperiodic	Multiple myeloma in ~ 18%, MGUS in some cases, less commonly B-cell lymphoma
Monoclonal immunoglobulin deposition disease (MIDD)	Mesangial nodules, thickened GBM, TBM	-	Monotypic light chains &/or monotypic heavy chains	Amorphous, dense, granular material GBM, TBM, mesangium	Dysproteinemia in > 70%, myeloma in ~ 40% of pure MIDD
Proliferative glomerulonephritis with monoclonal immunoglobulin deposits (PGNMID)	Acute, membranoproliferative (MPGN) or membranous glomerulonephritis (MGN)	-	Monotypic light chains, gamma heavy chain; C3, ± C1q	Usually amorphous, electron-dense "immune complex-type" deposits; subepithelial, subendothelial, mesangial	Dysproteinemia present in ~ 30%; myeloma rare
Type I cryoglobulinemia	MPGN, "pseudothrombi" in glomerular capillaries	-	Monotypic light chain and heavy chain	Fibrillary or tubular deposits, variable dimensions; occasionally amorphous	Chronic lymphocytic leukemia, Waldenström macroglobulinemia, other lymphoid-derived neoplasms
Light chain ("myeloma") cast nephropathy	Eosinophilic, PAS negative, fractured casts with giant cell reaction	-	Monotypic light/heavy chains	Granular, crystalline, or fibrillar casts	Multiple myeloma in ~ 90%
Light chain Fanconi syndrome (light chain proximal tubulopathy)	Crystalline structures within proximal tubular cytoplasm	-	Monotypic light chains in proximal tubular cytoplasm	Electron-dense crystalline structures within tubular epithelial cytoplasm	Multiple myeloma in ~ 50%, dysproteinemia in most
Light chain tubulopathy without crystals	Acute proximal tubular injury	±	Monotypic light chains in proximal tubular cytoplasm; may require pronase digestion of paraffin sections	Sometimes fibrillary aggregates in cytoplasm; Congo red positive (amyloid) or negative	> 90% with plasma cell dyscrasia but often unknown at time of biopsy
Diseases Sometimes Having Monotypic Immunoglobulin					
Immunotactoid glomerulopathy (GP)	Thickened GBM	-	Sometimes monotypic light chains	Tubular fibrils 20-80 nm	Monoclonal gammopathy in ~ 67%, myeloma in ~ 30%
Fibrillary GP	Thickened GBM, mesangial hypercellularity, crescents	-	Usually polyclonal; IgG4	Fibrils 10-30 nm	Monoclonal gammopathy in ~ 17%

- Sometimes revealed by IHC after antigen retrieval
- Rare forms show only heavy chain deposits

Electron Microscopy

- Organized vs. amorphous deposits, location of deposits helps distinguish different types of diseases

Laboratory Tests

- Serum or urine immunoelectrophoresis does not always detect monoclonal immunoglobulin
- Serum or urine free light chain assay is more sensitive technique

Ancillary Tests

- Bone marrow biopsy for monoclonal plasma cells
- Fat pad biopsy for amyloid deposits

SELECTED REFERENCES

1. Bridoux F et al: Diagnosis of monoclonal gammopathy of renal significance. Kidney Int. ePub, 2015
2. Nasr SH et al: Immunotactoid glomerulopathy: clinicopathologic and proteomic study. Nephrol Dial Transplant. 27(11):4137-46, 2012
3. Nasr SH et al: Renal monoclonal immunoglobulin deposition disease: a report of 64 patients from a single institution. Clin J Am Soc Nephrol. 7(2):231-9, 2012
4. Larsen CP et al: The morphologic spectrum and clinical significance of light chain proximal tubulopathy with and without crystal formation. Mod Pathol. 24(11):1462-9, 2011
5. Nasr SH et al: Fibrillary glomerulonephritis: a report of 66 cases from a single institution. Clin J Am Soc Nephrol. Epub ahead of print, 2011
6. Herrera GA et al: Renal diseases with organized deposits: an algorithmic approach to classification and clinicopathologic diagnosis. Arch Pathol Lab Med. 134(4):512-31, 2010
7. Markowitz GS: Dysproteinemia and the kidney. Adv Anat Pathol. 11(1):49-63, 2004
8. Lin J et al: Renal monoclonal immunoglobulin deposition disease: the disease spectrum. J Am Soc Nephrol. 12(7):1482-92, 2001

Congo Red With Polarization

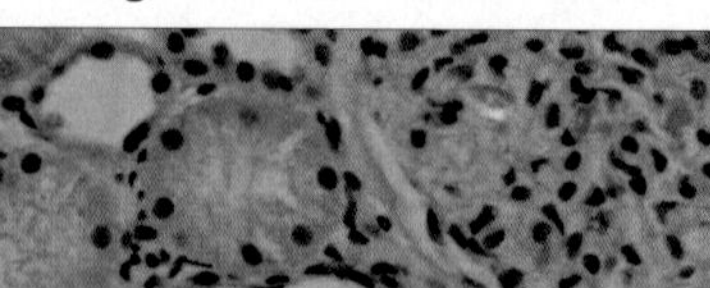

AL Amyloid With LIght Chain Restriction

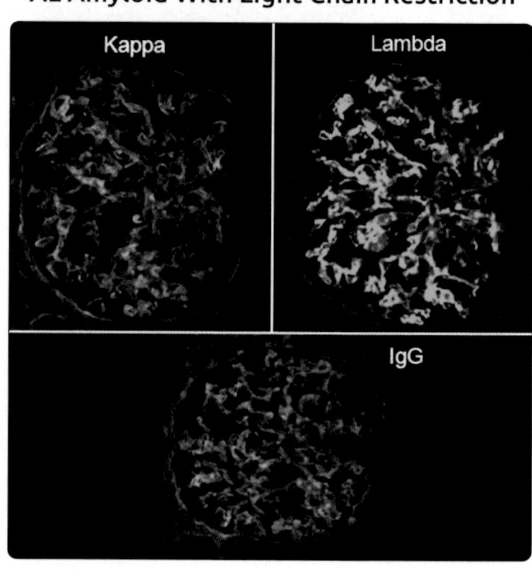

(Left) *Congo red stains many structures, and only the red and green birefringence under polarized light is specific for amyloid. (Courtesy I. Rosales, MD.)* **(Right)** *AL amyloid consists of monoclonal light chains, readily detected by immunofluorescence in frozen sections. If little or no light chains are detected or they are not restricted, search for other types of amyloidogenic proteins is done on frozen tissue. Monoclonal heavy chains can also form amyloid fibrils.*

Amyloid Fibrils 8-12 nm

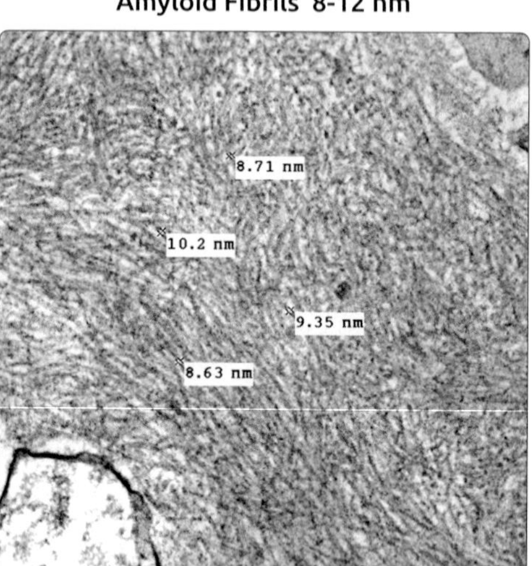

Immunotactoid Glomerulopathy

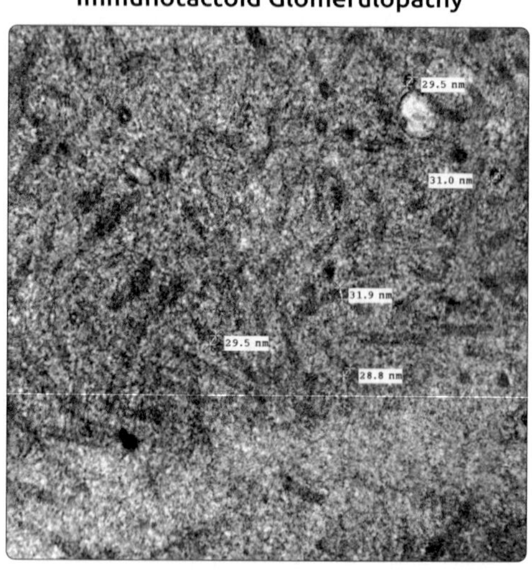

(Left) *Amyloid fibrils by electron microscopy are nonperiodic, nonbranching, and 8-12 nm in diameter. This overlaps with fibrillary glomerulopathy fibrils but the latter are Congo red negative.* **(Right)** *Immunotactoid glomerulopathy is characterized by EM by presence of abundant tubular fibrils typically around 30 nm in diameter (range: 17-52 nm), larger than the fibrils in amyloidosis and most cases of fibrillary glomerulopathy. About 70% have light chain restriction, as did this case (lambda).*

Fibrillary Glomerulopathy

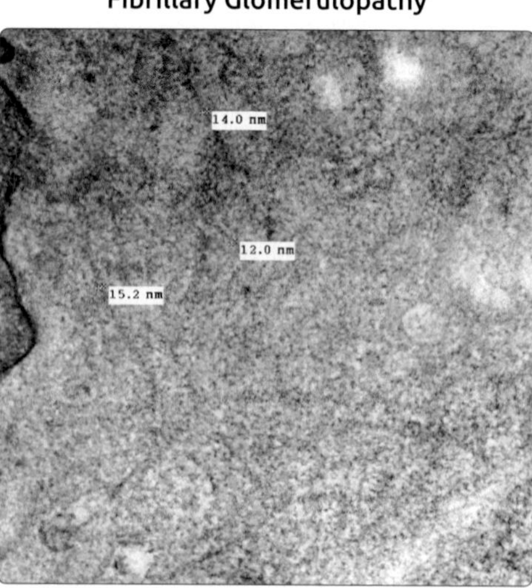

Fibrillary Glomerulopathy

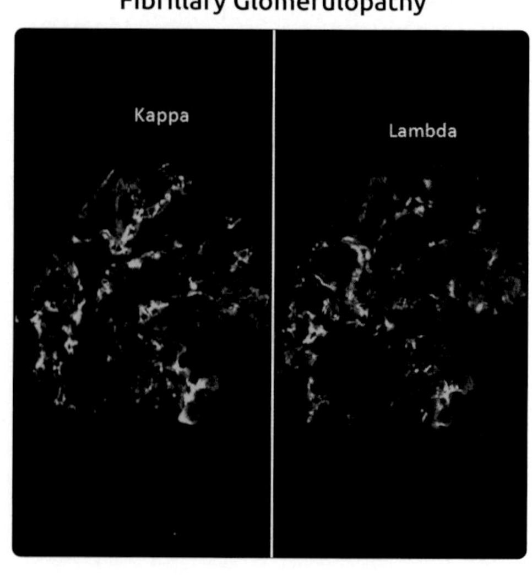

(Left) *Fibrillary glomerulopathy is characterized by abundant fibrils in the glomerular mesangium and glomerular basement membrane GBM that average 18 nm (range: 9-26 nm), overlapping somewhat with amyloid fibrils and immunotactoid glomerulopathy. A Congo red stain is necessary to exclude amyloid.* **(Right)** *Fibrillary glomerulopathy usually shows no light chain restriction (89%), as illustrated in this case. Most contain IgG4 and prominent C3 deposition.*

Monoclonal Immunoglobulin Deposition Disease (MIDD)

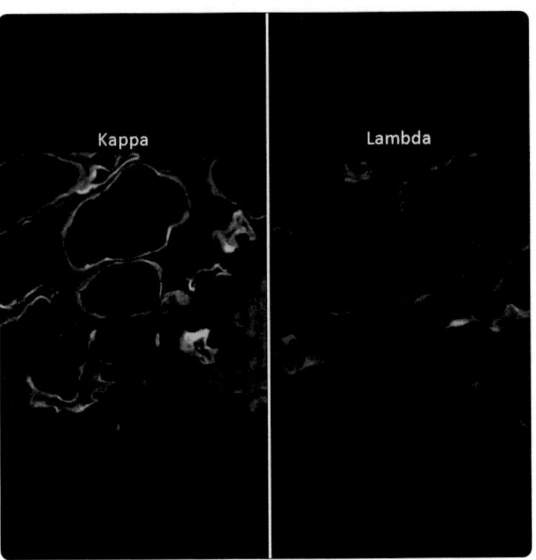

TBM Deposits in MIDD

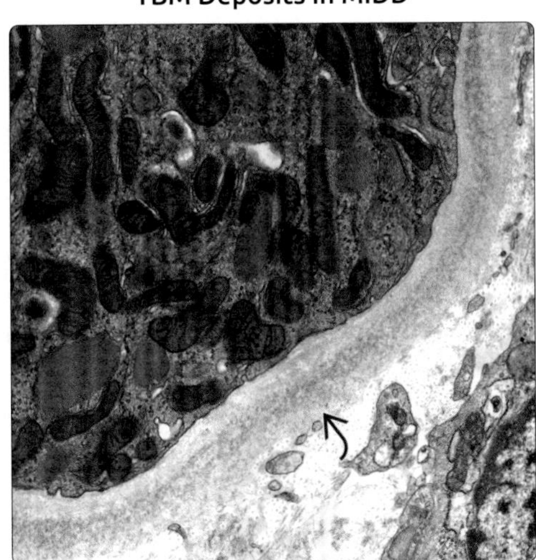

(Left) *The 1st suspicion of MIDD sometimes arises in the light chain restricted linear deposits along the tubular basement membrane, as in this case. Similar linear GBM staining was present. Heavy chain stains were negative.* **(Right)** *"Powdery" dense deposits ➔ in the tubular basement membrane correspond to the kappa light chain staining in this case of MIDD associated with myeloma and nodular glomerulopathy.*

Proliferative GN With Monoclonal IgG3

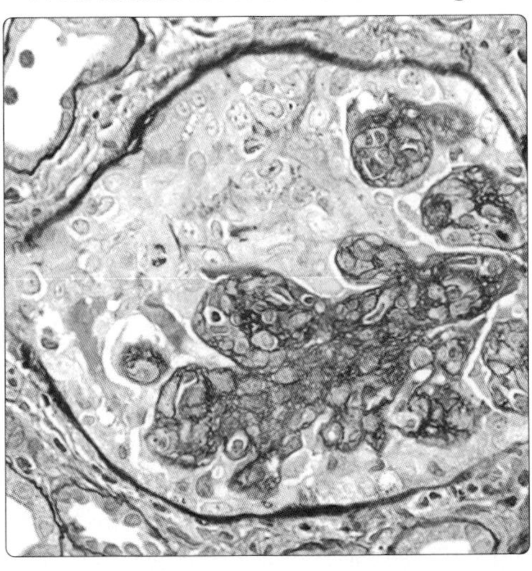

Subepithelial Amorphous Deposits

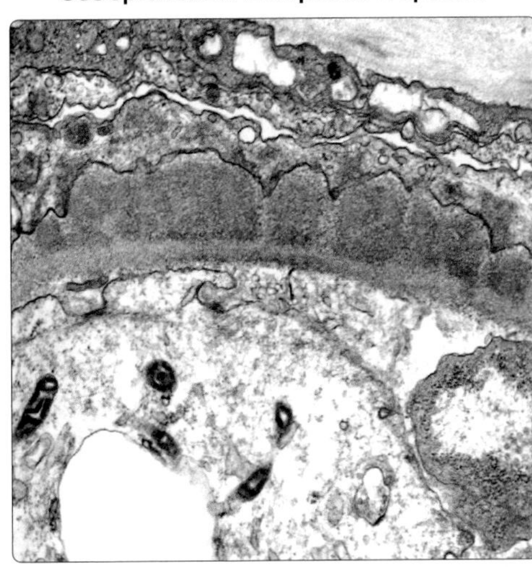

(Left) *Proliferative GN can occasionally be manifested by monoclonal immunoglobulin deposits, usually IgG3 subclass. This was in a 13-year-old boy with a 6-month history of fever and fatigue, proteinuria, and red cell casts.* **(Right)** *Proliferative GN with monoclonal immunoglobulin deposits look like immune complex GN because they usually are without substructure.*

Light Chain Restriction in Proliferative GN

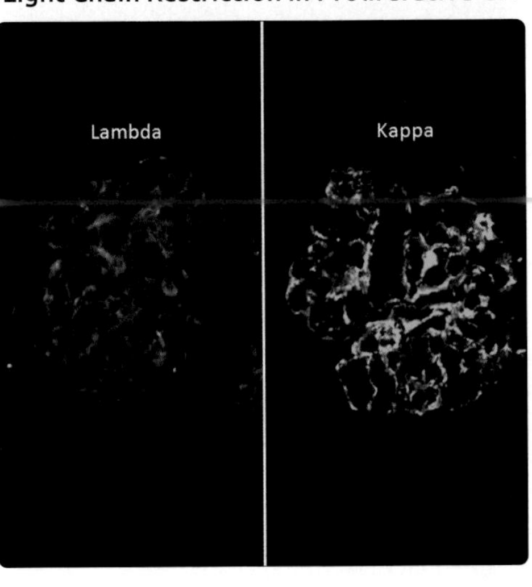

Proliferative GN With IgG3 Deposition

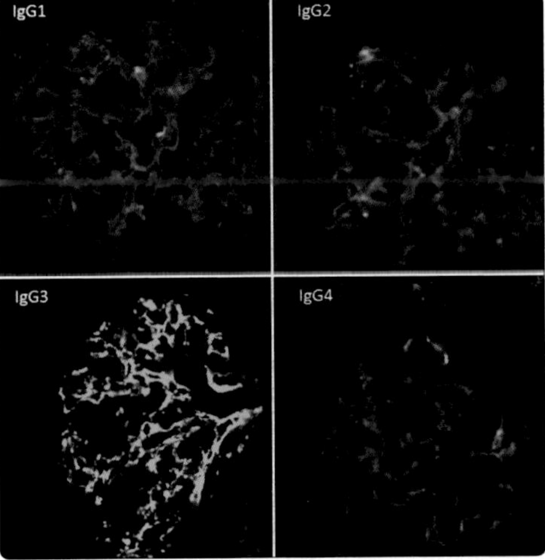

(Left) *Proliferative GN can occasionally be manifested by monoclonal immunoglobulin deposits, which can be detected by the routine use of light chain stains.* **(Right)** *Proliferative GN with monoclonal immunoglobulin deposits are usually of the IgG3 subclass. Subclass specific antibodies are commercially available and useful when indicated for diagnostic renal pathology.*

KEY FACTS

TERMINOLOGY

- Systemic, finely granular deposition of monoclonal immunoglobulins, including within glomerular basement membrane (GBM) and tubular basement membrane (TBM) and mesangium

CLINICAL ISSUES

- Nephrotic syndrome
- Acute or chronic renal failure
- Multiple myeloma diagnosed in ~ 40% of patients with pure MIDD
- Monoclonal protein in serum, urine, or both
  - ~ 15-20% have undetectable serum or urine paraprotein at time of diagnosis, even by immunofixation

MICROSCOPIC

- Nodular glomerulopathy
  - PAS-positive nodules, nonargyrophilic
- Interstitial inflammation
- Acute tubular injury
- TBM monoclonal immunoglobulin deposition
  - Kappa light chain in ~ 80% of LCDD
  - Linear basement membrane immunofluorescence staining (glomerular, tubular, vascular) for kappa or lambda light chain (LCDD), plus heavy chain (LHCDD) or heavy chain only (HCDD)
  - TBM thickening may be present
- By EM, finely granular, punctate, "powdery" electron-dense deposits distributed along basement membranes; nonfibrillary
- Concurrent light chain cast nephropathy in 1/3 with MIDD

TOP DIFFERENTIAL DIAGNOSES

- Nodular diabetic glomerulosclerosis
- Light chain deposition by immunofluorescence only
- Proliferative glomerulonephritis with monoclonal IgG deposits
- Dense deposit disease (DDD)

Nodular Glomerulosclerosis in Kappa LCDD

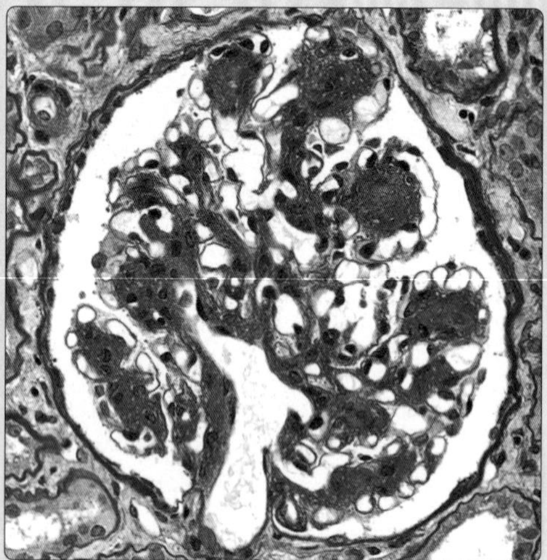

Light Chain Restriction in Kappa LCDD

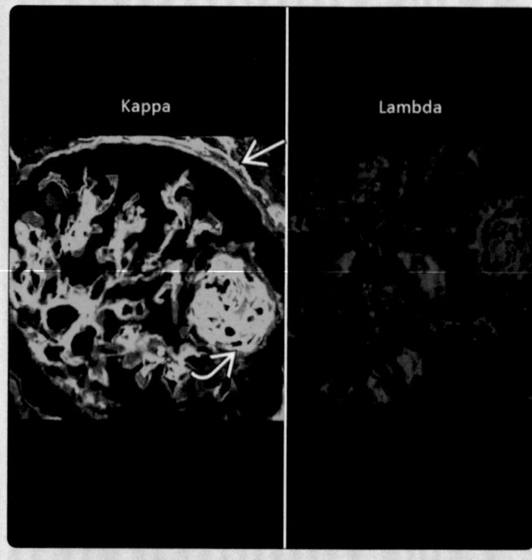

(Left) *Nodular expansion of the mesangium is characteristic of MIDD and closely resembles diabetic glomerulopathy by light microscopy.* **(Right)** *Stains for light chains are critical in the detection of MIDD. The light chains deposit in the GBM, TBM, mesangium ➡, and Bowman capsule ➡. Kappa is the most common light chain.*

Granular Deposits Along GBM in Kappa LCDD

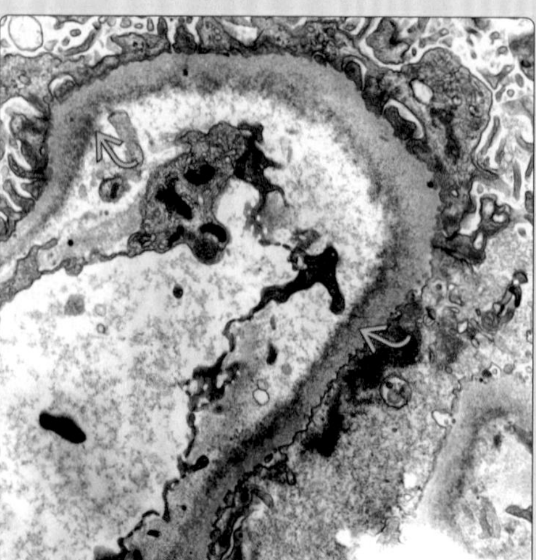

TBM Deposits in LCDD

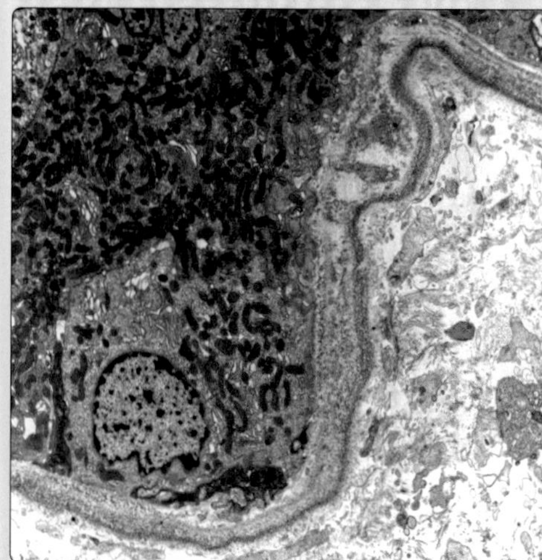

(Left) *Light chains deposit in a characteristic "powdery" finely granular dense pattern ➡ along the GBM by electron microscopy. The fine granularity allows distinction from DDD and also AL amyloidosis.* **(Right)** *The TBM is a common site of light chain deposition, which can be detected by electron microscopy as granular dense deposits, similar to those in the glomerulus and sometimes more prominent.*

TERMINOLOGY

Abbreviations

- Monoclonal immunoglobulin deposition disease (MIDD)
- Light chain deposition disease (LCDD)
- Heavy chain deposition disease (HCDD)
- Light and heavy chain deposition disease (LHCDD)

Synonyms

- Systemic light chain disease
- Nonamyloidogenic light chain deposition
- Monoclonal immunoglobulin deposition disease, Randall type

Definitions

- Systemic deposition of monoclonal immunoglobulin, including glomerular and tubular basement membranes and within mesangium
  - Characterized by linear GBM and TBM by immunofluorescence (IF) staining and finely granular deposits by electron microscopy (EM)

ETIOLOGY/PATHOGENESIS

Neoplastic

- Clonal proliferation of B cells/plasma cells
- Either malignant or benign

LCDD Deposits

- Differ from normal light chains in variable region, especially complementarity-determining regions and framework regions
- Glycosylated light chains larger than normal light chain

HCDD Deposits

- Deletion of CH1 constant domain of gamma heavy chain

CLINICAL ISSUES

Epidemiology

- Mean age: 56 years (36% < 50 years old)
- M:F = 2:1

Presentation

- Acute renal failure
- Chronic renal failure
- Proteinuria (58%; nonlight chain)
  - Nephrotic-range proteinuria (~ 40%)
- Multiple myeloma diagnosed in ~ 40% with pure MIDD (without concurrent cast nephropathy or amyloidosis)
- Hypocomplementemia
  - Present in gamma-HCDD with complement-fixing IgG subclass deposited (gamma-1 or gamma-3)

Laboratory Tests

- Monoclonal protein in serum, urine, or both
  - M spike on serum or urine protein electrophoresis in ~ 70% of patients with pure MIDD
  - Abnormal ratio of kappa or lambda free light chains in serum in 100% (even those with HCDD)
  - ~ 15-20% have undetectable serum or urine paraprotein at diagnosis by immunofixation
- Emerging test for free heavy chains in gamma heavy chain deposition disease
- Free light or heavy chain tests useful for monitoring response to therapy

Treatment

- Steroids, cyclophosphamide, melphalan/stem cell transplant, bortezomib
- None established, no controlled trials

Prognosis

- Mean renal survival: ~ 5 years
  - Myeloma cast nephropathy is poor prognostic feature of LCDD
  - Diabetes is risk factor for progression
- Recurs in transplants: ~ 75%

Other Organ Involvement

- Cardiac disease (~ 20-80%)
- Peripheral neuropathy (20%)
- Other: Gastrointestinal, liver, pulmonary nodules, muscle, skin, retina

MICROSCOPIC

Histologic Features

- Glomeruli
  - Nodular glomerulopathy in ~ 60%
    - 15% of patients with proteinuria < 0.5 g/d
    - PAS-positive nodules, nonargyrophilic
  - Rare cases show thick glomerular basement membranes with associated membranoproliferative pattern
    - Must show linear GBM and TBM monoclonal immunoglobulin deposits to be diagnosed as MIDD
  - Necrotizing and crescentic glomerulonephritis (rare)
    - More frequent in α-HCDD
- Tubules
  - Acute tubular injury
  - TBM thickening may be present
  - Concurrent light chain cast nephropathy present in ~ 30%
- Interstitium
  - Interstitial inflammation and edema
- Vessels
  - Normal by light microscopy
- Concurrent amyloidosis in 13% of MIDD cases

ANCILLARY TESTS

Immunohistochemistry

- Can detect glomerular and TBM deposits of light chains in paraffin-embedded tissue

Immunofluorescence

- Linear basement membrane staining (glomerular, tubular, vascular) for monoclonal immunoglobulin
  - ~ 75% LCDD
    - Usually monotypic kappa light chain in LCDD (73-91% kappa)
  - ~ 14% HCDD
    - Usually gamma heavy chain
    - All subclasses (1, 2, 3, and 4) reported
    - Minority due to α-HCDD

  - Rare delta heavy chain
- 11% LHCDD
  - 1 heavy and 1 light chain
  - Rarely, separate deposits of heavy and light chains
- May be present before deposits detectable by EM
- IF may be negative despite deposits by EM
  - Heavy chains may lack CH1
  - TBM deposits may be present in absence of GBM deposits, especially in patients with proteinuria < 0.5 g/day
- Smudgy staining of mesangium for monoclonal protein
- Staining for IgG subclasses helps determine monoclonal nature of deposits in gamma-HCDD

Electron Microscopy

- Finely granular, punctate, "powdery" electron-dense deposits distributed along GBM, TBM, and vascular basement membranes
  - Similar deposits in LCDD, LHCDD, and HCDD
- Monoclonal deposits may be seen by immunogold labeling

DIFFERENTIAL DIAGNOSIS

Light Chain Deposition by Immunofluorescence Only

- Monotypic light chain staining of GBM and TBM by IF, but no deposits detectable by EM and no changes by light microscopy
- Seen especially in cases of light chain cast nephropathy
- Uncertain significance
  - May be artifactual IF staining representative of monoclonal protein in urine

Proliferative Glomerulonephritis With Monoclonal IgG Deposits

- Proliferative glomerulonephritis pattern by light microscopy
- Monotypic IgG kappa or IgG lambda staining by IF; IgG is restricted to 1 subclass
- Amorphous electron-dense deposits in glomeruli by EM
- Absence of TBM deposits by IF and EM

Dense Deposit Disease (DDD)

- Some cases associated with serum paraprotein, which may have C3 nephritic factor activity
- DDD shows predominant C3 deposition, little Ig, and no light chain restriction
- Very electron-dense deposits, distinct from MIDD finely granular deposits

Nodular Diabetic Glomerulosclerosis

- Similar PAS-positive nodular glomerulopathy to MIDD but without IF (light chain) or EM findings of MIDD
- Linear GBM and TBM staining for IgG by IF; IgG subclass staining by IF can distinguish MIDD from gamma heavy chain deposition disease

Light Chain Tubulointerstitial Nephritis

- Acute tubulointerstitial nephritis without glomerulopathy
- Negative IF and EM for light chain-type deposits

Fibrillary or Immunotactoid Glomerulonephritis

- Fibrillary or tubular substructure of deposits by EM
- Usual absence of TBM deposits

Type 1 Cryoglobulinemic Glomerulonephritis or Waldenström Macroglobulinemic Glomerulonephritis

- Monoclonal immunoglobulin in glomeruli
- Membranoproliferative pattern of glomerular injury
- Absence of finely granular deposits along glomerular and TBMs

Amyloidosis

- Congo red positive
- Fibrillary structure by EM

IgA Nephropathy

- α-HCDD, in part due to its rarity, may be misdiagnosed as IgA nephropathy
- Like IgA nephropathy, α-HCDD may show necrotizing and crescentic glomerulonephritis
- Usual absence of TBM deposits in IgA nephropathy and presence of both light chains

DIAGNOSTIC CHECKLIST

Clinically Relevant Pathologic Features

- 31-45% of patients with pure MIDD have overt multiple myeloma at time of MIDD diagnosis
- 91% of patients with concurrent MIDD and cast nephropathy have multiple myeloma
- M spike on serum or urine protein electrophoresis in ~ 50% of patients with pure MIDD
- Hypocomplementemia
  - Present in gamma-HCDD with complement-fixing IgG subclass deposited (gamma-1 or gamma-3)

SELECTED REFERENCES

1. Bridoux F et al: Diagnosis of monoclonal gammopathy of renal significance. Kidney Int. ePub, 2015
2. Royal V et al: IgD heavy-chain deposition disease: detection by laser microdissection and mass spectrometry. J Am Soc Nephrol. 26(4):784-90, 2015
3. Sicard A et al: Light chain deposition disease without glomerular proteinuria: a diagnostic challenge for the nephrologist. Nephrol Dial Transplant. 29(10):1894-902, 2014
4. Darouich S et al: Light-chain deposition disease of the kidney: a case report. Ultrastruct Pathol. 36(2):134-8, 2012
5. Nasr SH et al: Renal monoclonal immunoglobulin deposition disease: a report of 64 patients from a single institution. Clin J Am Soc Nephrol. 7(2):231-9, 2012
6. Stratta P et al: Renal outcome and monoclonal immunoglobulin deposition disease in 289 old patients with blood cell dyscrasias: a single center experience. Crit Rev Oncol Hematol. 79(1):31-42, 2011
7. Herrera GA et al: Ultrastructural immunolabeling in the diagnosis of monoclonal light-and heavy-chain-related renal diseases. Ultrastruct Pathol. 34(3):161-73, 2010
8. Sethi S et al: Dense deposit disease associated with monoclonal gammopathy of undetermined significance. Am J Kidney Dis. 56(5):977-82, 2010
9. Alexander MP et al: Alpha heavy chain deposition disease: a comparison of its clinicopathological characteristics with gamma and mu heavy chain deposition disease. Mod Pathol. 20(Suppl. 2):270A, 2007
10. Salant DJ et al: A case of atypical light chain deposition disease--diagnosis and treatment. Clin J Am Soc Nephrol. 2(4):858-67, 2007
11. Gu X et al: Light-chain-mediated acute tubular interstitial nephritis: a poorly recognized pattern of renal disease in patients with plasma cell dyscrasia. Arch Pathol Lab Med. 130(2):165-9, 2006
12. Lin J et al: Renal monoclonal immunoglobulin deposition disease: the disease spectrum. J Am Soc Nephrol. 12(7):1482-92, 2001
13. Randall RE et al: Manifestations of systemic light chain deposition. Am J Med. 60(2):293-9, 1976

Nodular Glomerular Change in LHCDD

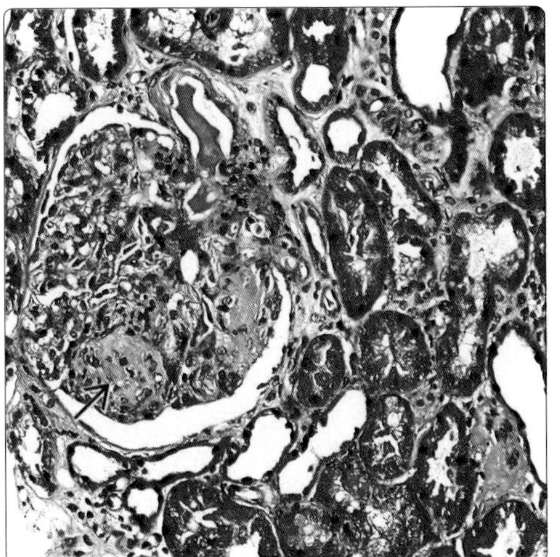

Light Chain Restriction in LHCDD

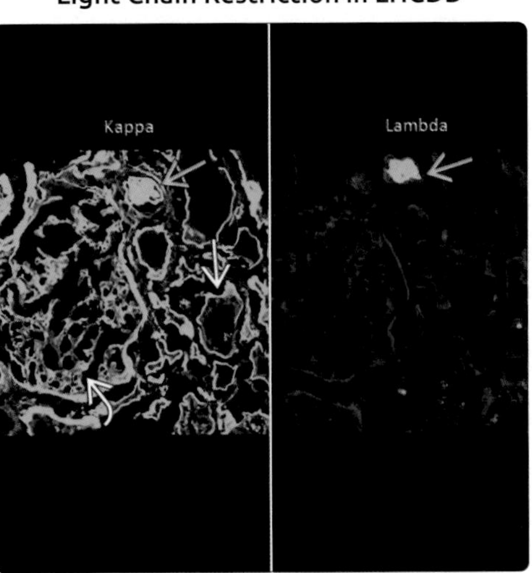

(Left) *This glomerulus has nodular expansion of the mesangium ⇒.* *Immunofluorescence showed bright linear staining of the glomerular and tubular basement membranes for IgG and kappa, without staining for lambda light chain.* **(Right)** *The GBM ⇒ and TBM ⇒ have bright linear staining for kappa but not lambda light chain. A cast is present, which stains equally for kappa and lambda ⇒.*

Linear IgG Along TBM and GBM in LHCDD

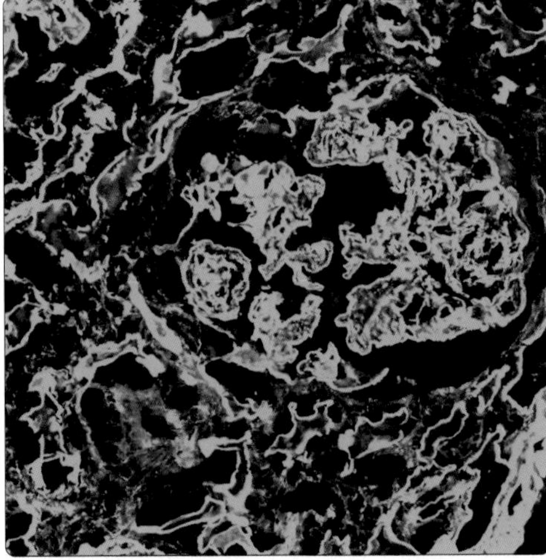

Subclass Restriction in LHCDD

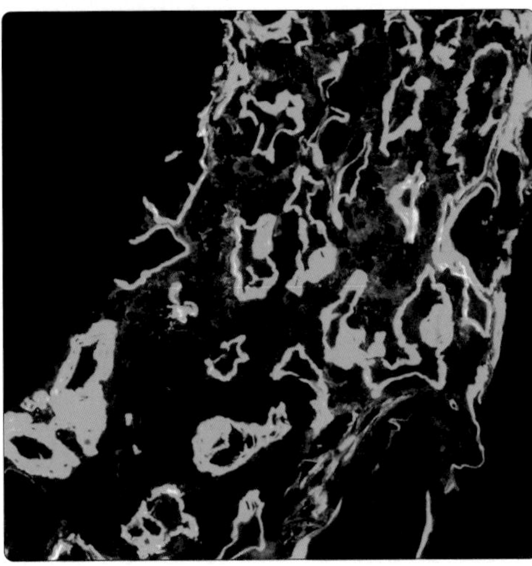

(Left) *Immunofluorescence staining for IgG shows bright linear glomerular and tubular basement membrane staining and smudgy mesangial staining. This appearance may also resemble IgG staining in diabetes.* **(Right)** *Immunofluorescence staining for the IgG3 subclass shows bright linear tubular basement membrane staining; glomeruli were also positive. Stains for IgG1, 2, and 4 were negative. The presence of staining for a single IgG subclass supports the diagnosis of HCDD or LHCDD.*

Finely Granular Electron-Dense Deposits in LHCDD

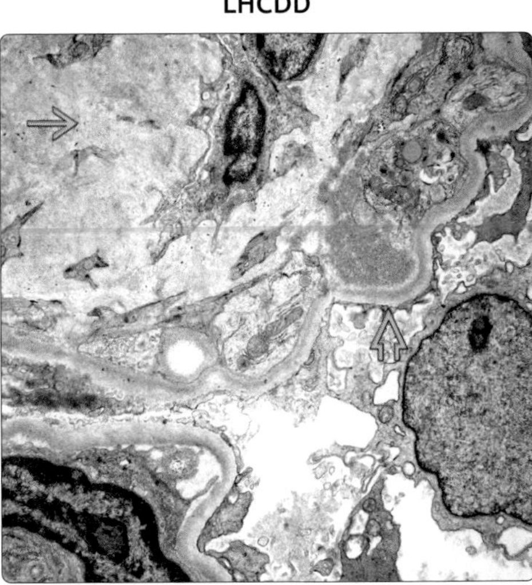

TBM Deposits in LHCDD

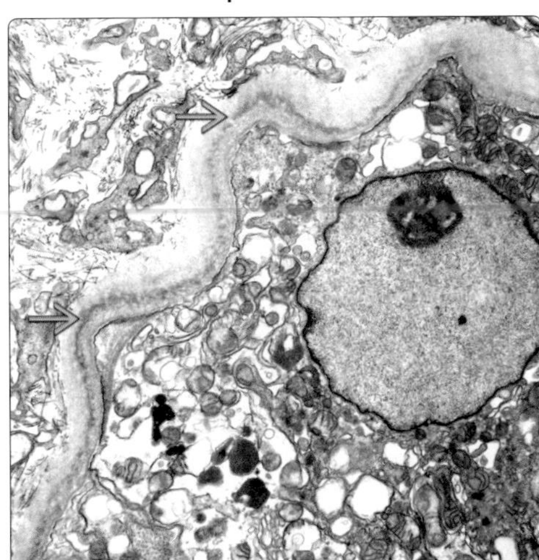

(Left) *Finely granular electron-dense deposits are seen in the mesangium ⇒ and in glomerular basement membranes ⇒.* **(Right)** *Finely granular electron-dense deposits ⇒ are present along the tubular basement membrane in this case of LHCDD.*

LCDD With Membranoproliferative Pattern

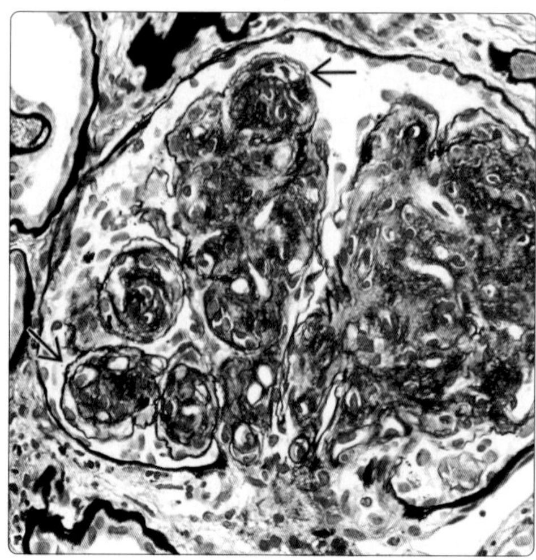

LCDD With Kappa Light Chains in GBM and TBM

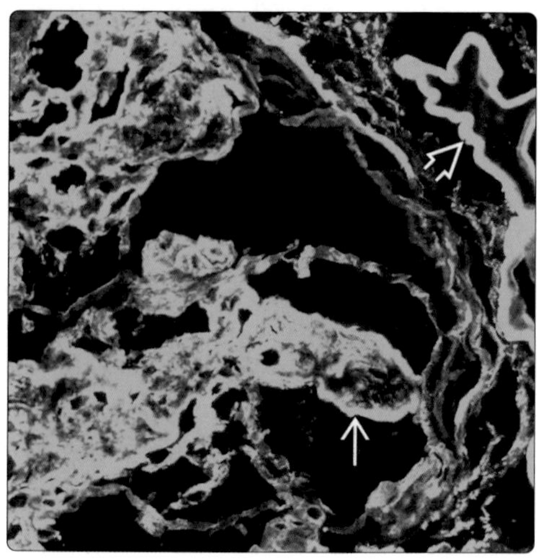

(Left) *Segmental glomerular basement membrane duplication* ➙*, a membranoproliferative feature, can be seen on a silver stain in this case of LCDD.* **(Right)** *Immunofluorescence reveals linear glomerular* ➙ *and tubular* ➙ *basement membrane staining and smudgy mesangial staining for kappa light chain.*

Minimal LCDD by Light Microscopy

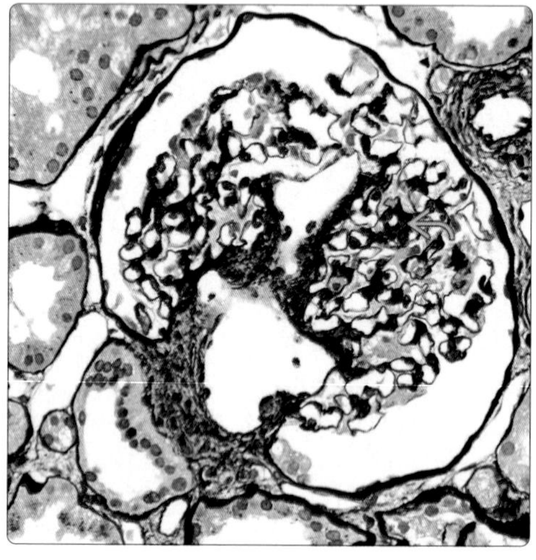

Acute Tubular Injury

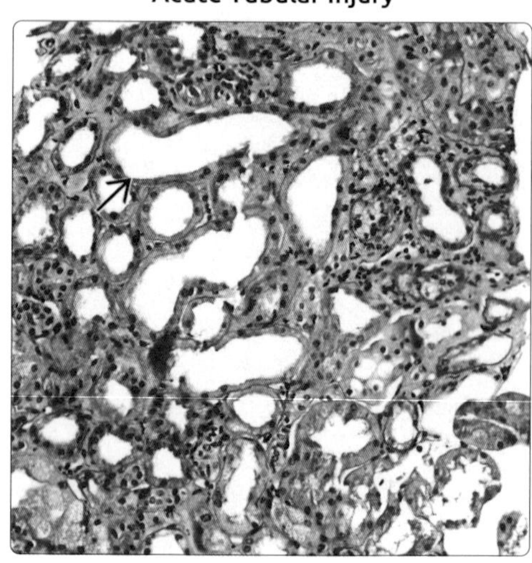

(Left) *A silver stain shows very mild mesangial expansion* ➙ *by nonargyrophilic material in a patient with light chain MIDD. The diagnosis would not be suspected without immunofluorescence demonstration of a single light chain and the electron-dense deposits by EM.* **(Right)** *Focal tubules show features of acute injury* ➙*, including dilatation of the tubules, flattening of the epithelium, and loss of the tubular brush border. There is very focal interstitial inflammation. (Courtesy S. Nasr, MD.)*

TBM Deposits in LCDD

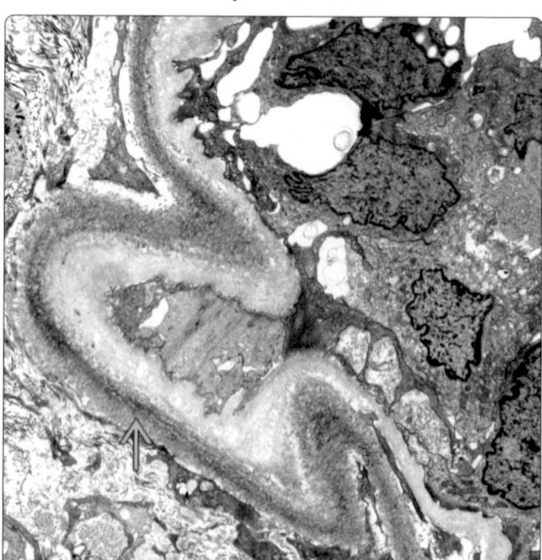

IF-Only MIDD

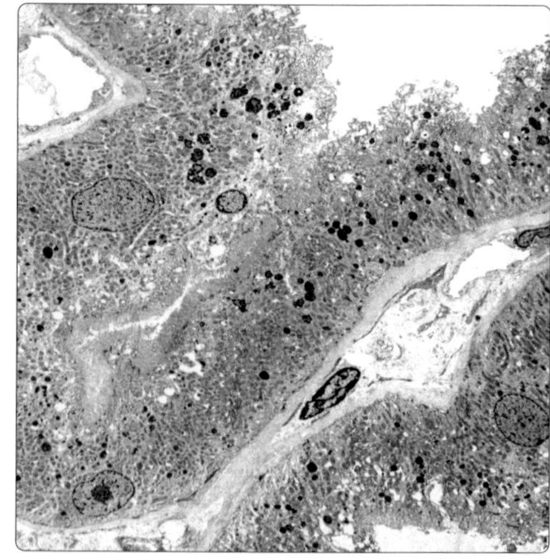

(Left) *Tubular basement membranes show finely granular electron-dense deposits* ➙*.* **(Right)** *MIDD "by immunofluorescence only" does not show evidence of tubular basement membrane deposits, despite bright staining by IF for IgG. The findings are of uncertain significance.*

α-HCDD With Segmental Necrosis

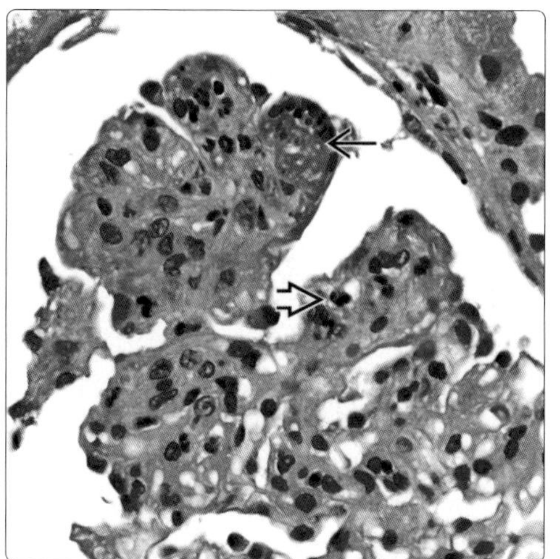

Nodular Glomerulosclerosis in α-HCDD

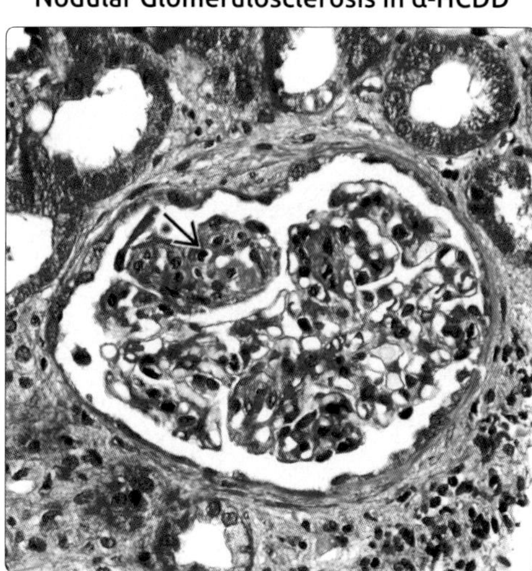

(Left) *Segmental necrosis of the glomerular tuft ⇒ is seen in α-HCDD. As opposed to gamma heavy chain or light chain deposition disease, it is not uncommon for α-HCDD to show glomerular necrosis or crescents. Segmental capillary loops contain neutrophils ⇒. (Courtesy S. Nasr, MD.)* **(Right)** *Trichrome stain shows nodular expansion of the glomerular mesangium ⇒ in α-HCDD. (Courtesy S. Nasr, MD.)*

α-HCDD After Pronase Digestion

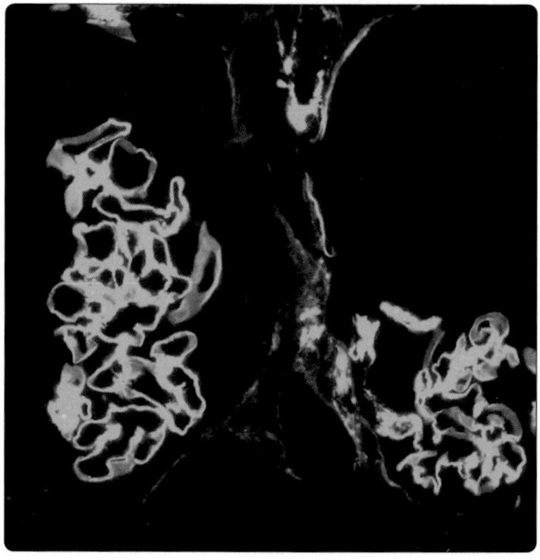

Gamma-HCDD Nodular Pattern

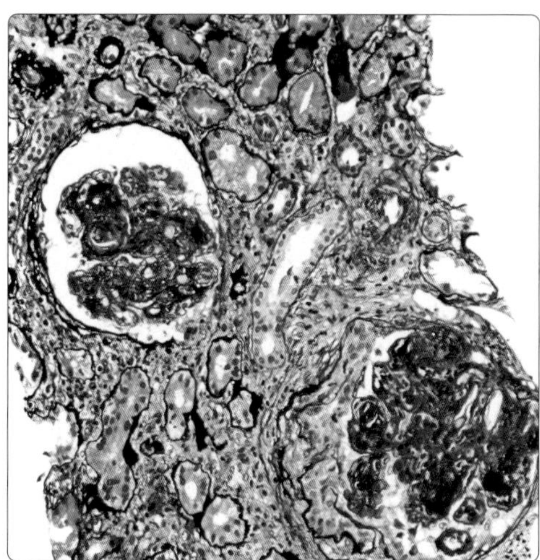

(Left) *Immunofluorescence on pronase-digested paraffin sections shows linear GBM and smudgy mesangial staining for IgA. No glomeruli were present on the tissue originally submitted for immunofluorescence; pronase-digested paraffin sections reveal this glomerular staining. (Courtesy S. Nasr, MD.)* **(Right)** *Nodular glomerulosclerosis is shown. Immunofluorescence showed bright linear glomerular and tubular basement membrane staining for IgG, without staining for light chains (silver stain).*

Gamma HCDD With Proliferative Pattern

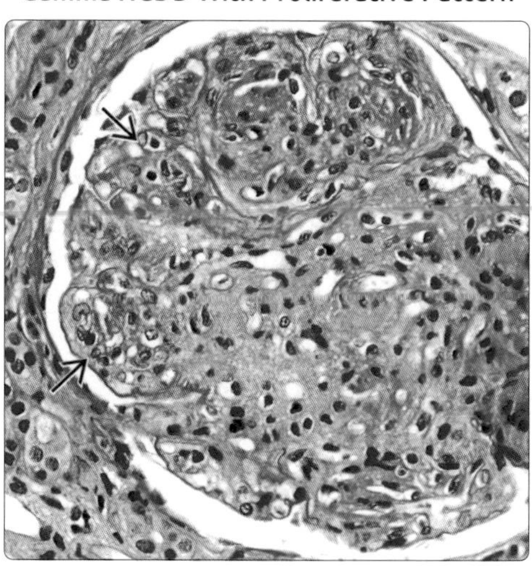

Gamma-HCDD

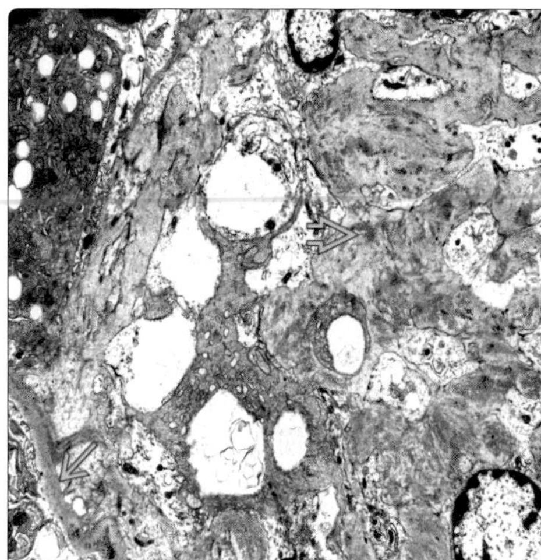

(Left) *A proliferative glomerular pattern is seen in this case of HCDD, with endocapillary hypercellularity ⇒ and segmental glomerular basement membrane duplication.* **(Right)** *Gamma heavy chain deposition disease shows finely granular electron-dense deposits present along the glomerular basement membranes ⇒ and within the mesangium ⇒, as in LCDD.*

(Left) *This case of LCDD has an unusual feature of granular, rather than linear, tubular basement membrane staining for monoclonal kappa light chain. The lambda light chain stain was negative.* **(Right)** *Despite granular rather than linear tubular basement membrane staining by immunofluorescence, tubular basement membranes by EM show finely granular electron-dense deposits.*

LCDD With Granular TBM Deposits

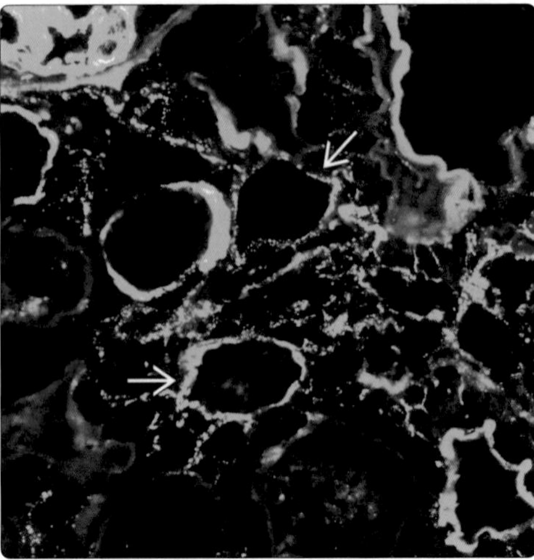

LCDD With Granular TBM Deposits

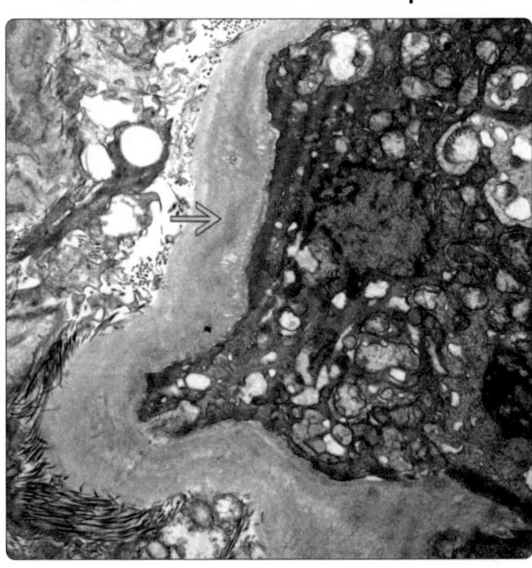

(Left) *DDD in a 48-year-old woman with a serum monoclonal protein shows very electron-dense amorphous deposits within the mesangium and within the GBM, not to be confused with MIDD. Some DDD cases have paraproteins with C3 nephritic factor activity.* **(Right)** *The apical surface of tubular epithelial cells shows unusual monotypic kappa light chain deposition. Tubular reabsorption droplets also showed monotypic kappa. TBMs are negative so this does not represent light chain deposition disease.*

Dense Deposit Disease

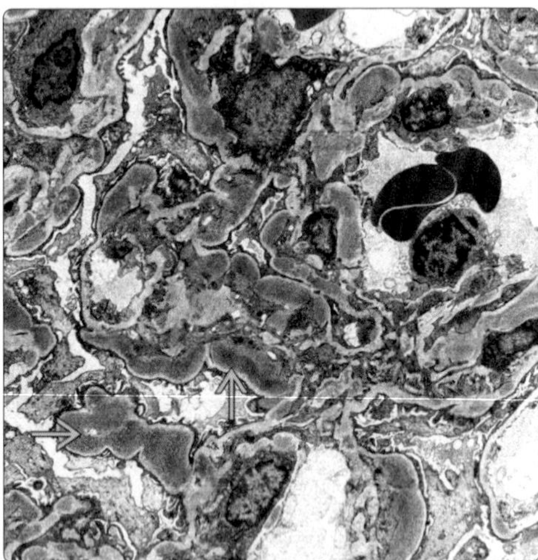

Kappa Tubulopathy

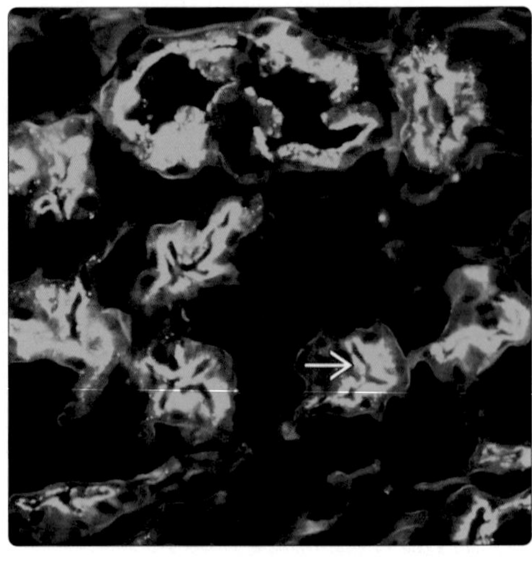

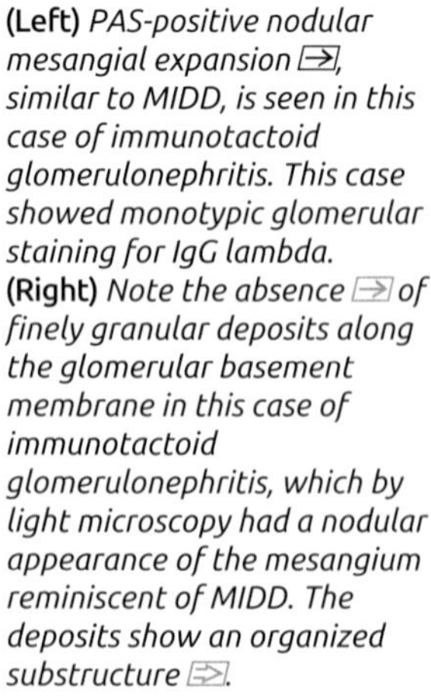

(Left) *PAS-positive nodular mesangial expansion, similar to MIDD, is seen in this case of immunotactoid glomerulonephritis. This case showed monotypic glomerular staining for IgG lambda.* **(Right)** *Note the absence of finely granular deposits along the glomerular basement membrane in this case of immunotactoid glomerulonephritis, which by light microscopy had a nodular appearance of the mesangium reminiscent of MIDD. The deposits show an organized substructure.*

Immunotactoid Glomerulopathy With Nodular Glomerular Lesions

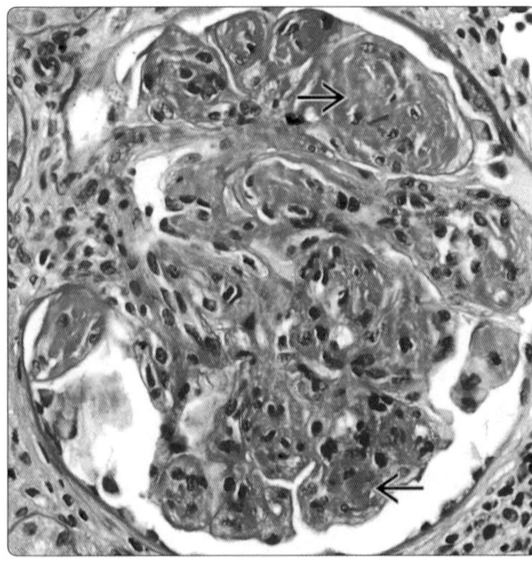

Immunotactoid Glomerulopathy

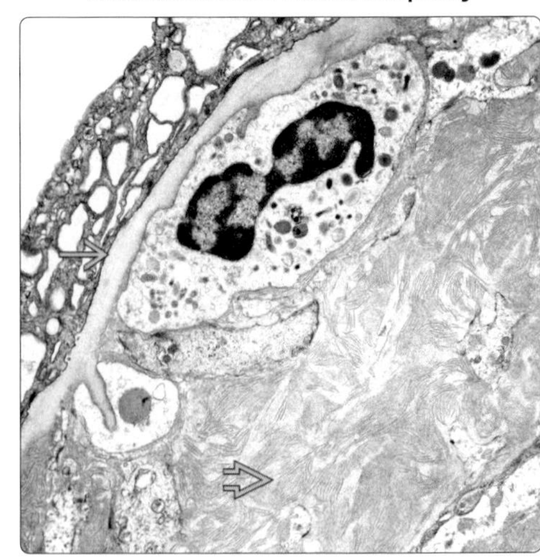

Myocyte Staining in MIDD

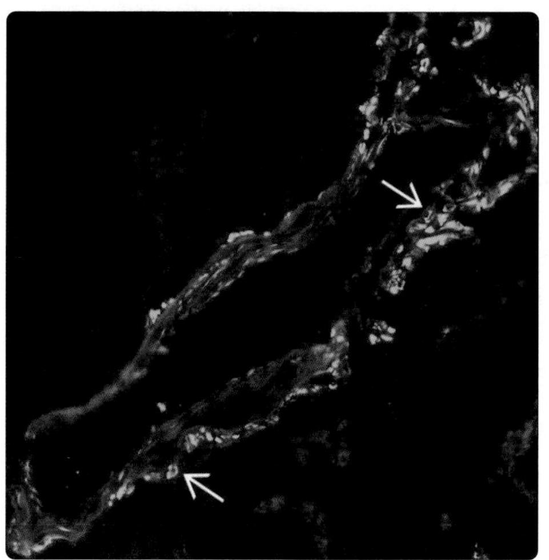

Myocyte Staining in MIDD

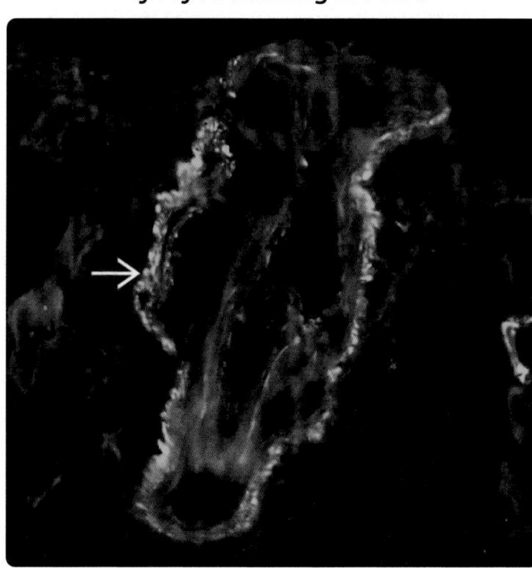

(Left) *An IF stain for IgG2 shows staining surrounding myocytes ➡ in an interlobular artery in light and heavy chain deposition disease. Similar positive staining was present for IgG and kappa light chain. Stains for IgG1, IgG3, IgG4, and lambda were negative.* **(Right)** *An IF stain for kappa light chain shows positive staining surrounding arterial myocytes ➡, a pattern in contrast to amyloidosis, which shows staining of amorphous material. A Congo red stain was negative in this case, including in reprocessed frozen tissue.*

Recurrent LCDD in Transplant

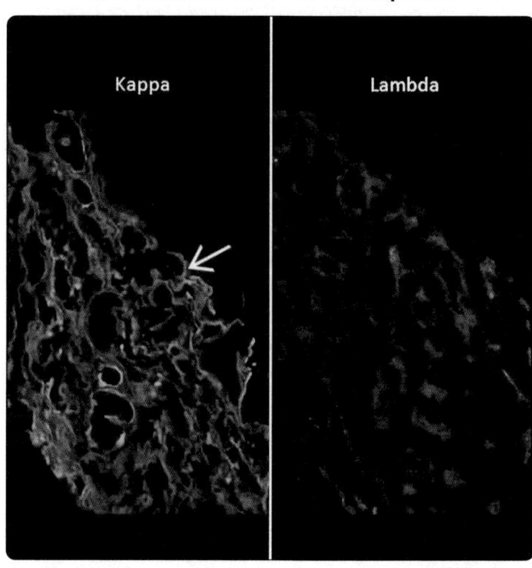

Recurrent LHCDD in Transplant

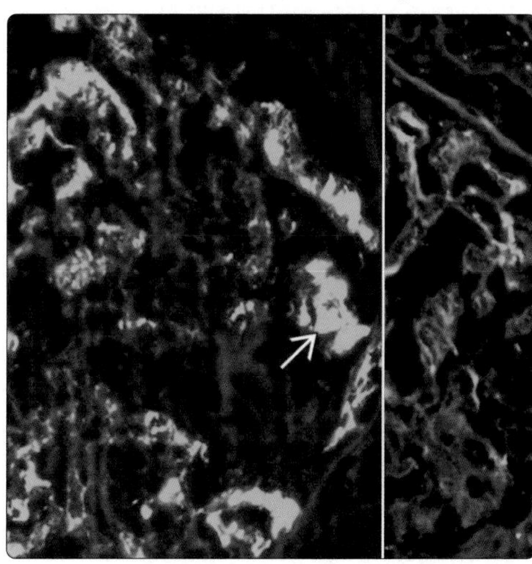

(Left) *Immunofluorescence staining for kappa light chain in a kidney transplant shows bright linear TBM staining for kappa light chain ➡. The stain for lambda is negative.* **(Right)** *Recurrent HL MIDD 28 days post transplant showed striking intracapillary deposits of κ ➡ (left) but not λ (right) light chains. γ heavy chain was also present. The native kidney had nodular glomerulosclerosis but reportedly did not stain for light or heavy chains.*

Recurrent LCDD in Renal Transplant

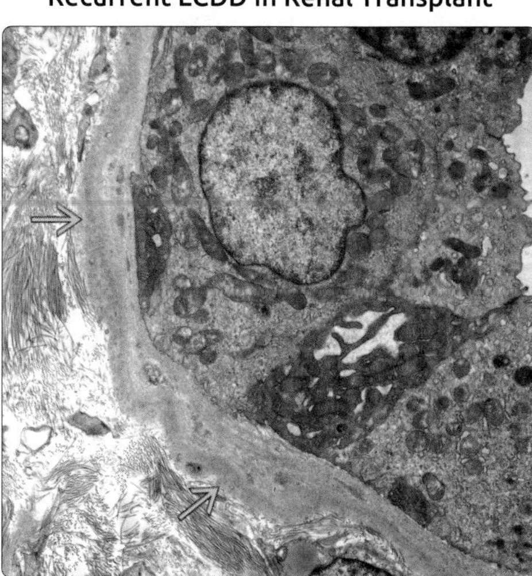

HCDD by Immunofluorescence Only

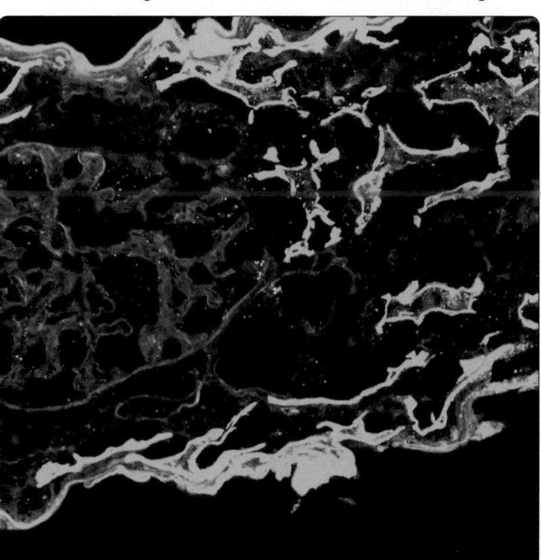

(Left) *EM shows early LCDD in a kidney 1.5 years post transplant. By IF, there was bright linear GBM and TBM staining for kappa light chain with negative lambda. Note the finely granular TBM deposits ⇨, which may be only focal by EM.* **(Right)** *MIDD "by immunofluorescence only" with linear TBM staining for IgG is seen on a protocol biopsy 5 years after kidney transplantation. Stains for kappa and lambda light chains were negative, and EM did not show deposits. The patient did not have a paraprotein by immunofixation.*

Proliferative Glomerulonephritis With Monoclonal IgG Deposits

KEY FACTS

TERMINOLOGY

- Proliferative glomerulonephritis with monoclonal IgG deposits (PGNMID); may have membranoproliferative, endocapillary, or membranous pattern

CLINICAL ISSUES

- Nephrotic-range proteinuria (~ 70%)
- Renal dysfunction (~ 65%)
- Rarely associated with multiple myeloma
- May recur in allograft
- Female predominance, 2:1

MICROSCOPIC

- Membranoproliferative pattern in 57%
- Endocapillary proliferative pattern in 35%
- Membranous or mesangial proliferative patterns less common
- ~ 30% show focal or diffuse crescents
- Focal segmental glomerulosclerosis may be present

ANCILLARY TESTS

- Single IgG subclass restriction, usually IgG3
  - Light chain restricted, usually kappa
- Predominantly mesangial and subendothelial, electron-dense deposits by EM
- Serum or urine monoclonal protein in ~ 30%
- Negative staining for IgA and IgM

TOP DIFFERENTIAL DIAGNOSES

- Membranoproliferative glomerulonephritis (with polyclonal deposits)
- Proliferative glomerulonephritis with monoclonal IgA
- Membranous glomerulonephritis (with polyclonal deposits)
- Membranous-like glomerulonephritis with masked IgG kappa deposits
- Light and heavy chain deposition disease
- Type 1 cryoglobulinemic glomerulonephritis
- Fibrillary or immunotactoid glomerulonephritis

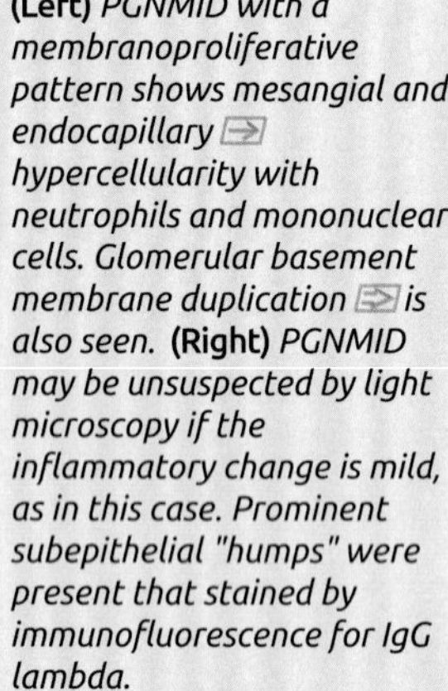

(Left) *PGNMID with a membranoproliferative pattern shows mesangial and endocapillary ➡ hypercellularity with neutrophils and mononuclear cells. Glomerular basement membrane duplication ➡ is also seen.* **(Right)** *PGNMID may be unsuspected by light microscopy if the inflammatory change is mild, as in this case. Prominent subepithelial "humps" were present that stained by immunofluorescence for IgG lambda.*

Endocapillary Hypercellularity

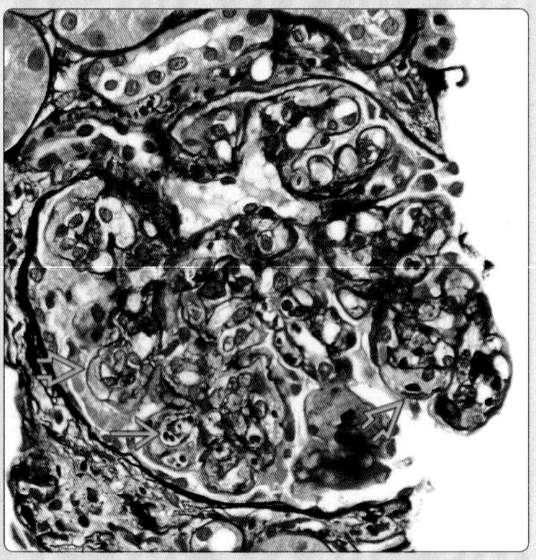

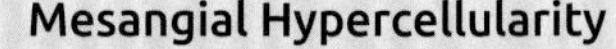

Mesangial Hypercellularity

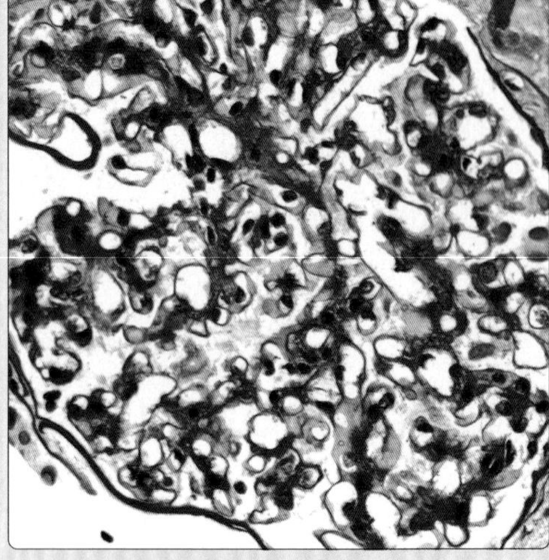

(Left) *Immunofluorescence staining reveals predominantly glomerular basement membrane ➡ granular staining for IgG3, here with a membranous pattern in areas. Staining of glomeruli was negative for IgG1, IgG2, and IgG4.* **(Right)** *Electron micrograph from a case of PGNMID with a membranoproliferative pattern shows subendothelial electron-dense deposits ➡ that appear almost intramembranous.*

IgG3

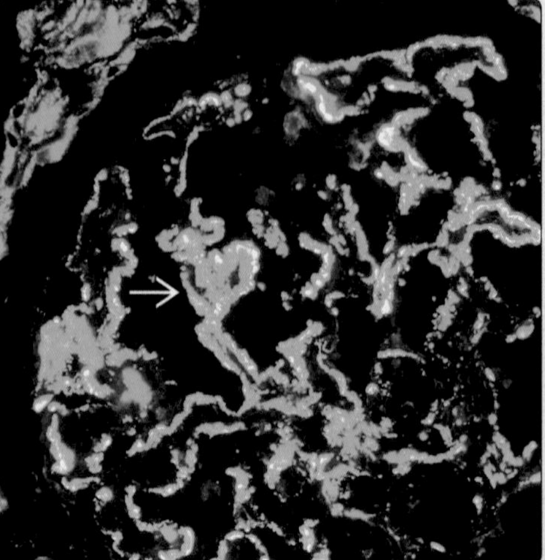

Subendothelial Deposits

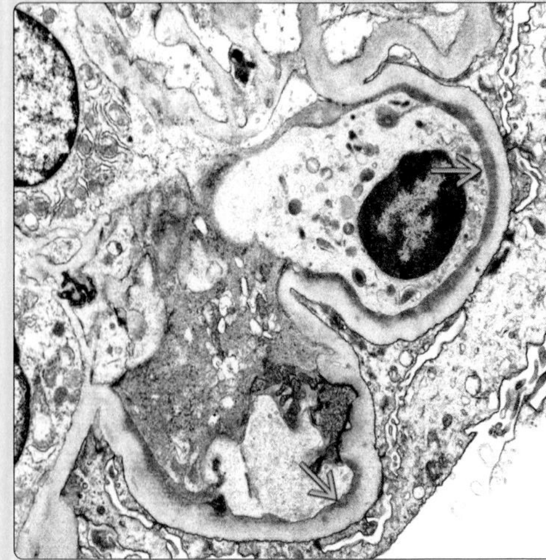

TERMINOLOGY

Synonyms

- Nasr glomerulopathy

Definitions

- Proliferative glomerulonephritis with monoclonal IgG deposits (PGNMID); may have membranoproliferative, endocapillary, or membranous pattern

ETIOLOGY/PATHOGENESIS

Monoclonal IgG Glomerular Deposition

- IgG3 kappa, typically
  - IgG3 highly complement fixing and may be more nephritogenic

CLINICAL ISSUES

Epidemiology

- Age
  - Average: 55 years; range: 20-81 years
- Sex
  - Female predominance, 2:1

Presentation

- Nephrotic-range proteinuria (~ 70%)
  - Nephrotic syndrome (~ 50%)
- Hematuria
- Renal dysfunction (~ 65%)
- Rarely associated with multiple myeloma
- May recur in allograft

Laboratory Tests

- Serum and urine monoclonal proteins in ~ 30%
- Negative for cryoglobulinemia
- Low C3 (± C4) in ~ 25%

Treatment

- Drugs
  - Steroids alone or with other immunosuppressive agents
  - Angiotensin-converting enzyme inhibitor or angiotensin II receptor blocker

Prognosis

- ~ 40% show partial or complete recovery
- ~ 20% progress to end-stage renal disease

MICROSCOPIC

Histologic Features

- Membranoproliferative pattern (57%)
  - Diffuse glomerular basement membrane duplication
  - Mesangial hypercellularity and matrix expansion
  - ± membranous or endocapillary proliferative patterns
- Endocapillary proliferative pattern (35%)
  - ± membranoproliferative or membranous patterns
- Membranous pattern in 5%
  - Global subepithelial immune deposits
  - Usually some proliferative features
- Mesangial proliferative pattern in 3%
- ~ 30% show focal or diffuse crescents
- Focal segmental glomerulosclerosis may be present

ANCILLARY TESTS

Immunofluorescence

- IgG subclass staining
  - IgG3 subclass restriction most common
  - IgG1 subclass 2nd most common
  - No IgG4 subclass restriction identified yet
  - Restriction of single IgG subclass required for diagnosis
- Monotypic IgG kappa or lambda staining
  - Kappa light chain restricted (73%)
- Granular mesangial and GBM staining
- C3 almost always present; C1q present in ~ 60%

Electron Microscopy

- Electron-dense deposits
  - Predominantly mesangial and subendothelial
  - Occasional subepithelial deposits (membranous pattern, segmentally)
  - Deposits mostly amorphous
    - Rare organized deposits present in some

DIFFERENTIAL DIAGNOSIS

Membranoproliferative Glomerulonephritis (MPGN)

- Polytypic deposits staining for kappa and lambda light chains

Membranous Glomerulonephritis (MGN)

- Polytypic deposits staining for kappa and lambda light chains
- Some PGNMID have predominantly membranous pattern
  - Usually some endocapillary proliferation

Proliferative GN Secondary to Monoclonal IgA

- Similar to PGNMID but with monoclonal IgA instead of IgG

Type 1 Cryoglobulinemic Glomerulonephritis

- Similar to PGNMID; type 1 cryoglobulin usually IgG3
- Intraluminal "pseudothrombi" in glomeruli
- Positive test for cryoglobulinemia

Membranous-Like Glomerulonephritis With Masked IgG Kappa Deposits

- Typically women ~ 25 years with autoimmune phenomena
- C3 staining by routine IF; IgG kappa deposits by pronase IF

Fibrillary or Immunotactoid Glomerulonephritis

- May show monotypic IgG kappa or lambda IF staining
- Fibrils or microtubules by electron microscopy (EM)

SELECTED REFERENCES

1. Larsen CP et al: Membranous-like glomerulopathy with masked IgG kappa deposits. Kidney Int. 86(1):154-61, 2014
2. Nasr SH et al: Proliferative glomerulonephritis with monoclonal IgG deposits recurs in the allograft. Clin J Am Soc Nephrol. 6(1):122-32, 2011
3. Nasr SH et al: Proliferative glomerulonephritis with monoclonal IgG deposits. J Am Soc Nephrol. 20(9):2055-64, 2009
4. Komatsuda A et al: Monoclonal immunoglobulin deposition disease associated with membranous features. Nephrol Dial Transplant. 23(12):3888-94, 2008
5. Nasr SH et al: Proliferative glomerulonephritis with monoclonal IgG deposits: a distinct entity mimicking immune-complex glomerulonephritis. Kidney Int. 65(1):85-96, 2004

(Left) *This example of PGNMID shows nodular mesangial expansion ⇨, mesangial hypercellularity, and glomerular basement membrane duplication ↷.* **(Right)** *Segmental glomerular basement membrane "spikes" → can be seen in this case of PGNMID with a mesangioproliferative and membranous pattern.*

MPGN Pattern

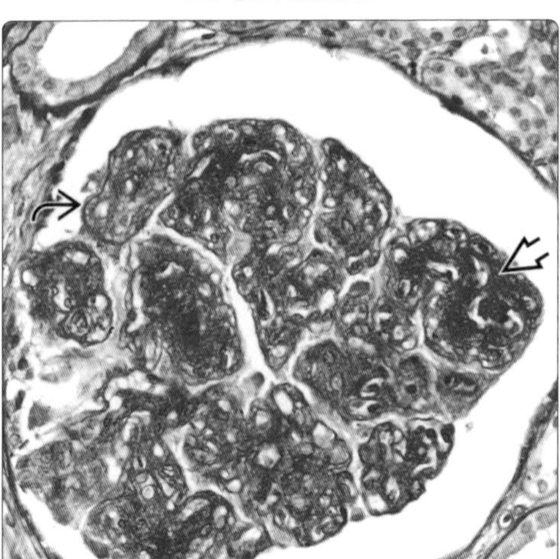

Segmental "Spike" Formation

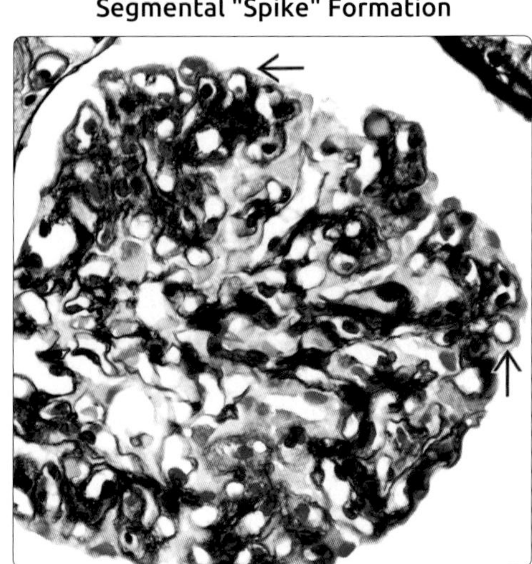

(Left) *Recurrent PGNMID 10 months post transplant shows diffuse endocapillary hypercellularity →, not to be confused with glomerulitis. The patient had proteinuria at 1.8 g/dL.* **(Right)** *Recurrent PGNMID 12 months post transplant shows progressively less endocapillary hypercellularity following treatment with cyclophosphamide; mesangial hypercellularity → is still present. The patient had only ~ 0.13 g/dL proteinuria.*

Endocapillary Hypercellularity

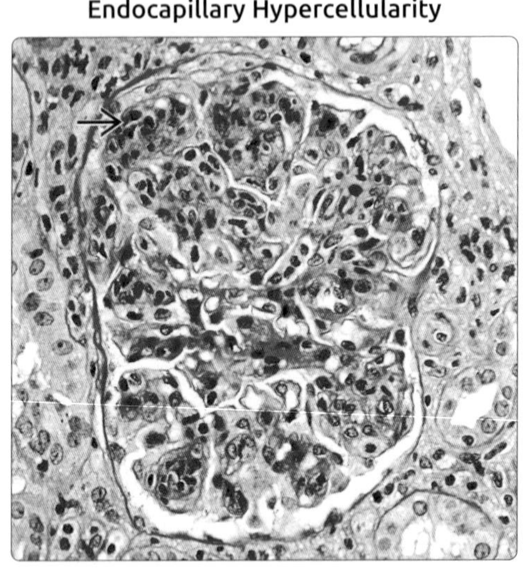

Mesangial Hypercellularity

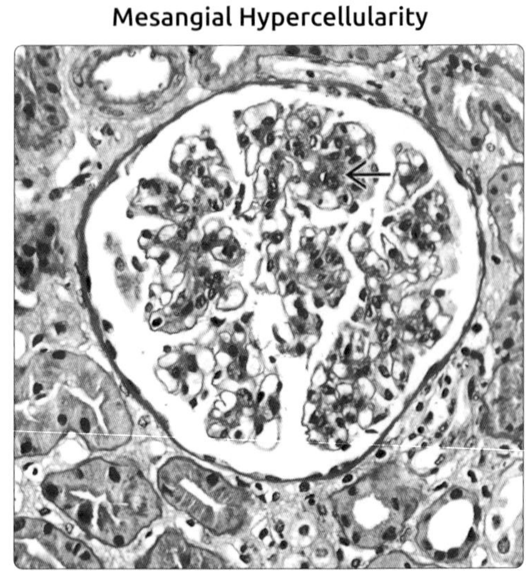

(Left) *PGNMID has a variable light microscopic appearance ranging from mild mesangial hypercellularity and inflammation (shown here) to full-blown acute glomerulonephritis. This case had IgG lambda deposits in subepithelial "humps."* **(Right)** *Immunofluorescence staining for IgG showed granular mesangial and segmental glomerular basement membrane staining. The same pattern was seen for IgG3 but with negative staining for IgG1, IgG2, or IgG4.*

Mild Mesangial Hypercellularity

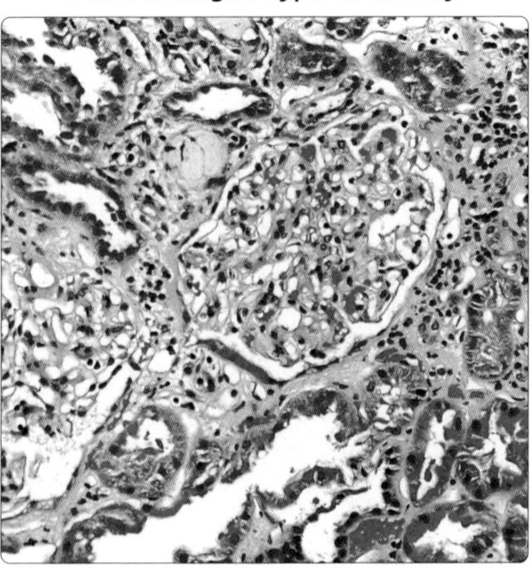

Immunofluorescence for IgG

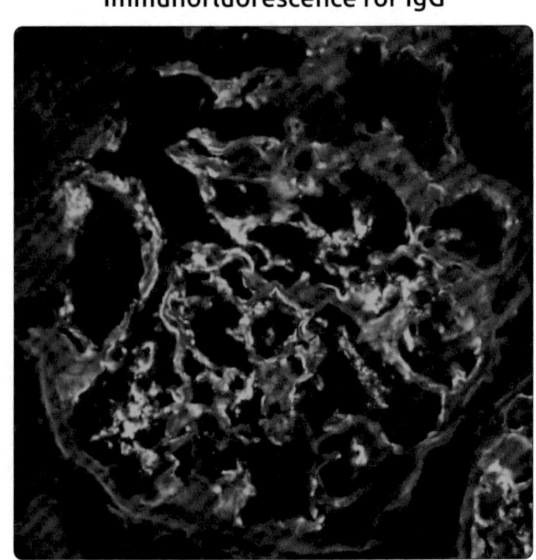

Crescent in PGNMID

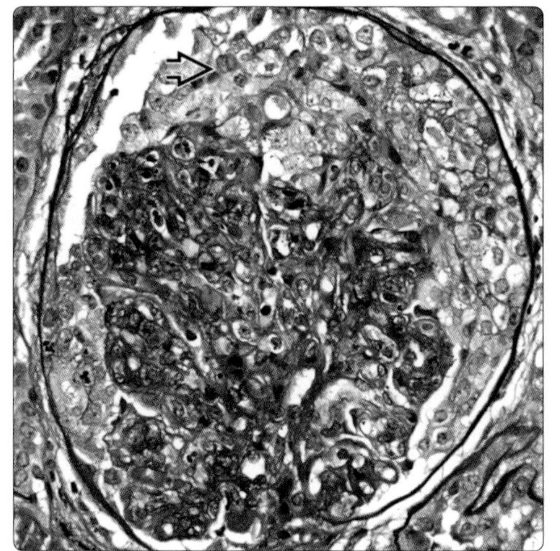

PGNMID With Chronic Lymphocytic Leukemia (CLL)

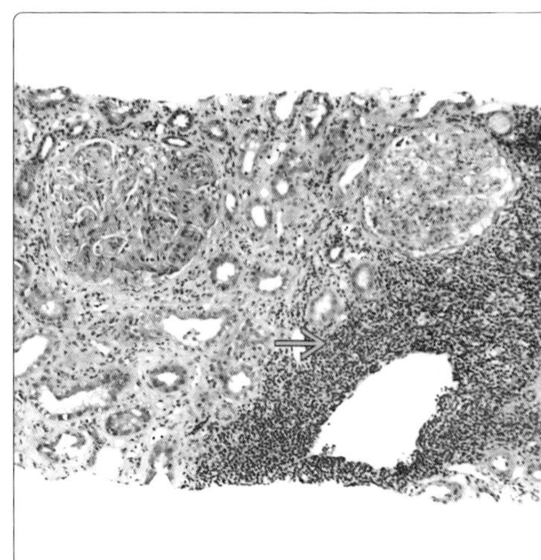

(Left) *This example of PGNMID showed crescents →, which are present focally or diffusely in ~ 30% of PGNMID. (Courtesy S. Nasr, MD.)* **(Right)** *In this case, PGNMID was present in glomeruli, and CLL → was present in the interstitium. Note the monomorphous small lymphocytes. (Courtesy S. Nasr, MD.)*

Mesangial Electron-Dense Deposits

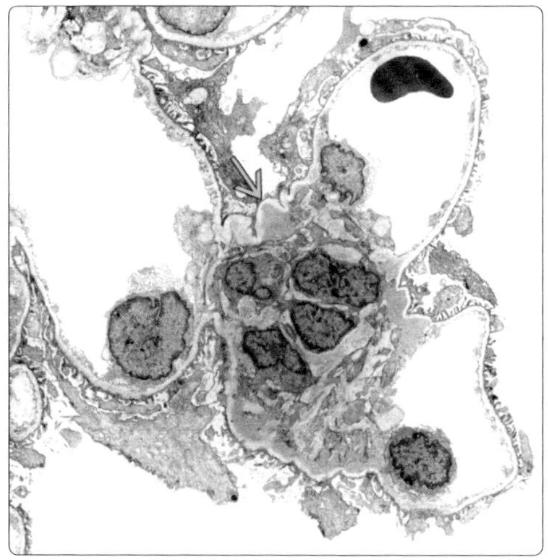

Subepithelial Electron-Dense Deposits

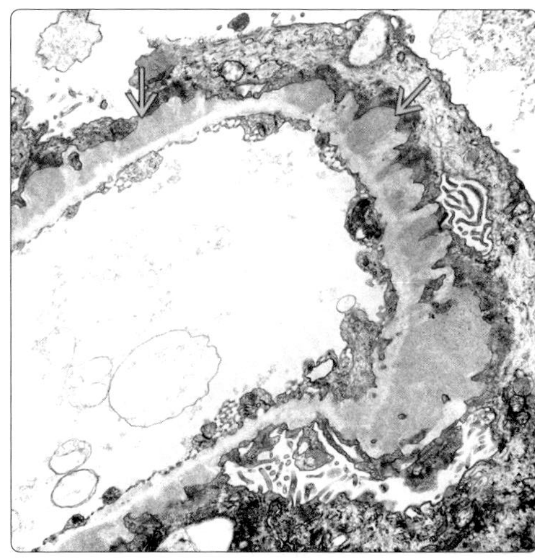

(Left) *Mesangioproliferative pattern of PGNMID shows mesangial hypercellularity and mesangial electron-dense deposits →. The glomerular capillary loops are largely free of deposits in this example.* **(Right)** *This case of PGNMID showed a predominantly membranous pattern with regularly spaced subepithelial, electron-dense deposits → with intervening basement membrane "spikes." By IF, the deposits showed staining for IgG2 kappa. There was rare endocapillary proliferation and a rare small cellular crescent by light microscopy.*

Subepithelial "Humps"

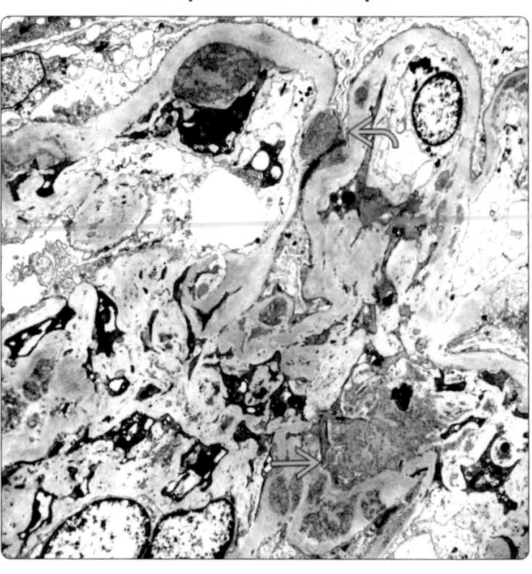

Subendothelial Electron-Dense Deposits

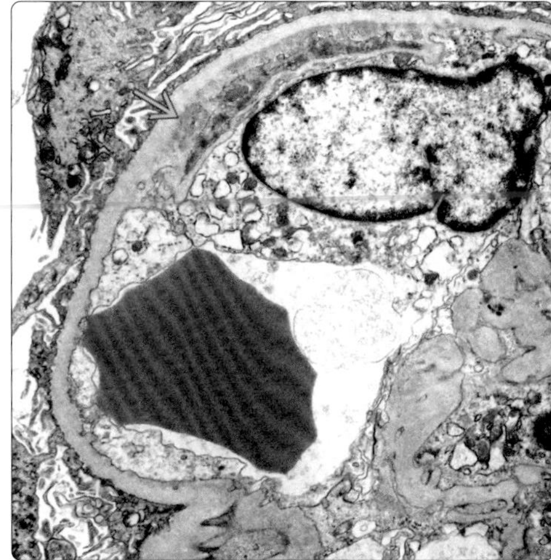

(Left) *Low-power EM shows widespread variegated deposits in the mesangium → and subepithelial "humps" → in a patient with PGNMID that stained for IgG lambda.* **(Right)** *An occasional subendothelial electron-dense deposit → is seen, with early glomerular basement membrane duplication, in early recurrent PGNMID in a transplant.*

Membranous Glomerulonephritis With Masked IgG Kappa Deposits

KEY FACTS

TERMINOLOGY

- Glomerular disease with subepithelial and mesangial immune complex-type deposits of IgG kappa type, which shows weak to no staining by routine immunofluorescence

CLINICAL ISSUES

- Most commonly affects young females (~ 25 years)
- Proteinuria in 100% and hematuria in ≥ 90%
- Renal insufficiency in ~ 20%
- > 50% show evidence of sytemic autoimmune disease
- SPEP and UPEP negative for paraprotein
- Normal complement studies in all patients

MICROSCOPIC

- Silver positive glomerular basement membrane (GBM) "spikes" or silver negative GBM "pin holes"
- No endocapillary proliferation
- ~ 20% of cases show cellular crescent formation
- Immunofluorescence
  - Routine IF on fresh tissue reveals predominantly C3 with little to no immunoglobulin
  - Paraffin IF (direct IF on pronase-digested paraffin-embedded tissue) shows strong staining for IgG and kappa
- Electron microscopy
  - Mesangial and subepithelial immune complex-type electron-dense deposits with no subendothelial deposits
  - 50% with hump-like deposits and 57% with hinge region deposits (a.k.a. mesangial waist region)

TOP DIFFERENTIAL DIAGNOSES

- C3 glomerulonephritis
- Infection-associated glomerulonephritis
- Proliferative glomerulonephritis with monoclonal IgG deposits
- Membranous glomerulopathy with monoclonal IgG deposits

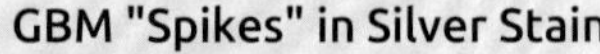

GBM "Spikes" in Silver Stain

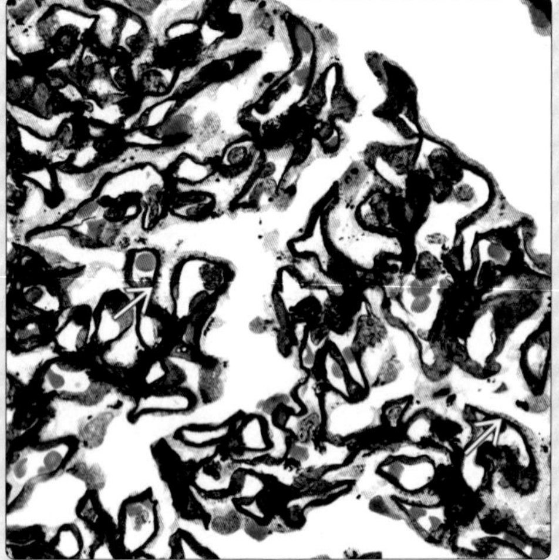

Subepithelial GBM Deposits in Trichrome Stain

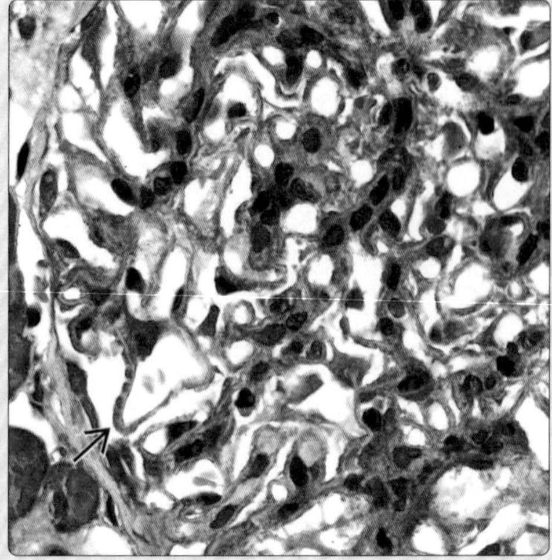

(Left) *"Spikes" are present along the glomerular basement membranes (GBM) by Jones methenamine sliver stain.* **(Right)** *Brightly fuschsinophilic subepithelial deposits are evident by Masson trichrome stain. This pattern is indistinguishable from idiopathic membranous glomerulopathy.*

Widespread IgG Deposits in GBM After Pronase

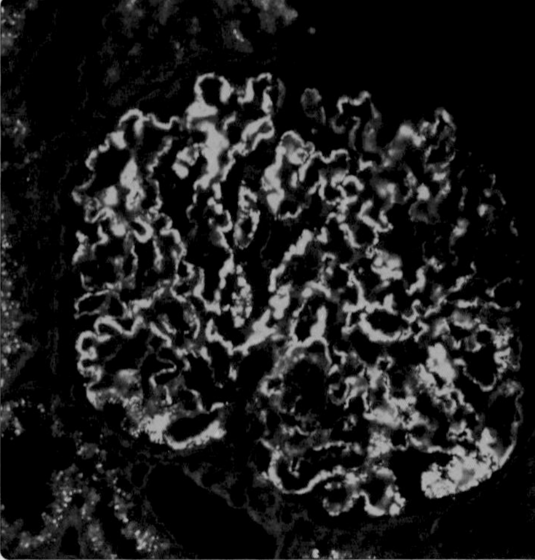

Subepithelial Deposits With GBM "Spikes"

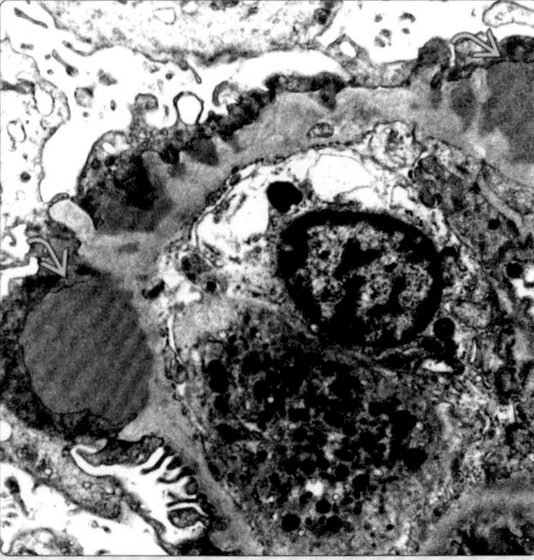

(Left) *Glomerulus with granular capillary loop IgG staining on pronase-digested tissue is shown. This biopsy had only C3 and no immunoglobulin detectable in the deposits in routine immunofluorescence. Kappa light chain showed a similar pattern and lambda light chain was negative.* **(Right)** *Large, amorphous subepithelial deposits along the GBM with surrounding "spikes" of basement membrane are typical of this disease, as are mesangial deposits (not shown).*

TERMINOLOGY

Abbreviations

- Membranous-like glomerulopathy with masked IgG kappa deposits (MGMID)

Synonyms

- Masked monoclonal membranous-like glomerulopathy (MMMG)

Definitions

- Glomerular disease with subepithelial and mesangial immune complex-type deposits of IgG kappa type, which shows weak to no staining by routine immunofluorescence

ETIOLOGY/PATHOGENESIS

Immunologic

- Posited to be autoimmune given the high incidence of other autoimmune phenomena and lack of infection
- Antigen unknown, but probably not PLA2R of idiopathic membranous glomerulopathy

CLINICAL ISSUES

Epidemiology

- Incidence < 1% of renal biopsies
- Average age: ~ 25 years
- F:M = 6:1

Presentation

- Proteinuria (100%)
    - Nephrotic (36%)
- Hematuria (> 90%)
- Renal insufficiency in ~ 20%
- Autoimmune findings in 62%
    - Weak ANA in ~ 42%
    - History of autoimmune disease in 36%
        - Hemolytic anemia 2/14; SLE 2/14, ITP 1/14
- ANCA-negative including those with crescents
- SPEP and UPEP negative for monoclonal immunoglobulins
- No evidence of infection
- Normal complement levels

Treatment

- Drugs
    - Not yet established, presumably similar to idiopathic membranous glomerulopathy

Prognosis

- Uncertain
- 6 of 9 patients with persistent kidney disease at mean of 14.9 months follow-up

MICROSCOPIC

Histologic Features

- Silver positive glomerular basement membrane (GBM) "spikes" or silver negative GBM "pin holes"
    - 36% segmental glomerular involvement
    - 64% global glomerular involvement
- Subepithelial deposits frequently visible on Masson trichrome staining
- Mesangial expansion and hypercellularity common
- ~ 20% of cases show cellular crescent formation
- No endocapillary proliferation
- GBM duplication not present

ANCILLARY TESTS

Immunofluorescence

- Routine IF on fresh tissue
    - Moderate to strong staining by C3 in 64% of cases
    - Weak to no staining for immunoglobulins and light chains by routine IF
        - ~ 82% negative IgG; 9% trace, 9% 1+ IgG
- Paraffin immunofluorescence (direct IF on pronase-digested paraffin-embedded tissue)
    - Strong mesangial and capillary loop staining for IgG and kappa (2-3+)
    - Negative staining for lambda light chains (100%)
- Reason for negative routine IF is unknown
- All cases lack PLA2R in deposits

Electron Microscopy

- Mesangial and subepithelial immune complex-type electron-dense deposits
- No subendothelial deposits
- 50% with hump-like deposits and 57% with hinge region deposits (a.k.a. mesangial waist region)

DIFFERENTIAL DIAGNOSIS

C3 Glomerulonephritis

- Little or no immunoglobulin by routine or by paraffin IF
- Clinical history of hypocomplementemia common

Infection-Associated Glomerulonephritis

- Typically endocapillary proliferation by LM
- Hypocomplementemia and history of recent infection common
- Immunoglobulin deposits in routine and paraffin IF

Proliferative Glomerulonephritis With Monoclonal IgG Deposits (PGNMID)

- IgG deposition with light chain restriction by routine IF
- Endocapillary proliferation by LM with subendothelial deposits by EM
- Typically affects elderly patients (mean age of 67.3 years vs. 25.7 for MGMID)

Membranous Glomerulopathy With Monoclonal IgG Deposits

- Immunoglobulins stain by routine and paraffin IF
- Elderly patients (mean age of 69.2 years vs. 25.7 for MGMID)

Membranous Glomerulopathy, Non-PLA2R

- Immunoglobulin in routine and paraffin IF

SELECTED REFERENCES

1. Larsen CP et al: Membranous-like glomerulopathy with masked IgG kappa deposits. Kidney Int. 86(1):154-61, 2014

(Left) *Representative glomerular photomicrograph shows a case of MGMID. Note the glomerular tuft with surrounding cellular crescent. Close examination reveals "spikes" along the capillary loops. Approximately 20% of MGMID cases have crescents on Jones methenamine silver stain.* **(Right)** *MGMID typically has strongly positive staining for C3 in mesangium and capillary loops by routine immunofluorescence. However, 7% have negative glomerular staining for C3, and only 1+ in 29%.*

Cellular Crescent

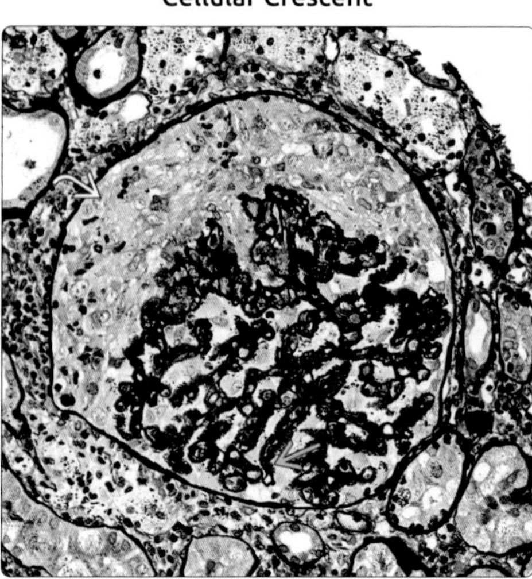

C3 Deposition in Routine IF

(Left) *Negative IgG stain by routine immunofluorescence in a glomerulus in a case of MGMID is shown. Tubular reabsorption droplets serve as a positive control.* **(Right)** *Glomerulus from the same case of MGMID shows strong granular capillary loop staining for IgG on the pronase-digested tissue.*

Negative IgG in Routine Frozen Section

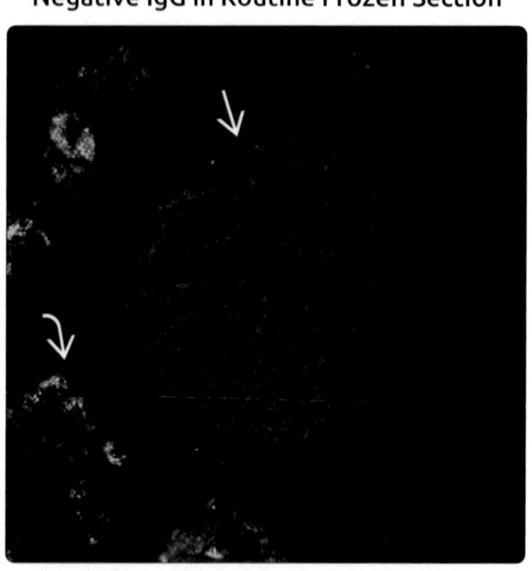

IgG Deposits Revealed After Pronase Digestion

(Left) *Representative glomerular photomicrograph shows a case of MGMID. Granular capillary loop staining by kappa is revealed after pronase-digestion of the paraffin embedded tissue. This stain was negative on routine frozen sections.* **(Right)** *Lambda light chain stain is negative in a glomerulus in the same patient even after pronase-digestion. The kappa stain was strongly positive in the same distribution as IgG.*

Kappa Light Chain Deposition After Pronase

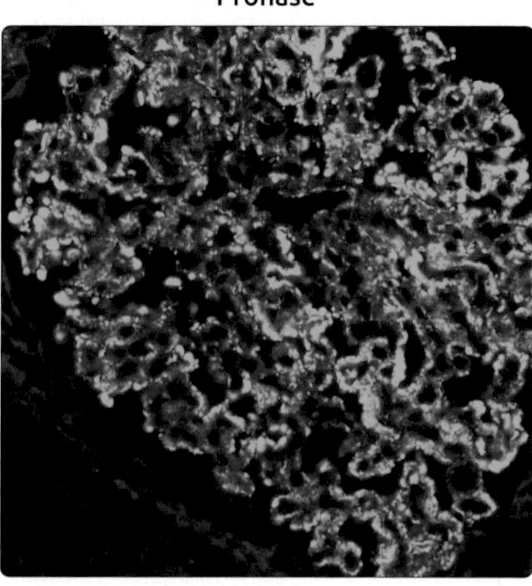

Negative Lambda Stain After Pronase

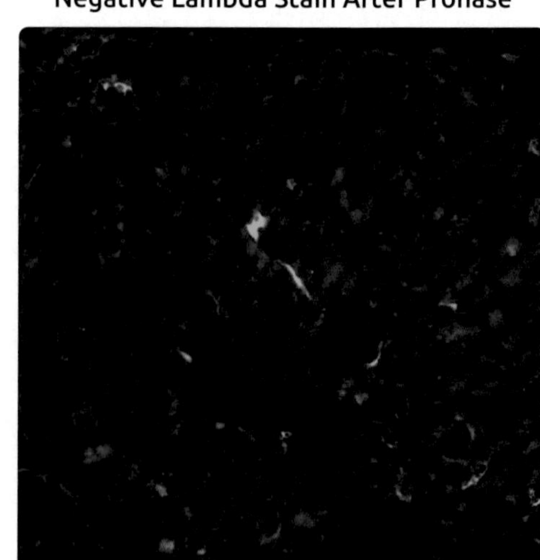

Subepithelial Deposits

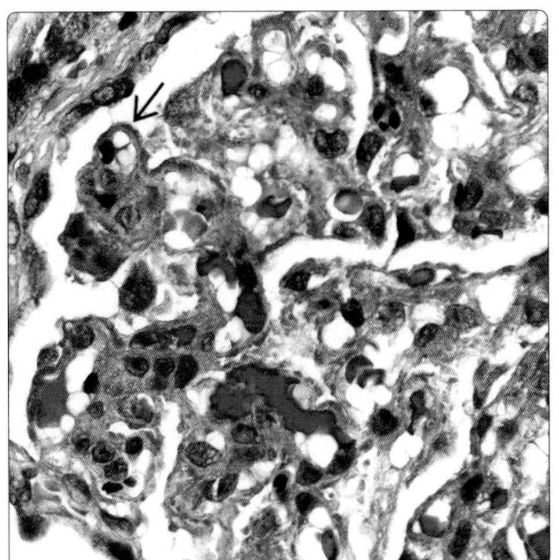

GBM "Spikes"

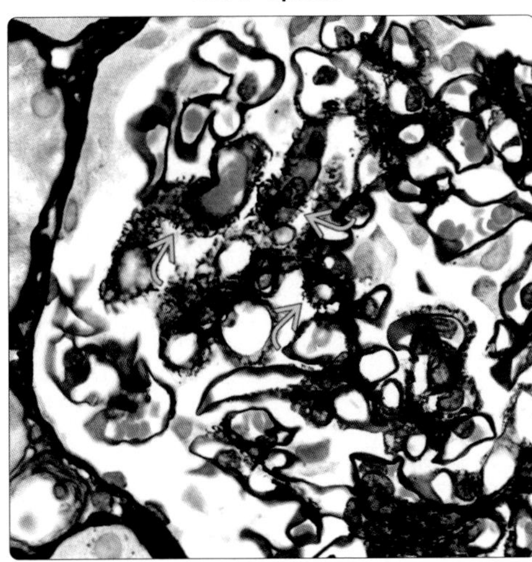

(Left) *Fuschsinophilic subepithelial deposits ⇨ can be seen by Masson trichrome stain.* **(Right)** *Glomerular basement membrane "spikes" are easily identified ⇨ in this case of MGMID by Jones methenamine sliver stain.*

Subepithelial Deposits

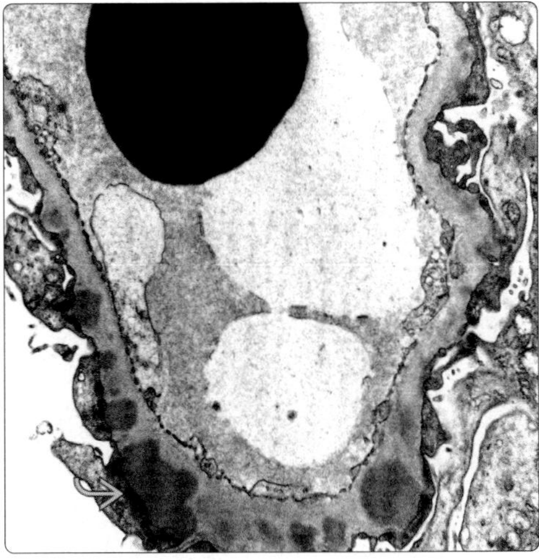

Hump-Like Deposits

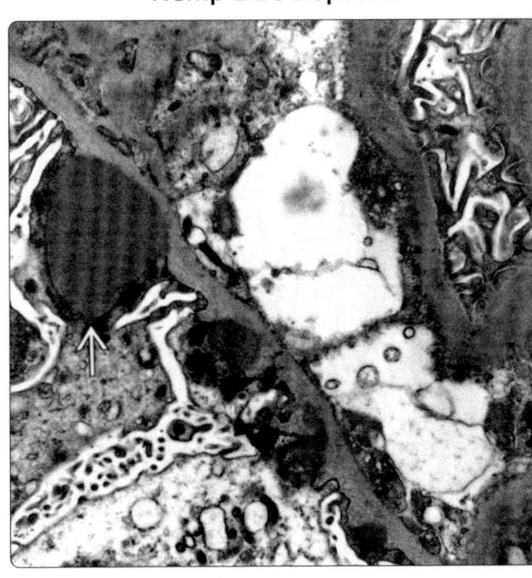

(Left) *Subepithelial deposits ⇨ typical of membranous glomerulopathy are seen in this case of MGMID. Tubuloreticular structures in endothelium, typical of lupus nephritis, are not present.* **(Right)** *Large, hump-like subepithelial deposits without "spikes" along the glomerular basement membranes ➡ are present in half of MGMID cases.*

Deposits in Hinge Region

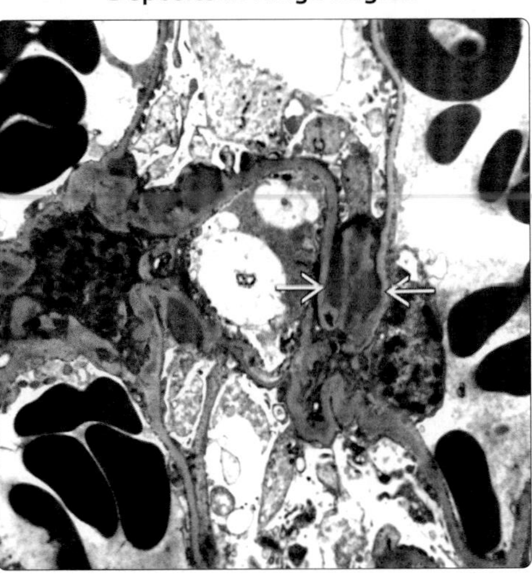

Mesangial Deposits

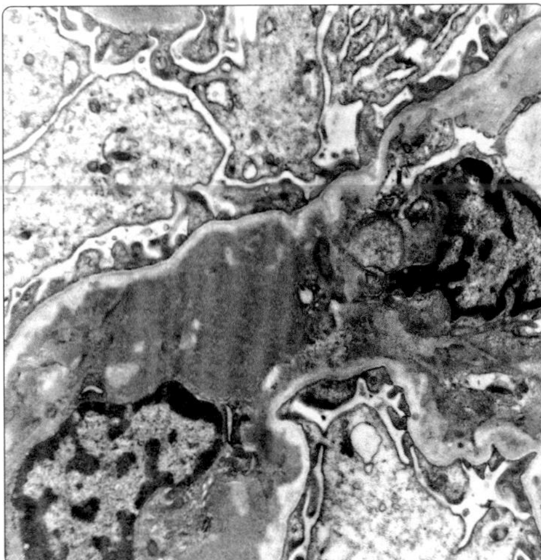

(Left) *Hinge region deposits, such as the ones pictured here ➡, are present in over half of MGMID cases.* **(Right)** *Mesangial deposits, such as the ones pictured here, are present in over 90% of MGMID cases.*

Type I Cryoglobulinemic Glomerulonephritis

KEY FACTS

TERMINOLOGY

- GN caused by monoclonal immunoglobulin cryoproteins

ETIOLOGY/PATHOGENESIS

- Intravascular precipitates obstruct blood flow, fix complement

CLINICAL ISSUES

- ~ 60% lymphoproliferative disease/40% MGUS
- 30% with symptomatic type I cryoglobulinemia develop renal disease
  - Nephrotic syndrome (70%)
  - Acute kidney injury (75%)
  - No extrarenal symptoms (45%)
- Cutaneous vasculitis, neuropathy, arthritis
- Serum/plasma cryoprecipitate at 4° C; monoclonal Ig
- Hypocomplementemia
- Partial remissions with cytoreduction, other agents
- Adverse risk factors: age > 60 years, malignancy

MICROSCOPIC

- Membranoproliferative GN
- Intracapillary pseudothrombi (hyaline thrombi)
- Congo red stain negative
- IF: Granular glomerular deposits stain for 1 light chain and 1 heavy chain, ±C3, C1q
  - > 90% kappa light chain and ~ 85% IgG
  - Pseudothrombi same pattern, fibrin negative
- EM: Fibrillary or microtubular deposits

TOP DIFFERENTIAL DIAGNOSES

- Type II mixed cryoglobulinemia
- Proliferative GN with monoclonal IgG deposits
- Fibrillary or immunotactoid glomerulonephritis
- Thrombotic microangiopathy

DIAGNOSTIC CHECKLIST

- Light chain stains essential in evaluation of GN
- PAS stain useful to highlight pseudothrombi

Pseudothrombi

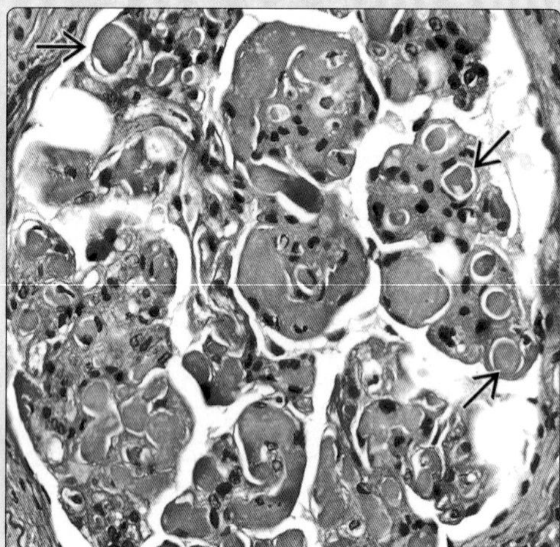

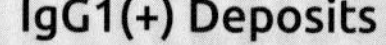

IgG1(+) Deposits

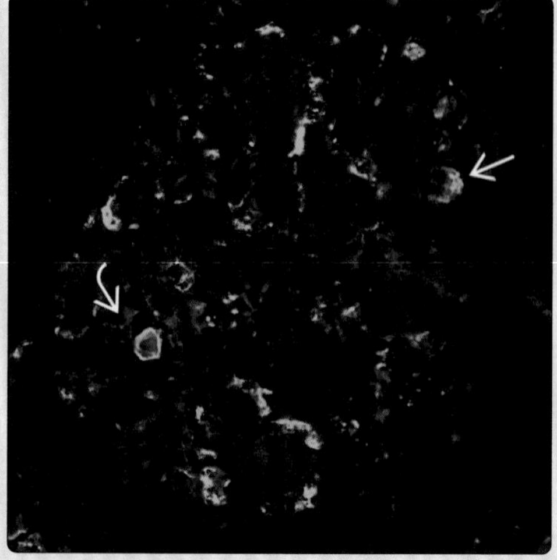

(Left) *Type I cryoglobulinemic GN shows occlusive deposition of monoclonal immunoglobuin ⇒ within glomerular capillary lumina, resembling thrombi. These are known as "pseudothrombi," since they do not consist of fibrin. These are best seen in PAS stains as in this image.* **(Right)** *Immunofluorescence shows pseudothrombi ➡ and subendothelial ➡ deposits stain predominantly for IgG1 in a patient with type I cryoglobulinemia. C3 and C1q were also strongly positive.*

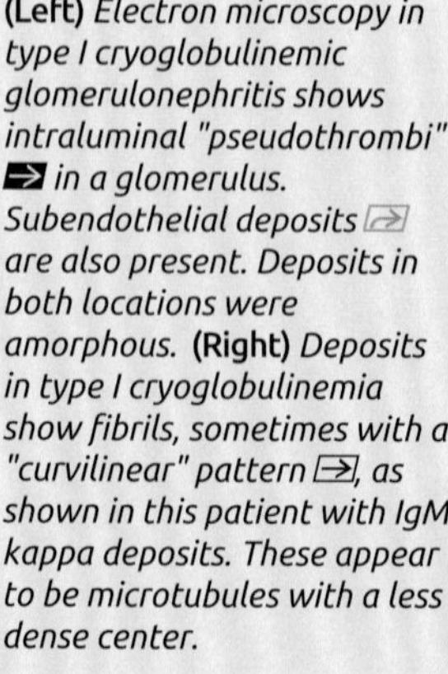

Pseudothrombi

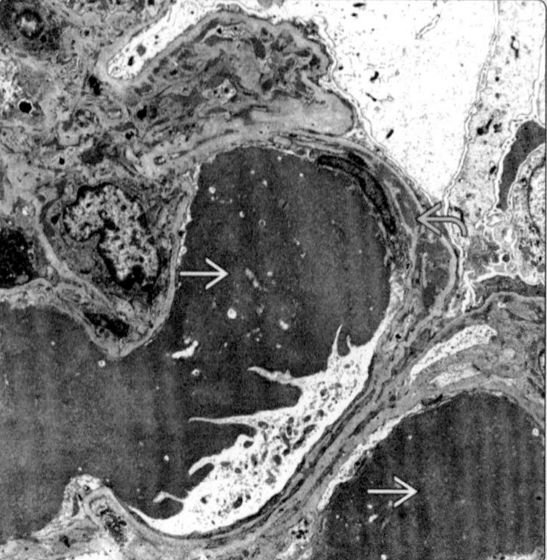

Curvilinear Structured Deposits

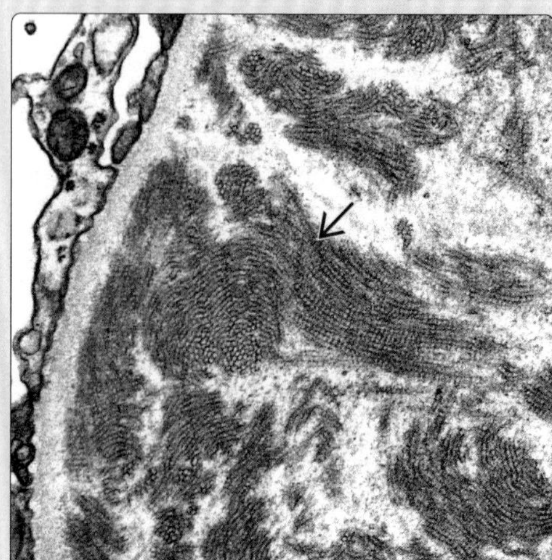

(Left) *Electron microscopy in type I cryoglobulinemic glomerulonephritis shows intraluminal "pseudothrombi" ➡ in a glomerulus. Subendothelial deposits ⇒ are also present. Deposits in both locations were amorphous.* **(Right)** *Deposits in type I cryoglobulinemia show fibrils, sometimes with a "curvilinear" pattern ⇒, as shown in this patient with IgM kappa deposits. These appear to be microtubules with a less dense center.*

TERMINOLOGY

Definitions

- Glomerulonephritis (GN) caused by cryoproteins derived from monoclonal immunoglobulins
- Cryoglobulins precipitate at 4° C in vitro, redissolve at 37° C

ETIOLOGY/PATHOGENESIS

Monoclonal Immunoglobulin Precipitation

- Aggregates obstruct blood flow, fix complement

Underlying B-Cell Clonal Proliferation

- Waldenström macroglobulinemia (25%)
- Multiple myeloma (16%)
- Low-grade non-Hodgkin B-cell lymphoma (15%)
- Chronic lymphatic leukemia (3%)
- Nonmalignant monoclonal gammopathy (MGUS) (41%)

CLINICAL ISSUES

Epidemiology

- Incidence
  - Rare (~ 1:1 million)
  - 10-20% of cryoglobulins are type I
    - Usually asymptomatic (84%)

Presentation

- 30% with symptoms have kidney involvement
  - Nephrotic syndrome (70%)
  - Acute kidney injury (75%)
  - No extrarenal involvement (45%)
- Purpura/cutaneous vasculitis/ulcers (86%)
- Peripheral neuropathy, Raynaud phenomenon (44%)
- Arthralgias/arthritis (28%)

Laboratory Tests

- Cryoprecipitate positive (0.1-10 g/L); monoclonal Ig
  - May have false-negative from pre-test cooling
- 81% low C4, 36% low C3

Treatment

- Cytoreduction, plasmapheresis, rituximab and other agents
- Cytoreduction therapy can precipitate symptoms

Prognosis

- 5-year survival 82-94%
- Adverse risk factors: Underlying malignancy, age > 60 years
- Nephropathy more severe with IgG than IgM

MICROSCOPIC

Histologic Features

- Glomeruli
  - Intracapillary PAS(+) pseudothrombi (hyaline thrombi)
  - Membranoproliferative GN
    - Mesangial hypercellularity, sometimes nodular
    - GBM duplication
  - Endocapillary hypercellularity
    - Monocytes/macrophages (CD68[+]) prominent
    - Swollen endothelial cells
  - Sometimes crescents
  - Congo red stain negative
- Interstitium and tubules
  - May be myeloma casts, rarely crystals
- Vessels
  - Vasculitis may be present, rarely crystals/thrombi

ANCILLARY TESTS

Immunofluorescence

- Granular GBM and mesangial deposits that stain for 1 light chain and 1 heavy chain, C3 and often C1q
  - 85% IgG (including IgG3), 15% IgM, rare IgA + IgG
  - > 90% kappa light chain
- Pseudothrombi have same IF pattern
  - Fibrin negative in contrast to true thrombi

Electron Microscopy

- Intracapillary, subendothelial, mesangial, &/or subepithelial deposits with substructure
  - Fibrillary (~ 50%) or microtubular (~ 25%) deposits
    - Straight, curved/aggregated in bundles, fingerprint or amorphous
    - Similar appearance in cryoprecipitate in vitro
  - Rarely intracytoplasmic crystals, "cryocrystalglobulinemia"
- Endothelial cells reactive; sometimes destroyed

DIFFERENTIAL DIAGNOSIS

Type II Mixed Cryoglobulinemia

- Both kappa and lambda in deposits
- Often HCV associated

Fibrillary and Immunotactoid GN

- Lack circulating cryoglobulins, pseudothrombi
- Some have monotypic light chains

Proliferative GN With Monoclonal IgG Deposits

- Lacks cryoglobulins, pseudothrombi
- Usually amorphous deposits

Thrombotic Microangiopathy

- Thrombi stain for fibrin; EM 22.5 nm periodicity
- No light chain restriction

DIAGNOSTIC CHECKLIST

Pathologic Interpretation Pearls

- PAS stain useful to highlight pseudothrombi
- Light chain stains essential in evaluation of GN

SELECTED REFERENCES

1. Gupta V et al: Crystalglobulin-Induced Nephropathy. J Am Soc Nephrol. ePub, 2014
2. Néel A et al: Long-term outcome of monoclonal (type 1) cryoglobulinemia. Am J Hematol. 89(2):156-61, 2014
3. Terrier B et al: The spectrum of type I cryoglobulinemia vasculitis: new insights based on 64 cases. Medicine (Baltimore). 92(2):61-8, 2013
4. Favre G et al: Membranoproliferative glomerulonephritis, chronic lymphocytic leukemia, and cryoglobulinemia. Am J Kidney Dis. 55(2):391-4, 2010
5. Karras A et al: Renal involvement in monoclonal (type I) cryoglobulinemia: two cases associated with IgG3 kappa cryoglobulin. Am J Kidney Dis. 40(5):1091-6, 2002

(**Left**) *"Pseudothrombi" are shown in type I CryoGN stain red on trichrome, similar to fibrin thrombi; however, they contain monotypic immunoglobulin.* (**Right**) *Type I CryoGN shows variable intracapillary hypercellularity, mostly due to mononuclear cells. Patient had chronic lymphocytic leukemia with an IgG kappa cryoprotein. Macrophages phagocytose the deposits in cryoglobulinemia, and few may be evident in a biopsy.*

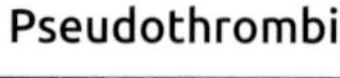

Pseudothrombi

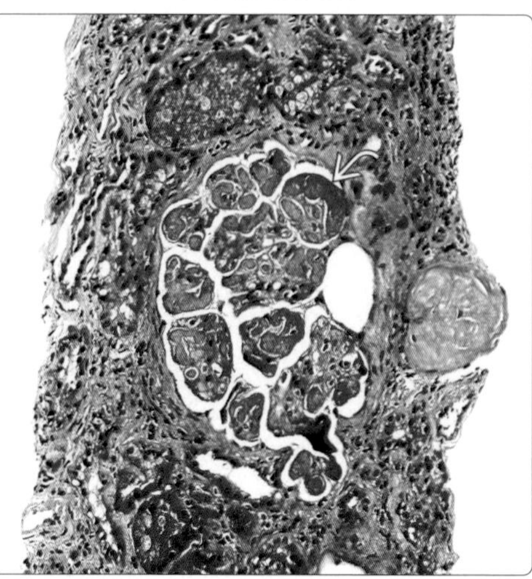

Endocapillary Hypercellularity (Macrophages)

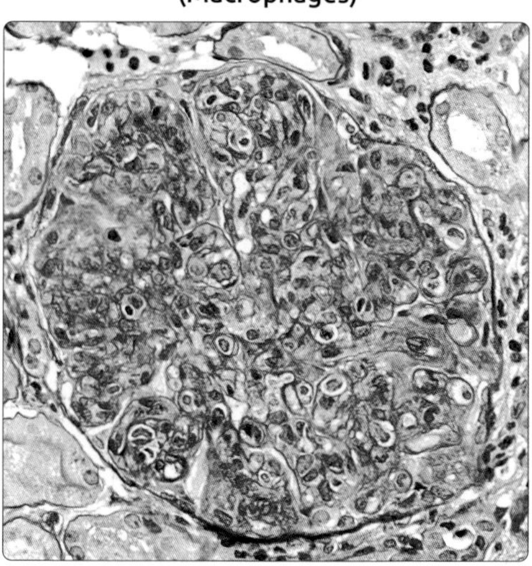

(**Left**) *The differential deposition of light chains is essential to demonstrate in the diagnosis of type I cryoglobulinemic GN. Shown here is immunofluorescence for kappa light chain staining with granular deposits along the GBM. Lambda was negative. The patient had CLL.* (**Right**) *In this case of type I cryoglobulinemic GN, the lambda light chain staining of glomeruli is negative except for rare speckles, but the deposits stained strongly for kappa light chain and gamma heavy chain (IgG).*

Positive Kappa Light Chain

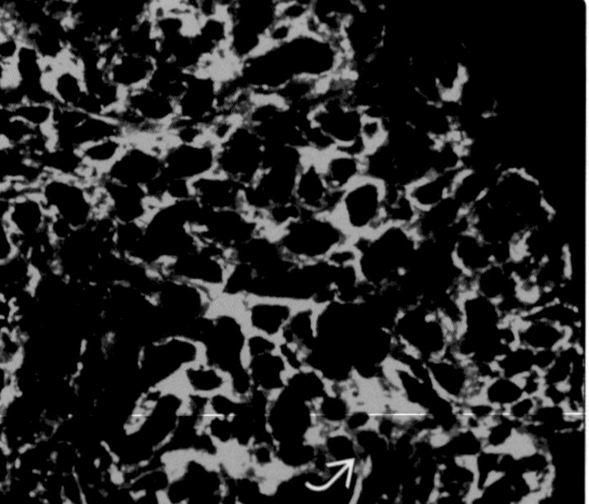

Negative Lambda Light Chain

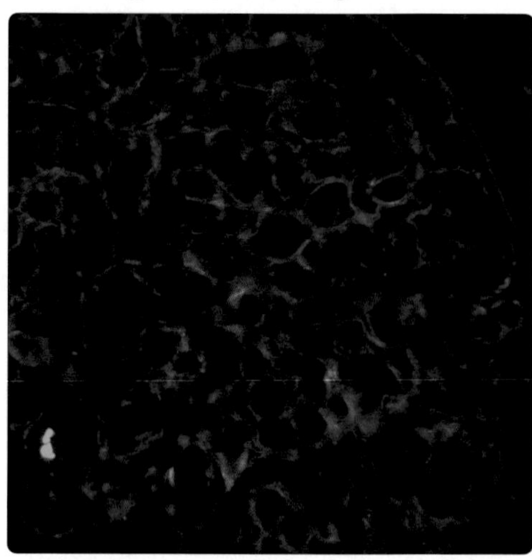

(**Left**) *Immunofluorescence shows a glomerulus in a patient with IgG kappa type I cryoglobulinemia, stained with IgG. Pseudothrombus stains prominently. Other deposits are along the capillary wall and in the mesangium. Underlying condition was MGUS.* (**Right**) *The deposits of type I cryoglobulinemia can fix complement and lead to prominent deposition of C1q (shown here) and C3 in a granular pattern along the GBM and in the mesangium. The glomeruli had an acute GN pattern by light microscopy.*

Pseudothrombus IgG Positive

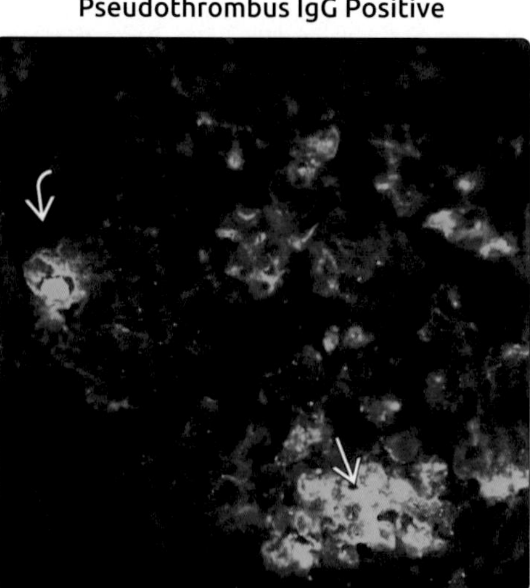

C1q Deposits

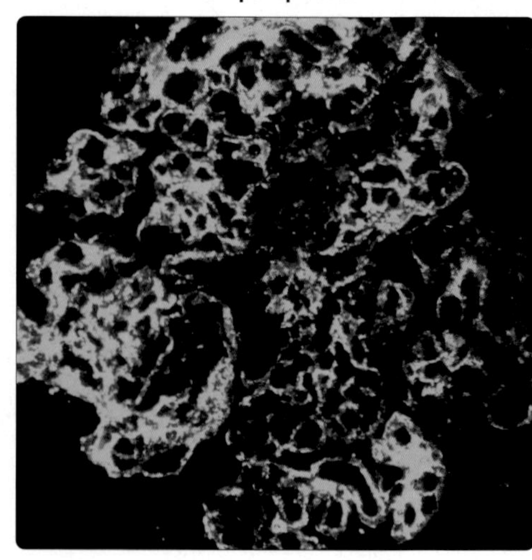

Subepithelial Deposits

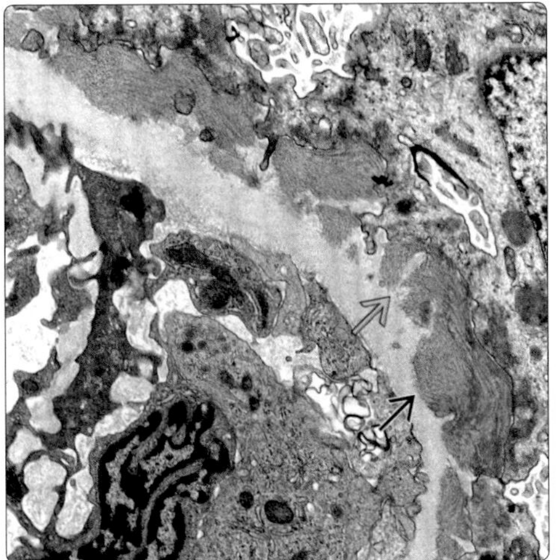

Fibrillary Substructure

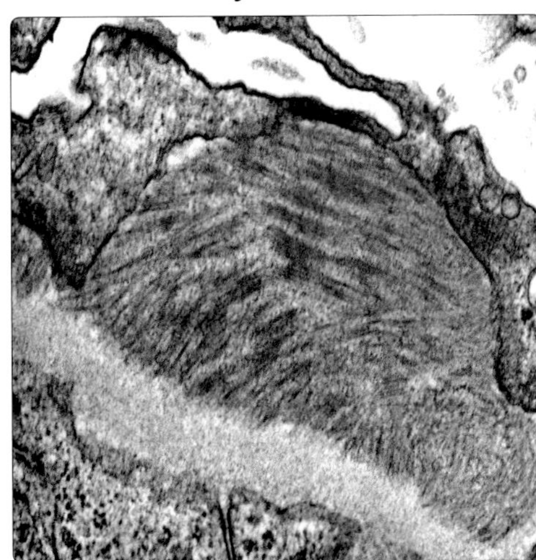

(Left) *Type I cryoglobulinemia can resemble membranous glomerulonephritis (MGN), with subepithelial deposits ➡ and "spikes" ➡. The presence of a single light chain and organized deposits distinguish it from the usual MGN.* **(Right)** *This electron micrograph shows type I cryoglobulinemia exhibiting the typical finding of organized deposits. These have a varied appearance but are usually fibrillar, as in this case with subepithelial deposits due to IgG kappa deposition.*

Pseudothrombi

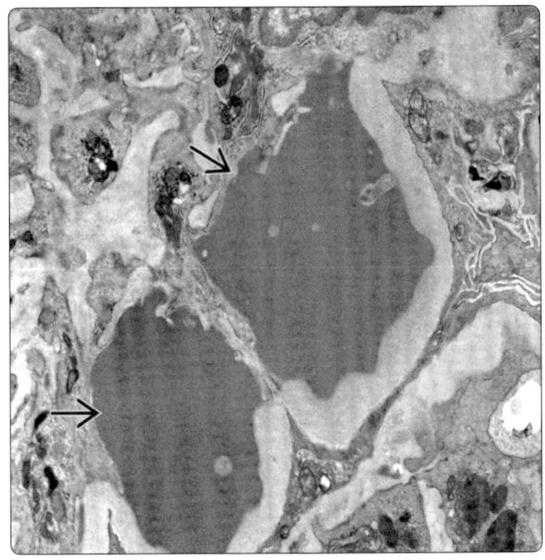

Endothelial Phagocytosis

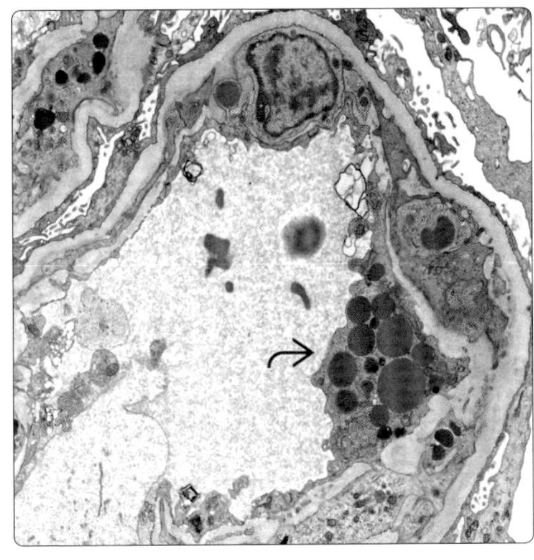

(Left) *Pseudothromb ➡ occlude glomerular capillary loops in patient with type I cryoglobulinemia. The endothelium is absent in these capillary loops.* **(Right)** *The secondary lysosomes ➡ of the endothelium of this glomerular capillary are filled with phagocytosed material derived from the cryoglobulin. Similar accumulations occur in macrophages and in types II and III cryoglobulinemias.*

Variant: Cryocrystalglobulinemia

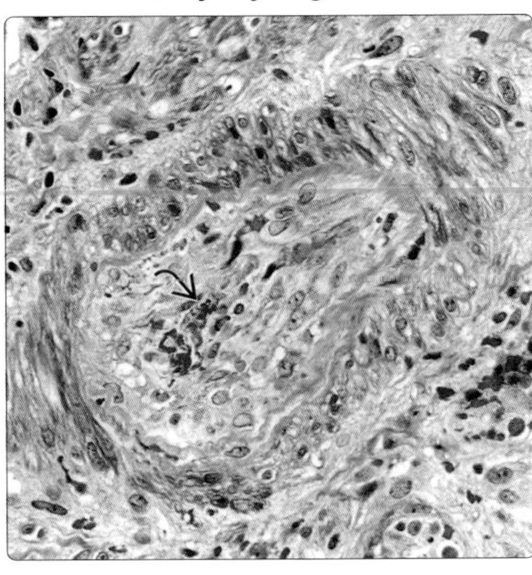

Crystals in Capillary Endothelium

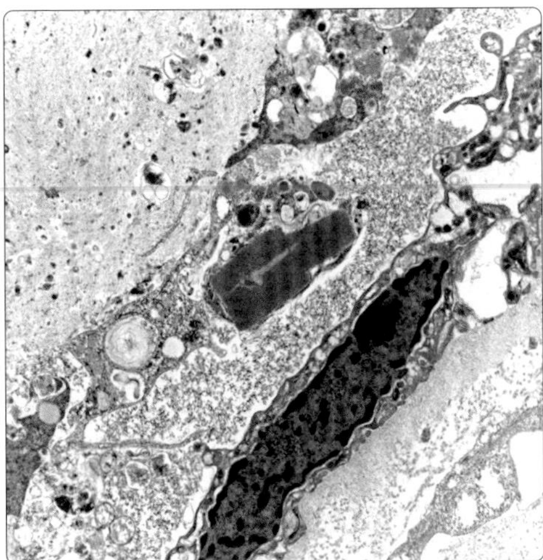

(Left) *A renal artery has crystals in the endothelium that stain red in trichrome stains ➡. Similar crystals were also in proximal tubules in this patient with type I cryoglobulinemia (IgG kappa) and MGUS. This condition has been termed "cryocrystal-globulinemia" or "crystal-globulinemia" if no cryoglobulin detected. (Courtesy E. Farkash, MD.)* **(Right)** *A peritubular capillary has rectangular crystals in the endothelium due to an IgG kappa MGUS, a variant termed cryocrystalglobulinemia. (Courtesy E. Farkash, MD.)*

Waldenström Macroglobulinemia

KEY FACTS

TERMINOLOGY

- Definition
  - Lymphoplasmacytic lymphoma (LPL) with bone marrow involvement and circulating IgM paraprotein
    - WM comprises subset of LPL

ETIOLOGY/PATHOGENESIS

- Postfollicular B cells may be cell of origin
  - Familial cases with younger age of onset reported

CLINICAL ISSUES

- Median age: > 60 years
  - Male > female
  - Caucasian predilection
- Proteinuria, nephrotic range
- Hyperviscosity syndrome
  - Reduced vision
  - Red blood cells with sludging and rouleaux formation

MICROSCOPIC

- Glomeruli: Spectrum of injury
  - Cryoglobulinemia
    - Proliferation, inflammation
- Spectrum of glomerular disease
  - Cryoglobulinemic glomerulonephritis (GN)
  - Amyloidosis
  - Minimal change disease
  - Membranous GN
- Other manifestations of monoclonal protein

ANCILLARY TESTS

- "Pseudothrombi" stain for IgM, kappa or lambda

TOP DIFFERENTIAL DIAGNOSES

- Other hematologic malignancies
- Cryoglobulinemic GN
- Thrombotic microangiopathy

Pseudothrombi

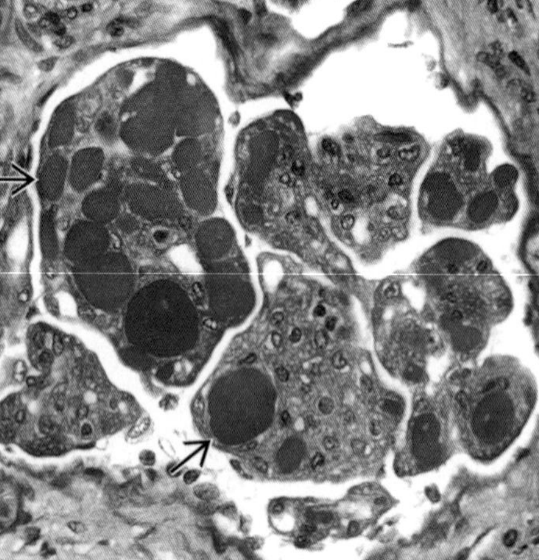

Pseudothrombi

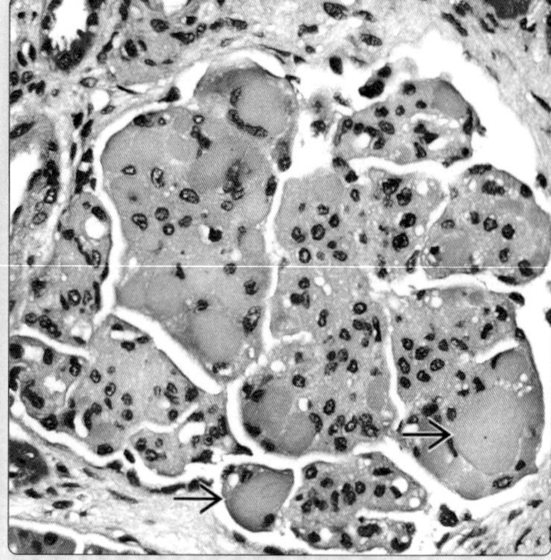

(Left) *Numerous hyaline "thrombi" or pseudothrombi occupy the glomerular capillaries in a patient with WM (PAS).* **(Right)** *Large aggregates of paraprotein ("pseudothrombi") fill the glomerular capillaries in a patient with circulating cryoglobulins due to WM (H&E).*

IgM Immunofluorescence

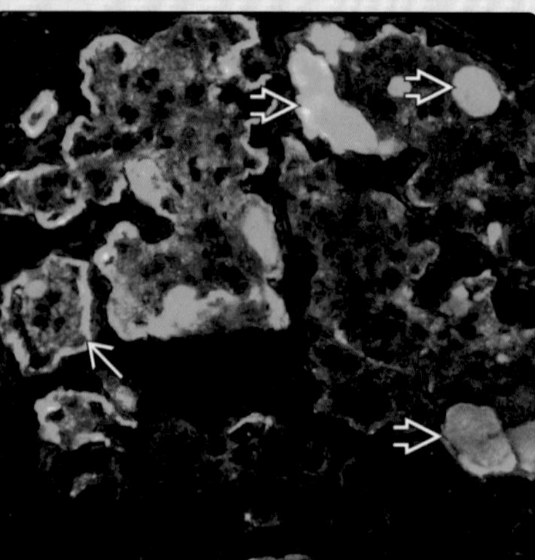

Electron Microscopy

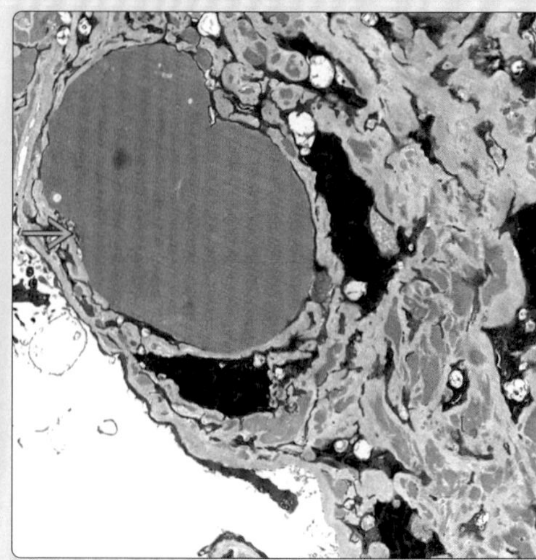

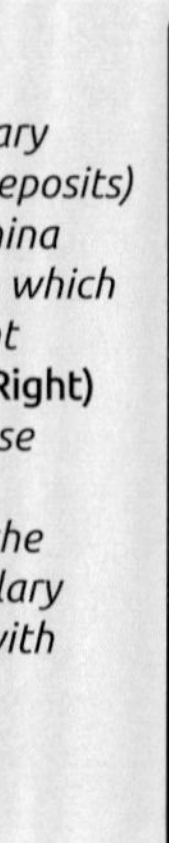

(Left) *IgM highlights prominent paraprotein deposition along capillary walls ("wire loop" deposits) and in the capillary lumina (hyaline "thrombi"), which correlates with the light microscopic findings.* **(Right)** *This large electron-dense deposit without substructure occupies the entire glomerular capillary lumen from a patient with WM.*

TERMINOLOGY

Abbreviations

- Waldenström macroglobulinemia (WM)

Definitions

- Subset of lymphoplasmacytic lymphoma (LPL) with bone marrow involvement and any circulating IgM paraprotein

ETIOLOGY/PATHOGENESIS

Neoplastic B Lymphocytes

- Postfollicular B cells may be cell of origin
  - Familial cases with younger age of onset reported

CLINICAL ISSUES

Epidemiology

- Incidence
  - 0.38/100,000 persons/year, increases with age
    - 2.85/100,000 80 years and older
- Age
  - Median: 73 years
- Sex
  - Male > female (2:1)
- Ethnicity
  - Whites > blacks (~ 2:1)

Presentation

- Renal involvement rare
  - Proteinuria, nephrotic-range (7-28%)
  - Light chain Fanconi syndrome
  - Acute renal failure
- Hyperviscosity syndrome in 10-30%
  - Reduced vision
  - Red blood cells with sludging and rouleaux formation
- May have autoantibody activity
  - Autoimmune hemolytic anemai, immune thrombocytopenia, von Willebrand disease, pemphigus, retinitis, peripheral neuropathy, protein-losing enteropathy
- 30% asymptomatic

Laboratory Tests

- Serum or urine protein electrophoresis
  - Detection of any monoclonal IgM protein
- Free light chains (can monitor response to therapy)
- Cryoglobulins (8-18%), type I or II
- Chromosomal deletion 6q in 40-50%

Treatment

- Rituximab
  - Can induce cryoglobulin flare and acute renal failure
- Chemotherapy
- Plasmapheresis for hyperviscosity or cryoglobulins

Prognosis

- Median survival: 5 years
- Adverse risk factors: age > 65 years, serum monoclonal protein > 7g/dl, hemoglobin ≤ 11.5 g/dL, platelet count ≤ 100,000/μL, β2 microglobulin > 3 mg/L

MICROSCOPIC

Histologic Features

- Glomeruli: Spectrum of injury
  - Cryoglobulinemia
    - Pseudothrombi (hyaline thrombi) in capillaries
    - Proliferation, inflammation
  - Rouleaux of RBCs in capillaries
  - Other manifestations of monoclonal protein
    - Amyloidosis (most common)
    - Monoclonal immunoglobulin deposition disease
  - Other pathology
    - Immune complex MPGN with hypocomplementemia
    - Minimal change disease
- Tubules
  - Acute tubular injury
    - Associated with cryoglobulin flare
  - Cast nephropathy, rare
- Interstitium
  - Interstitial infiltration by LPL may mimic renal or perirenal mass

ANCILLARY TESTS

Immunofluorescence

- Pseudothrombi stain for IgM and a monotypic light chain (kappa or lambda)
- Amyloid with monotypic light chains
- Immune complexes with multiple reactants in MPGN

Electron Microscopy

- "Pseudothrombi" and subendothelial deposits have microtubular/fibrillar substructure

DIFFERENTIAL DIAGNOSIS

Other Hematologic Malignancies

- Wide spectrum of B-cell malignancies can manifest with similar renal injuries, ranging from amyloidosis and cryoglobulinemic GN to cast nephropathy

Cryoglobulinemic GN

- Negative bone marrow biopsy

Thrombotic Microangiopathy

- Thrombi stain for fibrin rather than IgM

DIAGNOSTIC CHECKLIST

Pathologic Interpretation Pearls

- IgM paraproteins trigger work-up of monoclonal gammopathies
- Only the neoplastic infiltrate, if present, is specific for LPL
- WM diagnosis requires bone marrow biopsy and SPEP

SELECTED REFERENCES

1. Salviani C et al: Renal involvement in Waldenström's macroglobulinemia: case report and review of literature. Ren Fail. 36(1):114-8, 2014
2. Shaheen SP et al: Waldenström macroglobulinemia: a review of the entity and its differential diagnosis. Adv Anat Pathol. 19(1):11-27, 2012
3. Audard V et al: Renal lesions associated with IgM-secreting monoclonal proliferations: revisiting the disease spectrum. Clin J Am Soc Nephrol. 3(5):1339-49, 2008

Light Chain Cast Nephropathy

KEY FACTS

TERMINOLOGY

- Synonyms
  - Light chain cast nephropathy
  - Myeloma kidney
- Accumulation of monoclonal light chains may form casts (both cytotoxic and obstructive) in distal nephron segments

ETIOLOGY/PATHOGENESIS

- Precipitating factors for cast formation include
  - Dehydration
  - Hypercalcemia
  - Nonsteroidal anti-inflammatory drugs
- Certain light chains have affinity for Tamm-Horsfall protein; kappa:lambda = 3:1

CLINICAL ISSUES

- Acute renal failure
- 30-50% incidence among patients with multiple myeloma
- 5-year survival rate: 20-25%

MICROSCOPIC

- Tubular casts
  - Usually involve distal nephron segments (distal tubules and collecting ducts)
  - Sharp-edged or fractured appearance
  - Giant cell reaction to intratubular casts
  - Prominent intratubular aggregates of neutrophils can be present
- May have other lesions of monoclonal immunoglobulins (amyloidosis, light chain deposition disease)

ANCILLARY TESTS

- Immunofluorescence or immunohistochemistry shows light chain restriction

TOP DIFFERENTIAL DIAGNOSES

- Rhabdomyolysis-associated acute tubular injury
- Monoclonal immunoglobulin deposition disease
- Acute tubular injury

(Left) *H&E demonstrates a tubular cast that appears broken into 2 fragments with straight edges ➡ (or a fractured appearance). Scattered interstitial inflammatory cells ➡ with plasma cells are present, which can represent renal involvement by plasma cell dyscrasia.* **(Right)** *Several fragmented pieces ➡ of this tubular cast are enveloped by macrophages forming a prominent giant cell reaction ➡ that is characteristic of myeloma cast nephropathy.*

Fractured Cast

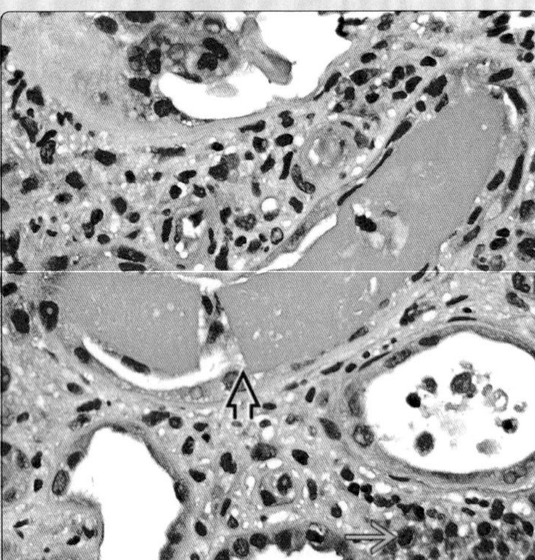

Giant Cell Cast Reaction

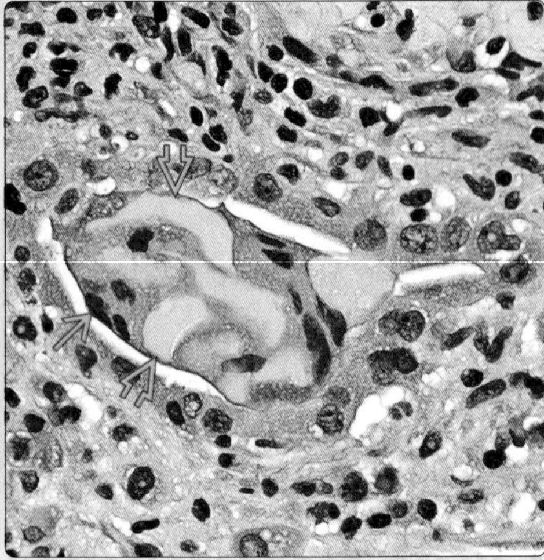

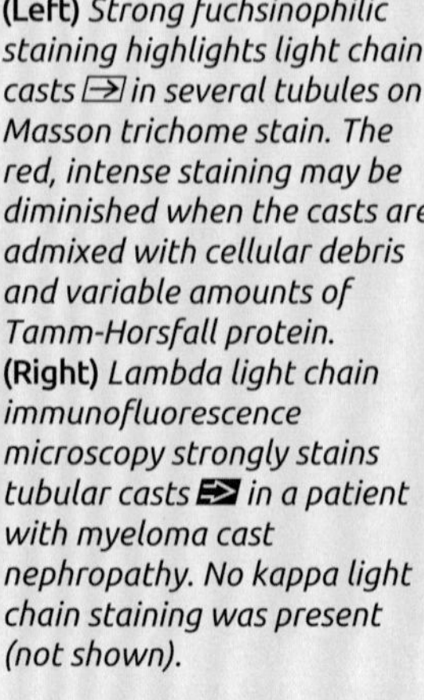

(Left) *Strong fuchsinophilic staining highlights light chain casts ➡ in several tubules on Masson trichome stain. The red, intense staining may be diminished when the casts are admixed with cellular debris and variable amounts of Tamm-Horsfall protein.* **(Right)** *Lambda light chain immunofluorescence microscopy strongly stains tubular casts ➡ in a patient with myeloma cast nephropathy. No kappa light chain staining was present (not shown).*

Myeloma Casts

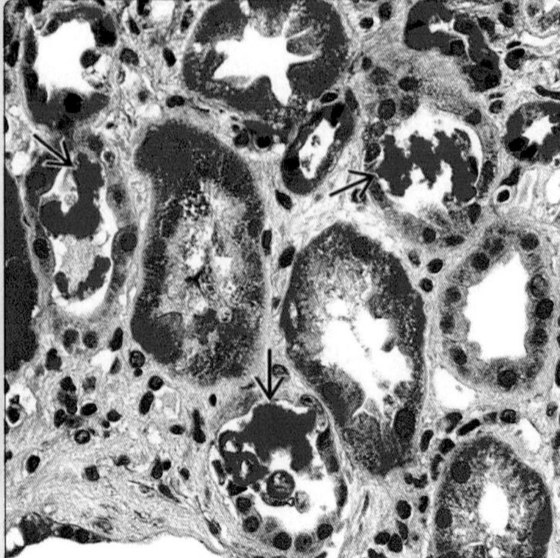

Monoclonal Light Chain IF Staining

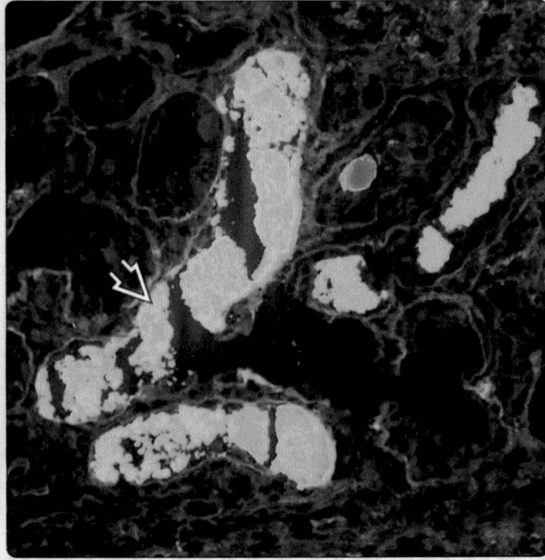

TERMINOLOGY

Abbreviations

- Myeloma cast nephropathy (MCN)

Synonyms

- Light chain cast nephropathy
- Bence Jones cast nephropathy
- Myeloma kidney

ETIOLOGY/PATHOGENESIS

Plasma Cell Dyscrasia

- Monoclonal light chain overproduction
  - Light chains (Bence Jones proteins) freely filtered by glomeruli
  - Certain monoclonal light chains are nephrotoxic
    - Kappa:lambda ~ 3:1
    - Correlated with sequence in complementarity determining region 3 (CDR3)
    - CDR3 consensus sequence LSADSSGSYLYV greatest affinity to Tamm-Horsfall protein (THP) (uromodulin)
  - Accumulation of Tamm-Horsfall protein and monoclonal light chains in distal nephron segments may lead to both obstruction and direct cytotoxicity
  - Precipitating factors for cast formation include
    - Dehydration, diuretics, hypercalcemia, nonsteroidal antiinflammatory druges, contrast media, infection

CLINICAL ISSUES

Epidemiology

- Incidence
  - 30-50% among patients with multiple myeloma
  - Most common biopsy finding in multiple myeloma (33%)
- Sex
  - Male > female

Presentation

- Acute renal failure and proteinuria

Laboratory Tests

- Serum &/or urine protein electrophoresis

Treatment

- Drugs
  - Treat underlying plasma cell dyscrasia, if present
    - Colchicine, thalidomide, bortezomib
- Hematopoietic stem cell transplantation
- Plasmapheresis

Prognosis

- 5-year survival rate: 20-25%

MICROSCOPIC

Histologic Features

- Tubular casts
  - Usually involve distal nephron segments (distal tubules and collecting ducts)
  - Sharp-edged or fractured appearance
  - Lined by flattened to reactive tubular epithelial cells
  - Giant cell reaction to intratubular casts may be present
  - Prominent intratubular aggregates of neutrophils can be present
  - Rare crystal appearance may be present
- Interstitial inflammation
- Interstitial neoplastic plasma cell infiltrates may be present
  - Monoclonal staining by immunofluorescence, in situ hybridization, or immunohistochemistry

ANCILLARY TESTS

Immunofluorescence

- Kappa > lambda with ratio ranging from 2:1 to 4:1
  - Paraffin tissue sections can yield good results

Electron Microscopy

- Monoclonal light chain tubular casts demonstrate spectrum of substructural organization
  - Nonspecific appearance to crystalline, granular, or even fibrillar substructure
- Immunogold labeling can be more sensitive than immunofluorescence or immunohistochemistry to demonstrate monoclonality

Immunohistochemistry

- Test κ and λ on paraffin tissue sections if tubular casts not present in immunofluorescence specimen

DIFFERENTIAL DIAGNOSIS

Rhabdomyolysis-Associated Acute Tubular Injury

- Pigmented tubular casts with granular consistency
  - Positive for myoglobin

mTOR Inhibitor Toxicity

- Reported in kidney transplant patients after using immunosuppressive regimen containing rapamycin
- Tubular casts with fractured appearance
  - Multinucleated giant cell reaction can be present
  - Casts may consist of myoglobin

End-Stage Kidney

- Hyaline casts in atrophic tubules may be fractured
  - Lined by flattened or atrophic tubular epithelial cells
  - Absence of giant cell reaction, PAS positive
  - Absence of monoclonal immunofluorescence staining

DIAGNOSTIC CHECKLIST

Pathologic Interpretation Pearls

- Careful evaluation of immunofluorescence specimen to exclude monoclonal staining of tubular casts
  - Some proteinaceous casts in atrophic tubules may stain strongly for both kappa and lambda, but other casts may demonstrate monoclonal staining
- Absence of renal medulla may lead to false-negative result

SELECTED REFERENCES

1. Leung N et al: Myeloma-related kidney disease. Adv Chronic Kidney Dis. 21(1):36-47, 2014
2. Ying WZ et al: Mechanism and prevention of acute kidney injury from cast nephropathy in a rodent model. J Clin Invest. 122(5):1777-85, 2012
3. Hutchison CA et al: The pathogenesis and diagnosis of acute kidney injury in multiple myeloma. Nat Rev Nephrol. 8(1):43-51, 2011

Acute Tubular Injury

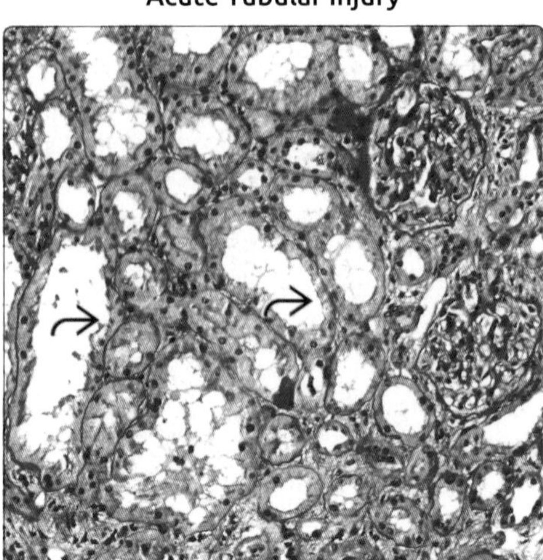

Atypical Myeloma Casts

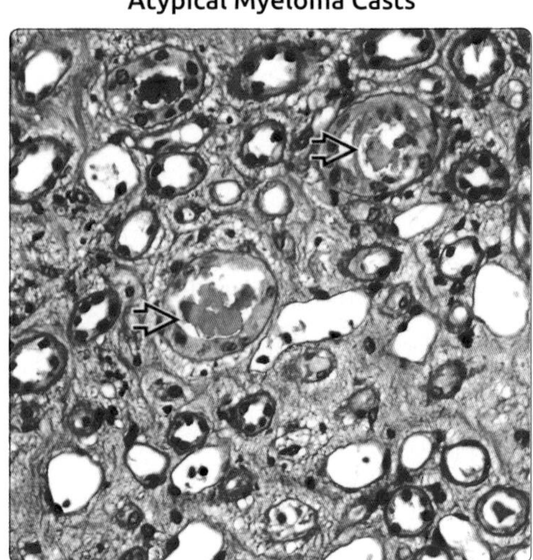

(Left) *Light chain cast nephropathy in a 48-year-old woman who presented with acute renal failure is shown. Many tubules in the cortex are dilated and show flattening or vacuolization of the epithelium, which are features of acute tubular injury ➡. The glomeruli appear normal on PAS.* **(Right)** *These atypical casts ➡ are PAS-negative and appear finely granular. These casts can be mistaken for intratubular cellular debris, which can be observed in the setting of acute tubular injury/necrosis.*

Myeloma Casts

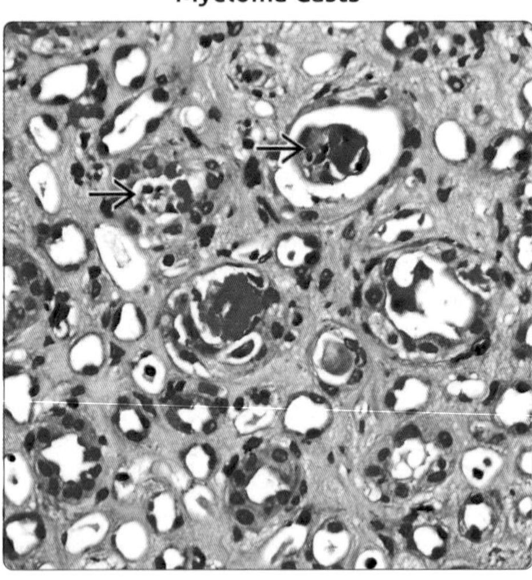

Myeloma Casts

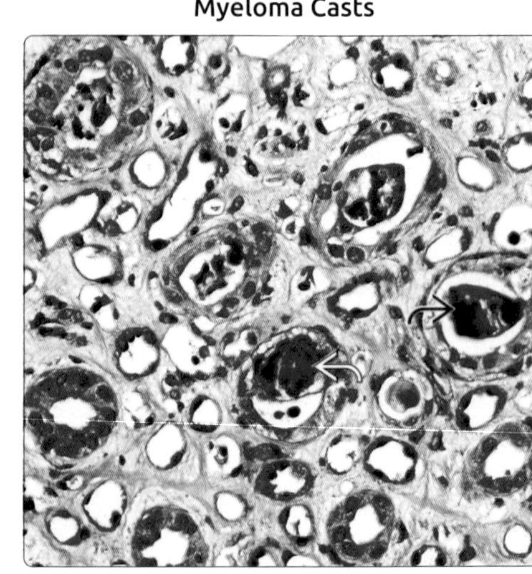

(Left) *Hypereosinophilic casts in the distal nephron segments are admixed with a few inflammatory cells ➡. Prominent neutrophilic reaction surrounding casts can occasionally be present (not shown).* **(Right)** *The "myeloma" casts in the renal medulla can reveal a spectrum of appearances that range from a strong red ➡ to a variegated red-blue ➡ appearance, as shown in this Masson trichrome stain.*

Kappa Light Chain

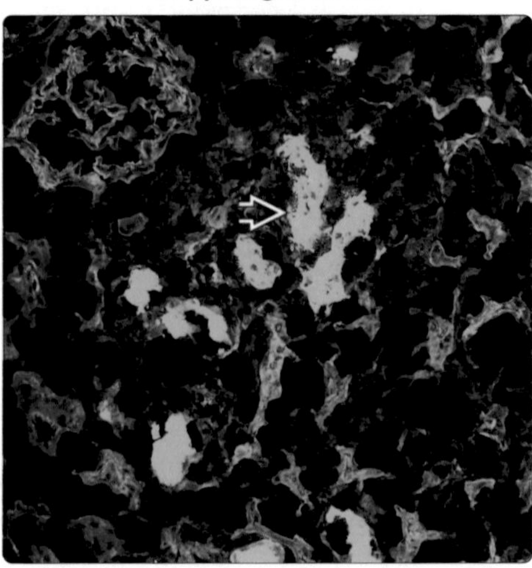

Lambda Light Chain

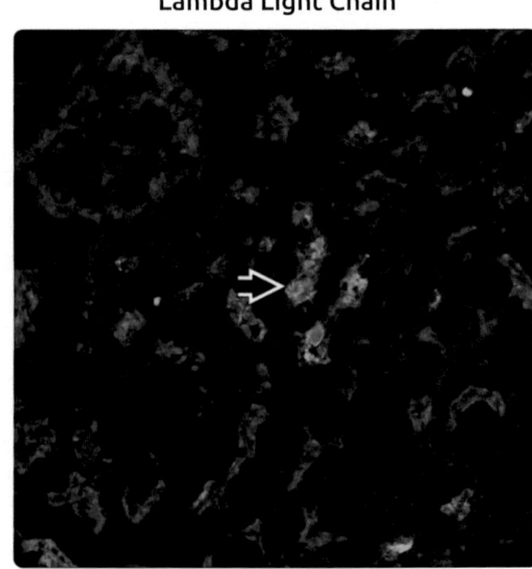

(Left) *Atypical casts are strongly positive for kappa light chain ➡. There is also confluent glomerular and tubular basement membrane staining (in this case dim) for kappa light chain but not for lambda light chain. This may be the earliest evidence of light chain deposition disease, which often occurs concurrently with myeloma cast nephropathy.* **(Right)** *These tubular casts are negative for lambda light chain ➡ but stain strongly for kappa light chain (not shown).*

Myeloma Cast

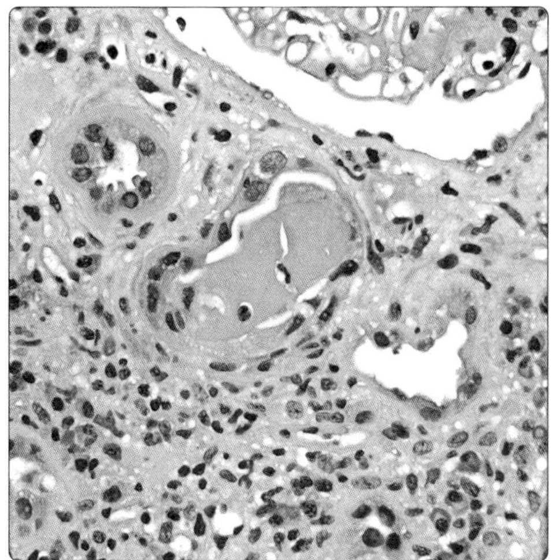

Myeloma Cast

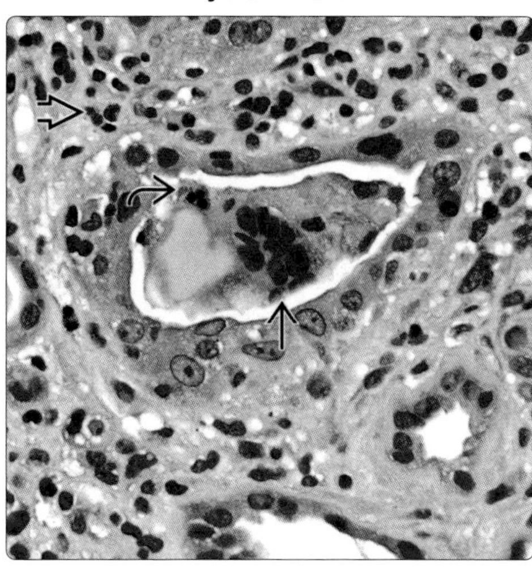

(Left) *"Myeloma" casts do not always reveal sharp edges or cellular reactions, but even irregular fractures should raise suspicion for the diagnosis.* **(Right)** *Prominent giant cell reaction → to the tubular cast is noted in the lumen on this tubule, and this feature alone is highly suggestive of myeloma cast nephropathy. Scattered inflammatory cells are noted in the interstitium → along with a few eosinophils → in the tubular lumen.*

Kappa Light Chain

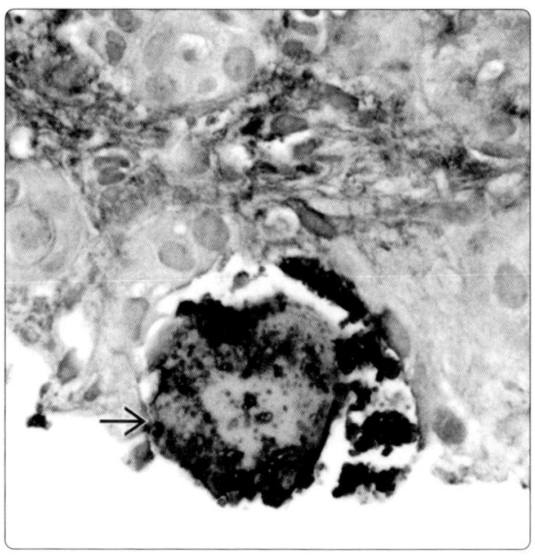

Lambda Light Chain

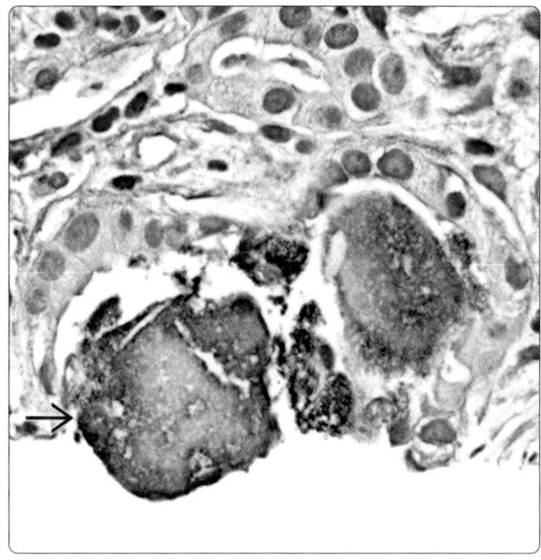

(Left) *Immunohistochemistry on the paraffin section for kappa light chain shows strong staining in this tubular cast → and a blush of interstitial staining.* **(Right)** *Tubular casts were not prominent in the sample submitted for immunofluorescence microscopy. Lambda light chain immunohistochemistry reveals no significant staining of this intratubular cast →. This finding, in conjunction with strong kappa light chain staining (not shown), supports the diagnosis of myeloma cast nephropathy.*

Atypical Myeloma Casts

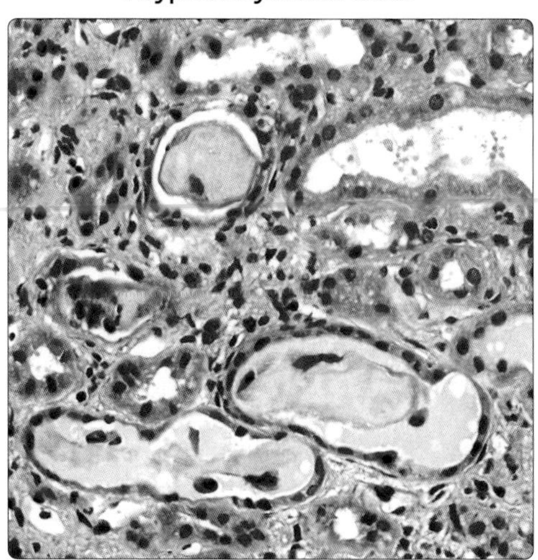

Myeloma Cast

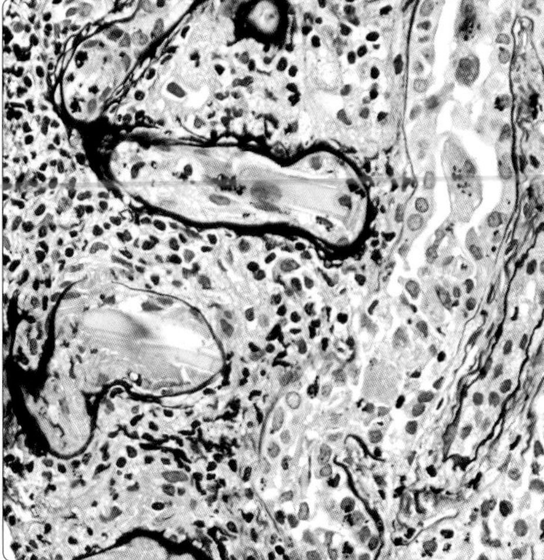

(Left) *These casts are atypical, but they do not have the hypereosinophilic appearance of usual light chain casts on H&E. By immunofluorescence, casts stained for lambda but not for kappa light chain.* **(Right)** *"Myeloma" casts are shown on Jones methenamine silver stain.*

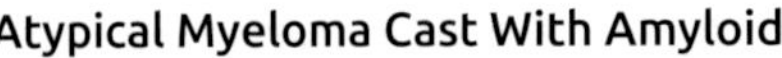
Atypical Myeloma Cast With Amyloid

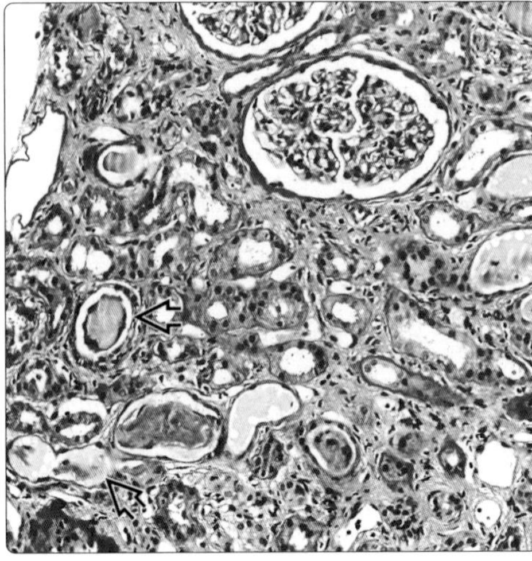

Atypical Myeloma Cast With Amyloid

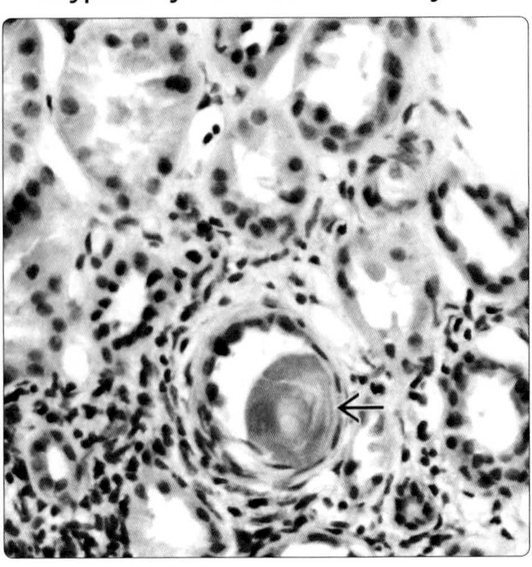

(Left) *Cast nephropathy and intratubular amyloid are present as a few tubules containing atypical, PAS-negative, or PAS-variable casts, some of which show a surrounding cellular reaction.* **(Right)** *A Congo red stain was positive in tubular casts, with apple green birefringence upon examination under polarized light. This is an unusual finding in myeloma cast nephropathy. No amyloid was present in other areas of the kidney biopsy, and the patient did not have systemic amyloidosis.*

Myeloma Cast

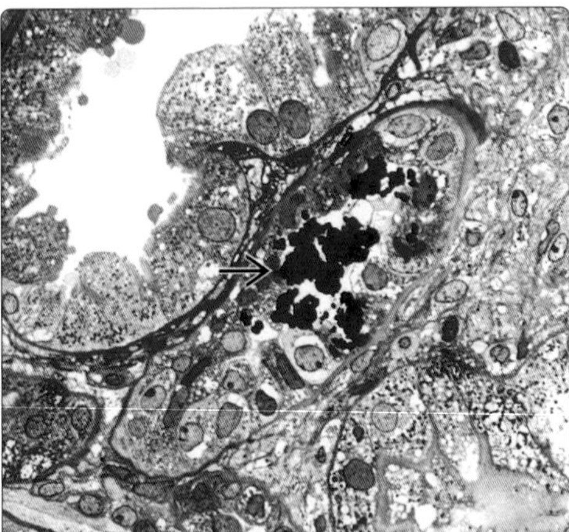

Atypical Myeloma Cast

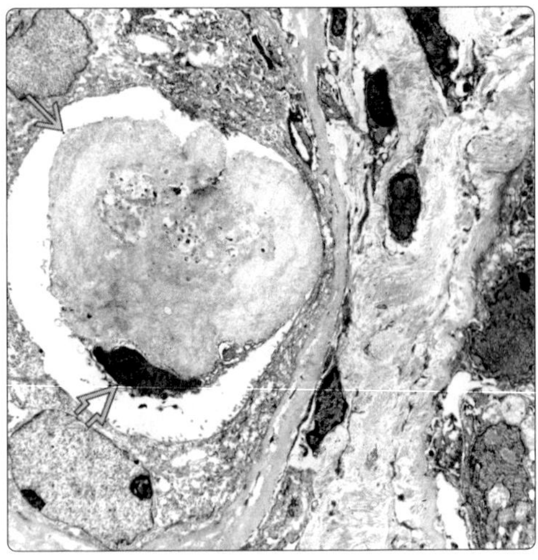

(Left) *The light chain casts in the tubules stain strongly blue with a granular and coarse appearance in the toluidine blue section submitted for electron microscopy.* **(Right)** *Electron micrograph of an atypical cast with an attached cell from myeloma cast nephropathy has a granular appearance. Some casts have substructural organization with a lattice framework (not shown), but the absence of this finding is not unusual.*

Ultrastructure of Cast

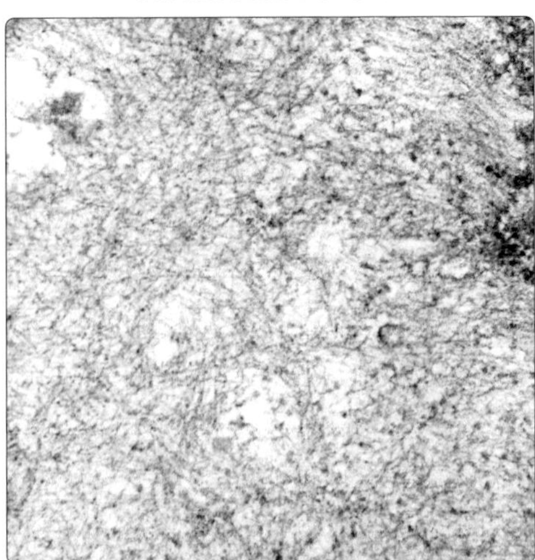

Myeloma Cast

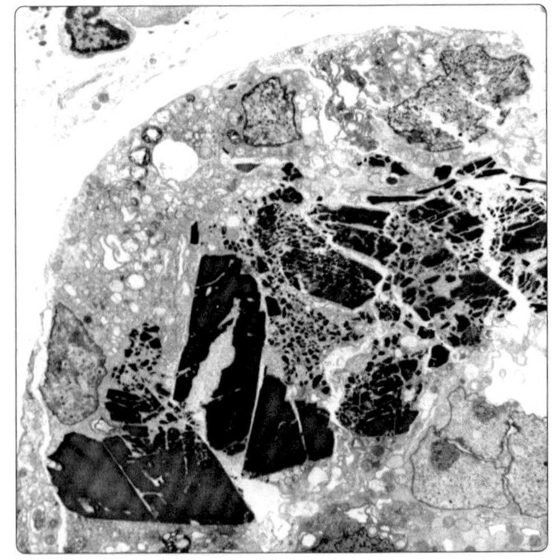

(Left) *At higher magnification, this tubular cast is composed of numerous randomly arranged fibrils, which can be observed in myeloma cast nephropathy whether or not the casts have amyloid.* **(Right)** *Crystalline structures formed from a lambda light chain paraprotein are shown within a tubule from myeloma cast nephropathy by electron microscopy.*

Cryocrystalglobulinemia

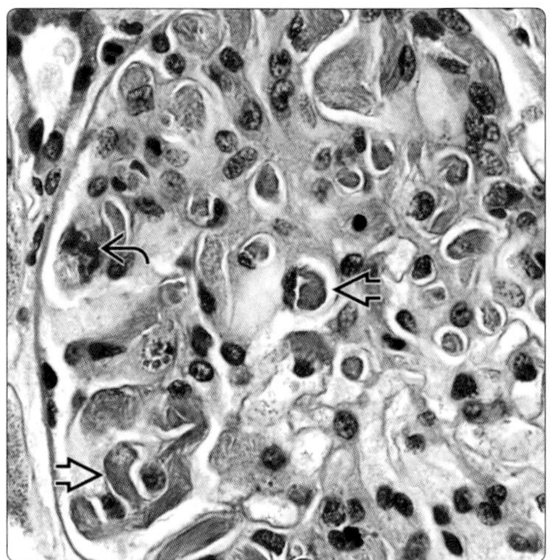

Cryocrystalglobulinemia

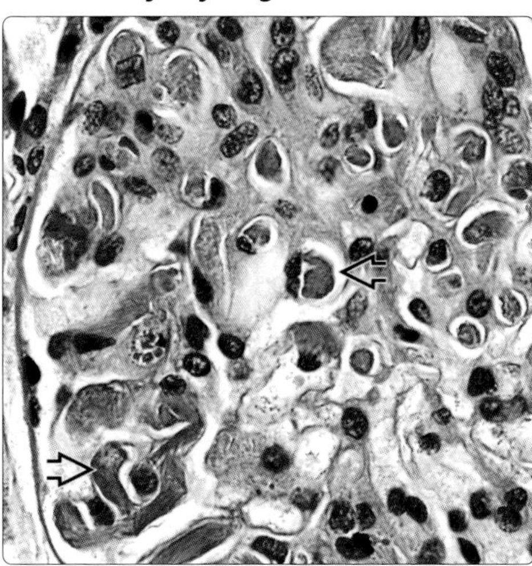

(Left) *Cryocrystalglobulinemia is shown with immunoglobulin "pseudothrombi" ⇨, some of which show a crystalline structure ↷, within glomerular capillary loops* **(Right)** *Cryocrystalglobulinemia is shown. Many immunoglobulin "pseudothrombi" ⇨, some of which show a crystalline structure, are within glomerular capillary loops on PAS stain.*

Casts, Tubulopathy, and Histiocytosis

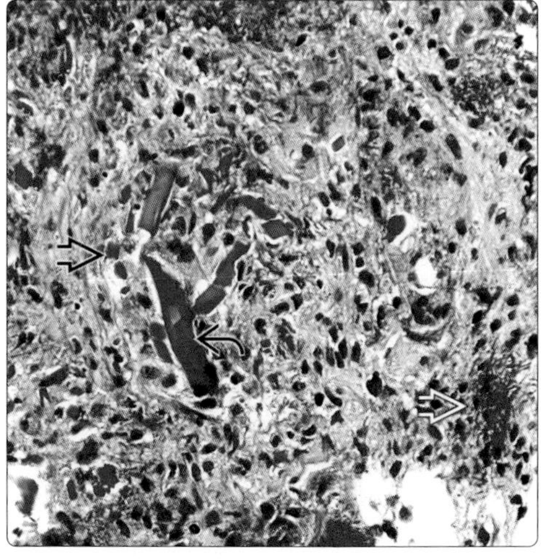

Cryocrystalglobulinemia

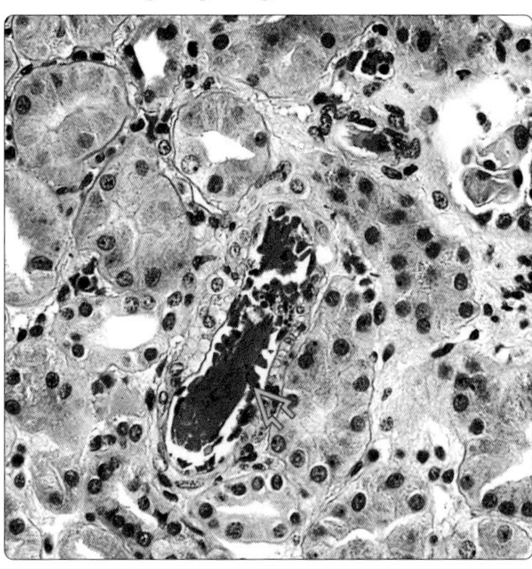

(Left) *An unusual case with 3 diagnoses related to a lambda paraprotein shows light chain cast nephropathy ↷, light chain proximal tubulopathy ⇨, and crystal-storing histiocytosis ➡. (Courtesy M. Fidler, MD.)* **(Right)** *A specimen with cryocrystalglobulinemia shows a crystalline structure within an arteriole ⇨ rather than a tubule. Note surrounding red blood cells. By immunofluorescence, these structures stained for kappa but not lambda light chain. (Courtesy A. Magil, MD.)*

Cryocrystalglobulinemia

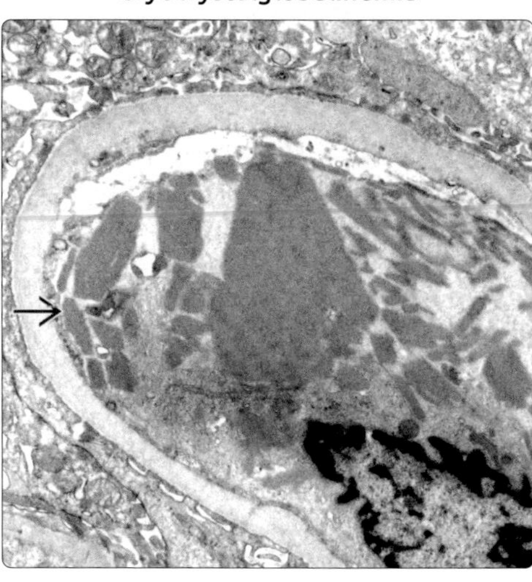

Cryocrystalglobulinemia

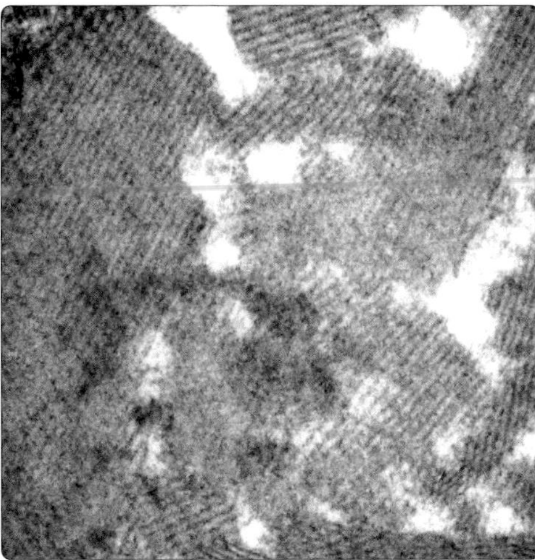

(Left) *This glomerular capillary lumen contains cryoglobulin deposits → with crystalline substructure. "Myeloma" casts are never present within glomerular capillaries.* **(Right)** *The cryoglobulin deposits within the glomerular capillaries demonstrate crystalline substructure with a periodicity at higher magnification. "Myeloma" casts may demonstrate a similar substructural organization by electron microscopy but are always located within the tubular lumina and not capillaries.*

Light Chain Proximal Tubulopathy With Crystals

KEY FACTS

TERMINOLOGY

- Chronic tubulointerstitial nephropathy caused by intracytoplasmic crystalline inclusions
  - Composed of monoclonal light chains present in proximal tubular epithelial cells

ETIOLOGY/PATHOGENESIS

- In LCPT, abnormal light chain, usually kappa (VK1 subgroup)
  - Resistant to enzymatic breakdown

CLINICAL ISSUES

- Fanconi syndrome
  - Normoglycemic glycosuria
  - Aminoaciduria, uricosuria
  - Hyperphosphaturia with hypophosphatemia
- Chronic renal failure, slowly progressive
- Monoclonal gammopathy

ANCILLARY TESTS

- Intracellular monotypic staining for kappa or lambda light chain
- Pronase-digested immunofluorescence sections increases sensitivity of staining in LCPT

TOP DIFFERENTIAL DIAGNOSES

- Acute tubular injury due to other causes
  - No light chains present in proximal tubular epithelial cytoplasm
- Light chain cast nephropathy
- Inflammatory tubulointerstitial nephritis associated with light chains
- Protein reabsorption droplets with monotypic light chain staining
  - Absence of intracytoplasmic crystalline material

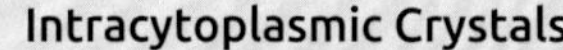

Intracytoplasmic Crystals

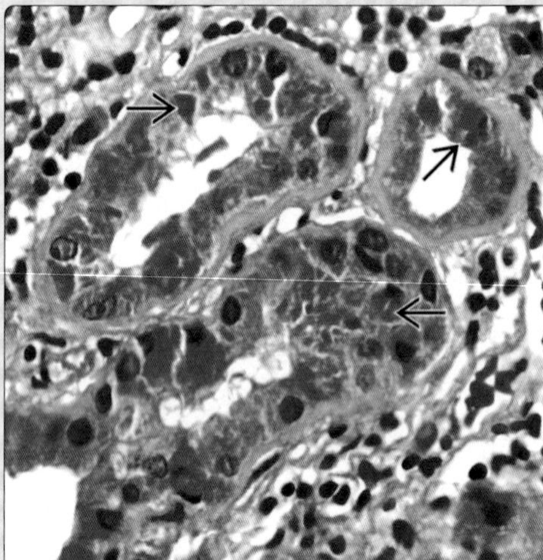

IF of Light Chain Proximal Tubulopathy

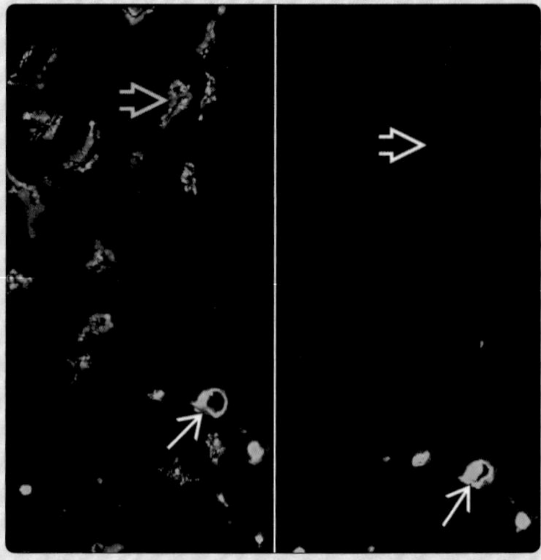

(Left) *Intracytoplasmic crystalline material that stained for monotypic light chain can be seen in the proximal tubules in this patient who had light chain Fanconi syndrome.* **(Right)** *IF of light chain proximal tubulopathy shows positive material within the tubular epithelial cell cytoplasm on an IF stain for kappa (left) with corresponding negative staining for lambda (right). Note the proteinaceous casts that stain for both kappa and lambda.*

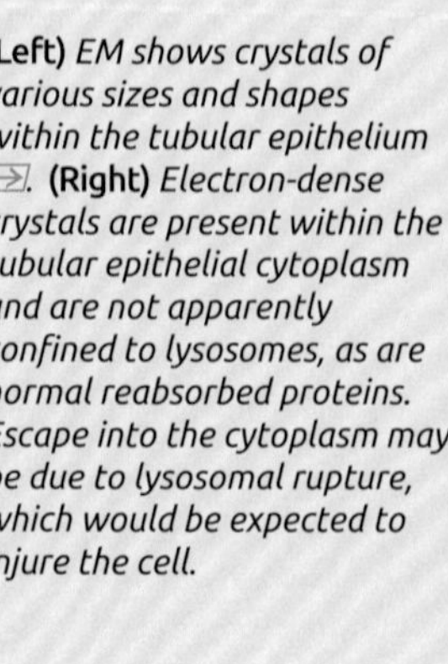

(Left) *EM shows crystals of various sizes and shapes within the tubular epithelium.* **(Right)** *Electron-dense crystals are present within the tubular epithelial cytoplasm and are not apparently confined to lysosomes, as are normal reabsorbed proteins. Escape into the cytoplasm may be due to lysosomal rupture, which would be expected to injure the cell.*

Rhomboid Crystals by EM

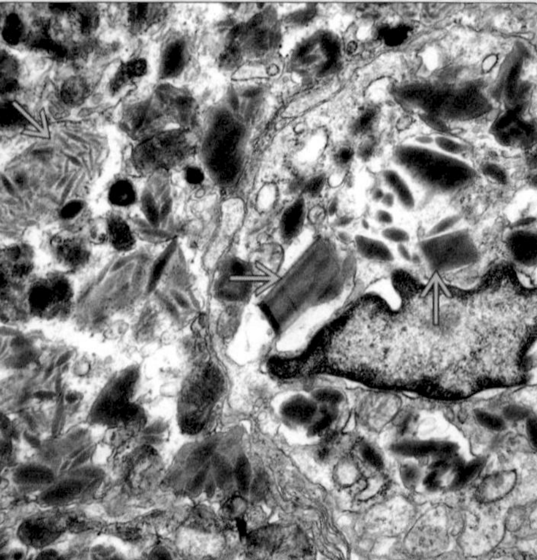

Free Crystals in Cytoplasm

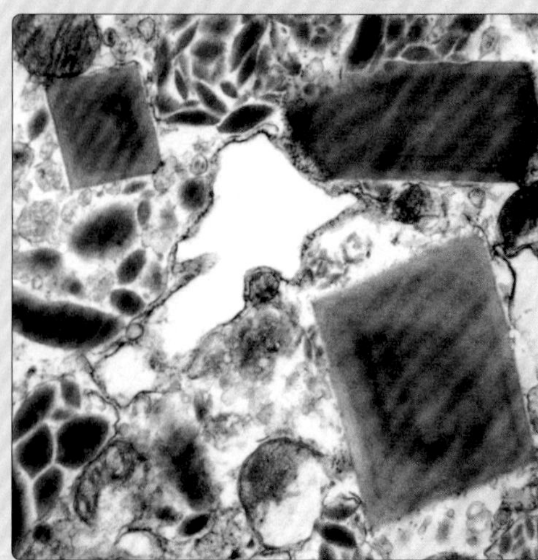

TERMINOLOGY

Abbreviations

- Light chain proximal tubulopathy (LCPT)

Synonyms

- Light chain Fanconi syndrome

Definitions

- Chronic tubulointerstitial nephropathy caused by intracytoplasmic crystalline inclusions
  - Composed of monoclonal light chains present in proximal tubular epithelial cells

ETIOLOGY/PATHOGENESIS

Monoclonal Immunoglobulin Light Chains

- Produced by clonal proliferation of plasma cells
  - Multiple myeloma (may be smoldering) or monoclonal gammopathy of undetermined significance (MGUS)
  - Also associated with Waldenström macroglobulinemia and B-cell lymphomas
- Normal light chains are reabsorbed by proximal tubule, where they are degraded
- In LCPT, abnormal light chain, usually kappa (VK1 subgroup)
  - Resistant to enzymatic breakdown
  - Nephrotoxic light chains crystallize or precipitate within lysosomes in proximal tubules

CLINICAL ISSUES

Epidemiology

- Incidence
  - Rare (~ 0.06% of renal biopsies) but may be overlooked

Presentation

- Fanconi syndrome (acquired)
  - Normoglycemic glycosuria, aminoaciduria, uricosuria, hyperphosphaturia with hypophosphatemia
  - Type II renal tubular acidosis
- Chronic renal failure, slowly progressive
- Monoclonal gammopathy or Bence Jones proteinuria
- Plasma cell dyscrasia or lymphoma
- Adult-acquired Fanconi syndrome with monoclonal light chains raises suspicion of LCPT

Treatment

- Treatment of underlying plasma cell dyscrasia or lymphoma
- In absence of myeloma, watchful waiting may be best approach

MICROSCOPIC

Histologic Features

- Tubules
  - Intracellular crystalline inclusions within proximal tubular epithelial cells
  - Acute and chronic tubular injury
- May show other manifestations of monoclonal protein deposition
  - Crystal-storing histiocytosis with monoclonal light chains
  - Myeloma cast nephropathy
  - Light chain deposition disease (in GBM and TBM)
- Interstitium
  - Commonly mononuclear inflammation, fibrosis

ANCILLARY TESTS

Immunohistochemistry

- Intracellular monotypic staining for κ or λ light chain
- Immunohistochemistry increases sensitivity of staining in LCPT when routine IF is negative

Immunofluorescence

- Intracellular monotypic staining for kappa light chain
  - Almost all cases positive for kappa; rare cases with lambda
- Routine IF often is negative in crystals
  - Increased kappa (+) protein reabsorption droplets in tubules may be a hint to look closely by light microscopy and EM, and perform immunostaining for light chains with an antigen-retrieval technique
- Pronase-digested IF staining increases sensitivity of staining in LCPT

Serologic Testing

- Monoclonal protein in serum, usually IgG kappa
- Bence Jones proteinuria, usually kappa light chain

Electron Microscopy

- Electron-dense crystalline structures within cytoplasm of proximal tubular epithelial cells

DIFFERENTIAL DIAGNOSIS

Acute Tubular Injury Due to Other Causes

- No light chain crystals in proximal tubular epithelial cytoplasm
- Note that light chains in LCPT are not always demonstrable by routine IF

Protein Reabsorption Droplets With Monotypic Light Chain Staining

- Absence of intracytoplasmic crystals by light microscopy and EM
- Light chain reflective of urinary monoclonal protein that does not cause renal disease

Light Chain (Myeloma) Cast Nephropathy

- Intratubular casts, rather than intracytoplasmic material, show monotypic staining for light chain
- Intratubular casts may have crystalline appearance and may show surrounding reactive tubular epithelial cells

Light Chain Deposition Disease

- Like LCPT, often shows tubular injury by light microscopy
- Linear glomerular and tubular basement membrane staining for monoclonal light chain by IF
- Finely granular, electron-dense deposits by EM along glomerular and tubular basement membranes

SELECTED REFERENCES

1. Gupta V et al: Crystalglobulin-Induced Nephropathy. J Am Soc Nephrol. ePub, 2014
2. Herlitz LC et al: Light chain proximal tubulopathy. Kidney Int. 76(7):792-7, 2009
3. Maldonado JE et al: Fanconi syndrome in adults. A manifestation of a latent form of myeloma. Am J Med. 58(3):354-64, 1975

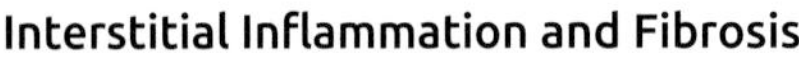

Interstitial Inflammation and Fibrosis

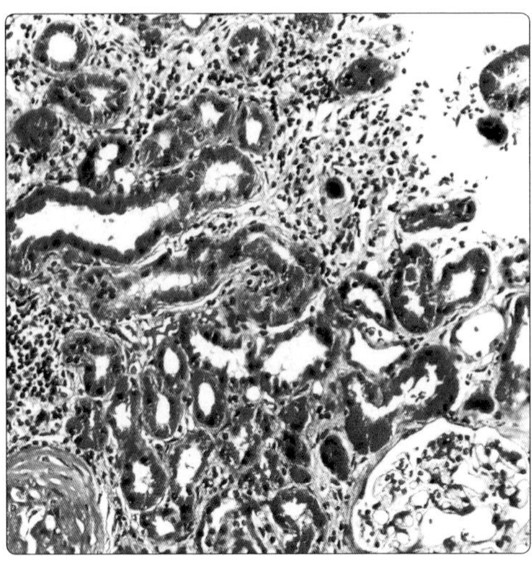

Intracytoplasmic Crystals

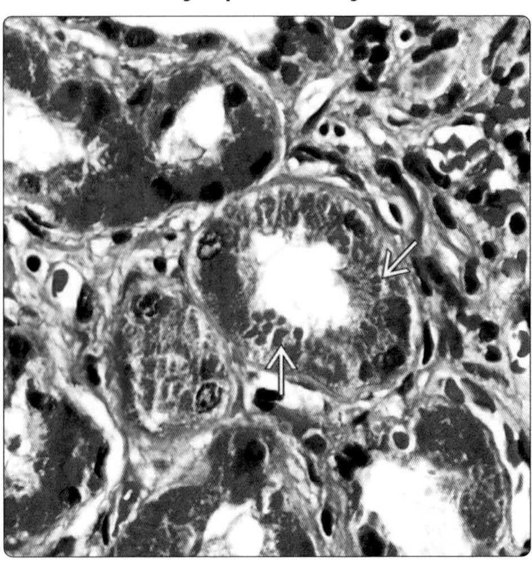

(Left) *Trichome stain shows focal interstitial inflammation and early fibrosis and tubular atrophy in a case of LCPT.* **(Right)** *High magnification reveals intracytoplasmic structures ➡ that are fuchsinophilic on a trichrome stain. The trichrome stain is usually the best stain for visualizing crystalline structures in LCPT.*

Intracytoplasmic Crystals

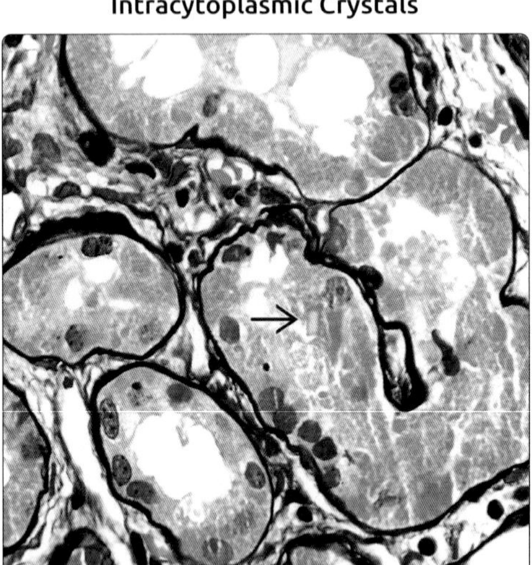

Crystalline Casts

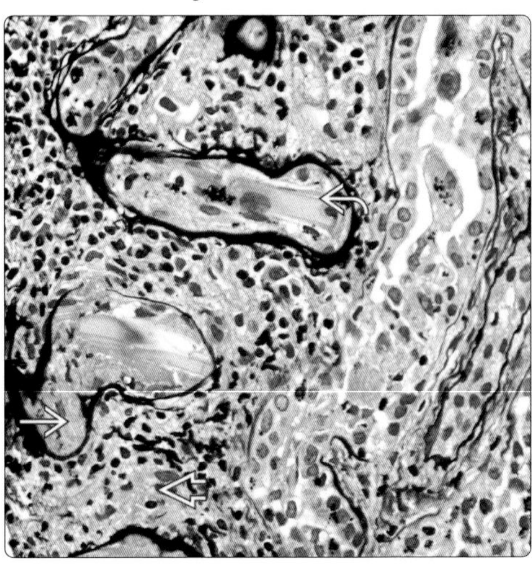

(Left) *Intracytoplasmic crystals are seen on a silver stain ➡.* **(Right)** *This case has 3 diagnoses: Light chain cast nephropathy with crystalline-shaped atypical casts ➡, light chain Fanconi syndrome with crystalline structures within proximal tubular epithelial cells ➡, and crystal-storing histiocytosis seen within the interstitium ➡. By immunofluorescence, the crystals stained for kappa light chain. (Courtesy M. Fidler, MD.)*

Light Chain Proximal Tubulopathy

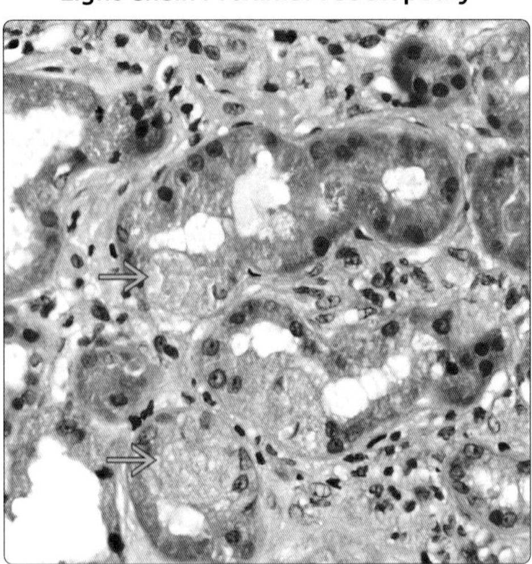

Kappa Positive Crystals by Pronase IF

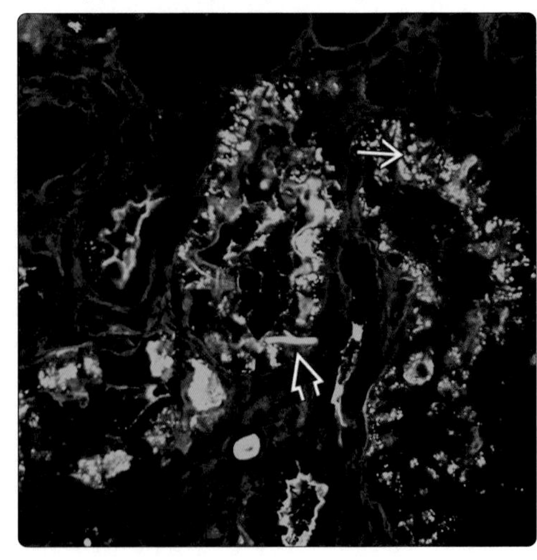

(Left) *In this case of LCPT, the proximal tubules on H&E stain show intracytoplasmic material ➡, which may initially be overlooked or attributed to acute tubular injury. Crystals may be identified by EM.* **(Right)** *Kappa (+) reabsorption granules ➡ and crystals ➡ are seen on this pronase-digested paraffin section stained for kappa light chain.*

Crystals in Proximal Tubule

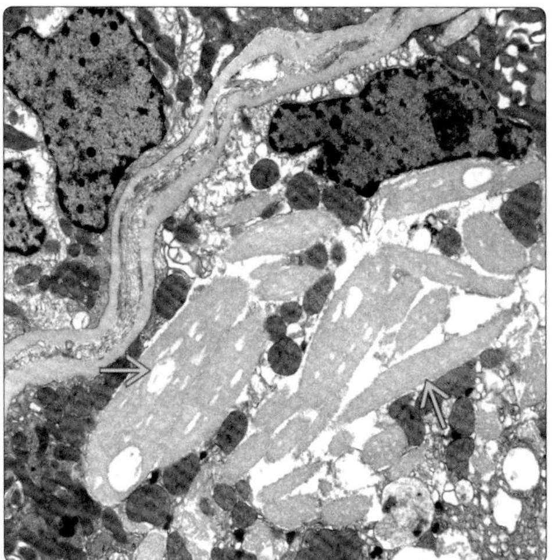

Crystals in Proximal Tubule

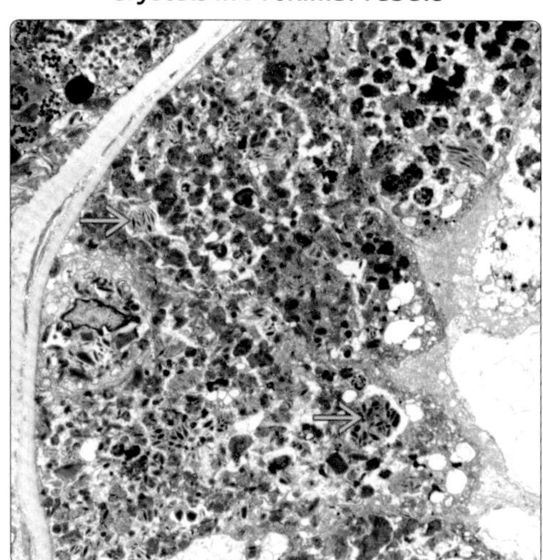

(Left) *Crystals* ⇨ *are seen within proximal tubular epithelial cells. By IF on pronase-digested paraffin sections, there was staining of this material for kappa light chain with negative staining for lambda light chain. Routine IF was negative for kappa and lambda.* **(Right)** *Electron micrograph shows a proximal tubule with crystalline structures within the cytoplasm* ⇨*. Lack of high-magnification electron micrographs of tubules may result in the diagnosis of light chain proximal tubulopathy being overlooked.*

Crystals in Atrophic Tubule

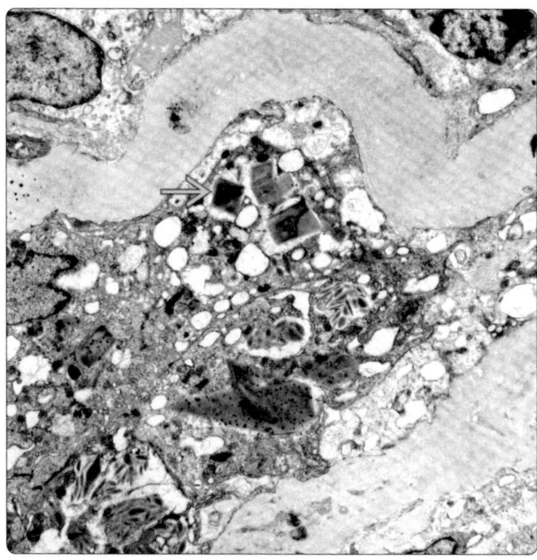

Rhomboid Crystals

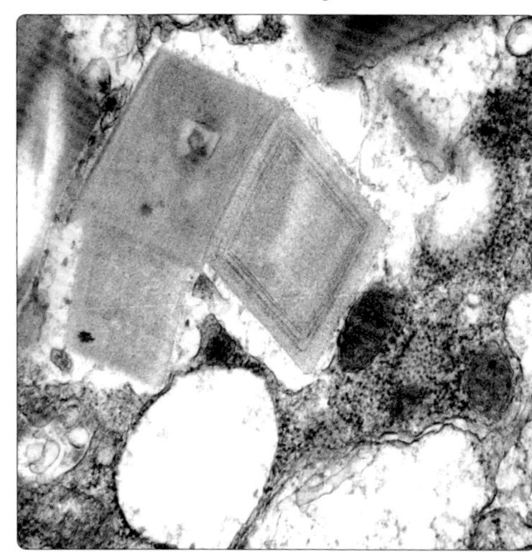

(Left) *EM shows crystalline structures* ⇨ *composed of light chains within the tubular cytoplasm. Note the absence of finely granular deposits along the basement membrane, which if present would indicate concurrent light chain deposition disease.* **(Right)** *Crystals have a rhomboid shape here but may have other patterns, probably dependent on the primary sequence of the protein.*

Rare Crystals in LCPT

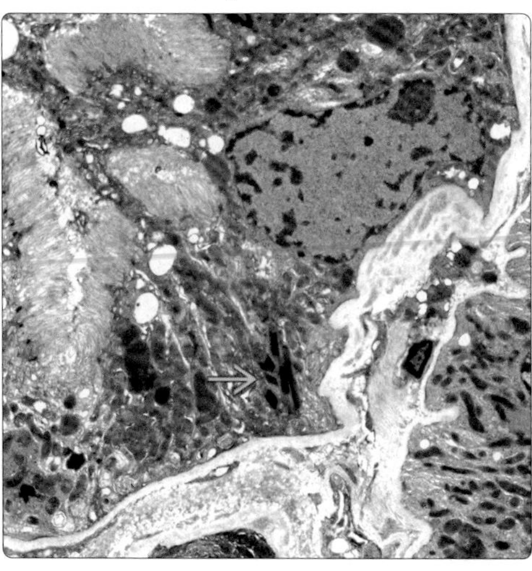

Normal Glomerulus

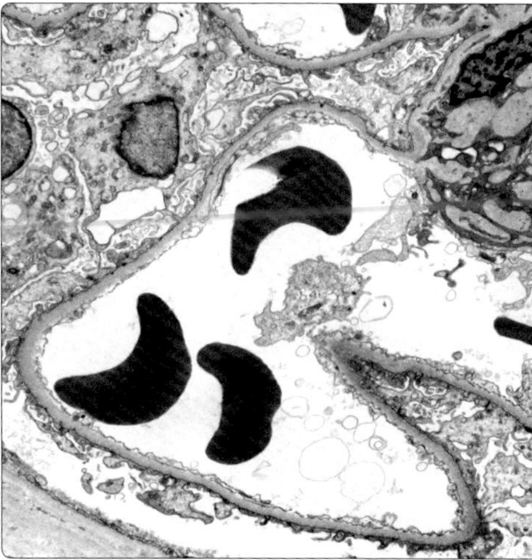

(Left) *In this biopsy performed for hematuria in a 37-year-old woman, there were only rare crystals* ⇨ *seen in focal tubular epithelial cells upon additional examination by EM. IF showed only mildly increased kappa (+) protein reabsorption droplets, not crystals. Three years after this biopsy, the patient was diagnosed with multiple myeloma.* **(Right)** *The glomerulus is unaffected in light chain Fanconi syndrome. The difference in localization of the monoclonal protein is probably related to its physiochemical properties.*

Proximal Tubulopathy Without Crystals

KEY FACTS

ETIOLOGY/PATHOGENESIS

- Proximal tubule injury secondary to excess of free light chains (FLC) accumulating in proximal tubule cytoplasm

CLINICAL ISSUES

- > 90% have plasma cell dyscrasia
  - Most patients will not carry this diagnosis at time of kidney biopsy
- Light chain proximal tubulopathy (LCPT) without organized deposits is controversial and may not always represent end organ damage

MICROSCOPIC

- 3 morphologic variants of LCPT without crystal formation
  - LCPT without organized deposits
    - Acute tubular injury by LM with proximal tubule cytoplasm light chain restriction by IF
    - Nonspecific EM findings
  - Amyloid proximal tubulopathy
    - Congo red-positive tubular inclusions by LM
      - Light chain restriction by IF
    - Intracytoplasmic aggregates of overlapping fibrils in proximal tubule cytoplasm by EM
  - Light chain proximal tubulopathy with large fibrillary aggregates
    - Intracytoplasmic textured inclusions in proximal tubules
      - Light chain restriction by IF
      - Congo red negative
      - Routine IF may show false-negative staining within aggregates
    - Tubular cytoplasm contains bundles of larger fibrils by EM

TOP DIFFERENTIAL DIAGNOSES

- Acute tubular injury
- Uromodulin storage disease
- Antiviral drug nephrotoxicity (e.g., tenofovir)

Acute Tubular Injury

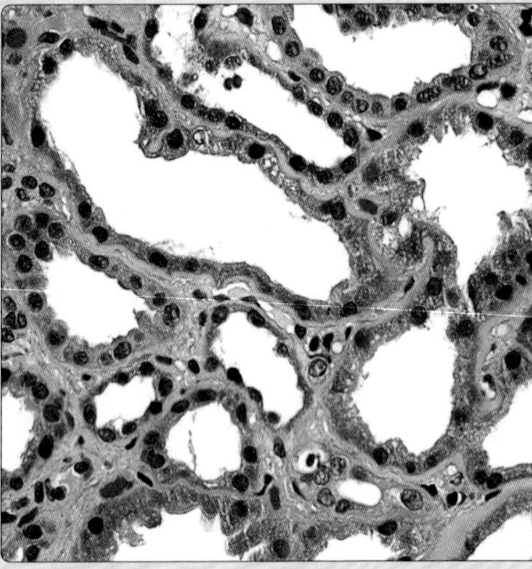

Mottled Lysosomes

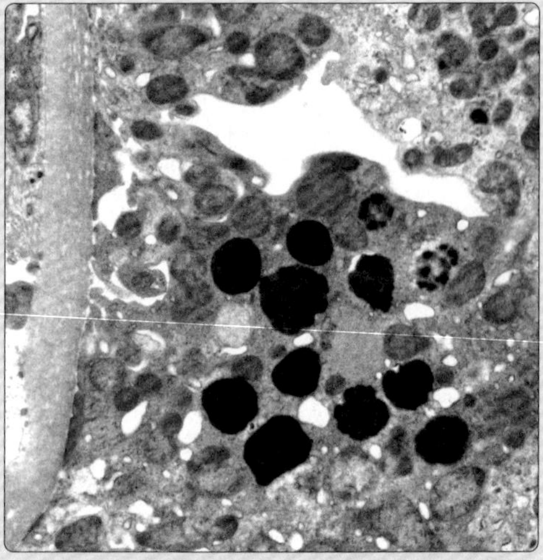

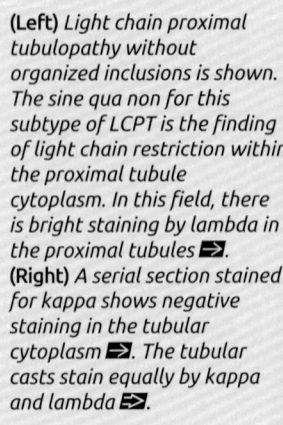

(Left) *Light chain proximal tubulopathy (LCPT) without organized inclusions is shown. This subtype of LCPT shows nonspecific acute tubular injury by light microscopy. In this field, the tubular epithelium shows reactive nuclei and cytoplasmic thinning.* **(Right)** *Transmission electron photomicrograph of proximal tubule cytoplasm shows lysozymes with an irregular mottled appearance and no evidence of crystal formation. This change is also nonspecific but commonly present in this subtype of LCPT.*

Positive Lambda in Tubular Cytoplasm

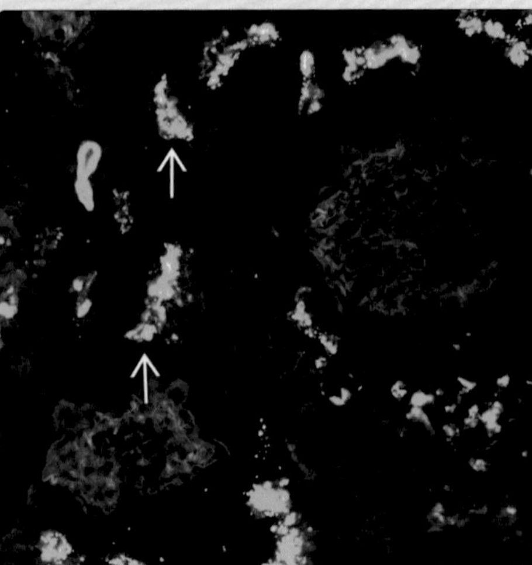

Negative Kappa in Tubular Cytoplasm

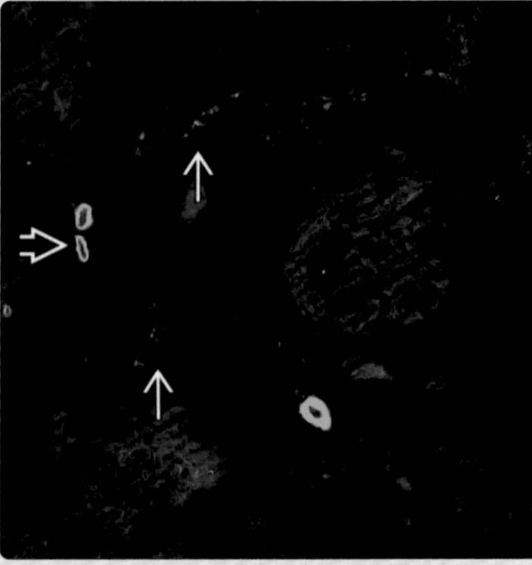

(Left) *Light chain proximal tubulopathy without organized inclusions is shown. The sine qua non for this subtype of LCPT is the finding of light chain restriction within the proximal tubule cytoplasm. In this field, there is bright staining by lambda in the proximal tubules ➡.* **(Right)** *A serial section stained for kappa shows negative staining in the tubular cytoplasm ➡. The tubular casts stain equally by kappa and lambda ➡.*

TERMINOLOGY

Abbreviations

- Light chain proximal tubulopathy (LCPT)

Definitions

- Injury secondary to monoclonal free light chains (FLC) accumulating in proximal tubule cytoplasm

ETIOLOGY/PATHOGENESIS

Injury Due to Excess Production of Free Light Chains

- Under normal conditions, FLCs degraded within proximal tubule lysosomes
- Plasma cell dyscrasia (PCD) results in excess FLC production and accumulation of FLC in proximal tubule cytoplasm
- Excessive FLC endocytosis induces spectrum of inflammatory effects that include
    - Activation of redox pathways
    - Increased transcription of inflammatory and pro-fibrotic cytokines

Clinical Significance of LCPT Without Organized Inclusions

- Controversial
- Free light chains are toxic to tubules and cause injury without forming organized inclusions visible by LM (e.g., crystals)
- Case by case clinicopathologic correlation required to determine whether this finding represents end-organ damage

CLINICAL ISSUES

Presentation

- Typically presents with slowly progressive renal failure or proteinuria
- > 90% have PCD
    - Most patients will not carry PCD diagnosis at time of kidney biopsy
- "Classic" finding of Fanconi syndrome absent in most patients

Treatment

- Treat underlying PCD or lymphoproliferative disorder

MICROSCOPIC

Histologic Features

- 3 variants of LCPT without crystal formation
    - Light chain proximal tubulopathy without organized inclusions
        - Light chain restriction within proximal tubule protein resorption droplets by IF is key finding
        - Nondescript acute tubular injury by LM
        - Nonspecific EM findings include increased lysosomes with irregular contours and mottled appearance
    - Amyloid proximal tubulopathy
        - Congo red-positive tubular inclusions by LM
        - Inclusions show light chain restriction by IF
        - EM shows intracytoplasmic membrane-bound inclusions containing overlapping fibrils in proximal tubule cytoplasm
    - Light chain proximal tubulopathy with large fibrillary aggregates
        - Intracytoplasmic textured inclusions in proximal tubules
            - Eosinophilic
            - Silver-negative on Jones methenamine silver
            - Fuchsinophilic on Masson trichrome stain
        - Congo red-negative inclusions show light chain restriction by IF
            - Some cases with false-negative routine IF staining require antigen retrieval to elicit staining
        - Bundles of larger fibrils present within tubular cytoplasm by EM

ANCILLARY TESTS

Immunohistochemistry

- LCPT with fibrillary aggregates may have false-negative light chain staining by routine immunofluorescence on frozen sections
    - Immunohistochemistry increases sensitivity for detection of light chain restriction due to antigen retrieval

Immunofluorescence

- Performed on paraffin-embedded sections after pronase digestion
    - Antigen retrieval allows demonstration of light chain restriction in cases with fibrillary aggregates that show false-negative staining by routine immunofluorescence on frozen sections

Serologic Testing

- Free light chain assay for demonstration of urine free light chains

DIFFERENTIAL DIAGNOSIS

Acute Tubular Injury

- No tubular cytoplasm inclusions or light chain restriction

Uromodulin Storage Disease

- Tubular cytoplasmic inclusions do not show light chain restriction

Antiviral Drug Nephrotoxicity (e.g., Tenofovir)

- Tubular megamitochondria, which resemble inclusions of LCPT
    - Do not show light chain restriction

SELECTED REFERENCES

1. Basnayake K et al: The biology of immunoglobulin free light chains and kidney injury. Kidney Int. 79(12):1289-301, 2011
2. Larsen CP et al: The morphologic spectrum and clinical significance of light chain proximal tubulopathy with and without crystal formation. Mod Pathol. 24(11):1462-9, 2011
3. Basnayake K et al: Immunoglobulin light chains activate tubular epithelial cells through redox signaling. J Am Soc Nephrol. 21(7):1165-73, 2010
4. Kapur U et al: Expanding the pathologic spectrum of immunoglobulin light chain proximal tubulopathy. Arch Pathol Lab Med. 2007 Sep;131(9):1368-72. Erratum in: Arch Pathol Lab Med. 132(1):13, 2008

(Left) *Amyloid proximal tubulopathy is shown. Proximal tubules have scattered cytoplasmic inclusions* ➡ *that stain blue on Masson trichrome stain.* **(Right)** *Cytoplasmic inclusions stain positive on Congo red* ➡ *and showed green birefringence upon polarization (not shown) in this example of amyloid proximal tubulopathy. This patient did not have amyloidosis deposition outside of the proximal tubule cytoplasm.*

Proximal Tubule Inclusions

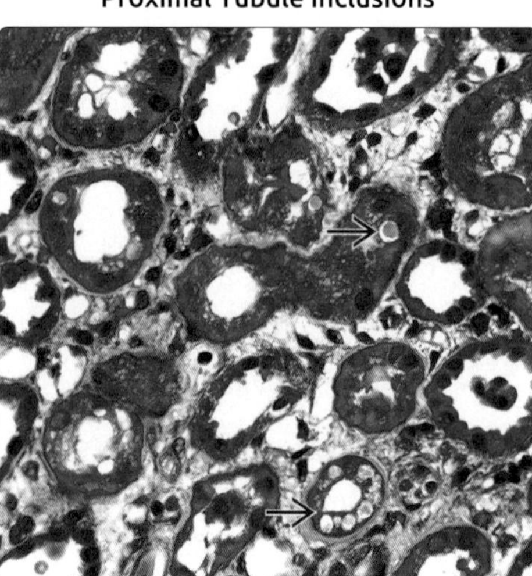

Positive Congo Red Staining

(Left) *Amyloid proximal tubulopathy is shown. Congo red-positive cytoplasmic inclusions are easily appreciated under red fluorescence* ➡. **(Right)** *Transmission electron photomicrograph shows an aggregate of fibrils in the proximal tubule cytoplasm of a case with amyloid proximal tubulopathy.*

Congo Red Staining Under Red Fluorescence

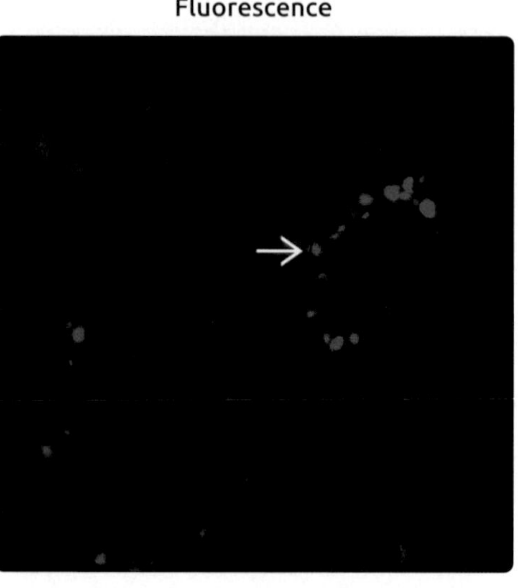

Fibrillary Aggregates in Tubular Cytoplasm

(Left) *Amyloid proximal tubulopathy is shown. Cytoplasmic inclusions stain positive for lambda* ➡ *by direct immunofluorescence on fresh tissue.* **(Right)** *Kappa is negative in the tubular cytoplasmic inclusions* ➡ *in this example of amyloid proximal tubulopathy.*

Inclusions Positive for Lambda

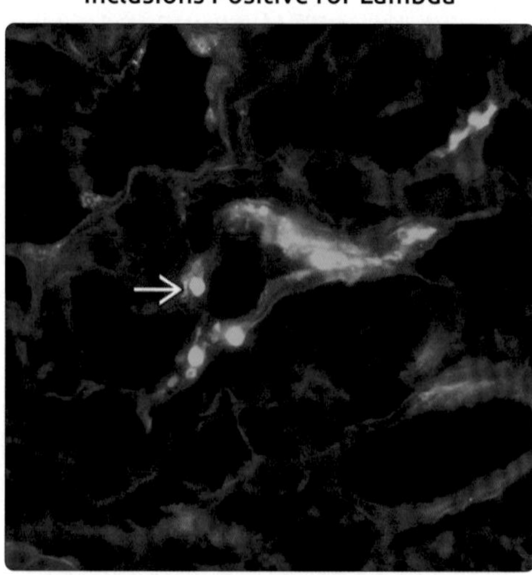

Inclusions Negative for Kappa

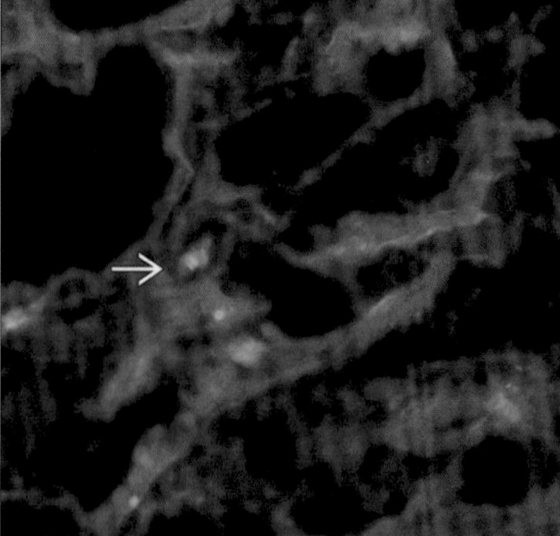

Textured Inclusions in PAS

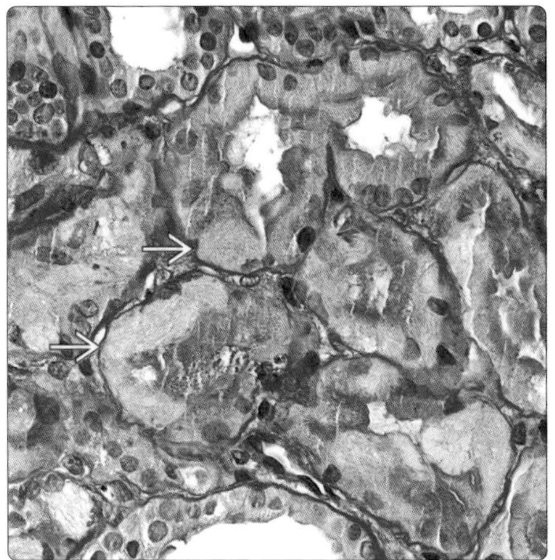

Fuchsinophilic Inclusions in Trichrome Stain

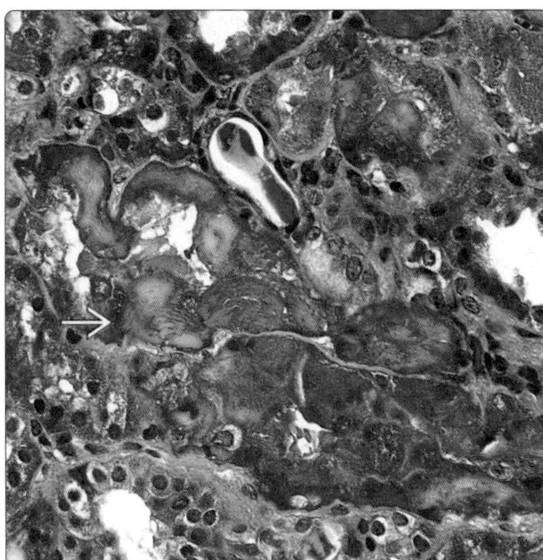

(Left) *Light chain proximal tubulopathy with fibrillary aggregates is shown. Proximal tubular intracytoplasmic textured inclusions* ➡ *stain negative on PAS. These same inclusions were negative by Congo red staining (not shown).* **(Right)** *The fibrillar inclusions are limited to the proximal tubule cytoplasm and stain brightly fuchsinophilic* ➡ *on Masson trichrome stain.*

Eosinophilic Inclusions in Silver Stain

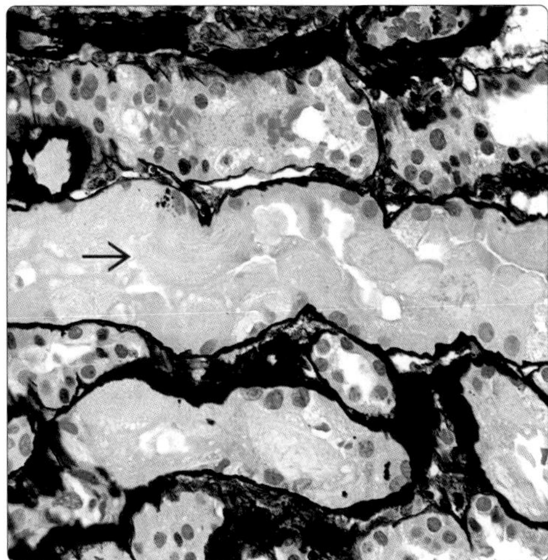

Kappa Restriction in Proximal Tubules

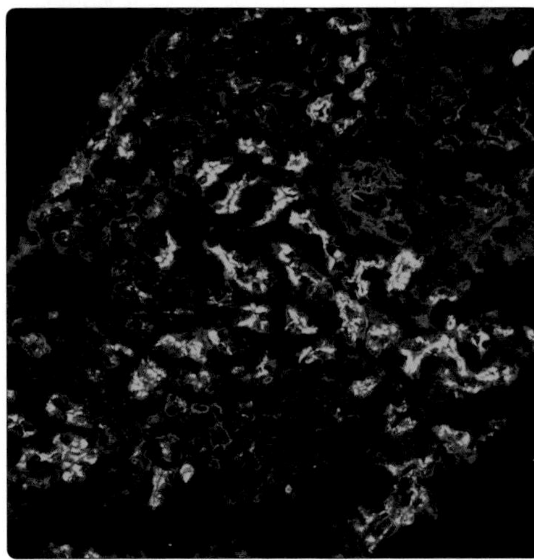

(Left) *Light chain proximal tubulopathy with fibrillary aggregates is shown. The fibrillar inclusions* ➡ *stain eosinophilic and silver negative on Jones methenamine silver.* **(Right)** *Immunofluorescence shows strong staining for kappa light chain within the proximal tubule cytoplasm. The lambda stain (not shown) was negative.*

Bundles of Large Fibrils

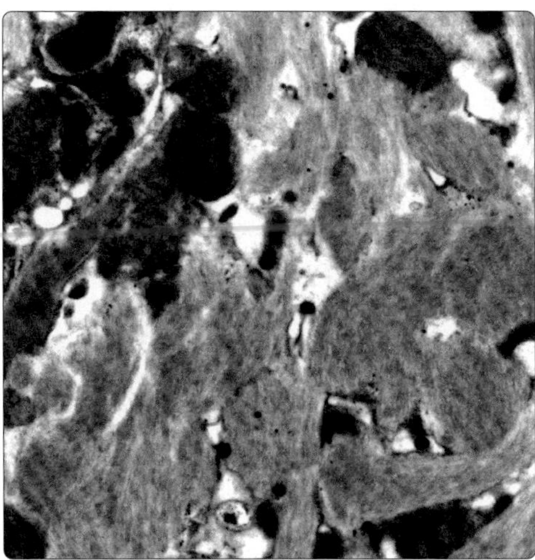

Bundles of Large Fibrils

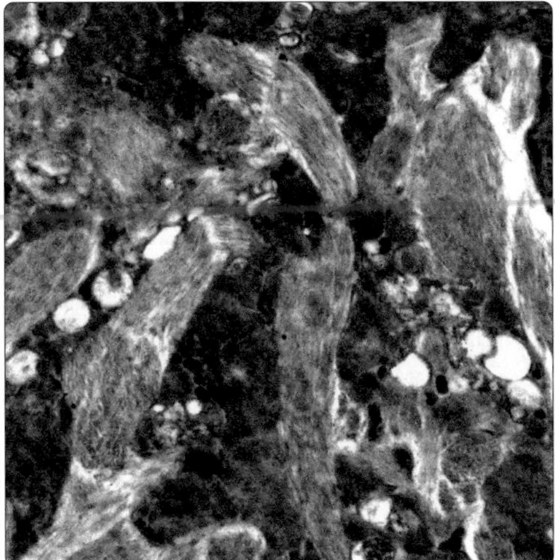

(Left) *Light chain proximal tubulopathy with fibrillary aggregates is shown. Bundles of larger fibrils are apparent by transmission electron microscopy.* **(Right)** *These bundles of fibrils are not obviously membrane bound and are therefore likely to not be restricted to the lysosomal compartment.*

TERMINOLOGY

Definitions

- Protein folding diseases characterized by accumulation of 7-12 nm diameter fibrils with β-pleated sheet structure that confers birefringence after staining with Congo red

EPIDEMIOLOGY

Age Range

- AL & AA amyloid: Typically 50-70 years old
- Familial forms: < 40 years old; AFib older

Gender

- M:F = 2:1 overall

Incidence

- 1.4/100,000 per person/year; all types (France)
- About 10% of cases are familial
- 1-5% of adult patients with nephrotic syndrome have some form of amyloidosis

ETIOLOGY/PATHOGENESIS

Amyloidogenic Proteins

- > 30 different precursor proteins
  - Clonal proliferation of plasma cells (AL/AH types)
  - Chronic inflammation (AA type)
  - Genetic (multiple proteins)
  - Failure of excretion (β2 microglobulin)
  - Localized forms
    - Islet amyloid polypeptide (AIAPP) in islets of Langerhans (type 2 diabetes mellitus)
    - Semenogelin 1 (ASem) in seminal vesicles (↑ with aging)
    - Lactadherin (AMed) in aortic media (↑ with aging)
    - Neoplasm (e.g., calcitonin [ACal] associated with medullary thyroid carcinoma)
- ~ 90% of renal amyloidosis cases are AL or AA

Pathogenesis

- Amyloidogenic proteins have antiparallel, β-pleated sheet tertiary structure (also termed cross β-sheets)
  - Structure determined by x-ray diffraction, which shows 2 reflections: Sharp one at ~ 4.7 & more diffuse one at ~ 8-12
  - Cross-β motif forms central structural spine of amyloid protofilaments
  - Structure accounts for Congo red staining & apple-green birefringence under polarized light since it enables anisotropic binding of Congo red molecules
  - Resistance to metabolic processing leads to accumulation & interference with physiologic functioning
- Amyloid deposits composed of amyloidogenic protein nonfibrillary glycoproteins serum amyloid P (SAP), apolipoprotein E, & glycosaminoglycans
  - Normal plasma proteins that bind all amyloid proteins
  - SAP present early & promotes deposits
  - Labeled SAP used to image amyloid in vivo

Renal Deposits

- Certain forms typically involve kidney (AL, AA, fibrinogen, Apo AI & AII, Alys)
- Glomerular mesangial amyloid accumulation often occurs 1st as mesangial cells lose usual smooth muscle phenotype & acquire macrophage phenotype
- Fibrils penetrate & aggregate in GBM, suggesting that they may be locally formed

CLINICAL IMPLICATIONS

Clinical Presentation

- Proteinuria
  - Present in virtually all with renal involvement
  - ~ 5% of adult cases of nephrotic syndrome
- Hematuria
  - Rarely a presenting feature
- Extrarenal manifestations
  - Congestive heart failure, arrhythmias, orthostatic hypotension

Pale PAS of Amyloid

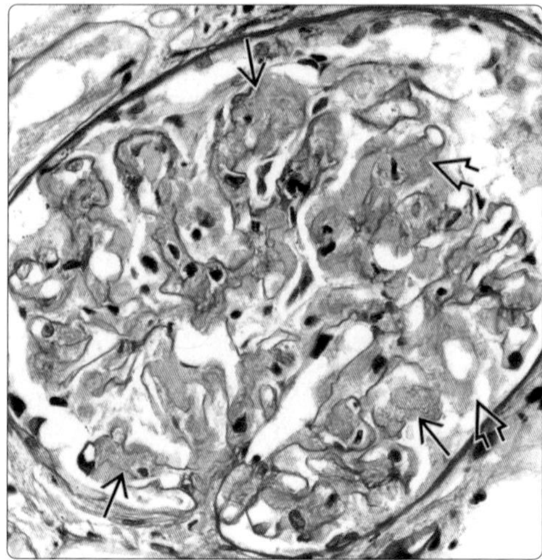

"Spicular" Amyloid Electron Microscopy

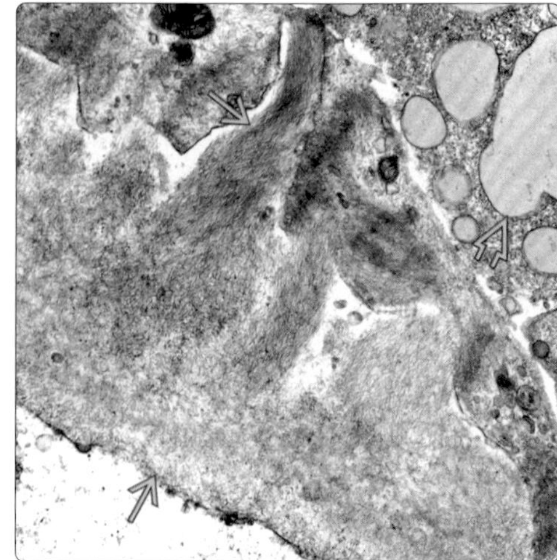

(Left) *The classic appearance of amyloid deposits is a pale amorphous accumulation in the mesangium ➡ and along the GBM ➡ in PAS stains without cellular proliferation or inflammation.* **(Right)** *EM reveals subepithelial "spicular" amyloid fibrils ➡ in the GBM. Fibrils are ~ 7-12 nm in diameter and are nonperiodic. Podocytes have effaced foot processes and reabsorption droplets ➡.*

- Dysesthesias
  - Bladder dysfunction
- ↑ organ size: Hepatomegaly/splenomegaly, macroglossia
- Carpal tunnel syndrome

MACROSCOPIC

General Features

- Enlarged, pale, firm, & with waxy appearance
- Cut surfaces remain firm & flat in contrast to normal kidney, which bulges after sectioning
- Lugol iodine stains glomeruli dark brown in cut surfaces (like starch)

MICROSCOPIC

General Features

- Glomeruli
  - Expansion of mesangium & thickening of capillary walls by amorphous eosinophilic material
    - Amorphous deposits are acidophilic, "salmon orange"
    - Usually less acidophilic than collagen (i.e., mesangial sclerosis, interstitial fibrosis)
    - Normal mesangial matrix, presumably destroyed by activated metalloproteinases, is replaced by amyloid fibrils
    - Nodular mesangial expansion can often be seen
    - Little or no hypercellularity
    - Amyloid is weakly PAS positive, less than GBM
  - Amyloid deposition can 1st be seen in mesangium & blood vessel walls
    - Early mesangial deposits may be quite small & subject to being overlooked, resulting in erroneous diagnosis of minimal change disease/glomerulopathy
  - Rare cases of AL & AA amyloid with crescents
  - Silver stains: Expanded mesangial areas but ↓ or no silver staining (i.e., "loss of argyrophilia")
    - GBMs also may be engulfed by the material, showing up as areas of complete GBM discontinuity
    - Subepithelial spikes in capillary loops ("cock's comb")
  - Eventually, ESRD kidneys with glomerulosclerosis from amyloid can be suspected by pale staining on JMS or PAS stains
    - Mesangial & subendothelial deposits eventually obliterate glomeruli
  - Trichrome stains blue in amyloid, usually paler than trichrome staining of collagen
- Tubulointerstitium
  - Congo red staining useful in identifying vascular & interstitial amyloid
  - Interstitial involvement often contiguous with involvement of TBMs & vessels
    - Eventually, IF & tubular atrophy (TA) may be extensive, admixed with interstitial inflammation
  - Tubular casts containing amyloid are sometimes present and, in rare case reports, are the only manifestation of amyloidosis
    - Material has fibrillar appearance characteristic of amyloid material on EM
  - Interstitium may be expanded by amyloid material
    - Mast cells may lead to IF in AA type

Immunofluorescence

- Pattern depends on type of amyloid

Electron Microscopy

- Fibrils
  - Nonbranching, nonperiodic, ~ 7-12 nm in diameter
    - Amorphous "cottony" appearance at ~ 5,000x
    - Electron-lucent core at ~ 100,000x
    - Internal references: Cell membrane 8.5 nm; actin: 5 nm
  - Randomly distributed in mesangium & GBM
  - Fibrils sometimes extend transmurally, replacing entire glomerular basement membrane
    - In subepithelial zone, fibrils align roughly perpendicular to GBM, producing "spike" formation or "cock's comb" (also called "spicular amyloid")
  - Podocyte foot processes often effaced, & cytoplasm has condensation of actin filaments
- Immunoelectron microscopy can be used for various amyloids, usually employing antibody probes conjugated with gold particles (immunogold)

Special Stains

- Congo red
  - Orangeophilic material on brightfield examination that has apple-green birefringence when examined with polarized light (i.e., crossed polars)
    - In contrast to fibrillar collagen, amyloid fibrils are only birefringent after Congo red stain
    - Important to have simultaneous positive control
    - Rather than "apple-green" birefringence, some advocate the term "anomalous colors"
  - Red without polarization (called "congophilia")
    - Elastic fibers are congophilic but not birefringent
  - Small amyloid quantities may make it difficult to demonstrate apple-green birefringence
    - Higher quality polarizing microscope will have greater sensitivity
    - 9 μm sections recommended for Congo red staining to maximize detection of small quantities of amyloid
    - Placing Congo red stains under green fluorescent light makes amyloid deposits appear bright red; sensitive but not specific
- Thioflavine T & S
  - Thioflavin T activated by blue light to emit yellow fluorescence; sensitive, not specific
  - Reports of ↑ sensitivity vs. Congo red if small quantities of amyloid present
  - Rarely used currently
- Crystal violet
  - Metachromatic stain not usually used in routine diagnostic work

Immunohistochemistry

- SAP (does not discriminate between types)
  - Used to compare with stains for specific protein
- Antibodies available for a variety of amyloid types

Pathologic Interpretation Pearls

- Quality of polarizing microscope is crucial determinant of sensitivity

Amyloid Types and Clinicopathologic Features

Amyloid Protein	Clinical Features	Tissue/Organ Distribution	Renal Pathology
Neoplastic/Clonal B Cell/Plasma Cell			
AL/AH (Ig light/heavy chain)	Most common renal amyloidosis cause; nephrotic syndrome common (40%); fatigue, weight loss, neuropathy, GI symptoms, hepatosplenomegaly, carpal tunnel	Widespread: Kidney, heart, GI, liver, spleen, nerves	Glomerular, interstitial, & arterial deposits (~ 10% lack glomerular deposits)
Chronic Inflammation			
AA amyloid; serum amyloid A protein; chronic infection or autoimmune disease	Chronic infection or inflammation; neoplasia; minority idiopathic (~ 10%); wide age range (~ 10-90 years); nephrotic syndrome or renal insufficiency	Widespread: Kidney almost always; GI, liver, spleen, thyroid, adrenal; less commonly heart	Glomerular deposits usually predominate; some cases with only tubulointerstitial &/or vascular deposits
AA amyloid; hereditary inflammatory syndromes	FMF, HIDS, FCU, & MWS; episodes of fevers, pain with peritonitis, pleuriits; onset of amyloidosis < 40 years old; nephrotic syndrome or renal insufficiency	Widespread, as above	Glomerular deposits usually predominate; prominent peritubular rings; sometimes primarily in medulla
Genetic Mutation			
AFib (fibrinogen Aα chain)	Onset 20s-70s, then rapid kidney failure (1-5 years); often no family history; recurs in transplants; at least 4 different mutations	Kidney, not heart or nerves	Exclusively glomerular deposits; stain positive for fibrinogen
AApoAI (apolipoprotein A-I)	Hypertension & renal failure without nephrotic syndrome	Liver, kidney, heart	Arterial & interstitial deposits
AApoAII (apolipoprotein A-II)	Slowly progressive renal insufficiency	Kidney, heart	Glomerular, arterial, & interstitial deposits
ACys (cystatin C)	Stroke, no renal disease	Cerebral vessels primarily	Arterial deposits
AFib (fibrinogen Aα-chain)	Onset 20s-70s, then rapid kidney failure (1-5 years); often no family history; recurs in transplants	Kidney; not heart or nerves	Exclusively glomerular deposits; stain positive for fibrinogen
AGel (gelsolin)	Cranial nerves, cornea, cutis laxa (Finnish hereditary amyloidosis)	Nerves, cornea, skin, kidney	Glomerular deposits
ALys (lysozyme)	Dermal petechiae, GI bleeding	Kidney, liver, spleen, skin, GI tract	Glomerular & arterial deposits
ATTR (transthyretin)	Congestive heart failure, peripheral neuropathy; > 100 different mutations; cardiac variant with wild-type AATR in elderly (senile systemic amyloidosis)	Heart & nerves; sometimes eye & kidney	Primarily glomerular deposits but sometimes limited to medullary interstitium
Decreased Excretion			
Aβ2m (β2-microgloblulin)	Osteoarthopathy & neuropathy in patients on chronic hemodialysis	Most organs, especially vascular deposits, juxtarticular cysts	Deposits present but not clinically significant
Unclassified			
ALECT2 (leukocyte chemotactic factor 2)	Proteinuria, nephrotic syndrome; no mutation yet identified; common SNP in *LECT2* gene (rs31517) in all sequenced cases	Kidney only	Diffuse involvement of glomeruli, arteries, & interstitium

FMF = familial Mediterranean fever; HIDS = hyper-IgD syndrome; FCU = familial cold urticaria; MWS = Muckle-Wells syndrome.

Adapted from Merlini G et al: Molecular mechanisms of amyloidosis. N Engl J Med. 349(6):583-96, 2003.

ANCILLARY TESTS FOR AMYLOID DETECTION

Mass Spectrometry (MS) & Proteomics

- Laser microdissection (LMD) & tandem mass spectrometry (MS)-based proteomic analysis useful in typing amyloidosis

Abdominal Fat Pad Fine-Needle Aspiration

- Sensitivity ~ 20-60%; specificity ~ 100%
- Core biopsy probably more sensitive

Rectal Biopsy

- Sensitivity & specificity likely varies based on amyloid form
    - For example: FMF biopsy studies indicate following sensitivities for amyloidosis: Renal (88%), testicular (87%), bone marrow (80%), rectal (75%), liver (48%), gingival (19%)

SELECTED REFERENCES

1. Sayed RH et al: Emerging treatments for amyloidosis. Kidney Int. 87(3):516-26, 2015
2. Westermark GT et al: AA amyloidosis: pathogenesis and targeted therapy. Annu Rev Pathol. 10:321-44, 2015
3. Gillmore JD et al: Pathophysiology and treatment of systemic amyloidosis. Nat Rev Nephrol. 9(10):574-86, 2013

Amyloid Fibrillogenesis

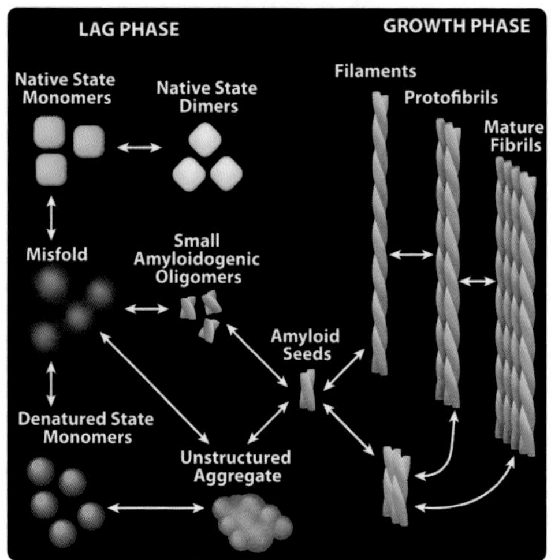

Amorphous Amyloid

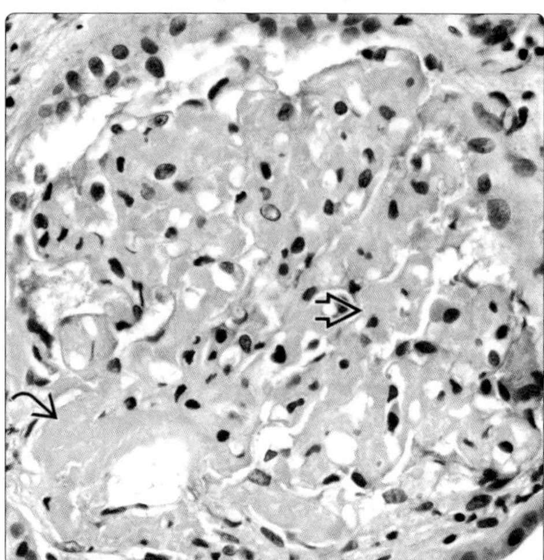

(Left) *Amyloid fibrillogenesis occurs in stages, proceeding through ordered self-assembly of unstable misfolded precursor proteins into protofilaments and culminating in mature fibrils with 3-6 filaments wrapped around each other.* **(Right)** *Relatively high power in a 68 year old with amyloidosis, proteinuria of 5 g/d, & creatinine of 1.3 mg/dL shows that there is accumulation of amorphous extracellular material in the mesangium ⇒ and in the arteriole entering the glomerulus ↷.*

Amyloid Pale on PAS

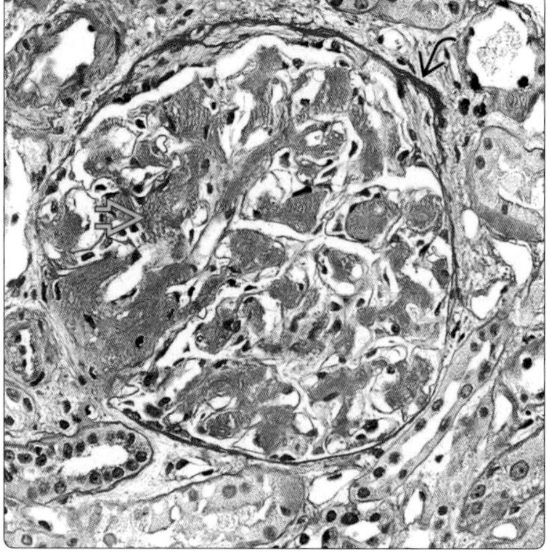

Nonargyrophilic Amyloid

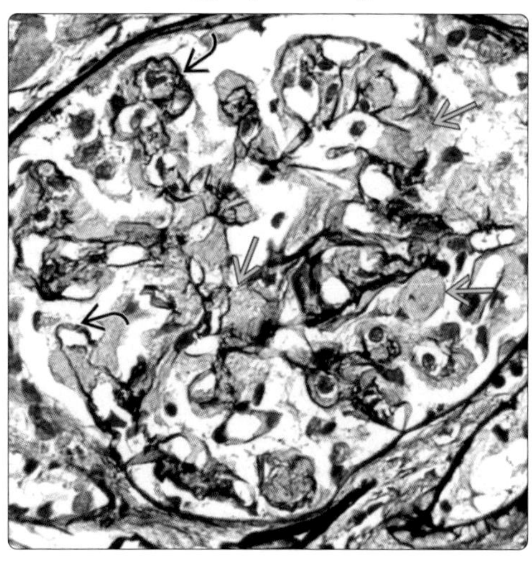

(Left) *Light microscopy shows accumulation of material in the mesangium ⇒, which stains less intensely by PAS stain than the basement membranes of the kidney (e.g., Bowman capsule ↷).* **(Right)** *Silver stains can be used to advantage in amyloidosis, in which they reveal the location of the pale-staining amyloid ⇒ that is less argyrophilic than the surrounding basement membranes ↷.*

Amyloid Trichrome Pale

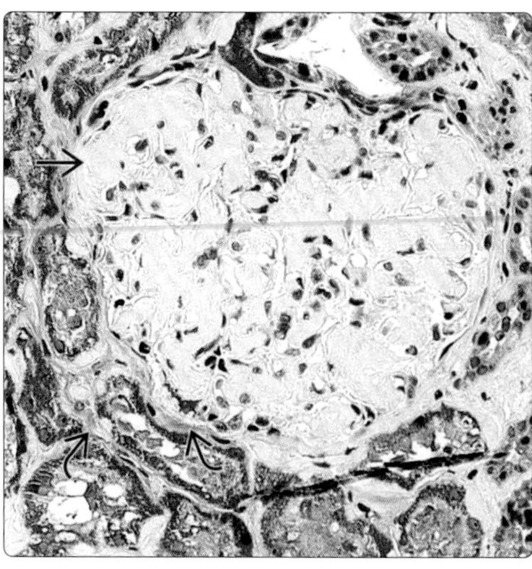

Vascular and Glomerular Amyloid

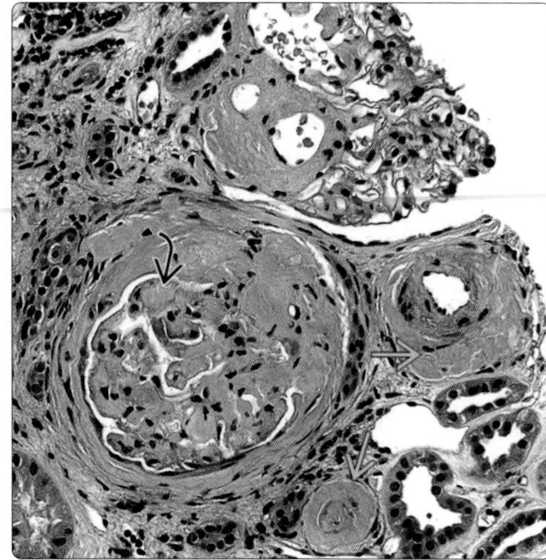

(Left) *On a trichrome stain, this glomerulus with amyloidosis shows that the amyloid material is pale blue ⇒, being less dark than the fibrous tissue "skeleton" ↷ of the surrounding kidney. Fibrillary GN, which has somewhat similar deposits by FM, is characteristically red on trichrome stain.* **(Right)** *By H&E, there is accumulation of amyloid in nearly sclerotic glomeruli ↷ and in vessels ⇒.*

(Left) *Examination of a case of amyloidosis using immunofluorescence for lambda shows extensive accumulation of lambda light chain in the glomerulus, primarily in the mesangium and also in the afferent arteriole.* (Right) *Immunofluorescence for lambda in a case of amyloidosis shows extensive amorphous accumulation in the interstitium.*

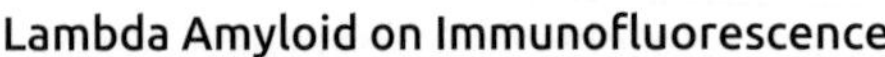

Lambda Amyloid on Immunofluorescence

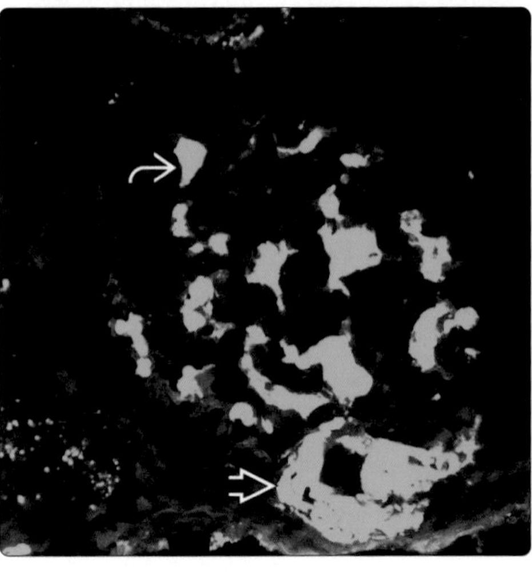

Interstitial Lambda Amyloid on Immunofluorescence

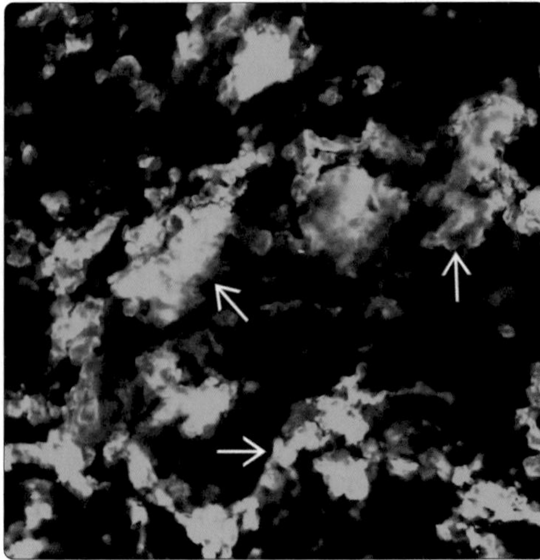

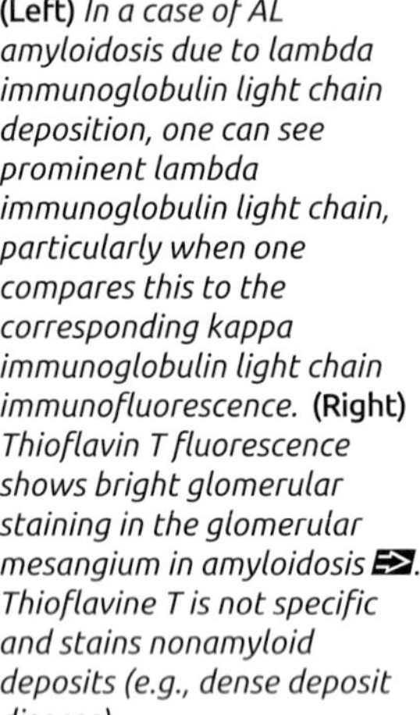

(Left) *In a case of AL amyloidosis due to lambda immunoglobulin light chain deposition, one can see prominent lambda immunoglobulin light chain, particularly when one compares this to the corresponding kappa immunoglobulin light chain immunofluorescence.* (Right) *Thioflavin T fluorescence shows bright glomerular staining in the glomerular mesangium in amyloidosis. Thioflavine T is not specific and stains nonamyloid deposits (e.g., dense deposit disease).*

Kappa vs. Lambda Immunofluorescence in Amyloidosis

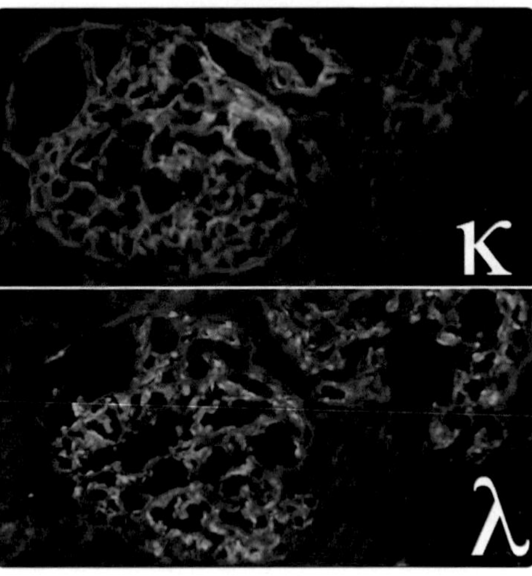

Thioflavin T Fluorescence

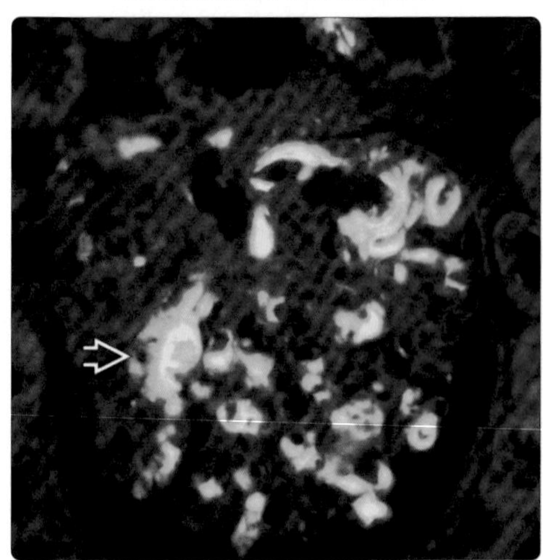

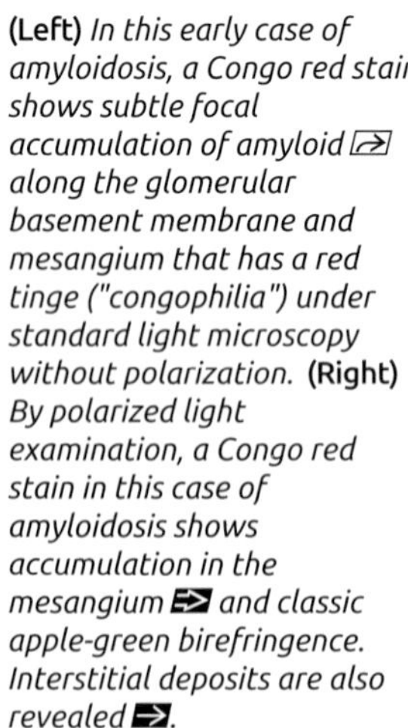

(Left) *In this early case of amyloidosis, a Congo red stain shows subtle focal accumulation of amyloid along the glomerular basement membrane and mesangium that has a red tinge ("congophilia") under standard light microscopy without polarization.* (Right) *By polarized light examination, a Congo red stain in this case of amyloidosis shows accumulation in the mesangium and classic apple-green birefringence. Interstitial deposits are also revealed.*

Congo Red(+) Amyloid

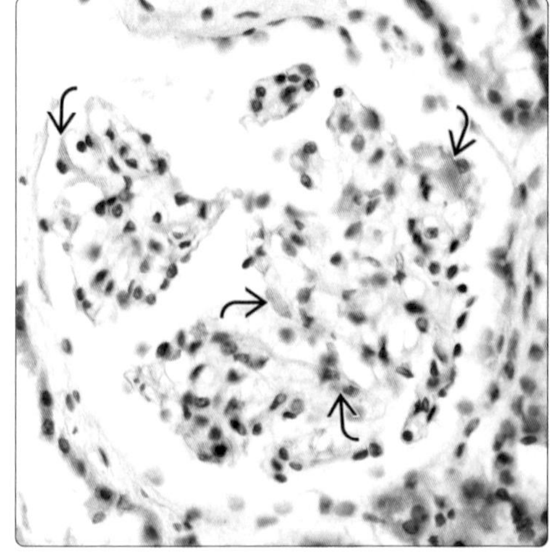

Apple-Green Birefringence of Amyloid

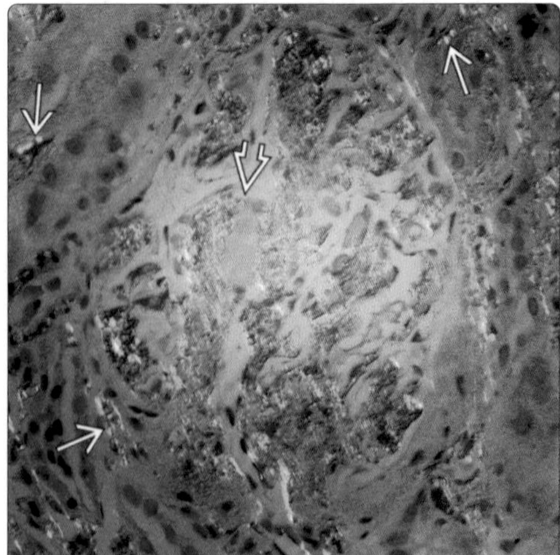

Congo Red(+) Interstitial Amyloid

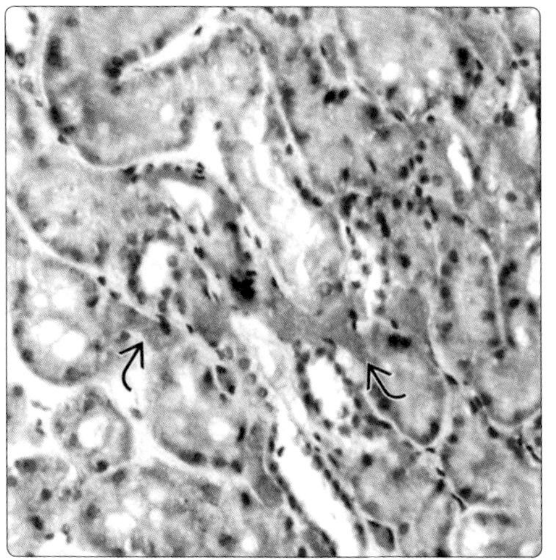

Congo Red(+) LECT2 Amyloid

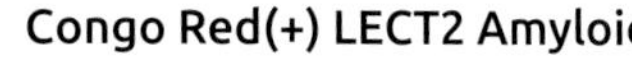

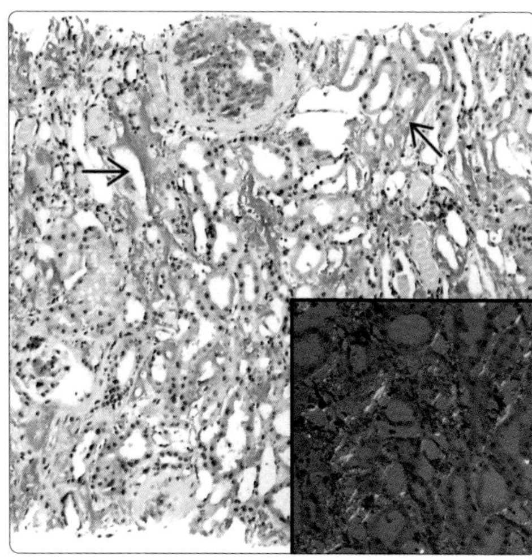

(Left) *In this case of amyloidosis, Congo red shows accumulation of amyloid in the interstitium between tubules* ↷*, staining red ("congophilic") under standard light microscopic examination without polarization.* **(Right)** *The interstitium stains positively by Congo red* →*. The Congo red(+) material shows apple-green birefringence under polarized light (insert). IF and AA amyloid staining were negative. Mass spectrometry confirmed LECT2 amyloidosis. (Courtesy M. Fidler, MD.)*

Glomerular Basement Membrane Amyloid on EM

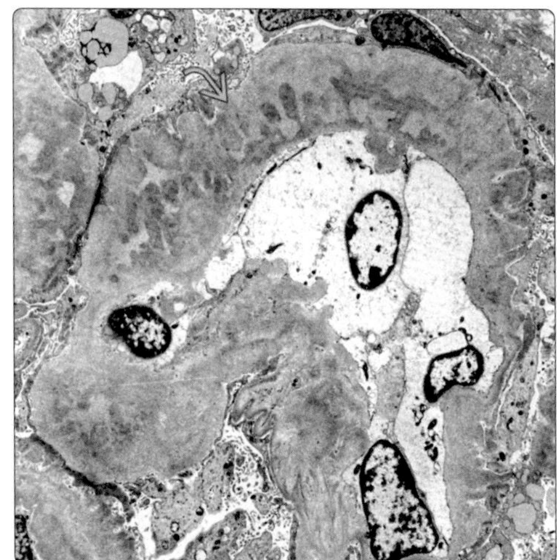

Small Vessel Amyloid

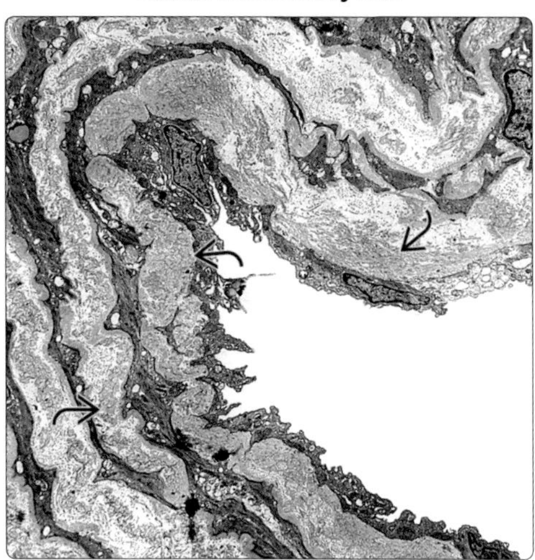

(Left) *EM of a glomerular capillary loop in a patient with amyloidosis and nephrotic syndrome shows marked thickening of the GBM* ⇨ *due to accumulation of amyloid fibrils, which appear amorphous at this power.* **(Right)** *In this case of amyloidosis, there is accumulation of amyloid material in a small blood vessel underneath the endothelium* ↷ *and between smooth muscle cells.*

Mesangial and GBM Amyloid

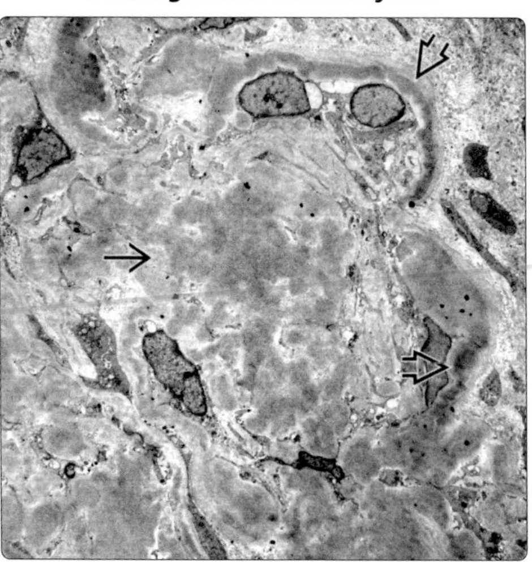

Amyloid Fibril Width

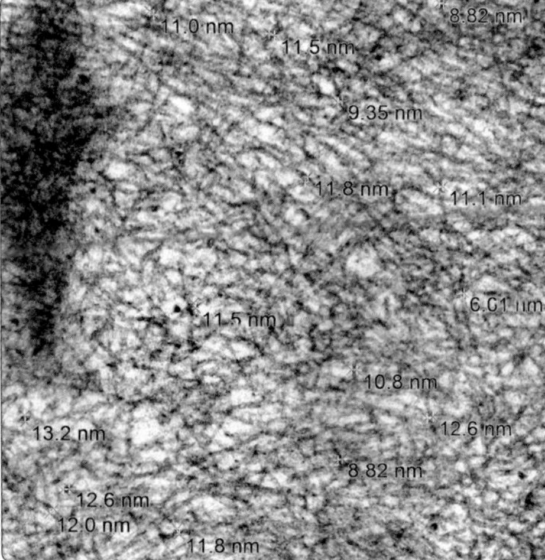

(Left) *An unusual case of amyloidosis resembles dense deposit disease by electron microscopy, with electron dense sausage-like deposits* ⇨ *along the glomerular basement membranes and within the mesangium* →*.* **(Right)** *Measurement of fibrils in fibrillar deposits can be useful in confirming that the deposits are amyloid since amyloid typically measures ~ 7-12 nm in diameter.*

AL/AH Amyloidosis

KEY FACTS

TERMINOLOGY

- Amyloidosis due to fibrils derived from immunoglobulin light (AL), heavy chain (AH), or combination (AHL)

ETIOLOGY/PATHOGENESIS

- AL amyloidosis is most common cause of renal amyloidosis in USA/western hemisphere
- Plasma cell dyscrasias or lymphoproliferative disorders

CLINICAL ISSUES

- Age: > 50 years old
- Proteinuria ± renal insufficiency
  - Nephrotic syndrome common
- Other organs affected including heart and GI tract
- Serum protein electrophoresis &/or free light chain assays may be useful
- Treatment: Myeloma chemotherapy, also bone marrow &/or renal transplantation

MICROSCOPIC

- Mesangial expansion by eosinophilic, weakly PAS(+) amorphous material
  - Congo red(+) deposits polarize
- GBM "spikes" on silver stains
- All renal compartments may have deposits

ANCILLARY TESTS

- IF: κ or λ deposition in AL amyloidosis or heavy chain in AH amyloidosis
- EM: Randomly arranged fibrils 7-12 nm in diameter in mesangium and GBM

TOP DIFFERENTIAL DIAGNOSES

- Other types of amyloidosis
- Fibrillary glomerulonephritis (GN)
- Minimal change disease

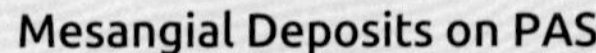

Mesangial Deposits on PAS

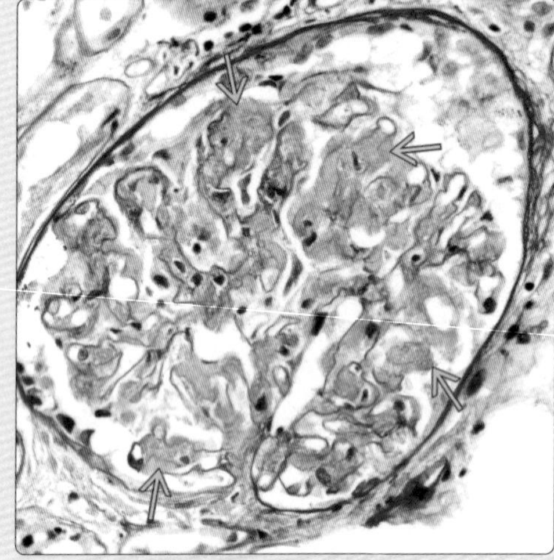

Unpolarized and Polarized Congo Red

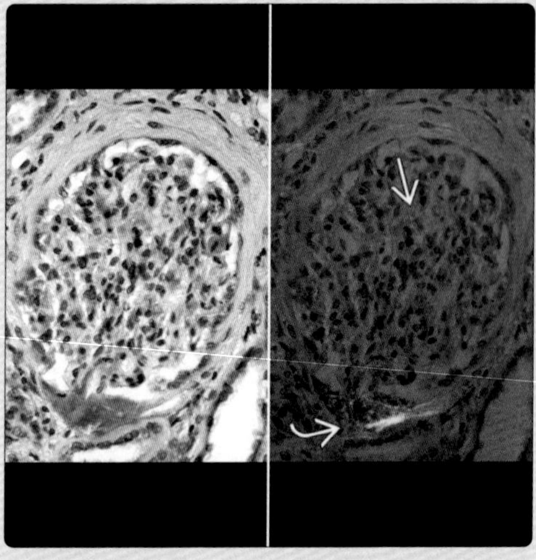

(Left) *Amyloid deposits are present as PAS-weak deposits → in a 68-year-old man with nephrotic-range proteinuria and a plasma cell dyscrasia with lambda immunoglobulin light chain restriction.* **(Right)** *Renal biopsy from a patient with AL amyloidosis (lambda) shows deposits in glomerulus that stain red with Congo red (left) and polarize red/green (right). The deposits in the arteriole are most prominent ➔, but faint birefringence is detectable in the mesangium ➔.*

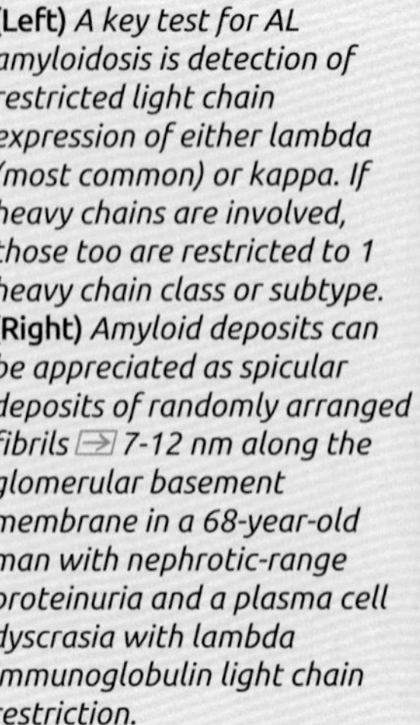

(Left) *A key test for AL amyloidosis is detection of restricted light chain expression of either lambda (most common) or kappa. If heavy chains are involved, those too are restricted to 1 heavy chain class or subtype.* **(Right)** *Amyloid deposits can be appreciated as spicular deposits of randomly arranged fibrils → 7-12 nm along the glomerular basement membrane in a 68-year-old man with nephrotic-range proteinuria and a plasma cell dyscrasia with lambda immunoglobulin light chain restriction.*

Light Chain Restriction

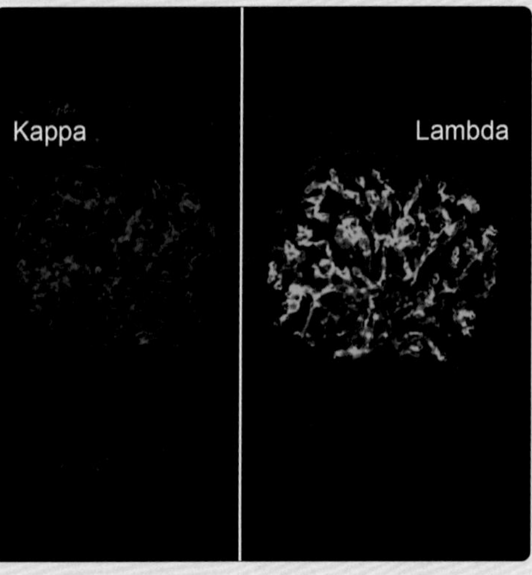

Spicular Amyloid Deposits in GBM

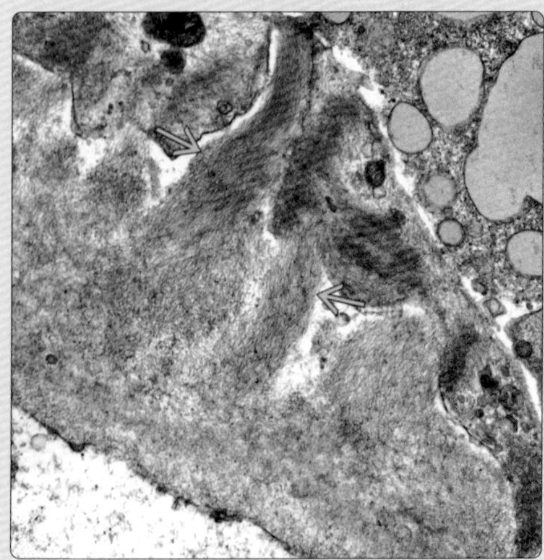

TERMINOLOGY

Abbreviations

- Amyloid light chain (AL)
- Amyloid heavy chain (AH)

Synonyms

- Primary amyloidosis
- Amyloidosis associated with multiple myeloma
- Immunoglobulin (Ig)-related amyloidosis

Definitions

- AL: Amyloid derived from immunoglobulin light chain
- AH: Amyloid derived from immunoglobulin heavy chain
- AHL: Amyloid derived from immunoglobulin heavy and light chain (also referred to by some as "AH + AL")

ETIOLOGY/PATHOGENESIS

AL Amyloid

- Most common renal amyloidosis in USA/western hemisphere
- Plasma cell dyscrasias or lymphoproliferative disorders
  - ~ 20% meet diagnostic criteria for multiple myeloma or leukemia/lymphoma when amyloidosis diagnosed
    - Some not until ≥ 15 years after amyloidosis diagnosis
  - ~ 75% lambda light chains
    - Often N-terminal of variable light chain region
  - 40% develop nephrotic syndrome
    - ~ 10% lack glomerular deposits

AH Amyloid

- Rare cases (~ 1.5% of Ig-related amyloid) composed of monoclonal Ig heavy chains
  - Most derived from Ig heavy chain variable region (VH) belonging to VH3 subgroup
  - No report of VH1 fragment deposition leading to AH amyloidosis
- Some composed of both light and heavy chain components (AL + AH)

AHL Amyloid

- Rare cases (~ 4% of Ig-related amyloid) composed of monoclonal heavy and light chains

Amyloidogenic Proteins

- Clonal proliferation of plasma cells (AL/AH types)
- Clathrin-mediated internalization of AL amyloid into mesangial cells that acquire macrophage phenotype
  - Mesangial fibrils extruded into mesangium
- Molecular differences resulting in amyloidogenic light chain
  - Amino acid sequence differences
  - Posttranslational modifications (e.g., glycosylation)

CLINICAL ISSUES

Epidemiology

- Incidence
  - Varies based on population
    - USA and Western world
      - ~ 74-85% of amyloidosis of AL type
    - 0.6-1.0/100,000 per person/year; AL type (Minnesota)
    - AA amyloid is most common type in developing countries
- Age
  - > 50 years
    - Uncommon in < 40 years old

Presentation

- Proteinuria ± renal insufficiency
  - Proteinuria most common presentation but variable extent
- Nephrotic syndrome
- Renal insufficiency
  - Patients with vascular-only AL amyloid in kidney present with higher creatinine than those with diffuse amyloid in kidney
- Hypotension
- General: Fatigue, weight loss, edema
- Visceral and soft tissue involvement: Hepatomegaly, gastrointestinal dysmotility/atony, diarrhea, malabsorption, neuropathy, carpal tunnel syndrome
  - 8% GI symptoms
  - 25% hepatic involvement
- Cardiovascular: Orthostatic hypotension, cardiac arrhythmias, congestive heart failure (2° to restrictive cardiomyopathy)

Laboratory Tests

- Serum protein electrophoresis and free light chain assays help demonstrate paraproteinemia

Treatment

- Drugs
  - Myeloma
    - Alkylating agents (e.g., melphalan), often given with steroids (e.g., dexamethasone)
      - May ↑ survival from 1- > 5 years
    - Proteosome inhibitors (e.g., bortezomib)
    - Immunomodulatory drugs (e.g., thalidomide & lenalidomide)
    - Aggresome inhibition (e.g., histone deacetylase [HDAC] inhibitors such as panobinostat)
- Bone marrow transplantation
- Renal transplantation
  - Recurs post-transplant (10-20%); graft failure in 33%
  - Outcome can be good in selected patients
    - AL in nonmyeloma patients without severe extrarenal disease

Prognosis

- Variable but generally poor
- Median survival: 2 years (Mayo series, 859 patients)

IMAGING

Radiographic Findings

- X-ray & other radiologic examination may show punched-out defects and generalized osteoporosis in myeloma patients
- Positron emission tomography-computed tomography (PET/CT) may be used in future to visualize amyloid deposits

- Antibody m11-1F4 labeled with iodine-125 is used with this PET/CT
  - Chimeric version of antibody is in clinical trials

MICROSCOPIC

Histologic Features

- All renal compartments may have amyloid deposits
- Glomeruli
  - 97% of immunoglobulin-related (AL/AH/AHL) amyloid cases have glomerular deposits
  - Amorphous, PAS-negative or PAS-weak deposits in mesangium and capillary loops
  - Glomerular basement membrane "spicules" present in ~ 70% of AL/AH/AHL amyloid
    - "Spicular" amyloid is also sometimes called eyelash sign
  - May have subtle glomerular involvement even in patients with heavy proteinuria
- Tubules
  - May have congophilic casts that polarize
  - Intracytoplasmic amyloid fibrils, rarely
- Interstitium
  - Amorphous material in interstitium
  - 58% of AL/AH/AHL cases have interstitial deposits
- Vessels
  - Amorphous material in arteries &/or arterioles
  - 85% of AL/AH/AHL cases have vascular deposits

ANCILLARY TESTS

Histochemistry

- Congo red stain shows orangeophilic material on bright-field microscopy
  - Apple-green birefringence under polarized light

Immunofluorescence

- Establish heavy chain, κ or λ predominance
- AH amyloid shows prominent Ig staining (IgG, IgA, or IgM)
  - Subclass staining to establish clonality of IgG heavy chain (e.g., IgG1, 2, 3, 4)
- Generally easier to interpret than IHC

Electron Microscopy

- Randomly arranged fibrils ~ 7-12 nm in diameter
- Present in mesangium & in GBM
- Often form spicules penetrating GBM

Mass Spectrometry

- Laser microdissection (LMD) & tandem mass spectrometry (MS) (LMD/MS) sensitive & specific
- Formalin-fixed paraffin-embedded tissue is used
- Serum amyloid P (SAP) and apolipoprotein E signatures detected, supporting presence of amyloidosis

DIFFERENTIAL DIAGNOSIS

Fibrillary Glomerulonephritis (GN)

- Congo red negative
- Usually larger (10-30 nm) but overlaps with amyloid fibrils (7-12 nm)
- ~ 10% have monotypic IgG and light chains
- May show "spicules" similar to amyloid
- Does not involve vessels
- Tubular basement membrane fibrillary deposits may be present

Minimal Change Disease

- Patients present with nephrotic syndrome in both minimal change disease and amyloid
- In adults with suspected minimal change disease, consider performing Congo red staining to evaluate for subtle amyloid
- Glomeruli can sometimes look normal by light microscopy but have amyloid detected on EM or Congo red stain

AA Amyloid

- Often shows nonspecific staining for heavy chains by IF
- Mass spectrometry & AA immunoperoxidase staining helpful to distinguish AA from AH or AHL amyloid

Amyloidogenic Cast Nephropathy

- Atypical casts of light chain cast nephropathy are Congo red(+)
- Clinical features similar to light chain cast nephropathy without amyloidogenic casts rather than systemic amyloidosis

DIAGNOSTIC CHECKLIST

Pathologic Interpretation Pearls

- Primary amyloidosis is term used for myeloma or paraproteinemia-associated amyloidosis
- Secondary amyloidosis is term used for other types (e.g., AA amyloidosis, familial/hereditary amyloidosis, dialysis-related amyloidosis, localized amyloid, etc.)

SELECTED REFERENCES

1. Fernández de Larrea C et al: A practical approach to the diagnosis of systemic amyloidoses. Blood. 125(14):2239-44, 2015
2. Huang X et al: The clinical features and outcomes of systemic AL amyloidosis: a cohort of 231 Chinese patients. Clin Kidney J. 8(1):120-6, 2015
3. Said SM et al: Renal amyloidosis: origin and clinicopathologic correlations of 474 recent cases. Clin J Am Soc Nephrol. 8(9):1515-23, 2013
4. Sethi S et al: Laser microdissection and proteomic analysis of amyloidosis, cryoglobulinemic GN, fibrillary GN, and immunotactoid glomerulopathy. Clin J Am Soc Nephrol. 8(6):915-21, 2013
5. Eirin A et al: Clinical features of patients with immunoglobulin light chain amyloidosis (AL) with vascular-limited deposition in the kidney. Nephrol Dial Transplant. 27(3):1097-101, 2012
6. Qian Q et al: De novo AL amyloidosis in the kidney allograft. Am J Transplant. 11(3):606-12, 2011
7. Sattianayagam PT et al: Solid organ transplantation in AL amyloidosis. Am J Transplant. 10(9):2124-31, 2010
8. Sethi S et al: Mass spectrometry-based proteomic diagnosis of renal immunoglobulin heavy chain amyloidosis. Clin J Am Soc Nephrol. 5(12):2180-7, 2010
9. Wall JS et al: Radioimmunodetection of amyloid deposits in patients with AL amyloidosis. Blood. 116(13):2241-4, 2010
10. Herrera GA: Renal lesions associated with plasma cell dyscrasias: practical approach to diagnosis, new concepts, and challenges. Arch Pathol Lab Med. 133(2):249-67, 2009
11. Osawa Y et al: Renal function at the time of renal biopsy as a predictor of prognosis in patients with primary AL-type amyloidosis. Clin Exp Nephrol. 8(2):127-33, 2004

Amyloid Spicules in GBM

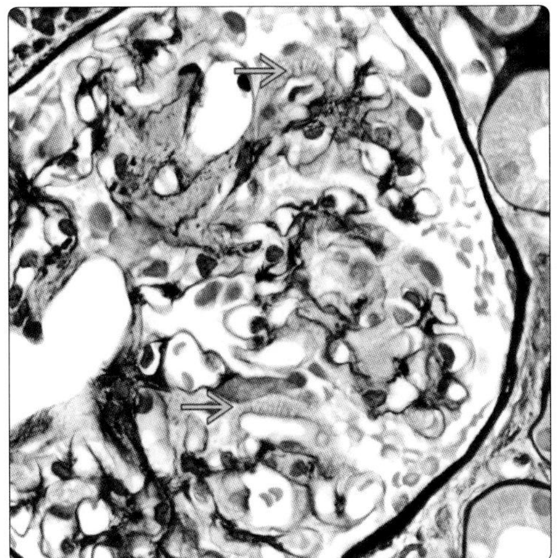

Amyloid Is Nonargyrophilic

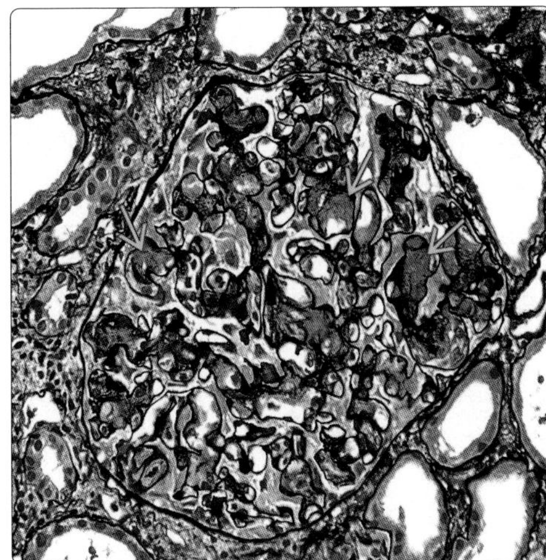

(Left) *Basement membrane spicules ⇒ are seen in a case of AL amyloidosis.* **(Right)** *Amyloid material is nonargyrophilic ⇒, which means that is seen only weakly on a silver stain in this case of AH + AL amyloidosis due to IgM and kappa deposition.*

Orangeophilic Deposits on Congo Red

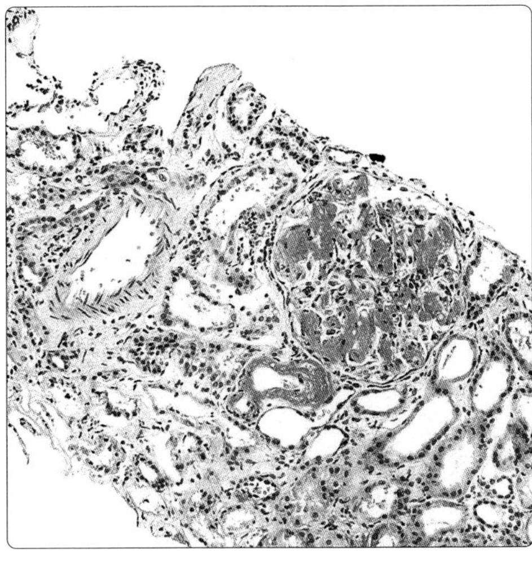

Minimal AL Amyloid

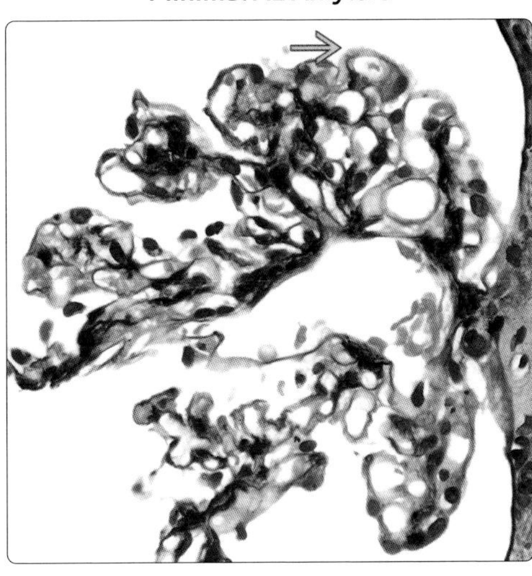

(Left) *Orangeophilic material is seen on a Congo red stain in a case of AH + AL amyloidosis due to IgM and kappa deposition.* **(Right)** *A glomerulus involved by AL amyloid appears nearly normal by light microscopy, with a few possible spicules ⇒. This glomerulus showed segmental positive staining by Congo red and was positive for lambda light chain by immunofluorescence.*

Congo Red Positive Cast

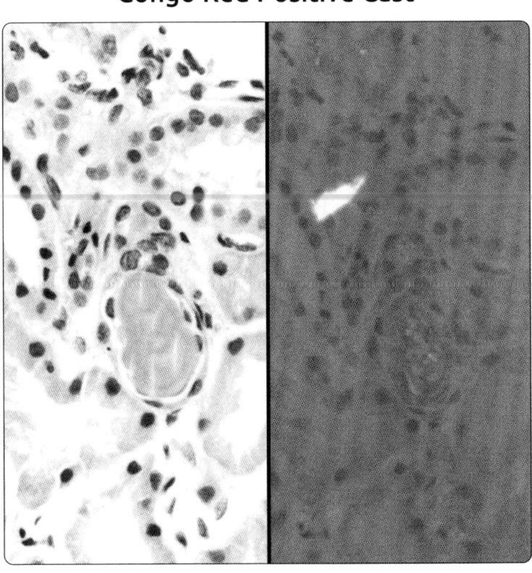

Amyloidogenic Cast

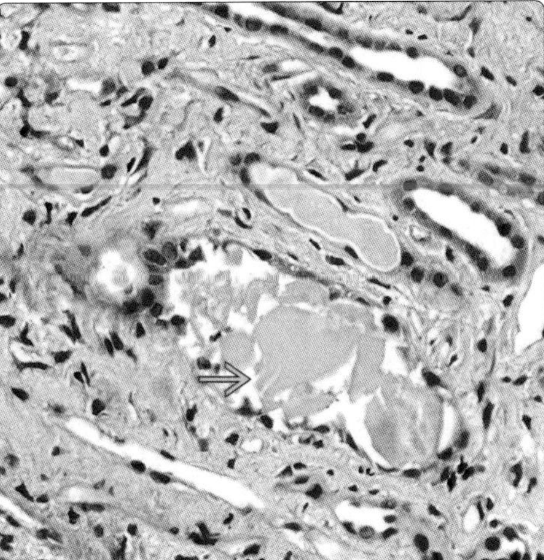

(Left) *This case of light chain cast nephropathy shows a Congo red(+) cast (left) with apple-green birefringence under polarized light (right). This is a variant of cast nephropathy, and the disease behaves more similarly to cast nephropathy than amyloidosis.* **(Right)** *On H&E stain, this amyloidogenic atypical cast ⇒ shows pale pink staining, similar to amyloid in other locations. In contrast, atypical casts that are not amyloidogenic are usually hypereosinophilic.*

(Left) *In a case of amyloidosis, extensive accumulation of λ light chain can be appreciated in the glomerulus → using immunofluorescence for lambda.* **(Right)** *Amorphous material due to amyloid deposition → can be seen in this case of AH + AL amyloidosis due to IgM and kappa deposition. The deposits are strongly PAS positive, probably due to the IgM heavy chain, which is rich in carbohydrates.*

Lambda Immunofluorescence in AL Amyloidosis

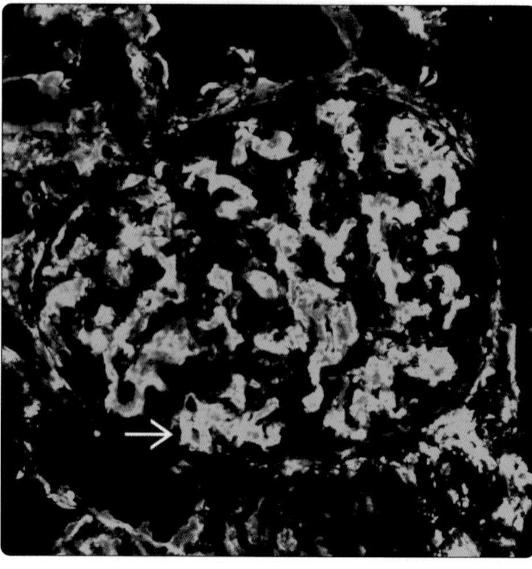

Amorphous Deposits in AH + AL Amyloidosis

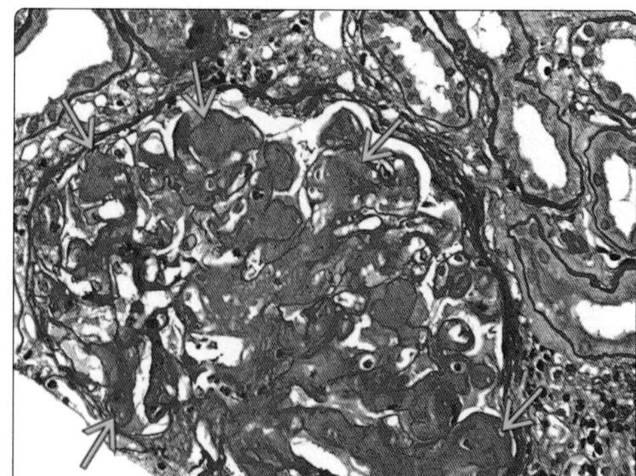

(Left) *Amyloid deposition manifests as amorphous material that stains pale blue → in a case of AH + AL amyloidosis due to IgM and kappa deposition.* **(Right)** *Glomeruli show bright staining of amorphous material for IgM (left) and λ (right). The κ stain was negative. AHL amyloid accounts for ~ 4% of immunoglobulin-related amyloid and is best confirmed by mass spectrometry, as IF may sometimes show nonspecific staining of amyloid.*

Amorphous Deposits in AH + AL Amyloidosis

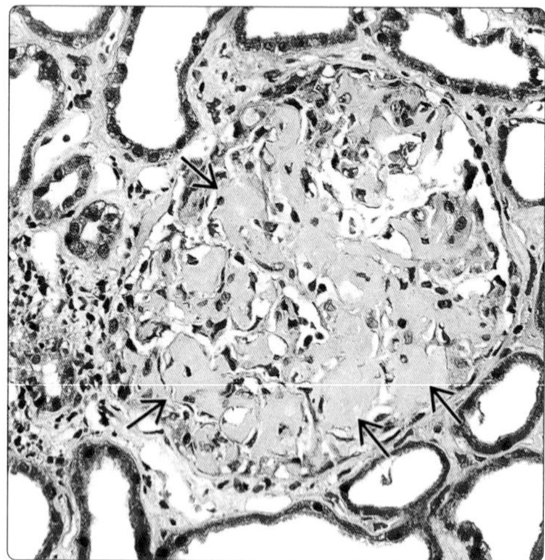

IgM Lambda AHL Amyloid

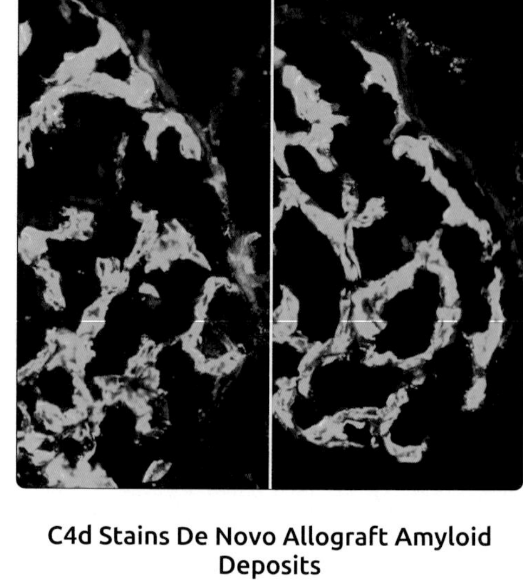

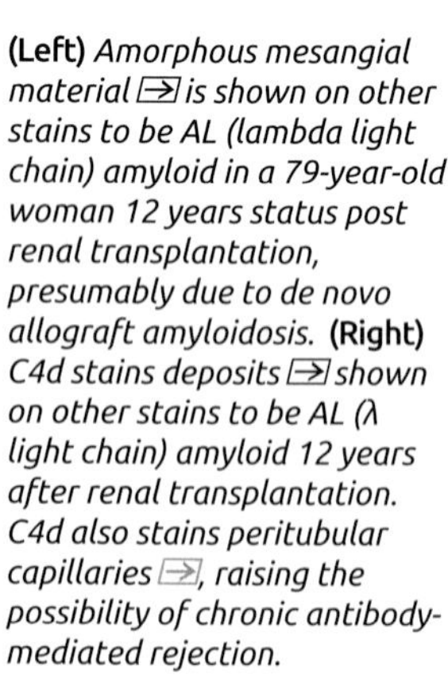

(Left) *Amorphous mesangial material → is shown on other stains to be AL (lambda light chain) amyloid in a 79-year-old woman 12 years status post renal transplantation, presumably due to de novo allograft amyloidosis.* **(Right)** *C4d stains deposits → shown on other stains to be AL (λ light chain) amyloid 12 years after renal transplantation. C4d also stains peritubular capillaries →, raising the possibility of chronic antibody-mediated rejection.*

De Novo Amyloidosis in Allograft

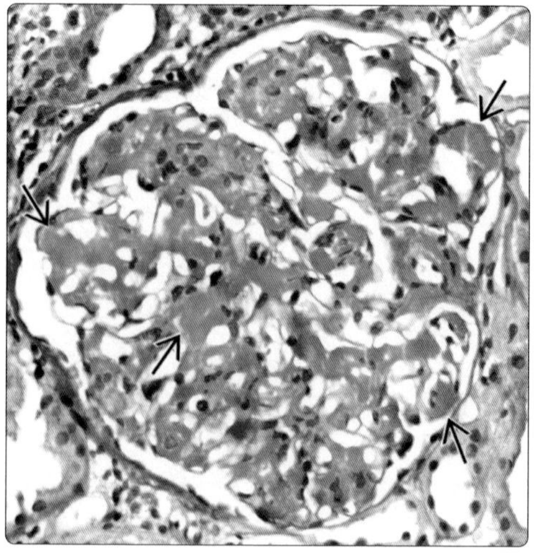

C4d Stains De Novo Allograft Amyloid Deposits

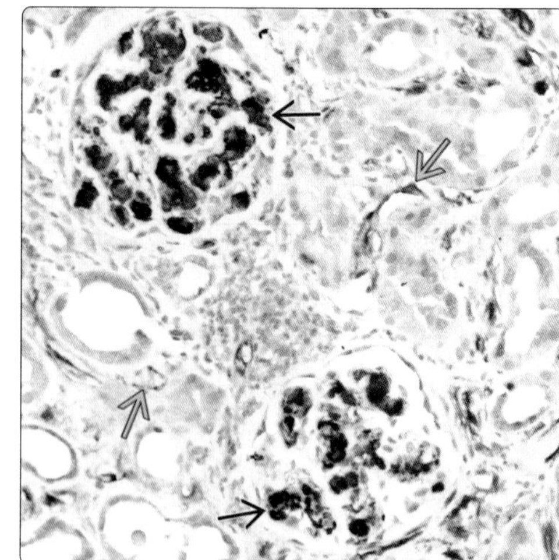

Extensive Amyloid Fibrils in Mesangium and GBM

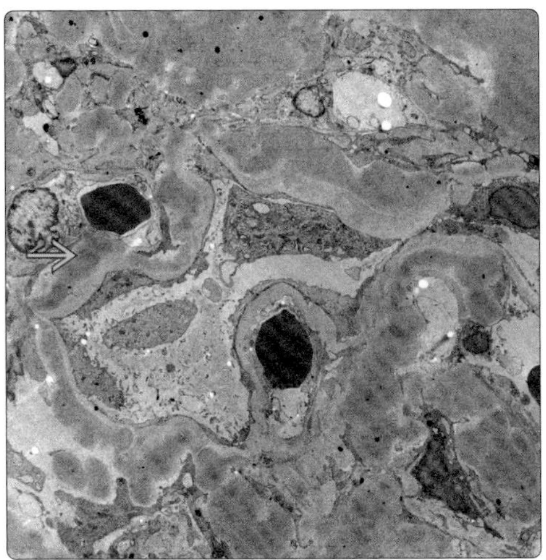

Subepithelial Fibrils in AH Amyloid

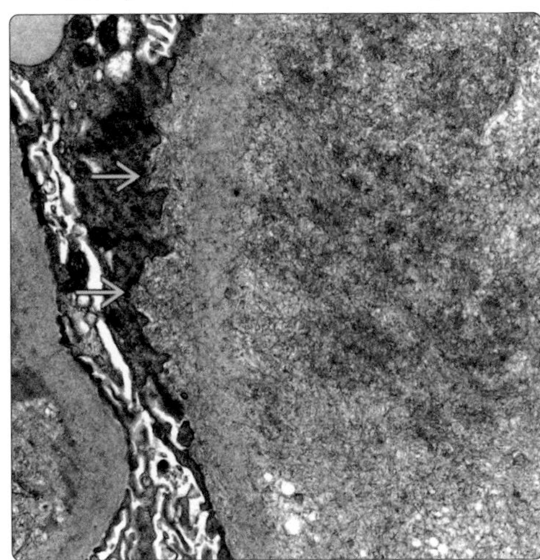

(Left) *This usual appearance of AL amyloid resembles dense deposit disease on EM, with electron-dense deposits along the basement membranes ⇒ and globular deposits in the mesangium. Higher magnification showed fibrillary deposits typical of amyloid; a Congo red stain was positive.* **(Right)** *In this example of AH (gamma) amyloid, fibrils are seen by electron microscopy, including "spicules" ⇒ in the basement membrane of a glomerulus. The ultrastructural appearance is identical to AL amyloid.*

Segmental Amyloid Fibrils in GBM

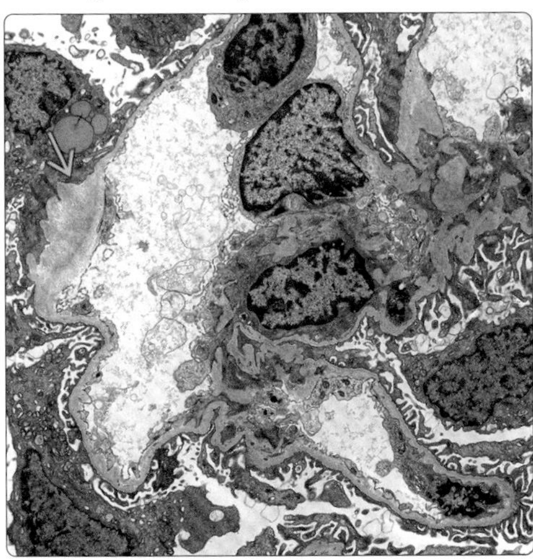

Intracytoplasmic Amyloid Fibrils

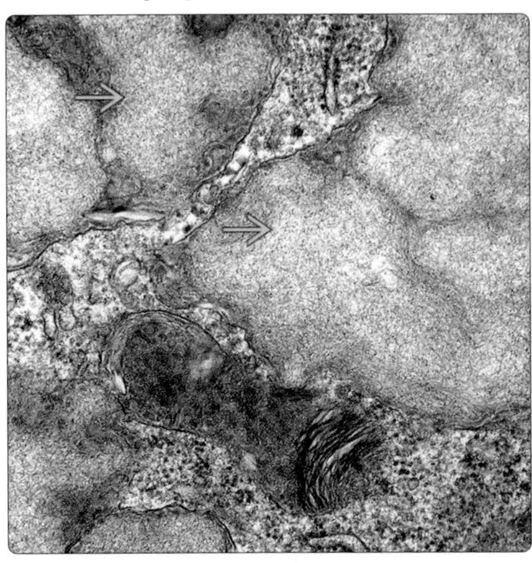

(Left) *EM of AL amyloidosis shows segmental glomerular basement membrane spicules ⇒. When segmental, amyloid may be overlooked and potentially misdiagnosed as minimal change disease or unsampled focal segmental glomerulosclerosis.* **(Right)** *A rare case of intracytoplasmic fibrillary material ⇒ in a tubule is shown. By immunofluorescence, this material stained for kappa light chain. The biopsy also showed light chain cast nephropathy.*

Spicules in Fibrillary Glomerulonephritis Resembling Amyloid Deposits

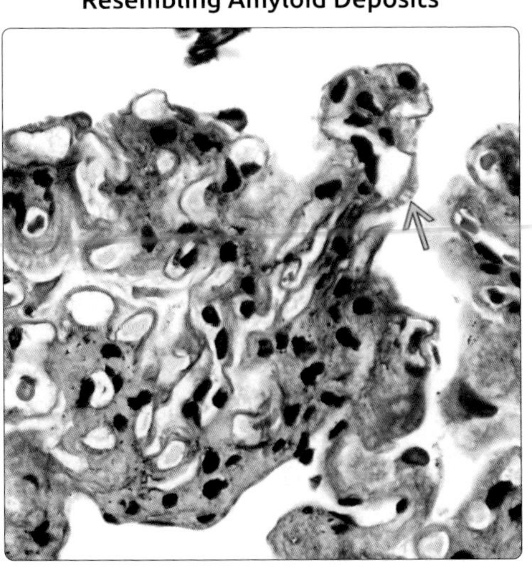

GBM Spicules in Fibrillary Glomerulonephritis

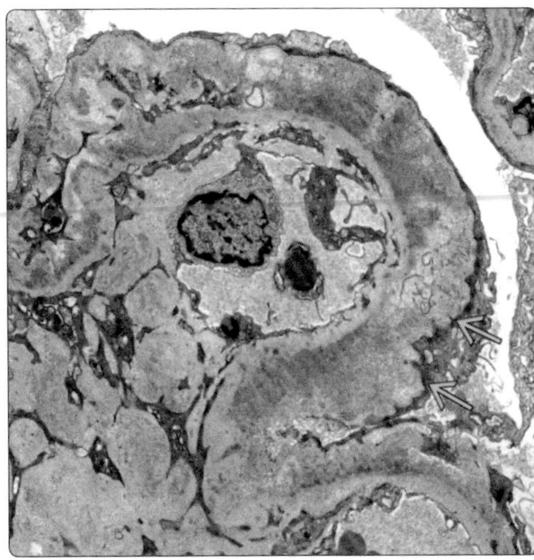

(Left) *Basement membrane "spicules" ⇒ can occasionally be seen in fibrillary GN, either by light or electron microscopy. This feature is not specific for amyloid.* **(Right)** *Ill-defined spicule ⇒ formation, not specific for amyloid, is seen by EM in this case of fibrillary GN. In contrast to amyloid, fibrillary GN tends to have fibrillary deposits "spread out" along the glomerular basement membranes in an intramembranous location.*

AA Amyloidosis

KEY FACTS

TERMINOLOGY

- Amyloid (AA amyloidosis) typically associated with chronic inflammation derived from proteolytic cleavage of serum amyloid A (SAA) protein, an acute phase reactant

ETIOLOGY/PATHOGENESIS

- Autoimmune disease and autoinflammatory disorders
  - Rheumatoid arthritis, ankylosing spondylitis, inflammatory arthritides, Behçet disease, inflammatory bowel disease (e.g., Crohn disease)
- Chronic infections
- Periodic fever syndrome
  - Monogenic autoinflammatory disease due to mutations in pyrin, cryopyrin, and tumor necrosis factor (TNF)
- Familial Mediterranean fever (FMF)
  - *MEFV* gene on short arm of chromosome 16 encodes pyrin and is responsible

CLINICAL ISSUES

- Presents with nephrotic syndrome or renal insufficiency ~ 90%
- Range: 11-87 years; median: 50 years
- ~ 45% of systemic amyloidoses

MICROSCOPIC

- Deposits begin in mesangium (particularly in FMF), spread to subendothelial space, and may replace glomerular tuft
- Tubulointerstitial and vascular involvement
- Extrarenal: GI tract and testes are most frequently involved; also spleen, liver, lungs, adrenal gland, and amyloid goiter

ANCILLARY TESTS

- AA protein detected by IF or IHC

TOP DIFFERENTIAL DIAGNOSES

- Other causes of amyloidosis
- Fibrillary glomerulopathy

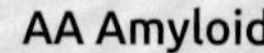
AA Amyloid

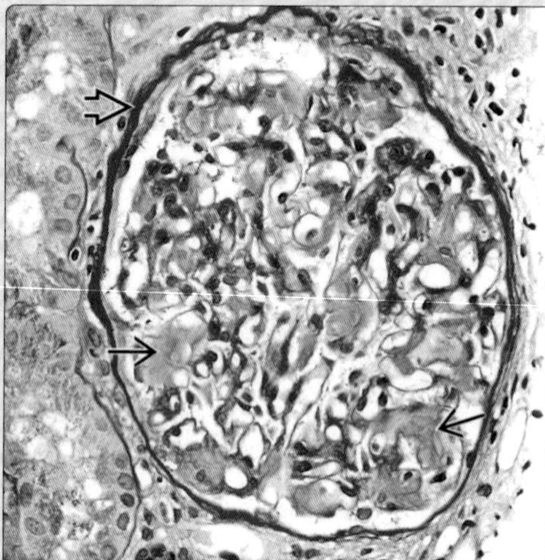

Nonargyrophilic Glomerular Amyloid Deposits

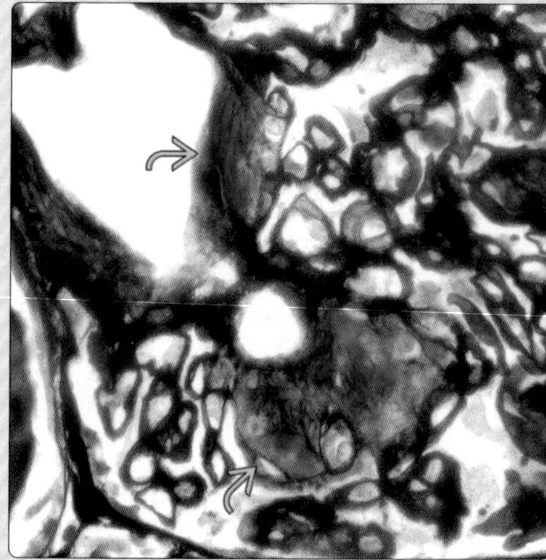

(Left) *Amyloid material within a glomerulus is PAS-negative ⇒ on a PAS-stained section is shown. Compare to the intensity of stain in the PAS-positive Bowman capsule ⇒.* **(Right)** *Glomerular amyloid deposits ⇒ are often nonargyrophilic, which means that they stain only weakly with a silver stain, as can be seen on this Periodic acid methenamine silver stain of a case of AA amyloidosis.*

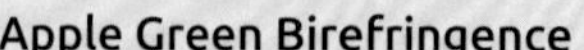
Congo Red Apple Green Birefringence

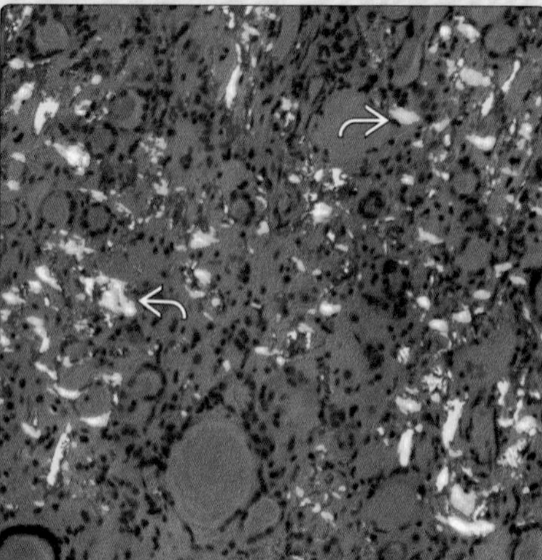

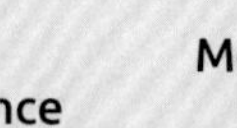
Mesangial Deposition of Serum Amyloid A Protein (SAA)

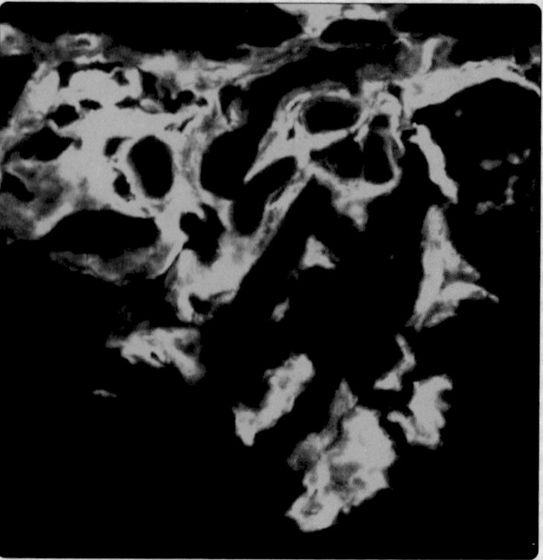

(Left) *In a 48-year-old man with familial Mediterranean fever and ESRD, there is extensive interstitial accumulation of apple green birefringent amyloid material ⇒ on polarized light examination of a Congo Red stain, shown in other studies to be AA amyloid.* **(Right)** *The definitive test for amyloid type is generally immunofluorescence. This image from a renal biopsy with AA amyloidosis shows predominantly mesangial deposition.*

TERMINOLOGY

Synonyms

- Formerly "secondary amyloidosis" or "reactive amyloidosis"

Definitions

- Amyloid associated with chronic inflammatory conditions
  - Derived from proteolytic cleavage of serum amyloid A (SAA) protein, acute phase reactant

ETIOLOGY/PATHOGENESIS

SAA

- SAA is precursor for amyloid A fibril protein
  - Acute phase reactant
  - Truncated apolipoprotein with unknown function
  - Secreted 104 amino acid protein primarily in α-helix structure
  - N-terminus amphipathic region facilitates interaction with HDL, determining fibril formation
    - Apolipoprotein AI (apo AI) and apolipoprotein E (apo E) present in SAA bound HDL fraction
  - Fibrils form due to defective degradation (not understood)
    - SAA transfers to lysosome where C-terminal portion cleaved
    - Remaining protein forms β-pleated sheet
    - Deposited amyloid with 66-76 amino acids
    - Fibrils deposit with amyloid P, proteoglycans, and glycosaminoglycans
      - Binding these components confers resistance to proteolysis and promotes deposition
  - 76-residue molecule is most common variant and frequently deposits in glomeruli
  - Rarer variant (~ 10%) consists of mixture of long (~ 100 residues) and short (~ 44 residues) N-terminal fragments of SAA
    - Deposit in renal medulla and blood vessel walls instead of glomeruli
    - Does not result in proteinuria and can be missed
    - Has stronger affinity for Congo red and stronger birefringence
- *SAA* genes located on human chromosome 11p15.1
  - *SAA1* and *SAA2* (acute-phase reactants) produced in liver
    - Proinflammatory cytokines (IL-6 in particular & also IL-1 & TNF-α)
    - ~ 80% of secreted SAA1 and SAA2 bound to lipoproteins
      - 90% bound to high-density lipoprotein (HDL)
    - Levels can ↑ > 1,000x during inflammation
    - Polymorphisms in *SAA1* gene with 3-7x ↑ risk to develop AA amyloidosis
    - Accounts for AA amyloidogenesis
  - *SAA3* is pseudogene and *SAA4* is constitutively expressed

Chronic Inflammation and Acute-Phase Response

- Autoimmune disease and autoinflammatory disorders
  - Behçet disease and sinus histiocytosis with massive lymphadenopathy (Rosai-Dorfman disease)
- Rheumatoid arthritis, ankylosing spondylitis, psoriatic arthritis, systemic juvenile arthritis, and other inflammatory arthritides
- Inflammatory bowel disease (e.g., Crohn disease)
  - Ulcerative colitis involvement rare
- Sarcoidosis and other granulomatous diseases
- Malignancies: Mesothelioma and Hodgkin disease
- Chronic infections
  - Tuberculosis, leprosy, human immunodeficiency virus, osteomyelitis, bronchiectasis, decubitus ulcers, and skin infections of IV drug abuse
- Idiopathic/unknown (~ 6%)

Hereditary Autoinflammatory Disease

- Repeated attacks of inflammation
  - Attacks may be unprovoked or stimulated by stress, trauma, or immunization
- Genetic disorders in innate immune system
  - Neutrophils and macrophages are components of innate immune systems
- Periodic fever syndromes
  - Monogenic autoinflammatory disease due to mutations in pyrin, cryopyrin, and tumor necrosis factor (TNF)
    - Autosomal dominant
      - Tumor necrosis factor receptor 1-associated periodic syndrome (TRAPS [originally identified in Irish and called "familial hibernian fever"])
      - Cryopyrin-associated periodic syndromes (CAPS)
    - Autosomal recessive
      - Hyperimmunoglobulinemia D syndrome (HIDS)
  - Arthritis, serositis, cutaneous rash, and ocular involvement
  - Prominent acute phase response (↑ c-reactive protein [CRP], erythrocyte sedimentation rate [ESR], and SAA)

FMF

- Most common nephropathic familial amyloidosis
- Mediterranean basin and descendants
  - Middle Eastern Arabs, non-Ashkenazi (Sephardic) Jews of North Africa or Middle Eastern descent, Turks, Armenians
    - Carrier frequency 1:3 to 1:10 in population-based studies
  - *MEFV* gene on short arm of chromosome 16 encodes pyrin/marenostrin and is responsible
    - Autosomal recessive inheritance, typically
      - Variable penetrance: Initial attack usually < age 20
    - > 60 mutations
      - 4 main mutations in Middle Eastern FMF populations: M680I, M694V, M694I, V726A
      - M680 and M694 give early onset FMF, ↑ severity, and ↑ amyloid deposition
    - In FMF, mutations result in activation of interleukin-1β pathway
- SAA level basally elevated 2-3x normal and may rise > 50x during febrile episodes

CLINICAL ISSUES

Epidemiology

- Incidence
  - Most common cause of amyloidosis in underdeveloped countries
    - Becoming less common in developed countries
    - ~ 45% of systemic amyloidoses worldwide are AA

- Age
  - Range of 11-87 years with median of 50 years
  - Most common cause in children
    - Many have autoinflammatory or infectious diseases
    - May affect children as young as 5 years old

Presentation

- Nephrotic syndrome or renal insufficiency (~ 90%)
- Proteinuria (~ 97%)
  - Albuminuria can be early finding
    - Periodic urinalysis in susceptible patients (e.g., FMF)
- FMF febrile episodes
  - Unpredictable and painful febrile episodes last 1-4 days and then resolve
  - Pleuritis, sterile peritonitis, synovitis, or erysipelas-lie erythema of lower extremities

Laboratory Tests

- SAA concentration can be followed
  - Favorable outcome noted with SAA concentration in low normal range (< 4 mg/L)

Natural History

- Takes years to develop
  - > 2 years in rheumatoid arthritis, with mean ~ 15 years

Treatment

- Drugs
  - Immunosuppressive agents for rheumatoid arthritis and other inflammatory conditions
    - Disease-modifying antirheumatic drugs (DMARDs) and biologic agents (anti-tumor necrosis factor)
  - Colchicine useful for FMF
    - Not as useful for other causes of AA amyloidosis
  - Anakinra (IL-1 receptor antagonist) may reduce clinical symptoms &/or acute phase reactants
  - Corticosteroids

Prognosis

- 5-year survival of patients with overt AA amyloidosis renal disease in ~ 40%
- Median survival after diagnosis is ~ 133 months
- Deposit regression shown in 60% of patients with median SAA concentration < 10 mg/L

MICROSCOPIC

Histologic Features

- Glomeruli
  - Main renal manifestation
  - Mesangiocapillary, mesangial segmental, mesangial nodular, and hilar involvement reported
  - Deposits begin in mesangium (particularly in FMF), spread to subendothelial space, and may replace glomerular tuft
  - Basement membrane "spicules" present in ~ 50% of cases
  - Rare cases of AA amyloidosis have crescents
- Tubules and interstitium
  - Mostly affects medulla
  - Can lead to tubular atrophy
- Vessels
  - May occur around blood vessels and can occur without glomerular involvement
- Other organ involvement
  - GI tract and testes most frequently involved
    - GI tract involvement (~ 20%) may correlate with renal deposition better than abdominal fat
    - Testicular involvement (~ 87%) may be associated with abnormal spermatogenesis and 2° infertility
  - Splenomegaly, hepatomegaly, lungs, adrenal gland, and amyloid goiter
    - Cardiac involvement rare

ANCILLARY TESTS

Histochemistry

- Congo red stain stains orange
  - Apple-green birefringence under polarized light
  - Does not polarize without Congo red (in contrast to collagen)
  - Elastin stains with Congo red but does not polarize

Immunohistochemistry

- Amyloid A protein positive

Immunofluorescence

- Amyloid A protein positive
- Variable nonspecific staining by IF, particularly for heavy chains

Electron Microscopy

- Randomly arranged fibrils ~ 7-12 nm in diameter

Mass Spectrometry

- Useful when IF shows nonspecific staining

DIFFERENTIAL DIAGNOSIS

AL, AH, or AHL Amyloidosis

- For AL amyloidosis, single light chain predominates; but for AA amyloidosis, usually neither or both light chains stain
- Heavy chain staining is present in AH and AHL amyloid; AA amyloid may show nonspecific heavy chain staining

Fibrillary Glomerulopathy

- Negative Congo red stain
- Sometimes >12 nm diameter

SELECTED REFERENCES

1. Westermark GT et al: AA amyloidosis: pathogenesis and targeted therapy. Annu Rev Pathol. 10:321-44, 2015
2. Said SM et al: Renal amyloidosis: origin and clinicopathologic correlations of 474 recent cases. Clin J Am Soc Nephrol. 8(9):1515-23, 2013
3. Obici L et al: Amyloidosis in autoinflammatory syndromes. Autoimmun Rev. 12(1):14-7, 2012
4. Nakamura T: Amyloid A amyloidosis secondary to rheumatoid arthritis: pathophysiology and treatments. Clin Exp Rheumatol. 29(5):850-7, 2011
5. Lachmann HJ et al: Natural history and outcome in systemic AA amyloidosis. N Engl J Med. 356(23):2361-71, 2007

Amyloid on Trichrome Stain

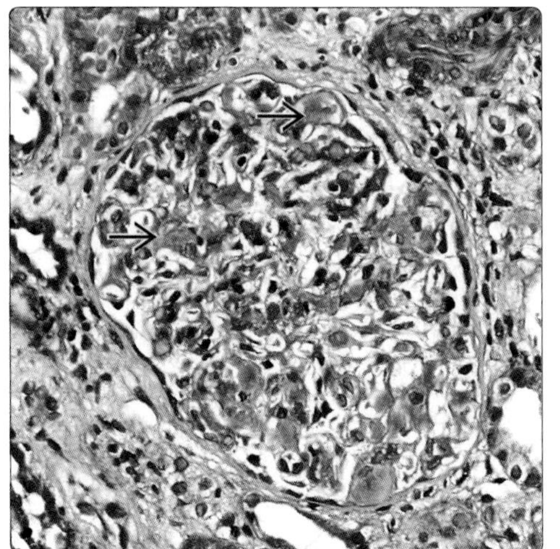

AA Immunohistochemistry

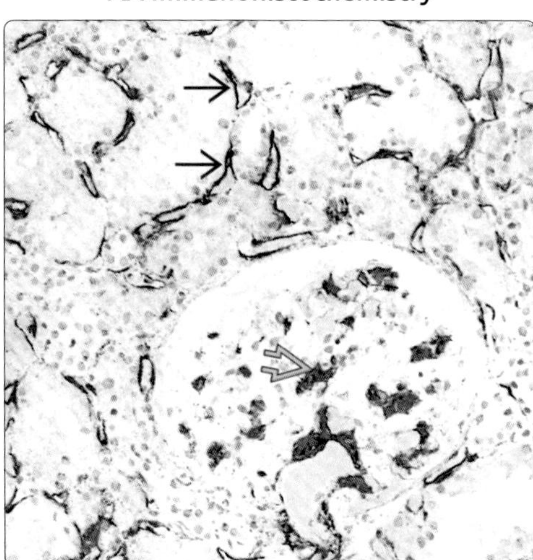

(Left) *Amyloid deposits often stain pale blue ⇨ on a trichrome stain, as seen in this case of AA amyloidosis.* **(Right)** *In this unusual case of recurrent AA amyloid in the transplant, the AA amyloid immunoperoxidase stain shows positivity in the mesangium ⇨ and in peritubular capillaries ⇨, the latter resembling a positive C4d stain.*

AA Amyloid Immunoperoxidase

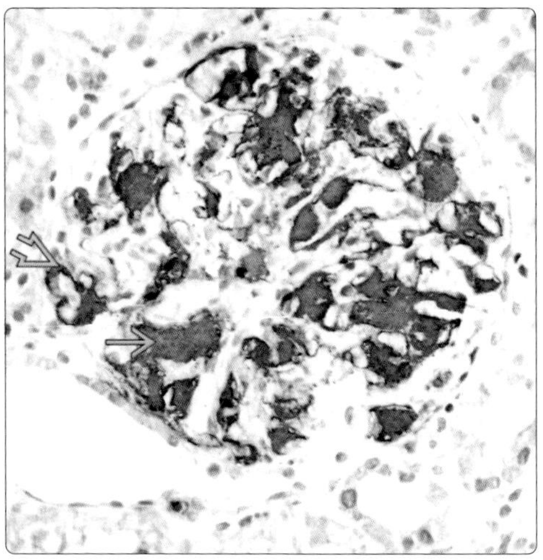

AA Amyloid Immunofluorescence

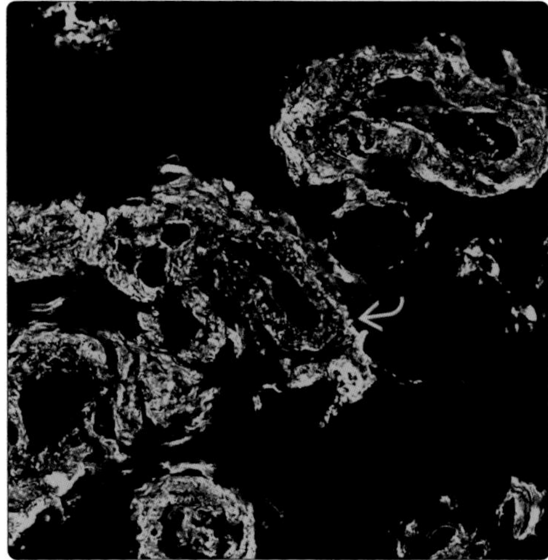

(Left) *An immunoperoxidase stain for AA amyloid shows positive staining in this glomerulus in the mesangium ⇨ and in segmental glomerular capillary loops ⇨.* **(Right)** *Identification of the amyloid protein is a necessary part of the pathology work-up. Immunofluorescence for AA amyloid shows extensive accumulation in vessels ⇨ in this case of renal amyloidosis due to AA amyloid.*

AA Amyloid

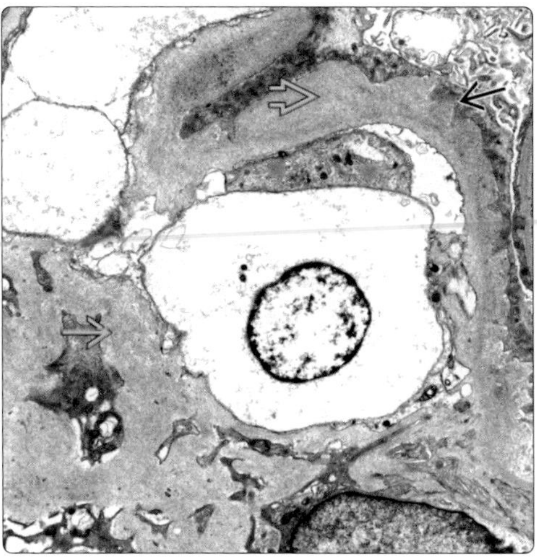

AA Amyloid

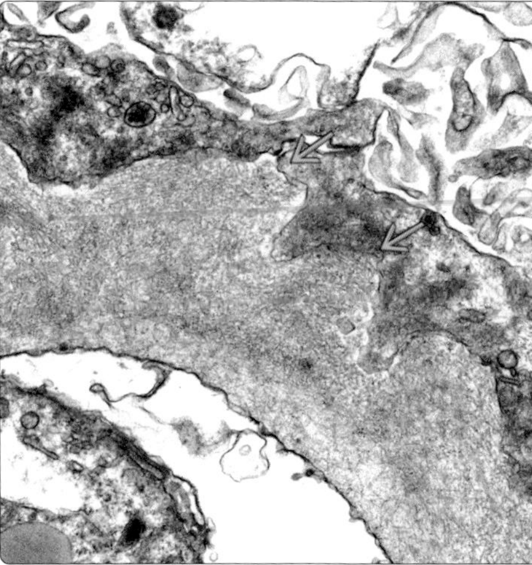

(Left) *Fibrillary material (visualized better at higher magnification) is present in the glomerular basement membranes ⇨ and in the expanded mesangium ⇨ in this case of AA amyloid. Ill-defined spicule formation is present ⇨.* **(Right)** *In this case of AA amyloid, fibrils form short, ill-defined "spicules" ⇨ along a glomerular capillary loop. Spicule formation is less common in AA amyloid compared to AL amyloid, but spicules are seen in ~ 50% of AA amyloid cases.*

ALECT2 Amyloidosis

KEY FACTS

TERMINOLOGY

- Leukocyte chemotactic factor 2 amyloidosis (ALECT2)

CLINICAL ISSUES

- 10% of renal biopsies with amyloidosis
- Primarily affects elderly (mean age at diagnosis: ~ 67)
- Commonly affects patients with Mexican ancestry though other ethnicities have been described as well
- Presents with chronic kidney disease
- Many without proteinuria
- > 75% show progressive renal failure after biopsy
- Siblings with disease have been described

MICROSCOPIC

- Light microscopy
  - Deposition of amorphous material with positive staining on Congo red that shows green birefringence upon polarization
  - Amyloid deposition primarily involves cortical interstitium
  - Deposition in glomeruli and arteries also commonly present
  - Medulla interstitial deposition is sparse to absent
- Immunofluorescence
  - Amyloid deposits negative for immunoglobulins, light chains, or fibrin/fibrinogen
- Electron microscopy
  - Typical randomly arranged fibrils (8-12 nm) of amyloid
- Extrarenal involvement rare

ANCILLARY TESTS

- LECT2 detected by immunohistochemistry or mass spectrometry

TOP DIFFERENTIAL DIAGNOSES

- Amyloidosis, AL or AA or other non-LECT2 amyloid
- Arterionephrosclerosis

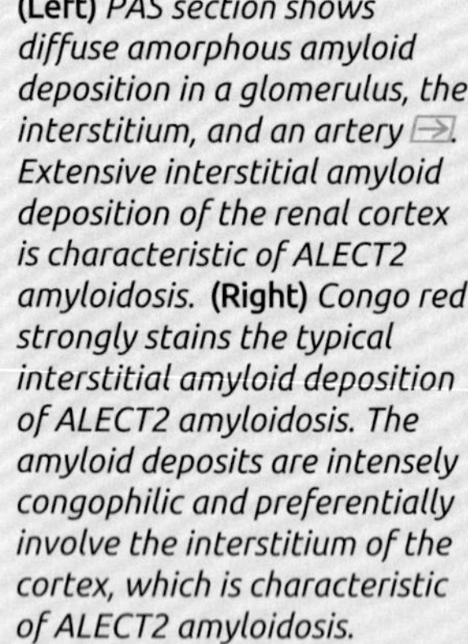

(Left) *PAS section shows diffuse amorphous amyloid deposition in a glomerulus, the interstitium, and an artery ⇒. Extensive interstitial amyloid deposition of the renal cortex is characteristic of ALECT2 amyloidosis.* **(Right)** *Congo red strongly stains the typical interstitial amyloid deposition of ALECT2 amyloidosis. The amyloid deposits are intensely congophilic and preferentially involve the interstitium of the cortex, which is characteristic of ALECT2 amyloidosis.*

Interstitial, Glomerular and Vascular Amyloid

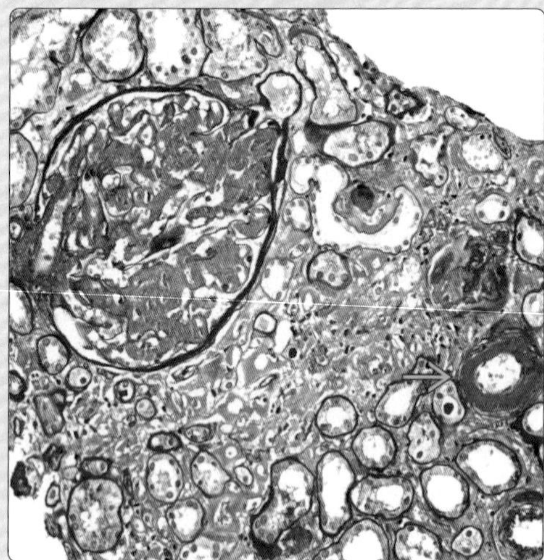

Congo Red In Renal Cortex

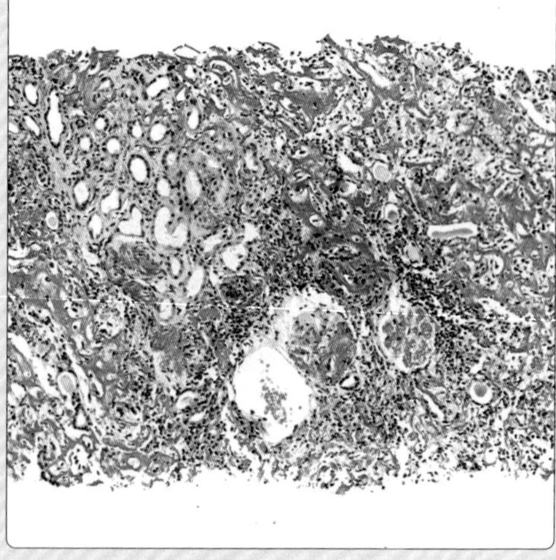

(Left) *High-power electron microscopic image from a case of LECT2 amyloidosis shows small, nonbranching, overlapping fibrils which are typical of amyloid (8-12 nm).* **(Right)** *Interstitial and glomerular amyloid deposits show strong reactivity to an anti-LECT2 antibody. All cases of amyloidosis should be typed by immunohistochemistry or immunofluorescence, because of therapeutic and prognostic implications.*

ALECT2 Amyloid Fibrils

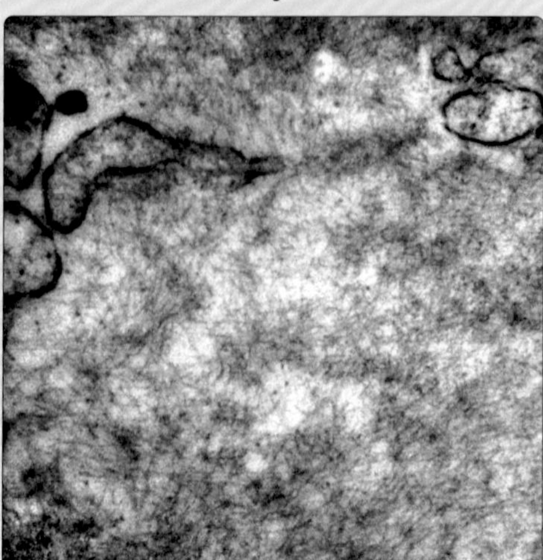

LECT2 Immunohistochemistry

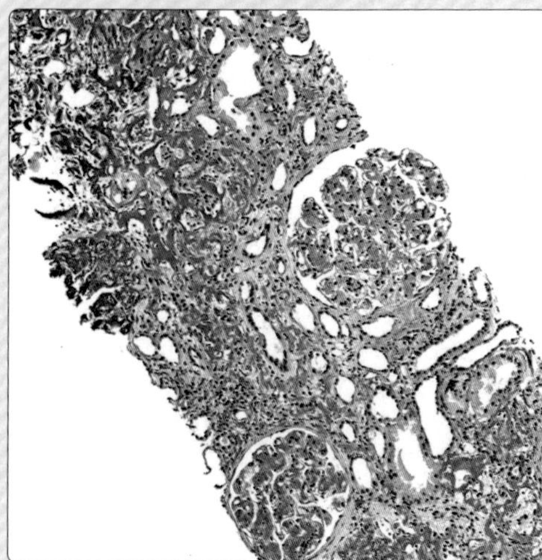

TERMINOLOGY

Abbreviations

- Leukocyte chemotactic factor 2 amyloidosis (ALECT2)

Synonyms

- Leukocyte cell-derived chemotaxin 2

Definitions

- Accumulation of insoluble LECT2 protein in the form of amyloid fibrils in tissue

ETIOLOGY/PATHOGENESIS

Deposition of LECT2

- LECT2
  - ~ 15 kD multifunctional cytokine in plasma produced in liver
- Increases phagocytosis and bacteriocidal activity of macrophages via CD209a receptor; protects from sepsis
- Deposition may result from hepatic overexpression or other mechanisms

Genetics

- No mutation in *LECT2* gene
- Common SNP in *LECT2* gene (rs31517) in all sequenced cases

CLINICAL ISSUES

Epidemiology

- Incidence
  - 10% of renal biopsies with amyloidosis (40/414)
- Age
  - Affects elderly (mean age at diagnosis: ~ 67)
- Sex
  - Equally affects males and females
- Ethnicity
  - In US, most common in patients with Mexican ancestry
  - Also reported in
    - Sudan, Israel, Middle East, Punjab, Native Americans in US, First Nations people in British Columbia
- Heredity
  - Siblings with disease described

Presentation

- Most common indication for renal biopsy is chronic kidney disease (67%) followed by proteinuria (33%)
- Many patients have no proteinuria
  - Rare nephrotic syndrome or hematuria
- Concurrent diabetes mellitus and hypertension common

Treatment

- Kidney transplantation
  - Rare recurrence in renal allograft

Prognosis

- 2 large case series with mean follow-up of 26 and 50 months
  - 21/85 (25%) with stable renal function
  - 33/85 (39%) with progressive renal failure
  - 31/85 (36%) progressed to end-stage renal disease (ESRD)
  - Mean eGFR decline of 0.5 mL/min/1.73 m^2 per month

MICROSCOPIC

Histologic Features

- Deposition of amorphous material with positive Congo red staining that shows green birefringence upon polarization
  - Primarily involves cortical interstitium
  - Deposition in glomeruli and arteries also common
  - Sparse to absent medullary interstitial deposition

Extrarenal Involvement Rare

- Liver
  - Hepatic sinusoids and periphery of portal tracts
  - Globular pattern highly distinctive for ALECT
- Spleen, adrenal glands, lungs, duodenum
- No cardiac involvement

ANCILLARY TESTS

Immunohistochemistry

- Amyloid typed with immunoperoxidase stain for LECT2

Immunofluorescence

- Amyloid deposits negative for immunoglobulins, light chains, or fibrin/fibrinogen

Electron Microscopy

- Randomly arranged overlapping 8-12 nm thick fibrils

Liquid Chromatography/Mass Spectrometry

- Proteomic analysis has high sensitivity and high specificity

DIFFERENTIAL DIAGNOSIS

Other Amyloid Types

- Most common amyloid types with overlapping histology include AA and AL amyloidosis
- Correct typing of amyloidosis is critical to avoid inappropriate treatment
- Amyloid typing should always be based on tissue diagnosis
  - Clinical findings (such as presence of monoclonal gammopathy of uncertain significance) can be misleading

Arterionephrosclerosis

- Nonspecific chronic injury if interstitial amyloid is not detected due to sampling

SELECTED REFERENCES

1. Chandan VS et al: Globular Hepatic Amyloid Is Highly Sensitive and Specific for LECT2 Amyloidosis. Am J Surg Pathol. ePub, 2015
2. Hutton HL et al: Renal Leukocyte Chemotactic Factor 2 (LECT2) Amyloidosis in First Nations People in Northern British Columbia, Canada: A Report of 4 Cases. Am J Kidney Dis. 64(5):790-2, 2014
3. Larsen CP et al: Clinical, morphologic, and genetic features of renal leukocyte chemotactic factor 2 amyloidosis. Kidney Int. 86(2):378-82, 2014
4. Said SM et al: Characterization and outcomes of renal leukocyte chemotactic factor 2-associated amyloidosis. Kidney Int. 86(2):370-7, 2014
5. Lu XJ et al: LECT2 protects mice against bacterial sepsis by activating macrophages via the CD209a receptor. J Exp Med. 210(1):5-13, 2013
6. Larsen CP et al: Prevalence and morphology of leukocyte chemotactic factor 2-associated amyloid in renal biopsies. Kidney Int. 77(9):816-9, 2010
7. Benson MD et al: Leukocyte chemotactic factor 2: A novel renal amyloid protein. Kidney Int. 74(2):218-22, 2008

AFib Amyloidosis

KEY FACTS

TERMINOLOGY

- AFib: Amyloidosis derived from fibrinogen A α-chain

ETIOLOGY/PATHOGENESIS

- ≥ 6 amyloidogenic mutations described in fibrinogen A α-chain
  - AFib E526V mutation is most common
  - AFib R554L mutation < < < E526V
- AFib protein
  - Coagulation cascade component but no coagulation abnormalities in AFib amyloidosis
  - Liver is source of aberrant amyloidogenic protein in AFib

CLINICAL ISSUES

- ~ 1.7% of amyloidosis
- Middle age to elderly (3rd-8th decade), median: 58 years
- Nephrotic syndrome/proteinuria & renal insufficiency
- Atheromatosis and hypertension
- Gut dysmotility and other visceral manifestations described
- Liver or combined liver/kidney transplantation
- Kidney failure: 1-5 years; median time from presentation to ESRD: 4.6 years

MICROSCOPIC

- Glomerular enlargement with almost complete replacement of glomeruli by amyloid
- No or little vascular or interstitial amyloid
- Congo red positive (birefringent)
- Other organs: Heart, GI, spleen, nerves

ANCILLARY TESTS

- IHC or IF: Positive fibrinogen stain
  - Mutation-dependent variability with commercial antibodies
- EM: 8-12 nm fibrils

TOP DIFFERENTIAL DIAGNOSES

- Other amyloidosis types

Mesangial Material

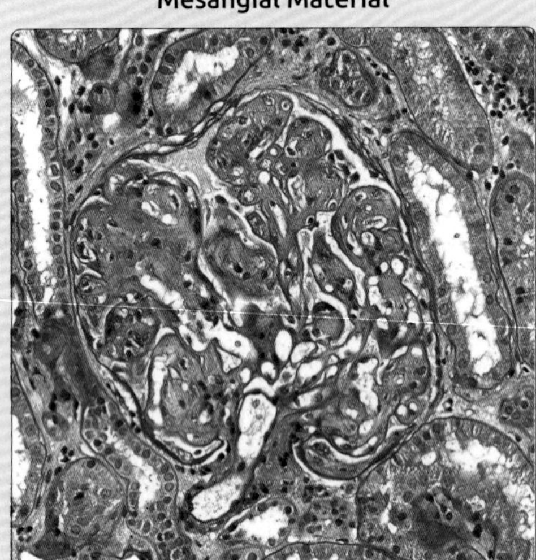

Antifibrinogen IHC

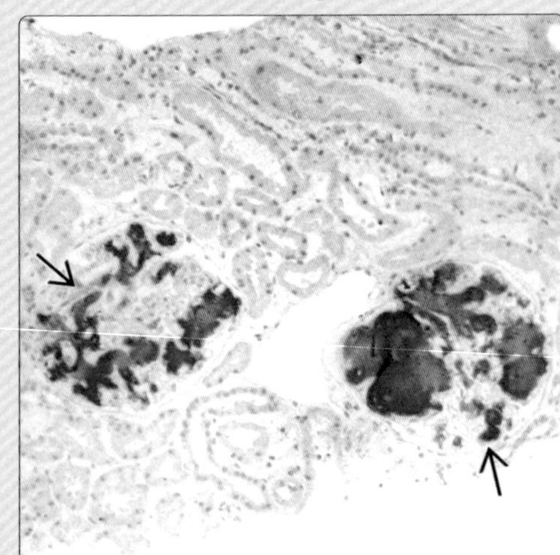

(Left) *Weakly PAS(+) mesangial material is shown to be fibrinogen in other studies, indicating AFib amyloidosis in a 55-year-old woman of northern European ancestry with nephrotic syndrome and no family history of renal disease. (Courtesy M. Picken, MD and R. Linke, MD.)* **(Right)** *Antifibrinogen IHC shows exclusively glomerular deposits ⇒ in AFib amyloidosis. (Courtesy M. Picken, MD and R. Linke, MD.)*

Fibrinogen Immunofluorescence

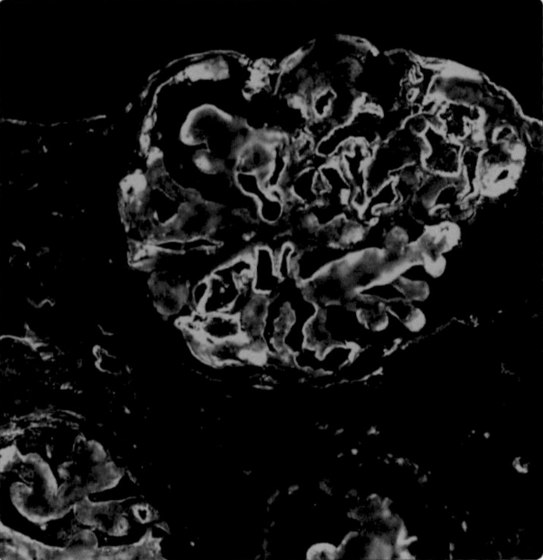

Ultrastructural Appearance

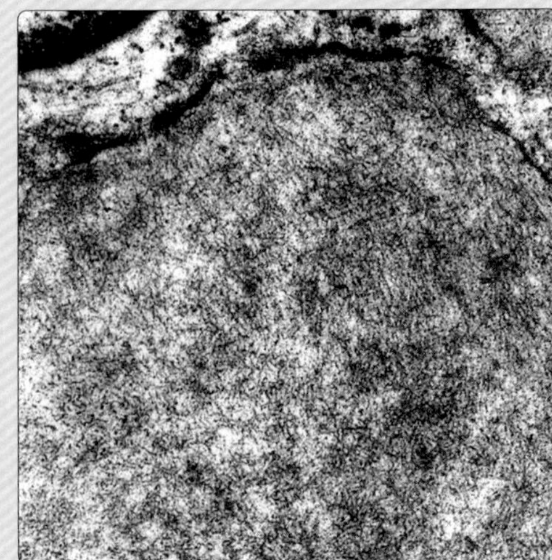

(Left) *AFib amyloidosis is identified by IF, as shown here with antibodies to fibrinogen. κ and λ light chains may also be present at low levels, confusing the diagnosis. (Courtesy M. Picken, MD.)* **(Right)** *AFib amyloid consists of randomly arranged fibrils. The fibrils have the typical size (7-12 nm) reported for amyloid. (Courtesy M. Picken, MD and R. Linke, MD.)*

TERMINOLOGY

Definitions

- Amyloid derived from mutant fibrinogen A α-chain (AFib)

ETIOLOGY/PATHOGENESIS

Fibrinogen α-Chain Gene (*AFib*) Mutations

- Described by Benson et al in 1993
- Autosomal dominant inheritance
- > 9 amyloidogenic mutations described
  - AFib Glu526Val (E526V) most common
    - Common in USA but probably originated in Germany
  - AFib R554L much less common than E526V mutation
  - Phenotype varies among different mutations
    - Also different progression and penetrance
- Penetrance variable
  - Family history of renal disease may be absent
  - Patients may be asymptomatic
  - However, high penetrance also reported
- De novo mutations documented, even in children

Fibrinogen

- Coagulation cascade component
  - No coagulation abnormalities observed
- Fibrinogen produced solely by liver
  - Source of amyloidogenic AFib protein
- C-terminal fragment of A α-chain incorporated into amyloid fibrils
  - Typically contains altered amino acid residues

CLINICAL ISSUES

Epidemiology

- Incidence
  - Rare
    - 1.7% of amyloidosis
- Age
  - 3rd-8th decade, median: 58 years

Presentation

- Nephrotic syndrome/proteinuria
- Renal insufficiency/azotemia
- Coronary atherosclerosis and systemic atheromatosis often
  - May precede proteinuria or renal insufficiency by years
  - Family history of coronary/vascular disease
- Hypertension
- Visceral involvement described
  - Gut dysmotility may be manifestation
- Hyperlipidemia can be present and possibly contributes to atheroma formation

Laboratory Tests

- DNA analysis by RFLP available for some mutations
- Direct nucleotide sequencing needed to determine genetic defect in many patients

Treatment

- Liver alone or combined liver and kidney transplantation
  - May stop progressive injury from amyloid deposition
    - Essentially curative
    - May even reverse organ dysfunction
    - Some argue for preemptive transplantation of liver alone
    - Explanted livers can be used for domino transplantation

Prognosis

- Kidney failure in 1-5 years with dialysis dependence
  - Median time to end-stage disease: 4.6 years
  - AFib amyloid deposition occurs slower than AL amyloid
- Median patient survival from presentation: 15.2 years
- Renal allografts (without liver transplantation) fail in 1-7 years with recurrent amyloidosis
  - 10-year graft survival for AFib: ~ 5.5%

MICROSCOPIC

Histologic Features

- Glomerular enlargement with complete replacement by amyloid
  - Clustering of glomeruli due to atrophy of intervening tubules
- No or little vascular or interstitial amyloid
- Extrarenal involvement
  - Cardiac and systemic vascular involvement
  - Autonomic, peripheral neuropathy, gastrointestinal, and splenic involvement reported

ANCILLARY TESTS

Histochemistry

- Congo red shows orangeophilic material on bright-field microscopy
  - Apple-green birefringence with polarized light

Immunofluorescence

- Fibrinogen demonstrates positivity, primarily in glomeruli

Electron Microscopy

- Randomly arranged fibrils ~ 7-12 nm in diameter

DIFFERENTIAL DIAGNOSIS

Other Amyloidosis Types

- AL/AH, AA, and AApoAI/AApoAII amyloidosis

SELECTED REFERENCES

1. Haidinger M et al: Hereditary amyloidosis caused by R554L fibrinogen Aα-chain mutation in a Spanish family and review of the literature. Amyloid. 20(2):72-9, 2013
2. Stangou AJ et al: Solid organ transplantation for non-TTR hereditary amyloidosis: report from the 1st International Workshop on the Hereditary Renal Amyloidoses. Amyloid. 19 Suppl 1:81-4, 2012
3. Gillmore JD et al: Hereditary fibrinogen A alpha-chain amyloidosis: clinical phenotype and role of liver transplantation. Blood. 115(21):4313; author reply 4314-5, 2010
4. Picken MM: Fibrinogen amyloidosis: the clot thickens! Blood. 115(15):2985-6, 2010
5. von Hutten H et al: Prevalence and origin of amyloid in kidney biopsies. Am J Surg Pathol. 33(8):1198-205, 2009
6. Benson MD et al: Hereditary renal amyloidosis associated with a mutant fibrinogen alpha-chain. Nat Genet. 3(3):252-5, 1993

AApoAI/II Amyloidosis

KEY FACTS

TERMINOLOGY

- Amyloid derived from apolipoprotein I (AApoAI) and apolipoprotein II (AApoAII)

ETIOLOGY/PATHOGENESIS

- ApoAI: 2nd most common systemic hereditary amyloidosis
  - ≥ 20 substitutions in coding region of *APOA1* gene
  - N-terminus mutations: Renal and hepatic and sometimes cardiac amyloidosis
  - C-terminus mutations: Cutaneous, laryngeal, and cardiac amyloid deposition
- ApoAII
  - Mutations in stop codon of *APOA2* gene resulting in C-terminal peptide extension of 21 amino acid residues

CLINICAL ISSUES

- Often presents with ↑ renal insufficiency without proteinuria and without ↓ in longevity

MICROSCOPIC

- Congo red: Apple-green birefringence under polarized light
- AApoAI
  - Interstitium and medulla most often affected, and glomeruli usually spared
  - Arterial involvement may be sole site (notably larger arteries)
- AApoAII
  - Glomerular, interstitial, and vascular involvement reported

ANCILLARY TESTS

- Positive apolipoprotein stain (ApoAI, ApoAII) by IF or IHC
- EM: Randomly arranged fibrils 7-12 nm in diameter

TOP DIFFERENTIAL DIAGNOSES

- AApo AIV
- Other amyloidosis types

(Left) *Abundant amorphous material → is present due to AApoAI amyloidosis in a 33-year-old woman with familial amyloidosis. Deposits were most prominent in the medulla and less appreciable toward the cortex ⇒.* **(Right)** *Abundant amorphous material → is present due to AApoAI amyloidosis in a 33-year-old woman. Her father had a liver and kidney transplant. A paternal grandfather and great-grandmother also had the disease, as well as several aunts and an uncle.*

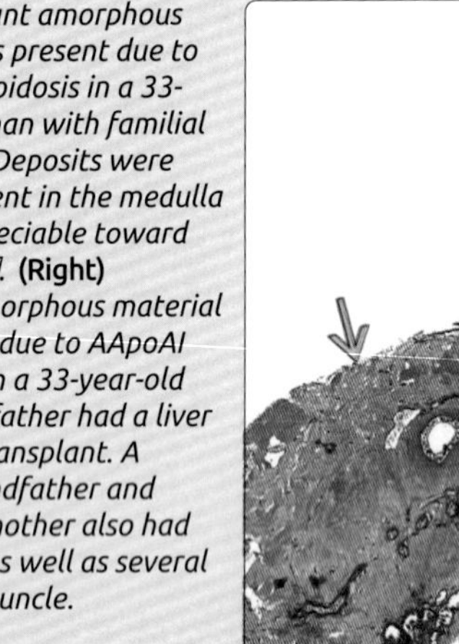

Medullary Amorphous Material Due to AApoAI Amyloidosis

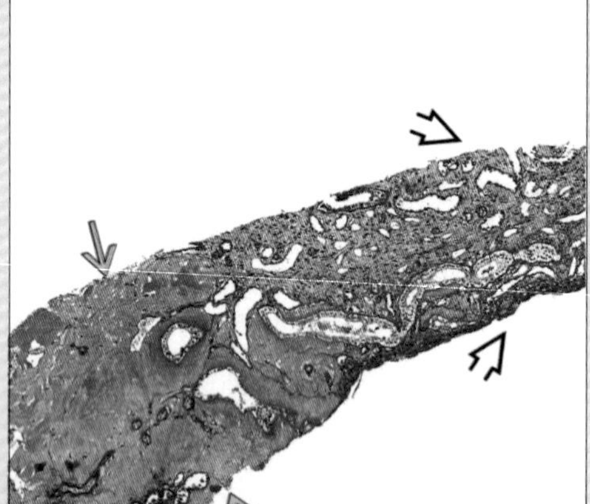

Amorphous Material Due to AApoAI Amyloidosis

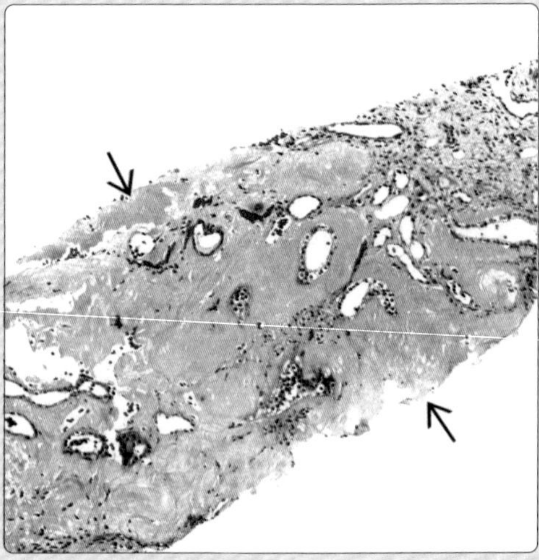

(Left) *Abundant amorphous material → is present due to AApoAI amyloidosis in a 33-year-old woman with familial amyloidosis. Her father had a liver and kidney transplant.* **(Right)** *In a case of AApoIV amyloidosis, abundant interstitial orangeophilic material can be seen on brightfield examination of a Congo red stain. The interstitial material has apple-green birefringence on polarized light examination →.*

Amorphous Material Due to AApoAI Amyloidosis

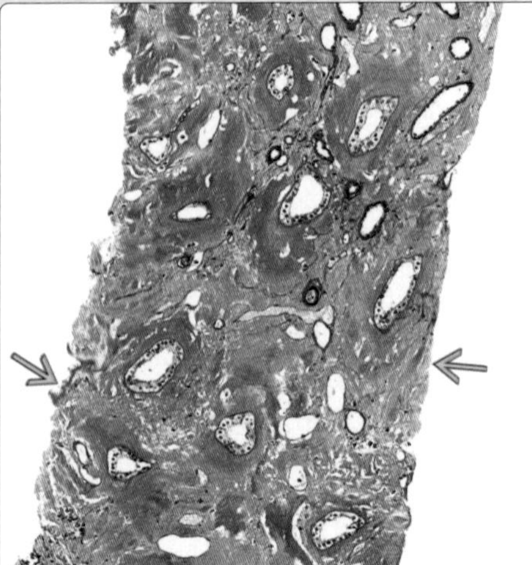

Congo Red of AApoIV Amyloidosis

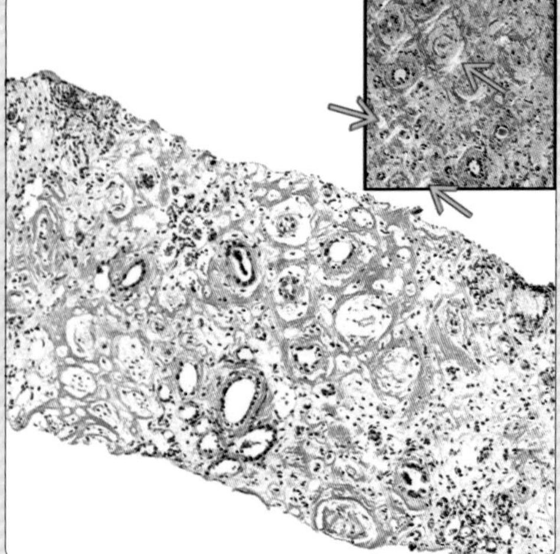

TERMINOLOGY

Abbreviations

- Amyloid derived from apolipoprotein I (ApoAI) and apolipoprotein II (ApoAII)

Definitions

- Familial systemic amyloidosis resulting from amino acid substitutions in ApoAI or ApoAII

ETIOLOGY/PATHOGENESIS

ApoAI Amyloidosis

- 2nd most common systemic hereditary amyloidosis
- ApoAI is 243-amino acid (28 kDa) protein
  - Synthesized in liver and small intestine
  - Located on chromosome 11q23-q24
  - ApoAI is major component of HDL
    - Helps form HDL cholesterol esters
- > 20 substitutions in *APOA1* gene identified
  - N-terminus associated with renal, hepatic, and sometimes cardiac amyloidosis
  - C-terminus associated with cutaneous, laryngeal, and cardiac amyloidosis
  - Most mutations familial but some de novo
    - Result in primary hypoalphalipoproteinemia (Tangier disease) or ApoAI amyloidosis
  - *APOA1* Leu64Pro and Leu75Pro cause renal amyloidosis
    - Slowly progressive renal impairment without shortened longevity
  - Gly26Arg (*G26R*) mutation
    - Associated with peripheral neuropathy

ApoAII Amyloidosis

- 77-amino acid (17.4 kDa) protein
- Located on chromosome 1p21-1qter
- Mutations in stop codon of *APOA2* gene extend C-terminus by 21 amino acids
- Also in senile amyloidosis due to wild-type protein deposition

CLINICAL ISSUES

Epidemiology

- Incidence
  - ApoAI or ApoAII account for 0.4% of amyloidosis
- Ethnicity
  - ApoAI amyloidosis identified in USA, UK, Germany, Italy, Spain, and South Africa

Presentation

- ApoAI often renal insufficiency without proteinuria
- ApoAII with rapidly progressive renal failure in absence of proteinuria
  - No neuropathy

Treatment

- Renal transplantation
  - Prolongs life by ≥ 10 years for ApoAII

Prognosis

- Frequently slow progression to hypertension and renal failure without nephrotic syndrome

MICROSCOPIC

Histologic Features

- AApoAI
  - Interstitium and medulla most often affected
  - Glomeruli usually spared
  - Arterial involvement may be sole site (notably larger arteries)
  - Other organs include liver, larynx, skin, and myocardium
    - Rarely adrenal glands and testes
- AApoAII
  - Glomerular, interstitial, and vascular involvement reported

ANCILLARY TESTS

Histochemistry

- Congo red shows orangeophilic material on brightfield microscopy
  - Apple-green birefringence under polarized light

Immunohistochemistry

- Positive apolipoprotein stain (ApoAI, ApoAII)

Immunofluorescence

- Positive apolipoprotein stain (ApoAI, ApoAII)
- Negative for immunoglobulins, κ, and λ

Electron Microscopy

- Randomly arranged fibrils 7-12 nm in diameter

Mass Spectrometry

- Identifies material as apolipoprotein

DIFFERENTIAL DIAGNOSIS

AApo AIV

- Systemic amyloidosis reported from wild-type apolipoprotein AIV
  - Renal involvement
    - Gradual loss in renal function without proteinuria
    - May be combined with cardiac involvement
    - Interstitium/medulla is 1° compartment affected, sometimes with large amounts of amyloid
    - Glomeruli and vessels not affected
  - Cardiac involvement reported first
  - No mutations reported in *APOA4* gene

Other Amyloidosis Types

- 5% of AA amyloidosis presents similar to ApoAI amyloidosis
  - Medullary deposits and ↑ renal insufficiency without proteinuria

SELECTED REFERENCES

1. Said SM et al: Renal amyloidosis: origin and clinicopathologic correlations of 474 recent cases. Clin J Am Soc Nephrol. 8(9):1515-23, 2013
2. Murphy CL et al: Renal apolipoprotein A-I amyloidosis associated with a novel mutant Leu64Pro. Am J Kidney Dis. 44(6):1103-9, 2004
3. Joy T et al: APOA1 related amyloidosis: a case report and literature review. Clin Biochem. 36(8):641-5, 2003
4. Magy N et al: Renal transplantation for apolipoprotein AII amyloidosis. Amyloid. 10(4):224-8, 2003
5. Yazaki M et al: Hereditary systemic amyloidosis associated with a new apolipoprotein AII stop codon mutation Stop78Arg. Kidney Int. 64(1):11-6, 2003

ATTR Amyloidosis

KEY FACTS

TERMINOLOGY

- Amyloidosis due to deposition of transthyretin (TTR)
- Senile systemic amyloidosis: Senile cardiac amyloidosis

ETIOLOGY/PATHOGENESIS

- TTR protein (also called prealbumin): Made mostly in liver
- Most common form of systemic hereditary amyloidosis
    - *TTR* gene on chromosome 18
        - Most common mutation is methionine substituted for valine at position 30
        - ~ 4% of recent African origin have isoleucine substituted for valine at position 122 (V122I)
            - ATTRV122I most notably affects heart
- Senile systemic amyloidosis due to wild-type TTR

CLINICAL ISSUES

- Hereditary ATTR: Clinically apparent middle to elderly age
- Senile systemic amyloidosis: 20-25% > 80 years old
- Males generally affected more than females
- Nephrotic proteinuria may be accompanied by renal dysfunction
    - Microalbuminuria can be 1st feature at presentation
- Cardiomyopathy & neuropathy are major clinical forms
- Treatment: Hemodialysis, liver transplantation

MICROSCOPIC

- Amyloid renal deposits in glomeruli & interstitial/medulla
    - Interstitial/medullary deposits can be involved in isolated manner
- Extrarenal: Peripheral nerves and myocardium typically affected
- Congo red positive (birefringent)

ANCILLARY TESTS

- TTR positive deposits
- EM: 8-12 nm fibrils

TOP DIFFERENTIAL DIAGNOSES

- Other types of amyloidosis

Interstitial ATTR Amyloid

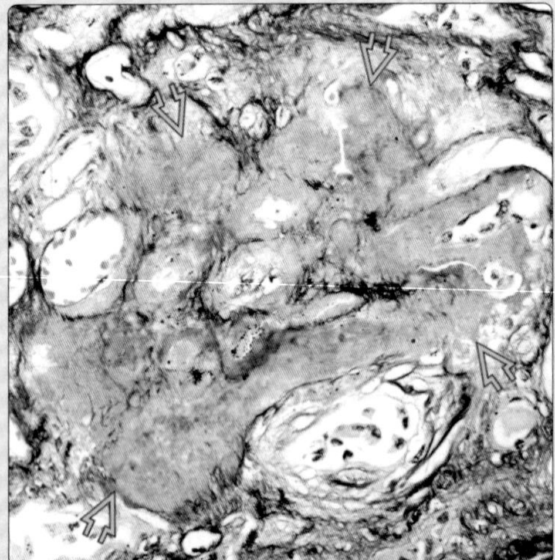

Nonargyrophilic Vascular Deposits

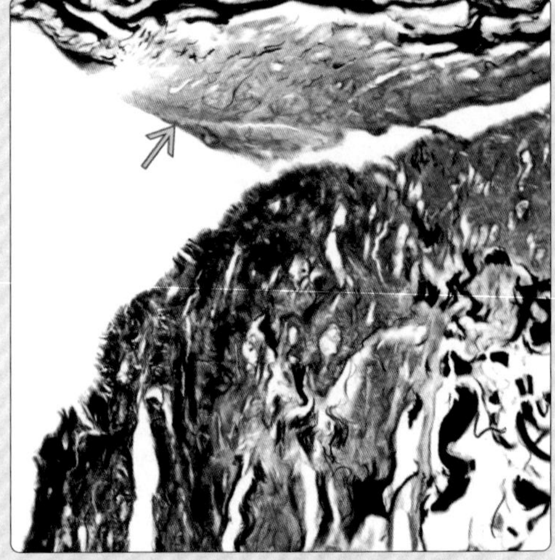

(Left) *There is abundant interstitial nonargyrophilic material* ⇒ *shown to be ATTR amyloid in a patient with familial amyloid polyneuropathy secondary to transthyretin-associated amyloid.* **(Right)** *There is nonargyrophilic material* ⇒ *within a blood vessel in a case of ATTR amyloidosis.*

TTR Immunofluorescence

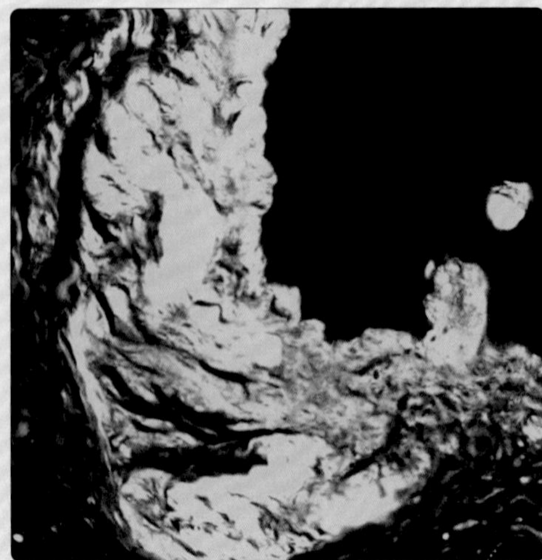

ATTR Amyloid Deposits

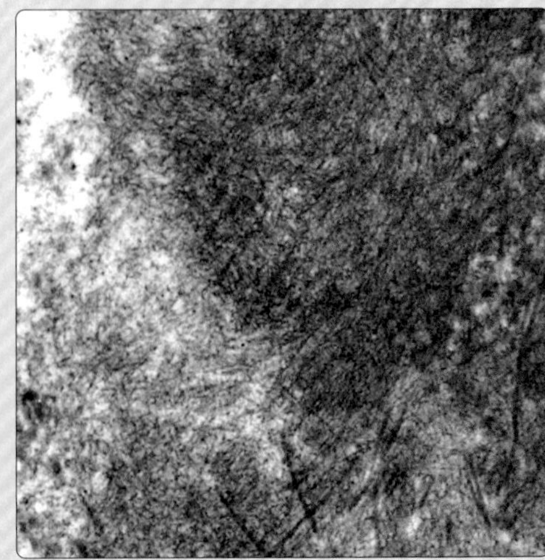

(Left) *Vascular material is positive on transthyretin (TTR), diagnostic of ATTR amyloidosis. Vascular deposits of TTR can be caused by mutations in TTR or by aging (senile amyloidosis).* **(Right)** *Electron microscopy shows a deposit of numerous randomly arranged fibrils in a case of ATTR amyloidosis. EM does not distinguish the different proteins that cause amyloidosis.*

TERMINOLOGY

Abbreviations

- Transthyretin amyloid (ATTR)

Synonyms

- "Familial amyloidotic polyneuropathy" (FAP) was original name for ATTR
- Senile systemic amyloidosis (SSA): Senile cardiac amyloidosis

Definitions

- Amyloidosis derived from transthyretin (TTR)

ETIOLOGY/PATHOGENESIS

Genetic Disorder

- ATTR is most common form of systemic hereditary amyloidosis
- TTR protein
  - Formerly called prealbumin
    - Migrates closer to anode than albumin on serum protein electrophoresis
  - Liver is primary site of synthesis
    - Small amounts synthesized in choroid plexus and retinal pigment epithelium
  - Carrier protein for thyroid hormone and retinol binding protein/vitamin A
    - 127 amino acids and 4 monomers form homotetramer
      - Circulates in blood as 56-kD transport protein
      - Tetramer has 2 binding sites for thyroxin
  - Mutant protein leads to misfolding of TTR forms that typically circulate as tetramers
    - Most mutations decrease TTR tetramer stability and increase dissociation
    - Tetramers dissociate as rate-limiting step
      - Monomers partially unfold, producing amyloidogenic intermediate
      - Intermediate is prone to aggregation and misassembly into fibrils and also spherical oligomers and amorphous aggregates
  - Mixed amyloid deposits derived from 2 proteins reported in heart with transthyretin and apolipoprotein IV
  - Deposition leads to degeneration primarily in postmitotic tissue
- *TTR* gene
  - On chromosome 18 & has 4 exons
  - > 100 transthyretin (*TTR*) mutations result in autosomal-dominant amyloidosis disease
    - Most common mutation is single amino-acid substitution of methionine for valine at position 30 (Val30Met [V30M])
      - Best described nephropathic variant
      - 1st mutation discovered
      - Associated principally with neuropathy
    - 4% of African-Americans have substitution of isoleucine for valine at position 122 (Val122Ile [V122I])
      - Mutation thought to originate on west coast of Africa
      - ATTRV122I affects heart most notably
    - Leu58His is another mutation common in USA that originated in Germany
    - Thr60Ala common in USA & originated in Ireland
    - Ser77Tyr discovered in USA & probably originated in Germany
    - Ile84Ser discovered in USA & probably originated in Switzerland
    - Low penetrance observed in carriers of mutations
      - Family history may be absent
      - Occasional sporadic ATTR cases reported
    - Almost always heterozygotes, thus tetramers generally composed of statistically distributed mutant &/or wild-type TTR subunits
- Senile systemic amyloidosis
  - Wild-type transthyretin forms amyloid, primarily in elderly individuals
    - 25% of octogenarians may be affected, males > females
    - 15% of males > 80 years of age
  - Heart failure eventually occurs but slower than in hereditary ATTR

CLINICAL ISSUES

Epidemiology

- Age
  - Hereditary ATTR: Not generally clinically apparent until middle to elderly age
  - Senile systemic amyloidosis: 20-25% of people > 80 years old
- Sex
  - Males > females
- Ethnicity
  - Well-established foci of familial ATTR in Japan, Sweden, and Portugal
    - Same Met30 variant produces later onset in Swedish and earlier onset in Portuguese

Presentation

- Cardiomyopathy and neuropathy are major clinical forms
  - Ocular forms also exist & "scalloped pupil" is uncommon pathognomonic finding 2° to amyloid deposition in ciliary nerves of eye
- Nephropathy most often affects patients with following characteristics
  - Peripheral neuropathy with late-onset neuropathy
  - Cardiomyopathy with cardiac dysrhythmias
  - May have low penetrance in affected family
  - Microalbuminuria can be 1st feature at presentation
    - Can occur before neuropathy
- Nephrotic range proteinuria is most frequent form of ATTR nephropathy and may be accompanied by renal dysfunction

Laboratory Tests

- Microalbuminuria may be 1st stage of clinical ATTR nephropathy & may precede neuropathy
- DNA analysis helps diagnose familial cases
  - Direct DNA sequencing of peripheral blood cells (e.g., white blood cells)
- Isoelectric focusing and mass spectrometry used to screen serum for variants of transthyretin

- Echocardiographic or electrocardiographic examination may be useful in identifying cardiac forms

Natural History

- End-stage renal disease may eventually develop in some patients

Treatment

- Hemodialysis
- Liver transplantation
  - Simultaneous liver-kidney transplantation to avoid nephropathy recurrence
- Tested therapies include compounds (e.g., tafamidis, diflunisal) that kinetically stabilize TTR tetramer
  - Slow dissociation into monomers and curtail aggregation
- Doxycycline used for ATTR and Aβ2M amyloidosis in Europe

Prognosis

- Poor survival in patients requiring hemodialysis

MICROSCOPIC

Histologic Features

- Amyloid renal deposits
  - Variable
    - Glomerular deposits are primary manifestation in some patients
    - Interstitial/medullary isolated deposits in some patients
- Peripheral nerves and myocardium typically affected
  - Heart most severely affected in ATTRV122I patients
  - Senile systemic amyloidosis mainly affects heart
    - Systemic involvement of other vessels and also lungs and carpal tunnel
  - Blood vessels in other tissues variably affected, including kidney, lung, gastrointestinal tract, liver, spleen, adrenal gland, urinary bladder, prostate, vitreous of eye, leptomeninges, and adipose tissue
    - Biopsies of other tissues sometimes performed (e.g., endomyocardial biopsies, peripheral nerve biopsies [e.g., sural nerve])

ANCILLARY TESTS

Histochemistry

- Congo red shows orangeophilic material on brightfield microscopy
  - Apple-green birefringence under polarized light

Immunohistochemistry

- TTR(+) deposits

Immunofluorescence

- TTR(+) deposits

Electron Microscopy

- Randomly arranged fibrils ~ 7-12 nm in diameter

DIFFERENTIAL DIAGNOSIS

AL/AH ("Primary") Amyloidosis

- Older patients may have ATTR senile amyloid and incidental MGUS
  - Immunofluorescence shows predominance of 1 light chain in AL amyloidosis monoclonal gammopathy of renal significance
    - In rare AH or AL+AH amyloidosis, immunofluorescence shows predominance of heavy chain
  - Some patients with MGUS will not have renal deposition of paraprotein
    - Important to determine if amyloid actually "senile" amyloid due to ATTR amyloidosis

DIAGNOSTIC CHECKLIST

Clinically Relevant Pathologic Features

- Endomyocardial biopsy may be needed in forms that primarily affect heart

SELECTED REFERENCES

1. Beirão JM et al: Impact of liver transplantation on the natural history of oculopathy in Portuguese patients with transthyretin (V30M) amyloidosis. Amyloid. 22(1):31-5, 2015
2. Quarta CC et al: The amyloidogenic V122I transthyretin variant in elderly black Americans. N Engl J Med. 372(1):21-9, 2015
3. Sekijima Y: Transthyretin (ATTR) amyloidosis: clinical spectrum, molecular pathogenesis and disease-modifying treatments. J Neurol Neurosurg Psychiatry. ePub, 2015
4. Herrera GA et al: Renal diseases associated with plasma cell dyscrasias, amyloidoses, and Waldenström's macroglobulinemia. In Jennette JC et al: Heptinstall's Pathology of the Kidney. 7th ed. Philadelphia, PA: Wolters Kluwer. 976-1014, 2015
5. Sekijima Y: Recent progress in the understanding and treatment of transthyretin amyloidosis. J Clin Pharm Ther. 39(3):225-33, 2014
6. Pinney JH et al: Senile systemic amyloidosis: clinical features at presentation and outcome. J Am Heart Assoc. 2(2):e000098, 2013
7. Bulawa CE et al: Tafamidis, a potent and selective transthyretin kinetic stabilizer that inhibits the amyloid cascade. Proc Natl Acad Sci U S A. 109(24):9629-34, 2012
8. Johnson SM et al: The transthyretin amyloidoses: from delineating the molecular mechanism of aggregation linked to pathology to a regulatory-agency-approved drug. J Mol Biol. 421(2-3):185-203, 2012
9. Lobato L et al: Transthyretin amyloidosis and the kidney. Clin J Am Soc Nephrol. 7(8):1337-46, 2012
10. Ruberg FL et al: Transthyretin (TTR) cardiac amyloidosis. Circulation. 126(10):1286-300, 2012
11. Benson MD: The hereditary amyloidoses. In Picken MM et al: Amyloid & Related Disorders: Surgical Pathology & Clinical Correlations. New York, NY: Humana Press, Springer Science + Business Media. 53-67, 2012
12. Ueda M et al: Clinicopathological features of senile systemic amyloidosis: an ante- and post-mortem study. Mod Pathol. 24(12):1533-44, 2011
13. Rapezzi C et al: Transthyretin-related amyloidoses and the heart: a clinical overview. Nat Rev Cardiol. 7(7):398-408, 2010
14. Benson MD: Aging, amyloid, and cardiomyopathy. N Engl J Med. 336(7):502-4, 1997
15. Jacobson DR et al: Variant-sequence transthyretin (isoleucine 122) in late-onset cardiac amyloidosis in black Americans. N Engl J Med. 336(7):466-73, 1997

Glomeruli Uninvolved in ATTR Amyloidosis

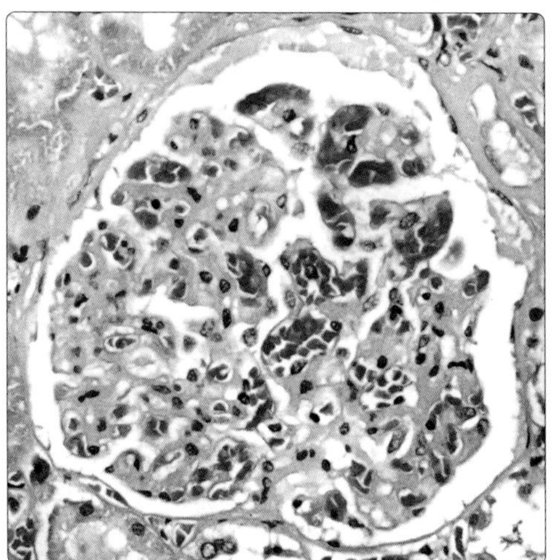

Glomeruli Uninvolved in ATTR Amyloidosis

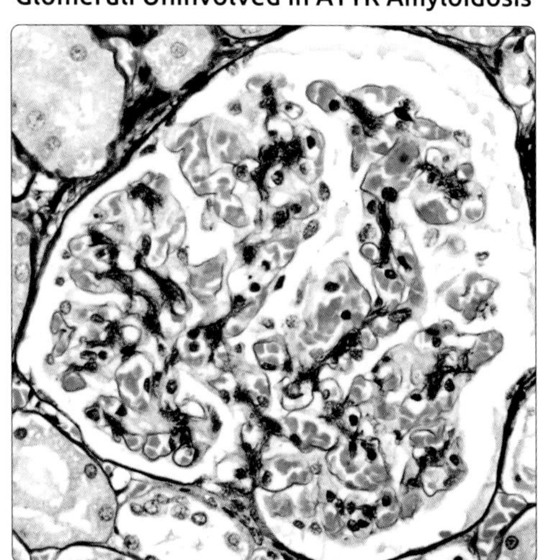

(Left) *In this case of ATTR amyloidosis, this glomerulus is not involved by amyloid deposition, which would show up as amorphous material on this H&E stain; this is typically the case in ATTR amyloidosis.* **(Right)** *This glomerulus in a case of ATTR amyloidosis is not involved by amyloid deposition, which would show up as nonargyrophilic material on this Jones silver stain; this is typically the case in ATTR amyloidosis.*

Interstitial ATTR Amyloid

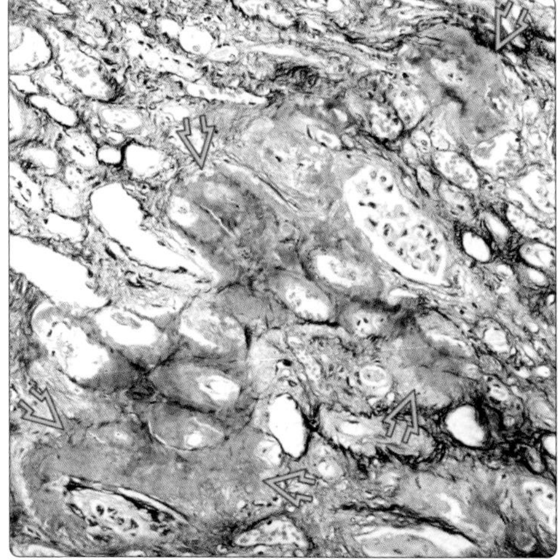

TTR Immunofluorescence

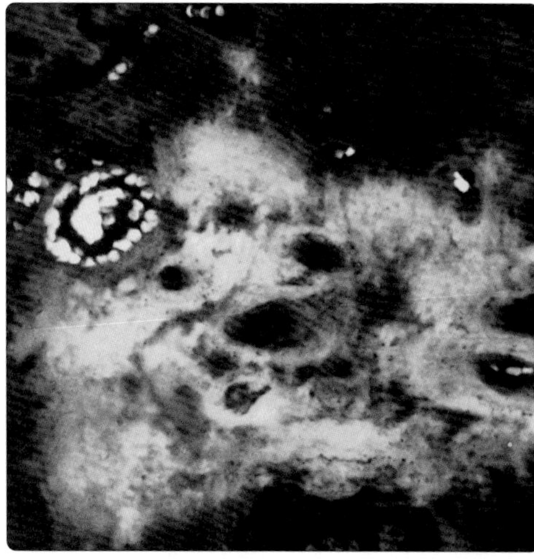

(Left) *There is abundant interstitial nonargyrophilic material ⇨ shown to be ATTR amyloid in a patient with familial amyloid polyneuropathy secondary to transthyretin-associated amyloid.* **(Right)** *Abundant interstitial material is positive on transthyretin (TTR) immunofluorescence, a definitive test for identifying ATTR amyloidosis.*

Glomeruli Uninvolved on TTR Immunofluorescence

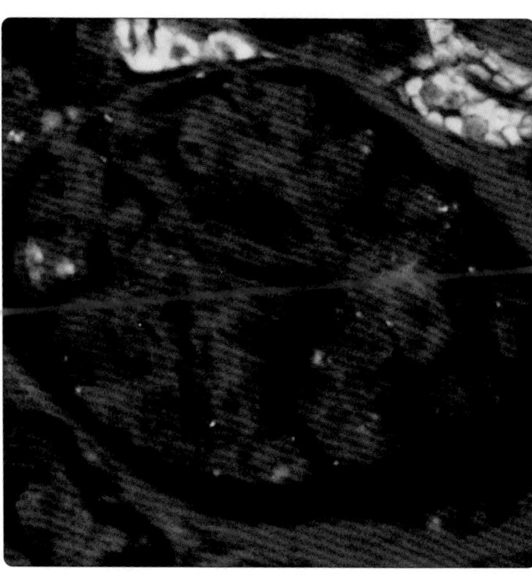

TTR Immunofluorescence Without Vascular Staining

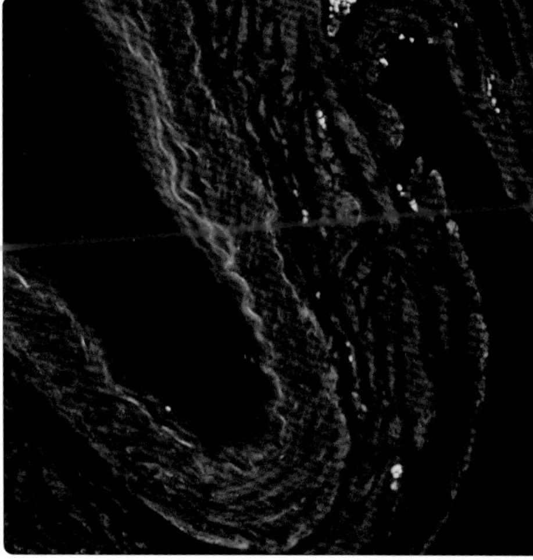

(Left) *In this case of ATTR amyloidosis, TTR immunofluorescence shows that there is essentially little or no deposition of amyloid within the glomeruli; this is the typical case in ATTR amyloidosis.* **(Right)** *TTR immunofluorescence shows that there is essentially little or no deposition of amyloid within this blood vessel in a patient with ATTR amyloidosis; this is sometimes the case in ATTR amyloidosis.*

INTRODUCTION

Approach

- Organized structures encountered by electron microscopy can provide key to diagnosis
- Identification of substance requires characterization of deposits by site, shape, size, periodicity, and composition

CHARACTERIZATION OF ORGANIZED DEPOSITS

Site

- Glomerulus (mesangium, glomerular basement membrane [GBM], capillary lumen, intracellular)
- Tubules (intracellular, TBM, casts)
- Vessels (endothelium, lumen)

Shape

- Fibrils
- Microtubules
- Paracrystalline arrays
- Spheroids
- Crystals

Size and Periodicity

- Modern electron microscopes have measurement software that can be applied directly to digital image
- Loupe is useful for measurement of images that have known magnification
- Without known magnification, useful guide is normal cell membrane lipid bilayer (~ 8 nm in cross section)

Techniques to Determine Composition

- Congo red stain
  - Amyloid has red-green birefringence in polarized light
  - Pitfalls
    - Small quantities may be negative even in thick sections
    - Quality of polarizer important
    - Other substances stain red, but do not polarize
      - Elastin in arteries
    - Other substances polarize without Congo red
      - Collagen fibers
    - Thioflavine T fluorescent dye
      - More sensitive but less specific
- Immunofluorescence
  - Standard panel to identify immunoglobulin heavy and light chains
  - Pitfalls
    - Some monoclonal immunoglobulin chains are nonreactive due to truncation (loss of constant region), crystal lattice, or unknown factors
    - Pronase digestion of paraffin tissue may unmask Ig reactivity
      - e.g., light chain Fanconi syndrome with crystals
  - Special panel for amyloid proteins
    - Serum amyloid A, fibrinogen, transthyretin, leukocyte chemotactic factor 2 (LECT2)
    - Best done in frozen sections rather than paraffin immunohistochemistry (lower background, more sensitive)
- Immunohistochemistry
  - Virus specific panel (polyomavirus, adenovirus, cytomegalovirus, and others)
  - Type III collagen
  - Pronase digestion reveals some occult immunoglobulin epitopes
- Mass spectrometry
  - General approach, useful when no standard test identifies composition
  - Able to type amyloid in 97% of cases
  - Can identify novel components (e.g., LECT2)
  - Applied to laser captured or isolated glomeruli
- Dispersive x-ray spectrometry/scanning electron microscopy
  - Used to identify mineral deposits
- Immunoelectron microscopy
  - Used largely in research to prove particular component is present in deposit
  - Best done with prospective sample preparation

Amyloid Fibrils

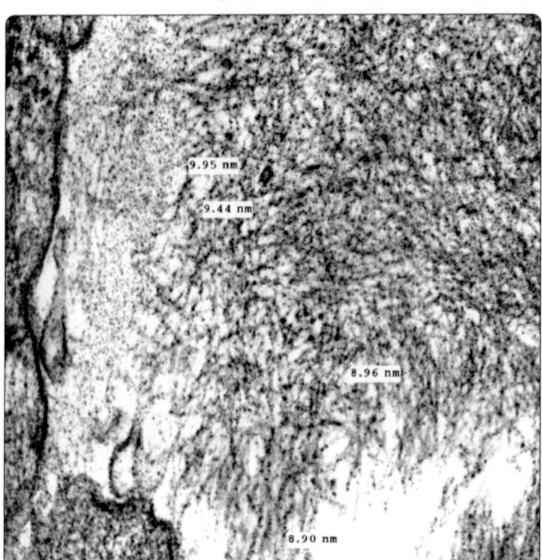

Cryoglobulin Type II

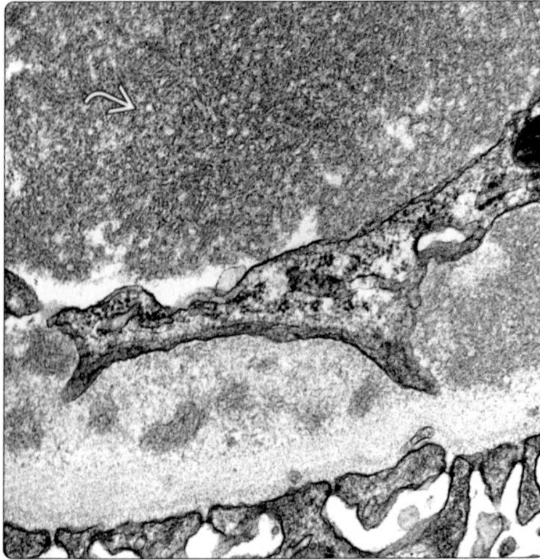

(Left) *Amyloid fibrils are typically 8-12 nm in diameter and have no obvious periodicity. All of the forms of amyloid have the same appearance and are Congo red positive. The protein composition can be identified by immunofluorescence or IHC. These deposits stained for serum amyloid A protein.* **(Right)** *The cryoglobulin "pseudothrombi" ➔ can contain curvilinear tubules characteristic of cryoglobulins. In this case with HCV and mixed cryoglobulinemia type II, they measure ~ 30 nm.*

Identification of Organized Deposits

Disease by Structure	Size (Diameter) and Appearance	Periodicity (nm)	Congo Red Stain	Location	Composition
Fibrils/Tubules					
Amyloidosis (all types)	8-12 nm, random fibrils	-	+	M, GBM, I, V	Light chains, serum amyloid protein and others
Fibrillary glomerulopathy	10-30 nm, random fibrils	-	-	M, GBM	IgG, rarely light chain restriction
Collagenofibrotic glomerulopathy	Curved, banded collagen fibrils	64 nm and minor bands	-	M, GBM	Type III collagen
Nail-patella syndrome (LXM1B mutation)	Discrete aggregates of collagen fibrils in GBM	64 nm and minor bands		GBM	Collagen, type uncertain
Immunotactoid glomerulopathy	20-90 nm, random tubules	-	-	M, GBM	IgG often light chain restriction
Fibronectin glomerulopathy	14-16 nm, Scattered fibrils	-	-	M, GBM	Fibronectin
Thrombotic microangiopathy	Fibrin tactoids	22 nm	-	Vascular lumen	Fibrin
Cryoglobulinemia	Microtubular, fibrillary or annular structures 10-30 nm, variable size and appearance	-	-	M, GBM, vascular lumen (pseudothrombi)	Type I: Ig with light chain restriction; type II IgM k predominant with other Ig and light chains; type III mixed Ig
Diabetic fibrillosis	5-25 nm, random	-	-	M	Unknown, often silver negative
Glomerulosclerosis, NOS	5-25 nm random	-	-	M	Unknown, often silver positive
Idiopathic	Microtubular/fibrillar, 5-25 nm	-	-	Subendothelial	Unknown
Crystals and Paracrystalline Deposits					
Systemic lupus erythematosus	Curved fingerprint pattern	20-25 nm	-	Within amorphous deposits	Unknown nature, may be immune complex with DNA/RNA or cryoprecipitate
Light chain Fanconi syndrome	Electron-dense rhomboid crystals	-	-	Proximal tubule cytoplasm	Monotypic light chain, usually kappa
Cryocrystalglobulinemia (variant of type I cryoglobulinemia)	Electron-dense rhomboid crystals	-	-	Endothelium, proximal tubules	Monotypic immunoglobulin
Spheroids					
Membranous glomerulonephritis	Round particles 15-20 nm, mimics nuclear pores	-	-	Subepithelial	IgG; cause of structure unknown
Viral particles	Round or elongated, regular size, 20-200 nm depending on agent; ± envelop, ± dense core,	-	-	Nuclear, cytoplasmic, or extracellular	Identified with virus-specific antibodies
Idiopathic	Aggregates of round particles ~ 20-50 nm	-	-	Subepithelial over mesangium or in TBM	Unknown, possible lipoproteins or cell membrane fragments

M = mesangium, GBM = glomerular basement membrane, I = interstitium, TBM = tubular basement membrane, V = vessel wall. Small molecule crystals are not included in this table. Some will be lost in processing and leave a void with the shape of the crystal (e.g., uric acid, cysteine, cholesterol). Lipids in the mesangium are prominent in liver disease.

SELECTED REFERENCES

1. Bridoux F et al: Diagnosis of monoclonal gammopathy of renal significance. Kidney Int. ePub, 2015
2. Said SM et al: Renal amyloidosis: origin and clinicopathologic correlations of 474 recent cases. Clin J Am Soc Nephrol. 8(9):1515-23, 2013
3. Sethi S et al: Mass spectrometry based proteomics in the diagnosis of kidney disease. Curr Opin Nephrol Hypertens. 22(3):273-80, 2013
4. Larsen CP et al: The morphologic spectrum and clinical significance of light chain proximal tubulopathy with and without crystal formation. Mod Pathol. 24(11):1462-9, 2011
5. Herrera GA et al: Renal diseases with organized deposits: an algorithmic approach to classification and clinicopathologic diagnosis. Arch Pathol Lab Med. 134(4):512-31, 2010
6. Howie AJ et al: Optical properties of amyloid stained by Congo red: history and mechanisms. Micron. 40(3):285-301, 2009
7. Alchi B et al: Collagenofibrotic glomerulopathy: clinicopathologic overview of a rare glomerular disease. Am J Kidney Dis. 49(4):499-506, 2007
8. Gonul II et al: Glomerular mesangial fibrillary deposits in a patient with diabetes mellitus. Int Urol Nephrol. 38(3-4):767-72, 2006
9. Kowalewska J et al: Membranous glomerulopathy with spherules: an uncommon variant with obscure pathogenesis. Am J Kidney Dis. 47(6):983-92, 2006

(Left) *The fibrils of fibrillary GN are usually larger (10-25 nm in diameter) but otherwise ultrastructurally similar to amyloid fibrils. In contrast to amyloid, these are Congo red negative and stain for IgG and C3, usually with both light chains.* **(Right)** *The deposits in immunotactoid glomerulopathy appear as tubules with a less dense center, typically about 30 nm in diameter (20-90 nm). They consist of IgG often with 1 light chain. The bar is 500 nm.*

Fibrillary Glomerulopathy

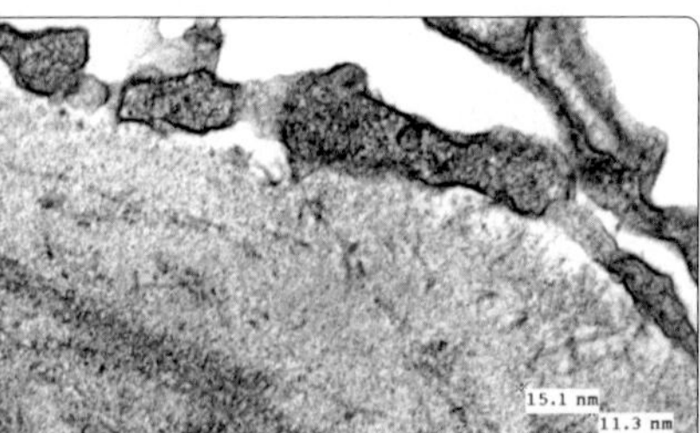

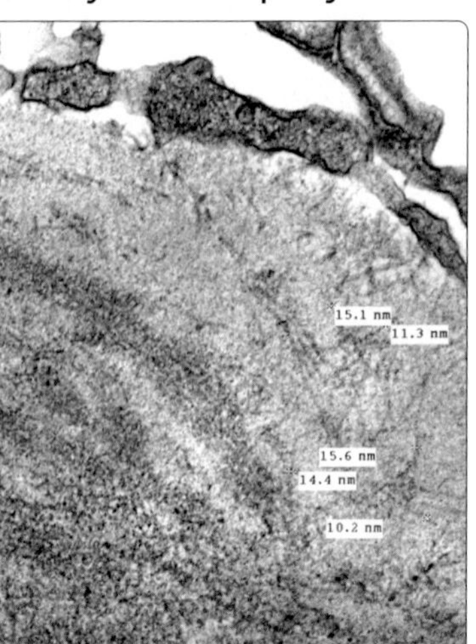

Immunotactoid Glomerulopathy

(Left) *Cryoglobulins vary in appearance by electron microscopy. The fibrils in the mesangium stained for IgG lambda in a patient with an IgG lambda cryoglobulin (type I cryoglobulinemia).* **(Right)** *In fibronectin glomerulopathy, mesangial deposits are rich in fibronectin. These appear mostly granular with foci of fibrils ➔ ~ 14-16 nm in diameter. The normal mesangium contains fibronectin by IF.*

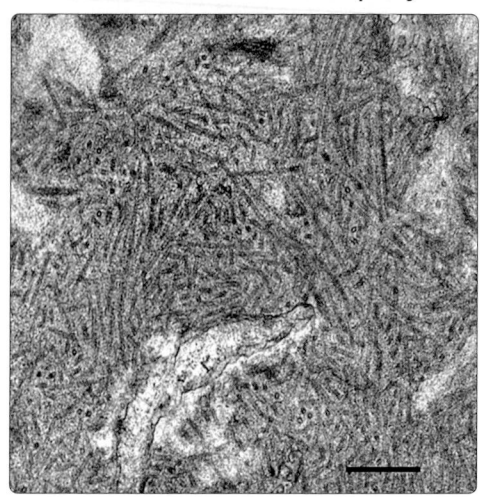

Cryoglobulinemia Type I

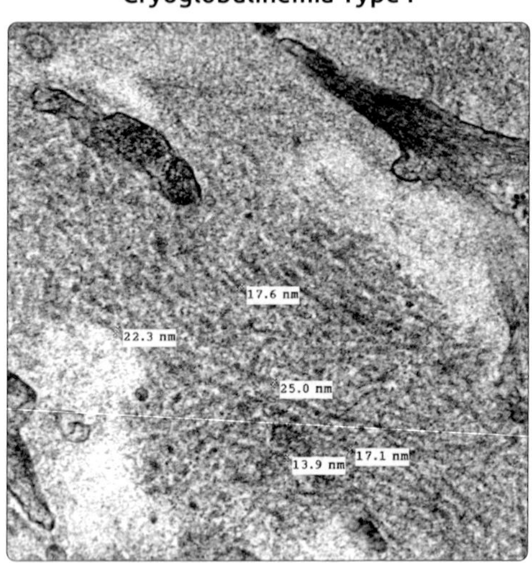

Fibronectin Glomerulopathy

(Left) *Fibrils with a vaguely microtubular structure can sometimes be prominent in nodular diabetic glomerulosclerosis. These are typically silver negative. Their nature is unknown. Congo red and IgG stains are negative, bar is 100 nm.* **(Right)** *Subendothelial fibrils are seen occasionally in renal biopsies without a clear explanation or identification. These are slightly thicker than the cell membrane (8 nm), a good reference point in this patient with nodular diabetic glomerulosclerosis.*

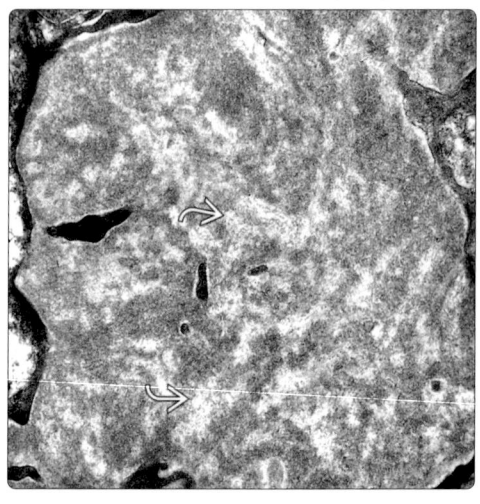

Diabetic Fibrillosis

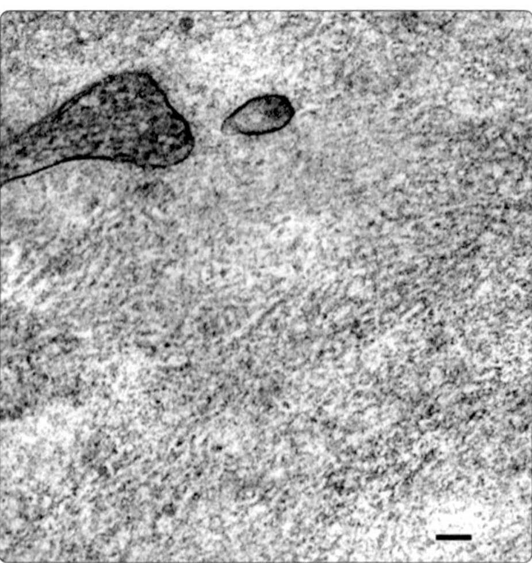

Subendothelial Fibrils of Undetermined Nature

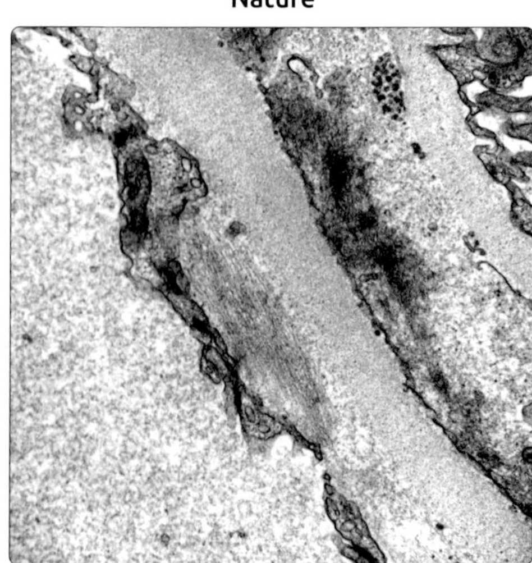

Type III Collagenopathy

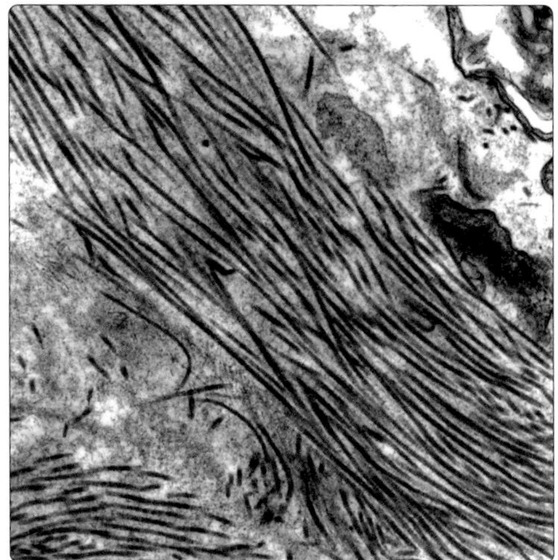

Nail-Patella Syndrome

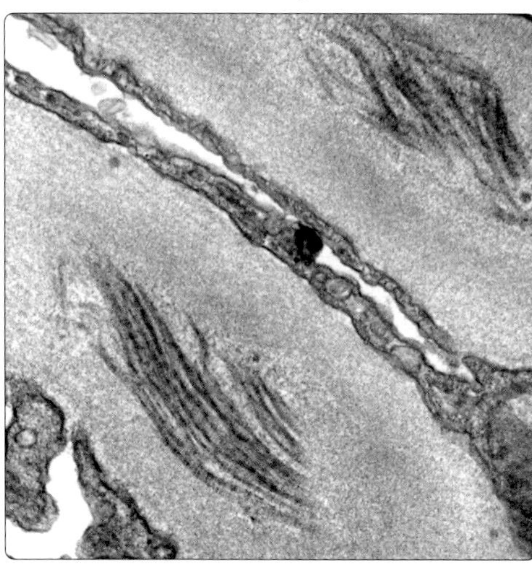

(Left) *Type III collagen accumulates in the glomerular mesangium in patients with collagenofibrotic glomerulopathy. The fibrils tend to be aligned and have the 64 nm periodicity of collagen with light and dark bands.* **(Right)** *Discrete aggregates of collagen bundles in the GBM are seen in patients with LMX1B mutations, whether or not they have the full nail-patella syndrome. Considerable searching may be required to find them. This patient had a mutation in LMX1B but had normal patella and nails.*

Fibrin

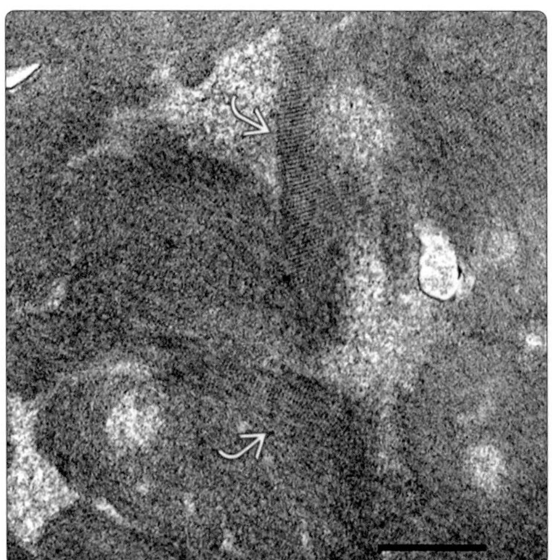

Fingerprint Deposits in Lupus Erythematosus

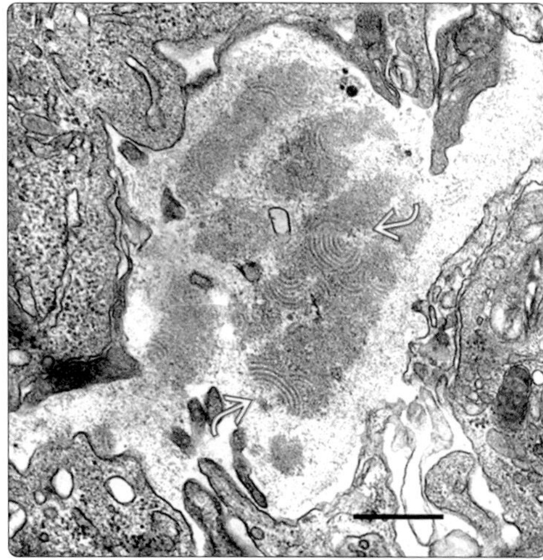

(Left) *Fibrin typically appears very electron dense, sometimes in tactoids. The characteristic periodicity is 22 nm ➡, but often the fibrin appears amorphous. Bar = 500 nm. This is an intracapillary thrombus in a thrombotic microangiopathy case.* **(Right)** *Within amorphous immune complex deposits in SLE, a curved, periodic fingerprint pattern ➡ can sometimes be discerned. Their nature is unknown, perhaps a cryoprecipitate or an immune complex with DNA/RNA. The periodicity is 20-25 nm.*

Spheroid Deposits in Membranous Glomerulonephritis

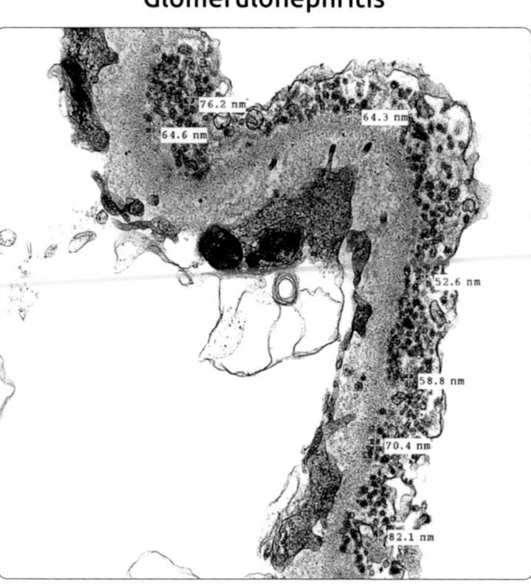

Subepithelial Particles of Uncertain Significance

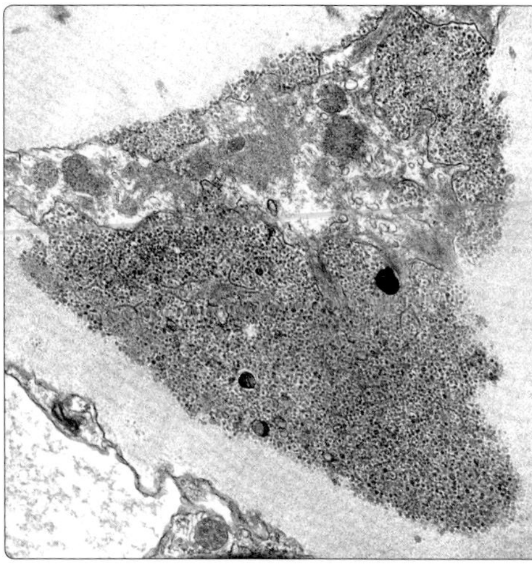

(Left) *Deposits in membranous glomerulonephritis (MGN) are occasionally a mass of spheroid particles. These resemble nuclear pores but do not have the relevant components. These stained for IgG, C3, and both light chains in the usual pattern of MGN.* **(Right)** *Aggregates of 30-50 nm diameter spherical particles can be found in renal biopsies, typically overlying mesangial areas between capillary loops. These should not be confused with viruses. This example was from a patient with nodular diabetic glomerulosclerosis.*

Fibrillary Glomerulopathy

KEY FACTS

TERMINOLOGY

- Fibrillary glomerulonephritis (FGN)

CLINICAL ISSUES

- Rare: < 1% of native kidney biopsies
- Associated with malignancy, dysproteinemia, and autoimmune disease
- Proteinuria (100%)
- Hematuria (~ 50%)
- 40-50% progress to end-stage renal disease (ESRD) within 2-4 years
- 35-50% recur in kidney allografts

MICROSCOPIC

- Diffuse mesangial expansion by eosinophilic material
  - Congo red negative
- Several histologic patterns
  - Mesangial proliferation
  - Membranoproliferative glomerulonephritis (GN)
  - Crescents in ~ 25%
  - Segmental &/or global glomerular scarring
- IF: IgG and C3 in mesangium and along GBM
  - Usually IgG4, rarely IgM and IgA
  - Usually kappa = lambda
- EM: Nonbranching, randomly arranged fibrils
  - Thicker than amyloid
  - Average: 20 nm; range: 10-30 nm

ANCILLARY TESTS

- TBM deposits by IF and EM (15%)

TOP DIFFERENTIAL DIAGNOSES

- Amyloidosis
- Immunotactoid glomerulopathy
- Cryoglobulinemic GN
- Fibronectin glomerulopathy

DIAGNOSTIC CHECKLIST

- IgG, kappa and lambda light chains strongly positive

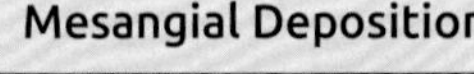

Mesangial Deposition

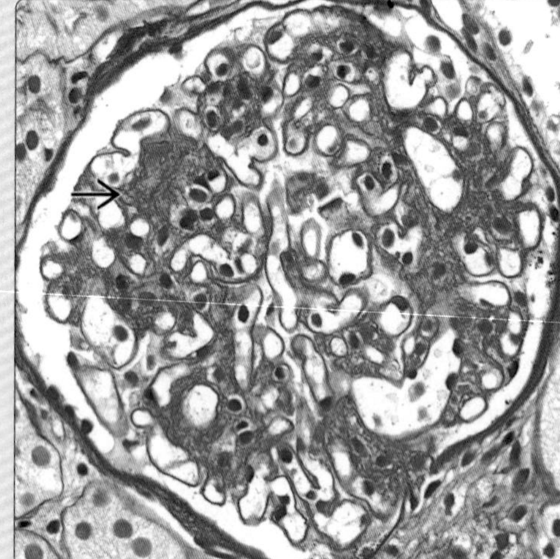

Mesangial Hypercellularity

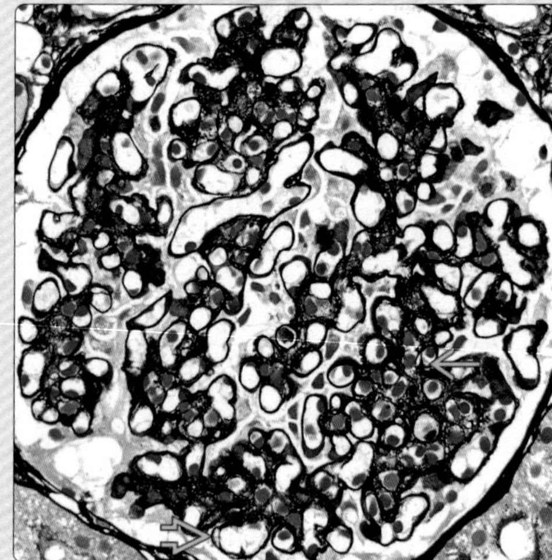

(Left) *Periodic acid-Schiff shows diffuse expansion of mesangial areas ➔ by eosinophilic material with normal glomerular basement membranes in a young woman with fibrillary glomerulonephritis (FGN).* **(Right)** *Jones methenamine silver reveals increased mesangial hypercellularity ➔ and focal duplication of the glomerular basement membrane ➔.*

IgG

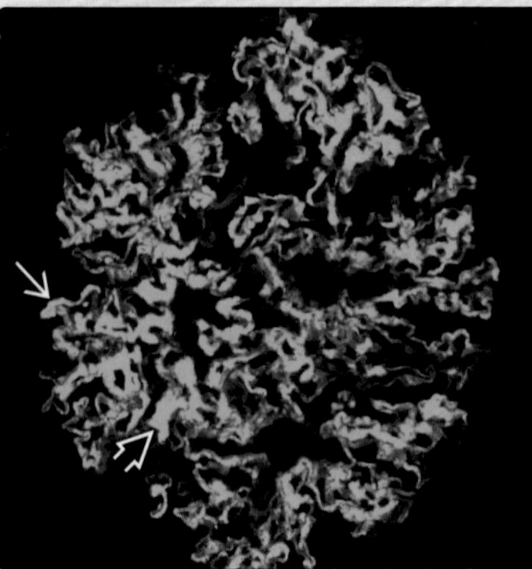

Fibrils

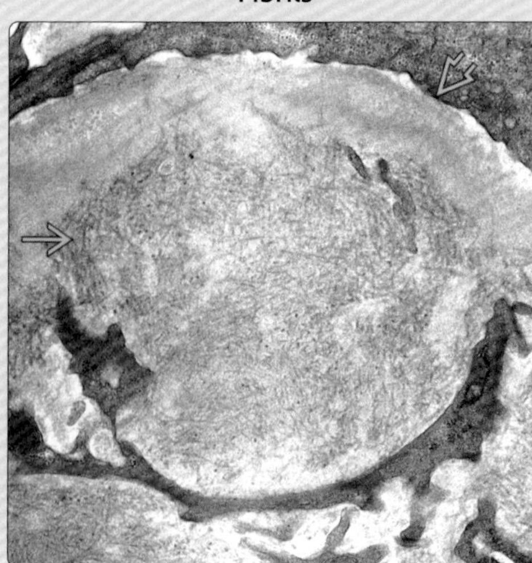

(Left) *Immunofluorescence microscopy for IgG shows strong mesangial ➔ staining with focal staining of glomerular capillary walls ➔, which correlates with the light microscopic alterations of the glomeruli.* **(Right)** *Electron micrograph shows numerous fibrillar deposits primarily limited to a subendothelial location ➔ without involvement of the overlying glomerular basement membrane ➔.*

TERMINOLOGY

Synonyms

- Fibrillary glomerulonephritis (FGN)

Definitions

- Glomerular disease characterized by nonamyloid, nonperiodic fibrillar deposits of immunoglobulin, 10-30 nm in diameter

ETIOLOGY/PATHOGENESIS

Unknown

- Fibrils contain IgG, usually IgG4 ± IgG1, with both light chains (polyclonal)
  - Occasional cases monotypic light chains (15%)
- Associations
  - Malignancy (23%)
  - Dysproteinemia (17%)
  - Autoimmune disease (15%), including systemic lupus erythematosus
  - Infection, including hepatitis C virus (3%)

CLINICAL ISSUES

Epidemiology

- Incidence
  - < 1% of native kidney biopsies
- Sex
  - Slight female predilection
- Ethnicity
  - Caucasian predilection (> 90%)

Presentation

- Proteinuria (100%)
  - Nephrotic (38%)
- Hematuria (52%)
- Hypertension (70%)
- Renal insufficiency

Laboratory Tests

- Normocomplementemic (97%)

Prognosis

- 40-50% progress to end-stage renal disease (ESRD) in 2-4 years
  - Occasional complete (5%) or partial (8%) remission
- Recurrence rate of 35-50% in kidney allografts

MICROSCOPIC

Histologic Features

- Glomeruli
  - Diffuse mesangial expansion by eosinophilic material
  - Mesangial sclerosis &/or hypercellularity pattern
    - Segmental &/or global glomerular scarring
    - Can manifest as nodular glomerulosclerosis
  - Membranoproliferative pattern
    - Focal GBM duplication
  - Marked subepithelial deposits may mimic membranous GN
  - Cellular crescents in ~ 25% of cases
    - Usually < 20% of glomeruli
  - Congo red negative
  - PAS positive and Jones silver stain negative (or weak)
- Tubules and interstitium
  - Interstitial fibrosis and tubular atrophy common
  - Interstitial inflammation may be prominent when tubular basement membrane (TBM) deposits present

ANCILLARY TESTS

Immunofluorescence

- Prominent IgG deposits in mesangium and along GBM
  - Often IgG4 (90%) with (80%) or without (10%) IgG1; rarely IgG1 alone (10%)
    - IgG4 heavy chains spontaneously reassociate, impairing detection of monotypic light chains
  - Kappa = lambda in most cases
    - 15% monotypic light chains (70% lambda)
- C3 almost always strongly positive (92%), often lesser C1q (60%)
- May have IgM (47%) or IgA (28%) but at lesser intensity than IgG
- TBM deposits of IgG (15%)

Electron Microscopy

- Randomly arranged fibrils deposited in mesangial areas and along GBM
  - Fibrils without hollow core or organized substructure
    - Average diameter: 18-20 nm; range: 10-30 nm
    - Resemble amyloid fibrils but usually larger diameter
  - Fibrils composed of immunoglobulins by immunogold labeling
- TBM with fibrillar deposits (15%)

DIFFERENTIAL DIAGNOSIS

Amyloidosis

- Congo red positive with apple-green birefringence under polarized light; 8-12 nm thick fibrils

Immunotactoid Glomerulopathy

- Microtubular substructure of deposits larger (30-50 nm thick fibrils)
- Usually (~ 80%) monotypic

Cryoglobulinemic Glomerulonephritis

- Serum cryoglobulins present
- Membranoproliferative pattern of injury with "pseudothrombi" on light microscopy

Fibronectin Glomerulopathy

- Mesangial and subendothelial deposition of PAS(+) material

SELECTED REFERENCES

1. Sethi S et al: Laser microdissection and proteomic analysis of amyloidosis, cryoglobulinemic GN, fibrillary GN, and immunotactoid glomerulopathy. Clin J Am Soc Nephrol. 8(6):915-21, 2013
2. Nasr SH et al: Fibrillary glomerulonephritis: a report of 66 cases from a single institution. Clin J Am Soc Nephrol. 6(4):775-84, 2011
3. Markowitz GS et al: Hepatitis C viral infection is associated with fibrillary glomerulonephritis and immunotactoid glomerulopathy. J Am Soc Nephrol. 9(12):2244-52, 1998
4. Iskandar SS et al: Clinical and pathologic features of fibrillary glomerulonephritis. Kidney Int. 42(6):1401-7, 1992

(Left) *H&E shows a prominent increase in eosinophilic material in mesangial areas →, which leads to an appearance of decreased patent glomerular capillaries.* **(Right)** *PAS shows mesangial expansion by eosinophilic material ⇨ that stains less pink than the glomerular basement membranes → and resembles amyloid but is distinct from diabetic nephropathy. The mesangial matrix in diabetic patients stains equally intense as the glomerular basement membranes.*

Diffuse Mesangial Deposition

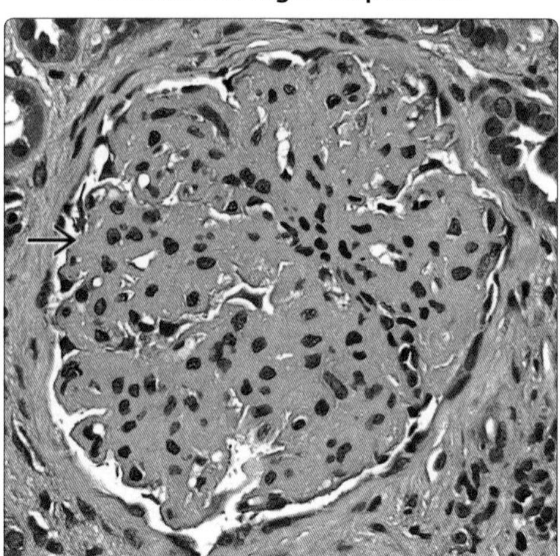

Mesangial Deposition

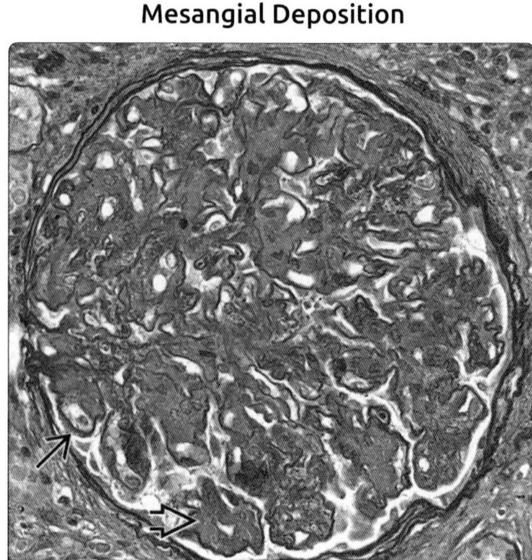

(Left) *A florid cellular crescent → compresses the remaining glomerular tufts ⇨. The collapsed glomerular tufts somewhat resemble collapsing glomerulopathy. Cellular crescents are found in about 20% of FGN.* **(Right)** *Masson trichrome shows segmental glomerular scarring → with loss of many glomerular capillary lumina and a fibrous attachment to Bowman capsule. This glomerular injury is common in advanced FGN.*

Cellular Crescent (PAS)

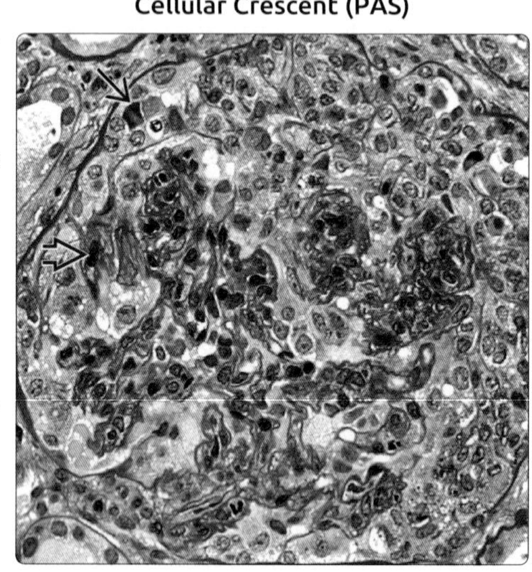

Segmental Glomerular Scarring

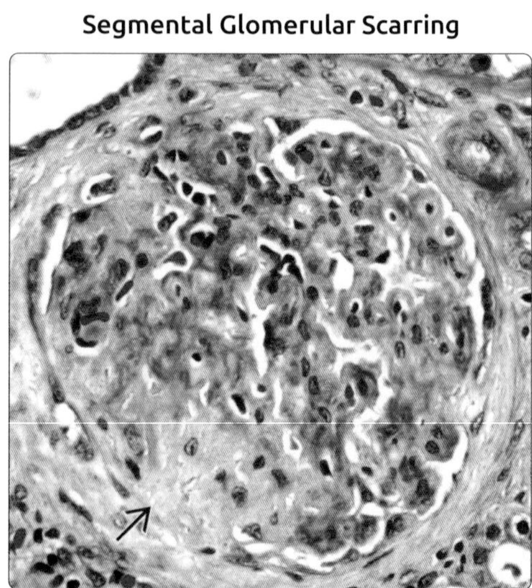

(Left) *Immunofluorescence for IgG of FGN with a crescent ↷ shows strong confluent staining of the capillary walls (pseudolinear pattern) → and mesangial regions. The confluent staining may resemble anti-glomerular basement membrane (GBM) disease, but the mesangial staining ⇨ excludes this diagnosis.* **(Right)** *Immunofluorescence shows C3 deposition in the glomerular mesangium → and along the glomerular capillary walls ⇨.*

IgG

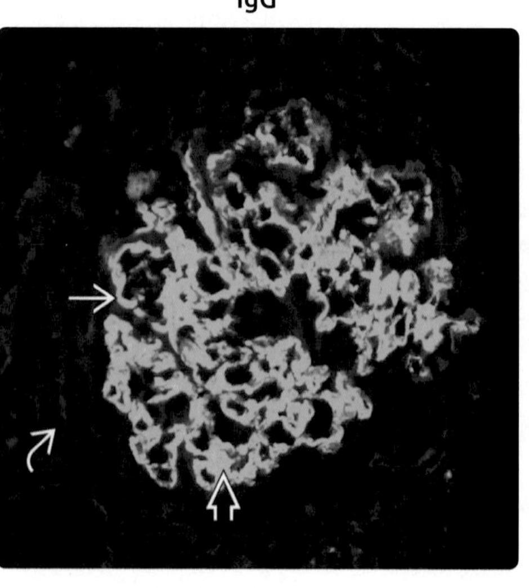

C3

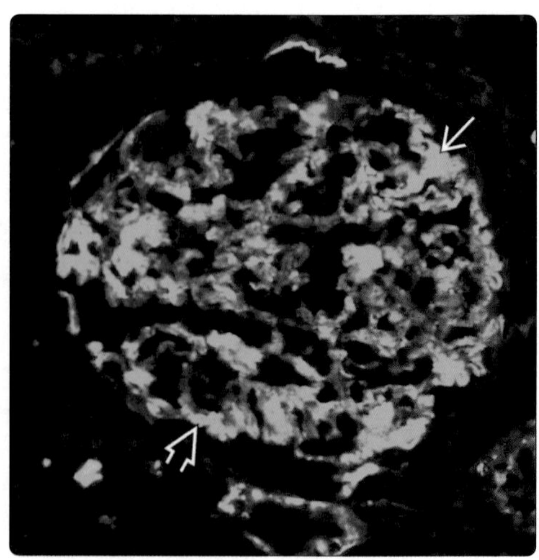

Kappa

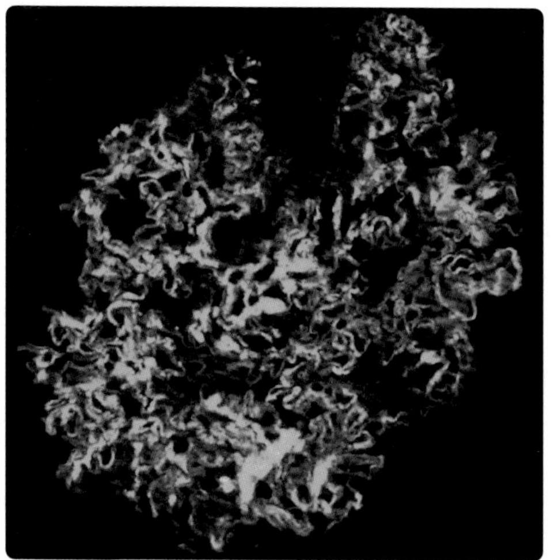

Tubular Basement Membranes (IgG)

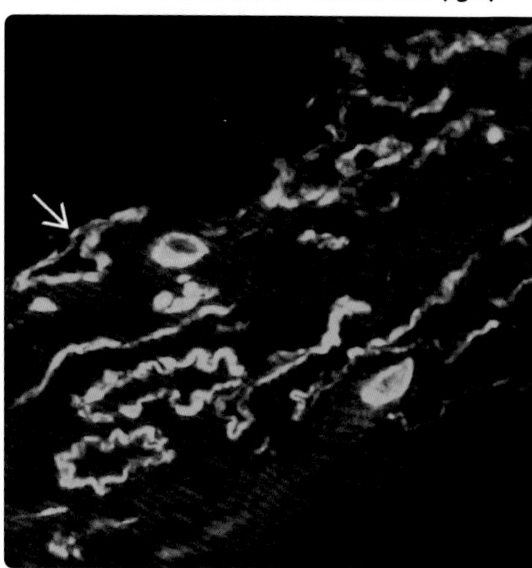

(Left) *Immunofluorescence microscopy for kappa light chain demonstrates a similar but less intense staining pattern to IgG and lambda light chains (not shown). Rare cases of monoclonal staining have been reported.* **(Right)** *Immunofluorescence microscopy shows that IgG staining of the tubular basement membranes* ➔ *can be observed in a subset of FGN. Prominent interstitial inflammation (not shown) was also noted by light microscopy.*

Fibrils

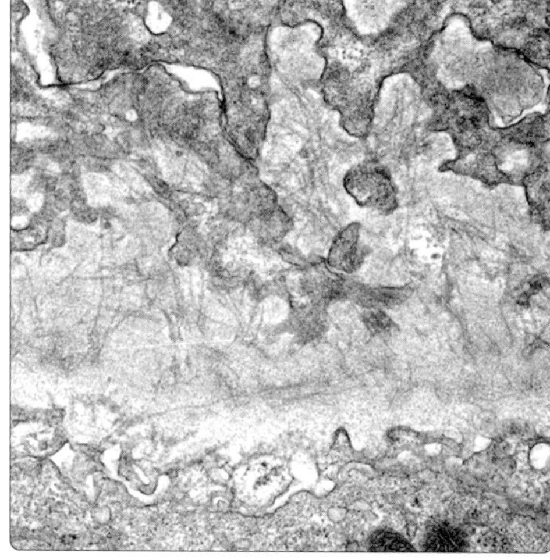

Fibrils

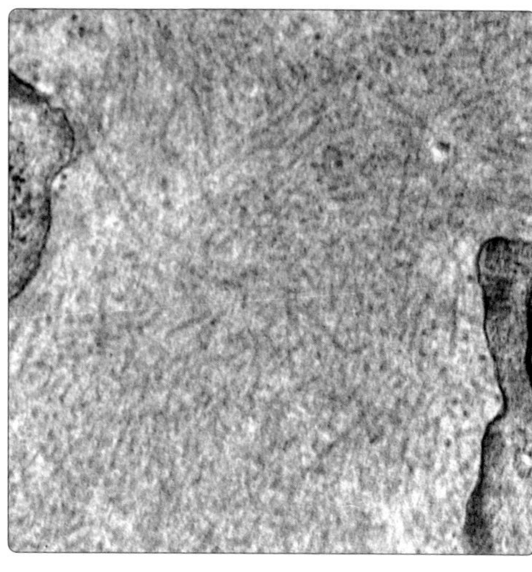

(Left) *Electron microscopy of FGN shows fibrils arranged in a haphazard pattern in the GBM and mesangial matrix. The Congo red stain was negative, and the diagnosis was further supported by the presence of characteristic polyclonal light chain IF staining.* **(Right)** *Numerous fibrils are distributed through the mesangium, which range in thickness from 16-24 nm. The absence of hollow cores distinguishes these from the microtubules of immunotactoid glomerulopathy.*

Subendothelial Fibrils

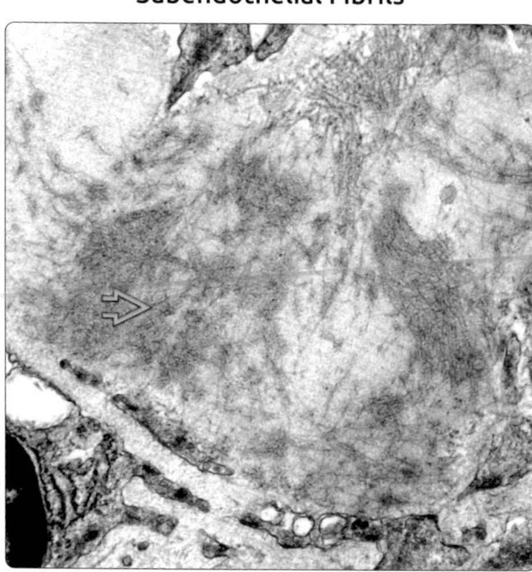

Fibrils in TBM

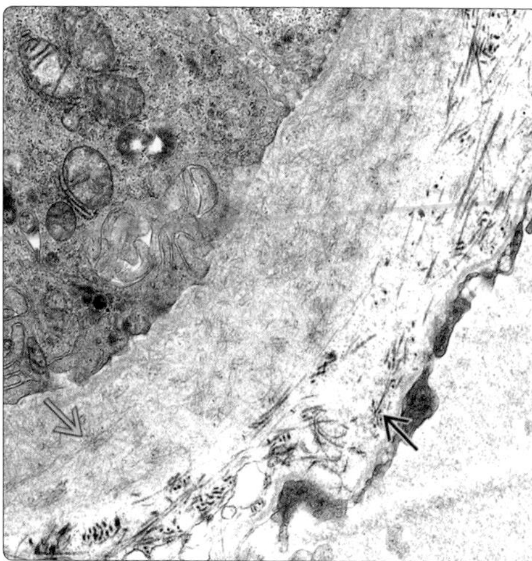

(Left) *Electron microscopy shows prominent accumulation of randomly arranged fibrils* ⇨ *in a subendothelial region. At low magnification, these aggregates of fibrils may resemble discrete immune complexes, but closer examination reveals their fibrillar substructure.* **(Right)** *Electron microscopy demonstrates many fibrils* ⇨ *within the tubular basement membrane that are clearly thinner than adjacent collagen fibrils* ➔ *in the interstitium.*

Immunotactoid Glomerulopathy

KEY FACTS

TERMINOLOGY

- Glomerulopathy with microtubular deposits of IgG, typically > 30 nm in diameter, arranged in parallel arrays and Congo red (-)

CLINICAL ISSUES

- Nephrotic syndrome, hematuria, and hypocomplementemia
- Associated with monoclonal gammopathy and hematologic malignancy
- Caucasian predilection

MICROSCOPIC

- Mesangial expansion with eosinophilic, PAS-positive material
- Mesangioproliferative, membranoproliferative, membranous, and endocapillary proliferative patterns
- Focal splitting and occasional "spikes" of basement membrane

ANCILLARY TESTS

- Congo red stain negative
- Immunofluorescence with predominant IgG, with some cases showing IgA or IgM
    - Majority have light chain restriction (70-90%)
    - IgG1 is most common subclass when monotypic deposits present
    - C3 usually positive, and C1q less frequently positive
- Electron microscopy shows microtubules organized in parallel arrays (> 30 nm) with hollow core

TOP DIFFERENTIAL DIAGNOSES

- Fibrillary glomerulopathy
- Cryoglobulinemic glomerulonephritis
- Fibronectin glomerulopathy
- Type III collagen glomerulopathy

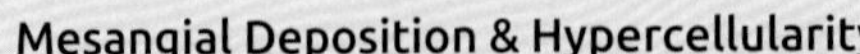

Mesangial Deposition & Hypercellularity

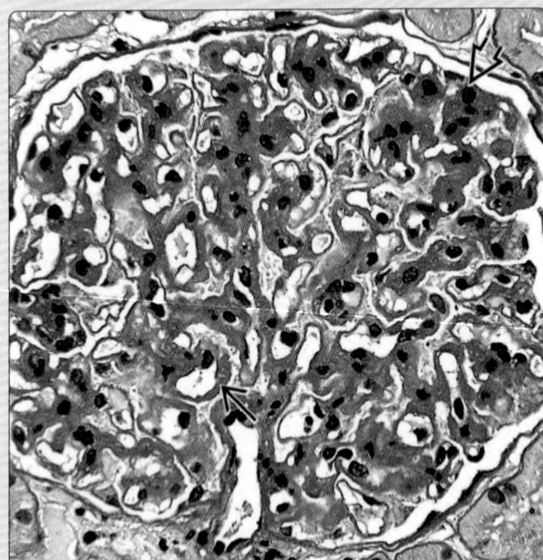

Mild Mesangial Hypercellularity

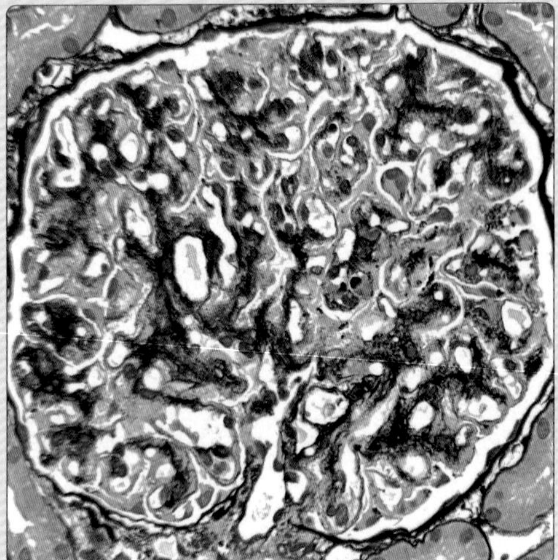

(Left) *PAS shows mild diffuse expansion of mesangial areas with focal hypercellularity → and irregular and segmental thickening of the glomerular basement membranes (GBMs) → due to the presence of immune deposits in this case of ITG. (Courtesy J. Kowalewska, MD.)* **(Right)** *Jones methenamine silver reveals that the immune deposits along the glomerular capillaries are mostly negative for silver staining in this case of ITG. (Courtesy J. Kowalewska, MD.)*

IgG

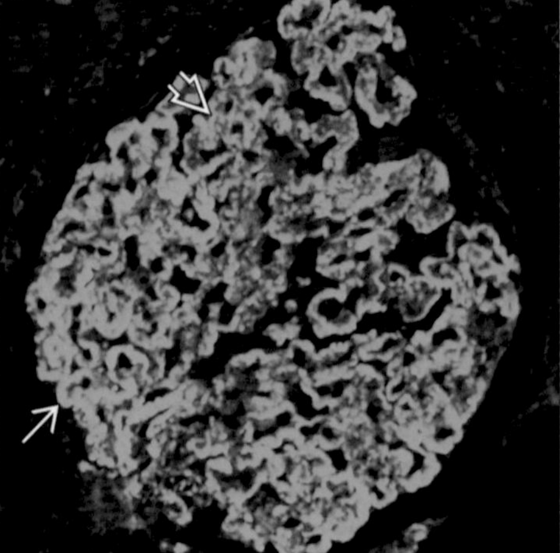

Microtubules With Hollow Cores

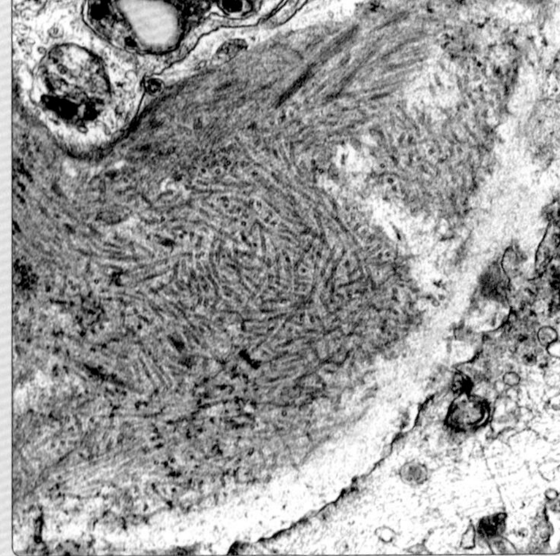

(Left) *Immunofluorescence microscopy for IgG shows strong staining along glomerular capillaries → and mesangial areas →. (Courtesy J. Kowalewska, MD.)* **(Right)** *The characteristic microtubular pattern of deposits in ITG is evident even in this medium-power electron micrograph.*

TERMINOLOGY

Abbreviations

- Immunotactoid glomerulopathy (ITG)

Definitions

- Glomerulopathy with microtubular deposits of IgG, typically > 30 nm in diameter, arranged in parallel arrays and Congo red (-)

ETIOLOGY/PATHOGENESIS

Unknown Mechanism

- Aggregration of immunoglobulins to form microtubules
- Activate complement

CLINICAL ISSUES

Epidemiology

- Incidence
  - < 0.1% of adult native kidney biopsies
- Age
  - 5th to 6th decade
- Sex
  - Slight female predilection
- Ethnicity
  - Caucasian predilection

Presentation

- Nephrotic syndrome in 86%
- Hematuria
- Hypocomplementemia (C3, C4) in 40%
- 63% with monoclonal gammopathy (serum M-spike)
- 38% with hematologic malignancy (myeloma in 13%, CLL in 19%, lymphoma in 13%)
- Occasional cases associated with HIV or HCV

Treatment

- Drugs
  - Chemotherapy for underlying lymphoproliferative disorder or plasma cell dyscrasia, if present

Prognosis

- Data limited
- 50% with partial remission; 17% progress to ESRD
- Clinical course depends on underlying lymphoproliferative disorder, if present
- Occasional response to chemotherapy
  - Repeat biopsies show loss of deposits in a minority
- Recurrence after kidney transplantation (~ 50%), more benign course

MICROSCOPIC

Histologic Features

- Glomerulus
  - Varied patterns: Mesangioproliferative, membranoproliferative (56%), membranous (31%) and endocapillary proliferation (13%)
    - Mesangial expansion by eosinophilic, PAS-positive material
    - Glomerular basement membrane (GBM) thickening, focal splitting and sometimes "spikes"
    - Focal crescents in 13%
- Tubular atrophy
- Interstitial fibrosis
- Extrarenal deposits rarely reported (e.g., peripheral nerve)
- Similar extrarenal deposits reported in cornea and stomach associated with monoclonal gammopathy

ANCILLARY TESTS

Immunofluorescence

- Predominantly IgG, with rare cases showing IgA or IgM
  - IgG1 is most common subclass when monotypic deposits present
- Kappa &/or lambda light chain
  - 69-93% of cases have light chain restriction, usually kappa
- C3 usually positive, and C1q less frequently positive

Electron Microscopy

- Microtubular deposits with electron-lucent lumen organized in parallel arrays
  - Typically > 30 nm in diameter (range: 20-90 nm)
- Subendothelial location in irregular, chunky pattern along capillary loops and mesangium
- Subepithelial and intramembranous deposits may be seen

DIFFERENTIAL DIAGNOSIS

Fibrillary Glomerulopathy

- Randomly arranged fibrils with average thickness of 20 nm without hollow core
- Polyclonal IF staining; commonly IgG4

Cryoglobulinemic Glomerulonephritis

- Serum positive for cryoglobulins; pseudothrombi

Fibronectin Glomerulopathy

- Fibrillar deposits < 30 nm; IgG negative
- Positive immunohistochemistry for fibronectin

Type III Collagen Glomerulopathy

- Periodic banded collagen fibrils by EM and type III collagen by IHC

Nail-Patella Syndrome

- Rare disorder with nail hypoplasia &/or bone abnormalities
- Periodic, sparse collagen fibrils by EM in GBM

DIAGNOSTIC CHECKLIST

Pathologic Interpretation Pearls

- Monoclonal immunoglobulin staining pattern
- Congo red (-) deposits with microtubular appearance and diameter typically > 30 nm

SELECTED REFERENCES

1. Nasr SH et al: Immunotactoid glomerulopathy: clinicopathologic and proteomic study. Nephrol Dial Transplant. 27(11):4137-46, 2012
2. Rosenstock JL et al: Fibrillary and immunotactoid glomerulonephritis: Distinct entities with different clinical and pathologic features. Kidney Int. 63(4):1450-61, 2003

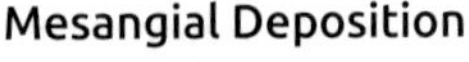

Mesangial Deposition

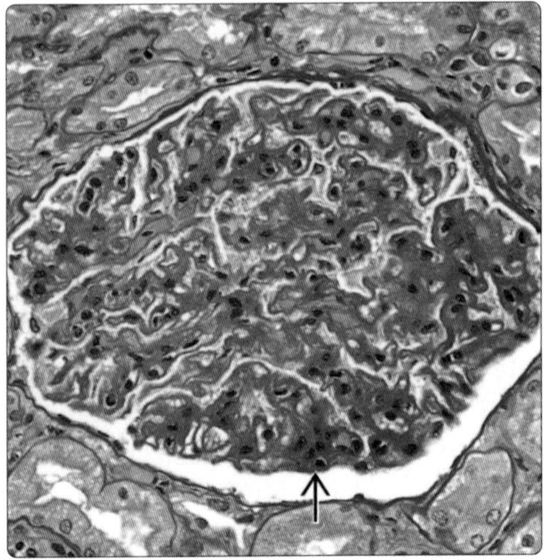

Segmental Sclerosis

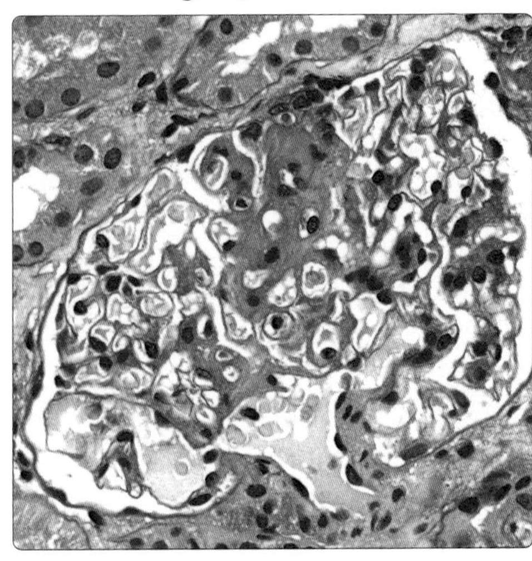

(Left) *Mesangial expansion by eosinophilic material with mild segmental hypercellularity* → *is present along with many neutrophils in the glomerular capillaries.* **(Right)** *PAS shows segmental increase of eosinophilic material in the mesangium with normal adjacent glomerular tufts, segmental sclerosis, and adhesion to Bowman capsule. The GBM is normal at this magnification.*

Eosinophilic Glomerular Deposits

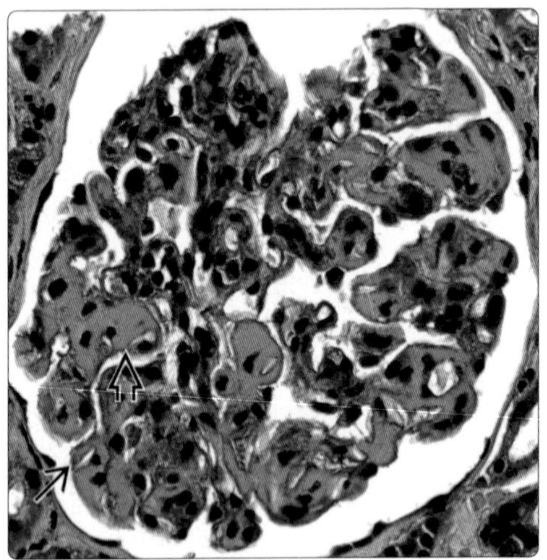

GBM "Spikes"

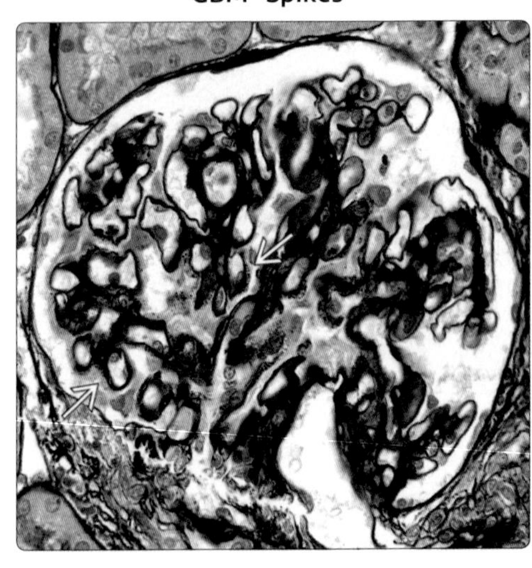

(Left) *H&E shows prominent deposition of refractile amorphous eosinophilic deposits along the capillary walls* → *and some mesangial areas* ⇒. **(Right)** *A membranous pattern of subepithelial deposits occurs in about 30% of ITG and shows segmental silver positive "spikes" along the GBM* ➡.

Kappa Light Chain

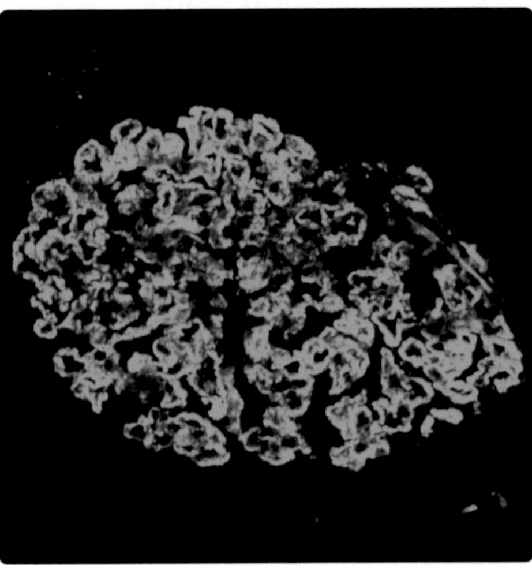

Lambda Light Chain

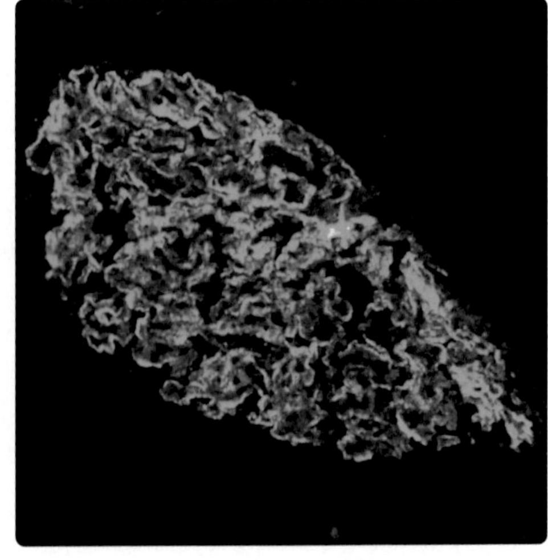

(Left) *IF for kappa light chain in ITG shows strong granular staining along the glomerular capillaries with a similar pattern to IgG and slightly less intensity. (Courtesy J. Kowalewska, MD.)* **(Right)** *Lambda light chain is similar to kappa but less intense in this polyclonal staining of the immune deposits. Among 18 cases in 2 series, 84% have a single predominant light chain (monoclonal), with kappa more common than lambda. (Courtesy J. Kowalewska, MD.)*

C3

Microtubules

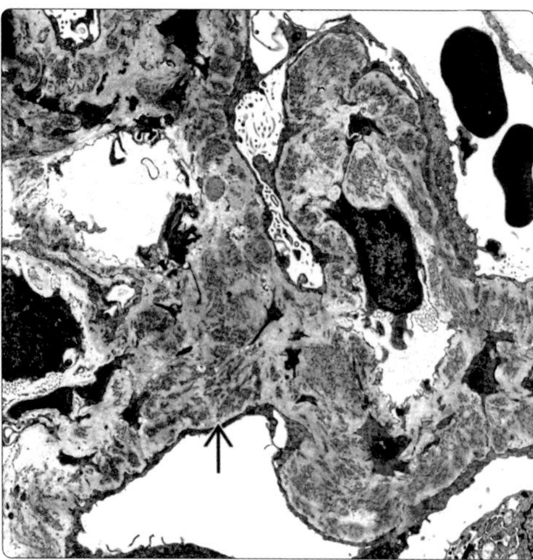

(Left) *IF for C3 shows strong staining of the glomerular capillaries ➡ and mesangial areas ➡ in a similar pattern as IgG. The location of the deposits correlates with the light microscopic findings. (Courtesy J. Kowalewska, MD.)* **(Right)** *Electron microscopy shows prominent thickening of the glomerular capillary walls due to the presence of microtubular deposits → that are randomly arranged and occasionally in parallel arrays. (Courtesy J. Kowalewska, MD.)*

Subepithelial Microtubular Deposits

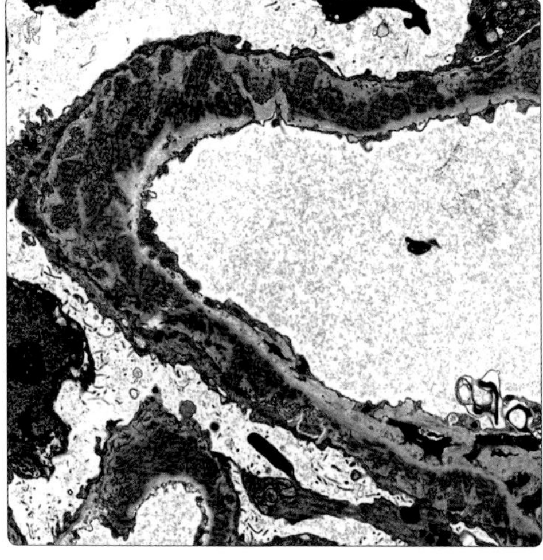

Subepithelial Deposits and "Spikes"

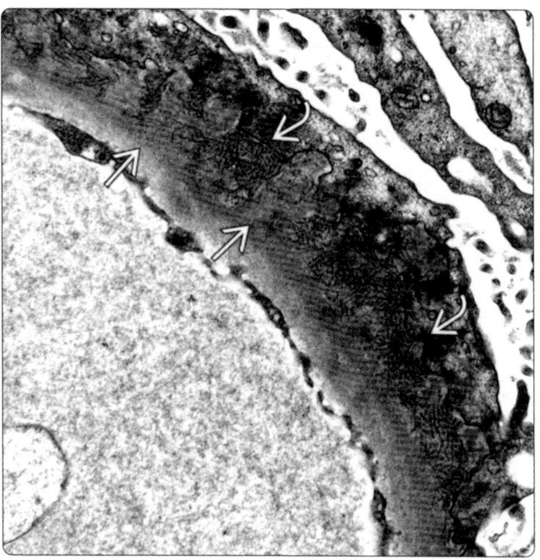

(Left) *Electron microscopy illustrates an advanced case of ITG with marked thickening of the GBM containing numerous microtubular deposits in subepithelial and intramembranous locations. (Courtesy J. Kowalewska, MD.)* **(Right)** *In this case of ITG, microtubular deposits ➡ are in a subepithelial location separated by GBM "spikes" ➡ , similar to idiopathic membranous glomerulonephritis.*

Subendothelial Deposits and Subepithelial Hump

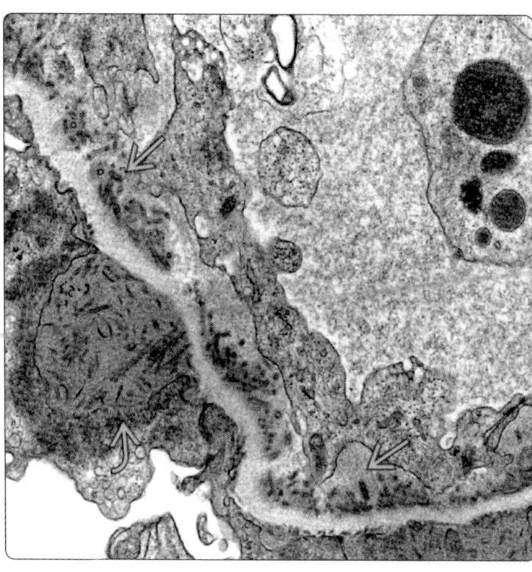

Microtubules With Hollow Cores

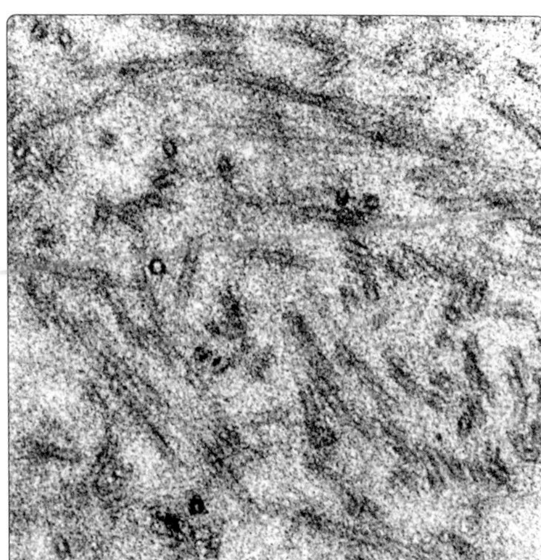

(Left) *Subendothelial tubular deposits → are seen in this case of ITG, along with a subepithelial hump →. Background amorphous material is also present in the deposits.* **(Right)** *The microtubules of ITG have a less dense core, best appreciated in the circular cross sections. (Courtesy J. Kowalewska, MD.)*

Fibronectin Glomerulopathy

KEY FACTS

TERMINOLOGY

- Non-immune lobular glomerulopathy with massive mesangial and subendothelial fibronectin (FN) deposits

ETIOLOGY/PATHOGENESIS

- Autosomal dominant inheritance with age-related penetrance
- Mutations in fibronectin *FN1* gene documented in ~ 40% of patients
  - *FN1* gene mapped to region in chromosome 2q34
  - Endothelial cell spreading and podocyte cytoskeletal reorganization impaired, resulting in proteinuria
  - Likely deposition of mutant plasma FN rather than local synthesis by mesangial cells

CLINICAL ISSUES

- Age at presentation: 2nd-4th decade of life
- Proteinuria, often in nephrotic range
- Microhematuria, hypertension
- Mild renal insufficiency or normal renal function
- Progression of renal insufficiency variable
- Can recur in transplanted kidney

MICROSCOPIC

- Glomeruli are diffusely enlarged with lobular accentuation and minimal hypercellularity
- Severe mesangial and variable subendothelial expansion by deposits
- Deposits stain with PAS and trichrome but not with methenamine silver or Congo red

ANCILLARY TESTS

- Deposits stain for fibronectin but not for immunoglobulins, C3, or C1q
- Granular deposits with focal fibrils on electron microscopy

DIAGNOSTIC CHECKLIST

- Family history cannot be elicited in some cases

(Left) *Renal biopsy in a patient with fibronectin (FN) glomerulopathy shows PAS-positive material ⇒ expanding the mesangium and subendothelium of an enlarged glomerulus.* **(Right)** *FN deposits ⇒ in the glomerulus fail to stain with methenamine silver, but the glomerular basement membrane ⇗ at the periphery is highlighted.*

Amorphous PAS(+) Fibronectin Deposits

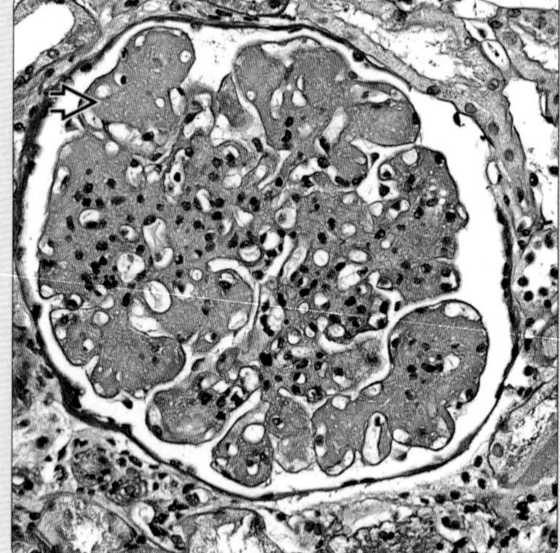

Silver Stain (-) Fibronectin Deposits

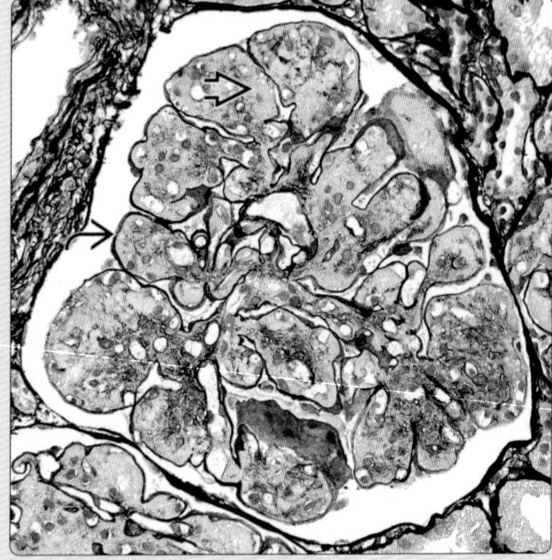

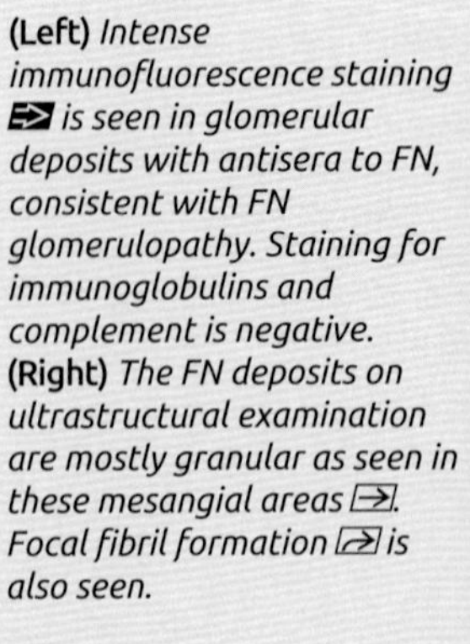

(Left) *Intense immunofluorescence staining ⇒ is seen in glomerular deposits with antisera to FN, consistent with FN glomerulopathy. Staining for immunoglobulins and complement is negative.* **(Right)** *The FN deposits on ultrastructural examination are mostly granular as seen in these mesangial areas →. Focal fibril formation ↷ is also seen.*

Fibronectin Immunofluorescence

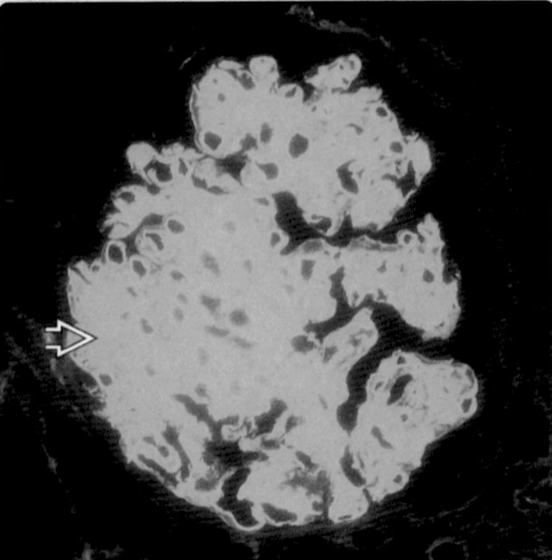

Granular Electron-Dense Fibronectin Deposits

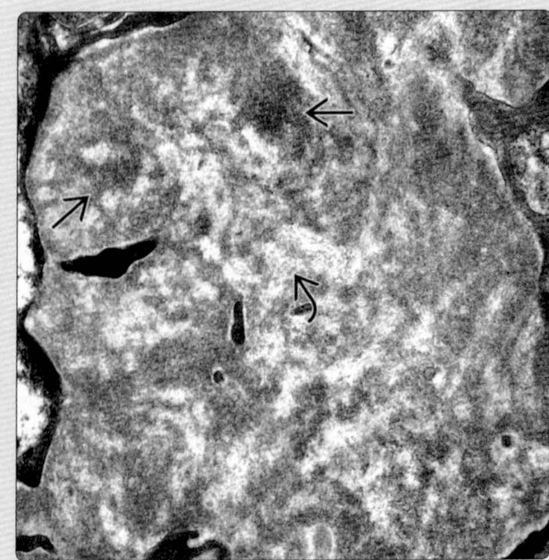

TERMINOLOGY

Abbreviations

- Fibronectin (FN) glomerulopathy

Definitions

- Non-immune lobular glomerulopathy with massive mesangial and subendothelial deposits composed of FN
  - Initially described as "familial lobular glomerulopathy"

ETIOLOGY/PATHOGENESIS

Fibronectin *FN1* Gene Mutation

- Mapped to chromosome 2q34
  - 3 heterozygous missense mutations (W1925R, L1974R, Y973C) affect heparin-binding domains of FN
    - Affect conformation and function of FN protein with potential increase in its affinity to heparin
      - Deficient binding to glomerular endothelial cells and podocytes
      - Endothelial cell spreading and podocyte cytoskeletal reorganization impaired, resulting in proteinuria
    - Assembly of FN fibrils also affected, with deposition of nonfibrillary protein in glomerular matrix
    - Unknown etiology of renal tubular acidosis seen in some patients
- Autosomal dominant inheritance pattern
  - Mutations identified in geographically diverse populations
  - Documented in 40% of patients
- Age-related penetrance
  - Family history negative in some instances
  - Unaffected family members may also harbor a mutation
- Other factors and additional genes may be involved
  - Abnormal accumulation of fibulin-1 and -5 along with FN identified by proteomic analysis
    - Fibulins are extracellular matrix (ECM) proteins that bind and regulate function of FN
  - No role of villin, desmin, or uteroglobin genes

Glomerular FN Deposition

- FN (ECM glycoprotein) involved in cellular proliferation, branching morphogenesis, phagocytosis, wound healing, and platelet adhesion
  - Occurs as soluble plasma form synthesized by hepatocytes and as insoluble cellular form in ECM
- FN composition of deposits 1st identified by Mazzucco et al
  - Deposition of plasma FN rather than local synthesis by mesangial cells
    - Absence of codeposition of other ECM proteins, such as tenascin and collagen IV, argues against local synthesis of abnormal FN
  - Recurrence in transplant kidney possibly due to abnormal circulating FN
  - Possible role of defective FN degradation by metalloproteinases
- Excess isolated FN deposition in FN glomerulopathy
  - Several glomerulopathies with mesangial sclerosis have increased FN deposits due to TGF-β activation
    - Other ECM proteins, such as tenascin and collagen IV, also increased in non-FN glomerulopathy

CLINICAL ISSUES

Epidemiology

- Age
  - Presentation in 2nd-4th decade of life
    - Wide age range (3-65 years)

Presentation

- Proteinuria
  - Often in nephrotic range
- Microhematuria
- Hypertension
- Mild renal insufficiency or normal renal function
- Type 4 renal tubular acidosis in some patients
- History of affected 1st-degree relatives

Treatment

- No specific treatment
  - Antihypertensives and proteinuria control with ACE inhibitors

Prognosis

- Progression of renal insufficiency variable
- Some progress to end-stage kidney over 15-20 years
- Can recur in transplanted kidney
  - Limited data due to rarity of disease
  - Biopsy-proven recurrence at 23 months and 14 years post transplantation

MICROSCOPIC

Histologic Features

- Glomeruli
  - Diffusely enlarged with lobular accentuation
  - Minimal hypercellularity
  - Severe mesangial and variable subendothelial expansion by deposits
    - Deposits stain intensely with PAS and red with trichrome but fail to stain with methenamine silver or Congo red
  - Glomerular basement membrane duplication typically absent
- Tubulointerstitium
  - No disease-specific changes in tubulointerstitium or vascular structures
  - Tubular atrophy, interstitial fibrosis seen in progressive renal disease

ANCILLARY TESTS

Immunohistochemistry

- FN
  - Positive within deposits

Immunofluorescence

- Immunoglobulin and complement usually show negative immunoreactivity
  - Less intense (1-2+) immunoglobulin and C3 deposits reported in some cases
- Antisera to FN highlight mesangial and subendothelial deposits (3+ intensity)

Electron Microscopy

- Massive electron-dense deposits replacing mesangium and in subendothelial spaces
  - Mostly amorphous deposits with focal filamentous structures, measuring 12-16 nm in diameter
- Glomerular basement membranes uninvolved

DIFFERENTIAL DIAGNOSIS

Immune Complex-Mediated Glomerulonephritis

- Characteristic immunofluorescence staining for immunoglobulins and complement, as in membranoproliferative glomerulonephritis, IgA nephropathy, lupus nephritis
- Intense staining for FN not identified

Amyloidosis

- Amorphous deposits weakly PAS positive and bluish purple on trichrome stain
- Congo red stain positive
- Immunoglobulin light or heavy chain restriction on immunofluorescence or amyloid A staining based on subtype
- Ultrastructural features characteristic of randomly oriented fibrils that are 8-12 nm thick

Fibrillary Glomerulopathy

- Immunoglobulin and complement deposition seen on immunofluorescence microscopy
  - Often polyclonal with rare monoclonal staining
- Ultrastructural features of nonbranching fibrils, 10-30 nm thick in mesangium, lamina densa, and, occasionally, in subepithelial spaces

Immunotactoid Glomerulopathy

- Immunoglobulin and complement deposition seen on immunofluorescence microscopy
  - Most cases monoclonal, but polyclonal staining can be observed
- Ultrastructural features of microtubules organized in parallel arrays (> 30 nm) with hollow core

Monoclonal Immunoglobulin Deposition Disease

- Immunofluorescence microscopy shows immunoglobulin light or heavy chain restriction
- Increased FN deposition may be seen due to fibrogenic monoclonal light chains stimulating TGF-β
- Granular electron-dense deposits in lamina rara interna in addition to mesangium

Type III Collagen Glomerulopathy

- Immunohistochemical staining for collagen III present
- Immunoglobulin and complement deposition absent on immunofluorescence microscopy
- Ultrastructural features of curved fibrils with distinct periodicity (43-65 nm)

Diabetic Nephropathy

- Characteristic Kimmelstiel-Wilson nodules may be seen
  - Mesangial sclerosis is PAS and silver stain positive and blue on trichrome
- Immunofluorescence microscopy negative for immune deposits
- Increase in mesangial matrix with focal fibrillosis on electron microscopy
- Increased FN deposition may be seen due to fibrogenic effects of hyperglycemia-driven advanced glycosylation mediated via TGF-β

DIAGNOSTIC CHECKLIST

Pathologic Interpretation Pearls

- Abundant FN deposits in absence of immunoglobulins or complement deposits
- Family history cannot be elicited in some cases

SELECTED REFERENCES

1. Chen H et al: Clinical and morphological features of fibronectin glomerulopathy: a report of ten patients from a single institution. Clin Nephrol. 83(2):93-9, 2015
2. Ertoy Baydar D et al: A case of familial glomerulopathy with fibronectin deposits caused by the Y973C mutation in fibronectin. Am J Kidney Dis. 61(3):514-8, 2013
3. Yoshino M et al: Clinicopathological analysis of glomerulopathy with fibronectin deposits (GFND): a case of sporadic, elderly-onset GFND with codeposition of IgA, C1q, and fibrinogen. Intern Med. 52(15):1715-20, 2013
4. Nadamuni M et al: Fibronectin glomerulopathy: an unusual cause of adult-onset nephrotic syndrome. Am J Kidney Dis. 60(5):839-42, 2012
5. Otsuka Y et al: A recurrent fibronectin glomerulopathy in a renal transplant patient: a case report. Clin Transplant. 26 Suppl 24:58-63, 2012
6. Satoskar AA et al: Characterization of glomerular diseases using proteomic analysis of laser capture microdissected glomeruli. Mod Pathol. 25(5):709-21, 2012
7. Brčić I et al: Fibronectin glomerulopathy in a 34-year-old man: a case report. Ultrastruct Pathol. 34(4):240-2, 2010
8. Herrera GA et al: Renal diseases with organized deposits: an algorithmic approach to classification and clinicopathologic diagnosis. Arch Pathol Lab Med. 134(4):512-31, 2010
9. Yong JL et al: Fibronectin non-amyloid glomerulopathy. Int J Clin Exp Pathol. 3(2):210-6, 2009
10. Castelletti F et al: Mutations in FN1 cause glomerulopathy with fibronectin deposits. Proc Natl Acad Sci U S A. 105(7):2538-43, 2008
11. Niimi K et al: Fibronectin glomerulopathy with nephrotic syndrome in a 3-year-old male. Pediatr Nephrol. 17(5):363-6, 2002
12. Gibson IW et al: Glomerular pathology: recent advances. J Pathol. 184(2):123-9, 1998
13. Gemperle O et al: Familial glomerulopathy with giant fibrillar (fibronectin-positive) deposits: 15-year follow-up in a large kindred. Am J Kidney Dis. 28(5):668-75, 1996
14. Hildebrandt F et al: Glomerulopathy associated with predominant fibronectin deposits: exclusion of the genes for fibronectin, villin and desmin as causative genes. Am J Med Genet. 63(1):323-7, 1996
15. Strøm EH et al: Glomerulopathy associated with predominant fibronectin deposits: a newly recognized hereditary disease. Kidney Int. 48(1):163-70, 1995

Lobular Accentuation With Amorphous Deposits

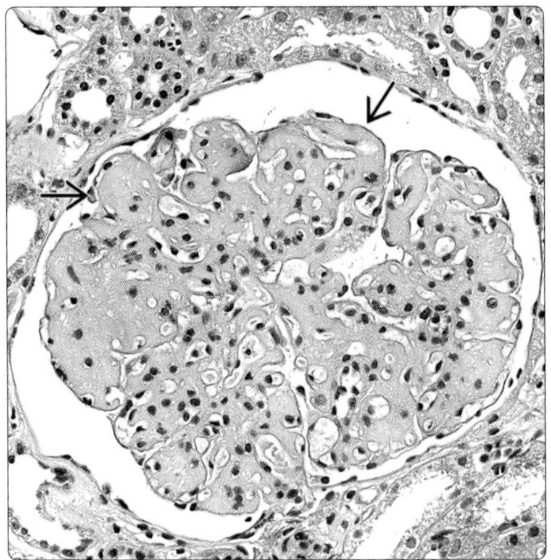

Fuchsinophilic Fibronectin Deposits

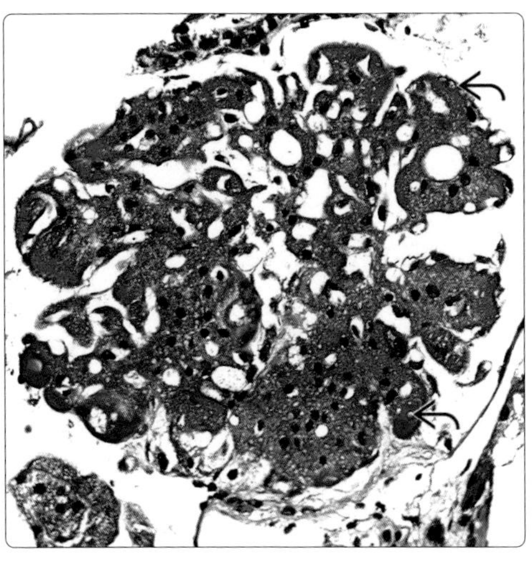

(Left) *Glomerular lobular accentuation due to abundant FN deposits ➡ is seen in the mesangial areas and along the capillary walls. The mesangial cellularity is only mildly increased.* **(Right)** *FN deposits ↪ in the mesangium and subendothelium stain red with trichrome.*

Massive Mesangial and Subendothelial Deposits on Silver Stain

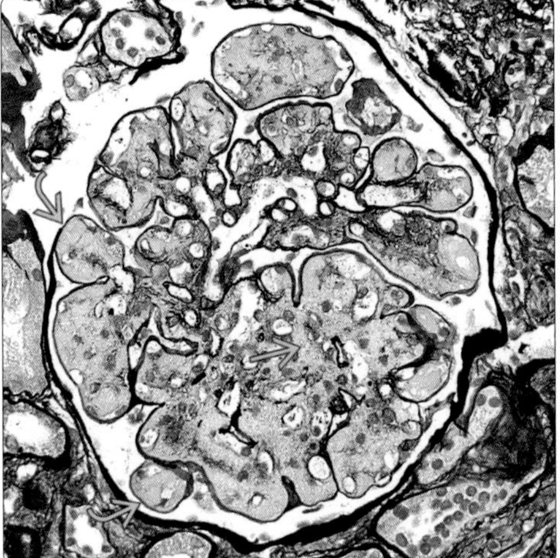

Lack of Immunoglobulin in Fibronectin Glomerulopathy

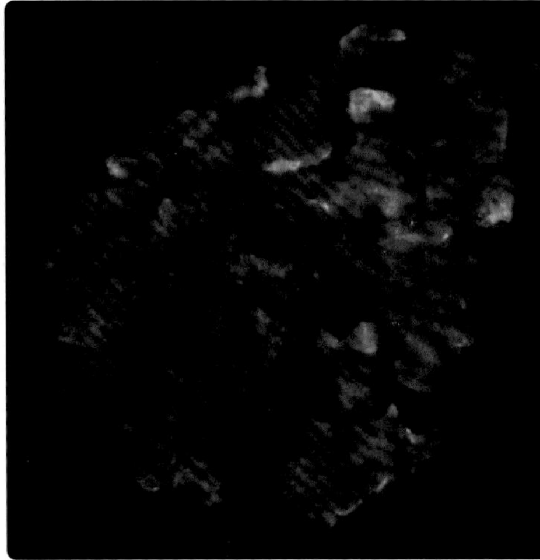

(Left) *Bulky FN deposits are seen in the mesangium ➡ and subendothelium ↪. These deposits fail to stain with methenamine silver in contrast to the glomerular basement membrane. There is no evidence of glomerular basement membrane double contours.* **(Right)** *The immunoglobulin and complement deposition is typically absent in FN glomerulopathy. The IgM staining here is segmental and weak (1+), in contrast to the 3+ intensity of FN staining.*

Mesangial and Subendothelial Fibronectin Deposits

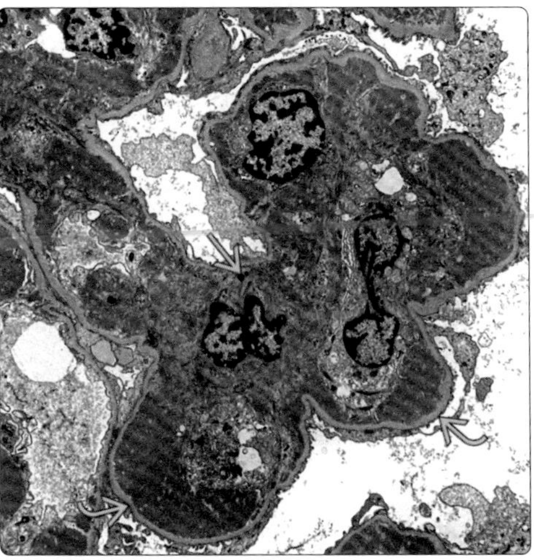

Granular Fibronectin Deposits With Focal Fibrils

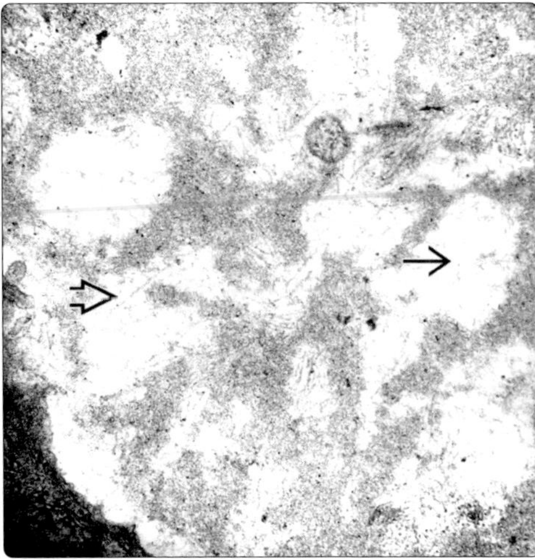

(Left) *Electron-dense deposits in FN glomerulopathy are large and typically in the mesangium ➡ and subendothelium ↪ with near occlusion of the capillary lumens. No significant hypercellularity is seen.* **(Right)** *On ultrastructural examination, FN deposits in the mesangium are mostly granular with focal fibrillar structures ⇨. Scattered electron-lucent areas ➡ are also seen.*

Diabetic Nephropathy

KEY FACTS

TERMINOLOGY

- Type 1 DM: Autoimmune destruction of pancreatic islets
- Type 2 DM: Insulin resistance due to obesity and other factors

ETIOLOGY/PATHOGENESIS

- Inadequate glycemic control is most important contributor to DN; judged by HbA1c
- Advanced glycosylated end products (AGE) are believed responsible for many DN features
- Multiple genetic loci and gene polymorphisms are implicated

CLINICAL ISSUES

- Most common cause of end-stage renal disease in USA
- DN develops typically after 10-15 years of DM
- Microalbuminuria is earliest sign and predicts loss of renal function
- Retinal microaneurysms correlate with nodular DN

MICROSCOPIC

- Mesangial hypercellularity and increased matrix
- Nodular mesangial sclerosis (Kimmelstiel-Wilson nodules)
- Mesangiolysis contributes to microaneurysms
- Hyaline insudation in glomeruli (fibrin cap, capsular drops) and arterioles
- Immunofluorescence: Linear IgG and albumin in GBM
- Electron microscopy
  - Diffuse thickening of otherwise normal-appearing GBM
  - Nodules contain cellular debris and matrix

TOP DIFFERENTIAL DIAGNOSES

- Idiopathic nodular glomerulosclerosis
- Monoclonal immunoglobulin deposition disease
- Membranoproliferative glomerulonephritis

DIAGNOSTIC CHECKLIST

- Biopsies from diabetic patients often show other superimposed renal diseases

(Left) *Prominent Kimmelstiel-Wilson nodules are seen in a glomerulus affected by diabetic nephropathy. The glomerular capillary lumina are obliterated, and an occasional foam cell is seen.* **(Right)** *The mesangium is normocellular but expanded by increased mesangial matrix deposition. The glomerular basement membranes are also diffusely thickened (> 700 nm) in DN.*

Nodular Glomerulosclerosis

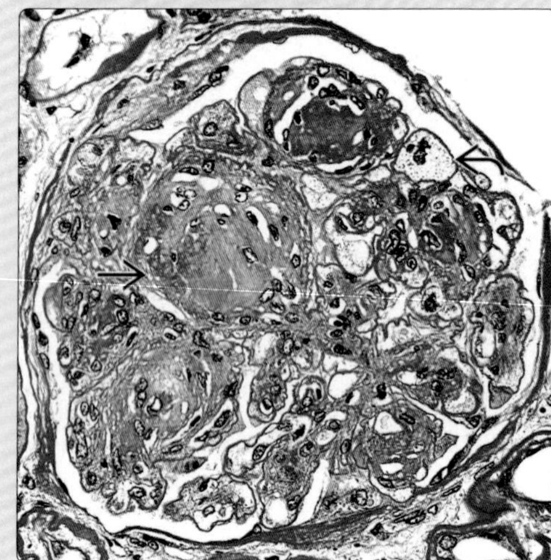

Diffusely Thickened GBM and Expanded Mesangium

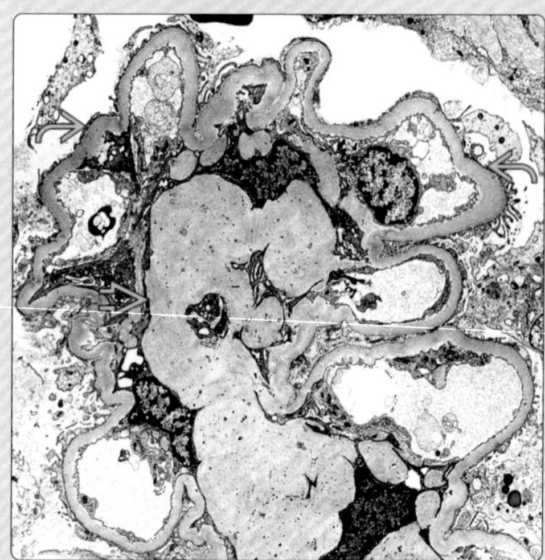

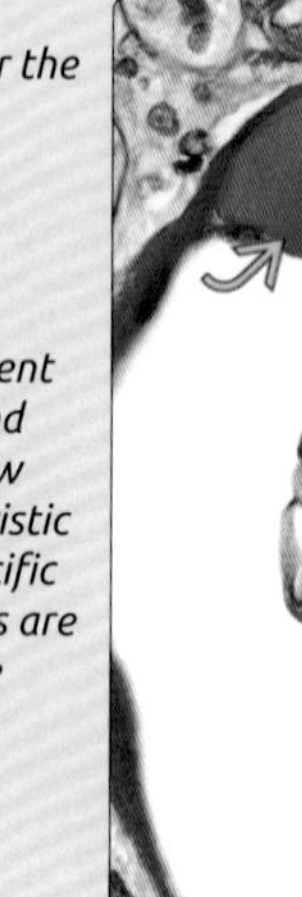

(Left) *Deposits of hyaline material are present under the parietal epithelium of Bowman capsule, forming "capsular drops" characteristic of diabetic nephropathy. Diffuse mesangial sclerosis is present.* **(Right)** *Afferent and efferent arterioles show hyaline deposits characteristic of, but not absolutely specific for, DN. Efferent arterioles are thinner and typically curve around the glomerulus.*

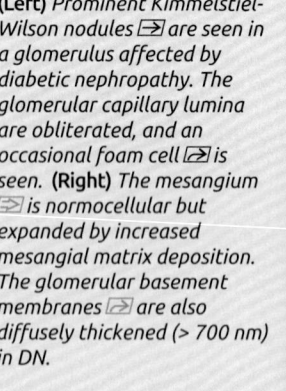

Capsular Drop

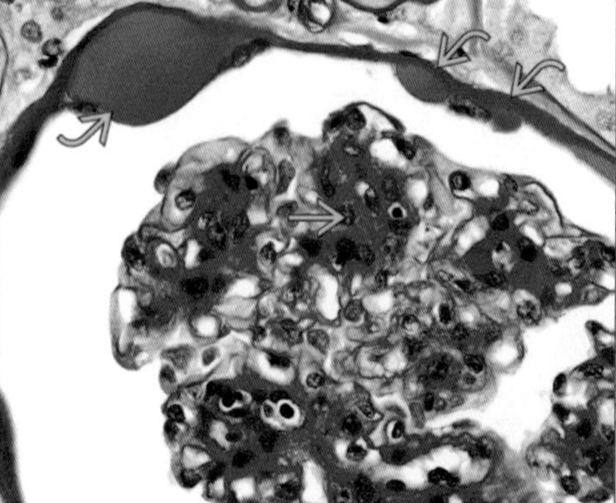

Afferent and Efferent Arteriolar Hyalinosis

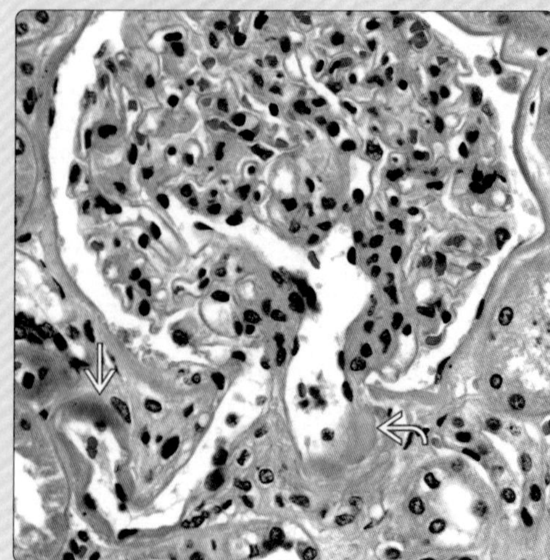

TERMINOLOGY

Abbreviations

- Diabetic nephropathy (DN)

Synonyms

- Diabetic glomerulosclerosis

Definitions

- Renal disease caused by diabetes mellitus (DM) types 1 and 2, including thickening of GBM, expansion of mesangium, nodular diabetic glomerulosclerosis, arteriolar hyalinosis, and arteriosclerosis

ETIOLOGY/PATHOGENESIS

Diabetes Mellitus

- Type 1 DM: Autoimmune disease that destroys pancreatic islets
- Type 2 DM: Insulin resistance, related to obesity and other factors
- Both lead to insulin deficiency and hyperglycemia
- DN is a multifactorial process, but inadequate glycemic control is most important contributor
  - Both initiation and maintenance of DN require hyperglycemia
  - Removal of hyperglycemic state as in successful pancreas transplantation can cause regression of DN lesions

Hyperglycemia

- Causes accumulation of advanced glycosylated end products (AGE) due to nonenzymatic glycosylation of proteins
  - Many proteins affected including GBM collagen and other matrix proteins
  - AGE result in injury and remodeling
    - Promote protein crosslinking
    - Stimulate synthesis of growth factors (TGF-β, IGF, VEGF) that cause increased extracellular matrix production
    - Binding of AGE to cell surface receptors (RAGE) increases intracellular oxidative stress
    - Podocytopenia via apoptosis
- Activates protein kinase C
  - Directly and via stimulation of aldol reductase, leading to increased sorbitol production, fructose, and diacylglycerol
  - Increases matrix production
- Induces defects in mitochondrial electron transport
  - Elevated nitric oxide and superoxide production results in vasodilatation and oxidation
  - Increased reactive oxygen species and oxidative stress

Genetic Factors

- Inherited factors may explain variable risk of developing DN regardless of glycemic control
  - Studies of siblings show high concordance rate of DN risk in both types 1 and 2 DM
  - Multiple genetic loci and gene polymorphisms have been implicated
    - Renin-angiotensin system genes such as angiotensin-converting enzyme, angiotensinogen, angiotensin II type 1 receptor
    - Insulin resistance (*ENPP1*, *PPARG2*, glucose transporter 1, apolipoprotein E)
    - Superoxide dismutase 1 gene, *CCR5*, *CNDP1* genes

Cardiovascular/Hemodynamic Factors

- Glomerular hyperfiltration observed in early DM promotes extracellular matrix accumulation and increased TGF-β1 expression
  - Loss of autoregulation in DM may predispose to hyperfiltration
  - Increased glomerular capillary pressure causes glomerulomegaly
  - Modulates progression of DN
- Systemic hypertension may aggravate progression of DN via angiotensin II
  - Angiotensin II increases glomerular capillary permeability via preferential constriction of efferent glomerular arteriole
  - Angiotensin II stimulates extracellular matrix proteins via TGF-β1 and increases AGE production
- Endothelial dysfunction
  - Due to oxidative and endoplasmic reticulum stress

Podocytopenia

- Causes include oxidative stress, AGE, fatty acids, peroxisome proliferator-activated receptors (PPARγ)
- Detected by WT-1 immunostain
- Correlates with proteinuria

Other Risk Factors

- Smoking, hyperlipidemia, obesity, and low vitamin D levels

Murine Models of DN

- Generally do not reproduce nodular glomerulosclerosis of human DN
- Type 1 DM: Islet cell destruction
  - Streptozotocin-induced diabetes (chemical)
  - NOD mouse (autoimmune)
- Type 2 DM: Insulin resistance
  - *db/db* mouse-leptin receptor deficient
  - BTBR-*ob/ob* mouse
    - Leptin deficient + other genetic predisposition
    - Full spectrum of pathology, including nodular DN

CLINICAL ISSUES

Epidemiology

- Incidence
  - 0.5% type 1, 5% type 2 DM in USA
  - Most common cause of ESRD in USA
  - Prevalence of DN increases with duration of DM
    - ~ 15% of patients with type 1 DM develop DN after 20 years
    - Prevalence is trending lower with improved treatment
- Ethnicity
  - Higher risk of DN in African Americans and Native Americans with type 2 DM

Presentation

- Microalbuminuria is earliest manifestation of DN
  - Defined as albuminuria of 30-300 mg/d (or μg/mg creatinine)
    - Not detected by standard urine dipstick method

- Typically occurs ≥ 5 years after onset of DM
- Predicts loss of renal function and is associated with progression to ESRD
- Proteinuria
  - Urine protein > 300 mg/d is detected by urine dipstick analysis
  - Indicates overt nephropathy that develops 20 years after onset of clinical DM although it may be much earlier in type 2 DM
  - Nephrotic-range proteinuria and nephrotic syndrome can develop
- Reduced renal function
  - Independent phenotype of early DN found in ~ 33% regardless of microalbuminuria
- Increased glomerular filtration rate (GFR)
  - Indicator of hyperfiltration and progressive DN
- Hypertension
- Retinopathy
  - Correlates with advanced DN
  - May be missed without fluorescein angiography
- Acute pyelonephritis and papillary necrosis may occur
- Microhematuria
  - Associated with papillary necrosis or nephrocalcinosis

Laboratory Tests

- Hemoglobin A1C levels indicate long-term glycemic control
- Cystatin C to monitor early renal function decline

Treatment

- Drugs
  - Strict glycemic control
    - Oral hypoglycemic agents and insulin therapy
  - Renin-angiotensin system blockade
    - Direct renoprotective effects in DN
    - Angiotensin-converting enzyme inhibitors and angiotensin II receptor blockers
  - Treatment of hypertension and hyperlipidemia
- Weight loss if obese

Prognosis

- Rate of progression is variable and is modulated by complex genetic and environmental factors, therapeutic interventions
- DN is associated with hypertension and increased cardiovascular disease
- DN can recur in a transplanted kidney due to persistent hyperglycemic state

MACROSCOPIC

General Features

- Kidneys are bilaterally enlarged
  - End-stage kidneys may be normal or slightly small
- Cortical scars may be present due to hypertensive renal disease or pyelonephritis
  - Loss of pyramids indicates papillary necrosis

MICROSCOPIC

Histologic Features

- Morphological changes in DN due to types 1 and 2 DN are similar
- Glomeruli
  - Earliest change is diffuse GBM thickening
    - Present even in absence of proteinuria
    - Detectable at light microscopy level only when ≥ 4x
  - Glomerulomegaly
    - Diameter > 50% of 400x field is a useful guide (220 μm)
  - Mesangial expansion and sclerosis
    - Diffuse mesangial hypercellularity in early phase
    - Accumulation of type IV and VI collagen, laminin, and fibronectin
  - Kimmelstiel-Wilson (KW) nodules
    - Round to oval mesangial lesions with acellular, matrix core with peripheral sparse crescent-shaped mesangial nuclei
    - Often variably sized and paucicellular
    - Matrix may be less dense, especially at periphery of these nodules, and is termed "mesangiolysis"
    - Stains positive for periodic acid-Schiff (PAS) and Jones methenamine silver (JMS), negative with Congo red
    - Often 1 or 2 per glomerular cross section and irregularly distributed
    - Progressive mesangial sclerosis results in obliterated capillary lumens
    - Described in autopsies by Paul Kimmelstiel and Clifford Wilson in 1936 who noted that all 7 patients had a clinical history of DM
    - Lesions seen in non-DM are related to hypertension and smoking
  - Microaneurysms
    - Mesangiolysis contributes to capillary lumen confluence and microaneurysms
    - Fragmented red cells are seen occasionally
    - Thrombi are rare
  - Hyaline insudation in glomerular capillary walls (fibrin cap)
  - Capsular drop observed between parietal epithelium and Bowman capsule
    - Probably represents tracking of plasma proteins from vascular pole to Bowman capsule
    - Characteristic but not specific for DN
      - Reported in ~ 5% of biopsies from non-DM
  - Segmental glomerulosclerosis
    - Likely initiated by podocyte loss and exposed GBM
    - Capillary tuft adhesions to Bowman capsules
    - Lesions ("tip lesions") at tubular pole result in atubular glomeruli
  - Global glomerulosclerosis increases progressive DN
    - Sclerosed glomeruli are enlarged with abundant hyaline insudation
  - No inflammatory change (neutrophils, necrosis)
  - Crescents rarely described
    - May be unusual response to heavy proteinuria
    - Collapsing glomerulopathy also mimics crescent formation
- Tubules
  - Prominent protein resorption and lipid droplets seen in proximal tubules in setting of severe proteinuria
  - Tubular atrophy and interstitial fibrosis progressively increase in advanced DN

- Tubular basement membranes (TBM) are thickened due to excessive collagen deposition
  - Both atrophic and nonatrophic tubules demonstrate TBM thickening
- In acute diabetic ketoacidosis, proximal tubules contain abundant clear vacuoles of glycogen
  - Termed Armann-Ebstein lesion
- Interstitium
  - Interstitial inflammation with eosinophils are prominent in ~ 40%, resembling drug-induced interstitial nephritis
    - Correlates with extent of fibrosis but not particular drugs
  - Prominent interstitial neutrophil infiltrates or neutrophil casts suggest acute pyelonephritis
    - Occasional interstitial neutrophils may not necessarily represent acute pyelonephritis
- Arteries
  - Larger arteries, including proximal interlobular and arcuate arteries, show intimal fibrosis
  - Atherosclerosis with lipid deposits in smaller arteries typical of severe DN
- Arterioles
  - Arteriolar hyalinosis
    - Hyaline (plasma protein) insudation in terminal interlobular arteries and arterioles
    - Present in intima and media or can be transmural
    - Arteriolar hyaline causes luminal occlusion with ischemic collapse and sclerosis of downstream glomeruli
  - Both afferent and efferent arterioles are affected
    - Efferent arteriolar hyalinosis strongly favors DN but is not pathognomonic
    - Afferent arterioles are thicker walled and more perpendicular to tuft
    - Efferent arterioles typically are thinner walled and curve around tuft
  - Nodular DN is rarely, if ever, observed in absence of prominent arteriolar hyalinosis

ANCILLARY TESTS

Immunofluorescence

- Diffuse linear staining (≥ 2+ intensity) of GBM and TBM for IgG and albumin
  - Due to nonimmunological trapping of proteins in thickened, abnormal basement membranes
  - No specific deposition of light chains in contrast to monoclonal immunoglobulin deposition disease
  - Linear IgG may mimic anti-GBM nephritis
- Segmental scars and insudative lesions in glomeruli/arterioles show nonspecific entrapment of IgM and C3
- No specific immune complexes are observed unless superimposed glomerulonephritis is present
- Protein reabsorption droplets in tubules stain for albumin and other plasma proteins

Electron Microscopy

- Diffuse thickening of otherwise normal-appearing GBM lamina densa
  - Segmental thinning may be observed near site of microaneurysms
  - Typically > 600 nm
- Increased deposition of mesangial matrix
  - Fine fibrillar quality (fibrillosis; 10 nm thick) typical of collagen
  - Lucent foci may be identified at periphery of mesangial sclerosis (mesangiolysis)
  - Nodules contain cellular debris but no amorphous deposits suggestive of immune complexes
- Foot process effacement is variable
  - Typically less extensive than in other causes of severe proteinuria such as minimal change disease
- Lucent foci may be identified at periphery of mesangial sclerosis, compatible with mesangiolysis
- Insudative lesions in glomeruli and arterioles are electron dense and admixed with lucent areas and basement membrane-like particles
- TBM is thickened and laminated

Immunohistochemistry

- WT1 immunostain used to document podocytopenia
- Nephronectin increased in mesangium and nodules in DN vs. other glomerular diseases

DIFFERENTIAL DIAGNOSIS

Monoclonal Immunoglobulin Deposition Disease (MIDD)

- Diffuse deposits of either kappa or lambda and, in rare cases, heavy chains on IF
- Fine granular dense deposits in mesangium, GBM, and TBM by EM
- Mesangial nodules in MIDD are often uniform in size and have less matrix on JMS stain

Membranoproliferative Glomerulonephritis (MPGN)

- Duplicated GBM is prominent (vs. DM)
- Immunofluorescence and electron microscopy reveal immune complexes &/or C3 deposits

Idiopathic Nodular Glomerulosclerosis

- Glomerular pathology mimics DN in all respects but is seen in patient with no clinical history of DM
- Possible etiologies include smoking and hypertension

Amyloidosis

- Amyloid nodules are Congo red positive and silver negative
- Characteristic ultrastructure with abundant fibrils 8-12 nm in diameter

Fibrillary and Immunotactoid Glomerulonephritis (GN)

- Immunofluorescence shows granular IgG and C3 in mesangium and capillary walls, sometimes with light chain restriction
- Characteristic ultrastructure with fibrils 10-30 nm (fibrillary) or microtubules 20-90 nm (immunotactoid)
- Rarely nodular; can have diffuse proliferative or membranoproliferative pattern

Metabolic Syndrome

- Obesity, glucose intolerance, hypertension, hyperlipidemia
- Increases risk for microalbuminuria and renal disease

Classification of Diabetic Glomerulopathy

Class	Name	Definition	5-Year Renal Survival
I	Isolated GBM thickening	GBM > 395 nm thick in females or > 430 nm thick in males; age ≥ 9 years	100%
II	Mesangial expansion	Width of mesangial matrix exceeds 2 mesangial cell nuclei in > 25% of mesangial areas	
IIa	Mild mesangial expansion	Mean mesangial area < capillary lumen	88%
IIb	Severe mesangial expansion	Mean mesangial area > capillary lumen	53%
III	Nodular sclerosis (Kimmelstiel-Wilson lesion)	≥ 1 convincing Kimmelstiel-Wilson lesion	36%
IV	Advanced diabetic glomerulosclerosis	Global glomerulosclerosis in > 50% of glomeruli; any lesions from class I-III	21%

Tervaert et al: Pathologic classification of diabetic nephropathy. J Am Soc Nephrol 21: 556, 2010. Mise et al: Renal prognosis a long time after renal biopsy on patients with diabetic nephropathy. Nephrol Dial Transplant 29: 109, 2014.

- Renal pathology: Interstitial fibrosis, global and segmental glomerulosclerosis and arteriosclerosis

Other Glomerular Diseases Superimposed on DN

- Approximately 33% of biopsies with DN have superimposed glomerular diseases
  - Membranous nephropathy
    - Diffuse glomerular capillary wall deposits of IgG and C3
    - GBM "spikes" and subepithelial deposits by EM
  - IgA nephropathy
    - Dominant IgA deposits
    - Widespread mesangial electron-dense deposits
  - Postinfectious glomerulonephritis
    - Diffuse endocapillary proliferative and exudative glomerulonephritis
    - Prominent granular GBM C3 and usually IgG deposits
      - Diabetic patients prone to develop IgA-dominant variant, likely due to IgA-rich immune responses
    - Mesangial deposits and subepithelial "humps" on EM
  - ANCA-mediated glomerulonephritis
    - Glomerular necrosis and crescents
    - No immune complexes or electron-dense deposits
  - Minimal change disease (MCD)
    - Abrupt onset of nephrotic syndrome favors MCD
    - Foot process effacement is diffuse in contrast to focal effacement usually seen in DN
  - Collapsing glomerulopathy
    - 5% of biopsies of diabetic nephropathy
    - Cytokeratin positive (CK18,19)
    - 75% develop ESRD within 7 months of biopsy
- Diabetics may have nondiabetic renal disease
  - 45% of biopsies in type 2 DM

DIAGNOSTIC CHECKLIST

Clinically Relevant Pathologic Features

- Class of glomerular lesions correlates with prognosis
- Severity of mesangial sclerosis, global glomerulosclerosis, and interstitial fibrosis correlates with progression of disease and reduced renal function
- Neutrophil casts and interstitial neutrophils should prompt evaluation of urine cultures

Pathologic Interpretation Pearls

- Diagnosis of DN unlikely unless there is prominent arteriolar hyalinosis
- Pronounced hyaline insudation in globally sclerosed glomeruli suggests DN
- Biopsies from diabetic patients often show other renal diseases, because it is uncommon to biopsy patients with typical presentation of DN

SELECTED REFERENCES

1. An Y et al: Renal histologic changes and the outcome in patients with diabetic nephropathy. Nephrol Dial Transplant. 30(2):257-66, 2015
2. Dai DF et al: Interstitial eosinophilic aggregates in diabetic nephropathy: allergy or not? Nephrol Dial Transplant. ePub, 2015
3. Luna J et al: Postmortem Diagnosis of Diabetic Ketoacidosis Presenting as the "Dead-in-Bed Syndrome". Endocr Pract. 20(7):e123-5, 2014
4. Mise K et al: Renal prognosis a long time after renal biopsy on patients with diabetic nephropathy. Nephrol Dial Transplant. 29(1):109-18, 2014
5. Salvatore SP et al: Collapsing glomerulopathy superimposed on diabetic nephropathy: insights into etiology of an under-recognized, severe pattern of glomerular injury. Nephrol Dial Transplant. 29(2):392-9, 2014
6. Harada K et al: Significance of renal biopsy in patients with presumed diabetic nephropathy. J Diabetes Investig. 4(1):88-93, 2013
7. Nakatani S et al: Nephronectin expression in glomeruli of renal biopsy specimens from various kidney diseases: nephronectin is expressed in the mesangial matrix expansion of diabetic nephropathy. Nephron Clin Pract. 122(3-4):114-21, 2012
8. Biesenbach G et al: Clinical versus histological diagnosis of diabetic nephropathy--is renal biopsy required in type 2 diabetic patients with renal disease? QJM. 104(9):771-4, 2011
9. Najafian B et al: Pathology of human diabetic nephropathy. Contrib Nephrol. 170:36-47, 2011
10. D'Agati V et al: RAGE, glomerulosclerosis and proteinuria: roles in podocytes and endothelial cells. Trends Endocrinol Metab. 21(1):50-6, 2010
11. Su J et al: Evaluation of podocyte lesion in patients with diabetic nephropathy: Wilms' tumor-1 protein used as a podocyte marker. Diabetes Res Clin Pract. 87(2):167-75, 2010
12. Tervaert TW et al: Pathologic classification of diabetic nephropathy. J Am Soc Nephrol. 21(4):556-63, 2010
13. Alexander MP et al: Kidney pathological changes in metabolic syndrome: a cross-sectional study. Am J Kidney Dis. 53(5):751-9, 2009
14. Perkins BA et al: Early nephropathy in type 1 diabetes: the importance of early renal function decline. Curr Opin Nephrol Hypertens. 18(3):233-40, 2009
15. Jefferson JA et al: Proteinuria in diabetic kidney disease: a mechanistic viewpoint. Kidney Int. 74(1):22-36, 2008
16. Alsaad KO et al: Distinguishing diabetic nephropathy from other causes of glomerulosclerosis: an update. J Clin Pathol. 60(1):18-26, 2007
17. Kimmelstiel P et al: Intercapillary lesions in the glomeruli of the kidney. Am J Pathol. 12(1):83-98, 1936

Mesangial Hypercellularity

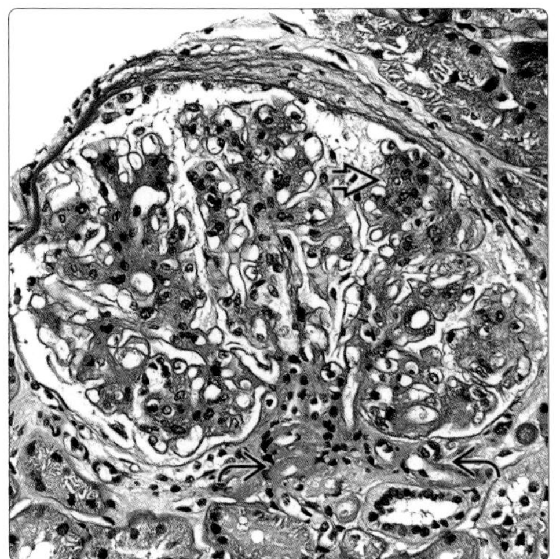

Mesangial Sclerosis

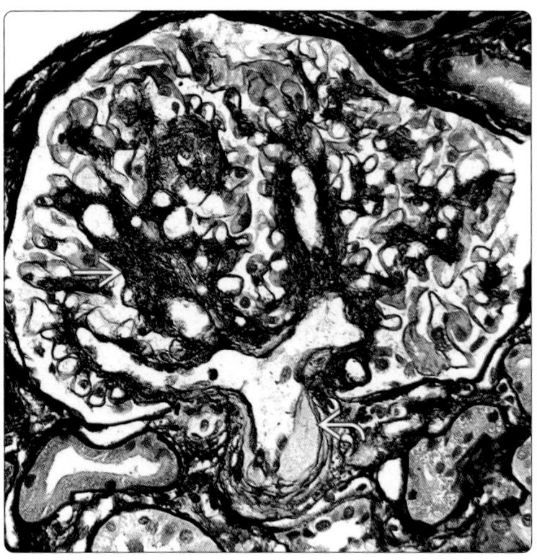

(Left) *The glomerulus is enlarged with diffuse mesangial sclerosis and moderate proliferation ➡. Mild arteriolar hyaline insudation is seen, a feature characteristic of DN. It is likely in both afferent and efferent limbs ➡.* **(Right)** *Moderate mesangial sclerosis ➡ in DN is highlighted by Jones methenamine silver stain. The glomerular basement membranes are mildly thickened, although this is best seen by electron microscopy. Arteriolar hyaline ➡ is at the vascular pole.*

Kimmelstiel-Wilson Nodules

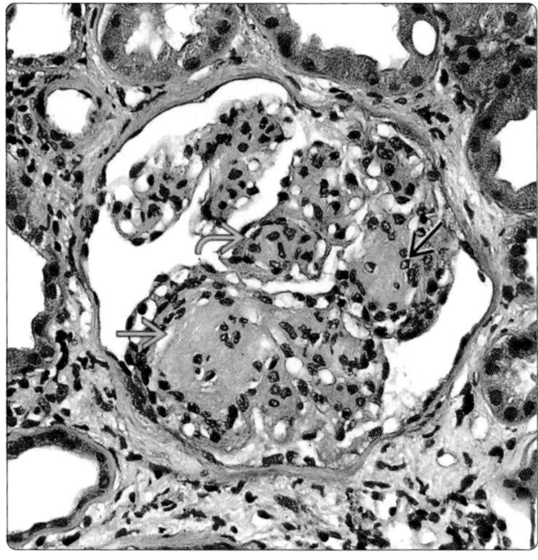

Thickened Tubular Basement Membrane

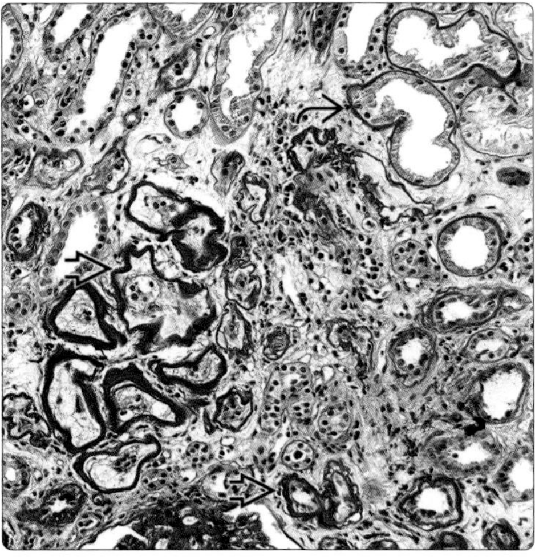

(Left) *Classic Kimmelstiel-Wilson (KW) nodules ➡ show a paucicellular center with peripheral elongated mesangial nuclei ➡ and a ring of capillaries. Foci of mesangial hypercellularity ➡ likely represent precursor lesions.* **(Right)** *Excessive deposition of extracellular matrix results in thickened tubular basement membranes in both atrophic ➡ and nonatrophic ➡ tubules. Mild interstitial inflammation is also seen (PAS stain).*

Acute Interstitial Nephritis

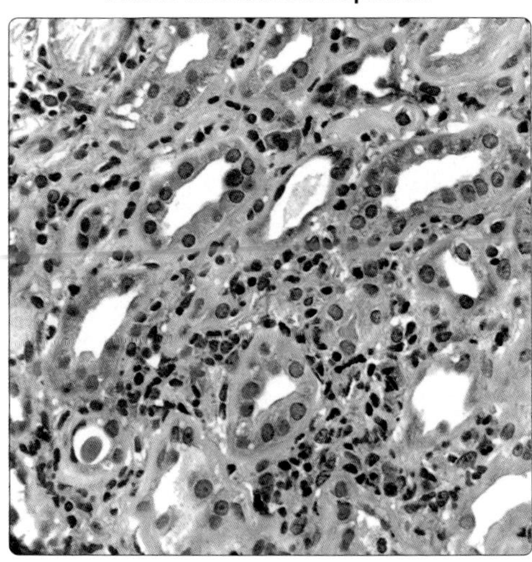

Armanni-Ebstein Lesion

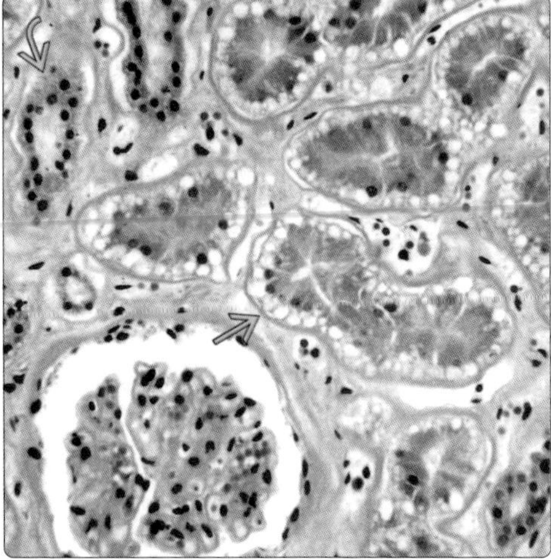

(Left) *Biopsies from patients with diabetic nephropathy often have substantial interstitial inflammation with eosinophils. Systematic studies have not found correlations with drug therapy, only with interstitial fibrosis and tubular atrophy.* **(Right)** *Armanni-Ebstein lesion is characteristic of diabetic ketoacidosis. The proximal tubules have basal vacuoles shown to contain lipid in this autopsy case ➡. Distal tubules are spared ➡. This can be a forensic clue in an unexplained death. (Courtesy C. Hebert, MD and R. Tanenberg, MD.)*

(Left) *A large KW nodule ➡ in a glomerulus, along with diffuse mesangial sclerosis, is typical of advanced DN. Arteriolar hyalinosis ➡ is seen at the vascular pole, and synechia at the tubular pole ➡ probably results in an atubular glomerulus.* **(Right)** *Mesangial nodules in DN stain for collagen on trichrome stain are shown. In this 58-year-old woman with nephrotic syndrome, many KW nodules are present, resembling membranoproliferative glomerulonephritis. However, duplication of the GBM was not present.*

Mesangial Nodule With Weak Silver Stain

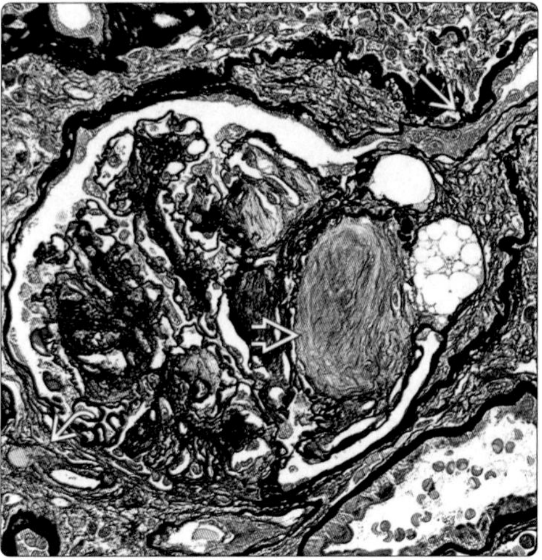

Collagen Deposition in Mesangium

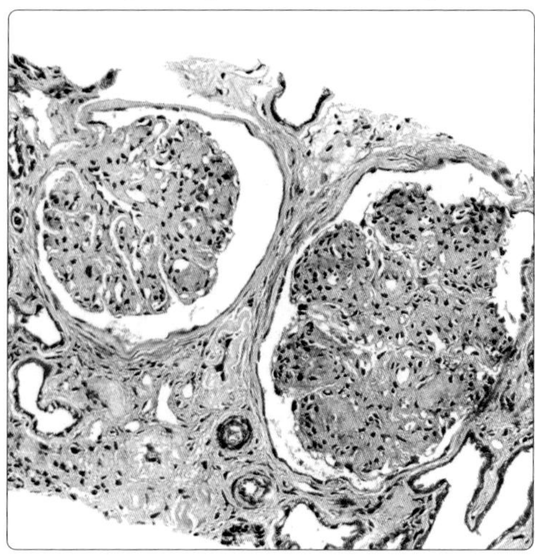

(Left) *Advanced DN is characterized by diffuse and nodular ➡ glomerulosclerosis and thickened glomerular and tubular basement membranes. Mesangiolysis at the periphery of a KW nodule ➡ and segmental adhesion to Bowman capsule are also seen ➡.* **(Right)** *Mesangiolysis ➡ with entrapped red blood cells is seen at the periphery of a KW nodule in DN. This degradation of mesangial matrix results in microaneurysms. A foam cell is seen in the adjacent capillary lumen ➡.*

Mesangiolysis and Aneurysm

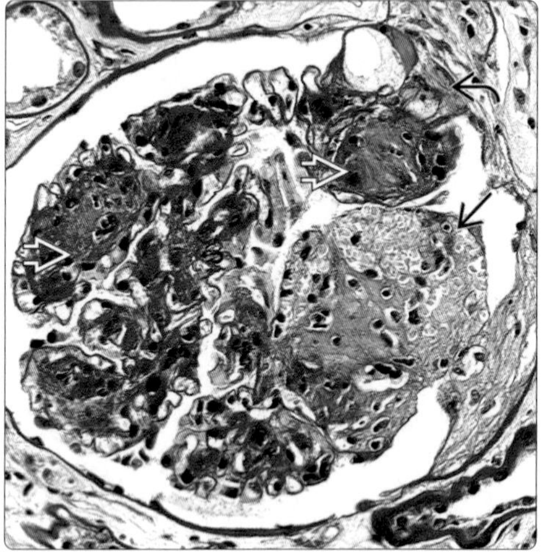

Mesangiolysis

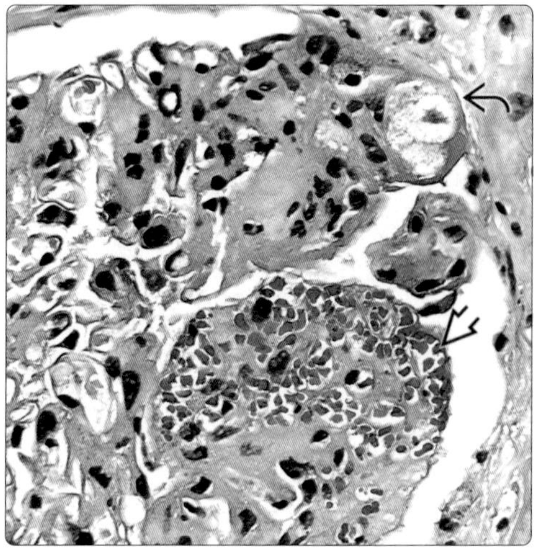

(Left) *Capillaries form a microaneurysm ➡ capping one of the mesangial nodules ➡. It is possible that thrombosis and organization of the microaneurysm are responsible for the nodule. Alternatively, the nodular lesion predisposes to the microaneurysm.* **(Right)** *The nodules are becoming acellular, with loss of podocytes and endothelial and mesangial cells. Vague laminations are evident in the nodules, suggesting recurrent episodes of injury and organization ➡.*

Microaneurysm

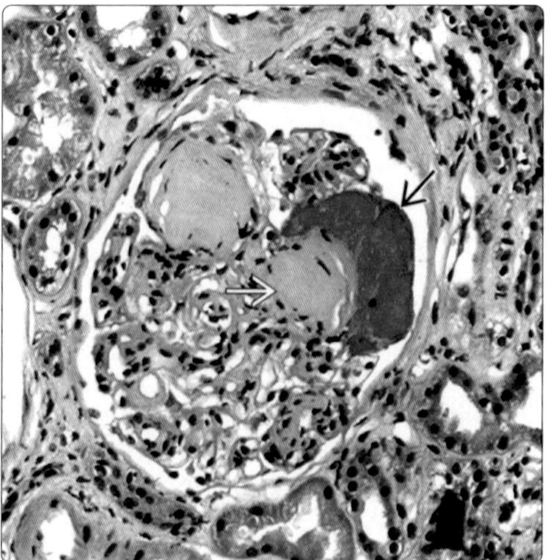

Late Stage of Nodular Glomerulosclerosis

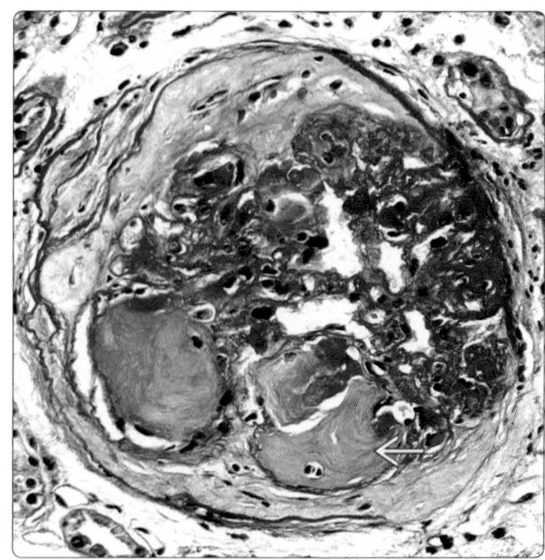

Linear IgG

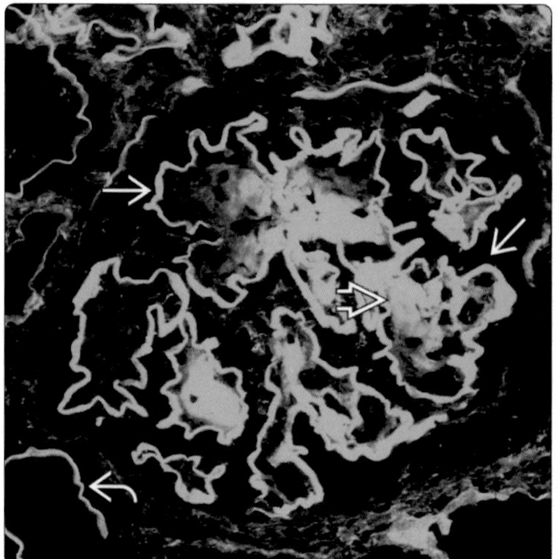

Nodular Glomerulosclerosis

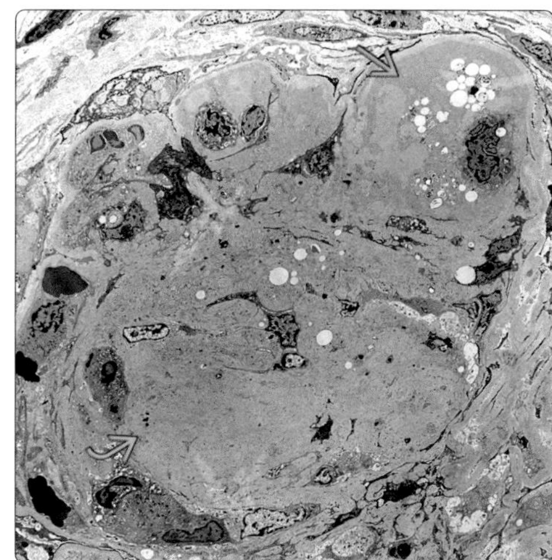

(Left) *Diffuse linear IgG staining is seen along the GBM ➡ and TBM ↪ in diabetic nephropathy due to nonimmunological trapping of immunoglobulin in the altered basement membranes and should not be confused with anti-GBM nephritis. In contrast to anti-GBM disease, albumin stains similarly. Nodules ➡ can also be seen.* **(Right)** *Late stage of DN shows nodular glomerulosclerosis ↪ and hyaline accumulation in capillaries → and almost global glomerulosclerosis. The thickened GBM and nodule are the only clues for DN.*

Diffusely Thickened GBM

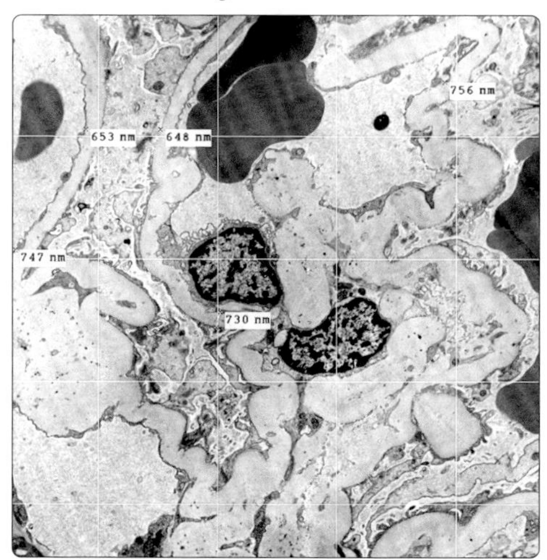

Intracapillary Leukocytes

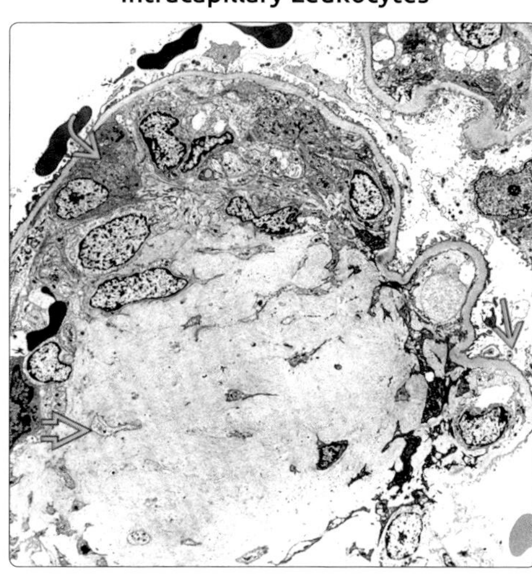

(Left) *Marked thickening of GBM and widespread foot process effacement are evident in a biopsy from a 52-year-old man with DM, 9 g/d proteinuria, and Cr 2.6 mg/dL. The effacement of foot processes is usually less extensive in DN.* **(Right)** *Nodular mesangial expansion is characteristic ⇨ of DN. The capillary lumina ↪ are obliterated by mesangial KW nodules and circulating inflammatory cells. The podocyte foot processes are only focally effaced → despite severe proteinuria.*

Matrix in Mesangium

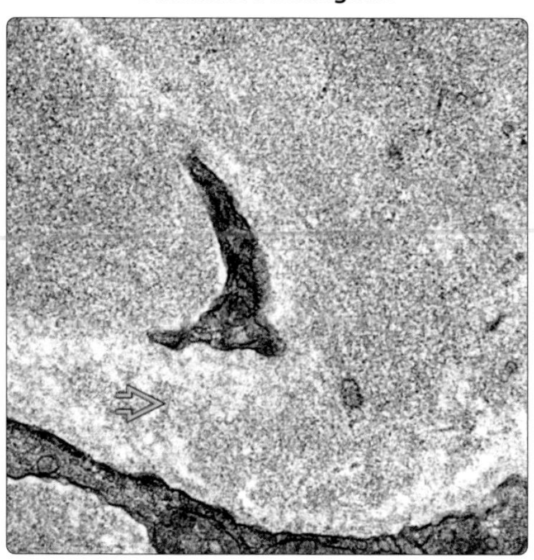

Arteriolar Hyalinosis

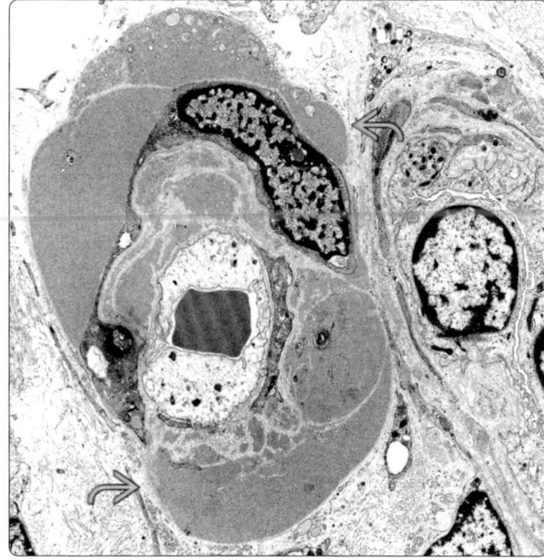

(Left) *Within the mesangium, sometimes accentuated mesangial matrix fibers ⇨ can be seen (termed diabetic fibrillosis). These fibers measure approximately 10 nm in diameter and are not composed of immunoglobulin or amyloid.* **(Right)** *Arteriolar hyalinosis ↪ in DN is characterized by plasma protein insudation under the endothelium and replacing the smooth muscle cells. Involvement of the efferent arteriole is considered specific for DN by some, although it may only reflect more severe hyalinosis.*

Class I Diabetic Glomerulopathy

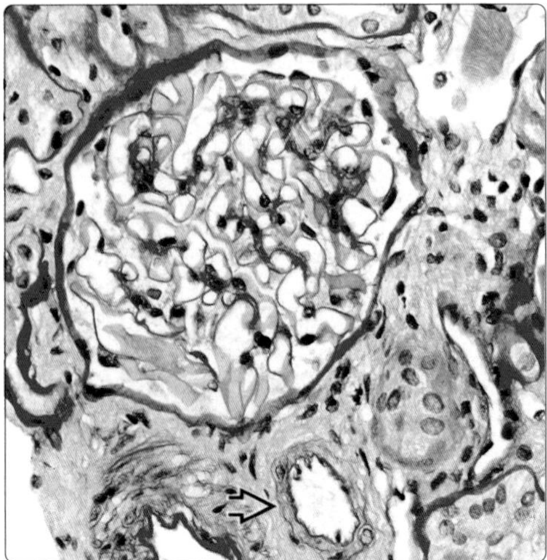

Class I

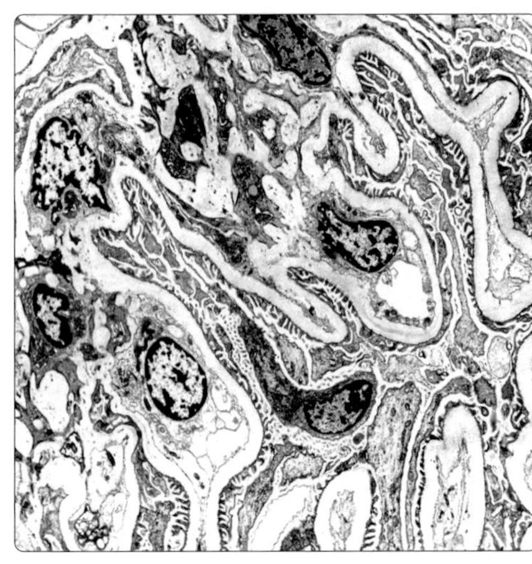

(Left) *Class I: Normal mesangium is seen in a 23-year-old man with type 1 DM for 17 years. Arterioles ➡ are normal, but GBM is thickened on electron microscopy (not appreciated by light microscopy). The patient had microalbuminuria, serum Cr 2.4 mg/dL, and no evidence of retinopathy.* **(Right)** *Class I: Thickened GBMs by electron microscopy measure 350-750 nm, averaging ~ 500 nm (upper limit of normal GBM is 430 nm in men and 395 nm in women). The podocytes are normal in this 23-year-old man with type 1 DM.*

Class IIa

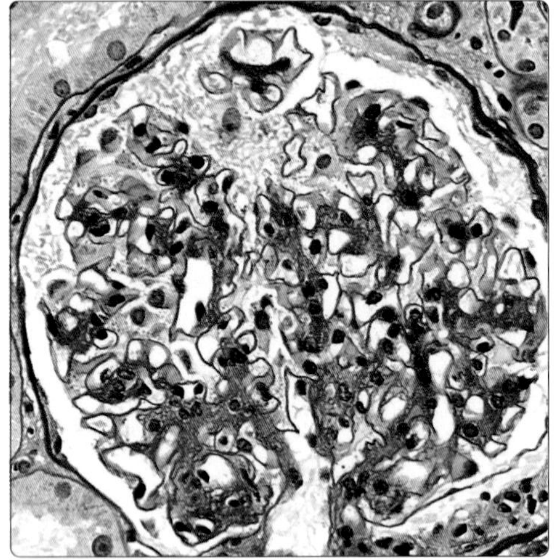

Class IIb

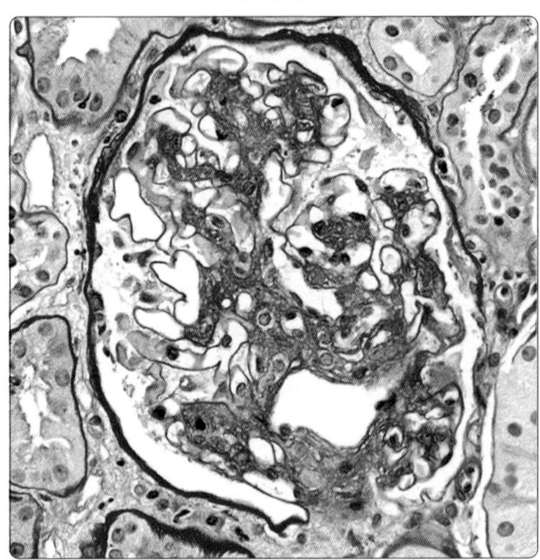

(Left) *Class IIa: Mild mesangial sclerosis is seen in which the width of the mesangium is < the average diameter of the glomerular capillaries. The distinction between IIa and IIb is likely to be poorly reproducible among different observers. Class II requires that no nodules are present and < 50% of glomeruli are globally sclerotic.* **(Right)** *Class IIb: Severe mesangial sclerosis is seen in which the width of the mesangium is > the average diameter of the glomerular capillaries (PAS stain).*

Class III

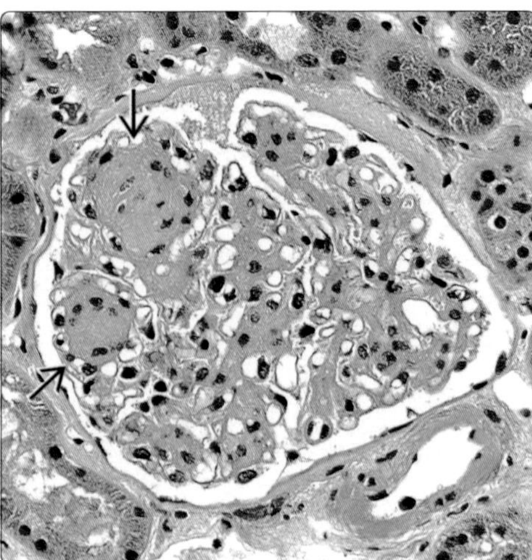

Class IV

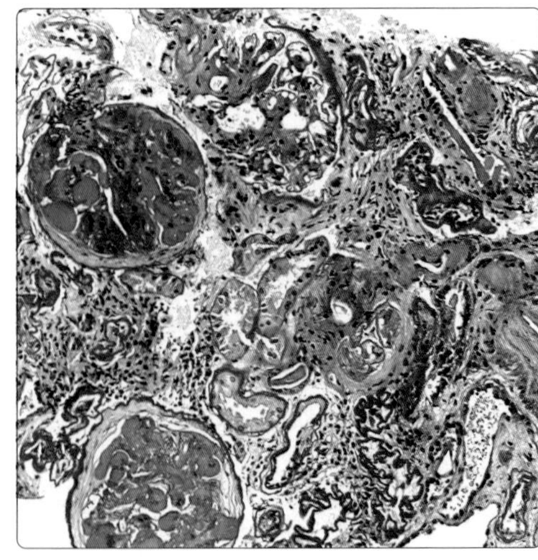

(Left) *Class III nodular diabetic glomerulosclerosis (Kimmelstiel-Wilson lesion): 2 mesangial nodules ➡ are present containing peripherally disposed mesangial cells surrounded by a necklace of capillary loops. Class III may not have > 50% global glomerulosclerosis (which would be class IV).* **(Right)** *Class IV: Advanced diabetic glomerulosclerosis with > 50% of globally sclerotic glomeruli is seen in this 53-year-old man with type 2 DM for 15 years (PAS stain).*

Superimposed Minimal Change Disease

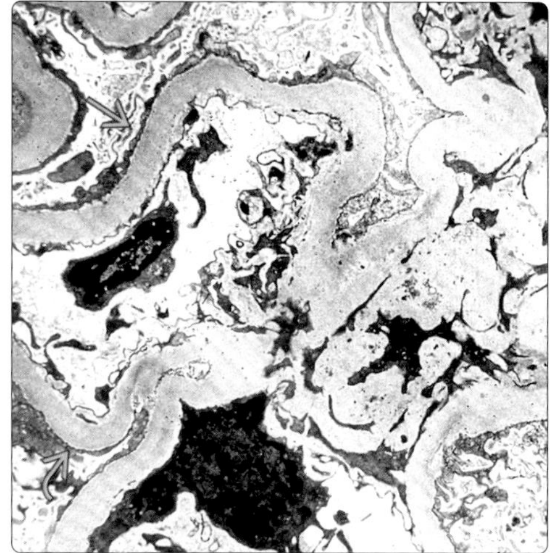

Thin Basement Membrane Disease (TBMD) in Diabetes

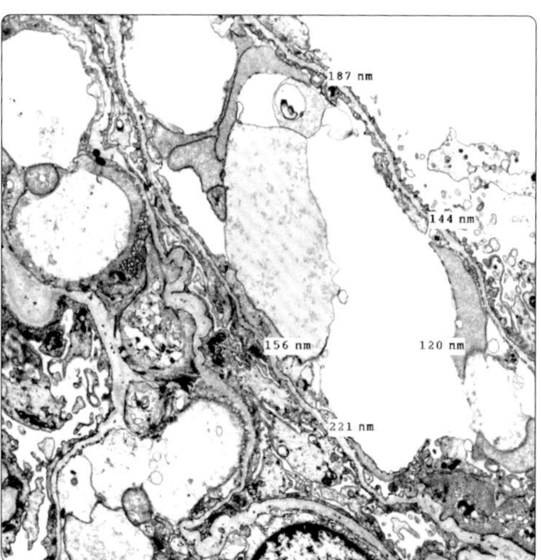

(Left) *Minimal change disease developed in a 51-year-old diabetic stung by a swarm of hornets who developed hemolytic anemia and nephrotic syndrome over 2 weeks. The podocytes show widespread effacement →, more extensive than in the usual DN. The GBM is diffusely thickened →.* **(Right)** *TBMD is present in this a 48-year-old woman with a 10-year history of type 2 DM, microhematuria, and mild proteinuria (400 mg/d) with Cr 0.7 mg/dL. DM does not necessarily thicken the GBM in TBMD.*

Superimposed ANCA Disease

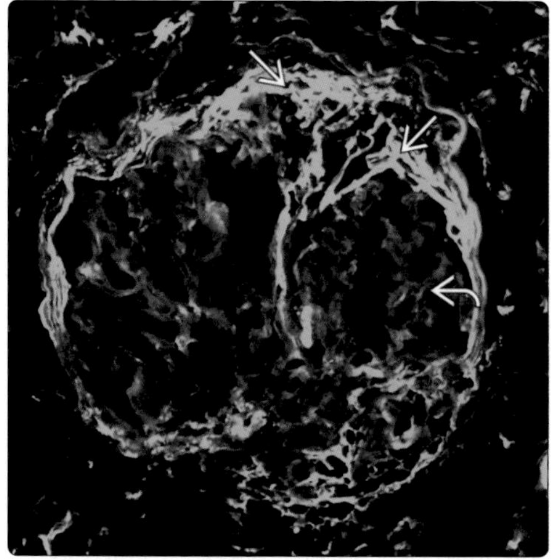

Superimposed IgA Nephropathy

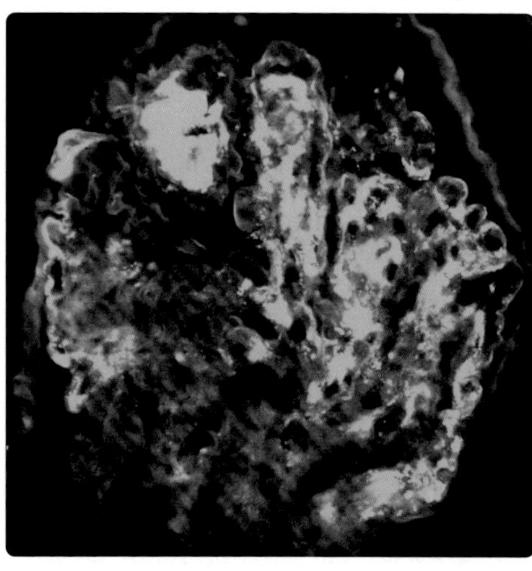

(Left) *Fibrin → stains the crescents around the KW nodules → in a 69-year-old woman with DM & c-ANCA positivity. The patient has pauci-immune glomerulonephritis superimposed on DN.* **(Right)** *IgA nephropathy superimposed on nodular DN is seen with granular mesangial IgA deposits. Patient had a longstanding history of microhematuria, an uncommon finding in uncomplicated DN.*

Superimposed Collapsing Glomerulopathy

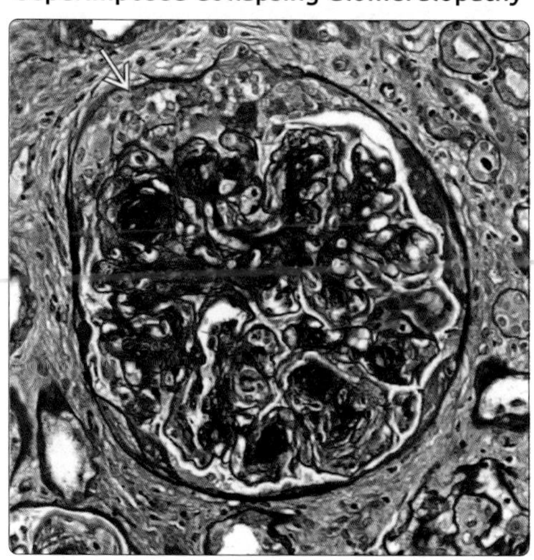

Collapsing Glomerulopathy (CK19)

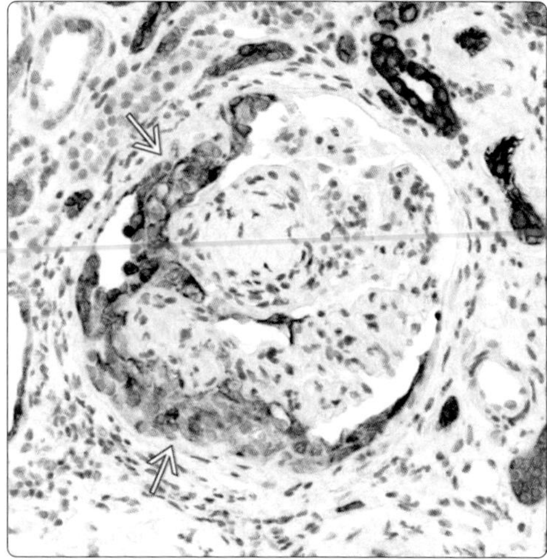

(Left) *Collapsing lesions → are found in ~5% of biopsies in diabetes and have a poor prognosis. The epithelial hypercellularity in Bowman space resembles crescents, but bridges to the GBM. Actual collapse is not conspicuous, perhaps due to the thickened GBM.* **(Right)** *Collapsing lesions → in diabetes are typically cytokeratin positive, similar to parietal epithelial cells and distinct from podocytes. Parietal cells are believed to bridge across to the GBM to replace lost podocytes.*

Idiopathic Nodular Glomerulopathy

KEY FACTS

TERMINOLOGY

- Idiopathic nodular glomerulopathy (ING)/glomerulosclerosis (GS)
- Smoking-associated nodular glomerulosclerosis (SANG)
- Nodular GS, associated with smoking &/or HTN without DM

ETIOLOGY/PATHOGENESIS

- Smoking leads to physiologic & molecular derangement (e.g., advanced glycation end product [AGE] production)
    - Pathologic processes include hypoxia, induction of oxidative stress, altered intrarenal hemodynamics, and angiogenesis
- Hypertension and obesity also closely linked to many cases, even without smoking history

CLINICAL ISSUES

- Renal dysfunction
- Nephrotic-range proteinuria
- Typically elderly, male, & white

MICROSCOPIC

- Rounded or nodular acellular PAS(+), Silver stain (+), Congo red (-) areas
- Minute endothelial-lined channels
- Glomerulomegaly
- Moderate to severe arteriosclerosis and arteriolosclerosis with hyalinosis

ANCILLARY TESTS

- No immune deposits by immunofluorescence or EM
- Segmental GBM thickening and mesangial matrix expansion by EM

TOP DIFFERENTIAL DIAGNOSES

- Diabetic glomerulosclerosis
- Monoclonal immunoglobulin deposition disease
- Amyloidosis
- MPGN, lobular variant
- Anti-glomerular basement membrane disease

(Left) *In ING, glomeruli have nodular mesangial expansion →, hypertrophy, and hypercellularity incidentally found in a nephrectomy for tumor in a 63-year-old woman with no history of diabetes.* **(Right)** *In a case of ING, there is a relatively acellular glomerular nodule →. Glomerular basement membranes → are possibly only segmentally thickened with no appreciable duplication.*

Nodular Glomerulosclerosis

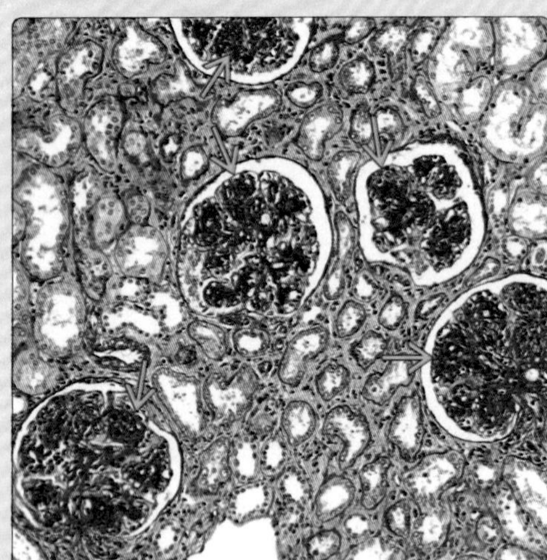

Nodular Glomerulosclerosis

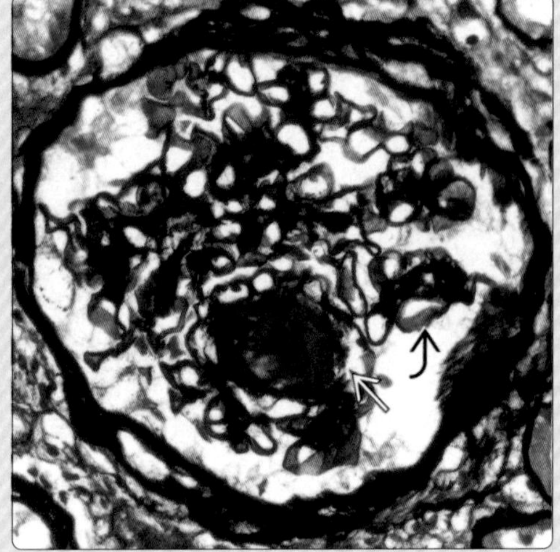

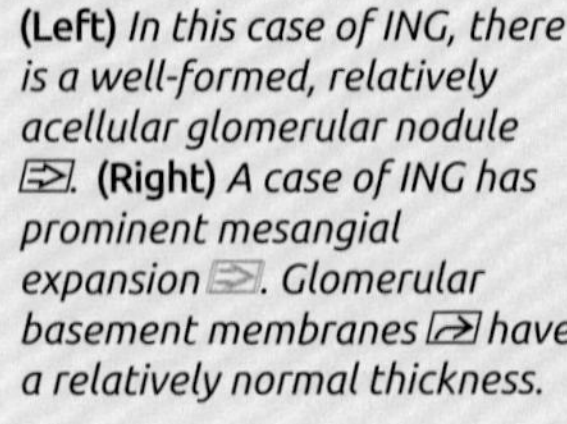

(Left) *In this case of ING, there is a well-formed, relatively acellular glomerular nodule →.* **(Right)** *A case of ING has prominent mesangial expansion →. Glomerular basement membranes → have a relatively normal thickness.*

Nodular Glomerulosclerosis

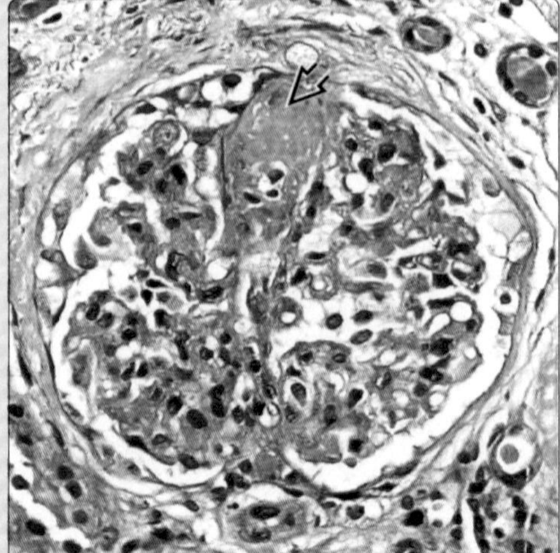

Mesangial Expansion

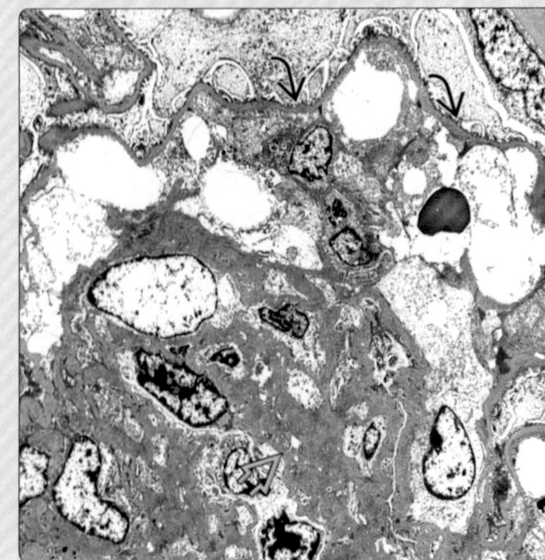

TERMINOLOGY

Abbreviations

- Idiopathic nodular glomerulopathy (ING)/glomerulosclerosis (GS)

Synonyms

- Smoking-associated nodular glomerulosclerosis (SANG)
- Idiopathic lobular glomerulonephritis
- Nodular mesangial sclerosis

Definitions

- Nodular GS, associated with smoking &/or hypertension (HTN) in absence of diabetes mellitus (DM)

ETIOLOGY/PATHOGENESIS

Environmental Exposure

- **Cigarette smoking**
  - Leads to microalbuminuria in healthy individuals
  - Risk factor for renal dysfunction
  - Advanced glycation end products (AGE) formation, oxidative stress, hypoxia, angiogenesis, & altered intrarenal hemodynamics
    - AGE alters extracellular matrix (ECM) by protein crosslinking and interaction with cell surface receptors such as receptor to AGE (RAGE)
    - Mediators include NF-κB, MAPK, JAK/STAT, Smad, TGF-β, IGF, VEGF, fibrogenic cytokines, PDGF, type IV collagen, laminin, heparan sulfate, & fibronectin
  - Chronic obstructive pulmonary disease (COPD)
    - Activates sympathetic & renin-angiotensin systems, leading to HTN & ECM production
  - Heavy smoking recorded in some (e.g., 52.9 pack-years in one series)
    - ING has also been seen in "reformed" smokers

Hypertension

- Smoking-induced renal injury probably more likely with preexisting sclerotic insult, such as hypertensive nephrosclerosis
- ING reported with only history of HTN in absence of smoking

Obesity

- Increased body mass index may also contribute to development and progression of ING
  - Likely overlap with obesity-related glomerulopathy (ORG) form of focal segmental glomerulosclerosis (FSGS)

CLINICAL ISSUES

Epidemiology

- Age
  - Elderly
- Sex
  - Male predominance
- Ethnicity
  - White predominance

Presentation

- Renal dysfunction (~ 80% of patients)
- Proteinuria
  - Nephrotic range (~ 70% of patients)
- Extrarenal vascular disease may be present

Laboratory Tests

- Normal blood glucose and hemoglobin A1c (HbA1c) values, supporting absence of diabetes

Treatment

- Drugs
  - Angiotensin II blockade

Prognosis

- End-stage renal disease (ESRD)
  - 35.3% over 14.2-month period in 1 series
  - Median time from biopsy to ESRD was 8.7 months in 1 series
- Factors predicting progression to ESRD
  - Severity of interstitial fibrosis and tubular atrophy
  - Smoking continuation
  - Lack of angiotensin II blockers

MICROSCOPIC

Histologic Features

- Glomeruli
  - Rounded/nodular acellular PAS(+), silver stain (+), Congo red (-) expansion of mesangium composed of lamellated matrix material
    - Nuclei often at periphery of nodules
  - Minute endothelial-lined channels present in and around nodules
    - Capillaries compressed or collapsed
    - Increased capillary density compared with normal controls
  - Glomerulomegaly
  - Segmental glomerular basement membrane (GBM) thickening
  - Little or no GBM duplication
  - Fibrin caps may be present
- Tubules and interstitium
  - Fibrosis and tubular atrophy common
- Vessels
  - Moderate to severe arteriosclerosis and arteriolar hyalinosis

ANCILLARY TESTS

Immunohistochemistry

- AGE demonstrable
  - Common marker is fluorescent derivative of ribose, pentosidine
  - Present in mesangial nodules and zones of interstitial fibrosis in ING and diabetic nephropathy
- Endothelial markers (e.g., CD31/34) stain glomerular capillaries at periphery of nodules

Immunofluorescence

- IgM and C3 staining in sclerotic areas, presumably due to entrapment and not immune deposits
- Linear IgG and albumin in glomerular and tubular basement membranes

Electron Microscopy

- No electron-dense immune-type deposits or fibrils
- GBM typically has moderate segmental thickening
- Mesangium segmentally expanded by increased matrix/sclerosis
- Foot process effacement variable
- Subendothelial expansion by electron-lucent fluffy material and GBM double contours sometimes seen resembling thrombotic microangiopathy
- Tubular basement membranes thickened

DIFFERENTIAL DIAGNOSIS

Diabetic Glomerulosclerosis

- Indistinguishable except by history of DM
  - GBM thickening more diffuse & dramatic in DM
  - Vascular disease usually more severe in DM
  - ING typically has more nodules in each glomerulus, and nodules are about same size

Monoclonal Immunoglobulin Deposition Disease

- Lobular pattern common
- Kappa/lambda light or heavy chain on IF & immune-type deposits on EM

Amyloidosis

- Nodular mesangial sclerosis may be prominent
- Congo red (+)

Membranoproliferative Glomerulonephritis

- Lobular, sclerosing variant resembles ING
- May represent "healing" or progressive sclerosis of longstanding GN that previously had mesangial hypercellularity
- Immune-type deposits usually found in MPGN (C3) but not ING

Chronic Thrombotic Microangiopathy (TMA)

- Nodules typically not prominent in TMA
- Chronic TMA shows GBM duplication
  - Can also be seen in ING
  - Suggests that SANG and chronic TMA share pathogenetic features

Anti-Glomerular Basement Membrane Disease

- Atypical form has similar nodules
- Serum Anti-GBM assay positive
- Small crescents may be present
- Also associated with smoking

Glomerulopathies Associated With Variety of Disorders Can Be Nodular

- Fibronectin glomerulopathy
- Fibrillary glomerulonephritis
- Immunotactoid glomerulonephritis
- Collagen type III glomerulopathy
- Takayasu arteritis
- Cyanotic congenital heart disease
- Cystic fibrosis

DIAGNOSTIC CHECKLIST

Pathologic Interpretation Pearls

- Smoking-associated nodular glomerulosclerosis possibly more appropriate term in some cases with prominent smoking history
  - Can occur with only hypertension in absence of smoking
- Correlate with blood glucose and HbA1c to exclude diabetes

SELECTED REFERENCES

1. Batal I et al: Nodular glomerulosclerosis with anti-glomerular basement membrane-like glomerulonephritis; a distinct pattern of kidney injury observed in smokers. Clin Kidney J. 7(4):361-366, 2014
2. Qian Q et al: Diagnosis and treatment of glomerular diseases in elderly patients. Adv Chronic Kidney Dis. 21(2):228-46, 2014
3. Wu J et al: Idiopathic nodular glomerulosclerosis in Chinese patients: a clinicopathologic study of 20 cases. Clin Exp Nephrol. 18(6):865-75, 2014
4. Raparia K et al: Renal morphologic lesions reminiscent of diabetic nephropathy. Arch Pathol Lab Med. 137(3):351-9, 2013
5. Kwok S et al: An unusual case of nephrotic syndrome and glucosuria. Am J Kidney Dis. 59(5):734-7, 2012
6. Kinoshita C et al: A case of idiopathic nodular glomerulosclerosis with fibrin caps. Clin Exp Nephrol. 15(6):937-41, 2011
7. Li W et al: Idiopathic nodular glomerulosclerosis: a clinicopathologic study of 15 cases. Hum Pathol. 39(12):1771-6, 2008
8. Liang KV et al: Nodular glomerulosclerosis: renal lesions in chronic smokers mimic chronic thrombotic microangiopathy and hypertensive lesions. Am J Kidney Dis. 49(4):552-9, 2007
9. Nasr SH et al: Nodular glomerulosclerosis in the nondiabetic smoker. J Am Soc Nephrol. 18(7):2032-6, 2007
10. Zhou XJ et al: Membranoproliferative glomerulonephritis. In Jennette JC: Heptinstall's Pathology of the Kidney. 6th ed. Philadelphia: Lippincott, Williams & Wilkins, 2007
11. Kuppachi S et al: Idiopathic nodular glomerulosclerosis in a non-diabetic hypertensive smoker–case report and review of literature. Nephrol Dial Transplant. 21(12):3571-5, 2006
12. Scholl-Bürgi S et al: Long-term outcome of renal glucosuria type 0: the original patient and his natural history. Nephrol Dial Transplant. 19(9):2394-6, 2004
13. Markowitz GS et al: Idiopathic nodular glomerulosclerosis is a distinct clinicopathologic entity linked to hypertension and smoking. Hum Pathol. 33(8):826-35, 2002
14. Herzenberg AM et al: Idiopathic nodular glomerulosclerosis. Am J Kidney Dis. 34(3):560-4, 1999
15. Schneider D et al: Hypercalciuria in children with renal glycosuria: evidence of dual renal tubular reabsorptive defects. J Pediatr. 121(5 Pt 1):715-9, 1992
16. Alpers CE et al: Idiopathic lobular glomerulonephritis (nodular mesangial sclerosis): a distinct diagnostic entity. Clin Nephrol. 32(2):68-74, 1989

Mesangial Expansion

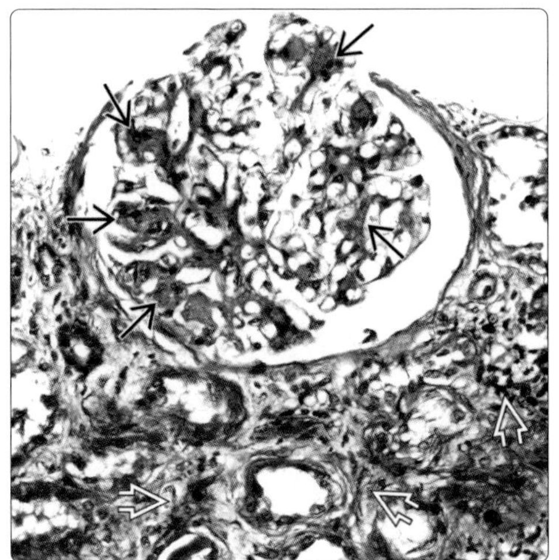

Nodular Glomerulosclerosis

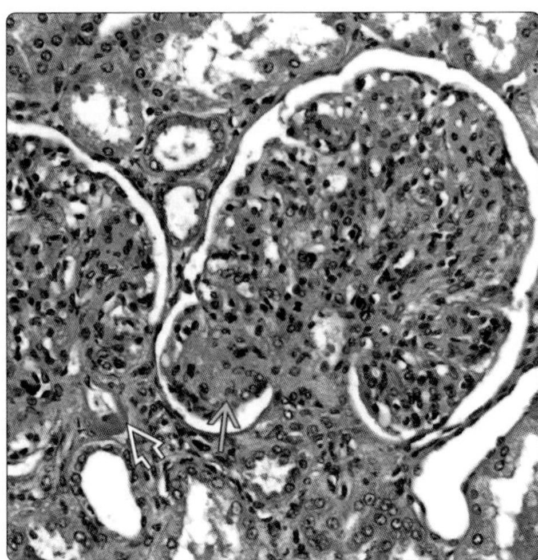

(Left) *A case of ING has prominent mesangial expansion ➙. Interstitial fibrosis ➙ is also present.* **(Right)** *A case of ING has prominent mesangial expansion leading to nodule formation ➙. Arteriolar hyalinosis ➙ is also present.*

Nodular Glomerulosclerosis

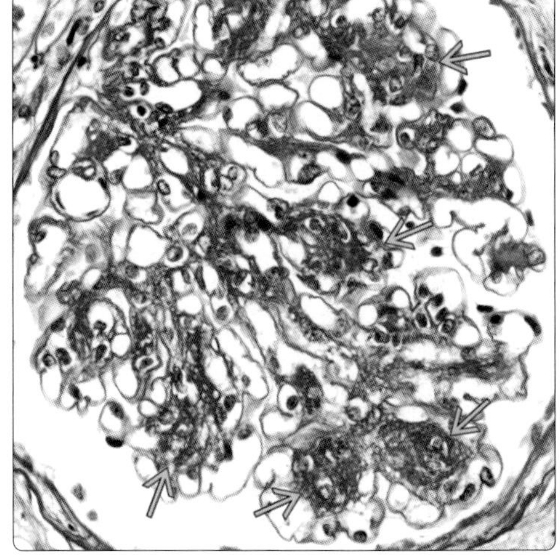

Nodular Glomerulosclerosis

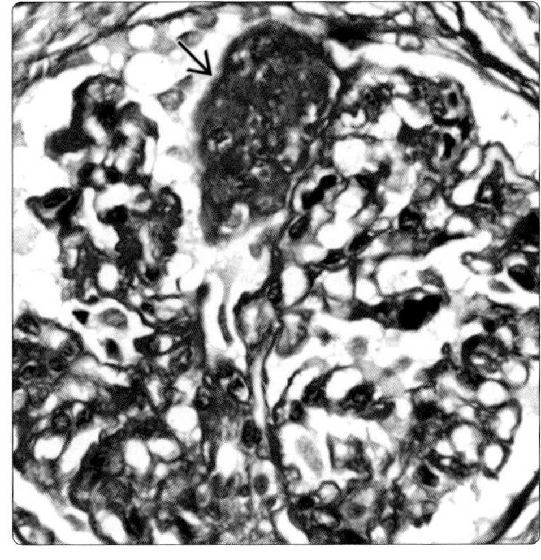

(Left) *PAS(+) nodule formation ➙ is present due to the prominent mesangial expansion/sclerosis in a case of ING.* **(Right)** *This PAS stain in a case of ING shows a relatively acellular nodule ➙ that stains PAS(+).*

Mesangial Expansion

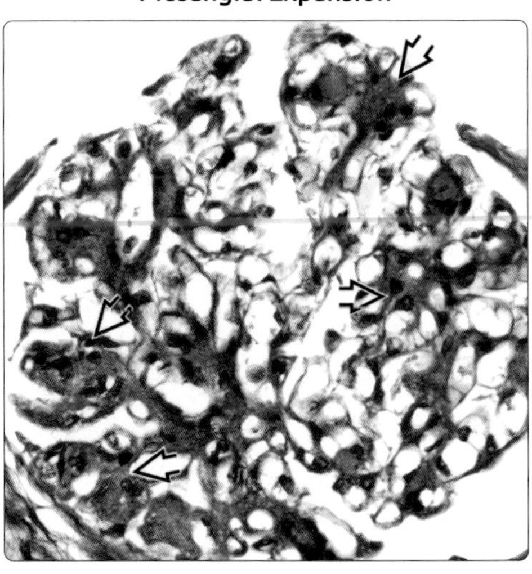

Organizing Capillary Loop Occlusion

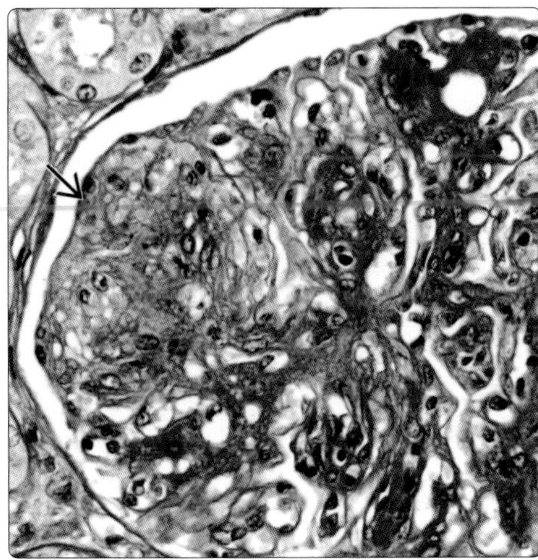

(Left) *Prominent mesangial expansion ➙ is present in a case of ING.* **(Right)** *ING sometime shows features of thrombotic microangiopathy, as in this case with an apparent organizing occlusion of a glomerular capillary ➙. This may be the origin of the mesangial nodules.*

(Left) *This glomerulus from a patient with ING has hemorrhage and congestion in glomerular capillaries with loss of endothelial nuclei →, suggestive of localized severe endothelial injury.* **(Right)** *This glomerulus from a patient with ING shows segmental duplication of the GBM →, a feature not common in diabetes, which is more typical of thrombotic microangiopathy.*

Congestion of Glomerular Capillary Loop

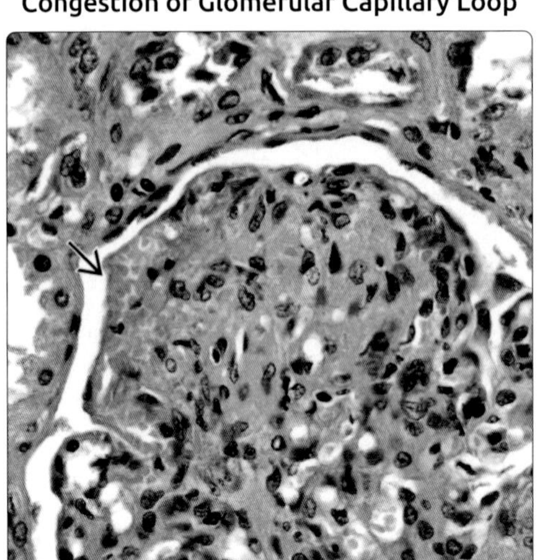

GBM Duplication

(Left) *In an ING case, there is a well-formed, relatively acellular glomerular nodule →.* **(Right)** *In this case of ING, there is arteriolar hyalinosis →, a feature also seen in diabetes and hypertension, but here there was no history of diabetes. Mesangial expansion → is also present, compatible with early glomerular nodule formation, and well-formed nodules were present in other glomeruli. In addition, there was proteinuria; proteinaceous casts → can be identified.*

Nodular Glomerulosclerosis

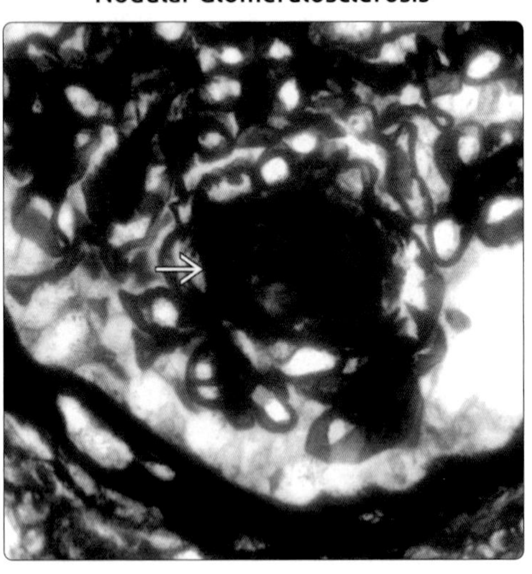

Mesangial Sclerosis and Arteriolar Hyalinosis

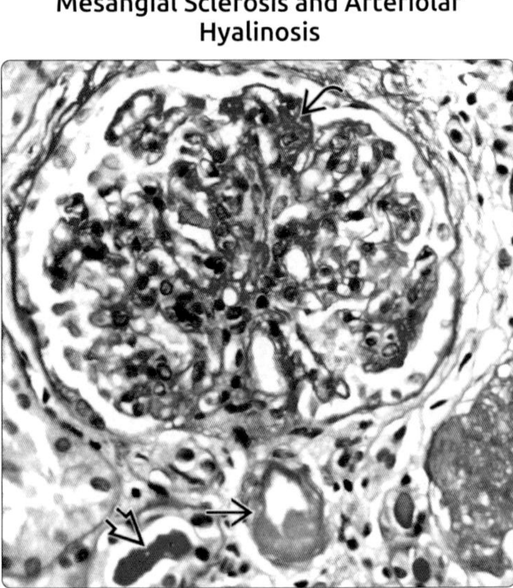

(Left) *In this case of ING, trichrome staining reveals foci of arteriolar hyalinosis →, a feature associated with diabetes and hypertension (and calcineurin inhibitor use in renal transplants); however, there was no diabetes history here.* **(Right)** *In a case of ING, CD34 immunohistochemistry stains the endothelium of capillaries at the periphery of glomerular nodules →.*

Arteriolar Hyalinosis

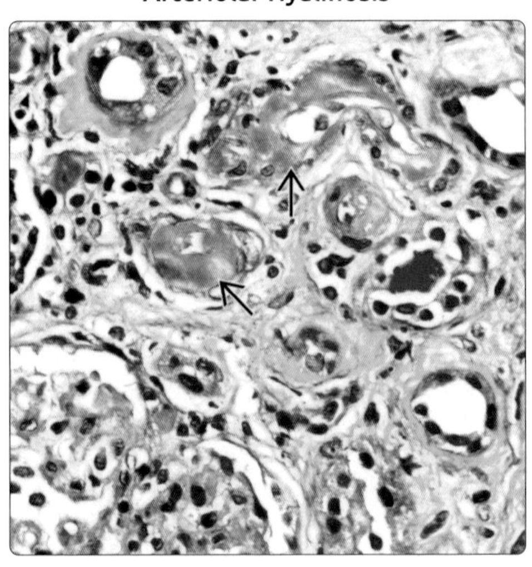

Capillaries at Nodule Periphery

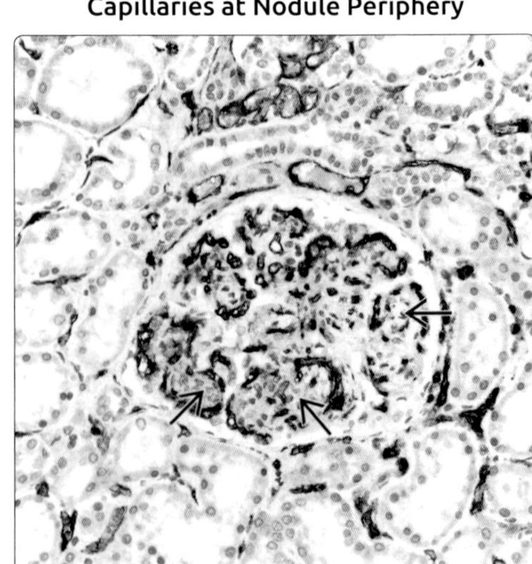

Capillaries Surrounding Nodules

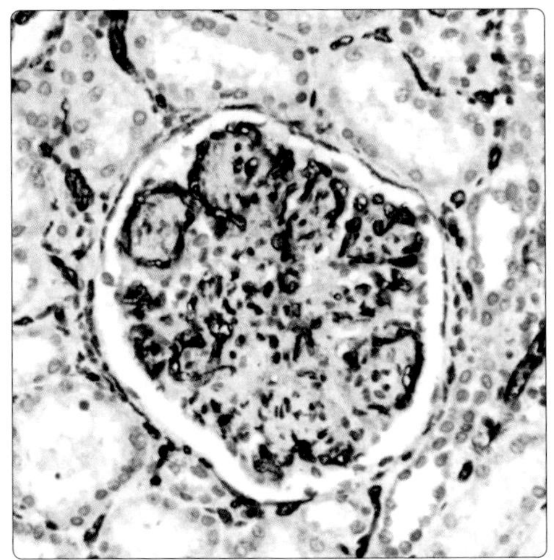

Capillaries Surrounding Nodules

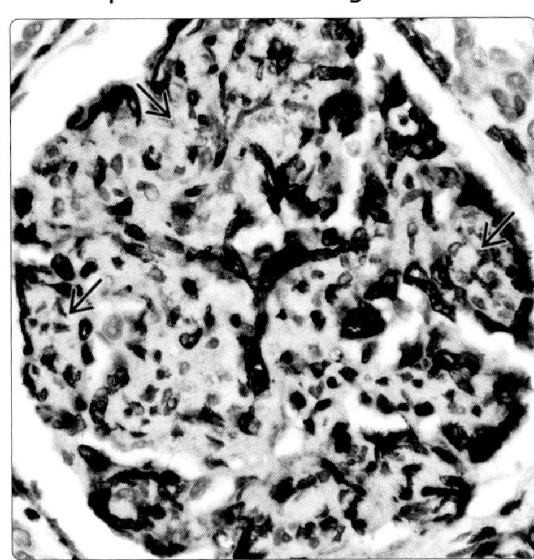

(Left) *A ring of CD34(+) capillaries surround the mesangial nodules in ING, with an increase in the overall numbers of capillaries compared with normal glomeruli.* **(Right)** *CD31 immunohistochemistry stains the endothelium of increased numbers of small capillaries at the periphery of glomerular nodules ⇨ in a case of ING.*

Mesangial Sclerosis

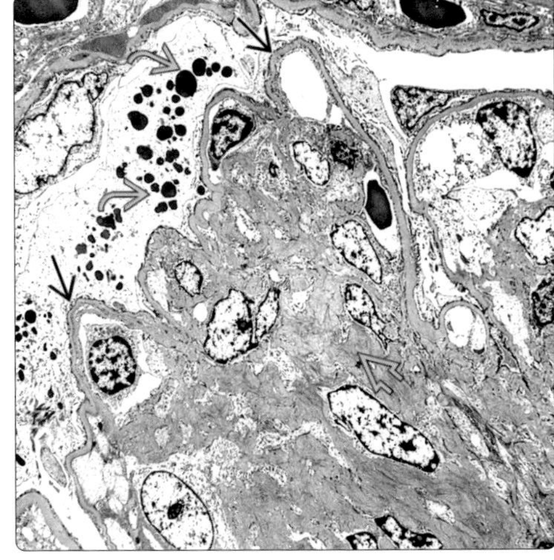

Mesangial Nodule

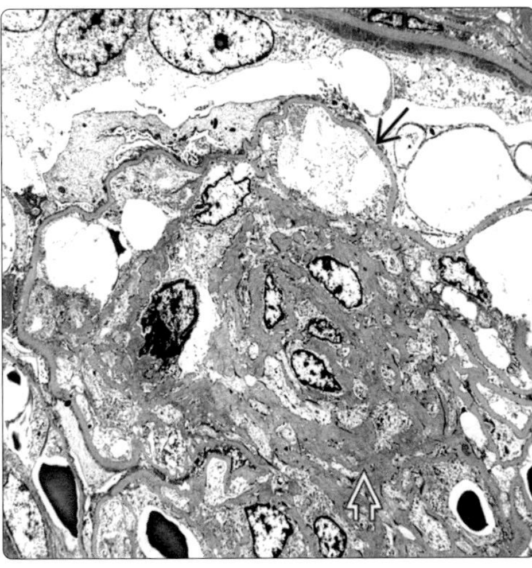

(Left) *Electron microscopy shows glomerular basement membranes ⇨ with a relatively normal thickness and a mesangial nodule ⇨ at the center of the glomerular capillaries in a case of ING. Prominent proteinaceous resorption droplets ⇨ are present within podocytes.* **(Right)** *Electron microscopy shows glomerular basement membranes ⇨ with a relatively normal thickness and a mesangial nodule ⇨ at the center of the glomerular capillaries in a case of ING.*

Mesangial Nodule

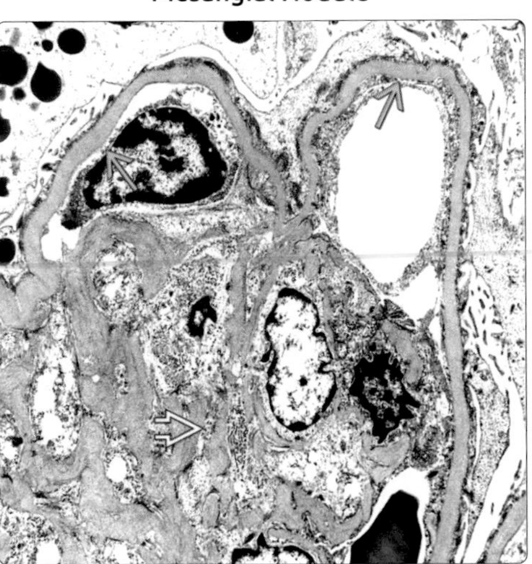

Thickened Glomerular Basement Membranes

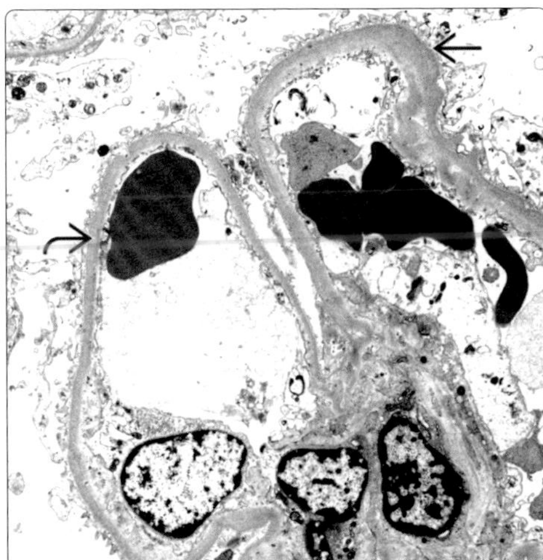

(Left) *Electron microscopy shows glomerular basement membranes ⇨ with slight thickening and a mesangial nodule ⇨ at the center of the collection of glomerular capillaries in a case of ING.* **(Right)** *Segmental glomerular basement membrane thickening is present ⇨ in this case of ING; in general, however, the remainder of glomerular basement membranes ⇨ have a relatively normal thickness.*

TERMINOLOGY

Abbreviations

- Postinfectious glomerulonephritis (PIGN); infection-related GN (IRGN); membranoproliferative GN (MPGN)

Definitions

- Spectrum of glomerular diseases arising from extrarenal infection by a variety of microorganisms

EPIDEMIOLOGY

Incidence

- Sporadic and epidemic
- Poststreptococcal and poststaphylococcal glomerulonephritis (GN) most common
  - Developed countries: 6/100,000 adults; 0.3/100,000 children
  - Developing countries: 24.3/100,000 adults; 2/100,000 children

ETIOLOGY/PATHOGENESIS

Host Susceptibility Factors

- Impaired immunity
  - Alcoholism, underlying chronic disease (e.g., diabetes mellitus), human immunodeficiency virus (HIV) infection

Pathogenic Microorganisms

- Bacteria, viruses, fungi, parasites, and protozoa

Pathogenetic Mechanisms

- Direct infection
  - Colonization: Detectable infectious organisms without inflammation
  - Infection: Infectious organisms with tissue injury, necrosis, and inflammatory exudation
  - Capillary collapse and podocyte infection with hypertrophy and hyperplasia in HIV
- Immune complex-mediated injury (e.g., IRGN, PIGN, MPGN, and membranous GN)
  - Glomerular deposition of preformed circulating antigen-antibody (Ag-Ab) complexes
  - Glomerular in situ immune complex formation (theoretical)
    - Trapped nephritogenic Ag = planted Ag
    - Ab binds planted Ag and cross reactive intrinsic glomerular Ag
  - Complement activated by aggregated immunoglobulins and directly by lectins from pathogens
  - Complement C5a and C3a, and locally produced cytokines and chemokines have chemotaxic effects
  - Leukocyte (neutrophil and monocyte) Fcγ receptors link immune complex deposition and cellular infiltrates
  - Leukocyte activation and exocytosis contribute to glomerular injury
- Cryoglobulins in MPGN
  - Specific Ag bound by IgG (e.g., hepatitis C virus [HCV] core protein)
  - Monotypic (type II) or polytypic (type III) antiglobulin reaction: IgM or IgG
  - Deposition of large complexes in subendothelium seen as "wire loops"
  - May accumulate in large amounts and occlude capillaries forming hyaline (pseudo)thrombi
  - Complement activated by classical pathway
  - Endothelial injury with detachment and repair by neomembrane formation resulting in double contours
  - May cause necrotizing vasculitis
- Vasculitic injury in crescentic GN
  - Local complement, neutrophil, and macrophage activation
  - Fibrinoid necrosis, capillary basement membrane perforation
  - Exudation to Bowman space initiates crescent formation
  - Possible contribution of antineutrophil cytoplasmic autoantigen (ANCA)-mediated injury
- Thrombotic microangiopathy
  - Shiga toxin binds globotriaosylceramide (CD77) on endothelium, mesangial cells, and epithelium

Cytomegalovirus (CMV) Glomerulopathy

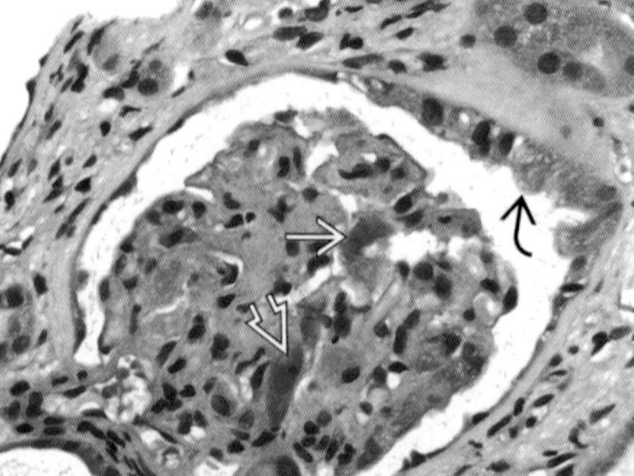

Collapsing Glomerulopathy in HIV

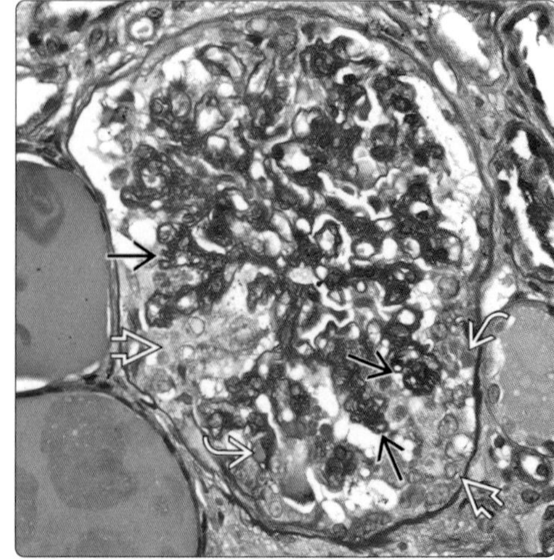

(Left) *Endocapillary ➡ and possible extracapillary ➡ cells have CMV cytopathic changes associated with hypercellularity and few open capillaries. CMV can infect endothelium and epithelium. There is tubularization of parietal Bowman capsule ➡.* **(Right)** *HIV can infect podocytes and tubular epithelium. HIV-associated nephropathy characteristically has glomerular capillary collapse ➡, podocyte hyperplasia and hypertrophy ➡, and cytoplasmic hyaline droplets ➡.*

- Endocytosis of toxin inactivates ribosomes resulting in cellular injury, and triggers apoptosis
- IgM autoantibodies to the T-cryptantigan exposed by *Streptococcus pneumoniae* derived neuraminidase injures endothelium and binds platelets

- Fibril deposition in AA amyloidosis and HCV-associated fibrillary GN (rare)

CLINICAL IMPLICATIONS

Clinical Presentation

- Glomerular disease may arise during or after infection
- Clinical and laboratory evidence of infection is crucial for diagnosis
  - GN follows a latency of ~ 2 weeks after initial infection in postinfectious GN
  - GN arises with concurrent infection in infection-related GN
- Acute renal dysfunction
  - Nephritic syndrome
  - Rapidly progressive nephritic syndrome
  - Acute kidney dysfunction with hemolysis and thrombosis
- Nephrotic syndrome: Acute or gradual onset
- Chronic renal dysfunction with hematuria and proteinuria
- Potential sites of infection
  - Upper respiratory tract and lungs
  - Heart valves, viscera
  - Skin, bones, and teeth
  - Indwelling vascular catheters and shunts

MACROSCOPIC

General Features

- Kidney enlargement in acute phase of GN and thrombotic microangiopathy (TMA) ± hemorrhage and infarction

MICROSCOPIC

Patterns of Glomerular Injury

- Direct infection
  - Viral inclusions, collapsing glomerulopathy, parasites in capillaries or mesangium
  - Microorganisms may be observed in injured glomeruli: Especially fungi and parasites
- Acute GN
  - Diffuse or focal exudative and proliferative GN ± crescent formation
    - Exudation of neutrophils & monocytes/macrophages
- Mesangial proliferative GN
  - > 3 cells per mesangial area; resolving phase of acute GN sometimes
- MPGN
  - Hypercellularity and increased lobularity of glomeruli ± hyaline pseudothrombi and "wire loop" thickening
  - Capillary basement membrane double contours and mesangial sclerosis in later phases
- Necrotizing and crescentic GN
  - Focal segmental fibrinoid necrosis, basement membrane perforation, and extracapillary hypercellularity
- Membranous GN
  - Open capillaries, subepithelial projections of neomembrane ("spikes")
- Collapsing glomerulopathy
  - Segmental or global capillary collapse with hypertrophy and hyperplasia of podocytes
- Thrombotic microangiopathy
  - Fibrin-platelet thrombi, endothelial injury, subendothelial widening, mesangiolysis
- Amyloid AA nephropathy
  - Mesangial and capillary matrix deposits; nodular glomerulosclerosis; Congo red positive

Immunofluorescence

- Granular immunoglobulin (Ig) and complement (C) deposits in glomeruli in GN
  - C3 and IgG in poststreptococcal GN
  - IgA and C3 in poststaphylococcal GN
  - IgM, IgG, C3 in MPGN with cryoglobulinemia
- Scant or no immune deposits in pauci-immune crescentic GN
- Fibrinogen and IgM in TMA
- AA amyloid detectable by immunohistochemistry or mass spectrometry

Electron Microscopy

- Viral inclusions in cytomegalovirus (CMV) glomerulopathy and others
- Tubuloreticular inclusions and nuclear bodies in HIV-associated nephropathy
- Discrete electron-dense deposits in immune complex GN
  - Subepithelial "humps" in PIGN or IRGN
  - Subendothelial deposits with basement membrane double layering in MPGN
  - Subendothelial deposits with curved tubular substructure in cryo GN ± pseudothrombi
  - Subepithelial deposits ± spike-like basement membrane projections in MGN
  - Mesangial deposits in mesangial proliferative GN
- Endothelial swelling with subendothelial widening in TMA
- Fibrils in AA amyloid ~ 10 nanometers

DIAGNOSIS

Clinical Features of Infection

- History of recent or current infection

Laboratory Evidence of Infection

- Microbiology: Pathogen isolation by culture of body fluids
- Molecular diagnostics: Detection of pathogen DNA or RNA by polymerase chain reaction assays
- Serology: Specific IgM or IgG; cryoglobulins; pathogen antigens (e.g. hepatitis B core Ag)

Pathology

- Spectrum of acute and chronic glomerulopathy ± immune complex deposition

SELECTED REFERENCES

1. Couser WG et al: The etiology of glomerulonephritis: roles of infection and autoimmunity. Kidney Int. 86(5):905-14, 2014
2. Stratta P et al: New trends of an old disease: the acute post infectious glomerulonephritis at the beginning of the new millenium. J Nephrol. 27(3):229-39, 2014
3. Nasr SH et al: Bacterial infection-related glomerulonephritis in adults. Kidney Int. 83(5):792-803, 2013

Infectious Causes of Acute GN

Bacteria	Viruses, Fungi, Parasites
Streptococcus pyogenes and *Streptococcus viridans*	Dengue virus
Staphylococus aureus MRSA, MSSA; *Streptococcus epidermidis*	Varicella zoster
Pseudomonas aeruginosa	Hantavirus
Haemophilus influenzae	Influenza virus
Escherichia coli	Human immunodeficiency vIrus
Proteus mirabilis	Coxsackie virus (A-4, B-5)
Klebsiella pneumoniae	Parvovirus B19
Enterobacter cloacae	
Serratia marcescens	*Candida albicans*
Mycobacterium leprae	*Histoplasma capsulatum*
Mycoplasma pneumoniae	*Coccidioides immitis*
Treponema pallidum	
Bartonella henselae	*Leishmania donovani*
Coxiella burnetii and *Rickettsia rickettsii*	*Entamoeba histolytica*
Borrelia burgdorferi	*Filaria*
Chlamydia pneumoniae	

Acute GN is defined as acute exudative and proliferative GN, ± crescents.

Infectious Causes of Thrombotic Microangiopathy

Enteric Pathogens	Nonenteric Pathogens
E. coli O157:H7	*Streptococcus pneumoniae*
E. coli O104:H4	*Mycoplasma pneumoniae*
Campylobacter jejuni	*Legionella* spp
Yersinia	Coxsackie A and B
Shigella and *Salmonella*	HIV

Infectious Causes of Membranoproliferative Glomerulonephritis

Bacteria	Viruses, Parasites
Staphylococci and *Streptococci*	Hepatitis B and C
Mycoplasma pneumoniae	HIV
Mycobacterium leprae	*Plasmodium malariae* and *Plasmodium falciparum*
Propionibacterium acnes	*Schistosoma hematobium, mansoni, japonicum*
Neisseria meningitidis	*Leishmania donovani*
Borrelia burgdorferi	*Wuchereria bancrofti*
Nocardia	
Coxiella burnetii	

Membranoproliferative GN is associated with chronic antigenemic states.

Infectious Causes of Membranous Glomerulonephritis

Bacteria, Viruses	Parasites
Yersinia enterocolitica	*Plasmodium malariae*
Treponema pallidum	*Leishmania donovani*
Hepatitis B and C	*Schistosoma hematobium, mansoni, japonicum*
HIV	*Strongyloides* and *Loa loa*

Acute GN of Infection

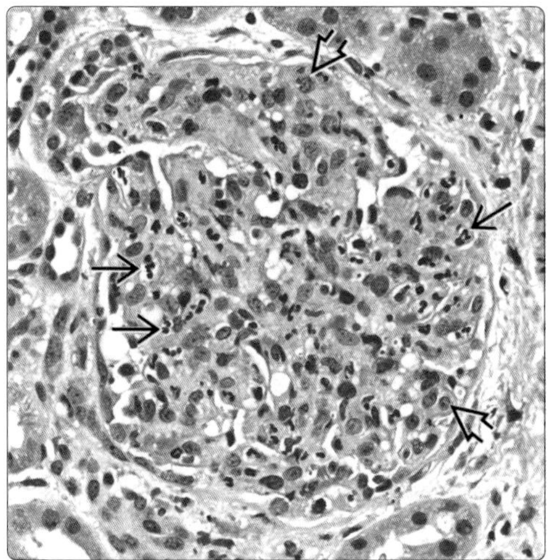

Subepithelial "Humps" in Postinfectious GN

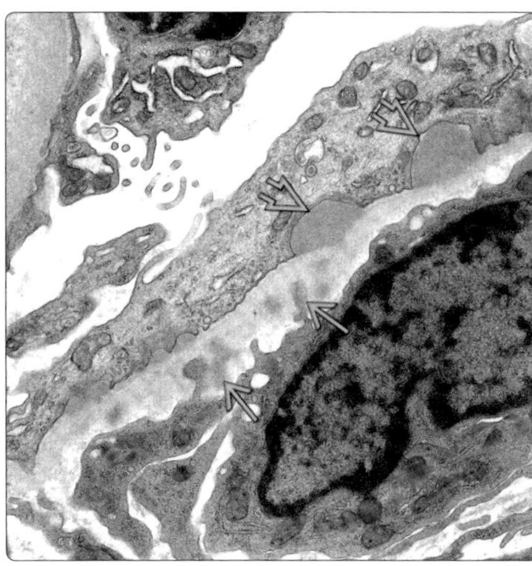

(Left) *The glomerulus has endocapillary hypercellularity with neutrophils ➔ and mononuclear cells ➯ that consist of exudating monocytes, proliferating endothelial and mesangial cells. These are classical features of acute infection-related GN and acute postinfectious GN.* **(Right)** *Subepithelial hump-like deposits ➯ are characteristic of postinfectious GN. Intramembranous dense deposits ➔ are also typical. The endothelial cell has cytoplasmic swelling.*

MPGN With Hyaline Thrombi

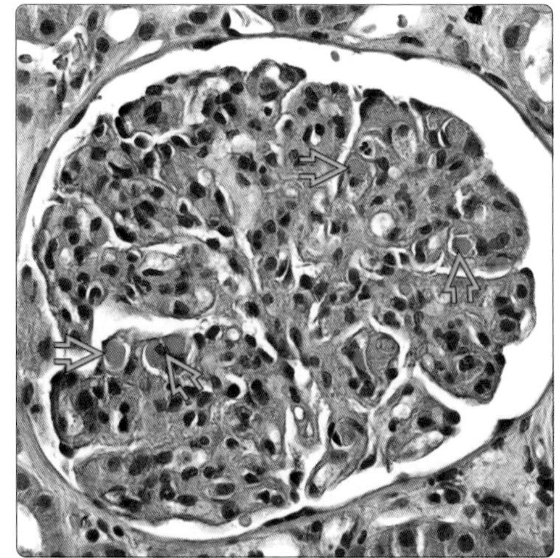

Subepithelial Deposits in Syphilis

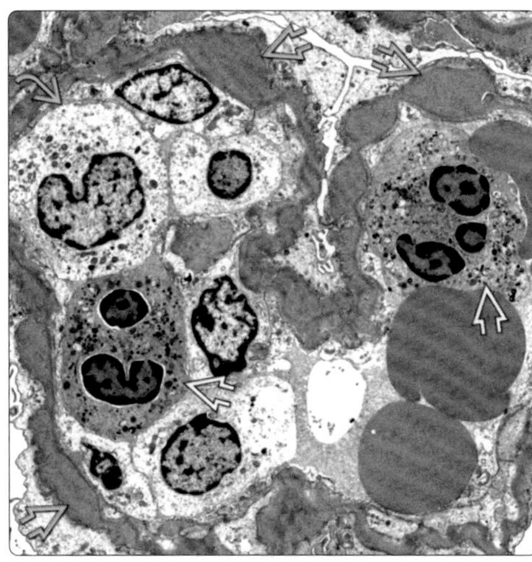

(Left) *There is global endocapillary hypercellularity and numerous intracapillary eosinophilic hyaline pseudothrombi ➯. These are characteristic of cryoglobulinemic MPGN, most frequently caused by hepatitis C virus infection.* **(Right)** *Subepithelial immune complex electron-dense deposits ➯ are apparent in membranous GN in a patient with tertiary Treponema pallidum infection. Neutrophils ➡ and monocytes ➚ are in the capillary lumen.*

Thrombotic Microangiopathy

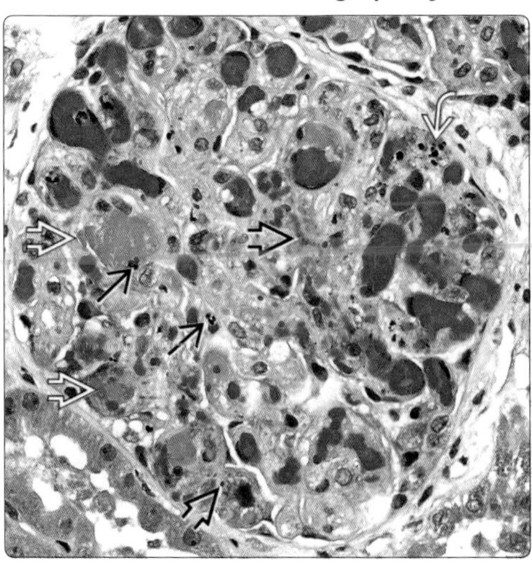

AA Amyloidosis in Chronic Osteomyelitis

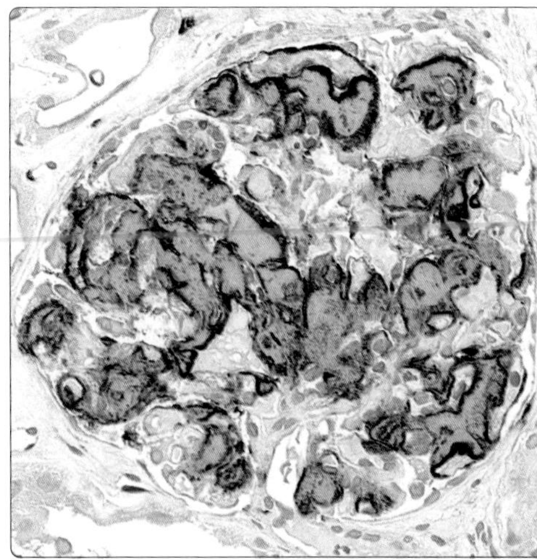

(Left) *Thrombi ➡ occlude the capillaries in this glomerulus from a patient with Shiga toxin-associated TMA from infectious colitis due to E. coli O157:H7. Capillaries are congested, with erythrocytolysis ➯, and there are neutrophils ➔ and karyorrhexis ➡.* **(Right)** *Chronic bacterial infections (e.g., osteomyelitis, empyema, bronchiectasis) are associated with secondary AA amyloid deposits in the glomeruli, interstitium, and blood vessels.*

Acute Poststreptococcal Glomerulonephritis

KEY FACTS

TERMINOLOGY

- Acute diffuse proliferative ("exudative") GN with clinical history of streptococcal infection

ETIOLOGY/PATHOGENESIS

- *Streptococcus pyogenes*, group A, β-hemolytic
  - Subset of strains are nephritogenic, by M protein type
- Acute immune complex disease
- Primarily activate alternative complement pathway

CLINICAL ISSUES

- Gross hematuria in 30-60%; smoky, brown urine
- Nephrotic syndrome (5-10%)
- Hypertension (85%), azotemia (60%)
- Low C3 (90%); normal C4
- Positive ASO or anti-DNAse B (95%)
- Majority of children spontaneously resolve
- Minority have abnormalities in alternative complement pathway

MICROSCOPIC

- Diffuse hypercellularity
  - Numerous neutrophils within capillary tufts
  - Mesangial hypercellularity
- Glomerular capillaries are not thickened or duplicated
- Typically no necrosis
- Crescents, if present, are poor prognostic feature
- Interstitial inflammation & edema, red cell casts
- May be superimposed on other diseases, such as diabetes
- IF shows "starry sky," "garland," or mesangial pattern of IgG and C3, usually no C1q or IgA
- EM shows "humps" without surrounding BM reaction
  - Occasional subendothelial, intramembranous, & mesangial deposits

TOP DIFFERENTIAL DIAGNOSES

- Nonstreptococcal postinfectious GN
- C3 glomerulopathies
- Proliferative GN with monoclonal immunoglobulin deposits

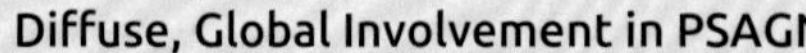

Diffuse, Global Involvement in PSAGN

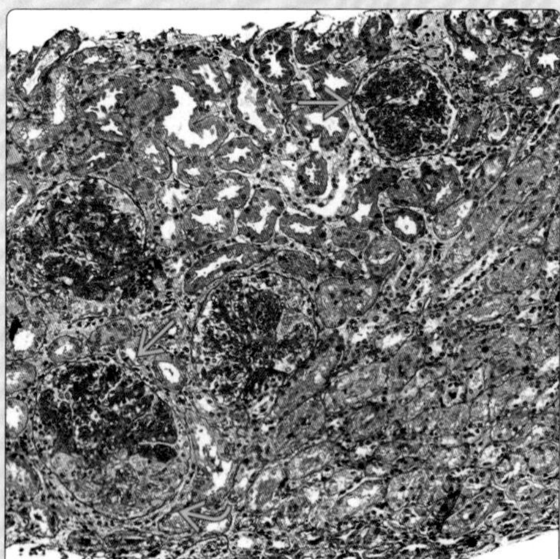

Exudative Proliferation With Neutrophils

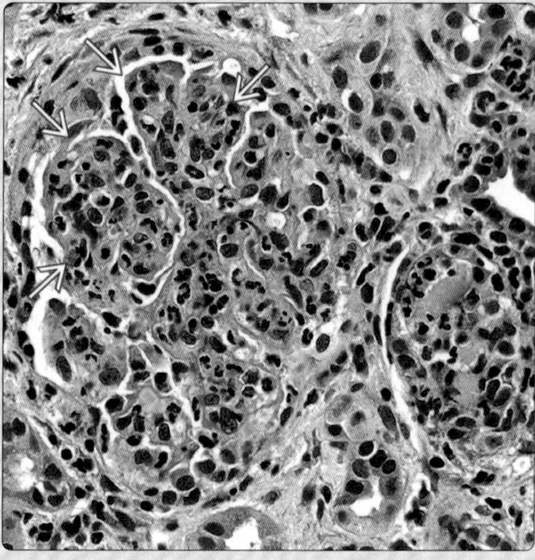

(Left) *Low-power magnification (PAS) of the cortex in poststreptococcal acute glomerulonephritis (PSAGN) reveals that glomeruli ➡ are most prominently affected. All glomeruli are typically involved (diffuse), and entire glomerular tufts are affected (global). Crescents may occur ➡.* **(Right)** *PSAGN is often characterized by glomeruli with accentuated lobularity ➡ containing abundant neutrophils in what is termed an exudative proliferative pattern.*

"Starry Sky" C3

"Hump" Deposit

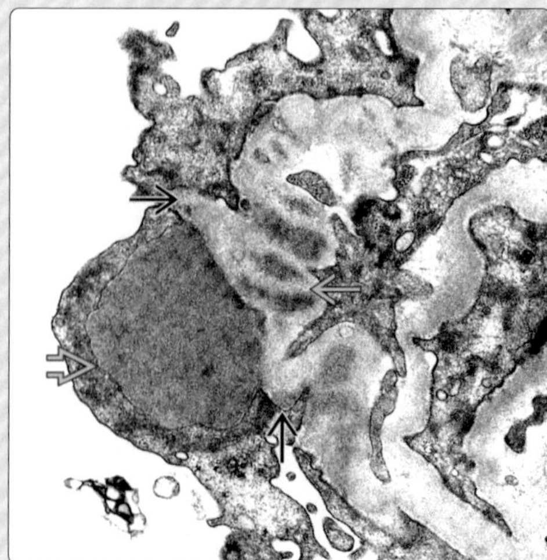

(Left) *Positive immunofluorescence for C3 shows a diffusely scattered, granular pattern (resembling a starry sky) of staining of the glomerular basement membrane in acute poststreptococcal GN.* **(Right)** *EM shows subepithelial "hump" ➡ on the GBM ➡ with little or no surrounding basement membrane reaction in a case of PSAGN. Intramembranous dense deposits are present ➡.*

TERMINOLOGY

Abbreviations

- Poststreptococcal acute glomerulonephritis (PSAGN)

Synonyms

- Diffuse proliferative & exudative glomerulonephritis

Definitions

- AGN that follows *Streptococcus* infection

ETIOLOGY/PATHOGENESIS

Infectious Agents

- *Streptococcus pyogenes*, group A, β-hemolytic
  - Usually pharyngitis or skin infection (pyoderma)
    - Less commonly mastoiditis & otitis media
- Only certain strains nephritogenic
  - Typed by surface M protein (virulence factor)
  - Different M-type strains cause rheumatic fever
- Virulence factors provoke antibodies, useful for diagnosis, but not relevant to immune complex formation
  - DNase, hyaluronidase, streptokinase, NADase, proteinases, & hemolysins streptolysins-O & -S
- *Streptococcus zooepidemicus*
  - Unpasteurized milk and cheese

Acute Immune Complex Disease

- Delayed onset after infection (1-3 weeks)
- Deposition of antibody-antigen complexes in glomerulus
  - Complement fixed in glomerular capillaries, predominantly alternate pathway
  - Attracts neutrophils & monocytes
  - Digestion of GBM, endothelial injury
- Many target antigens proposed
  - Streptococcal pyrogenic exotoxin B (SPEB)
    - Cationic secreted protein that binds plasmin
    - Colocalizes with IgG & C3 present in "humps"
    - However, some nephritogenic strains lack gene
  - Nephritis-associated plasmin receptor
    - Promotes plasmin activity
    - Does not colocalize with C3
  - Other strep antigens and autoantigens postulated

Animal Models

- 1 IV dose of foreign serum protein (e.g., bovine serum albumin in rabbits)
  - Mimics all features, including GN, "humps," and ↓ C3
- No good *S. pyogenes* GN model in animals

Direct Activation of Complement

- Lectin pathway activated by *S. pyogenes*
- Neuromidase activates alternate pathway

CLINICAL ISSUES

Epidemiology

- Incidence
  - ~ 500,000 cases/year worldwide; 95% in less developed countries
    - Developed countries ~ $3/10^6$/year; less developed ~ $26/10^6$/year
    - Incidence underestimated due to subclinical cases
  - ~ 1:1,000 develop PSAGN after *Strep* pharyngitis
    - ↑ in epidemics of nephritogenic strains
    - Individual risk factors not defined
- Age
  - Peak at age 6-8 years; rare < 2 years
  - Up to 33% are > 40 years old
- Sex
  - Male:female ~ 2:1

Presentation

- Subclinical in ~ 20%
- Abrupt onset 1-4 weeks after infection (average: ~ 10 days)
- Hematuria (almost universal)
  - Gross hematuria (~ 60% children, 30% adults)
    - Smoky, Coca-Cola-, tea-, or coffee-colored urine
- Proteinuria (nephrotic syndrome in 5-10%)
- Edema: Typically sudden onset of periorbital edema
- Acute renal failure & oliguria/anuria
  - ~ 60% elevated BUN
- Hypertension (85%)
  - Largely 2° to sodium & fluid retention
- Anemia

Laboratory Tests

- Evidence of preceding *Streptococcus* group A infection required for diagnosis
  - Throat and skin cultures negative in ~ 75% at presentation
- Antistreptolysin O (ASO) serology best for pharyngitis, anti-DNase-B for pyoderma
  - 2 together are 95% sensitive; false-positive due to ubiquity of *Strep* infections
- ↓ C3 (90%), precedes onset of hematuria; normal C4
- Rare reports of superimposed ANCA or anti-GBM

Treatment

- Drugs
  - Antibiotics if active infection

Prognosis

- Usually, spontaneous resolution in children
  - C3 returns to normal within 8 weeks
  - Microscopic hematuria may persist up to 5 years
  - < 1% of children have decreased GFR after 10 years
  - 20% have persistent signs (proteinuria, hypertension, or microhematuria)
- Renal abnormalities persist in 1/3 adults > 60 years old
  - Comorbidities contribute to outcome
- Repeated PSAGN attacks rare
- *CFH* mutations risk factor for persistent GN (C3 glomerulopathies)

MACROSCOPIC

General Features

- Soft, pale with petechiae & surface bulges 2° to edema
- Sometimes 25-50% > normal weight

MICROSCOPIC

Histologic Features

- Glomeruli

- Diffuse ↑ cellularity mostly 2° to leukocytes in capillaries
  - Neutrophils, monocytes, lymphocytes
  - ± eosinophils, particularly in tropical cases
  - Mesangial hypercellularity & ↑ mesangial area/matrix
  - Accentuated glomerular lobularity with clubbed appearance
  - Glomerular capillary lumina variably occluded due to endocapillary hypercellularity and endothelial swelling
  - All glomeruli affected (diffuse) in global pattern
- Subepithelial "humps" visible in trichrome stain
  - Tiny nodules on epithelial side of GBM
- Cellular, but not fibrous, crescents may be present
  - > 50% of glomeruli present in up to 40% of recent biopsied cases
  - Associated with poorer outcome
- Necrosis rare
- GBM duplication, if present, suggests other diagnosis

- Interstitium
  - Monocytes, lymphocytes, neutrophils, eosinophils
  - Little or no fibrosis with admixed edema
  - Inflammation may be prominent without glomerular disease mimicking drug-induced acute interstitial nephritis
- Tubules
  - Red cell casts in distal nephron
    - Compacted, hemolyzed, fragmented
    - Later in course, pigmented casts appear
  - Protein resorption droplets
  - Acute tubular injury & later atrophy
- Vessels
  - Vasculitis rare; suggests other diagnoses
- Late biopsies
  - Resolving PSAGN not well defined
  - Mesangial hypercellularity without inflammation

ANCILLARY TESTS

Immunofluorescence

- Primarily IgG and C3 in 1 of 3 patterns
  - "Starry sky" or "lumpy bumpy": Fine, irregular, granular deposits in capillary walls & mesangium; seen early in disease course
  - "Garland": Densely packed, thick, elongated, & confluent capillary wall deposits; seen in patients with crescents and nephrotic-range proteinuria; seen early in disease course; may have worse prognosis
  - Mesangial: Granular, with sparing of capillary loops (C3 more common than IgG) noted later
- IgM > 50%; IgA rare (suggests *S. aureus* AGN)
- C3 present without IgG in ~ 30% suggesting C3 glomerulopathy
  - C1q & C4 usually lacking, supporting role of alternative complement pathway
- Fibrin in mesangium & crescents
- Properdin, C5b-9, factor B present in GBM & mesangium
- Variably reported *Streptococcus* antigens (e.g., SpeB virulence factor)

Electron Microscopy

- Immune complex deposits
  - Subepithelial deposits ("humps") on surface of GBMs
    - Without surrounding GBM reaction ("spikes")
    - Deposits may become confluent
  - Mesangial subepithelial deposits common
  - Intramembranous deposits may resemble dense deposit disease
  - Subendothelial deposits less common
- Foot process effacement over "humps"
- Swollen endothelial cells & sometimes disrupted endothelium

DIFFERENTIAL DIAGNOSIS

Nonstreptococcal Postinfectious GN

- More common than PSAGN in developed world
- Pathology similar if not identical
- IgA prominence prompts consideration of *Staph* infection

C3 Glomerulopathy

- Prominent subendothelial and intramembranous deposits
- Hyperdense intramembranous deposits (DDD)
- Suspect if persistent low C3

Proliferative GN With Monoclonal Immunoglobulin Deposits

- Light chain restriction by IF

Membranoproliferative GN (MPGN), Type I

- Duplication of GBM favors MPGN
  - Subendothelial deposits more prominent in MPGN

DIAGNOSTIC CHECKLIST

Clinically Relevant Pathologic Features

- Crescents and interstitial inflammation increase risk of ESRD in adults
- Complete recovery with > 50% cellular crescents reported in children

Pathologic Interpretation Pearls

- PSAGN can be superimposed on other diseases, such as IgA nephropathy
- Biopsy series biased for atypical or severe course

SELECTED REFERENCES

1. Prasto J et al: Streptococcal infection as possible trigger for dense deposit disease (C3 glomerulopathy). Eur J Pediatr. 173(6):767-72, 2014
2. Kambham N: Postinfectious glomerulonephritis. Adv Anat Pathol. 19(5):338-47, 2012
3. Vernon KA et al: Acute presentation and persistent glomerulonephritis following streptococcal infection in a patient with heterozygous complement factor H-related protein 5 deficiency. Am J Kidney Dis. 60(1):121-5, 2012
4. Eison TM et al: Post-streptococcal acute glomerulonephritis in children: clinical features and pathogenesis. Pediatr Nephrol. 26(2):165-80, 2011
5. Nadasdy T et al: Infection-related glomerulonephritis: understanding mechanisms. Semin Nephrol. 31(4):369-75, 2011
6. Nasr SH et al: Postinfectious glomerulonephritis in the elderly. J Am Soc Nephrol. 22(1):187-95, 2011
7. Rodriguez-Iturbe B et al: The current state of poststreptococcal glomerulonephritis. J Am Soc Nephrol. 19(10):1855-64, 2008

Lobular Glomeruli in PSAGN

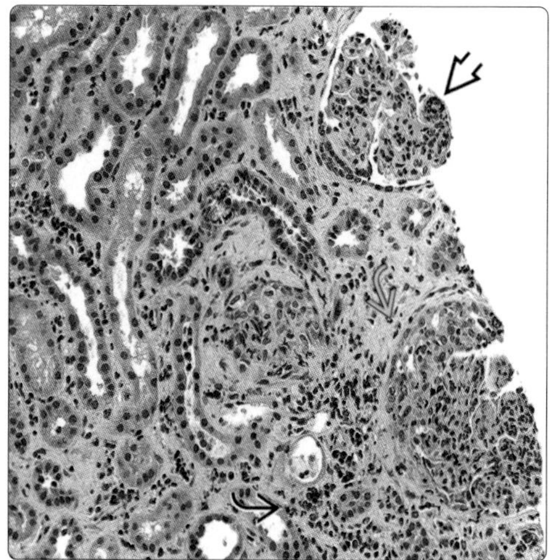

Exudative Pattern With Neutrophils

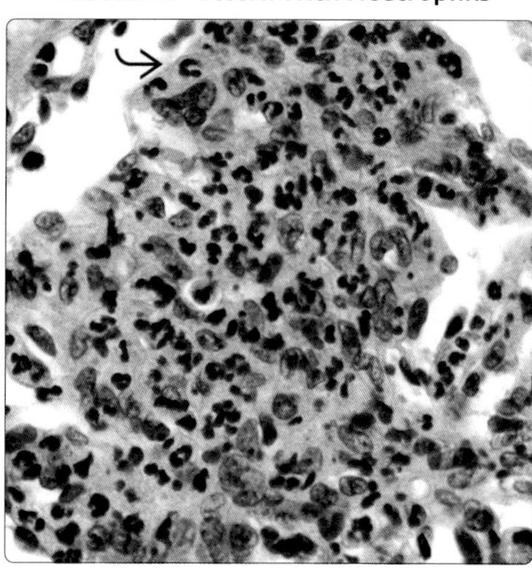

(Left) *Low-power H&E image shows hypercellular glomeruli with a lobular architecture ➲ (sometimes referred to as club-shaped) and an interstitial inflammatory infiltrate ➲ in a case of PSAGN. A cellular crescent ➲ is present.* **(Right)** *High-power view of a glomerulus in a case of PSAGN reveals striking hypercellularity with numerous neutrophils ➲, the presence of which makes this an "exudative" GN.*

Neutrophils, Eosinophils, & Endocapillary Hypercellularity

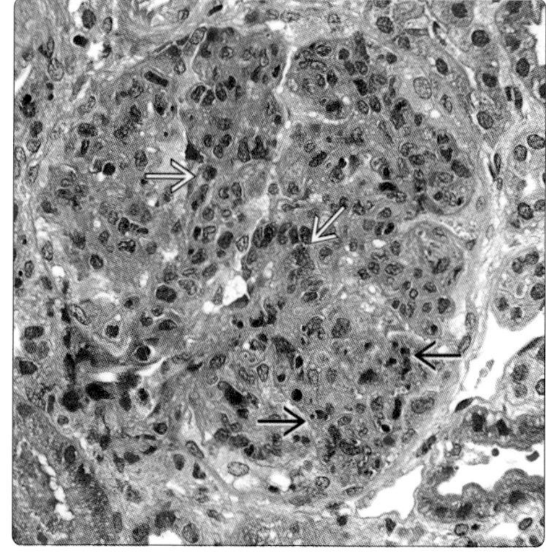

Cellular Crescent

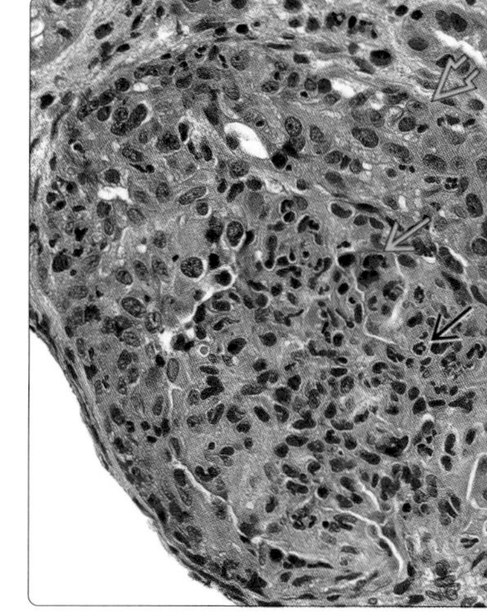

(Left) *PSAGN characteristically has endocapillary hypercellularity with a loss of open capillary loops. Neutrophils ➲, as well as occasional eosinophils ➲, can be seen in glomerular capillaries.* **(Right)** *A cellular crescent ➲ is present in a case of PSAGN. The glomerulus is also hypercellular with neutrophils ➲ and eosinophils ➲ in glomerular capillary loops. About 30% of biopsied cases have > 50% crescents, a poor prognostic finding in adults but probably not in children.*

Hypercellular Glomerulus & Tubular Casts

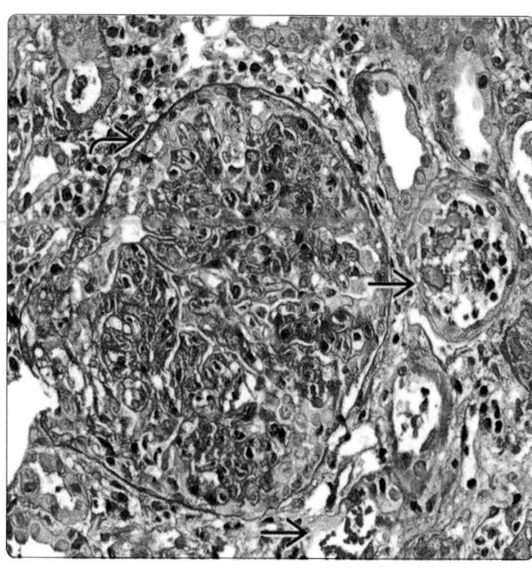

Subepithelial "Humps"

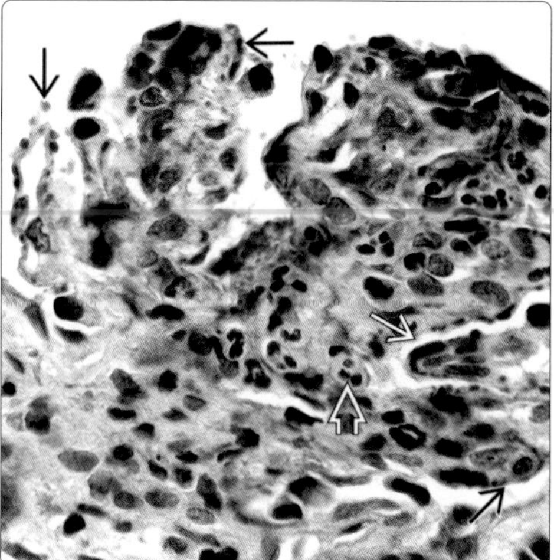

(Left) *A 9-year-old girl has acute poststreptococcal GN, and high power of a PAS stain shows a lobular hypercellular glomerulus with crescent formation ➲ & adjacent tubules ➲ containing proteinaceous cast material. Red cell casts are not readily appreciated in PAS-stained sections.* **(Right)** *Subepithelial deposits ➲ along the glomerular basement membrane stain red or blue in trichrome stains. Elongated intramembranous deposits are also seen ➲. Neutrophils ➲ are in glomerular capillary loops.*

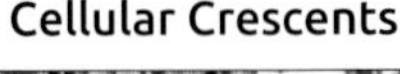

Cellular Crescents

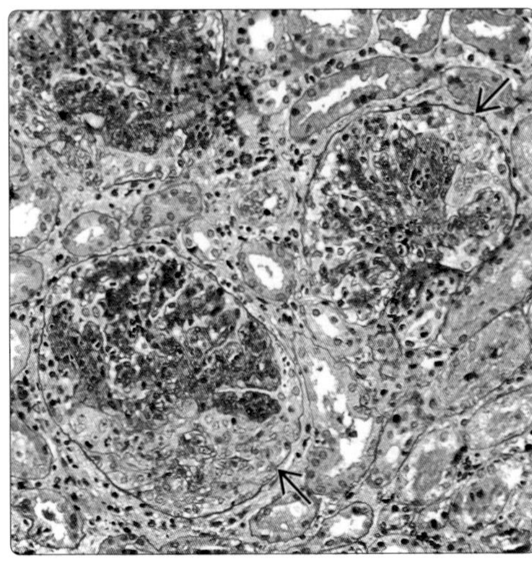

Crescent & Hypercellular Glomerulus

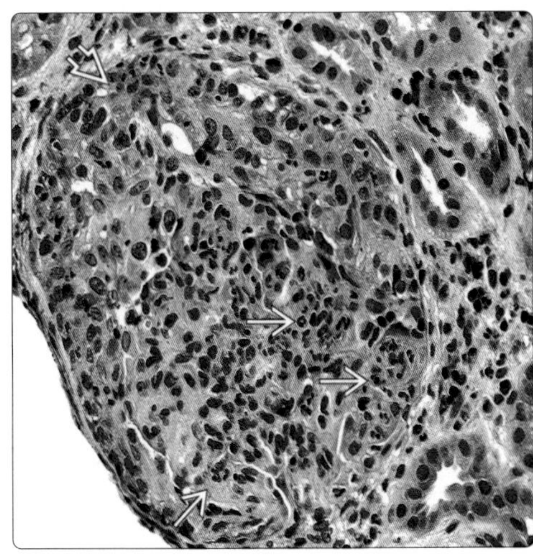

(Left) *Prominent cellular crescents → are seen in a child with PSAGN. Patient presented with sudden onset of gross hematuria, hypertension, low C3 (25 mg/dL), normal C4, pneumonia, 10 g/d proteinuria, & positive anti-DNAse B antibodies.* **(Right)** *Hypercellular, lobulated glomerulus shows numerous neutrophils → and a cellular crescent → in a child with PSAGN. Capillary loops are characteristically not patent due to endocapillary hypercellularity and endothelial swelling.*

Hump-Like Subepithelial Deposits

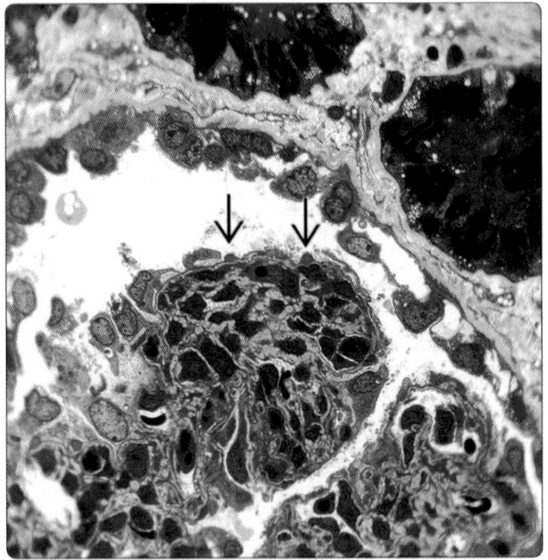

Red Blood Cell Casts

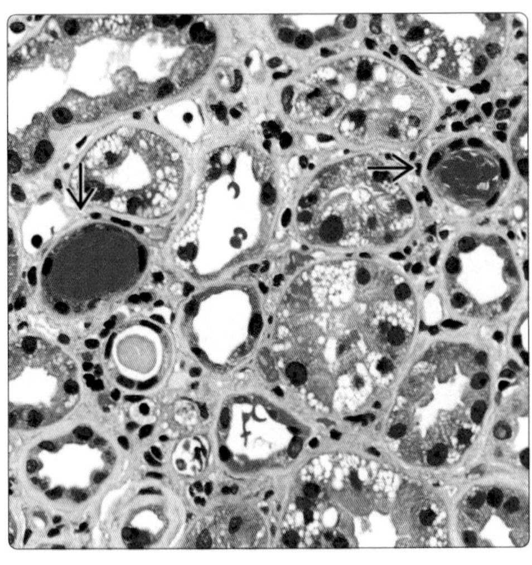

(Left) *In PSAGN, toluidine blue-stained, semi-thin "scout" sections prepared for EM can reveal subepithelial, hump-like deposits → along the glomerular capillary loops. Glomerular capillary loops are hypercellular.* **(Right)** *H&E shows red cell casts → in the medulla. These can be distinguished from artifactual bleeding from the biopsy procedure by their compaction & mixing with proteinaceous material. Another useful feature is hemolysis & fragmentation.*

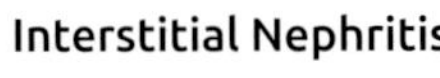

Interstitial Nephritis

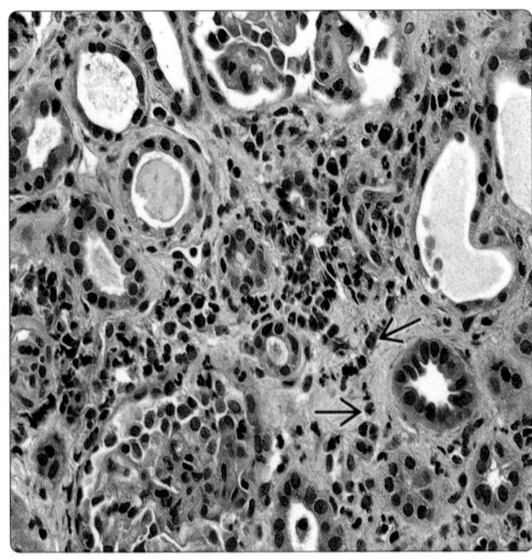

Interstitial Inflammation, Including Eosinophils

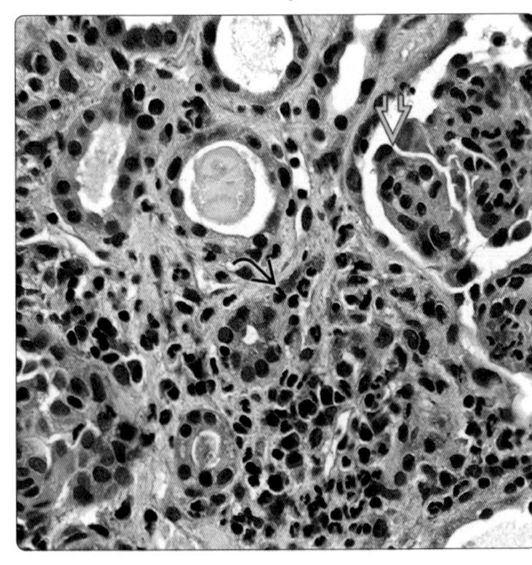

(Left) *Prominent interstitial inflammation with a mixed infiltrate of mononuclear cells, neutrophils, & eosinophils → can be seen in PSAGN, and sometimes is present in the absence of glomerular involvement.* **(Right)** *In a child with PSAGN, there is an expansion of the interstitium by edema & an inflammatory infiltrate, including occasional eosinophils →. This can be mistaken for a drug reaction if glomerular involvement is slight. A portion of a hypercellular glomerulus → can be seen.*

"Garland" Pattern of IgG Deposition

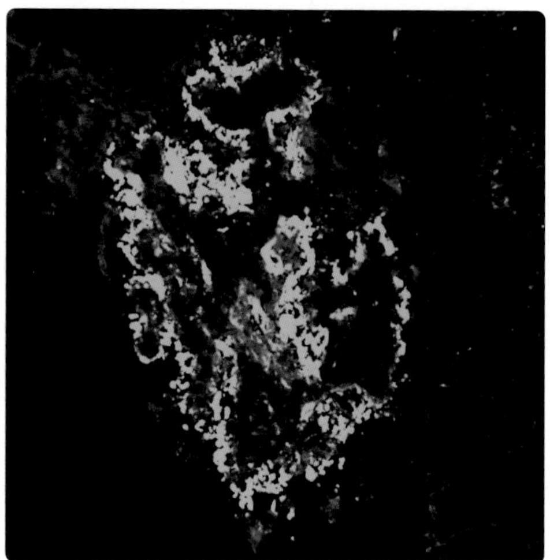

"Lumpy Bumpy" IgG

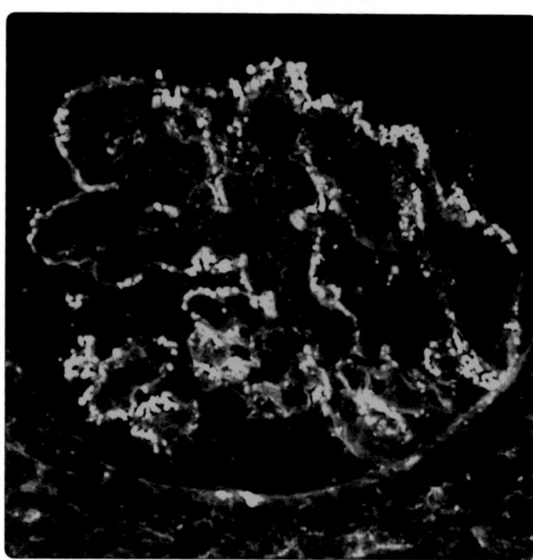

(Left) *Immunofluorescence for IgG shows characteristic granular staining in a continuous band (or "garland" pattern) along the glomerular basement membrane in PSAGN.* **(Right)** *Immunofluorescence for IgG shows coarsely granular, "lumpy bumpy" staining of the glomerular basement membrane in acute poststreptococcal GN, corresponding to the subepithelial "humps" seen by EM.*

Mesangial and GBM IgG Deposits

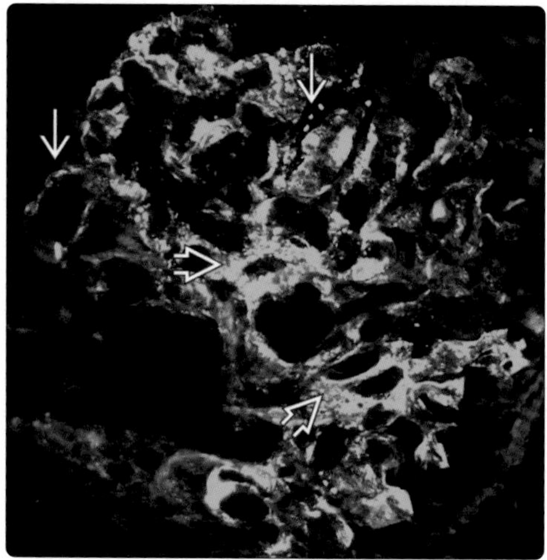

"Starry Sky" Pattern

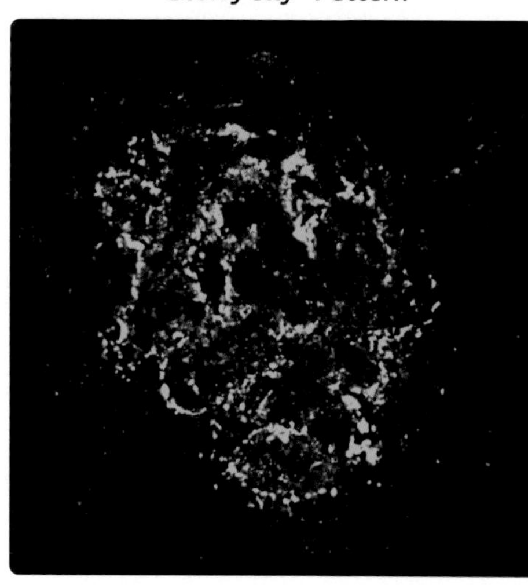

(Left) *PSAGN with a mesangial dominant pattern ➔ of IgG deposition is shown in a 62-year-old man presenting with Cr 1.6, hypertension, 5 g/d proteinuria, low C3 & C4, positive ASO, & anti-DNAse. Scattered granular deposits along the GBM can also be seen ➔.* **(Right)** *In this case, C1q is deposited in a granular, starry sky-type pattern along the glomerular basement membrane in acute PSAGN. C1q is not commonly seen and should prompt consideration of other GNs such as lupus nephritis.*

"Lumpy Bumpy" Kappa

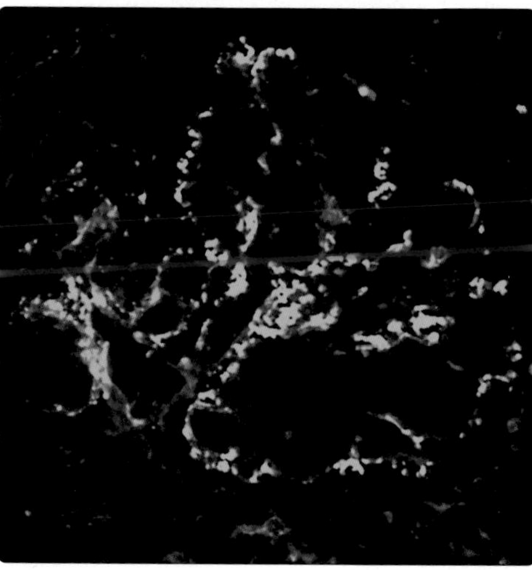

"Garland" Kappa

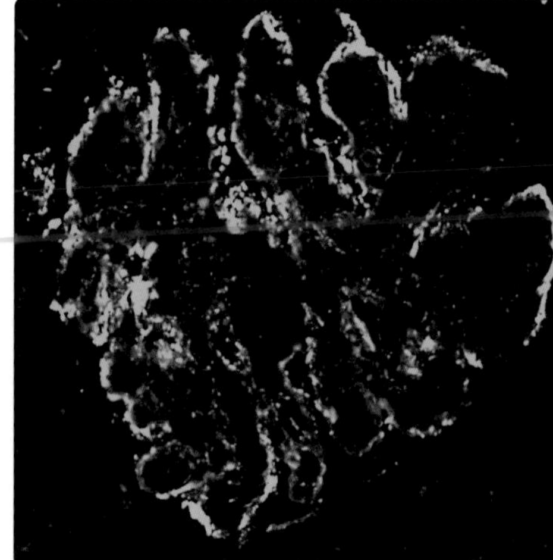

(Left) *Immunofluorescence shows a coarsely granular, "lumpy bumpy" pattern of staining along the glomerular basement membrane for kappa in PSAGN. Kappa and lambda stain equally in PSAGN.* **(Right)** *Immunofluorescence shows a band-like pattern of staining ("garland") along the glomerular basement membrane for kappa in acute poststreptococcal GN. Kappa was equal to lambda.*

(Left) *In a child with PSAGN, there are numerous subepithelial deposits along the GBM, some of which are confluent. A number of the confluent deposits produce the "garland" pattern visible on FM.* **(Right)** *EM shows PSAGN with neutrophil in the glomerular capillary loop infiltrating under the endothelium near subepithelial "humps" & in direct contact with the GBM. Neutrophils are attracted by C5a & other chemokines & cause injury by digesting the GBM.*

Subepithelial Deposits

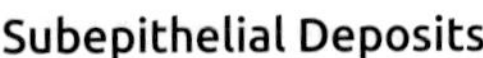

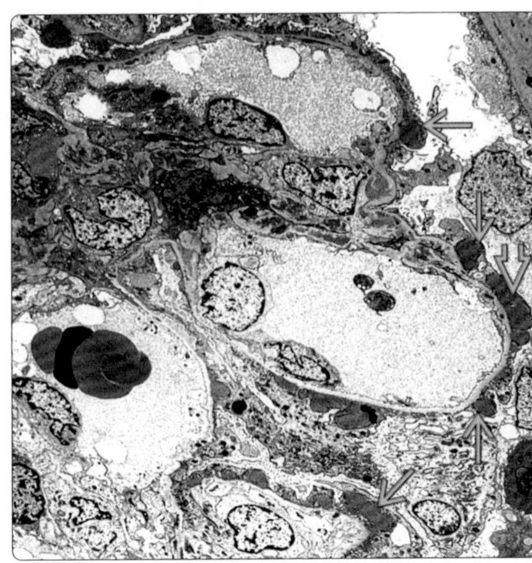

Neutrophil and Subepithelial "Humps"

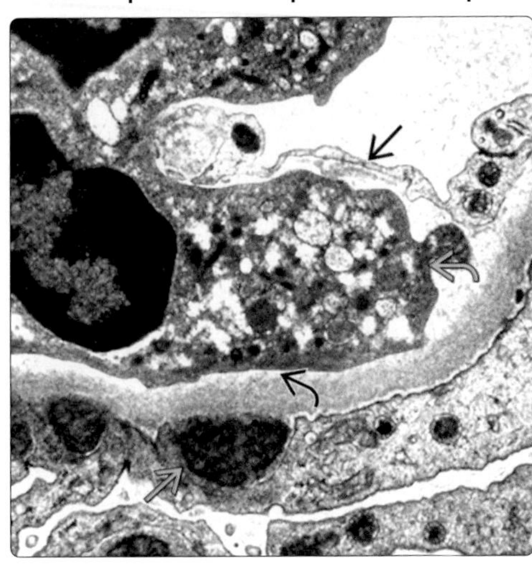

(Left) *Relatively dense, variegated subepithelial deposit in PSAGN is seen. There is no cupping of the deposits in contrast to membranous glomerulonephritis.* **(Right)** *Sometimes "humps" erode the GBM in continuity with intramembranous deposits. Loss of GBM integrity is probably the basis of hematuria. This biopsy is from 3-year-old girl with hypertension, "Coca-Cola" urine, 3+ protein & blood on urinalysis, Cr 2.1 mg/dL, anti-DNase B 240, & negative Strep culture.*

Hump-Like Deposit

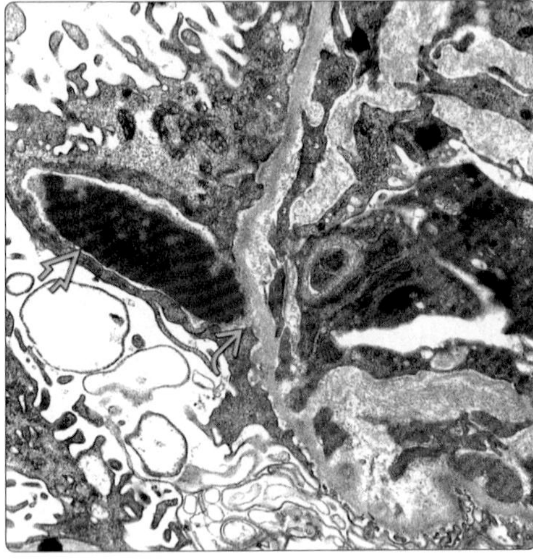

GBM Erosion by Hump-Like Deposits

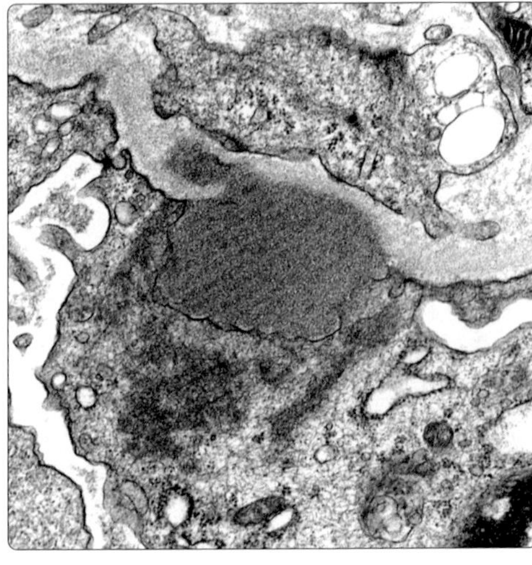

(Left) *PSAGN can have prominent mesangial deposits in addition to the characteristic "humps," as in this child with acute renal failure, hypocomplementemia, & elevated anti-DNAse B.* **(Right)** *Subendothelial deposits are also focally present in PSAGN in addition to the "hump" deposits.*

Mesangial Deposits

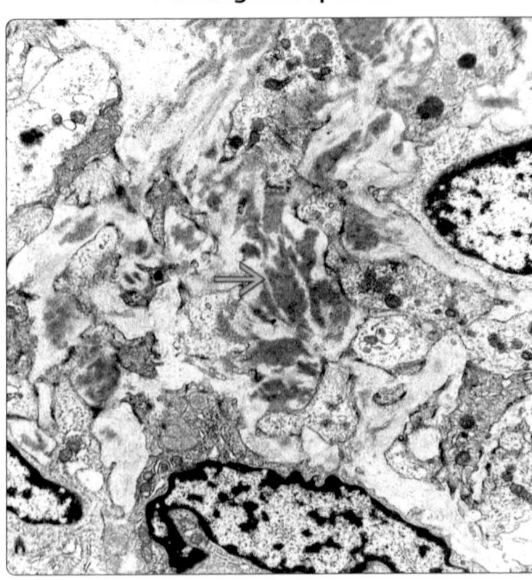

Subendothelial and Hump Deposits

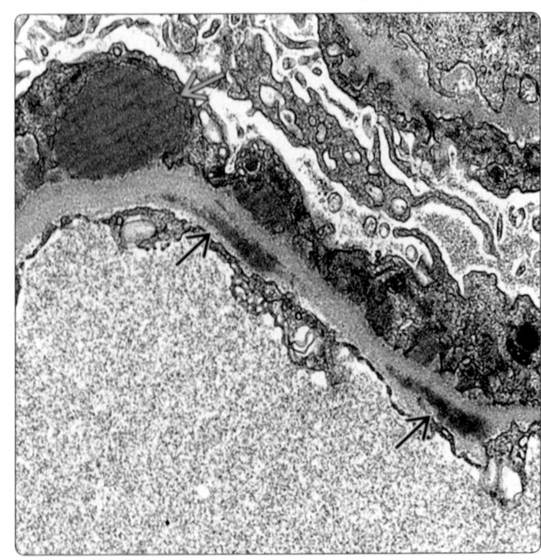

Variegated Deposits

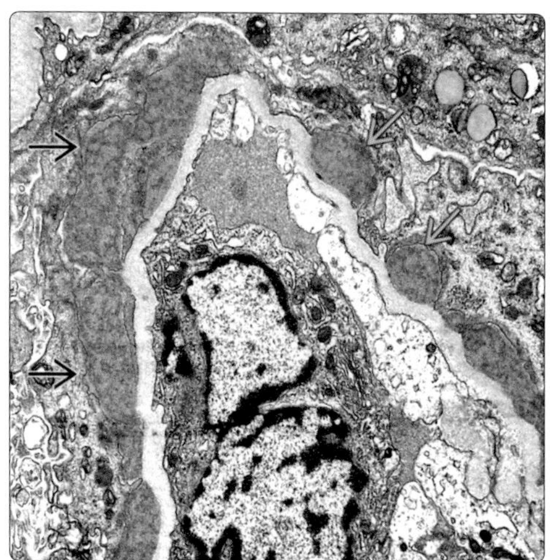

Intramembranous Deposits

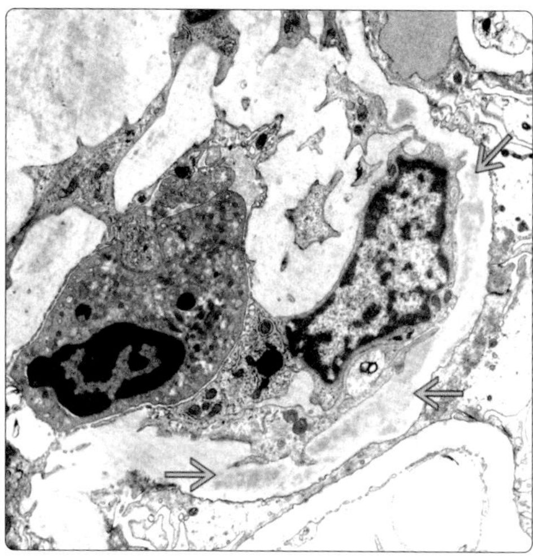

(Left) *EM shows confluent subepithelial deposits ➡ in a 3 year old with PSAGN. Typical "humps" with the same texture are also seen ➡. These deposits have a variegated appearance, which is not unusual.* **(Right)** *Intramembranous dense deposits ➡ are sometimes conspicuous in PSAGN and raise the question of C3 glomerulopathy, including dense deposit disease (DDD). Some patients with PSAGN have dysregulation of the alternative complement pathway and PSAGN can precipitate DDD.*

Acute Glomerulonephritis Superimposed on Diabetic Glomerulopathy

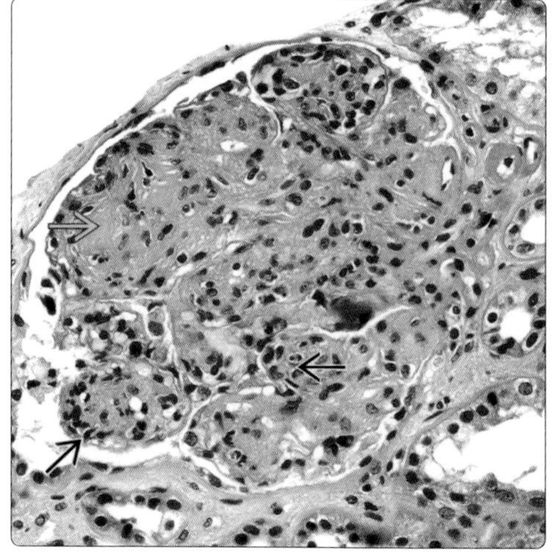

Granular Deposits in AGN Superimposed on Diabetic Glomerulopathy

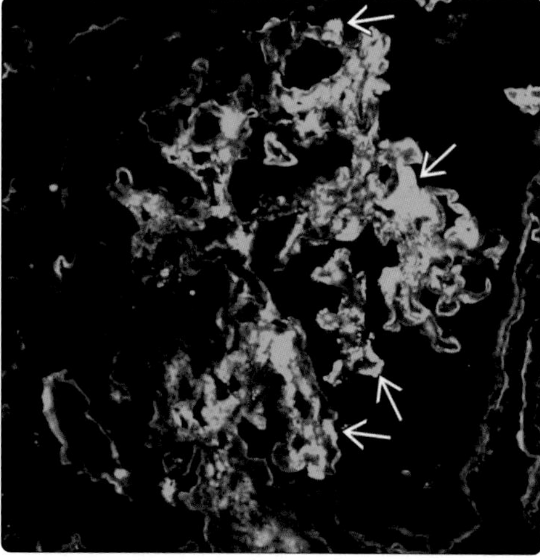

(Left) *Acute postinfectious glomerulonephritis superimposed on diabetic glomerulopathy in a 55 year old is shown. Nodules are evident ➡, but the neutrophils ➡ in capillaries indicate an additional process. This pattern can be associated with staphylococcal or streptococcal infections.* **(Right)** *Sparse granular deposits ➡ of IgG along the GBM are shown in a patient with postinfectious AGN superimposed on nodular diabetic glomerulosclerosis in addition to the linear IgG seen in diabetes. IgA was negative.*

"Humps" in Postinfectious AGN and Diabetes

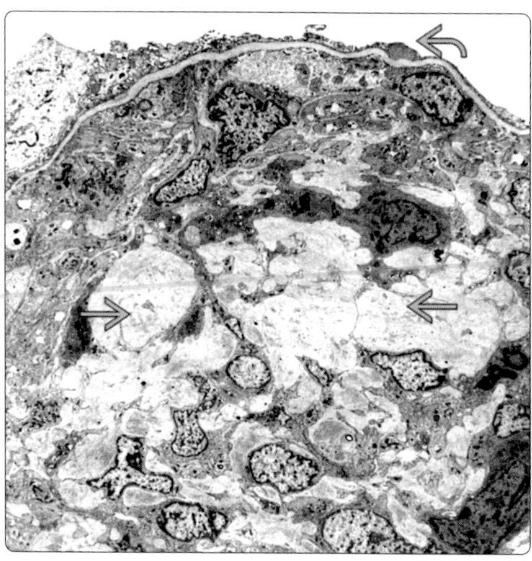

Acute Interstitial Nephritis in PSAGN

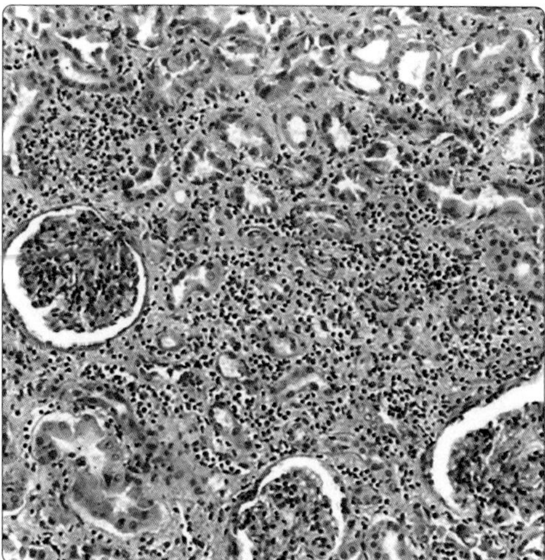

(Left) *Nodular mesangial expansion ➡ and rare "humps" ➡ are present in this diabetic patient with acute glomerulonephritis after a toe infection. The organism in this case was not proved.* **(Right)** *Acute interstitial nephritis (AIN) without significant glomerulonephritis was described in the preantibiotic era. This child died after a streptococcal infection & was reported as a clinicopathologic case in 1929 by Cabot and Mallory. This cannot be distinguished from drug-induced AIN.*

Acute Postinfectious Glomerulonephritis, Nonstreptococcal

KEY FACTS

TERMINOLOGY

- Acute GN occurring after exposure to an infectious agent other than group A *Streptococcus*

ETIOLOGY/PATHOGENESIS

- Called "postinfectious" to differentiate from GN related to chronic infection
- Variety of infections (bacterial, viral, parasitic, mycotic, etc.)
- Infectious Ag/Ab interactions and circulating immune complexes likely play role
- *Staphylococcus* notably appear in elderly

CLINICAL ISSUES

- Hematuria, hypocomplementemia, ± RF, ± cryoglobulins
- Classically described in pediatrics but recently more in elderly
- ~ 90% resolve spontaneously but worse prognosis in elderly

MICROSCOPIC

- Diffuse proliferative, mesangial proliferative, focally proliferative
- Diffuse proliferative form most common and often exudative, with neutrophils
- May be superimposed on diabetic nephropathy

ANCILLARY TESTS

- IF: Scattered fine, large, or chunky deposits along GBM
  - Typically stain with IgG & even more prominently with C3
- EM: Deposits in subepithelial location
  - Have hump-shaped configuration, overlying basement membrane without surrounding GBM reaction

TOP DIFFERENTIAL DIAGNOSES

- IgA nephropathy
- C3 glomerulonephritis
- Dense deposit disease (DDD)
- Membranoproliferative GN (MPGN)

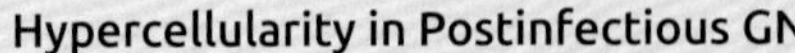

Hypercellularity in Postinfectious GN

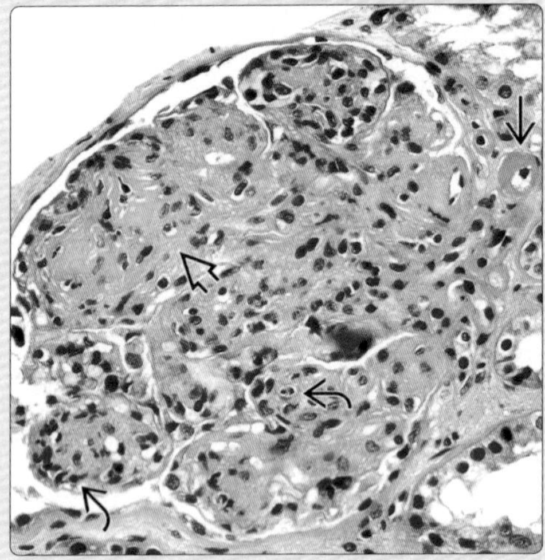

Neutrophils in Postinfectious GN Superimposed on Diabetes

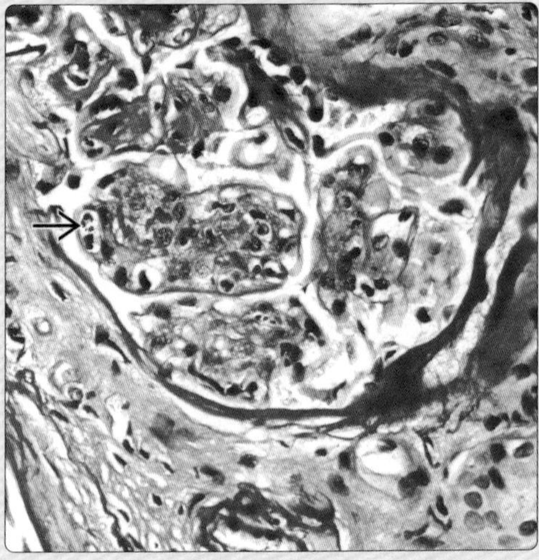

(Left) *In a diabetic with postinfectious GN and a recently infected toe amputation, there is glomerular intracapillary ↑ cellularity, including neutrophils* ➢*, ↑ mesangium* ➢*, and arteriolar hyalinosis* ➢*.* **(Right)** *In a case of diabetic glomerulosclerosis and concurrent postinfectious GN, scattered neutrophils* ➢ *can be seen within glomerular capillary loops. This is an important clue that there is more than just diabetic glomerulopathy.*

Granular Deposits of IgG along GBM

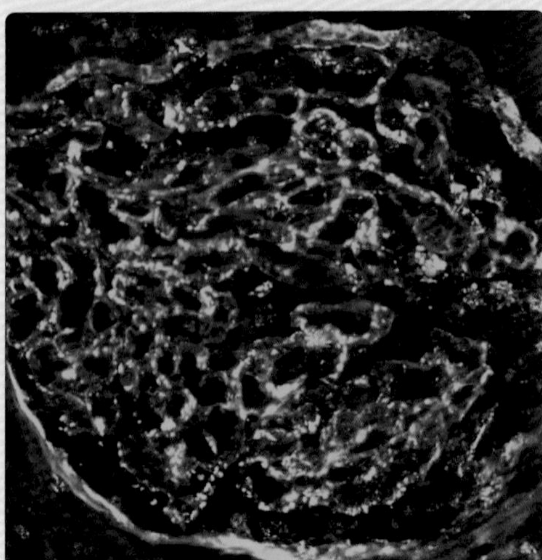

Hump-Like Deposits in Postinfectious GN

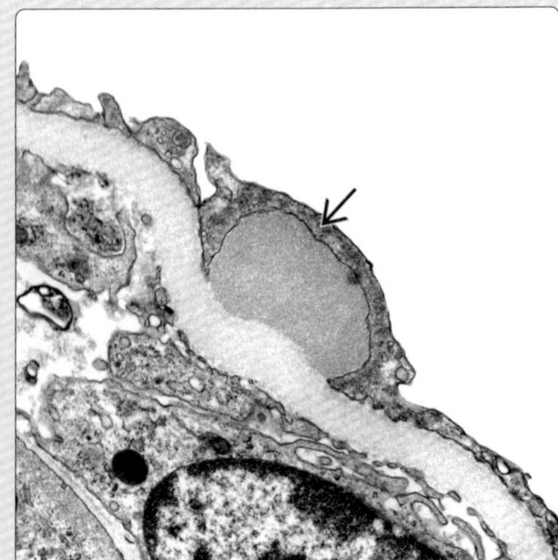

(Left) *Acute postinfectious GN usually has prominent IgG along the GBM corresponding to the humps seen by electron microscopy. Some cases will have C3 dominance similar to C3 glomerulopathy.* **(Right)** *Electron microscopy shows hump-like subepithelial electron-dense deposits* ➢ *scattered along the glomerular basement membrane in postinfectious GN affecting a diabetic patient.*

TERMINOLOGY

Synonyms

- Acute diffuse intracapillary proliferative (exudative) glomerulonephritis (GN)

Definitions

- Acute GN that occurs after exposure to microbe other than group A *Streptococcus*
  - Differentiated from MPGN typical of chronic infections

ETIOLOGY/PATHOGENESIS

Infectious Agents

- Bacteria
  - *Staphylococcus* (coagulase positive and negative)
    - Most common cause in elderly (~ 50%)
  - *Streptococcus pneumoniae* (pneumococcus)
  - Group D *streptococcus*
  - Gram-negative bacilli
    - *Escherichia coli, Pseudomonas, Salmonella, Proteus, Klebsiella*
  - Others
    - *Treponema pallidum, Brucella, Campylobacter, Nocardia, Legionella, Actinobacillus actinomycetem-comitans, Yersinia, Borrelia burgdorferi, Bartonella henselae, Propionibacterium acnes, Mycobacterium*
- Viruses
  - Adenovirus, measles, mumps, coxsackievirus, varicella, Cytomegalovirus, Epstein-Barr, influenza, hepatitis B and C, ECHO, parvovirus B19, vaccina virus, herpes, polyomavirus
- Other
  - Rickettsiae (Q fever [*Coxiella burnetii*]), fungi (*Candida*), parasites (malaria, *Schistosoma*)

Sites of Infection

- Infective endocarditis, lung infections, wound infections, appendix abscesses, osteomyelitis (including mastoiditis), valvular and vascular Dacron prostheses

Pathogenesis

- Microbial antigens demonstrated in glomeruli of some affected patients
  - Believed to be circulating immune complexes that deposit in glomeruli
- Alternatively, antigens may traverse GBM and bind to glomerular sites
- Immunologic activation thought to ensue, stimulating antibody and complement activation

Host Factors

- Alcoholism, diabetes, and intravenous drug use
- Defective regulation of alternative complement pathway documented in a few patients

CLINICAL ISSUES

Epidemiology

- Age
  - Children and young adults classically affected, but recent literature has focused on elderly
    - Most common cause in elderly is *Staphylococcus* (~ 50%)
    - Associated with diabetes and malignancy
- Sex
  - M:F ~ 2:1

Presentation

- Hematuria
  - Acute nephritic syndrome
- Hypertension
- Oliguria
- Hypocomplementemia
  - Described in some, including patients with staphylococcal GN superimposed on diabetic nephropathy

Laboratory Tests

- Circulating immune complexes
  - Disappear when infection treated
- Rheumatoid factor (RF) may be positive
- Cryoglobulins, usually type 3 (mixed)

Treatment

- Surgical approaches
  - Abscesses and other deep-seated infections often surgically treated
- Drugs
  - Antibiotics typically most effective therapy

Prognosis

- ~ 90% of cases resolve in weeks
  - Microhematuria or proteinuria may persist after apparent recovery of renal function
- Less favorable prognosis in adults with ~ 2/3 of patients recovering
  - If infections and GN persist (~ 1/3 of patients), renal failure may require dialysis

MICROSCOPIC

Histologic Features

- Glomeruli
  - Mesangial proliferative, focally proliferative, diffuse proliferative
    - Diffuse, exudative, proliferative GN is most classic pattern of injury
      - Endocapillary proliferation with numerous neutrophils
    - Hump-shaped deposits sometimes seen on silver, trichrome, and toluidine blue stains
    - Crescents in severe cases (up to 33%) and may predict worse prognosis
  - Late changes
    - Glomerulosclerosis 3-15 years from onset on rebiopsy
    - Mesangial hypercellularity and capillary wall thickening may also remain
- Tubules and Interstitium
  - Focal interstitial inflammation
  - Little or no interstitial fibrosis or tubular atrophy unless other cause or chronic infection
- Vessels
  - No specific findings

- Many cases not biopsied; therefore, biopsy findings may overrepresent severe lesions

ANCILLARY TESTS

Immunofluorescence

- Scattered deposits with fine, large, or chunky appearance along GBM
  - Typically stain with IgG and even more prominently with C3
  - Patterns described include starry sky, garland, and mesangial
    - Starry sky and garland patterns reportedly seen early in disease course
    - Mesangial deposits seen later
- IgM and IgA staining absent or minimal, except in recently identified cases of IgA-dominant postinfectious GN
- Concurrent diabetic nephropathy may be present with linear staining for IgG and albumin along GBMs and TBMs

Electron Microscopy

- Deposits in subepithelial location have hump shape and overlying basement membrane without surrounding GBM reaction
  - Numerous deposits or "humps" in acute phase and may be variegated
  - Hump-shaped deposits may be present in subepithelial area overlying mesangium between folds of GBM (a.k.a. "notch" or "waist" area)
    - Notably described by Haas in diabetic patients with postinfectious GN
  - Clinically silent postinfectious GN results in healed, "incidental" postinfectious lesions, indicated by presence of subepithelial deposits by EM
- Occasional mesangial and subendothelial deposits
  - Chronically, mesangial deposits predominate
- Rare, hump-like, subepithelial deposits suggest infectious etiology of immune complex GN
- Duplication of the GBM if present indicates chronic process and most likely infection of longer duration

DIFFERENTIAL DIAGNOSIS

IgA Nephropathy

- Typically predominance of mesangial deposits and absence of well-formed subepithelial hump-like deposits
- Difficult to distinguish IgA nephropathy from postinfectious GN if there is diffuse proliferative GN and unknown history of preceding infection

C3 Glomerulonephritis

- Stain predominantly for C3 with mild or absent immunoglobulin (except for faint IgM or C1q)
- Some cases of postinfectious GN may have a component of C3 glomerulonephritis manifested as abnormal regulation of alternative complement pathway
- Evidence of chronicity (e.g., duplication of the GBM) would be against acute postinfectious GN
- Distribution of deposits more often subendothelial but not very discriminating: Both can have subepithelial deposits

Dense Deposit Disease (DDD)

- Hyperdense intramembranous deposits by EM in GBM and TBM; may be segmental
- Predominance of C3 deposition
  - Postinfectious GN typically has some immunoglobulin

Membranoproliferative GN (MPGN) Related to Infection

- GBM duplication, mesangial matrix expansion, glomerulosclerosis indicative of a chronic process
- Associated with chronic infection (e.g., shunts, abscesses, parasitic diseases)

Systemic Lupus Erythematosus (SLE)

- Physical findings (e.g., rashes and arthralgias)
- Serologies (e.g., ANA, anti- ds-DNA)
- "Full house" immunofluorescence (IgG, IgM, IgA, C1q, and C3)
- Tubuloreticular structures and TBM deposits favor lupus

Cryoglobulinemic GN

- Glomerular capillary hyaline "thrombi"/"pseudothrombi"

DIAGNOSTIC CHECKLIST

Pathologic Interpretation Pearls

- Intracapillary inflammatory cells may provide clue to presence of postinfectious GN in setting of diabetes
- Chronic glomerular changes such as GBM duplication indicate chronic, ongoing process rather than acute GN
- Susceptibility to postinfectious GN may be influenced by underlying abnormalities in alternative complement pathway

SELECTED REFERENCES

1. Alsaad KO et al: Acute diffuse proliferative post-infectious glomerulonephritis in renal allograft–a case report and literature review. Pediatr Transplant. 18(3):E77-82, 2014
2. Stratta P et al: New trends of an old disease: the acute post infectious glomerulonephritis at the beginning of the new millenium. J Nephrol. 27(3):229-39, 2014
3. Nasr SH et al: Bacterial infection-related glomerulonephritis in adults. Kidney Int. 83(5):792-803, 2013
4. Nasr SH et al: Postinfectious glomerulonephritis in the elderly. J Am Soc Nephrol. 22(1):187-95, 2011
5. Wen YK et al: Discrimination between postinfectious IgA-dominant glomerulonephritis and idiopathic IgA nephropathy. Ren Fail. 32(5):572-7, 2010
6. Kanjanabuch T et al: An update on acute postinfectious glomerulonephritis worldwide. Nat Rev Nephrol. 5(5):259-69, 2009
7. Haas M et al: IgA-dominant postinfectious glomerulonephritis: a report of 13 cases with common ultrastructural features. Hum Pathol. 39(9):1309-16, 2008
8. Nasr SH et al: Acute postinfectious glomerulonephritis in the modern era: experience with 86 adults and review of the literature. Medicine (Baltimore). 87(1):21-32, 2008
9. Nasr SH et al: Acute poststaphylococcal glomerulonephritis superimposed on diabetic glomerulosclerosis. Kidney Int. 71(12):1317-21, 2007
10. Haas M: Incidental healed postinfectious glomerulonephritis: a study of 1012 renal biopsy specimens examined by electron microscopy. Hum Pathol. 34(1):3-10, 2003
11. Nasr SH et al: IgA-dominant acute poststaphylococcal glomerulonephritis complicating diabetic nephropathy. Hum Pathol. 34(12):1235-41, 2003

Diabetes With Postinfectious GN and Interstitial Inflammation

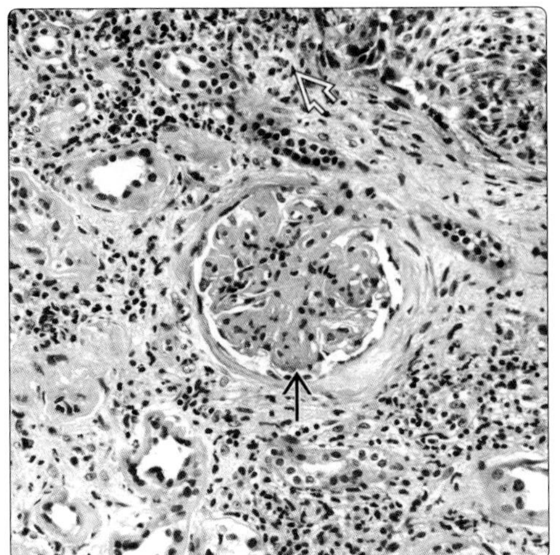

Inflammatory Cells in Postinfectious GN

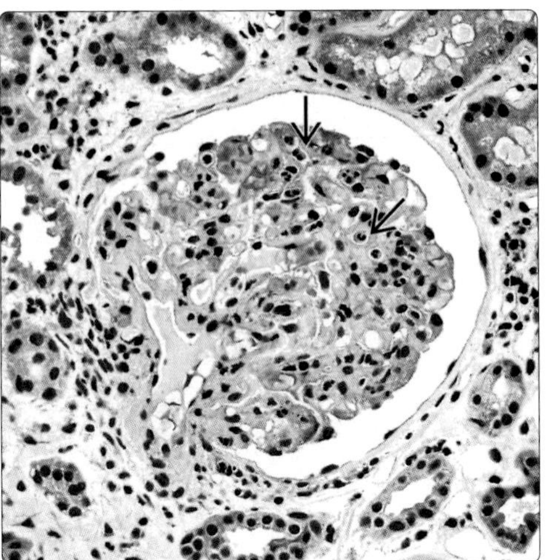

(Left) *A glomerulus displays a nodule → in diabetic glomerulosclerosis concurrently affected by postinfectious GN in a 55-year-old diabetic patient with a history of the recent amputation of an infected toe. The interstitium contains an inflammatory infiltrate, including scattered eosinophils →.* **(Right)** *This glomerulus in a case of postinfectious GN shows hypercellularity, including intracapillary neutrophils →.*

Hypercellularity in Postinfectious GN

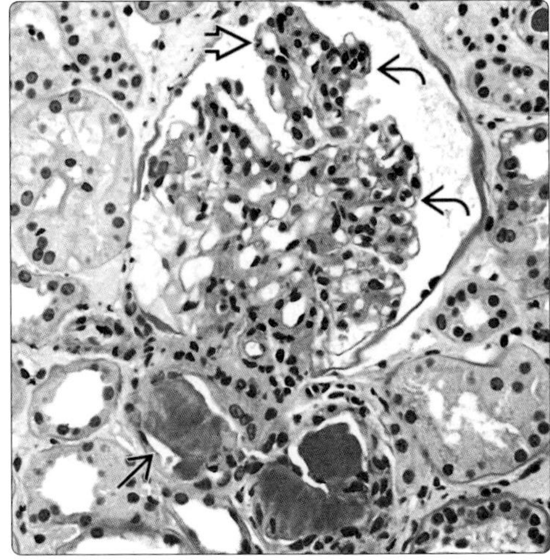

Nodule in Diabetic Glomerulosclerosis Superimposed on Postinfectious GN

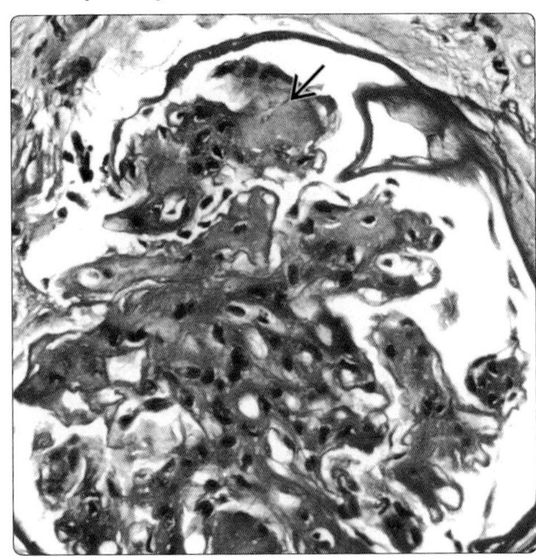

(Left) *In this case of postinfectious GN, the glomerulus appears hypercellular and has vague lobules with glomerular basement membrane thickening → and occasional increases in endocapillary cellularity →. Proteinaceous casts are present in the renal tubules →.* **(Right)** *In this case of diabetic glomerulosclerosis and concurrent postinfectious GN, a glomerular nodule → can be seen.*

Lobules in Postinfectious GN

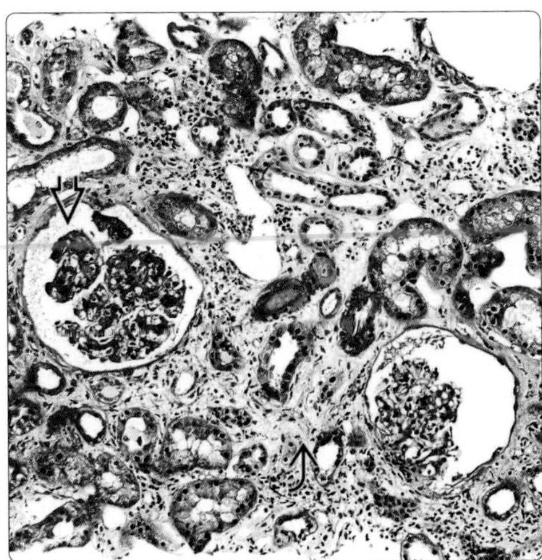

Pigmented Cast in Postinfectious GN

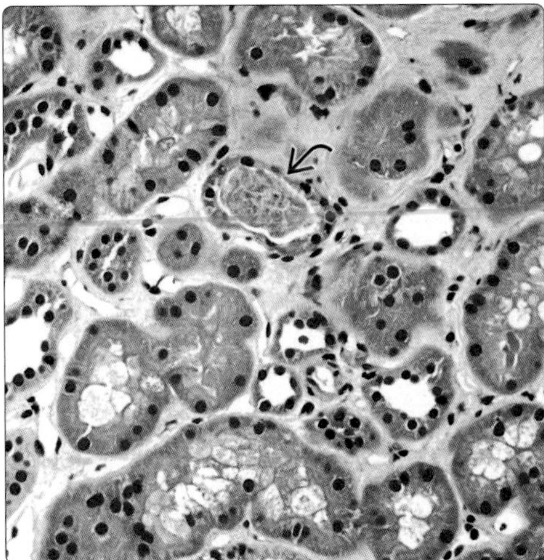

(Left) *In this case of postinfectious GN, the glomeruli appear hypercellular and have vague lobules →. The interstitium is expanded by inflammation, loose fibrosis, and admixed edema →.* **(Right)** *In this case of postinfectious GN, the tubules are injured with tubular epithelial cell flattening → and contain pigmented cast material.*

(Left) *In this case of postinfectious GN, there is prominent granular staining for C3 ➡ in a starry sky pattern.* **(Right)** *In this case of postinfectious GN, there is prominent granular staining for C3 in a lumpy-bumpy pattern ↪.*

"Starry Sky" C3 in Postinfectious GN

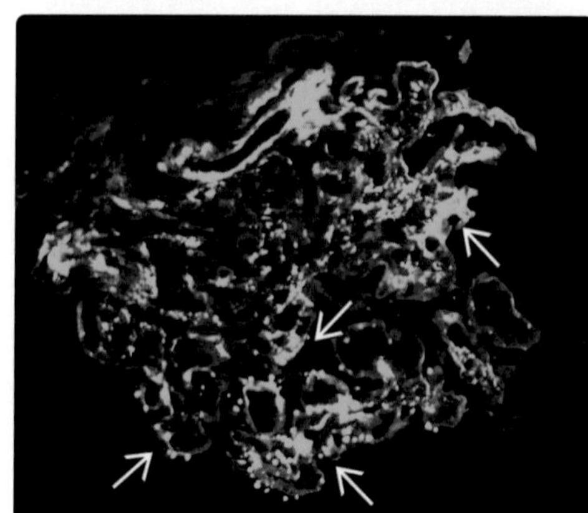

Lumpy-Bumpy C3 in Postinfectious GN

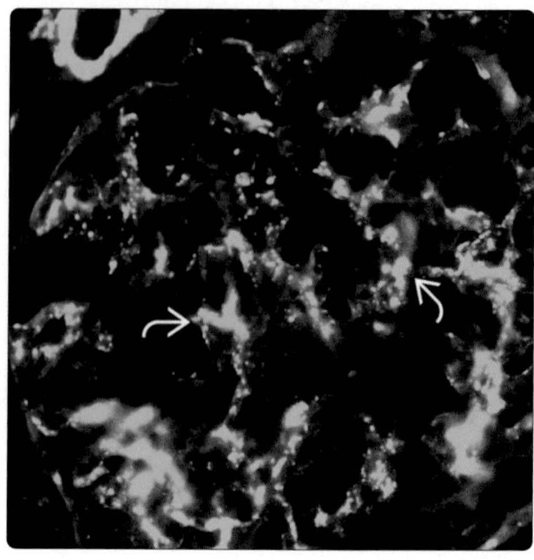

(Left) *In this case of postinfectious GN and concurrent diabetes mellitus, there is staining for IgG along the periphery of glomerular capillary loops ➡ with an absence of staining in the center of glomerular nodules ↪.* **(Right)** *There is staining for C3 along the periphery of glomerular capillary loops ➡ with an absence of staining in the center of glomerular nodules ↪ in postinfectious GN with concurrent diabetes mellitus.*

Granular IgG in Postinfectious GN

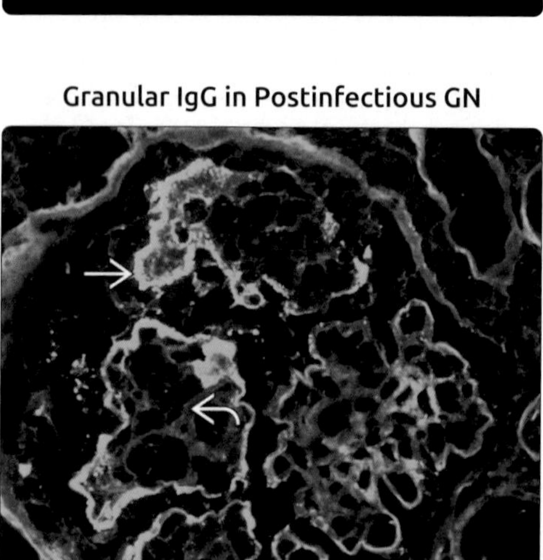

C3 in Postinfectious GN With Concurrent Diabetes

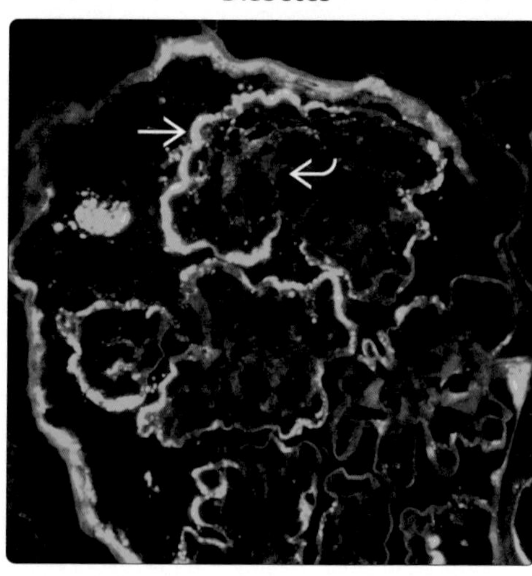

(Left) *In this case of diabetes mellitus with concurrent postinfectious GN, there is broad mesangial staining for fibrin, including in well-formed nodules ↪ with focal intense staining ➡, a finding not associated with nodular type diabetic glomerulosclerosis.* **(Right)** *In diabetes mellitus with concurrent postinfectious GN, there is broad mesangial staining for C3 ➡, which is focally brighter than what would typically be seen in nodular-type diabetic glomerulosclerosis ↪.*

Mesangial Fibrin in Postinfectious GN and Concurrent Diabetes

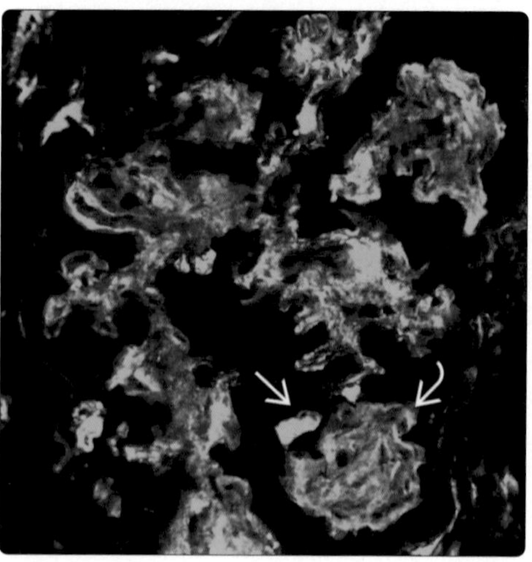

Mesangial C3 in Postinfectious GN

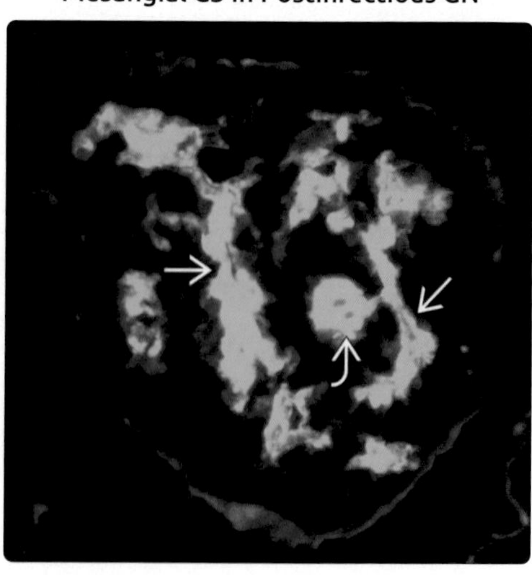

"Notch" Postinfectious Deposits

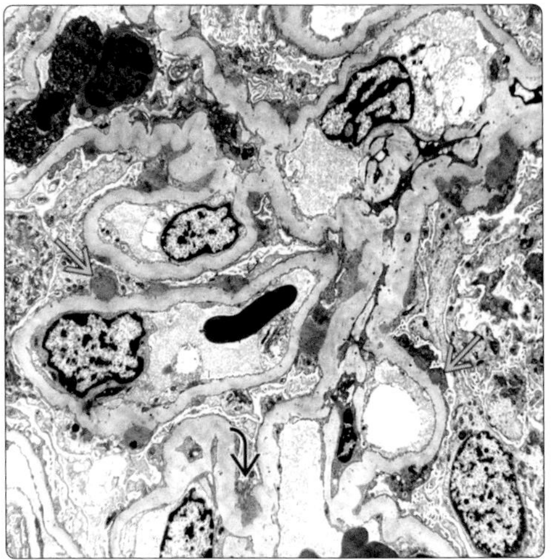

Hump-Like Postinfectious Deposits

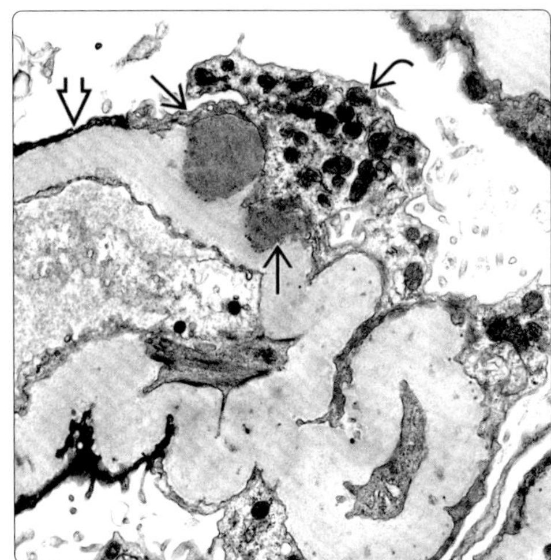

(Left) *By electron microscopy (EM) there are well-formed, subepithelial, hump-like, electron-dense deposits* ⇒ *in a case of postinfectious GN as well as electron-dense deposits* ⇒ *at the reflection (or "notch") of the glomerular basement membrane.* **(Right)** *In this case of postinfectious GN, there are frequent subepithelial, hump-like, electron-dense deposits* ⇒*. Overlying podocytes* ⇒ *that are effaced and reactive contain increased numbers of cytoplasmic organelles* ⇒*.*

"Notch" Deposits in Postinfectious GN

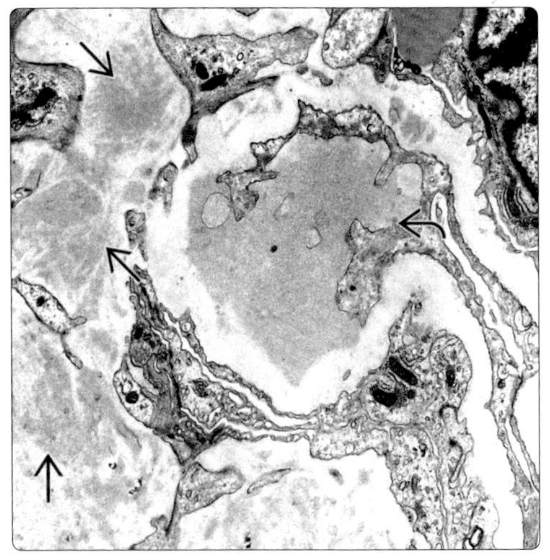

Mesangial Nodule Postinfectious Deposits

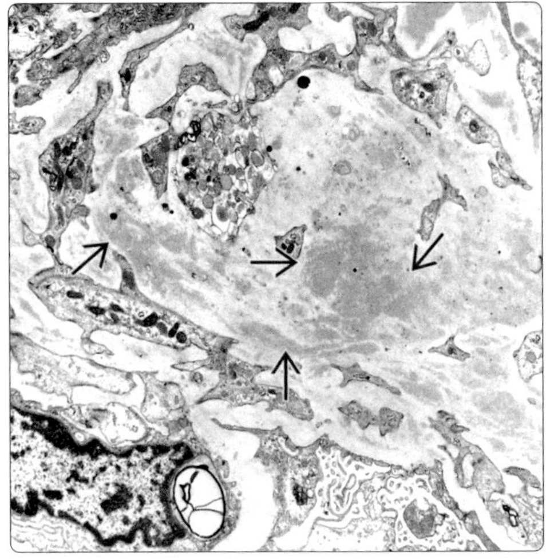

(Left) *In this case of postinfectious GN in a diabetic patient, there are scattered, mesangial, electron-dense deposits* ⇒ *as well as electron-dense subepithelial deposits overlying the mesangium* ⇒ *at a GBM fold in what is referred to as the "notch" region.* **(Right)** *In this case of postinfectious GN and concurrent diabetic glomerulosclerosis, a mesangial nodule of the type in diabetes can be observed containing scattered, electron-dense mesangial deposits* ⇒*, which are not normally seen in diabetic glomerulopathy.*

Hump-Like Postinfectious Deposits

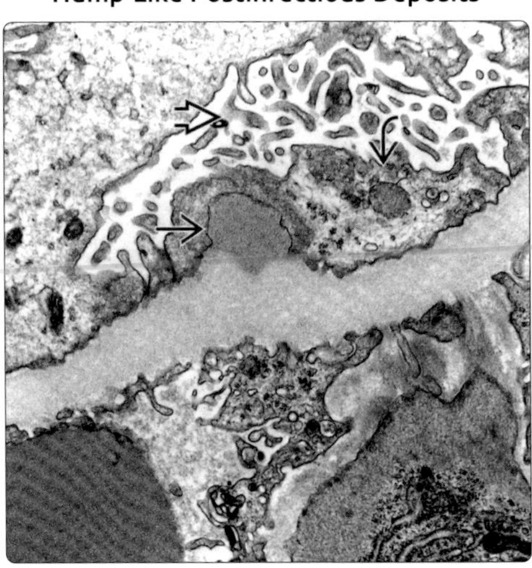

Variegated Subepithelial Deposits

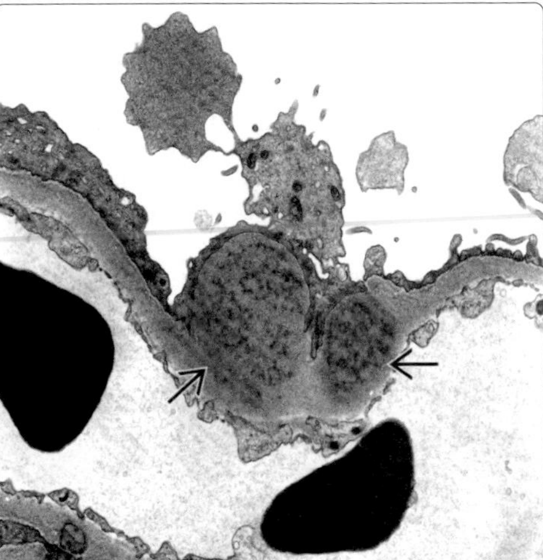

(Left) *In this case of postinfectious GN, there are hump-like, subepithelial, electron-dense immune-type deposits* ⇒*. Podocytes show effacement* ⇒ *and foci of microvillus change* ⇒*.* **(Right)** *In this case of postinfectious GN, there are a couple of subepithelial electron-dense deposits with a vaguely variegated appearance* ⇒ *but without a clear substructure.*

IgA Acute Glomerulonephritis Associated With *Staphylococcus aureus*

KEY FACTS

ETIOLOGY/PATHOGENESIS

- *Staphylococcus aureus*, coagulase positive, often MRSA
- Increased risk with diabetes mellitus, neoplasia, old age
- Occurs during infection, typically of several weeks duration

CLINICAL ISSUES

- Infection, septicemia
- Acute renal failure
- Proteinuria, nephrotic range (20-80%)
- Purpura resembling Henoch-Schönlein purpura in 22%
- ~ 25% of biopsies with acute postinfectious glomerulonephritis (GN)
- Hypocomplementemia in 70%

MICROSCOPIC

- Glomerular involvement varies from mild mesangial hypercellularity to marked acute inflammation with crescents
- Red cell casts common
- Focal interstitial nephritis

ANCILLARY TESTS

- IgA sole, dominant or codominant immunoglobulin, mostly mesangial
  - C3 always present and often > IgA
  - Variable IgG, IgM, C1q
  - Lambda > kappa
- EM deposits primarily mesangial and paramesangial
  - Occasional subendothelial, intramembranous or subepithelial deposits ("humps")
  - "Humps" sometimes have "cups" in contrast to postinfectious GN

TOP DIFFERENTIAL DIAGNOSES

- IgA nephropathy
- Henoch-Schönlein purpura
- Acute glomerulonephritis from other causes

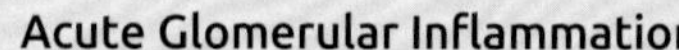

Acute Glomerular Inflammation

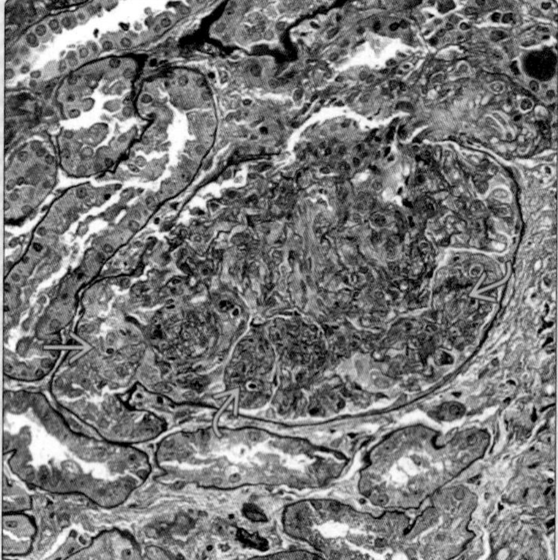

IgA Deposition

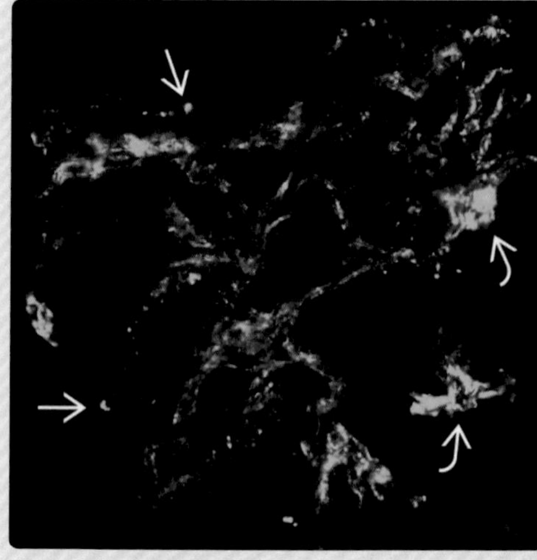

(Left) *S. aureus-associated acute GN has features ranging from mild glomerulitis with occasional neutrophils to proliferative GN with crescents. This glomerulus has endocapillary hypercellularity with loss of patency of capillary loops. Epithelial proliferation is present that is probably a nascent crescent.* **(Right)** *IgA deposition is principally in the mesangium, similar to IgA nephropathy and HSP. Punctate deposits along the GBM correspond to subepithelial "humps".*

Mesangial Deposits

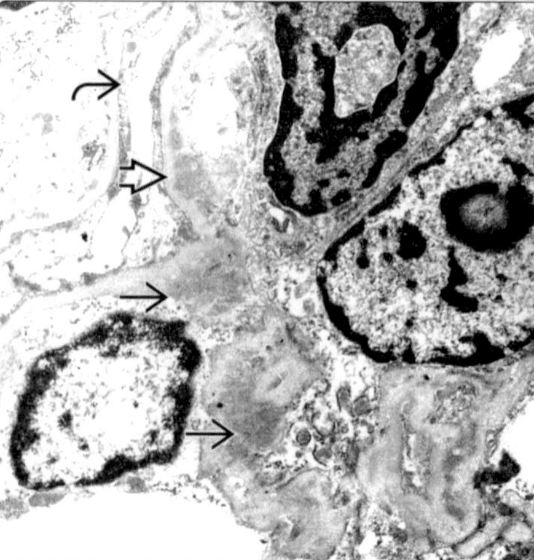

Subepithelial "Humps"

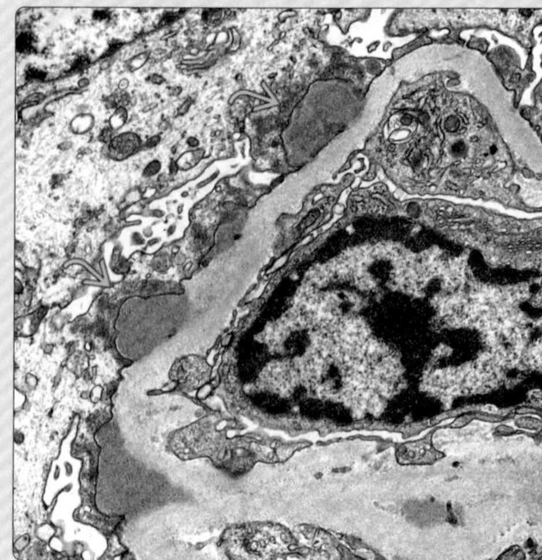

(Left) *The amorphous, electron-dense deposits are primarily in the mesangium in S. aureus-associated acute glomerulonephritis (AGN). Some are paramesangial, as in idiopathic IgA nephropathy. Podocyte foot processes show extensive effacement.* **(Right)** *Subepithelial "humps" are often seen in IgA dominant acute glomerulonephritis associated with S. aureus. This patient had diabetes and an methicillin-resistant Staphylococcus aureus (MRSA) infection of a vertebral disc.*

IgA Acute Glomerulonephritis Associated With *Staphylococcus aureus*

TERMINOLOGY

Definitions

- IgA dominant acute glomerulonephritis (GN) due to *Staphylococcus aureus* infection

ETIOLOGY/PATHOGENESIS

Infectious Agents

- *S. aureus*, coagulase positive, often methicillin resistant (MRSA)
  - Osteomyelitis, pneumonia, septic arthritis, discitis, soft tissue abscess, empyema, sinusitis, endocarditis, septicemia
  - Occurs **during** infection (not postinfectious)
    - Average duration of infection 5 weeks
- Rarely *Staphylococcus epidermidis*

Host Factors

- Diabetes mellitus, neoplasia, old age, alcoholism

Immune Response

- IgA antibodies to *S. aureus* cell membrane antigen
- *S. aureus* enterotoxins may act as superantigens, stimulating T cells leading to polyclonal B-cell activation
- SSL7 protein binds Fc of IgA, blocking FcR activity

CLINICAL ISSUES

Presentation

- Acute renal failure
- Proteinuria, nephrotic range (20-80%)
- Hematuria
- Hypertension
- Hypocomplementemia (70%)
- Lower extremity rash mimics Henoch-Schönlein purpura (HSP) (22%)

Treatment

- Antibiotics and renal support
- Anecdotal reports of steroids/immunosuppression

Prognosis

- Recovery possible if infection successfully treated
- Range from complete recovery to end-stage renal disease (ESRD)
  - Underlying disease and age are important factors

Prevalence

- ~ 25% of renal biopsies with postinfectious acute glomerulonephritis (AGN)

MICROSCOPIC

Histologic Features

- Glomerulus
  - Varies from mild mesangial hypercellularity to marked acute inflammation with crescents
  - Leukocytes in capillaries
    - Neutrophils and mononuclear cells
    - Usually not prominent
  - Mesangial hypercellularity
  - Normal glomerular basement membrane (GBM)
  - Rare "pseudothrombi" due to cryoglobulins
- Tubules
  - Red cell casts common
  - May be active inflammation and tubular damage
- Interstitium
  - Focal interstitial mononuclear cells and scattered neutrophils and eosinophils
- Vessels:
  - Skin may have vasculitis if HSP-like rash

ANCILLARY TESTS

Immunofluorescence

- IgA sole (~ 50%) dominant (44%), or codominant (6%) immunoglobulin, mostly mesangial
  - Lambda > kappa in majority, similar to IgA nephropathy
  - Rarely *S. aureus* GN has absent IgA or pauci-immune
- IgG present ~ 50%; IgM usually not conspicuous
- C3 present (~ 100%) and often brighter than IgA
- C1q positive in ~ 16%
- *S. aureus* cell envelope antigen reported in 68%

Electron Microscopy

- Amorphous, electron-dense deposits
  - Primarily mesangial and paramesangial
  - Occasional subepithelial deposits
    - In contrast with postinfectious GN, "humps" may have "cupping" reaction
  - Occasional subendothelial and intramembranous deposits
- Foot process effacement

DIFFERENTIAL DIAGNOSIS

IgA Nephropathy

- Chronic disease (vs. acute onset)
- Normal complement levels

Henoch-Schönlein Purpura

- Absence of staphylococcal infection
- Not associated with old age or diabetes
- More often crescents

Acute Glomerulonephritis From Other Causes

- IgA dominance in some cases related to *Streptococcus* and gram-negative organisms

DIAGNOSTIC CHECKLIST

Pathologic Interpretation Pearls

- "Humps" sometimes have "cups" in contrast to poststreptococcal GN

SELECTED REFERENCES

1. Stratta P et al: New trends of an old disease: the acute post infectious glomerulonephritis at the beginning of the new millenium. J Nephrol. 27(3):229-39, 2014
2. Satoskar AA et al: Henoch-Schönlein purpura-like presentation in IgA-dominant Staphylococcus infection - associated glomerulonephritis - a diagnostic pitfall. Clin Nephrol. 79(4):302-12, 2013
3. Nasr SH et al: IgA-dominant postinfectious glomerulonephritis: a new twist on an old disease. Nephron Clin Pract. 119(1):c18-25; discussion c26, 2011
4. Nasr SH et al: Acute postinfectious glomerulonephritis in the modern era: experience with 86 adults and review of the literature. Medicine (Baltimore). 87(1):21-32, 2008

IgA Acute Glomerulonephritis Associated With *Staphylococcus aureus*

Mesangial Hypercellularity and Red Cell Casts

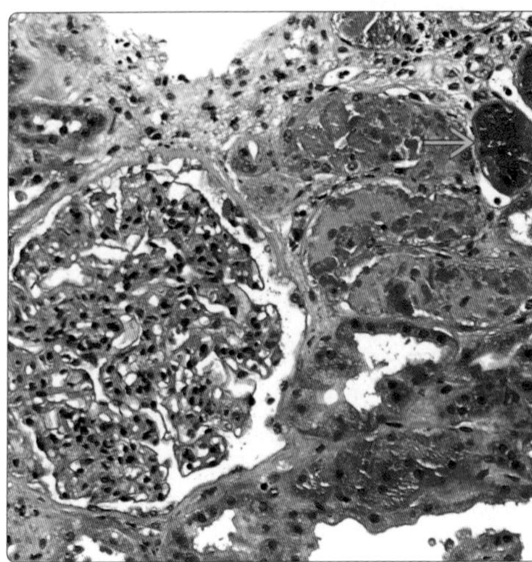

Mesangial Hypercellularity and Mild Interstitial Nephritis

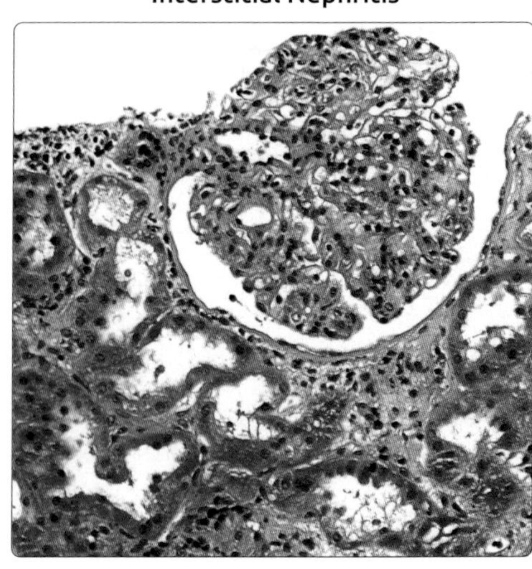

(Left) *Glomerular mesangial hypercellularity is prominent in this case of S. aureus-associated IgA GN. Red cell casts ➔ are frequent.* **(Right)** *Glomerulitis and mesangial hypercellularity are present in S. aureus glomerulonephritis associated with IgA deposits. A mild interstitial nephritis is also evident with occasional neutrophils and eosinophils.*

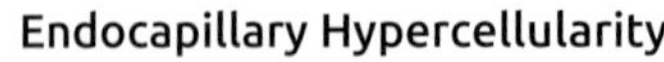

Endocapillary Hypercellularity

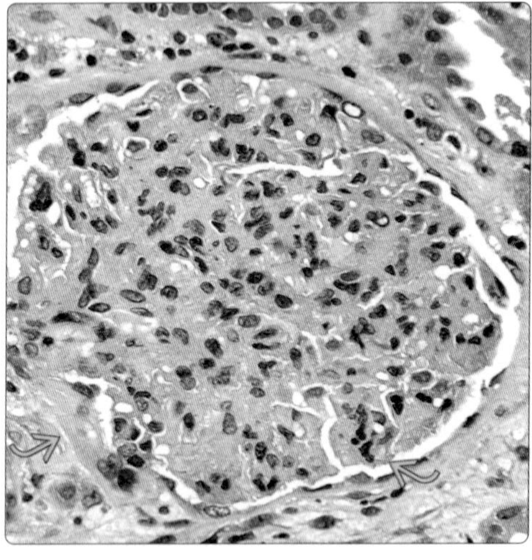

Mesangial IgA

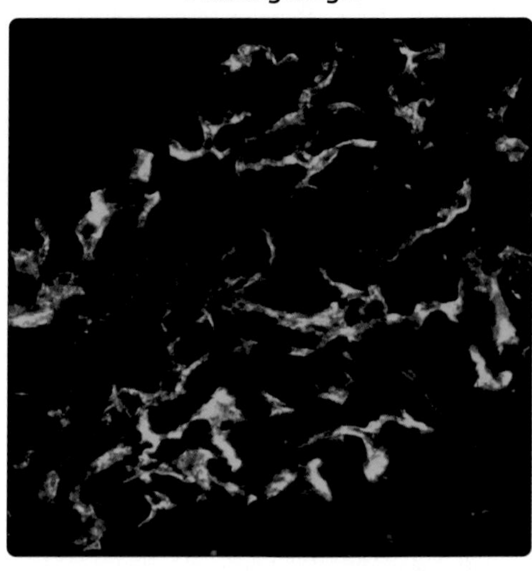

(Left) *Mesangial and endocapillary hypercellularity ➔ are evident with loss of patent capillaries in this diabetic patient who had S. aureus infection of vertebral disc.* **(Right)** *AGN associated with S. aureus infection typically has prominent mesangial IgA deposits, which resemble IgA nephropathy or HSP.*

Mesangial IgG

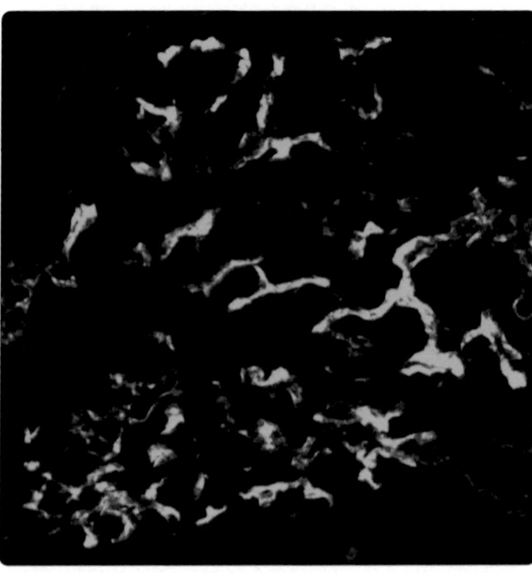

Lambda Light Chain Predominant

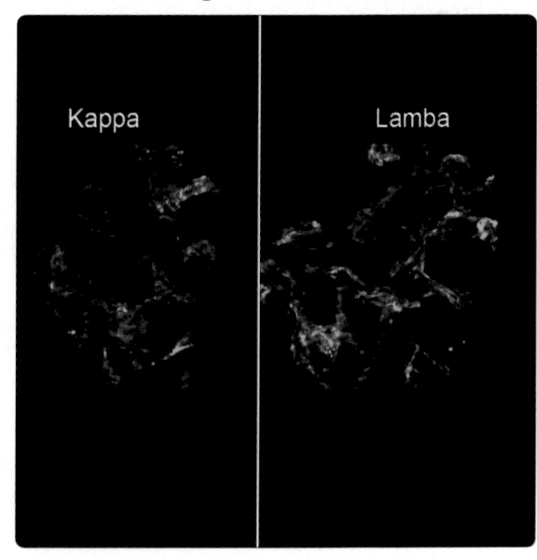

(Left) *IgG with a predominately mesangial pattern commonly accompanies IgA in S. aureus-associated AGN. The differential diagnosis includes idiopathic IgA nephropathy, HSP, and lupus nephritis.* **(Right)** *Lambda light chain is typically more prominent than kappa in IgA dominant AGN, similar to IgA nephropathy and HSP, however both are present.*

Mesangial C3

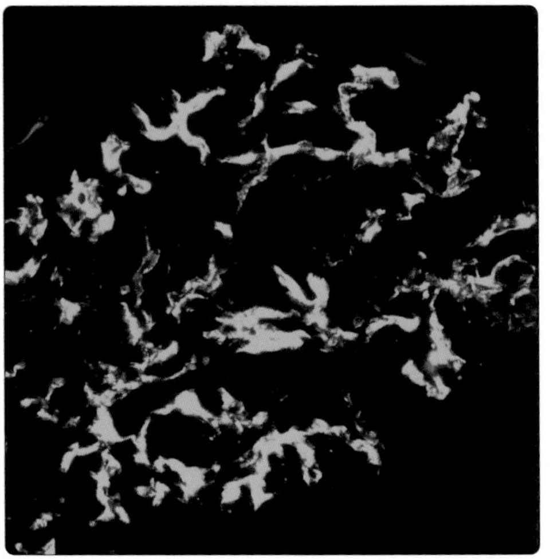

Mesangial C1q

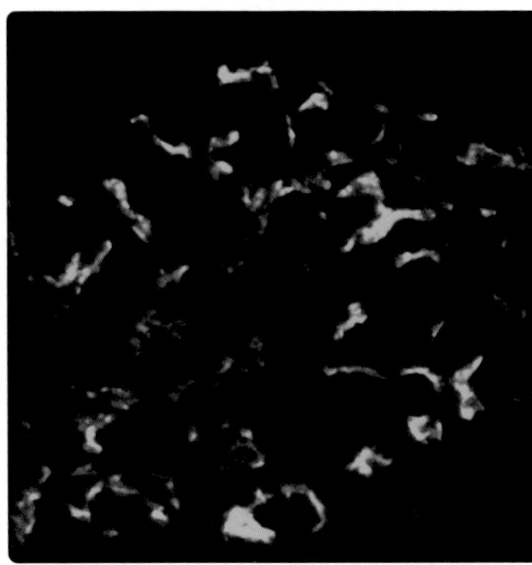

(Left) *AGN associated with S. aureus septicemia and probably vertebral osteomyelitis is shown. Prominent C3 is present primarily in the mesangium and was accompanied by IgA and IgG. C3 is usually more intense than IgA in this condition, in contrast to IgA nephropathy.* **(Right)** *C1q is present in ~ 16% of S. aureus-associated AGN, somewhat more often than in IgA nephropathy (6-10%). If C1q is prominent, a diagnosis of lupus should be considered.*

Mesangial Deposits

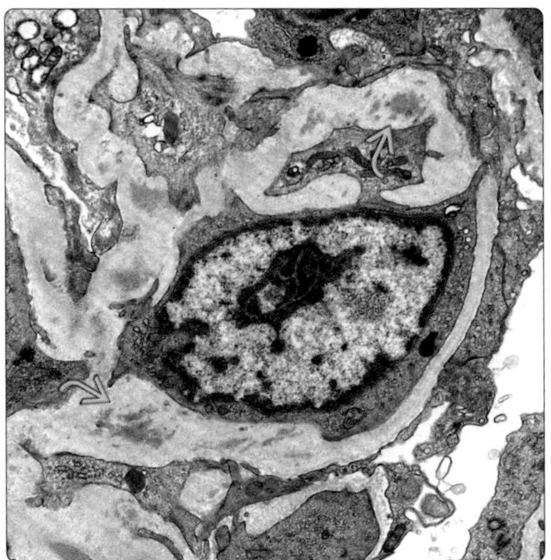

Intramembranous and Subepithelial Deposits

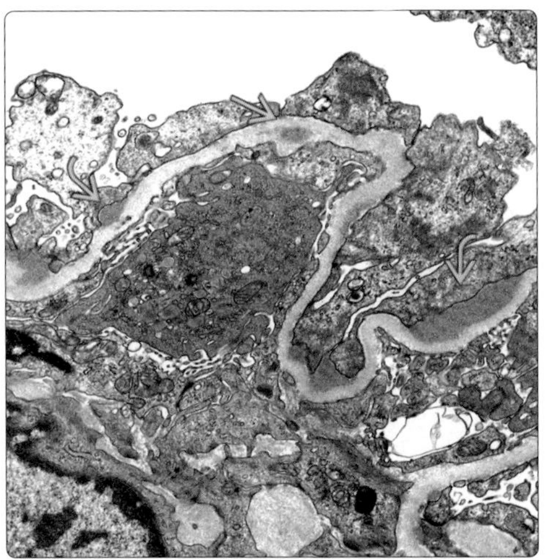

(Left) *Amorphous mesangial deposits ➔ are diffusely present in IgA dominant AGN associated with S. aureus. This patient had diabetes and S. aureus infection of a vertebral disc.* **(Right)** *Intramembranous ➔ and subepithelial ➔ "humps" are often seen in IgA-dominant AGN associated with S. aureus. These findings are seen in other AGN-related to other infections.*

Subepithelial Deposit

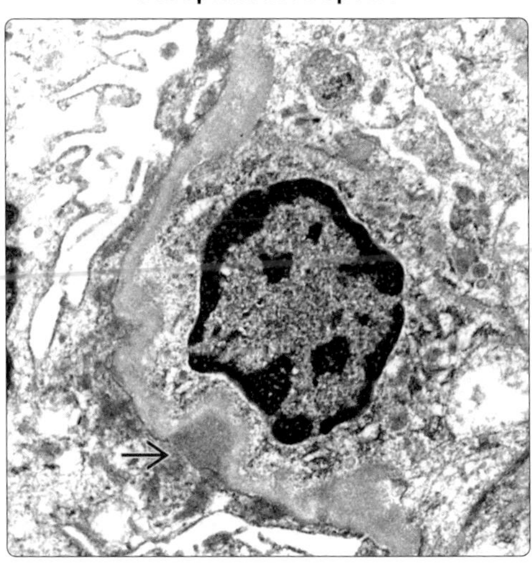

Subepithelial Deposit With Cupping

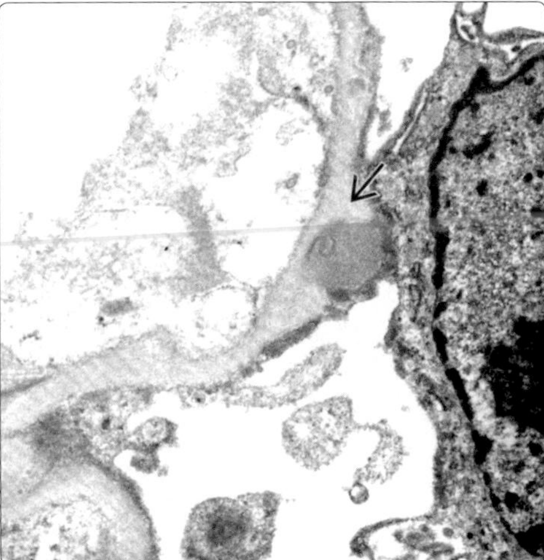

(Left) *Subepithelial deposits are found in S. aureus-associated AGN, but they may not form typical "humps" ➔. Subepithelial deposits also occur sporadically in idiopathic IgA nephropathy.* **(Right)** *Subepithelial deposits can be sometimes found in S. aureus-associated AGN, but they may not form typical "humps." "Humps" in poststreptococcal GN do not have surrounding "spikes" or "cups" of basement membrane as this case does ➔. This pattern has been described as "ball-in-cup" and is also seen in HIV-associated immune complex disease.*

Glomerulonephritis of Chronic Infection Including Shunt Nephritis

KEY FACTS

TERMINOLOGY

- Chronic visceral infection glomerulonephritis (CVI-GN)/shunt nephritis (SN): GN from bacterial infection of cerebrospinal shunts or visceral abscess
- Ventriculoatrial (VA), ventriculojugular (VJ), and less common ventriculoperitoneal (VP) shunts

ETIOLOGY/PATHOGENESIS

- SN: Mostly *Staphylococcus epidermidis* (75% of cases) & *S. albus*
- Chronic visceral infection (abscess): *Staphylococcus aureus* most common pathogen

CLINICAL ISSUES

- Proteinuria/hematuria, acute or chronic renal failure, ↓ complement
- Fever, malaise, arthralgias, purpura
- Treatment: Removal of shunt, drainage of abscess, antibiotics

MICROSCOPIC

- 3 major glomerular patterns
  - MPGN, type 1 with GBM duplication
  - Focal/diffuse proliferative GN &/or mesangial proliferation
  - Crescentic GN (particularly in visceral abscesses)
- Immunofluorescence microscopy
  - Deposits band-like or granular
  - SN: C3 in > 90%; IgM & IgG in > 60%
  - Visceral abscess: C3 in 100%; IgM & IgG negative in 67%
- Electron microscopy
  - Mesangial & subendothelial immune complex deposits
  - GBM duplication with mesangial cell interposition

TOP DIFFERENTIAL DIAGNOSES

- Cryoglobulinemic GN (HCV)
- MPGN, type I

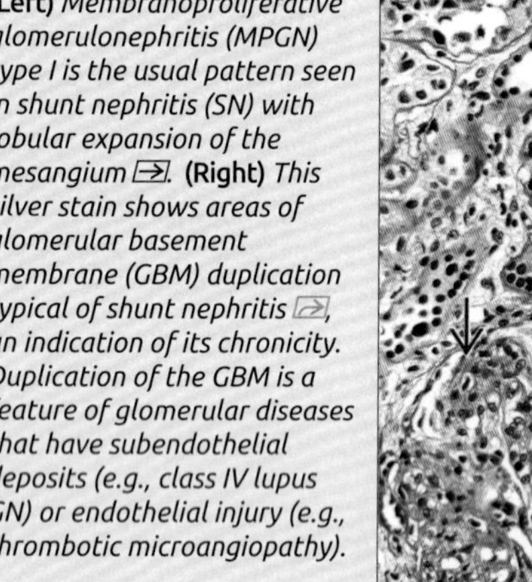

(Left) *Membranoproliferative glomerulonephritis (MPGN) type I is the usual pattern seen in shunt nephritis (SN) with lobular expansion of the mesangium.* **(Right)** *This silver stain shows areas of glomerular basement membrane (GBM) duplication typical of shunt nephritis, an indication of its chronicity. Duplication of the GBM is a feature of glomerular diseases that have subendothelial deposits (e.g., class IV lupus GN) or endothelial injury (e.g., thrombotic microangiopathy).*

Membranoproliferative Glomerulonephritis

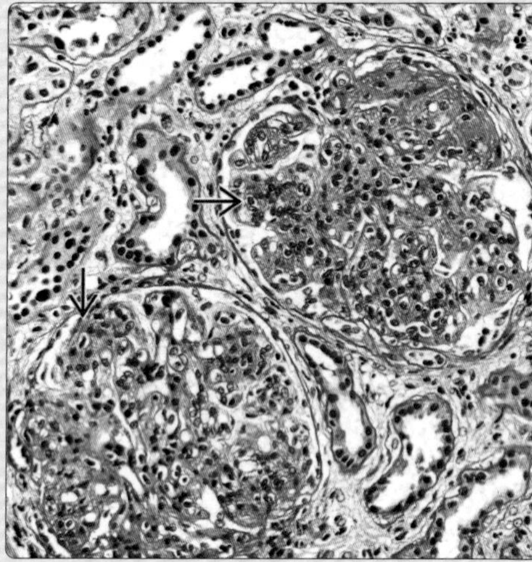

Duplication of the GBM and Mesangial Expansion

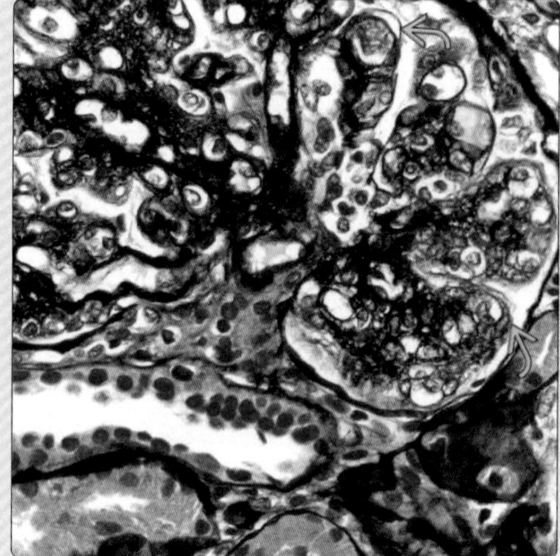

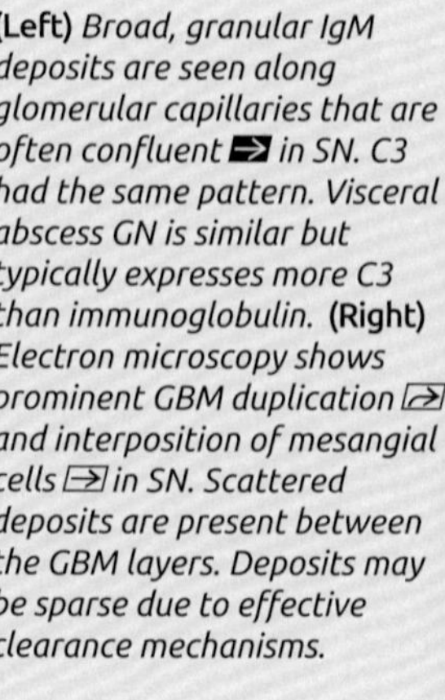

(Left) *Broad, granular IgM deposits are seen along glomerular capillaries that are often confluent in SN. C3 had the same pattern. Visceral abscess GN is similar but typically expresses more C3 than immunoglobulin.* **(Right)** *Electron microscopy shows prominent GBM duplication and interposition of mesangial cells in SN. Scattered deposits are present between the GBM layers. Deposits may be sparse due to effective clearance mechanisms.*

IgM Deposition

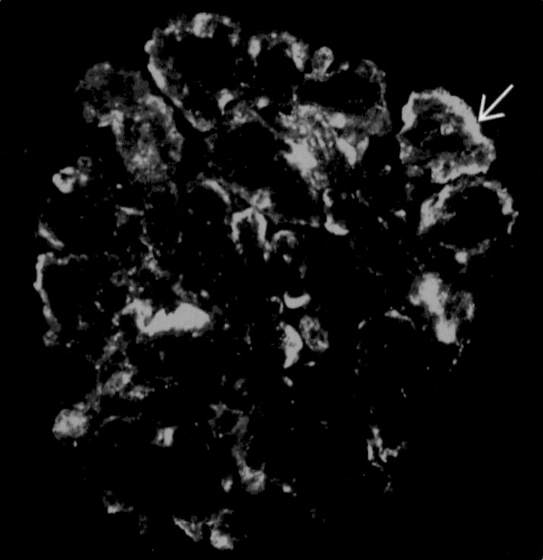

GBM Duplication and Deposits

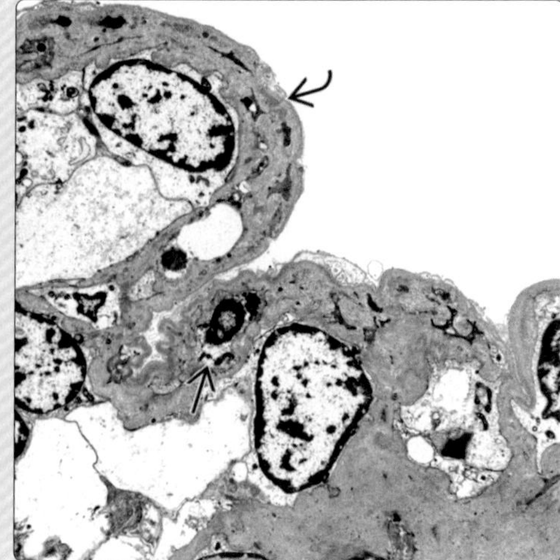

TERMINOLOGY

Definitions

- GN from chronic bacterial infection of cerebrospinal fluid (CSF) shunt, or visceral abscess

ETIOLOGY/PATHOGENESIS

Infectious Agents

- Shunt nephritis (SN)
  - Cerebral ventricle CSF shunt to atrium, jugular vein or peritoneum
  - Bacteria adhere to plastic shunt and form biofilm, protecting them from antibiotics and immune system
    - Low-grade bacteremia in 4-5% of patients
  - Typically low virulence bacteria
    - *Staphylococcus epidermidis* (75% of all cases)
    - Less often: *Staphylococcus albus*, *Acinetobacter*, *Bacillus*, *Corynebacterium*, *Listeria*, *Propionibacterium*, *Pseudomonas*, *Peptococcus*, and *Micrococcus*
- Glomerulonephritis of CVI-GN
  - Visceral abscesses: Lung, rectum, appendix, septic abortion
  - Bone (osteomyelitis), subcutaneous, periodontal abscesses
  - Prostheses: Valvular, vascular, other
  - Vascular device-associated infection (e.g., injection reservoirs, indwelling catheters)
  - *S. aureus* most common pathogen

Chronic Immune Complex GN

- Shedding of bacterial antigens, not bacteria
- Trigger low-grade, persistent inflammation

CLINICAL ISSUES

Presentation

- Proteinuria, hematuria seen in virtually all cases
  - Nephrotic syndrome ~ 25%
- Acute or chronic renal failure
- Usually signs of infection: Fever, malaise, arthralgias, anemia, hepatosplenomegaly
- May have purpura, if cryoglobulinemia
- Symptoms related to increased intracranial pressure (SN) or visceral abscess
- Donor kidney with SN has been transplanted with reversal in SN

Laboratory Tests

- Often hypocomplementemia (↓ C3 & C4), cryoglobulinemia, rheumatoid factor
- Hypergammaglobulinemia: IgM and variably IgG
- ↑ C-reactive protein (CRP)
- Occasional cases with positive ANA or ANCA (proteinase 3)

Treatment

- Removal of shunt, drainage of abscess, antibiotics

Prognosis

- Most recover with treatment of shunt infection
  - ~ 25% develop end-stage renal disease (ESRD) or die from complications
  - ~ 25% have persistent proteinuria and azotemia

MICROSCOPIC

Histologic Features

- SN: 3 patterns
  - Membranoproliferative GN (MPGN), mostly type I; > 60%
  - Global glomerular endocapillary hypercellularity (~ 33%)
    - < 10% exclusively mesangial proliferation without GBM thickening
  - Crescents & necrosis apparently uncommon
- Visceral abscess
  - 3 patterns
    - Diffuse, MPGN-like in ~ 33%
    - Focal or isolated mesangial proliferation in ~ 33%
    - Pure extracapillary proliferation (crescents) in ~ 33%
  - Crescents common (~ 75%); glomerular necrosis common (~ 65%)
- Biopsy after infection resolution
  - Mild residual hypercellularity, fibrous crescents, global sclerosis
  - Deposits disappear by EM and IF

ANCILLARY TESTS

Immunofluorescence

- Band-like or granular along GBM &/or mesangium
- Immunoglobulins more prominent in SN than in visceral infections
  - SN: IgM (> 80%) > IgG (~ 67%) > IgA
  - Visceral abscess: IgM, IgG, IgA negative in ~ 67%
- C3 prominent in > 90% of visceral abscess cases and SN
  - SN has C1q & C4 (25-33%)

Electron Microscopy

- Mesangial and subendothelial deposits most common as well as hump-like deposits in minority
- Mesangial interposition with new GBM formation
- Focal podocyte foot process effacement

DIFFERENTIAL DIAGNOSIS

MPGN, Type I

- Pathologically similar; distinguished by presence of chronic infection

Cryoglobulinemic GN

- Morphology similar to SN but has intraluminal PAS(+) "pseudothrombi"
- Often associated with hepatitis C virus (HCV)

Portosystemic Shunt-Associated GN

- IgA-dominant MPGN vs. IgM dominance in SN

SELECTED REFERENCES

1. Burström G et al: Subacute bacterial endocarditis and subsequent shunt nephritis from ventriculoatrial shunting 14years after shunt implantation. BMJ Case Rep. 2014, 2014
2. Franchi-Abella S et al: Complications of congenital portosystemic shunts in children: therapeutic options and outcomes. J Pediatr Gastroenterol Nutr. 51(3):322-30, 2010
3. Haffner D et al: The clinical spectrum of shunt nephritis. Nephrol Dial Transplant. 12(6):1143-8, 1997

Endocarditis

KEY FACTS

TERMINOLOGY

- Glomerulonephritis (GN) following infection of heart valves

ETIOLOGY/PATHOGENESIS

- Subacute bacterial endocarditis (SBE)
  - e.g., *Streptococcus viridans* infecting rheumatic heart
- Acute bacterial endocarditis (ABE)
  - e.g., *Staphylococcus aureus* infecting previously normal heart, as in intravenous drug abuser

CLINICAL ISSUES

- Hematuria and proteinuria
- Renal dysfunction: ↑ blood urea nitrogen (BUN) and creatinine (mostly with diffuse GN)
- Hypocomplementemia
- Antineutrophil cytoplasmic antibody (ANCA) positivity has been described

MICROSCOPIC

- Diffuse or focal proliferative GN ~ 50%
  - Necrotizing and crescentic GN can be seen
  - Neutrophils and nuclear fragments in glomeruli
- Membranoproliferative glomerulonephritis (MPGN), type I pattern ~ 50%
  - Lobular mesangial hypercellularity, duplicated glomerular basement membrane (GBM)
- IF: Usually IgG, IgM, and C3 (subendothelial and mesangial); sometimes IgA
- EM: Mesangial and subendothelial amorphous deposits

TOP DIFFERENTIAL DIAGNOSES

- Postinfectious GN, other site
- MPGN, type I
- Lupus nephritis
- ANCA-related GN
- IgA nephropathy

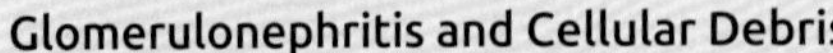

Glomerulonephritis and Cellular Debris

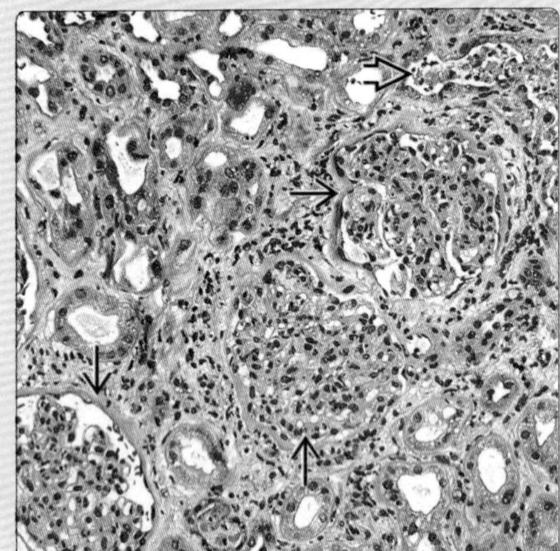

Cellular Crescent

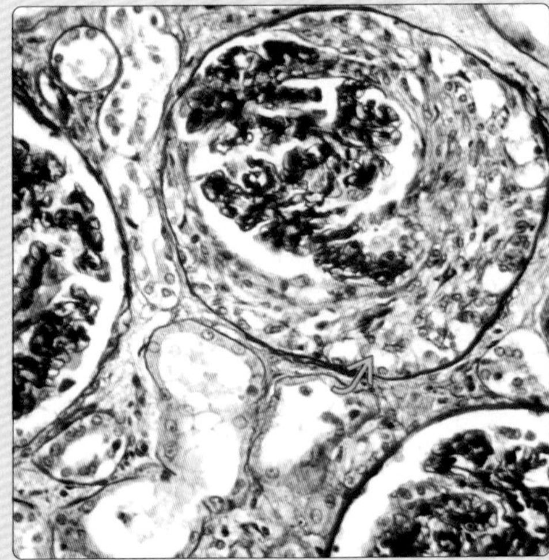

(Left) *Renal biopsy from a 68-year-old man with staphylococcal endocarditis shows necrotic cellular debris ➡ and hypercellular glomeruli ➡.* **(Right)** *Cellular crescent ➡ is shown in a patient who died with nongroupable, nonhemolytic streptococcal infection of a calcified aortic valve. ANCA reactivity has been associated with some cases of endocarditis and may augment the glomerular inflammatory injury.*

Granular Deposits of C3

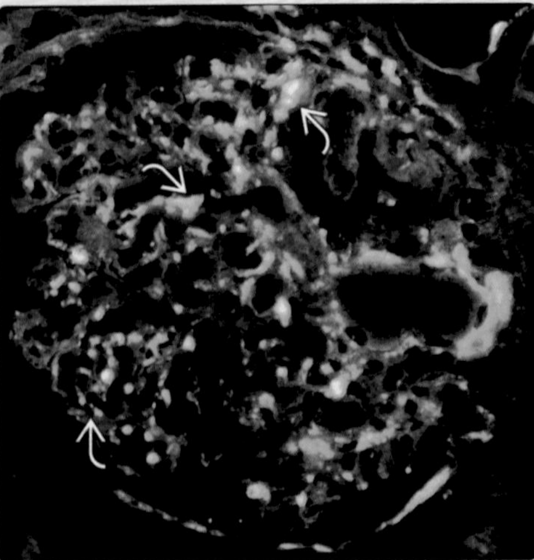

Subepithelial Hump

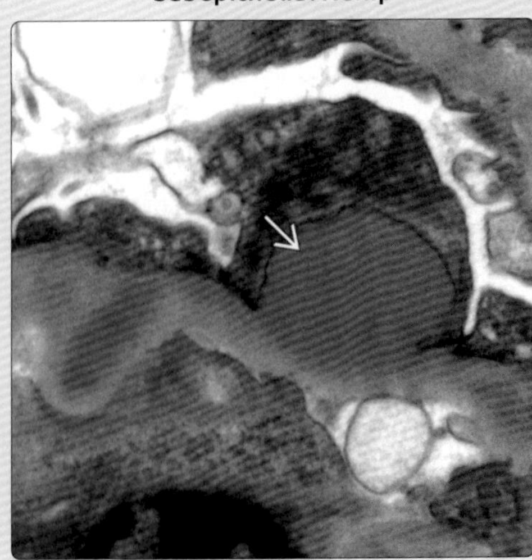

(Left) *Immunofluorescence of C3 shows granular positivity ➡ in a 68-year-old man with staphylococcal endocarditis.* **(Right)** *Electron microscopy of a renal biopsy from a 68-year-old man with a history of staphylococcal endocarditis shows a well-formed, subepithelial, electron-dense deposit (hump) ➡.*

TERMINOLOGY

Abbreviations

- Subacute bacterial endocarditis (SBE)
- Acute bacterial endocarditis (ABE)

Synonyms

- Embolic nonsuppurative focal nephritis
- Focal embolic nephritis
- Focal and segmental proliferative, necrotizing, or sclerosing glomerulonephritis (GN)

Definitions

- GN following infection of heart valves (i.e., endocarditis)

ETIOLOGY/PATHOGENESIS

Infectious Agents

- SBE: *Streptococcus viridans* group bacteria infecting rheumatic heart (classic example) and others
  - Coagulase-negative staphylococci, including *Staphylococcus epidermis*
  - *Actinobacillus actinomycetemcomitans, Enterococcus, Streptococcus mitis, Haemophilus influenzae, Neisseria gonorrhea, Chlamydophila psittaci, Bartonella henselae, Coxiella burnetii*
    - *Streptococcus bovis* and *Neisseria subflava* bacteremia reported with concurrent high antineutrophil cytoplasmic antibody (ANCA) (anti-proteinase-3) titer
- ABE: *Staphylococcus aureus* infecting previously normal heart (e.g., intravenous drug abuser) is classic example
  - Bacterial endocarditis-associated GN caused by *S. aureus* increasing
    - > 50% of all cases and > 1/3 of fatal cases
    - 40-70% of intravenous drug abusers with acute endocarditis from *S. aureus* have GN
- Immunologic injury thought to be primary mechanism of endocarditis-associated GN
  - Presence of glomerular immune complexes is evidence
    - Circulating immune complexes demonstrated
  - Decreased serum complement levels also indicate process involving immune system
  - Associated with activation of classical complement pathway in many patients
    - ± classical pathway activation by bacterial cell wall antigens (e.g., staphylococcal) in nonimmune manner
  - Eluates from kidney with focal GN associated with endocarditis react with bacteria cultured from patient's blood
- Comorbidities include intravenous drug use, cardiac valve disease, hepatitis C virus, and diabetes
  - Cardiac valves involved include tricuspid, mitral, and aortic (43%, 33%, and 29%, respectively)

CLINICAL ISSUES

Epidemiology

- Incidence
  - Endocarditis-associated GN: 2-60%
    - Difficult to measure accurately
    - Antibiotics have decreased incidence

Presentation

- Renal disease is presenting feature in 20% of patients
- Hematuria
  - Macroscopic hematuria
    - May be associated with GN or renal infarction from "septic" emboli
- Proteinuria
  - Usually mild
  - Nephrotic syndrome (rare)
- Urinary casts
- Renal dysfunction
  - Blood urea nitrogen (BUN) and creatinine elevations typically associated with diffuse form of GN
  - Uremia in 5-10% of patients before epoch of antibiotics, 3-4% after advent of antibiotics
- Retinal hemorrhages (Roth spots)
- Anemia
- Hepatosplenomegaly
- Purpura

Laboratory Tests

- Hypocomplementemia (56%)
  - Low C3 (53%), low C4 (19%)
- ANCA (28%), PR3 or MPO (or both)
- Rheumatoid factor may be positive
- Cryoglobulins (mixed [type III]) reported

Treatment

- Surgical approaches
  - Valve replacement
- Drugs
  - Antibiotics may resolve mild cases
    - Prophylaxis in patients at risk for endocarditis
  - Corticosteroids
    - Brief course may resolve nephritis without exacerbating endocarditis

Prognosis

- Necrotizing and crescentic GN indicates worse prognosis

MACROSCOPIC

General Features

- Abscesses in severe cases
- Infarction (50-57% according to early studies) in severe cases
  - Single or multiple, of size associated with arcuate or large interlobular arteries
  - Typically due to embolism of valve vegetations and not immune-mediated vasculitis
- Petechial hemorrhages ("flea-bitten") in 2/3 of patients studied by Heptinstall

Size

- Enlarged or normal-sized kidneys ± petechiae
- Renal infarction may be present

MICROSCOPIC

Histologic Features

- Largely based on biopsy series (n=49) reported by Boils (2015)

- Glomeruli
  - Crescentic GN (53%)
    - Polymorphonuclear leukocytes and nuclear fragments in glomeruli
    - Focal necrosis (77%)
    - Diffuse inflammation (62%)
    - May contain intracapillary thrombi in addition to fibrinoid necrosis
    - Segmental or lobular hypercellularity or sclerosis
  - Diffuse proliferative GN (33%)
    - Diffuse endocapillary hypercellularity sometimes present, narrowing or occluding glomerular capillaries
    - Little increase in mesangial matrix
  - Mild mesangial hypercellularity (10%)
    - Resolving phase often shows only mesangial proliferation
  - Focal proliferative pattern (4%)
  - Membranoproliferative pattern (rare)
    - Diffuse endocapillary hypercellularity, duplicated GBM, and lobular mesangial expansion
    - Subendothelial fuchsinophilic deposits
  - Chronic lesions (autopsy)
    - Advanced or scarred lesions commonly found in chronic cases and nonbacterial endocarditis (Libman-Sacks endocarditis)
    - Adhesion or synechia between Bowman capsule and sclerotic lesion
  - Organisms not present unless septic emboli
- Tubules
  - Acute tubular injury (86%)
  - Red cell casts (64%)
  - Tubular atrophy
- Interstitium
  - Inflammation (88%)
    - Even in treated patients with quiescent disease
- Arteries
  - Intimal thickening (nonspecific)
  - Vasculitis rare

Other Diseases

- Secondary amyloidosis rare complication of longstanding endocarditis
- Interstitial nephritis may be induced by antibiotic and other drug therapy

ANCILLARY TESTS

Immunofluorescence

- Immunoglobulin and complement show widespread granular deposition along glomerular capillaries and sometimes mesangium, even though lesions may be focal by light microscopy
  - C3 almost universally present (94%)
    - 37% C3 only
  - IgG, IgA, and/or IgM in 27-37%
  - Dominant IgA in ~ 12%
  - IgG and IgM may be seen in large subendothelial deposits
  - Linear pattern described but not indicative of anti-GBM antibody formation
- No significant deposition of Ig or C3 in 6%
- Bacterial antigens sometimes detected

Electron Microscopy

- Subendothelial, subepithelial, &/or mesangial deposits (90%)
  - Subepithelial dense deposits ("humps") in 14%, associated with diffuse proliferative GN
  - Subendothelial deposits in 45%
  - Mesangial deposits in 84%, typically near endothelium of glomerular capillary
  - Capillary wall deposits are lost 1st after effective treatment
    - Mesangial dense deposits may persist ≥ 6 months
- Pure necrotizing cases may have no dense deposits
- Extensive foot process effacement in 55%

DIFFERENTIAL DIAGNOSIS

Postinfectious Glomerulonephritis, Other Site

- Variety of infections give similar biopsy findings (e.g., osteomyelitis, abscesses, shunts, and infected catheters)
- Clinical correlation helps determine infection source

IgA Nephropathy

- Necrosis, thrombi, and subendothelial deposits more common in endocarditis

ANCA-Associated Pauci-Immune Necrotizing Glomerulonephritis

- Lack of deposits favor ANCA disease triggered by infection
- May be indistinguishable from endocarditis-associated necrotizing GN

Lupus Nephritis

- Usually more extensive Ig deposits

Membranoproliferative Glomerulonephritis

- Conspicuous necrosis often indicates possibility of endocarditis GN

DIAGNOSTIC CHECKLIST

Pathologic Interpretation Pearls

- Clinical history of endocarditis critical in suspecting GN mediated by endocarditis

SELECTED REFERENCES

1. Boils CL et al: Update on endocarditis-associated glomerulonephritis. Kidney Int. ePub, 2015
2. Khalighi MA et al: Bartonella endocarditis-associated glomerulonephritis: a case report and review of the literature. Am J Kidney Dis. 63(6):1060-5, 2014
3. Mankongpaisarnrung C et al: Renal infarction as a presentation of Austrian syndrome: thromboembolic phenomenon of pneumococcal endocarditis. Am J Med Sci. 344(3):251-4, 2012
4. Uh M et al: Positive cytoplasmic antineutrophil cytoplasmic antigen with PR3 specificity glomerulonephritis in a patient with subacute bacterial endocarditis. J Rheumatol. 38(7):1527-8, 2011
5. Morel-Maroger L et al: Kidney in subacute endocarditis. Pathological and immunofluorescence findings. Arch Pathol. 94(3):205-13, 1972

"Flea Bitten" Kidney

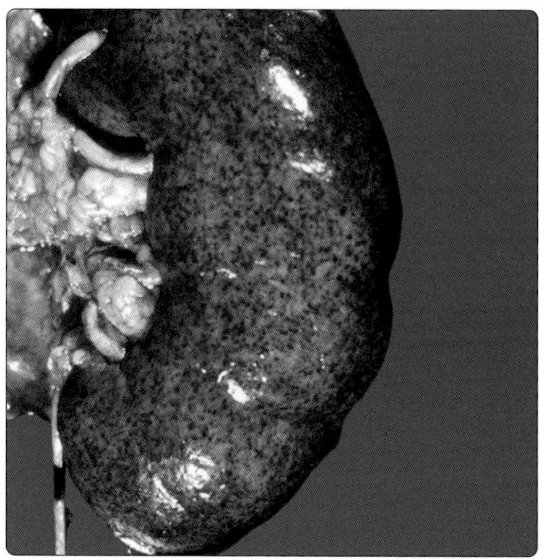

Hypercellular Glomerulus

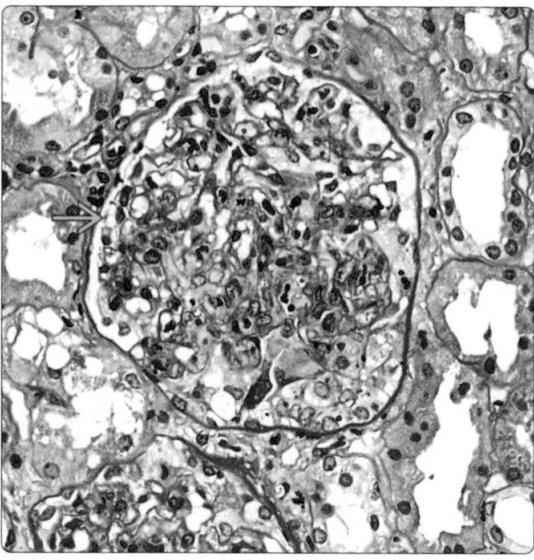

(Left) *The surface of the kidney has innumerable red spots resembling flea bites in a patient with endocarditis due to nongroupable, nonhemolytic streptococcal infection of a calcified aortic valve. These are probably due to blood in the tubules.* **(Right)** *A glomerulus ⇒ has ↑ cellularity in a 78-year-old man with serum Cr 3.7 mg/dL, 3.7 g/d proteinuria, hematuria, petechial rash, gastrointestinal ulcers, and Staphylococcus aureus on blood culture secondary to endocarditis.*

Hypercellular Glomeruli and Tubular Injury in Endocarditis

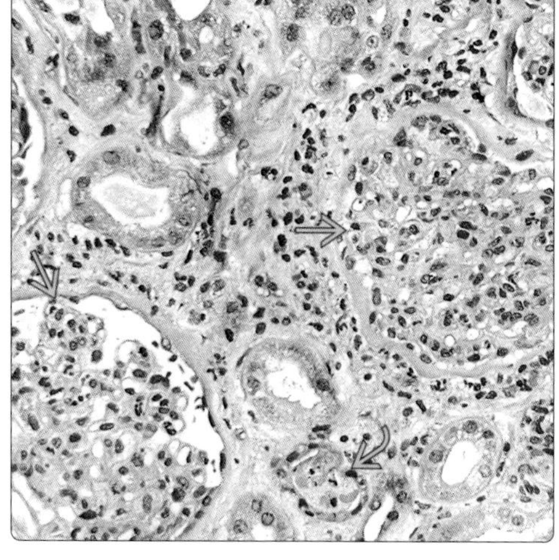

Segmental Glomerular Hypercellularity

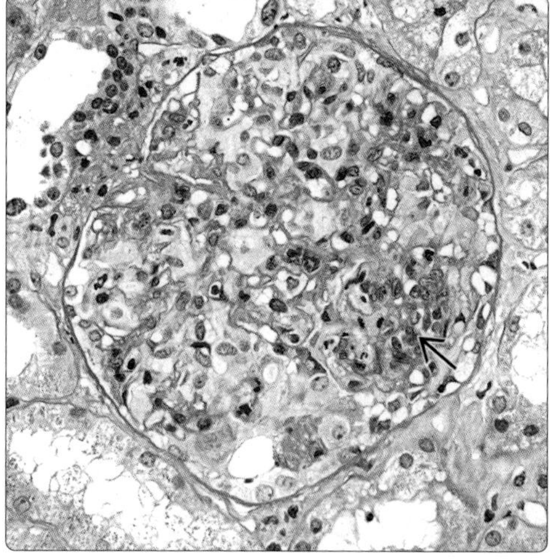

(Left) *In glomerulonephritis associated with endocarditis, hypercellular glomeruli ⇒ and tubular debris ⇗ can be seen.* **(Right)** *PAS stain shows a hypercellular glomerulus in glomerulonephritis associated with endocarditis that is particularly noteworthy in 1 segment of the glomerulus ⇒.*

Fibrinoid Necrosis

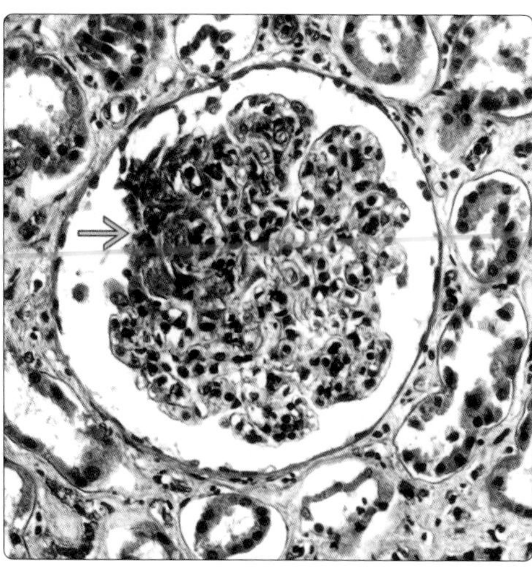

Glomerular Capillary Thrombus

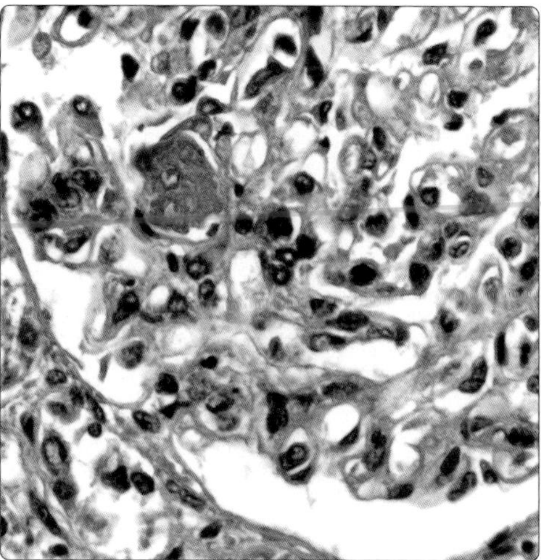

(Left) *Segmental fibrinoid necrosis ⇒ in a glomerulus due to endocarditis (bacteroides) is shown. This pattern can resemble ANCA-related glomerulonephritis.* **(Right)** *A glomerular capillary from a patient with endocarditis has a fibrin thrombus. This feature led to the view that glomerular lesions of endocarditis were "embolic," however, the glomerulonephritis is now known to be largely mediated by immune complexes.*

Syphilis

KEY FACTS

TERMINOLOGY

- Acute or chronic infection caused by *Treponema pallidum* subspecies *pallidum*, with tissue invasion and immunopathology

ETIOLOGY/PATHOGENESIS

- Direct kidney infection
- Immune complex-mediated nephritis in untreated disease
  - Immune complex deposits contain treponemal antigens and antitreponemal IgG
  - Usually manifests in tertiary or less frequently in secondary stages of disease
  - Renal lesions resolve with antibiotic therapy
- Onset of treatment: Immunologic reaction to released treponemal antigens

CLINICAL ISSUES

- Acquired adult syphilis: 2.4-3.7 per 100,000 population
  - Kidney disease (rare)
  - Secondary/tertiary stages nephrotic syndrome; nephritic syndrome is uncommon
- Congenital syphilis: Nephrotic syndrome, nephritic syndrome or hematuria
- Treatment-related nephropathy: Nephrotic syndrome or azotemia with hematuria after antisyphilitic therapy
- Typically disease eliminated within 3-6 weeks of therapy

MICROSCOPIC

- Membranous nephropathy most common lesion of congenital and acquired syphilis
  - IgG and C3 deposits in subepithelium and mesangium
- Tubulointerstitial nephritis ± gumma formation
- Histologic resolution of renal lesions demonstrated 1-6 months after treatment
- AA amyloidosis

TOP DIFFERENTIAL DIAGNOSES

- Other causes of membranous GN and postinfectious GN

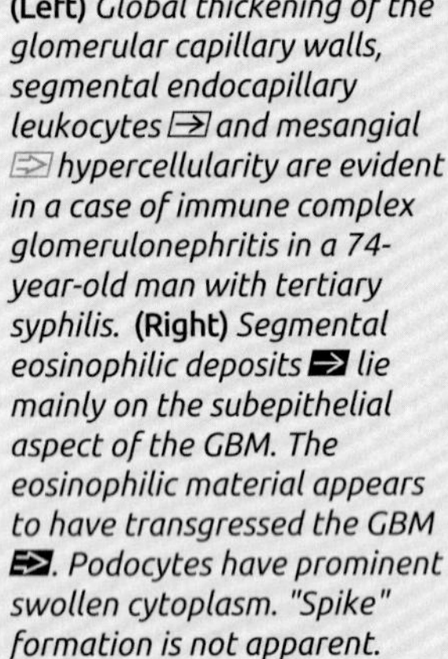

(Left) *Global thickening of the glomerular capillary walls, segmental endocapillary leukocytes* ⇨ *and mesangial* ⇨ *hypercellularity are evident in a case of immune complex glomerulonephritis in a 74-year-old man with tertiary syphilis.* **(Right)** *Segmental eosinophilic deposits* ➡ *lie mainly on the subepithelial aspect of the GBM. The eosinophilic material appears to have transgressed the GBM* ➡*. Podocytes have prominent swollen cytoplasm. "Spike" formation is not apparent.*

Secondary Membranous Nephropathy

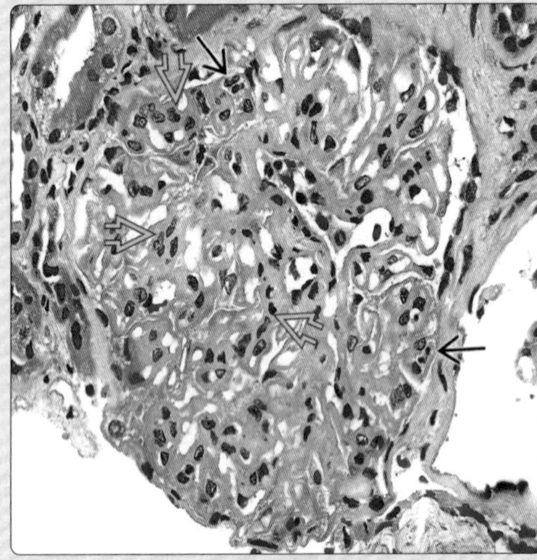

Subepithelial Eosinophilic Deposits

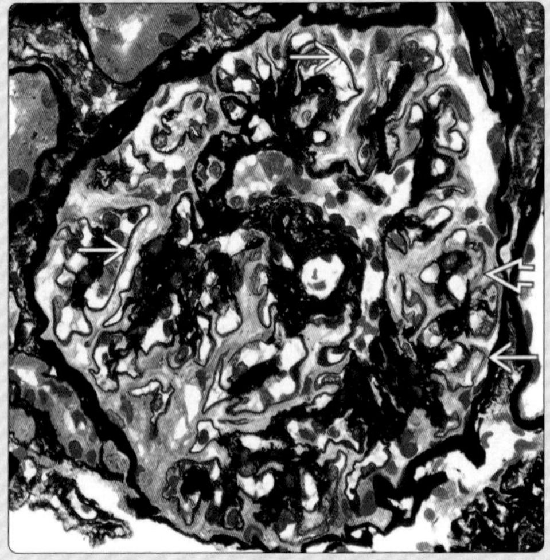

(Left) *Global granular and band-like staining of the capillary walls for IgG is seen in a case of GN associated with tertiary syphilis. This atypical pattern contrasts with the discrete granularity of IgG in idiopathic and other forms of membranous GN.* **(Right)** *Confluent and discrete* ⇨ *subepithelial electron-dense deposits associated with tertiary syphilis are shown. The pattern of deposits is atypical for both membranous and postinfectious glomerulonephritis.*

Capillary Wall IgG Immune Deposits

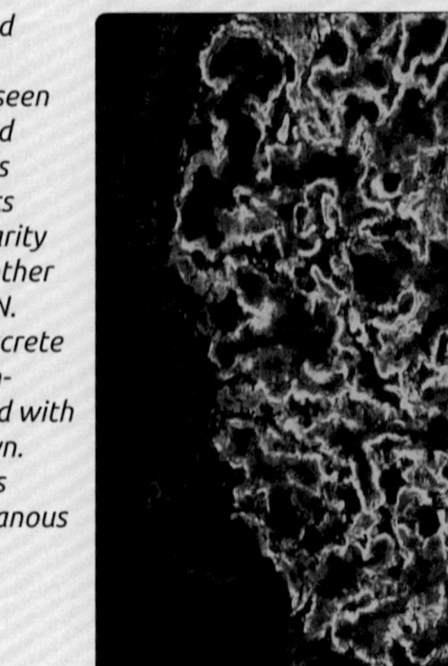

Subepithelial Immune Deposits in Syphilis

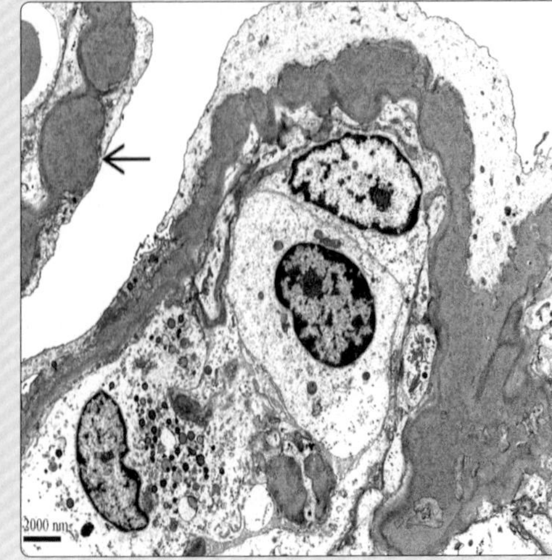

TERMINOLOGY

Synonyms

- Lues, luetic infection, syphilitic nephrosis or nephritis

Definitions

- Acute and chronic infection with tissue invasion and immunopathology caused by *Treponema pallidum* subspecies *pallidum*

ETIOLOGY/PATHOGENESIS

Infectious Agents

- *T. pallidum* subspecies *pallidum* is a microaerophilic spirochete venereally or vertically transmitted
- Kidney disease in syphilis may arise in 4 ways
  - Direct infection by spirochetes
  - Immune complex-mediated nephritis in untreated disease
    - Usually manifests in tertiary or less frequently in secondary or latent stages of disease
  - Immune complex nephritis in response to antibiotic therapy (rare)
    - Destruction of *T. pallidum* releases bacterial antigens and incites immune complex formation and deposition (Jarisch-Herxheimer reaction)
  - Fibril deposition in secondary AA amyloidosis

CLINICAL ISSUES

Epidemiology

- Incidence
  - Congenital syphilis rare in developed countries
    - Renal involvement in up to 46% of cases
  - Acquired adult syphilis: 2.4-3.7 per 100,000
    - Prevalence: 7.7-12 per 100,000
    - Rare renal disease with estimated prevalence at 0.3%
- Age
  - Congenital infection seen in infants from 2 weeks to 18 months, with median of 3 months
  - Acquired infection at any age

Presentation

- Primary syphilis characterized by painless ulcer (chancre) with regional lymphadenopathy
- 25% of untreated primary disease progresses to secondary syphilis in weeks to months
- 20-40% of untreated secondary syphilis progresses to tertiary syphilis in 1-30 years after primary infection
- Congenital: Nephrotic syndrome, nephritic syndrome, or hematuria
- Acquired: Latent, secondary, or tertiary stages may have nephrotic syndrome; nephritic syndrome uncommon
- Treatment-related: Nephrotic syndrome or azotemia with hematuria after antisyphilitic therapy

Laboratory Tests

- Organisms detected by silver stains, dark field microscopy, immunofluorescence, or PCR
- Treponemal antibody tests: *T. pallidum* hemagglutination assay (TPHA) and fluorescent treponemal antibody absorption test (FTA-Abs)

Treatment

- Drugs
  - Benzathine penicillin G or ceftriaxone

Prognosis

- Disease eliminated within 3-6 weeks of therapy

MICROSCOPIC

Histologic Features

- Congenital syphilis
  - Membranous nephropathy ± mesangial hypercellularity
  - Tubulointerstitial nephritis in stillborn (spirochetes Warthin-Starry or Steiner positive)
- Acquired syphilis
  - Membranous nephropathy ± mesangial hypercellularity
  - Diffuse proliferative glomerulonephritis ± crescents
  - Minimal change disease
  - Tubulointerstitial nephritis with plasma cells; gumma formation (late feature)
- Histologic resolution of renal lesions demonstrated 1-6 months after treatment
- AA amyloidosis

ANCILLARY TESTS

Immunofluorescence

- Granular IgG and C3 in capillary walls and mesangium
- Treponemal antigen and antibody may be demonstrable in immune complexes

Electron Microscopy

- Subepithelial electron-dense deposits with spike and dome pattern in membranous nephropathy
- Subepithelial "humps" in proliferative postinfectious-like glomerulonephritis

DIFFERENTIAL DIAGNOSIS

Other Causes of Membranous GN and Postinfectious GN

- Resolved by serology and history
- PLA2R negative in syphilitic membranous GN
- Congenital syphilis should be considered in infants with membranous GN

DIAGNOSTIC CHECKLIST

Pathologic Interpretation Pearls

- *T. pallidum* antigen may be identifiable in immune deposits in syphilitic GN

SELECTED REFERENCES

1. Viecelli AK et al: Spiralling into the nephrotic syndrome. Med J Aust. 200(11):673-4, 2014
2. Scheid LM et al: A 17-year-old male with nephrotic syndrome and diffuse adenopathy: questions. Pediatr Nephrol. 27(10):1889-90, 1891-3, 2012
3. Havill JP et al: The Case An age-old enemy should not be forgotten. Kidney Int. 79(8):924-5, 2011
4. Bani-Hani S et al: Renal disease in AIDS: it is not always HIVAN. Clin Exp Nephrol. 14(3):263-7, 2010
5. Satoskar AA et al: An uncommon cause of membranous glomerulonephritis. Am J Kidney Dis. 55(2):386-90, 2010

Lyme Disease

KEY FACTS

TERMINOLOGY

- Glomerulonephritis, typically with membranoproliferative glomerulonephritis (MPGN) pattern, associated with *Borrelia burgdorferi* infection

ETIOLOGY/PATHOGENESIS

- *B. burgdorferi* infection causes chronic antigenemia and immune complex formation
- Immunity against self-antigens may be precipitated by molecular mimicry of *Borrelia* organisms

CLINICAL ISSUES

- Most common tick-borne infection in USA
- Early symptoms after tick bite include fever, fatigue, and characteristic skin rash, erythema migrans
- Lyme disease glomerulonephritis rarely documented in humans
- Microscopic hematuria and proteinuria if renal involvement
- Diagnostics: ELISA, Western Blot, PCR
- Treatment
  - Antibiotic therapy directed against spirochete
  - Immunosuppressive therapy may be indicated

MICROSCOPIC

- MPGN pattern with peripheral capillary wall double contours and prominent C3; IgG
- Focal mesangioproliferative GN with IgA predominance
- Interstitial foam cells may be observed

ANCILLARY TESTS

- Dominant C3 staining in mesangium and capillary walls
- Subendothelial and mesangial electron dense deposits

TOP DIFFERENTIAL DIAGNOSES

- MPGN due to other causes/C3 glomerulopathy
- IgA nephropathy
- High level of clinical suspicion is needed for diagnosis of MPGN due to Lyme disease

Lyme Disease MPGN

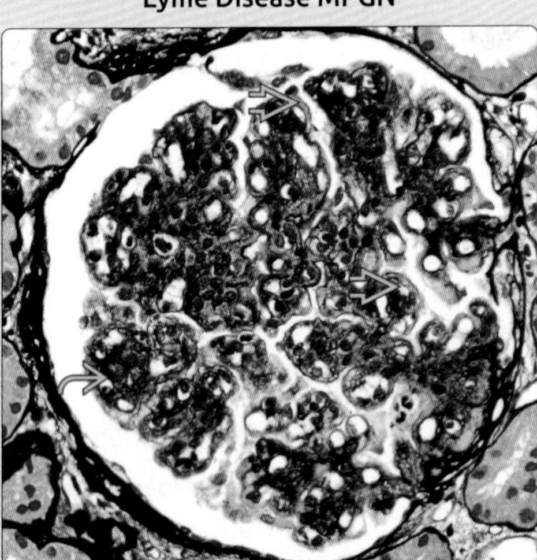

Lyme Disease

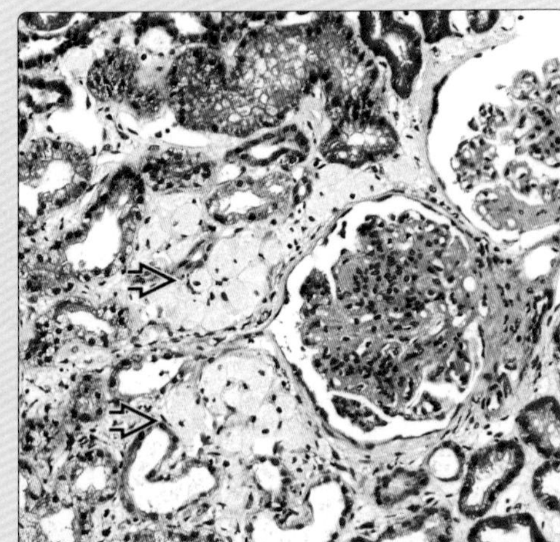

(Left) *Renal biopsy from a 13-year-old girl demonstrates mesangial proliferation ⇨ with extensive basement membrane double contours ⇨. Extensive work-up revealed positive Lyme disease screen.* **(Right)** *Biopsy shows scattered collections of interstitial foam cells ⇨ in a young girl with MPGN due to a Borrelia burgdorferi spirochete infection. The patient presented with nephrotic-range proteinuria and hematuria.*

IF: Lyme Disease

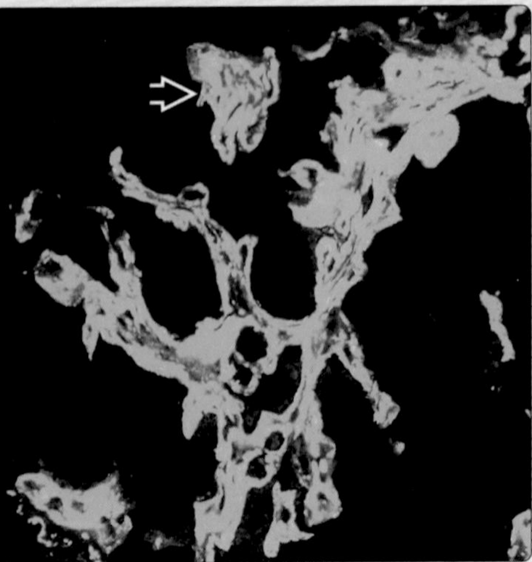

EM: Lyme Disease

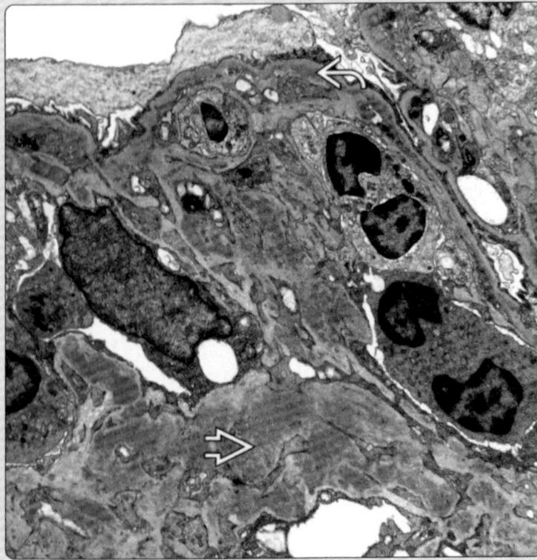

(Left) *Immunofluorescence with antisera to C3 shows granular deposits in the mesangium and capillary walls ⇨. The renal biopsy findings of Membranoproliferative glomerulonephritis (MPGN), type 1 were associated with B. burgdorferi infection.* **(Right)** *Electron micrograph reveals mesangial ⇨ and subendothelial ⇨ deposits seen in MPGN due to Lyme disease.*

TERMINOLOGY

Definitions

- Glomerulonephritis (GN), typically with membranoproliferative glomerulonephritis (MPGN) pattern, associated with *Borrelia burgdorferi* infection

ETIOLOGY/PATHOGENESIS

Infectious Agents

- Lyme disease is caused by *B. burgdorferi,* a spirochete, transmitted by ticks of genus *Ixodes*

Immune Complex Formation

- *B. burgdorferi* infection causes chronic antigenemia and immune complex formation
- Circulating immune complexes deposited in glomeruli, with resultant glomerulonephritis

Autoimmunity

- Immunity against self-antigens may be precipitated by molecular mimicry of *Borrelia* organisms

CLINICAL ISSUES

Epidemiology

- Incidence
  - Most common tick-borne infection in USA
    - Highest incidence in Northeast and Wisconsin
  - Lyme disease GN rarely documented in humans

Presentation

- Early symptoms after tick bite include fever, fatigue, and characteristic skin rash, erythema migrans
- Manifestations of untreated disease include arthritis and neurologic and cardiac abnormalities
- Microscopic hematuria and proteinuria, if renal involvement
  - Nephrotic syndrome
- Typically has remissions and exacerbations with variable organ involvement

Laboratory Tests

- Serological tests
  - ELISA for detection of IgM and IgG anti-*B. burgdorferi* antibodies is sensitive
    - High false-positive rate, and careful clinical evaluation needed to determine validity
    - May be negative in early infection due to slow development of immune response
    - May remain positive after antibiotic therapy
  - Confirmatory serological test is Western blot
- PCR
  - *B. burgdorferi* DNA can be detected in blood, urine, joint fluid, or CSF
  - Not clinically validated; susceptible to false-positive/false-negative results
- Low C3 level (may be normal)

Treatment

- Drugs
  - Oral doxycycline 14-28 days, longer for chronic disease
  - Steroids, IVIG, and plasmapheresis used for MPGN

Prognosis

- With adequate therapy, complete resolution of MPGN manifestations documented in literature

MICROSCOPIC

Histologic Features

- Glomeruli
  - MPGN pattern
    - Diffuse and global glomerular hypercellularity seen with lobular accentuation typical of MPGN, type I
    - Mesangial and endocapillary proliferation with endocapillary lymphocytes and monocytes
    - Glomerular basement membrane (GBM) double contours with mesangial cell interposition
    - Deposits on trichrome stain
  - Mesangioproliferative pattern
    - Focal proliferation, little or no duplication of GBM
    - May have small cellular crescents
- Interstitium and tubules
  - Varying degrees of interstitial inflammation, tubular atrophy, and interstitial fibrosis are seen
  - In setting of chronic nephrotic-range proteinuria, interstitial foam cells may be observed

ANCILLARY TESTS

Immunofluorescence

- Dominant C3 staining in mesangium and capillary walls
- IgG in similar distribution; weak IgM, IgA, and C1q
- Rare cases with prominent IgA (mesangioproliferative pattern)
- No light chain restriction

Electron Microscopy

- Amorphous, electron-dense deposits in predominantly subendothelial but also mesangial distribution
- Few subepithelial deposits
- GBM duplication identified
- Mesangial cell interposition

DIFFERENTIAL DIAGNOSIS

MPGN Due to Other Causes/C3 Glomerulopathy

- Clinical and serological evidence of other causes
- Positive evidence of Lyme disease

IgA Nephropathy

- Clinical history; Lyme serology/PCR

SELECTED REFERENCES

1. Rolla D et al: Post-infectious glomerulonephritis presenting as acute renal failure in a patient with Lyme disease. J Renal Inj Prev. 3(1):17-20, 2014
2. Branda JA et al: Performance of United States serologic assays in the diagnosis of Lyme borreliosis acquired in Europe. Clin Infect Dis. 57(3):333-40, 2013
3. Mc Causland FR et al: Lyme disease-associated glomerulonephritis. Nephrol Dial Transplant. 26(9):3054-6, 2011
4. Aguero-Rosenfeld ME: Lyme disease: laboratory issues. Infect Dis Clin North Am. 22(2):301-13, vii, 2008
5. Kirmizis D et al: MPGN secondary to Lyme disease. Am J Kidney Dis. 43(3):544-51, 2004
6. Kelly B et al: Lyme disease and glomerulonephritis. Ir Med J. 92(5):372, 1999

Hepatitis B Virus

KEY FACTS

TERMINOLOGY

- Hepatitis B virus (HBV)

CLINICAL ISSUES

- High prevalence in Asia and Africa
  - Perinatal transmission results in > 90% chronic infection without acute response
- Low prevalence in Western countries
  - Acquired during adolescence or early adulthood
  - Acute hepatitis with rare chronic progression
- Antiviral agents
  - Lamivudine
  - Interferon-α

MICROSCOPIC

- Membranous glomerulonephritis (MGN)
  - Normal to thick glomerular basement membranes, depending on stage
  - ± "spikes" on PAS or silver stain
- Membranoproliferative GN (MPGN)
  - Lobular accentuation of glomerular tufts
  - Duplication of glomerular basement membranes (GBM) (tram track appearance)
- Cryoglobulinemic GN
  - Lobular accentuation of glomerular tufts with "wire loop" or hyaline "thrombi" deposits
- Polyarteritis nodosa

TOP DIFFERENTIAL DIAGNOSES

- Primary MGN
- Primary MPGN
- Type I cryoglobulinemic glomerulonephritis, non-HBV-associated
- IgA nephropathy
- Bile cast nephropathy
- Vasculitis, non-HBV-associated

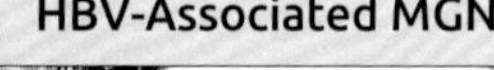

HBV-Associated MGN

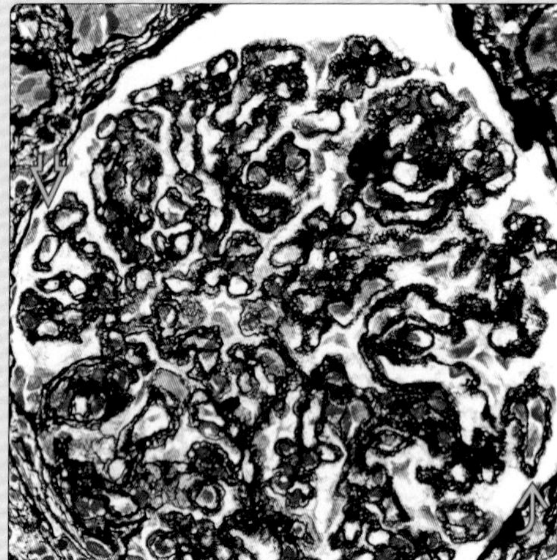

HBsAg Immunofluorescence

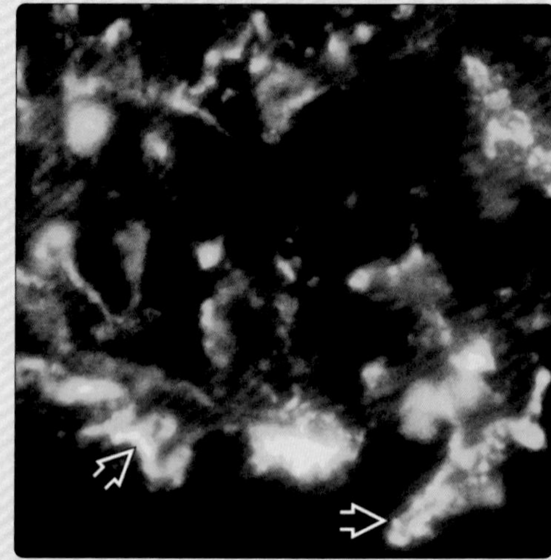

(Left) *Jones methenamine silver stain reveals a prominent, vacuolated appearance with "spike" formation involving the glomerular basement membranes in the glomeruli of a patient with HBV-associated MGN.* **(Right)** *Immunofluorescence microscopy for HBV surface antigen reveals granular staining along the glomerular capillaries in locations where there are subepithelial immune complexes in an HBV-associated case of MGN.*

HBV-Associated MPGN

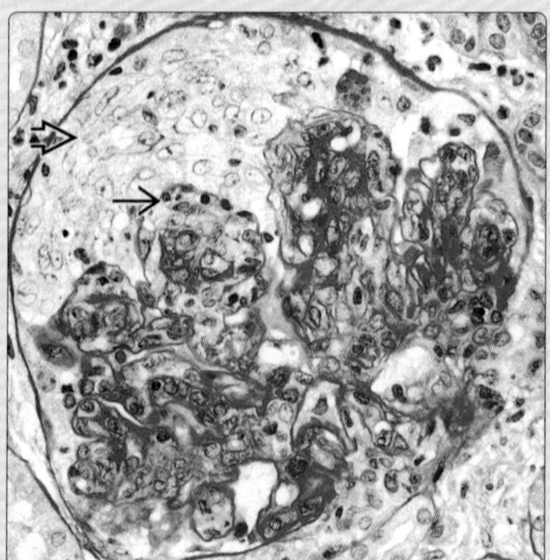

C3

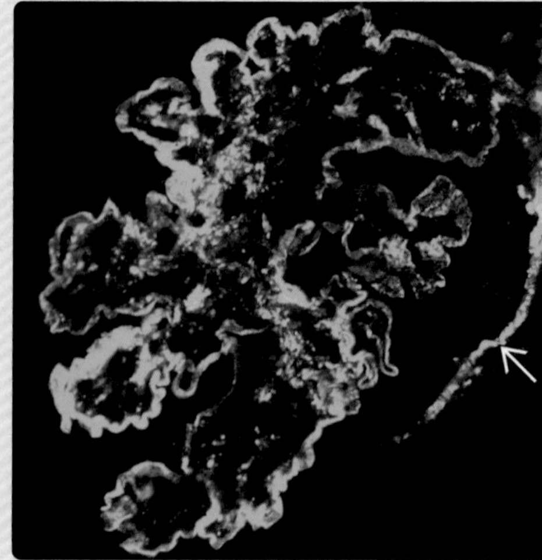

(Left) *Endocapillary hypercellularity with increased inflammatory cells is present in the glomerular tufts in this patient with MPGN associated with HBV infection, but the cellular crescent occupying and compressing the residual glomerulus obscures some of these alterations.* **(Right)** *Granular C3 staining along the glomerular capillaries and mesangial areas is prominent in this glomerulus with MPGN associated with hepatitis B infection. Note focal Bowman capsule staining.*

TERMINOLOGY

Abbreviations

- Hepatitis B virus (HBV)

Definitions

- Immune complex-mediated renal injury associated with hepatitis B virus (HBV) infection

ETIOLOGY/PATHOGENESIS

Infectious Agents

- Hepatitis B virus
  - Hepadnavirus family
    - Strong preference for infection of liver cells
    - DNA also detectable in kidney, pancreas, and mononuclear cells
  - Modes of transmission include
    - Percutaneous
    - Sexual
    - Perinatal or vertical (mother to child)
- Possible pathogenic mechanisms of kidney diseases
  - Circulating immune complexes of HBV antigen and antibodies
  - Cryoglobulins

CLINICAL ISSUES

Epidemiology

- Incidence
  - High prevalence in Asia and Africa
    - Perinatal transmission results in > 90% chronic infection without acute response
  - Low prevalence in Western countries
    - Acquired during adolescence or early adulthood
    - Acute hepatitis with rare chronic progression
    - 1.5 per 100,000 in United States infected with HBV
- Sex
  - Males have slight higher risk of death from liver disease

Laboratory Tests

- HBV serology
  - HBV surface antigen (HBsAg)
    - Marker of active viral replication
    - Hepatitis B surface Ab (Anti-HBs)
  - HBV core antigen (HBcAg)
  - HBe antigen
    - Loss or seroconversion in inactive carriers
- HBV PCR test

Natural History

- Asymptomatic
  - Majority of HBV infections
- Chronic HBV infection
  - < 5%
- Cirrhosis
  - Develops in 20% of chronic HBV infections
    - 100x ↑ risk for hepatocellular carcinoma compared with noncarriers of HBV
  - 40% lifetime risk of death

Treatment

- Drugs
  - Lamivudine
  - Interferon-α
- Plasma exchange
  - Consider for cryoglobulinemic glomerular nephritis (GN) and polyarteritis nodosa
- HBV vaccine
  - Not useful for active infection
  - Should decrease future disease burden

Prognosis

- HBV genotype A more responsive to interferon

MICROSCOPIC

Histologic Features

- Glomerular patterns of injury
  - Membranous glomerulonephritis (MGN)
    - Normal to thick GBMs
      - Depends on stage of subepithelial immune complex deposition
    - Mesangial hypercellularity may be present
  - Membranoproliferative GN (MPGN)
    - Lobular accentuation of glomerular tufts
    - Duplication of GBMs ("tram track" appearance)
    - Interposition of cells between duplicated basement membranes
  - Cryoglobulinemic GN
    - MPGN pattern common
    - Immune complex deposition in form of "wire-loop" or hyaline "thrombi" (intraluminal cryoglobulins)
  - Hepatic glomerulosclerosis (or secondary IgA nephropathy)
    - Usually in setting of cirrhosis
    - Mesangial to membranoproliferative pattern of glomerular injury
    - May show "full-house" immunofluorescence staining
      - Can mislead one to consider lupus nephritis
- Bile/bilirubin casts may be present if jaundiced or cirrhotic
  - May have eosinophilic appearance
  - Affect distal nephron segments and, if severe, proximal tubules
- Vasculitis
  - Often negative antineutrophil cytoplasmic antibody (ANCA) titer
  - Fibrinoid necrosis of arteries without crescentic GN
    - Consistent with polyarteritis nodosa
  - When chronic, pseudoaneurysms or thrombosis can occur

ANCILLARY TESTS

Immunohistochemistry

- HBcAg stains subepithelial immune complexes along glomerular capillaries

Immunofluorescence

- MGN
  - Granular glomerular capillary wall staining for IgG, C3 (variable), and κ and λ

- Mesangial staining also present
- Phospholipase A2 receptor (PLA2R) positive (67%)
- MPGN
  - Coarse to granular glomerular capillary wall staining for IgG, C3 (variable), and κ and λ
- Cryoglobulinemic GN
  - Coarse to granular glomerular capillary wall staining for IgG &/or IgM, κ and λ

Electron Microscopy

- MGN
  - Subepithelial immune deposits
  - Mesangial immune deposits
- MPGN
  - Subendothelial immune deposits
  - Mesangial immune deposits
  - Duplication of GBMs
  - Subepithelial deposits variably present
- Cryoglobulinemic GN
  - Subendothelial immune deposits
  - Mesangial immune deposits
  - Substructural organization of deposits may be present
- Tubuloreticular inclusions in endothelial cells may be present
- HBV virions not demonstrable

DIFFERENTIAL DIAGNOSIS

Primary MGN

- Subepithelial without prominent mesangial immune deposits
- PLA2R positive

Primary MPGN

- Similar pathologic features to HBV-associated MPGN

Type I Cryoglobulinemic Glomerulonephritis, Non-HBV-Associated

- Appears identical to HBV-associated cryoglobulinemic GN
- Absence of HBV infection

IgA Nephropathy

- Concurrent IgA nephropathy with HBV-associated MGN reported
  - Consider possibility of hepatic glomerulosclerosis
    - May be secondary to severe hepatobiliary disease

Bile Cast Nephropathy

- Red to dark green tubular casts
  - Severity correlates with duration of jaundice and total bilirubin levels
- Severe renal dysfunction
- Concurrent hepatic glomerulosclerosis, if cirrhosis present

Vasculitis, Non-HBV-Associated

- Fibrinoid necrosis of arteries
- Absence of HBV infection
- No glomerular injury

DIAGNOSTIC CHECKLIST

Pathologic Interpretation Pearls

- Need clinical correlation to establish HBV-associated immune complex disease

SELECTED REFERENCES

1. Hernández-Rodríguez J et al: Diagnosis and classification of polyarteritis nodosa. J Autoimmun. 48-49:84-9, 2014
2. Dienstag JL: Hepatitis B virus infection. N Engl J Med. 359(14):1486-500, 2008
3. Chuang TW et al: Complete remission of nephrotic syndrome of hepatitis B virus-associated membranous glomerulopathy after lamivudine monotherapy. J Formos Med Assoc. 106(10):869-73, 2007
4. Kusakabe A et al: Virological features of hepatitis B virus-associated nephropathy in Japan. J Med Virol. 79(9):1305-11, 2007
5. Rodrigues RG: Membranous glomerulonephropathy in a child with hepatitis B. Int J Clin Pract. 61(5):878-9, 2007
6. Dede F et al: Efficient treatment of crescentric glomerulonephritis associated with hepatitis B virus with lamivudin in a case referred with acute renal failure. Nephrol Dial Transplant. 21(12):3613-4, 2006
7. Herberth J et al: Hepatitis B infection as a possible cause of focal segmental glomerulosclerosis (FSGS). Clin Nephrol. 65(5):380-4, 2006
8. Izzedine H et al: Lamivudine and HBV-associated nephropathy. Nephrol Dial Transplant. 21(3):828-9, 2006
9. Kim SE et al: Study on hepatitis B virus pre-S/S gene mutations of renal tissues in children with hepatitis B virus-associated membranous nephropathy. Pediatr Nephrol. 21(8):1097-103, 2006
10. Ren J et al: Gene expression profile of transgenic mouse kidney reveals pathogenesis of hepatitis B virus associated nephropathy. J Med Virol. 78(5):551-60, 2006
11. Tang S et al: Hepatitis B-related membranous nephropathy should be treated with a specific anti-viral agent. Kidney Int. 70(4):818, 2006
12. Wen YK et al: Remission of hepatitis B virus-associated membranoproliferative glomerulonephritis in a cirrhotic patient after lamivudine therapy. Clin Nephrol. 65(3):211-5, 2006
13. Passarino G et al: Histopathological findings in 851 autopsies of drug addicts, with toxicologic and virologic correlations. Am J Forensic Med Pathol. 26(2):106-16, 2005
14. Sakallioglu O et al: Hepatitis B complicated focal segmental glomerulosclerosis. J Nephrol. 18(4):433-5, 2005
15. Tang S et al: Lamivudine in hepatitis B-associated membranous nephropathy. Kidney Int. 68(4):1750-8, 2005
16. Bhimma R et al: Hepatitis B virus-associated nephropathy. Am J Nephrol. 24(2):198-211, 2004
17. Ganem D et al: Hepatitis B virus infection--natural history and clinical consequences. N Engl J Med. 350(11):1118-29, 2004
18. Ozdamar SO et al: Hepatitis-B virus associated nephropathies: a clinicopathological study in 14 children. Pediatr Nephrol. 18(1):23-8, 2003
19. Stokes MB et al: Combined membranous nephropathy and IgA nephropathy. Am J Kidney Dis. 32(4):649-56, 1998
20. Collins AB et al: Hepatitis B immune complex glomerulonephritis: simultaneous glomerular deposition of hepatitis B surface and e antigens. Clin Immunol Immunopathol. 26(1):137-53, 1983

HBV-Associated MGN

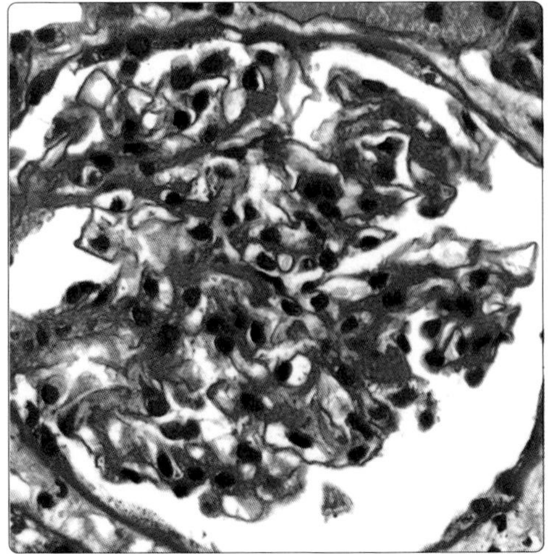

HBcAg Immunohistochemistry

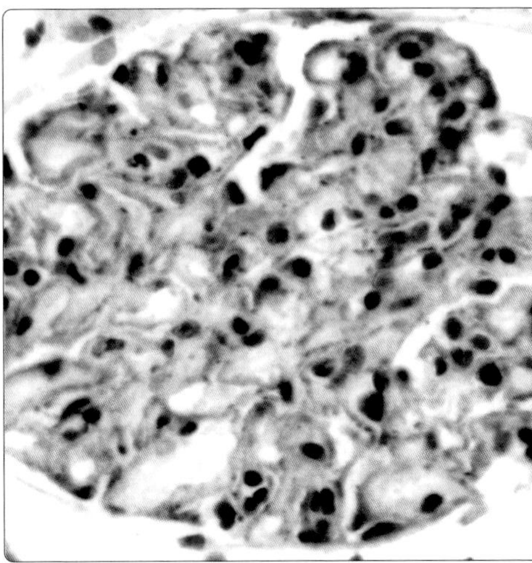

(Left) *PAS reveals a normal glomerulus from a patient with MGN associated with HBV infection.* **(Right)** *Immunohistochemistry for HBcAg shows strong and diffuse granular staining along the glomerular capillaries where subepithelial immune complexes are located in this patient with MGN associated with HBV infection.*

HBV-Associated MGN

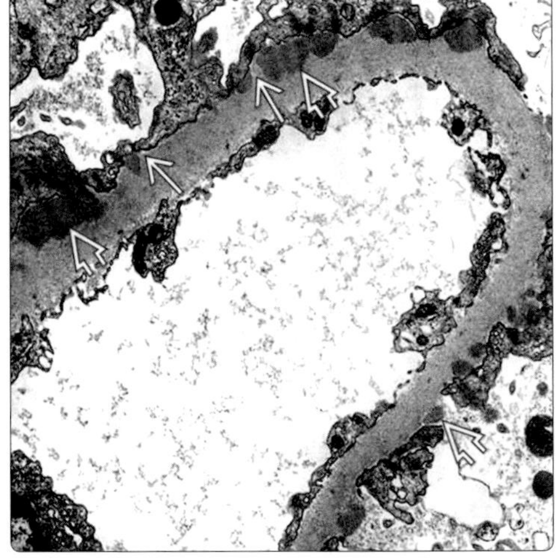

Polyarteritis Nodosa and Infarction

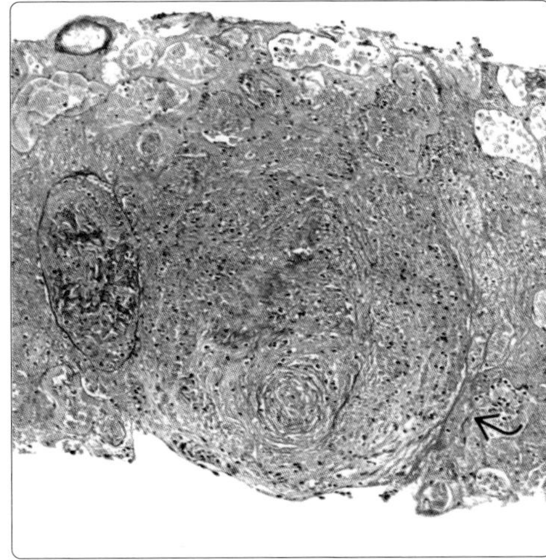

(Left) *Electron microscopy reveals many variably sized, subepithelial, electron-dense deposits ➡ with intervening basement membrane "spikes" ➡ between and surrounding most deposits. Extensive effacement of the podocyte foot processes correlates with the presence of nephrotic-range proteinuria.* **(Right)** *Renal biopsy from a patient with HBV shows an interlobular artery with old arteritis and thrombosis. The adjacent kidney had an infarction. The elastin stain was used to detect the disrupted elastic layers ➢.*

Membranoproliferative GN

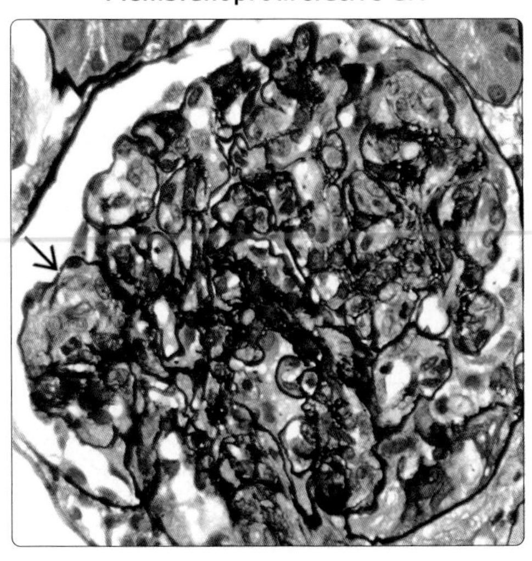

HBV-Associated MPGN

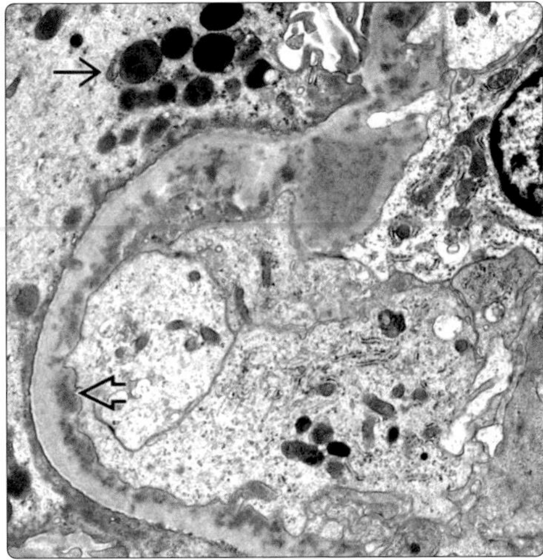

(Left) *Increased endocapillary cellularity in this glomerulus is noted. Focal duplication of the GBMs ➡ is also present, which is characteristic of MPGN associated with HBV infection.* **(Right)** *Numerous small, electron-dense deposits accumulate in a subendothelial region ➡ along and within the GBM. Similar deposits in other cases have contained HBe antigens. Protein reabsorption droplets ➡ are noted in an adjacent podocyte with extensive foot process effacement.*

Hepatitis C Virus

KEY FACTS

TERMINOLOGY

- Hepatitis C virus (HCV)
- Wide spectrum of immune complex-mediated glomerular injuries associated with HCV infection

CLINICAL ISSUES

- > 200 million people worldwide infected
- Infected children have high rate of spontaneous resolution
- Young females may spontaneously resolve
  - Cirrhosis or hepatocellular carcinoma (HCC) less likely
- 17-55% of HCV-infected patients progress to cirrhosis
  - 2-23% develop HCC
- Males progress to end-stage liver disease faster
- New therapies curative, even in advanced stages

MICROSCOPIC

- Spectrum of glomerular injury
  - Membranoproliferative glomerulonephritis (MPGN)
  - Cryoglobulinemic GN
  - Membranous glomerulonephritis (MGN)
  - Fibrillary GN
  - Immunotactoid glomerulopathy
  - IgA nephropathy
- Polyarteritis nodosa

TOP DIFFERENTIAL DIAGNOSES

- HCV-associated focal segmental glomerulosclerosis
- Hepatitis B virus-associated immune complex disease
- Lupus nephritis
- HIV-associated immune complex disease
- Vasculitis, non-HCV-associated

DIAGNOSTIC CHECKLIST

- No pathognomonic features for HCV infection
- Coinfection with HIV common
- Bile cast nephropathy can occur concurrently
  - If cirrhosis or jaundice present

HCV-Associated MGN

HCV-Associated MPGN

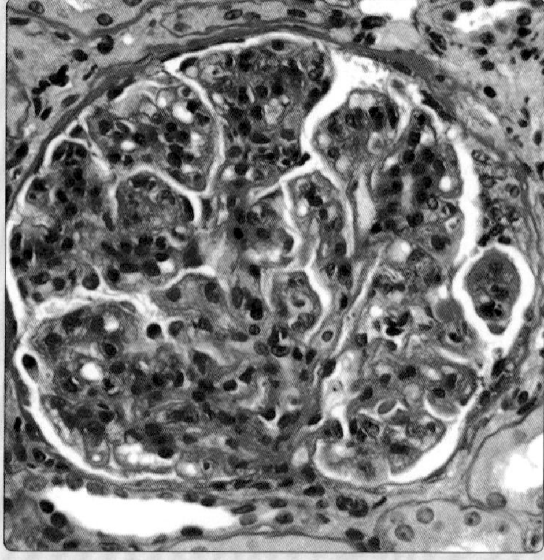

(Left) *Jones methenamine silver demonstrates prominent subepithelial "spikes" and vacuoles → along all of the glomerular capillary basement membranes that are diagnostic of membranous GN. Correlation with clinical and laboratory data is necessary to confirm the association with hepatitis C infection.* **(Right)** *Periodic acid-Schiff reveals increased cellularity that highlights the lobularity of the glomerular tufts, which is characteristic of a membranoproliferative injury pattern.*

HCV-Associated Cryoglobulinemic GN

IgG and Cryoglobulinemic GN

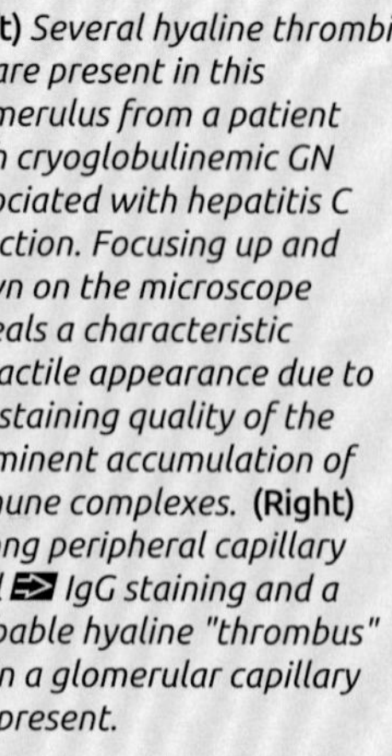

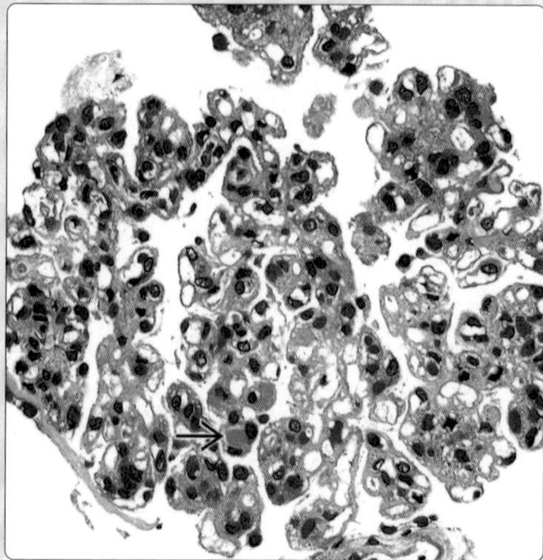

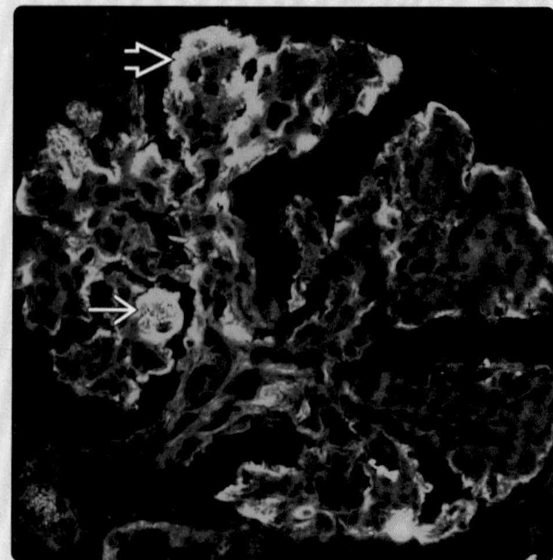

(Left) *Several hyaline thrombi → are present in this glomerulus from a patient with cryoglobulinemic GN associated with hepatitis C infection. Focusing up and down on the microscope reveals a characteristic refractile appearance due to the staining quality of the prominent accumulation of immune complexes.* **(Right)** *Strong peripheral capillary wall → IgG staining and a probable hyaline "thrombus" → in a glomerular capillary are present.*

TERMINOLOGY

Abbreviations

- Hepatitis C virus (HCV)

Definitions

- Wide spectrum of immune complex-mediated glomerular injuries in association with HCV infection

ETIOLOGY/PATHOGENESIS

Infectious Agents

- HCV
  - RNA virus: Single-stranded, positive sense
  - Infects hepatocytes and B lymphocytes
  - Blood-to-blood with rare sexual transmission
- Possible pathogenic mechanism of kidney diseases
  - Circulating immune complexes of HCV antigen and antibodies
  - Cryoglobulins

CLINICAL ISSUES

Epidemiology

- Incidence
  - > 200 million people worldwide infected
- Age
  - Children have high rate of spontaneous resolution
- Sex
  - Young females may spontaneously resolve
  - Males progress to end-stage liver disease faster

Presentation

- Proteinuria
- Hematuria
- Renal failure

Natural History

- 17-55% of HCV-infected patients progress to cirrhosis
  - 2-23% develop HCC

Treatment

- Drugs
  - Sofosbuvir
  - Simeprevir
  - Ribavirin
- Kidney &/or liver transplantation

Prognosis

- New drugs are curative, even in advanced disease
  - HCV genotype 2A and 3A have high cure rates
  - Secondary consequences, such as mixed cryoglobulinemia, can persist after viral cure

MICROSCOPIC

Histologic Features

- Membranoproliferative glomerulonephritis (MPGN)
  - Accentuation of glomerular tuft/lobules
  - Duplication of glomerular basement membranes or "tram track"
  - Interposition of cells or cell processes between duplicated GBMs
- Cryoglobulinemic GN
  - Endocapillary hypercellularity
  - Duplication of GBMs
  - "Wire loop" or hyaline "thrombi" deposits
    - PAS positive
- Membranous glomerulonephritis (MGN)
  - Thickened glomerular basement membranes with subepithelial "spike" formation
  - Mesangial hypercellularity
- Fibrillary or immunotactoid glomerulopathy
  - Mesangial expansion
  - Variable global &/or segmental glomerular scarring
- IgA nephropathy/hepatic glomerulosclerosis
  - Variable mesangial hypercellularity
- Polyarteritis nodosa
  - Fibrinoid necrosis of small arteries

DIFFERENTIAL DIAGNOSIS

HCV-Associated Focal Segmental Glomerulosclerosis

- Segmental sclerosis of glomeruli
- Absence of immune complex deposition

Hepatitis B Virus-Associated Immune Complex Disease

- Pathologically identical to HCV-associated immune complex disease

Lupus Nephritis

- Spectrum of glomerular injury mimics HCV-associated immune complex disease

HIV-Associated Immune Complex Disease

- Spectrum of glomerular injury mimics HCV-associated immune complex disease
- Requires laboratory tests to establish presence of HIV infection

DIAGNOSTIC CHECKLIST

Pathologic Interpretation Pearls

- No pathognomonic features for HCV infection
- Coinfection with HIV common
- Bile cast nephropathy can occur concurrently
  - If cirrhosis or jaundice present

SELECTED REFERENCES

1. Cornella SL et al: Persistence of mixed cryoglobulinemia despite cure of hepatitis C with new oral antiviral therapy including direct-acting antiviral sofosbuvir: A case series. Postgrad Med. 1-5, 2015
2. Fabrizi F et al: Hepatitis C virus infection, mixed cryoglobulinemia, and kidney disease. Am J Kidney Dis. 61(4):623-37, 2013
3. Perico N et al. Hepatitis C infection and chronic renal diseases. Clin J Am Soc Nephrol. 4(1):207-20, 2009
4. Seeff LB: The history of the "natural history" of hepatitis C (1968-2009). Liver Int. 29 Suppl 1:89-99, 2009
5. Kamar N et al: Hepatitis C virus-related kidney disease: an overview. Clin Nephrol. 69(3):149-60, 2008
6. Alpers CE et al: Emerging paradigms in the renal pathology of viral diseases. Clin J Am Soc Nephrol. 2 Suppl 1:S6-12, 2007
7. Barsoum RS: Hepatitis C virus: from entry to renal injury–facts and potentials. Nephrol Dial Transplant. 22(7):1840-8, 2007
8. Markowitz GS et al: Hepatitis C viral infection is associated with fibrillary glomerulonephritis and immunotactoid glomerulopathy. J Am Soc Nephrol. 9(12):2244-52, 1998

(Left) *Prominent subepithelial "spikes" are noted in this membranous GN case associated with HCV infection.* **(Right)** *Immunofluorescence microscopy for IgG reveals strong granular staining of the glomerular capillaries with faint granular staining of the mesangial areas. Mesangial staining suggests a secondary form of membranous GN, but establishing the presence of hepatitis C infection requires other lab tests.*

MGN

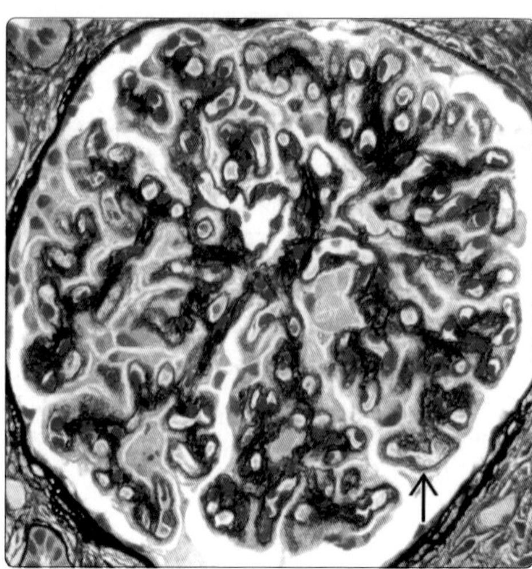

MGN and IgG

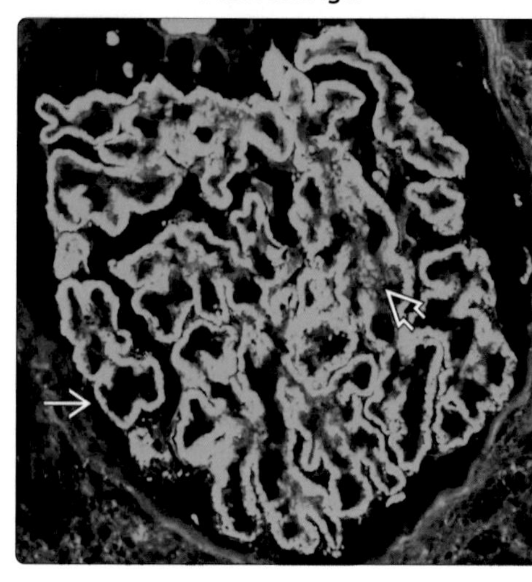

(Left) *Electron microscopy reveals numerous subepithelial electron-dense deposits with basement membrane reaction between and surrounding some of the deposits. The podocyte foot processes show extensive effacement.* **(Right)** *A cellular crescent occupies the urinary space and surrounds the remaining glomerulus, which has a membranoproliferative pattern of injury characterized by endocapillary proliferation and a lobular appearance of the glomerular tufts.*

Subepithelial Deposits

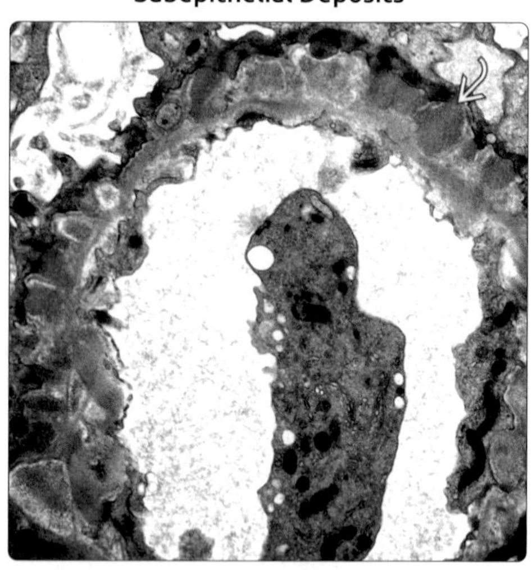

MPGN With Crescent

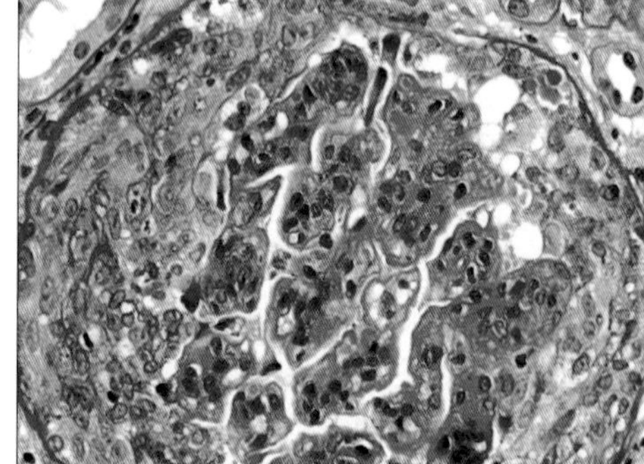

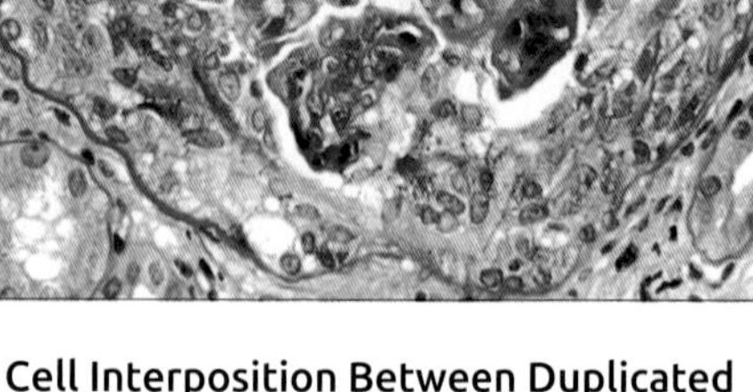

(Left) *IgG staining of the glomerular capillaries and mesangial areas is characteristic for membranoproliferative GN. This staining pattern is not specific for HCV-associated MPGN and is identical to that seen in idiopathic MPGN.* **(Right)** *Interposition of cells between the duplicated GBMs is a characteristic finding of MPGN as identified in this patient with hepatitis C infection. Occasional subepithelial deposits are seen in this case with features of type III MPGN.*

MPGN and IgG

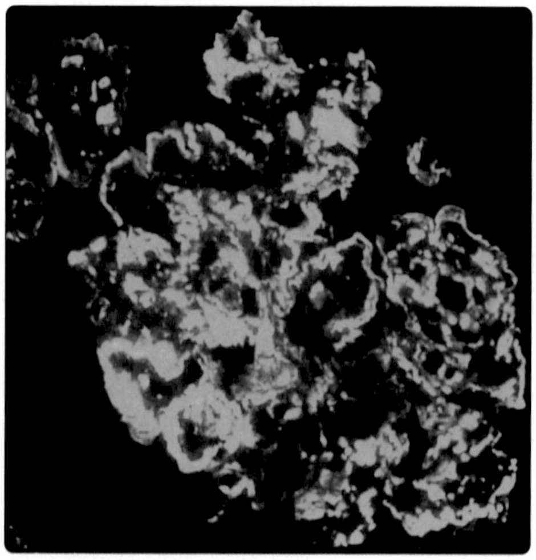

Cell Interposition Between Duplicated GBMs

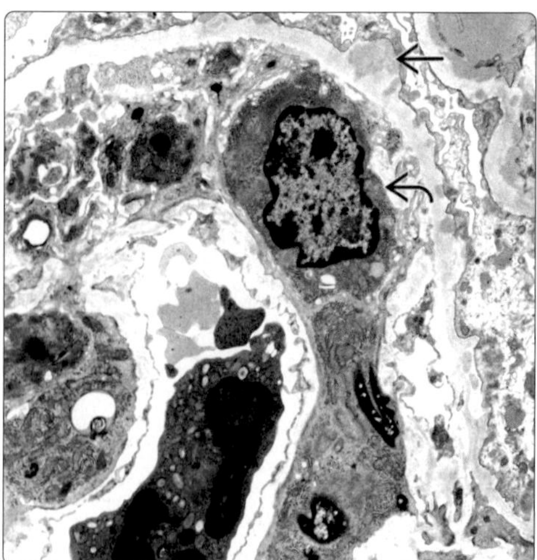

Cryoglobulinemic GN

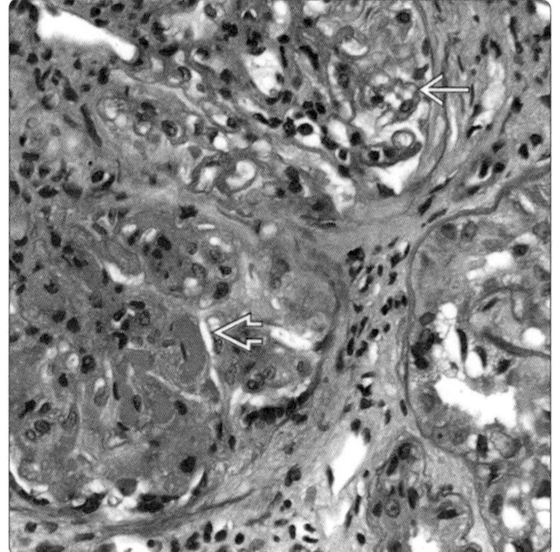

IgM

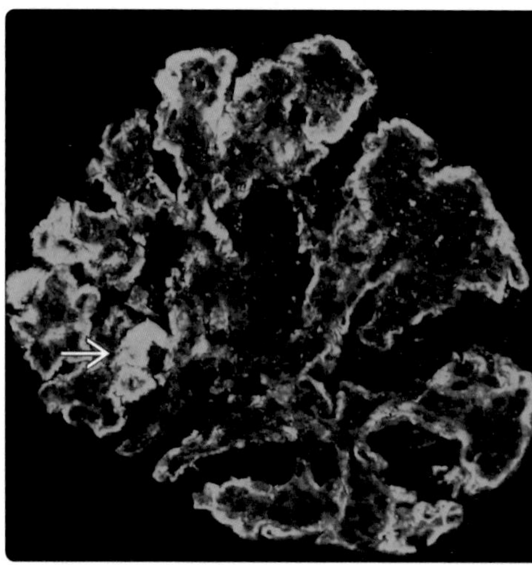

(Left) *Numerous hyaline thrombi ➡ are present in the glomerular capillaries. The alterations in an adjacent glomerulus ➡ are not as noticeable.* **(Right)** *IgM demonstrates strong staining of the peripheral glomerular capillaries with a hyaline thrombus ➡ in 1 glomerular capillary. HCV should be considered as a potential etiologic agent in almost any form of immune complex glomerulonephritis.*

Cryoglobulinemic GN EM Substructure

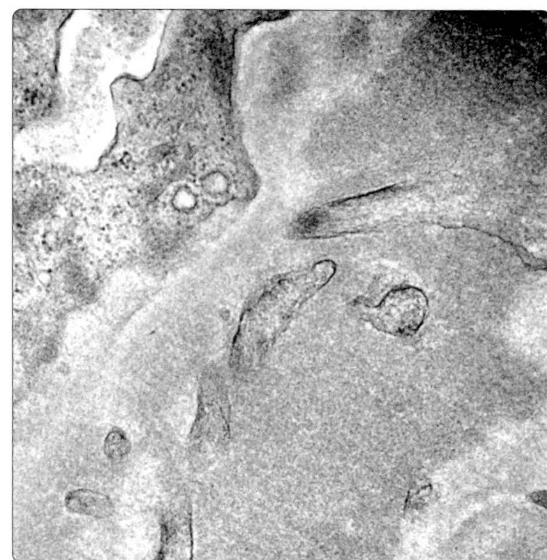

Fibrillary GN

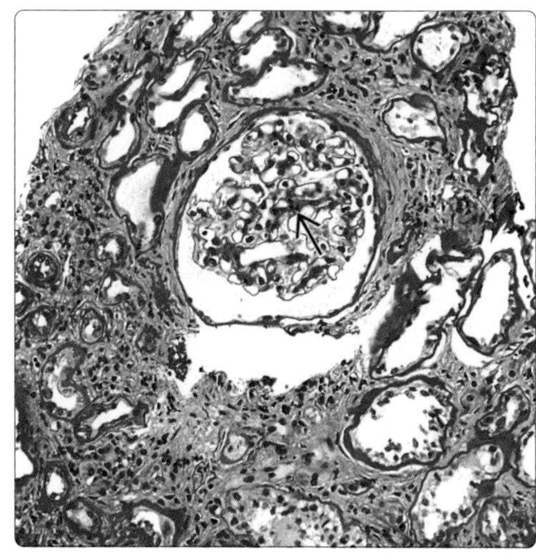

(Left) *At high magnification, a vague substructure of the electron-dense deposits can be seen, but the presence or absence of this finding is not diagnostic for cryoglobulinemic GN.* **(Right)** *This case of fibrillary GN in a 50-year-old woman with chronic kidney disease, hypertension, and hepatitis C infection reveals extensive global glomerulosclerosis (not shown), interstitial fibrosis, and tubular atrophy. A rare intact glomerulus shows very mild mesangial hypercellularity and mesangial matrix expansion ➡.*

Fibrillary GP and IgG

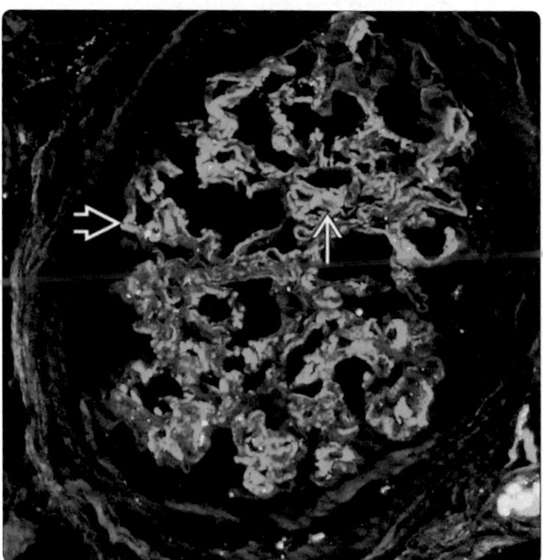

Fibrillary GN

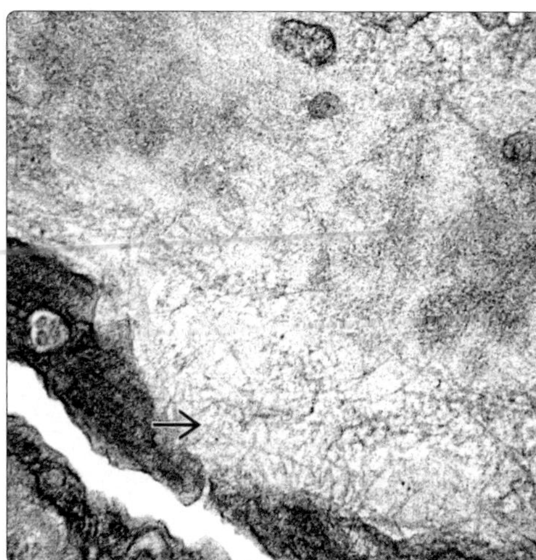

(Left) *Immunofluorescence reveals smudgy mesangial ➡ and glomerular capillary loop ➡ staining for IgG. Polyclonal staining for kappa and lambda light chains (not shown) helps support the diagnostic consideration of fibrillary GN.* **(Right)** *Electron microscopy at high magnification reveals many randomly arranged fibrils ➡ that each measure approximately 17 nm in diameter.*

HIV-Associated Nephropathy

KEY FACTS

TERMINOLOGY

- Characteristic renal disease developing in setting of HIV infection, manifested by nephrotic-range proteinuria and collapsing glomerulopathy

ETIOLOGY/PATHOGENESIS

- *APOL1* polymorphisms predispose to HIV-associated nephropathy (HIVAN) but not HIV-immune complex kidney disease

CLINICAL ISSUES

- 90% occur in African Americans, mostly male
- Rapid progression to end-stage renal disease (ESRD)
- Hypertension uncommon (< 50%)
- Nephrotic-range proteinuria & ↑ creatinine
- Treatment: HAART, ACE inhibitors

MICROSCOPIC

- Global or segmental collapse of capillary tufts without mesangial matrix increase
  - Hyperplasia of visceral epithelium
  - May resemble crescents
- Microcystic tubular dilatation (30-40% of cases)
- Mononuclear cells (including lymphocytes & monocytes) & plasma cells
- Interstitial inflammation & edema

ANCILLARY TESTS

- IF: IgM, C3, & C1q in capillary walls in segmental distribution
- EM
  - Podocyte foot process effacement & multilamination of subepithelial glomerular basement membrane
  - Tubuloreticular inclusions (TRIs) in endothelial cells, lymphocytes, & monocytes

TOP DIFFERENTIAL DIAGNOSES

- Idiopathic collapsing glomerulopathy
- HIV-associated, lupus-like GN & other immune complex GN
- Diffuse mesangial hypercellularity

Visceral Epithelial Hyperplasia

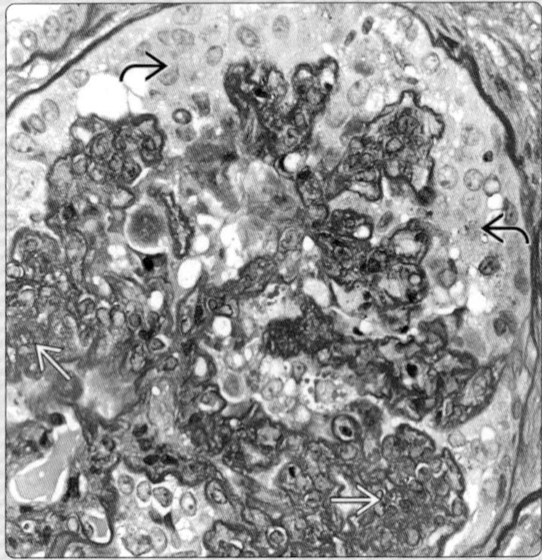

Segmental C3

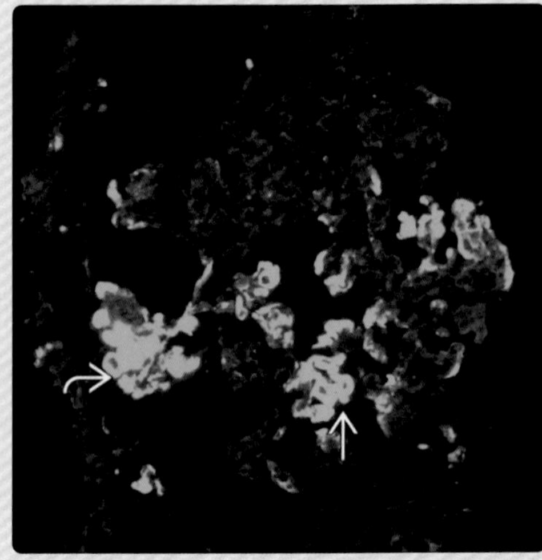

(Left) *Classic appearance of HIVAN with glomerular collapse ➡ & proliferation of overlying podocytes ⮕ is well demonstrated by PAS stains in this HIV(+) man. The podocyte hypercellularity mimics a crescent.* **(Right)** *In a 46-year-old man with HIV, 11 g/d proteinuria, & Cr 4.5, recently started on HAART, there is peripheral glomerular capillary loop staining for C3 by immunofluorescence along glomerular basement membranes ➡ and in collapsed glomerular capillary loops ⮕.*

Cisternae and Tubuloreticular Structures

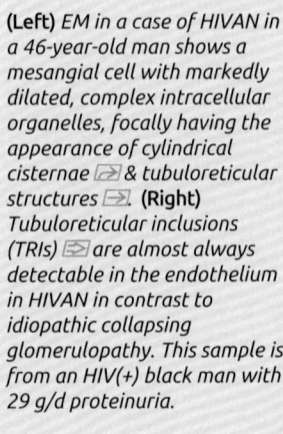

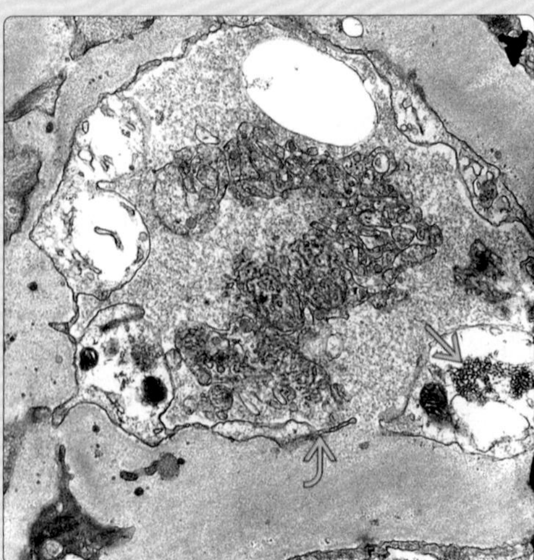

Tubuloreticular Inclusions

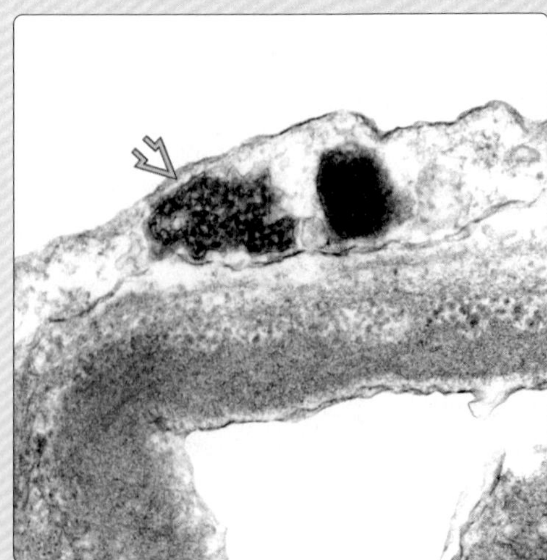

(Left) *EM in a case of HIVAN in a 46-year-old man shows a mesangial cell with markedly dilated, complex intracellular organelles, focally having the appearance of cylindrical cisternae ⮕ & tubuloreticular structures ⮕.* **(Right)** *Tubuloreticular inclusions (TRIs) ⮕ are almost always detectable in the endothelium in HIVAN in contrast to idiopathic collapsing glomerulopathy. This sample is from an HIV(+) black man with 29 g/d proteinuria.*

TERMINOLOGY

Synonyms

- HIV-associated nephropathy (HIVAN)
- HIV-associated collapsing glomerulopathy

Definitions

- Characteristic renal disease developing in setting of HIV infection, manifested by nephrotic-range proteinuria and collapsing glomerulopathy

ETIOLOGY/PATHOGENESIS

Infectious Agents

- Kidney may be HIV "reservoir"
  - HIV genome demonstrated in glomerular visceral & tubular epithelial cells in HIVAN
- Others suggest direct viral infection of tubular & glomerular epithelial cells & viral gene expression in kidney
  - HIV enters tubule cells via DEC205 & podocytes via DCSIGN
  - HIV tat protein enters podocytes via lipid rafts
  - Viral contributing factors include HIV proteins, Nef & Vpr
- Researchers failed to find direct action of infectious pathogen on renal parenchyma (i.e., glomeruli)
- Abnormal immunophenotype of podocytes demonstrated
- Cytokines may have role (e.g., transforming growth factor-β [TGF-β], basic fibroblast growth factor [bFGF], interleukin, & others)
- AIDS not required for condition to occur

Genetic Factors

- Higher risk with African ancestry (except Ethiopian)
  - *APOL1* polymorphisms predispose to HIVAN but not HIV-immune complex kidney disease

CLINICAL ISSUES

Epidemiology

- Incidence
  - Highest rates in East Coast of USA
  - Acute kidney injury: 2.7 episodes per 100 person-years
    - Higher in first 3 months: 19.3 episodes per 100 person-years
- Sex
  - ~ 70% male
- Ethnicity
  - 90% African Americans
  - Less common in whites (essentially absent in Swiss-Europeans & Thai populations)

Presentation

- Proteinuria, nephrotic range
  - Severe, averaging 6-7 g/d
  - Edema, hypoalbuminemia, & hypercholesterolemia (nephrotic syndrome) uncommon
- Renal dysfunction: Creatinine at diagnosis ~ 5 mg/dL
- Hypertension: < 50%
- Microhematuria

Laboratory Tests

- ± granular casts; red blood cells on urinalysis
- CD4 count does not correlate with HIVAN development
- Hypercholesterolemia uncommon, possibly due to ↓ hepatic lipoprotein synthesis in AIDS patients

Treatment

- Drugs
  - Highly active antiretroviral therapy (HAART)
    - May reverse tubular microcysts & slow HIVAN
  - Angiotensin-converting enzyme (ACE) inhibitors
- Hemodialysis
- Renal transplantation

Prognosis

- Rapid progression, with end-stage renal disease (ESRD) developing in months
  - Early in AIDS epidemic, mean time to dialysis < 2 months & median survival of renal disease to death was 4.5 months
- Does not recur in renal transplants, which have good outcomes

IMAGING

Ultrasonographic Findings

- Enlarged, highly echogenic kidneys

MACROSCOPIC

General Features

- Pale cortex
- 0.5-1 mm cysts in cortex or corticomedullary junction

Size

- Enlarged
  - Mean combined weight up to 500 g in adults
- 1.2-1.3x normal weight in children

MICROSCOPIC

Histologic Features

- Collapsing glomerulopathy ± glomerular enlargement
  - Global or segmental collapse of capillary tufts without mesangial matrix increase
    - Shrunken, global glomerulosclerosis ± enlarged Bowman space may represent advanced phase of collapsing injury
  - ± marked podocyte hyperplasia, protein resorption droplets, & mitoses
    - Contrary to prior belief that podocytes could not proliferate
  - Hyperplastic/hypertrophic podocytes
    - May mimic crescent
    - Termed visceral glomerular epitheliosis
- Tubules
  - Microcystic tubular dilatation (30-40% of cases)
    - ± scalloped tubular outline
    - ± PAS(+) proteinaceous casts (fuchsin[+] on trichrome) in renal tubules
  - Patchy epithelial injury, regeneration/mitosis, degeneration, necrosis, & eventual tubular atrophy
    - Tubular resorption droplets prominent
- Interstitium
  - Interstitial inflammation & edema

- Mononuclear cells (including lymphocytes & monocytes) & plasma cells
  - Interstitial fibrosis typically present
- Vessels typically unremarkable
  - Rare cases of thrombotic microangiopathy

ANCILLARY TESTS

Immunofluorescence

- Segmental IgM, C3, & C1q
  - ± IgM & C3 granular positivity
- Resorption droplets in podocytes & proximal tubules stain for multiple plasma proteins

Electron Microscopy

- Glomeruli
  - Podocytes enlarged with ≥ 1 dense, round secondary lysosome & enlarged vacuoles
    - Foot processes completely effaced
    - Cell detachment from original glomerular basement membrane (GBM) forming new basement membrane material
      - BM-type material may eventually occlude capillary loops in segmental sclerosing/collapsing-type process
    - Nuclear bodies: Nuclear inclusions with broad morphologic variety
  - Subepithelial deposits sometimes seen in superimposed immune complex kidney disease with "ball-in-cup" architectural pattern
    - Deposits can be large & associated with GBM reaction & GBM holes
    - Associated crescent formation can be found
    - Investigators suggest these deposits overlap with postinfectious & membranous glomerulopathy
      - Such cases may represent HIV immune complex kidney disease (HIVICK)
      - Some suggest that these contain viral particles
      - Others have seen such "ball-in-cup" lesions outside of HIV setting (in lupus nephritis, postinfectious GN prior to HIV era, & lecithin cholesterol acyltransferase deficiency)
      - "Ball-in-cup" lesions typical but not specific for HIVICK
  - ± small nonspecific deposits in mesangium, correlating to mesangial IgM & C3
  - Tubuloreticular inclusions (TRIs) in endothelial cells, lymphocytes, & monocytes
    - Measure ~ 25 nm & found in dilated endoplasmic reticulum cisternae as anastomosed tubular structures
    - Most easily identified in glomerular endothelium
      - Also, infiltrating leukocytes or arterial peritubular capillary or interstitial capillary endothelium
    - Less common than in HIVAN initial description due to ↓ with HAART therapy, likely due to ↓ viral burden
    - Also referred to as interferon (IFN) footprints or myxovirus-like inclusions; seen in other settings, e.g., systemic lupus erythematosus (SLE), multiple sclerosis (MS), & IFN-α therapy
    - Cylindrical confronting cisternae: Fused membranous lamellae forming long cylinders (known as test tube & ring-shaped forms) occur in cells with TRIs (monocytes & lymphocytes) (also seen in SLE, MS, & IFN-α therapy)
- Tubules & other cells sometimes have granular or granulofibrillar nuclear changes
  - Granular: Coarsely granular material disrupting nuclear membrane
  - Granulofibrillar: Chromatin replaced by material with coarse or fine granularity, primarily seen post mortem
- HIV not definitively observed in renal cells by standard EM methods

Immunohistochemistry

- IHC shows CD4(+) & CD8(+) cells & ↓ CD4/CD8 ratio
- HLA-DR on inflammatory & parenchymal cells (endothelial, glomerular mesangial, & visceral epithelial)
- Minor B-cell & macrophage component

DIFFERENTIAL DIAGNOSIS

Idiopathic Collapsing Glomerulopathy

- HIV negative
- TRIs more often in HIVAN
- Other etiologies of collapsing glomerulopathy to be considered
  - Viruses (parvovirus B19, cytomegalovirus, & Epstein-Barr virus)
  - Drug toxicity, thrombotic microangiopathy, and others

Idiopathic/Primary Focal Segmental Glomerulosclerosis (FSGS)

- Glomerular hyalinosis is common feature in idiopathic FSGS but not HIVAN
- Collapsing FSGS with prominent hyperplastic podocytes more typical of HIVAN
- TRIs much more common in HIVAN

Heroin-Associated Nephropathy (HAN)

- Difficult to distinguish from HIVAN if both risk factors present
- Glomerulosclerosis in HAN more typical of idiopathic form of FSGS, displaying hyalinosis
- Prominent collapsing glomerulopathy with microcystic tubular dilatation more common in HIVAN

Diffuse Mesangial Hypercellularity (DMH) & Minimal Change Disease (MCD)

- Usually milder than HIVAN & present with nephrotic syndrome & normal renal function (i.e., normal GFR)
- Typical HIVAN accounts for ≤ 50% of HIV-related glomerulopathies in children
  - DMH almost as common as HIVAN
  - Minimal change disease also quite common
- Rapid renal failure course favors HIVAN

SELECTED REFERENCES

1. Rosenberg AZ et al: HIV-associated nephropathies: epidemiology, pathology, mechanisms and treatment. Nat Rev Nephrol. 11(3):150-160, 2015
2. Mohan S et al: The changing pattern of glomerular disease in HIV and hepatitis C co-infected patients in the era of HAART. Clin Nephrol. 79(4):285-91, 2013
3. Ahmed S et al: Evolving spectrum of HIV-associated nephropathy. Nephron Clin Pract. 121(3-4):c131-5, 2012

Podocyte Resorption Droplets

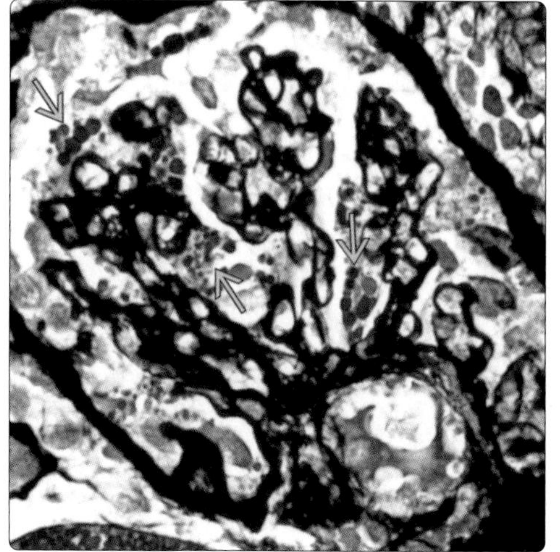

Collapsed Glomerulus

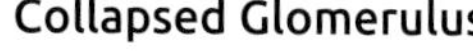

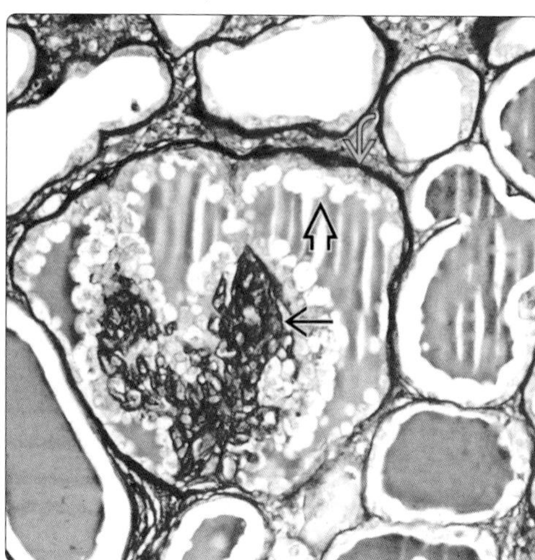

(Left) *Prominent podocyte resorption droplets → are present. This finding alone should prompt careful searching for focal segmental glomerulosclerosis and additional level sections should be ordered if needed.* **(Right)** *Higher power shows that the collapsed glomerulus in a case of HIVAN → is surrounded by a dilated Bowman space → with scalloping of proteinaceous cast material at the periphery →.*

Glomerular Collapse & Bowman Space Dilatation

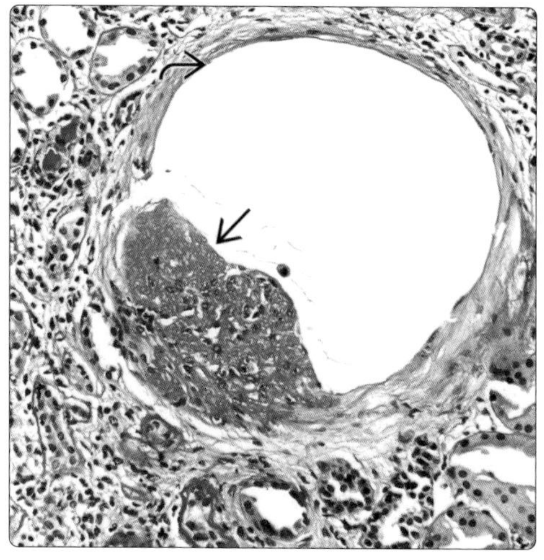

Collapsed Glomerulus

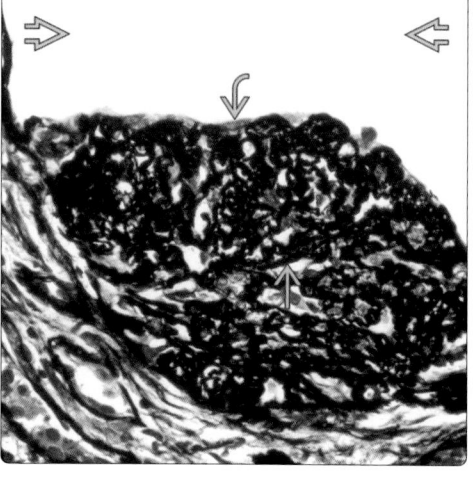

(Left) *Collapsed glomerulus → with a dilated Bowman space → is shown in a case of HIVAN in a 58-year-old man not on HAART with CD4 count < 200, Cr 3.7, and > 3 g/d proteinuria.* **(Right)** *Higher power shows a completely collapsed glomerulus → with a dilated Bowman space → in a 58-year-old man with HIVAN. The Jones silver stain allows the appreciation of the residual GBM →.*

Ki-67 Proliferative Glomerular Epithelial Cells

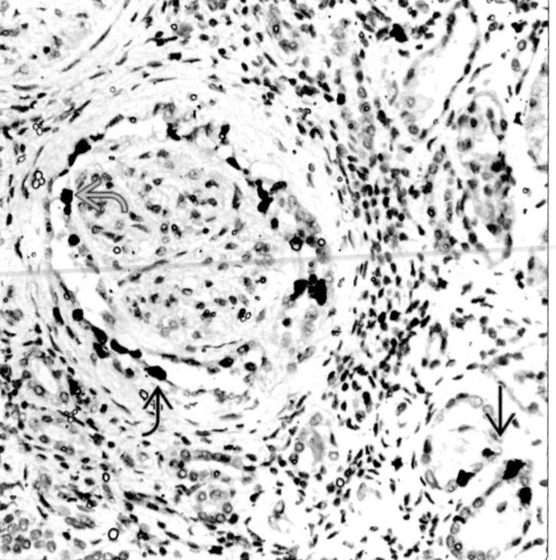

Segmental IgM

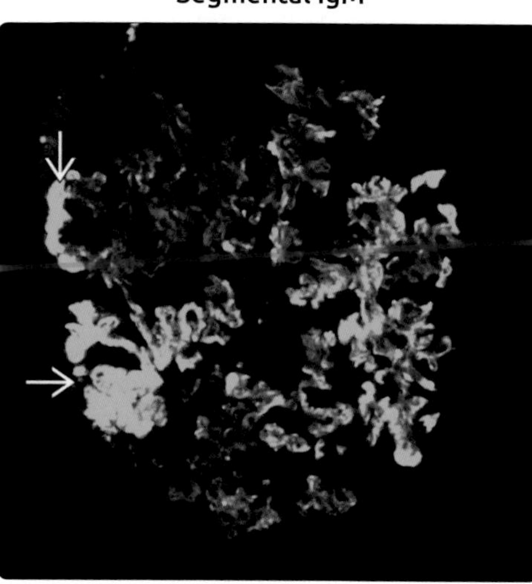

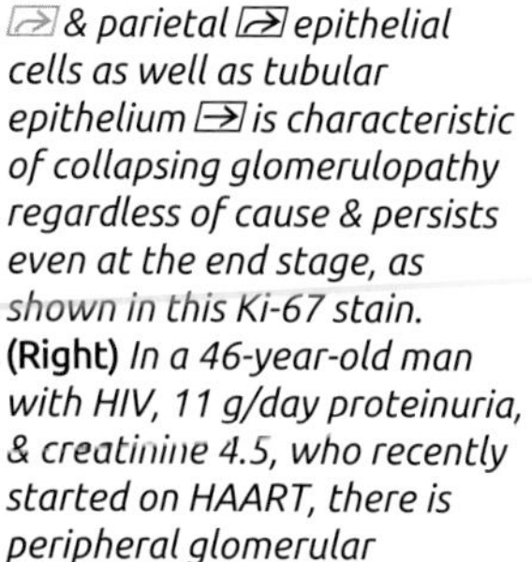

(Left) *Proliferation of visceral → & parietal → epithelial cells as well as tubular epithelium → is characteristic of collapsing glomerulopathy regardless of cause & persists even at the end stage, as shown in this Ki-67 stain.* **(Right)** *In a 46-year-old man with HIV, 11 g/day proteinuria, & creatinine 4.5, who recently started on HAART, there is peripheral glomerular capillary loop staining for IgM → by immunofluorescence.*

(Left) *Massively dilated tubules are a characteristic of collapsing glomerulopathy in HIVAN as well as in other causes. Interstitial inflammation is also a typical feature.* **(Right)** *At relatively low power, glomerular basement membrane wrinkling & collapse can be appreciated. There is also tubular cystic change with accumulation of proteinaceous casts.*

Tubular Dilatation

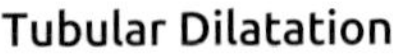

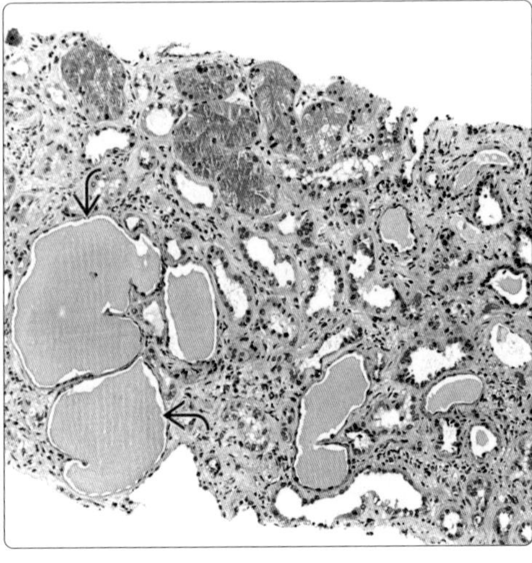

Glomerular Collapse & Cystic Tubular Change

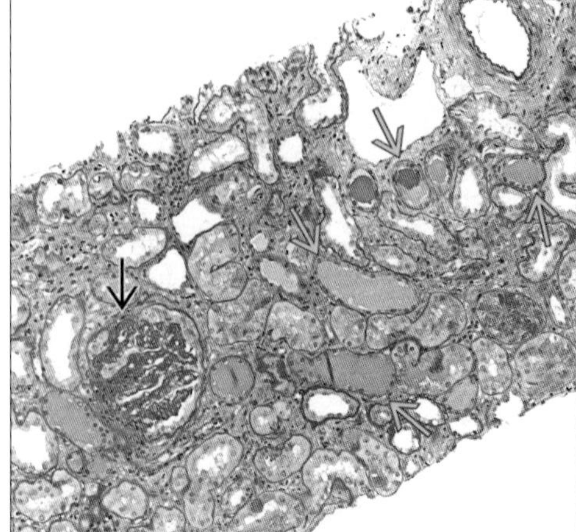

(Left) *Glomerular capillary loop collapse is present & is accompanied by cystic tubular dilatation with prominent proteinaceous casts.* **(Right)** *In the tubulointerstitium of a 58-year-old man with HIVAN, CD4 count < 200, Cr 3.7, & > 3 g/d proteinuria, there is tubular injury with evident mitotic activity & an inflammatory infiltrate composed of mononuclear cells & plasma cells.*

Glomerular Collapse & Cystic Tubular Change

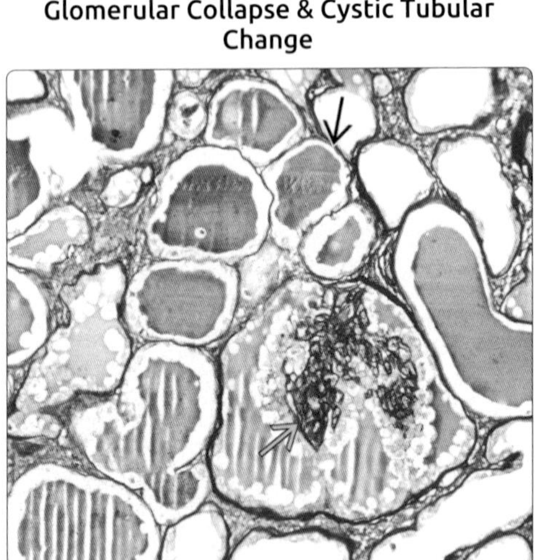

Tubular Injury & Mitotic Activity

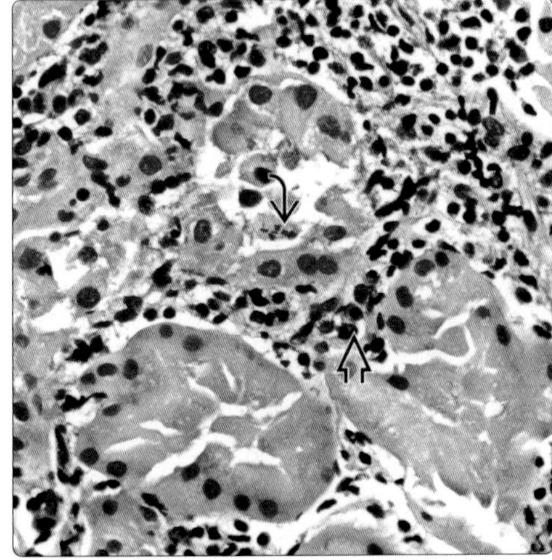

(Left) *Renal tubules are injured, as evidenced by patchy nuclear loss and apoptotic activity.* **(Right)** *HAART has reduced HIVAN incidence considerably; however, the inhibitory effects of antireverse transcriptase on mtDNA can cause a mitochondriopathy, diagnosed by abnormally shaped and enlarged mitochondria by EM and revealed by light microscopy, which leads to interstitial fibrosis & tubular atrophy.*

Tubular Injury & Apoptotic Activity

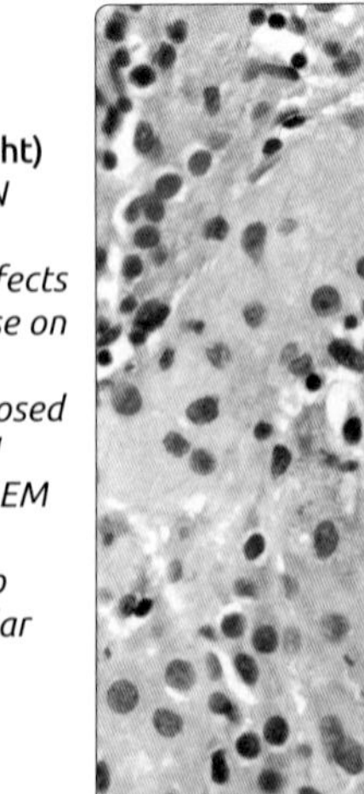

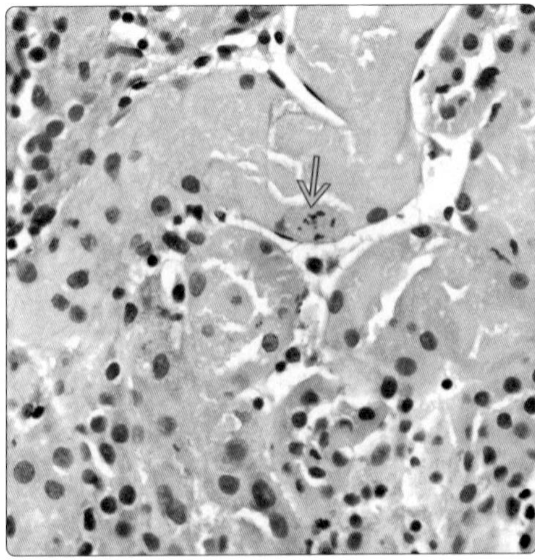

Mitochondrial Abnormalities in HIVAN

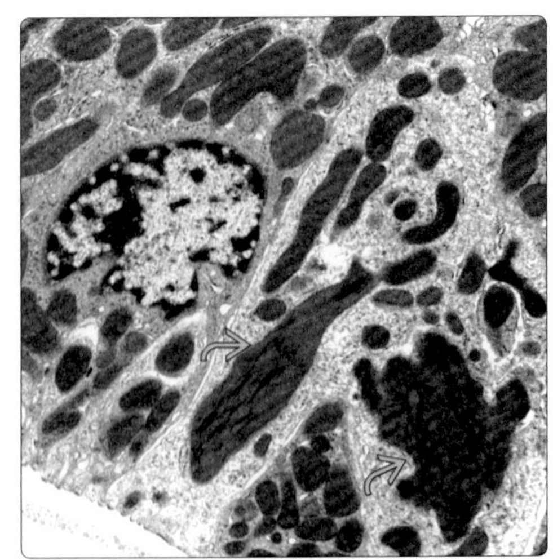

Podocyte Foot Process Effacement in HIVAN

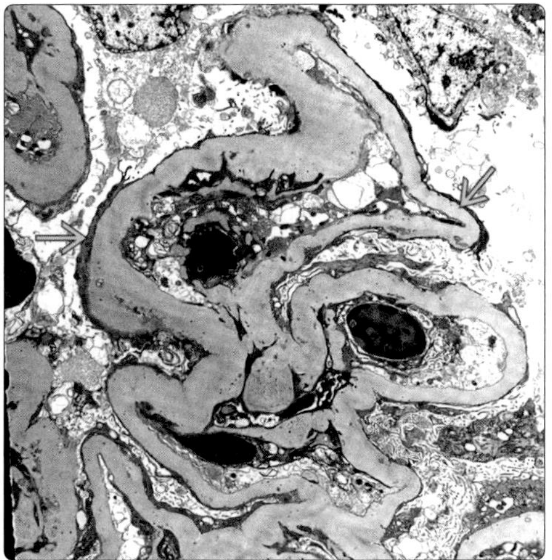

New GBM-Associated With Podocyte Foot Process Effacement

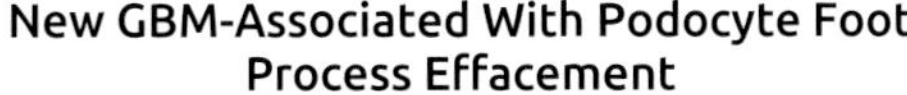

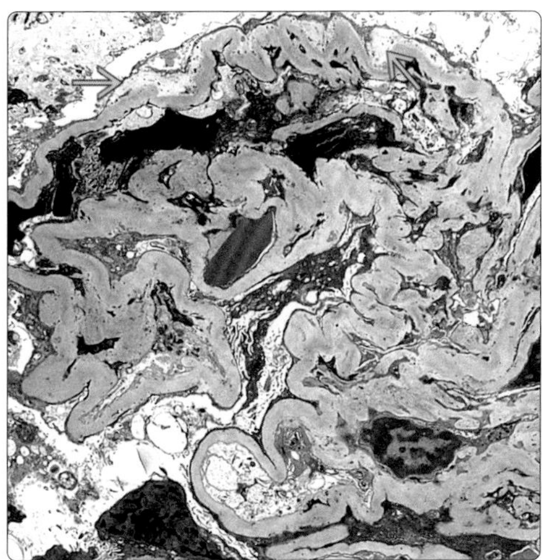

(Left) *In a case of HIVAN in a 46-year-old man with HIV, 11 g/d proteinuria, & Cr 4.5, who recently started on HAART, EM shows collapsed glomerular capillary loops with completely effaced podocyte foot processes.* **(Right)** *One of the characteristic features of collapsing glomerulopathy, whether due to HIV or other causes, is the separation of podocytes from the GBM by multilaminated new basement membrane, originally described in heroin nephropathy.*

Parietal Epithelial Cells Replacing Podocytes

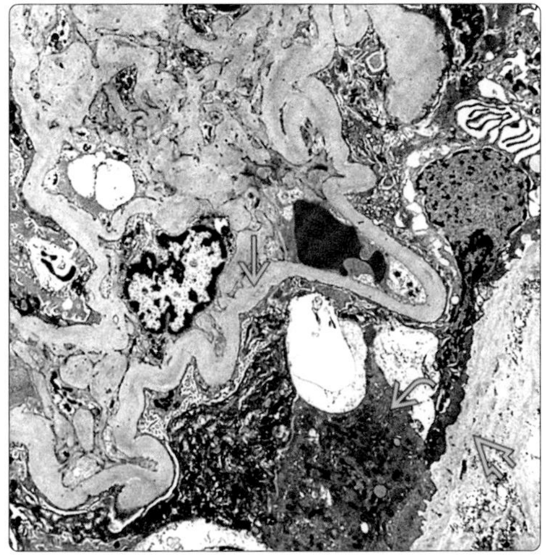

Podocyte Hyperplasia in HIVAN

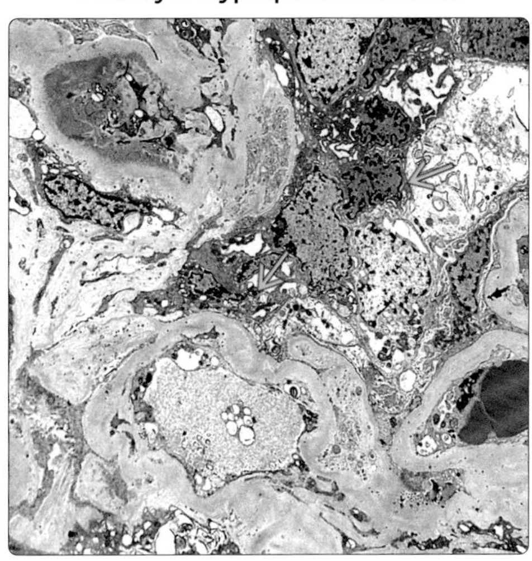

(Left) *One of the debates in collapsing glomerulopathy is the nature of the proliferating epithelial cells. This image from a case of HIVAN shows a cell bridging between Bowman capsule and the GBM, consistent with replacement of podocytes by parietal epithelium.* **(Right)** *In HIVAN, the podocytes are hyperplastic and have complete loss of foot processes. The podocytes lose expression of many markers of differentiation, such as WT1 and synaptopodin.*

Tubuloreticular Inclusions (TRIs) in HIVAN

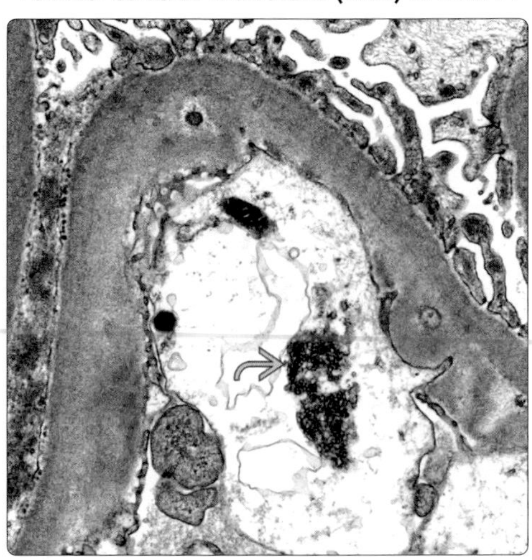

Tubuloreticular Inclusions

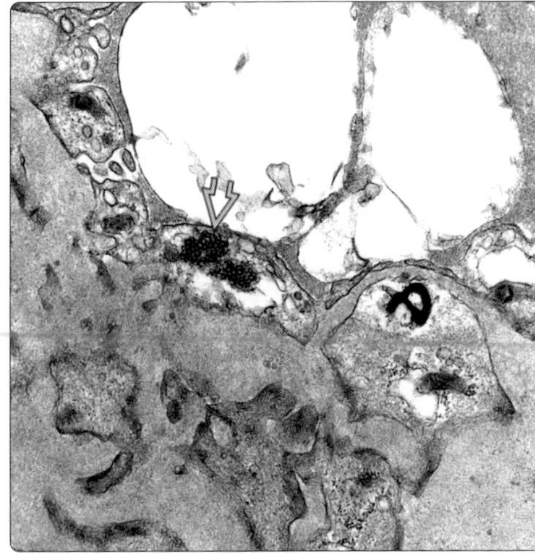

(Left) *In this biopsy from a 58-year-old HIV(+) man not on HAART with a CD4 count < 200, Cr 3.7, and > 3 g/d proteinuria, there are TRIs in glomerular endothelium.* **(Right)** *In this case of collapsing glomerulopathy secondary to HIV infection, a tubuloreticular inclusion is present at the periphery of a glomerular capillary loop within a cell that is likely an activated glomerular endothelial cell.*

TERMINOLOGY

Abbreviations

- HIV-associated renal diseases (HIV-ARD)

Definitions

- Diseases in HIV patients other than collapsing glomerulopathy (HIV-associated nephropathy [HIVAN]), due to direct effect on kidney, altered immune system, or drug toxicity

HIV-ASSOCIATED LUPUS-LIKE GLOMERULONEPHRITIS

Terminology

- Immune complex disease with LM, IF, and EM features of lupus nephritis in HIV-infected patients without systemic lupus erythematosus
  - Described by Haas et al and Nochy et al

Pathogenesis

- Probably related to immune dysregulation
- Loss of CD4(+) T regulatory cells causes autoimmune disease
- Role of infectious agent not excluded
- *APOL1* genetic variants confer risk for HIVAN but not HIV-immune-complex kidney disease

Incidence

- 3% in series of > 100 biopsies for glomerular disease in HIV(+) patients
  - Possibly 2nd most common form of glomerular lesions (after HIVAN) in HIV patients undergoing biopsy
  - Most were blacks in US (93%) (Haas)
  - Equal number of whites and blacks in Europe (Nochy)

Presentation

- Hematuria
- Proteinuria/nephrotic syndrome
- Other features such as anemia, leukopenia, multiorgan involvement, and serositis

Laboratory Tests

- ± ANA and anti-dsDNA and ↓ complement C3, C4
  - Assessment complicated because some HIV patients have low-titer ANAs
    - Screening of > 150 AIDS patients found 19 ANA(+) but only 2 at high titer and all anti-dsDNA Ab(-)

Treatment

- Corticosteroids, ACE inhibitors, highly active antiretroviral therapy (HAART)

Prognosis

- Poor, because most with advanced disease
- Recurrence after transplantation reported

Microscopic Pathology

- Focal/diffuse proliferative or membranous glomerulonephritis

Immunofluorescence

- "Full house" pattern of IgG, IgA, IgM, C3, and C1q

Electron Microscopy

- Tubuloreticular inclusions
- Most common combination with mesangial, subendothelial, subepithelial, and intramembranous deposits

Differential Diagnosis

- Lupus nephritis
  - HIV-associated lupus-like GN less commonly has positive lupus serologies (ANA, dsDNA) and nonrenal manifestations
  - "Full house" immunofluorescence staining pattern more common in lupus than HIV
  - Tubuloreticular inclusions may be seen in both lupus nephritis and HIV

Glomerular Hypercellularity in Lupus-Like GN in HIV

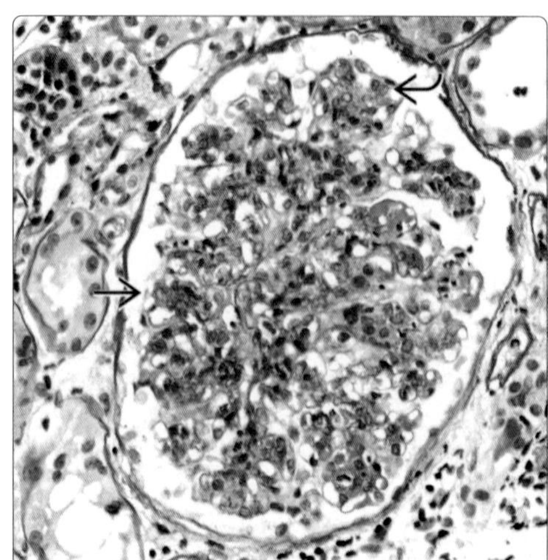

Thickened GBMs in Lupus-Like GN in HIV

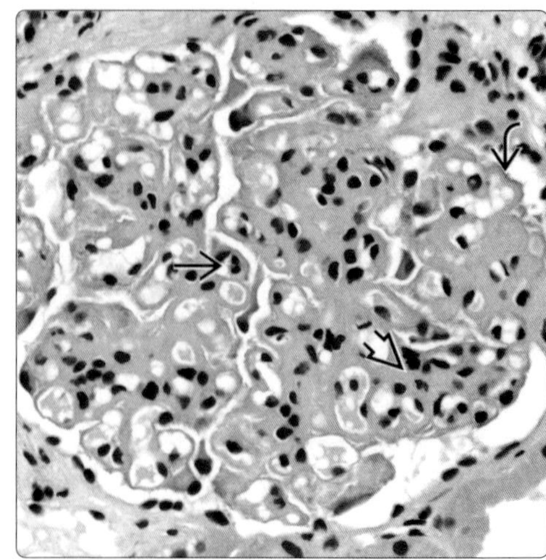

(Left) *In a 56-year-old woman with HIV, hepatitis C, decreased C3, low normal C4, and hypertension, there is a marked increase in glomerular cellularity* ➔ *in a lupus-like glomerulonephritis (GN). The glomerulus also appears enlarged with vague lobules* ➚. **(Right)** *Lupus-like GN is one of the more frequent diseases associated with HIV, typically showing a markedly expanded mesangium* ⇨, *thickened capillary walls* ➚, *and inflammatory cells in glomerular capillary loops* ➔.

IgA NEPHROPATHY

Terminology

- IgA(+) glomerular disease arising in HIV(+) patients has similar clinical and pathologic aspects to idiopathic IgA nephropathy
  - Reports included Henoch-Schönlein purpura (HSP) nephritis

Pathogenesis

- Deposits eluted from glomeruli have specificity for HIV envelope (e.g., gp41, gp120, gp160) or core proteins (e.g., p24) (Kimmel)

Incidence

- Higher incidence of IgA nephropathy in white HIV patients reported in several series
- Some studies indicate high prevalence of IgA deposits, but without increased IgA nephropathy

Presentation

- Hematuria and low-grade proteinuria common
- May present with HSP (rash, leukocytoclastic angiitis of skin)

Laboratory Tests

- Associated with IgA-containing cryoglobulins
- ↑ IgA levels, IgA-containing circulating immune complexes, and IgA-rheumatoid factor

Treatment

- ACE inhibitors may be useful

Prognosis

- Same as IgA nephropathy in non-HIV-infected patients

Histologic Features

- Similar to conventional IgA nephropathy in absence of HIV
  - Mesangial proliferation ± collapsing glomerulosclerosis (if coexisting HIVAN)

Immunofluorescence

- Shows mesangial IgA deposits like conventional IgA nephropathy seen in absence of HIV

Electron Microscopy

- Tubuloreticular structures provide clue to presence of HIV in contrast with idiopathic IgA nephropathy

HIV IMMUNE COMPLEX KIDNEY DISEASE

Terminology

- Infection-related immune complex GN, also referred as HIV immune complex kidney disease (HIVICK)

Etiology

- Some cases have identifiable postinfectious association
  - Recent series indicate *Staphylococcus* is important cause in HIV patients

Epidemiology

- Many reports originate from South Africa
- In HIV-positive populations of European origin, HIVICK is dominant glomerular disease and HIVAN is less common

Prognosis

- End-stage renal disease (ESRD) progression less likely in HIVICK than HIVAN
- May recur in transplants

Histologic Features

- May have patterns of typical postinfectious GN
- Acute
  - Diffuse segmental to global endocapillary hypercellularity with mostly neutrophils
  - EM shows primarily subepithelial deposits in "notch" configuration and sometimes "humps"
  - ± resorption along with rare intramembranous, mesangial, and subendothelial deposits
- Healed
  - ± endocapillary hypercellularity with mostly mononuclear cells, if present
  - EM shows "notch" and rare "hump" deposits, sometimes with numerous intramembranous, mesangial, and subendothelial deposits, all of which can show evidence of resorption
- Persistent
  - Focal segmental endocapillary hypercellularity with mostly mononuclear cells
  - EM shows "humps" and "notch" deposits with at least some resorption ± intramembranous, mesangial, and subendothelial deposits
  - Immune complexes seen on EM may have "ball-in-cup" configuration, with a subepithelial deposit surrounded by a cup of GBM.
    - Described in South African cases
    - Found in other settings such as lupus nephritis

THROMBOTIC MICROANGIOPATHY

Terminology

- Thrombotic microangiopathy (TMA) associated with HIV infection
- Thrombotic thrombocytopenic purpura (TTP) and hemolytic uremic syndrome (HUS)

Pathogenesis

- Etiology not known
  - HIV injury to endothelium or infection of megakaryocytes may be involved
  - Role attributed to CMV infection, cryptosporidiosis, AIDS-related neoplasia, drugs, and antiphospholipid antibodies
  - ADAMTS13 level not ↓ in HIV-associated TMA as with TTP
  - *Escherichia coli* 0157:H7 not involved
- Animal model
  - 6/27 (22.2%) pig-tailed macaques (*Macaca nemestrina*) acutely infected with HIV-2 developed histological and EM features of renal TMA such as glomerular capillary platelet thrombi and mesangiolysis

Incidence

- French study (Peraldi et al) attributed rapid renal function decline to HUS-type syndrome in 32 of 92 patients
- Multicenter autopsy study showed 15 (7%) of 214 patients with deaths attributable to AIDS had evidence of TMA

Presentation

- Acute renal failure ± proteinuria and hematuria
- Microangiopathic hemolytic anemia and thrombocytopenia
- May be classified as either HUS or TTP (neurologic symptoms and fever)

Laboratory Tests

- ± thrombocytopenia ± schistocytosis

Treatment

- Treatment of underlying HIV
- Plasmapheresis and fresh frozen plasma
- Rituximab and corticosteroids
- Hemodialysis may be needed

Prognosis

- Higher mortality in HIV-infected than non-HIV-infected patients

Histologic Features

- Pathologic findings similar to those of TMA in non-HIV-infected patients
  - Mucoid arterial intimal hyperplasia and intraluminal thrombi may be observed
  - Fragmented intramural RBCs in vessels
- May coexist with HIVAN

Immunofluorescence

- As in other TMA, fibrinogen/fibrin may be found in glomerular capillary walls, in mesangium, and in arteriolar/arterial walls, corresponding to intravascular thrombi
- Glomerular capillary walls may show IgM, C3, IgG, and rarely IgA
- IgM may be seen in arteriolar/arterial walls

Electron Microscopy

- Tubuloreticular structures may be only clue to presence of HIV

Differential Diagnosis

- Hypertensive nephrosclerosis
  - If vascular changes mild, then disease may be hypertension-related nephrosclerosis
  - Since HAART, patients with RNA levels of HIV-1 < 400 copies/mL are more likely to have hypertensive nephrosclerosis than HIVAN

OTHER IMMUNE COMPLEX DISEASES

Membranoproliferative GN (MPGN)

- Seen in HIV patients coinfected with hepatitis C virus (HCV)
- Type I or III MPGN or cryoglobulinemic-type GN
- Mainly Caucasian but also African patients
- 10% had MPGN in series of > 100 biopsies for glomerular disease in HIV(+) patients,

Membranous GN

- May be present in HIV-infected patients, particularly those co-infected with HCV
- Of those infected with HCV and HIV, 80% had MPGN and 20% had membranous nephropathy
  - Clinical course in this study associated with rapid progression to renal failure or death (median: 5.8 months)

Hepatitis C Virus (HCV)

- HCV-associated immune complex GN common in HIV(+) patients
- HCV and HIV have common risk factors, such as intravenous drug use

Fibrillary and Immunotactoid GN

- Fibrillary GN: Glomerular deposition of fibrils 15-25 nm long
  - Fibrillary GN rarely reported in HIV, except in those coinfected with HCV
- Immunotactoid GN: Electron-dense microtubules in glomeruli, having hollow core, arranged in parallel arrays
  - Microtubules as small as 20 nm but usually 30-40 nm in diameter
  - Reported in ~ 4% of HIV-positive biopsies; occurs ± HCV(+)

TUBULOINTERSTITIAL DISEASE

Drug-Induced Mitochondriopathy

- Not uncommon after HAART
  - Nucleotide reverse transcriptase inhibitors impair mitochondrial replication through DNA polymerase-γ inhibition
- May present with markedly elevated creatinine, subnephrotic proteinuria, and normoglycemic glycosuria
- Eosinophilic inclusions of tubular epithelial cells seen
- Electron microscopy
  - Giant mitochondria (2 μm diameter or greater)
  - Abnormal shapes and small number of broken, distorted cristae
    - Enlarged mitochondria may be totally devoid of cristae
    - Changes resemble mitochondrial DNA (mtDNA) depletion syndromes

Other Drug Toxicity

- ATN and myoglobulinuria associated with pentamidine and zidovudine
- Indinavir therapy can produce characteristic intratubular crystals, yielding tubular injury

Acute Interstitial Nephritis

- Diffuse infiltrative lymphocytosis syndrome (DILS)
  - May occur in absence of HIVAN
  - May involve multiple organs
    - Parotid gland enlargement, bilateral
    - Xerostomia
  - Unknown whether directly related to HIV infection or secondary viral infection
- Immune reconstitution inflammatory syndrome (IRIS)
  - Recent initiation of HAART
    - Exaggerated immune response

Viral Infections

- Polyomavirus
- Cytomegalovirus (CMV)
  - May produce hematuria and proteinuria

- Epstein-Barr virus (EBV) causes some cases of acute interstitial nephritis

Bacterial Infections

- Syphilis
  - Often overlooked since recent resurgence after progressive decline in 1990s
  - Presents with proteinuria, nephrotic syndrome, acute nephritic syndrome, acute renal failure, and chronic progressive renal failure
  - Serology positive for syphilis
  - Manifests as proliferative GN, crescentic GN, membranous glomerulopathy, minimal change disease, interstitial nephritis, amyloidosis, and gumma formation
- Mycobacterial infections
  - May produce ill-defined granulomatous inflammation

Fungal Infections

- Disseminated *Pneumocystis jirovecii* (*carinii*)
- Systemic candidiasis and cryptococcosis in 5-10% of patients at autopsy
- *Histoplasma capsulatum*
  - Southern and midwestern parts of USA along Mississippi and Ohio River valleys
- Mucormycosis may be aggressive and mass-forming
- Acute kidney injury or nephrotic syndrome with preserved renal function
- Diagnosis confirmed by blood or urine culture or by biopsy
  - Biopsy shows noncaseating granulomas, interstitial inflammation, and acute tubular injury
  - GMS(+) or PAS(+) yeast forms

RENAL NEOPLASMS

Lymphomas

- Usually B-cell origin (i.e., diffuse large B-cell lymphoma and Burkitt lymphoma)
- Angiocentric and intravascular lymphoma may occur (both are usually T cell in origin)
- Usually whitish or white-gray grossly as opposed to renal cell carcinoma, which is yellow
- Commonly composed of large immunoblast-type lymphoid cells with prominent nucleoli having a B-cell or Burkitt phenotype
- Some lymphomas are EBV-associated, which can be detected by EBV-encoded RNA (EBER) in situ hybridization (ISH)

Kaposi Sarcoma

- Purple-red lesion(s) in cortex
- Malignant spindle cells with slit-like endothelial spaces and extravasated red blood cells
- Immunohistochemistry can identify presence of human herpesvirus-8 (HHV-8), which is diagnostic

Angiosarcoma

- Not frequent
- Highly malignant vascular proliferation
- Positive for vascular markers (CD31, CD34) but negative for HHV-8

Renal Cell Carcinoma

- Not frequent
- Displays usual renal cell carcinoma subtypes seen in non-HIV-infected individuals

DIAGNOSTIC CHECKLIST

Pathologic Interpretation Pearls

- HIVICK and non-collapsing forms of focal segmental glomerulosclerosis reported more in post-antiretroviral era
- HIV-associated immune complex glomerulonephritis with lupus-like features possibly 2nd most common glomerulopathy in adults with HIV
- HIV leads to variety of other glomerular, tubulointerstitial, and vascular disorders

SELECTED REFERENCES

1. Rosenberg AZ et al: HIV-associated nephropathies: epidemiology, pathology, mechanisms and treatment. Nat Rev Nephrol. 11(3):150-160, 2015
2. Murakami CA et al: The clinical characteristics and pathological patterns of postinfectious glomerulonephritis in HIV-infected patients. PLoS One. 9(10):e108398, 2014
3. Chandran S et al: Recurrent HIV-associated immune complex glomerulonephritis with lupus-like features after kidney transplantation. Am J Kidney Dis. 62(2):335-8, 2013
4. Melica G et al: Acute interstitial nephritis with predominant plasmacytic infiltration in patients with HIV-1 infection. Am J Kidney Dis. 59(5):711-4, 2012
5. Ray PE: HIV-associated nephropathy: a diagnosis in evolution. Nephrol Dial Transplant. 27(11):3969-72, 2012
6. Swanepoel CR et al: The evolution of our knowledge of HIV-associated kidney disease in Africa. Am J Kidney Dis. 60(4):668-78, 2012
7. Wearne N et al: The spectrum of renal histologies seen in HIV with outcomes, prognostic indicators and clinical correlations. Nephrol Dial Transplant. 27(11):4109-18, 2012
8. Wyatt CM et al: Recent progress in HIV-associated nephropathy. Annu Rev Med. 63:147-59, 2012
9. Papeta N et al: APOL1 variants increase risk for FSGS and HIVAN but not IgA nephropathy. J Am Soc Nephrol. 22(11):1991-6, 2011
10. Arendse CG et al: The acute, the chronic and the news of HIV-related renal disease in Africa. Kidney Int. 78(3):239-45, 2010
11. Bani-Hani S et al: Renal disease in AIDS: it is not always HIVAN. Clin Exp Nephrol. 14(3):263-7, 2010
12. Herlitz LC et al: Tenofovir nephrotoxicity: acute tubular necrosis with distinctive clinical, pathological, and mitochondrial abnormalities. Kidney Int. 78(11):1171-7, 2010
13. Strøm EH et al: The 'ball-in-cup' lesion is not specific for human immunodeficiency virus-related glomerulonephritis. Kidney Int. 78(11):1189; author reply 1190, 2010
14. Nebuloni M et al: Glomerular lesions in HIV-positive patients: a 20-year biopsy experience from Northern Italy. Clin Nephrol. 72(1):38-45, 2009
15. Park YA et al: ADAMTS13 activity levels in patients with human immunodeficiency virus-associated thrombotic microangiopathy and profound CD4 deficiency. J Clin Apher. 24(1):32-6, 2009
16. Brecher ME et al: Is it HIV TTP or HIV-associated thrombotic microangiopathy? J Clin Apher. 23(6):186-90, 2008
17. Cohen SD et al: Immune complex renal disease and human immunodeficiency virus infection. Semin Nephrol. 28(6):535-44, 2008
18. Fine DM et al: Thrombotic microangiopathy and other glomerular disorders in the HIV-infected patient. Semin Nephrol. 28(6):545-55, 2008
19. Gerntholtz TE et al: HIV-related nephropathy: a South African perspective. Kidney Int. 69(10):1885-91, 2006
20. Haas M et al: HIV-associated immune complex glomerulonephritis with "lupus-like" features: a clinicopathologic study of 14 cases. Kidney Int. 67(4):1381-90, 2005
21. Haas M et al: Fibrillary/immunotactoid glomerulonephritis in HIV-positive patients: a report of three cases. Nephrol Dial Transplant. 15(10):1679-83, 2000

Mesangial Expansion in Lupus-Like GN

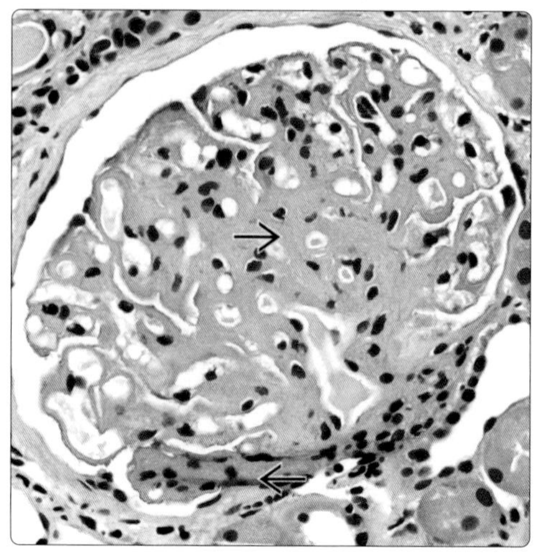

Mesangial Expansion in Lupus-Like GN

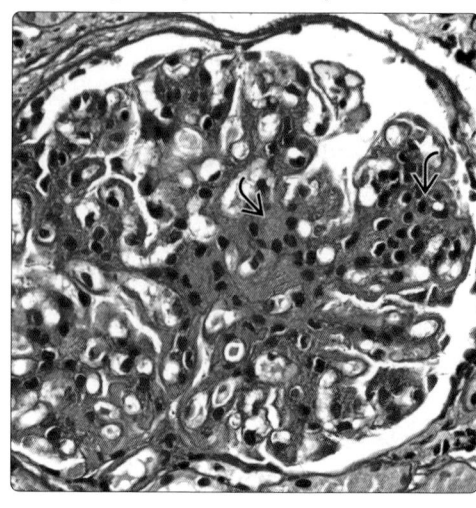

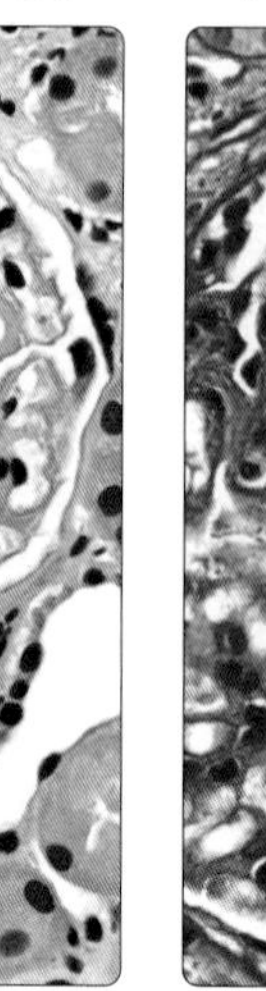

(Left) *In a 37-year-old man with HIV, 4+ proteinuria, creatinine 2.36 mg/dL, and a lupus-like GN, there is a marked expansion of mesangial matrix and cellularity →.* **(Right)** *Higher power view of a glomerulus in the same patient shows marked expansion of mesangial matrix and cellularity →.*

Glomerular Hypercellularity in Lupus-Like GN

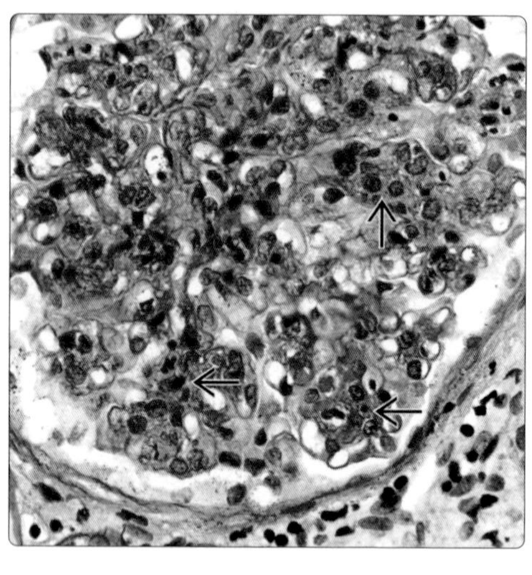

Subendothelial Deposits in Lupus-Like GN

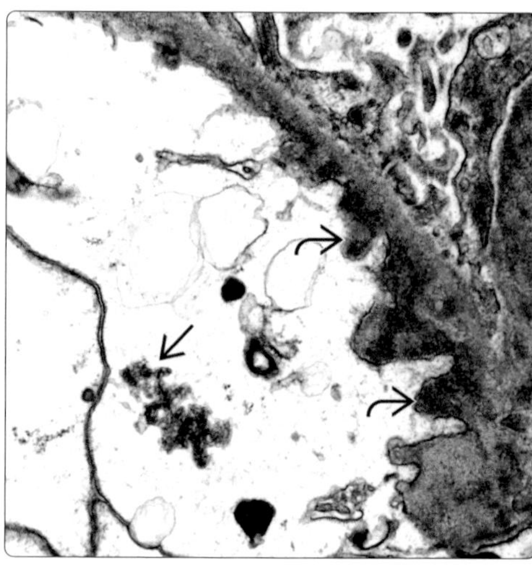

(Left) *A 56-year-old woman with HIV, hepatitis C, decreased C3, low normal C4, and hypertension shows a marked increase in glomerular cellularity → in a lupus-like GN.* **(Right)** *Tubuloreticular inclusions can be seen → along with occasional subendothelial electron-dense deposits → in the same patient.*

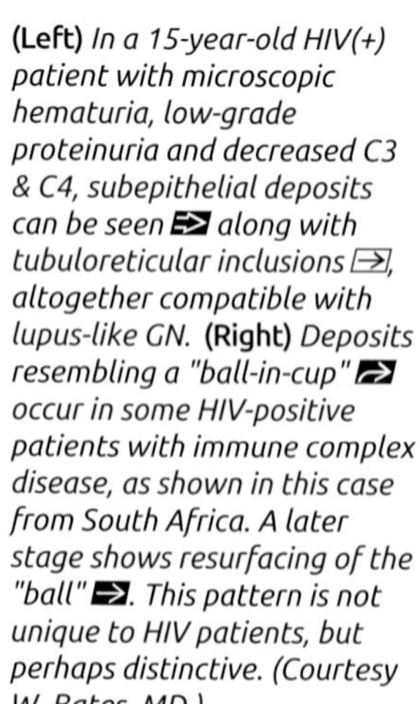

Tubuloreticular Inclusions and Subendothelial Deposits in Lupus-Like GN

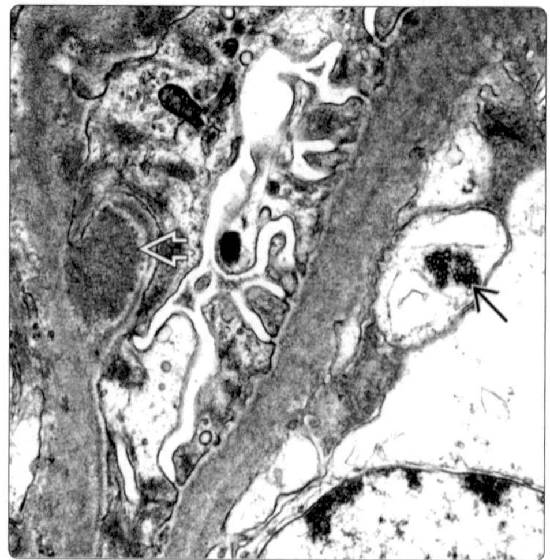

Ball-in-Cup Deposit

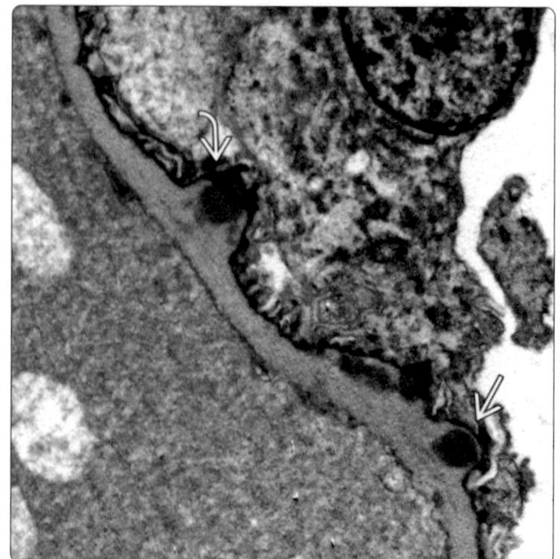

(Left) *In a 15-year-old HIV(+) patient with microscopic hematuria, low-grade proteinuria and decreased C3 & C4, subepithelial deposits can be seen → along with tubuloreticular inclusions →, altogether compatible with lupus-like GN.* **(Right)** *Deposits resembling a "ball-in-cup" → occur in some HIV-positive patients with immune complex disease, as shown in this case from South Africa. A later stage shows resurfacing of the "ball" →. This pattern is not unique to HIV patients, but perhaps distinctive. (Courtesy W. Bates, MD.)*

IgA Deposits in HIV-Associated IgA Nephropathy

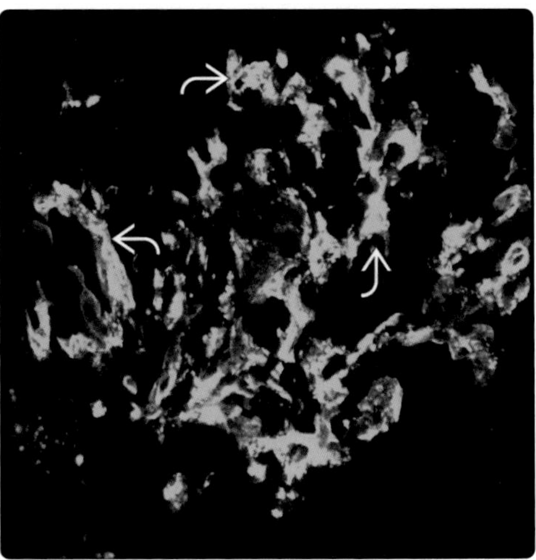

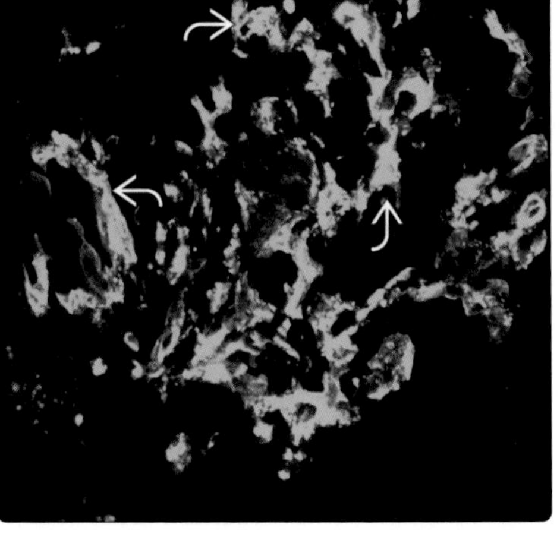

C3 Deposits in HIV-Associated IgA Nephropathy Correlate With IgA Deposits

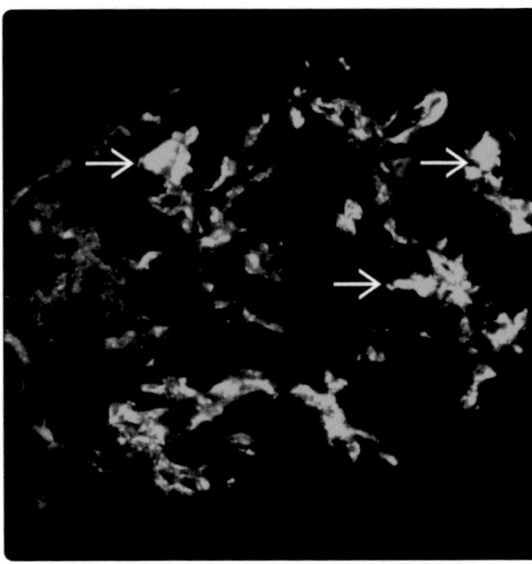

(Left) *In a 38-year-old woman with a history of HIV and HCV, bright IgA deposits can be seen in the mesangium in a dendritic pattern, which together with light and electron microscopic findings of typical IgA nephropathy justified the diagnosis of HIV-associated IgA nephropathy.* **(Right)** *Mesangial C3 deposits can be seen in the same location as the IgA deposits in the same patient.*

Mesangial Deposits in HIV-Associated IgA Nephropathy

Tubuloreticular Inclusions in HIV-Associated IgA Nephropathy

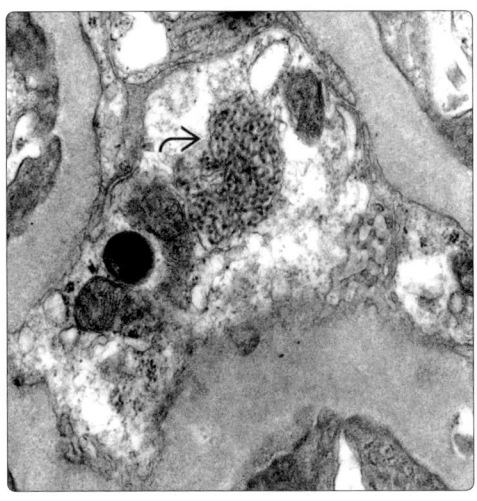

(Left) *In a 38-year-old woman with a history of HIV, HCV, and bright mesangial IgA deposits, EM shows mesangial deposits closely associated with reactive-appearing mesangial cells, compatible with the diagnosis of HIV-associated IgA nephropathy.* **(Right)** *There are tubuloreticular structures in the same patient, which otherwise would have made this case virtually indistinguishable from IgA nephropathy not associated with HIV.*

Fibrillary GN in HIV

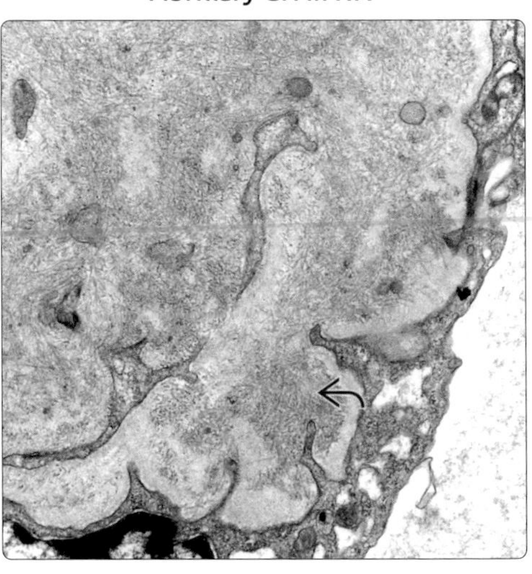

Mitochondrial Abnormalities in HIVAN

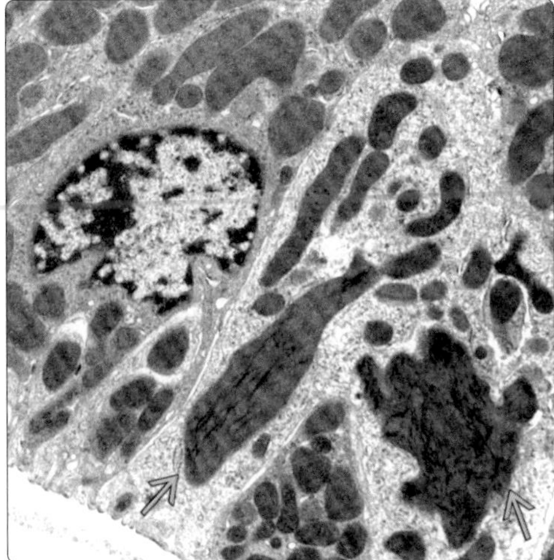

(Left) *Fibrillary GN is one glomerular disease associated with HIV infection. Fibrils are evident in the GBM in an electron micrograph from a 50-year-old HIV(+), HCV(+) man with 11 g/d proteinuria. Congo red stain was (-).* **(Right)** *HAART has reduced HIVAN incidence considerably; however, the inhibitory effects of anti-reverse transcriptase on mtDNA can cause a mitochondriopathy, diagnosed by abnormally shaped and enlarged mitochondria by EM and manifested by LM by leading to interstitial fibrosis and tubular atrophy.*

KEY FACTS

TERMINOLOGY

- *Schistosoma* parasitic infection-related renal disease

ETIOLOGY/PATHOGENESIS

- *S. mansoni* migrates to mesenteric vessels, causes GI symptoms and manifestations of portal hypertension
  - Glomerulonephritis due to humoral host response to parasitic antigen
- *S. haematobium* migrates to perivesical venous plexus and causes genitourinary tract and colonic symptoms
  - Fibrosis and calcified tissue-trapped ova in lower urinary tract lead to stricture, reflux, and infection
- Intermediate host is freshwater snail
- Cercariae in water penetrate human skin

CLINICAL ISSUES

- Endemic in Africa, Middle East (*S. mansoni, S. haematobium*), South America (*S. mansoni*), and Asia (*S. japonicum*)
- Antiparasitic drugs and immunosuppressive therapy do not affect glomerulonephritis

MICROSCOPIC

- Membranoproliferative glomerulonephritis (MPGN)
  - Mesangial and endocapillary proliferation, thickening of glomerular capillary walls with double contours
- Membranous nephropathy
- Cortical scar in reflux nephropathy
- Amyloid AA deposition in glomeruli and arterial walls

ANCILLARY TESTS

- Characteristic ova in urine (*S. haematobium* with terminal spine), stools (*S. mansoni* with lateral spine), or tissues
- Mesangial and capillary wall C3-dominant deposits in MPGN
  - Schistosomal circulating anodic antigen demonstrated in immune complexes
- Electron-dense deposits in mesangium and subendothelium in MPGN

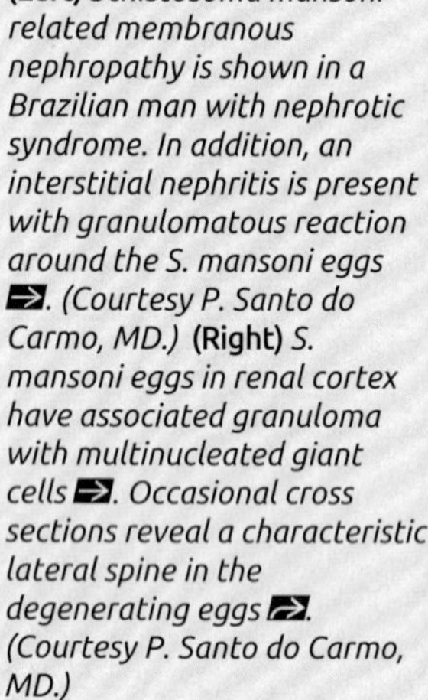

(Left) *Schistosoma mansoni-related membranous nephropathy is shown in a Brazilian man with nephrotic syndrome. In addition, an interstitial nephritis is present with granulomatous reaction around the S. mansoni eggs. (Courtesy P. Santo do Carmo, MD.)* **(Right)** *S. mansoni eggs in renal cortex have associated granuloma with multinucleated giant cells. Occasional cross sections reveal a characteristic lateral spine in the degenerating eggs. (Courtesy P. Santo do Carmo, MD.)*

Membranous Glomerulonephritis and Interstitial Nephritis

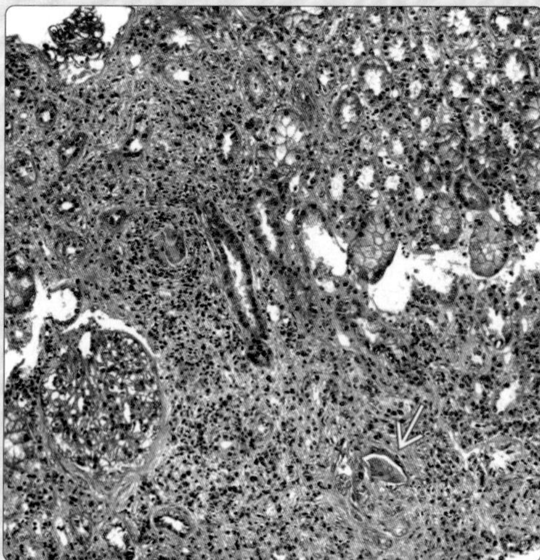

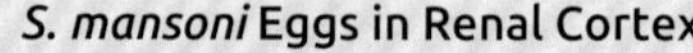

***S. mansoni* Eggs in Renal Cortex**

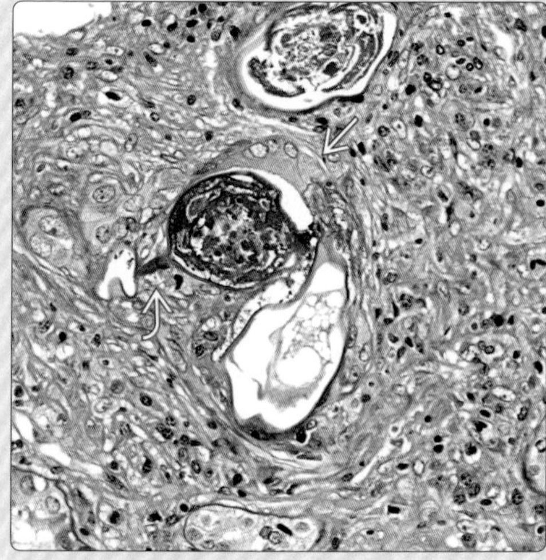

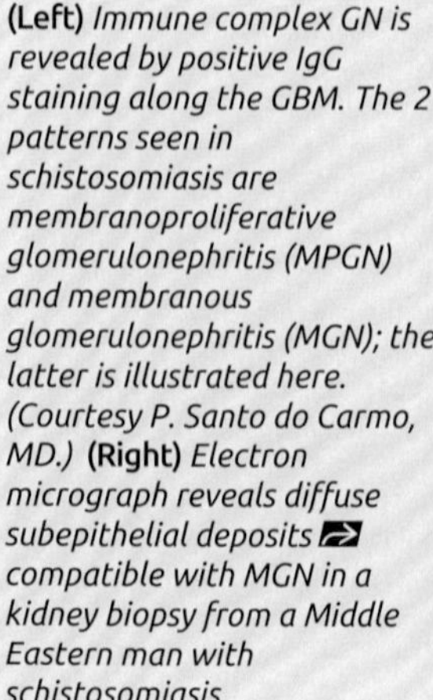

(Left) *Immune complex GN is revealed by positive IgG staining along the GBM. The 2 patterns seen in schistosomiasis are membranoproliferative glomerulonephritis (MPGN) and membranous glomerulonephritis (MGN); the latter is illustrated here. (Courtesy P. Santo do Carmo, MD.)* **(Right)** *Electron micrograph reveals diffuse subepithelial deposits compatible with MGN in a kidney biopsy from a Middle Eastern man with schistosomiasis.*

Granular IgG along GBM

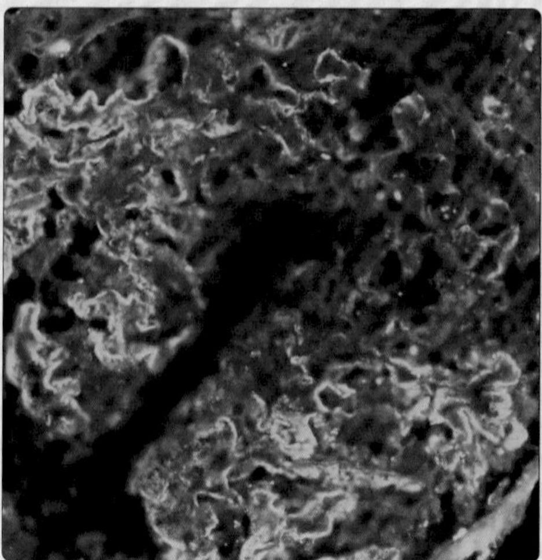

Subepithelial Deposits

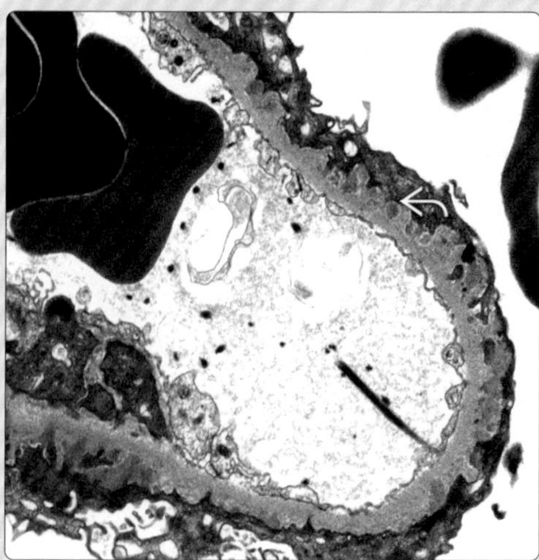

TERMINOLOGY

Definitions

- *Schistosoma* parasitic infection-related renal disease

ETIOLOGY/PATHOGENESIS

Infectious Agents

- *Schistosoma mansoni*
  - Parasite migrates to mesenteric vessels
  - Causes gastrointestinal symptoms and manifestations of portal hypertension
  - Causes glomerulonephritis
    - Circulating anodic antigen within gut epithelium of adult worm may elicit immune response
    - Immune complexes due to humoral host response
- *Schistosoma haematobium*
  - Migrates to perivesical venous plexus and causes genitourinary tract and colonic symptoms
  - Fibrosis and calcified tissue-trapped ova in lower urinary tract lead to stricture, reflux, and infection
  - Glomerulonephritis less common
- *Schistosoma japonicum*
  - Causes hepatosplenomegaly and cirrhosis
  - Glomerulonephritis described only in animals

Source of Infection

- Intermediate host is freshwater snail
- Cercariae in water penetrate human skin

Role of Coinfection

- *Salmonella* coinfection causes severe glomerulonephritis
- Hepatitis C virus infection may cause increased disease manifestations in endemic areas

CLINICAL ISSUES

Epidemiology

- Incidence
  - Affects 200 million people worldwide
  - Endemic in Africa, Middle East (*S. mansoni, S. haematobium*), South America (*S. mansoni*), and Asia (*S. japonicum*)
  - Glomerulonephritis uncommon
- Age
  - Children and young adults in endemic areas

Presentation

- Hematuria, proteinuria
- Dysuria and polyuria with hydronephrosis or chronic pyelonephritis
- Nephrotic syndrome may be seen

Treatment

- Drugs
  - Praziquantel (antiparasitic drug)

Prognosis

- Antiparasitic drugs and immunosuppressive therapy do not affect glomerulonephritis
  - Prolonged antiparasitic therapy may reduce urinary tract morbidity

MICROSCOPIC

Histologic Features

- Glomeruli
  - Membranoproliferative glomerulonephritis (MPGN) most common (~ 50%)
    - Mesangial and endocapillary proliferation, thickening of glomerular capillary walls with double contours
  - Membranous glomerulonephritis (MGN)
    - Glomerular basement membrane "spikes"
  - Focal segmental glomerulosclerosis
  - Amyloid AA deposition in glomeruli and arterial walls
- Interstitium and tubules
  - Interstitial nephritis
    - Egg granuloma may be present
  - Cortical scar with chronic inflammation may suggest reflux nephropathy due to *S. hematobium* infection
    - Neutrophil casts suggest acute pyelonephritis

ANCILLARY TESTS

Immunofluorescence

- Mesangial and capillary wall C3-dominant deposits in MPGN
  - IgM and IgG deposits can also be seen
  - Mesangial IgA may be present in membranoproliferative and focal segmental sclerosis forms
- Glomerular capillary wall IgG staining in MGN
- Schistosomal antigens demonstrated in immune complexes in 50% of cases

Electron Microscopy

- Electron-dense deposits in mesangium and subendothelium in MPGN
- Subepithelial deposits in MGN
- Randomly oriented fibrils (8-11 nm thick) in amyloidosis

Identification of Ova

- In urine (*S. hematobium* with terminal spine), stools (*S. mansoni* with lateral spine), or tissues

DIFFERENTIAL DIAGNOSIS

Nonschistosomal Glomerulonephritis

- Clinical and travel history may be helpful

SELECTED REFERENCES

1. dos-Santos WL et al: Schistosomal glomerulopathy and changes in the distribution of histological patterns of glomerular diseases in Bahia, Brazil. Mem Inst Oswaldo Cruz. 106(7):901-4, 2011
2. Gryseels B et al: Human schistosomiasis. Lancet. 368(9541):1106-18, 2006
3. Barsoum R: The changing face of schistosomal glomerulopathy. Kidney Int. 66(6):2472-84, 2004
4. Mahmoud KM et al: Impact of schistosomiasis on patient and graft outcome after renal transplantation: 10 years' follow-up. Nephrol Dial Transplant. 16(11):2214-21, 2001
5. Barsoum R et al: Immunoglobulin-A and the pathogenesis of schistosomal glomerulopathy. Kidney Int. 50(3):920-8, 1996
6. Abensur H et al: Nephrotic syndrome associated with hepatointestinal schistosomiasis. Rev Inst Med Trop Sao Paulo. 34(4):273-6, 1992
7. Martinelli R et al: Schistosoma mansoni-induced mesangiocapillary glomerulonephritis: influence of therapy. Kidney Int. 35(5):1227-33, 1989
8. Lambertucci JR et al: Glomerulonephritis in Salmonella-Schistosoma mansoni association. Am J Trop Med Hyg. 38(1):97-102, 1988
9. Sobh MA et al: Characterisation of kidney lesions in early schistosomal-specific nephropathy. Nephrol Dial Transplant. 3(4):392-8, 1988

Filariasis

KEY FACTS

TERMINOLOGY

- Kidney infection caused by filarial nematodes, a.k.a. threadworms, which are arthropod-transmitted parasites

ETIOLOGY/PATHOGENESIS

- Infectious agents
  - *Wuchereria bancrofti, Loa loa, Onchocerca volvulus*
- Role of blood-feeding flies and several kinds of mosquitos in parasite transmission and completion of life cycle
- Renal injury by direct invasion or indirectly via immune complex-mediated glomerulonephritis or podocyte injury

CLINICAL ISSUES

- Endemic in Africa, Southeast Asia, South America
- Most common presentation is nephrotic syndrome
- Lymphatic obstruction manifests by hydrocele, lymphedema, &/or chyluria
- Diagnosis
  - ELISA or test for circulating microfilaria antigens
  - Parasite isolation from infected tissues or body fluids
- Treatment
  - Drugs/antiparasitic agents
  - Dietary modifications to minimize chyle production

MICROSCOPIC

- Spectrum of glomerular lesions
  - Immune complex-mediated glomerulonephritis
    - Mesangioproliferative glomerulonephritis
    - Membranous glomerulopathy
    - Membranoproliferative glomerulonephritis
    - Acute eosinophilic glomerulonephritis
  - Podocyte injury
    - Minimal change disease
    - Collapsing glomerulopathy

TOP DIFFERENTIAL DIAGNOSES

- Other causes of glomerular disease (infectious, autoimmune, idiopathic) or chyluria

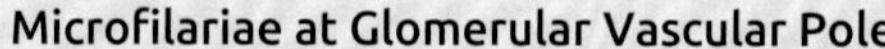

Microfilariae at Glomerular Vascular Pole

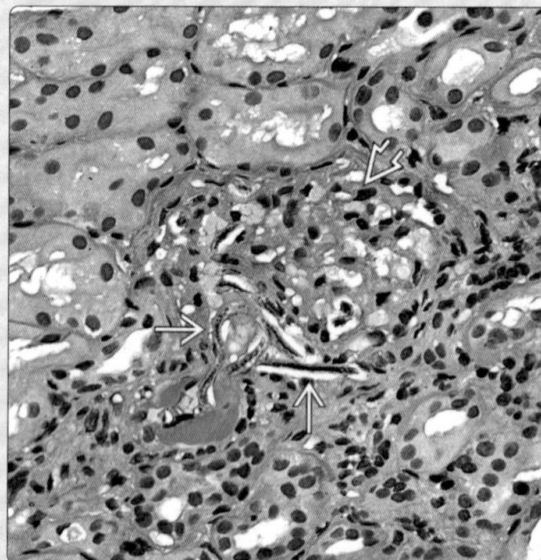

Direct Invasion of Glomerulus by Microfilariae

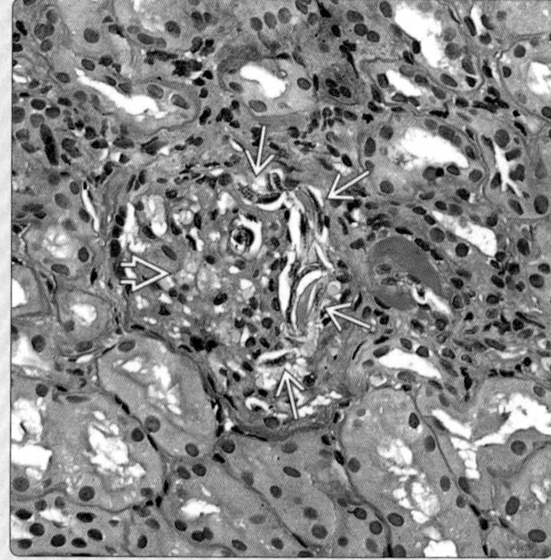

(Left) *Microfilariae* ➡ *are noted at the glomerular vascular pole. The glomerular tuft* ➡ *shows no mesangial expansion, endocapillary hypercellularity, or crescent formation. Electron microscopy revealed extensive epithelial foot process effacement, and the patient was diagnosed with minimal change disease secondary to filariasis.* **(Right)** *Direct invasion of a glomerulus* ➡ *by microfilariae* ➡ *is shown, with sections noted at the vascular pole and within capillary lumina.*

Microfilariae Within Arteriolar Lumen

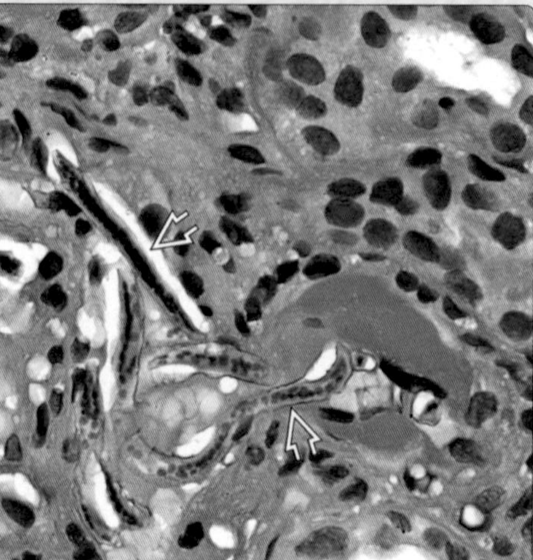

Microfilariae Within Arteriolar and Capillary Lumina

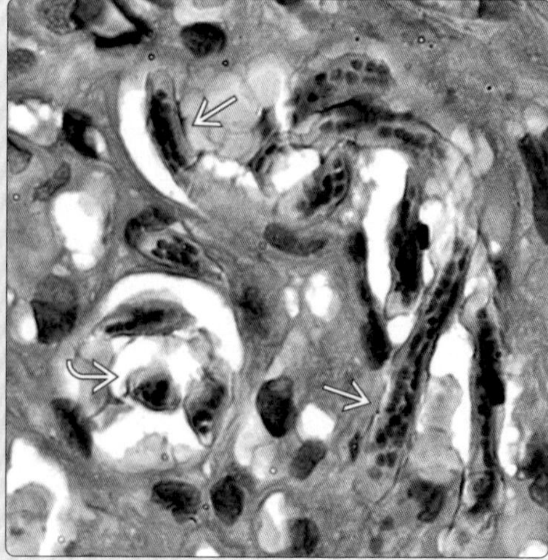

(Left) *Curved and elongated sections of microfilariae are shown within the arteriolar lumen of a glomerulus. Note the column of nuclei* ➡ *throughout the central portion of the microfilariae.* **(Right)** *Microfilariae are shown directly invading this glomerulus. Several curved and elongated longitudinal* ➡ *and cross sections* ➡ *of the microorganisms are noted within the arteriolar and capillary lumina.*

TERMINOLOGY

Synonyms

- *Wuchereria bancrofti* (bancroftian filariasis, elephantiasis)
- *Loa loa* (loiasis, loaiasis, African eyeworm)
- *Onchocerca volvulus* (onchocerciasis, river blindness)

Definitions

- Kidney infection caused by filarial nematodes
  - a.k.a. threadworms
  - Arthropod-transmitted parasites

ETIOLOGY/PATHOGENESIS

Infectious Agents

- Of 8 filarial nematodes, 3 associated with renal disease in humans
  - *W. bancrofti*
  - *L. loa*
  - *O. volvulus*

Pathogenesis

- Role of blood-feeding flies and several kinds of mosquitos in parasite transmission and completion of life cycle
- Larvae, known as microfilariae, circulate within blood for some species
- Mechanisms of renal injury
  - Direct invasion
  - Indirect via immune complex-mediated glomerulonephritis (GN) or podocyte injury

CLINICAL ISSUES

Epidemiology

- Rare in North America
- Endemic in geographic regions
  - Africa and Southeast Asia (bancroftian filariasis)
  - South America and tropical sub-Saharan Africa (onchocerciasis)
  - West Central Africa (loiasis)

Presentation

- Nephrotic syndrome (most common)
- Nephritic syndrome
- Lymphatic obstruction, manifested by hydrocele, lymphedema, &/or chyluria

Laboratory Tests

- ELISA or test for circulating microfilaria antigens
- Parasite isolation from infected tissues or body fluids
- Test for chyluria by estimation of urine triglycerides

Treatment

- Drugs/antiparasitic agents
  - Diethylcarbamazine (DEC) (Hetrazan, Benocide)
- Dietary modifications to minimize chyle production
  - Fat-free, high-protein diet
  - Medium chain triglyceride (coconut oil) supplementation
- Management of chyluria
  - Renal pelvic instillation sclerotherapy using 0.2% povidone-iodine (Betadine) injected into renal pelvis
  - Sclerosants induce inflammatory reaction within lymphatic vessels to scar communicating lymphatics

MICROSCOPIC

Histologic Features

- Spectrum of glomerular lesions
  - Immune complex-mediated GN
    - Mesangioproliferative GN
    - Membranous GN
    - Membranoproliferative GN
    - Acute eosinophilic GN
  - Podocyte injury
    - Minimal change disease
    - Collapsing glomerulopathy
- Direct invasion by microfilariae
  - *L. loa*
    - Microfilariae measure 240 x 7 μm
    - Sheath (clear halo) can be observed surrounding microorganism
    - 4-6 nuclei evenly spaced at tail tip and extends to end, while cephalic region is devoid of nuclei
  - *W. bancrofti*
    - Sheathed, microfilariae measure 250 x 8 μm
    - Round cephalic region and pointed tail devoid of nuclei
  - *O. volvulus*
    - Unsheathed, microfilariae measure 300 x 8 μm
    - No nuclei in tail tip

ANCILLARY TESTS

Immunofluorescence

- Granular deposits of IgG &/or IgM and C3 in mesangium &/or capillary walls in GN

Electron Microscopy

- Mesangial &/or capillary loop electron-dense deposits (subepithelial &/or subendothelial) in GN
- Severe epithelial foot process effacement without deposits in minimal change disease or collapsing glomerulopathy

DIFFERENTIAL DIAGNOSIS

Differential for Glomerular Pathology

- Other infections including HIV or bacterial coinfection, autoimmune, idiopathic

Differential for Chyluria (Milky White Urine)

- Phosphaturia (clears with 10% acetic acid)
- Amorphous urates
- Severe pyuria
- Lipiduria secondary to fat embolism
- Pseudochylous urine and casseousuria due to renal tuberculosis

SELECTED REFERENCES

1. Barsoum RS: Parasitic kidney disease: milestones in the evolution of our knowledge. Am J Kidney Dis. 61(3):501-13, 2013
2. Sundar S et al: Filariasis, with chyluria and nephrotic range proteinuria. J Assoc Physicians India. 61(7):487-9, 2013

Leishmaniasis

KEY FACTS

TERMINOLOGY

- Infection caused by *Leishmania*, an obligate intracellular protozoa

ETIOLOGY/PATHOGENESIS

- *Leishmania donovoni, Leishmania infantum*
- Transmitted by infected female sandfly bites
- Tropical, subtropical, and all Mediterranean countries
- Immunodeficiency predisposes

CLINICAL ISSUES

- Malaise, fever, weight loss, papular rash
- Hepatosplenomegaly, jaundice
- Proteinuria
- Hematuria
- Acute renal failure

MICROSCOPIC

- Mesangial and endocapillary hypercellularity
- Glomerular endothelial cells and podocytes may contain amastigotes
- AA amyloid deposition reported
- May have acute tubular injury related to drug toxicity
- Mixed inflammatory infiltrate of lymphocytes, macrophages, and plasma cells
- Amastigotes in peritubular capillary endothelium

ANCILLARY TESTS

- Glomerular deposition of IgG, C3
- Intramembranous, amorphous deposits in GBM

TOP DIFFERENTIAL DIAGNOSES

- Membranoproliferative glomerulonephritis
- HIV nephropathies
- Transplant glomerulopathy
- Microsporidiosis

DIAGNOSTIC CHECKLIST

- Amastigotes in capillary endothelium and macrophages

(Left) *Diffuse mesangial and endocapillary hypercellularity is evident in this PAS-stained glomerulus. Duplication of the GBM is also segmentally present ⇨. (Courtesy K. Amann, MD.)* **(Right)** *Leishmania amastigotes, a.k.a. Leishman bodies, are seen in tubular epithelial cells ➯. The amastigotes can also be seen in capillary endothelial cells and macrophages. The dark staining kinetoplast ⇨ helps identify these as amastigotes in this PAS-stained slide. Giemsa stains are also useful. (Courtesy K. Amann, MD.)*

Membranoproliferative GN

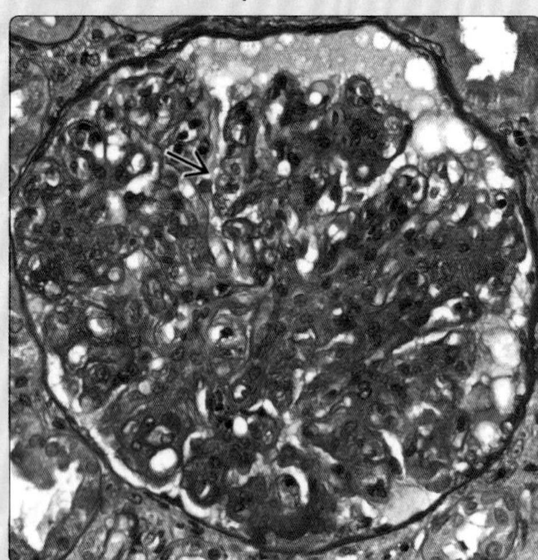

Leishmania Amastigotes in Peritubular Capillary

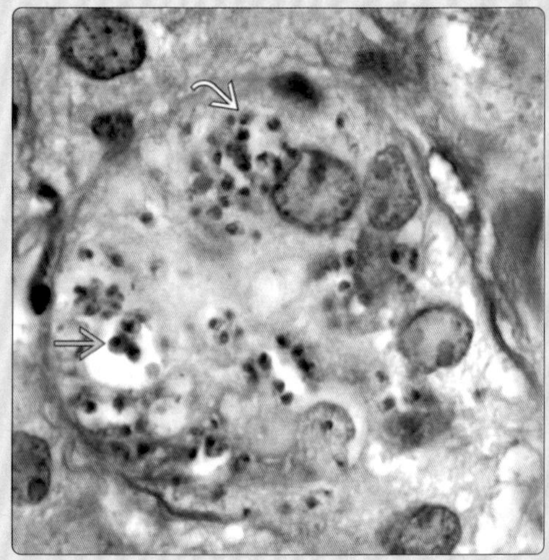

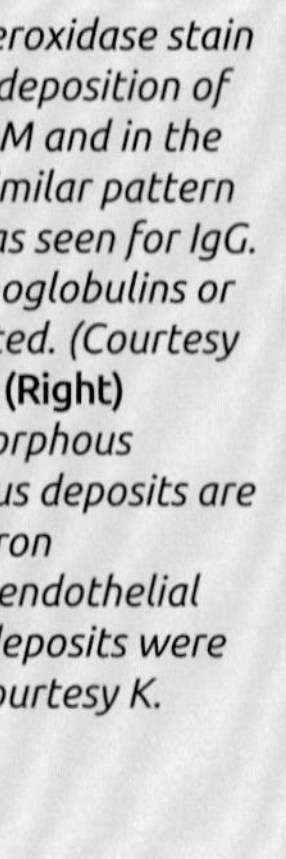

(Left) *Immunoperoxidase stain shows granular deposition of C3 along the GBM and in the mesangium. A similar pattern of deposition was seen for IgG. No other immunoglobulins or C1q were detected. (Courtesy K. Amann, MD.)* **(Right)** *Widespread amorphous intramembranous deposits are evident by electron microscopy. Subendothelial and mesangial deposits were also present. (Courtesy K. Amann, MD.)*

C3 Deposition

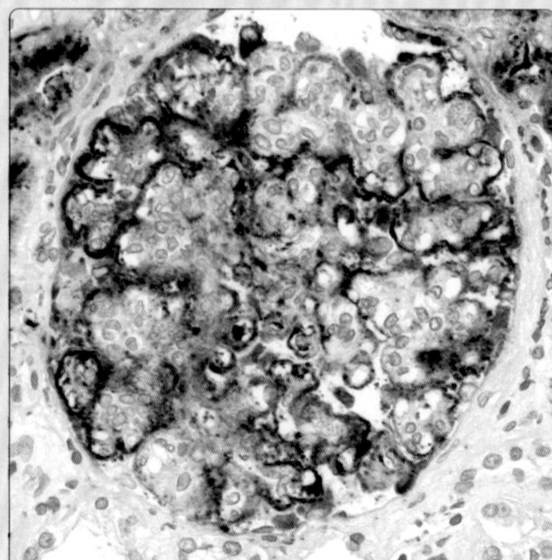

Glomerular Deposits

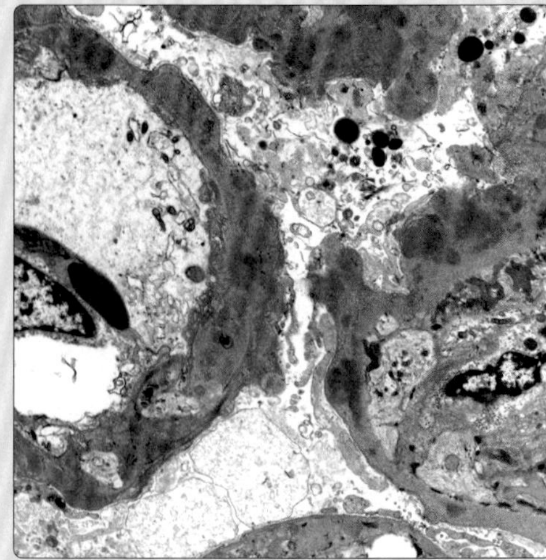

TERMINOLOGY

Synonyms

- Visceral leishmaniasis (a.k.a. kala-azar)

Definitions

- Infection caused by *Leishmania*, an obligate intracellular protozoa

ETIOLOGY/PATHOGENESIS

Infectious Agents

- Visceral leishmaniasis caused by *Leishmania donovoni* or *Leishmania infantum*
- Cutaneous leishmaniasis caused by *Leishmania braziliensis*
- Transmitted by infected female sandfly bites
  - Promastigote from sandfly infects cells of reticuloendothelial system
  - Intracellular transformation into amastigote form with kinetoplast
- Immunodeficiency predisposes
  - HIV infection, immunosuppressive drugs

Immune Complex Deposition

- Contain *Leishmania* antigens
- Documented in animal studies, especially dogs

Autoantibodies

- ANA, anti-Sm RNP, SS-B, intermediate filaments

CLINICAL ISSUES

Epidemiology

- 500,000 cases per year worldwide
- Tropical, subtropical, and all Mediterranean countries

Presentation

- Malaise, fever, weight loss, papular rash
- Hepatosplenomegaly, jaundice, pancytopenia
- Proteinuria (~ 50%)
  - Nephrotic syndrome
- Hematuria (~ 50%)
  - Acute glomerulonephritis
- Acute renal failure (~ 37%)

Treatment

- Miltefosine, liposomal amphotericin B, paromomycin
- Potential renal toxicity

Prognosis

- 95% fatal without treatment
- Relapsing course in immunodeficient patients

MICROSCOPIC

Histologic Features

- Glomerulus: 5 patterns described
  - Membranoproliferative glomerulonephritis (MPGN): Most common
    - Mesangial and endocapillary hypercellularity
    - Thickening and duplication of GBM
    - Amastigotes occasionally in endothelium, mesangial cells, or podocytes
  - Mesangial proliferation without GBM changes
  - Collapsing glomerulopathy
  - Necrotizing and crescentic glomerulonephritis
  - AA amyloidosis
- Tubules
  - May have acute tubular injury related to drug toxicity
  - Tubular atrophy variable
  - Tubular cells may have amastigotes
- Interstitium
  - Mixed inflammatory infiltrate of lymphocytes, macrophages, and plasma cells
    - May be present without glomerular lesions
  - Interstitial fibrosis variable
- Vessels
  - Peritubular capillary endothelium swollen with amastigotes best shown on PAS or Giemsa stains

ANCILLARY TESTS

Immunofluorescence

- MPGN form: Glomerular capillary wall and mesangial deposition of IgG, C3; ± IgM ± IgA; little or no C1q
- Collapsing form: Negative IgG, C3

Electron Microscopy

- MPGN form: Amorphous intramembranous, subendothelial, and mesangial deposits
- Podocyte foot process effacement
- Amyloid fibrils

DIFFERENTIAL DIAGNOSIS

Membranoproliferative Glomerulonephritis

- No amastigotes
- Other known infections (HCV, schistosomiasis and others)

HIV Nephropathies

- No amastigotes

Transplant Glomerulopathy

- Immune complexes by immunofluorescence and electron microscopy

Microsporidiosis

- Microsporidia primarily in tubular epithelium

DIAGNOSTIC CHECKLIST

Pathologic Interpretation Pearls

- Amastigotes in capillary endothelium and macrophages

SELECTED REFERENCES

1. Silva Junior GB et al: Kidney involvement in leishmaniasis–a review. Braz J Infect Dis. 18(4):434-40, 2014
2. Amann K et al: Renal leishmaniasis as unusual cause of nephrotic syndrome in an HIV patient. J Am Soc Nephrol. 23(4):586-90, 2012
3. Suankratay C et al: Autochthonous visceral leishmaniasis in a human immunodeficiency virus (HIV)-infected patient: the first in thailand and review of the literature. Am J Trop Med Hyg. 82(1):4-8, 2010
4. Kumar PV et al: Leishmania in the glomerulus. Arch Pathol Lab Med. 128(8):935-6, 2004

TERMINOLOGY

Definitions

- Next-generation sequencing (NGS): Various high throughput technologies to sequence regions of genome or whole genome instead of 1 DNA strand at a time
- Single nucleotide polymorphism (SNP): Common single nucleotide change observed at particular location in > 1 % in population
- Rare variant: Single nucleotide change observed at < 1% frequency

CLASSIFICATION CATEGORIES

Inheritance Pattern or Genetics

- Autosomal Dominant
- Autosomal Recessive
- X-linked
- Syndromes

Clinical Presentation

- Nephrotic syndrome or proteinuria
    - Genes posing risk to develop steroid resistant nephrotic syndrome (SRNS), focal segmental glomerulosclerosis (FSGS)
- Nephritic
    - Genes implicated in IgA nephropathy, Alport syndrome, thin basement membrane nephropathy

Therapeutic Response

- Steroid Resistant
    - Often congenital nephrotic syndromes
    - Mutations in one of podocyte genes
    - Very rare
- Steroid Responsive

Anatomy or Physiology

- Primary glomerular
    - Podocytes (many causes of FSGS, SRNS)
        - Extracellular matrix/glomerular basement membrane (GBM)
        - Slit diaphragm interacting proteins
        - Cytoskeleton
        - Cell signaling
        - Mitochondrial function
        - Nucleic acid regulation (DNA/RNA)
        - Lysosomal
    - GBM (Alport syndrome, thin basement membrane disease)
    - Mesangium (IgA nephropathy)
    - Endothelium (aHUS, thrombotic microangiopathy)
- Secondary glomerular (defects in urinary tract but not glomerulus)
    - Congenital obstructive or reflux nephropathy (CAKUT genes)
- Systemic diseases affecting glomeruli
    - Diabetic nephropathy in type 1 diabetes
    - Diabetic nephropathy in type 2 diabetes
    - Fabry disease
    - Lipoprotein glomerulopathy

Pathology (1 or More Present in Same Glomerulus)

- FSGS
    - Many gene defects can exhibit FSGS (*NPHS1*, *COL4A3*, *UPKIII* in CAKUT, such as reflux)
- Thickened GBM
    - Seen in diabetic nephropathy (*ELMO1*), Alport syndrome (*COL4A3*)
- Thin basement membranes
    - Mutations in *COL4A3*, *4*, *5* in Alport or in thin basement membrane disease can show thin basement membranes (less than 250 nm)
- Glomerular cysts
    - Seen in *HNF1B* mutations (MODY), *PKD1*, *PKD2* (ADPKD), *PKHD1* (ARPKD) mutations
- Mesangial hypercellularity or sclerosis
    - *IGAN1* (IgA nephropathy), *CFH* (aHUS)
    - *PLCE1*, *WT1*, *LAMB2* (SRNS)
- Thrombotic microangiopathy
    - *DGKE* (aHUS), *ADAMTS13* (TTP), *APOE* (lipoprotein glomerulopathy)

FSGS in Atypical Alport

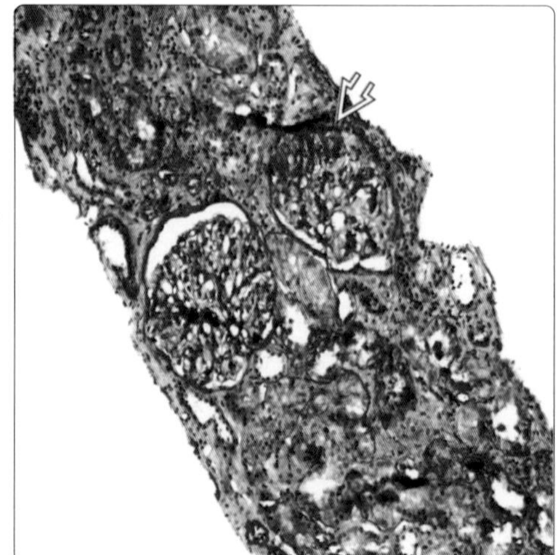

Next Generation Sequencing Confirms Alport in a Patient With FSGS

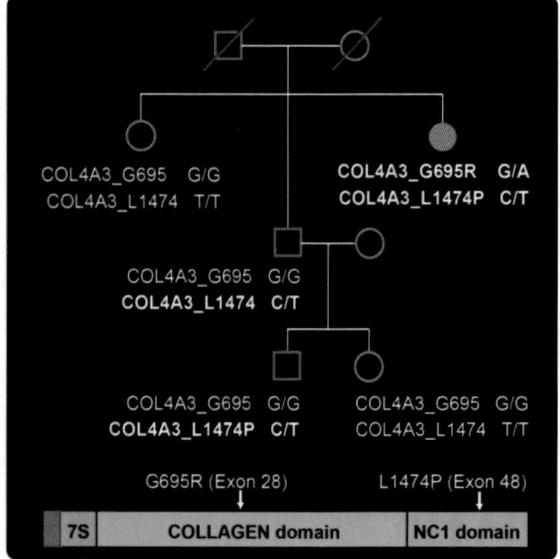

(Left) *Biopsy from a 50-year-old Caucasian woman shows FSGS ➲. She has history of recurrent UTIs, hydronephrosis, and 3+ proteinuria for 5 years, initially partially responsive to steroids. There is no hematuria or family history of renal disease.* **(Right)** *Targeted exome sequencing of the same patient (arrow) described in left reveals 2 COL4A3 mutations. COL4A3_G695R is a de novo mutation, presence of both mutations appear to be causative.*

ETIOLOGY/PATHOGENESIS

Primary Glomerular Genetic Diseases

- Podocyte function
  - Typically cause SRNS
  - Almost 70% of SRNS present in first 3 months of life due to mutations in *NPHS1, NPHS2, WT1, PLCE1*
  - Mutations in genes important in slit diaphragm (*NPHS1*), podocyte-podocyte or podocyte-GBM interactions (*PLCE1*) or mitochondrial function (*COQ2*)
- GBM function
  - Alport syndrome, thin basement membrane disease
  - Genes encoding proteins, such as laminins or collagen 4 alpha 3, 4, 5 chains, may be abnormally expressed by podocytes disrupting integrity of GBM structure and supporting vascular network (*LAMB2, COL4A3*)
  - Defect may cause increased ER stress due to accumulation of abnormal polypeptides in ER
- Mesangium function
  - IgA nephropathy
  - Possibly causative mutations in *IGAN1*
  - Anti-IgA IgG antibodies increased due to increased mutagenicity of IgA and defective O-glycosylation
- Endocapillary function
  - Atypical hemolytic uremic syndrome (aHUS), thrombotic microangiopathy
  - ~ 50% caused by various genetic defects of complement system, including
    - *CFH, CF1, ADAMTS13, THBD*
  - Dysregulation of complement system

Secondary Glomerular Genetic Diseases

- Defects in urinary tract can lead to glomerular dysfunction
  - Genes that cause CAKUT especially obstruction or reflux can manifest as FSGS (*UPK3A, ROBO2*)

Systemic Diseases With Genetic Risk to Glomeruli

- Diabetic nephropathy: *SLC12A3* (in Japanese), *ELMO1, TCF7L2* (type 2), *FRMD3, CARS* (type 1)
- Lipoprotein glomerulopathy: *APOE*
- Fabry disease: *GLA*
- Glycogen storage disease: *G6PC*

CLINICAL IMPLICATIONS

Clinical Risk Factors

- Presence of 2 of G1 or G2 APOL1 risk variants (in any combination: G1G1 or G2G2 or G1G2) in African Americans poses risk to develop FSGS
- Mutations in *NPHS1, NPHS2, WT1, PLCE1* identify 70% of SRNS in children with proteinuria 0-3 months of age and ~ 20% in late onset
- Causative mutations in gene associated with congenital nephrotic syndrome can render
  - Resistance to steroid treatment
  - Recurrence of FSGS in allografts post transplant
- Susceptibility to diabetic nephropathy associated with SNPs in *CNDP1, GCK1*

Diagnostic Modalities

- G1 or G2 *APOL1* risk allele status in African American patients or donors
  - TaqMan analysis (especially if large number of patients)
  - Sanger sequencing
- Known or clinically well established or to rule out Alport syndrome or thin basement membrane nephropathy
  - Targeted panel for *COL4A3, 4, 5*
    - PCR amplification then NGS
    - Targeted capture using baits then NGS
    - Multiplex ligation-dependent probe amplification (MLPA) for exon deletions
- SRNS
  - Targeted panel of ~ 30 podocyte genes (scalable) for capture or amplicon based NGS
- FSGS pattern on biopsy
  - Proteinuria without other congenital kidney defect
    - Targeted panel of SRNS, Alport genes for sequencing
  - Proteinuria with other congenital defects
    - Targeted panel with SRNS with Alport with CAKUT or ciliopathy or nephrolithiasis genes for exome NGS
    - Scalable, up to 1000 genes
- Hematuria (glomerular origin)
  - Targeted panel Alport, IgAN
- aHUS/TTP
  - Targeted panel of complement and clotting factors for amplicon based or targeted exome based NGS
- For novel genes and in atypical cases not explained by any genes above
  - Whole exome or genome sequencing, prefer simultaneous analysis of parents and functional proof

MICROSCOPIC

General Features

- FSGS
- Glomerular cysts
- GBM abnormalities
- Mesangial thickening or proliferation
- Thrombi

SELECTED REFERENCES

1. Fogo AB: Causes and pathogenesis of focal segmental glomerulosclerosis. Nat Rev Nephrol. ePub, 2014
2. Chatterjee R et al: Targeted exome sequencing integrated with clinicopathological information reveals novel and rare mutations in atypical, suspected and unknown cases of Alport syndrome or proteinuria. PLoS One. 8(10):e76360, 2013
3. Lemaire M et al: Recessive mutations in DGKE cause atypical hemolytic-uremic syndrome. Nat Genet. 45(5):531-6, 2013
4. Parsa A et al: APOL1 risk variants, race, and progression of chronic kidney disease. N Engl J Med. 369(23):2183-96, 2013
5. Agrawal S et al: Genetic contribution and associated pathophysiology in end-stage renal disease. Appl Clin Genet. 3:65-84, 2010
6. Chiang CK et al: Glomerular diseases: genetic causes and future therapeutics. Nat Rev Nephrol. 6(9):539-54, 2010
7. Hildebrandt F: Genetic Kidney Diseases. Lancet. 375: 1287-1295, 2010

Classification of Podocyte Genetic Disorders Based on Cell Biology

Defect	Protein, Function	Disease	Pathology	Inheritance
Extracellular Matrix/Glomerular Basement Membrane				
COL4A3	α3 (type IV collagen), GBM component	Alport syndrome, thin basement nephropathy	FSGS, absence α3-5 GBM	AR, AD
COL4A4	α4 (type IV collagen), GBM component	Alport syndrome, thin basement nephropathy	FSGS, absence α3-5 GBM	AR, AD
COL4A5	α5 (type IV collagen), GBM component	Alport syndrome	FSGS, absence α3-5 GBM	XD
COL4A6	α6 (type IV collagen), parietal layer of glomerulus	Alport syndrome with leiomyomatosis	absence α5α6 parietal	XD
LAMB2	Laminin β2, links GBM to actin via α3β1 integrin	Pierson syndrome	FSGS, mesangial sclerosis	AR
Slit Diaphragm (SD) or Interacting Proteins				
NPHS1	NEPHRIN anchors SD to cytoskeleton	SRNS1 (CNS Finnish Type)	FSGS, minimal change	AR
NPHS2	PODOCIN links cell membrane-cytoskeleton	SRNS2 (CNS type2), SRNS (adult onset)	FSGS, minimal change	AR
CD2AP	Anchors SD to actin	SRNS4 (CNS with *CD2AP* mutations)	FSGS	AR
PTPRO	Receptor-type tyrosine-protein phosphatase O	Childhood FSGS	FSGS	AR
MYO1E	Unconventional myosin 1E, actin function	Early onset FSGS	FSGS	AR
Cytoskeleton				
ACTN4	α actinin 4, cross links actin filaments	SRNS (adult onset)	FSGS	AD
MYH9	Non-muscle type myosin, cell morphology	Epstein, Fechner syndrome	FSGS	Varies
ARHGAP24	Rho GTPase activating protein 24, actin remodeling	Familial FSGS	FSGS	AD
INF2	Inverted formin-2, actin regulation	Adult FSGS	FSGS	AD
ARGDIA	Rho GDP-dissociation inhibitor 1	Early onset nephrotic syndrome, FSGS	FSGS	AR
Cell Signaling				
TRPC6	Nonselective transient receptor potential calcium channel 6	SRNS (adult onset)	FSGS	AD
PLCE1	phospholipase Cε1, cell junction, podocyte differentiation	SRNS3, glomerular development	FSGS, mesangial sclerosis	AR
IGB4	Integrin β4, Cell–matrix adhesion	FSGS	FSGS	AR
DNA Repair, Transcription				
LMX1B	regulates NPHS1, 2, CD2AP and COL4A3, 4	Nail-patella syndrome, isolated proteinuria	FSGS	AD
WT1	Wilms tumor 1, transcription factor	Frasier syndrome, Denys-Drash syndrome	FSGS, minimal change	AD
SMARCAL1	SWI/SNF-related matrix-associated actin-dependent regulator of chromatin subfamily A-like protein 1	SRNS, Schimke immuno-osseous dystrophy	FSGS	AR
NEIL1	Nei endonuclease VIII-like 1, DNA glycosylation	SRNS	FSGS	AR
Mitochondria				
NXF5	Nuclear RNA Export Factor 5	FSGS	FSGS	XR
COQ2	Polyprenyl transferase, electron transport, deficient coenzyme Q10	Early onset SRNS, CoQ10 deficiency	FSGS	AR
COQ6	Ubiquinone biosynthesis monooxygenase COQ6, Ubiquinone biosynthesis	FSGS, CoQ10 deficiency	FSGS	AR
MTTL1	Mitochondrially encoded tRNA leucine 1	SRNS, progressive nephropathy	FSGS	Mother
PDSS2	Decaprenyl diphosphate synthase subunit 2, CoQ10	SRNS, CoQ10 deficiency	FSGS, collapsing FSGS	AR
Lysosomal				
SCARB2	Scavenger receptor class B member 2	SRNS, CKD, action myoclonus	FSGS, collapsing FSGS	AR

SRNS = steroid resistant nephrotic syndrome; CNS = congenital nephrotic syndrome; AR = autosomal recessive; AD = autosomal dominant; XD = X-linked dominant; FSGS = focal segmental glomerulosclerosis.

Major Cell Structures Where Gene Defects Can Lead to Primary Glomerular Diseases

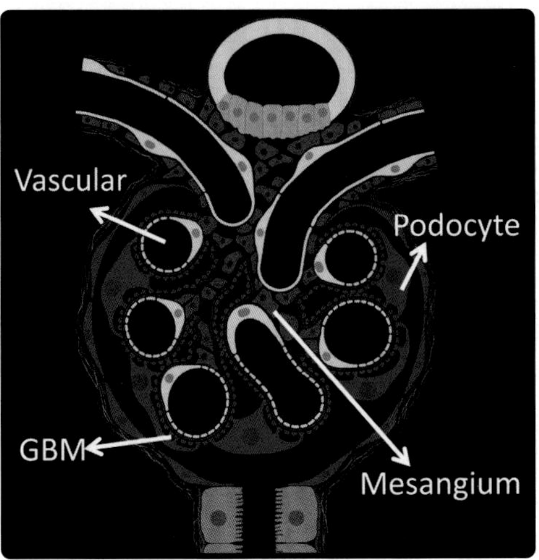

Single Genes and Gene Interactions Can Cause FSGS

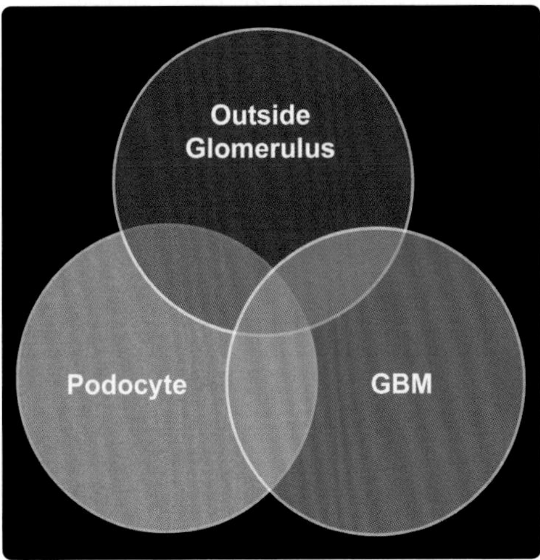

(Left) *Illustration shows 4 main glomerular regions where genetic mutations have been identified as a cause of glomerular pathology.* **(Right)** *The diagram illustrates that single genetic defects as well as interactions in genes important in podocyte or GBM function or outside the glomerulus can determine FSGS phenotype. For example, mutations in MYH9 and COL4A3 have been detected in proteinuria.*

APOL1 Risk Alleles in Young African American Patients With Hypertension

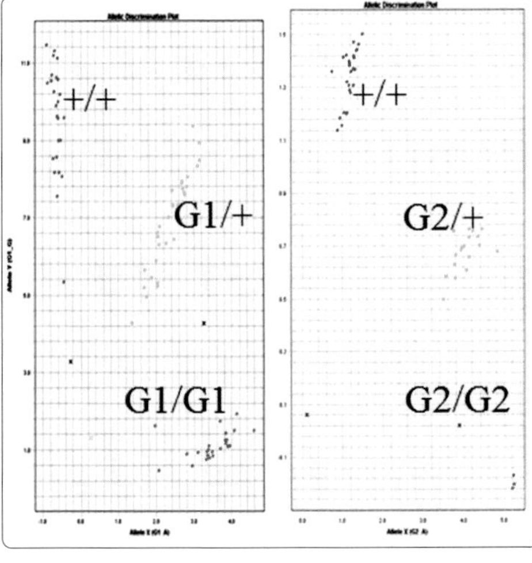

NPHS2 Mutations in a Child With SRNS

	Nucleotide	Nucleic acid
NPHS2	413G > A	R138Q
NPHS2	586C > T	R196*STOP*

(Left) *Allele discrimination plots using TaqMan assay show genotyping of G1, G2 APOL1 risk alleles in African American children with hypertension and family history of hypertension attributable ESRD. Harboring 2 alleles increases the odds to develop ESRD. Each colored spot is a patient.* **(Right)** *PCR bases sequencing in a 2-year-old child with steroid resistant nephrotic syndrome (SRNS) reveals 2 NPHS2 mutations, suggesting compound recessive mechanism. The biopsy showed MPGN.*

Mouse Model of Pierson Syndrome

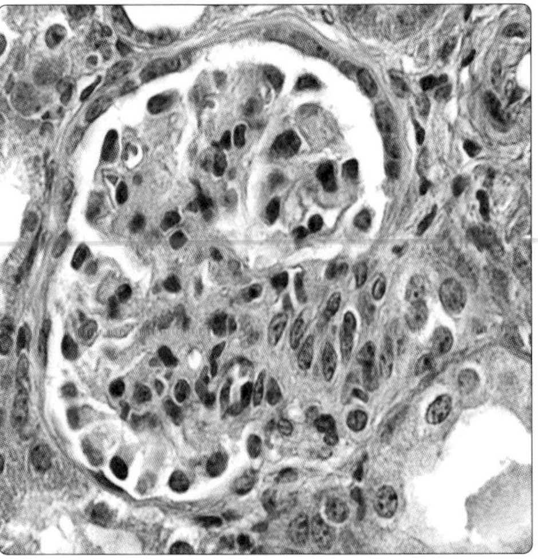

Pierson Syndrome Model in Transgenic Mice

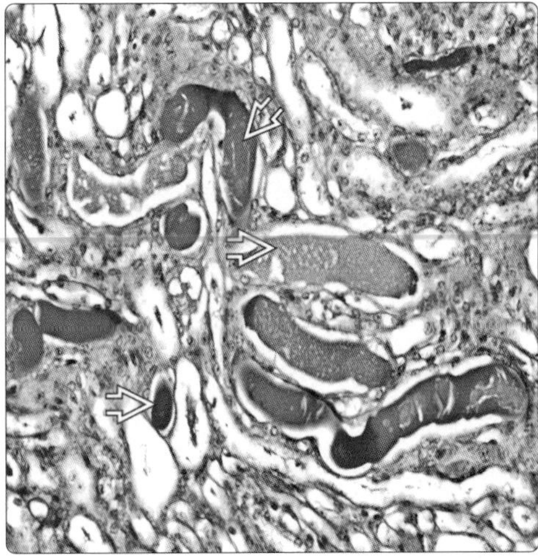

(Left) *The image shows a glomerulus from a transgenic mouse expressing the mutant LAMB2 C321R protein. This same mutation was found in a Pierson syndrome patient. These mutant mice exhibit heavy proteinuria as seen in patients with Pierson syndrome.* **(Right)** *Image shows protein casts ➡ in the tubules in LAMB2-C321R mutant mice. (Courtesy M. Chen, MD, PhD.)*

Alport Syndrome

KEY FACTS

TERMINOLOGY

- Inherited disease secondary to mutations in genes encoding α3, α4, or α5 chains of type IV collagen
- Classically characterized by hematuria, progressive renal insufficiency, neurosensory deafness, and lenticonus

ETIOLOGY/PATHOGENESIS

- ~ 85% X-linked inheritance of mutations in *COL4A5*
- ~ 10% autosomal recessive *COL4A3, COL4A4*
- ~ 5% autosomal dominant *COL4A3, COL4A4*

CLINICAL ISSUES

- Presentation
  - Hematuria, proteinuria, sensorineural deafness, hypertension, eye abnormalities
- 90% of X-linked males and 12% of X-linked carrier females develop ESRD by age 40
- Genetic testing definitive, especially by next generation sequencing

MICROSCOPIC

- Early: Minimal glomerular changes, mesangial hypercellularity, interstitial foamy macrophages
- Late: Thick capillary loops, FSGS, global sclerosis, tubular atrophy, interstitial fibrosis
- GBM multilamellation, microparticles, scalloping, and thin GBM by EM
- Decreased staining for α3, α4, α5 (IV) collagen in GBM and TBM
  - X-linked male AS: α5(IV) absent in BC
  - X-linked female heterozygotes: Mosaic loss
  - Autosomal recessive: α5(IV) present in BC
  - Epidermal BM: X-linked form
    - Absent α5(IV) in men, mosaic loss in women

TOP DIFFERENTIAL DIAGNOSES

- Thin basement membrane disease
- Focal segmental glomerulosclerosis
- Segmental lamination of GBM from repair in other diseases

Almost Normal Glomeruli in Early AS

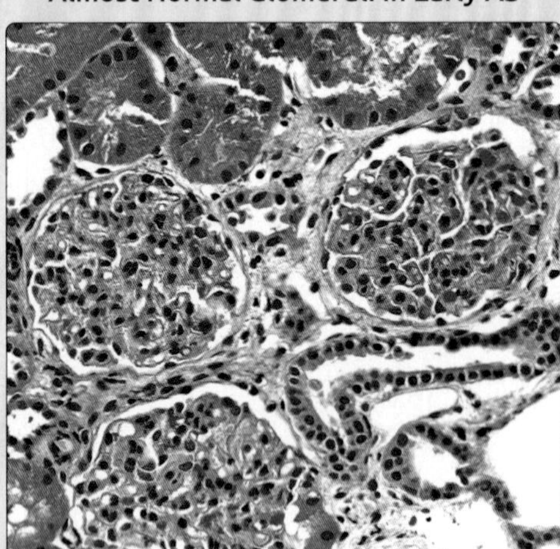

α5(IV) Chain: AS vs. Normal Kidney

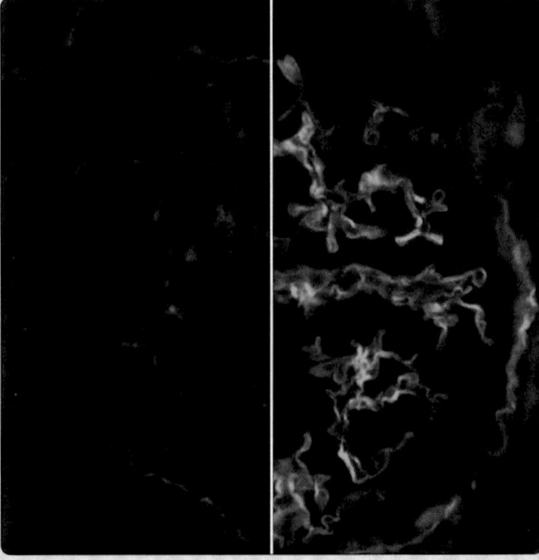

(Left) *This kidney biopsy is from a 2-year-old boy who presented with proteinuria and a family history of X-linked Alport syndrome. The glomeruli show mild mesangial hypercellularity but are generally unremarkable.* **(Right)** *The left half of this image shows the loss of GBM and Bowman capsule immunofluorescence staining for the α5 chain of type IV collagen in a boy with X-linked AS. The right half is a normal kidney stained and photographed in the same way. Loss of BC α5(IV) occurs in X-linked form of AS.*

Laminated and Thin GBM

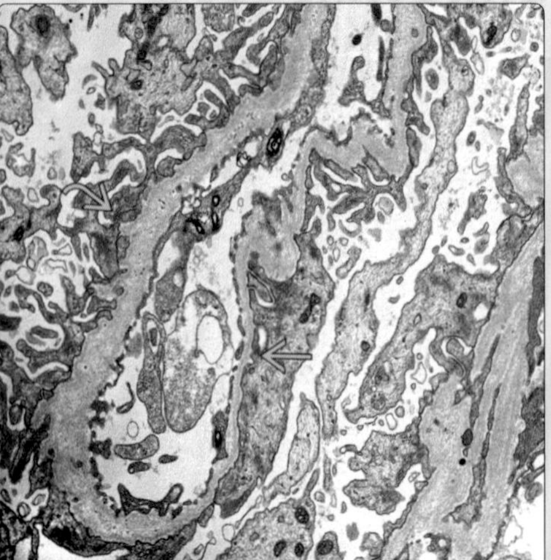

Multilamellation and Microparticles in GBM

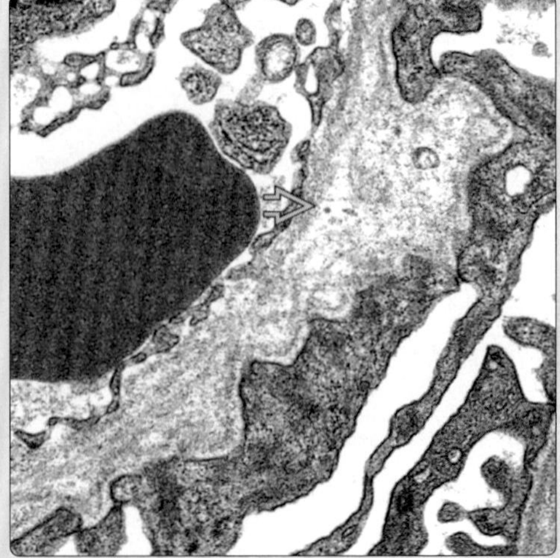

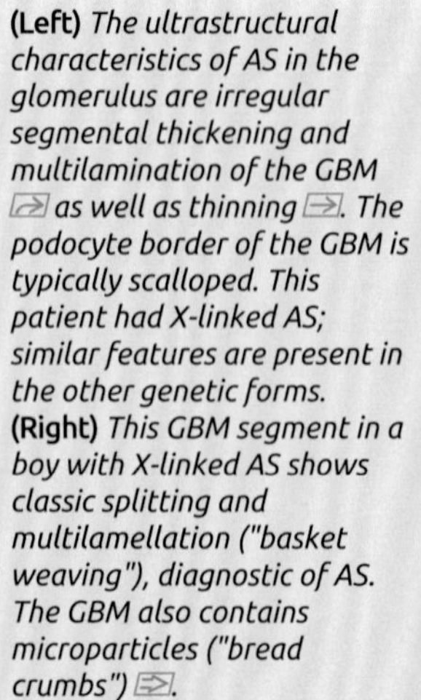

(Left) *The ultrastructural characteristics of AS in the glomerulus are irregular segmental thickening and multilamination of the GBM ⇨ as well as thinning ⇨. The podocyte border of the GBM is typically scalloped. This patient had X-linked AS; similar features are present in the other genetic forms.* **(Right)** *This GBM segment in a boy with X-linked AS shows classic splitting and multilamellation ("basket weaving"), diagnostic of AS. The GBM also contains microparticles ("bread crumbs") ⇨.*

TERMINOLOGY

Abbreviations

- Alport syndrome (AS)

Synonyms

- Hereditary nephritis

Definitions

- Spectrum of inherited diseases caused by mutations in genes encoding the α3, α4, or α5 chains of type IV collagen (*COL4A3/A4/A5*)
- Classically manifested by childhood onset hematuria, progressive renal insufficiency, sensorineural deafness, and lenticonus

ETIOLOGY/PATHOGENESIS

Genetics

- *COL4A5*
  - Encodes α5 type IV collagen chain
  - X-linked inheritance
    - Large gene, 53 exons; maps to chromosome Xq26-48
  - 80-85% of AS patients
    - Female carriers may show disease depending on degree of mosaicism following lyonization
  - > 1,900 different mutations recorded in database (2014)
    - Widely distributed over gene
    - 77% substitutions, 16% deletions, 5% insertions/duplications
      - Most frequent missense mutation affects glycine in canonical Gly-X-X collagen repeat
      - Cysteine in NC domain also commonly affected
    - 10-15% are de novo mutations (no family history)
    - 29% no known pathogenicity
  - Mutations in adjacent *COL4A6* gene result in diffuse leiomyomatosis
- Nature of mutation influences phenotype in males
  - Truncating mutation: Early-onset ESRD (mean: 25 years)
  - Splice site mutations: Intermediate-onset ESRD (mean: 28 years)
  - Missense mutations: Late-onset ESRD (mean: 37 years)
    - Lower incidence and later onset of deafness (50% at age 20 years)
  - Mutation at 5' end with earlier onset and more extrarenal manifestations
- No clear correlation of genotype and phenotype in female carriers
- *COL4A3* and *COL4A4*
  - Encode α3 and α4 chains of type IV collagen, respectively
    - Large genes (48 and 52 exons); adjacent on chromosome 2q35-37
  - Autosomal recessive inheritance
    - 10-15% of AS patients
    - Homozygous or compound heterozygous mutations
    - Onset of ESRD: 10-44 years
  - Variable phenotype in heterozygotes
    - Usually just recurrent hematuria (thin basement membrane disease)
    - Minority present as autosomal dominant AS
  - Autosomal dominant inheritance
    - ~ 5% AS patients historically
    - Higher prevalence with next generation sequencing (NGS) (20-30% of AS patients)
    - Progression to ESRD less common (~ 25%) and later (mean age: 56 years old) than homozygotes
    - May have hearing loss only; lenticonus rare
    - Hearing loss later and mild, parallels loss of renal function
- May be other genes involved
  - 10-45% of suspected AS patients have no detected *COL4A3*, *COL4A34*, or *COL4A35* mutation by NGS

Pathogenesis

- Normal GBM and distal TBM composed primarily of α3α4α5 trimeric collagen IV molecules
  - Deficiency in any 1 of 3 chains leads to failure of formation of trimer and lack of other 2 chains
  - Bowman capsule contains α5α5α6 trimers, so expression of α5 not dependent on α3 or α4
  - α1α1α2 collagen IV chains, minimally present in subendothelial side of normal GBM, increased in AS
- Mutations may result in protein misfolding, truncation, or absence of chain
  - Protein misfolding leads to unfolded protein response and degradation of α3α4α5 type IV collagen

CLINICAL ISSUES

Epidemiology

- Incidence
  - 1:5,000-1:10,000 gene frequency in USA
  - Cause of 3% of ESRD in children
  - Associated with 1-2% of ESRD in Western countries
  - No associations with race or ethnicity
- Age
  - X-linked males (hemizygotes)
    - Median: 33 years
  - X-linked female heterozygote carriers
    - Median: 37 years
  - Autosomal recessive
    - Median: 35 years

Presentation

- Hematuria
  - Males typically present with gross hematuria
  - Females typically present with microscopic hematuria
  - Tends to be persistent in males and intermittent in females
  - Exacerbated by exercise, infection
- Proteinuria, 1-2 g/d
  - Tends to develop later in disease course
  - Variable in X-linked AS
  - Common in autosomal recessive AS
    - Nephrotic syndrome in 30%
- Sensorineural deafness
  - Precedes ESRD by 5-10 years
  - 90% of X-linked hemizygotes by age 40
  - 10% of X-linked heterozygotes by age 40
  - 67% of AR homozygotes before age 20
- Hypertension
- Eye abnormalities

- Anterior lenticonus in ~ 22% of patients < 25 years old
  - Pathognomonic of AS
  - Associated with rapid ESRD and hearing loss
- Retinal flecks in ~ 37% of patients < 25 years old
- Leiomyomatosis (rare)
  - Mutations in exons 1-2 of *COL4A6* and *COL4A5*
- Thoracic aorta aneurysm and dissection reported in X-linked AS in males

Treatment

- None available to reverse, but combination of antihypertensive and new drugs targeting slow progression are gaining popularity
- Transplantation for ESRD
  - Anti-GBM disease develops post transplant in ~ 2.5% of X-linked AS
    - Associated with large deletions

Prognosis

- X-linked males
  - 90% develop ESRD by age 40
- X-linked carrier females
  - 12% develop ESRD by age 40
  - 60% develop ESRD by age 60
- Autosomal recessive
  - Earlier and more rapid progression to ESRD
- Autosomal dominant
  - Slower progression to ESRD

MICROSCOPIC

Histologic Features

- Glomeruli
  - Minimal changes early
    - Mild mesangial hypercellularity
    - Small capillary diameter
    - Lamination of GBM hard to appreciate by light microscopy (LM)
  - Late changes
    - Focal segmental glomerulosclerosis (FSGS)
    - Global glomerulosclerosis
- Interstitium and tubules
  - Interstitial fibrosis and tubular atrophy
  - Interstitial foamy macrophages
- Vessels
  - Arteriosclerosis

ANCILLARY TESTS

Immunohistochemistry

- Loss of α3(IV) and α5(IV) in basement membranes
  - Panel of monoclonal antibodies to α3(IV), α5(IV), and α1(IV) (control)
  - Immunofluorescence or immunohistochemistry on frozen tissue
- Normal distribution
  - α5(IV) in GBM, Bowman capsule (BC), distal TBM, collecting duct BM, and EBM of skin
  - α3(IV) and α4(IV) in GBM and distal TBM
  - α1(IV) is abundant in GBM during development; decreases with normal GBM maturation
- X-linked AS: Male
  - Absent α5(IV) staining in GBM, TBM, BC
  - Absent α3(IV) staining GBM, TBM
  - α1(IV) increased in GBM
  - ~ 10% stain normally (missense and intron mutations)
- X-linked AS: Female (heterozygote)
  - α5(IV) and α3(IV) expression may be preserved, decreased, or may show mosaic pattern in GBM and TBM
- Autosomal recessive AS (homozygote)
  - Absent or severely decreased α3(IV) and α5(IV) staining in GBM and distal TBM
  - Preserved α5(IV) staining in BC
- Autosomal dominant AS (heterozygote)
  - Normal α5(IV) and α3(IV) reported in 8 cases
- Skin biopsy EBM
  - X-linked AS in males: Absent α5(IV)
  - X-linked AS in female heterozygotes:mosaic α5(IV)
    - Segmental loss of α5(IV) occasionally even when kidney biopsy shows normal α5(IV)
  - Autosomal recessive or dominant AS: Normal α5(IV)

Immunofluorescence

- No specific deposition of IgG, IgA, IgM, C3, C1q, kappa, or lambda
- Segmental IgM and C3 typical in FSGS lesions

Genetic Testing

- Gold standard in AS diagnostics
  - Validate biopsy results in classic or atypical clinical presentation (e.g., no family history) and when biopsy is inconclusive
  - Not all mutations have clinical significance
  - Biopsy needed to access pathological consequences of mutation
  - Sensitivity of linkage analysis reported to be ~ 60%
- Next generation sequencing (NGS) and web-based sequence visualization tools evaluate all 3 *COL4A3-5* genes simultaneously and increase the sensitivity of detecting Alport mutations to > 90%
  - Can reveal new mutations, new combinations of mutations, and heterogeneity within a family
  - Autosomal dominant Alport detected more frequently
  - Advantageous when mode of inheritance is difficult to determine
  - Will become cheaper as new technology becomes more widely available
- AS mutations can coexist with mutations in other renal genes, e.g., *NPHS2* and *APOL1*

Electron Microscopy

- Similar GBM changes in all genetic forms of AS
- Multilamellation of GBM lamina densa imparting basket weave appearance
  - Increases with age in males, not in females
  - Segmental lesions in females, little change with age
- GBM microparticles or "bread crumbs" between laminations
- Irregular, variable GBM thick and thin segments
- Thin GBM only lesion in some cases of classic X-linked AS regardless of age
  - Identical to thin basement membrane disease in *COL4A3* or *COL4A4* mutation heterozygotes
  - X-linked carrier females

Collagen IV α1, α3, and α5 Staining Patterns

AS Variant	α1(IV) Chain	α3(IV) Chain	α5(IV) Chain
Normal	GBM(±), BC(+), DT(+)	GBM(+), DT(+)	GBM(+), DT(+), BC(+) CD(+)
X-linked (male)	GBM(+), BC(+), DT(+)	Absent GBM,* DT	Absent GBM, DT, BC, EBM
X-linked heterozygote (female)	GBM(+), BC(+), DT(+)	Mosaic or decreased GBM, DT	Mosaic or decreased GBM, DT, BC, EBM
Autosomal recessive	GBM(+), BC(+), DT(+)	Absent or decreased GBM, DT	Absent or decreased GBM, DT; present BC and EBM
Thin basement membrane disease	GBM(±), BC(+), DT(+)	May be weaker than normal in GBM; normal in DT	May be weaker than normal in GBM; normal in BC, DT

*GBM = glomerular basement membrane; BC = Bowman capsule; DT = distal tubule basement membrane; CD = collecting duct; EBM = epidermal basement membrane. *~ 10% have normal or minimal decrease.*

  - Typically have milder clinical course
  - Most common in missense mutations
  - Combined with FSGS in autosomal dominant AS
- Scalloping or "outpouching" of subepithelial surface of GBM
- Generally concordant lesions within families
- Podocyte foot process effacement

DIFFERENTIAL DIAGNOSIS

Thin Basement Membrane Nephropathy

- Normal or slightly weak collagen IV α3 and 5(IV) staining pattern
- Generally no structural damage to glomeruli
- May be manifestation of AS

Epstein and Fechtner Syndromes

- Hereditary nephritis, deafness, macrothrombocytopenia (Epstein) or cataracts, blue leukocyte inclusions (Fechtner)
- GBM EM changes resemble AS
- Mutation in *MYH9*; normal expression of α3-5(IV) chains

Denys-Drash Syndrome

- GBM laminations resemble AS
- Onset < 2 years; ambiguous genitalia; Wilms tumor
- *WT1* mutation

IgA Nephropathy

- Segmental GBM laminations from repair may resemble AS
- Mesangial IgA deposits prominent
- Normal expression of α3-5(IV)

Focal Segmental Glomerulosclerosis

- Primary FSGS lacks widespread laminations of GBM and has normal α3 and α5(IV) staining
- 10% of familial FSGS patients have heterozygous mutations in *COL4A3* or *COL4A3*
  - These lack classic EM GBM changes of AS

DIAGNOSTIC CHECKLIST

Clinically Relevant Pathologic Features

- Global GBM multilamellation/thickening has worse prognosis

Pathologic Interpretation Pearls

- Carriers of either X-linked or AR forms may show only GBM thinning
- Immunofluorescence of collagen IV α3 and α5 chains cannot always distinguish AS from TBMD, but in most cases can differentiate autosomal recessive AS from X-linked AS
- Segmental lamination of GBM can also be seen in repair in other diseases such as IgA nephropathy

SELECTED REFERENCES

1. Fallerini C et al: Unbiased next generation sequencing analysis confirms the existence of autosomal dominant Alport syndrome in a relevant fraction of cases. Clin Genet. 86(3):252-7, 2014
2. International Alport Mutation Consortium et al: DNA variant databases improve test accuracy and phenotype prediction in Alport syndrome. Pediatr Nephrol. 29(6):971-7, 2014
3. Malone AF et al: Rare hereditary COL4A3/COL4A4 variants may be mistaken for familial focal segmental glomerulosclerosis. Kidney Int. 86(6):1253-9, 2014
4. Morinière V et al: Improving mutation screening in familial hematuric nephropathies through next generation sequencing. J Am Soc Nephrol. 25(12):2740-51, 2014
5. Wang Y et al: Clinical and genetic features in autosomal recessive and X-linked Alport syndrome. Pediatr Nephrol. 29(3):391-6, 2014
6. Chatterjee R et al: Targeted exome sequencing integrated with clinicopathological information reveals novel and rare mutations in atypical, suspected and unknown cases of Alport syndrome or proteinuria. PLoS One. 8(10):e76360, 2013
7. Liapis H et al: The interface of genetics with pathology in alport nephritis. J Am Soc Nephrol. 24(12):1925-7, 2013
8. Storey H et al: COL4A3/COL4A4 mutations and features in individuals with autosomal recessive Alport syndrome. J Am Soc Nephrol. 24(12):1945-54, 2013
9. Bekheirnia MR et al: Genotype-phenotype correlation in X-linked Alport syndrome. J Am Soc Nephrol. 21(5):876-83, 2010
10. Haas M: Alport syndrome and thin glomerular basement membrane nephropathy: a practical approach to diagnosis. Arch Pathol Lab Med. 133(2):224-32, 2009
11. Heidet L et al: The renal lesions of Alport syndrome. J Am Soc Nephrol. 20(6):1210-5, 2009
12. Marcocci E et al: Autosomal dominant Alport syndrome: molecular analysis of the COL4A4 gene and clinical outcome. Nephrol Dial Transplant. 24(5):1464-71, 2009
13. White RH et al: The Alport nephropathy: clinicopathological correlations. Pediatr Nephrol. 20(7):897-903, 2005
14. Jais JP et al: X-linked Alport syndrome: natural history in 195 families and genotype- phenotype correlations in males. J Am Soc Nephrol. 11(4):649-57, 2000

(Left) *Glomeruli show mild expansion of the mesangium. The abnormalities in the GBM are difficult to appreciate by light microscopy, although a few loops have apparent thickening &/or duplication ➡.* **(Right)** *Glomeruli in Alport syndrome sometimes show abnormally small capillary loops, as shown here in a 66-year-old woman with hematuria and proteinuria whose 2 brothers died of kidney disease.*

Mild Glomerular Lesions in AS

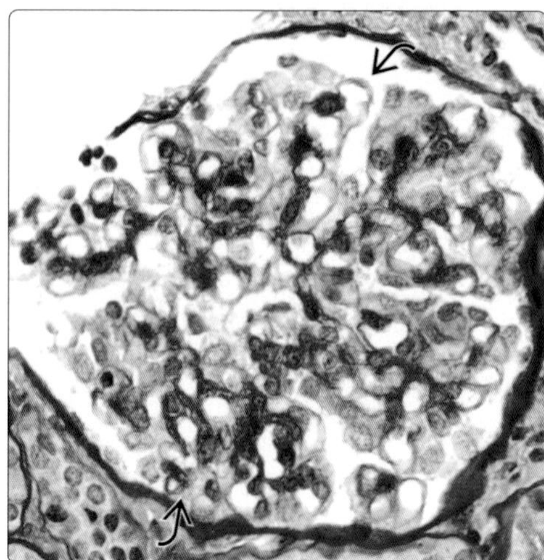

Glomerulus With Small Capillary Loops

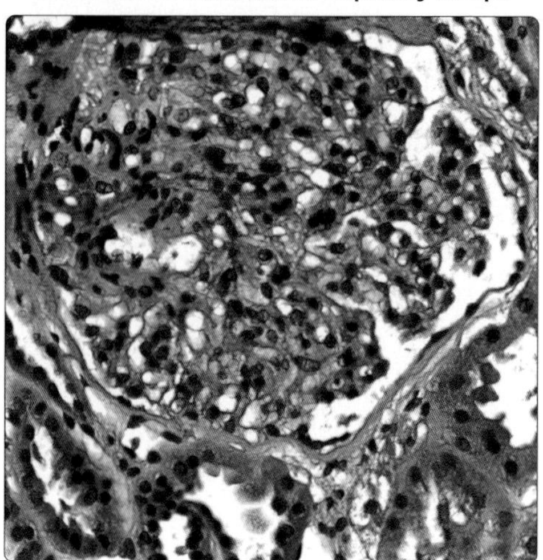

(Left) *Focal segmental glomerulosclerosis (FSGS) ➡ in this biopsy led to an initial diagnosis of FSGS. However, based on GBM abnormalities seen on EM, AS was suggested.* **(Right)** *Alport syndrome may be mistaken for idiopathic FSGS by LM. This glomerulus shows a segmental scar and adhesion ➡ (toluidine blue stain). The diagnosis was made by EM and demonstration of diminished α3, α5 (IV) collagen staining.*

Focal Segmental Glomerulosclerosis in AS

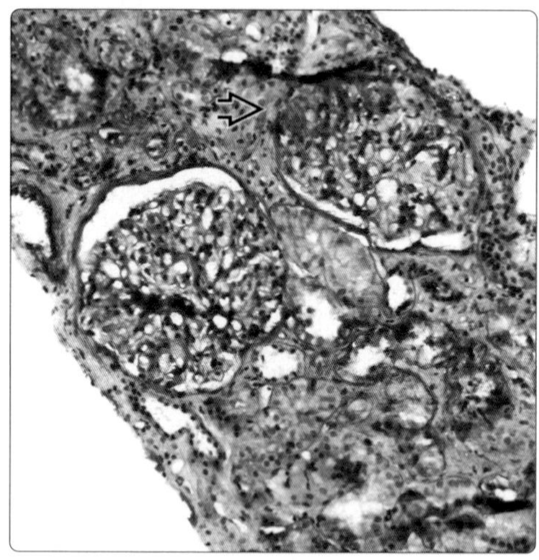

FSGS in AS

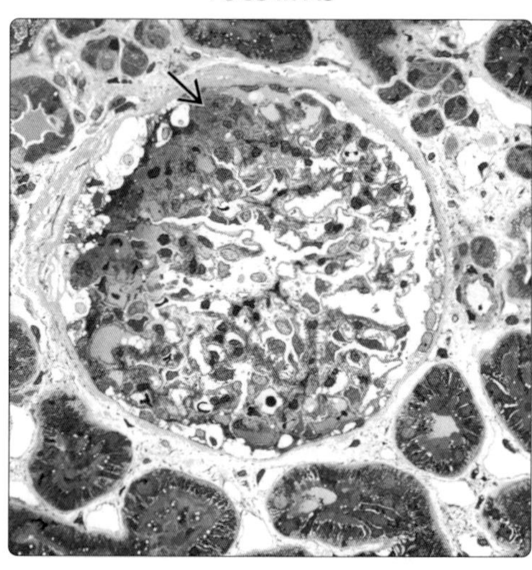

(Left) *H&E shows interstitial foamy macrophages ➡ in a biopsy from a 51-year-old woman with hematuria, recent & worsening proteinuria, & sensorineural deafness. Interstitial foamy macrophages, once thought specific for AS, are now seen in biopsies from patients with nephrotic syndrome of a variety of diagnoses.* **(Right)** *Red cell cast ➡ in tubule in a patient with AS is shown. Sometimes this is the only light microscopic clue for AS as in this 8-year-old girl.*

Interstitial Foamy Macrophages

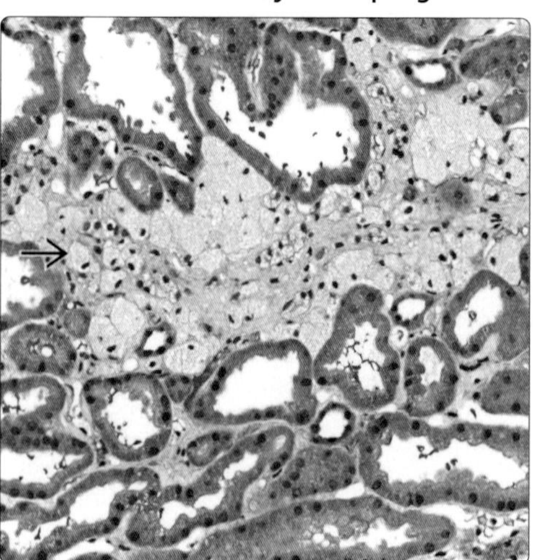

Red Cell Cast in AS

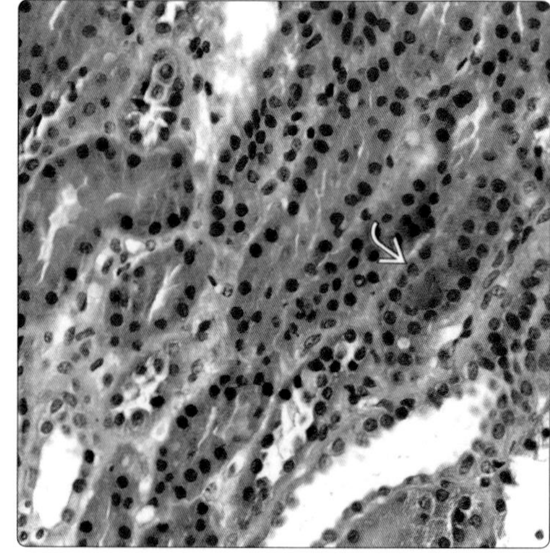

Normal Glomerular α3(IV)

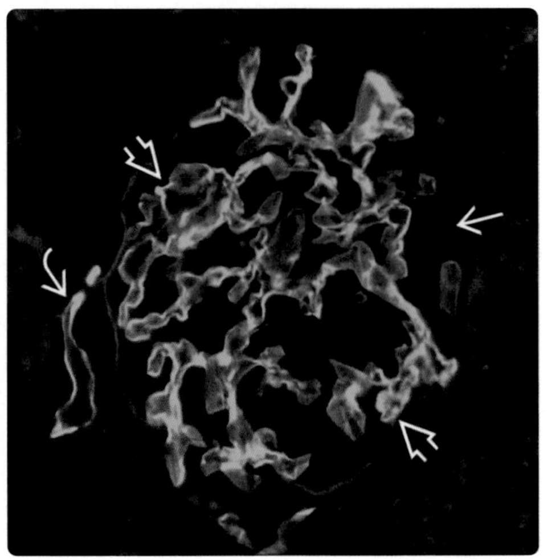

Diminished Glomerular α3(IV) X-Linked AS

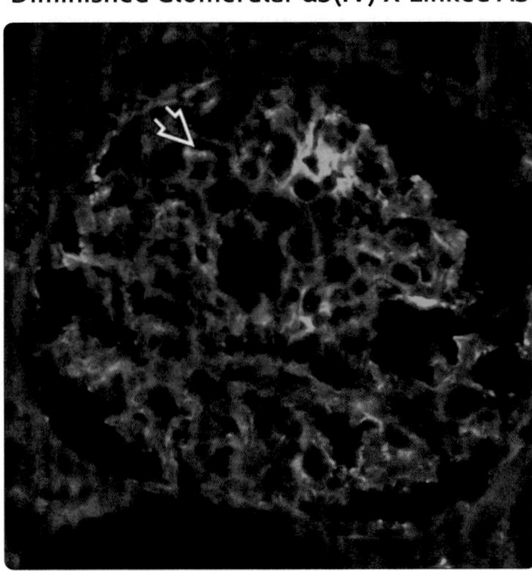

(Left) *Normal kidneys stained with a monoclonal antibody to α3(IV) collagen show bright linear staining of the GBM ➡ and distal TBM ➡, which contain α3, 4, 5 (IV) collagen chains. Bowman capsule ➡ is negative.* **(Right)** *Glomerulus from a 9-year-old boy with X-linked AS shows very weak, focal staining for α3(IV) collagen in the GBM ➡ compared with the normal control. X-linked AS has a mutation in the α5(IV) collagen gene, but α3(IV) collagen requires α5 chain (and α4) to be deposited in the GBM.*

Normal Distribution of α5(IV)

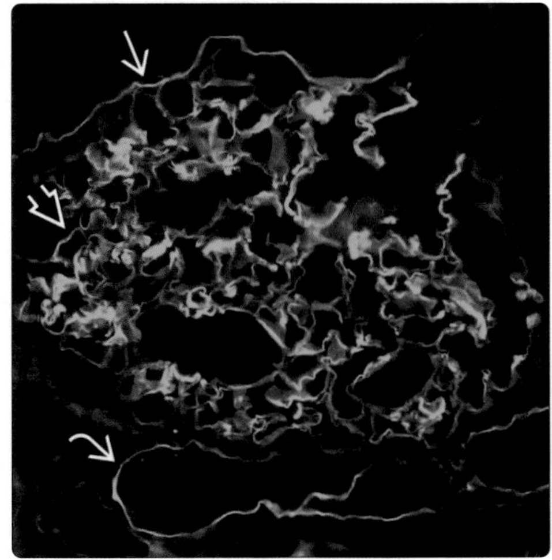

Loss of α5(IV) in AS

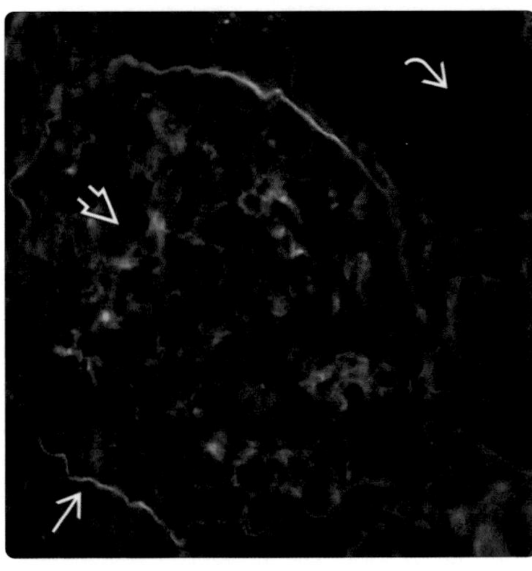

(Left) *The normal human kidney has α5(IV) collagen in the GBM ➡, distal TBM ➡, and Bowman capsule ➡. The bright linear staining pattern is typical.* **(Right)** *In X-linked AS there is negative staining for α5(IV) collagen in GBM ➡, as well as Bowman capsule ➡, and distal TBM ➡. Renal biopsy is from an 3-year-old boy with Alport syndrome; α3(IV) was also negative. Absent α5(IV) in Bowman capsule distinguishes X-linked from autosomal recessive AS.*

Loss α5(IV) in Male X-Linked AS

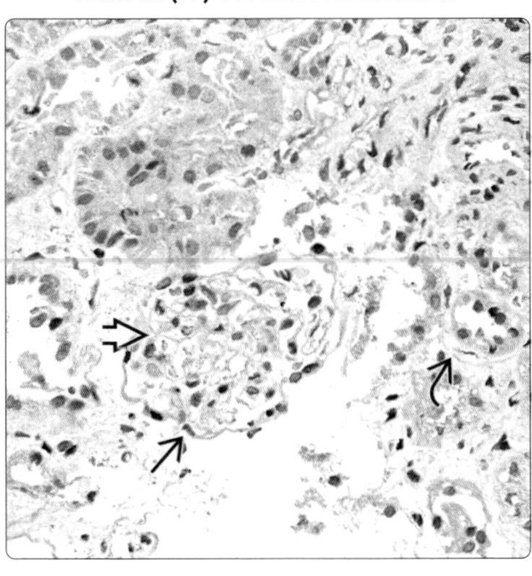

Equivocal α5(IV) Stain in AS

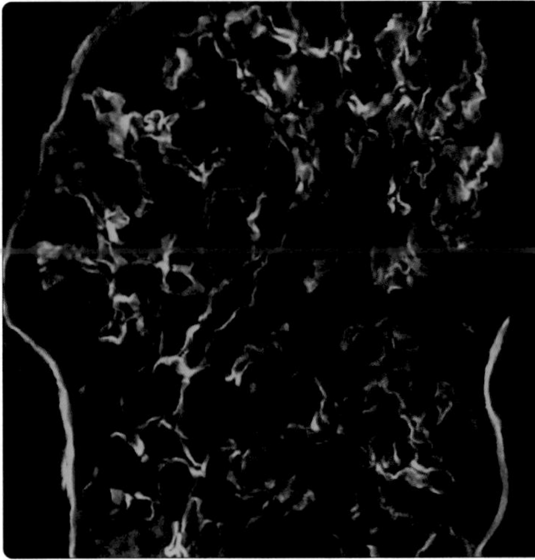

(Left) *This biopsy from a male with X-linked AS is entirely negative for α5(IV) collagen chains in glomeruli ➡, Bowman capsule ➡, and distal tubules ➡, structures that are normally α5(IV) collagen positive.* **(Right)** *This stain from a 21-year-old man with deafness, maternal grandfather with ESRD, and classic AS EM changes in the GBM shows that α5(IV) chain is present in the GBM and BC, although it is weak in spots. About 15% of AS patients have normal or weak staining for α5(IV), related to missense or intron mutations.*

(Left) *Normal control kidney stained with a monoclonal antibody to α3(IV) collagen chain shows bright linear GBM and distal TBM staining but no staining of Bowman capsule.* **(Right)** *This biopsy is from a 64-year-old woman with hematuria. Her mother, brother, and sister also had hematuria. A stain for α3(IV) collagen chains reveals decreased staining with segmental loss in the GBM and distal TBM, which is highly suggestive of X-linked AS in a female heterozygote.*

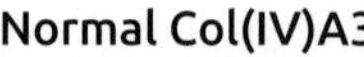

Normal Col(IV)A3

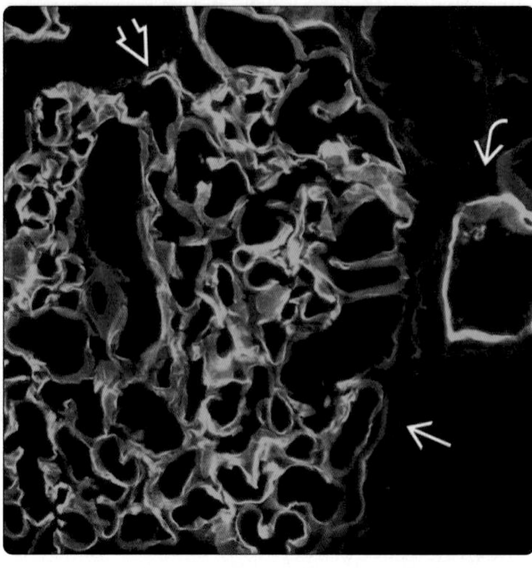

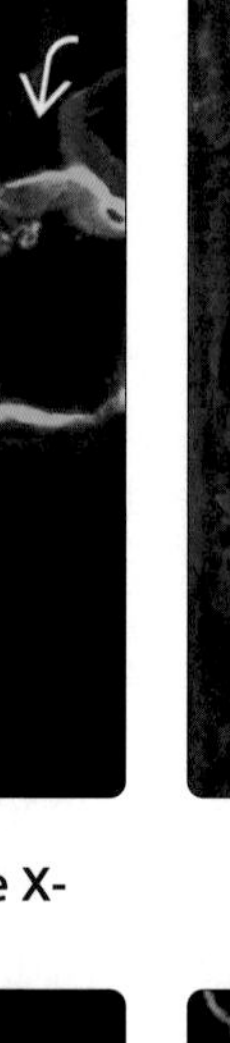

Segmental Loss of α3(IV) in Female X-Linked AS

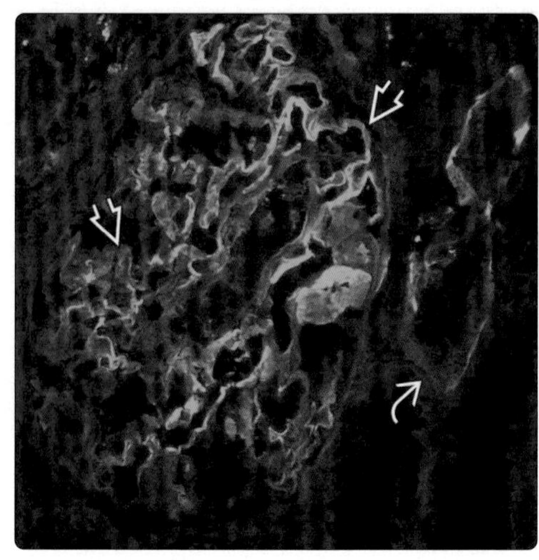

(Left) *IF for α3(IV) collagen shows interrupted (mosaic) GBM staining in a biopsy from a woman diagnosed with FSGS 5 years previously. She had marked GBM changes by EM (thick and thin areas).* **(Right)** *Positive collagen α1(IV) in a woman with X-linked Alport syndrome shows increased accumulation of α1(IV) in the glomerulus, where it is normally limited to the subendothelium and mesangium. This stain is useful to confirm that irregular staining for α3, 5 (IV) is not an artifact.*

Segmental Loss of α3(IV) in Female X-Linked AS

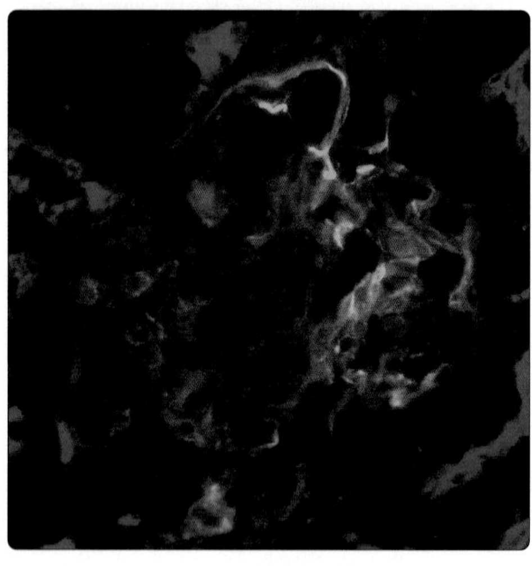

Increased α1(IV) in Female X-Linked AS

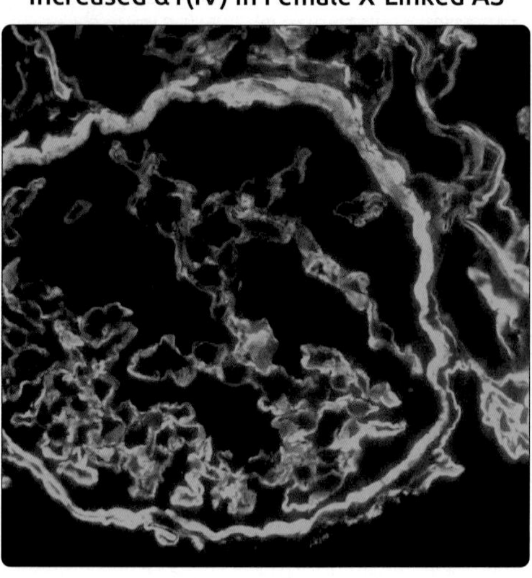

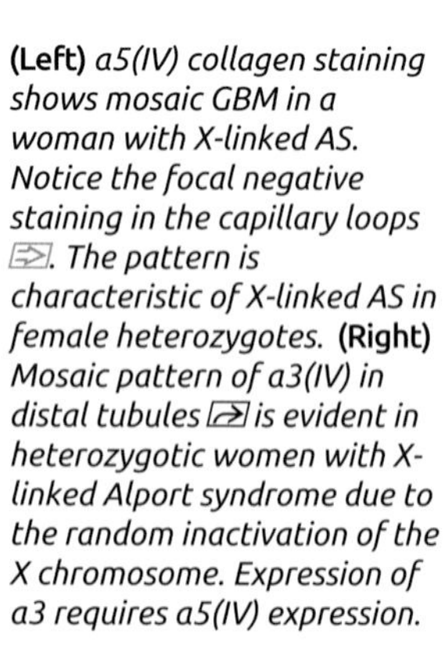

(Left) *α5(IV) collagen staining shows mosaic GBM in a woman with X-linked AS. Notice the focal negative staining in the capillary loops. The pattern is characteristic of X-linked AS in female heterozygotes.* **(Right)** *Mosaic pattern of α3(IV) in distal tubules is evident in heterozygotic women with X-linked Alport syndrome due to the random inactivation of the X chromosome. Expression of α3 requires α5(IV) expression.*

Segmental Loss of α3(IV) in Female X-Linked AS

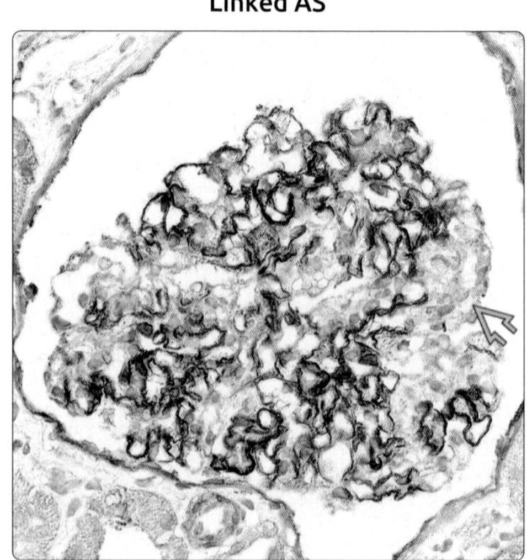

Segmental Loss of α3(IV) in Female X-Linked AS

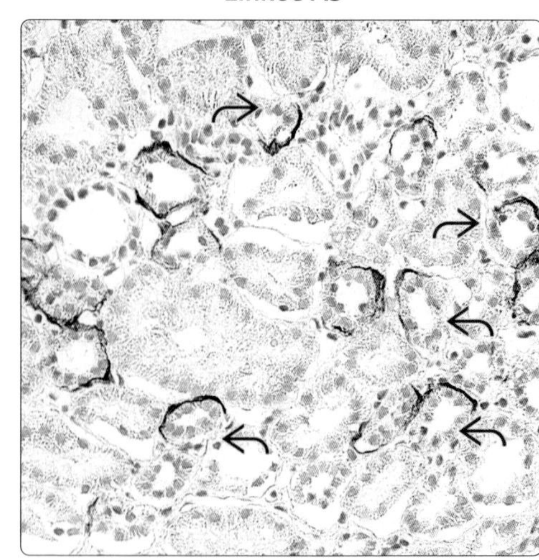

Autosomal Recessive AS α5(IV)

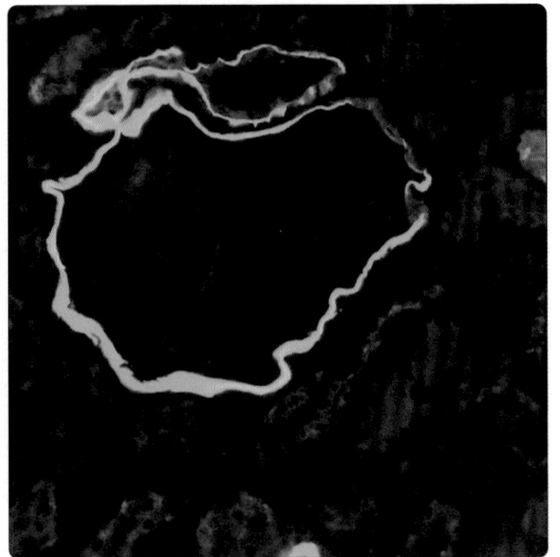

Autosomal Recessive AS α3(IV)

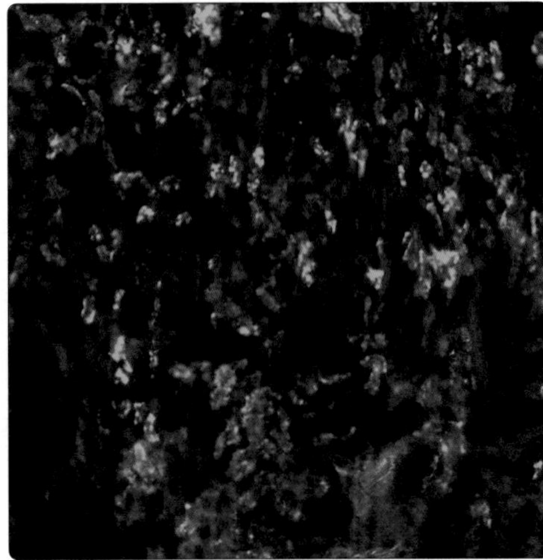

(Left) *α5(IV) shows absent staining in the GBM and positive staining of Bowman capsule. This pattern is seen in autosomal recessive AS. Bowman capsule contains α5.α5.α6(IV) trimers and does not require α3 or α4 collagen to express α5, in contrast to the GBM and distal TBM, which contain α3.α4.α5(IV) trimers.* **(Right)** *In autosomal recessive AS, α3(IV) collagen is entirely negative in the GBM and distal TBM, sites where α3(IV) collagen is normally expressed. This pattern is similar to that in men with X-linked AS.*

Normal Skin α1(IV) Collagen

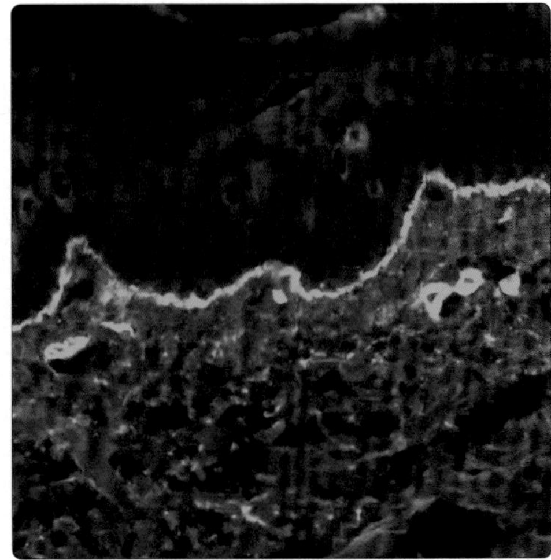

Normal Skin α5(IV) Collagen

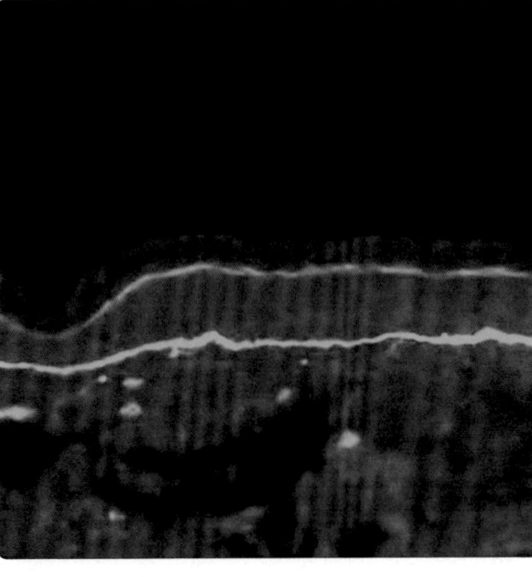

(Left) *Immunofluorescence of normal skin shows bright linear staining for α1(IV) collagen chains in the epidermal and vascular basement membranes. The EBM contains collagen α1(IV), α2(IV), α5(IV), and α6(IV) chains but no α3(IV) or α4(IV).* **(Right)** *Staining of skin with α5(IV) is a screening test for X-linked AS. Shown here is normal skin in which the antibody to α5(IV) collagen highlights the epidermal basement membrane (EBM).*

Loss of α5(IV) in Male X-Linked AS

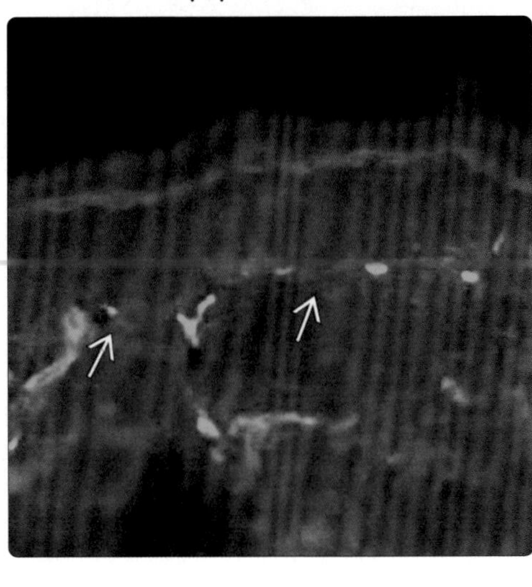

Segmental Loss of α5(IV) in Female X-Linked AS

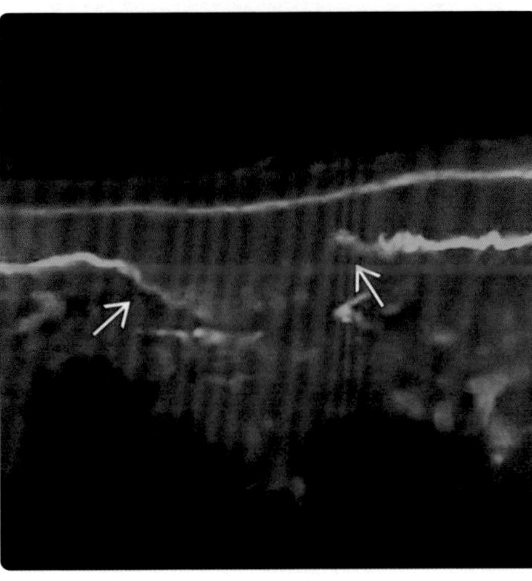

(Left) *This skin biopsy is from a boy with proteinuria and a family history of AS. The skin shows absent α5(IV) collagen chain in the epidermal basement membrane ➡, diagnostic of X-linked AS. Patients with autosomal recessive AS have normal α5(IV) staining in the skin.* **(Right)** *This skin biopsy is from a woman with X-linked AS. The epidermal basement membrane shows interrupted (mosaic) α5(IV) collagen staining ➡ due to random inactivation of the X chromosome.*

(**Left**) *EM from a 41-year-old man shows markedly irregular subendothelial GBM surface with splitting & scalloping, typical of AS. Foot process effacement is prominent. a3, a5 (IV) collagen chains were reduced by immunofluorescence.* (**Right**) *EM shows diffusely abnormal GBM, with loss of density and fine laminations in a man with X-linked AS. The particles are not conspicuous in this case, which had typical reduction of a3, a5 (IV) collagen chains reduced by IF.*

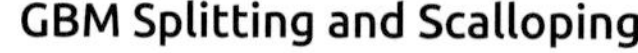

GBM Splitting and Scalloping

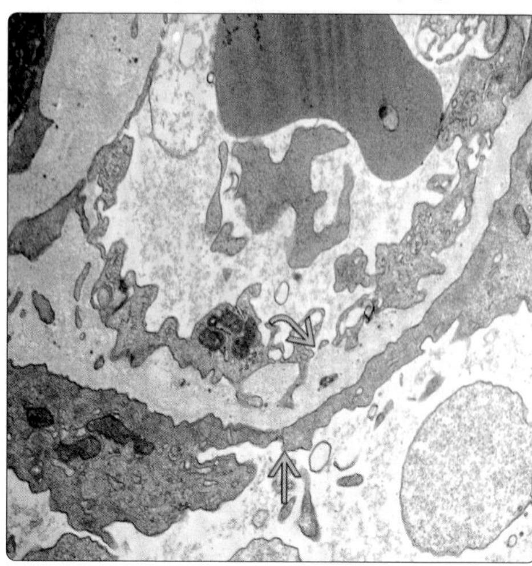

Loss of GBM Density and Fine Lamellation

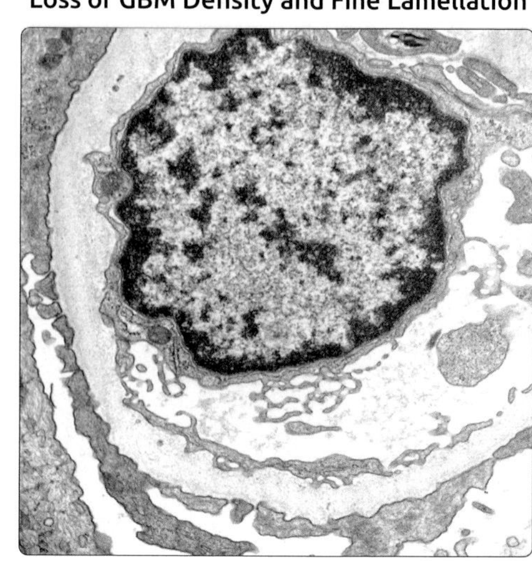

(**Left**) *AS may show segmentally thin GBM, as illustrated here. AS might be confused with thin basement membrane disease (TBMD); however, other GBM segments had reticulated laminated GBM, and a3, 5 (IV) collagen chains were reduced by IF.* (**Right**) *This glomerular capillary in a 41-year-old man with X-linked AS shows irregular thickening of the GBM and scalloping on the subepithelial side of the GBM, typical of AS.*

Segmentally Thin GBM

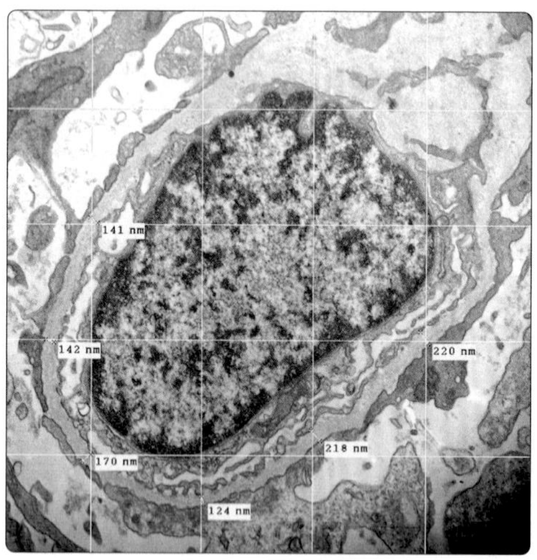

Irregular GBM Thickening and Scalloping

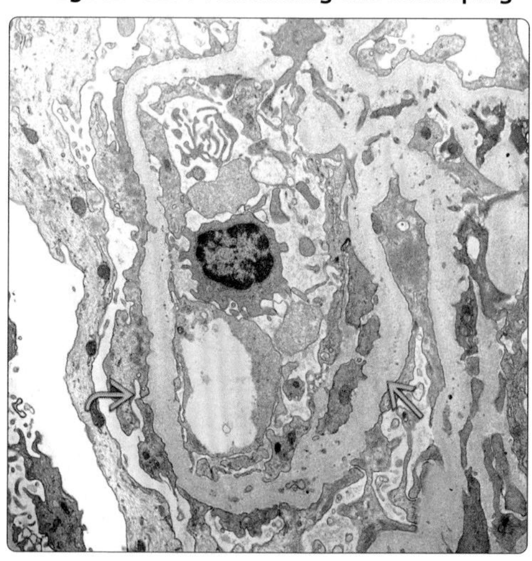

(**Left**) *EM shows a thin GBM segment from a woman with AS. In other glomerular capillaries, the GBM was thickened. Collagen IV a3-5 stains were decreased. Early AS may manifest by GBM thinning before the characteristic basket weave pattern develops.* (**Right**) *Tubular basement membrane may also show "bread crumbs" &/or multilamellation in AS.*

Thin GBM in a Woman With AS

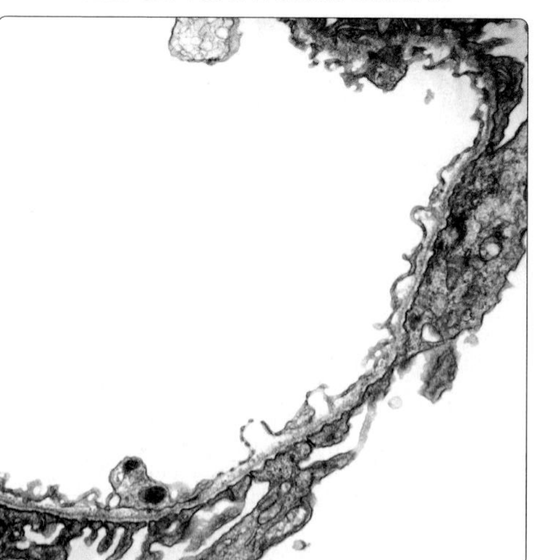

"Bread Crumbs" in Tubular Basement Membrane

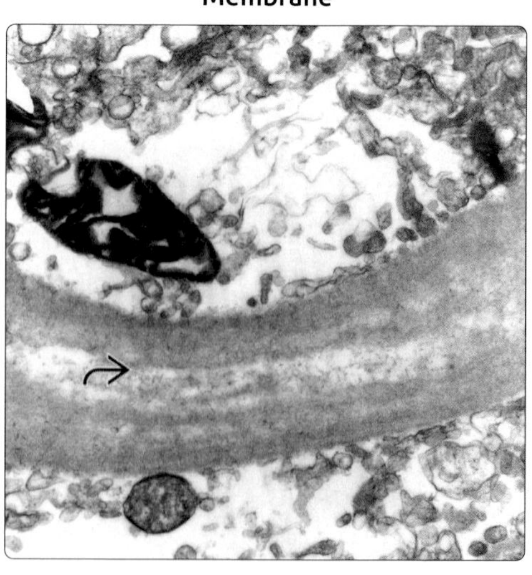

Foot Process Effacement

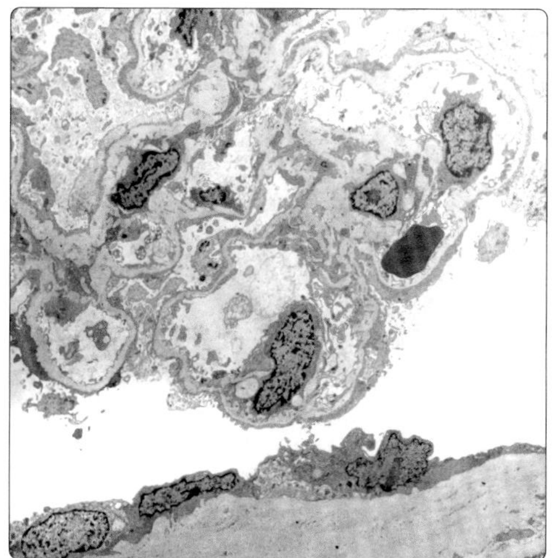

GBM Outpouching

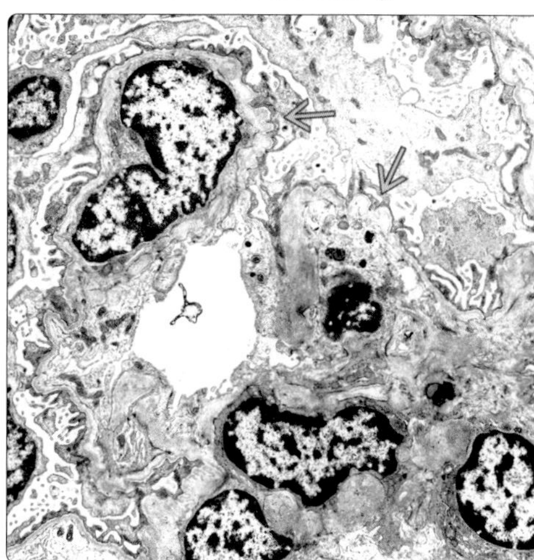

(Left) *EM shows a 41-year-old Brazilian man with recurrent hematuria, proteinuria, and mild renal insufficiency. The daughter and aunt also had hematuria and proteinuria. Diffuse, irregular thickening of the GBM is evident with effacement of foot processes. Stains for α3 and α5 (IV) collagen chains confirmed the diagnosis.* **(Right)** *A characteristic feature of AS is GBM outpouching ➙. This biopsy was from a middle-aged woman with hematuria and proteinuria. Collagen α3 and α5 (IV) chains were decreased.*

"Bread Crumbs"

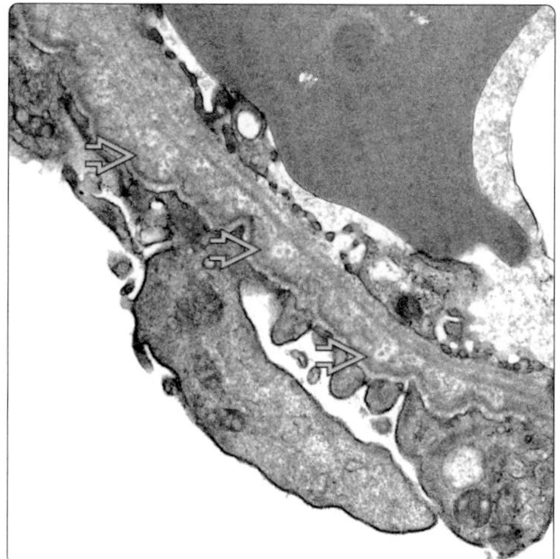

GBM Splitting

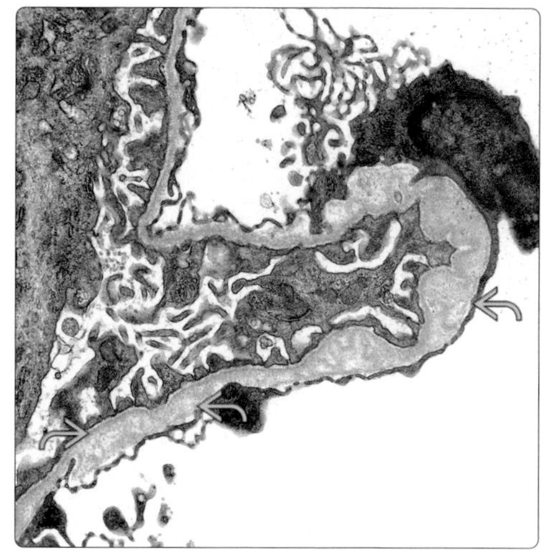

(Left) *An 8-year-old girl, daughter of a woman with Alport syndrome, shows GBM "basket weaving" and "bread crumbs" ➙. These are features of collagen IV α3-5 triplex degeneration.* **(Right)** *This electron micrograph of a kidney biopsy from a 35-year-old woman with a family history of AS shows segmental GBM thickening alternating with thin segments. Notably, GBM splitting is focal ➙. Her 8-year-old daughter also had typical Alport syndrome findings.*

GBM Scalloping

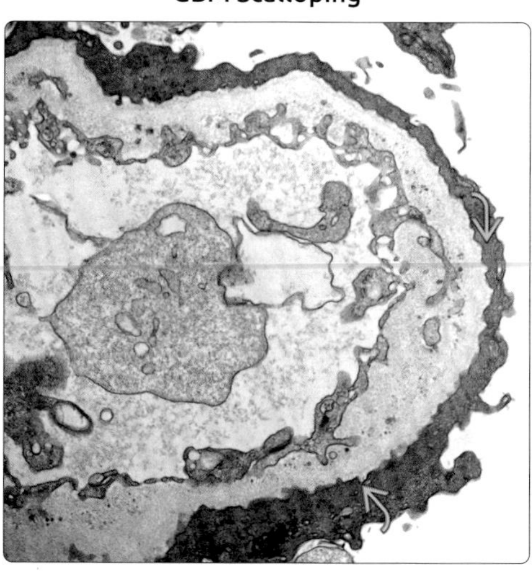

Mild GBM Lesions in Female With X-Linked AS

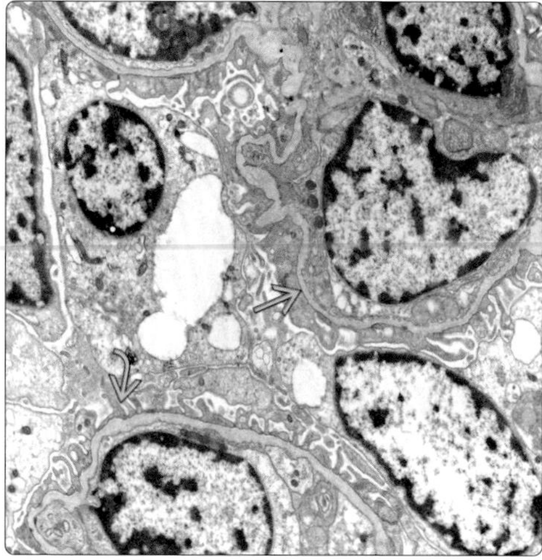

(Left) *Scalloping of the subepithelial GBM is characteristic of AS ➙. Normally, the GBM has a smooth subepithelial surface.* **(Right)** *EM shows an 8 year old with recurrent gross hematuria and proteinuria and segmental loss of α3 and α4 (IV) along the GBM. Some segments are thin ➙, and some have mild lamination ➙. IF was essential for validating the diagnosis.*

(**Left**) *Biopsy from a 23-year-old Caucasian woman with nephrotic syndrome shows global glomerulosclerosis* ➡, *podocyte hypertrophy/hyperplasia, and focal segmental glomerulosclerosis with an adhesion to Bowman capsule* ↷. (**Right**) *Other glomeruli from the same biopsy appear relatively unremarkable. Foci of interstitial foam cells are present* ↷.

AS Presenting as FSGS

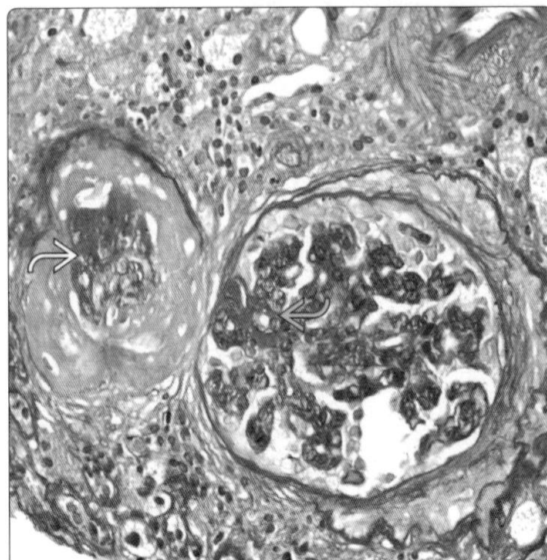

Atypical AS Presentation

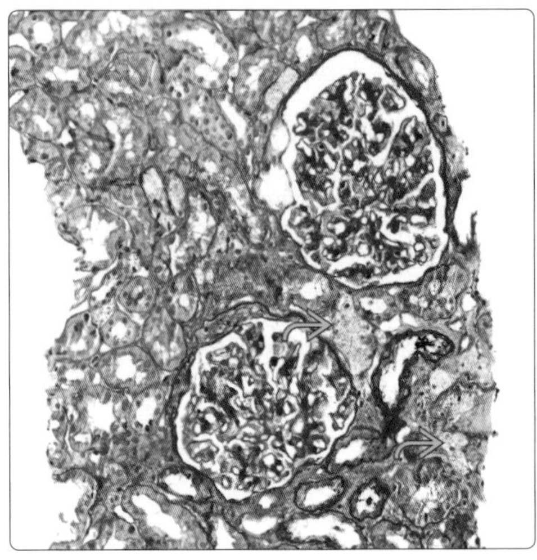

(**Left**) *Complete absence of glomerular staining for α5(IV) collagen was seen in the renal biopsy of the young woman with FSGS shown on the left image.* (**Right**) *Electron microscopic examination of the GBM from the same biopsy shows multilamellation and microparticulate "bread crumbs"* ↷, *characteristic of AS.*

Absence of Glomerular α5(IV)

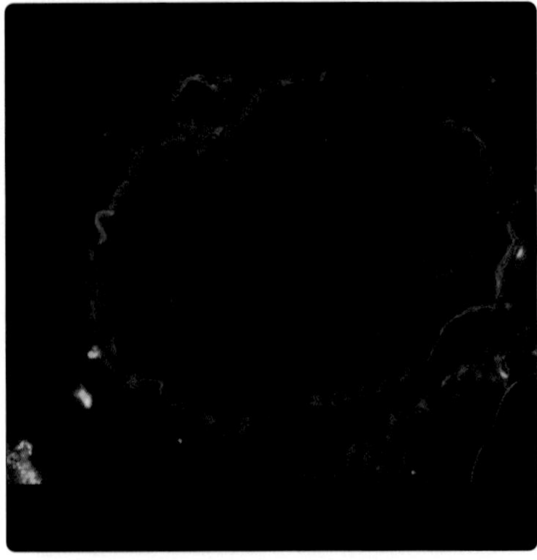

Multilamination

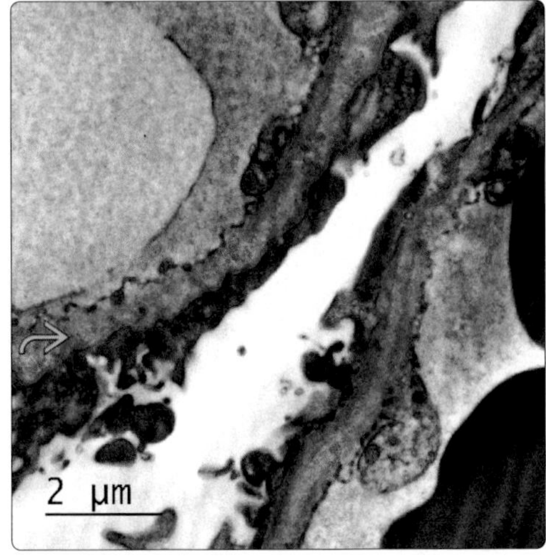

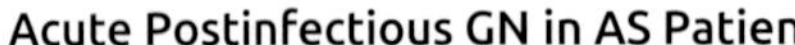

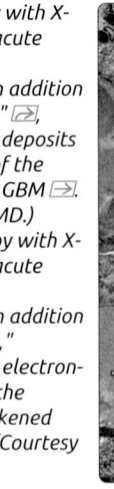

(**Left**) *11-year-old boy with X-linked AS developed acute postinfectious glomerulonephritis. In addition to the typical "humps"* ↷, *extensive amorphous deposits filled the interstices of the thickened lamellated GBM* ➡. *(Courtesy I. Rosales, MD.)* (**Right**) *11-year-old boy with X-linked AS developed acute postinfectious glomerulonephritis. In addition to the typical "humps," extensive amorphous electron-dense deposits filled the interstices of the thickened lamellated GBM* ➡. *(Courtesy I. Rosales, MD.)*

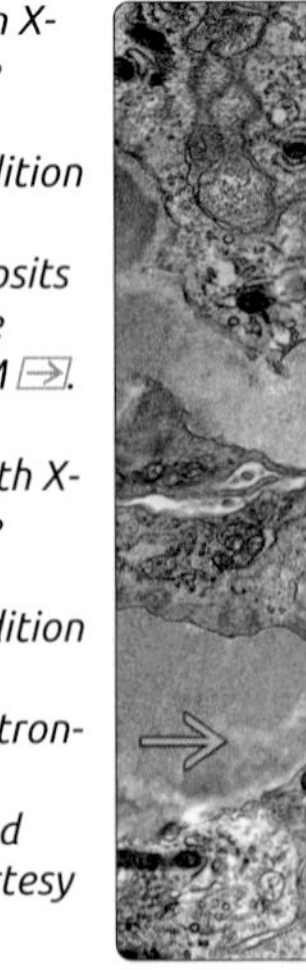

Acute Postinfectious GN in AS Patient

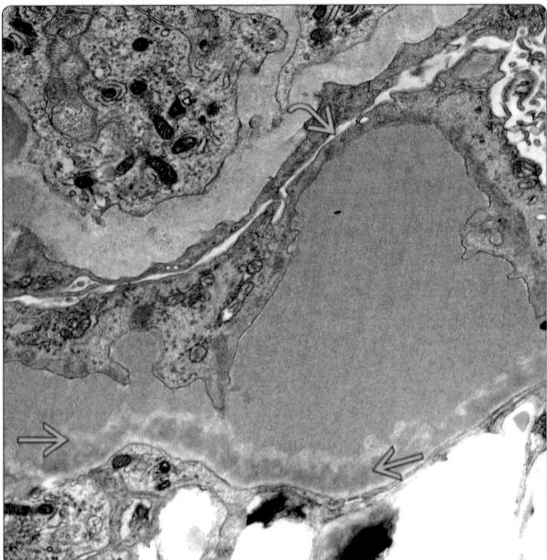

Acute Postinfectious GN in AS Patient

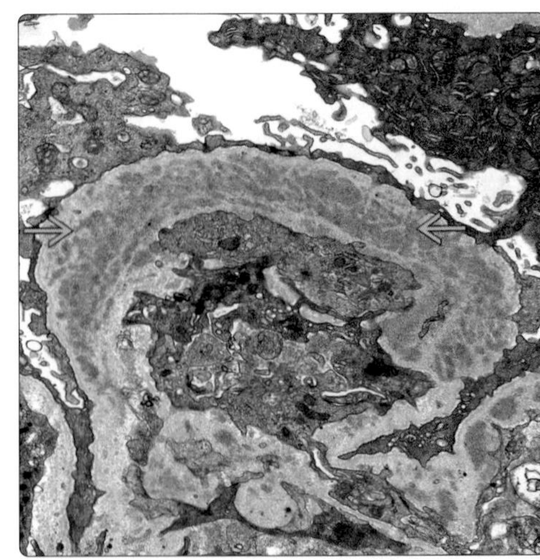

IgA Nephropathy Can Mimic AS

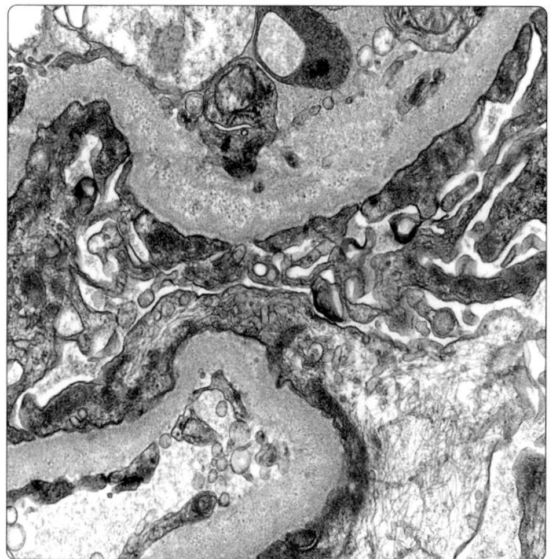

IgA Nephropathy Can Mimic AS

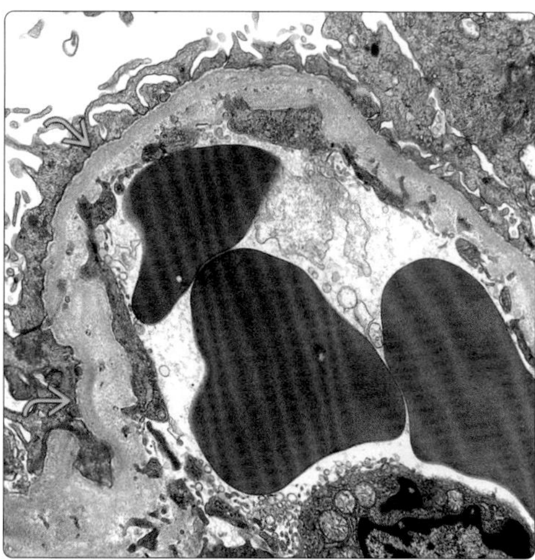

(Left) *EM shows lamination and particles in the GBM in a patient with IgA nephropathy. Focal multilamination can be seen as a repair process in glomerulonephritis and without other evidence is not sufficient for the diagnosis of AS.* **(Right)** *Focal lamination and particles in the GBM in IgA nephropathy are shown. Other segments of the GBM were normal. A clue that is against AS is the presence of normal subepithelial GBM ➢. In AS, the entire thickness of the GBM is abnormal.*

Diffusely Thin GBM in AS

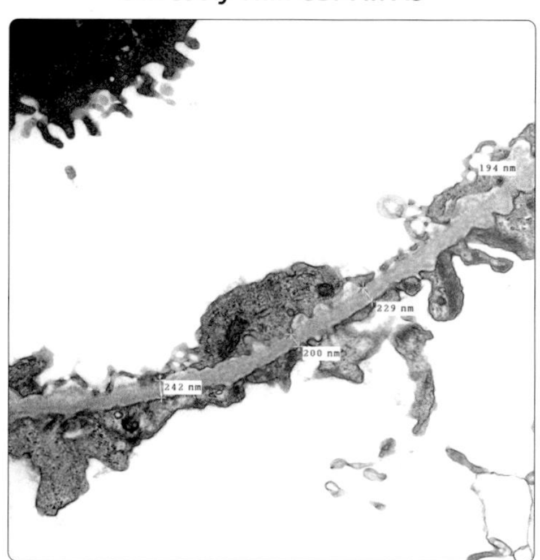

α5(IV) in Thin Basement Membrane Disease

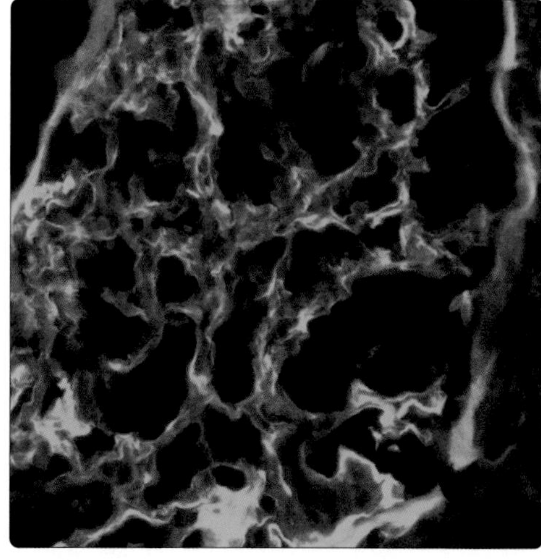

(Left) *EM shows diffusely thin GBM in a woman with X-linked AS. Ruling out TBMD without genetic analysis or IF for collagen chains is not possible in some patients, particularly if family history is unclear.* **(Right)** *TBMD can have reduced staining for collagen components due to the thin GBM, as shown here in a biopsy stained for α5(IV) collagen from a woman with recurrent hematuria and normal renal function. Bowman capsule stains normally, which is a useful clue.*

Thin Basement Membrane Disease vs. AS

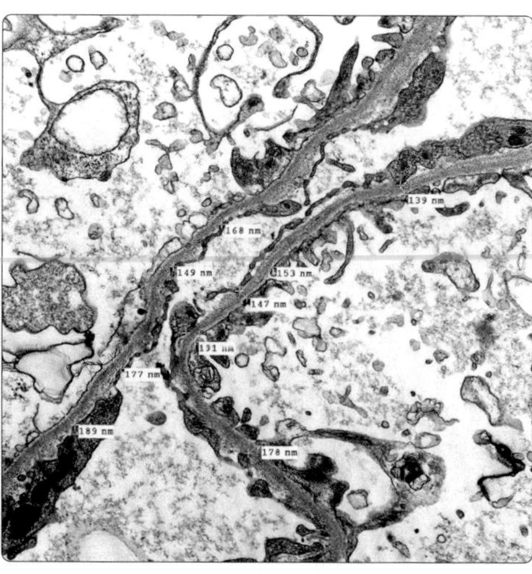

AS Ultrastructure Lesions With Normal Collagen Stains

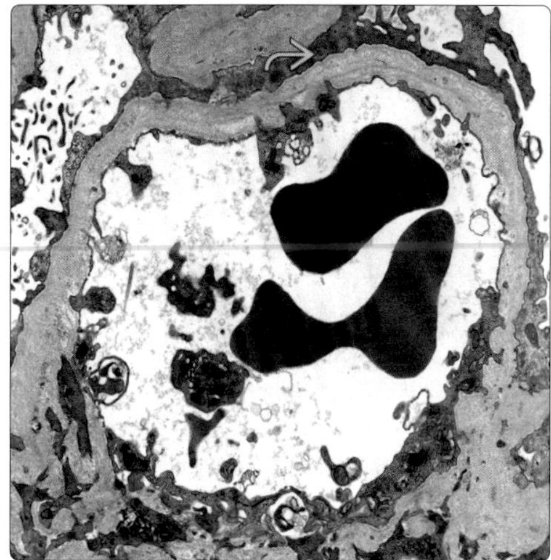

(Left) *Apparent TBMD in a 49-year-old man with global glomerulosclerosis & chronic renal failure is shown. Though there was no GBM multilamellation, this may be AS masquerading as TBMD since TBMD typically does not cause significant glomerulosclerosis.* **(Right)** *This biopsy is from a 44-year-old woman with hematuria & proteinuria. The GBM is focally thickened with splitting ➢, strongly suggestive of AS. α3, α5(IV) chains were present by IF. Genetic analysis is required for confirmation in cases with disparate IF and EM.*

Thin Basement Membrane Disease

KEY FACTS

TERMINOLOGY

- Autosomal dominant disorder presenting with asymptomatic microscopic hematuria characterized by diffuse glomerular basement membrane (GBM) thinning

ETIOLOGY/PATHOGENESIS

- 40% of patients with GBM thinning have mutations in *COL4A3* or *COL4A4* genes

CLINICAL ISSUES

- Presents with persistent microscopic hematuria
- 1-5% of population
- Autosomal dominant inheritance
  - 40% mutations in *COL4A3* or *COL4A4* genes

MICROSCOPIC

- Normal glomeruli by light microscopy
- Red cell casts

ANCILLARY TESTS

- Immunofluorescence
  - Normal or slightly reduced GBM staining for α-3, α-4, and α-5 chains of type IV collagen
  - Normal expression does not definitively exclude Alport syndrome
- Electron microscopy
  - Uniform GBM thinning (< 200 nm) by morphometry
    - Multilamination of GBM not present
  - Measure between base of podocyte foot process and edge of endothelial cells
  - Only measure the peripheral capillaries
  - Alternatively use harmonic mean and grid method

TOP DIFFERENTIAL DIAGNOSES

- Alport syndrome
- IgA nephropathy

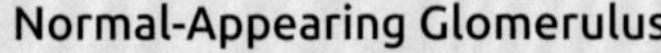

Normal-Appearing Glomerulus

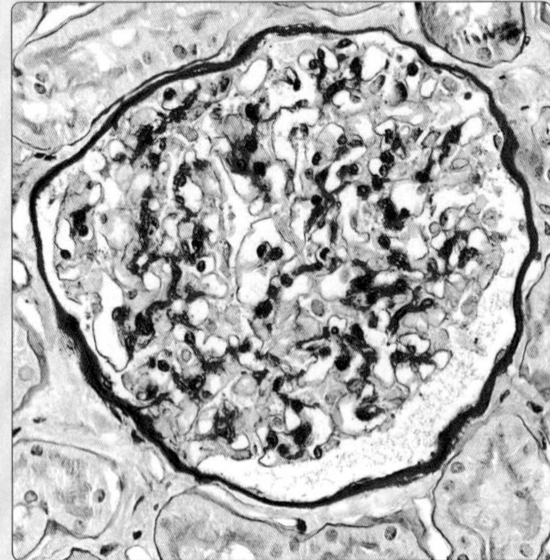

Thin Basement Membranes

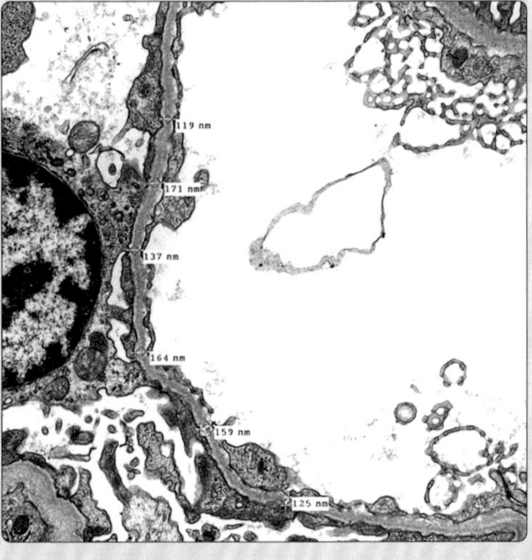

(Left) *This PAS-stained slide from a woman with thin basement membrane disease (TBMD) shows a normal glomerulus, typical of TBMD by light microscopy. The GBM averaged 230 nm by electron microscopy.* **(Right)** *Electron microscopy in TBMD reveals a diffusely thin but otherwise unremarkable GBM that measures < 200 nm in average thickness (normal is 320 ± 50 nm in women and 370 ± 50 nm in men). Morphometry is recommended to assess the thickness of the GBM.*

Interstitial Fibrosis and Tubular Atrophy

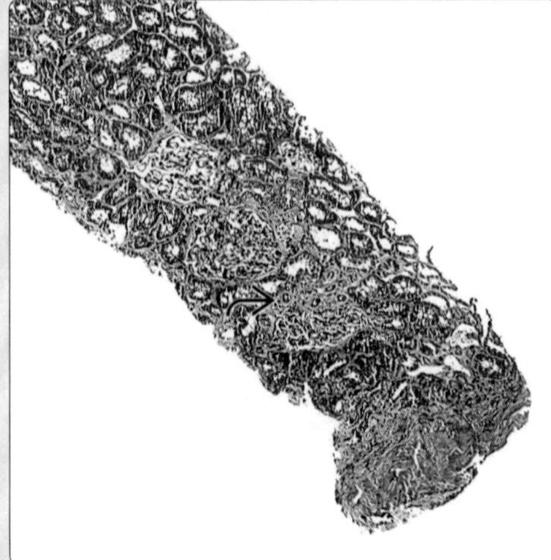

Collagen IV Alpha 5 Immunofluorescence

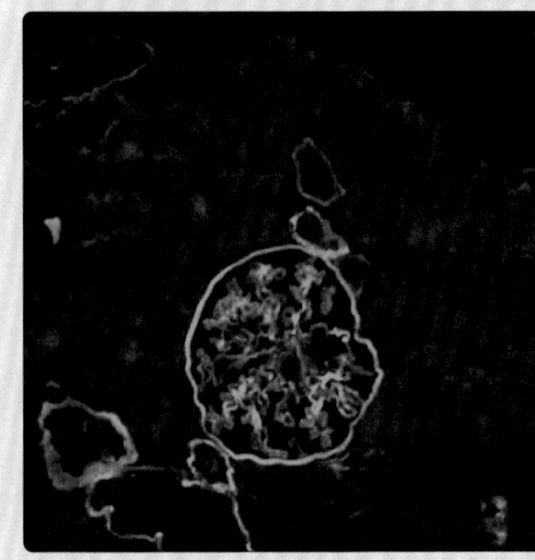

(Left) *Biopsy from an adult woman with recurrent hematuria and thin basement membrane disease shows focal interstitial fibrosis and tubular atrophy ➙.* **(Right)** *Immunofluorescence for collagen IV alpha 5 chain from a patient with thin basement membrane disease shows preserved expression in Bowman capsule and the glomerular basement membrane.*

TERMINOLOGY

Abbreviations

- Thin basement membrane disease (TBMD)

Synonyms

- Benign familial hematuria (BFH)
- Thin basement membrane nephropathy

Definitions

- Autosomal dominant disorder presenting with asymptomatic microscopic hematuria characterized by diffuse glomerular basement membrane (GBM) thinning

ETIOLOGY/PATHOGENESIS

Genetics

- Autosomal dominant in majority of BFH
- 40% of patients with GBM thinning have mutations in *COL4A3* or *COL4A4* genes
  - Encode α-3 and α-4 chains of type IV collagen, respectively
  - Heterozygotes, typically women
  - Autosomal recessive Alport syndrome (ARAS)

CLINICAL ISSUES

Epidemiology

- Incidence
  - 1-5% of population
- Age
  - All ages
- Sex
  - Some studies indicate slight female predominance, but this is inconclusive

Presentation

- Persistent microscopic hematuria
  - Dysmorphic RBCs and RBC casts
- Macroscopic hematuria (5-22%)
- Flank pain (7-31%)
- Proteinuria, subnephrotic (rare)

Laboratory Tests

- Gene sequencing *COL4A3*, *COL4A4*, *COL4A5*

Treatment

- No specific treatment
- Close monitoring for HTN, proteinuria, elevated creatinine

Prognosis

- Excellent except for heterozygous Alport presenting as TBMD

MICROSCOPIC

Histologic Features

- Glomeruli
  - Generally within normal limits
  - Mild mesangial hypercellularity
  - Rare cases associated with focal segmental glomerulosclerosis (FSGS)
- Tubules
  - Red cell and pigment casts

ANCILLARY TESTS

Immunofluorescence

- No specific IF findings
  - Nonspecific IgM, C3, and C1q occasionally seen
- Normal or slightly reduced staining for α-3, α-4, and α-5 chains of type IV collagen
  - Normal expression does not exclude Alport syndrome

Electron Microscopy

- Uniform (> 50%) thinning of GBM measuring < 200 nm in thickness
- Normal GBM thickness
  - Adult males: 370 ± 50 nm
  - Adult females: 320 ± 50 nm
  - 150 nm at birth, 200 nm at 1 year, gradually increases to adult thickness at 11 years of age

Morphometry for GBM Thickness

- Simple method
  - Distance between base of podocyte foot processes and edge of endothelial cells
  - Only measure peripheral capillaries
  - Calculate mean and standard deviation
- Alternative method with grid
  - Measure where grid crosses GBM
  - Calculate harmonic mean to reduce effect of nonperpendicular measurements
  - Normal adult male 373 ± 84 nm; female 326 ± 90 nm (mean ± 2 s.d.)

DIFFERENTIAL DIAGNOSIS

Alport Syndrome (AS)

- More likely to have proteinuria and hypertension
- GBM multilamellation
- Absent α3 and α5 (IV) collagen by IF
- X-linked AS may initially present with thin GBM
- Genetic testing for *COL4A3*, *COL4A4*, and *COLA5* gene mutations for complex cases

IgA Nephropathy

- Some cases of IgA nephropathy also have TBMD
- Does not alter prognosis of IgA nephropathy

SELECTED REFERENCES

1. Savige J et al: Expert guidelines for the management of Alport syndrome and thin basement membrane nephropathy. J Am Soc Nephrol. 24(3):364-75, 2013
2. Kashtan CE et al: Genetic disorders of glomerular basement membranes. Nephron Clin Pract. 118(1):c9-c18, 2011
3. Haas M: Alport syndrome and thin glomerular basement membrane nephropathy: a practical approach to diagnosis. Arch Pathol Lab Med. 133(2):224-32, 2009
4. Tryggvason K et al: Thin basement membrane nephropathy. J Am Soc Nephrol. 17(3):813-22, 2006
5. Norby SM et al: Thin basement membrane nephropathy associated with other glomerular diseases. Semin Nephrol. 25(3):176-9, 2005
6. Savige J et al: Thin basement membrane nephropathy. Kidney Int. 64(4):1169-78, 2003
7. Liapis H et al: Histopathology, ultrastructure, and clinical phenotypes in thin glomerular basement membrane disease variants. Hum Pathol. 33(8):836-45, 2002

Pierson Syndrome

KEY FACTS

TERMINOLOGY

- Congenital nephrotic syndrome, neurologic defects, and microcoria due to *LAMB2* mutations

ETIOLOGY/PATHOGENESIS

- Decreased/absent expression of laminin β2 in glomerular basement membrane (GBM) and other sites
- Other laminins intact

CLINICAL ISSUES

- Severe phenotype (truncating mutations)
  - Ocular abnormalities, characteristically microcoria
- Milder phenotype (missense mutations)
  - May or may not have ocular abnormalities

IMAGING

- Large, hyperechogenic kidneys at 15 weeks

MICROSCOPIC

- Diffuse mesangial sclerosis with severe phenotype
- Fetal glomeruli seen with milder phenotype
- Diffuse mesangial sclerosis not specific
  - May present with focal segmental glomerulosclerosis
  - May present with diffuse mesangial hypercellularity

ANCILLARY TESTS

- IF: Negative staining for laminin β2
- EM Diffuse podocyte foot process effacement
  - Irregular lamellation and wrinkling of GBM
- Molecular genetic testing for *LAMB2* mutations

TOP DIFFERENTIAL DIAGNOSES

- Denys-Drash syndrome (diffuse mesangial sclerosis, *WT1*)
- Frasier syndrome (focal segmental glomerulosclerosis [FSGS], *WT1*)
- Congenital nephrotic syndrome of the Finnish type (*NPHS1*)
- CoQ2 deficiency
- Galloway-Mowat Syndrome
- Diffuse mesangial sclerosis, other causes

Fetal-Appearing Glomeruli

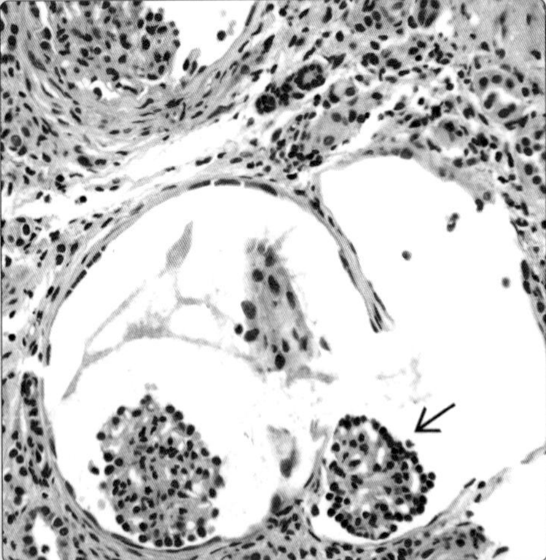

Focal Segmental Glomerulosclerosis

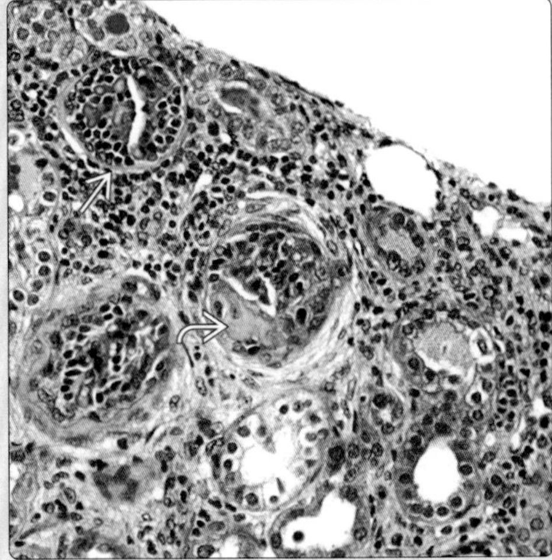

(Left) *Glomeruli in Pierson syndrome show mesangial hypercellularity or prominent podocytes forming a corona over the capillary loops, often called fetal glomeruli. Segmental glomerulosclerosis is also present.* **(Right)** *Kidney shows some glomeruli with focal segmental glomerulosclerosis and others with fetal pattern of closely packed podocytes resembling collapsing glomerulopathy.*

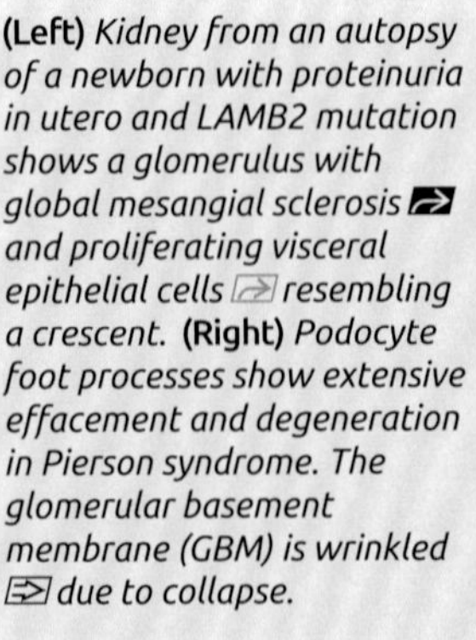

(Left) *Kidney from an autopsy of a newborn with proteinuria in utero and LAMB2 mutation shows a glomerulus with global mesangial sclerosis and proliferating visceral epithelial cells resembling a crescent.* **(Right)** *Podocyte foot processes show extensive effacement and degeneration in Pierson syndrome. The glomerular basement membrane (GBM) is wrinkled due to collapse.*

Pseudocrescent

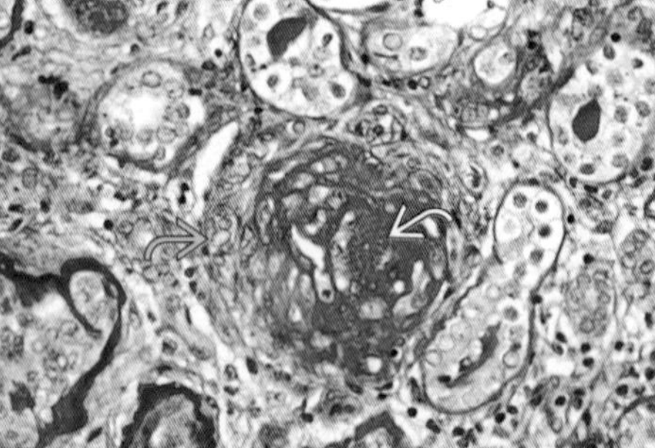

Foot Process Effacement and GBM Collapse

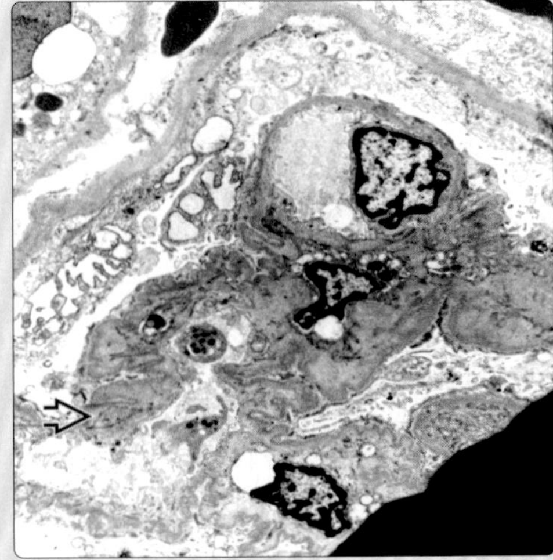

TERMINOLOGY

Definitions

- Congenital nephrotic syndrome, neurologic defects, and microcoria due to *LAMB2* mutations

ETIOLOGY/PATHOGENESIS

LAMB2 Mutations

- Encodes laminin β2 subunit
  - Normal component of glomerular basement membrane (GBM), anterior eye, and neuromuscular junction
  - Maps to chromosome 3p
- Laminins are family of 16 heterotrimeric glycoproteins
  - Major noncollagenous component of basement membranes
    - Organize and stabilize basement membranes
    - Promote cell adhesion
- Autosomal recessive inheritance
  - Truncating mutations cause severe disease
  - Missense mutations have milder clinical course
    - Result in protein misfolding, disrupted trafficking, impaired excretion

CLINICAL ISSUES

Epidemiology

- Incidence
  - 2.5% of nephrotic syndrome cases in 1st year of life
- Age
  - Truncating mutations: < 3 months
  - Missense mutations: 3 months to 10 years

Presentation

- Proteinuria, edema
- Neurodevelopmental abnormalities
- Ophthalmologic findings
  - Truncating mutations associated with microcoria, posterior lenticonus
  - Missense mutations associated with milder phenotype
    - Retinal detachment, posterior synechiae, hypopigmented fundus or no eye abnormalities
- Prenatal findings: Oligohydramnios, enlarged placenta

Laboratory Tests

- Increased amniotic α-fetoprotein
- Mutational analysis for *LAMB2* on chromosome 3

Treatment

- None curative

Prognosis

- Severe phenotype die within 1st year of life
- Milder phenotype progresses to end-stage renal disease (ESRD) at 1-10 years of age

IMAGING

Ultrasonographic Findings

- Large, hyperechogenic kidneys detectable by 15 weeks of gestation

MICROSCOPIC

Histologic Features

- Truncating mutations → severe phenotype
  - Increased mesangial matrix identical to idiopathic diffuse mesangial sclerosis
  - Global glomerulosclerosis with obliteration of capillaries
  - Closely packed podocytes in coronal (fetal) pattern
  - May show glomerulocystic changes with retraction of glomerular tuft towards vascular pole
- Missense mutations → milder phenotype
  - Variable findings
    - Focal segmental glomerulosclerosis, minimal changes, diffuse mesangial hypercellularity

ANCILLARY TESTS

Immunofluorescence

- Negative staining for laminin β2
- Other laminins, such as γ1 and α2, intact

Electron Microscopy

- Diffuse podocyte foot process effacement
- Irregular lamellation and wrinkling of GBM

DIFFERENTIAL DIAGNOSIS

Denys-Drash Syndrome

- Diffuse mesangial sclerosis
- Male gonadal dysgenesis
- Mutations in exons 8 or 9 of *WT1*

Frasier Syndrome

- Focal segmental glomerulosclerosis
- Female external genitalia, streak gonads, XY karyotype
- Mutations in intron 9 of *WT1*

Galloway-Mowat Syndrome

- *WDR73* mutation in some families
- Microcephaly, seizures

Congenital Nephrotic Syndrome of the Finnish Type

- Minimal changes and cystic dilatation of tubules on light microscopy
- Absent slit diaphragms on electron microscopy
- Mutations in *NPHS1*

PLCE1 Mutation

- Diffuse mesangial sclerosis
- Autosomal recessive

SELECTED REFERENCES

1. Aydin B et al: A novel mutation of laminin β-2 gene in Pierson syndrome manifested with nephrotic syndrome in the early neonatal period. Genet Couns. 24(2):141-7, 2013
2. Chen YM et al: Laminin β2 gene missense mutation produces endoplasmic reticulum stress in podocytes. J Am Soc Nephrol. 24(8):1223-33, 2013
3. Chen YM et al: A missense LAMB2 mutation causes congenital nephrotic syndrome by impairing laminin secretion. J Am Soc Nephrol. 22(5):849-58, 2011
4. Matejas V et al: Mutations in the human laminin beta2 (LAMB2) gene and the associated phenotypic spectrum. Hum Mutat. 31(9):992-1002, 2010
5. Choi HJ et al: Variable phenotype of Pierson syndrome. Pediatr Nephrol. 23(6):995-1000, 2008
6. Liapis H: Molecular pathology of nephrotic syndrome in childhood: a contemporary approach to diagnosis. Pediatr Dev Pathol. 11(4):154-63, 2008

(Left) *Early changes in a renal biopsy from an infant with Pierson syndrome reveal small, immature (fetal)-appearing glomeruli with prominent clustering podocyte nuclei.* **(Right)** *Chronic lesions in Pierson syndrome are shown. Glomeruli are globally or partially sclerosed, and some are fetal appearing ⇨. Periglomerular fibrosis is evident ⇨. The interstitium has an extensive infiltrate of mononuclear cells. The tubules are markedly atrophic.*

Early Changes of Pierson Syndrome

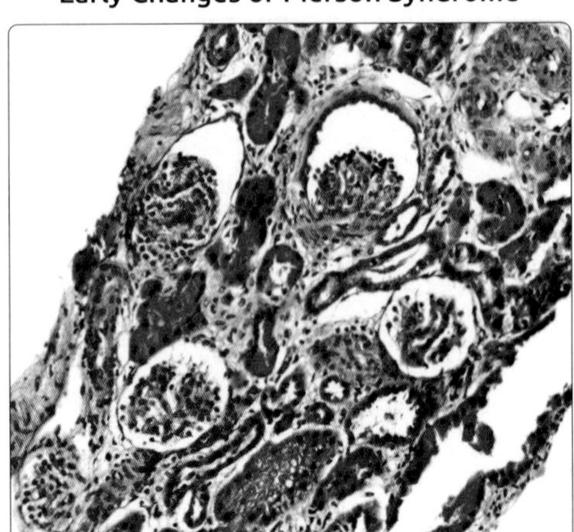

Advanced Chronic Lesions

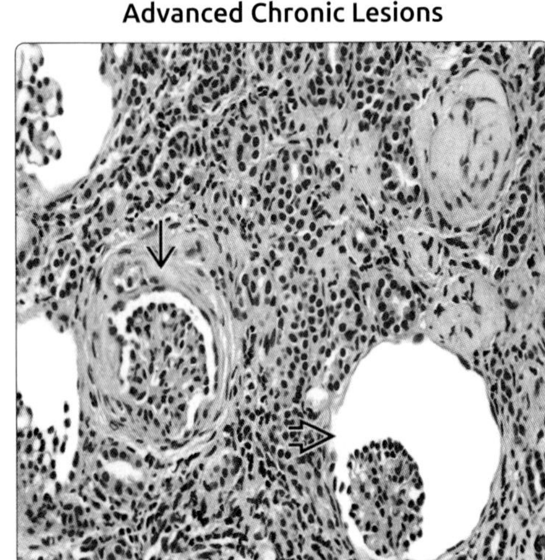

(Left) *Normal human neonatal kidneys show prominent laminin β2 in glomeruli ➡. Tubular basement membranes and vessels are negative.* **(Right)** *On rhodamine immunofluorescence, this biopsy from a patient with Pierson syndrome demonstrates no staining with mouse anti-human laminin β2 antibody.*

Normal Laminin β2 in Control Glomeruli

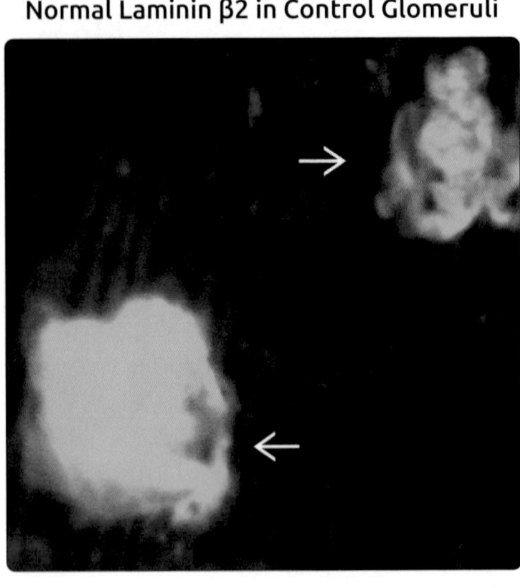

Absent Laminin β2 in Pierson Syndrome

(Left) *Normal mouse podocytes on scanning electron microscopy show interdigitating foot processes ⇗. (Courtesy G. Jarad, MD.)* **(Right)** *Podocytes from mice with a genetic knock out of LAMB2 on scanning electron microscopy show villiform transformation of the foot processes. (Courtesy G. Jarad, MD.)*

Normal Mouse Kidney

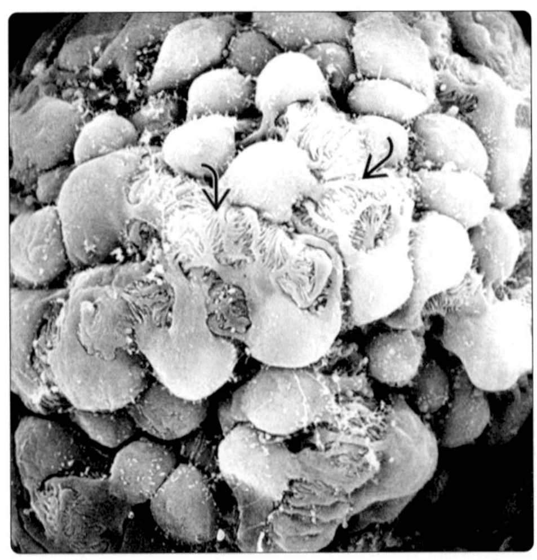

Mouse Deficient in *LAMB2*

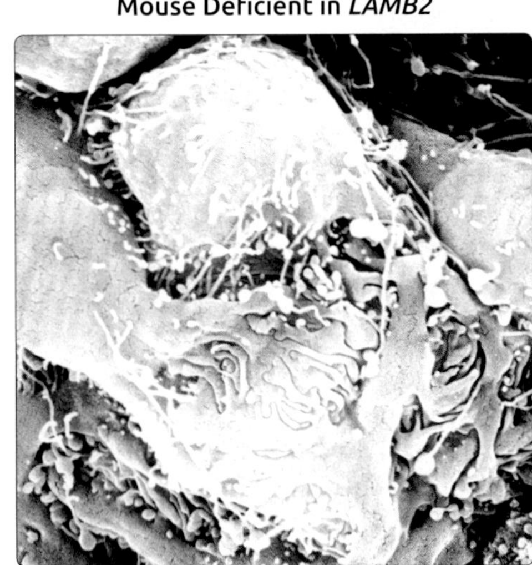

Electron Microscopy of Patient With Novel *LAMB2* Mutation

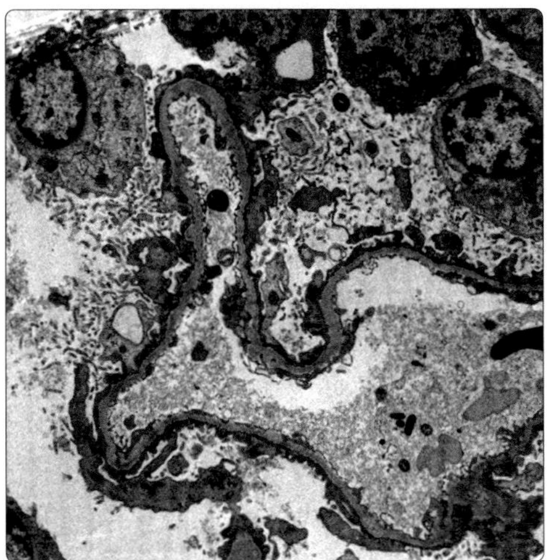

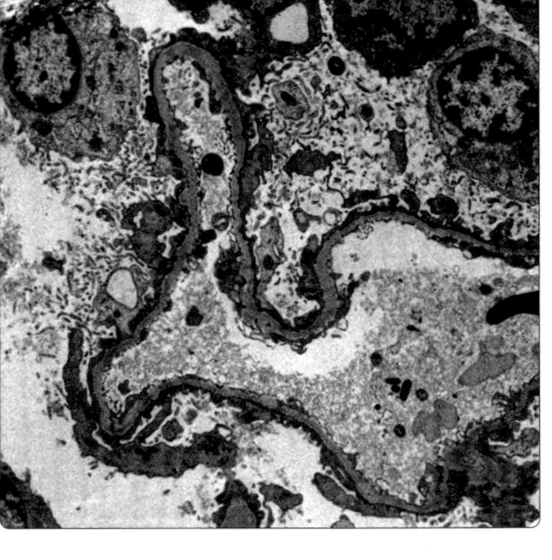

Electron Microscopy in Pierson Syndrome

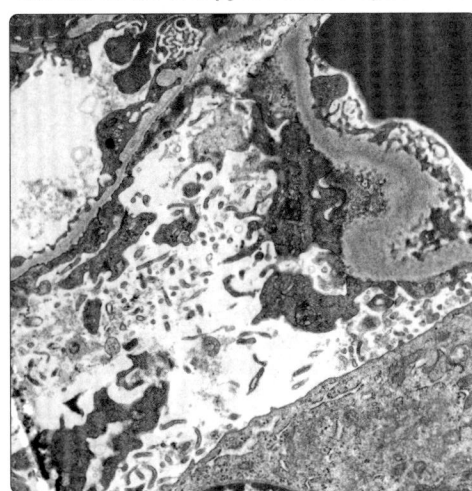

(Left) *There is diffuse degeneration and fragmentation of the podocyte cytoplasm. Podocytes are densely spaced as seen in fetal glomeruli.* **(Right)** *Same case shows foot process effacement and microvillous transformation. These findings are nonspecific and can be seen in severe nephrotic syndrome irrespective of underlying etiology.*

Electron Microscopy of Advanced Glomerular Lesions in Pierson Syndrome

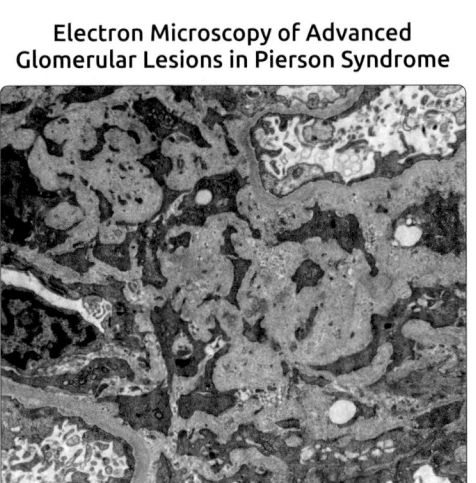

Electron Microscopy in Pierson Syndrome

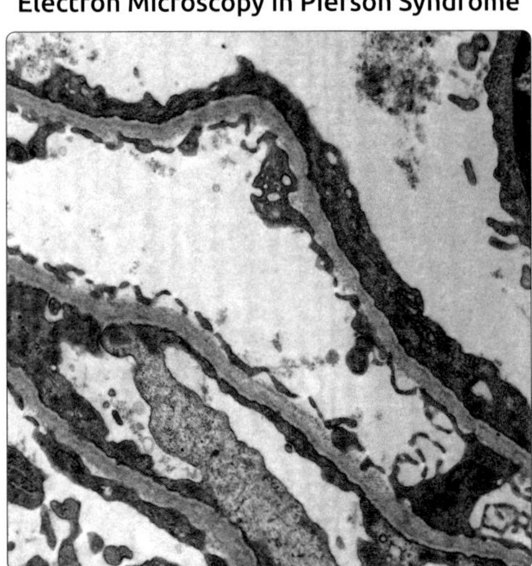

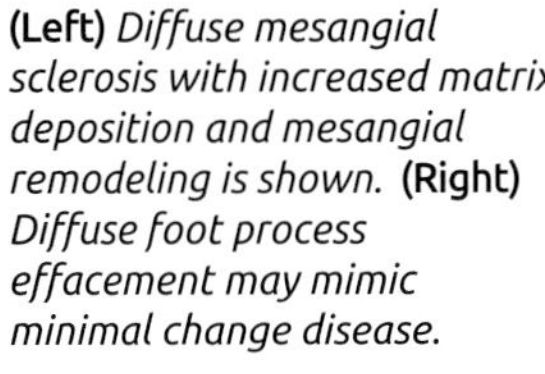

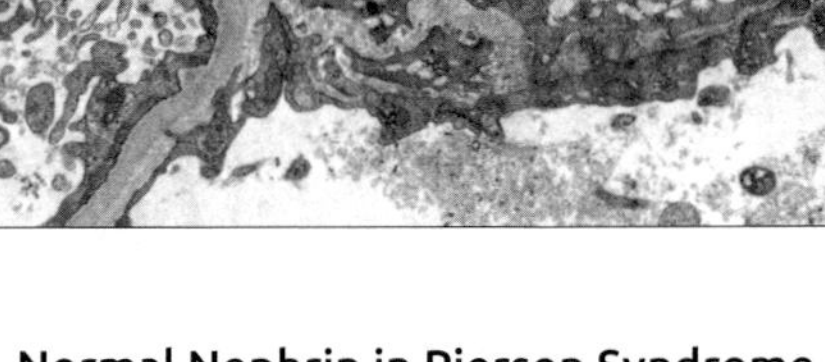

(Left) *Diffuse mesangial sclerosis with increased matrix deposition and mesangial remodeling is shown.* **(Right)** *Diffuse foot process effacement may mimic minimal change disease.*

Normal Nephrin in Pierson Syndrome

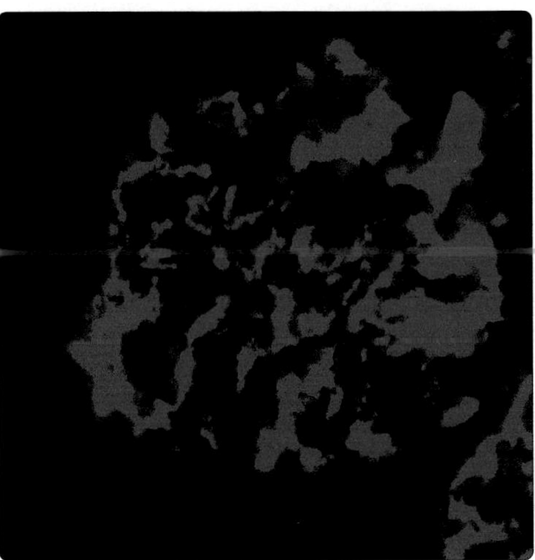

Normal Synaptopodin Pierson Syndrome

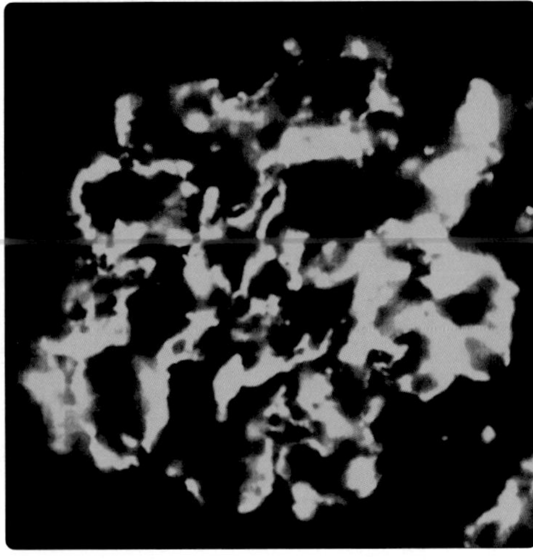

(Left) *Normal nephrin positivity on rhodamine immunofluorescence in a patient with congenital nephrotic syndrome rules out Finnish nephropathy.* **(Right)** *Normal synaptopodin expression in Pierson syndrome is shown by FITC immunofluorescence.*

Congenital Nephrotic Syndrome of the Finnish Type

KEY FACTS

TERMINOLOGY

- Congenital nephrotic syndrome due to mutations in gene-encoding nephrin (*NPSHS1*)

ETIOLOGY/PATHOGENESIS

- Nephrin is major structural protein of glomerular filtration slit diaphragm, linking foot processes of podocytes
- Absent or mutant nephrin results in absent slit diaphragms and massive proteinuria

CLINICAL ISSUES

- Presents at birth or shortly after (< 3 months of age) steroid-resistant nephrotic syndrome
- Prognosis depends on nature of *NPHS1* mutation
- Autosomal recessive inheritance
- Elevated AFP in amniotic fluid and maternal serum
- Mean time to ESRD: 32 months
- Variable rate of progression
- Fin-major have earliest onset and most rapid course
- Fin-minor have later onset and delayed progression

MICROSCOPIC

- Minimal glomerular changes early
- Microcystic dilation of proximal and distal tubules
- Interstitial fibrosis in progressive disease
- Focal and global glomerulosclerosis in advanced stages

ANCILLARY TESTS

- Absent slit diaphragms by EM
- Routine IF stains negative
- Negative nephrin staining
- Mutational analysis of *NPHS1*

TOP DIFFERENTIAL DIAGNOSES

- Podocin deficiency
- Diffuse mesangial sclerosis (various causes)
- Minimal change disease
- Focal segmental glomerulosclerosis, idiopathic

Schematic of Foot Process Slit Diaphragm

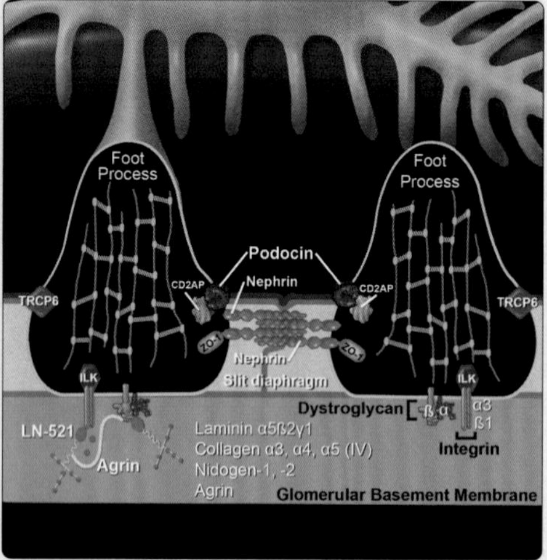

Absent Slit Diaphragms by Electron Microscopy

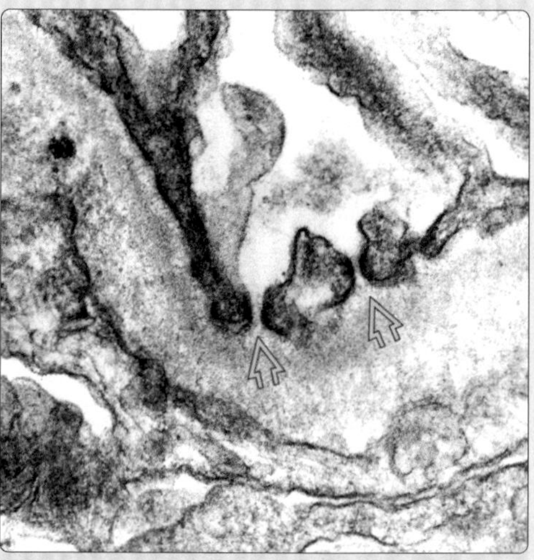

(Left) *Nephrin, a key component of the slit diaphragm, is mutated in patients with FN. Podocin mutations present with similar clinical symptoms and pathologic findings of FSGS.* **(Right)** *The diagnostic feature in congenital nephrosis of the Finnish type is absence of slit diaphragms ➡ between the podocyte foot processes, as shown in biopsy from a newborn.*

Minimal Glomerular Histologic Changes

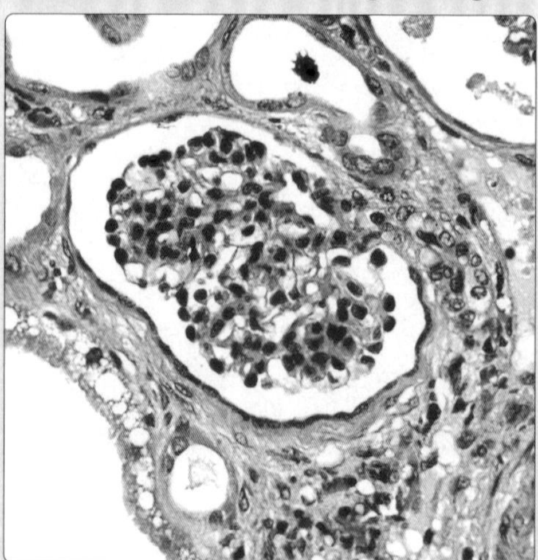

Lack of Nephrin by Immunofluorescence

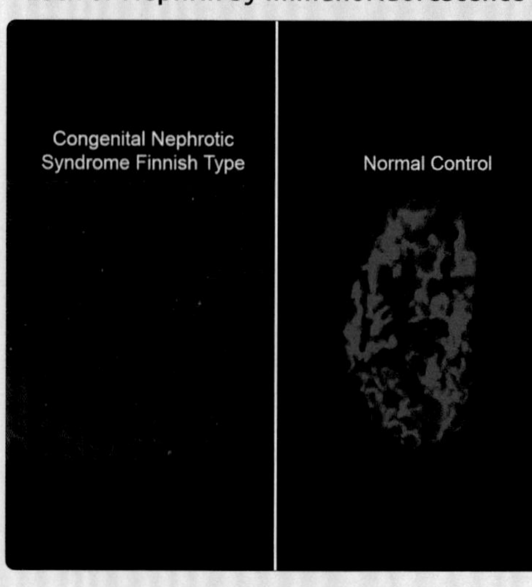

(Left) *Light microscopy of this glomerulus from a newborn with congenital nephrotic syndrome of the Finnish type demonstrates prominent podocytes and mild mesangial hypercellularity. Tubules are dilated (microcystic).* **(Right)** *Glomeruli show no staining with an antibody to nephrin in a patient with congenital nephrotic syndrome of the Finnish type (L), a marked contrast to glomeruli from a normal patient (R).*

TERMINOLOGY

Abbreviations

- Finnish nephropathy (FN)

Synonyms

- Microcystic kidney disease

Definitions

- Steroid-resistant nephrotic syndrome in neonates < 3 months of age due to nephrin (*NPHS1*) gene mutations

ETIOLOGY/PATHOGENESIS

Genetics

- Autosomal recessive disease
- Homozygous mutation in *NPHS1*
  - Maps to chromosome 19q13.1
  - Encodes protein nephrin
    - Transmembrane protein, immunoglobulin (Ig) superfamily with 8 extracellular Ig-like domains with N-glycosylated sites
    - N-glycosylation important for protein folding, slit diaphragm, GBM localization
    - Forms "zipper" structure of slit diaphragm
  - > 70 mutations identified in Finland and worldwide
  - Fin-major
    - 19q13.1 frameshift mutation
    - Absent slit diaphragms without nephrin expression
  - Fin-minor
    - Exon 26 nonsense mutations
    - Truncated/nonfunctioning nephrin
- Compound heterozygous *NPHS1* mutations rare
  - May present as adult onset focal segmental glomerulosclerosis (FSGS)
- Heterozygotes with 1 normal *NPHS1* allele (carriers) are normal after birth
  - In utero may have transient deficiency of nephrin during podocytogenesis
  - Can lead to false-positive α-fetoprotein (AFP) test in amniotic fluid and maternal serum

CLINICAL ISSUES

Epidemiology

- Incidence
  - Finland highest incidence
    - 1:10,000-80,000 births (gene frequency 1:200)
    - Fin-major (exon 2; truncated at 90 amino acids)
      - 78% of Finnish cases
    - Fin-minor (exon 26; truncated at 1109 amino acids)
      - 22% of Finnish cases
  - Occurs worldwide at lower frequency
    - 61% of nephrotic syndrome in 1st 3 months of life
    - Novel mutations in ~ 50% (non-Fin) with variable effects on nephrin structure
    - Homozygous or compound heterozygous
- Age
  - Onset < 3 months: Homozygous mutation
  - Onset 6 months to 5 years: Compound heterozygous mutation
  - Rare adult-onset FSGS attributed to *NPHS1* mutations

Presentation

- Massive proteinuria-nephrotic syndrome
- Elevated AFP in amniotic fluid and maternal serum
  - Fetal proteinuria

Laboratory Tests

- AFP elevated in maternal plasma and amniotic fluid (in utero nephrotic syndrome)
- Anti-nephrin antibodies post transplant

Treatment

- Supportive therapy
- Transplantation after patient weight > 8 kg
  - 30% rate of recurrent nephrotic syndrome post transplant
    - Secondary to antinephrin antibodies
      - Plasmapheresis, cyclophosphamide, and methylprednisolone prolong graft survival
      - Poor response to cyclophosphamide may respond to anti-CD20 (rituximab) therapy

Prognosis

- Mean time to ESRD: 32 months
  - Variable rate of progression
    - Slower in females (40 months) than males (21 months)
    - Fin-major have earliest onset and most rapid course
    - Fin-minor have later onset and delayed progression
- Many severely affected infants with FN die from infection
- Compound heterozygotes develop ESRD later at 6-15 years of age
- Carriers of *NPHS1* mutations live normally

IMAGING

Ultrasonographic Findings

- Echogenic kidneys with symmetric microcysts
- Nuchal translucency

MACROSCOPIC

General Features

- Slightly enlarged, edematous kidneys
  - Diffuse microcystic change on cross sections

MICROSCOPIC

Histologic Features

- Glomerulus
  - Minimal glomerular changes early
    - Mesangial hypercellularity
    - Immature glomeruli
  - Focal and global glomerulosclerosis in advanced stages
- Tubules
  - Reabsorption droplets
    - α-fetoprotein in reabsorption droplets in utero
  - Microcystic dilation of proximal and distal tubules
  - Tubular atrophy in progressive disease
- Interstitium
  - Interstitial fibrosis in progressive disease
  - Chronic interstitial inflammation, variable
- Vessels

Congenital Nephrotic Syndrome Pathology, Proteins, and Genes

Pathology	Mode of Inheritance	Protein	Disease/Gene
Minimal change	Autosomal recessive	Nephrin	Finnish/*NPHS1*
Minimal change	Autosomal recessive	Lamβ2	Pierson syndrome/*LAMβ2*
Diffuse mesangial sclerosis	Autosomal dominant	WT1	DDS/*WT1*
Diffuse mesangial sclerosis	Autosomal recessive	Lamβ2	Pierson syndrome/*LAMβ2*
Diffuse mesangial sclerosis	Autosomal recessive	Plcε-1	DMS/*PLCE1*
Minimal change or FSGS	Autosomal recessive	Podocin	SRNS/*NPHS2* mutations

Immunohistochemistry is most helpful when mutations are truncating, resulting in loss of protein expression. FSGS = focal segmental glomerulosclerosis; Lamβ2 = laminin β2; DMS = diffuse mesangial sclerosis; DDS = Denys-Drash syndrome; Plcε-1 = phospholipase C epsilon 1; SRNS = steroid resistant nephrotic syndrome.

  - Arterial wall thickening
  - May be normal

ANCILLARY TESTS

Immunofluorescence

- Immunoglobulin negative
  - IgM and C3 highlight focal segmental glomerulosclerotic lesions
- Negative nephrin staining with Fin-major or Fin-minor mutations
  - Entirely absent nephrin not seen in all, particularly those with point mutations

Genetic Testing

- *NPHS1* gene sequencing for known and novel mutations

Electron Microscopy

- Podocyte foot process effacement
  - Absent slit diaphragms
  - Variable villous transformation
- Mesangial expansion
- Endothelial blebs (endotheliosis)
  - Normal fenestrations and attachment to GBM
- Normal glomerular basement membrane

DIFFERENTIAL DIAGNOSIS

Podocin Deficiency

- Mutations in *NPHS2*, encodes podocin
- May be histologically indistinguishable from FN when it affects neonates
- Accounts for 15% of nephrotic syndrome in 1st 3 months of life

Early Diffuse Mesangial Sclerosis (DMS) Including Pierson Syndrome

- Early idiopathic DMS and Pierson syndrome may present with minimal changes, mimicking FN histologically
- Mutations in *WT1*, *PCLE1*, or *LAMB2* account for ~ 5.6% of nephrotic syndrome in 1st 3 months

Minimal Change Disease (MCD)

- Even with widespread foot process effacement, occasional filtration slit diaphragms can be found (and some nephrin staining)

Focal Segmental Glomerulosclerosis (FSGS), Idiopathic

- Occasional familial and sporadic childhood and adult onset FSGS with documented homozygous or compound heterozygous *NPHS1* mutations

DIAGNOSTIC CHECKLIST

Clinically Relevant Pathologic Features

- Microcystic tubular dilatation
- Glomerulosclerosis and interstitial fibrosis in late stages

Pathologic Interpretation Pearls

- Minimal glomerular changes on light microscopy
- Absent slit diaphragms on electron microscopy
- Negative nephrin staining
- *NPHS1* mutations occasionally in adults with FSGS

SELECTED REFERENCES

1. Holmberg C et al: Congenital nephrotic syndrome and recurrence of proteinuria after renal transplantation. Pediatr Nephrol. 29(12):2309-17, 2014
2. Kari JA et al: Clinico-pathological correlations of congenital and infantile nephrotic syndrome over twenty years. Pediatr Nephrol. 29(11):2173-80, 2014
3. Ovunc B et al: Mutation analysis of NPHS1 in a worldwide cohort of congenital nephrotic syndrome patients. Nephron Clin Pract. 120(3):c139-46, 2012
4. Machuca E et al: Genetics of nephrotic syndrome: connecting molecular genetics to podocyte physiology. Hum Mol Genet. 18(R2):R185-94, 2009
5. Santín S et al: Nephrin mutations cause childhood- and adult-onset focal segmental glomerulosclerosis. Kidney Int. 76(12):1268-76, 2009
6. Liapis H: Molecular pathology of nephrotic syndrome in childhood: a contemporary approach to diagnosis. Pediatr Dev Pathol. 11(4):154-63, 2008
7. Philippe A et al: Nephrin mutations can cause childhood-onset steroid-resistant nephrotic syndrome. J Am Soc Nephrol. 19(10):1871-8, 2008
8. Hinkes BG et al: Nephrotic syndrome in the first year of life: two thirds of cases are caused by mutations in 4 genes (NPHS1, NPHS2, WT1, and LAMB2). Pediatrics. 119(4):e907-19, 2007
9. Patari-Sampo A et al: Molecular basis of the glomerular filtration: nephrin and the emerging protein complex at the podocyte slit diaphragm. Ann Med. 38(7):483-92, 2006

Gross Pathology

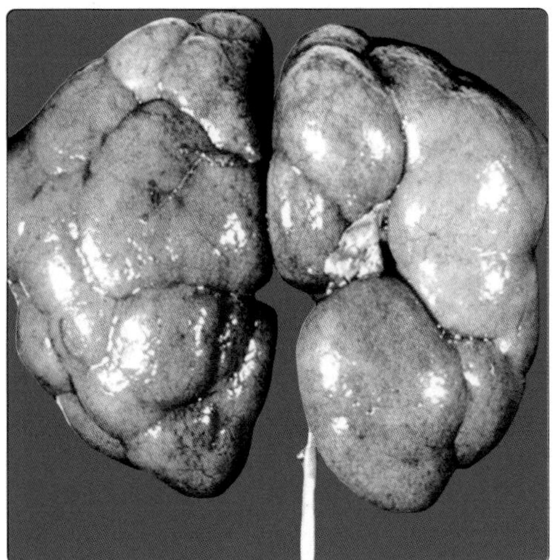

Microcystic Kidney from Patient With FN

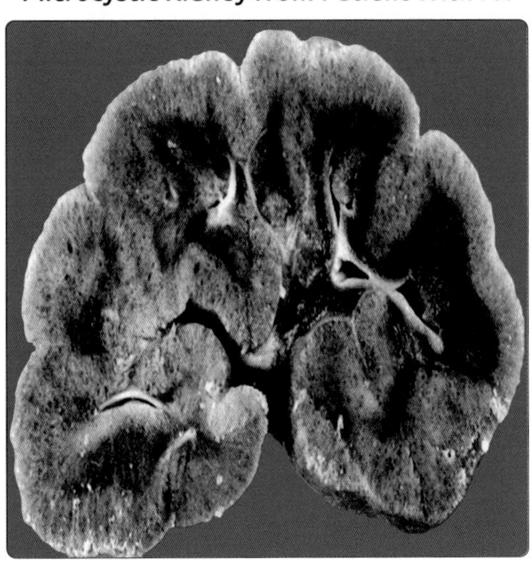

(Left) *Gross kidney appearance from newborn with FN shows edematous kidneys with fetal lobulations.* **(Right)** *Bisected kidney from a patient with FN demonstrates diffuse minute cysts.*

Light Microscopy

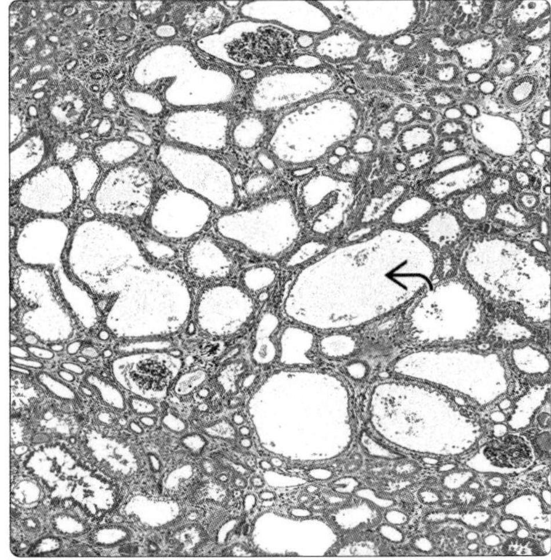

Cystically Dilated Tubules

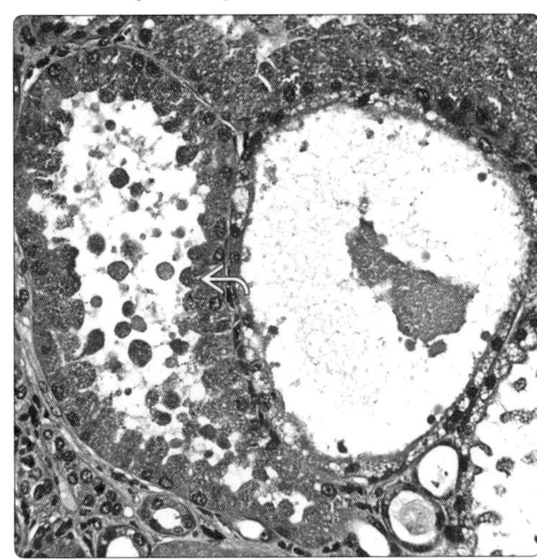

(Left) *H&E shows nephrectomy specimen from a patient with FN. Sections show diffuse tubular microcystic dilatation ➔ and mild interstitial fibrosis.* **(Right)** *High-power view shows cystic tubules. Tubular epithelial cell cytoplasm is edematous and fragmented due to massive proteinuria ➔.*

Normal-Appearing Glomerulus

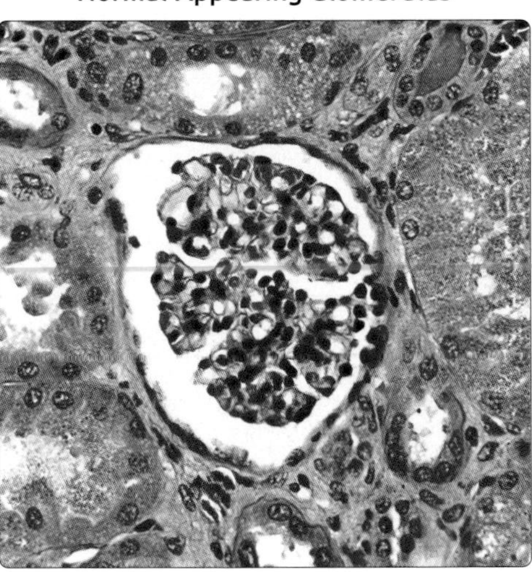

Mild Mesangial Hypercelularity

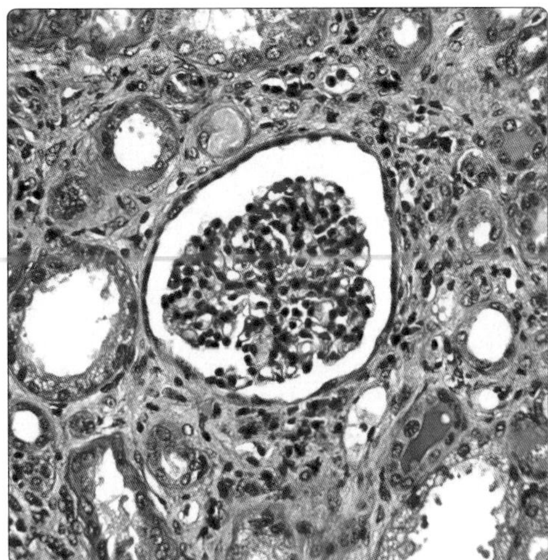

(Left) *H&E shows glomerulus with minimal histopathological changes in a renal biopsy from a newborn baby with FN.* **(Right)** *Mild mesangial hypercellularity is among the light microscopic findings of FN.*

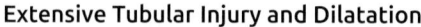

(Left) *Trichrome stain shows advanced FN with occasional globally sclerosed glomeruli and extensive microcystic tubular dilatation.* **(Right)** *This trichrome-stained section from a patient with FN shows fetal (immature)-appearing glomeruli with prominent podocytes* ➡. *This feature is also seen in congenital nephrotic syndrome of other causes, including DMS and Pierson syndrome. Mild interstitial inflammation and moderate fibrosis are also present.*

Extensive Tubular Injury and Dilatation

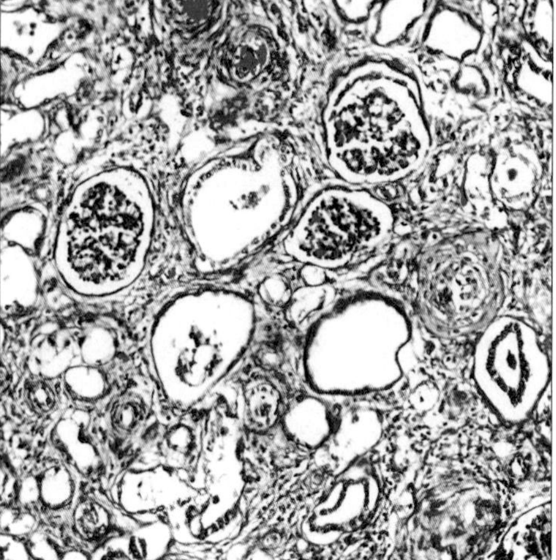

Fetal Glomeruli

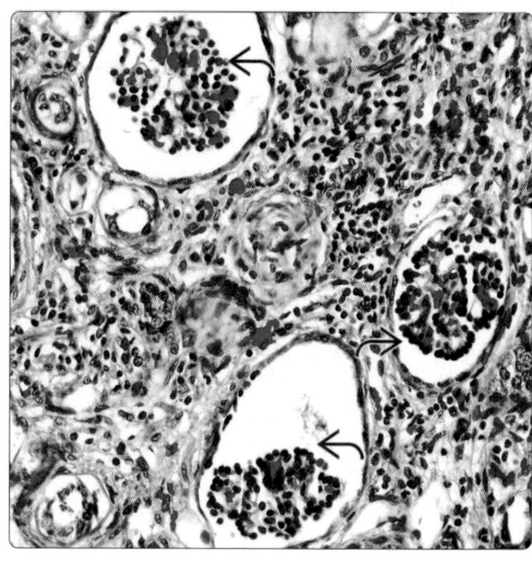

(Left) *IF with antibody to synaptopodin highlights the GBM in this patient with congenital nephrotic syndrome of the Finnish type (FN). This stain is used here as a positive control.* **(Right)** *Double staining in the glomerulus in an infant with FN with antibody to nephrin is entirely negative. Absent nephrin expression is typical of severe mutations leading to abolished protein production (IF).*

Synaptopodin Immunofluorescence (FITC)

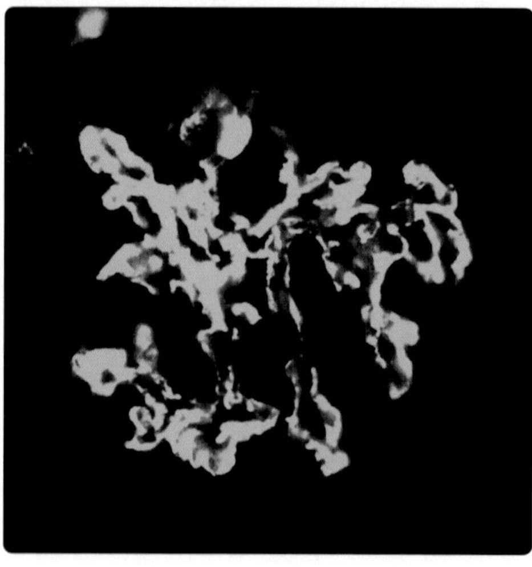

Nephrin Stain is Negative (Texas Red Label)

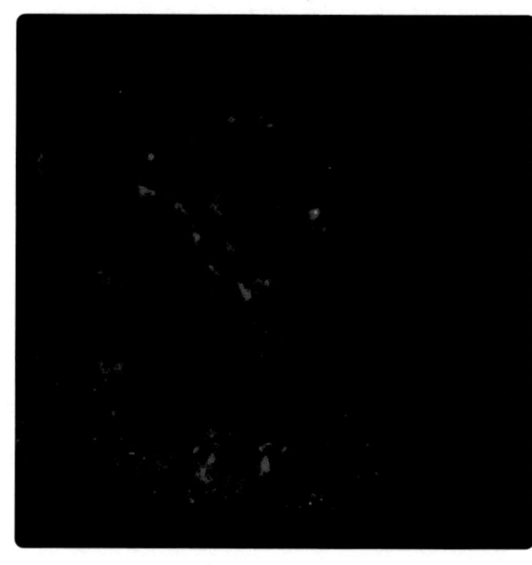

(Left) *IF shows glomeruli from a 2-month-old baby with congenital nephrotic syndrome of the Finnish type. Synaptopodin highlights the GBM.* **(Right)** *In an atypical case of FN, double staining with antibody to nephrin (rhodamine label) in the glomerulus shows nephrin antigen is present. Some NPH1 mutations allow for nephrin antigen synthesis in spite of significant proteinuria and presumably defective slit diaphragms. Thus, a positive nephrin stain does not rule out FN.*

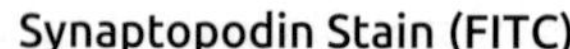

Synaptopodin Stain (FITC)

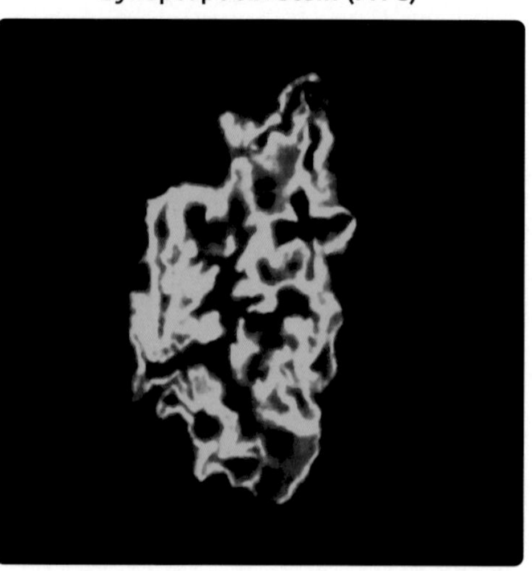

Nephrin Stain (Texas Red)

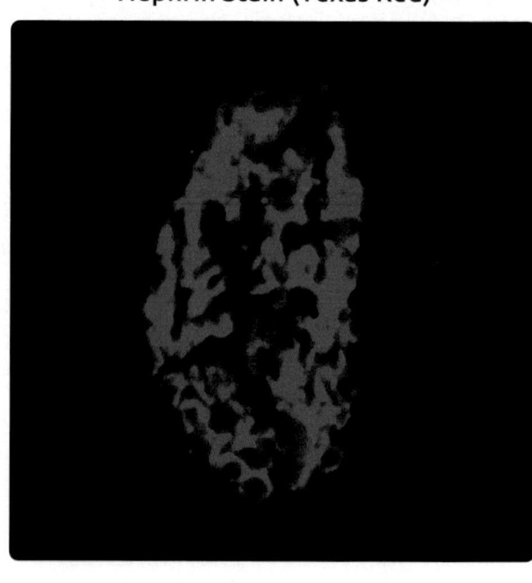

Slit Diaphragms Appear as Linear Bridges

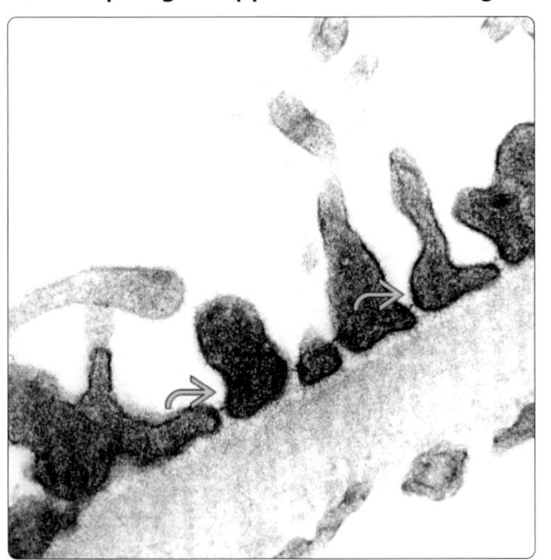

Absent Slit Diaphragm in FN

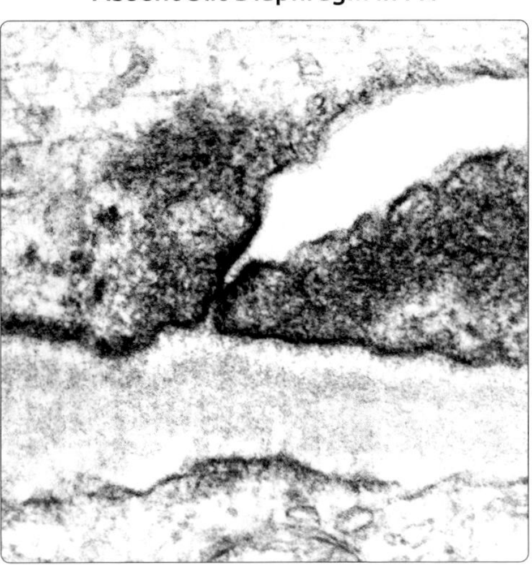

(Left) *Slit diaphragms* ➔ *in a normal human glomerulus consist of bridge-like structures extending between adjacent foot processes.* **(Right)** *High-magnification view of a pore between 2 podocyte foot processes shows that the slit diaphragm is absent in a patient with congenital nephrotic syndrome of the Finnish type.*

Nephrin Molecule

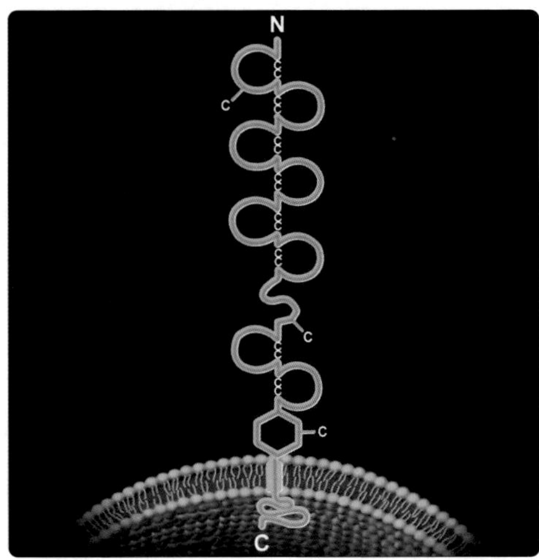

Slit Diaphragm as Seen With Freeze Fracture EM

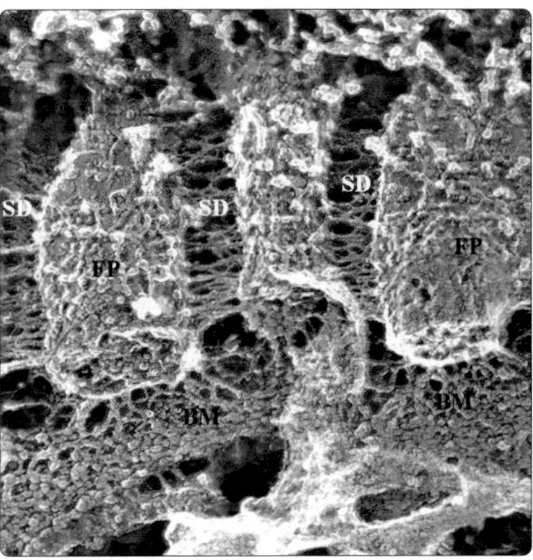

(Left) *The nephrin molecule is a transmembrane protein with an extracellular domain that forms noncovalent bonds with a 2nd nephrin molecule extending from an adjacent podocyte foot process. Four nephrin molecules from adjacent podocytes are required for 1 slit diaphragm formation.* **(Right)** *This freeze fracture EM shows how interlacing nephrin molecules compose the slit diaphragm (SD). Thread-like connections extend from foot processes (FP) to GBM (BM). (Courtesy G. Jarad, MD.)*

Scanning EM of Normal Foot Processes

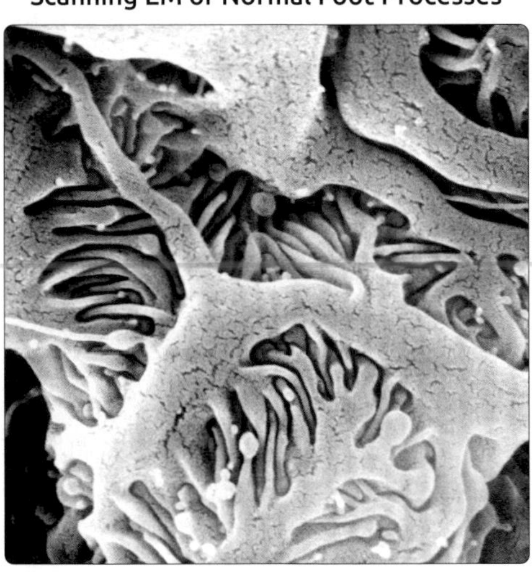

Scanning EM of Foot Processes in Proteinuria

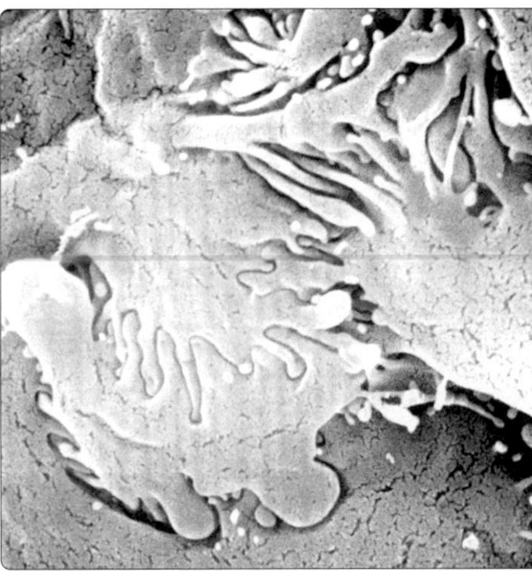

(Left) *Scanning electron microscopy shows podocyte cell body and interdigitating foot processes from normal mouse kidney. (Courtesy G. Jarad, MD.)* **(Right)** *Podocytes from a mouse with congenital nephrotic syndrome show wide foot processes and loss of the interdigitating distribution pattern. (Courtesy G. Jarad, MD.)*

Podocin Deficiency

KEY FACTS

ETIOLOGY/PATHOGENESIS

- Steroid-resistant nephrotic syndrome caused by mutations in *NPHS2*, which encodes podocin and results in defective slit diaphragm and podocyte signaling

CLINICAL ISSUES

- Autosomal recessive inheritance pattern
- ~ 10% of familial focal segmental glomerulosclerosis (FSGS), rarely cause of sporadic FSGS in adults
- Proteinuria, may be nephrotic range
- Steroid-resistant nephrotic syndrome
- 90% of familial cases progress to end-stage renal disease (ESRD) within ~ 6 years
- 35% of sporadic cases progress to ESRD within ~ 6 years

MICROSCOPIC

- Focal and segmental glomerulosclerosis (50%)
- Minimal changes (50%)
- Mesangial hypercellularity without FSGS
- Electron microscopy shows podocyte foot process effacement
- No unique features noted except loss of podocin by immunohistochemistry

ANCILLARY TESTS

- Immunohistochemistry with antibody to human podocin show loss of podocin in podocytes
- Sequencing *NPHS2* gene
  - R229Q mutation: Onset at age < 18 years
  - R138Q mutation: Onset at ~ age 1 year

TOP DIFFERENTIAL DIAGNOSES

- Idiopathic FSGS
- Other inherited forms of FSGS
- Minimal change disease

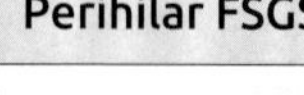

Perihilar FSGS

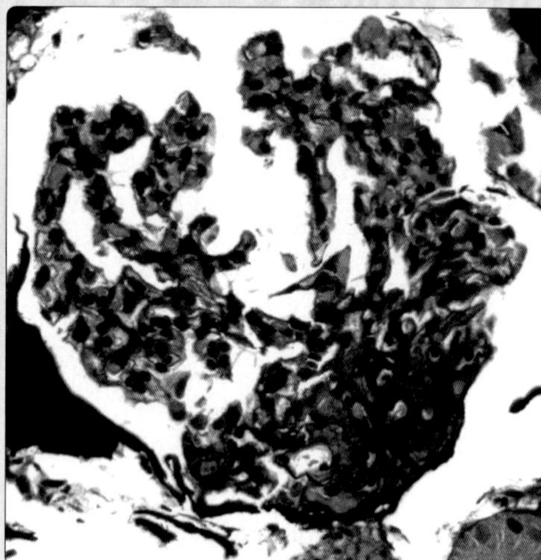

Electron Microscopy

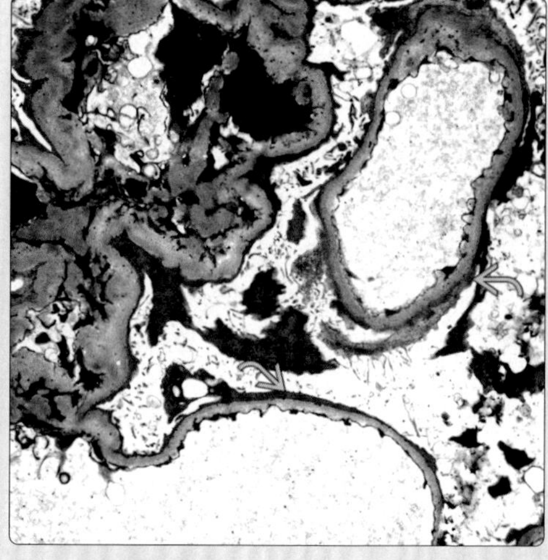

(Left) *A 10-year-old boy previously diagnosed with minimal change disease had persistent proteinuria of 3 g/d. A repeat biopsy showed perihilar focal segmental glomerulosclerosis (FSGS). Podocin was undetectable by immunofluorescence.* **(Right)** *In this case of podocin deficiency, the glomerular capillary loops show diffuse foot process effacement ➢. (Courtesy L. Barisoni-Thomas, MD.)*

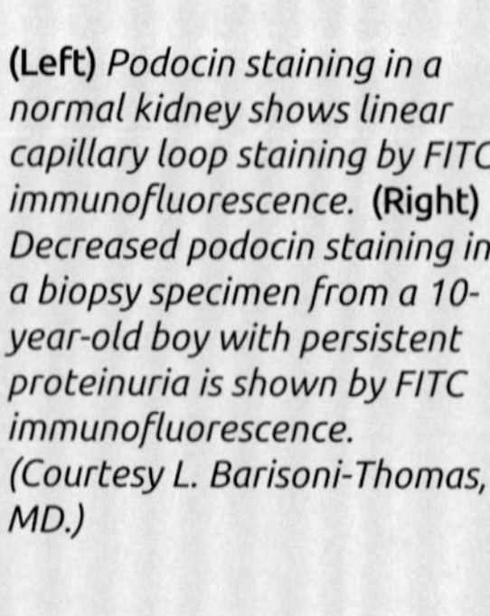

Podocin Staining in Control Normal Kidney

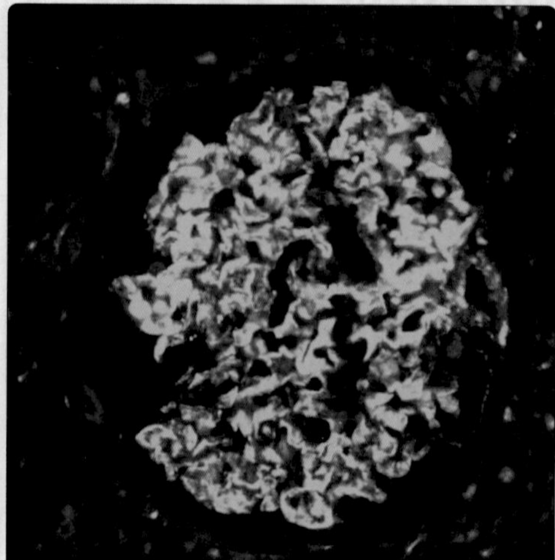

Decreased Podocin Expression

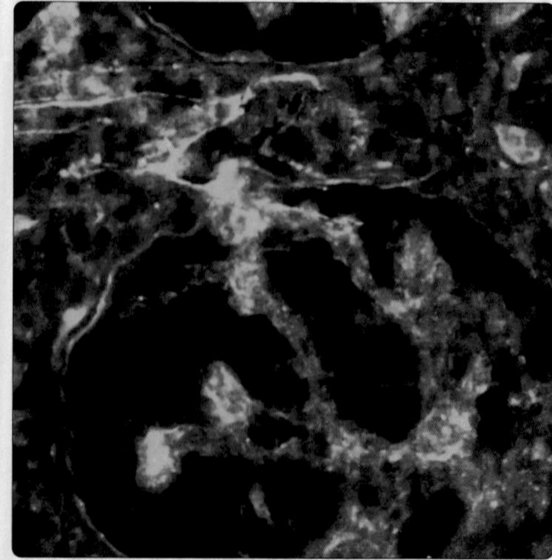

(Left) *Podocin staining in a normal kidney shows linear capillary loop staining by FITC immunofluorescence.* **(Right)** *Decreased podocin staining in a biopsy specimen from a 10-year-old boy with persistent proteinuria is shown by FITC immunofluorescence. (Courtesy L. Barisoni-Thomas, MD.)*

TERMINOLOGY

Definitions

- Inherited or sporadic steroid-resistant nephrotic syndrome secondary to mutations in *NPHS2* gene

ETIOLOGY/PATHOGENESIS

Genetics

- Mutation in *NPHS2*
  - Encodes podocin
    - Important for maintaining podocyte foot process structure and signaling
    - Interacts with nephrin and CD2AP to form part of slit diaphragm
  - Autosomal recessive inheritance
    - Maps to chromosome 1q25-q31
    - > 50 mutations reported to date
- Some cases have mutations in other glomerular genes, e.g., *NPHS1*

CLINICAL ISSUES

Epidemiology

- Incidence
  - *NPHS2* mutations account for ~ 10-15% of familial steroid-resistant nephrotic syndrome
  - *NPHS2* mutations account for ~ 7% of cases of sporadic steroid-resistant nephrotic syndrome in children
  - Rare cause of adult-onset steroid-resistant nephrotic syndrome
- Age
  - Truncation mutations onset at median of 1.7 years
  - Missense mutations onset at median of 4.7 years
  - R229Q mutation: Adult onset (> 18 years)
  - R138Q mutation: Very early onset (12 ± 3 months)
- Sex
  - M:F = 1:1

Presentation

- Proteinuria, may be nephrotic range
- Nephrotic syndrome

Treatment

- Surgical approaches
  - Transplantation
    - 9% recurrence rate post transplant
- Drugs
  - Cyclosporine

Prognosis

- 90% of familial cases progress to end-stage renal disease (ESRD) within 73 months (median)
- 35% of sporadic cases progress to ESRD within 76 months (median)
- Recurrence post transplant
  - 7.7% of patients with homozygous or compound heterozygous mutations
  - 62.5% of patients with heterozygous mutations

MICROSCOPIC

Histologic Features

- Glomeruli: Various patterns
  - Focal and segmental glomerulosclerosis (FSGS) (50%)
  - Minimal changes (50%)
  - Mesangial hypercellularity without FSGS
  - No distinctive feature described by light microscopy compared with nongenetic FSGS
- Tubules and interstitium
  - Variable fibrosis, tubular atrophy

ANCILLARY TESTS

Immunofluorescence

- C3 deposits occasionally present
- Antipodocin antibodies show decreased, granular staining of capillary loops

Genetic Testing

- Sequencing *NPHS2* gene

Electron Microscopy

- Effacement of podocyte foot processes
- Segmental adhesion

DIFFERENTIAL DIAGNOSIS

Primary (Idiopathic, Nonhereditary) FSGS

- Diffuse podocyte foot process effacement
- Normal podocin immunoreactivity

Other Inherited Forms of FSGS

- Includes inherited mutations in *WT1*, *NPHS1*, *LAMB2*, *PLCE1*, *TRPC6*, and *CD2AP*
- Normal podocin immunoreactivity

Minimal Change Disease

- Normal podocin immunoreactivity
- Negative family history

DIAGNOSTIC CHECKLIST

Pathologic Interpretation Pearls

- Distinction among various genetic causes of FSGS depends on demonstration of lack of relevant protein or mutation in relevant gene

SELECTED REFERENCES

1. Bouchireb K et al: NPHS2 mutations in steroid-resistant nephrotic syndrome: a mutation update and the associated phenotypic spectrum. Hum Mutat. 35(2):178-86, 2014
2. Giglio S et al: Heterogeneous Genetic Alterations in Sporadic Nephrotic Syndrome Associate with Resistance to Immunosuppression. J Am Soc Nephrol. ePub, 2014
3. Sadowski CE et al: A Single-Gene Cause in 29.5% of Cases of Steroid-Resistant Nephrotic Syndrome. J Am Soc Nephrol. ePub, 2014
4. Caridi G et al: Clinical features and long-term outcome of nephrotic syndrome associated with heterozygous NPHS1 and NPHS2 mutations. Clin J Am Soc Nephrol. 4(6):1065-72, 2009
5. Machuca E et al: Clinical and epidemiological assessment of steroid-resistant nephrotic syndrome associated with the NPHS2 R229Q variant. Kidney Int. 75(7):727-35, 2009
6. Hinkes B et al: Specific podocin mutations correlate with age of onset in steroid-resistant nephrotic syndrome. J Am Soc Nephrol. 19(2):365-71, 2008
7. Tonna SJ et al: NPHS2 variation in focal and segmental glomerulosclerosis. BMC Nephrol. 9:13, 2008

Alpha-Actinin-4 Deficiency

KEY FACTS

TERMINOLOGY

- Autosomal dominant focal segmental glomerulosclerosis (FSGS) caused by *ACTN4* gene mutations

ETIOLOGY/PATHOGENESIS

- Mutations in *ACTN4* gene encoding α-actinin-4
  - Cause increased α-actinin-4 aggregation and loss of normal function
  - Widely expressed actin binding protein
    - Localized to podocyte foot processes
  - Maps to chromosome 19q13
  - Highly but not fully penetrant, thereby affecting disease severity

CLINICAL ISSUES

- Subnephrotic-range proteinuria (most common)
  - May present in teenagers
- Accounts for ~ 2% of familial FSGS
- No association with ESRD in nondiabetic African Americans

MICROSCOPIC

- FSGS
  - Perihilar segmental sclerosis characteristic
- Arteriolar hyalinosis of perihilar arteriole

ANCILLARY TESTS

- Electron microscopy
  - Podocyte electron-dense aggregates
  - Segmental foot process effacement
- Antibodies to α-actinin-4 show decreased glomerular capillary staining
- Genetic testing
  - Sequencing exon 8 of *ACTN4* gene
  - Whole exome sequencing technologies

TOP DIFFERENTIAL DIAGNOSES

- Primary FSGS
- Secondary FSGS
- Other inherited forms of FSGS

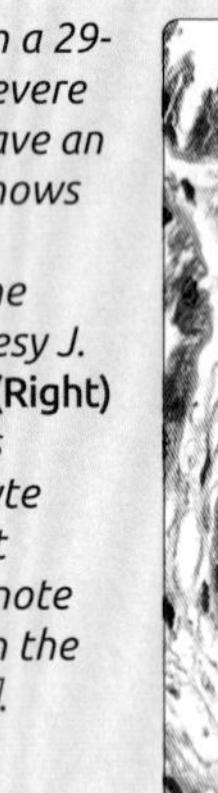

(Left) *Renal biopsy from a 29-year-old woman with severe proteinuria, found to have an α-actinin-4 mutation, shows focal segmental glomerulosclerosis in the perihilar region. (Courtesy J. Henderson, MD, PhD.)* **(Right)** *Segmental foot process effacement and podocyte lifting off the basement membrane are shown; note the electron densities in the podocyte cytoplasm* ➯.

Segmental Sclerosis

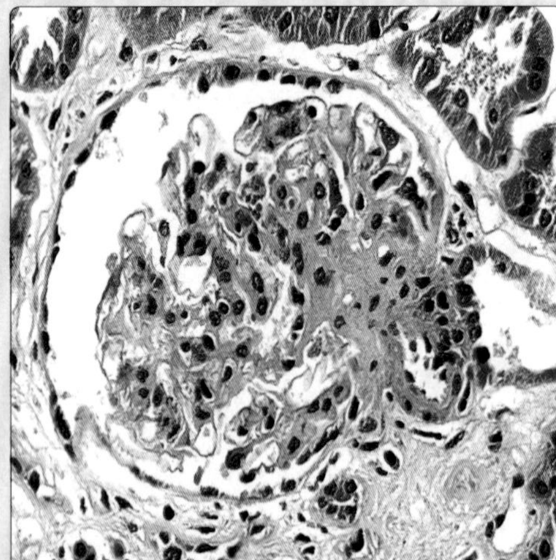

Segmental Foot Process Effacement

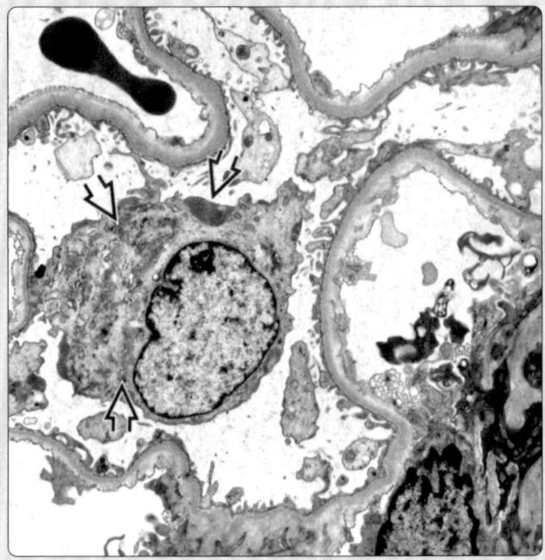

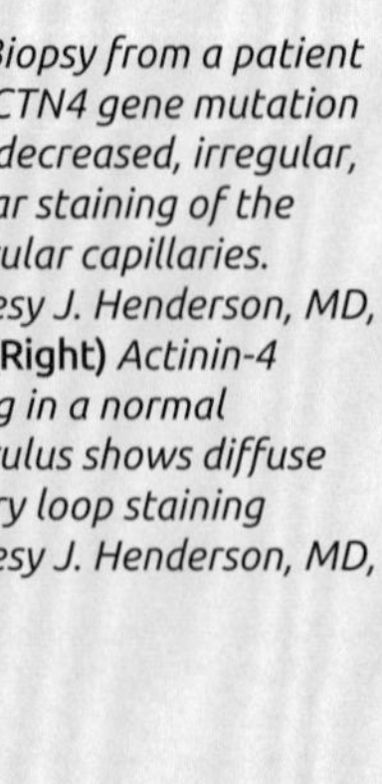

(Left) *Biopsy from a patient with ACTN4 gene mutation shows decreased, irregular, granular staining of the glomerular capillaries. (Courtesy J. Henderson, MD, PhD.)* **(Right)** *Actinin-4 staining in a normal glomerulus shows diffuse capillary loop staining (Courtesy J. Henderson, MD, PhD.)*

ACTN4 Immunohistochemistry

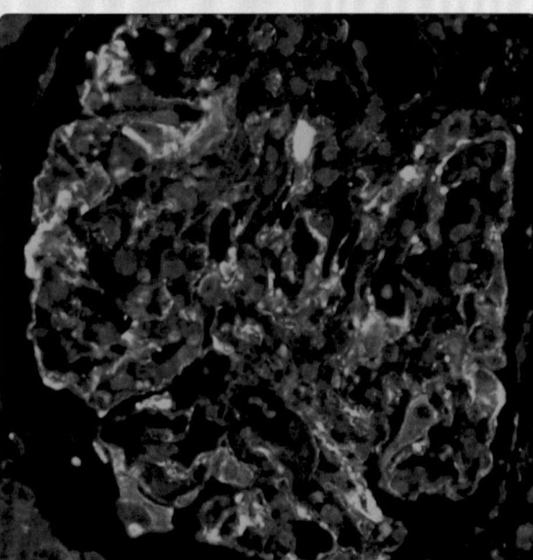

Normal ACTN4 Expression

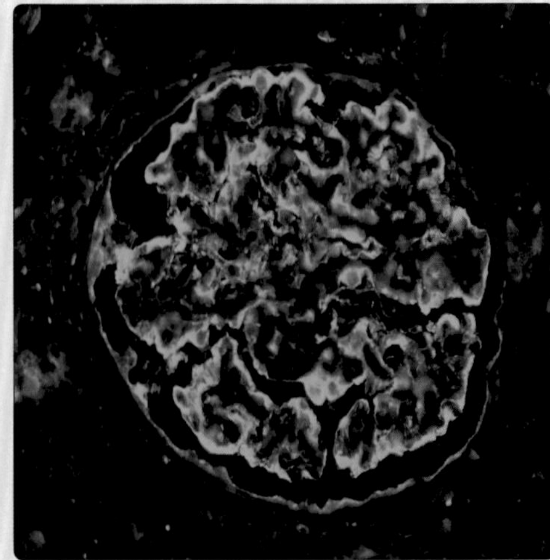

TERMINOLOGY

Definitions

- Familial focal segmental glomerulosclerosis (FSGS) caused by *ACTN4* gene mutations

ETIOLOGY/PATHOGENESIS

Genetics

- *ACTN4* mutations
  - Encodes α-actinin-4
    - In kidney, localized to podocyte; predominantly in foot processes
    - Widely expressed actin binding protein
  - Mutations in exon 8
    - Cause increased α-actinin-4 aggregation
      - May have direct toxic podocyte effects, causing loss of α-actinin-4 function
  - Autosomal dominant inheritance
  - Maps to chromosome 19q13
  - Highly but not fully penetrant, thereby affecting disease severity

CLINICAL ISSUES

Epidemiology

- Incidence
  - Very rare
    - Accounts for ~ 2% of familial FSGS
- Age
  - 16-56 years
  - Mild proteinuria may begin in teenage years
- Sex
  - M:F = 1:1
- Ethnicity
  - Not associated with ESRD in African Americans

Presentation

- Subnephrotic-range proteinuria (most common)
- Nephrotic syndrome
- Hematuria (rare)

Prognosis

- Slowly progressive renal failure in some individuals

MICROSCOPIC

Histologic Features

- Glomeruli
  - Focal, segmental glomerulosclerosis
    - Perihilar variant common
- Tubules
  - Tubular atrophy
- Interstitium
  - Variable interstitial fibrosis
- Vessels
  - Arteriolar hyalinosis
  - Variable degrees of arteriosclerosis

ANCILLARY TESTS

Immunofluorescence

- Segmental deposition of IgM and C3 in glomerular scars
  - Similar to other forms of FSGS
- Reduced podocyte staining for α-actinin-4

Genetic Testing

- Sequencing exon 8 of *ACTN4* gene
- Whole exome sequencing technologies

Electron Microscopy

- Podocytes
  - Electron-dense aggregates within cytoplasm
  - Segmental foot process effacement
  - Microvillous degeneration
  - Cytoplasmic vacuolization
- Segmental GBM thickening and thickening
- Vague mesangial electron-dense deposits
- Subendothelial edema and loss of fenestrae

DIFFERENTIAL DIAGNOSIS

Primary (Idiopathic Nonhereditary) FSGS

- Extensive podocyte foot process effacement
- Lack of podocyte electron-dense aggregates
- Normal α-actinin-4 expression

FSGS Secondary to Hypertension

- Prominent arteriolar hyalinosis
- Prominent arteriosclerosis
- Segmental podocyte foot process effacement affecting < 50% of total glomerular surface area
- Lack of podocyte electron-dense aggregates
- Normal α-actinin-4 expression

Other Inherited Forms of FSGS

- Includes inherited mutations in *WT1, NPHS1, NPHS2, LAMB2, PLCE1, TRPC6, CD2AP, INF2, APOL1*
- Segmental podocyte foot process effacement
- Lack of podocyte electron-dense aggregates
- Normal α-actinin-4 expression

SELECTED REFERENCES

1. Laurin LP et al: Podocyte-associated gene mutation screening in a heterogeneous cohort of patients with sporadic focal segmental glomerulosclerosis. Nephrol Dial Transplant. 29(11):2062-9, 2014
2. Lipska BS et al: Genetic screening in adolescents with steroid-resistant nephrotic syndrome. Kidney Int. 84(1):206-13, 2013
3. Henderson JM et al: Patients with ACTN4 mutations demonstrate distinctive features of glomerular injury. J Am Soc Nephrol. 20(5):961-8, 2009
4. Choi HJ et al: Familial focal segmental glomerulosclerosis associated with an ACTN4 mutation and paternal germline mosaicism. Am J Kidney Dis. 51(5):834-8, 2008
5. Lee SH et al: Crystal structure of the actin-binding domain of alpha-actinin-4 Lys255Glu mutant implicated in focal segmental glomerulosclerosis. J Mol Biol. 376(2):317-24, 2008
6. Michaud JL et al: FSGS-associated alpha-actinin-4 (K256E) impairs cytoskeletal dynamics in podocytes. Kidney Int. 70(6):1054-61, 2006
7. Weins A et al: Mutational and Biological Analysis of alpha-actinin-4 in focal segmental glomerulosclerosis. J Am Soc Nephrol. 16(12):3694-701, 2005
8. Kos CH et al: Mice deficient in alpha-actinin-4 have severe glomerular disease. J Clin Invest. 111(11):1683-90, 2003
9. Michaud JL et al: Focal and segmental glomerulosclerosis in mice with podocyte-specific expression of mutant alpha-actinin-4. J Am Soc Nephrol. 14(5):1200-11, 2003

Autosomal Dominant FSGS Due to *INF2* Mutations

KEY FACTS

TERMINOLOGY

- Podocytopathy manifested by proteinuria and focal segmental glomerulosclerosis (FSGS), caused by mutation in *INF2* gene, also causing Charcot-Marie-Tooth disease (CMT), a demyelinating peripheral neuropathy

ETIOLOGY/PATHOGENESIS

- Mutation in *INF2* gene
- Formin protein INF2 accelerates actin polymerization and depolymerization
- Mechanism postulated to be altered actin dynamics in podocyte
- Expressed in Schwann cells

CLINICAL ISSUES

- Most common cause of autosomal dominant FSGS (9-17% of families)
- Rarely mutated in sporadic FSGS (~ 0.7%)
- Proteinuria onset childhood-7th decade
- ~ 12% with mutation have Charcot-Marie-Tooth disease
- ESRD develops at 13-67 years old

MICROSCOPIC

- Focal segmental glomerulosclerosis (FSGS)
- Usually not otherwise specified (NOS) pattern
- Collapsing FSGS (1 case)
- Patchy tubular atrophy
- Patchy interstitial fibrosis

ANCILLARY TESTS

- Normal expression of α3 and α5 chains of type IV collagen
- Only segmental effacement of podocyte foot processes more typical of adaptive FSGS
- Foot processes described as "irregular, jagged" with prominent actin bundles

TOP DIFFERENTIAL DIAGNOSES

- Other causes of FSGS
- Alport syndrome

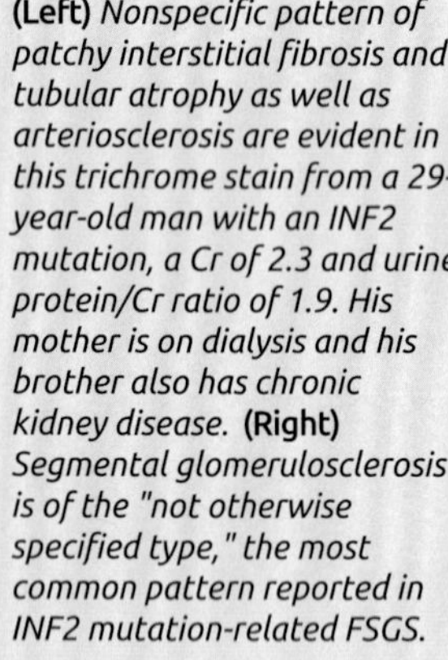

(Left) *Nonspecific pattern of patchy interstitial fibrosis and tubular atrophy as well as arteriosclerosis are evident in this trichrome stain from a 29-year-old man with an INF2 mutation, a Cr of 2.3 and urine protein/Cr ratio of 1.9. His mother is on dialysis and his brother also has chronic kidney disease.* **(Right)** *Segmental glomerulosclerosis is of the "not otherwise specified type," the most common pattern reported in INF2 mutation-related FSGS.*

FSGS With Interstitial Fibrosis

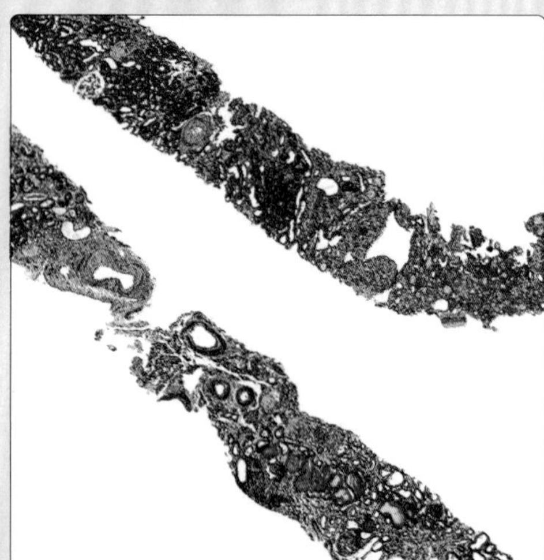

FSGS, Not Otherwise Specified (NOS)

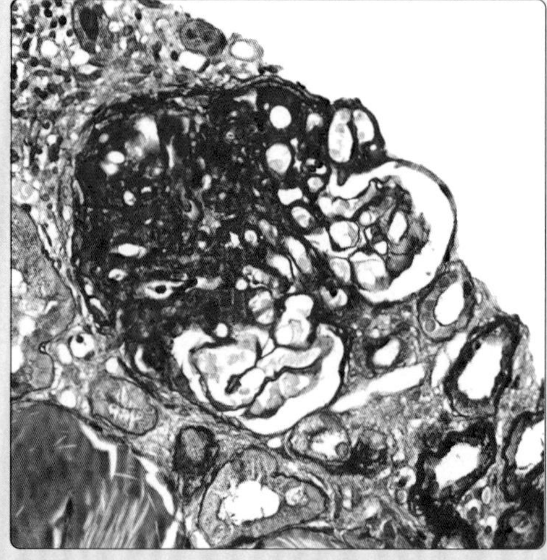

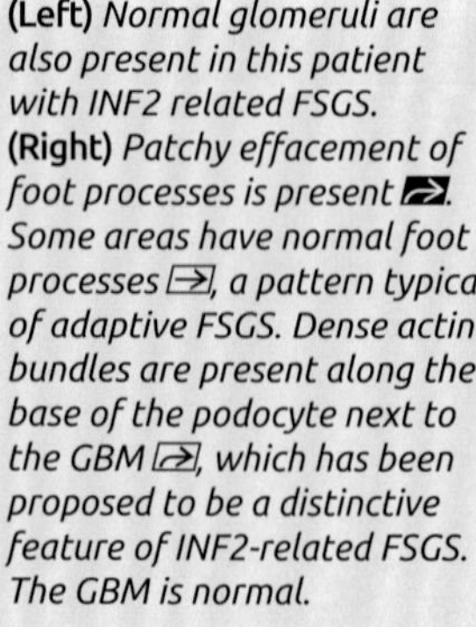

(Left) *Normal glomeruli are also present in this patient with INF2 related FSGS.* **(Right)** *Patchy effacement of foot processes is present ➙. Some areas have normal foot processes ➙, a pattern typical of adaptive FSGS. Dense actin bundles are present along the base of the podocyte next to the GBM ➙, which has been proposed to be a distinctive feature of INF2-related FSGS. The GBM is normal.*

Normal Glomerulus

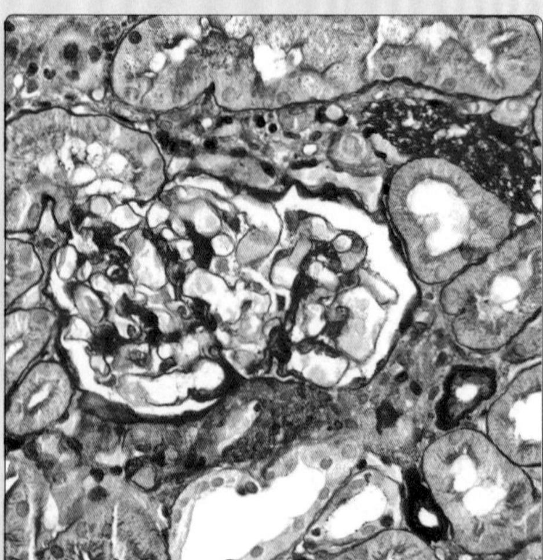

Effacement of Foot Processes

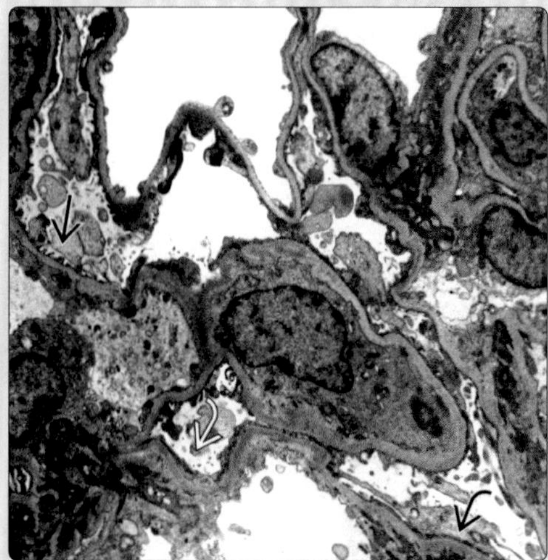

TERMINOLOGY

Abbreviations

- Inverted formin 2 (INF2)

Definitions

- Podocytopathy manifested by proteinuria and focal segmental glomerulosclerosis (FSGS)
  - Caused by *INF2* gene mutation
    - Also causing Charcot-Marie-Tooth disease (CMT), a demyelinating peripheral neuropathy

ETIOLOGY/PATHOGENESIS

Genetic

- Mutation in *INF2* gene
  - Missense mutations in exons 2,3,4,5 (diaphanous inhibitory domain)
- Formin protein INF2 accelerates actin polymerization and depolymerization
- INF2 mRNA and protein expressed in podocyte and some tubular cells
  - Colocalizes with nephrin
  - Mechanism postulated to be altered actin dynamics in podocyte
- Expressed in Schwann cells
  - Interacts with myelin and lymphocyte protein (MAL)

CLINICAL ISSUES

Epidemiology

- Ethnicity
  - Caucasian
  - Recent African descent
  - Mexican
- Most common cause of autosomal dominant FSGS (9-17% of families)
  - Rarely mutated in sporadic FSGS (~ 0.7%)

Presentation

- Proteinuria onset childhood-7th decade
  - Variable proteinuria even in same family
  - Sometimes nephrotic syndrome
- Variable penetrance
  - Some affected family members with only asymptomatic proteinuria or rarely no proteinuria
- ~ 12% with mutation have Charcot-Marie-Tooth (CMT) disease
  - Peripheral neuropathy precedes glomerular disease
  - Motor and sensory neurons affected

Prognosis

- Indolent course to ESRD (~ 20 years or more)
  - ESRD develops at 13-67 years old
- More rapid progression to ESRD if associated with CMT (typically 5 years)

MICROSCOPIC

Histologic Features

- Glomeruli
  - Focal segmental glomerulosclerosis (FSGS)
    - Usually not otherwise specified (NOS) pattern
    - Collapsing FSGS (1 case)
  - Global glomerulosclerosis
  - No glomerular hypertrophy
- Tubules
  - Patchy tubular atrophy
- Interstitium
  - Patchy interstitial fibrosis
- Vessels
  - No specific changes

ANCILLARY TESTS

Immunofluorescence

- Limited reports: Presumed negative except for IgM and C3 in scarred glomeruli
- Normal expression of α3 and α5 chains of type IV collagen

Electron Microscopy

- Segmental effacement of podocyte foot processes, more typical of adaptive FSGS
  - Foot processes described as "irregular, jagged"
  - Prominent longitudinal actin bundles in foot processes described in 1 report
- Focal thinning and lamellation of GBM
- No electron dense deposits

DIFFERENTIAL DIAGNOSIS

Other Causes of FSGS

- Family history of proteinuria suggests genetic component
- Genetic testing definitive

Alport Syndrome

- Decreased expression of α3 and α5 chains of type IV collagen
- Extensive lamination and scalloping of GBM

DIAGNOSTIC CHECKLIST

Pathologic Interpretation Pearls

- No distinctive pathologic features yet documented that distinguish this genetic cause of FSGS

SELECTED REFERENCES

1. Caridi G et al: Novel INF2 mutations in an Italian cohort of patients with focal segmental glomerulosclerosis, renal failure and Charcot-Marie-Tooth neuropathy. Nephrol Dial Transplant. 29 Suppl 4:iv80-6, 2014
2. Park HJ et al: A novel INF2 mutation in a Korean family with autosomal dominant intermediate Charcot-Marie-Tooth disease and focal segmental glomerulosclerosis. J Peripher Nerv Syst. 19(2):175-9, 2014
3. Barua M et al: Mutations in the INF2 gene account for a significant proportion of familial but not sporadic focal and segmental glomerulosclerosis. Kidney Int. 83(2):316-22, 2013
4. Gbadegesin RA et al: Inverted formin 2 mutations with variable expression in patients with sporadic and hereditary focal and segmental glomerulosclerosis. Kidney Int. 81(1):94-9, 2012
5. Boyer O et al: Mutations in INF2 are a major cause of autosomal dominant focal segmental glomerulosclerosis. J Am Soc Nephrol. 22(2):239-45, 2011
6. Ireland R: Genetics: INF2 mutations often implicated in autosomal dominant focal segmental glomerulosclerosis. Nat Rev Nephrol. 7(4):181, 2011
7. Pei Y: INF2 is another piece of the jigsaw puzzle for FSGS. J Am Soc Nephrol. 22(2):197-9, 2011
8. Brown EJ et al: Mutations in the formin gene INF2 cause focal segmental glomerulosclerosis. Nat Genet. 42(1):72-6, 2010

Diffuse Mesangial Sclerosis

KEY FACTS

TERMINOLOGY

- Pattern of glomerular disease early in life with mesangial matrix accumulation and podocyte proliferation due to many causes

ETIOLOGY/PATHOGENESIS

- Most cases idiopathic (genetic basis, if any, unknown)
- Six known causal genetic mutations
  - *WT1, LAMB2, PLCE1, WDR73, PMM2, NPHS1*

CLINICAL ISSUES

- Nephrotic syndrome
  - Presents early, usually under 2 years of age
  - Steroid resistant
- Progression to ESRD in 3 years
  - Slower progression if no mutation identified
- Renal transplantation when patient weight > 8 kg
  - Post-transplant recurrence of DMS not yet described

MICROSCOPIC

- Early glomerular changes resemble fetal glomeruli
- Late glomerular changes consist of replacement of mesangium by fibrillar matrix and mesangial consolidation
- Pseudocrescents
- Tubules dilated with hyaline casts
- Electron microscopy
  - Wide, lamellated GBM
  - Podocyte proliferation

ANCILLARY TESTS

- Sequencing *WT1*, *PLCE1*, and *LAMB2* genes
- Karyotyping to rule out male pseudohermaphroditism (Frasier syndrome)

TOP DIFFERENTIAL DIAGNOSES

- Denys-Drash syndrome
- Frasier syndrome
- Pierson syndrome

Solidified Glomerulus

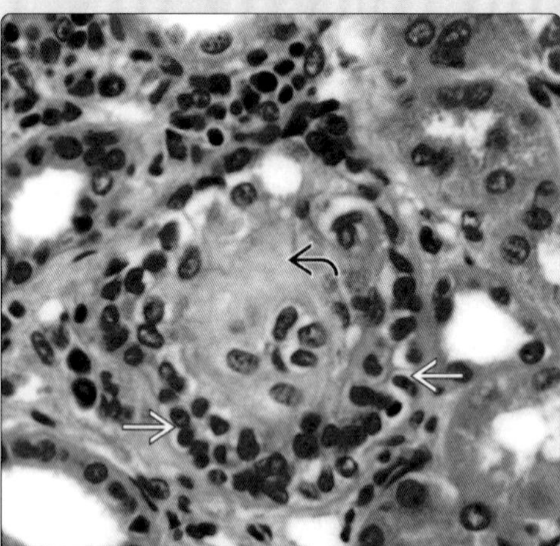

Collapsed Glomeruli

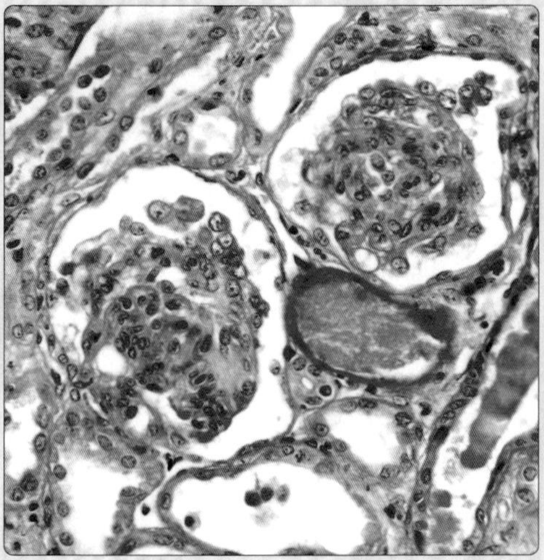

(Left) *Classic late diffuse mesangial sclerosis (DMS) shows solidified glomeruli with obliterated capillaries replaced by mesangial matrix ➙. Proliferation of podocytes forms a pseudocrescent ➙.* **(Right)** *H&E shows DMS with ball-like glomeruli with proliferating podocytes. The pattern resembles collapsing glomerulopathy.*

Crowd of Podocytes

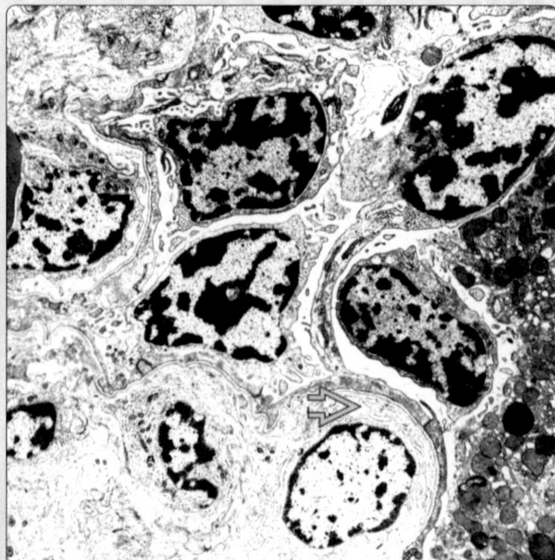

Podocyte Detachment

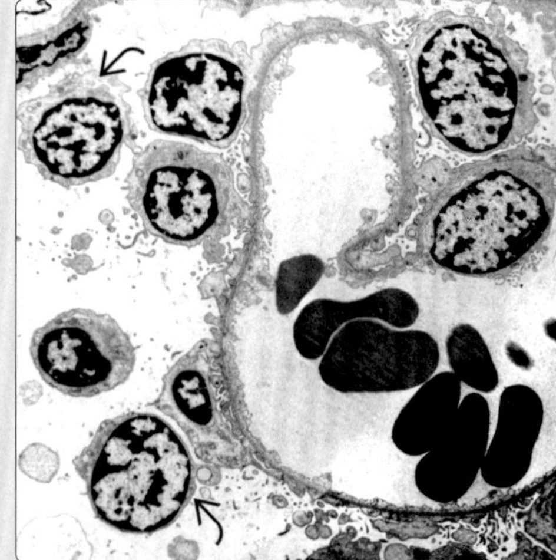

(Left) *Podocytes appear crowded. Segmental GBM multilamination is a common feature of DMS ➙. Formation of glomerular capillaries is halted.* **(Right)** *This electron micrograph shows proliferation and detachment of podocytes into Bowman space ➙.*

TERMINOLOGY

Abbreviations

- Diffuse mesangial sclerosis (DMS)

Definitions

- Pattern of glomerular disease early in life with mesangial matrix accumulation and podocyte proliferation due to many causes

ETIOLOGY/PATHOGENESIS

Genetic Factors

- *WT1* (Denys-Drash, Frasier Syndromes)
  - Encodes Wilms tumor-1 on chromosome 11p13
    - Zinc finger transcription factor regulates cell proliferation and gonad and podocyte differentiation
  - Exon 9 mutations typical of Denys-Drash syndrome
    - Hot spot in exon 9 R394W/Q/L
  - Intron 9 mutations typical of Frasier syndrome
  - Mutations in exons 8 and 9 may be associated with sporadic DMS
- *PLCE1* (Familial steroid resistant nephrotic syndrome)
  - Encodes phospholipase C enzyme (PLCε1) on chromosome 10q
  - Truncating mutations associated with DMS
  - Nontruncating missense mutations associated with FSGS
  - Autosomal recessive inheritance pattern
- *WDR73* (Galloway-Mowat syndrome)
- *LAMB2* (Pierson syndrome)
- *PMM2* (type 1 carbohydrate-deficient glycoprotein syndrome)
- *NPHS1* (Congenital nephrotic syndrome, Finnish type)

Infectious Agents

- Cytomegalovirus (CMV)
  - DMS associated with CMV inclusions in newborns with congenital nephrotic syndrome

Idiopathic

- Most cases, genetic basis, if any, unknown

CLINICAL ISSUES

Presentation

- Nephrotic syndrome
  - < 2 years of age but may be as late as 4 years
  - Steroid resistant

Laboratory Tests

- α-fetoprotein may be elevated

Treatment

- Surgical approaches
  - Bilateral nephrectomy to prevent massive protein loss, hypertension, and Wilms tumors
  - Renal transplantation when patient weight > 8 kg
- Drugs
  - IVIG, ACE inhibitors, corticosteroids, cyclosporine
  - Ganciclovir for DMS associated with CMV

Prognosis

- Typically progresses to ESRD within 3 years
- Absence of identified mutations with milder clinical course
- Post-transplant recurrence of DMS not yet described

MICROSCOPIC

Histologic Features

- Early glomerular changes
  - Prominent, closely spaced podocytes create fetal (immature)-looking glomeruli without DMS
  - Pseudocrescents composed of proliferating visceral podocytes and parietal epithelial cells
- Late glomerular changes
  - Mesangial consolidation
  - Fibrillar mesangial matrix increase
- Early tubular changes
  - May be dilated with hyaline casts secondary to heavy proteinuria

ANCILLARY TESTS

Immunofluorescence

- IgM, C1q, and C3 may stain sclerotic mesangial areas

Genetic Testing

- *WT1*, *PLCE1*, and *LAMB2* gene mutation analysis
- Karyotyping to rule out male pseudohermaphroditism

Electron Microscopy

- Podocyte proliferation
- Increased mesangial matrix
- Wide, lamellated GBM

DIFFERENTIAL DIAGNOSIS

Denys-Drash Syndrome

- Male gonad dysgenesis
- Autosomal dominant mutations in *WT1* exon 9
- Association with Wilms tumor and gonadoblastoma

Frasier Syndrome

- DMS or FSGS associated with *WT1* intron 9 mutations
- Male pseudohermaphroditism

Pierson Syndrome

- Ocular abnormalities (microcoria)
- DMS associated with *LAMB2* mutations
- Autosomal recessive

DIAGNOSTIC CHECKLIST

Pathologic Interpretation Pearls

- Fetal-appearing glomeruli
- Solidified glomerular mesangium

SELECTED REFERENCES

1. Martínez Mejía S et al: Renal transplantation in children with nephrotic syndrome in the first year of life. Transplant Proc. 47(1):38-41, 2015
2. Lipska BS et al: Genotype-phenotype associations in WT1 glomerulopathy. Kidney Int. 85(5):1169-78, 2014
3. Gbadegesin R et al: Mutations in PLCE1 are a major cause of isolated diffuse mesangial sclerosis (IDMS). Nephrol Dial Transplant. 23(4):1291-7, 2008
4. Liapis H: Molecular pathology of nephrotic syndrome in childhood: a contemporary approach to diagnosis. Pediatr Dev Pathol. 11(4):154-63, 2008
5. Niaudet P et al: WT1 and glomerular diseases. Pediatr Nephrol. 21(11):1653-60, 2006

(Left) *DMS can be mistaken for crescentic glomerulonephritis. Unlike true crescents, pseudocrescents do not contain fibrin or inflammatory cells.* **(Right)** *WT1 immunohistochemistry of a case of DMS demonstrates strong nuclear staining of the majority of proliferating cells, which represent podocytes filling Bowman space. No inflammatory cells, fibrin deposits, or ruptured capillary loops are seen in these pseudocrescents, in contrast to the crescents seen in vasculitis.*

Pseudocrescent

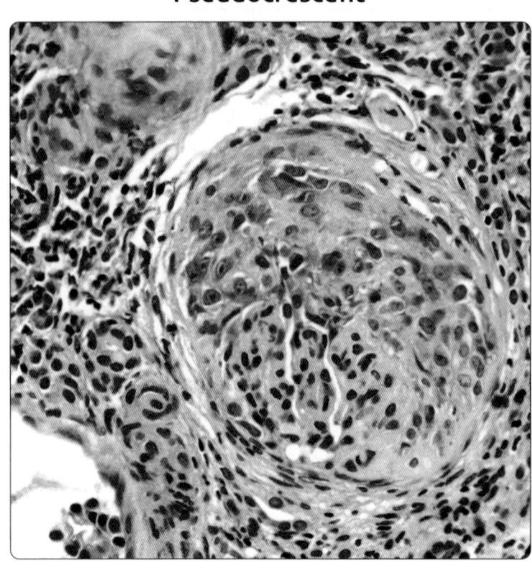

WT1

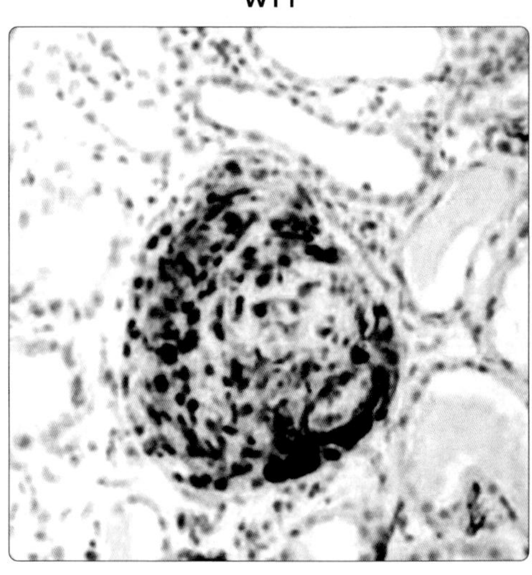

(Left) *Early DMS is characterized by prominent podocytes, giving the glomeruli a fetal appearance ➢.* **(Right)** *Immunofluorescence for laminin β2 shows diffuse glomerular capillary loop staining in a biopsy from a patient with DMS. These findings exclude the diagnosis of Pierson syndrome in which laminin β2 is absent.*

Prominent Podocytes

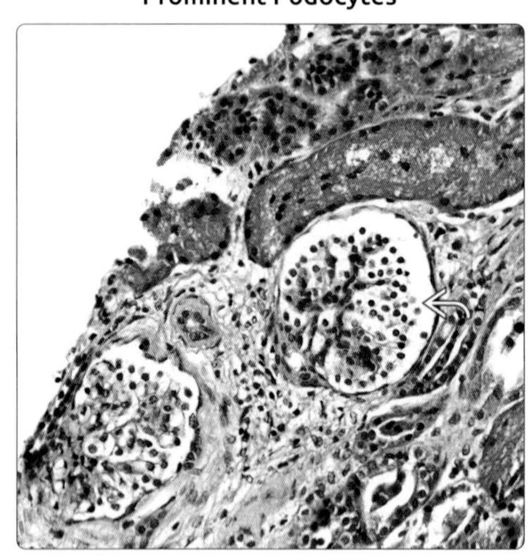

Laminin β2

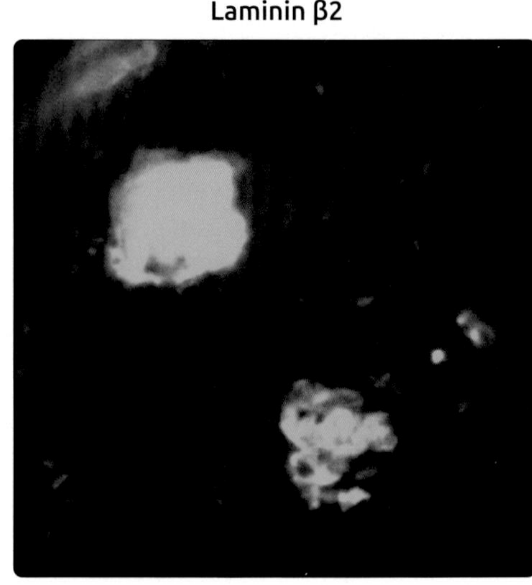

(Left) *Electron microscopy shows DMS foot process effacement and GBM multilamination. The latter resembles Alport syndrome, which must be excluded. A red blood cell is in a glomerular capillary ➢, which is bounded by reactive endothelial cells.* **(Right)** *This electron micrograph demonstrates extensive podocyte proliferation and detachment ➢.*

GBM Alterations

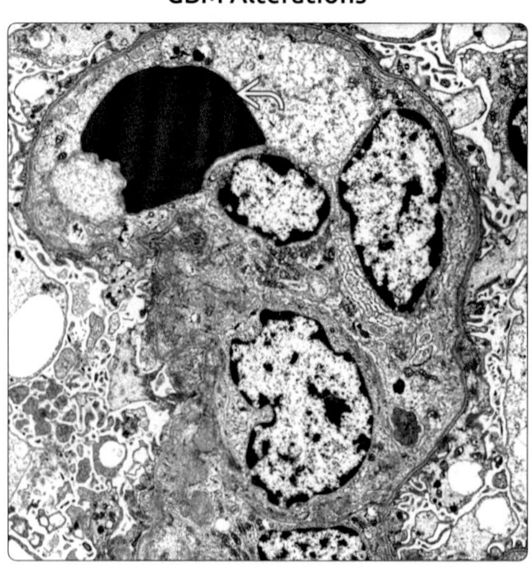

Podocyte Alterations

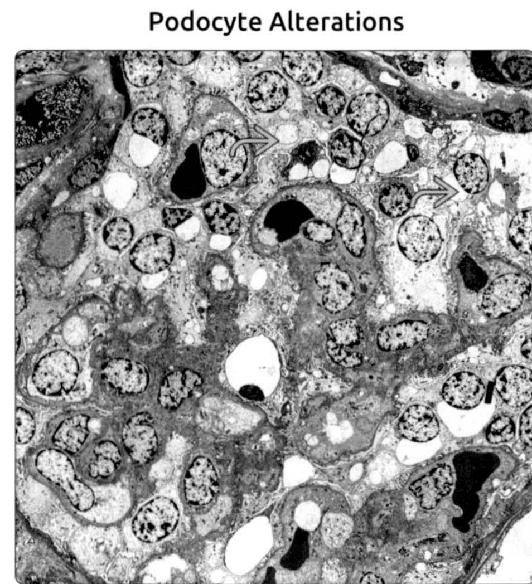

DMS in Congenital NS

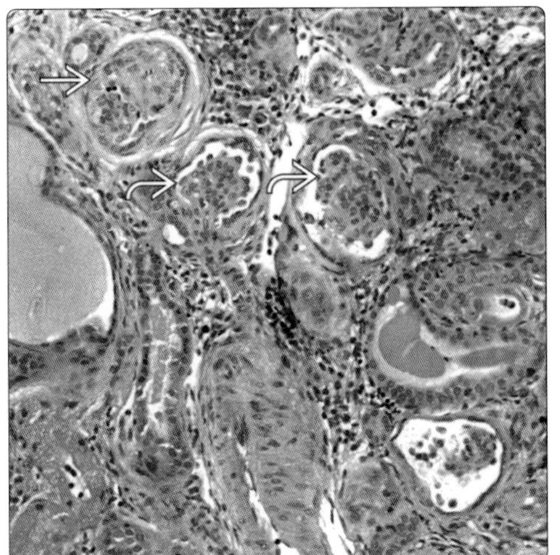

DMS in Congenital Nephrotic Syndrome

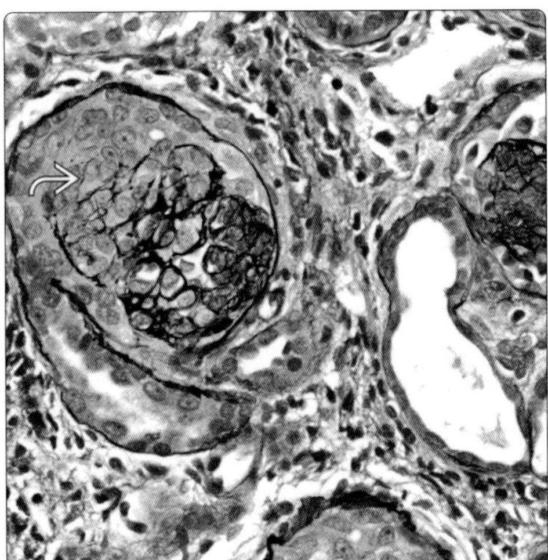

(Left) *Glomeruli appear small with no capillary lumens ➡ in this 16-day-old full term neonate with congenital nephrotic syndrome. Some glomeruli are partially sclerotic ➡. Tubules are focally dilated. Arterioles appear thick.* **(Right)** *Silver stain shows an S-shaped glomerulus ➡, which is an abnormal finding in itself since in a normal term infant glomerulogenesis is compete at birth.*

Solidified Glomerulus

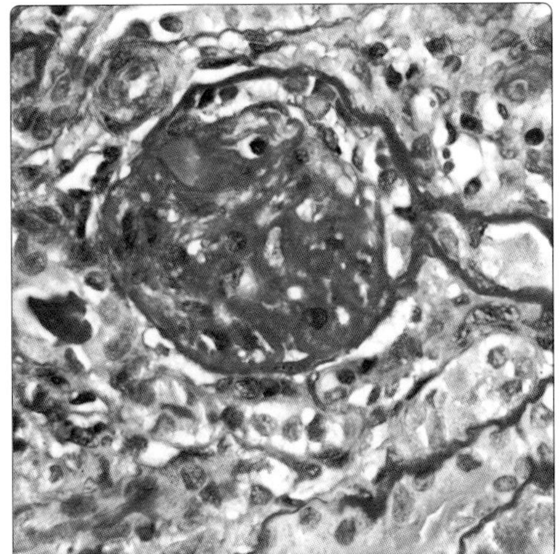

DMS and Dilated Tubules

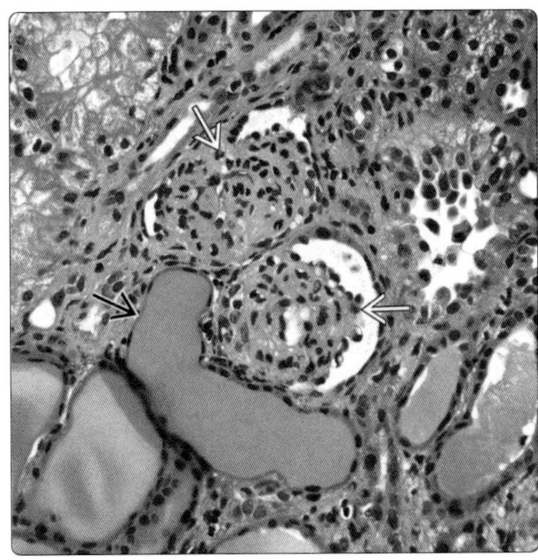

(Left) *PAS stain shows a solidified glomerulus with some prominence of adjacent epithelial cells and loss of patent capillary lumina.* **(Right)** *Prominent tubular microcysts ➡ with proteinaceous casts are seen adjacent to 2 glomeruli with increased mesangial matrix and cells ➡. There is also prominence of adjacent podocytes and loss of capillary lumina.*

Mesangial Hypercellularity

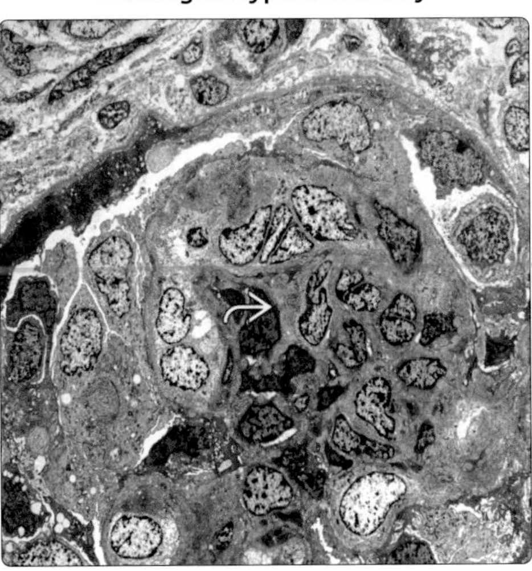

DMS

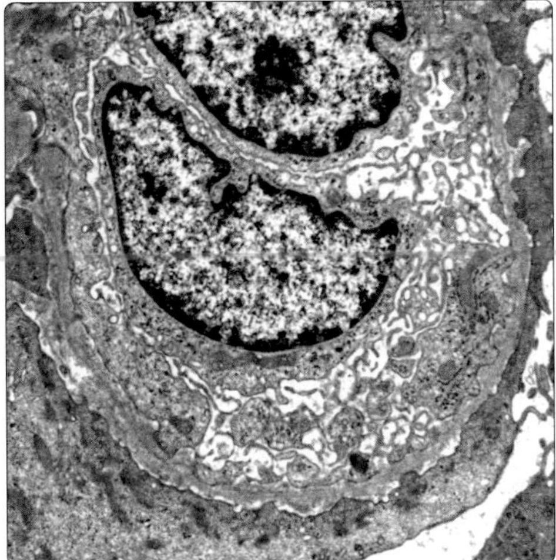

(Left) *Electron microscopy shows no patent capillary loop lumina without any red blood cells present. Mesangial cell nuclei are also increased in number ➡.* **(Right)** *High magnification shows diffuse effacement of foot processes, prominent endothelial cells, and obscured capillary lumen with an irregular GBM.*

Denys-Drash Syndrome

KEY FACTS

TERMINOLOGY

- Triad syndrome
  - Male pseudohermaphroditism
  - Steroid-resistant nephrotic syndrome due to diffuse mesangial sclerosis
  - Risk of Wilms tumor

ETIOLOGY/PATHOGENESIS

- *WT1* exon 9 mutations
- Most occur sporadically as de novo mutation

CLINICAL ISSUES

- Rapid progression to renal failure in 2-3 years
- Wilms tumor at early age, often bilateral

MICROSCOPIC

- Mesangial sclerosis and capillary loop collapse
- Hyperplastic epithelial cells
- Tubulointerstitial scarring

ANCILLARY TESTS

- Gene sequencing for *WT1* mutation
- Glomerular basement membrane ultrastructural abnormalities
  - Thick, irregular and multilayered
  - Electron-dense and lucent foci

TOP DIFFERENTIAL DIAGNOSES

- Sporadic diffuse mesangial sclerosis
  - Consider incomplete Denys-Drash syndrome
  - Risk of Wilms tumor
- Sporadic Wilms tumor
  - Consider incomplete form of Denys-Drash syndrome
  - Examine nonneoplastic cortex
- Frasier syndrome
  - Develop FSGS rather than diffuse mesangial sclerosis
  - Risk of gonadoblastoma rather than Wilms tumor
- Pierson syndrome
  - Diffuse mesangial sclerosis and ocular abnormalities

(Left) *The glomerular alterations of diffuse mesangial sclerosis in DDS show a broad spectrum of abnormalities. This glomerulus from a 1 year old with DDS demonstrates mild mesangial matrix increase ⇨ and normal-appearing podocytes.* **(Right)** *This glomerulus from a 3-month-old with DDS shows advanced sclerosis with a compacted glomerular tuft and expanded mesangial matrix ⇨. The capillary loops are obliterated with exuberant epithelial cell hyperplasia ⇨.*

Mild Mesangial Matrix Increase

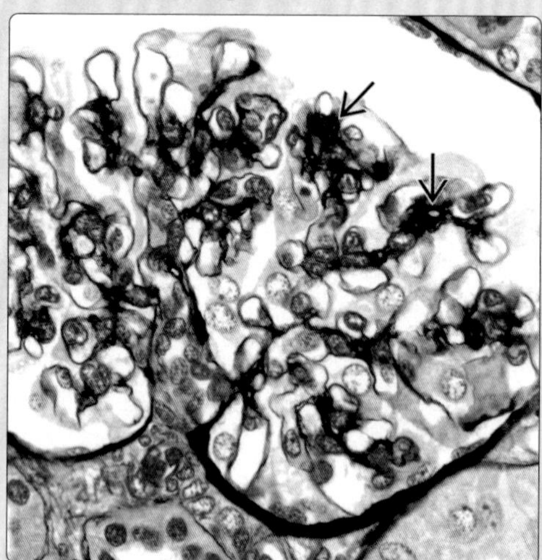

Advanced Mesangial Sclerosis

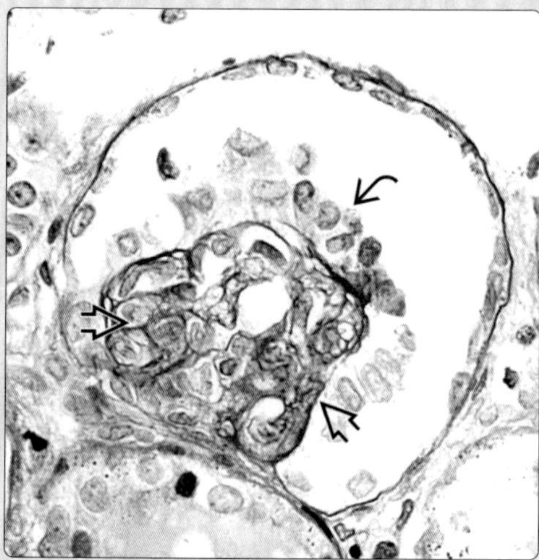

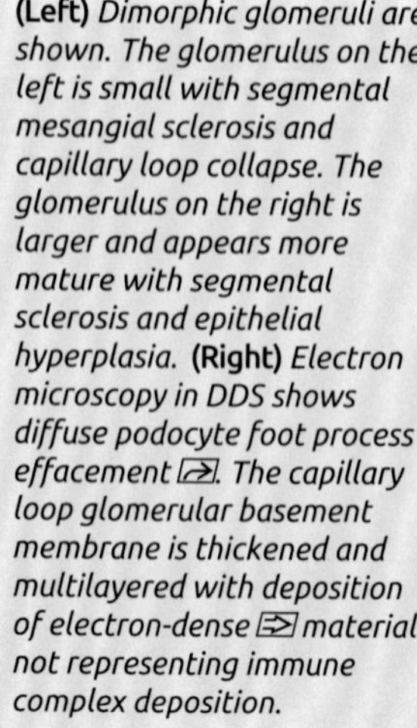

(Left) *Dimorphic glomeruli are shown. The glomerulus on the left is small with segmental mesangial sclerosis and capillary loop collapse. The glomerulus on the right is larger and appears more mature with segmental sclerosis and epithelial hyperplasia.* **(Right)** *Electron microscopy in DDS shows diffuse podocyte foot process effacement ⇨. The capillary loop glomerular basement membrane is thickened and multilayered with deposition of electron-dense ⇨ material not representing immune complex deposition.*

Dimorphic Glomeruli

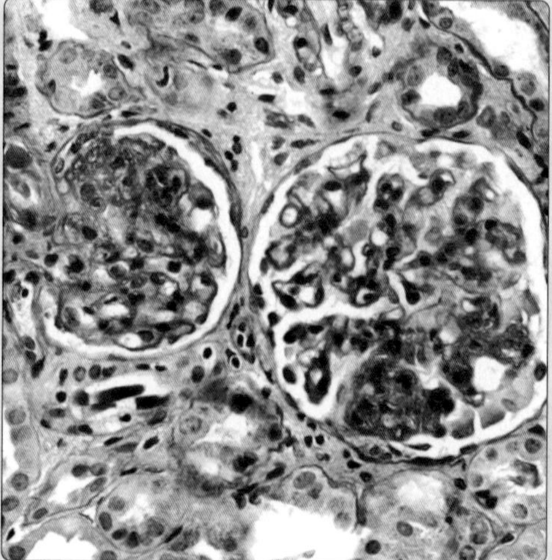

Marked GBM Abnormalities

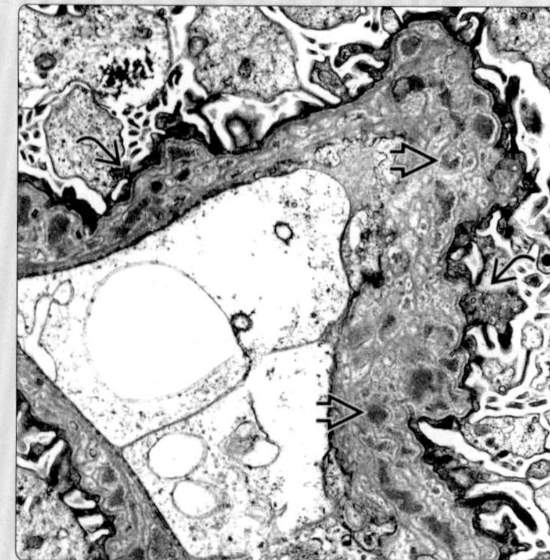

TERMINOLOGY

Abbreviations

- Denys-Drash syndrome (DDS)
- Diffuse mesangial sclerosis (DMS)

Definitions

- Triad syndrome due to *WT1* mutation
  - Male pseudohermaphroditism
  - Nephropathy due to DMS
  - Risk of Wilms tumor (WT)
- Incomplete forms occur
  - Nephropathy is the one constant component
    - Nephropathy and Wilms tumor
    - Nephropathy and male pseudohermaphroditism

ETIOLOGY/PATHOGENESIS

Genetic Factors

- Autosomal dominant
- *WT1* mutation
  - WT1 protein: Transcription factor that regulates podocyte proliferation and differentiation
  - Mutation: Chromosome 11p13, exon 9
    - Hot spot in exon 9 R394W/Q/L is common in DDS

CLINICAL ISSUES

Presentation

- Steroid-resistant nephrotic syndrome
  - Onset usually before age 2
- Ambiguous genitalia with XY karyotype
  - Up to 40% phenotypically female
- Wilms tumor
  - Younger onset (median: 9 months) compared with sporadic WT
  - 30% bilateral compared with 5% in sporadic WT
  - Nephrogenic rests in 80% compared with 25% in sporadic WT

Laboratory Tests

- Gene sequencing of *WT1* gene

Treatment

- Wilms tumor associated with DDS
  - Chemotherapy
  - Nephron-sparing surgery with bilateral disease
- Renal transplantation for ESRD or bilateral nephrectomy

Prognosis

- DMS rapid progression to renal failure in 2-3 years
- WT outcomes similar to sporadic WT

MICROSCOPIC

Histologic Features

- Glomeruli: Diffuse mesangial sclerosis
  - Early glomerular changes
    - Immature glomerulus with hyperplastic podocytes
    - Mesangial matrix increase ± hypercellularity
  - Late glomerular changes
    - Collapsing features and hyperplastic epithelial cells
    - Solidified glomerulus ± mesangial hypercellularity
- Tubules
  - Tubular ectasia leading to atrophy with interstitial fibrosis

ANCILLARY TESTS

Immunohistochemistry

- Podocytes cytokeratin(+) and Ki67(+) and are WT1(-), similar to collapsing glomerulopathy

Immunofluorescence

- IgM and C3 deposition is scarred areas, without other immunoglobulin or complement components

Electron Microscopy

- GBM irregularly thickened and multilayered
- GBM lucent foci &/or electron-dense material
- Diffuse podocyte foot process effacement
- Mesangial matrix increase ± hypercellularity

DIFFERENTIAL DIAGNOSIS

Sporadic DMS

- GBM is ultrastructurally normal
- Must always consider incomplete forms of DDS

Sporadic Wilms Tumors

- Must always consider incomplete form of DDS
- Examine nonneoplastic kidney for DMS

Frasier Syndrome

- Normal female external genitalia and streak gonads
- Focal segmental glomerulosclerosis
- *WT1* mutation usually in donor splice site of intron 9 rather than exons 8 and 9, as in DDS

Pierson Syndrome

- Ocular abnormalities (microcoria)
- Diffuse mesangial sclerosis or fetal glomeruli
- Mutations in *LAMB2* gene

Collapsing Glomerulopathy

- Rarely occurs before age 2
- No association with pseudohermaphroditism or Wilms tumor

DIAGNOSTIC CHECKLIST

Pathologic Interpretation Pearls

- DMS on biopsy, consider syndromic diseases

SELECTED REFERENCES

1. Nso Roca AP et al: Evolutive study of children with diffuse mesangial sclerosis. Pediatr Nephrol. 24(5):1013-9, 2009
2. Niaudet P et al: WT1 and glomerular diseases. Pediatr Nephrol. 21(11):1653-60, 2006
3. Yang AH et al: The dysregulated glomerular cell growth in Denys-Drash syndrome. Virchows Arch. 445(3):305-14, 2004
4. Natoli TA et al: A mutant form of the Wilms' tumor suppressor gene WT1 observed in Denys-Drash syndrome interferes with glomerular capillary development. J Am Soc Nephrol. 13(8):2058-67, 2002
5. McTaggart SJ et al: Clinical spectrum of Denys-Drash and Frasier syndrome. Pediatr Nephrol. 16(4):335-9, 2001
6. Mueller RF: The Denys-Drash syndrome. J Med Genet. 31(6):471-7, 1994

(Left) *Biopsy from a 10-day-old infant with DDS shows two glomeruli with end-stage DMS. The glomerular tuft is small and consolidated with clusters of central mesangial cells ⇒ and no discernible glomerular capillaries.* **(Right)** *This sclerotic glomerulus from a 10 day old shows abundant mesangial matrix and mesangial cells ⇒. Capsular adhesions are not present, distinguishing this from focal segmental glomerulosclerosis. The epithelial cells are prominent but are not hyperplastic.*

Advanced Glomerosclerosis

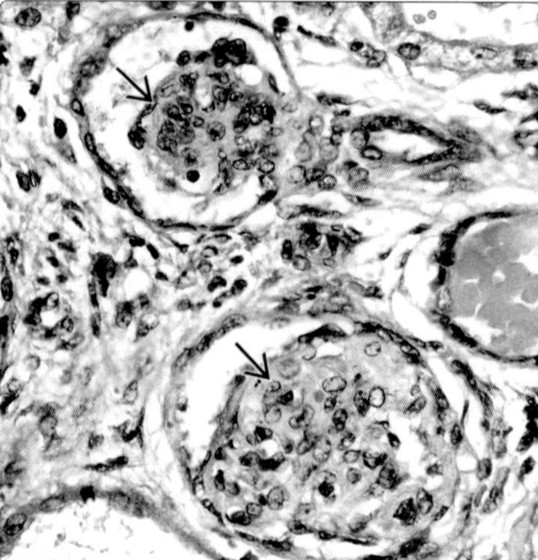

Advanced Glomerulosclerosis

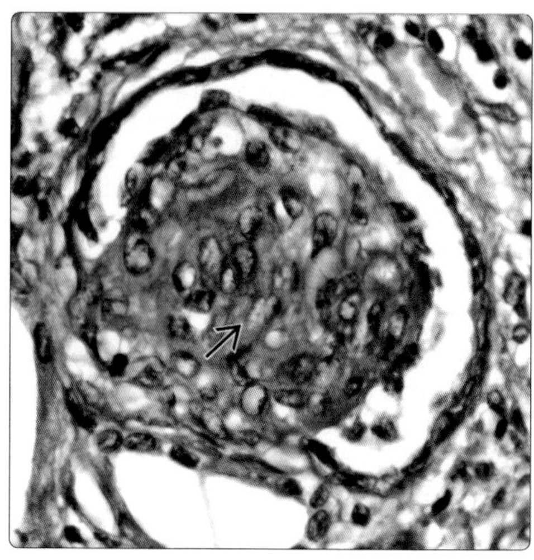

(Left) *This glomerulus from a 10 day old shows prominent epithelial proliferation ⇒ and glomerular obliteration resembling collapsing glomerulopathy. The glomerular tuft is small, suggesting developmental abnormalities in addition to the sclerosing process.* **(Right)** *In addition to glomerulosclerosis ⇒, there is extensive interstitial fibrosis with mild nonspecific inflammation. The tubular cell attenuation ⇒ likely represents tubules in an agonal phase destined for atrophy.*

Epithelial Hyperplasia

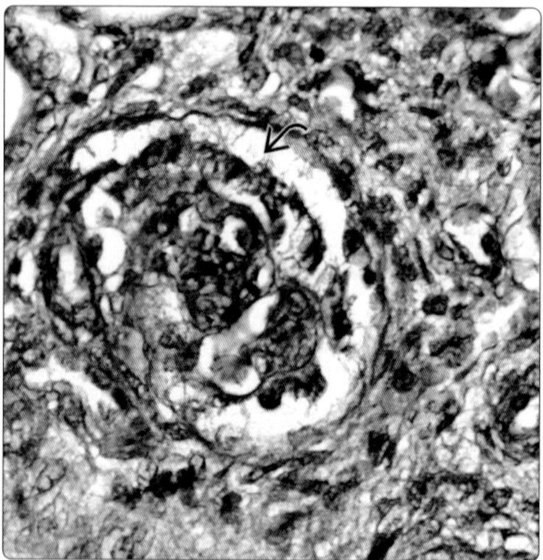

Advance Tubulointerstitial Scarring

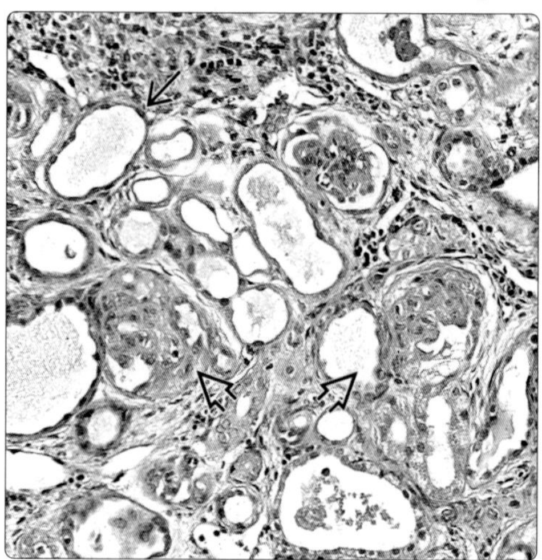

(Left) *This glomerulus shows central mesangial hypercellularity ⇒. The capillary loops are difficult to resolve. There is mild epithelial cell proliferation, vacuolization, and hypertrophy present ⇒.* **(Right)** *This glomerulus shows a mesangial sclerosis and hypercellularity with capillary loop obliteration and prominent epithelial proliferation ⇒. Capsular adhesions are not present, distinguishing this from focal segmental glomerulosclerosis.*

Hyperplastic Epithelium and Mesangium

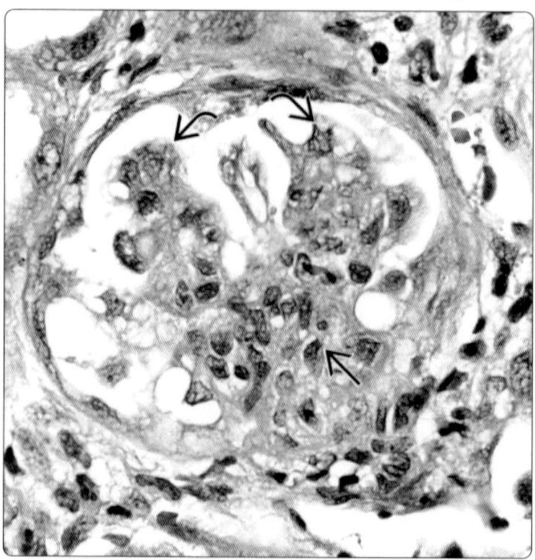

Mesangial and Epithelial Hyperplasia

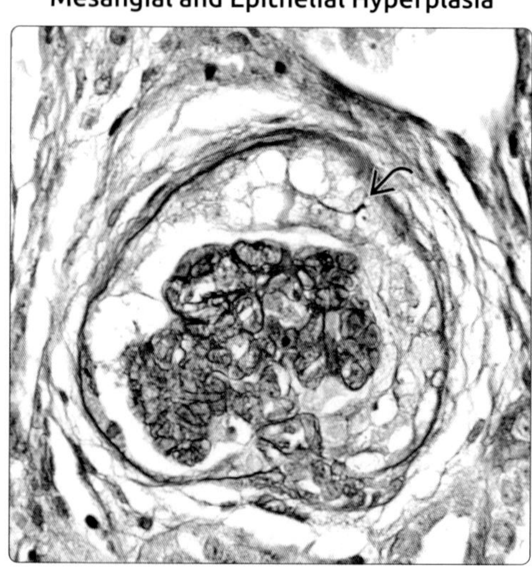

Small Glomerulus With Mesangial Increase

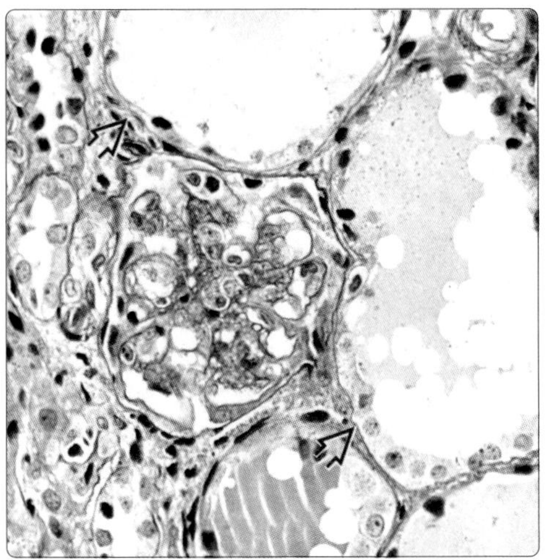

Mesangial and Epithelial Hyperplasia

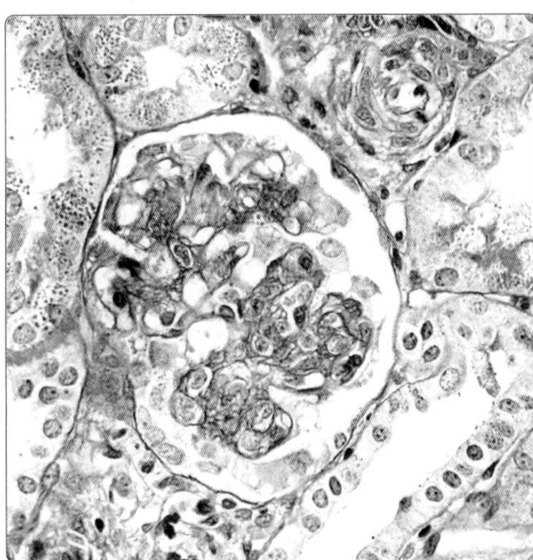

(Left) *Biopsy from a 3-month-old infant with DDS shows a small glomerulus with mesangial matrix increase with capillary loop irregularity and prominent podocytes. The adjacent tubules show ectasia ⇨ and cell attenuation.* **(Right)** *This glomerulus from a 3 month old with DDS shows a few open capillary loops associated with mesangial cell and matrix increase and epithelial cell proliferation. The cellularity could suggest immune complex disease, but immunofluorescence studies were negative.*

Mesangial Hypercellularity and Sclerosis

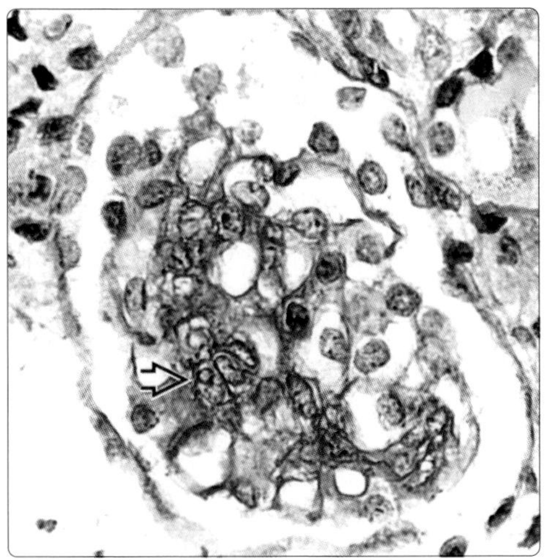

Minimal Glomerular Abnormalities

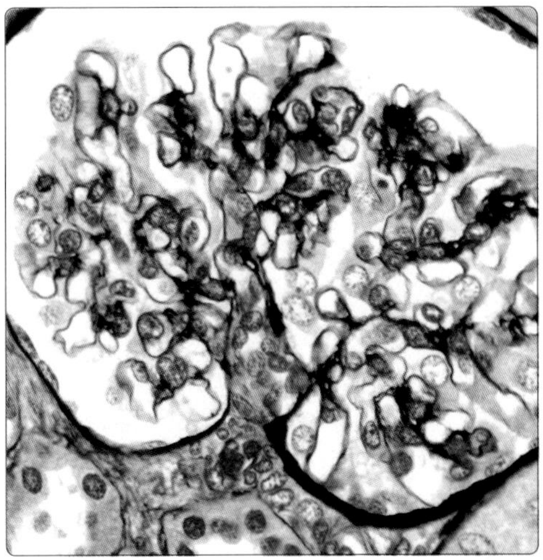

(Left) *This glomerulus in a 3 month old with DDS appears small with only a few open capillary loops. There is extensive mesangial matrix increase and mild hypercellularity ⇨. The podocytes are prominent but not greatly enlarged.* **(Right)** *This glomerulus in a 1 year old with DDS shows a well-developed glomerulus with minimal mesangial expansion and normal-appearing podocytes.*

Marked Epithelial Hyperplasia and Hypertrophy

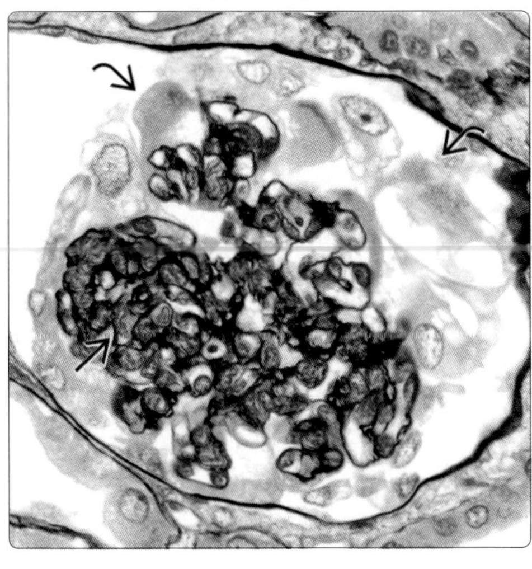

Mesangial and Capillary Loop Sclerosis

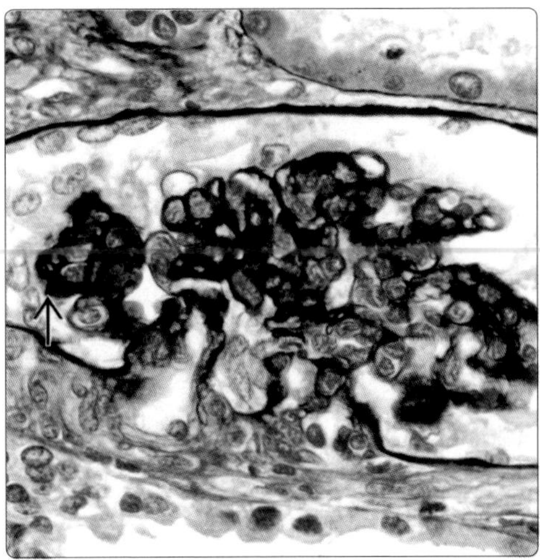

(Left) *Glomerulus in the same patient shows an impressive mesangial matrix increase ➙ with numerous mesangial cells. There is also capillary loop obliteration and impressive large, vacuolated epithelial cells ⇗ enveloping the glomerular tuft. Other glomeruli resembled MCD.* **(Right)** *This markedly abnormal glomerulus in the same patient has extensive capillary loop obliteration ➙.*

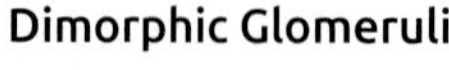

(Left) *Biopsy from a 2 year old with DDS shows a dimorphic glomerular population. One glomerulus is small and immature-appearing with closely spaced podocytes ➩. The 2 larger glomeruli appear more mature.* **(Right)** *Biopsy from a 2 year old with DDS shows ectatic tubules. The glomerulus shows epithelial cell hypertrophy with numerous vacuoles and protein droplets ➩. The immature glomeruli elsewhere in this biopsy and the tubular changes prompt consideration of Finnish-type congenital nephrotic syndrome.*

Dimorphic Glomeruli

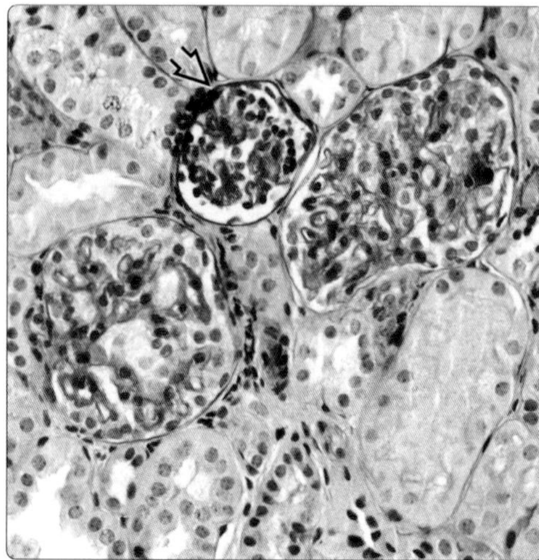

Vacuolated Epithelial Cells

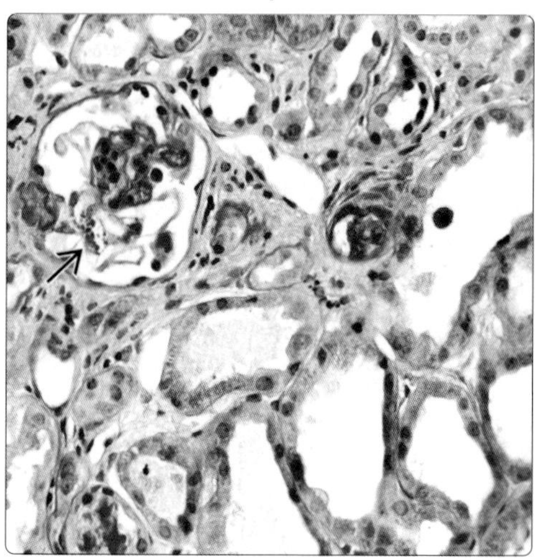

(Left) *In this 2 year old with DDS, the glomerulus shows mesangial matrix increase ➩ and hypercellularity with a capsular adhesion ➩. The capillary loop is thickened ➩ and irregular. The podocytes have protein resorption droplets ➩.* **(Right)** *In this 2 year old with DDS, the glomerulus shows segmental mesangial matrix increase ➩ and mild hypercellularity with exuberant epithelial proliferation ➩ overlying the sclerotic portion. The remainder of the glomerulus is minimally affected.*

Capillary Loop Sclerosis

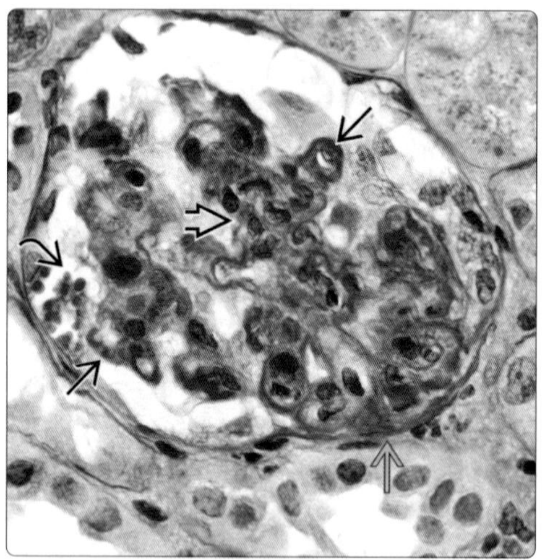

Epithelial Hypercellularity

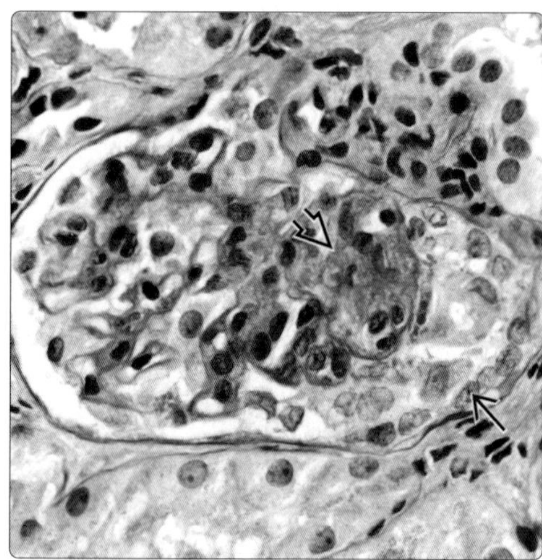

(Left) *This section is from a nephrectomy performed for florid nephrotic syndrome prior to transplant in a 7 year old with DDS. There is advanced nephrosclerosis. Biopsy at age 2 showed DMS.* **(Right)** *This nephrectomy specimen performed prior to transplant in a 7 year old with DDS shows persistent mesangial hypercellularity. The advanced sclerosis with hyaline deposits ➩ and capsular adhesions make recognition of underlying diffuse mesangial sclerosis as the primary disease difficult to recognize.*

Progressive Nephrosclerosis

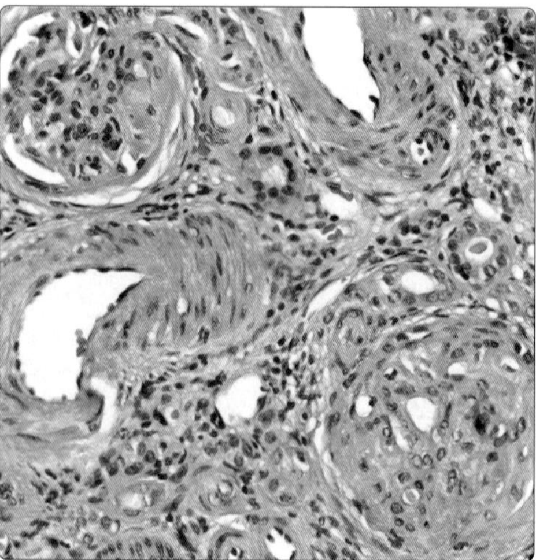

Progressive Sclerosis and Hyalinosis

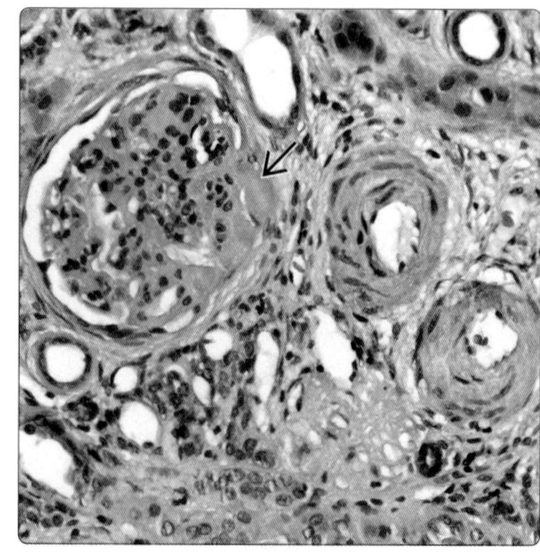

Effaced Foot Processes, GBM Irregularities

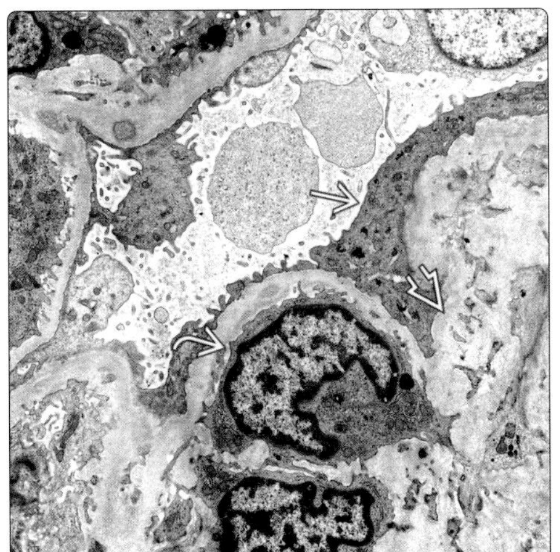

Effaced Foot Processes, GBM Irregularities

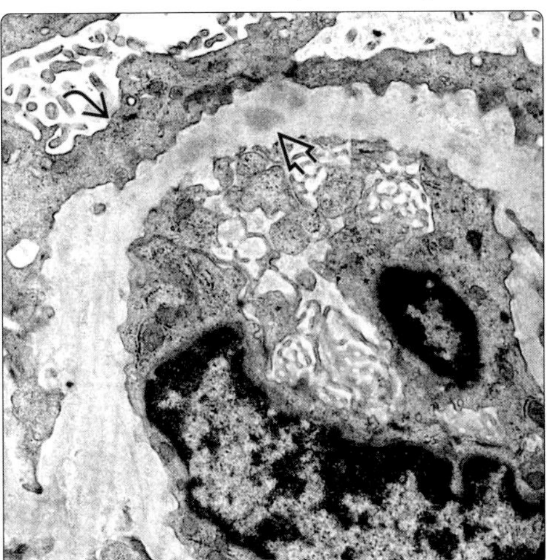

(Left) *This electron micrograph shows diffuse podocyte foot process effacement. The glomerular basement membranes are thick and irregular with electron densities that are not immune deposits. There is also mesangial hypercellularity and matrix increase.* **(Right)** *This glomerular capillary loop shows diffuse podocyte foot process effacement. The GBM is thickened and irregular with small deposits of electron-dense material not representing immune complex deposits.*

Mesangial Expansion

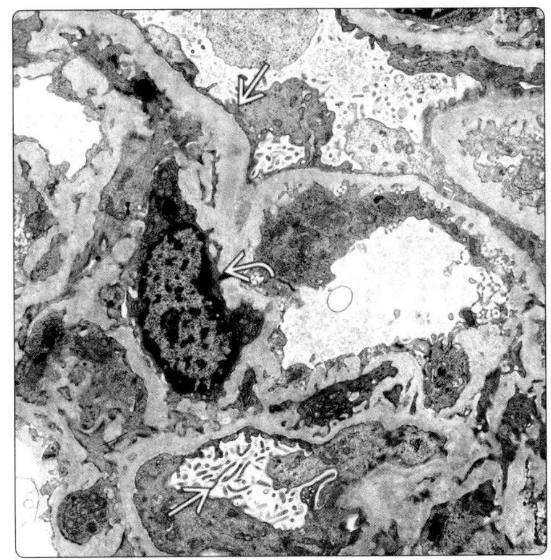

GBM Irregularities and Electron Densities

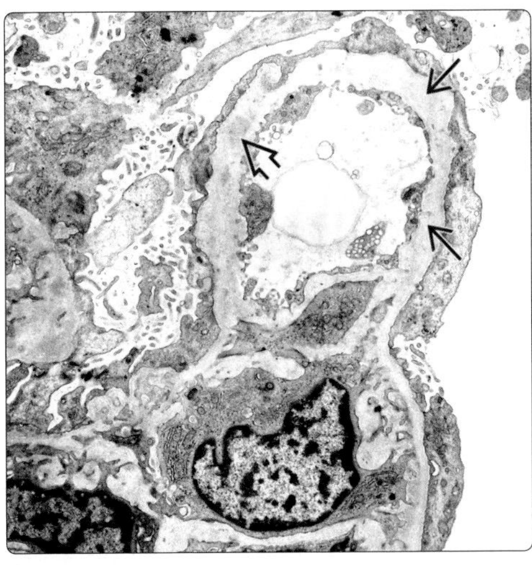

(Left) *This EM shows diffuse podocyte foot process effacement and microvillous transformation with mesangial expansion and hypercellularity.* **(Right)** *This EM from a 2 year old with Denys-Drash syndrome shows diffuse podocyte foot process effacement. There is prominent irregularity and thickening of the capillary loop basement membrane, which contains electron-dense deposits. These should not be misinterpreted as immune complexes.*

GBM Lamellations and Electron Densities

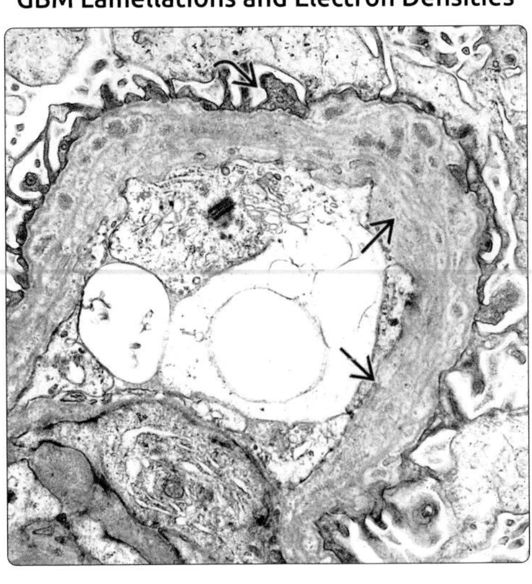

GBM Lamellations and Electron Densities

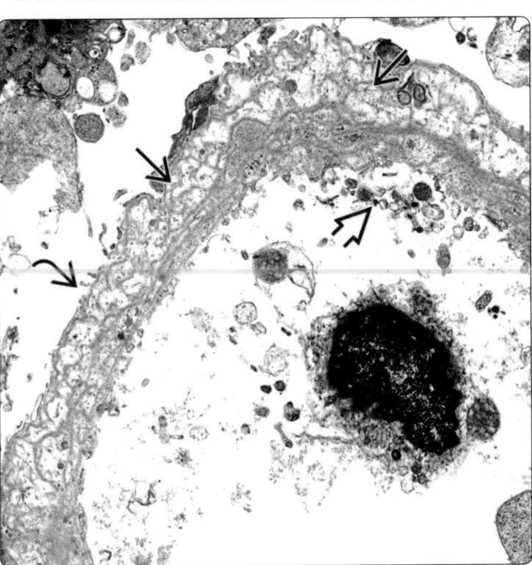

(Left) *This electron micrograph shows podocyte foot process effacement. The markedly thickened capillary loop GBM is extensively lamellated and strongly resembles alterations that occur in Alport hereditary nephritis.* **(Right)** *This electron micrograph shows a complex reticulated and multilayered alteration of the capillary loop basement membrane with numerous lucent foci. The endothelial cells and epithelial cells show marked artifactual autolysis.*

KEY FACTS

TERMINOLOGY

- Triad syndrome
  - Steroid-resistant nephrotic syndrome
  - Male pseudohermaphroditism
  - Gonadal dysgenesis with streak gonads

ETIOLOGY/PATHOGENESIS

- *WT1* mutation

CLINICAL ISSUES

- Male pseudohermaphroditism
- Steroid-resistant nephrotic syndrome
- Slow progression to renal failure
- Risk of gonadoblastoma

MICROSCOPIC

- Normal glomeruli to focal segmental glomerulosclerosis
- Ultrastructural glomerular basement membrane abnormalities

ANCILLARY TESTS

- Sequencing of *WT1* gene shows intron 9 mutation

TOP DIFFERENTIAL DIAGNOSES

- Denys-Drash syndrome
  - Male pseudohermaphroditism
  - Diffuse mesangial sclerosis
- Podocin mutation
  - Normal external genitalia
  - Minimal change disease or focal segmental glomerulosclerosis
- Alport syndrome
  - Normal external genitalia
  - Normal glomeruli to focal segmental glomerulosclerosis
  - ± collagen IV α-chain immunohistochemical abnormalities
  - Glomerular basement membrane abnormalities with thinning ± scalloping and lamellations

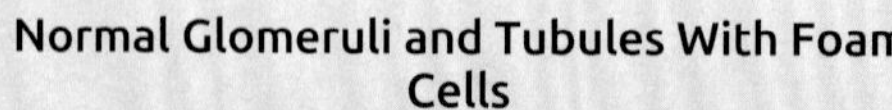

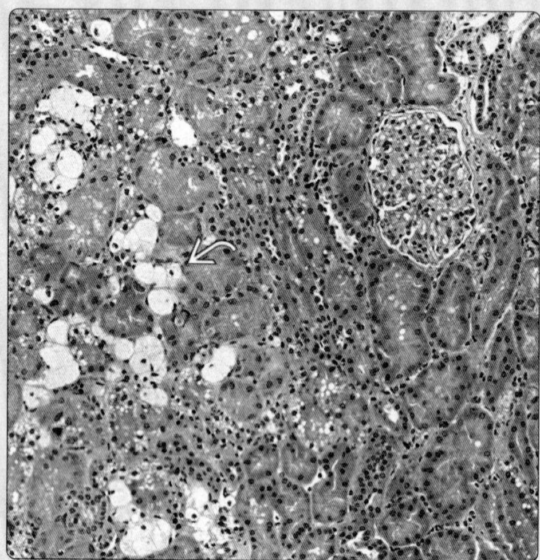

Thick and Irregular Glomerular Basement Membranes

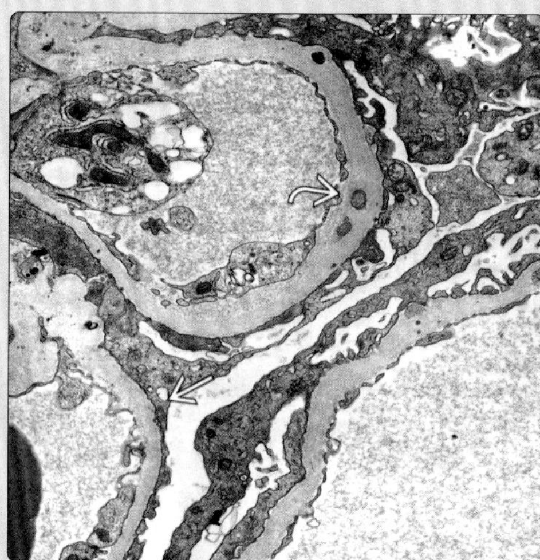

(Left) *Biopsy from a 3 year old with genetically confirmed Frasier syndrome shows a normal glomerulus and tubules. There are also numerous clusters of interstitial foam cells without interstitial fibrosis, a feature seen in other causes of nephrotic syndrome.* **(Right)** *The glomerular basement membranes in this 3 year old with Frasier syndrome show generalized thickening with irregularities and several electron densities. There is also diffuse podocyte foot process effacement.*

Segmental Glomerulosclerosis With Foam Cells

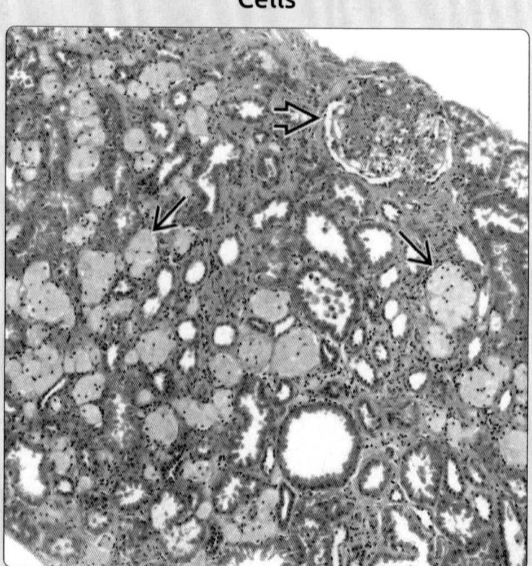

GBM Irregularities

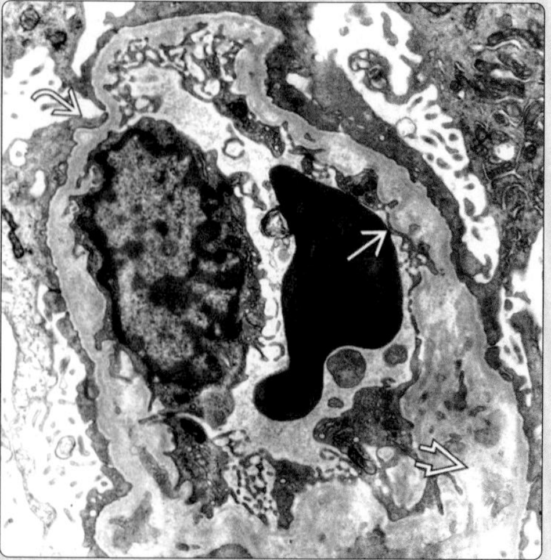

(Left) *Biopsy from a 13 year old with Frasier syndrome shows segmental glomerulosclerosis. There is interstitial fibrosis and large numbers of interstitial foam cells. Immunofluorescence studies showed that IgM and C3 were present in areas of sclerosis. (Courtesy T. Cook, MD.)* **(Right)** *There is diffuse podocyte foot process effacement in this 13 year old with Frasier syndrome. The capillary loop basement membranes are irregularly thickened with lucencies and vague, nonspecific mesangial hyaline deposits.*

TERMINOLOGY

Abbreviations

- Frasier syndrome

Definitions

- Triad syndrome due to mutations of *WT1* gene
  - Steroid-resistant nephrotic syndrome
  - Male pseudohermaphroditism
  - Gonadal dysgenesis with streak gonads

ETIOLOGY/PATHOGENESIS

Genetic Factors

- *WT1* mutation 11p13
  - Encodes for Wilms tumor protein
    - Zinc transcription factor
    - Regulates cell proliferation and podocyte differentiation
- Genotype-phenotype correlation
  - Mutations in donor splice site intron 9 (KTS)
    - Steroid-resistant nephrotic syndrome
    - Risk of gonadoblastoma

CLINICAL ISSUES

Presentation

- Childhood onset (usually 2-6 years) to young adult
- Steroid-resistant nephrotic syndrome
- Slow progression to renal failure by 2nd-3rd decade
- Male pseudohermaphroditism
  - Female XY karyotype
  - Streak gonads, small uterus and primary amenorrhea
  - Absent pubertal development
- Rarely XX phenotypic female
- Rarely XY phenotypic male
- Gonadoblastoma
- Rarely Wilms tumor

Laboratory Tests

- *WT1* gene sequencing
  - Mutations in donor splice site in intron 9
  - Rarely, DDS may present with intron 9 mutation

Treatment

- Surgical approaches
  - Prophylactic gonadectomy to prevent gonadoblastoma
  - Renal transplantation for renal failure
  - Nephron-sparing surgery for the rare Wilms tumor

Prognosis

- Slowly progressive renal failure by 2nd-3rd decade

MICROSCOPIC

Histologic Features

- Glomeruli
  - Early presentation glomeruli are histologically normal
  - Later present with focal segmental glomerulosclerosis
    - Segmental capillary loop sclerosis, hyaline, adhesion
    - Mesangial matrix increase ± hypercellularity
- Tubules and interstitium
  - Early presentation tubules and interstitium are normal
  - Later presentation shows tubulointerstitial scarring
  - Interstitial foams cells
- Rarely, diffuse mesangial sclerosis is present

ANCILLARY TESTS

Immunohistochemistry

- Decreased WT1 staining, but limited experience

Immunofluorescence

- Nonspecific IgM, C3 and light chains in segmental scars
- IgG, IgA, C1q, and fibrinogen are usually negative
  - Occasionally immune deposits present

Electron Microscopy

- GBM normal or irregular thinning and thickening
- Podocyte foot process effacement
- Mesangial matrix expansion

DIFFERENTIAL DIAGNOSIS

Denys-Drash Syndrome

- Autosomal recessive
- *WT1* in mutations in exons 8 and 9
- Male pseudohermaphroditism
- Rapid progression to renal failure
- Diffuse mesangial sclerosis
- Risk of Wilms tumor

Podocin Mutation

- Autosomal recessive
- Normal external genitalia and karyotype
- No neoplastic diathesis
- Variable age of onset (<3 months to young adult)
- Focal segmental glomerulosclerosis on biopsy

Alport Syndrome

- X-linked (rarely autosomal recessive or dominant)
- Normal external genitalia
- GBM thinning and irregular thickening with lamellations
- Collagen type IV α5 (rarely α3 or α4) mutation

SELECTED REFERENCES

1. Bache M et al: Frasier syndrome, a potential cause of end-stage renal failure in childhood. Pediatr Nephrol. 25(3):549-52, 2010
2. Chernin G et al: Genotype/phenotype correlation in nephrotic syndrome caused by WT1 mutations. Clin J Am Soc Nephrol. 5(9):1655-62, 2010
3. Auber F et al: Management of Wilms tumors in Drash and Frasier syndromes. Pediatr Blood Cancer. 52(1):55-9, 2009
4. Nso Roca AP et al: Evolutive study of children with diffuse mesangial sclerosis. Pediatr Nephrol. 24(5):1013-9, 2009
5. Liapis H: Molecular pathology of nephrotic syndrome in childhood: a contemporary approach to diagnosis. Pediatr Dev Pathol. 11(4):154-63, 2008
6. Leatherdale ST et al: The tobacco control community of tomorrow: a vision for training. Can J Public Health. 98(1):30-2, 2007
7. Niaudet P et al: WT1 and glomerular diseases. Pediatr Nephrol. 21(11):1653-60, 2006
8. Ito S et al: Alport syndrome-like basement membrane changes in Frasier syndrome: an electron microscopy study. Am J Kidney Dis. 41(5):1110-5, 2003
9. Demmer L et al: Frasier syndrome: a cause of focal segmental glomerulosclerosis in a 46,XX female. J Am Soc Nephrol. 10(10):2215-8, 1999

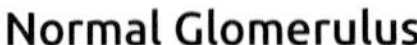

(Left) *The glomerulus is normal with open capillary loops and has an inconspicuous PAS-positive mesangium ➡ in this 3 year old with Frasier syndrome.* (Right) *Podocyte foot process effacement and mild glomerular basement membrane irregularity in the same patient are shown. The mesangium ⮫ contains electron-dense deposits. Immunofluorescence was positive for IgG and C3, likely representing a second abnormality unrelated to Frasier syndrome.*

Normal Glomerulus

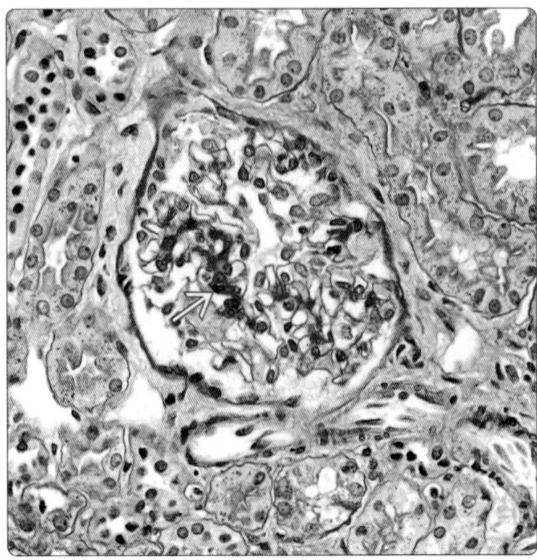

Mesangial Electron-Dense Deposits

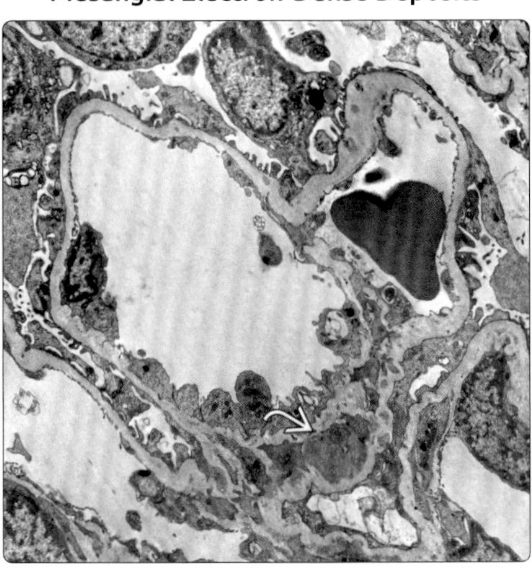

(Left) *The same patient had mesangial IgG immune deposits on direct immunofluorescence. This was in addition to the characteristic glomerular basement membrane ultrastructural abnormalities seen previously.* (Right) *The basement membrane of this capillary loop contains tiny electron densities ⮫ and is markedly thickened for a 3 year old (same patient). It also shows irregularities ➡ along its inner and outer aspects. The podocyte foot processes are effaced.*

Mesangial IgG Deposits

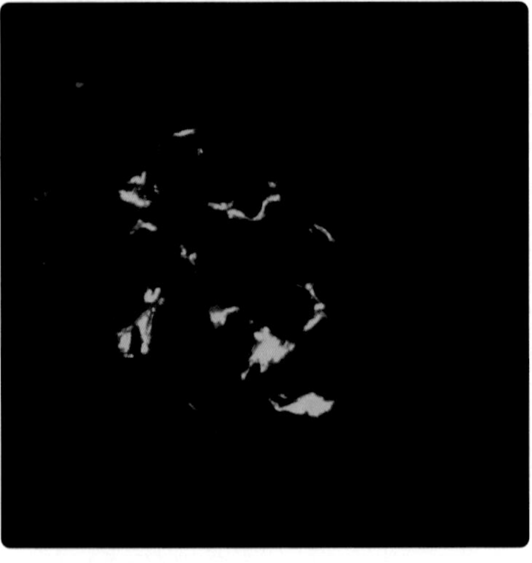

Irregularly Thickened GBM

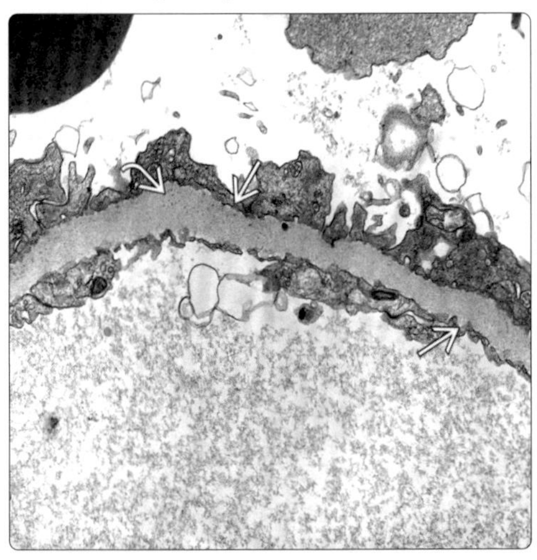

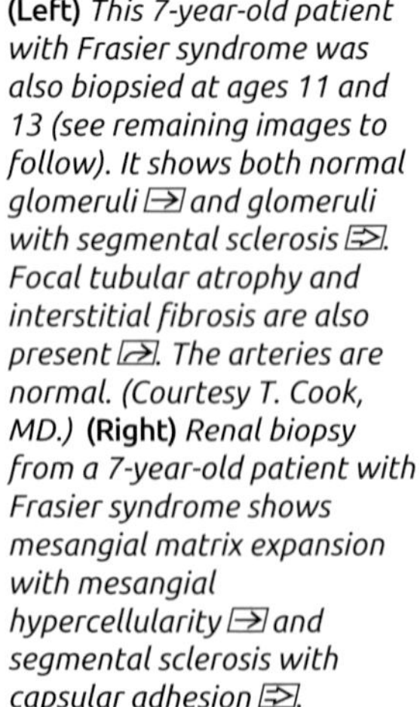

(Left) *This 7-year-old patient with Frasier syndrome was also biopsied at ages 11 and 13 (see remaining images to follow). It shows both normal glomeruli ➡ and glomeruli with segmental sclerosis ⇨. Focal tubular atrophy and interstitial fibrosis are also present ⮫. The arteries are normal. (Courtesy T. Cook, MD.)* (Right) *Renal biopsy from a 7-year-old patient with Frasier syndrome shows mesangial matrix expansion with mesangial hypercellularity ➡ and segmental sclerosis with capsular adhesion ⇨.*

Segmental Sclerosis and Interstitial Fibrosis

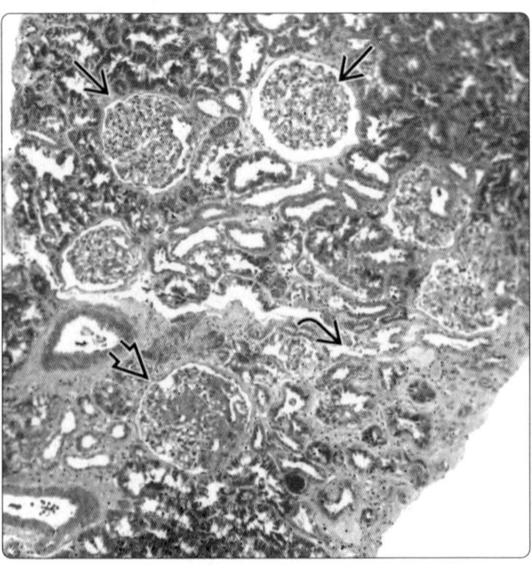

Segmental Capillary Loop Sclerosis

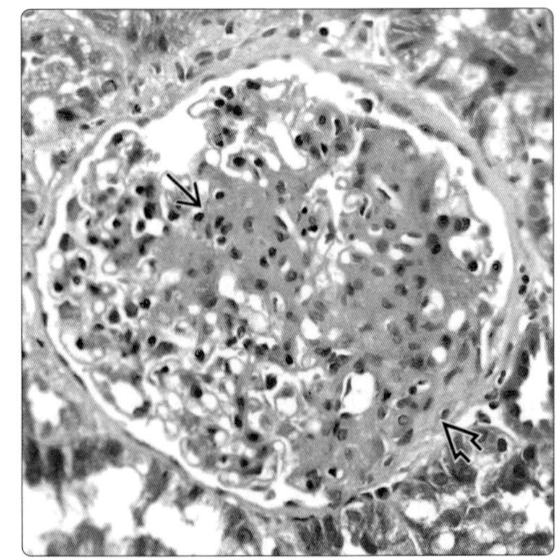

Thin Irregular GBM

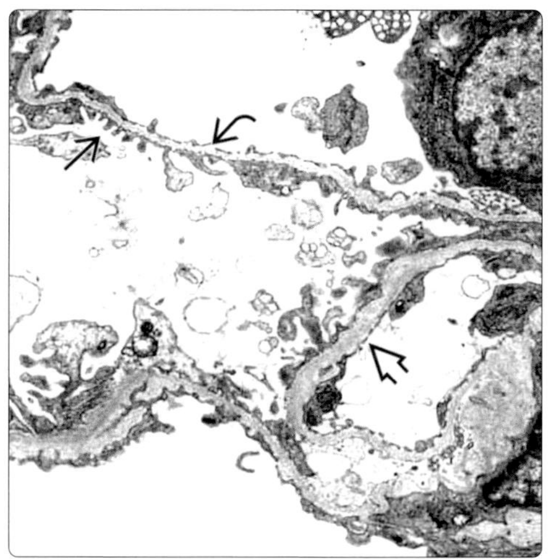

Segmental Glomerulosclerosis

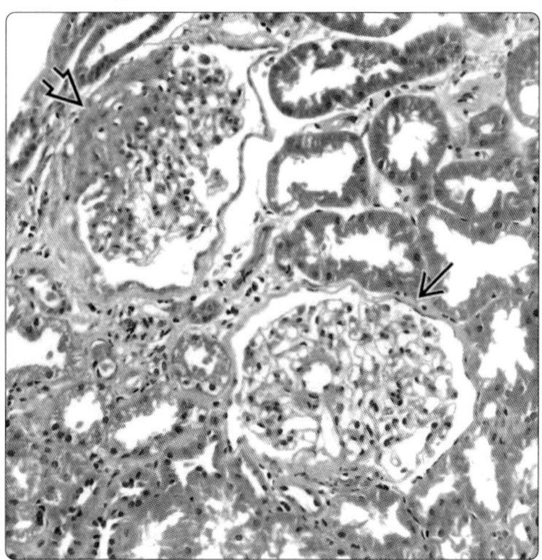

(Left) *Diffuse podocyte foot process effacement with a short segment of foot process preservation ➡ is shown in a 7 year old with Frasier syndrome. The capillary loop basement membranes range from thin ➡ to irregularly thickened ➡ segments.* **(Right)** *Biopsy from the same patient four years later (at age 11) shows that segmental sclerosis is still present ➡. The sclerotic segment appears to be hilar in location. The 2nd glomerulus ➡ appears normal. (Courtesy T. Cook, MD.)*

GBM Irregularities

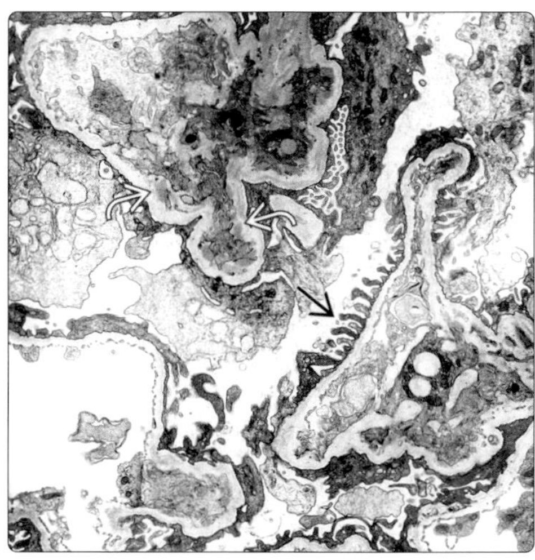

Segmental Sclerosis and Interstitial Foam Cells

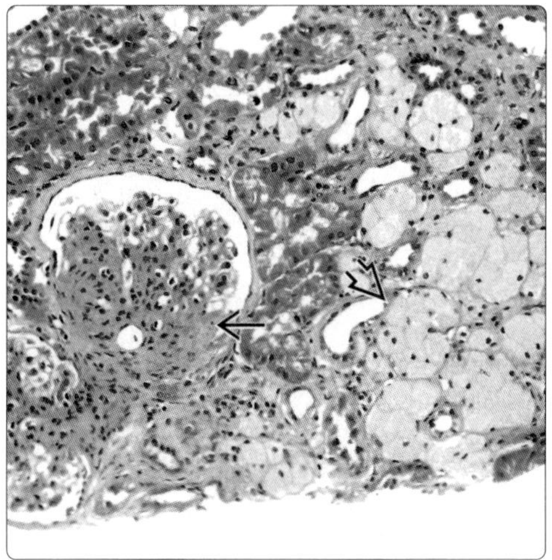

(Left) *Biopsy from an 11 year old with Frasier syndrome shows extensive podocyte foot process effacement with a short segment of preservation ➡. The mesangium contains electron-dense deposits ➡ that by IF showed IgA, IgM, and C1q deposition, not typical of Frasier syndrome.* **(Right)** *Biopsy from a 13-year-old patient shows perihilar segmental sclerosis ➡ and generalized mesangial matrix increase. There are large collections of interstitial foam cells ➡. (Courtesy T. Cook, MD.)*

Podocyte Foot Process Effacement

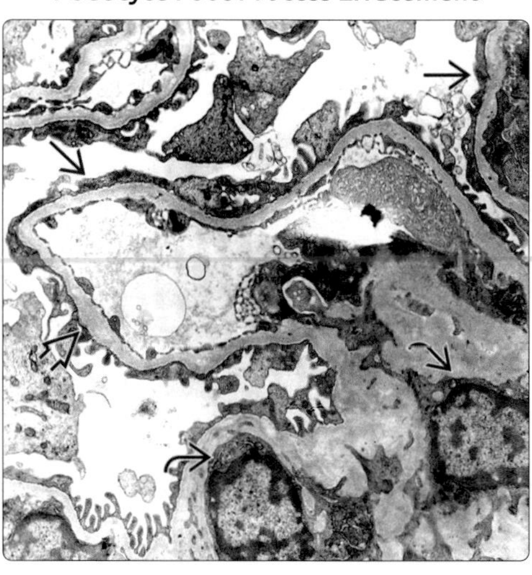

Mesangial Sclerosis With Nonspecific Hyaline material

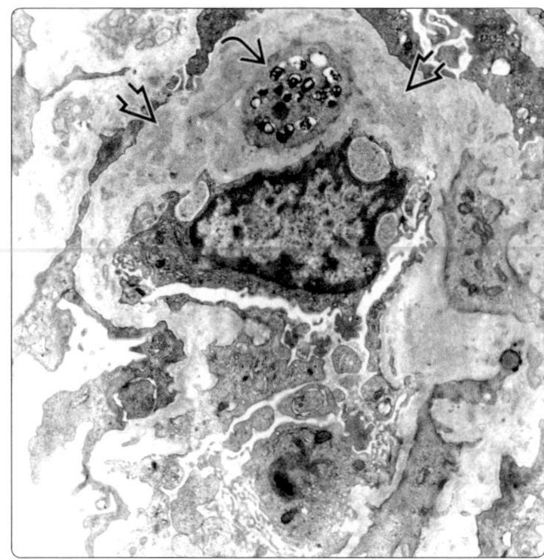

(Left) *Note the diffuse effacement of podocyte foot processes ➡. The mesangial matrix is increased. Two mesangial cells ➡ are visible in this portion of the mesangium. There is persistent mild irregularity in GBM thickness ➡.* **(Right)** *Diffuse effacement of podocyte foot processes is evident over mesangial areas. This portion of the glomerulus contains prominent mesangial hyaline deposition ➡. Mesangial cells also contain intracellular lipochrome deposits ➡.*

APOL1-Related Glomerular Disease

KEY FACTS

TERMINOLOGY

- Kidney diseases associated with genetic variants of *APOL1* gene; can be superimposed on other diseases
- Disease spectrum includes
  - Collapsing glomerulopathy in
    - HIV, SLE, membranous glomerulonephritis
  - Focal segmental glomerulosclerosis (FSGS) other types
  - Chronic kidney disease that mimics hypertension-related nephropathy clinically and histologically

ETIOLOGY/PATHOGENESIS

- *APOL1* risk alleles associated with African ancestry
  - Protection against trypanosomiasis
  - G1 variant: 2 single nucleotide polymorphisms
  - G2 variant: 6 base pair in-frame deletion
- 2 risk alleles (G1/G1, G2/G2, or G1/G2) ↑ odds of renal disease 7-29x; present in ~ 12% of African Americans
  - Donor kidneys with 2 *APOL1* variants have 2x increased risk of allograft failure

CLINICAL ISSUES

- Presentation varies from nephrotic syndrome (collapsing glomerulopathy) to chronic progressive renal insufficiency (global glomerulosclerosis)

MICROSCOPIC

- Collapsing glomerulopathy
- Global glomerulosclerosis with solidified or disappearing patterns
- Segmental glomerulosclerosis, a nonspecific finding
- Tubulointerstitial changes
  - Microcystic tubular dilatation
  - Thyroidization-pattern of tubular atrophy

TOP DIFFERENTIAL DIAGNOSES

- Hypertensive nephrosclerosis and primary FSGS

DIAGNOSTIC CHECKLIST

- *APOL1* genotyping required to exclude *APOL1* nephropathy

HIV-Associated Nephropathy

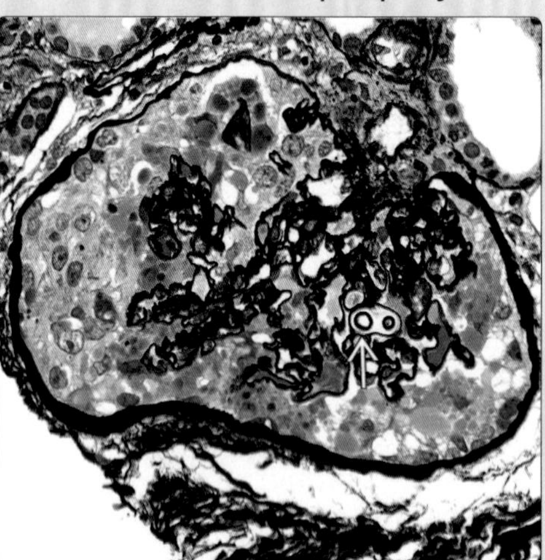

Microcystic Tubular Dilatation

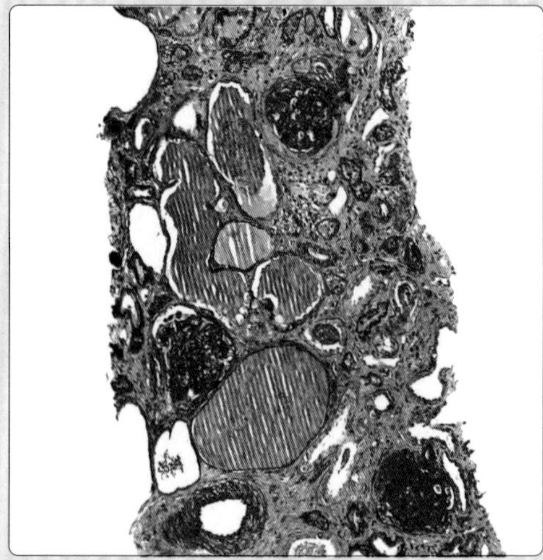

(Left) *The most well-known type of APOL1-associated renal disease is HIV-associated nephropathy. This case shows the characteristic collapsing glomerular lesion that is seen in this disease. Close inspection also reveals intraluminal Cryptococcus organisms ➡ in 1 of the glomerular capillary loops.* **(Right)** *Tubular dilatation with large intraluminal hyaline casts (microcystic tubular dilatation) is significantly more common in all types of APOL1-associated nephropathy.*

Interstitial Inflammation and Dilated Proximal Tubules

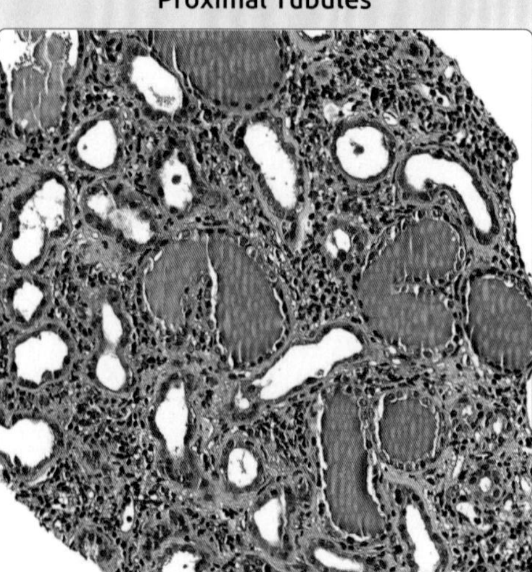

APOL1-Associated Chronic Kidney Disease

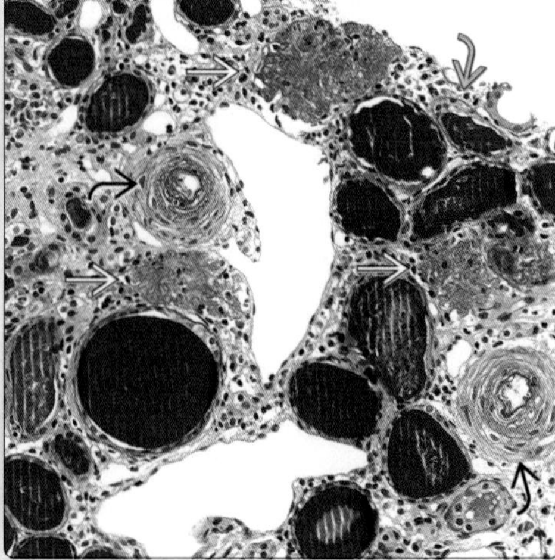

(Left) *Interstitial edema with a prominent inflammatory infiltrate as well as dilated proximal tubules and tubular injury are commonly present in cases with collapsing glomerulopathy.* **(Right)** *APOL1-associated chronic kidney disease (CKD) typically shows glomeruli ➡ with a disappearing pattern of global glomerulosclerosis and thyroidization-type tubular atrophy ⇨. This patient presented with progressive renal failure and was found to have 2 copies of the APOL1 risk alleles. Severe arteriolar thickening is also present ⇗.*

TERMINOLOGY

Abbreviations

- Apolipoprotein L1 (APOL1)

Definitions

- Group of kidney diseases associated with G1 and G2 coding risk variants of *APOL1* gene; may be superimposed on other kidney diseases
- Disease spectrum includes
  - Collapsing glomerulopathy in variety of settings including
    - HIV-associated nephropathy
    - SLE-associated collapsing glomerulopathy
    - Membranous glomerulopathy
  - Focal segmental glomerulosclerosis (FSGS)
  - Progressive chronic kidney disease that mimics hypertension-related nephropathy clinically and histologically

ETIOLOGY/PATHOGENESIS

Overexpression of APOL1

- Absence of kidney disease in individuals with null mutations in *APOL1* suggests risk alleles confer a detrimental gain-of-function
- APOL1 overexpression is harmful to cells in vitro
  - APOL1 risk variants more injurious to these cells than wild-type APOL1
- Innate immune pathways via interferons and toll-like receptors induce APOL1 overexpression
- In normal kidneys APOL1 protein most abundant in podocytes by IF thought be both uptake and synthesis
  - APOL1 mRNA detected in podocytes, tubular epithelial cells, endothelium, and arterial media
  - Validated antibody 3245-1 from Epitomics, Burlingame, CA

Infection

- Viruses associated with collapsing variant of APOL1-associated nephropathy include HIV, HCV, CMV, HTLV-1, and parvovirus B19

CLINICAL ISSUES

Epidemiology

- Genetics
  - *APOL1* risk alleles associated with African ancestry
    - G1 variant consists of 2 single nucleotide polymorphisms
      - c.1024A>G; p.Ser342Gly (rs73885319)
      - c.1152T>G; p.Ile384Met (rs60910145)
    - G2 variant has a 6 base pair in-frame deletion
      - c.1164_1169delTTATAA; p.Asn388_Tyr389del (rs71785313)
  - Inheritance of 2 risk alleles (G1/G1, G2/G2, or G1/G2) confers 7-29x increased risk for renal disease
    - ~ 12% of African Americans have 2 risk alleles
    - Donor kidneys with 2 *APOL1* variants have increased risk of allograft failure (~ 2x), recipient variants had no effect
- G1 and G2 variants protect against trypanosomiasis
  - *Trypanosoma brucei rhodesiense* produces serum resistance factor (SRA) that neutralizes the trypanolytic effect of wild-type APOL1
    - G1 and G2 variants are not neutralized by SRA, leading to resistance in heterozygotes

Presentation

- Heterogeneous
- Depends on type of APOL1-associated nephropathy
  - Nephrotic syndrome with collapsing glomerulopathy
  - Slowly progressive renal failure with minimal or absent proteinuria that mimics hypertension-related nephropathy clinically and histologically

Treatment

- Drugs
  - No specific treatments available
  - Prevention of disease in setting of HIV by effective antiretroviral therapy

MICROSCOPIC

Histologic Features

- Segmental glomerulosclerosis
  - Common nonspecific finding
- Collapsing glomerulopathy
  - Typical with sudden onset of nephrotic syndrome
- Solidified and disappearing patterns of global glomerulosclerosis associated with chronic kidney disease presentation
- Tubulointerstitial changes associated with APOL1-associated nephropathy
  - Microcystic tubular diltation
  - Thyroidization-pattern of tubular atrophy

DIFFERENTIAL DIAGNOSIS

Hypertensive Nephrosclerosis

- Obsolescent pattern of global glomerulosclerosis more likely
- "Thyroidization" pattern of tubular atrophy less likely
- Definitive diagnosis requires APOL1 genotyping

Primary FSGS

- Definitive diagnosis requires APOL1 genotyping

SELECTED REFERENCES

1. Larsen CP et al: Histopathologic findings associated with APOL1 risk variants in chronic kidney disease. Mod Pathol. ePub, 2014
2. Larsen CP et al: Histopathologic effect of APOL1 risk alleles in PLA2R-associated membranous glomerulopathy. Am J Kidney Dis. 64(1):161-3, 2014
3. Ma L et al: Localization of APOL1 protein and mRNA in the human kidney: nondiseased tissue, primary cells, and immortalized cell lines. J Am Soc Nephrol. ePub, 2014
4. Nichols B et al: Innate immunity pathways regulate the nephropathy gene Apolipoprotein L1. Kidney Int. ePub, 2014
5. Larsen CP et al: Apolipoprotein L1 risk variants associate with systemic lupus erythematosus-associated collapsing glomerulopathy. J Am Soc Nephrol. 24(5):722-5, 2013
6. Reeves-Daniel AM et al: The APOL1 gene and allograft survival after kidney transplantation. Am J Transplant. 11(5):1025-30, 2011
7. Genovese G et al: Association of trypanolytic ApoL1 variants with kidney disease in African Americans. Science. 329(5993):841-5, 2010

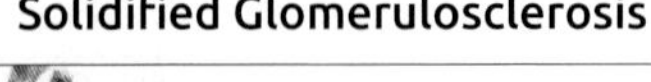
Solidified Glomerulosclerosis

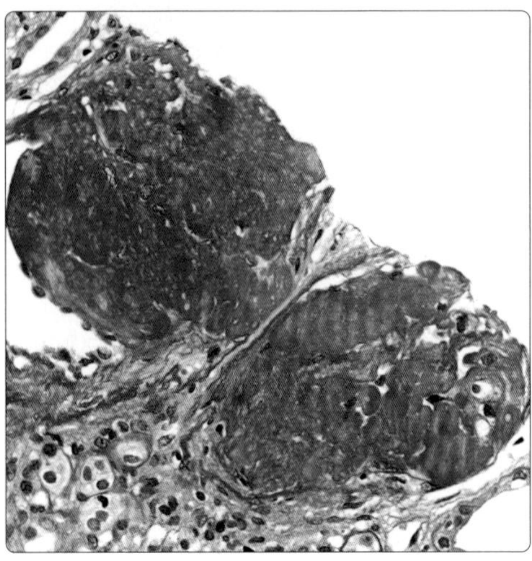

Disappearing Glomerulosclerosis

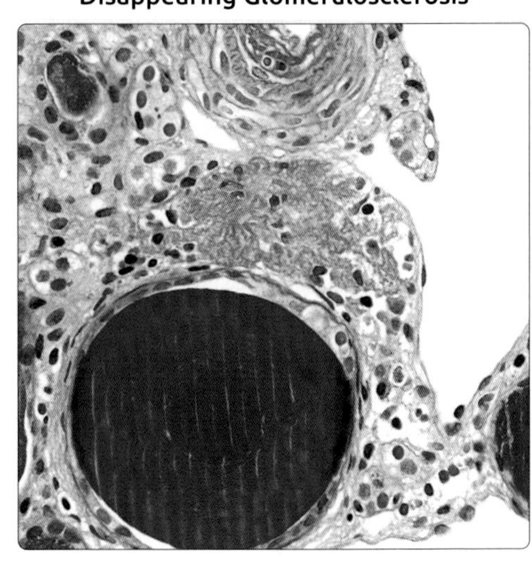

(Left) *Glomerulosclerosis of the solidified type, in which the sclerotic tuft is not contracted and fills Bowman space, is associated with the presence of 2 risk alleles in African American patients with CKD.* **(Right)** *Disappearing glomerulosclerosis is characterized by disappearance of Bowman capsule and the sclerotic tuft begins to blend in with background fibrosis. This type is also associated with the presence of 2 risk alleles in African Americans with CKD.*

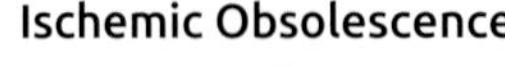
Ischemic Obsolescence

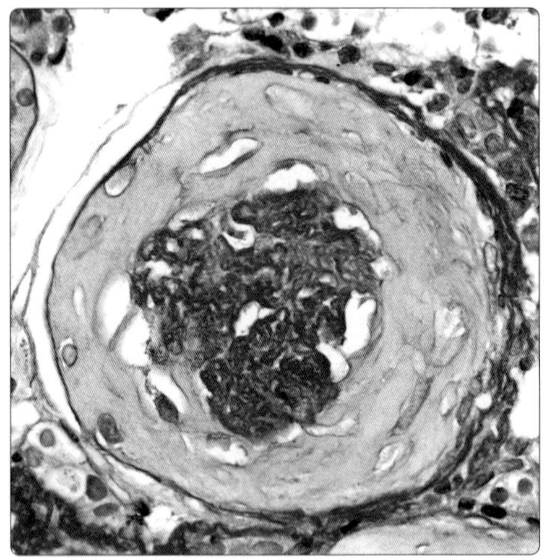

Thyroidization-Type Tubular Atrophy

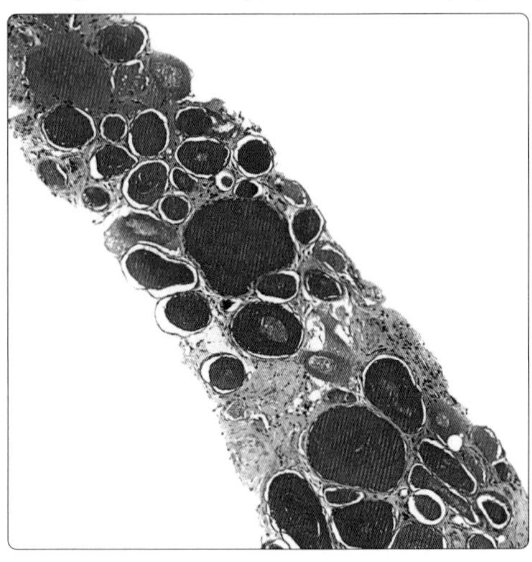

(Left) *Ischemic obsolescent pattern of glomerulosclerosis with a contracted sclerotic tuft surrounded by fibrosis in Bowman space is shown. This is commonly seen in hypertension and is not associate with APOL1 variants.* **(Right)** *Microcystic, atrophic tubules have luminal hyaline casts surrounded by simplified epithelium. This pattern of tubular atrophy was associated with the presence of 2 APOL1 risk alleles in African Americans with CKD.*

FSGS

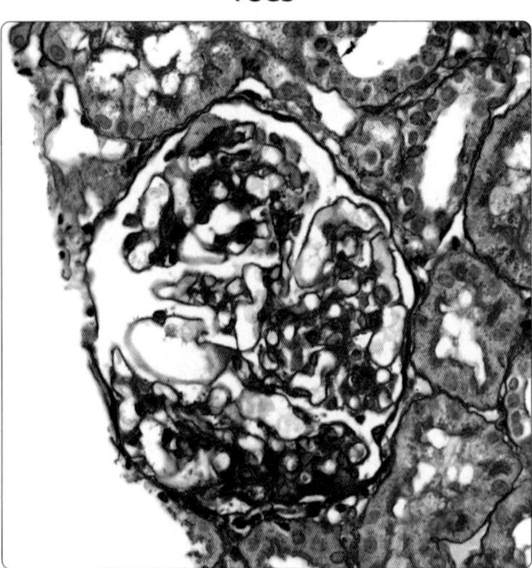

Foot Process Effacement

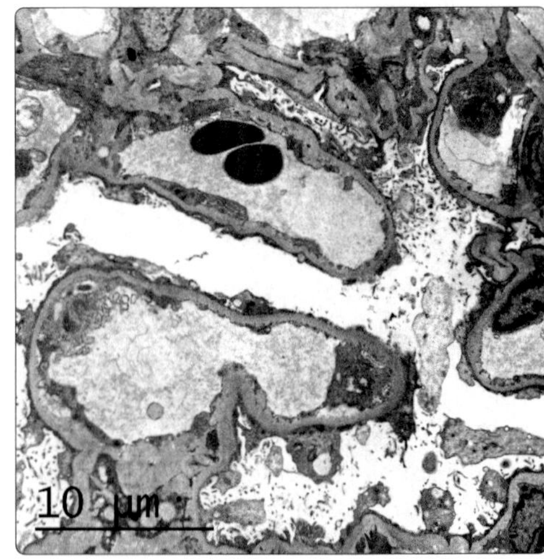

(Left) *While collapsing glomerulopathy is the most characteristic type of FSGS seen in the APOL1-associated disease spectrum, the not otherwise specified (NOS) variant of FSGS is actually the most common. This glomerulus is from a 10-year-old African American with 2 APOL1 risk alleles.* **(Right)** *Widespread foot process effacement is often present in cases of APOL1-associated FSGS.*

Membranous GN With Glomerular Collapse

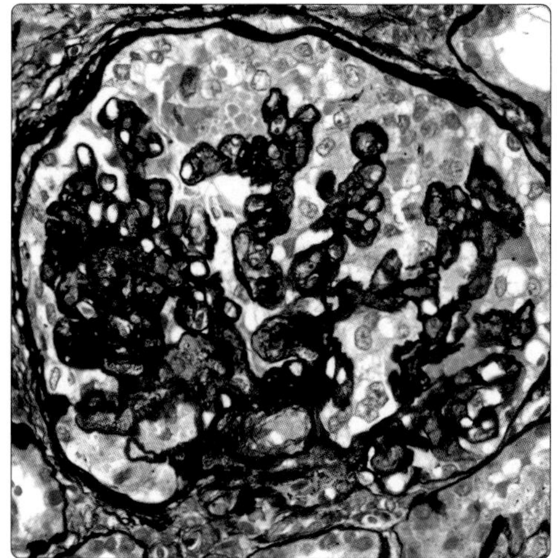

IgG

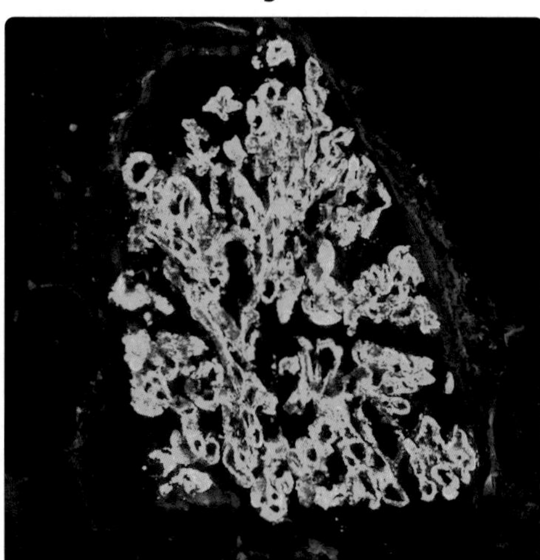

(Left) *A glomerulus from a patient with idiopathic membranous glomerulonephritis with tuft collapse and overlying epithelial hypertrophy and hyperplasia. Collapsing lesions in idiopathic membranous are associated with the presence of 2 APOL1 risk alleles.* **(Right)** *Glomerulus from the same case shows the typical immunofluorescence findings of membranous glomerulopathy with granular capillary loop staining for IgG.*

APOL1 in Podocytes

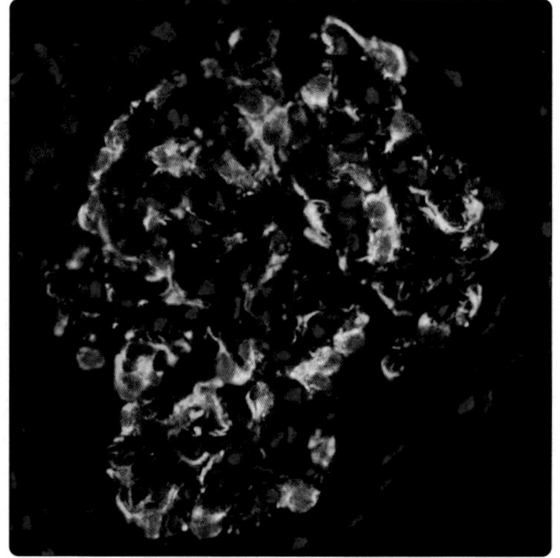

SLE-Associated Collapsing GP

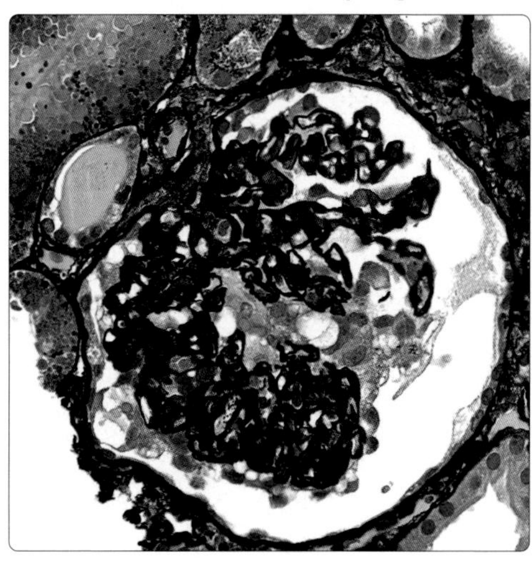

(Left) *APOL1 is in podocytes in normal glomeruli. Cryosections stained with antibodies to APOL1 (red) and WT1 (green) show colocalization (yellow). Nuclei are counterstained with DAPI (blue). (Courtesy L. Ma, MD, PhD and B. Freedman, MD.)* **(Right)** *Glomerulus from a patient with lupus shows tuft collapse with overlying epithelial hyperplasia. Representative photomicrographs of the immunofluorescence and electron microscopy from this case are pictured below.*

IgG in SLE-Associated Collapsing GP

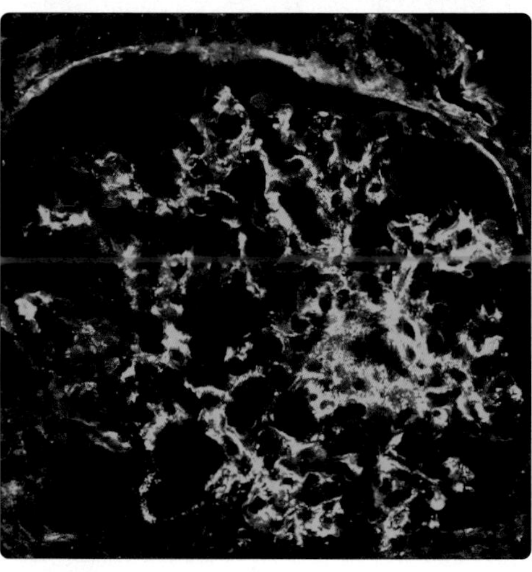

SLE-Associated Collapsing

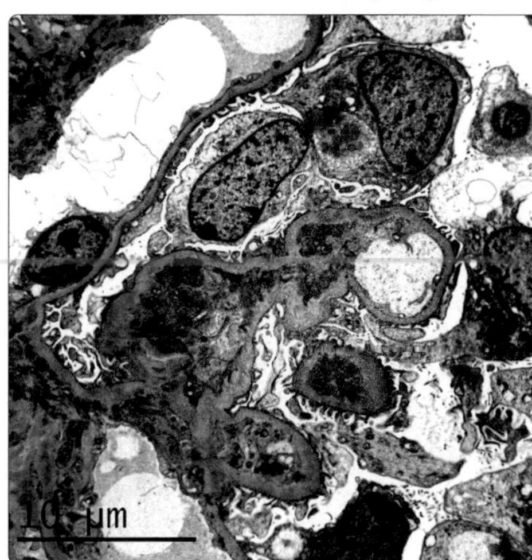

(Left) *Glomerulus from a patient who had SLE-associated collapsing glomerulopathy on light microscopy shows predominantly mesangial IgG staining by immunofluorescence.* **(Right)** *Mesangial deposits are evident by electron microscopy in this patient with SLE-associated collapsing glomerulopathy.*

Lecithin-Cholesterol Acyltransferase Deficiency

KEY FACTS

TERMINOLOGY

- Autosomal recessive renal disease caused by complete or partial lecithin-cholesterol acyltransferase (LCAT) deficiency
  - Familial LCAT deficiency (complete)
  - Fish eye disease (partial)

ETIOLOGY/PATHOGENESIS

- Mutation of *LCAT* gene on chromosome 16q22
- Defect in LCAT-mediated cholesterol ester formation

CLINICAL ISSUES

- Very rare autosomal recessive disease
- Corneal opacities and cataracts
- Hemolytic anemia
- Proteinuria, may begin in childhood
- Renal failure in 4th decade

MICROSCOPIC

- Mesangial expansion with vacuolated matrix
- Capillary loop thickening with spikes, vacuoles, duplication
- Tubular atrophy, interstitial fibrosis, and foam cells
- Lipid deposits in liver, spleen, and bone marrow

ANCILLARY TESTS

- Laboratory tests
  - Low LCAT activity in plasma
  - Reduced plasma total cholesterol
  - Decreased HDL cholesterol
  - Increased free cholesterol-phospholipid vesicles (LpX)
- Electron microscopy
  - Extracted lipid with residual rounded granular and lamellar dense material in GBM and mesangium

TOP DIFFERENTIAL DIAGNOSES

- Hepatic glomerulopathy
- Alagille syndrome
- Autoantibody-related acquired LCAT deficiency

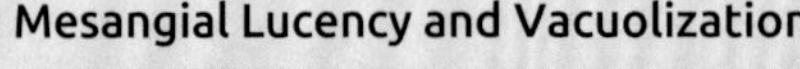

Mesangial Lucency and Vacuolization

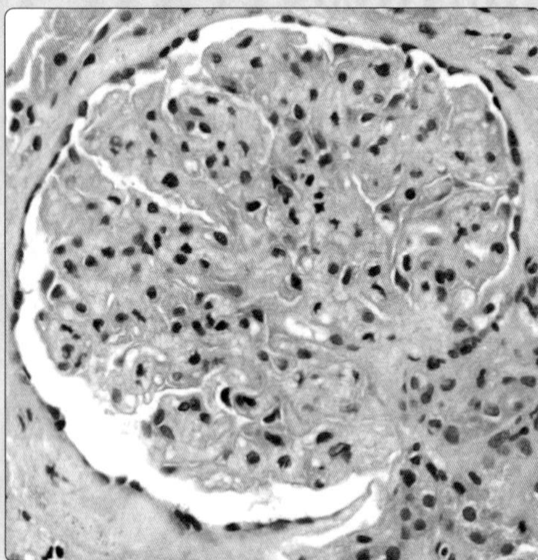

Mesangial Vacuolization

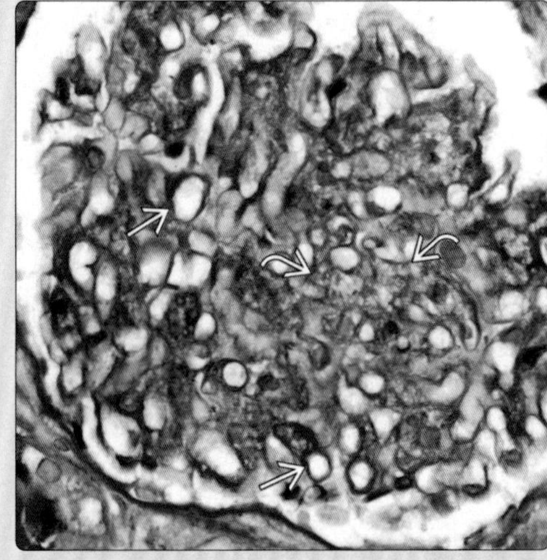

(Left) *This glomerulus in a patient with LCAT deficiency shows glomerular tuft expansion and diffuse pallor. The pallor is due to prominent mesangial vacuolization. There is mild matrix increase without hypercellularity. There is also capillary loop thickening with open loops.* **(Right)** *The right side of this glomerulus nicely demonstrates mesangial vacuolization ↷. There is marked mesangial matrix expansion but no appreciable mesangial hypercellularity. The capillary loops are open →.*

Marked Capillary Loop Basement Membrane Abnormalities

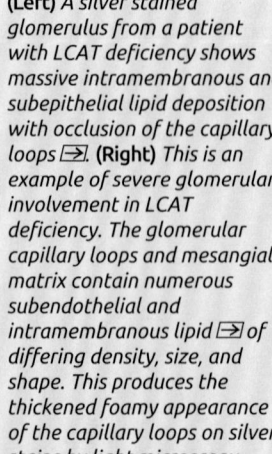

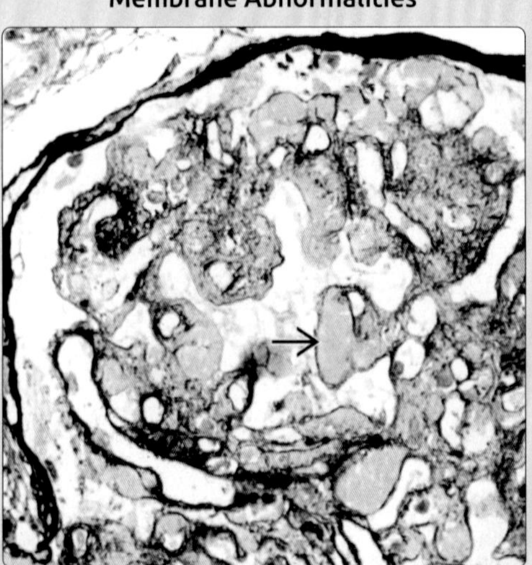

Capillary Loop Lipid With Duplication

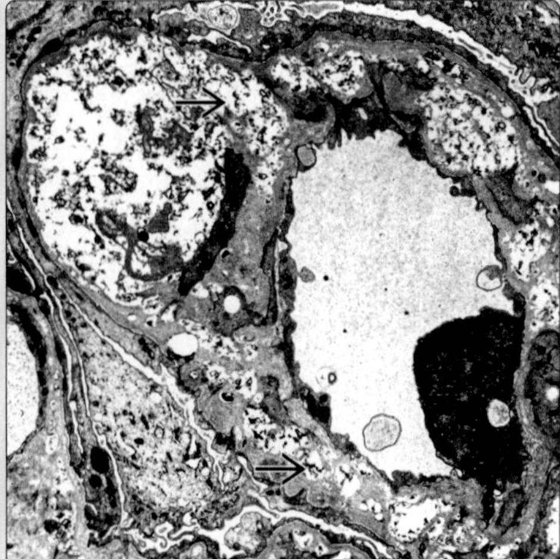

(Left) *A silver stained glomerulus from a patient with LCAT deficiency shows massive intramembranous and subepithelial lipid deposition with occlusion of the capillary loops →.* **(Right)** *This is an example of severe glomerular involvement in LCAT deficiency. The glomerular capillary loops and mesangial matrix contain numerous subendothelial and intramembranous lipid → of differing density, size, and shape. This produces the thickened foamy appearance of the capillary loops on silver stains by light microscopy.*

TERMINOLOGY

Abbreviations

- Lecithin-cholesterol acyltransferase (LCAT) deficiency

Synonyms

- Phosphatidylcholine-sterol o-acyltransferase deficiency

Definitions

- 2 diseases caused by LCAT deficiencies
  - Familial LCAT deficiency: Low or undetectable LCAT
  - Fish eye disease: LCAT activity on LDL maintained

ETIOLOGY/PATHOGENESIS

Genetic Disorder

- Autosomal recessive
- Mutation of *LCAT* gene on chromosome 16q21-22
  - > 70 mutations described
- Defect in LCAT-mediated cholesterol ester formation
- Failure to secrete active LCAT into plasma
  - Unesterified cholesterol deposits in kidneys, liver, cornea

CLINICAL ISSUES

Epidemiology

- Incidence
  - Rare cases reported worldwide
    - 60 with complete and 20 partial LCAT deficiency
- Ethnicity
  - Initially reported in Norway, now widely distributed

Presentation

- **Familial LCAT deficiency**
  - Corneal cataracts
  - Hemolytic anemia
  - Proteinuria, may begin in childhood
  - Renal insufficiency by 4th decade
- **Fish eye disease**
  - Corneal opacities
  - No overt renal disease

Laboratory Tests

- Low LCAT activity in plasma
- Reduced HDL cholesterol
- Increased unesterified cholesterol
- Increased free cholesterol-phospholipid vesicles (LpX)

Treatment

- Low-fat and low-calorie diet may delay progression
- Corneal transplantation
- Dialysis and transplantation for renal failure

Prognosis

- Renal failure by 4th decade
- Renal transplantation moderately successful
  - Lipid deposits recur early, days to weeks

MICROSCOPIC

Histologic Features

- Glomeruli
  - Mesangial expansion ± hypercellularity and foam cells
    - Mesangium appears bubbly or vacuolated
  - Capillary loop thickening
    - Silver stain shows GBM "spikes," vacuoles, duplication
    - Subendothelial deposits can occlude capillaries
- Tubules and interstitium
  - Tubular atrophy, interstitial fibrosis and foam cells

Other Organs Involved

- Cornea, liver, spleen, and bone marrow

ANCILLARY TESTS

Immunofluorescence

- Negative for immunoglobulins and complement

Electron Microscopy

- Glomerular capillary loop contains largely extracted lipid deposits
  - Intramembranous with GBM "spikes" and vacuolization
  - Subendothelial expansion with GBM duplication
- Mesangial matrix expansion with densities and lucencies
- Interstitial foam cells
- Lipid deposits in vascular endothelial and smooth muscle cells

Glomerular Lipid Characterization

- Contain ApoB and ApoE lipoproteins by immunohistochemistry
  - Positive acid-hematin staining for phospholipids
  - Positive for oxidized phosphocholine
- Negative Nile blue and oil red O stains

DIFFERENTIAL DIAGNOSIS

Hepatic Glomerulopathy

- Glomerular IgA deposits usually present
- Lipid deposition, mostly mesangial

Alagille Syndrome

- Mesangial vacuolization
- GBM membranous glomerulopathy-like "spikes"
- Glomerular deposits oil red O positive

Autoantibody-Related Acquired LCAT Deficiency

- Biopsy resembles familial LCAT deficiency
- Associated with membranous nephropathy
  - Contains subepithelial LCAT and IgG immune deposits

SELECTED REFERENCES

1. Hirashio S et al: Characteristic kidney pathology, gene abnormality and treatments in LCAT deficiency. Clin Exp Nephrol. 18(2):189-93, 2014
2. Strøm EH et al: Lecithin: Cholesterol Acyltransferase (LCAT) Deficiency: renal lesions with early graft recurrence. Ultrastruct Pathol. 35(3):139-45, 2011
3. Horina JH et al: Long-term follow-up of a patient with lecithin cholesterol acyltransferase deficiency syndrome after kidney transplantation. Transplantation. 56(1):233-6, 1993
4. Lager DJ et al: Lecithin cholesterol acyltransferase deficiency: ultrastructural examination of sequential renal biopsies. Mod Pathol. 4(3):331-5, 1991
5. Hovig T et al: Familial plasma lecithin: cholesterol acyltransferase (LCAT) deficiency. Ultrastructural aspects of a new syndrome with particular reference to lesions in the kidneys and the spleen. Acta Pathol Microbiol Scand A. 81(5):681-97, 1973

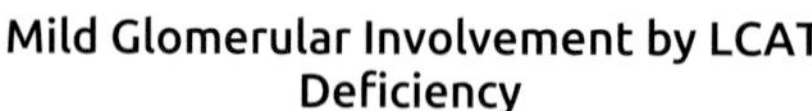

Mild Glomerular Involvement by LCAT Deficiency

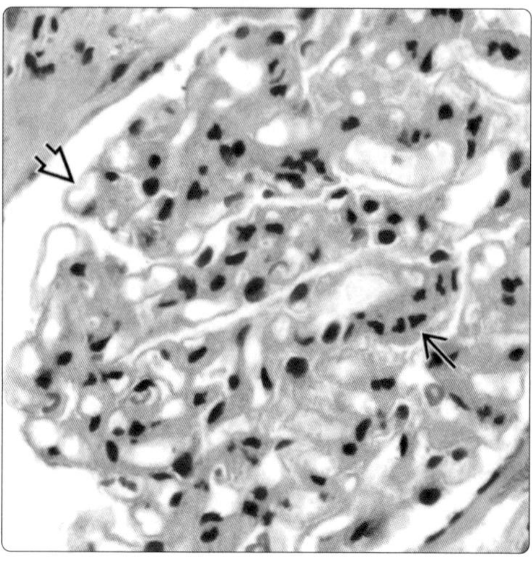

Mild Glomerular Involvement by LCAT Deficiency

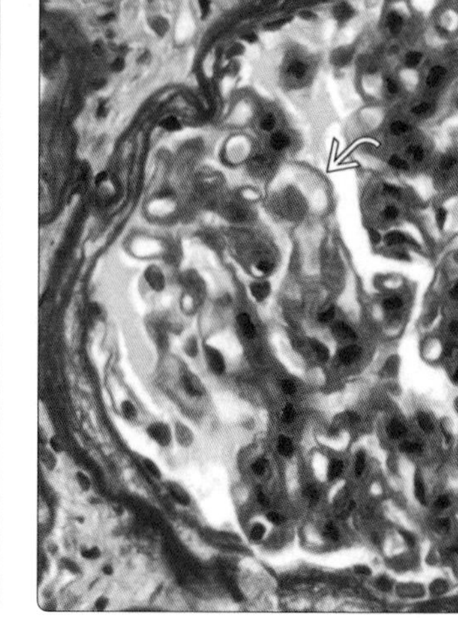

(Left) *This patient with familial LCAT deficiency shows mild glomerular involvement. There is mild mesangial matrix expansion and a mild increase in mesangial hypercellularity without obvious vacuolization. The capillary loops are minimally thickened.* **(Right)** *This PAS stain highlights the thickened glomerular capillary loop basement membranes in a patient with LCAT deficiency. There is mild mesangial matrix expansion without obvious vacuolization or hypercellularity.*

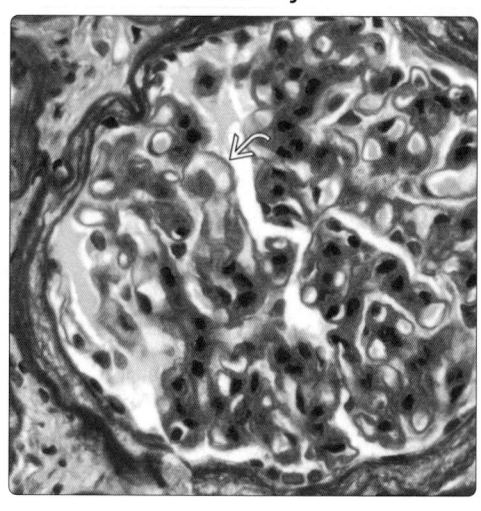

Membranous Glomerulopathy-Like Changes

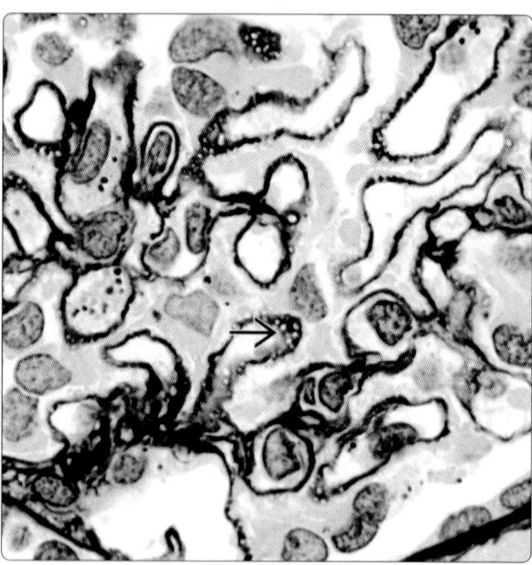

Severe Glomerular Involvement With Vacuolated Mesangial Matrix

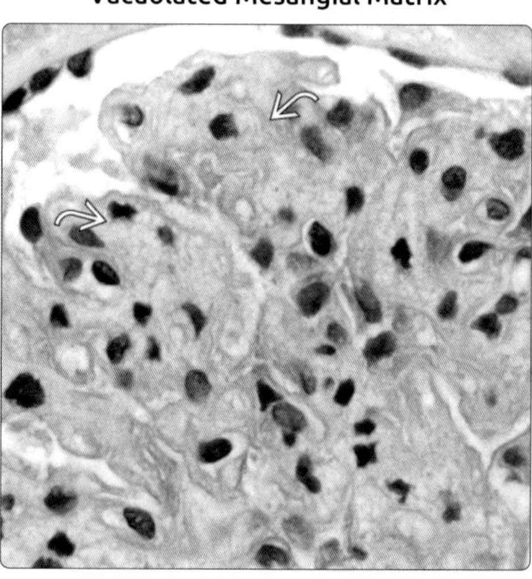

(Left) *This silver stained glomerulus in LCAT deficiency shows vacuolated capillary loops and "spikes" due to accumulation of lipid. This mimics membranous glomerulonephritis. However, in LCAT deficiency, the immunofluorescence studies would be negative for immune reactants.* **(Right)** *The mesangial matrix is prominently expanded. Notice its vacuolated appearance. This is due to extraction of the lipid deposits during processing for paraffin embedding.*

Severe Mesangial Lipid Deposition

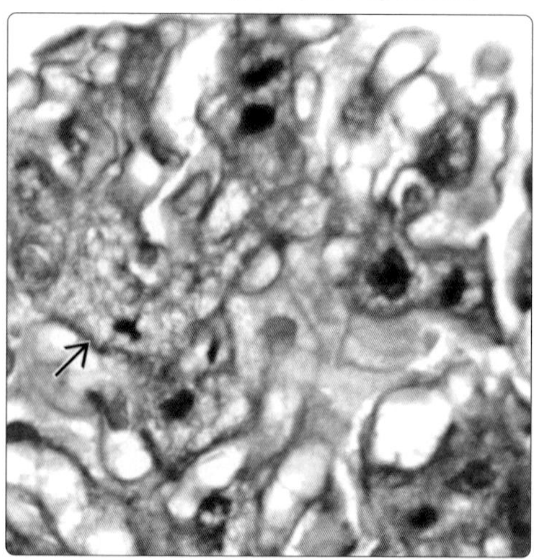

Faintly Stained Lipid Deposits

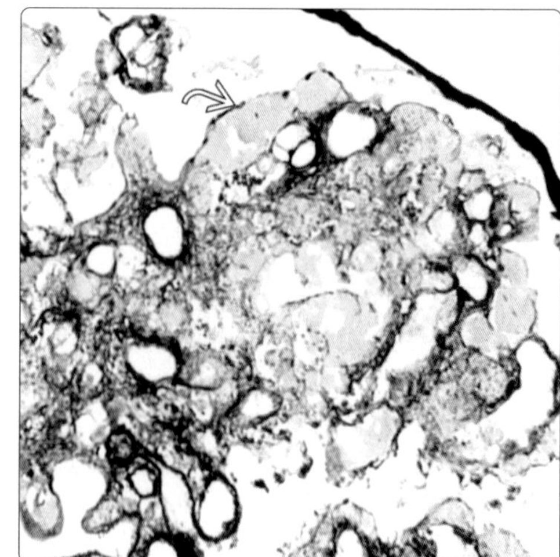

(Left) *There is prominent mesangial matrix expansion and vacuolization. The lipids deposited in LCAT deficiency are extracted by solvents employed in tissue processing. This results in a vacuolated appearance to the mesangial matrix and capillary loop basement membranes.* **(Right)** *There is marked mesangial expansion and capillary loop duplication. Although the mesangial and subendothelial lipid deposits, in this case, stain faintly, most often they will not stain.*

Marked Mesangial Lipid Deposition

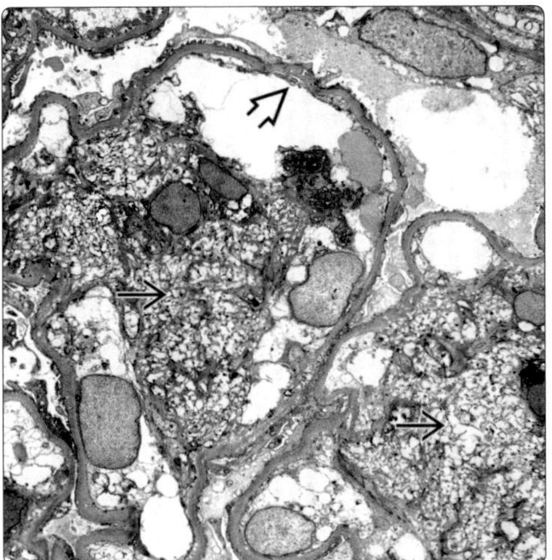

Mesangial Lipid Deposition

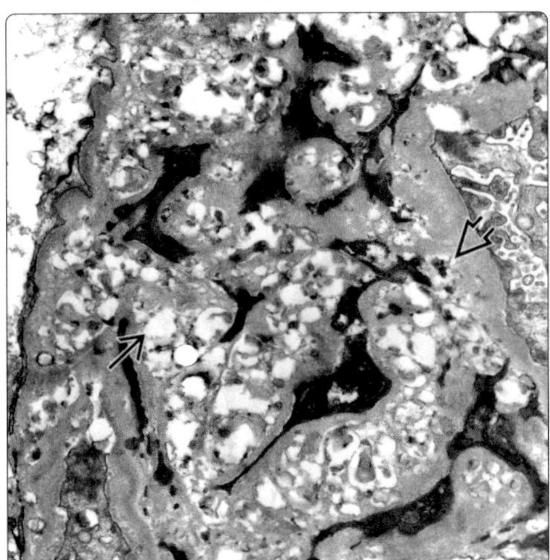

(Left) *This is an electron micrograph of a glomerulus from a patient with mild LCAT deficiency. It shows electron-dense lamellar structures ➡ within the expanded mesangium. The capillary loops ➡ are open and do not contain lipid deposits. There is focal podocyte foot process effacement.* **(Right)** *This electron micrograph shows partially extracted lipid deposits in LCAT deficiency. The matrix contains electron dense lamellar material ➡ and lucencies ➡ resulting from incomplete lipid extraction.*

Mesangial Lipid With Open Capillary Loops

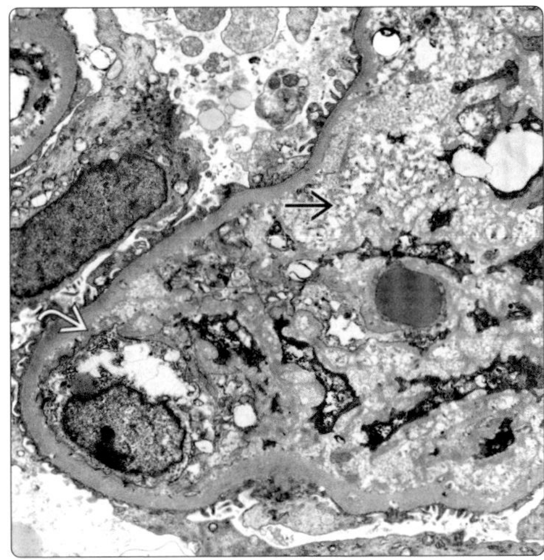

Capillary Loop Lipid Deposition

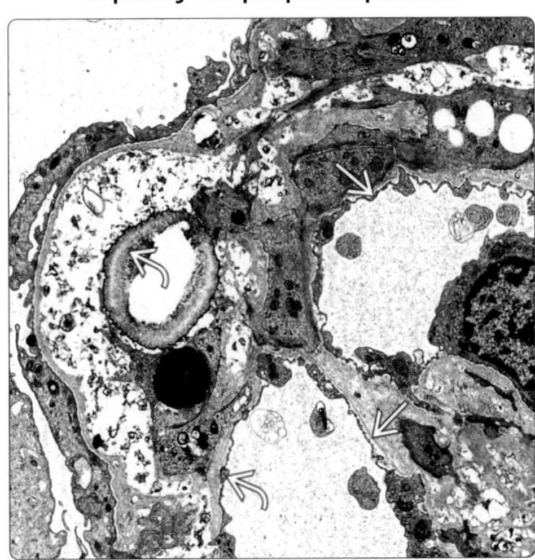

(Left) *This electron micrograph shows the characteristic lipid deposits ➡ diagnostic of LCAT deficiency. The mesangial matrix has a vacuolated appearance with lucent and lamellar material. The accumulated material imparts a "honeycomb" quality to the mesangium. There is no capillary loop involvement ➡.* **(Right)** *The lipid in this capillary loop is primarily subendothelial and has elicited basement membrane duplication ➡. Despite the marked capillary loop thickening the lumen ➡ remains patent.*

Lipid Obliterates Capillary Lumen

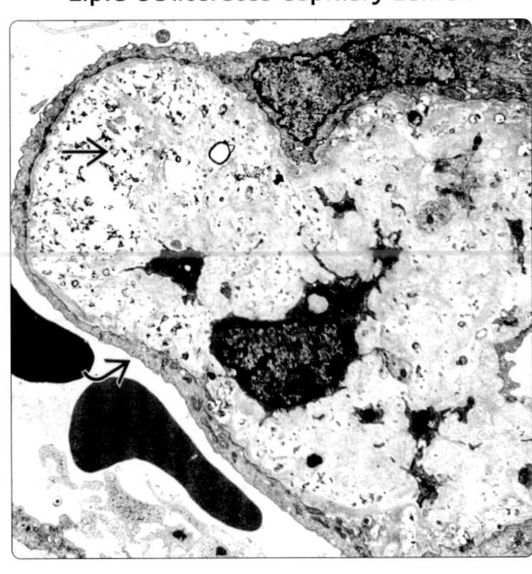

Unusually Electron Dense Lipid Deposits

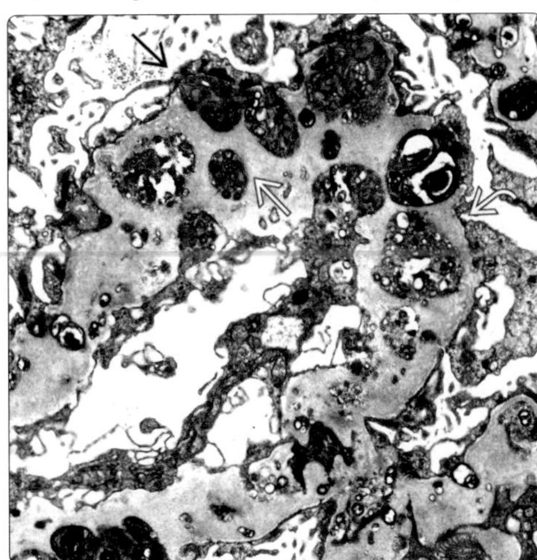

(Left) *In this electron micrograph of LCAT deficiency, there is massive subendothelial lipid deposition ➡. The capillary loop is nearly occluded. There is complete podocyte foot process effacement ➡.* **(Right)** *There is massive intramembranous ➡ and subepithelial ➡ lipid deposition in the capillary loops of this patient with LCAT deficiency. The rounded deposits are solid or have a lamellar substructure and are unusually electron dense. There is podocyte foot process effacement ➡.*

APOE Lipoprotein Glomerulopathy

KEY FACTS

TERMINOLOGY

- Glomerular disease characterized by glomerular capillary lipoprotein thrombi, proteinuria, and progressive renal failure

ETIOLOGY/PATHOGENESIS

- *APOE* gene mutation
  - Autosomal recessive trait
- ApoE is component of chylomicrons and intermediate density lipoprotein (IDL) particles
  - Mutation results in defective lipoprotein receptor binding
  - Hyperlipoproteinemia results (type III)

CLINICAL ISSUES

- Rare; < 80 cases reported
- Majority of cases reported in patients of Asian ancestry
- Proteinuria, mild to severe
- 50% of patients progress to renal failure
- Intensive lipid-lowering therapy has been shown to result in clinical and pathologic remission

MICROSCOPIC

- Glomerular intracapillary lipoprotein thrombi
- Oil red O positive thrombi
- Foam cells in glomeruli or interstitium
- EM shows glomerular capillaries contain variably sized granules and vacuoles forming lamellated structures

ANCILLARY TESTS

- Elevated serum apolipoprotein E to ~ 2x upper normal range
- *APOE* gene sequencing
- Immunohistochemistry with antibodies to B or E apolipoproteins

TOP DIFFERENTIAL DIAGNOSES

- Fat emboli

Lipoprotein "Thrombi"

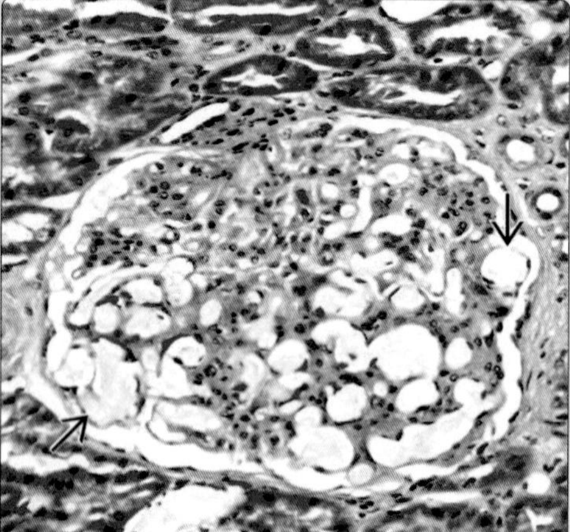

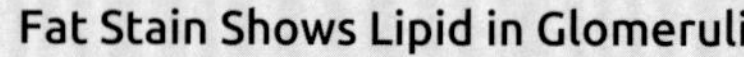

Fat Stain Shows Lipid in Glomeruli

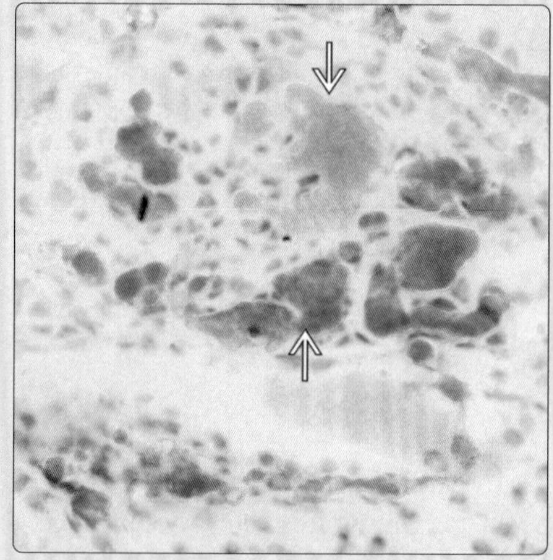

(Left) *In lipoprotein glomerulopathy, glomeruli have segmentally dilated capillaries filled with pale-staining lipid material ⇨ that is not well preserved in routine paraffin sections.* **(Right)** *The lipid thrombi ➡ distend glomerular capillaries in lipoprotein glomerulopathy are well preserved in fresh frozen tissue and positive with oil red O.*

Lipid "Thrombi"

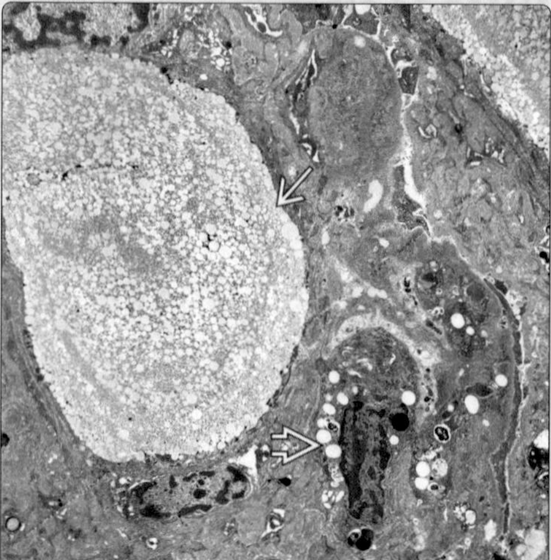

Lipoprotein Particles

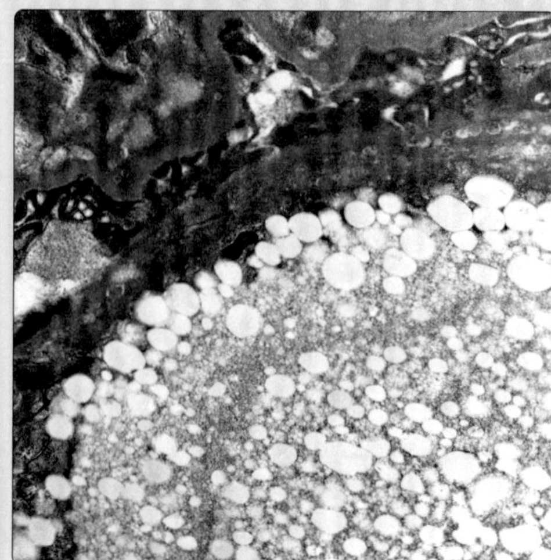

(Left) *In lipoprotein glomerulopathy, glomerular capillaries are filled with vacuolated lipoprotein thrombi ➡. Mesangial and subendothelial cells contain lipid vacuoles ➡.* **(Right)** *High magnification of intracapillary thrombi in lipoprotein glomerulopathy shows vacuolated lipoprotein particles.*

APOE Lipoprotein Glomerulopathy

TERMINOLOGY

Abbreviations

- Lipoprotein glomerulopathy (LPG)

Definitions

- Glomerular disease characterized by capillary lipoprotein thrombi, proteinuria, and progressive renal failure

ETIOLOGY/PATHOGENESIS

Genetics

- *APOE* gene mutation
  - Encodes apolipoprotein E (ApoE)
    - Major component of chylomicrons and intermediate density lipoprotein (IDL) particles that transport triglycerides
    - Cleared from circulation by receptor-mediated endocytosis in liver
  - Autosomal recessive trait
    - Chromosome 19
    - Mutation results in defective lipoprotein receptor binding
    - Hyperlipoproteinemia results (type III)
- 2 major loci of mutations
  - Exon 3
    - Kyoto mutation Cys25Arg
    - Gln3Lys
  - Exon 4 (LDL receptor binding site)
    - Tokyo Leu141-Lys143 del
    - Sendai Arg145Pro
    - Arg147Pro
    - Arg150Gly
    - Arg150Pro
    - Las Vegas Ala152Asp
    - Gln156-Lys173 del
- Macrophage Fc receptor deficiency enhances disease in mouse models

CLINICAL ISSUES

Epidemiology

- Incidence
  - Rare; < 80 cases reported
- Age
  - 4-69 years; mean: 32 ± 2.2 years
- Sex
  - M:F = 3:2
- Ethnicity
  - Predominantly Japanese, Taiwanese, and Chinese
  - Occasionally reported in Caucasians/Europeans

Presentation

- Proteinuria, mild to severe
- Elevated serum apolipoprotein E to ~ 2x upper normal range
- Elevated very low-density lipoprotein
- Elevated intermediate-density lipoprotein
- May be associated with IgA, membranous, or lupus nephritis
- May be associated with psoriasis vulgaris

Laboratory Tests

- *APOE* gene sequence analysis

Treatment

- Drugs
  - Fibrates
  - Niceritrol
  - Probucol

Prognosis

- 50% progress to renal failure
- Intensive lipid-lowering therapy may result in clinical and pathologic remission

MICROSCOPIC

Histologic Features

- Marked dilatation of glomerular capillary loops with pale substance
- Foam cells in glomeruli or interstitium

ANCILLARY TESTS

Frozen Sections

- Oil red O stain shows lipid thrombi in glomerular capillaries

Immunohistochemistry

- Antibodies to apolipoproteins B or E highlight intraglomerular thrombi

Immunofluorescence

- No specific deposition of immunoglobulin or complement

Electron Microscopy

- Glomerular capillaries contain variably sized granules and vacuoles forming lamellated structures
  - Clusters of circulating IDLs ~ 24-35 nm
- Lipid droplets in mesangial and endothelial cells

DIFFERENTIAL DIAGNOSIS

Fat Emboli

- Round globules of fat
- Little or no apolipoprotein component
- No finely vacuolated pattern on electron microscopy

Focal Segmental Glomerulosclerosis, Tip or Cellular Variant

- Glomerular capillary foam cells

SELECTED REFERENCES

1. Hu Z et al: Hereditary features, treatment, and prognosis of the lipoprotein glomerulopathy in patients with the APOE Kyoto mutation. Kidney Int. 85(2):416-24, 2014
2. Toyota K et al: A founder haplotype of APOE-Sendai mutation associated with lipoprotein glomerulopathy. J Hum Genet. 58(5):254-8, 2013
3. Bomback AS et al: A new apolipoprotein E mutation, apoE Las Vegas, in a European-American with lipoprotein glomerulopathy. Nephrol Dial Transplant. 25(10):3442-6, 2010
4. Han J et al: Common apolipoprotein E gene mutations contribute to lipoprotein glomerulopathy in China. Nephron Clin Pract. 114(4):c260-7, 2010
5. Zhang B et al: Clinicopathological and genetic characteristics in Chinese patients with lipoprotein glomerulopathy. J Nephrol. 21(1):110-7, 2008
6. Rovin BH et al: APOE Kyoto mutation in European Americans with lipoprotein glomerulopathy. N Engl J Med. 357(24):2522-4, 2007

Type III Collagen Glomerulopathy

KEY FACTS

TERMINOLOGY

- Idiopathic glomerular disease defined by accumulation of mesangial and subendothelial type III collagen

CLINICAL ISSUES

- Rare (< 0.1% of biopsies)
- Presents with proteinuria and microscopic hematuria
- Hemolytic uremic syndrome and thrombotic microangiopathy can be seen in children
- Variable disease course
- Increased serum and urine procollagen III peptide

MICROSCOPIC

- Lobular glomeruli without inflammation
- Thickened capillary walls
- Mesangial and capillary wall expansion with pale eosinophilic material
- Electron microscopy
    - Mesangial and subendothelial curvilinear fibrils
    - Fibers tend to be frayed and curved, ~ 60 nm periodicity
- Immunohistochemical staining for type III collagen positive in mesangium and GBM

TOP DIFFERENTIAL DIAGNOSES

- Nail-patella syndrome
- Hereditary multiple exostoses
- Fibronectin glomerulopathy
- Amyloidosis
- Fibrillary glomerulopathy
- Diabetic fibrillosis

DIAGNOSTIC CHECKLIST

- Diagnosis made by demonstration of banded collagen in glomeruli by EM
- Confirmation by immunohistochemical staining for type III collagen
- Must exclude nail-patella syndrome clinically

(Left) *Type III collagen glomerulopathy shows mesangial expansion by homogeneous, pale material and segmental hypercellularity.* **(Right)** *Jones silver stain shows frequent double contour formation by interposition of pale material ⇨.*

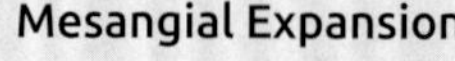

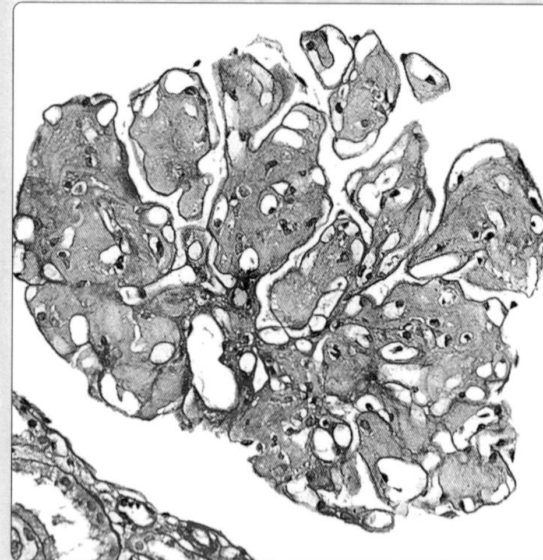

Double Contours on Silver Stain

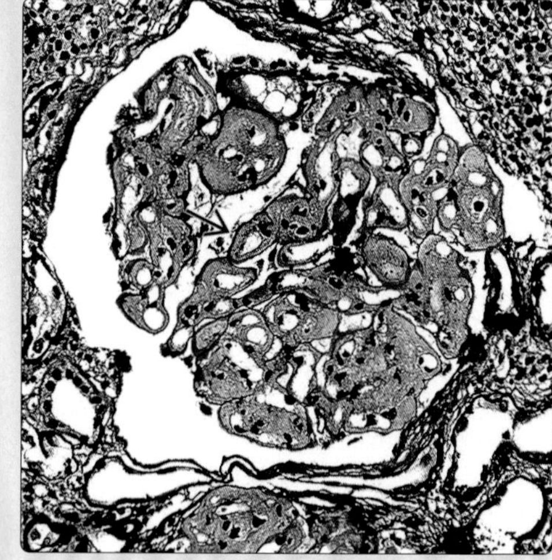

(Left) *Immunohistochemical stain for collagen III shows deposits of collagen III in the GBM and mesangium in a case of type III collagen glomerulopathy. Normal glomeruli have no detectable type III collagen.* **(Right)** *Trichrome stain shows mesangial → and capillary wall ⇨ expansion by pale, blue staining material. (Courtesy A. Abraham, MD.)*

Type III Collagen Staining

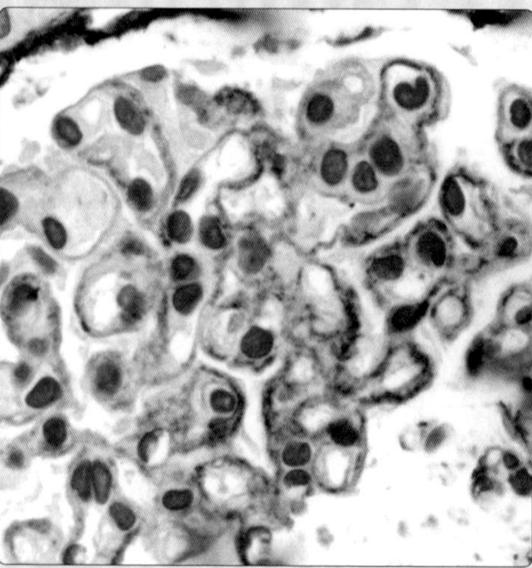

Trichrome Stain With Mesangial Expansion

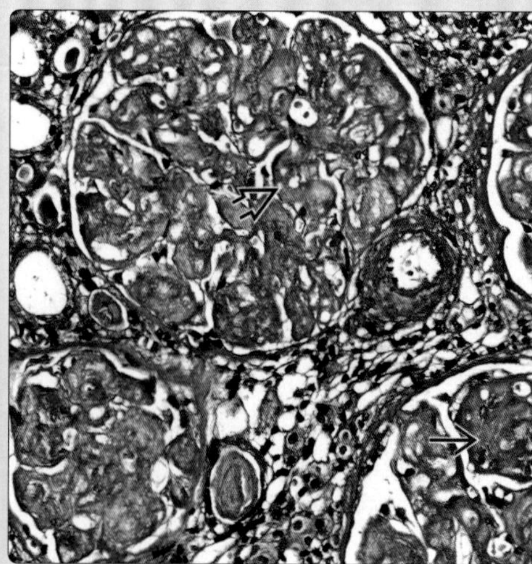

TERMINOLOGY

Synonyms

- Collagenofibrotic glomerulopathy

Definitions

- Idiopathic glomerular disease defined by accumulation of type III collagen in mesangium and subendothelial space
  - Initially described by Arakawa and colleagues in 1979

ETIOLOGY/PATHOGENESIS

Unknown

- Controversy whether this represents systemic or primary glomerular disease
  - Underlying defect in type III collagen synthesis/production postulated
    - Genetic basis if any not identified
- Accumulation of type III collagen in mesangial and subendothelial space
  - Site and extent of type III collagen production unknown
    - Type III collagen virtually absent in normal glomeruli
  - Co-deposition of types I and V collagen with type III also reported
- N-terminal procollagen type III peptide (PIIINP)
  - Markedly increased quantities reported in urine of those with type III collagen glomerulopathy
    - Not specific to type III collagen glomerulopathy and can be seen in advanced renal disease

Animal Models

- Canine autosomal recessive disorder
  - Does **not** involve *Col3A1* gene

CLINICAL ISSUES

Epidemiology

- Incidence
  - Rare (~ 0.1% of biopsies)
- Age
  - All ages; rarely reported after age 60
- Sex
  - M:F = 1:1
- Ethnicity
  - Majority of cases from Japan where disease first described
    - Also reported in USA, Europe, India, South America, China
  - Increased incidence reported in southern/western India

Presentation

- Proteinuria
- Edema
- Microscopic hematuria
- Hypertension
- Childhood onset
  - Frequent family history of nephropathy, especially in siblings
  - Autosomal recessive inheritance suggested, but genetic basis unknown
  - Earliest report is 3 months of age
  - Superimposed hemolytic uremic syndrome common
  - Hemolytic anemia
  - Poorly defined respiratory disease
  - Rare association with hypocomplementemia and complement factor H deficiency
- Adult onset
  - Typically sporadic without family history of renal disease
  - Can occur at any age
    - Most frequently reported in 30s and 40s
    - Rarely reported in patients over 60 (oldest 79)
  - Anemia may be present
    - Especially those with chronic kidney disease
  - Rare association with Hodgkin lymphoma and hepatic perisinusoidal fibrosis

Laboratory Tests

- 10-100x increase in serum and urine PIIINP
  - Not specific to type III collagen glomerulopathy
- 1,000x increase in serum hyaluronan

Treatment

- Drugs
  - No clinical trials performed to evaluate efficacy of treatments
  - No specific treatment advocated currently
  - Steroid therapy reported to slow disease progression

Prognosis

- Variable disease course, limited data
  - ~ 35% of adults progress to end-stage renal disease
    - Most have slow consistent decline in renal function
  - ~ 90% of children progress to end-stage renal disease
    - May progress rapidly, especially if superimposed hemolytic uremic syndrome present

MICROSCOPIC

Histologic Features

- Glomeruli
  - Lobular accentuation
    - Nodular pattern may resemble diabetic glomerulopathy
    - Less pronounced cases resemble membranoproliferative GN
  - Mesangial expansion and variable hypercellularity
    - Expansion by pale to segmentally eosinophilic material on PAS stain
      - Usually silver negative but can be variably argyrophilic
      - Pale, light blue staining by trichrome
  - GBM thickening
    - Variable double contour formation with intervening pale, silver negative material
    - Some show predominantly double contour formation with only minor mesangial expansion
  - Rare endocapillary foam cells may be present
  - Thrombi (may be pseudothrombi)
- Tubules
  - No specific changes
- Interstitium
  - Foci of interstitial foam cells may be present
- Vessels

- No specific changes
- Other organs
  - Deposition of collagen III along sinusoids in liver
    - Deposits also in spleen, myocardium, and thyroid gland

ANCILLARY TESTS

Immunohistochemistry

- Staining for type III collagen confirms presence of abnormal collagen in mesangium or GBM
  - Case reports with accumulation of collagen type I or V

Immunofluorescence

- Glomerular accumulation of pale material shows no significant immune complex deposition
  - Nonspecific trapping of IgM and C3 may be seen

Electron Microscopy

- Mesangial and subendothelial fibrillar collagen deposits
  - Morphology of collagen differs depending on method of fixation
  - In routine prepared and paraffin-retrieved EM, collagen forms stacked bundles that show irregular, frayed edges and mild curvilinear morphology
    - Irregular bundles on longitudinal sectioning
    - Collagen fibers have characteristic ~ 60 nm periodicity (banded pattern bundles)
    - Collagen bundles occur on background of electron-lucent, expanded mesangium and subendothelial space
    - Subepithelial and intramembranous deposition not typically seen
  - When tannic acid-lead or phosphotungstic acid employed, similar collagen bundles seen, however
    - Superior detail with more pronounced curvilinear structure
- GBM lamina densa of normal thickness
- Foot process effacement variable

DIFFERENTIAL DIAGNOSIS

Nail-Patella Syndrome

- Characteristic bone and nail abnormalities may be absent
- Collagen deposits in GBM sparse and discrete
- Absence of curvilinear bundles of collagen by EM
- Presence of characteristic moth-eaten appearance of GBM

Hereditary Multiple Exostoses

- Absence of IHC staining for type III collagen
- Absence of curvilinear bundles of collagen by EM
- Presence of mesangial and subendothelial collagen deposition

Fibronectin Glomerulopathy

- Absence of IHC staining for type III collagen
- Absence of curvilinear bundles of collagen by EM
- Presence of granular, fibrillary electron-dense deposits measuring 9-16 nm in diameter
- Presence of glomerular fibronectin deposits by IF or IHC

Fibrillary Glomerulopathy

- Presence of capillary wall and mesangial smudgy to granular staining for IgG, C3, kappa, and lambda
- Presence of random, 10-30 nm fibrils in mesangium and capillary walls
- Absence of curvilinear bundles of collagen by EM
- Absence of IHC staining for type III collagen

Diabetic Fibrillosis

- Presence of densely packed, randomly oriented, non-branching microfibrils measuring 10-25 nm on electron microscopy
- Presence of diabetic glomerulopathy
- Absence of curvilinear bundles of collagen by EM
- Absence of IHC staining for type III collagen

Membranoproliferative Glomerulonephritis

- Presence of immune complex deposition by immunofluorescence
- Presence of immune complex deposition by electron microscopy
- Absence of curvilinear bundles of collagen by EM
- Absence of IHC staining for type III collagen

Amyloidosis

- Presence of Congo red positive deposits
- Presence of random, 8-12 nm non-banded fibrils in mesangium and capillary walls
- Absence of curvilinear bundles of collagen by EM
- Absence of IHC staining for type III collagen

DIAGNOSTIC CHECKLIST

Pathologic Interpretation Pearls

- Diagnosis by EM demonstration of collagen type III in glomeruli
  - Confirmed by immunohistochemical staining for type III collagen

SELECTED REFERENCES

1. Bao H et al: Clinical and morphological features of collagen type III glomerulopathy: a report of nine cases from a single institution. Histopathology. ePub, 2015
2. Goto S et al: Marked elevation of serum hyaluronan levels in collagenofibrotic glomerulopathy. Intern Med. 53(16):1801-4, 2014
3. Cohen AH: Collagen Type III Glomerulopathies. Adv Chronic Kidney Dis. 19(2):101-6, 2012
4. Rørtveit R et al: A canine autosomal recessive model of collagen type III glomerulopathy. Lab Invest. 92(10):1483-91, 2012
5. Khubchandani SR et al: Banded collagen in the kidney with special reference to collagenofibrotic glomerulopathy. Ultrastruct Pathol. 34(2):68-72, 2010
6. Ferreira RD et al: Collagenofibrotic glomerulopathy: three case reports in Brazil. Diagn Pathol. 4:33, 2009
7. Alchi B et al: Collagenofibrotic glomerulopathy: clinicopathologic overview of a rare glomerular disease. Am J Kidney Dis. 49(4):499-506, 2007
8. Yasuda T et al: Collagenofibrotic glomerulopathy: a systemic disease. Am J Kidney Dis. 33(1):123-7, 1999
9. Vogt BA et al: Inherited factor H deficiency and collagen type III glomerulopathy. Pediatr Nephrol. 9(1):11-5, 1995
10. Gubler MC et al: Collagen type III glomerulopathy: a new type of hereditary nephropathy. Pediatr Nephrol. 7(4):354-60, 1993
11. Arakawa M et al: [Idiopathic mesangio-degenerative glomerulopathy]. Jpn J Nephrol 21:914-5, 1979

Mesangial Type III Collagen Bundles

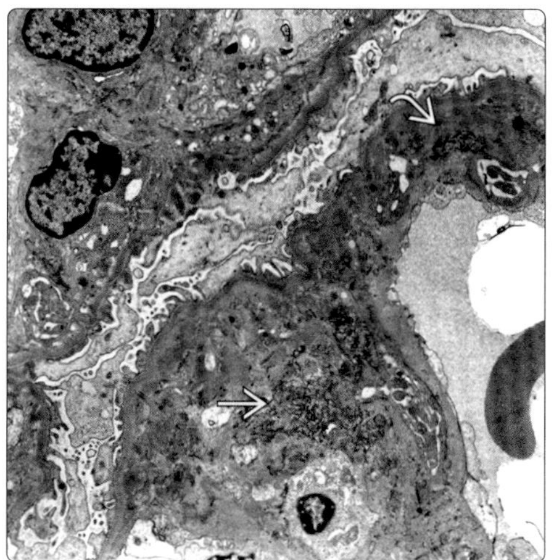

Curvilinear Type III Collagen

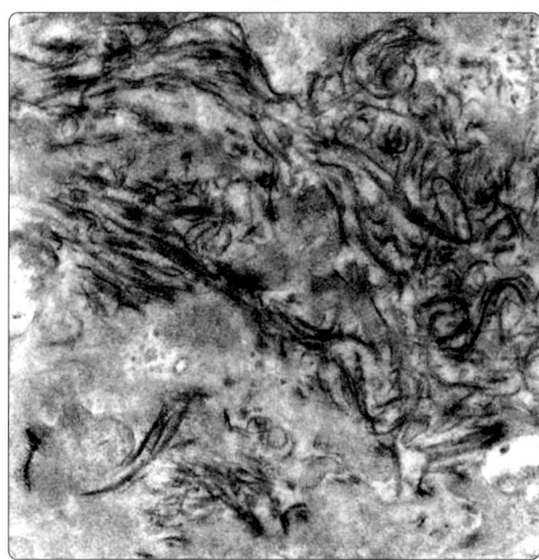

(Left) *This example of type III collagen glomerulopathy demonstrates characteristic curvilinear fibrils of collagen in the mesangium →, GBM ↗, and the subendothelial space.* **(Right)** *This specimen was stained with tannic acid-lead and processed for electron microscopy. The tannic acid highlights the randomly arranged, curved, and banded collagen fibers within the mesangium.*

Positive Type III Collagen Stain

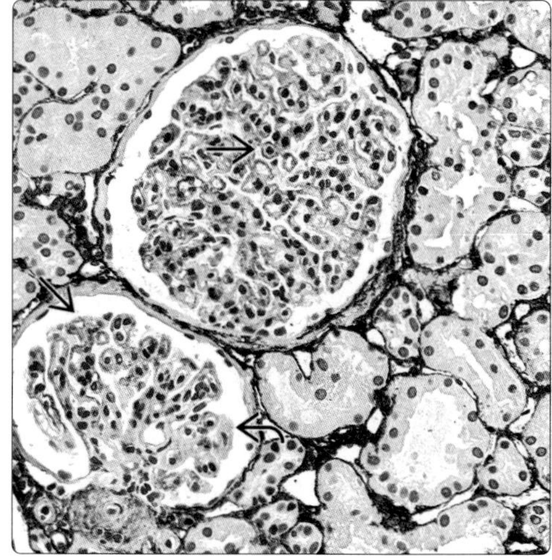

Negative Type III Collagen Stain

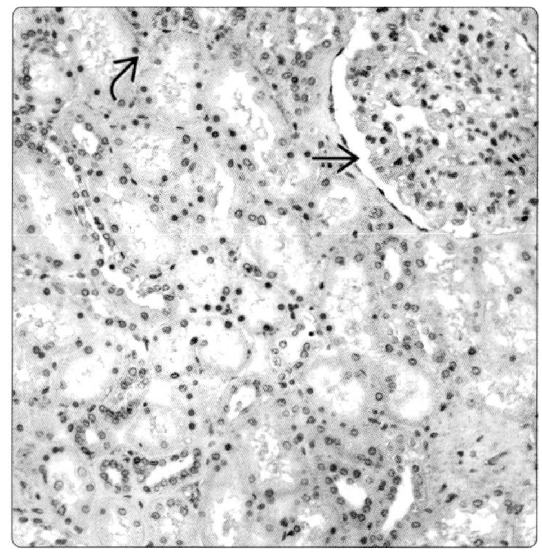

(Left) *An immunohistochemical stain for collagen III (BioGenex MU167-UC) shows prominent GBM → and mesangial deposits of collagen III. Some capillaries are negative ↗. The interstitium also stains, but this is a normal feature of interstitial fibrosis.* **(Right)** *In contrast, a normal kidney stained with antibody to collagen III shows no glomerular immunoreactivity →. Small amounts are, however, seen in the interstitium ↗.*

Fibrillary Glomerulopathy

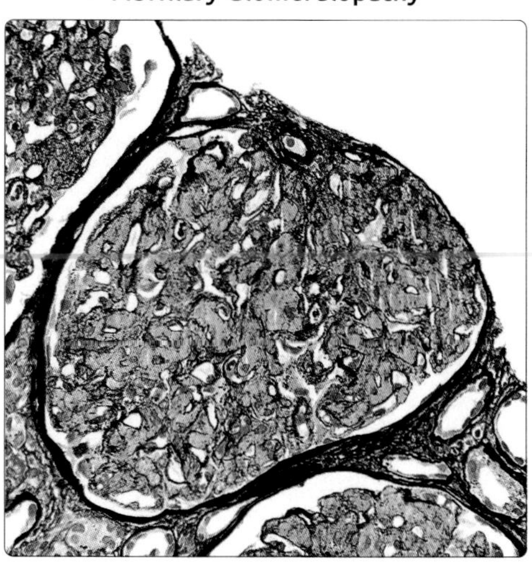

Fibrils in Fibrillary Glomerulopathy

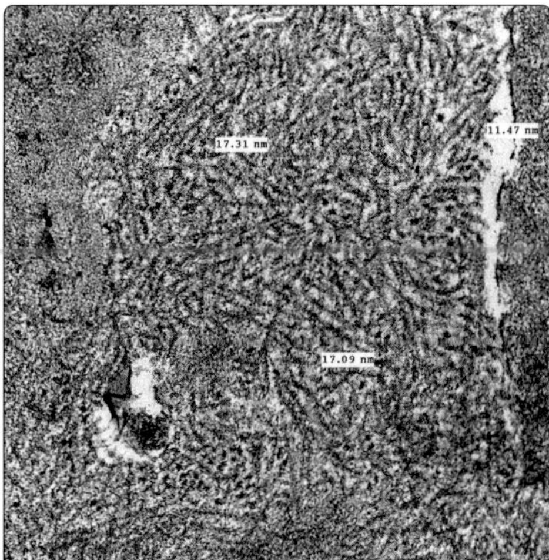

(Left) *Fibrillary GN can resemble collagen III glomerulopathy by light microscopy but is readily distinguished by immunofluorescence as the deposits consist of IgG, not collagen (silver stain).* **(Right)** *For comparison, fibrils in fibrillary glomerulopathy lack periodicity and are thinner, measuring less than half the size of fibrillar collagen, 15-25 nm in diameter.*

KEY FACTS

TERMINOLOGY

- Autosomal recessive disorder, manifested by early onset nephrotic syndrome, hiatal hernia, and microcephaly

ETIOLOGY/PATHOGENESIS

- Genetic basis may be heterogeneous
  - *WDR73* mutation identified in 2 families

CLINICAL ISSUES

- Clinically heterogeneous
- Diverse neurological symptoms
- Steroid-resistant nephrotic syndrome leading to renal failure by 6 years
- Fatal in early childhood

MICROSCOPIC

- Diffuse mesangial sclerosis (DMS)
  - Capillary loop collapse
  - Epithelial cell hyperplasia
  - Mesangial matrix increase ± hypercellularity
  - Podocyte foot process effacement
  - Glomerular basement membrane abnormalities
- Focal segmental glomerulosclerosis (FSGS)
  - Segmental sclerosing lesions
  - Podocyte foot process effacement abnormalities
  - No glomerular basement membrane abnormalities
- Minimal change disease
  - Seen in early biopsies but evolve into FSGS or DMS

TOP DIFFERENTIAL DIAGNOSES

- Diffuse mesangial sclerosis
  - Denys-Drash syndrome; *WT1* mutation
  - Pierson syndrome; *LAMB2* mutation
  - Lowe syndrome; *OCRL1* mutation
- Focal segmental glomerulosclerosis
  - Frasier syndrome; *WT1* mutation
  - Nail-patella syndrome; *LMX1B* mutation

Diffuse Mesangial Sclerosis in Galloway-Mowat Syndrome

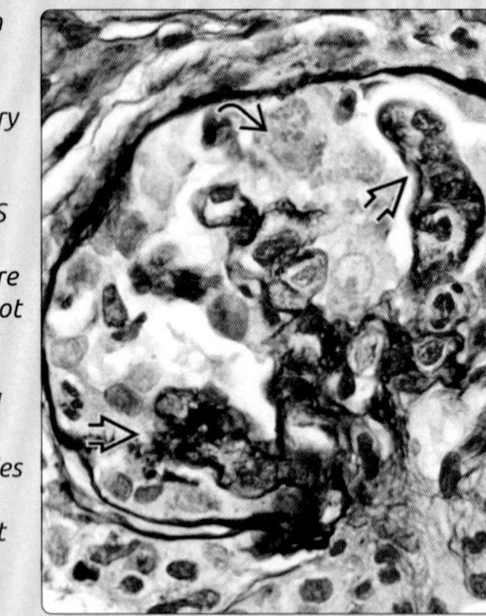

Glomerular Basement Membrane Abnormalities

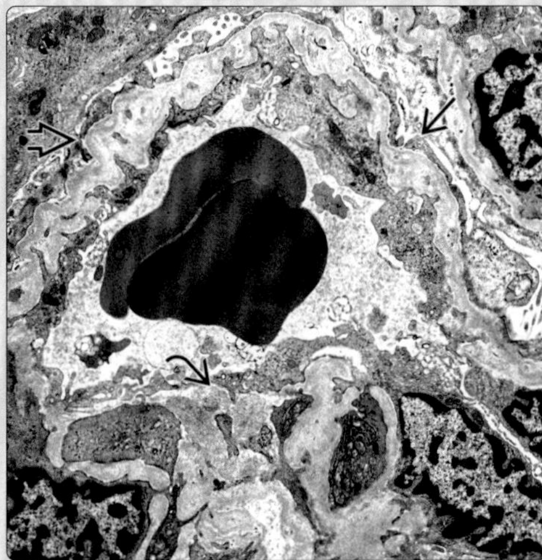

(Left) *This glomerulus is from a 3 year old with GMS. It shows diffuse mesangial matrix expansion and capillary loop collapse ➡. Prominent epithelial hyperplasia ➡ is a characteristic feature of DMS and resembles collapsing glomerulopathy.* **(Right)** *There is effacement of podocyte foot processes ➡. The capillary loop basement membrane shows marked thickening ➡ and irregularity with basement membrane lucencies that contain tiny cell remnants. There is prominent mesangial matrix expansion ➡.*

Focal Segmental Glomerulosclerosis in Galloway-Mowat Syndrome

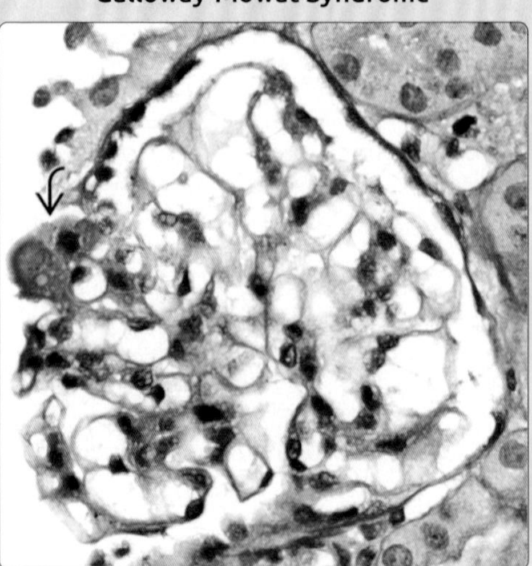

Segmental Sclerosis With Capsular Adhesion

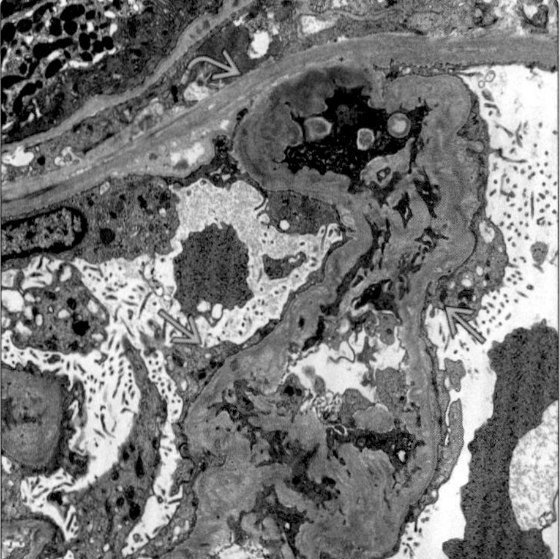

(Left) *This glomerulus from a 2 year old with GMS shows focal segmental glomerulosclerosis. There is a small segmental sclerosing lesion ➡ with hyaline accumulation and tiny lipid droplets. The remainder of the glomerulus is essentially normal.* **(Right)** *This electron micrograph shows a small area of segmental sclerosis with a small amount of hyaline and lipid and adhesion to Bowman capsule ➡. There is diffuse podocyte foot process effacement with microvillus transformation ➡.*

Galloway-Mowat Syndrome

TERMINOLOGY

Abbreviations

- Galloway-Mowat syndrome (GMS) glomerulopathy

Synonyms

- Nephrosis-microcephaly syndrome

Definitions

- Autosomal recessive disorder, manifested by early onset nephrotic syndrome, hiatal hernia, and microcephaly

ETIOLOGY/PATHOGENESIS

Developmental Anomaly

- Autosomal recessive
- Genetic basis may be heterogeneous
  - *WDR73* mutation identified in 2 families
  - WDR73 protein associated with microtubules and expressed in developing glomerular podocytes

CLINICAL ISSUES

Presentation

- Clinically heterogeneous
- Wide spectrum of neurological manifestations
  - Microcephaly; most common feature
  - Seizures and psychomotor delay often occur
- Steroid-resistant nephrotic syndrome in 1st months of life
  - Diffuse mesangial sclerosis (DMS)
  - Focal segmental glomerulosclerosis/minimal change disease
- Hiatal hernia in some cases
- May have dysmorphic facial features
  - Micrognathia
  - Ocular abnormalities
  - Receding forehead
  - Large floppy ears

Treatment

- No known treatment

Prognosis

- Often fatal in childhood, inevitable by 6 years
- Progresses to end-stage renal disease in 2-3 years

MACROSCOPIC

General Features

- Dysmorphic craniofacial features
- Deformities of extremities
- Ocular abnormalities
- Abnormal gyri and sulci in brain
- Cerebellar atrophy

MICROSCOPIC

Histologic Features

- Diffuse mesangial sclerosis
  - Glomerular capillary loop collapse
  - Epithelial hyperplasia overlying collapsed loops
    - Resembles collapsing glomerulopathy
  - Mesangial matrix increase ± hypercellularity
  - Tubular ectasia and tubulointerstitial scarring
  - Immunofluorescence
    - Negative for immune reactants
    - IgM and C3 in areas of sclerosis
  - Electron microscopy
    - Irregular glomerular basement membrane thickening
    - Lucent foci and lamina densa splitting
    - Diffuse podocyte foot process effacement
- Focal segmental glomerulosclerosis
  - Segmental sclerosing lesions
  - Immunofluorescence
    - Negative for immune reactants
    - IgM and C3 in areas of sclerosis
  - Electron microscopy
    - Glomerular basement membrane normal
    - Podocyte foot process effacement
- Minimal change disease
  - May evolve into diffuse mesangial sclerosis
  - May evolve into focal segmental glomerulosclerosis
- Other glomerular lesions described
  - Diffuse mesangial hypercellularity
    - May subsequently evolve into DMS or FSGS
    - GBM changes resembling DMS must be absent
  - Focal segmental glomerulosclerosis with collapsing features

DIFFERENTIAL DIAGNOSIS

Syndromic Forms of DMS

- Denys-Drash syndrome
  - *WT1* mutation
- Pierson syndrome
  - *LAMB2* mutation
- Lowe syndrome
  - *OCRL1* mutation

Syndromic Forms of FSGS

- Frasier syndrome
  - *WT1* mutation
- Nail-patella syndrome
  - *LMX1B* mutation

DIAGNOSTIC CHECKLIST

Pathologic Interpretation Pearls

- In congenital and infantile nephrotic syndrome, knowledge of syndromic features is essential to diagnosis

SELECTED REFERENCES

1. Colin E et al: Loss-of-function mutations in WDR73 are responsible for microcephaly and steroid-resistant nephrotic syndrome: Galloway-Mowat syndrome. Am J Hum Genet. 95(6):637-48, 2014
2. Sartelet H et al: Collapsing glomerulopathy in Galloway-Mowat syndrome: a case report and review of the literature. Pathol Res Pract. 204(6):401-6, 2008
3. Lin CC et al: Galloway-Mowat syndrome: a glomerular basement membrane disorder? Pediatr Nephrol. 16(8):653-7, 2001
4. Kucharczuk K et al: Additional findings in Galloway-Mowat syndrome. Pediatr Nephrol. 14(5):406-9, 2000
5. Sano H et al: Microcephaly and early-onset nephrotic syndrome–confusion in Galloway-Mowat syndrome. Pediatr Nephrol. 9(6):711-4, 1995
6. Cohen AH et al: Kidney in Galloway-Mowat syndrome: clinical spectrum with description of pathology. Kidney Int. 45(5):1407-15, 1994

(**Left**) *These glomeruli from a patient with GMS show early DMS. The glomerulus on the left shows mild mesangial matrix increase with mild mesangial hypercellularity. Overall, these features would be regarded as minimal change disease except that GBM changes on EM indicate DMS.* (**Right**) *This glomerulus shows minimal abnormalities. There is mesangial matrix increase and a cluster of prominent podocytes. No evidence of capillary loop collapse is present.*

Galloway-Mowat Syndrome With Minimal Glomerular Abnormalities

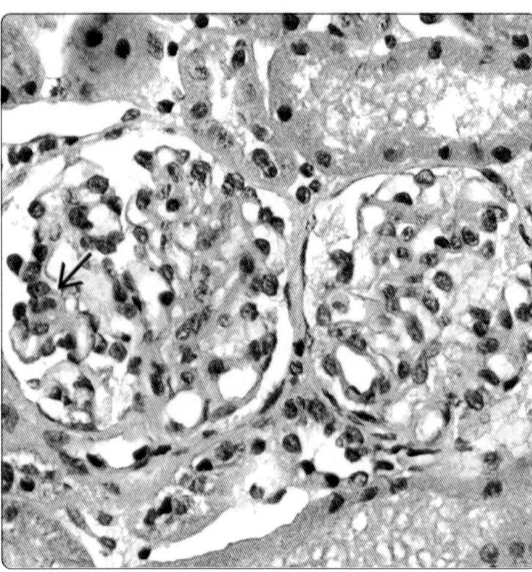

Galloway-Mowat Syndrome With Minimal Glomerular Abnormalities

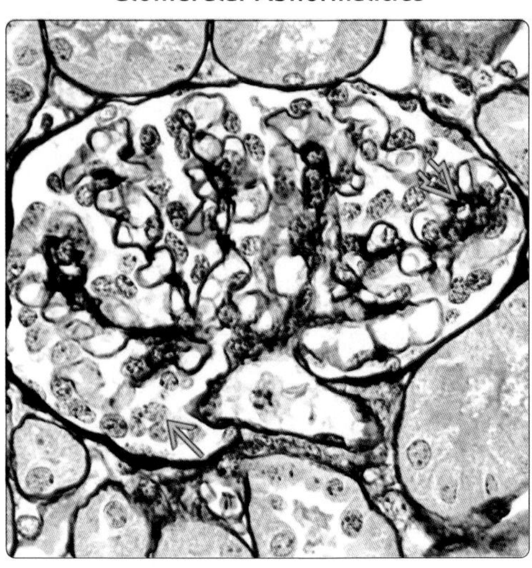

(**Left**) *This glomerulus in GMS is nearly normal. However, it does show mild mesangial hypercellularity without capillary loop alterations. The podocytes are more prominent than normal but would not in themselves be diagnostic.* (**Right**) *This EM in GMS shows diffuse effacement of podocyte foot processes. The capillary loop basement membrane shows mild thickening with mild lucency and subtle lamellations of the GBM similar to early changes encountered in Alport syndrome.*

Mild Mesangial Hypercellularity

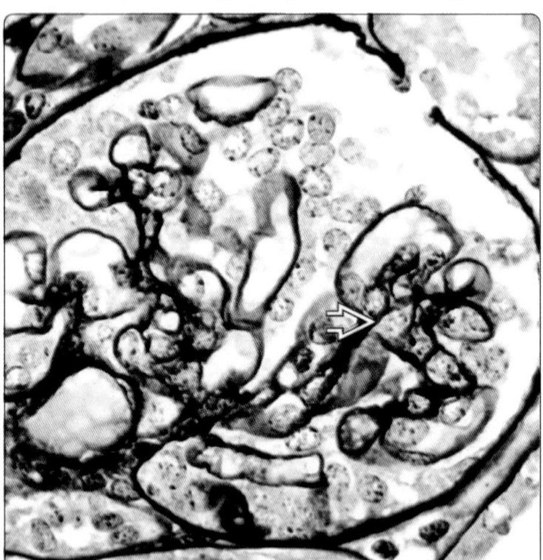

Mild Glomerular Basement Membrane Abnormalities

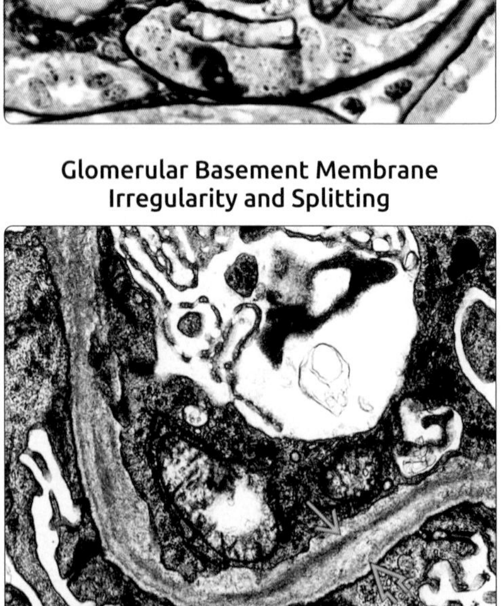

(**Left**) *This capillary loop in GMS with DMS shows diffuse podocyte foot process effacement. There is a complete sheet of cytoplasm covering the capillary loop. The basement membrane is diffusely thickened and "split" resulting in a double lamina densa layer.* (**Right**) *In DMS of GMS, the capillary loop basement membrane may be markedly abnormal. There is impressive irregularity and thickening of the lamina rara interna and lamina rara externa. The lamina densa is irregularly thickened and splayed.*

Glomerular Basement Membrane Irregularity and Splitting

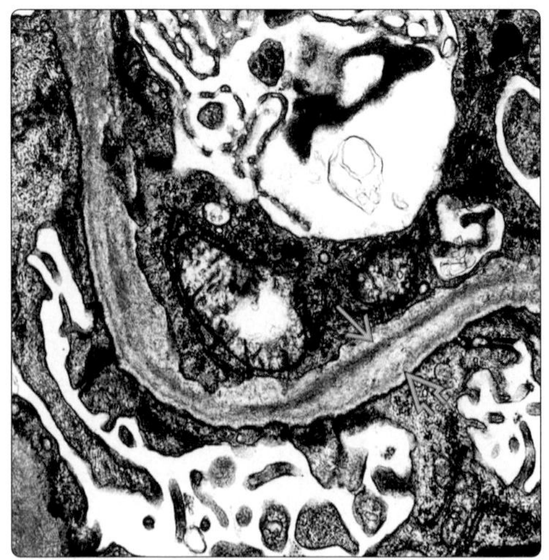

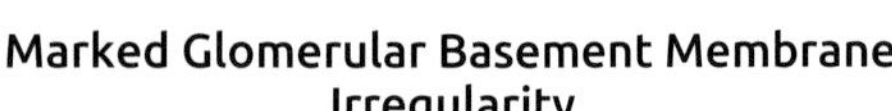

Marked Glomerular Basement Membrane Irregularity

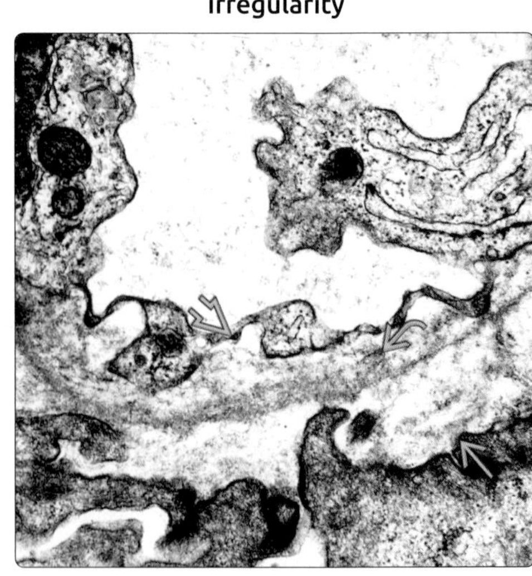

Mesangial Matrix Expansion in Galloway-Mowat Syndrome

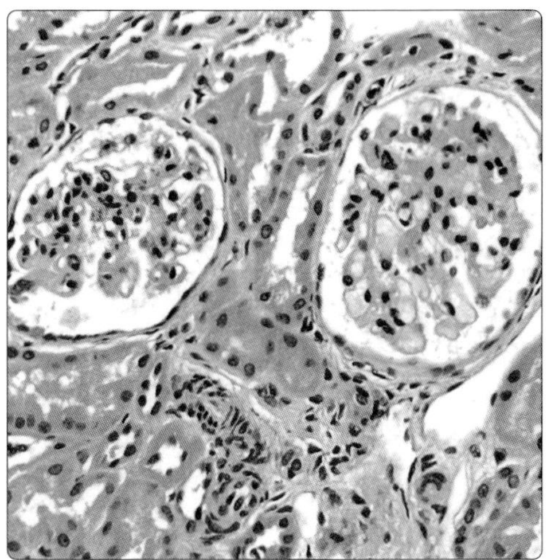

Variability in Mesangial Matrix Expansion in Galloway-Mowat Syndrome

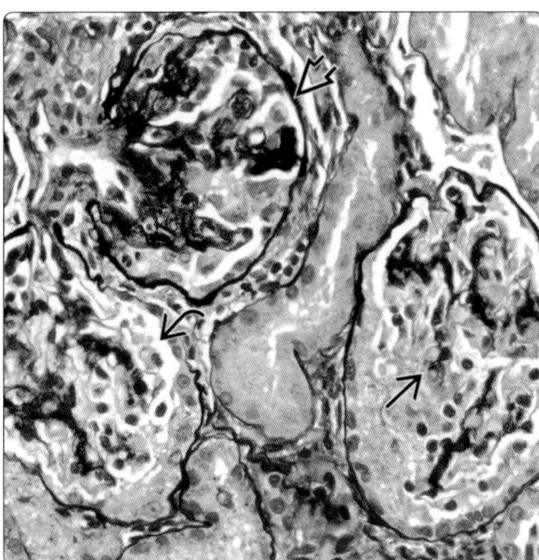

(Left) *These 2 glomeruli in a 3 year old with GMS and diffuse mesangial sclerosis show variable degrees of mesangial matrix increase. There is also mild mesangial hypercellularity in the glomerulus on the left.* **(Right)** *This cluster of 3 glomeruli illustrates variable severity of involvement. One glomerulus ➩ shows pronounced mesangial matrix increase and capillary loop collapse. A 2nd glomerulus shows mild mesangial sclerosis ➩, and the 3rd appears essentially normal ➩.*

Marked Variability in Mesangial Matrix

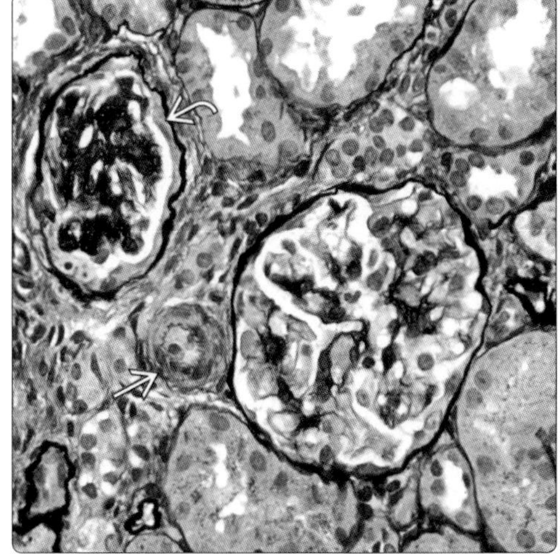

Severe Mesangial Sclerosis

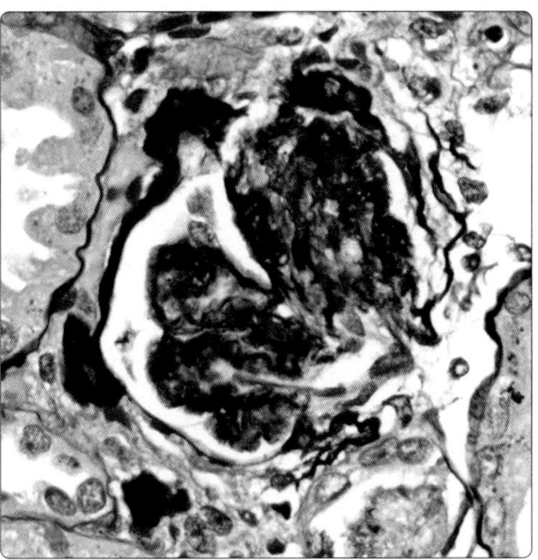

(Left) *This 3 year old with Galloway-Mowat syndrome and diffuse mesangial sclerosis shows a severely affected glomerulus ➩ and a minimally affected glomerulus. There is a markedly thickened arteriole present ➩ with a few adjacent atrophic tubules.* **(Right)** *This glomerulus is completely sclerotic. There is severe mesangial matrix increase and total capillary loop obliteration. Epithelial hyperplasia is absent, possibly because of the terminal stage of the process.*

Mesangial Matrix Expansion and Segmental Sclerosis

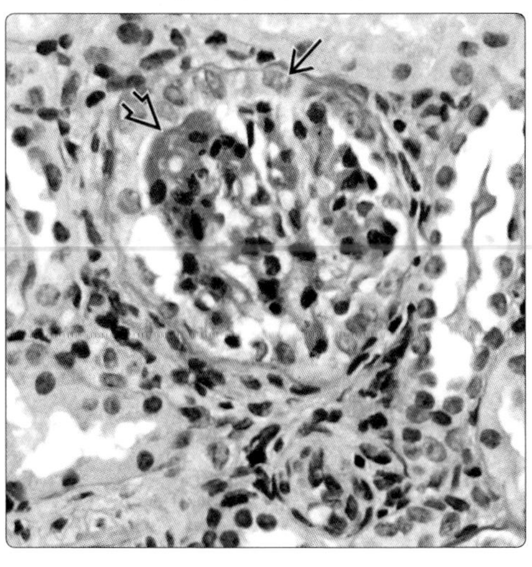

Mesangial Sclerosis and Capillary Loop Collapse

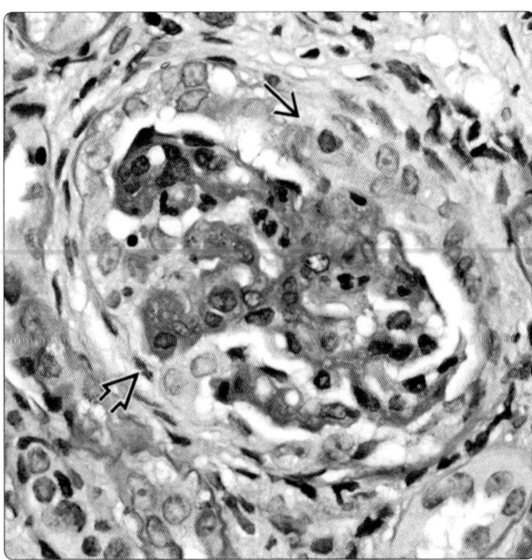

(Left) *This glomerulus shows mild mesangial sclerosis and segmental collapse with hyalinosis similar to FSGS ➩. There is generalized epithelial cell hyperplasia that includes both the parietal ➩ and visceral epithelial cells.* **(Right)** *This glomerulus shows advanced mesangial and capillary loop sclerosis with a capsular adhesion ➩ and disruption of Bowman capsule. There is very prominent epithelial cell hyperplasia involving both parietal ➩ and visceral epithelial cells.*

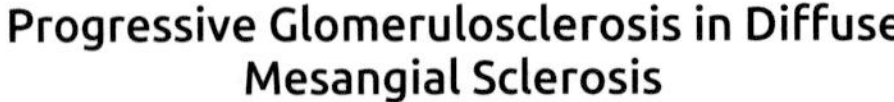

Progressive Glomerulosclerosis in Diffuse Mesangial Sclerosis

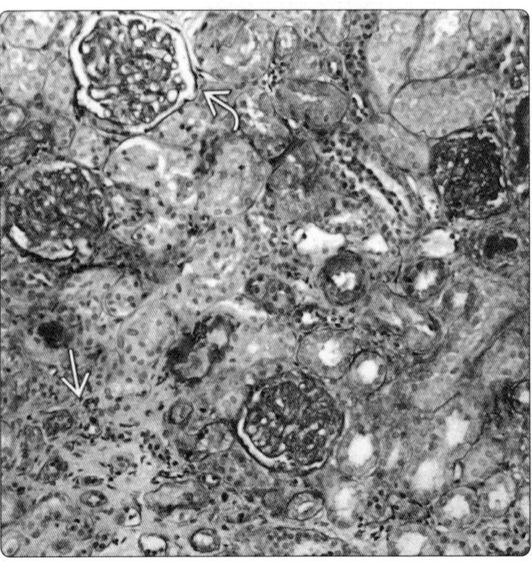

Glomerulosclerosis in Diffuse Mesangial Sclerosis

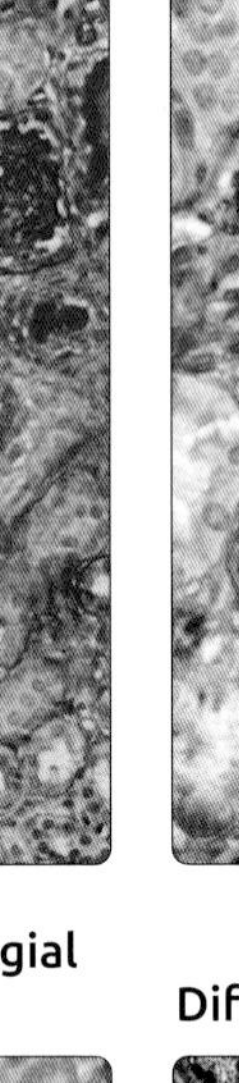

(Left) *This 5-year-old patient with GMS and DMS shows 1 relatively normal glomerulus, while 3 other glomeruli show severe, but somewhat variable, degrees of mesangial sclerosis. Tubulointerstitial scarring is also developing.* **(Right)** *This 5 year old with GMS shows advanced, approaching end-stage, diffuse mesangial sclerosis. One glomerulus shows severe mesangial matrix increase and diffuse capillary loop collapse. The other glomerulus shows mesangial sclerosis with residual, but compromised, capillary loops.*

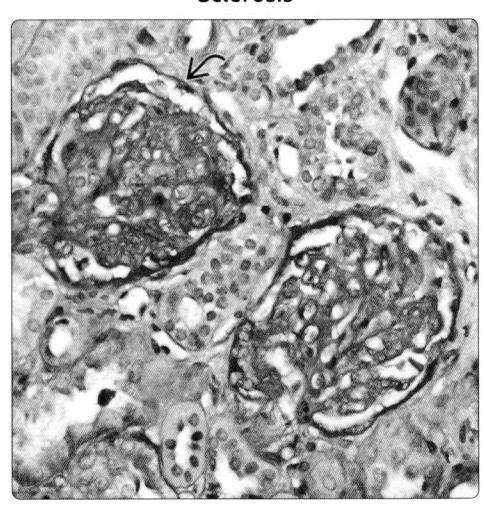

Glomerulosclerosis in Diffuse Mesangial Sclerosis

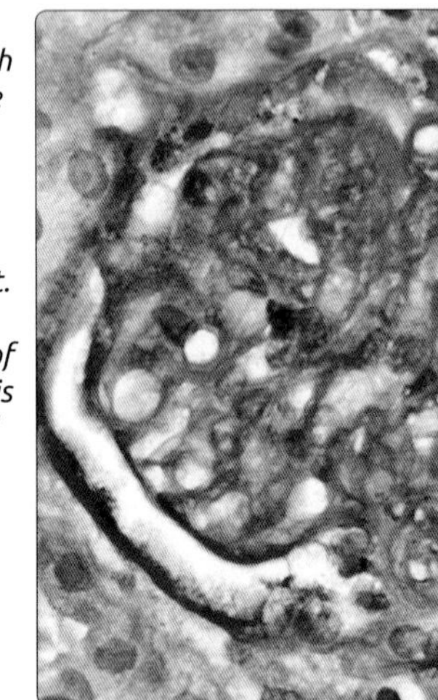

Diffuse Podocyte Foot Process Effacement

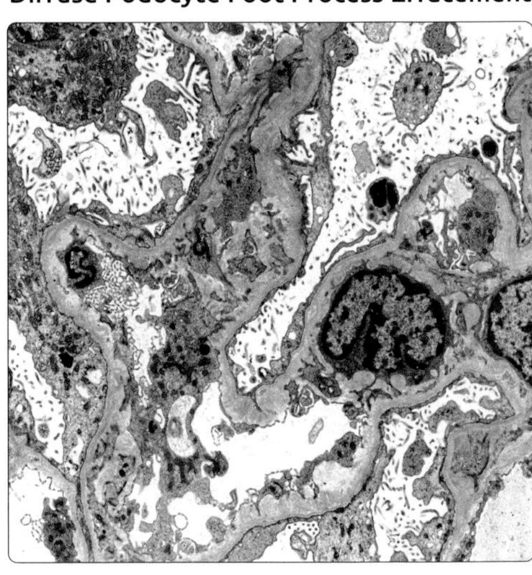

(Left) *This is another glomerulus in a 5 year old with GMS and DMS. There is severe mesangial sclerosis. Most of the capillary loops are completely obliterated with extensive capsular adhesions. Hypercellularity is not present.* **(Right)** *Electron microscopy shows complete effacement of podocyte foot processes in this glomerulus. There is also mild variability in the thickness of the capillary loop basement membrane with prominent scalloping along the inner surface of the capillary loop.*

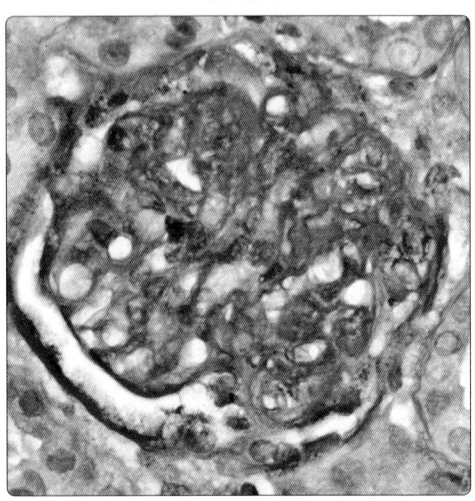

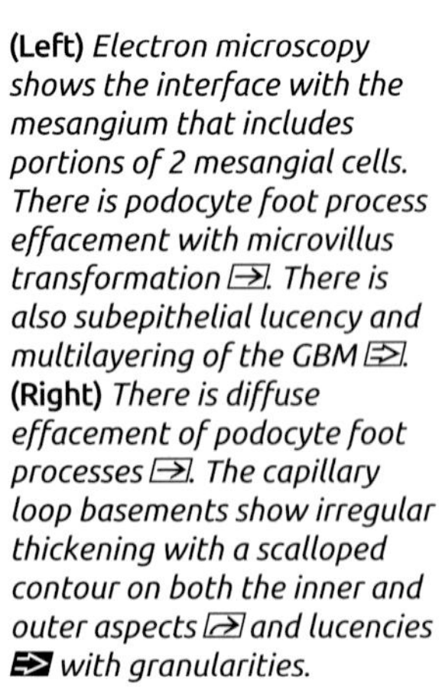

Subepithelial Basement Membrane Abnormalities

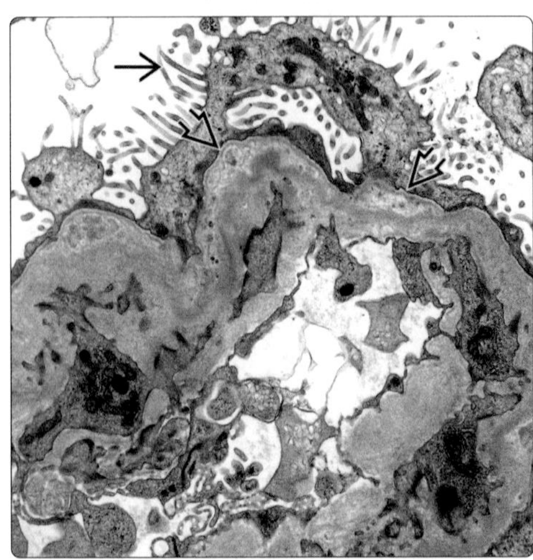

Subepithelial Basement Membrane Abnormalities

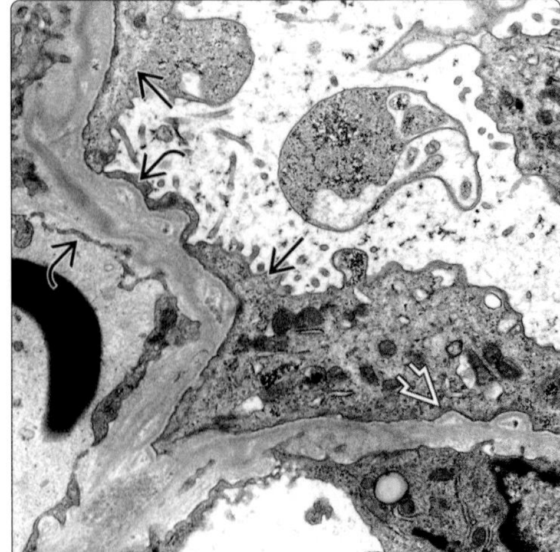

(Left) *Electron microscopy shows the interface with the mesangium that includes portions of 2 mesangial cells. There is podocyte foot process effacement with microvillus transformation. There is also subepithelial lucency and multilayering of the GBM.* **(Right)** *There is diffuse effacement of podocyte foot processes. The capillary loop basements show irregular thickening with a scalloped contour on both the inner and outer aspects and lucencies with granularities.*

Mild Mesangial Hypercellularity in Galloway-Mowat Syndrome

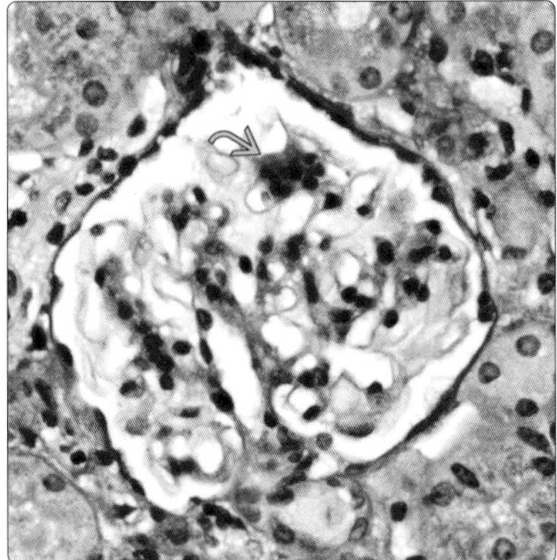

Early Segmental Sclerosis With Epithelial Hyperplasia in Galloway-Mowat Syndrome

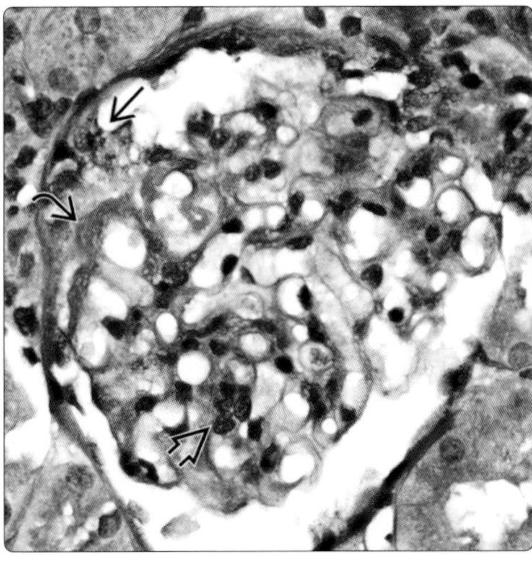

(Left) *This 2 year old with GMS and focal segmental glomerulosclerosis shows the usual spectrum of glomerular lesions associated with that diagnostic entity. This glomerulus shows mild segmental mesangial hypercellularity ⬀, which occurs in FSGS. The capillary loops remain patent.* **(Right)** *This glomerulus shows mild segmental mesangial hypercellularity ⇒ and segmental sclerosis ⬀. The segmental sclerosing lesion contains hyaline and lipid with overlying epithelial hyperplasia ⇒.*

Segmental Sclerosis With Capsular Adhesion in Galloway-Mowat Syndrome

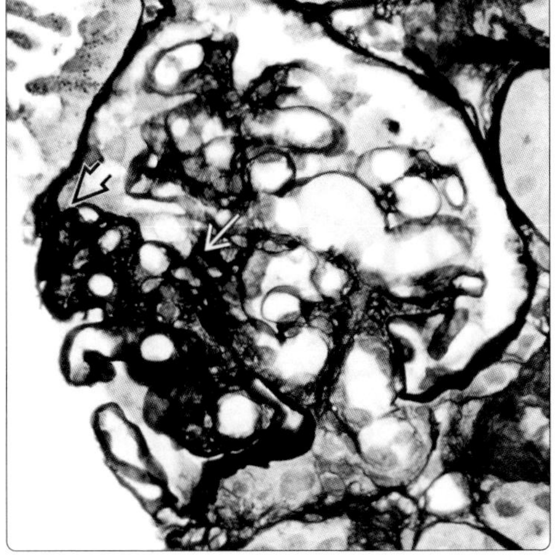

Sclerotic Glomerulus in Galloway-Mowat Syndrome

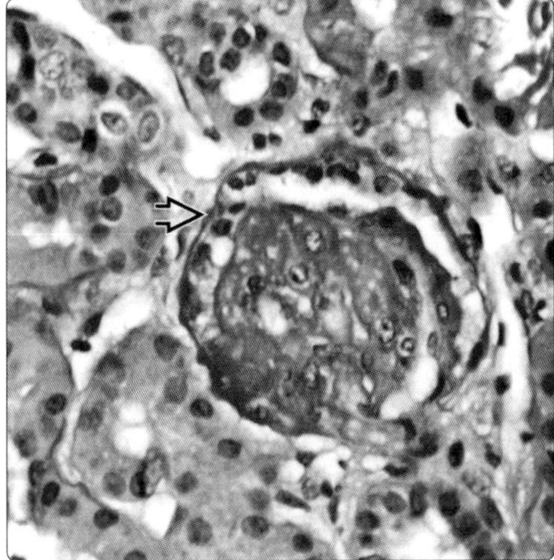

(Left) *This is another segmental sclerosing lesion ➡. This lesion is larger than the previous lesion. It contains hyaline, which stains black on silver stain, and a capsular adhesion ⇒. The upper left portions of the glomerulus appears normal.* **(Right)** *This glomerulus shows the end stage of segmental sclerosis in which the entire glomerulus is sclerotic, known as global glomerulosclerosis. There is residual mild epithelial cell hyperplasia ⇒, a feature that will disappear over time. There is no glomerular tuft hypercellularity.*

Podocyte Foot Process Effacement

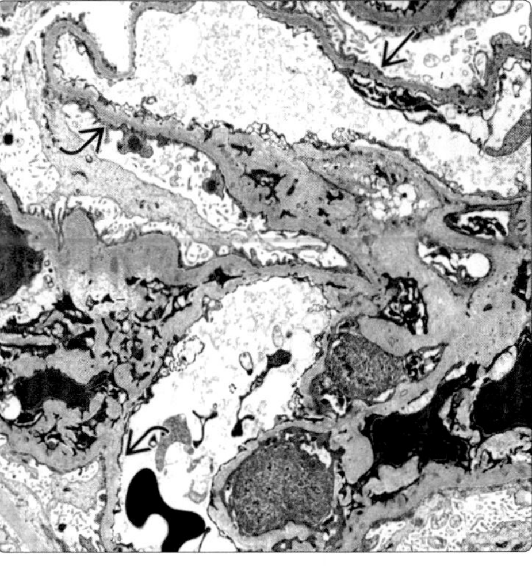

Segmental Sclerosis With Synecheal Capsular Adhesion

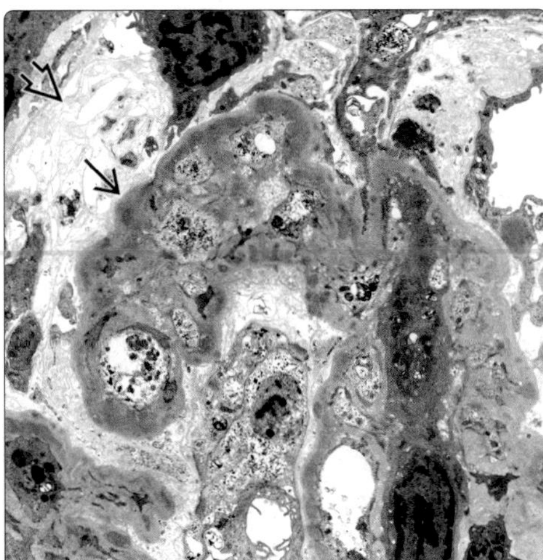

(Left) *This glomerulus shows diffuse effacement of podocyte foot processes ⇒ by EM. There is mild mesangial matrix increase, far less than in DMS. The capillary loop basement membrane is fairly uniform in thickness, but mild irregularity is present ⬀.* **(Right)** *EM shows capillary loop collapse and sclerosis. There is an adhesion composed of strands of matrix material ⇒ that connects the collapsed capillary loop ⇒ to the Bowman capsule. Embedded within the adhesion are trapped epithelial cells.*

Fabry Disease

KEY FACTS

TERMINOLOGY

- Lysosomal storage disease caused by genetic deficiency in α-galactosidase A enzyme (αGal), leading to accumulation of globotriaosylceramide (GL3) in many cell types
  - Affects function of kidney, heart, sweat gland, nerves

ETIOLOGY/PATHOGENESIS

- X-linked recessive
- Symptoms and signs vary with mutation and consequent functional level of αGal (more severe with deletion or termination mutations)
  - > 500 different mutations
  - 5% spontaneous mutations
- GL3 accumulates in endothelial and smooth muscle cells, podocytes, distal tubules, and many other cells

CLINICAL ISSUES

- ~ 0.3% of patients on dialysis
- Renal dysfunction: Age 15-40 years
- Often misdiagnosed clinically
- Females vary from asymptomatic to renal failure

MICROSCOPIC

- Podocyte-expanded cytoplasm appears pale and lacy due to lipid deposits
- EM demonstrates diagnostic feature of laminated, electron-dense lipid deposits in podocytes, endothelial cells, and distal tubular cells
- 1 μm Epon-embedded tissue reveals dense lipid granules by light microscopy
- Female heterozygotes have patchy distribution of podocyte lipid
- FSGS may develop

TOP DIFFERENTIAL DIAGNOSES

- Chloroquine toxicity
- Focal segmental glomerulosclerosis (FSGS)
- I-cell disease

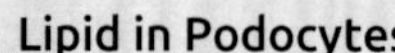

Lipid in Podocytes

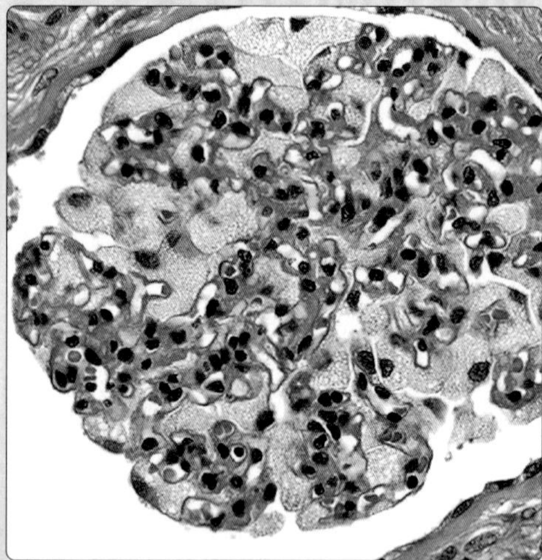

Lacy Lipid Inclusions in Podocytes

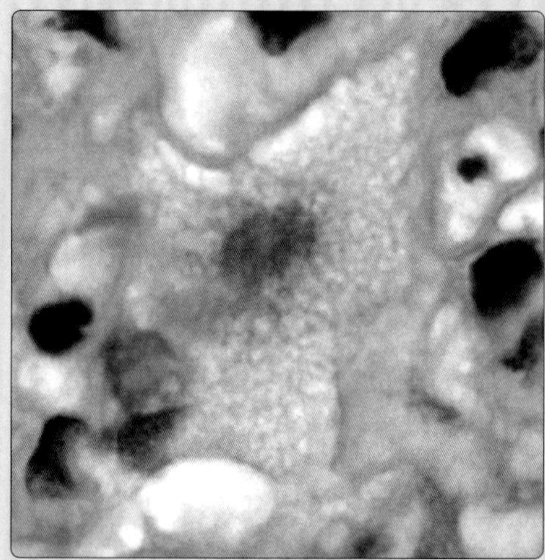

(Left) *The characteristic podocytes have clear, lacy cytoplasm in Fabry disease. The lipid consists of globotriasolylceremide (GL3), which accumulates in the podocyte more than in other renal structures.* **(Right)** *High power shows a podocyte in a biopsy from a patient with Fabry disease. The podocyte has an enlarged lacy clear cytoplasm, filled with lipid that has been dissolved in processing. This is often the most conspicuous change in routine stains that raises the question of Fabry disease.*

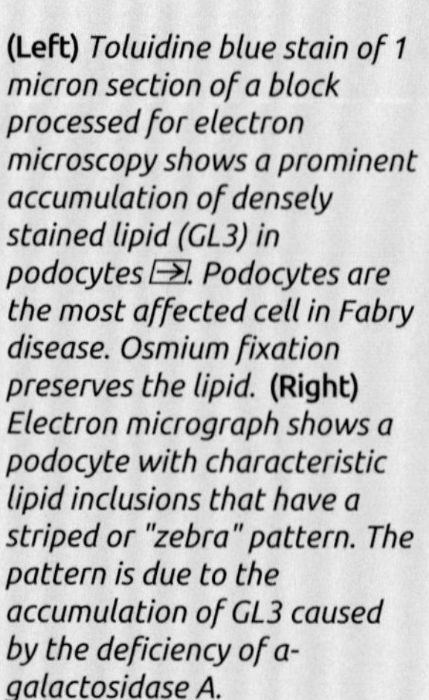

(Left) *Toluidine blue stain of 1 micron section of a block processed for electron microscopy shows a prominent accumulation of densely stained lipid (GL3) in podocytes* ⇨*. Podocytes are the most affected cell in Fabry disease. Osmium fixation preserves the lipid.* **(Right)** *Electron micrograph shows a podocyte with characteristic lipid inclusions that have a striped or "zebra" pattern. The pattern is due to the accumulation of GL3 caused by the deficiency of a-galactosidase A.*

Lipid Inclusions in 1 μm Section

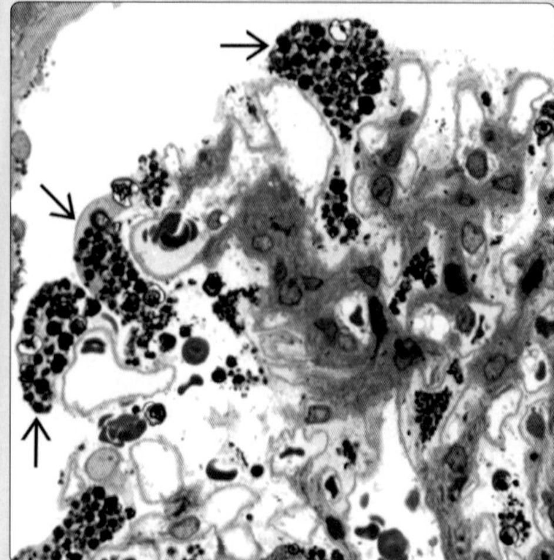

Zebra Pattern of Lipid Inclusion by EM

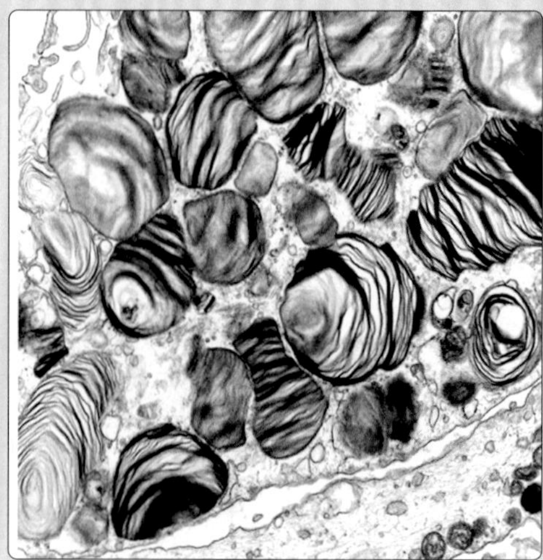

TERMINOLOGY

Synonyms

- Anderson-Fabry disease
- Angiokeratoma corporis diffusum

Definitions

- Lysosomal storage disease caused by genetic deficiency in α-galactosidase A enzyme (αGal), leading to globotriaosylceramide (GL3) accumulation in many cell types
  - Affects function of kidney, heart, sweat gland, and nerves

ETIOLOGY/PATHOGENESIS

Genetic Disease

- X-linked recessive trait
- Mutation in α-galactosidase A gene (*GLA*) on long arm of X chromosome (Xq22.1)
  - > 500 different mutations
    - 5% spontaneous mutations
  - Symptoms and signs vary with consequent functional level of αGal
    - More severe with deletion or termination mutations

Pathophysiology

- α-galactosidase A enzyme deficiency in lysosomes
  - Cleaves glycosphingolipids, including globotriaosylceramide, galabiosylceramide (podocytes), and blood group B substance
- GL3 accumulates in endothelial and smooth muscle cells, podocytes, distal tubular cells, collecting ducts, sweat glands, cardiac myocytes, macrophages, dorsal root ganglia, perineurium, cornea stroma, and other cells
  - Endothelial involvement leads to microvascular obstruction
    - Proinflammatory and procoagulant effects
    - Global and segmental glomerular sclerosis, interstitial fibrosis, tubular atrophy
    - Smooth muscle loss, nodular hyalinosis

Experimental Model

- *GLA* knockout mice
  - GL3 lipid inclusions in tubular epithelium and Bowman capsules
  - Minimal podocyte inclusions without endothelial cell inclusions
    - Do not develop renal disease
      - Argues for role of podocyte &/or endothelial lipid in pathogenesis of renal disease

CLINICAL ISSUES

Epidemiology

- Incidence
  - Mutation prevalence 1:40,800 (UK)
  - Symptomatic disease prevalence 1:64,600 (UK)
  - Pathogenic mutation in newborn screening: 1:7,057 (Japan)
  - Often misdiagnosed (mean time to diagnosis: 20 years)
- Sex
  - Dialysis patients: 0.33% of males, 0.1% of females

Presentation

- Vary depending on severity of enzyme deficiency
  - Type 1: Males present in childhood or adolescence with acroparesthesias, hypohidrosis, angiokeratomas, and corneal dystrophy; later development of progressive renal, cardiac, and cerebrovascular disease
    - Little or no αGal activity (< 1% normal)
    - Acroparesthesia: Age 5-25 years
      - Burning sensation in hands
    - Renal dysfunction: Age 15-40 years; renal failure (median age: 40 years)
    - CNS disease (stroke) > 25 years
    - Cardiac disease > 35 years
  - Type 2: Males present after 4th decade with renal and cardiac disease
    - Residual αGal activity
    - Renal variant
      - Signs and symptoms restricted to kidney
      - 1.2% of male dialysis patients (Japan)
      - Lack classic features: Angiokeratoma, acroparesthesias, hypohidrosis, corneal opacities
    - Cardiac variant
      - Occurs in males with partial αGal activity
      - Hypertrophic cardiomyopathy
      - Prominent cardiomyocyte lipid
      - No endothelial GL3
      - No renal failure, neurological disease, or skin lesions
- Female heterozygotes variable manifestation
  - Asymptomatic to renal failure (Fabry Registry, n = 1077)
    - 30% asymptomatic
    - 19% eGFR < 60 mL/min/1.73m^2
    - 2.2% ESRD
      - ~ 1/6 as frequent as in males in Registry

Treatment

- Drugs
  - Enzyme replacement therapy (ERT)
    - Recombinant αGal
      - Agalsidase-α (Replagal)
      - Agalsidase-β (Fabrazyme)
  - Other drugs in clinical trials
- Dialysis
  - Survival worse than nondiabetics
    - 60-63% 3-year survival
- Transplantation
  - Deposits may recur in minor amounts in endothelium, not in podocytes
  - Graft survival similar to non-Fabry patients
    - Rare graft loss attributed to recurrent Fabry disease Increased mortality from other causes
  - Heterozygote female donor kidneys show mosaic podocyte lipid; does not progress

Prognosis

- ERT benefits pain and quality of life
  - Reduces lipid storage in endothelium of kidney, heart, skin < 6 months
    - Reduction of podocyte lipid in 4/6 patients at 54 months
  - Improvement of hypertension and cardiac hypertrophy

- Reduced rate of loss of renal function vs. historical controls
- Long-term effect of ERT on renal function and survival to be determined
  - Retrospective evidence of reduced proteinuria in women with mild disease
  - Renal function continues decline in males with advanced disease
- Leading causes of death prior to ERT (pre-2001)
  - Renal failure in males (42%) and cerebrovascular disease in females (25%)
- Leading causes of death after ERT (post-2001)
  - Cardiac disease in males (34%) and females (57%)
- Proteinuria is most predictive risk factor for progressive renal failure
  - In males, urinary protein/Cr > 1.5 has mean eGFR slope of -5.6 mL/min per 1.73 m^2/year

MACROSCOPIC

Biopsy Appearance

- Diagnosis may be suspected on renal biopsy
- Glomeruli are paler and whiter compared with non-Fabry cases

MICROSCOPIC

Histologic Features

- Glomeruli
  - Podocyte cytoplasm appears expanded, foamy, pale, and lacy due to lipid deposits dissolved in processing
    - Lipid granules stain with Luxol fast blue
  - Female heterozygotes have patchy distribution of podocyte lipid due to random inactivation of X chromosome
  - Mesangium can be expanded and mildly hypercellular
    - Contain lipid, but not easily appreciated in routine sections
  - Endothelial cells appear normal in routine sections although they also contain lipid
  - Focal segmental glomerulosclerosis (FSGS) can be present with adhesion to Bowman capsule and segmental scars
    - Some glomeruli show collapsing glomerulopathy
- Tubules
  - Distal tubules have abundant lipid deposits, which make them pale and vacuolated in routine sections
  - Tubular atrophy is common
- Interstitium
  - Commonly affected by increased fibrosis with sparse infiltrate
  - Fibroblasts in interstitium also contain lipid
  - Granulomatous interstitial nephritis (rare)
- Vessels
  - Endothelium of all vessels accumulate lipid
    - Not visible in capillary endothelium in routine sections
    - Sometimes appreciated in arteries as lacy, vacuolated cytoplasm
    - Intimal fibrosis can be prominent
  - Lipid in arterial smooth muscle makes them appear pale in routine sections
  - Arteriolar hyalinosis may present as peripheral nodular replacement of smooth muscle, indistinguishable from calcineurin inhibitor toxicity
- Plastic-embedded section
  - Glutaraldehyde/paraformaldehyde-fixed tissue for routine EM ideal to detect lipid
  - Lipid granules most conspicuous as dense granules filling podocytes and distal tubular epithelium
  - High power (100x oil) useful to detect lipid droplets in endothelium
    - Endothelial lipid varies from rare granules to large aggregates that bulge into lumen
      - Similar lipid deposits in endothelium of other organs
  - Podocyte lipid decreased in areas of segmental sclerosis, adhesion, or collapse
    - Possibly due to increased local podocyte turnover, yielding "young" podocytes with less lipid
- Type 1 (classic) vs. type 2 (late onset) Fabry disease
  - Type 2 lacks endothelial and mesangial lipid droplets
    - Lipid in podocytes, tubular epithelium, and smooth muscle cells
- Superimposed diseases reported
  - Minimal change disease superimposed on Fabry disease
  - IgA nephropathy (may be incidental)
  - Crescentic glomerulonephritis (± ANCA)

ANCILLARY TESTS

Immunohistochemistry

- Monoclonal antibody to GL3 (CD77) detects residual GL3 in paraffin-embedded tissue (podocytes, tubules, smooth muscle cells, endothelium)

Immunofluorescence

- Generally negative, except IgM and C3 in segmental scars
- Incidental IgA deposition observed in protocol biopsies

Electron Microscopy

- Diagnostic feature of laminated, electron-dense lipid deposits in podocytes, endothelial cells, mesangial cells, smooth muscle cells, distal tubules, and interstitial fibroblasts
- Dense, variegated granules without lamination also present
- Foot process effacement and podocyte lipid accumulation seen in protocol biopsies in 75% of children ≤ 16 years old before detectable proteinuria
- Females have mosaic expression of mutated gene
  - Among 12 women, 51% of podocytes per glomerulus had lipid (range: 0-87%)
  - % of podocytes with lipid ↓ with age, suggesting disproportionate loss

Fluorescence Microscopy

- Fabry lipid inclusions autofluorescence yellow in UV light

Morphometry

- Primary endpoint in clinical trials are extent and severity of lipid inclusions in capillary endothelium
  - 1 μm Epon embedded tissues, toluidine blue stain
  - Examined at 100x oil in microscopy or scanned whole slide images

- Scored 0-4 (Genzyme) or actual counts of granules (Barisoni)
- Comprehensive scoring system developed by International Study Group of Fabry Nephropathy
  - Incorporates scoring of glomerulosclerosis, interstitial fibrosis, and vascular lesions

DIFFERENTIAL DIAGNOSIS

Chloroquine Toxicity

- Lipids that accumulate with lysosomal inhibitor (chloroquine) therapy are indistinguishable from Fabry disease
- History of chloroquine therapy may not be known, but this possibility should be raised
- Diagnosis of Fabry disease requires ancillary studies (GL3 blood levels or genetic testing)

Focal Segmental Glomerulosclerosis (FSGS)

- Fabry patients commonly develop FSGS due to either direct lipid effect on podocyte or decreased nephron mass
- Lipid in podocytes are best clue but can be overlooked in light microscopy
  - EM is best method to detect lipid
    - Readily detected in podocytes

I-Cell Disease

- Podocyte deposits positive for colloidal iron

Arteriosclerosis

- Vascular disease in Fabry disease similar to usual arteriosclerosis in hypertension
- If lipid in podocytes (or other sites) not appreciated, diagnosis may be missed

Subclinical Fabry Disease (in Patients With Other Renal Diseases)

- Lipid deposits may be "incidental" finding in biopsies for other diseases (e.g., crescentic glomerulonephritis, IgA nephropathy, myeloma)

DIAGNOSTIC CHECKLIST

Clinically Relevant Pathologic Features

- Loss of lipid in microvascular circulation can be surrogate measure of ERT effectiveness

Pathologic Interpretation Pearls

- 1 μm plastic sections (100x oil) best for evaluating lipid by light microscopy
- Lipid may be inconspicuous in later stages and may be overlooked
- Diagnosis suggested by pale white bulging glomeruli on macroscopic inspection of biopsy core
- Kidney biopsy with EM analysis required to confirm Fabry disease in ambiguous cases with gene variants of uncertain pathogenicity

SELECTED REFERENCES

1. Bangari DS et al: α-galactosidase A knockout mice: progressive organ pathology resembles the type 2 later-onset phenotype of Fabry disease. Am J Pathol. 185(3):651-65, 2015
2. Pokuri VK et al: Synchronous presentation of monoclonal gammopathy and Fabry nephropathy; diagnostic renal biopsy obviates initiation of myeloma therapy. Ann Hematol. ePub, 2015
3. Tøndel C et al: Foot process effacement is an early marker of nephropathy in young classic Fabry patients without albuminuria. Nephron Physiol. 129(1):16-21, 2015
4. van der Tol L et al: Chronic kidney disease and an uncertain diagnosis of Fabry disease: Approach to a correct diagnosis. Mol Genet Metab. 114(2):242-7, 2015
5. Brennan P et al: Case-finding in Fabry disease: experience from the North of England. J Inherit Metab Dis. 37(1):103-7, 2014
6. Inoue T et al: Newborn screening for Fabry disease in Japan: prevalence and genotypes of Fabry disease in a pilot study. J Hum Genet. 58(8):548-52, 2013
7. Rombach SM et al: Long term enzyme replacement therapy for Fabry disease: effectiveness on kidney, heart and brain. Orphanet J Rare Dis. 8:47, 2013
8. Barisoni L et al: Novel quantitative method to evaluate globotriaosylceramide inclusions in renal peritubular capillaries by virtual microscopy in patients with fabry disease. Arch Pathol Lab Med. 136(7):816-24, 2012
9. Feriozzi S et al: The effectiveness of long-term agalsidase alfa therapy in the treatment of Fabry nephropathy. Clin J Am Soc Nephrol. 7(1):60-9, 2012
10. Valbuena C et al: Immunohistochemical diagnosis of Fabry nephropathy and localisation of globotriaosylceramide deposits in paraffin-embedded kidney tissue sections. Virchows Arch. 460(2):211-21, 2012
11. Fogo AB et al: Scoring system for renal pathology in Fabry disease: report of the International Study Group of Fabry Nephropathy (ISGFN). Nephrol Dial Transplant. 25(7):2168-77, 2010
12. Linthorst GE et al: Screening for Fabry disease in high-risk populations: a systematic review. J Med Genet. 47(4):217-22, 2010
13. Marchesoni CL et al: Misdiagnosis in Fabry disease. J Pediatr. 156(5):828-31, 2010
14. Mignani R et al: Dialysis and transplantation in Fabry disease: indications for enzyme replacement therapy. Clin J Am Soc Nephrol. 5(2):379-85, 2010
15. Ramaswami U et al: Assessment of renal pathology and dysfunction in children with Fabry disease. Clin J Am Soc Nephrol. 5(2):365-70, 2010
16. Wanner C et al: Prognostic indicators of renal disease progression in adults with Fabry disease: natural history data from the Fabry Registry. Clin J Am Soc Nephrol. 5(12):2220-8, 2010
17. Zarate YA et al: A case of minimal change disease in a Fabry patient. Pediatr Nephrol. 25(3):553-6, 2010
18. Abaterusso C et al: Unusual renal presentation of Fabry disease in a female patient. Nat Rev Nephrol. 5(6):349-54, 2009
19. Hirashio S et al: Renal histology before and after effective enzyme replacement therapy in a patient with classical Fabry's disease. Clin Nephrol. 71(5):550-6, 2009
20. Mehta A et al: Enzyme replacement therapy with agalsidase alfa in patients with Fabry's disease: an analysis of registry data. Lancet. 374(9706):1986-96, 2009
21. Mehta A et al: Natural course of Fabry disease: changing pattern of causes of death in FOS - Fabry Outcome Survey. J Med Genet. 46(8):548-52, 2009
22. Wilcox WR et al: Females with Fabry disease frequently have major organ involvement: lessons from the Fabry Registry. Mol Genet Metab. 93(2):112-28, 2008
23. Germain DP et al: Sustained, long-term renal stabilization after 54 months of agalsidase beta therapy in patients with Fabry disease. J Am Soc Nephrol. 18(5):1547-57, 2007
24. Fischer EG et al: Fabry disease: a morphologic study of 11 cases. Mod Pathol. 19(10):1295-301, 2006
25. Nakao S et al: Fabry disease: detection of undiagnosed hemodialysis patients and identification of a "renal variant" phenotype. Kidney Int. 64(3):801-7, 2003
26. Thurberg BL et al: Globotriaosylceramide accumulation in the Fabry kidney is cleared from multiple cell types after enzyme replacement therapy. Kidney Int. 62(6):1933-46, 2002
27. Eng CM et al: Safety and efficacy of recombinant human alpha-galactosidase A–replacement therapy in Fabry's disease. N Engl J Med. 345(1):9-16, 2001

(Left) *Low-power view of a renal biopsy from a patient with Fabry disease shows nonspecific findings of interstitial fibrosis and glomerulosclerosis. Demonstration of the lipid accumulation is best shown by electron microscopy or 1 μm sections.* **(Right)** *Increased size of the podocytes with pale cytoplasm → is suggested in a patient with Fabry disease. Diffuse fine interstitial fibrosis is present and commonly accompanied by patchy tubular atrophy.*

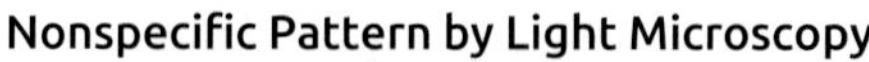

Nonspecific Pattern by Light Microscopy

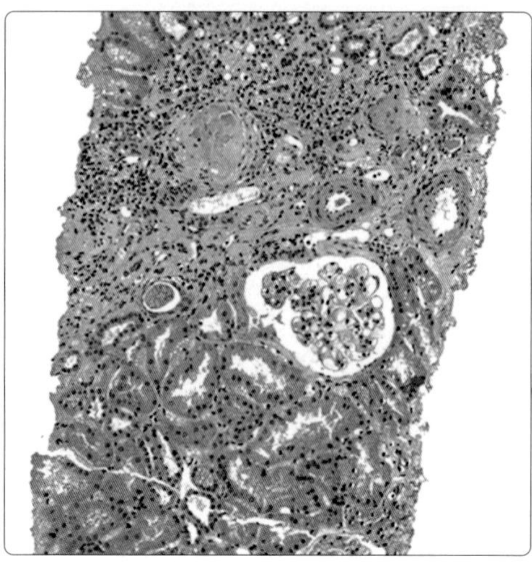

Pale Cytoplasm of Podocytes

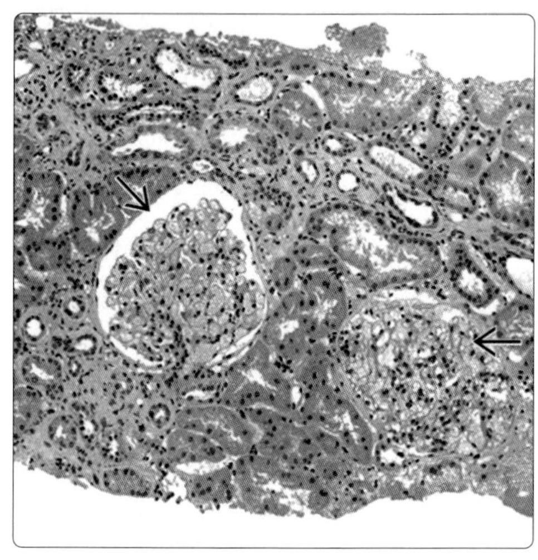

(Left) *Periodic acid-Schiff stain of a biopsy from a patient with Fabry disease shows characteristic lacy cytoplasm in the podocytes. The GL3 lipid in the inclusions is dissolved by processing.* **(Right)** *Fabry disease may be deceptively nonspecific on light microscopy, as in this case, which appears to be focal segmental glomerulosclerosis. A careful search for lipid-filled podocytes is generally helpful, and EM is most definitive.*

Lacy Podocyte Cytoplasm

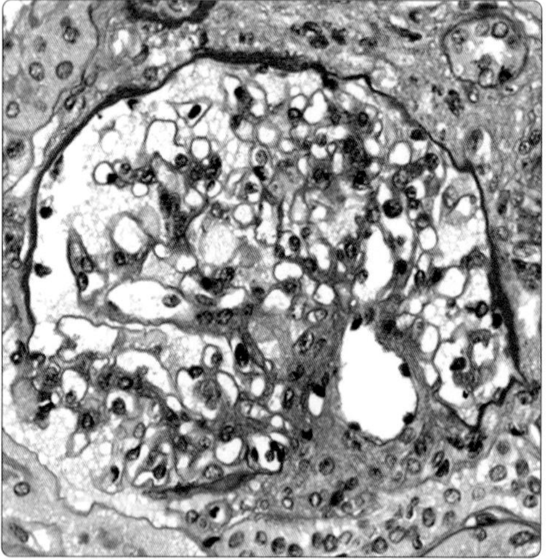

Focal Segmental Glomerulosclerosis

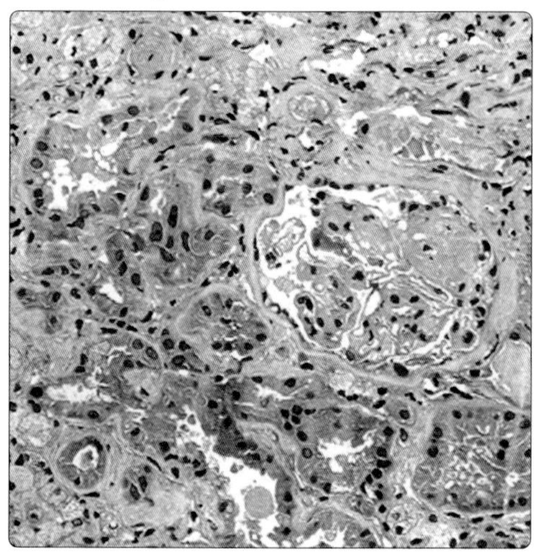

(Left) *Renal biopsy from a heterozygous female with Fabry disease shows variable lipid inclusion in podocytes; some are markedly affected → and some are normal → due to the random inactivation of the X chromosome.* **(Right)** *End-stage renal disease occasionally develops in women with Fabry disease, as in this case. Lipid is evident even at low power in glomeruli → and tubules →. Collapsing focal sclerosis is also present →.*

Heterogenous Podocytes in Female With Fabry Disease

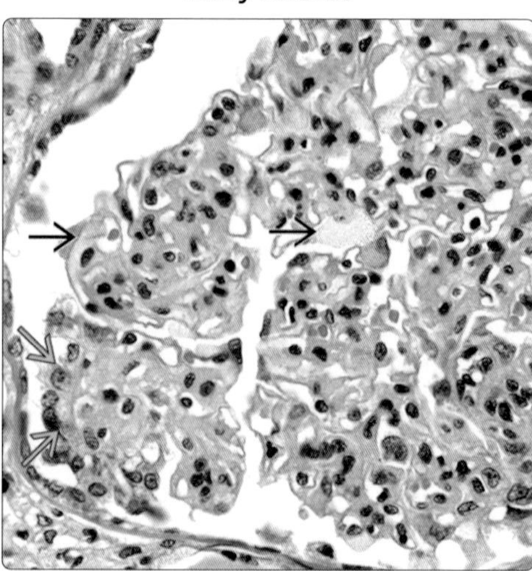

Advanced Disease

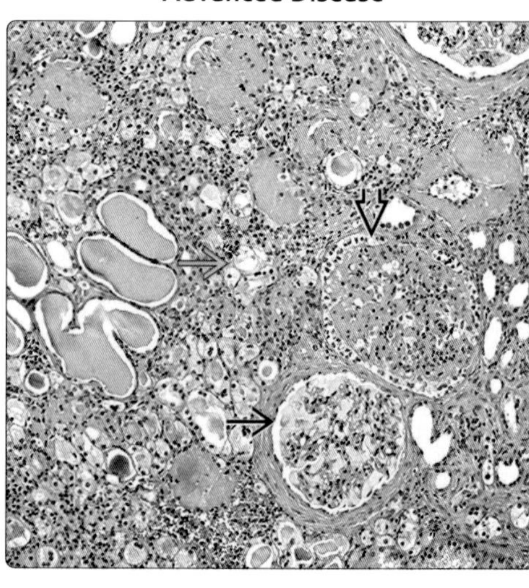

Characteristic Lipid Granules

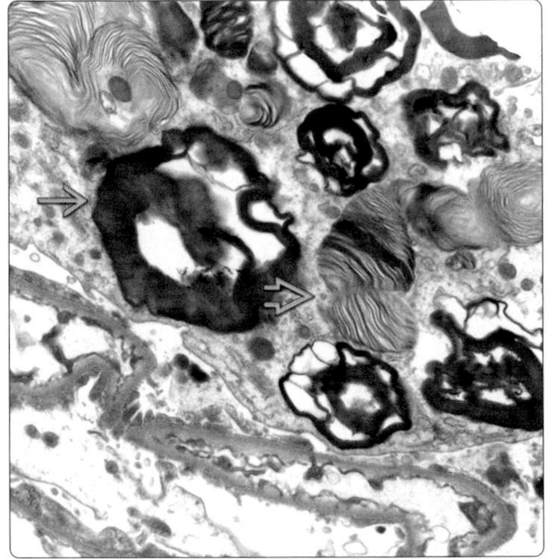

Myelin Figure Pattern of Lipid

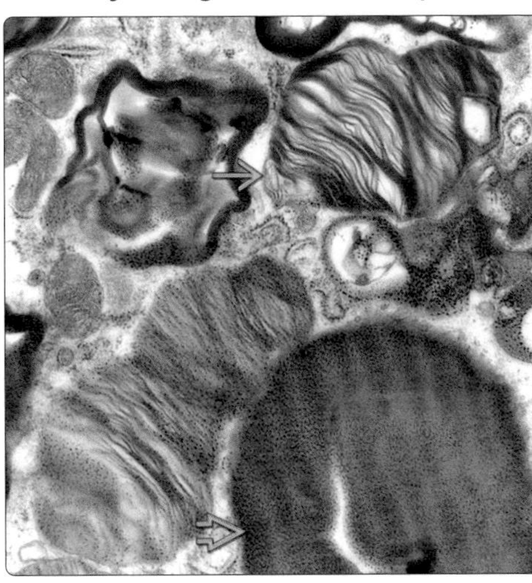

(Left) *Electron micrograph of a podocyte shows characteristic laminated lipid deposits in the cytoplasm ➡. Other coarser, dense deposits of lipid are also present ➡. These deposits are dissolved in lipid solvents in routine formalin/xylene/paraffin processing.* **(Right)** *Electron micrograph at high power shows lipid storage deposits with a myelin figure pattern ➡ in a podocyte in Fabry disease. Some lipid deposits have no substructure ➡.*

Endothelial Lipid Inclusions

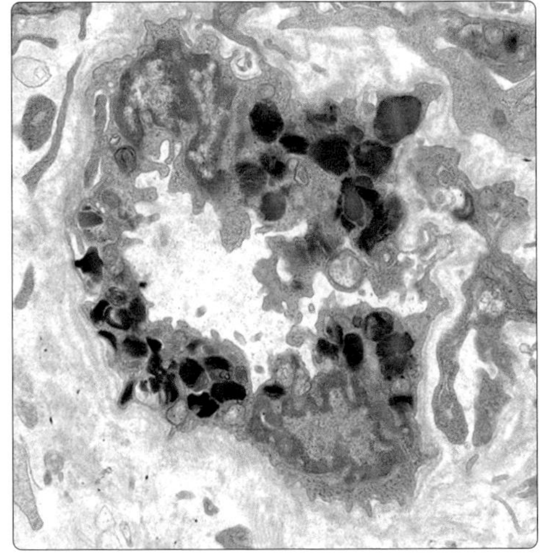

Lipid in Peritubular Capillary Endothelium

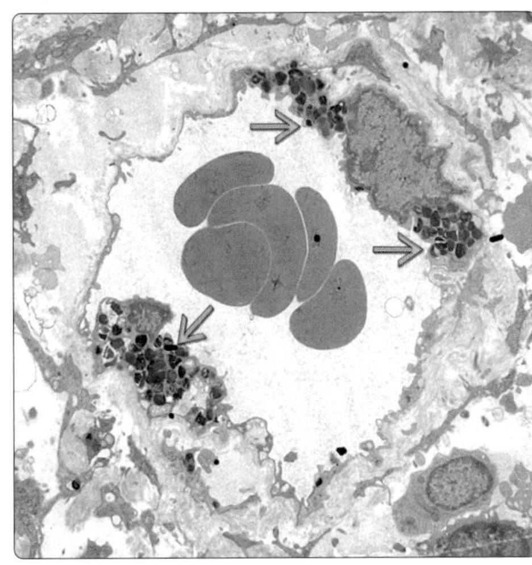

(Left) *Electron micrograph of a peritubular capillary shows extensive lipid droplets in the endothelium. This accumulation may affect luminal patency and promote a proinflammatory and procoagulant response and lead to ischemic injury to the affected organ.* **(Right)** *This electron micrograph shows a peritubular capillary from a patient with Fabry disease. The lipid droplets are typically in a perinuclear location ➡.*

Lipid in Endothelium

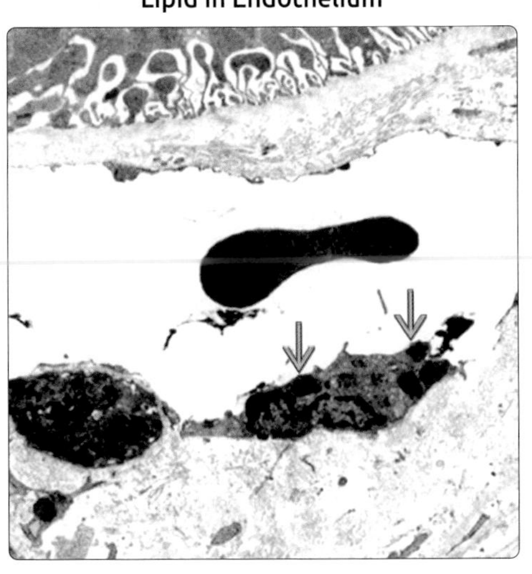

Distal Tubule Lipid Inclusions

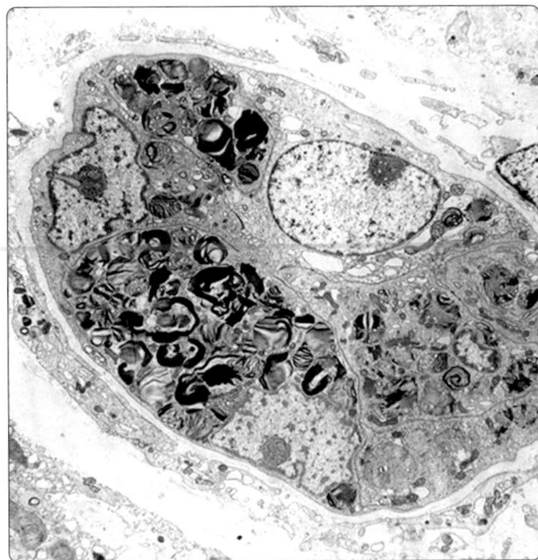

(Left) *Electron micrograph of a peritubular capillary from a patient with Fabry disease shows a few lipid droplets near the nucleus ➡.* **(Right)** *Electron micrograph of a distal tubule from a patient with Fabry disease shows typical laminated lipid deposits in the cytoplasm. The distal tubules and collecting ducts are the most severely affected of the kidney tubules.*

Lipid in Media and Endothelium

Lacy Endothelium in Artery

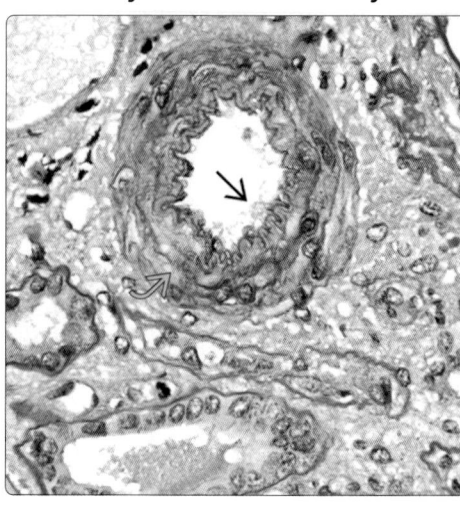

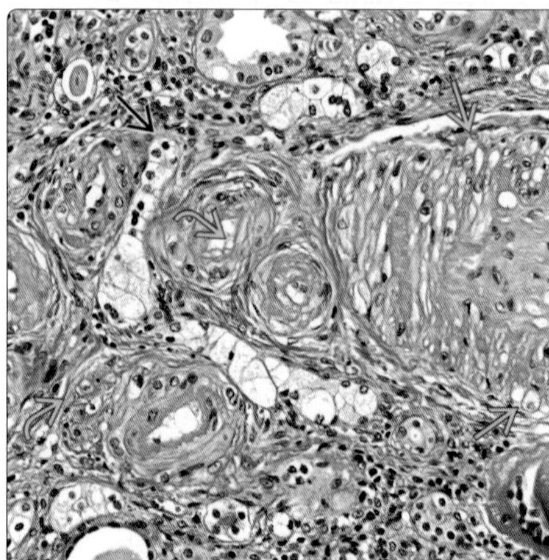

(Left) *Lipid accumulates in the endothelium and smooth muscle cells of arteries and arterioles. In routine paraffin-embedded material, most of the lipid dissolves and the cells appear vacuolated. Distal tubules also have abundant lipid.* **(Right)** *The arterial endothelium accumulates GL3 lipid in Fabry disease. The endothelial cells show lacy vacuolization on routine paraffin-processed material, which can be easily overlooked. Lipid also accumulates in smooth muscle cells, which makes the cytoplasm less dense.*

Dense Granules in Toluidine Blue-Stained 1 µm Sections

Arteriolar Endothelial and Smooth Muscle Lipid

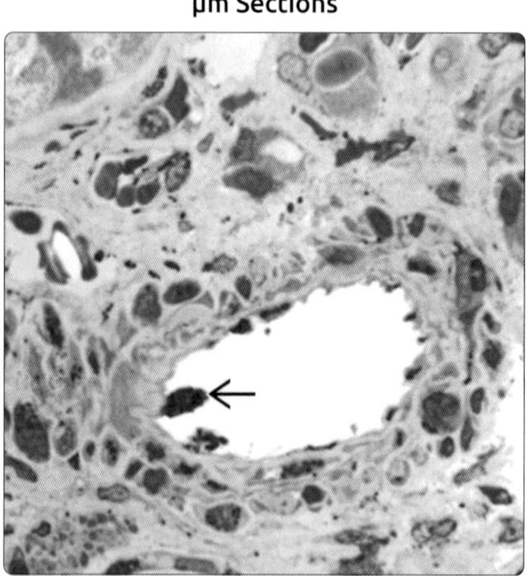

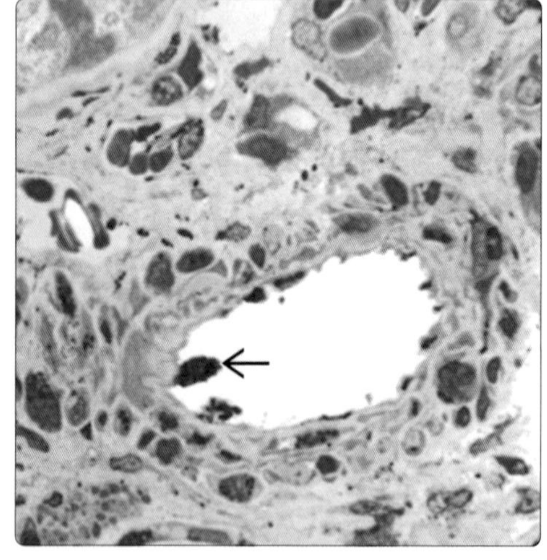

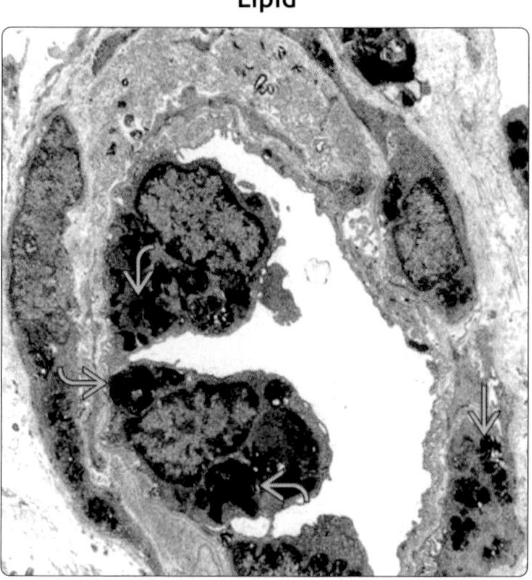

(Left) *Toluidine blue stain shows a 1 µm section with densely stained granules in arterial endothelial cells, which bulge into the lumen.* **(Right)** *Electron-dense lipid granules in arterioles are prominent in untreated Fabry disease, as shown in this electron micrograph. Lipid is also present in the smooth muscle.*

Dense Granules in Toluidine Blue-Stained 1 µm Sections

Loss of Lipid After Enzyme Replacement Therapy

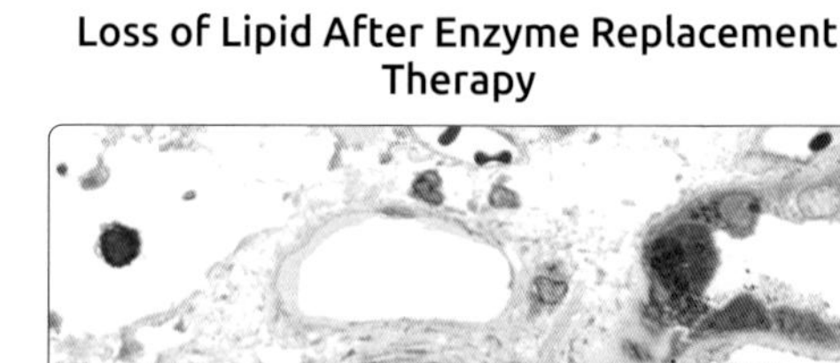

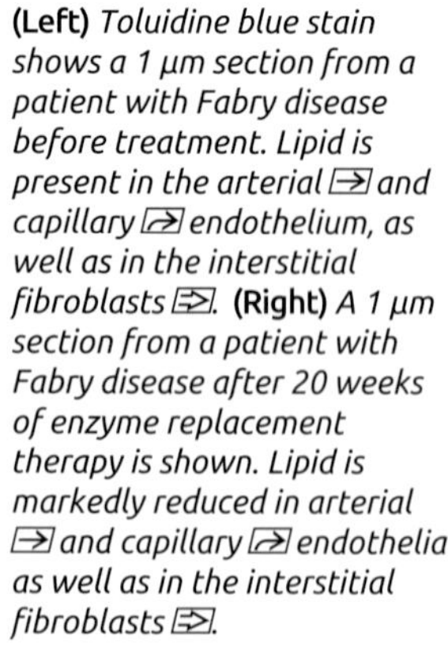

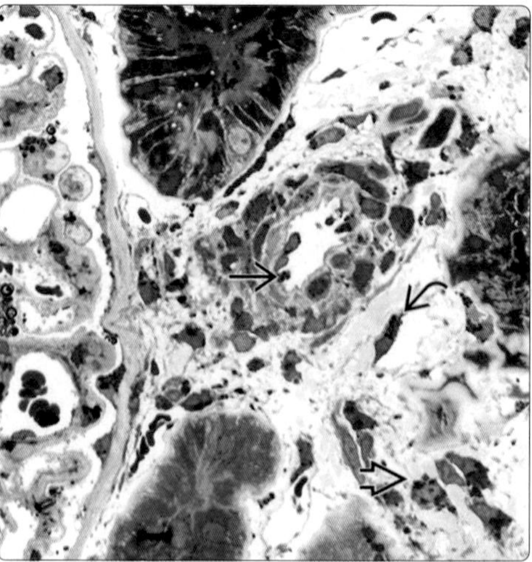

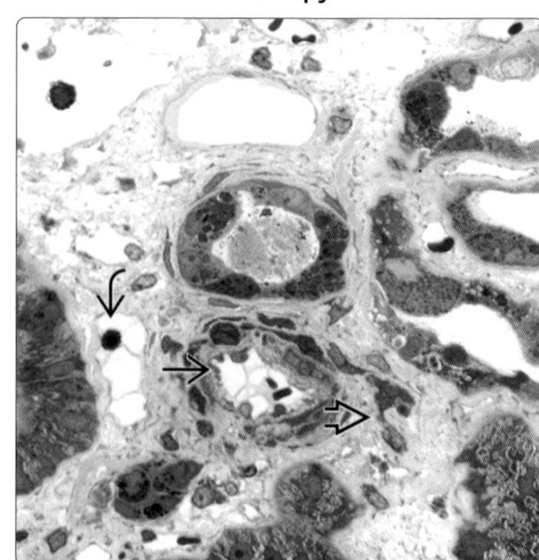

(Left) *Toluidine blue stain shows a 1 µm section from a patient with Fabry disease before treatment. Lipid is present in the arterial and capillary endothelium, as well as in the interstitial fibroblasts.* **(Right)** *A 1 µm section from a patient with Fabry disease after 20 weeks of enzyme replacement therapy is shown. Lipid is markedly reduced in arterial and capillary endothelia as well as in the interstitial fibroblasts.*

Collapsing Variant of FSGS

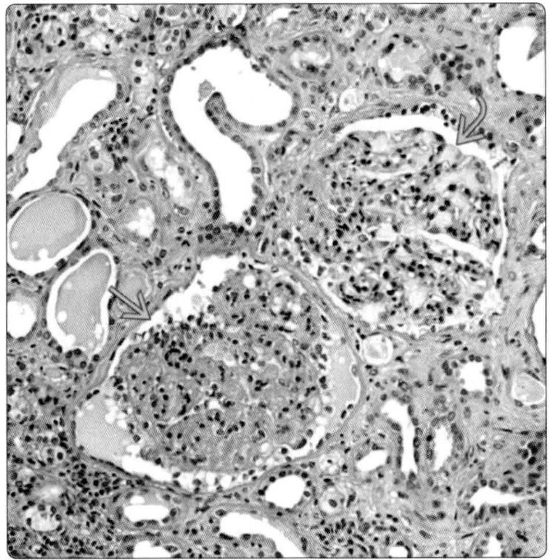

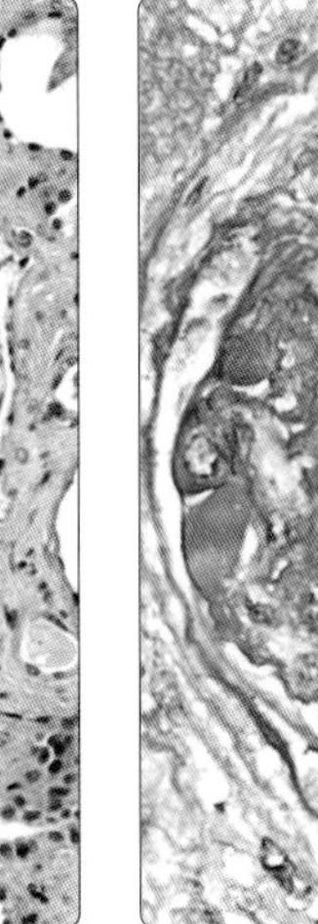

Focal Segmental Glomerulosclerosis

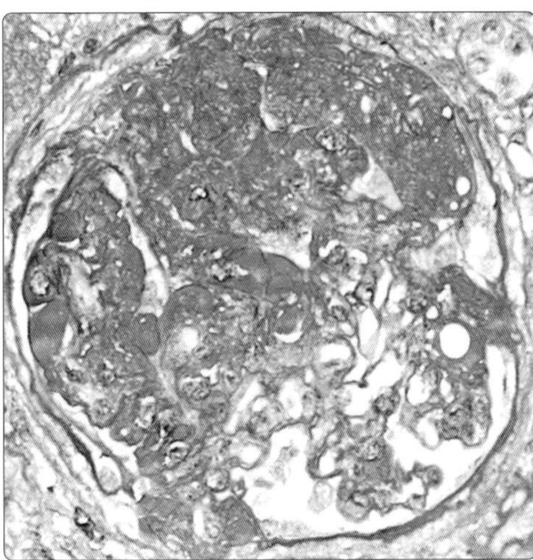

(Left) *This end-stage kidney from a woman with Fabry disease shows 2 patterns of glomerular involvement, lipid-filled podocytes → and collapsing FSGS →. The visceral epithelial cells in the collapsing lesion have less lipid that in the more intact glomerulus, consistent with either increased turnover or replacement with parietal epithelium.* **(Right)** *Periodic acid-Schiff stain of a glomerulus from a patient with Fabry disease shows focal, segmental glomerulosclerosis, not otherwise specified.*

Lack of Lipid in Visceral Epithelial Cells in FSGS

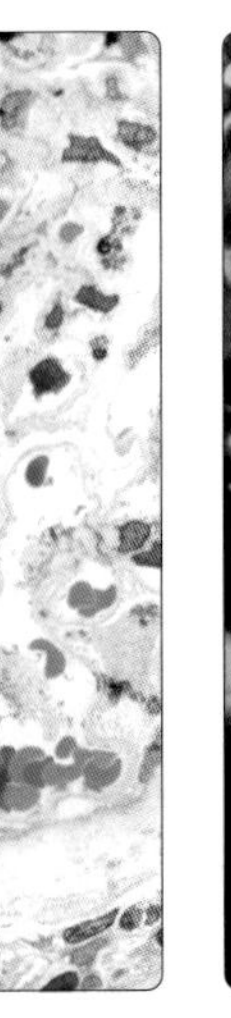

Autofluorescence of Lipid

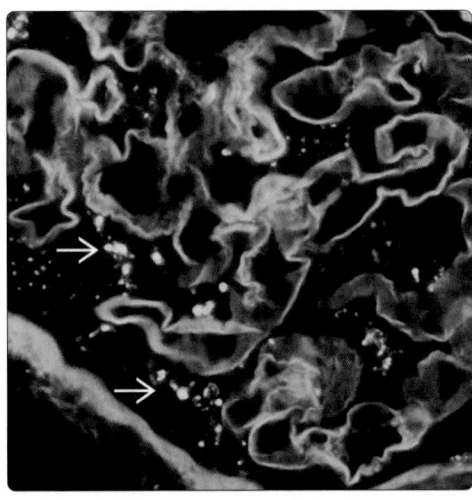

(Left) *Epon-embedded tissue from a patient with Fabry disease shows focal, segmental glomerulosclerosis. Visceral epithelial cells near the adhesion are relatively free of lipid → compared with podocytes in the normal loops →, consistent with either increased turnover or replacement with parietal epithelium.* **(Right)** *Immunofluorescence of a glomerulus from a patient with Fabry disease shows characteristic yellow autofluorescence of the lipid droplets in podocytes →. (Courtesy V. D'Agati.)*

Donor Fabry Disease

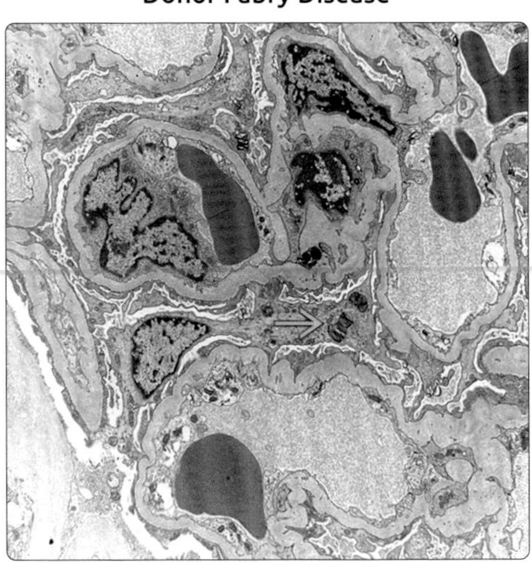

Inclusion in Podocyte in Donor Kidney

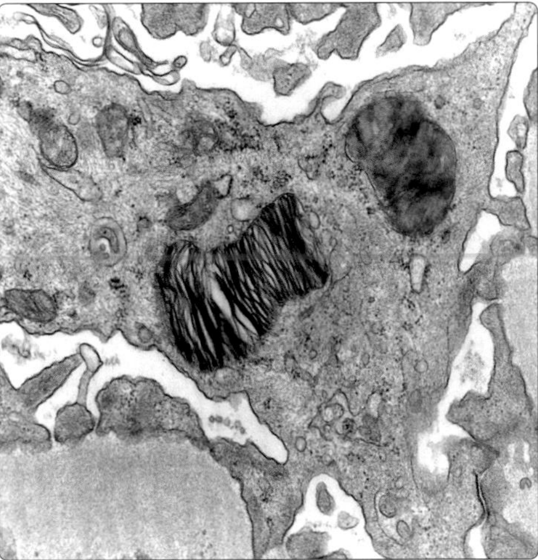

(Left) *Electron micrograph of a transplant kidney from a heterozygous Fabry female shows lipid deposits present in occasional podocytes →.* **(Right)** *High power shows the occasional laminated lipid inclusion in podocytes in this transplanted kidney from a heterozygous female. No lipid was detected in the endothelium as the patient was on enzyme replacement therapy.*

KEY FACTS

TERMINOLOGY

- Autosomal recessive lysosomal storage disease caused by mutation in GBA, which encodes glucocerebrosidase

ETIOLOGY/PATHOGENESIS

- Glucosylceramide accumulation 2° to ↓ lysosomal glucosylceramidase activity
  - Glucosylceramidase typically catalyzes hydrolysis of glucosylceramide into glucose & ceramide
    - Sphingolipids are components of lipid rafts in plasma membranes

CLINICAL ISSUES

- Most common inherited lipid storage disease
- Varied presentation: Hepatosplenomegaly, anemia, thrombocytopenia, neurological signs and bony involvement
  - Type I: Classic adult form with hepatic and splenic involvement but central nervous system (CNS) spared
  - Type II: CNS involved, leading to childhood death
  - Type III: Late form
- Clinical renal involvement rare but has been described after splenectomy or with comorbidities (diabetes, myeloma)
  - Proteinuria, hematuria, nephrotic syndrome

MICROSCOPIC

- Gaucher cells (monocyte/macrophage-type cells) in glomerular capillaries, mesangium, interstitium
  - PAS(+), Sudan black (+), oil red O (+)
  - "Wrinkled paper" inclusions
- EM: Gaucher cells have membrane-bound, elongated bodies and tubules with 60-80 nm diameter fibrils
- No specific IF findings

TOP DIFFERENTIAL DIAGNOSES

- Fabry disease
- Type III hyperlipoproteinemia

Wrinkled Paper Gaucher Cell in Glomerulus

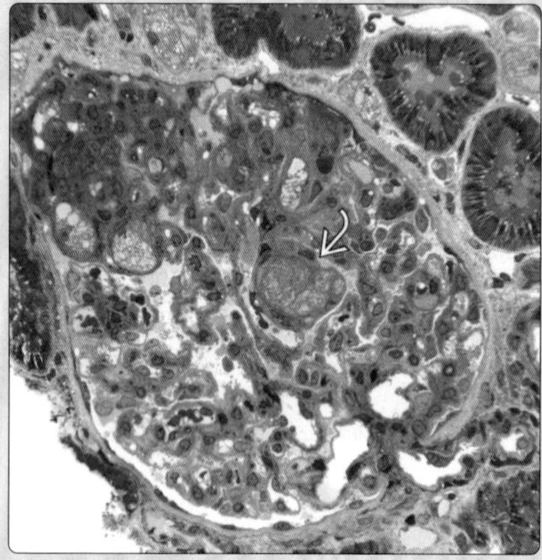

Gaucher Cell in Glomerular Capillary

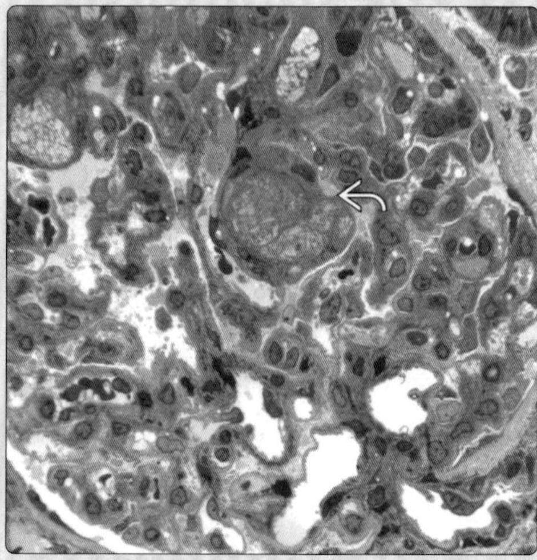

(Left) *In a 54-year-old woman with Gaucher disease, a glomerular capillary loop contains a large Gaucher cell ➡, which displays a cytoplasmic wrinkled paper appearance. (Courtesy A. Cohen, MD.)* **(Right)** *This 54 year old with Gaucher disease has a large Gaucher cell ➡ with a wrinkled paper, laminated appearance in the cytoplasm. (Courtesy A. Cohen, MD.)*

Gaucher Cell Cytoplasmic Inclusions

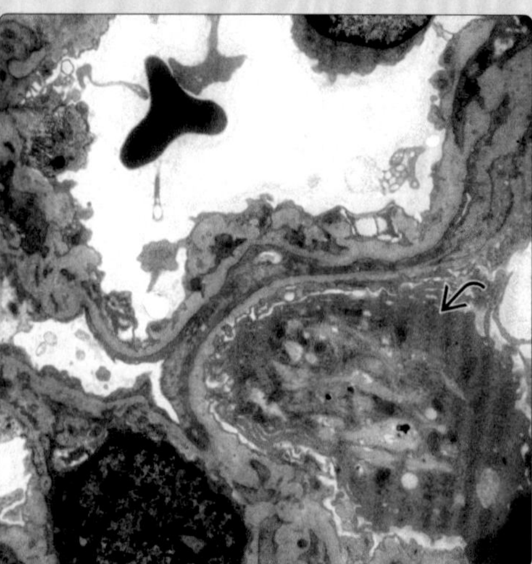

Gaucher Cell Cytoplasmic Inclusions Resembling Microtubules

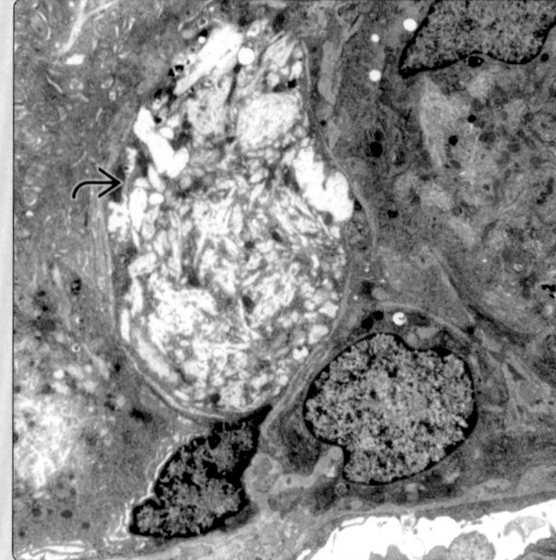

(Left) *A Gaucher cell ➡ with intracytoplasmic inclusions is seen in a circulating monocyte in the glomerular capillary lumen.* **(Right)** *A Gaucher cell ➡ occluding a glomerular capillary lumen has numerous cytoplasmic inclusions, some of which resemble the microtubular structures classically described in Gaucher cells. (Courtesy A. Cohen, MD.)*

TERMINOLOGY

Definitions

- Autosomal recessive lysosomal storage disease caused by mutation in GBA, which encodes glucocerebrosidase
- Glucosylceramide lipid accumulates in many cell types, including macrophages

ETIOLOGY/PATHOGENESIS

Genetic Lysosomal Storage Disease

- Mutation in *GBA*
  - Located on chromosome 1q22
  - Encodes glucocerebrosidase (acid β-glucosidase)
    - Catalyzes hydrolysis of glucosylceramide into glucose & ceramide
  - Accumulation of glucosylceramide (GlcCer) and glucocerebroside
  - Macrophages full of lipid termed "Gaucher cells" for Phillipe Gaucher who first described them in 1882 as a medical student
- Renal disease mainly occurs after splenectomy

CLINICAL ISSUES

Epidemiology

- Incidence
  - Most common inherited lipid storage disease
  - Type I: Classic adult form with hepatic & splenic involvement but central nervous system (CNS) spared
    - 1 in 50,000 people for type I disease (notably in Ashkenazi Jews)
  - Type II: CNS involved, leading to childhood death
    - 1 in 100,000
  - Type III: Late form
    - 1 in 100,000

Presentation

- Varied presentation
- Hepatosplenomegaly, anemia, thrombocytopenia, neurological signs, and bony involvement
- Clinical renal involvement rare but has been described after splenectomy or with comorbidities (e.g., diabetes, myeloma)
- Proteinuria
  - Nephrotic syndrome
- Hematuria

Treatment

- Drugs
  - Macrophage-targeted recombinant human glucocerebrosidase enzyme replacement therapy
    - Proteinuria may disappear
  - GlcCer synthesis blocking drugs being tested

Prognosis

- Gaucher cells 1st accumulate in liver, spleen, and bone marrow reticuloendothelial cells
  - Also accumulate in other tissues (heart and lungs, with eventual respiratory compromise)

MICROSCOPIC

Histologic Features

- Glomeruli
  - Gaucher cells in capillaries and mesangia
    - Inclusions in linear configuration, giving wrinkled paper appearance
    - Belong to monocyte/macrophage lineage
    - Storage material is
      - PAS(+) (2° to glucosyl moiety) and may reveal PAS(+) rod-like inclusions
      - Sudan black (+)
      - Oil red O (+)
    - Identical to those in other organs (e.g., spleen & liver)
- Interstitium
  - Gaucher cells may also accumulate

ANCILLARY TESTS

Immunofluorescence

- No specific findings
- ± granular deposits of IgA & IgM
  - Usually only trace if pure Gaucher disease

Electron Microscopy

- Gaucher cells
  - Endothelial cells/monocytes
  - Contain membrane-bound, elongated bodies
    - Tubular structures consisting of fibrils 60-80 nm in diameter with twisted arrangement
- Sometimes nonspecific intramembranous dense deposits

DIFFERENTIAL DIAGNOSIS

Fabry Disease

- α-galactosidase A deficiency leads to accumulation of glycosphingolipids
- Foamy cells in tubules, interstitium, and glomeruli
- Podocytes display osmiophilic inclusions
- Zebra bodies seen by EM, consisting of whorled cytoplasmic inclusions
- Myelin inclusions/figures in cytoplasm of arterial endothelial cells & myocytes of small arteries

Type III Hyperlipoproteinemia

- Capillary loop foam cells
  - Lamellated, electron-dense material
  - Cholesterol clefts

Other Renal Diseases in Gaucher Patients

- Membranoproliferative GN, focal and segmental glomerulosclerosis, amyloidosis, and others reported
  - Likely coincidental and unrelated to Gaucher disease

SELECTED REFERENCES

1. Merscher S et al: Podocyte pathology and nephropathy - sphingolipids in glomerular diseases. Front Endocrinol (Lausanne). 5:127, 2014
2. Nagral A: Gaucher disease. J Clin Exp Hepatol. 4(1):37-50, 2014
3. Boot RG et al: CCL18: a urinary marker of Gaucher cell burden in Gaucher patients. J Inherit Metab Dis. 29(4):564-71, 2006
4. Becker-Cohen R et al: A comprehensive assessment of renal function in patients with Gaucher disease. Am J Kidney Dis. 46(5):837-44, 2005
5. Santoro D et al: Gaucher disease with nephrotic syndrome: response to enzyme replacement therapy. Am J Kidney Dis. 40(1):E4, 2002

I-Cell Disease (Mucolipidosis II)

KEY FACTS

TERMINOLOGY

- Autosomal recessive lysosomal storage disease secondary to N-acetylglucosamine-phosphotransferase deficiency

ETIOLOGY/PATHOGENESIS

- Mutation of *GNPTAB* gene on chromosome 12q23.3
- N-acetylglucosamine-phosphotransferase fails to form mannose-6-phosphate necessary for trafficking of enzymes to lysosomes

CLINICAL ISSUES

- Usually no renal symptoms
- Rarely, proximal tubular dysfunction manifested by low-grade proteinuria, hyperphosphaturia, hypercalcuria, and aminoaciduria
- Increased serum levels of lysosomal enzymes

MICROSCOPIC

- Diffuse podocyte vacuolization
- Vacuole contents can be stained in paraffin sections
    - Hale colloidal iron stain positive
    - Alcian blue-PAS pH 2.5 stain positive
    - Sudan black stain positive
- Renal tubule and interstitial cells are rarely affected

ANCILLARY TESTS

- Electron microscopy
    - Podocyte cytoplasm distended by vacuoles
    - Vacuoles largely empty but may contain fibrillogranular or lamellar material
    - Endothelial cells and mesangial cells not affected

TOP DIFFERENTIAL DIAGNOSES

- Fabry disease
- GM1 gangliosidosis
- Nephrosialidosis

Enlarged Podocytes With Foamy Cytoplasm

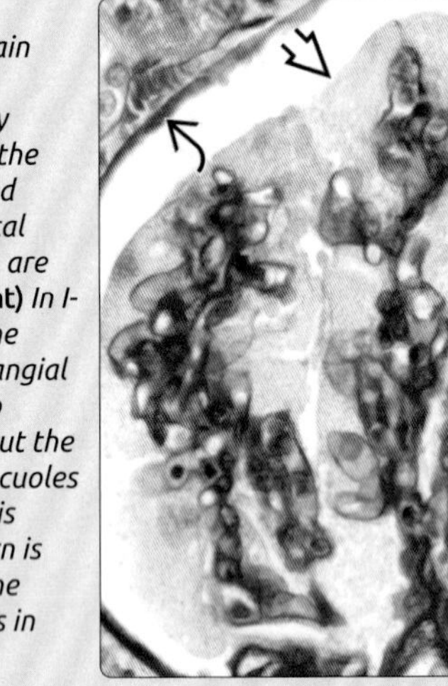

Enlarged Podocytes With Foamy Cytoplasm

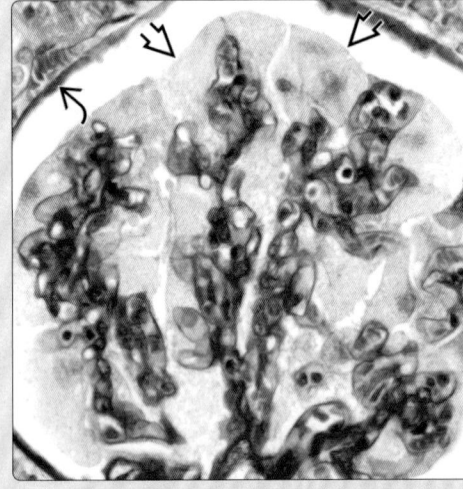

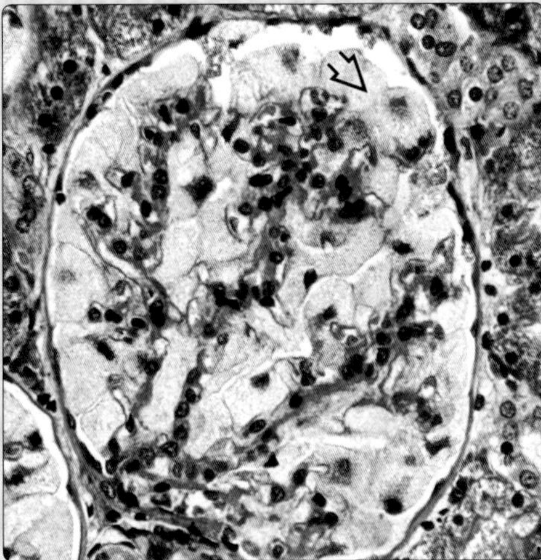

(Left) *In I-cell disease (mucolipidosis II), PAS stain highlights the mesangial matrix and open capillary loops but does not stain the enlarged, pale vacuolated podocytes ⇨. The parietal epithelial cells, however, are not vacuolated ⇨.* **(Right)** *In I-cell disease, the trichrome stain highlights the mesangial matrix and capillary loop basement membranes, but the podocyte cytoplasmic vacuoles ⇨ remain unstained. This podocyte staining pattern is indistinguishable from the appearance of podocytes in Fabry disease.*

Colloidal Iron Positive Podocytes

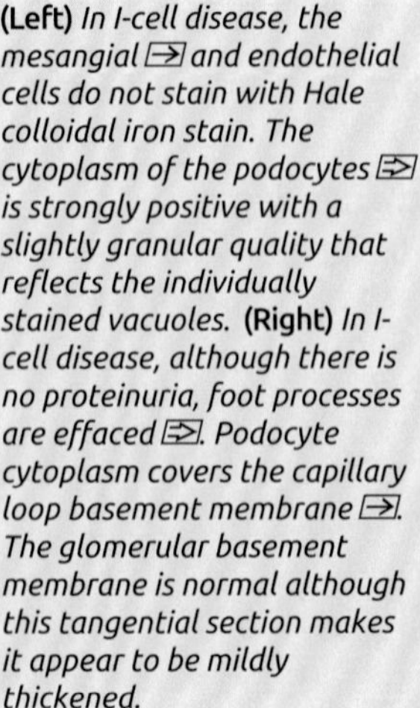

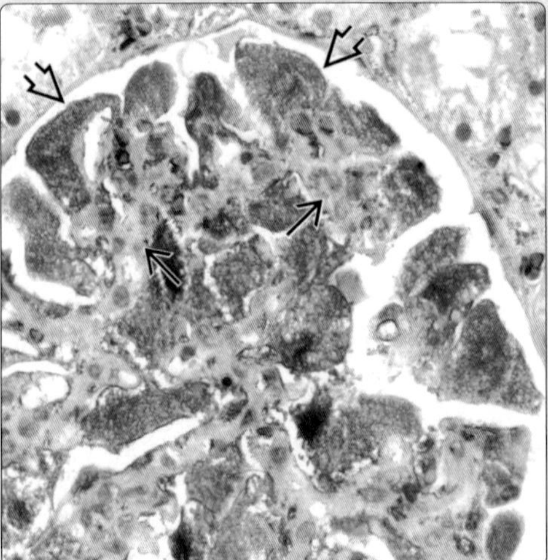

Podocyte Vacuoles With Membranous Remnants

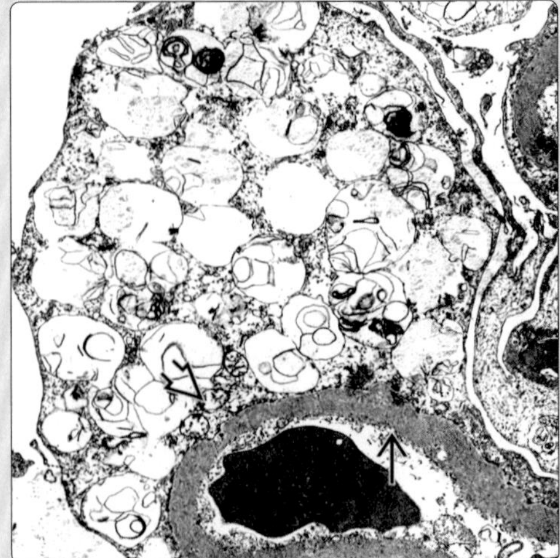

(Left) *In I-cell disease, the mesangial → and endothelial cells do not stain with Hale colloidal iron stain. The cytoplasm of the podocytes ⇨ is strongly positive with a slightly granular quality that reflects the individually stained vacuoles.* **(Right)** *In I-cell disease, although there is no proteinuria, foot processes are effaced ⇨. Podocyte cytoplasm covers the capillary loop basement membrane →. The glomerular basement membrane is normal although this tangential section makes it appear to be mildly thickened.*

TERMINOLOGY

Abbreviations

- Mucolipidosis II (MLII)

Synonyms

- Inclusion cell (I-cell) disease
- Mucolipidosis II α/β

Definitions

- Sialyl oligosaccharide storage disease secondary to N-acetylglucosamine-phosphotransferase deficiency

ETIOLOGY/PATHOGENESIS

Genetic Factors

- Autosomal recessive disorder
- 2 disease-causing mutations of *GNPTAB* gene on chromosome 12q23.3 are responsible
  - Encodes Golgi enzyme, N-acetylglucosamine-phosphotransferase
  - Failure to form mannose-6-phosphate, necessary for trafficking of enzymes to lysosome

CLINICAL ISSUES

Presentation

- Hurler-like syndrome presenting at birth
  - Psychomotor retardation
  - Coarse facial features and thickened skin
  - Large joint contractures and deformed long bones
  - Hypertrophic gingiva
- Mitral and aortic valve insufficiency
- Respiratory insufficiency
- Renal abnormalities are usually absent
  - Proximal tubular dysfunction may be present with low-grade proteinuria, hyperphosphaturia, hypercalcuria, and aminoaciduria

Laboratory Tests

- Genetic testing for *GNPTAB* mutation
  - Partial or whole gene deletions or duplications
- Increased activity 5-20x of all lysosomal hydrolases (B-D-hexosaminidase, B-D-glucuronidase, B-N-galactosidase and α-l-fucosidase) in plasma and other body fluids
- Increased urinary excretion of oligosaccharides

Treatment

- Symptomatic
- Bone marrow or hematopoietic stem cell transplantation

Prognosis

- Slowly progressive with fatal outcome in early childhood

IMAGING

Radiographic Findings

- Skeletal radiographs show dysostosis multiplex

MICROSCOPIC

Histologic Features

- Podocyte cytoplasmic ballooning
  - Clear vacuoles distend cytoplasm
- Podocyte vacuoles do not stain with renal biopsy stains
  - PAS negative
  - Trichrome negative
  - Methenamine silver negative
- Vacuolar glycolipids and acidic glycosaminoglycans can be stained in paraffin-embedded tissue
  - Hale's colloidal iron positive
  - Alcian blue-PAS pH 2.5 positive
  - Sudan black positive
  - Oil red O positive in frozen sections
- Rarely vacuoles in proximal tubules and interstitial cells

ANCILLARY TESTS

Electron Microscopy

- Podocyte cytoplasm is enlarged and vacuolated
  - Most vacuoles appear empty
  - Membranous or lamellar material in some vacuoles
- Endothelial cells and mesangial cells free of vacuoles
- Peripheral blood lymphocytes contain vacuoles
- Mesenchymal cells of any organ contain vacuolated cells

DIFFERENTIAL DIAGNOSIS

Storage Diseases Primarily Affecting Podocytes

- Fabry disease
  - Storage material extracted by solvents during preparation cannot be stained
  - Podocyte cytoplasm stains dark blue with toluidine blue in plastic-embedded sections for EM
  - Ultrastructural examination reveals vacuoles filled with whirled lamellar myeloid bodies
- GM1 gangliosidosis
  - No clinical evidence of renal disease like in I-cell disease
  - Storage material extracted by solvents during preparation cannot be stained
  - EM reveals vacuoles that contain small amount of membranous or lamellar material
- Nephrosialidosis
  - Storage material causes vacuolated podocytes, parietal epithelium, endothelium, tubules, and interstitial cells
  - Storage material is Hale's colloidal iron positive

DIAGNOSTIC CHECKLIST

Pathologic Interpretation Pearls

- Impressive podocyte vacuolization but no renal disease
- Podocyte lipid not removed by routine processing

SELECTED REFERENCES

1. Cathey SS et al. Phenotype and genotype in mucolipidoses II and III alpha/beta: a study of 61 probands. J Med Genet. 47(1):38-48, 2010
2. Kudo M et al: Mucolipidosis II (I-cell disease) and mucolipidosis IIIA (classical pseudo-hurler polydystrophy) are caused by mutations in the GlcNAc-phosphotransferase alpha/beta -subunits precursor gene. Am J Hum Genet. 78(3):451-63, 2006
3. Renwick N et al: Foamy podocytes. Am J Kidney Dis. 41(4):891-6, 2003
4. Koga M et al: Histochemical and ultrastructural studies of inclusion bodies found in tissues from three siblings with I-cell disease. Pathol Int. 44(3):223-9, 1994
5. Leroy JG, Cathey S, Friez MJ. Mucolipidosis II. 1993-, 2008

Enlarged Podocytes With Foamy Cytoplasm

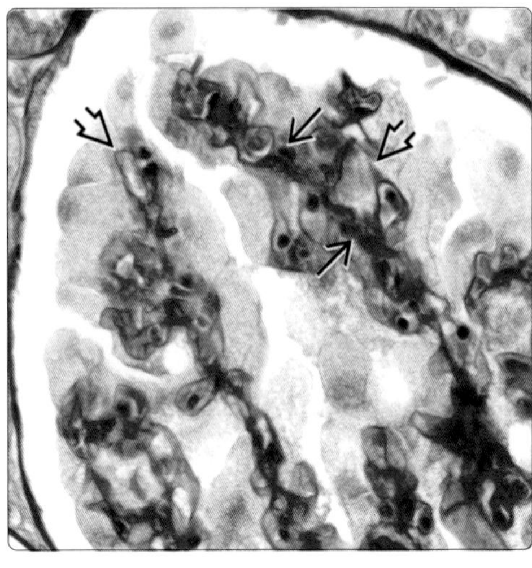

Enlarged Podocyte With Foamy Cytoplasm

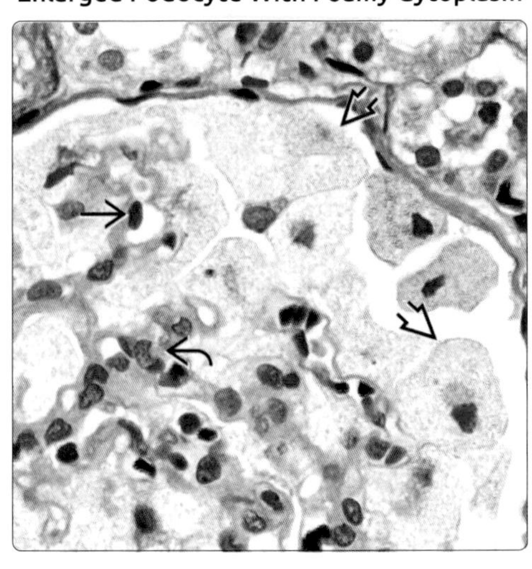

(Left) *In I-cell disease, PAS stain highlights the inconspicuous mesangial matrix → and small and patent capillary loops → but not the enlarged vacuolated podocytes. The endothelial cells and mesangial cells do not contain vacuoles and are difficult to identify.* **(Right)** *The podocyte vacuoles → do not stain with Luxol fast blue in I-cell disease. The mesangium is scant and the capillary loops are open but small. The mesangial → and endothelial → cells are not vacuolated.*

Fabry Disease With Enlarged Podocytes With Foamy Cytoplasm

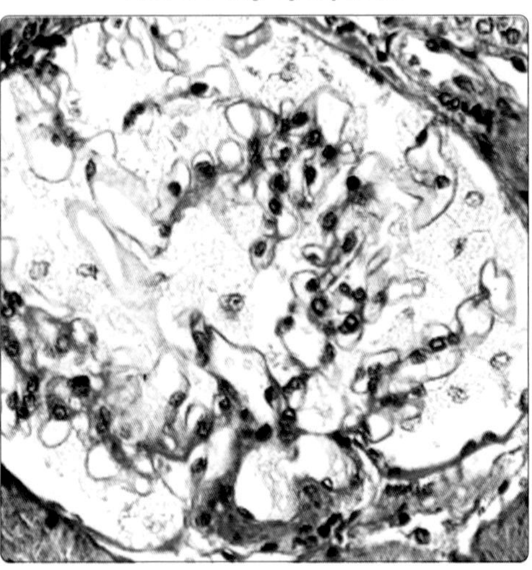

Colloidal Iron Positive Podocytes

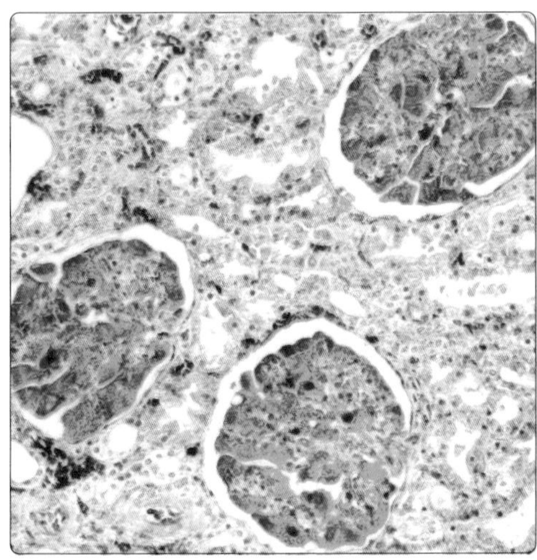

(Left) *This trichrome-stained glomerulus is from a patient with Fabry disease. It is shown for comparison with I-cell disease. In both diseases, the glomeruli show impressive podocyte cytoplasmic expansion by clear vacuoles. There is no endothelial cell or mesangial cell involvement.* **(Right)** *In I-cell disease, Hale's colloidal iron stain brilliantly stains the cytoplasm of every podocyte but shows no appreciable staining of other cell types within glomeruli. The renal tubules and interstitial cells are also negative.*

Colloidal Iron Positive Podocytes

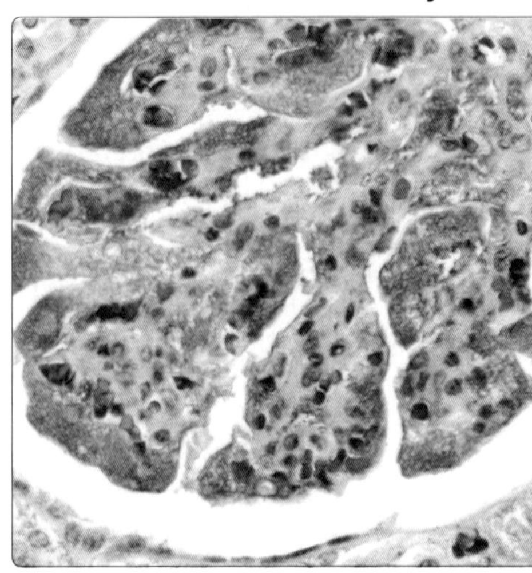

Mitral Valve With Foamy Macrophages

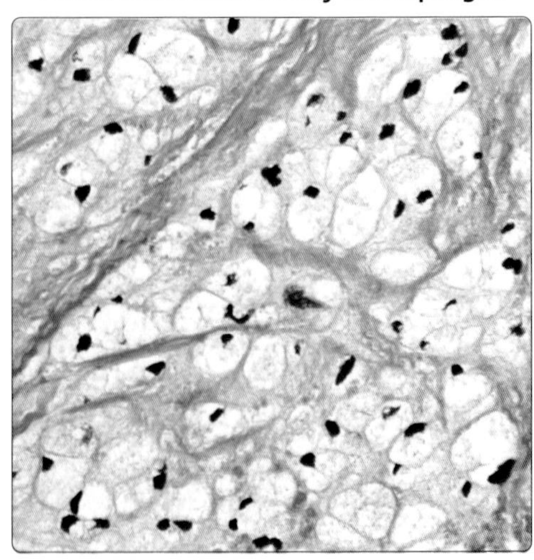

(Left) *The podocytes are markedly enlarged and densely stained with Hale's colloidal iron stain. The inconspicuous mesangium and capillary loops appear compressed by comparison.* **(Right)** *Sialyl oligosaccharide storage products accumulate in other organs in I-cell disease. This section from a mitral valve shows clusters of macrophages with foamy cytoplasm very similar to podocytes. Although there is no cellular or stromal reaction to this accumulation, valve thickening and insufficiency result.*

Podocytes Distended by Cytoplasmic Vacuoles

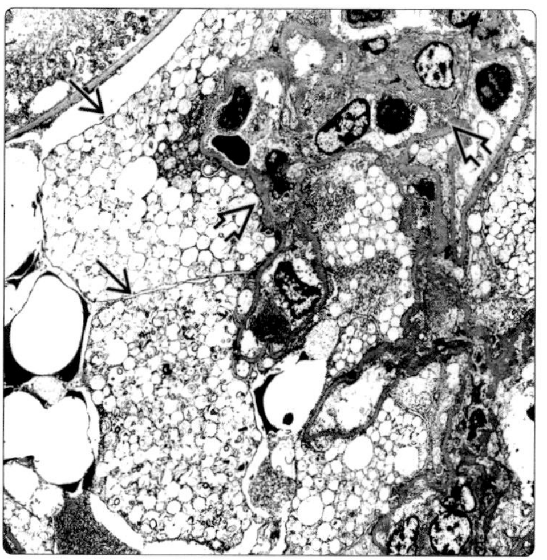

Endothelial Cells Lack Vacuoles

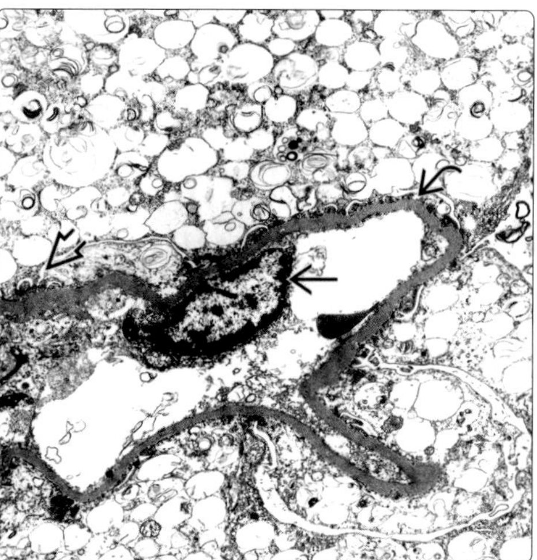

(Left) *The cytoplasm of every podocyte is distended by large vacuoles* ➞. *The vacuoles vary in size and are largely empty. The endothelial cells and mesangial cells lack cytoplasmic vacuoles* ➞. **(Right)** *In I-cell disease, the podocyte cytoplasm is distended by largely empty vacuoles. There is preservation of some podocyte foot processes* ➞, *but others are widened or effaced. The endothelial cells* ➞ *lining the capillary loop are not affected, and the capillary loop basement membrane* ➞ *is normal.*

Podocyte Vacuoles Are Largely Empty

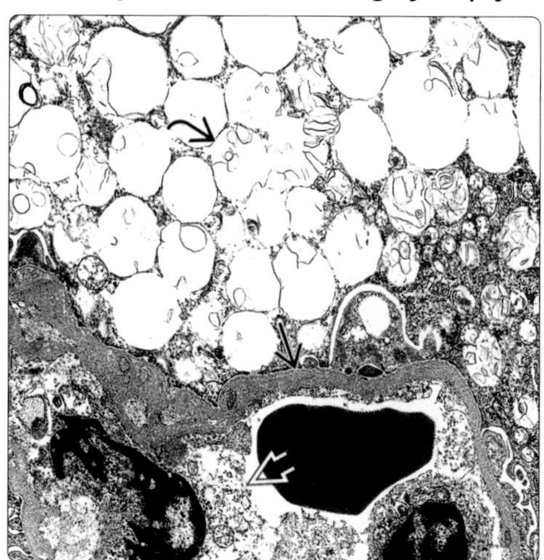

Podocyte Vacuoles Contain Membranous Material

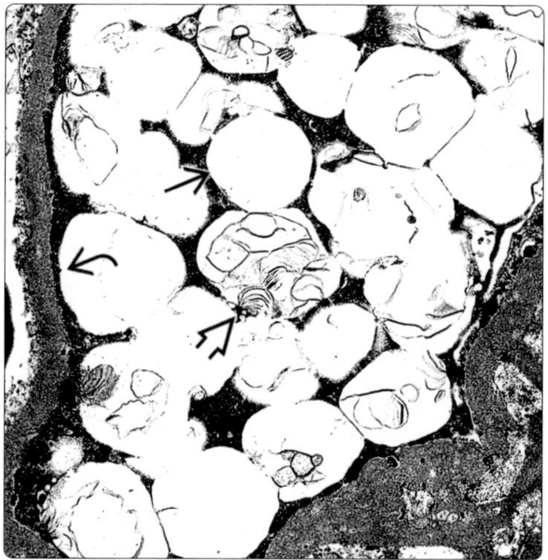

(Left) *The podocyte vacuoles are largely empty. However, characteristically they contain strands* ➞ *of membranous to lamellar material of unknown composition. The glomerular basement membrane* ➞ *is normal and the endothelial cells* ➞ *lack vacuoles.* **(Right)** *Some podocyte vacuoles are empty* ➞, *at least in this plane of section. Other vacuoles contain scant lamellar or membranous material* ➞. *There is diffuse effacement of foot processes with a sheet-like covering of the capillary loop basement membranes* ➞.

Podocyte Vacuoles With Abundant Membranous Material

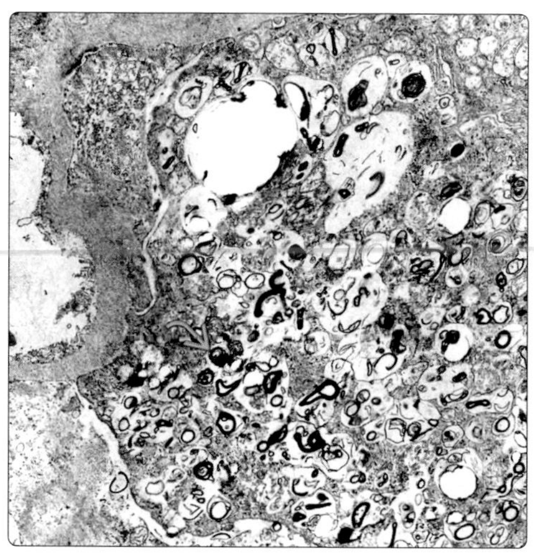

Membranous Remnants Can Resemble Fabry Inclusions

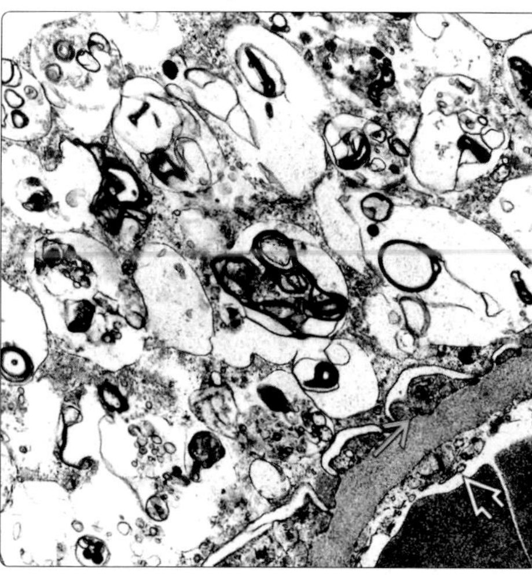

(Left) *The podocyte vacuoles in this patient with I-cell disease contain more abundant lamellar and membranous material* ➞ *than typical, reflecting variability in solvent extraction during the dehydration step of tissue processing.* **(Right)** *The membranous and lamellar material is more irregular in structure and distribution in I-cell disease than in Fabry disease. There is widening of podocyte foot processes* ➞ *without complete effacement. The endothelial cell is not affected* ➞.

Alagille Syndrome

KEY FACTS

TERMINOLOGY

- Arteriohepatic dysplasia
- Syndrome characterized by paucity of intrahepatic bile ducts with at least 3 of the following
  - Chronic cholestasis
  - Cardiac abnormalities
  - Eye abnormalities (commonly posterior embryotoxon)
  - Skeletal abnormalities (usually butterfly vertebrae)
  - Characteristic facies

ETIOLOGY/PATHOGENESIS

- *JAG1* mutation
  - Jagged-1 protein, a notch ligand
  - Autosomal dominant inheritance pattern
  - > 90% of patients with Alagille syndrome have this mutation
- *NOTCH2* mutation

CLINICAL ISSUES

- Chronic renal insufficiency
- Proteinuria

MACROSCOPIC

- Renal dysplasia (60%) is most common renal abnormality

MICROSCOPIC

- Mesangial and GBM lipidosis
- Tubular basement membrane lipidosis
- Glomerular basement membrane "spikes" or vacuolated appearance
- Global and segmental glomerulosclerosis

TOP DIFFERENTIAL DIAGNOSES

- Lecithin-cholesterol acyltransferase deficiency
- Membranous GN
- Renal dysplasia
- Bile cast nephropathy

GBM Lipidosis

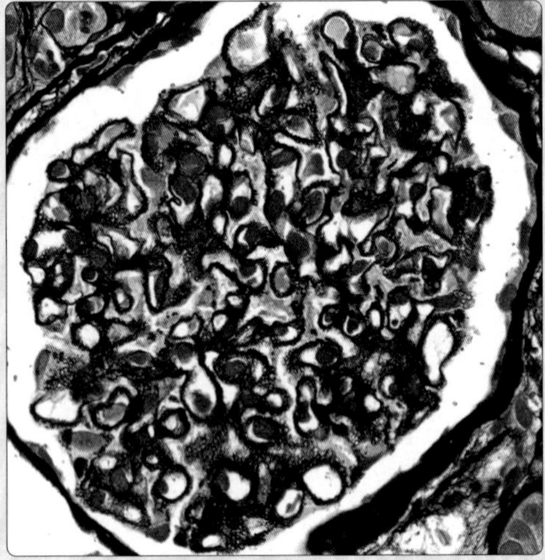

Bile Casts and Renal Dysplasia

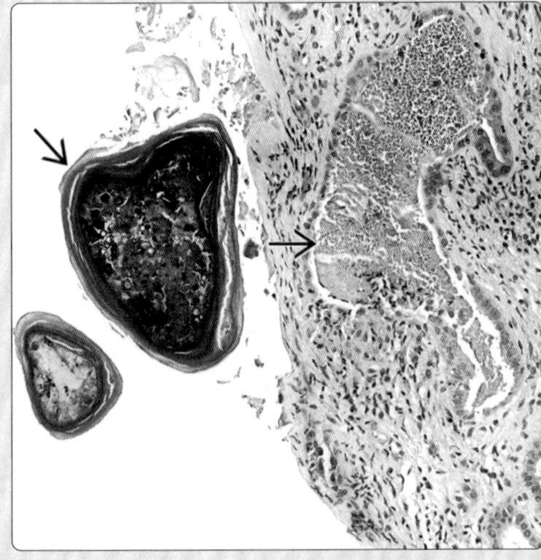

(Left) *Prominent "spike" formation and a vacuolated appearance are shown along the glomerular basement membranes in a 19-year-old man with Alagille syndrome.* **(Right)** *Large bile casts* → *are present in several tubules surrounded by undifferentiated mesenchyme in a region of renal dysplasia, which appeared to be segmental in distribution, even within a single needle core biopsy.*

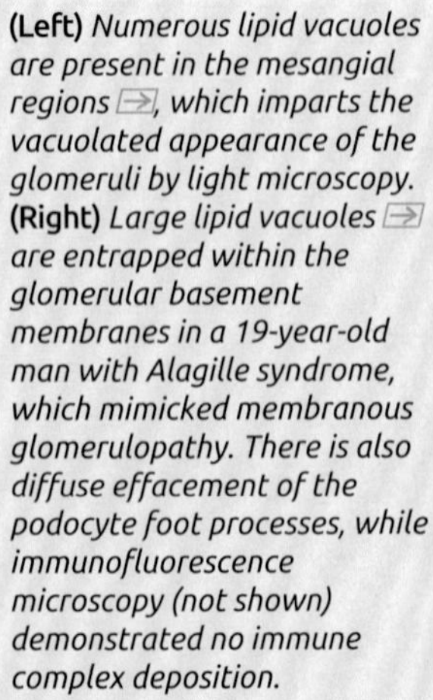

(Left) *Numerous lipid vacuoles are present in the mesangial regions* →*, which imparts the vacuolated appearance of the glomeruli by light microscopy.* **(Right)** *Large lipid vacuoles* → *are entrapped within the glomerular basement membranes in a 19-year-old man with Alagille syndrome, which mimicked membranous glomerulopathy. There is also diffuse effacement of the podocyte foot processes, while immunofluorescence microscopy (not shown) demonstrated no immune complex deposition.*

Mesangial and GBM Lipidosis

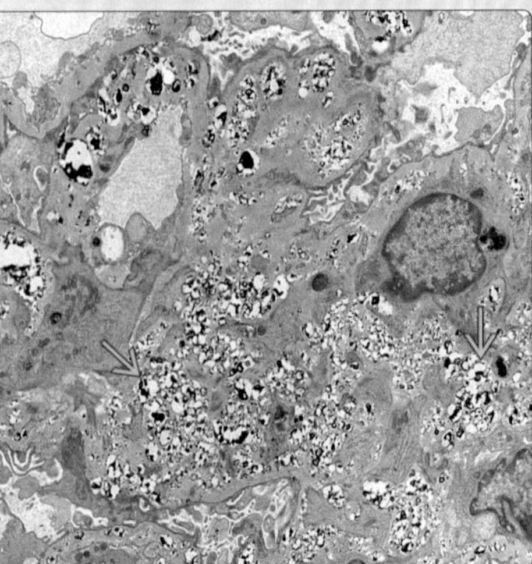

GBM Lipidosis

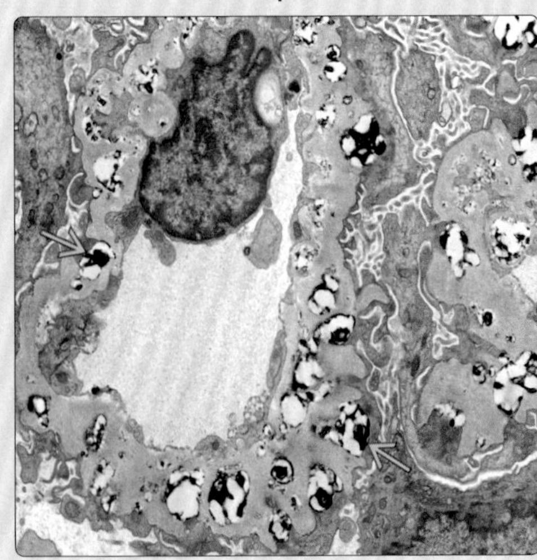

TERMINOLOGY

Synonyms

- Alagille-Watson syndrome
- Arteriohepatic dysplasia

Definitions

- Syndrome characterized by paucity (absence or hypoplasia) of intrahepatic bile ducts with at least 3 of the following major features
  - Chronic cholestasis
  - Cardiac abnormalities
    - Peripheral pulmonary stenosis (76%)
    - Tetralogy of Fallot (12%)
  - Skeletal abnormalities (usually butterfly vertebrae)
  - Eye abnormalities (commonly posterior embryotoxon)
  - Characteristic facies
  - Renal abnormalities
    - Proposed as 6th criterion for Alagille syndrome
    - 40% of Alagille syndrome patients
- First described in 1969 by Daniel Alagille (French hepatologist)

ETIOLOGY/PATHOGENESIS

Developmental Anomaly

- *JAG1* mutation
  - Jagged-1 protein, a notch ligand
    - Required for kidney development in mice
  - Autosomal dominant inheritance pattern
    - High degree of penetrance with variable manifestations
  - > 90% of patients with Alagille syndrome have this mutation
  - > 430 mutations identified
- *NOTCH2* mutation
  - Associated with increased renal involvement

CLINICAL ISSUES

Epidemiology

- Incidence
  - 1 in 30,000 live births

Presentation

- Chronic renal insufficiency
- Proteinuria
  - Often subnephrotic range
- Hypertension
- Renal tubular acidosis
- Cholestasis
- Conjugated hyperbilirubinemia

Treatment

- Surgical approaches
  - Liver transplantation for end-stage liver disease in 15-20% of children
  - Kidney transplantation

MACROSCOPIC

General Features

- Abnormalities reported in Alagille syndrome include
  - Renal dysplasia ± cysts (60%)
    - Most common abnormality
  - Renal agenesis or hypoplasia
  - Renal artery stenosis
  - Duplicated ureters
  - Horseshoe kidney

MICROSCOPIC

Histologic Features

- Glomeruli
  - Mesangial lipidosis
  - GBM lipodosis
    - Glomerular basement membrane "spikes" or vacuolated appearance
      - Advanced stages mimic membranous nephropathy
  - Global and segmental glomerulosclerosis
  - Bile pigment in podocyte cytoplasm
- Tubules and interstitium
  - Tubular basement membrane lipidosis
  - Renal dysplasia
  - Bile cast nephropathy

ANCILLARY TESTS

Electron Microscopy

- Lipid vacuoles within mesangial cells and glomerular basement membranes

DIFFERENTIAL DIAGNOSIS

Lecithin-Cholesterol Acyltransferase Deficiency

- Renal lipidosis
- Autosomal recessive inheritance pattern

Membranous GN

- Subepithelial immune complex deposition

Renal Dysplasia

- Primitive collecting ducts with smooth muscle collarettes
- May be cystic

Bile Cast Nephropathy

- Greenish-yellow tubular casts

SELECTED REFERENCES

1. Kamath BM et al: Renal involvement and the role of Notch signalling in Alagille syndrome. Nat Rev Nephrol. 9(7):409-18, 2013
2. Kamath BM et al: Renal anomalies in Alagille syndrome: a disease-defining feature. Am J Med Genet A. 158A(1):85-9, 2012
3. Salem JE et al: Hypertension and aortorenal disease in Alagille syndrome. J Hypertens. 30(7):1300-6, 2012
4. Davis J et al: Glomerular basement membrane lipidosis in Alagille syndrome. Pediatr Nephrol. 25(6):1181-4, 2010
5. Shrivastava R et al: An unusual cause of hypertension and renal failure: a case series of a family with Alagille syndrome. Nephrol Dial Transplant. 25(5):1501-6, 2010
6. Jacquet A et al: Alagille syndrome in adult patients: it is never too late. Am J Kidney Dis. 49(5):705-9, 2007

Glomerulopathy of Hereditary Multiple Exostoses

KEY FACTS

TERMINOLOGY

- Autosomal dominant inherited condition resulting in osteochondromas and abnormal glomerular collagen deposition secondary to *EXT1* gene mutations

ETIOLOGY/PATHOGENESIS

- *EXT1* encodes protein exostosin-1
- Complex with product of *EXT2* gene
  - Forms glycosyl transferase for heparin sulfate glycosaminoglycan synthesis
- Defective exostosin-1 results in deficient heparan sulfate glycosaminoglycans
- Response to steroids suggests that steroids facilitate alternative heparin sulfate synthesis

CLINICAL ISSUES

- Steroid-sensitive nephrotic syndrome
- Multiple osteochondromas
  - Distal femur (90%)
- Hearing abnormalities

MICROSCOPIC

- Nonspecific changes
- Mild mesangial hypercellularity
- Pauci-immune pattern with crescents in 1 case
- Electron microscopy
  - GBM and mesangial collagen fibril deposition
  - Diffuse mesangial fibrillar collagen deposition
  - Moderate podocyte foot process effacement

ANCILLARY TESTS

- Gene sequencing *EXT1* gene

TOP DIFFERENTIAL DIAGNOSES

- Nail-patella syndrome
- Collagen type III glomerulopathy
- Fibronectin glomerulopathy
- Fibrillary glomerulopathy

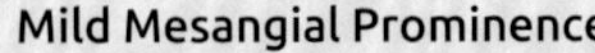

Mild Mesangial Prominence

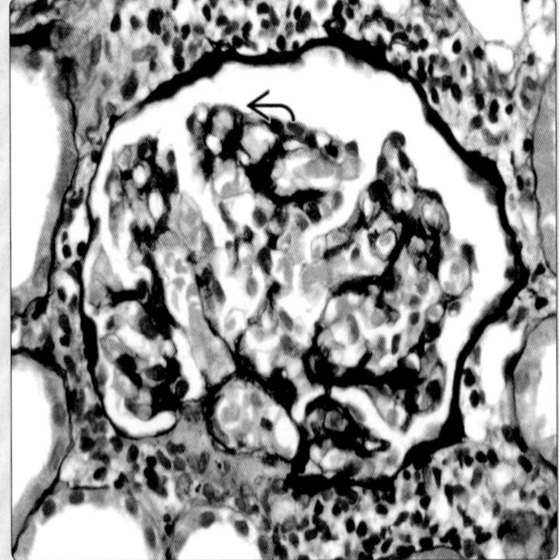

Fibrillar Collagen in GBM

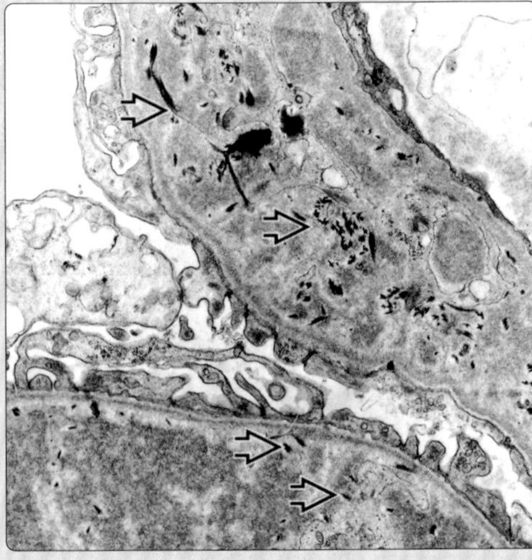

(Left) *Renal biopsy from a 37-year-old woman with nephrotic-range proteinuria and hereditary multiple exostoses shows mild mesangial matrix increase and focal capillary loop thickening ➙. (Courtesy I. Roberts, MD.)* **(Right)** *Fibrillar collagen deposits in lamina densa and subendothelial areas ➙ are characteristic of hereditary multiple exostoses involving the kidney. (Courtesy I. Roberts, MD.)*

Mesangial Fibrillar Collagen

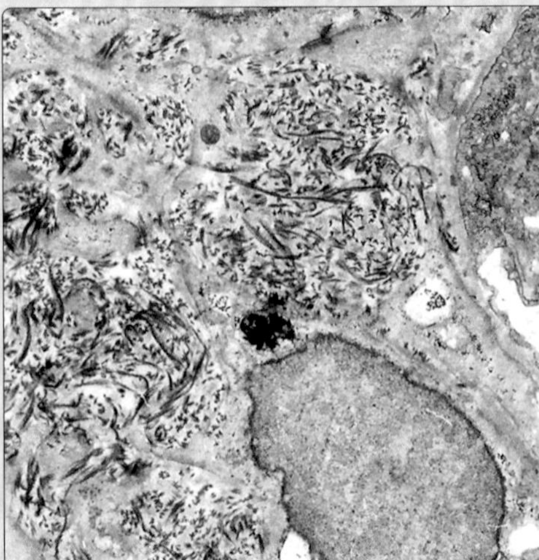

Enhanced Contrast With Phosphotungstic Acid

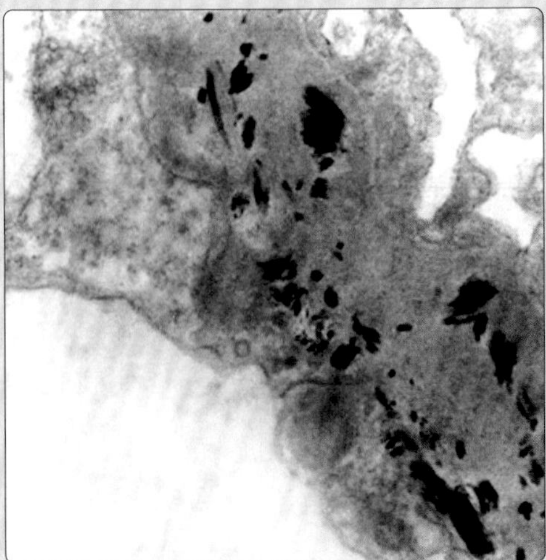

(Left) *Mesangial and GBM fibrillar collagen deposits are shown from a biopsy of a 37-year-old woman with HME who presented with nephrotic syndrome. (Courtesy I. Roberts, MD.)* **(Right)** *This phosphotungstic acid-stained section shows lamina densa collagen bundles characteristic of nail-patella syndrome.*

TERMINOLOGY

Abbreviations

- Hereditary multiple exostoses (HME)

Definitions

- Autosomal dominant inherited condition resulting in osteochondromas and abnormal glomerular collagen deposition secondary to *EXT1* gene mutations

ETIOLOGY/PATHOGENESIS

Genetics

- *EXT1* and *EXT2* account for 80% of cases
  - *EXT1* encodes exostosin-1 protein
    - Localized to Golgi apparatus
    - Complex with product of *EXT2* gene
      - Forms glycosyl transferase for heparin sulfate glycosaminoglycan synthesis
  - Frameshift mutation 238 del A in *EXT1*
  - Maps to chromosome 8q24.11-q24.13
- Autosomal dominant
- Exostoses deficient in heparan sulfate and perlecan and accumulate collagen I and X
  - Postulated to be similar process in glomerulus
- Response to steroids suggests that steroids facilitate alternative heparin sulfate synthesis

Pathophysiology

- Defective exostosin-1 results in deficient heparan sulfate glycosaminoglycans
- Heparan sulfate deficiency alters podocyte structure and function
- Mechanism leading to proteinuria and collagen accumulation in glomerulus unclear

CLINICAL ISSUES

Epidemiology

- Incidence
  - Very rare (5 cases, 1 family)
- Age
  - Hearing impairment in infancy
  - Osteochondromas develop in childhood
  - Renal symptoms develop in adulthood

Presentation

- Steroid-sensitive nephrotic syndrome
- Hearing abnormalities
- Multiple osteochondromas
  - Benign, metaphyseal, cartilage-capped bone tumors
  - Distal femur (90%)
  - Proximal tibia (84%)
  - Fibula (76%)
  - Humerus (72%)

Laboratory Tests

- Sequencing *EXT1* gene

Treatment

- Drugs
  - Steroids

Prognosis

- Steroids reported effective, but experience limited

MICROSCOPIC

Histologic Features

- Glomeruli
  - Mild mesangial hypercellularity
  - Mild increase in mesangial matrix
  - Focal capillary wall thickening
  - Pauci-immune pattern with crescents (1 case)
- Tubules, interstitium, and vessels
  - No specific changes described

ANCILLARY TESTS

Immunofluorescence

- Negative IgG, IgA, IgM, C3, & C1q

Electron Microscopy

- Diffuse mesangial fibrillar collagen deposition
- GBM and mesangial collagen fibril deposition
  - Associated with focal GBM duplication and mesangial interposition
- Moderate podocyte foot process effacement

DIFFERENTIAL DIAGNOSIS

Nail-Patella Syndrome

- Autosomal dominant inherited defect in *LMX1B* gene
- Presents with proteinuria ± hematuria
  - Nephrotic syndrome, atypical
- Mild glomerular changes
- Nail and bone abnormalities
- Irregular type III collagen within GBM
- Characteristic moth-eaten appearance of GBM

Collagen Type III Glomerulopathy

- Abundant subendothelial and mesangial collagen fibrils
- Collagen fibrils are curved, ~ 60 nm periodicity
- Autosomal recessive inheritance pattern

Fibronectin Glomerulopathy

- Lobular glomeruli, with expanded mesangial matrix
- 9-16 nm, granular, fibrillary electron-dense deposits

Fibrillary Glomerulopathy

- Random 10-30 nm fibrils in mesangium and GBM
- IgG and C3 in deposits

SELECTED REFERENCES

1. Jennes I et al: Multiple osteochondromas: mutation update and description of the multiple osteochondromas mutation database (MOdb). Hum Mutat. 30(12):1620-7, 2009
2. Chen S et al: Loss of heparan sulfate glycosaminoglycan assembly in podocytes does not lead to proteinuria. Kidney Int. 74(3):289-99, 2008
3. Nadanaka S et al: Heparan sulphate biosynthesis and disease. J Biochem. 144(1):7-14, 2008
4. Roberts IS et al: Familial nephropathy and multiple exostoses with exostosin-1 (EXT1) gene mutation. J Am Soc Nephrol. 19(3):450-3, 2008
5. McCormick C et al: The putative tumor suppressors EXT1 and EXT2 form a stable complex that accumulates in the Golgi apparatus and catalyzes the synthesis of heparan sulfate. Proc Natl Acad Sci U S A. 97(2):668-73, 2000
6. Schmale GA, Wuyts W, Chansky HA, Raskind WH. Hereditary Multiple Osteochondromas. 1993-, 2000

Type III Hyperlipoproteinemia

KEY FACTS

TERMINOLOGY

- Hypercholesterolemia and hypertriglyceridemia associated with homozygous apolipoprotein-E2 allele

ETIOLOGY/PATHOGENESIS

- Autosomal recessive
- *APOE* chromosome 19q13.2
  - 3 alleles: E2, E3, E4
  - ~ 5% of *APOE2* homozygotes develop type III hyperlipidemia

CLINICAL ISSUES

- Males more commonly affected
- Nephrotic syndrome
- Premature vascular disease
- Palmar and tuberous xanthomas
- Hypercholesterolemia (> 300 mg/dL)
  - VLDL/TG ratio > 0.3
- Hypertriglyceridemia (> 300 mg/dL)

MICROSCOPIC

- Glomeruli
  - Endothelial and mesangial foamy macrophage aggregates
  - Segmental glomerulosclerosis
- Interstitium
  - Foamy macrophages
  - Fibrosis as disease progresses
- Electron microscopy
  - Glomeruli
    - Capillary loop foam cells
    - Lamellated electron-dense material
    - Cholesterol clefts
    - Extensive podocyte foot process effacement
  - Mesangial, endothelial, and tubular lipid vacuoles

TOP DIFFERENTIAL DIAGNOSES

- Lipoprotein glomerulopathy
- FSGS

Lipid-Filled Macrophages in Capillaries

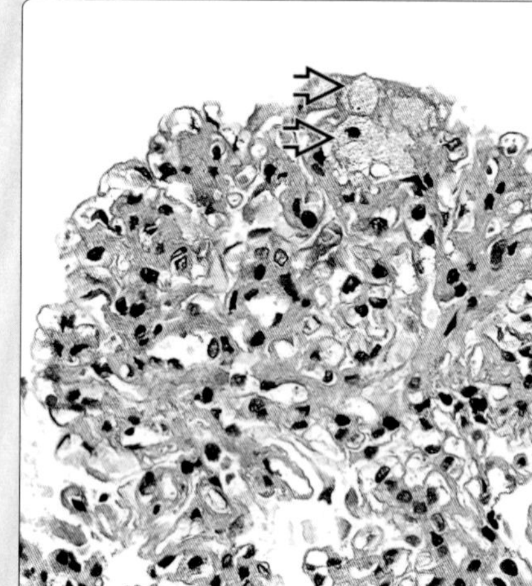

Lipid in Macrophages

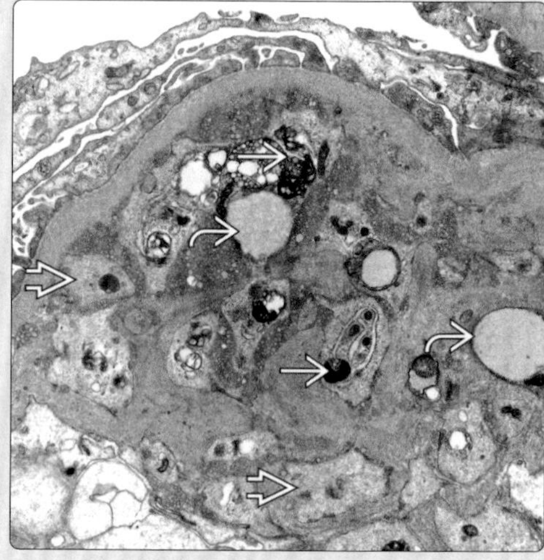

(Left) *Foamy macrophages are seen in this glomerulus from biopsy of a 55-year-old man with nephrotic syndrome and type III hyperlipoproteinemia (cholesterol 559 mg/dL and triglycerides 2169 mg/dL). (Courtesy J. Churg, MD.)* **(Right)** *Glomerular capillary lumen is obliterated by a mixture of foamy cells, lipid vacuoles, and dark-staining membrane-bound particles and lysosomes. (Courtesy J. Churg, MD.)*

Subendothelial Lipid

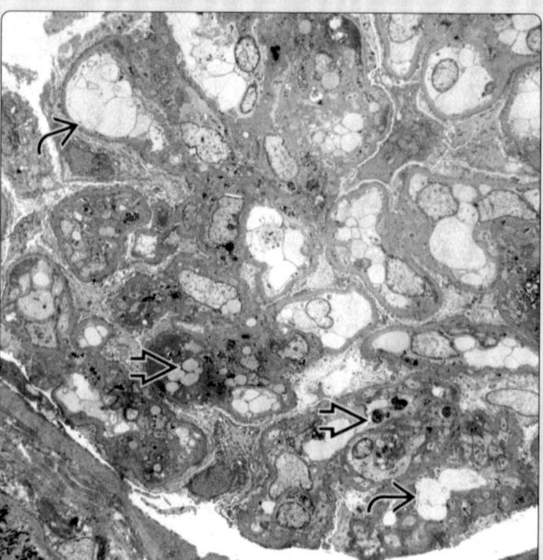

Lipid in GBM

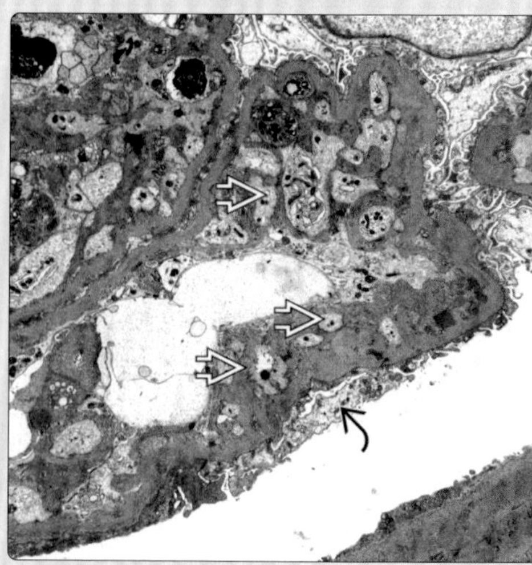

(Left) *At this low magnification, the glomerulus shows diffuse capillary loop thickening and subendothelial lipid accumulation. Lumens are filled with lipid vacuoles and lysosomal particles.* **(Right)** *High magnification of the glomerular capillary reveals foot process effacement and lipid in the thickened GBM. (Courtesy J. Churg, MD.)*

TERMINOLOGY

Synonyms

- Type III hyperlipidemia

Definitions

- Hypercholesterolemia and hypertriglyceridemia associated with apolipoprotein-E2 allele

ETIOLOGY/PATHOGENESIS

Genetics

- *APOE*
  - Encodes apolipoprotein E
  - Maps to chromosome 19q13.2
  - 3 alleles: E2, E3, E4
    - E2 is least common (~ 5% frequency)
    - E3 is most common (> 60% frequency)
- Autosomal recessive
  - Approximately 5% of *APOE2* homozygotes develop type III hyperlipidemia
  - Secondary genetic &/or environmental factors implicated
- *APOE2* carriers also prone to developing type III hyperlipidemia
- Rare variant mutations result in autosomal dominant inheritance pattern

Pathogenesis

- ApoE2 proteins bind ineffectively to the low-density lipoprotein (LDL) receptor, leading to ineffective clearance of lipoproteins and accumulation in plasma

CLINICAL ISSUES

Epidemiology

- Incidence
  - 0.02% of population; worldwide distribution
- Age
  - Children and adults affected
- Sex
  - Males more commonly affected

Presentation

- Nephrotic-range proteinuria
- Hyperlipidemia (turbid plasma)
- Nephrotic syndrome
- Palmar and tuberous xanthomas
- Hepatomegaly and splenomegaly
- Premature vascular disease
- Ascites

Laboratory Tests

- Lipid profile: Type III hyperlipidemia
  - Hypercholesterolemia (> 300 mg/dL)
    - Very low-density lipoprotein (VLDL):triglyceride ratio > 0.3
    - Normal high-density lipoprotein (HDL)
    - Decreased LDL
  - Hypertriglyceridemia (> 300 mg/dL)
- ApoE genotyping
  - *APOE2* homozygosity

Treatment

- Drugs
  - Lipid-lowering agents, ACE inhibitors
- Plasmapheresis
- Dietary modifications

MICROSCOPIC

Histologic Features

- Glomeruli
  - Endothelial and mesangial foamy macrophage aggregates
  - Segmental sclerosis
  - Mesangial hypercellularity
- Tubules
  - Atrophy as disease progresses
- Interstitium
  - Foamy macrophages
  - Fibrosis as disease progresses
  - Lymphocytic infiltrates
- Vessels
  - Thickening

ANCILLARY TESTS

Electron Microscopy

- Capillary loop foam cells
  - Lamellated electron-dense material
  - Cholesterol clefts
- Mesangial, endothelial, and tubular lipid vacuoles
- Extensive podocyte foot process effacement
- Increased mesangial matrix

DIFFERENTIAL DIAGNOSIS

Lipoprotein Glomerulopathy

- Lipoprotein thrombi in glomerular capillary loops
- Typically associated with unique *APOE* gene mutations
- Rarely associated with type III hyperlipidemia
- Absent xanthoma

Focal Segmental Glomerulosclerosis (FSGS)

- Glomerular capillary, tubular, and interstitial foam cells can be seen in FSGS and other diseases with nephrotic syndrome
  - Lack abundant aggregates of foam cells seen in type III hyperlipidemia
- Associated with type IIa, IIb, and IV hyperlipidemia

DIAGNOSTIC CHECKLIST

Pathologic Interpretation Pearls

- Aggregates of glomerular and interstitial foam cells with FSGS should prompt lipid analysis

SELECTED REFERENCES

1. Matsunaga A et al: Apolipoprotein E mutations: a comparison between lipoprotein glomerulopathy and type III hyperlipoproteinemia. Clin Exp Nephrol. 18(2):220-4, 2014
2. Eichner JE et al: Apolipoprotein E polymorphism and cardiovascular disease: a HuGE review. Am J Epidemiol. 155(6):487-95, 2002
3. Ellis D et al: Atypical hyperlipidemia and nephropathy associated with apolipoprotein E homozygosity. J Am Soc Nephrol. 6(4):1170-7, 1995

Nail-Patella Syndrome

KEY FACTS

TERMINOLOGY

- Inherited syndrome with nail, skeletal abnormalities, and proteinuria secondary to *LMX1B* gene mutations
- Variant without extrarenal signs

ETIOLOGY/PATHOGENESIS

- Autosomal dominant inheritance
- *LMX1B*: Chromosome 9q34.1 (ABO linkage)
  - Encodes LIM homeodomain transcription factor
    - Expressed in podocytes

CLINICAL ISSUES

- Rare (~ 1/50,000)
- 30-60% have renal involvement
  - Proteinuria, 10% progress to ESRD
- Iliac horns pathognomonic (70%)
- Absent, hypoplastic, or dystrophic nails
- Small, irregularly shaped, or absent patellae
- Glaucoma, cataracts, deafness

MICROSCOPIC

- Glomeruli
  - Focal segmental glomerulosclerosis
  - Normal appearance by light microscopy
  - Focal thickening of capillary loops
- Tubules, interstitium, vessels: No specific changes

ANCILLARY TESTS

- Collagen fibrils in GBM with characteristic ~ 60 nm periodicity by EM
  - Phosphotungstic acid enhances contrast
- "Moth-eaten" GBM classically described
- *LMX1B* gene sequencing
  - 85% of mutations in exons/introns 2 through 6

TOP DIFFERENTIAL DIAGNOSES

- Type III collagen glomerulopathy
- Fibronectin glomerulopathy
- Glomerulopathy of hereditary multiple exostoses

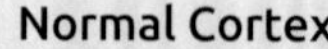

Normal Cortex

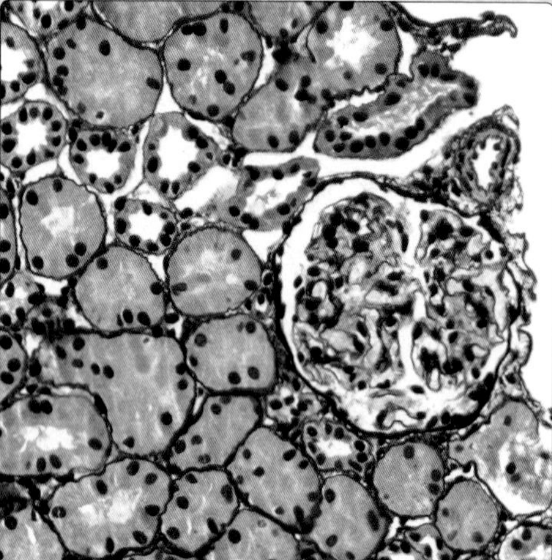

"Moth-Eaten" GBM

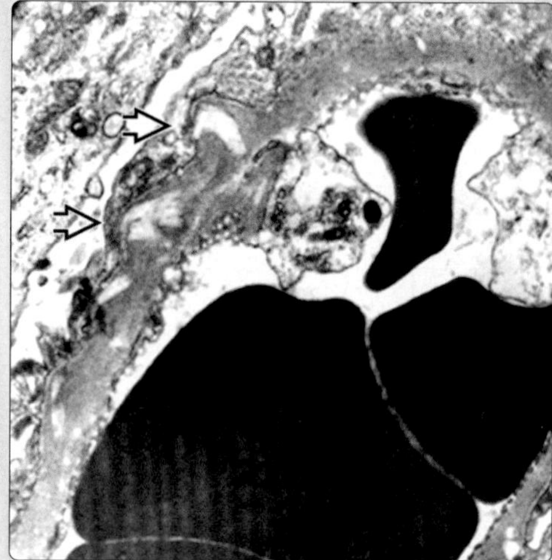

(Left) *In this case of nail-patella syndrome (NPS), glomeruli, tubules, and interstitium are unremarkable.* **(Right)** *"Moth-eaten" GBM appearance ➡ in areas corresponding to fibrillar collagen deposits is the clue to the diagnosis by electron microscopy with uranyl nitrate staining.*

Collagen Bundles

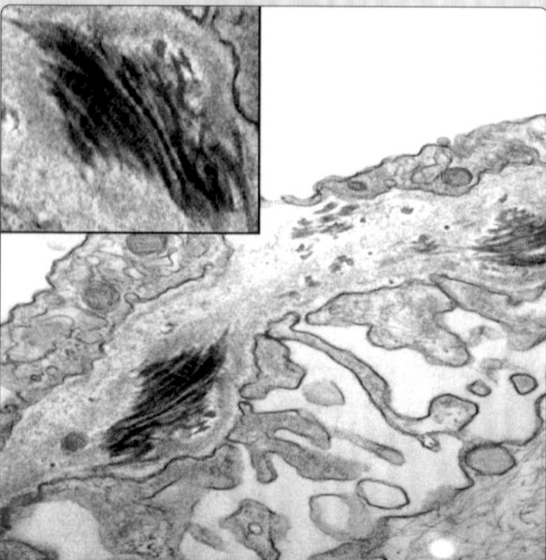

Collagen in GBM Without Extrarenal Signs

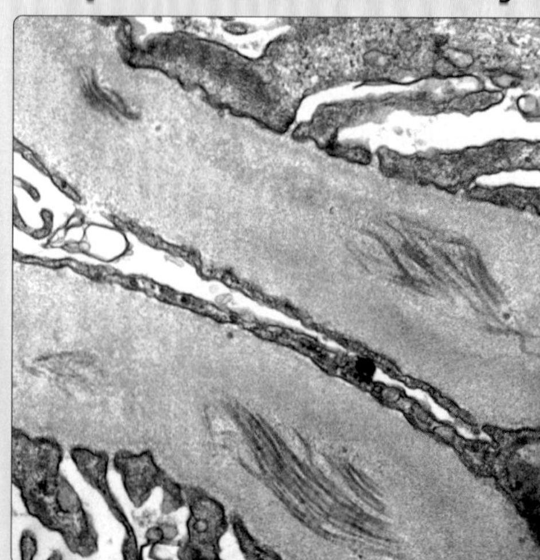

(Left) *Characteristic fibrillar collagen bundles display the axial packing arrangement of positive and negative-staining pattern, known as periodicity, seen after phosphotungstic acid staining.* **(Right)** *This 18-year-old girl had no extrarenal signs but had characteristic focal deposition of banded collagen in the GBM in routine EM studies. She had no detectable LMX1B mutation on genetic analysis, suggesting other potential causes of this finding.(Courtesy I. Rosales, MD.)*

TERMINOLOGY

Abbreviations

- Nail-patella syndrome (NPS)

Synonyms

- Hereditary onychoosteodysplasia (HOOD) syndrome
- Nail-patella-like renal disease
  - Renal manifestations without nail or skeletal findings

Definitions

- Inherited syndrome with nail, skeletal abnormalities, and proteinuria secondary to *LMX1B* gene mutations

ETIOLOGY/PATHOGENESIS

Genetics

- *LMX1B* gene mutations
  - Maps to chromosome 9q34.1 (ABO linkage)
    - Autosomal dominant inheritance
      - Variable phenotype
  - Encodes LIM homeodomain transcription factor
    - Expressed in podocytes
    - Critical for limb development
    - Regulates transcription of α3 and α4 of collagen IV, CD2AP, and podocin
    - Homeodomain region mutations associated with proteinuria
  - Mutation c.737G.A, p.R246Q associated with FSGS without extrarenal signs

CLINICAL ISSUES

Epidemiology

- Incidence
  - Rare (~ 1/50,000)

Presentation

- Renal manifestations (30-60%)
  - Proteinuria (~ 20%)
    - May develop nephrotic syndrome
  - Microscopic hematuria (~ 10%)
  - May have renal involvement (FSGS) without extrarenal signs
- Hypoplastic, dystrophic, or absent nails (98%)
- Small, irregularly shaped, or absent patella (74%)
- Limited extension, pronation, supination of elbow (70%)
- Iliac horns (70%)
  - Posterior, bilateral bony processes
  - Considered pathognomonic
- Glaucoma, cataracts
- Hearing defects
- Renal artery aneurysms

Treatment

- No specific therapy
- Recurrence in transplant not reported
- Not associated with post-transplant antiglomerular basement membrane (GBM) disease

Prognosis

- ~ 10% progress to end-stage renal disease

MICROSCOPIC

Histologic Features

- Glomeruli
  - Normal appearance by light microscopy
  - Focal thickening of capillary loops
  - Focal segmental glomerulosclerosis
    - Can occur without extrarenal signs with certain mutation
- Tubules, interstitium, vessels
  - No specific changes

ANCILLARY TESTS

Immunofluorescence

- IgM and C3 in sclerotic glomerular lesions
- Superimposed disease (IgA, anti-GBM) described

Genetic Testing

- Sequencing *LMX1B* exons and introns 2 through 6
  - 85% of mutations in this region

Electron Microscopy

- Focal banded collagen fibrils in GBM with characteristic periodicity (~ 60 nm)
  - Enhanced by phosphotungstic acid-stain
- "Moth-eaten" GBM
- Irregular thickening of GBM

DIFFERENTIAL DIAGNOSIS

Type III Collagen Glomerulopathy

- Also has mesangial collagen fibers
- Abundant curvilinear collagen fibrils

Fibronectin Glomerulopathy

- Lobular glomeruli with expanded mesangial matrix
- 14-16 nm, granular, fibrillary electron-dense deposits

Glomerulopathy of Hereditary Multiple Exostoses

- Mesangial and subendothelial collagen
- Multiple osteochondromas

DIAGNOSTIC CHECKLIST

Pathologic Interpretation Pearls

- Intramembranous banded collagen fibrils on EM

SELECTED REFERENCES

1. Edwards N et al: A novel LMX1B mutation in a family with end-stage renal disease of 'unknown cause'. Clin Kidney J. 8(1):113-9, 2015
2. Isojima T et al: LMX1B mutation with residual transcriptional activity as a cause of isolated glomerulopathy. Nephrol Dial Transplant. 29(1):81-8, 2014
3. Zhou TB et al: LIM homeobox transcription factor 1B expression affects renal interstitial fibrosis and apoptosis in unilateral ureteral obstructed rats. Am J Physiol Renal Physiol. 306(12):F1477-88, 2014
4. Boyer O et al: LMX1B mutations cause hereditary FSGS without extrarenal involvement. J Am Soc Nephrol. 24(8):1216-22, 2013
5. Kamath S et al: Nail-patella syndrome with an emphasis on the risk of renal and ocular findings. Pediatr Dermatol. 27(1):95-7, 2010
6. Lemley KV: Kidney disease in nail-patella syndrome. Pediatr Nephrol. 24(12):2345-54, 2009
7. Miner JH et al: Transcriptional induction of slit diaphragm genes by Lmx1b is required in podocyte differentiation. J Clin Invest. 109(8):1065-72, 2002
8. Sweeney E, Hoover-Fong JE, McIntosh I. Nail-Patella Syndrome. 1993-, 2003

C1q Nephropathy

KEY FACTS

TERMINOLOGY

- Dominant or codominant C1q staining (≥ 2+ intensity) in mesangium without evidence of SLE or MPGN

ETIOLOGY/PATHOGENESIS

- No definite pathogenetic mechanism, but 4 possibilities include
  - Immune complex formation due to binding of C1q and immunoglobulin
  - Direct binding of C1q to mesangial cell C1q receptors
  - Increased synthesis of C1q by macrophages and dendritic cells
  - Nonspecific entrapment of C1q in severe proteinuria

CLINICAL ISSUES

- Prevalence: 0.2-2.5% of renal biopsies
- Studies have documented higher rates of resistance to steroid therapy, but prognosis seems largely based on histology
- Nephrotic syndrome, asymptomatic hematuria &/or proteinuria, or chronic renal insufficiency

MICROSCOPIC

- Heterogeneity of glomerular changes
  - No glomerular abnormalities, resembling MCD
  - Mesangial proliferative glomerulonephritis
  - Focal segmental glomerulosclerosis
- Predominately mesangial C1q with C3, IgG, IgA, and IgM in various combinations
- Amorphous electron-dense deposits in mesangium
  - Occasionally subendothelial; rarely, subepithelial deposits

DIAGNOSTIC CHECKLIST

- Glomerular pathology and degree of tubular atrophy and interstitial fibrosis are prognostic
- Strict adherence to threshold of ≥ 2+ intensity of C1q staining prevents overdiagnosis

FSGS Pattern

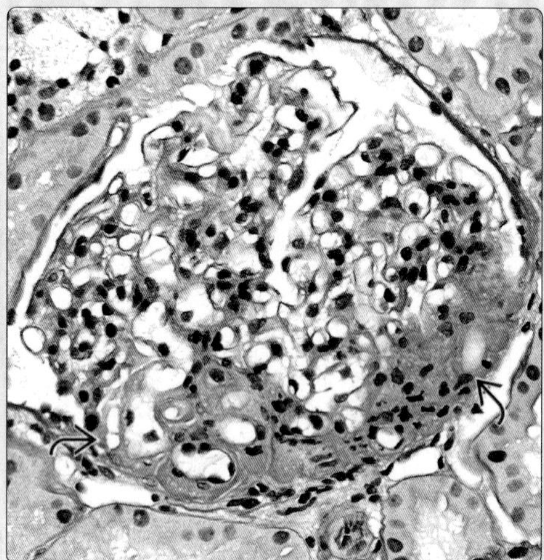

3+ Mesangial C1q

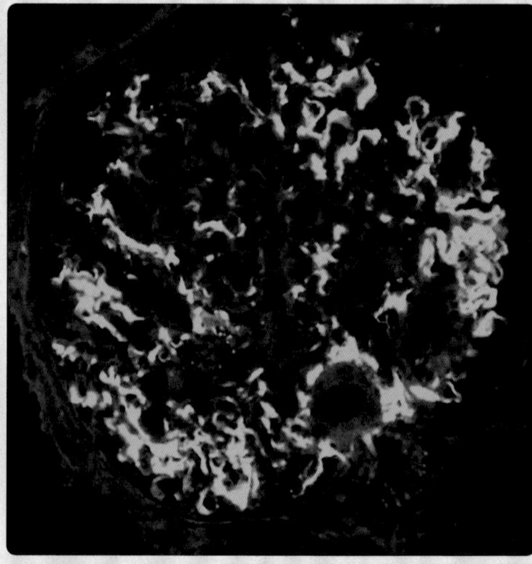

(Left) *A biopsy from a 12-year-old girl with nephrotic syndrome due to C1q nephropathy is shown. Focal segmental glomerulosclerosis (FSGS)* ➡*, a common histologic pattern in C1q nephropathy, is evident.* **(Right)** *C1q nephropathy is characterized by dominant or codominant C1q deposits of ≥ 2+ intensity, seen in this 15-year-old boy with microhematuria and proteinuria. IgG staining was 2+, and lupus serologies were negative.*

Mild Mesangial Proliferation Pattern

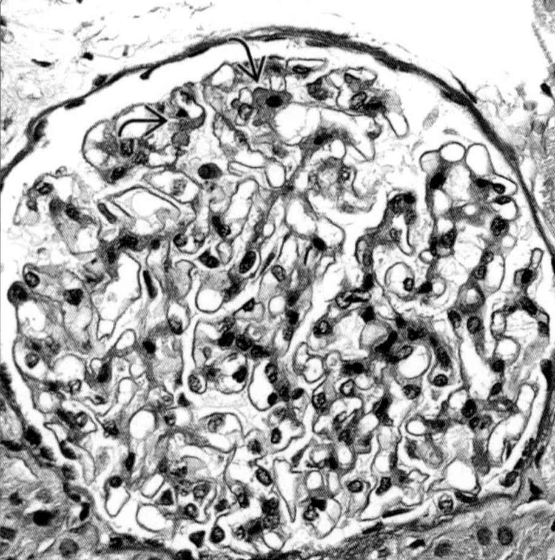

Amorphous Mesangial Electron Dense Deposits

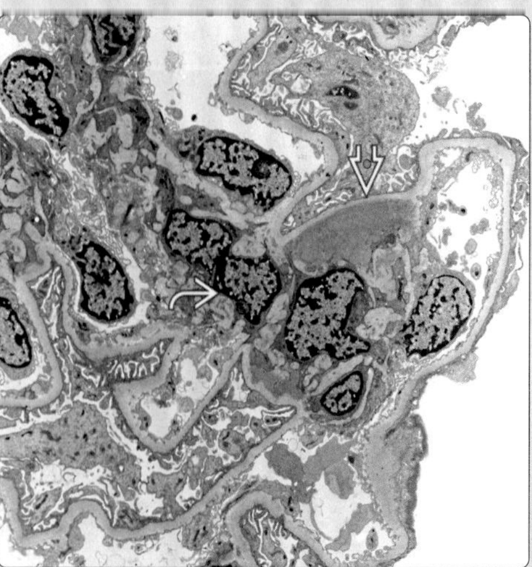

(Left) *10-year-old boy with asymptomatic proteinuria and a biopsy diagnosis of C1q nephropathy. There is no glomerular proliferation, but paramesangial deposits* ➡ *are evident on light microscopy in this PAS stained slide.* **(Right)** *Electron-dense deposits in C1q nephropathy are typically paramesangial* ➡ *in location. This biopsy from a 10-year-old boy with 2 g/d of proteinuria shows mild mesangial hypercellularity* ➡*.*

TERMINOLOGY

Definitions

- Idiopathic glomerular disease characterized by dominant or codominant C1q staining (≥ 2+ intensity) primarily in mesangium in patients without evidence of systemic lupus erythematosus (SLE), membranoproliferative glomerulonephritis, or infection
  - Originally described by Jennette and Hipp in 1985
  - Controversy remains whether it is a distinct entity

ETIOLOGY/PATHOGENESIS

Idiopathic

- No definitive pathogenetic mechanism identified; speculation on 4 leading possibilities

Immune Complex Formation

- C1q is component of classical complement activation pathway and links innate immunity to IgG/IgM-mediated acquired immunity
  - Classical pathway activated when C1q binds to Fc portion of immunoglobulin
    - C1q binding strongest with IgM, IgG1, and IgG3
- Deposits may alter course of minimal change disease (MCD) and focal segmental glomerulosclerosis (FSGS)

Direct Binding of C1q

- C1q receptors expressed on monocytes, macrophages, platelets, neutrophils, lymphocytes, endothelial cells, and mesangial cells
  - C1q can bind mesangial cells through C1q receptors
- C1q also binds polyanionic substances, such as DNA, RNA, lipopolysaccharides, and viral and bacterial proteins
  - C1q triggers phagocytosis of bacteria and neutralization of retroviruses
  - C1q nephropathy reported in BK polyoma nephritis and CMV infection

Increased Synthesis of C1q

- Macrophages and dendritic cells synthesize C1q
- Inflammatory cytokines upregulate C1q production

Nonspecific Entrapment of C1q

- Increased glomerular protein trafficking in severe proteinuria causes nonspecific entrapment of immunoglobulin in mesangium
- C1q fixes entrapped immunoglobulin
  - May not represent true immune complexes
  - Hypothesis may be best applicable to MCD/FSGS clinicopathological subset of C1q nephropathy

CLINICAL ISSUES

Epidemiology

- Incidence
  - Prevalence of C1q glomerulopathy ranges from 0.2-2.5% of renal biopsies from adults and children
    - Higher prevalence in biopsies from children (6%), especially those with nephrotic syndrome (16.5%)
  - Subclinical C1q ≥ 2+ in ~ 7% of asymptomatic donor kidneys
- Age
  - Often seen in older children and young adults
- Sex
  - No consistent gender predisposition
- Ethnicity
  - African Americans have frequent nephrotic syndrome presentation with FSGS histology

Presentation

- Nephrotic syndrome (NS) (> 50%)
  - Abrupt onset is most common
  - Often correlates with MCD/FSGS histology
- Subnephrotic proteinuria (15-20%)
- Asymptomatic hematuria (10-15%)
  - Reports include incidental detection in Japanese children, who undergo routine urine screen
- Isolated hematuria and proteinuria (5-10%)
- Chronic renal insufficiency (15-20%)
  - Frequent presentation of mesangioproliferative GN
  - Hematuria and proteinuria may be present
- Gross hematuria (< 5%)

Laboratory Tests

- Serological studies supportive of lupus, such as ANA, anti-ds DNA, and anti-C1q antibodies are negative
  - Remain negative even after several years of follow-up
- Normal serum complement levels, rarely low C1q
- HIV-negative

Treatment

- Drugs
  - Corticosteroids
  - Cyclosporine or rituximab in steroid-resistant NS
  - No treatment needed for asymptomatic hematuria and proteinuria

Prognosis

- Largely based on histology
  - Long term outcomes identical to MCD without C1q deposits (0% ESRD) unless FSGS develops (3%)
    - Some studies show more relapses in C1q+ patients
  - Mesangial proliferative histology has good treatment response and renal outcome (0% ESRD)
  - FSGS associated with poorer outcomes and progression (27% ESRD)
- Children diagnosed with C1q nephropathy after urine screen may normalize urinalysis even without therapy

MICROSCOPIC

Histologic Features

- 3 glomerular patterns
  - No glomerular abnormalities by light microscopy ~ 40% of cases (range: 0-100%)
    - Resembles MCD
  - Mesangial proliferation ~ 20% of cases (range: 0-75%)
    - Usually mild to moderate
    - Occasional cases show segmental endocapillary proliferation or focal crescents (~ 7%)
  - Focal segmental glomerulosclerosis ~ 40% of cases (range: 0-90%)
    - ~ 50% associated with mesangial proliferation

- FSGS lesions characterized by Bowman capsular adhesions and hyaline insudation
- Collapsing and cellular variants of FSGS described
- Occasionally, MCD evolves into FSGS on follow-up biopsy
- C1q nephropathy may also be variant of FSGS
  - Incidental finding
    - Present in 7% of transplant donor kidneys
    - Occasionally with other diseases, such as thin basement membrane disease, interstitial nephritis, polycystic kidneys, global sclerosis
  - Relative frequency of histological findings varies based on study cited
  - Membranoproliferative histology generally considered exclusion criterion
- Acute tubular injury with loss of brush borders and simplified epithelium seen in severe proteinuria
- Variable tubular atrophy and interstitial fibrosis
- Small vessel vasculitis rare (~ 3%)

ANCILLARY TESTS

Immunofluorescence

- Dominant or codominant C1q staining (≥ 2+ intensity) in mesangium and occasionally along capillary loops
  - Paramesangial deposits may have comma-shaped appearance
- Most cases have IgG (67%), IgM (81%), IgA (47%), and C3 (83%) deposits, but of lesser intensity than C1q
  - "Full house" (IgG, IgA, IgM, C1q, C3) in ~ 30%
  - C4 staining (35%), usually minimal or trace
- C1q deposits may disappear on follow-up biopsies, even with FSGS histology
- De novo C1q deposits in renal allografts have no apparent clinical significance

Electron Microscopy

- Mesangial amorphous electron-dense deposits in ~ 90% (range: 45-100%)
  - Lack of electron-dense deposits in a few cases probably due to segmental distribution of deposits
  - Usually paramesangial (near GBM reflection)
- Occasional subendothelial deposits (7-44%)
- Rare subepithelial deposits (0-17%)
- Podocyte foot process effacement ranges from mild to extensive and correlates with degree of proteinuria
- Endothelial cell tubuloreticular inclusions rare (0-6%)

DIFFERENTIAL DIAGNOSIS

Lupus Nephritis

- Clinical and serological evidence of SLE
- More common subepithelial and subendothelial deposits
  - Deposits may have substructure
  - Tubuloreticular inclusions in endothelial cells
- Deposits in tubular basement membrane common
- Glomerular inflammation, necrosis, crescents more common

IgA Nephropathy

- Dominant or co-dominant glomerular IgA deposits
- C1q typically scant or absent
- When C1q present, worse outcome

Minimal Change Disease

- More responsive to steroids and fewer relapses than MCD with C1q deposits
- Long term outcome and presentation similar to MCD with C1q deposits

Focal Segmental Glomerulosclerosis

- Some believe C1q nephropathy is variant of FSGS
- Abundant mesangial deposits typical of C1q nephropathy

Membranoproliferative Glomerulonephritis With Immunoglobulin Deposits

- Usually C3 dominant
- Prominent subendothelial deposits and GBM duplication
- Hypocomplementemia

DIAGNOSTIC CHECKLIST

Clinically Relevant Pathologic Features

- Glomerular histologic lesion predicts outcome and treatment response
  - Better with MCD and mesangial proliferation than FSGS
- Degree of tubular atrophy and interstitial fibrosis are prognostic

Pathologic Interpretation Pearls

- Strict adherence to threshold of ≥ 2+ intensity of C1q staining prevents overdiagnosis

SELECTED REFERENCES

1. Gunasekara VN et al: C1q nephropathy in children: clinical characteristics and outcome. Pediatr Nephrol. 29(3):407-13, 2014
2. Vintar Spreitzer M et al: Do C1q or IgM nephropathies predict disease severity in children with minimal change nephrotic syndrome? Pediatr Nephrol. 29(1):67-74, 2014
3. Sinha A et al: Resolution of clinical and pathologic features of C1q nephropathy after rituximab therapy. Clin Exp Nephrol. 15(1):164-70, 2011
4. Said SM et al: C1q deposition in the renal allograft: a report of 24 cases. Mod Pathol. 23(8):1080-8, 2010
5. Wenderfer SE et al: C1q nephropathy in the pediatric population: pathology and pathogenesis. Pediatr Nephrol. 25(8):1385-96, 2010
6. Mii A et al: Current status and issues of C1q nephropathy. Clin Exp Nephrol. 13(4):263-74, 2009
7. Roberti I et al: A single-center study of C1q nephropathy in children. Pediatr Nephrol. 24(1):77-82, 2009
8. Hisano S et al: Clinicopathologic correlation and outcome of C1q nephropathy. Clin J Am Soc Nephrol. 3(6):1637-43, 2008
9. Vizjak A et al: Pathology, clinical presentations, and outcomes of C1q nephropathy. J Am Soc Nephrol. 19(11):2237-44, 2008
10. Fukuma Y et al: Clinicopathologic correlation of C1q nephropathy in children. Am J Kidney Dis. 47(3):412-8, 2006
11. Lau KK et al: Pediatric C1q nephropathy and incidental proteinuria. Pediatr Nephrol. 21(6):883; author reply 884, 2006
12. Nishida M et al: C1q nephropathy with asymptomatic urine abnormalities. Pediatr Nephrol. 20(11):1669-70, 2005
13. Markowitz GS et al: C1q nephropathy: a variant of focal segmental glomerulosclerosis. Kidney Int. 64(4):1232-40, 2003
14. Jennette JC et al: C1q nephropathy: a distinct pathologic entity usually causing nephrotic syndrome. Am J Kidney Dis. 6(2):103-10, 1985

Mesangial Proliferative Pattern

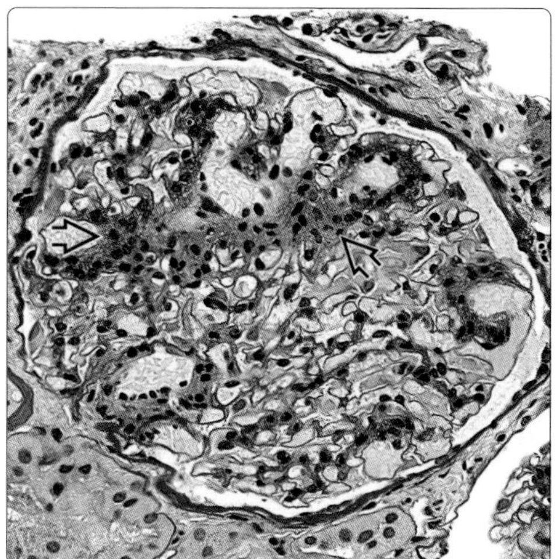

MInimal Change Disease Pattern

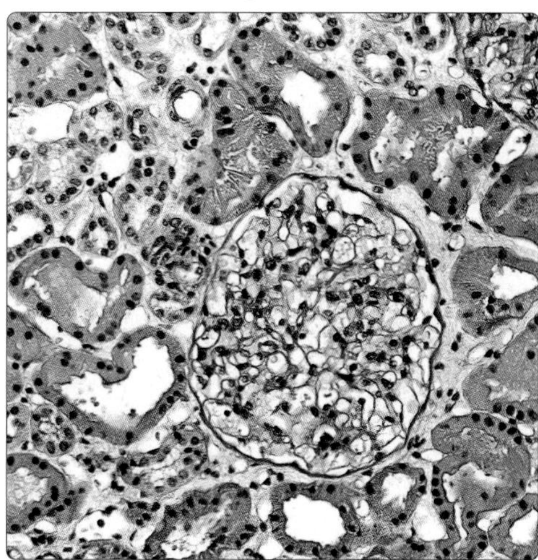

(Left) *A 15-year-old boy with microscopic hematuria and non-nephrotic proteinuria was diagnosed with C1q nephropathy on immunofluorescence microscopy. Mild segmental mesangial proliferative glomerulonephritis ➡ is seen on light microscopy.* **(Right)** *A 26-year-old man with abrupt onset of nephrotic syndrome showed normal kidney on light microscopy. Immunofluorescence microscopy was compatible with C1q nephropathy.*

Tubular Protein Reabsorption Droplets

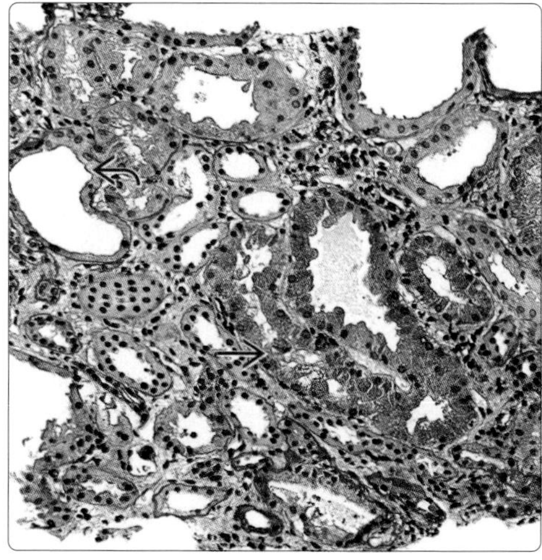

Focal Segmental Glomerulosclerosis Pattern

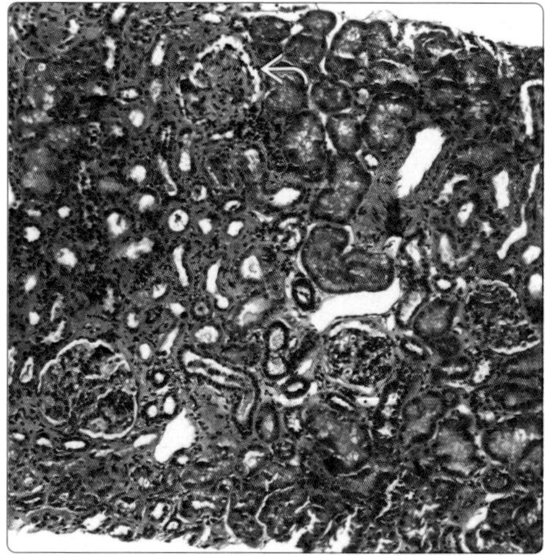

(Left) *C1q nephropathy can present as an MCD phenotype with abrupt onset of nephrotic syndrome. Prominent protein resorption droplets ➡ are seen in the proximal tubules. Mild acute tubular injury is evident with simplified epithelium ➡.* **(Right)** *C1q nephropathy has a variety of light microscopic patterns. One of the most common is focal segmental glomerulosclerosis ➡, illustrated in this biopsy from a 14-year-old boy with nephrotic syndrome and negative lupus serologies.*

FSGS Pattern

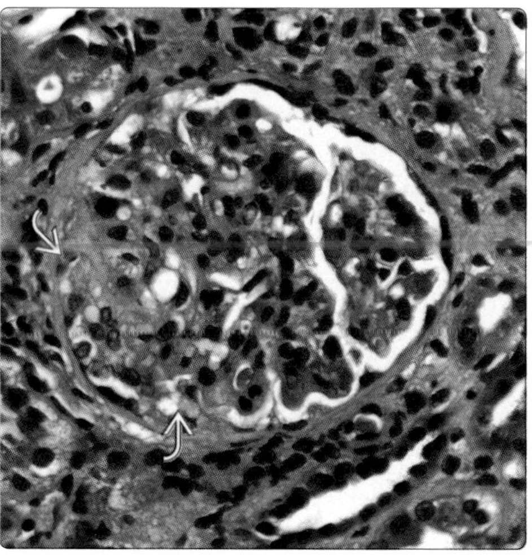

Advanced FSGS Pattern

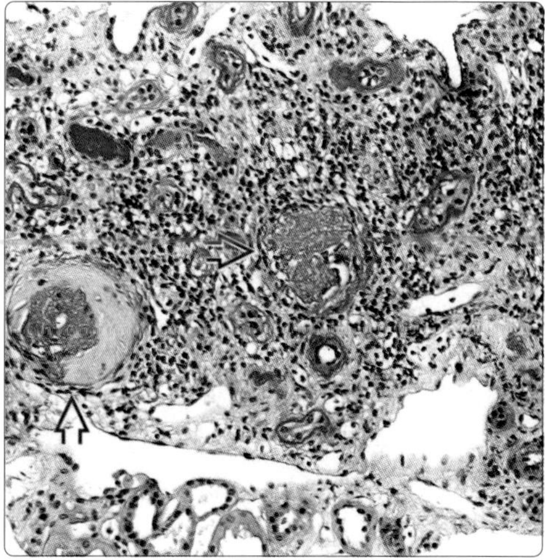

(Left) *C1q nephropathy often shows segmental sclerosis and adhesions (FSGS) ➡. The glomeruli in this case, from a 14-year-old patient with nephrotic syndrome, had a full-house pattern by immunofluorescence, resembling lupus; however, ANA and anti-dsDNA antibodies were negative.* **(Right)** *Globally sclerotic glomeruli ➡ are seen in this case of NS and C1q nephropathy with FSGS in a 9-year-old African American boy. Cases with extensive tubular atrophy have a poorer prognosis.*

(Left) *This is the 1st of 6 images from a 14-year-old boy with C1q nephropathy. This sample displays 2+ granular C1q staining, primarily in the mesangium. The IF pattern resembles lupus in that IgG, IgA, IgM, C3, and C1q are present ("full house"). C1q nephropathy is defined as dominant or codominant C1q in glomeruli of ≥ 2+ intensity in a patient without SLE.* **(Right)** *IgG is similar to C1q in intensity (2+) and distribution in this case of C1q nephropathy.*

Mesangial C1q

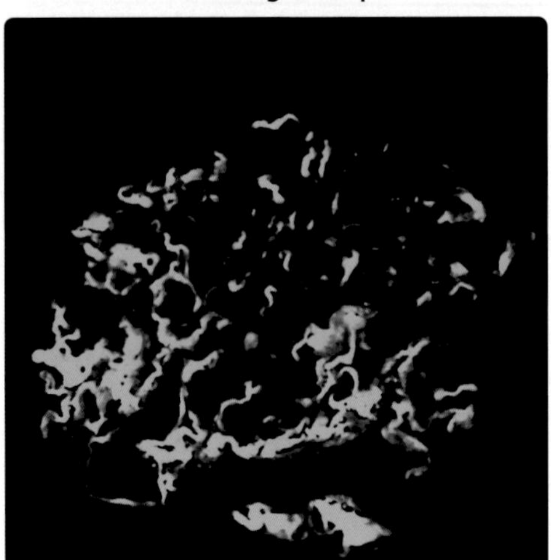

Mesangial IgG

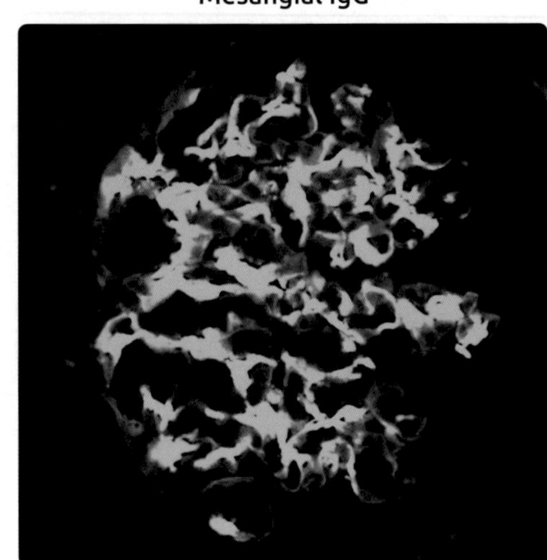

(Left) *IgM is present primarily in the mesangium in a similar distribution to C1q although not as intense (1+). This distribution corresponds to the location of the amorphous electron-dense deposits seen by electron microscopy.* **(Right)** *IgA is present in the deposits in the mesangium in this case of C1q nephropathy, similar to C1q, although of lesser intensity (1+). Kappa and lambda stains were similar (1-2+) and equal.*

Mesangial IgM

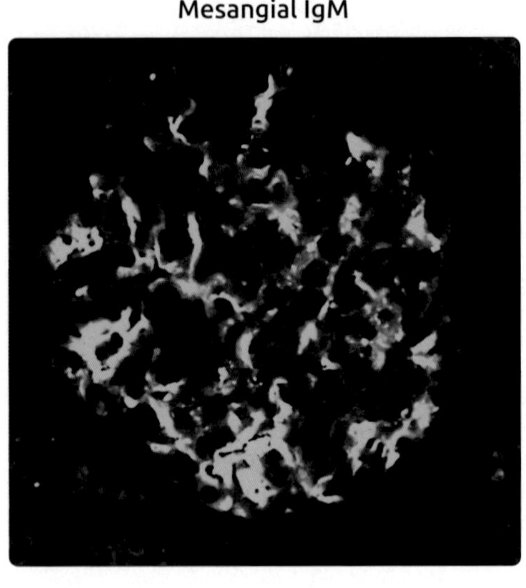

Mild IgA Mesangial Deposits

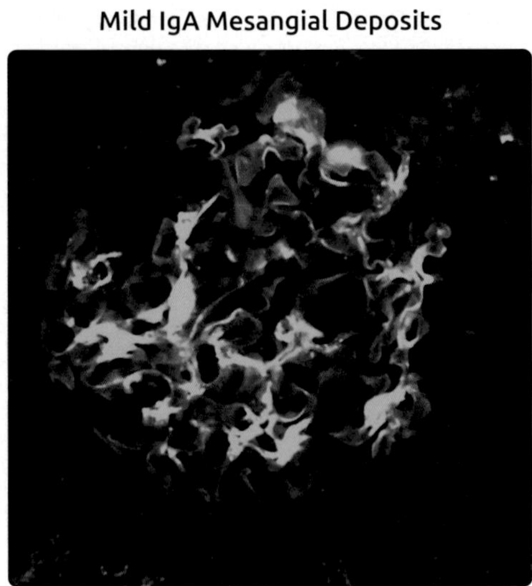

(Left) *C3 is present in this case at a level similar to C1q (1-2+).* **(Right)** *Glomerular segments with sclerosis commonly stain for C3 ➡ and IgM, as shown in this case of C1q nephropathy. This universal pattern in focal segmental glomerulosclerosis is presumed to be nonspecific. It is also possible that IgM &/or C3 is reacting with products released from damaged cells.*

C3 Deposition

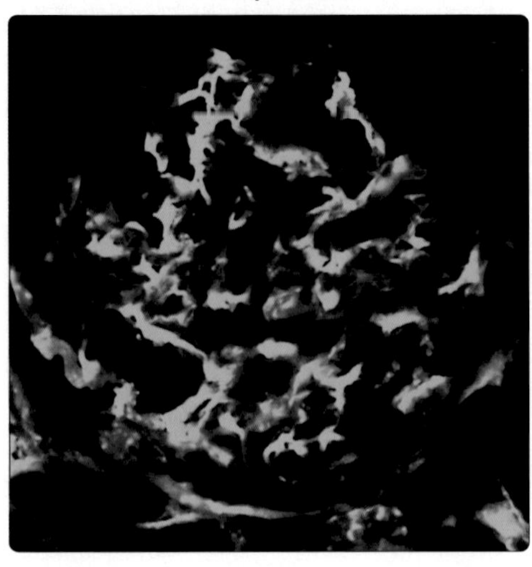

C3 in Sclerotic Segment

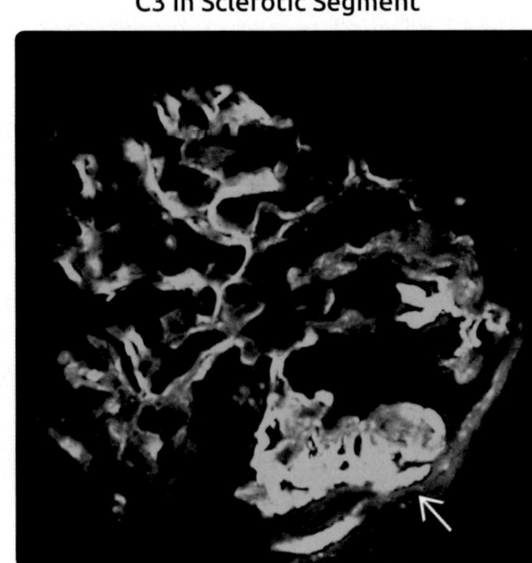

Abundant Mesangial Deposits

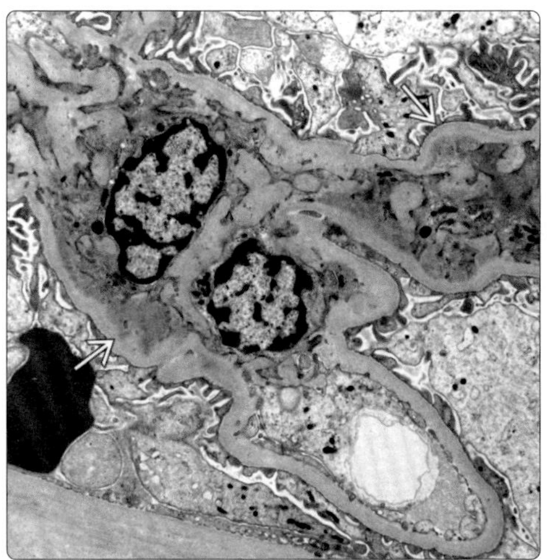

Normal GBM and Mesangial Deposits

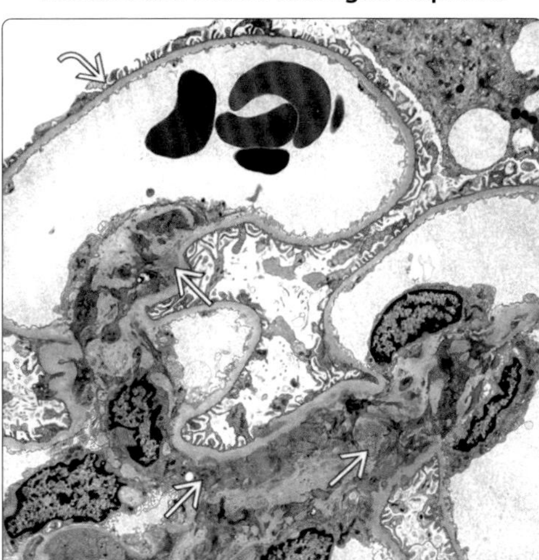

(Left) *The biopsy is from a 33-year-old woman with nephrotic-range proteinuria and intermittent mild pedal edema. The C1q deposits seen on immunofluorescence correspond to the mesangial electron dense deposits.* **(Right)** *Low-power view of C1q nephropathy shows the normal GBM and amorphous electron-dense deposits primarily in the mesangium.*

Amorphous Deposits

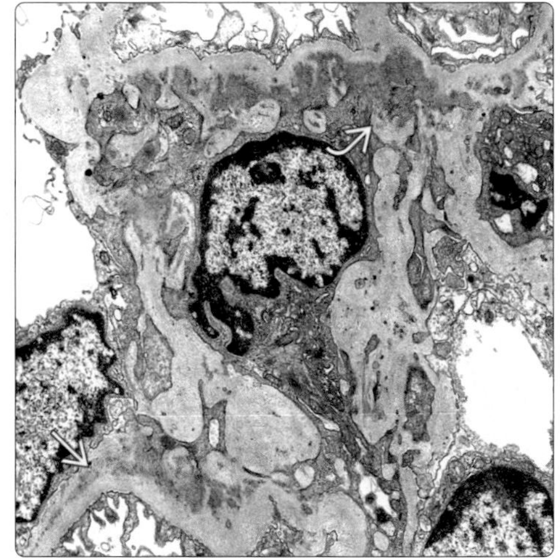

Intramembranous Deposits

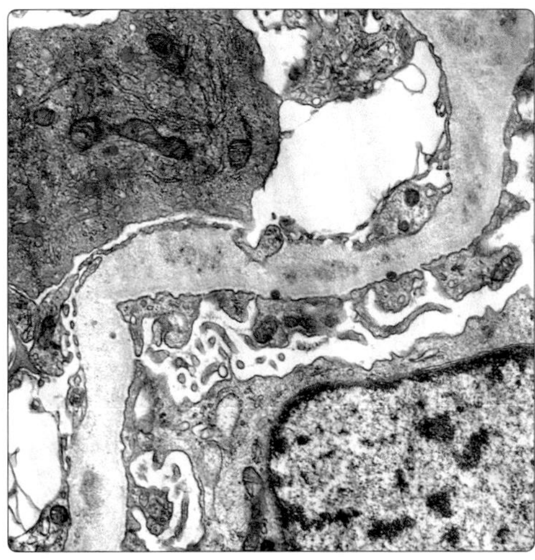

(Left) *Abundant mesangial and paramesangial deposits in a case of C1q nephropathy are shown. The deposits "hug" the mesangial cells, similar to those in IgA nephropathy. No substructure is evident, in contrast to some cases of lupus nephritis.* **(Right)** *Deposits in C1q nephropathy are sometime found in the GBM and as subendothelial deposits, similar to lupus. Rare subepithelial deposits have also been reported. Tubuloreticular structures, typical of lupus nephritis, are rarely present.*

Subendothelial Deposits

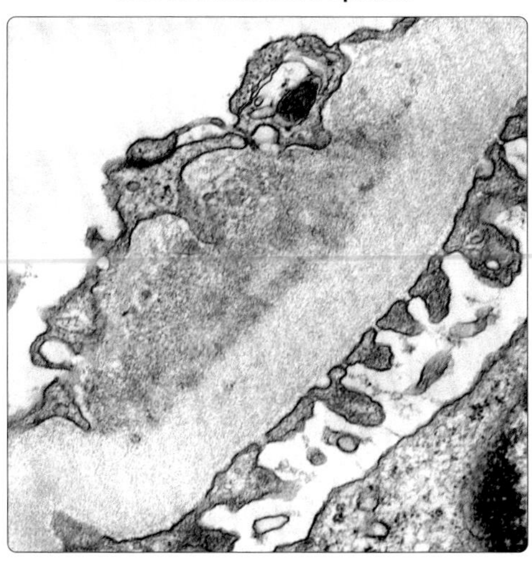

Segmental Glomerulosclerosis

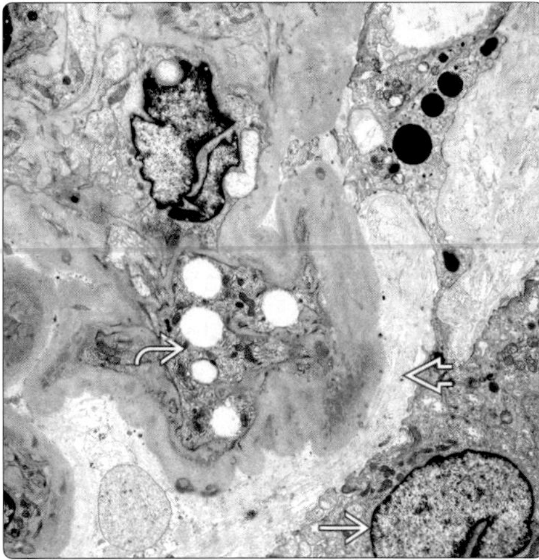

(Left) *Subendothelial deposits in a 14-year-old boy with nephrotic syndrome due to C1q nephropathy are shown. No substructure is evident, and no tubuloreticular structures were found, which help distinguish this from lupus nephritis.* **(Right)** *A 9-year-old African American boy with NS has dominant C1q deposits on IF, consistent with C1q nephropathy. Segmental glomerulosclerosis with lipid in mesangial is seen with overlying detached podocyte and neobasement membrane layers.*

KEY FACTS

TERMINOLOGY

- Idiopathic glomerular disease with dominant diffuse IgM immune deposits (≥ 2+ intensity by definition) in nonsclerotic glomeruli

CLINICAL ISSUES

- Nephrotic syndrome is most common presentation, often with steroid dependence or resistance
  - Presentation similar to MCD but with greater frequency of hypertension and hematuria
  - Microhematuria can be isolated with no significant proteinuria
- Good long-term prognosis of steroid-responsive cases
- Few cases demonstrate evolution to FSGS on repeat biopsies, suggesting pathogenic link

MICROSCOPIC

- Light microscopy
  - Glomeruli may appear entirely normal (~ 35%)
  - Mild segmental mesangial hypercellularity (~ 32%)
  - Mild mesangial sclerosis (~ 35%)
  - Global sclerosis (~ 15%)
- Immunofluorescence
  - IgM mesangial deposits of ≥ 2+ intensity
  - C3 mesangial deposits often identified
- Electron microscopy
  - Diffuse foot process effacement
  - ~ 50% amorphous, mesangial electron-dense deposits

TOP DIFFERENTIAL DIAGNOSES

- Minimal change disease
- Focal segmental glomerulosclerosis
- Immune complex-mediated diseases

DIAGNOSTIC CHECKLIST

- FSGS must be excluded
- MCD with ≥ 2+ IgM behaves similarly to MCD without IgM

(Left) *Most cases of IgM nephropathy have normal glomeruli by light microscopy. This biopsy from a child with nephrotic syndrome had 3+ IgM staining on immunofluorescence microscopy.* **(Right)** *Mild segmental mesangial hypercellularity → may be seen in IgMN as demonstrated in this biopsy specimen with ~ 20% of glomeruli affected.*

Normal Glomerular Morphology

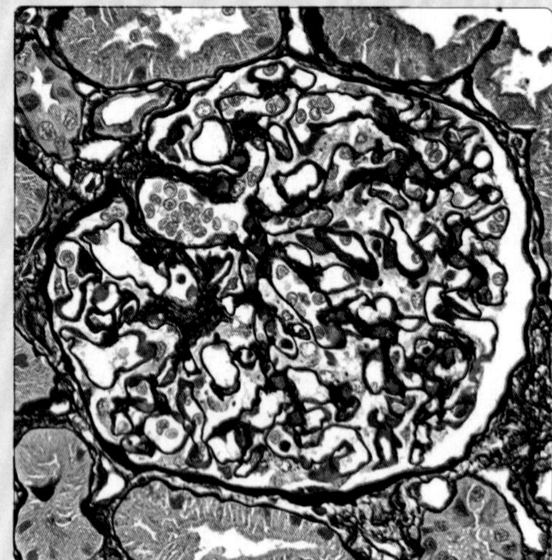

Mild Segmental Mesangial Hypercellularity

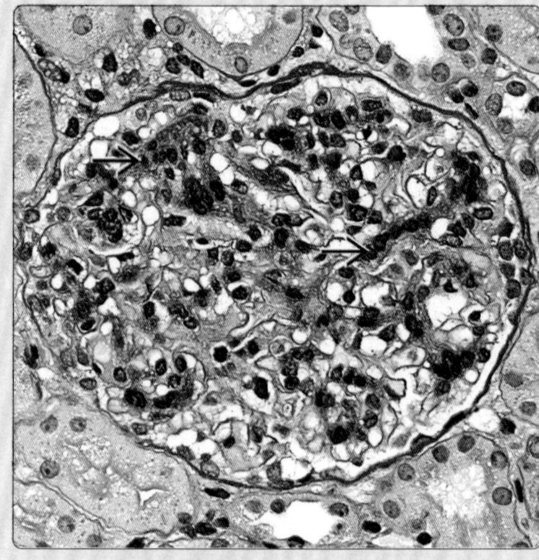

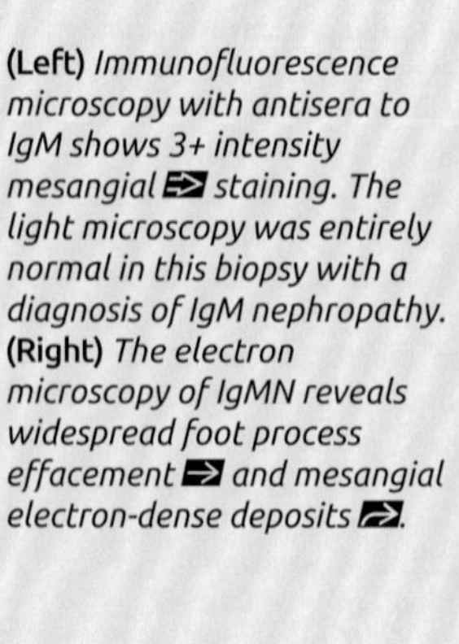

(Left) *Immunofluorescence microscopy with antisera to IgM shows 3+ intensity mesangial → staining. The light microscopy was entirely normal in this biopsy with a diagnosis of IgM nephropathy.* **(Right)** *The electron microscopy of IgMN reveals widespread foot process effacement → and mesangial electron-dense deposits →.*

Dominant Mesangial IgM Deposits

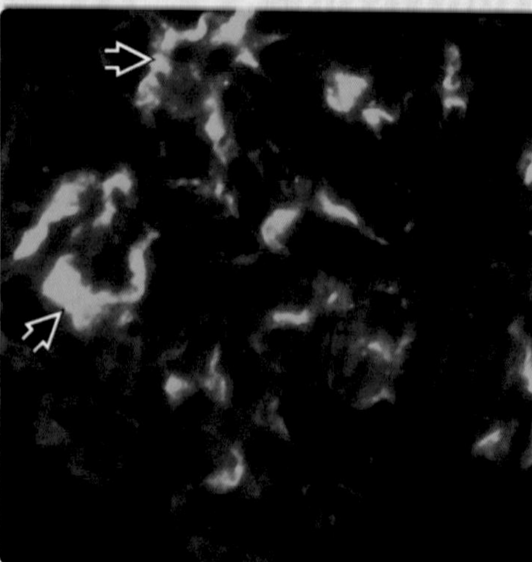

Ultrastructural Features of IgM Nephropathy

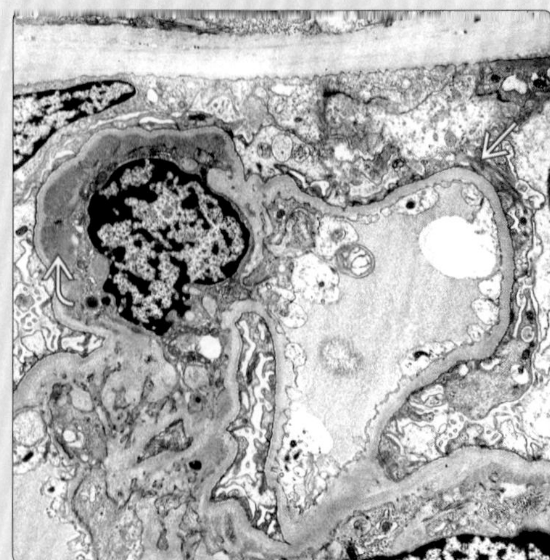

TERMINOLOGY

Abbreviations

- IgM nephropathy (IgMN)

Definitions

- Idiopathic glomerular disease with dominant diffuse mesangial IgM deposits (≥ 2+) in nonsclerotic glomeruli
  - Described independently in 1978 by Cohen and Bhasin
  - Relationship to minimal change disease (MCD) and focal segmental glomerulosclerosis (FSGS) debated

ETIOLOGY/PATHOGENESIS

Presumed Immunologic Pathogenesis

- Dysregulated T-lymphocyte response with altered proportions of T-cell subsets
- Impaired B lymphocyte IgM to IgG switch in vitro
  - Elevated IgM levels
  - Elevated IgM circulating immune complexes
- Defective clearance of immune deposits by mesangial cells

CLINICAL ISSUES

Epidemiology

- Incidence
  - Unknown due to lack of uniform diagnostic criteria and indication for biopsy
    - 5% of medical kidney biopsies (1 series)
- Age
  - 1-75 years old; mean: 29 years
- Sex
  - Men present with NS, while women present predominantly with isolated hematuria

Presentation

- Nephrotic syndrome
  - Presentation similar to MCD but with greater frequency of hypertension and hematuria
- Microhematuria
  - Can be isolated with no significant proteinuria

Natural History

- Few cases demonstrate evolution to FSGS on repeat biopsies, suggesting pathogenic link

Treatment

- Drugs
  - Up to 50% steroid dependent or steroid resistant
  - Cyclosporine or cyclophosphamide if steroid-resistant
  - Isolated case reports of rituximab response
- Recurs in transplants

Prognosis

- Good prognosis of steroid-responsive cases
- ~ 17% progress to chronic kidney disease

MICROSCOPIC

Histologic Features

- Glomeruli
  - Normal by light microscopy (~ 35%)
  - Mild segmental mesangial hypercellularity (~ 32%)
  - Mild mesangial sclerosis (~ 35%)
  - Global sclerosis (~ 15%)
- Tubulointerstitium
  - Tubular atrophy in minority (~ 20%)
  - Acute tubular injury
  - Interstitial fibrosis or inflammation in minority (~ 7%)
- Vessels: Hyalinosis (~ 20%), intimal fibrosis (~ 5%)

ANCILLARY TESTS

Immunofluorescence

- IgM mesangial deposits of ≥ 2+ intensity
- C3 mesangial deposits often identified
- Low intensity (trace to 1+) IgG, IgA, and C1q staining can be observed due to nonspecific entrapment

Electron Microscopy

- Diffuse foot process effacement
- Mesangial, electron-dense deposits in ~ 50%

DIFFERENTIAL DIAGNOSIS

Minimal Change Disease

- Segmental low-intensity mesangial IgM may be observed in MCD due to nonspecific entrapment
- IgMN reserved for cases with ≥ 2+ IgM

Focal Segmental Glomerulosclerosis

- Minority of FSGS have ≥ 2+ IgM staining
- FSGS diagnosis should supersede IgMN

Immune Complex-Mediated Diseases

- IgA Nephropathy
  - Dominant or codominant IgA deposits
- Mesangioproliferative lupus nephritis
  - IgG dominant with IgA, IgM, C3, C1q ("full house")

Diffuse Mesangial Hypercellularity

- > 4 cells/mesangial area involving > 80% of glomeruli
- Occasional cases have IgM and C3 deposits

DIAGNOSTIC CHECKLIST

Pathologic Interpretation Pearls

- MCD with ≥ 2+ IgM behaves similarly to MCD without IgM
- FSGS must be excluded

SELECTED REFERENCES

1. Vintar Spreitzer M et al: Do C1q or IgM nephropathies predict disease severity in children with minimal change nephrotic syndrome? Pediatr Nephrol. 29(1):67-74, 2014
2. Betjes MG et al: Resolution of IgM nephropathy after rituximab treatment. Am J Kidney Dis. 53(6):1059-62, 2009
3. Swartz SJ et al: Minimal change disease with IgM+ immunofluorescence: a subtype of nephrotic syndrome. Pediatr Nephrol. 24(6):1187-92, 2009
4. Silverstein DM et al: Mesangial hypercellularity in children: presenting features and outcomes. Pediatr Nephrol. 23(6):921-8, 2008
5. Myllymäki J et al: IgM nephropathy: clinical picture and long-term prognosis. Am J Kidney Dis. 41(2):343-50, 2003
6. O'Donoghue DJ et al: IgM-associated primary diffuse mesangial proliferative glomerulonephritis: natural history and prognostic indicators. Q J Med. 79(288):333-50, 1991
7. Helin H et al: IgM-associated glomerulonephritis. Nephron. 31(1):11-6, 1982
8. Bhasin HK et al: Mesangial proliferative glomerulonephritis. Lab Invest. 39(1):21-9, 1978
9. Cohen AH et al: Nephrotic syndrome with glomerular mesangial IgM deposits. Lab Invest. 38(5):610-9, 1978

KEY FACTS

TERMINOLOGY

- Glomerular disease related to cirrhosis or portal hypertension, manifested by accumulation of IgA and lipid debris in mesangium; excludes HCV immune complex diseases

ETIOLOGY/PATHOGENESIS

- Systemic shunting of blood bypasses liver Kupffer cells
- Accumulation of IgA immune complexes
- Lipid cell debris

CLINICAL ISSUES

- End-stage liver disease or portal hypertension of any etiology
  - Highest in alcoholic cirrhosis (~ 70%)
- Asymptomatic hematuria, proteinuria
- Remission with correction of portal hypertension
- Outcome after liver transplantation not documented

MICROSCOPIC

- Glomeruli usually show mild mesangial expansion
  - MPGN type I
  - Normal glomeruli
- Immunofluorescence microscopy
  - Mesangial deposits of IgA
  - With or without IgG, IgM, C3, C1q
  - Occasionally lambda light chain restriction
- Electron microscopy
  - Electron-dense lipid granules, lucencies in mesangium
  - Amorphous electron-dense deposits

TOP DIFFERENTIAL DIAGNOSES

- IgA nephropathy
- HCV glomerulonephritis
- LCAT deficiency

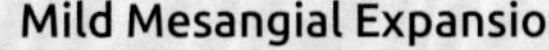

Mild Mesangial Expansion

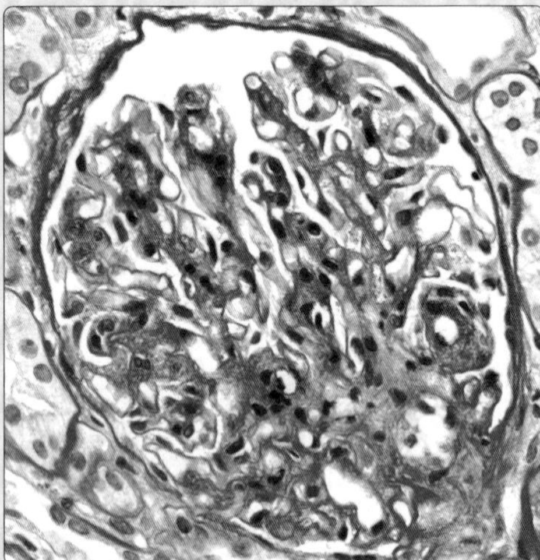

IgA Predominance

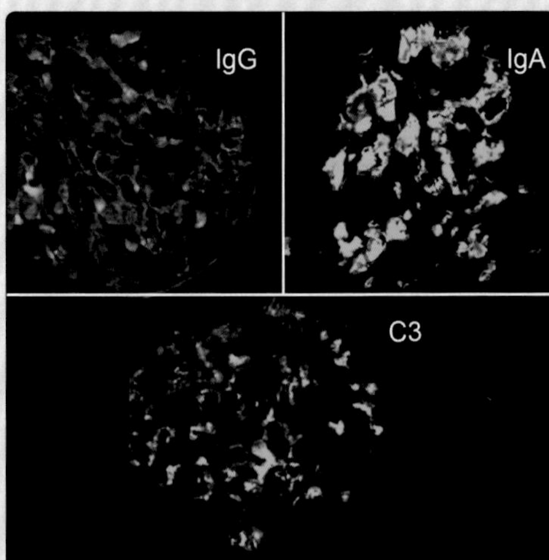

(Left) *Mesangial matrix expansion with minimal GBM changes and no glomerular inflammation is the usual pattern of HGS (PAS stain).* **(Right)** *By immunofluorescence, prominent IgA deposits are present in the expanded mesangium in HGS. The pattern resembles IgA nephropathy, although inflammatory changes are absent. C3 is also present but there is little or no IgG.*

Lipid Granules and Lucencies in Mesangium

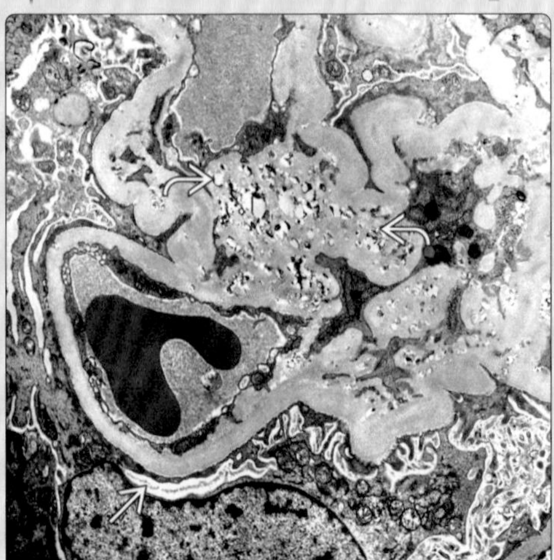

Mesangial and Subendothelial Deposits

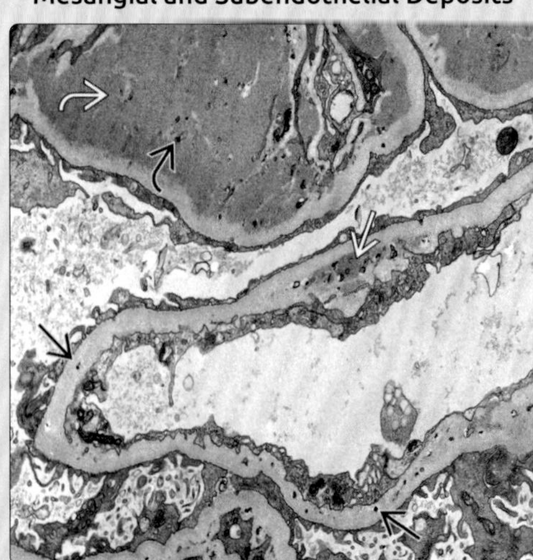

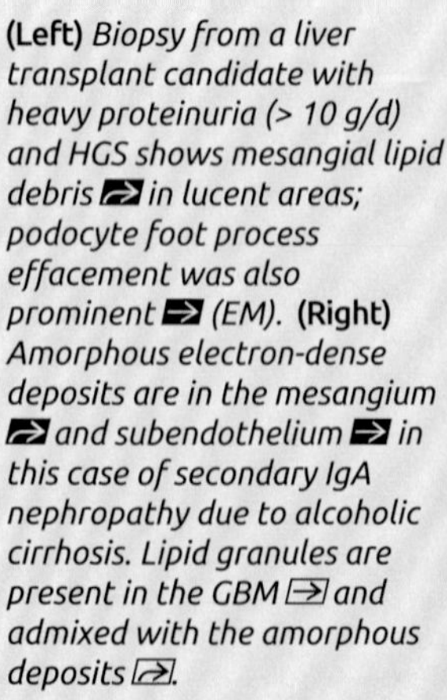

(Left) *Biopsy from a liver transplant candidate with heavy proteinuria (> 10 g/d) and HGS shows mesangial lipid debris in lucent areas; podocyte foot process effacement was also prominent (EM).* **(Right)** *Amorphous electron-dense deposits are in the mesangium and subendothelium in this case of secondary IgA nephropathy due to alcoholic cirrhosis. Lipid granules are present in the GBM and admixed with the amorphous deposits.*

TERMINOLOGY

Abbreviations

- Hepatic glomerulosclerosis (HGS)

Synonyms

- Cirrhotic glomerulosclerosis

Definitions

- Glomerular disease related to cirrhosis or portal hypertension, manifested by accumulation of IgA and lipid debris in mesangium; excludes HCV-related GN

ETIOLOGY/PATHOGENESIS

Failure of Normal Liver Clearance Mechanisms

- Systemic shunting of blood bypasses liver Kupffer cells
  - HGS occurs with portal hypertension without cirrhosis
- Accumulation of IgA immune complexes
- Lipid cell debris

Abnormal IgA Glycosylation

- Galactose deficiency and decreased sialylation of IgA1 similar to primary IgA nephropathy

CLINICAL ISSUES

Epidemiology

- Incidence
  - ~ 60% prevalence of glomerular IgA deposits in cirrhotics at autopsy
  - ~ 35% at time of liver transplantation

Presentation

- End-stage liver disease or portal hypertension of any etiology
  - Highest in alcoholic cirrhosis (~ 70%)
- Usually asymptomatic
- Hematuria (~ 9%) and proteinuria
  - Nephrotic-range proteinuria (~ 2%)
  - Rarely acute renal failure due to red cell casts

Prognosis

- Uncommonly leads to ESRD by itself but has limited data
- Remission of nephrotic proteinuria and hematuria with correction of portal hypertension reported
- Hematuria diminished after liver transplantation
  - Did not recur by 10 weeks in liver-kidney transplant recipient

MICROSCOPIC

Histologic Features

- Glomeruli show varied patterns
  - Normal
  - Mild to moderate mesangial expansion
    - Typical in asymptomatic patients
  - Prominent mesangial expansion, duplication of GBM, and mesangial interposition
    - More common in biopsies for cause
    - Seen in association with HCV & cryoglobulinemia
  - Crescents (rare)
- Tubules
  - May show acute injury (hepatorenal syndrome)
  - Bile-stained casts
- Interstitium
  - No specific features
- Arteries
  - Intimal fibrosis common

ANCILLARY TESTS

Immunofluorescence

- Variable IgA deposits, primarily in mesangium
  - Segmentally along GBM
  - Rarely monoclonal (4 cases)
  - IgA1 subclass
- IgA usually accompanied by less intense deposits of IgG, IgM, C3, C1q, and, occasionally, fibrin
  - C3 in 50-80%
  - C1q in 50-70%
- About 55% have no IgA pre-liver transplant

Electron Microscopy

- Electron-dense lipid granules in mesangium
  - Uncertain provenance, independent of IgA deposits
  - Sometimes seen as dense granules in rounded lucencies, 50-150 nm
  - Honeycomb pattern of lucencies in mesangium with lipid deposits
  - Similar lipid deposits segmentally in GBM
- Amorphous electron-dense deposits in mesangium
  - Typical of immune complex deposits in other diseases
- Subendothelial deposits segmentally
  - Mesangial cell interposition

DIFFERENTIAL DIAGNOSIS

IgA Nephropathy

- Lacks characteristic lipid debris in mesangium
- C1q less common (0-14%) and C3 more common (83-100%)

Hepatis C Virus-Associated Immune Complex Glomerulonephritis

- More striking subendothelial IgG and IgM deposits
- Pseudothrombi

Lecithin-Cholesterol Acyltransferase Deficiency (LCAT)

- Far more extensive lipid deposits in mesangium and GBM
- No IgA association

SELECTED REFERENCES

1. Ujire MP et al: A simultaneous liver kidney transplant recipient with IgA nephropathy limited to native kidneys and BK virus nephropathy limited to the transplant kidney. Am J Kidney Dis. 62(2):331-4, 2013
2. Tissandié E et al: Both IgA nephropathy and alcoholic cirrhosis feature abnormally glycosylated IgA1 and soluble CD89-IgA and IgG-IgA complexes: common mechanisms for distinct diseases. Kidney Int. 80(12):1352-63, 2011
3. Trawalé JM et al: The spectrum of renal lesions in patients with cirrhosis: a clinicopathological study. Liver Int. 30(5):725-32, 2010
4. Wadei HM et al: Kidney allocation to liver transplant candidates with renal failure of undetermined etiology: role of percutaneous renal biopsy. Am J Transplant. 8(12):2618-26, 2008

Chloroquine Toxicity

KEY FACTS

TERMINOLOGY
- Iatrogenic phospholipidosis due to chloroquine exposure

ETIOLOGY/PATHOGENESIS
- Chloroquine is lysosomotropic, cationic, and amphiphilic
  - Inhibits activity of numerous enzymes including α-galactosidase A in lysosomes
- ↓ α-galactosidase A enzymatic activity → accumulation of globotriaosylceramide, sphingolipid

CLINICAL ISSUES
- Toxicity manifested by proteinuria ± declining renal function

MICROSCOPIC
- Glomerular capillary and mesangial cells with vacuolated, foamy cytoplasm
- Podocytes have foamy cytoplasm

ANCILLARY TESTS
- Electron microscopy
  - Capillary lumens and mesangium have vacuolated cells with granular, electron-dense inclusions
  - Some podocytes have myelin figures

TOP DIFFERENTIAL DIAGNOSES
- Fabry disease
- Other lipidoses
  - Gaucher disease
  - Infantile nephrosialidosis, I-cell disease, ceroid lipofuscinosis, Hurler syndrome, Niemann-Pick disease, Farber disease, GM1 gangliosidosis
  - Lecithin cholesterol acyltransferase deficiency
- Drugs and toxins
  - Amiodarone, ranolazine, and silicon

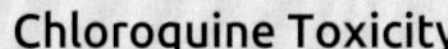

Chloroquine Toxicity

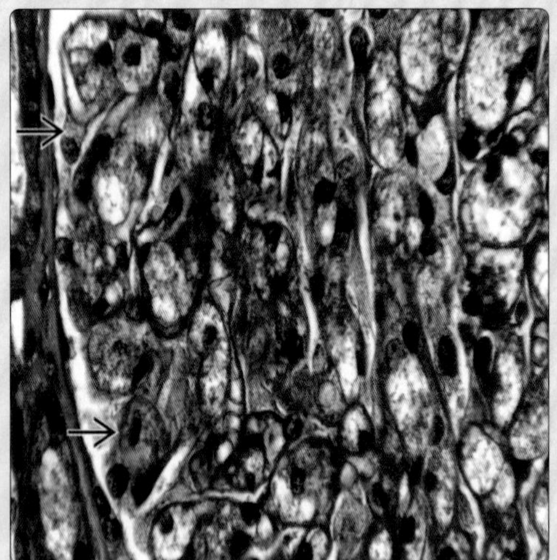

Chloroquine Toxicity Myelin Figures

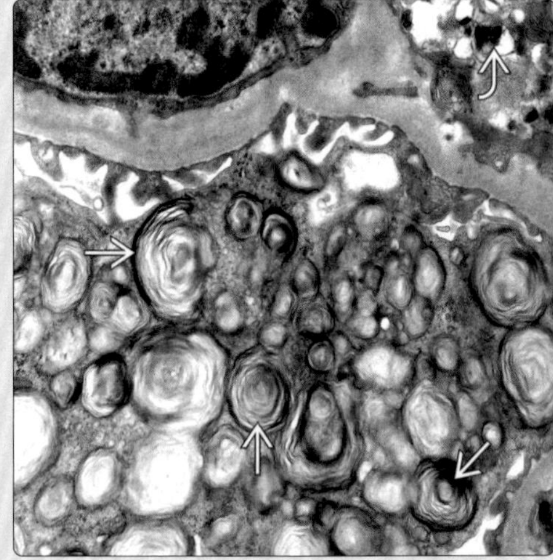

(Left) *This glomerulus has many vacuolated endocapillary foam cells, which appear to partially occlude capillary lumens. Swollen, finely vacuolated podocytes are also evident →. (Courtesy A. Cohen, MD.)* **(Right)** *This podocyte has myelin figures → in abundance. Mesangium also has vacuolated cells with electron-dense granules →. (Courtesy A. Cohen, MD.)*

Chloroquine Toxicity With Giant Lysosomes

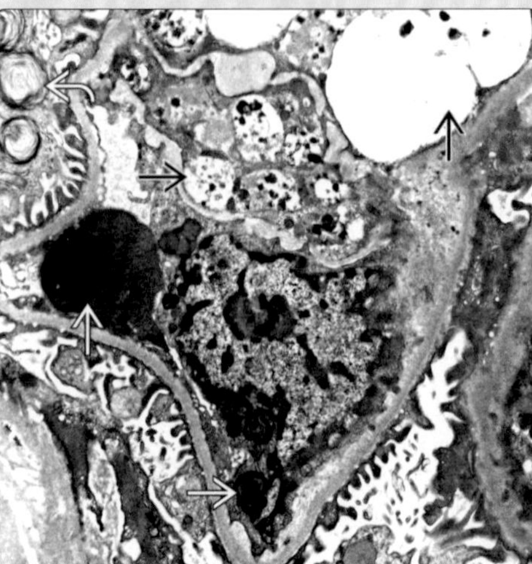

Hydroxychloroquine Toxicity

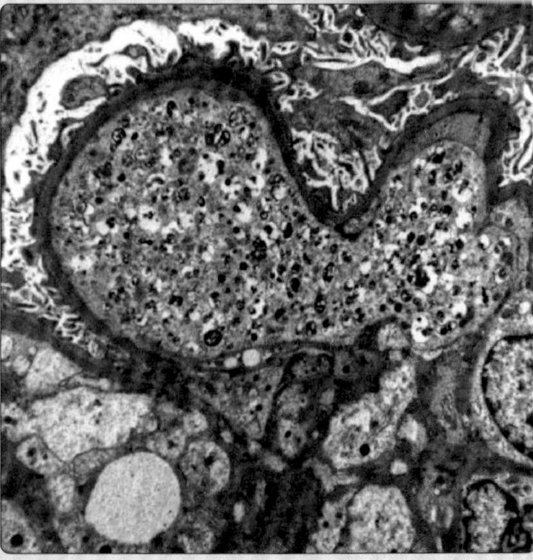

(Left) *EM shows mesangial cytoplasmic vacuoles → with granular debris of variable density. Endothelium has large, electron-dense lysosomes →. Myelin figures are in podocytes →. (Courtesy A. Cohen, MD.)* **(Right)** *Glomerular endothelial cells are filled with lipid in a patient who received chronic hydroxychloroquine treatment for lupus erythematosus. (Courtesy S. Khubchandani, MD.)*

TERMINOLOGY

Abbreviations

- Chloroquine toxicity (CT)

Synonyms

- Chloroquine-induced (phospho)lipidosis

Definitions

- Iatrogenic phospholipidosis characterized by nephropathy due to chloroquine or hydroxychloroquine exposure

ETIOLOGY/PATHOGENESIS

Chloroquine or Hydroxychloroquine

- Cationic, amphiphilic, and lysosomotropic
  - Inhibits activity of numerous enzymes, including α-galactosidase A, in lysosomes
- ↓ α-galactosidase A enzymatic activity → accumulation of globotriaosylceramide, sphingolipid
  - Accumulates in endothelium, podocytes, smooth muscle, and tubular epithelium

CLINICAL ISSUES

Presentation

- Indications for chloroquine and hydroxychloroquine treatment
  - Malaria, extraintestinal amebiasis, rheumatoid arthritis, lupus erythematosus, and others
- Toxicity
  - Renal toxicity: Proteinuria, declining renal function
  - Cardiac conduction defects, cardiomyopathy; proximal myopathy, retinopathy, keratopathy, hearing loss

Treatment

- Cessation of chloroquine exposure

Prognosis

- Proteinuria and reduced glomerular filtration rate potentially reversible after chloroquine cessation

MICROSCOPIC

Histologic Features

- Glomerular capillaries and mesangium have cells with vacuolated, foamy cytoplasm
  - Some but not all podocytes have swollen foamy cytoplasm
- Proximal and distal tubules may have fine cytoplasmic vacuolization
- Toluidine blue-stained sections have vacuolated endocapillary cells, and cytoplasmic azurophilic granules in podocytes, proximal and distal tubular cells

ANCILLARY TESTS

Electron Microscopy

- Podocytes have whorled lipid inclusions, called myelin figures or "zebra bodies," and may have curvilinear bodies and variable foot process effacement
- Glomerular capillaries and mesangium have vacuolated cells with granular, electron-dense inclusions
- Myelin figures and vacuoles evident in smooth muscle cells and endothelium of glomeruli, peritubular capillaries, arterioles, and arteries

DIFFERENTIAL DIAGNOSIS

Hereditary Disorders of Lipid Storage

- Fabry disease
  - Hereditary X-linked mutation of α-galactosidase A gene with accumulation of globotriaosylceramide
    - Myelin figures in podocytes, endothelium, mesangial cells, distal tubules, smooth muscle
  - Capillary lumens not occluded by vacuolated cells, and curvilinear bodies are not seen in podocytes
  - Plasma and leukocyte α-galactosidase A activity decreased or absent, but can be normal
  - Mutational analysis by DNA sequencing needed to exclude this diagnosis
- Gaucher disease
  - Gaucher cells in capillary lumens and mesangium
    - PAS and oil red O positive material in cytoplasm
    - Podocytes spared
  - By electron microscopy, elongated lysosomes contain irregular branching fibrils (60-80 nm in diameter)
- Other lipidoses
  - Infantile nephrosialidosis, I-cell disease, ceroid lipofuscinosis, Hurler syndrome, Niemann-Pick disease, Farber disease, GM1 gangliosidosis
    - Vacuolated podocytes mainly; Niemann-Pick disease may have vacuolated intracapillary cells
    - Differential diagnosis resolved by DNA mutational analysis
  - Lecithin cholesterol acyltransferase deficiency
    - Vacuolated cells and extracellular vacuolated structures in glomerular capillaries and mesangium

Drugs and Toxins

- Hydroxychloroquine, amiodarone, ranolazine, and silicon nephropathies
  - Pathologic features may be identical to chloroquine toxicity; diagnosis established by clinical history

DIAGNOSTIC CHECKLIST

Clinically Relevant Pathologic Features

- Pathologic features not specific and require clinical and molecular correlation, especially to exclude Fabry disease

Pathologic Interpretation Pearls

- Segmental podocyte involvement and curvilinear bodies are helpful clues

SELECTED REFERENCES

1. Khubchandani SR et al: Hydroxychloroquine-induced phospholipidosis in a case of SLE: the wolf in zebra clothing. Ultrastruct Pathol. 37(2):146-50, 2013
2. Bracamonte ER et al: Iatrogenic phospholipidosis mimicking Fabry disease. Am J Kidney Dis. 48(5):844-50, 2006
3. Albay D et al: Chloroquine-induced lipidosis mimicking Fabry disease. Mod Pathol. 18(5):733-8, 2005
4. Müller-Höcker J et al: Chloroquine-induced phospholipidosis of the kidney mimicking Fabry's disease: case report and review of the literature. Hum Pathol. 34(3):285-9, 2003

Intravascular Large B-Cell Lymphoma

KEY FACTS

CLINICAL ISSUES

- Median age: 6th-7th decade
- Western variant
  - Central nervous system (CNS) and cutaneous involvement common
- Asian variant
  - B-cell symptoms (fever, night sweats, weight loss)
  - Fatigue
  - Hemophagocytic syndrome
  - Poor prognosis
    - Death often occurs within short time of presentation
    - Vague signs and symptoms delay diagnosis
- Cutaneous variant or renal limited variant
  - More responsive to therapy

MACROSCOPIC

- Kidney enlargement

MICROSCOPIC

- Malignant large lymphoid cells
  - Preferential involvement of glomerular and peritubular capillaries
  - Large vesicular nuclei
  - Prominent nucleoli
  - Mitotic figures

ANCILLARY TESTS

- CD20(+)
- CD34 outlines blood vessels and capillaries
- Podocyte foot process effacement seen by electron microscopy
  - Often diffuse

TOP DIFFERENTIAL DIAGNOSES

- Other B-cell lymphomas
- Acute interstitial nephritis

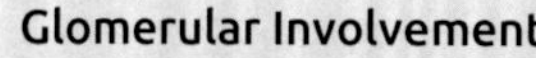

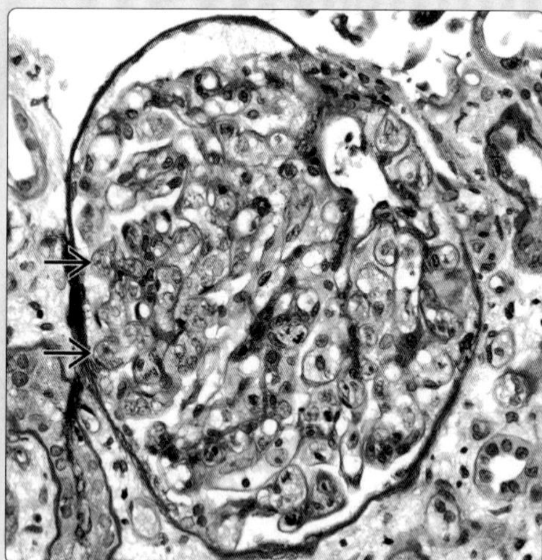

Intravascular Large B-Cell Lymphoma

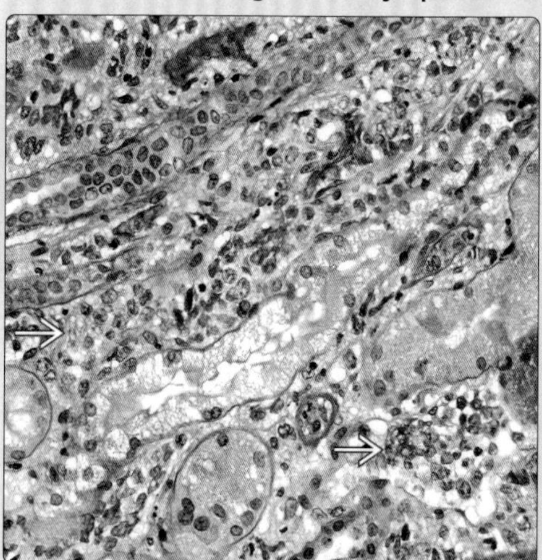

(Left) *Numerous malignant monotonous lymphoid cells ⇨ are plugging the capillaries in this glomerulus, which is characteristic of intravascular large B-cell lymphoma.* **(Right)** *Prominent aggregates of monotonous malignant lymphoid cells ➡ are packed into several peritubular capillaries. The patient died shortly after the diagnosis of intravascular large B-cell lymphoma was established.*

CD20

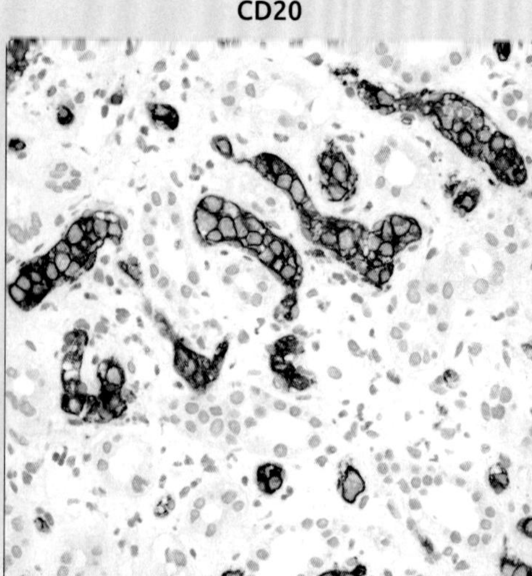

pax-5

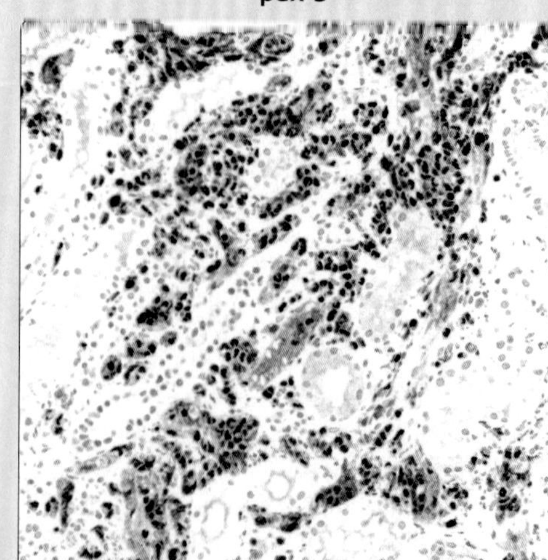

(Left) *CD20 immunohistochemistry outlines the clusters of malignant B cells clogging the peritubular capillaries in this kidney involved by intravascular large B-cell lymphoma.* **(Right)** *Strong nuclear pax-5 staining highlights the numerous malignant lymphoid B cells within the peritubular capillaries.*

TERMINOLOGY

Synonyms

- Angiotropic large cell lymphoma
- Intravascular lymphomatosis
- Angioendotheliomatosis proliferans systemisata
- Malignant angioendotheliomatosis

Definitions

- Subtype of extranodal large B-cell lymphoma with characteristic involvement of lymphoma cells in small vessel lumina, especially capillaries

CLINICAL ISSUES

Epidemiology

- Incidence
  - Rare
- Age
  - Median: 6th-7th decade
- Sex
  - No predilection
- Ethnicity
  - Western variant
    - Central nervous system (CNS) and cutaneous involvement common
  - Asian variant
    - Hemophagocytic syndrome
    - Hepatosplenomegaly
    - Anemia
    - Thrombocytopenia
    - Fever
    - Night sweats
    - Weight loss

Site

- CNS
- Skin
- Lung
- Kidney

Presentation

- Fatigue
- Proteinuria
  - Mild
  - Nephrotic syndrome occasionally
- Hypertension
- Hypercalcemia (rare)

Treatment

- CHOP chemotherapy
  - Cyclophosphamide
  - Doxorubicin
  - Leurocristime
  - Prednisone
- Rituximab

Prognosis

- Poor
  - Death often occurs within short time of presentation
  - Vague signs and symptoms delay diagnosis
- Good
  - Cutaneous variant or renal limited variant
    - More responsive to therapy

MACROSCOPIC

General Features

- Kidney enlargement

MICROSCOPIC

Histologic Features

- Malignant large lymphoid cells
  - Preferential involvement of glomerular and peritubular capillaries

Cytologic Features

- Malignant large lymphoid cells
  - Large vesicular nuclei
  - Prominent nucleoli
  - Mitotic figures
  - Abundant cytoplasm

ANCILLARY TESTS

Immunohistochemistry

- CD20(+)
- pax-5(+)
- MUM1(+)
- Ki-67(+)
- Bcl-2(+)
- Bcl-6(+)
- CD34 outlines endothelial cells in blood vessels

Immunofluorescence

- No glomerular or tubulointerstitial deposits

Electron Microscopy

- Podocyte foot process effacement
  - Often diffuse
- No electron dense deposits

DIFFERENTIAL DIAGNOSIS

Other B-Cell Lymphomas

- Diffuse large B-cell lymphoma

Acute Interstitial Nephritis

- No glomerular involvement by inflammatory cells

SELECTED REFERENCES

1. Akpinar TS et al: Isolated renal intravascular lymphoma: a case report and review of the literature. Ren Fail. 36(7):1125-8, 2014
2. Bilgili SG et al: Intravascular large B-cell lymphoma presenting with anasarca-type edema and acute renal failure. Ren Fail. 35(8):1163-6, 2013
3. Zhu J et al: Mild proteinuria in a patient with glomerular limited intravascular large B-cell lymphoma. Clin Nephrol. 80(4):286-92, 2013
4. Bai X et al: Intravascular large B-cell lymphoma of the kidney: a case report. Diagn Pathol. 6:86, 2011
5. Chinen Y et al: Intravascular B-cell lymphoma with hypercalcemia as the initial presentation. Int J Hematol. 94(6):567-70, 2011
6. Kameoka Y et al: Kidney-limited intravascular large B cell lymphoma: a distinct variant of IVLBCL? Int J Hematol. 89(4):533-7, 2009
7. Sepandj F et al: Renal manifestations of angiotrophic lymphoma: clinicopathological features. Nephrol Dial Transplant. 12(1):190-4, 1997
8. D'Agati V et al: Angiotropic large cell lymphoma (intravascular malignant lymphomatosis) of the kidney: presentation as minimal change disease. Hum Pathol. 20(3):263-8, 1989

SECTION 3

Vascular Diseases

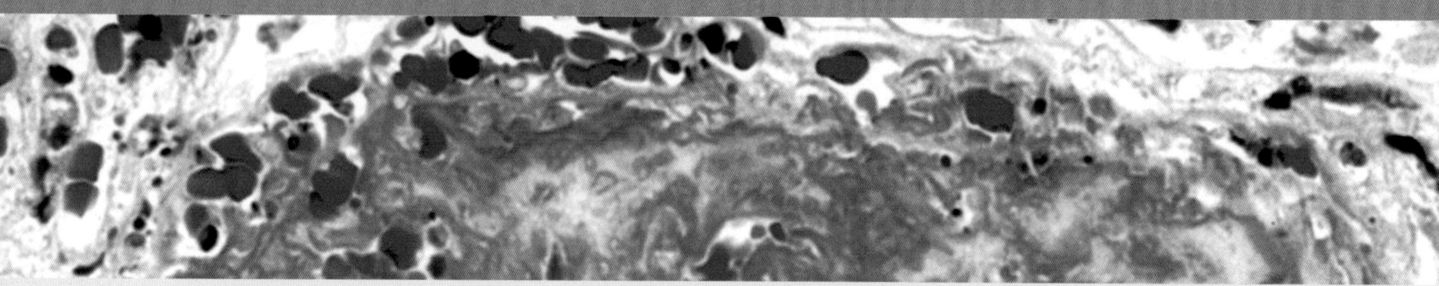

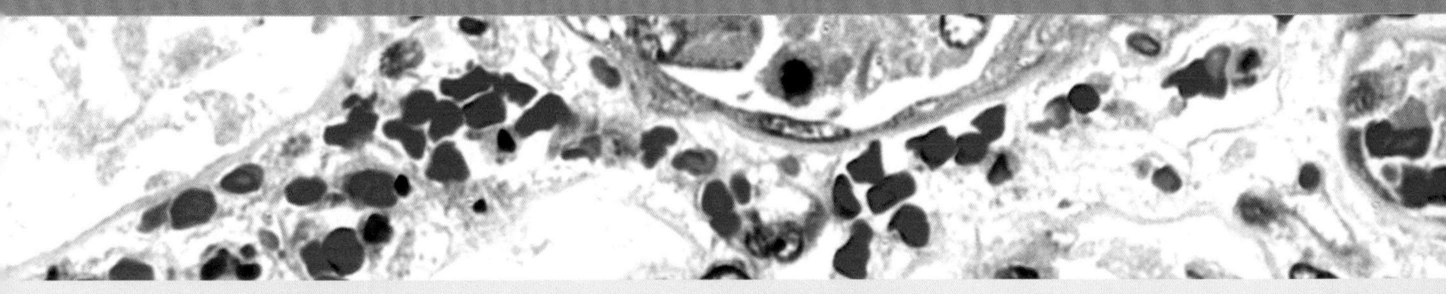

Hypertensive Renal Disease

Thrombotic and Embolic Disease

TERMINOLOGY

Synonyms

- Primary systemic vasculitides

Definitions

- Pathological
  - Vasculitis defined as inflammation of blood vessels with demonstrable structural injury, such as disruption of elastic lamina ± fibrinoid necrosis
  - Occlusive changes due to inflammatory infiltrate or thrombosis often evident
- Clinical
  - Clinical definition not possible due to organ-specific or multisystemic disease
  - Rapid or prolonged evolution of clinical features over time may impede or delay definitive diagnosis
  - Thorough correlation with pathophysiologic mechanisms, serology, and imaging studies essential

History

- Vasculitis 1st described by Kussmaul and Maier in 1866
  - Termed "periarteritis nodosa"
- Giant cell arteritis described by Hutchinson (1890)
- Multiple vessel involvement and transmural arterial inflammation led to term "polyarteritis nodosa" by Ferrari (1903) and Dickson (1908)
- Takayasu arteritis described by Takayasu (1909)
- Granulomatosis with polyangiitis (Wegener) described by Klinger (1931) and Wegener (1934)
- Eosinophilic granulomatosis with Polyangiitis described by Churg and Strauss (1951), as allergic type
- Introduction of term "necrotizing angiitis" and attempt to classify vasculitis by Zeek in 1952
- Vasculitis and mucocutaneous lymph node syndrome described by Kawasaki in 1966
- "Microscopic polyangiitis" introduced in 1994 by Jennette and colleagues

CHCC Schematic of Systemic Vasculitides 2012

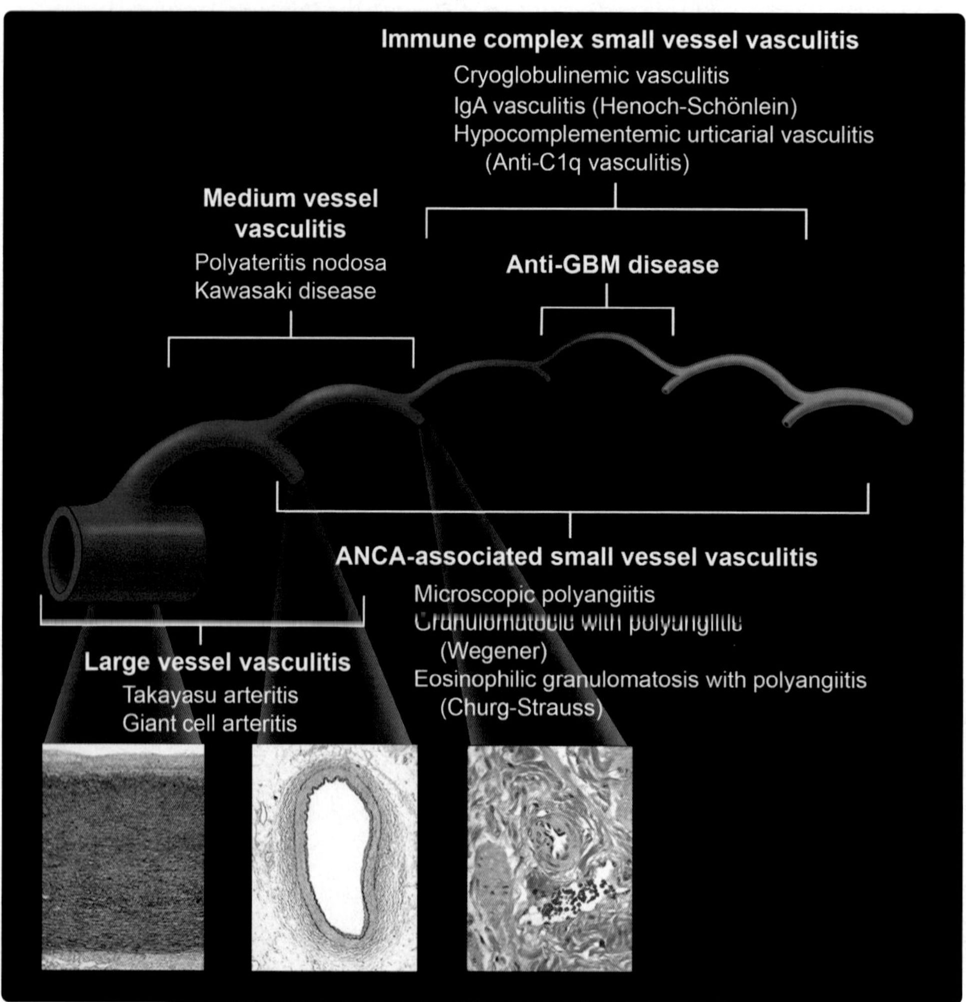

This schematic shows the predominant range of vascular involvement by different vasculitides, as described in the Chapel Hill Consensus Conference (CHCC) on Nomenclature of Systemic Vasculitis (2012). Those that affect capillaries are most likely to cause glomerulonephritis (modified from Jennette JC et al, CHCC 2012).

Classification Considerations

- Vasculitides may be primary or secondary to systemic disease
- Vasculitides can localize to 1 organ or affect multiple organ systems
- Consensus classifications and criteria based on demographics, clinical characteristics, and pathology
- Progess toward classification based on etiology and pathogenesis

CHAPEL HILL CONSENSUS CONFERENCE NOMENCLATURE OF SYSTEMIC VASCULITIDES (1994 AND REVISED 2012)

General

- Developed definitions and standardized diagnostic terminology
- Categorization based on etiology, pathogenesis, pathology, and clinical characteristics
- Classification based on size of arterial vessel involved and type of inflammatory reaction
- Introduction of new terms in small vessel vasculitis to replace those with eponyms
- Division of small vessel vasculitis into ANCA-associated vasculitis (AAV) and immune complex (SVV)
- Emphasize role of ANCA (MPO-ANCA, PR3-ANCA) in pauci-immune small vessel vasculitis and crescentic glomerulonephritis
- Pathological correlation with clinical and laboratory features may identify specific therapeutic groups
- Pulmonary renal syndromes of pauci-immune small vessel vasculitides may have similarities and be distinguished by ANCA serology
- Inclusion of variable vessel vasculitis (2012)
- Inclusion of secondary form of vasculitis (2012)
- Disease in single organ may progress to systemic vasculitis

Large Vessel Vasculitis (LVV)

- Giant cell (temporal) arteritis (GCA)
  - Granulomatous arteritis of aorta and its major branches
  - Common in extracranial branches of carotid artery
  - Usually occurs in patients > 50 years
  - Often associated with polymyalgia rheumatica
- Takayasu arteritis (TAK)
  - Granulomatous inflammation of aorta and its major branches usually in patients < 50 years

Medium-Sized Vessel Vasculitis (MVV)

- Polyarteritis nodosa (PAN)
  - Necrotizing inflammation of medium-sized or small arteries without glomerulonephritis or vasculitis in arterioles, capillaries, or venules
- Kawasaki disease (KD)
  - Arteritis involving large, medium-sized and small arteries
    - Associated with mucocutaneous lymph node syndrome
  - Coronary arteries often involved
  - Aorta and veins may be involved
  - Usually occurs in children

Small Vessel Vasculitis Including Capillaries, Venules, Arterioles, and Arteries (SVV)

- Antineutrophil cytoplasmic antibodies (ANCA) associated vasculitis (AAV)
  - Granulomatosis with polyangiitis (Wegener) (GPA)
    - Granulomatosis inflammation involving respiratory tract and necrotizing vasculitis affecting small to medium-sized vessels
    - Necrotizing glomerulonephritis is common
  - Eosinophilic granulomatosis with polyangiitis (EGPA) (Churg-Strauss)
    - Eosinophil-rich and granulomatous inflammation involving respiratory tract and necrotizing vasculitis affecting small to medium-sized vessels; associated with asthma and eosinophilia
    - Crescentic glomerulonephritis when ANCA present
  - Microscopic polyangiitis (microscopic polyarteritis)
    - Necrotizing vasculitis with few or no immune deposits, affecting small and medium-sized vessels
    - Necrotizing glomerulonephritis very common
    - Pulmonary capillaritis often occurs
- Immune complex vasculitis
  - Vasculitis with moderate to marked vessel wall deposits of immunoglobulins &/or complement components
  - Predominantly affects small vessels: Capillaries, arterioles, venules, small arteries
  - Glomerulonephritis frequent
- Antiglomerular basement membrane (anti-GBM) disease
  - Vasculitis affecting glomerular capillaries, pulmonary capillaries, or both
  - GBM deposition of anti-GBM autoantibodies
  - Lung involvement causes pulmonary hemorrhage
- IgA vasculitis (Henoch-Schönlein) (IgAV)
  - Vasculitis with IgA-dominant immune deposits, affecting small vessels
  - Typically involves skin, gut, and glomeruli, and associated with arthralgias or arthritis
- Cryoglobulinemic Vasculitis
  - Small vessel vasculitis with cryoglobulin immune deposits
  - Associated with serum cryoglobulins
  - Skin, glomeruli and peripheral nerves often involved
- Hypocomplementemic urticarial vasculitis (HUV) (anti-C1q vasculitis)
  - Vasculitis with urticaria and hypocomplementemia
  - Affects small vessels
  - Associated with anti-C1q antibodies
  - Glomerulonephritis, arthritis, obstructive pulmonary disease, ocular inflammation common

Variable Vessel Vasculitis (VVV) Affecting Any Size Vessel

- Behçet disease (BD)
  - Vasculitis can affect arteries or veins
  - Recurrent oral &/or genital aphthous ulcers
  - Inflammatory lesions in cutaneous, ocular, articular, gastrointestinal, &/or central nervous system
  - SVV, thromboangiitis, thrombosis, arterial aneurysms
- Cogan syndrome (CS)
  - Ocular inflammatory lesions
  - Inner ear disease

- Arteritis of all sizes, aortitis/aneurysms, aortic and mitral valvulitis

Single Organ Vasculitis (SOV)

- Vasculitis of arteries or veins of any size in single organ
- Skin, central nervous system, isolated aortitis
- Unifocal or multifocal
- May progress to septic vasculitis

Vasculitis Associated With Systemic Disease

- Rheumatoid vasculitis
- Lupus vasculitis
- Sarcoid vasculitis

Vasculitis Associated With Probable Etiology

- Drug induced vasculitis e.g., hydralazine
- Infection related vasculitis
- Hepatitis C virus-associated cryoglobulinemic vasculitis
- Hepatitis B virus-associated vasculitis
- Syphilis-associated aortitis
- Drug-associated immune-complex vasculitis
- Drug-associated ANCA-associated vasculitis
- Cancer-associated vasculitis

OTHER CLASSIFICATION SYSTEMS

American College of Rheumatology (1990) (ACR)

- Criteria for diagnosis of vasculitides
  - Clinical criteria developed to standardize cohorts of patients in almost all primary systemic vasculitides
  - ≥ 3 criteria associated with high degree of sensitivity and specificity for diagnosis in appropriate context
  - Application of criteria for individual patients may not be entirely helpful
  - ANCA not used in this classification process

EULAR/PRES Classification of Pediatric Vasculitis (European League Against Rheumatism/Pediatric Rheumatology European Society)

- Predominantly large vessel
  - Takayasu arteritis
- Predominantly medium vessel
  - Childhood polyarteritis nodosa
  - Cutaneous polyarteritis
  - Kawasaki disease
- Predominantly small vessel
  - Granulomatous
    - Granulomatosis with polyangiitis (Wegener)
    - Eosinophilic granulomatosis with polyangiitis (Churg-Strauss)
  - Nongranulomatous
    - Microscopic polyangiitis
    - Henoch-Schönlein purpura
    - Isolated cutaneous leukocytoclastic vasculitis
    - Hypocomplementemic urticarial vasculitis
- Other
  - Behçet disease
  - Vasculitis secondary to infection, malignancy, drugs
  - Isolated vasculitis of central nervous system
  - Cogan syndrome
  - Unclassified

EPIDEMIOLOGY

Incidence

- Depends on specific types of vasculitis and associated primary or secondary systemic diseases

Ethnicity and Distribution

- Takayasu arteritis and Kawasaki disease most common in Asia and Far East countries
- Granulomatosis with polyangiitis and eosinophilic granulomatosis and polyangiitis have predilection for North America and Northern Europe, mainly in Caucasians
- Higher incidence of microscopic polyangiitis in Asia

Age Range

- Adults: Age range depends on type of disease
- Children at or below 18 years old
  - Annual incidence: 53.3/100,000
- Geographical variations of diseases may reflect environmental and ethnic influences

ETIOLOGY/PATHOGENESIS

Etiology

- Immune complexes
  - Mixed cryoglobulinemia
  - Lupus erythematosus
  - Henoch-Schönlein purpura (IgA Vasculitis)
- Autoantibodies
  - ANCA
    - Microscopic polyangiitis
    - Granulomatosis with polyangiitis (Wegener)
    - Eosinophilic granulomatosis with polyangiitis (Churg-Strauss)
  - Possibly other forms of vasculitides
- Idiopathic
  - Takayasu arteritis
  - Kawasaki disease
  - Giant cell arteritis
- Other factors
  - Infections
    - Bacteria, viruses, fungi, rickettsia, parasites
  - Drug reaction

CLINICAL IMPLICATIONS

Clinical Presentation

- General constitutional symptoms are common with all forms of vasculitis in initial or acute stage
- Specific signs and symptoms depend on several factors
  - Single or multiple organ system involvement
  - Size and type of vessel involved
  - Pathogenetic mechanisms
  - Pathological findings
  - Severity of disease
- Specific presenting symptoms of complications of vasculitis
  - Vascular stenosis, occlusion, aneurysm, hemorrhage
- Symptoms can be acute, subacute, or chronic
- Clinical features of vasculitis can mimic vasculitis-like diseases, vasculopathies, and, rarely, nonvascular diseases
- Renal findings in vasculitis

- Hematuria, subnephrotic proteinuria
- Rapidly progressive renal failure
- Chronic renal failure
- Benign or malignant hypertension

Laboratory Findings

- Acute phase response associated with active vasculitis
- Complete blood counts
  - Varied granulocytosis or lymphocytosis
  - Thrombocytosis
  - Anemia
- Specific organ function tests
  - Kidney, lung, heart, liver, pancreas, endocrine
- Serologic tests
  - Various types of infections
  - Autoantibodies
    - Antineutrophil cytoplasmic antibodies
    - Antinuclear antibodies
    - Rheumatoid factor
    - Antiglomerular basement membrane
    - Other less frequent but specific antibodies
  - Complement levels
    - C3, C4, C1q
  - Urinalysis
    - Hematuria, proteinuria, casts, cells

Imaging Findings

- Most useful in large and medium-sized vessel vasculitides
- Each diagnostic category has several vascular patterns
- Variety of imaging modalities may be used
  - Plain x-ray
  - Angiography
    - Computed tomogram
    - Magnetic resonance
  - Doppler studies
  - Tc-99m DMSA scanning

Prognosis

- Vasculitides range from self-limiting to relapsing disease
- Significant diagnostic delays occur due to frequent clinical overlap and nonspecific findings leading to worse prognosis
- Varied morbidity and mortality
  - Specific organ involvement
  - Severity of vasculitis
  - Complications
- Sequelae of vasculitis contribute to further organ damage
- Infectious complications due to immunosuppression

Treatment

- Ideally, therapeutic approaches should be based on etiology &/or pathophysiology of the vasculitides
  - Corticosteroid therapy alone useful for giant cell arteritis and eosinophilic granulomatosis with polyangiitis without renal involvement
- Clinical heterogeneity and varied immune-mediated pathogenetic mechanisms prompt empirical initial therapy
- Number of treatment protocols used for primary and secondary vasculitides
  - Cyclophosphamide and steroids in small vessel vasculitides
  - Plasmapheresis and anti-CD20 antibody in severe disease
  - Oral steroids, methotrexate, and azathioprine employed for maintenance of remission
  - New biological agents being tested

MACROSCOPIC

General Features

- Large and medium-sized vessel vasculitides display distinctive gross characteristics from specimens obtained following excision during surgery or autopsy specimen
- Renal vasculitides of all sizes may result in segmental/total infarction and parenchymal atrophy in renal artery stenosis
- Cortical petechial hemorrhages in small vessel vasculitides

MICROSCOPIC

General Features

- Types of vascular inflammation in vasculitis can be
  - Neutrophil, eosinophil, or lymphocyte rich
  - Granulomatous
  - Necrotizing
  - Can be focal, segmental, or circumferential in distribution
- Other findings
  - Endothelial injury and necrosis
  - Disruption of internal &/or external elastic lamina
  - Focal medial laminar lysis of elastic fibers
  - Medial and adventitial inflammation
  - Intravascular thrombosis
  - Tissue infarction
  - Fibromyointimal thickening of healed lesions
- Organ-specific changes
  - Kidneys showing crescentic glomerulonephritis and medullary angiitis
  - Alveolar capillaritis and lung hemorrhage
  - Leukocytoclastic vasculitis in skin
  - Myocardial inflammation and valvulitis

CONDITIONS THAT MIMIC VASCULITIS

Large Arteries

- Fibromuscular dysplasia
- Extensive atherosclerosis
- Other forms of aortitis

Medium-Sized Arteries

- Embolic phenomena

Small Vessel Disease

- Atheroemboli
- Bacterial endocarditis
- Thrombotic microangiopathy
  - Antiphospholipid antibody syndrome
- Atrial myxoma
- Amyloid angiopathy

SELECTED REFERENCES

1. Flores-Suárez LF et al: Critical appraisal of classification criteria for vasculitides. Curr Rheumatol Rep. 16(6):422, 2014
2. Jennette JC: Overview of the 2012 revised International Chapel Hill Consensus Conference nomenclature of vasculitides. Clin Exp Nephrol. 17(5):603-6, 2013

Differential Diagnosis

Type	Clinical Features	Serology	Pathologic Features	Glomerular Lesion
Large Vessel Vasculitis (Large, Aorta and Major Branches)				
Giant cell arteritis: Usually > 50 years, M:F 1:2-6	Polymyalgia rheumatica (50%), mostly head and neck symptoms	ANCA(-)	Commonly temporal arteritis, mononuclear infiltration with multinucleated giant cells	Ischemic changes; amyloidosis
Takayasu arteritis: Usually 30-50 years, M:F = 1:8	Initial nonspecific symptoms, later ischemic effects of tissues	ANCA(-)	Granulomatous panarteritis with multinucleated giant cells	Ischemic changes; mesangial or focal proliferative GN
Medium-Sized Vessel Vasculitis (Medium-Sized Arteries)				
Polyarteritis nodosa: Peak 40-60 years, M:F = 2:1	Multisystem, hypertension, organ ischemic symptoms	Rarely MPO+; Hepatitis B virus (+)	Fibrinoid necrotizing arteritis, transmural, healed lesions, stenosis, aneurysms	Ischemic changes; rare pauci-immune crescentic GN
Kawasaki disease: < 3 years in most cases; M:F = 5:1	Mucocutaneous lymph node syndrome; coronary artery vasculitis	Systemic atypical cytoplasmic ANCA(+)	Depending on stage: Acute neutrophilic arteritis, aneurysm formation, chronic inflammation, and scarring	Rare mesangial proliferative GN; patchy interstitial inflammation
Small Vessel Vasculitis (Small Arteries, Arterioles, Venules, Capillaries)				
Microscopic polyangiitis: Any age, peak: 50 years; M = F	Multisystemic, kidney (90-100%), nephritic syndrome, rapidly progressive renal failure, no asthma	MPO ANCA (+) 60%, PR3 ANCA (+) 15%	Fibrinoid necrotizing vasculitis	Pauci-immune crescentic GN
Granulomatosis with polyangiitis: Any age, peak: 30-50 years, M > F	Multisystemic, upper airway, lung and kidneys (90%), rapidly progressive renal failure, no asthma	PR3 ANCA (+) > 75%, MPO ANCA (+) < 25%	Necrotizing, vascular or extravascular granulomatous inflammation	Pauci-immune crescentic GN, acute, subacute, and chronic
IgA vasculitis: 90% before 10 years; M > F; adult/secondary	Multisystemic, kidney, lung, gastrointestinal tract	↑ serum IgA, normal complement, ANCA(-)	Leukocytoclastic vasculitis, dominant IgA and C3 deposits	Mesangial or endocapillary proliferation ± crescents and IgA deposits
Eosinophilic granulomatosis with polyangiitis: Peak: 40-60 years; M = F	Multisystemic, asthma, eosinophilia, renal manifestations in < 30% of cases	ANCA(+) (40-70%), mostly anti-MPO	Eosinophil-rich fibrinoid necrotizing vasculitis and granulomatous inflammation	Commonly mesangial, occasional pauci-immune, proliferation, focal GN with crescents
Cryoglobulinemic vasculitis: Adults	Multisystemic, skin and kidney frequently involved	Elevated monoclonal IgM κ RF, 90% HCV(+)	Leukocytoclastic vasculitis with cryoprecipitates, IgM κ, IgG, and C3 deposits	Membranoproliferative GN ± crescents and cryo deposits
Systemic lupus erythematosus: Any age, M:F = 1:9	Multisystemic, skin and kidney (90%)	ANA(+), dsDNA(+), sometimes ANCA(+)	Necrotizing vasculitis	Immune complex GN ± crescents; rarely, pauci-immune crescentic GN

Vascular Diseases Mimicking Vasculitis

Disease	Location	Pathology	Inflammation	Pathogenesis
Antiphospholipid antibody syndrome	All calibers of arteries and veins, capillaries	Fibrin or organizing vascular thrombi, focal recanalization	Rare or none	Antiphospholipid antibodies or lupus anticoagulant
Thrombotic microangiopathy	Small arteries, arterioles, capillaries	Endothelial swelling, mucoid change, fibrin, thrombi; intact elastic lamina	Minimal mononuclear	Abnormalities of ADAMTS13; immune complexes; drug induced
Atheroembolism	All calibers of arteries up to capillaries	Luminal occlusion by crystalline cholesterol clefts ± thrombosis	Giant cell reaction in older lesions	Embolic phenomenon from atheromas of larger arteries
Amyloid angiopathy	Medium and small arteries, arterioles, and capillaries	Congo red positive, amorphous, acellular, vascular amyloid	None	AL amyloid; rarely other forms of amyloid
Atrial myxoma (intracardiac tumor)	Small arteries, arterioles, and capillaries	Luminal occlusion by fragments of myxoma	None	Emboli from cardiac tumor
Bacterial endocarditis	Small arteries, arterioles, and capillaries	Local ischemic changes, focal glomerulonephritis	Sometimes	Emboli from valvular vegetations, bland or septic

Giant Cell (Temporal) Arteritis

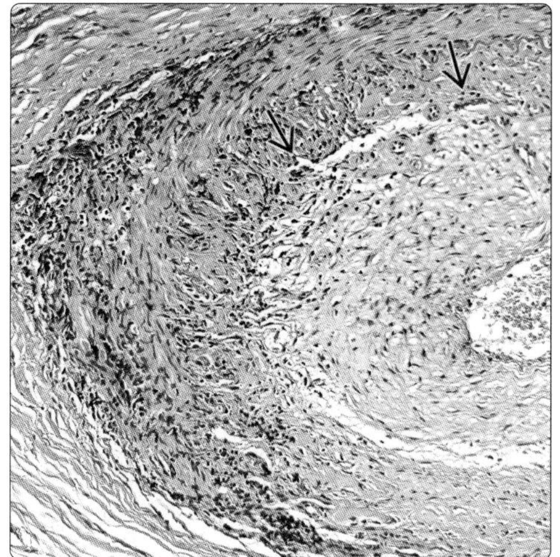

Takayasu Arteritis

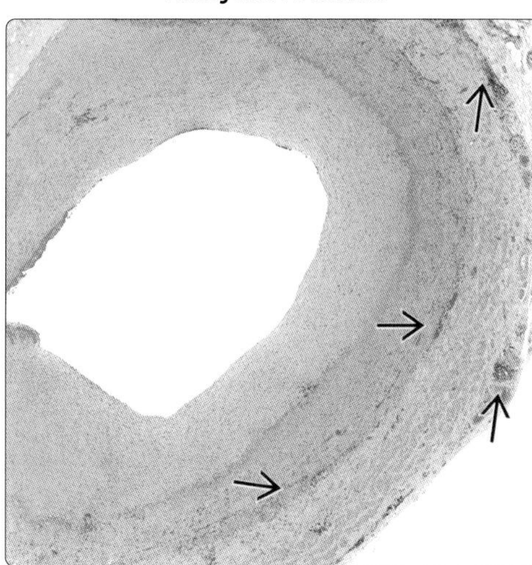

(Left) *Segment of temporal artery with giant cell arteritis shows transmural arteritis with inflammatory cell infiltration in the adventitia and the media with marked fibromyointimal thickening. Rare multinucleated giant cells are noted ➙.* **(Right)** *Cross section of a thickened large artery from a young female with Takayasu arteritis shows myointimal proliferation with inflammation and focal medial and adventitial inflammation ➙. (Courtesy J.C. Jennette, MD.)*

Polyarteritis Nodosa

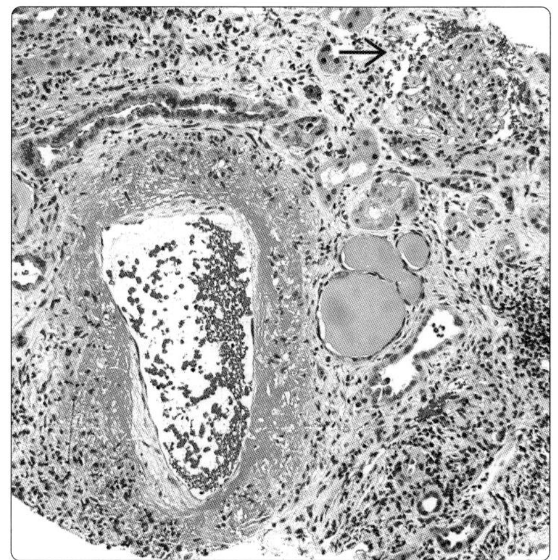

Kawasaki Disease, Coronary Artery

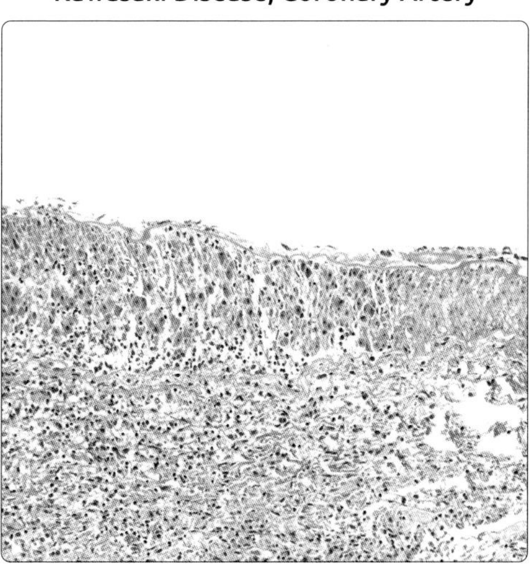

(Left) *A renal artery larger than interlobular type with polyarteritis nodosa shows circumferential, transmural fibrinoid necrosis accompanied by primarily neutrophilic infiltrate. An uninvolved glomerulus is seen ➙.* **(Right)** *Microscopic section of a coronary artery from a patient with Kawasaki disease shows medial and intimal mixed inflammatory cell infiltrate without significant fibrinoid necrosis. (Courtesy J.C. Jennette, MD.)*

Granulomatous Arteritis

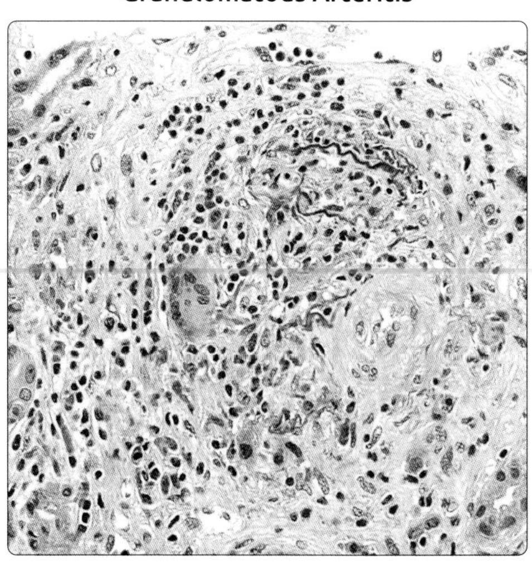

Necrotizing Interstitial Granulomatous Inflammation in GPA

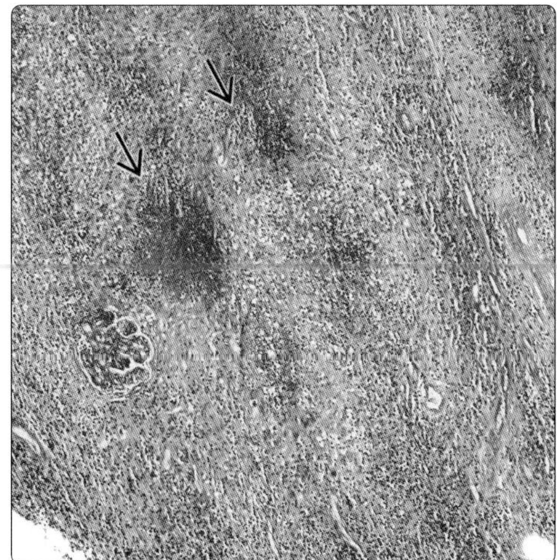

(Left) *Case of GPA with organizing granulomatous arteritis showing disruption and fragmentation of the elastic lamina by GMS stain.* **(Right)** *PAS-stained kidney section with granulomatosis with polyangiitis (Wegener) shows typical irregular necrotizing granulomatous inflammation with a neutrophilic center ➙. An adjacent glomerulus with ischemic change is noted. (Courtesy W. Travis, MD.)*

(Left) *A specimen from a patient with high-titer MPO-ANCA shows full-thickness necrotizing vasculitis of a small intrarenal artery surrounded by active neutrophilic and lymphocytic infiltrate with loss of elastic lamina, consistent with microscopic polyangiitis. There is interstitial inflammation and tubulitis.* **(Right)** *Glomerulus from a patient with PR3-ANCA(+) shows a large, almost circumferential cellular crescent. Part of the Bowman capsule is disrupted by periglomerular inflammatory infiltrate →.*

Necrotizing Vasculitis in Intrarenal Artery of MPA

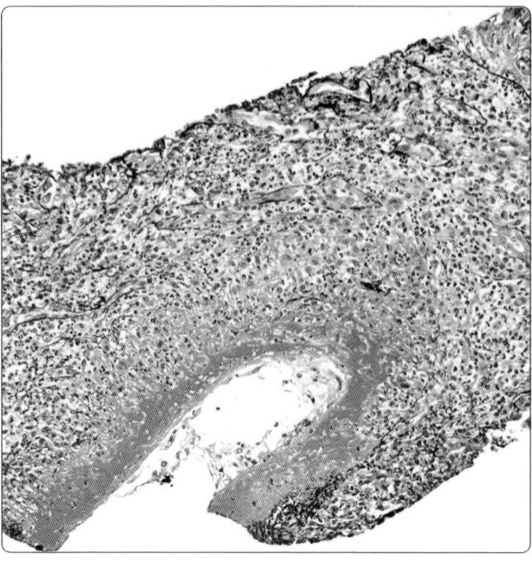

Glomerulus With Circumferential Cellular Crescent

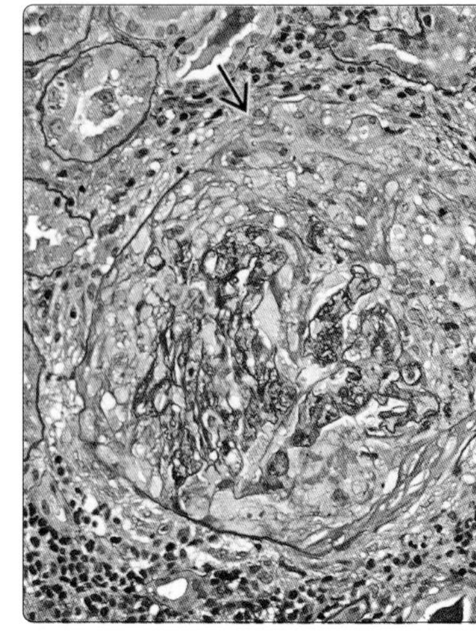

(Left) *Subcutaneous, medium-sized artery from a patient with eosinophilic granulomatosis with polyangiitis (EGPA) (Churg-Strauss) shows segmental transmural inflammation with many eosinophils.* **(Right)** *Detailed diagram of the arterial vessels involved by large, medium, and small vessel vasculitides as proposed by The Chapel Hill Consensus Conference 2012.*

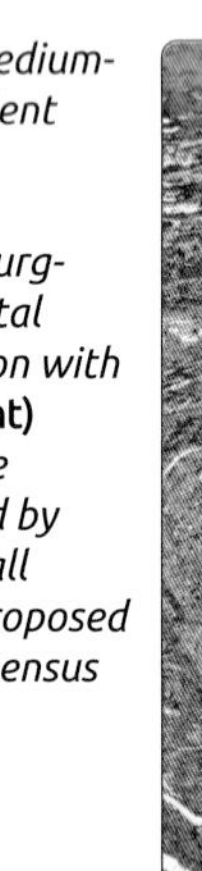

EGPA (Churg-Strauss) in a Subcutaneous Artery

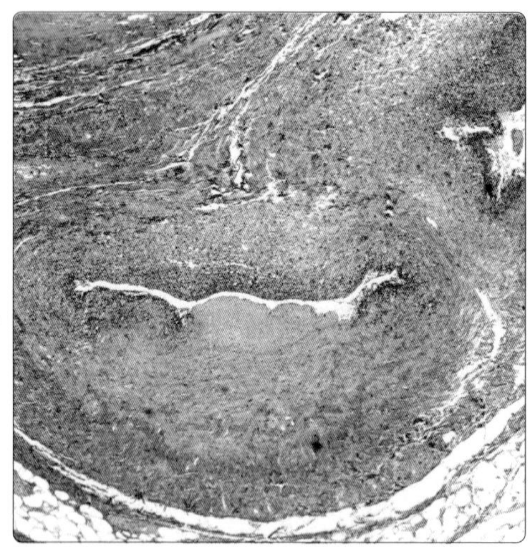

Diagrams Representing Large, Medium and Small Vessels Associated With Kidney

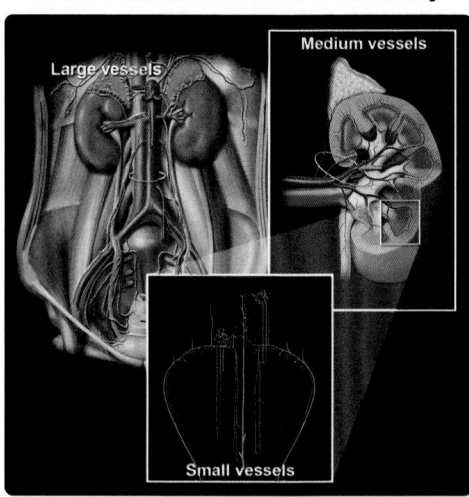

(Left) *p-ANCA (perinuclear) pattern → due to MPO IgG antibodies is demonstrated by indirect IF with a patient's serum incubated on alcohol-fixed normal neutrophils. The cytoplasm is not visible. A negative eosinophil is also present ↶. (Courtesy A.B. Collins, BS.)* **(Right)** *The c-ANCA (cytoplasmic) pattern → due to PR3 antibodies is demonstrated by indirect IF with a patient's serum incubated on an alcohol-fixed smear of normal neutrophils. (Courtesy A.B. Collins, BS.)*

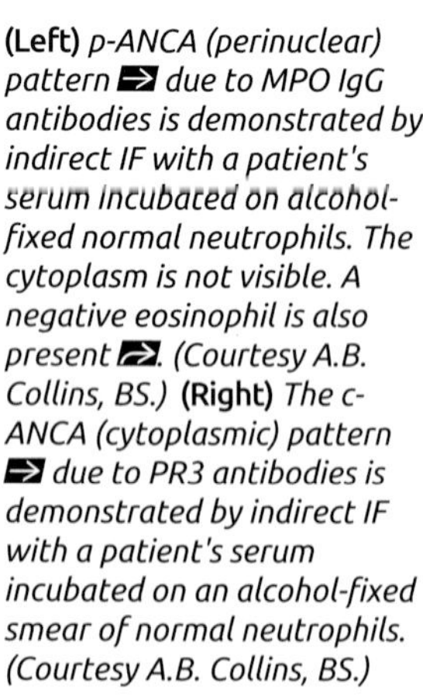

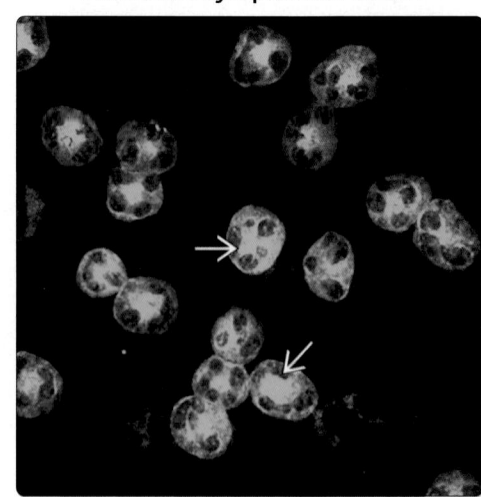

MPO-ANCA (Perinuclear) Pattern

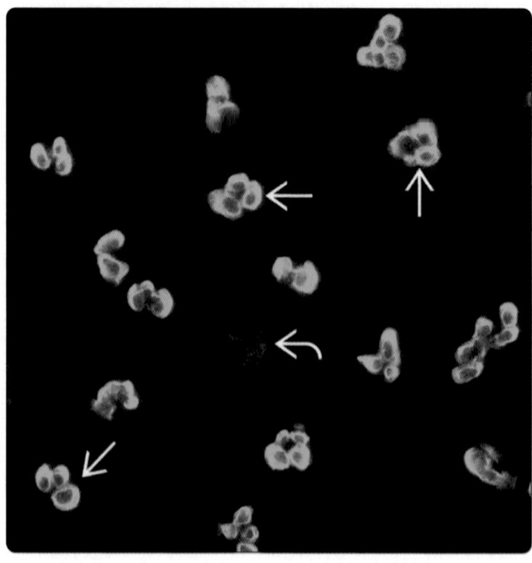

PR3-ANCA Cytoplasmic Pattern

Global Proliferative Glomerulonephritis in HUVS

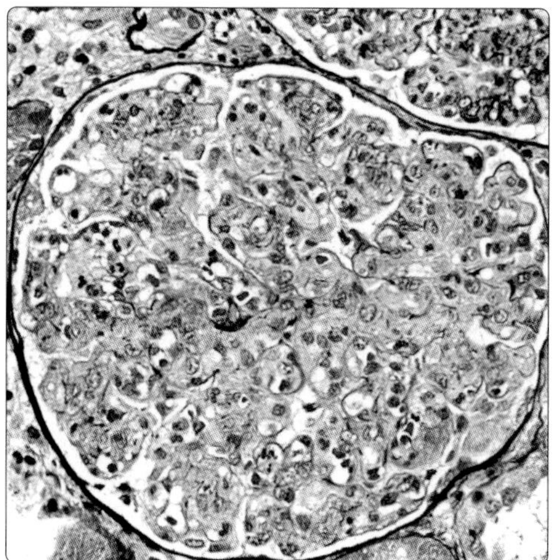

Global Mesangial Proliferative GN in HUVS

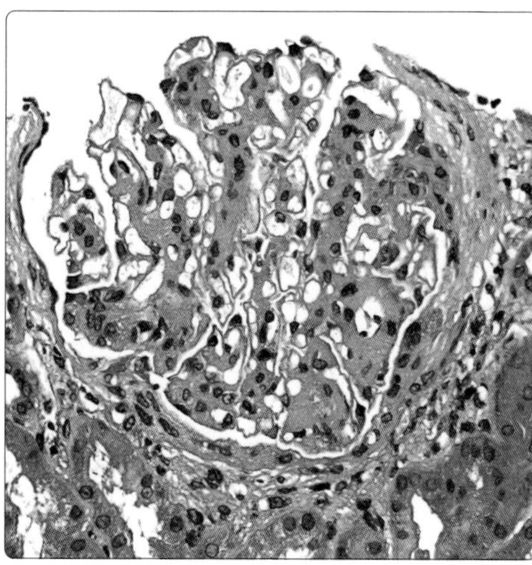

(Left) *Glomerular capillaries are filled with leukocytes, including neutrophils and mononuclear cells. The glomerular basement membrane appears normal, without duplication. The mesangium is hypercellular. (Courtesy S. Florquin, MD.)* **(Right)** *A case of HUVS showing diffuse mesangial proliferation and segmental capsular adhesion containing increased mesangial immune complex deposits. The peripheral capillary walls appear mostly uninvolved. (Courtesy D. Ferluga, MD.)*

Global Capillary Wall IgG Deposits

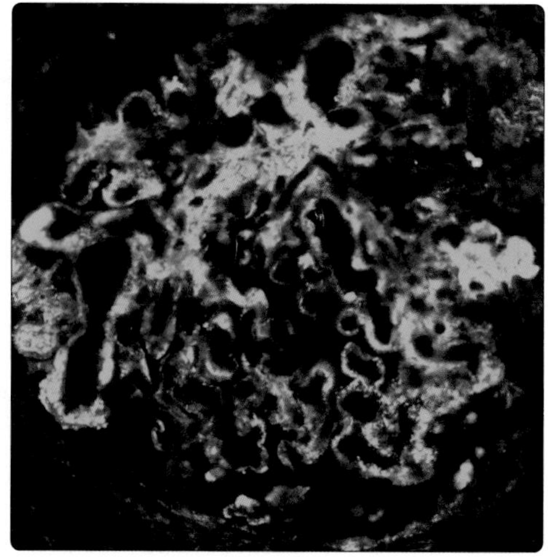

Mesangial GN With Necrotizing Small Vessel Vasculitis

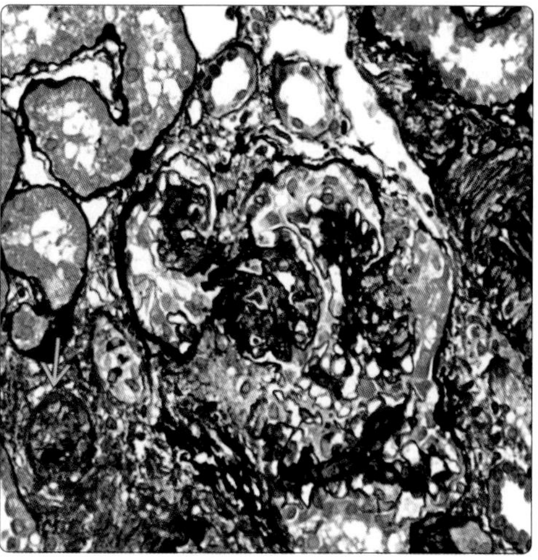

(Left) *A case of hypocomplementemic urticarial vasculitis with glomerulonephritis showing granular 3+ IgG deposits within the glomerular capillary walls and mesangial areas in global distribution along with C1q deposits in the same areas. (Courtesy A. Vizjak, PhD.)* **(Right)** *This case of HUVS shows a focus of small vessel vasculitis with thrombosis* ➙ *and mesangial proliferative glomerulonephritis with capsular adhesion. (Courtesy D. Ferluga, MD.)*

Immune Complex Glomerulonephritis With Crescent

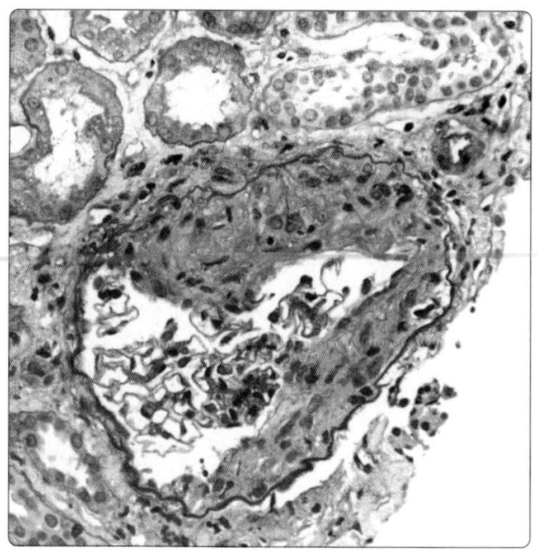

Global Mesangial and Capillary Wall Immune Deposits

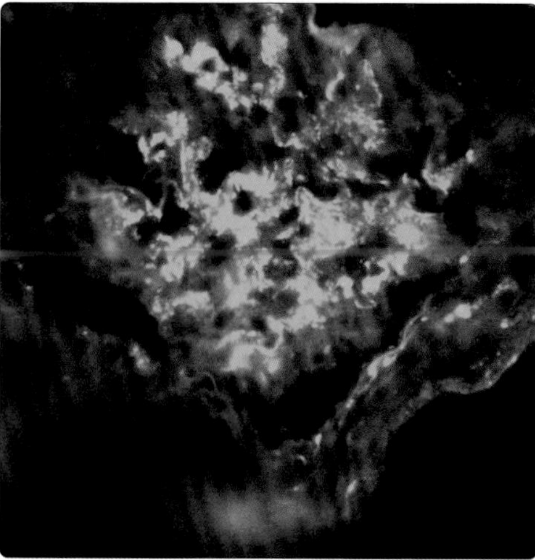

(Left) *A case of Behcet disease presented with nephritic syndrome and immune complex glomerulonephritis with crescents. This image shows a fibrocellular crescent. (Courtesy B. Fyfe, MD.)* **(Right)** *Image from the same case shows mild proliferative and crescentic glomerulonephritis with deposits composed of polyclonal IgG, IgM and C3. (Courtesy B. Fyfe, MD.)*

Necrotizing Lupus Vasculitis Resembling MPA

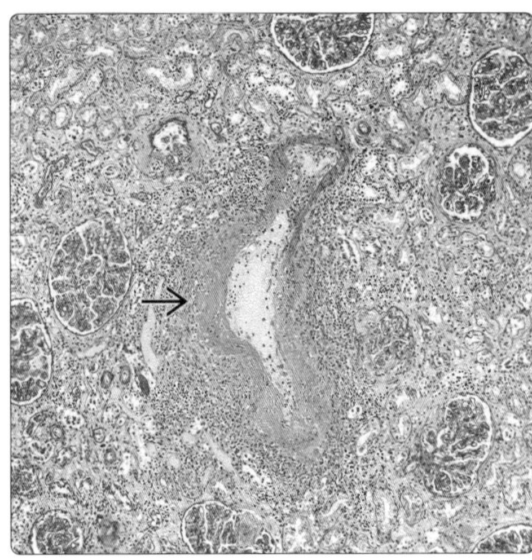

Cryoglobulinemic Vasculitis

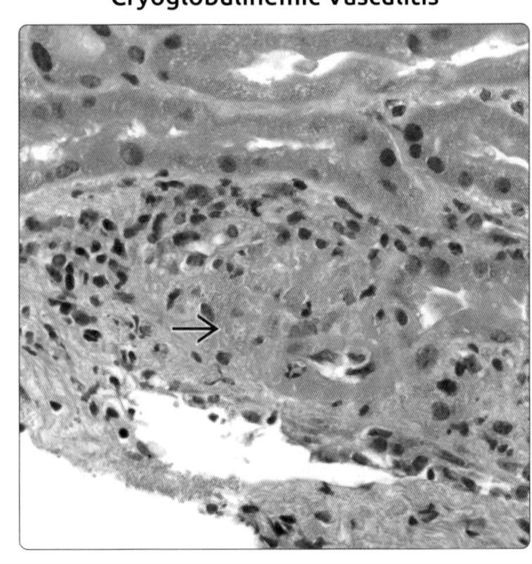

(Left) *Florid arteritis in an SLE patient is manifested by an interlobular artery with transmural fibrinoid necrosis* ⇒ *and inflammatory infiltrate of neutrophils and lymphocytes. (Courtesy B. Fyfe, MD.)* **(Right)** *SVV in mixed cryoglobulinemia with eosinophilic material resembles fibrin* ⇒ *composed of precipitated immune complexes of monoclonal IgM rheumatoid factor and IgG. In contrast to fibrin, these deposits are rounded, PAS(+), and stain for IgM and IgG.*

Cryoglobulinemic Vasculitis in HCV Patient

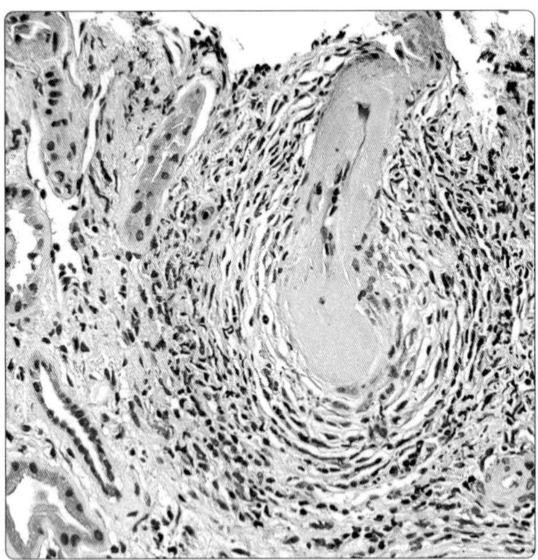

IF of Skin With IgM Cryoglobulin Deposits

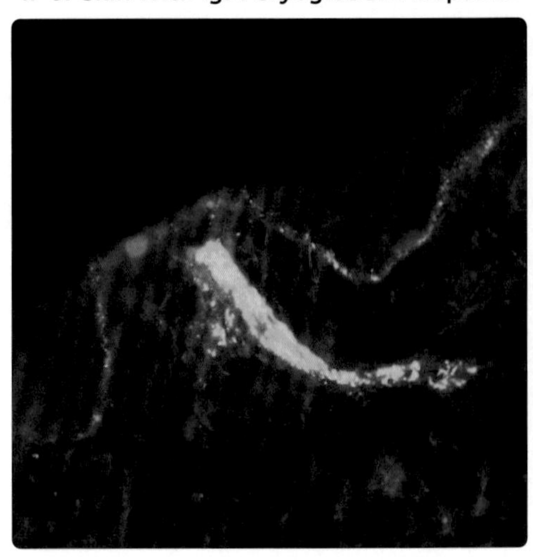

(Left) *Cryoglobulin-associated small vessel vasculitis typically has amorphous pale eosinophilic vascular cryoglobulin deposits. Here, they narrow the lumen in a kidney biopsy from a patient with HCV and cryoglobulinemic glomerulonephritis.* **(Right)** *Immunofluorescence microscopy of skin shows positive cryoglobulin deposits that stain for IgM within the dermal vessels. These deposits also stain for IgG and C3. The IgM is a monoclonal (kappa) rheumatoid factor.*

Skin Biopsy With IgA Leukocytoclastic Vasculitis

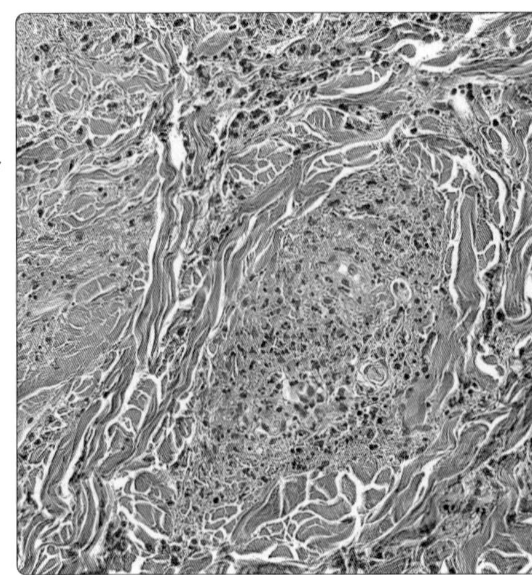

Skin Biopsy With IgA Vasculitis

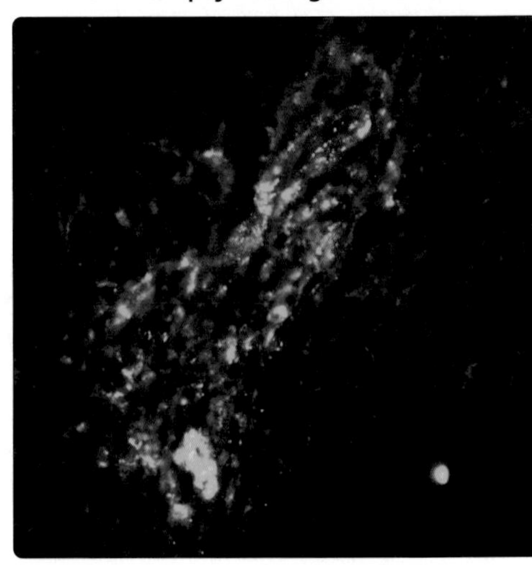

(Left) *Skin biopsy shows leukocytoclastic vasculitis and extravasation of red blood cells in a patient with Henoch-Schönlein purpura (HSP).* **(Right)** *Immunofluorescence of skin biopsy from a patient with Henoch-Schönlein purpura shows dominant granular staining for IgA in the vascular and perivascular areas enabling the diagnosis of HSP to be made.*

Intrarenal Arterial Atheroemboli

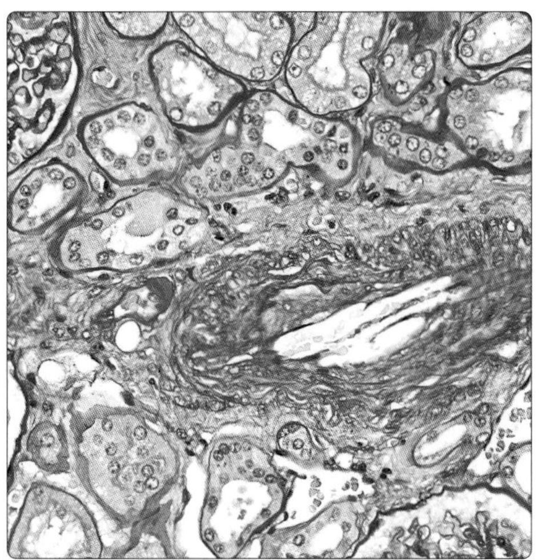

Glomerular Hilar Arteriole With Atheroemboli

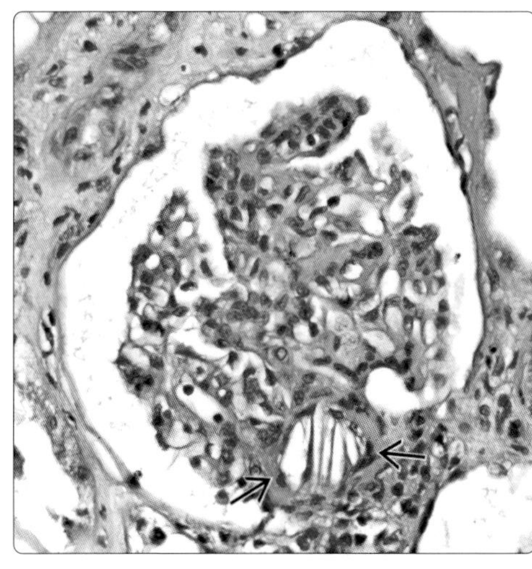

(Left) *A biopsy from an elderly patient presenting with acute renal failure, skin rash, and early gangrenous changes of digits in the foot shows atheroemboli within an interlobular artery characterized by needle-shaped spaces signifying cholesterol crystals washed off during processing of the tissue.* **(Right)** *A glomerulus shows needle-shaped atheroemboli ➔ within the hilar arteriole that led to mild to moderate ischemic collapse of the capillary tuft. (Courtesy L. Barisoni, MD.)*

Renal Arteriolar and Capillary Amyloid Deposits

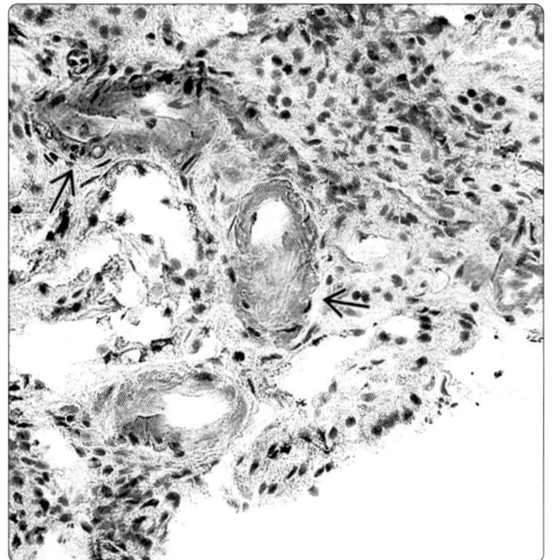

Phospholipid Antibody Syndrome With Microvascular Thrombi

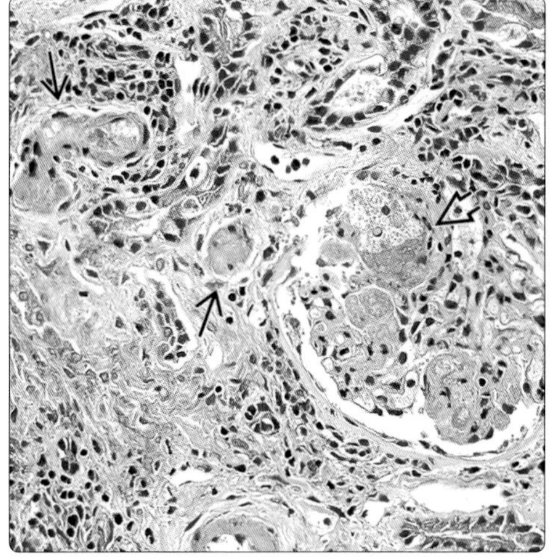

(Left) *Amyloid angiopathy is shown. Kidney biopsy from an older patient presenting with heart and liver disease and progressive renal failure with minimal proteinuria shows exclusively vascular and microvascular ➔ amyloid deposits by Congo red.* **(Right)** *A kidney biopsy from a patient with antiphospholipid antibody syndrome having livedo reticularis, stroke, and acute renal failure shows noninflammatory microvascular thrombi within the arterioles ➔ and glomerulus ➡.*

Thrombotic Microangiopathy in a Glomerulus

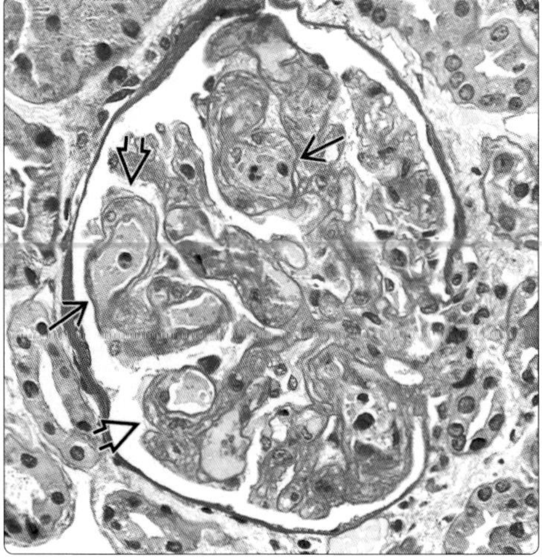

Renal Arteriole With Thrombotic Microangiopathy

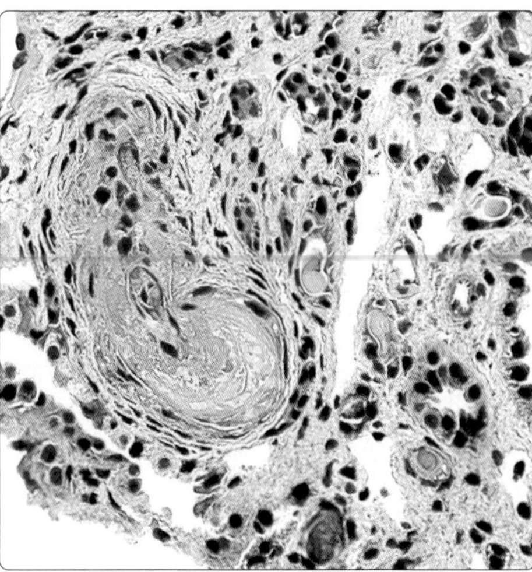

(Left) *Glomerulus in a patient with thrombotic thrombocytopenic purpura shows focal intracapillary microthrombi ➔ and thickening of the peripheral capillary wall with segmental double contours ➡.* **(Right)** *Renal biopsy from a patient with thrombotic thrombocytopenic purpura shows noninflammatory endothelial injury of an arteriole with detachment, subendothelial widening, and accumulation of a fibrin thrombus. Focal trapped fragmented RBCs are noted.*

ANCA-Related Glomerulonephritis

KEY FACTS

TERMINOLOGY

- Crescentic GN related to ANCA
- Can be renal-limited pauci-immune GN or with systemic vasculitis (GPA, MPA, EGPA)

ETIOLOGY/PATHOGENESIS

- Autoantibody to lysosomal components in neutrophils and monocytes
  - MPO (p-ANCA) and PR3 (c-ANCA)
  - Anti-LAMP2, plasminogen, Moesin antibodies
- ANCA activates neutrophils, injuring endothelium
- Classified as MPO-AAV and PR3-AAV and crescentic GN

CLINICAL ISSUES

- Rapidly progressive renal failure
  - Hematuria, proteinuria
- Systemic signs of vasculitis present in majority
- Poor prognostic factors: Higher creatinine level, proteinuria fewer normal glomeruli, higher chronic histologic indices
- ANCA testing: 80% sensitive and 96% specific for crescentic GN

MICROSCOPIC

- Focal, necrotizing glomerulonephritis with crescents
  - Renal vasculitis (5-35%), variable interstitial inflammation
- IF: Little or no immunoglobulin or complement deposits
- EM: Scant or no immune-complex type deposits

TOP DIFFERENTIAL DIAGNOSES

- ANCA-negative crescentic GN
- Anti-GBM disease
- Immune complex-mediated crescentic GN
- ANCA superimposed on other diseases

DIAGNOSTIC CHECKLIST

- Histopathologic classification correlates with outcome
  - Adverse risk factors: ≥ 50% global sclerosis, fibrous crescents, tubular atrophy/interstitial fibrosis

Diffuse, Necrotizing Crescentic Glomerulonephritis

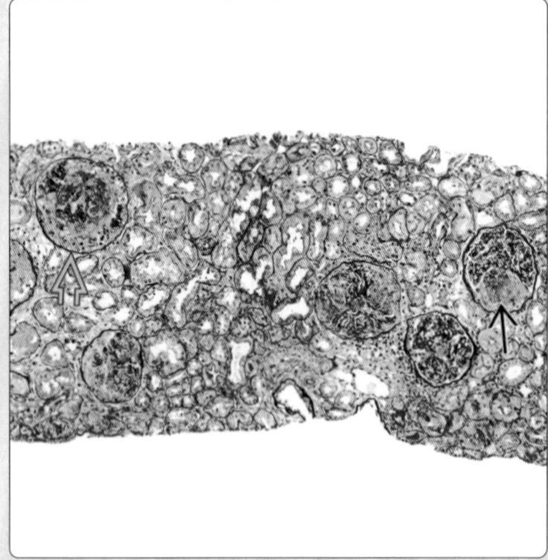

Glomerular Necrosis and Crescent

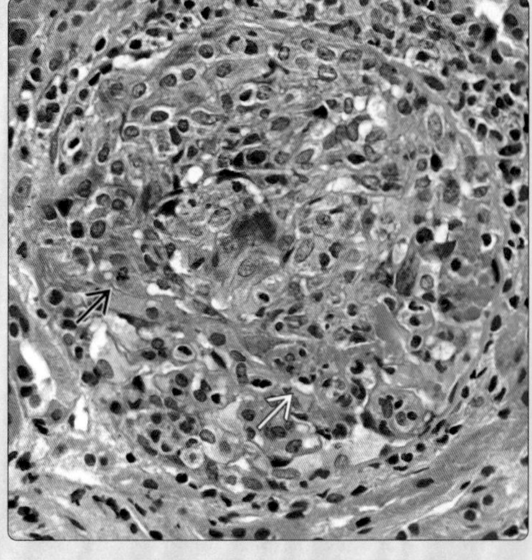

(Left) *ANCA-mediated glomerulonephritis shows segmental necrotizing lesions ⇒ along with segmental or circumferential ⇒ cellular crescents variably compressing the underlying glomerular capillary tuft.* **(Right)** *ANCA-related glomerulonephritis (GN) typically has focal necrosis and crescents. Here, the cellular crescent fills most of the Bowman capsule and contains a mitotic figure ⇒. Neutrophils ➡ and fibrin are present.*

Sparse IgG Deposits (Pauci-Immune)

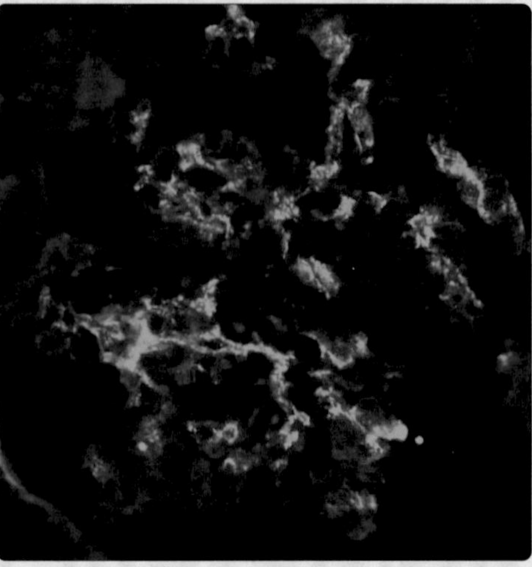

Medullary Capillaritis and Necrosis

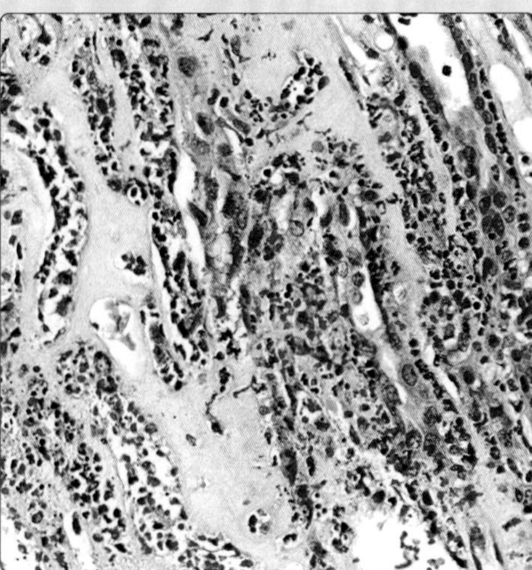

(Left) *Although ANCA-GN usually has little or no immunoglobulin, sometimes scattered immune complex deposits are noted, as seen in this case stained for IgG. In addition, 1+ or lower IgM, C3, and even IgA can be seen.* **(Right)** *Medullary capillaritis with neutrophils in an 84-year-old woman shows positive cANCA and an elevated Cr that rose from 2.7 to 4.0 over 2 weeks. Necrotizing glomerulonephritis with crescents was also present. This can mimic acute pyelonephritis. (Courtesy I. Rosales, MD.)*

TERMINOLOGY

Abbreviations

- Glomerulonephritis related to antineutrophil cytoplasmic antibodies (ANCA-GN)

Synonyms

- Pauci-immune glomerulonephritis (PIGN)
- Pauci-immune crescentic glomerulonephritis
- ANCA-associated vasculitis (AAV)

Definitions

- Glomerulonephritis related to or caused by ANCA, usually with prominent crescents and little or no immunoglobulin deposition (pauci-immune)
- May occur as isolated glomerular disease or part of systemic ANCA vasculitis syndrome
- History
  - Autoantibody to neutrophil cytoplasmic antigen(s) detected in segmental necrotizing GN (1982)
  - ANCA reported in granulomatosis with polyangiitis (GPA, Wegener) (1985)
  - Perinuclear antigen (p-ANCA) identified as anti-myeloperoxidase (MPO) in patients with pauci-immune necrotizing GN ± vasculitis (1988)
  - Cytoplasmic antigen (c-ANCA) identified as proteinase 3 (PR3) (1989)

ETIOLOGY/PATHOGENESIS

Autoimmune Disease

- Autoantibodies to neutrophil and monocyte lysosomal components
  - T cells also play role
- Trigger for ANCA production generally unknown
  - Presumed immune dysregulation (Th17/Treg)
  - Microbial factors and molecular mimicry
  - Can be precipitated by drugs
    - Propothiouracil, hydralazine, penicillamine, minocycline
- Suggested risk factors
  - Distinct HLA class II associations for MPO and PR3-ANCA
  - Leptin receptor gene (*LEPR*) polymorphism
  - CD226, leukocyte-endothelial adhesion molecule
  - Epigenetic control of MPO and PR3 expression, both neutrophil cytoplasmic enzymes

ANCA

- Mechanism of action
  - Autoantibodies react to either PR3 or MPO, constituents of lysosomal proteins in neutrophils and monocytes
    - Occur as anti-MPO or anti-PR3, but rarely both (~ 6%)
  - Action on neutrophil
    - ANCA-initiated signal transduction pathways for cell activation, FcR participation
    - Neutrophils activate alternative complement pathway
    - Leukocyte activation → adhesion to primed endothelial cells, resulting in subsequent damage
  - ANCA can be present without overt disease
    - Infection as trigger for neutrophil activation
- Measurement of ANCA titers useful in management
- May be other targets, since up to 20% of PIGN is ANCA(-)
  - Plasminogen antibodies in 25% of ANCA(+) patients
  - Lysosomal-associated membrane protein-2 (LAMP-2)
    - Anti-LAMP-2 reported in most patients with vasculitis
    - Less frequently noted with PIGN

Animal Models

- Adoptive transfer of anti-MPO antibodies precipitates crescentic GN and vasculitis in immunodeficient mice (RAG-1 knockout), proving ANCA pathogenic
  - Requires neutrophils as target
  - Enhanced by activation of alternate complement pathway
- No animal models with anti-PR3 antibodies yet developed that cause granulomatous inflammation
  - Additional cofactors may be necessary
- Transfer of GN and vasculitis to rats with anti-LAMP-2

Human Data

- Pregnant female with PIGN and positive ANCA titer delivered baby that developed acute renal failure and pulmonary hemorrhage
- 2 reports of ANCA(+) pregnant females with normal deliveries

CLINICAL ISSUES

Epidemiology

- Incidence
  - Crescentic GN occurs in 70-80% in GPA and PR3-ANCA
  - Nearly 100% in MPA and MPO-ANCA
  - ~ 60% of patients with crescentic GN (> 50% crescents) are ANCA(+)
  - ~ 60% of pulmonary-renal syndrome are ANCA(+)
- Age
  - Mean: ~ 60 years (increased incidence > 60 years)
  - Higher with MPA (> 60 years)
  - Lower with GPA (< 60 years)
  - Occasionally in children (as young as 2 years)
- Sex
  - No gender predilection
- Ethnicity
  - Geographic variation of anti-MPO and PR3-ANCA

Presentation

- Hematuria with cellular and RBC casts, proteinuria, usually nonnephrotic range associated with immune deposits
- Rapidly progressive renal failure
- Flu-like syndrome common at onset
  - Fever, arthralgia, myalgia
- Signs of extrarenal vasculitis in ~ 75%
  - Specific features lead to diagnosis of granulomatosis with polyangiitis, microscopic polyangiitis, or eosinophilic granulomatosis with polyangiitis

Laboratory Tests

- Positive ANCA test by indirect immunofluorescence plus ELISA
  - Sensitivity of 80% and specificity of 96% for PIGN
  - Negative ANCA in ~ 20% of PIGN
- Type of ANCA does not permit specific diagnosis
  - MPO ANCA most common in PIGN, MPA, and EGPA (50-60%)

- PR3 ANCA most common in GPA (~ 75%)
- Other ("atypical") ANCA specificities described
  - React with lactoferrin, elastase, and P-cathepsin-G
  - Found in variety of conditions with chronic inflammation or infection
- Negative ANCA associated with absence of disease activity
- Normal complement levels

Treatment

- Drugs
  - Cyclophosphamide and prednisolone to induce remission
  - Maintenance therapy with less toxic drugs such as mycophenolate mofetil, azathioprine
  - Plasmapheresis or plasma exchange in refractory cases
  - Rituximab (anti-CD20) for induction or relapses

Prognosis

- ~ 75% achieve remission
- ~ 30% relapse, frequently with PR3-ANCA
- 60-75% 5-year patient and kidney survival
  - Risk factors for early death and ESRD
    - Higher serum creatinine or dialysis dependence at onset
    - Female gender
    - Age > 65 years

Pathological Prognostic Features

- Number of normal glomeruli (strong predictor of renal function)
- Active glomerular necrosis and crescents, higher in GPA
- Degree of tubulitis and interstitial inflammation
- Tubular atrophy and interstitial fibrous
- Glomerulosclerosis higher in MPA &/or MPO-ANCA than in GPA &/or PR3-ANCA patients
- Sclerosis of crescents
- Arteriosclerosis
- Chronic damage indices higher in MPA

MACROSCOPIC

General Features

- Flea-bitten appearance due to blood in tubules and Bowman space

MICROSCOPIC

Histologic Features

- Glomeruli
  - Focal fibrinoid necrosis with neutrophils
    - GBM is disrupted in areas of necrosis
    - Segmental to global pattern of involvement
  - Crescents prominent, typically > 50% of glomeruli
    - Crescents contain proliferating parietal epithelial cells, neutrophils, and macrophages
    - Age of crescents (cellular, fibrocellular, fibrous)
  - Active necrosis and crescents, higher in GPA
  - Active periglomerular inflammation and rupture of Bowman capsule
  - Sometimes periglomerular granulomatous inflammation
  - Normal glomeruli usually present
- Tubules and interstitium
  - Varying degrees of active interstitial inflammation
    - Neutrophil, eosinophil, or plasma cell rich
  - Necrotizing medullary capillaritis
- Vessels
  - Renal vasculitis in 5-35%
    - Involves small arteries, arterioles, capillaries, venules
    - Leukocytoclastic vasculitis pattern (neutrophils, fibrinoid necrosis)
    - Fibrinoid necrotizing arteritis with neutrophils
    - Disruption of elastic lamina
    - Rarely transmural lymphocytic arteritis
    - Associated with elevated C-reactive protein
- Later stages
  - Global glomerulosclerosis and progressive interstitial fibrosis and tubular atrophy
  - Arterial vessels heal by sclerosis and narrowing of lumina

ANCILLARY TESTS

Immunofluorescence

- Pauci-immune glomerular pattern
  - Typically ≤ 1+ granular staining for IgG, IgM, IgA, C3, and C1q (60%)
  - Sclerotic lesions: Nonspecific IgM and C3
- If > 1+ Ig, consider immune complex GN as underlying cause with superimposed ANCA
  - Immune complex GN with granular mesangial/capillary wall immunoglobulin and complement staining (24%)
- If > 1+ linear staining of GBM, probably anti-GBM GN concurrent with ANCA-GN
  - Anti-GBM antibody GN with linear glomerular IgG (15%)
- Active crescents and fibrinoid necrosis stain for fibrin

Electron Microscopy

- Glomerular endothelial swelling, injury, and loss
- Neutrophils, fibrin in capillaries
- Disrupted GBM in necrotic segments associated with crescents
- Scant or no immune-complex deposits
  - May be scattered mesangial and even subepithelial deposits of uncertain significance

DIFFERENTIAL DIAGNOSIS

ANCA-Negative Crescentic GN

- 10-30% of pauci-immune crescentic GN
- Relatively younger groups
- Have fewer extrarenal symptoms hence delay in diagnosis
- More chronic glomerular and tubulointerstitial lesions

Anti-GBM Disease

- Bright, linear staining of GBM for IgG
- Vasculitis absent
- ~ 30-40% also positive for ANCA

Immune Complex-Mediated Crescentic GN

- ~ 30-40% of crescentic GN
- 2+ or greater of Ig and complement
  - Immune complex deposits in mesangium and GBM
- Some due to specific diseases such as lupus, cryoglobulinemia, IgA nephropathy, MPGN

Frequency of MPO-ANCA & PR3-ANCA by Clinicopathologic Syndromes

	Granulomatosis With Polyangiitis	Microscopic Polyangiitis	Eosinophilic Granulomatosis With Polyangiitis	Renal-Limited Crescentic GN
MPO-ANCA	20%	50%	40%	70%
PR3-ANCA	75%	40%	5%	20%
ANCA(-)	5%	10%	55%	10%

Adapted from Jennette JC et al: Pauci-immune and antineutrophil cytoplasmic autoantibody mediated crescentic glomerulonephritis and vasculitis. In Jennette JC et al: Heptinstall's Pathology of the Kidney. 7th ed. Philadelphia: Lippincott Williams & Wilkins. 686-713, 2015.

Comparison Between MPO-ANCA & PR3-ANCA Pauci-Immune Crescentic GN

	MPO-ANCA	PR3-ANCA
Extrarenal disease	Lower	Higher
Glomerular lesion	Diffuse	Focal
Chronic renal parenchymal change	Higher	Lower
Intrarenal granulomata	5.5% of cases	2.7% of cases
Kidney survival at 5 years	60%	65%
Patient survival at 5 years	67%	75%
Normal glomeruli	Less	More
Immunofluorescence	More C3 deposition	Less C3 deposition
Genetic predisposition	HLA-DQ, CTLA-4	HLA-DPB1, PRTN3, HLA-DRB15

Adapted from Vizjak A et al: Am J Kidney Dis. 41(3):539-49, 2003, Hilhorst M et al: J Am Soc Nephrol 26: 2015.

IgA Vasculitis (Henoch-Schönlein)

- Prominent IgA in mesangium
- Mesangial hypercellularity
- Segmental or global endocapillary proliferation

Acute Postinfectious GN

- Prominent endocapillary hypercellularity
- Prominent granular IgG and C3 along GBM
- Numerous subepithelial "humps" by EM

ANCA Superimposed on Other Diseases

- MGN, IgA nephropathy, lupus nephritis may have crescents and necrosis due to superimposed ANCA-GN

DIAGNOSTIC CHECKLIST

Clinically Relevant Pathologic Features

- Pathological classification of ANCA-GN (Berden 2010)
  - Focal
    - > 50% normal glomeruli
    - Glomerular lesions in < 50%
    - Normal = no segmental sclerosis, synechiae, or extensive splitting of Bowman capsule, and > 1 layer of parietal epithelium
      - May have < 4 leukocytes/glomerulus, segmental GBM wrinkling, slight collapse of tuft
  - Crescentic
    - > 50% cellular or fibrocellular crescents
    - Crescents containing > 10% cellularity included
    - Fibrous crescents not counted
  - Mixed
    - Heterogeneous glomerular lesions, none predominating as > 50%
  - Sclerotic
    - > 50% global glomerulosclerosis
      - Defined as > 80% of capillary tuft
- Prognostic significance
  - 5-year renal survival
    - 93% focal
    - 76% crescentic
    - 61% mixed
    - 50% sclerotic

Pathologic Interpretation Pearls

- Extensive crescents and fibrinoid necrosis with scant immune deposits almost always due to ANCA
- Glomerular pathology does not discriminate various clinicopathologic conditions caused by ANCA (isolated PIGN, GPA, MPA, CSS)
- % normal glomeruli correlates with outcome at 5 years

SELECTED REFERENCES

1. Hilhorst M et al: Proteinase 3-ANCA vasculitis versus myeloperoxidase-ANCA vasculitis. J Am Soc Nephrol. ePub, 2015
2. Jennette JC et al: ANCAs are also antimonocyte cytoplasmic autoantibodies. Clin J Am Soc Nephrol. 10(1):4-6, 2015
3. Zhao L et al: M2 macrophage infiltrates in the early stages of ANCA-associated pauci-immune necrotizing GN. Clin J Am Soc Nephrol. 10(1):54-62, 2015
4. Ford SL et al: Histopathologic and clinical predictors of kidney outcomes in ANCA-associated vasculitis. Am J Kidney Dis. 63(2):227-35, 2014
5. Jennette JC et al: Pathogenesis of antineutrophil cytoplasmic autoantibody-mediated disease. Nat Rev Rheumatol. 10(8):463-73, 2014
6. Kallenberg CG: Key advances in the clinical approach to ANCA-associated vasculitis. Nat Rev Rheumatol. 10(8):484-93, 2014

(**Left**) *A case of GPA with PR3-ANCA shows pauci-immune segmental necrotizing glomerulonephritis with disruption of the capillary basement membranes by silver stain and fibrin deposits.* (**Right**) *Segmental destruction ⇒ of the glomerulus in ANCA-GN is seen here, with sparing of a portion on the left. Note the marked periglomerular inflammatory response ➡ associated with the segmental necrosis.*

Segmental, Fibrinoid Necrotizing Glomerulonephritis

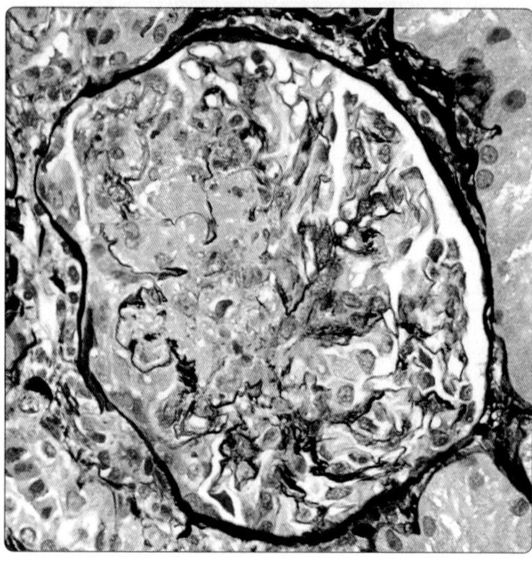

Segmental Glomerular Capillary Destruction

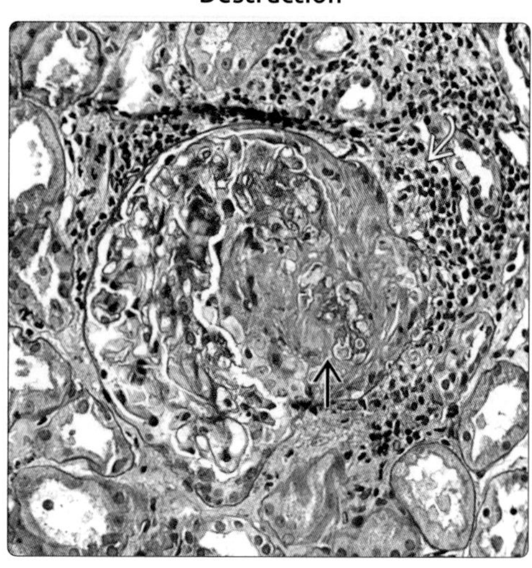

(**Left**) *Anti-MPO-related GN with destruction of the Bowman capsule is accompanied by a marked granulomatous reaction with multinucleated giant cells ⇒. Giant cells are also sometimes encountered in anti-GBM nephritis.* (**Right**) *A fibrocellular crescent in a patient with ANCA-GN is seen. A Bowman capsule disruption is evident in this PAS stain ⮐. The epithelium has attempted to "recanalize" ⇒ the crescent. In animal studies, it takes only a few weeks to reach this stage.*

Destruction of Bowman Capsule

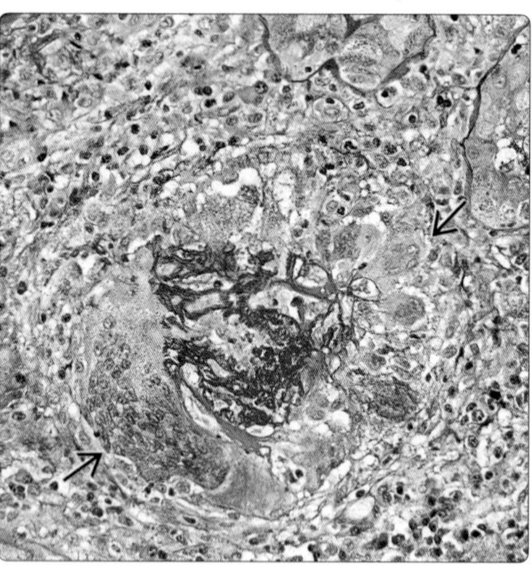

Fibrocellular Crescent

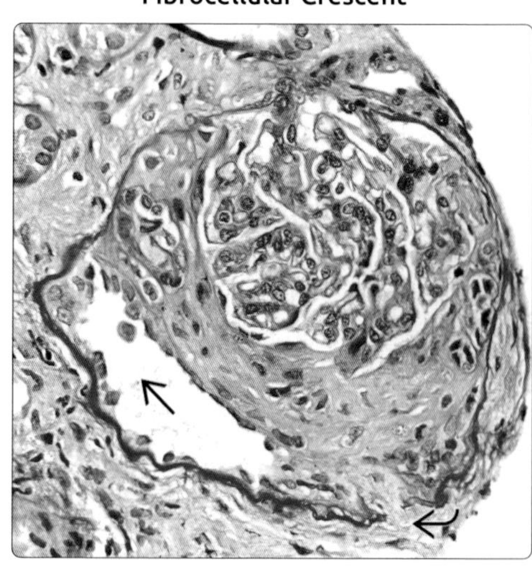

(**Left**) *A case of microscopic polyangiitis with high titer MPO-ANCA shows necrotizing vasculitis of an intralobular artery along with a large cellular crescent in the adjacent glomerulus with significant compression of the tuft.* (**Right**) *In the same patient, predominantly necrotizing arteriolitis are at the glomerular hilum leading to ischemic glomerular collapse. This is surrounded by active interstitial inflammation. This case shows necrotizing SVV in a small artery, arteriole, and glomerular capillaries.*

Necrotizing Arteritis and Crescentic GN

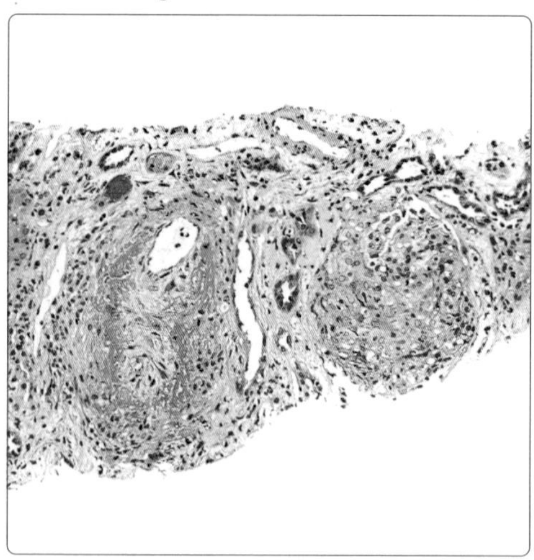

Necrotizing Arteriolitis

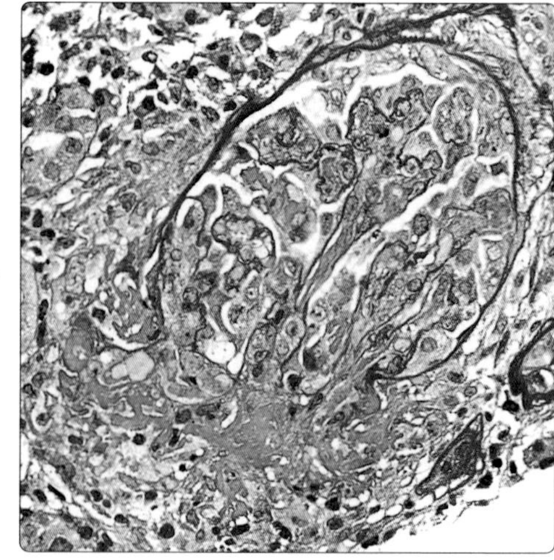

Fibrin in Crescent

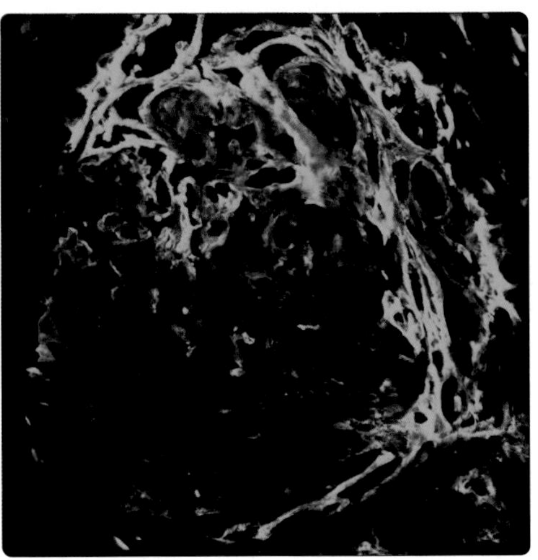

Sparse Electron-Dense Deposits

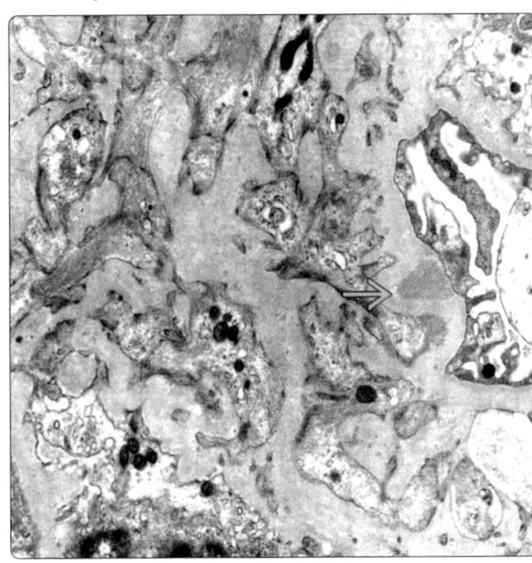

(Left) *Fibrin or fibrinogen is a characteristic feature of the active crescents in ANCA-GN, as shown here in a p-ANCA(+) case with isolated GN (no documented vasculitis).* **(Right)** *Just as sparse deposits can be seen by IF in ANCA disease, scattered electron-dense deposits can sometimes be seen by EM, as seen here in the subepithelial space ⇒. Their significance, if any, is unknown.*

Glomerular Crescent Rich in Macrophages

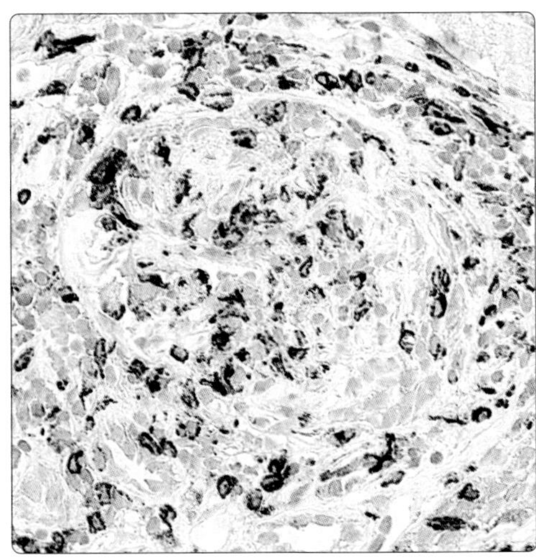

Parietal Epithelial Cells in Glomerular Crescent

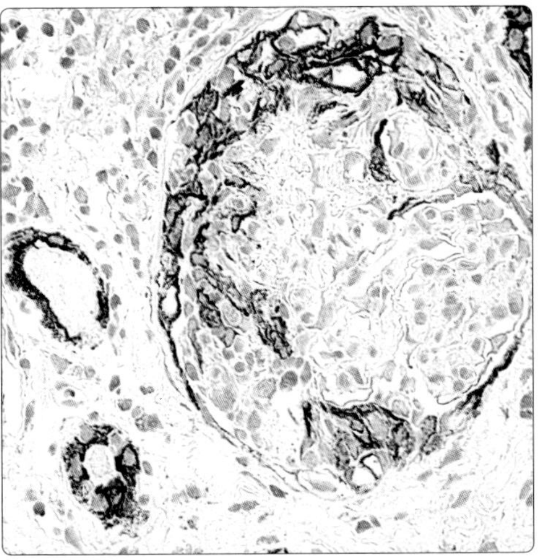

(Left) *A case of ANCA-associated crescentic glomerulonephritis shows significant CD68-positive macrophage infiltration (brown-stained cells) within the cellular crescent along with T lymphocytes (not shown here).* **(Right)** *A case of ANCA-associated crescentic glomerulonephritis shows participation of cytokeratin positive parietal epithelial cells mixed with inflammatory cells in the formation of the cellular crescent.*

Acute, Subacute, and Chronic Crescentic GN, ANCA(-)

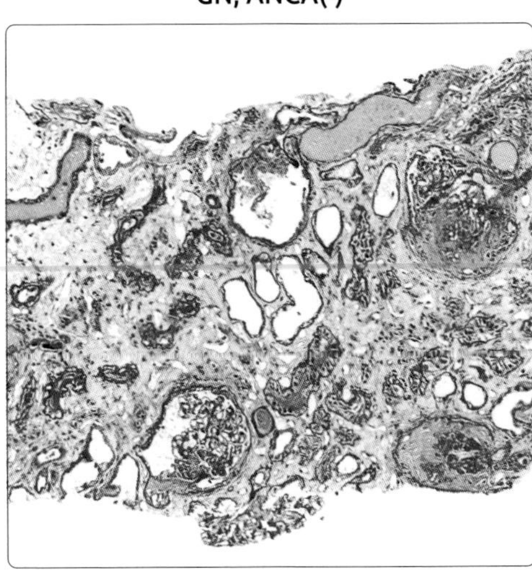

Segmental and Circumferential Cellular Crescents, ANCA(-)

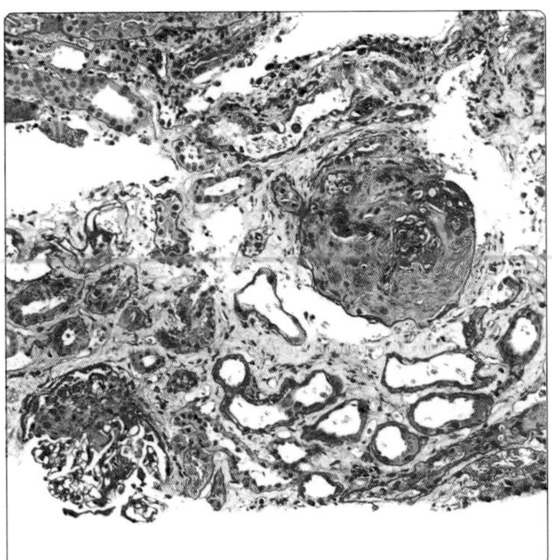

(Left) *A case of ANCA-negative, pauci-immune crescentic glomerulonephritis shows glomerular lesions of all stages as well as a normal glomerulus in the background of significant chronic tubulointerstitial disease.* **(Right)** *In the same patient, active necrosis and segmental and circumferential cellular crescents are shown. ANCA-negative GN occurs at a younger age with less systemic involvement and more chronic renal lesions.*

Microscopic Polyangiitis

KEY FACTS

TERMINOLOGY

- Necrotizing vasculitis, with few or no immune deposits, affecting small arteries (capillaries, venules, or arterioles)
- Necrotizing glomerulonephritis is common

ETIOLOGY/PATHOGENESIS

- ANCA-mediated small vessel vasculitis
  - p-ANCA/anti-myeloperoxidase positive (60%)
  - c-ANCA/anti-PR3 positive (15%)
  - Subset are ANCA(-) renal-limited necrotizing crescentic glomerulonephritis
- Cell-mediated immune mechanism
- Anti-hLAMP and moesin antibodies

CLINICAL ISSUES

- Renal (90-100%), lung (25-55%) involvement
  - Rapidly progressive or oliguric acute renal failure
  - Pulmonary hemorrhage
- Renal-limited vasculitis

MICROSCOPIC

- Crescentic glomerulonephritis with fibrinoid necrosis
- Vasculitis, small vessel
  - Not always present, even in multiple levels
  - Healed vascular lesions show loss of elastic lamina
- Active tubulointerstitial inflammation
- No significant granulomatous inflammation
- IF: Fibrin in crescents but little or no IgG, IgA, or IgM
  - Linear IgG in GBM indicates concurrent anti-GBM disease
- Small vessel vasculitis and capillaritis may be seen in skin, lung, and other organs
- Concomitant thrombotic microangiopathy confers poor prognosis

TOP DIFFERENTIAL DIAGNOSES

- Granulomatosis with polyangiitis and eosinophilic granulomatosis with polyangiitis
- Immune complex-mediated glomerulonephritis
- Anti-GBM disease

(Left) *Medium magnification shows several glomeruli with different stages of healing of crescents. Cellular and fibrocellular crescents → and fibrous crescents ⇨ are present.* **(Right)** *Two glomeruli show segmental pauci-immune-type glomerulonephritis with small cellular crescents ↷ in the Bowman space. The remaining portions of the glomeruli are unremarkable.*

Crescents

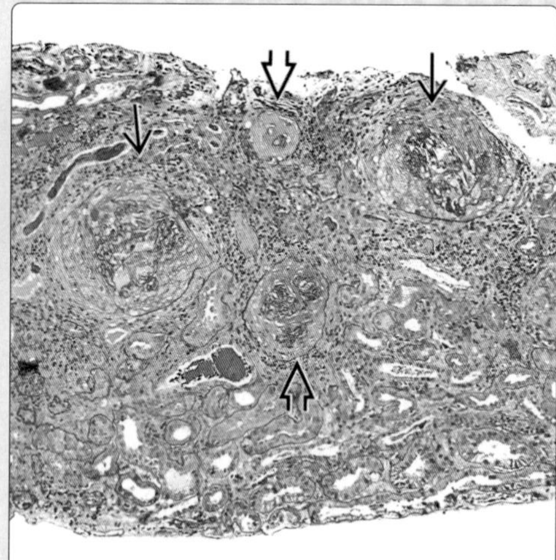

Segmental Crescents

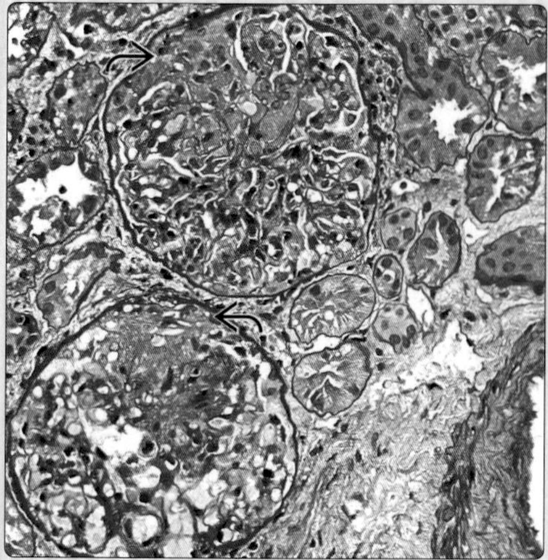

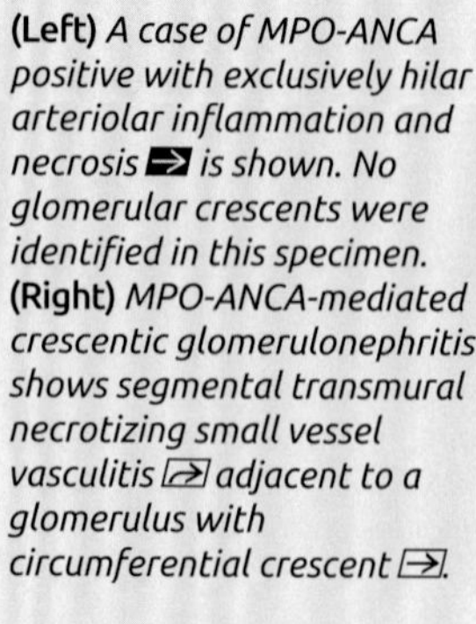

(Left) *A case of MPO-ANCA positive with exclusively hilar arteriolar inflammation and necrosis ➡ is shown. No glomerular crescents were identified in this specimen.* **(Right)** *MPO-ANCA-mediated crescentic glomerulonephritis shows segmental transmural necrotizing small vessel vasculitis ↷ adjacent to a glomerulus with circumferential crescent →.*

Destruction of Hilar Vessels

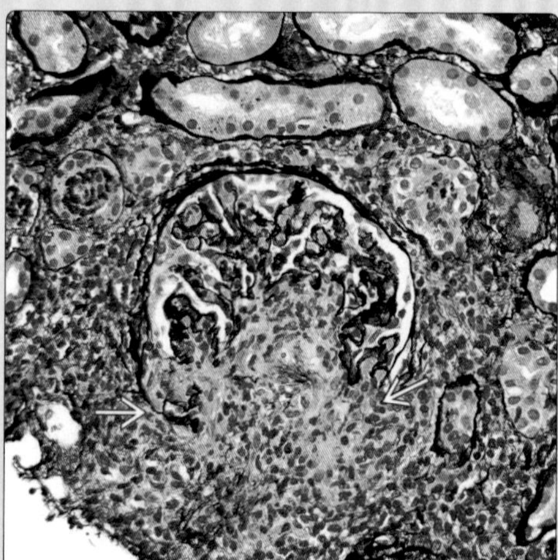

Transmural Necrotizing Arteritis

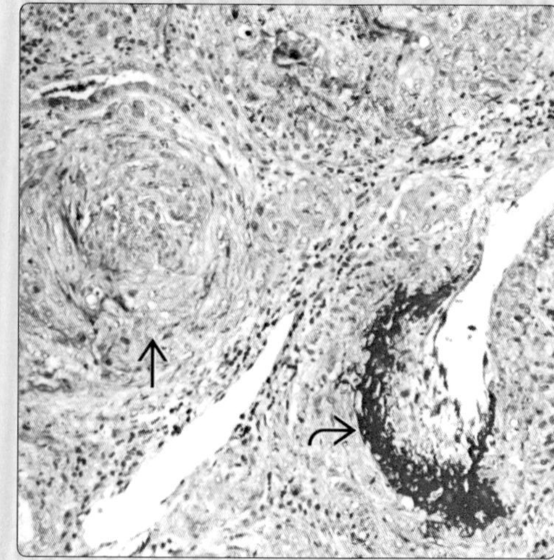

TERMINOLOGY

Abbreviations

- Microscopic polyangiitis (MPA)

Synonyms

- Microscopic polyarteritis
- p-ANCA/MPO-ANCA-mediated small vessel vasculitis
- Systemic or renal limited crescentic glomerulonephritis

Definitions

- Chapel Hill Consensus Conference 2012
  - Necrotizing vasculitis, with few or no immune deposits, predominantly affecting small vessels (i.e., capillaries, venules, or arterioles)
  - Necrotizing arteritis involving small and medium-sized arteries may be present
  - Necrotizing glomerulonephritis is very common
  - Pulmonary capillaritis often occurs

ETIOLOGY/PATHOGENESIS

Environmental Exposure

- Higher rate of onset in winter than summer
- Silica exposure-associated ANCA vasculitis

Pathogenesis

- Anti-neutrophil cytoplasmic antibody (ANCA)-mediated small vessel vasculitis
  - Mainly autoantibodies to myeloperoxidase (p-ANCA)
  - Minority have autoantibodies to proteinase 3 (c-ANCA)
  - Autoantibodies to human lysosome-associated membrane protein-2 (90% of ANCA vasculitis)
  - Subset of MPO-ANCA small vessel vasculitis is renal-limited necrotizing crescentic glomerulonephritis
  - Subset are ANCA-negative renal-limited necrotizing crescentic glomerulonephritis
- Cell-mediated immune mechanism with T-lymphocytes, neutrophils, and histiocytes are necessary for development of crescentic glomerulonephritis
  - Abnormal formation and disordered regulation of neutrophil extracellular traps (NET)
  - ANCA-activated neutrophils tend to adhere to activated microvascular endothelium to initiate injury
  - Alternate pathway of complement initiates and enhances endothelial injury and vasculitis
  - Inflammatory response enhanced by anti-moesin antibodies by stimulating cytokine production

CLINICAL ISSUES

Epidemiology

- Incidence
  - Varies with geographic locations
    - 1-8/1 million in Europe and United States
    - 10-24/1 million in Asian and Arab countries
- Age
  - All ages affected
  - Average age at onset is 50 years, older in Japan
- Ethnicity
  - Geographic variations may be related to ethnic background

Presentation

- General
  - Pulmonary renal syndrome
  - Constitutional symptoms (up to 75%)
    - Fever, weakness, weight loss
    - Arthralgias, myalgias (25-50%)
    - Hypertension
- Renal (90-100%)
  - Hematuria
  - Proteinuria
  - Renal insufficiency
  - Rapidly progressive or oliguric acute renal failure
- Skin
  - Purpuric rash, palpable (45%)
- Lung (25-55%), higher in Japan
  - Hemoptysis
  - Dyspnea
  - Pulmonary hemorrhage
  - Lung infiltrates
- Gastrointestinal (50%)
  - Abdominal pain
    - Severe form with bowel perforation
  - Hepatomegaly
- Neurologic (30%)
  - Peripheral neuropathy less frequent than PAN
  - Central nervous system
- Ear, nose, throat (30-35%)
  - Mouth ulcers, epistaxis, sinusitis

Laboratory Tests

- p-ANCA/anti-myeloperoxidase positive (60%)
- c-ANCA/anti-PR3 positive (15%)
- Elevated BUN and serum creatinine
- Urinalysis
  - Red cells and RBC casts
  - Varying degrees of proteinuria
- Anemia (normochromic normocytic)
- Leukocytosis and thrombocytosis
- Elevation of acute phase proteins: ESR, CRP
- Rheumatoid factor (39-50%)
- Antinuclear antibodies (21-33%)

Treatment

- Remission induction, remission maintenance, and relapse treatment are 3 phases of therapy
- Corticosteroids combined with cyclophosphamide is most common induction protocol
- Other forms of immunosuppressive therapy in refractory cases (10%)
- Oral cyclophosphamide, mycophenolate mofetil, or azathioprine used for remission maintenance

Prognosis

- Severe form of glomerular disease with aggressive course
- 1-year mortality rate of untreated cases: 80%
- Early deaths are usually due to fulminant renal disease and lung hemorrhage in MPA
- Frequent relapses occur (25-35%)
  - Different or new organs may be involved during relapses
  - Often associated with rash and arthralgias

- Generally less severe
- Induction protocol
  - Improvement in > 90% of patients
  - Complete remission in > 75%
- Independent factors that correlate with worse prognosis are older age, higher initial serum creatinine, and pulmonary hemorrhage
- Pathologic parameters representative of recovery of renal function include percentage of normal glomeruli at initial biopsy, fewer glomerular crescents, and interstitial inflammation
  - Concomitant overlap with polyarteritis nodosa (PAN)
  - Concomitant renal thrombotic microangiopathy
  - High chronicity index determines poor prognosis

MACROSCOPIC

General Features

- Normal or mildly increased kidney size
- Infarcts when present are small
- Petechial hemorrhages
  - Focal or diffuse
  - Represent glomerular necrosis; hemorrhage in Bowman space or within tubular lumina

MICROSCOPIC

Histologic Features

- Glomeruli
  - Pauci-immune crescentic glomerulonephritis
    - Segmental or, rarely, global glomerular necrosis (80-100%)
    - Disruption of glomerular basement membranes with accumulation of eosinophilic/fuchsinophilic fibrinoid
    - Majority of glomeruli have crescents (average: 45-55%), which frequently accompany necrosis
    - Segmental to extensive lysis of Bowman capsule in severe necrotizing glomerular lesions
    - Sometimes mild to moderate endocapillary hypercellularity with neutrophils and macrophages
  - Active periglomerular inflammation of varying intensity
    - Periglomerular granulomatous reaction is unlike that seen in granulomatosis with polyangiitis (Wegener)
  - Subacute or chronic glomerular lesions display fibrocellular or fibrous crescents
    - Segmental and global glomerular necrosis heals by sclerosis
    - Sclerosing glomerular changes are accompanied by tubular atrophy and interstitial fibrosis
- Tubules and interstitium
  - Active disease often associated with acute tubulointerstitial inflammation
  - Rare isolated tubulointerstitial inflammation is noted without glomerular lesions in kidney biopsy
  - No significant granulomatous inflammation is noted
- Renal and extrarenal vessels
  - Interlobular arteries, smaller arteries, arterioles, capillaries, and venules are affected
    - Segmental or circumferential fibrinoid necrosis
    - Palisading mild to intense active inflammatory reaction around necrotic areas
    - Inflammatory cells include neutrophils, activated lymphocytes, and variable eosinophils
    - Focal renal medullary capillaritis with fibrinoid necrosis
  - Healed vascular lesions show intimal thickening, narrowing of lumen, and variable loss of elastic lamina
  - Small vessel vasculitis and capillaritis may be seen in skin, lung, and other organs
    - Intrarenal small vessel vasculitis often not observed in renal biopsies

ANCILLARY TESTS

Immunofluorescence

- Necrotizing lesions and active crescents stain for fibrinogen
- Pauci-immune glomerular lesions with minimal or no deposits
  - Low-intensity staining of < 1-2+ may be observed for immunoglobulins and complement components
- Intense global, linear IgG staining along GBM indicates concurrent anti-GBM disease

Electron Microscopy

- Earliest change seen in glomeruli is endothelial swelling and widened subendothelial areas
- Later endothelial detachment from basement membranes and microthrombi formation with fibrin tactoids
- On occasion, rare small deposits are noted

DIFFERENTIAL DIAGNOSIS

Granulomatosis With Polyangiitis (GPA) and Eosinophilic Granulomatosis With Polyangiitis (EGPA)

- Renal histopathological changes are similar to those seen in granulomatosis with polyangiitis (Wegener) (GPA) (i.e., pauci-immune crescentic glomerulonephritis)
- Granulomatous inflammation (GPA), asthma, and eosinophilia (EGPA) are useful if seen

Immune Complex-Mediated Glomerulonephritis With Crescents &/or Small Vessel Vasculitis

- Clinical features, appropriate serology, and immunohistochemistry useful for differentiation

Anti-Glomerular Basement Membrane Antibody Disease (Goodpasture)

- Need serology, immunofluorescence for differentiation

SELECTED REFERENCES

1. Chen SF et al: Clinicopathologic characteristics and outcomes of renal thrombotic microangiopathy in anti-neutrophil cytoplasmic autoantibody-associated glomerulonephritis. Clin J Am Soc Nephrol. 10(5):750-8, 2015
2. Carney EF: Vasculitis: Potential role of an anti-moesin autoantibody in MPO-AAV. Nat Rev Nephrol. 10(2):65, 2014
3. Endo A et al: Significance of small renal artery lesions in patients with antineutrophil cytoplasmic antibody-associated glomerulonephritis. J Rheumatol. 41(6):1140-6, 2014
4. Furuta S et al: Comparison of phenotype and outcome in microscopic polyangiitis between Europe and Japan. J Rheumatol. 41(2):325-33, 2014
5. Kallenberg CG: The diagnosis and classification of microscopic polyangiitis. J Autoimmun. 48-49:90-3, 2014
6. Sun L et al: Clinical and pathological features of microscopic polyangiitis in 20 children. J Rheumatol. 41(8):1712-9, 2014
7. Suzuki K et al: A novel autoantibody against moesin in the serum of patients with MPO-ANCA-associated vasculitis. Nephrol Dial Transplant. 29(6):1168-77, 2014

Small Vessel Vasculitides (Pauci-Immune Types)

	MPA	GPA	EGPA
Clinical features	Multisystemic	Multisystemic	Multisystemic, associated with asthma or allergy
Serology	ANCA(+) (90%), mainly anti-MPO(+) (50%), PR3(+) (40%)	ANCA(+) (95%), mainly anti-PR3(+) (75%), anti-MPO(+) (20%)	ANCA(+) (50%), mostly anti-MPO(+) (60%)
Organs affected	Thoracic and abdominal viscera, skin, infrequently cerebral vessels	Upper and lower respiratory tract, abdominal viscera, kidney, heart, skin	Upper and lower respiratory tract, kidney, and rarely heart, skin, and brain
Size of vessel involved	Small arteries, arterioles, capillaries	Small arteries and veins, arterioles, capillaries, and venules	Small arteries, veins, arterioles, and rarely capillaries
Pathology of vasculitis	Necrotizing type, polymorphous inflammatory infiltrate and some eosinophils	Necrotizing or granulomatous type, polymorphous inflammatory infiltrate, mild eosinophils	Necrotizing or granulomatous type, eosinophil-rich, inflammatory infiltrate
Other vascular and nonvascular features	Renal limited form seen	Extravascular granulomatous inflammation with "geographic" pattern	Extravascular necrotizing granulomatous inflammation with prominent eosinophils
Glomerular pathology	Acute and chronic forms of crescentic glomerulonephritis and vasculitis, pauci-immune type	Acute and chronic crescentic glomerulonephritis, pauci-immune type	Less frequent crescentic glomerulonephritis, pauci-immune type
Relapse	++	+++	-/+

MPA = microscopic polyangiitis; GPA = granulomatosis with polyangiitis (Wegener); CSS = Churg-Strauss syndrome.

Comparison of Anti-GBM and ANCA-Associated Diseases

Clinical	ANCA	aGBM + ANCA	aGBM
Age	63 ± 12.7	64 ± 8.7	52 ± 20.6
Gender	PR3 - M > F MPO - F > M	F ≈ M	Younger males, older females
Antecedent events	Possible infection	Unknown	Possible smoking, hydrocarbon exposure
Lung hemorrhage	++	+	+
Renal involvement	100%	90%	100%
Multisystemic disease	Yes	20-50%	0
Systemic vasculitis	Yes	10-15%	0
Serology	PR3 or MPO	PR3 or MPO+ aGBM	aGBM
Serum creatinine	+	++	+++
Active urine sediment	+	+	+
Pathology (Crescentic GN)			
Distribution	Focal/diffuse	90-100%	75-100%
Stage of crescents	Acute/subacute/chronic	Mostly acute, some chronic	All acute/1 stage
Severity of glomerular necrosis	Segmental	Segmental/global	Segmental/global
Periglomerular granulomatous inflammation	+	+	-
Prognosis			
Relapse	Frequent	+	Rare
1-year survival			
Renal	~ 50%	~ 10%	~ 40%
Patient	~ 85%	~ 55%	~ 75%

8. Wilke L et al: Microscopic polyangiitis: a large single-center series. J Clin Rheumatol. 20(4):179-82, 2014
9. Hendricks AR et al: Renal medullary angiitis: a case series from a single institution. Hum Pathol. 44(4):521-5, 2013
10. Jennette JC et al: 2012 revised International Chapel Hill Consensus Conference Nomenclature of Vasculitides. Arthritis Rheum. 65(1):1-11, 2013
11. Chen M et al: ANCA-negative pauci-immune crescentic glomerulonephritis. Nat Rev Nephrol. 5(6):313-8, 2009
12. Rutgers A et al: Coexistence of anti-glomerular basement membrane antibodies and myeloperoxidase-ANCAs in crescentic glomerulonephritis. Am J Kidney Dis. 46(2):253-62, 2005

(Left) *Glomerulus in a p-ANCA(+) patient shows early intraglomerular thrombosis or fibrinoid change* → *prior to a fully developed necrotizing lesion.* **(Right)** *Glomerulus shows partial necrosis of the capillary tuft with a cellular crescent and fuchsinophilic fibrinoid material.*

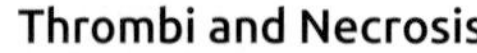

Thrombi and Necrosis

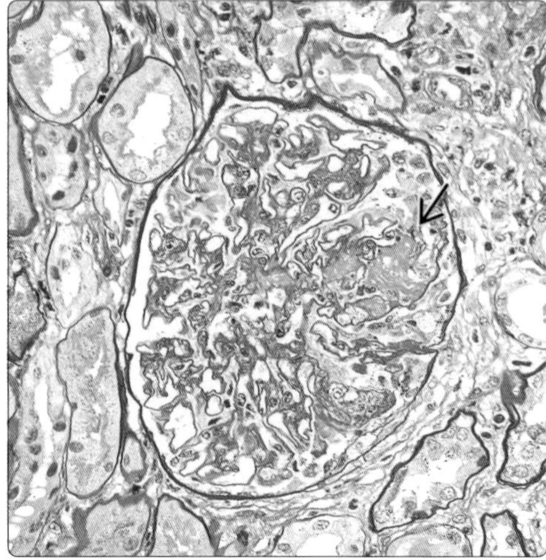

Glomerular Necrosis

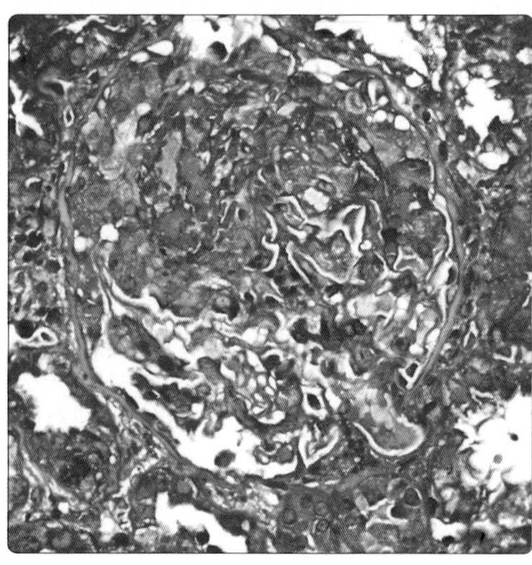

(Left) *Glomerulus shows segmental crescentic features with capillary necrosis and disruption of the basement membranes* →. **(Right)** *Scanning electron microscopy of glomerular capillary basement membrane from a patient with ANCA-mediated crescentic glomerulonephritis shows a frayed and fenestrated appearance, i.e., the GBM is broken, allowing crescent formation.*

Disruption of GBM

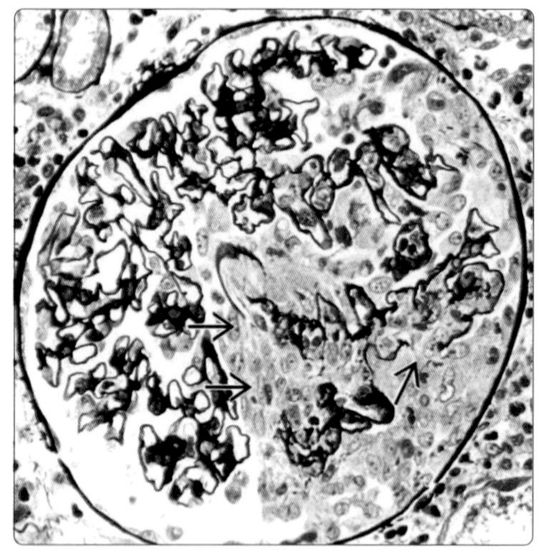

Scanning EM of GBM

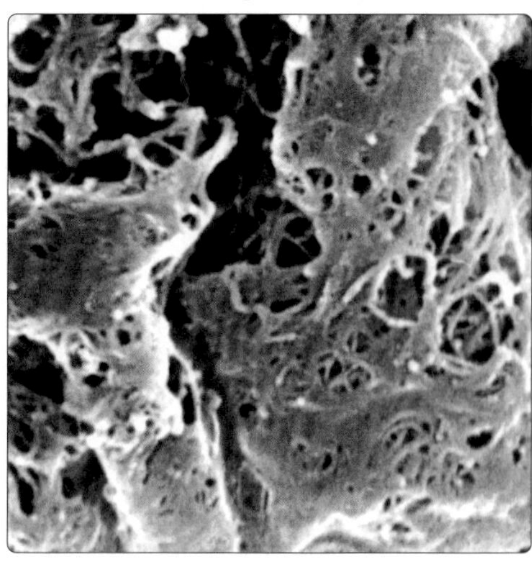

(Left) *Crescentic glomerulonephritis with strong staining for fibrinogen is shown within the crescent in the Bowman space. Fibrin is characteristically present in active crescents, regardless of cause.* **(Right)** *Pauci-immune crescentic glomerulonephritis typically has little or no immunoglobulin deposits in the glomeruli. Illustrated here is a minor degree of segmental positive IgG staining in the glomerulus, compatible with the diagnosis.*

Crescent With Fibrin

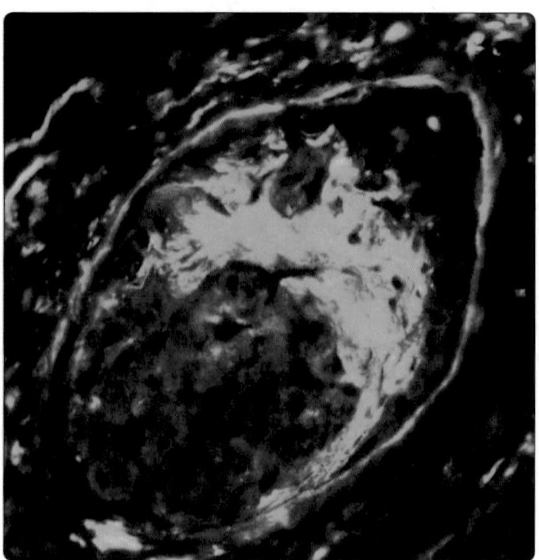

Scant IgG

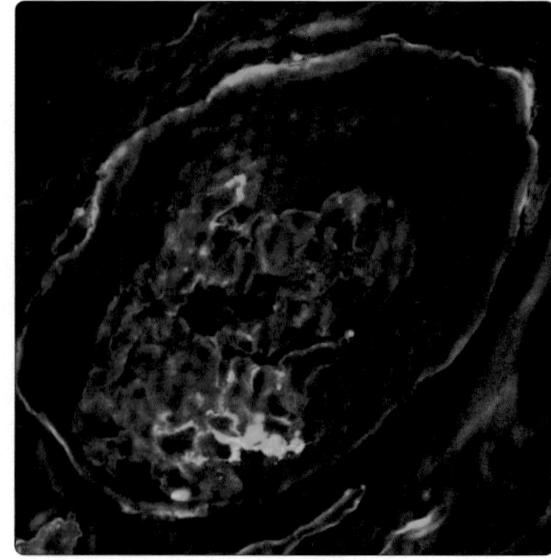

Disruption of Arterial Wall

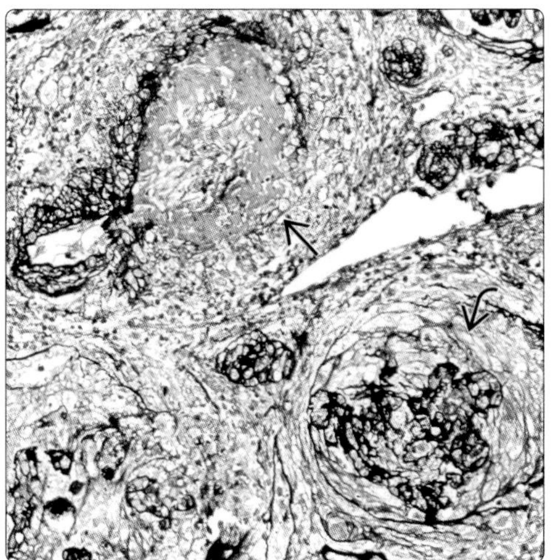

Necrotizing Arteritis and Crescent

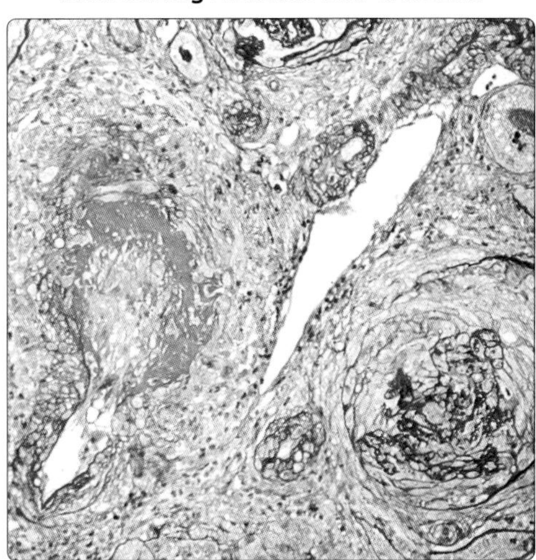

(Left) *An artery with necrotizing arteritis shows disruption of silver positive elastic lamina ➔ in the area of necrosis. A nearby glomerulus has a fibrocellular crescent ➔.* **(Right)** *Crescentic glomerulonephritis accompanied by necrotizing arteritis in a segmental distribution is shown.*

Granulomatous Change in Glomerulus

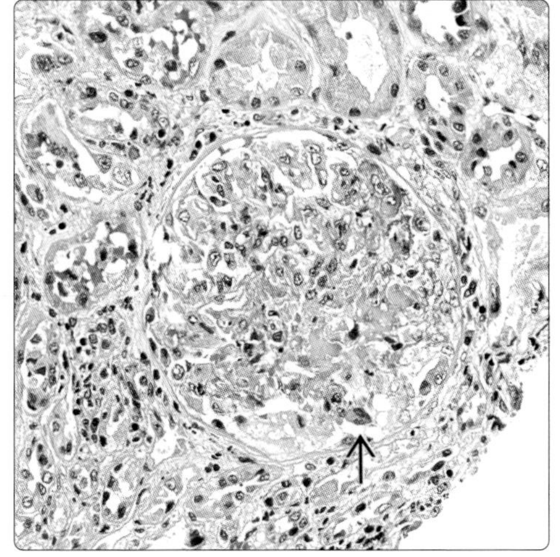

Sparse Electron-Dense Deposits

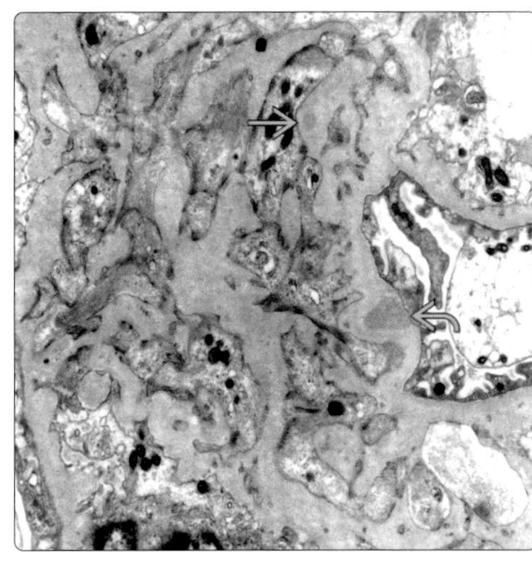

(Left) *Glomerulus with segmental fibrinoid necrotizing lesion shows occasional large cells and 1 multinucleated giant cell ➔. Granulomatous changes in crescentic glomerulonephritis are not unusual.* **(Right)** *In polyangiitis associated with ANCA, occasional mesangial ➔ and subepithelial ➔ deposits of uncertain significance can be seen. This does not change the diagnosis. The GBM may also show areas of disruption in glomeruli with crescents.*

Medullary Capillaritis

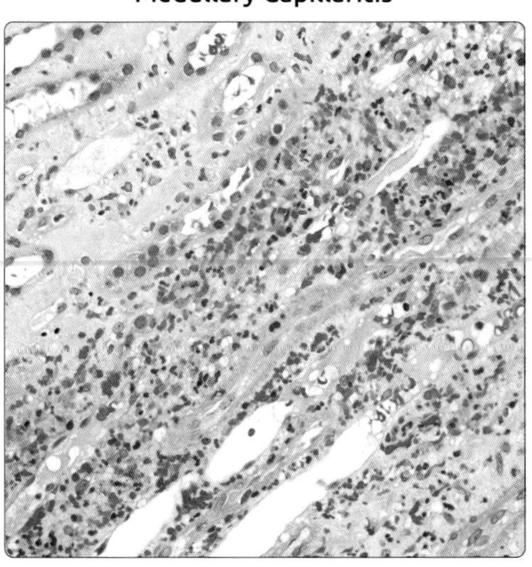

Arteriolitis

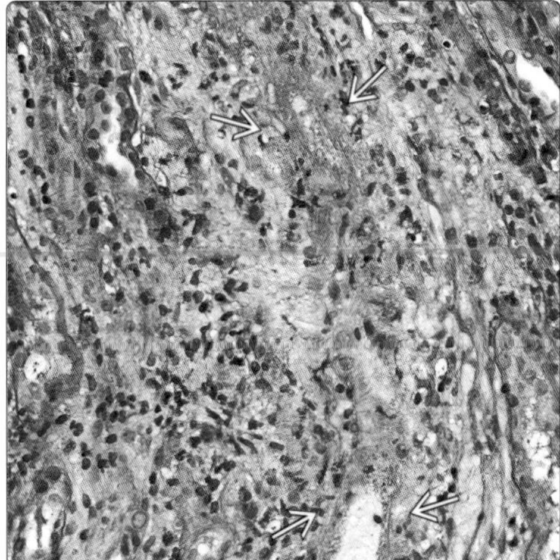

(Left) *A case of MPO-ANCA-mediated focal crescentic glomerulonephritis shows isolated patchy medullary capillaritis with mainly neutrophils and interstitial hemorrhage. (Courtesy B. Fyfe, MD.)* **(Right)** *MPO-ANCA-positive case shows predominantly glomerular hilar arteriolitis and medullary capillaritis with fibrinoid change ➔.*

(Left) *A case of ANCA-negative crescentic glomerulonephritis in a 52-year-old man shows segmental and circumferential cellular glomerular crescents with fibrinoid necrosis.* **(Right)** *Same case as the previous image shows a fibrocellular crescent partially compressing the glomerular capillary tuft.*

Crescents With Necrosis

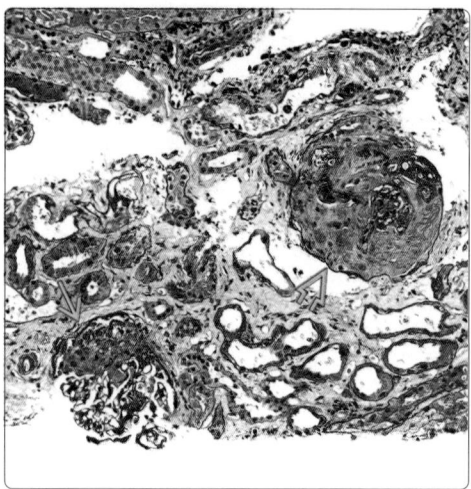

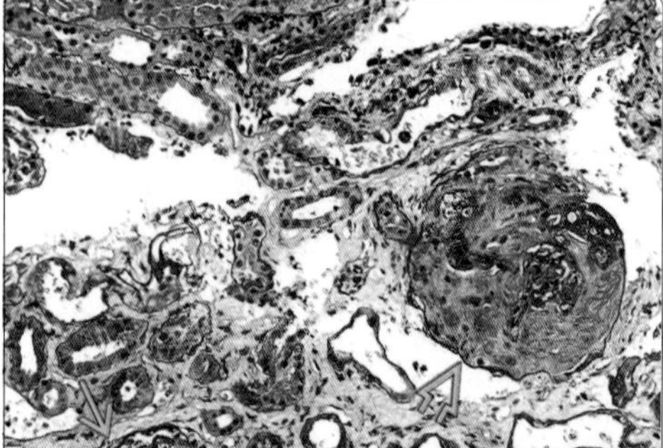

Fibrocellular Crescent

(Left) *A case of MPA with MPO-ANCA with microhematuria and proteinuria shows segmental sclerosing lesion with a small fibrous crescent and capsular adhesion.* **(Right)** *Glomerulus shows a circumferential fibrocellular crescent along with a pseudotubular space lined by epithelial cells within the Bowman space.*

Segmental Crescent

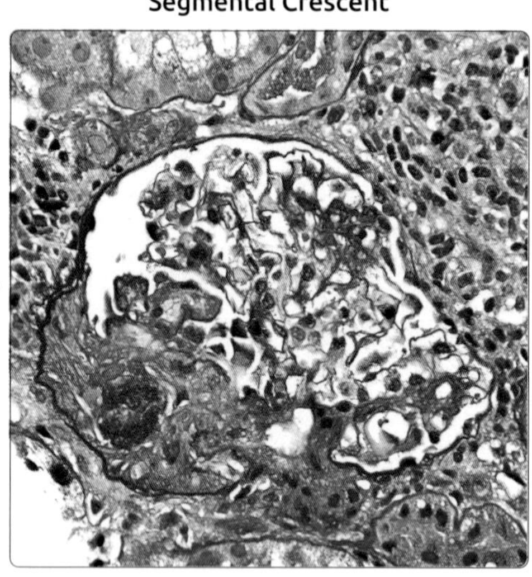

Circumferential Crescent

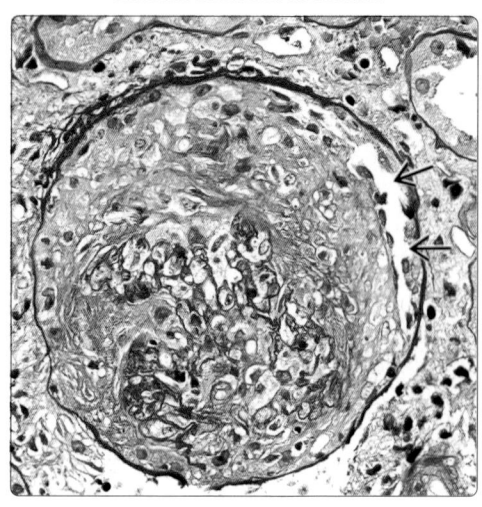

(Left) *Intrarenal small vessel necrotizing vasculitis is shown, with transmural and circumferential fibrinoid change accompanied by active inflammation. Intimal and medial layers are not visualized.* **(Right)** *Elastic stain from the autopsy kidney of a known case of fulminant polyangiitis shows a healed small artery with fibrointimal thickening, narrowing of the lumen, and almost complete disappearance of internal and external elastic lamina. An adjacent glomerulus is noted.*

Fibrinoid Necrosis

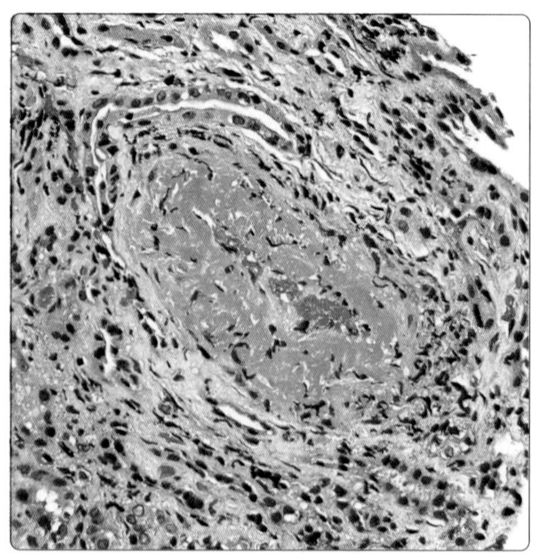

Disappearance of Internal Elastica

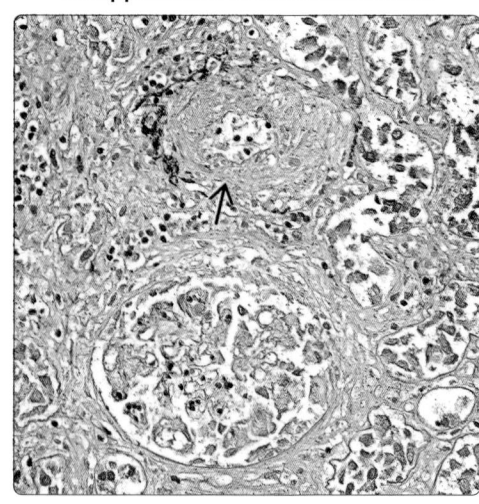

Underlying Diabetic Glomerulopathy

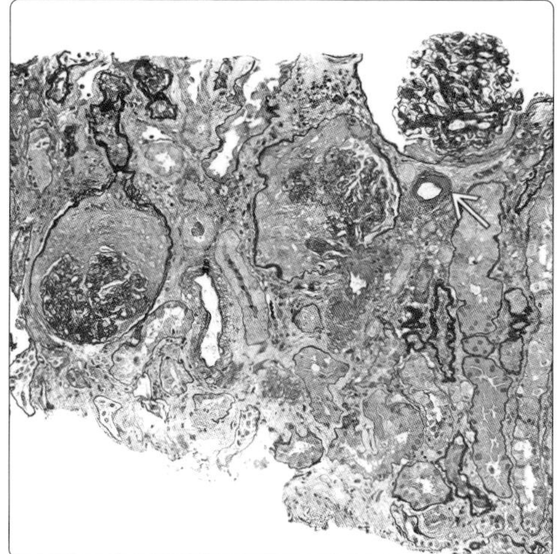

Membranous GN With ANCA-Related Crescents

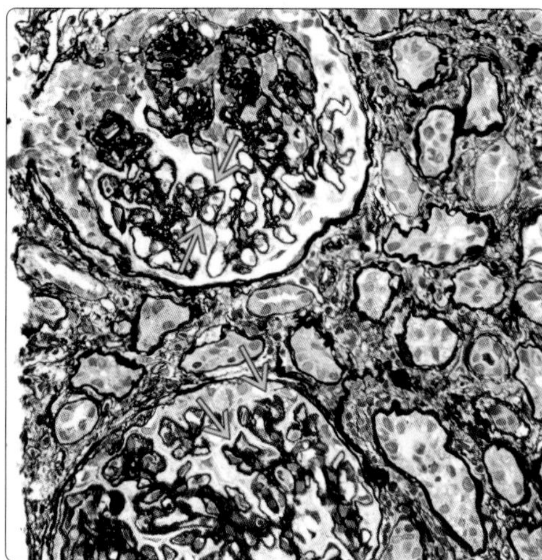

(Left) *Diabetic nephropathy with MPO-ANCA(+) serology superimposed by fibrocellular crescents overlying diabetic glomerular changes shows arteriolar hyalinosis ➡ & thickening of the tubular basement membranes.* **(Right)** *Idiopathic membranous glomerulonephritis stage III superimposed by MPO-ANCA crescentic disease is shown. The uninvolved glomerular capillary walls & portion of the glomerulus below show irregular thickening of the basement membranes ➡.*

Purpura

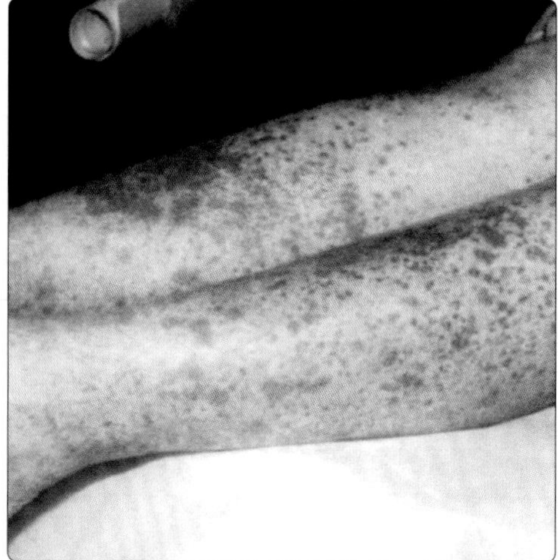

Dermal Vasculitis

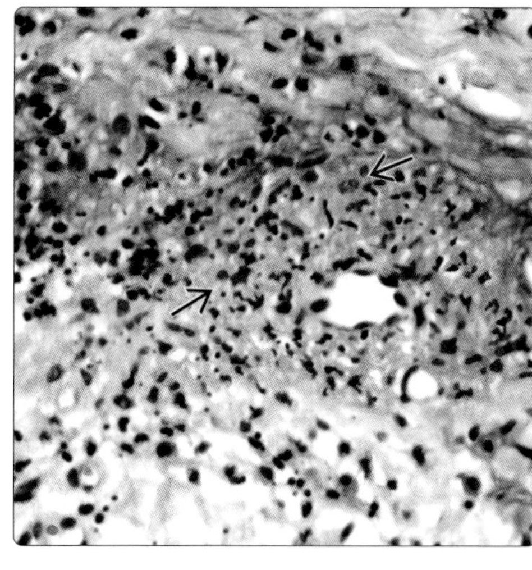

(Left) *Clinical photo shows purpuric rash in a patient with microscopic polyangiitis having multisystemic symptoms of lung hemorrhage and acute renal failure.* **(Right)** *Dermal capillaries show leukocytoclastic vasculitis ➡.*

Disruption of Bowman Capsule

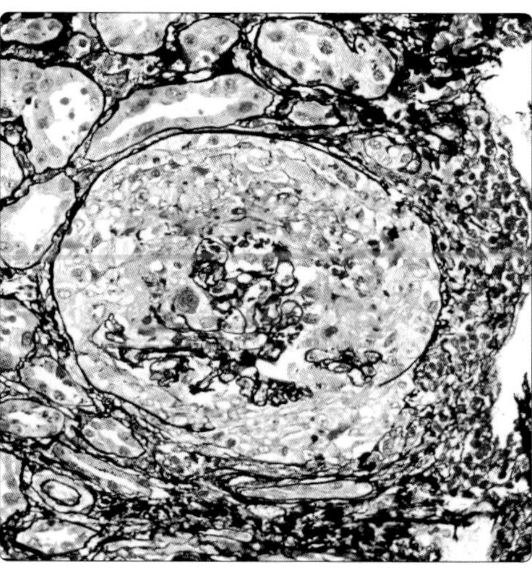

Linear IgG (Anti-GBM + ANCA)

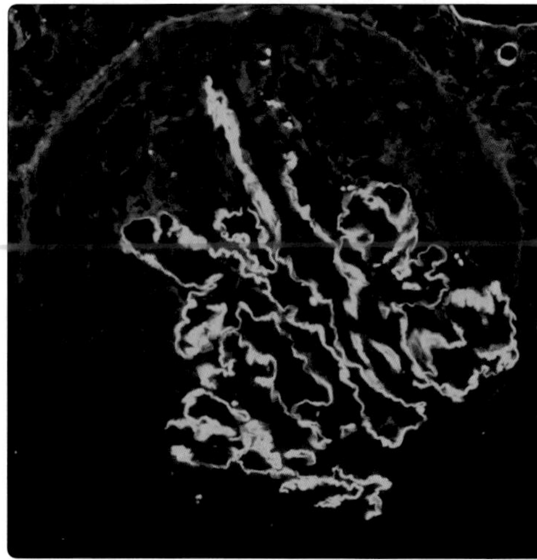

(Left) *Silver-stained glomerulus almost completely compressed by a large cellular crescent in the Bowman space is shown in a case dual positive for anti-GBM antibody and MPO-ANCA.* **(Right)** *Global, linear glomerular capillary basement membrane fluorescence for IgG is shown, partly compressed by a crescent in a patient with positive serology for ANCA-MPO and anti-GBM antibody.*

Granulomatosis With Polyangiitis (Wegener)

KEY FACTS

TERMINOLOGY

- Granulomatous inflammation of respiratory tract and necrotizing vasculitis of small to medium-sized vessels, commonly with necrotizing glomerulonephritis with little or no immune deposits (pauci-immune)

ETIOLOGY/PATHOGENESIS

- Primary role of antineutrophil cytoplasmic antibodies (ANCA)
  - ~ 75% anti-PR3 antibodies, ~ 25% MPO

CLINICAL ISSUES

- Peak age at onset: 50-70 years
- Kidney, upper airway, and lung involvement in 90% of cases
- Acute or rapidly progressive renal failure
- Steroids combined with cyclophosphamide; rituximab beneficial in relapses
- Poor prognostic factors: High initial Cr, lung disease, frequent relapses

MICROSCOPIC

- Glomeruli: Fibrinoid necrosis, crescents, periglomerular inflammation due to disruption of Bowman capsule
- Interstitium: Necrotizing neutrophilic granulomatous inflammation, mass lesion
- Vessels: Vasculitis, interlobular and smaller arteries
- Medullary capillaritis
- IF, EM: Little or no immunoglobulin or complement component deposits

TOP DIFFERENTIAL DIAGNOSES

- ANCA(+) vasculitides (Churg-Strauss syndrome, microscopic polyangiitis), anti-GBM disease, HSP, drug-induced vasculitis

DIAGNOSTIC CHECKLIST

- Good prognostic features: High number of preserved glomeruli, low number of cellular crescents, absence of fibrinoid necrosis, little tubular atrophy, fibrosis

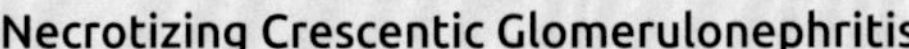

Necrotizing Crescentic Glomerulonephritis

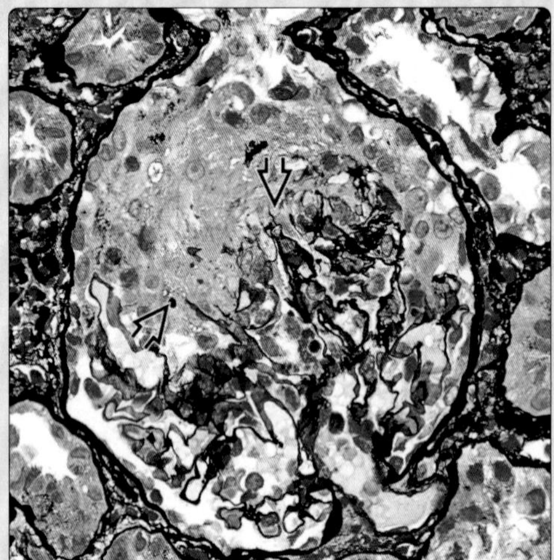

Stages of Crescentic Glomerulonephritis

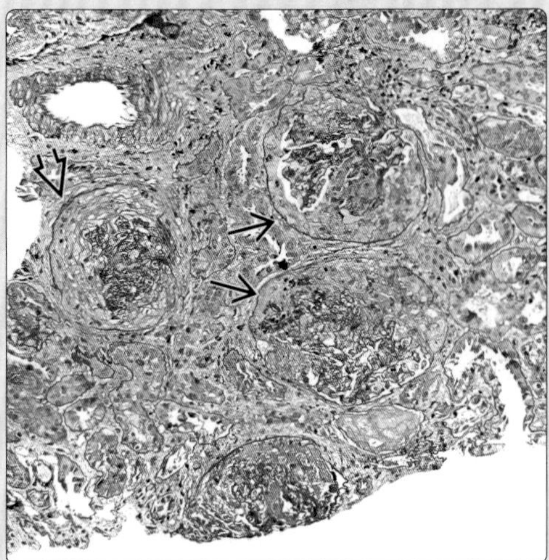

(Left) *Silver methenamine-stained glomerulus shows segmental fibrinoid necrotizing lesion with focal disruption of silver-positive basement membranes → and accumulation of pink fibrinoid material covered by a cellular crescent.* **(Right)** *Low magnification of PAS-stained section with 4 glomeruli shows various stages of crescentic glomerulonephritis having fibrinoid necrosis, cellular crescents →, and a fibrocellular crescent →.*

Necrotizing Granulomatous Interstitial Inflammation

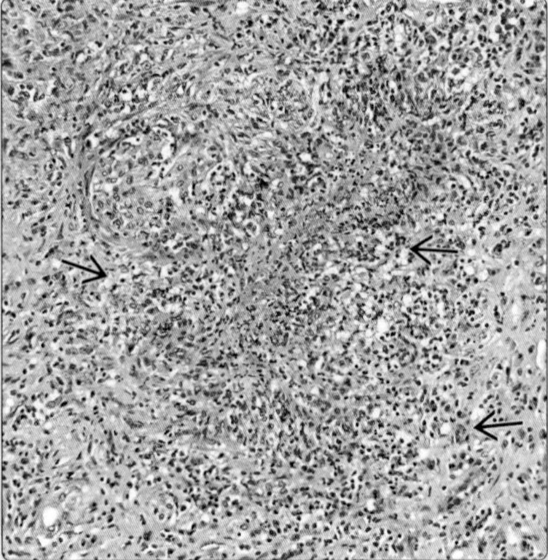

Necrotizing Vasculitis

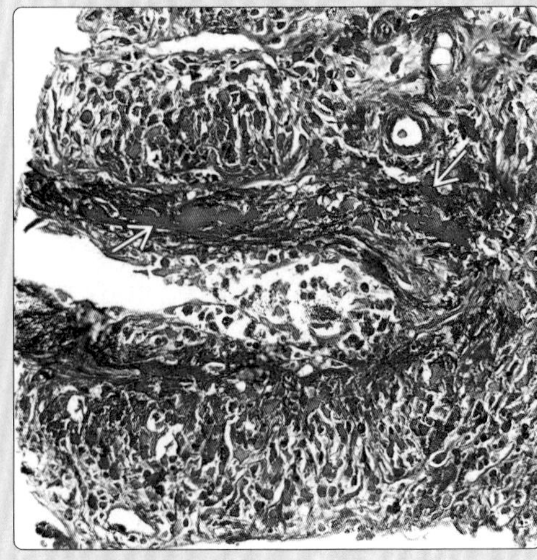

(Left) *GPA in a kidney shows irregular necrotizing granulomatous inflammation with palisading and giant cells → and a neutrophil-rich infiltrate with lymphocytes and epithelioid cells.* **(Right)** *Trichrome-stained interlobular artery shows acute transmural fibrinoid necrotizing vasculitis, where the fibrin is strongly fuchsinophilic →.*

TERMINOLOGY

Abbreviations

- Granulomatosis with polyangiitis (GPA)

Synonyms

- Wegener granulomatosis (WG)

Definitions

- Chapel Hill Consensus Conference 2012
  - GPA is granulomatous inflammation of respiratory tract and necrotizing vasculitis of small to medium-sized vessels (capillaries, venules, arterioles, and arteries), commonly with necrotizing glomerulonephritis (GN) with no or very few deposits (pauci-immune crescentic GN)
- Americal College of Rheumatology (ACR) criteria
  - Nasal or oral inflammation or oral ulcers
  - Abnormal chest radiograph
    - Cavitating or noncavitating nodules
    - Infiltrates
  - Abnormal urinary finding (e.g., microhematuria)
  - Granulomatous inflammation in vessel wall, perivascular or interstitial locations
  - ≥ 2 criteria above have high diagnostic specificity and sensitivity
- EULAR/PRINTO/PRES Criteria, childhood GPA
  - Upper airway involvement
  - Pulmonary involvement
  - Laryngo-tracheobronchial involvement
  - ANCA positivity: MPO or PR3
  - Any 3 of above have high diagnostic specificity and sensitivity

ETIOLOGY/PATHOGENESIS

Antineutrophil Cytoplasmic Antibody (ANCA)-Mediated Small Vessel Vasculitis

- Autoantibodies to proteinase 3 (PR3) in > 75%
  - PR3: Serine proteinase related to neutrophil elastase
  - ANCAs react to peptide sequences in complementary PR3-molecule (cPR3)
    - Significant homology with infectious agents, e.g., *Staphylococcus*
  - < 25% have antimyeloperoxidase (MPO) ANCA with mild renal involvement
  - Antibodies against lysosome-associated membrane protein-2 (LAMP-2) via molecular mimicry
    - Activate neutrophils and induce apoptoses of microvascular endothelium
    - 100% homology to bacterial adhesion protein
  - Autoantibodies to plasminogen and tissue plasminogen activator (25%)
  - Neutrophil activation via feedback loop with ANCA
    - Toll-like receptor TLR2 and TLR9 stimulation triggers neutrophil activation
    - Activated neutrophils express PR3 on surface
    - Neutrophils and macrophages activated via binding of ANCA
    - Release of oxygen radicals, lytic enzymes, inflammatory cytokines, neutrophil extracellular trap products (NET-derived)
    - Dendritic cell activation by NET-derived products
    - Alternative pathway complement activation to form terminal complement complex (C5b-9)
  - Increased adhesion of neutrophils and NK cells to activated endothelium and transmigration
    - Mediate endothelial damage and vascular inflammation
  - Disease activity related to inhibition of PR3-α-1-antitrypsin complex formation
- T cells, autoreactive B cells promote autoimmune response
  - T cells responsive to cPR3 antigen, T helper 17 activation producing IL-17
  - Decreased T-regulatory cells and activation

Genetic Risk Factors

- MHC class II gene *HLA-DPB1*0401* in Caucasians
- MHC class II gene *HLA-DRB1*15* in African Americans
- Retinoid X receptor B polymorphism
- Other associated gene polymorphisms: *DNAM 1* (CD226), *SERPINA1* (α-1-antitrypsin), TNF-α, *CTLA-4, INFγ*, IL-10, *PTPN22* (protein tyrosine phosphatase), *PD 1* gene (also Kawasaki disease), *FCGR3B* (FcγRIIIb)
- Genetic polymorphisms share susceptibility loci with rheumatoid arthritis

Potential Triggers of Autoantibody Response

- Include infections (bacteria, viral, fungal, mycobacterial)
  - GPA onset more common in winter
- Exposure to allergens
- Exposure to dust, heavy metal, respiratory toxins

Animal Model

- Different animal models fail to demonstrate pathogenic role of PR3-ANCA-associated GPA

CLINICAL ISSUES

Epidemiology

- Incidence
  - 30-60/1,000,000
  - Higher prevalence in Caucasians, among North America and northern Europe; lower in Asia, southern Europe
- Age
  - GPA can develop at any age
  - Peak age at onset: 50-70 years
  - Mean: 60 years
  - Can also occur in children and elderly
- Sex
  - Slight male predominance
- Ethnicity
  - Geographic variations may be related to ethnic background

Presentation

- Multisystemic involvement, often preceded by constitutional symptoms
  - Kidney, upper airway, and lung involvement in 90% of cases, also skin and other organs
  - Pulmonary renal syndrome
- 2 disease phases
  - Granulomatous disease of upper respiratory tract
  - Vasculitic phase
- Renal

- Renal disease symptoms (40-80%) in GPA
- Macroscopic or microscopic hematuria
- Red blood cell casts
- Oliguria
- Rapidly progressive or acute renal failure
- Sometimes insidious onset of renal insufficiency with proteinuria &/or hematuria
- Mass lesion (rare)
- Occasionally presents with renal mass

Laboratory Tests

- Hematuria, proteinuria, elevated BUN, Cr
- Anemia, elevated ESR
- ~ 95% positive for ANCA
  - ELISA: Anti-PR3 ANCA (~ 75%) or anti-MPO (~ 25%)
  - Indirect IF: c-ANCA (PR3) or p-ANCA (MPO)
- Rheumatoid factor positive (20-30%)

Treatment

- Steroids combined with cyclophosphamide
- Plasmapheresis beneficial in severe disease
- Maintenance therapies have oral cyclophosphamide, cyclosporine, azathioprine, or mycophenolate mofetil
- Rituximab targets B cells, prevents relapses
- Blocking tumor necrosis factor-α
- Adjuvant therapy: Prophylactic antibiotics

Prognosis

- 20% renal morbidity and end-stage renal disease
  - Lack of treatment or late diagnosis leads to ESRD
- Trend toward improved renal and patient survival
- Clinical factors of poor prognosis
  - Older age
  - High creatinine level at initial presentation
  - High serum titer of ANCA (anti-PR3)
  - Severity of initial vascular damage
  - Multisystem involvement
    - Concomitant lung involvement or hemorrhage
    - Concomitant thrombotic microangiopathy
  - Increased relapse rate (10-50%)
- Clinical factors of good prognosis
  - Close to normal baseline renal function

Renal Transplantation

- Both renal and extrarenal relapses occur after renal transplantation (though uncommon)
  - Recurrent disease or relapses are managed effectively by cyclophosphamide therapy

IMAGING

Radiographic Findings

- Single or multiple nodular lung lesions
- Diffuse pulmonary infiltrates suggesting hemorrhage
- Occasional mass-like lesions in kidneys

MACROSCOPIC

Kidney

- Usually normal in size or slightly enlarged
- In acute phase, small scattered infarcts and petechial hemorrhages in cortex and medulla
- Larger vessels appear grossly normal
- Aneurysms or thrombi rare
- Focal or diffuse papillary necrosis

MICROSCOPIC

Histologic Features

- Glomeruli
  - Wide range and extent of glomerular lesions with crescents
  - Segmental to severe capillary tuft thrombosis
    - Fibrinoid necrosis with rupture of basement membranes
    - Accumulation of neutrophils and karyorrhexis of cells in areas of necrosis
  - Crescents in different stages of healing (such as cellular, fibrocellular, and fibrous types) may be in same biopsy
    - Cellular crescent composed of mainly parietal epithelial cells and exuded inflammatory cells (> 2-3 layers thick)
    - Segmental/small to large, sometimes circumferential cellular crescents
    - Few crescents acquire granulomatous appearance with epithelioid and giant cells
    - Varying degrees of glomerular tuft compression
  - Acute and subacute periglomerular inflammation due to disruption of Bowman capsule
  - No intraglomerular cell proliferation
  - Segmental and global glomerulosclerosis, residual disruption of Bowman capsule
- Tubules
  - Active tubulitis and epithelial cell injury
  - Tubular red blood cells and RBC casts
  - Tubular atrophy and interstitial fibrosis
- Interstitium
  - Mild to marked active interstitial inflammation may accompany glomerular crescentic lesions
    - May be neutrophil- or eosinophil-rich
    - Plasma cells (IgG4[+] in > 30%) can be prominent
  - Focal microscopic interstitial hemorrhages
  - Sometimes necrotizing neutrophilic granulomatous interstitial nephritis with palisading histiocytes (geographic pattern) or mass lesion
    - Interstitial granulomas with mixed inflammatory infiltrates
    - Epithelioid macrophages and giant cells
    - T and B lymphocytes with partial follicular organization
- Vessels
  - Interlobular arteries usually site affected by vasculitis
    - Segmental or circumferential fibrinoid necrosis
    - Cellular reaction composed of neutrophils, histiocytes, and sometimes prominent eosinophils
    - Occasional granulomatous inflammation
  - Smaller arteries down to pre- and postglomerular arterioles and venules involved with vasculitis
  - Progressive vascular sclerosis with variable loss of elastic lamina by EVG stain
  - Peritubular capillaritis
    - Isolated or concomitant medullary inflammation, capillaritis, and interstitial hemorrhages

Other Organs

- Lung
  - Pulmonary (nodular), extravascular granulomatous inflammation is hallmark lesion
  - Usually shows irregular necrosis with neutrophilic infiltrate
  - Progressive, irregular expansion of granuloma affecting bronchial tree and vasculature
  - Vasculitis can be characterized by fibrinoid necrosis or granulomatous inflammation
  - Pulmonary capillaritis leads to pulmonary hemorrhage (in 1/3 of cases)
- Skin
  - Leukocytoclastic vasculitis of dermal capillaries
  - Granulomatous vasculitis with neutrophilic center
  - May be accompanied by extravascular palisading granulomatous inflammation
- Sinuses
  - Necrotizing granulomata and vasculitis
- Other genitourinary lesions
  - Ureteral stenosis
  - Prostatitis, orchitis, epididymitis
  - Penile ulceration

ANCILLARY TESTS

Immunofluorescence

- Strong fibrinogen/fibrin staining noted in capillary lumina, active necrotizing lesions, or in Bowman space in crescents
- Usually negative glomeruli for immunoglobulins (IgG, IgA, IgM) and complement components (C3, C1q)
  - Sometimes scant, randomly distributed glomerular immunoglobulin and complement deposits of < 2+ intensity may be localized
- Presence of unequivocal or significant glomerular deposits leads to overlap of autoimmune or infection-related GN

Electron Microscopy

- Glomerular basement membrane (GBM) and mesangium contain rare or no deposits (pauci-immune)
- GBM can be disrupted by necrotizing lesions
- Fibrin in capillaries and crescents
- Endothelial cells may be reactive (loss of fenestrations)

DIFFERENTIAL DIAGNOSIS

ANCA(+) Vasculitides (Eosinophilic Granulomatosis With Polyangiitis, Microscopic Polyangiitis)

- Necrotizing granuloma, sinus involvement more common in GPA than in microscopic polyangiitis
- Eosinophilia/asthma in EGPA

Anti-GBM Glomerulonephritis

- Linear IgG in GBM distinctive, crescents of same age
- Some patients have both ANCA and anti-GBM

Drug-Induced Granulomatous Interstitial Nephritis and Vasculitis

- History of drug intake
- Skin rash
- Noncaseating granulomata
- Eosinophilia and tissue infiltration in some cases

Sarcoidosis

- Mediastinal lymphadenopathy and lung involvement
- Compact nonnecrotizing granuloma
- Rare: Granulomatous angiitis and crescentic glomerulonephritis
- Elevated angiotensin converting enzyme levels

Henoch-Schönlein Purpura (HSP)

- IgA prominent in glomerular deposits

IgG4-Related Tubulointerstitial Disease

- Multisystemic or renal limited
- Elevated IgG4 level
- No crescentic glomerulonephritis
- Nodular plasma cell-rich infiltrates; 20-30% IgG4(+) cells

DIAGNOSTIC CHECKLIST

Clinically Relevant Pathologic Features

- Pathology features of poor prognosis
  - Number of fibrous glomerular crescents and fibrinoid necrosis at renal biopsy
  - Extra vascular granulomas, necrotizing and nonnecrotizing
  - Extent of tubular atrophy and interstitial fibrosis
- Renal factors of good prognosis
  - High number of preserved glomeruli
  - Low number of cellular crescents
  - Absence of fibrinoid necrosis

Pathologic Interpretation Pearls

- GPA can have only interstitial inflammation/capillaritis without glomerular involvement (possibly due to sampling)
- Negative ANCA does not exclude GPA

SELECTED REFERENCES

1. Chen SF et al: Clinicopathologic characteristics and outcomes of renal thrombotic microangiopathy in anti-neutrophil cytoplasmic autoantibody-associated glomerulonephritis. Clin J Am Soc Nephrol. 10(5):750-8, 2015
2. Watts RA et al: HLA allele variation as a potential explanation for the geographical distribution of granulomatosis with polyangiitis. Rheumatology (Oxford). 54(2):359-62, 2015
3. Lutalo PM et al: Diagnosis and classification of granulomatosis with polyangiitis (aka Wegener's granulomatosis). J Autoimmun. 48-49:94-8, 2014
4. Tognarelli S et al: Tissue-specific microvascular endothelial cells show distinct capacity to activate NK cells: implications for the pathophysiology of granulomatosis with polyangiitis. J Immunol. 192(7):3399-408, 2014
5. Chang SY et al: IgG4-positive plasma cells in granulomatosis with polyangiitis (Wegener's): a clinicopathologic and immunohistochemical study on 43 granulomatosis with polyangiitis and 20 control cases. Hum Pathol. 44(11):2432-7, 2013
6. Csernok E et al: Current understanding of the pathogenesis of granulomatosis with polyangiitis (Wegener's). Expert Rev Clin Immunol. 9(7):641-8, 2013
7. Furuta S et al: Antineutrophil cytoplasmic antibody-associated vasculitis: recent developments. Kidney Int. 84(2):244-9, 2013
8. Holl-Ulrich K: L18. Granuloma formation in granulomatosis with polyangiitis. Presse Med. 42(4 Pt 2):555-8, 2013
9. Holle JU et al: Toll-like receptor TLR2 and TLR9 ligation triggers neutrophil activation in granulomatosis with polyangiitis. Rheumatology (Oxford). 52(7):1183-9, 2013
10. Jennette JC et al: 2012 revised International Chapel Hill Consensus Conference Nomenclature of Vasculitides. Arthritis Rheum. 65(1):1-11, 2013
11. Mueller A et al: Granuloma in ANCA-associated vasculitides: another reason to distinguish between syndromes? Curr Rheumatol Rep. 15(11):376, 2013

(Left) *H&E-stained glomerulus shows segmental, intracapillary fibrinoid material with early necrosis. The rest of the glomerulus has a normal appearance.* **(Right)** *A trichrome-stained glomerulus shows segmental fibrinoid (fuchsinophilic) necrosis overlaid by a cellular crescent. Mild periglomerular inflammatory infiltrate adjacent to the area of the necrotizing lesion is noted.*

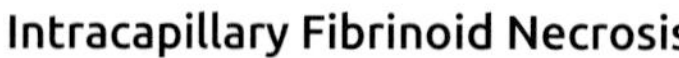

Intracapillary Fibrinoid Necrosis

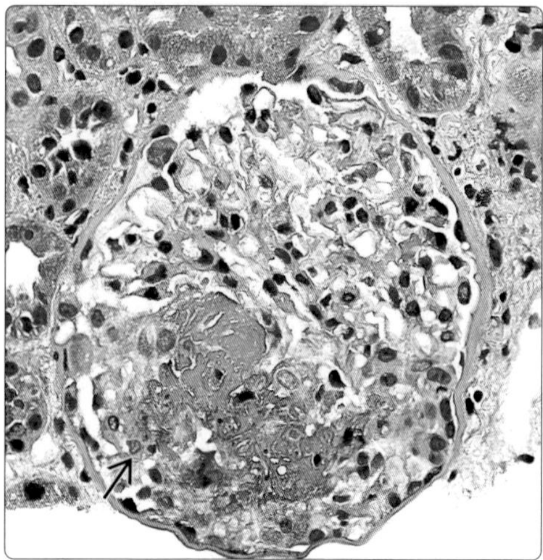

Fuchsinophilic Fibrinoid Material

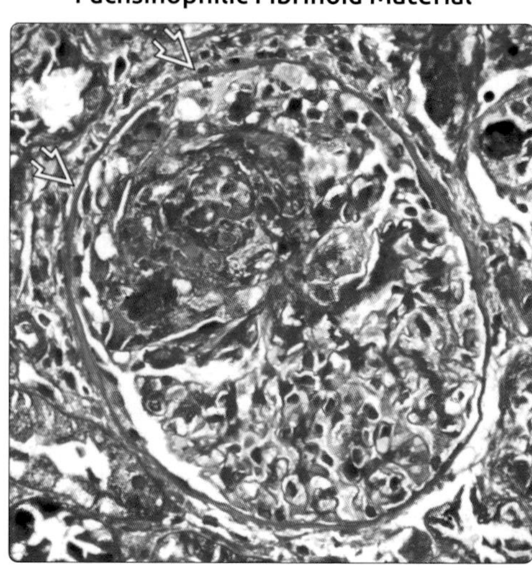

(Left) *Glomerulus in GPA with segmental fibrinoid necrotizing lesion and a small cellular crescent are located at the tubular pole of the glomerulus. This can be differentiated from a glomerular tip lesion of focal segmental sclerosis where foam cells and sclerosing changes may predominate.* **(Right)** *Glomerulus (PAS stain) shows a larger cellular crescent with an only minimal fibrin deposit in the center.*

Segmental Fibrinoid Necrosis

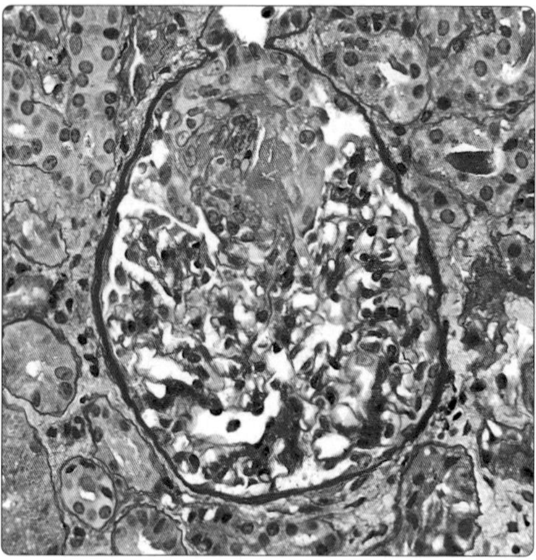

Cellular Crescent

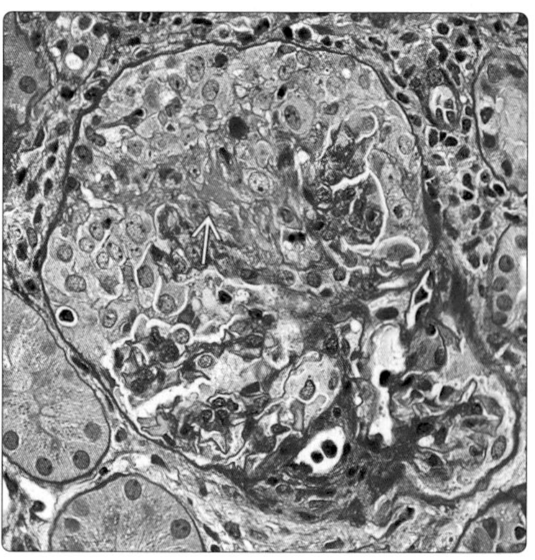

(Left) *PAS shows glomerular tuft mostly compressed by a cellular crescent in the Bowman space mixed with inflammatory cells, typical lesion of GPA, and other ANCA-mediated vasculitides.* **(Right)** *Silver-stained section shows extensive glomerular fibrinoid necrosis with residual compressed glomerular capillaries and portion of a cellular crescent. The GBM has been disrupted by the inflammatory process, and fragments are disconnected from the tuft.*

Circumferential Cellular Crescent

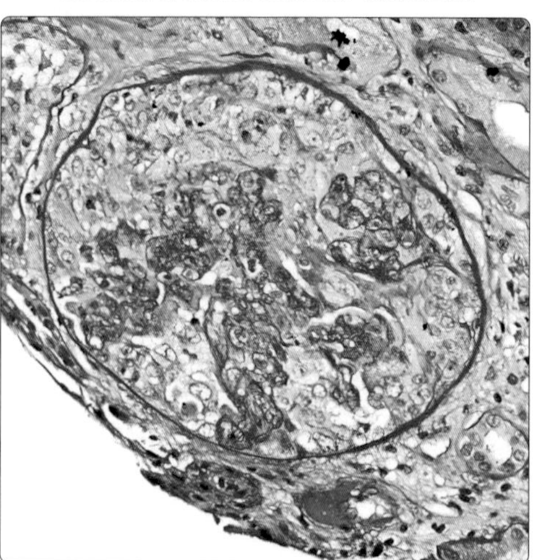

Extensive Glomerular Fibrinoid Necrosis

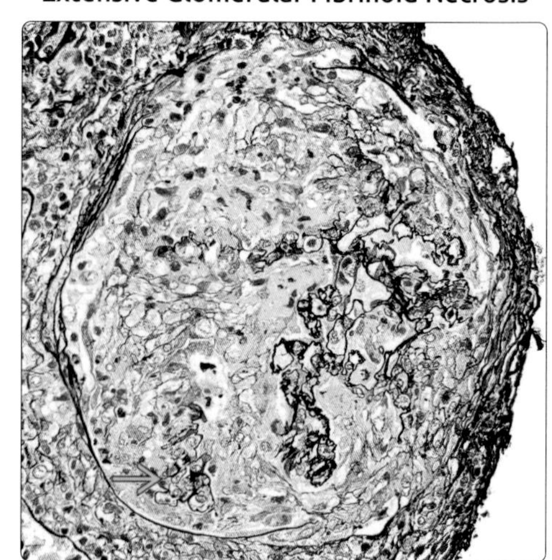

Stages of Organizing Crescents

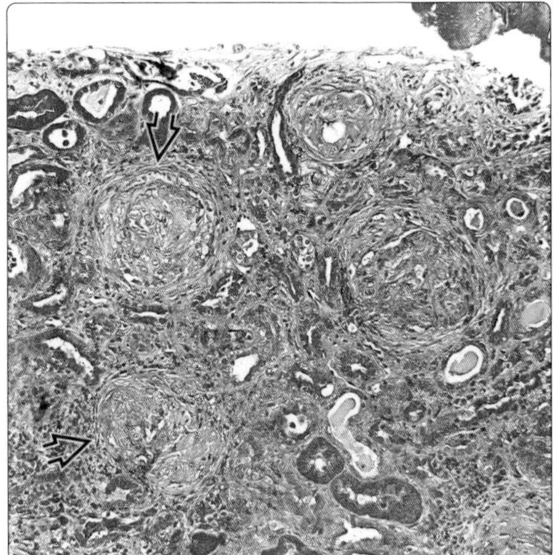

Extensive Intracapillary Fibrinoid Thrombosis

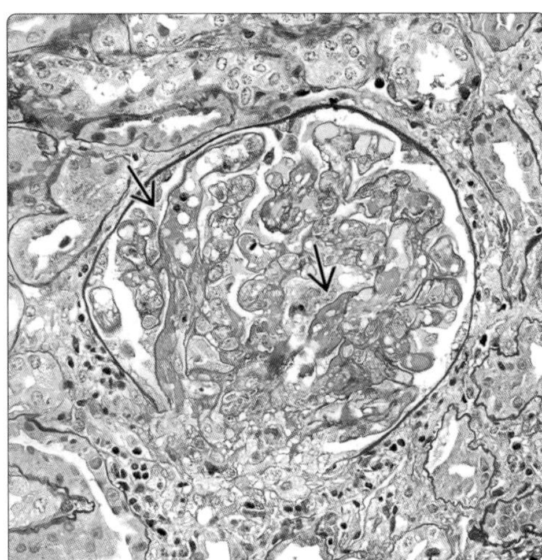

(Left) *Low-magnification trichrome stain shows glomeruli with varying stages of organizing crescents with fibrosis (blue color)* ⇨. **(Right)** *Glomerulus shows extensive intracapillary fibrinoid thrombosis* ⇨ *without capillary disruption or inflammation, resembling thrombotic microangiopathy.*

Negative IgG Staining

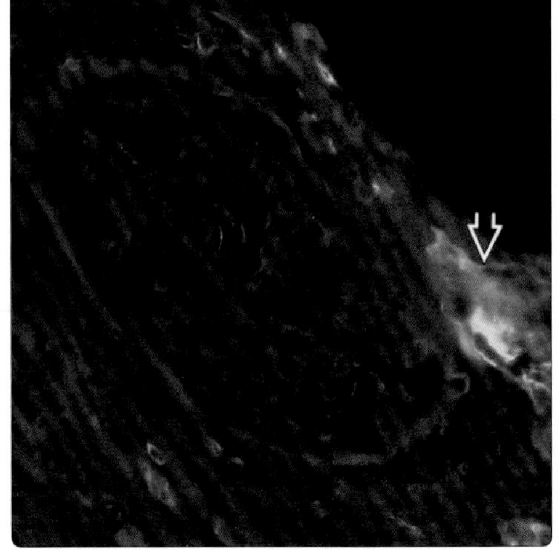

Strong Fibrinogen Stain

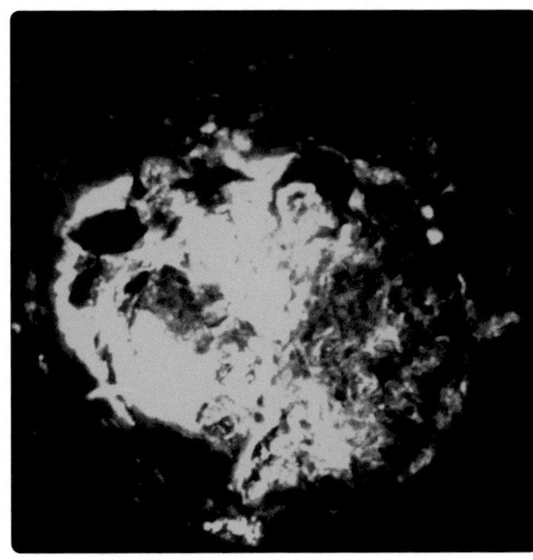

(Left) *Immunofluorescence of glomerulus shows no staining for IgG within the capillary tuft and is positive in the hilar arteriole* ⇨ *in this patient with pauci-immune crescentic glomerulonephritis.* **(Right)** *Glomerulus with necrotizing lesions shows strong immunofluorescence localization of fibrin.*

Rupture of GBM With Cellular Crescent

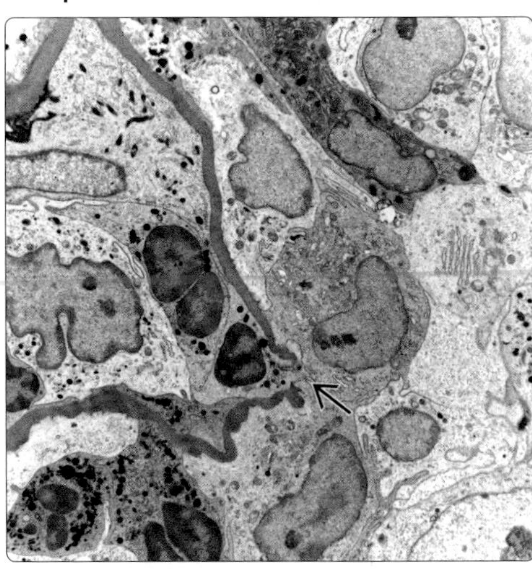

Normal Glomerulus

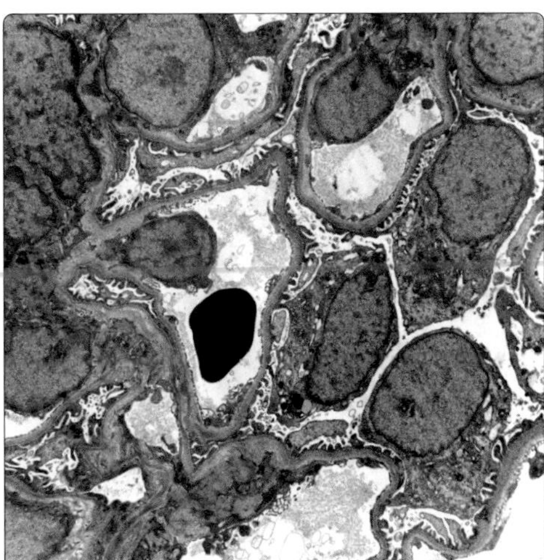

(Left) *Electron micrograph shows a glomerular capillary loop with disruption/break* ⇨ *with margination of neutrophils and monocytes in the lumen overlaid by an inflammatory cellular crescent. Breaks in the GBM are a common feature in glomerulonephritis with crescents of any etiology.* **(Right)** *Electron micrograph shows an uninvolved glomerulus with no significant changes or deposits in this patient with pauci-immune crescentic glomerulonephritis.*

(Left) *CT scan shows a renal mass → thought to be neoplastic, an uncommon presentation of GPA. A biopsy showed necrotizing granulomatosis interstitial nephritis.* **(Right)** *Needle biopsy of a renal mass identified by CT scan in GPA reveals diffuse destruction of tubules and infiltration of the cortex with lymphocytes, plasma cells, and focal necrosis ➡. Glomeruli → were spared. Patient had sinusitis, a saddle nose deformity, and tracheal stenosis. ANCA was negative (~ 10% of GPA).*

Nodular Necrotizing Granulomatosis

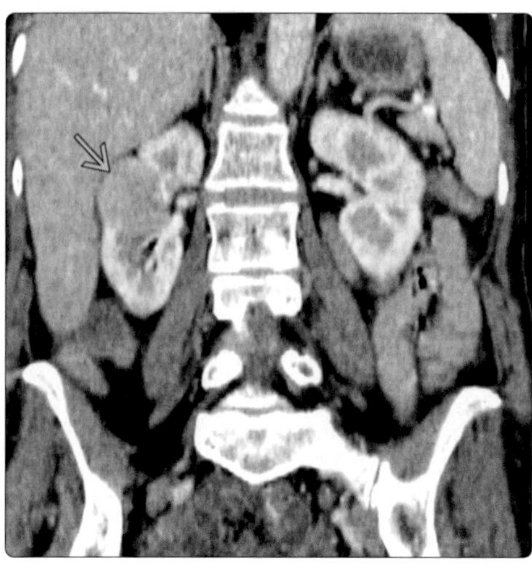

Nodular Necrotizing Granulomatosis

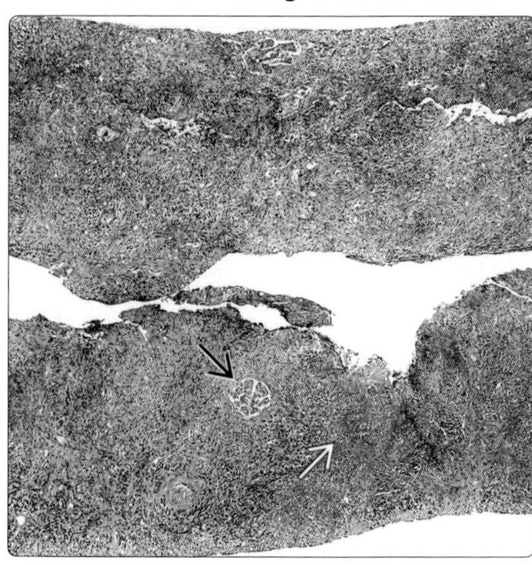

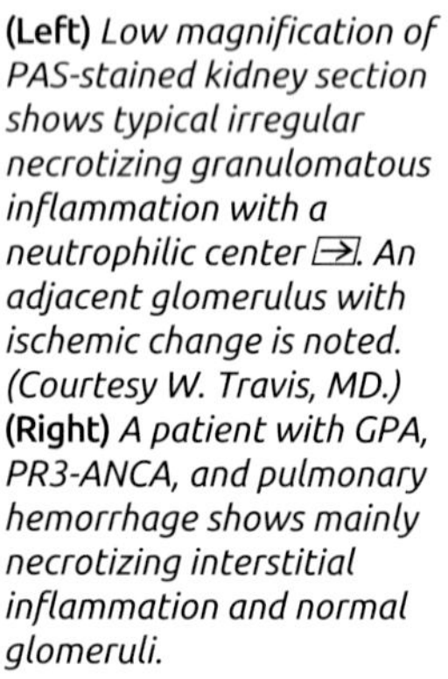

(Left) *Low magnification of PAS-stained kidney section shows typical irregular necrotizing granulomatous inflammation with a neutrophilic center →. An adjacent glomerulus with ischemic change is noted. (Courtesy W. Travis, MD.)* **(Right)** *A patient with GPA, PR3-ANCA, and pulmonary hemorrhage shows mainly necrotizing interstitial inflammation and normal glomeruli.*

Irregular Necrotizing Granulomatous Inflammation

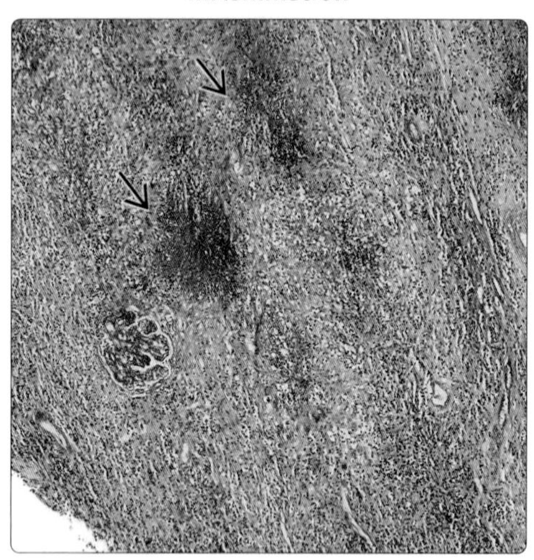

Necrotizing Granulomatous Inflammation

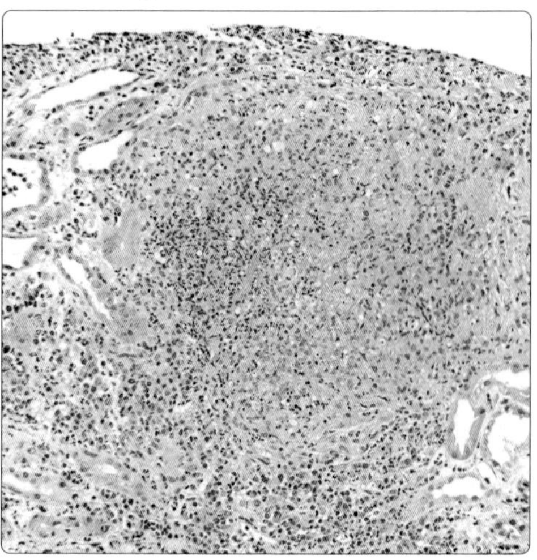

(Left) *A patient with GPA, PR3-ANCA, and pulmonary hemorrhage shows multiple irregular granulomatous inflammatory infiltrates in the interstitial and normal glomeruli.* **(Right)** *Same case shows increased IgG4(+) plasma cells within the granulomatous inflammation.*

Necrotizing Granulomatous Inflammation

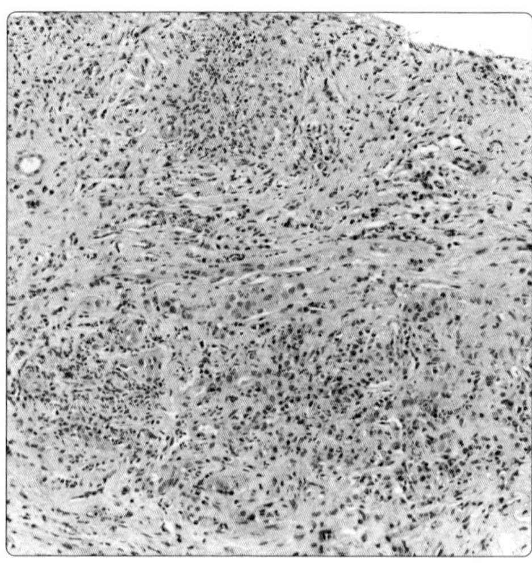

Increased IgG4(+) Cells

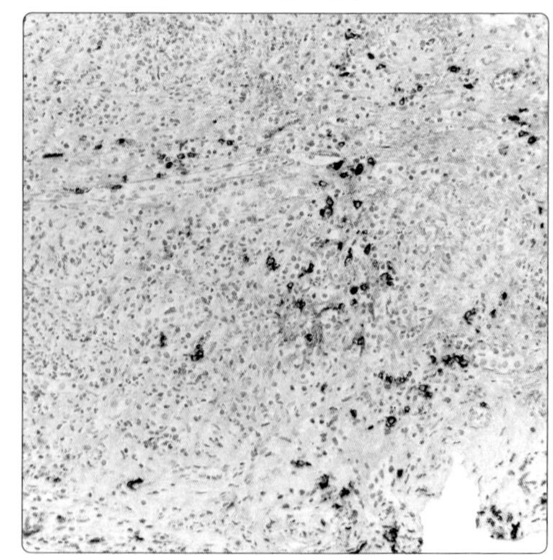

Nonspecific, Active Interstitial Inflammation

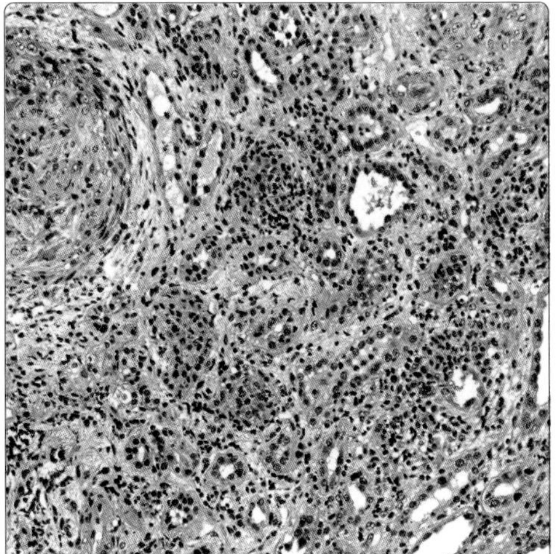

Nonnecrotizing Granuloma

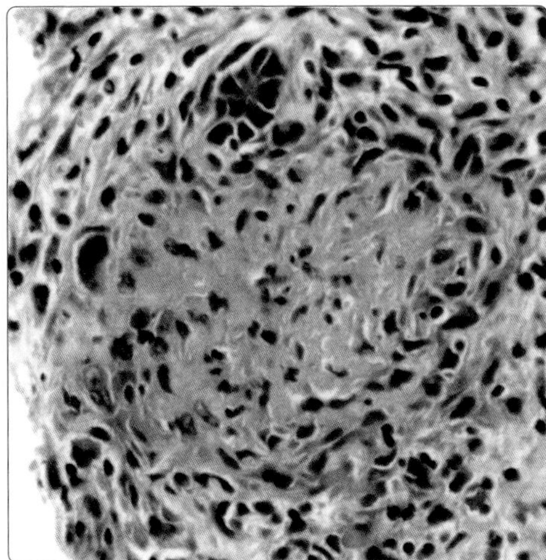

(Left) *Diffuse, active, nonspecific interstitial inflammation with edema is associated with crescentic GN composed of neutrophils, eosinophils, and lymphocytes.* **(Right)** *H&E shows a well-developed, small, interstitial, nonnecrotizing granuloma with epithelioid and rare giant cells at the periphery in a patient with GPA.*

Necrotizing Granulomatous Vasculitis

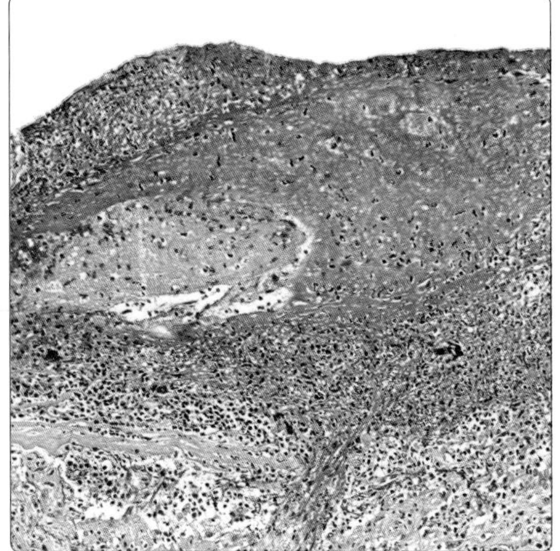

Fibrinoid Necrotizing Arteritis

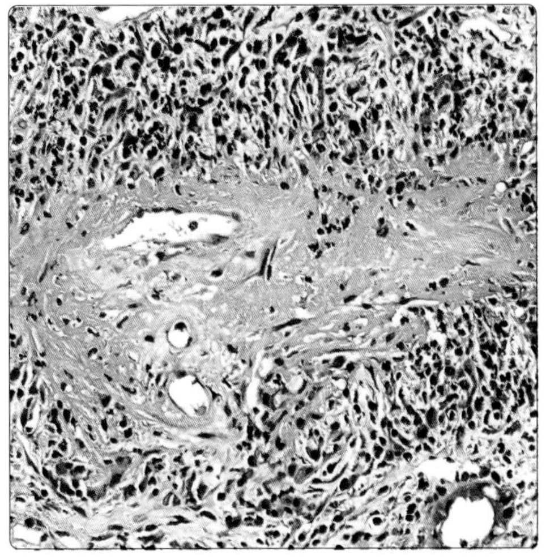

(Left) *A case of GPA, PR3-ANCA, and acute renal failure shows extensive, fibrinoid necrosis of an interlobular artery with multiple multinucleated giant cells at the periphery.* **(Right)** *A case of GPA shows interlobular artery with marked arteriosclerosis affected by active vasculitis composed of lymphocytes and neutrophils with focal granulomatous features.*

Medullary Capillaritis and Hemorrhage

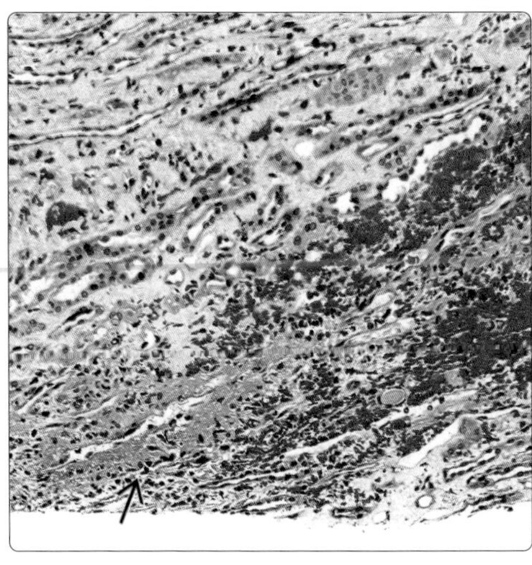

Medullary Capillaritis and Hemorrhage

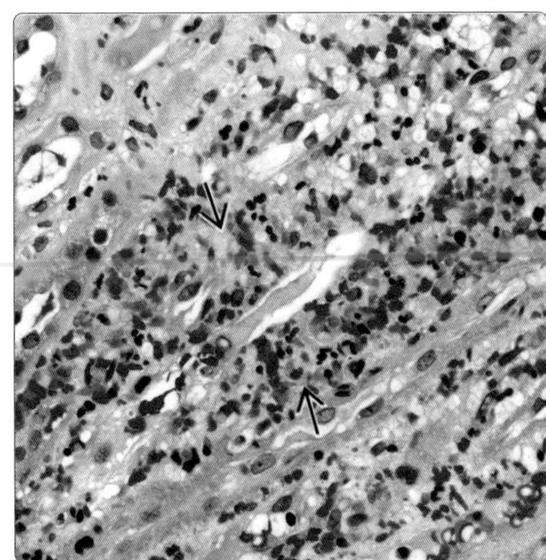

(Left) *Fibrinoid necrotizing capillaritis ➡ with interstitial hemorrhages is shown in the renal medulla of a patient with c-ANCA(+) GPA.* **(Right)** *H&E shows active medullary capillaritis ➡ with extravasation of red cells in the interstitium in a patient with GPA.*

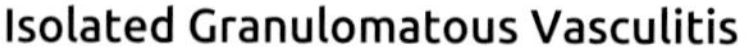

Isolated Granulomatous Vasculitis

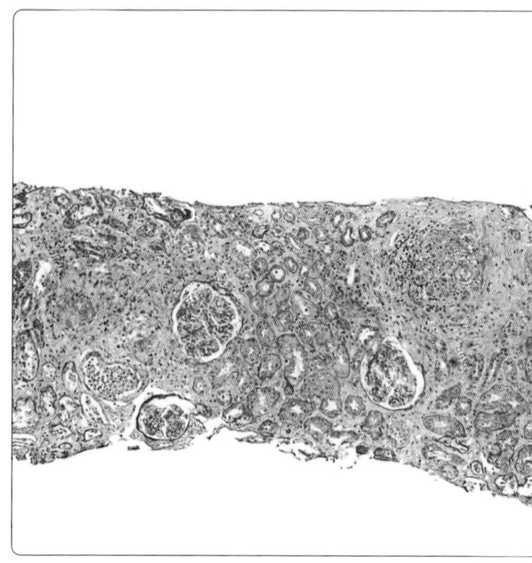

Arteritis With Disruption of Elastic Lamina

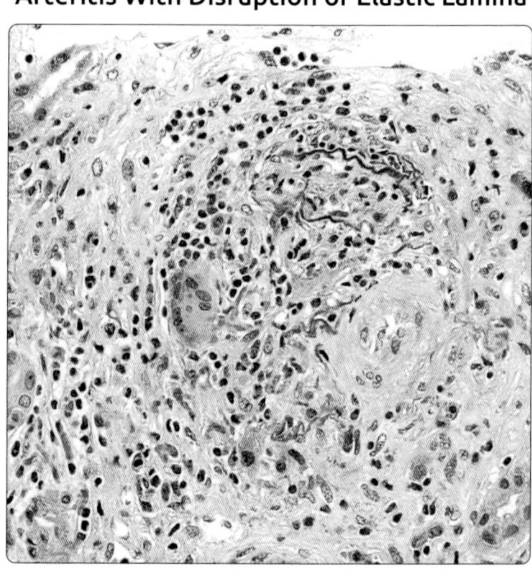

(Left) *A case of GPA shows isolated organizing granulomatous vasculitis and normal glomeruli without crescents.* **(Right)** *The same case shows organizing granulomatous arteritis with disruption and fragmentation of the elastic lamina by Jones silver staining.*

Granulomatous Arteritis

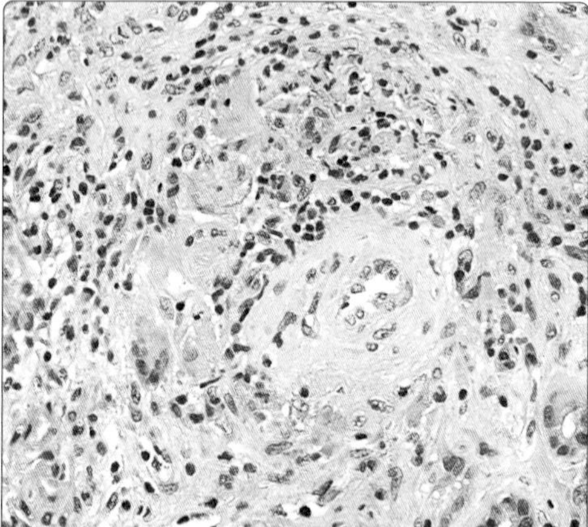

Granulomatous Arteritis

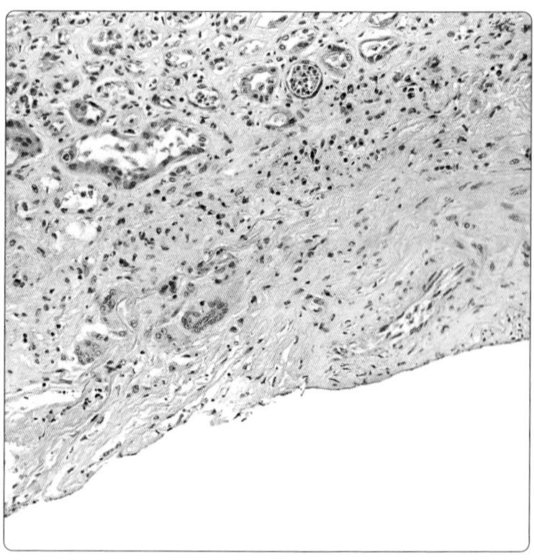

(Left) *In the same case, organizing granulomatous arteritis with narrowing of the lumina is seen.* **(Right)** *This image from the same case shows organizing granulomatous arteritis with obliterative luminal changes.*

Necrotizing Granulomatous Vasculitis

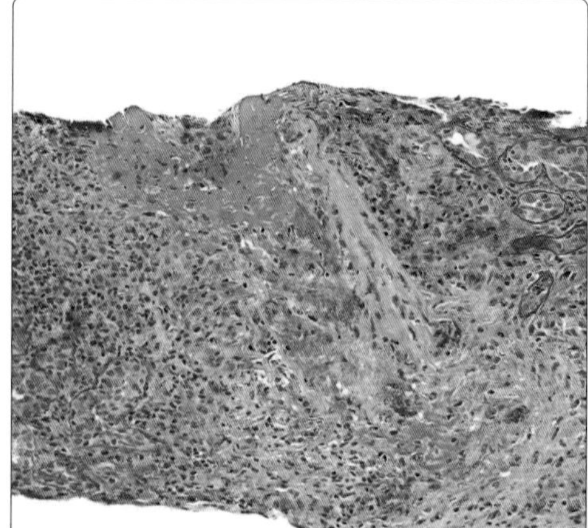

Necrotizing Granulomatous Vasculitis

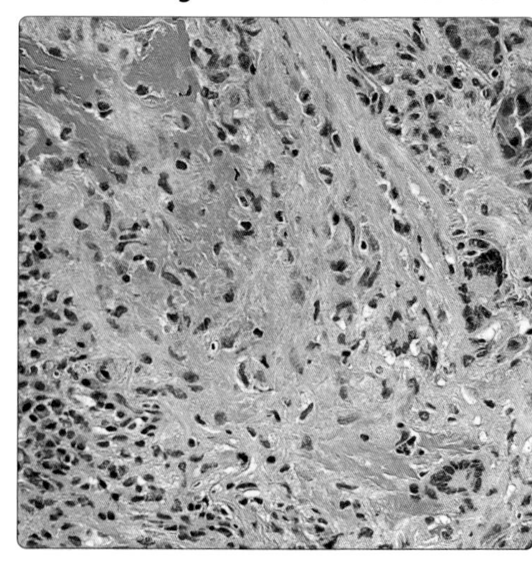

(Left) *A case of GPA shows necrotizing granulomatous vasculitis of an interlobular artery with a few multinucleated giant cells. Focal glomerular crescents were present in this case.* **(Right)** *A case of GPA shows necrotizing granulomatous vasculitis of an interlobular artery with a few multinucleated giant cells. Focal glomerular crescents were present in this case.*

Healed Arteritis With Disruption of Elastica

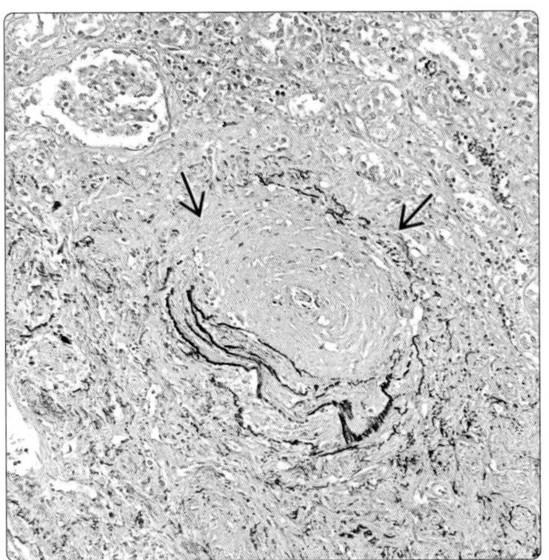

Leukocytoclastic Vasculitis

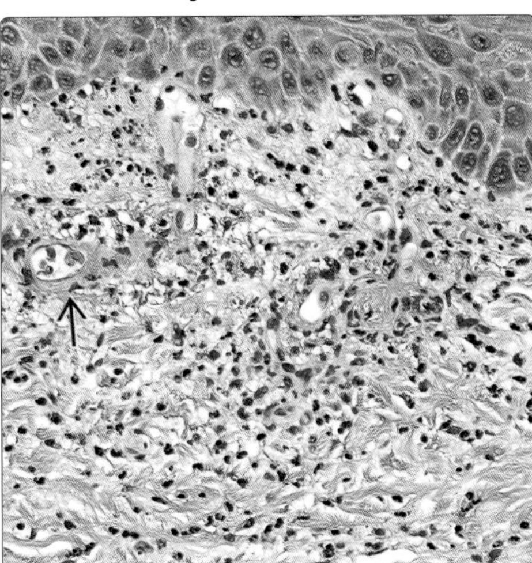

(Left) *Elastic (EVG) stain shows partial loss of internal elastic lamina of an interlobular artery ➡ following necrotizing vasculitis in a patient with GPA. An elastic stain is useful to detect old arteritis because the disrupted elastica persists in the fibrous scar.* **(Right)** *Skin in GPA shows dermal leukocytoclastic vasculitis of the capillaries, with one showing an early fibrinoid change ➡.*

Granulomatous Vasculitis

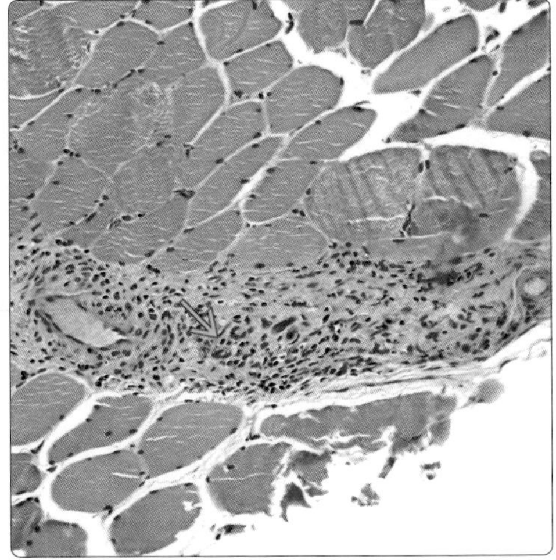

Granulomatous Vasculitis

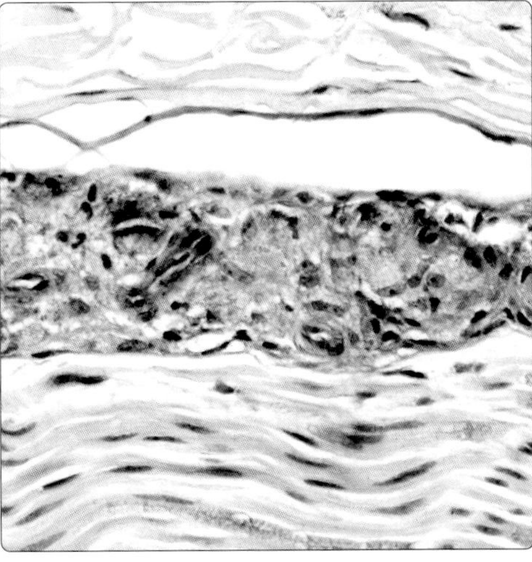

(Left) *Skeletal muscle biopsy shows granulomatous inflammation ➡ of an arteriole in the perimysial tissue.* **(Right)** *Nerve biopsy shows granulomatous arteriolitis associated with acute peripheral neuropathy.*

Pulmonary Hemorrhage and Capillaritis

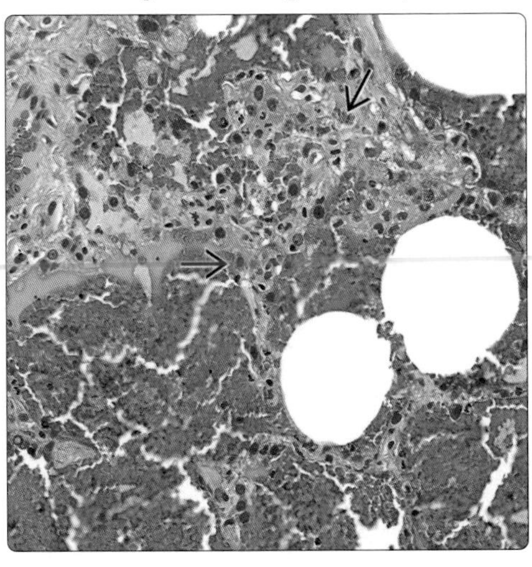

Pulmonary Necrotizing Granulomatous Inflammation

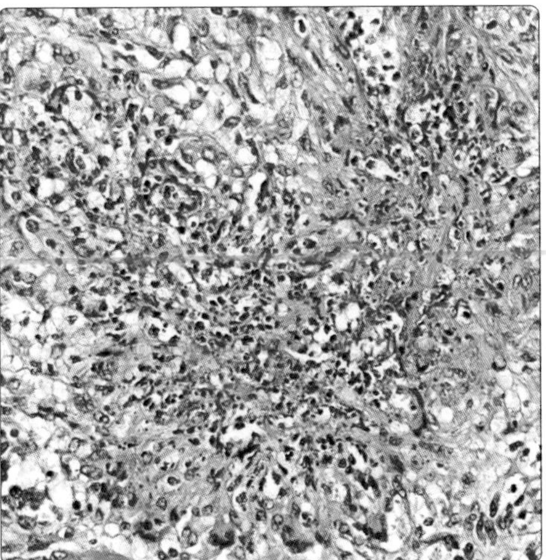

(Left) *Section of lung shows extensive alveolar hemorrhage adjacent to capillaritis with neutrophils ➡. This is believed to be an early lesion in GPA.* **(Right)** *Irregular, necrotizing granulomatous inflammation with palisading of epithelioid and giant cells with neutrophilic center are shown in the lung of a patient with GPA.*

KEY FACTS

TERMINOLOGY

- Allergic granulomatosis and angiitis manifested by asthma, eosinophilia, extravascular eosinophil infiltration, pulmonary infiltrates, ANCA(+) and pauci-immune glomerulonephritis

ETIOLOGY/PATHOGENESIS

- Triggers: Allergens, vaccines, drugs
- T-helper cell and eosinophil activation

CLINICAL ISSUES

- Occurs in any age, mostly 40-60 years
- Asthma, granulomatous inflammation
- Peripheral eosinophilia (10-20%)
- Positive MPO-ANCA (40-70%)
  - High renal incidence in ANCA(+) cases
  - Rapid renal failure, mild renal impairment, hematuria
- Remission after initial treatment (90%)
- Typically relapsing (35-74%)
- Cyclophosphamide in steroid-resistant or relapsing disease

MICROSCOPIC

- Acute, subacute, &/or chronic crescentic GN, pauci-immune
- Occasional isolated eosinophilic interstitial nephritis
- Small vessel vasculitis, fibrinoid necrotizing and granulomatous types, eosinophil rich
- Necrotizing granuloma with eosinophils, necrotic eosinophilic cellular debris, scattered multinucleated giant cells, and epithelioid macrophages in palisading layer

ANCILLARY TESTS

- Negative IF and nonspecific EM
- No immune deposits

TOP DIFFERENTIAL DIAGNOSES

- Granulomatosis with polyangiitis (Wegener) with renal involvement
- Drug-induced vasculitis
- Systemic parasitic infestation

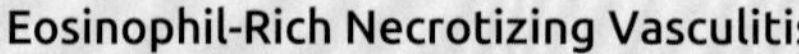
Eosinophil-Rich Necrotizing Vasculitis

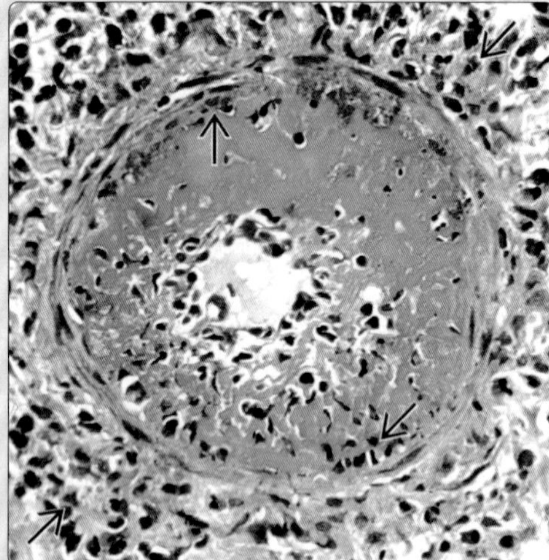

Necrotizing and Crescentic Glomerulonephritis

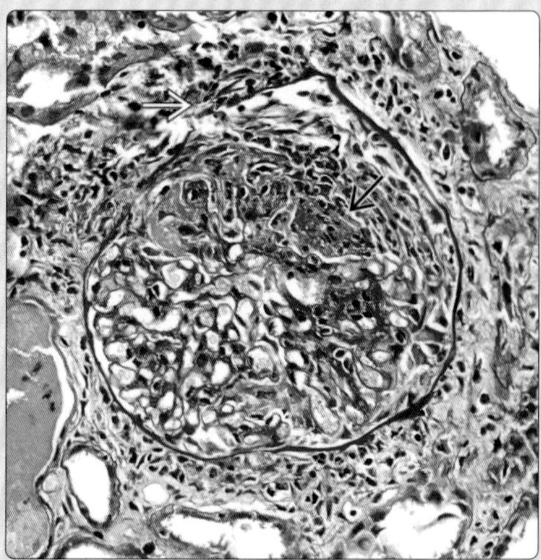

(Left) *Renal biopsy from a patient with EGPA (CS) shows circumferential, transmural necrotizing arteritis surrounded by numerous eosinophils and by lymphocytes. Eosinophils invade the media* ⇨. **(Right)** *Periodic acid-Schiff stain of a glomerulus in EGPA (CS) reveals segmental necrosis* ⇨, *a cellular crescent in Bowman space, and rupture of Bowman capsule* ➡ *with periglomerular inflammation.*

Granulomatous Interstitial Inflammation

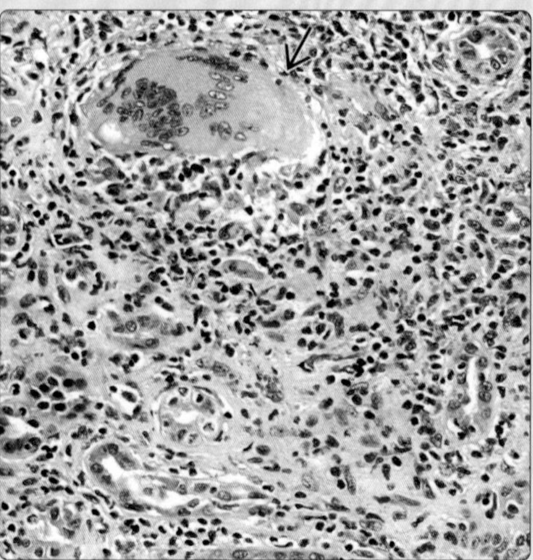

Eosinophil-Rich Interstitial Inflammation

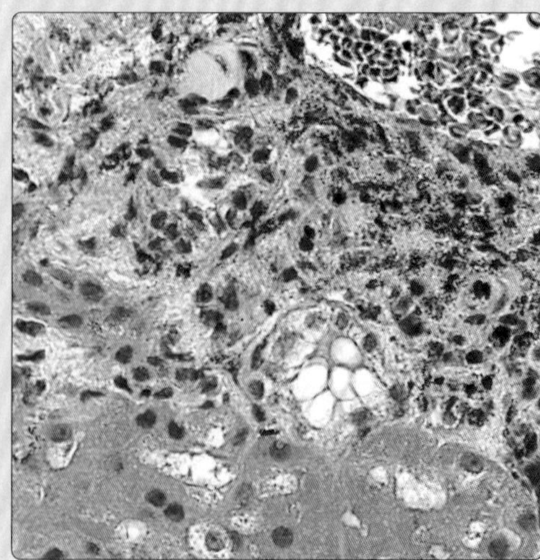

(Left) *Active interstitial inflammation contains eosinophils sometimes admixed with multinucleated giant cells* ⇨ *in EGPA (CS) renal disease, giving it a granulomatous appearance.* **(Right)** *This case of EGPA (CS) shows intense renal interstitial eosinophil infiltration and tubulitis with early necrosis. Eosinophilic infiltration of affected tissue is a hallmark of EGPA (CS).*

TERMINOLOGY

Abbreviations

- Eosinophilic granulomatoses with polyangiitis (EGPA)

Synonyms

- Allergic granulomatosis and angiitis
- Churg-Strauss syndrome (CSS)

Definitions

- American College of Rheumatology (ACR) criteria differentiate various forms of vasculitides once diagnosis of vasculitis is made
  - EGPA diagnosis requires 4 of 6 following features
    - Asthma
    - Eosinophilia > 10%
    - Extravascular eosinophil infiltration
    - Pulmonary infiltrates
    - Paranasal sinus changes
    - Peripheral neuropathy
- Chapel Hill Consensus Conference 2012
  - Eosinophil-rich and necrotizing granulomatous inflammation involving the respiratory tract
  - Eosinophil-rich necrotizing vasculitis affecting small to medium-sized vessels
  - Associated with asthma and peripheral eosinophilia
  - ANCA is frequent when glomerulonephritis is present
- Diagnostic criteria of EGPA proposed by the European Respiratory Society CSS-Task Force
  - Asthma
  - Blood eosinophils > 1.5 G/L or > 10% of leukocytes
  - Vasculitis (or surrogates), which includes necrotizing vasculitis of any organ (kidney, lung, skin, heart, peripheral nerve), positive MPO-ANCA or PR3-ANCA ± systemic manifestations considered to be related to eosinophilic disease

ETIOLOGY/PATHOGENESIS

Environmental Exposure

- Allergens, vaccinations, drugs or infectious agents

Genetic

- Positive association with *HLA-DRB1* gene

Pathogenesis

- Primarily cell-mediated tissue and vascular injury
  - CD4(+) T cells secrete interferon-gamma (Th-1 cytokine), promoting granulomatous inflammation
  - Eosinophil activation via IL-4, IL-5, and IL-13 secretion and CD95-CD95L pathway
  - Crucial role for B cells
  - Tissue damage by eosinophils due to release of cytotoxic eosinophilic cationic and major basic protein
  - Eotaxin-3 from endothelial cells and CCL17 are chemotactic for eosinophils
- ANCA is positive in up to 40%
  - ANCA titers correlate with disease activity and renal lesions

CLINICAL ISSUES

Epidemiology

- Incidence
  - 11-13/1 million worldwide
  - 16-27% have renal involvement, up to 50%
  - 35-65/10^6 in asthmatic population
  - Lesser frequency and milder disease than other small vessel vasculitides involving kidney
- Age
  - Peak age: 40-60 years; mean: 50 years
  - Younger adults may also be affected
- Sex
  - No gender predilection
- Ethnicity
  - No ethnic predisposition

Presentation

- Multisystemic disease
- 4 phases
  - **Allergic**
    - Constitutional symptoms: Fever, malaise, weight loss
    - Asthma
    - Rhinitis
  - **Eosinophilic**
    - Peripheral eosinophilia
    - Tissue eosinophil infiltration (e.g., gastrointestinal, sinusitis)
    - Heart
  - **Vasculitic**
    - Skin purpuric rash
    - Peripheral neuropathy
    - Cerebral vessels
    - Lung
    - Kidney
  - **Postvasculitic**
    - Sequelae related to major organ damage and hypertension
- Renal disease
  - Kidney involvement varies from 8-50%; median: 18% of EGPA
  - High incidence in ANCA(+) cases
    - No renal disease in 25% EGPA with ANCA
    - Any renal disease in 75% with ANCA
    - Necrotizing glomerulonephritis in 100% with ANCA
  - Progressive renal insufficiency
  - Acute renal failure (less frequent)
  - Hematuria (mild to severe)
  - Asymptomatic (isolated) urinary abnormalities
  - Obstructive uropathy caused by ureteral stenosis
- Polyangiitis overlap syndrome
  - EGPA may coexist with GPA or MPA
- ANCA(-) cases
  - Increased proportion of cardiac, gastrointestinal, and pulmonary involvement

Laboratory Tests

- Anemia, leukocytosis
- Peripheral eosinophilia (10-20%) (> 1-1.5 g/l)

- May be lower or normal in patients previously treated with steroids for asthma
- Elevated erythrocyte sedimentation rate
- ANCA (30-40% positive)
    - Mainly p-ANCA (antimyeloperoxidase antibodies [MPO]); rarely c-ANCA or atypical
- Rheumatoid factor (up to 50% positive)
- Elevated serum IgE levels and immune complexes containing IgE
- Renal dysfunction
    - Elevated creatinine
    - Hematuria
    - Proteinuria

Treatment

- Drugs
    - Immunosuppressive therapy used to treat severe, multisystemic disease manifestations, particularly vasculitis or ANCA(+) cases
        - Good response to high-dose corticosteroids
        - Cyclophosphamide in steroid-resistant or relapsing disease
        - Rituximab anti-CD20 antibody in refractory and relapsing disease
        - Mycophenolate mofetil
    - Maintenance: Oral cyclophosphamide or azathioprine

Prognosis

- Typically relapsing disease (35-74%)
- Remission after initial treatment (90%)
- Renal flares are rare, and long-term prognosis is favorable; overall survival: 97%
- 5 factors of poor prognosis from French Vasculitis Study Group
    - Heart, gastrointestinal, central nervous system involvement
    - Proteinuria > 1 g/24 hours
    - Creatinine > 1.5 mg/dL
- Rare: Severe renal vasculitic or crescentic glomerulonephritis and chronic renal failure

MICROSCOPIC

Histologic Features

- **Glomeruli** (mild to severe involvement)
    - Focal glomerulonephritis, pauci-immune
        - Segmental necrotizing lesions
        - Cellular crescents/extracapillary proliferation (5-50% of glomeruli)
        - Crescents in varying stages of healing: Fibrocellular and fibrous types (5-50% of glomeruli)
        - Focal segmental glomerulosclerosis
        - Global glomerulosclerosis, if chronic
    - Mesangial hypercellularity
        - Mild to moderate
    - Focal eosinophil or neutrophil infiltration
    - No endocapillary proliferation or capillary wall abnormalities
- **Tubulointerstitium**
    - Focal eosinophil-rich interstitial infiltrate
    - Tissue eosinophils best seen on H&E and trichrome-stained sections
    - Isolated acute tubulointerstitial nephritis
    - Focal granuloma formation, rare
    - Necrotizing granuloma with eosinophils, necrotic eosinophilic cellular debris, scattered multinucleated giant cells, and epithelioid macrophages in a palisading layer
        - Healing of granuloma spontaneous or following treatment
    - Free red blood cells, RBC casts, and hemosiderin casts in tubular lumina in acute cases
    - Tubular atrophy, interstitial fibrosis, and chronic inflammation
- **Vessels**
    - Interlobular (commonly), arcuate, and large branches of renal artery (sometimes) affected
        - Necrotizing fibrinoid necrosis involves endothelium and intima 1st and extends to media
        - Eosinophils, predominant cell infiltration
        - Focal granulomatous change may be seen
    - Small vessel vasculitis &/or venulitis
- **Lower urinary tract**
    - Renal pelvis, ureter, or prostate
        - Eosinophilic and granulomatous inflammation
    - Healed lesions lead to
        - Obstructive uropathy
        - Cause of renal functional impairment
- **Lung and other organs**
    - Pulmonary capillaritis with hemorrhage
    - Small vessel vasculitis &/or venulitis; other organs and skin with prominent eosinophils

ANCILLARY TESTS

Immunofluorescence

- Generally, no deposits of immunoglobulins (IgG, IgM, IgA) or complement (C3, C1q)
- Strong fibrinogen staining in necrotizing glomerular and vascular lesions

Electron Microscopy

- Glomerular epithelial (parietal and visceral) cell injury in active crescentic lesions
- Variable foot process effacement depending on visceral cell injury
- Normal thickness, contour, and texture of glomerular basement membranes (GBM)
- Variable collapse of capillary tuft due to presence of crescent
- Mild to moderate mesangial hypercellularity and increased matrix
- No immune complex type of electron-dense deposits

DIFFERENTIAL DIAGNOSIS

Granulomatosis With Polyangiitis (Wegener)

- No history of asthma
- Mild or no eosinophilia
- Higher incidence of crescentic GN (90%)
- Almost always c-ANCA positive
- Mild to moderate eosinophil infiltration

- More striking granulomatous inflammation

Drug-Induced Vasculitis and Interstitial Nephritis

- History of drug intake
- No history of asthma
- Small proportion associated with MPO-ANCA (hydralazine, antithyroid drugs)
- Less severe eosinophilia (< 10%)
- Rarely, crescentic glomerulonephritis
- Sometimes indistinguishable from CSS

Systemic or Renal Parasitic Infestation

- History of parasitic infection
- Travel to parasite endemic area
- Not associated with positive ANCA serology
- No crescentic glomerulonephritis
  - Rare small vessel vasculitis or capillaritis, sometimes varied forms of immune-complex glomerular lesions
- Eosinophil-rich tubulointerstitial nephritis with occasional evidence of parasitic eggs or larvae
- May have episodes of asthma

Allergic Bronchopulmonary Aspergillosis

- Absence of systemic vasculitis
- Absence of ANCA
- Lower response to steroids

DIAGNOSTIC CHECKLIST

Pathologic Interpretation Pearls

- Vasculitis with prominent eosinophils and clinical history of asthma should raise possibility of CSS

SELECTED REFERENCES

1. Greco A et al: Churg-Strauss syndrome. Autoimmun Rev. 14(4):341-348, 2015
2. Boita M et al: The molecular and functional characterization of clonally expanded CD8+ TCR BV T cells in eosinophilic granulomatosis with polyangiitis (EGPA). Clin Immunol. 152(1-2):152-63, 2014
3. Kim MY et al: Clinical features and prognostic factors of Churg-Strauss syndrome. Korean J Intern Med. 29(1):85-95, 2014
4. Mahr A et al: Eosinophilic granulomatosis with polyangiitis (Churg-Strauss): evolutions in classification, etiopathogenesis, assessment and management. Curr Opin Rheumatol. 26(1):16-23, 2014
5. Mouthon L et al: Diagnosis and classification of eosinophilic granulomatosis with polyangiitis (formerly named Churg-Strauss syndrome). J Autoimmun. 48-49:99-103, 2014
6. Sokolowska BM et al: ANCA-positive and ANCA-negative phenotypes of eosinophilic granulomatosis with polyangiitis (EGPA): outcome and long-term follow-up of 50 patients from a single Polish center. Clin Exp Rheumatol. 32(3 Suppl 82):S41-7, 2014
7. Uematsu H et al: Polyangiitis overlap syndrome of granulomatosis with polyangiitis (Wegener's granulomatosis) and eosinophilic granulomatosis with polyangiitis (Churg-Strauss syndrome). BMJ Case Rep. 2014, 2014
8. Comarmond C et al: Eosinophilic granulomatosis with polyangiitis (Churg-Strauss): clinical characteristics and long-term followup of the 383 patients enrolled in the French Vasculitis Study Group cohort. Arthritis Rheum. 65(1):270-81, 2013
9. Cordier JF et al: L5. Eosinophilic granulomatosis with polyangiitis (Churg-Strauss). Presse Med. 42(4 Pt 2):507-10, 2013
10. Gendelman S et al: Childhood-onset eosinophilic granulomatosis with polyangiitis (formerly Churg-Strauss syndrome): a contemporary single-center cohort. J Rheumatol. 40(6):929-35, 2013
11. Hara T et al: Eosinophilic myocarditis due to Churg-Strauss syndrome with markedly elevated eosinophil cationic protein. Int Heart J. 54(1):51-3, 2013
12. Jennette JC et al: 2012 revised International Chapel Hill Consensus Conference Nomenclature of Vasculitides. Arthritis Rheum. 65(1):1-11, 2013
13. Llewellyn R et al: Lesson of the month. (1). What lies beneath the surface? Diagnosis. Churg-Strauss syndrome. Clin Med. 13(1):103-5, 2013
14. Roufosse F: L4. Eosinophils: how they contribute to endothelial damage and dysfunction. Presse Med. 42(4 Pt 2):503-7, 2013
15. Thiel J et al: Rituximab in the treatment of refractory or relapsing eosinophilic granulomatosis with polyangiitis (Churg-Strauss syndrome). Arthritis Res Ther. 15(5):R133, 2013
16. Vaglio A et al: Eosinophilic granulomatosis with polyangiitis (Churg-Strauss): state of the art. Allergy. 68(3):261-73, 2013
17. Zwerina J et al: Can ANCA differentiate eosinophilic granulomatosis with polyangiitis (Churg-Strauss) from idiopathic hypereosinophilic syndrome? Clin Exp Rheumatol. 31(6):989-90, 2013
18. Sinico RA et al: Antineutrophil cytoplasmic autoantibodies and clinical phenotype in patients with Churg-Strauss syndrome. J Allergy Clin Immunol. 130(6):1440; author reply 1440-1, 2012
19. Vaglio A et al: Churg-Strauss syndrome. Kidney Int. 76(9):1006-11, 2009
20. Sinico RA et al: Renal involvement in Churg-Strauss syndrome. Am J Kidney Dis. 47(5):770-9, 2006
21. Sablé-Fourtassou R et al: Antineutrophil cytoplasmic antibodies and the Churg-Strauss syndrome. Ann Intern Med. 143(9):632-8, 2005
22. Sinico RA et al: Prevalence and clinical significance of antineutrophil cytoplasmic antibodies in Churg-Strauss syndrome. Arthritis Rheum. 52(9):2926-35, 2005
23. Keogh KA et al: Churg-Strauss syndrome: clinical presentation, antineutrophil cytoplasmic antibodies, and leukotriene receptor antagonists. Am J Med. 115(4):284-90, 2003
24. Kikuchi Y et al: Glomerular lesions in patients with Churg-Strauss syndrome and the anti-myeloperoxidase antibody. Clin Nephrol. 55(6):429-35, 2001
25. Holloway J et al: Churg-Strauss syndrome associated with zafirlukast. J Am Osteopath Assoc. 98(5):275-8, 1998
26. Jennette JC et al: Nomenclature of systemic vasculitides. Proposal of an international consensus conference. Arthritis Rheum. 37(2):187-92, 1994
27. Vogel PS et al: Churg-Strauss syndrome. J Am Acad Dermatol. 27(5 Pt 2):821-4, 1992
28. Clutterbuck EJ et al: Renal involvement in Churg-Strauss syndrome. Nephrol Dial Transplant. 5(3):161-7, 1990
29. Lanham JG et al: Systemic vasculitis with asthma and eosinophilia: a clinical approach to the Churg-Strauss syndrome. Medicine (Baltimore). 63(2):65-81, 1984
30. Chumbley LC et al: Allergic granulomatosis and angiitis (Churg-Strauss syndrome). Report and analysis of 30 cases. Mayo Clin Proc. 52(8):477-84, 1977
31. Churg J et al: Allergic granulomatosis, allergic angiitis, and periarteritis nodosa. Am J Pathol. 27(2):277-301, 1951

(Left) *In EGPA (CS), often some degree of mesangial proliferation/hypercellularity may be noted in the glomeruli, in contrast to anti-GBM disease.* **(Right)** *This glomerulus from a patient with EGPA (CS) is scarcely recognizable due to intraglomerular fibrinoid necrosis ⇨, infiltrating eosinophils ⇨, and lymphocytes. (Courtesy R. Wieczorek, MD.)*

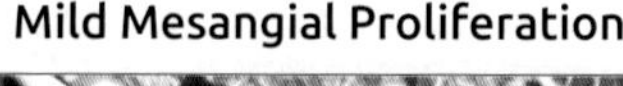

Mild Mesangial Proliferation

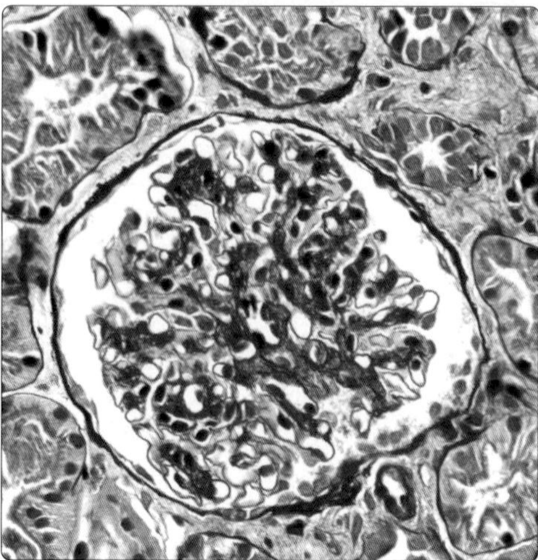

Fibrinoid Necrosis With Eosinophils

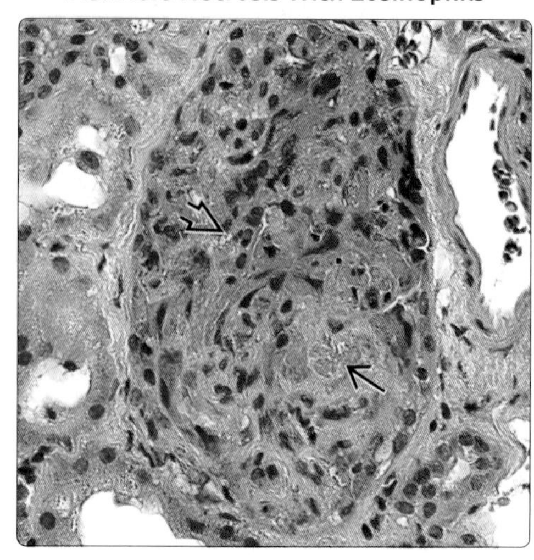

(Left) *Periodic acid-Schiff stain of a glomerulus with a fibrocellular crescent ⇨ and periglomerular inflammation is partially compressing the glomerulus with rupture of Bowman capsule ➡, typical of crescents of whatever etiology.* **(Right)** *PAS-stained glomerulus shows segmental sclerosing lesion with a fibrous crescent and capsular adhesion. Various stages of healing of crescentic GN may be seen in the same renal biopsy as in ANCA disease.*

Small Fibrocellular Crescent

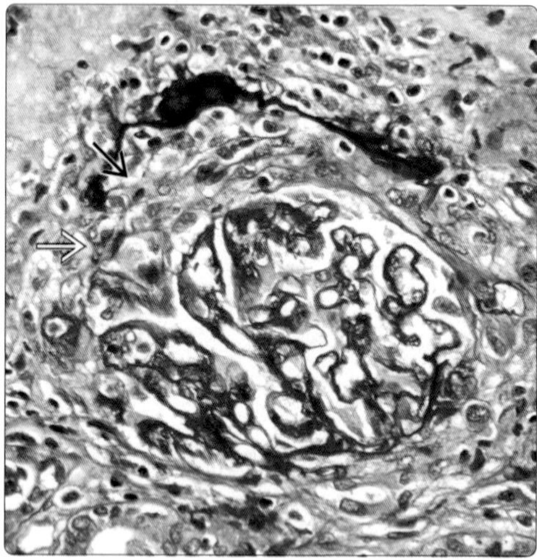

Segmental Sclerosis With Fibrous Crescent

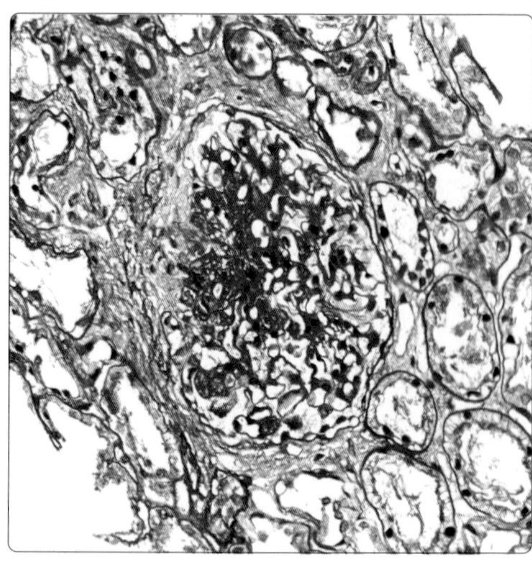

(Left) *45-year-old woman with positive anti-MPO antibodies, asthma, and eosinophilia with chronic sclerosing glomerulonephritis shows fibrocellular crescents. (Courtesy J. Pullman, MD.)* **(Right)** *In the same case with EGPA (CS) and positive anti-MPO antibodies and chronic sclerosing glomerulonephritis shows fibrocellular crescent and active interstitial inflammation. (Courtesy J. Pullman, MD.)*

Segmental Sclerosis With Fibrocellular Crescents

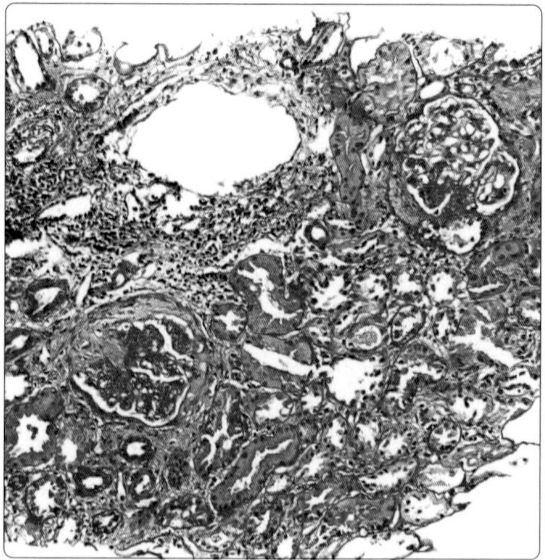

Segmental Sclerosis With Fibrocellular Crescent

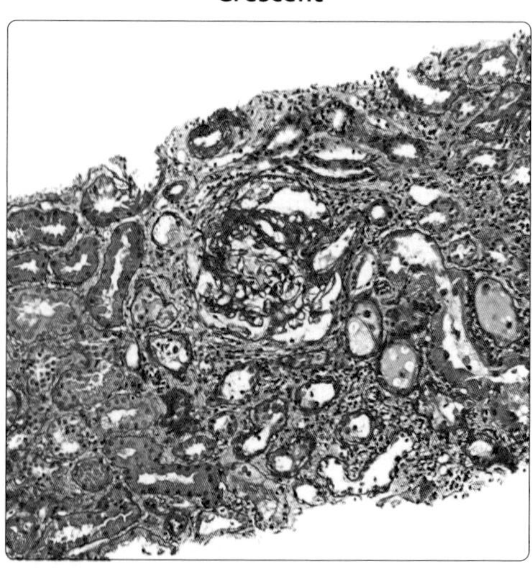

Active Interstitial Inflammation

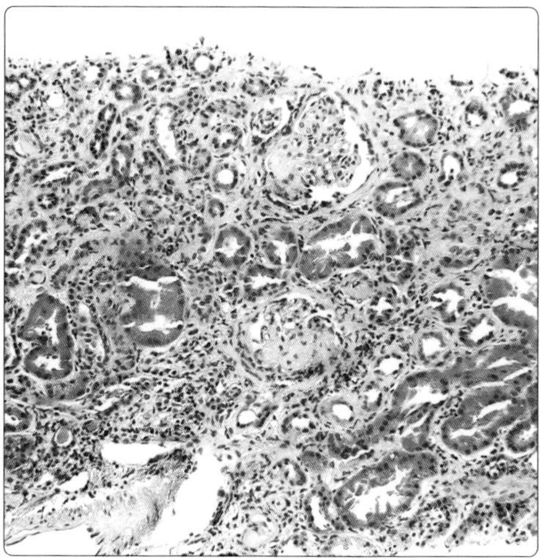

Eosinophil-Rich Interstitial Inflammation

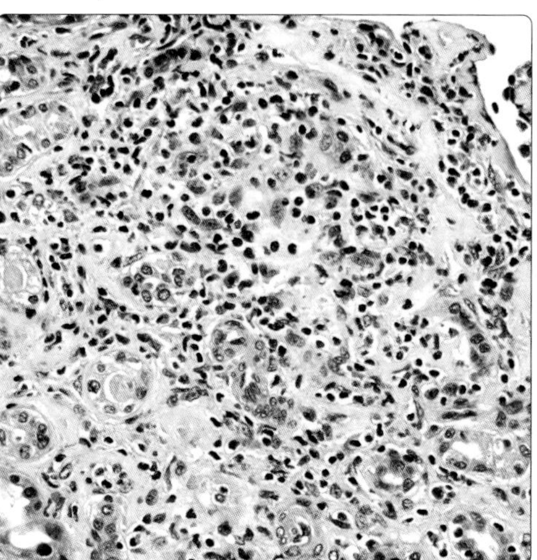

(Left) *45-year-old woman with EGPA (CS), MPO antibodies, and a nephritic syndrome shows segmental sclerosing glomerulonephritis along with moderate active interstitial inflammatory infiltrate with a few eosinophils. (Courtesy J. Pullman, MD.)* **(Right)** *H&E-stained renal biopsy shows an isolated eosinophil-rich tubulointerstitial inflammation in a patient with EGPA (CS) and a recent rise in creatinine. Without the glomerular or arterial lesions, this might be mistaken for a drug reaction.*

Sclerosing Granulomatous Inflammation

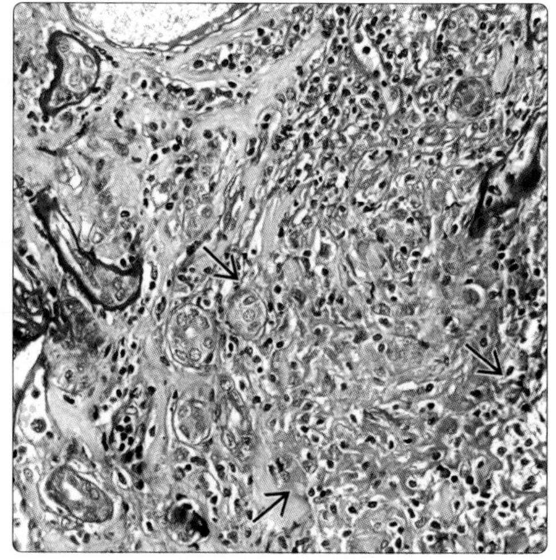

Granulomatous Inflammation

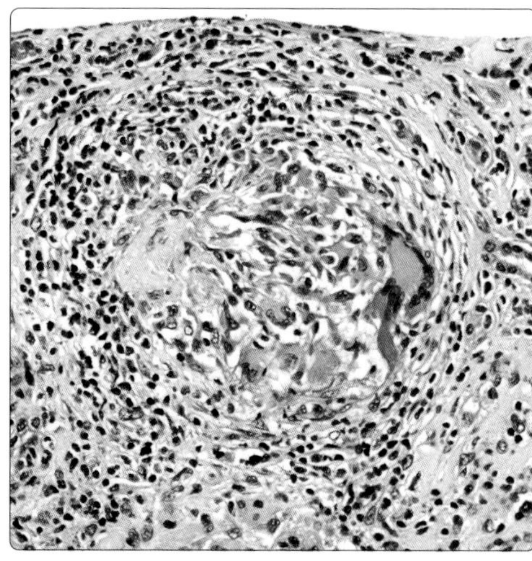

(Left) *EGPA (CS) patient with mild chronic insufficiency and previously treated with steroids shows a focus of sclerosing granulomatous inflammation ⇨ with residual lymphocytic infiltrate and interstitial fibrosis.* **(Right)** *Kidney biopsy from a EGPA (CS) patient with progressive renal failure reveals circumscribed interstitial granulomatous inflammation surrounded by a cuff of lymphocytes and eosinophils.*

Granulomatous Inflammation

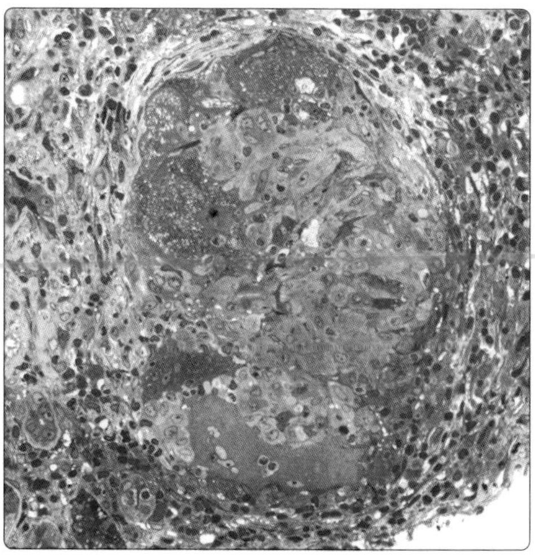

Small Vessel Vasculitis in Skin

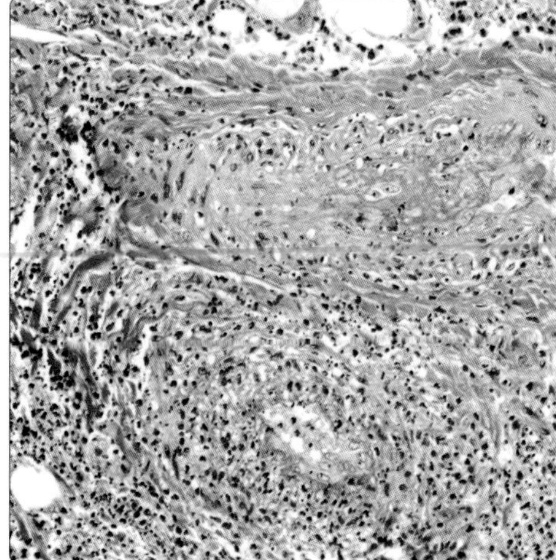

(Left) *A toluidine blue-stained, Epon-embedded section of a kidney biopsy from a EGPA (CS) patient shows a well-developed nonnecrotizing interstitial granuloma with giant cells. Granulomatous interstitial nephritis can be caused by drugs, sarcoidosis, certain infections, and granulomatosis with polyangiitis (Wegener).* **(Right)** *Palpable purpuric leg rash in an EGPA (CS) patient shows subcutaneous transmural arteritis and venulitis. ANCA-related diseases typically involve vasculitis in both arteries and veins.*

Drug-Induced ANCA Vasculitis

KEY FACTS

TERMINOLOGY

- ANCA-related vasculitis caused by an idiosyncratic autoimmune reaction to a drug

ETIOLOGY/PATHOGENESIS

- Most common drugs
  - Propylthiouracil, hydralazine, minocycline, anti-TNFα agents and levamisole (cocaine)
- Antimyeloperoxidase: ANCA (~ 90%)
- Antiproteinase 3: ANCA (< 10%)

CLINICAL ISSUES

- Fever, arthralgia, myalgia, rash, weight loss
- Skin involvement common: Purpura, ulcerations, ecchymotic lesions (Levamisole)
- Kidney affected in ~ 15% of DAV
  - Hematuria, proteinuria
  - Rapidly progressive renal failure
- Treatment: Discontinuation of drug

MICROSCOPIC

- Pauci-immune (necrotizing) crescentic glomerulonephritis
- Renal vasculitis, rare
- Cutaneous leukocytoclastic vasculitis, 60-80%
- Polyarteritis nodosa (minocycline)

ANCILLARY TESTS

- Pauci-immune pattern: Little or no IgG, IgA, IgM, C3, or C1q
- Little or no immune complex deposits by EM

TOP DIFFERENTIAL DIAGNOSES

- ANCA-related glomerulonephritis
- Lupus nephritis

DIAGNOSTIC CHECKLIST

- Dual positivity for MPO and PR3 is a strong clue for levamisole/cocaine DAV
- Outcome correlated with severity of vasculitis and crescentic GN

(Left) *45-year-old woman with Graves disease treated with propylthiouracil for 25 months presented with acute nephritic syndrome and renal failure. Kidney biopsy shows acute, subacute, and chronic crescentic GN. IF stains were pauci-immune.* **(Right)** *Propylthiouracil-induced ANCA GN shows segmental fibrinoid necrotizing glomerulonephritis with a cellular crescent. The adjacent glomerulus is unremarkable.*

Propylthiouracil-Induced ANCA-GN

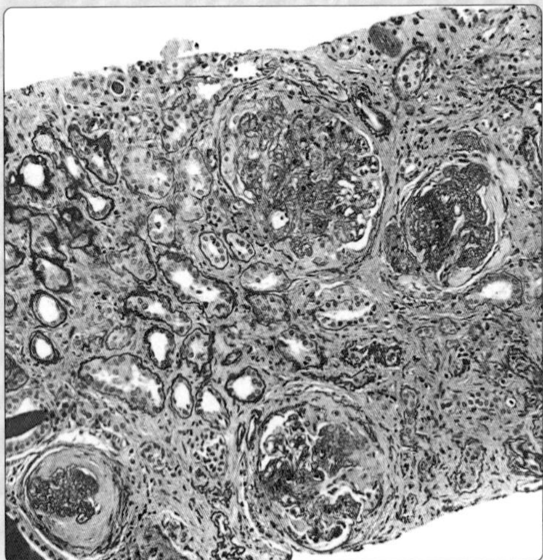

Segmental Necrotizing Crescentic GN

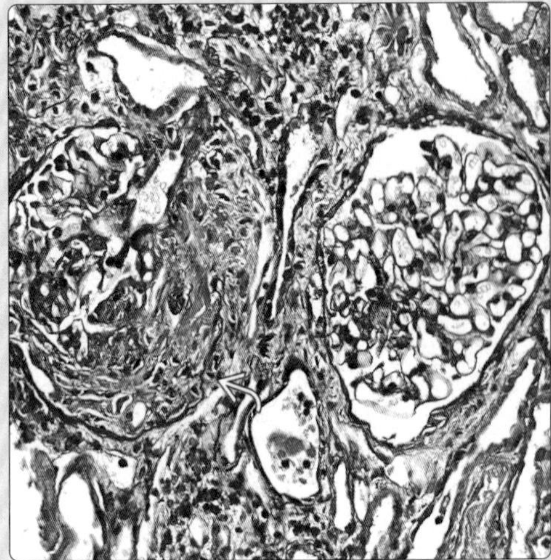

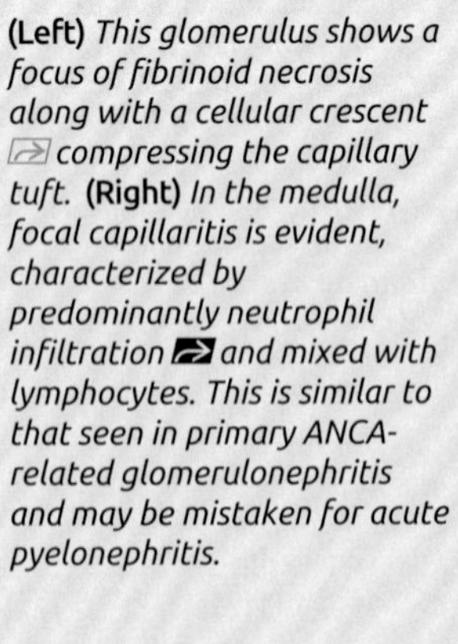

(Left) *This glomerulus shows a focus of fibrinoid necrosis along with a cellular crescent compressing the capillary tuft.* **(Right)** *In the medulla, focal capillaritis is evident, characterized by predominantly neutrophil infiltration and mixed with lymphocytes. This is similar to that seen in primary ANCA-related glomerulonephritis and may be mistaken for acute pyelonephritis.*

Hydralazine-Induced ANCA-GN

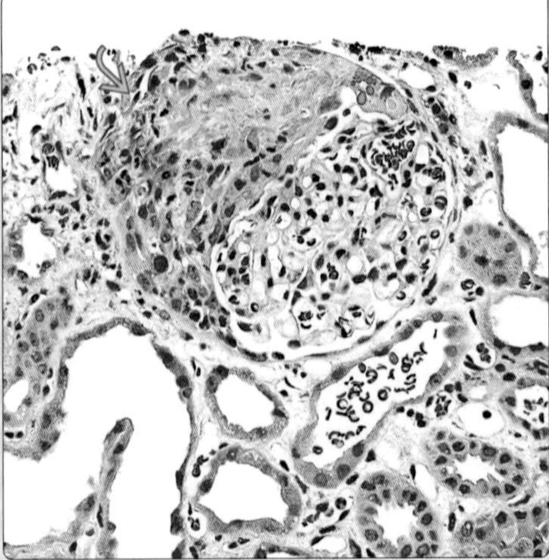

Hydralazine DAV With Medullary Capillaritis

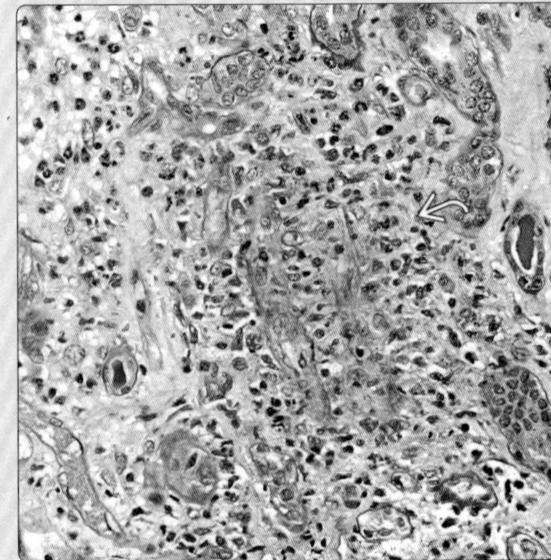

TERMINOLOGY

Abbreviations

- Drug-induced antineutrophil cytoplasmic antibodies (ANCA) vasculitis (DAV)

Definitions

- ANCA-related vasculitis caused by an idiosyncratic autoimmune reaction to a drug

ETIOLOGY/PATHOGENESIS

Autoimmune Response

- Immune system activation by drug or its metabolites
- Autoantibodies to ANCA and other targets
  - ANA, dsDNA, histone, phospholipids
  - Exact mechanisms are not understood, probably idiosyncratic
- Most common drugs
  - Propylthiouracil, hydralazine, minocycline, levamisole (cocaine), antitumor necrosis factor-α (TNFα) agents
- Variable risk with regard to dose and duration of each drug

ANCA

- Antimyeloperoxidase: ANCA (~ 90%)
- Antiproteinase 3: ANCA (< 10%)
- Other ANCA specificities: Elastase, lactoferrin, cathepsin G, bactericidal permeability increasing protein (BPI)

Drug-Specific Features

- Propylthiouracil (PTU)
  - 20-60% of patients on PTU develop high titers of MPO-ANCA
    - Restricted MPO epitope specificity and IgG subclass
  - 15-20% of ANCA(+) patients develop vasculitis
  - ↓ C4
  - Oxidation of PTU by MPO forming sulfonate metabolite
  - 91% have antiendothelial antibodies (AECA)
    - AECA correlates with disease activity
  - Other autoantibodies (ANA, dsDNA)
- Hydralazine
  - Dose and duration dependent in slow acetylators
  - Hydralazine reverses epigenetic silencing of PR3 and MPO in neutrophils to break tolerance
  - Stimulate aberrant neutrophil autoantigens causing MPO-ANCA and other p-ANCA specifities to elastase and lactoferrin
  - Renal involvement more common in hydralazine-DAV than in lupus-like syndrome caused by hydrolyze
- Anti-TNFα
  - Biological agents use to treat rheumatic and autoimmune diseases
    - Etanercept, adalimumab, infliximab, golimumab
  - Increase risk of autoimmune phenomena, single organ and multisystemic disease
  - MPO, PR3, antinuclear antibodies, anti-dsDNA antibodies
  - 15% develop clinical renal involvement
- Levamisole
  - Antihelminthic drug commonly added to illicit cocaine
  - Known immunomodulating agent
  - Characteristically, dual ANCA specificities (MPO and PR3)
    - Both MPO-ANCA (100%) and PR3-ANCA(50%) are formed
  - Other ANCA autoantigens: Elastase, cathepsin G, lactoferrin
- Minocycline
  - Used to treat acne and tick-borne diseases
  - MPO-ANCA
  - Polyarteritis nodosa
  - Kidney involvement rare

Other Drugs Implicated in DAV

- Antithyroid drugs: Methimazole, carbimazole, benzylthiouracil
- Antibiotics: Sulfasalazine, quinine, tetracycline, isoniazid
- Antihypertensive agents: Enalapril
- NSAID: Indomethacin, benoxaprofen
- Psychoactive drugs: Clozapine, thioridazine
- Interferons: Interferon beta, interferon alpha
- Miscellaneous: D-penicillamine, allopurinol, phenytoin

CLINICAL ISSUES

Epidemiology

- Mostly younger women affected with PTU DAV
- Older patients with hydralazine

Presentation

- Cutaneous leukocytoclastic vasculitis
  - Purpura, ulcerations, ecchymotic lesions (Levamisole)
- Renal
  - Kidney affected in ~ 15% of drug-induced ANCA cases
  - Rapidly progressive renal failure
  - Occasional acute and chronic renal disease
- Frequently preceded by constitutional symptoms
  - Fever, arthralgia, myalgia, rash, weight loss
- Other systems
  - Lung: Pleural inflammation, alveolar capillaritis and inflammation

Laboratory Tests

- Serology: ANA, ANCA usually p-ANCA or MPO-ANCA, antihistone antibodies, anti-ds (DNA [rare])
- ↑ C-reactive proteins, ESR

Treatment

- Discontinuation of drug
- Contraindicated in future

Prognosis

- Reversal or improvement with drug withdrawal
- Factors of poor prognosis
  - High titers of ANCA, particularly anti-MPO
  - Severity of vasculitis and crescentic GN
  - Lung involvement

MICROSCOPIC

Histologic Features

- Glomeruli
  - Focal glomerulitis
  - Necrotizing crescentic glomerulonephritis
- Tubulointerstitial lesions

Comparison of Primary and Drug-Induced ANCA Vasculitis

Parameter	Primary ANCA Vasculitis	Drug-Induced ANCA Vasculitis
Fever, malaise, arthralgias, rash	Similar	Similar
Age	Usually older	Younger (PTU)
Organ involvement	Multisystem	Multisystem
Renal involvement	Common (> 60%)	Relatively rare (15%)
Renal histopathology	More severe	Less severe or mild
Treatment	Immunosuppression	Withdrawal of drug
Renal survival	Worse	Better (Propylthiouracil)
Serology		
ANCA specificity	MPO or PR-3	MPO or PR-3
Dual ANCA reactivity	Rare	Common with levamisole (MPO+PR3 ANCA)
Other ANCA antigens	Rare	Common (elastase, lactoferrin, cathepsin G, BPI)
ANA	Rare positive	Often positive with lupus-like disease

Chen YX et al, 2012; Gao Y et al, 2009; Bonaci-Nikolic B et al, 2005.

- Active or chronic interstitial inflammation
- Vascular lesions
  - Medullary capillaritis
  - Other renal vasculitis rare
- Other organs
  - Cutaneous leukocytoclastic vasculitis, 60-80%
  - Polyneuropathy, 50%
  - Pulmonary capillaritis and alveolar hemorrhage
  - Polyarteritis nodosa (minocycline)

ANCILLARY TESTS

Immunofluorescence

- Pauci-immune pattern: Little or no IgG, IgA, IgM, C3, or C1q
- Fibrin/fibrinogen in crescents and areas of necrosis

Electron Microscopy

- Capillary wall disruption
- Little or no immune complex deposits

DIFFERENTIAL DIAGNOSIS

Primary ANCA-Related Vasculitis

- No history of drug use
- Absence of other autoantibody specificities

Lupus Nephritis

- Several of the drugs that cause ANCA also cause lupus autoantibodies and glomerulonephritis
- Immune complex deposition prominent by IF and EM

DIAGNOSTIC CHECKLIST

Clinically Relevant Pathologic Features

- Diagnosis of DAV is based on temporal relationship between onset of vasculitis and exposure to suspected drug
- Dual positivity for MPO and PR3 is a strong clue for levamisole/cocaine DAV

SELECTED REFERENCES

1. Markowitz GS et al: Drug-Induced Glomerular Disease: Direct Cellular Injury. Clin J Am Soc Nephrol. ePub, 2015
2. Agur T et al: Minocycline-induced polyarteritis nodosa-like vasculitis. Isr Med Assoc J. 16(5):322-3, 2014
3. Pendergraft WF 3rd et al: Trojan horses: drug culprits associated with antineutrophil cytoplasmic autoantibody (ANCA) vasculitis. Curr Opin Rheumatol. 26(1):42-9, 2014
4. Piga M et al: Biologics-induced autoimmune renal disorders in chronic inflammatory rheumatic diseases: systematic literature review and analysis of a monocentric cohort. Autoimmun Rev. 13(8):873-9, 2014
5. Tan CD et al: Systemic necrotizing vasculitis induced by isoniazid. Cardiovasc Pathol. 23(3):181-2, 2014
6. Xiao X et al: Diagnosis and classification of drug-induced autoimmunity (DIA). J Autoimmun. 48-49:66-72, 2014
7. Mavrakanas TA et al: Carbimazole-induced, ANCA-associated, crescentic glomerulonephritis: case report and literature review. Ren Fail. 35(3):414-7, 2013
8. Perez-Alvarez R et al: Biologics-induced autoimmune diseases. Curr Opin Rheumatol. 25(1):56-64, 2013
9. Chen YX et al: Propylthiouracil-induced antineutrophil cytoplasmic antibody (ANCA)-associated renal vasculitis versus primary ANCA-associated renal vasculitis: a comparative study. J Rheumatol. 39(3):558-63, 2012
10. Espinoza LR et al: Cocaine-induced vasculitis: clinical and immunological spectrum. Curr Rheumatol Rep. 14(6):532-8, 2012
11. Kermani TA et al: Polyarteritis nodosa-like vasculitis in association with minocycline use: a single-center case series. Semin Arthritis Rheum. 42(2):213-21, 2012
12. Pearson T et al: Vasculopathy related to cocaine adulterated with levamisole: A review of the literature. Dermatol Online J. 18(7):1, 2012
13. Radić M et al: Drug-induced vasculitis: a clinical and pathological review. Neth J Med. 70(1):12-7, 2012
14. McGrath MM et al: Contaminated cocaine and antineutrophil cytoplasmic antibody-associated disease. Clin J Am Soc Nephrol. 6(12):2799-805, 2011
15. Csernok E et al: Clinical and immunological features of drug-induced and infection-induced proteinase 3-antineutrophil cytoplasmic antibodies and myeloperoxidase-antineutrophil cytoplasmic antibodies and vasculitis. Curr Opin Rheumatol. 22(1):43-8, 2010
16. Parekh K et al: Onset of Wegener's granulomatosis during therapy with golimumab for rheumatoid arthritis: a rare adverse event? Rheumatology (Oxford). 49(9):1785-7, 2010
17. Gao Y et al: Review article: Drug-induced anti-neutrophil cytoplasmic antibody-associated vasculitis. Nephrology (Carlton). 14(1):33-41, 2009
18. Bonaci-Nikolic B et al: Antineutrophil cytoplasmic antibody (ANCA)-associated autoimmune diseases induced by antithyroid drugs: comparison with idiopathic ANCA vasculitides. Arthritis Res Ther. 7(5):R1072-81, 2005

Necrotizing GN

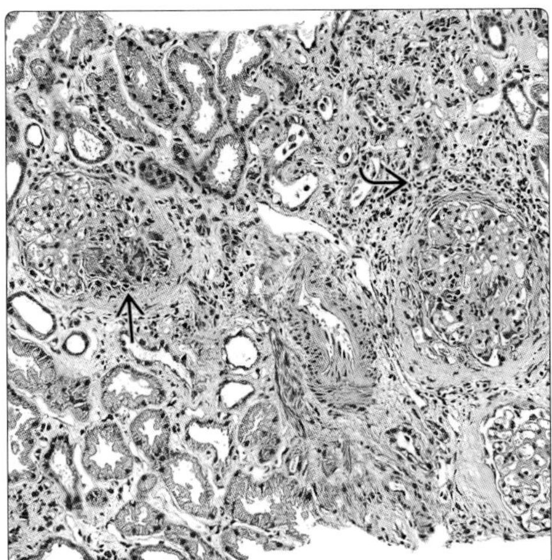

Early Segmental Glomerulitis

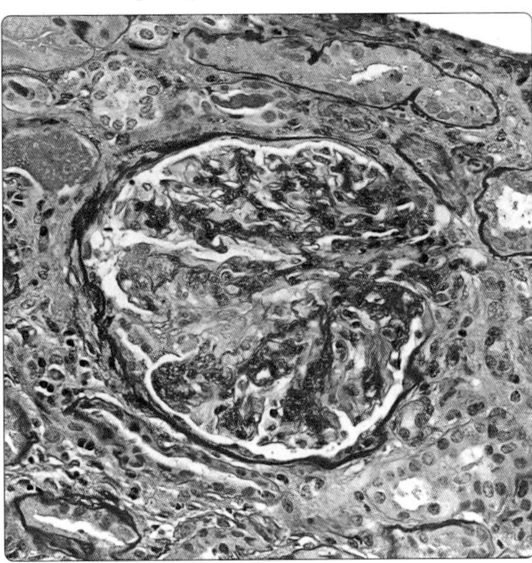

(Left) *A biopsy from a 25 year old treated with propylthiouracil for hyperthyroidism shows segmental necrotizing GN → and a patchy mononuclear interstitial nephritis →.* **(Right)** *A 50-year-old diabetic patient treated with hydralazine for 2 years presented with hematuria and mild renal insufficiency. This glomerulus shows diabetic changes superimposed by early segmental necrotizing glomerulitis. Drug-induced ANCA glomerulonephritis (GN) is often mild compared with primary ANCA-related GN.*

Segmental Necrotizing GN

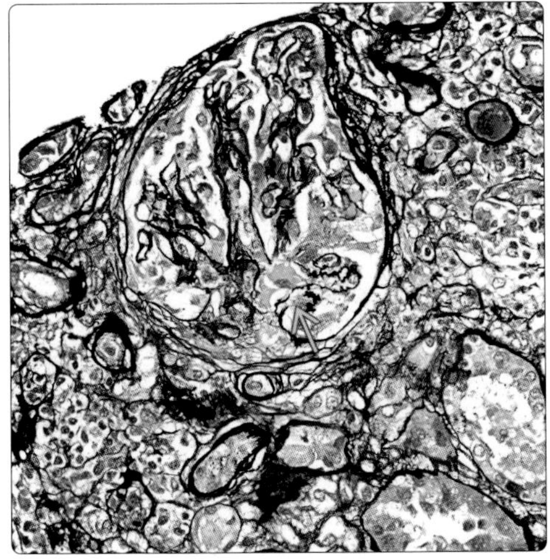

Crescentic GN Secondary to Anti-TNFα Therapy

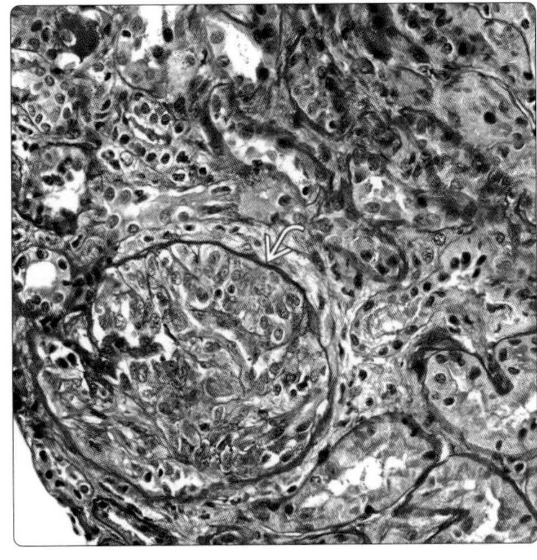

(Left) *An 80-year-old woman with recent hydralazine therapy for hypertension presented with acute renal failure. This glomerulus shows segmental fibrinoid necrosis → without a cellular crescent, surrounded by active interstitial inflammation.* **(Right)** *A 55-year-old woman with infliximab for rheumatoid arthritis presented with acute renal failure and positive high titer of MPO-ANCA. A large cellular crescent → fills Bowman space and obscures the architecture of the glomerular capillary tuft.*

Pauci-Immune Pattern of Immunofluorescence

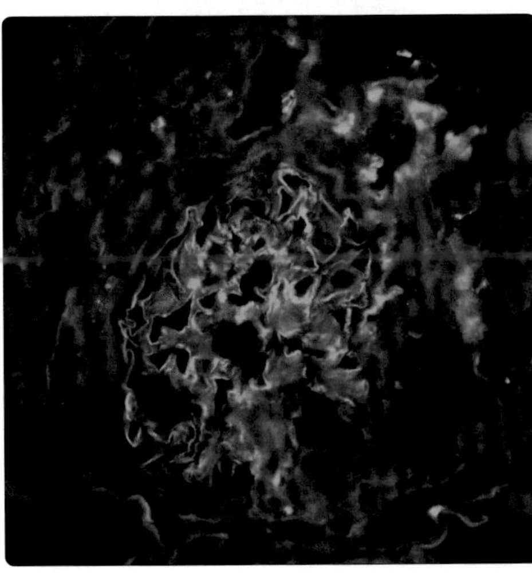

Levamisole-ANCA-Associated Skin Lesions

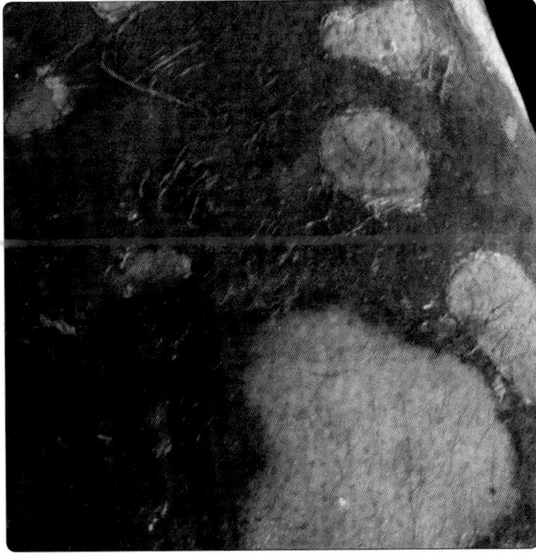

(Left) *A case of hydralazine-induced, MPO ANCA-mediated, crescentic glomerulonephritis shows no significant immune deposit for IgG within the glomerulus, characteristic of the pauci-immune GN related to ANCA.* **(Right)** *The lower extremity of this patient with MPO ANCA has areas of ecchymosis and necrotic ulceration. Patients ingesting illicit levamisole-contaminated cocaine can develop skin lesions associated with ANCA (not uncommonly to both MPO and PR3).*

Polyarteritis Nodosa

KEY FACTS

TERMINOLOGY

- Necrotizing inflammation of medium-sized or small arteries without glomerulonephritis or vasculitis in arterioles, capillaries, or venules

ETIOLOGY/PATHOGENESIS

- Idiopathic in majority
- Hepatitis B virus, hepatitis C virus
- Mutation in *CECR1* (autosomal recessive)

CLINICAL ISSUES

- HBV association in ~ 36% of PAN cases, endemic areas
- Adult: Peak at 3rd to 6th decade; children: 7-11 years
- Multisystemic involvement
- ANCA negative
- Kidney frequently involved (70-80%)
- New-onset hypertension, sometimes malignant range
- Cyclophosphamide and steroids, 90% remission rate

IMAGING

- Angiography localizes microaneurysms and stenosis

MICROSCOPIC

- Intralobar, arcuate, and, rarely, interlobular arteries affected (medium-sized vessels)
- Fibrinoid necrosis and transmural and periarterial inflammation
- Neutrophilic and mononuclear inflammatory infiltrate
- Late arterial lesions include aneurysms and stenosis
- Normal glomeruli located away from vasculitis
- Disruption of internal and external elastic laminae
- Intravascular thrombosis with occlusion

TOP DIFFERENTIAL DIAGNOSES

- Kawasaki disease
- ANCA-related small vessel vasculitides
- Systemic lupus erythematosus
- Fibromuscular dysplasia

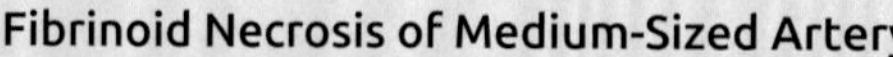

Fibrinoid Necrosis of Medium-Sized Artery

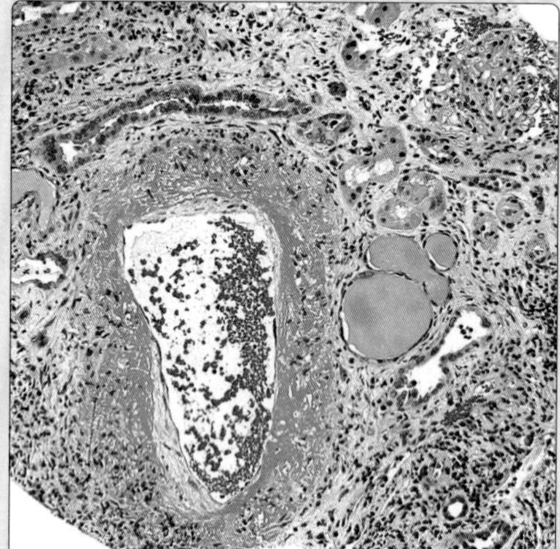

Disruption of Elastica

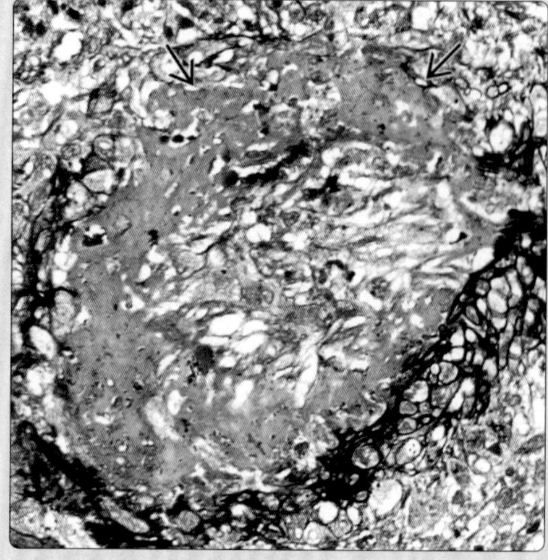

(Left) *Kidney biopsy in polyarteritis nodosa (PAN) shows circumferential, transmural fibrinoid necrosis and active inflammatory infiltrate composed of neutrophils and lymphocytes.* **(Right)** *High magnification shows an artery with fibrinoid necrosis and segmental loss of elastic lamina → in a case of PAN. Elastin stains increase sensitivity to detect old lesions of arteritis.*

Circumferential Fibrinoid Necrosis

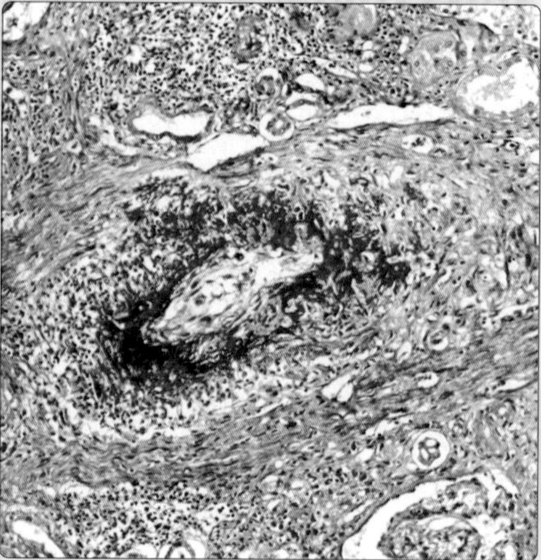

Ischemic Changes

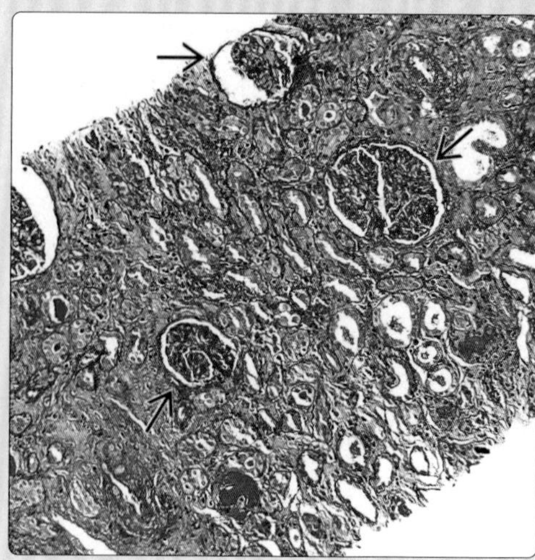

(Left) *An interlobular artery in the kidney shows circumferential fibrinoid necrosis (fuchsinophilic) in a trichrome-stained section surrounded by active transmural inflammatory infiltrate.* **(Right)** *Low magnification of a kidney biopsy shows mainly mild to moderate ischemic collapse without evidence of crescentic GN →. Ischemic simplification of tubules and mild interstitial inflammation is noted.*

TERMINOLOGY

Abbreviations

- Polyarteritis nodosa (PAN)

Definitions

- Chapel Hill Consensus Conference criteria 2012
  - Necrotizing arteritis of medium-sized or small arteries without GN or vasculitis in arterioles, capillaries, or venules
    - Not associated with antineutrophil cytoplasmic antibodies
- American College of Rheumatology criteria
  - Weight loss ≥ 4 kg, livedo reticularis, testicular pain or tenderness, myalgias, weakness or leg tenderness, mono- or polyneuropathy, diastolic BP > 90 mm Hg, elevated BUN or creatinine, hepatitis B virus, biopsy diagnosis of small or medium-sized arteries, arteriography with aneurysms or occlusions in visceral arteries
    - ≥ 3 of above criteria have high sensitivity and specificity for diagnosis
- EULAR/PRINTO/PRES criteria for childhood PAN
  - Necrotizing vasculitis, angiographic abnormalities, and either skin involvement, myalgia/muscle tenderness, hypertension, peripheral neuropathy, or renal involvement

ETIOLOGY/PATHOGENESIS

Infectious Agents

- Hepatitis B virus (HBV)
- Possibly other viral infections
  - Hepatitis C virus (HCV)
    - Most also infected with HBV
    - ~ 20% of HCV(+) vasculitis is PAN
  - Rarely HIV, parvovirus B-19, cytomegalovirus

Genetic

- Mutation in *CECR1* (autosomal recessive)
- Encodes adenosine deaminase 2
  - Major extracellular enzyme for inactivating adenosine
  - Also acts as growth factor
- Israeli (Georgian heritage), Germans, and Turks
  - 10% carrier frequency in Georgian Jews in Israel

Other Triggers

- Exposure to silica-containing compounds
- In majority, etiology unknown

Pathogenesis

- Immunologically mediated
  - Chronic immune-complex-mediated disease with HBV
  - Antigen-specific T-cell-mediated immune mechanisms with CD4 T cells and dendritic cells
  - May be microbial or autoantigen in vessel wall
- Participation of neutrophils and macrophages
  - Weakness in vessel wall leads to thrombosis or fibrosis and microaneurysm formation
- Chronic, cyclic insults support presence of different stages of vasculitis in tissue and relapses

CLINICAL ISSUES

Epidemiology

- Incidence
  - 1-2/million in Europe and USA
    - Prevalence: Up to 31/million
  - Up to 77/million in endemic areas for HBV infection, accounting for 36% of PAN cases
  - < 5% of PAN patients HBV(+) in developed countries
- Age
  - Adults: Peak at 3rd to 6th decade
  - Children: 7-11 years
- Sex
  - Male predilection (M:F = 2:1)
- Ethnicity
  - Involves all ethnic groups
  - HLA B27, B39 associated

Presentation

- Multisystemic clinical symptoms related to ischemia and dependent on organ involved and disease severity
- Constitutional symptoms: Fever, malaise, weight loss, myalgia, abdominal pain, arthralgia
- Renal
  - Kidney frequently involved (70-80%)
    - Focal renal infarction (~ 30%)
    - Microaneurysms (~ 65%)
    - Hematuria, proteinuria (~ 20%)
    - Loin pain
    - Acute renal failure
  - New-onset hypertension, sometimes malignant range
  - Rare: Rupture of kidney with perirenal hematoma
  - Massive retroperitoneal and peritoneal hemorrhage
- Heart
  - Ischemic heart disease
- Neurologic (10%)
  - Hemiplegia, visual loss, mononeuritis multiplex
- Skin
  - Varied lesions: Palpable purpura, necrotic with peripheral gangrene, livedo reticularis, ulcers
  - Subcutaneous nodules
- Skeletal muscle and mesentery (30%)
- Gastrointestinal, peripheral nerves (50%)

Laboratory Tests

- Anemia, leukocytosis, thrombocytosis
- Elevation of ESR and C-reactive protein
- Positive HBV serology in some cases
- No specific serologic tests
- No significant association with ANCA
- Rarely, ANCA positive (usually perinuclear) by indirect IF only, when overlap with microscopic polyangiitis

Treatment

- Steroids are 1st-line therapy; remission in 50%
- Cyclophosphamide/steroids for severe cases; remission in 90%
- Plasma exchange/plasmapheresis in refractory cases
- HBV-associated PAN needs antiviral therapy

Prognosis

- Fulminant disease with < 5-year survival
- 40% of patients relapse
- 5 factor score (FFS) estimates prognosis
  - Scores renal (Cr > 1.6 mg/dL, proteinuria > 1 gm/24 hr), GI, cardiac, and CNS involvement
  - Lower score correlates with better 5-year survival
  - 3x risk of mortality with renal involvement

IMAGING

Ultrasonographic Findings

- Pulsed and color Doppler ultrasonography
  - Localization of microaneurysm (seen in 50-60%)

Computed Tomography Angiography

- Microaneurysms (1-5 mm) at artery bifurcations
- Stenotic lesions
- Tc-99m DMSA uptake scanning detects patchy renal parenchymal disease

MICROSCOPIC

Histologic Features

- Glomeruli
  - Mostly varying degrees of ischemic collapse
  - Global glomerulosclerosis in cortical scars
  - Normal glomeruli located away from vasculitis
  - Rarely, focal crescentic GN (pauci-immune type)
    - Suggests overlap of PAN and microscopic polyangiitis
- Tubules and interstitium
  - Acute ischemic infarction along distribution of affected artery
  - Tubular injury, atrophy, and mild interstitial fibrosis
  - Active &/or chronic interstitial and periarterial inflammation
  - Granulomatous inflammation absent
- Arteries
  - Intralobar, arcuate, and, rarely interlobular artery (medium-sized vessels)
    - Small arterioles and capillaries lacking muscular coat not affected
  - Obliterative arteritis (acute, subacute, or chronic)
  - Transmural fibrinoid necrosis and inflammation
    - Fuchsinophilic/eosinophilic amorphous fibrinoid material in areas of necrosis
    - Destruction of medial smooth muscle
    - Disruption of internal and external elastic laminae
  - Moderate to intense inflammatory infiltrate
    - Neutrophils, eosinophils with karyorrhexis
    - Activated T lymphocytes and macrophages
    - Increased expression of matrix metalloproteinase-1, tumor necrosis factor α, and decreased smoothelin
  - Varying degrees of luminal narrowing, neoangiogenesis
  - Intravascular thrombosis with occlusion
  - Acute and chronic/healed lesions can coexist in same vessel
  - Healed lesions show progressive fibrotic change, obliterative arteriopathy, and intimal hyperplasia
    - Late lesions include arterial aneurysms
    - Progressive scarring can lead to stenosis

DIFFERENTIAL DIAGNOSIS

Kawasaki Disease

- Mucocutaneous lymph node syndrome
- Mononuclear infiltrate
- Less fibrinoid necrosis

ANCA-Related Small Vessel Vasculitides

- Multisystemic microscopic polyangiitis
- Granulomatosis with polyangiitis (Wegener)
- Churg-Strauss syndrome (CSS)

Fibromuscular Dysplasia

- Lesions lack fibrinoid necrosis
- No inflammation
- Disorganized media

Systemic Lupus Erythematosus

- Eosinophils in CSS
- PAN-like pauci-immune vasculitis
- Positive serology for SLE

DIAGNOSTIC CHECKLIST

Clinically Relevant Pathologic Features

- Arkin classification
  - Stages I and II: Acute arterial inflammatory lesion
  - Stages III and IV: Chronic arterial lesions
- Medium artery aneurysm seen on imaging studies
- Focal and patchy involvement of medium-sized or (rarely) small arteries with necrotizing inflammation
- No ANCA or crescentic GN
- Biopsy from affected area (e.g., skin, skeletal muscle) or organ improves diagnostic yield

Pathologic Interpretation Pearls

- Absence of vasculitic lesion (usually larger vessel) does not exclude diagnosis due to sampling

SELECTED REFERENCES

1. Hernández-Rodríguez J et al: Diagnosis and classification of polyarteritis nodosa. J Autoimmun. 48-49:84-9, 2014
2. Navon Elkan P et al: Mutant adenosine deaminase 2 in a polyarteritis nodosa vasculopathy. N Engl J Med. 370(10):921-31, 2014
3. Eleftheriou D et al: Systemic polyarteritis nodosa in the young: a single-center experience over thirty-two years. Arthritis Rheum. 65(9):2476-85, 2013
4. Jennette JC et al: 2012 revised International Chapel Hill Consensus Conference Nomenclature of Vasculitides. Arthritis Rheum. 65(1):1-11, 2013
5. Masuda M et al: Pathological features of classical polyarteritis nodosa: analysis of 19 autopsy cases. Pathol Res Pract. 209(3):161-6, 2013
6. Saadoun D et al: Hepatitis C virus-associated polyarteritis nodosa. Arthritis Care Res (Hoboken). 63(3):427-35, 2011
7. Dillon MJ et al: Medium-size-vessel vasculitis. Pediatr Nephrol. 25(9):1641-52, 2010
8. Ozen S et al: EULAR/PRINTO/PRES criteria for Henoch-Schönlein purpura, childhood polyarteritis nodosa, childhood Wegener granulomatosis and childhood Takayasu arteritis: Ankara 2008. Part II: Final classification criteria. Ann Rheum Dis. 69(5):798-806, 2010
9. Pagnoux C et al: Clinical features and outcomes in 348 patients with polyarteritis nodosa: a systematic retrospective study of patients diagnosed between 1963 and 2005 and entered into the French Vasculitis Study Group Database. Arthritis Rheum. 62(2):616-26, 2010
10. Ruperto N et al: EULAR/PRINTO/PRES criteria for Henoch-Schönlein purpura, childhood polyarteritis nodosa, childhood Wegener granulomatosis and childhood Takayasu arteritis: Ankara 2008. Part I: Overall methodology and clinical characterisation. Ann Rheum Dis. 69(5):790-7, 2010

Infarct: External Surface

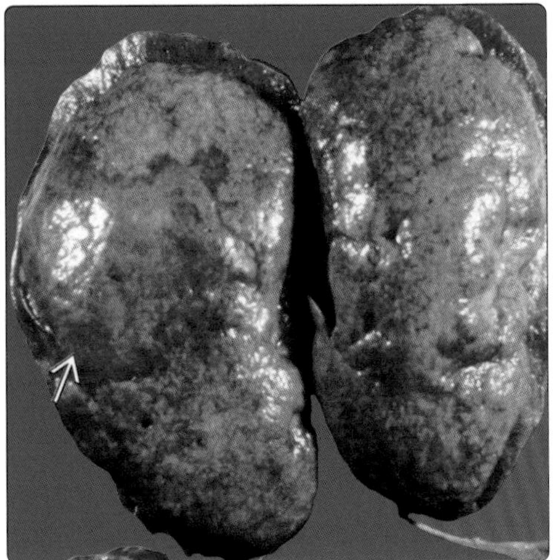

Infarct: Cross Section

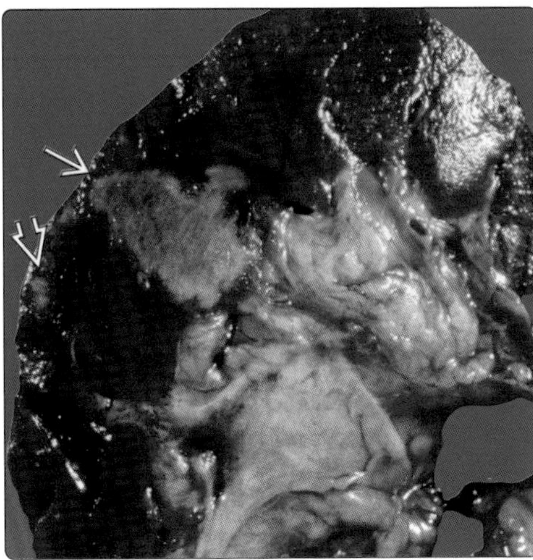

(Left) *Gross photograph shows autopsy kidneys from a patient with widespread PAN. Note a large, paler area of the left-sided kidney with a hemorrhagic border representing an infarct* ➡*.* **(Right)** *Cut section from the kidney shows large, pale (ischemic) infarct* ➡ *with a hemorrhagic border. Smaller pale areas* ➡ *are also noted in the cortex adjacent to the large infarct, suggesting additional cortical infarcts.*

Fibrinoid Necrosis

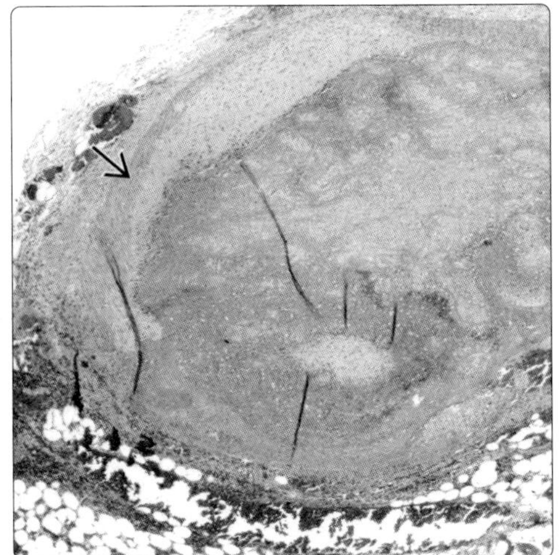

Cortical Infarct

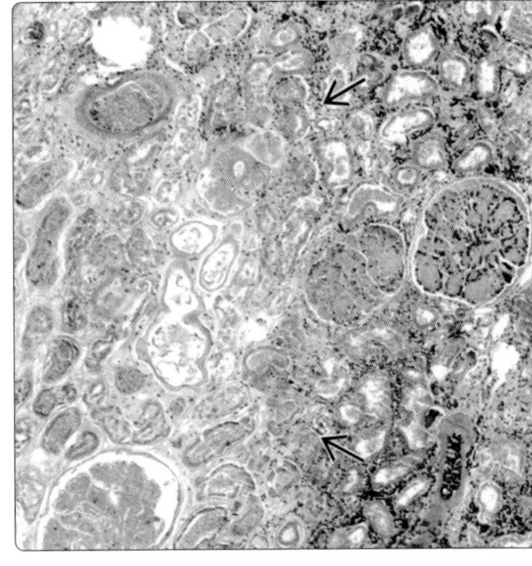

(Left) *Section of a large renal artery in the pelvis shows arterial inflammation* ➡*, fibrinoid necrosis, and thrombosis filling the lumen. This leads to areas of cortical and medullary infarction.* **(Right)** *Microscopic section from a kidney shows ischemic infarction of the renal cortex with a hemorrhagic border and congestion seen on the right side* ➡*.*

Thrombosis

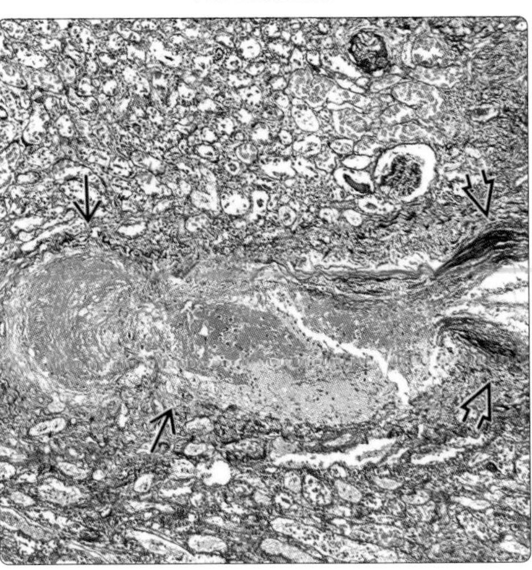

Microaneurysms

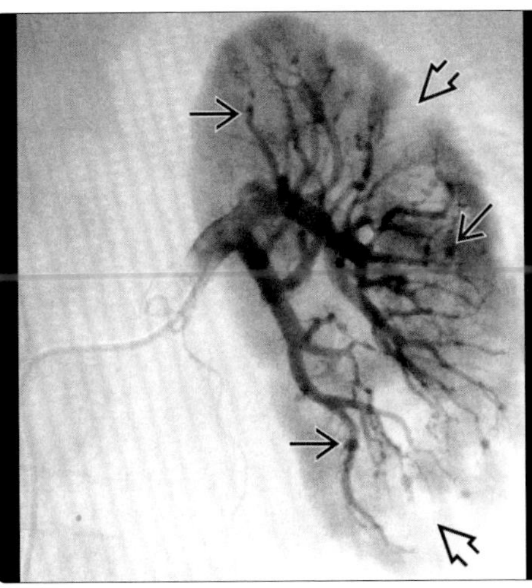

(Left) *The artery is stained with EVG, showing lack of elastic lamina* ➡ *in areas of fibrinoid necrosis and thrombosis. A preserved portion of the artery* ➡ *shows multiple layers of elastic lamina consistent with arteriosclerosis.* **(Right)** *Digital subtraction angiogram shows characteristic multiple microaneurysms* ➡*. There are also areas within the kidney parenchyma with decreased perfusion consistent with infarcts* ➡*. Infarcts may represent necrosis or thrombosis. Hemorrhage may occur if aneurysms rupture.*

(Left) *A medium-sized artery from the subcutaneous tissue (EVG stain) shows residual transmural inflammatory infiltrate along with obliterative arteriopathy and segmental disruption of the elastic lamina. The elastin stain is particularly useful in chronic lesions.* **(Right)** *A medium-sized artery (arcuate type) in the kidney from a patient with PAN shows no evidence of vasculitis with preserved internal and external elastic lamina. The duplication of the internal elastica (fibroelastosis) ➡ is typical of hypertension.*

Fragmented Elastica

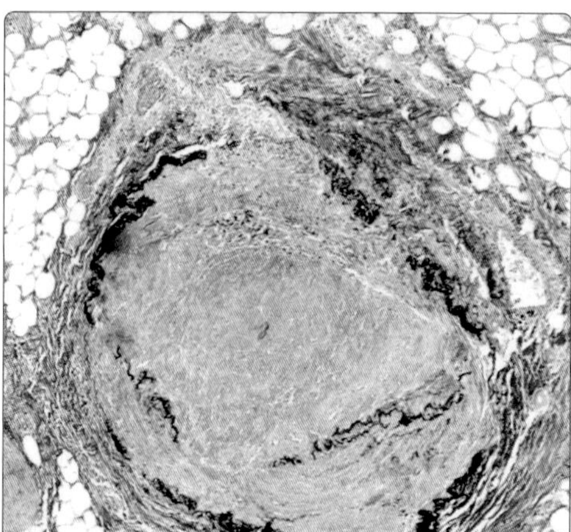

Artery With Fibroelastosis

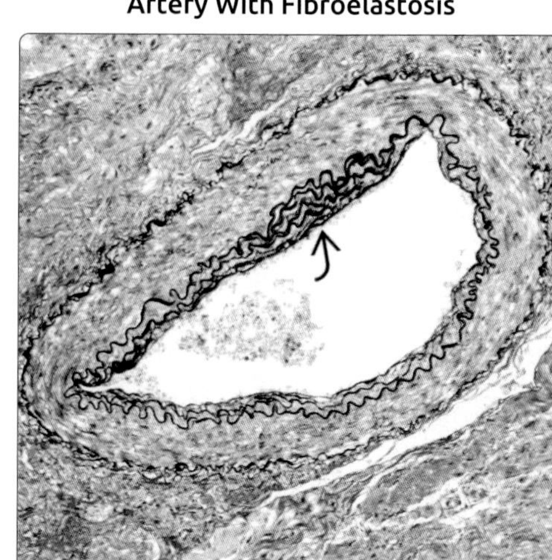

(Left) *Trichrome-stained low-magnification kidney section shows 2 medium-sized vessels with obliterative features ➡ following acute PAN. The multiple glomeruli are spared aside from ischemic changes and show no crescents.* **(Right)** *EVG-stained low-magnification kidney section shows interruption and extensive loss of elastic lamina within the obliterated vessel walls.*

Obliterative Arteritis and Fibrosis

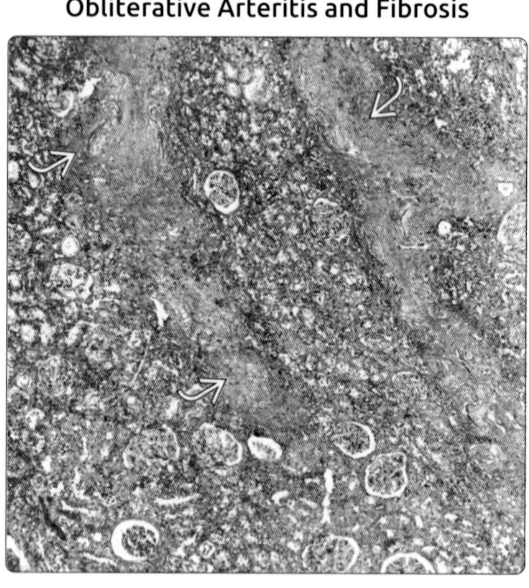

Fragmented Elastica in Old Arteritis

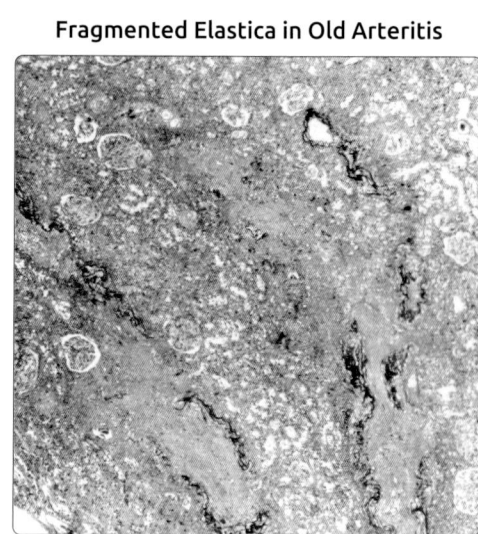

(Left) *In addition to a generally unremarkable but ischemic glomerulus, some of the small arteries show evidence of sclerosis and are surrounded by sparse inflammatory infiltrate without significant vasculitis ➡.* **(Right)** *An overlapping form of PAN and microscopic polyangiitis with a rare glomerulus shows fibrocellular crescents ➡. An adjacent glomerulus is uninvolved.*

Arteriosclerosis

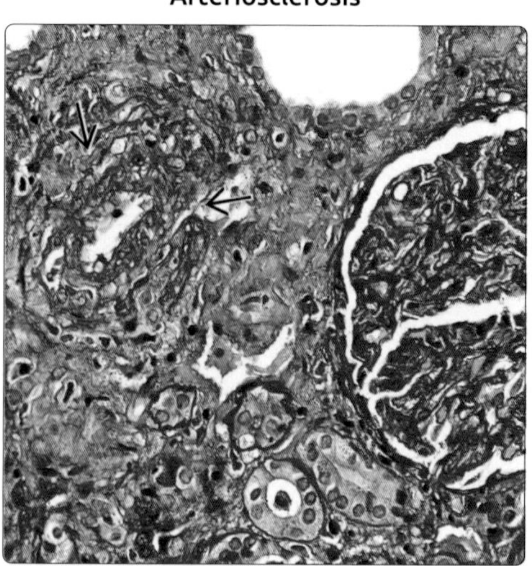

Fibrocellular Crescent

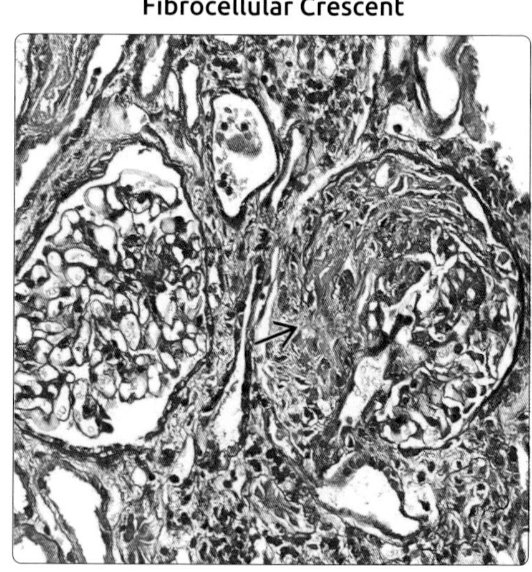

Circumferential Fibrinoid Necrosis

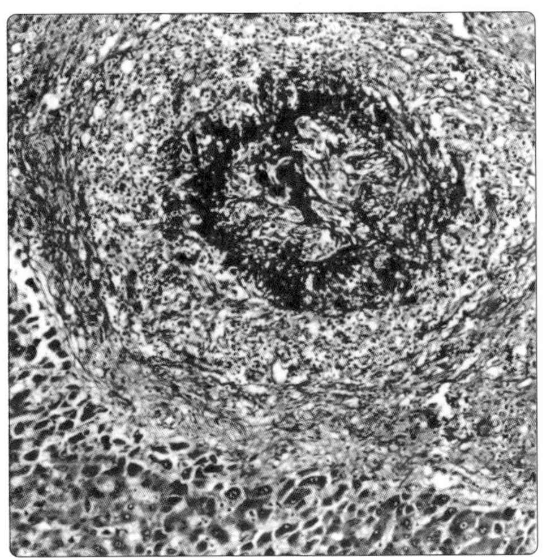

Transmural Arteritis

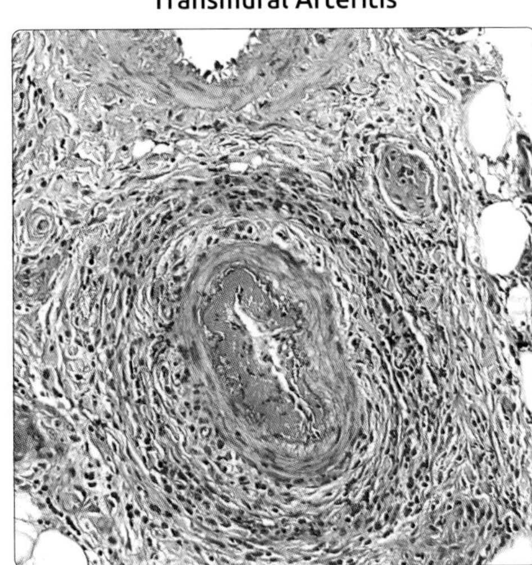

(Left) *A medium-sized artery in the liver parenchyma shows circumferential fibrinoid necrosis along with active inflammatory infiltrate.* **(Right)** *A medium-sized artery adjacent to the pancreas from the same autopsy case of PAN shows fibrinoid intimal necrosis and transmural and severe adventitial inflammation and arteritis.*

Fibrinoid Necrosis

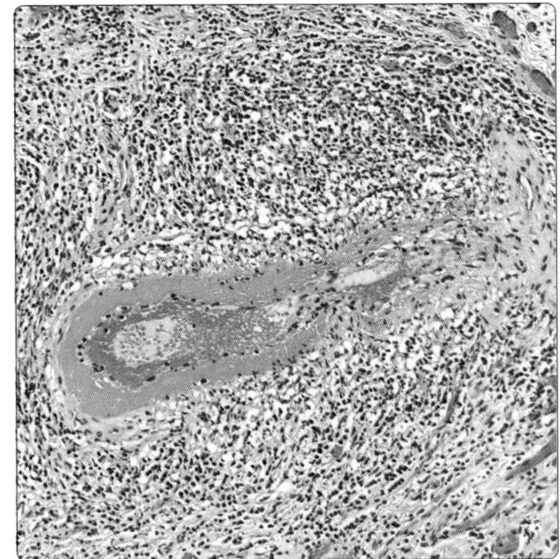

Microaneurysm and Thrombosis

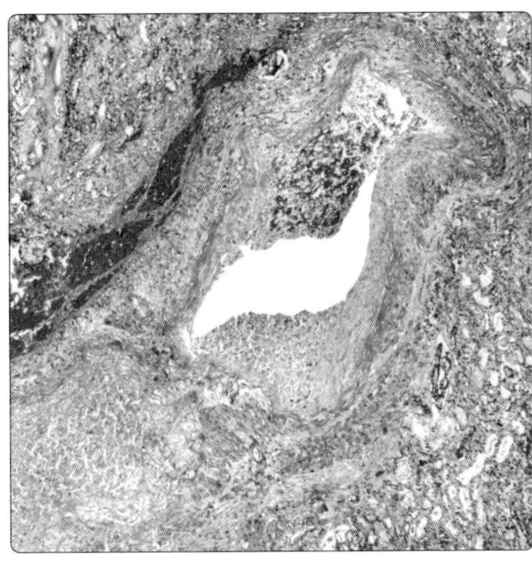

(Left) *The colonic adventitia layer shows circumferential fibrinoid necrosis surrounded by intense active inflammatory infiltrate without evidence of preserved media or adventitia.* **(Right)** *Trichrome-stained kidney section shows a healing PAN of a medium-sized vessel with focal thrombosis and early microaneurysm formation. It is common to have both active and healed lesions in PAN.*

Transmural Arteritis in Muscle

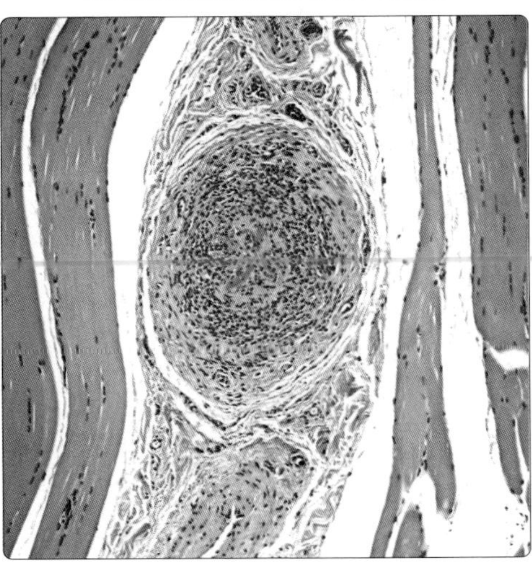

Livedo Reticularis

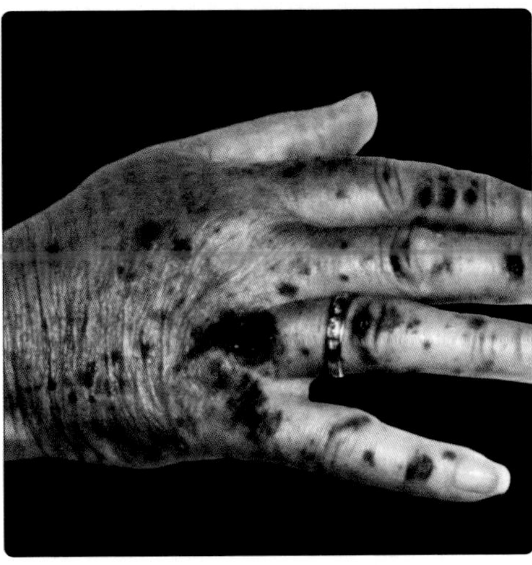

(Left) *Low-magnification view of a medium-sized artery in the perimysial area of skeletal muscle shows marked transmural arteritis with central fibrinoid necrosis.* **(Right)** *Clinical photo shows livedo reticularis along with palpable purpuric rash with occasional nodules in the skin.*

Kawasaki Disease

KEY FACTS

TERMINOLOGY

- Arteritis involves large, medium-sized, and small arteries and is associated with mucocutaneous lymph node syndrome and coronary arteritis

ETIOLOGY/PATHOGENESIS

- Activation of cells of innate and adaptive immunity likely caused by an exogenous trigger
- Role for antiendothelial antibodies

CLINICAL ISSUES

- High incidence in Japan (epidemic and endemic)
- 9-11 months of age in Japanese, 1.5-2 years in North Americans; M:F = 5:1
- Renal disease: Acute nephritic syndrome, acute renal failure
- Proteinuria
- Leukocytosis (17,000 ± 900 mm^3)
- Thrombocytosis, 600,000 to 1.5 million/mm^3
- Combination of aspirin and intravenous gamma-globulin therapy is mainstay
- Tumor necrosis factor inhibition

IMAGING

- Angiography (arteritis, dilatation, aneurysm, stenosis)
- DMSA renal SPECT (parenchymal inflammation and scarring)

MICROSCOPIC

- Panarteritis (commonly coronary arteries) involving intima and adventitial layer, with disruption of internal and external elastic lamina
- Arteritis, thrombosis, microaneurysms
- Focal/patchy or diffuse interstitial inflammation or scarring
- Glomerular lesions: Normal glomeruli, immune complex GN, thrombotic microangiopathy

TOP DIFFERENTIAL DIAGNOSES

- Polyarteritis nodosa in childhood

Transmural Renal Artery Inflammation

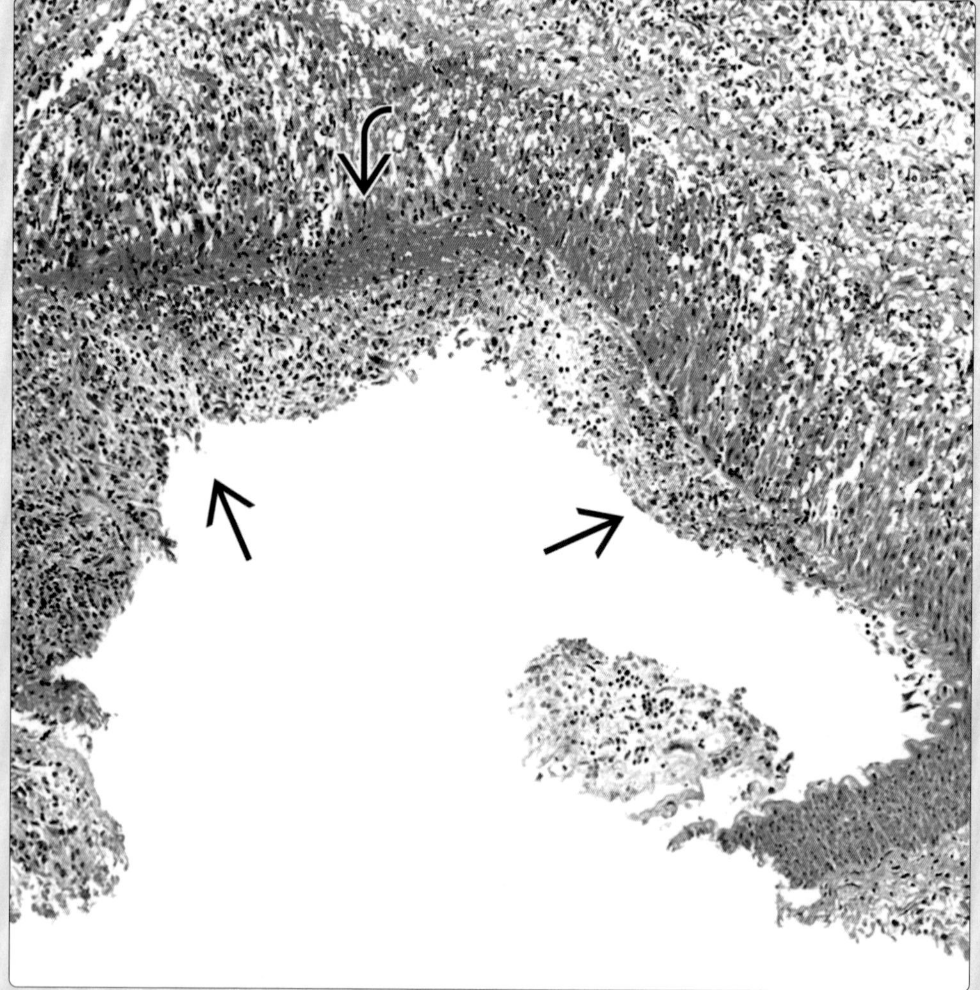

Renal artery branch in Kawasaki disease shows transmural acute inflammation ➔ with dilatation of the lumen, aneurysm formation, and focal fibrinoid necrosis ➔. (Courtesy J.C. Jennette, MD.)

TERMINOLOGY

Abbreviations

- Kawasaki disease (KD)

Synonyms

- Kawasaki syndrome
- Kawasaki disease arteritis

Definitions

- Chapel Hill Consensus Conference 2012
  - Arteritis involves medium and small arteries and is associated with mucocutaneous lymph node syndrome (MCLNS)
  - Coronary arteries are often involved
  - Aorta and veins may be involved
  - Usually occurs in infants and children
- Japan Kawasaki Disease Research Committee Criteria
  - Fever of unknown etiology for 5 days or more (95%)
  - Bilateral congestion of ocular conjunctivae (88%)
  - Reddening of lips and oropharyngeal mucosa and strawberry tongue (at least 1 finding) (90%)
  - Reddening, edema, and desquamation of digits in peripheral extremities (at least 1 finding) (90%)
  - Polymorphous exanthema of body trunk without vesicles or crusts (92%)
  - Acute nonpurulent swelling of cervical lymph nodes of 1.5 cm or more in diameter

ETIOLOGY/PATHOGENESIS

Environmental Exposure

- Exposure to an infectious agent is suggested based on epidemiologic considerations
- Susceptibility in infants with minimal or no immunity having an abnormal immune response
- Bacterial superantigen or viral infection

Genetic

- Interleukin 18 promoter gene polymorphism
- *HLA-Bw22* in Japanese, *Bw51* or combined *A2*, *B44*, *Cw5* in North Americans, *IL-21R* in Koreans

Pathogenesis

- Activation of cells (monocytes, T lymphocytes) regulatory T-cell dysfunction
- Inflammatory cytokines and chemokines activate endothelial cells, leading to vascular inflammation
- Possible role for antiendothelial antibodies
- Vasoactive (endothelin, nitric oxide) and growth factors (VEGF, PDGF) promote vascular permeability and myointimal proliferation
- Oligoclonal IgA response

Animal Model

- Candida albicans water-soluble fraction induces severe coronary arteritis with typical histologic features of KD

CLINICAL ISSUES

Epidemiology

- Incidence
  - Highest in Japan, Korea (239-105/100,000) in children under 5 years of age
  - Lower in Europe and North America (5-20/100,000)
  - Global sporadic or epidemic occurrence
  - Seasonal incidence, winter and early spring months
- Age
  - Almost exclusively children
    - 70% of all cases occur < 3 years of age
    - Peaks at age 9-11 months in Japanese
    - Other populations peak at age 1.5-2 years (e.g., North Americans)
- Sex
  - Male predominance (5:1)
- Ethnicity
  - Japanese and Koreans > Chinese > Polynesians > whites and blacks
  - All racial backgrounds may be affected with lesser frequency (5/100,000 in North Americans)

Presentation

- General constitutional symptoms in the acute phase
- Systemic disease involving skin, mucous membranes, and lymph nodes
- Phases of disease: Acute, subacute, convalescent
- Associated with medium-sized vessel arteritis, frequently affecting coronary arteries (15-25%)
- Exacerbation and recrudescence of symptoms during acute and subacute stages
- Renal
  - Hypertension related to renal artery disease
  - Usually mild and clinically silent
  - Sterile pyuria and proteinuria (β2 microglobulin)
  - Microscopic hematuria, acute nephritic syndrome
  - Mild renal insufficiency or acute renal failure

Laboratory Tests

- Generally nonspecific and nondiagnostic
- Reflect systemic inflammatory process
  - Cultures for infective agents are negative
  - Leukocytosis (17,000 ± 900 mm^3), anemia
  - Increased ESR and acute phase proteins
  - Thrombocytosis (600,000 to 1.5 million/mm^3)
  - Elevated liver enzymes
  - Diffuse cytoplasmic ANCA pattern, atypical
  - Elevated serum/urine filamin C and Meprin A

Treatment

- Combination of aspirin and intravenous gamma-globulin therapy is mainstay
  - For inflammatory symptoms and to reduce coronary artery complications
  - Aimed toward symptomatic relief and prevention of serious consequences (e.g., cardiac and coronary involvement)
- Tumor necrosis factor inhibition
- Corticosteroids contraindicated due to increased incidence of coronary aneurysms
- Transcatheter coronary intervention thrombolysis

Prognosis

- Factors related to poor prognosis

Medium-Sized Vessel Vasculitides

	Polyarteritis Nodosa	Kawasaki Disease
Age of onset	Adults, children	Infants (> 6 months), children (up to 3 years)
Organ system involved	Multisystemic	Mainly heart & coronary arteries; rarely systemic
Mucocutaneous lymph node involvement	No	Yes
Level of arterial involvement	Before and after entrance into organ	Before entrance into organ
Size of vessel	Small and medium-sized arteries	Medium-sized arteries
Pathogenesis	Cell mediated	Cell mediated, antibody mediated
Histopathology	Acute, subacute, and chronic lesions in same organ	All same-stage lesions (acute, subacute, or chronic) in organ affected or may appear in different stages in same artery
Fibrinoid necrosis	Yes	Rare
Vascular infiltrate	Mainly neutrophils and later mononuclear cells	Mainly mononuclear cells (lymphocytes, macrophages)
ANCA serology	Rarely positive ANCA titers	Atypical ANCA or ANCA negative

  - Coronary arteries (arteritis, thrombosis, aneurysms)
  - Heart (acute interstitial myocarditis and valvulitis)
  - Recurrence rate of KD (4%) between 5-24 months
  - Mortality rate with appropriate treatment (0.04%)
  - Peripheral medium-sized arteritis with infarction (e.g., extremities, central nervous system, small and large intestines)

IMAGING

Radiographic Findings

- Heart and coronary arteries
  - 2-dimensional echocardiography
    - Proximal aneurysms of coronary artery
  - Coronary angiography (arteritis, dilatation, or aneurysm)
- Kidney
  - Ultrasound (increased size, echogenicity)
  - DMSA renal SPECT (inflammation and scarring)
  - Renal Doppler study (flow pattern and vasculitis)
  - Renal angiography (arterial stenosis)

MICROSCOPIC

Histologic Features

- Arterial changes can be a consequence of acute clinical disease, subclinical continued activity, recurrent acute attacks, or clinically inapparent disease
- Divided into 4 stages
  - Initiation of arteritis (6-8 days after onset)
  - Aneurysm formation (8-12 days)
  - Persistent arterial inflammation (2-6 weeks)
  - Scarring (> 6 weeks)
- > 1 stage may be observed in different arteries or within different segments of same artery
- Medium-sized arteritis (coronary, renal, intestinal)
  - Panarteritis: Intima and adventitial layer, with disruption of internal and external elastic lamina
  - Early neutrophilic infiltration, peak 10 days
  - Macrophages and lymphocytes after 2 weeks
  - Damage to smooth muscle cells of media
  - Loss of α-smooth muscle actin and type IV collagen
  - Rare: Fibrinoid necrosis
- Microaneurysm formation with thrombosis
- Vascular fibrosis and recanalization of thrombi
- Renal parenchyma
  - Focal or diffuse interstitial inflammation, edema or scarring
    - Lymphocytes, plasma cells, neutrophils
  - Normal glomeruli, rarely podocytopathy
    - Rare: Mesangial proliferative GN with immune complexes
    - Rare: Interlobular and small arterial vasculitis
  - Rare: Thrombotic microangiopathy

DIFFERENTIAL DIAGNOSIS

Polyarteritis Nodosa in Childhood

- Differentiated from Kawasaki disease by absence of mucocutaneous lymph node syndrome
- Pathologic findings of vasculitis frequently show fibrinoid necrotizing features

SELECTED REFERENCES

1. Dimitriades VR et al: Kawasaki disease: pathophysiology, clinical manifestations, and management. Curr Rheumatol Rep. 16(6):423, 2014
2. Ni FF et al: Regulatory T cell microRNA expression changes in children with acute Kawasaki disease. Clin Exp Immunol. 178(2):384-93, 2014
3. Sánchez-Manubens J et al: Diagnosis and classification of Kawasaki disease. J Autoimmun. 48-49:113-7, 2014
4. Jamieson N et al: Kawasaki Disease: A Clinician's Update. Int J Pediatr. 2013:645391, 2013
5. Jennette JC et al: 2012 revised International Chapel Hill Consensus Conference Nomenclature of Vasculitides. Arthritis Rheum. 65(1):1-11, 2013
6. Kentsis A et al: Urine proteomics for discovery of improved diagnostic markers of Kawasaki disease. EMBO Mol Med. 5(2):210-20, 2013
7. Kim MH et al: Interleukin-21 receptor gene polymorphisms in kawasaki disease. Korean Circ J. 43(1):38-43, 2013
8. Watanabe T: Kidney and urinary tract involvement in kawasaki disease. Int J Pediatr. 2013:831834, 2013
9. Wang JN et al: Renal scarring sequelae in childhood Kawasaki disease. Pediatr Nephrol. 22(5):684-9, 2007

Patchy Perivascular Infiltrate

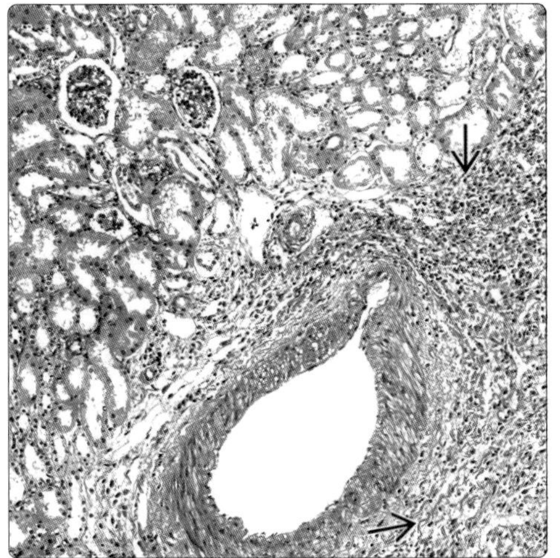

Normal Glomerulus

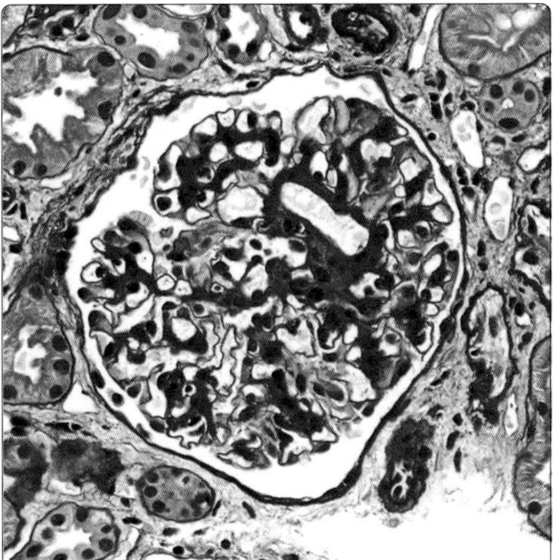

(Left) *Low-magnification image of kidney tissue shows an arcuate artery and patchy active interstitial inflammation and edema ➙. The glomeruli are unremarkable. (Courtesy J.C. Jennette, MD.)* **(Right)** *Glomerulus from a 2-year-old girl shows mild, nonspecific mesangial hypercellularity without a significant increase in matrix in an acute case of KD. No immune deposits are localized (PAS).*

Segmental Transmural Inflammation

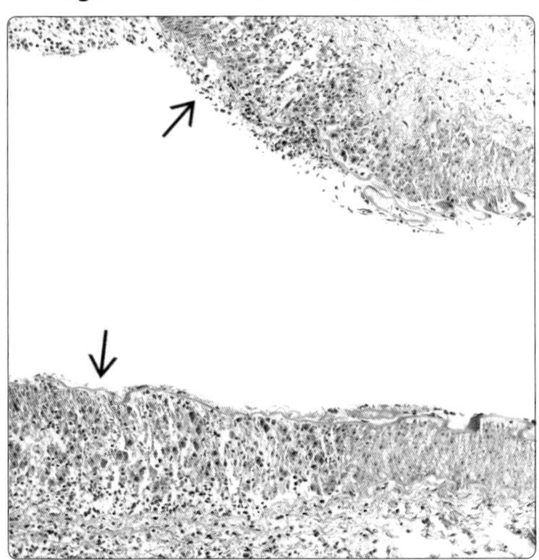

Mononuclear Inflammation

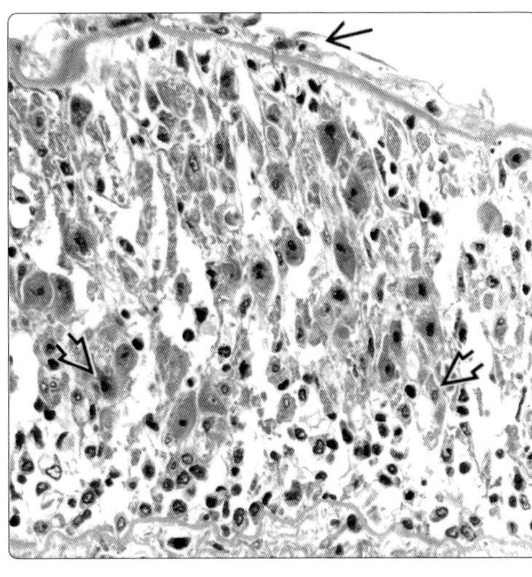

(Left) *Dilated portion of a renal artery shows segmental transmural inflammation ➙. (Courtesy J.C. Jennette, MD.)* **(Right)** *High magnification of a renal artery in Kawasaki disease shows mild to moderate transmural mononuclear inflammatory infiltrate from tunica intima ➙, media to adventitia ➙, and intercellular edema of the media. (Courtesy J.C. Jennette, MD.)*

Coronary Artery Aneurysms

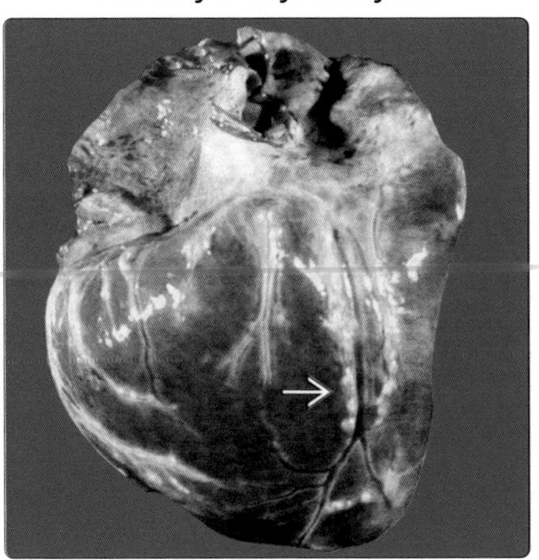

Old Scarring Small Artery Vasculitis

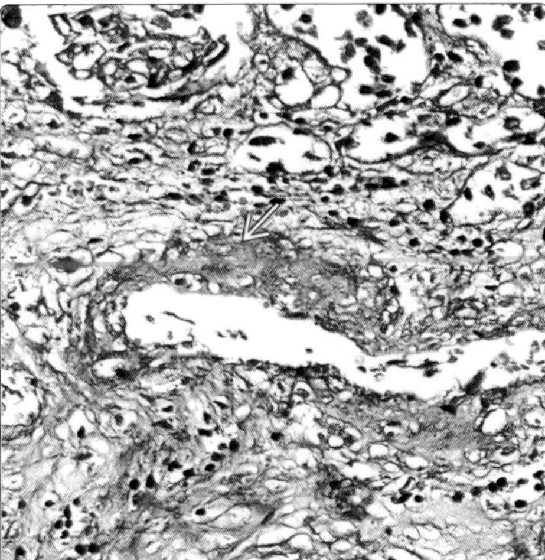

(Left) *Gross photograph at autopsy shows the heart of a young patient with Kawasaki disease. Multiple small aneurysms are seen in the left anterior descending coronary artery ➙. (Courtesy J. Fallon, MD.)* **(Right)** *On rare occasion, intrarenal healing small vessel vasculitis with obliterative changes ➙ may be seen in Kawasaki disease.*

Giant Cell Arteritis

KEY FACTS

TERMINOLOGY

- Granulomatous arteritis of aorta and its major branches

ETIOLOGY/PATHOGENESIS

- Possible triggers include exposure to several upper respiratory disease pathogens
- Associated with *HLA-DRB1* and *HLA-DR4* gene alleles
- Cell-mediated immune mechanism
- Auto-antibodies to ferritin

CLINICAL ISSUES

- Usually > 50 years
- Female predilection (M:F = 1:2-6)
- Symptoms of polymyalgia rheumatica (50-75%)
- Elevation of acute phase reactants in active disease
- Rapid response to steroid treatment
- Microscopic hematuria &/or proteinuria with increased disease activity

IMAGING

- MR angiography and high spatial configuration
- Angiography of aorta and great vessels

MICROSCOPIC

- Granulomatous inflammation from media to intima and adventitia with disruption of elastic lamina by giant cells
- Crescentic GN

TOP DIFFERENTIAL DIAGNOSES

- Takayasu arteritis
- Rheumatoid aortitis
- Atherosclerotic arterial disease
- Fibromuscular dysplasia
- Calcinosis of temporal or larger arteries
- Drug-induced large vessel vasculitis

DIAGNOSTIC CHECKLIST

- Biopsy diagnosis obligatory to confirm diagnosis of GCA

Temporal Artery With Transmural Inflammation

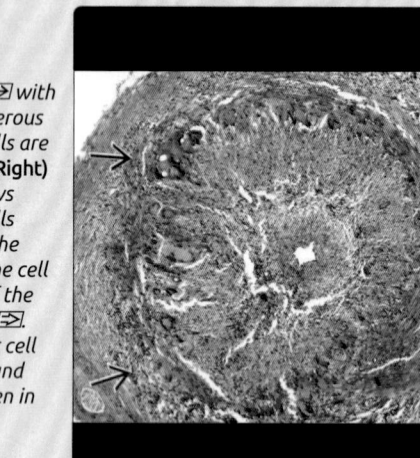

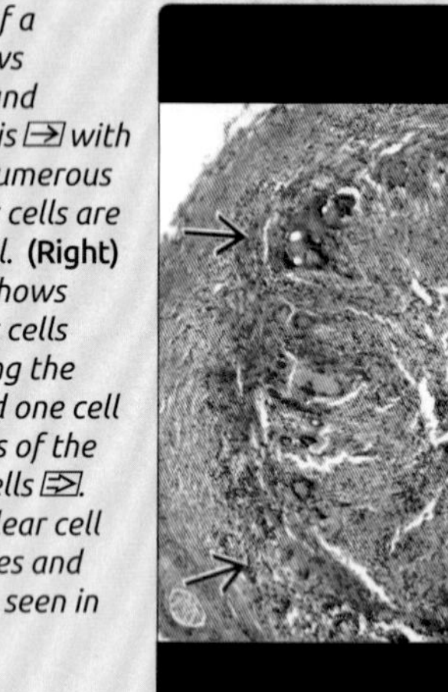

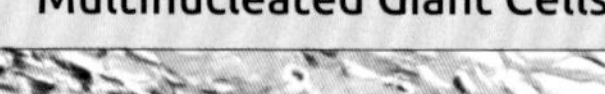

Multinucleated Giant Cells

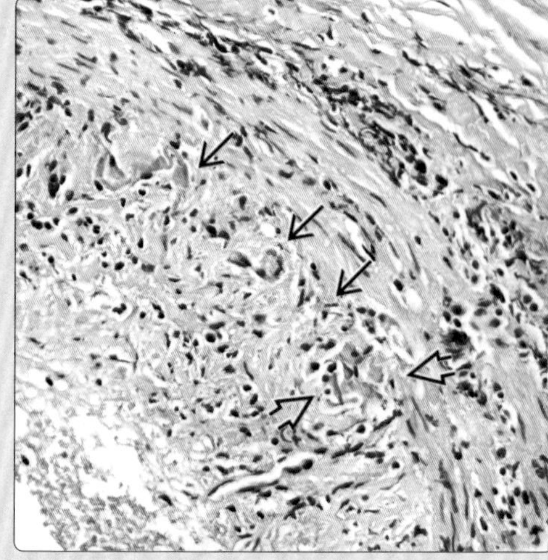

(Left) *Cross section of a temporal artery shows adventitial, medial, and intimal active arteritis → with occlusive changes. Numerous multinucleated giant cells are noted within the wall.* **(Right)** *High magnification shows multinucleated giant cells disrupting and eroding the elastic lamina → and one cell containing fragments of the elastica within the cells ⇨. Significant mononuclear cell infiltrate (lymphocytes and macrophages) is also seen in the adventitial layer.*

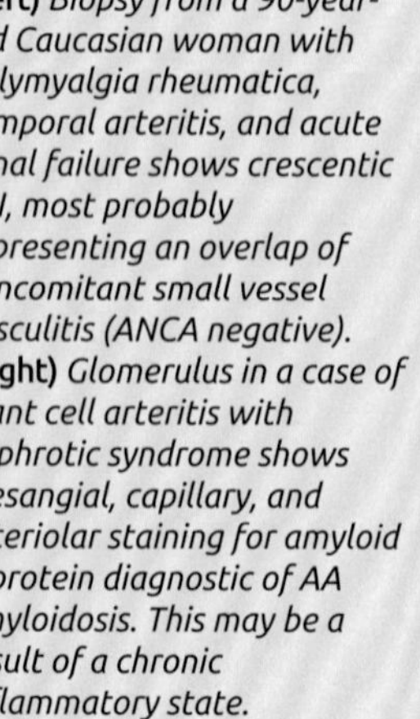

Crescentic Glomerulonephritis

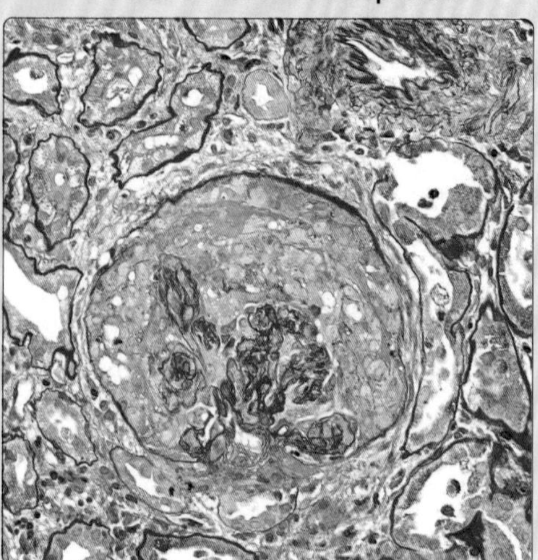

AA Amyloid

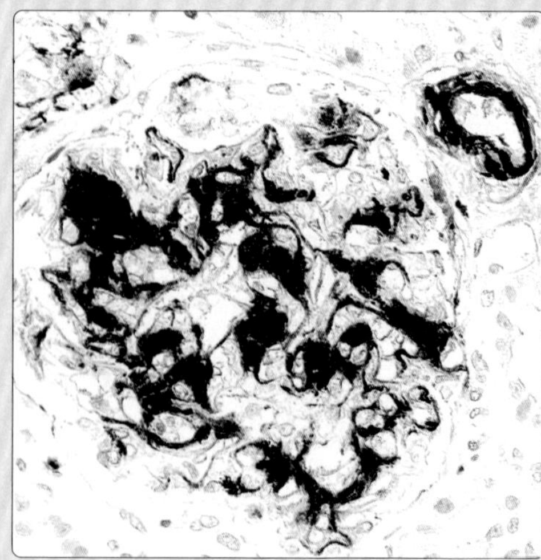

(Left) *Biopsy from a 90-year-old Caucasian woman with polymyalgia rheumatica, temporal arteritis, and acute renal failure shows crescentic GN, most probably representing an overlap of concomitant small vessel vasculitis (ANCA negative).* **(Right)** *Glomerulus in a case of giant cell arteritis with nephrotic syndrome shows mesangial, capillary, and arteriolar staining for amyloid A protein diagnostic of AA amyloidosis. This may be a result of a chronic inflammatory state.*

TERMINOLOGY

Abbreviations

- Giant cell arteritis (GCA)

Synonyms

- Temporal (cranial) arteritis, Horton syndrome

Definitions

- Chapel Hill Consensus Conference 2012
  - Granulomatous arteritis of aorta and its major branches; predilection for extracranial branches of carotid and vertebral arteries; includes temporal artery
  - Usually occurs in patients > 50 years of age and is often associated with polymyalgia rheumatica
- American College of Rheumatology Criteria
  - Age ≥ 50 years
  - New onset of localized headache
  - Temporal artery tenderness or decreased temporal artery pulse
  - Elevated ESR ≥ 50 mm/hr
  - Biopsy of artery with necrotizing arteritis with mononuclear infiltrates or granulomatous process
  - Presence of any 3 or more of above yields high sensitivity and specificity

ETIOLOGY/PATHOGENESIS

Environmental Exposure

- Etiology unknown
- Possible triggers include exposure to several upper respiratory disease pathogens
  - *Mycoplasma/Chlamydia pneumoniae*
  - Parvovirus B19, human parainfluenza virus type I
  - Herpes simplex virus

Genetic

- Associated with *HLA-DRB1* and *HLA-DR4* gene alleles
- *ICAM-1* gene polymorphism (R241)

Pathogenesis

- Autoimmune cell-mediated mechanism
  - T-cell mediated process
    - CD4(+) T-helper cells via IL-6
    - Interferon γ production
  - Dendritic antigen presenting cells, macrophages
  - Destructive vascular inflammation
  - Vaso-occlusive intimal proliferation
  - Aneurysm formation
- Humoral-mediated immunity
  - Elevated serum immunoglobulins
  - Circulating immune complexes with rare deposits
  - Autoantibodies to ferritin (92%)

CLINICAL ISSUES

Epidemiology

- Incidence
  - 15-25/100,000 in patients > 50 years of age
  - Low incidence in the Mediterranean, rare in Asians and African Americans
- Age
  - Usually > 50 years
  - Peaks at 75-85 years
- Sex
  - Female predilection (M:F = 1:2-6)
- Ethnicity
  - Highest in patients of northern European descent

Presentation

- Wide variability of clinical symptoms
- Fever, malaise, weight loss, paresthesias
- Symptoms of polymyalgia rheumatica (50-75%)
  - Proximal muscle ache, stiffness, and weakness
  - Bursitis and tenosynovitis
- Vascular
  - Visual disturbance/blindness (optic nerve or retinal ischemia)
  - Jaw claudication, temporal tenderness ± pulsation, headache
  - Peripheral vascular stenotic or occlusive symptoms
    - With decreased pulses in extremities
    - Carotid or subclavian artery bruits
    - Vessels outside head and neck (10-15% of cases)
- Renal
  - Renal manifestations occur infrequently
  - Associated hypertension is uncommon
  - Microscopic hematuria, particularly with increased disease activity
  - Proteinuria or, rarely, nephrotic syndrome
  - Impaired renal function or acute renal insufficiency
  - Glomerular disease, anecdotal

Laboratory Tests

- Elevation of acute phase reactants in active disease (ESR, CRP)
- Anemia, thrombocytosis
- Elevated liver enzymes (50%)
- Serologic studies for autoimmune diseases are negative, including ANCA

Treatment

- Rapid response to steroid treatment
- Immunosuppressive drugs in refractory cases

Prognosis

- Generally self-limiting disease
- Long-term complications
  - Sometimes relapsing-remitting course
  - Thoracic aortic aneurysm (17x risk)
  - Abdominal aortic aneurysm (2x risk)
  - Aortic dissection
  - Myocardial infarction
  - Large artery stenosis

IMAGING

General Features

- Findings similar to Takayasu arteritis except in older age groups
- Pre- and post-contrast MR findings
  - T2 identified mural thickening associated with edema and active vasculitis
  - MR angiography and high spatial configuration

- Identifies flow direction and end-organ perfusion
- Stenosis or occlusion

MICROSCOPIC

Kidney

- Glomeruli
  - Concomitant or isolated pauci-immune crescentic glomerulonephritis with fibrinoid necrosis
  - Secondary amyloidosis
  - Rare: Membranous glomerulonephritis
- Tubules and Interstitium
  - No specific findings
- Arteries
  - Large vessel vasculitis ± granulomatous features
    - Ischemic renal parenchymal lesions
  - Occasionally, small vessel vasculitis with fibrinoid necrosis occurs

Nonrenal

- Giant cell arteritis is characterized by
  - Inflammatory infiltrate seen initially in media and extending to intima and adventitia
  - Disruption or fragmentation of internal and external elastic lamina is associated with inflammation
  - Mainly mononuclear cell infiltration composed of mainly T lymphocytes, macrophages, and dendritic cells is seen
  - Variable number of multinucleated giant cells present (50% of cases), particularly at elastic lamina
  - Occasionally, fibrinoid necrosis of wall is observed
  - Intimal findings include fibroblastic and myointimal cell proliferation, edema, and inflammation
  - Range of healing lesions of intimal and medial fibrosis accompanies active lesions, leading to narrowing or occlusion of lumina
- Temporal arteries
  - Commonly affected
  - Unilateral or bilateral involvement
  - Typically focal and segmental in distribution

DIFFERENTIAL DIAGNOSIS

Takayasu Arteritis

- Similar vessel size and pathology
- Occurs at younger age (≤ 30-50)
- High incidence in Asian population
- Aortic involvement is frequent

Rheumatoid Aortitis

- Positive rheumatoid serology
- Features suggestive of rheumatoid arthritis
- Typical bone and hand lesions

Atherosclerotic Arterial Disease

- Some (older) age group and radiographic findings
- Clinical symptoms in active disease and polymyalgia rheumatica may help in GCA

Other Systemic Vasculitides

- Primary angiitis of central nervous system
- Polyarteritis nodosa
  - More in small and medium-sized vessels
  - Fibrinoid necrotizing vasculitis by pathology
  - Involvement of kidneys

Fibromuscular Dysplasia

- Younger patients
- No acute constitutional symptoms
- Commonly affects renal and carotid arteries
- Distinct radiographic changes
- Genetic or familial background

Other Causes

- Calcinosis of temporal or larger arteries
  - Age related
  - Calciphylaxis secondary to chronic renal disease
- Drug-induced large vessel vasculitis

DIAGNOSTIC CHECKLIST

Clinically Relevant Pathologic Features

- Biopsy diagnosis obligatory to confirm diagnosis of GCA
  - Multiple levels of sections suggested for focal lesions

SELECTED REFERENCES

1. El-Dairi MA et al: Diagnostic Algorithm for Patients With Suspected Giant Cell Arteritis. J Neuroophthalmol. ePub, 2015
2. Alba MA et al: Relapses in patients with giant cell arteritis: prevalence, characteristics, and associated clinical findings in a longitudinally followed cohort of 106 patients. Medicine (Baltimore). 93(5):194-201, 2014
3. Nesher G: The diagnosis and classification of giant cell arteritis. J Autoimmun. 48-49:73-5, 2014
4. Jennette JC et al: 2012 revised International Chapel Hill Consensus Conference Nomenclature of Vasculitides. Arthritis Rheum. 65(1):1-11, 2013
5. Ness T et al: The diagnosis and treatment of giant cell arteritis. Dtsch Arztebl Int. 110(21):376-85; quiz 386, 2013
6. Awwad ST et al: Calciphylaxis of the temporal artery masquerading as temporal arteritis. Clin Experiment Ophthalmol. 38(5):511-3, 2010
7. Burke AP: Takayasu arteritis and giant cell arteritis. Pathol Case Rev 12(5):186-92, 2007
8. Powers JF et al: High prevalence of herpes simplex virus DNA in temporal arteritis biopsy specimens. Am J Clin Pathol. 123(2):261-4, 2005
9. Müller E et al: Temporal arteritis with pauci-immune glomerulonephritis: a systemic disease. Clin Nephrol. 62(5):384-6, 2004
10. Hamidou MA et al: Temporal arteritis associated with systemic necrotizing vasculitis. J Rheumatol. 30(10):2165-9, 2003
11. Nuenninghoff DM et al: Incidence and predictors of large-artery complication (aortic aneurysm, aortic dissection, and/or large-artery stenosis) in patients with giant cell arteritis: a population-based study over 50 years. Arthritis Rheum. 48(12):3522-31, 2003
12. Weyand CM et al: Medium- and large-vessel vasculitis. N Engl J Med. 349(2):160-9, 2003
13. Nasher G: Giant cell arteritis and polymyalgia rheumatica. In Vasculitis. Ball G et al, eds. Oxford: Oxford University Press. 255-277, 2002
14. Burke A et al: Temporal artery biopsy of giant cell arteritis. Pathol Case Rev 6(6): 265-73, 2001
15. Escribá A et al: Secondary (AA-type) amyloidosis in patients with polymyalgia rheumatica. Am J Kidney Dis. 35(1):137-40, 2000
16. Salvarani C et al: Intercellular adhesion molecule 1 gene polymorphisms in polymyalgia rheumatica/giant cell arteritis: association with disease risk and severity. J Rheumatol. 27(5):1215-21, 2000
17. Strasser F et al: Giant cell arteritis "causing" AA-amyloidosis with rapid renal failure. Schweiz Med Wochenschr. 130(43):1606-9, 2000
18. Lie JT: The vasculitides. In Biopsy Diagnosis of Rheumatoid Diseases. Tokyo: Igaku-Shoin. 61-106, 1997
19. Montoliu J et al: Lessons to be learned from patients with vasculitis. Nephrol Dial Transplant. 12(12):2781-6, 1997
20. Jennette JC et al: The pathology of vasculitis involving the kidney. Am J Kidney Dis. 24(1):130-41, 1994
21. Canton CG et al: Renal failure in temporal arteritis. Am J Nephrol. 12(5):380-3, 1992
22. Hunder GG et al: The American College of Rheumatology 1990 criteria for the classification of giant cell arteritis. Arthritis Rheum. 33(8):1122-8, 1990

Disruption of Internal Elastica

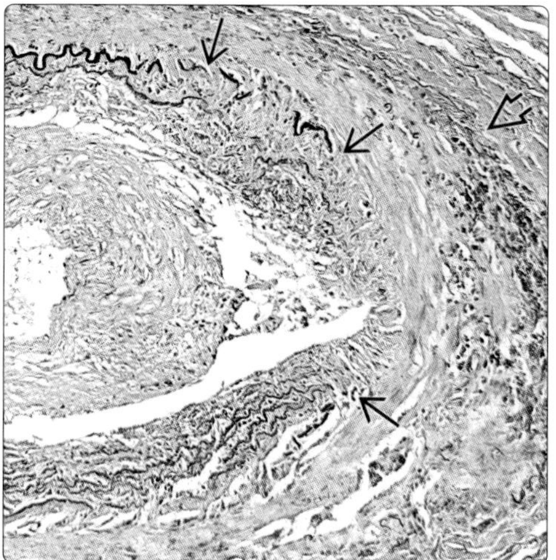

Intimal Fibrosis

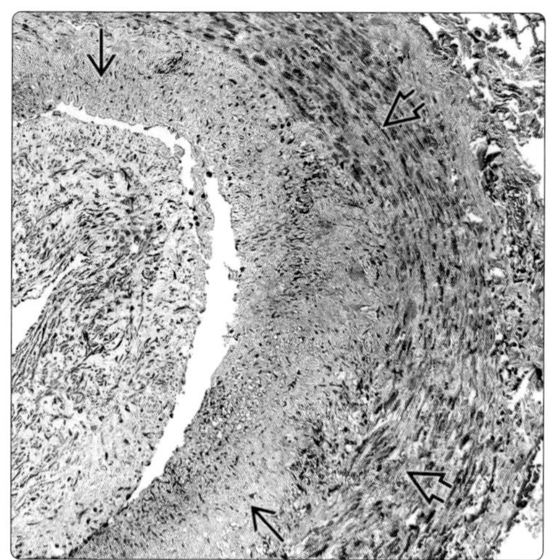

(Left) *Section of a temporal artery shows disruption of the elastic lamina and extensive loss of the internal ⇒ and external ⇒ elastic lamina along with intimal and medial inflammatory infiltrate. Marked fibromyointimal thickening, leading to narrowing of the lumen, is noted.* **(Right)** *Segment of the temporal artery shows moderate fibrosing changes within the intima ⇒ and early fibrocollagenous deposits in the media separating the smooth muscle cells ⇒.*

T-Cell Infiltrates (CD3+) in Artery

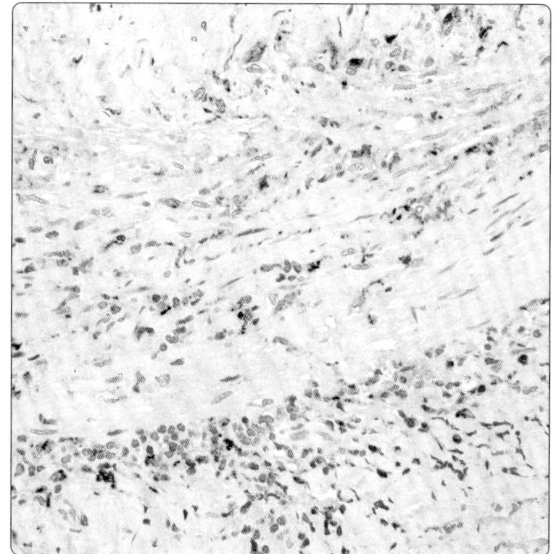

Macrophages (CD68[+]) in Artery

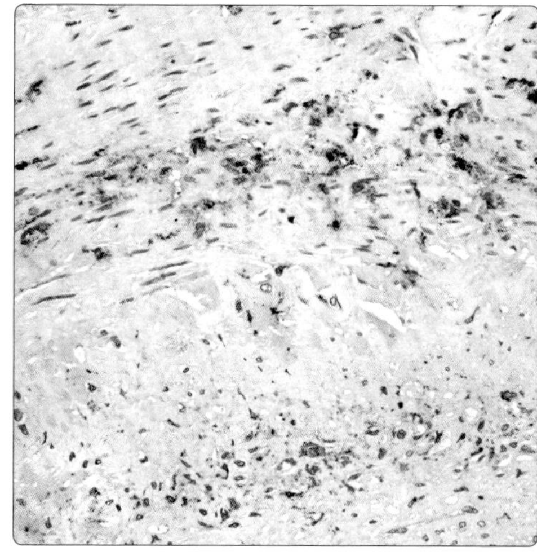

(Left) *Segment of temporal artery shows full thickness arteritis (intimal and medial layer) with increased CD3(+) T lymphocyte infiltration.* **(Right)** *Segment of temporal artery shows full-thickness arteritis (intimal and medial layer) with increased CD68(+) macrophage infiltration.*

Advanced Crescentic Glomerulonephritis

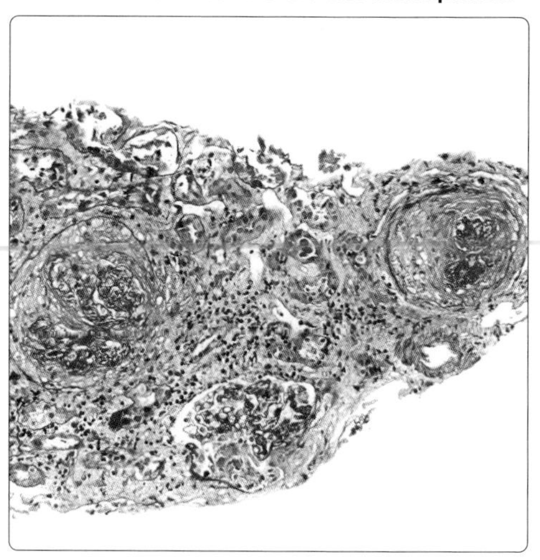

Stenotic Carotid Artery

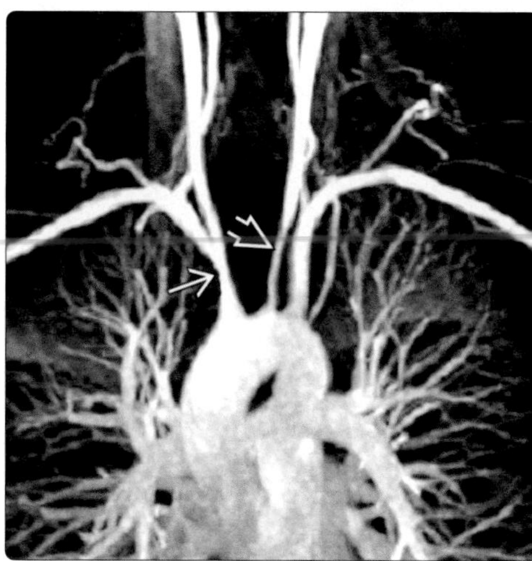

(Left) *Biopsy from a 78-year-old woman with temporal arteritis and acute renal failure shows subacute crescentic GN with fibrocellular crescents and one small cellular crescent (ANCA negative).* **(Right)** *MR angiogram shows an irregular, long-segment stenosis of the left common carotid artery ⇒ and brachiocephalic artery stenosis ➡ due to mural thickening. These findings are typical of GCA.*

Takayasu Arteritis

KEY FACTS

TERMINOLOGY

- Granulomatous inflammation of aorta and its major branches

ETIOLOGY/PATHOGENESIS

- Cell and antibody-mediated immune mechanism

CLINICAL ISSUES

- Common in Asia (6/1,000) compared with USA (1-3/1,000)
- Patients usually < 30 years (90%)
- Pain of involved vessels and bruits
- Renovascular hypertension
- Steroid therapy as primary form
- Complications mainly due to hypertension and stroke
- Elevated acute phase protein, pentraxin-3
- Predominantly female (F:M = 8:1)
- Steroid therapy as primary form of therapy
- Complications mainly due to hypertension and stroke

IMAGING

- Disease classified by abnormalities of aorta or main branches using angiography (gold standard)
- Aneurysmal dilatation may alternate with stenosis

MICROSCOPIC

- Granulomatous panarteritis with variable number of multinucleated giant cells
- Multifocal disruption of the medial elastic fibers
- Adventitial and marked intimal thickening
- Mainly mesangial proliferative glomerulonephritis
- Full-thickness arterial walls or entire endarterectomy specimens essential for histological examination

TOP DIFFERENTIAL DIAGNOSES

- Isolated granulomatous aortitis
- Giant cell arteritis
- Atherosclerosis
- Fibromuscular dysplasia

(Left) *Segment of aortic wall in Takayasu arteritis (TAK) shows adventitia* ⇨ *and a band of medial granulomatous inflammatory infiltrate* ⇨. **(Right)** *EVG stain shows focal disruption of the external elastic lamina enclosing the media. Note also the fragmentation of the elastic fibers within the media in the upper 1/3 of the picture. (Courtesy J.C. Jennette, MD.)*

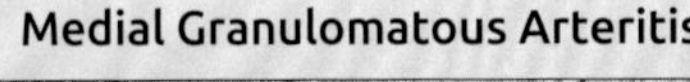

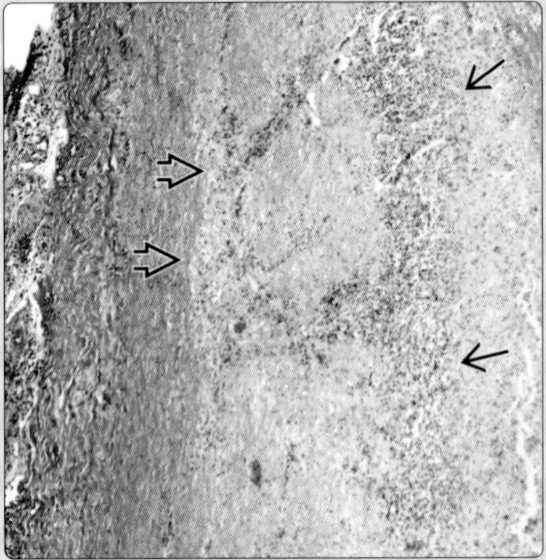

Disruption of Medial Elastic Lamina and Fibers

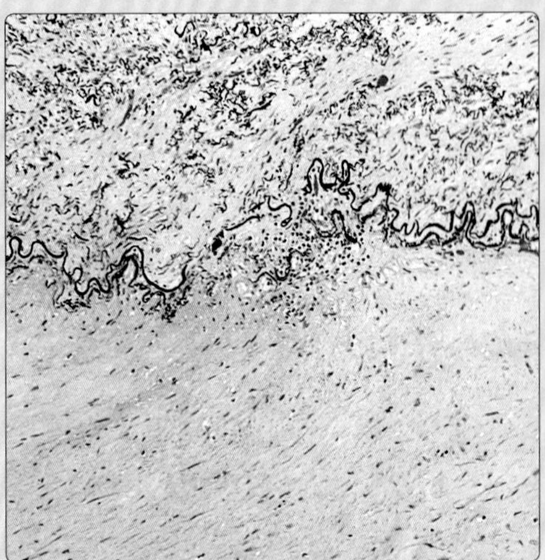

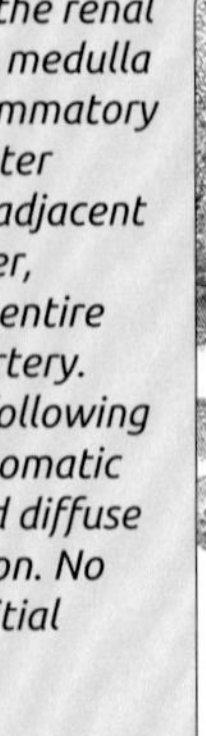

(Left) *Large artery in the renal pelvis adjacent to the medulla shows a band of inflammatory infiltrate* ⇨ *in the outer portion of the media adjacent to the adventitial layer, almost encircling the entire cross section of the artery.* **(Right)** *Renal biopsy following active TA and asymptomatic hematuria shows mild diffuse mesangial proliferation. No chronic tubulointerstitial changes were seen.*

Renal Medial Arteritis

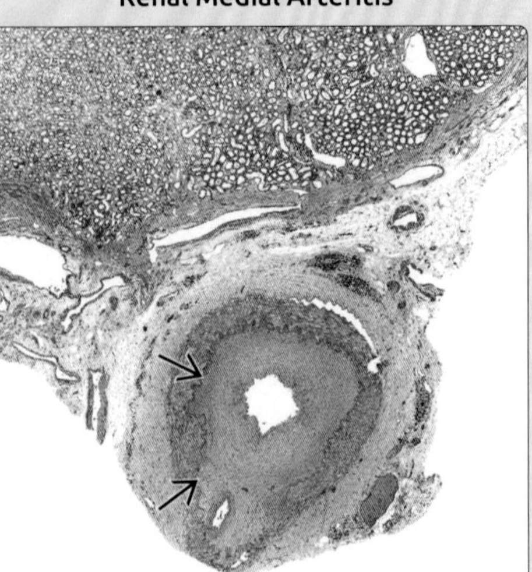

Mild Mesangial Proliferation

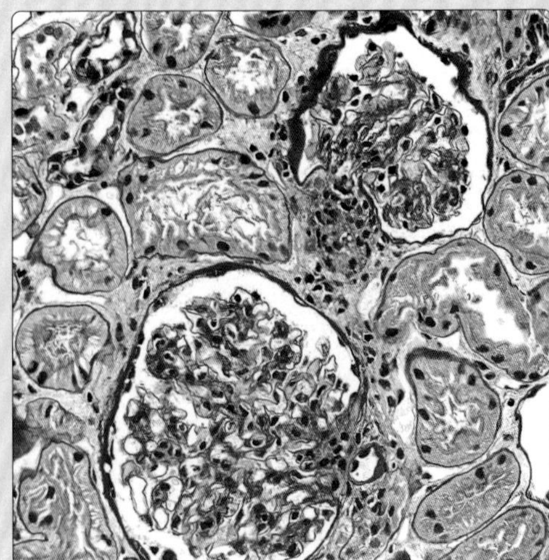

TERMINOLOGY

Abbreviations

- Takayasu arteritis (TAK)

Synonyms

- Takayasu disease/syndrome
- Pulseless disease
- Aortoarteritis
- Idiopathic medial aortopathy and arteriopathy

Definitions

- Chapel Hill Consensus Conference 2012
  - TAK is granulomatous inflammation of aorta and its major branches
  - Usually occurs in patients < 50 years of age
- American College of Rheumatology criteria
  - Age ≤ 40 years
  - Claudication of extremity
  - Decreased brachial artery pulse
  - Systolic blood pressure difference > 10 mm Hg (between arms)
  - Bruit over subclavian arteries or aorta
  - Angiographic abnormalities (narrowing or occlusion)
  - Any 3 of above fulfills diagnosis of TAK with high sensitivity and specificity
- Definitive diagnosis may be problematic and delayed due to slow evolution and low activity of disease

ETIOLOGY/PATHOGENESIS

Etiology

- Unknown, autoimmune disease

Genetic

- HLA-B52 antigen, in 44% of Japanese patients with TAK
- ILI2B: Beyond ethnicity
- HLA-B22, HLA-DQB1/HLA-DRB1

Pathogenesis

- Cell-mediated, autoimmune mechanisms
  - T-lymphocytes (γ δ cells, CD4, CD8), natural killer cells, macrophages, dendritic cells, and B cells
- Autoantibodies: Anti-aortic antibody, antiendothelial antibodies, circulating immune complexes
- Participation of TNF-ά, IL-6, IL-12, TLR 2 and 4
- Inflammation causes aortic and arterial wall damage
- Elevated acute phase protein, pentraxin-3 in active disease phase

CLINICAL ISSUES

Epidemiology

- Incidence
  - Asian women more common (Japan, India, Korea)
  - Annual incidence around world: 0.4-3/10^6 per year
  - Highest prevalence in Japan: 40 cases/10^6
  - Japan: Higher aortic arch involvement
  - India: Higher thoracic and abdominal aorta
  - USA: Higher great vessel involvement
- Age
  - Patients usually < 30 years (90%)
  - Common in 2nd and 3rd decades of life
- Sex
  - Commonly female (F:M = 8:1), except India (M:F = 2:1)
- Ethnicity
  - Pattern of disease varies by geographic area

Presentation

- 2 phases of disease
  - Early inflammatory phase
    - Constitutional symptoms of fever, myalgias, arthralgias, weight loss, anemia
    - Pain of involved vessels
    - Hypertension
    - Bruits over great vessels
    - Aortic valve insufficiency
    - Ischemic effects: Stroke, claudication, mesenteric ischemia
  - Late occlusive or pulseless phase
  - May coexist with other autoimmune diseases (≤ 10%)
    - Rheumatoid arthritis
    - Systemic lupus erythematosus
    - Inflammatory bowel disease (Crohn disease)
  - Initial nonspecific symptomatology may delay definitive diagnosis for months or years
  - Renal
    - Renovascular hypertension (60%) due to obstructive abdominal aortic disease involving renal artery ostia
    - Renal artery stenosis
    - Evidence of glomerular disease (hematuria, proteinuria), anecdotal
    - Progressive renal insufficiency

Treatment

- Steroid therapy as primary form of therapy
- Addition of other immunosuppressants or methotrexate in severe/refractory cases or relapse
- Biologic agents
  - Antitumor necrosis factor alpha
  - Anti-IL-6R (Tocilizumab)
  - Anti-B cell: Rituximab
- Angioplasty or surgical bypass when disease activity quiescent
- Renal lesions according to type and frequency of specific lesion

Prognosis

- Complications mainly due to hypertension and stroke
- Mortality mainly due to congestive heart failure
- 15-year survival: 90-95%
- Some have monophasic disease

IMAGING

General Features

- Disease classified by abnormalities of aorta or main branches using angiography (gold standard)
  - Computerized tomography
  - Magnetic resonance imaging
  - Fluorodeoxy glucose positron emission tomography/CT
- Smooth narrowing of aorta and major vessels
- Patchy distribution of disease

Large Vessel Vasculitis

	Giant Cell Arteritis	Takayasu Arteritis
Age	> 50 years (peak: 75-85 years)	< 50 years (peak: 15-25 years)
Gender	M:F = 1:2	80% women
Ethnicity	Northern European	Asian
Vessels, symmetric	Carotid arteries, more axillary, aorta	Aorta, more carotid, mesenteric
Clinical	Polymyalgia rheumatica, localized headache	Nonspecific constitutional symptoms
Pathology	Giant cell arteritis, mainly medial layer	Giant cell arteritis, full thickness, nonnecrotizing
Sequelae	Stenosis, ischemia, CNS symptoms, medial necrosis	Stenosis, dilatation, aneurysm formation, thrombosis
Serology	Negative	Negative
Pathogenesis	CD4, CD8, macrophages, antigen unknown	CD4, CD8, macrophages, genetic basis

- Aneurysmal dilatation may alternate with stenosis
- Symmetrical great vessel distribution
- 5 patterns of aorta and large vessel involvement seen by angiography
  - Type I: Branches of aortic arch (pulseless disease)
  - Type IIa: Ascending aorta, aortic arch, branches from the aortic arch
  - Type IIb: Ascending aorta, arch, branches, and thoracic descending aorta
  - Type III: Thoracic descending aorta, abdominal aorta, &/or renal arteries (most common, 60%)
  - Type IV: Abdominal aorta &/or renal arteries
  - Type V: Combination of stages IIb and IV

MACROSCOPIC

General Features

- Ridged "tree bark" intimal surface when very advanced
  - Thickened intimal and medial layers, patchy

MICROSCOPIC

Histologic Features

- Glomeruli
  - Nonspecific ischemic glomerular lesions
  - Mesangial proliferative, focal proliferative GN
  - Membranoproliferative and crescentic GN
  - Amyloidosis (rare)
- Tubules and interstitium
  - Tubulointerstitial scarring
- Renal artery
  - Affected by obliterative inflammatory process
  - Early adventitial inflammation and cuffing of vasa vasorum
  - Granulomatous panarteritis with variable number of multinucleated giant cells
    - Rare: Lymphoplasmacytic arteritis without giant cells
  - Mainly medial and adventitial inflammation
    - Multifocal disruption of medial elastic fibers
  - Late phase
    - Thickening and occlusive intimal scarring
    - Adventitial and external medial fibrosis

Aorta and Large Vessels

- Generally elastic arteries affected
- Biopsy diagnosis or confirmation of TAK with tissues obtained at surgery
- Full-thickness arterial walls or entire endarterectomy specimens essential for histological examination
  - Typically involves subclavian vessels and various parts of aorta; different radiographic and clinical patterns
- Autoimmune aortic lymphoplasmacytic valvulitis

DIFFERENTIAL DIAGNOSIS

Isolated Granulomatous Aortitis

- Predilection for ascending aorta
- Medial (cystic) necrosis, less adventitial and intimal fibrosis
- Increased risk of aortic dissection
- Occasionally associated with Marfan syndrome

Giant Cell Arteritis

- Age of onset > 50 years, polymyalgia rheumatica (50%)
- Frequent temporal artery involvement, similar pathology

Atherosclerosis

- In older individuals
- Focal mural inflammation, eccentric wall involvement
- Primarily intimal disease with atheromatous deposits

Fibromuscular Dysplasia

- Young females
- Multiple arteries involved (frequently renal and carotid) with beaded appearance
- Aorta not affected

SELECTED REFERENCES

1. Chatterjee S et al: Clinical diagnosis and management of large vessel vasculitis: Takayasu arteritis. Curr Cardiol Rep. 16(7):499, 2014
2. Clifford A et al: Recent advances in the medical management of Takayasu arteritis: an update on use of biologic therapies. Curr Opin Rheumatol. 26(1):7-15, 2014
3. de Souza AW et al: Diagnostic and classification criteria of Takayasu arteritis. J Autoimmun. 48-49:79-83, 2014
4. Terao C et al: Recent advances in Takayasu arteritis. Int J Rheum Dis. 17(3):238-47, 2014
5. Chaudhry MA et al: Takayasu's arteritis and its role in causing renal artery stenosis. Am J Med Sci. 346(4):314-8, 2013
6. Isobe M: Takayasu arteritis revisited: current diagnosis and treatment. Int J Cardiol. 168(1):3-10, 2013
7. Grayson PC et al: Distribution of arterial lesions in Takayasu's arteritis and giant cell arteritis. Ann Rheum Dis. Epub ahead of print, 2012

Internal Mammary Arteritis

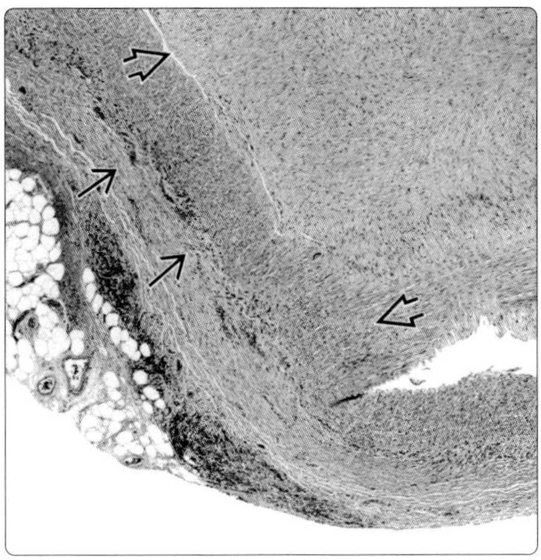

Healing Renal Arteritis With Obliterative Changes

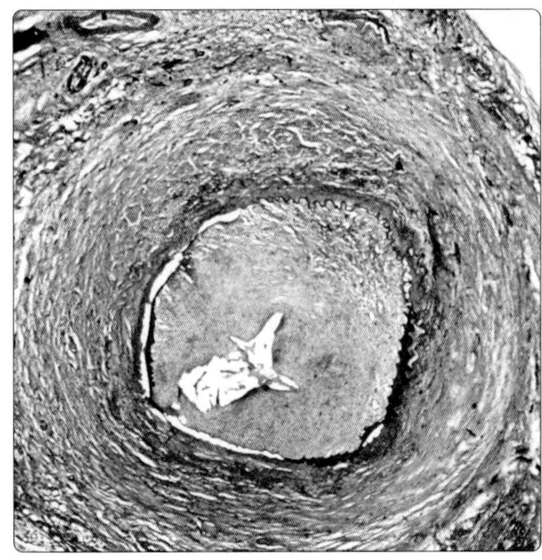

(Left) H&E shows a segment of an internal mammary artery from a 30-year-old Asian woman with chest pain and tenderness. Note the adventitial and outer medial inflammatory infiltrate → with marked intimal sclerosis ⇒. **(Right)** *Cross section of a renal artery with TAK shows focal adventitial and areas of perimedial and medial inflammation along with fibrointimal thickening and sclerosis leading to narrowing of the lumen. (Courtesy L. Salinas, MD.)*

Aortic Granulomatous Inflammation With Giant Cells

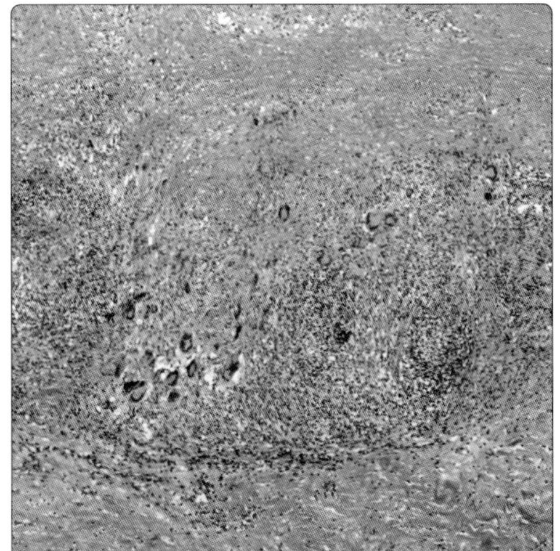

Aortic Granulomatous Inflammation With Giant Cells

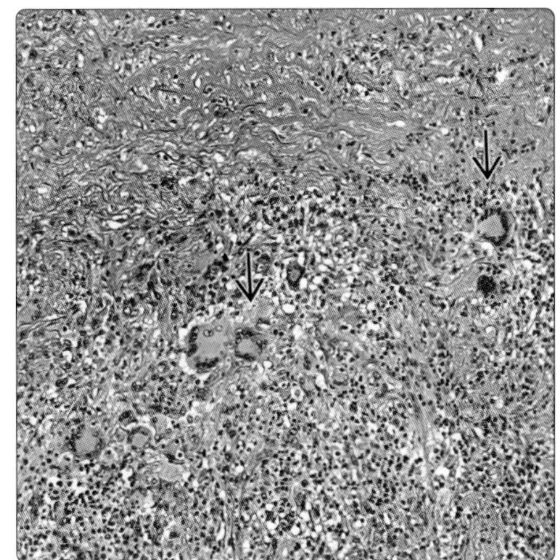

(Left) *Segment of an aortic wall shows active medial and adventitial granulomatous inflammation with infiltration of large aggregates of inflammatory cells. (Courtesy A. Shimizu, MD and R. Ohashi, MD.)* **(Right)** *High magnification shows frequent multinucleated giant cells → along with other mononuclear cell infiltrates disrupting the medial architecture. (Courtesy A. Shimizu, MD and R. Ohashi, MD.)*

Membranoproliferative GN

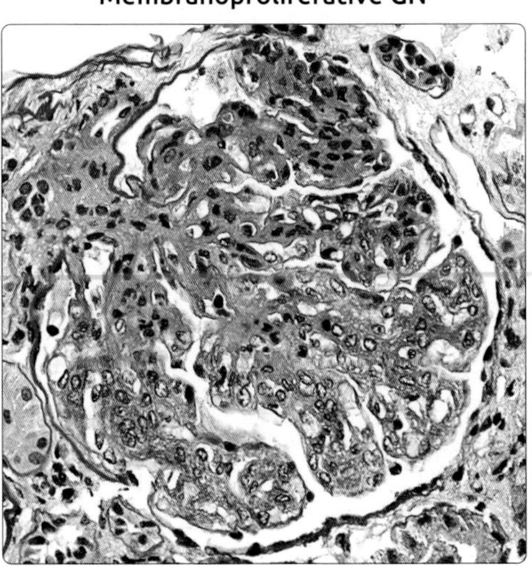

Glomerular Fibrocellular Crescent

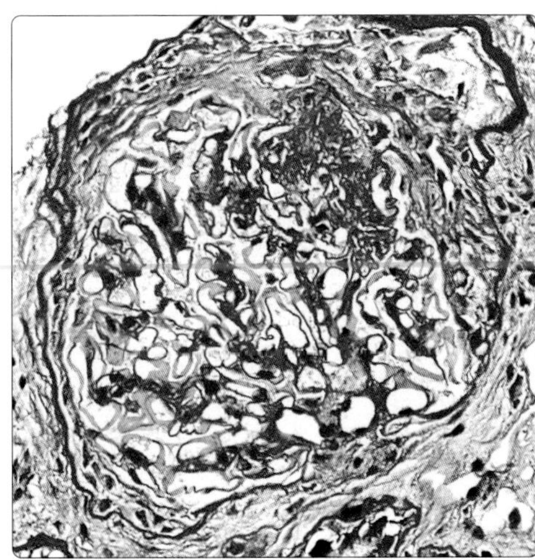

(Left) *Glomerulus shows membranoproliferative pattern of injury with a lobulated appearance and hypercellularity. Scant deposits were identified by electron microscopy.* **(Right)** *A case of TAK with hematuria and proteinuria shows focal crescentic glomerulonephritis with a fibrocellular crescent in this glomerulus.*

Hypocomplementemic Urticarial Vasculitis (Anti-C1q Vasculitis)

KEY FACTS

TERMINOLOGY

- Syndrome with hypocomplementemia (C1, C4, C3), chronic recurrent urticaria and often detectable anti-C1q autoantibodies; associated with variable other manifestations, including glomerulonephritis

ETIOLOGY/PATHOGENESIS

- Anti-C1q antibodies detected in ~ 55%
- Immune complex deposition in microvasculature
- Occurs as an isolated disease (50-75%) or in association with SLE, Sjögren syndrome, or monoclonal gammopathy

CLINICAL ISSUES

- Predominantly females (74%)
- Mean age: 45 years (range: 15-83 years)
- Recurrent urticaria over at least 6 months
- Fever, weight loss, uveitis, scleritis
- Glomerulonephritis (12%) (26% in those with C1q antibodies)
- Low C1q (88%) (100% of those with C1q antibodies)
- ANA positive (51%), anti-dsDNA (18%)
- Responds to steroids (58%) and immunosuppressive agents (74%)

MICROSCOPIC

- Endocapillary hypercellularity (neutrophils, mononuclear cells)
- Mesangial hypercellularity and matrix expansion
- Crescents and segmental necrosis in some cases
- May have focal necrotizing vasculitis

ANCILLARY TESTS

- Often "full house" (IgG, IgM, IgA, C3, C1q) and C4d
- Subendothelial and mesangial amorphous electron-dense deposits

TOP DIFFERENTIAL DIAGNOSES

- Systemic lupus erythematosus
- Membranoproliferative GN, type I

Endocapillary Hypercellularity

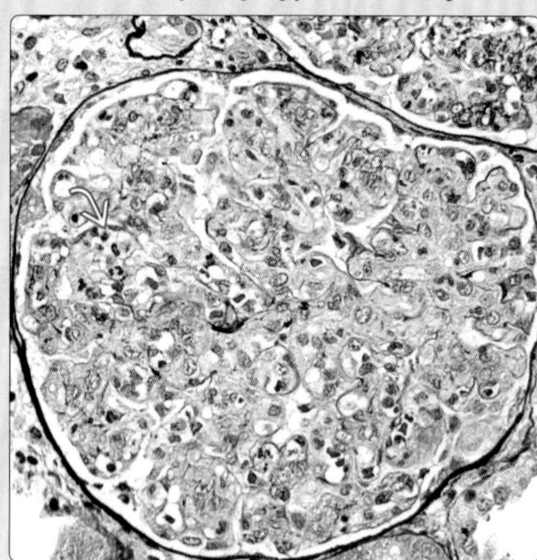

Granular Deposition of IgG in Mesangium and Along GBM

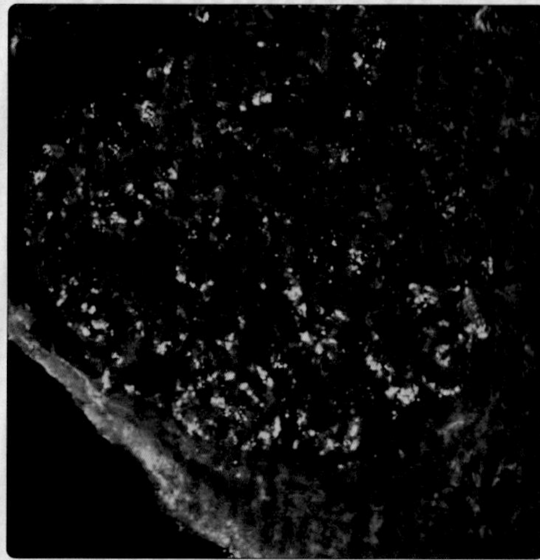

(Left) *Glomerular capillaries are filled with leukocytes, including neutrophils ➡ and mononuclear cells. The glomerular basement membrane appears normal, without duplication. The mesangium is hypercellular. (Courtesy S. Florquin, MD.)* **(Right)** *Coarse granular deposits of IgG are present in most reported cases of HUV. A full-house pattern is typical similar to SLE (IgG, IgA, IgM, C3, C1). (Courtesy S. Florquin, MD.)*

Endocapillary Leukocytes and Endothelial Activation

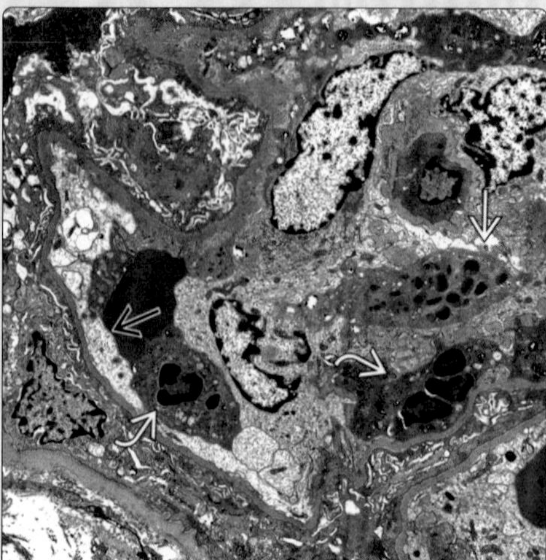

Subendothelial Deposit

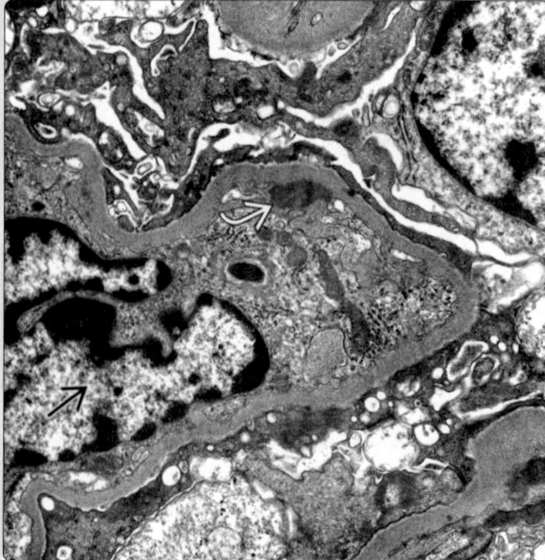

(Left) *The glomerular capillary is filled with leukocytes including neutrophils ➡ and an eosinophil ➡. The GBM is unremarkable but the endothelium is reactive, with loss of fenestrations ➡.* *(Courtesy S. Florquin, MD.)* **(Right)** *Subendothelial ➡ and mesangial amorphous deposits are usually described in HUV. The endothelium ➡ is activated with loss of fenestrations and increased ribosomes. (Courtesy S. Florquin, MD.)*

TERMINOLOGY

Abbreviations

- Hypocomplementemic urticaria vasculitis (HUV)

Synonyms

- Anti-C1q vasculitis
- McDuffie syndrome (when no associated disease)

Definitions

- Syndrome with hypocomplementemia (C1, C4, C3), chronic recurrent urticaria and often detectable anti-C1q autoantibodies
  - Associated with variable other manifestations, including glomerulonephritis, often associated with SLE
- Termed HUV syndrome, if unassociated with other diseases

ETIOLOGY/PATHOGENESIS

Activation of Classic Complement Pathway

- Anti-C1q antibodies detected in ~ 55%
  - Bind to collagen-like domain of immobilized C1q
  - Same antibodies in ~ 35% of SLE patients
- Immune complex deposition in microvasculature
  - Antigen unknown other than C1q
- 25-50% meet criteria for SLE
- Minority with with Sjögren syndrome, monoclonal gammopathy

DNASE1L3 Loss of Function Mutation in Familial HUV

- Encodes endo-nuclease associated with SLE
- All had GN typical of SLE

CLINICAL ISSUES

Epidemiology

- Predominantly females (74%)
- Mean age: 45 years (range: 15-83 years)

Presentation

- Recurrent urticaria over ≥ 6 months
  - Also angioedema, purpura, livedo reticularis
- Fever, weight loss (56%)
- Arthritis, arthralgias, myalgia (82%)
- Uveitis, scleritis (56%)
- Glomerulonephritis (12%) (26% in those with C1q antibodies)
  - May be more common in children (limited data)

Laboratory Tests

- Low C1q (88%) (100% of those with C1q antibodies)
  - Low CH50 (96%), low C3, C4
  - Normal C1 inhibitor
- ANA positive (51%), anti-dsDNA (18%)

Treatment

- Drugs
  - Steroids, dapsone, immunosuppressive agents

Prognosis

- Responds to steroids (58%); immunosuppressive agents (74%)
- Recurrence after transplant described in 1 case

MICROSCOPIC

Histologic Features

- Glomeruli
  - Endocapillary hypercellularity (neutrophils, mononuclear cells)
  - Crescents and segmental necrosis in some cases
  - Mesangial hypercellularity and matrix expansion
  - Duplication of GBM not prominent
  - Segmental and global glomerulosclerosis
- Tubules
  - Atrophy in chronic/recurrent cases
- Interstitium
  - Fibrosis in chronic/recurrent cases
- Vessels
  - May have focal necrotizing vasculitis
- Skin: Leukocytoclastic vasculitis with immune complexes

ANCILLARY TESTS

Immunofluorescence

- Granular deposits in mesangium and along GBM
  - Often "full house" (IgG, IgM, IgA, C3, C1q) and C4d
    - Rare cases without IgG or IgM
  - May have light chain restriction (rare)
- Similar deposits in vasculitis lesions
- TBM deposits not reported, except in asssociation with SLE

Electron Microscopy

- Subendothelial and mesangial amorphous electron-dense deposits
- Fingerprint pattern of deposits and tubuloreticular strucures reported in association with SLE

DIFFERENTIAL DIAGNOSIS

Systemic Lupus Erythematosus

- HUV occurs in patients with SLE
- Similar renal pathology
- Criteria to distinguish primary HUV from SLE associated HUV not established

Membranoproliferative GN, Type I

- No C1q antibodies, urticaria, vasculitis

SELECTED REFERENCES

1. Jachiet M et al: The clinical spectrum and therapeutic management of hypocomplementemic urticarial vasculitis: data from a French nationwide study of fifty-seven patients. Arthritis Rheumatol. 67(2):527-34, 2015
2. Park C et al: Membranoproliferative glomerulonephritis presenting as arthropathy and cardiac valvulopathy in hypocomplementemic urticarial vasculitis: a case report. J Med Case Rep. 8:352, 2014
3. Pasini A et al: Renal involvement in hypocomplementaemic urticarial vasculitis syndrome: a report of three paediatric cases. Rheumatology (Oxford). 53(8):1409-13, 2014
4. Ozçakar ZB et al: DNASE1L3 mutations in hypocomplementemic urticarial vasculitis syndrome. Arthritis Rheum. 65(8):2183-9, 2013
5. Buck A et al: Hypocomplementemic urticarial vasculitis syndrome: a case report and literature review. J Clin Aesthet Dermatol. 5(1):36-46, 2012
6. Grimbert P et al: Renal transplantation in a patient with hypocomplementemic urticarial vasculitis syndrome. Am J Kidney Dis. 37(1):144-148, 2001
7. Cadnapaphornchai MA et al: Hypocomplementemic urticarial vasculitis: report of a pediatric case. Pediatr Nephrol. 14(4):328-31, 2000

TERMINOLOGY

Abbreviations

- Thrombotic microangiopathy (TMA)

Definitions

- TMA is characterized by microvascular endothelial injury and thrombosis

ETIOLOGY/PATHOGENESIS

Hemolytic Uremic Syndrome (HUS)

- Predominantly due to endothelial injury and activation with secondary prothrombotic state
- Typical HUS
  - Shiga-like and Shiga toxins produced by enteric pathogens
  - May be genetic susceptibility in minority of cases
- Atypical HUS (and other related TMA)
  - Multifactorial

Thrombotic Thrombocytopenic Purpura (TTP)

- Predominantly due to increased thrombosis and secondary endothelial injury
- Deficiency of ADAMTS13 (**A** **D**isintegrin **A**nd **M**etallopeptidase with **T**hrombo**S**pondin type 1 motif, member **13**)
  - ADAMTS13 (zinc metalloproteinase) synthesized predominantly in liver
    - Required for cleavage of vWF multimers
      - vWF is glycoprotein synthesized by endothelial cells and megakaryocytes
      - After secretion, vWF normally proteolyzed to smaller units by ADAMTS13
      - In absence of ADAMTS13, large vWF multimers promote platelet aggregation in microvessels
  - Genetic deficiency of ADAMTS13 (Upshaw-Schulman syndrome)
    - Rare autosomal recessive inheritance results in ADAMTS13 levels < 5% of normal levels
    - Homozygous or compound heterozygous mutations of *ADAMTS13* allele cause clinical disease
    - Heterozygous mutations result in ADAMTS13 levels approximately 1/2 of normal and lack clinical disease
  - Autoantibodies against ADAMTS13
    - IgG or IgM antibodies act as inhibitors against ADAMTS13
    - Seen in approximately 30-80% of acquired idiopathic TTP
    - Autoimmunity triggered by environmental or endogenous factors (infections, cytokines, drugs) in susceptible host

CLINICAL IMPLICATIONS

Clinical Presentation

- Varies in HUS and TTP and also based on etiology
  - Shiga toxin-associated HUS typically affects children < 5 years of age
  - Patients with *DGKE*, *CFH*, *THBD* mutations and Cobalamin C disease present during infancy
  - Patients with anti-factor H antibodies present 9-13 years of age
  - Hereditary TTP typically presents in children
    - Environmental triggers may precipitate disease in adults
  - Acquired ADAMTS13 deficiency-mediated TTP occurs in adults (18-50 years)
    - More often in African Americans and females
- Atypical HUS etiologically different from TTP but has significant clinical overlap
  - Hence, clinical syndrome often referred as atypical HUS/TTP

Acute Presentation

- Typical HUS
  - Watery diarrhea followed by bloody diarrhea
  - Fever
  - Renal insufficiency
  - Acute renal failure more common in adults
  - Hypertension

Arteriolar "Onion-Skinning" Changes in TMA

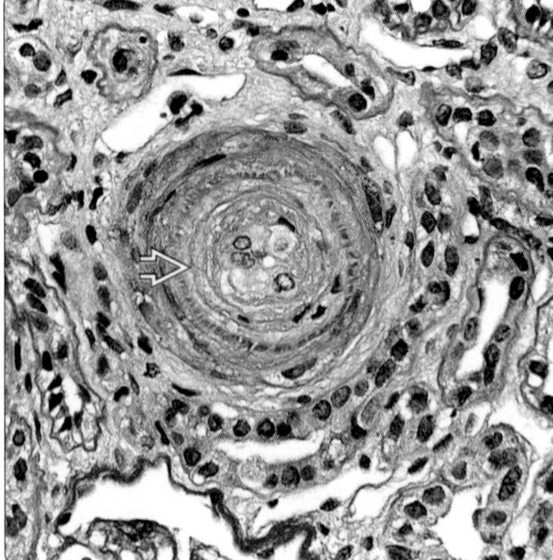

GBM Duplication in Chronic TMA

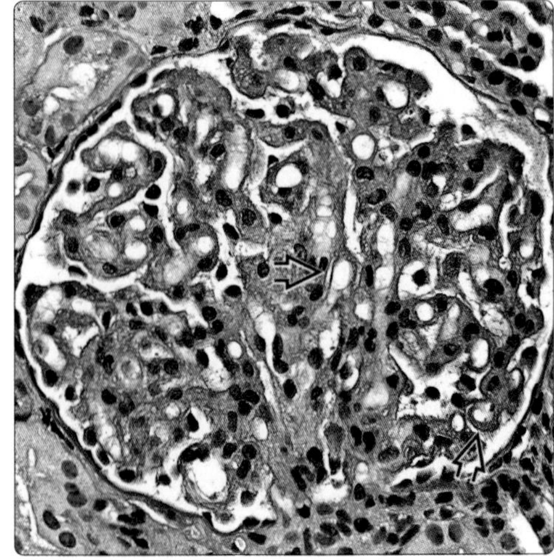

(Left) *Acute TMA shows classic arteriolar narrowing due to intimal edema and lamination (i.e., "onion skinning") ➡ in this 30-year-old woman with acute renal failure and dilated cardiomyopathy.* **(Right)** *Chronic (or recurrent) TMA is classically manifested by thickened, duplicated GBMs ➡ as seen in this biopsy from a 4 year old with recurrent atypical HUS and a normal serum complement level.*

- Other systemic manifestations less common
- Subset of atypical HUS
  - Catastrophic antiphospholipid antibody syndrome and scleroderma renal crisis
    - Abrupt onset of symptoms
    - No prodrome of diarrhea

Chronic/Insidious Presentation

- TTP and subset of atypical HUS
  - Fever
  - Hypertension
  - Mild proteinuria
  - Microscopic hematuria
  - Chronic renal insufficiency
  - Neurological symptoms predominate in TTP
  - Recurrences and relapses may occur with TTP

LABORATORY INVESTIGATIONS

Microangiopathic Hemolytic Anemia

- Blood flow through injured or narrowed blood vessels causes erythrocyte fragmentation and platelet consumption
  - Anemia
  - Thrombocytopenia
  - Schistocytes on peripheral smear
  - Elevated serum lactate dehydrogenase
  - Reduced haptoglobin levels
  - Negative Coombs test
  - Normal prothrombin and partial thromboplastin time
- Leukocytosis, especially in typical HUS

Determination of Etiology

- Stool cultures to confirm enteric bacterial infection
- Antiphospholipid antibodies
- Serum complement C3, C4 levels
- ANA, anti-dsDNA for systemic lupus erythematosus (SLE)
- ADAMTS13 autoantibodies
- Anti-topoisomerase 1 and anti-RNA polymerase (I & III) antibodies
  - If systemic sclerosis suspected
- Plasma levels of complement factors H and I recommended in all aHUS cases, as are MCP levels on mononuclear cells, and screening for anti-CFH antibodies
- Genetic testing for specific gene mutations and deletions
  - *ADAMTS13*, *CFH* (including recombination with *CFHR* gene), *CFI*, *MCP (CD46)*, Thrombomodulin, *CFB*, *C3*, *DGKE*, deletion of *CFHR1* and *CFHR3* genes

MACROSCOPIC

General Features

- Enlarged kidneys in acute phase
- Petechial hemorrhages usually seen on external surface
- Patchy cortical necrosis can occur
- In chronic phase, small kidneys with granular cortical surface

MICROSCOPIC

Acute TMA

- Glomeruli
  - Bloodless appearance
  - Apparent thickening of capillary wall due to subendothelial expansion
  - Mesangiolysis
  - Endothelial swelling
  - Thrombi, hilum or glomerular capillaries
    - Nuclear debris present but no significant inflammation
    - Some initial data suggested HUS thrombi are fibrin rich, and TTP thrombi are platelet rich
      - Not reliable feature and not possible to differentiate histologically
    - Fibrinoid necrosis may be present
  - Rare crescents seen in occasional cases
  - Fragmented RBCs entrapped in thrombi, subendothelium, and mesangium
  - In presence of arteriolar changes, downstream glomeruli demonstrate ischemic collapse of capillary tufts
    - Segmental sclerosis with collapsing features may be observed
- Tubulointerstitium
  - Acute tubular injury characterized by simplified epithelium, nuclear reactive atypia
  - Interstitial edema
  - Cortical necrosis in severe cases
- Blood vessels
  - Arterioles near vascular pole affected frequently
    - Endothelial swelling and luminal occlusion
    - Intimal mucoid edema with entrapped schistocytes
    - Thrombi
      - Fibrinoid necrosis may be present without evidence of inflammatory infiltrate
  - Interlobular and arcuate arteries show similar changes

Chronic TMA

- Changes may be seen within days of acute onset of TMA
- Glomeruli
  - GBM duplication and double contours
    - Due to endothelial cell injury
  - Mesangial expansion with features of mesangiolysis
  - Variable focal segmental and global glomerulosclerosis
- Tubulointerstitium
  - Tubular atrophy and interstitial fibrosis
- Arterioles and small arteries
  - Intimal fibrosis with narrowed lumina
  - Concentric lamination of intimal fibrosis causes "onion skin" appearance
  - Recanalized thrombi may be identified

Immunofluorescence Microscopy

- Thrombi in glomeruli and blood vessels stain for fibrinogen
- Nonspecific entrapment of C3 and IgM in glomeruli
- No immune complexes unless associated with connective tissue disorder like SLE

Electron Microscopy

- Acute TMA
  - Endothelial swelling and loss of fenestrations
  - Expansion of subendothelial space by electron-lucent material

- Entrapped schistocytes and fibrin tactoids in subendothelium
  - Mesangial matrix also lucent (mesangiolysis)
  - Podocyte foot process effacement common
  - Thrombi show mixture of platelets, fibrin, and erythrocytes
  - Myocyte degeneration may be seen in affected arterioles
- Chronic TMA
  - Increased matrix in mesangium and subendothelium
  - Depolymerized fibrin may be identified
  - Duplication of glomerular basement membranes
  - Mesangial cell interposition
  - Podocyte foot processes often effaced

DIAGNOSTIC CHECKLIST

Clinically Relevant Pathological Features

- Isolated involvement of glomeruli associated with better prognosis than when arterioles also affected
- Cortical necrosis is poor prognostic factor

Pathologic Interpretation Pearls

- Etiology cannot be distinguished based on biopsy findings
- Anemia, thrombocytopenia, and schistocytes may be absent in mild disease
- Latency period between exposure to radiation and TMA can be very long
- Biopsy with TMA due to malignant hypertension often shows hypertensive arteriopathy
- Significant thrombosis in absence of TMA or arterial remodeling should raise suspicion for antiphospholipid antibody syndrome

SELECTED REFERENCES

1. Hamaguchi Y et al: Clinical and Immunologic Predictors of Scleroderma Renal Crisis in Japanese Systemic Sclerosis Patients With Anti-RNA Polymerase III Autoantibodies. Arthritis Rheumatol. 67(4):1045-52, 2015
2. Kayser C et al: Autoantibodies in systemic sclerosis: unanswered questions. Front Immunol. 6:167, 2015
3. George JN et al: Syndromes of thrombotic microangiopathy. N Engl J Med. 371(7):654-66, 2014
4. Hofer J et al: Complement factor H-antibody-associated hemolytic uremic syndrome: pathogenesis, clinical presentation, and treatment. Semin Thromb Hemost. 40(4):431-43, 2014
5. Riedl M et al: Spectrum of complement-mediated thrombotic microangiopathies: pathogenetic insights identifying novel treatment approaches. Semin Thromb Hemost. 40(4):444-64, 2014
6. Rosove MH: Thrombotic microangiopathies. Semin Arthritis Rheum. 43(6):797-805, 2014
7. Usui J et al: Clinicopathological spectrum of kidney diseases in cancer patients treated with vascular endothelial growth factor inhibitors: a report of 5 cases and review of literature. Hum Pathol. 45(9):1918-27, 2014
8. Legendre CM et al: Terminal complement inhibitor eculizumab in atypical hemolytic-uremic syndrome. N Engl J Med. 368(23):2169-81, 2013
9. Mehrazma M et al: Prognostic value of renal pathological findings in children with atypical hemolytic uremic syndrome. Iran J Kidney Dis. 5(6):380-5, 2011
10. Said SM et al: Myeloproliferative neoplasms cause glomerulopathy. Kidney Int. 80(7):753-9, 2011
11. Batal I et al: Scleroderma renal crisis: a pathology perspective. Int J Rheumatol. 2010:543704, 2010
12. Benz K et al: Thrombotic microangiopathy: new insights. Curr Opin Nephrol Hypertens. 19(3):242-7, 2010
13. Izzedine H et al: VEGF signalling inhibition-induced proteinuria: Mechanisms, significance and management. Eur J Cancer. 46(2):439-48, 2010
14. Ruiz-Irastorza G et al: Antiphospholipid syndrome. Lancet. 376(9751):1498-509, 2010
15. Satoskar AA et al: De novo thrombotic microangiopathy in renal allograft biopsies-role of antibody-mediated rejection. Am J Transplant. 10(8):1804-11, 2010
16. Sánchez-Corral P et al: Advances in understanding the aetiology of atypical Haemolytic Uraemic Syndrome. Br J Haematol. 150(5):529-42, 2010
17. Zipfel PF et al: DEAP-HUS: deficiency of CFHR plasma proteins and autoantibody-positive form of hemolytic uremic syndrome. Pediatr Nephrol. 25(10):2009-19, 2010
18. Zipfel PF et al: Thrombotic microangiopathies: new insights and new challenges. Curr Opin Nephrol Hypertens. 19(4):372-8, 2010
19. Changsirikulchai S et al: Renal thrombotic microangiopathy after hematopoietic cell transplant: role of GVHD in pathogenesis. Clin J Am Soc Nephrol. 4(2):345-53, 2009
20. Gigante A et al: Antiphospholipid antibodies and renal involvement. Am J Nephrol. 30(5):405-12, 2009
21. Moake J: Thrombotic thrombocytopenia purpura (TTP) and other thrombotic microangiopathies. Best Pract Res Clin Haematol. 22(4):567-76, 2009
22. Noris M et al: Atypical hemolytic-uremic syndrome. N Engl J Med. 361(17):1676-87, 2009
23. Copelovitch L et al: The thrombotic microangiopathies. Pediatr Nephrol. 23(10):1761-7, 2008
24. Fine DM et al: Thrombotic microangiopathy and other glomerular disorders in the HIV-infected patient. Semin Nephrol. 28(6):545-55, 2008
25. Stokes MB et al: Glomerular disease related to anti-VEGF therapy. Kidney Int. 74(11):1487-91, 2008
26. Zheng XL et al: Pathogenesis of thrombotic microangiopathies. Annu Rev Pathol. 3:249-77, 2008
27. Chang A et al: Spectrum of renal pathology in hematopoietic cell transplantation: a series of 20 patients and review of the literature. Clin J Am Soc Nephrol. 2(5):1014-23, 2007
28. Desch K et al: Is there a shared pathophysiology for thrombotic thrombocytopenic purpura and hemolytic-uremic syndrome? J Am Soc Nephrol. 18(9):2457-60, 2007
29. Fakhouri F et al: Does hemolytic uremic syndrome differ from thrombotic thrombocytopenic purpura? Nat Clin Pract Nephrol. 3(12):679-87, 2007
30. Fischer MJ et al: The antiphospholipid syndrome. Semin Nephrol. 27(1):35-46, 2007
31. Franchini M et al: Reduced von Willebrand factor-cleaving protease levels in secondary thrombotic microangiopathies and other diseases. Semin Thromb Hemost. 33(8):787-97, 2007
32. Schneider M: Thrombotic microangiopathy (TTP and HUS): advances in differentiation and diagnosis. Clin Lab Sci. 20(4):216-20, 2007
33. Izzedine H et al: Gemcitabine-induced thrombotic microangiopathy: a systematic review. Nephrol Dial Transplant. 21(11):3038-45, 2006
34. Tsai HM: The molecular biology of thrombotic microangiopathy. Kidney Int. 70(1):16-23, 2006
35. Lian EC: Pathogenesis of thrombotic thrombocytopenic purpura: ADAMTS13 deficiency and beyond. Semin Thromb Hemost. 31(6):625-32, 2005
36. Lowe EJ et al: Thrombotic thrombocytopenic purpura and hemolytic uremic syndrome in children and adolescents. Semin Thromb Hemost. 31(6):717-30, 2005
37. Zakarija A et al: Drug-induced thrombotic microangiopathy. Semin Thromb Hemost. 31(6):681-90, 2005
38. Denton CP et al: Scleroderma–clinical and pathological advances. Best Pract Res Clin Rheumatol. 18(3):271-90, 2004
39. Medina PJ et al: Drug-associated thrombotic thrombocytopenic purpura-hemolytic uremic syndrome. Curr Opin Hematol. 8(5):286-93, 2001
40. Ray PE et al: Pathogenesis of Shiga toxin-induced hemolytic uremic syndrome. Pediatr Nephrol. 16(10):823-39, 2001
41. Tsai HM et al: Antibodies to von Willebrand factor-cleaving protease in acute thrombotic thrombocytopenic purpura. N Engl J Med. 339(22):1585-94, 1998
42. Boyce TG et al: Escherichia coli O157:H7 and the hemolytic-uremic syndrome. N Engl J Med. 333(6):364-8, 1995
43. Myers KA et al: Thrombotic microangiopathy associated with Streptococcus pneumoniae bacteremia: case report and review. Clin Infect Dis. 17(6):1037-40, 1993

Causes of Thrombotic Microangiopathy

Etiology	Mechanism of Action
Typical Hemolytic Uremic Syndrome (HUS)	
Enteropathogenic infections (*Escherichia coli, Shigella dysenteriae*)	Shiga-like toxin causes endothelial damage by binding to Gb3 receptors; reported cases with complement gene mutations
Atypical HUS (& Other Forms of TMA; Clinical Overlap With TTP)	
Nonenteric infections (e.g., *Streptococcus pneumoniae*, HIV, *Mycoplasma pneumoniae*, Coxsackie A & B)	Neuraminidase produced by *S. pneumoniae* exposes cryptic antigens on erythrocytes, platelets, & glomerular endothelial cells with resultant immunological damage;
Genetic defects in complement activation & regulation (mutations in genes *CFH, MCP* (*CD46*), *CFI, CFB, C3*	Uncontrolled activation of alternate complement pathway causes endothelial damage & prothrombotic state; environmental triggers act as "2nd hit" to precipitate HUS; low C3 levels in aHUS may indicate genetic component
Genetic defects in cobalamin metabolism & coagulation pathway	Homozygous or compound heterozygous mutations in *MMACHC* gene; genetic abnormalities of thrombomodulin, plasminogen & *DGKE* genes affect the coagulation cascade
Drugs (cyclosporine, tacrolimus, sirolimus, anti-VEGF therapy, mitomycin-C, cisplatin, quinine, vaccines)	Either idiosyncratic reaction or dose-dependent toxicity; potential mechanisms depend on drug, including drug-dependent antibodies, direct endothelial injury, & inhibition of VEGF
Bone marrow transplantation	Endothelial injury due to chemotherapy, radiation, drugs, or manifestation of graft-vs.-host disease (GVHD); genetic predisposition may play a role
Radiation	Direct endothelial injury, delayed effect
Pregnancy & post partum	Increased susceptibility to HUS during post partum; genetic mutations in complement system appear to have a role
Systemic sclerosis	Endothelial injury due to antiendothelial antibodies
Autoimmune (antiphospholipid antibody syndrome, SLE, anti-factor H autoantibodies)	Antiphospholipid antibodies cause endothelial damage & hypercoagulability; CFH antibodies interfere with complement regulation
Malignant hypertension	Endothelial injury due to shear stress
Antibody-mediated rejection in transplantation	Endothelial injury mediated by donor specific antibodies
Neoplasms such as adenocarcinomas (especially mucin producing) &, rarely, myeloproliferative neoplasms, leukemia & lymphoma	Causes include tumor emboli or procoagulants, impaired fibrinolysis, & low ADAMTS13; may be triggered by chemotherapeutic agents & radiation; TMA associated with myeloproliferative neoplasm is probably mediated by cytokines & chemokines
Idiopathic	Unknown cause
Thrombotic Thrombocytopenic Purpura (TTP)	
Familial	Mutations in gene encoding ADAMTS13, a vWF cleaving protease; large vWF multimers cause increased platelet aggregation
Autoimmune	Autoantibodies against ADAMTS13 result in large vWF multimers
Drugs (Ticlopidine, Clopidogrel)	Deficiency of ADAMTS13 due to autoantibodies in a subset
Hereditary	Homozygous or compound heterozygous *ADAMTS13* gene mutations

Clinical Parameters of Typical HUS & TTP: Two Ends of a Spectrum

Parameter	Typical HUS	TTP
Age at presentation	Infants & young children	Middle age
Gender predilection	None	More frequent in women
Seasonal variation	Epidemic form usually occurs in summer months	None
Prodrome of diarrhea	Present	Absent
Predisposing factors	Intake of contaminated food or fecal-oral transmission	Nondietary factors
Renal involvement	Present in all cases	Often mild, so patients infrequently undergo renal biopsy
Hemorrhagic colitis	Usually present	Rare
Systemic involvement	Severe cases have systemic manifestations, including neurological	Neurological symptoms predominate with multiorgan involvement
Treatment	Supportive therapy; antibiotics often contraindicated	Plasmapheresis
Morbidity & mortality	Low; most children recover completely	High; can recur in 20-30% of patients
Recurrence after transplant	Rare	Frequency unknown due to clinical overlap with aHUS

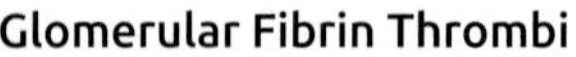

Glomerular Fibrin Thrombi

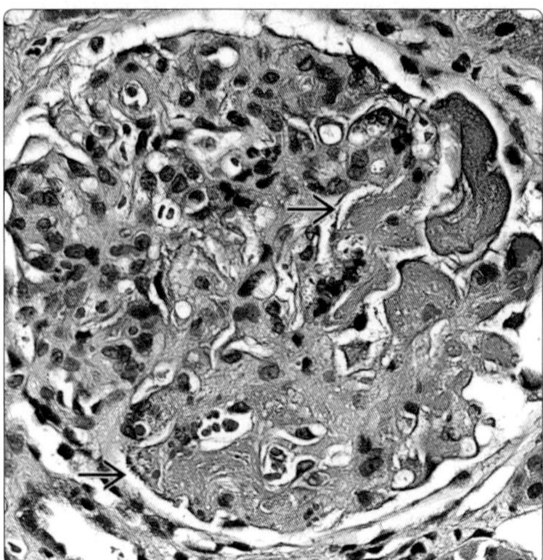

Fragmented RBCs in Acute TMA

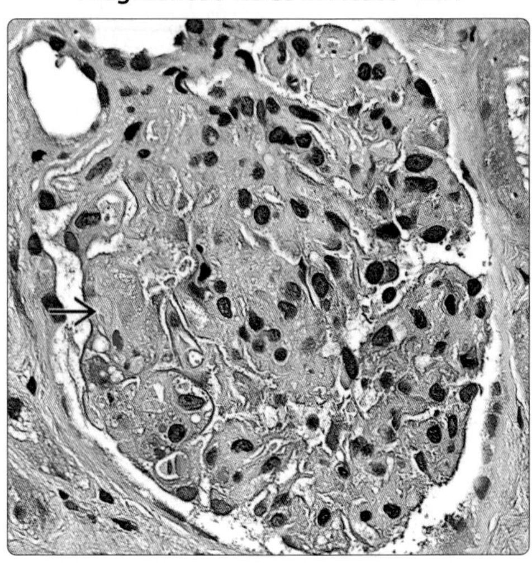

(Left) *Glomerular fibrin thrombi ➡ are seen with entrapped RBCs, compatible with acute TMA. The biopsy is from a 25-year-old woman with acute renal failure, congestive heart failure, and schistocytes on peripheral smear. Etiology of TMA is undetermined.* **(Right)** *Acute TMA is seen with glomerular thrombi ➡ and fragmented RBCs. Patient is 4 months post bone marrow transplantation for follicular lymphoma and has evidence of skin GVHD. Cyclosporine had been discontinued a month prior.*

Acute Tubular Injury in TMA

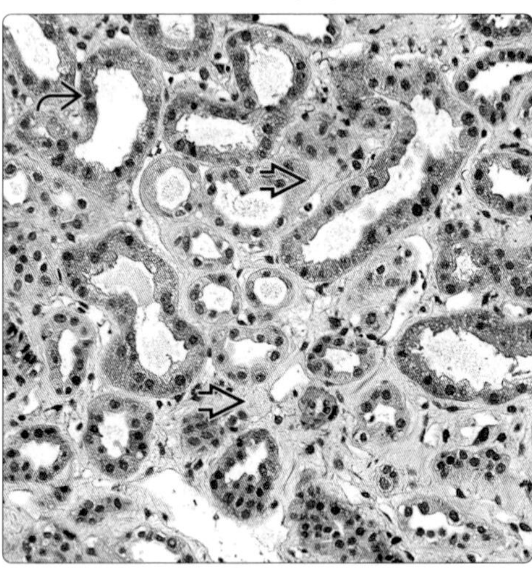

Arteriolar Changes in Malignant HTN

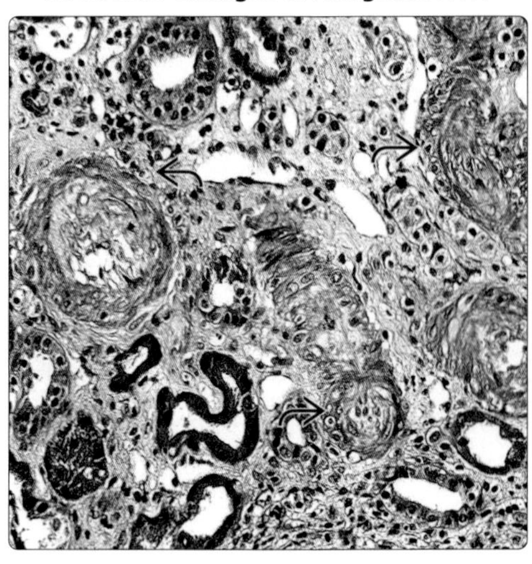

(Left) *The interstitium is expanded by edema ➡, and the proximal tubules ➡ are ectatic with simplified epithelium. The patient was clinically diagnosed with TTP, and renal biopsy showed TMA.* **(Right)** *Several cross sections of interlobular arteries ➡ show intimal edema and narrowed lumina. In this case, TMA changes are due to malignant hypertension. This patient is a 27 year old with a 2-year history of uncontrolled hypertension and noncompliance to medications.*

GBM Double Contours in Chronic TMA

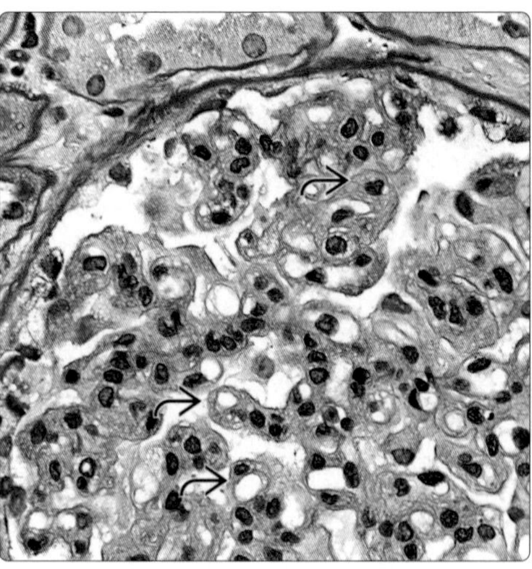

Chronic TMA in Genetic Atypical HUS

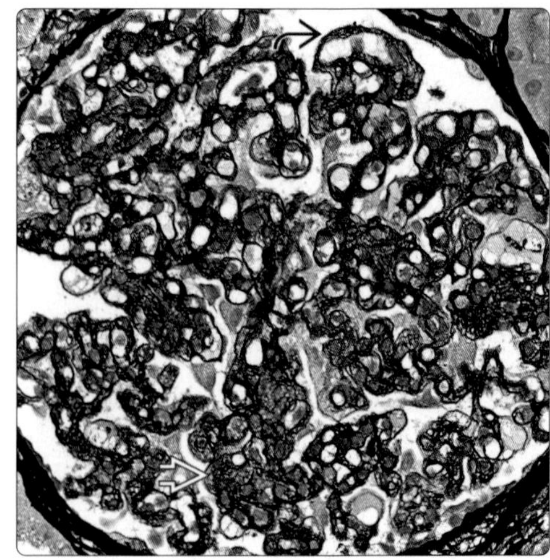

(Left) *Chronic TMA is characterized by extensive duplication of GBM due to remodeling and mesangial cell interposition ➡. This patient is a 19 year old with recurrent atypical HUS. A limited work-up at the time of biopsy revealed low C3 and normal factor H levels.* **(Right)** *Extensive double contours ➡ and mesangial expansion ➡ are seen in chronic TMA due to recurrent atypical HUS. This patient is a 19-year-old woman with low serum C3 levels, suggestive of a genetic component.*

Chronic TMA and Segmental Sclerosis

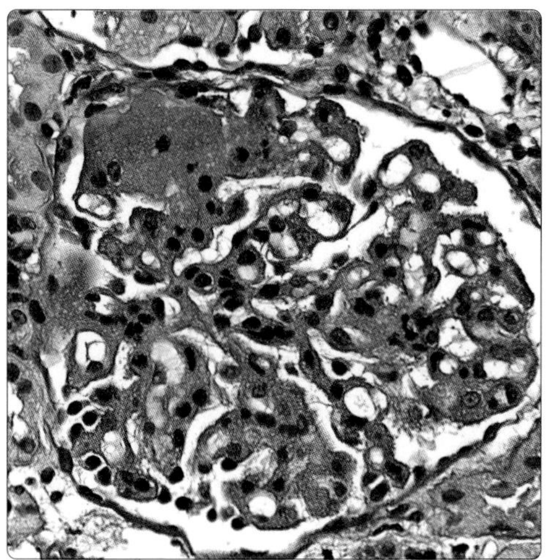

Arterial Mucoid Intimal Edema

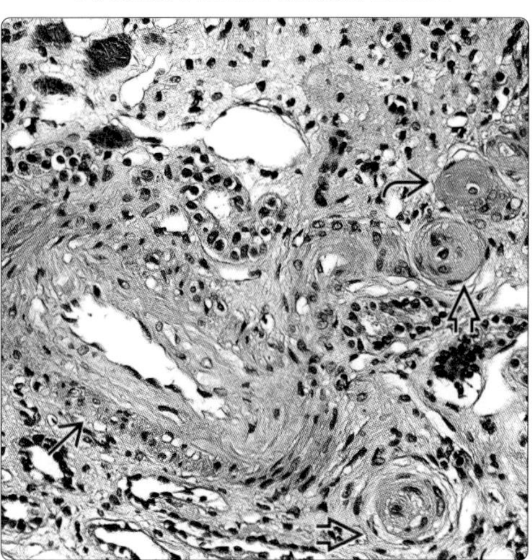

(Left) *Segmental glomerulosclerosis is seen along with GBM thickening due to chronic TMA. GBMs appear thickened due to subendothelial expansion and basement membrane remodeling in this 4 year old with recurrent atypical HUS.* **(Right)** *Malignant hypertension shows hypertensive arteriosclerosis in the background. An interlobular artery ➡ has mucoid intimal change and arteriolar hyaline ➡ is seen. Arterioles ➡ are edematous with narrowed lumina, consistent with TMA.*

Subendothelial Electron-Lucent Material

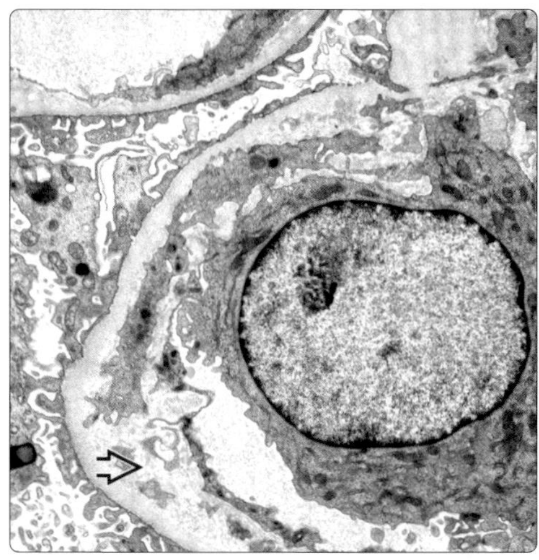

Acute TMA With Fibrin Tactoids

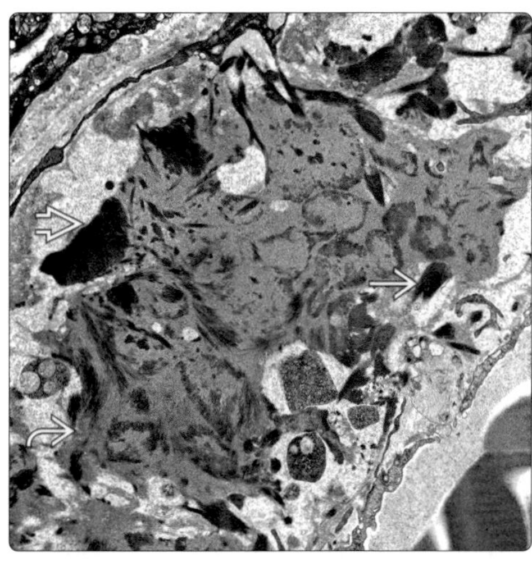

(Left) *In TMA, endothelial cells are detached from GBM, and subendothelium is expanded ➡ by electron-lucent material. Patient presented with fever, microangiopathic hemolytic anemia, and acute renal failure. Clinical diagnosis was TTP. Serological tests included were normal (ANA, C3, anticardiolipin antibody[-], serum C3).* **(Right)** *Note fibrin thrombus ➡, fibrin tactoids ➡, and entrapped fragmented erythrocytes ➡ in capillary lumen in acute TMA.*

Glomerular Ischemia in Acute TMA

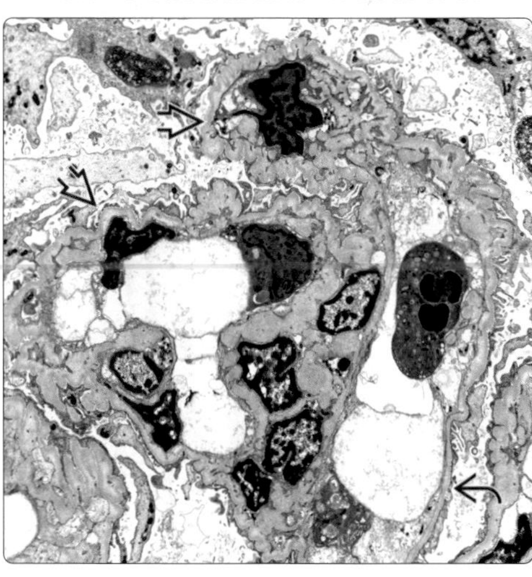

Arteriolar Luminal Narrowing in TMA

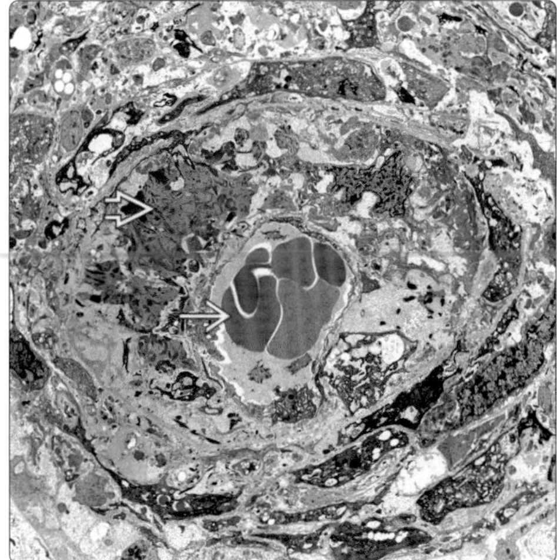

(Left) *The GBM shows extensive wrinkling ➡, and podocyte foot processes are effaced ➡ in this biopsy of a patient with acute TMA. Arteriolar thrombosis and necrosis result in capillary tuft collapse of downstream glomeruli.* **(Right)** *Prominent subendothelial edema is seen in this arteriole with luminal narrowing ➡. Fibrin and cellular debris ➡ are seen in subendothelial space, compatible with acute arteriolar TMA. No inflammatory infiltrate is present to suggest vasculitis.*

Hemolytic Uremic Syndrome, Infection Related

KEY FACTS

TERMINOLOGY

- D+HUS caused by enteropathogenic bacteria and associated with prodrome of diarrhea

ETIOLOGY/PATHOGENESIS

- *Escherichia coli* infection in ~ 90%
- *E. coli* (STEC) producing Shiga-like toxin (Stx) or subtilase cytotoxin (SubAB)
  - Endothelial damage by Stx causes prothrombotic state, hemorrhagic enteritis, and thrombotic microangiopathy
  - Activation of alternative complement pathway by Stx
- Nonenteric pathogens usually result in atypical HUS
- Complement gene mutations rarely detected

CLINICAL ISSUES

- 5-10% of patients with *E. coli* O157:H7 infection develop HUS, mainly infants and young children
- Acute renal failure and microangiopathic anemia develop abruptly ~ 1 week after onset of diarrhea
- Most patients (especially children) recover completely with supportive care
  - Antibiotics contraindicated in STEC infections
- Eculizumab (anti-C5) beneficial in uncontrolled studies

MICROSCOPIC

- Fibrinoid necrosis and thrombosis in glomeruli and arterioles
- Mesangiolysis
- Glomerular endothelial swelling and injury
- Cortical necrosis in severe cases

TOP DIFFERENTIAL DIAGNOSES

- Thrombotic microangiography due to other causes
- Vasculitis

DIAGNOSTIC CHECKLIST

- Isolated glomerular involvement has better prognosis than if blood vessels are affected
- Cause of HUS cannot be distinguished by renal pathology

(Left) *The glomerular capillary lumen near the vascular pole is occluded by an organizing thrombus. This biopsy is from a 37-year-old man with documented Escherichia coli O157:H7-associated HUS.* **(Right)** *Arteriolar lumen is occluded by intimal edema with entrapped RBCs and fuchsinophilic fibrin. Acute tubular injury is also seen with simplified epithelium and nuclear atypia.*

Organizing Thrombus in Vascular Pole

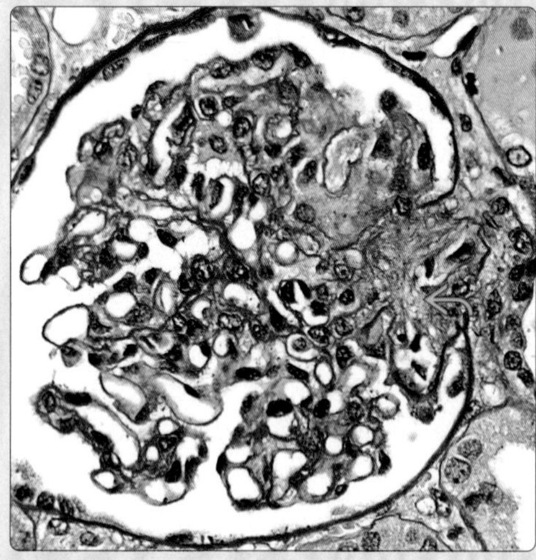

Arterial Intimal Edema and Trapped Erythrocytes

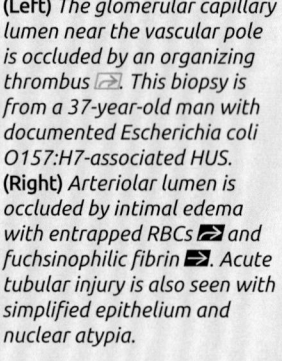

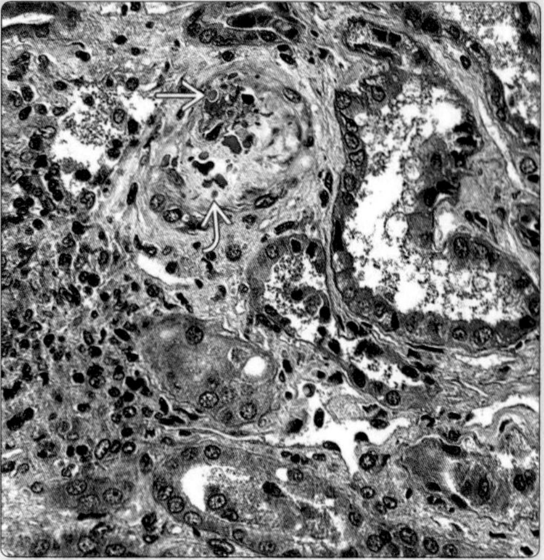

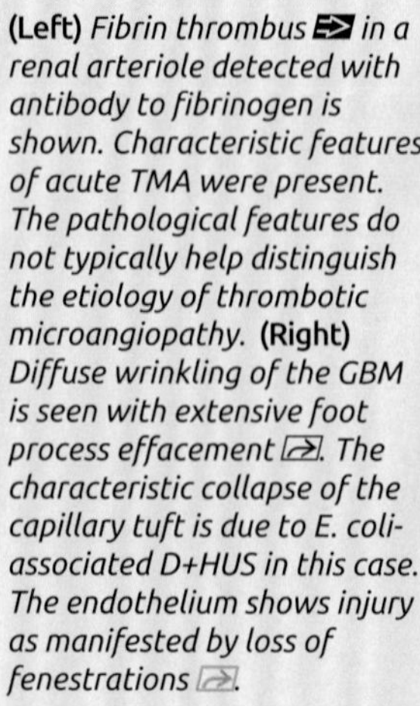

(Left) *Fibrin thrombus in a renal arteriole detected with antibody to fibrinogen is shown. Characteristic features of acute TMA were present. The pathological features do not typically help distinguish the etiology of thrombotic microangiopathy.* **(Right)** *Diffuse wrinkling of the GBM is seen with extensive foot process effacement. The characteristic collapse of the capillary tuft is due to E. coli-associated D+HUS in this case. The endothelium shows injury as manifested by loss of fenestrations.*

Fibrin in Arteriole

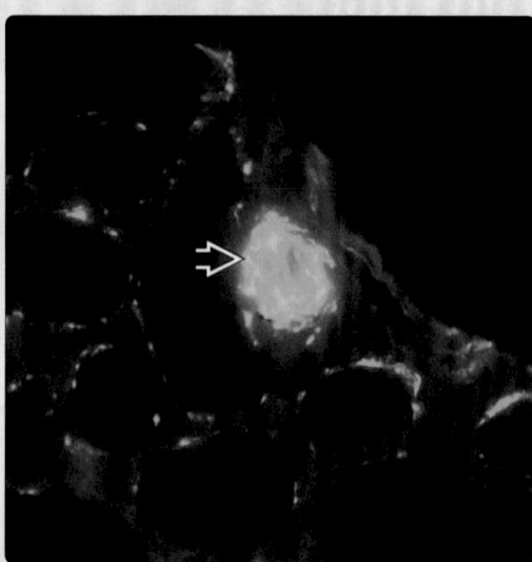

Wrinkling of GBM and Endothelial Injury

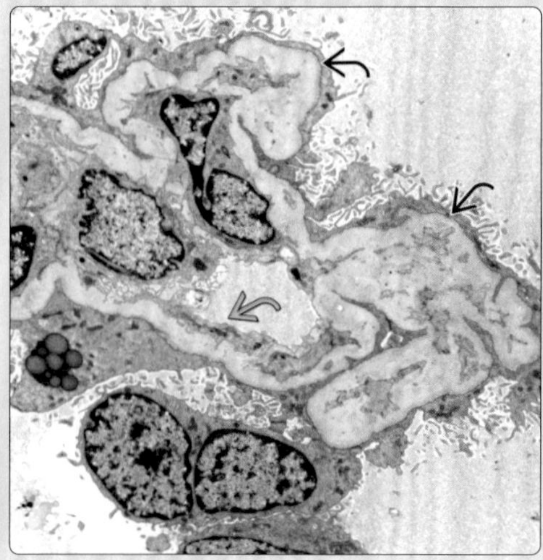

TERMINOLOGY

Abbreviations

- Diarrhea-associated hemolytic uremic syndrome (D+HUS)

Synonyms

- Epidemic form of HUS, classic HUS

Definitions

- HUS caused by enteropathogenic infectious organisms
  - Associated with prodrome of diarrhea

ETIOLOGY/PATHOGENESIS

Infectious Agents

- *Escherichia coli* infection accounts for > 90% of D+HUS in children in USA
  - Route of infection
    - Ingestion of contaminated undercooked hamburgers, raw vegetables, raw milk, or drinking water
    - Animal fecal contact (petting zoos, fairs)
    - Fecal-oral contact, as in child care centers
  - Shiga toxigenic *E. coli* (STEC) or enterohemorrhagic *E. coli* capable of producing Shiga-like toxins (Stx1 and Stx2)
    - Majority of D+HUS in North America and Europe caused by O157:H7 strain of STEC
    - Genes encoding Stx1 and Stx2 located on bacteriophages infecting bacteria
    - After colonization of gut epithelium by STEC, locally produced Stx crosses intestinal barrier and enters circulation
  - Shiga toxin (a.k.a. verotoxin) has 1 A and 5 B subunits
    - Stx B subunit binds to glycoprotein receptors, globotriaosylceramide (Gb3)
    - Gb3 receptors expressed in highest concentration in microvascular endothelial cells of kidney, gut, pancreas, and brain and in renal tubular epithelial cells
  - Internalized Stx A subunit in cells has RNA-N-glycosidase activity
    - Inhibits host cell protein synthesis and causes apoptosis
    - Endothelial damage by Stx causes prothrombotic state, ischemia-induced hemorrhagic enteritis, and thrombotic microangiopathy
      - Microangiopathic anemia caused by shear stress as erythrocytes traverse injured arterioles and glomeruli
  - Activation of alternative complement pathway
    - Stx2 directly activates complement leading to formation of terminal complement complex
    - Stx2 binds factor H (FH), reducing cofactor activity on cell surface
    - Stx2 downregulates membrane bound complement regulator CD59 on glomerular endothelial cells
- Other STEC virulence factors
  - Subtilase cytotoxin (SubAB)
    - Causes proteolytic cleavage of essential endoplasmic reticulum chaperone molecule and triggers stress response leading to apoptosis
    - SubAB receptor is glycan chain terminating in sialic acid (Neu5Gc), a glycoprotein not synthesized by humans due to evolutionary loss
    - Neu5Gc synthesized in nonhuman primates and present abundantly in red meat and dairy products
    - Neu5Gc from dietary sources can be incorporated metabolically into surfaces of human endothelium and intestinal epithelium
  - Locus of enterocyte effacement (LEE) encodes capacity to adhere to enterocytes and cause effacement of microvilli
  - High pathogenicity island (HPI) contributes to STEC survival
  - Large plasmids encode hemolysin, a pore-forming cytolysin

Other Organisms

- *Shigella dysenteriae* produces Shiga toxin
  - Most common cause of D+HUS in Asia and Africa
  - *Shigella* directly invades intestinal epithelium and induce apoptosis
- Other enteric infectious agents include *Salmonella*, *Campylobacter*, and *Yersinia*
- Nonenteric pathogens usually result in atypical HUS (without prodrome of diarrhea)
  - Examples include human immunodeficiency virus (HIV), *Streptococcus pneumoniae*, *Mycoplasma pneumoniae*, Coxsackie A and B viruses, *Legionella* infection, histoplasmosis, and brucellosis
  - *S. pneumoniae* produces neuraminidase that cleaves N-acetyl neuraminic acid from cell surfaces and exposes Thomsen-Friedenreich (T) antigen, causing hemolysis

Host Risk Factors

- Genetic factors
  - Complement gene mutations rarely detected
    - Reported mutations in *CFH*, *CFI*, and *CD46*
  - Polymorphisms of genes involved in coagulation, complement activation, and renin angiotensin systems may influence susceptibility or severity
- Nongenetic factors
  - Gb3 receptors
    - More abundantly expressed in young children
    - Upregulated by cytokines and lipopolysaccharides
    - Upregulated by HIV in renal tubules
  - Consumption of red meat and dairy products primes target cells with SubAB receptors

CLINICAL ISSUES

Epidemiology

- Incidence
  - ~ 5-10% of patients with *E. coli* O157:H7 infection develop HUS
  - 1-3 cases per 100,000 per year in USA
  - Epidemic *E. coli* outbreaks often in summer months in North America and Europe
- Age
  - Mainly in infants, young children, and elderly
- Sex
  - Slightly more common in males
- Ethnicity
  - Rare in African Americans

Presentation

- Diarrhea initially watery and subsequently becomes bloody
  - Acute renal failure develops ~ 1 week after onset of diarrhea
    - Oliguria or anuria
    - Hematuria and proteinuria
- Pallor, melena, hematemesis, and petechiae due to anemia and bleeding tendencies
- Hypertension
- Severe disease may have congestive heart failure, acute pancreatitis, headaches, seizures, and visual changes
- *Shigella* infection often more severe systemic symptoms: Fever, bacteremia, and severe hemolysis

Laboratory Tests

- Microangiopathic hemolytic anemia
  - Schistocytes on peripheral smear
  - Elevated serum LDH and reduced haptoglobin levels
  - Thrombocytopenia
  - Coombs test negative
- Stool cultures confirm enteric bacterial infection
- Elevated sC5b-9 and Bb, normal C3 and C4

Treatment

- Drugs
  - Eculizumab (anti-C5) appears beneficial in uncontrolled studies
- Supportive care and dialysis as needed

Prognosis

- Most patients (especially children) recover completely
- Prognosis of D+HUS vastly better than D-HUS
- Approximately 3-5% die during acute phase of illness due to cardiovascular or neurological complications
- About 1/3 of D+HUS patients have persistent mild proteinuria &/or renal insufficiency
  - Poor prognostic factors include marked leucocytosis and older age at onset

MICROSCOPIC

Histologic Features

- Glomeruli
  - Glomerular endothelial swelling and congestion
    - Mesangiolysis
    - Mesangial hypercellularity
  - Thrombi
    - Ischemic collapse
  - Glomerular necrosis, often contiguous with fibrinoid necrosis in hilar arterioles
    - Apoptotic debris and fragmented erythrocytes in foci of fibrinoid necrosis
    - infiltration of neutrophils documented
  - GBM duplication in chronic phase
- Tubules and interstitium
  - Acute tubular injury with simplified epithelium and reactive nuclear atypia
  - Cortical necrosis and infarction in severe cases
- Arteries
  - Fibrinoid necrosis and thrombosis of arterioles
  - Arteriolar endothelial swelling and mucoid intimal change (seen with Alcian Blue stain)
  - Arteriolar thrombi at hilum and in interlobular arteries
- Other organs
  - Microvascular endothelial damage also occurs in gastrointestinal tract, brain, pancreas, and liver

ANCILLARY TESTS

Immunofluorescence

- Nonspecific entrapment of C3 and IgM in affected glomeruli and blood vessels
- Thrombi highlighted on fibrinogen stain
- Fibrinogen in mesangium

Electron Microscopy

- Endothelial swelling and expansion of subendothelial zone by flocculent material
- Glomerular and arteriolar thrombi show platelets and fibrin tactoids with entrapped fragmented erythrocytes
- Foot process effacement (variable)
- No electron-dense deposits

DIFFERENTIAL DIAGNOSIS

Thrombotic Microangiopathy Due to Other Causes

- Seek evidence for genetic predisposition, autoantibodies, neoplasm, and drug history

Vasculitis

- Fibrinoid necrosis accompanied by transmural inflammatory infiltrate
- Crescents common

DIAGNOSTIC CHECKLIST

Clinically Relevant Pathologic Features

- Isolated glomerular involvement associated with better prognosis than if blood vessels affected

Pathologic Interpretation Pearls

- Cause of HUS cannot be distinguished by pathological features

SELECTED REFERENCES

1. Ferraris JR et al: Activation of the alternative pathway of complement during the acute phase of typical hemolytic uremic syndrome. Clin Exp Immunol. ePub, 2015
2. Mele C et al: Hemolytic uremic syndrome. Semin Immunopathol. 36(4):399-420, 2014
3. Orth-Höller D et al: Role of complement in enterohemorrhagic Escherichia coli-Induced hemolytic uremic syndrome. Semin Thromb Hemost. 40(4):503-7, 2014
4. Alberti M et al: Two patients with history of STEC-HUS, posttransplant recurrence and complement gene mutations. Am J Transplant. 13(8):2201-6, 2013
5. Kemper MJ: Outbreak of hemolytic uremic syndrome caused by E. coli O104:H4 in Germany: a pediatric perspective. Pediatr Nephrol. 27(2):161-4, 2012
6. Constantinescu AR et al: Non-enteropathic hemolytic uremic syndrome: causes and short-term course. Am J Kidney Dis. 43(6):976-82, 2004
7. Chaisri U et al: Localization of Shiga toxins of enterohaemorrhagic Escherichia coli in kidneys of paediatric and geriatric patients with fatal haemolytic uraemic syndrome. Microb Pathog. 31(2):59-67, 2001
8. Inward CD et al: Renal histopathology in fatal cases of diarrhoea-associated haemolytic uraemic syndrome. British Association for Paediatric Nephrology. Pediatr Nephrol. 11(5):556-9, 1997

Organizing Thrombus at Vascular Pole

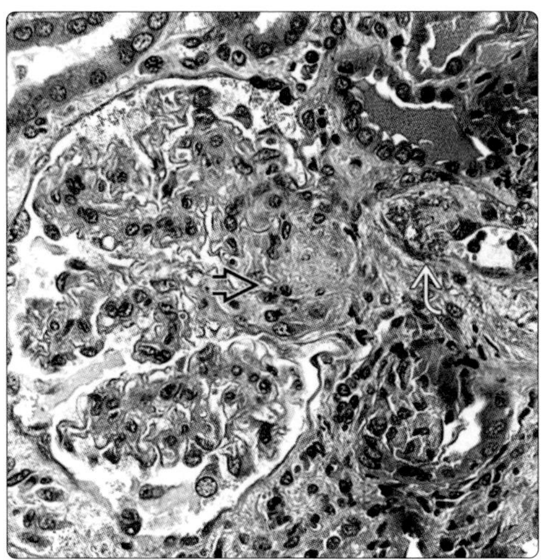

Thrombus at Vascular Pole

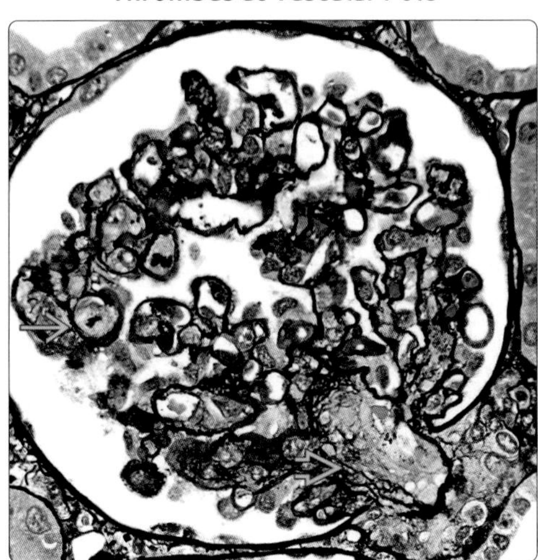

(Left) *Typical D+HUS due to E. coli results in glomerular and arteriolar thrombosis. The glomerular organizing thrombus near the vascular pole* ⇨ *is in continuity with the arteriolar fibrin thrombus* ↪*. Fibrin in the arteriole is red on trichrome stain.* **(Right)** *Diffuse glomerular endothelial swelling* → *is seen associated with capillary luminal occlusion. Thrombosis is also present near the vascular pole* ⇨ *in this biopsy with HUS due to a documented E. coli infection.*

Arterial Fibrinoid Necrosis

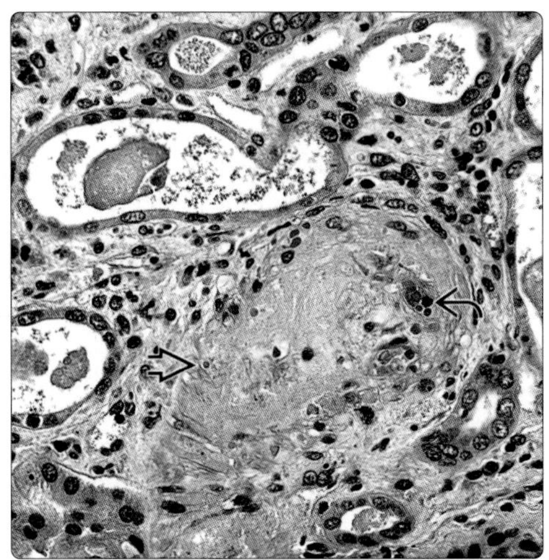

Arterial Thrombosis and Intimal Edema

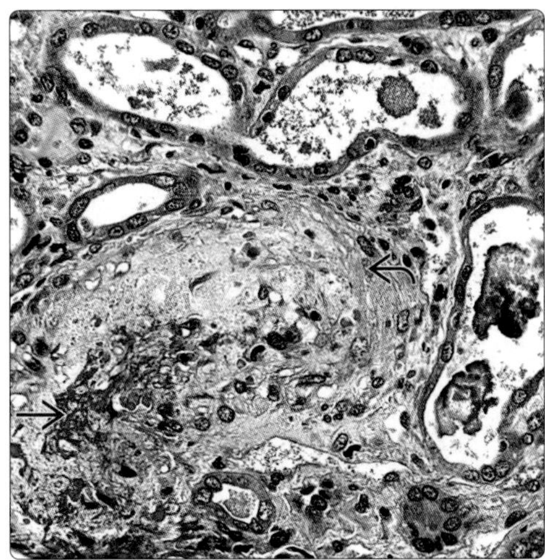

(Left) *Fibrinoid necrosis and thrombosis* ⇨ *of an interlobular artery in a 37-year-old man with E. coli O157:H7 infection is shown. The vessel is expanded and lumen is occluded by fibrin with entrapped erythrocytes. Focal apoptotic debris* ↪ *is seen, but inflammatory infiltrate is characteristically absent.* **(Right)** *Acute thrombotic microangiopathy is seen with thrombosis and intimal edema in an interlobular artery* ↪*. The fibrin* → *within the thrombus stains bright red on trichrome.*

Late Arterial Lesions in HUS

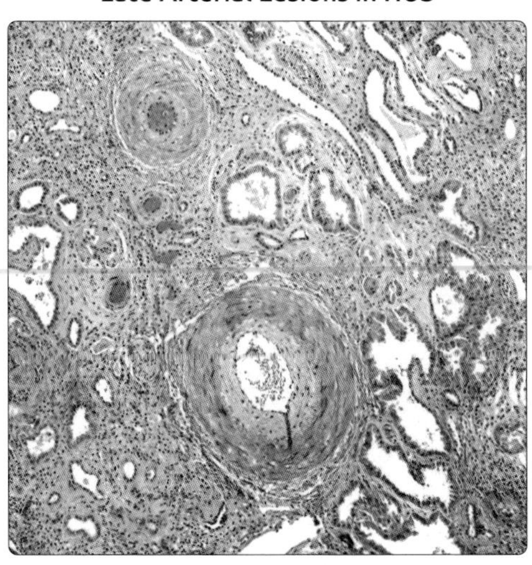

ESRD Due to HUS

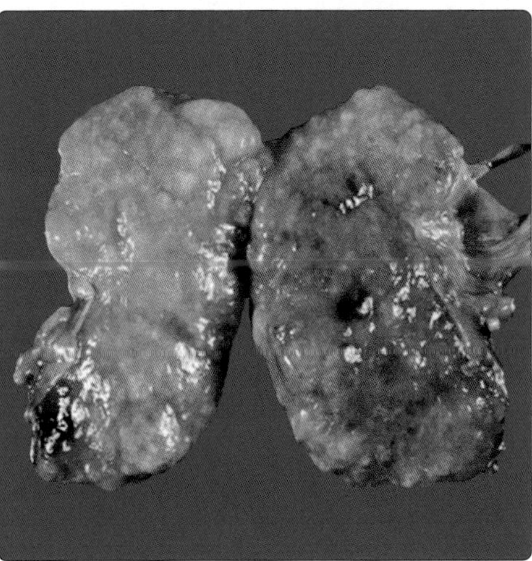

(Left) *This kidney is from a 5-year-old girl who developed HUS after an episode of diarrhea due to E. coli 2 years previously. Marked intimal fibrosis is evident in the medium-sized arteries. There was no evidence of active HUS.* **(Right)** *This kidney shows coarse irregular scarring on the cortical surface, typical of disease of medium-sized arteries. This is from a 5-year old-girl who developed ESRD after an episode of diarrhea due to E. coli infection. HUS did not recur after transplantation.*

KEY FACTS

TERMINOLOGY

- aHUS caused or predisposed by genetic factors

ETIOLOGY/PATHOGENESIS

- Mutations in alternate complement pathway account for 50-60% of aHUS cases
  - Mutations in *CFH, CFHR1-5, MCP, CFI, CFB, C3*
  - Certain high-risk haplotypes
  - Environmental triggers precipitate aHUS
- Mutations in Cobalamin metabolism genes (*MMACHC*)
- Mutations in coagulation protein genes (*THBD, DGKE*)

CLINICAL ISSUES

- Insidious onset of hypertension and renal manifestations
  - Genetic aHUS often presents in children and adolescents
  - Environmental triggers precipitate aHUS in middle age
- Low C3 levels in some patients
  - Genotyping of complement genes recommended even if serum levels are normal
- Initiation of plasma exchange, consider anti-C5 therapy
- End-stage renal disease in > 50% of patients
- Renal outcomes vary based on underlying genetic mutation
- Recurrence rate high after renal transplantation
- Parenteral hydroxycobalamin for cobalamin C disease

MICROSCOPIC

- Glomerular fibrinoid necrosis
- Arterial mucoid intimal thickening
- Fibrin thrombi
- Subendothelial zone expansion by EM
  - No electron-dense deposits

TOP DIFFERENTIAL DIAGNOSES

- Thrombotic microangiopathy due to other causes
- Pauci-immune crescentic glomerulonephritis

DIAGNOSTIC CHECKLIST

- Low C3 levels in patient with aHUS should raise suspicion for genetic causes

Arteriolar Intimal Thickening With RBCs

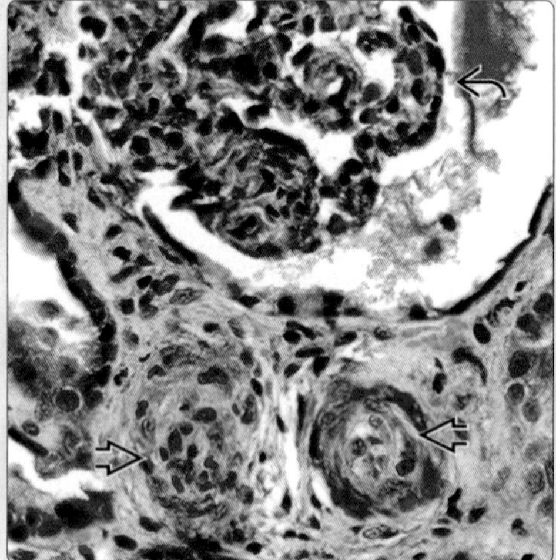

Arterial Occlusion in TMA

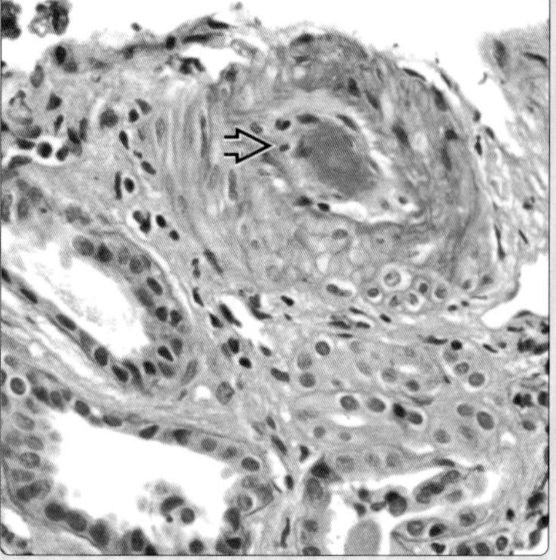

(Left) *Renal biopsy from a 13-year-old boy with factor H mutation shows arterioles occluded by loose intimal fibrosis with trapped red cells ⇨. The glomerulus ⇨ demonstrates ischemic collapse.* **(Right)** *Kidney biopsy from a patient with CFH mutation shows cross section of the interlobular artery with intimal fibrosis ⇨ and central luminal occlusion.*

Fibrin Thrombi With Factor VIII in Genetic aHUS

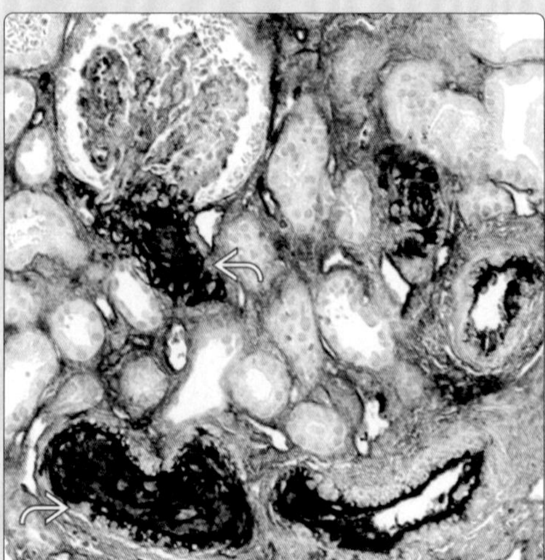

Subendothelial Flocculent Material

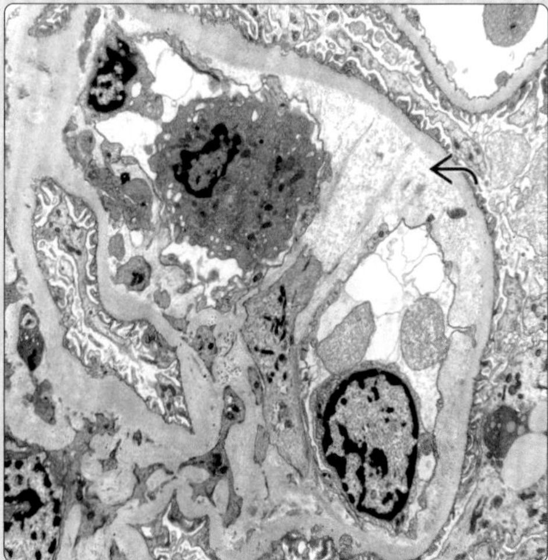

(Left) *Numerous fibrin thrombi with factor VIII ➡ are seen in arterioles and interlobular arteries (compatible with TMA) in an adolescent patient with atypical hemolytic uremic syndrome (aHUS) due to a complement factor H mutation.* **(Right)** *Prominent expansion of the subendothelial space by electron-lucent flocculent material is seen ⇨ in a renal biopsy from an adolescent boy with aHUS due to a missense mutation in the CFH gene.*

TERMINOLOGY

Abbreviations

- Atypical hemolytic uremic syndrome (aHUS)

Definitions

- aHUS caused or predisposed by genetic factors

ETIOLOGY/PATHOGENESIS

Genetic Defects in Alternative Complement Pathway

- Complement factor H (CFH) mutations (chromosome 1q32)
  - Factor H is plasma protein that competes with factor B for C3b enhancing dissociation of C3 convertase
    - Downregulates alternative pathway activation
    - N-terminal complement regulatory domain binds C3b
    - C-terminal end bind to cell surface of endothelium and other cells
      - Most *CFH* mutations that cause TMA are at C-terminus
  - 40-45% of familial aHUS and 10-20% of sporadic "idiopathic" aHUS
    - Majority of *CFH* mutations are heterozygous
      - In heterozygous mutations, mutant factor H interacts and impairs normal factor H binding to endothelial cells, thus exacerbating defective cofactor activity
      - Defective binding to platelets predisposes to platelet activation
    - Homozygous mutations result in quantitative factor H deficiency and low C3 levels
  - Complement factor H-related proteins (*CFHR1-5*) mutations
    - 3-5% of aHUS patients
    - CFHR1 inhibits C5 convertase and membrane insertion of terminal complement complex
    - CFHR1 and factor H share identical surface binding region
      - Competes with CFH for ligand
    - Children with homozygous deletions of *CFHR1* and *3* genes develop autoimmune reaction against CFHR1 and 3 in heterozygous mother
      - DEAP-HUS (**DE**ficiency of CFHR plasma proteins and **A**utoantibody **P**ositive **HUS**) proposed term for these patients
- Membrane cofactor protein (MCP, CD46) mutations
  - Expressed on most cell surfaces, including kidney
    - Cofactor for factor I
    - Prevents complement activation on endothelium
  - *MCP* mutations account for 10-15% of aHUS
    - Most heterozygous, but homozygous and compound heterozygous forms described
  - Mutant MCP result in low expression levels, low C3b binding or cofactor activity
- Complement factor I (CFI) mutations
  - Serine protease circulates in plasma
    - Cleaves C3b and C4b
  - Heterozygous mutations in *CFI* account for 4-10% of aHUS cases
  - Mutant forms result in low serum CFI levels or disrupt cofactor activity
- Complement factor B (CFB) mutations
  - Mutations in *CFB* occur in 1-2% of patients with aHUS
  - Mutant forms have more affinity to C3b and form hyperactive C3 convertase resistant to dissociation
  - Increased C3b formation results in chronic activation of alternate complement pathway
- Complement C3 mutations
  - Heterozygous *C3* mutations occur in 4-10% of aHUS patients
  - Mutant C3 forms have reduced C3b binding to CFH and MCP impairing its degradation
  - Serum C3 levels often low

Disease-Modifying Genes

- Single nucleotide polymorphisms in *CFH* and *MCP*, copy number variations in *CFHR1* and *CFHR3* genes, fusion genes of *CFHR* region with *CFH* reported in aHUS patients with complement genes mutations
  - May account for variability in genetic penetrance among family members

Superimposed Precipitating Factors

- Penetrance among carriers of *CFH*, *MCP*, and *CFI* mutations only 40-50%
  - Individuals predisposed to environmental triggers that may cause in aHUS
- Precipitating factors include infections, pregnancy, transplantation, oral contraceptive pills, and other drugs
  - Associated inflammation and complement activation override multiple protective complement regulators, causing aHUS
  - Complement gene mutations detected in de novo thrombotic microangiopathy after kidney or hematopoietic stem cell transplantation and in Shiga-toxin associated HUS

Cobalamin Metabolism Gene Mutations (Cobalamin C Disease)

- Homozygous or compound heterozygous mutations in *MMACHC*
- Cause TMA in infants and rarely adults
  - Platelet activation, reactive oxygen species, endothelial dysfunction, and coagulation activation
  - Infants have developmental abnormalities, hyperhomocysteinemia, methylmalonic aciduria, and reduced plasma methionine levels

Coagulation Protein Gene Mutations

- Thrombomodulin
  - Membrane-bound glycoprotein on endothelium with anticoagulant and anticomplement properties
  - Heterozygous mutations in *THBD* (gene encoding thrombomodulin) identified in 5% of aHUS
  - Facilitates C3b inactivation by CFI and CFH
- Diacylglycerol kinase mutations ε (DGKE)
  - Expressed in endothelium, platelets and podocytes
  - Homozygous or compound heterozygous mutations
  - Causes protein kinase C activation
    - Leads to prothrombotic state and complex interaction between coagulation and complement systems
    - Protein kinase C downregulates VEGF function causing podocyte injury

CLINICAL ISSUES

Epidemiology

- Age
  - Genetic aHUS often presents in children and adolescents
  - Exogenous triggers can precipitate aHUS in middle age
  - Cobalamin C disease, *DGKE* and some *CFH* mutations present during infancy

Presentation

- Hypertension and renal insufficiency
- Mild hematuria and proteinuria
- Diarrhea may precede genetic aHUS precipitated by infections

Laboratory Tests

- Schistocytes in peripheral smear
- Low platelet counts
- Elevated lactate dehydrogenase
- Low C3 and normal C4 levels suggest activation of alternate complement pathway
- Plasma levels of complement factors H, I, and B, CFHR, and MCP are recommended in all cases of aHUS
- Genetic analysis of complement genes
- Plasma homocysteine and methionine levels and urinary methylmalonic acid levels

Treatment

- Plasma exchange within 24 hours after diagnosis
  - Since MCP is membrane protein, plasma exchange does not replenish MCP and is ineffective
- Monoclonal antibody against complement C5
  - Switch to anti-C5 therapy suggested after lack of response to five days of plasma exchange
- Renal transplantation
  - Living-related donor contraindicated due to high risk of recurrence and possible carrier status of donor
  - Peritransplant plasma exchange helps prevent ischemia-reperfusion trigger of complement cascade
- Liver transplantation
  - Factor H, I, B and C3 synthesized in liver
  - Combined liver-kidney transplantation may benefit patients with *CFH*, *CFI*, and *CFB* mutations
- Cobalamin C disease
  - Hydroxycobalamin

Prognosis

- Incidence of ESRD varies with cause
  - 70-80% of patients with *CFH*, *CFI*, C3 and *CFB* mutations
  - 10-20% of patients with *MCP* mutations
- *DGKE* mutation patients have multiple recurrences with variable response to plasma infusions and anti-C5 therapy
  - Progress to ESRD in 2nd decade of life
- Cobalamin C disease patients have neurological sequelae
  - End-stage renal disease develops if not treated with hydroxycobalamin
- aHUS recurs in transplant recipients with *CFH* (80-90%), *CFI* (70-80%), or *MCP* (15-20%) mutations
  - Transplanted kidney has normal MCP

MICROSCOPIC

Histologic Features

- Glomeruli
  - Fibrinoid necrosis with fragmented RBCs
  - "Bloodless" tuft, collapse
  - Duplicated GBM in subacute or chronic stages
- Tubules
  - Acute tubular injury
  - Tubular atrophy (late)
- Interstitium
  - Edema
  - Fibrosis (late)
- Arterioles/small arteries
  - Fibrin thrombi and intimal mucoid edema
  - Intimal fibrosis, hyalinosis (late)

ANCILLARY TESTS

Immunofluorescence

- Granular C3, IgM, and fibrinogen in affected glomeruli and arterioles

Electron Microscopy

- Endothelial swelling in glomerular capillaries and arterioles
- Expanded subendothelial zones by flocculent material
  - Fibrin tactoids, fragmented erythrocytes, and platelets are seen in subendothelial zone
- Increased electron lucency of mesangial matrix
- Podocyte foot process effacement

DIFFERENTIAL DIAGNOSIS

Thrombotic Microangiopathy Due to Other Causes

- Clinical presentation and serological tests help identify cause of thrombotic microangiopathy

Pauci-Immune Crescentic Glomerulonephritis

- Glomerular necrosis and crescents associated with basement membrane rupture and leukocyte infiltration
- ANCA serology positive in most cases

DIAGNOSTIC CHECKLIST

Pathologic Interpretation Pearls

- Low C3 levels in patient with aHUS presentation should raise suspicion for genetic causes

SELECTED REFERENCES

1. Koenig JC et al: Nephrotic syndrome and thrombotic microangiopathy caused by cobalamin C deficiency. Pediatr Nephrol. 30(7):1203-6, 2015
2. Noris M et al: Dynamics of complement activation in aHUS and how to monitor eculizumab therapy. Blood. 124(11):1715-26, 2014
3. Rodríguez de Córdoba S et al: Genetics of atypical hemolytic uremic syndrome (aHUS). Semin Thromb Hemost. 40(4):422-30, 2014
4. Kavanagh D et al: Atypical hemolytic uremic syndrome. Semin Nephrol. 33(6):508-30, 2013
5. Noris M et al: STEC-HUS, atypical HUS and TTP are all diseases of complement activation. Nat Rev Nephrol. 8(11):622-33, 2012
6. Noris M et al: Relative role of genetic complement abnormalities in sporadic and familial aHUS and their impact on clinical phenotype. Clin J Am Soc Nephrol. 5(10):1844-59, 2010

Endothelial Swelling in Genetic aHUS

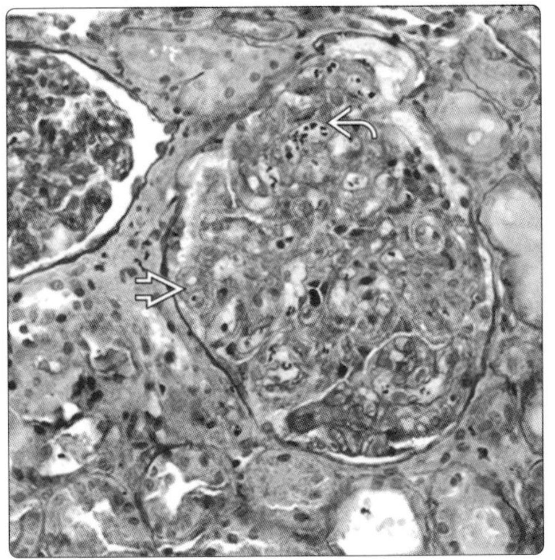

Arterial Intimal Mucoid Edema

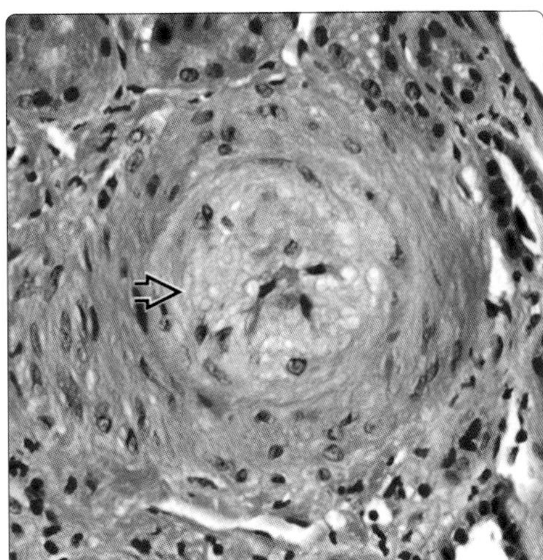

(Left) *The glomerulus shows typical features of thrombotic microangiopathy with diffuse endothelial swelling and mesangiolysis ➡. Focal karyorrhectic debris is seen ↩, but there is no significant leukocyte infiltration in this patient with genetic form of aHUS.* **(Right)** *Severe mucoid intimal edema ➡ is observed in an interlobular artery. These changes of thrombotic microangiopathy in an adolescent boy with seizures and hypertension were determined to be due to genetic aHUS.*

Endothelial Swelling and Endothelialitis

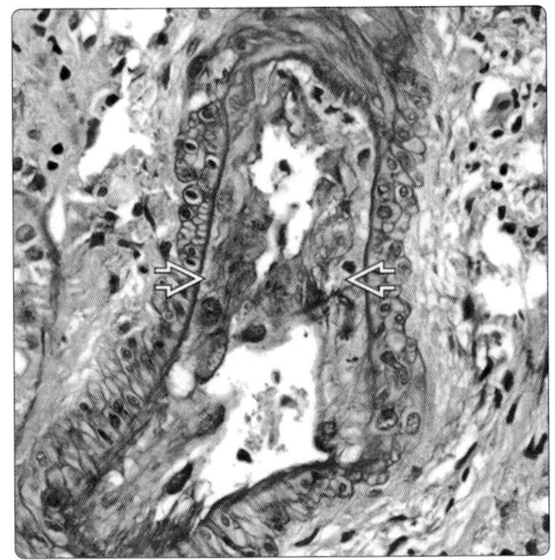

Fibrin in Arteriole

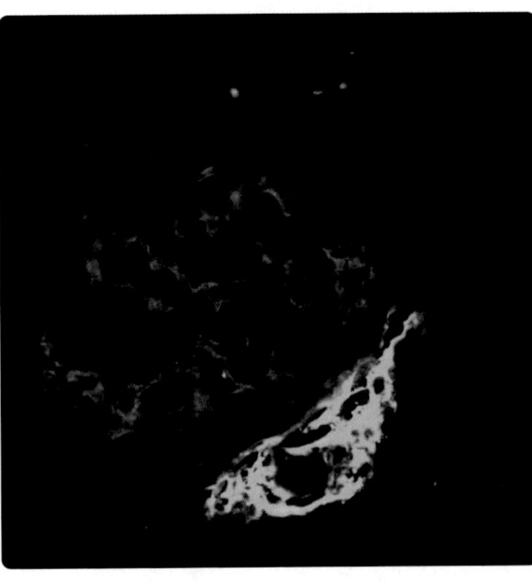

(Left) *Prominent endothelial swelling ➡ and inflammation are seen in an interlobular artery. Other blood vessels had fibrin thrombi occluding the lumina, compatible with thrombotic microangiopathy due to CFH mutation. This mimics endarteritis in an allograft.* **(Right)** *Fibrin in an arteriole is shown from a patient with TMA due to mutation in methylenetetrahydrofolate reductase gene (MTHFR), causing homocysteinemia.*

Ischemic Glomerular Collapse in aHUS

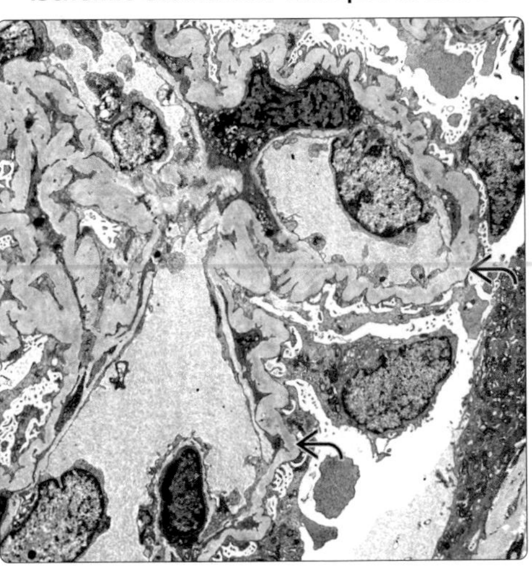

Loss of Endothelial Fenestrations

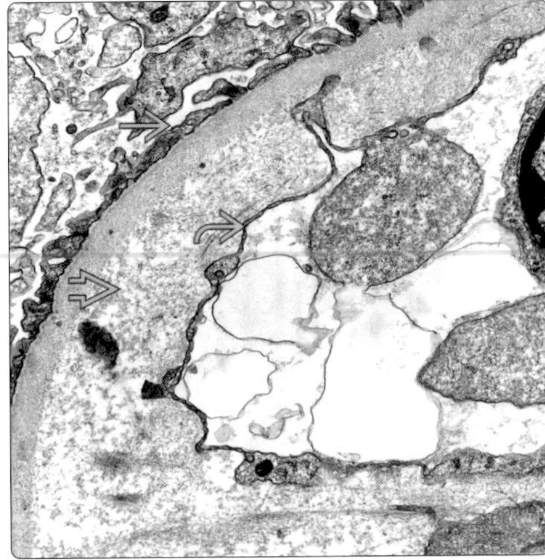

(Left) *Extensive glomerular basement membrane wrinkling ↩ is seen in this glomerulus with ischemic collapse. Characteristic features of thrombotic microangiopathy were seen elsewhere in this biopsy with genetic form of aHUS.* **(Right)** *Electron micrograph shows expanded subendothelial space ➡, loss of endothelial cell fenestration ↩, and podocyte foot process effacement ➡. The aHUS in this patient was determined to be due to missense mutation in CFH gene.*

Thrombotic Microangiopathy, Autoimmune

KEY FACTS

TERMINOLOGY
- TMA due to autoantibodies affecting coagulation system

ETIOLOGY/PATHOGENESIS
- Autoantibodies
  - Lupus anticoagulant (phospholipids)
  - Anticardiolipin antibodies and anti-β2GPI antibodies
  - ADAMTS13 autoantibodies
    - ADAMTS13 deficiency causes vWF multimers to promote platelet aggregation
  - Complement factor H autoantibodies
    - Inhibit CFH regulatory activity
    - Strongly associated with deletion of *CFHR1* gene

CLINICAL ISSUES
- CFH autoantibodies in children 5-13 years of age
  - Presents as severe multisystemic disease
- TTP more common in adult women; neurological symptoms predominate
- Acute or chronic renal failure
- Proteinuria, hematuria, hypertension
- Systemic thrombosis in APLS

MICROSCOPIC
- Acute TMA: Glomerular and arterial thrombi, endothelial swelling and mesangiolysis
- Chronic TMA
  - GBM duplication and arterial intimal thickening
  - Organized arterial thrombi and vessels in APLS
- EM: Endothelial swelling, subendothelial flocculent material, duplication of GBM (chronic)
  - No deposits unless associated with lupus nephritis

TOP DIFFERENTIAL DIAGNOSES
- Infection (STEC) associated HUS
- TMA due to other causes

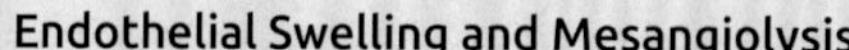

Endothelial Swelling and Mesangiolysis

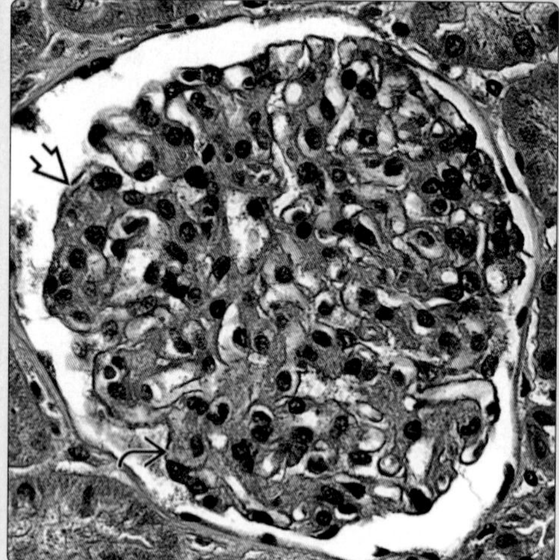

Lupus Nephritis With Arterial Thrombi

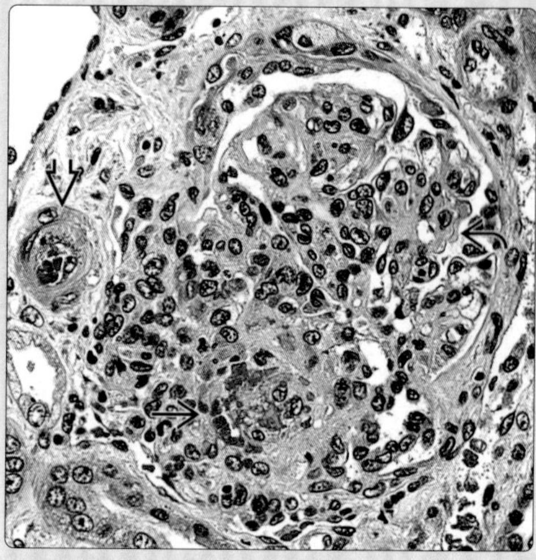

(Left) *Bloodless glomerulus shows very segmental endothelial swelling ⇨ and mesangiolysis ➩. The patient presented with catastrophic APLS with positive aPLs but negative ANA and normal C3 and C4.* **(Right)** *Glomerulus demonstrates endocapillary proliferation ➩ and segmental necrosis ⇨. An adjacent arteriole ⇨ has characteristic TMA features of endothelial swelling and luminal fibrin. The patient is 27 years old with proliferative lupus nephritis and detectable aCL.*

Arterial Intimal Edema and Fibrin in Lupus

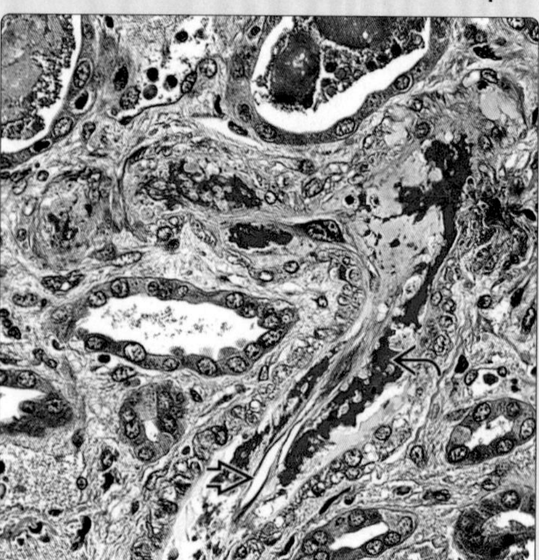

Subendothelial Flocculent Material

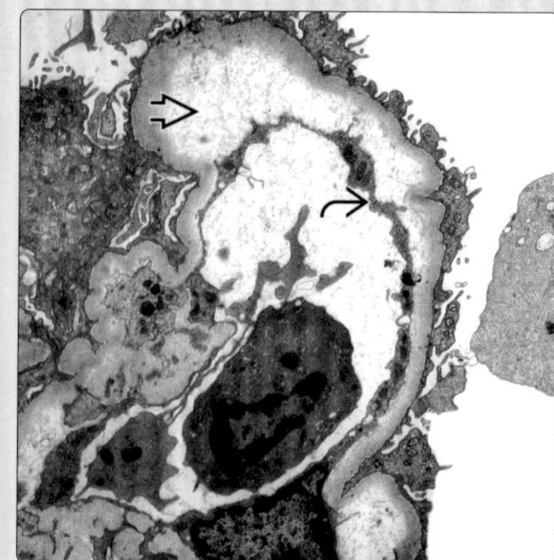

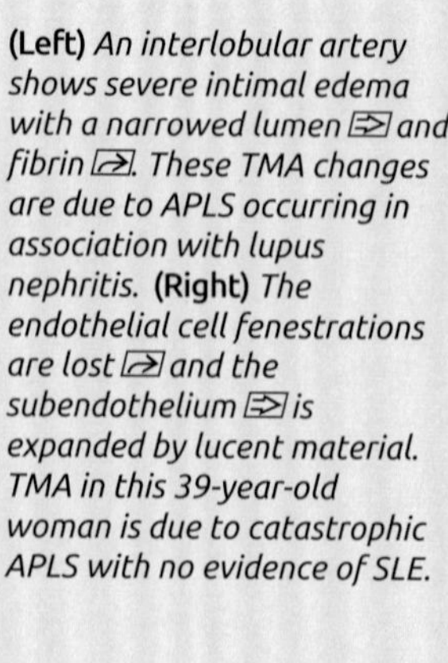

(Left) *An interlobular artery shows severe intimal edema with a narrowed lumen ⇨ and fibrin ➩. These TMA changes are due to APLS occurring in association with lupus nephritis.* **(Right)** *The endothelial cell fenestrations are lost ➩ and the subendothelium ⇨ is expanded by lucent material. TMA in this 39-year-old woman is due to catastrophic APLS with no evidence of SLE.*

TERMINOLOGY

Abbreviations

- Thrombotic microangiopathy (TMA)

Definitions

- TMA due to autoantibodies affecting coagulation system

ETIOLOGY/PATHOGENESIS

Antiphospholipid Autoantibodies (aPLs)

- Autoantibodies directed against broad range of antigens recognizing phospholipids and phospholipid-binding proteins
  - Subsets of aPLs determined by detection method used
    - Both methods recommended to increase sensitivity of aPL detection
  - Lupus anticoagulant (AL)
    - Functional coagulation assay to detect prolonged clotting times
    - Despite name, causes prothrombotic state due to inhibition of anticoagulant pathways
  - Anticardiolipin antibodies (aCL) and anti-β2GPI antibodies
    - Immunoassay detects binding to anionic phospholipids or phospholipid-binding proteins
- Hypercoagulability in all vascular beds causing antiphospholipid antibody syndrome (APLS)
  - Thrombosis in large-caliber vessels and TMA in microvasculature
  - Antibodies interfere with phospholipid-binding proteins involved in coagulation pathways
  - Endothelial cell activation by aPLs causes cytokine secretion and alteration of prostacyclin metabolism
  - Low-density lipoproteins cross react with aPLs, causing oxidant-mediated injury of endothelium
- APLS can be primary (no autoimmune disease) or secondary
  - Infectious organisms trigger aPLs by molecular mimicry
  - Secondary APLS in systemic lupus erythematosus (SLE) or other connective tissue disorders
    - aPLs can precede clinical onset of SLE by 7-8 years
    - Renal prognosis in SLE patients worsened by presence of aPLs
    - aPLs can be induced by interferon therapy

ADAMTS13 Autoantibodies

- ADAMTS13 (**A D**isintegrin **A**nd **M**etalloprotease with **T**hrombo**S**pondin type 1 motif, member 13)
  - Cleaves von Willebrand factor (vWF) multimers
- Autoantibodies cause severe deficiency of ADAMTS13 (plasma levels < 5%)
  - In absence of ADAMTS13, unchecked vWF multimers cause platelet aggregation, thrombi, and consequent end organ damage
  - Known autoantibody triggers include drugs and infections
- Idiopathic thrombotic thrombocytopenic purpura (TTP)
  - IgG or IgM autoantibodies in 30-80%
  - Clinical response after plasmapheresis despite persistent autoantibodies in subset, suggesting alternate pathogenetic mechanism
  - Antibodies against platelet glycoprotein IV (CD36) reported in some
- Drug-induced TTP
  - Ticlopidine and clopidogrel
    - ADAMTS13 antibodies detected more frequently in ticlopidine-associated TMA
  - Interferon-α and interferon-β
    - Anti-ADAMTS13 IgG antibody reported with interferon-β therapy

Complement Factor H Autoantibodies

- Present in up to 4% of healthy adults
- ~ 6% of atypical HUS (aHUS) belong to this subgroup
  - Predominant subtype in an Indian cohort (56%)
- Antibodies bind to various functional domains of CFH
  - Inhibit alternate complement regulatory activity of CFH
  - Multiple pathogenic antibody binding sites
    - Predominantly C-terminal portion of CFH, which binds host cell surfaces and protect against complement-mediated lysis
  - Can cross-react with CFHR1 and sometimes with CFHR2
- Presence of CFH antibodies strongly associated with deletion of *CFHR1* gene
  - Homozygous deletion of *CFHR1* gene seen in 84% of aHUS patients with CFH autoantibodies
    - DEAP-HUS (**DE**ficiency of CFHR plasma proteins and **A**utoantibody **P**ositive for **HUS**) proposed for this condition
    - Identified in children with homozygous deletions of CFHR1 and 3 genes
      - Developed autoimmune reaction against maternal heterozygous CFHR1 and 3
  - CFHR1 expression may be needed to induce tolerance against CFH
  - *CFHR1* gene deletion occurs normally in 2% of Caucasians and 16% of African population
    - Other genetic factors such as specific HLA alleles may predispose to develop autoimmune aHUS
    - Other triggers may include infections, possibly pathogen acquisition of CFH and loss of tolerance to CFH
- CFH antibodies described in patients with other complement gene mutations (*CFH, C3, CD46, CFI*)
- Anti-CFH antibodies reported in TMA associated with hematopoietic stem cell transplantation and occasionally in systemic lupus erythematosus, rheumatoid arthritis, and lupus anticoagulant (+) patients

Complement Factor I Autoantibodies

- Rare in aHUS patients, who also had functionally significant mutations in *CFH*
- Significance of antibodies unclear, likely epiphenomenon

TMA Associated With Autoimmune Disease

- SLE and APLS, mainly
  - SLE-TMA without aPLs may be induced by many autoantibodies, including antiendothelial antibodies
  - Subset have ADAMTS13 antibodies
- Multicentric Castleman disease
  - Usually associated with plasma cell histological variant

- Reported in scleroderma, mixed connective tissue disorder, rheumatoid arthritis, adult Still disease, ANCA vasculitis, Sjögren syndrome, Behçet disease, ulcerative colitis, and myasthenia gravis

CLINICAL ISSUES

Epidemiology

- Age
  - CFH autoantibodies mainly in children 5-13 years of age (mean age: 8 years)
  - TTP more common in adult women (18-50 years of age)

Presentation

- Mild renal insufficiency or acute renal failure
- Proteinuria, hematuria, hypertension
- Neurological symptoms predominate and severe acute injury less common in TTP
- Evidence of systemic thrombosis in APLS
- aHUS associated with CFH antibodies presents as severe multisystemic disease
  - Often with sudden diarrhea, abdominal pain and may even have gastrointestinal infection with enterohemorrhagic *E. coli*
  - Can develop cardiovascular, hepatic, and neurological symptoms in addition to acute renal failure

Laboratory Tests

- Assay for autoantibodies
  - Cardiolipin, β2GPI, lupus anticoagulant, ADAMTS13, CFH
  - CFH-antibody titers correlate with disease activity
- Schistocytes on peripheral smear
- Thrombocytopenia
  - Platelets can be particularly low in CFH-antibody associated aHUS and TTP
- Thrombocytopenia, elevated LDH
- Low C3 levels in 40-60% of CFH-antibody associated aHUS
  - Inversely correlated with CFH IgG antibody titers in CFH-antibody associated aHUS
    - No correlation between CFH plasma levels and anti-CFH IgG titers

Treatment

- Plasma infusion and exchange in TTP, CFH antibody associated aHUS
- Anticoagulation is mainstay of therapy in APLS
- Immunosuppression to inhibit autoantibodies
  - CFH antibody associated aHUS may benefit from eculizumab, Rituximab, IVIG and maintenance therapy of corticosteroids, MMF, azathioprine

Prognosis

- Mortality high in untreated TTP or catastrophic APLS
- TTP may be chronic or relapsing
- aHUS due to CFH antibodies has highly relapsing course, especially < 2 years after disease onset
  - ESRD in 20-35% of patients and mortality rate of 10%
  - High serum creatinine, high CFH antibody titers at onset, low C3, delayed plasma exchange, acute cortical necrosis are adverse prognostic factors
  - Monitoring CFH antibodies and prophylactic pretransplant treatment may reduce post-transplant recurrence

MICROSCOPIC

Histologic Features

- Acute TMA
  - Glomerular and arterial thrombi
  - Endothelial swelling, fibrinoid necrosis, and mesangiolysis
  - Acute tubular injury and interstitial edema
- Chronic TMA
  - GBM duplication and arterial intimal thickening
  - Arterial thrombi of varying ages and recanalized lumens in APLS
  - Variable tubular atrophy and interstitial fibrosis

ANCILLARY TESTS

Immunofluorescence

- Glomerular and arterial thrombi stain for fibrinogen
- Immune complexes if associated with lupus nephritis

Electron Microscopy

- Endothelial swelling and subendothelial expansion by flocculent material
- Fibrin tactoids, fragmented red blood cells
- No deposits unless associated with lupus nephritis

DIFFERENTIAL DIAGNOSIS

TMA Due to Other Causes

- Histologically indistinguishable
- Clinical information and family history may suggest etiology

SELECTED REFERENCES

1. Hofer J et al: Complement factor H-antibody-associated hemolytic uremic syndrome: pathogenesis, clinical presentation, and treatment. Semin Thromb Hemost. 40(4):431-43, 2014
2. Sinha A et al: Prompt plasma exchanges and immunosuppressive treatment improves the outcomes of anti-factor H autoantibody-associated hemolytic uremic syndrome in children. Kidney Int. 85(5):1151-60, 2014
3. Lee JP et al: Successfully treated multicentric Castleman's disease with renal thrombotic microangiopathy using rituximab and corticosteroid. Clin Nephrol. 75(2):165-70, 2011
4. Dragon-Durey MA et al: Clinical features of anti-factor H autoantibody-associated hemolytic uremic syndrome. J Am Soc Nephrol. 21(12):2180-7, 2010
5. Zipfel PF et al: Thrombotic microangiopathies: new insights and new challenges. Curr Opin Nephrol Hypertens. 19(4):372-8, 2010
6. Gigante A et al: Antiphospholipid antibodies and renal involvement. Am J Nephrol. 30(5):405-12, 2009
7. Shelat SG et al: Inhibitory autoantibodies against ADAMTS-13 in patients with thrombotic thrombocytopenic purpura bind ADAMTS-13 protease and may accelerate its clearance in vivo. J Thromb Haemost. 4(8):1707-17, 2006
8. Lian EC: Pathogenesis of thrombotic thrombocytopenic purpura: ADAMTS13 deficiency and beyond. Semin Thromb Hemost. 31(6):625-32, 2005

Mesangiolysis and Arterial Occlusive Edema

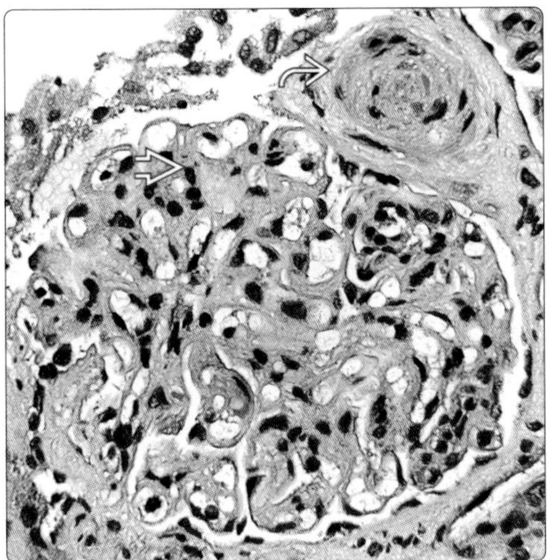

Arteriolar Fibrinoid Necrosis and Thrombosis

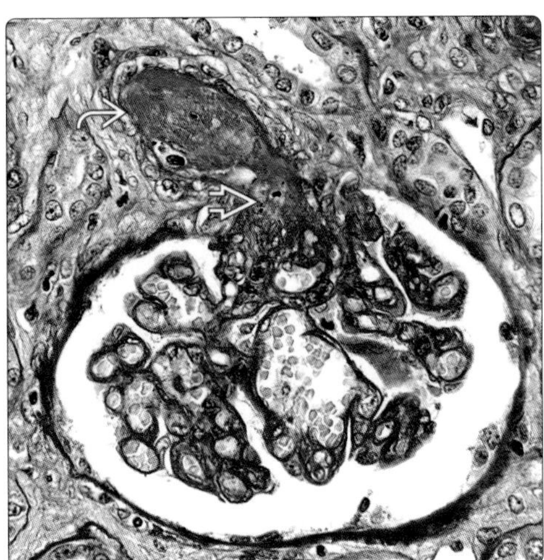

(Left) *The capillary tuft is mildly retracted, and mesangiolysis* ➡ *is seen. An adjacent arteriole* ➡ *shows TMA features of intimal edema and luminal occlusion. The patient is a 27-year-old man with Still disease and positive aCL.* **(Right)** *Biopsy from a 20-year-old woman with relapsing TTP shows an arteriolar luminal thrombus* ➡ *extending into the vascular pole. Focal apoptotic debris* ➡ *is present, but there is no vascular inflammation.*

Fragmented RBCs in Arterial Wall

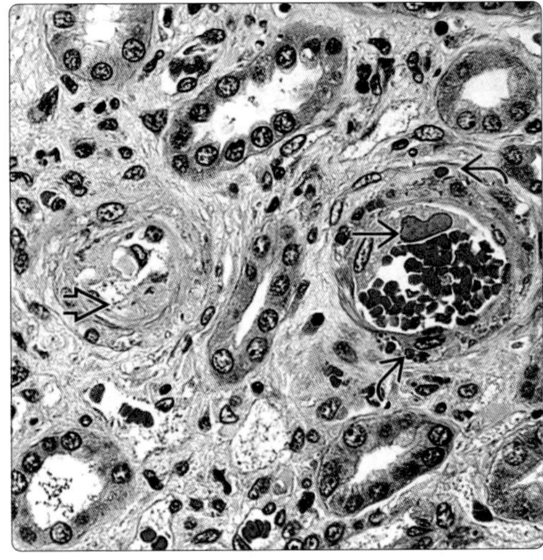

Glomerular Ischemia and GBM Duplication

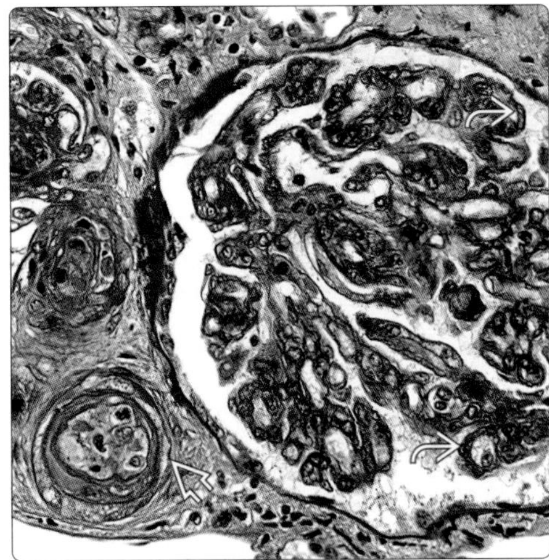

(Left) *Cross sections of arterioles show intimal edema* ➡ *and focal luminal thrombus* ➡*. Fragmented RBCs* ➡ *are also seen within the arteriolar wall. These features are characteristic of acute TMA and in this case are due to TTP.* **(Right)** *Endothelial swelling is seen in an arteriole* ➡ *with luminal occlusion and mononuclear inflammatory cells. Adjacent glomerulus shows ischemic collapse and also extensive GBM duplication* ➡*. TMA changes in this patient are attributed to idiopathic TTP.*

Arterial Thrombus and Fragmented Red Cells

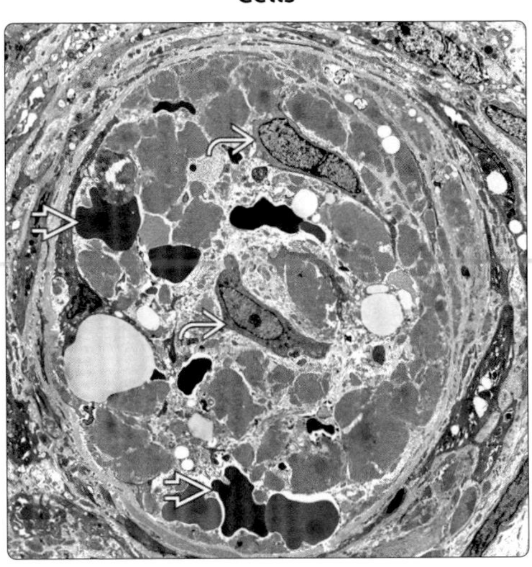

Subendothelial Cellular Debris and Fibrin

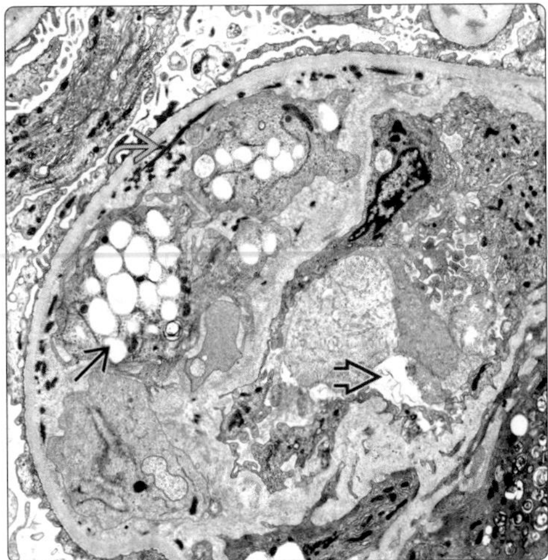

(Left) *The arteriolar lumen is occluded by electron-dense deposits, cellular debris, edema, and fragmented RBCs* ➡*. The endothelial nuclei* ➡ *are nearly detached. The patient has proliferative lupus nephritis and secondary APLS.* **(Right)** *The capillary lumen* ➡ *is severely occluded by a swollen endothelial cell. The subendothelium is expanded by cells* ➡*, likely macrophages and focal fibrin tactoids* ➡*, consistent with a diagnosis of acute TMA.*

Thrombotic Microangiopathy, Drug Induced

KEY FACTS

ETIOLOGY/PATHOGENESIS

- Direct endothelial injury or immune mediated
- > 60 drugs reportedly associated with TMA but often difficult to establish causative role
  - Chemotherapeutic agents
  - Anti-vascular endothelial growth factor (VEGF) therapy
    - Transmembrane communication between podocyte and endothelium via VEGF signaling disrupted by anti-VEGF therapy
  - Immunomodulators (CNi, mTORi)
  - Antiplatelet drugs of thienopyridine family
    - ADAMTS13 levels can be severely deficient (< 5%), or ADAMTS13 inhibitor detected
  - Quinine

CLINICAL ISSUES

- Proteinuria ranges from mild to nephrotic
- Mild renal insufficiency or acute renal failure
- Worsening hypertension
- Treatment
  - Withdrawal of offending drug
  - Plasma exchange helpful in some settings
  - Better prognosis if TMA limited to kidney
- Diagnosis
  - Thrombocytopenia
  - Schistocytes on peripheral smear
  - Serum lactate dehydrogenase may be elevated
  - ADAMTS13 levels may be low in TMA due to thienopyridines

MICROSCOPIC

- Fibrin thrombi and endothelial swelling in glomeruli and arterioles
- Reduplicated GBM in chronic phase

TOP DIFFERENTIAL DIAGNOSES

- TMA due to other causes
- Antibody-mediated rejection in renal allografts

Endothelial Swelling in TMA Due to Sirolimus

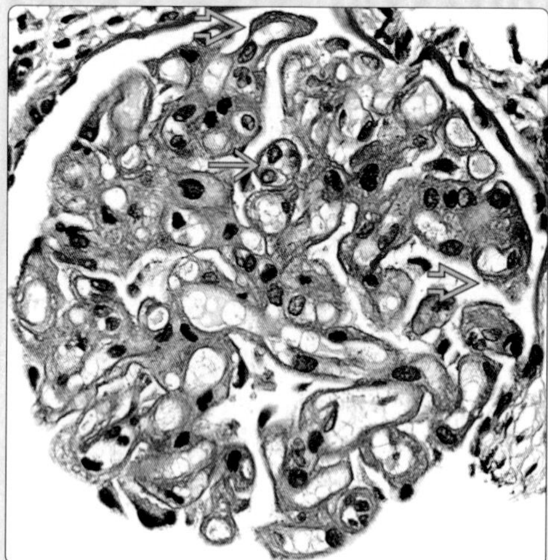

Subendothelial Expansion in TMA

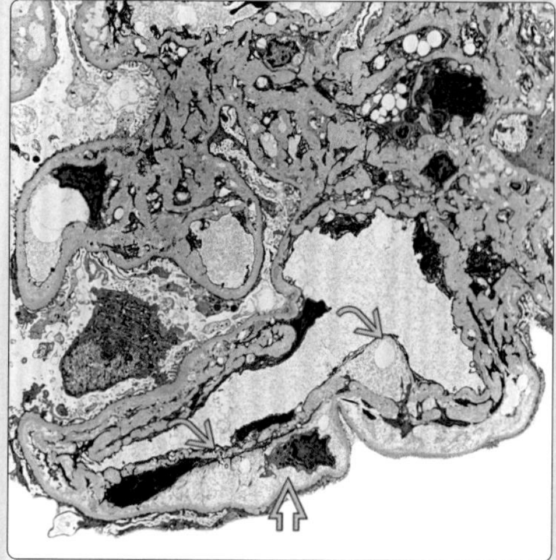

(Left) *The glomerulus demonstrates extensive duplication of basement membranes ⇨ associated with endothelial swelling ⇨ and mild mesangiolysis. TMA in this 13 year old with renal allografts is attributed to sirolimus.* **(Right)** *TMA is characterized by expansion of the subendothelial space as seen in this biopsy. The endothelial membrane ⇨ is lifted off the GBM with subendothelial cells and flocculent material ⇨. TMA in this case is due to aflibercept, a VEGF trap.*

Fibrin Thrombi in Cyclosporine Toxicity

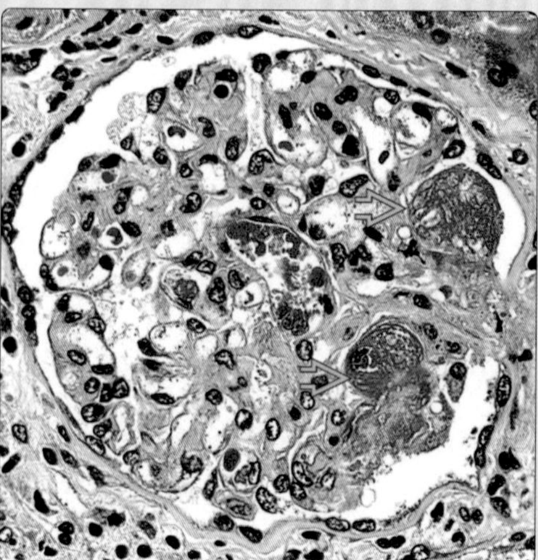

GBM Duplication in Anti-VEGF Therapy

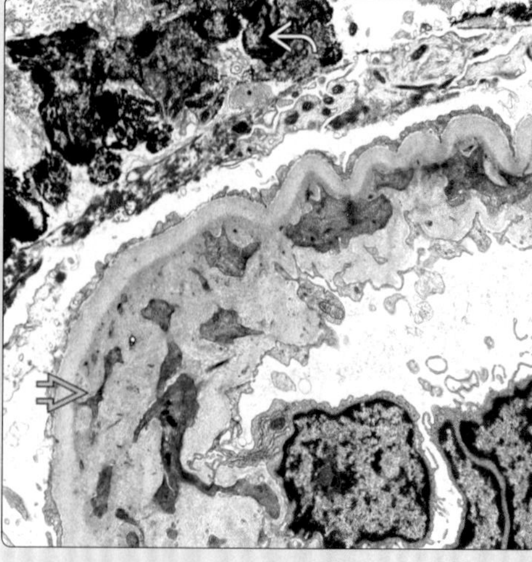

(Left) *A 39-year-old woman, 3 weeks post renal transplantation, presented with acute renal failure. Fibrin thrombi ⇨ are seen in the capillary lumens, and TMA is attributed to cyclosporine toxicity.* **(Right)** *GBM duplication and mesangial cell interposition ⇨ is seen in a 64 year old with TMA. The patient received aflibercept (VEGF trap) for prostate carcinoma. Fibrin ➡ is also seen in the urinary space.*

TERMINOLOGY

Abbreviations

- Thrombotic microangiopathy (TMA)

Definitions

- Atypical hemolytic uremic syndrome (HUS) caused by drugs

ETIOLOGY/PATHOGENESIS

Mechanism of TMA Induction

- Direct endothelial injury due to dose-related toxicity
  - Gradual onset of renal failure over weeks or months
- Immune-mediated dose-unrelated idiosyncratic reaction
  - Sudden onset of severe systemic symptoms with anuric acute renal failure

Implicated Drugs

- > 60 drugs reportedly associated with TMA
  - Often difficult to establish causative role
- Chemotherapeutic agents
  - Mitomycin-C
    - Dose-dependent endothelial toxicity
    - Median time from last dose to development of TMA is 75 days
  - Gemcitabine
    - Endothelial damage causes TMA
    - Median time from initiation of therapy to development of TMA is 6-8 months
    - Withdrawal of drug resolves TMA in > 50%
  - Other agents include bleomycin, cisplatin, daunorubicin, vinblastine, deoxycoformycin
    - Mutation in complement gene *CD46* reported in cisplatin-induced HUS
- Anti-vascular endothelial growth factor (VEGF) therapy
  - Bevacizumab is anti-VEGF monoclonal antibody and aflibercept/VEGF trap is decoy VEGF receptor
    - TMA most common pathology, occurring in ~ 50%
      - Transmembrane communication between podocyte and endothelium via VEGF signaling disrupted by anti-VEGF therapy
      - Also disrupts endothelial cell synthesis of nitric oxide, vasodilator, resulting in endothelial injury and hypertension
      - TMA due to endothelial damage can occur 1 week to 9 months after initiation of therapy
      - Symptoms can occur after discontinuation of drug
      - Some biopsies show associated focal segmental glomerulonephritis (FSGS)
      - Mild proteinuria common with bevacizumab (21-63%)
      - Nephrotic-range proteinuria occurs only in 1-2%
    - VEGF synthesis by podocytes needed for survival of glomerular endothelial cells that express VEGF receptors
    - Other less common pathology (either alone or superimposed on TMA) includes
      - Collapsing glomerulopathy
      - Mesangioproliferative glomerulonephritis
      - Cryoglobulinemic glomerulonephritis
      - Immune-complex mediated focal proliferative glomerulonephritis
      - IgA nephropathy
  - Tyrosine kinase inhibitors that inhibit VEGF receptors (sunitinib, sorafenib, pazopanib)
    - Endothelial damage causes TMA
    - Other pathology FSGS, minimal change disease
      - Likely related arterial thrombosis-related ischemia and hypertension
- Immunomodulators
  - Calcineurin inhibitors (CNi)
    - Cyclosporine and tacrolimus associated with TMA
    - Direct endothelial toxicity due to reduced prostacyclin synthesis or reduced formation of activated protein C
    - Cyclosporine shown to reduce protein expression of clusterin, a fluid phase regulator of terminal complement complex formation
    - Toxicity often seen in first 6 months after transplantation
    - In most, cyclosporine or tacrolimus can be resumed after resolution of TMA or patients may tolerate switching of drug
  - mTORi (mammalian target of rapamycin inhibitors)
    - Sirolimus and everolimus can cause post-transplant de novo TMA and increase risk of recurrent atypical HUS
    - mTOR regulates VEGF production and affects cell cycle
    - Inhibition of VEGF results in endothelial damage
    - Toxicity exacerbated by concomitant calcineurin inhibitors
- Antiplatelet drugs of thienopyridine family
  - Ticlopidine and clopidogrel
    - TMA occurs < 1 month (or even 1 week) of exposure
    - Cause direct endothelial toxicity
    - ADAMTS13 levels can be severely deficient (< 5%), and inhibitor to ADAMTS13 has been detected
    - At risk polymorphisms in *CFH* gene reported in ticlopidine-induced TTP
- Miscellaneous drugs
  - Quinine
    - Treatment of malaria and nocturnal leg cramps
    - Found in herbal supplements and tonic water
    - Patients develop antibodies to platelet glycoprotein Ib/IX or IIb/IIIa complexes
    - TMA not dose related, can occur after years of intake, and recurs after reexposure
  - α-interferon, β-interferon,
    - Antiphospholipid antibodies or anti-ADAMTS13 antibodies can be induced
  - Cocaine
  - Simvastatin
  - Aprotinin
  - Valacyclovir
  - H2-receptor antagonists
  - NSAIDs
  - Vaccines
  - Several antibiotics
  - Hormone supplements

CLINICAL ISSUES

Presentation

- Proteinuria ranges from mild to nephrotic

- Microscopic hematuria
- Mild renal insufficiency or acute renal failure
- Worsening hypertension

Laboratory Tests

- Thrombocytopenia
- Schistocytes may be present on peripheral smear
- Serum lactic acid dehydrogenase may be elevated
- ADAMTS13 levels may be low in TMA due to thienopyridines
- Serum complement and genetic testing maybe helpful in some patients

Treatment

- Withdrawal of offending drug
- Plasma exchange helpful in some settings

Prognosis

- Variable but usually associated with high morbidity and mortality
- Better prognosis if TMA limited to kidney as can occur in renal transplantation

MICROSCOPIC

Histologic Features

- Glomeruli
  - Fibrin thrombi and endothelial swelling
  - Ischemic collapse of capillary tuft
  - Mesangiolysis
  - Duplicated GBM in chronic phase
- Tubulointerstitium
  - Acute tubular injury with degenerating epithelium
  - Tubular atrophy and interstitial fibrosis maybe related underlying chronic kidney disease
- Arterioles and interlobular arteries
  - Endothelial swelling and fibrinoid necrosis
  - No associated arterial inflammation

ANCILLARY TESTS

Immunofluorescence

- Fibrin in glomerular and arterial thrombi
- Nonspecific entrapment of C3, IgM in glomeruli and vessels
- No evidence of immune complexes

Electron Microscopy

- Glomeruli
  - Endothelial swelling and subendothelial expansion by lucent material
    - Loss of endothelial fenestrations
  - Platelets and fibrin in capillary lumens
  - No electron-dense deposits
  - Podocyte foot processes generally well preserved
    - Effacement in sunitinib toxicity associated with severe proteinuria

DIFFERENTIAL DIAGNOSIS

TMA Due to Other Causes

- Rule out: Malignant hypertension, infections, postpartum HUS, scleroderma, HUS/TTP
- Clinical history and serological evidence of autoantibodies help determine etiology

Antibody-Mediated Rejection

- C4d stain and donor-specific antibodies usually positive
- Difficult to distinguish in renal allograft biopsy
- Glomerulitis, tubulointerstitial inflammation, and peritubular capillaritis helpful if present

DIAGNOSTIC CHECKLIST

Clinically Relevant Pathologic Features

- Isolated kidney involvement has favorable outcome compared to systemic involvement
- Biopsy features of isolated glomerular TMA associated with favorable prognosis than when arterioles involved

Pathologic Interpretation Pearls

- Etiology cannot be determined on biopsy findings alone
- Thrombocytopenia and peripheral smear schistocytes may not be evident in mild disease

SELECTED REFERENCES

1. Izzedine H et al: Kidney diseases associated with anti-vascular endothelial growth factor (VEGF): an 8-year observational study at a single center. Medicine (Baltimore). 93(24):333-9, 2014
2. Riedl M et al: Spectrum of complement-mediated thrombotic microangiopathies: pathogenetic insights identifying novel treatment approaches. Semin Thromb Hemost. 40(4):444-64, 2014
3. Ruebner RL et al: Nephrotic syndrome associated with tyrosine kinase inhibitors for pediatric malignancy: case series and review of the literature. Pediatr Nephrol. 29(5):863-9, 2014
4. Usui J et al: Clinicopathological spectrum of kidney diseases in cancer patients treated with vascular endothelial growth factor inhibitors: a report of 5 cases and review of literature. Hum Pathol. 45(9):1918-27, 2014
5. Yahata M et al: Immunoglobulin A nephropathy with massive paramesangial deposits caused by anti-vascular endothelial growth factor therapy for metastatic rectal cancer: a case report and review of the literature. BMC Res Notes. 6:450, 2013
6. Takahashi D et al: Sunitinib-induced nephrotic syndrome and irreversible renal dysfunction. Clin Exp Nephrol. 16(2):310-5, 2012
7. Broughton A et al: Thrombotic microangiopathy induced by long-term interferon-β therapy for multiple sclerosis: a case report. Clin Nephrol. 76(5):396-400, 2011
8. Costero O et al: Inhibition of tyrosine kinases by sunitinib associated with focal segmental glomerulosclerosis lesion in addition to thrombotic microangiopathy. Nephrol Dial Transplant. 25(3):1001-3, 2010
9. Eremina V et al: VEGF inhibition and renal thrombotic microangiopathy. N Engl J Med. 358(11):1129-36, 2008
10. Stokes MB et al: Glomerular disease related to anti-VEGF therapy. Kidney Int. 74(11):1487-91, 2008
11. Roncone D et al: Proteinuria in a patient receiving anti-VEGF therapy for metastatic renal cell carcinoma. Nat Clin Pract Nephrol. 3(5):287-93, 2007
12. Zakarija A et al: Drug-induced thrombotic microangiopathy. Semin Thromb Hemost. 31(6):681-90, 2005
13. Robson M et al: Thrombotic micro-angiopathy with sirolimus-based immunosuppression: potentiation of calcineurin-inhibitor-induced endothelial damage? Am J Transplant. 3(3):324-7, 2003
14. Saikali JA et al: Sirolimus may promote thrombotic microangiopathy. Am J Transplant. 3(2):229-30, 2003
15. Schwimmer J et al: De novo thrombotic microangiopathy in renal transplant recipients: a comparison of hemolytic uremic syndrome with localized renal thrombotic microangiopathy. Am J Kidney Dis. 41(2):471-9, 2003

Glomerular Fibrin in Sirolimus Therapy

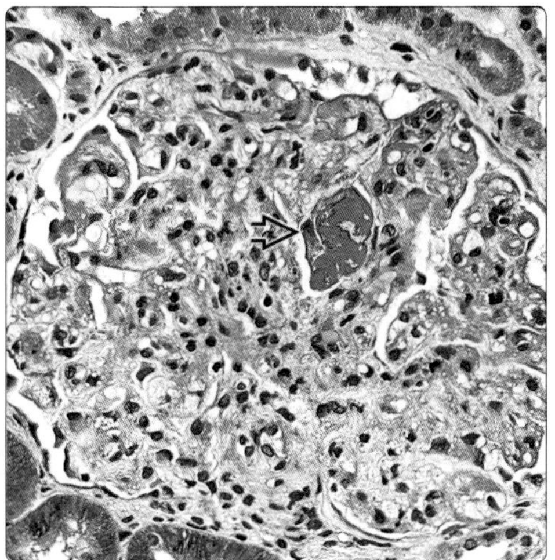

Arteriolar Endothelial Swelling

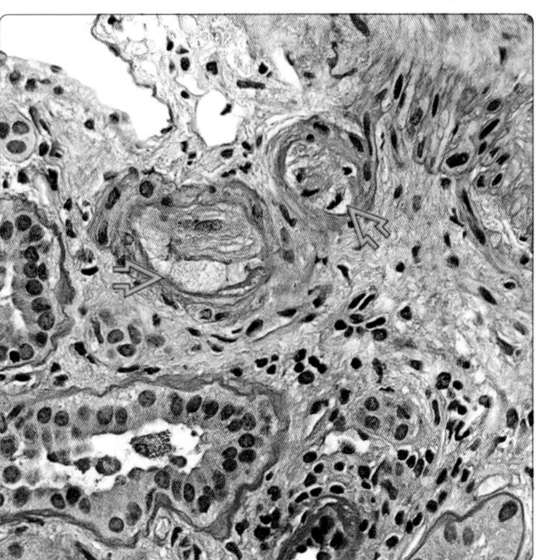

(Left) *Glomerular fibrin thrombus* ➔ *stains red on trichrome in this biopsy with TMA. Histological features do not help distinguish the etiology of TMA, and in this case, it is clinically attributed to sirolimus toxicity.* **(Right)** *An interlobular artery shows severe intimal edema* ➔ *with luminal occlusion. No inflammatory infiltrate is seen to suggest vasculitis. The arteriolar TMA changes in this post transplantation biopsy are due to sirolimus.*

Fibrinoid Necrosis in Arterioles

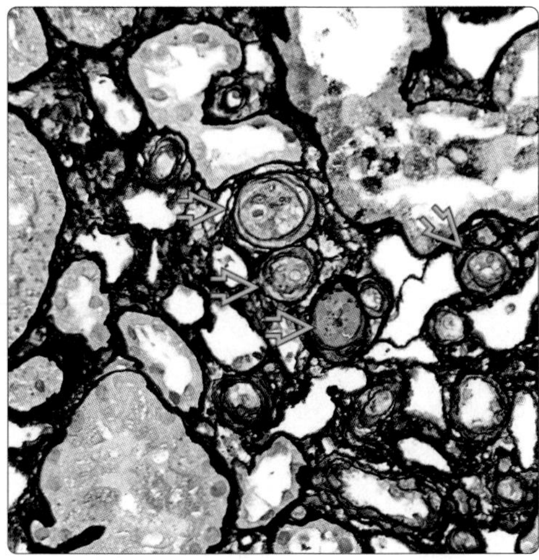

Ischemic Collapse of Glomerular Capillaries

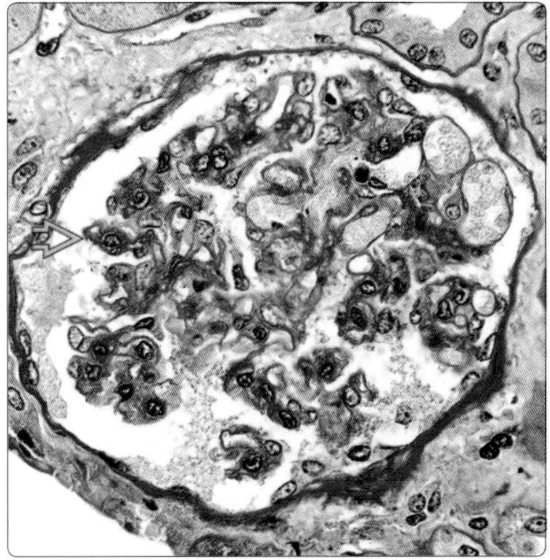

(Left) *Cross sections of arterioles show endothelial swelling* ➔ *with entrapped erythrocytes and apoptotic debris. These TMA changes are due to VEGF trap therapy the patient received for metastatic prostate carcinoma.* **(Right)** *The glomerulus shows collapse of the capillary tuft with wrinkling of the GBM* ➔. *Characteristic features of TMA with arteriolar and glomerular fibrin thrombi are seen elsewhere in this biopsy from a patient with cyclosporine toxicity.*

Fibrin Thrombi With Bevacizumab

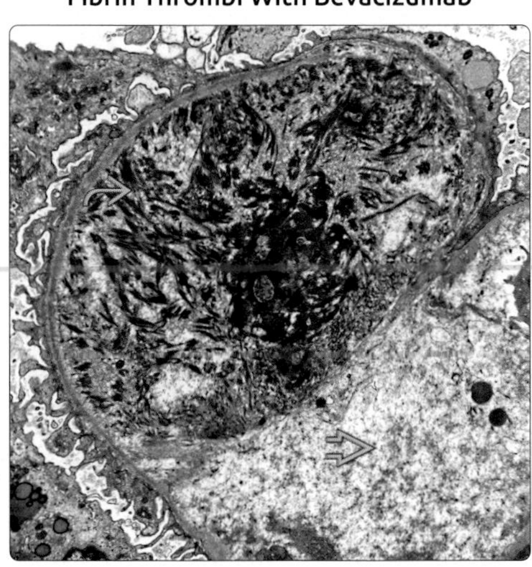

TMA With Proteinuria and TMA Due to Sunitinib

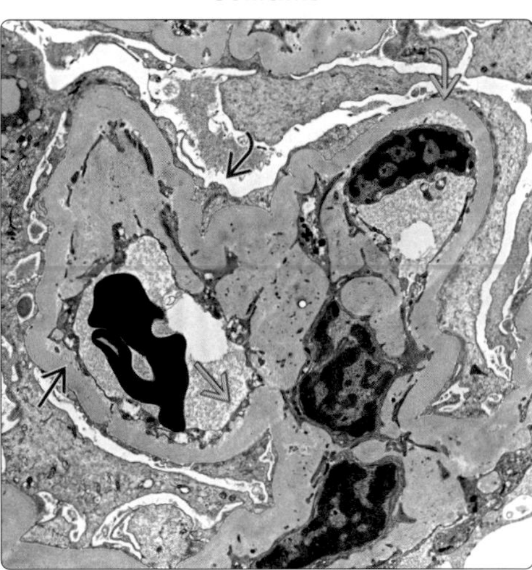

(Left) *A glomerular capillary is occluded with fibrin tactoids* ➔ *and depolymerized fibrin* ➔. *The endothelium is absent. This patient on bevacizumab for neuroendocrine carcinoma presented with proteinuria and TMA.* **(Right)** *This diabetic patient developed proteinuria on sunitinib for ~ 10 months. Glomerular endothelial cells show loss of fenestrations* ➔, *detachment* ➔, *vacuolization, and subendothelial lucency* ➔. *Extensive foot process effacement is present* ➔. *The thickened GBM is due to diabetes.*

Postpartum Hemolytic Uremic Syndrome

KEY FACTS

TERMINOLOGY

- HUS in postpartum period, characterized by microangiopathic hemolytic anemia, thrombocytopenia, and acute renal failure

ETIOLOGY/PATHOGENESIS

- Many have mutations in genes encoding factor H, factor I, C3, and membrane cofactor protein
- Single-nucleotide polymorphisms and haplotype blocks of complement genes increase susceptibility
- Antepartum protective mechanisms compromised in immediate postpartum period in susceptible individuals

CLINICAL ISSUES

- Presentation postpartum within 24 hours to several weeks
- Laboratory testing with schistocytes in peripheral smear, elevated LDH, low platelets
- Complement screening and genetic screening for mutational analysis recommended
- Plasma exchange and steroids may be beneficial
- Eculizumab used successfully in pHUS

MICROSCOPIC

- Glomerular endothelial swelling, fragmented RBCs, and fibrin thrombi
    - Lobulated accentuation and double contours predominate in chronic phase
- Fibrin thrombi and mucoid intimal edema in arterioles
- Cortical necrosis and infarction in severe cases
- Subendothelial expansion by electron-lucent flocculent material and mesangiolysis
- No electron-dense deposits

TOP DIFFERENTIAL DIAGNOSES

- Thrombotic thrombocytopenic purpura (TTP)
- Preeclampsia and HELLP syndrome
- Thrombotic microangiopathy due to other causes

(Left) *The glomerulus shows endothelial swelling and denudation along with capillary lumen fibrin thrombi in pHUS. The patient underwent a C-section for HELLP syndrome 6 days prior.* **(Right)** *A 27-year-old woman with preeclampsia, 1 week postpartum, underwent a kidney biopsy for acute renal failure. Diffuse endothelial swelling is seen, and focal fibrin thrombi were observed in arterioles, compatible with pHUS.*

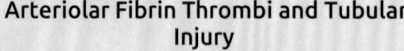

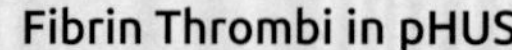

Fibrin Thrombi in pHUS

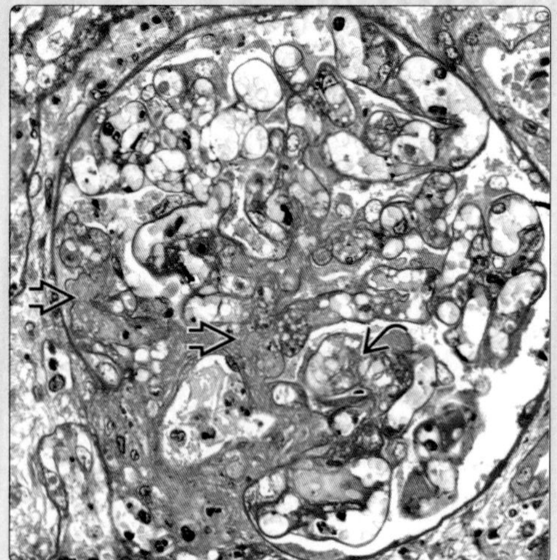

Diffuse Glomerular Endothelial Swelling

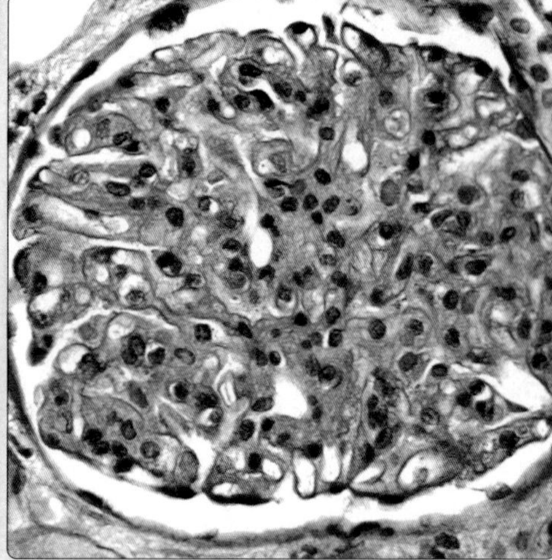

(Left) *Arteriolar fibrin thrombi are seen with entrapped RBCs in a biopsy with pHUS. Fibrin strands are also observed within adjacent tubular lumens. Features of cortical necrosis were present in the biopsy.* **(Right)** *Ultrastructurally, pHUS shows accumulation of electron-lucent material in the subendothelium and mesangium. Glomerular and arteriolar fibrin thrombi were also seen in the biopsy.*

Arteriolar Fibrin Thrombi and Tubular Injury

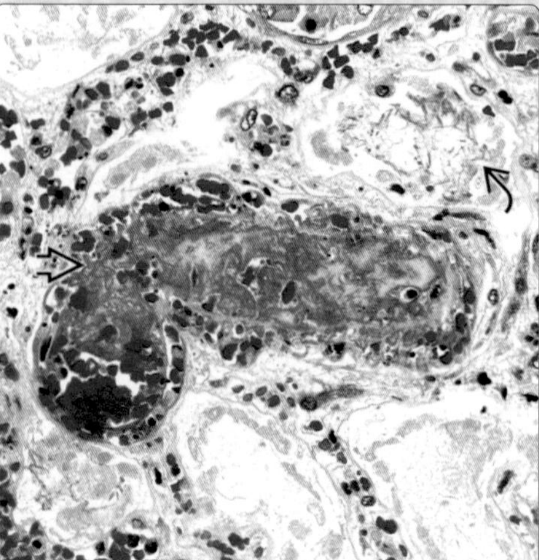

Subendothelial Electron-Lucent Material

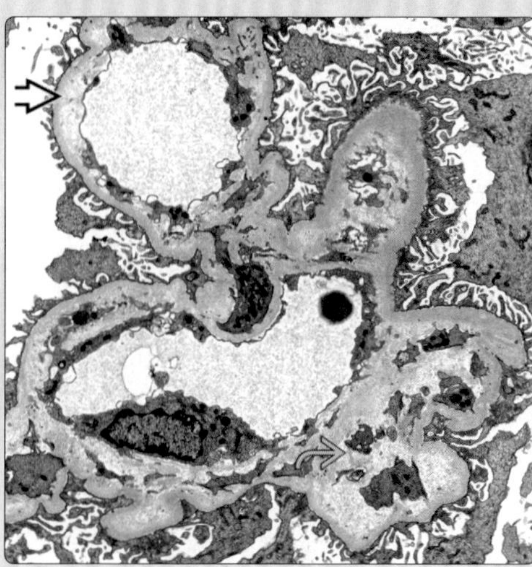

TERMINOLOGY

Abbreviations

- Postpartum hemolytic uremic syndrome (pHUS)

Definitions

- HUS in postpartum period, characterized by microangiopathic hemolytic anemia, thrombocytopenia, and acute renal failure
  - Vast majority categorized as atypical HUS
    - Occasional infection-related (verotoxin) classic HUS forms reported in postpartum period

ETIOLOGY/PATHOGENESIS

Genetic Abnormalities in Complement System

- High incidence of mutations in complement genes (86% in 1 series)
  - Mutations in genes encoding factor H (*CFH*), factor I (*CFI*), C3 (*C3*), membrane cofactor protein (*CD46*)
    - Normal regulation of alternate complement pathway cascade via effects on C3 convertase
    - Mutations cause quantitative deficiencies or impaired binding to C3b
      - As a result, C3 convertase causes persistent activation of alternate complement pathway
    - Mutations most common in CFH
      - Loss of function mutations in *CFH*, *CFI*, and *CD46*, while *C3* mutations are gain of function
      - 14% in 1 series had > 1 mutation
  - Excessive complement activation causes endothelial injury and prothrombotic state
    - Fenestrated endothelium of glomerular capillaries may be more susceptible
  - Mutation alone insufficient to develop atypical HUS
    - Genetic complement abnormalities cause increased frequency of preeclampsia and fetal loss
- Single-nucleotide polymorphisms and haplotype blocks of *CFH*, *CD46*, and *CFHR1* genes increase susceptibility to disease
  - Homozygosity for high risk-associated haplotypes of *CFH* and *CD46* genes in > 50% of patients
    - At-risk haplotypes identified thus far are CFH TGTGT and MCP GGAAC
      - Increase risk of atypical HUS by 3-4x
- Incomplete penetrance explains disease heterogeneity in affected individuals
  - 50% nonpenetrance rate
  - > 50% with postpartum HUS had uneventful previous pregnancies
  - Additional triggers, such as pregnancy, infections, drugs, autoimmune conditions, transplantation, etc., result in manifestation of atypical HUS

Increased Susceptibility During Postpartum Period

- Physiological mechanisms protect fetus from maternal complement-mediated immunological attack
  - Complement regulatory factors such as membrane cofactor protein, decay accelerating factor, and CD59 expressed on trophoblasts
  - Factor H may be synthesized by trophoblasts
  - Fetus also benefit from paternally inherited complement regulatory factors
  - All these mechanisms downregulate C3 convertase, preventing complement activation
- Antepartum protective mechanisms may be compromised in immediate postpartum period in susceptible individuals
  - Sudden lack of complement regulatory factors
  - Peripartum inflammation, infections, and hemorrhage potentially activate alternate complement pathway

Other

- Other etiologies include infections and anticardiolipin antibodies
- Thrombotic thrombocytopenic purpura (TTP) can occur postpartum, although more frequent in late 2nd and 3rd trimesters

CLINICAL ISSUES

Epidemiology

- Incidence
  - Postpartum subtype accounts for ~ 15% of atypical HUS
    - pHUS risk highest during 2nd pregnancy
    - 80% of atypical HUS associated with pregnancy occurs in postpartum period
      - May also occur during pregnancy

Presentation

- Symptoms manifest postpartum within 24 hours to several weeks
  - Acute renal failure
  - Hematuria, proteinuria
  - Fever, severe hypertension
- May have preceding preeclampsia, acute fatty liver of pregnancy, or HELLP syndrome
  - Persistent and severe renal abnormalities postpartum suggest atypical HUS

Laboratory Tests

- Schistocytes in peripheral smear
- Coombs test negative
- Elevated lactate dehydrogenase
- Thrombocytopenia
- Complement screening
  - Serum levels of C3, C4, factor F, factor I, anti-factor H autoantibodies
  - ADAMTS13 protease levels normal (> 10%) and anti-ADAMTS13 autoantibodies absent
    - Testing done to exclude pregnancy-associated TTP
- Genetic screening for mutational analysis

Treatment

- Plasma exchange and steroids may be beneficial
  - Empiric therapy started prior to results of complement tests and genetic tests
  - Failure to induce TMA remission in 5 days may prompt treatment with eculizumab
- Eculizumab, recombinant humanized monoclonal antibody directed against C5
  - Used safely and successfully during pregnancy and postpartum with documented *CFH* and *CFI* mutations
  - Associated with high risk of meningococcal infections

- Challenges include prohibitive cost and lack of guidelines on treatment duration

Prognosis

- Frequent progression to end-stage kidney disease
  - Occurs in 76% despite receiving plasma exchange
- Can recur in renal allograft
  - 80% with known factor H mutations lose allograft to recurrent disease
  - Factor H deficiency can be corrected by combined liver-kidney transplantation
    - Complement factors synthesized by liver
    - Transplantation can itself be trigger and hence may need empiric plasma exchange perioperatively

MICROSCOPIC

Histologic Features

- Glomeruli
  - Glomerular endothelial swelling
  - Fragmented red blood cells
  - Fibrin thrombi
    - Lobulated accentuation and double contours predominate in chronic phase
- Tubules and interstitium
  - Acute tubular injury with loss of brush borders and simplified epithelium
  - Cortical necrosis and infarction in severe cases
- Vessels
  - Fibrin thrombi and mucoid intimal edema in arterioles

ANCILLARY TESTS

Immunofluorescence

- No immune complexes
  - Nonspecific entrapment of IgM and C3 along GBM
- Fibrin thrombi in arterioles stain for fibrinogen

Electron Microscopy

- Glomeruli
  - Subendothelial expansion by electron-lucent flocculent material and mesangiolysis
  - Fibrin tactoids and depolymerized fibrin in capillary lumens or subendothelial areas
  - GBM remodeling with neobasement membrane formation in chronic phase
  - No electron-dense deposits
- Vessels
  - Fibrin tactoids and depolymerized fibrin
  - Fragmented red blood cells

DIFFERENTIAL DIAGNOSIS

Thrombotic Thrombocytopenic Purpura (TTP)

- Due to ADAMTS13 deficiency or autoantibodies directed against it
- Pregnancy may be initial presentation or exacerbate recurrence in patients with known TTP
  - Vulnerability during pregnancy due to progressive physiological decrease in ADAMTS13
- Often presents in late 2nd or 3rd trimesters (23-26 weeks)
- Renal involvement often mild, and neurological symptoms predominate
- Treatment includes plasma exchange, steroids, rituximab

Preeclampsia and HELLP Syndrome

- Occurs in late pregnancy (> 20 weeks), but may also manifest in immediate postpartum
- Treatment includes antihypertensive therapy, magnesium sulfate, and delivery or pregnancy termination

Thrombotic Microangiopathy Due to Other Causes

- Antiphospholipid antibody syndrome can occur frequently during pregnancy and postpartum period
- Clinical and serological tests may identify potential causes, such as drugs, infections, neoplasms, or autoimmune diseases

SELECTED REFERENCES

1. Kourouklaris A et al: Postpartum thrombotic microangiopathy revealed as atypical hemolytic uremic syndrome successfully treated with eculizumab: a case report. J Med Case Rep. 8:307, 2014
2. Riedl M et al: Spectrum of complement-mediated thrombotic microangiopathies: pathogenetic insights identifying novel treatment approaches. Semin Thromb Hemost. 40(4):444-64, 2014
3. Abudiab M et al: Differentiating scleroderma renal crisis from other causes of thrombotic microangiopathy in a postpartum patient. Clin Nephrol. 80(4):293-7, 2013
4. Ardissino G et al: Eculizumab for atypical hemolytic uremic syndrome in pregnancy. Obstet Gynecol. 122(2 Pt 2):487-9, 2013
5. Zschiedrich S et al: Successful treatment of the postpartum atypical hemolytic uremic syndrome with eculizumab. Ann Intern Med. 159(1):76, 2013
6. Brown JH et al: Postpartum aHUS secondary to a genetic abnormality in factor H acquired through liver transplantation. Am J Transplant. 12(6):1632-6, 2012
7. Fakhouri F et al: Pregnancy-associated hemolytic uremic syndrome revisited in the era of complement gene mutations. J Am Soc Nephrol. 21(5):859-67, 2010
8. Goodship TH et al: Pulling the trigger in atypical hemolytic uremic syndrome: the role of pregnancy. J Am Soc Nephrol. 21(5):731-2, 2010
9. Magee CC et al: Case records of the Massachusetts General Hospital. Case 2-2008. A 38-year-old woman with postpartum visual loss, shortness of breath, and renal failure. N Engl J Med. 358(3):275-89, 2008
10. Martin JN Jr et al: Thrombotic thrombocytopenic purpura in 166 pregnancies: 1955-2006. Am J Obstet Gynecol. 199(2):98-104, 2008
11. Sánchez-Luceros A et al: von Willebrand factor-cleaving protease (ADAMTS13) activity in normal non-pregnant women, pregnant and post-delivery women. Thromb Haemost. 92(6):1320-6, 2004
12. Vesely SK et al: ADAMTS13 activity in thrombotic thrombocytopenic purpura-hemolytic uremic syndrome: relation to presenting features and clinical outcomes in a prospective cohort of 142 patients. Blood. 102(1):60-8, 2003
13. Banatvala N et al: The United States National Prospective Hemolytic Uremic Syndrome Study: microbiologic, serologic, clinical, and epidemiologic findings. J Infect Dis. 183(7):1063-70, 2001
14. Shemin D et al: Clinical outcome in three patients with postpartum hemolytic uremic syndrome treated with frequent plasma exchange. Ther Apher. 2(1):43-8, 1998
15. Segonds A et al: Postpartum hemolytic uremic syndrome: a study of three cases with a review of the literature. Clin Nephrol. 12(5):229-42, 1979

Fragmented Entrapped RBCs in Mesangium

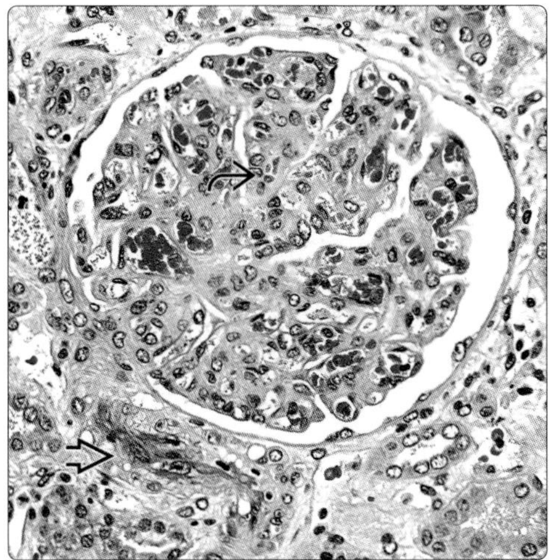

Nonspecific IgM Deposition in Glomerulus

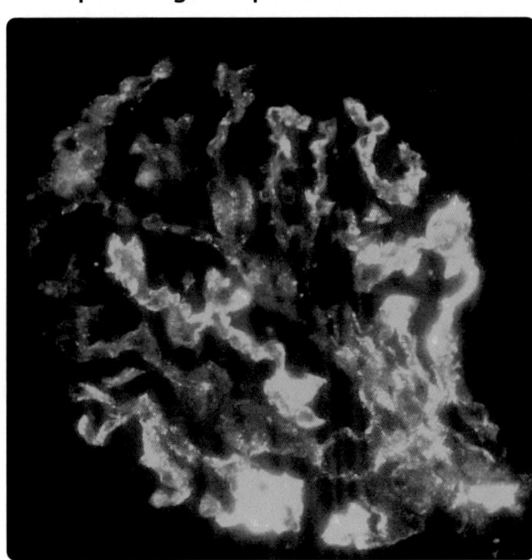

(Left) *The patient developed acute renal failure 1 week postpartum, concerning for pHUS. Fibrin thrombus is seen in the arteriole ⇒, and the glomerulus had entrapped RBCs ⇗ in the mesangium.* **(Right)** *Nonspecific entrapment of IgM within the glomerulus is seen on immunofluorescence. This biopsy is from a young woman who was 1 week postpartum and had persistently elevated levels of serum creatinine. The light microscopy was compatible with thrombotic microangiopathy.*

Glomerular Fibrin Postpartum

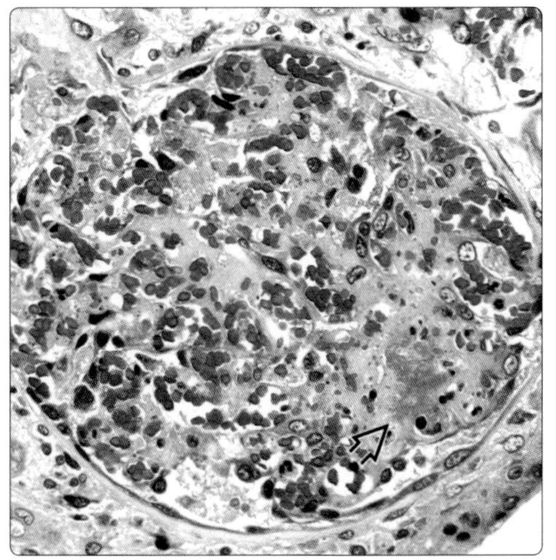

Cortical Necrosis in pHUS

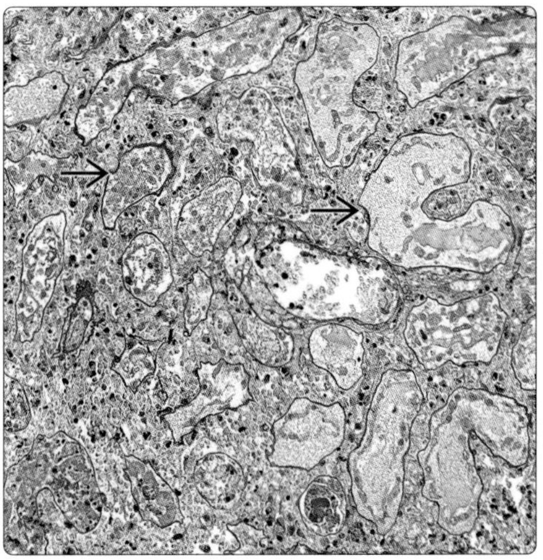

(Left) *A 33-year-old woman underwent a C-section at 25 weeks gestation for presumed HELLP syndrome. Within a few days, the patient developed acute renal failure, and renal biopsy showed glomerular fibrin thrombi ⇒, compatible with pHUS. Extensive cortical necrosis was also present.* **(Right)** *Extensive cortical necrosis can be observed in severe pHUS. Fibrin thrombi identified in several arterioles likely precipitated cortical necrosis. Only outlines of the tubules → are observed within the infarcted parenchyma.*

Platelet Aggregation in Glomerulus

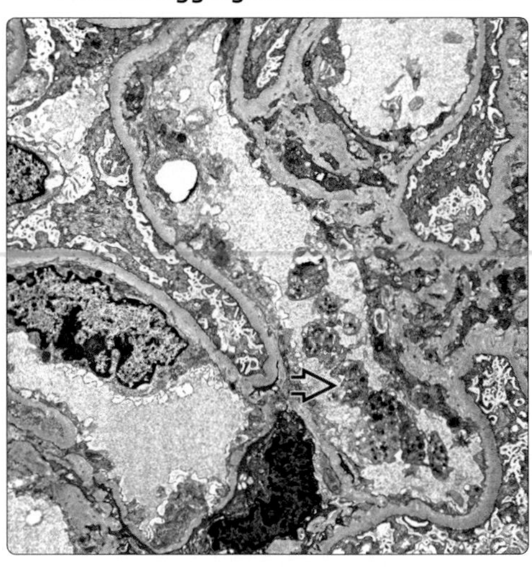

Glomerular Basement Membrane Duplication

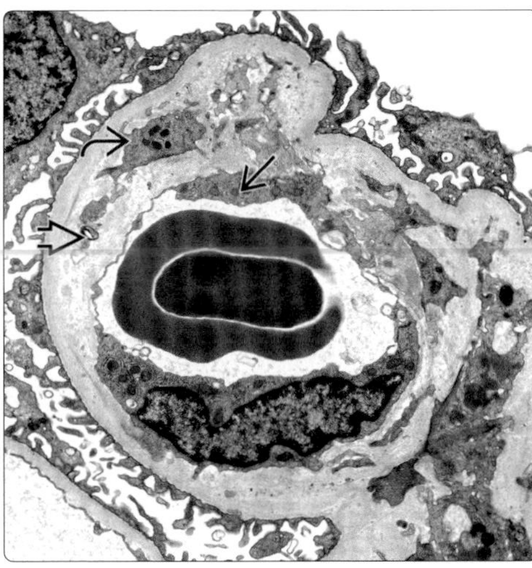

(Left) *An aggregate of platelets ⇒ is seen in the glomerular capillary lumen. Characteristic features of thrombotic microangiopathy were observed on light microscopy in this 27-year-old woman with acute renal failure and pHUS.* **(Right)** *The subendothelial zone ⇒ is expanded by lucent flocculent material in pHUS. The endothelial cells are reactive and have lost fenestrations →. Duplication of the glomerular basement membrane is observed with an entrapped platelet ⇗.*

Scleroderma Renal Disease

KEY FACTS

TERMINOLOGY

- Idiopathic systemic disease manifested by fibrosis microvascular pathology of skin (sclerodactyly, telangiectasia, Raynaud phenomenon), kidney (scleroderma renal crisis), and other organs (lung, heart, GI tract)

ETIOLOGY/PATHOGENESIS

- Idiopathic
- Endothelial &/or fibroblast autoantibodies in > 50%
  - Increased synthesis of matrix components
  - ↑ vascular permeability, endothelial apoptosis intimal edema, and platelet aggregation
- 5-31% RNA polymerase III
  - Increased risk of scleroderma renal crisis (SRC)

CLINICAL ISSUES

- Scleroderma renal crisis
  - 25% present without preceding diagnosis of SS
  - Acute renal failure
  - New onset malignant hypertension (10% normotensive)
  - Headaches, fever, malaise, convulsions, visual disturbances, dyspnea, or arrhythmias
- Therapy: Angiotensin-converting enzyme inhibitors

MICROSCOPIC

- Arcuate and interlobular arteries affected by TMA
  - Intimal mucoid edema and endothelial swelling result in onion skin concentric appearance
  - Luminal occlusion and fragmented RBCs
  - Fibrin thrombi and fibrinoid necrosis
- Ischemic collapse of glomerular capillary tufts
- Immunofluorescence: Fibrin, IgM, C3 in vessel walls
- Electron microscopy
  - Endothelial swelling, loss, and reactive changes
  - GBM duplication, no immune deposits

TOP DIFFERENTIAL DIAGNOSES

- Other causes of thrombotic microangiopathy

Thrombotic Microangiopathy

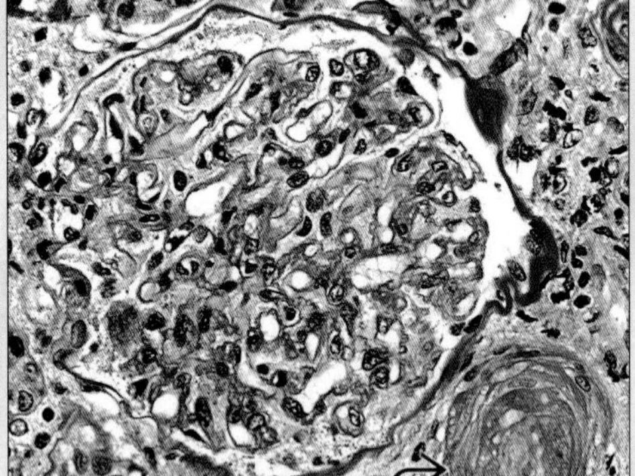

Reactive Glomerular Endothelial Cells

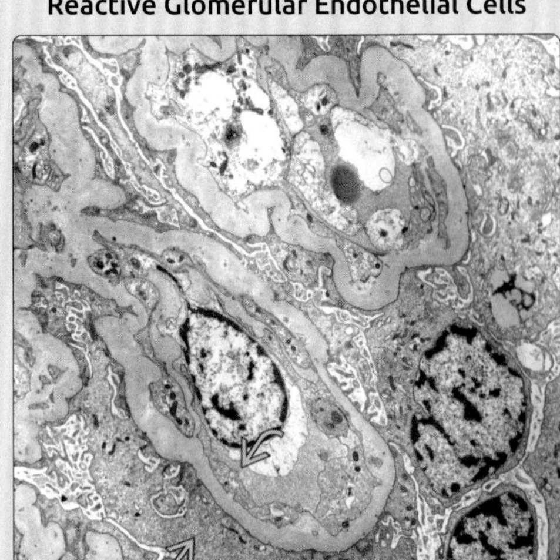

(Left) *The glomeruli are relatively spared in SRC, as seen in this 37-year-old woman with Raynaud phenomenon and features of scleroderma. An adjacent arteriole with thrombotic microangiopathy ➡ has an onion skin appearance.* **(Right)** *The endothelial cells of the glomerulus show extensive loss of fenestrations and expansion of cytoplasm ⇨, signs of injury and reactive change. Podocytes have extensive foot processes effacement ⇨. The GBM is normal except for wrinkling due to the arterial disease.*

Acute Arterial Lesions

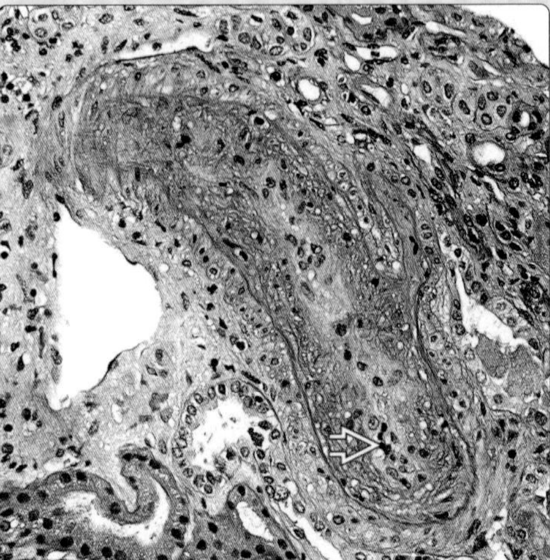

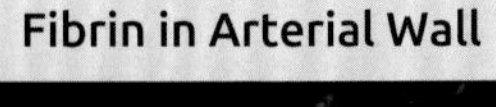

Fibrin in Arterial Wall

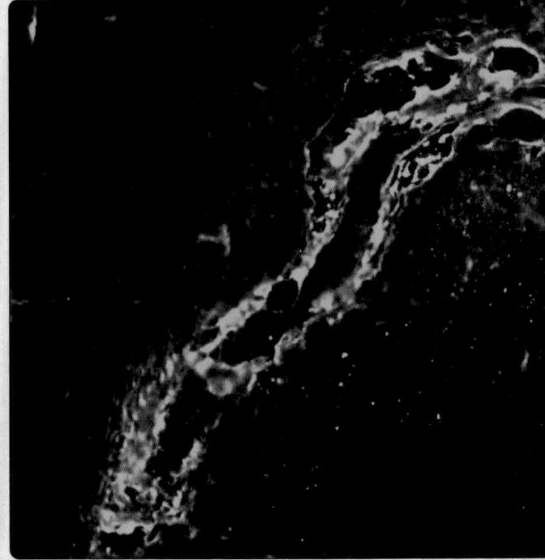

(Left) *Arterial and arteriolar changes predominate in thrombotic microangiopathy due to SRC. An interlobular artery is completely occluded by intimal edema ➡ and proliferation, resembling endarteritis in allografts.* **(Right)** *The acutely injured arteries show deposition of fibrin in the wall. IgM and C3 are also commonly deposited putatively due to nonspecific trapping.*

TERMINOLOGY

Abbreviations

- Scleroderma renal crisis (SRC)

Synonyms

- Systemic sclerosis (SS)

Definitions

- Idiopathic systemic disease manifested by fibrosis microvascular pathology of skin (sclerodactyly, telangiectasia, Raynaud phenomenon) and other organs (kidney, lung, heart, GI tract)
- Scleroderma renal crisis is acute renal injury characterized by features of thrombotic microangiopathy

ETIOLOGY/PATHOGENESIS

Idiopathic

- Current evidence points to endothelial cells and fibroblasts as targets of autoimmune mechanisms

Vascular Injury

- ↑ vascular permeability, endothelial apoptosis intimal edema, and platelet aggregation
- ↑ endothelin-1 (ET-1)/vasoconstriction
- Endothelial autoantibodies in 44-84%
  - Associated with more severe vasculopathy
  - Induces apoptosis in vitro
  - Specificity unknown

Fibroblasts

- Increased synthesis of matrix components
  - Increased mRNA for collagen I in skin
- Increased fibroblast expression of TGF-β receptors
- ↑ platelet-derived growth factor, connective tissue growth factor
- Autoantibodies to fibroblasts
  - Anti-fibrillin-1
    - Detected in > 50% of SS
    - Activate fibroblasts in vitro
      - Increased matrix production, including collagen I
      - Release TGFb from matrix
      - Increase MMP-1
  - Anti-MMP1, anti-MMP3
    - Inhibit matrix degradation

Autoantibodies to Intracellular Components

- > 90% antinuclear antibodies
- Mechanism by which these autoantibodies to intranuclear components contribute to pathogenesis is unclear; nonetheless, they are useful predictors of outcome
- Some highly specific for SS and correlate with phenotype but not clearly linked to pathogenesis
  - 5-31% RNA polymerase III
    - Speckled antinuclear antibody pattern
    - ~ 20x higher risk of SRC
  - 15-42% antitopoisomerase-1 (scl70)
    - 90-100% with antibody have SS
    - Increased risk of lung and heart involvement and poor prognosis
    - Not consistently associated with SRC
  - 20-38% anticentromere (HEp2 cells)
    - Correlates with limited form and better prognosis
    - Also found in SLE, primary biliary cirrhosis, Sjögren and Raynaud syndromes
  - 4-10% antifibrillarin (U3RNP)
    - More frequent in patients of recent African descent
    - Associated with SRC and cardiac involvement
- Once considered mutually exclusive
  - Multiplex tests show ~ 17% have > 1 autoantibody

T-Cell Mediation

- Th2 responses by activated T cells increase fibrosis
- SS resembles chronic graft-vs.-host disease
- Mixed chimerism post pregnancy demonstrated

Scleroderma Renal Crisis

- Severe vascular lesions can precede hypertension
- Arterial luminal narrowing triggers renin production and exacerbates hypertension
- Certain polymorphisms of ET-1 receptors increase risk
- Corticosteroids are known to precipitate SRC

CLINICAL ISSUES

Epidemiology

- Incidence
  - 10-20% of patients with diffuse SS develop SRC; ~ 6-7% with limited SS
- Sex
  - F:M = 3:1
- Ethnicity
  - African Americans at risk for developing SRC

Presentation

- Diffuse or limited cutaneous forms
  - Diffuse has widespread cutaneous fibrosis and higher prevalence of organ involvement
  - Limited form affects distal extremities, later and milder organ involvement
    - Synonym: CREST (calcinosis, Raynaud phenomenon, esophageal hypomotility, sclerodactyly, telangiectasia)
- Skin lesions
  - Telangiectasia
  - Sclerodactyly
  - Raynaud phenomenon
- Scleroderma renal crisis
  - 25% present without preceding diagnosis of SS
  - New onset malignant hypertension
    - 10% normotensive
  - Elevated serum Cr and acute renal failure
  - Headaches, fever, malaise, convulsions, visual disturbances, dyspnea, or arrhythmias
  - 50% schistocytes, thrombocytopenia, ↑ LDH
- Other kidney diseases uncommon
  - Membranous glomerulonephritis or ANCA-related glomerulonephritis secondary to D-penicillamine
- Other organs
  - Dysphagia (esophageal involvement)
  - Dyspnea (pulmonary involvement)

Treatment

- Angiotensin converting enzyme (ACE) inhibitor

- ET-1 receptor antagonist (bosentan) in clinical trials
- Dialysis, transplantation

Prognosis

- ~ 50% require dialysis
  - ~ 50% recover enough renal function to go off dialysis
- 10-year survival rate with ACE inhibitors (60-70%)

MICROSCOPIC

Histologic Features

- Scleroderma renal crisis
  - Glomeruli
    - Fibrin thrombi, endothelial swelling, and fibrinoid necrosis
    - Ischemic collapse
    - GBM duplication, mesangiolysis in chronic cases
    - Usually little mesangial or endocapillary hypercellularity
    - Crescents not common and raise possibility of associated ANCA disease
  - Tubules
    - Acute tubular injury
  - Arteries
    - Arcuate and interlobular arteries more often affected
      - Luminal occlusion and fragmented RBCs
      - Fibrin thrombi and fibrinoid necrosis
    - Intimal mucoid edema and endothelial swelling result in onion skin concentric appearance
      - Duplication of internal elastic lamina and adventitial fibrosis seen in chronic cases
      - No associated vessel wall inflammation
- Late (chronic) changes
  - Increased arterial intimal fibrosis
  - Increased tubular atrophy and interstitial fibrosis
  - Recanalization of arteries
- Superimposed diseases
  - ANCA-related glomerulonephritis, ± penicillamine therapy
  - Membranous glomerulonephritis, penicillamine associated

ANCILLARY TESTS

Immunohistochemistry

- C4d in granular pattern has been described in paraffin-embedded renal tissue
  - Associated with poor prognosis
- ET-1 increased in glomeruli and arteries

Immunofluorescence

- IgM, C3, and fibrinogen in glomeruli and arteries

Electron Microscopy

- Endothelial swelling, loss of fenestrations, and expanded subendothelial space by electron-lucent material
- GBM duplication, wrinkling, and mesangial cell interposition in chronic phase

DIFFERENTIAL DIAGNOSIS

Thrombotic Microangiopathy, Other Causes

- SRC may present without skin lesions
- Clinical and serological data help differentiate
  - Anti-RNA polymerase III usually positive in SCR

ANCA-Related Glomerulonephritis

- Secondary to penicillamine therapy
- Crescents, necrosis suggest ANCA disease

Membranous Glomerulonephritis

- Secondary to penicillamine therapy
- GBM immune complexes distinguish it from SRC

DIAGNOSTIC CHECKLIST

Clinically Relevant Pathologic Features

- Features that increase risk of irreversible renal failure
  - Vascular thrombosis
  - Severe glomerular ischemic collapse
  - Granular C4d deposition in peritubular capillaries
  - Mucoid intimal thickening in interlobular arteries &/or fibrinoid necrosis in arterioles

SELECTED REFERENCES

1. Hamaguchi Y et al: Clinical and immunologic predictors of scleroderma renal crisis in Japanese systemic sclerosis patients with anti-RNA polymerase III autoantibodies. Arthritis Rheumatol. 67(4):1045-52, 2015
2. Kayser C et al: Autoantibodies in systemic sclerosis: unanswered questions. Front Immunol. 6:167, 2015
3. Logee KM et al: Scleroderma renal crisis as an initial presentation of systemic sclerosis: a case report and review of the literature. Clin Exp Rheumatol. ePub, 2015
4. Bhavsar SV et al: Anti-RNA polymerase III antibodies in the diagnosis of scleroderma renal crisis in the absence of skin disease. J Clin Rheumatol. 20(7):379-82, 2014
5. Bose N et al: Scleroderma renal crisis. Semin Arthritis Rheum. ePub, 2014
6. Kumar RP et al: D-penicillamine-induced membranous nephropathy. Indian J Nephrol. 24(3):195-6, 2014
7. Steen VD: Kidney involvement in systemic sclerosis. Presse Med. 43(10 Pt 2):e305-14, 2014
8. Toescu SM et al: Steroid-induced scleroderma renal crisis in an at-risk patient. BMJ Case Rep. 2014, 2014
9. Maruyama A et al: Glucocorticoid-induced normotensive scleroderma renal crisis: a report on two cases and a review of the literature in Japan. Intern Med. 52(16):1833-7, 2013
10. Penn H et al: Targeting the endothelin axis in scleroderma renal crisis: rationale and feasibility. QJM. 106(9):839-48, 2013
11. Op De Beéck K et al: Antinuclear antibody detection by automated multiplex immunoassay in untreated patients at the time of diagnosis. Autoimmun Rev. 12(2):137-43, 2012
12. Batal I et al: Scleroderma renal crisis: a pathology perspective. Int J Rheumatol. 2010:543704, 2010
13. Batal I et al: Renal biopsy findings predicting outcome in scleroderma renal crisis. Hum Pathol. 40(3):332-40, 2009
14. Penn H et al: Diagnosis, management and prevention of scleroderma renal disease. Curr Opin Rheumatol. 20(6):692-6, 2008
15. Arnaud L et al: ANCA-related crescentic glomerulonephritis in systemic sclerosis: revisiting the "normotensive scleroderma renal crisis". Clin Nephrol. 68(3):165-70, 2007
16. Penn H et al: Scleroderma renal crisis: patient characteristics and long-term outcomes. QJM. 100(8):485-94, 2007

Thrombi in Arteries

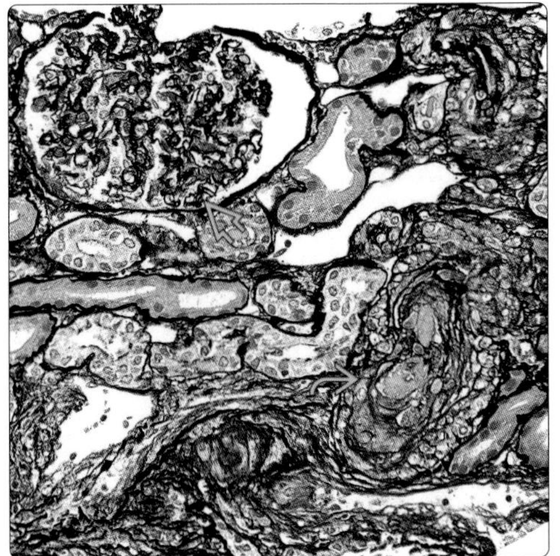

Basophilic Intima With Red Cell Fragments

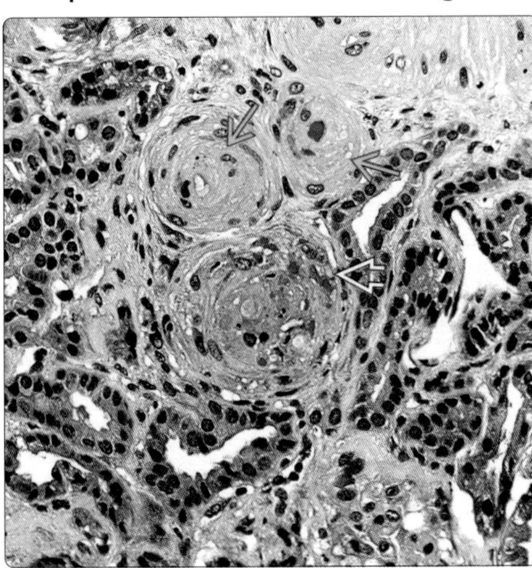

(Left) *A 46-year-old woman with dermatomyositis and features suggestive of SS presented with acute renal failure. The interlobular arteries demonstrate intimal edema with luminal fibrin thrombi ➙, while the adjacent glomerulus ➙ shows mild ischemic collapse.* **(Right)** *Cross sections of interlobular arteries show basophilic intimal thickening ➙, karyorrhexis, and entrapped fragmented red cells (schistocytes) ➙. Based on the clinical history of SS, these characteristic features of TMA are attributed to SRC.*

"Onion Skinning"

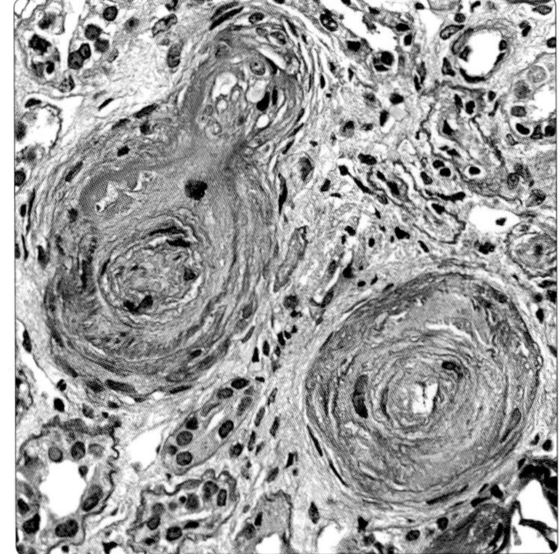

Mucoid Intimal Edema

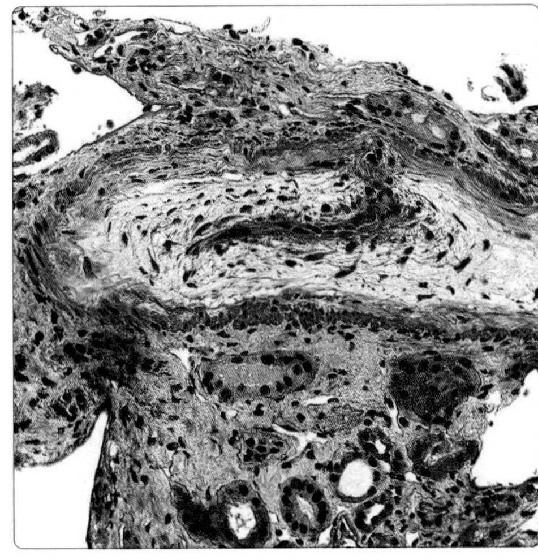

(Left) *The interlobular arterial walls show concentric lamination with associated edema and severe narrowing of the lumina ("onion skinning"). Arcuate arteries are also similarly affected in SRC.* **(Right)** *Severe mucoid intimal edema is seen in this cross section of an arcuate caliber artery. The patient, a 64-year-old man with SS, was biopsied for rapidly progressive renal failure. Almost all arteries sampled in the biopsy were affected.*

Cellular Intimal Proliferation

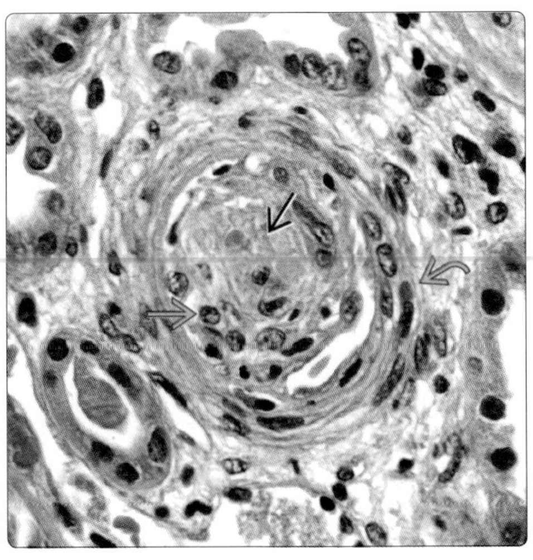

Artery With Edema and Red Cells in Intima

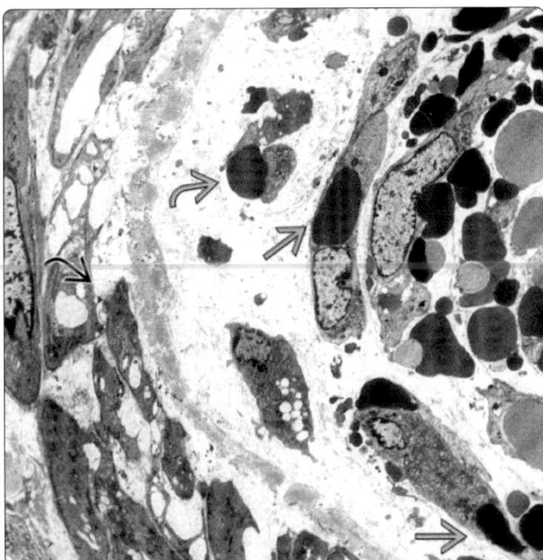

(Left) *This artery has increased cellularity in the intima ➙ and occlusion of the lumen ➙. There is no obvious endothelial lining. A red cell is trapped in the media ➙.* **(Right)** *Electron microscopy reveals red cells ➙ trapped in an edematous intima and phagocytosed ➙ by cells in a small intrarenal artery. There is no apparent endothelium. Smooth muscle cells show vacuoles, suggesting injury ➙.*

(Left) *The glomerulus appears ischemic and "bloodless" in this 63-year-old man with SS and acute renal failure. Thrombi are occasionally seen* ➩*. All interlobular and arcuate arteries sampled in the biopsy had characteristic features of acute thrombotic microangiopathy due to SRC.* **(Right)** *The artery shows transmural fibrinoid necrosis* ➩*, while the nearby glomerulus has loss of endothelial cell nuclei and fibrin in capillaries* ➡*. Another glomerulus is hypocellular with thrombi* ➩*.*

Acute Ischemic Injury

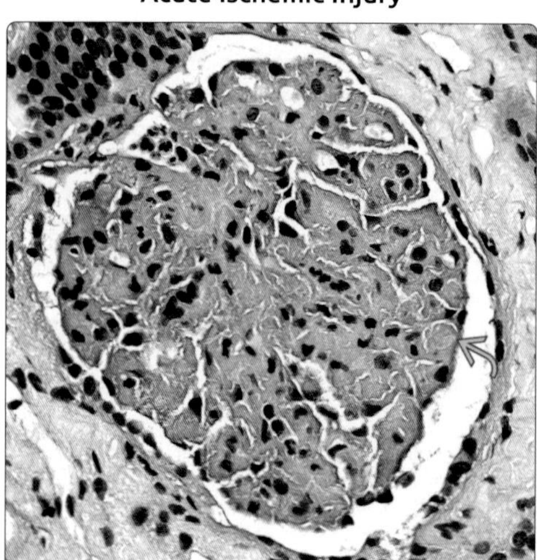

Necrosis of Artery and Glomerulus

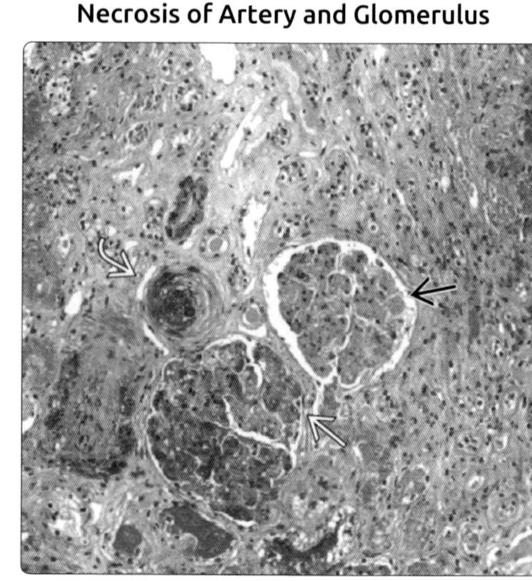

(Left) *The principal immunoreactant seen in SRC is fibrin in glomerular capillaries and in the walls of arteries. IgM and C3 sometimes are also present in affected glomeruli and arteries, thought to be nonspecific.* **(Right)** *Electron-lucent flocculent material* ➩ *is seen in the mesangium and subendothelium, compatible with acute TMA. Some capillary loops have lost their endothelium and collapsed* ➩ *in this 37-year-old woman with SS and acute renal failure.*

Fibrin Thrombi in Glomeruli

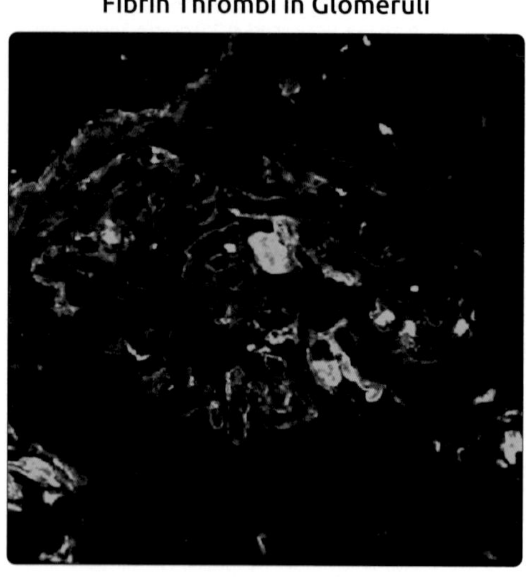

Flocculent Subendothelial Material

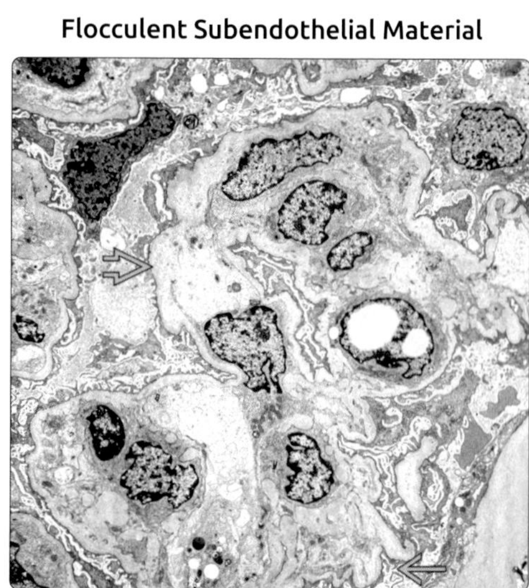

(Left) *The glomerular basement membrane shows extensive wrinkling* ➩ *with a collapsed capillary tuft. The podocytes demonstrate foot process effacement* ➩*, and electron-dense deposits are observed. The arteries in the biopsy had classic features of SRC-related TMA.* **(Right)** *A platelet thrombus* ➩ *is seen within the capillary lumen. The biopsy is from an SS patient with acute renal failure. Endothelial injury in SRC causes altered vascular permeability, intimal edema, and platelet aggregation.*

GBM Wrinkling

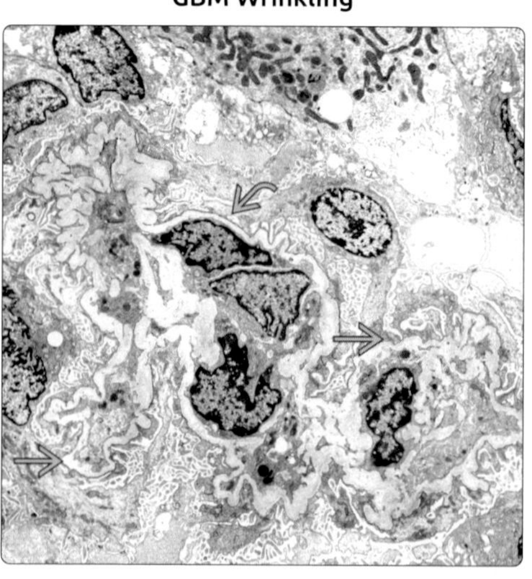

Platelet Thrombus in Glomerulus

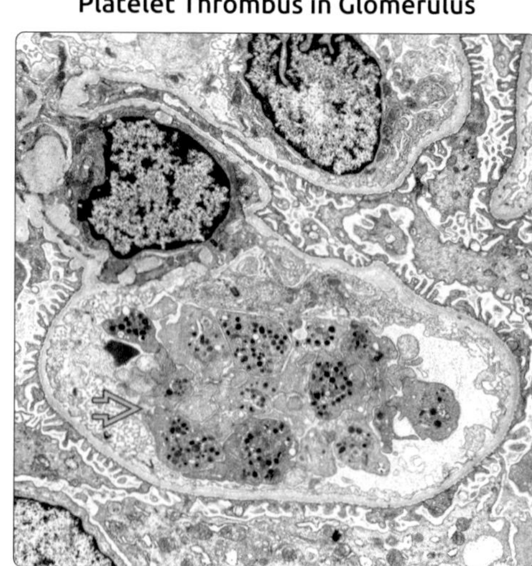

Chronic Changes: GBM Duplication

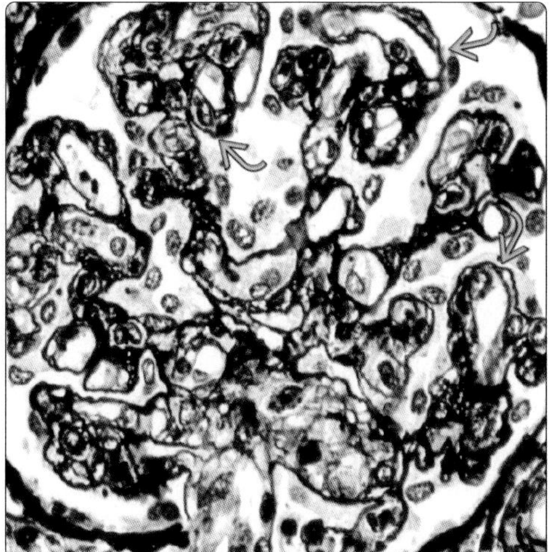

GBM Duplication on EM

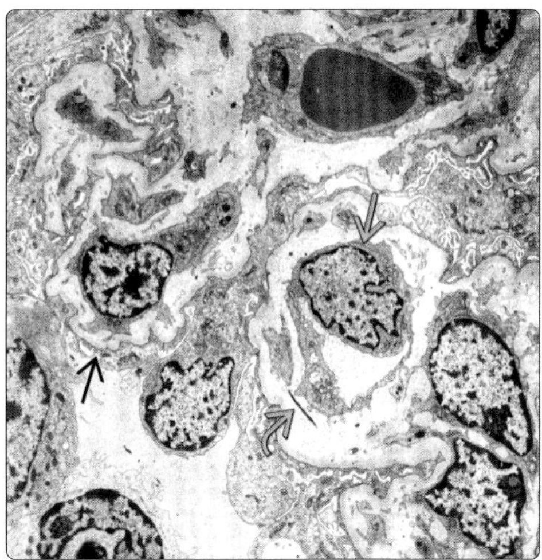

(Left) *Later changes of SRC include duplication of the GBM ➡, shown here in a silver stain. This is a manifestation of endothelial injury and repair.* **(Right)** *Duplication of the GBM is seen by EM, with lucent material between the GBM layers, sometimes with fibrin tactoids ➡. The endothelial cells show reactive changes, including loss of fenestrations and increased cytoplasmic organelles ➡. Some capillaries have a wrinkled GBM and collapse with no evident lumen ➡.*

Glomerular Ischemia and Tubular Atrophy

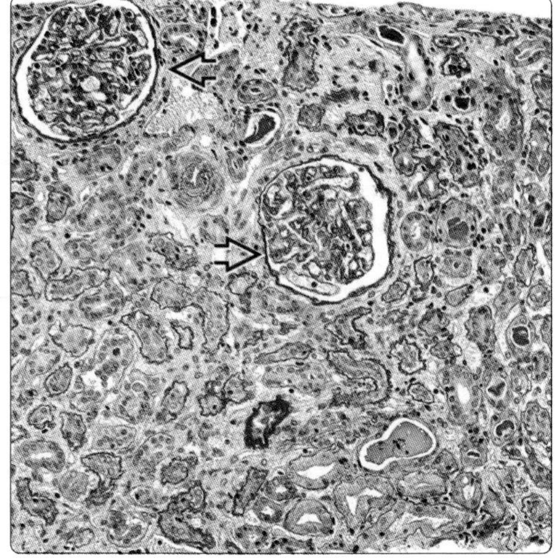

Recanalization of Artery

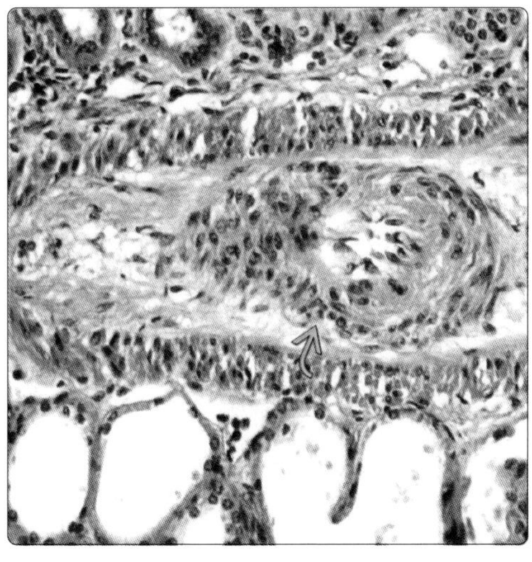

(Left) *Extensive glomerular ischemic retraction ➡ and tubular atrophy are seen in this kidney biopsy. Characteristic arterial wall changes were seen elsewhere in this biopsy from a 36-year-old woman with SRC.* **(Right)** *Late changes show evidence of repair, with restoration of the arterial lumen by recanalization and neomedia ➡, giving the artery a bull's eye appearance.*

Occlusion of Artery

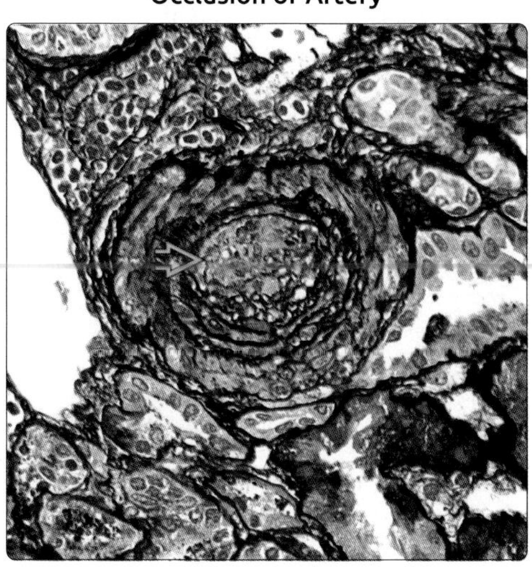

Skin Biopsy

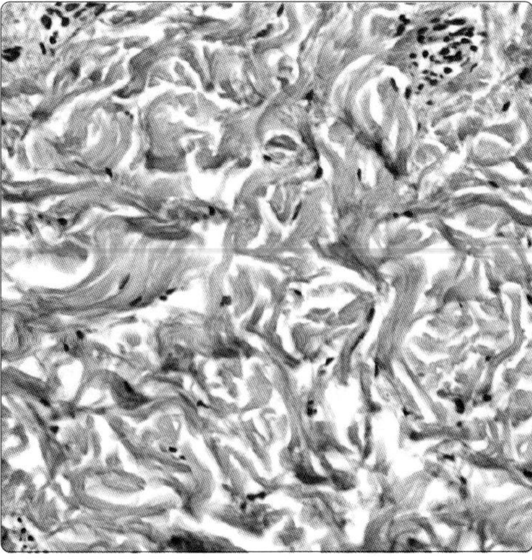

(Left) *A 36-year-old woman with mixed connective tissue disorder and SS presented with malignant hypertension and nephrotic-range proteinuria. Luminal cellular occlusion ➡ and intimal concentric lamination are seen within an interlobular artery.* **(Right)** *The skin in scleroderma shows dermal hypocellularity and thickened bands of collagen with increased eosinophilia in the dermis that extend into the subcutaneous tissue entrapping sweat glands (not shown).*

Preeclampsia, Eclampsia, HELLP Syndrome

KEY FACTS

TERMINOLOGY

- Toxemia of pregnancy
- Pregnancy-induced hypertension
- Preeclampsia is characterized by hypertension, proteinuria, and edema
- Eclampsia is characterized by seizures or convulsions along with signs and symptoms of preeclampsia

ETIOLOGY/PATHOGENESIS

- Placental factor
  - Upregulation of soluble fms-like tyrosin kinase-1 (sFlt-1)
    - Receptor for vascular endothelial growth factor (VEGF)

CLINICAL ISSUES

- Preeclampsia
  - 5-8% of pregnancies
- HELLP syndrome
  - 4-12% of preeclampsia patients
- Hypertension
- Headache

MICROSCOPIC

- "Bloodless" appearance due to occlusion by swollen endothelial cells
- Duplication of glomerular basement membranes
- Mesangiolysis
- Focal segmental glomerulosclerosis
- Glomerular endotheliosis
- Thrombotic microangiopathy

TOP DIFFERENTIAL DIAGNOSES

- Other causes of TMA
  - Atypical hemolytic uremic syndrome
    - Mutations in factors C3, B, H, I, or MCP (CD46)
    - TMA with pregnancy in 20% with these mutations
  - Thrombotic thrombocytopenic purpura
  - Anti-phospholipid antibody syndrome

Bloodless Glomerulus

Arteriolar Thrombus

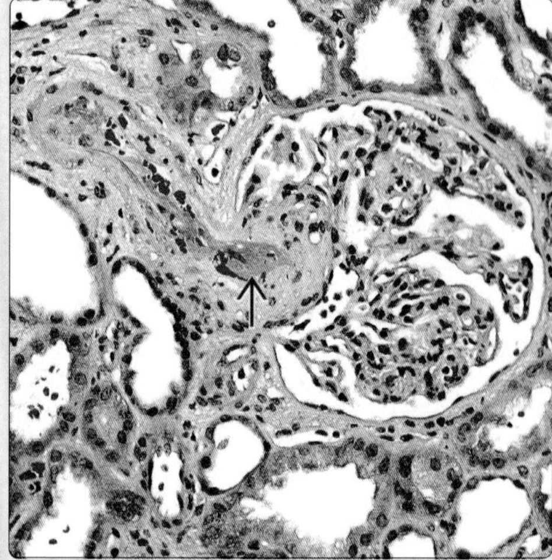

(Left) *Preeclampsia manifests glomeruli with a "bloodless" appearance due to prominent swelling of endothelial cells. The glomerular capillary lumina are obscured, which results in a substantial decrease in glomerular filtration.* **(Right)** *Hematoxylin & eosin reveals an arteriolar thrombus → with entrapped red blood cells and red blood cell fragments from a pregnant woman with HELLP syndrome.*

Mucoid Intimal Change

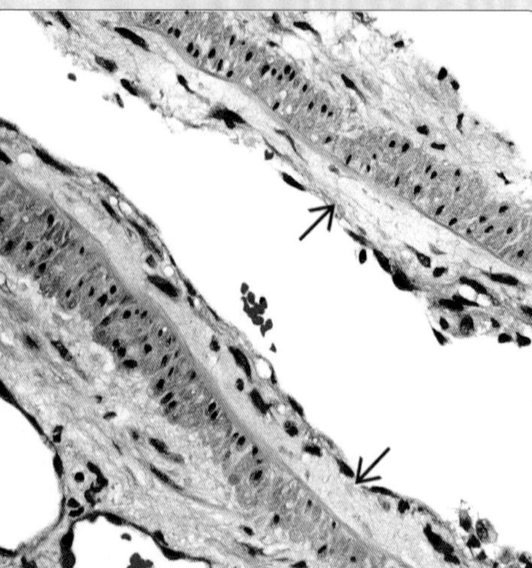

Endotheliosis

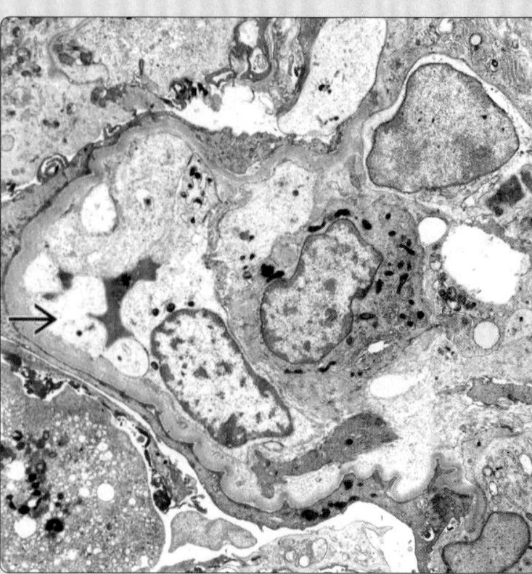

(Left) *Hematoxylin & eosin shows marked mucoid intimal change → in an intrarenal artery of a patient with HELLP syndrome. This intimal alteration of the artery can also be observed in scleroderma and malignant hypertension.* **(Right)** *Electron microscopy reveals prominent swelling → of the endothelial cells (also termed "endotheliosis"), which decreases the effective glomerular capillary lumen. There is also diffuse effacement of the overlying podocyte foot processes.*

TERMINOLOGY

Abbreviations

- Hemolysis, elevated liver enzymes, low platelets (HELLP) syndrome

Synonyms

- Toxemia of pregnancy

Definitions

- Preeclampsia: Hypertension and proteinuria during pregnancy
- Eclampsia: Seizures and neurologic symptoms in addition

ETIOLOGY/PATHOGENESIS

Proposed Mechanism for Preeclampsia/Eclampsia

- Placental factor
  - Upregulation of soluble fms-like tyrosine kinase-1 (sFlt-1)
    - Receptor for vascular endothelial growth factor (VEGF)
  - Endothelial cell injury
  - Glomerular endothelium is dependent on podocyte for high local levels of VEGF
  - Symptoms resolve with delivery of placenta
- Anti-VEGF monoclonal antibody therapy causes proteinuria

Proposed Mechanism for HELLP Syndrome

- May be related to pregnancy-associated atypical hemolytic uremic syndrome
  - Mutations in complement factors C3, B, H, I, or membrane cofactor protein (MCP)
  - Acquired autoantibodies to complement factor H

Animal Models

- Heterozygous deletion of VEGF leads to glomerular endotheliosis mimicking human preeclampsia/eclampsia

CLINICAL ISSUES

Epidemiology

- Incidence
  - Preeclampsia 5-8% of pregnancies
    - HELLP syndrome 4-12% of preeclampsia patients
    - Low risk after normal first pregnancy (1%)
  - Eclampsia ~ 0.05% pregnancies
  - Multiple gestations, molar pregnancies, and preexisting renal disease are risk factors

Presentation

- Onset after the 20th week of pregnancy in 1st pregnancy
- Hypertension
- Proteinuria
- Acute kidney injury (rare)

Treatment

- Blood pressure control
- Emergent delivery or termination of pregnancy if life-threatening symptoms present

Prognosis

- Preeclampsia recurs in ~ 20% of subsequent pregnancies
- 2% death rate from eclampsia

MICROSCOPIC

Histologic Features

- Glomeruli
  - Glomerular endotheliosis
    - "Bloodless" appearance due to occlusion by swollen endothelial cells
  - Mesangiolysis
  - Focal segmental glomerulosclerosis
  - Collapsing glomerulopathy (rare)
  - Rare crescents
  - Duplication of glomerular basement membranes
- Tubules
  - Ischemic changes
- Vessels
  - Thrombotic microangiopathy (TMA) may involve glomerular capillaries or arterioles

ANCILLARY TESTS

Immunohistochemistry

- Activated parietal epithelial cells (Ki-67[+] CD44[+])

Immunofluorescence

- Fibrin or fibrinogen deposition in thrombi, if present
  - IgM may be entrapped in similar distribution as fibrin/fibrinogen

Electron Microscopy

- Reactive endothelium
  - Swelling of endothelial cells
  - Loss of endothelial fenestrations
- Mesangial cell swelling
- Focal effacement of foot processes may be present
- Subendothelial space widening by electron-lucent material

DIFFERENTIAL DIAGNOSIS

Other Causes of TMA

- Atypical hemolytic uremic syndrome
  - Mutations in factors C3, B, H, I, or MCP (CD46)
  - TMA with pregnancy in 20% with these mutations
- Thrombotic thrombocytopenic purpura
- Anti-phospholipid antibody syndrome

DIAGNOSTIC CHECKLIST

Pathologic Interpretation Pearls

- Clinical correlation is required to distinguish preeclampsia, eclampsia, HELLP syndrome and other etiologies of TMA
- Endotheliosis is highly specific and possibly pathognomonic for preeclampsia, but beware of artifactual endothelial swelling due to poor fixation

SELECTED REFERENCES

1. Penning ME et al: Association of preeclampsia with podocyte turnover. Clin J Am Soc Nephrol. 9(8):1377-85, 2014
2. Fakhouri F et al: Factor H, membrane cofactor protein, and factor I mutations in patients with hemolysis, elevated liver enzymes, and low platelet count syndrome. Blood. 112(12):4542-5, 2008
3. Stillman IE et al: The glomerular injury of preeclampsia. J Am Soc Nephrol. 18(8):2281-4, 2007

Radiation Nephropathy

KEY FACTS

TERMINOLOGY

- Renal injury due to radiation exposure, typically therapeutic radiation for malignancy

ETIOLOGY/PATHOGENESIS

- Total body irradiation dosage
  - 20-25 Gy over > 1 month leads to radiation nephropathy
- Graft-vs.-host disease
  - Possible risk factor for developing thrombotic microangiopathy

CLINICAL ISSUES

- 20-40% of patients receiving significant radiation
- Higher susceptibility in pediatric patients
- Renal dysfunction
- Proteinuria
- Hypertension

MICROSCOPIC

- Mesangiolysis
- Thrombi
- GBM duplication, if chronic
- Global or segmental glomerulosclerosis
- Interstitial edema
- Interstitial fibrosis and tubular atrophy
- Mucoid intimal change
- Arteriolar hyalinosis

TOP DIFFERENTIAL DIAGNOSES

- Thrombotic microangiopathy, various causes
- Graft-vs.-host glomerulopathies

DIAGNOSTIC CHECKLIST

- Clinical history of hematopoietic cell (bone marrow) transplantation
- Chemotherapy often is used in combination with radiation, and both can result in thrombotic microangiopathic injuries

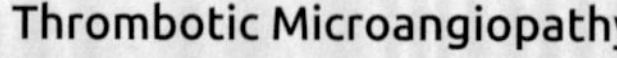

Thrombotic Microangiopathy

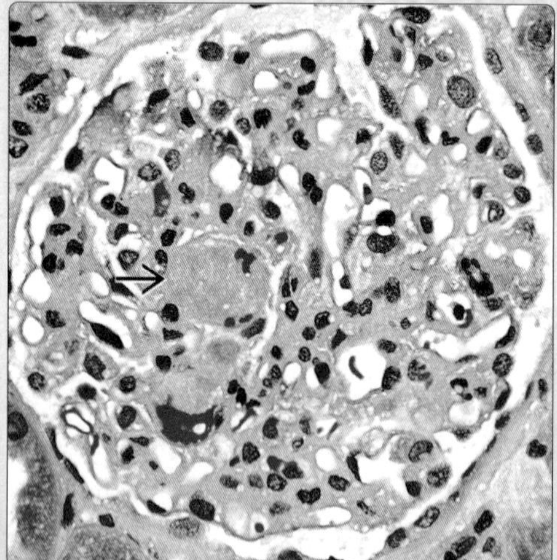

Hilar Thrombus

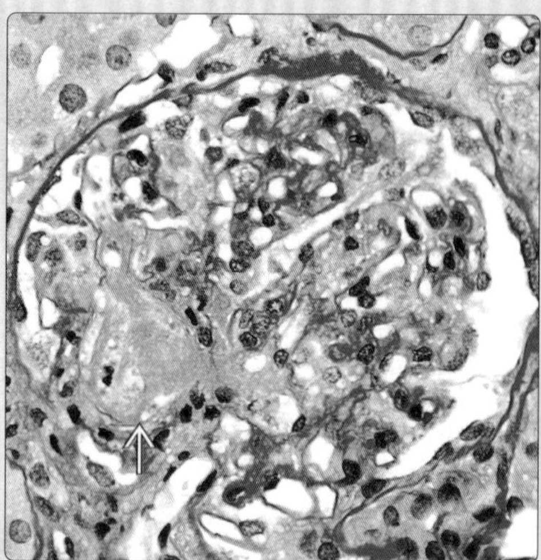

(Left) *H&E shows a thrombus with a few entrapped red blood cells distending a glomerular capillary in a patient with a history of radiation therapy and hematopoietic cell transplantation due to acute myeloid leukemia.* **(Right)** *Periodic acid-Schiff is not the ideal stain for identification of thrombi, but this large thrombus is easily noted due to the prominent distention of the hilar arteriole.*

CD61

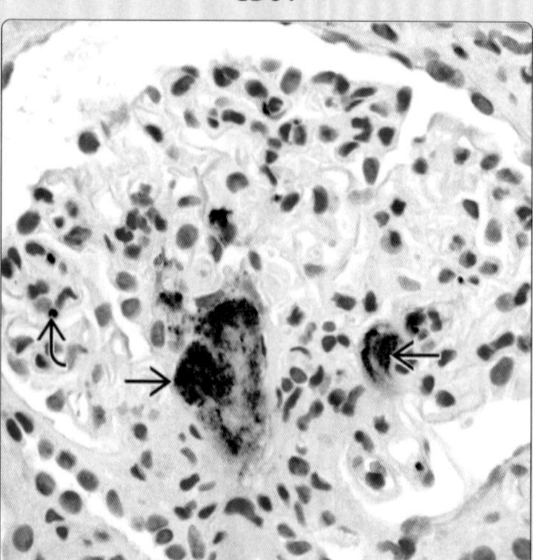

Chronic Radiation Nephropathy

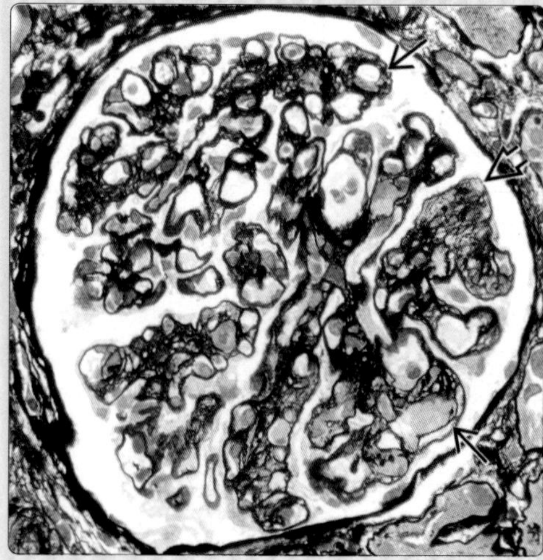

(Left) *CD61 highlights the glomerular thrombi. Masson trichrome stain (not shown) can also be useful for identifying thrombi. Normal circulating platelets are also noted.* **(Right)** *Jones methenamine silver demonstrates focal mesangiolysis. There is also frequent duplication of the glomerular basement membranes, which is a manifestation of chronic endothelial cell injury.*

TERMINOLOGY

Synonyms

- Radiation nephritis
- Bone marrow transplant nephropathy
- Hematopoietic stem cell transplant-associated thrombotic microangiopathy

Definitions

- Renal injury due to radiation exposure

ETIOLOGY/PATHOGENESIS

Irradiation Dosage

- 20-25 Gy to kidneys over > 1 month leads to radiation nephropathy
  - 5% incidence of nephrotoxicity with 9.8 Gy in absence of nephrotoxic drugs

Graft-vs.-Host Disease

- Possible risk factor for developing thrombotic microangiopathy

Additional Risk Factors

- Chemotherapeutic agents may increase risk of developing radiation nephropathy

CLINICAL ISSUES

Epidemiology

- Incidence
  - 20-40% of patients receiving significant radiation
- Age
  - Higher susceptibility in pediatric patients

Presentation

- Renal dysfunction
- Hypertension
- Proteinuria
- Anemia

Prognosis

- Variable
  - Dependent on total radiation dosage

MICROSCOPIC

Histologic Features

- Glomeruli
  - Mesangiolysis
  - Capillary thrombi
  - Duplication of GBM
  - Global or segmental glomerular sclerosis
  - Foam cells in glomerular capillaries may be noted
- Interstitium and tubules
  - Interstitial edema
  - Interstitial fibrosis and tubular atrophy
- Arteries and arterioles
  - Mucoid intimal change
  - Thrombi
  - Hyalinosis

ANCILLARY TESTS

Histochemistry

- Masson trichrome
  - Reactivity: If present, thrombi stain strongly red

Immunohistochemistry

- CD61 highlights thrombi, if present

Immunofluorescence

- Fibrinogen highlights thrombi, if present
- IgM and C3 may demonstrate nonspecific trapping along glomerular basement membranes (GBM) and arterioles

Electron Microscopy

- Separation of endothelial cells from GBM with widening of subendothelial space by electron-lucent material
- Duplication of GBM when injury is chronic

DIFFERENTIAL DIAGNOSIS

Thrombotic Microangiopathy, Drugs

- Chemotherapeutic agents

Thrombotic Microangiopathy, Autoimmune

- Autoantibodies targeting phospholipids or phospholipid-binding proteins, ADAMTS13, or complement regulators

Thrombotic Microangiopathy, Genetic

- Genetic defects in alternative pathway of complement activation and regulation

Thrombotic Thrombocytopenic Purpura/Hemolytic Uremic Syndrome

- Correlation with clinical history necessary

Graft-vs.-Host Glomerulopathies

- May occur concurrently with radiation nephropathy

DIAGNOSTIC CHECKLIST

Pathologic Interpretation Pearls

- Clinical history of hematopoietic cell (bone marrow) transplantation
- Chemotherapy often is used in combination with radiation, and both can result in thrombotic microangiopathic injuries

SELECTED REFERENCES

1. Burton JO et al: A delayed case of radiation nephropathy. Kidney Int. 86(5):1063, 2014
2. Singh N et al: Kidney complications of hematopoietic stem cell transplantation. Am J Kidney Dis. 61(5):809-21, 2013
3. Esiashvili N et al: Renal toxicity in children undergoing total body irradiation for bone marrow transplant. Radiother Oncol. 90(2):242-6, 2009
4. Chang A et al: Spectrum of renal pathology in hematopoietic cell transplantation: a series of 20 patients and review of the literature. Clin J Am Soc Nephrol. 2(5):1014-23, 2007
5. Lawton CA et al: Long-term results of selective renal shielding in patients undergoing total body irradiation in preparation for bone marrow transplantation. Bone Marrow Transplant. 20(12):1069-74, 1997
6. Cassady JR: Clinical radiation nephropathy. Int J Radiat Oncol Biol Phys. 31(5):1249-56, 1995
7. Cohen EP et al: Bone marrow transplant nephropathy: radiation nephritis revisited. Nephron. 70(2):217-22, 1995
8. Luxton RW: Radiation nephritis. A long-term study of 54 patients. Lancet. 2(7214):1221-4, 1961

Hereditary Endotheliopathy, Retinopathy, Nephropathy, and Stroke

KEY FACTS

TERMINOLOGY

- Systemic disease causing vascular endothelial injury in brain, retina, kidney, and other sites due to mutation in *TREX1*

ETIOLOGY/PATHOGENESIS

- *TREX1* encodes 3'-5' DNA exonuclease
- Mechanism unknown, probably involving endothelial cell damage/injury and thrombotic microangiopathy

CLINICAL ISSUES

- Onset in middle age with neuropsychiatric, retinal, and renal symptoms
- Proteinuria, asymptomatic
- Chronic renal failure
- Dementia and mood disorders
- Migraine headaches, strokes
- Progressive dementia, visual loss, and renal dysfunction over 3-4 years
- Uniformly fatal neurological disease over 5-10 years

MICROSCOPIC

- Irregularly thickened capillary walls
- Glomerular basement membrane thickening
- Subendothelial arteriolar hyaline and replacement of smooth muscle cells with hyaline
- Thickened arterial intima with fibrosis
- Endothelial activation described in brain, with enlarged cells, hyperchromatic nuclei, and prominent nucleoli
- Electron microscopy
  - Subendothelial multilaminated basement membranes in glomerular and peritubular capillaries and arteries
  - Activation of glomerular endothelial cells with loss of fenestrations
  - Similar lesions in other organs

TOP DIFFERENTIAL DIAGNOSES

- Chronic thrombotic microangiopathy
- Chronic antibody-mediated rejection in renal transplant

Lamination of Glomerular Basement Membrane (GBM)

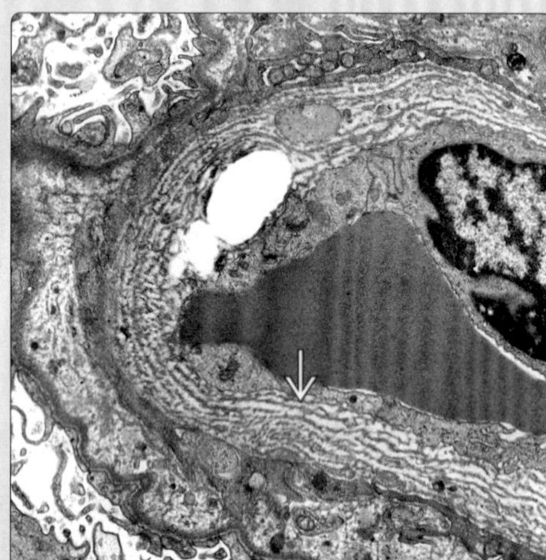

GBM Lamination

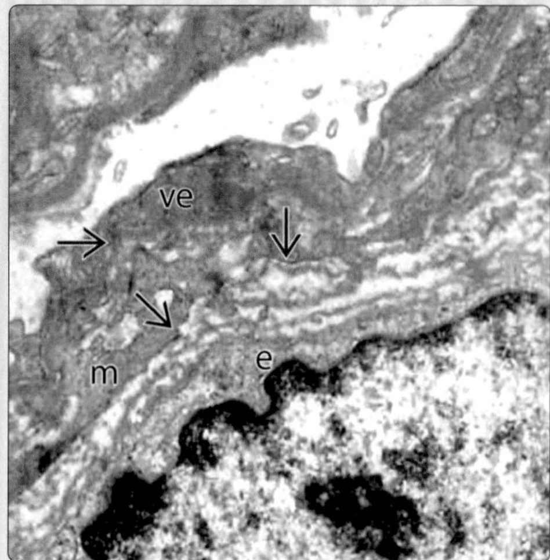

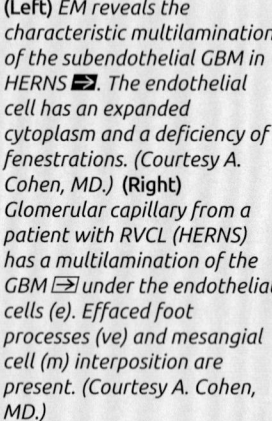

(Left) *EM reveals the characteristic multilamination of the subendothelial GBM in HERNS ➡. The endothelial cell has an expanded cytoplasm and a deficiency of fenestrations. (Courtesy A. Cohen, MD.)* **(Right)** *Glomerular capillary from a patient with RVCL (HERNS) has a multilamination of the GBM ➙ under the endothelial cells (e). Effaced foot processes (ve) and mesangial cell (m) interposition are present. (Courtesy A. Cohen, MD.)*

Lamination of Peritubular Capillary Basement Membrane

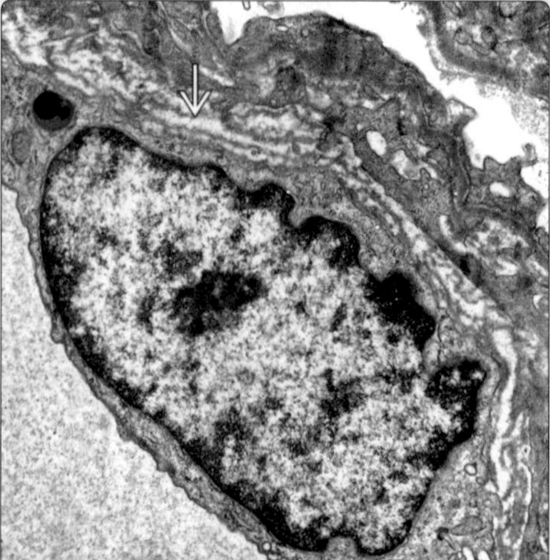

Peritubular Capillary Lamination

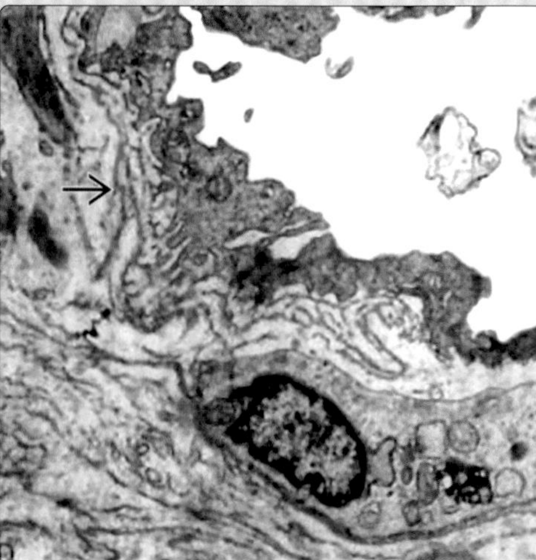

(Left) *Hereditary endotheliopathy (HERNS) renal biopsy is shown. Electron microscopy of a peritubular capillary demonstrates several layers of new basement membrane ➡. (Courtesy A. Cohen, MD.)* **(Right)** *PTC shows multilamination of the basement membrane ➙. The endothelium appears "activated" with increased cytoplasm, organelles and loss of fenestrations. (Courtesy A. Cohen, MD.)*

TERMINOLOGY

Synonyms

- Retinal vasculopathy and cerebral leukodystrophy (RVCL) is preferred term for 4 formerly separate syndromes
  - Hereditary endotheliopathy with retinopathy, nephropathy, and stroke (HERNS)
  - Cerebroretinal vasculopathy
  - Vascular retinopathy
  - Hereditary systemic angiopathy

Definitions

- Systemic disease causing vascular endothelial injury in brain, retina, kidney, and other sites due to 3-prime repair exonuclease mutation (TREX1)
  - Previously termed DNAse III

ETIOLOGY/PATHOGENESIS

Genetic

- Autosomal dominant trait
- *TREX1* gene on chromosome 3p21
  - Encodes *TREX1*, most abundant DNA 3'-5' exonuclease
  - Carboxyterminal frameshift mutation
    - Becomes diffusely distributed in cytoplasm vs. normal perinuclear space, but exonuclease activity retained
- 3 generations of Chinese family with 11 affected members
- Other mutations of *TREX1* reported in Aicardi-Goutieres syndrome, familial chilblain lupus, and 3% of systemic lupus erythematosus

Mechanism

- Unknown, probably involving endothelial cell damage/injury
- May involve thrombotic microangiopathy

CLINICAL ISSUES

Presentation

- Proteinuria, asymptomatic
- Chronic renal failure
- Dementia and mood disorders
- Migraine headaches
- Visual field defects due to retinopathy
  - Retinal telangiectasias
  - Macular edema
- Strokes

Natural History

- Onset in middle age
- Progressive dementia, visual loss, and renal dysfunction over 3-4 years

Prognosis

- Uniformly fatal neurological disease over 5-10 years

IMAGING

MR Findings

- Brain: Multiple high T2 and gadolinium-enhancing lesions

MICROSCOPIC

Histologic Features

- Glomeruli
  - Irregularly thickened capillary walls
  - Slightly widened mesangium
- Arteries
  - Subendothelial hyaline and replacement of smooth muscle cells with hyaline
  - Thickened intima with fibrosis
  - Resembles calcineurin inhibitor arteriolopathy
- Endothelial activation described in brain, with enlarged cells, hyperchromatic nuclei, and prominent nucleoli

ANCILLARY TESTS

Electron Microscopy

- Glomeruli
  - Thickened capillary walls
  - Subendothelial multilamination of glomerular basement membrane (GBM)
    - Original GBM appears normal
  - Mesangial cell interposition
- Peritubular capillaries
  - Multilaminated basement membrane
- Arteries and arterioles
  - Multilaminated basement membrane
- Tubules
  - No distinctive changes in basement membrane
  - Normal mitochondria
- Cerebral vessels
  - Multilamination of capillary basement membrane

DIFFERENTIAL DIAGNOSIS

Chronic Thrombotic Microangiopathy

- Thrombi more evident
- Capillaries not affected by multilamination

Chronic Antibody-Mediated Rejection (Transplant Kidney)

- Positive C4d in peritubular capillaries (PTC)
- Limited to kidney transplant

SELECTED REFERENCES

1. Kolar GR et al: Neuropathology and genetics of cerebroretinal vasculopathies. Brain Pathol. 24(5):510-8, 2014
2. Kavanagh D et al: New roles for the major human 3'-5' exonuclease TREX1 in human disease. Cell Cycle. 7(12):1718-25, 2008
3. Winkler DT et al: Hereditary systemic angiopathy (HSA) with cerebral calcifications, retinopathy, progressive nephropathy, and hepatopathy. J Neurol. 255(1):77-88, 2008
4. Richards A et al: C-terminal truncations in human 3'-5' DNA exonuclease TREX1 cause autosomal dominant retinal vasculopathy with cerebral leukodystrophy. Nat Genet. 39(9):1068-70, 2007
5. Jen J et al: Hereditary endotheliopathy with retinopathy, nephropathy, and stroke (HERNS). Neurology. 49(5):1322-30, 1997

Sickle Cell Nephropathy

KEY FACTS

TERMINOLOGY
- Sickle cell disease (SCD)

ETIOLOGY/PATHOGENESIS
- β-globin gene mutation
  - Chromosome 11p15.5
  - Single nucleotide change leads to a switch in amino acid sequence from glutamic acid to valine

CLINICAL ISSUES
- Presentation
  - Proteinuria
  - Chronic kidney disease

MACROSCOPIC
- Papillary necrosis
- Vascular congestion of vasa recta in renal medulla

MICROSCOPIC
- Glomerular hypertrophy
- Glomerular sclerosis
  - Global
  - Segmental
- Duplication of glomerular basement membranes
- Hemosiderosis
- Peritubular capillary thrombi can be only manifestation in some sickle cell trait patients
- Sickled red blood cells

ANCILLARY TESTS
- Electron microscopy
  - Cytoplasmic rod-like inclusions of polymerized hemoglobin in red blood cells

TOP DIFFERENTIAL DIAGNOSES
- Focal segmental glomerulosclerosis
- Chronic thrombotic microangiopathy
- Membranoproliferative glomerulonephritis/C3 nephropathy

Segmental Sclerosis

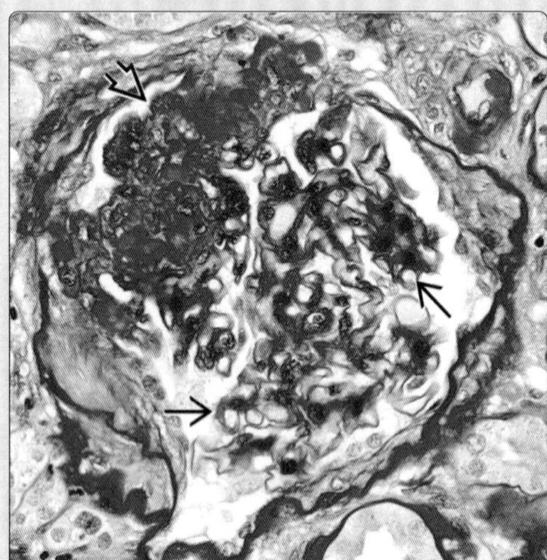

Sickled Red Blood Cells and GBM Duplication

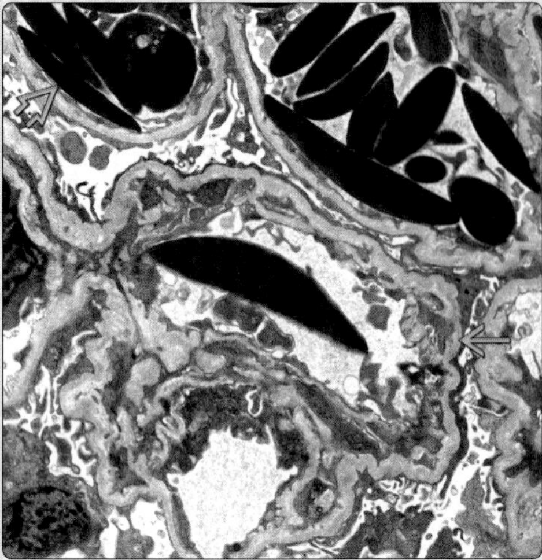

(Left) *Segmental sclerosis ⇨ and duplication of the GBM ⇨ are common findings in advanced cases of sickle cell nephropathy. This patient had significant proteinuria and a papillary renal cell carcinoma.* **(Right)** *Electron micrograph shows numerous sickled red blood cells ⇨ within the glomerular capillaries of a patient with sickle cell disease and nephropathy. Focal duplication of the glomerular basement membranes ⇨ is noted in some capillaries.*

Hemosiderosis

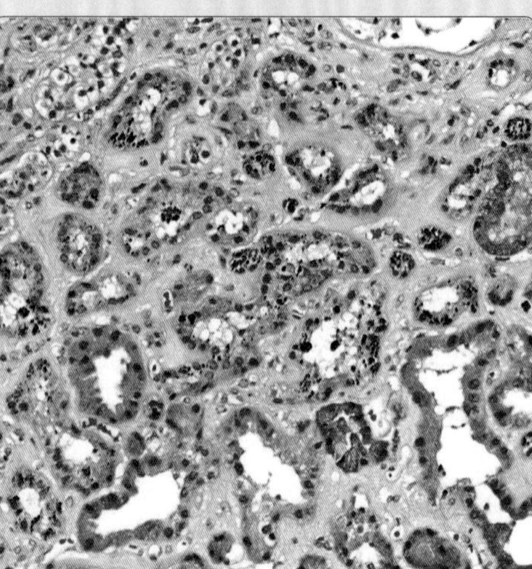

Congestion of Vasa Recta

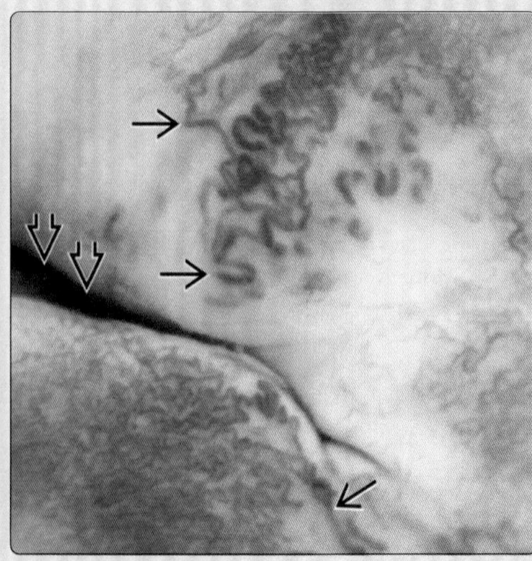

(Left) *Hematoxylin & eosin shows marked hemosiderosis of the tubular epithelial cells, which is a diagnostic clue that should raise the consideration of sickle cell nephropathy.* **(Right)** *Gross photograph shows marked congestion of the vasa recta ⇨ in the renal pyramid with prominent scarring of the renal papilla ⇨, as shown by the deep horizontal divot. (Courtesy C. Abrahams, MD.)*

TERMINOLOGY

Definitions

- Renal diseases due to sickle cell disease (SCD), which is caused by a mutation in β-globin gene

ETIOLOGY/PATHOGENESIS

β-globin Gene Mutation

- Chromosome 11p15.5, gene *HBB*
- Single nucleotide substitution changes β-globin amino acid glutamic acid to valine: Hemoglobin SS (HbSS)
- Homozygous mutations cause sickle cell anemia
  - Variants when combined with thalassemia gene mutations or other globulin mutations
- Heterozygous mutation causes sickle cell trait

Pathogenesis

- Sickling of red cells is promoted by hypoxia
- Obstruction of capillaries leads to ischemia in many organs
- Sickle cell crisis increases risk of renal disease

CLINICAL ISSUES

Epidemiology

- Incidence
  - Most common in blacks: HbSS in 1 in 601 African American births
    - Chronic kidney disease in 4-18%
  - Sickle cell trait in ~ 8% of blacks
- Age
  - 3rd to 5th decade

Presentation

- Hyposthenuria, earliest sign of renal disease (children)
- Microalbuminuria ~ 68% adults; begins in childhood
- Nephrotic syndrome (5%)
- Hematuria
  - Non-dysmorphic red cells

Laboratory Tests

- Hemoglobin electrophoresis

Treatment

- Drugs
  - Hydroxyurea
  - Transfusion
  - Angiotensin-converting enzyme inhibitors
  - Analgesics

Prognosis

- Average life expectancy: 48 years
- Increased risk of medullary renal carcinoma in sickle cell trait

MACROSCOPIC

General Features

- Papillary necrosis
  - 15-36% incidence by imaging studies
- Vascular congestion of vasa recta in renal medulla
  - Hypoxic milieu enables sickling of red blood cells

MICROSCOPIC

Histologic Features

- Glomeruli
  - Enlarged glomeruli engorged with sickled red cells
  - 4 patterns reported
    - Hypertrophy
      - More prominent in juxtamedullary glomeruli
    - Focal global or segmental glomerulosclerosis (FSGS)
      - Usually perihilar or NOS; may have tip lesion
      - Collapsing glomerulopathy (rare)
    - Membranoproliferative glomerulonephritis
      - Duplication of GBM
      - No immune complex deposition
      - May be a result of chronic thrombotic microangiopathy
    - Chronic thrombotic microangiopathy
      - Mesangiolysis, duplication of GBM, swollen endothelial cells
  - Hemosiderin accumulation
- Tubules and Interstitium
  - Prominent hemosiderin deposition
  - Confirmed by Prussian blue iron stain
  - Interstitial fibrosis and tubular atrophy
  - Papillary necrosis
- Vessels
  - Sickled red blood cells, thrombi
  - Peritubular capillary thrombi can be only manifestation in sickle cell trait

ANCILLARY TESTS

Immunofluorescence

- Minimal or no immunoglobulin or complement, except IgM and C3 in scarred glomeruli; may have fibrin in mesangium and thrombi

Electron Microscopy

- Sickle-shaped red blood cells with polymerized hemoglobin forming cytoplasmic rod-like inclusions
- Widening of subendothelial space, loss of endothelial fenestrations, duplication of GBM

DIFFERENTIAL DIAGNOSIS

Focal Segmental Glomerulosclerosis (FSGS)

- No hemosiderin deposition or sickled cells

Membranoproliferative Glomerulonephritis/C3 Nephropathy

- Prominent C3 deposition with or without immunoglobulin
- No hemosiderin deposition or sickled cells

Other Causes of Thrombotic Microangiopathy

- No hemosiderin deposition or sickled cells

SELECTED REFERENCES

1. Dedeken L et al: Haematopoietic stem cell transplantation for severe sickle cell disease in childhood: a single centre experience of 50 patients. Br J Haematol. 165(3):402-8, 2014

(Left) *Glomerular hypertrophy ⇒ is frequently observed as an early feature. A rough rule of thumb for hypertrophy is whether the glomerulus is > 50% of a 40x field. Note hemosiderosis of adjacent tubular epithelial cells ⇒.* **(Right)** *Typical features of sickle cell nephropathy are duplication of the GBM ⇒, mesangial cell interposition ⇒, and little or no deposits. The endothelium shows loss of fenestrations ⇒, a sign of injury in this 38-year-old woman with a recent sickle cell crisis trace proteinuria and a Cr 3.6.*

Glomerular Hypertrophy

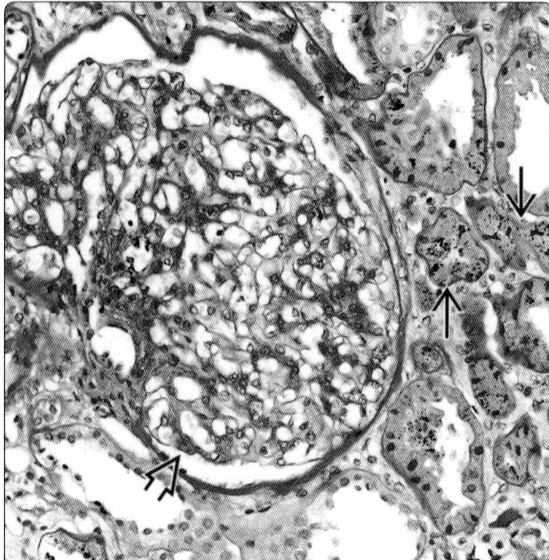

GBM Duplication

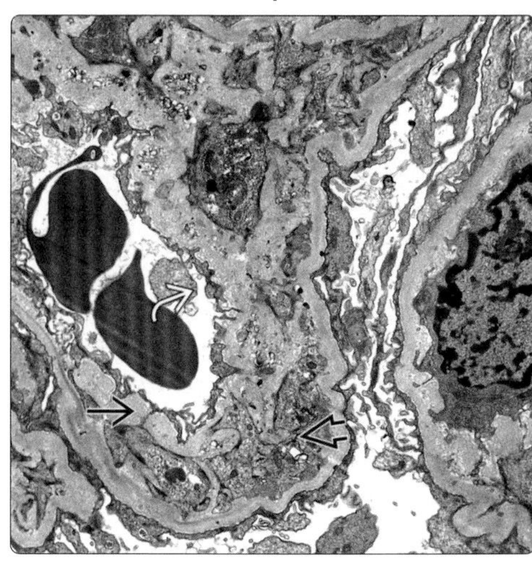

(Left) *Periodic acid-Schiff demonstrates segmental sclerosis in 1/2 of this glomerulus ⇒. There is substantial interstitial fibrosis ⇒ and tubular atrophy ⇒ surrounding the scarred glomerulus.* **(Right)** *Periodic acid-Schiff shows segmental sclerosis with accumulation of matrix ⇒ and foam cells ⇒ and focal prominence of adjacent visceral epithelial cells (or podocytes) ⇒.*

Segmental Sclerosis

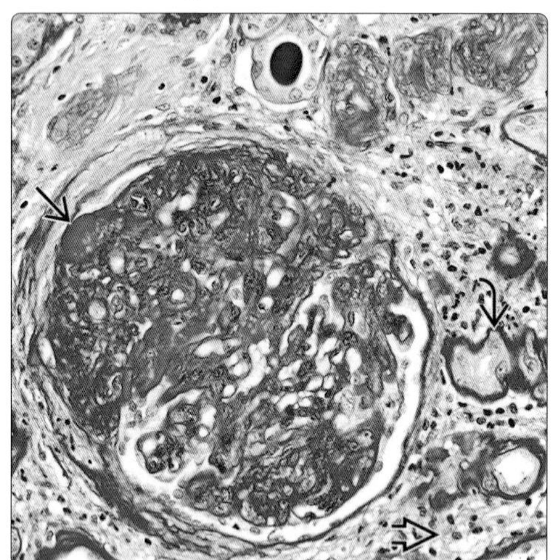

Segmental Sclerosis

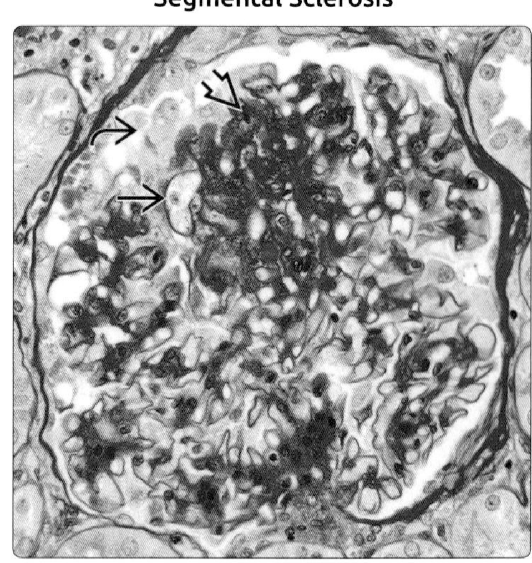

(Left) *Jones methenamine silver demonstrates collapsing glomerulopathy, which can rarely occur in sickle cell disease patients. Focal duplication ⇒ of the glomerular basement membranes is noted. (Courtesy S. Nasr, MD.)* **(Right)** *Peritubular capillary thrombi ⇒ and congestion of the peritubular capillaries by red blood cells were the only hints of sickle cell nephropathy in this sickle cell trait patient.*

Collapsing Glomerulopathy

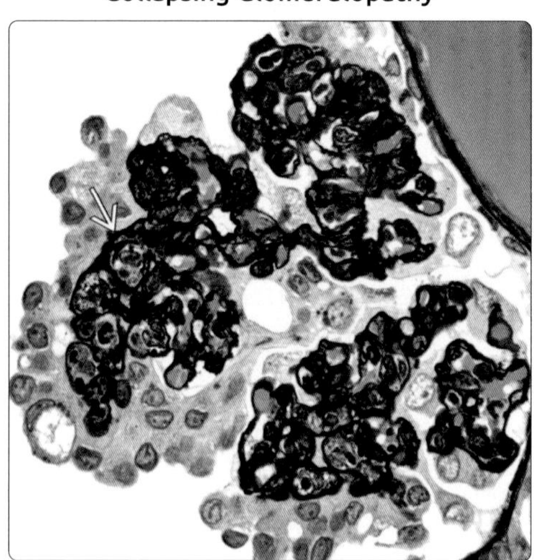

Peritubular Capillary Thrombus

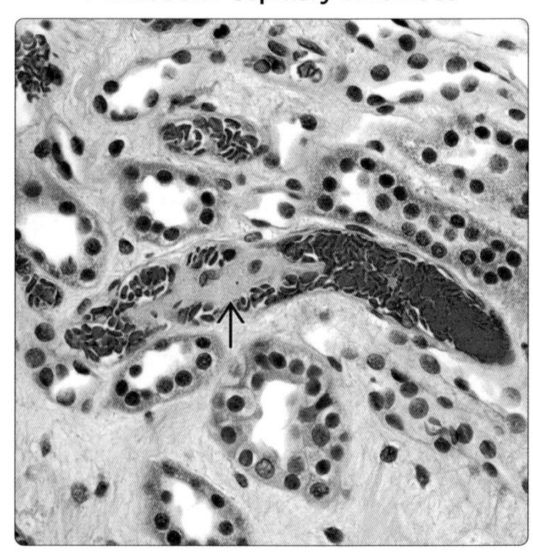

Polymerized Hemoglobin

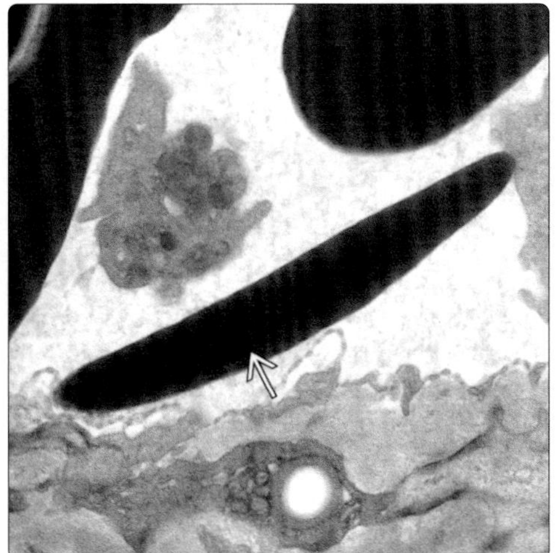

Polymerized Hemoglobin

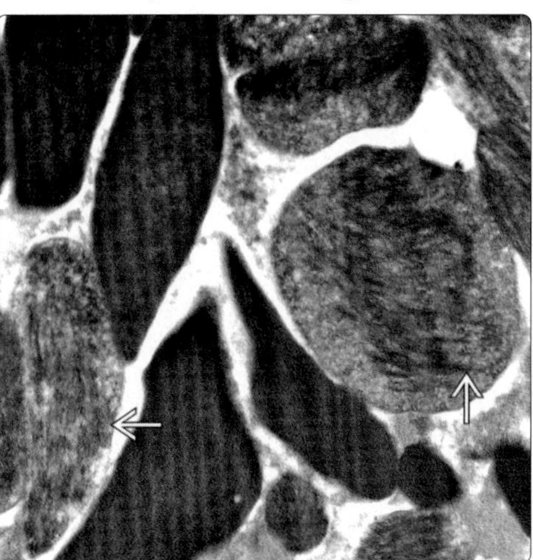

(Left) *Electron microscopy at high magnification shows a sickle-shaped red blood cell in a glomerular capillary with cytoplasmic rod-like inclusions* →*, which represents polymerized hemoglobin.* **(Right)** *Electron microscopy at high magnification reveals numerous rod-like inclusions* → *that represent polymerized hemoglobin within the cytoplasm of several red blood cells in a sickle cell disease patient.*

Hemosiderosis

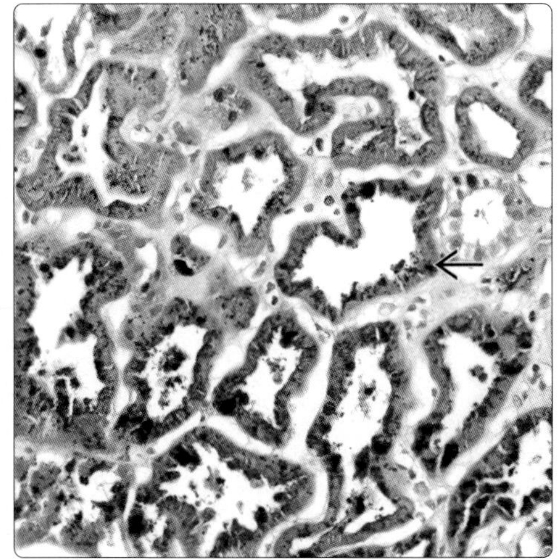

Hemosiderin Granules

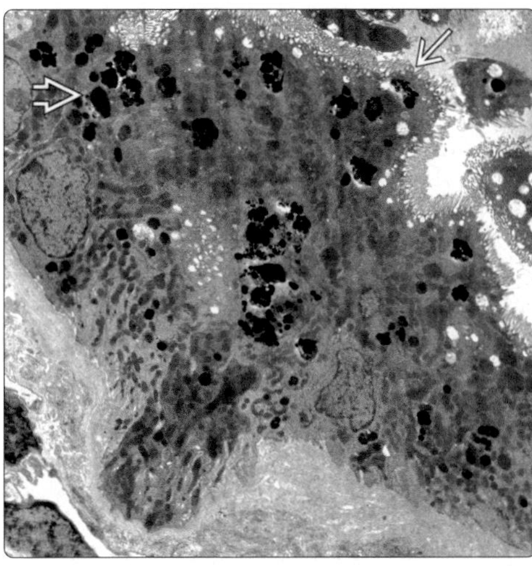

(Left) *Prussian blue stain reveals widespread blue granules* → *in proximal tubular epithelial cells. This identifies the pigment as iron.* **(Right)** *Electron microscopy of the proximal tubular epithelial cells, characterized by their brush border* → *and numerous mitochondria, reveals prominent electron-dense hemosiderin granules* → *within the cytoplasm.*

Papillary Scarring

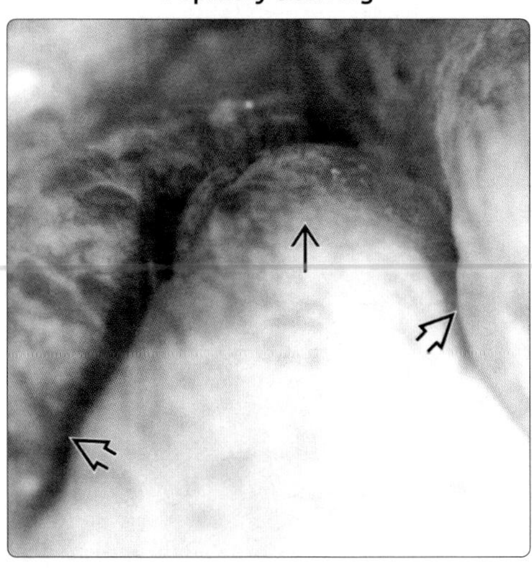

Papillary Scarring

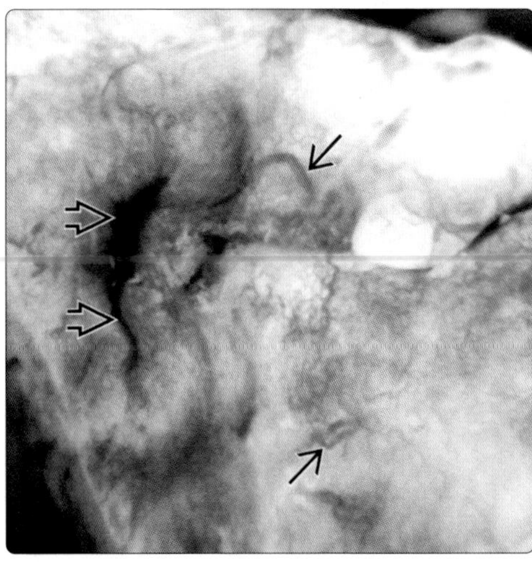

(Left) *Gross photograph shows congestion of the vasa recta* → *in the renal medulla with marked scarring of the renal papilla* → *in a sickle cell disease patient with papillary necrosis. (Courtesy C. Abrahams, MD.)* **(Right)** *Gross photograph of a kidney after formalin fixation shows the consequences of papillary necrosis with severe pitting and scarring of the renal papilla* → *and marked congestion of the vasa recta in the renal medulla* →*. (Courtesy C. Abrahams, MD.)*

KEY FACTS

TERMINOLOGY

- Vascular and glomerular disease 2° to hypertension

CLINICAL ISSUES

- ~ 30% of American adults have hypertension (HTN)
  - 95% due to "essential HTN" (without known cause)
- Major cause of ESRD (~ 25%)
- Effective drug therapy ameliorates renal sequelae

MACROSCOPIC

- Finely granular cortical surface
- Petechiae in malignant HTN

MICROSCOPIC

- Subcapsular sclerotic scars with sclerotic glomeruli, thickened arterioles, and atrophic tubules
- Global or segmental glomerulosclerosis
- Arterial intimal fibrosis and arteriolar hyalinosis
- "Onion skinning," endothelial swelling, and fibrinoid necrosis of arterioles in accelerated HTN
- Hyperplastic juxtaglomerular apparatus (JGA) can be seen in renal artery stenosis and Bartter syndrome
- IF may show glomerular and arteriolar IgM, C3, fibrin
- EM: Wrinkled GBMs, and in malignant HTN, may show subendothelial expansion and fibrinoid necrosis

TOP DIFFERENTIAL DIAGNOSES

- Diabetic nephropathy
- Renal atheroembolization or severe atherosclerosis from hyperlipidemia
- Primary FSGS
- Renal artery stenosis leading to renal atrophy
- Thrombotic microangiopathy, any cause
- Systemic sclerosis

(Left) *Nephrectomy in a case of hypertensive renovascular disease shows a characteristic coarsely granular, "flea-bitten" surface with scattered petechial hemorrhages ➡.* **(Right)** *This PAS stain shows arterioles ➡ with plump endothelial cells and muscular hypertrophy in a case of hypertensive renovascular disease.*

Hypertensive Nephrosclerosis

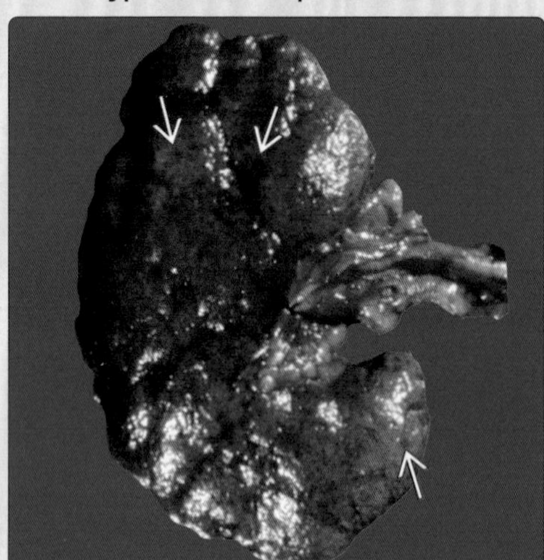

Arteriolosclerosis

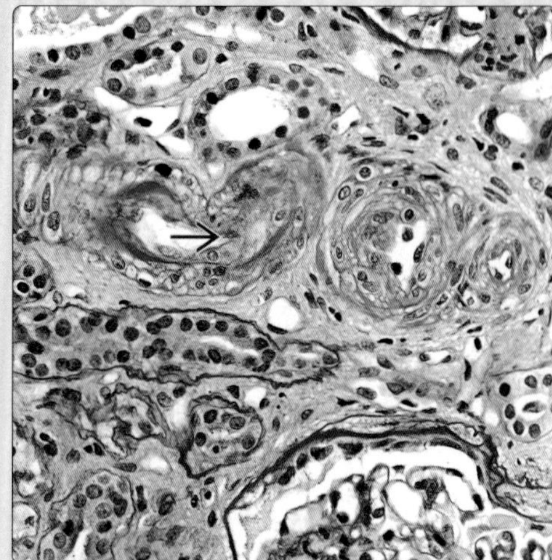

(Left) *Arteriole with hyalinization ➡ is commonly found in a number of disorders, including HTN, diabetes, and calcineurin inhibitor toxicity.* **(Right)** *IF for fibrin shows deposition in arterioles in hypertensive renovascular disease.*

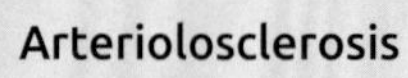

Arteriolosclerosis

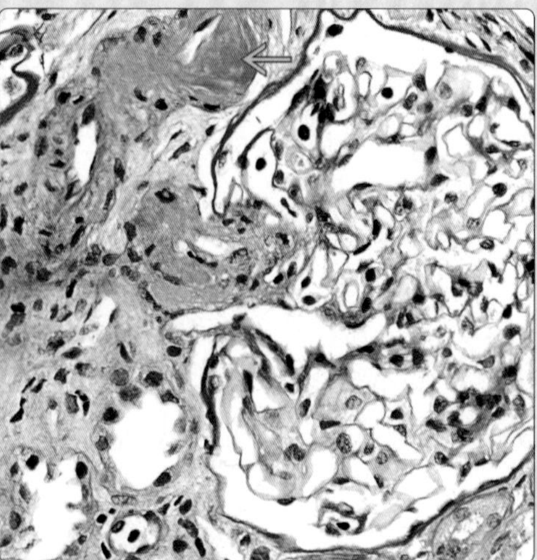

Arteriolar Fibrin

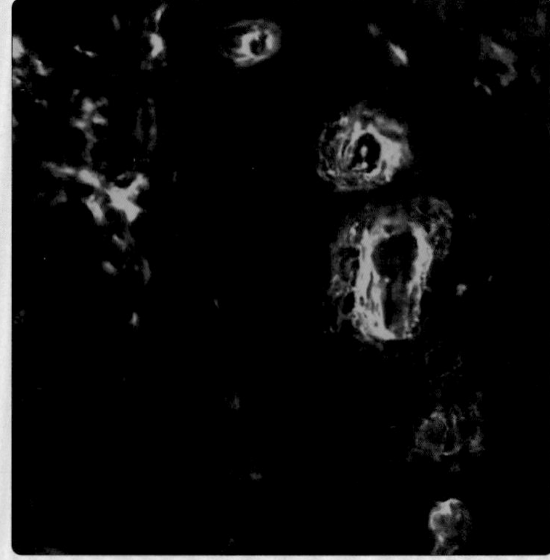

TERMINOLOGY

Abbreviations

- Hypertension (HTN)
- Arterionephrosclerosis (ANS)

Synonyms

- Arterio-/arteriolonephrosclerosis
- Hypertensive nephrosclerosis
- Benign nephrosclerosis
- Malignant nephrosclerosis

Definitions

- Renal vascular and glomerular disease 2° to HTN (blood pressure [BP] > 120/80 mmHg)
- Accelerated HTN, mean BP > 140 mmHg, papilledema, retinal hemorrhage

ETIOLOGY/PATHOGENESIS

Essential HTN

- 95% of cases
- Evidence for multigenic basis plus environmental factors
- Risk factors include obesity, lack of exercise, salt intake, black race
- Other factors: Low birth weight, ↓ nephron number, dysmetabolic syndrome

Secondary Causes of HTN

- 5% of cases
- Renal artery stenosis
  - Atherosclerosis, dysplasia, vasculitis, dissection
  - ↑ production of renin by ischemic kidney
- Neoplasia
  - Pheochromocytoma, adrenal cortical tumors, renin-producing tumors
- Chronic renal disease, end-stage renal disease (ESRD)
- Cocaine abuse
- Hypercoagulable states

Malignant HTN

- May be 1° or 2°
- Renin release causes cycle of vascular injury followed by ↑ renin release
- Features of thrombotic microangiopathy

Effect of HTN on Arteries and Arterioles

- HTN precedes renal vascular disease
  - Seen in early series of Castleman and Smithwick
  - More severe renal vascular disease leads to ↓ glomerular filtration rate and renal blood flow
  - Vascular disease is result, rather than cause, of HTN
- Involves direct injury to endothelium
- Plasma (and fibrin) insudates into vascular walls
- Arterial stiffening and ↑ pulse pressure conducted to afferent arteriolar level eventually leads to hyalinosis
- Severe HTN causes renal vascular fibrinoid necrosis (Goldblatt)

CLINICAL ISSUES

Epidemiology

- Incidence
  - ~ 30% of adult Americans have HTN
  - HTN accounts for ~ 25% of ESRD
  - Malignant nephrosclerosis as result of malignant HTN occurs at rate of 1-2 cases/100,000 per year
- Age
  - HTN appears mostly between mid 40s and mid 50s
    - Renal damage and dysfunction take years to develop and manifest
- Sex
  - Males have predisposition
- Ethnicity
  - Disproportionately affects black race

Presentation

- Hypertension
- Proteinuria, asymptomatic
  - Related to severity of HTN
- Renal dysfunction
- Accelerated (malignant) HTN if mean BP > 160 mmHg
  - Papilledema, retinal hemorrhage
  - Congestive heart failure
  - Stroke, encephalopathy
  - Renal insufficiency
  - Microangiopathic hemolytic anemia (MAHA)

Treatment

- Drugs
  - Antihypertensive agents
    - Diuretics, mineralocorticoid receptor antagonists
    - ACE inhibitors, vasopeptidase inhibitors, renin inhibitors
    - Smooth muscle dilators, endothelin antagonists
    - β-adrenergic blockers, α-adrenoceptor blockers
  - Optimal BP control ↓ progression to renal insufficiency and may reverse hypertensive nephrosclerosis

Prognosis

- ESRD develops in mean of 6 years from onset of azotemia
- Factors that predispose to renal failure include
  - Increasing age
  - Poor serum glucose control in diabetic patients
  - Level of systolic BP, high diastolic BP
  - Male gender
  - Black race
  - Elevated uric acid and triglycerides
- **Malignant hypertension**
  - If left untreated, survival is poor (20% 1-year survival)
  - Long-term survival is > 90% if BP controlled

MACROSCOPIC

General Features

- May be normal or slightly ↓ in size and weight
- Capsular surface is usually finely granular
- Cortical scars and simple cysts may be present
- Cortex may be thinned
- **Malignant hypertension**
  - Weight normal or increased to as high as 400 g
  - Petechial hemorrhages 2° to arteriolar necrosis gives "flea-bitten" appearance
  - ± mottled yellow and red if infarcts arise

MICROSCOPIC

Histologic Features

- Glomeruli
  - ± swollen endothelial cells and may thus appear "bloodless" and consolidated
  - ± glomerular basement membrane duplication
  - ± glomerular mesangial matrix increase
  - Global glomerulosclerosis
    - Solidified type: Global solidification without collagenous material in Bowman space
    - Obsolescent type: Glomerular tuft sclerosed and Bowman space filled with collagenous material
  - Segmental glomerulosclerosis
    - Secondary focal segmental glomerulosclerosis (FSGS) may occur, typically with GBM corrugation and periglomerular fibrosis and subtotal foot process effacement
  - Glomerular hypertrophy (compensatory) in spared areas
- Interstitium and tubules
  - Subcapsular scars
    - Composed of sclerotic glomeruli, thickened arterioles, and atrophic tubules
    - Result in granular surface of kidney
    - Bulging areas between depressed scars contain spared and hypertrophied nephrons
  - Interstitial fibrosis and mononuclear inflammation
  - ± tubular atrophy and tubular hypertrophy in spared areas
- Vessels
  - Medium-sized arteries
    - Intimal fibrosis
    - Internal elastic lamina becomes multilayered (fibroelastosis); best seen on elastic stains
    - Smooth muscle hyperplasia
    - ↓ vascular lumen size
  - Arterioles
    - Hyaline arteriolosclerosis
      - Afferent arteriolar media is replaced by homogeneous eosinophilic material positive on PAS or Masson trichrome
      - Begins under endothelial layer and eventually replaces entire media
- Malignant hypertension
  - Glomeruli
    - Segmental necrosis of glomeruli
    - Ischemic retraction of glomeruli with corrugation of GBM
  - Small arteries
    - Mucoid (myxoid) intimal change, concentric medial smooth muscle hypertrophy/hyperplasia & endothelial swelling in arterioles, a.k.a. "onion skinning"
    - Fibrinoid necrosis
    - Karyorrhectic debris
    - Occasional neutrophils within endothelium
    - Fibrin thrombi
  - Arterioles
    - Arteriolar occlusion by endothelial swelling/edema-type change
    - ± fibrinoid necrosis &/or fibrin thrombi
- Treated malignant hypertension
  - As shown by Pickering and Heptinstall
    - Acute lesions of fibrinoid necrosis and mucoid intimal thickening resolve with adequate treatment
    - Intima becomes fibrous with increased cellularity and elastic fibers

ANCILLARY TESTS

Immunofluorescence

- ± IgM and C3 in hyaline layers of arterioles
- ± C3 in absence of immunoglobulins
- Fibrinogen is most common reactant seen on IF in malignant HTN (in areas of fibrinoid necrosis and glomerular capillary loops)

Electron Microscopy

- Glomerulli
  - ± thickened or wrinkled glomerular capillary basement membranes
  - No electron-dense immune-type deposits in glomeruli (or in vessels or other compartments)
  - Foot process effacement may be present but is usually only segmental
- Arterioles
  - Thickening and duplication of arteriolar basement membranes
  - Arteriolar hyalinosis
- **Malignant hypertension**
  - Expanded lamina rara interna (subendothelial expansion) and prominent corrugation of GBM
  - Fibrinoid necrosis

DIFFERENTIAL DIAGNOSIS

Diabetic Nephropathy

- Hyaline arteriosclerosis
  - Afferent and efferent arterioles characteristically involved
- Nodular diabetic glomerulosclerosis
  - Diffuse thickening of GBM

Hyperlipidemia

- May also have hyaline arteriosclerosis
- Relative lack of medium-sized arterial fibroelastosis

Primary FSGS

- HTN preceding other manifestations of renal disease useful in favoring 2° etiology of segmental glomerulosclerosis rather than 1° FSGS
- Foot process effacement more extensive and widespread

Renal Atrophy Due to Ipsilateral Renal Artery Stenosis

- Tubular atrophy can be of endocrine type with little fibrosis
- May be little intimal fibrosis and arteriolar hyalinosis due to protection from HTN
- ± hyperplastic juxtaglomerular apparatus (JGA) in kidney affected by stenosis

Causes of Hypertensive Renovascular Disease

Category	Associated Etiologies
Primary	
	Benign (essential) HTN
	Malignant HTN
Secondary	
	Renal artery stenosis (e.g., from fibromuscular dysplasia, arterio-/atherosclerosis, etc.)
	Glomerulonephritis (similar picture is typically produced by chronic glomerulonephritis)
	Neoplasms (renin-producing tumors, adrenal cortical tumors, pheochromocytoma)
	Endocrine abnormalities (thyrotoxicosis, adrenal cortical hyperplasia, hyperparathyroidism, oral contraceptives)
	Neurogenic disorders
	Thrombotic microangiopathy (TMA) (e.g., hemolytic uremic syndrome [HUS] or thrombotic thrombocytopenic purpura [TTP])
	Antiphospholipid antibody syndrome (APS)
	Preeclampsia
	Systemic sclerosis
	Miscellaneous vascular etiologies (vasculitis or coarctation of aorta)

Renal Atheroembolization (Cholesterol Crystal Embolization)

- Cholesterol clefts can be identified in vascular lumina upon thorough examination
- ± atheromatous debris, thrombosis, leukocytes, or giant cells reacting to atheroemboli
- Interstitial fibrosis can be present

Renal Infarct

- ± similar gross appearance to hypertensive renovascular disease with subcapsular scarring
- Infarcts usually larger than subcapsular scars of hypertensive renovascular disease
- Usually single or may be multiple but do not diffusely affect kidney as in hypertensive renovascular disease
- PAS stain shows collapsed, condensed glomeruli without collagenous tissue in Bowman space that is seen in benign nephrosclerosis

Primary or Secondary Glomerulonephritis

- Usually has appropriate clinical history of proteinuria &/or hematuria early in course
- Usually, specific features are present that identify glomerular diagnosis
  - Affects glomeruli diffusely throughout cortex rather than in subcapsular areas, which show accentuation in nephrosclerosis from hypertensive renovascular disease
  - Difficult to identify in late stage

Bartter Syndrome

- Children with hypokalemia, alkalosis, hypercalciuria, hyperreninemia, high angiotensin II, and hyperaldosteronemia
- Have normal BP due to mutation in genes involved with salt resorption in thick ascending limb of Henle
- Hyperplastic JGA; widespread, macula densa expansion prominent
  - ↑ number of cells with renin granules, particularly in afferent arterioles

Thrombotic Microangiopathy, Any Cause

- Vascular and glomerular lesions similar to malignant HTN
- Distinguished by clinical correlation
  - Severe HTN precedes renal failure in hypertensive renovascular disease

Systemic Sclerosis

- Extrarenal and serologic features of systemic sclerosis usually present
- 5% of systemic sclerosis patients present with renal disease before extrarenal manifestations

SELECTED REFERENCES

1. Hughson MD et al: Hypertension, glomerular hypertrophy and nephrosclerosis: the effect of race. Nephrol Dial Transplant. 29(7):1399-409, 2014
2. Hill GS: Hypertensive nephrosclerosis. Curr Opin Nephrol Hypertens. 17(3):266-70, 2008
3. Marcantoni C et al: A perspective on arterionephrosclerosis: from pathology to potential pathogenesis. J Nephrol. 20(5):518-24, 2007
4. Senitko M et al: An update on renovascular hypertension. Curr Cardiol Rep. 7(6):405-11, 2005
5. Fogo AB: Mechanisms in nephrosclerosis and hypertension-beyond hemodynamics. J Nephrol. 14 Suppl 4:S63-9, 2001
6. Kashgarian M: Pathology of small blood vessel disease in hypertension. Am J Kidney Dis. 5(4):A104-10, 1985
7. Sommers SC et al: Histologic studies of kidney biopsy specimens from patients with hypertension. Am J Pathol. 34(4):685-715, 1958
8. Pickering GW et al: The reversibility of malignant hypertension. Lancet. 2:952-6, 1952
9. Castleman B et al: The relation of vascular disease to the hypertensive state; the adequacy of the renal biopsy as determined from a study of 500 patients. N Engl J Med. 239(20):729-32, 1948
10. Talbott JH et al: Renal biopsy studies correlated with renal clearance observations in hypertensive patients treated by radical sympathectomy. J Clin Invest. 22(3):387-94, 1943

(Left) *Typical vascular changes of hypertensive nephrosclerosis include intimal fibrosis of an arcuate-sized artery ⇨ and arteriolar hyalinosis ⇨. The internal elastica, the border between the intima and media, is indicated ⇨. Secondary features are interstitial fibrosis, tubular atrophy, and global glomerulosclerosis ⇨.* **(Right)** *PAS stain shows a prominent JGA ⇨, a finding that can be seen in hypertensive renovascular disease.*

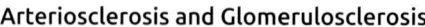

Arteriosclerosis and Glomerulosclerosis

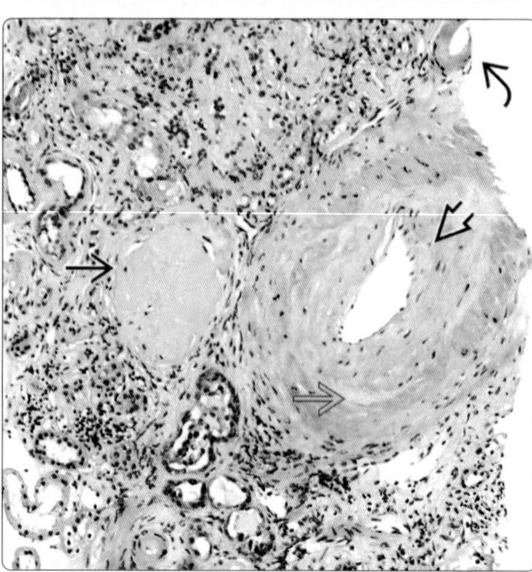

Juxtaglomerular Apparatus Hyperplasia

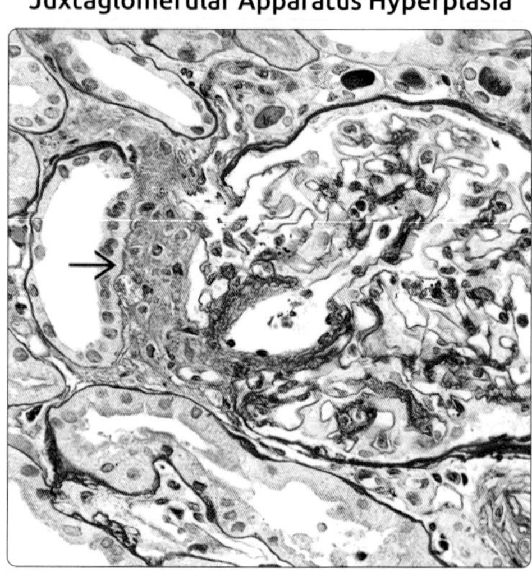

(Left) *Jones methenamine silver shows hyperplasia of the juxtaglomerular apparatus with renin granules ⇨; this feature can sometimes be found in hypertensive renovascular disease.* **(Right)** *Jones methenamine silver stain shows a prominent juxtaglomerular apparatus with granular consistency, accounted for by renin granules ⇨, a finding that can be seen in hypertensive renovascular disease.*

Juxtaglomerular Apparatus Hyperplasia

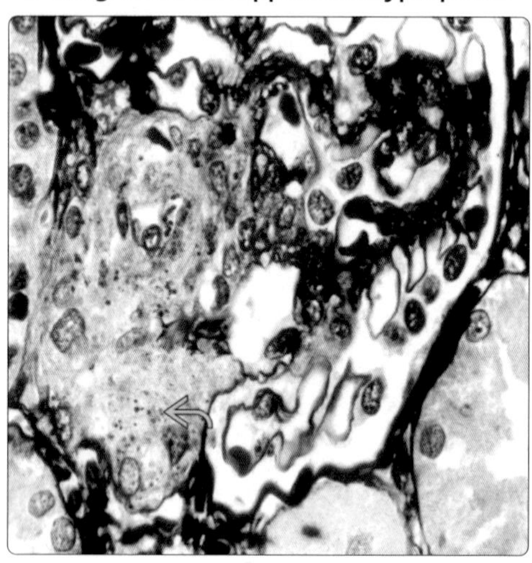

Juxtaglomerular Apparatus Renin Granules

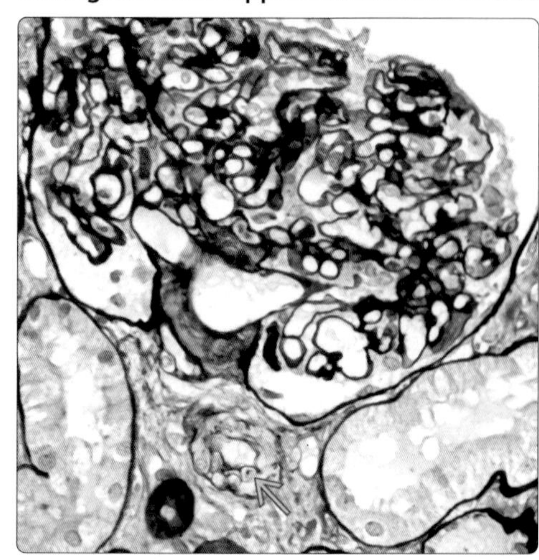

(Left) *Enlarged juxtaglomerular apparatus (JGA) ⇨ in a case of Bartter syndrome, which is characterized by hypotension or normal BP despite morphologic, biochemical, and hormonal changes, suggests that HTN could be present (Trichrome stain).* **(Right)** *Renal artery stenosis ⇨ is an important secondary cause of hypertension as seen on this magnetic resonance angiography image.*

Bartter Syndrome With Enlarged JGA

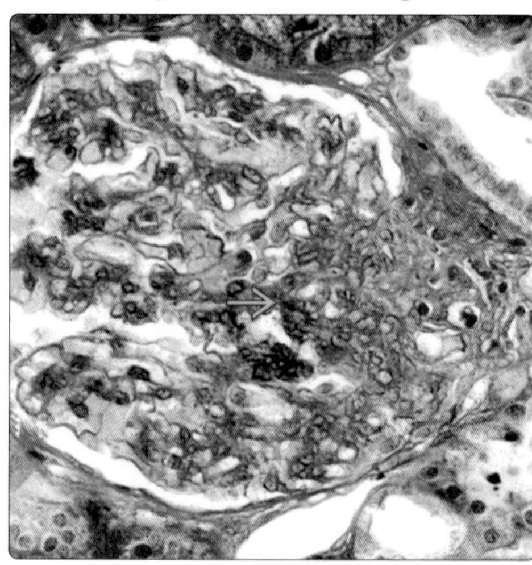

Renal Artery Stenosis

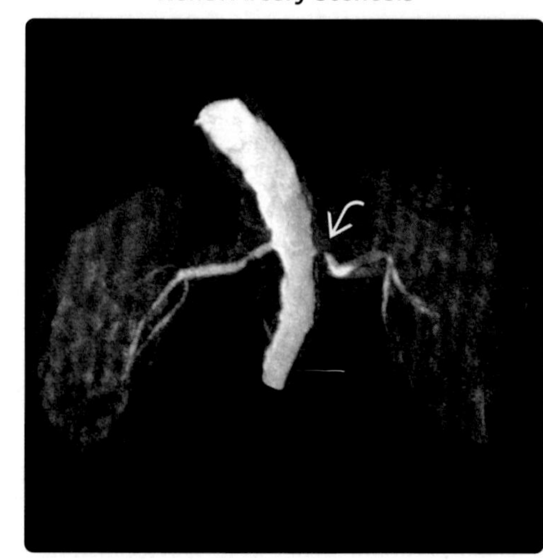

Intimal Fibroplasia

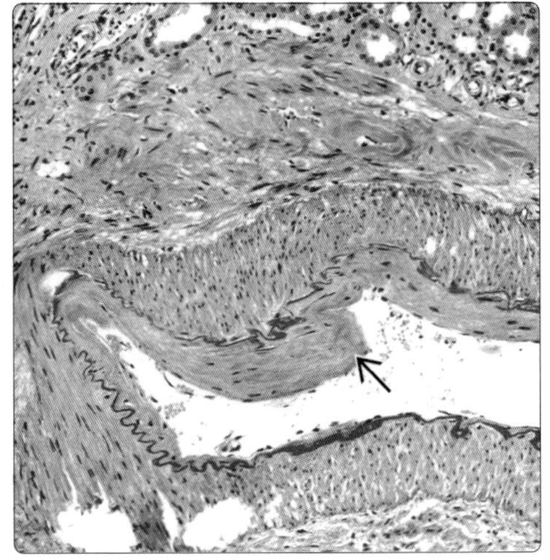

Arteriosclerosis

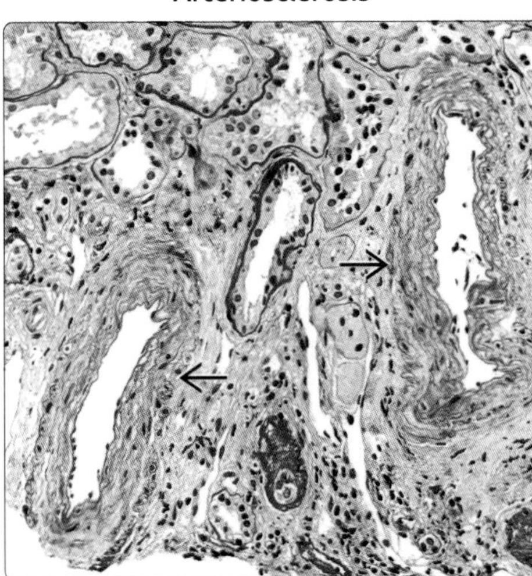

(Left) *Intimal fibroplasia ⇨ is present in an interlobar-sized artery, and this change can often be found in hypertensive renovascular disease.* **(Right)** *PAS stain shows thickening and lamellation (reduplication) of the elastic lamellae ⇨ of interlobar-sized arteries in a case of hypertensive renovascular disease.*

Arteriosclerosis

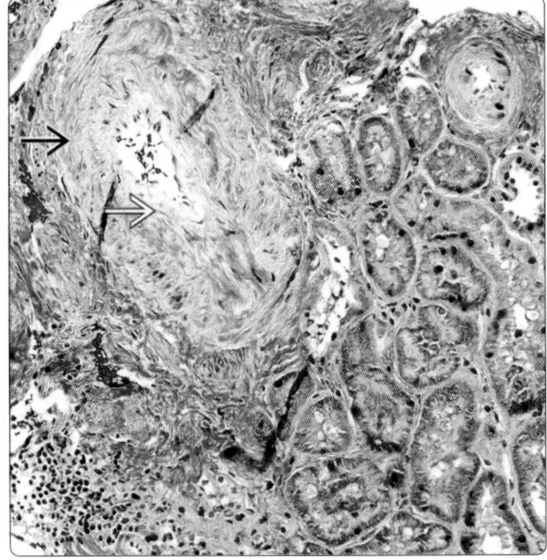

Arteriosclerosis

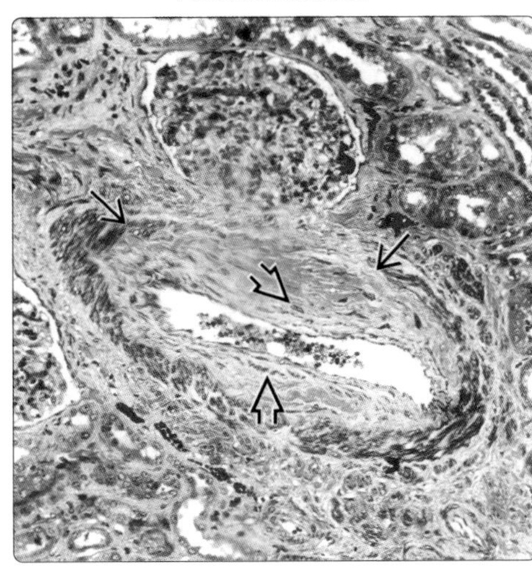

(Left) *Trichrome stain shows an interlobar-sized artery with arterial intimal thickening ➡ and medial smooth muscle layer thinning ⇨ in hypertensive renovascular disease.* **(Right)** *In an interlobar-sized artery, trichrome stain shows arterial medial thinning ⇨ with thickening of the arterial intima ⇨ in hypertensive renovascular disease. There is a migration of fuchsinophilic medial muscle cells into the intima, a process called intimal fibroplasia.*

Medial Hypertrophy

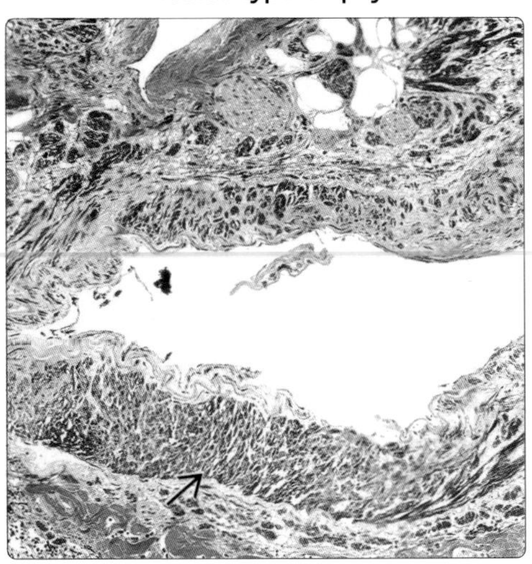

Fibroelastosis

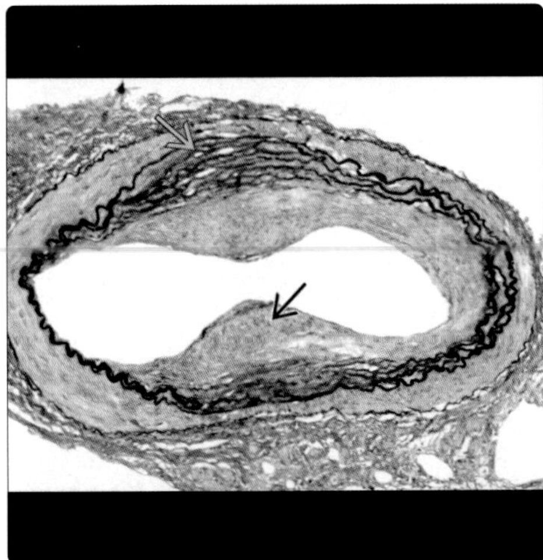

(Left) *In a case of hypertensive renovascular disease, a trichrome stain shows thickening of the arterial media ⇨.* **(Right)** *Elastic van Gieson stain shows duplication of the internal elastic lamina ⇨ and fibrous intimal thickening ⇨ in a case of hypertensive renovascular disease.*

GBM Thickening and Foot Process Effacement

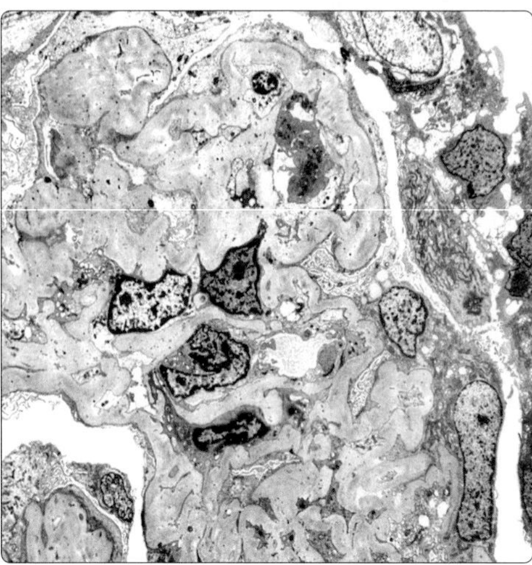

Glomerular Endothelial Cell Swelling and Platelet Accumulation

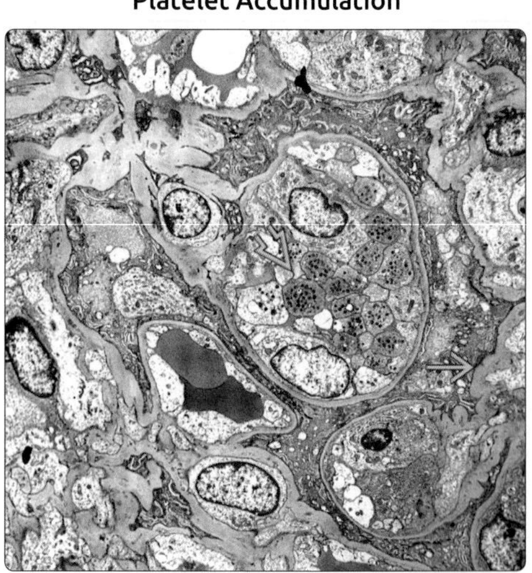

(Left) *EM from a patient with HTN and 2 g/d proteinuria shows widespread wrinkling and mild thickening of the GBM and effacement of foot processes, more than is usually seen in HTN alone. It is difficult to determine the primary disease in this setting.* **(Right)** *EM shows numerous platelets ➲ in a glomerular capillary loop in a patient with hypertensive renovascular disease. Glomerular capillary loops are wrinkled and variably thickened ➲. Endothelial cells are swollen.*

Activated Glomerular Endothelial Cells

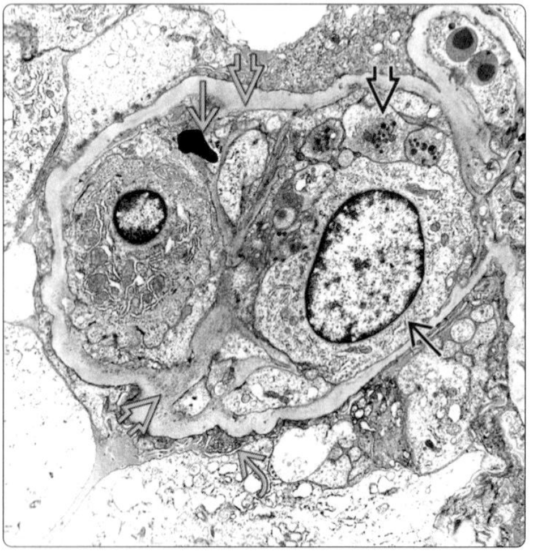

Ischemic Collapse

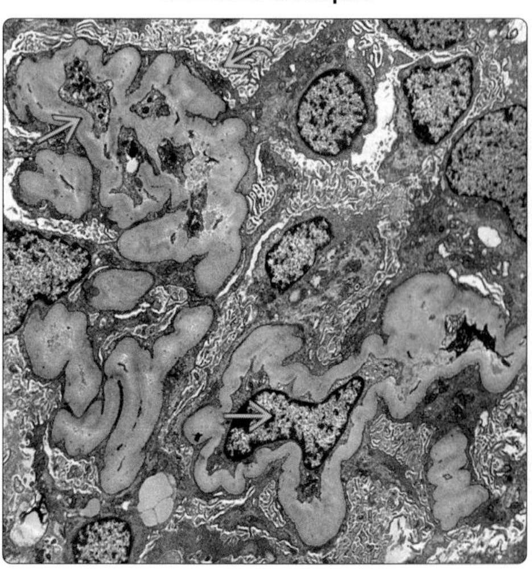

(Left) *EM shows swollen endothelial cells ➲, fragmented red blood cells ➲, and platelets ➲ in the glomerular capillary loops in a case of hypertensive renovascular disease. There is focal foot process effacement ➲. There is also widening of the subendothelial zone ➲.* **(Right)** *In severe hypertension, vasoconstriction and endothelial injury lead to collapse of the glomerular tuft and secondary podocyte injury manifested as extensive loss of foot processes ➲ and villous hypertrophy. Capillary loops appear occluded ➲.*

Glomerular IgM

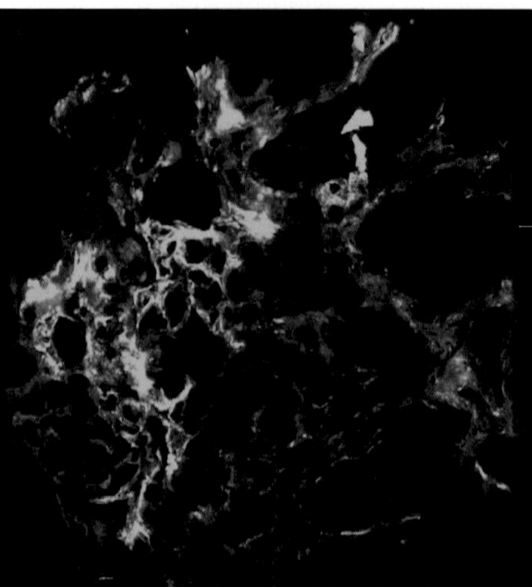

Glomerular C3

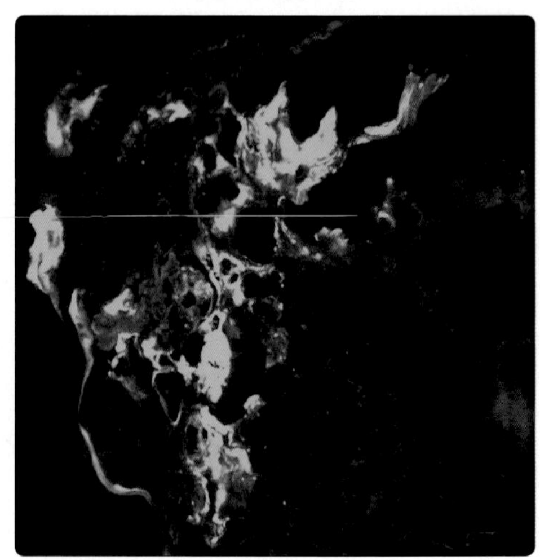

(Left) *In a case of hypertensive renovascular disease, IF for IgM shows segmental deposition in a glomerulus.* **(Right)** *IF for C3 shows segmental deposition in a glomerulus in a case of hypertensive renovascular disease.*

Myointimal Thickening

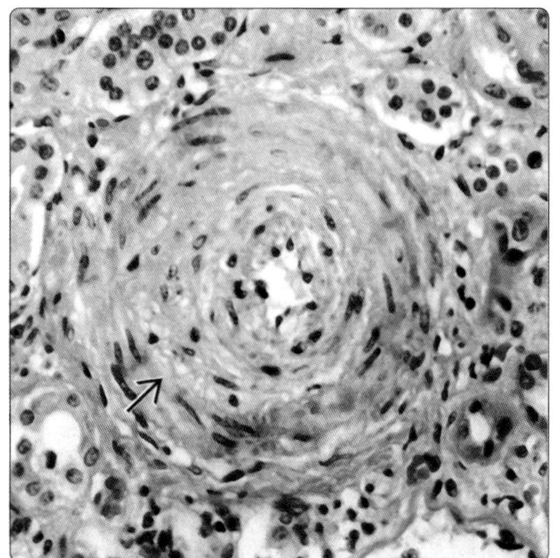

Hyperplastic Arteriolosclerosis ("Onion Skinning")

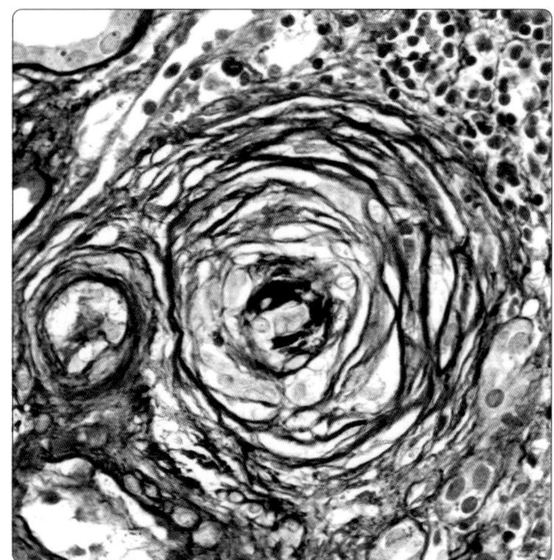

(Left) *Higher power image of this renal vessel shows the "onion skin" ⇒ change in a vessel wall due to concentric myointimal thickening.* **(Right)** *Jones silver stain shows lamination ("onion skin" changes) of an arteriolar wall with near obliteration of the arteriolar lumen, a process that has been referred to as hyperplastic arteriolosclerosis in malignant HTN. (Courtesy R. Hennigar, MD.)*

Vascular IgM

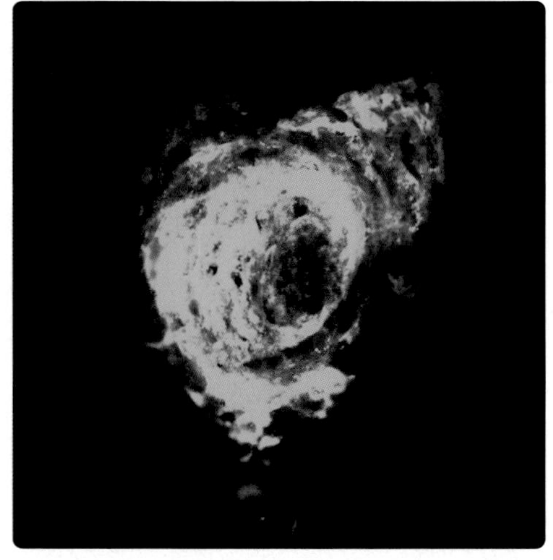

Vascular Fibrin

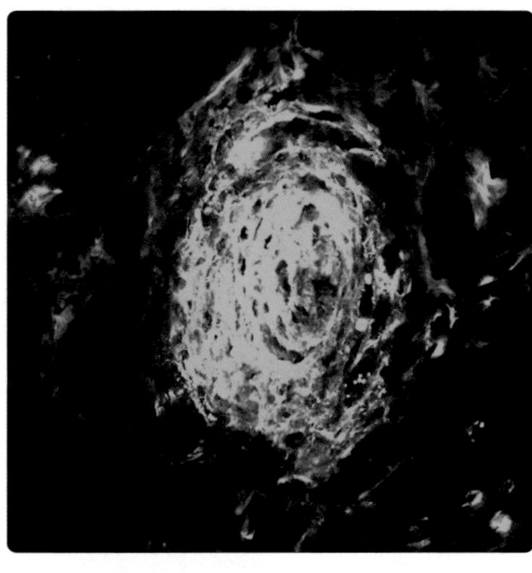

(Left) *Immunofluorescence stain for IgM shows accumulation of material in a small artery in a case of severe hypertensive renovascular disease. This should not be confused with vasculitis.* **(Right)** *Immunofluorescence for fibrinogen shows accumulation of fibrin in the intima of the small intrarenal artery in severe hypertensive renovascular disease. A similar pattern can be seen in any type of thrombotic microangiopathy.*

Fragmented Red Cells in Capillary

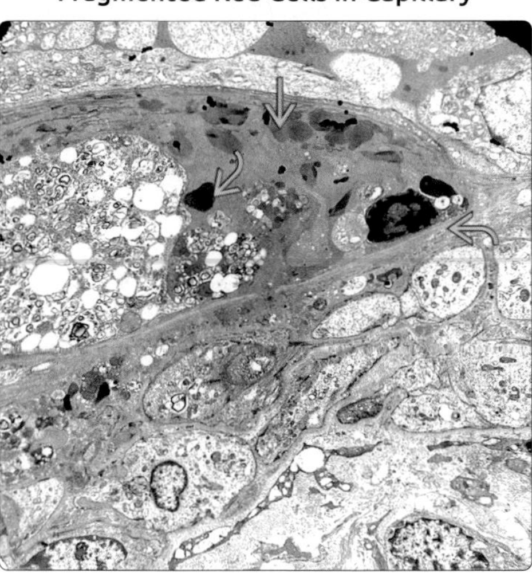

Arterial Matrix Accumulation

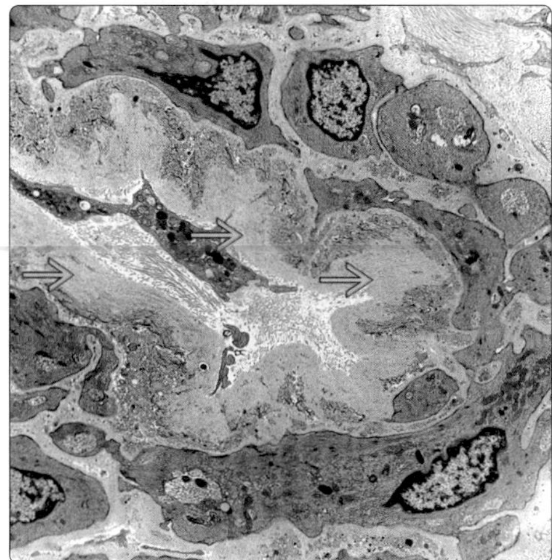

(Left) *Electron micrograph shows a capillary with fragmented red blood cells (schistocytes) ⇒ in a severe case of hypertensive renovascular disease. The endothelium is severely injured and shows ballooning of the cytoplasm and apoptotic nuclei ⇒.* **(Right)** *Electron micrograph of a small renal artery shows accumulation of amorphous material between the endothelium and the media ⇒, probably the residua of "onion skin" thickening.*

Renal Artery Stenosis

KEY FACTS

ETIOLOGY/PATHOGENESIS

- Renal artery stenosis from variety of potential causes results in ischemic atrophy

CLINICAL ISSUES

- Atherosclerosis is most common etiology
- Other causes include fibromuscular dysplasia, arteritis, neurofibromatosis, coarctation of aorta
- Hypertension
- Renal dysfunction
- Proteinuria secondary to FSGS

MACROSCOPIC

- Kidneys small from ischemic atrophy

MICROSCOPIC

- Ischemic glomerular changes
  - GBM wrinkling
  - Intracapsular fibrosis
  - Atubular glomeruli
  - ± hyperplasia of juxtaglomerular apparatus (JGA)
- Tubular atrophy with small atrophic simplified epithelial cells resembling parathyroid (endocrine change) with little fibrosis if "pure" RAS
- Intrarenal vessels spared if protected from hypertension
- Intrarenal arteriosclerosis or arteriolohyalinosis if hypertension preceded RAS
  - Coarse interstitial fibrosis and interstitial inflammation, thyroid pattern of tubular atrophy
- Secondary changes due to loss of nephrons
  - Focal segmental and global glomerulosclerosis (FSGS)

TOP DIFFERENTIAL DIAGNOSES

- Atherosclerosis and atheromatous emboli
- Neurofibromatosis
- Takayasu arteritis and other arteritides
- Fibromuscular dysplasia
- Other causes of JGA hyperplasia

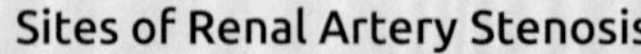

Sites of Renal Artery Stenosis

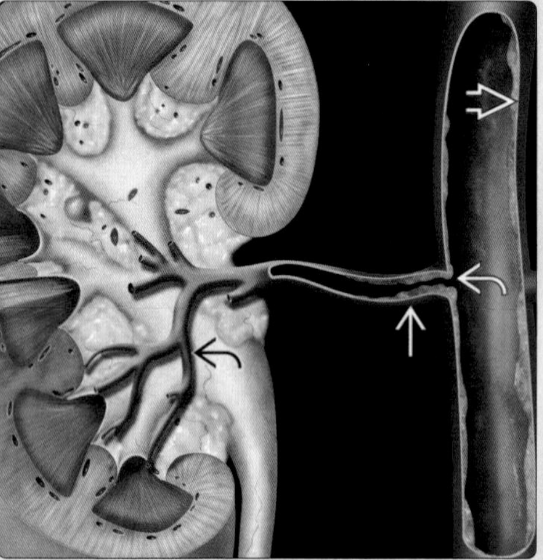

Atherosclerotic RAS

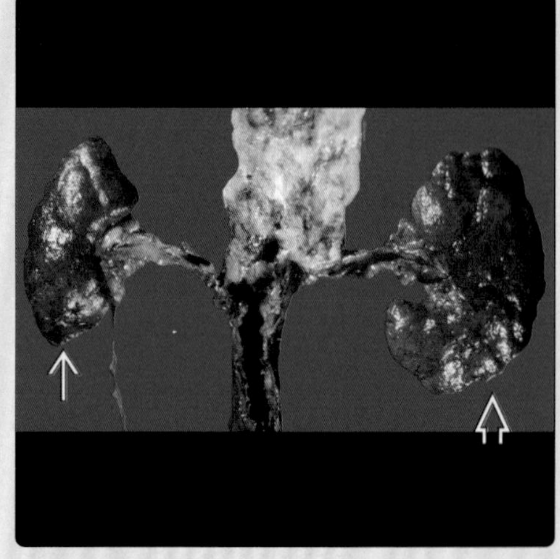

(Left) *Graphic illustrates the common sites of stenosis, which most often occurs in the aorta, renal artery, its ostium, or one of the renal artery branches.* **(Right)** *Shown here are a shrunken kidney affected by renal artery stenosis and a granular kidney affected by hypertension, likely stimulated by renin production by the shrunken kidney.*

Tubular Atrophy Due to RAS

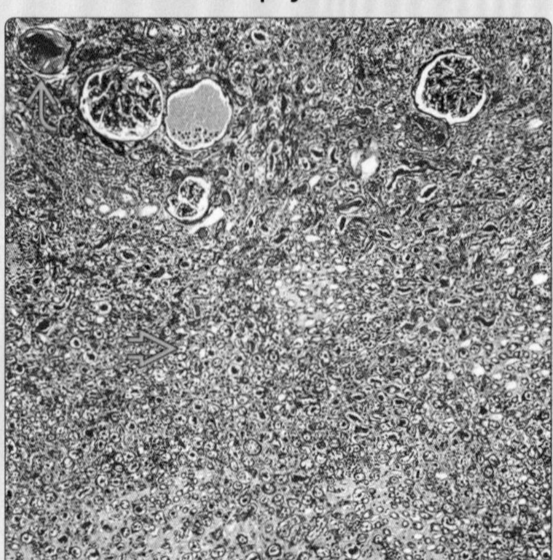

Juxtaglomerular Apparatus Hyperplasia

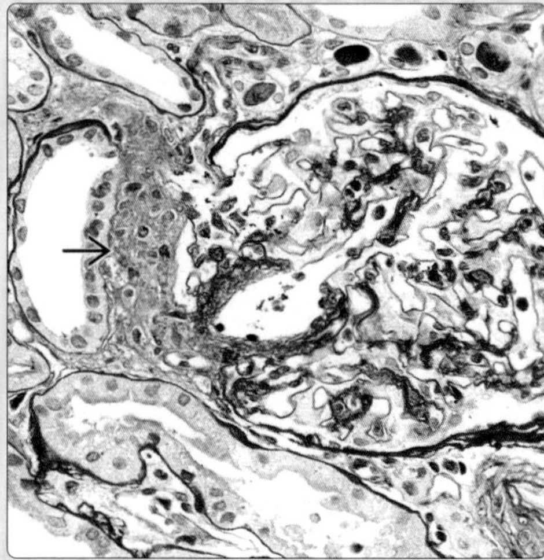

(Left) *PAS stain of a kidney affected by renal artery stenosis shows global glomerulosclerosis and prominent tubular atrophy.* **(Right)** *This kidney affected by RAS shows an enlarged hypercellular juxtaglomerular apparatus (JGA), not always detectable in RAS. Other causes of JGA hyperplasia include salt loss (diuretics, diarrhea) and Bartters syndrome.*

TERMINOLOGY

Abbreviations

- Renal artery stenosis (RAS)
- Hypertension (HTN)

Definitions

- Narrowing of renal artery lumen sufficient to cause ischemic changes in kidney and hypertension

ETIOLOGY/PATHOGENESIS

Causes of RAS

- Atherosclerosis
  - Most common cause of occlusion/stenosis of large renal arteries (70-90% of RAS)
    - Up to 50% of patients with extensive peripheral vascular disease have RAS
    - Anatomical RAS in 5-42% of patients at autopsy
    - 33-39% bilateral
      - Higher incidence of renal failure
  - Patients often have multifocal occlusive vascular disease
    - Injury is conceptually semiepisodic, leading to "layers" of injury with vessels that are not able to autoregulate, eventually leading to "critical stenosis"
  - Atheromatous plaques
    - More common with age and in those with risk factors (cigarette smoking, HTN, diabetes, hyperlipidemia)
  - Atheroemboli (cholesterol emboli)
    - May occur immediately after or within months of angiographic or surgical procedures involving vessels
    - 0.1-0.8% frequency of symptomatic cholesterol emboli after angiography
    - Incidence of 0.1-3.3% in renal vessels
    - ~ 31% of patients with aortic aneurysms
    - ~ 77% after abdominal aortic surgery at autopsy
- Other causes
  - Fibromuscular dysplasia, neurofibromatosis, coarctation of aorta, Moyamoya disease, Takayasu arteritis and other arteritides, dissecting aneurysms of aorta or renal artery, neonatal umbilical artery catheterization, irradiation, retroperitoneal fibrosis, compression by tumor, arteriovenous fistula, trauma

Ischemic Renal Disease/Ischemic Nephropathy

- Fundamental mechanism of injury in RAS
- Occurs when renal artery has 70-80% or greater stenosis

Goldblatt Kidney

- Unilateral RAS experimental model developed by Goldblatt has revealed pathophysiology
- Causes HTN by activation of renal-angiotensin-aldosterone system
  - Ischemic kidney produces renin
  - Increased angiotensin II
    - Increased aldosterone production is stimulated
    - Leads to volume retention, hypervolemia, and increased cardiac output
  - Systemic HTN results
    - Ischemic kidney is protected from effects of HTN
    - Contralateral kidney suffers from effects of HTN (arterial and arteriolar nephrosclerosis)

CLINICAL ISSUES

Epidemiology

- Age
  - Varies with cause
  - Atherosclerotic RAS primarily affects older patients
- Sex
  - Varies with cause
  - 2:1 = M:F in atherosclerotic RAS

Presentation

- Hypertension
- Chronic renal insufficiency
  - Increased serum creatinine and blood urea nitrogen
- Proteinuria
  - Usually of low or moderate degree
  - Especially in patients with secondary focal segmental glomerulosclerosis (FSGS)
- Retinopathy
- Abdominal or flank bruits
- Hypokalemia sometimes present

Treatment

- Surgical approaches
  - Percutaneous transluminal angioplasty
    - Used more often than stent placement
  - Bypass grafts
    - Particularly useful when stenosis is at renal artery ostium, where angioplasty has higher failure rate
- Drugs
  - Antihypertensive agents
    - ACE inhibitors, beta blockers, calcium channel blockers

Prognosis

- With 70-80% narrowing of renal artery lumen, ischemic renal disease may occur and rapidly progress to failure of affected kidney
  - Around 1/2 progress within 2 years

IMAGING

Radiographic Findings

- Intraarterial digital subtraction is gold standard
  - If renal artery narrowing, there may be poststenotic dilatation
- Other useful radiographic imaging modalities include MR, CT angiography, color-aided duplex ultrasonography, aortic angiography
- Renal functional measurements useful in determining contribution of each kidney

MACROSCOPIC

General Features

- Narrowing of major renal artery
  - 50% of cases involve origin from aorta
    - Aorta may override renal artery ostium
- Affected kidney is small, most < 50% of normal weight
  - Thin renal cortex, with smooth capsular surface, unless intrarenal vessels affected
  - Large cortical scars if intrarenal arteries diseased
  - Granular capsular surface if intrinsic arteriolosclerosis

MICROSCOPIC

Histologic Features

- Glomeruli
  - Changes of ischemia
    - GBM wrinkling
      - Sometimes referred to as accordion-like
    - Contraction of tuft toward vascular pole ("simplified"), leading to relative increase in Bowman space
    - Glomeruli close together due to tubular atrophy
    - Collagen deposition in Bowman space
      - Perihilar 1st, extending toward urinary pole
      - Distinguish from fibrous crescents by lack of disruption of Bowman capsule
  - Atubular glomeruli may be present in fibrotic scars
    - Open capillary loops are not attached to tubules on serial sectioning, and mean glomerular volume tends to be larger than in controls
    - May be useful prognostic sign (irreversible)
  - FSGS and global glomerulosclerosis
    - FSGS occurs as secondary (adaptive) form, typically perihilar
    - Usually little hypertrophy
  - Hyperplasia juxtaglomerular apparatus
    - Usually only mild to moderate
    - Increased granules are not usually found in setting of prolonged renal artery stenosis, severe atrophy, and scarring
- Tubules
  - Classic pattern of pure RAS is endocrine change form of tubular atrophy
    - Cuboidal epithelial cells, with clear cytoplasm resemble parathyroid
    - Decreased tubular diameter with narrowed or inconspicuous lumina
    - Little fibrosis
    - Often occur in clusters
  - Atrophic tubules due to scarring and disruption of architecture
    - Thickened tubular basement membranes
    - Decrease in cellular organelles
    - Thyroidization, dilated tubule cysts filled with proteinaceous casts
  - Compensatory dilated tubules (super tubules)
  - Fibrosis
  - Tubular atrophy can be potentially reversible
    - Reversal of atrophy can be accomplished with reestablishment of blood flow in rat model of RAS
- Interstitium
  - Fibrosis may be diffuse and fine, demonstrable with connective tissue stains
  - Interstitial fibrosis and inflammation may be more severe in hypertensive nephrosclerosis than in RAS
- Vessels
  - Extrarenal vessel with stenosis
    - Atherosclerosis
    - Fibromuscular dysplasia
    - Arteritis
  - Intrarenal vessels on stenotic side
    - Arteries and arterioles may be normal, because they are protected from HTN
    - Hyaline arteriolosclerosis and arterial intimal fibrosis may be present if HTN preceded RAS
    - Atheromatous emboli common if cause of RAS is atherosclerosis
- If only segmental branch of renal artery is involved, only that portion of that kidney will be affected
- Unprotected contralateral kidney (nonstenotic artery)
  - Severe arterial and arteriolar sclerosis and nephrosclerosis
  - May show changes of malignant HTN

ANCILLARY TESTS

Electron Microscopy

- GBM are often wrinkled in ischemic pattern, sometimes with collapsing glomerulopathy pattern
- Segmental foot process effacement in secondary FSGS
- Renin granules may be increased in afferent arteriolar granular myoepithelial cells, and these cells may be increased in number
- Atrophic proximal tubular cells have reduced number of microvilli and organelles and reduced basolateral interdigitations

DIFFERENTIAL DIAGNOSIS

Fibromuscular Dysplasia

- Distinguished by changes in renal arteries
- Narrowing of artery typically concentric as opposed to atheromas, which are typically eccentric
- Alternating constrictions and aneurysmal dilatations may be present
- Accounts for 10-30% of cases of RAS in published series
- Most common in young women

Renal Artery Aneurysms and Dissection

- 92% in extrarenal portion of renal artery in saccular or fusiform shape, sometimes with dissection
- Medial hyperplasia and calcifications can be seen
- Sometimes associated with polyarteritis nodosa

Aortic Dissection

- May extend into renal artery
- HTN and flank pain may result, sometimes suddenly, eventually followed by renal failure
- May be spontaneous or associated with trauma or renal artery catheterization

Takayasu Arteritis

- Inflammatory process in aorta &/or major branches
- Granulomatous arteritis in media and adventitia composed of lymphocytes, plasma cells, histiocytes, and sometimes giant cells
- Elastic lamellae may be disrupted

Giant Cell Aortitis

- Gives similar microscopic appearance to Takayasu disease

Neurofibromatosis

- Common cause of renovascular HTN in children and adolescents

Differential Diagnosis of Renal Artery Stenosis (RAS)

Diagnosis	Useful Distinguishing Features in Artery	Useful Distinguishing Features in Kidney
Atherosclerosis	Aortic &/or renal artery atherosclerotic disease with marked narrowing of renal artery or ostium	Cholesterol clefts in vascular lumina and tubular atrophy on affected side; glomerulosclerosis, arterial intimal fibrosis, and arteriolar hyalinosis more severe on contralateral side
Dissecting aneurysm	Plane of dissection in main renal artery	
Fibromuscular dysplasia	Intimal, medial, and perimedial fibroplasia	Larger intrarenal arteries may be affected by dysplastic process; best shown on trichrome and elastin stains
Neurofibromatosis	Occlusion by Schwann cells, fibrosis, smooth muscle cells, and mesodermal dysplasia 1st appearing in adolescent age group	Smaller intrarenal vessels may be affected
Takayasu aortitis	Granulomatous arteritis in media and adventitia with giant cells	
Giant cell aortitis	Granulomatous arteritis in media and adventitia; typically includes giant cells	
Moyamoya disease	Net-like formations with fibrointimal thickening, medial thinning, and sometimes intimal fibroplasia	
Renal artery aneurysm/dissection	Sometimes due to polyarteritis nodosa	Larger intrarenal arteries may have arteritis; best shown with trichrome and elastin stains
Coarctation of aorta	Aorta itself affected	
Thrombosis	Thrombus in artery, usually organized	May be distal emboli, infarction; can occur in infants with umbilical artery catheterization
Radiation	Intimal fibrosis, periarterial fibrosis	Tubular atrophy and fibrosis increased in field of radiation

- Due to renal artery stenosis or aortic coarctation
  - Commonly secondary to compression to Schwann cell proliferation and accompanying fibrosis, usually in adventitia but sometimes in intima
  - Mesodermal dysplasia can be seen in media or intima of smaller vessels, a process whereby cells have nodular proliferation, shown to be smooth muscle cells by electron microscopy and immunohistochemistry
- Pheochromocytomas can be cause of HTN in these patients also

Moyamoya Disease

- 1st described in Japan, typically in carotid artery and branches
- Renovascular HTN in 8.3% of children with moyamoya disease
- Stenosis of vessels through net-like formations, fibrointimal thickening, medial thinning, and sometimes intimal fibroplasia

Other Causes of JGA Hyperplasia

- Chronic salt loss (diuretics, diarrhea, Addison disease)
- ATII receptor antagonists, calcineurin inhibitors
- Bartters syndrome
- Cardiac failure

DIAGNOSTIC CHECKLIST

Pathologic Interpretation Pearls

- Longitudinal sections of renal artery can be more revealing than cross sections
  - Atherosclerotic disease has multiple atheromas
  - Fibromuscular dysplasia has ridges of hyperplastic tissue

SELECTED REFERENCES

1. Kwon SH et al: Atherosclerotic renal artery stenosis: current status. Adv Chronic Kidney Dis. 22(3):224-231, 2015
2. Weber BR et al: Renal artery stenosis: epidemiology and treatment. Int J Nephrol Renovasc Dis. 7:169-81, 2014
3. Seddon M et al: Atherosclerotic renal artery stenosis: review of pathophysiology, clinical trial evidence, and management strategies. Can J Cardiol. 27(4):468-80, 2011
4. Plouin PF et al: Diagnosis and treatment of renal artery stenosis. Nat Rev Nephrol. 6(3):151-9, 2010
5. Aggarwal A et al: Prevalence and severity of atherosclerosis in renal artery in Northwest Indian population: an autopsy study. Surg Radiol Anat. 31(5):349-56, 2009
6. Dworkin LD et al: Clinical practice. Renal-artery stenosis. N Engl J Med. 361(20):1972-8, 2009
7. Gröne HJ et al: Characteristics of renal tubular atrophy in experimental renovascular hypertension: a model of kidney hibernation. Nephron. 72(2):243-52, 1996
8. Marcussen N: Atubular glomeruli in renal artery stenosis. Lab Invest. 65(5):558-65, 1991
9. Selye H et al: Pathogenesis of the cardiovascular and renal changes which usually accompany malignant hypertension. J Urol. 56:399-419, 1946
10. Goldblatt H et al: Studies on experimental hypertension : I. The production of persistent elevation of systolic blood pressure by means of renal ischemia. J Exp Med. 59(3):347-79, 1934

(Left) *Maximum-intensity projection (MIP) from a contrast-enhanced MR angiogram shows mild right* ⇨ *and high-grade left* ↪ *renal artery stenoses, particularly at the left renal artery origin. There is also aortic ectasia.* **(Right)** *An atrophic kidney with a tortuous, stenotic renal artery is shown. Atrophy purely due to RAS imparts a smooth surface with no parenchymal scarring. When hypertension damages the kidney before the stenosis, a granular surface due to subcapsular scars is evident.*

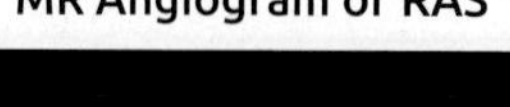

MR Angiogram of RAS

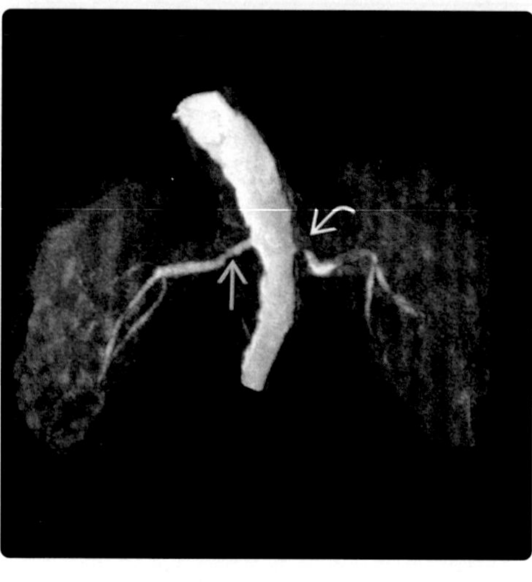

Tortuous, Stenotic Renal Artery

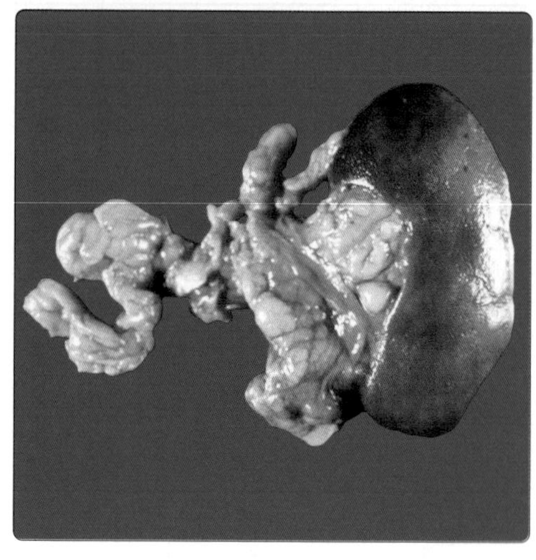

(Left) *There are numerous sclerotic, closely approximated glomeruli* ➡ *and tubular atrophy in a thyroidization pattern* ➡ *in this kidney affected by renal artery stenosis.* **(Right)** *This higher power image of a PAS stain shows prominent tubular atrophy with a focal endocrinization-type pattern* ⇨*, resembling parathyroid tissue, proteinaceous casts* ➡*, and thickened, wrinkled tubular basement membranes* ↪*.*

Glomerulosclerosis and Thyroidization of Tubules

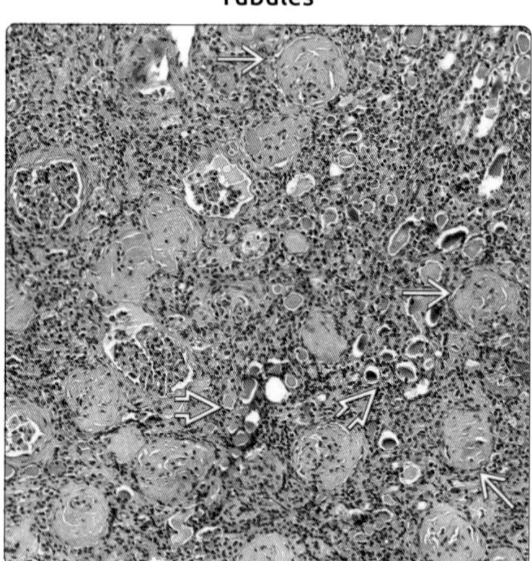

Parathyroidization Tubular Atrophy Due to RAS

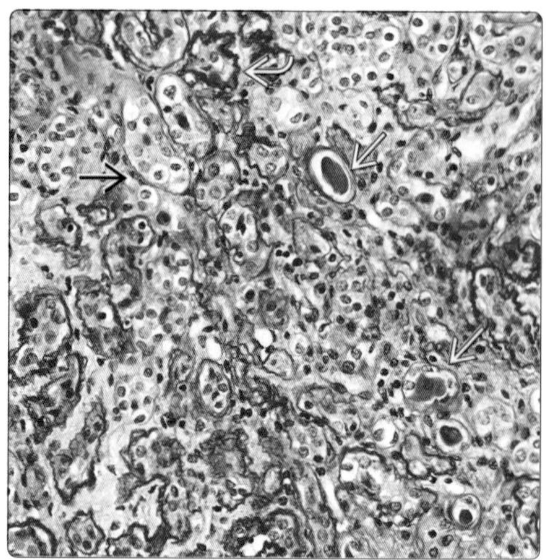

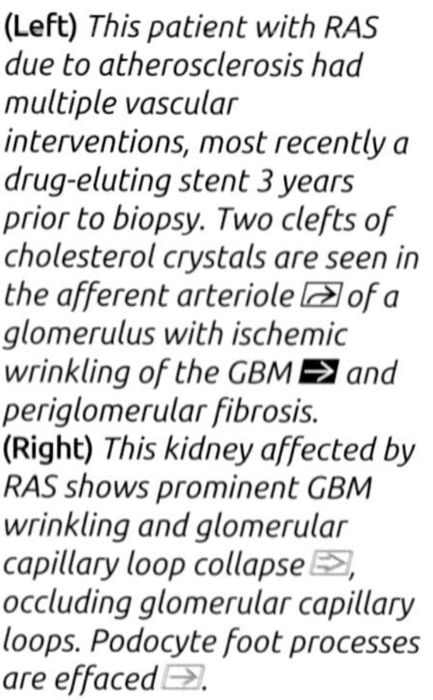

(Left) *This patient with RAS due to atherosclerosis had multiple vascular interventions, most recently a drug-eluting stent 3 years prior to biopsy. Two clefts of cholesterol crystals are seen in the afferent arteriole* ↪ *of a glomerulus with ischemic wrinkling of the GBM* ➡ *and periglomerular fibrosis.* **(Right)** *This kidney affected by RAS shows prominent GBM wrinkling and glomerular capillary loop collapse* ⇨*, occluding glomerular capillary loops. Podocyte foot processes are effaced* ⇨*.*

Cholesterol Embolus, Wrinkling of GBM

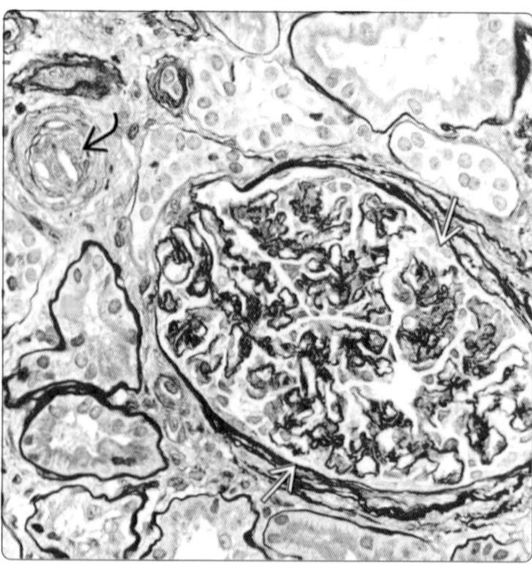

Glomerular Collapse and Foot Process Effacement

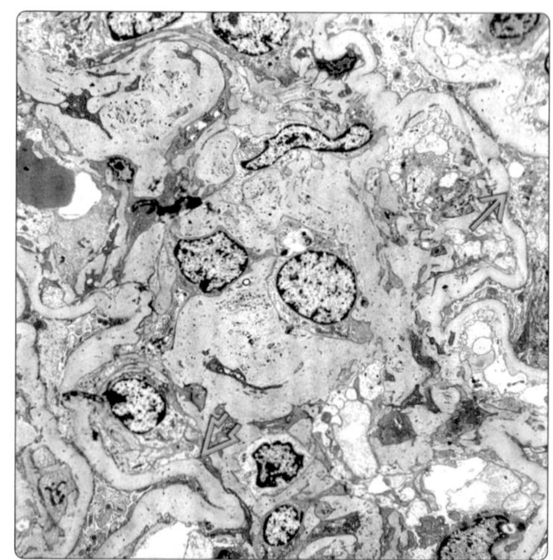

Decreased Kidney Perfusion Due to RAS

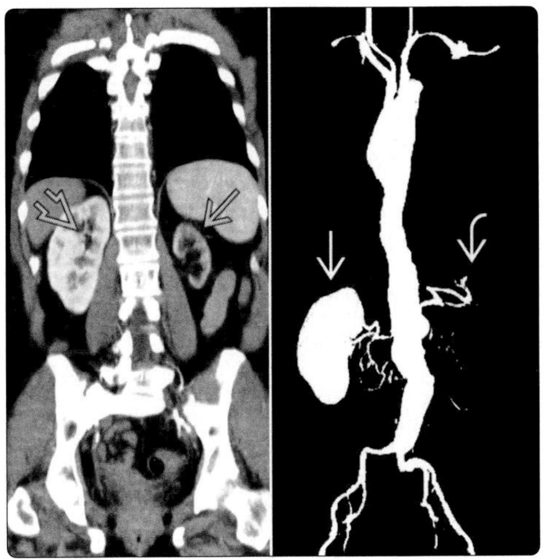

RAS Due to Atherosclerosis

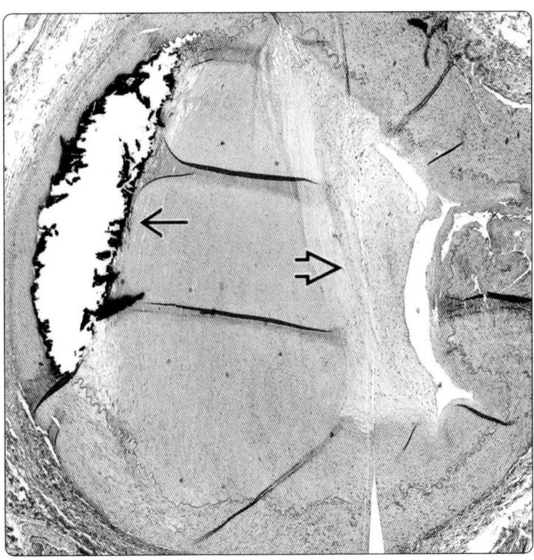

(Left) *Coronal CT (left) shows a shrunken kidney ⇒ compared with the contralateral kidney ⇒. Angiography (right) shows that the shrunken kidney essentially has no blood supply. The tortuous renal arteries effectively terminate where the kidney is expected to appear ➡, compared with the contralateral kidney ➡.* **(Right)** *A section of the renal artery shows atherosclerotic disease with intimal thickening by an atheromatous plaque ⇒ and calcification ⇒.*

Intimal Fibrosis

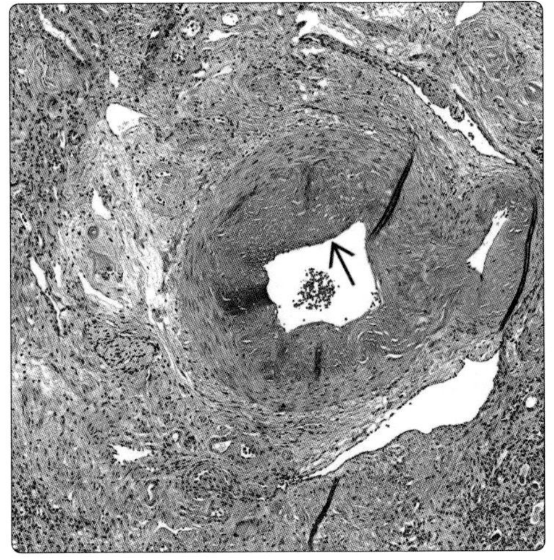

Juxtaglomerular Apparatus Renin Granules

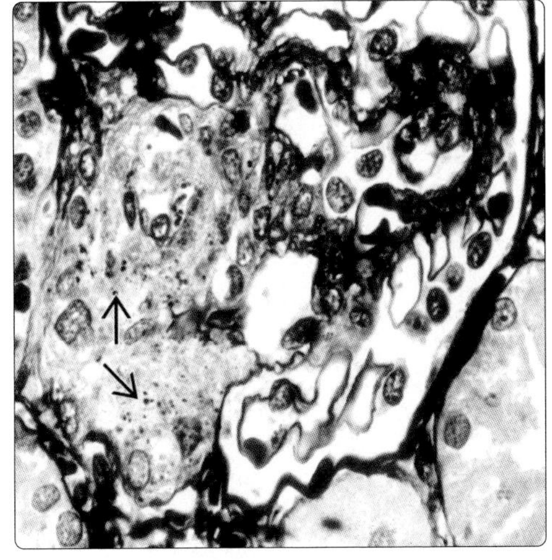

(Left) *An artery in a kidney affected by RAS has intimal fibrosis ⇒, compatible with arteriosclerosis, likely due to preexisting vascular disease, since RAS protects distal arteries from the effects of hypertension.* **(Right)** *Renin granules ⇒ can be appreciated in the hyperplastic juxtaglomerular apparatus of this kidney affected by renal artery stenosis.*

Juxtaglomerular Apparatus Renin Granules

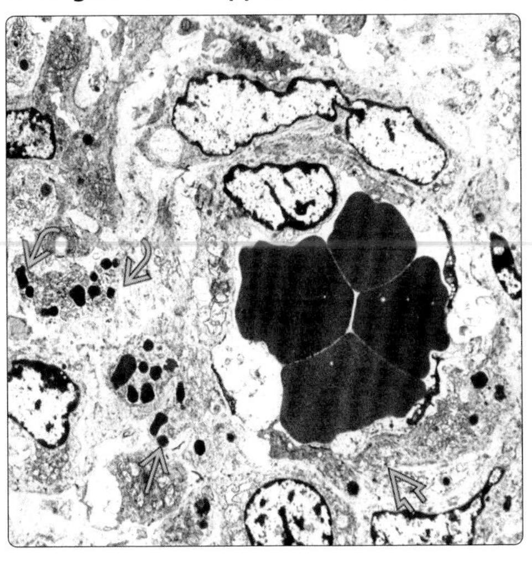

Renin Granules in Juxtaglomerular Apparatus

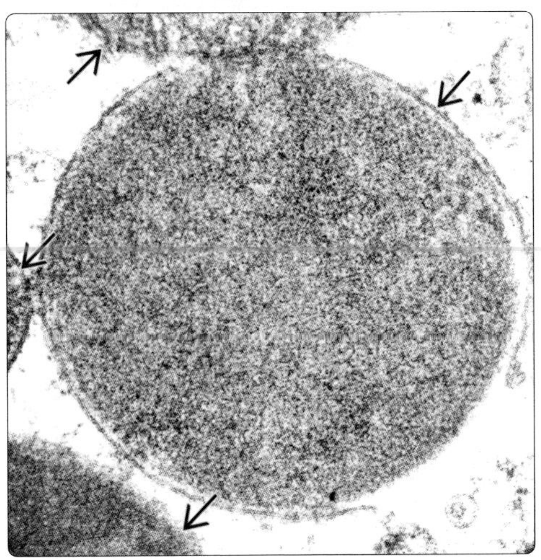

(Left) *The juxtaglomerular apparatus in a case of RAS shows numerous renin granules in the specialized smooth muscle cells derived from the afferent arteriole ⇒, which appear homogeneous and electron dense and either rhomboid ⇒ or round ⇒.* **(Right)** *High-power electron micrograph of the cells in the juxtaglomerular apparatus shows the ultrastructural characteristics of mature secretory renin granules ⇒, which have no substructure and are bound by a lipid bilayer membrane. Immature granules are rhomboid.*

Fibromuscular Dysplasia

KEY FACTS

TERMINOLOGY

- Nonatherosclerotic, noninflammatory fibrous, and fibromuscular proliferation of artery, typically leading to stenosis

CLINICAL ISSUES

- Mostly young and female
- Smoking is risk factor
- 60-90% involve renal artery, 50% bilateral
  - Commonly present with hypertension
  - May be asymptomatic
- Percutaneous transluminal renal angioplasty is treatment of choice

IMAGING

- "String of beads" pattern on angiography

MICROSCOPIC

- Intimal
  - Intimal hyperplasia resembles atherosclerosis but without lipid deposition
- Medial
  - Medial fibroplasia with abnormally oriented smooth muscle and aneurysms most common
  - Perimedial fibroplasia with fibrous band in outer media
  - Medial hyperplasia with hyperplastic but otherwise normal media
- Periarterial (adventitial) fibroplasia
  - Circumferential adventitial fibrosis, normal media and intima
- Inflammation typically absent

TOP DIFFERENTIAL DIAGNOSES

- Atherosclerosis
- Vasculitis
- Dissecting aneurysm

Fibromuscular Dysplasia Variants

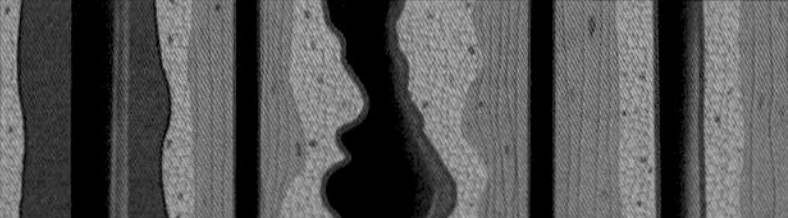

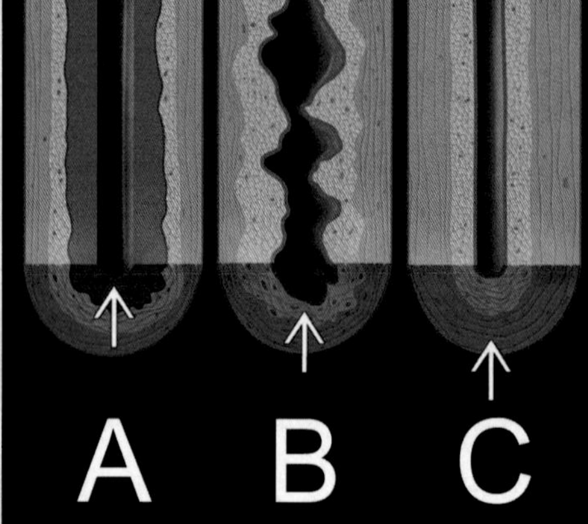

Arteriogram of Fibromuscular Dysplasia

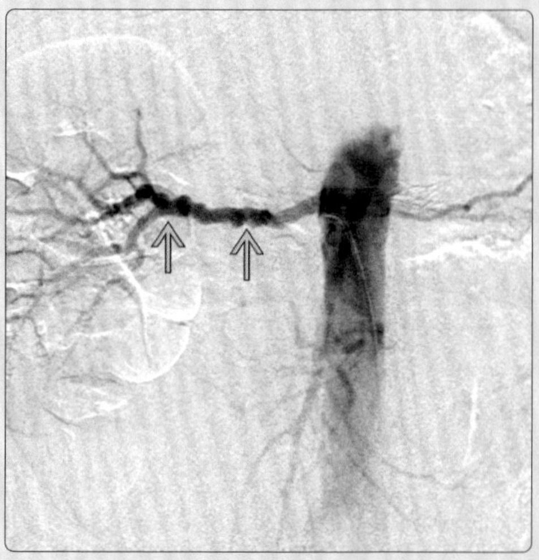

(Left) *Fibromuscular dysplasia occurs in 3 main varieties: (A) intimal fibroplasia, (B) medial fibroplasia, and (C) periarterial (adventitial) fibroplasia. A, B, and C identify the portion of the artery that is abnormal* ➡. **(Right)** *A renal arteriogram shows a "string of beads" with multiple stenotic regions* ⇨*, consistent with fibromuscular dysplasia.*

Perimedial Fibroplasia

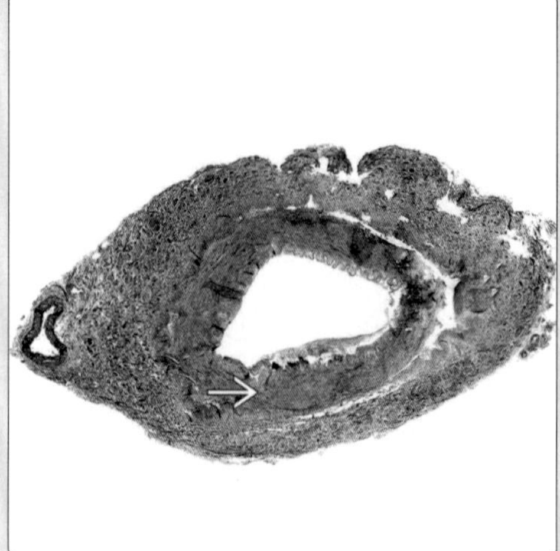

Fibrous Tissue in Perimedial Fibroplasia

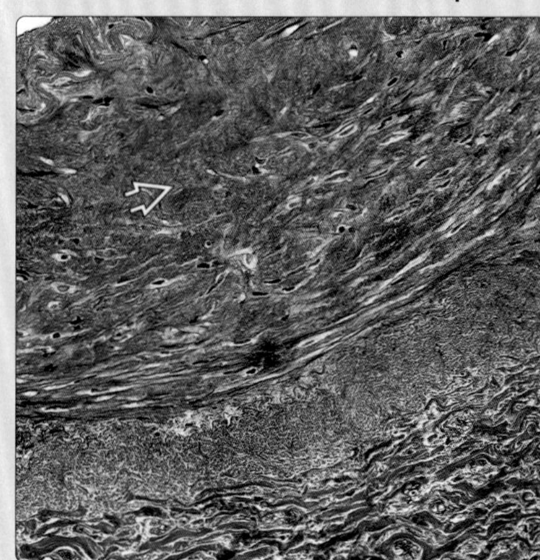

(Left) *Low-power view of the renal artery with perimedial fibroplasia shows that the outer media is occupied by a layer of blue-staining fibrous tissue* ➡*, as highlighted on this trichrome stain.* **(Right)** *Higher power view of a trichrome stain in a case of perimedial fibroplasia shows that the majority of the renal artery wall is composed of variably staining fibrous tissue* ➡.

TERMINOLOGY

Abbreviations

- Fibromuscular dysplasia (FMD)

Synonyms

- Arterial fibrodysplasia
- Fibromuscular hyperplasia
- Intimal or periarterial (adventitial) fibroplasia

Definitions

- Idiopathic, segmental, noninflammatory, nonatherosclerotic small and medium-sized artery diseases causing stenosis and aneurysms
- 3 major categories
  - Medial
  - Intimal
  - Periarterial (adventitial)

ETIOLOGY/PATHOGENESIS

Genetic

- Sibling affected in 11% of patients
- Medial fibroplasia may be congenital since it appears to be from a malformation
- Occasionally, associated with Ehlers-Danlos syndrome type IV or Marfan syndrome
- 1 report of increased prevalence of angiotensin-converting enzyme (ACE) I allele

Environment

- Smoking

Female Gender

- No link to estrogens or oral contraceptives

CLINICAL ISSUES

Epidemiology

- Incidence
  - Estimated 4/1,000 for symptomatic renal FMD
    - Medial: 60-85%
    - Intimal: 1-5%
    - Periarterial: < 1%
  - 10-20% of patients with renal artery stenosis
- Age
  - Younger (15-50 years) for fibromuscular dysplasia
  - Older (> 50 years) for fibrotic forms
- Sex
  - Female predominance (medial form)
    - 85% affect women under 50 years old
  - Male predominance (intimal form)

Site

- Renal arteries (60-90%)
  - 50% bilateral
  - Distal 2/3 of renal artery
  - Extends into arcuate and interlobular arteries
    - May account for continued hypertension after correction of extrarenal stenosis
  - May have associated aneurysm
- May involve multiple vascular beds
  - Carotid arteries (26%)
  - Mesenteric/intestinal arteries (9%)
  - Popliteal, hepatic, coronary, and subclavian arteries (9%)
  - Iliac arteries (5%)
  - Less commonly, aorta and brachial, superficial femoral, tibial, and peroneal arteries

Presentation

- Hypertension
- Asymptomatic
- Associated with hypertrophic cardiomyopathy

Laboratory Tests

- Renin levels elevated

Treatment

- Surgical approaches
  - Surgery curative in ~ 70%
  - Percutaneous transluminal renal angioplasty with balloon is treatment of choice
  - Complex reconstruction, such as aortorenal bypass, required in difficult cases
  - Stents may be needed
- Drugs
  - Hypertension may respond to ACE inhibitors but not most other antihypertensive agents
  - Antiplatelet drugs

Prognosis

- Good, if corrected
- If untreated, progressive narrowing may occur
  - Obstruction, dissecting aneurysms, and emboli
  - Sudden death, particularly in FMD of cardiac arteries (e.g., artery supplying the sinus node)
- Renal failure (rare)

IMAGING

CT Findings

- CT and catheter angiography to identify stenosis or classical "string of beads" appearance

MACROSCOPIC

General Features

- Beaded pattern of aneurysms and stenosis in renal artery branches

Size

- Kidney may show cortical thinning

MICROSCOPIC

Histologic Features

- **Medial fibroplasia**
  - Fibrous and muscular ridges may alternate with marked thinning and even aneurysm formation
  - Aneurysms form from loss of smooth muscle and deficient elastic lamina
  - Renal infarcts more common with this than other types of FMD
  - Rare thrombosis or rupture
  - Medial dissection in 5-10% of cases
    - Channel forms in outer 1/3 of vessel wall

Fibromuscular Dysplasia Types

Type	General Features	Pathologic Features
Medial		
Medial fibroplasia	Most common variant (60-85%); young women; "string of beads" appearance	Fibrous expansion of media, fibromuscular ridges, thrombosis, and aneurysms
Perimedial fibroplasia	10-25%; severe or complete stenosis; women and men ages 15-30 years	Hyperplasia of muscle, usually circumferential, particularly inner media, with fibrous tissue in outer media, thrombosis
Medial hyperplasia	1-15%; severe stenosis	Smooth muscle hyperplasia devoid of fibrosis
Intimal	Uncommon (1-5%); severe or total stenosis	Circumferential or eccentric hyperplasia of intima
Periarterial (adventitial)	Rare (< 1%)	Collagenous fibroplasia encircles adventitia and may extend into surrounding tissue

– Intimal fibroplasia may occur in area of dissection

- **Perimedial fibroplasia**
  - Dense, pale fibrous tissue in outer media demarcated from hypertrophied circular muscle of inner media
    - Cellular fibrous tissue may extend transmurally
    - Adventitial fibrosis may extend into adjacent adipose and connective tissue, causing constriction (rare)
  - External elastic lamina outside fibrous zone may be replaced
    - Outer medial border may have circumferential aggregates of elastic tissue
      - Appears like dense collagen on light microscopy, but EM shows to be elastin
  - Thrombosis more common in this form than other types of renal artery dysplasia
  - Multifocal stenoses produce irregular beading
    - Beads smaller than vessel diameter on radiographic examination
- **Medial hyperplasia**
  - Medial smooth muscle hyperplasia devoid of fibrosis showing normal orientation
  - Intima, elastica, and adventitia normal
  - Angiographic appearance similar to intimal fibroplasia
- **Intimal fibroplasia**
  - Affects major branches of aorta
  - Often bilateral
  - Irregular, long tubular stenosis in young
  - Smooth, focal stenosis in elderly
  - Circumferential or eccentric intimal fibrosis
    - Intimal proliferation of loose, moderately cellular fibrous tissue inside internal elastic lamina without lipid or inflammatory cells
    - Internal elastic lamina present
    - Media and adventitia normal
- **Periarterial (adventitial) fibroplasia**
  - Collagenous fibroplasia encircles adventitia and extends into surrounding periarterial fibroadipose tissue
  - Few mononuclear cells present
  - Intima, internal elastic lamina, external elastic lamina, and media usually normal
- **Parenchymal lesions, affected side**
  - Atrophy of tubules
    - Small, back-to-back tubules with simple epithelium and little interstitial fibrosis
  - Prominent juxtaglomerular apparatus
  - Small arteries spared changes of hypertension
- **Parenchymal lesions, contralateral side**
  - Compensatory hypertrophy of tubules and glomeruli
  - Vascular lesions related to hypertension
    - Intimal fibrosis of arcuate-sized arteries
    - Arteriolar hyalinosis

DIFFERENTIAL DIAGNOSIS

Atherosclerosis

- Resembles intimal form
- Lipid-laden cells, foam cells, and often lymphocytes present

Macroscopic Polyarteritis (Polyarteritis Nodosa)

- Can resemble perimedial fibroplasia or adventitial form
- Typically eccentric scarring, disruption of elastica, and no hyperplasia

Dissecting Aneurysm

- Healed lesions resemble perimedial fibroplasia
- Longer continuous involvement

Normal Artery

- Occasionally, normal arteries may have disoriented smooth muscle
- Elastin stains reveal normal layers of elastic lamina

DIAGNOSTIC CHECKLIST

Pathologic Interpretation Pearls

- Elastin stains valuable for evaluation and classification

SELECTED REFERENCES

1. Alhaj EK et al: Fibromuscular dysplasia of the renal artery: an underdiagnosed cause of severe hypertension. Int J Cardiol. 167(6):e159-60, 2013
2. Pontes Tde C et al: Fibromuscular dysplasia: a differential diagnosis of vasculitis. Rev Bras Reumatol. 52(1):70-4, 2012
3. Sperati CJ et al: Fibromuscular dysplasia. Kidney Int. 75(3):333-6, 2009
4. Davies MG et al: The long-term outcomes of percutaneous therapy for renal artery fibromuscular dysplasia. J Vasc Surg. 48(4):865-71, 2008
5. Olin JW et al: Contemporary management of fibromuscular dysplasia. Curr Opin Cardiol. 23(6):527-36, 2008
6. Olin JW: Recognizing and managing fibromuscular dysplasia. Cleve Clin J Med. 74(4):273-4, 277-82, 2007
7. Plouin PF et al: Fibromuscular dysplasia. Orphanet J Rare Dis. 2:28, 2007
8. Carmo M et al: Surgical management of renal fibromuscular dysplasia: challenges in the endovascular era. Ann Vasc Surg. 19(2):208-17, 2005
9. Slovut DP et al: Fibromuscular dysplasia. N Engl J Med. 350(18):1862-71, 2004

Layers of Perimedial Fibroplasia

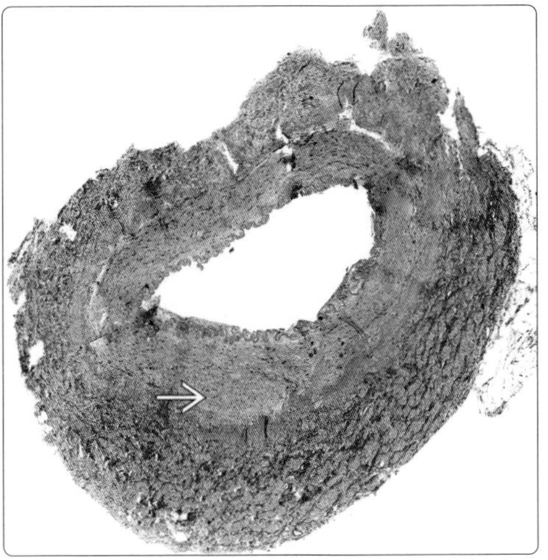

Heterogeneous Medial Layers in Fibromuscular Dysplasia

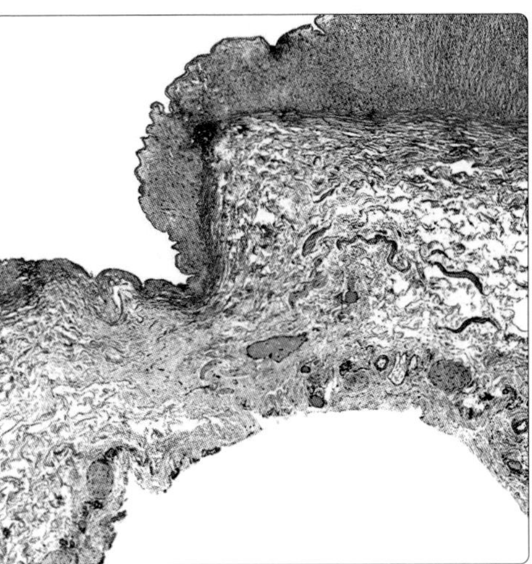

(Left) *Low-power view shows perimedial fibroplasia of the renal artery in which the outer media is occupied by a layer of fibrous tissue ➡ that is paler than the smooth muscle in this H&E stain.* **(Right)** *Hematoxylin & eosin of the renal artery shows pale-staining loose fibrous tissue in the outer media and darker staining dense fibrous tissue in the inner media in a case of perimedial fibroplasia of the renal artery.*

Loose and Dense Fibrous Tissue in Perimedial Fibroplasia

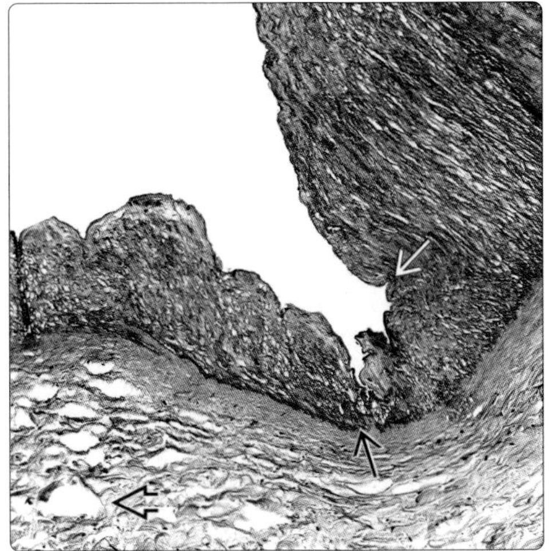

Spindled and Epithelioid Cells in Perimedial Fibroplasia

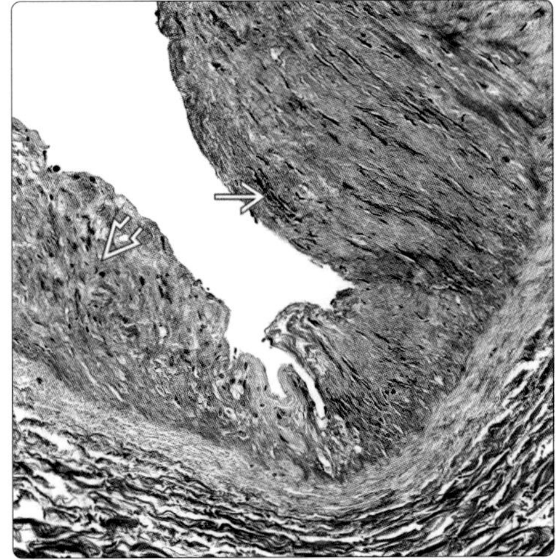

(Left) *PAS stain of the renal artery shows pale-staining loose fibrous tissue in the outer media ➡ and denser fibrous tissue admixed with smooth muscle in the inner media ➡ and loose connective tissue in the adventitia ➡ in a case of perimedial fibroplasia of the renal artery.* **(Right)** *Higher power trichome stain of perimedial fibroplasia of the renal artery shows dense fibrous tissue between smooth muscle cells. Some smooth muscle cells are spindled ➡, and others simulate an epithelioid morphology ➡.*

Aneurysm-Type Formation in Fibromuscular Dysplasia

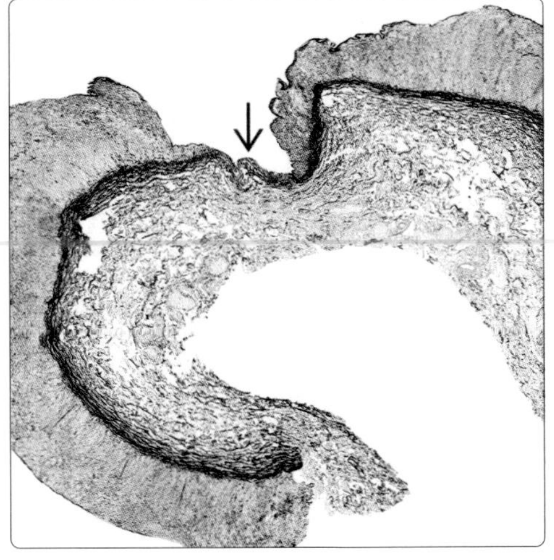

Elastic Fiber Heterogeneity in Aneurysm-Type Change

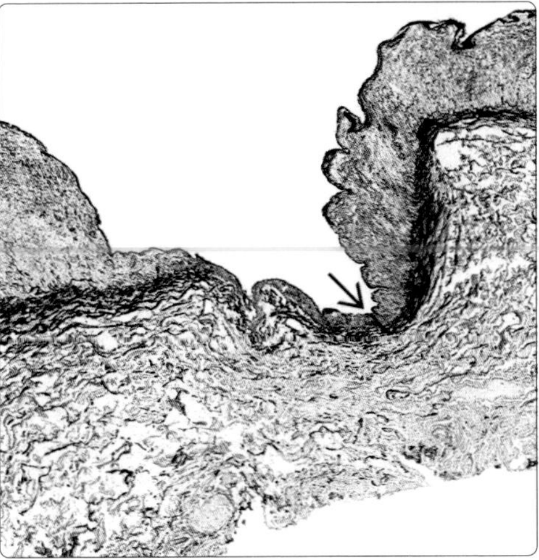

(Left) *An elastic stain of the renal artery involved by fibromuscular dysplasia shows pale-staining fibrous tissue filling the outer media with the inner media being filled by a darker layer, which alternates between thick and thin, focally simulating aneurysm ➡ formation.* **(Right)** *Elastic stain of an artery with FMD shows an abnormally thin region of the media, which was probably dilated in vivo, forming an aneurysm ➡. The outer media has dense bands of elastic fibers.*

(Left) *Higher power image of fibromuscular dysplasia of the renal artery stained with PAS shows dense fibrous tissue → between smooth muscle cells and disoriented smooth muscle cells.* **(Right)** *Medium-power view shows fibromuscular dysplasia due primarily to perimedial fibroplasia, consisting of a proliferation in which loose, moderately cellular fibrous tissue leads to narrowing of the renal artery.*

Smooth Muscle Disarray

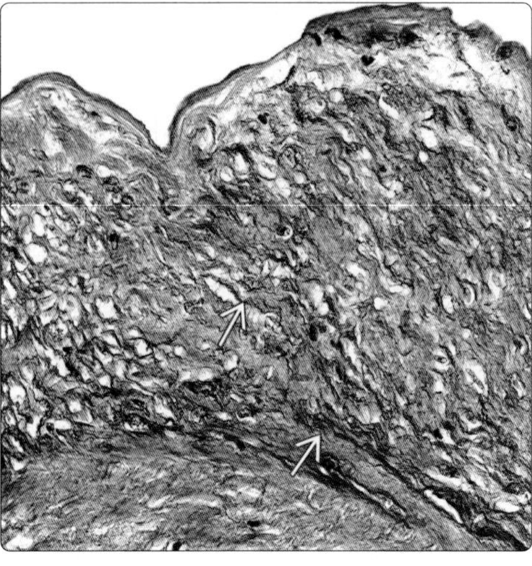

Loose Cellular Fibrous Tissue

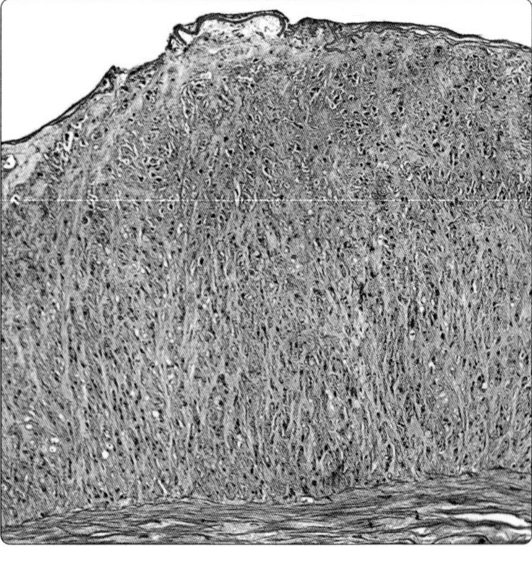

(Left) *High-power H&E of perimedial fibroplasia with "secondary" intimal fibroplasia shows loose, cellular fibrous tissue expanding the media and extending into the intima, leading to renal artery stenosis. Due to the admixed variety of cells, some of which resemble lymphocytes →, this may simulate "endarteritis" seen in other contexts.* **(Right)** *Higher power view of a PAS stain of the renal artery in FMD shows dense fibrous tissue between smooth muscle cells.*

Loose Cellular Fibrous Tissue Simulating Endarteritis

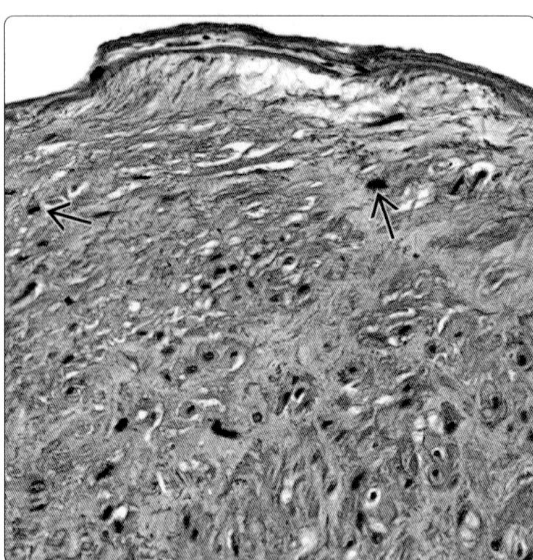

Dense Fibrous Tissue in Fibromuscular Dysplasia

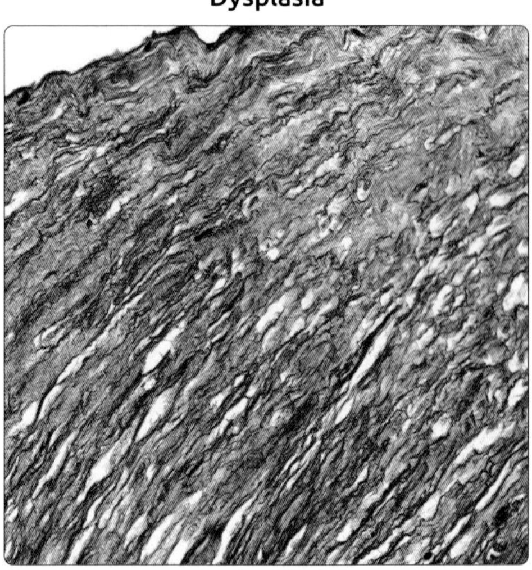

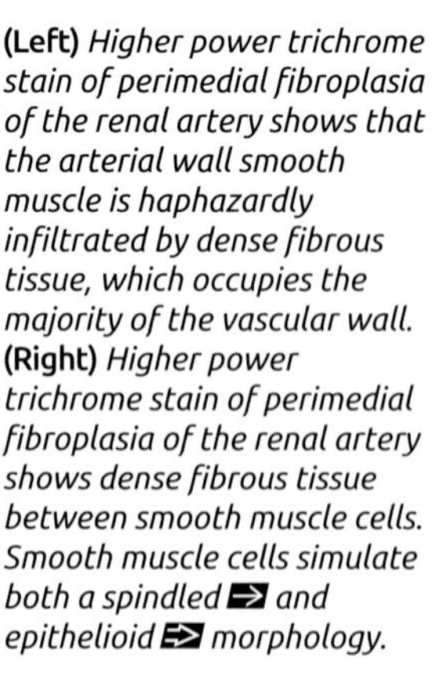

(Left) *Higher power trichrome stain of perimedial fibroplasia of the renal artery shows that the arterial wall smooth muscle is haphazardly infiltrated by dense fibrous tissue, which occupies the majority of the vascular wall.* **(Right)** *Higher power trichrome stain of perimedial fibroplasia of the renal artery shows dense fibrous tissue between smooth muscle cells. Smooth muscle cells simulate both a spindled → and epithelioid → morphology.*

Haphazard Infiltration of Dense Fibrous Tissue

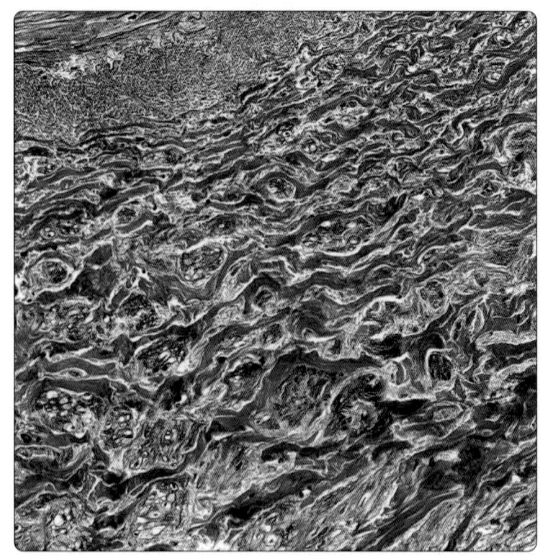

Spindled and Epithelioid Cells in Perimedial Fibroplasia

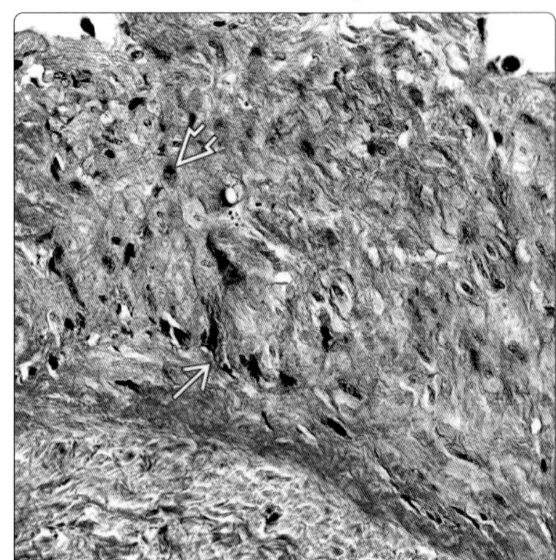

Spindling in Perimedial Fibroplasia

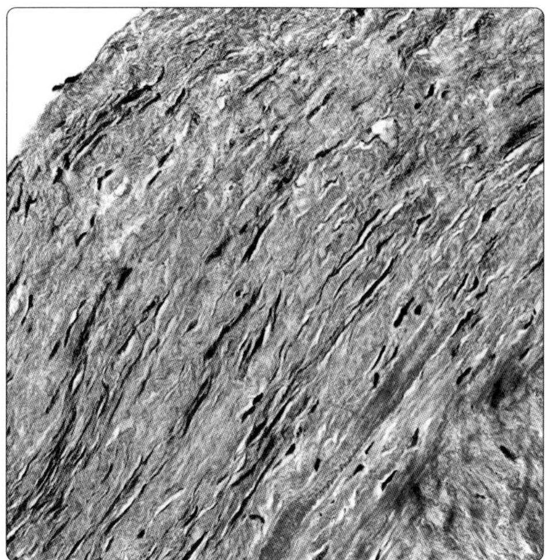

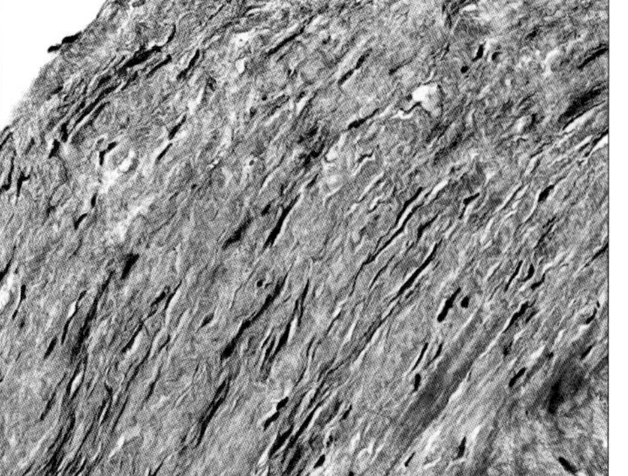

Chondroid-Type Change in Fibromuscular Dysplasia

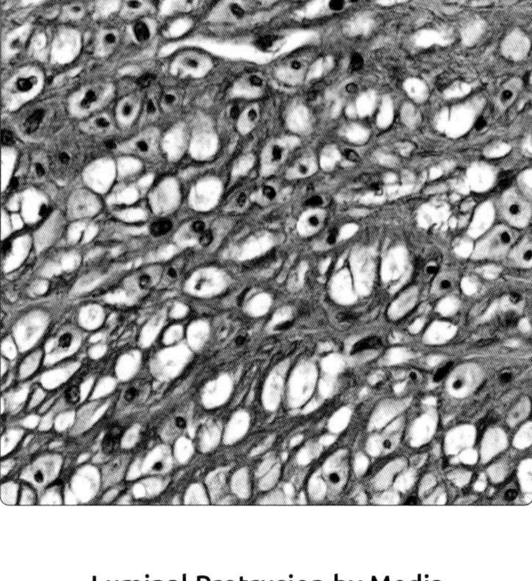

(Left) *Higher power trichrome stain of perimedial fibroplasia of the renal artery shows dense fibrous tissue between smooth muscle cells, which have acquired a spindled morphology.* **(Right)** *Higher power view of perimedial fibroplasia of the renal artery stained with PAS shows dense fibrous tissue between smooth muscle cells. The smooth muscle cells in this case acquire a clear cell appearance that superficially resembles cartilage.*

Disoriented Muscle in Fibromuscular Dysplasia

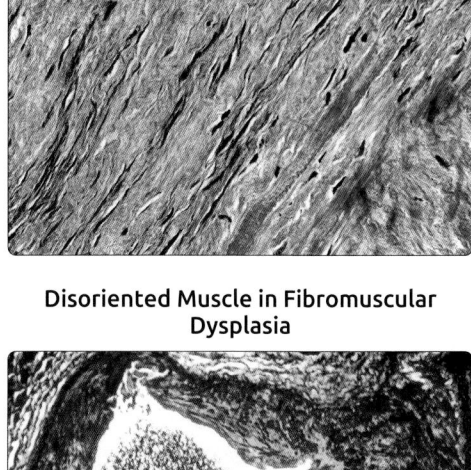

Luminal Protrusion by Media

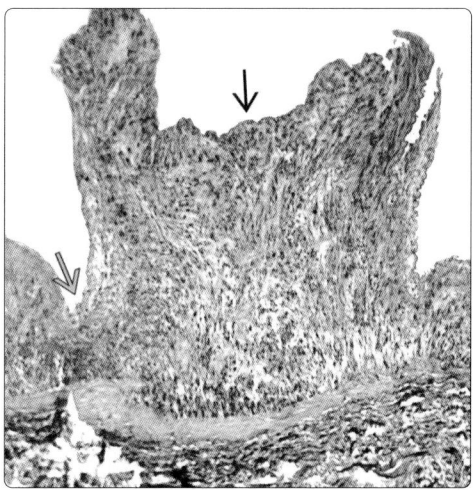

(Left) *The medial fibroplasia form shows disoriented medial smooth muscle that protrudes into the lumen of the renal artery highlighted with this trichrome stain.* **(Right)** *Disoriented medial smooth muscle cells protrude into the lumen of a renal artery alternating with abnormally thin regions, typical of the medial fibroplasia variant of fibromuscular dysplasia. This form is probably a congenital malformation.*

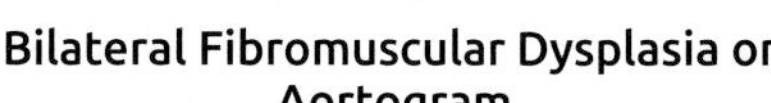

Bilateral Fibromuscular Dysplasia on Aortogram

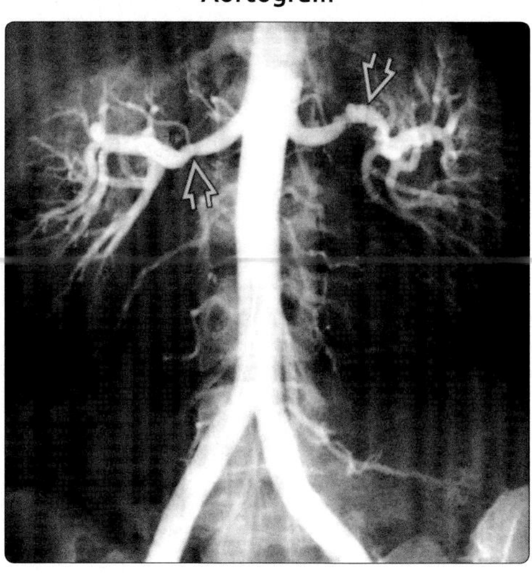

Fibromuscular Dysplasia Patterns

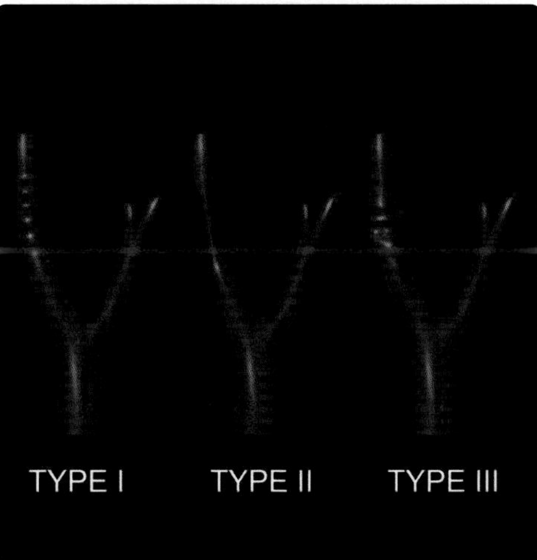

(Left) *Abdominal aortogram shows bilateral involvement of the renal arteries with fibromuscular dysplasia with the classic "string of beads" appearance.* **(Right)** *A diagram shows the 3 patterns of fibromuscular dysplasia as seen on angiography: I) "string of beads" appearance, II) tubular stenosis along a segment of the artery, and III) unifocal abnormality/stenosis.*

Neurofibromatosis

KEY FACTS

TERMINOLOGY

- Neurofibromatosis type 1: von Recklinghausen disease
- Neurofibromatosis type 2: Central neurofibromatosis

ETIOLOGY/PATHOGENESIS

- Neurofibromatosis type 1
  - Mutation of *NF1* gene on 17q11.2
- Neurofibromatosis type 2
  - Mutation of *NF2* gene on 22q12

CLINICAL ISSUES

- Autosomal dominant
- Hypertension most common renal presentation
- Life-threatening hemorrhage if rupture occurs

IMAGING

- Intimal stenosis, ± beading, ± aneurysmal dilatation
- Arterial-venous malformation
- Extravascular neurofibroma with NF2

MACROSCOPIC

- Arterial stenosis ± aneurysm
- Arterial-venous malformation
- Extraarterial mass representing neurofibroma

MICROSCOPIC

- Intimal &/or medial myxoid spindle cell foci
- Aneurysm with smooth muscle attenuation or loss and disruption of elastica
- Luminal thrombosis, organization and hemorrhage
- Renal sclerosing peritubular nodules: NF2

TOP DIFFERENTIAL DIAGNOSES

- Sporadic fibromuscular dysplasia
- Takayasu arteritis

DIAGNOSTIC CHECKLIST

- Consider NF1 vasculopathy with clusters of intimal or medial spindled cells within myxoid matrix

(Left) *In NF1, large arteries are more prone to aneurysm formation compared to small arteries. This interlobar artery shows occlusive intimal fibromuscular dysplasia with secondary aneurysm formation, and luminal thrombosis and organization.* **(Right)** *Elastic stain of this arcuate artery shows florid fibroblastic intimal thickening, segmental absence of medial smooth muscle and multifocal disruptions of the elastica with early aneurysm formation. The arterial branch has intimal thickening.*

Arterial Aneurysm

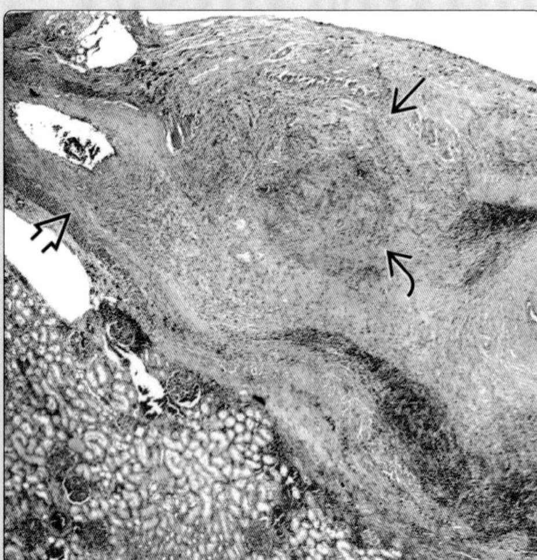

Arterial Aneurysm

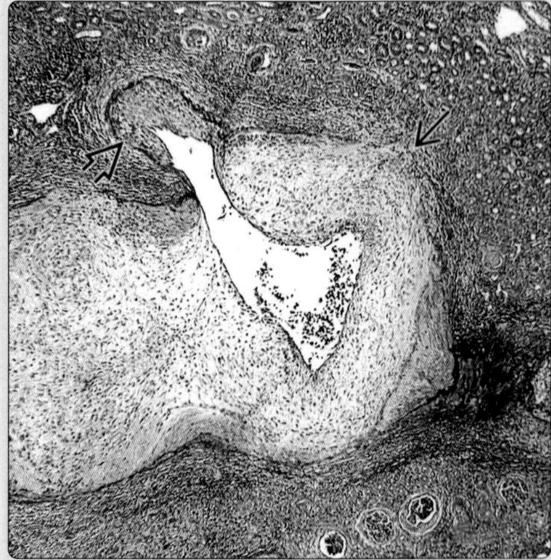

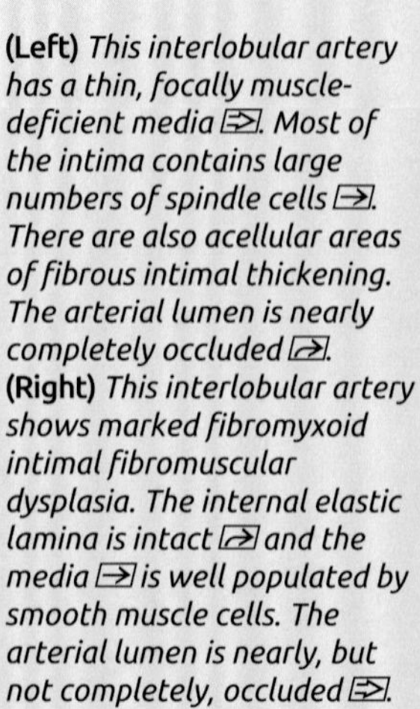

(Left) *This interlobular artery has a thin, focally muscle-deficient media. Most of the intima contains large numbers of spindle cells. There are also acellular areas of fibrous intimal thickening. The arterial lumen is nearly completely occluded.* **(Right)** *This interlobular artery shows marked fibromyxoid intimal fibromuscular dysplasia. The internal elastic lamina is intact and the media is well populated by smooth muscle cells. The arterial lumen is nearly, but not completely, occluded.*

Cellular Fibrointimal Thickening

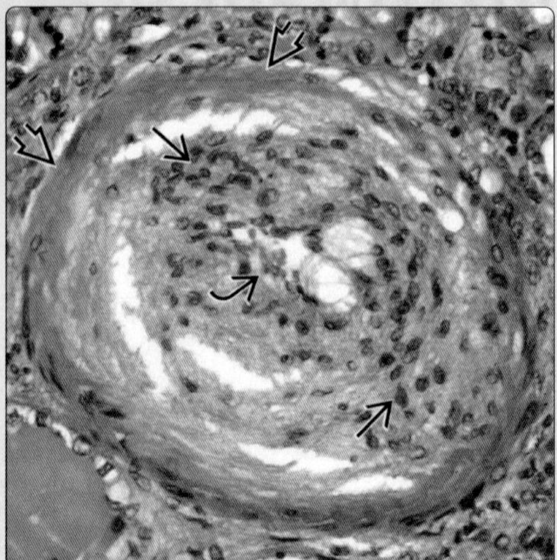

Cellular Fibrointimal Thickening

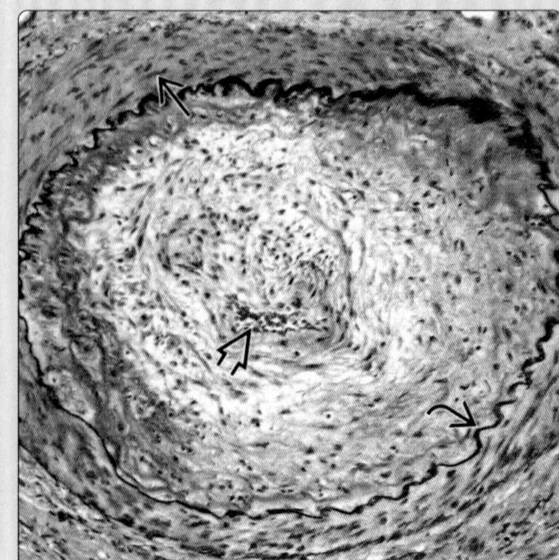

TERMINOLOGY

Abbreviations

- Neurofibromatosis type 1 (NF1)
- Neurofibromatosis type 2 (NF2)

Synonyms

- NF1: von Recklinghausen disease
- NF2: Central neurofibromatosis

Definitions

- NIH consensus statement requires 2 diagnostic criteria
  - ≥ 6 café au lait macules
  - ≥ 2 neurofibromas
  - Axillary freckling
  - ≥ 2 Lisch nodules (iris hamartomas)
  - Splenoid dysplasia or thinning of long bones
  - 1st-degree relative with NF1
- NF1 vasculopathy: Stenoses, aneurysms, arteriovenous malformations or arterial compression by neurofibroma
  - Much more common in NF1 than NF2

ETIOLOGY/PATHOGENESIS

Genetic Mutations

- *NF1*
  - Autosomal dominant, 1:3,000
  - Chromosome 17q11.2
    - Neurofibromin, GTPase-activating protein for *RAS* oncogene
      - Mutation increases mitogenic signaling (MAPK) in neural, endothelial, and smooth muscle cells
- *NF2*
  - Autosomal dominant, 1:40-50,000
  - Chromosome 22q12
    - Merlin, structurally similar to cytoskeletal proteins
      - Regulates membrane receptor signaling and contact growth inhibition

CLINICAL ISSUES

Presentation

- Renovascular hypertension due to renal artery stenosis
  - Most common in pediatric NF1 patients

Treatment

- Surgical repair or bypass if main renal artery affected
- Nephrectomy if intrarenal vessels affected

Prognosis

- Surgical cure of hypertension achieved in most
- Recurrent disease not uncommon
- Sudden death if rupture of large artery aneurysm or AVM

IMAGING

General Features

- Stenosis of main renal artery or segmental branches (90%)
- Stenosis of intraparenchymal arteries (12%)
- Bilateral disease (30%)

Radiographic Findings

- Angiography: Intimal stenosis, occasionally with beading or poststenotic aneurysmal dilatation
- Reduced renal size

MACROSCOPIC

General Features

- Arterial stenosis: Most common in NF1
- Arterial or venous aneurysm: Most common in NF1
- Arterial-venous malformation: Most common in NF1
- Periarterial neurofibroma: NF 1 and NF2

MICROSCOPIC

Histologic Features

- Arterial fibromuscular dysplasia
  - Intimal proliferation with myxoid stroma
  - Intimal or medial clusters of bland spindle cells
  - Thrombosis, organization, hemorrhage
- Arterial or venous aneurysmal dilatation
  - Medial attenuation or absence
  - Disruption of internal and external elastica
  - Thrombosis, organization, extravascular hemorrhage
- Neurofibroma
  - Disordered proliferation of Schwann cells and fibroblasts
- Renal sclerosing peritubular nodules (NF2)
  - Concentric peritubular spindle cells with myofibroblastic differentiation and collagen

DIFFERENTIAL DIAGNOSIS

Fibromuscular Dysplasia

- Most common cause of RAS of young adults and children
- Angiography indistinguishable from NF1 vasculopathy

Takayasu Arteritis

- Most common cause of renovascular hypertension in Asians

Other Causes of Secondary Hypertension

- Pheochromocytoma, ~ 4% have NF1
- Coarctation of aorta, minority have NF1

DIAGNOSTIC CHECKLIST

Pathologic Interpretation Pearls

- NF1 vasculopathy: Clusters of intimal or medial spindled cells in myxoid matrix ± aneurysm formation

SELECTED REFERENCES

1. Srinivasan A et al: Spectrum of renal findings in pediatric fibromuscular dysplasia and neurofibromatosis type 1. Pediatr Radiol. 41(3):308-16, 2011
2. Gökden N et al: Renal sclerosing peritubular nodules in a patient with neurofibromatosis type 2: a case report with immunohistochemical and electron microscopic studies. Hum Pathol. 40(11):1650-4, 2009
3. Oderich GS et al: Vascular abnormalities in patients with neurofibromatosis syndrome type I: clinical spectrum, management, and results. J Vasc Surg. 46(3):475-484, 2007
4. Westenend PJ et al: A 4-year-old boy with neurofibromatosis and severe renovascular hypertension due to renal arterial dysplasia. Am J Surg Pathol. 18(5):512-6, 1994
5. Finley JL et al: Renal vascular smooth muscle proliferation in neurofibromatosis. Hum Pathol. 19(1):107-10, 1988

(Left) *This is an arcuate artery affected by an aneurysm that has thrombosed and is undergoing organization. There is disruption of the media ⇨ with a vigorous proliferation of spindled cells associated with organization.* **(Right)** *Cellular fibrointimal proliferation is shown within a myxoid stroma in an arcuate artery, typical of NF1.*

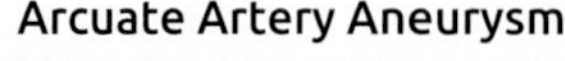

Arcuate Artery Aneurysm

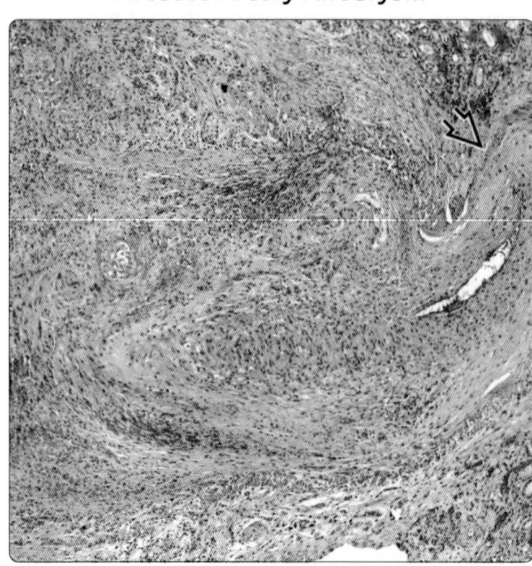

Cellular Fibrointimal Proliferation

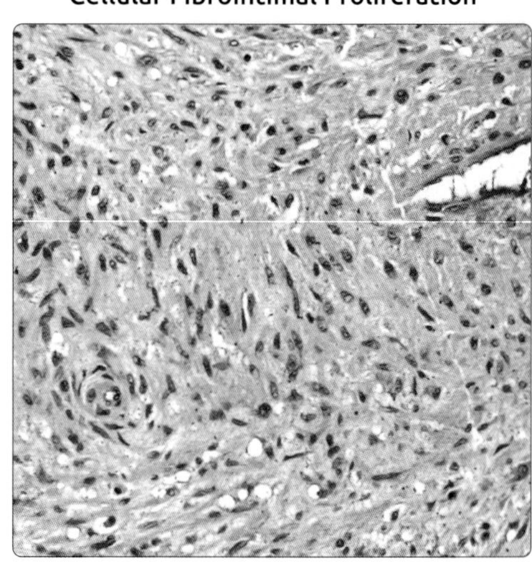

(Left) *This arcuate artery aneurysm is contained by the elastic lamina → whereas the aneurysm lumen is largely filled by loose, edematous paucicellular tissue ⇨. The arcuate arterial intima is fibrotic and shows marked elastosis and luminal compromise.* **(Right)** *This arcuate artery is affected by early aneurysm formation. The media abruptly terminates ↪, and the elastica → is focally absent or disrupted. The lumen of the aneurysm and the artery are filled with loose edematous tissue, hemorrhage and scattered spindle cells.*

Arcuate Artery Aneurysm

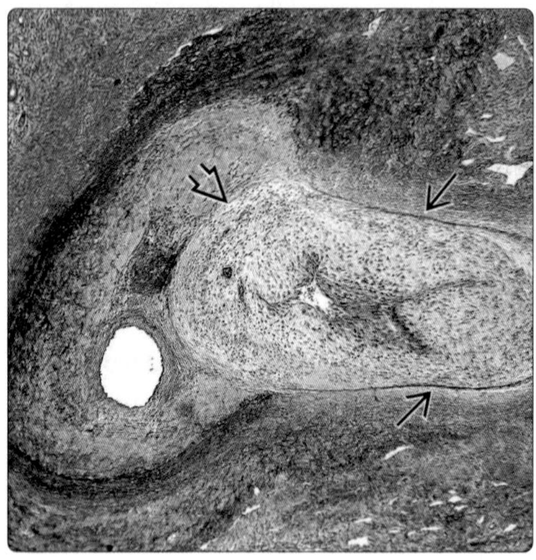

Arcuate Artery Aneurysm

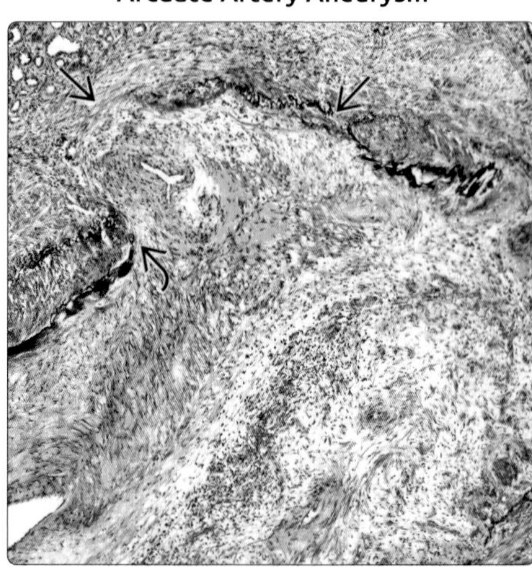

(Left) *This arcuate artery has loose paucicellular intimal tissue with small clusters of palisading spindle cells → that suggested neural derivation in early reports. EM and immunoperoxidase studies of spindle cells demonstrate fibrous and myoid features.* **(Right)** *This arcuate artery shows dense, acellular, fibrotic intimal thickening ⇨. In two regions, the medial smooth muscle layer is completely absent → with only a single interrupted layer of elastica remains. These would be sites for aneurysm formation if the intima wasn't so fibrotic.*

Intimal Thickening With Palisading Cells

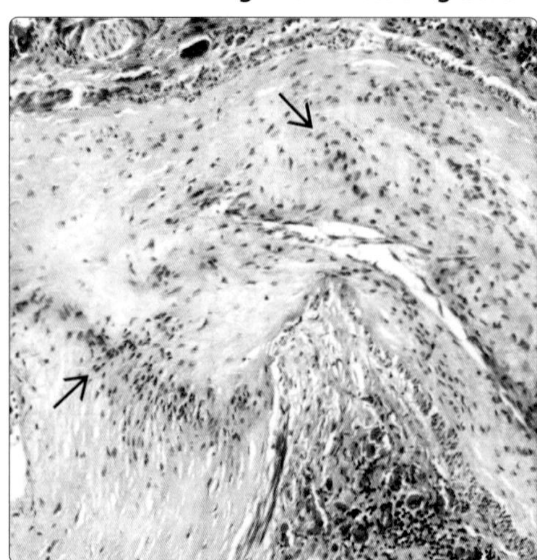

Dense Intimal Fibrosis

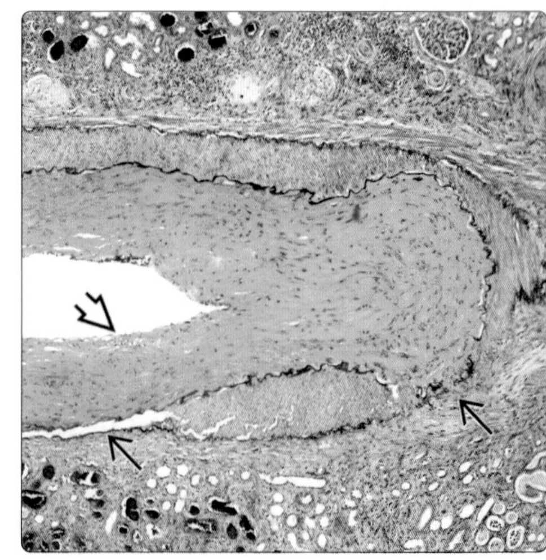

Cellular Fibrointimal Thickening

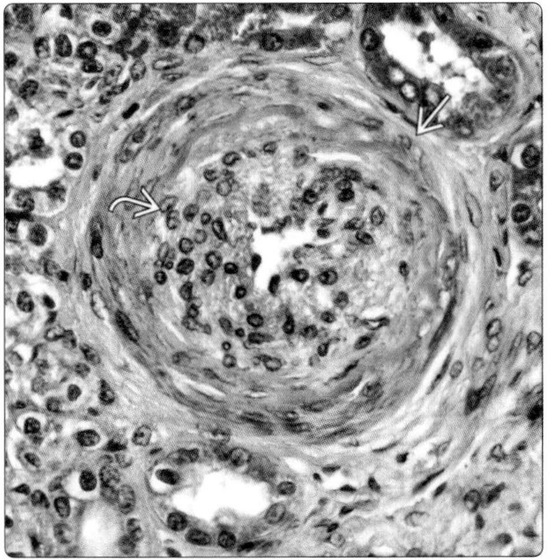

Paucicellular Fibrointimal Thickening

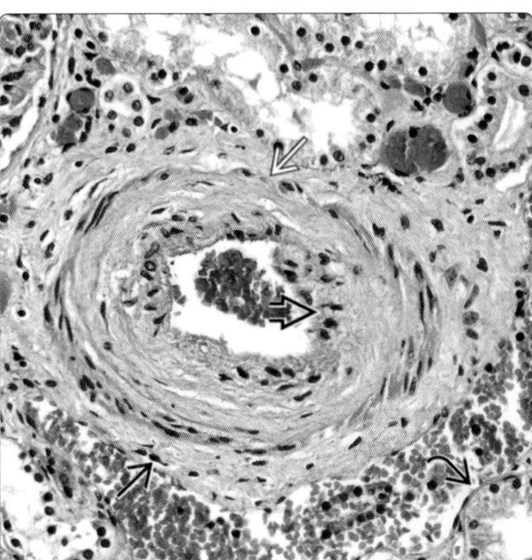

(Left) *This peripheral interlobular artery shows loose but cellular, intimal thickening ➡ with marked luminal compromise. The medial smooth muscle cell layer ➡ appears attenuated. The elastic lamina has been lost.* **(Right)** *This intralobular artery has a very thin ➡ to interrupted media and loose, largely acellular intimal thickening ⇨. There is a similar loose paucicellular alteration of the adventitia ⇨. The adjacent vein ⇨ is normal. Notice that the cortical vein lacks a smooth muscle media.*

Renal Sclerosing Peritubular Nodule

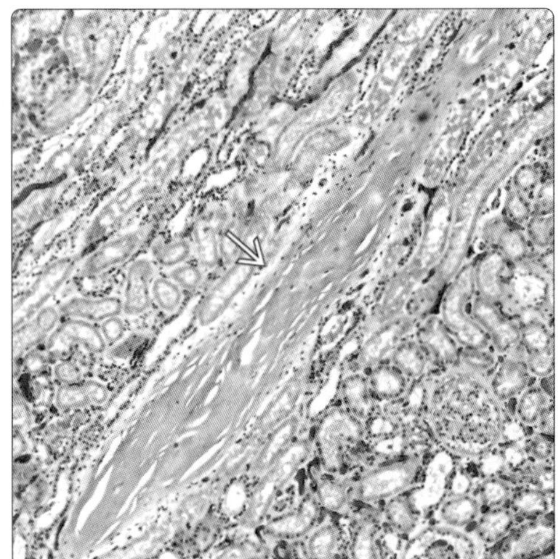

Renal Sclerosing Peritubular Nodule

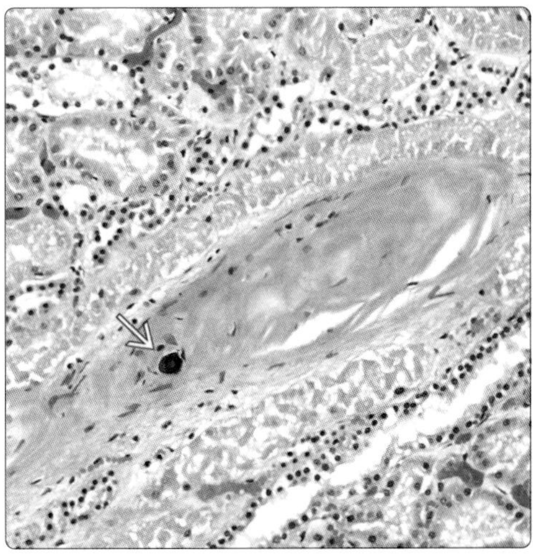

(Left) *Renal sclerosing peritubular nodules ➡ are very rare and have only been described as case reports in neurofibromatosis 2. They are mainly cortical lesions but also occur in the outer stripe of the outer medulla. They are not associated with renal arteries. (Courtesy N. Gokden, MD.)* **(Right)** *The early lesions of renal sclerosing peritubular nodules have been reported to contain a central tubule not present in this more advanced lesion. Focal calcification ➡ with scant spindled cells is common in advanced lesions.*

Renal Sclerosing Peritubular Nodule

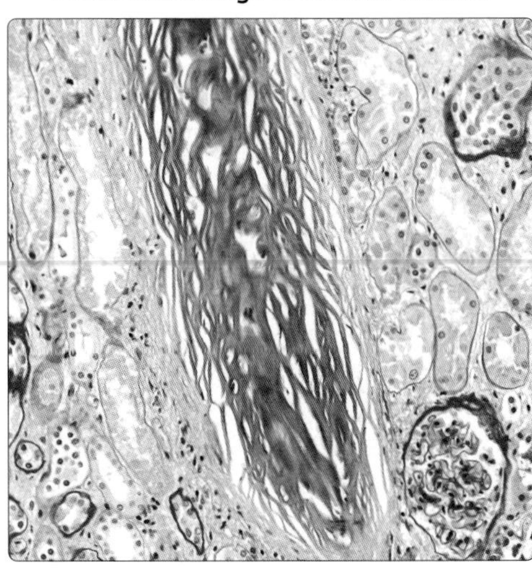

Renal Sclerosing Peritubular Nodule

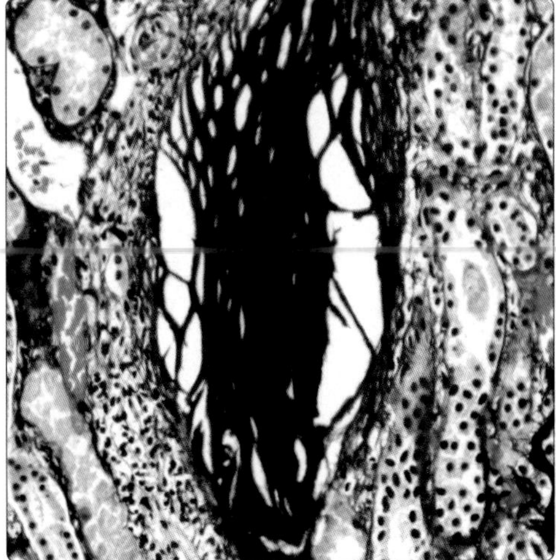

(Left) *PAS-stained section of a renal sclerosing peritubular nodule shows no evidence of any preexisting structure such as a renal tubule. It does, however, stain prominently despite its largely connective tissue composition. The glomeruli, tubules, and interstitium are otherwise normal. The splitting of the nodule is likely due to shrinkage during tissue processing.* **(Right)** *This renal sclerosing peritubular nodule stains intensely on Jones methenamine silver. It does not show evidence of any preexisting structure.*

Renal Vein Thrombosis

KEY FACTS

TERMINOLOGY

- Renal vein thrombosis (RVT)
  - Thrombus involving main renal vein

ETIOLOGY/PATHOGENESIS

- Risk factors
  - Nephrotic syndrome
    - Most common in membranous glomerulonephritis
    - Loss of antithrombin III
  - Neoplasm
    - Renal cell carcinoma with renal vein invasion
  - Coagulopathy
    - Factor V Leiden
    - Antiphospholipid syndrome
  - Trauma, dehydration, infection

CLINICAL ISSUES

- Treatment
  - Anticoagulation or fibrinolytic therapy
- Does not affect prognosis in nephrotic syndrome
- 60% mortality rate in neonates with main renal vein involvement

MICROSCOPIC

- Thrombi in veins and glomeruli
- Glomerular and peritubular capillary dilatation
- Glomerular capillaritis or glomerulitis
- Interstitial edema
- Acute tubular injury
- Frequent endothelial cell swelling by electron microscopy

TOP DIFFERENTIAL DIAGNOSES

- Thrombotic microangiopathy
- Renal artery thrombosis
- Hydronephrosis

DIAGNOSTIC CHECKLIST

- May have little histologic change on biopsy

(Left) *CT scan demonstrates a large opacity leading into the right kidney ➡ that represents a large thrombus in the right renal vein.* **(Right)** *A thrombus ➡ is slightly detached from a renal venule ➡ at the edge of this kidney biopsy. This finding may be observed in some patients with nephrotic syndrome.*

Renal Vein Thrombus

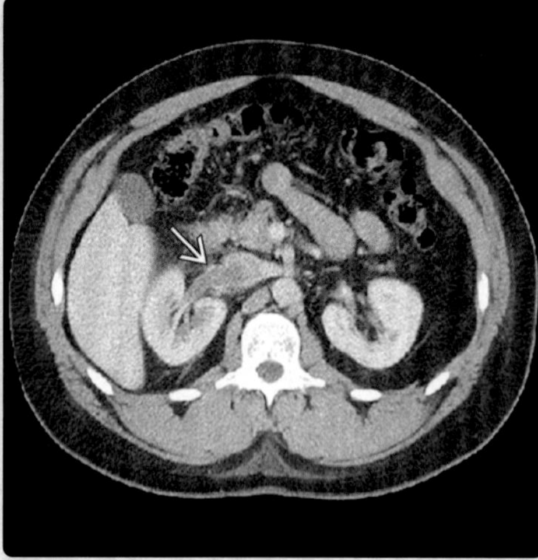

Venular Thrombus

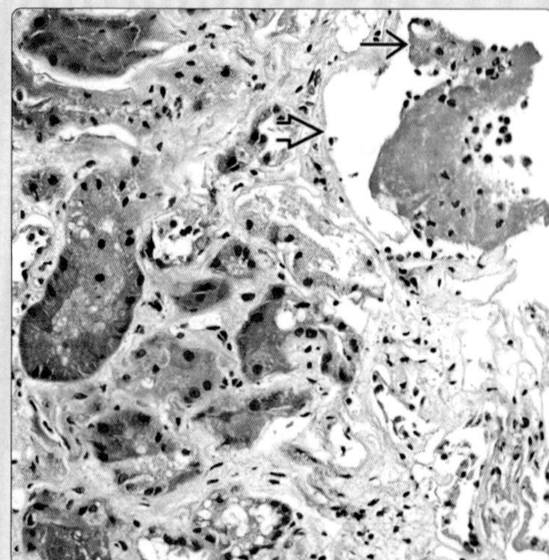

(Left) *Hematoxylin & eosin demonstrates a thrombus ➡ within a portion of the lumen of a renal venule ➡ in a patient with nephrotic syndrome due to minimal change disease.* **(Right)** *Hematoxylin & eosin demonstrates increased numbers of neutrophils ➡ within the glomerular capillaries of this glomerulus in a patient with renal vein thrombosis.*

Thrombus

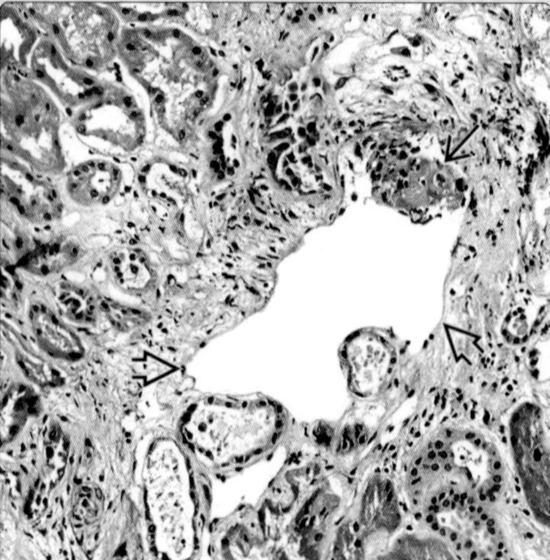

Glomerular Capillaritis

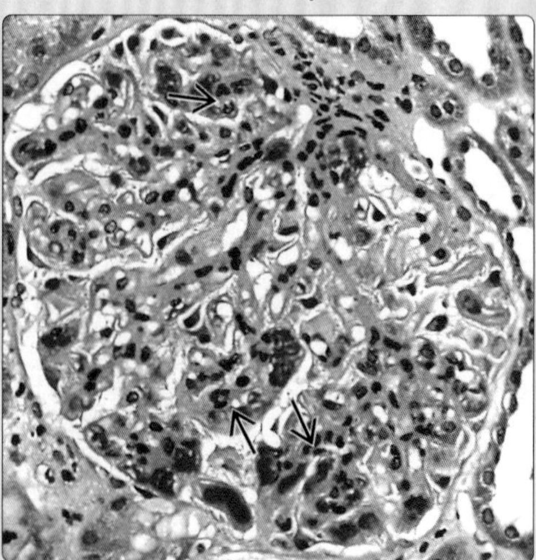

TERMINOLOGY

Abbreviations

- Renal vein thrombosis (RVT)

Definitions

- Thrombus involving main renal vein

ETIOLOGY/PATHOGENESIS

Risk Factors

- Nephrotic syndrome
  - Loss of anti-thrombin III
- Coagulopathy
  - Antiphospholipid antibody syndrome
  - Factor V Leiden (including newborn)
- Neoplasm
- Renal vein entrapment (nutcracker syndrome)
- Infection, trauma, surgery, immobilization, dehydration, diuretics, renal transplantation, sickle cell trait

CLINICAL ISSUES

Epidemiology

- Incidence
  - RVT in nephrotic syndrome
    - More common in adults (27%) than children (2.8%)
    - Usually occurs < 12 months of nephrotic syndrome onset
    - Incidence by glomerular disease
      - Membranous glomerulonephritis (37%)
      - Membranoproliferative glomerulonephritis (26%)
      - Minimal change disease (24%)
      - Focal segmental glomerulosclerosis (19%)
      - Congenital nephrotic syndrome (10%)
    - Increased incidence of pulmonary embolism and deep vein thrombosis
    - Hypoalbuminemia is risk factor (< 2.8 g/dl)

Presentation

- Proteinuria, nephrotic range
  - RVT usually asymptomatic (~ 90%)
  - Flank pain (8%)
  - Hematuria (5%)
- Renal failure
- Scrotal pain
  - More common on left than right (2:1)

Treatment

- Surgical approaches
  - Thrombectomy (rare option)
- Drugs
  - Anticoagulation
  - Fibrinolytic therapy

Prognosis

- Does not affect prognosis in nephrotic syndrome
- 60% mortality rate in neonates

MICROSCOPIC

Histologic Features

- Pathology reports limited
- Glomeruli
  - Capillary dilatation
  - Glomerular capillaritis or glomerulitis
    - Leukocyte or neutrophil congestion within glomerular capillaries
    - Thrombi
  - Swelling or prominence of podocytes
  - Other lesions if concurrent glomerular disease is present
    - Membranous glomerulonephritis, focal segmental glomerulosclerosis
- Tubules
  - Acute tubular injury or atrophy
- Interstitium
  - Disproportionate edema, fibrosis
  - Focal hemorrhage
- Vessels
  - Thrombi
    - Renal vein, venules
    - Thrombi stain red in Masson trichrome
  - Peritubular capillary dilation

ANCILLARY TESTS

Immunohistochemistry

- CD61
  - Platelet marker (glycoprotein IIIa) highlights thrombi

Electron Microscopy

- Frequent endothelial cell swelling
  - Increased numbers of mitochondria, ribosomes, and endoplasmic reticulum

DIFFERENTIAL DIAGNOSIS

Thrombotic Microangiopathy

- Typically does not involve veins or venules

Renal Artery Thrombosis

- Hemorrhagic necrosis and infarct

Hydronephrosis

- Dilatation of distal nephron segments

DIAGNOSTIC CHECKLIST

Pathologic Interpretation Pearls

- May have little histologic change on biopsy

SELECTED REFERENCES

1. Zhang LJ et al: Pulmonary Embolism and Renal Vein Thrombosis in Patients with Nephrotic Syndrome: Prospective Evaluation of Prevalence and Risk Factors with CT. Radiology. 273(3):897-906, 2014
2. Barbour SJ et al: Disease-specific risk of venous thromboembolic events is increased in idiopathic glomerulonephritis. Kidney Int. 81(2):190-5, 2012
3. Kerlin BA et al: Epidemiology and pathophysiology of nephrotic syndrome-associated thromboembolic disease. Clin J Am Soc Nephrol. 7(3):513-20, 2012
4. Rosenmann E et al: Renal vein thrombosis in the adult: a clinical and pathologic study based on renal biopsies. Medicine (Baltimore). 47(4):269-335, 1968

Renal Artery Thrombosis

KEY FACTS

ETIOLOGY/PATHOGENESIS

- Risk factors
  - Fibromuscular dysplasia
  - Renal artery or abdominal aortic aneurysm
  - Trauma
    - Motor vehicle accident (MVA)
    - Complication of surgical procedure or instrumentation
  - Hypercoagulable state
    - Antiphospholipid antibody syndrome
    - Factor V Leiden homozygous mutation
    - Protein C or S deficiency
  - Inflammation
    - Takayasu arteritis
    - Kawasaki disease
  - Infection
    - Syphilis
    - Sepsis

MACROSCOPIC

- Hemorrhagic necrosis
- Wedge infarct

MICROSCOPIC

- Arterial thrombus
  - Lines of Zahn
  - Distension of renal artery
- Diffuse cortical necrosis
- Interstitial hemorrhage
- Acute tubular injury

TOP DIFFERENTIAL DIAGNOSES

- Thrombotic microangiopathy
- Renal vein thrombosis
- Atheromatous emboli
- Renal artery stenosis
- Acute tubular necrosis

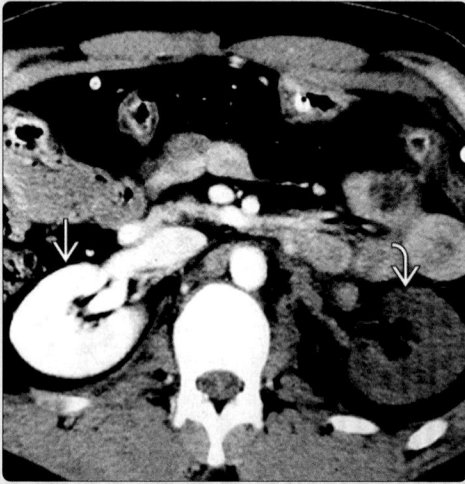

(Left) *Contrast-enhanced CT shows normal enhancement of the right kidney ➡ with no enhancement of the left kidney ↷, indicating acute thrombosis of the left renal artery. This patient was involved in an MVA.* **(Right)** *Hematoxylin & eosin reveals a thrombus → at the bifurcation of this large renal artery from a nephrectomy specimen in a female patient with numerous thrombi throughout her vasculature.*

Renal Artery Thrombus

Acute Thrombus

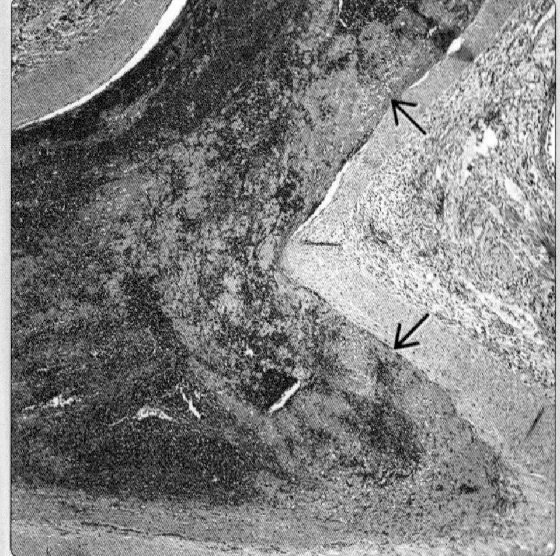

(Left) *Hematoxylin & eosin demonstrates prominent leukocyte infiltration of the intima → and loose intimal thickening in a segment of a renal artery downstream from a renal artery thrombus.* **(Right)** *Hematoxylin & eosin reveals diffuse cortical necrosis → with interstitial hemorrhage ➡ in this young female with a renal artery thrombus.*

Arterial Intimal Changes

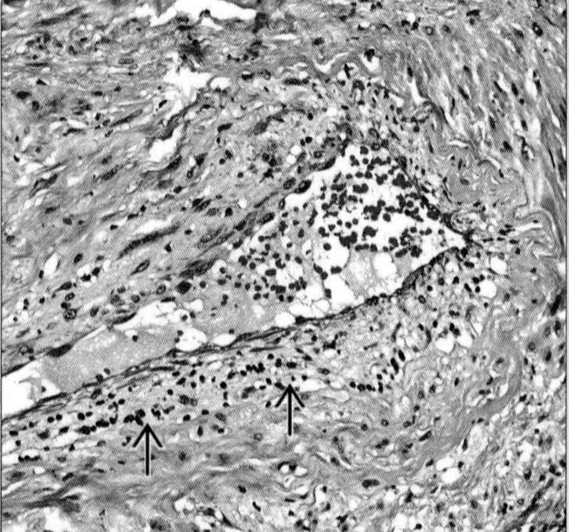

Hemorrhagic Necrosis

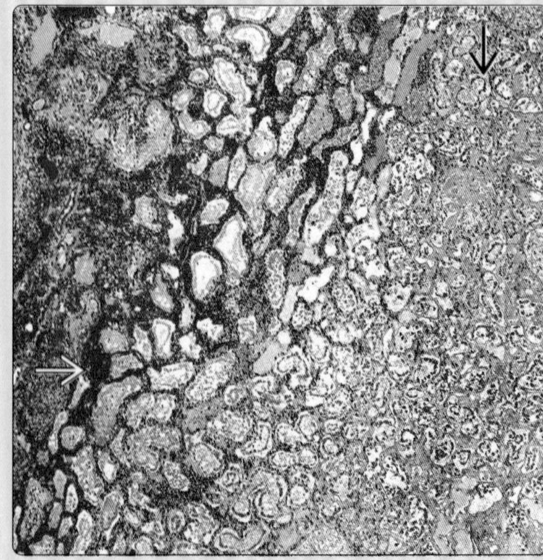

TERMINOLOGY

Definitions

- Thrombus of main renal artery

ETIOLOGY/PATHOGENESIS

Risk Factors

- Renal artery stenosis
  - Rupture of atherosclerotic plaques can lead to renal artery thrombosis
- Fibromuscular dysplasia
- Renal artery or abdominal aortic aneurysm
- Trauma
  - Motor vehicle accident (MVA)
  - Complication of surgical procedure or instrumentation
- Hypercoagulable state
  - Antiphospholipid antibody syndrome
  - Factor V Leiden homozygous mutation
  - Protein C deficiency
  - Protein S deficiency
  - Heparin-induced thrombocytopenia
- Inflammation
  - Takayasu arteritis
  - Kawasaki disease
  - Polyarteritis nodosa
- Infection
  - Syphilis
  - Sepsis
- Cocaine use
- Nephrotic syndrome
  - Rare

CLINICAL ISSUES

Epidemiology

- Incidence
  - Dependent on underlying disease or predisposing risk factors

Presentation

- Acute renal failure
- Flank pain
- Hypertension
- Hematuria

Laboratory Tests

- Serologic tests
  - Work-up for hypercoagulable state

Treatment

- Surgical approaches
  - Surgical exploration
  - Thrombectomy
- Drugs
  - Anticoagulation
  - Fibrinolytic therapy

IMAGING

CT Findings

- Occlusion of renal artery with nonenhancement of involved kidney
  - Kidney will infarct and become smaller over time

MACROSCOPIC

General Features

- Hemorrhagic necrosis
- Wedge infarct

MICROSCOPIC

Histologic Features

- Arterial thrombus
  - Distension of renal artery
  - Lines of Zahn
    - Indicates thrombus formed gradually in flowing blood
    - Layers of platelets/fibrin alternating with red blood cells
- Diffuse cortical necrosis
- Interstitial hemorrhage
- Acute tubular injury

DIFFERENTIAL DIAGNOSIS

Thrombotic Microangiopathy

- Thrombi involving arteries, arterioles, or glomerular capillaries

Renal Vein Thrombosis

- Thrombi in vein, venules, or glomerular capillaries
- Glomerular or peritubular capillary dilatation

Renal Artery Stenosis

- Hypertension
- Marked narrowing of main renal arterial lumen

Atheromatous Emboli

- Presence of cholesterol clefts within occluded artery

Acute Tubular Injury/Necrosis

- Prominent tubular injury with loss of proximal tubular brush borders or cell sloughing into tubular lumina

SELECTED REFERENCES

1. Tektonidou MG: Renal involvement in the antiphospholipid syndrome (APS)-APS nephropathy. Clin Rev Allergy Immunol. 36(2-3):131-40, 2009
2. Balci YI et al: Nonstroke arterial thrombosis in children: Hacettepe experience. Blood Coagul Fibrinolysis. 19(6):519-24, 2008
3. Tsugawa K et al: Renal artery thrombosis in a pediatric case of systemic lupus erythematosus without antiphospholipid antibodies. Pediatr Nephrol. 20(11):1648-50, 2005
4. Nishimura M et al: Acute arterial thrombosis with antithrombin III deficiency in nephrotic syndrome: report of a case. Surg Today. 30(7):663-6, 2000
5. Klinge J et al: Selective thrombolysis in a newborn with bilateral renal venous and cerebral thrombosis and heterozygous APC resistance. Nephrol Dial Transplant. 13(12):3205-7, 1998
6. Le Moine A et al: Acute renal artery thrombosis associated with factor V Leiden mutation. Nephrol Dial Transplant. 11(10):2067-9, 1996
7. Farkas JC et al: Arterial thrombosis: a rare complication of the nephrotic syndrome. Cardiovasc Surg. 1(3):265-9, 1993

Atheromatous Emboli

KEY FACTS

TERMINOLOGY

- Vascular disease caused by embolization of dislodged components, atheromatous plaques

ETIOLOGY/PATHOGENESIS

- Severe atherosclerosis
- Precipitating causes
  - Invasive vascular procedure
  - Cardiopulmonary resuscitation
  - Anticoagulant or thrombolytic therapy
  - Trauma
  - ~ 24% spontaneous

CLINICAL ISSUES

- Clinical presentation
  - Acute renal failure
  - Hypertension
  - Proteinuria, hematuria
  - Eosinophilia
- Treatment
  - HMG-CoA reductase inhibitors
  - Avoidance of anticoagulation

MACROSCOPIC

- Nobbled surface due to vascular scars

MICROSCOPIC

- Atheroembolus
  - Cholesterol clefts: Crystals dissolved by formalin fixation
  - Acute lesion surrounded by red blood cells, fibrin, or leukocytes
  - Chronic lesion embedded within intimal fibrosis
  - Multinucleated giant cell reaction may be present

TOP DIFFERENTIAL DIAGNOSES

- Thrombotic microangiopathy
- Arteriosclerosis
- Vasculitis
- Tissue artifact

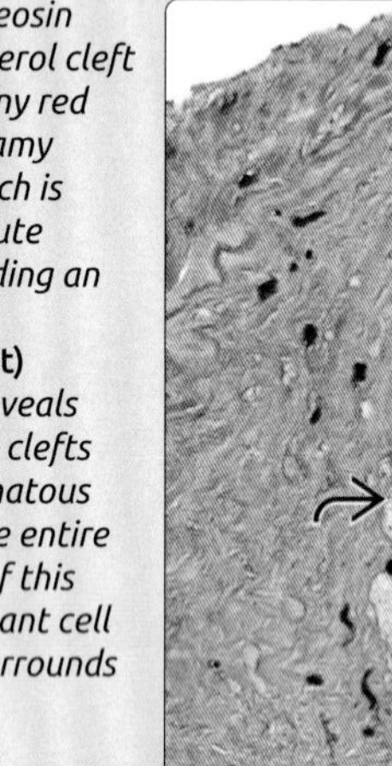

(Left) *Hematoxylin & eosin shows a large cholesterol cleft → surrounded by many red blood cells → and foamy macrophages →, which is consistent with an acute atheroembolus occluding an artery with severe atherosclerosis.* **(Right)** *Periodic acid-Schiff reveals numerous cholesterol clefts → of a large atheromatous embolus occluding the entire longitudinal section of this interlobar artery. A giant cell histiocytic reaction surrounds the individual clefts.*

Acute Atheroembolus

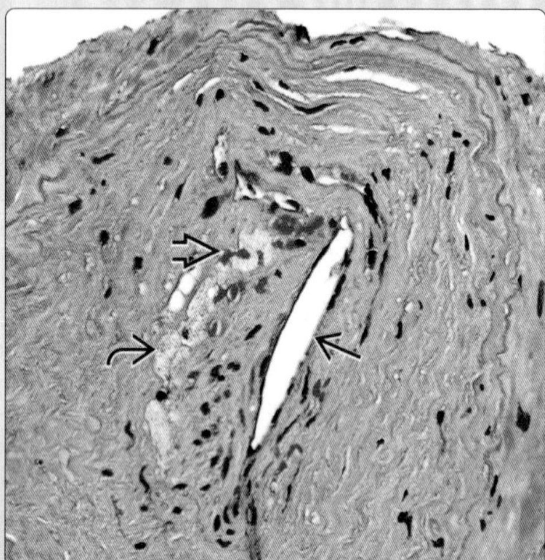

Large Atheroembolus

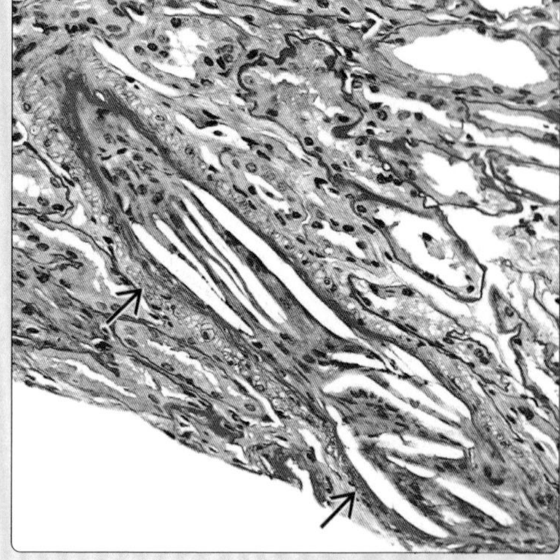

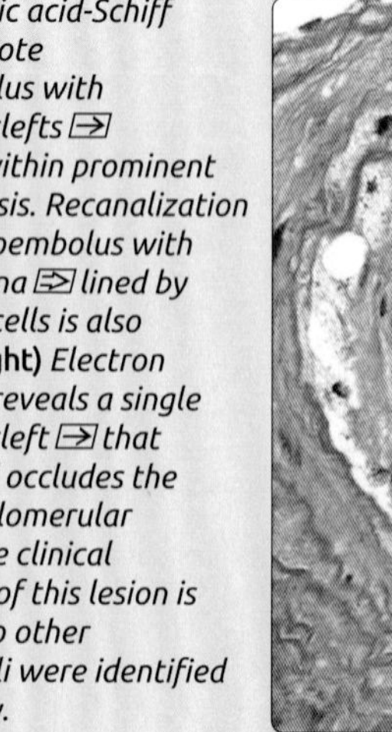

(Left) *Periodic acid-Schiff shows a remote atheroembolus with cholesterol clefts → embedded within prominent intimal fibrosis. Recanalization of the atheroembolus with slit-like lumina → lined by endothelial cells is also present.* **(Right)** *Electron micrograph reveals a single cholesterol cleft → that distends and occludes the lumen of a glomerular capillary. The clinical significance of this lesion is unclear as no other atheroemboli were identified in this biopsy.*

Chronic Atheroembolus

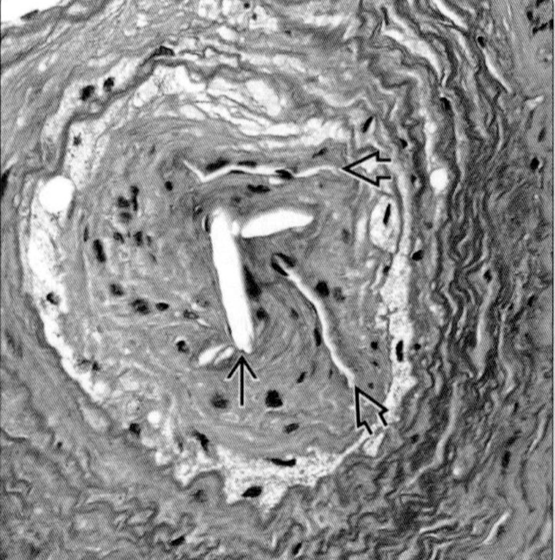

Glomerular Capillary Atheroembolus

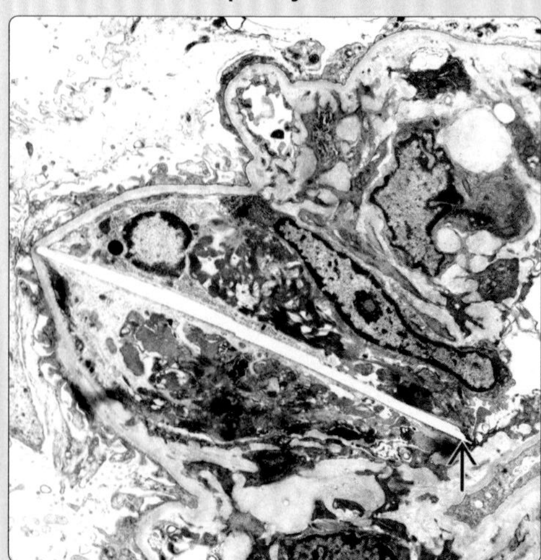

TERMINOLOGY

Synonyms

- Atheroembolic renal disease
- Cholesterol crystal emboli

Definitions

- Vascular disease caused by embolization of dislodged components, atheromatous plaques

ETIOLOGY/PATHOGENESIS

Risk Factors

- Severe atherosclerosis
    - Hypertension, diabetes mellitus, smoking, hypercholesterolemia

Precipitating Event: Plaque Disruption

- Iatrogenic (~ 76% of cases)
    - Invasive vascular procedure
        - Coronary artery bypass
        - Aortic aneurysm repair
        - Angioplasty or angiography
    - Cardiopulmonary resuscitation
    - Anticoagulant or thrombolytic therapy
- Spontaneous (~ 24% of cases)
- Trauma

Embolization

- Elicits inflammatory response, thrombosis, ischemia

CLINICAL ISSUES

Epidemiology

- Incidence
    - 5-10% of acute renal failure cases
    - 77% of abdominal aortic aneurysm repairs
    - 0.5-2% of tumor nephrectomies
    - 0.8-4.4% of autopsies
- Age
    - > 60 years old

Presentation

- Acute renal failure (20-30%)
- Subacute or chronic renal failure (70-80%)
- Skin lesions (35-90%)
    - Livedo reticularis, blue toe, gangrene, palpable purpura
- Eosinophilia (22-73%), transient
- GI signs (10-33%)
- Retinal emboli (7-25%); Hollenhorst plaques
- Proteinuria usually minimal
    - May be nephrotic range in association with diabetes or focal segmental glomerulosclerosis
- Fever, myalgia, weight loss
- Hypertension

Treatment

- Drugs
    - HMG-CoA reductase inhibitors to stabilize plaques
    - Steroids controversial
    - Avoidance of anticoagulation

Prognosis

- 33-61% require dialysis; 21-39% recover function
- 13-81% 1-year mortality
- Hypertension or preexisting renal disease predict poor outcome

MACROSCOPIC

General Features

- Nobbled surface due to vascular scars, infarcts

MICROSCOPIC

Histologic Features

- Glomeruli
    - Ischemic global or segmental glomerulosclerosis
    - Rare cholesterol emboli
- Tubules and interstitium
    - Acute tubular injury
    - Interstitial fibrosis and tubular atrophy
- Arteries/arterioles
    - Atheroemboli
        - Slit-like cholesterol clefts
            - Crystals dissolved by formalin fixation
        - Acute lesion surrounded by red blood cells, fibrin, neutrophils, eosinophils
        - Chronic lesion embedded within cellular intimal fibrosis
        - Multinucleated giant cell reaction often present
        - Recanalization of vessels may occur
    - Intimal fibrosis/elastosis

ANCILLARY TESTS

Immunofluorescence

- Fibrin in arteries affected

Electron Microscopy

- Podocyte foot process effacement may be present
- Rare cholesterol crystals in glomerular capillaries

DIFFERENTIAL DIAGNOSIS

Artifact

- Arterioles and small arteries may have slit-like lumen that mimic cholesterol clefts
- Artifact due to compression, forceps, or tissue processing

Arteriosclerosis

- Severe intimal fibrosis
- No cholesterol clefts in severely narrowed lumen

Thrombotic Microangiopathy

- Thrombi without cholesterol clefts

Vasculitis

- Clinical presentation can suggest vasculitis
- Inflammation extends through wall

SELECTED REFERENCES

1. Scolari F et al: Atheroembolic renal disease. Lancet. 375(9726):1650-60, 2010
2. Mittal BV et al: Atheroembolic renal disease: a silent masquerader. Kidney Int. 73(1):126-30, 2008

SECTION 4
Tubulointerstitial Diseases

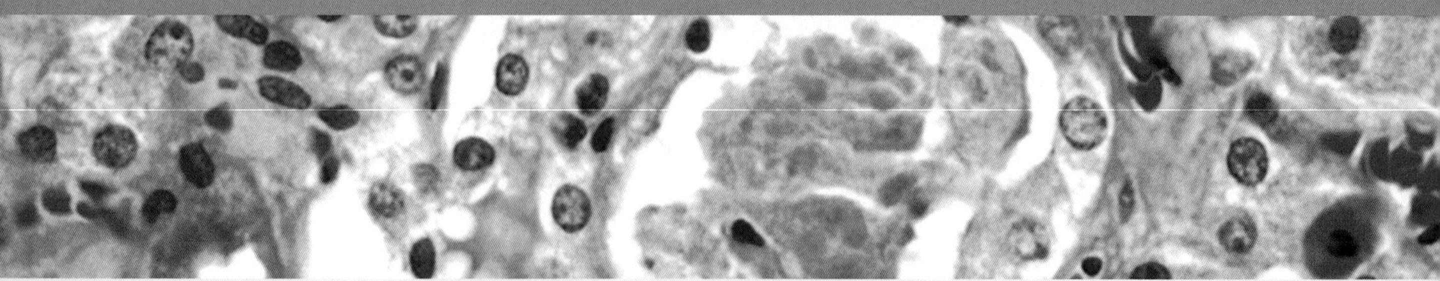

Ischemic Injury

Drug-Induced Tubulointerstitial Diseases

Toxic Injury

Immunologic Tubular Disease

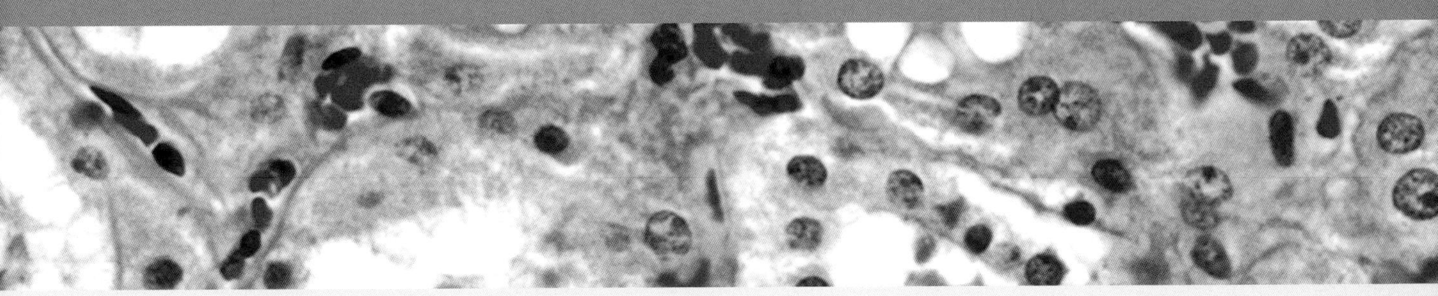

Autosomal Dominant Tubulointerstitial Kidney Disease

Genetic Crystal Depostion Diseases

Genetic Transport Diseases

Other Genetic Diseases Affecting Tubules

Miscellaneous Tubulointerstitial Diseases

TERMINOLOGY

Abbreviations

- Acute interstitial nephritis (AIN)
- Chronic interstitial nephritis (CIN)
- Acute tubular injury (ATI)

Synonyms

- Tubulointerstitial nephritis
- Interstitial nephritis

Definitions

- Group of diseases primarily manifested by inflammation &/or injury of renal tubules and interstitium

APPROACH TO DIAGNOSIS OF TUBULOINTERSTITIAL DISEASES

Biopsy

- Appearances often similar despite varied mechanisms
- Search for etiologic agent (organisms) or distinctive pathologic features (granulomata, eosinophils, plasma cells, neutrophils, antibody/immune complex deposition, crystals, viral inclusions)
- General tools
  - Light microscopy
    - Special stains (PAS, silver methenamine, Giemsa, Brown-Breen, acid fast)
    - Granuloma (sarcoid, drug allergy, infection, polyangiitis with granulomatosis, gout, idiopathic)
    - Polarized light for crystals, also processing in nonaqueous solutions (urates)
    - Immunohistochemistry or in situ hybridization for organisms (polyomavirus, adenovirus, CMV, EBER)
    - Casts (myoglobin, hemoglobin, bile/bilirubin, light chain)
  - Immunofluorescence microscopy
    - IgG, IgA, IgM, C3, C1q, fibrinogen, kappa, lambda
    - TBM: Immune complexes, anti-TBM antibodies, monoclonal light chain deposition
  - Electron microscopy
    - Organisms (viruses, bacteria, microsporidia) or distinctive deposits (immune complexes in TBM, light chains, crystals)

Clinical Information

- Careful clinical history may provide clues
  - Drug exposure, work, family history, travel, rash, fever, other systemic symptoms
  - Over the counter drugs or herbal supplements may not be mentioned by patient

Laboratory Tests

- Blood tests for autoantibodies (Sjögren, anti-TBM), IgG4, functional tests for enzymes, electrolyte and metabolite levels, genetic screen
- Screening for organisms, molecular tests, cultures, antibodies
- Urinalysis for organisms, crystals, leukocytes, eosinophils, and casts

Radiologic Studies

- Evidence of hydronephrosis, obstruction, perfusion, kidney size, stones

SELECTED REFERENCES

1. Praga M et al: Changes in the aetiology, clinical presentation and management of acute interstitial nephritis, an increasingly common cause of acute kidney injury. Nephrol Dial Transplant. ePub, 2014
2. Raghavan R et al: Acute interstitial nephritis - a reappraisal and update. Clin Nephrol. 82(3):149-62, 2014
3. Airy M et al: Tubulointerstitial nephritis and cancer chemotherapy: update on a neglected clinical entity. Nephrol Dial Transplant. 28(10):2502-9, 2013
4. Hodgkins KS et al: Tubulointerstitial injury and the progression of chronic kidney disease. Pediatr Nephrol. 27(6):901-9, 2012
5. Praga M et al: Acute interstitial nephritis. Kidney Int. 77(11):956-61, 2010
6. Colvin RB et al: Interstitial nephritis. In Tisher CC et al: Renal Pathology. 2nd ed. Philadelphia: JB Lippincott. 723-68, 1994
7. Cameron JS: Immunologically mediated interstitial nephritis: primary and secondary. Adv Nephrol Necker Hosp. 18:207-48, 1989
8. Papper S: Interstitial nephritis. Contrib Nephrol. 23:204-19, 1980
9. Heptinstall RH: Interstitial nephritis. A brief review. Am J Pathol. 83(1):213-36, 1976
10. Councilman WT: Acute Interstitial Nephritis. J Exp Med. 3(4-5):393-420, 1898

Tubulitis

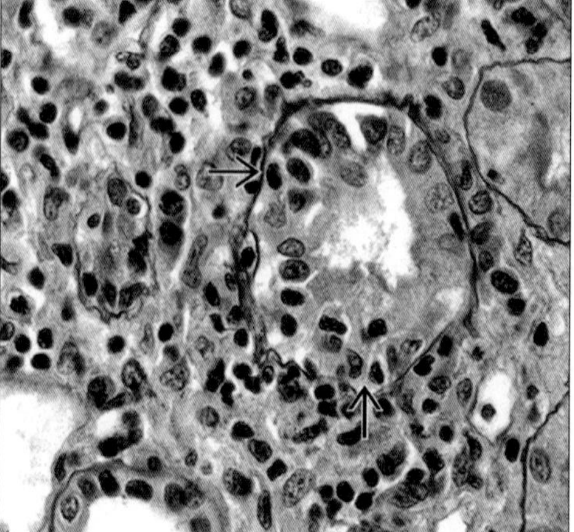

Cast

(Left) *Tubulitis, invasion of tubules by lymphocytes →, is a common finding in immunologically mediated tubulointerstitial disease, as illustrated in this example associated with uveitis (TINU syndrome).* **(Right)** *Casts may reveal an etiology, as in this case of rhabdomyolysis due to a statin drug. The granular material stained for myoglobin by immunohistochemistry, but looks identical to hemoglobin or bile casts.*

Etiologic Classification of Tubulointerstitial Diseases (With Selected Examples)	
Genetic	
	Ciliopathies (e.g., nephronophthisis group)
	Autosomal dominant tubulointerstitial kidney diseases (*UMOD, MUC1, HNF1β*)
	Mitochondrionopathies
	Adenine phosphoribosyl transferase deficiency
Infection	
Direct infection	Polyomavirus nephropathy
	Acute pyelonephritis
	Tuberculosis
	Brucellosis
Indirect effects	Streptococcal infection
Immunologic	
Exogenous antigen	Drug-induced interstitial nephritis
Auto-antigen	Sjögren syndrome
	Anti-TBM disease
	Anti-brush border antibody disease
Allogeneic antigen	Acute cellular allograft rejection
Unknown antigen	Sarcoidosis
	IgG4-Systemic disease
	Tubulo-interstitial nephritis with uveitis (Dobrin syndrome)
	Idiopathic hypocomplementemic interstitial nephritis
Toxic	
	Lithium nephropathy
	Calcineurin inhibitor toxicity
	Chemotherapy
	Aristolochic acid nephropathy (Balkan and Chinese herb nephropathies)
	Spice (recreational drug)
	Heavy metal poisoning
Metabolic	
	Nephrocalcinosis
	Acute phosphate nephropathy
	Gouty (Urate) nephropathy
	Secondary oxalosis
	Bile cast nephropathy
Ischemia	
	Acute tubular injury (e.g., shock)
	Rhabdomyolysis
Obstruction	
	Benign prostatic hypertrophy
Radiation	
	Radiation interstitial nephritis
Neoplastic	
	Myeloma cast nephropathy
	Light chain tubulopathy
Idiopathic	
	Behçet disease
	Karyomegalic interstitial nephritis

Differential Diagnosis of Acute Interstitial Nephritis

KEY FACTS

TERMINOLOGY

- Acute interstitial inflammation, commonly also involving tubules, due to variety of causes

ETIOLOGY/PATHOGENESIS

- Drugs
  - May account for 60-70% of AIN cases
- Autoimmune
- Infection
- Hereditary/toxic/metabolic

CLINICAL ISSUES

- ~ 15-27% of renal biopsies for acute renal failure show AIN
- Treatment: Discontinuation of causative drug in drug-related AIN; corticosteroids (controversial)

MICROSCOPIC

- Interstitial inflammation with lymphocytes, monocytes/macrophages, eosinophils, plasma cells
- High number of eosinophils suggestive of allergic AIN but not specific
- Tubulitis
- Interstitial fibrosis may be present

TOP DIFFERENTIAL DIAGNOSES

- Drug-induced interstitial nephritis
- Sarcoidosis
- IgG4-related systemic disease
- Light chain deposition disease
- Infection
- Acute cellular rejection in renal allograft
- Interstitial inflammation associated with glomerular disease
- Hematopoietic neoplasm

Acute Allergic Interstitial Nephritis

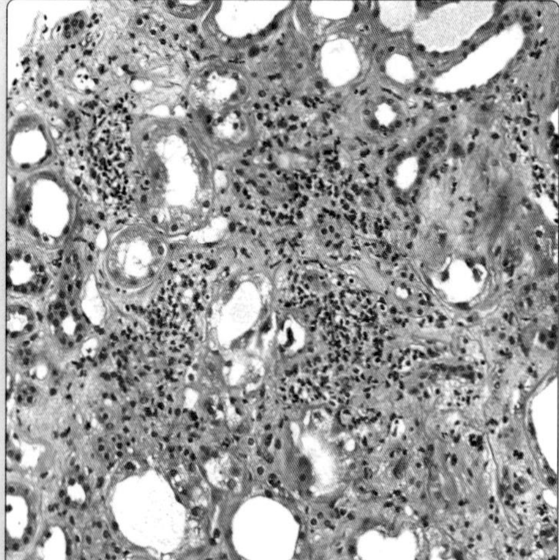

Acute Allergic Interstitial Nephritis

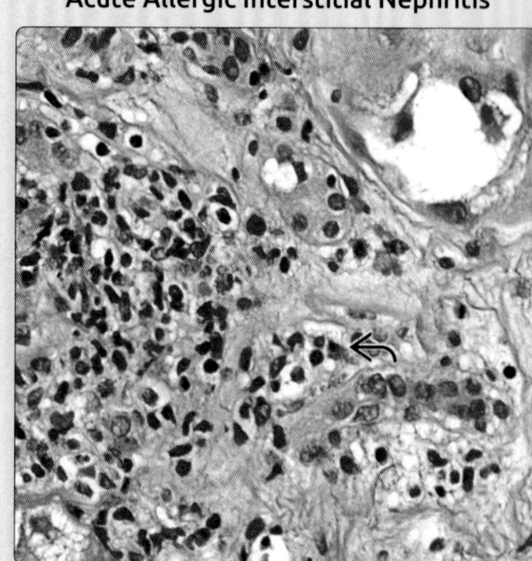

(Left) *Acute interstitial nephritis is a heterogeneous group of diseases. This case in a 78-year-old man with acute renal failure was due to a recent exposure to antibiotics.* **(Right)** *Eosinophilic tubulitis ➾ is seen in a case of acute allergic interstitial nephritis due to antibiotics, regarded as a useful sign of drug-induced AIN, although the specificity has not been proven.*

BK Polyomavirus

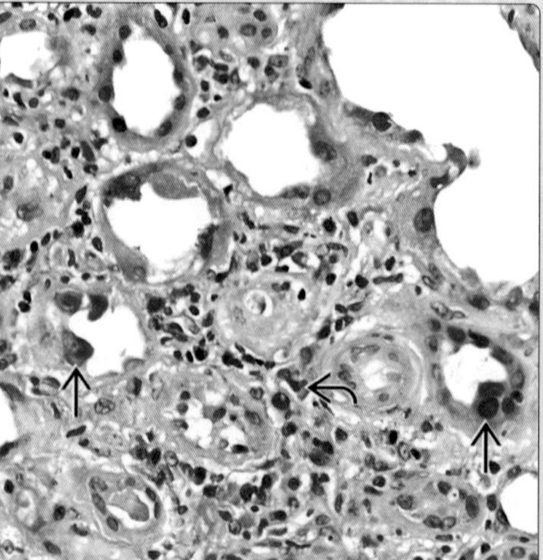

BK Polyomavirus

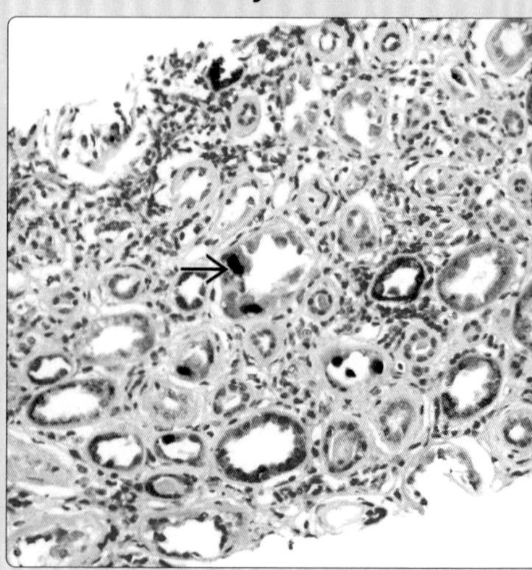

(Left) *BK polyomavirus tubulointerstitial nephritis shows interstitial inflammation with increased plasma cells ➾ in an allograft. Some tubular epithelial cells show viral cytopathic effect ➙.* **(Right)** *In situ hybridization for BK polyomavirus reveals several tubules with positive epithelial cell nuclei ➙. Polyoma can also be readily detected by immunohistochemistry, using an antibody to the large T antigen.*

ETIOLOGY/PATHOGENESIS

Drugs

- May account for 60-70% of acute interstitial nephritis (AIN)
- Allergic (e.g., antibiotics, proton pump inhibitors, nonsteroidal anti-inflammatory drugs [NSAIDs])
- Toxic (e.g., cisplatinum, lithium, NSAIDs)

Autoimmune

- Primary in kidney
  - e.g., anti-tubular basement membrane (TBM) disease
- Associated with systemic disease
  - e.g., Sjögren syndrome, tubulointerstitial nephritis with uveitis (TINU) syndrome, IgG4-related systemic disease

Infection

- Direct infection
  - Bacteria (e.g., pyelonephritis), mycobacteria
  - Virus (e.g., BK polyomavirus tubulointerstitial nephritis)
  - Other, including parasites
- Reaction to distant infection (e.g., poststreptococcal GN)

Hereditary/Toxic/Metabolic

- e.g., hyperoxaluria, gout, heavy metal toxicity
- Typically chronic injury, less inflammation

Idiopathic

- Accounts for ~ 25% of cases

CLINICAL ISSUES

Epidemiology

- Incidence
  - ~ 15-27% of biopsies for acute renal failure show AIN

Presentation

- Acute or subacute renal failure
- Proteinuria, subnephrotic
- Microhematuria
- Pyuria
- Eosinophiluria
- In drug-related AIN, renal failure may be accompanied by rash, fever, arthralgias, and eosinophilia
- Clinical history important to determine cause of AIN
  - Recent (a week to months) exposure to new drug may suggest allergic AIN
  - Longer period of exposure prior to AIN associated with NSAID use

Treatment

- Drugs
  - Corticosteroids
    - May be of benefit in some cases with more acute onset of AIN
  - Cytotoxic drugs (e.g., cyclophosphamide) and plasmapheresis may be used in anti-TBM disease
- Discontinuation of causative drug in drug-related AIN

MICROSCOPIC

Histologic Features

- Interstitial inflammation with lymphocytes, macrophages, plasma cells, and eosinophils
  - High number of eosinophils suggest allergic AIN but not specific
  - Increased plasma cells suggest autoimmune AIN but not specific
- Interstitial edema
- Tubulitis
- Acute tubular injury
- Granulomatous AIN
  - Nonnecrotizing granulomas in sarcoidosis and drug-related AIN
  - Poorer prognosis in drug-related AIN
- Interstitial fibrosis / tubular atrophy when chronic

Immunofluorescence

- Granular TBM deposits in some cases of autoimmune interstitial nephritis
- Linear TBM deposits in anti-TBM disease

Electron Microscopy

- Amorphous, electron-dense deposits in TBMs in some cases of autoimmune interstitial nephritis

DIFFERENTIAL DIAGNOSIS

Diverse Causes of AIN Pattern on Biopsy

- AIN may be due to drugs, autoimmune disease, infection, hereditary/toxic/metabolic, idiopathic

Granulomatous AIN

- Type of AIN; most commonly allergic drug reactions or sarcoidosis
- Rarely direct infection (e.g., tuberculosis)

Interstitial Inflammation Associated With Glomerular Disease

- Glomerulonephritis (GN)
  - Pauci-immune necrotizing and crescentic GN
  - IgA nephropathy
  - Acute postinfectious GN
  - Other
- Focal segmental glomerulosclerosis, collapsing variant

Neoplasm

- Infiltrating lymphoid neoplasm or plasma cell myeloma

Light Chain Deposition Disease (Monoclonal Immunoglobulin Deposition Disease)

- Interstitial inflammation and acute tubular injury
- Linear glomerular and tubular basement membrane immunofluorescence staining by monoclonal protein
- Finely granular, electron-dense deposits in basement membranes seen by electron microscopy

Acute Cellular Rejection in Renal Allograft

- May be indistinguishable from AIN

SELECTED REFERENCES

1. Dai DF et al: Interstitial eosinophilic aggregates in diabetic nephropathy: allergy or not? Nephrol Dial Transplant. ePub, 2015
2. Muriithi AK et al: Biopsy-proven acute interstitial nephritis, 1993-2011: a case series. Am J Kidney Dis. 64(4):558-66, 2014
3. Perazella MA et al: Drug-induced acute interstitial nephritis. Nat Rev Nephrol. 6(8):461-70, 2010
4. Praga M et al: Acute interstitial nephritis. Kidney Int. 77(11):956-61, 2010

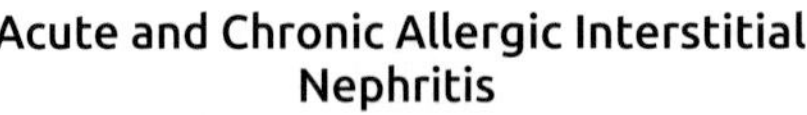

Acute and Chronic Allergic Interstitial Nephritis

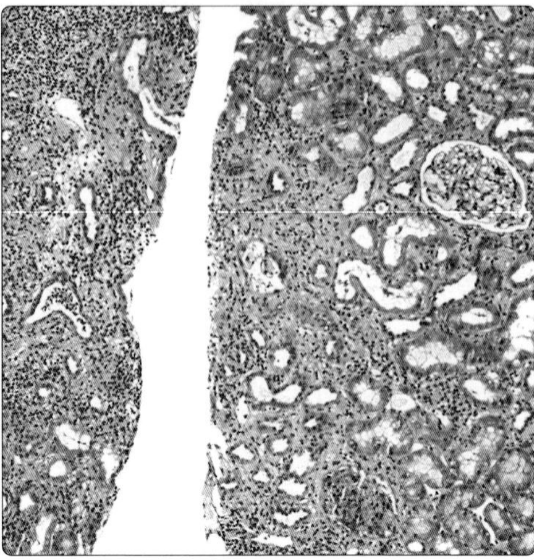

Acute and Chronic Interstitial Nephritis

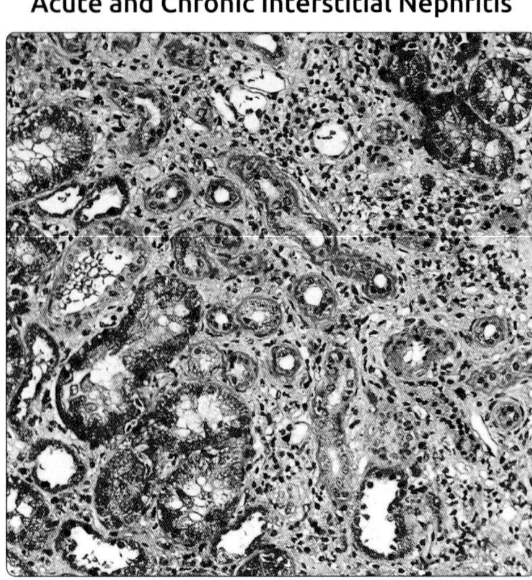

(Left) *H&E shows acute and chronic allergic tubulointerstitial nephritis with diffuse interstitial inflammation. This patient had been taking a number of herbal preparations for many months, after which she was found to have an elevated serum creatinine. Immunofluorescence staining was negative.* **(Right)** *This case of AIN also showed areas of interstitial fibrosis with inflammation. The fibrosis is indicative of a chronic component of the interstitial nephritis (trichome stain).*

Acute Pyelonephritis

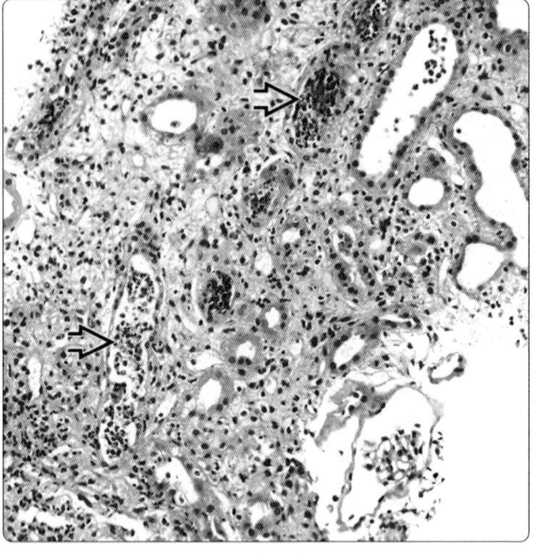

Acute Pyelonephritis

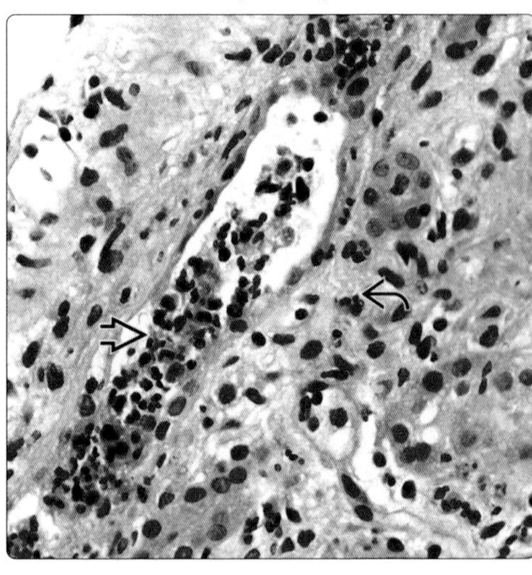

(Left) *Acute interstitial inflammation with mononuclear cells and neutrophils is seen in a case of acute pyelonephritis. Neutrophilic casts are present ➾. This biopsy is from a renal transplant patient who had laboratory evidence of a urinary tract infection.* **(Right)** *A neutrophilic cast ➾ within a tubule is seen in acute pyelonephritis. Neutrophils are also present within the interstitium ↶. Occasional neutrophil casts can be seen for no apparent reason in end-stage kidneys.*

Diabetic Glomerulosclerosis and Allergic AIN

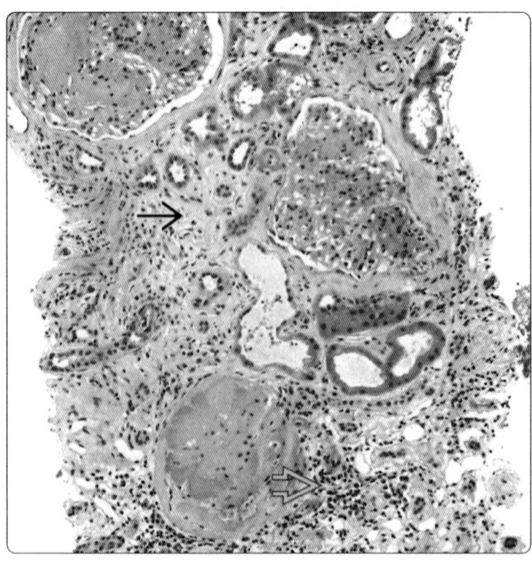

Diabetic Glomerulosclerosis and Allergic AIN

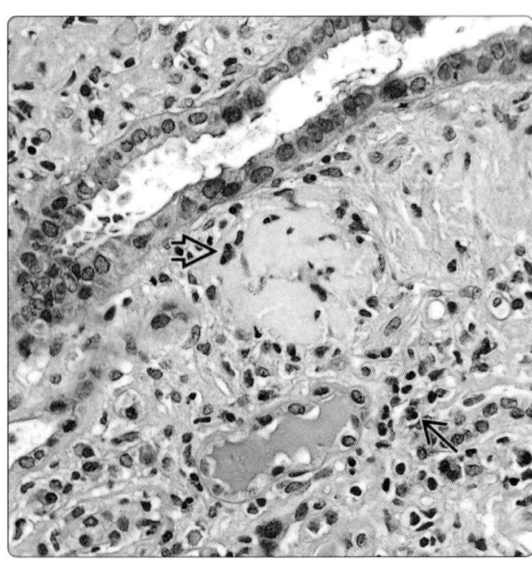

(Left) *This biopsy shows nodular diabetic glomerulosclerosis as well as interstitial edema → and increased inflammation ➾.* **(Right)** *This example of diabetic glomerulosclerosis and AIN shows eosinophils in the interstitium → and embedded within proteinaceous cast material ➾. This patient had acute renal failure and recent exposure to antibiotics. Increased eosinophils have been observed in patients with diabetes, but patients with diabetes may also develop allergic AIN.*

Sjögren Syndrome

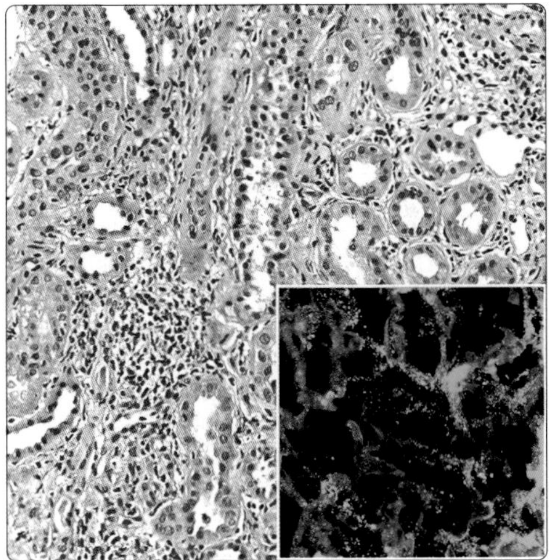

Sarcoidosis

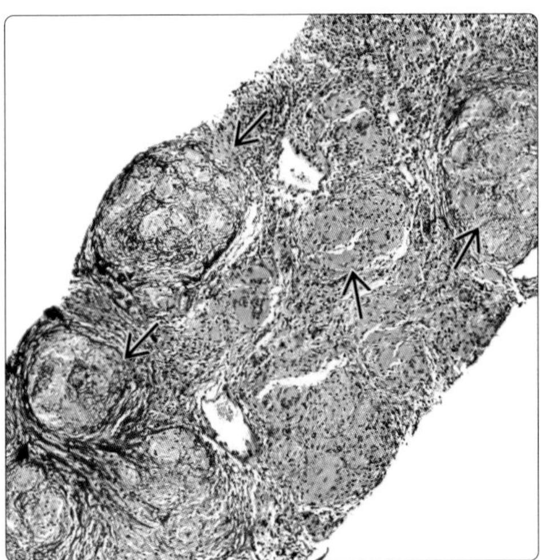

(Left) *Tubulointerstitial nephritis with mononuclear cells and plasma cells is seen in Sjögren syndrome. Tubular basement membrane immune complex deposits (inset, immunofluorescence staining for IgG) aid in the diagnosis of an autoimmune interstitial nephritis.* **(Right)** *Renal biopsy is shown from a 50-year-old man with a history of sarcoidosis and progressive renal failure over several months. This case shows extensive involvement by nonnecrotizing granulomatous inflammation ➙.*

TINU Syndrome

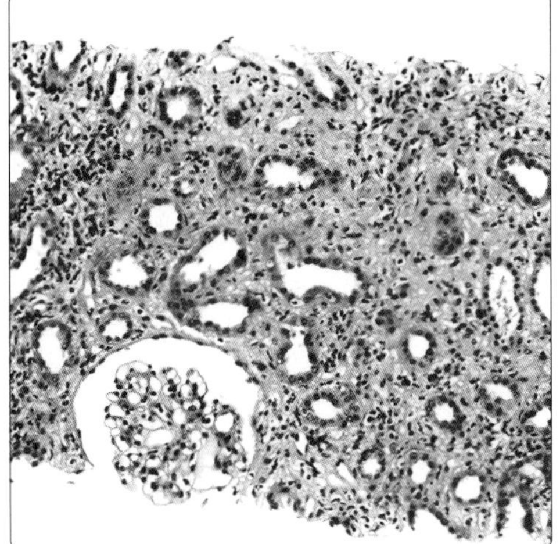

TINU Syndrome

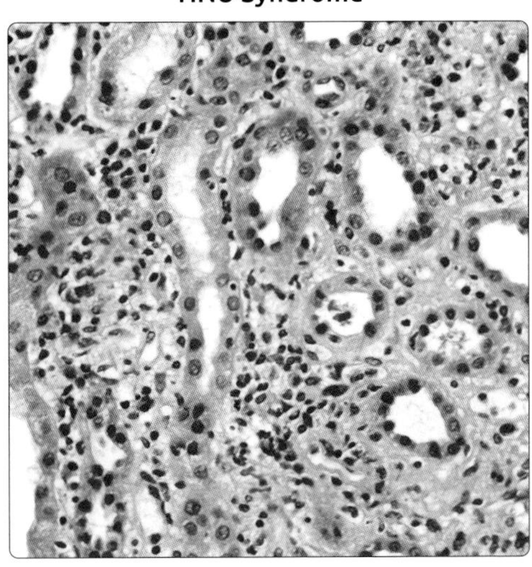

(Left) *AIN is seen in a 10-year-old girl who presented with acute renal failure. Several weeks prior, she had a cough and fever; no antibiotics were given. Four months later, the patient developed uveitis and was diagnosed with tubulointerstitial nephritis-uveitis (TINU) syndrome.* **(Right)** *The infiltrate in this case of TINU syndrome is composed of mononuclear cells, plasma cells, and eosinophils, mimicking drug-induced AIN, but this patient was on no medications.*

IgG4-Related Tubulointerstitial Nephritis

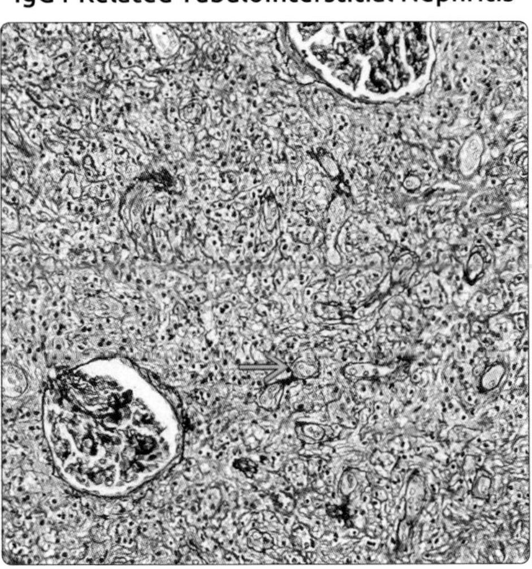

IgG4(+) Plasma Cells

(Left) *This example of IgG4-related tubulointerstitial nephritis shows interstitial plasma cell-rich inflammation with "storiform" fibrosis. Residual tubular basement membranes ➙ are seen on this silver stain.* **(Right)** *In IgG4-related tubulointerstitial nephritis, there is a marked increase (> 30 cells/HPF) in IgG4(+) plasma cells.*

(Left) *Hyperoxaluria related to gastric bypass shows interstitial fibrosis and tubular atrophy with interstitial mononuclear cell inflammation ⇨. Focal tubules contain calcium oxalate crystals ↪. Usually this condition does not have a florid inflammatory component, in contrast to the usual AIN.* **(Right)** *A form of hereditary interstitial nephritis/nephropathy is shown with chronic tubulointerstitial nephritis ⇨ in a patient with a mutation in the gene for renin.*

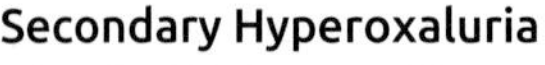

Secondary Hyperoxaluria

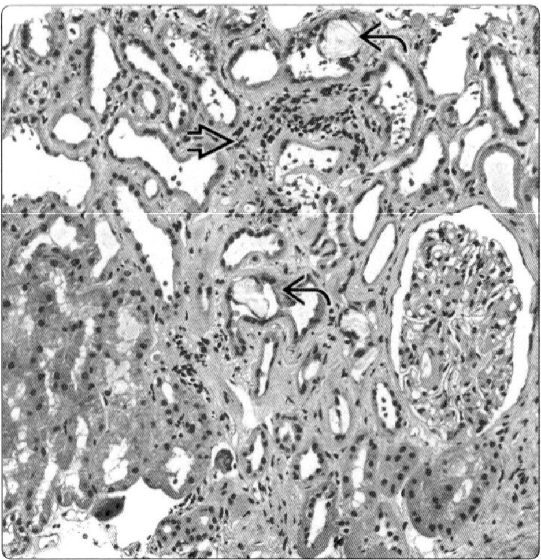

Hereditary Interstitial Nephritis/Nephropathy

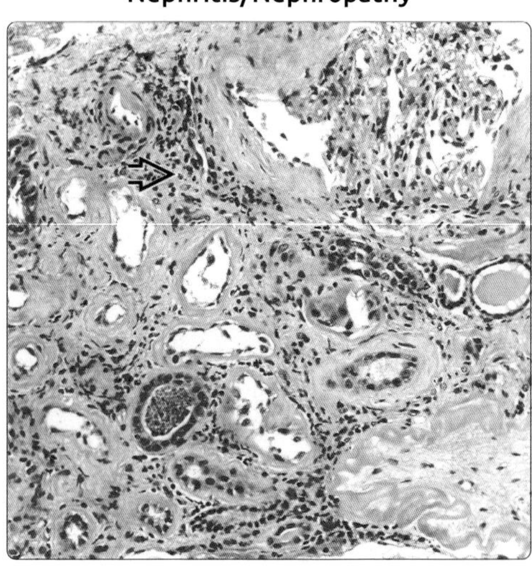

(Left) *Urate nephropathy shows interstitial inflammation ⇨ surrounding dissolved urate crystals ↪ in a patient with a history of gout and chronic renal failure.* **(Right)** *Acute postinfectious glomerulonephritis often shows focal interstitial inflammation, including several neutrophils ⇨ as shown here. A glomerulus shows an acute exudative glomerulonephritis ⇾.*

Urate Nephropathy

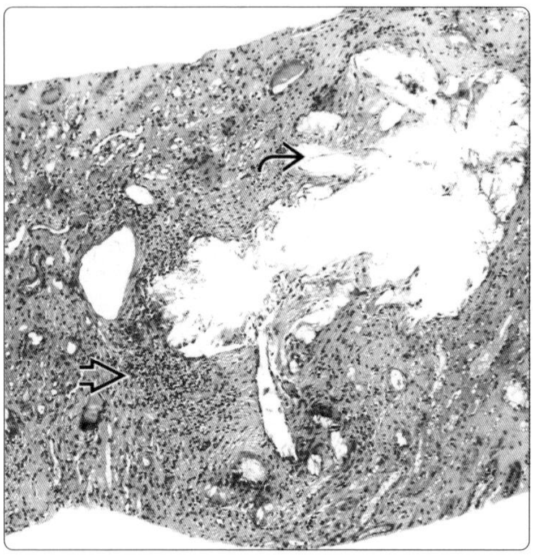

Interstitial Inflammation Secondary to Glomerulonephritis

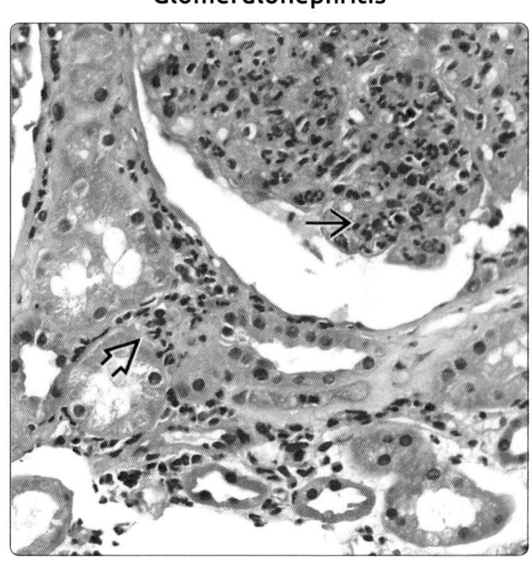

(Left) *Interstitial inflammation ⇨ is seen in a case of light chain deposition disease (LCDD). A glomerulus shows a nodular glomerulosclerosis ↪.* **(Right)** *This case showed bright linear glomerular and tubular basement membrane staining for lambda light chain but not kappa light chain by IF, although most cases of LCDD show kappa light chain. Electron microscopy showed finely granular glomerular and tubular basement membrane deposits.*

Light Chain Deposition Disease

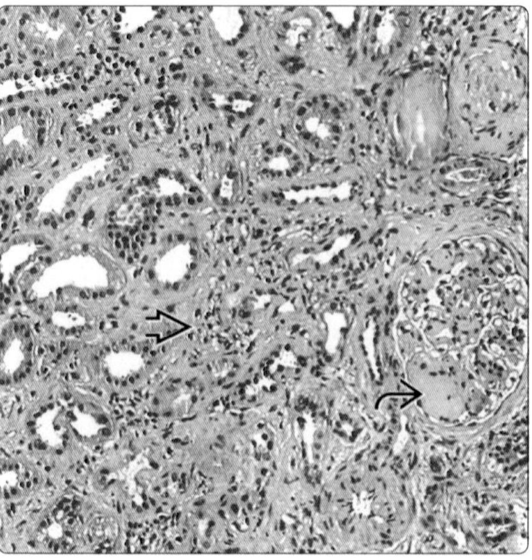

Light Chain Deposition Disease

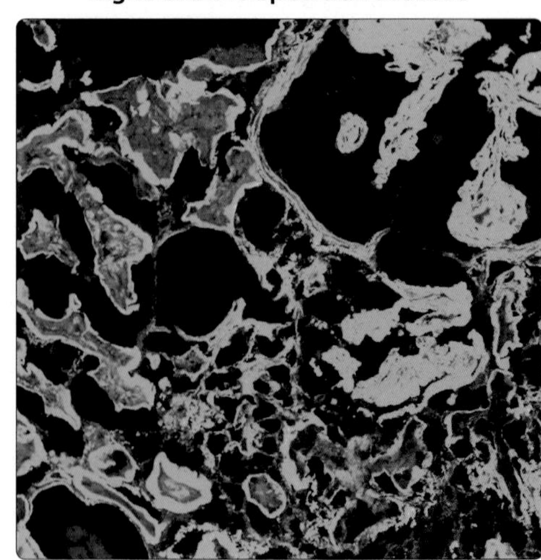

Extramedullary Hematopoiesis

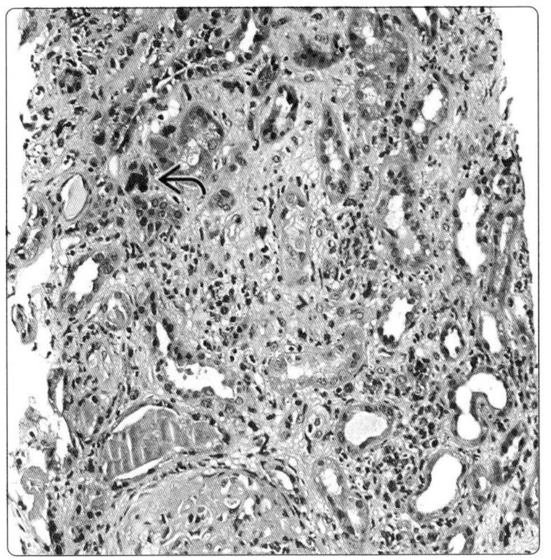

Extramedullary Hematopoiesis

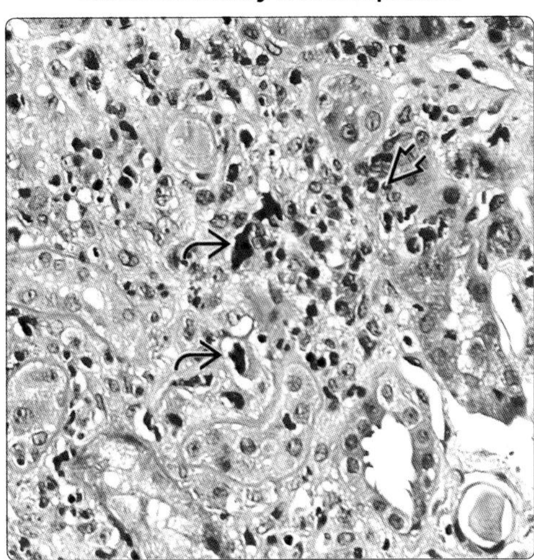

(Left) *Extramedullary hematopoiesis shows an interstitial infiltrate at medium magnification. A few cells with large, irregular nuclei stand out ➔. The biopsy is from a 77-year-old man with renal failure and a history of myelofibrosis.* **(Right)** *Extramedullary hematopoiesis can be confused with AIN. The larger cells can be recognized as megakaryocytes ➔, confirming the diagnosis. Eosinophil and neutrophil precursors are also present ➔.*

Acute Myeloid Leukemia

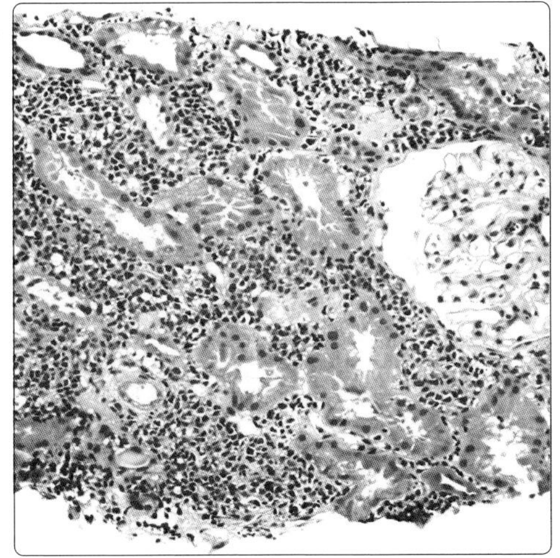

Acute Myeloid Leukemia

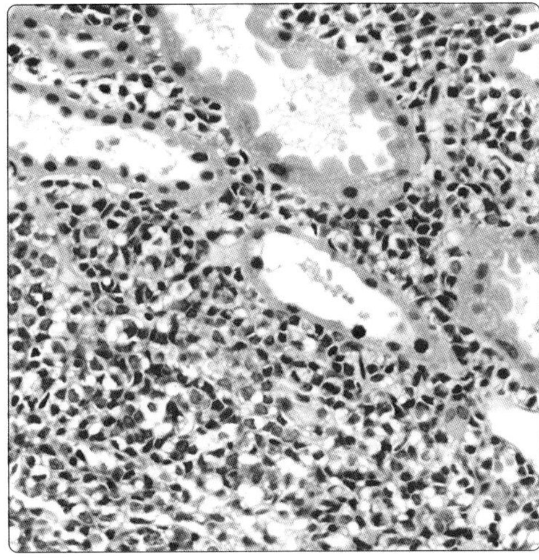

(Left) *Acute myeloid leukemia (AML) involving the kidney can resemble AIN. This case has extensive interstitial infiltration by leukocytes. This patient had a history of treated AML and then developed acute renal failure and markedly enlarged kidneys.* **(Right)** *On higher magnification in this case of AML, atypical cells are seen to be large and monomorphic. Immunohistochemistry revealed blasts positive for CD33 and CD34 and negative for CD3 and CD20.*

Plasma Cell Myeloma

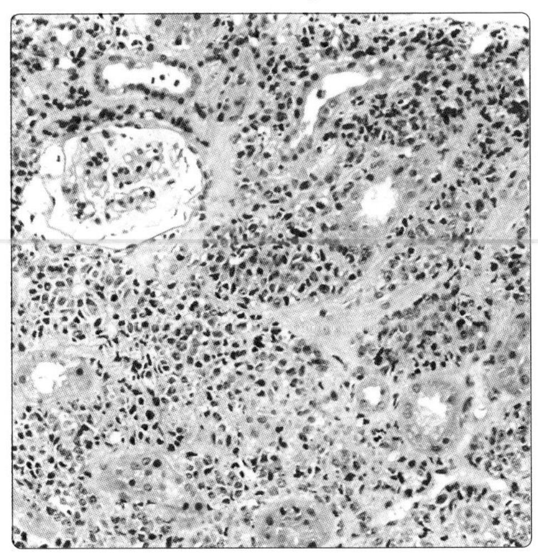

Plasma Cell Myeloma

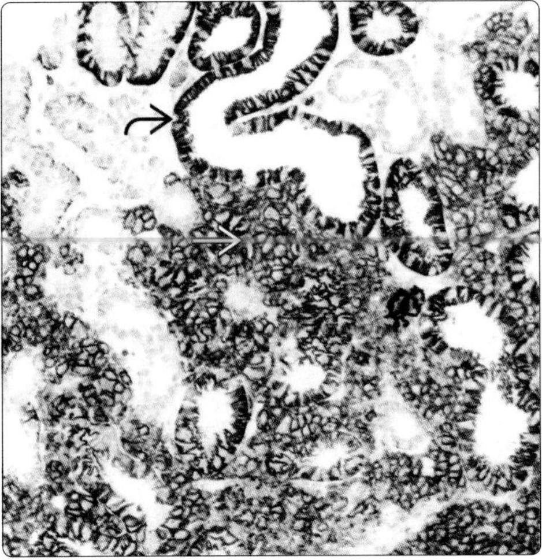

(Left) *Plasma cell myeloma in an allograft is shown. Atypical cells are infiltrating the interstitium. No mass lesion was detected; the biopsy was performed for renal dysfunction.* **(Right)** *Infiltrating cells ➔ are positive for the plasma cell marker CD138, as are some tubular epithelial cells ➔ (a normal finding).*

KEY FACTS

TERMINOLOGY

- Acute renal failure caused by acute tubular epithelial injury due to either ischemia or toxins

ETIOLOGY/PATHOGENESIS

- Hypovolemia, reduced perfusion pressure (90%)
- Direct toxicity of drugs, exogenous toxins or endogenous substances (10%)

CLINICAL ISSUES

- Deterioration of glomerular filtration rate occurs over hours to days
- Urinary microscopy reveals muddy brown casts and sloughed epithelium

MICROSCOPIC

- Tubular epithelial cells have apical cytoplasmic loss, reduced brush border, open lumens
- Necrosis is sparse except in toxins
- Interstitial edema may be prominent, but minimal inflammatory infiltrate
- Casts of necrotic cells, cell debris, and lipofuscin pigment

TOP DIFFERENTIAL DIAGNOSES

- Acute interstitial nephritis
- Autolysis
- Cortical necrosis

DIAGNOSTIC CHECKLIST

- Important to determine the cause of the ATI
- Casts, pigments, epithelial cytoplasmic changes and nuclear features may provide clues to etiology
- Glomerular neutrophils, monocytes, and sparse thrombi in sepsis
- Ischemia shows little or no overt necrosis in contrast to toxins
- Histologic changes can be subtle despite severe dysfunction

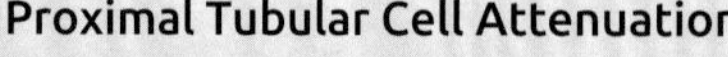

Proximal Tubular Cell Attenuation

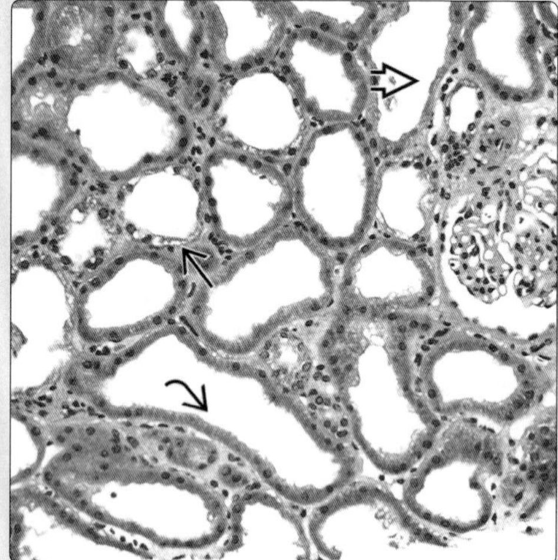

Apoptosis

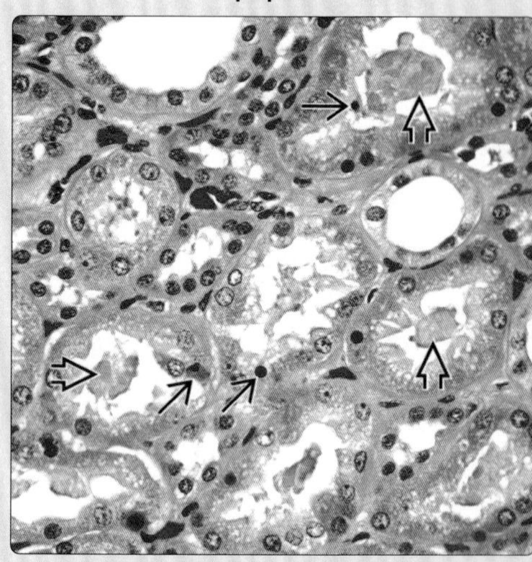

(Left) *The proximal tubules have epithelial attenuation with loss of apical cytoplasm ⇨ and markedly open lumens. Loss of cells can be inferred by the loss of nuclei ↗. Distal tubular epithelial cells have cytoplasmic vacuolization ↘.* **(Right)** *Early cellular injury in ATI is seen as cytoplasmic debris in tubular lumens ⇨ and focal apoptotic bodies →. Frank necrosis is not commonly conspicuous in ischemic acute tubular injury, which is why many prefer that term over acute tubular necrosis.*

Distal Tubular Pigmented Cast

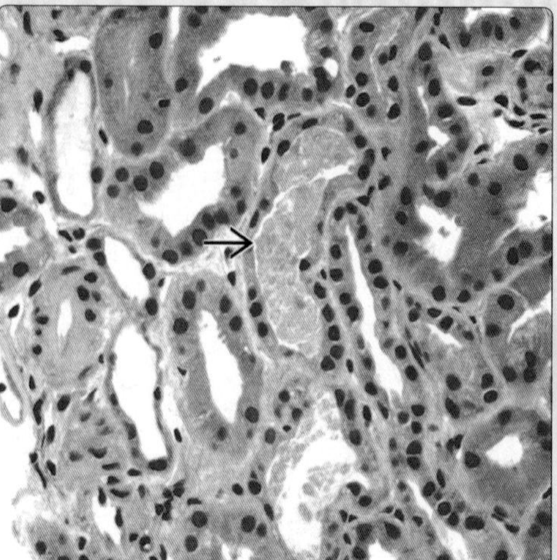

Tubular Cell Mitoses

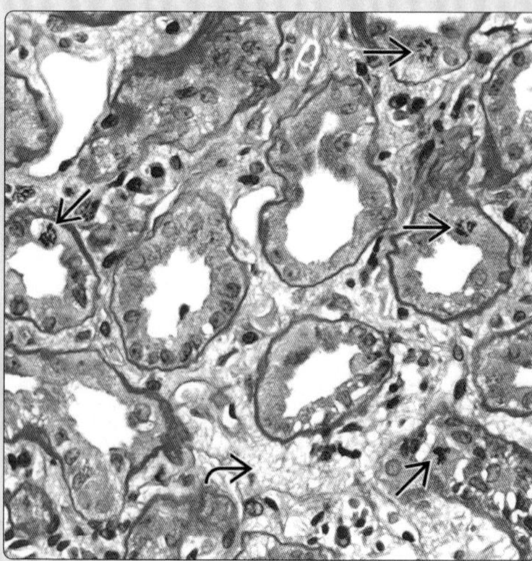

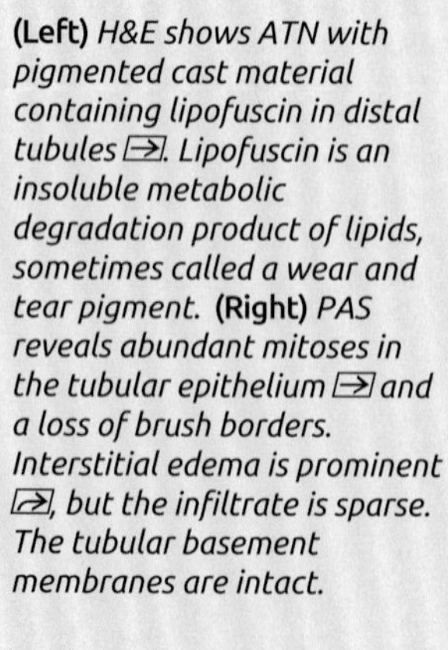

(Left) *H&E shows ATN with pigmented cast material containing lipofuscin in distal tubules →. Lipofuscin is an insoluble metabolic degradation product of lipids, sometimes called a wear and tear pigment.* **(Right)** *PAS reveals abundant mitoses in the tubular epithelium → and a loss of brush borders. Interstitial edema is prominent ↗, but the infiltrate is sparse. The tubular basement membranes are intact.*

TERMINOLOGY

Abbreviations

- Acute tubular injury (ATI)

Synonyms

- Acute tubular necrosis (ATN)

Definitions

- Acute renal failure caused by acute tubular epithelial injury due to either ischemia or toxins

ETIOLOGY/PATHOGENESIS

Etiology

- Renal ischemia due to reduced renal perfusion (~ 90%)
  - Hypovolemia
    - Blood loss (trauma, surgery, peripartum hemorrhage)
    - External fluid loss (burns, sweat, diarrhea)
    - 3rd space fluid loss (hypoalbuminemia, bowel obstruction, pancreatitis)
  - Decreased perfusion pressure
    - Systemic: Cardiac failure, cardiac tamponade, myocardial infarction, arrhythmia
    - Local: Renal artery stenosis, malignant hypertension, cholesterol atheroembolism
  - Reduced effective intravascular volume
    - Sepsis, hepatorenal syndrome, anaphylaxis, vasodilator drugs
- Nephrotoxins (~ 10%)
  - Drugs
    - Antibiotics (e.g., aminoglycosides, vancomycin, amphotericin)
    - Antiviral agents (e.g., tenofovir, acyclovir, indinavir)
    - Chemotherapeutic agents (e.g., cisplatin, ifosfamide)
    - Nonsteroidal anti-inflammatory agents (NSAIDs)
    - Calcineurin inhibitors (cyclosporine, tacrolimus)
    - Inhibitors of mTOR (rapamycin/sirolimus)
    - Angiotensin-converting enzyme (ACE) inhibitors
    - Anesthetics (halothane)
    - Radiologic contrast agents
    - Traditional herbal preparations (Africa, Asia)
  - Organic solvents: Ethylene glycol, carbon tetrachloride
  - Heavy metals: Hg, Pb, Bi, Ur, Pt
  - Endogenous substances
    - Hemoglobin (hemolysis, transfusion reactions)
    - Myoglobin (crush injury, statin drugs)
    - Monoclonal immunoglobulin light chains
    - Intratubular crystals (calcium oxalate, urates)
    - Bile casts (± hepatorenal syndrome)

Pathogenesis

- Ischemic or toxic insult to tubular epithelium
  - Spectrum of injury from sublethal cellular injury to necrosis and apoptosis
- Tubular injury and dysfunction
  - Altered epithelial transport reduces resorption of NaCl
  - Increased NaCl at macula densa activates tubulo-glomerular feedback, reducing GFR
  - Loss of tubular cell adhesion allows leak of glomerular filtrate into interstitium, reducing effective GFR
  - Exfoliated epithelium and Tamm-Horsfall protein form luminal casts that obstruct flow
- Hemodynamic changes
  - Afferent arteriolar vasoconstriction reduces glomerular hydrostatic pressure
  - Mesangial contraction in tubuloglomerular feedback reduces effective surface area for filtration
  - Endothelial activation increases adhesion molecule expression and procoagulant activity

CLINICAL ISSUES

Presentation

- Acute renal failure: Decrease of GFR, elevation of serum creatinine and blood urea nitrogen over hours to days
- Clinical phases
  - Oliguric: Days to weeks; low GFR and urine output < 400 mL/day
  - Early diuretic: Days to weeks; low GFR and increased urinary output
  - Late diuretic: Weeks; normalization of GFR and increased urinary output
- Acute Kidney Injury Network (AKIN) stages
  - Stage 1: ↑ serum Cr 1.5-2.0 x from baseline (or ≥ 0.3 mg/dL)
  - Stage 2: ↑ serum Cr > 2.0-3.0 x from baseline
  - Stage 3: ↑ serum Cr > 3.0 x from baseline or ≥ 4.0 with acute rise of ≥ 0.5 mg/dL

Laboratory Tests

- Muddy brown casts and sloughed epithelial cells in urine
- Elevated markers of injury in urine (e.g., KIM-1, NGAL, IL-18) or blood (NGAL, cystatin C)

Treatment

- Ischemia
  - Restoration of intravascular volume
- Toxin
  - Cessation of exposure and removal of toxin (dialysis, chelation)
- Restoration of electrolyte balance and pH

Prognosis

- 5-16% of patients with ischemic ATN have irreversible renal failure
- Mortality is ~ 50% and as high as 79% in critically ill patients with ATN requiring dialysis
  - Infection: Sepsis causes death in 30-70%
  - Cardiovascular: Congestive heart failure, pulmonary edema, hypertension, arrhythmia
  - Gastrointestinal: Hemorrhage (10-30%)
  - Neurologic: Encephalopathy, seizures

MACROSCOPIC

General Features

- Kidneys are enlarged and weigh up to ~ 130% of normal
- Cut surface reveals bulging pale cortex with red medulla

MICROSCOPIC

Histologic Features

- Glomeruli

- Glomeruli generally unremarkable
- Fibrin thrombi, monocytes and neutrophils in sepsis
- Cuboidal parietal epithelium (tubularization) in regeneration
- Tubules
  - Epithelial injury prominent in early phase
    - Thinning and loss of apical cytoplasm, open lumen
    - Reduced or absent brush borders on PAS
    - Necrosis or apoptosis of individual cells
    - Loss of nuclei, loss of adhesion, denudation of tubular basement membrane
    - Patchy distribution of changes with variable thickness of tubular epithelium
    - Distal tubular casts of necrotic cells and cell debris often with lipofuscin pigment
  - Regeneration in later phases: Increased cytoplasmic basophilia, nucleoli, mitoses
  - Dystrophic calcium phosphate or apatite may be evident ± oxalate
  - Tubulocapillary anastomosis may form due to ruptured tubules and cause red cell casts
  - Ischemic injury: Vast majority of tubular cells have non-necrotizing sublethal injury
  - Toxic injury: Cell necrosis common, most prominent in proximal tubule
- Interstitium
  - Interstitial edema with sparse mononuclear infiltrates, most marked at vasa recta
- Vessels
  - Arteries and arterioles generally unremarkable
  - Vasa recta may have luminal leukocytes, ± extramedullary hematopoiesis
- Often subtle histologic changes despite severe dysfunction

ANCILLARY TESTS

Immunohistochemistry

- Increased tubular cell proliferation (Ki-67)
- Kidney injury molecule-1 (KIM-1), expressed in injured tubules, may be useful to define extent of tubular injury
- Increased tubular expression of vimentin, CD24

Immunofluorescence

- Generally negative, may have increased C3 along tubular basement membranes and fibrin in interstitium

Electron Microscopy

- Tubular cell injury
  - Loss of brush borders, apical blebs and shedding, increased phagolysosomes, cell swelling, mitochondrial condensation, nuclear fragmentation, detachment of cells

Gene Expression

- Decreased transporter protein mRNA
- Increased C3 mRNA

DIFFERENTIAL DIAGNOSIS

Causes of ATN

- Ischemia: Tubular injury without necrosis
- Rhabdomyolysis: Eosinophilic globular luminal casts (myoglobin positive by IHC)
- Hemoglobinuria/hemolysis: Eosinophilic granular and globular casts (hemoglobin A positive by IHC)
- Bile cast nephropathy: Green bile casts seen in distal tubules (Hall stain positive)
- Lead and bismuth toxicity: Tubular nuclear eosinophilic inclusions
- Antiviral agents (e.g., tenofovir, adefovir): Tubular nucleomegaly and pleomorphism, megamitochondria
- Cisplatin and other DNA synthesis inhibitors: Tubular nucleomegaly with pleomorphism
- Calcineurin inhibitor toxicity: Isometric vacuolization of flattened tubular epithelium
- Ethylene glycol toxicity: Calcium oxalate crystals
- Radiocontrast agents: Isometric vacuolization of swollen tubular epithelium
- Sulfonamides, acyclovir, indinavir: Drug crystals in tubules

Mimics of ATN

- Acute interstitial nephritis
  - Interstitial inflammation and tubulitis more prominent
- Autolysis
  - No pigment casts, thinned cytoplasm or mitoses
  - Kidney weight not increased
  - Negative vimentin, KIM-1, Ki-67
- Cortical necrosis
  - All elements affected by necrosis, including glomeruli and vessels

DIAGNOSTIC CHECKLIST

Pathologic Interpretation Pearls

- Ischemia has little or no overt necrosis vs. toxins
- Most epithelial cells have sublethal injury with simplification and open lumens
- Histologic changes can be subtle despite severe dysfunction

SELECTED REFERENCES

1. Kumar S et al: Defining the Acute Kidney Injury and Repair Transcriptome. Semin Nephrol. 34(4):404-417, 2014
2. Sabbisetti VS et al: Blood kidney injury molecule-1 is a biomarker of acute and chronic kidney injury and predicts progression to ESRD in type I diabetes. J Am Soc Nephrol. 25(10):2177-86, 2014
3. McCullough JW et al: The role of the complement system in acute kidney injury. Semin Nephrol. 33(6):543-56, 2013
4. Takasu O et al: Mechanisms of cardiac and renal dysfunction in patients dying of sepsis. Am J Respir Crit Care Med. 187(5):509-17, 2013
5. Sharfuddin AA et al: Pathophysiology of ischemic acute kidney injury. Nat Rev Nephrol. 7(4):189-200, 2011
6. Ricci Z et al: Classification and staging of acute kidney injury: beyond the RIFLE and AKIN criteria. Nat Rev Nephrol. 7(4):201-8, 2011
7. Rosen S et al: Acute tubular necrosis is a syndrome of physiologic and pathologic dissociation. J Am Soc Nephrol. 19(5):871-5, 2008

Loss of Brush Borders in ATI

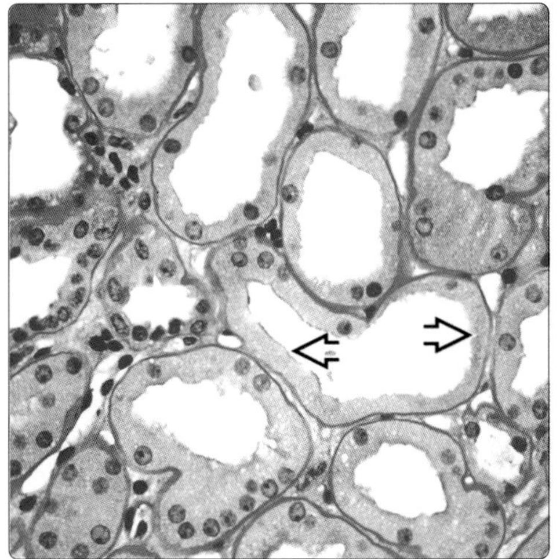

Normal Brush Borders

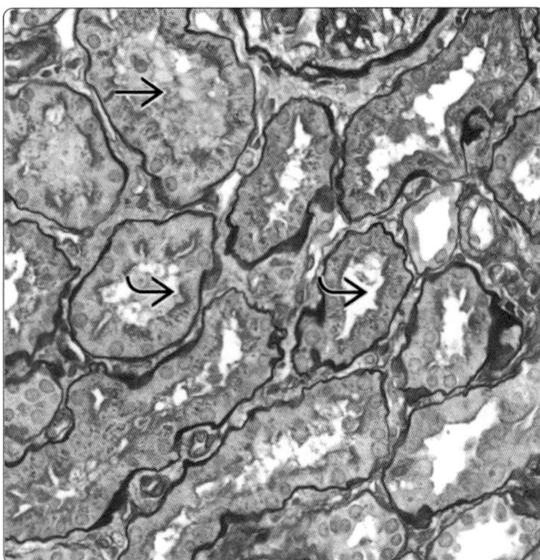

(Left) *Compare the normal appearance with the reduction or absence of brush border (a "crew cut") seen in ATI, which is demonstrated by this PAS stain. The lumina appear dilated but in fact are about the same diameter. Notice the loss of nuclei in some areas, indicating that some cells have sloughed* ⇨. **(Right)** *PAS stain shows proximal tubular brush borders* ⮫ *in a normal kidney. Notice that most lumina are "full"* ⇨ *or closed and the tubules are back to back without interstitial edema.*

Coarse Cytoplasmic Vacuolization

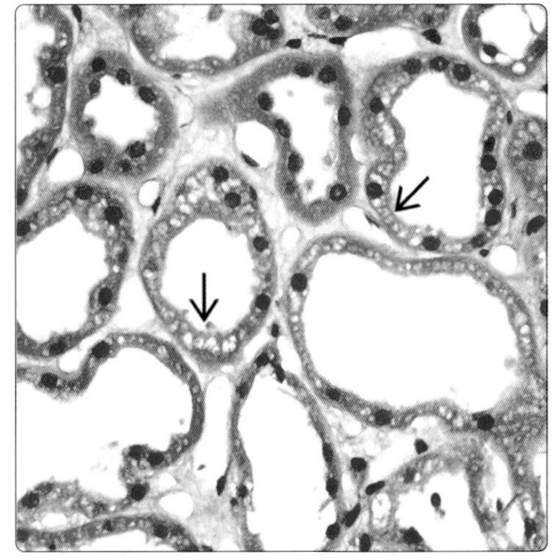

Dystrophic Calcification

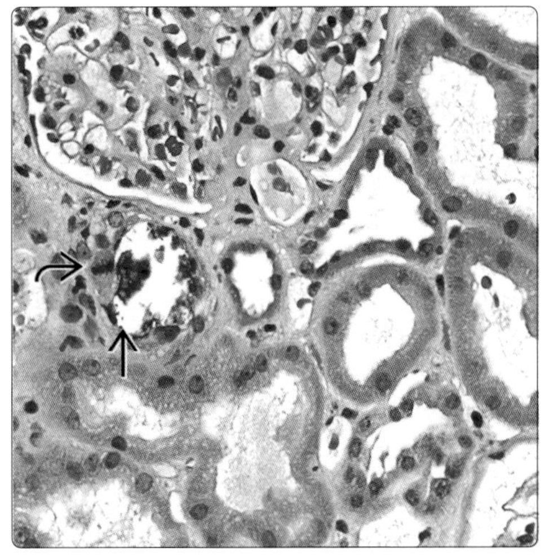

(Left) *These tubules with marked cytoplasmic attenuation have extensive coarse vacuolization* ⇨. *This can be seen in ischemic injury, and therefore is not necessarily due to drugs such as calcineurin inhibitors, contrast agents, or osmotic agents. Interstitial edema is slight.* **(Right)** *Dystrophic calcification* ⇨ *and an adjacent epithelial mitosis* ⮫ *are seen in this tubular profile. The dystrophic calcification was probably formed from the debris of necrotic cells. The glomerulus is unremarkable.*

Intraepithelial Calcium Oxalate

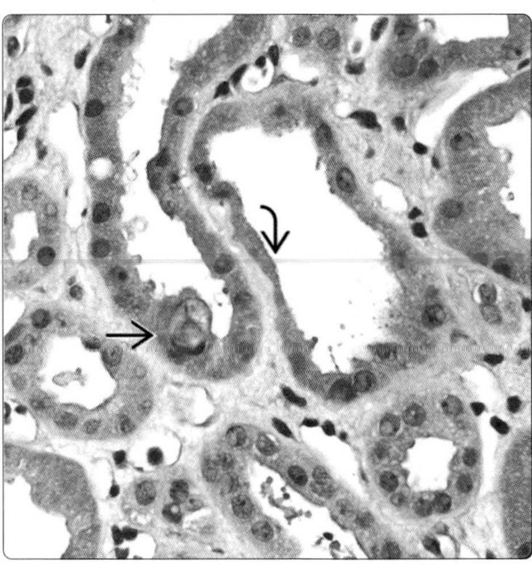

Vimentin in Proximal Tubules

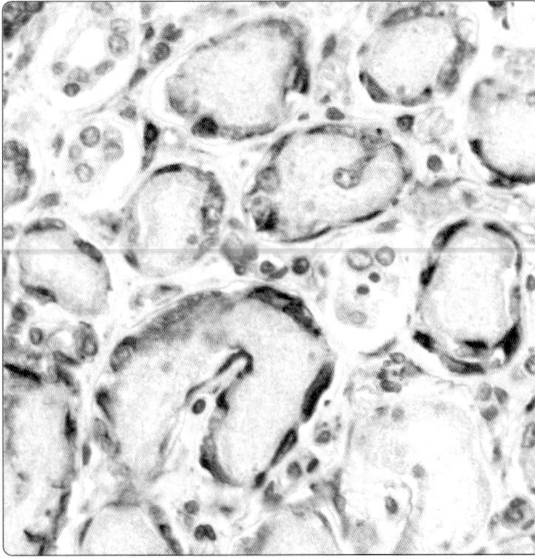

(Left) *An intracellular calcium oxalate crystal* ⇨ *is evident in an injured tubule. The cytoplasm of the tubular cells is basophilic, indicating increased ribosomal content, a sign of regeneration. Thinning and loss of nuclei are evident* ⮫, *as well as interstitial edema.* **(Right)** *Proximal tubules in ATI increase expression of vimentin ("dedifferentiate"). Other markers that increase are Ki-67 (proliferation) and KIM-1. Autolysis does not cause increased vimentin.*

(Left) *Electron microscopy shows tubular epithelium in ATI with loss of surface microvilli and separation of the cells due to the loss of intercellular adhesion ➙. Mitochondria are also sparser than normal, and the cell has lost its basolateral folds.* **(Right)** *Electron microscopy shows a distal tubular segment in ATI with luminal necrotic debris ➙. Phagolysosomes are prominent in some of the cells ↪. The nuclei have an open chromatin pattern, which suggests regeneration.*

Loss of Microvilli and Intercellular Adhesion

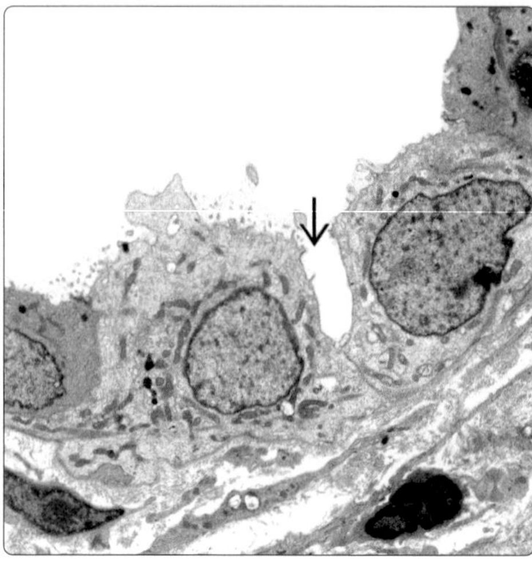

Luminal Necrotic Debris and Phagolysosomes

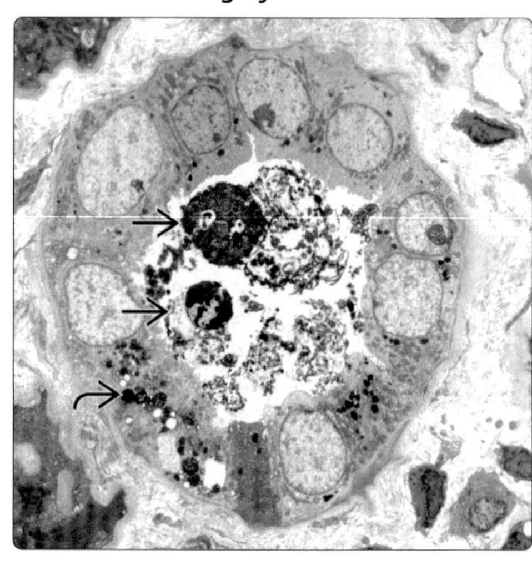

(Left) *An autopsy kidney with ATI shows tubular luminal necrotic cellular debris ⇨ and autolysis ➙. Congestion of peritubular capillaries is prominent.* **(Right)** *A pigmented cast ⇨ in a distal tubule is shown in an autopsy kidney. The presence of pigment casts is a valuable sign that the injury occurred in vivo. Mitoses are usually not frequent in autopsy kidneys with ATI. Autolysis with separation of the epithelium from the basement membrane is seen in adjacent tubules ➙.*

Sloughed Necrotic Tubular Cells

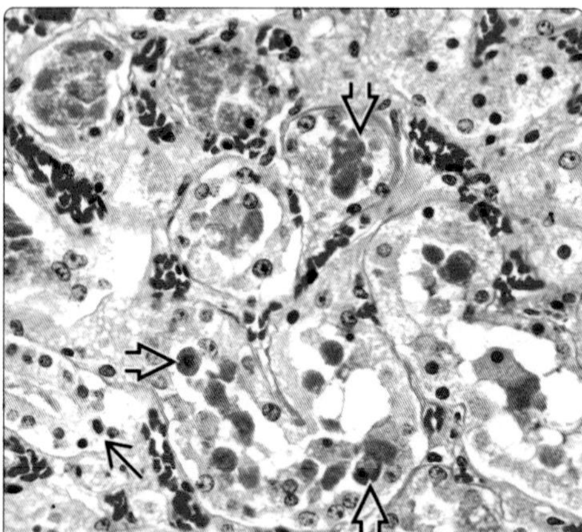

Pigmented Cast

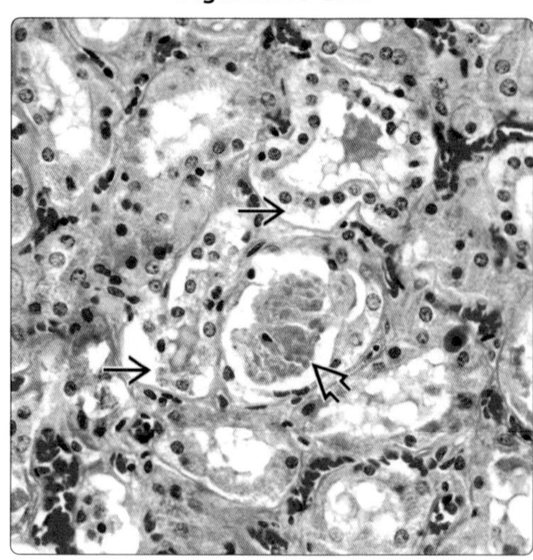

(Left) *Medullary vasa recta contain mononuclear granulocytic and erythroid precursors, a characteristic feature of ATI, presumably caused by production of hematopoietic growth factors by the injured kidney.* **(Right)** *Proximal tubules are filled with debris ↪ and distal tubular cells are detached ➙ due to autolysis in this autopsy kidney. In contrast to premortem ATI, there is no thinning of cytoplasm, pigmented casts, or vimentin expression. (Courtesy A. Shih, MD.)*

Extramedullary Hematopoiesis

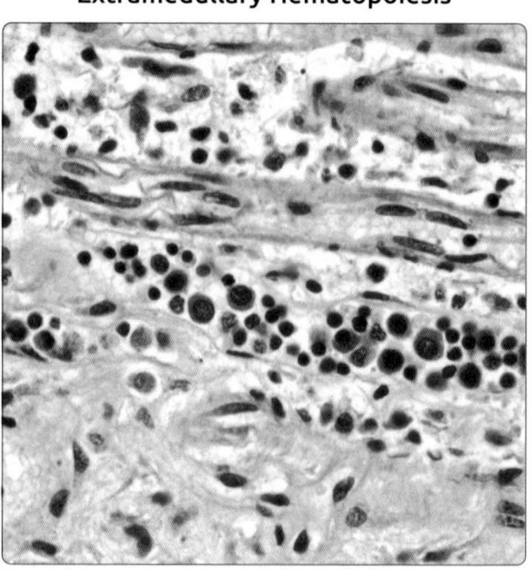

Autolysis

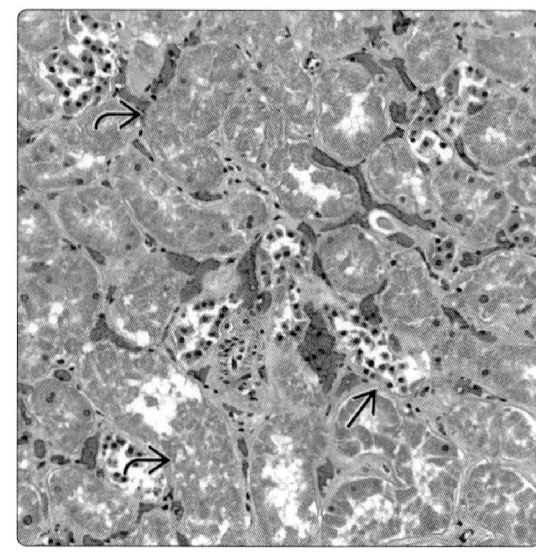

March Hemoglobinuria With ATI

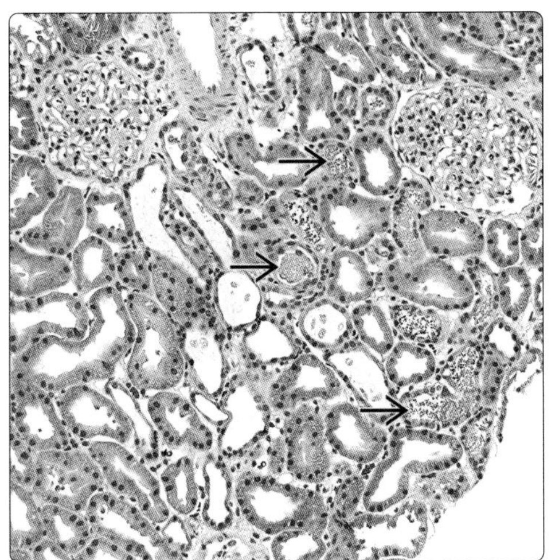

Hemoglobin Casts

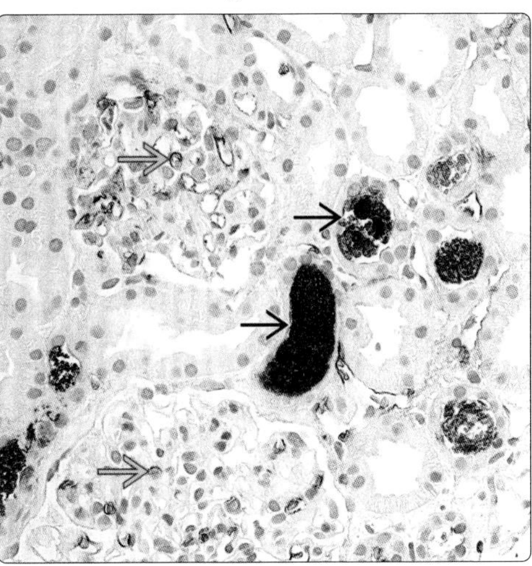

(Left) *Granular and pigmented casts ⇒ are seen mainly in distal tubules in this biopsy from a 16-year-old male who developed ATI with hemolysis, attributable to hours of strenuous exercise in 90°F conditions and probable dehydration. Glomeruli are unremarkable.* **(Right)** *Intratubular casts ⇒ stain for hemoglobin A in a 16-year-old male with march hemoglobinuria. The casts did not stain for myoglobin. Intracapillary erythrocytes ⇒ also stain for hemoglobin, providing an internal control.*

Myoglobin Casts With ATI

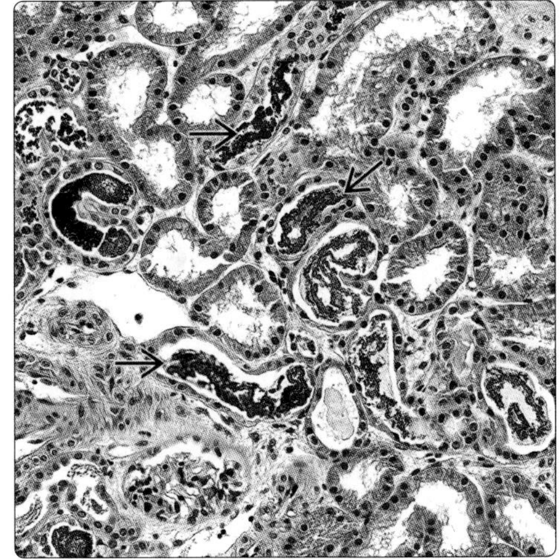

Myoglobin Casts

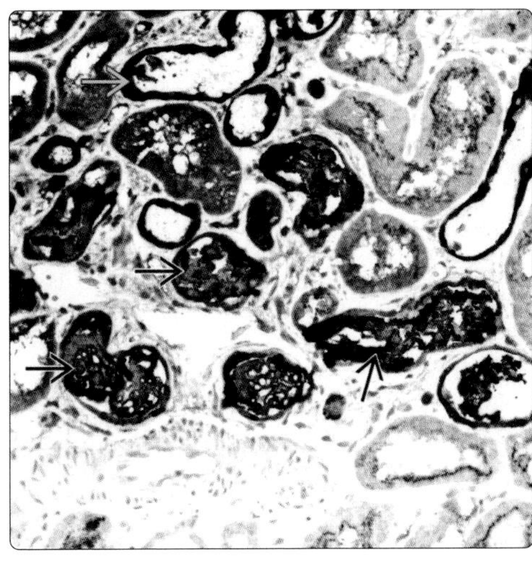

(Left) *Eosinophilic globular casts ⇒ are seen mainly in distal tubular segments in this biopsy from a 34-year-old man with acute kidney injury. Myoglobinuria was due to severe muscle exertion and the plasma creatine kinase level was 30,000 U/L.* **(Right)** *Staining for myoglobin is present in tubular luminal casts ⇒ and in tubular epithelium ⇒ by immunohistochemistry. The casts did not stain for hemoglobin.*

Bile Cast Nephropathy

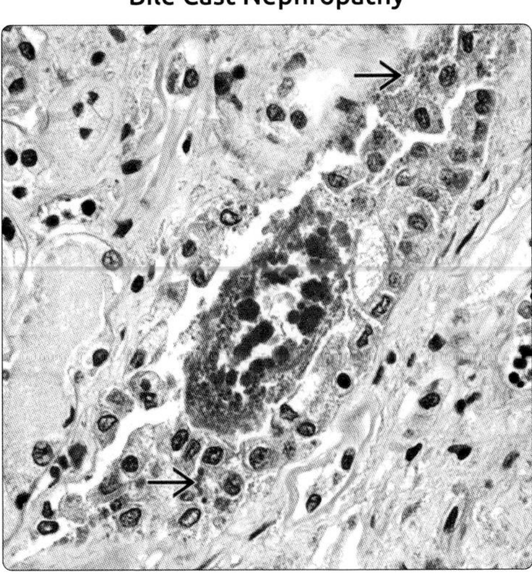

Lead Toxicity

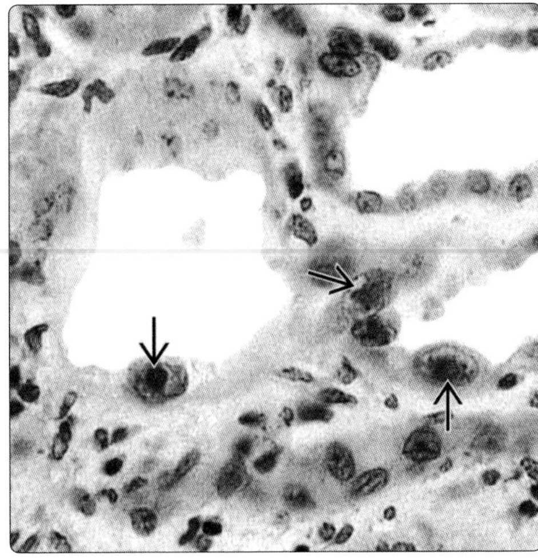

(Left) *A distal tubular bile cast is seen in this autopsy specimen from a patient with jaundice due to alcoholic cirrhosis and acute tubular injury. The cast has a brown rather than green hue. Similar colored material is seen in the epithelial cytoplasm ⇒.* **(Right)** *H&E stain in lead toxicity shows attenuated epithelium with the characteristic eosinophilic nuclear inclusions in proximal tubules ⇒. These are fuchsinophilic on Ziehl-Neelsen stains. The diagnosis is confirmed by elevated blood or tissue Pb levels.*

Renal Cortical Necrosis

KEY FACTS

TERMINOLOGY

- Bilateral, multifocal, or diffuse coagulative necrosis of renal cortex

ETIOLOGY/PATHOGENESIS

- Distribution of blood flow: Cortex (80%), medulla (20%)
- High metabolic demand of cortex increases susceptibility to ischemic injury
- Outer 1-2 mm of cortex receives blood supply from capsular vessels and spared in CN
- Obstetric complications ~ 50-60% of cases
- Sepsis ~ 30-40% of cases
- Thrombotic microangiopathy (HUS/TTP)
- Shock associated with any cause
- Antibody-mediated renal allograft rejection

CLINICAL ISSUES

- Prolonged oliguria or anuria
- 20% of ARF in pregnancy due to CN
- Duration of oliguria and extent of CN determine renal survival
- ~ 50% develop chronic renal failure

MACROSCOPIC

- Early: Yellow cortex with subcapsular and juxtamedullary congestion
- Late: Irregular scarring with calcification

MICROSCOPIC

- Multifocal or diffuse coagulative necrosis of cortex
- Subcapsular cortex (1-2 mm), juxtamedullary cortex, and medulla spared
- Thrombi in glomeruli, arterioles, venules, and veins
- Nonnecrotic tubules have acute tubular injury

TOP DIFFERENTIAL DIAGNOSES

- Renal Infarction
- Toxins
- Autolysis Autopsy)

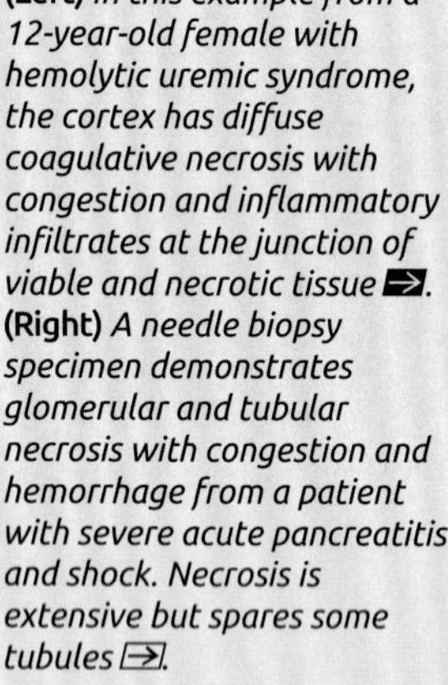
(Left) *In this example from a 12-year-old female with hemolytic uremic syndrome, the cortex has diffuse coagulative necrosis with congestion and inflammatory infiltrates at the junction of viable and necrotic tissue ➡.* **(Right)** *A needle biopsy specimen demonstrates glomerular and tubular necrosis with congestion and hemorrhage from a patient with severe acute pancreatitis and shock. Necrosis is extensive but spares some tubules ➡.*

Cortical Necrosis in HUS

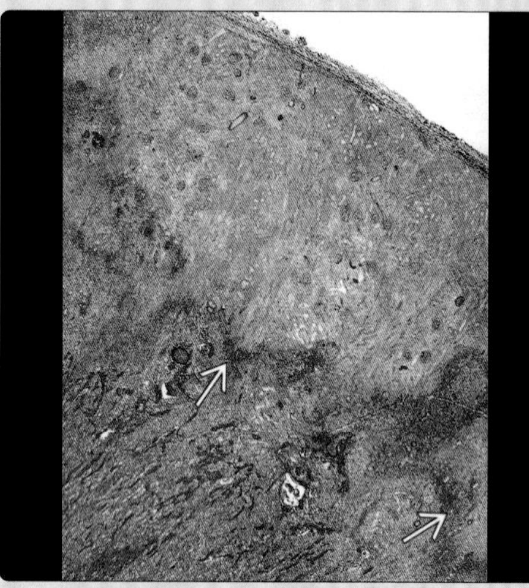

Cortical Necrosis in a Needle Biopsy

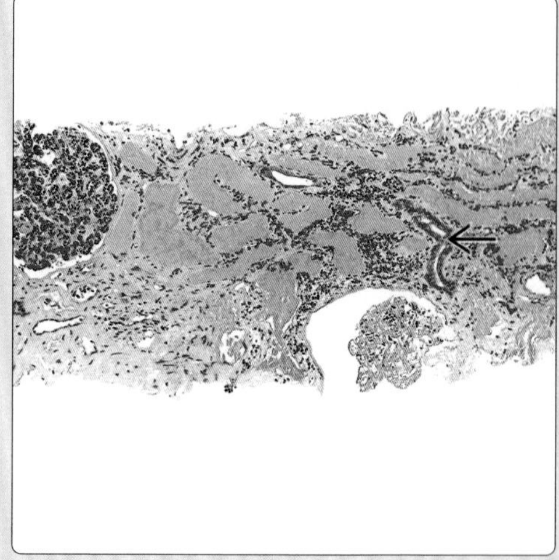

(Left) *Severe septicemia and shock led to cortical necrosis and graft loss 4 days after allograft transplantation. An interlobular artery ➡ has intimal fibrin and luminal mononuclear cells. Arterioles have occlusive thrombi ➡. The cortex has diffuse necrosis and hemorrhage.* **(Right)** *The junction of necrotic and viable tissue ➡ has congestion and hemorrhage. There is arterial fibrinoid necrosis ➡ consistent with antibody-mediated rejection of a kidney transplant.*

Cortical Necrosis in a Renal Allograft

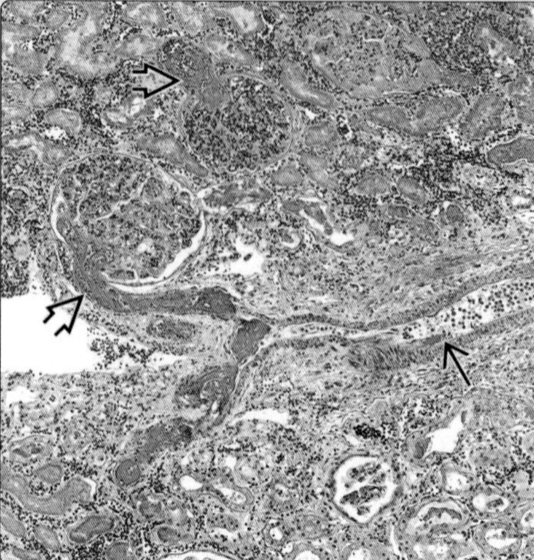

Cortical Necrosis in Antibody-Mediated Rejection

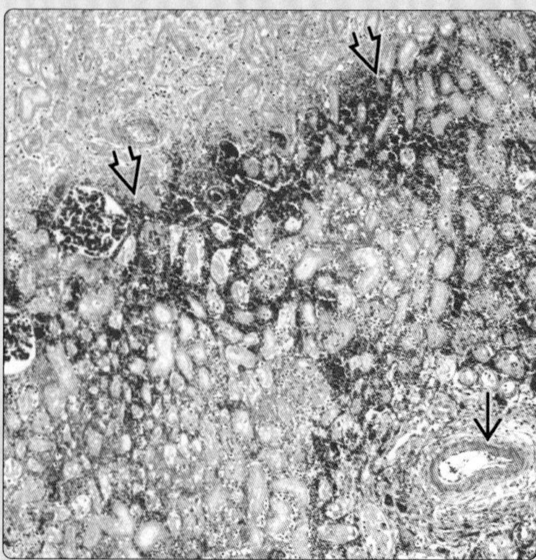

Renal Cortical Necrosis

TERMINOLOGY

Abbreviations

- Renal cortical necrosis (CN)

Definitions

- Bilateral, multifocal, or diffuse coagulative necrosis of cortex

ETIOLOGY/PATHOGENESIS

Obstetric Complications

- ~ 50-60% of cases
  - Placental abruption with hemorrhage
  - Placenta previa with hemorrhage
  - Puerperal sepsis with placental retention
  - Amniotic fluid embolism
  - Severe eclampsia

Sepsis

- ~ 30-40% of all cases
  - Bacterial infections: *E. coli*, *Klebsiella*
  - Infantile gastroenteritis

Toxins

- Diethylene glycol
- Snake venom

Miscellaneous Causes

- Shock associated with acute pancreatitis, diabetic ketoacidosis, blood loss, transfusion reaction, burns
- Thrombotic microangiopathy associated with hemolytic uremic syndrome or thrombotic thrombocytopenic purpura
- Atheroembolism
- Acute antibody-mediated rejection

Pathogenesis

- Distribution of blood flow: Cortex (80%), medulla (20%)
- High metabolic demand of cortex increases susceptibility to ischemic injury
- Outer 1-2 mm of cortex receives blood supply from capsular vessels and spared in CN
- Widespread thrombosis and vascular spasm of intrarenal vessels results in occlusion, ischemia, and tissue necrosis
  - May also occur secondary to hypertension or shock

CLINICAL ISSUES

Presentation

- Prolonged oliguria or anuria without diuresis
- Acute renal failure (ARF) in pregnancy
  - 20% of ARF in pregnancy due to CN

Treatment

- Supportive: Renal replacement therapy
- Correct underlying cause

Prognosis

- ~ 50% develop chronic renal failure
- Duration of oliguria and extent of CN determine renal survival
- Recovery may be complicated by hypertension
- In pregnancy, 77% renal recovery rate reported

IMAGING

CT Findings

- Narrow interlobular arteries with prominence of subcapsular vessels
- Dystrophic calcification late in disease

MACROSCOPIC

General Features

- Acute phase: Yellow cortex with subcapsular and juxtamedullary congestion
- Late phase: Irregular scarring with thin cortex and calcification

MICROSCOPIC

Histologic Features

- Glomeruli
  - Thrombi
- Tubules
  - Multifocal or diffuse coagulative necrosis of cortex
  - Subcapsular cortex (1-2 mm), juxtamedullary cortex, and medulla spared
  - Nonnecrotic tubules have acute tubular injury
- Interstitium
  - Usually little inflammation; hemorrhage at edges
- Vessels
  - Thrombi, arterioles, venules, and veins

DIFFERENTIAL DIAGNOSIS

Renal Infarction

- Segmental involvement of cortex, with arterial thrombosis or arteritis

Toxins

- Proximal tubule affected predominantly

Autolysis (Autopsy)

- Does not spare outer cortex

DIAGNOSTIC CHECKLIST

Clinically Relevant Pathologic Features

- Duration of oliguria proportional to extent of CN
- Extent of necrosis correlates with renal survival

SELECTED REFERENCES

1. Pourreau F et al: Bilateral renal cortical necrosis with end-stage renal failure following envenoming by Proatheris superciliaris: a case report. Toxicon. 84:36-40, 2014
2. Yap DY et al: Cortical necrosis in a kidney transplant recipient due to leptospirosis. Nephrology (Carlton). 19(4):257-8, 2014
3. Kim JO et al: Bilateral acute renal cortical necrosis in SLE-associated antiphospholipid syndrome. Am J Kidney Dis. 57(6):945-7, 2011
4. Prakash J et al: Decreasing incidence of renal cortical necrosis in patients with acute renal failure in developing countries: a single-centre experience of 22 years from Eastern India. Nephrol Dial Transplant. 22(4):1213-7, 2007
5. Alfonzo AV et al: Acute renal cortical necrosis in a series of young men with severe acute pancreatitis. Clin Nephrol. 66(4):223-31, 2006
6. Chugh KS et al: Acute renal cortical necrosis–a study of 113 patients. Ren Fail. 16(1):37-47, 1994
7. Kleinknecht D et al: Diagnostic procedures and long-term prognosis in bilateral renal cortical necrosis. Kidney Int. 4(6):390-400, 1973

Bile Cast Nephropathy

KEY FACTS

TERMINOLOGY

- Acute &/or chronic kidney injury with bile-containing casts

ETIOLOGY/PATHOGENESIS

- Elevated blood bilirubin and bile acid levels lead to intratubular bile casts
  - Direct toxicity to tubular epithelial cells by bilirubin and bile salts and subsequent acute tubular injury
  - Distal nephron obstruction
- Circulatory disturbance causing decreased perfusion of kidney

CLINICAL ISSUES

- Jaundice
- Occurs in both pediatric and adult patients
- Occurs with cirrhotic or noncirrhotic liver injuries

MACROSCOPIC

- Yellow when unfixed; green when fixed
- Pigment most prominent in renal pyramids

MICROSCOPIC

- Intratubular yellow-green pigmented casts
  - Hall stain highlights bile casts
- Dark red and some green-yellowish discoloration of sloughed cells
- Acute tubular injury

TOP DIFFERENTIAL DIAGNOSES

- Rhabdomyolysis
- Hemoglobinuria
- Acute tubular injury/acute tubular necrosis
- Myeloma cast nephropathy

DIAGNOSTIC CHECKLIST

- Identification of red to yellow-green tubular casts
  - Correlates with presence of jaundice
  - Hall stain is insensitive and a negative result does not exclude bile cast nephropathy (BCN)

(Left) *Gross photograph shows the cut surface of a formalin-fixed kidney with prominent green discoloration, accentuated in the renal pyramids ➡ where bile and bile casts are present in greater numbers and higher concentration compared with the renal cortex. The green color is due to biliverdin.* **(Right)** *Gross photograph of a cross section of renal medulla shows plugging of nephrons by bile casts ➡ in a patient with end-stage liver disease. Some of these bile casts ➡ are red. (Courtesy C. Abrahams, MD.)*

Green Kidney

Nephrons Plugged by Bile Casts

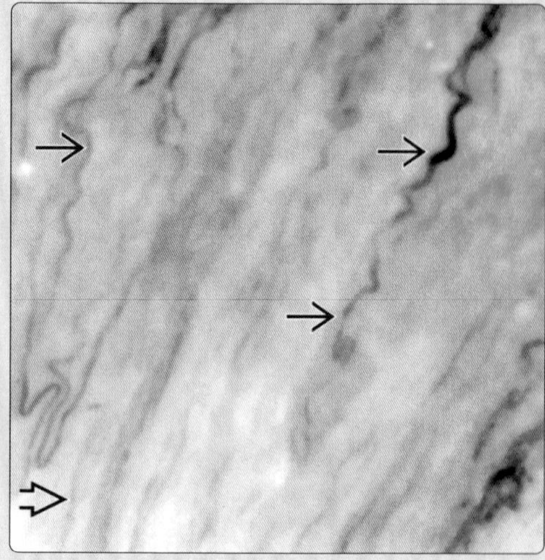

(Left) *Hematoxylin & eosin stain of the medulla shows numerous green-yellow ➡ casts within the distal tubules and collecting ducts of the renal medulla with vasa recta ➡ congested by red blood cells in a patient with end-stage liver disease.* **(Right)** *Hematoxylin & eosin stain of the medulla at high power shows green-yellowish red casts with granular and irregular edges within a collecting duct ➡.*

Bile Casts in Medulla

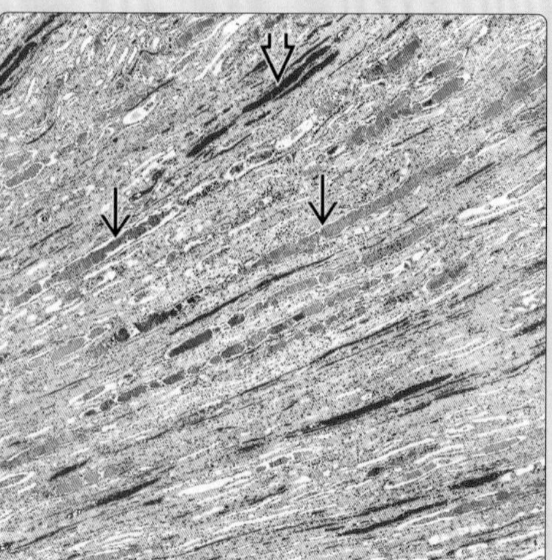

Bile Casts

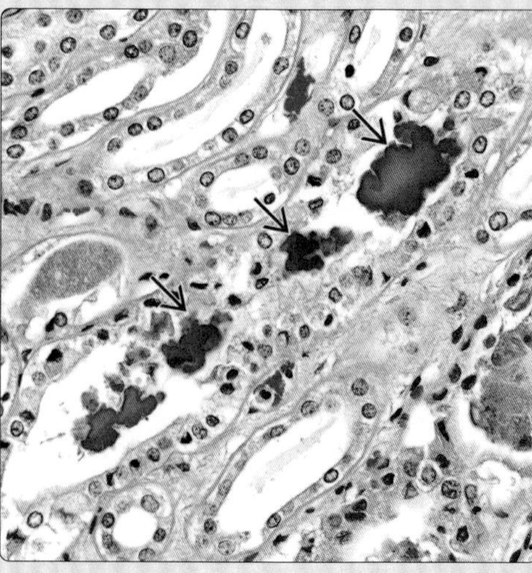

TERMINOLOGY

Synonyms

- Bile acid nephropathy
- Cholemic nephrosis or bile nephrosis

Definitions

- Bile cast nephropathy (BCN): Acute &/or chronic kidney injury with bile-containing casts
- Hepatorenal syndrome (HRS): Renal failure with cirrhosis
  - Type 1: Rapid reduction of renal function
  - Type 2: Slowly progressive loss of renal function
  - Lack of benefit from volume expansion
  - Absence of other causes

ETIOLOGY/PATHOGENESIS

Proposed Mechanisms of Injury

- Distal nephron casts containing bilirubin and bile acids
  - Direct toxicity to tubular epithelium by bile acids and bilirubin
  - Obstruction in distal nephron
    - Propensity of distal nephron due to admixture of Tamm-Horsfall protein with bile components
- Can be observed in HRS but is not restricted to this specific condition

CLINICAL ISSUES

Presentation

- Hepatic failure
  - Total bilirubin levels often > 20 mg/dL
  - Jaundice
- Severe cholestasis
- Acute &/or chronic renal failure
  - Concentrated urine, low Na

Treatment

- Surgical approaches
  - Liver transplantation if cause of liver failure is irreversible
- Drugs
  - Vasopressors for type 1 HRS
- Supportive therapy
  - Renal replacement therapy

Prognosis

- Dependent on reversibility of liver failure
- Reduction of bilirubin and bile acids leads to recovery of renal function

MACROSCOPIC

General Features

- Yellow kidneys before fixation (bilirubin)
- Green kidneys after formalin fixation (biliverdin)
  - More prominent in pyramids than cortex due to more frequent bile casts in renal medulla

MICROSCOPIC

Histologic Features

- Intratubular yellow-green to red pigmented casts
  - Localized predominantly in distal tubules and collecting ducts
  - Sloughed tubular epithelial cells may be admixed with bile casts
  - Hall stain highlights bile by converting bilirubin to biliverdin but is an insensitive test
- Acute tubular injury
  - Loss or attenuation of proximal tubular brush borders
  - Sloughed cells and cell cytoplasm accumulate within tubular lumina
  - Cellular debris within distal nephron segments admixed with bile and bile salts
- Calcium oxalate crystal deposition
  - Bile stained crystals **not** to be mistaken for bile casts
  - Localized to distal nephron segments

DIFFERENTIAL DIAGNOSIS

Rhabdomyolysis

- Pigmented granular eosinophilic casts in distal nephron
  - IHC of casts positive for myoglobin

Hemoglobinuria

- Pigmented granular eosinophilic casts in distal nephron
  - IHC of casts positive for hemoglobin

Acute Tubular Injury/Acute Tubular Necrosis

- Lack of bile-stained tubular casts
  - Hall stain negative and clinical absence of jaundice
- Granular tubular casts (cell debris)

Myeloma Cast Nephropathy

- Intratubular casts with sharp edge or fractured appearance
  - Casts polychromatic on trichome stain
  - Multinucleated giant cell reaction around casts
  - Monoclonal light chains by IHC or IF

DIAGNOSTIC CHECKLIST

Pathologic Interpretation Pearls

- Red to yellow-green tubular casts
- Bile casts can mimic myoglobinuria or hemoglobinuria
  - Negative myoglobin immunohistochemistry should always raise consideration of BCN
- Hepatorenal syndrome may occur with little bile accumulation

SELECTED REFERENCES

1. Adebayo D et al: Renal dysfunction in cirrhosis is not just a vasomotor nephropathy. Kidney Int. ePub, 2014
2. Luciano RL et al: Bile acid nephropathy in a bodybuilder abusing an anabolic androgenic steroid. Am J Kidney Dis. 64(3):473-6, 2014
3. Fickert P et al: Bile acids trigger cholemic nephropathy in common bile-duct-ligated mice. Hepatology. 58(6):2056-69, 2013
4. van Slambrouck CM et al: Bile cast nephropathy is a common pathologic finding for kidney injury associated with severe liver dysfunction. Kidney Int. 84(1):192-7, 2013
5. Betjes MG et al: The pathology of jaundice-related renal insufficiency: cholemic nephrosis revisited. J Nephrol. 19(2):229-33, 2006
6. Thompson LL et al: The renal lesion in obstructive jaundice. Am J Med Science. 199:305-312, 1940

(Left) *Gross photograph shows the capsular surface of an autopsy kidney from a 32-year-old man with cirrhosis. The green discoloration of the kidney is accentuated after formalin fixation.* **(Right)** *Gross photograph of a cross section of the renal medulla in a jaundiced patient demonstrates numerous bile casts ➔ within the renal tubules. (Courtesy C. Abrahams, MD.)*

Green Kidney

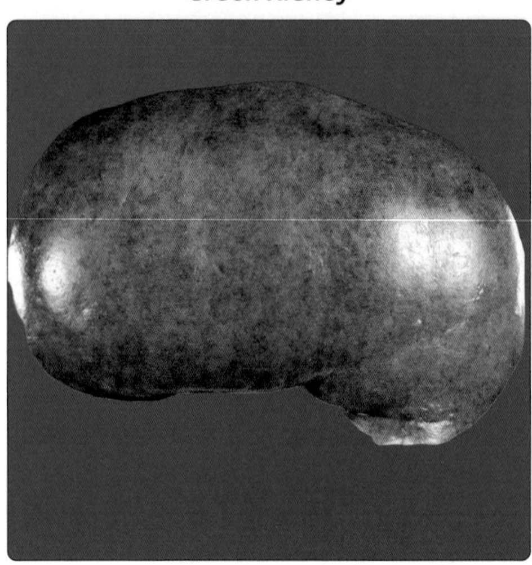

Bile Casts

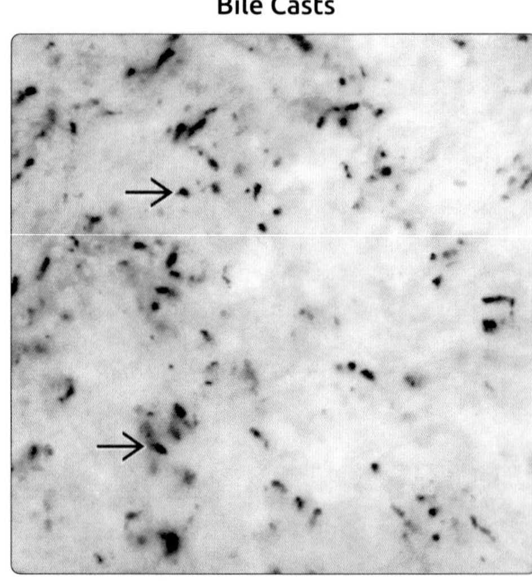

(Left) *Many large bile casts ➔ are noted in this kidney with renal dysplasia from a teenage male with Alagille syndrome.* **(Right)** *Bile casts ➔ initially form within the distal nephron segments. The adjacent proximal tubules ➩ are free of bile casts but they can be involved in severe cases of bile cast nephropathy. Correlation with clinical and lab data confirms the the diagnosis of BCN.*

Bile Casts (H&E)

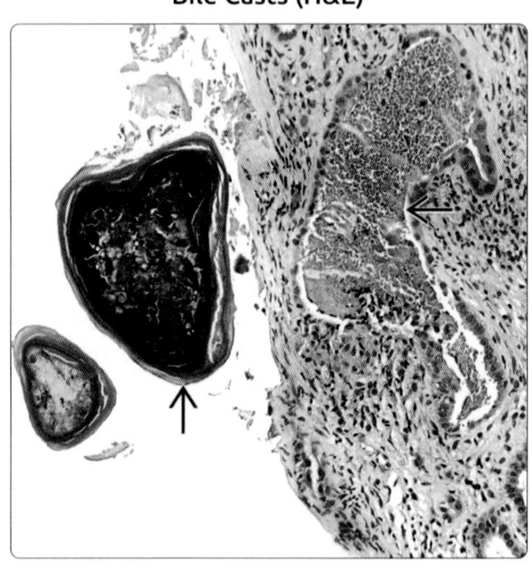

Bile Casts (H&E)

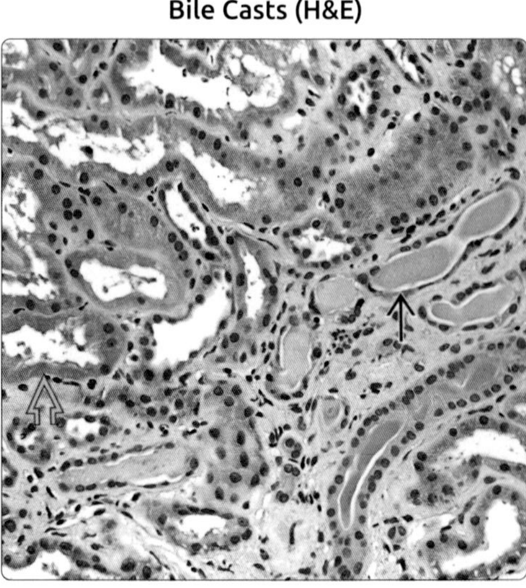

(Left) *Granular red intratubular casts ➔ occupy many tubular lumina in a jaundiced patient at autopsy. These casts mimic myoglobin and hemoglobin casts. A Hall stain is not required in this context to diagnose bile cast nephropathy.* **(Right)** *Hematoxylin & eosin stain shows a calcium oxalate crystal ➔ that is tinged green with bile and should not be confused with a bile cast. Calcium oxalate crystals are uncommon and, when noted, may also be found in distal nephron segments similar to the bile casts.*

Bile Casts (H&E)

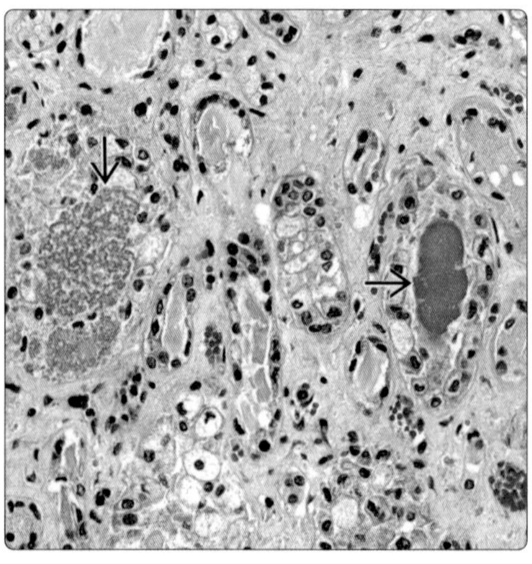

Bile-Stained Calcium Oxalate Crystal

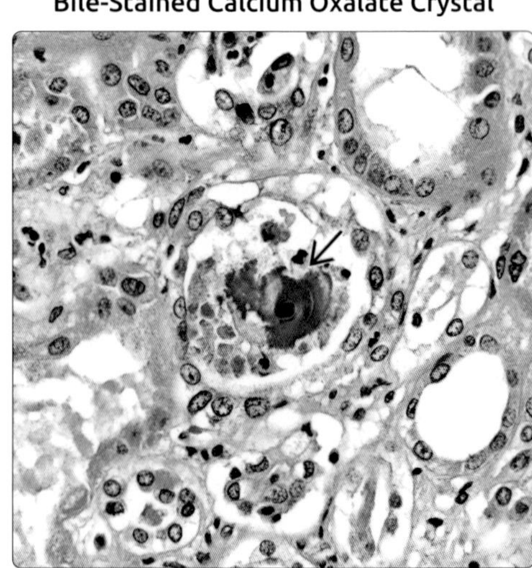

Bile Cast

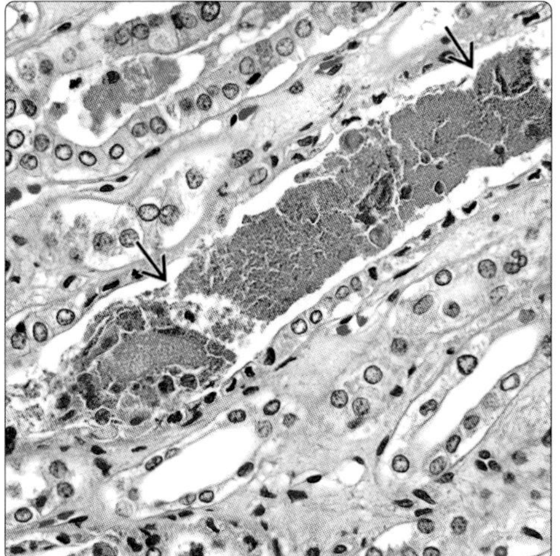

Bile Cast (Hall Stain)

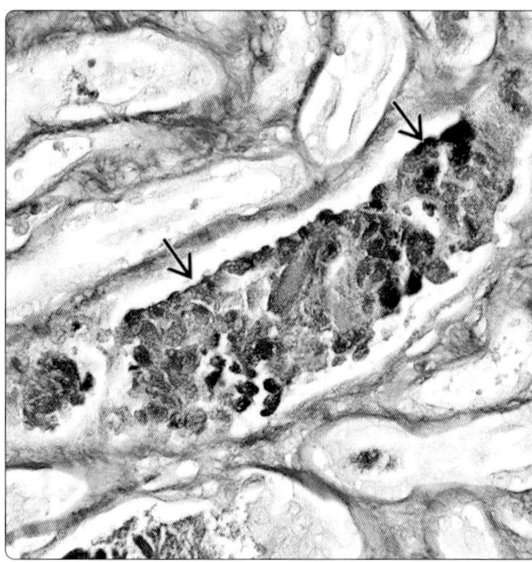

(Left) *Hematoxylin & eosin stain shows a dark red cast* ⇒ *within a distal nephron segment that consists of sloughed cells and granular cellular debris. Immunohistochemistry for myoglobin was negative in the tubular casts.* **(Right)** *Hall stain confirms the presence of bile within the pigmented granular casts* ⇒ *with abundant cellular debris. Bile cast formation in the distal nephron segments may be due in part to the increased concentration of bile and bile salts.*

Bile Cast (PAS)

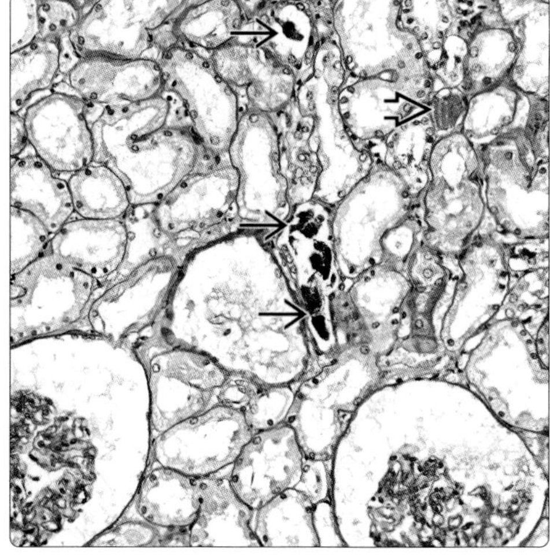

Bile Cast

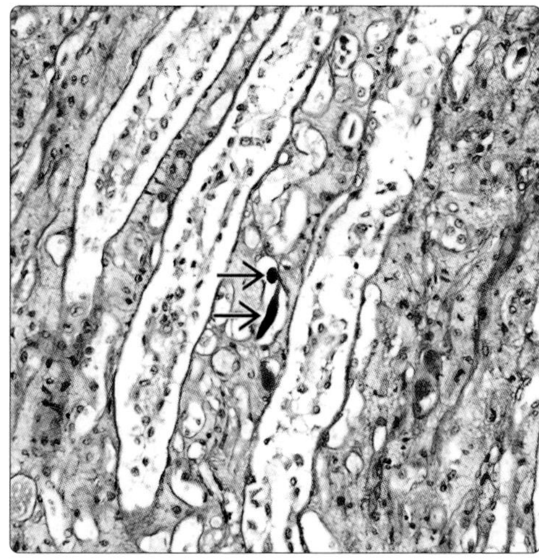

(Left) *Periodic acid-Schiff stain reveals bile casts* ⇒ *that have a dark red staining quality, which contrasts with Tamm-Horsfall protein* ⇛ *in a nearby tubule that has a much lighter and uneven pink color.* **(Right)** *Periodic acid-Schiff stain reveals a fragmented intratubular bile cast* ⇒ *that has a dark red staining quality and retracted edge. Bile casts do not fill up the entire tubular lumen, which contrasts to intratubular accumulation of Tamm-Horsfall protein.*

Myoglobin Casts (H&E)

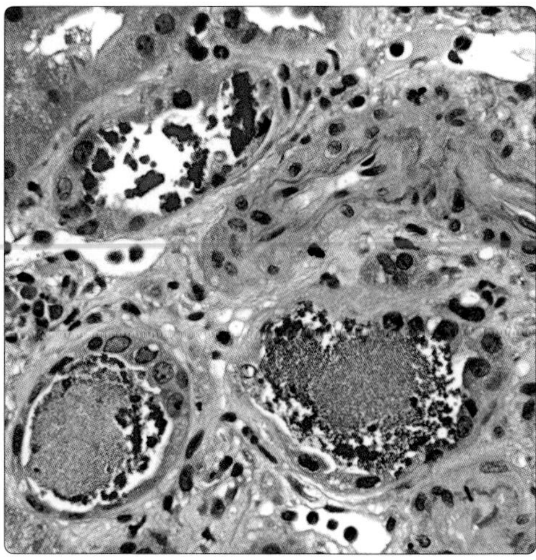

Hemoglobin Casts (H&E)

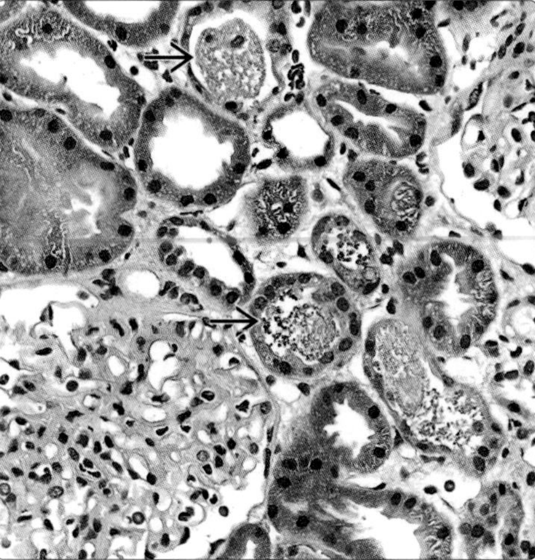

(Left) *Pigmented granular eosinophilic casts may mimic bile casts, but immunohistochemistry for myoglobin will strongly stain these casts to confirm rhabdomyolysis-associated acute tubular injury.* **(Right)** *Granular red casts* ⇒ *due to hemoglobinuria can mimic bile or myoglobin casts, but immunohistochemistry for hemoglobin and a history of hemolysis exclude the diagnosis of BCN.*

Drug-Induced Acute Interstitial Nephritis

KEY FACTS

TERMINOLOGY

- Acute tubulointerstitial inflammation due to allergic reaction to a drug

ETIOLOGY/PATHOGENESIS

- T-cell-mediated hypersensitivity reaction
- Idiosyncratic reaction, not dose dependent

CLINICAL ISSUES

- Triad of fever, rash, eosinophilia in < 50%
- Urine eosinophils
- Subnephrotic range proteinuria
- Recovery of renal function in 60-90%

MICROSCOPIC

- Interstitial inflammation with tubulitis, usually with eosinophils
- Other features variably present
  - Granulomas
  - Fibrosis and atrophy with prolonged drug exposure
  - Minimal change disease: NSAIDs and others
  - Papillary necrosis: NSAIDs

ANCILLARY TESTS

- EM may show foot process effacement
- TBM deposits by IF rarely

TOP DIFFERENTIAL DIAGNOSES

- Acute tubular injury
- Autoimmune AIN
- Acute pyelonephritis
- Granulomatous AIN due to infection or sarcoidosis

DIAGNOSTIC CHECKLIST

- Adverse prognostic features: Fibrosis, granulomas, marked diffuse inflammation

Interstitial Inflammation and Normal Glomerulus

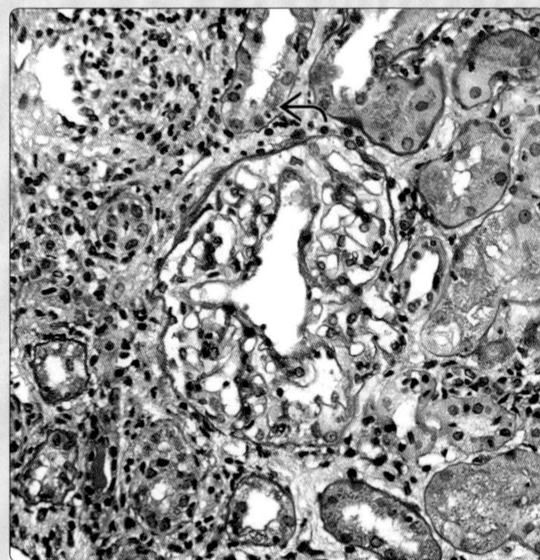

Medullary Interstitial Inflammation

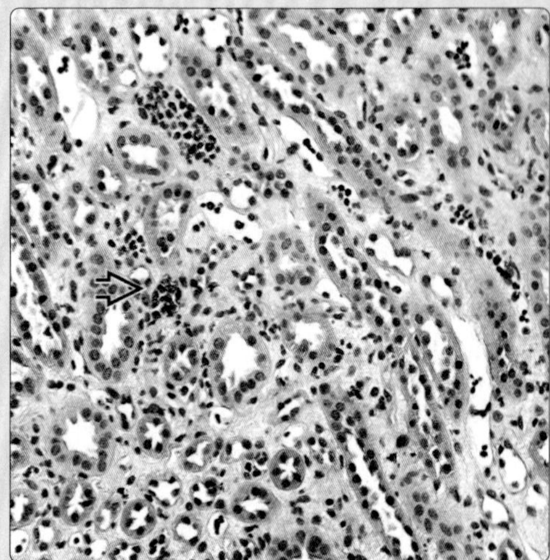

(Left) *Periodic acid-Schiff shows interstitial infiltrate of mononuclear cells and intraepithelial lymphocytes in tubules ⮫. The glomerulus is well preserved with no evidence of proliferation or inflammation.* **(Right)** *Hematoxylin & eosin of a biopsy from a patient treated with naproxen shows a small collection of eosinophilic infiltrate ➾ within the medulla. Patients with NSAID-induced acute interstitial nephritis can have only sparse interstitial inflammation.*

Interstitial Granulomas

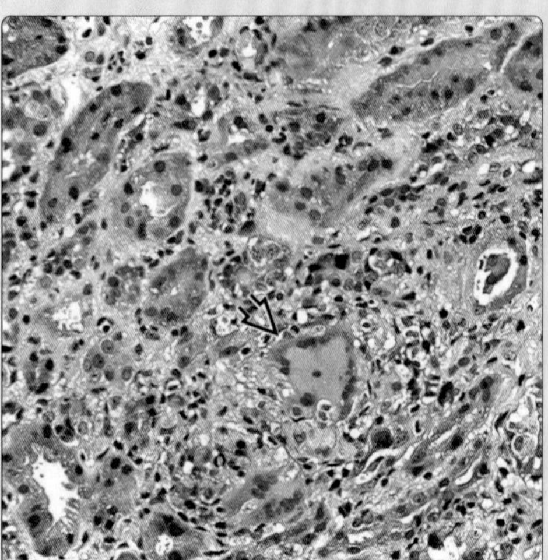

EM of Tubulitis

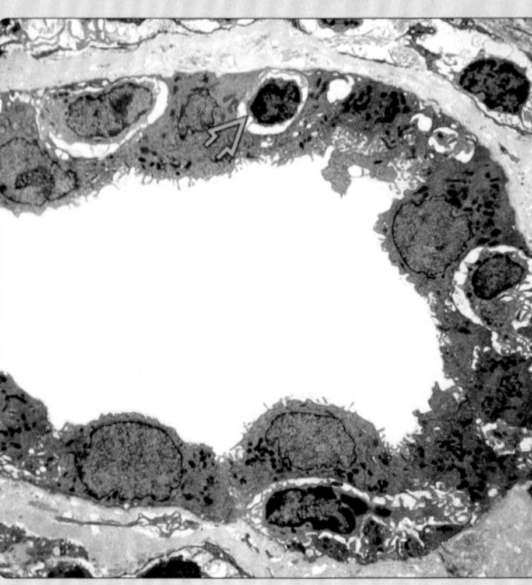

(Left) *Hematoxylin & eosin shows AIN with interstitial mononuclear infiltrate presumably due to a drug. Although well-formed granulomas were absent, scattered multinucleated giant cells were identified ➾.* **(Right)** *Electron micrograph of a biopsy with clinical and histological features of drug-induced AIN shows infiltrating intraepithelial lymphocytes ➾ within a tubule.*

TERMINOLOGY

Abbreviations

- Acute interstitial nephritis (AIN)

Synonyms

- Drug-induced acute tubulointerstitial nephritis

Definitions

- Acute tubulointerstitial inflammation due to allergic reaction to a drug

ETIOLOGY/PATHOGENESIS

Hypersensitivity Reaction

- T-cell-mediated reaction
- Idiosyncratic reaction, not dose dependent
  - Exacerbated response seen with reexposure
- Often associated with systemic hypersensitivity manifestations
- Cross-reactivity with similar class of drugs

Cell-Mediated/Delayed Hypersensitivity Reaction

- Positive skin tests to drug "haptens" seen in some patients
- Oligoclonal T-cell reactivity to drug in vitro
- Granuloma formation within interstitium
- Drug molecules act as "haptens" and elicit immunological reaction
- Drugs bind covalently to tubular basement membranes (TBM) or tubular epithelial cell components and alter or cross react with endogenous antigens

Antigen/Antibody-Mediated Process (Immune Complexes)

- Subset of cases have circulating antibodies to inciting drug (e.g., rifampin)
- Anti-TBM autoantibodies occasionally identified

IgE Mediated

- IgE antibodies to drugs identified in some cases

Drug Classes Implicated

- All drug classes have been implicated in AIN
  - Most common specific drugs in one series (Muriithi): Omeprazole (12%), amoxicillin (8%), ciprofloxacin (8%)
- Antibiotics (~ 50%)
  - Penicillins, cephalosporins, sulfonamides, vancomycin, rifampin, tetracyclines, erythromycin and most others (if not all)
- Proton pump inhibitors (~ 14%)
- NSAIDs (~ 11%)
  - Both COX-1 and COX-2 inhibitors
  - AIN can occur after long-term exposure to NSAIDs
    - Prolonged use can cause analgesic nephropathy
  - Nonallergic mechanism of injury
    - Inhibit renal prostaglandin (vasodilator) synthesis
    - Nephrotoxicity greater with advancing age, dehydration, preexisting renal disease, cirrhosis
  - Can cause minimal change disease (secondary)
- Diuretics
  - Thiazides, furosemide, triamterene
- Antiviral drugs
  - Acyclovir, foscarnet, indinavir
- Miscellaneous drugs
  - Phenytoin, allopurinol, cimetidine, diphenylhydantoin, captopril, lithium, valproate, warfarin, interferon-α, lamotrigine
- Herbal remedies
  - Aristolochic acid ("Chinese herb nephropathy"), kudzu root juice

Other Possible Lesions of Drug-Induced Kidney Disease

- Granulomatous interstitial nephritis
  - Penicillins, polymyxin, rifampin, spiramycin, sulfonamides, vancomycin, acyclovir, thiazides, triamterene, NSAIDs, allopurinol, captopril, heroin, lamotrigine
- Papillary necrosis
  - NSAIDs (fenoprofen, ibuprofen, indomethacin) and acetaminophen
- Podocytopathy (minimal change disease or focal segmental glomerulosclerosis)
  - Mechanism unknown
  - NSAIDs, penicillins, rifampin, celecoxib, diphenylhydantoin, lithium, interferon-α
- Membranous glomerulonephritis
  - NSAIDs, gold, penicillamine

CLINICAL ISSUES

Epidemiology

- Incidence varies with drug
  - Epidemiology study of AIN from proton pump inhibitor found incidence of 12/100,000 persons/year

Presentation

- Maculopapular rash (~ 25% of drug-induced AIN)
  - Onset usually few days to weeks after drug exposure
  - Predominantly involves trunk and proximal extremities
  - Represents systemic manifestation of hypersensitivity reaction
  - Rash may be absent in NSAID-induced AIN
- Fever (~ 40%)
- Arthralgias
- Oliguria may be seen
- Acute renal failure
  - Often nonoliguric
  - Older patients more susceptible
- Hypertension and pedal edema occasionally

Laboratory Tests

- Blood
  - Elevated BUN and serum creatinine
  - Eosinophilia (~ 35% > 500/mm^3)
  - Serological studies usually negative or normal (ANA, anti-DNA antibodies, ANCA, complement)
- Urine
  - Sterile pyuria
  - WBC casts
  - Eosinophils in urine
    - Typical, but not specific to AIN
  - Proteinuria
    - Usually subnephrotic range, < 1 g/day
    - Nephrotic-range proteinuria may be seen with NSAIDs

- Microscopic hematuria may be seen
- Fractional excretion of sodium > 1%
- Urine cultures negative
- Evidence of proximal and distal tubular defects
  - Aminoaciduria, glucosuria, phosphaturia, hyperkalemia, urine concentration defects

Natural History

- Acute tubular injury and acute renal failure
- Subset of untreated cases can progress to chronic renal failure

Treatment

- Drugs
  - Removal of offending drug is 1st line of therapy
  - Steroid therapy may improve recovery of renal function, especially if started early
- Supportive measures for acute renal insufficiency or renal failure

Prognosis

- Excellent recovery of renal function in most cases (60-90%) within 1-12 months
- Subset of patients are at risk for chronic renal insufficiency
  - Especially with prolonged intake of offending drug prior to diagnosis, as with over-the-counter NSAIDs
- Minimal change disease resolves on discontinuance of drug but may recur on reexposure to same or similar drug

IMAGING

Ultrasonographic Findings

- Enlarged kidneys may be seen in presence of interstitial edema

MACROSCOPIC

General Features

- Nephrectomy uncommon
  - Diagnosis based on kidney biopsy
- Enlarged kidneys due to interstitial edema

MICROSCOPIC

Histologic Features

- Interstitial inflammation
  - Predominantly mononuclear cells, plasma cells, and fewer neutrophils
  - Eosinophils usually present
  - Inflammation may be sparse in NSAID-induced AIN
- Tubulitis with infiltrating mononuclear inflammatory cells
  - Disruption of TBM may be seen on PAS stain
  - Reactive epithelial changes with sloughing, loss of brush border
  - Eosinophils in tubules
- Interstitial edema
- Granulomas in interstitium not uncommon
  - Noncaseating granulomas with epithelioid histiocytes
  - Occasional multinucleated giant cells may be seen
  - Admixed with interspersed interstitial infiltrate
  - Drug hypersensitivity causes 45% of granulomatous interstitial nephritis in biopsies
- Medullary angiitis
- Glomeruli and blood vessels usually spared
- Prominent tubular protein droplets
  - May be observed in cases of NSAID-induced coexistent minimal change disease
- Chronic changes may be seen with prolonged use of offending drug
  - Mild interstitial fibrosis
  - Thickening of TBMs and tubular atrophy
- Ureteral inflammation observed in nephrectomy specimens

ANCILLARY TESTS

Histochemistry

- Acid-fast bacteria and Gomori methenamine silver
  - Reactivity: Negative
  - Staining Pattern: Organisms may be identified in presence of mycobacterial or fungal infections

Immunohistochemistry

- Rarely necessary
- Inflammatory infiltrate usually mixed and reactive, predominantly T cells
- κ and λ immunohistochemistry or in situ hybridization reveals polyclonal plasma cell infiltrate

Immunofluorescence

- Interstitial fibrin accumulates in edema, as in delayed hypersensitivity reactions in skin
- Linear IgG stain along TBMs seen rarely
  - Reported in cases with methicillin and rifampin-induced AIN
- Tubular protein reabsorption droplets may be seen with NSAID-induced minimal change disease on albumin stain

Electron Microscopy

- Tubular epithelial changes such as loss of brush border may be seen
- Normal glomeruli in most cases
- Diffuse podocyte injury and foot process effacement may be observed
  - Seen in NSAID-induced minimal change disease
- Small, discrete TBM deposits may rarely be seen (probably of no significance)

DIFFERENTIAL DIAGNOSIS

Acute Tubular Injury

- Less interstitial inflammation and tubulitis
- Loss of tubular cell nuclei in areas without inflammation

Glomerulonephritis-Associated Interstitial Inflammation

- Interstitial inflammation can accompany any type of glomerulonephritis, but particularly in crescentic GN
- ANCA-mediated glomerulonephritis can show severe interstitial inflammation including eosinophils
  - If inadequate glomerular sampling, can be mistaken for AIN
- Presence of RBC casts should raise concern for "missed" crescentic lesions

Acute Pyelonephritis

- Neutrophils may predominate in setting of bacterial infections
- Neutrophil casts may be observed
- Infectious etiology should be ruled out with urine and blood cultures

Toxic Tubular Injury

- More necrosis of tubules, less inflammation

Granulomatous Interstitial Nephritis Due to Infection or Autoimmunity

- Caseating necrosis in granulomas may be present in mycobacterial and fungal infections
- Nonnecrotizing granulomas can be seen in sarcoidosis or granulomatosis with polyangiitis (Wegener)
- Clinical history, presence of glomerular crescents, and special stains (AFB, GMS) are helpful

Lupus Nephritis

- May have predominant tubulointerstitial inflammation
- Immune complex deposits may be seen on immunofluorescence microscopy (granular TBM deposits and interstitial deposits) and electron microscopy

IgG4-Related Tubulointerstitial Nephritis

- Increased IgG4(+) plasma cells, tubular basement membrane immune complex deposits

Sjögren Syndrome

- Clinical renal manifestations may include distal tubular acidosis, impaired urinary concentration ability, Fanconi syndrome
- Serological manifestations include anti-Ro/SSA, anti-La/SSB antibodies, hypergammaglobulinemia, and in some cases ANA
- Tubulointerstitial nephritis is active but may appear more chronic with varying degrees of tubular atrophy and interstitial fibrosis

Giant Cell Tubulitis With Tubular Basement Membrane Deposits

- Peritubular giant cell reaction
- Tubular basement membrane immune complex deposition

Tubulointerstitial Nephritis With Uveitis (Dobrin Syndrome)

- Rare in adults and reported mainly in children
- Clinical manifestations include Fanconi syndrome, renal insufficiency, proteinuria
- Ocular symptoms due to uveitis may precede or follow renal presentation

Antitubular Basement Membrane Antibody Nephritis

- Immunofluorescence microscopy shows linear staining along tubular basement membranes with IgG and often with C3

Lymphoma

- Monomorphic lymphocyte interstitial infiltrates or plasma cell infiltrate
- Evidence of monoclonal population of lymphocytes or plasma cells by immunohistochemistry or in situ hybridization

Diabetic Nephropathy

- Focal infiltrates rich in eosinophils are found in ~ 40% of biopsies with diabetic nephropathy
- Correlated with extent of fibrosis, but not with drugs or allergies

DIAGNOSTIC CHECKLIST

Clinically Relevant Pathologic Features

- Adverse prognostic features
    - Marked interstitial inflammation
    - Granulomas
    - Tubular atrophy and interstitial fibrosis

Pathologic Interpretation Pearls

- Rule out coincidental pathological changes such as IgA nephropathy or diabetic nephropathy that might explain inflammation
- Diagnosis usually requires detailed clinical history, including all drugs and serologies for autoimmune diseases
- Eosinophils in tubules may be detected
    - May have diagnostic value

SELECTED REFERENCES

1. Dai DF et al: Interstitial eosinophilic aggregates in diabetic nephropathy: allergy or not? Nephrol Dial Transplant. ePub, 2015
2. Blank ML et al: A nationwide nested case-control study indicates an increased risk of acute interstitial nephritis with proton pump inhibitor use. Kidney Int. 86(4):837-44, 2014
3. Muriithi AK et al: Biopsy-proven acute interstitial nephritis, 1993-2011: a case series. Am J Kidney Dis. 64(4):558-66, 2014
4. Hendricks AR et al: Renal medullary angiitis: a case series from a single institution. Hum Pathol. 44(4):521-5, 2013
5. Jung JM et al: Acute interstitial nephritis following kudzu root juice ingestion. Clin Nephrol. 80(4):298-300, 2013
6. González E et al: Early steroid treatment improves the recovery of renal function in patients with drug-induced acute interstitial nephritis. Kidney Int. 73(8):940-6, 2008
7. Cornell LD et al: Pseudotumors due to IgG4 immune-complex tubulointerstitial nephritis associated with autoimmune pancreatocentric disease. Am J Surg Pathol. 31(10):1586-97, 2007
8. Nadasdy T et al: Acute and chronic tubulointerstitial nephritis. In Jennette JC et al: Heptinstall's Pathology of the Kidney. 6th ed. Philadelphia: Lippincott Williams & Wilkins. 1083-1109, 2007
9. Bijol V et al: Granulomatous interstitial nephritis: a clinicopathologic study of 46 cases from a single institution. Int J Surg Pathol. 14(1):57-63, 2006
10. Spanou Z et al: Involvement of drug-specific T cells in acute drug-induced interstitial nephritis. J Am Soc Nephrol. 17(10):2919-27, 2006
11. Rossert J: Drug-induced acute interstitial nephritis. Kidney Int. 60(2):804-17, 2001
12. Whelton A: Nephrotoxicity of nonsteroidal anti-inflammatory drugs: physiologic foundations and clinical implications. Am J Med. 106(5B):13S-24S, 1999
13. De Vriese AS et al: Rifampicin-associated acute renal failure: pathophysiologic, immunologic, and clinical features. Am J Kidney Dis. 31(1):108-15, 1998
14. Michel DM et al: Acute interstitial nephritis. J Am Soc Nephrol. 9(3):506-15, 1998
15. Kleinknecht D: Interstitial nephritis, the nephrotic syndrome, and chronic renal failure secondary to nonsteroidal anti-inflammatory drugs. Semin Nephrol. 15(3):228-35, 1995
16. Ten RM et al: Acute interstitial nephritis: immunologic and clinical aspects. Mayo Clin Proc. 63(9):921-30, 1988
17. Adler SG et al: Hypersensitivity phenomena and the kidney: role of drugs and environmental agents. Am J Kidney Dis. 5(2):75-96, 1985
18. Laberke HG et al: Acute interstitial nephritis: correlations between clinical and morphological findings. Clin Nephrol. 14(6):263-73, 1980
19. Colvin RB et al: Letter: Penicillin-associated interstitial nephritis. Ann Intern Med. 81(3):404-5, 1974
20. Baldwin DS et al: Renal failure and interstitial nephritis due to penicillin and methicillin. N Engl J Med. 279(23):1245-52, 1968

(Left) *Hematoxylin & eosin shows sparse interstitial infiltrates of lymphocytes and eosinophils ➩ along with mild interstitial edema. The patient was previously treated with sulphonamide (Bactrim).* **(Right)** *Periodic acid-Schiff stain of a biopsy with AIN shows predominantly lymphocytic interstitial inflammation ➩ with a few plasma cells. The history was compatible with a drug-induced process. Acute tubular injury is evident with reactive epithelial changes and mitoses ➩.*

Aggregates of Eosinophils

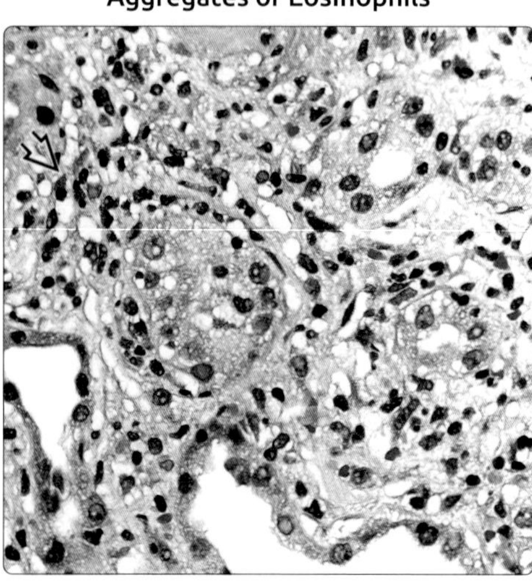

Interstitial Inflammation

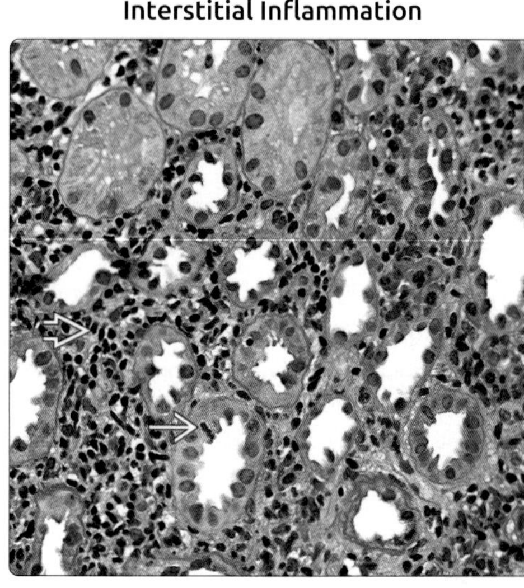

(Left) *A case of granulomatous drug-induced AIN due to moxifloxacin has a few noncaseating granulomas ➩ within the interstitium along with lymphocytes and eosinophils ➩. Multinucleated giant cells are seen in the granuloma.* **(Right)** *Perivascular granuloma consisting of epithelioid histiocytes and lymphocytes is seen in a case of drug-induced interstitial nephritis. About 45% of cases of granulomatous interstitial nephritis are caused by drugs.*

Granulomatous Interstitial Nephritis

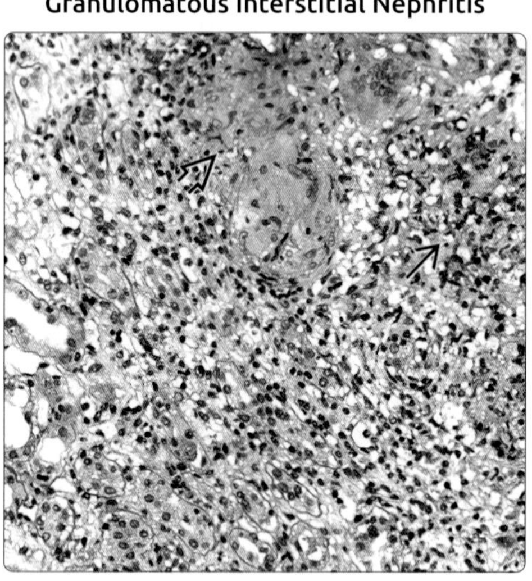

Perivascular Granuloma

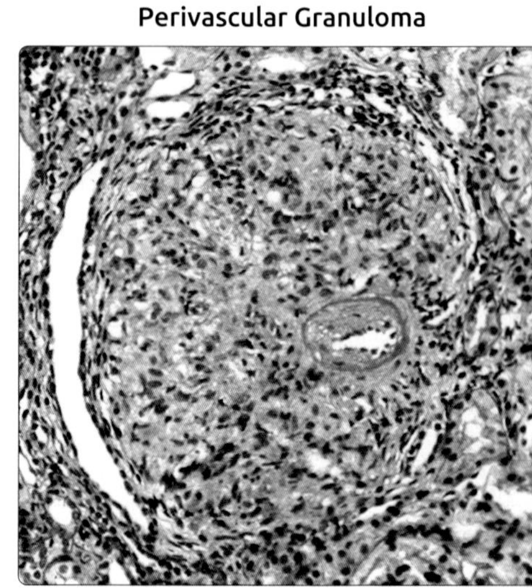

(Left) *A biopsy with acute interstitial nephritis shows predominant plasma cell infiltrate ➩ along with lymphocytes and rare eosinophils. The patient was on multiple potentially nephrotoxic drugs.* **(Right)** *Infiltrating intraepithelial lymphocytes are seen within nonatrophic tubules (tubulitis) ➩ in a biopsy with AIN. There is evidence of proximal tubular injury with loss of brush borders ➩.*

Plasma Cell Aggregates

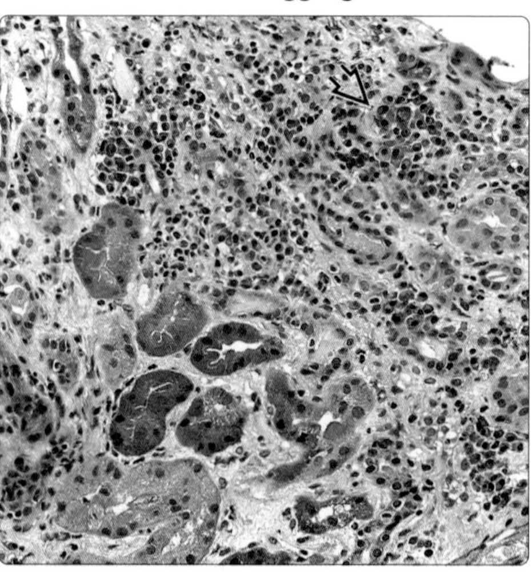

Tubulitis

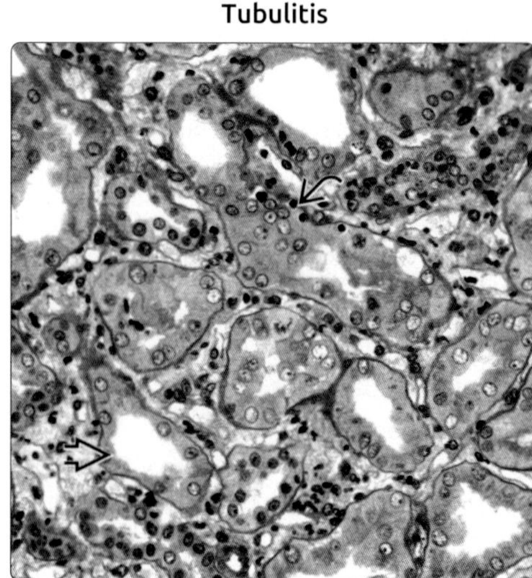

Acute Tubular Injury

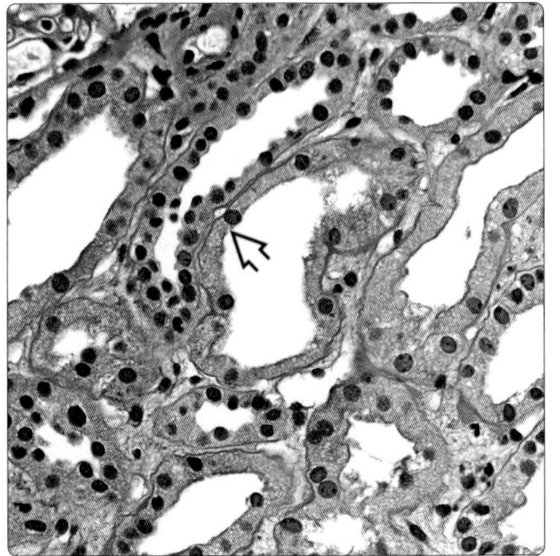

Chronic Interstitial Nephritis

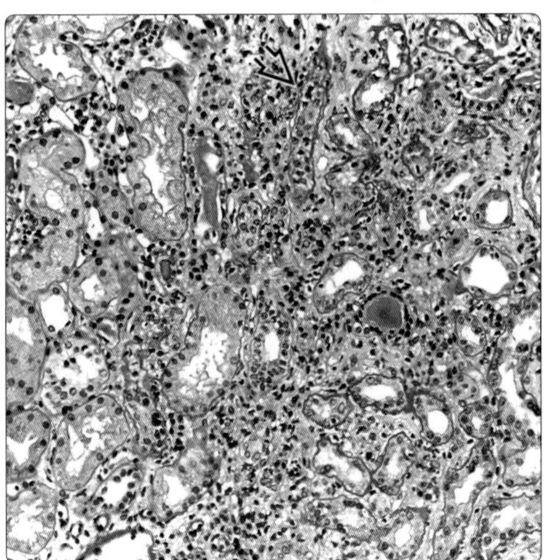

(Left) *Periodic acid-Schiff shows mild acute tubular injury characterized by loss of brush borders ➡ in the proximal tubules. The patient presented with acute renal insufficiency subsequent to NSAID treatment. Sparse interstitial infiltrate was seen elsewhere.* **(Right)** *The patient had been on furosemide for a few months prior to biopsy. Chronic tubulointerstitial damage is evident with TBM thickening in atrophic tubules ➡. In the absence of other pathology, these changes were attributed to progression of furosemide-induced AIN.*

Eosinophilic Inflammatory Infiltrate

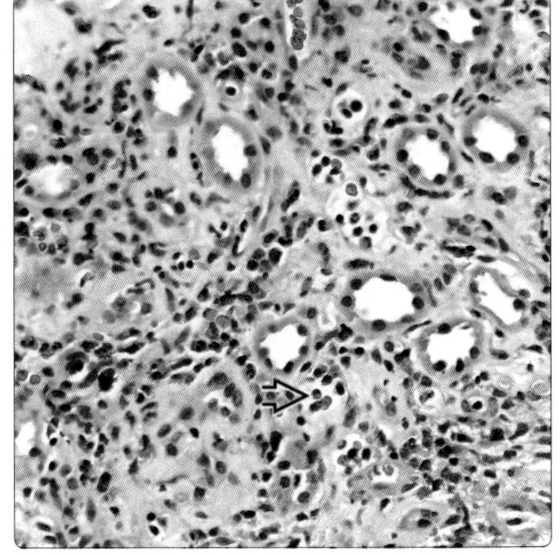

Red Blood Cell Casts

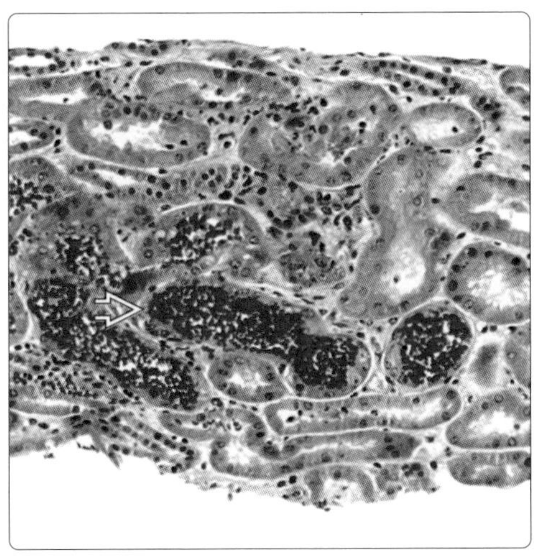

(Left) *Pauci-immune glomerulonephritis can have prominent eosinophilic infiltrate ➡ in interstitium, reminiscent of AIN. Patient presented with acute renal failure, and urinalysis revealed RBC casts, which would be unusual in AIN.* **(Right)** *Presence of RBC casts ➡ in a suspected case of AIN (clinically and histologically) should raise concern for unsampled crescents in pauci-immune glomerulonephritis. Patient was subsequently found to have positive ANCA serologies.*

Acute Interstitial Nephritis in Diabetes

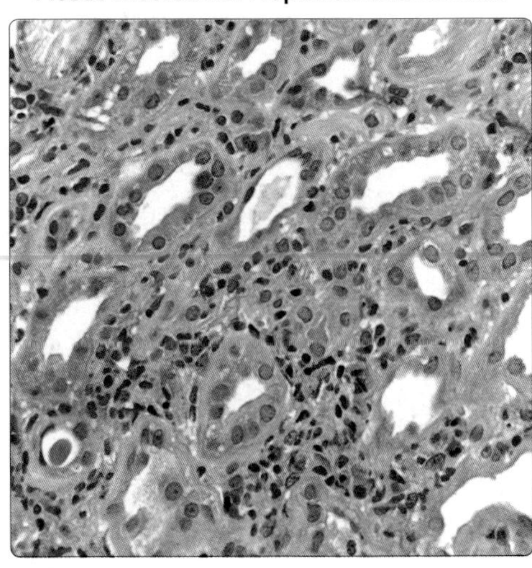

Low-Grade Lymphoma

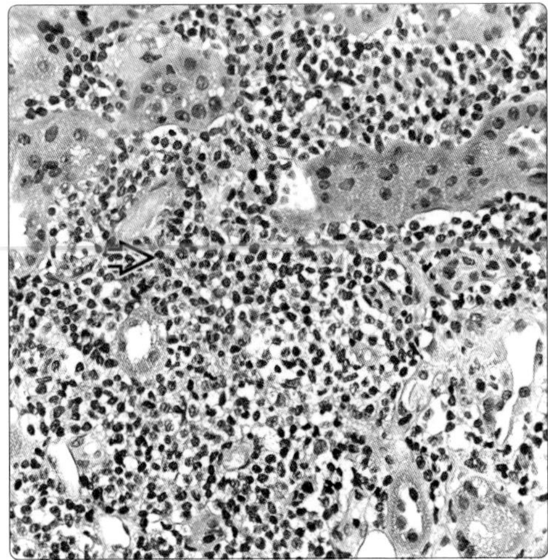

(Left) *This field shows prominent eosinophils in a mixed interstitial infiltrate in a patient with diabetes. No specific drug or infection could be implicated. Renal biopsies with diabetic nephropathy often show mild interstitial nephritis with eosinophils, without a clear etiology.* **(Right)** *Prominent interstitial monomorphic lymphocytic infiltrate ➡ is seen, atypical for AIN. Immunohistochemical analysis confirmed the presence of a low-grade lymphoma (CD5 and CD10 negative).*

KEY FACTS

TERMINOLOGY

- Coagulative necrosis of papillary tips of medulla

ETIOLOGY/PATHOGENESIS

- Medullary ischemia
  - Vasoconstriction by NSAIDs
  - Luminal occlusion of small arteries and arterioles
    - Diabetic arteriopathy, sickle hemoglobinopathy, transplant arteriopathy
- Concentration of nephrotoxic agents in medulla
- Infection
- Urinary outflow obstruction
- Volume depletion exacerbates risk

CLINICAL ISSUES

- > 60 years at presentation
- More common in women, diabetics
- Subacute presentation more common
  - Lumbar pain, hematuria
  - Fever, chills
- Bilateral in 65-70% of cases
- Long history of analgesic use

MICROSCOPIC

- Inner zone of medulla and papillary tip
- Papillae with coagulative necrosis
  - Loss of outlines of tubules and blood vessels
- Necrotic area rimmed by neutrophils in tubules and interstitium
- No inflammatory cells within necrotic area

TOP DIFFERENTIAL DIAGNOSES

- Parenchymal infarction
  - Area of involvement not limited to medullary tip

DIAGNOSTIC CHECKLIST

- Histological features may suggest causative factor
- Shed papilla in urine identified with periodic acid-Schiff stain

Papillary Necrosis in Analgesic Abuse

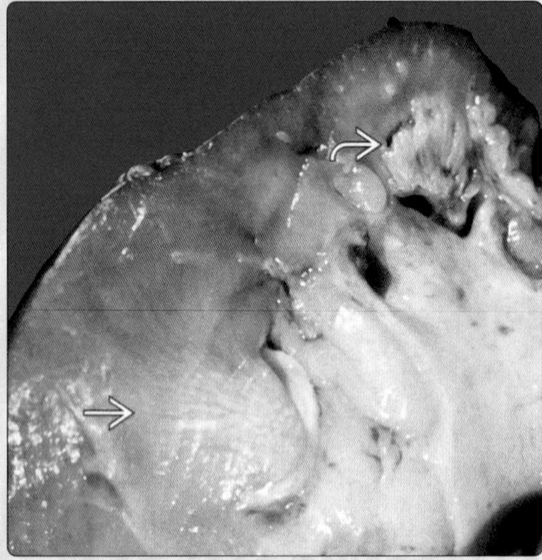

Necrotic Papillary Tip With Adjacent Inflammation

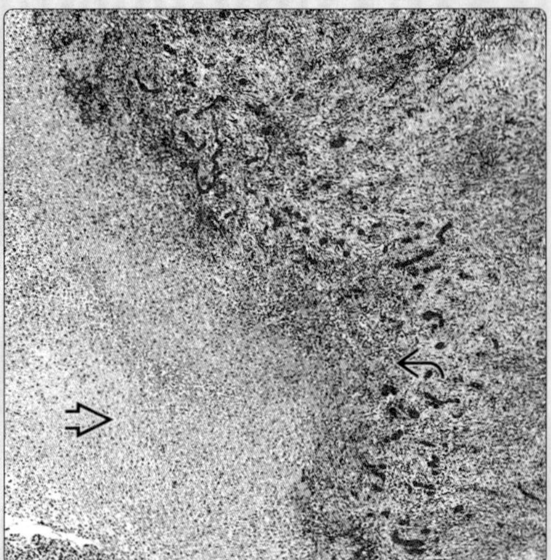

(Left) *Gross photograph of a kidney shows necrotic papilla ➲ and corresponding atrophic cortex due to analgesic abuse. The line of demarcation of the necrosis is evident. One papilla with its overlying cortex is normal ➡.* **(Right)** *Hematoxylin and eosin of the papillary tip of the renal medulla shows extensive necrosis ⇨ with scant inflammation. The periphery of this necrotic area shows intense inflammatory infiltrate ➲.*

Acute Pyelonephritis Involving Papillary Tip

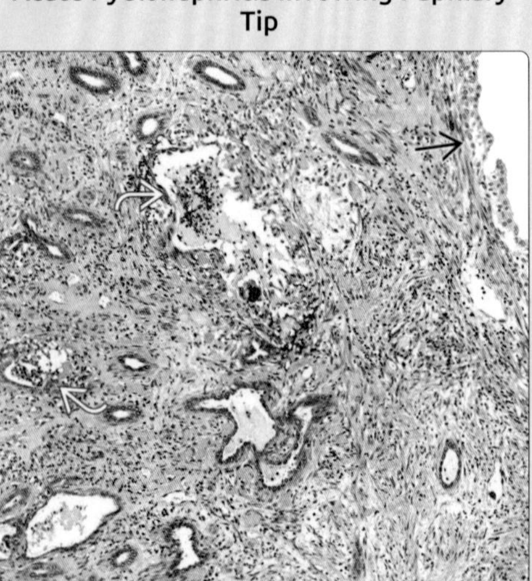

Papilla Shed in Urine

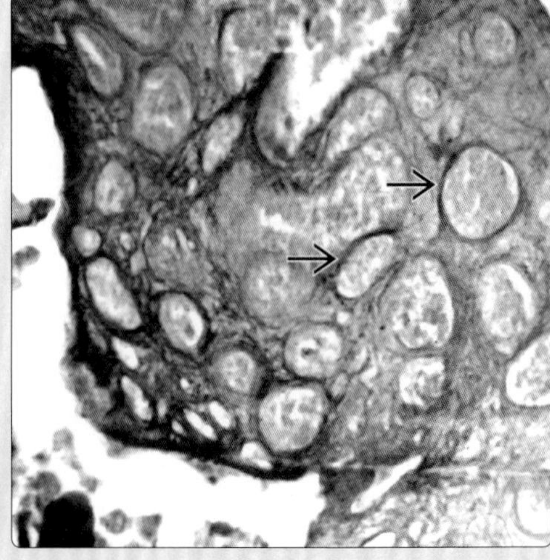

(Left) *Hematoxylin and eosin shows accumulation of neutrophils in dilated collecting ducts ➲ at papillary tip. Adjacent pelvic urothelium ➡ is seen. The patient has ureteral stricture, hydronephrosis, and acute pyelonephritis. Necrotic papillae were seen elsewhere in the kidney.* **(Right)** *Periodic acid-Schiff, applied to shed papilla recovered in the urine, highlights the tubular basement membranes ➡. No cellular elements are preserved.*

TERMINOLOGY

Abbreviations

- Papillary necrosis (PN)

Synonyms

- Medullary necrosis
- Necrotizing papillitis

Definitions

- Coagulative necrosis of papillary tips of medulla

ETIOLOGY/PATHOGENESIS

Medullary Ischemia

- Medulla receives 8-10% of total renal blood flow
- Rich vascular plexus of vasa recta contribute mainly to countercurrent mechanism
- Nutrient supply for medulla is limited, blood vessels are mostly terminal
- Aggravating factors
  - Luminal occlusion of small arteries and arterioles
    - Diabetic arteriopathy
    - Sickle hemoglobinopathy
    - Transplanted kidney with arteriopathy
    - Age-related arteriolosclerosis
  - Vasoconstrictor effect due to prostaglandin inhibition
    - Nonsteroidal anti-inflammatory drugs (NSAIDs)
  - Volume depletion
    - Dehydration, congestive heart failure

Concentration of Nephrotoxic Agents in Medulla

- Tubular concentration of solute in medulla promotes water reabsorption
- Potentially nephrotoxic agents concentrated in medulla
  - Phenacetin, NSAIDs (ibuprofen, indomethacin, naproxen, tolmetin, benoxaprofen)

CLINICAL ISSUES

Epidemiology

- Incidence
  - Uncommon in absence of predisposing factors
  - Reduced incidence with improved therapeutic options for aggressive control of predisposing factors, such as diabetes mellitus and acute pyelonephritis
    - Affected patients often have > 1 causative factor for PN, such as diabetes mellitus, infection, or analgesic abuse
- Age
  - > 60 years old
  - Occurs at younger age in sickle hemoglobinopathies
- Sex
  - More common in women

Site

- Inner zone of medulla and papillary tip
- Bilateral in 65-70% of cases

Presentation

- Subacute presentation more common
  - Lumbar pain
  - Hematuria
  - Fever, chills
  - Inability to concentrate urine with resultant polyuria and nocturia
  - Renal insufficiency if several papillae affected
- Acute onset (rare)
  - Acute renal failure
  - Sepsis
- Asymptomatic passage of necrotic papillary material

Laboratory Tests

- Difficult to diagnose
- Strain urine for necrotic papillae

Treatment

- Options, risks, complications
  - Complications
    - Acute or chronic renal failure
    - Infection and septicemia as necrotic papilla forms nidus for infection
    - Severe hematuria
    - Obstruction of urinary tract by sloughed papillae
- Surgical approaches
  - Relieve urinary tract obstruction, if present
- Adjuvant therapy
  - Removal of offending factor
    - Avoidance of analgesics
    - Treatment of sickle cell crisis
    - Blood glucose control in diabetics
  - Control aggravating factors for medullary injury
    - Control of hypertension
    - Avoidance of antihypertensives that reduce renal blood flow, such as β-blockers
    - Avoidance of volume depletion and dehydration
- Drugs
  - Antimicrobial therapy for acute pyelonephritis, if present
  - Adequate glycemic control in diabetes mellitus

Prognosis

- Variable based on early identification of causative factors and prompt treatment

IMAGING

Radiographic Findings

- Retrograde pyelogram can show calyceal blunting
- Imaging studies may identify evidence of urinary tract obstruction

MACROSCOPIC

General Features

- Kidneys may be enlarged in diabetes mellitus
- Edematous kidneys may be seen in acute pyelonephritis
- Yellowish red, sharply defined areas in papillae with congested borders
- Cortical atrophy restricted to lobes with papillary necrosis

MICROSCOPIC

Histologic Features

- Papillae with coagulative necrosis and loss of outlines of tubules

Clinical Conditions Associated With Renal Papillary Necrosis

Condition	Frequency of Cause	Comments
Diabetes mellitus	50-60%	PN is 5x more prevalent in diabetic than nondiabetic patients (autopsy series); urinary tract infection always concurrent complication
Urinary tract obstruction	10-40%	Urinary outflow obstruction can reduce medullary blood flow, mediated by cytokines released from infiltrating monocytes
Analgesic abuse (analgesic nephropathy)	15-20%	More common with phenacetin use and its removal from the market > 20 years ago resulted in dramatic decline in diagnosis
Sickle hemoglobinopathy	10-15%	Can occur in both sickle cell anemia and trait; often present with hematuria
Acute pyelonephritis	5%	More often in diabetic patients with severe acute pyelonephritis and urinary tract obstruction
Renal transplantation	< 5%	Allograft arteriopathy can predispose to medullary ischemia
Other reported conditions associated with papillary necrosis include tuberculosis, chronic liver disease, and systemic vasculitis.		

- No inflammatory cells within necrotic area in early phase
- Necrotic area rimmed by neutrophils in interstitium
- Calcification of rim of necrotic area or tubular basement membranes
- Features of predisposing factors may be seen
  - Diabetic nephropathy with diffuse and nodular mesangial sclerosis, hyalinosis
  - Analgesic nephropathy with
    - Interstitial fibrosis
    - Tubular atrophy
    - Capillary sclerosis
  - Sickle cell disease with sickled red cells within capillaries (often peritubular)
  - Acute pyelonephritis with neutrophil casts

ANCILLARY TESTS

Immunofluorescence

- Negative with no evidence of immune complexes

Electron Microscopy

- No electron-dense deposits
- Nonspecific glomerular changes in acute pyelonephritis and analgesic nephropathy
- Diabetic nephropathy features, such as mesangial sclerosis, thickened basement membranes may be seen

DIFFERENTIAL DIAGNOSIS

Parenchymal Infarction

- Nonviable parenchyma with outlines of glomeruli, tubules, and blood vessels
- No acute inflammation in area of infarction, but inflammatory infiltrate may be at periphery
- Can occur in thromboembolism
  - Thrombi may be in blood vessels
  - No evidence of transmural inflammatory infiltrate to suggest vasculitis
- Can occur in vasculitis
  - Transmural inflammation of arteries/arterioles with necrosis
  - Glomerular involvement may be present with proliferation &/or crescents
- Can occur in thrombotic microangiopathy
  - Thrombi and fragmented red blood cells in arterioles &/or glomeruli
  - No evidence of vasculitis
- Clinical history and serological testing help determine cause of thromboembolism, vasculitis, or thrombotic microangiopathy
- Area of involvement not limited to medullary tip but can include glomeruli and blood vessels
- Usually results in wedge-shaped cortical infarcts

DIAGNOSTIC CHECKLIST

Clinically Relevant Pathologic Features

- Extent of necrosis
- Histological features may suggest causative factor

Pathologic Interpretation Pearls

- Shed necrotic papilla in urine can be identified with periodic acid-Schiff stain

SELECTED REFERENCES

1. Gupta KL et al: Mucormycosis of the transplanted kidney with renal papillary necrosis. Exp Clin Transplant. 11(6):554-7, 2013
2. Saravu K et al: Candidal renal papillary necrosis conquered. J Assoc Physicians India. 61(8):573-4, 2013
3. Bansal R et al: An unusual cause of renal allograft dysfunction: graft papillary necrosis. J Nephrol. 20(1):111-3, 2007
4. Olson JL et al: Diabetic nephropathy. In Jennette JC et al: Heptinstall's Pathology of the Kidney. 6th ed. Philadelphia: Lippincott Williams & Wilkins. 840-1, 2007
5. Mihatsch MJ et al: Obituary to analgesic nephropathy–an autopsy study. Nephrol Dial Transplant. 21(11):3139-45, 2006
6. Eknoyan G et al: Renal papillary necrosis. In Greenberg A et al: Primer on Kidney Disease. 4th ed. San Diego: National Kidney Foundation. 385-8, 2005
7. Ducloux D et al: Renal papillary necrosis in a marathon runner. Nephrol Dial Transplant. 14(1):247-8, 1999
8. Whelton A: Nephrotoxicity of nonsteroidal anti-inflammatory drugs: physiologic foundations and clinical implications. Am J Med. 106(5B):13S-24S, 1999
9. Fong P et al: Idiopathic acute granulomatous interstitial nephritis leading to renal papillary necrosis. Nephrol Dial Transplant. 12(5):1043-5, 1997
10. Patterson JE et al: Bacterial urinary tract infections in diabetes. Infect Dis Clin North Am. 11(3):735-50, 1997
11. Griffin MD et al: Renal papillary necrosis–a sixteen-year clinical experience. J Am Soc Nephrol. 6(2):248-56, 1995
12. Eknoyan G et al: Renal papillary necrosis: an update. Medicine (Baltimore). 61(2):55-73, 1982

Multiple Necrotic Papillae

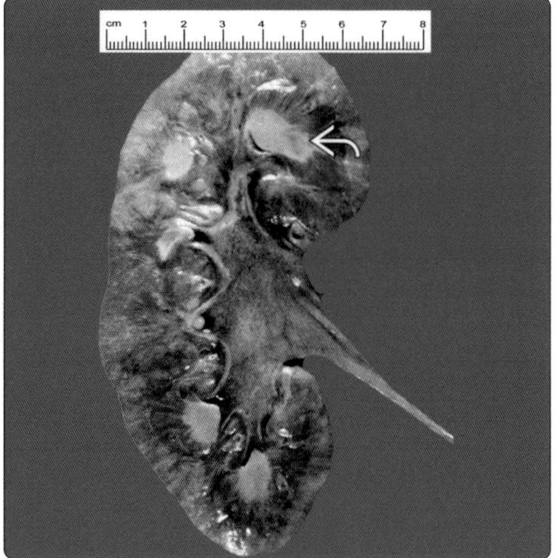
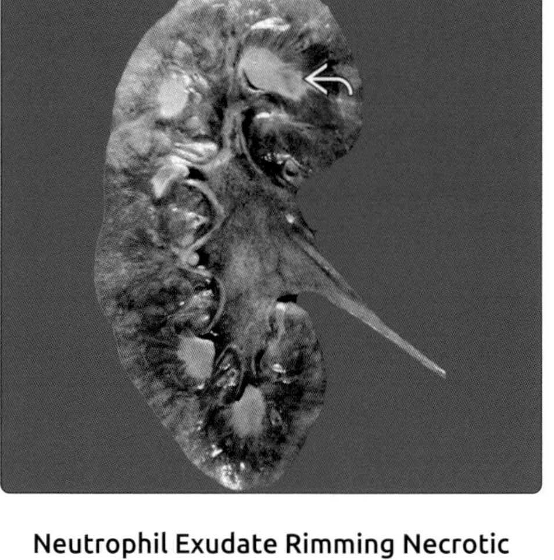

Renal Papillary Necrosis

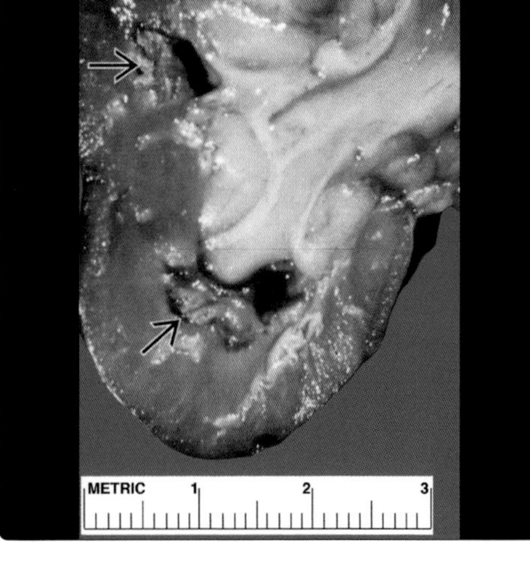

(Left) *A kidney is shown with multiple necrotic papillae ➡ that are pale and distinctly demarcated from the overlying cortex. The etiology of renal papillary necrosis in this instance was acute pyelonephritis. (Courtesy L. Fajardo, MD.)* **(Right)** *The necrotic papillae ➡ in this nephrectomy specimen are soft and friable. The etiology of renal papillary necrosis is acute pyelonephritis. (Courtesy L. Fajardo, MD.)*

Neutrophil Exudate Rimming Necrotic Papillae

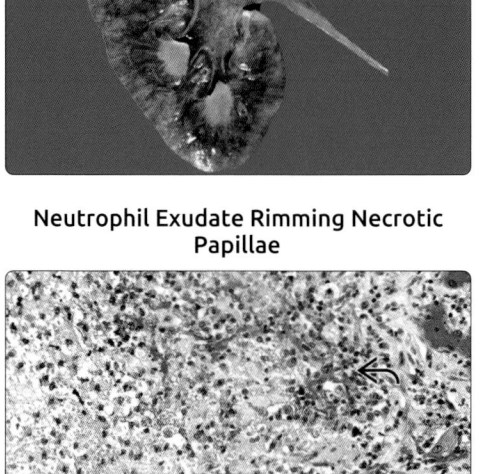

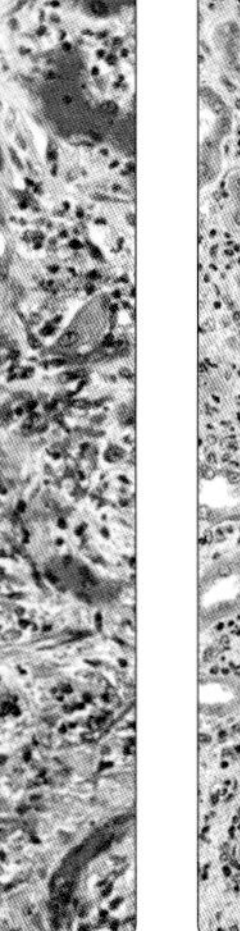

Neutrophil Casts in Acute Pyelonephritis

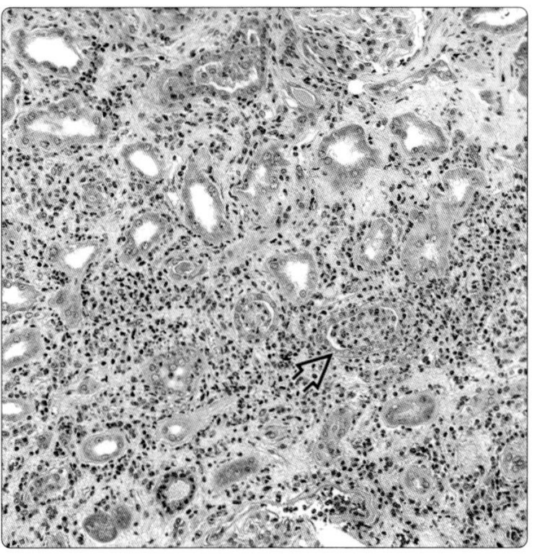

(Left) *Hematoxylin and eosin shows an area of necrotic papillae with acellular debris rimmed by neutrophils ➡. Mild chronic inflammation and granulation tissue reaction are seen at the periphery ➡.* **(Right)** *Hematoxylin and eosin shows acute pyelonephritis with interstitial edema and inflammation composed of neutrophils and lymphocytes. Focal neutrophil casts are also seen ➡. The patient was diabetic, and there was evidence of papillary necrosis elsewhere in the kidney.*

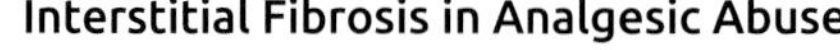

Interstitial Fibrosis in Analgesic Abuse

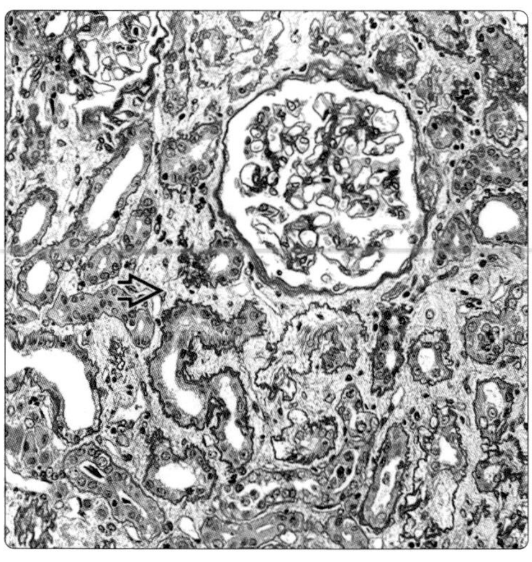

Diabetic Nephropathy and Acute Pyelonephritis

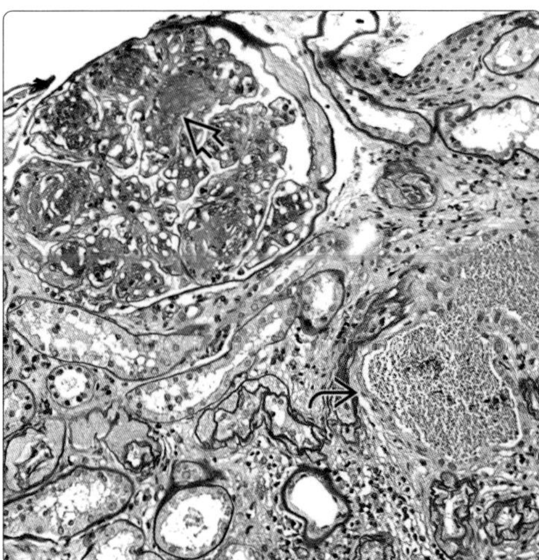

(Left) *Diffuse interstitial fibrosis and tubular atrophy are seen ➡, although the glomeruli are relatively spared in a patient with prolonged use of analgesics and anti-inflammatory drugs. Analgesic abuse may be associated with papillary necrosis.* **(Right)** *Biopsy specimen shows nodular sclerosing diabetic nephropathy ➡ with adjacent tubular debris and neutrophil casts ➡. Diabetes mellitus is a predisposing factor for acute pyelonephritis and papillary necrosis.*

KEY FACTS

TERMINOLOGY

- Acute renal failure associated with pigmented tubular casts due to either myoglobinuria or hemoglobinuria

ETIOLOGY/PATHOGENESIS

- Rhabdomyolysis (injury to skeletal muscle) releases myoglobin, an iron-containing skeletal muscle protein
  - Trauma, drugs, toxins, inherited metabolic disorders
  - Predisposing factors include dehydration, fasting, hypo- or hyperthermia, hypoxia, hypokalemia
- Intravascular hemolysis
  - Mismatched blood transfusions, infections
- Kidney susceptible to toxicity of heme proteins via vasoconstriction and tubular cytotoxicity
- Reduced urinary pH promotes promotes cast formation
- Distal tubular obstruction by pigmented casts and sloughed cells prolongs exposure to denatured heme proteins

CLINICAL ISSUES

- Acute renal failure
- Elevated creatine kinase (CK-MM, often > 100,000 IU/L)
  - Peaks within 48 hours after rhabdomyolysis with half-life of 48 hours
- Treatment is supportive with hydration

MICROSCOPIC

- Brown pigmented casts of hemoglobin or myoglobin, especially in distal tubules
- Acute tubular injury

ANCILLARY TESTS

- Myoglobin and hemoglobin immunohistochemistry

TOP DIFFERENTIAL DIAGNOSES

- Bile cast nephropathy
- Myeloma cast nephropathy
- Acute ischemic or toxic tubular injury

Pigmented Casts and Acute Tubular Injury

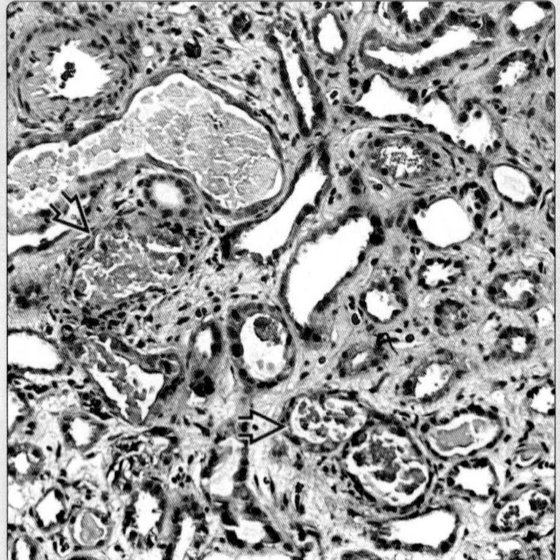

Pigmented Tubular Casts

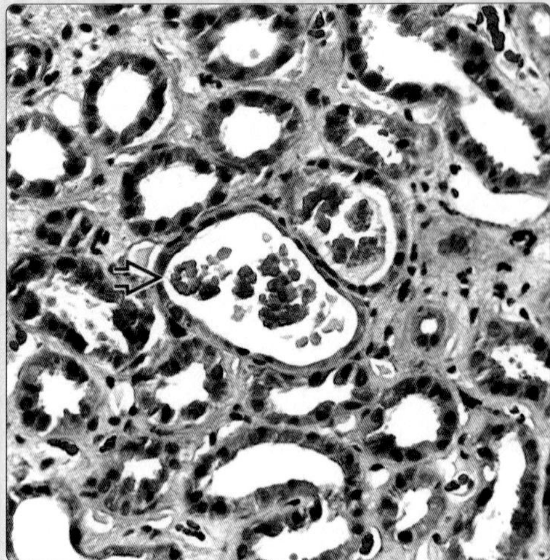

(Left) *In rhabdomyolysis, light brown pigmented casts* ⇨ *can be seen within renal tubules. Other tubules show acute injury with simplified epithelium and ectatic lumens separated by interstitial edema.* **(Right)** *This renal biopsy is from a patient with acute renal failure after a motor vehicle accident. Pigmented casts due to myoglobin are present* ⇨. *Features of acute tubular injury are also seen with loss of brush borders, dilated lumens, and basophilic cytoplasm.*

Myoglobin Casts on Immunohistochemistry

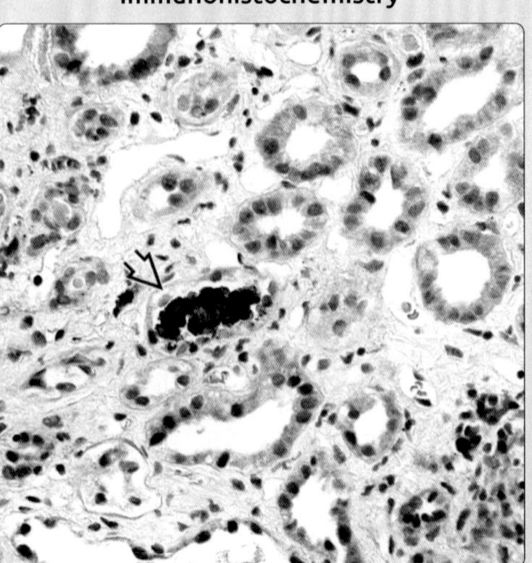

Ultrastructure of Myoglobin Casts

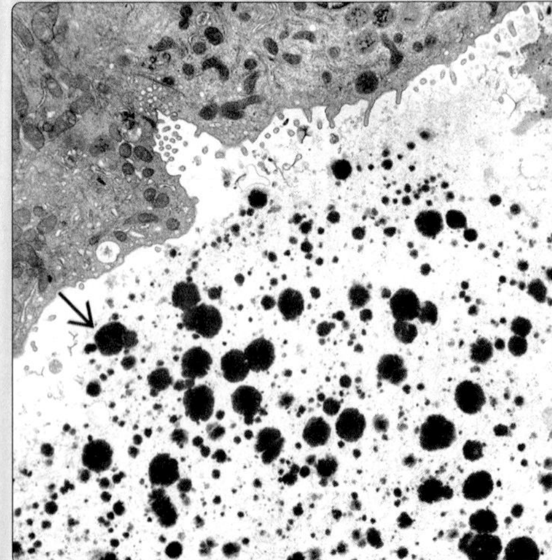

(Left) *Myoglobin immunohistochemistry stains the myoglobin casts* ⇨. *Myoglobin, released by rhabdomyolysis, is excreted in the glomerular filtrate and forms tubular casts. (Courtesy M. Troxell, MD, PhD.)* **(Right)** *On electron microscopy, the tubular pigmented cast is composed of electron-dense myoglobin globules* ➔.

TERMINOLOGY

Definitions

- Acute renal failure associated with pigmented tubular casts due to either myoglobinuria or hemoglobinuria

ETIOLOGY/PATHOGENESIS

Myoglobinuria

- Rhabdomyolysis (injury to skeletal muscle) releases myoglobin, an iron-containing skeletal muscle protein
  - Trauma, such as intense physical exercise, grand mal seizures, pressure injury
  - Drugs, such as cocaine, heroin, amphetamines, HMG-CoA inhibitors (statins)
  - Toxins, such as snake venom, clostridial toxin
  - Inflammation, as in polymyositis
  - Inherited metabolic myopathies
- Precipitating and exacerbating factors for muscle injury
  - Dehydration, fasting, hypo- or hyperthermia, hypoxia, hypokalemia

Hemoglobinuria

- Intravascular hemolysis
  - Mismatched blood transfusions
  - Infections, such as falciparum malaria, *Mycoplasma pneumoniae*
  - Free hemoglobin that exceeds capacity of binding protein haptoglobin filtered by glomerulus

Mechanisms of Renal Injury by Myoglobin and Hemoglobin

- Myoglobin smaller than hemoglobin (16,700 vs. 64,500 daltons), more easily filtered by glomerulus
- Heme proteins promote vasoconstriction and ischemic tubular injury
- Heme proteins have cytotoxic effects
  - Breakdown product heme and iron are toxic to cell organelles and cause oxidative stress
- Reduced urinary pH promotes cast formation
- Distal tubular obstruction by pigmented casts and sloughed cells prolongs exposure to denatured heme proteins

CLINICAL ISSUES

Epidemiology

- Sex
  - Men more susceptible to exertional rhabdomyolysis

Presentation

- Acute renal failure
  - Abrupt onset of oliguria
  - Cola-colored urine
- Muscle swelling, bruising, stiffness

Laboratory Tests

- Urinalysis
  - Dipstick + for heme protein, but no erythrocytes
  - Dark pigmented casts on urine microscopy
- Blood tests
  - ↑ creatine kinase (CK-MM isoform, often > 100,000 IU/L)
    - Peaks within 48 hours after rhabdomyolysis with half-life of 48 hours
    - False negative with very high levels
  - ↑ serum Cr (BUN: Cr ratio < 5:1)
  - Hyperkalemia, hyperphosphatemia, hypocalcemia, hyperuricemia

Treatment

- Supportive
  - Hydration, alkalinization of urine, mannitol, correction of electrolyte imbalances, dialysis
- Elimination of cause (drug, toxin, trauma, infection)

Prognosis

- Recovery with prompt diagnosis and treatment

MICROSCOPIC

Histologic Features

- Brown pigmented casts of hemoglobin or myoglobin, especially in distal tubules
- Acute tubular injury
  - Loss of brush borders, sloughed epithelial cells, dilated lumens
  - Hyaline, cellular, and granular casts may be seen
- Interstitial edema without significant interstitial inflammation
- Glomeruli spared
- No evidence of deposits on light microscopy, immunofluorescence, or electron microscopy

ANCILLARY TESTS

Immunohistochemistry

- Myoglobin positive in myoglobin casts
- Hemoglobin positive in hemoglobin casts

Electron Microscopy

- Casts contain electron-dense granules

DIFFERENTIAL DIAGNOSIS

Bile Cast Nephropathy

- Severe liver dysfunction, usually with jaundice
- Casts appear identical to myoglobin or hemoglobin

Myeloma Cast Nephropathy

- Fractured casts, which are light chain restricted on immunofluorescence microscopy

Acute (Ischemic or Toxic) Tubular Necrosis

- Pigmented casts from mitochondrial cytochromes lack myoglobin or hemoglobin

SELECTED REFERENCES

1. Khalighi MA et al: Intratubular hemoglobin casts in hemolysis-associated acute kidney injury. Am J Kidney Dis. 65(2):337-41, 2015
2. Zimmerman JL et al: Rhabdomyolysis. Chest. 144(3):1058-65, 2013
3. Pelletier R et al: Acute renal failure following kidney transplantation associated with myoglobinuria in patients treated with rapamycin. Transplantation. 82(5):645-50, 2006
4. Zager RA: Rhabdomyolysis and myohemoglobinuric acute renal failure. Kidney Int. 49(2):314-26, 1996
5. Knochel JP: Mechanisms of rhabdomyolysis. Curr Opin Rheumatol. 5(6):725-31, 1993
6. Gabow PA et al: The spectrum of rhabdomyolysis. Medicine (Baltimore). 61(3):141-52, 1982

Cisplatin Nephrotoxicity

KEY FACTS

TERMINOLOGY

- Nephropathy due to toxicity of platinum compounds

ETIOLOGY/PATHOGENESIS

- *Cis*-diamminedichloroplatinum (II)
  - Potent inhibitor of nuclear and mitochondrial DNA synthesis
    - 1/3 develop acute kidney injury after dose of 2 mg/kg
  - Nephrotoxicity may be detectable after a single dose
    - Dose dependent severity
  - Exposure in cancer chemotherapy

CLINICAL ISSUES

- Acute kidney injury within days of exposure
- Majority receiving low dose CDDP have reversible kidney injury
  - Small proportion develop chronic kidney disease (< 5%)
- Hydration as prophylaxis
- Cessation of CDDP exposure

MICROSCOPIC

- Acute tubular necrosis may be marked and affects proximal, distal, and collecting tubules
- Regeneration characterized by nuclear atypia and polypoid epithelial proliferations
- Necrosis and tubular nuclear atypia may persist for months

TOP DIFFERENTIAL DIAGNOSES

- Heavy metal toxicity: Mercury, lead, and copper
- Drugs: Antiretroviral reverse transcriptase agents; busulfan (rare)
- Viral infections: Polyomavirus, adenovirus, HIV
- Karyomegalic interstitial nephritis

Acute Tubular Injury

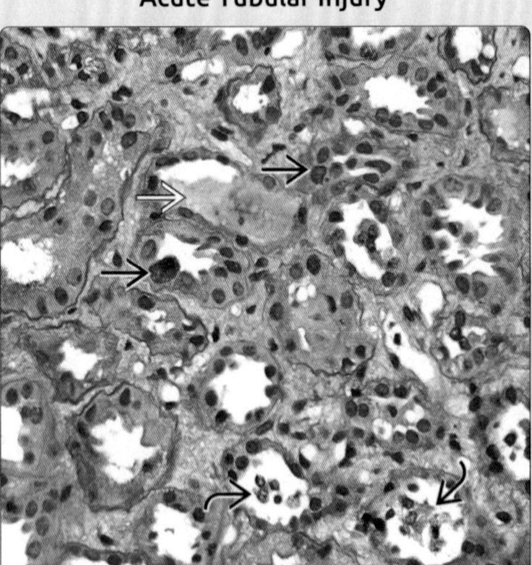

Dilated Distal Tubules in CDDP Toxicity

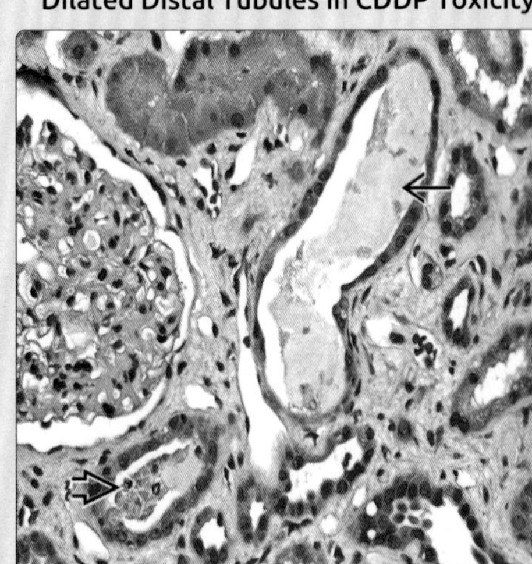

(Left) *The renal cortex in recent cisplatin nephrotoxicity demonstrates luminal cellular debris ➪, distal tubular casts ➡, regenerative nuclear atypia ➙, and interstitial edema, features of acute tubular injury/necrosis.* **(Right)** *Kidney cortex shows dilated distal tubular segments with luminal cast material ➙ and cellular debris ➪ from a patient with recent cisplatin exposure. The interstitium is edematous.*

Acute Tubular Injury and Regeneration

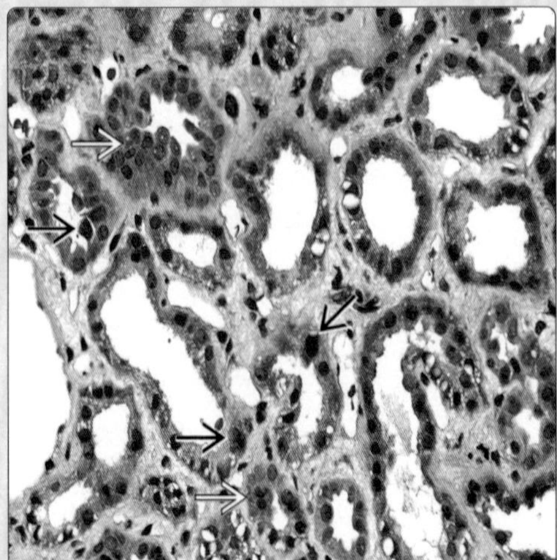

Tubular Nuclear Atypia

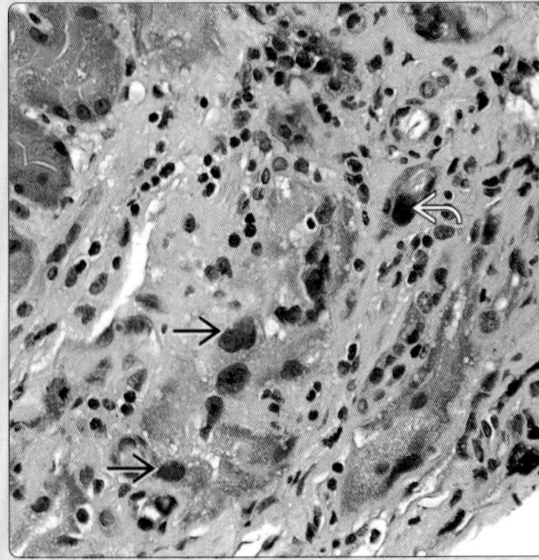

(Left) *Acute tubular injury in cisplatin toxicity is shown with open lumens and atypical nuclei ➙. Hypercellular collecting ducts ➡ are a feature of regeneration after acute tubular injury/necrosis.* **(Right)** *Remote exposure to cisplatin may be associated with interstitial mononuclear inflammation, fibrosis, and marked nuclear atypia in proximal ➙ and distal ➡ tubular segments.*

TERMINOLOGY

Abbreviations

- *Cis*-diamminedichloroplatinum (II) (CDDP)

Synonyms

- Platinum nephrotoxicity
- Cisplatinum nephrotoxicity
- Cis-platinum nephrotoxicity
- CDDP nephrotoxicity

Definitions

- Nephropathy due to toxic effects of platinum compounds

ETIOLOGY/PATHOGENESIS

Cis-diamminedichloroplatinum (II)

- Heavy metal and potent inhibitor of DNA synthesis
  - Intracellular transporters of CDDP
    - OCT2 (SLC22A2)
    - Ctr1
  - Concentrated in kidney tissue and excreted in urine
  - Human exposure in cancer chemotherapy
  - Nephrotoxicity mediated in part by p53
- Nephrotoxicity may be detectable after single dose with dose-dependent severity
  - 1/3 develop acute kidney injury after dose of 2 mg/kg
- Toxicity initially reversible, but repeat doses increase irreversibility

CLINICAL ISSUES

Presentation

- Acute kidney injury
  - Increased serum creatinine within days after administration
  - Serum creatinine peaks at about 10 days (8-12)
  - Recovery may take weeks or months
- Subnephrotic-range proteinuria
- Hypomagnesemia due to decreased tubular reabsorption
- Impaired urinary concentrating ability with polyuria

Treatment

- Hydration as prophylaxis
- Cessation of CDDP exposure
- Amifostine
  - FDA approved to reduce nephrotoxicity in advanced ovarian carcinoma

Prognosis

- Majority receiving low-dose CDDP have reversible kidney injury
  - Small proportion develop chronic kidney disease (< 5%)
  - Underlying kidney disease predisposes to irreversible injury
- Unknown risk of renal carcinoma

MACROSCOPIC

Gross Examination

- Kidneys with acute injury are enlarged with pale cortex and red, congested medulla

MICROSCOPIC

Histologic Features

- Acute tubular injury and necrosis affect proximal, distal, and collecting tubules
  - Multifocal attenuated epithelium ± vacuoles, desquamation, coagulative necrosis
    - Cellular, granular or hyaline casts
    - Distal tubular dilation
    - Necrosis of medullary collecting ducts
  - Necrosis may persist for months
- Regenerative tubular nuclear atypia arises after 10 days and persists for months
  - Nuclear enlargement and hyperchromasia prominent in collecting ducts
    - Regenerative epithelial proliferation often polypoid
- Mild interstitial edema and mononuclear infiltrate
  - Interstitial nephritis uncommon
- Glomeruli and vessels have no specific abnormalities
  - Rare reports of thrombotic microangiopathy

ANCILLARY TESTS

Electron Microscopy

- Proximal tubules
  - Mitochondrial vacuolar changes in 2 days
  - Loss of surface microvilli in about 3 days
  - Platinum particles undetectable even by electron probe x-ray analysis

DIFFERENTIAL DIAGNOSIS

Tubular Necrosis With Nuclear Atypia

- Heavy metal toxicity: Mercury, lead, and copper
- Drugs: Antiretroviral reverse transcriptase agents; busulfan (rare)
- Viral infections: Polyomavirus, adenovirus, HIV
- Karyomegalic interstitial nephritis

DIAGNOSTIC CHECKLIST

Clinically Relevant Pathologic Features

- Tubular necrosis and regenerative atypia persist for months

Pathologic Interpretation Pearls

- Tubular epithelial necrosis affects all nephron segments
- Regeneration with nuclear atypia and epithelial polypoid proliferations

SELECTED REFERENCES

1. Peres LA et al: Acute nephrotoxicity of cisplatin: molecular mechanisms. J Bras Nefrol. 35(4):332-40, 2013
2. Miller RP et al: Mechanisms of Cisplatin nephrotoxicity. Toxins (Basel). 2(11):2490-518, 2010
3. Ries F et al: Nephrotoxicity induced by cancer chemotherapy with special emphasis on cisplatin toxicity. Am J Kidney Dis. 8(5):368-79, 1986
4. Tanaka H et al: Histopathological study of human cisplatin nephropathy. Toxicol Pathol. 14(2):247-57, 1986
5. Madias NE et al: Platinum nephrotoxicity. Am J Med. 65(2):307-14, 1978
6. Gonzales-Vitale JC et al: The renal pathology in clinical trials of cis-platinum (II) diamminedichloride. Cancer. 39(4):1362-71, 1977

Osmotic Tubulopathy

KEY FACTS

TERMINOLOGY

- Tubular epithelial swelling and isometric vacuolization associated with exposure to parenteral carbohydrate solutions or contrast media and acute kidney injury

ETIOLOGY/PATHOGENESIS

- Parenteral infusion of hyperosmolar agents
  - Carbohydrate: Dextrans, mannitol, sucrose
  - Contrast agents
- Mechanism includes direct toxic and ischemic tubular injury

CLINICAL ISSUES

- Acute oliguric renal failure
- Diagnosis established by kidney biopsy

MICROSCOPIC

- Diffuse or focal clear cell change with cytoplasmic swelling
  - Proximal tubules have luminal narrowing
- Uniform isometric vacuolization of proximal tubular epithelium
- Preservation of brush border on PAS staining
- Cellular necrosis and sloughed cells are uncommonly seen
- Distal tubules and collecting ducts unaffected

TOP DIFFERENTIAL DIAGNOSES

- Tubular calcineurin inhibitor toxicity
- Ischemic acute tubular injury
- Tubulopathy associated with nephrotic syndrome
- Glycosuria in diabetes mellitus

DIAGNOSTIC CHECKLIST

- Cell swelling with luminal narrowing or obliteration rather than attenuation
- Widespread isometric vacuolar changes
- Electron microscopy reveals endosomes and lysosomes and preserved surface microvilli

Isometric Vacuolization of Pars Recta and Convoluta

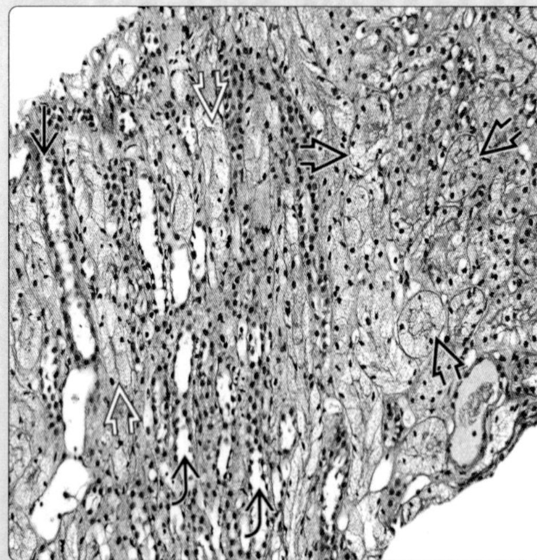

Proximal Tubule Isometric Vacuolization

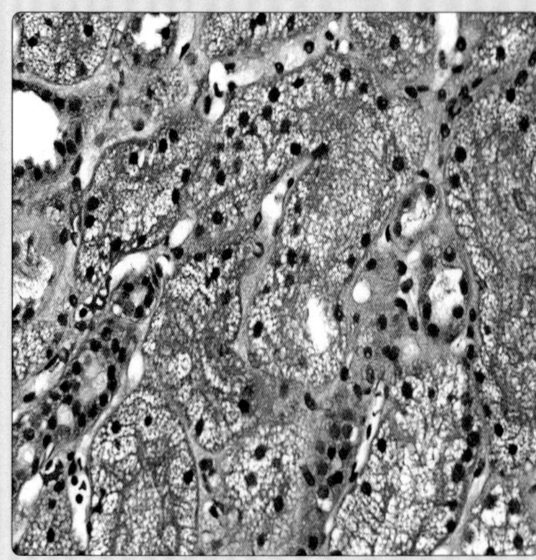

(Left) *Osmotic tubulopathy arising in a kidney transplant due to intravenous immunoglobulin (IVIg) exposure demonstrates vacuolar changes in pars recta* ➡ *and pars convoluta* ⇨*, with sparing of collecting ducts* → *and loops of Henle* ⇗*.* **(Right)** *This kidney transplant has proximal tubular cytoplasmic swelling, luminal obliteration, and abundant small isometric vesicles. The changes arose after IVIg exposure.*

Radiocontrast Osmotic Tubulopathy

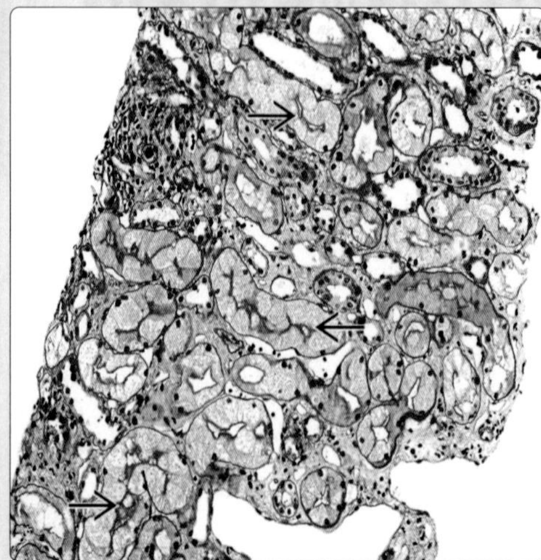

Osmotic Tubulopathy of Perfusion Preservation

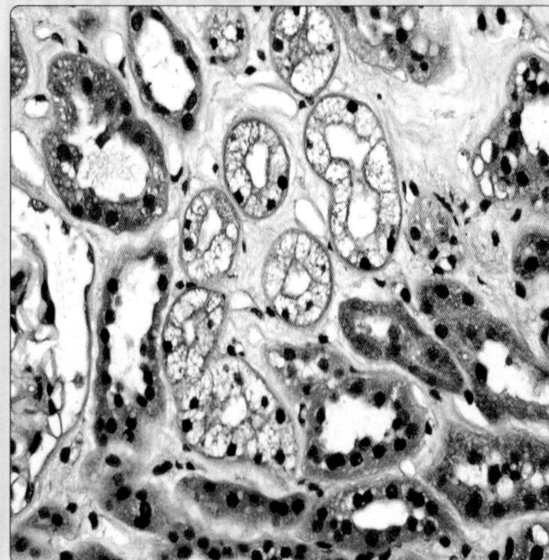

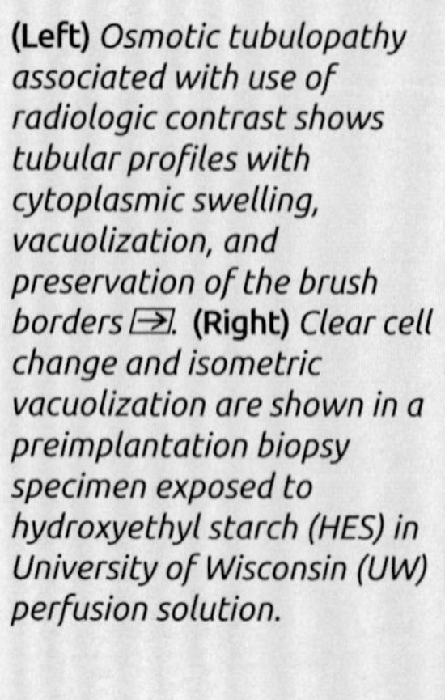

(Left) *Osmotic tubulopathy associated with use of radiologic contrast shows tubular profiles with cytoplasmic swelling, vacuolization, and preservation of the brush borders* →*.* **(Right)** *Clear cell change and isometric vacuolization are shown in a preimplantation biopsy specimen exposed to hydroxyethyl starch (HES) in University of Wisconsin (UW) perfusion solution.*

TERMINOLOGY

Synonyms

- Osmotic nephrosis
- Contrast nephropathy
- Intravenous immunoglobulin-associated tubular toxicity

Definitions

- Tubular epithelial swelling and isometric vacuolization associated with exposure to parenteral carbohydrate solutions or contrast media and acute kidney injury

ETIOLOGY/PATHOGENESIS

Parenteral Infusion of Hyperosmolar Agents

- Parenteral carbohydrate solutions
  - Mannitol: Used as plasma expander and to treat cerebral edema
  - Dextran: Used as plasma expander
  - Hydroxyethyl starch (HES): Plasma expander and perfusion of kidney transplants (University of Wisconsin [UW] solution)
    - Lesions may be evident in preimplantation donor kidneys after perfusion preservation
  - Glucose, sucrose, and maltose: Stabilizing agents
    - Intravenous immunoglobulin (IVIg)
  - Radiologic contrast agents: Iodine-containing agents, ionic or nonionic, high and low osmolality

Pathogenesis

- Hyperosmotic solution filtered and absorbed by proximal tubules through pinocytosis
  - Solute retained in endosomes and not broken down
    - Intracellular oncotic gradient thus created
  - Dose-related accumulation of pinocytotic vesicles
- Water absorption causes hydropic swelling of cytoplasm
- Vacuoles arise by fusion of vesicles with lysosomes
  - Experimentally, vacuolar change appears in minutes and disappears in days after exposure
- Direct cellular toxicity
  - Disruption of cellular integrity
  - Oxidative injury
- Reduced glomerular filtration rate due to afferent arteriolar vasoconstriction
- Experimental evidence for RIP1-kinase mediation of radiocontrast induced tubulopathy

Risk Factors

- Age > 65 years
- Preexisting chronic kidney disease and diabetic nephropathy
- Concurrent exposure to nephrotoxic agents
- Coexistent ischemic or hypoxic renal injury, especially in kidney transplants
- Dehydration
- Quantity and osmolarity of administered solution, especially for contrast media and mannitol

CLINICAL ISSUES

Epidemiology

- Incidence
  - Incidence varies with agent administered and presence of associated risk factors

Presentation

- Acute deterioration of function of native and transplanted kidneys with exposure to inciting agents
  - Begins within days of infusion and reverses after cessation
- Renal failure may develop and resolve without clinical symptoms or signs
  - Typically oliguric
- Persistent impairment (rare)
- High osmolal gap (measured: Calculated osmolality)
- Diagnosis established by kidney biopsy

Treatment

- Dialysis necessary in ~ 40% of patients
- Plasma exchange for removal of dextran

Prognosis

- Recovery typically takes days to weeks
- Prolonged renal failure over months may be observed
  - Increased mortality associated with acute renal failure
- End-stage renal failure (rare)

MACROSCOPIC

Gross Examination

- Enlarged and pale kidneys

MICROSCOPIC

Histologic Features

- Glomeruli
  - Vacuolization of parietal epithelium of Bowman capsule and podocytes
- Tubules
  - Diffuse or focal clear cell transformation with lumInal narrowing or solidification of proximal tubules
  - Uniform isometric vacuolization of proximal tubular epithelium of convoluted and straight segments
  - Vacuoles impinge on nuclear membrane imparting scalloped appearance
    - 1-4 microns in diameter and appear empty
    - Earliest vacuoles in cell apex
    - May persist with protracted renal failure
  - Preservation of brush border on PAS staining
  - Cellular necrosis and sloughed cells are uncommonly seen
  - Distal tubules and collecting ducts unaffected
- Interstitium
  - Interstitial foam cells may be seen
  - Mild cortical interstitial edema with scattered inflammatory cells may be evident

Cytologic Features

- Foamy epithelial cells in urine cytology

ANCILLARY TESTS

Immunofluorescence

- Negative
  - Immune complex deposits not seen with IVIg usage

Frequency and Natural History

Agent	Frequency	Time to ARF	Duration of ARF	Persistent ARF	ESRD
Contrast media	2-15%	1-5 days	Days-weeks	Uncommon	Uncommon
IVIg	1-7%	3 days (range: 1-10 days)	14 days (range: 2-60 days)	Up to 20%	Uncommon
Hydroxyethyl starch	42-80%	10 days (range: 2-30 days)	Weeks-months	Uncommon	Uncommon
Mannitol	Up to 50%	3 days (range: 2-6 days)	Days-weeks	Rare	Not reported
Dextran	Up to 85%	4 days (range: 3-6 days)	Days-weeks	Uncommon	Uncommon
ARF = acute renal failure; ESRD = end-stage renal disease; IVIg = intravenous immunoglobulin					

Differential Diagnosis of Osmotic Tubulopathy

Diagnosis	Distinguishing Features	Other Helpful Features
Tubular calcineurin inhibitor toxicity	Focal vacuolization, often in medullary rays	Arteriolopathy; dilated endoplasmic reticulum by EM
Ischemic acute tubular injury	Coarse vacuolization, flattened epithelium, necrosis, cellular casts	Loss of brush border on PAS and EM
Nephrotic syndrome	Focal, often basal vacuoles, interstitial foam cells	Glomerular cause of nephrosis
Ethylene glycol toxicity	Coarse large vacuoles, not isometric; calcium oxalate crystals	Mild tubulointerstitial inflammation
Methanol toxicity	No distinguishing features; may see myoglobin casts	
Potassium depletion	Proximal tubules have single well-defined vacuoles	Medullary interstitial cells with PAS(+) granules
Armanni-Ebstein tubulopathy	Outer medullary clear cell change; PAS(+) and glycogen	
Light chain proximal tubulopathy	Rare diffuse fine vacuolization of proximal tubules; monoclonal light chain IF staining	
Xanthogranulomatous pyelonephritis	Interstitial foamy macrophages, mixed neutrophilic and mononuclear inflammatory infiltrate	
Alport nephropathy	Clusters of interstitial foam cells; Alport glomerulopathy	
Intrarenal ectopic adrenal gland	Organoid zonal layers; typically subcapsular	

Electron Microscopy

- Swollen cytoplasm
- Abundant cytoplasmic vacuoles and lysosomes
- Surface microvilli preserved

DIFFERENTIAL DIAGNOSIS

Calcineurin Inhibitor Toxicity

- Focal distribution; rarely, if ever, diffuse
- Isometric vacuolization affects mainly proximal straight segments (medullary rays)

Ischemic Acute Tubular Injury

- Vacuolization typically coarse and irregular
- Epithelial flattening rather than swelling

Nephrotic Syndrome

- Lipid vacuoles often focal, basally located in proximal epithelium
- PAS(+) protein reabsorption droplets
  - Stain for albumin and immunoglobulins by IF

Hyperglycemia (Armanni-Ebstein Tubulopathy)

- Clear cells are PAS(+) and diastase digestible indicating glycogen
- Clear cell change mainly in outer medulla

DIAGNOSTIC CHECKLIST

Pathologic Interpretation Pearls

- In contrast to acute tubular injury, no attenuation or cellular necrosis
- EM reveals endosomes and lysosomes; preserved microvilli

SELECTED REFERENCES

1. Nomani AZ et al: Osmotic nephrosis with mannitol: review article. Ren Fail. 36(7):1169-76, 2014
2. Wiedermann CJ et al: Accumulation of hydroxyethyl starch in human and animal tissues: a systematic review. Intensive Care Med. 40(2):160-70, 2014
3. Linkermann A et al: The RIP1-kinase inhibitor necrostatin-1 prevents osmotic nephrosis and contrast-induced AKI in mice. J Am Soc Nephrol. 24(10):1545-57, 2013
4. Dickenmann M et al: Osmotic nephrosis: acute kidney injury with accumulation of proximal tubular lysosomes due to administration of exogenous solutes. Am J Kidney Dis. 51(3):491-503, 2008
5. Soares SM et al: Impairment of renal function after intravenous immunoglobulin. Nephrol Dial Transplant. 21(3):816-7, 2006
6. Haas M et al: Isometric tubular epithelial vacuolization in renal allograft biopsy specimens of patients receiving low-dose intravenous immunoglobulin for a positive crossmatch. Transplantation. 78(4):549-56, 2004

Differential Diagnosis: Calcineurin Inhibitor Toxicity

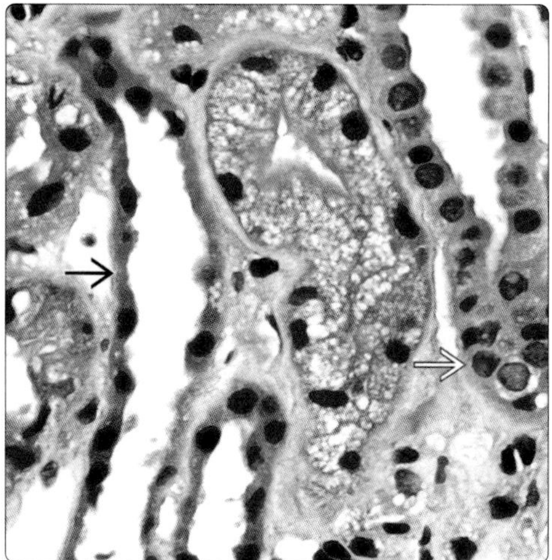

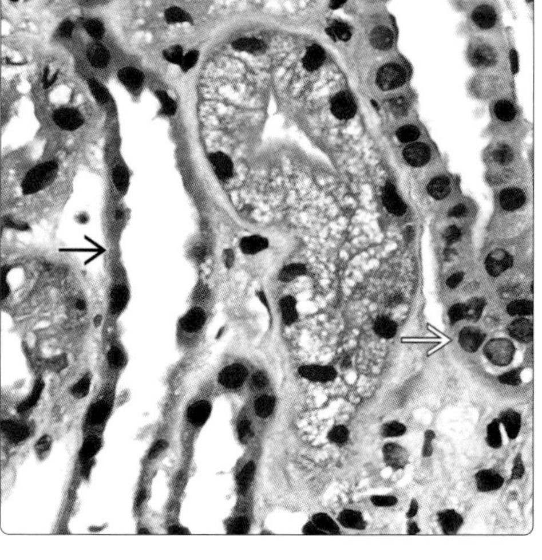

Differential Diagnosis: Ischemic Acute Tubular Injury

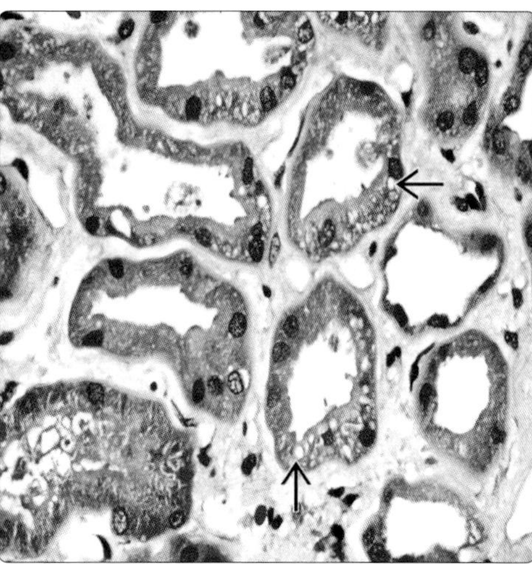

(Left) *Focal isometric vacuolization in a straight segment of a proximal tubule from a kidney transplant with tubular calcineurin inhibitor toxicity. Other tubular segments, including a loop of Henle* ⇨ *and a collecting duct* ➡*, are spared.* **(Right)** *Acute ischemic tubular injury in the native nontransplant kidney with coarse irregular vacuolization of the proximal tubular cytoplasm* ⇨ *shows that the interstitium has mild edema with scattered inflammatory cells (lower middle).*

Differential Diagnosis: Coarse Vacuoles in Ischemic Injury

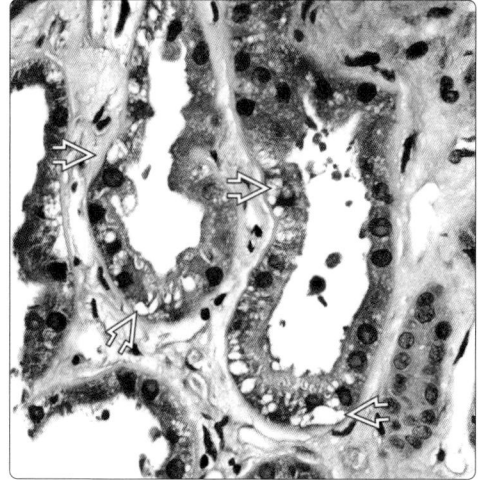

Differential Diagnosis: Hypokalemia

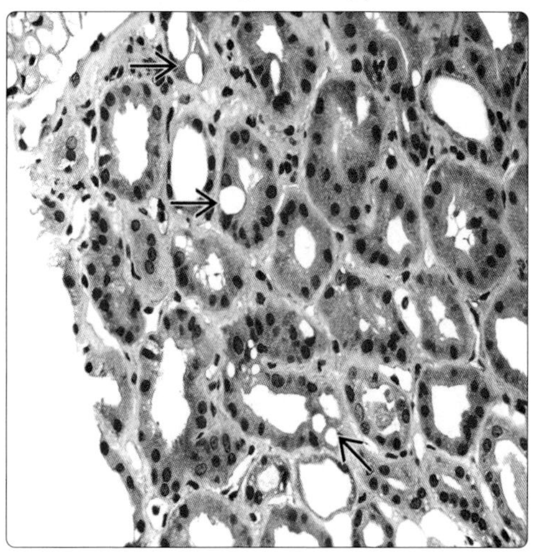

(Left) *Coarse irregular cytoplasmic vacuolization of proximal tubules* ➡ *is seen in a native nontransplant kidney with ischemic acute tubular injury. Cell debris is evident in the tubular lumen on the right.* **(Right)** *H&E shows single "punched out" coarse vacuoles in the proximal tubules* ⇨ *of a kidney transplant patient with acute tubular injury and severe hypokalemia.*

Differential Diagnosis: Nephrotic Syndrome

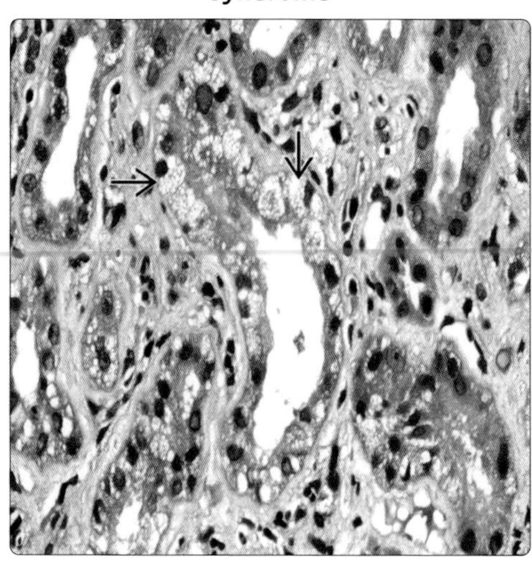

Differential Diagnosis: Interstitial Foam Cells in Nephrotic Syndrome

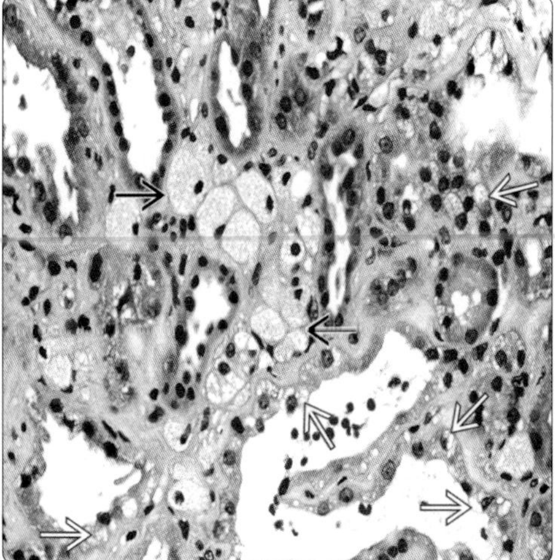

(Left) *Tubular cytoplasmic vacuolization without hydropic change associated with lipiduria in nephrotic syndrome is shown. Small, even-sized vacuoles are mainly basal in distribution, but they fill the cytoplasm in some instances* ⇨*.* **(Right)** *In this case of interstitial foam cells associated with the nephrotic syndrome, collections of interstitial foam cells* ⇨ *are seen in a patient with IgA nephropathy and nephrotic-range proteinuria. Focal tubular epithelial vacuoles are also evident* ➡*.*

Antiviral Drug Nephrotoxicity

KEY FACTS

TERMINOLOGY

- Kidney dysfunction due to exposure to antiviral agents

ETIOLOGY/PATHOGENESIS

- Direct tubular toxicity: Tenofovir, adefovir, acyclovir, cidofovir
- Tubulointerstitial nephritis (TIN): Indinavir, atazanavir, abacavir, efavirenz, foscarnet
- Crystal nephropathy: Acyclovir, indinavir, foscarnet
- Glomerulopathy: Foscarnet, valacyclovir, acyclovir, enfuvirtide

MICROSCOPIC

- Acute tubular injury or necrosis ± TIN
  - Karyomegaly + megamitochondria
  - Proximal tubules are most severely affected
- TIN: Acute and chronic
- Crystal nephropathy: Intrarenal precipitation of crystallized salts of antiviral agent (indinavir and foscarnet)
- Glomerular crystals (foscarnet), thrombotic microangiopathy (acyclovir)

ANCILLARY TESTS

- Mitochondrial enlargement, dysmorphism, distortion of cristae; mitochondrial depletion on electron microscopy
- Infrared spectroscopy allows definitive identification of crystal composition

TOP DIFFERENTIAL DIAGNOSES

- Acute tubular injury: Ischemic, toxic
- TIN: Infection, nonantiviral drugs, allograft rejection
- Tubular nuclear atypia: Viral infections, chemotherapeutic agents, karyomegalic interstitial nephropathy
- Crystal nephropathy: Sulfadiazine, ciprofloxacin, hyperoxaluria, uric acid nephropathy

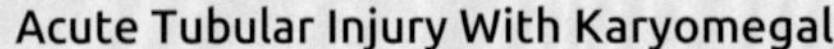

Acute Tubular Injury With Karyomegaly

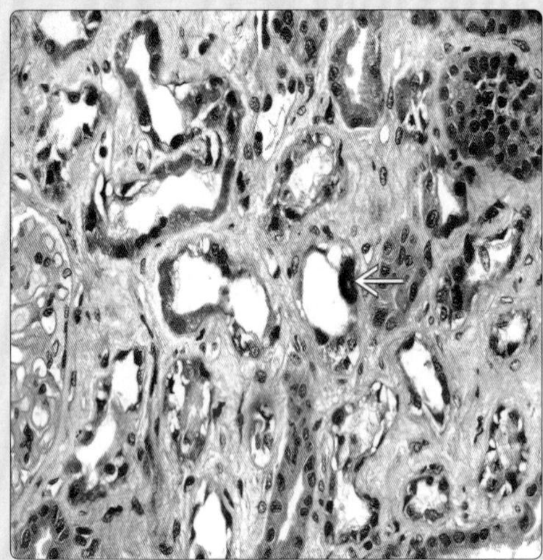

Megamitochondria

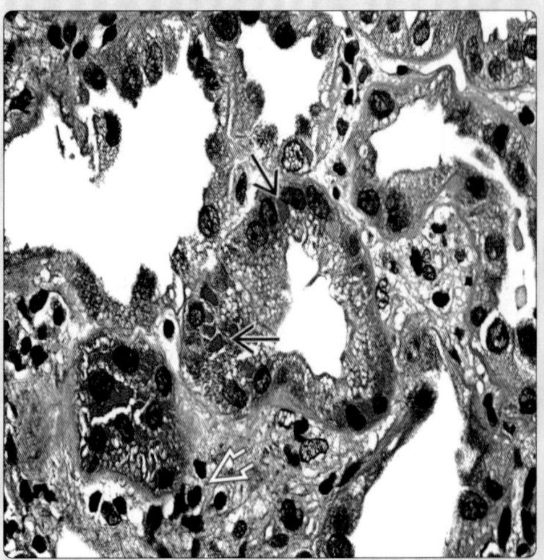

(Left) *Tubular karyomegaly ➡, coarse vacuoles, and acute tubular injury are evident in this biopsy specimen from a patient with tenofovir toxicity. The interstitium has extensive fibrosis.* **(Right)** *Megamitochondria may be seen singly and in clusters ➡ in tubular epithelium in tenofovir toxicity. There is acute tubular injury and interstitial mononuclear inflammation ➡. (Courtesy L. Herlitz, MD.)*

Acute Tubulointerstitial Nephritis

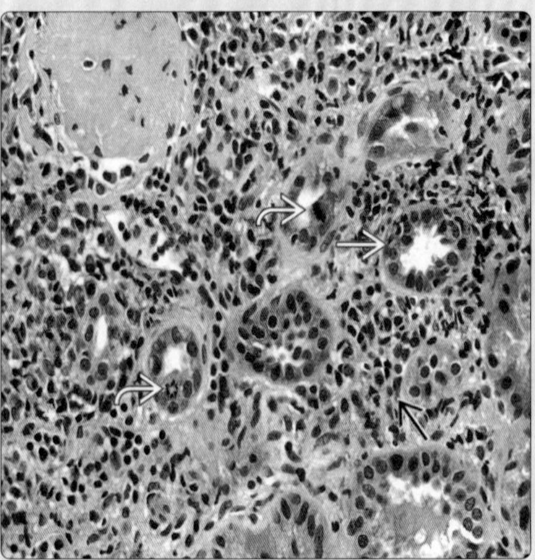

Crystal Tubulopathy

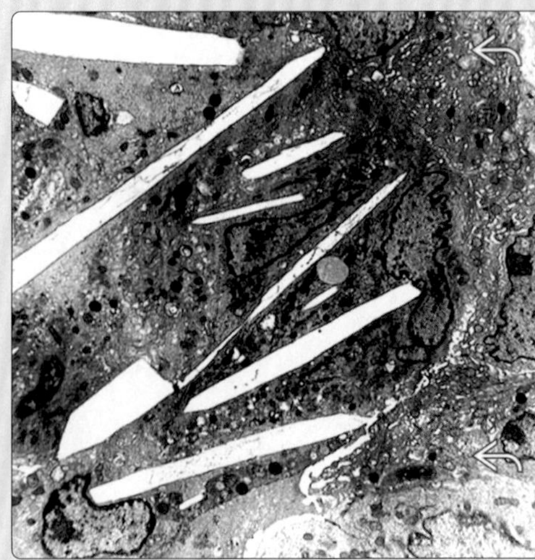

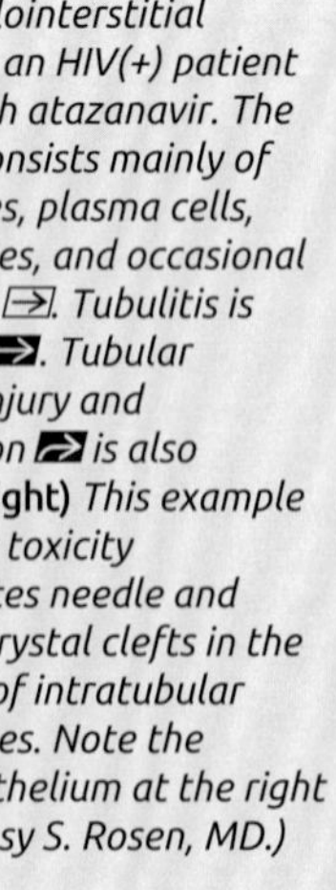

(Left) *Tubulointerstitial nephritis in an HIV(+) patient treated with atazanavir. The infiltrate consists mainly of lymphocytes, plasma cells, macrophages, and occasional eosinophils ➡. Tubulitis is prominent ➡. Tubular epithelial injury and regeneration ➡ is also evident.* **(Right)** *This example of indinavir toxicity demonstrates needle and rhomboid crystal clefts in the cytoplasm of intratubular macrophages. Note the tubular epithelium at the right ➡. (Courtesy S. Rosen, MD.)*

TERMINOLOGY

Synonyms

- Antiviral nephrotoxicity

Definitions

- Kidney dysfunction due to exposure to antiviral agents

ETIOLOGY/PATHOGENESIS

Environmental Exposure

- Antiviral agents with known nephrotoxicity
  - Nucleoside analogs (reverse transcriptase inhibitors): Acyclovir, valacyclovir, ganciclovir, abacavir, lamivudine, zidovudine, stavudine, didanosine
  - Nucleotide analogs (reverse transcriptase inhibitors): Tenofovir, adefovir, cidofovir
  - Peptide analogs (protease inhibitors): Indinavir, ritonavir, atazanavir
  - Pyrophosphate analogs: Foscarnet (trisodium phosphonoformate)
  - Fusion or entry inhibitors: Enfurtivide
  - Other agents: Intravenous immunoglobulin, interferon-α
- Risk factors for nephrotoxicity
  - Kidney
    - Drugs are concentrated in specific nephron segments; proximal tubules are at greatest risk of injury
    - Organic anion transporter system concentrates tenofovir and cidofovir in proximal tubules
  - Patient
    - Infection, e.g., HIV, hepatitis B
    - Underlying chronic kidney disease and dehydration
    - Pharmacogenetics and immune response genes
  - Drug
    - Dose dependent: High dose increases risk of renal injury
    - Solubility: Concentration and pH dependent
    - Immune stimulatory potential
      - Drug hypersensitivity
      - Immune reconstitution inflammatory syndrome (IRIS)
- Pathogenesis
  - Direct tubular toxicity: Tenofovir, adefovir, acyclovir, cidofovir
    - Mitochondrial toxicity: Antiviral nucleoside and nucleotide analogs (ANA) act as competitive alternative substrate for mitochondrial thymidine kinase
    - ANA triphosphate inhibits mitochondrial DNA polymerase-γ, resulting in altered mitochondrial DNA
    - Both mitochondrial DNA depletion and mitochondrial depletion are associated with tenofovir, adefovir, and cidofovir
  - Tubulointerstitial nephritis (TIN)
    - Hypersensitivity reaction to drugs
      - Indinavir, atazanavir, abacavir, efavirenz, foscarnet
    - IRIS may cause TIN
    - Dysfunction associated with inflammatory injury
    - Injury may be precipitated by tubular injury or idiosyncratic immunologic reactions ± effects of HIV infection
  - Crystal nephropathy: Acyclovir, indinavir
    - Crystals may be toxic to epithelium and may obstruct tubules
    - Crystal precipitation is often associated with interstitial nephritis
  - Glomerulopathy: Foscarnet, valacyclovir, acyclovir, enfuvirtide
    - Glomerular crystal deposition

CLINICAL ISSUES

Presentation

- Proximal tubulopathy and Fanconi syndrome: Cidofovir, tenofovir, adefovir, foscarnet, stavudine, lamivudine
  - Frequency: Tenofovir (0.3-2%), adefovir (up to 50% at high dose)
- Distal tubular acidosis: Foscarnet
- Nephrogenic diabetes insipidus: Foscarnet, didanosine, abacavir
- Acute renal failure/kidney injury: Acyclovir, ganciclovir, cidofovir, indinavir, tenofovir, adefovir, foscarnet
  - Frequency: Tenofovir (0.5-1.5%), acyclovir (10%)
- Crystalluria, lithiasis: Acyclovir, indinavir
  - Frequency: Indinavir (10-20%), acyclovir (12-48% with intravenous infusions), atazanavir (< 1%)
  - Crystalluria may be associated with acute kidney injury
- Proteinuria: Cidofovir, foscarnet, interferon-α
- Chronic renal failure: Cidofovir, indinavir, tenofovir

Treatment

- Drug withdrawal or substitution
- Hydration and restoration of high urinary output

Prognosis

- Most acute dysfunction due to antiviral agents is reversible
  - Most acute kidney injuries and acute crystal nephropathies are reversible
  - TIN ± crystal deposits are reversible if interstitial fibrosis is limited
  - Lesions have limited reversibility if there is extensive scarring on biopsy
- Anecdotal reports of end-stage renal failure due to cidofovir and foscarnet toxicity
- Causes of death in patients on anti-retroviral therapy (ART)
  - Mycobacterium tuberculosis, other bacterial and fungal infections
  - IRIS contributory in > 70%

MICROSCOPIC

Histologic Features

- Acute tubular injury or necrosis may be caused by most antiviral agents
  - Proximal tubules are most severely affected
    - Loss of apical cytoplasm, brush border, karyomegaly, large nucleoli
    - Megamitochondria are rounded eosinophilic cytoplasmic inclusions; fuchsinophilic on trichrome stain; PAS negative
      - Tenofovir, cidofovir, adefovir, lamivudine, and stavudine

- Distal tubular segments and collecting ducts injury with regeneration
- Interstitial fibrosis
  - Myoglobinuric acute tubular necrosis has been described with use of didanosine and zidovudine in HIV infection
  - Osmotic tubulopathy with intravenous immunoglobulin
- Crystal nephropathy: Intrarenal precipitation of crystallized salts of antiviral agent
  - Crystal deposits on air-dried or alcohol-fixed frozen sections
  - Crystal nephropathy is accompanied by TIN
  - Acyclovir: Distal tubular crystals and mild tubulointerstitial inflammation
  - Foscarnet: Rhomboid and clustered polyhedral yellow crystals; birefringent
    - Luminal macrophages, giant cells, and tubular injury, all with cytoplasmic crystal clefts
    - Crystal clefts in glomerular capillaries, associated with fibrin deposition and, rarely, crescent formation
    - Crystals are von Kossa positive
    - Infrared spectroscopy reveals trisodium foscarnet and calcium phosphate salts containing foscarnet
  - Indinavir: Polyhedric, rectangular, or needle-shaped crystals; birefringent
    - Cellular casts composed of macrophages containing sharp-ended clefts in cytoplasm
    - Distal tubular and collecting ductal crystal deposits associated with tubular injury, inflammation, and fibrosis
    - Infrared spectroscopy reveals indinavir monohydrate
  - Nephrolithiasis is associated with acyclovir, indinavir, atazanavir
- TIN
  - Described in foscarnet, atazanavir, abacavir, efavirenz, and indinavir toxicity
  - Interstitial inflammation, edema, and focal tubulitis
    - Infiltrates of mononuclear cells and polymorphonuclear neutrophils
  - Tubular nuclear atypia/karyomegaly is common
  - Interstitial fibrosis and tubular atrophy variable
- Glomerular disorders
  - Glomerular crystal deposits in foscarnet toxicity; may be associated with crescent formation
  - Thrombotic microangiopathy: Acyclovir, valacyclovir
  - Membranoproliferative glomerulonephritis: Enfurtivide
  - Focal segmental glomerulosclerosis rarely associated with interferon-α therapy for hepatitis C infection

ANCILLARY TESTS

Electron Microscopy

- Acute tubular injury in tenofovir and cidofovir toxicity
  - Mitochondrial enlargement, dysmorphism, distortion of cristae; mitochondrial depletion
- Crystal clefts in glomerular capillaries and mesangium, in tubules in foscarnet toxicity
- Crystal clefts in intratubular macrophages in indinavir toxicity

Infrared Spectroscopy

- Allows definitive identification of crystal composition

Immunofluorescence

- Nonspecific

DIFFERENTIAL DIAGNOSIS

Acute Tubular Injury

- Tubular injury can be caused by many therapeutic agents
- Megamitochondria also in calcineurin inhibitor toxicity and mitochondrial cytopathies
- HIV infection can have renal tubular injury and mitochondrial dysmorphism in absence of exposure to antiretroviral agents

Tubulointerstitial Nephritis (TIN)

- TIN can be caused by many different agents; specific cause difficult to determine
- Reactive tubular nuclear karyomegaly/atypia
  - Viral infections (adenovirus, polyomavirus, HIV), cisplatinum/busulfan/ifosfamide toxicity, and karyomegalic interstitial nephropathy must be excluded

Crystal Nephropathy

- Oxalate nephropathy
- Uric acid nephropathy
- Other drugs: Sulfadiazine, triamterene, ampicillin, methotrexate, vitamin C, ciprofloxacin, orlistat
- Intratubular precipitates of cholesterol crystals in nephrotic states

DIAGNOSTIC CHECKLIST

Clinically Relevant Pathologic Features

- Acute tubular necrosis, TIN, and intratubular crystal deposition are most common causes of acute kidney injury

Pathologic Interpretation Pearls

- Megamitochondria are characteristic of tenofovir and cidofovir toxicity
- Intratubular crystals in indinavir toxicity and glomerular crystals in foscarnet toxicity

SELECTED REFERENCES

1. Philipponnet C et al: Intravascular foscarnet crystal precipitation causing multiorgan failure. Am J Kidney Dis. 65(1):152-5, 2015
2. Zaidan M et al: Tubulointerstitial nephropathies in HIV-infected patients over the past 15 years: a clinico-pathological study. Clin J Am Soc Nephrol. 8(6):930-8, 2013
3. Wong EB et al: Causes of death on antiretroviral therapy: a post-mortem study from South Africa. PLoS One. 7(10):e47542, 2012
4. Herlitz LC et al: Tenofovir nephrotoxicity: acute tubular necrosis with distinctive clinical, pathological, and mitochondrial abnormalities. Kidney Int. 78(11):1171-7, 2010
5. Justrabo E et al: Irreversible glomerular lesions induced by crystal precipitation in a renal transplant after foscarnet therapy for cytomegalovirus infection. Histopathology. 34(4):365-9, 1999
6. Martinez F et al: Indinavir crystal deposits associated with tubulointerstitial nephropathy. Nephrol Dial Transplant. 13(3):750-3, 1998

Acute Tubular Injury

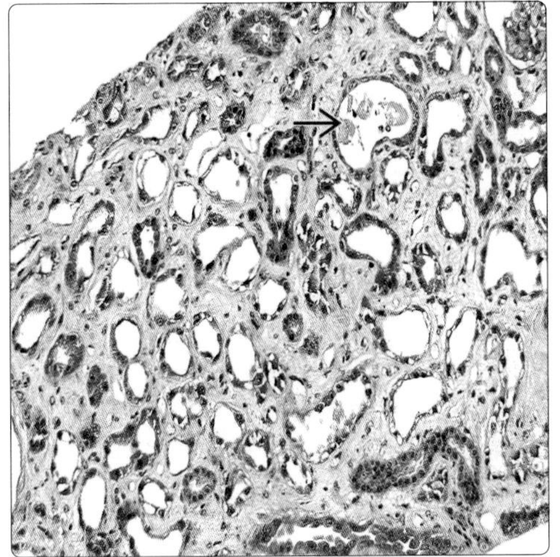

Megamitochondria and Acute Tubular Injury

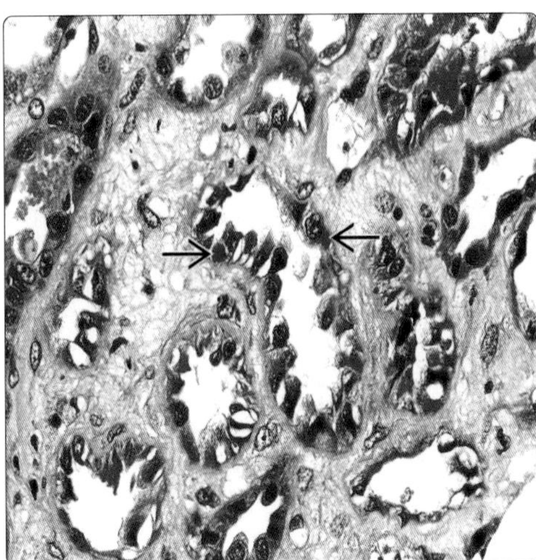

(Left) *Acute tubular injury with severe attenuation of the epithelium, luminal widening, and necrotic debris ➙ is seen in this biopsy from an HIV(+) patient exposed to tenofovir. There is also diffuse interstitial fibrosis.* **(Right)** *Markers of antiviral nephrotoxicity include megamitochondria ➙ often present in tubules with other features of acute injury. Coarse cytoplasmic vacuolization and karyomegaly are also apparent. The interstitium is edematous with early fibrosis.*

Megamitochondria in Antiviral Toxicity

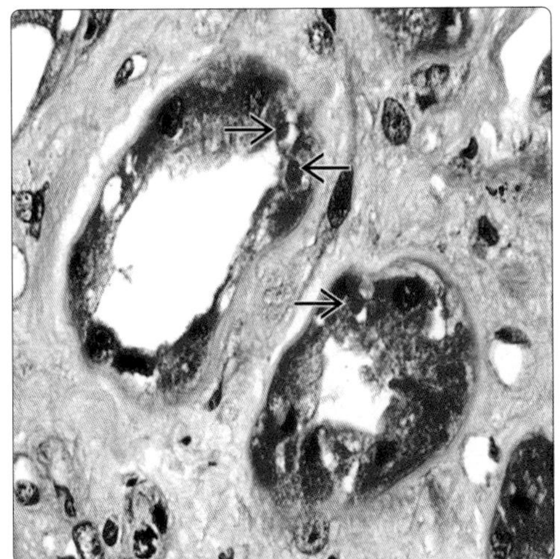

Megamitochondria in Tenofovir Toxicity

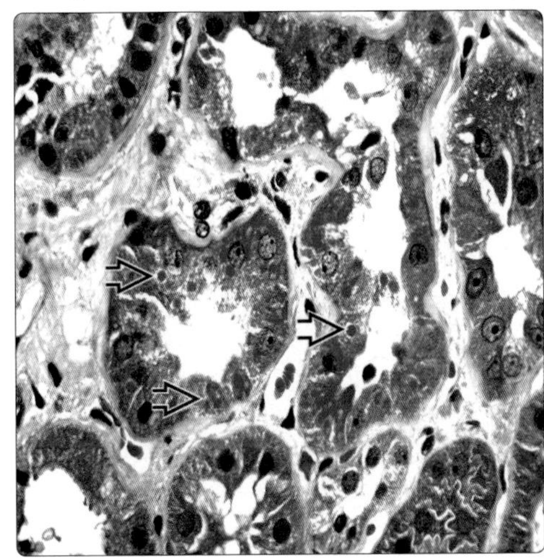

(Left) *Megamitochondria may be quite subtle and require careful search for their identification ➙. These were identified in an HIV(+) patient treated with tenofovir. These proximal segments are shrunken, and there is background fibrosis.* **(Right)** *Acute tubular injury with prominent brightly fuchsinophilic megamitochondria ➙ are seen in this trichrome stain of a biopsy specimen from a patient with hepatitis B infection treated with tenofovir. (Courtesy L. Herlitz, MD.)*

Megamitochondria in Tenofovir Toxicity

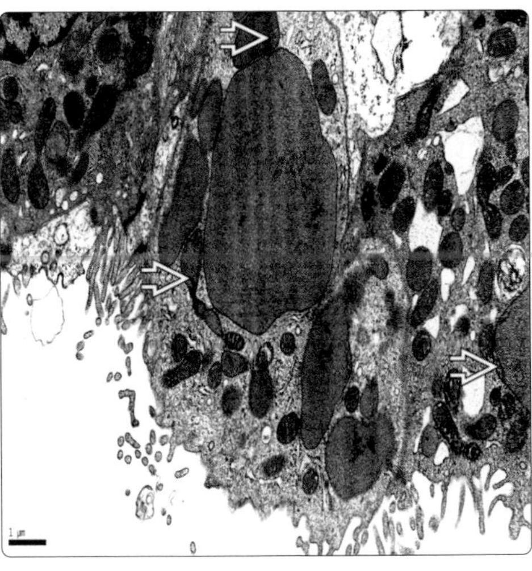

Megamitochondria in Tenofovir Toxicity

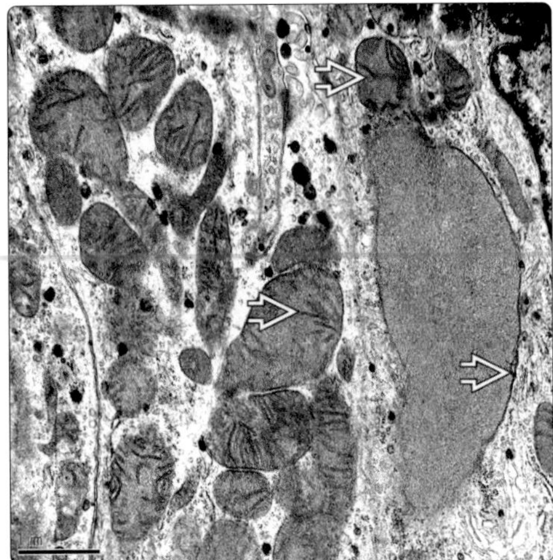

(Left) *EM shows enlarged dysmorphic mitochondria with shrunken and misshapen cristae ➙ in this injured proximal tubular epithelial cell from a patient treated with tenofovir for hepatitis B infection. (Courtesy L. Herlitz, MD.)* **(Right)** *A cluster of dysmorphic mitochondria with varied sizes and shapes and distorted cristae ➙ are evident in the proximal tubular epithelium of a patient with HIV infection and tenofovir toxicity (EM).*

ATN in Foscarnet Toxicity

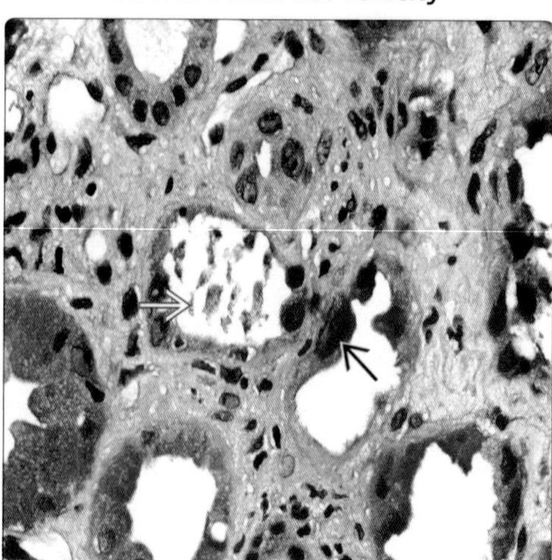

Foscarnet Toxicity With Nuclear Atypia

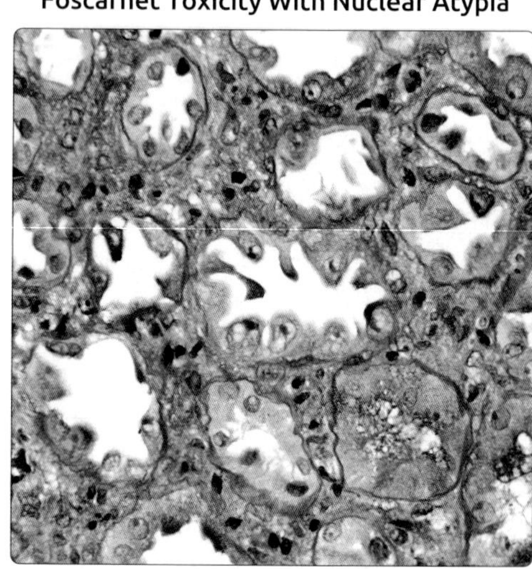

(Left) *Acute tubular epithelial injury with attenuation of epithelium, karyomegaly* ⇨, *and luminal basophilic crystalline material in the tubule* ➡ *is seen in a biopsy from a patient with foscarnet exposure. This material may contain foscarnet salts. There is interstitial fibrosis and mononuclear infiltrate.* **(Right)** *Periodic acid-Schiff shows large atypical tubular epithelial nuclei and a luminal sawtooth pattern in tubular injury associated with the use of foscarnet.*

Foscarnet Acute TIN

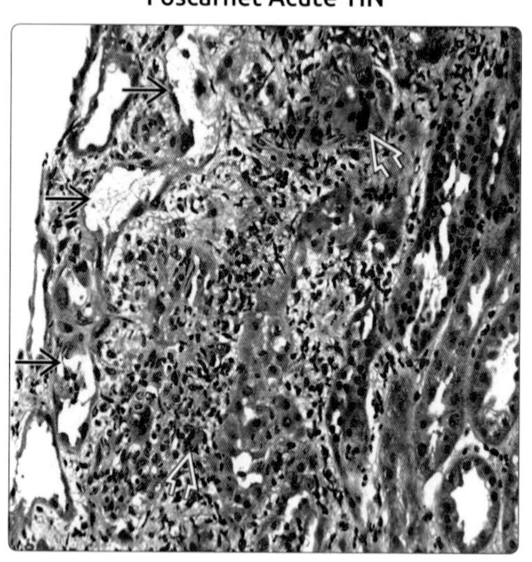

Foscarnet Chronic TIN

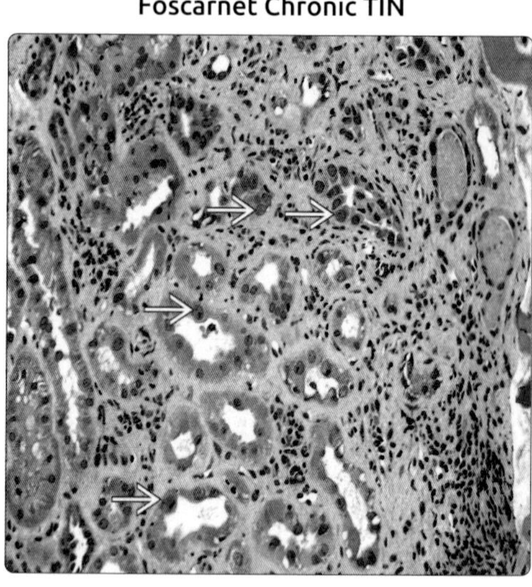

(Left) *Active acute interstitial nephritis associated with foscarnet exposure is seen in a renal transplant biopsy from a patient with systemic cytomegalovirus infection. The inflammatory infiltrate is composed of mononuclear cells, granulocytes, and giant cells* ➡*. There is acute tubular injury* ⇨*.* **(Right)** *Chronic tubulointerstitial nephritis associated with foscarnet exposure is shown. Tubules have nuclear atypia* ➡*. There is interstitial fibrosis, tubular atrophy, and mononuclear inflammation.*

Antiviral Agent TIN

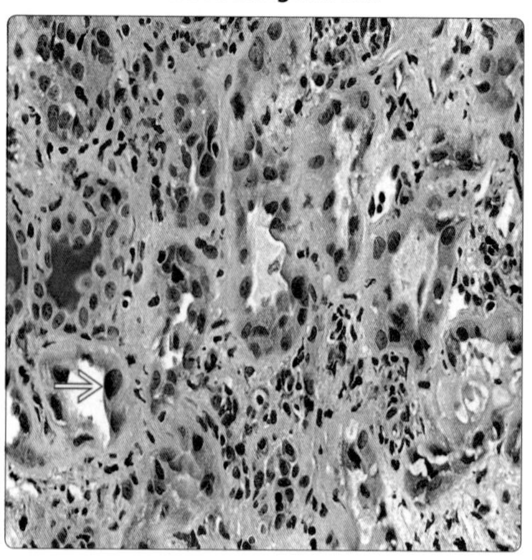

Nuclear Atypia in HIV-Associated Nephropathy

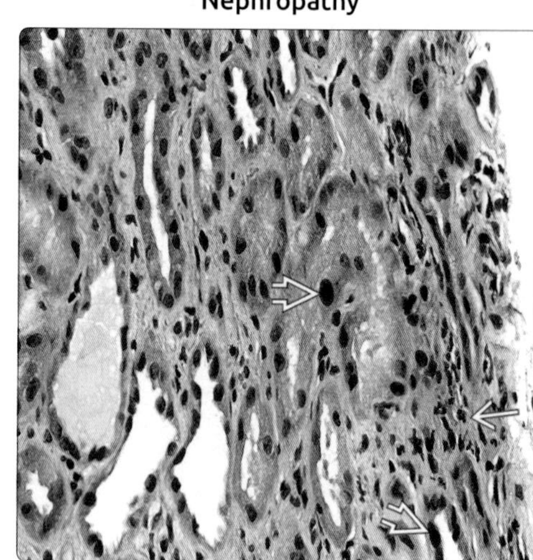

(Left) *Acute tubulointerstitial nephritis in HIV nephropathy with exposure to tenofovir, lamivudine, and efavirenz for ~ 3 months. Nuclear atypia is evident* ➡*. The relative contribution of drug toxicity and infection is difficult to resolve.* **(Right)** *HIV-associated nephropathy may have TIN, tubular injury, and enlarged hyerpchromatic atypical tubular epithelial nuclei* ➡ *unrelated to exposure to antiretroviral agents. Interstitial inflammatory cells are also evident* ➡*.*

Foscarnet Toxicity With Crescentic Glomerulonephritis

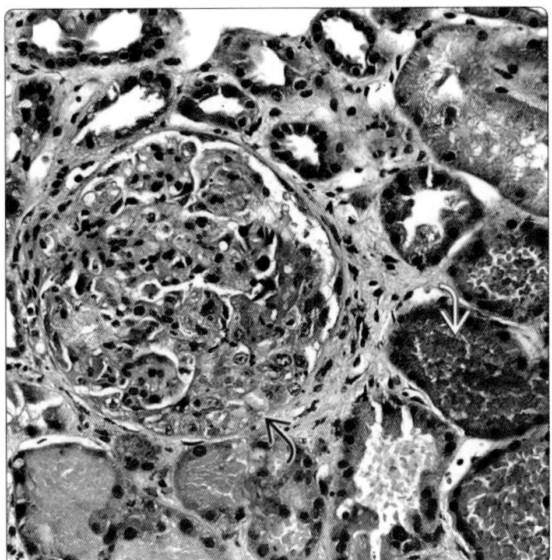

Glomerular Foscarnet Crystal Deposition

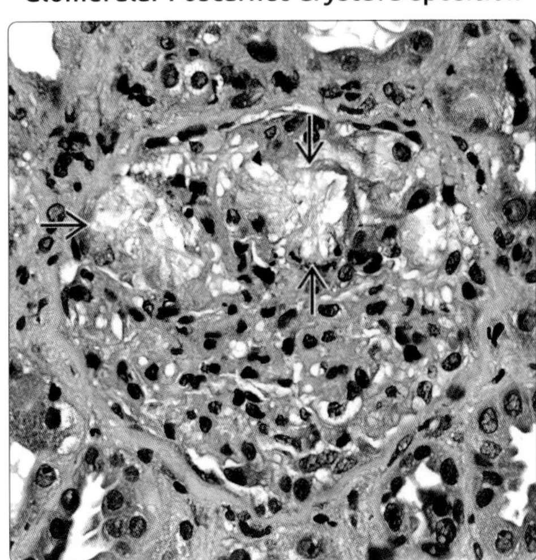

(Left) *Crescentic glomerulonephritis is shown in this example of foscarnet toxicity. Crescents* ⇨ *and red cell casts* ➡ *were prominent in this biopsy, mimicking glomerulonephritis, but they were caused by crystals lodging in glomerular capillaries. Crystals appear as clear spaces in capillaries and are difficult to identify at medium power.* **(Right)** *H&E shows glomerular crystalline clefts* ⇨ *in a biopsy specimen from a patient with CMV infection treated with foscarnet.*

Glomerular Foscarnet Crystals

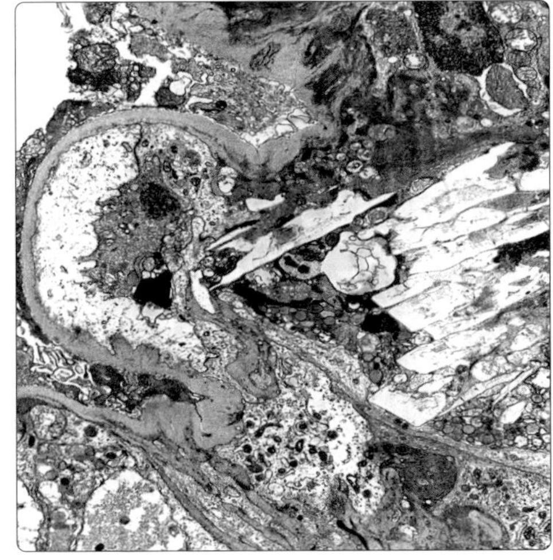

Indinavir Crystal Deposition

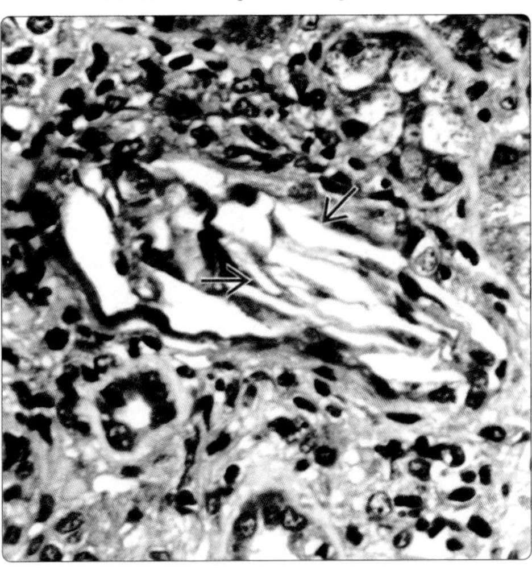

(Left) *EM shows angulated cytoplasmic crystal clefts in a mesangial phagocyte associated with foscarnet toxicity. Foscarnet salts are an uncommon but characteristic of toxicity from this agent.* **(Right)** *This intratubular cellular cast composed of macrophages contains needle-like clefts* ⇨*. Crystals of indinavir salts were washed out in tissue preparation. There is mononuclear inflammation and fibrosis in the interstitium. (Courtesy S. Rosen, MD.)*

TIN in Antiviral Nephrotoxicity

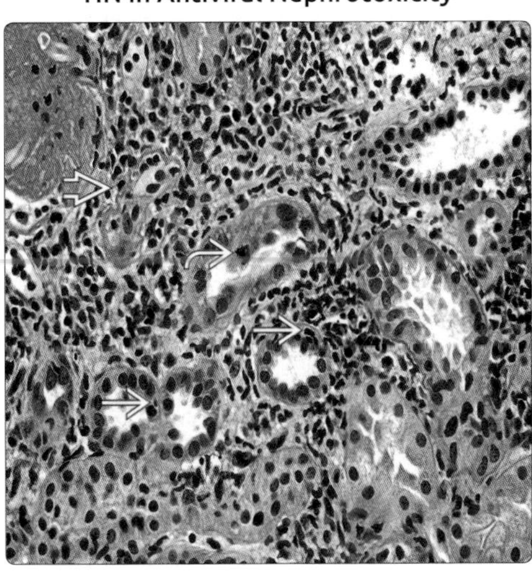

TIN in Foscarnet Toxicity

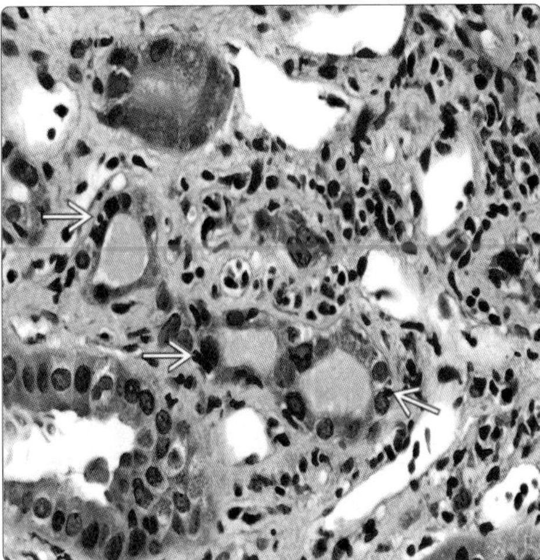

(Left) *TIN may arise in patients with HIV infection and exposure to atazanavir, ritonavir, abacavir, and lamivudine. Tubulitis* ➡*, mitoses* ➡*, and tubular atrophy* ➡ *indicate active and chronic TIN.* **(Right)** *Tubulointerstitial nephritis in a patient exposed to foscarnet for treatment of cytomegalovirus infection. There is tubulitis* ➡*, reactive tubular nuclear changes, interstitial mononuclear infiltrate, and early interstitial fibrosis.*

Acute Phosphate Nephropathy

KEY FACTS

TERMINOLOGY

- Acute tubular injury or atrophy due to abundant intratubular calcium phosphate precipitates

ETIOLOGY/PATHOGENESIS

- Oral sodium phosphate (OSP) ingestion as part of bowel preparation for colonoscopy
- Risk factors for phosphate nephropathy with OSP use
  - Inadequate hydration while receiving OSP
  - Use of angiotensin converting enzyme inhibitor or angiotensin receptor blocker or diuretics

CLINICAL ISSUES

- Acute or chronic renal failure
- Renal function may improve after initial insult
- May be discovered months to > 1 year following exposure to OSP
- Prevention by aggressive hydration before, during, and after OSP administration

MICROSCOPIC

- Calcium phosphate crystals within tubular lumens
  - Deposits within distal tubules and collecting ducts
  - Positive (black) on von Kossa stain
  - Nonpolarizable
- Tubular atrophy and interstitial fibrosis
- EM shows electron-dense, radially oriented crystals around central nidus

TOP DIFFERENTIAL DIAGNOSES

- Nephrocalcinosis
- Oxalate nephropathy
- Other crystalline nephropathies
  - e.g., drug crystals

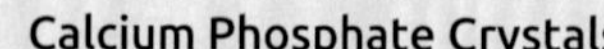

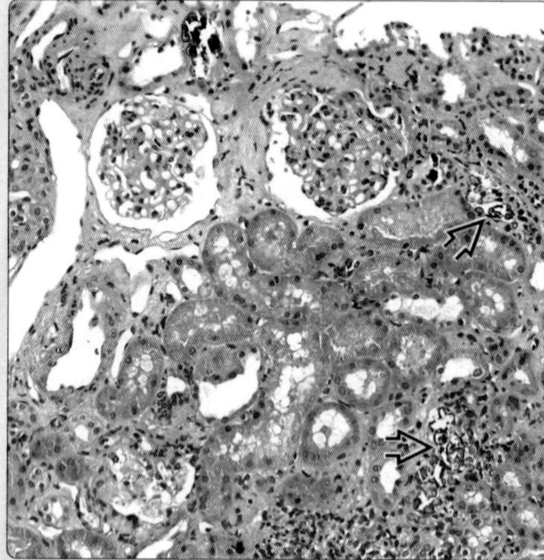

Calcium Phosphate Crystals

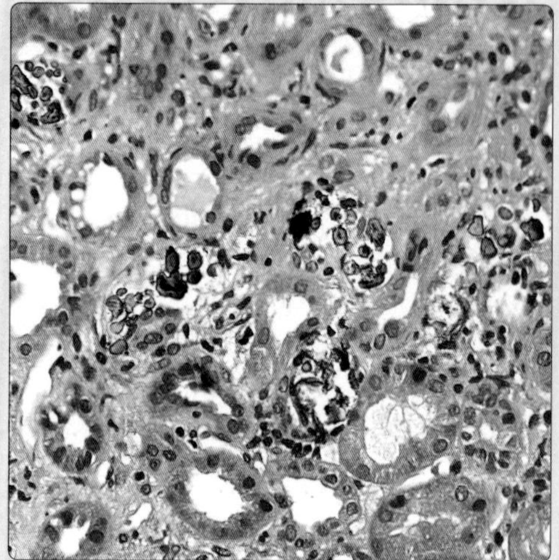

(Left) *Calcium phosphate precipitates ➡ are seen within tubular lumina in a case of acute phosphate nephropathy related to ingestion of oral sodium phosphate solution for bowel preparation. Proximal tubules are relatively spared of crystals.* **(Right)** *Numerous calcium phosphate crystals appear to be present in the interstitium, but likely originated within distal nephron segments, and now the tubules have atrophied and completely disappeared.*

von Kossa

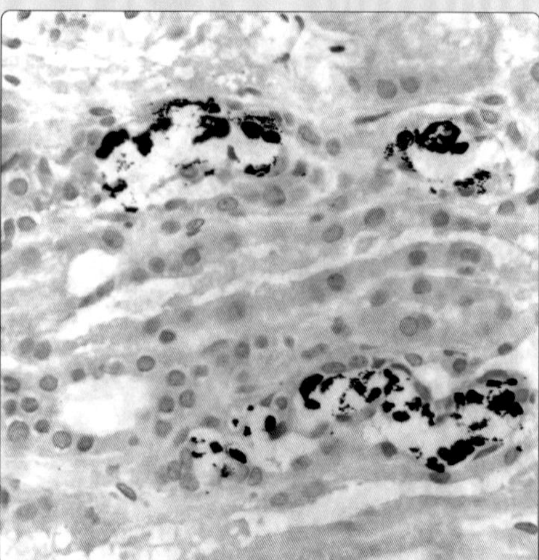

Calcium Phosphate Crystals

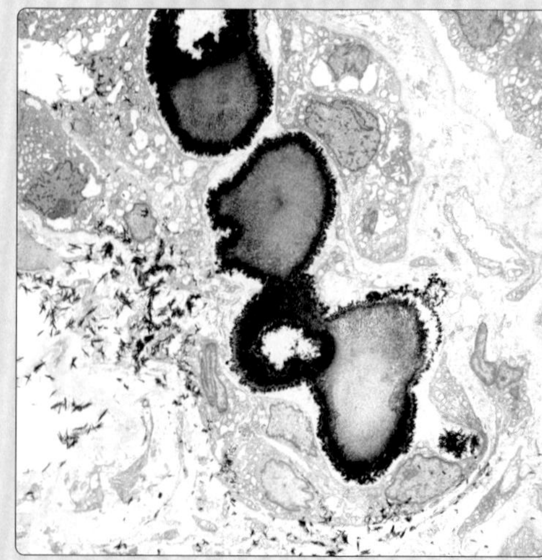

(Left) *Calcium phosphate crystals stain positively (black) on a von Kossa stain, which detects phosphate.* **(Right)** *Electron microscopy shows calcium phosphate precipitates present within the tubular lumina. The crystals are electron-dense and appear radially oriented around a central nidus.*

TERMINOLOGY

Synonyms

- Phosphate-induced nephrocalcinosis

Definitions

- Acute tubular injury or atrophy due to abundant intratubular calcium phosphate precipitates

ETIOLOGY/PATHOGENESIS

Calcium Phosphate Precipitation in Tubules

- Elevated calcium phosphate product (CPP) within distal tubules and collecting ducts
  - Exacerbated by volume depletion

Clinical Causes of Phosphate Nephropathy

- Oral sodium phosphate (OSP) ingestion for colonoscopy bowel preparation
  - Phospho-soda solution or Visicol (sodium phosphate) tablets
    - Decreased phosphate content in more recent formulations
  - Risk factors for phosphate nephropathy with OSP use
    - Inadequate hydration while receiving OSP
    - Hypertension
    - Angiotensin converting enzyme inhibitor or angiotensin receptor blocker or diuretics
    - Older age
    - Female gender
  - Increased risk of acute renal failure with OSP than polyethylene glycol bowel preparation
    - Incidence: 1:1,000-5,000 receiving OSP bowel preparation
- Phosphate supplementation in renal transplant patients
  - Post-transplant hyperparathyroidism and hypophosphatemia in early post-transplant period
  - Allograft biopsies may show calcium phosphate precipitates within tubular lumens
- Nephrocalcinosis in children with hypophosphatemic rickets
  - Calcium phosphate deposition in kidney associated with oral vitamin D and phosphate administration

CLINICAL ISSUES

Presentation

- Acute renal failure
  - Renal function may improve after initial insult
    - Most develop some degree of chronic renal failure
- Chronic renal failure
  - May be discovered months to > 1 year following recognized exposure to OSP

Prognosis

- High risk for chronic renal failure

Prevention

- Prevention by aggressive hydration before, during, and after OSP administration

MICROSCOPIC

Histologic Features

- Calcium phosphate crystals within tubular lumens
  - Deposits within distal tubules and collecting ducts
    - Appear purple on H&E stained sections
    - Nonpolarizable crystals
    - Calcium phosphate deposits positive (black) on von Kossa stain
  - Interstitial calcium phosphate deposits as residua of atrophic tubule
- Acute tubular injury
- Tubular atrophy and interstitial fibrosis
- Focal mild interstitial inflammation
- No specific glomerular or vascular involvement, except as related to underlying hypertensive disease

ANCILLARY TESTS

Electron Microscopy

- Electron-dense, radially oriented crystals around central nidus

Laboratory Testing

- Serum calcium and phosphorus levels usually normal
  - Serum phosphorus levels may be transiently elevated at time of OSP administration
    - If elevated, levels return to normal within days after administration

DIFFERENTIAL DIAGNOSIS

Nephrocalcinosis

- Occurs in setting of chronic hypercalcemia
  - e.g., hyperparathyroidism, malignancy, granulomatous disorders, milk alkali syndrome, vitamin D intoxication, and some medications
- No history of oral sodium phosphate ingestion
- May have tubular basement membrane calcium phosphate deposits along with tubular lumen and interstitial deposits

Oxalate Nephropathy

- Calcium oxalate crystals within tubular lumens
  - Calcium oxalate crystals are clear and polarizable on H&E-stained sections

Other Crystalline Nephropathies

- e.g., drug crystals

SELECTED REFERENCES

1. Weiss J et al: Acute phosphate nephropathy: a cause of chronic kidney disease. BMJ Case Rep. 2011
2. Agrawal N et al: Unrecognized acute phosphate nephropathy in a kidney donor with consequent poor allograft outcome. Am J Transplant. 9(7):1685-9, 2009
3. Manfro RC et al: Acute phosphate nephropathy in a kidney transplant recipient with delayed graft function. Transplantation. 87(4):618-9, 2009
4. Markowitz GS et al: Acute phosphate nephropathy. Kidney Int. 76(10):1027-34, 2009
5. Hurst FP et al: Association of oral sodium phosphate purgative use with acute kidney injury. J Am Soc Nephrol. 18(12):3192-8, 2007
6. Bhan I et al: Post-transplant hypophosphatemia: Tertiary 'Hyper-Phosphatoninism'? Kidney Int. 70(8):1486-94, 2006
7. Markowitz GS et al: Acute phosphate nephropathy following oral sodium phosphate bowel purgative: an underrecognized cause of chronic renal failure. J Am Soc Nephrol. 16(11):3389-96, 2005

Lithium-Induced Renal Disease

KEY FACTS

ETIOLOGY/PATHOGENESIS

- Principal cells of collecting ducts are primary target of lithium toxicity
- Exposure > 10 years

CLINICAL ISSUES

- 40% develop nephrogenic diabetes insipidus
- 0.5-1% of patients develop end-stage renal disease
- Proteinuria, bland sediment
- Treatment
  - Reduction or discontinuation of lithium therapy
  - Amiloride targets and inhibits ENaC, which may reduce lithium nephrotoxic effects
- Sequelae
  - Chronic kidney disease
  - Hypercalcemia
  - Increased risk of renal tumors

MACROSCOPIC

- Small to normal-sized kidneys with numerous 2-5 mm cysts

MICROSCOPIC

- Renal microcysts
  - Lined by collecting duct cells
- Tubular dilation
  - Hobnail appearance of tubular epithelial cells may be present
- Interstitial inflammation, fibrosis, tubular atrophy
- Glomerulosclerosis, focal, segmental
- Foot process effacement

TOP DIFFERENTIAL DIAGNOSES

- Other forms of FSGS or minimal change disease
- Other forms of cystic and tubulointerstitial disease

DIAGNOSTIC CHECKLIST

- Fibrosis correlates inversely with concurrent and later GFR

(Left) *Axial T2-weighted MR shows innumerable tiny bright lesions ➡ throughout both kidneys, which represent fluid in microcysts (a typical feature of lithium-induced nephropathy). The patient had long-term lithium use.* **(Right)** *This kidney from a patient on long term lithium therapy reveals numerous cysts ➡ with marked atrophy of the cortex ⇨ and dilated calices ⇨.*

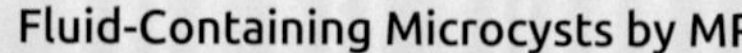

Fluid-Containing Microcysts by MR

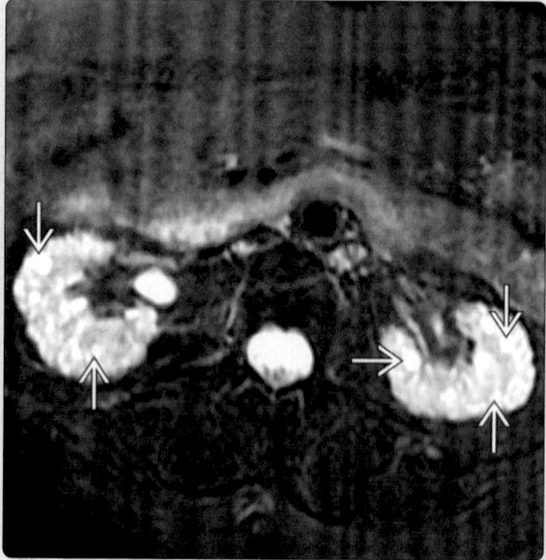

Multiple Microcysts and Atrophy

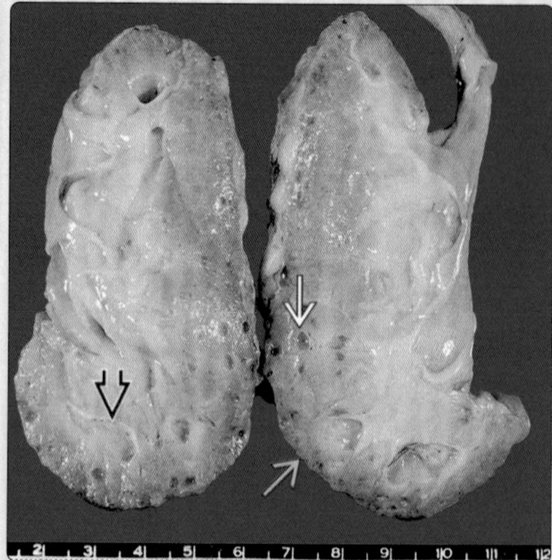

(Left) *The cortex from a 50 year old with renal failure after long-term lithium therapy for bipolar disorder shows many cysts ⇨, as well as 1 elongated space that is probably an ectatic collecting duct ➡.* **(Right)** *Periodic acid-Schiff shows a nonspecific pattern of lithium-associated chronic tubulointerstitial nephritis, with mononuclear cells ⇨, atrophic tubules ➡, and diffuse interstitial fibrosis. Glomeruli are normal, except for periglomerular fibrosis ➡.*

Cortical Cysts, Tubular Atrophy, and Interstitial Fibrosis

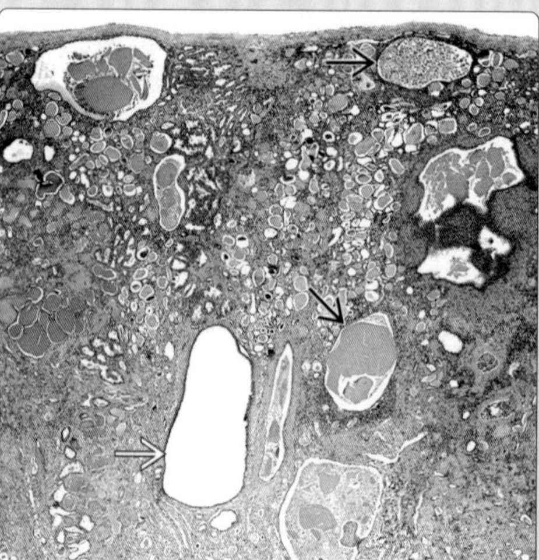

Interstitial Inflammation and Tubular Atrophy

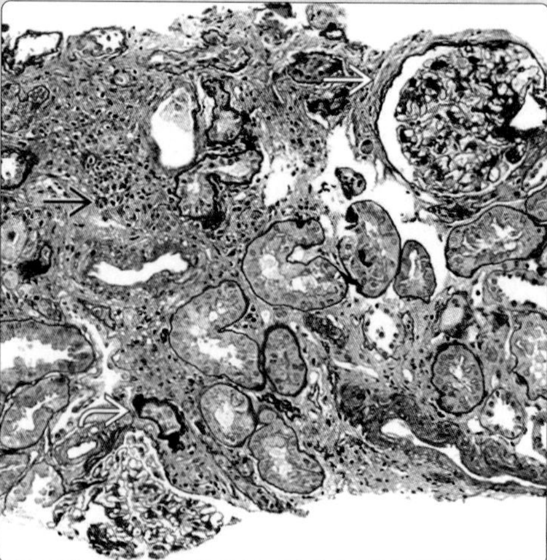

TERMINOLOGY

Definitions

- Disease affecting tubules, glomeruli, &/or interstitium related to chronic lithium (Li) treatment

ETIOLOGY/PATHOGENESIS

Nephrogenic Diabetes Insipidus

- Primary targets of lithium toxicity are principal cells of collecting ducts
  - Epithelial sodium channel (ENaC) in apical surface
    - Permeable to only sodium and lithium
  - Marked downregulation of aquaporin-2 expression, which controls water permeability and leads to nephrogenic diabetes insipidus
- Increased rate of proliferation
  - G2/M phase arrest results in decreased principal:intercalated cell ratio
  - May increase sensitivity to other tubular injury

Chronic Tubulointerstitial Nephritis and Cyst Formation

- Mechanism(s) unknown
- Other drugs/toxins or genetic factors may contribute since ESRD affects small minority of patients

CLINICAL ISSUES

Epidemiology

- Incidence
  - Increased incidence of Li-related ESRD from 0.14 to 0.78/million/year in Australia (1991-2011)
  - 1.2% of Swedish Li-treated patients have Cr > 150 μM/L
    - 0.53% develop end-stage renal disease
    - 6x risk compared with general population
  - Nephrogenic diabetes insipidus
    - 40% of all patients treated with lithium
    - 80% of patients with lithium nephrotoxicity

Presentation

- Nephrogenic diabetes insipidus
  - Polydipsia, polyuria
- Chronic kidney disease
- Proteinuria, nephrotic range 25%

Natural History

- Chronic kidney disease
  - Occurs after 10-20 years of lithium use
  - Can develop up to 10 years after lithium use is stopped
- Hypercalcemia
- 7-14x increased risk of renal tumors

Treatment

- Reduction or discontinuation of lithium therapy
  - Not effective when cystic change and glomerular and tubulointerstitial scarring present
- Amiloride, inhibits ENaC, may reduce lithium nephrotoxicity

Prognosis

- 0.5-1% of patients on lithium progress to ESRD
  - Average of 20 years of lithium therapy

MACROSCOPIC

Gross

- Small to normal-sized kidneys with numerous 2-5 mm cysts

MICROSCOPIC

Histologic Features

- Glomeruli
  - Segmental glomerulosclerosis
  - Global glomerulosclerosis
  - Glomerular hypertrophy
  - Mesangial hypercellularity &/or sclerosis
- Tubules and Interstitium
  - Interstitial fibrosis and tubular atrophy (85%)
  - Interstitial inflammation
  - Cysts and dilation (ectasia) of collecting ducts
    - Contain Tamm-Horsfall protein and cellular debris
    - Hobnail appearance of collecting duct cells
- Vessels: Moderate arteriosclerosis (85%)

Tumors

- Oncocytoma (~ 30%), clear cell carcinoma (~ 30%); papillary carcinoma (14%), and angiomyolipoma (14%)

ANCILLARY TESTS

Immunofluorescence

- IgM and C3 in segmental glomerular scars

Electron Microscopy

- Podocyte foot process effacement: Common
- Tubules have mitochondrial abnormalities (small, very dense; large, less dense) and increased autophagic lysosomes

DIFFERENTIAL DIAGNOSIS

Other Forms of FSGS or Minimal Change Disease

- Lack ectatic collecting ducts, hobnail cells

Other Forms of Cystic or Tubulointerstitial Disease

- Lack ectatic collecting ducts, hobnail cells

DIAGNOSTIC CHECKLIST

Clinically Relevant Pathologic Features

- Fibrosis and cysts correlate with cumulative Li dose
- Fibrosis correlates inversely with concurrent and later GFR

SELECTED REFERENCES

1. de Groot T et al: Lithium causes G2 arrest of renal principal cells. J Am Soc Nephrol. 25(3):501-10, 2014
2. Roxanas M et al: Renal replacement therapy associated with lithium nephrotoxicity in Australia. Med J Aust. 200(4):226-8, 2014
3. Zaidan M et al: Increased risk of solid renal tumors in lithium-treated patients. Kidney Int. 86(1):184-90, 2014
4. Grünfeld JP et al: Lithium nephrotoxicity revisited. Nat Rev Nephrol. 5(5):270-6, 2009
5. Presne C et al: Lithium-induced nephropathy: Rate of progression and prognostic factors. Kidney Int. 64(2):585-92, 2003
6. Markowitz GS et al: Lithium nephrotoxicity: a progressive combined glomerular and tubulointerstitial nephropathy. J Am Soc Nephrol. 11(8):1439-48, 2000

(Left) *This ectatic collecting duct ⇨ is a characteristic feature of chronic lithium nephrotoxicity. This patient required a renal transplant.* **(Right)** *A large tubular cyst filled with Tamm-Horsfall protein admixed with cellular debris and lined by collecting duct type epithelium is seen. Microcysts 1-2 mm in diameter are common in the late stages of lithium nephrotoxicity and appear to be derived from the distal nephron, especially the collecting ducts.*

Cysts and Tubulointerstitial Scarring

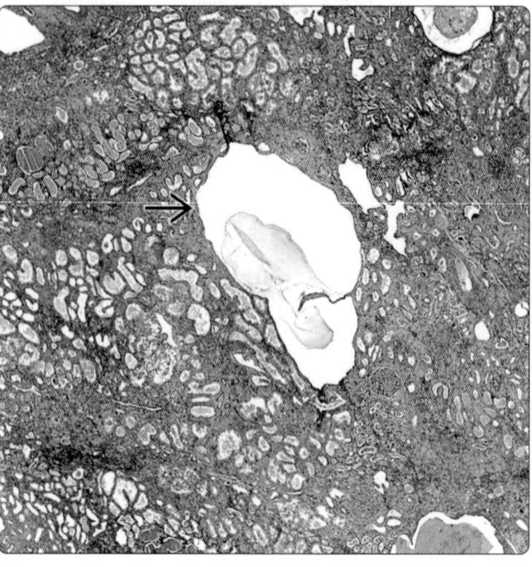

Collecting Duct Cysts

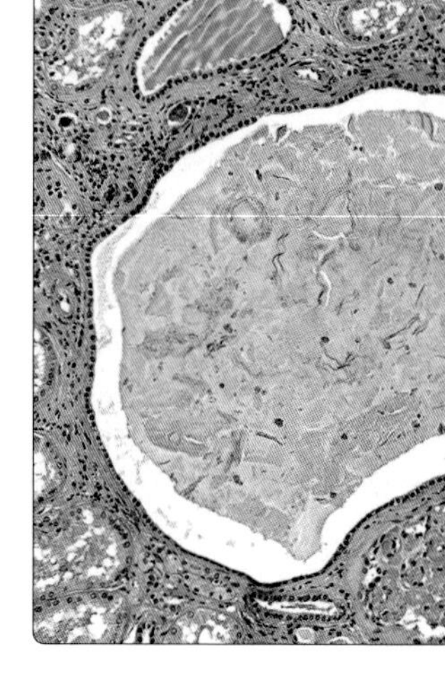

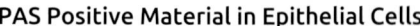

(Left) *Portions of 2 separate cysts ⇨ from a patient with lithium nephrotoxicity shows that the cells are simple cuboidal cells without brush borders or prominent mitochondria, suggesting a collecting duct origin. It is not common to see an entire cyst within a percutaneous kidney biopsy.* **(Right)** *Periodic acid-Schiff shows acute tubular injury in lithium toxicity. Tubular epithelial cells have a hobnailed appearance ⇨ and PAS(+) reabsorption droplets. Other tubules have cell debris in their lumen ➡ and thinned cytoplasm.*

Cyst Epithelium Suggests Collecting Duct Cells

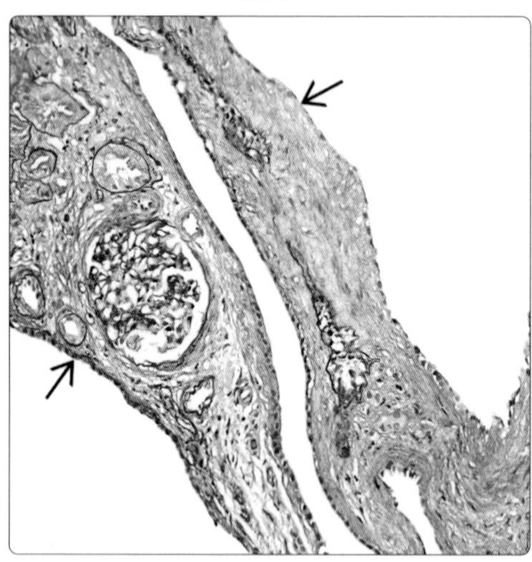

Tubular Epithelial Cell Injury

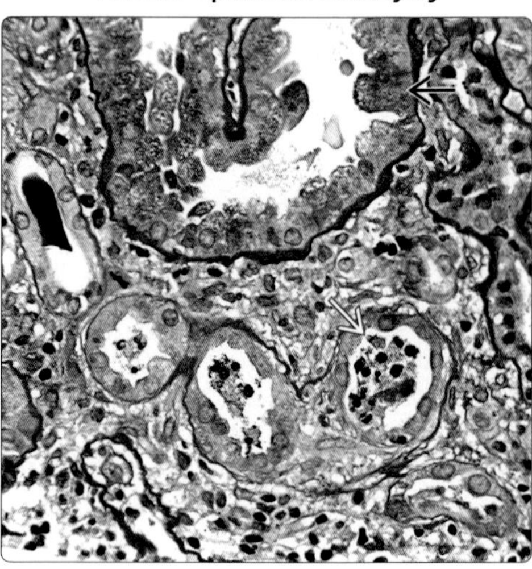

(Left) *Periodic acid-Schiff demonstrates prominent interstitial inflammation with a mixture of lymphocytes, eosinophils, and plasma cells among many atrophic tubules.* **(Right)** *PAS(+) material in distal and collecting duct cells and cells lining cysts have been reported in patients currently on lithium but not in patients who have discontinued the drug. The nature of the material is uncertain, reportedly glycogen.*

Interstitial Inflammation

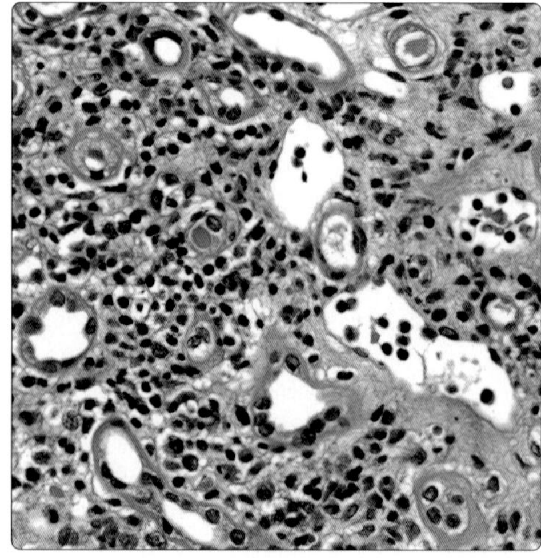

PAS Positive Material in Epithelial Cells

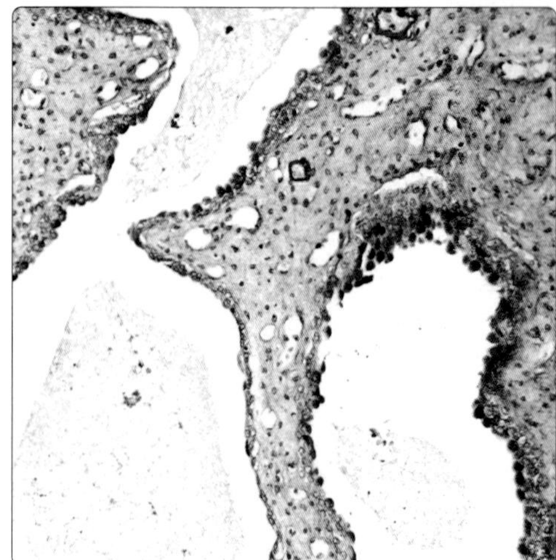

Partial Cyst Lining

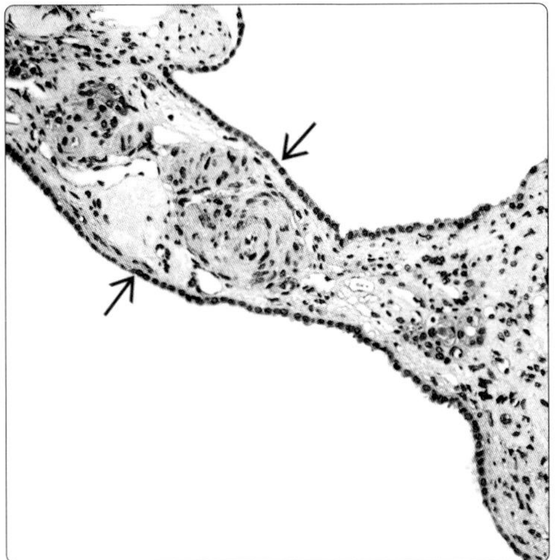

Glomerular Hypertrophy and Focal Segmental Sclerosis

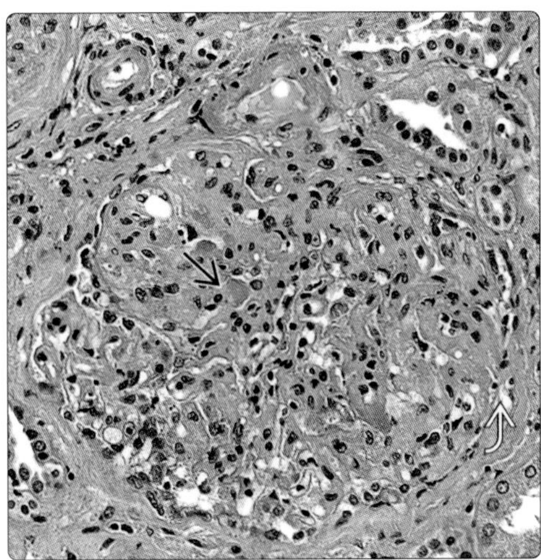

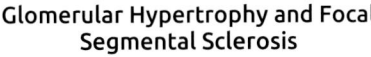

(Left) *Complete cysts may not be present in needle core biopsies, but careful examination may reveal a significant length of tubular epithelial cells lining basement membranes, such as these 2 partial cysts →.* **(Right)** *H&E shows focal segmental glomerulosclerosis (FSGS) in a patient on long-term lithium. Glomerular hypertrophy, hyaline →, and adhesions ↷ are also present.*

Autophagic Lysosomes in Tubular Epithelium

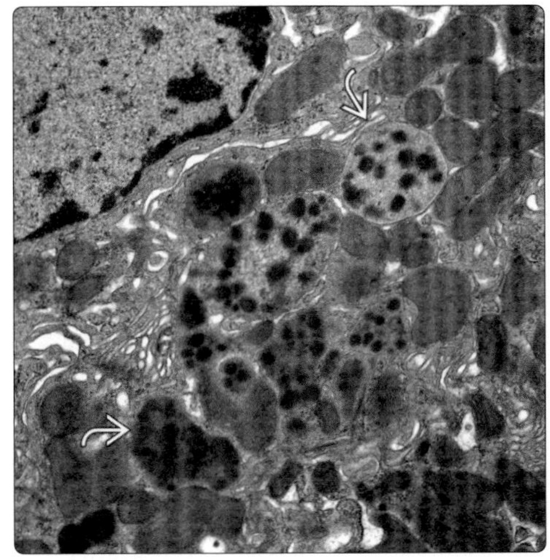

Mitochondriopathy

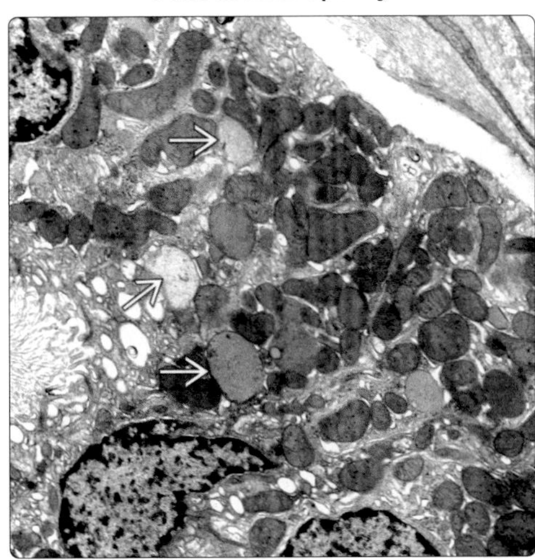

(Left) *Lithium stimulates autophagocytosis by decreasing intracellular myo-inositol-1,4,5-triphosphate levels. The autophagic lysosomes ↷ contain remnants of cytoplasmic organelles.* **(Right)** *Abnormal mitochondria have been described in chronic lithium nephrotoxicity in the form of abnormally large, less-dense mitochondria →. The reproducibility and relevance to the pathophysiology is unknown.*

Podocyte Foot Process Effacement

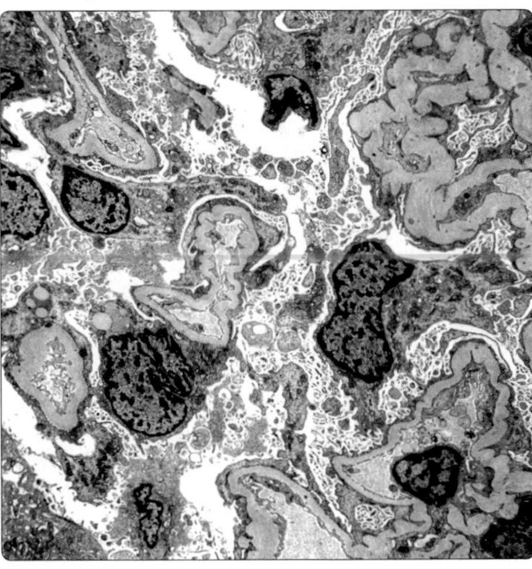

Oncocytoma

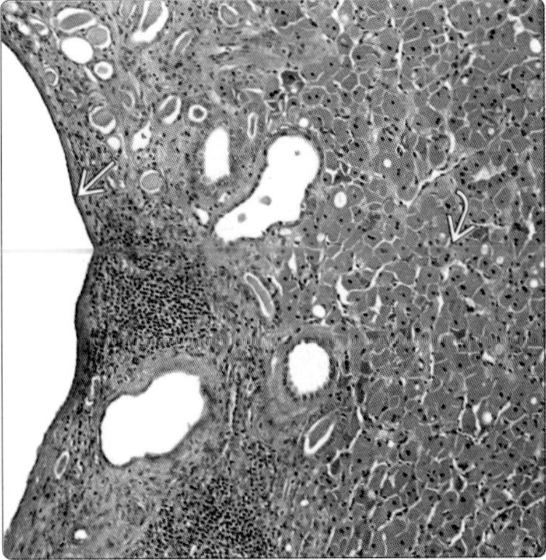

(Left) *Widespread effacement of foot processes and villous hypertrophy of podocytes are seen in this patient on lithium with nephrotic syndrome and FSGS. Minimal change disease is also associated with lithium therapy.* **(Right)** *Patients with lithium nephrotoxicity have an increased risk for certain benign and malignant renal tumors, including oncocytoma ↷. Oncocytomas arise from the intercalated cells of the collecting duct, which proliferate in lithium nephrotoxicity. Collecting duct microcysts are present →.*

Calcineurin Inhibitor Toxicity

KEY FACTS

TERMINOLOGY

- Kidney dysfunction attributable to injury from calcineurin inhibitor immunosuppressive agents

ETIOLOGY/PATHOGENESIS

- Transplanted and native kidneys affected by calcineurin inhibitor toxicity (CNIT)
- CNIT is dose related, with variable individual susceptibility
- Functional CNIT: Reversible acute renal dysfunction associated with afferent arteriolar vasoconstriction
- Structural CNIT: Tubular and vascular direct toxicity

CLINICAL ISSUES

- Acute or chronic elevation of serum creatinine
- Elevated blood or serum levels of CNI
- Correlation of structural tissue injury and blood levels is not strong

MICROSCOPIC

- Tubular toxicity
  - Acute: Acute tubular injury with focal isometric vacuolization of proximal tubular segments
  - Chronic: Striped interstitial fibrosis and tubular atrophy with microcalcifications
- Vascular toxicity
  - Acute arteriolopathy: Smooth muscle loss and expansion of intima and media by loose matrix
  - Chronic arteriolopathy: Nodular medial hyalinization
  - Thrombotic microangiopathy (TMA): Acute and chronic

DIAGNOSTIC CHECKLIST

- Exposure to CNI is a sine qua non for diagnosis
  - Elevated blood levels of CNI and long-term exposure increase certainty of diagnosis
- Absence of pathologic lesions in kidney biopsy does not exclude functional CNIT
- Observation of combined tubulopathy and vasculopathy increases diagnostic certainty
- No single histologic lesion is specific or pathognomonic

Acute Tubular Toxicity

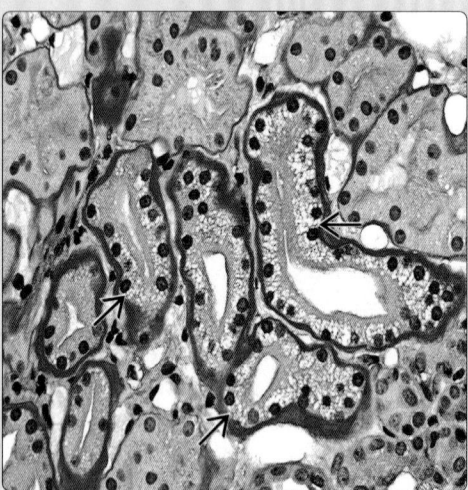

Chronic Tubular Toxicity

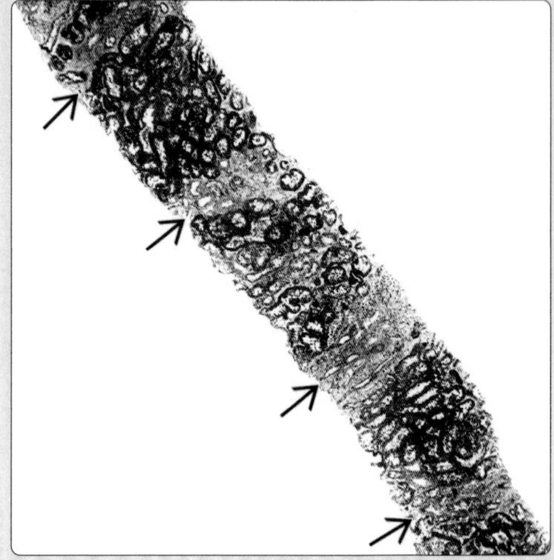

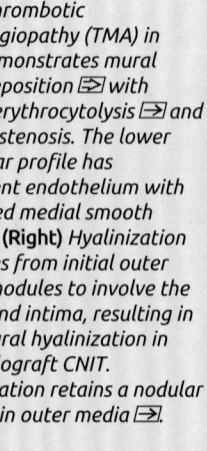

(Left) *Focal tubular isometric vacuolization → is evident in a renal transplant biopsy with calcineurin inhibitor toxicity (CNIT) due to tacrolimus. The affected tubules have thickened basement membranes, a nonspecific finding.* **(Right)** *The striped pattern of fibrosis → in chronic tubular CNI toxicity is probably a result of both chronic ischemia in "watershed" zones of the medullary rays, from hyaline arteriolosclerosis and direct tubular toxicity.*

Acute Vascular Toxicity

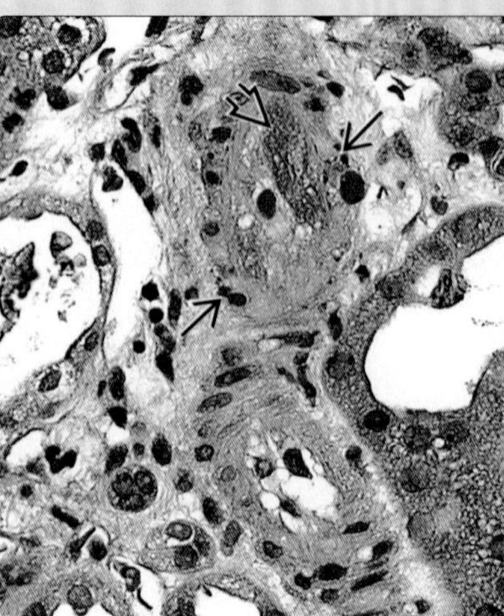

Chronic Vascular Toxicity

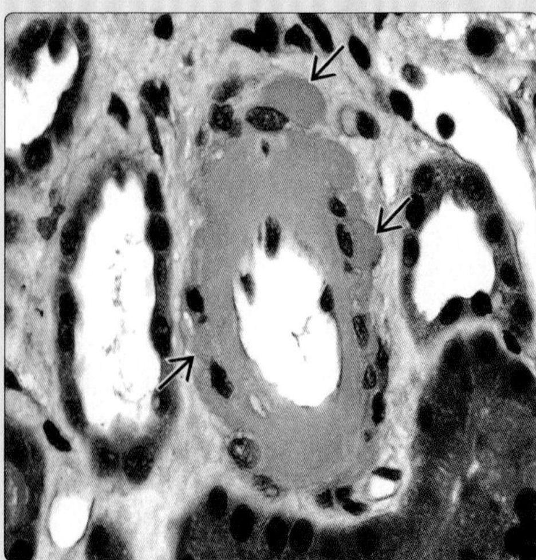

(Left) *Thrombotic microangiopathy (TMA) in CNIT demonstrates mural fibrin deposition ⇨ with medial erythrocytolysis → and luminal stenosis. The lower arteriolar profile has prominent endothelium with preserved medial smooth muscle.* **(Right)** *Hyalinization increases from initial outer medial nodules to involve the media and intima, resulting in transmural hyalinization in renal allograft CNIT. Hyalinization retains a nodular pattern in outer media →.*

TERMINOLOGY

Abbreviations

- Calcineurin inhibitor toxicity (CNIT)

Synonyms

- Cyclosporine toxicity, cyclosporine A (CsA or CyA) toxicity, tacrolimus toxicity, FK506 toxicity

Definitions

- Acute or chronic kidney dysfunction attributable to direct injury from calcineurin inhibitor immunosuppressive agents

ETIOLOGY/PATHOGENESIS

Types of CI Toxicity

- Functional CNIT: Reversible acute renal dysfunction associated with afferent arteriolar vasoconstriction
- Structural CNIT: Characterized by cellular injury and matrix remodeling
  - Tubular CNIT: Acute tubular injury with vacuolization of epithelium
  - Vascular CNIT: Direct toxic injury to endothelium and smooth muscle of arterioles
    - Thrombotic microangiopathy (TMA) or chronic hyaline arteriolopathy
    - Glomerular endothelial injury also a feature
- Tubular and vascular toxicity typically coexist
- Native and transplanted kidneys develop CNIT and histologic manifestations are similar

Mechanisms

- Histologic lesions are dose related
  - Acute CNIT with markedly elevated blood levels of CNI
  - Chronic CNIT with long-term exposure to CNI
- Dose-independent susceptibility factors, e.g., genes for enzymes that metabolize arachidonic acid
- CsA and tacrolimus bind intracellular receptors called immunophilins
  - Immunophilin/CI complexes bind and inhibit calcineurin
  - Calcineurin is T-cell activator via nuclear factors of activated T cells (NFAT)
  - NFAT activate transcription of inflammatory mediators like interleukin-2, interferon γ, and tumor necrosis factor α
- Immunosuppressive potency and renal toxicity of CI are pharmacologically inseparable
- Renal toxic effects of CsA and tacrolimus are identical
- CNIT affects endothelium, vascular smooth muscle, and tubular epithelium
  - Endothelium: Increased thromboxane A2, endothelin-1, superoxide and peroxynitrite, decreased prostaglandin and prostacyclin, apoptosis, necrosis
  - Smooth muscle: Vacuolization, necrosis, apoptosis, hyalinization
  - Tubular epithelium: Vacuolization, megamitochondria, calcification, necrosis

CLINICAL ISSUES

Epidemiology

- Incidence
  - Kidney transplants
    - TMA in 2-5%
    - Chronic CNIT in 60-70% at 2 years and > 90% at 10 years

Presentation

- Acute or chronic elevation of serum creatinine
  - CNIT may arise at any time after initiation of therapy
- Elevated trough blood levels of CNI may confirm diagnosis, but correlation of structural tissue injury and blood level is not strong
- TMA may be localized to kidney (40%) or may be systemic

Treatment

- Dose reduction or cessation of CI therapy

Prognosis

- Acute CNIT is typically reversible and associated with resolution of histologic changes
- Chronic CNIT is less likely to be reversible
  - Resolution of arteriolopathy possible with cessation of CNI

MICROSCOPIC

Histologic Features

- Functional CNIT
  - No morphologic tissue injury by definition
- Tubular CNIT
  - Acute
    - Focal proximal tubular epithelial isometric vacuolization in straight > convoluted segments
    - Vacuolar changes may be accompanied by acute tubular injury ± dystrophic microcalcification
    - Large eosinophilic cytoplasmic granules are megamitochondria (CsA toxicity) or lysosomes (tacrolimus toxicity)
  - Chronic
    - Striped fibrosis characterized by radial fibrosis of cortical medullary rays with intervening nonscarred parenchyma ± tubular microcalcification
      - Result of chronic ischemia from arteriolopathy and direct tubular toxicity
- Vascular CNIT
  - Acute and chronic vasculopathy may be present in same biopsy
  - Acute arteriolopathy: Focal lesion
    - Loss of definition of smooth muscle cells, cytoplasmic vacuolization and dropout
    - Clear or basophilic medial or intimal loose matrix accumulation with separation of myocytes
    - Intimal or medial platelet insudates (CD61[+])
  - TMA
    - Arteriolar thrombi, intimal and medial fibrinoid change ± erythrocytolysis, platelets (CD61+)
    - Obliterative arteriolopathy has stenosis, intimal and medial hypercellularity ("onion skinning")
    - Arteries may have intimal myxoid thickening
  - Chronic arteriolopathy
    - Early lesions have hyaline replacement of individual outer medial smooth muscle cells
    - Nodular hyalinization of outer media imparts an eosinophilic, PAS(+) beaded necklace appearance

- Over months to years, entire vessel wall is hyalinized
- Hyalinization mainly affects afferent arterioles but can involve vasa recta and small arteries
- Striped interstitial fibrosis, tubular atrophy, calcification, and glomerular sclerosis may be present
- Glomerulopathy and CNIT
  - Acute TMA
    - Capillary thrombi; glomerular hilar thrombi (so-called "pouch lesions")
    - Capillary double contours and mesangiolysis
  - Chronic TMA and other chronic lesions
    - Capillary basement membrane double contours
    - Ischemic collapse, obsolescence, and focal segmental glomerular sclerosis
- Immunohistology
  - Acute arteriolopathy and TMA
    - Immunofluorescence: Arteriolar and glomerular IgM, C3, and fibrinogen
    - Immunoperoxidase staining: CD61 or CD62 positive platelet deposits in arterioles and glomeruli
  - Chronic arteriolopathy
    - IgM, C3, and C1q in hyaline deposits; no platelets
- Electron microscopy
  - Tubules: Dilated endoplasmic reticulum; multiple large lysosomes, megamitochondria, endocytotic vesicles
  - Arterioles and glomeruli
    - Endothelial swelling, cytoplasmic vacuolization, detachment from basal lamina and apoptosis or necrosis
      - Capillary double contours and interposition
    - Myocyte vacuoles, disruption of myofibrils, detachment from basal lamina, apoptosis
    - Electron-dense hyaline material replaces smooth muscle

DIFFERENTIAL DIAGNOSIS

Tubulopathy

- Osmotic tubulopathy associated with exposure to parenteral carbohydrates, intravenous immunoglobulin, or radiocontrast agents
  - Diffuse cytoplasmic vacuolization, swollen epithelium, preserved brush border
    - Vacuoles are endosomes and phagolysosomes
- Ischemic acute tubular injury
  - Coarse irregular vacuoles
- Tubulopathy associated with lipiduria in nephrotic syndrome
  - Vacuoles are isometric, focal, and contain lipid, ± interstitial foam cells
  - PAS(+) protein droplets in tubules; stain for Ig and albumin by immunofluorescence
  - Causal glomerulopathy is typically identified

Vasculopathy

- Lesions outlined below affect native and transplant kidneys, with exception of humoral rejection
- TMA
  - Acute antibody mediated (humoral) rejection
    - Transplant glomerulitis, peritubular capillaritis, each with neutrophils, and C4d positive
    - Donor-specific antibodies
  - Malignant hypertension: Clinical history
  - Hemolytic uremic syndrome/thrombotic thrombocytopenic purpura
    - Diffuse in contrast to focal distribution in CI toxicity
  - Antiphospholipid nephropathy: Antiphospholipid or anticardiolipin antibodies
- Acute arteriolopathy
  - Indistinguishable changes seen in severe hypertensive arteriolosclerosis
- Hyaline arteriolosclerosis of diabetic nephropathy and hypertension
  - Initial lesions classically intimal rather than medial
  - Peripheral nodular medial hyalinization may be seen rarely
  - Transmural hyalinization in advanced disease, making determination of etiology difficult
  - Hyaline deposits in afferent and efferent vessels in diabetic arteriolopathy
- Amyloid vasculopathy deposits are not typically nodular and are Congo red positive

Focal Segmental Glomerulosclerosis (FSGS)

- Widespread effacement of foot processes in primary FSGS
- Less conspicuous arteriolar hyalinosis
- CNIT may have collapsing variant of FSGS

DIAGNOSTIC CHECKLIST

Clinically Relevant Pathologic Features

- Absence of pathologic lesions in kidney biopsy does not exclude CNIT
- Exposure to CNI inhibitors is a sine qua non for diagnosis of CNIT
- Observation of combined tubulopathy and vasculopathy increases diagnostic certainty

Pathologic Interpretation Pearls

- Acute CNIT: Tubulopathy with isometric vacuolization, acute tubular injury, acute arteriolopathy, and TMA
- Chronic CNIT: Nodular arteriolar hyalinization, striped fibrosis, calcifications, global and segmental glomerular sclerosis
- No single histologic lesion is pathognomic

SELECTED REFERENCES

1. Bröcker V et al: Arteriolar lesions in renal transplant biopsies: prevalence, progression, and clinical significance. Am J Pathol. 180(5):1852-62, 2012
2. Jacobson PA et al: Genetic and clinical determinants of early, acute calcineurin inhibitor-related nephrotoxicity: results from a kidney transplant consortium. Transplantation. 93(6):624-31, 2012
3. Snanoudj R et al: Specificity of histological markers of long-term CNI nephrotoxicity in kidney-transplant recipients under low-dose cyclosporine therapy. Am J Transplant. 11(12):2635-46, 2011
4. Nankivell BJ et al: Calcineurin inhibitor nephrotoxicity: longitudinal assessment by protocol histology. Transplantation. 78(4):557-65, 2004
5. Mihatsch MJ et al: The side-effects of ciclosporine-A and tacrolimus. Clin Nephrol. 49(6):356-63, 1998
6. Mihatsch MJ et al: Histopathology of cyclosporine nephrotoxicity. Transplant Proc. 20(3 Suppl 3):759-71, 1988

Normal Arteriole

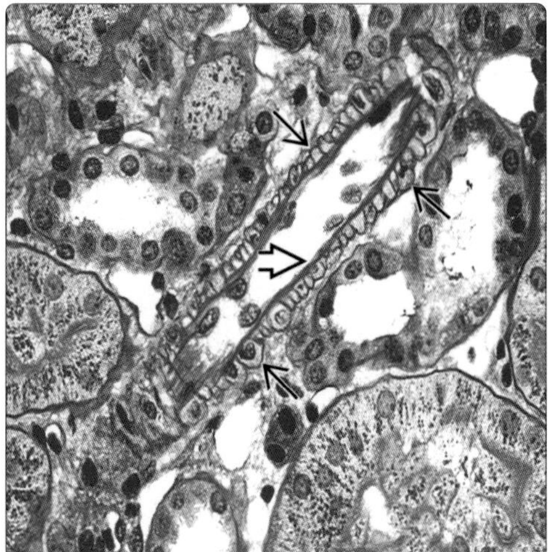

Acute Vascular Toxicity

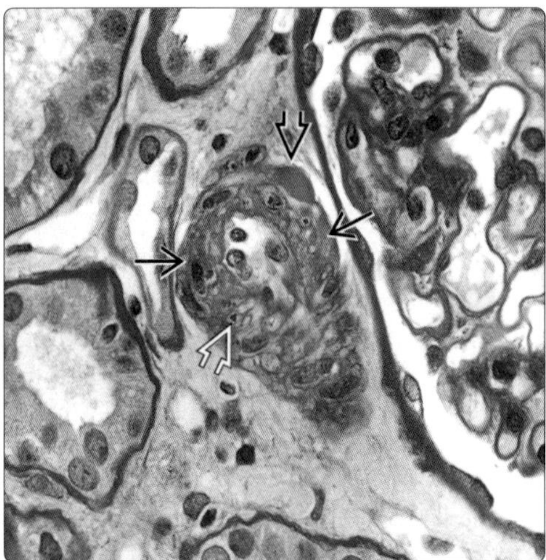

(Left) *The profile of a normal-appearing arteriole is seen, with PAS highlighting the basal lamina of the medial smooth muscle cells* ➙. *The endothelial basal lamina is also evident* ➙. **(Right)** *In early vascular CNI toxicity, the medial smooth muscle cells lose their discrete definition* ➙ *and may acquire PAS(+) granules* ➙. *The discrete, well-delineated appearance of outer medial hyalin nodules* ➙ *indicates hyaline replacement of myocytes within the confines of the basal lamina.*

Chronic Vascular Toxicity

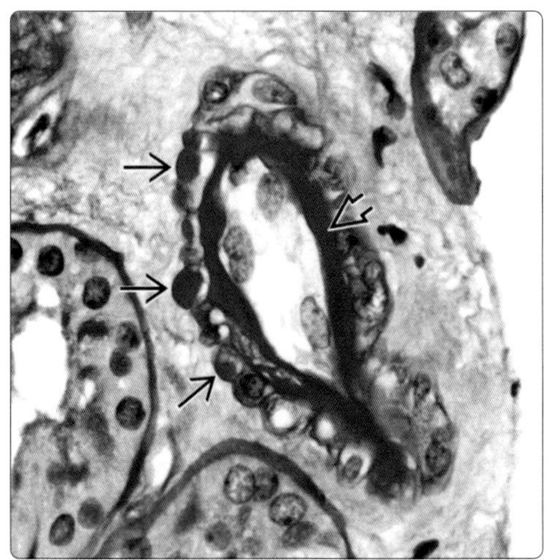

Hyaline Replacing Myocyte

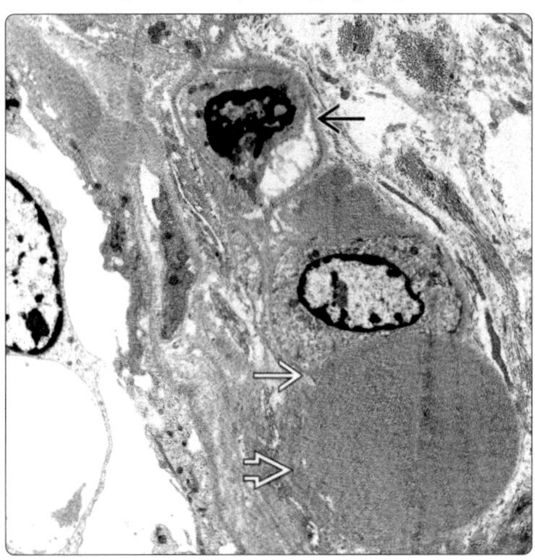

(Left) *Nodular outer medial hyalinization* ➙ *with a discrete beaded appearance is evident in this biopsy from a patient with chronic CNIT. Prominent intimal hyalinization with thickening of the endothelial basal lamina is also evident* ➙. **(Right)** *EM shows nodular hyaline arteriolosclerosis in a kidney transplant with CIT. Upper myocyte shows shrinkage & detachment from basal lamina* ➙. *Rounded amorphous hyaline material* ➙ *fills the basal lamina, replacing the myocyte and compressing adjacent cell* ➙.

Arteriolar Hyalinosis Vasa Recta

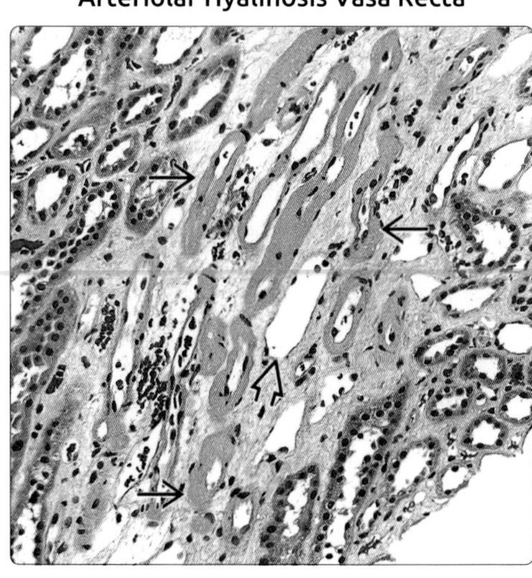

Peripheral Nodular Hyalinosis

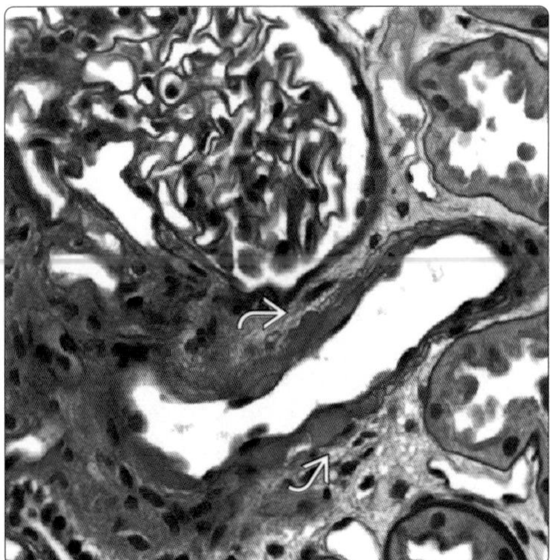

(Left) *Vasa recta are also prone to chronic CNI toxicity. This is an example of extensive transmural hyalinization of the arteriolar vasa in a renal transplant with chronic CI toxicity* ➙. *Venules are unaffected* ➙. **(Right)** *Multiple peripheral nodular hyaline deposits are present in this afferent arteriole from a donor biopsy* ➙. *Occasionally, this pattern of hyalinosis can be seen without a history of CNI administration.*

Myxoid Matrix

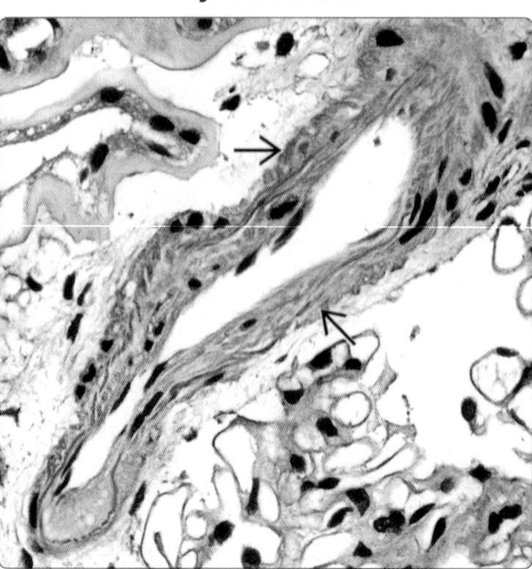

CD61 Deposition

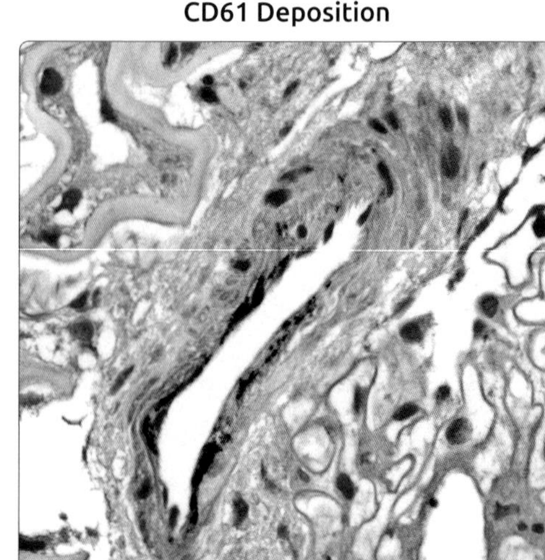

(Left) *Myxoid matrix accumulation is shown in the media and intima of an arteriole from a kidney transplant with CNI toxicity. There is segmental absence of smooth muscle cell nuclei* ⮕. **(Right)** *Immunohistochemical staining for CD61 may reveal unexpected platelet insudation in the intima or media of arterioles with myxoid changes by light microscopy. The tissue is a biopsy from a renal transplant with CNI toxicity.*

Obliterative Arteriolopathy

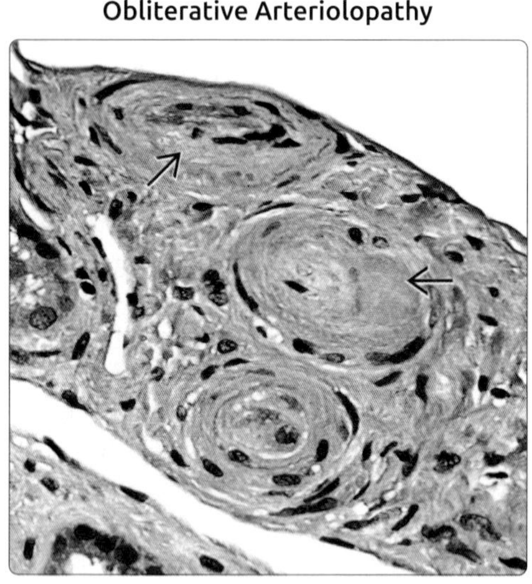

CD61 Deposits Suggest TMA

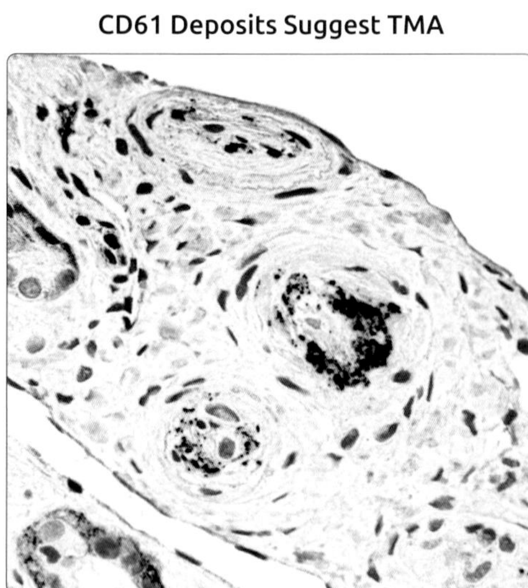

(Left) *A kidney transplant biopsy with severe obliterative arteriolopathy from CNIT is shown. The arterioles have luminal obliteration, loss of smooth muscle, and matrix accumulation* ⮕*, and were observed in the context of greatly elevated blood levels of tacrolimus.* **(Right)** *Obliterative arteriolopathy attributable to CNIT may have unrecognized mural platelet deposits. Immunostaining for CD61 reveals granular platelets and platelet microparticles in the intima and media.*

Glomerular Thrombi

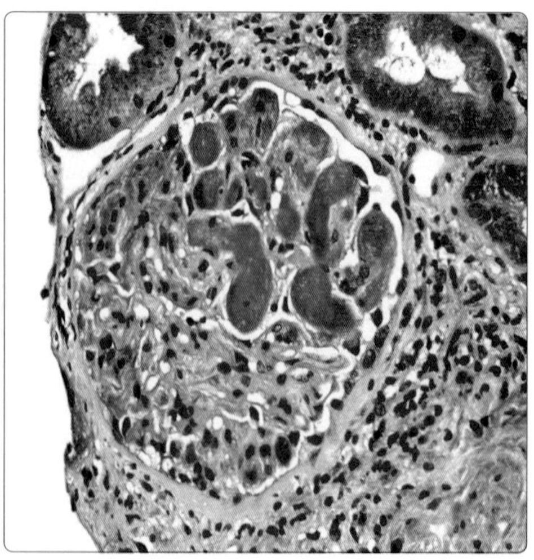

Platelet CD61 in Thrombi

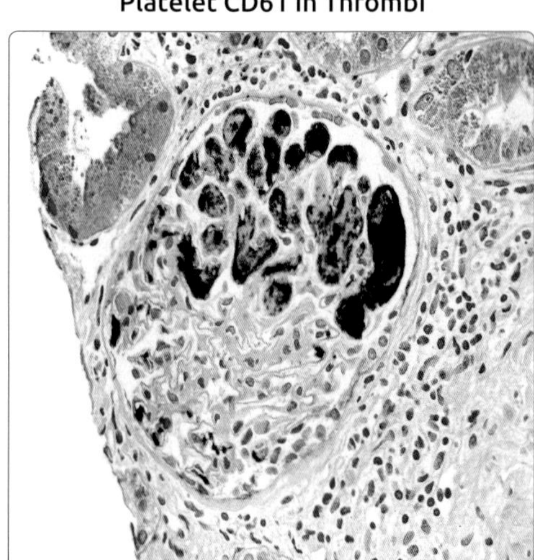

(Left) *This glomerulus has segmental occlusive glomerular capillary fibrin-platelet thrombi from a kidney transplant with CNIT and TMA. Pericapsulitis is nonspecific.* **(Right)** *Immunohistochemical staining for CD61, a marker of platelets, reveals occlusive glomerular capillary thrombi in a renal allograft with CI toxicity and thrombotic microangiopathy.*

Chronic Vascular Toxicity

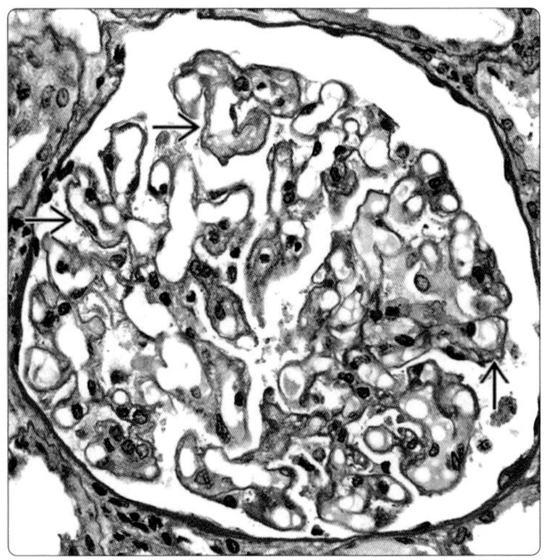

Endothelial Injury in CNIT

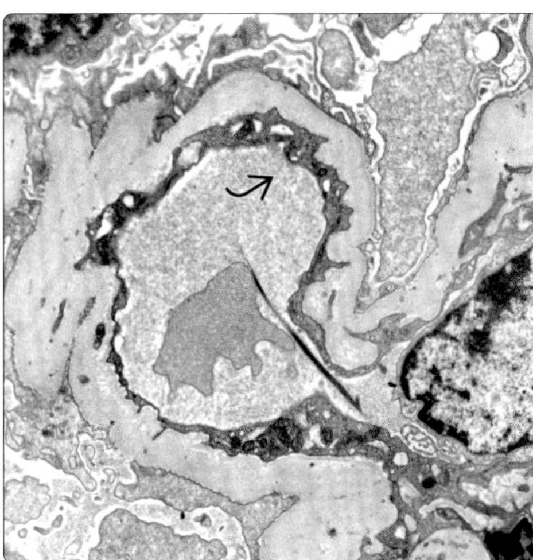

(Left) *Glomeruli in chronic TMA due to CNIT have segmental or global double contours of the GBM ➡. These lesions represent repair of endothelial injury and must be distinguished from transplant glomerulopathy. Thrombi may be absent from glomeruli with these lesions.* **(Right)** *Electron microscopy of a native kidney with thrombotic microangiopathy due to CNI reveals marked endothelial injury manifested by loss of fenestrations ➡ in this glomerular capillary from a liver transplant recipient*

Focal Segmental Glomerulosclerosis

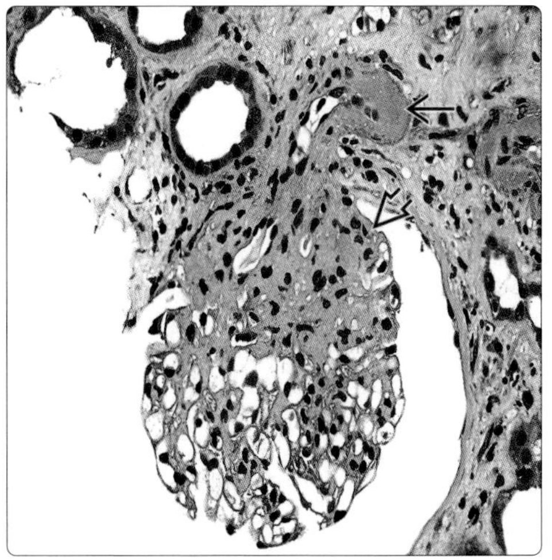

Collapsing Glomerulopathy

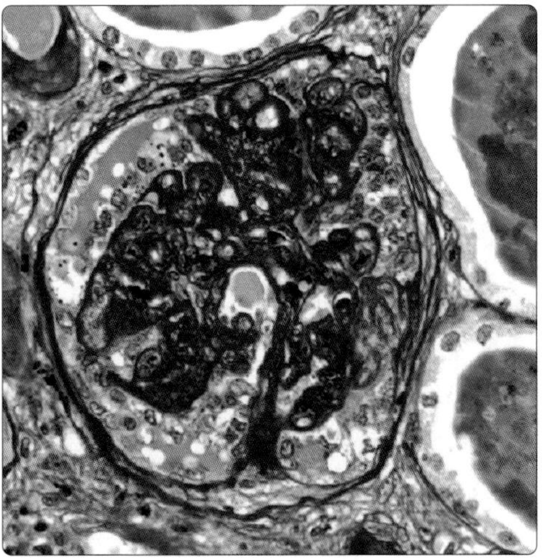

(Left) *Perihilar focal segmental glomerulosclerosis ➡ associated with arteriolar hyalinization ➡ in a renal allograft is shown in a patient with exposure to CNI for more than 7 years.* **(Right)** *Collapsing glomerulopathy is shown in a native kidney of a heart-lung transplant recipient on CNI for 10 years. Severe arteriolar hyalinosis due to CNI was also present. Severe microvascular disease is a known cause of collapsing glomerulopathy.*

Acute Tubular Toxicity

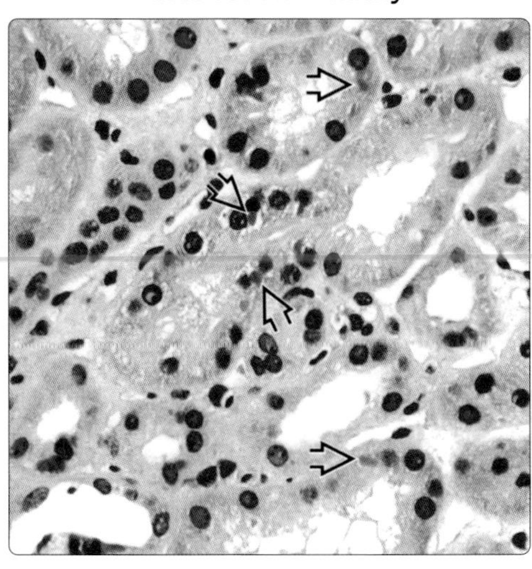

Chronic Tubular Toxicity: Striped Fibrosis

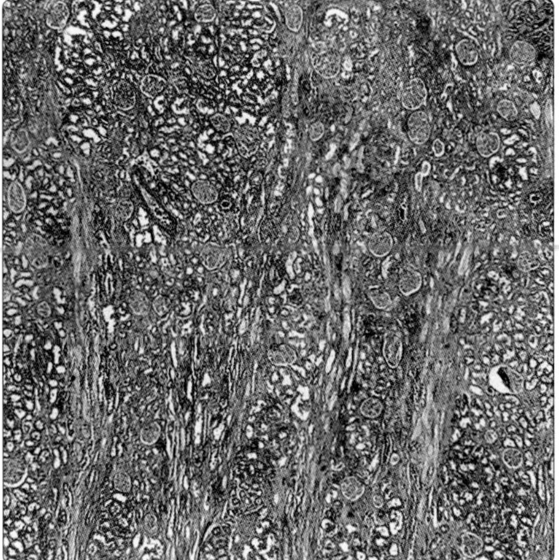

(Left) *Megamitochondria appear as irregularly shaped eosinophilic globules ➡ in the epithelial cytoplasm in tubular CI toxicity.* **(Right)** *The pattern of striped fibrosis is due to ischemia in the watershed areas of the cortex, the medullary rays, here illustrated in a trichrome stain of a native kidney from a lung transplant recipient. (Courtesy S. Rosen, MD.)*

KEY FACTS

ETIOLOGY/PATHOGENESIS

- mTOR drugs
  - Inhibit tubular epithelial cell proliferation and apoptosis in setting of acute injury
  - Decreases VEGF synthesis, related to development of focal segmental glomerulosclerosis (FSGS)

CLINICAL ISSUES

- Acute renal failure, delayed graft function (acute toxicity)
- Proteinuria (chronic toxicity)

MICROSCOPIC

- Acute mTOR inhibitor toxicity
  - Severe acute tubular injury
  - Epithelial cell necrosis
  - Atypical, eosinophilic PAS(-) casts reminiscent of myeloma cast nephropathy
    - Stain for cytokeratin by immunohistochemistry
  - Myoglobin-appearing casts; stain for myoglobin by immunohistochemistry
  - Thrombotic microangiopathy (TMA)
- Chronic mTOR inhibitor toxicity
  - Focal segmental glomerulosclerosis
  - Abnormal podocyte phenotype, suggestive of podocyte dedifferentiation

TOP DIFFERENTIAL DIAGNOSES

- Acute mTOR inhibitor toxicity
  - Severe acute tubular necrosis
  - Acute humoral rejection
  - Light chain (myeloma) cast nephropathy
  - Rhabdomyolysis
- Chronic mTOR inhibitor toxicity
  - FSGS due to other factors

Acute Tubular Injury

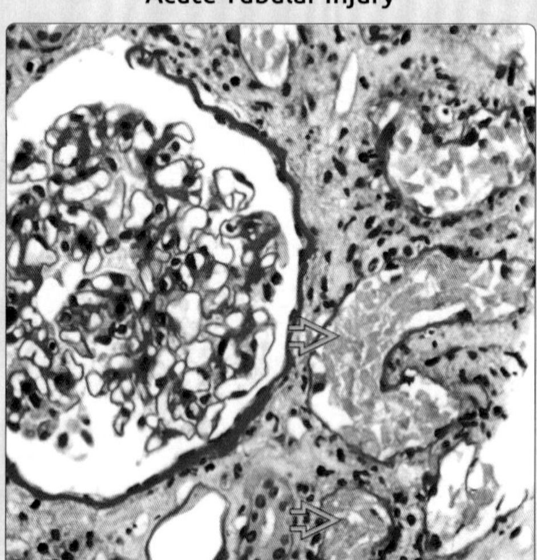

FSGS

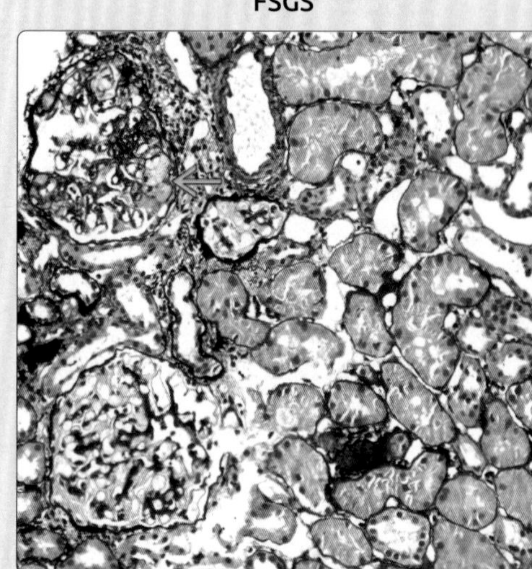

(Left) *PAS shows acute rapamycin toxicity with PAS(-) casts ➡ and severe acute tubular injury. The material consists of cytoplasmic debris from damaged tubular epithelial cells.* **(Right)** *De novo FSGS ➡ due to chronic mTOR inhibitor toxicity is present in a 58-year-old man with 425 mg/day of proteinuria 2.5 years after transplantation. He had never been treated with calcineurin inhibitors.*

Thrombus

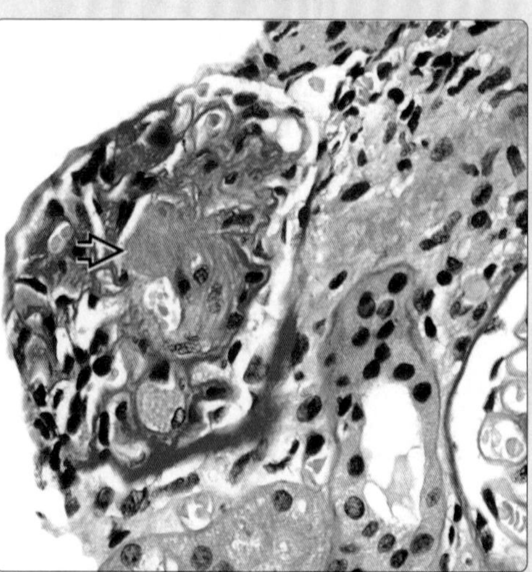

Myoglobin

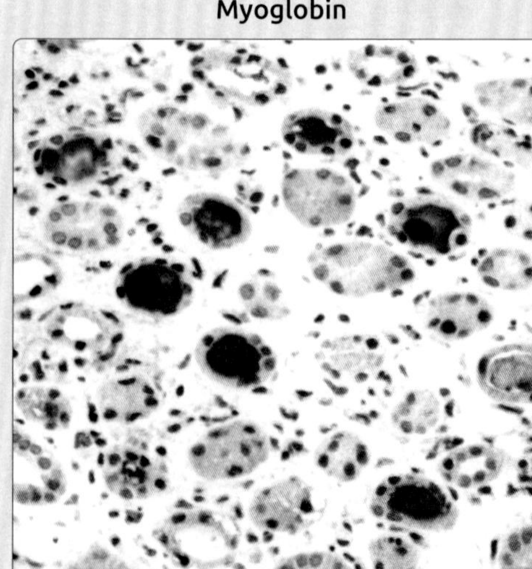

(Left) *Acute mTOR inhibitor toxicity shows a glomerular thrombus ➡ in a renal transplant patient on sirolimus and tacrolimus. Either sirolimus or tacrolimus by itself may cause TMA; there is greater risk of TMA in combined sirolimus and tacrolimus therapy than in sirolimus without a calcineurin inhibitor.* **(Right)** *Tubular casts can stain for myoglobin by immunohistochemistry in mTOR inhibitor toxicity, similar to those in rhabdomyolysis. This is presumptive evidence of muscle injury.*

TERMINOLOGY

Abbreviations

- Mammalian target of rapamycin (mTOR)

Definitions

- mTOR inhibitors used in renal transplantation
  - Rapamycin (sirolimus)
  - Everolimus
    - Similar structure to sirolimus; shorter half-life

ETIOLOGY/PATHOGENESIS

mTOR Inhibitor (Rapamycin/Sirolimus): Drug Effects

- Sirolimus binds FK506 binding protein-12 to form sirolimus effector protein (SEP) complex
- SEP complex inhibits mTOR pathway
  - Sirolimus blocks cytokine-mediated signal transduction, affecting T-cell cycle progression
  - Decreases lymphocyte proliferation
- mTOR expressed in kidney, e.g., tubular epithelial cells
  - Repair response to acute tubular injury requires tubular epithelial cell turnover and proliferation
    - Sirolimus inhibits tubular epithelial cell proliferation and apoptosis
- Decreases VEGF synthesis
  - Mechanism of thrombotic microangiopathy

mTOR Inhibitor Effect on Podocyte

- Focal segmental glomerulosclerosis (FSGS) lesions show abnormal podocyte phenotype, suggestive of podocyte dedifferentiation
  - PAX2 and cytokeratin expression in proliferating podocytes
  - Loss of synaptopodin and VEGF expression
  - Downregulated nephrin expression in podocytes
    - Similar pattern in sirolimus-related FSGS and other types of FSGS
- In vitro decreased VEGF synthesis and Akt phosphorylation by podocytes in presence of sirolimus and decreased synthesis of WT1, protein required for podocyte integrity

CLINICAL ISSUES

Presentation

- Delayed graft function (DGF)
  - More common in mTOR inhibitor treatment (25%) than without (9%)
  - Correlates with mTOR inhibitor dose
- Acute renal failure (acute mTOR inhibitor toxicity)
- Proteinuria (chronic mTOR inhibitor toxicity)

Treatment

- Drugs
  - Discontinuation or reduced dose of mTOR inhibitor
  - Initiation of alternative immunosuppressive therapy

MICROSCOPIC

Histologic Features

- Acute mTOR inhibitor toxicity
  - Severe acute tubular injury
    - Dilatation of tubules, epithelial flattening, loss of tubular brush border
    - Epithelial cell necrosis
  - Casts
    - Atypical, eosinophilic PAS(-) casts
      - Stain for cytokeratin by immunohistochemistry
    - Irregular, sharply demarcated cast edges
    - Casts may appear "fractured"
    - Casts may have surrounding cellular reaction
      - Reminiscent of myeloma cast nephropathy
    - Myoglobin-appearing casts; stain for myoglobin by immunohistochemistry
  - Histologic resolution upon sirolimus removal
  - Thrombotic microangiopathy (TMA)
    - Increased risk in patients on both sirolimus and cyclosporine
    - Some associated with lab evidence of acute TMA: Thrombocytopenia, anemia, low haptoglobin levels
- Chronic mTOR inhibitor toxicity
  - FSGS
    - May have collapsing pattern
    - Some have proteinuria without FSGS

DIFFERENTIAL DIAGNOSIS

Severe Acute Tubular Necrosis

- Due to causes other than an mTOR inhibitor

Rhabdomyolysis

- Myoglobin casts present in both rhabdomyolysis and mTOR inhibitor toxicity

Acute Humoral Rejection

- C4d-positive peritubular capillaries
- May show acute tubular necrosis &/or TMA

Light Chain (Myeloma) Cast Nephropathy

- Monotypic light chain immunolocalization
- Serum or urine paraprotein usually detectable
- Unusual in renal allograft

Focal Segmental Glomerulosclerosis

- Recurrent or de novo in allograft
- FSGS pattern may be result of chronic calcineurin inhibitor (CNI) toxicity
  - Arteriolar hyalinosis also present in chronic CNI toxicity

SELECTED REFERENCES

1. Shihab F et al: Focus on mTOR inhibitors and tacrolimus in renal transplantation: pharmacokinetics, exposure-response relationships, and clinical outcomes. Transpl Immunol. 31(1):22-32, 2014
2. Vollenbröker B et al: mTOR regulates expression of slit diaphragm proteins and cytoskeleton structure in podocytes. Am J Physiol Renal Physiol. 296(2):F418-26, 2009
3. Letavernier E et al: High sirolimus levels may induce focal segmental glomerulosclerosis de novo. Clin J Am Soc Nephrol. 2(2):326-33, 2007
4. Pelletier R et al: Acute renal failure following kidney transplantation associated with myoglobinuria in patients treated with rapamycin. Transplantation. 82(5):645-50, 2006
5. Izzedine H et al: Post-transplantation proteinuria and sirolimus. N Engl J Med. 353(19):2088-9, 2005
6. Sartelet H et al: Sirolimus-induced thrombotic microangiopathy is associated with decreased expression of vascular endothelial growth factor in kidneys. Am J Transplant. 5(10):2441-7, 2005

Warfarin Nephropathy

KEY FACTS

TERMINOLOGY

- Warfarin-related nephropathy is defined as unexplained increase in serum creatinine in patients supratherapeutic on warfarin therapy (defined as INR > 3)

ETIOLOGY/PATHOGENESIS

- Warfarin is thought to cause acute kidney injury by inducing glomerular hematuria leading to tubular obstruction by red blood cell casts and subsequent acute tubular injury

CLINICAL ISSUES

- Patients present with acute rise in serum creatinine after becoming supratherapeutic on warfarin

MICROSCOPIC

- RBCs in Bowman space, tubular lumens, and acute tubular injury with numerous occlusive RBC casts
- Occlusive RBC casts preferentially involve distal nephron

TOP DIFFERENTIAL DIAGNOSES

- Glomerulonephritis with RBC casts
  - RBC casts are not specific for warfarin nephropathy
  - Number of RBC casts is disproportionate to degree of glomerular lesions in warfarin nephropathy (e.g., mild mesangial immune complex deposition with acute kidney injury and numerous RBC casts)
  - Diagnosis of warfarin nephropathy requires clinical correlation
- Red blood cells in tubular lumens due to biopsy artifact
  - Tubular injury and flattening/compression of epithelial cells not present in artifact
  - RBCs typically seen around edges of biopsy specimen if artifactual
  - RBC casts preferentially involve distal nephron in warfarin nephropathy

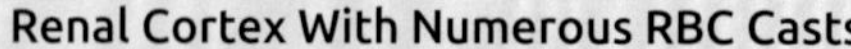

Renal Cortex With Numerous RBC Casts

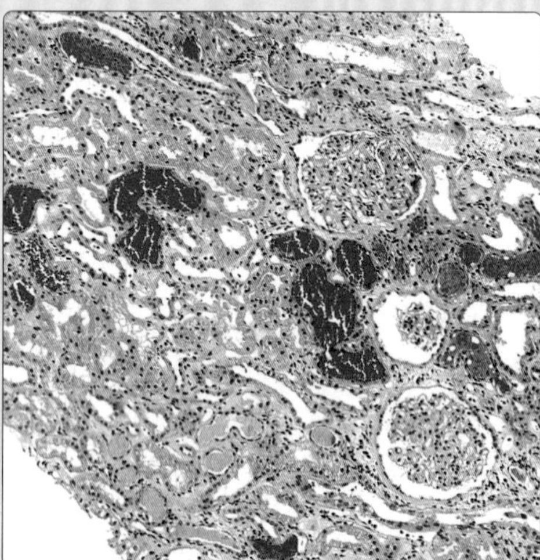

Glomerular Hemorrhage

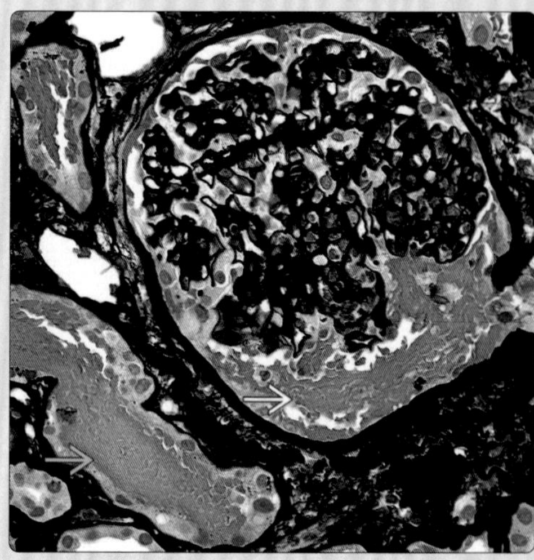

(Left) *Many of the tubular lumina show RBC casts and glomeruli show mild mesangial expansion. This biopsy is from a patient with atrial fibrillation who was recently supratherapeutic on warfarin. The glomeruli had mild mesangial IgA deposition without crescents or endocapillary proliferation by light microscopy.* **(Right)** *Higher power view from the same case shows numerous RBCs in the Bowman space ➔ and tubular injury with flattening of the tubular epithelium by an RBC cast ➔.*

Medulla With RBC Casts

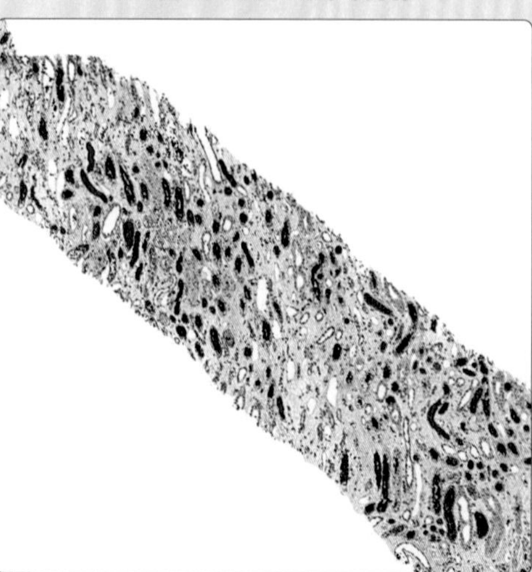

RBC Casts

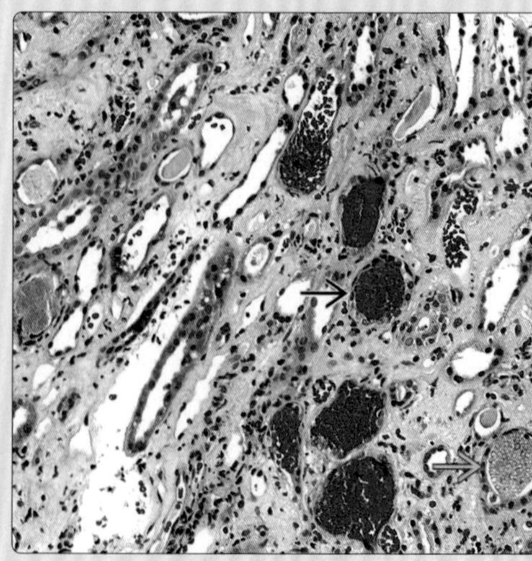

(Left) *Numerous obstructive RBC casts are present within the tubular lumina in the medulla. This patient presented with acute renal failure and was found to be supratherapeutic on warfarin 2 weeks prior to biopsy.* **(Right)** *Higher power view from the same case shows RBC casts of varying ages, including fresh bright red casts ➔ as well as older casts with a more faded appearance ➔.*

TERMINOLOGY

Synonyms

- Anticoagulation-related nephropathy

Definitions

- Warfarin-related nephropathy is defined as unexplained increase in serum creatinine in patients supratherapeutic on warfarin therapy (defined as INR > 3)

ETIOLOGY/PATHOGENESIS

Anticoagulation With Warfarin (Coumadin)

- Warfarin is thought to cause acute kidney injury by inducing glomerular hematuria, leading to tubular obstruction by red blood cell casts and subsequent acute tubular injury
- Associated with high level of anticoagulation (INR > 3)

Animal Models

- Warfarin, brodifacoum, or dabigatran administration to rats with 5/6 nephrectomy
- Relative lack in normal controls argues glomerular hypertension may be a risk factor

CLINICAL ISSUES

Epidemiology

- Warfarin is most commonly used anticoagulant, with > 30 million prescriptions filled annually
- Large retrospective analysis showed warfarin-related nephropathy occurred in 20.5% of patients within 1 week of developing INR > 3, including 16.5% of nonchronic kidney disease and 33% of chronic kidney disease cohort
- Other risk factors for warfarin-related nephropathy include age, diabetes mellitus, cardiovascular disease, and hypertension

Presentation

- Patients present with an acute rise in serum creatinine after becoming supratherapeutic on warfarin

Treatment

- Prevent by carefully monitoring INR in patients on warfarin therapy, especially those with chronic kidney disease
- Stop warfarin treatment until INR is normalized

Prognosis

- Mortality significantly increased in patients with warfarin-related nephropathy
- Hazard for death in warfarin-related nephropathy was highest within1st week after developing INR > 3 (hazard ratio at 1 week = 3.65)

MICROSCOPIC

Histologic Features

- Warfarin nephropathy is often superimposed on chronic kidney disease, in which case those pathological changes are present in glomeruli, tubules, interstitium, and vessels
- Changes related to anticoagulation
  - Glomeruli
    - Red blood cells in Bowman space
    - Little or no glomerular pathology by LM
  - Tubules
    - Occlusive red blood cell casts preferentially involve distal nephron
    - Acute tubular injury
  - Interstitium and vessels
    - No specific findings

DIFFERENTIAL DIAGNOSIS

IgA Nephropathy With Extensive Red Blood Cell Casts

- Sometimes presents with acute renal failure due to abundant red blood cell casts
- Prominent IgA deposition in glomeruli
- History of hematuria/proteinuria

Glomerulonephritis With Red Blood Cell Casts

- Generally fewer red blood cell casts
- In warfarin nephropathy, number of red blood cell casts are disproportionate to degree of glomerular lesions (e.g., mild mesangial immune complex deposition with acute kidney injury and numerous red blood cell casts)
- Diagnosis of warfarin nephropathy requires clinical correlation

Red Blood Cells in Tubular Lumina Due to Biopsy Artifact

- Tubular injury and flattening/compression of epithelial cells not present in artifact
- Red blood cells typically seen around edges of biopsy specimen if artifactual
- Red blood cell casts preferentially involve distal nephron in warfarin nephropathy

SELECTED REFERENCES

1. Ryan M et al: Warfarin-related nephropathy is the tip of the iceberg: direct thrombin inhibitor dabigatran induces glomerular hemorrhage with acute kidney injury in rats. Nephrol Dial Transplant. 29(12):2228-34, 2014
2. Brodsky SV et al: Warfarin-related nephropathy occurs in patients with and without chronic kidney disease and is associated with an increased mortality rate. Kidney Int. 80(2):181-9, 2011
3. Rizk DV et al: Warfarin-related nephropathy: another newly recognized complication of an old drug. Kidney Int. 80(2):131-3, 2011
4. Brodsky SV et al: Acute kidney injury during warfarin therapy associated with obstructive tubular red blood cell casts: a report of 9 cases. Am J Kidney Dis. 54(6):1121-6, 2009

KEY FACTS

TERMINOLOGY

- Sepsis defined as systemic inflammatory response associated with infection, commonly associated with acute kidney injury (AKI)

ETIOLOGY/PATHOGENESIS

- Septic kidney injury is multifactorial
- Hemodynamic instability, inflammatory mediators, DIC, tubular obstruction, drug toxicity

CLINICAL ISSUES

- 20 million cases of sepsis per year worldwide
- Renal insufficiency occurs in 30-60% of septic patients
- When kidney injury occurs in sepsis, mortality is high
- Sepsis is leading cause of death in noncoronary intensive care units

MICROSCOPIC

- Tubules show dilatation, epithelial simplification, cytoplasmic blebbing
- Proximal tubular coarse vacuolization is common and associated with mitochondrial damage
- Isometric tubular vacuolization may be seen and correlates with swollen lysosomes
- Coagulative-type tubular necrosis rare and typically focal, when occurs
- Interstitial chronic inflammation common, but typically mild
- Circulating nucleated red blood cells may be seen in medulla, associated with poor prognosis
- Glomeruli may show intracapillary fibrin thrombi (DIC)

ANCILLARY TESTS

- KIM-1 IHC assists in assessing tubular injury and distinguishing injury from autolysis
- Ki-67 labeling index increased in corticomedullary junction tubular cells

TOP DIFFERENTIAL DIAGNOSES

- Acute tubular injury from other causes
- Autolysis

(Left) *Acute tubular injury is demonstrated in this image by epithelial simplification, cytoplasmic blebbing, and cell sloughing . Granular cytoplasmic and cellular debris is seen within tubular lumina .* **(Right)** *This glomerulus shows prominent expansion of the capillary loops by intracapillary fibrin thrombi . This finding is rare,but may be encountered in septic patients with diffuse intravascular coagulation.*

Tubular Injury

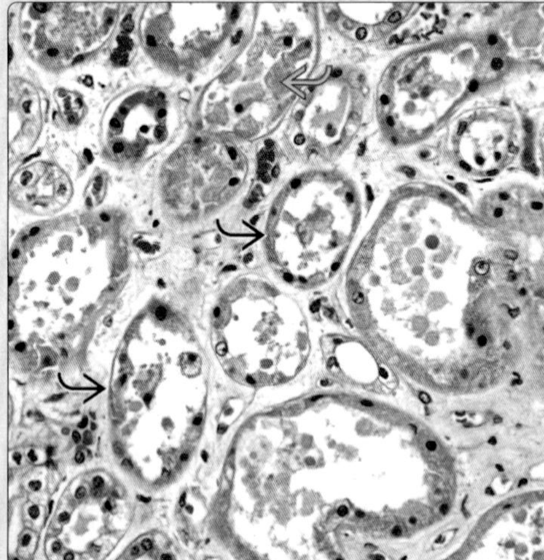

Glomerular Fibrin Thrombi

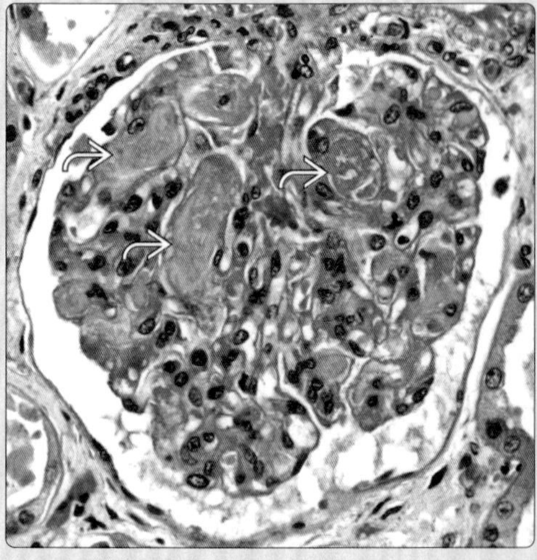

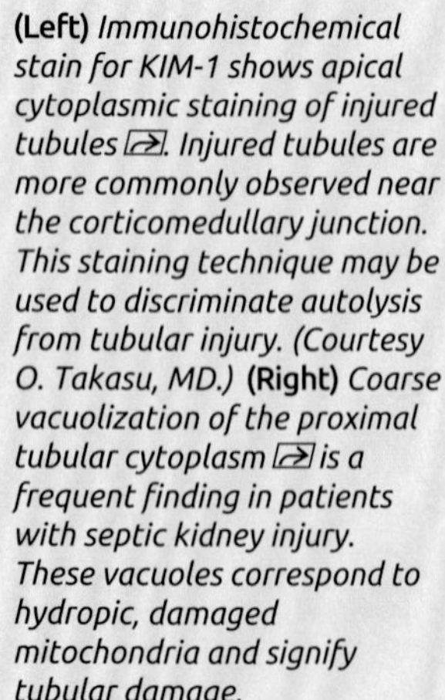

(Left) *Immunohistochemical stain for KIM-1 shows apical cytoplasmic staining of injured tubules . Injured tubules are more commonly observed near the corticomedullary junction. This staining technique may be used to discriminate autolysis from tubular injury. (Courtesy O. Takasu, MD.)* **(Right)** *Coarse vacuolization of the proximal tubular cytoplasm is a frequent finding in patients with septic kidney injury. These vacuoles correspond to hydropic, damaged mitochondria and signify tubular damage.*

KIM-1 Immunohistochemistry

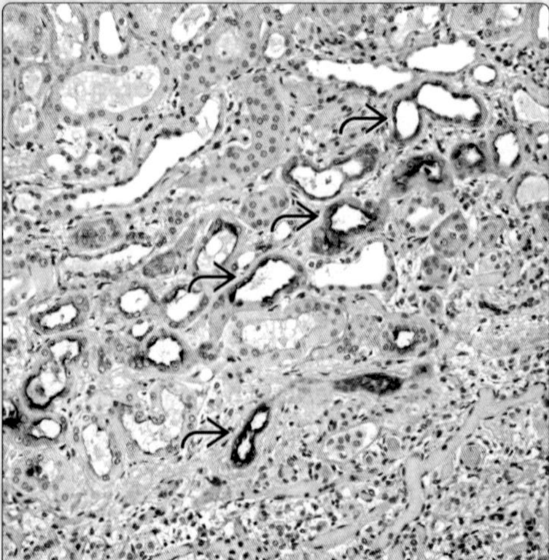

Tubular Injury

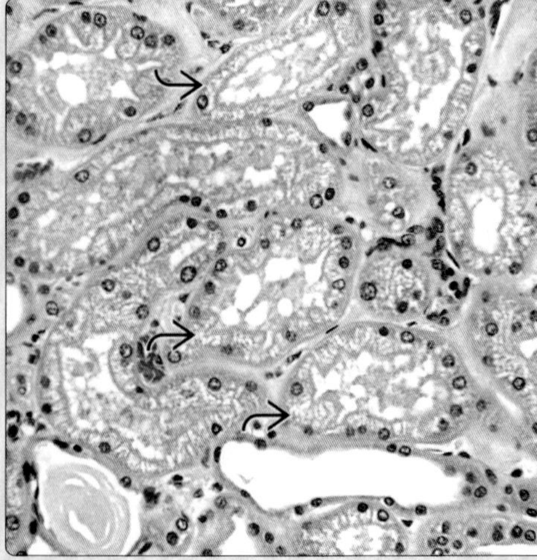

TERMINOLOGY

Synonyms

- Sepsis

Definitions

- Sepsis defined as systemic inflammatory response associated with infection, commonly associated with acute kidney injury (AKI)

ETIOLOGY/PATHOGENESIS

Pathophysiology

- Initial proinflammatory response results in hypotension and organ dysfunction
- Followed by anti-inflammatory response resulting in immune depression
- Multifactorial kidney injury
  - Hemodynamic instability
  - Diffuse intravascular coagulation (DIC)
  - Inflammatory mediators
  - Tubular obstruction
  - Iatrogenic causes (drugs, intravenous contrast, etc.)

CLINICAL ISSUES

Epidemiology

- 20 million cases of sepsis per year worldwide
  - 1 million cases per year in USA
- Sepsis is leading cause of death in noncoronary intensive care units
  - > 210,000 deaths/year in USA
- Renal insufficiency occurs in 30-60% of septic patients
- Septic kidney injury patients with ~ 70% mortality

Presentation

- Systemic inflammatory response in setting of confirmed infection
  - Hypothermia
  - Tachycardia
  - Tachypnea
  - Hypocapnia
  - Leukopenia or leukocytosis
- Severe sepsis occurs with systemic inflammatory response syndrome (SIRS) plus organ dysfunction
- Septic shock occurs in setting of sepsis with
  - Persistent arterial hypotension
  - Hypoperfusion despite fluid administration

MICROSCOPIC

Histologic Features

- Glomeruli
  - Capillary loop thrombi, rare and focal
    - May occur in cases with DIC
- Tubules
  - Mild degree of tubular injury
    - Disproportionate to degree of renal dysfunction
  - Dilatation/epithelial simplification
  - Cell sloughing/detachment
  - Cytoplasmic blebbing
  - Coarse vacuolization
  - Proximal tubule cytoplasmic fine isometric vacuolization in cases complicated by osmotic nephrosis
  - Calcium phosphate and calcium oxalate crystals, focal
- Interstitium
  - Patchy, mild, chronic interstitial inflammation in majority of cases
- Vessels
  - Circulating nucleated red blood cells may be in medullary capillaries

ANCILLARY TESTS

Immunohistochemistry

- Increased kidney injury molecule-1 (KIM-1) expression in proximal tubule cells
- Increased Ki-67 labeling of corticomedullary junction tubular cells

Immunofluorescence

- Negative

Electron Microscopy

- Proximal tubules
  - Enlarged, hydropic mitochondria
  - Increased numbers of lysosomes and autophagosomes

DIFFERENTIAL DIAGNOSIS

Autolysis

- Tubular epithelial cells appear detached from underlying basement membrane
- KIM-1 immunohistochemistry is negative

Acute Tubular Injury Due to Other Etiologies

- Similar histopathologic findings
- Requires clinical correlation

DIAGNOSTIC CHECKLIST

Clinically Relevant Pathologic Features

- Glomerular fibrin thrombi may rarely occur in setting of DIC
- Coarse tubular vacuolization correlates with mitochondrial damage
- Tubular injury typically mild and focal, despite severe renal functional impairment

SELECTED REFERENCES

1. Parikh SM et al: Mitochondrial function and disturbances in the septic kidney. Semin Nephrol. 35(1):108-19, 2015
2. Langenberg C et al: Renal histopathology during experimental septic acute kidney injury and recovery. Crit Care Med. 42(1):e58-67, 2014
3. Angus DC et al: Severe sepsis and septic shock. N Engl J Med. 369(9):840-51, 2013
4. Takasu O et al: Mechanisms of cardiac and renal dysfunction in patients dying of sepsis. Am J Respir Crit Care Med. 187(5):509-17, 2013
5. Dickenmann M et al: Osmotic nephrosis: acute kidney injury with accumulation of proximal tubular lysosomes due to administration of exogenous solutes. Am J Kidney Dis. 51(3):491-503, 2008
6. Schrier RW et al: Acute renal failure and sepsis. N Engl J Med. 351(2):159-69, 2004
7. Hotchkiss RS et al: The pathophysiology and treatment of sepsis. N Engl J Med. 348(2):138-50, 2003

Fine, Isometric Vacuolization

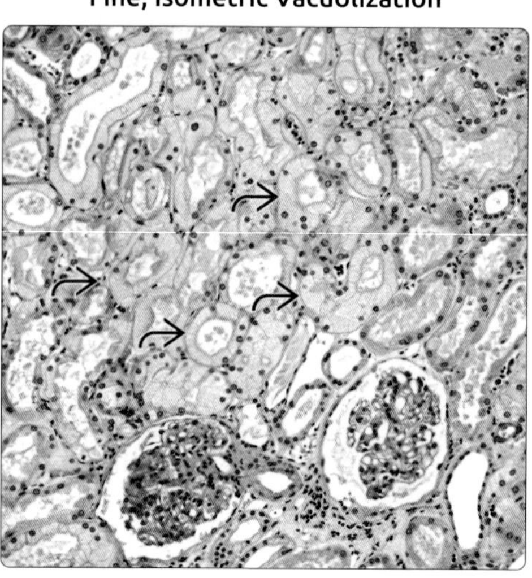

Coarse Vacuolization

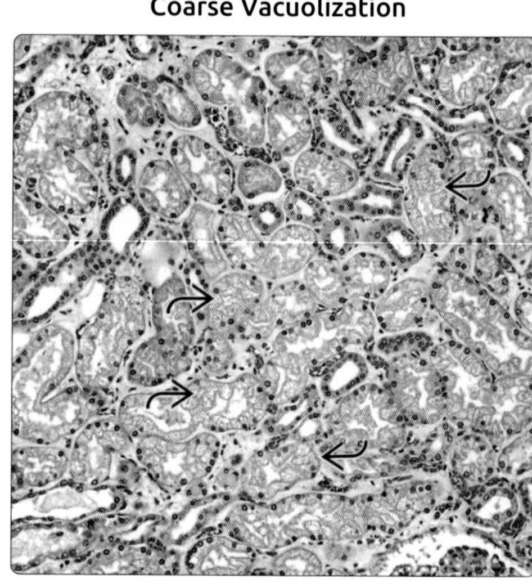

(Left) *Isometric, fine vacuolization of the proximal tubules* ➡ *may be focal or diffuse. This change is also referred to as osmotic nephrosis and corresponds to swollen lysosomes by electron microscopy.* **(Right)** *In contrast to the fine, isometric vacuoles, coarse vacuolization* ➡ *may also be seen in septic AKI. This form of tubular injury is common in such patients and corresponds to mitochondrial damage. Similar changes have been described in animal models of septic AKI.*

Coagulative Necrosis

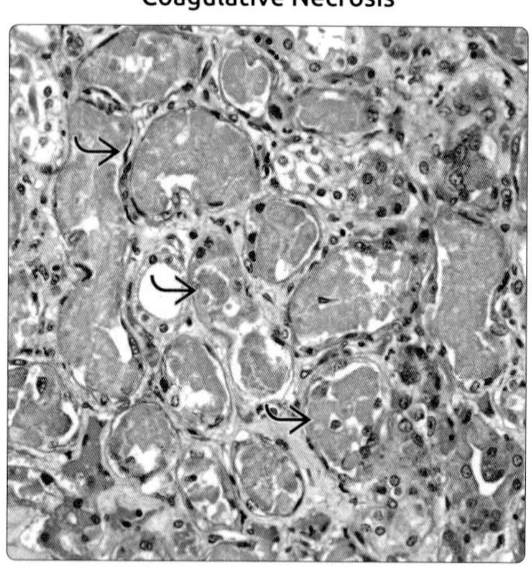

Tubular Injury and Necrosis

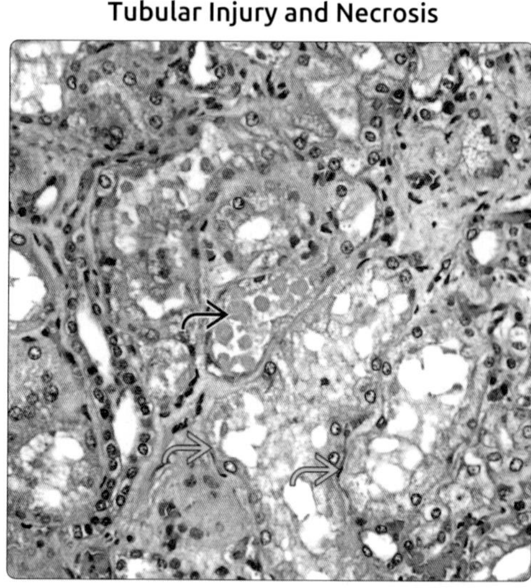

(Left) *True coagulative-type of necrosis* ➡ *is rare in septic AKI. When this is seen, it is typically focal. As in other examples of coagulative necrosis, the cells appear as anucleate ghosts. The dead cells are shed into the tubular lumens.* **(Right)** *Coagulative-type necrosis* ➡ *may be seen alongside other manifestations of tubular injury, including epithelial simplification, cytoplasmic blebbing, and coarse vacuolization* ➡*.*

Tubular Injury and Cell Sloughing

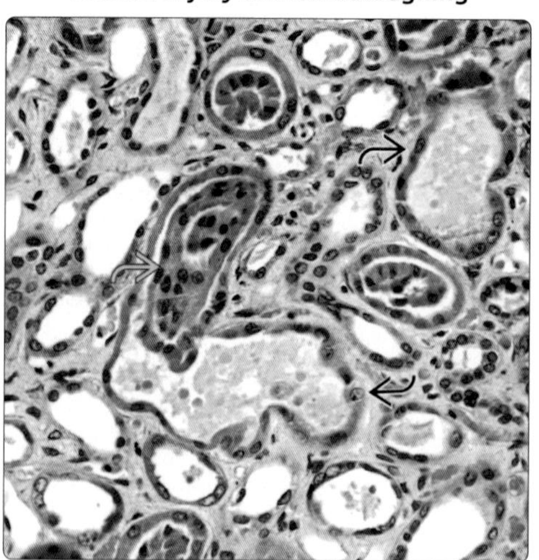

Nucleated Red Blood Cells

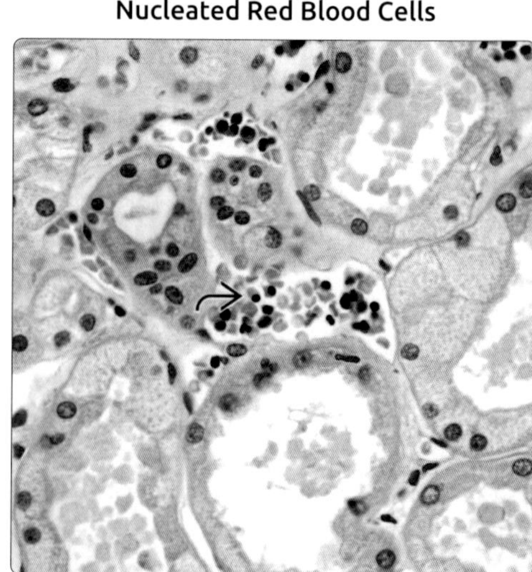

(Left) *These damaged tubules show prominent dilatation and epithelial simplification* ➡ *with cell sloughing. It appears that the tubular epithelium has shed an entire intact layer into the lumen* ➡*.* **(Right)** *The peritubular capillaries contain numerous circulating nucleated red blood cells* ➡*. Increased nucleated red blood cells in the circulation of septic patients has been associated with a poor prognosis.*

KIM-1 Immunohistochemistry

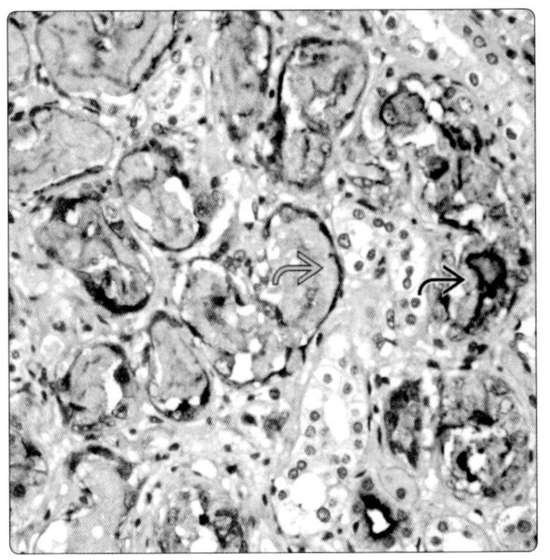

KIM-1 Immunohistochemistry

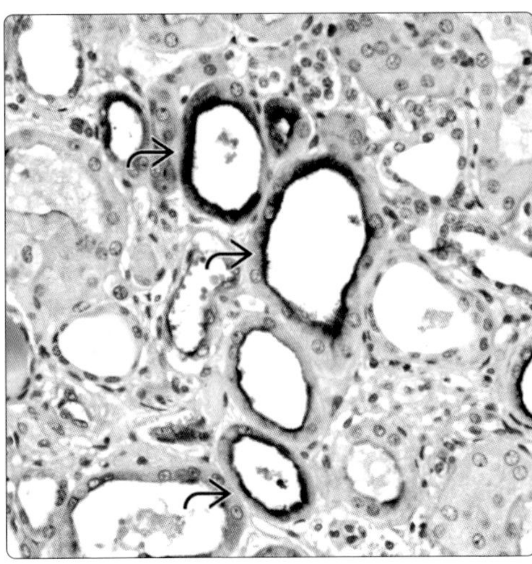

(Left) *Coagulative type necrosis is evident in this case of septic kidney injury; KIM-1 staining outlines the simplified epithelium that remains ➡. Some of the damaged, sloughed cells also show focal staining ➡. (Courtesy O. Takasu, MD.)* **(Right)** *Immunohistochemical staining for KIM-1 shows concentrated staining of the apical cytoplasm ➡ in damaged proximal tubular epithelium. The damaged tubules may demonstrate dilatation and epithelial simplification. (Courtesy O. Takasu, MD.)*

Calcium Phosphate Crystals

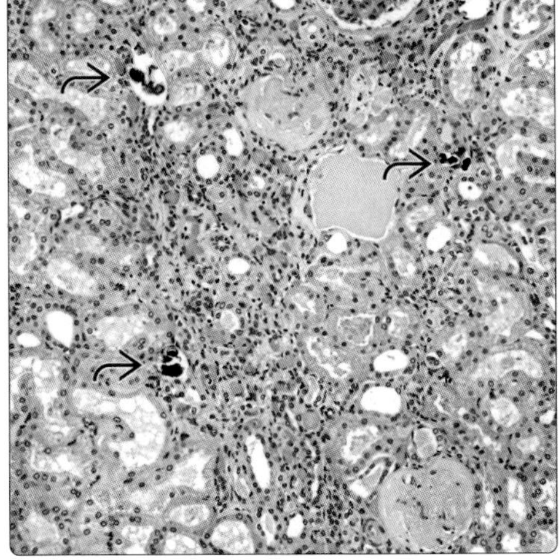

Calcium Oxalate Crystals

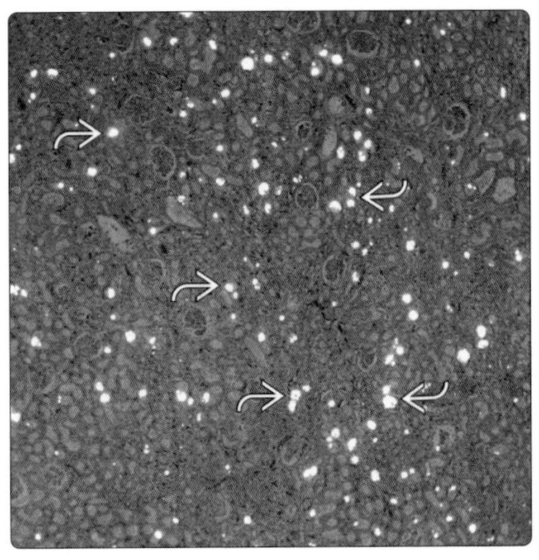

(Left) *Scattered calcium phosphate crystals ➡ within the tubulointerstitium may be observed. These likely represent the sequelae of prior tubular damage.* **(Right)** *In contrast to the more common calcium phosphate crystals, calcium oxalate crystals are rarely observed in septic kidney injury. When seen, particularly in large numbers, oxalate nephropathy should be considered. In this polarized image, crystals are seen throughout the tubulointerstitium ➡. This patient had prior gastric bypass surgery.*

Damaged Mitochondria

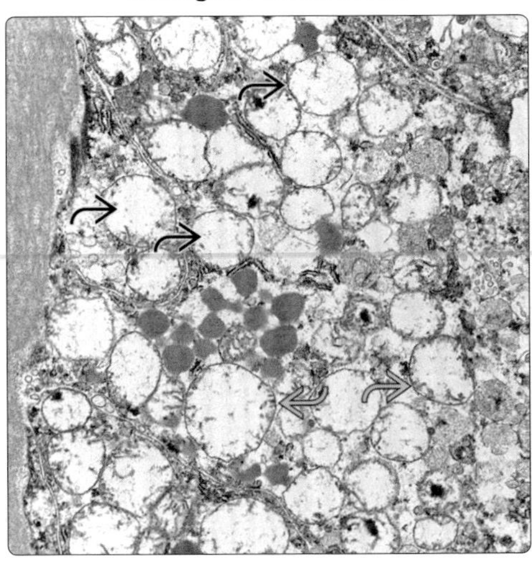

Dilated Lysosomes

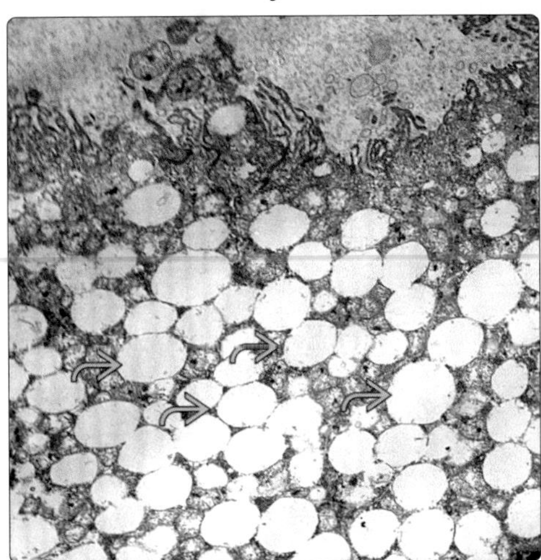

(Left) *This electron photomicrograph demonstrates hydropic, damaged mitochondria ➡. Remnants of mitochondrial cristae are seen at the periphery ➡. This finding corresponds to coarse vacuolization seen on routine light microscopy.* **(Right)** *Electron photomicrograph depicts enlarged, swollen lysosomes ➡. This corresponds to the finely vacuolated cells observed on light microscopy. Injury of this type may occur in the setting of hydroxyethyl starch and other resuscitative agents.*

Lead and Other Heavy Metal Toxins

KEY FACTS

TERMINOLOGY

- Renal disease due to toxic effects of lead and other metals

ETIOLOGY/PATHOGENESIS

- Principal toxic metals encountered include lead (Pb), mercury (Hg), gold (Au), and cadmium (Cd)
- Direct tubular toxicity may be acute (high-dose toxicity) or chronic (low-dose prolonged toxicity)
- Membranous glomerulopathy in Hg and Au toxicity due to immune complex deposition

CLINICAL ISSUES

- History of recent or past exposure to toxic metals critical for diagnosis
- Blood and urinary levels of toxic metals elevated in acute nephropathy

MICROSCOPIC

- Acute nephropathy: Acute tubular injury
  - Eosinophilic nuclear inclusions (lead, bismuth) or pigment (iron, copper)
  - Hg and Au particles in proximal tubules by EM
- Nonspecific chronic tubulointerstitial nephritis
- Membranous glomerulonephritis in Hg and Au toxicity
- Radiographic fluorescence or spectroscopy may be used to quantify metal content in tissues

TOP DIFFERENTIAL DIAGNOSES

- Acute tubular injury/necrosis from drugs and infection
- Chronic tubulointerstitial diseases (lithium, Balkan, aristolochic acid nephropathies)
- Membranous glomerulonephritis and chronic TIN (lupus nephritis, nonsteroidal anti-inflammatory agent nephritis)

Acute Lead Nephropathy

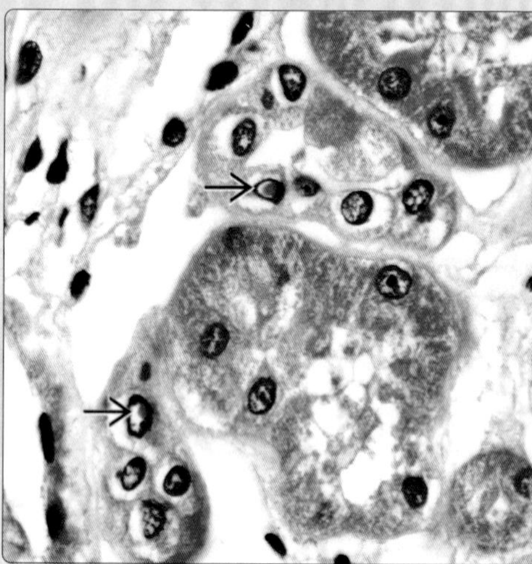

Acute Lead Nephropathy With Prominent Eosinophilic Nuclear Inclusions

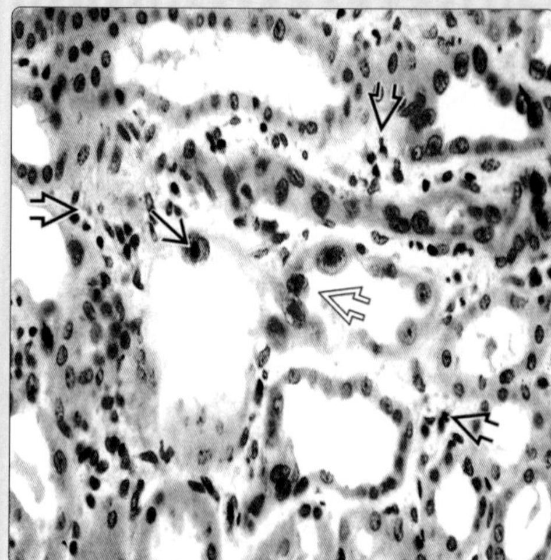

(Left) *Acute lead nephropathy is characterized by bright eosinophilic nuclear inclusions ➔ in the proximal tubular nuclei. (Courtesy A. Cohen, MD.)* **(Right)** *Acute tubular injury with prominent eosinophilic nuclear inclusions ➔, 3 in 1 tubular profile ➔, is characteristic of acute lead nephropathy from a nonhuman primate, as in this example. There is mild interstitial edema and inflammatory exudate ➔.*

Nuclear Inclusions in Acute Lead Nephropathy

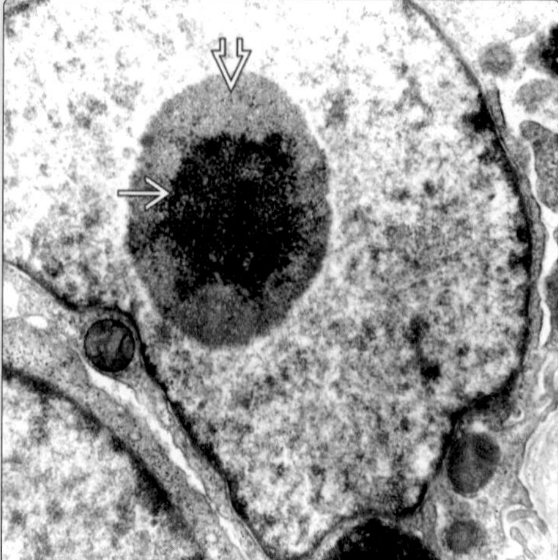

Lead Nephrotoxicity

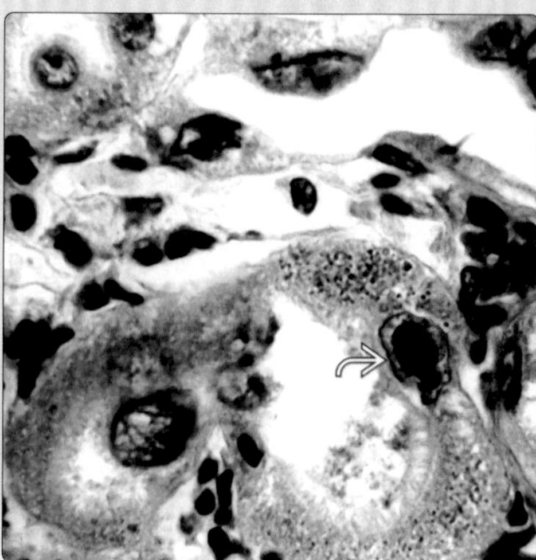

(Left) *Acute lead nephropathy has nuclear inclusions composed of central, electron-dense spicules ➔ and a halo of less electron-dense material ➔ by electron microscopy. (Courtesy A. Cohen, MD.)* **(Right)** *H&E staining (black and white photo) shows proximal tubule nuclear inclusion ➔ in a case of lead nephrotoxicity. The inclusion is typically slightly eosinophilic and nearly fills the nucleus, somewhat resembling Cytomegalovirus. These inclusions are infrequent in chronic lead nephropathy. (Courtesy M. Mihatsch, MD.)*

Lead and Other Heavy Metal Toxins

TERMINOLOGY

Definitions

- Group of disorders characterized by renal dysfunction due to toxic effects of lead and other metals

ETIOLOGY/PATHOGENESIS

Toxic Renal Injury

- Principal toxic metals encountered include lead (Pb), mercury (Hg), gold (Au), cadmium (Cd), uranium (U), platinum (Pt), copper (Cu), chromium (Cr), bismuth (Bi), antimony (Sb), arsenic (As), iron (Fe), and lithium (Li)
- Exposure may be environmental, occupational, iatrogenic, or secondary to metabolic and hematologic disease states
- Routes of entry include ingestion, inhalation, and absorption through skin
  - Environmental exposure
    - Ingestion: Contamination of water supplies in lead pipes or lead soldered joints, moonshine stills, lead paint, contaminated foods
      - Mercuric chloride and colloidal bismuth ingestion in suicide
    - Inhalation: Lead, mercury, and cadmium vapors, fumes, or dust
    - Topical: Mercury-containing skin lightening products
  - Occupational exposure
    - Paint manufacture and spraying, plumbing, welding, smelting, mining, pesticides, thermometer and fluorescent light manufacture, and others
  - Iatrogenic exposure
    - Gold therapy for rheumatoid arthritis
    - Colloidal bismuth for treatment of peptic ulcer and syphilis
    - Copper intrauterine contraceptive devices
    - Lithium for bipolar disorders
    - Platinum in cancer chemotherapy
    - Iron for deficiency states
  - Metabolic and hematologic diseases
    - Hemochromatosis
    - Wilson disease
    - Hemolysis
- Metals may be absorbed through gastrointestinal tract, lungs, or skin
- Circulating metals filtered, reabsorbed and secreted, before final excretion
- 3 principal mechanisms of renal injury
  - Direct tubular injury
    - High-dose leads to acute nephropathy
    - Low-dose prolonged exposure leads to chronic nephropathy
  - Podocytopathy may also occur
  - Glomerular immune complex deposition results in membranous glomerulopathy
    - Associated with gold and mercury toxicity
      - Neither metal detected in immune deposits

CLINICAL ISSUES

Presentation

- Acute nephropathy
  - Toxic metal exposures to Pb, Hg, Au, Cd, Cu, Cr, Bi, Sb, U, Pt, Fe can be associated with acute kidney injury
  - Proximal tubulopathy often early manifestation
    - Aminoaciduria, glycosuria, phosphaturia (Fanconi syndrome), and increased urinary β2-microglobulin excretion
  - Blood and urinary levels of toxic metals elevated
- Chronic nephropathy
  - Lead
    - Hyperuricemia and (saturnine) gout, chronic renal failure, hypertension, positive calcium-EDTA mobilization test
  - Mercury and gold
    - Chronic renal failure and proteinuria
  - Cadmium
    - Chronic renal failure, hypercalciuria, nephrolithiasis, osteomalacia
  - Lithium
    - Chronic renal failure and proteinuria
- History of recent or past exposure to toxic metals critical for diagnosis

Treatment

- Cessation of toxic exposure; chelation therapy; dialysis

Prognosis

- Acute tubular necrosis generally reversible
- Reversibility of chronic nephropathy depends on extent of renal scarring
- Membranous glomerulonephritis: Recovery of function occurs in most patients after months or years

MACROSCOPIC

Gross Findings

- Acute nephropathy: Diffuse enlargement with cortical swelling
- Chronic nephropathy: Bilateral shrunken kidneys with granular outer surface
- Cadmium toxicity: Calcium phosphate stones

MICROSCOPIC

Histologic Features

- Lead
  - Acute nephropathy
    - Acute tubular injury with nuclear inclusions in proximal tubules and loops of Henle
      - Inclusions: Variable size and shape, eosinophilic, positive on periodic acid-Schiff, acid-fast, and Giemsa staining
  - Chronic nephropathy
    - Mild chronic tubulointerstitial nephritis; rare inclusions
    - Gouty tophi in renal medulla
    - Hypertensive vascular sclerosis
- Mercury
  - Acute nephropathy
    - Acute tubular necrosis with most severe involvement of straight proximal tubule
    - Hg particles detectable by electron microscopy in injured tubular cytoplasm
  - Chronic nephropathy

    - Membranous glomerulonephritis, typically Ehrenreich and Churg stage I-II
    - Tubular epithelial flattening and atrophy; interstitial fibrosis
- Gold
  - Acute nephropathy
    - Membranous glomerulonephritis, typically Ehrenreich and Churg stage I-II
    - Acute tubular necrosis with gold inclusions in proximal tubules
  - Chronic nephropathy
    - Membranous glomerulonephritis
    - Minimal change disease
    - Mesangial proliferative glomerulonephritis
    - Chronic tubulointerstitial nephritis (TIN)
- Cadmium
  - Chronic tubulointerstitial nephritis
    - Bland outer cortical interstitial fibrosis and tubular atrophy
  - Calcium phosphate stones
- Arsenic
  - Acute tubular necrosis with hemoglobin casts secondary to hemolysis
  - Cortical necrosis
  - Chronic tubulointerstitial nephritis
- Iron
  - Acute tubular injury with iron in tubular epithelium by Prussian blue stain
- Copper
  - Acute tubular injury with copper in tubular epithelium using Rubeanic acid stain

ANCILLARY TESTS

Immunofluorescence

- Glomerular capillary wall IgG and C3 in membranous glomerulonephritis associated with mercury and gold toxicity

Electron Microscopy

- Lead
  - Tubular nuclei: Inclusions of electron-dense spicules in matrix
  - Tubular cytoplasm: Abundant lysosomes with electron-dense material containing lead
- Mercury
  - Tubules have cytoplasmic clusters of electron-dense, particulate matter containing mercury
  - Glomerular subepithelial electron-dense deposits ± "spikes"
- Gold
  - Tubules have clustered spicular material in cytoplasm associated with lysosomes
  - Glomerular subepithelial electron-dense deposits ± "spikes"
- Cadmium
  - Proximal tubular cytoplasmic lysosomes with electron-dense material containing cadmium
- Bismuth
  - Tubular nuclear inclusions are rounded and uniformly electron dense
  - Tubular mitochondria have small, rounded, smooth electron densities containing bismuth

Imaging

- Radiographic fluorescence or spectroscopy may be useful to quantify metal content in tissues

DIFFERENTIAL DIAGNOSIS

Acute Tubular Necrosis With Inclusions

- Cytomegalovirus, polyomavirus, adenovirus nephropathy

Acute Tubular Necrosis With Nuclear Atypia

- Busulphan and ifosfamide toxicity
- Karyomegalic interstitial nephritis
- Foscarnet, tenofovir, adefovir, and other antiretroviral agents
- Viral infections: Polyomavirus, adenovirus

Acute Tubular Necrosis With Pigmentation

- Acute tubular necrosis (ATN) with lipofuscinosis
- ATN with metastatic melanoma

Chronic Tubulointerstitial Nephropathy

- Histologic features generally nonspecific
  - Aristolochic acid and Balkan nephropathy
  - Collecting duct cysts and focal segmental glomerulosclerosis (FSGS) in lithium nephropathy
- Membranous glomerulonephritis and chronic TIN
  - Lupus nephritis
  - Nonsteroidal anti-inflammatory agents

DIAGNOSTIC CHECKLIST

Clinically Relevant Pathologic Features

- ATN
  - With nuclear inclusions: Lead or bismuth toxicity
  - With cytoplasmic pigment: Copper or iron toxicity

Pathologic Interpretation Pearls

- Nuclear inclusions in acute lead and bismuth nephropathy
- Gold and mercury particles in tubular cytoplasm by EM in acute nephropathy
- Membranous nephropathy ± chronic TIN suggests gold or mercury toxicity

SELECTED REFERENCES

1. Sabath E et al: Renal health and the environment: heavy metal nephrotoxicity. Nefrologia. 32(3):279-86, 2012
2. Evans M et al: Chronic renal failure from lead: myth or evidence-based fact? Kidney Int. 79(3):272-9, 2011
3. Li SJ et al: Mercury-induced membranous nephropathy: clinical and pathological features. Clin J Am Soc Nephrol. 5(3):439-44, 2010
4. Brewster UC et al: A review of chronic lead intoxication: an unrecognized cause of chronic kidney disease. Am J Med Sci. 327(6):341-7, 2004
5. Goyer RA: Mechanisms of lead and cadmium nephrotoxicity. Toxicol Lett. 46(1-3):153-62, 1989
6. Bennett WM: Lead nephropathy. Kidney Int. 28(2):212-20, 1985

Mercury-Induced Acute Tubular Necrosis

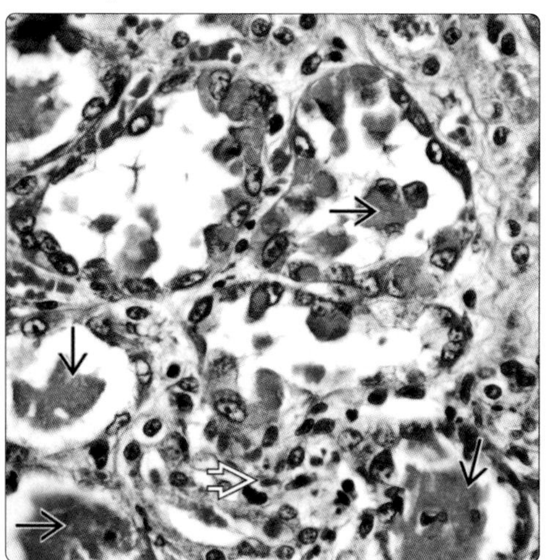

Gold Nephrotoxicity

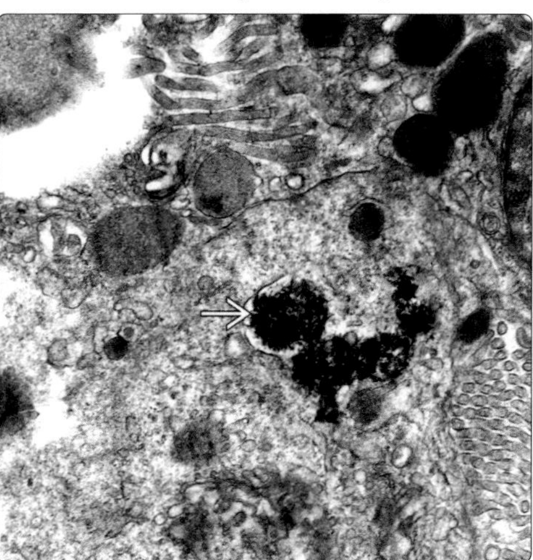

(Left) *Mercury ingestion leads to acute tubular necrosis affecting all segments, but proximal straight segments are affected most severely. Tubules have markedly flattened epithelium & luminal cell debris* ➙. *Mild interstitial inflammation is also apparent* ➙. *(Courtesy A. Cohen, MD.)* **(Right)** *Cytoplasmic spicular gold particles* ➙ *may be seen in acute gold nephrotoxicity. Glomeruli in such cases may have membranous glomerulopathy, although this is more commonly a feature of chronic gold toxicity. (Courtesy A. Cohen, MD.)*

Hemosiderosis

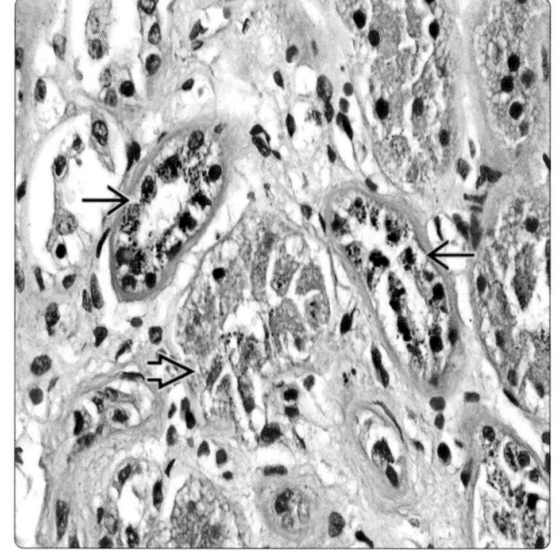

Hemosiderosis

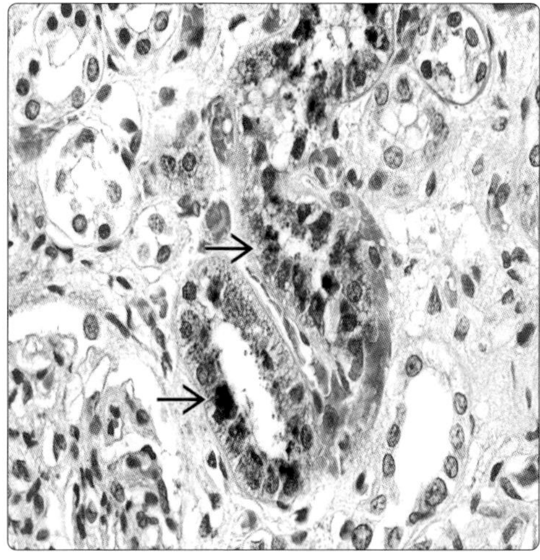

(Left) *Tubular hemosiderosis in a patient with hemochromatosis has granular brown hemosiderin deposits in the epithelium of the proximal* ➙ *and distal* ➙ *tubules. Heavy deposits of iron may cause acute tubular necrosis.* **(Right)** *A Prussian blue stain for iron highlights granular deposits in the tubular epithelial cytoplasm* ➙ *in hemosiderosis. This patient had symptomatic primary hemochromatosis.*

Secondary Membranous Glomerulonephritis

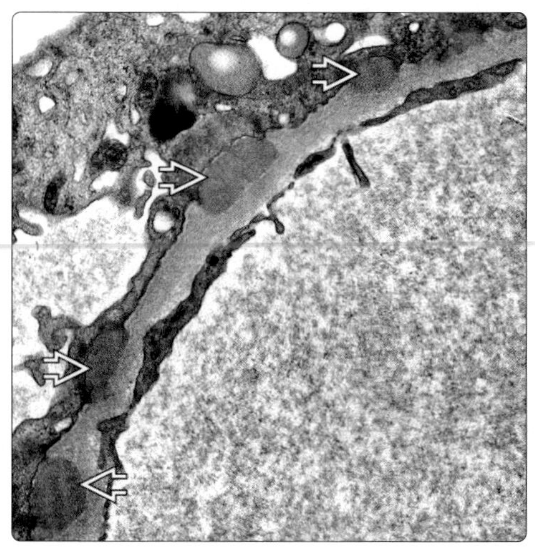

Minimal Change Disease

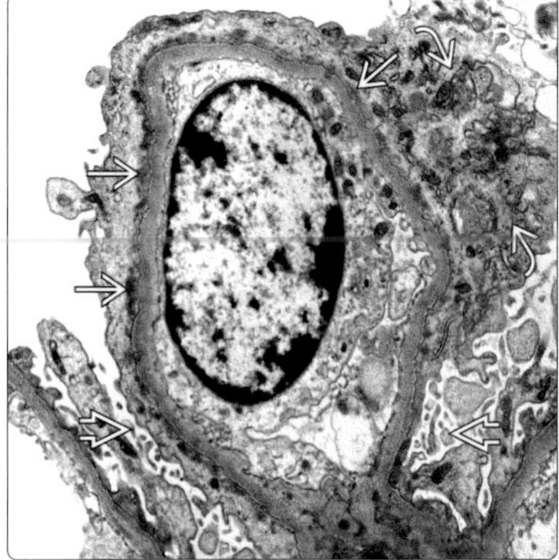

(Left) *Proteinuria, often nephrotic range, is a feature of gold and mercury toxicity. Membranous glomerulonephritis is the most common cause. Glomerular capillary subepithelial deposits* ➙ *are often of early stage, Ehrenreich and Churg stage I-II.* **(Right)** *Proteinuria due to gold and mercury toxicity is occasionally explained by podocytopathy with diffuse effacement of the foot processes, cytoplasmic swelling, increased vesicles* ➙, *microvilli* ➙, *and basal condensation of filaments* ➙.

Aristolochic Acid Nephropathy

KEY FACTS

TERMINOLOGY

- Progressive tubulointerstitial nephropathy and urothelial carcinoma related to aristolochic acid (AA) in herbal remedies

ETIOLOGY/PATHOGENESIS

- History of intake of herbal preparations containing AA
- Severity of renal injury is dose dependent
- Aristolactams, derived from reduction of AA, bind adenine and guanine residues on DNA, forming DNA-adducts
  - Adducts cause activation of H-ras and p53, and carcinogenesis

CLINICAL ISSUES

- Acute renal failure/acute kidney injury
- Tubular dysfunction
- Chronic renal failure
- History of intake of herbal preparations for weight loss
- Risk of progression to ESRD proportional to exposure
- Renal failure progresses after cessation of AA exposure
- Increased risk of urothelial carcinoma

MICROSCOPIC

- Early lesions have acute tubular injury with interstitial myxoid change and scattered mononuclear cell infiltrates
- Late interstitial fibrosis tends to be paucicellular and most pronounced in outer cortex
- Urothelial carcinoma in pelvis, ureter, or bladder
- Aristolochic acid-DNA adducts can be detected in tissue

TOP DIFFERENTIAL DIAGNOSES

- Balkan endemic nephropathy (same toxin)
- Analgesic nephropathy, associated with papillary necrosis
- Advanced chronic tubulointerstitial nephritis associated with infection or drugs

DIAGNOSTIC CHECKLIST

- Paucicellular interstitial fibrosis, most pronounced in outer cortex, is an initial clue to diagnosis

Acute AAN

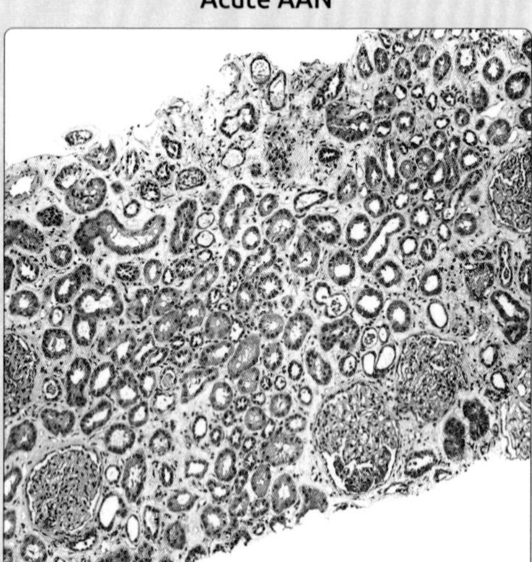

Acute AAN

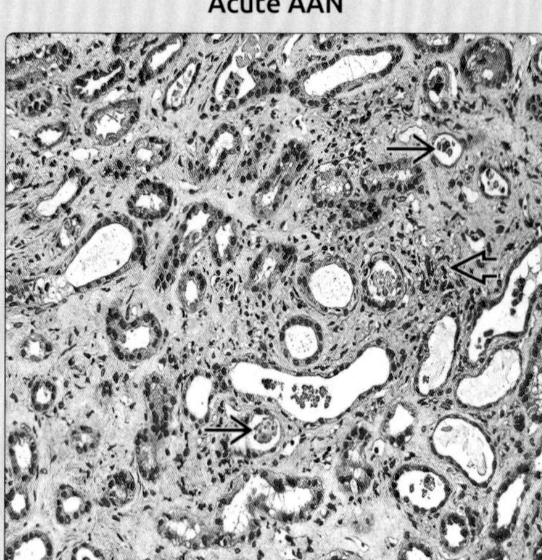

(Left) *Early features of aristolochic acid nephropathy (AAN) include acute tubular injury, early tubular atrophy, and diffuse fine interstitial fibrosis with little inflammation. Glomeruli are spared. The changes are usually most pronounced in the outer cortex.* **(Right)** *The predominant lesion is myxoid interstitial fibrosis, but tubular injury with necrotic casts* → *and scattered mononuclear infiltrates* ⇨ *are also described.*

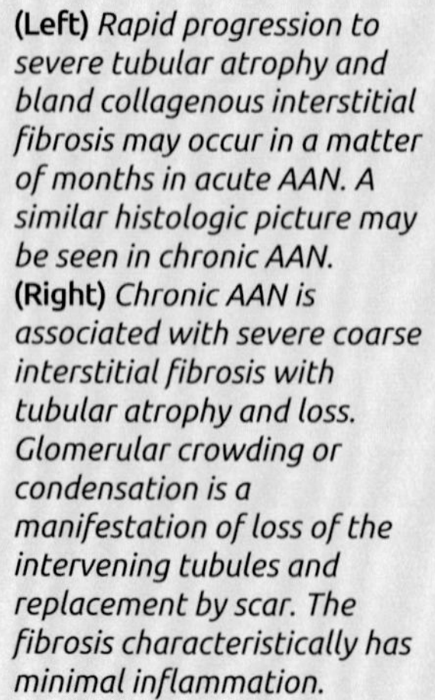

(Left) *Rapid progression to severe tubular atrophy and bland collagenous interstitial fibrosis may occur in a matter of months in acute AAN. A similar histologic picture may be seen in chronic AAN.* **(Right)** *Chronic AAN is associated with severe coarse interstitial fibrosis with tubular atrophy and loss. Glomerular crowding or condensation is a manifestation of loss of the intervening tubules and replacement by scar. The fibrosis characteristically has minimal inflammation.*

AAN With Severe Tubular Atrophy

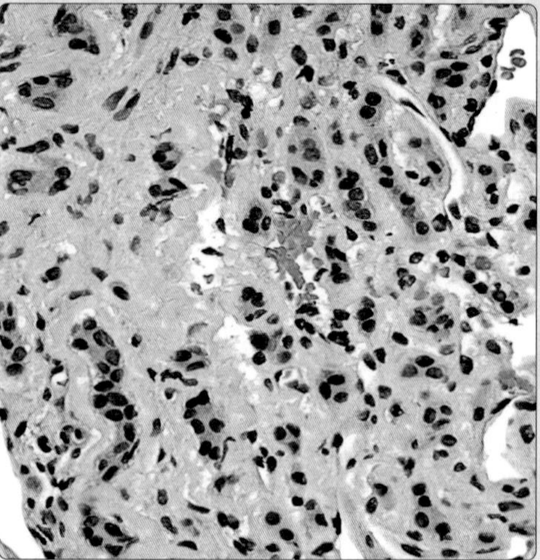

Chronic AAN With Tubular Loss

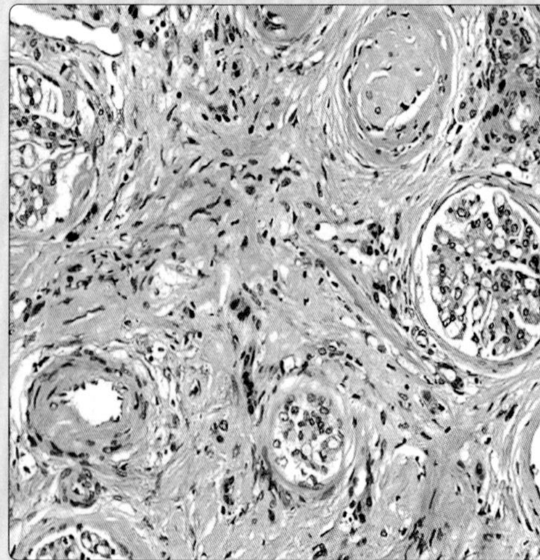

TERMINOLOGY

Abbreviations

- Aristolochic acid nephropathy (AAN)

Synonyms

- Chinese herb nephropathy

Definitions

- Tubulointerstitial nephropathy and urothelial carcinoma associated with exposure to aristolochic acid (AA) in herbal remedies

ETIOLOGY/PATHOGENESIS

Toxin From Plant Genus *Aristolochia* (~ 500 Species)

- Used in traditional Chinese, Indian, and European medical preparations
- AA containing herbs banned by FDA in 2000 but herbal preparations (~ 25%) marketed via internet in USA have detectable AA (as reported in 2014)
- Aristolactams, derived from reduction of AA
  - Bind adenine and guanine residues on DNA, forming DNA-adducts
    - Adducts cause activation of H-ras and p53, and may be important in carcinogenesis
      - A:T → T:A transversions are signature p53 mutations from AA exposure
  - Proximal tubule most affected in experimental studies
- Severity of renal injury cumulative dose dependent
  - > 100 g associated with chronic renal failure
  - > 200 g associated with ESRD and urothelial carcinoma
- Toxicity confounded by simultaneous exposure to appetite suppressants in original Belgian cohort
- Balkan nephropathy also caused by AA due to wheat contamination with *Aristolochia clematitis*

CLINICAL ISSUES

Presentation

- Acute renal failure/acute kidney injury
  - Progression to end-stage renal disease in months
  - Daily intake of ~ 0.04 g over weeks to months
- Tubular dysfunction
  - Glycosuria, tubular proteinuria, renal tubular acidosis, decreased osmolarity
  - Daily intake of ~ 0.02 g over months
- Slowly progress chronic renal failure
  - Daily intake of ~ 0.5 mg over years

Prognosis

- Risk of progression to end-stage disease proportional to duration of exposure
- Renal failure tends to be progressive even after cessation of AA-containing compounds
- Increased risk of urothelial carcinoma (46%)

MACROSCOPIC

General Features

- Papillary or papular urothelial lesions in pelvis, ureter, or bladder
- Asymmetrically shrunken kidneys

MICROSCOPIC

Histologic Features

- Glomeruli unaffected initially
  - Progressive global sclerosis in chronic disease
- Tubules and interstitium
  - Early: Acute (mainly proximal) tubular injury with interstitial myxoid change and scattered mononuclear cell infiltrates
  - Late: Marked interstitial fibrosis and tubular atrophy
    - Most pronounced in outer cortex
    - Paucicellular fibrosis with some mast cells
- Arteriosclerosis with intimal fibrosis
- Urothelium
  - Highest frequency of urothelial carcinoma in upper urinary tract
  - Hyperplasia, dysplasia, in situ or invasive carcinoma
    - Dysplastic nuclei are p53 positive by immunohistochemistry
- Electron microscopy and immunofluorescence findings are nonspecific

ANCILLARY TESTS

DNA Adduct Analysis

- ^{32}P-postlabelling of DNA extracts can detect AA-DNA adducts

DIFFERENTIAL DIAGNOSIS

Cortical Interstitial Fibrosis and Tubular Atrophy

- Chronic renal ischemia: Hypertensive renovascular disease
- Advanced chronic tubulointerstitial nephritis associated with infection or drugs

Cortical Interstitial Fibrosis, Tubular Atrophy, and Urothelial Carcinoma

- Balkan endemic nephropathy (same toxin)
- Analgesic nephropathy, associated with papillary necrosis

DIAGNOSTIC CHECKLIST

Pathologic Interpretation Pearls

- Outer cortical paucicellular interstitial fibrosis is characteristic
- Exposure to AA containing compounds is sine qua non

SELECTED REFERENCES

1. Anandagoda N et al: Preventing aristolochic Acid nephropathy. Clin J Am Soc Nephrol. 10(2):167-8, 2015
2. Vaclavik L et al: Quantification of aristolochic acids I and II in herbal dietary supplements by ultra-high-performance liquid chromatography-multistage fragmentation mass spectrometry. Food Addit Contam Part A Chem Anal Control Expo Risk Assess. 31(5):784-91, 2014

Balkan Endemic Nephropathy

KEY FACTS

TERMINOLOGY

- Chronic tubulointerstitial nephropathy with high risk of urothelial carcinoma, endemic in specific regions of Balkan countries, Romania, Croatia, and Bulgaria

ETIOLOGY/PATHOGENESIS

- Aristolochic acid (AA)
  - Present in weeds (*Aristolochia* sp) in wheat fields
  - AA metabolites form DNA adducts; may induce mutations of p53 with A:T → T:A transversions
  - Chromosomal breakage in several bands, most frequently 3q25, containing oncogenes *src* and *raf-1*
  - Also responsible for Chinese herb nephropathy
- Tubulopathy is earliest lesion
  - Proximal tubules are probably major site of renal injury

CLINICAL ISSUES

- Tubular dysfunction early in course
- Slowly progressive renal failure in 30-50 year olds
  - Impaired concentrating ability and salt wasting, Fanconi syndrome later
  - Copper-toned skin, orange palms and soles, weight loss, anemia - late
- Urothelial carcinoma develops in 30-50%
- Survival varies from months to more than 10 years

MICROSCOPIC

- Interstitial fibrosis and tubular atrophy
  - Begins in outer cortex later extending to deep cortex
  - Scanty inflammatory infiltrate
- Urothelial dysplasia and papillomas
  - Malignancy develops in up to 50%
- Urothelial carcinomas affect mainly pelvis and ureter

TOP DIFFERENTIAL DIAGNOSES

- Chinese herb nephropathy
- Chronic tubulointerstitial nephritis, any cause

Kidney Atrophy

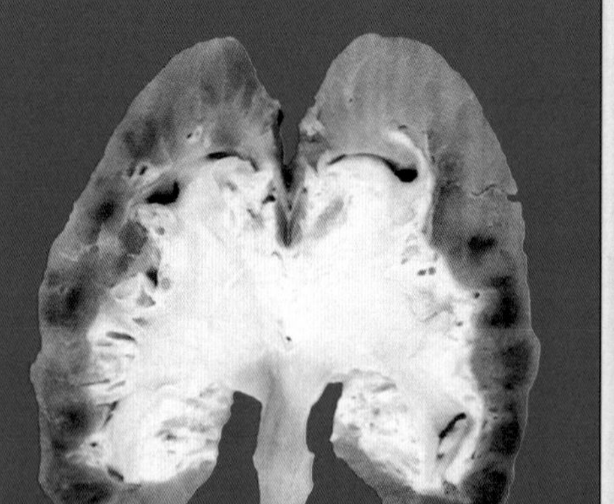

Outer Cortical Zonal Fibrosis

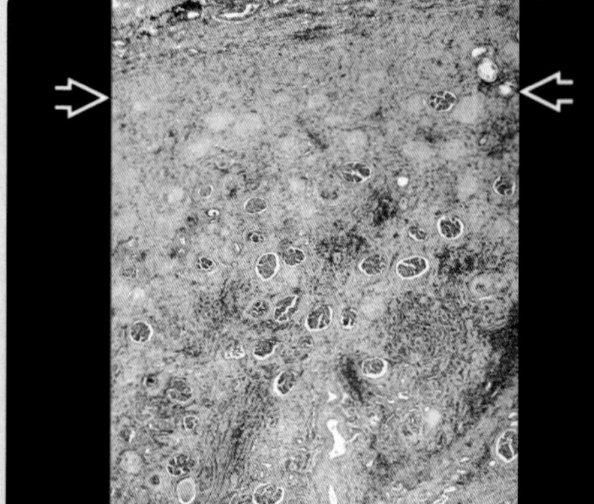

(Left) *This atrophic kidney (7 cm in length) shows the typical features of Balkan endemic nephropathy (BEN) with marked thinning of the cortex and a smooth capsular surface. (Courtesy D. Ferluga, MD.)* **(Right)** *BEN characteristically has a zonal distribution, with progressively increasing severity of interstitial fibrosis and glomerular sclerosis from the juxtamedullary* ➡ *to the subcapsular cortex* ➡*. (Courtesy D. Ferluga, MD.)*

Bland Interstitial Fibrosis

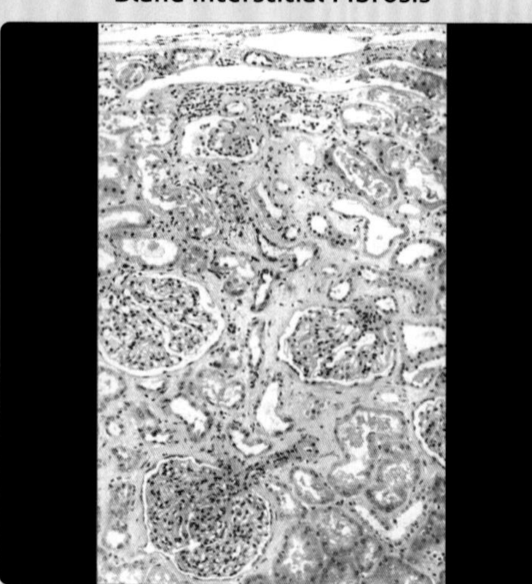

Papillary Urothelial Carcinoma

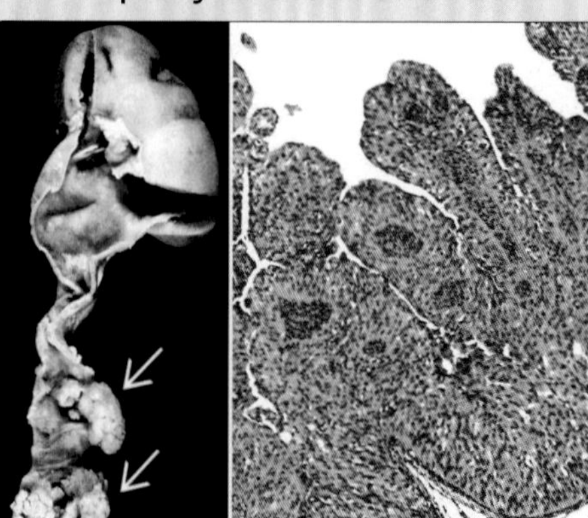

(Left) *BEN characteristically has hypocellular interstitial fibrosis and tubular atrophy, with sparing of glomeruli. (Courtesy D. Ferluga, MD.)* **(Right)** *Multifocal exophytic ureteral tumors* ➡ *and hydronephrosis are shown in BEN with a papillary pattern on histology. (Courtesy D. Ferluga, MD.)*

TERMINOLOGY

Abbreviations

- Balkan endemic nephropathy (BEN)

Synonyms

- Yugoslavian chronic endemic nephropathy
- Southeastern Europe endemic nephropathy
- Danubian endemic familial nephropathy

Definitions

- Chronic tubulointerstitial nephropathy with high risk of urothelial carcinoma, endemic in specific regions of Balkan countries, Romania, Croatia, and Bulgaria

ETIOLOGY/PATHOGENESIS

Aristolochic Acid (AA)

- Present in weeds (*Aristolochia* sp) in wheat fields
- AA metabolites form DNA adducts; may induce mutations of p53 with A:T → T:A transversions
- Specific p53 mutations frequent in urothelial carcinomas
- DNA adducts detected in kidney tissue
- Also responsible for Chinese herb nephropathy
- Proximal tubulopathy thought to be earliest lesion
- Chromosomal breakage in several bands, most frequently 3q25, containing oncogenes *src* and *raf-1*
  - Possibly reflect environmentally induced DNA injury
- Ochratoxin A causes porcine nephropathy pathologically similar to BEN
  - No clear examples of human kidney disease

CLINICAL ISSUES

Epidemiology

- Incidence
  - Up to 10% in endemic areas
  - Discrete geographic distribution
    - Farming populations most affected
    - Familial clustering but not hereditary
  - Immigrants to endemic areas at risk after 15-20 years

Presentation

- Tubular dysfunction early
  - Impaired concentrating ability and salt wasting
  - Tubular proteinuria: Increased urinary β2-microglobulin
- Slowly progressive renal failure beginning at 30-50 years
- Late features
  - Copper-toned skin, orange palms and soles, weight loss, anemia, Fanconi syndrome

Prognosis

- Survival varies from months to > 10 years
  - 33% progression to end-stage kidney disease in 15 years (1 study)
  - Mortality of 43% in Bulgaria (1961-1970)
  - A few studies indicate mortality rate of 50% within 2 years of diagnosis
- Urothelial carcinoma develops in 30-50% with BEN

MACROSCOPIC

Bilateral Shrunken Kidneys

- Finely granular surface and smooth contour
- Down to 20 grams in advanced disease
- Obstructive hydronephrosis with urothelial carcinoma

MICROSCOPIC

Histologic Features

- Glomeruli
  - Spared early in disease
  - Global glomerular sclerosis in advanced disease
    - Focal segmental glomerular sclerosis (FSGS) and focal GBM duplication described
- Tubules and interstitium
  - Interstitial fibrosis and tubular atrophy
    - Begins in outer cortex and extends to inner cortex over years
    - Scanty inflammatory infiltrates
  - Early tubular dysfunction may have normal histology
- Blood vessels
  - Hyalin arteriolosclerosis and arteriosclerosis
- Urothelium
  - Urothelial dysplasia and papillomas of pelvis and ureter
  - Malignancy develops in up to 50%
  - Squamous carcinoma rarely
- IF and EM are nonspecific

DIFFERENTIAL DIAGNOSIS

Chinese Herb Nephropathy

- Also caused by AA (typically less exposure)

Chronic Tubulointerstitial Nephritis, Any Cause

- Especially chronic pyelonephritis, obstructive uropathy, and radiation nephropathy

Chronic Renal Ischemia

- Ischemic glomerulopathy, with intrarenal or extrarenal vascular stenosis

DIAGNOSTIC CHECKLIST

Pathologic Interpretation Pearls

- Outer cortical interstitial fibrosis and upper urinary tract urothelial carcinoma in a patient from an endemic area

SELECTED REFERENCES

1. Jelaković B et al: Chronic dietary exposure to aristolochic Acid and kidney function in native farmers from a croatian endemic area and bosnian immigrants. Clin J Am Soc Nephrol. 10(2):215-23, 2015
2. Jelaković B et al: Consensus statement on screening, diagnosis, classification and treatment of endemic (Balkan) nephropathy. Nephrol Dial Transplant. 29(11):2020-7, 2014
3. Bukvic D et al: Today Balkan endemic nephropathy is a disease of the elderly with a good prognosis. Clin Nephrol. 72(2):105-13, 2009
4. Grollman AP et al: Role of environmental toxins in endemic (Balkan) nephropathy. October 2006, Zagreb, Croatia. J Am Soc Nephrol. 18(11):2817-23, 2007
5. Ferluga D et al: Renal function, protein excretion, and pathology of Balkan endemic nephropathy. III. Light and electron microscopic studies. Kidney Int Suppl. 34:S57-67, 1991
6. Hall PW 3rd et al: Investigation of Chronic Endemic Nephropathy in Yugoslavia. II. Renal Pathology. Am J Med. 39:210-7, 1965

Ethylene Glycol Toxicity

KEY FACTS

TERMINOLOGY

- Toxicity due to ethylene glycol ingestion

ETIOLOGY/PATHOGENESIS

- Acute toxicity by oral ingestion
  - Suicides and homicides
  - Contamination
- Metabolized in liver to glycoaldehyde by alcohol dehydrogenase
  - Glycoaldehyde → glycolic acid → glyoxylic acid → oxalic acid + calcium → calcium oxalate
- Renal injury due to calcium oxalate deposition and other toxins like glycolic acid
- Epithelial injury with balloon vacuoles may be due to glycolic acid

CLINICAL ISSUES

- Phase 1: Neurologic (0.5-12 hours after ingestion)
- Phase 2: Cardiopulmonary (12-24 hours)
- Phase 3: Renal (24-72 hours)
- Diagnosis
  - Altered mental state with high anion gap metabolic acidosis
  - Urinary calcium oxalate crystals on microscopy
  - Increased serum EG and glycolic acid levels more specific
- Permanent renal insufficiency uncommon in nonfatal cases
- May have history of alcoholism, depression

MICROSCOPIC

- Acute tubular injury and necrosis
- Proximal tubular cytoplasmic ballooning vacuolization
- Tubular calcium oxalate crystals

TOP DIFFERENTIAL DIAGNOSES

- Primary and secondary oxalosis
- Acute tubular injury

Ethylene Glycol Nephrotoxicity

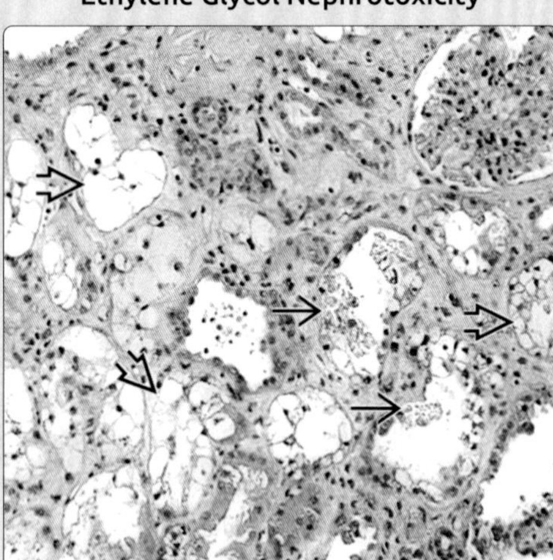

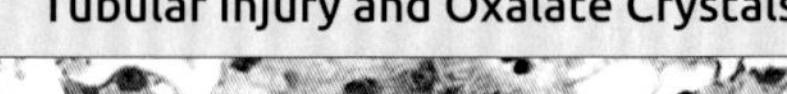

Tubular Injury and Oxalate Crystals

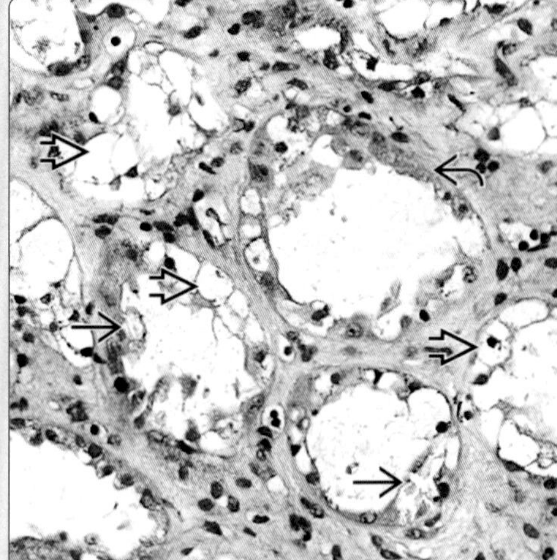

(Left) *Cortex is shown with intratubular, refractile, pale yellow, crystalline calcium oxalate →, epithelial injury with macrovesicular (ballooning) vacuolization ⇨, and interstitial edema with scattered inflammation. (Courtesy T. Nadasdy, MD.)* **(Right)** *Refractile, pale yellow crystals of calcium oxalate accumulate in the cytoplasm of proximal tubular cells → in ethylene glycol toxicity. Crystals are associated with severe tubular injury ↶ and ballooning epithelial cytoplasmic vacuoles ⇨. (Courtesy T. Nadasdy, MD.)*

Oxalate Deposits in Polarized Light

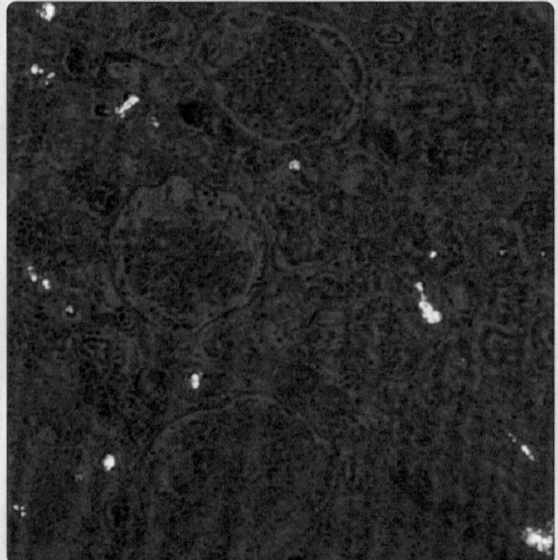

Tubular Vacuolization and Regeneration

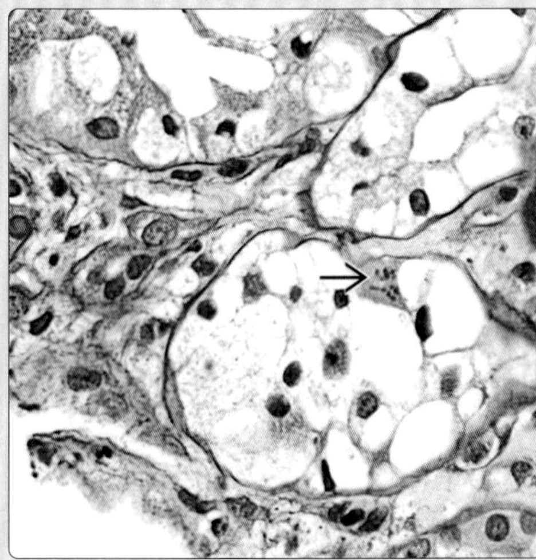

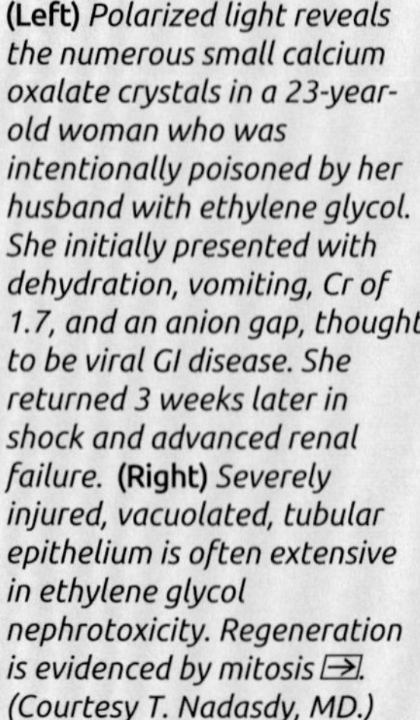

(Left) *Polarized light reveals the numerous small calcium oxalate crystals in a 23-year-old woman who was intentionally poisoned by her husband with ethylene glycol. She initially presented with dehydration, vomiting, Cr of 1.7, and an anion gap, thought to be viral GI disease. She returned 3 weeks later in shock and advanced renal failure.* **(Right)** *Severely injured, vacuolated, tubular epithelium is often extensive in ethylene glycol nephrotoxicity. Regeneration is evidenced by mitosis →. (Courtesy T. Nadasdy, MD.)*

TERMINOLOGY

Abbreviations

- Ethylene glycol (EG)

Definitions

- Toxicity including acute renal failure due to EG ingestion

ETIOLOGY/PATHOGENESIS

Toxic Exposure

- EG is colorless, odorless fluid with bittersweet flavor
  - Common component of antifreeze radiator fluid, hydraulic brake fluid, de-icing solutions, lacquers, and polishes
- Acute toxicity by oral ingestion
  - Deliberate in suicides and homicides
  - Inadvertent in contamination cases
- EG rapidly absorbed with peak serum concentration in 1-4 hours
  - Minimum lethal dose for adults is 1-1.5 mL/kg
- Metabolized in liver to glycoaldehyde by alcohol dehydrogenase
  - Glycoaldehyde → glycolic acid → glyoxylic acid → oxalic acid + calcium → calcium oxalate
  - Glycolic acid and glyoxylic acid contribute to metabolic acidosis
- Calcium oxalate deposits in kidneys, myocardium, vasculature, brain, liver, and spleen
- Renal injury attributed to calcium oxalate deposition
  - Severe tubular injury with balloon vacuoles may be due to other toxins like glycolic acid

CLINICAL ISSUES

Presentation

- Pattern of presentation depends on EG ingested dose
  - Phase 1: Neurologic (0.5-12 hours after ingestion)
    - Inebriation, altered mental status, seizures, coma
  - Phase 2: Cardiopulmonary (12-24 hours)
    - Tachycardia, congestive heart failure, respiratory distress syndrome
  - Phase 3: Renal (24-72 hours)
    - Oliguric acute renal failure, flank pain, hematuria, crystalluria
- Diagnosis
  - Inebriation or altered mental state with high anion gap and metabolic acidosis
  - Urinary calcium oxalate crystals on microscopy
    - Octahedral- or tent-shaped crystals typical of calcium oxalate dihydrate more specific for ethylene glycol-oxalosis (EGO)
  - Urinary fluorescence in Wood light indicates excretion of sodium fluorescein (component of antifreeze)
  - Increased serum EG and glycolic acid levels more specific

Treatment

- Intravenous fluids for shock and sodium bicarbonate for acidosis
- Hemodialysis for acute renal failure and removal of EG
- Antidotes include ethanol and fomepizole
  - Competitive inhibitors of alcohol dehydrogenase reduce formation of toxic metabolites

Prognosis

- Permanent renal insufficiency uncommon in nonfatal cases

MACROSCOPIC

Gross Examination

- Enlarged swollen kidneys with bulging cut surface and gritty texture
- Imprint or "scrimp" specimens reveal calcium oxalate crystals on polarization microscopy

MICROSCOPIC

Histologic Features

- Glomeruli
  - Unremarkable
- Tubules
  - Acute tubular injury and necrosis
  - Cytoplasmic vacuolization (macrovesicular or ballooning or hydropic) in proximal tubules
  - Refractile calcium oxalate in proximal tubules
    - Birefringent in polarized light
  - Rare findings include crystals with multinucleated giant cells and cortical necrosis
- Interstitium
  - Edema with mild inflammation
- Vessels
  - Unremarkable

ANCILLARY TESTS

Uncalled For

- IF and EM do not add diagnostic information

DIFFERENTIAL DIAGNOSIS

Primary and Secondary Oxalosis

- Intratubular and interstitial calcium oxalate with foreign body giant cell reaction and inflammation
- Severe acute tubular injury with macrovesicles not a feature of this group of disorders

Acute Tubular Injury

- Oxalate crystals sometimes prominent

DIAGNOSTIC CHECKLIST

Pathologic Interpretation Pearls

- Calcium oxalate and ballooning vacuoles are typical
- Severe acute tubular injury, large vacuoles, intraepithelial and intraluminal calcium oxalate

SELECTED REFERENCES

1. Latus J et al: Ethylene glycol poisoning: a rare but life-threatening cause of metabolic acidosis-a single-centre experience. Clin Kidney J. 5(2):120-3, 2012
2. Porter WH: Ethylene glycol poisoning: quintessential clinical toxicology; analytical conundrum. Clin Chim Acta. 413(3-4):365-77, 2012
3. Goodkin DA: Urinalysis in ethylene glycol poisoning. Am J Kidney Dis. 54(4):780, 2009
4. Ting SM et al: Early and late presentations of ethylene glycol poisoning. Am J Kidney Dis. 53(6):1091-7, 2009

Argyria

KEY FACTS

TERMINOLOGY

- Systemic disease caused by accumulation of silver (Ag) or silver salts in skin and other tissues due to chronic exposure to silver colloid or salts

ETIOLOGY/PATHOGENESIS

- Silver salts or colloid ingestion
- Silver colloid available as over-the-counter drug promoted in alternative medicine
- Deposits are elemental silver, Ag_2S, or Ag-protein complexes

CLINICAL ISSUES

- Slate gray discoloration of light-exposed skin and conjunctiva
- Usually no other systemic manifestations
- No effective treatment to remove systemic deposits

MACROSCOPIC

- Renal biopsy cores have prominent black glomeruli

MICROSCOPIC

- Granular black deposits along glomerular basement membrane (GBM)
- Also described in peritubular capillary BM and arteries
- Marked accumulation in sclerotic glomeruli
- Membranous glomerulonephritis described
- Skin: Black silver deposits in dermis, macrophages

ANCILLARY TESTS

- Electron microscopy (EM)
- Dense black grains about 100-200 nm in GBM and mesangium
- Deposited primarily along subendothelial side of GBM
- Energy filtered transmission EM: Identifies elements in tissue deposits

TOP DIFFERENTIAL DIAGNOSES

- Ochronosis
- Lecithin-cholesterol acyltransferase deficiency

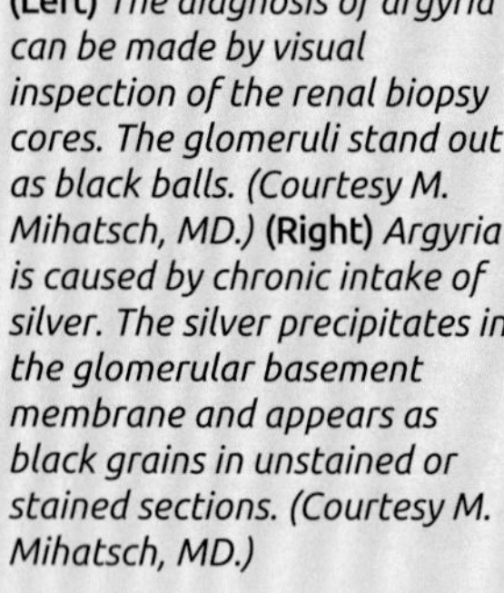

(Left) *The diagnosis of argyria can be made by visual inspection of the renal biopsy cores. The glomeruli stand out as black balls. (Courtesy M. Mihatsch, MD.)* **(Right)** *Argyria is caused by chronic intake of silver. The silver precipitates in the glomerular basement membrane and appears as black grains in unstained or stained sections. (Courtesy M. Mihatsch, MD.)*

Glomeruli Appear Black in Biopsy Without Staining

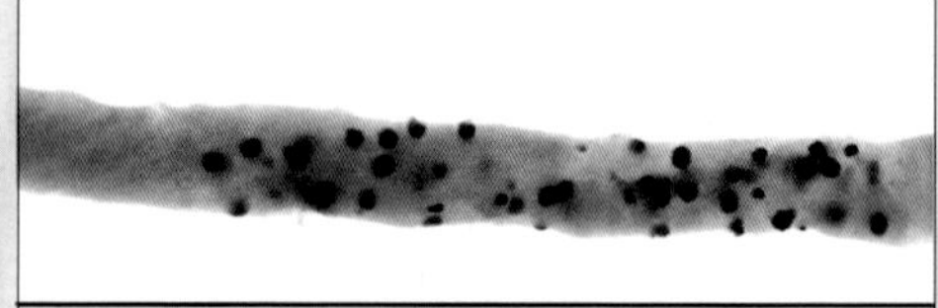

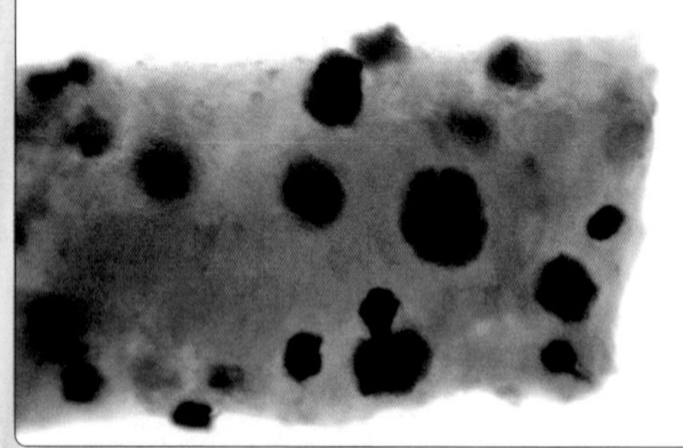

Black Silver Deposits in GBM

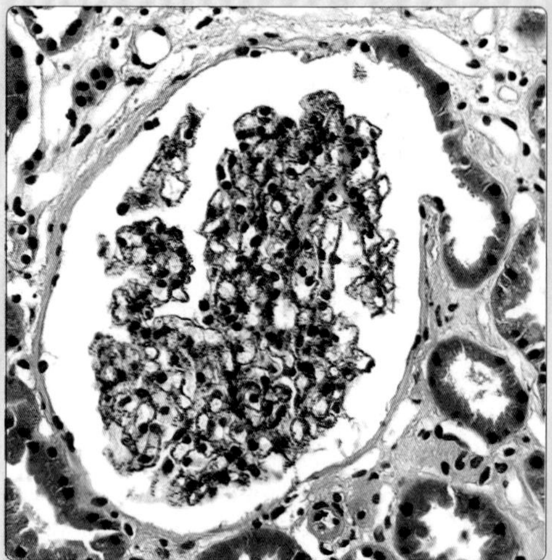

(Left) *In this case of argyria, electron microscopy reveals the characteristic electron-opaque silver deposits along the endothelial side of the GBM → and in the mesangium ↪. (Courtesy M. Mihatsch, MD.)* **(Right)** *Macrophages in the interstitium accumulate the silver particles over time, similar to a tattoo. This patient was 75 years old and had received silver supplements as a child for a ventriculo-peritoneal shunt; she had slate blue skin. Kidney biopsy also had AL amyloidosis.*

Electron-Opaque Silver Deposits in GBM and Mesangium

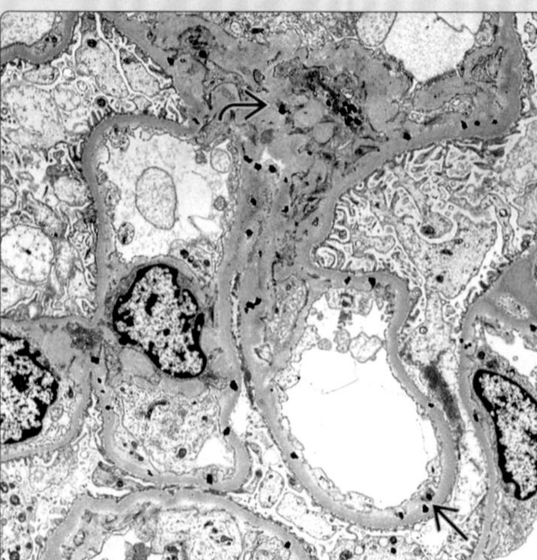

Silver in Interstitial Macrophages

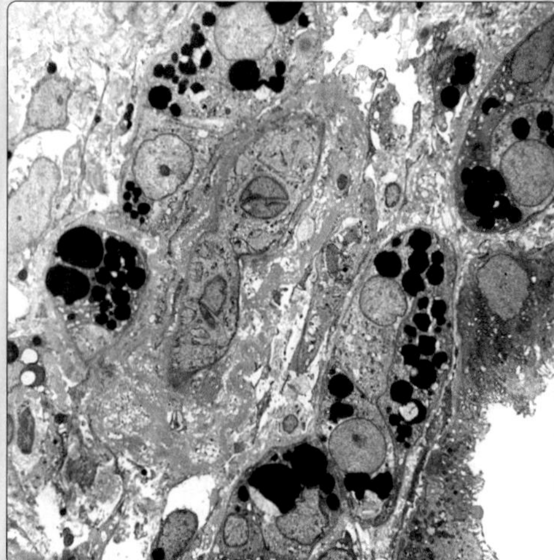

TERMINOLOGY

Synonyms

- Argyrosis (pigmentation of conjunctiva)

Definitions

- Systemic disease caused by accumulation of silver (Ag) or silver salts in skin and other tissues due to chronic exposure to silver colloid or salts
  - Localized form due to topical silver exposure

ETIOLOGY/PATHOGENESIS

Environmental Exposure

- Silver salts or colloid ingestion
  - Silver salts used as antibacterial agent
    - Ag+ bacteriocidal (not metallic Ag)
    - Declining use of silver salts and colloids as antibiotic
    - Silver colloid available as over-the-counter drug promoted in alternative medicine
    - Nanoparticles of Ag used as coating of materials
- Exposure measured in years

Silver Precipitates in Tissues

- Deposits are elemental silver, Ag_2S or Ag-protein complexes
  - Ag+ binds to sulfhydryl (e.g., glutathione), amino, carboxyl, phosphate, and imidazole groups
  - Light catalyzes reduction of Ag+ to silver metal (as in photographic film)
  - Ag oxidized in tissue to Ag_2S
- Debatable evidence that renal disease is caused by silver deposition alone
  - Some patients with chronic renal dysfunction had exposure to heavy metals, solvents, or other nephrotoxins

Animal Models

- Heavy oral exposure to silver nitrate (mice, rats) or 56 nm nanoparticles of silver shows GBM deposition, but no renal disease
- Used to show turnover of GBM in vivo

CLINICAL ISSUES

Presentation

- Slate gray discoloration of light-exposed skin and conjunctiva
- Usually no other systemic manifestations
  - Questionable link to silver deposition
    - Variable loss of renal function
    - Nephrotic syndrome
    - Hypertension

Treatment

- Laser treatment of skin
- No effective treatment to remove systemic deposits

MACROSCOPIC

General Features

- Renal biopsy cores have prominent black glomeruli easily visible to naked eye

MICROSCOPIC

Histologic Features

- Glomeruli
  - Granular black deposits along glomerular basement membrane (GBM)
  - Marked accumulation in sclerotic glomeruli
  - Membranous glomerulonephritis described
- Tubules and interstitium
  - No silver deposition in tubular basement membrane (TBM)
  - Peritubular capillary basement membrane (BM) deposits of silver
  - Macrophages take up silver particles
- Vessels
  - Deposits along internal elastica of arteries described at autopsy
  - Some cases with arteriosclerosis
    - Not clearly related to silver deposition

ANCILLARY TESTS

Electron Microscopy

- Dense black grains about 100-200 nm in GBM and mesangium
  - Deposited primarily along subendothelial side of GBM
- No obvious effect on podocytes, endothelial cells

Energy-Filtered Transmission Electron Microscopy

- Able to identify elements in tissue deposits
  - Higher resolution than energy dispersive x-ray scanning electron microscopy
- Deposits have energy spectrum of silver

Skin Biopsy

- Black silver deposits in dermis, macrophages

DIFFERENTIAL DIAGNOSIS

Ochronosis

- Black pigmented kidney
- Deposits of homogentisic acid in tubules/casts, not glomeruli

Lecithin-Cholesterol Acyltransferase Deficiency

- Osmophilic lipid deposits in GBM may be confused with silver deposits by electron microscopy (EM)
- No pigment on light microscopy

DIAGNOSTIC CHECKLIST

Pathologic Interpretation Pearls

- Black glomeruli in renal biopsy core

SELECTED REFERENCES

1. Mayr M et al: Argyria and decreased kidney function: are silver compounds toxic to the kidney? Am J Kidney Dis. 53(5):890-4, 2009
2. Stepien KM et al: Unintentional silver intoxication following self-medication: an unusual case of corticobasal degeneration. Ann Clin Biochem. 46(Pt 6):520-2, 2009
3. Schroeder JA et al: Ultrastructural evidence of dermal gadolinium deposits in a patient with nephrogenic systemic fibrosis and end-stage renal disease. Clin J Am Soc Nephrol. 3(4):968-75, 2008
4. Drake PL et al: Exposure-related health effects of silver and silver compounds: a review. Ann Occup Hyg. 49(7):575-85, 2005

Tubulointerstitial Nephritis With Uveitis

KEY FACTS

TERMINOLOGY

- Tubulointerstitial nephritis with uveitis (TINU)
    - a.k.a. Dobrin syndrome

ETIOLOGY/PATHOGENESIS

- Autoimmune, infectious, environmental, & genetic
    - Most likely cause in most cases is autoimmune

CLINICAL ISSUES

- Mostly children
    - Females affected more than males
- Uveitis & other eye abnormalities
- Renal dysfunction: Proteinuria & Fanconi syndrome
- Multitude of signs/symptoms (e.g., fever, weight loss, anorexia)
- Laboratory abnormalities such as anemia, increased creatinine, increased ESR, proteinuria, urinary leukocytes, normoglycemic glucosuria, hematuria
- Spontaneous remission can occur but recovery is usually facilitated with steroids
- Permanent renal dysfunction may persist

MICROSCOPIC

- Tubulointerstitial nephritis with mononuclear cells (lymphocytes & macrophages), plasma cells, eosinophils, & neutrophils
    - Centered on proximal tubules, sometimes arranged in circular arrays
- Acute tubular injury
- Noncaseating granulomata in kidneys, bone marrow, & lymph nodes

TOP DIFFERENTIAL DIAGNOSES

- Drug-induced acute interstitial nephritis
- Sarcoidosis
- Sjögren syndrome
- IgG4-related systemic disease

Interstitial Inflammation and Fibrosis

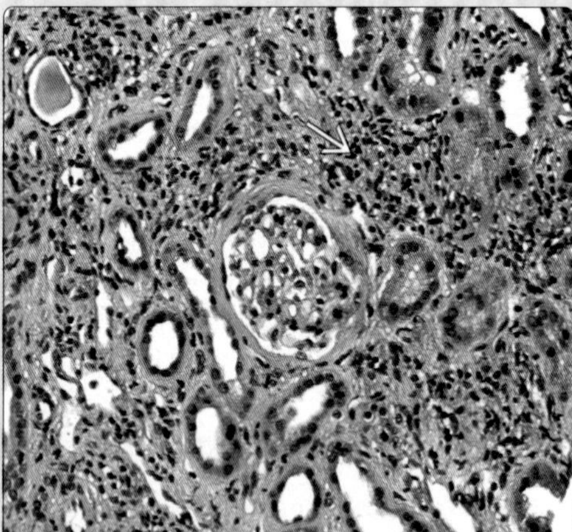

Tubulitis

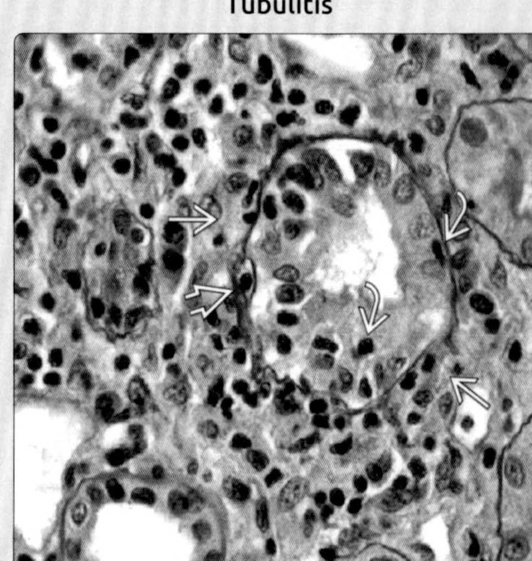

(Left) *A diffuse interstitial infiltrate ➡ with interstitial fibrosis and tubular atrophy is typical of cases of tubulointerstitial nephritis with uveitis (TINU), indicating a chronic, active process* **(Right)** *Proximal tubule is shown with invasion of lymphocytes into the tubule ➡ (tubulitis). Many lymphocytes are applied to the outer surface of the tubular basement membrane (TBM) ➡. One appears to be in between layers of the TBM ➡.*

Destructive Tubulitis

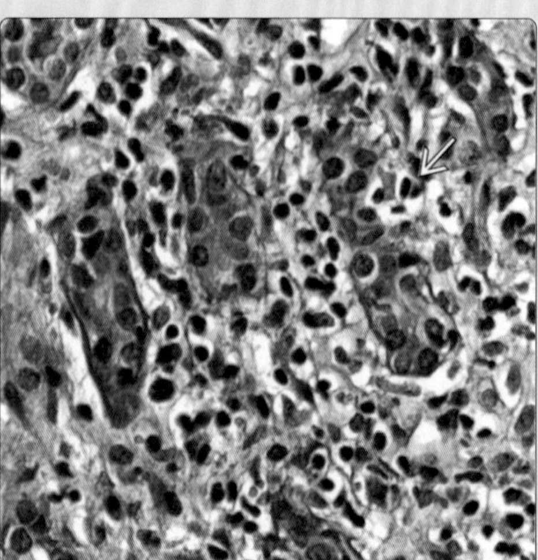

Granuloma

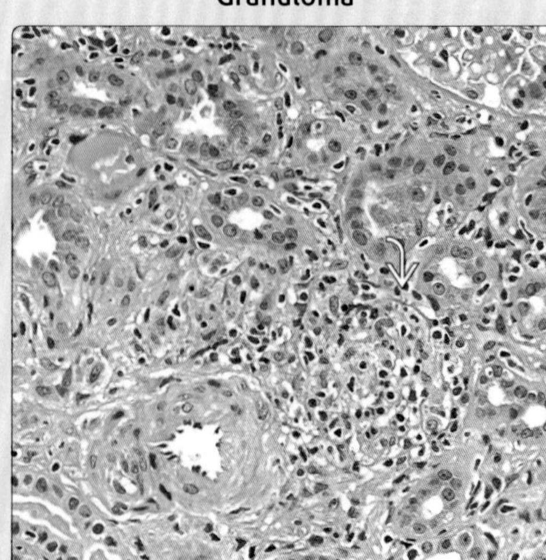

(Left) *Periodic acid-Schiff shows a tubulointerstitial nephritis with a focus of tubulitis ➡ in a case of TINU.* **(Right)** *H&E in a 56-year-old woman with renal failure (Cr 11.9) due to TINU shows a granuloma in the interstitium ➡, seen in ~ 13% of patients. She also had anterior uveitis with Koeppe's nodules (granulomas on the inner margin of the iris) and elevated IgG levels.*

TERMINOLOGY

Definitions

- Idiopathic autoimmune disease characterized by tubulointerstitial nephritis & anterior uveitis

ETIOLOGY/PATHOGENESIS

Autoimmune

- Appears to be T-cell mediated
- Lymphocyte reactivity & circulating antibodies to renal tubular epithelia
- Antibodies may also be directed against uveal cells
- No IgG4-related autoimmune disease association

Genetic

- Occurrence in identical twins & siblings with identical HLA haplotypes suggest genetic component

Other

- Insect bites, herpes zoster, Epstein-Barr virus, *Klebsiella, Chlamydia, Mycoplasma, Toxoplasma*

CLINICAL ISSUES

Epidemiology

- Incidence
  - ~ 5% of tubulointerstitial nephritis biopsies
- Age
  - Median onset: 15 years (range: 9-74 years)
- Sex
  - F:M = 3:1

Presentation

- Anterior uveitis (85% bilateral); eye pain or redness (32%)
  - 20% precedes, 65% follows renal involvement (2-14 months)
- Proteinuria & sometimes form of Fanconi syndrome (proximal tubule dysfunction)
- Fever (53%), weight loss (47%), anorexia (28%)
- Fatigue, malaise (44%) &/or weakness, asthenia (28%)
- Abdominal or flank pain (28%), arthralgias/myalgias (17%)
- Uncommonly: Rash (1%) and lymphadenopathy (1%)

Laboratory Tests

- Anemia (96%), increased creatinine (90%)
- ↑ erythrocyte sedimentation rate (ESR) (89%), ↑ IgG (83%)
- Urine: Protein (86%), leukocytes (55%), normoglycemic glucosuria (47%), microscopic hematuria (42%), urinary eosinophils (3%), aminoaciduria (3%)
- Negative for ANA & RF
- Elevated urinary β2-microglobulin

Treatment

- Drugs
  - Corticosteroids
- Spontaneous remission can occur

Prognosis

- Renal disease usually responds to steroids
  - ~ 2% develop ESRD
- Uveitis less steroid responsive
  - Persists in 23% of children, recurs in 35%
- Recurrence after transplantation reported

MICROSCOPIC

Histologic Features

- Glomeruli: No specific features
- Tubules
  - Acute tubular injury: Flattened, irregular tubular epithelium
  - Mononuclear tubulitis
  - Thickened and multilaminated TBM
  - Tubular atrophy
- Interstitium
  - Mononuclear cells: Frequent lymphocytes (CD4[+] & CD8[+] T cells) with fewer plasma cells and macrophages
    - Centered on proximal tubules, sometimes arranged in circular arrays
    - Eosinophils (34%) & neutrophils (25%)
  - Granulomas ~ 13%
  - Interstitial fibrosis commonly present
- Vessels: No vasculitis
- Other organs: ~ 1% granuloma bone marrow or lymph nodes

ANCILLARY TESTS

Immunohistochemistry

- Inflammatory cells mostly

Immunofluorescence

- No specific findings (no immune complexes)

Electron Microscopy

- No specific findings

DIFFERENTIAL DIAGNOSIS

Drug-Induced Acute Interstitial Nephritis

- Pathology similar or indistinguishable
- History of drug exposure, rash, lack of uveitis

Sarcoidosis

- Granulomas with multinucleated cells more prominent than in TINU

Sjögren Syndrome

- Xerostomia, xerophthalmia, & positive ANA

IgG4-Related Systemic Disease

- More prominent plasma cells, IgG4(+); TBM immune complex deposits

DIAGNOSTIC CHECKLIST

Pathologic Interpretation Pearls

- Often more chronic injury/atrophy of tubules with TBM thickening than in typical drug-related interstitial nephritis

SELECTED REFERENCES

1. Matsumoto K et al: A report of an adult case of tubulointerstitial nephritis and uveitis (TINU) syndrome, with a review of 102 Japanese cases. Am J Case Rep. 16:119-23, 2015
2. Saarela V et al: Tubulointerstitial nephritis and uveitis syndrome in children: a prospective multicenter study. Ophthalmology. 120(7):1476-81, 2013

(Left) *There is severe interstitial nephritis in this case of TINU with an inflammatory infiltrate composed of mononuclear cells, many of which appear to be macrophage-type cells. Tubules contain proteinaceous cast material ⇒.* **(Right)** *Prominent tubulointerstitial nephritis with frequent eosinophils is seen in this case of TINU. Eosinophils can be quite prominent, also a feature of drug-induced acute interstitial nephritis.*

Interstitial Nephritis and Proteinaceous Casts

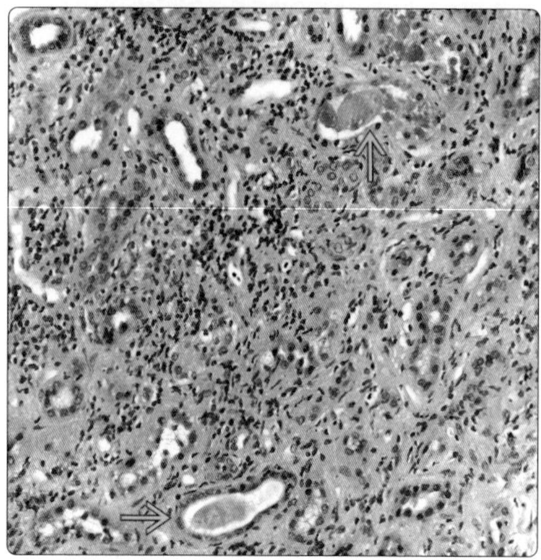

Prominent Eosinophils

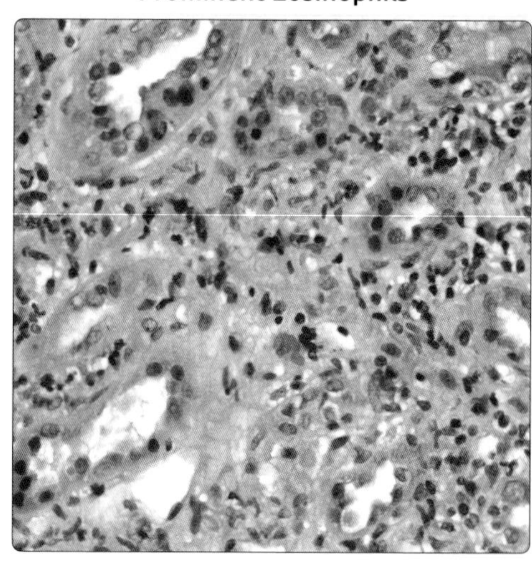

(Left) *Prominent tubulointerstitial nephritis is present in this case of TINU with a predominantly mononuclear infiltrate composed primarily of lymphocytes and macrophage-type cells. Tubules appear injured and contain proteinaceous cast material.* **(Right)** *This patient presented with uveitis and acute renal failure. The biopsy showed diffuse mononuclear interstitial nephritis with tubulitis ➔ and acute tubular injury. A mitotic figure is present in a tubular cell ➔.*

Acute Tubular Injury

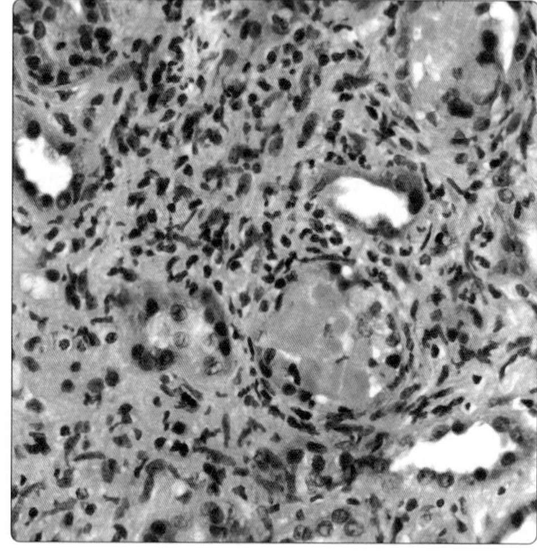

Severe Tubular Injury and Tubulitis

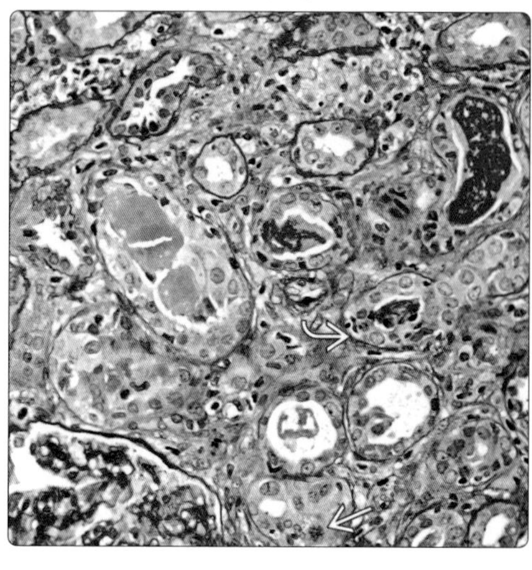

(Left) *Periodic acid-Schiff stain shows markedly disrupted tubules in a case of TINU. Ring-like duplication of the TBM is evident ➔, indicative of chronic or repeated tubular damage and repair.* **(Right)** *Trichrome stain shows severe fibrosis & tubular atrophy with a predominantly mononuclear lymphoid infiltrate in a case of TINU. Tubules contain proteinaceous cast material.*

Lamination of TBM and Tubular Atrophy

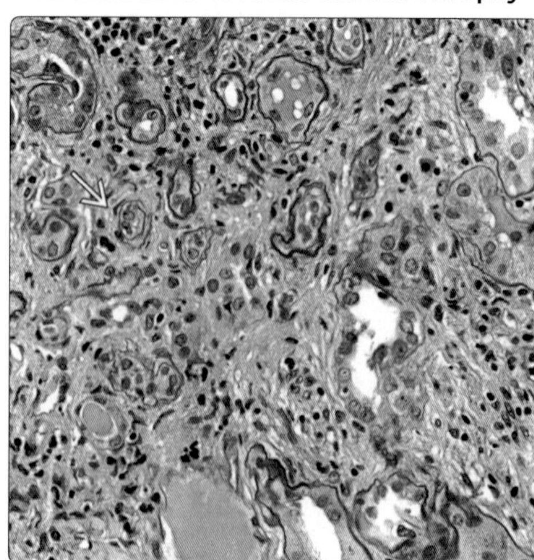

Interstitial Fibrosis and Tubular Atrophy

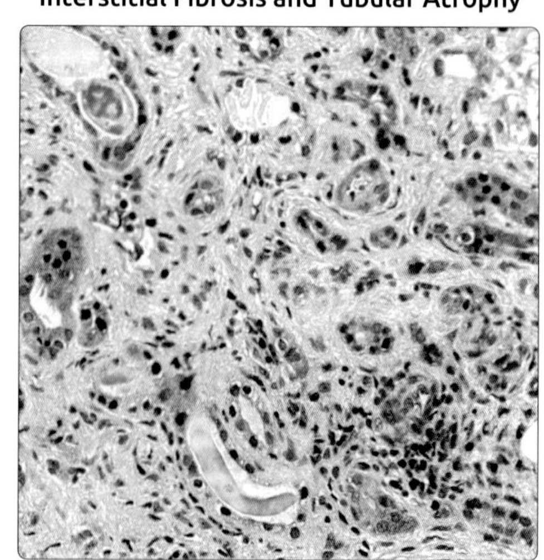

Interstitial Mononuclear Cells

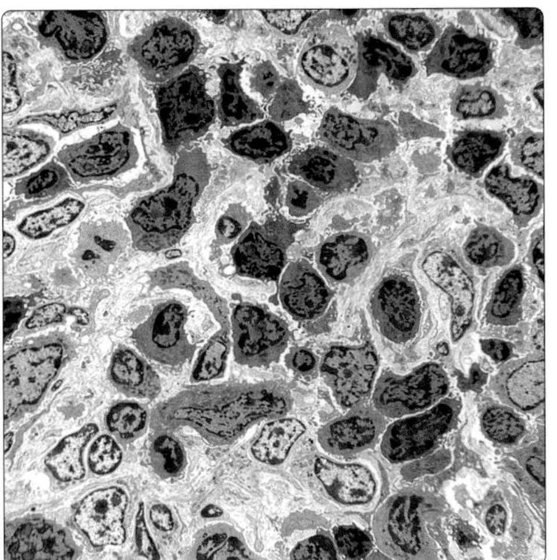

CD3(+) Cells in Interstitium and Tubule

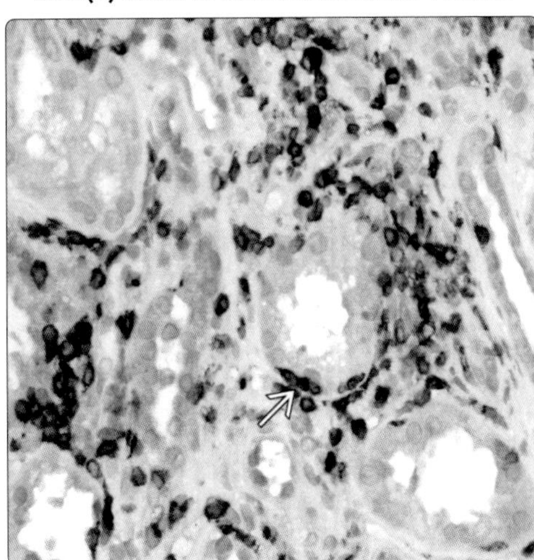

(Left) *Electron micrograph shows a dense infiltrate of mononuclear cells in a case of TINU, which includes mostly small, activated lymphocytes.* **(Right)** *CD3 immunohistochemical stain shows numerous CD3(+) lymphocytes with foci of tubulitis ➡ in TINU. Tubulitis with intratubular T cells is seen in other forms of acute interstitial nephritis, such as that due to drugs and allograft rejection.*

CD4(+) Cells

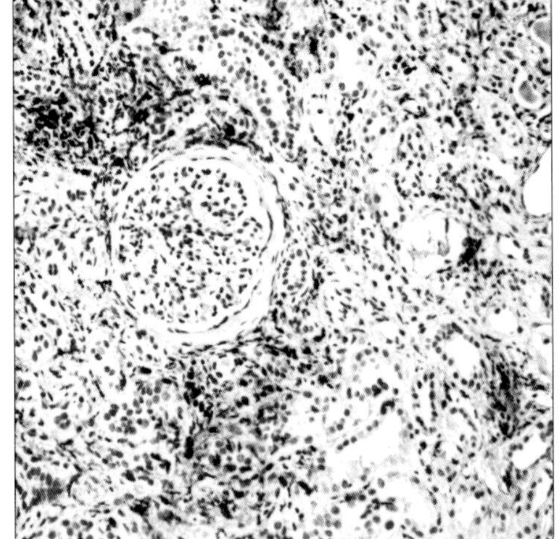

CD8(+) Cells

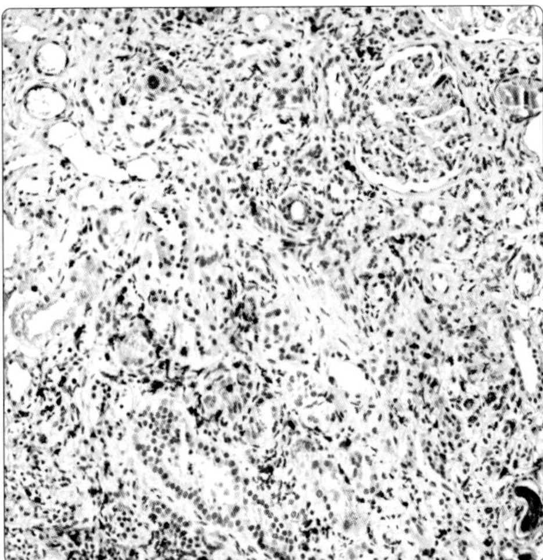

(Left) *Numerous lymphocytes are CD4(+) in this case of TINU.* **(Right)** *A minority of the lymphocytes in TINU are CD8(+), as demonstrated in this CD8 immunohistochemical stain.*

Increased Interstitial Smooth Muscle Actin in TINU

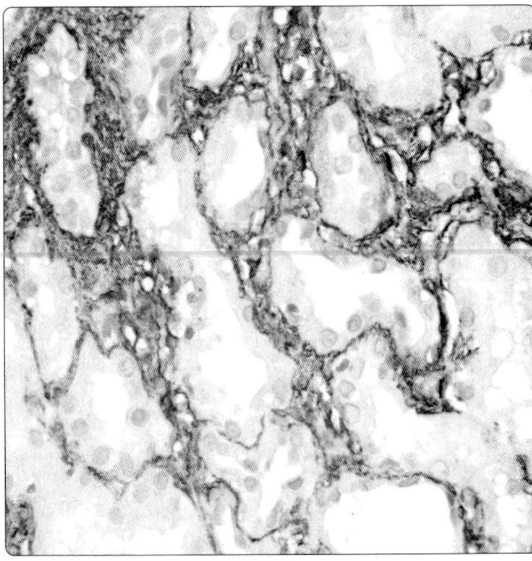

Minor Foot Process Effacement

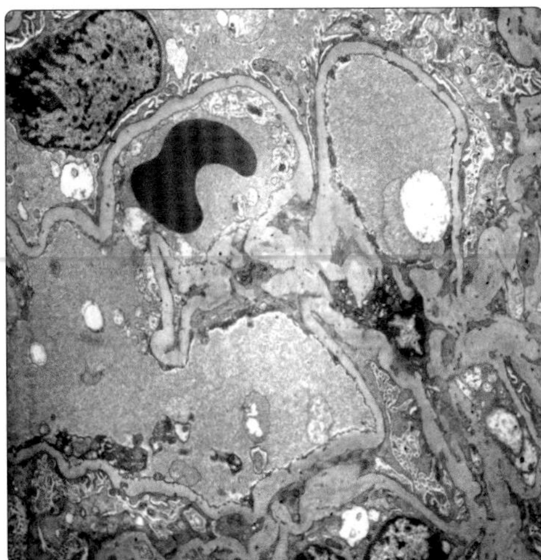

(Left) *α-smooth muscle actin is increased in the expanded, fibrotic interstitium. Expression of α-smooth muscle actin is indicative of active fibrosis with myofibroblasts.* **(Right)** *Glomeruli in TINU do not appear to be involved, aside from a minor degree of foot process effacement and occasional features of endothelial injury with loss of fenestrations.*

Sjögren Syndrome

KEY FACTS

TERMINOLOGY

- Progressive autoimmune disorder involving exocrine glands, particularly salivary and lacrimal glands
- May be primary or component of other autoimmune disorders

CLINICAL ISSUES

- Female predominance; age range: 45-55
- Keratoconjunctivitis and xerostomia most common
- Renal disease
  - Renal failure
  - Renal tubular acidosis
  - Proteinuria and hematuria
- Risk of non-Hodgkin, typically B-cell, lymphoma
- Cutaneous vasculitis
  - Cryoglobulins in 30%
  - SS most common cause of non-hepatitis C virus-related mixed cryoglobulinemia

MICROSCOPIC

- Chronic tubulointerstitial nephritis
  - Plasma cell-rich infiltrate
  - Tubular atrophy and interstitial fibrosis
- Acute tubulointerstitial nephritis
  - Active tubulitis and edema
- Glomerulonephritis
  - Many forms described,most commonly MPGN and membranous GN

TOP DIFFERENTIAL DIAGNOSES

- IgG4-related systemic disease
- Drug-induced allergic interstitial nephritis
- Sarcoidosis

DIAGNOSTIC CHECKLIST

- If plasma cell-rich interstitial nephritis, think SS

Acute Tubulointerstitial Nephritis

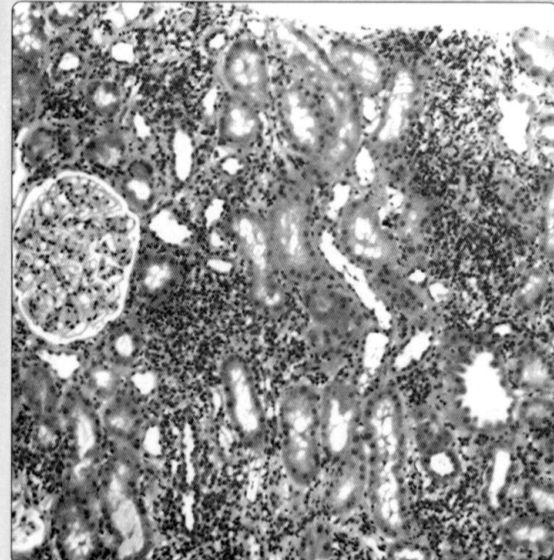

Interstitial Inflammation With Plasma Cells

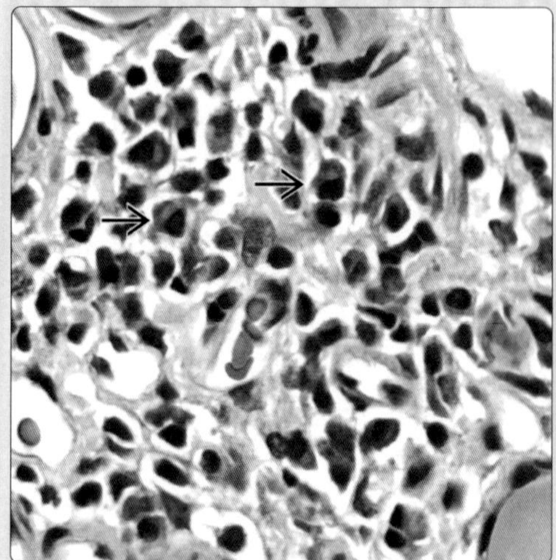

(Left) *Renal biopsy in Sjögren syndrome typically shows a patchy but heavy tubulointerstitial inflammatory infiltrate. The glomeruli are usually normal. The infiltrate forms broad sheets of cells that separate the tubules.* **(Right)** *This biopsy in Sjögren syndrome shows the plasma cell-rich ➔ nature of the inflammatory infiltrate. The paranuclear "hoff" is visible in several cells representing the Golgi apparatus. The interstitium is greatly expanded and tubular atrophy and interstitial fibrosis has developed.*

Normal Glomerulus

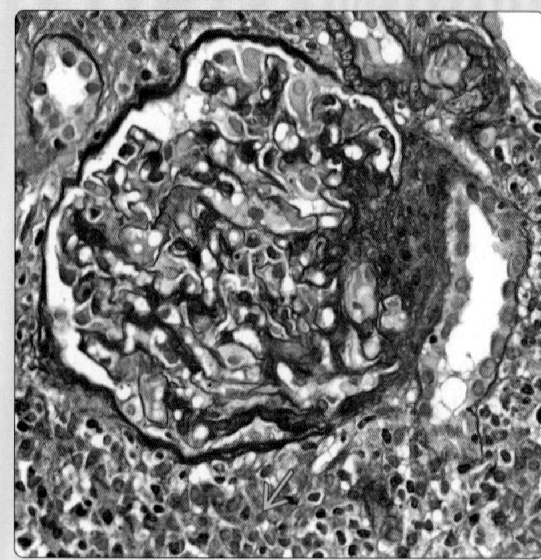

Cryoglobulinemic Glomerulonephritis

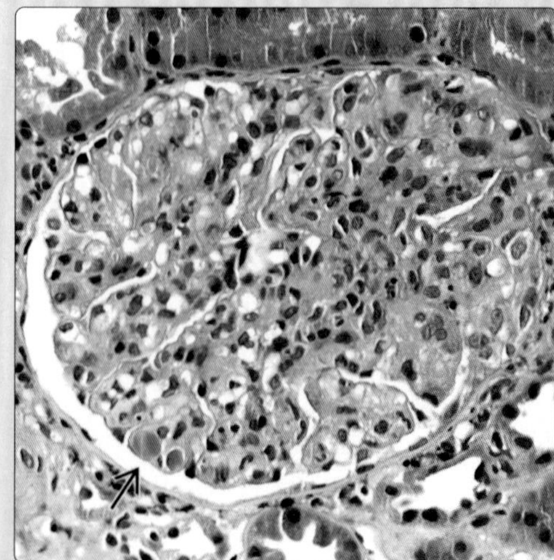

(Left) *A normal glomerulus is present in this biopsy showing chronic tubulointerstitial nephritis ➔. Although various forms of glomerulonephritis have been described in Sjögren syndrome, glomerular involvement is less common.* **(Right)** *Membranoproliferative glomerulonephritis with capillary loop hyaline thrombi ➔, consistent with cryoglobulinemic glomerulonephritis, is shown here. MPGN (± features of cryoglobulinemia) is the most common glomerulonephritis present in Sjögren syndrome.*

TERMINOLOGY

Abbreviations

- Sjögren syndrome (SS)

Synonyms

- Sicca syndrome

Definitions

- Autoimmune disorder involving exocrine glands, particularly salivary and lacrimal glands
  - May be primary (70%) or component of other autoimmune disorders

ETIOLOGY/PATHOGENESIS

Etiology Not Clear

- May be multifactorial, genetic susceptibility
- Initiation by exogenous factor, possibly viral
- Lymphoplasmacytic inflammation with atrophy of eccrine, salivary, and lacrimal glands
  - T-lymphocyte response
  - B-lymphocyte hyper-reactivity
    - Autoantibodies: Rheumatoid factor (RF), SS-A (Ro), and SS-B (La)

CLINICAL ISSUES

Epidemiology

- Age
  - 45-55 years
- Sex
  - Female predominance (F:M = 9:1)

Presentation

- Renal disease in ~ 5%
  - Tubulointerstitial disease
    - Distal renal tubular acidosis: 70-80%
    - Renal failure: 25-30%
    - Tubular proteinuria: 20%
  - Glomerulonephritis: 5-15%
    - Proteinuria (occasionally nephrotic) &/or hematuria
- Keratoconjunctivitis (dry eyes): > 95%
- Xerostomia (dry mouth): > 95%
- Cutaneous vasculitis: 10-30%
  - Associated with cryoglobulins in 30%
- Lymphoma 40x increased risk

Laboratory Tests

- 50-90% have SS-A antibodies
  - ANA, anti-SS-B, and RF often positive
- Hypergammaglobulinemia
- Cryoglobulins
  - Most common cause of non-hepatitis C virus-related mixed cryoglobulinemia
- Low C4, C3 (9%)

Treatment

- Immunosuppression: Corticosteroids, rituximab

Prognosis

- Tubulointerstitial disease an early manifestation
- Glomerulonephritis develops later
- Renal function and proteinuria improves with treatment in most

MICROSCOPIC

Histologic Features

- Glomeruli
  - Involved in minority (25-30%)
    - Membranoproliferative glomerulonephritis
      - Cryoglobulinemic glomerulonephritis
    - Membranous glomerulonephritis
    - Mesangial proliferative glomerulonephritis
    - Crescentic glomerulonephritis
- Tubules and interstitium
  - Chronic tubulointerstitial nephritis: 40-50%
    - Dense, patchy, plasma cell and lymphocytic infiltrate
    - Eosinophils usually absent
    - Tubular atrophy and interstitial fibrosis
  - Acute tubulointerstitial nephritis: 25%
    - Active tubulitis and interstitial edema

ANCILLARY TESTS

Immunofluorescence

- Usually negative unless glomerulonephritis present
- Rarely TBM or interstitial deposits of IgG and C3

Electron Microscopy

- Usually no detectable deposits in interstitium or TBM
- Mesangial &/or capillary loop electron-dense deposits if glomerulonephritis present

DIFFERENTIAL DIAGNOSIS

IgG4-Related Systemic Disease

- Prominent IgG4(+) plasma cells
- Immune deposits in TBM

Drug-Induced Allergic Interstitial Nephritis

- Prominent eosinophils typically

Sarcoidosis

- Presence of granulomas, nephrocalcinosis

DIAGNOSTIC CHECKLIST

Pathologic Interpretation Pearls

- If plasma cell-rich interstitial nephritis, think SS

SELECTED REFERENCES

1. Anand A et al: Sjögren Syndrome and Cryoglobulinemic Glomerulonephritis. Am J Kidney Dis. ePub, 2015
2. Kidder D et al: Kidney biopsy findings in primary Sjogren syndrome. Nephrol Dial Transplant. ePub, 2015
3. Bogdanović R et al: Renal involvement in primary Sjogren syndrome of childhood: case report and literature review. Mod Rheumatol. 23(1):182-9, 2013
4. Maripuri S et al: Renal involvement in primary Sjögren's syndrome: a clinicopathologic study. Clin J Am Soc Nephrol. 4(9):1423-31, 2009
5. Ren H et al: Renal involvement and followup of 130 patients with primary Sjögren's syndrome. J Rheumatol. 35(2):278-84, 2008
6. Bossini N et al: Clinical and morphological features of kidney involvement in primary Sjögren's syndrome. Nephrol Dial Transplant. 16(12):2328-36, 2001
7. Winer RL et al: Sjögren's syndrome with immune-complex tubulointerstitial renal disease. Clin Immunol Immunopathol. 8(3):494-503, 1977

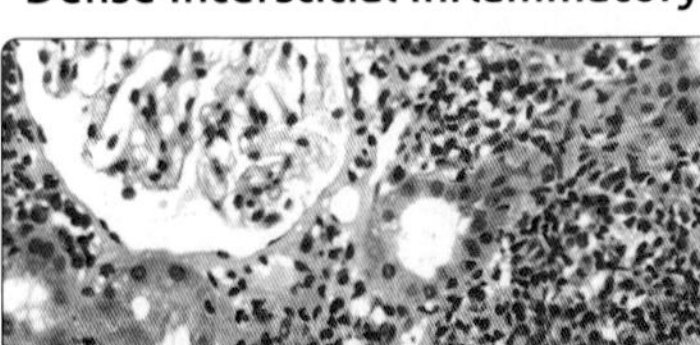

(Left) *The interstitial inflammatory infiltrate in Sjögren syndrome is broad, widely separating the tubules. This pattern of infiltration simulates a malignant lymphoma involving the kidney. The cytologic features are usually sufficient to resolve any diagnostic concern.* **(Right)** *This interstitial infiltrate consists of lymphocytes and numerous plasma cells. A typical drug-induced tubulointerstital nephritis would be more polymorphous, showing fewer plasma cells and including eosinophils, not present here.*

Dense Interstitial Inflammatory Infiltrate

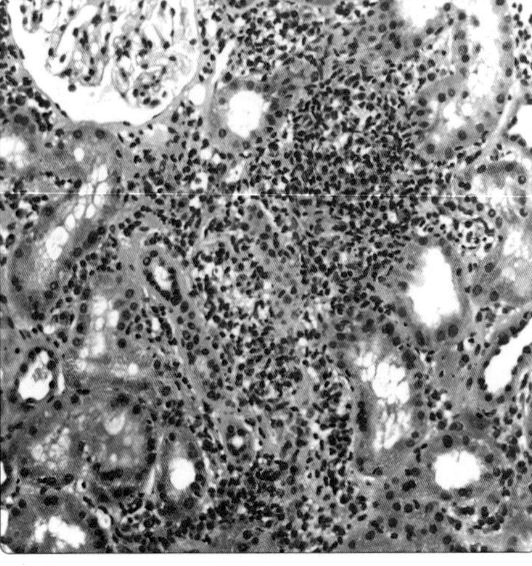

Plasma Cell-Rich Inflammatory Infiltrate

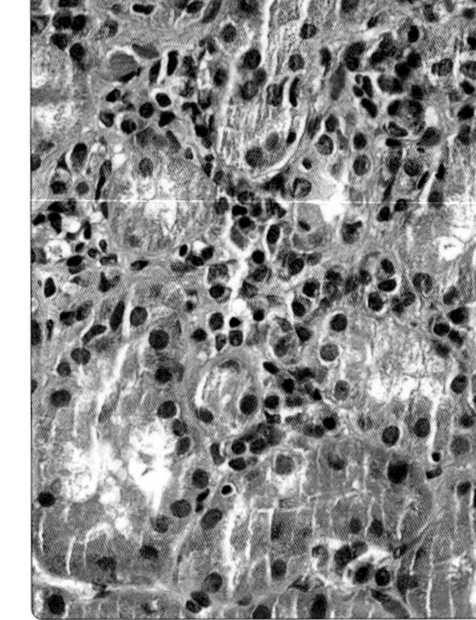

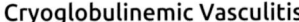

(Left) *Tubulitis is shown; although the interstitial infiltrate is primarily composed of plasma cells ➡, the cells within the tubules are lymphocytes ⇨, likely T cells. There is interstitial expansion due to edema.* **(Right)** *Patient with Sjögren syndrome has developed progressive renal injury. There is diffuse interstitial fibrosis & tubular atrophy with persistent inflammation. The severe tubulointerstitial disease has resulted in glomerular injury with periglomerular fibrosis → and focal global sclerosis ↗.*

Acute Tubulointerstitial Nephritis With Tubulitis

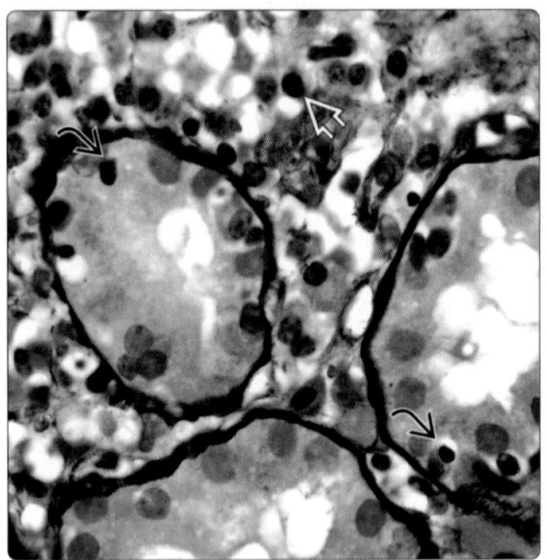

Chronic Tubulointerstitial Nephritis

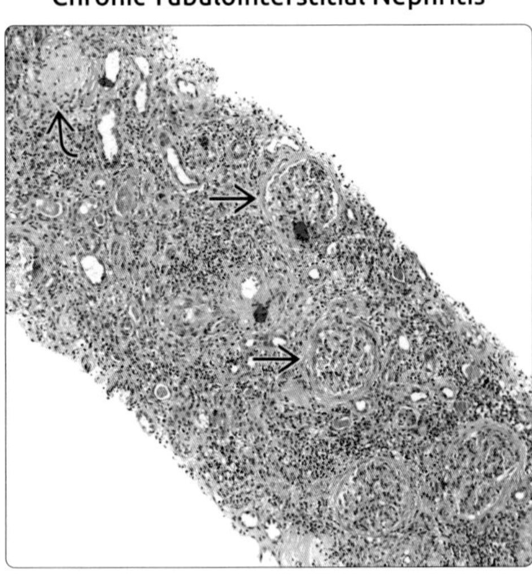

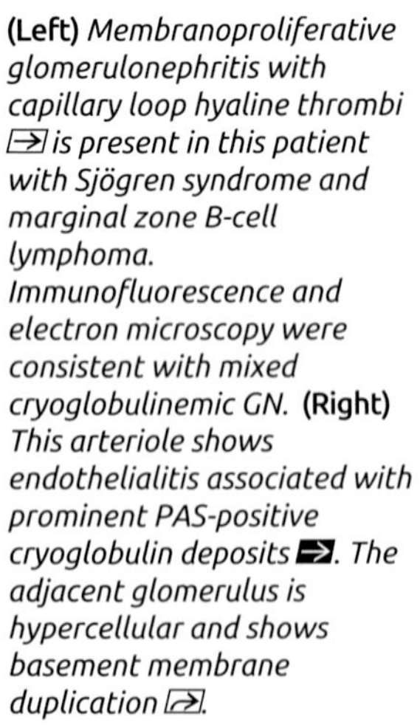

(Left) *Membranoproliferative glomerulonephritis with capillary loop hyaline thrombi → is present in this patient with Sjögren syndrome and marginal zone B-cell lymphoma. Immunofluorescence and electron microscopy were consistent with mixed cryoglobulinemic GN.* **(Right)** *This arteriole shows endothelialitis associated with prominent PAS-positive cryoglobulin deposits ➡. The adjacent glomerulus is hypercellular and shows basement membrane duplication ↗.*

Membranoproliferative Glomerulonephritis With Hyaline Thrombi

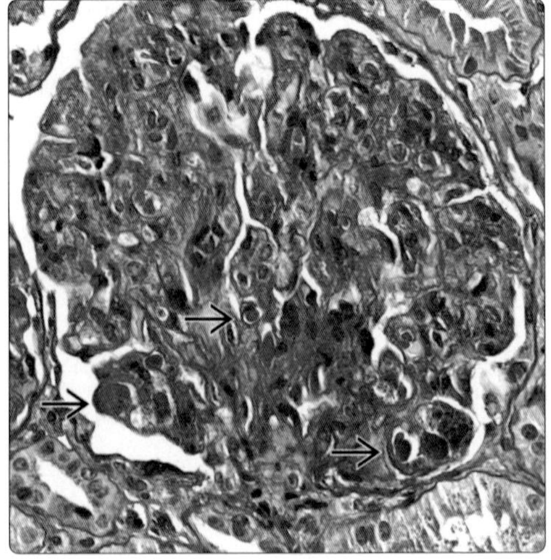

Cryoglobulinemic Vasculitis

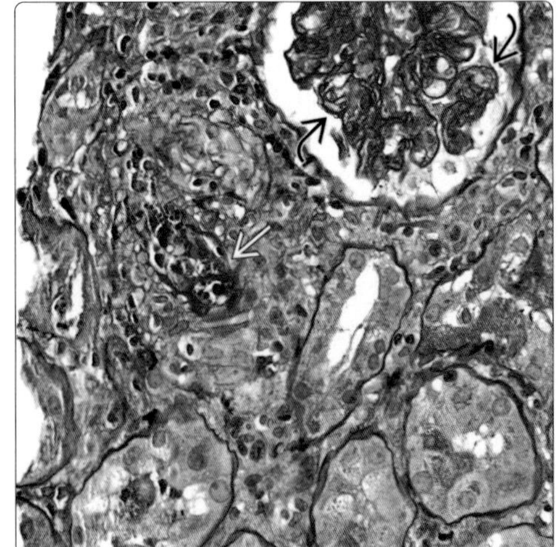

Membranous Glomerulonephritis

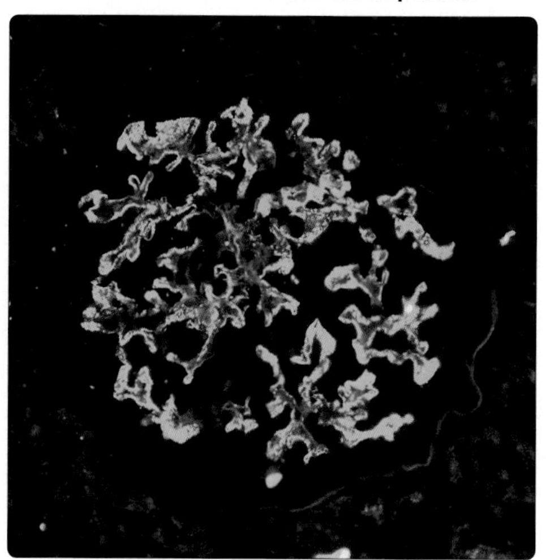

Cryoglobulinemic Glomerulonephritis

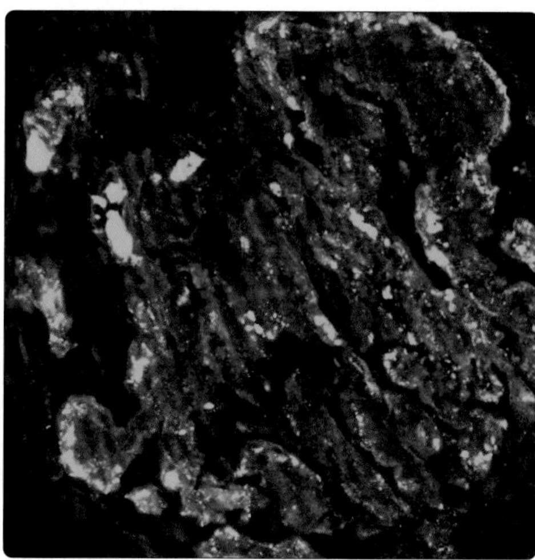

(Left) *Membranous glomerulonephritis has also been reported in patients with Sjögren syndrome. This glomerulus shows global, finely granular, IgG capillary loop staining in a membranous pattern.* **(Right)** *This glomerulus shows peripheral accentuation of the capillary loops by IgM with milder mesangial staining. Several capillary loops show strong luminal staining by IgM, consistent with the hyaline thrombi seen by light microscopy. IgG was also positive in this case of mixed cryoglobulinemia.*

Lymphocytic Tubulitis

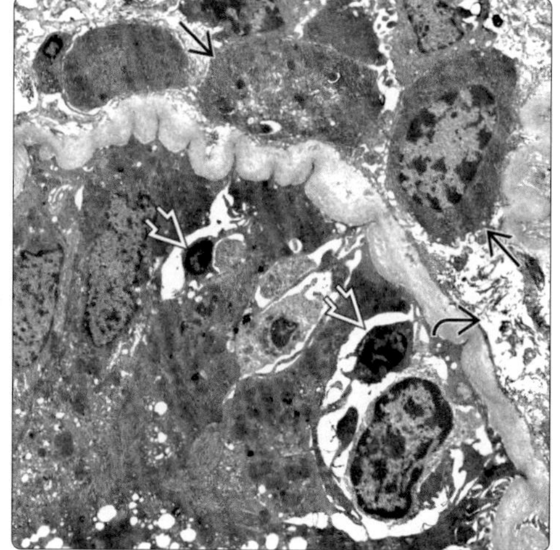

Interstitial Plasma Cells

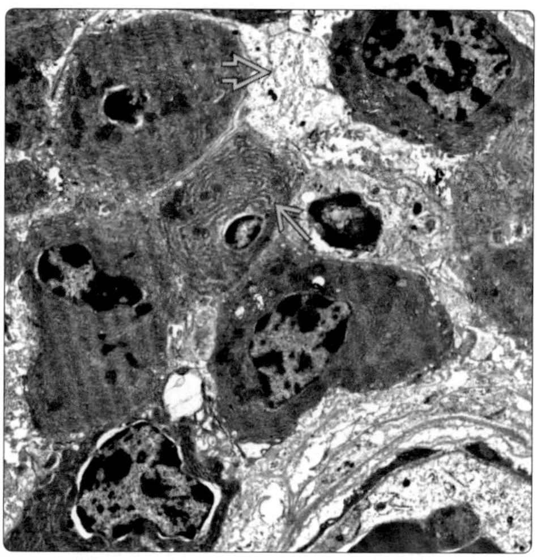

(Left) *This tubule shows lymphocytic tubulitis. Notice that there are lymphocytes ➔ on the inside of the tubular basement membrane and between tubular epithelial cells. The interstitium shows edema ➔, and all of the interstitial cells are plasma cells ➔.* **(Right)** *This electron micrograph shows interstitial edema ➔ and a cluster of plasma cells. Plasma cells are distinctive because their cytoplasm is filled with rough endoplasmic reticulum ➔.*

Normal Glomerulus

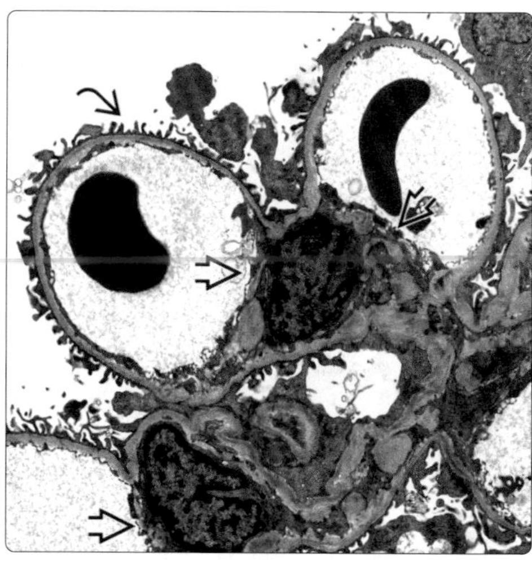

Mild Glomerular Immune Complex Deposition

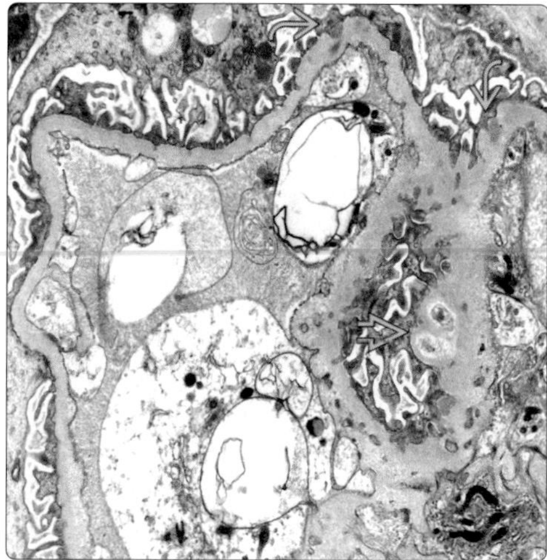

(Left) *In most cases of Sjögren syndrome, the glomerulus is normal, as shown in this case. There is preservation of the podocyte foot processes ➔, no deposits, and the mesangium ➔ is not expanded.* **(Right)** *Notice the scattered subepithelial deposits ➔ in this EM from a patient with Sjögren syndrome. Some are undergoing reabsorption ➔. This is an immune complex disease, perhaps a forme fruste of membranous glomerulonephritis occasionally seen in Sjögren syndrome.*

KEY FACTS

TERMINOLOGY

- IgG4-related disease (IgG4-RD) refers to systemic fibroinflammatory disease that can affect nearly any organ
- IgG4-related kidney disease (IgG4-RKD) refers to any pattern of kidney involvement by IgG4-RD
  - May include IgG4-TIN, IgG4-related membranous glomerulonephritis, and IgG4 plasma cell arteritis
  - IgG4-TIN is immune-mediated TIN with increased IgG4(+) plasma cells and often tubulointerstitial immune complex deposits

ETIOLOGY/PATHOGENESIS

- Renal involvement by systemic immune-mediated disease, now called IgG4-related disease
- Immune-mediated systemic disease, unknown antigen
- IgG4 is anti-inflammatory IgG subclass

CLINICAL ISSUES

- Renal mass(es)
- Acute or chronic renal failure
- Steroid therapy usually effective

MICROSCOPIC

- Plasma cell-rich interstitial inflammation
  - Increased IgG4(+) plasma cells (polyclonal)
- Granular TBM immune complex deposits by IF
  - Contain IgG, IgG4, C3, kappa and lambda light chains
- Glomeruli negative by IF unless concurrent immune complex glomerulonephritis
- Amorphous electron-dense deposits within tubular basement membranes and in interstitium by EM

TOP DIFFERENTIAL DIAGNOSES

- Granulomatosis with polyangiitis (Wegener)
- Drug-induced acute interstitial nephritis
- Lymphoma or leukemia
- Inflammation may be misinterpreted as nondiagnostic in biopsy taken for "mass"

IgG4-TIN

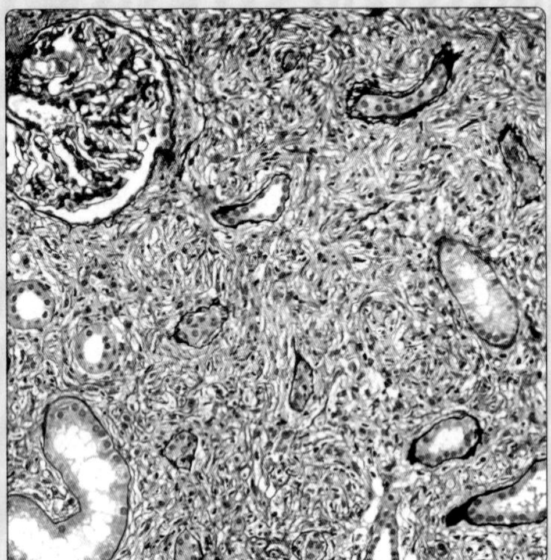

IgG4-TIN

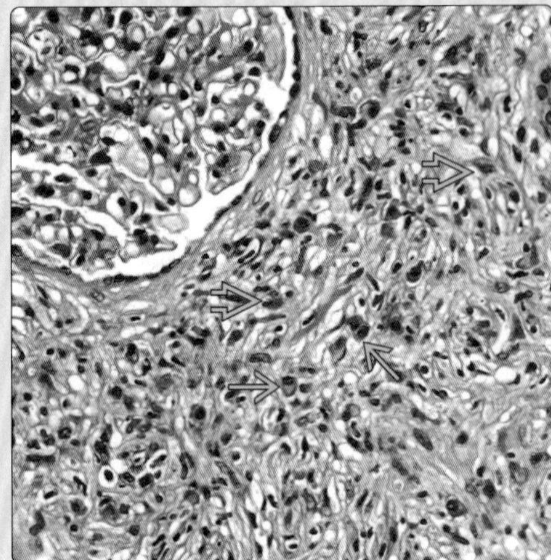

(Left) *IgG4-TIN shows expansile interstitial fibrosis with a storiform pattern that pushes apart the tubules.* **(Right)** *The interstitial inflammatory infiltrate is composed of plasma cells ⇨, eosinophils ⇨, and mononuclear cells.*

Tubulointerstitial Immune Complex Deposits

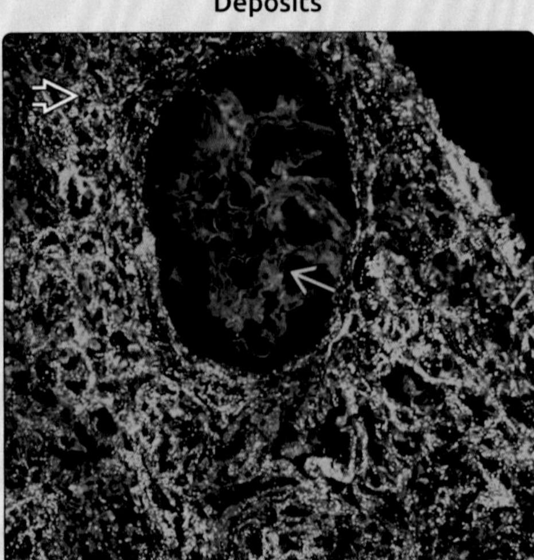

IgG4(+) Plasma Cells in IgG4-TIN

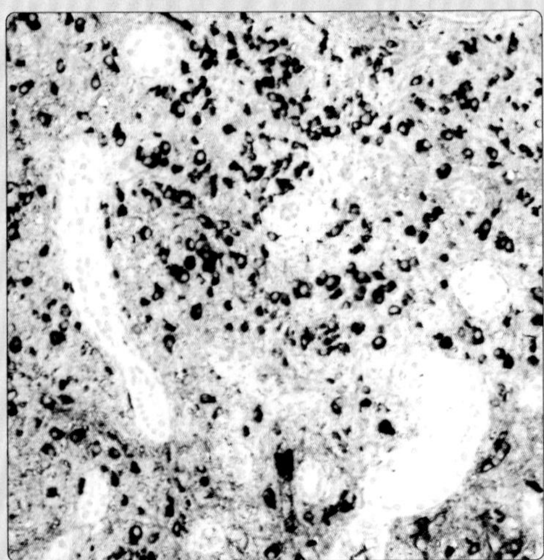

(Left) *Immunofluorescence for IgG shows striking tubular basement membrane, interstitial ➡, and Bowman capsule granular staining, with conspicuous lack of staining of the glomerulus ⇨.* **(Right)** *This case of IgG4-TIN shows a marked increase (> 30 cells/40x field) in IgG4(+) plasma cells.*

TERMINOLOGY

Abbreviations

- IgG4-related tubulointerstitial nephritis (IgG4-TIN)

Synonyms

- IgG4-related disease (IgG4-RD)
  - Systemic immune-mediated disease that can affect nearly any organ
- IgG4-related kidney disease (IgG4-RKD)
  - Includes IgG4-TIN, IgG4-related membranous glomerulonephritis, and IgG4 plasma cell arteritis

Definitions

- Immune-mediated TIN with increased IgG4(+) plasma cells and often tubulointerstitial immune complex deposits; usually associated with systemic fibroinflammatory disease

ETIOLOGY/PATHOGENESIS

Systemic Autoimmune Disease

- Renal involvement by systemic immune-mediated disease, now called IgG4-related disease
- Affected organs include pancreas, liver, kidney, lung, salivary glands, thyroid, lymph nodes

Proposed Etiology/Autoantigens

- Clonal expansion of CD19(+), CD27(+), CD20(-), CD38(hi) plasmablasts in peripheral blood of active IgG4-RD patients
- No definite antigen identified; some antigens proposed
  - Plasminogen-binding protein (PBP) peptide
    - Homologue of PBP of *Helicobacter pylori* and of ubiquitin-protein ligase E3 component n-recognin 2
      - Enzyme expressed in pancreatic acinar cells
    - PBP peptide antibodies in 95% of autoimmune pancreatitis (AIP) patients
      - May include patients with other forms of AIP, not only IgG4-related AIP (type 1)
  - Carbonic anhydrase-II and -IV
  - Lactoferrin
  - Pancreatic secretory trypsin inhibitor
  - α-fodrin
- In IgG4-MGN, negative phospholipase A2 receptor (PLA2R) staining, implying secondary MGN

IgG4 Distinctive Subclass of IgG

- Weaker interchain disulfide bridges
  - IgG4 immunoglobulin half-molecules dissociate and reassociate with other IgG4 half-molecules, including those with different antigen specificities
- Does not fix complement
  - Serve as anti-inflammatory antibodies
  - May block antigen binding site for more pathogenic IgG1 or IgE
- Rheumatoid factor activity via Fc-Fc interactions

Propensity to Form Mass Lesions

- May be due to anti-inflammatory cytokines, including IL-10, tumor necrosis factor-α, and fibrogenic IL-13, and resultant expansion of IgG4-secreting plasma cells

CLINICAL ISSUES

Presentation

- Renal mass(es), enlarged kidneys, or heterogeneous appearance on CT scan
- Acute or chronic renal failure
- Other organ involvement may be present concurrently, previously, or may emerge in future
  - AIP type 1, IgG4-related AIP
  - Sclerosing cholangitis
  - Sialadenitis/Mikulicz disease
  - Inflammatory aortic aneurysm
  - Retroperitoneal fibrosis
  - Lymphadenopathy
  - Orbital pseudolymphoma
  - Inflammatory masses in liver, lung, breast, heart, prostate, pituitary, other organs
  - Often patients have history of allergy
- Not all cases of IgG4-TIN have extrarenal involvement
- Proteinuria
  - Due to IgG4-related membranous glomerulonephritis (IgG4-MGN)
- Obstruction due to IgG4-related retroperitoneal fibrosis

Laboratory Tests

- Hypergammaglobulinemia
  - Typically no monoclonal protein
- Elevated serum IgG4 or total IgG in ~ 80%
  - Elevated serum IgG4 in 70-75% of AIP patients
  - Prozone effect in ~ 30% of IgG4-RD patients by routine IgG4 serum laboratory test
    - Need dilutions with nephelometry or mass spectrometry to evaluate for IgG4 serum excess
- Increased circulating plasmablasts by flow cytometry in patients with active IgG4-RD
- Hypocomplementemia (50%)
- Eosinophilia (~ 30%)

Treatment

- Drugs
  - Steroids
    - Glucocorticoids are 1st-line treatment unless contraindicated
    - ~ 90% sensitive to steroid therapy but high rate of relapse
    - Steroid responsiveness is 1 diagnostic criterion for AIP
  - Rituximab
    - Anti-CD20 drug used with success in IgG4-RD and IgG4-TIN
  - Mycophenolate mofetil
    - Used with steroids in some IgG4-TIN cases
  - Optimal treatment for IgG4-related MGN may differ from inflammatory manifestations of IgG4-RD

IMAGING

Ultrasonographic Findings

- Enlarged kidneys in some IgG4-TIN

CT Findings

- Radiographic abnormalities in some IgG4-TIN

- Single or multiple low-attenuation lesions, usually bilateral, in renal cortex
- Findings suggestive of vasculitis, lymphoma, or other tumor mass(es)
- Inflammatory lesions may extend beyond kidney
- Masses in other organs (e.g., pancreas, liver, lung) may give clue to renal diagnosis

MICROSCOPIC

Histologic Features

- Glomeruli
  - Membranous glomerulonephritis (MGN)
    - ~ 8% of cases in one IgG4-TIN series
    - May be present without or with little interstitial inflammation
    - Subepithelial deposits also IgG4 dominant
  - IgA nephropathy
    - May be coincidental, particularly in reports of IgG4-RD from Asia
  - Mild mesangial immune complex glomerulonephritis
    - Mild mesangial proliferation in some cases with IgG deposits, no specific diagnosis
  - Diabetic glomerulosclerosis
    - May be coincidental, or diabetes may be secondary to IgG4-related autoimmune pancreatitis (AIP) with resultant kidney disease
  - Minimal change disease
- Tubules and interstitium
  - Plasma cell-rich interstitial inflammation
    - Eosinophils often present and may be prominent
    - Paucity of neutrophils
  - Tubulitis with mononuclear cells, plasma cells, and eosinophils
  - Interstitial fibroinflammatory process, expansile interstitial fibrosis
  - Tubular atrophy and destruction of tubules by interstitial fibrosis
  - Thickened tubular basement membranes
  - Range of appearances
    - Some show more interstitial inflammation and less fibrosis
      - Acute interstitial nephritis pattern may be present but unusual
    - Other cases show more fibrosis and less inflammation
      - Cases with less inflammation often show fewer IgG4(+) plasma cells, but still > 10/HPF in most concentrated areas
      - IgG4/IgG(+) plasma cell ratio useful for cases with less inflammation and more fibrosis
  - Fibroinflammatory process may extend outside of kidney and involve surrounding organs
  - Presence of granulomatous inflammation or necrosis **excludes** diagnosis of IgG4-TIN
- Vessels
  - IgG4 plasma cell arteritis
    - Transmural inflammation with plasma cells (many IgG4[+])
    - Absence of fibrinoid necrosis
  - Obliterative phlebitis present in other organs affected by IgG4-RD, but not observed yet in kidneys

ANCILLARY TESTS

Immunohistochemistry

- Increased IgG4(+) plasma cells
  - At least moderate increase: > 10 IgG4(+) cells/40x field in most concentrated area
  - Some cases show marked increase, > 30 IgG4(+) cells/40x field
  - IgG4 staining ~ 100% sensitive and ~ 92% specific for detecting TIN related to IgG4(+) TIN vs. other types of plasma cell-rich interstitial nephritis
    - False-positives in interstitial infiltrate associated with pauci-immune necrotizing and crescentic glomerulonephritis
- Increased IgG4/IgG(+) plasma cell ratio
  - Ratio typically > 30% in IgG4-RD
    - Useful when fewer plasma cells present with more fibrosis or in treated patients
- Increased IgG4(+) plasma cells or high IgG4/IgG(+) plasma cell ratio not necessary for diagnosis, however, in presence of typical diagnostic histologic features
- Kappa and lambda immunoperoxidase or in situ hybridization reveal polytypic plasma cell population

Immunofluorescence

- Granular tubular basement membrane (TBM) immune complex deposits in > 80% of cases
  - IgG, C3, kappa and lambda light chains; accompanying IgM, IgA, &/or C1q present in ~ 10% of cases
  - IgG4(+) deposits; other IgG subclasses also variably present
  - Deposits may be focal; present in most but not all cases
  - Deposits present in areas of interstitial inflammation and fibrosis
  - TBM deposits typically **not** present in cases with histologic pattern of acute interstitial nephritis
- Granular interstitial deposits may be present
- Glomeruli usually negative by IF unless concurrent MGN or other immune complex glomerulonephritis

Electron Microscopy

- Amorphous electron-dense deposits within tubular basement membranes and in interstitium
- Thickened and laminated TBM
- Normal glomeruli unless concurrent immune complex glomerulonephritis

DIFFERENTIAL DIAGNOSIS

Pauci-Immune Necrotizing and Crescentic Glomerulonephritis/Granulomatosis With Polyangiitis

- May be mass-forming
- 25% of cases show at least moderate increase in IgG4(+) plasma cells in interstitial infiltrate
- Areas of necrosis in interstitial infiltrate may be present in granulomatosis with polyangiitis (Wegener)
  - Necrosis not present in IgG4-associated TIN
- Most cases ANCA(+)
- Absence of tubulointerstitial immune complex deposits

Drug-Induced Acute Interstitial Nephritis

- Both IgG4-TIN and allergic TIN can show numerous eosinophils
- IgG4-TIN shows more plasma cells and characteristic storiform fibrosis

Idiopathic Hypocomplementemic Tubulointerstitial Nephritis With Deposits

- Most cases of this entity represent IgG4-TIN and show increased IgG4(+) plasma cells

Sjögren Syndrome-Associated Tubulointerstitial Nephritis

- May be related to IgG4-associated autoimmune disease
- Usually no increase in IgG4(+) plasma cells
- Tubulointerstitial immune complex deposits
- Both IgG4-TIN and TIN secondary to Sjögren syndrome may have salivary gland involvement

Giant Cell Tubulitis With Tubular Basement Membrane Immune Deposits

- Probably represents allergic drug reaction
- Giant cells surrounding tubules
- TBM deposits

Tubulointerstitial Lupus Nephritis

- Usually biopsies show glomerular disease with glomerular immune deposits along with TBM or interstitial immune deposits
- Many IgG4-RD patients have low-titer positive ANA

Chronic Pyelonephritis

- May have appearance of mass on imaging studies
- Neutrophils in infiltrate in addition to plasma cells; neutrophilic casts may also be present
- Evidence of urinary tract bacterial infection

Lymphoma

- May be mass on radiographic studies
- Atypical and monotypic cellular infiltrate
- Rare cases show TBM immune complex deposits by IF
- Immunohistochemical studies can confirm monoclonal infiltrate

Interstitial Inflammation With TBM Deposits Associated With Glomerular Disease

- Minority of MGN or other immune complex GN show TBM immune complex deposits

Monoclonal Immunoglobulin Deposition Disease (MIDD)

- Linear vs. granular TBM deposits in MIDD
- Monoclonal immune deposits by IF

Renal Neoplasm

- Imaging studies often suggest neoplasm
- Inflammation may be misinterpreted as missing the tumor

Membranous Glomerulonephritis (Primary or Secondary)

- MGN may be secondary to systemic lupus erythematosus or other autoimmune diseases

DIAGNOSTIC CHECKLIST

Pathologic Interpretation Pearls

- Needle biopsy sometimes performed for renal mass
  - Inflammatory process may be misinterpreted as reaction around tumor, and specimen considered inadequate for diagnosis
- Exclusion of ANCA-related inflammation necessary

SELECTED REFERENCES

1. Khosroshahi A et al: International consensus guidance statement on the management and treatment of IgG4-related disease. Arthritis Rheumatol. ePub, 2015
2. Wallace ZS et al: Plasmablasts as a biomarker for IgG4-related disease, independent of serum IgG4 concentrations. Ann Rheum Dis. 74(1):190-5, 2015
3. Kamisawa T et al: IgG4-related disease. Lancet. ePub, 2014
4. Khosroshahi A et al: Brief report: spuriously low serum IgG4 concentrations caused by the prozone phenomenon in patients with IgG4-related disease. Arthritis Rheumatol. 66(1):213-7, 2014
5. Mattoo H et al: De novo oligoclonal expansions of circulating plasmablasts in active and relapsing IgG4-related disease. J Allergy Clin Immunol. 134(3):679-87, 2014
6. Alexander MP et al: Membranous glomerulonephritis is a manifestation of IgG4-related disease. Kidney Int. 83(3):455-62, 2013
7. Rispens T et al: Fc-Fc interactions of human IgG4 require dissociation of heavy chains and are formed predominantly by the intra-chain hinge isomer. Mol Immunol. 53(1-2):35-42, 2013
8. Sharma SG et al: IgG4-related tubulointerstitial nephritis with plasma cell-rich renal arteritis. Am J Kidney Dis. 61(4):638-43, 2013
9. Cornell LD: IgG4-related kidney disease. Curr Opin Nephrol Hypertens. 21(3):279-88, 2012
10. Deshpande V et al: Consensus statement on the pathology of IgG4-related disease. Mod Pathol. 25(9):1181-92, 2012
11. Stone JH et al: Recommendations for the nomenclature of IgG4-related disease and its individual organ system manifestations. Arthritis Rheum. 64(10):3061-7, 2012
12. Stone JH et al: IgG4-related disease. N Engl J Med. 366(6):539-51, 2012
13. Raissian Y et al: Diagnosis of IgG4-related tubulointerstitial nephritis. J Am Soc Nephrol. 22(7):1343-52, 2011
14. Sah RP et al: Serologic issues in IgG4-related systemic disease and autoimmune pancreatitis. Curr Opin Rheumatol. 23(1):108-13, 2011
15. Cheuk W et al: IgG4-related sclerosing disease: a critical appraisal of an evolving clinicopathologic entity. Adv Anat Pathol. 17(5):303-32, 2010
16. Saeki T et al: Clinicopathological characteristics of patients with IgG4-related tubulointerstitial nephritis. Kidney Int. 78(10):1016-23, 2010
17. Aalberse RC et al: Immunoglobulin G4: an odd antibody. Clin Exp Allergy. 39(4):469-77, 2009
18. Cornell LD et al: Pseudotumors due to IgG4 immune-complex tubulointerstitial nephritis associated with autoimmune pancreatocentric disease. Am J Surg Pathol. 31(10):1586-97, 2007
19. Deshpande V et al: Autoimmune pancreatitis: a systemic immune complex mediated disease. Am J Surg Pathol. 2006 Dec;30(12):1537-45. Erratum in: Am J Surg Pathol. 31(2):328, 2007
20. Aalberse RC et al: IgG4 breaking the rules. Immunology. 105(1):9-19, 2002
21. Kambham N et al: Idiopathic hypocomplementemic interstitial nephritis with extensive tubulointerstitial deposits. Am J Kidney Dis. 37(2):388-99, 2001

(Left) In IgG4-TIN, partially atrophic tubules are pushed apart by fibroinflammatory tissue. "Storiform" fibrosis ➡ is present in the interstitium. (Right) A biopsy from a case of IgG4-TIN shows a dense interstitial infiltrate with plasma cells and eosinophils ➡ as well as a lymphoid follicle ➡.

IgG4-TIN

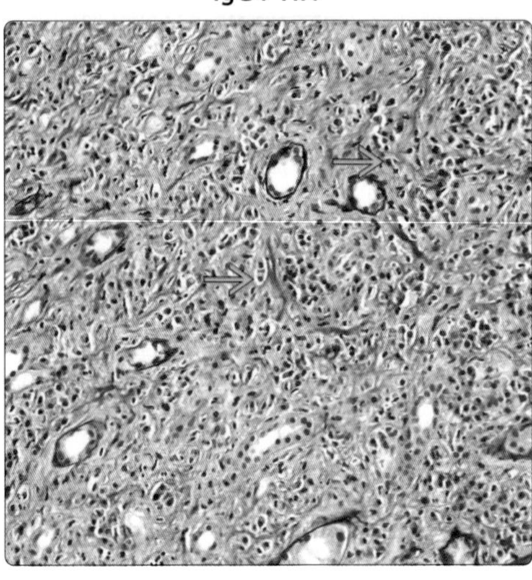

Lymphoid Follicle in IgG4-TIN

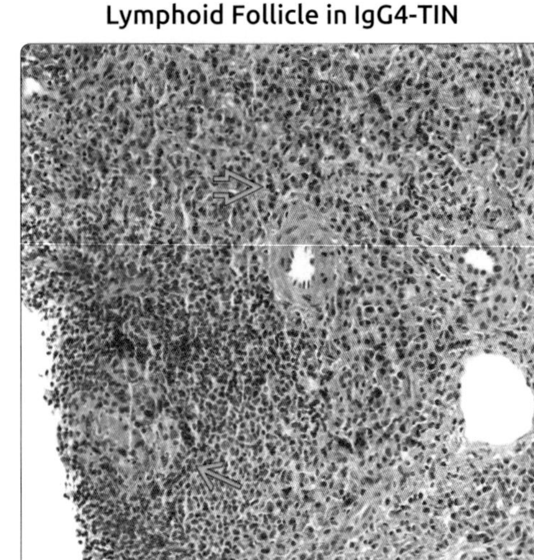

(Left) This biopsy came from a 72-year-old man with chronic renal failure and heterogeneous renal masses; he had elevated serum IgG levels and a history of primary biliary cirrhosis. The biopsy reveals a diffuse, expansile interstitial nephritis within the cortex. (Right) In IgG4-TIN, a plasma cell-rich, expansile interstitial nephritis is characteristic and shows fibrosis and destruction of the tubules. Scattered eosinophils ➡ are present and do not imply an allergic drug reaction.

IgG4-TIN

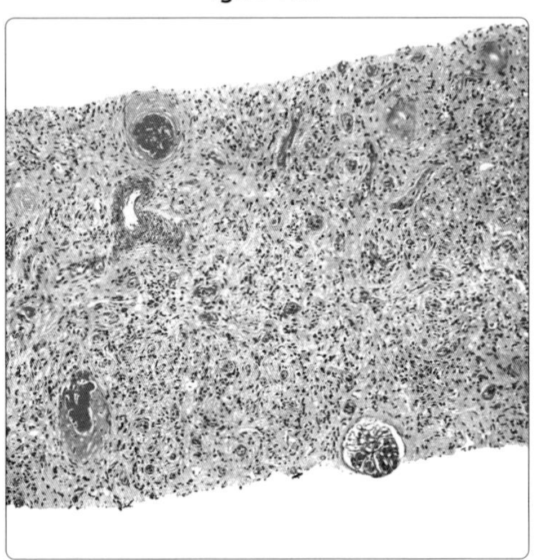

IgG4-TIN

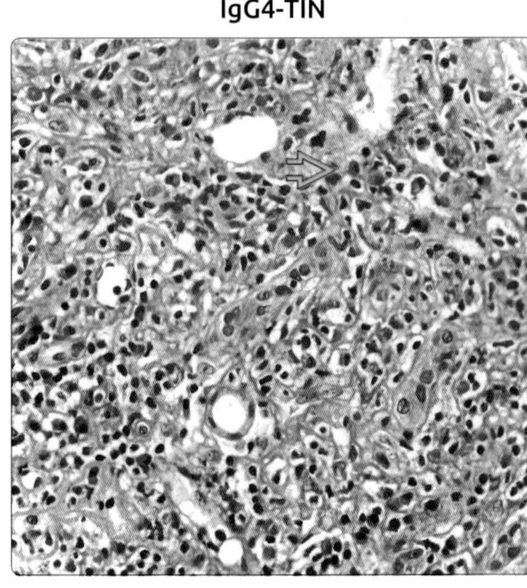

(Left) A nephrectomy specimen shows a mass-forming lesion composed of a fibroinflammatory infiltrate. Note the increased inflammation (darker blue areas) on the edge ➡ of the lesion, with more fibrosis in the center ➡. Glomeruli ➡ are present scattered throughout the mass lesion. (Right) A nephrectomy performed for a mass lesion shows dense fibrosis ➡ closer to the center of the mass, with increased inflammation ➡ and lymphoid follicles ➡ closer to the edge of the lesion.

Mass Lesion in IgG4-TIN

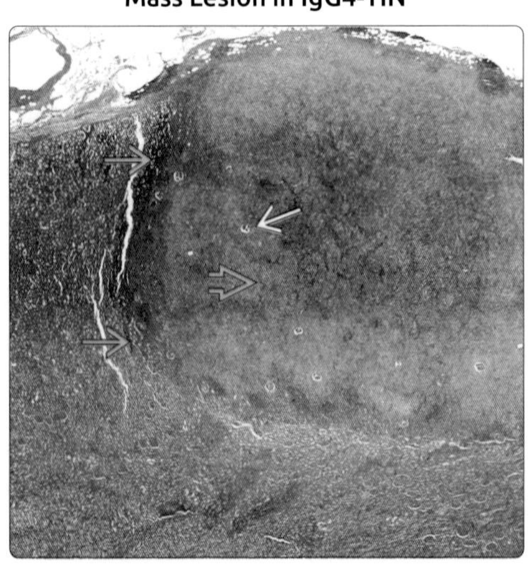

Mass Lesion in IgG4-TIN

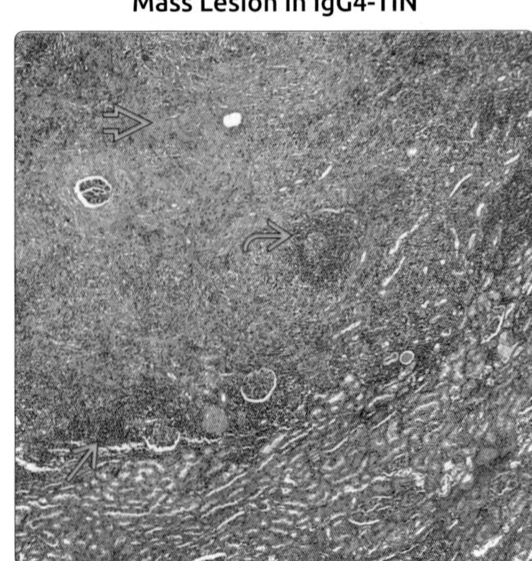

IgG4-TIN With Increased IgG4(+) Plasma Cells

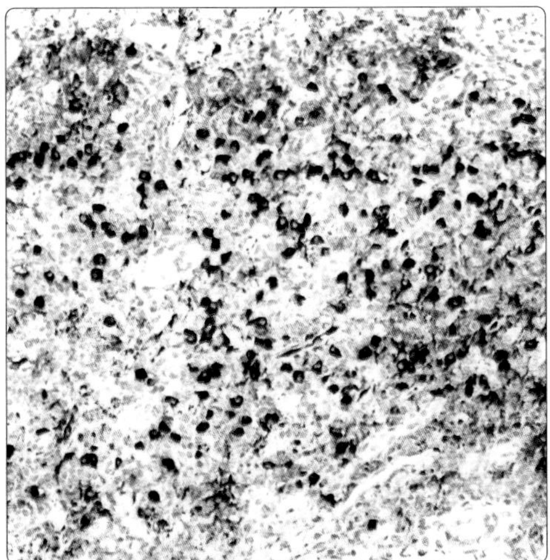

IgG4(+) TBM Deposits

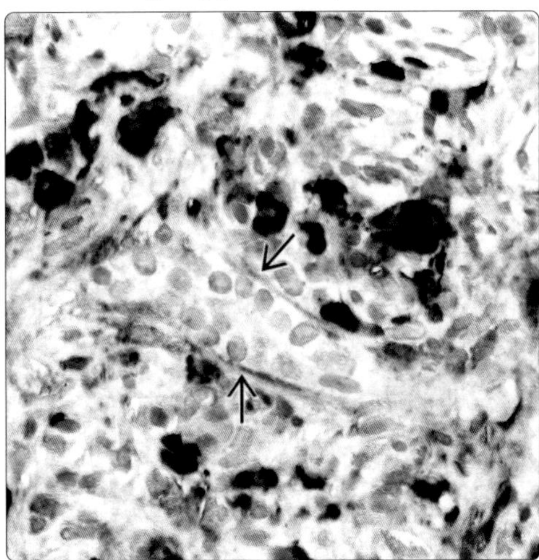

(Left) *An immunohistochemical stain for IgG4 reveals numerous (> 30/40x field) IgG4-positive plasma cells, a feature that helps to distinguish IgG4-TIN from other types of TIN, although an increase in IgG4(+) cells is not specific for IgG4-TIN.* **(Right)** *Tubular basement membrane granular deposits ➡ can be seen in this IgG4 immunohistochemical stain. The densely stained cells are IgG4(+) plasma cells. Of note, immunoperoxidase staining is less sensitive than immunofluorescence for detection of TBM deposits.*

IgG4(+) Cells in Lymphoid Follicle

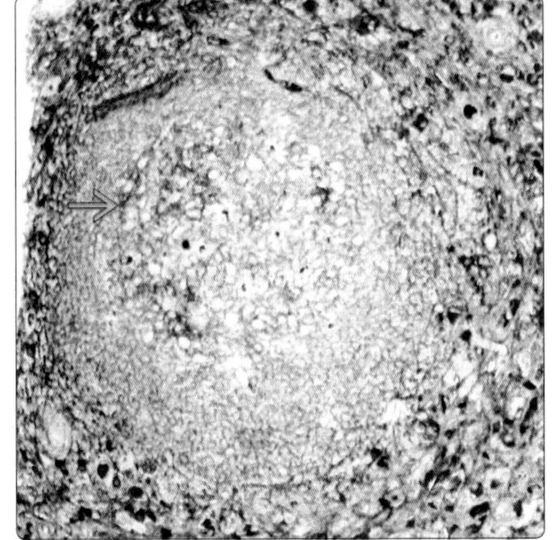

IgG4-TIN With Few IgG4(+) Plasma Cells

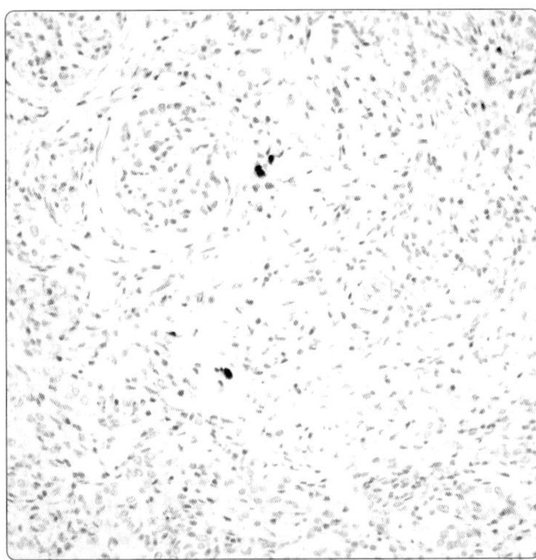

(Left) *A lymphoid follicle in this case of IgG4-TIN shows IgG4(+) cells polarized ➡ on 1 side of the follicle.* **(Right)** *Despite a renal mass lesion and typical histology on this specimen, there were very few IgG4(+) plasma cells. A diagnosis of IgG4-TIN may still be made with typical histology and other supporting clinical and laboratory features.*

IgG4(+) Plasma Cells in IgG4-TIN

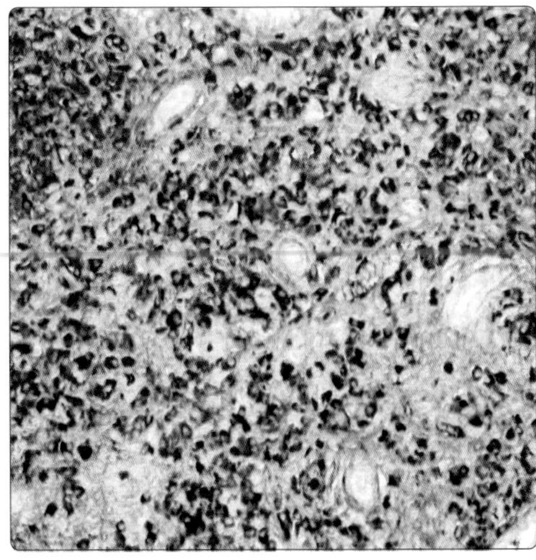

IgG(+) Plasma Cells in IgG4-TIN

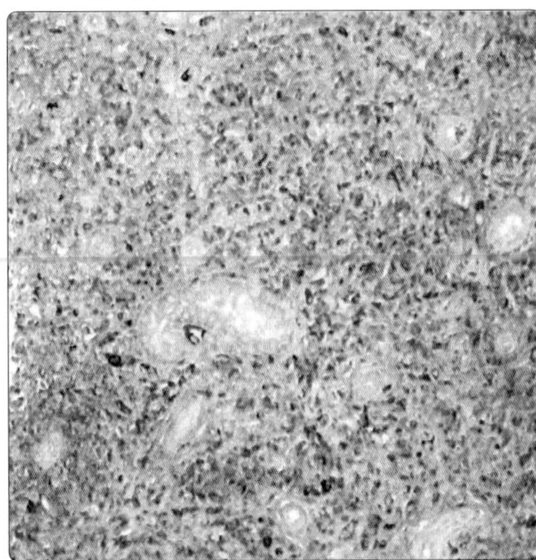

(Left) *Immunoperoxidase stain for IgG4 shows a marked increase in IgG4(+) plasma cells in this case of IgG4-TIN.* **(Right)** *Immunoperoxidase stain for IgG shows numerous IgG(+) plasma cells; this biopsy showed a very high IgG4/IgG(+) plasma cell ratio.*

IgG4-TIN With Few IgG4(+) Plasma Cells

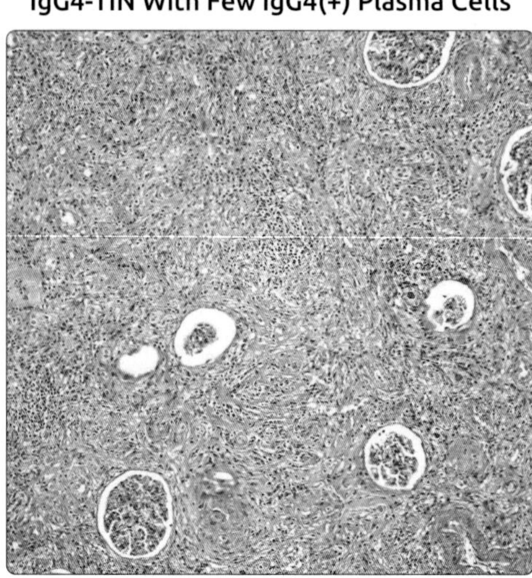

IgG4-TIN

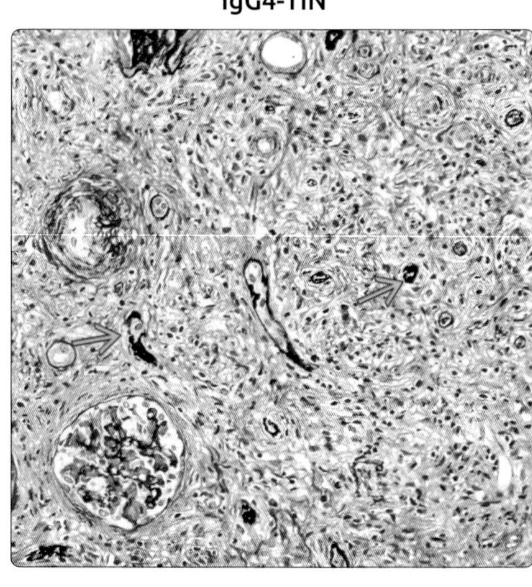

(Left) *A nephrectomy specimen performed for a mass shows mass-forming tubulointerstitial nephritis with increased plasma cells and storiform fibrosis. Despite typical histology, few IgG4(+) plasma cells were present on the immunoperoxidase stain, and there was a low IgG4/IgG(+) plasma cell ratio.* **(Right)** *A silver stain nicely highlights the residual basement membranes ➡ of destroyed tubules. Glomeruli show only secondary changes of periglomerular fibrosis and global glomerulosclerosis.*

Interstitial Crescent in IgG4-TIN

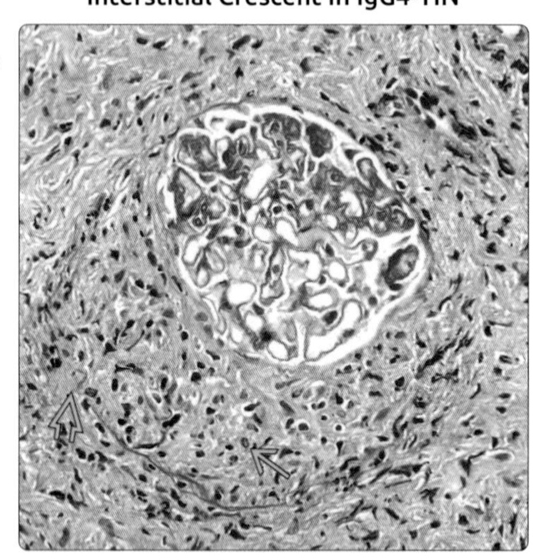

Interstitial Crescent in IgG4-TIN

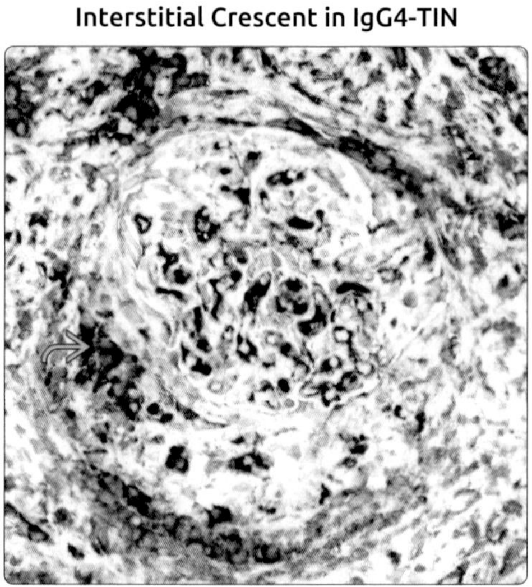

(Left) *Sometimes in IgG4-TIN, the fibroinflammatory process involves Bowman capsule similarly to the TBMs. Here, a crescent-like structure ➡ is seen, but in the absence of glomerulonephritis and without necrosis. Bowman capsule is disrupted ➡ by the process.* **(Right)** *An interstitial crescent in IgG4-TIN shows infiltrating IgG4(+) plasma cells ➡.*

Storiform Fibrosis in IgG4-TIN

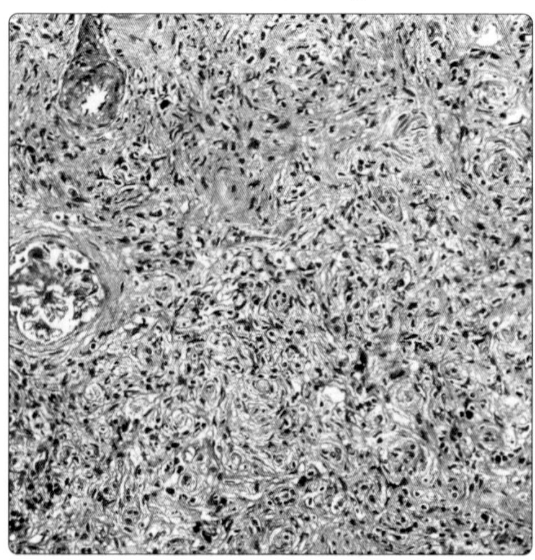

Fibrosis in Kidney Transplant

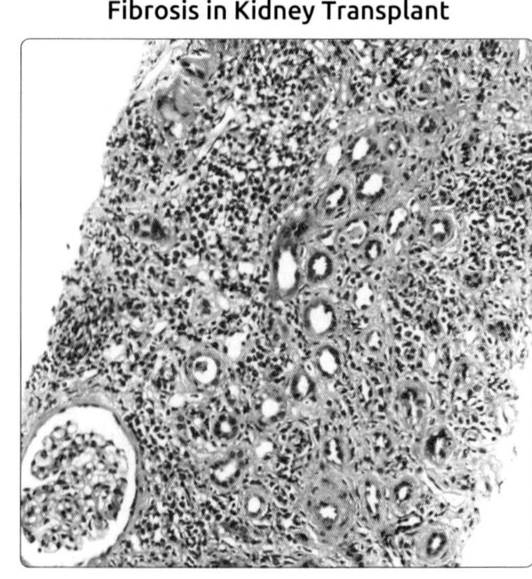

(Left) *A trichrome stain reveals extensive interstitial fibrosis, which was present diffusely throughout the cortex, and profound loss of tubules. This fibrosis is expansile and pushes apart the tubules and the glomeruli.* **(Right)** *As opposed to the expansile and storiform fibrosis seen in IgG4-TIN, this example of fibrosis with inflammation in a kidney transplant recipient shows tubules that are compressed together.*

TBM Immune Complex Deposits

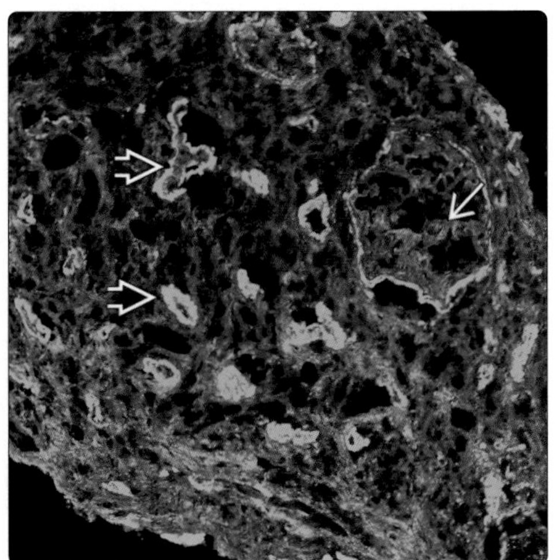

TBM Deposits for C3 in IgG4-TIN

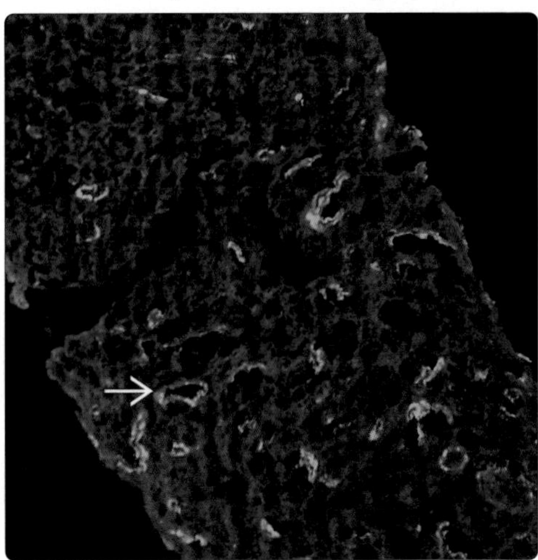

(Left) *Immunofluorescence for IgG reveals granular tubular basement membrane* ➡ *and Bowman capsule deposits. Similar staining was seen for C3, kappa, and lambda. The glomerular tuft is negative* ➡. *Staining was similar for kappa and lambda light chains.* **(Right)** *Immunofluorescence staining for C3 often shows less bright staining of TBMs* ➡ *compared to IgG, kappa, and lambda.*

TBM Deposits in IgG4-TIN

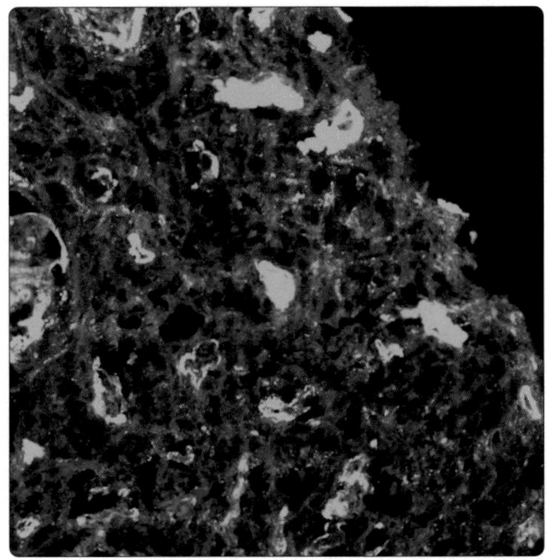

TBM Deposits in IgG4-TIN

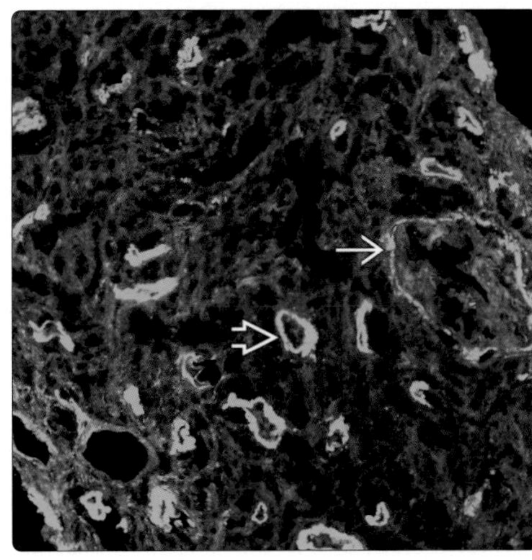

(Left) *Immunofluorescence for kappa light chain shows the same staining pattern as IgG, with granular tubular basement membrane staining, and was equal to lambda staining.* **(Right)** *Immunofluorescence for lambda light chain shows the same staining pattern as IgG and kappa light chain* ➡. *Note the glomerulus that shows Bowman capsule staining but no glomerular tuft staining* ➡.

TBM Deposits in IgG4-TIN

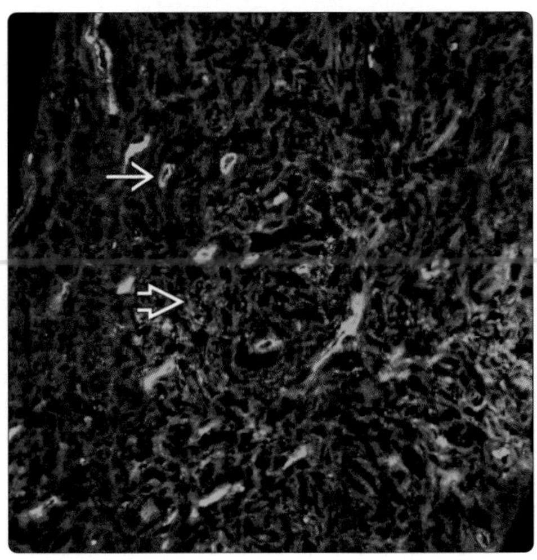

TBM Deposits in IgG4-TIN

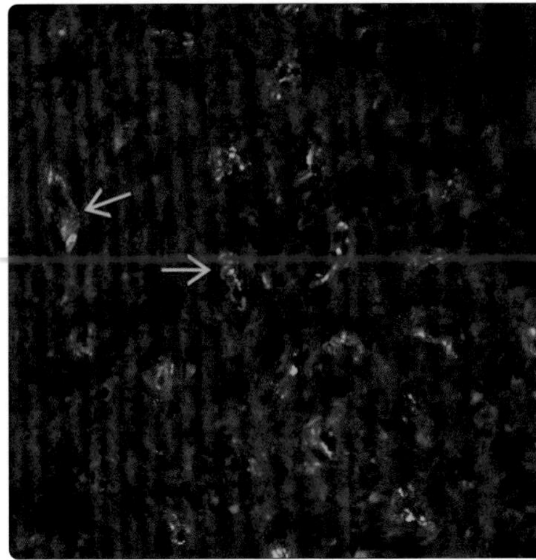

(Left) *Immunofluorescence for IgG4 shows bright staining of TBM* ➡ *and interstitial* ➡ *deposits. Other IgG subclasses were also variably present.* **(Right)** *In ~ 10% of cases of IgG4-TIN, the TBMs show granular staining for C1q* ➡, *which is usually dim.*

(Left) *CT scan in a patient with IgG4-TIN shows bilateral mass lesions ⇒ in the kidneys. On biopsy, these lesions show tubulointerstitial nephritis.* (Right) *Massive immune deposits ⇒ within and surrounding a tubular basement membrane are evident in this case and were seen in trichrome stains by light microscopy.*

Renal Mass Lesions in IgG4-TIN

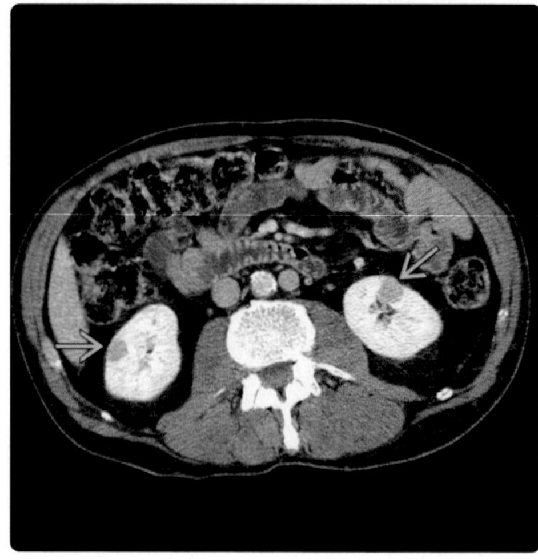

TBM Deposits in IgG4-TIN

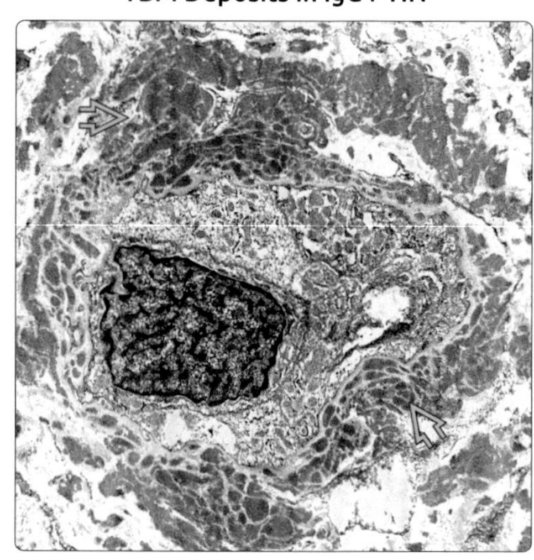

(Left) *Electron microscopy reveals interstitial leukocytes, increased collagen deposition in the interstitium, and a few residual tubular basement membranes containing immune deposits ⇒.* (Right) *This residual destroyed tubule shows a markedly thickened basement membrane that contains electron-dense immune deposits ⇒.*

TBM Immune Complex Deposits

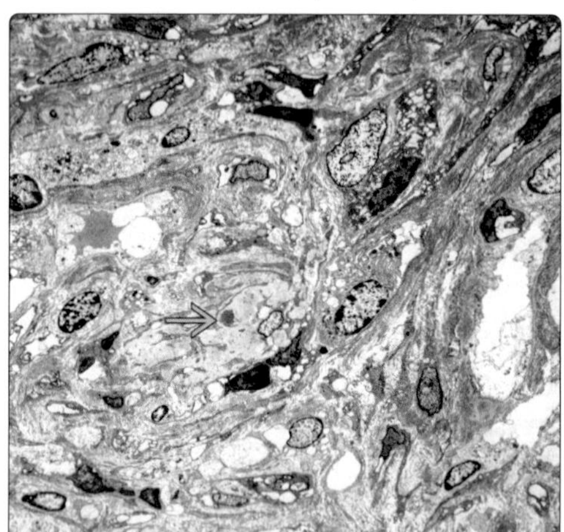

Electron-Dense TBM Deposits

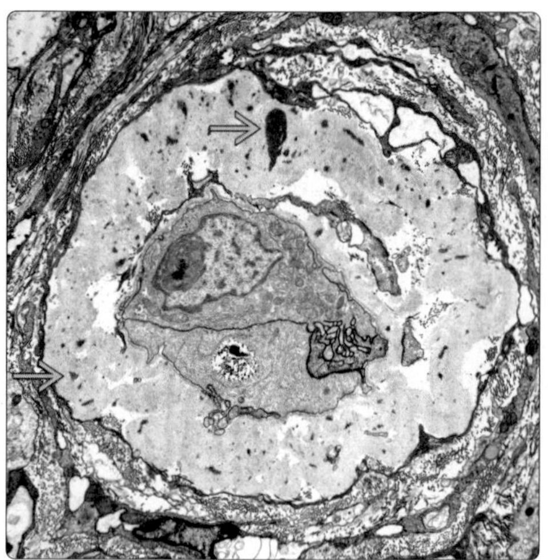

(Left) *Amorphous electron-dense deposits ⇒ are seen in a thickened tubular basement membrane.* (Right) *In IgG4-TIN, glomeruli usually do not show immune deposits. Rare cases of IgG4-associated tubulointerstitial nephritis have been associated with membranous glomerulonephritis. This glomerulus appears ischemic and shows basement membrane wrinkling.*

TBM Deposits

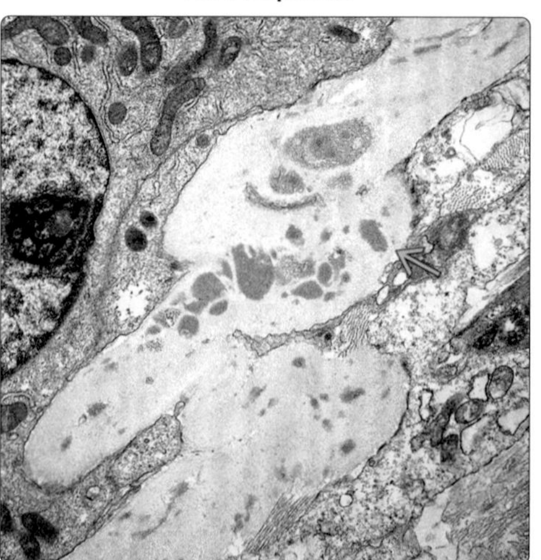

Glomerulus in IgG4-TIN

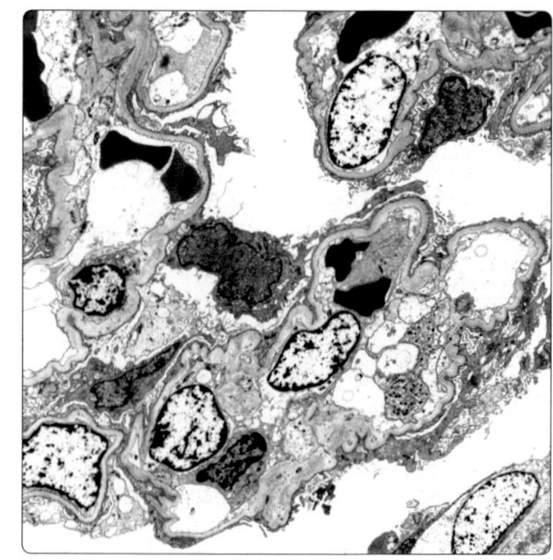

IgG4-MGN Without TIN

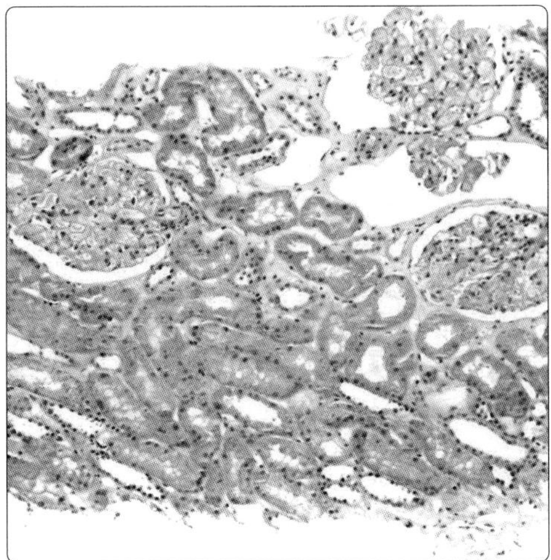

MGN in IgG4-RD

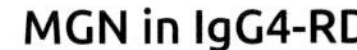

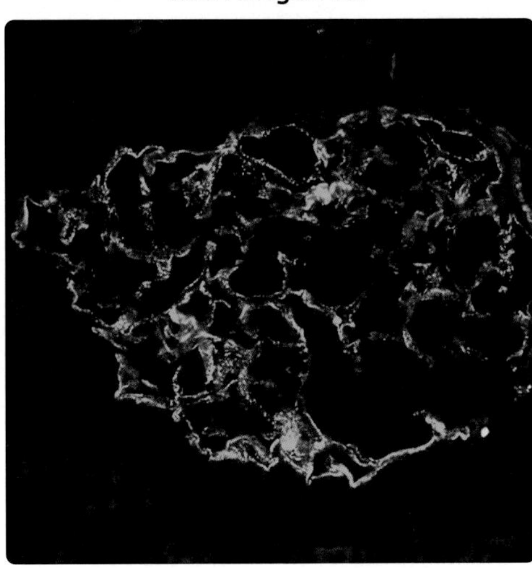

(Left) *This biopsy from a patient with nephrotic syndrome shows normal-appearing glomeruli by light microscopy and no interstitial inflammation. The patient had a history of IgG4-RD, with autoimmune pancreatitis and sclerosing cholangitis. Immunofluorescence showed MGN.* **(Right)** *Immunofluorescence staining for IgG shows global granular glomerular basement membrane staining with subepithelial deposits (membranous pattern) in a patient with concurrent IgG4-TIN on the kidney biopsy.*

Subepithelial Deposits in MGN

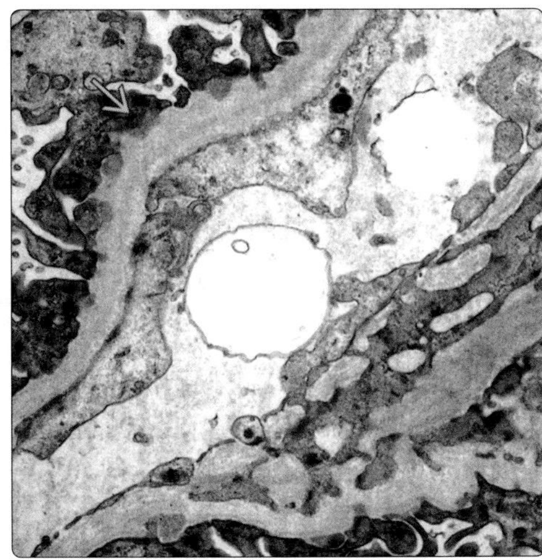

MGN and Diabetes in IgG4-RD

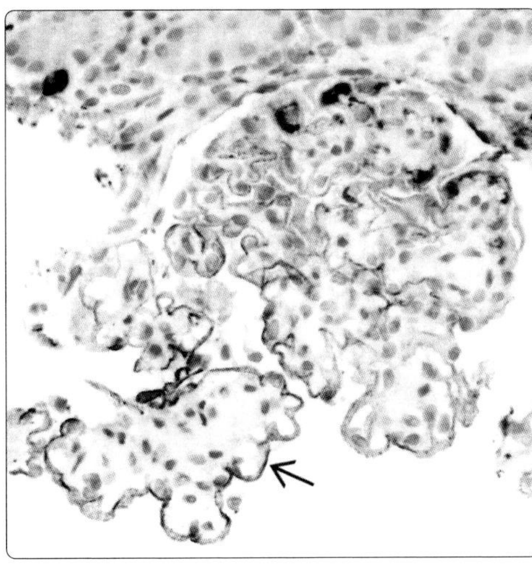

(Left) *By electron microscopy, subepithelial deposits ⇨ are seen along the glomerular basement membranes in this case of MGN associated with IgG4-RD. The electron-dense deposits do not show substructure.* **(Right)** *An immunoperoxidase stain for IgG4 shows granular staining along glomerular basement membranes ⇨ in this case of IgG4-RD with MGN and diabetic glomerulosclerosis. IgG4-TIN was also present. Immunoperoxidase staining is less sensitive than immunofluorescence for detection of these deposits.*

IgG4 Plasma Cell Arteritis

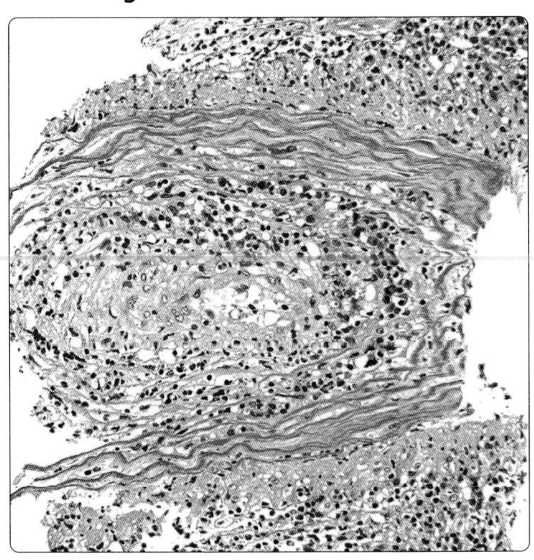

IgG4 Plasma Cell Arteritis

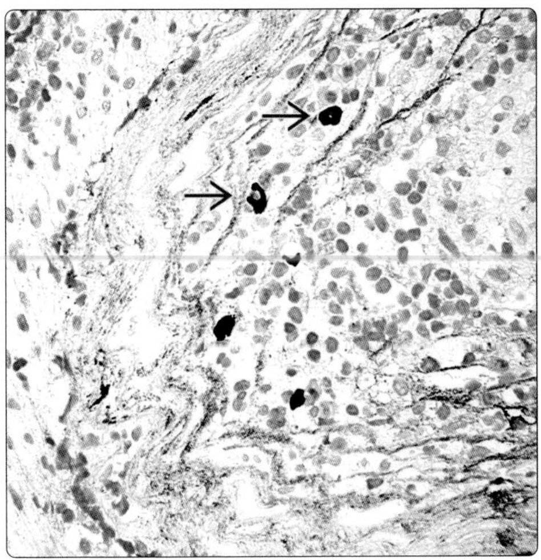

(Left) *Plasma cells, including IgG4(+) plasma cells, infiltrate the walls of this artery in a kidney biopsy specimen showing IgG4-TIN. No fibrinoid necrosis is present. (Courtesy V.D. D'Agati, MD and S. Sharma, MD.)* **(Right)** *IgG4(+) plasma cells ⇨ are present in the walls of this artery in a kidney biopsy specimen that showed IgG4-TIN. (Courtesy V.D. D'Agati, MD and S. Sharma, MD.)*

KEY FACTS

TERMINOLOGY

- Tubulointerstitial nephritis with polyclonal tubular basement membrane (TBM) deposits and hypocomplementemia

CLINICAL ISSUES

- Average ~ 65 years
- Male predominance (M:F = 7:1 in 1 series)
- Renal dysfunction with little proteinuria
  - Improvement with immunosuppressive therapy
- Low serum complement levels
- No history of Sjögren syndrome or SLE
  - Negative or low-titer positive ANA

MICROSCOPIC

- Prominent tubulointerstitial nephritis
  - Lymphocytes, plasma cells, and sometimes eosinophils
- Destruction of tubules and interstitial fibrosis
- Glomeruli relatively spared

ANCILLARY TESTS

- Granular TBM and interstitial deposits of IgG and C3
  - IgG in all cases; often C3 deposits
  - IgE(+) TBM deposits may be present
  - Kappa and lambda equal
  - Glomeruli usually negative
- TBM and interstitial deposits by EM
  - Usually amorphous; few cases with fingerprint substructure
  - No glomerular deposits

TOP DIFFERENTIAL DIAGNOSES

- IgG4-related tubulointerstitial nephritis
- Sjögren syndrome
- Giant cell tubulitis with TBM immune deposits
- Lupus nephritis
- Anti-TBM nephritis
- Monoclonal immunoglobulin deposition disease
- TIN associated with glomerular disease

Interstitial Inflammation

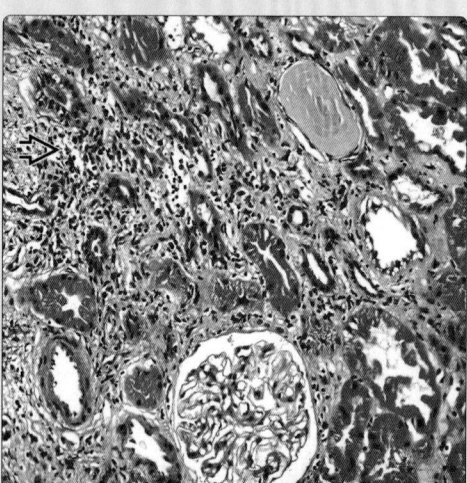

Masson Trichrome

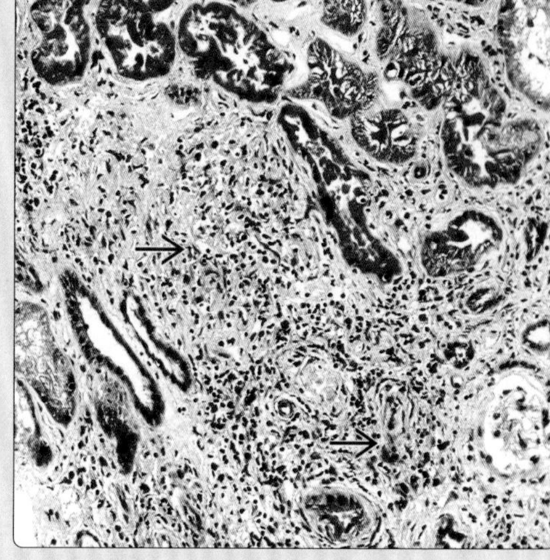

(Left) *The predominant lesion in hypocomplementemic tubulointerstitial nephritis (HTIN) is focal interstitial inflammation ⇨ with tubular damage and fibrosis; glomeruli are relatively spared. This specimen is from a 69-year-old man who had progressive chronic renal failure, a low-titer ANA, and no clinical evidence of liver disease, pancreatitis, or systemic lupus.* **(Right)** *In HTIN, a trichrome stain highlights the interstitial fibrosis, areas of which show inflammation and tubular destruction. Remnants of tubules are evident →.*

IgG

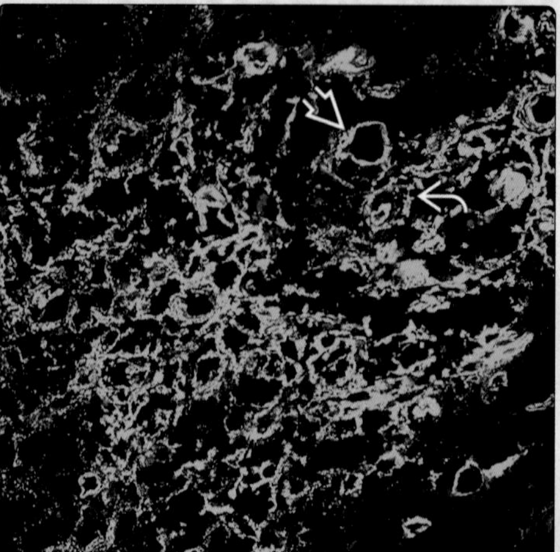

TBM Deposits

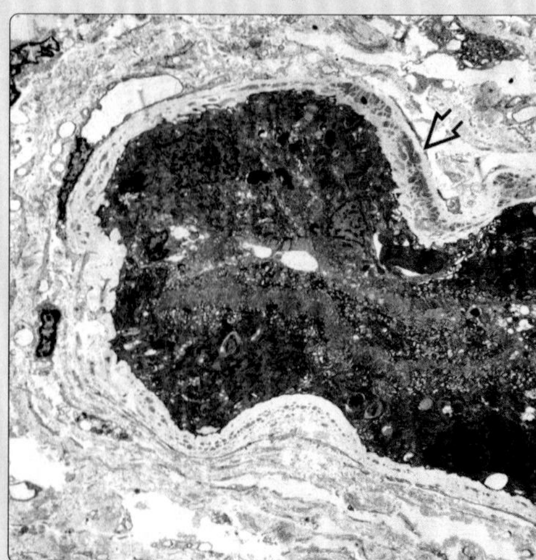

(Left) *Immunofluorescence staining for IgG in HTIN reveals prominent granular tubular basement membrane ⇨ and interstitial deposits ↩.* **(Right)** *By electron microscopy, the tubular basement membranes are thickened and duplicated. Electron-dense, immune-type deposits are widespread in the tubular basement membrane (TBM) ⇨.*

TERMINOLOGY

Abbreviations

- Hypocomplementemic tubulointerstitial nephritis (HTIN)

Definitions

- Tubulointerstitial nephritis with polyclonal tubular basement membrane (TBM) deposits and hypocomplementemia

ETIOLOGY/PATHOGENESIS

Antibody Deposition in TBM

- Immune complexes formed, probably locally
  - Antigen unknown
- Local complement fixation
  - Promotion of inflammation, tubular injury

CLINICAL ISSUES

Epidemiology

- Age
  - Average ~ 65 years
- Sex
  - Male predominance (M:F = 7:1 in 1 series)

Presentation

- Renal dysfunction
- No significant proteinuria or hematuria
- No history of Sjögren syndrome or SLE
- Hypocomplementemia

Laboratory Tests

- Low serum complement levels
- Negative ANA or low-titer positive ANA

Treatment

- Drugs
  - May respond to prednisone

Prognosis

- Improvement with immunosuppressive therapy

IMAGING

Radiographic Findings

- No cases forming masses, in contrast to IgG4-associated TIN

MICROSCOPIC

Histologic Features

- Glomeruli
  - No specific findings
  - Secondary glomerulosclerosis in advanced cases
- Tubules
  - Tubulitis, mononuclear
  - Thickened TBM
  - Destruction and atrophy of tubules in advanced cases
- Interstitium
  - Marked mononuclear inflammation
    - Polytypic infiltrate
    - T cells, B cells, plasma cells
      - Eosinophils sometimes present
    - Lymphocytes may appear atypical, suggesting extranodal marginal zone B-cell lymphoma

ANCILLARY TESTS

Immunofluorescence

- Granular TBM and interstitial deposits of immunoglobulin and complement components
  - IgG and complement in all cases; usually C3 and C1q
  - Variable IgM staining; rare IgA staining
  - Kappa and lambda equal
- Sometimes mesangial deposits with same reactants

Genetic Testing

- B cells and T cells usually polyclonal

Electron Microscopy

- TBM and interstitial immune complex deposits
  - Usually amorphous; few with fingerprint substructure
- No glomerular deposits

DIFFERENTIAL DIAGNOSIS

IgG4-Related Tubulointerstitial Nephritis (IgG4-TIN)

- Systemic disease: Autoimmune pancreatitis, sclerosing cholangitis, inflammatory lesions in other organs
  - May be mass forming on radiographic studies
- Increased IgG4(+) plasma cells in infiltrate
- Elevated serum IgG4
- May also have hypocomplementemia
  - May be related to hypocomplementemic TIN
- Probably most or all cases of hypocomplementemic TIN represent IgG4-TIN

Sjögren Syndrome

- May show hypocomplementemia and tubulointerstitial immune complex deposits

Giant Cell Tubulitis With Tubular Basement Membrane Immune Deposits

- Multinucleated giant cells surrounding tubules

Anti-TBM Disease

- Linear polyclonal TBM immunoglobulin deposits

Lupus Nephritis

- Rare cases of lupus TIN without glomerular deposits

SELECTED REFERENCES

1. Kidder D et al: The case. Idiopathic hypocomplementemic interstitial nephritis. Diagnosis: Idiopathic hypocomplementemic tubulointerstitial nephritis. Kidney Int. 87(2):485-6, 2015
2. Saeki T et al: Clinicopathological characteristics of patients with IgG4-related tubulointerstitial nephritis. Kidney Int. 78(10):1016-23, 2010
3. Cornell LD et al: Pseudotumors due to IgG4 immune-complex tubulointerstitial nephritis associated with autoimmune pancreatocentric disease. Am J Surg Pathol. 31(10):1586-97, 2007
4. Vaseemuddin M et al: Idiopathic hypocomplementemic immune-complex-mediated tubulointerstitial nephritis. Nat Clin Pract Nephrol. 3(1):50-8, 2007
5. Mihindukulasuriya JC et al: Idiopathic hypocomplementemic interstitial nephritis with extensive tubulointerstitial deposits: Reversal of subacute renal failure with mycophenolate mofetil and corticosteroids [Abstract]. J Am Soc Nephrol 14: 800A, 2003
6. Kambham N et al: Idiopathic hypocomplementemic interstitial nephritis with extensive tubulointerstitial deposits. Am J Kidney Dis. 37(2):388-99, 2001

Anti-Tubular Basement Membrane Disease

KEY FACTS

TERMINOLOGY

- Renal disease caused by autoantibodies to TBM; antibodies arise as primary or secondary event

ETIOLOGY/PATHOGENESIS

- Primary idiopathic disease (rare)
- Associated with other diseases
  - Familial MGN anti-TBM syndrome
  - Drug-induced tubulointerstitial nephritis
  - Renal allograft rejection
  - Kimura disease
  - Oxalosis post-jejunoileal bypass
  - Aristolochic acid (Chinese herb nephropathy)

CLINICAL ISSUES

- Chronic renal failure
- Polyuria, polydipsia, proteinuria

MICROSCOPIC

- Mononuclear infiltrate, rarely giant cells
- Tubulitis
- Tubular atrophy and fibrosis
- Immunofluorescence shows linear staining of proximal TBM for IgG and C3
  - No linear GBM staining

TOP DIFFERENTIAL DIAGNOSES

- Tubulointerstitial nephritis with uveitis
- Sjögren syndrome
- Immune complex-mediated tubulointerstitial nephritis

DIAGNOSTIC CHECKLIST

- Requires linear IgG along TBM: C3 alone is commonly present in TBM as nonspecific finding
- Serum anti-TBM activity detected by indirect IF on normal kidney (proximal tubule TBM[+], distal TBM and GBM [-])

(Left) *Linear staining of the proximal tubular basement membrane (TBM) is the 1st clue that anti-TBM antibodies are present. This case was associated with methicillin interstitial nephritis.* **(Right)** *Methicillin hypersensitivity with aTBM antibodies is shown. An extensive infiltrate is present, which focally invades the tubules ➡.*

Linear TBM IgG Deposition

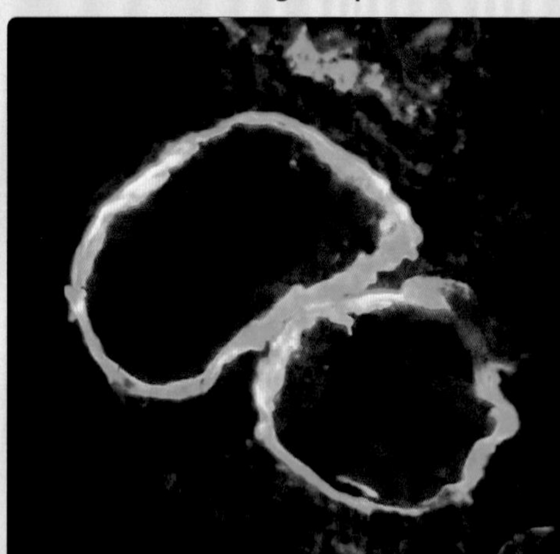

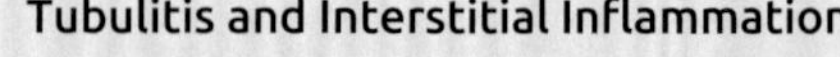

Tubulitis and Interstitial Inflammation

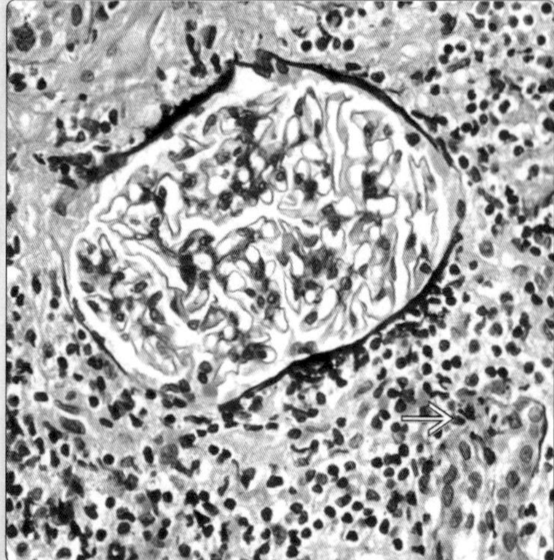

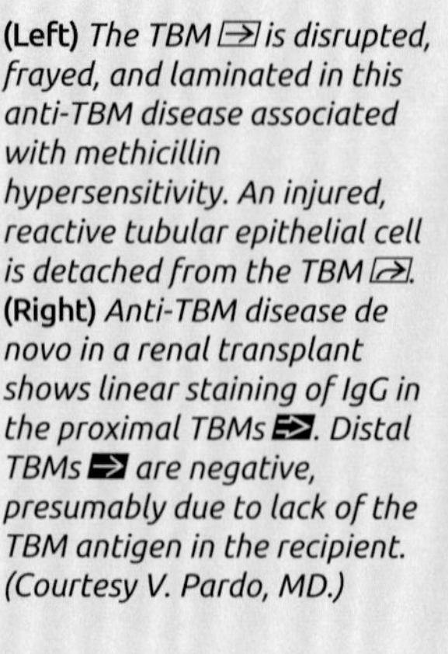

(Left) *The TBM → is disrupted, frayed, and laminated in this anti-TBM disease associated with methicillin hypersensitivity. An injured, reactive tubular epithelial cell is detached from the TBM ↗.* **(Right)** *Anti-TBM disease de novo in a renal transplant shows linear staining of IgG in the proximal TBMs ➡. Distal TBMs ➡ are negative, presumably due to lack of the TBM antigen in the recipient. (Courtesy V. Pardo, MD.)*

Disrupted TBM

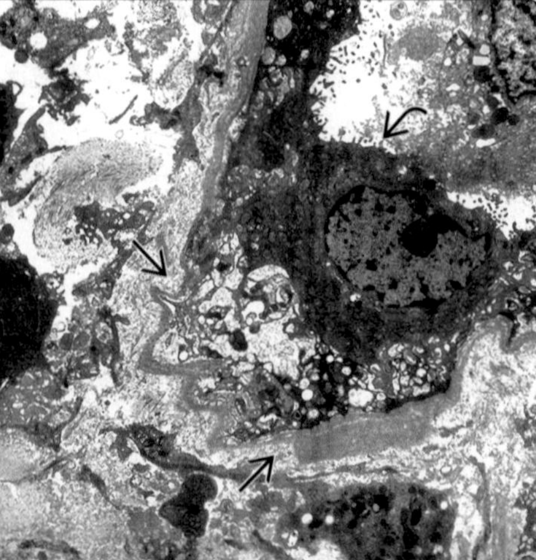

Renal Transplant With Anti-TBM Disease

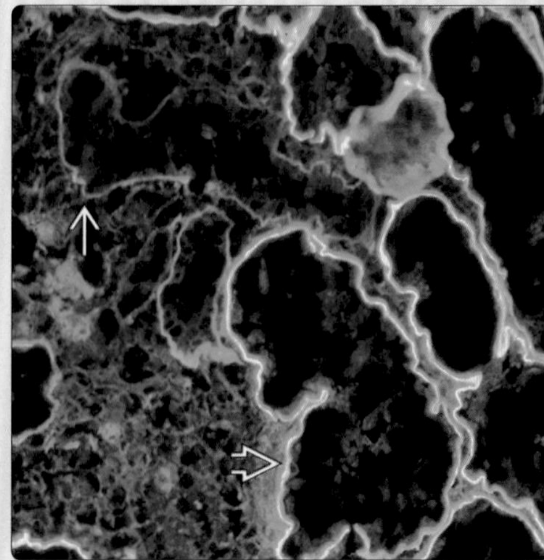

TERMINOLOGY

Abbreviations

- Anti-TBM (aTBM) disease

Definitions

- Renal disease caused by autoantibodies to tubular basement membrane (TBM); antibodies arise as primary or secondary event

ETIOLOGY/PATHOGENESIS

Antibody-Mediated Disease

- TBM antigen
  - Noncollagenous 54-58 kD protein in proximal tubular basement membranes
  - Expressed only in kidneys (adult and fetal)
    - Chromosome 6p11.2-12
    - Homology to follistatin, agrin, osteonectin/SPARC; laminin-α-1, vitronectin
  - Reduced or absent expression in some cases of juvenile nephronophthisis

Conditions Anti-TBM Antibodies Arise

- Primary diseases
  - Idiopathic tubulointerstitial nephritis
  - Membranous glomerulonephritis (MGN) in children, familial
- Secondary to other renal diseases
  - Drug-induced tubulointerstitial nephritis
  - Aristolochic acid (Chinese herb nephropathy)
  - Kimura disease
  - Oxalosis post-jejunoileal bypass
- Renal allografts
  - Presumably due to lack of TBM alloantigen in recipient

Cell-Mediated Component

- Mononuclear cells likely contribute to damage

Animal Models

- Strain 13 guinea pigs immunized with autologous TBM develop interstitial nephritis over several weeks
- Lewis rats lack TBM antigen and develop aTBM disease in allografts from Fisher 344 strain

CLINICAL ISSUES

Epidemiology

- Rare

Presentation

- Polyuria, polydipsia
- Chronic renal failure
- Microhematuria
- Proteinuria
  - Nephrotic in those with MGN

Treatment

- Steroids often used
- Stop drug use if disease is drug associated

Prognosis

- Outcome uncertain; can lead to renal failure

MICROSCOPIC

Histologic Features

- Glomeruli normal, unless other disease
- Tubules
  - Tubulitis, atrophy
  - Destruction of TBM on PAS stains
- Interstitium
  - Mononuclear infiltrate
    - T cells, macrophages
    - Eosinophils usual in setting of drug-induced interstitial nephritis
    - Fibrosis
    - Rarely giant cells
- Vessels have no specific changes

ANCILLARY TESTS

Immunofluorescence

- Linear staining of proximal tubules for IgG and C3
  - Occasionally other reactants, IgA, C4, IgM
- No glomerular staining unless superimposed on glomerular disease (such as MGN)
- Test serum for anti-TBM activity by indirect immunofluorescence (IF)
  - Reacts with normal proximal TBM, not GBM or distal tubules
  - Anti-type IV collagen antibodies in Goodpasture syndrome that react with GBM and distal TBM

DIFFERENTIAL DIAGNOSIS

Tubulointerstitial Nephritis With Uveitis

- No linear TBM staining

Sjögren Syndrome

- No linear TBM staining

Immune Complex-Mediated Tubulointerstitial Nephritis

- Granular deposits of Ig in TBM
- Amorphous electron-dense deposits in TBM by EM

DIAGNOSTIC CHECKLIST

Pathologic Interpretation Pearls

- Requires linear IgG along TBM: C3 alone is commonly present in TBM as nonspecific finding
- Must demonstrate anti-TBM activity in serum (indirect IF with normal kidney)

SELECTED REFERENCES

1. Dixit MP et al: Kimura disease with advanced renal damage with anti-tubular basement membrane antibody. Pediatr Nephrol. 19(12):1404-7, 2004
2. Iványi B et al: Childhood membranous nephropathy, circulating antibodies to the 58-kD TIN antigen, and anti-tubular basement membrane nephritis: an 11-year follow-up. Am J Kidney Dis. 32(6):1068-74, 1998
3. Lindqvist B et al: The prevalence of circulating anti-tubular basement membrane-antibody in renal diseases, and clinical observations. Clin Nephrol. 41(4):199-204, 1994
4. Katz A et al: Role of antibodies to tubulointerstitial nephritis antigen in human anti-tubular basement membrane nephritis associated with membranous nephropathy. Am J Med. 93(6):691-8, 1992

Anti-Brush Border Autoantibody Tubulointerstitial Nephritis

KEY FACTS

TERMINOLOGY

- Chronic tubulointerstitial nephritis (TIN) mediated by autoantibodies targeting proximal tubule brush border

ETIOLOGY/PATHOGENESIS

- Target antigen in brush border of proximal tubule
  - Nature of antigen unknown

CLINICAL ISSUES

- Extremely rare
- Acute renal failure
- Slowly progressive renal failure
- Little or no proteinuria
- Bland sediment
- Normal complement levels
- Recurs in transplant

MICROSCOPIC

- Diffuse loss of proximal tubule brush borders on PAS stains
- Blebs, vacuoles, regenerative changes
- Tubulitis, focal
- Infiltrate of lymphocytes, plasma cells, few eosinophils

ANCILLARY TESTS

- Widespread granular deposits along tubular basement membrane (TBM) that stain for IgG and C3
- Prominent amorphous electron-dense deposits in TBM
  - Sometimes abutting basal plasma membrane of tubular epithelium
- Little or no detectable deposits in glomeruli
- Glomerular deposits resemble membranous glomerulonephritis, but of very limited extent

TOP DIFFERENTIAL DIAGNOSES

- Systemic lupus erythematosus
- IgG4-related systemic disease
- Idiopathic hypocomplementemic TIN

(Left) *Biopsy from patient with ABBA-TIN shows focally intense mononuclear interstitial infiltrate. Some proximal tubules are dilated with loss of normal brush border ➡, others in areas of inflammation are small and atrophic ➡. Glomeruli are normal by light microscopy ➡.* **(Right)** *Granular deposits of IgG are shown along the TBM of proximal tubules. These deposits also stain for C3 and both light chains. Deposits are not detected by IF in glomeruli or distal tubules.*

Diffuse Interstitial Infiltrate

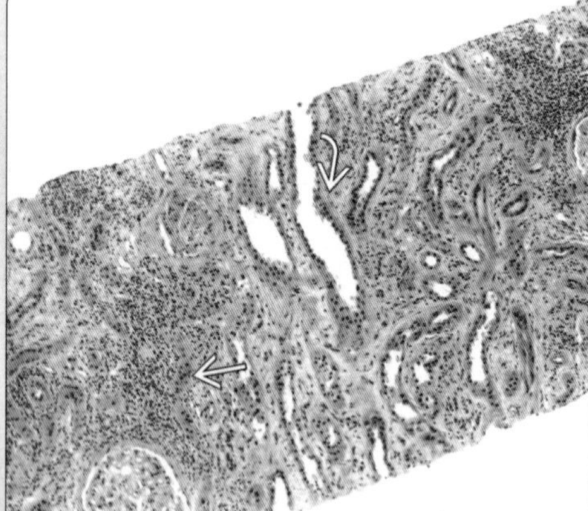

Deposits of IgG Along TBM

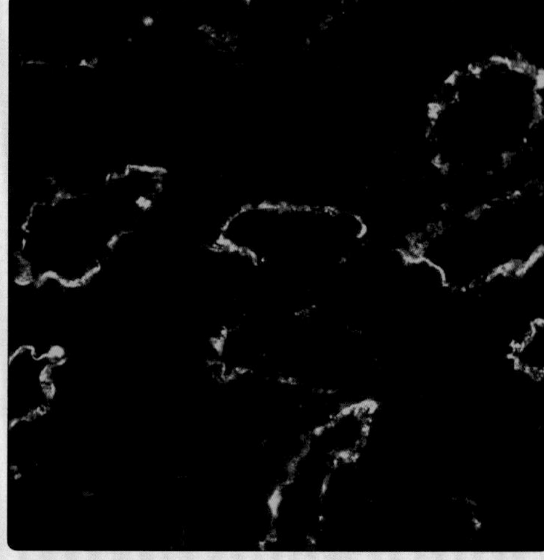

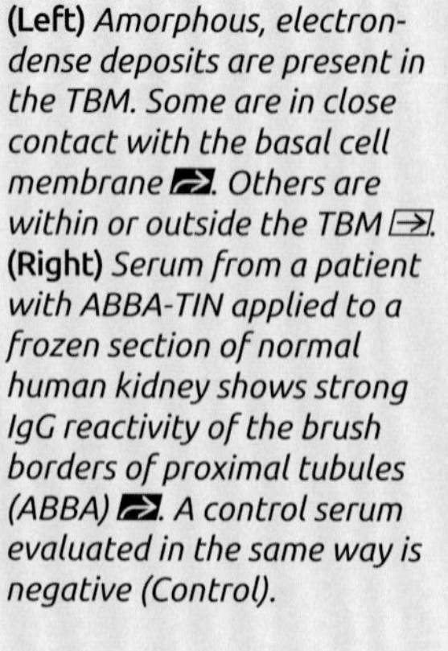

(Left) *Amorphous, electron-dense deposits are present in the TBM. Some are in close contact with the basal cell membrane ➡. Others are within or outside the TBM ➡.* **(Right)** *Serum from a patient with ABBA-TIN applied to a frozen section of normal human kidney shows strong IgG reactivity of the brush borders of proximal tubules (ABBA) ➡. A control serum evaluated in the same way is negative (Control).*

TBM Deposits

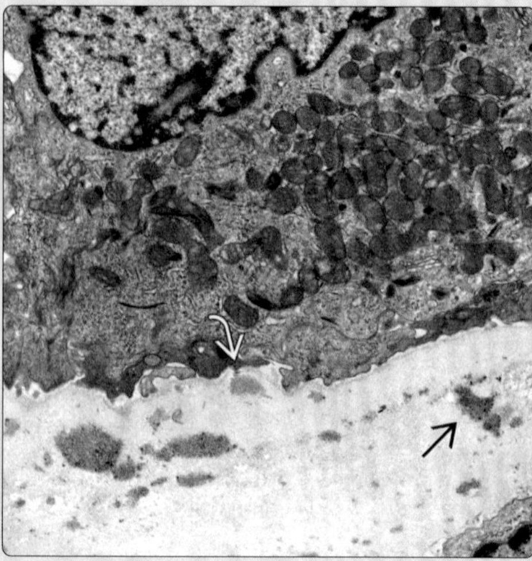

Serological Assay for Anti-Brush Border Antibody

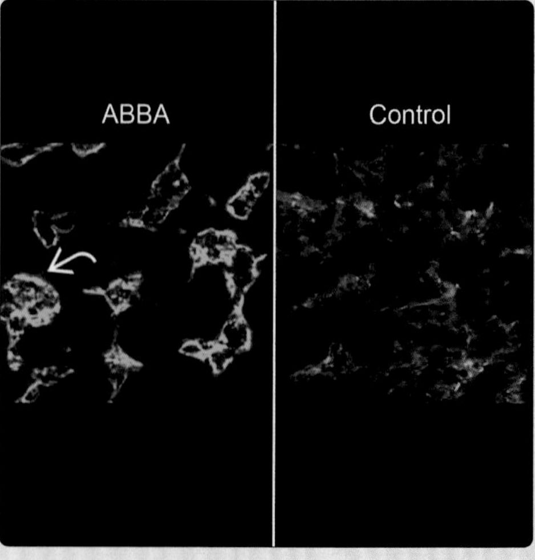

TERMINOLOGY

Abbreviations

- Anti-brush border antibody tubulointerstitial nephritis (ABBA-TIN)

Definitions

- Chronic TIN mediated by autoantibodies targeting proximal tubule brush border

ETIOLOGY/PATHOGENESIS

Autoimmune Disease

- Target antigen in brush border of proximal tubule
  - May have limited expression in podocyte
  - Nature of antigen unknown
- Stimulus for autoantibody response unknown
  - May be associated with other autoimmune diseases (e.g., myasthenia gravis)

Animal Model

- Immunization of rabbits with nonglomerular kidney extract causes ABBA-TIN
  - ABBA could be eluted from affected kidneys

CLINICAL ISSUES

Epidemiology

- Incidence
  - Extremely rare
- Age
  - 59-73 years
- Sex
  - Males

Presentation

- Acute renal failure
- Slowly progressive renal failure
- Little or no proteinuria
- Bland sediment

Laboratory Tests

- Normal complement levels

Treatment

- Immunosuppression
  - Rituximab tried without success
- Transplantation
  - Recurs in transplant

Prognosis

- End-stage renal disease over months
  - Based on very limited data

MICROSCOPIC

Histologic Features

- Glomeruli
  - Varied from normal to mild glomerular basement membrane (GBM) thickening
- Tubules
  - Diffuse loss of proximal tubule brush borders on PAS stains
    - Blebs, vacuoles, regenerative changes
  - Tubular atrophy
  - Tubulitis, focal
- Interstitium
  - Infiltrate of lymphocytes, plasma cells, few eosinophils
- Vessels
  - No specific changes

ANCILLARY TESTS

Immunofluorescence

- Little or no IgA, IgM, C1q
- Widespread granular deposits along tubular basement membrane (TBM)
  - Stain for IgG, C3, and C4d
  - One case had IgG1, IgG2, and IgG4, but no IgG3
- Equal light chain staining
- Little or no detectable deposits in glomeruli

Electron Microscopy

- Prominent amorphous electron-dense deposits in TBM
  - Sometimes abutting basal plasma membrane of tubular epithelium
- Glomerular deposits resemble membranous glomerulonephritis, but of very limited extent

Serologic Tests

- Serum IgG reacts with normal brush border antigens as shown by indirect immunofluorescence

DIFFERENTIAL DIAGNOSIS

Systemic Lupus Erythematosus (SLE)

- TBM immune complex deposits common (~ 60%)
  - Rare cases have TBM deposits with little or no glomerular involvement
- Serologies and other evidence of SLE make diagnosis
- No ABBA

IgG4-Related Systemic Disease

- IgG4 is predominant immunoglobulin in deposits
- IgG4 dominant plasma cells in infiltrate
- May have extrarenal signs
- No ABBA

Idiopathic Hypocomplementemic TIN

- Low complement level
- No ABBA

SELECTED REFERENCES

1. Rosales I et al: Immune complex tubulointerstitial nephritis due to autoantibodies to the proximal tubule brush border. Am J Soc Nephrol. In press, 2015
2. Morrison EB et al: Primary tubulointerstitial nephritis caused by antibodies to proximal tubular antigens. Am J Clin Pathol. 75(4):602-9, 1981
3. Klassen J et al: Studies of the antigens involved in an immunologic renal tubular lesion in rabbits. Am J Pathol. 88(1):135-44, 1977

Sarcoidosis

KEY FACTS

TERMINOLOGY

- Idiopathic noncaseating granulomatous inflammation that involves multiple organs, including lymph nodes, spleen, kidney, and other sites

ETIOLOGY/PATHOGENESIS

- Unclear etiology; disordered immune regulation
- Renal dysfunction related to nature and extent of involvement

CLINICAL ISSUES

- 3-10x more common in blacks than whites
- Peripheral and hilar lymphadenopathy
- Fever, hepatosplenomegaly, rash, uveitis
- Kidney involved in 10-20%
  - Tubular dysfunction due to aberrant Ca metabolism
  - Polyuria
  - Acute or chronic renal failure
  - Proteinuria > 1 gm/d in ~ 33%
- Elevated ACE and serum and urine calcium levels aid in diagnosis
- Responds to steroids but frequent relapse

MICROSCOPIC

- Tubulointerstitial nephritis with well-formed noncaseating granulomas
- Nephrocalcinosis
- Interstitial fibrosis and tubular atrophy in chronic recurrent disease
- Glomerulonephritis rarely occurs, most commonly membranous GN
- Special stains for organisms negative

TOP DIFFERENTIAL DIAGNOSES

- Hypersensitivity (drug-induced) tubulointerstitial nephritis
- Granulomatous infections
- Granulomatosis with polyangiitis

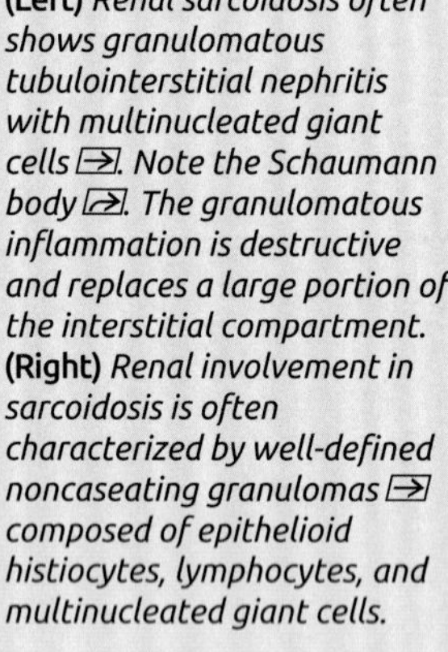

(Left) *Renal sarcoidosis often shows granulomatous tubulointerstitial nephritis with multinucleated giant cells ➔. Note the Schaumann body ➔. The granulomatous inflammation is destructive and replaces a large portion of the interstitial compartment.* **(Right)** *Renal involvement in sarcoidosis is often characterized by well-defined noncaseating granulomas ➔ composed of epithelioid histiocytes, lymphocytes, and multinucleated giant cells.*

Granulomatous Tubulointerstitial Nephritis With Giant Cells

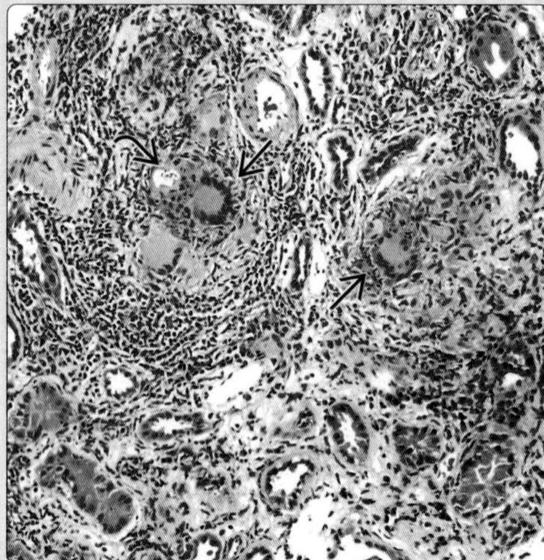

Sharply Delineated, Noncaseating Granulomas

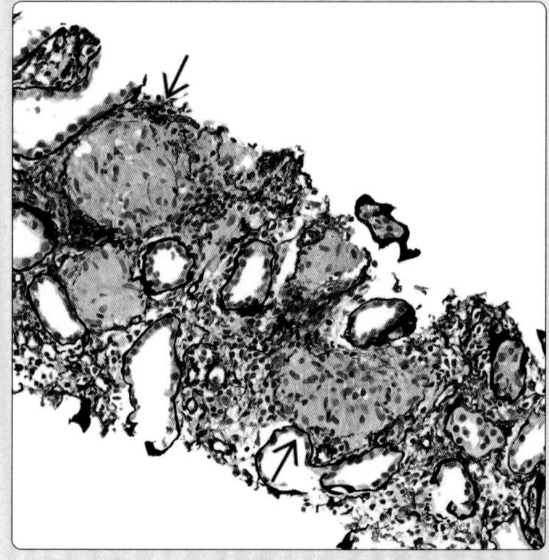

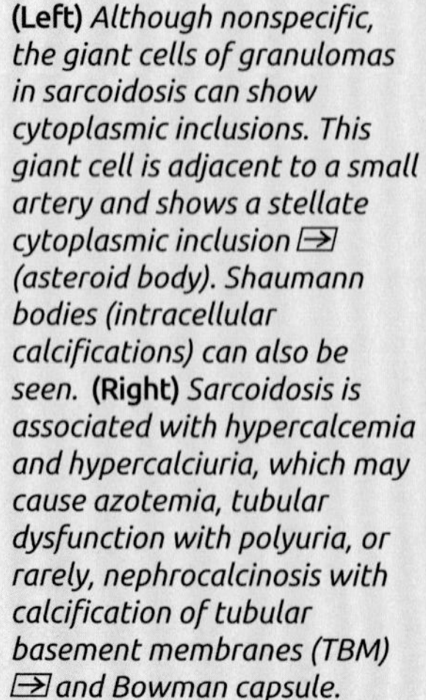

(Left) *Although nonspecific, the giant cells of granulomas in sarcoidosis can show cytoplasmic inclusions. This giant cell is adjacent to a small artery and shows a stellate cytoplasmic inclusion ➔ (asteroid body). Shaumann bodies (intracellular calcifications) can also be seen.* **(Right)** *Sarcoidosis is associated with hypercalcemia and hypercalciuria, which may cause azotemia, tubular dysfunction with polyuria, or rarely, nephrocalcinosis with calcification of tubular basement membranes (TBM) ➔ and Bowman capsule.*

Giant Cell With Asteroid Body

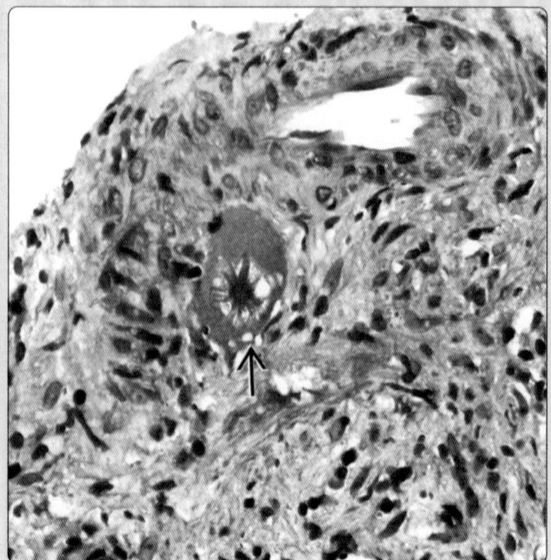

Nephrocalcinosis With Calcification of TBM

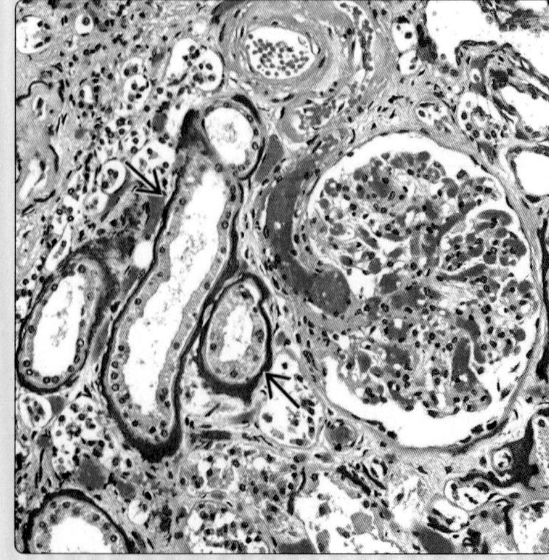

TERMINOLOGY

Definitions

- Systemic granulomatous disorder of unknown etiology

ETIOLOGY/PATHOGENESIS

Unknown

- Possibly multifactorial
  - Disordered immune regulation affecting T cells and macrophages leading to tissue injury
  - Genetic susceptibility &/or environmental factors

CLINICAL ISSUES

Epidemiology

- Incidence
  - 1-40 per 100,000 population
- Age
  - Most common in 2nd-4th decades
- Sex
  - More common in males than females
- Ethnicity
  - 3.5-10x higher in blacks than whites

Presentation

- Cough, dyspnea, fever
- Lymphadenopathy, hepatosplenomegaly
- Uveitis, arthritis, rash
- Kidney involved in 10-20%
  - Tubular dysfunction due to aberrant Ca metabolism
    - Nephrocalcinosis and nephrolithiasis
    - Urine concentration defect with polyuria
  - Acute or chronic renal failure
  - Hydronephrosis from retroperitoneal lymphadenopathy
  - Proteinuria > 1 gm/d in ~ 33% of published cases

Laboratory Tests

- Hypercalcemia (10-20%) and hypercalciuria (50-60%)
- Elevated angiotensin-converting enzyme (ACE) level

Treatment

- Drugs
  - Corticosteroids

Prognosis

- Good response to steroids, though relapses are frequent
  - Worse outcome in African Americans and elderly
- Rare recurrence in transplanted kidney

IMAGING

Radiographic Findings

- Bilateral hilar adenopathy

MICROSCOPIC

Histologic Features

- Glomeruli
  - Glomerular disease rare (frequency not established)
    - Precedes sarcoidosis diagnosis in 20-40%
    - Membranous glomerulonephritis (MGN) (42%)
    - IgA nephropathy (23%)
    - Focal segmental glomerulosclerosis (FSGS) (15%)
    - Minimal change disease (12%)
- Tubules
  - Tubular atrophy and interstitial fibrosis
  - Nephrocalcinosis
- Interstitium
  - Noncaseating granulomatous tubulointerstitial nephritis
  - Well-formed, sharply defined granulomas
    - Epithelioid histiocytes and multinucleated giant cells
    - Schaumann bodies (intracellular calcific bodies)
  - Active tubulointerstitial inflammation
    - Lymphoplasmacytic infiltrate, eosinophils rare
    - Tubular injury and interstitial edema
- Vessels
  - No specific findings

ANCILLARY TESTS

Immunofluorescence

- Negative in tubulointerstitial nephritis alone
- Granular deposits of IgG in GBM and mesangium in MGN
  - PLA2R positive, correlates with disease activity

Electron Microscopy

- Mesangial &/or capillary loop electron-dense deposits in glomerulonephritis
- Foot process effacement (MGN and FSGS)
- Calcific deposits in tubular basement membranes

DIFFERENTIAL DIAGNOSIS

Granulomatous Drug/Hypersensitivity Reaction (Most Common)

- Granulomas less distinct
- Eosinophils more numerous

Granulomatous Infections

- Acid-fast bacterial infection
- Fungal infection

Granulomatous Angiitis

- Granulomatosis with polyangiitis
- Giant cell arteritis

DIAGNOSTIC CHECKLIST

Pathologic Interpretation Pearls

- Discrete noncaseating granulomas: Think drugs and sarcoidosis
  - Rule out infection and systemic vasculitis

SELECTED REFERENCES

1. Gedalia A et al: Childhood sarcoidosis: Louisiana experience. Clin Rheumatol. ePub, 2015
2. Bagnasco SM et al: Sarcoidosis in native and transplanted kidneys: incidence, pathologic findings, and clinical course. PLoS One. 9(10):e110778, 2014
3. Goldsmith S et al: Sarcoidosis manifesting as a pseudotumorous renal mass. J Radiol Case Rep. 7(5):23-34, 2013
4. Stehlé T et al: Clinicopathological study of glomerular diseases associated with sarcoidosis: a multicenter study. Orphanet J Rare Dis. 8:65, 2013
5. Shah R et al: Diagnostic utility of kidney biopsy in patients with sarcoidosis and acute kidney injury. Int J Nephrol Renovasc Dis. 4:131-6, 2011
6. Mahévas M et al: Renal sarcoidosis: clinical, laboratory, and histologic presentation and outcome in 47 patients. Medicine (Baltimore). 88(2):98-106, 2009

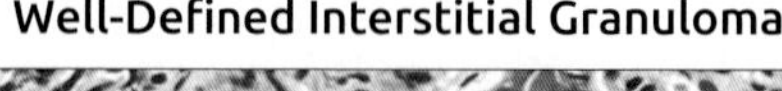

Well-Defined Interstitial Granuloma

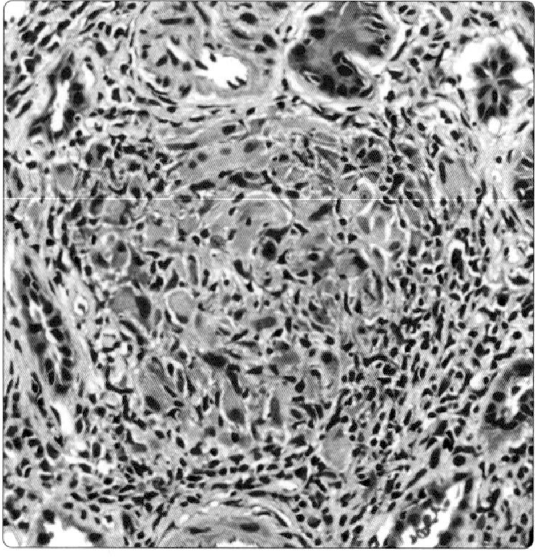

Interstitial Granuloma

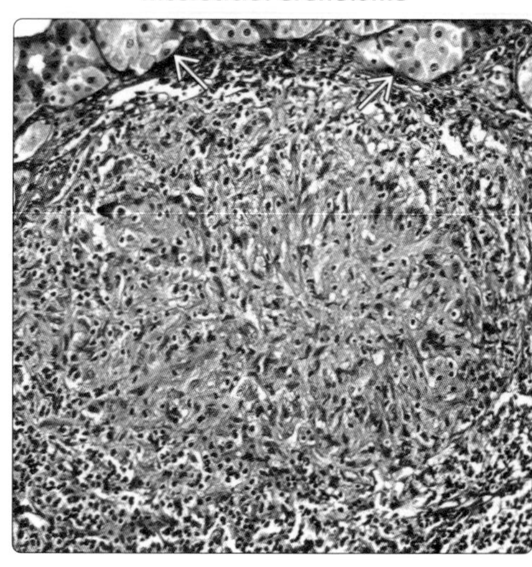

(Left) *This granuloma is composed of histiocytes without multinucleated giant cells. Numerous lymphocytes are present but no eosinophils are identified. The discrete granuloma and lack of eosinophils make a drug-induced/hypersensitivity reaction unlikely.* **(Right)** *This granuloma, composed of histiocytes and lymphocytes, was present in a nephrectomy performed for a renal neoplasm. The cells* ➡ *above the granuloma are tumor cells and the tumor is a benign oncocytoma.*

Tubular Calcium Phosphate Deposition

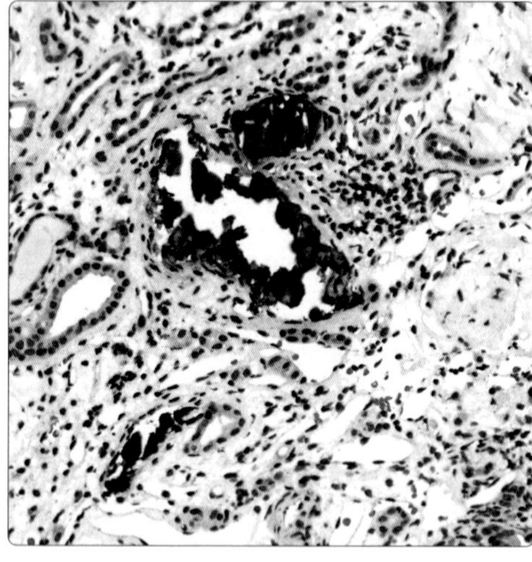

Chronic Tubulointerstitial Nephritis

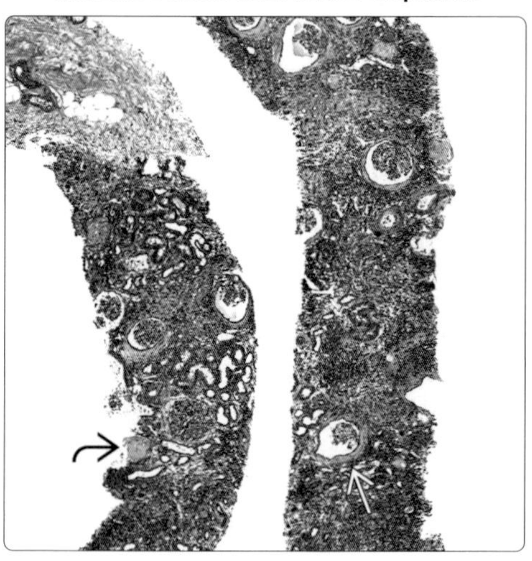

(Left) *Hypercalciuria is common in sarcoidosis and may lead to nephrocalcinosis and nephrolithiasis. As such, focal tubular calcium phosphate deposition is not infrequently present.* **(Right)** *Some patients with sarcoidosis have recurrent episodes of renal involvement or steroid-resistant disease. This can result in severe interstitial fibrosis and tubular atrophy, as seen here, with persistent inflammation. Secondary glomerular injury is also present with periglomerular fibrosis* ➡*, retraction of the tuft, and global sclerosis* ⇨*.*

Calcified Cast and Mild Interstitial Fibrosis

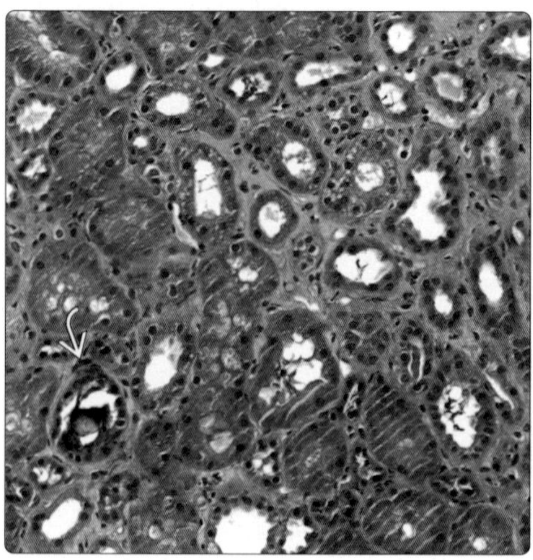

Normal Glomerulus

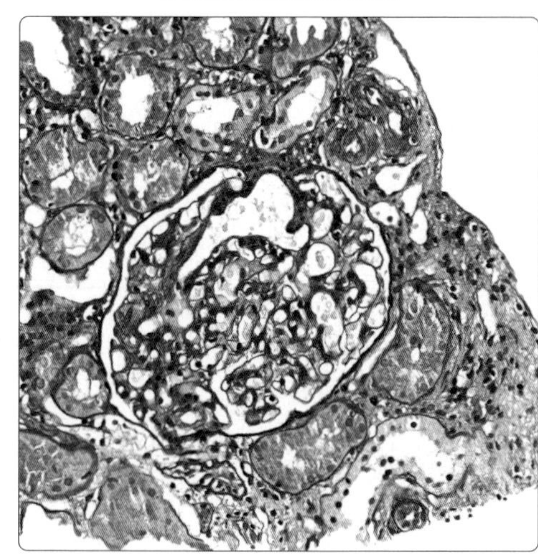

(Left) *In this case of sarcoidosis, no granulomas were found in a kidney biopsy, only occasional calcified casts* ↪ *and mild diffuse interstitial fibrosis and tubular atrophy. Sarcoidosis should be in the differential in any biopsy with prominent calcium/phosphate deposition.* **(Right)** *Glomerular involvement in sarcoidosis is uncommon. A normal glomerulus is seen here and is uninvolved by the acute tubulointerstitial nephritis present.*

Differential Diagnosis: Renal Tuberculosis

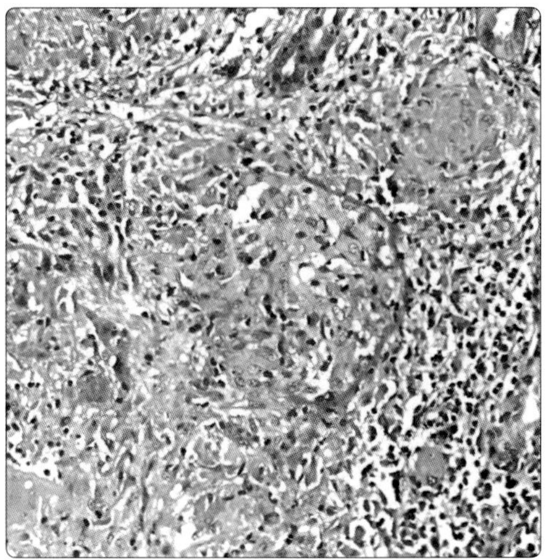

Differential Diagnosis: Renal Tuberculosis

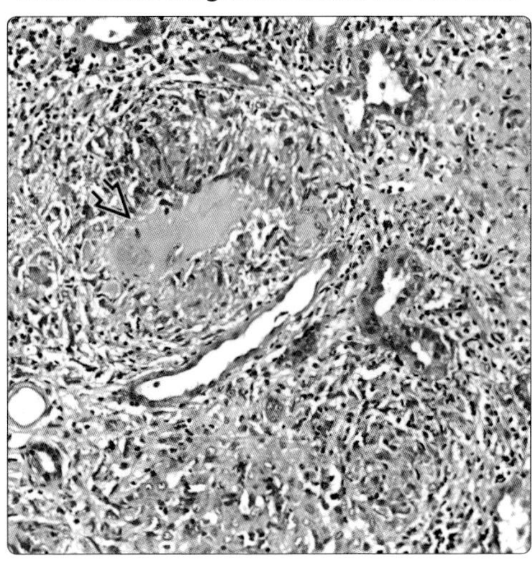

(Left) *Renal sarcoidosis needs to be distinguished from other forms of granulomatous tubulointerstitial nephritis, such as infection, drug-induced, and granulomatous angiitis. This micrograph from a case of renal TB shows active granulomatous inflammation. Although caseous necrosis is not present, special stains for organisms must be performed.* **(Right)** *This is a case of renal TB. The granuloma shows central caseous necrosis ➾, making an infectious etiology likely.*

Differential Diagnosis: Drug-Induced Tubulointerstitial Nephritis

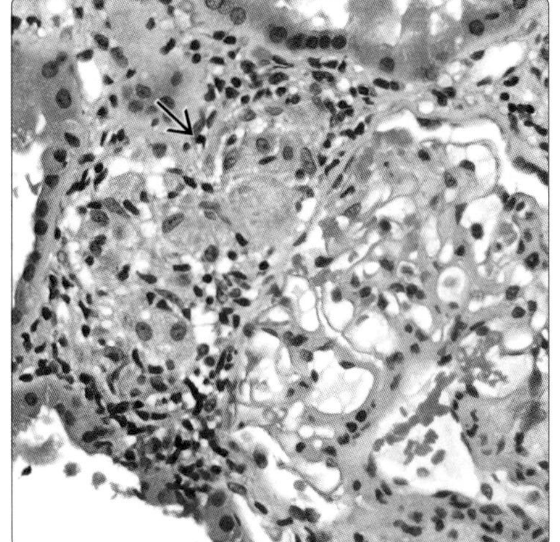

Differential Diagnosis: Drug-Induced Tubulointerstitial Nephritis

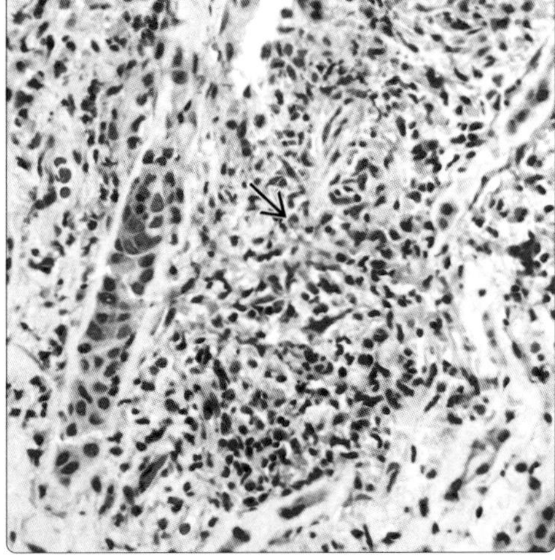

(Left) *Drug-induced/hypersensitivity reactions are the most common cause of granulomatous tubulointerstitial nephritis. In this situation, the granulomas are often less distinct. This micrograph shows a drug-induced tubulointerstitial nephritis with a small granuloma ➾.* **(Right)** *This antibiotic-induced tubulointerstitial nephritis shows a cluster of histiocytes ➾ without a well-defined granuloma. Numerous lymphocytes, plasma cells, and eosinophils are also present.*

Differential Diagnosis: ANCA-Related Granulomatous Angiitis

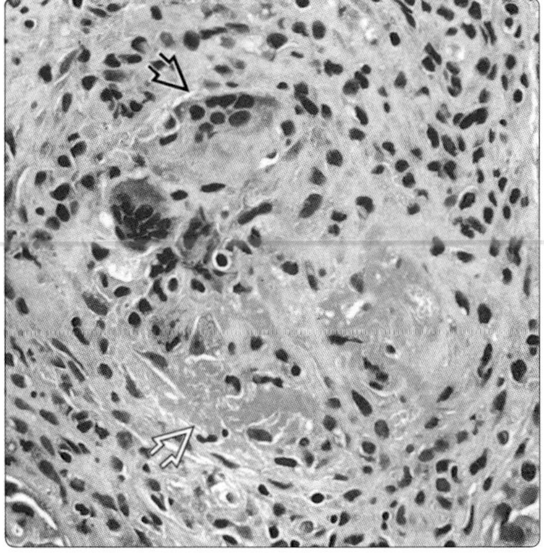

Differential Diagnosis: Granulomas in Giant Cell Arteritis

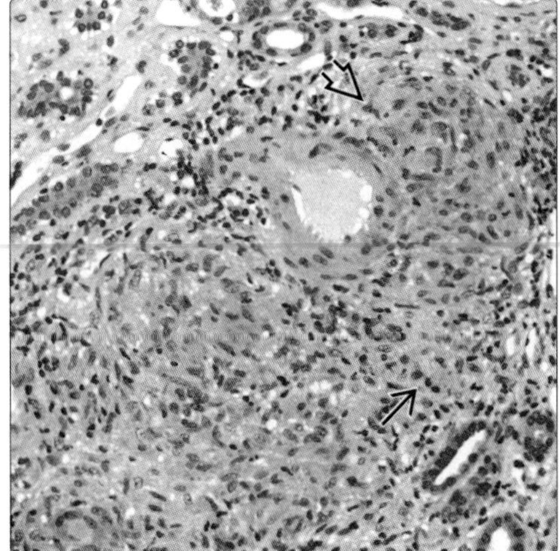

(Left) *ANCA-associated necrotizing and granulomatous arteritis may involve renal arteries. This is a case of granulomatosis with polyangiitis with necrotizing arteritis that includes multinucleated giant cells ➾ associated with fibrinoid necrosis ➾ of the arterial wall.* **(Right)** *This is a case of organ-isolated giant cell arteritis. There are numerous granulomas ➾ centered on small arteries and arterioles. There is also acute tubulointerstitial nephritis associated with eosinophils ➾.*

Giant Cell Tubulitis With TBM Deposits

KEY FACTS

TERMINOLOGY

- Acute tubulointerstitial nephritis with tubular basement membrane (TBM) immune complex deposition and multinucleated peritubular macrophages

ETIOLOGY/PATHOGENESIS

- Suspected drug reaction
  - Aprotinin
    - Used in complex cardiac and liver surgeries
- Lupus nephritis
  - Case report in patient after cardiac surgery

MICROSCOPIC

- Granulomatous interstitial inflammation
  - Multinucleated giant cells surrounding TBM
  - Disruption of TBM
- Prominent interstitial inflammation
  - Lymphocytes, plasma cells, eosinophils

ANCILLARY TESTS

- Immunofluorescence microscopy
  - Granular staining of tubular basement membranes
    - IgG, kappa/lambda light chains
    - C3 much less intense than IgG
- Electron microscopy
  - Discrete electron-dense deposits in TBM with associated macrophages

TOP DIFFERENTIAL DIAGNOSES

- IgG4 tubulointerstitial nephritis
- Idiopathic hypocomplementemic tubulointerstitial nephritis
- Lupus tubulointerstitial nephritis
- Anti-TBM disease
- Sjögren syndrome
- Monoclonal immunoglobulin deposition disease

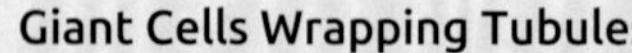

Giant Cells Wrapping Tubules

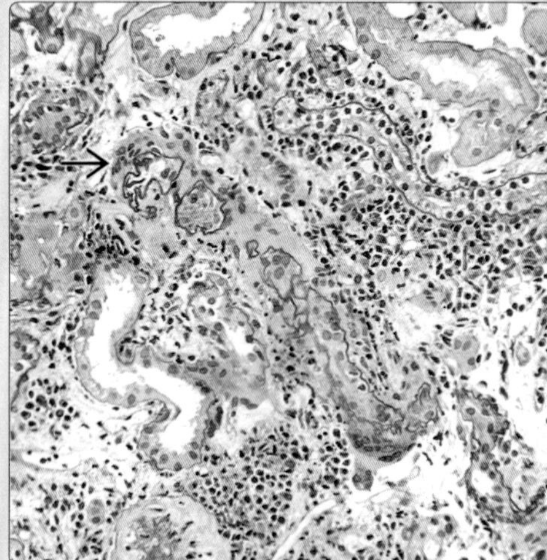

Peritubular Multinucleated Giant Cells

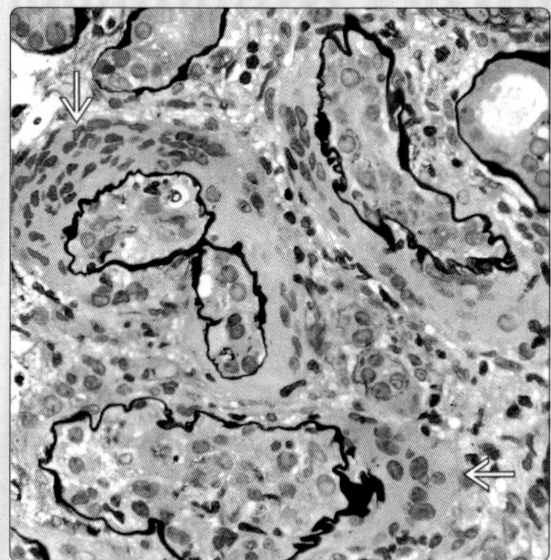

(Left) *Prominent interstitial inflammation consisting of lymphocytes, plasma cells, and eosinophils is admixed with several multinucleated giant cells ⇒ wrapped around several atrophic tubules (PAS).* **(Right)** *Several large, multinucleated giant cells ⇒ are intimately wrapped around tubular basement membranes.*

IgG

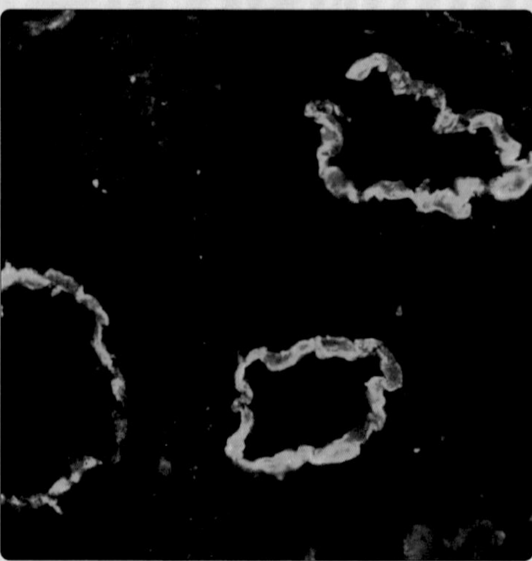

TBM Electron-Dense Deposits

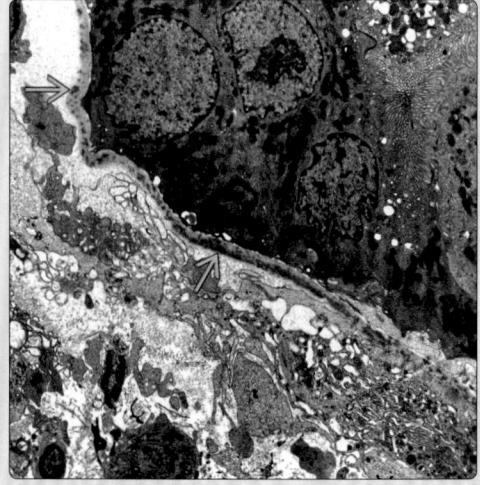

(Left) *Prominent IgG deposition is present in several tubules, which has a nearly confluent appearance due to the nearly continuous deposition of immune complexes.* **(Right)** *Numerous small, electron-dense deposits ⇒ are present within a segment of tubular basement membrane, which is focally quite prominent.*

Giant Cell Tubulitis With TBM Deposits

TERMINOLOGY

Synonyms

- Giant cell interstitial nephritis

Definitions

- Acute tubulointerstitial nephritis with tubular basement membrane (TBM) immune complex deposition and multinucleated peritubular macrophages

ETIOLOGY/PATHOGENESIS

Possible Pathogenic Mechanisms

- Drug reaction
  - Aprotinin
    - Suspected pharmacologic agent
    - Slows fibrinolysis
    - Used in complex cardiac and liver surgeries
    - Temporarily withdrawn worldwide in 2007
      - Increased risk of mortality compared to aminocaproic acid
- Lupus tubulointerstitial nephritis
  - Case report in patient after cardiac surgery

CLINICAL ISSUES

Epidemiology

- Incidence
  - Rare
    - Only 5 reported cases

Presentation

- Acute kidney injury
- Hematuria
- Proteinuria

Treatment

- Withdrawal of potential offending drug if known

MICROSCOPIC

Histologic Features

- Glomeruli
  - Normal
- Tubulointerstitium
  - Granulomatous interstitial inflammation
    - Multinucleated giant cells adjacent and surrounding tubular basement membranes
    - Disruption of tubular basement membranes
  - Prominent interstitial inflammation
    - Lymphocytes
    - Plasma cells
    - Eosinophils
  - Interstitial fibrosis/tubular atrophy
- Vessels
  - Age-related changes

ANCILLARY TESTS

Immunofluorescence

- Granular to confluent staining of tubular basement membranes
  - IgG
  - C3 less intense than IgG
  - Kappa/lambda light chains equal

Electron Microscopy

- Discrete electron-dense deposits in TBM
  - Macrophages adjacent to TBM with electron-dense deposits

DIFFERENTIAL DIAGNOSIS

IgG4 Tubulointerstitial Nephritis

- Prominent tubulointerstitial inflammation with IgG4 immune complex deposition
- No peritubular giant cell reaction

Idiopathic Hypocomplementemic Tubulointerstitial Nephritis

- TBM and interstitial immune complex deposition
- No peritubular giant cell reaction

Anti-TBM Disease

- Negative serum indirect immunofluorescence on normal kidney

Sjögren Syndrome

- No peritubular giant cell reaction

Lupus Tubulointerstitial Nephritis

- Rare reports of predominantly tubulointerstitial without glomerular immune complex deposition
- Single case report with peritubular giant cell reaction

Amyloidosis

- Congo red positive amorphous deposits
- Randomly arranged, nonbranching fibrils
- Rare cases with peritubular and perihilar multinucleated giant cells

Fibrillary Glomerulopathy

- Characteristic fibrils by EM
  - Thinner and without periodicity compared to adjacent collagen fibrils

Monoclonal Immunoglobulin Deposition Disease

- Rare cases with peritubular multinucleated giant cells
- Monoclonal immunofluorescence staining of both glomeruli and tubulointerstitium

SELECTED REFERENCES

1. Troxell ML et al: Light chain renal amyloidosis with prominent giant cells. Am J Kidney Dis. 62(6):1193-7, 2013
2. Lee L et al: Giant cell tubulitis and tubular basement membrane immune deposits. Pathology. 43(4):383-6, 2011
3. Hodgin JB et al: Giant cell tubulitis with immune complex deposits in a patient with lupus nephritis. Am J Kidney Dis. 53(3):513-7, 2009
4. Tong JE et al: Drug-induced granulomatous interstitial nephritis in a pediatric patient. Pediatr Nephrol. 22(2):306-9, 2007
5. Chang A et al: Giant cell tubulitis with tubular basement membrane immune deposits: a report of two cases after cardiac valve replacement surgery. Clin J Am Soc Nephrol. 1(5):920-4, 2006
6. Yamashita F et al: Light chain nephropathy with remarkable accumulation of multinucleated giant cells in the kidney. Nihon Jinzo Gakkai Shi. 36(11):1276-81, 1994

Mucin-1-Related Kidney Disease

KEY FACTS

TERMINOLOGY

- Autosomal dominant kidney disease due to *MUC1* mutation
  - Characterized by tubulointerstitial nephritis ± cysts
    - Progressive renal failure in adulthood
  - Formerly, medullary cystic kidney disease-1 (MCKD-1)

ETIOLOGY/PATHOGENESIS

- Mucin-1 expressed in distal tubule and collecting ducts
- Mutation in GC rich VNTR domain inserts cytosine
- Leads to truncated protein lacking transmembrane and intracellular domains

CLINICAL ISSUES

- Slowly progressive renal failure in adulthood
- Bland urinary sediment
- Gout absent
- Family history of renal disease absent in ~ 15%

IMAGING

- Corticomedullary cysts not an early or typical sign

MICROSCOPIC

- Nonspecific chronic tubulointerstitial nephritis
  - Diffuse interstitial fibrosis and chronic inflammation
  - Tubular atrophy
  - Dilation of distal tubules and collecting ducts
  - 12% microcysts in biopsy
- Global or segmental glomerulosclerosis

TOP DIFFERENTIAL DIAGNOSES

- Uromodulin-related kidney disease
- Renin mutation with tubulointerstitial nephritis
- HNF1β-related tubulointerstitial nephritis
- Nephronophthisis

DIAGNOSTIC CHECKLIST

- Diagnosis often overlooked due to nonspecific features

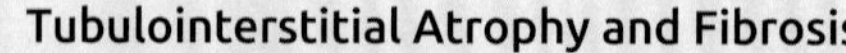

Tubulointerstitial Atrophy and Fibrosis

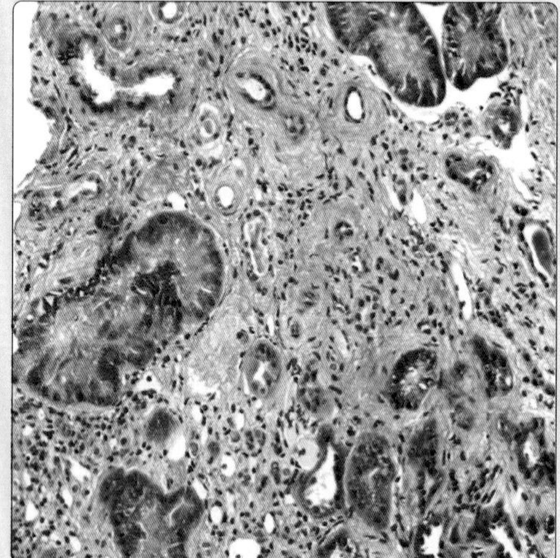

Glomerulosclerosis and Tubular Atrophy

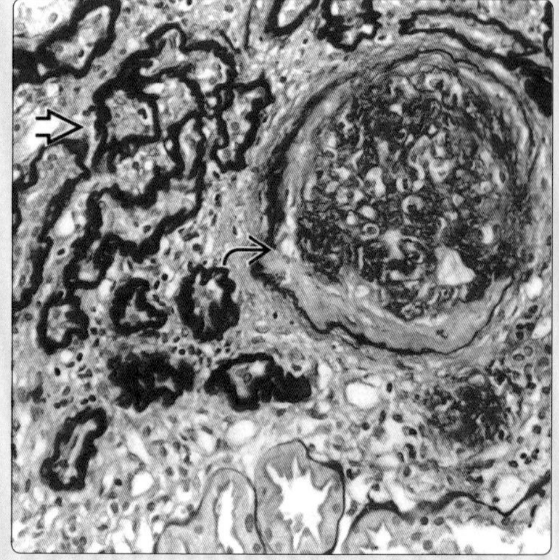

(Left) *Tubulointerstitial atrophy and fibrosis are the most common findings in ADTKD-MUC1. Light microscopy is not diagnostic.* **(Right)** *Biopsy from 56-year-old man with ADTKD-MUC1 (MCKD1) shows tubular atrophy with typical basement membrane thickening. The glomerulus shows periglomerular fibrosis (PAS). (Courtesy I. Zouvani, MD.)*

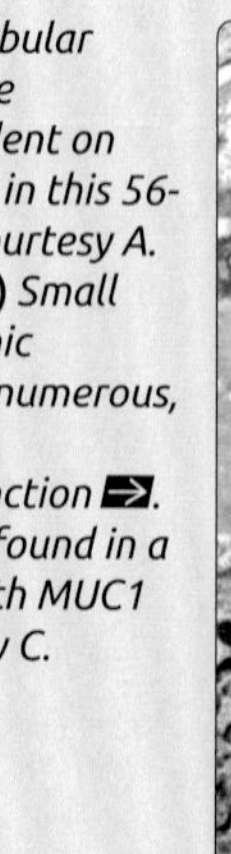

Tubular Basement Membrane Thickening

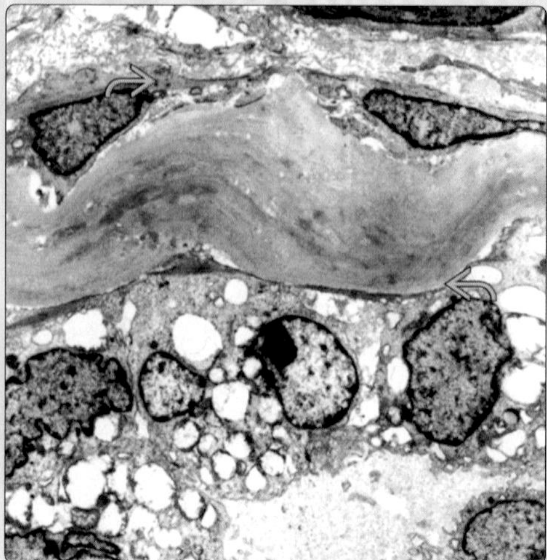

Cysts by Ultrasound

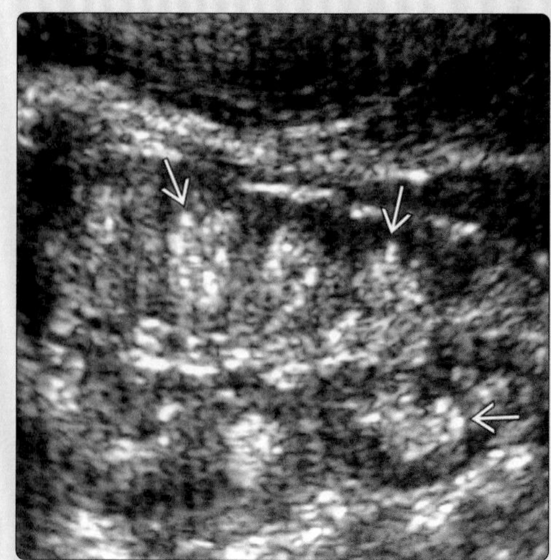

(Left) *Nonspecific tubular basement membrane thickening is evident on electron microscopy in this 56-year-old patient. (Courtesy A. Pieridis, MD.)* **(Right)** *Small kidney with echogenic pyramids caused by numerous, tiny cysts at the corticomedullary junction. Medullary cysts are found in a minority of cases with MUC1 mutations. (Courtesy C. Menias, MD.)*

TERMINOLOGY

Definitions

- Autosomal dominant kidney disease due to mutation in *MUC1*, characterized by tubulointerstitial nephritis ± cysts, and progressive renal failure in adulthood (OMIM 174000)
- Formerly termed medullary cystic kidney disease, type 1 (MDKD1)
  - Now termed autosomal dominant tubulointerstitial kidney diseases (ADTKD) due to mutations in *UMOD*, *REN*, or *HNF1β*

ETIOLOGY/PATHOGENESIS

Genetics

- *MUC1*
  - Encodes mucin-1
  - Autosomal dominant inheritance
    - Maps to chromosome 1q21
  - Variable number tandem repeat (VNTR) domain
    - ~ 1.5-5 kb GC-rich sequence of 60 nt that repeats 20-125 times
    - Encodes serine-threonine glycosylation sites responsible for mucinous properties of mucin-1
    - Mutations insert single cytosine in sequence of 7 cytosines
      - Create novel stop codon eliminating mucin-1 transmembrane and intracellular domains
      - Site varies in different families
      - Missed by massively parallel sequencing
  - May be dominant negative mutation
    - MUC1 deficient mice have no renal disease
- Mucin-1
  - Also known as epithelial membrane antigen (EMA)
  - Expressed on apical surface of epithelium of Henle's loop, distal tubule, and collecting duct
    - Also epithelium of breast, skin, GI, lung, ovary, pancreas, salivary glands
  - Protects epithelial surfaces from bacteria
  - Increased in kidney during hypoxia
    - May be involved in HIFα signaling
  - Overexpressed in neoplasia

CLINICAL ISSUES

Epidemiology

- Age
  - Onset of ESRD 16-81 years
  - Variable within families

Presentation

- Progressive chronic kidney failure
- No hematuria
- Proteinuria minimal
- Gout absent or late (24%), no polyuria
- No extrarenal disease
- ~ 15% no family history (presumed de novo mutation)

Laboratory Tests

- Difficult to detect VNTR mutations
- Probe-extension assay used in research studies

Treatment

- Dialysis and renal transplantation

IMAGING

Ultrasonographic Findings

- Corticomedullary cysts not an early or typical sign
  - 17% had ≥ 2 cysts, none in medulla (Bleyer)

MICROSCOPIC

Histologic Features

- Glomeruli
  - Glomerulosclerosis 20-50%
- Tubules
  - Tubulointerstitial atrophy and fibrosis
  - Tubular basement membrane disruption with duplication and thickening
  - Dilation of distal tubules and collecting ducts
  - 12% microcysts in biopsy
- Interstitium
  - Diffuse fibrosis and mild inflammation
- Vessels
  - No specific findings

ANCILLARY TESTS

Immunohistochemistry

- Antibody to mutant VNTR peptide positive in distal tubules and collecting ducts (Kirby)

Electron Microscopy

- Thickening, splitting, and duplication of tubular basement membrane

DIFFERENTIAL DIAGNOSIS

Uromodulin-Related Kidney Disease (ADTKD-UMOD)

- Uromodulin deposits accumulate in distal tubules
- Hyperuricemia

Renin Mutation With Tubulointerstitial Nephritis (ADTKD-REN)

- Hyperuricemia, hyperkalemia, anemia

Nephronophthisis

- Autosomal recessive, polyuria

DIAGNOSTIC CHECKLIST

Pathologic Interpretation Pearls

- Suspected in biopsy in only 6% of confirmed cases

SELECTED REFERENCES

1. Eckardt KU et al: Autosomal dominant tubulointerstitial kidney disease: diagnosis, classification, and management-A KDIGO consensus report. Kidney Int. ePub, 2015
2. Bleyer AJ et al: Variable clinical presentation of an MUC1 mutation causing medullary cystic kidney disease type 1. Clin J Am Soc Nephrol. 9(3):527-35, 2014
3. Kirby A et al: Mutations causing medullary cystic kidney disease type 1 lie in a large VNTR in MUC1 missed by massively parallel sequencing. Nat Genet. 45(3):299-303, 2013

KEY FACTS

TERMINOLOGY

- Autosomal dominant tubulointerstitial disease with chronic renal failure and hyperuricemia
  - Progressive interstitial fibrosis and tubular atrophy ± tubular cysts and epithelial inclusions
- Current preferred designation is ADTKD-*UMOD*
- Formerly
  - Uromodulin-associated kidney disease; uromodulin storage disease
  - Familial juvenile hyperuricemic nephropathy
  - Medullary cystic kidney disease type 2; familial glomerulocystic kidney disease

ETIOLOGY/PATHOGENESIS

- Multiple uromodulin (*UMOD*) gene mutations
  - Located on chromosome 16p12
- Missense mutations in > 50% associated with cysteine indels
- Protein folding disorder
  - Misfolds in mutated protein impair intracellular trafficking
  - *UMOD* not secreted and accumulates in endoplasmic reticulum
  - Intraepithelial retention leads to cell injury, inflammation, and scarring

CLINICAL ISSUES

- ADTKD-*UMOD*
  - Hyperuricemia in childhood; teenage gout
  - Progressive chronic renal failure
  - Renal cysts in 40%
- Family history of chronic renal failure (CRF)

MICROSCOPIC

- Tubular atrophy and interstitial fibrosis
  - UMOD(+) inclusions in TALH
  - Bundles of ER and dilated ER by EM
  - Distal nephron microcysts; glomerular cysts rare

TALH Inclusions in ADTKD-UMOD

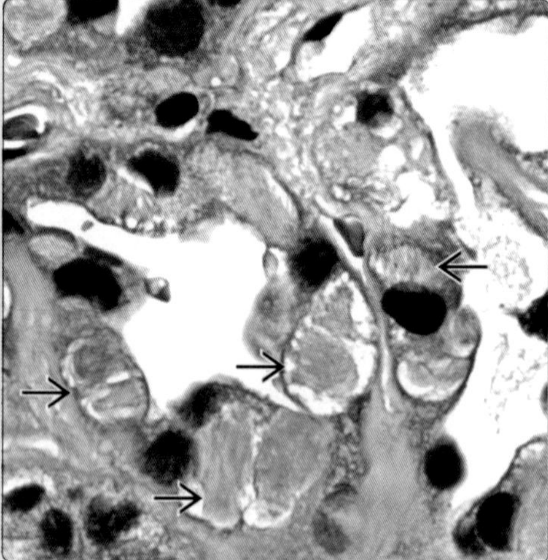

TALH Inclusions in ADTKD-UMOD

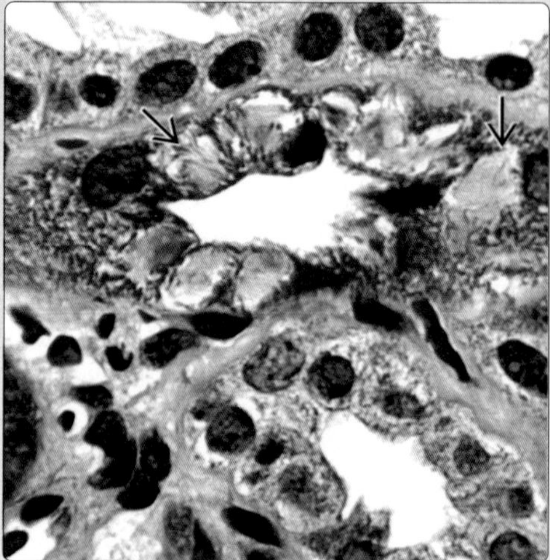

(Left) *Hematoxylin & eosin staining shows characteristic intracytoplasmic fibrillar or fluffy inclusions ➡ in the thick ascending loop of Henle (TALH). (Courtesy S. Nasr, MD and V. D'Agati, MD.)* **(Right)** *Masson trichrome stain shows fibrillar or "fluffy" inclusions ➡ in the epithelial cytoplasm of TALH. This unique finding is characteristic of ADTKD-UMOD (Courtesy S. Nasr, MD and V. D'Agati, MD.)*

Uromodulin Accumulation in TALH

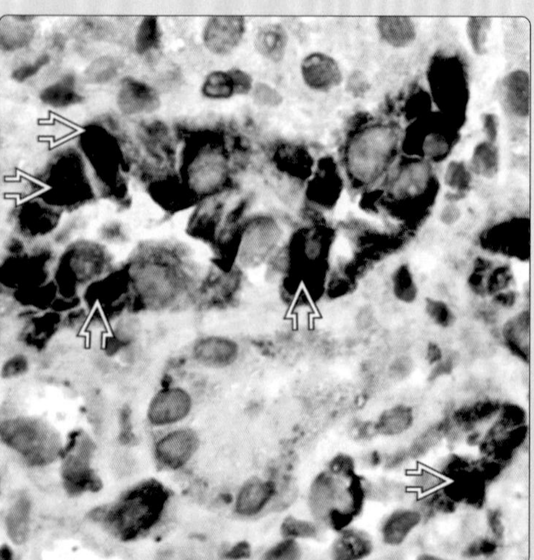

ER Changes in ADTKD-UMOD

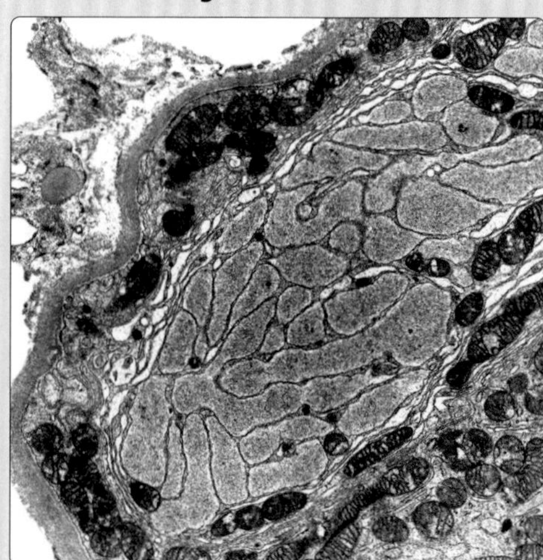

(Left) *Cytoplasmic aggregates of UMOD ➡ are identified using anti-UMOD IHC in the cells of the thick ascending loops of Henle. Misfolded mutated UMOD cannot exit from the endoplasmic reticulum (Courtesy S. Nasr, MD and V. D'Agati, MD.)* **(Right)** *Electron micrograph shows dilated endoplasmic reticulum with UMOD accumulations seen as granular amorphous material. (Courtesy S. Nasr, MD and V. D'Agati, MD.)*

TERMINOLOGY

Abbreviations

- Autosomal dominant tubulointerstitial kidney disease (ADTKD)
- Uromodulin (UMOD)

Synonyms

- Current preferred designation is ADTKD-*UMOD*
  - Formerly: Uromodulin-associated kidney disease; uromodulin storage disease; familial juvenile hyperuricemic nephropathy (sometimes type 1); medullary cystic kidney disease type 2; familial glomerulocystic kidney disease

Definitions

- Rare monogenic disorder characterized by
  - Autosomal dominant inheritance
  - Slowly progressive chronic renal failure (CRF) ± early onset gout
  - Progressive interstitial fibrosis and tubular atrophy ± tubular cysts and epithelial inclusions

ETIOLOGY/PATHOGENESIS

Genetic Disorder

- *UMOD* gene mutations
  - Located on chromosome 16p12
  - Autosomal dominant inheritance with heterogeneity
  - Missense mutations in > 50% associated with cysteine indels
  - Present in 30% of ADTKD

Pathogenesis

- Protein folding disorder
  - Misfolding impairs intracellular trafficking
  - UMOD not secreted and accumulates in endoplasmic reticulum
    - Intraepithelial retention leads to cell injury, inflammation, and scarring

CLINICAL ISSUES

Presentation

- Hyperuricemia in childhood; teenage gout
- Hyposthenuria; minimal or no proteinuria
- Renal cysts in ~ 40% by radiologic imaging
- Progressive CRF; family history of CRF

Laboratory Tests

- Gene sequencing identifies specific mutations

Treatment

- No specific therapy; xanthine oxidase inhibitors for gout
- Supportive for end-stage renal failure

Prognosis

- End-stage renal failure at 20-70 years; median 54 years

MACROSCOPIC

General Features

- Normal-sized or small kidneys ± cysts
- Cysts: Cortex, medulla, and corticomedullary junction
  - Medullary cysts uncommon despite former name

MICROSCOPIC

Histologic Features

- Tubular atrophy and interstitial fibrosis
  - Tubular basement membrane lamellation
- Distal nephron cysts in cortex, corticomedullary junction, medulla
- Eosinophilic "fluffy" inclusions in thick ascending loop of Henle (TALH)
  - Bundled and cystic endoplasmic reticulum by EM
  - Cytoplasmic UMOD(+) aggregates in TALH by IHC
- No tophi or uric acid crystal deposits
- Glomerular cysts very rare

DIFFERENTIAL DIAGNOSIS

ADTKD-MUC1

- Slowly progressive CRF and hypertension; family history of CRF
- No hyperuricemia or gout in early phases

ADTKD-HNF1B

- Renal cysts with chronic renal failure; family history of CRF
- Pancreatic dysplasia with early onset diabetes; genital malformations; intrahepatic ductopenia; early onset gout

Cystic Kidney Disease

- Polycystic kidney disease (dominant or recessive), others

Interstitial Fibrosis and Tubular Atrophy With Cytoplasmic Inclusions

- Light chain crystals: Light chain tubulopathy
- Mitochondria: Calcineurin inhibitor or antiretroviral agent nephrotoxicity

DIAGNOSTIC CHECKLIST

Pathologic Interpretation Pearls

- Interstitial fibrosis and tubular atrophy, with inclusions or cysts in young patient with gout and family history of CRF

SELECTED REFERENCES

1. Eckardt KU et al: Autosomal dominant tubulointerstitial kidney disease: diagnosis, classification, and management-A KDIGO consensus report. Kidney Int. ePub, 2015
2. Ekici AB et al: Renal fibrosis is the common feature of autosomal dominant tubulointerstitial kidney diseases caused by mutations in mucin 1 or uromodulin. Kidney Int. 86(3):589-99, 2014
3. Bollée G et al: Phenotype and outcome in hereditary tubulointerstitial nephritis secondary to UMOD mutations. Clin J Am Soc Nephrol. 6(10):2429-38, 2011
4. Nasr SH et al: Uromodulin storage disease. Kidney Int. 73(8):971-6, 2008
5. Vylet'al P et al: Alterations of uromodulin biology: a common denominator of the genetically heterogeneous FJHN/MCKD syndrome. Kidney Int. 70(6):1155-69, 2006
6. Dahan K et al: A cluster of mutations in the UMOD gene causes familial juvenile hyperuricemic nephropathy with abnormal expression of uromodulin. J Am Soc Nephrol. 14(11):2883-93, 2003

Renin Mutation With Tubulointerstitial Nephritis

KEY FACTS

TERMINOLOGY

- Autosomal dominant tubulointerstitial nephropathy due to renin gene mutation

ETIOLOGY/PATHOGENESIS

- Renin normally expressed in juxtaglomerular apparatus
- Heterozygous gene mutation in signal sequence of renin causes chronic kidney disease
- Reduced production of renin in juxtaglomerular cells
- Intracellular accumulation of unfolded preprorenin may lead to accelerated apoptosis, nephron loss, and progressive chronic kidney disease
- Mutations affect endoplasmic reticulum (ER) cotranslational translocation and post-translational processing, resulting in accumulation of nonglycosylated preprorenin in the cytoplasm; or affect protein insertion in ER membrane

CLINICAL ISSUES

- Chronic kidney disease
- Hyperuricemia
- Anemia
- Hypoaldosteronism

MICROSCOPIC

- Interstitial fibrosis and tubular atrophy
- Tubular basement membrane thickening and duplication
- Mild interstitial inflammation with mononuclear cells

TOP DIFFERENTIAL DIAGNOSES

- Familial juvenile hyperuricemic nephropathy (uromodulin storage disease)
- Chronic tubulointerstitial nephropathy, not otherwise specified
  - Genetic cause may be monogenic or multifactorial

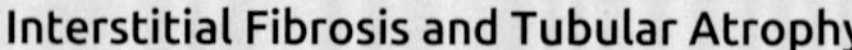

Interstitial Fibrosis and Tubular Atrophy

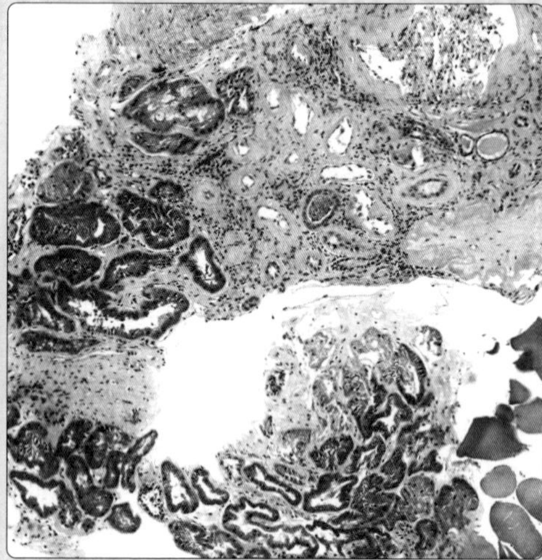

Tubular Atrophy

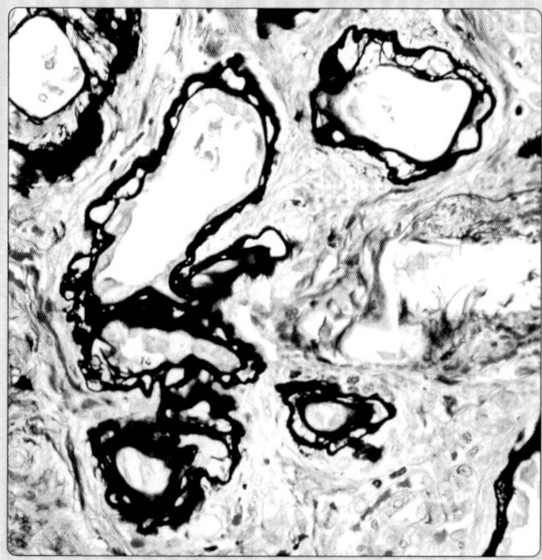

(Left) *Biopsy from a patient with chronic kidney disease and a renin mutation shows interstitial fibrosis and tubular atrophy, which is nonspecific.* **(Right)** *Atrophic tubules show basement membrane duplication, also a nonspecific feature.*

Interstitial Inflammation

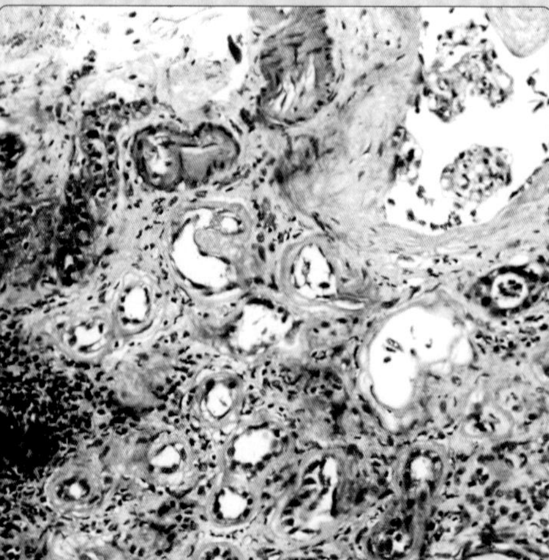

Ischemic Glomerulus

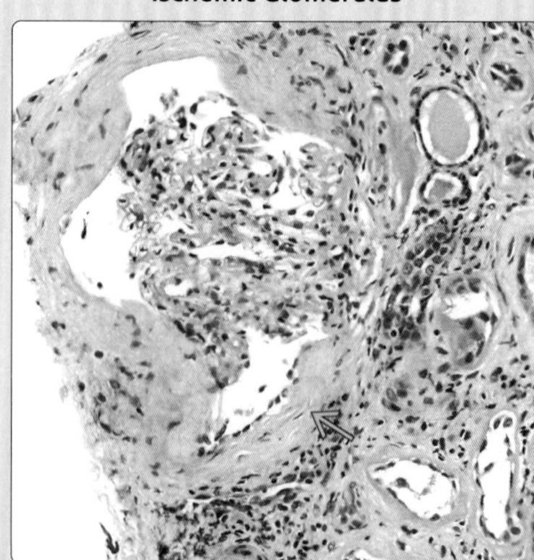

(Left) *There is mild interstitial inflammation in areas of marked tubular atrophy and interstitial fibrosis.* **(Right)** *A glomerulus shows features of ischemia, with a thickened and frayed Bowman capsule ⇒. Juxtaglomerular apparatus hyperplasia was not apparent.*

TERMINOLOGY

Abbreviations

- Renin (*REN*) gene

Definitions

- Autosomal dominant tubulointerstitial kidney disease (ADTKD) due to *REN* gene mutation

ETIOLOGY/PATHOGENESIS

Renin

- Synthesized as preprorenin
  - Preprorenin translocated to endoplasmic reticulum (ER), then processed into prorenin, an inactive precursor
- Enzyme cleaves angiotensinogen to angiotensin I
- Expressed in juxtaglomerular apparatus

REN Gene Mutations

- *REN* gene composed of 10 exons and spans ~ 1.7 kb on chromosome 1q32
- Heterozygous mutation in signal sequence of renin causes chronic kidney disease
  - 2 categories of causative mutations identified
    - One affects polar C-terminal (c-region) portion of preprorenin signal sequence
      - Substitution of cysteine for arginine (p.Cys20Arg)
      - Affects ER cotranslational translocation and post-translational processing, resulting in cytoplasmic accumulation of nonglycosylated preprorenin
      - Prevents renin granule formation
    - Other involves hydrophobic portion (h-region) of renin signal sequence
      - Deletion (p.Leu16del) or amino acid exchange (p.Leu16Arg) of single leucine residue
      - Affects protein insertion in ER membrane
  - Reduced production of renin in juxtaglomerular cells
  - Intracellular accumulation of unfolded preprorenin may lead to accelerated apoptosis, nephron loss, and progressive chronic kidney disease
  - Anemia due to involvement of renin-angiotensin system in erythropoiesis
- Homozygous mutations in REN cause renal tubular dysgenesis
  - 11 mutations identified
  - Prenatal or immediate postnatal death

CLINICAL ISSUES

Presentation

- Chronic renal failure
- Anemia
- Hyperuricemia
- Hypoaldosteronism
- Mild hypokalemia
- Decreased plasma renin levels
- Polyuria (p.Cys20Arg mutation)

Treatment

- Drugs
  - Fludrocortisone in some patients
    - Improved renal function in child with hyporeninemic hypoaldosteronism and kidney disease
    - Did not affect renal function in 2 adults with more advanced kidney disease

MICROSCOPIC

Histologic Features

- Glomeruli
  - May show ischemic changes (periglomerular fibrosis)
  - No specific features identified in juxtaglomerular apparatus
- Tubules
  - Tubular basement membrane thickening and duplication
  - Absence of tubular epithelial cytoplasmic inclusions
  - Atrophy
- Interstitium
  - Fibrosis
  - Mild interstitial inflammation with mononuclear cells
- Vessels: No specific findings

ANCILLARY TESTS

Immunofluorescence

- Negative staining of glomeruli, tubules, and interstitium

Electron Microscopy

- Distention of intercellular spaces between tubular epithelial cells (may be nonspecific)

DIFFERENTIAL DIAGNOSIS

ADTKD-UMOD

- Tubulointerstitial nephropathy due to uromodulin (*UMOD*) gene mutation
- Autosomal dominant inheritance pattern and hyperuricemia
- Intracytoplasmic fibrillar inclusions in tubular epithelial cells in thick ascending limb of loop of Henle

Chronic Tubulointerstitial Nephropathy, Not Otherwise Specified

- Autosomal dominant inheritance pattern with yet unidentified genetic cause
- Genetic cause may be monogenic or multifactorial

Autosomal Recessive Renal Tubular Dysgenesis

- Due to *REN* gene mutation, but at different loci
- Severe phenotype, prenatal or immediate postnatal death
- Autosomal recessive inheritance pattern

SELECTED REFERENCES

1. Eckardt KU et al: Autosomal dominant tubulointerstitial kidney disease: diagnosis, classification, and management-A KDIGO consensus report. Kidney Int. ePub, 2015
2. Gribouval O et al: Spectrum of mutations in the renin-angiotensin system genes in autosomal recessive renal tubular dysgenesis. Hum Mutat. 33(2):316-26, 2012
3. Bleyer AJ et al: Clinical and molecular characterization of a family with a dominant renin gene mutation and response to treatment with fludrocortisone. Clin Nephrol. 74(6):411-22, 2010
4. Zivná M et al: Dominant renin gene mutations associated with early-onset hyperuricemia, anemia, and chronic kidney failure. Am J Hum Genet. 85(2):204-13, 2009

Kidney Disease Due to Mutations in *HNF1B*

KEY FACTS

TERMINOLOGY

- Kidney disease caused by mutations in *HNF1B*, manifested by varied pathology including tubulointerstitial disease with cysts, hypodysplasia, or unilateral agenesis and associated with early onset diabetes

ETIOLOGY/PATHOGENESIS

- Autosomal dominant trait
- Mutation in *HNF1B*, which encodes HNF1β
- Homeodomain containing transcription factor predominantly expressed in kidney and pancreas epithelium and liver

CLINICAL ISSUES

- 10-30% of congenital abnormalities of kidney and urinary tract (CAKUT) are associated with *HNF1B* mutations
- 9% of adults with chronic renal failure of unknown origin with positive family history or renal structural abnormalities
- Chronic renal failure (neonatal to adult)
- Little or no proteinuria (< 1 gm/d) and no hematuria
- Macroscopic cysts (60-80%)
- Hypomagnesemia 25-60%
- 3-15% develop ESRD

MACROSCOPIC

- Varied pathology: Hypoplasia/dysplasia, solitary kidney, horseshoe kidney, hydronephrosis, cortical atrophy, cysts

MICROSCOPIC

- Spreading of glomerular tufts along cystic Bowman capsule
- Glomerular hypertrophy, oligomeganephronia
- Paucity of proximal and distal tubules
- Fibrosis, tubular atrophy

TOP DIFFERENTIAL DIAGNOSES

- Adults: *UMOD*, *MUC1*, or *REN* mutations
- Fetuses and young children: Other causes of hypodysplasia or cystic disease
- Genetic testing required for definitive diagnosis

(Left) *This kidney from a fetus (23 weeks) with an HNF1B mutation shows widespread cysts with a paucity of convoluted tubules and medullary dysplasia. Glomerulogenesis is evident in the subcortical zone ➙. Glomerular tufts can be seen in a few of the cysts ↶. (Courtesy M.C. Gubler, MD.)* **(Right)** *The kidney from this fetus with an HNF1B mutation shows dysmorphic glomeruli, with spreading or duplication of glomerular tufts ⇗ along Bowman capsule, and a paucity of convoluted tubules. (Courtesy M.C. Gubler, MD.)*

Fetal Kidney With Prominent Cysts

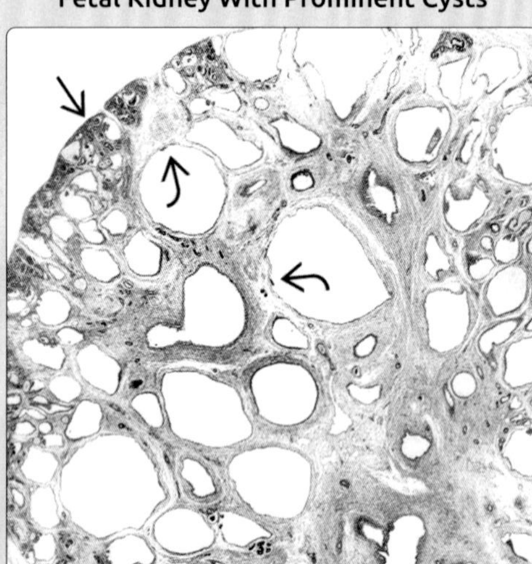

Dysmorphic Glomeruli

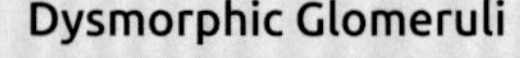

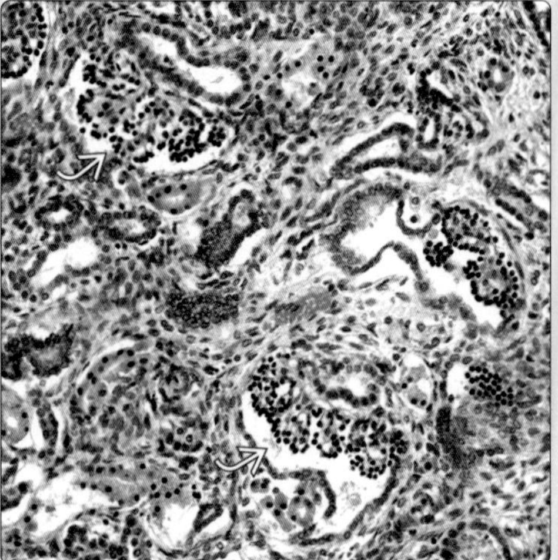

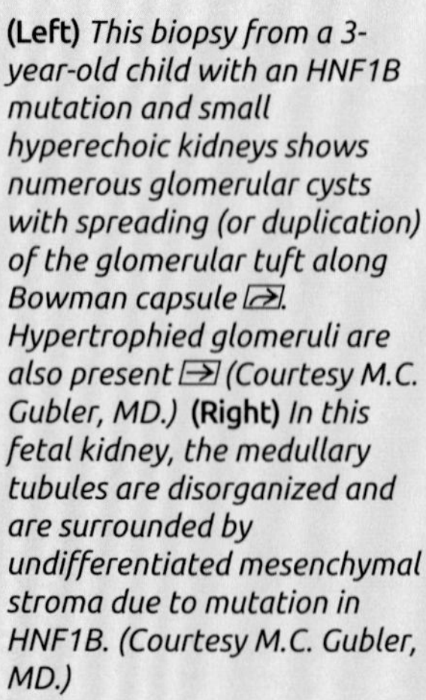

(Left) *This biopsy from a 3-year-old child with an HNF1B mutation and small hyperechoic kidneys shows numerous glomerular cysts with spreading (or duplication) of the glomerular tuft along Bowman capsule ↶. Hypertrophied glomeruli are also present ➙ (Courtesy M.C. Gubler, MD.)* **(Right)** *In this fetal kidney, the medullary tubules are disorganized and are surrounded by undifferentiated mesenchymal stroma due to mutation in HNF1B. (Courtesy M.C. Gubler, MD.)*

Glomerular Cysts in Renal Biopsy

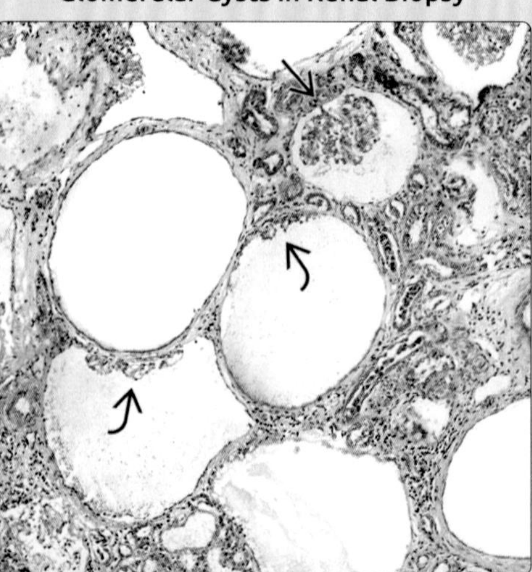

Medullary Dysplasia

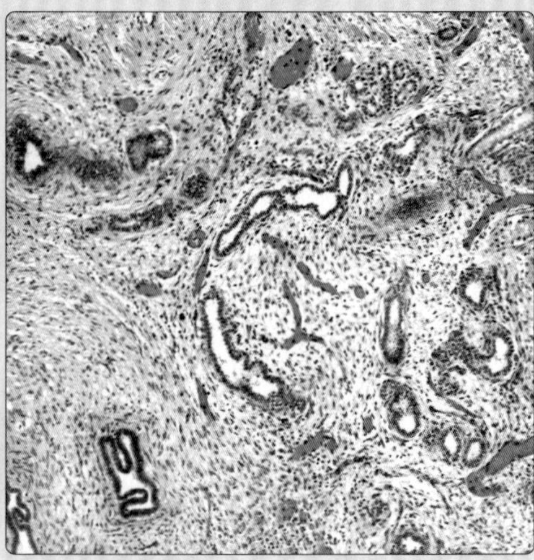

TERMINOLOGY

Abbreviations

- Hepatocyte nuclear factor 1β (HNF1β)

Synonyms

- Autosomal dominant tubulointerstitial kidney disease due to mutations in *HNF1B* (ADTKD-HNF1β)
- Maturity onset diabetes mellitus of the young, type 5

Definitions

- Kidney disease caused by mutations in *HNF1B*, variously manifested by tubulointerstitial disease with cysts, hypoplastic glomerulocystic kidney disease, unilateral multicystic dysplasia, hypodysplasia, unilateral agenesis, horseshoe kidney, hydronephrosis, or oligomeganephronia and associated with early-onset diabetes (OMIM 137920)

ETIOLOGY/PATHOGENESIS

Genetic Cause

- Autosomal dominant trait
- Mutation in *HNF1B* gene on chromosome 17
  - Encodes hepatocyte nuclear factor 1β
  - *HNF1B* is flanked by areas of duplication and thereby susceptible to recurrent rearrangement
  - ~ 50% complete or partial deletion
  - ~ 50% heterozygous mutations coding region/splice site
  - Spontaneous mutations ~ 50% (no family history)

HNF1β Transcription Factor

- Homeodomain containing transcription factor expressed in kidney and pancreas epithelium and liver; wolffian and müllerian ducts
  - Essential for embryogenesis of these organs
- Binds to DNA elements in *UMOD*, *PKDH1*, *PKD2*, *FXYD2*

Mouse Model (Massa)

- *Hnf1b* mutation effect depends on developmental timing
- Inactivation of *Hnf1b* in metanephric mesenchyme
  - Absence of proximal, distal, and Henle loop segments
  - Glomeruli in dilated Bowman space are directly connected to collecting ducts

CLINICAL ISSUES

Epidemiology

- 5-31% of congenital abnormalities of kidney and urinary tract (CAKUT) are associated with *HNF1B* mutations
- ~ 9% of adults with chronic renal failure of unknown origin with positive family history or renal structural abnormalities
  - 0.7% of patients with chronic kidney disease
  - Average age at diagnosis: 24 years

Presentation

- Chronic renal failure (adult)
  - Little or no proteinuria (< 1 gm/d) and no hematuria
- CAKUT in fetuses and young children
  - Fetal hyperechogenic kidneys (~ 30% *HNF1B* mutation)
  - Macroscopic cysts (60-80%)
- Pancreatic hypoplasia, agenesis
  - Insulin-dependent diabetes mellitus (~ 45%)
- Hypomagnesemia (25-60%)
- Absent vas deferens; absent or bicoronal uterus

Treatment

- Supportive
- Does not recur in transplants

Prognosis

- 3-15% develop ESRD

MACROSCOPIC

Varied Features

- Cortical atrophy, fibrosis, cysts
- Hypoplasia/dysplasia
- Solitary kidney, horseshoe kidney
- Hydronephrosis

MICROSCOPIC

Histologic Features

- Glomeruli
  - Glomerular cysts
    - Spreading of glomerular tufts along Bowman capsule
  - Glomerular hypertrophy, oligomeganephronia
- Tubules and interstitium
  - Paucity of proximal and distal tubules
  - Chronic tubulointerstitial nephritis
  - Fibrosis, tubular atrophy
- Vessels: No specific findings
- Other microscopic appearances
  - Cystic dysplasia (cartilage, smooth muscle)
  - Normal structure (unilateral agenesis, horseshoe kidney)
  - Obstructive uropathy

DIFFERENTIAL DIAGNOSIS

Fetuses and Young Children

- Other causes of hypodysplasia or cystic diseases

Adults

- Mutation in *UMOD*
  - Accumulation of uromodulin in distal tubule
- Mutation in *MUC1*
  - No extrarenal disease
  - Dilation of distal tubules and collecting ducts
- Mutation in *REN*
  - Hyperuricemia, anemia

DIAGNOSTIC CHECKLIST

Clinically Relevant Pathologic Features

- Genetic testing required for definitive diagnosis

SELECTED REFERENCES

1. Clissold RL et al: HNF1B-associated renal and extra-renal disease-an expanding clinical spectrum. Nat Rev Nephrol. 11(2):102-112, 2015
2. Ekici AB et al: Renal fibrosis is the common feature of autosomal dominant tubulointerstitial kidney diseases caused by mutations in mucin 1 or uromodulin. Kidney Int. 86(3):589-99, 2014
3. Musetti C et al: Chronic renal failure of unknown origin is caused by HNF1B mutations in 9% of adult patients: a single centre cohort analysis. Nephrology (Carlton). 19(4):202-9, 2014
4. Raaijmakers A et al: Criteria for HNF1B analysis in patients with congenital abnormalities of kidney and urinary tract. Nephrol Dial Transplant. ePub, 2014

Primary Hyperoxaluria

KEY FACTS

TERMINOLOGY

- Oxalate overproduction due to gene mutations affecting enzymes that catalyze glyoxylate breakdown manifested by renal and systemic calcium oxalate deposition and urolithiasis

ETIOLOGY/PATHOGENESIS

- Autosomal recessive mutations of genes that encode
  - Alanine glyoxylate aminotransferase (*AGXT*) 80%
  - Glyoxalate reductase (*GR*) ~ 10%
  - 4-hydroxy-2-oxoglutarate aldolase (*HOGA*) ~ 10%

CLINICAL ISSUES

- PH1 (*AGXT*): Urolithiasis, hyperoxaluria (> 100 mg/d), increased urinary glycolate, renal failure frequent
- PH2 (*GR*): Urolithiasis, hyperoxaluria, increased urinary L-glyceric acid, renal failure 20%
- PH3 (*HOGA*): Early childhood urolithiasis, rarely renal failure
- Diagnosis by assay of enzyme activity in liver tissue
  - Gene sequencing identifies specific mutation

MACROSCOPIC

- Stones > 95% calcium oxalate monohydrate (whewellite)
- Shrunken, scarred kidney with gritty texture on cut surface
- Dilated pelvicalyceal system with crystalline stone material

MICROSCOPIC

- Extensive tubulointerstitial crystal deposits with giant cell reaction and fibrosis
- Arteries have mural oxalate deposits (characteristic but uncommon)

TOP DIFFERENTIAL DIAGNOSES

- Secondary hyperoxaluria
- 2,8-Dihydroxyadeninuria

DIAGNOSTIC CHECKLIST

- Extensive tubulointerstitial and vascular calcium oxalate deposits in young patient

(Left) *Partially polarized light shows abundant anisotropic calcium oxalate in the cortex of a 4-month-old male with primary hyperoxaluria type 1. The crystals are largely in giant cells ➡ and there is interstitial inflammation and fibrosis.* **(Right)** *Refractile, pale yellow calcium oxalate crystals, in sheaves and rosettes, are present mainly in giant cells ➡ in the renal cortex. The interstitium is inflamed and tubules are atrophic.*

Primary Hyperoxaluria Type 1

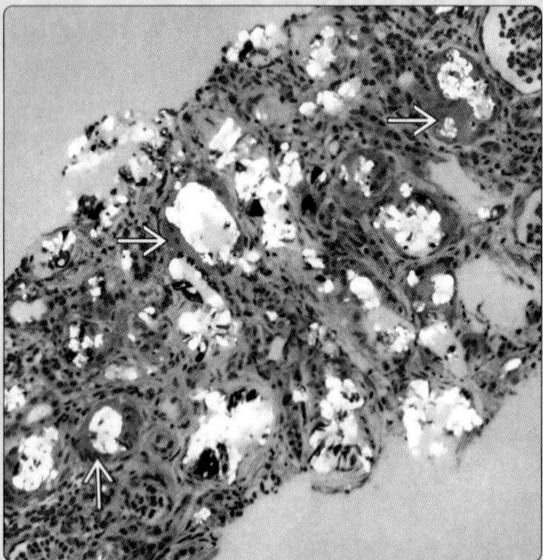

Primary Hyperoxaluria

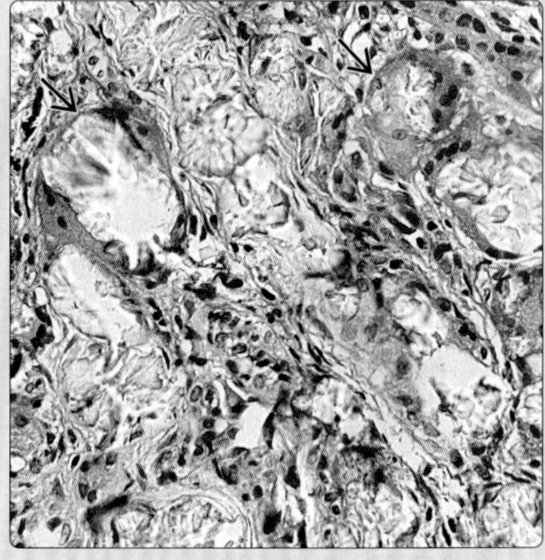

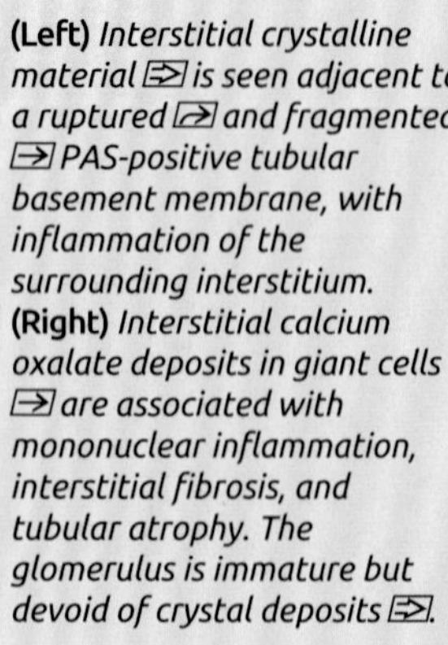

(Left) *Interstitial crystalline material ➡ is seen adjacent to a ruptured ➡ and fragmented ➡ PAS-positive tubular basement membrane, with inflammation of the surrounding interstitium.* **(Right)** *Interstitial calcium oxalate deposits in giant cells ➡ are associated with mononuclear inflammation, interstitial fibrosis, and tubular atrophy. The glomerulus is immature but devoid of crystal deposits ➡.*

Crystal Deposits With Tubular Rupture

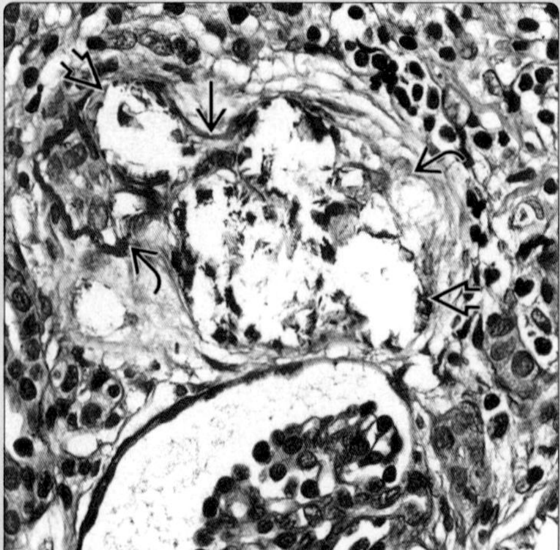

Interstitial Calcium Oxalate

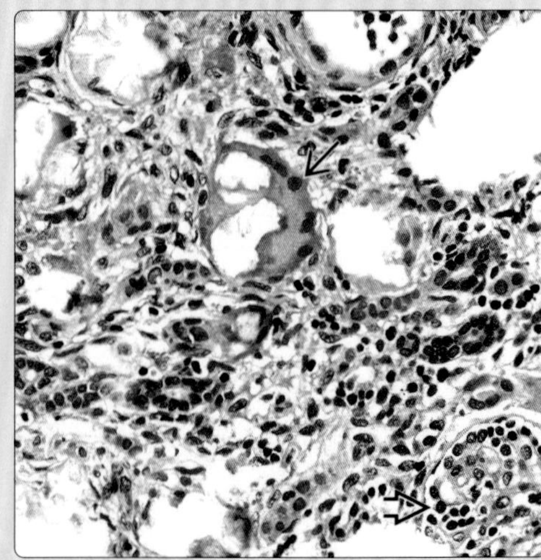

TERMINOLOGY

Abbreviations

- Primary hyperoxaluria (PH)
  - Type 1 (PH1), type 2 (PH2), type 3 (PH3)

Definitions

- Oxalate overproduction due to gene mutations affecting enzymes that catalyze glyoxylate breakdown with
  - Hyperoxaluria and stone formation
  - Renal and systemic calcium oxalate deposition

ETIOLOGY/PATHOGENESIS

Hereditary Disorders of Hepatocyte Enzymes

- Autosomal recessive mutations
  - Alanine glyoxylate aminotransferase (*AGXT*) gene in PH1 (80%)
    - Located on chromosome 2q37.3
    - Converts glyoxylate to glycine in peroxisomes
  - Glyoxalate reductase (*GR*) gene in PH2 (~ 10%)
    - Located on chromosome 9q11
    - GR converts glyoxylate to glycolate in cytoplasm
  - 4-hydroxy-2-oxoglutarate aldolase (*HOGA*) gene in PH3 (~ 10%)
    - Located on chromosome 10q24.2
    - Converts 4-hydroxy-2-oxoglutarate to glyoxalate and pyruvate in mitochondria
- Multiple mutations (178 for *AGXT*, 28 for GR,19 for *HOGA1* to date)
  - Result in variable clinical presentation
- Loss of function results in excess glyoxylate
  - Converted to oxalate by lactate dehydrogenase
- Hyperoxalemia leads to widespread calcium oxalate deposition in tissues (oxalosis)
- Excess urinary excretion predisposes to renal oxalate deposition and lithiasis
  - Stones composed of > 95% calcium oxalate monohydrate (whewellite)

CLINICAL ISSUES

Presentation

- PH1: Urolithiasis, nephrocalcinosis, and renal failure begin in childhood
  - Marked hyperoxaluria (> 100 mg/d, normal 20-55 mg/d), ↑ urinary glycolate
- PH2: Urolithiasis, marked hyperoxaluria, ↑ urinary L-glyceric acid, mild renal impairment
- PH3: Recurrent urolithiasis in early childhood
  - Abates after 6 years of age; no end-stage renal failure
- Renal oxalate deposition causes renal failure and compounds systemic oxalosis
  - Systemic oxalosis: Retinopathy, neuropathy, osteoarthropathy, cardiomyopathy, and bone marrow deposits with pancytopenia
- Diagnosis made by assay of enzyme activity in liver tissue
  - Gene sequencing identifies specific mutations

Treatment

- Hydration, pyridoxine (vitamin B6), pyridoxamine, citrate
- Combined liver and kidney transplantation for PH1
  - Rapid recurrence in kidney transplant if not combined with liver

Prognosis

- End-stage renal failure frequent in PH1; 20% PH2
- PH3 milder and rarely causes end-stage renal failure

MACROSCOPIC

Stones

- Rounded, white or pale yellow with smooth surface
  - Ultrastructure: 50 μm plates that aggregate to form rounded structures resembling balls of wool

Kidney

- Shrunken, scarred kidney with gritty texture on cut surface
- Dilated pelvicalyceal system with crystalline stone material

MICROSCOPIC

Histologic Features

- Early: Intratubular yellow, birefringent calcium oxalate crystal deposits in rosettes and sheaves
- Later: Extensive crystal deposits in cortical and medullary tubules
  - Injured and necrotic tubular epithelium
  - Tubular rupture with extrusion of crystals and giant cell reaction
  - Tubulointerstitial inflammation and fibrosis
- Arteries have mural oxalate deposits (characteristic but uncommon)
- Glomeruli devoid of crystal deposits but may have segmental or global sclerosis in advanced disease

DIFFERENTIAL DIAGNOSIS

Secondary Hyperoxaluria

- Excess ingestion: Ethylene glycol toxicity
- Excess enteric absorption: Inflammatory bowel disease, ileal resection or bypass
- Oxalosis in chronic renal failure from other causes

2,8-Dihydroxyadeninuria

- Brownish hue of crystals

DIAGNOSTIC CHECKLIST

Pathologic Interpretation Pearls

- Extensive tubulointerstitial and vascular calcium oxalate deposits in young patient

SELECTED REFERENCES

1. Hopp K et al: Phenotype-Genotype Correlations and Estimated Carrier Frequencies of Primary Hyperoxaluria. J Am Soc Nephrol. ePub, 2015
2. Rumsby G et al: Primary hyperoxaluria. N Engl J Med. 369(22):2163, 2013
3. Hoppe B: An update on primary hyperoxaluria. Nat Rev Nephrol. 8(8):467-75, 2012
4. Asplin JR: Hyperoxaluric calcium nephrolithiasis. Endocrinol Metab Clin North Am. 31(4):927-49, 2002

2,8-Dihydroxyadeninuria

KEY FACTS

TERMINOLOGY

- Autosomal recessive trait caused by genetic deficiency in adenine phosphoribosyltransferase (APRT)

ETIOLOGY/PATHOGENESIS

- Autosomal recessive, *APRT* gene located on 16q24
- Increased production and renal excretion of 2,8-DHA as stones &/or intratubular crystals

CLINICAL ISSUES

- Underdiagnosed
  - 2,8-DHA stones are radiolucent
  - May be confused with uric acid stones
- Nephrolithiasis, recurrent
- Chronic renal failure
- Renal transplantation: In patients with undiagnosed 2,8-DHA, original diagnosis may be made when disease recurs in allograft

MICROSCOPIC

- Birefringent intratubular crystals under polarized light
  - Reddish brown-tinged crystals on H&E-stained sections
- Very fine deposits within tubular epithelial cells
- Numerous 2,8-DHA crystals in tubular lumens, tubular epithelial cell cytoplasm, and interstitium
- Crystals may show foreign body giant cell reaction

TOP DIFFERENTIAL DIAGNOSES

- Oxalate crystals/oxalate nephropathy

DIAGNOSTIC CHECKLIST

- Red-brown color distinguishes 2,8-DHA crystals from oxalates

(Left) *2,8-DHA crystals have a brown-tinged appearance on H&E stain* ⇒ *and are birefringent under polarized light, which may lead the pathologist to misinterpret them as calcium oxalate crystals.* **(Right)** *Strongly birefringent 2,8-DHA crystals* ↷ *are seen under partially polarized light. Numerous additional small crystals are appreciable* ➡ *that are not initially apparent.*

2,8-DHA Crystals

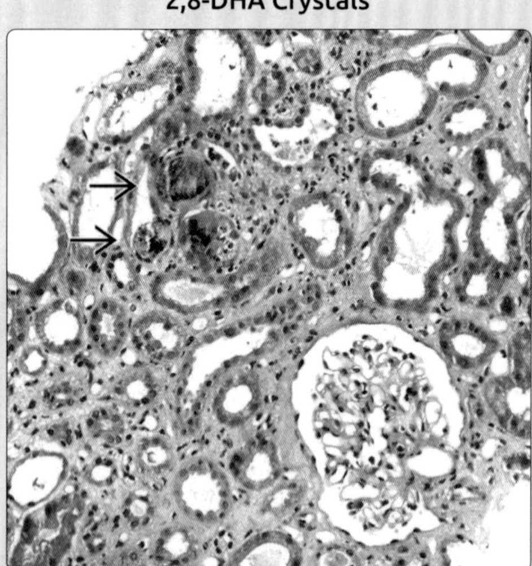

Birefringent 2,8-DHA Crystals

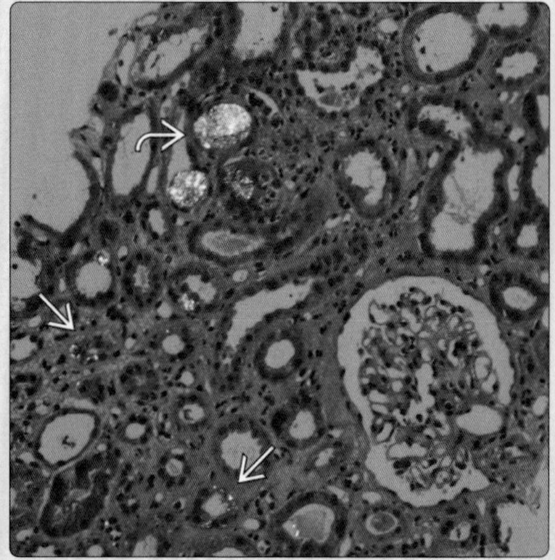

(Left) *High-power view shows an intratubular cast of brown 2,8-DHA crystals with a vague radial and ring pattern.* **(Right)** *Crystals are seen within tubules by electron microscopy, appearing as radiating spicules within cells and free in the lumen* ➡.

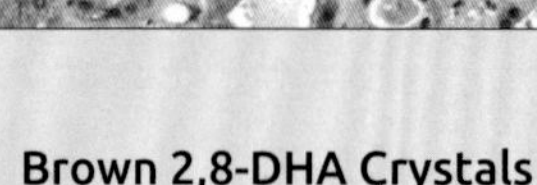

Brown 2,8-DHA Crystals

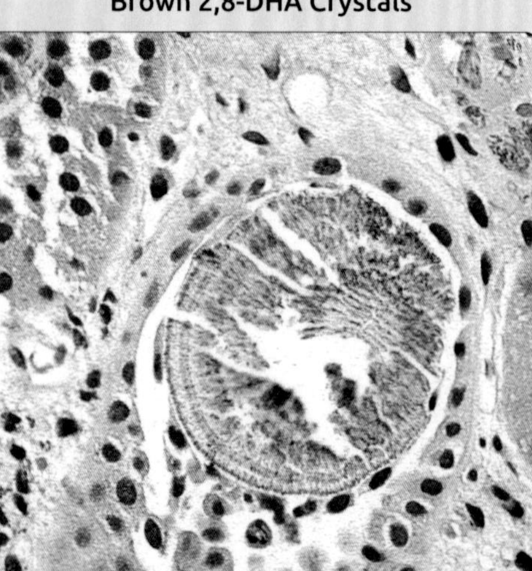

2,8-DHA Crystals by EM

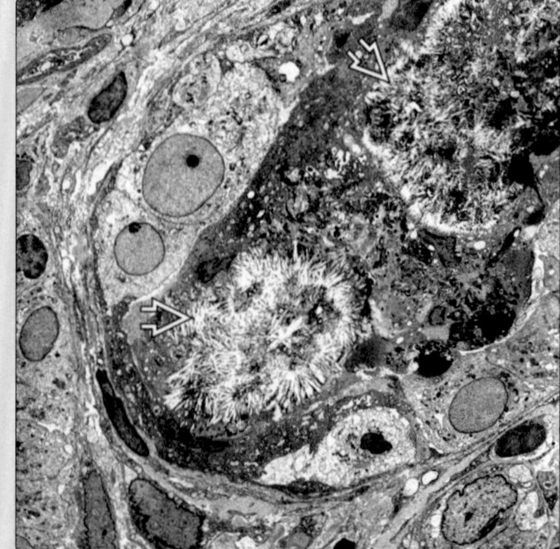

TERMINOLOGY

Abbreviations

- 2,8-dihydroxyadeninuria (2,8-DHA)

Synonyms

- Adenine phosphoribosyltransferase (APRT) deficiency

Definitions

- Autosomal recessive trait caused by genetic deficiency in APRT

ETIOLOGY/PATHOGENESIS

Genetic Basis

- Autosomal recessive, *APRT* gene located on 16q24
- 2 forms with complete in vivo deficiency of APRT
  - Type I complete in vitro deficiency of APRT (APRT*QO)
    - Commonest form in Caucasians
    - Heterogeneous mutations
      - Missense
      - Nonsense
      - Insertion or deletion
    - Most common (40%) in France: Mutation in intron 4 splice donor site
      - Results in truncated protein (IVS4 + 2insT)
    - Most common (100%) in Iceland: D65V
  - Type II: Some in vitro activity of APRT (APRT*J)
    - Commonest in Japanese
    - Single missense mutation in *APRT* (M136T)

Metabolic Pathway

- APRT is purine salvage enzyme
- Converts adenine to 5'-AMP from 5-phosphoribosyl-1-pyrophosphate
- Adenine normally transformed into adenosine monophosphate
  - In disease state, oxidized into 2,8-DHA
- 2,8-DHA poorly soluble and crystallizes in water (and urine) over wide range of pH
  - Protein-bound in plasma
- Increased production and renal excretion of 2,8-DHA as stones &/or intratubular crystals

CLINICAL ISSUES

Epidemiology

- Incidence
  - Estimated frequency of heterozygosity at APRT locus 0.4-1.1% in whites
    - Suggests homozygosity of 1 in 50,000 to 1 in 100,000 Fewer cases diagnosed
    - May be due to patients being asymptomatic, unrecognized, or misdiagnosed

Site

- Kidney and urinary tract
  - No known extrarenal manifestations of APRT deficiency

Presentation

- Variable clinical presentation with wide age range
  - Often diagnosed in adults (> 30 years old) with chronic kidney disease
  - May be diagnosed in children as well
    - Median age of diagnosis was 3 years in pediatric cohort (< 16 years)
  - Variable phenotype even among patients with same *APRT* gene mutation
- Nephrolithiasis, recurrent (90%)
  - 2,8-DHA stones are radiolucent
    - May be misdiagnosed as uric acid stones
  - Patients do not always have history of nephrolithiasis
- Chronic kidney disease (31%)
- Acute kidney injury (18%)
- Chronic kidney disease with radiolucent stones
  - Radiolucent stones most common clinical manifestation of APRT deficiency in children
    - Uric acid stones (also radiolucent) are uncommon in children
- Infection, urinary tract
- Urinary tract obstruction
- Hematuria
- Renal transplant recipient with idiopathic graft dysfunction (15%)
- Crystalluria
  - 2,8-DHA insoluble in urine at physiologic pH
- May be asymptomatic in children and diagnosed via screening after diagnosis of sibling

Laboratory Tests

- 2,8-DHA crystals detected by urine microscopy
  - Regular and polarized light microscopy
  - In normal individuals, no 2,8-DHA crystals identified in urine
  - 2,8-DHA crystals may be difficult to identify in oliguric patients due to decreased crystal clearance
- APRT enzyme activity in erythrocytes
- Elevated oxalate levels in blood
  - To lesser degree than primary hyperoxaluria
- 2,8-DHA crystals identified by infrared and ultraviolet spectrophotometry &/or X-ray crystallography
  - Biochemical stone analysis does not distinguish 2,8-DHA from uric acid crystals
- *APRT* gene mutation

Treatment

- Drugs
  - Xanthine analog (allopurinol) therapy to block formation of 2,8-dihydroxyadenine
    - Prevents stone formation and crystal deposition in kidneys
    - Renal function may improve
    - Febuxostat, another xanthine dehydrogenase inhibitor, is newer drug
      - Can be used in patients not able to tolerate allopurinol
- Low purine diet
- Sufficient fluid intake
- Renal transplantation
  - If not treated, disease recurs in transplant
    - Diagnosis may be first made with recurrence

Prognosis

- Excellent if started on allopurinol before renal failure develops

Radiographic Studies

- Radiolucent stones
- Stones detectable by ultrasonography

MICROSCOPIC

Histologic Features

- Numerous 2,8-DHA crystals in tubular lumens, tubular epithelial cell cytoplasm, and interstitium
  - Very fine deposits within tubular epithelial cells
  - Most crystals in renal cortex
    - Needle, rod, or rhomboid-shaped crystals
    - Range from single crystals to small aggregates to large aggregates
      - Reddish brown-tinged on H&E and PAS
      - Light blue on trichrome
      - Black on silver stains
      - Birefringent under polarized light
- Acute tubular injury in nonatrophic tubules
- Interstitial fibrosis and tubular atrophy
- Mild to moderate interstitial inflammation
  - Crystals may show foreign body giant cell reaction
  - Lymphocytes and monocytes
    - No significant eosinophilic infiltrate

DIFFERENTIAL DIAGNOSIS

Oxalate Crystals/Oxalate Nephropathy

- Calcium oxalate crystals are colorless
- 2,8-DHA crystals are red-brown

Phosphate Nephropathy

- Intratubular calcium phosphate deposits
  - Appear purple/blue on H&E-stained sections, rather than brown 2,8-DHA crystals
  - Do not polarize

Urate Nephropathy/Uric Acid Stone Disease

- Urates dissolve in routine processing (need alcohol-fixed tissue)
  - Needle-like, colorless crystals
- Both uric acid stones and 2,8-DHA stones are radiolucent
- Uric acid stones uncommon in children

Cystinosis

- Crystals dissolve in routine processing (need alcohol-fixed tissue)
  - Hexagonal, colorless crystals, often in cells
- Multinucleated podocytes

DIAGNOSTIC CHECKLIST

Pathologic Interpretation Pearls

- Red-brown color distinguishes 2,8-DHA crystals from oxalates

SELECTED REFERENCES

1. Ceballos-Picot I et al: 2,8-Dihydroxyadenine urolithiasis: a not so rare inborn error of purine metabolism. Nucleosides Nucleotides Nucleic Acids. 33(4-6):241-52, 2014
2. Kaartinen K et al: Adenine phosphoribosyltransferase deficiency as a rare cause of renal allograft dysfunction. J Am Soc Nephrol. 25(4):671-4, 2014
3. Valaperta R et al: Adenine phosphoribosyltransferase (APRT) deficiency: identification of a novel nonsense mutation. BMC Nephrol. 15:102, 2014
4. Edvardsson VO et al: Hereditary causes of kidney stones and chronic kidney disease. Pediatr Nephrol. 28(10):1923-42, 2013
5. Harambat J et al: Adenine phosphoribosyltransferase deficiency in children. Pediatr Nephrol. 27(4):571-9, 2012
6. Marra G et al: Adenine phosphoribosyltransferase deficiency: an underdiagnosed cause of lithiasis and renal failure. JIMD Rep. 5:45-8, 2012
7. Sharma SG et al: 2,8-dihydroxyadeninuria disease. Kidney Int. 82(9):1036, 2012
8. Bollée G et al: Phenotype and genotype characterization of adenine phosphoribosyltransferase deficiency. J Am Soc Nephrol. 21(4):679-88, 2010
9. Nasr SH et al: Crystalline nephropathy due to 2,8-dihydroxyadeninuria: an under-recognized cause of irreversible renal failure. Nephrol Dial Transplant. 25(6):1909-15, 2010
10. Edvardsson V et al: Clinical features and genotype of adenine phosphoribosyltransferase deficiency in iceland. Am J Kidney Dis. 38(3):473-80, 2001
11. Brown HA: Recurrence of 2,8-dihydroxyadenine tubulointerstitial lesions in a kidney transplant recipient with a primary presentation of chronic renal failure. Nephrol Dial Transplant. 13(4):998-1000, 1998
12. Sahota A et al: Missense mutation in the adenine phosphoribosyltransferase gene causing 2,8-dihydroxyadenine urolithiasis. Hum Mol Genet. 3(5):817-8, 1994
13. Edvardsson VO et al: Adenine phosphoribosyltransferase deficiency, 1993
14. Ceballos-Picot I et al: 2,8-Dihydroxyadenine urolithiasis, an underdiagnosed disease. Lancet. 339(8800):1050-1, 1992
15. Simmonds H et al: 2,8-Dihydroxyadenine urolithiasis. Lancet. 339(8804):1295-6, 1992

Recurrent 2,8-DHA in Transplant

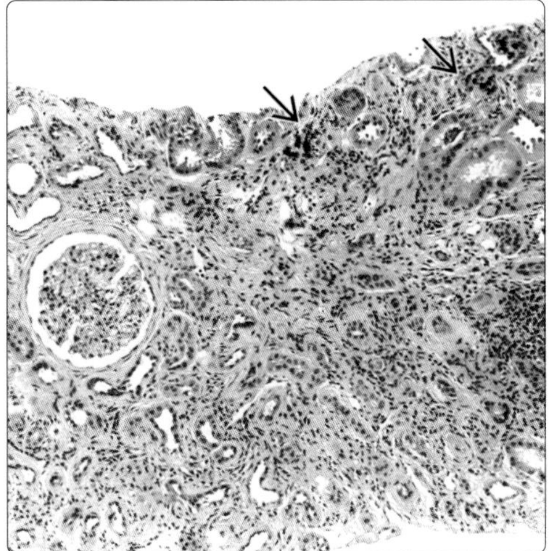

Fine Brown Crystals

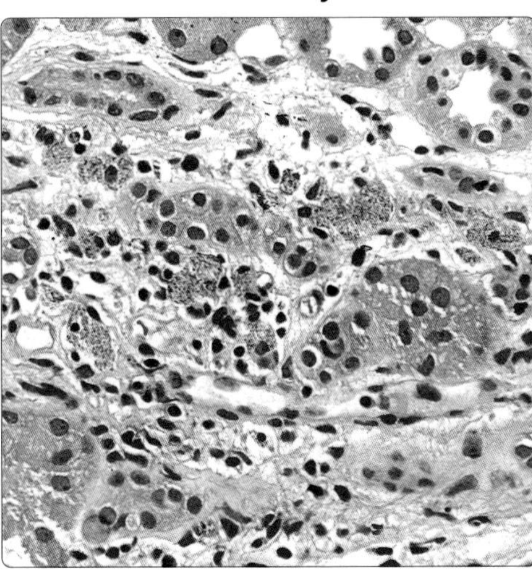

(Left) *Recurrent 2,8-DHA deposition is seen in a renal transplant recipient. The disease was first diagnosed in this patient at the time of recurrence, 8 months after transplant. The interstitium has marked fibrosis and the tubules are atrophic. A few foci of brown crystals are present ➙.* **(Right)** *Fine brown crystals of 2,8-DHA are seen in the interstitium of the cortex, probably in macrophages.*

2,8-DHA Crystals

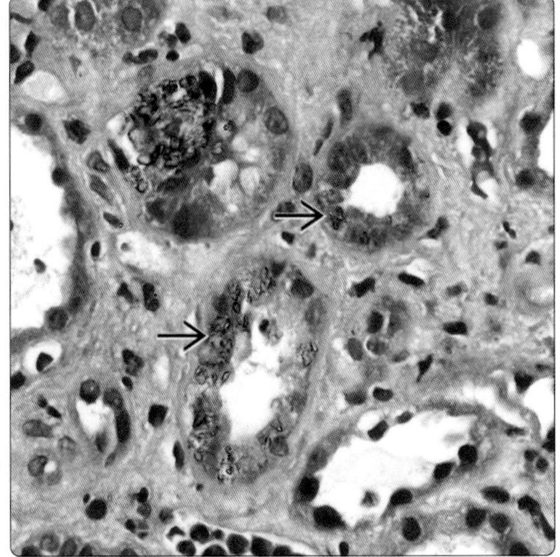

2,8-DHA Crystals

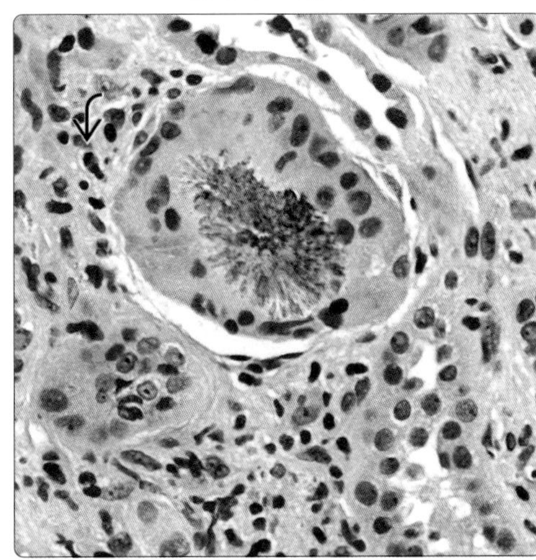

(Left) *Clear to brown-tinged small crystals are seen within the tubular epithelial cell cytoplasm ➙. The interstitium has a fine fibrosis with minimal inflammation.* **(Right)** *Intratubular 2,8-DHA crystals in a patient with APRT deficiency sometimes provoke a giant cell response and inflammation, as shown in this field. An eosinophil is also present ➙.*

2,8-DHA Crystals

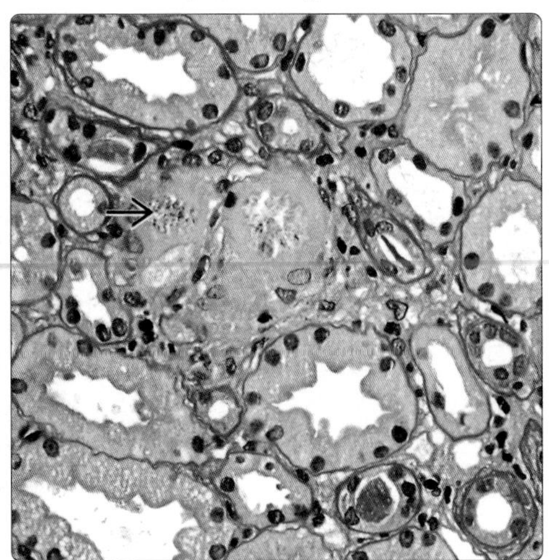

2,8-DHA Crystals

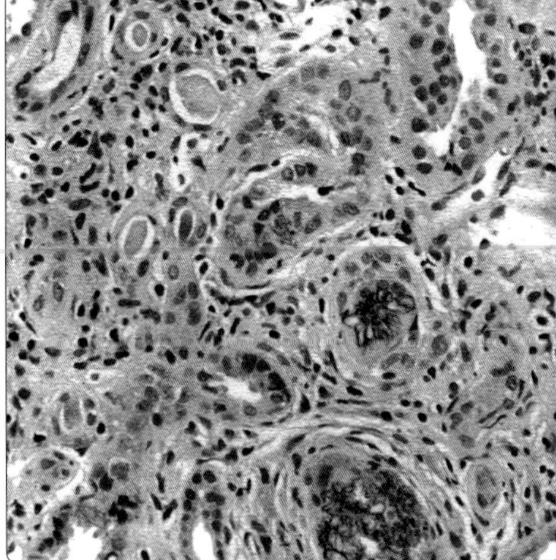

(Left) *A few small crystals ➙ are visualized on this PAS-stained section. Proximal tubules appear generally normal and there is no fibrosis. The diagnosis could easily be missed on this sample.* **(Right)** *By light microscopy 2,8-DHA crystals resemble calcium oxalate, except for the brown color. Here the crystals are primarily in tubules, with an accompanying interstitial inflammation and fibrosis.*

Cystinosis

KEY FACTS

TERMINOLOGY

- Autosomal recessive lysosomal storage disease secondary to mutations in *CTNS* gene resulting in intralysosomal accumulation of cystine and multiorgan damage

ETIOLOGY/PATHOGENESIS

- *CTNS* gene mutations
- 75% of European patients homozygous for 57 kb deletion

CLINICAL ISSUES

- 3 types
  - Infantile type presents with Fanconi syndrome
    - Progress to ESRD by age 10
  - Juvenile type slowly progressive
    - Presents with proteinuria
  - Adult type: Presents with ocular disease
- > 1 nmol cystine/mg protein in peripheral blood neutrophils
- Treat with cysteamine
- Transplantation extends life of patients with juvenile form

MICROSCOPIC

- Podocyte and tubular epithelial multinucleation
- Atubular glomeruli
- Proximal tubule "swan neck" deformity, atubular glomeruli
- Polarizable cystine crystals on frozen section

ANCILLARY TESTS

- Electron microscopy
  - Intracellular spaces (plate, hexagon) where crystals located

TOP DIFFERENTIAL DIAGNOSES

- Oxalosis
- Fabry disease
- Cystinuria

DIAGNOSTIC CHECKLIST

- Multinucleated podocytes pathognomic

Multinucleated Podocytes

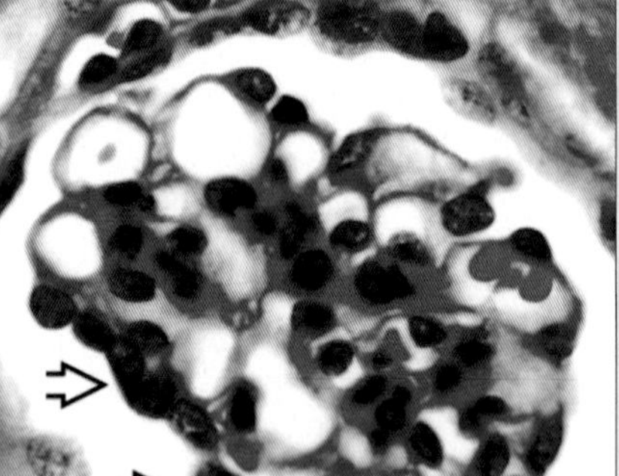

Cystine Crystals

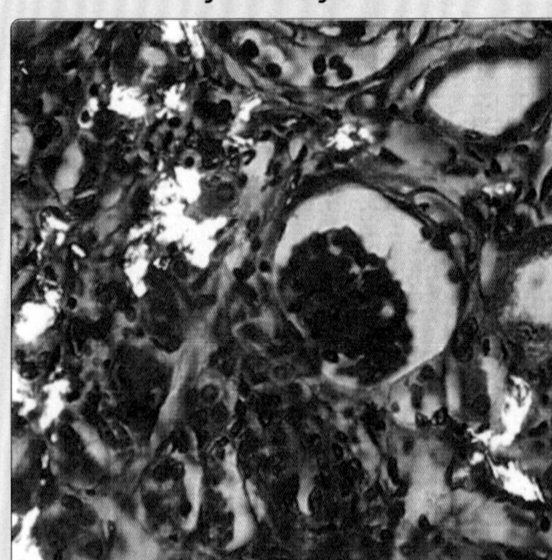

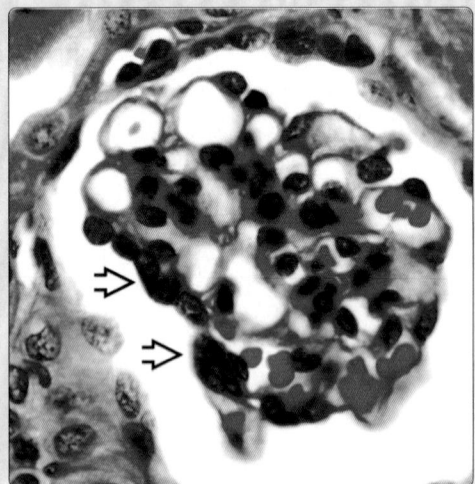

(Left) *Multinucleated podocytes* ➡ *are characteristic of cystinosis even in the absence of Fanconi syndrome. Pathogenesis may involve aberrant podocyte division without cytokinesis.* **(Right)** *Cystine crystals are water soluble and dissolve with formalin fixation; rhomboid or polymorphous are best seen on frozen sections under polarized light. (Courtesy J. Bernstein, MD.)*

Cystine Crystals

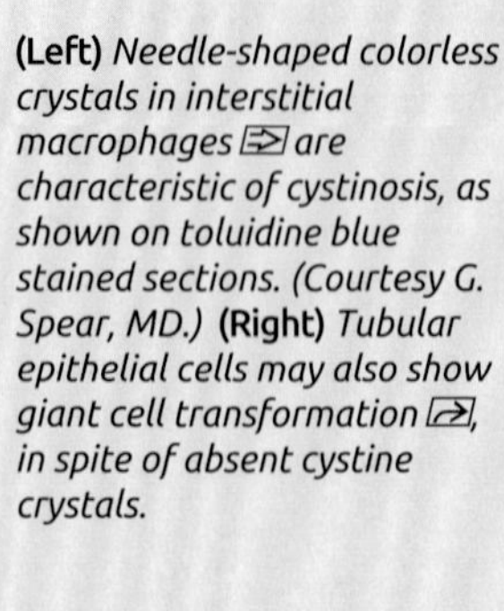

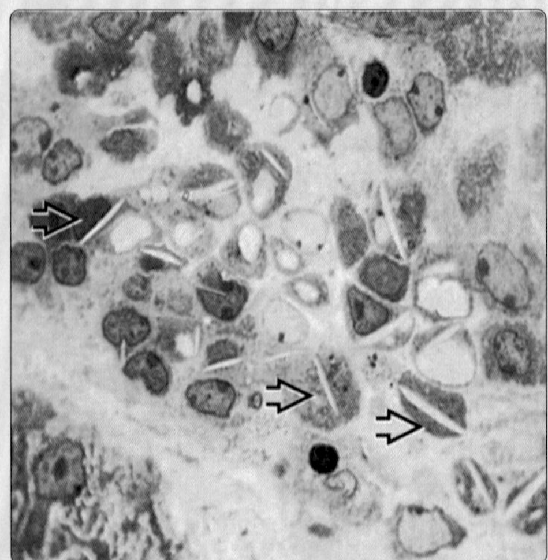

Multinucleated Tubular Epithelial Cell

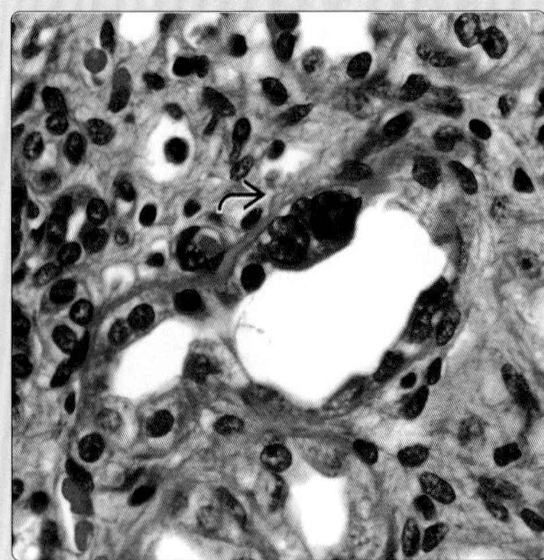

(Left) *Needle-shaped colorless crystals in interstitial macrophages* ➡ *are characteristic of cystinosis, as shown on toluidine blue stained sections. (Courtesy G. Spear, MD.)* **(Right)** *Tubular epithelial cells may also show giant cell transformation* ↗*, in spite of absent cystine crystals.*

TERMINOLOGY

Definitions

- Autosomal recessive lysosomal storage disease secondary to mutations in *CTNS* gene resulting in intralysosomal accumulation of cystine and multiorgan damage

ETIOLOGY/PATHOGENESIS

Genetics

- *CTNS*
  - Encodes cystinosin, a lysosomal membrane cystine transporter
  - Maps to chromosome 17p13
  - > 90 mutations reported
  - Infantile form
    - 75% homozygous 57 kb deletion (Europe)
    - Eliminates protein expression
  - Juvenile and adult forms
    - Point or missense mutations affecting transmembrane loops or N-terminus

Pathophysiology

- Defective cystine transport and accumulation in lysosomes
- Cystine-induced injury of proximal tubular cells thought due to
  - ↓ ATP
  - ↓ glutathione
  - ↑ apoptosis
- Mitochondria in cystinotic proximal tubules contain ↓ ATP and ↓ glutathione
  - Tubular cell apoptosis increased
- Multinucleated podocytes may reflect newly recognized form of podocyte cell death called mitotic catastrophe

CLINICAL ISSUES

Epidemiology

- Incidence
  - Infantile form: 1 in 100,000-200,000 live births
  - Juvenile and adult forms: 5% of cystinosis cases
- Age
  - Infantile form: Presents at 6-12 months
  - Juvenile and adult forms: Onset of symptoms at 3-50 years

Presentation

- Fanconi syndrome (infantile)
  - Polyuria, polydipsia, electrolyte abnormalities, dehydration, rickets, growth retardation
  - Not always present in juvenile and adult forms
- Hypothyroidism: 5-10 years
- Retinopathy, corneal deposits (only adults), pulmonary dysfunction: 21-40 years; male hypogonadism, swallowing abnormalities, myopathy

Laboratory Tests

- Cystine levels in blood polymorphonuclear leukocytes
  - Tandem mass spectrometry most sensitive
    - Homozygotes: > 1 nmol cystine/mg protein
    - Heterozygotes: 0.14-0.57 nmol cystine/mg protein
    - Normal range: 0.04-0.16 nmol cystine/mg protein

Treatment

- Drugs
  - Cysteamine, aminothiol
- Transplantation
- Stem cell and gene therapy approaches evolving

Prognosis

- Infantile form
  - If untreated, ESRD develops at mean of 9.2 years
  - Diagnosis frequently delayed, which worsens prognosis
- Juvenile form
  - May progress to ESRD, but at later age (12-28 years)

MICROSCOPIC

Histologic Features

- Glomeruli
  - Podocyte multinucleation
  - FSGS, typically seen in juvenile form
  - Endothelial and podocyte cystine crystals
  - Atubular glomeruli prominent
- Tubules
  - Cystine crystal deposition
    - Polarizable, hexagonal, rhomboid, or polymorphous
    - Water soluble, best seen in froze0n sections under polarized light
  - Proximal tubule "swan neck" deformity
    - Shortened, atrophic early proximal tubule after 6 months of age
  - Epithelial multinucleation
- Interstitium
  - In allografts, infiltrating macrophages contain hexagonal crystals

DIFFERENTIAL DIAGNOSIS

Oxalosis

- Fan-shaped, needle-like polarizable crystals
  - Preserved after formalin fixation

Fabry Disease

- Lacey podocytes
- Laminated deposits by EM

Cystinuria

- Recurrent nephrolithiasis without intracellular accumulation

DIAGNOSTIC CHECKLIST

Pathologic Interpretation Pearls

- Multinucleated podocytes pathognomic

SELECTED REFERENCES

1. Emma F et al: Nephropathic cystinosis: an international consensus document. Nephrol Dial Transplant. 29 Suppl 4:iv87-94, 2014
2. Ivanova E et al: Cystinosis: clinical presentation, pathogenesis and treatment. Pediatr Endocrinol Rev. 12 Suppl 1:176-84, 2014
3. Surendran K et al: Lysosome dysfunction in the pathogenesis of kidney diseases. Pediatr Nephrol. 29(12):2253-61, 2014
4. Liapis H et al: New insights into the pathology of podocyte loss: mitotic catastrophe. Am J Pathol. 183(5):1364-74, 2013
5. Larsen CP et al: The incidence of atubular glomeruli in nephropathic cystinosis renal biopsies. Mol Genet Metab. 101(4):417-20, 2010

Uric Acid Nephropathy/Gout

KEY FACTS

TERMINOLOGY

- Intrarenal precipitation of uric acid associated with hyperuricemia

ETIOLOGY/PATHOGENESIS

- Decreased uric acid excretion (75-90%)
- Overproduction of uric acid (10-25%)

CLINICAL ISSUES

- Acute uric acid nephropathy (UAN): Acute oliguric or anuric renal failure
- Chronic UAN: Chronic renal failure and hypertension

MACROSCOPIC

- Acute UAN: Medullary and papillary yellow radial striations
- Chronic UAN: Medullary yellow flecks corresponding to tophi or microtophi
- Uric acid stones

MICROSCOPIC

- Acute UAN: Birefringent urate crystals in collecting ducts forming linear streaks, acute tubular injury
- Chronic UAN: Medullary foreign body-type granulomas containing needle-like urate crystals or crystal clefts (= microtophus)

TOP DIFFERENTIAL DIAGNOSES

- Acute tubular injury with crystal deposits: Indinavir, acyclovir, sulfadiazine, light chain proximal tubulopathy
- Chronic nephropathy with granulomas: Cholesterol granulomas, oxalate nephropathy, indinavir or acyclovir nephropathy, sarcoidosis

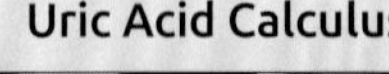

Uric Acid Calculus

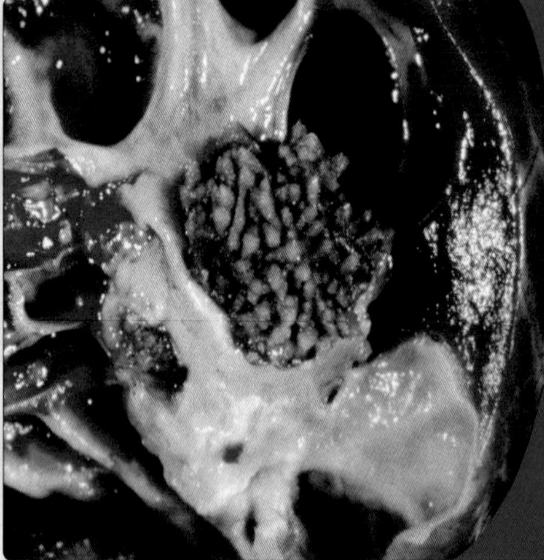

Acute Uric Acid Nephropathy

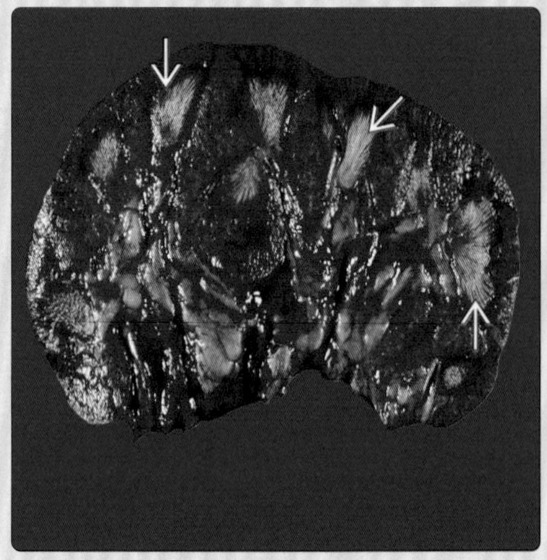

(Left) *Gross photograph reveals a brown calculus with a rough surface in the renal pelvis. There is marked calyceal dilation, pyramidal effacement, and parenchymal thinning. (Courtesy V. Nickeleit, MD.)* **(Right)** *Gross photograph reveals distinct yellow striae in the medulla* ➔*, with congestion at the corticomedullary junction, of a kidney with acute uric acid nephropathy. (Courtesy V. Nickeleit, MD.)*

Medullary Tubular Urate Crystals

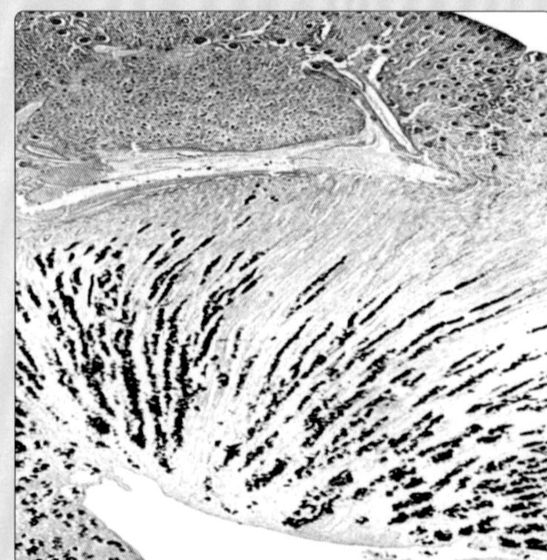

Histochemical Stain for Uric Acid

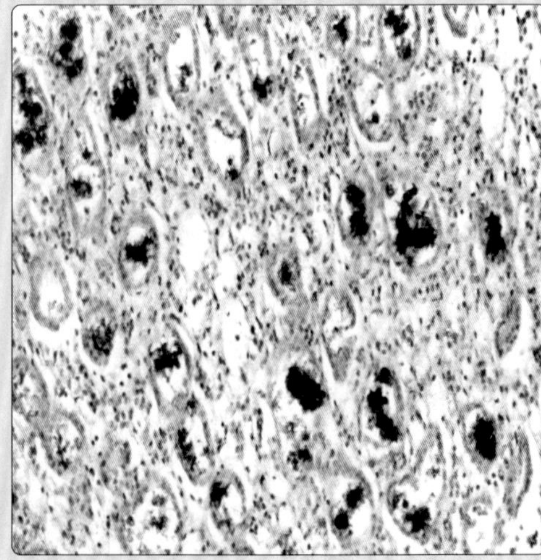

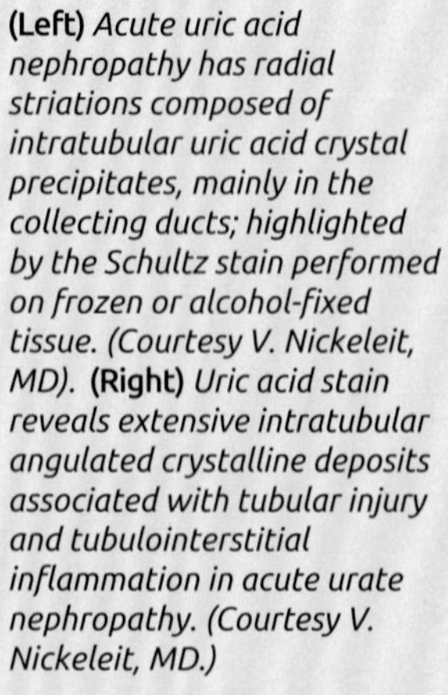

(Left) *Acute uric acid nephropathy has radial striations composed of intratubular uric acid crystal precipitates, mainly in the collecting ducts; highlighted by the Schultz stain performed on frozen or alcohol-fixed tissue. (Courtesy V. Nickeleit, MD).* **(Right)** *Uric acid stain reveals extensive intratubular angulated crystalline deposits associated with tubular injury and tubulointerstitial inflammation in acute urate nephropathy. (Courtesy V. Nickeleit, MD.)*

TERMINOLOGY

Abbreviations

- Uric acid nephropathy (UAN)

Synonyms

- Urate nephropathy, gouty nephropathy, gout nephropathy

Definitions

- Intrarenal precipitation of uric acid associated with hyperuricemia or hyperuricosuria

ETIOLOGY/PATHOGENESIS

Normal Metabolism

- Uric acid is final degradation product of purine metabolism
- Sources: Endogenous from adenine or guanine nucleotides; exogenous from diet
- Uric acid is generated in all cells but most markedly by hepatocytes
- Urate is filtered freely, reabsorbed, secreted, and there is post-secretory reabsorption in proximal tubules
- 10% of filtered load is excreted in urine

Hyperuricemia

- Defined as plasma uric acid > 7 mg/dL
    - Decreased excretion (75-90%); overproduction (10-25%)
- Decreased tubular secretion/increased reabsorption
    - Idiopathic
    - Drugs: Thiazide diuretics, cyclosporine A, low dose salicylates
    - Chronic heavy metal toxicity: Lead (saturnine gout), beryllium
    - Metabolic: Ketoacidosis, lactic acidosis, dehydration, Bartter syndrome, chronic renal failure
    - Endocrine: Hypothyroidism, hyperparathyroidism
    - Genetic: Familial juvenile hyperuricemic nephropathy (uromodulin storage disease)
    - Miscellaneous: Sickle cell anemia, Down syndrome, sarcoidosis, eclampsia
- Overproduction/excessive release
    - Idiopathic (60%)
    - Massive tissue destruction
        - Hematologic diseases: Leukemia, lymphoma, myeloma, polycythemia
        - Tumor lysis syndrome: Treatment of leukemia, lymphoma, myeloma, and solid tumors with cytotoxic agents or radiation
        - Crush injury, rhabdomyolysis, seizures (prolonged, severe)
    - Hereditary enzyme deficiencies
        - X-linked: Hypoxanthine guanine phosphoribosyl transferase deficiency; complete (Lesch-Nyhan syndrome) or partial
        - Autosomal recessive: Glucose-6-phosphatase deficiency in glycogen storage disease type 1

Hyperuricemia and Kidney Disease

- Tissue deposits are monosodium urate monohydrate or (rarely) ammonium urate
    - Doubly refractile on polarization microscopy
- Kidney is involved in 3 ways
    - Intratubular uric acid deposits: Acute UAN
    - Interstitial deposits: Chronic UAN
    - Lithiasis: Uric acid or mixed uric acid and calcium oxalate stones
- Severe hyperuricemia (plasma levels 20-50 mg/dL)
    - Urinary solubility exceeded with resultant precipitation
    - Compounded by acidic urine, high urinary calcium phosphate
    - Usually associated with acute UAN
- Kidney injury in acute UAN has at least 4 potential contributing mechanisms
    - Intrarenal tubular obstruction: Precipitated uric crystals in lumens of collecting ducts
    - Direct toxicity to tubular epithelium: Release of lysosomal contents resulting in epithelial injury
    - Indirect tubular epithelial injury: Release of chemokines with secondary inflammation
    - Vasoconstriction, impaired autoregulation, and renal ischemia

CLINICAL ISSUES

Presentation

- Acute UAN
    - Acute oliguric or anuric renal failure
    - Severe hyperuricemia (> 15 mg/dL)
    - Urinalysis reveals birefringent uric acid crystals
    - Typically arises in tumor lysis syndrome or crush injury
    - Flank pain if nephrolithiasis
- Chronic UAN (classical gouty nephropathy)
    - Arises in patients with gout, chronic hyperuricemia, and hypertension
    - Chronic renal failure is uncommonly caused by pure chronic UAN (1.5% in 1 series)
    - Significantly increased odds of developing chronic renal failure with chronic UAN (odds ratio 4:6)
- Uric acid calculi
    - May arise in acute UAN
    - Are identified in 15-20% of patients with gout
        - Associated with hyperuricemia, low urinary pH, and low fractional excretion of uric acid
        - Chronic obstructive pyelonephritis may be significant cause of chronic renal failure

Treatment

- Acute UAN: Prevention is mainstay of treatment in acute disease
    - Volume expansion, loop diuretics
    - Allopurinol; recombinant urate oxidase
    - Hemodialysis to remove uric acid load
- Chronic UAN
    - Hydration
    - Uricosuric agents: Probenecid, sulfinpyrazone

Prognosis

- Acute UAN
    - High rates of reversal of acute renal failure with full recovery if treated early
- Chronic UAN
    - No therapy: 40% develop chronic renal failure and 10% develop uremia

- Gouty nephropathy is rare with uricosuric therapy
- < 1% of end-stage renal failure is attributable to chronic UAN

MACROSCOPIC

Gross Examination

- Acute UAN: Medullary yellow striations converging on papilla
- Chronic UAN: Medullary yellow flecks corresponding to tophi
- Chronic renal disease with reduced renal mass, cortical thinning, and surface granularity
- Uric acid stones
  - Yellow-brown, hard, rough or smooth, multiple, small (2 cm or less)
  - Dilated pelvis or ureter
  - 6-25% with chronic UAN have features of pyelonephritis

MICROSCOPIC

Histologic Features

- Acute UAN
  - Intraluminal clusters of birefringent urate crystals in collecting ducts forming linear streaks
  - Acute tubular injury; mild interstitial inflammation
  - Tubular rupture with extrusion of uromodulin
  - Glomeruli usually are unremarkable and rarely have a lobular form of glomerulopathy
  - Needle-like birefringent crystals of monosodium urate seen in alcohol-fixed or frozen tissue
  - De Galantha and Schultz stains identify uric acid in tissue
  - Electron microscopy reveals injured epithelial cells with cytoplasmic angulated crystals in collecting ducts
- Chronic UAN
  - Tophi are granulomas containing birefringent, needle-like sodium urate crystals or crystal clefts
    - Syncytial giant cells, epithelioid macrophages, lymphocytes, and eosinophils
    - Intratubular or interstitial
    - Mainly medullary; cortical tophi are uncommon
  - Interstitial fibrosis and tubular atrophy are variable
  - Glomerular changes include mesangial sclerosis and capillary double contours
  - Pyelonephritis may also be evident if there are calculi

DIFFERENTIAL DIAGNOSIS

Acute Tubular Injury With Crystal Deposits

- Distinction from other crystal deposits based on clinical drug exposure and spectroscopic analysis
- Drugs: Antivirals and antibiotics
  - Indinavir and acyclovir
    - Acute tubular injury, interstitial inflammation, and granulomas
    - Cortical and medullary collecting duct crystals
  - Sulfadiazine
    - Collecting duct crystals mixed with secreted protein and cell debris
    - Acute tubulointerstitial nephritis, eosinophils, granulomas
- Light chain proximal tubulopathy (Fanconi syndrome)
  - Proximal tubular needle-like crystals or crystal clefts in epithelial cytoplasm (kappa > lambda)

Chronic Nephropathy With Granulomas

- Cholesterol granulomas: Associated with nephrotic syndrome
- Oxalate nephropathy: Characteristic birefringent crystals on polarization microscopy
- Indinavir or acyclovir nephropathy
  - Needle-like birefringent crystals with granulomas and fibrosis
  - Indinavir sulfate lithiasis
- Sarcoidosis
  - Noncaseating "tight" granulomas ± Schaumann bodies (psammomatous calcium phosphate) or asteroid bodies (eosinophilic stellate inclusions) in cytoplasm of giant cells

DIAGNOSTIC CHECKLIST

Clinically Relevant Pathologic Features

- Acute UAN
  - Linear intratubular precipitates of uric acid crystals in medullary collecting ducts
  - Acute tubular injury with interstitial inflammation
  - Acute renal failure associated with
    - Toxic tubular injury
    - Tubular obstruction
    - Tubulointerstitial inflammation
    - Secondary ischemia associated with hyperuricemia
- Chronic UAN
  - Medullary tubulointerstitial microtophi
  - Interstitial fibrosis, tubular atrophy, and glomerular sclerosis
  - Glomerular mesangial sclerosis and double contours

Pathologic Interpretation Pearls

- Acute UAN: Massive intratubular deposits of uric acid with acute tubular injury, ectasia, and inflammation
- Chronic UAN: Noncaseating granulomas with radial clefts or needle-like crystals, localized to medulla
  - Often accompanied by interstitial fibrosis, tubular atrophy, and vascular sclerosis
- De Galantha or Schultz stains identify uric acid deposits in alcohol fixed or frozen sections

SELECTED REFERENCES

1. Wilson FP et al: Tumor lysis syndrome: new challenges and recent advances. Adv Chronic Kidney Dis. 21(1):18-26, 2014
2. Wilson FP et al: Onco-nephrology: tumor lysis syndrome. Clin J Am Soc Nephrol. 7(10):1730-9, 2012
3. Shimada M et al: A novel role for uric acid in acute kidney injury associated with tumour lysis syndrome. Nephrol Dial Transplant. 24(10):2960-4, 2009
4. Nickeleit V et al: Uric acid nephropathy and end-stage renal disease–review of a non-disease. Nephrol Dial Transplant. 12(9):1832-8, 1997
5. Robinson RR et al: Acute uric acid nephropathy. Arch Intern Med. 137(7):839-40, 1977
6. Kanwar YS et al: Leukemic urate nephropathy. Arch Pathol. 99(9):467-72, 1975

Medullary Tophus

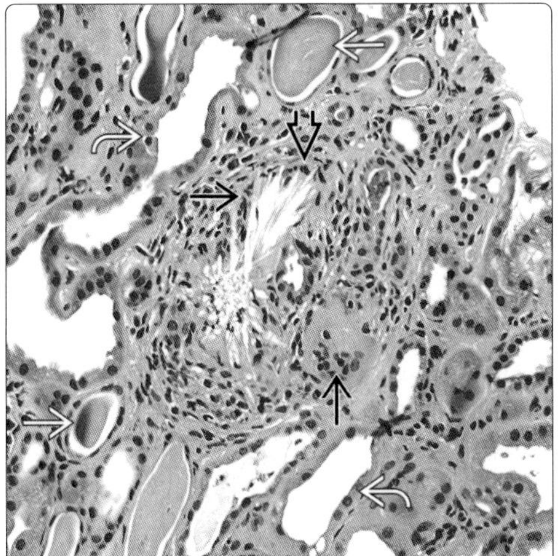

Gouty Tophus

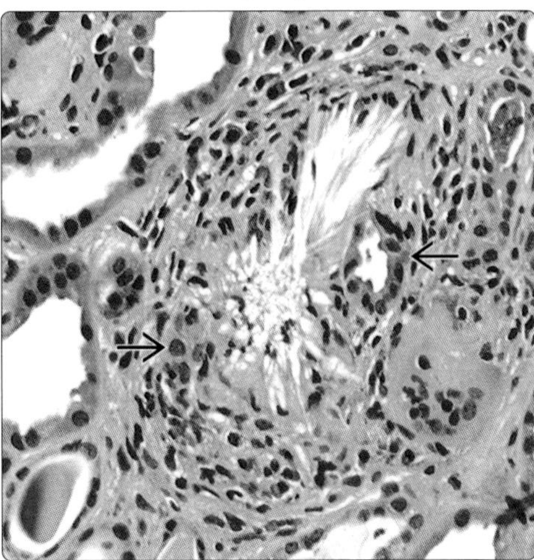

(Left) *A discrete medullary interstitial microtophus is composed of a collection of macrophages and foreign body giant cells ➙, some of which contain needle-like clefts ➙, with lymphocytes, plasma cells, and eosinophils. Surrounding tubules have epithelial flattening ➙ and casts ➙.* **(Right)** *A high-power view reveals radial needle-like clefts, giant cells, mononuclear and eosinophilic infiltrates, and atrophic tubular profiles ➙ within the granuloma.*

Multiple Medullary Tophi

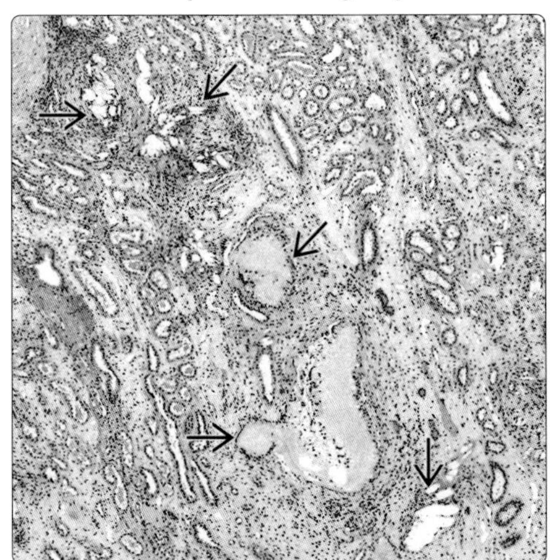

Crystalline Clefts in a Medullary Tophus

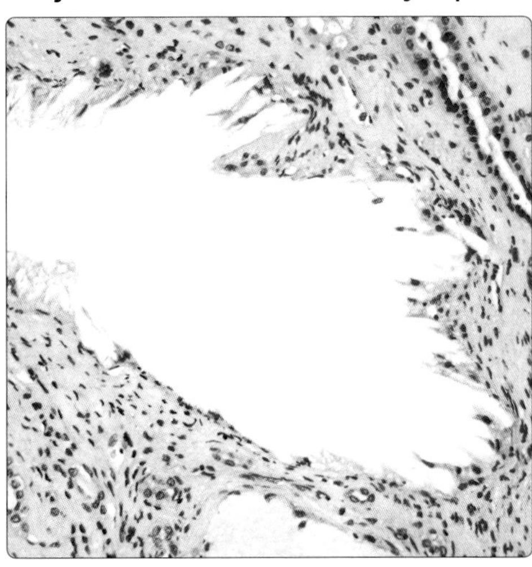

(Left) *Multiple tophi are evident in the medulla of this kidney specimen, both with and without crystal clefts ➙. There is interstitial fibrosis, mononuclear inflammation, and tubular loss in the surrounding medulla.* **(Right)** *A medullary interstitial microtophus is shown with cleft-like spaces remaining after dissolution of urate crystals during formalin fixation. There is fibrosis and mild mononuclear inflammation in the surrounding medulla.*

Calcium Oxalate Crystal Deposits

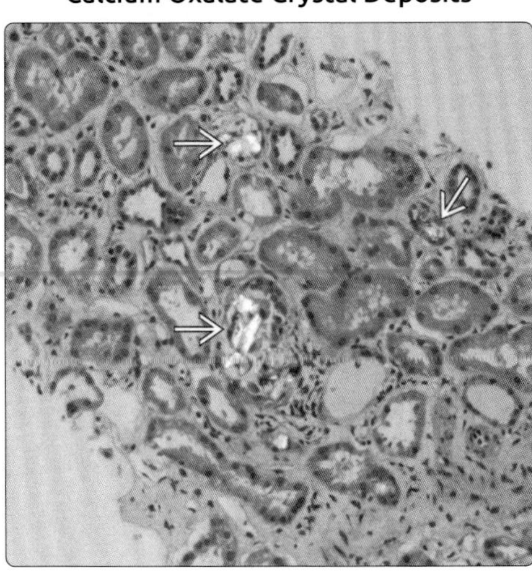

Cholesterol Clefts in Tubules and Interstitium

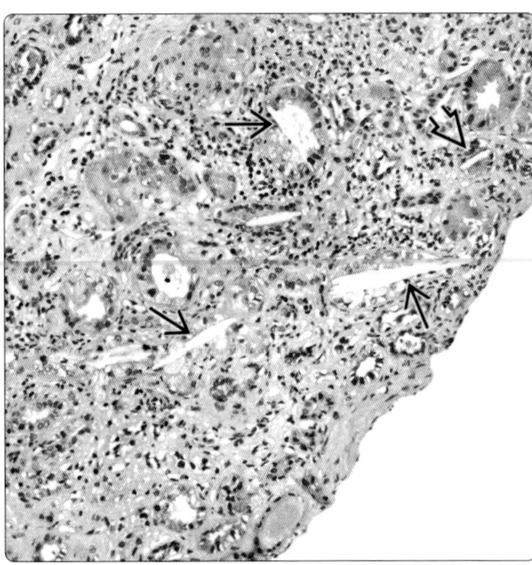

(Left) *Calcium oxalate crystal deposits are retained in tissue after fixation and processing. Crystals are localized to tubules in this instance ➙ but may also be interstitial. They have characteristic birefringence when viewed in partially polarized light.* **(Right)** *Cholesterol clefts are evident in tubules ➙ and in the interstitium ➙. Interstitial crystals are in macrophages and can form granulomas that are easy to misinterpret as tophi. Such cholesterol deposits are associated with the nephrotic syndrome.*

Bartter Syndrome

KEY FACTS

TERMINOLOGY

- Syndrome of hypokalemia, alkalosis, elevated renin and aldosterone and normal or low blood pressure, due to autosomal recessive mutations in tubular ion channels/transporters

ETIOLOGY/PATHOGENESIS

- 6 genetic mutations affecting ion channels in TALH
  - Type I: *NKCC2* gene for NKCC2 (a Na-K-Cl cotransporter)
  - Type II: *KCNJ1* gene for ROMK (renal outer medullary K channel)
  - Type III: *CLCNKB* gene for ClCKB (Cl channel)
  - Type IV A: *BSND* gene for barttin (Cl channel)
  - Type IV B: *CLCNKA+B* genes for ClC-Ka+b (Cl channel)
  - Type V: *CASR* gene encoding CaSR (calcium sensor)

CLINICAL ISSUES

- Neonatal forms (types I, II, IV)
  - Early onset, severe
  - Polyhydramnios, polyuria, growth retardation, hypercalciuria, nephrocalcinosis
- Classic form (type III)
  - Presents in infancy or childhood
  - Failure to thrive, growth retardation, dehydration
- Bartter syndrome with sensorineural deafness (type IV)

MICROSCOPIC

- Diffuse enlargement of JGA with increased renin
- Clusters of sclerotic and immature glomeruli in outer cortex
- Hypertrophy and hyperplasia of medullary interstitial cells

TOP DIFFERENTIAL DIAGNOSES

- Drugs: ATII receptor antagonists, cyclosporine, diuretics
- Addison disease
- Chronic renal ischemia

Juxtaglomerular Apparatus Enlargement

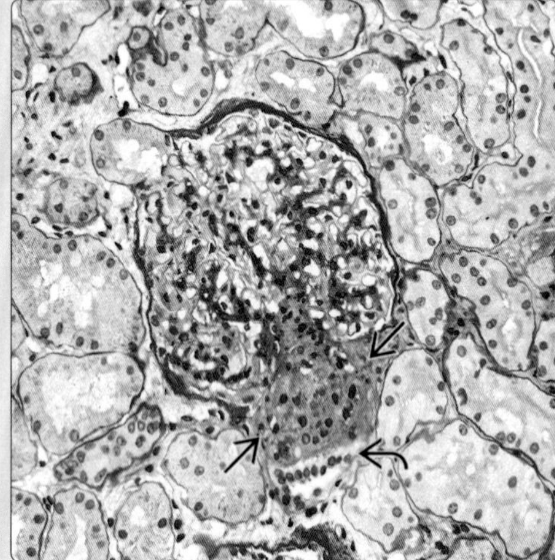

JGA Cytoplasmic Granules

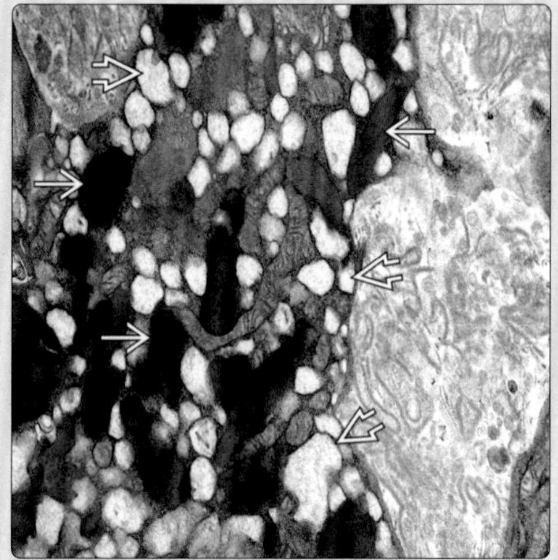

(Left) *Bartter syndrome is characterized by hyperplasia and hypertrophy of the juxtaglomerular apparatus → with prominent macula densa ↶. This reaction to Na loss is the primary histologic feature in Bartter syndrome.* **(Right)** *By electron microscopy juxtaglomerular cells demonstrate membrane-bound granules of varying electron density → and numerous vesicles ⇨.*

Outer Cortical Glomerulosclerosis

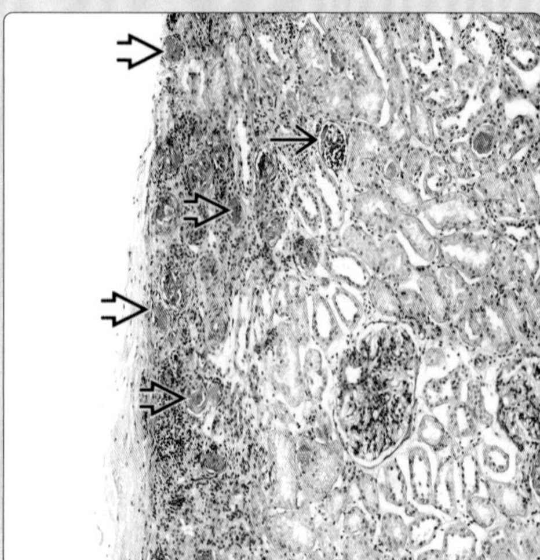

Medullary Interstitial Cell Hyperplasia

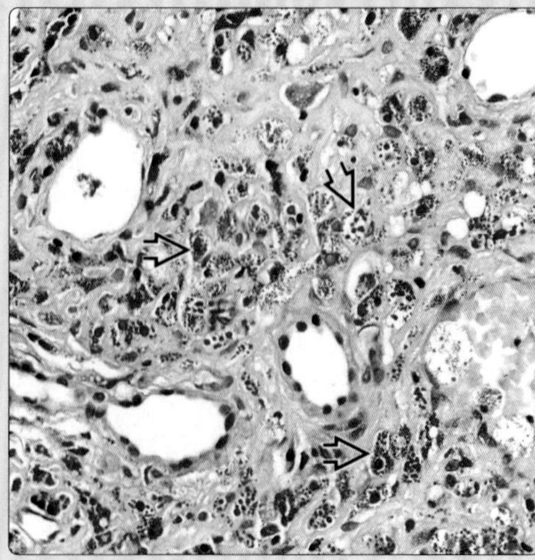

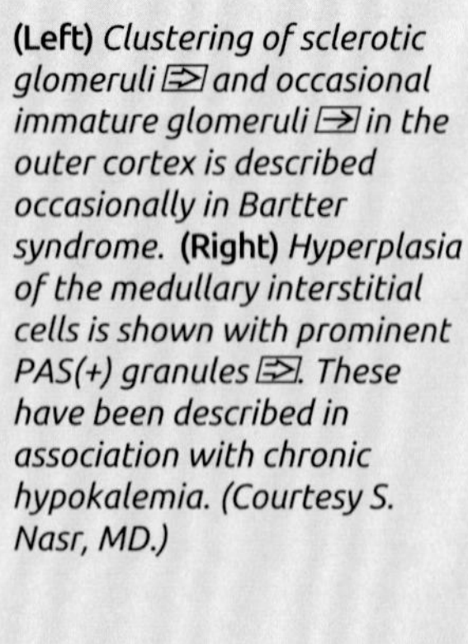

(Left) *Clustering of sclerotic glomeruli ⇨ and occasional immature glomeruli → in the outer cortex is described occasionally in Bartter syndrome.* **(Right)** *Hyperplasia of the medullary interstitial cells is shown with prominent PAS(+) granules ⇨. These have been described in association with chronic hypokalemia. (Courtesy S. Nasr, MD.)*

TERMINOLOGY

Definitions

- Group of salt-losing tubulopathies characterized by
  - Genetic mutations of Na and Cl membrane channels in the loop of Henle
  - Salt and water loss with hypokalemic alkalosis
  - Hyperreninemic secondary hyperaldosteronism
  - Hyperplasia of juxtaglomerular apparati

ETIOLOGY/PATHOGENESIS

Genetic Disorders

- 5 loss-of-function mutations: Autosomal recessive
  - Type I: *NKCC2* gene for NKCC2 (Na-K-Cl cotransporter)
  - Type II: *KCNJ1* gene for ROMK (renal outer medullary K channel)
  - Type III: *CLCNKB* gene for ClCKB (Cl channel)
  - Type IV A: *BSND* gene for barttin (Cl channel)
  - Type IV B: *CLCNKA+B* for ClC-Ka+b (Cl channel)
- 1 gain-of-function mutation: Autosomal dominant
  - Type V: *CASR* gene encoding CaSR (calcium sensor)

Pathophysiology

- Mutations mainly affect NaCl membrane channels in thick ascending loop of Henle
  - Reduced NaCl reabsorption
  - Delivers excess NaCl to distal tubule and collecting duct
  - Promotes NaCl loss, volume depletion, K, and acid secretion
- Electrolyte and water depletion with hypovolemia
  - Activates renin-angiotensin-aldosterone (RAA) system
  - Aldosterone promotes further K loss
  - Angiotensin II (ATII) promotes prostaglandin synthesis (especially PGE2) and may influence interstitial cell hyperplasia
  - Prolonged RAA activation leads to hyperplasia of juxtaglomerular apparatus (JGA)

CLINICAL ISSUES

Presentation

- Neonatal forms (types I, II, IV)
  - Early onset, severe
  - Polyhydramnios, polyuria, growth retardation, hypercalciuria, nephrocalcinosis
- Classic form (type III)
  - Presents in infancy or childhood (in type V also)
  - Failure to thrive, growth retardation, dehydration
- Bartter syndrome with sensorineural deafness (type IV)
  - Onset in infancy or childhood
  - Polyuria, hypochloremia, hypomagnesemia, deafness, chronic renal failure

Treatment

- Drugs
  - Nonsteroidal anti-inflammatory agents and potassium-sparing diuretics
  - Potassium and sodium replacement

Prognosis

- Limited data suggests chronic renal functional impairment occurs in ~ 20% of patients

MICROSCOPIC

Histologic Features

- Glomeruli and blood vessels
  - Diffuse hypertrophy and hyperplasia of JGA
    - JGA cells and arteriolar myocytes have granular cytoplasm
      - Periodic acid-Schiff and silver stain positive
      - Renin localized to granules by IHC
  - Clusters of sclerotic and immature glomeruli in outer cortex
  - Most glomeruli normal
    - Rarely focal segmental glomerulosclerosis or C1q nephropathy
  - Afferent arterioles may be hyalinized
- Tubules and interstitium
  - Hypertrophy and hyperplasia of medullary interstitial cells
    - Cytoplasmic vacuoles and PAS(+) granules
  - Proximal tubular coarse vacuoles (secondary to hypokalemia)
  - Medullary nephrocalcinosis in types I & II
- Immunofluorescence findings nonspecific
- Electron microscopy
  - JGA and arteriolar myocytes
    - Electron-dense secretory granules, some rhomboid forms
  - Hyperplastic medullary interstitial cells
    - Cytoplasmic, membrane-bound granules and myelin figures

DIFFERENTIAL DIAGNOSIS

Juxtaglomerular Apparatus Hyperplasia

- Chronic renal ischemia
  - Renal artery stenosis
  - Cardiac failure
  - Intrarenal vascular sclerosis: Hypertension, chronic thrombotic microangiopathies
- Drugs: ATII receptor antagonists, cyclosporine, diuretics
- Addison disease

DIAGNOSTIC CHECKLIST

Pathologic Interpretation Pearls

- Enlarged JGA in neonates, infants, and children

SELECTED REFERENCES

1. Bhat YR et al: Antenatal bartter syndrome: a review. Int J Pediatr. 2012:857136, 2012
2. Park CW et al: Renal dysfunction and barttin expression in Bartter syndrome Type IV associated with a G47R mutation in BSND in a family. Clin Nephrol. 75 Suppl 1:69-74, 2011
3. Shaer AJ: Inherited primary renal tubular hypokalemic alkalosis: a review of Gitelman and Bartter syndromes. Am J Med Sci. 322(6):316-32, 2001
4. Bartter FC et al: Hyperplasia of the juxtaglomerular complex with hyperaldosteronism and hypokalemic alkalosis. A new syndrome. Am J Med. 33:811-28, 1962

KEY FACTS

TERMINOLOGY

- X-linked tubulopathy manifested by low molecular weight proteinuria, hypercalciuria, nephrocalcinosis, nephrolithiasis, and progressive renal failure

ETIOLOGY/PATHOGENESIS

- *CLCN5* gene, Dent disease 1
  - Mutation in 2/3 of Dent disease patients
  - Encodes electrogenic chloride/proton exchanger ClC-5
- *OCRL1* gene, Dent disease 2
  - Encodes protein (OCRL1) with phosphatidylinositol-4, 5-bisphosphate 5-phosphatase activity
  - Lowe syndrome, a related disease, also has mutation in *OCRL1* gene
    - More severe phenotype than Dent disease 2
- *CLCN5* and *OCRL1* genes, both located on X chromosome

CLINICAL ISSUES

- Nephrolithiasis
- Hypercalciuria
- Low molecular weight proteinuria
- Chronic renal failure
- Dent disease is likely underdiagnosed
  - Should be suspected in young males with nephrolithiasis and any degree of proteinuria

MICROSCOPIC

- Interstitial fibrosis and tubular atrophy
- Focal global or segmental glomerulosclerosis

ANCILLARY TESTS

- Urinary retinol binding protein

TOP DIFFERENTIAL DIAGNOSES

- Other causes of partial Fanconi syndrome
- Focal glomerulosclerosis due to other causes
- Nephrolithiasis

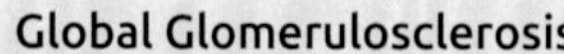

Global Glomerulosclerosis

Normal Glomerulus

(Left) *Focal glomeruli show global glomerulosclerosis. No segmental scars were identified in this case, although focal segmental glomerulosclerosis may be seen in Dent disease.* **(Right)** *A nonglobally sclerotic glomerulus appears normal by light microscopy.*

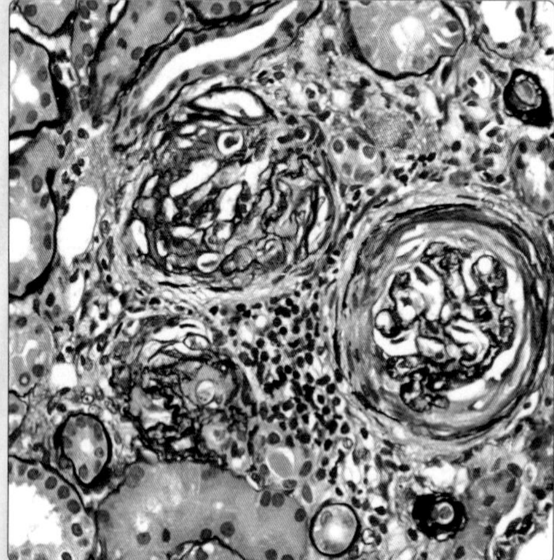

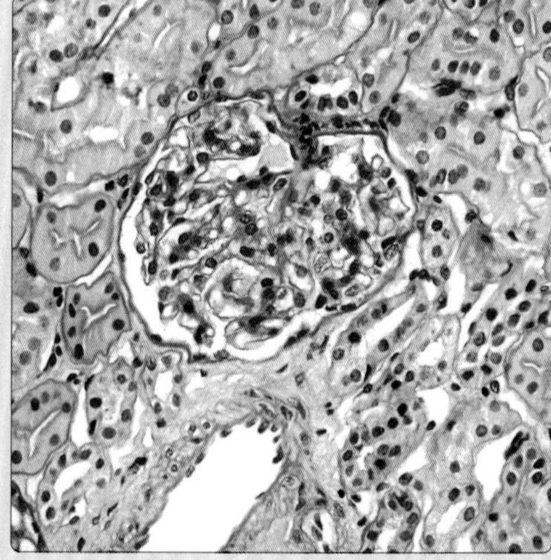

Focal Interstitial Fibrosis/Tubular Atrophy

Segmental Foot Process Effacement

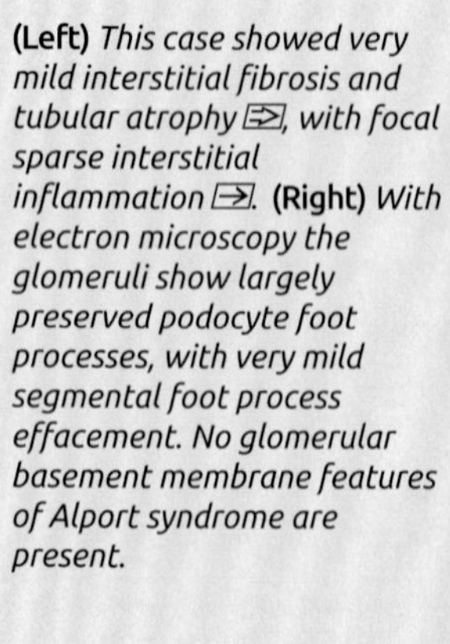

(Left) *This case showed very mild interstitial fibrosis and tubular atrophy ⇨, with focal sparse interstitial inflammation ➔.* **(Right)** *With electron microscopy the glomeruli show largely preserved podocyte foot processes, with very mild segmental foot process effacement. No glomerular basement membrane features of Alport syndrome are present.*

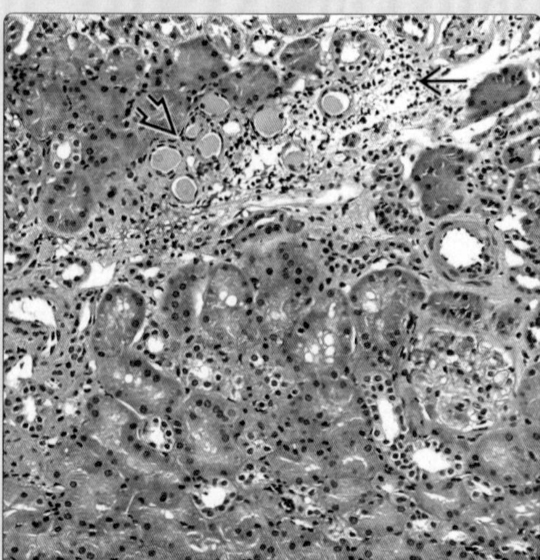

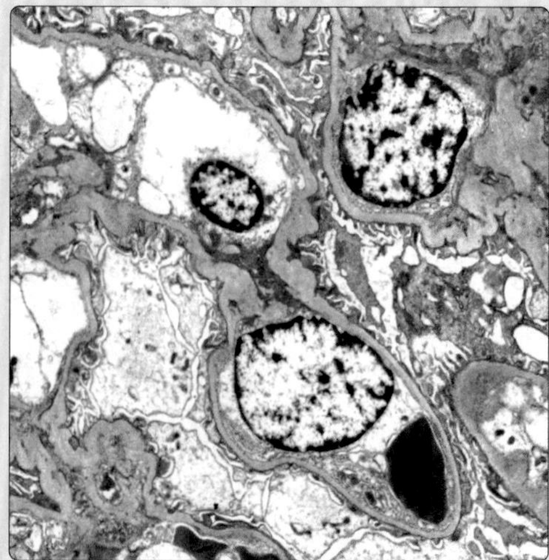

TERMINOLOGY

Synonyms

- Dent-Wrong disease
- X-linked recessive nephrolithiasis
- X-linked recessive hypophosphatemic rickets

Definitions

- X-linked tubular disease manifested by low molecular weight proteinuria, hypercalciuria, nephrocalcinosis, nephrolithiasis, and progressive renal failure

ETIOLOGY/PATHOGENESIS

Gene Mutations

- *CLCN5* gene, Dent disease 1
  - Mutation in 2/3 of Dent disease patients
  - Encodes electrogenic chloride/proton exchanger ClC-5
    - Deficiency alters membrane trafficking via receptor-mediated endocytic pathway in proximal tubular epithelial cells
- *OCRL1* gene, Dent disease 2
  - Encodes protein (OCRL1) with phosphatidylinositol-4,5-bisphosphate 5-phosphatase activity
    - Present on clathrin-coated intermediates, early endosomes, and Golgi apparatus
    - May facilitate trafficking between these compartments in tubular epithelial cells
  - Lowe syndrome, a related disease, also has mutation in *OCRL1* gene
    - More severe phenotype than Dent disease 2
- Both identified genes located on X chromosome
- Some patients with Dent disease phenotype have neither mutation
- No known clinical disease in female carriers
  - May have low molecular weight proteinuria

CLINICAL ISSUES

Presentation

- Usually presents in childhood
- Nephrocalcinosis
- Nephrolithiasis
- Hypercalciuria
  - Normal serum calcium level
- Proteinuria, asymptomatic
  - Usually < 2 g/day total proteinuria
  - Low molecular weight proteinuria (100%)
- Proximal tubular dysfunction, partial Fanconi syndrome
  - Glycosuria, aminoaciduria, concentrating defect
  - Rickets (uncommon)
- Hematuria
- Chronic renal failure
  - Age: 25-50 years

Treatment

- Surgical approaches
  - Kidney transplantation for end-stage renal disease
    - Disease not known to recur in allograft
- Drugs
  - Thiazide diuretics stimulate calcium reabsorption in distal tubules
- Other
  - Restrict dietary sodium intake
    - Sodium excretion promotes calcium excretion
  - Dietary calcium restriction reduces calciuria
    - Increases risk of bone disease

MICROSCOPIC

Histologic Features

- Glomeruli
  - Focal global glomerulosclerosis
  - Focal segmental glomerulosclerosis
- Tubules
  - Atrophy
- Interstitium
  - Focal deposition of calcium phosphate or calcium oxalate
  - Focal inflammation

Electron Microscopy

- Mild segmental podocyte foot process effacement
- No specific features in tubules

ANCILLARY TESTS

Genetic Testing

- Dent disease-specific mutations in *CLCN5* or *OCRL1*

Urine Testing

- Retinol binding protein
- β2-microglobulin
- α1-microglobulin

DIFFERENTIAL DIAGNOSIS

Other Causes of Partial Fanconi Syndrome

- Heavy metal toxicity
- Interstitial nephritis/nephropathy
- Cystinosis
- Mitochondriopathy
- Lowe syndrome

Focal Segmental Glomerulosclerosis (FSGS)

- Some cases may be familial

Nephrolithiasis

- Calcium phosphate &/or calcium oxalate stones
- If low molecular weight proteinuria present, suspect Dent disease

DIAGNOSTIC CHECKLIST

Pathologic Interpretation Pearls

- May be overlooked as cause of FSGS in males

SELECTED REFERENCES

1. Mansour-Hendili L et al: Mutation Update of the Clcn5 Gene Responsible for Dent Disease 1. Hum Mutat. ePub, 2015
2. Solano A et al: Dent-Wrong disease and other rare causes of the Fanconi syndrome. Clin Kidney J. 7(4):344-7, 2014
3. Claverie-Martín F et al: Dent's disease: clinical features and molecular basis. Pediatr Nephrol. Epub ahead of print, 2010
4. Hodgin JB et al: Dent disease presenting as partial Fanconi syndrome and hypercalciuria. Kidney Int. 73(11):1320-3, 2008
5. Copelovitch L et al: Hypothesis: Dent disease is an underrecognized cause of focal glomerulosclerosis. Clin J Am Soc Nephrol. 2(5):914-8, 2007

KEY FACTS

TERMINOLOGY

- Disease triad due to mutations in *OCRL*, manifested by renal proximal tubulopathy, congenital cataracts, and cognitive impairment

ETIOLOGY/PATHOGENESIS

- *OCRL* encodes OCRL1 protein
  - Inositol polyphosphate 5-phosphatase
  - Affects membrane trafficking and actin cytoskeletal organization

CLINICAL ISSUES

- X-linked disorder; 1:200,000-1:500,000 births
- Hypotonia and cataracts at birth
- Severe mental retardation (~ 33%)
- Renal proximal tubular dysfunction
  - Aminoaciduria
  - Hypercalciuria
  - Not Fanconi syndrome, no glycosuria, mild phosphaturia

MICROSCOPIC

- Nonspecific tubulointerstitial abnormalities most frequent
  - Dilated tubules with proteinaceous casts
  - Tubular atrophy and interstitial fibrosis
  - Medullary nephrocalcinosis
- Glomerular disease is rare
  - Diffuse mesangial sclerosis
  - Glomerulosclerosis secondary to tubular injury

ANCILLARY TESTS

- EM: Dilated proximal tubule infolding, TBM lamellation, mitochondrial swelling and irregularity
- OCRL1 activity of cultured skin fibroblasts

TOP DIFFERENTIAL DIAGNOSES

- Dent disease
- Cystinosis
- Fanconi syndrome
- Hypophosphatemic rickets

Nonspecific Interstitial Fibrosis and Tubular Atrophy

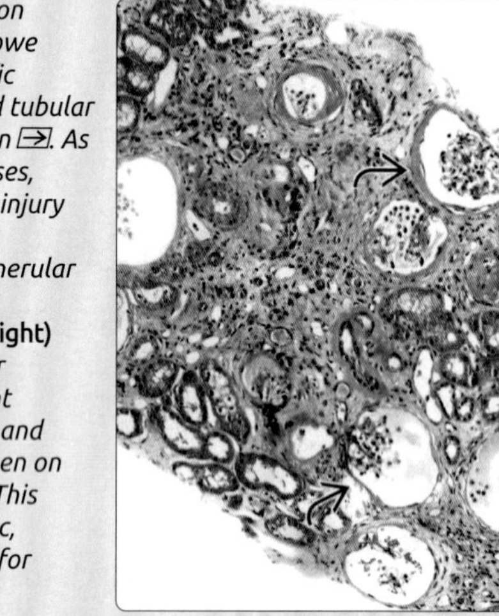

Tubular Atrophy With Lamellar Thickening of Basement Membranes

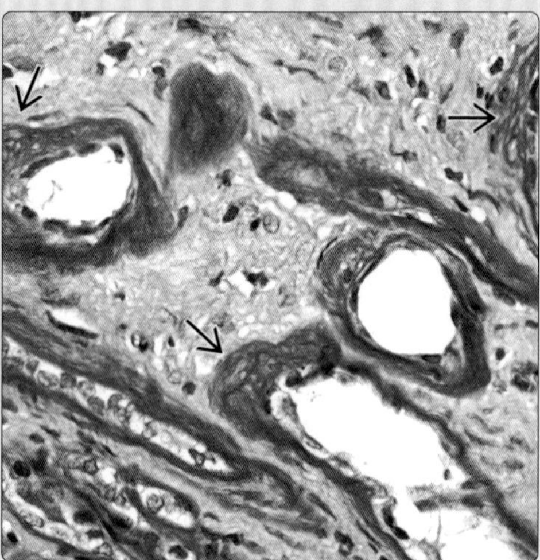

(Left) *The most common histologic finding in Lowe syndrome is nonspecific interstitial fibrosis and tubular atrophy with dilatation. As tubular injury progresses, secondary glomerular injury ensues with atubular glomeruli, periglomerular fibrosis, and glomerulosclerosis.* **(Right)** *There is severe tubular atrophy with basement membrane thickening and lamellation best seen on PAS and silver stains. This finding is characteristic, although not specific, for Lowe syndrome.*

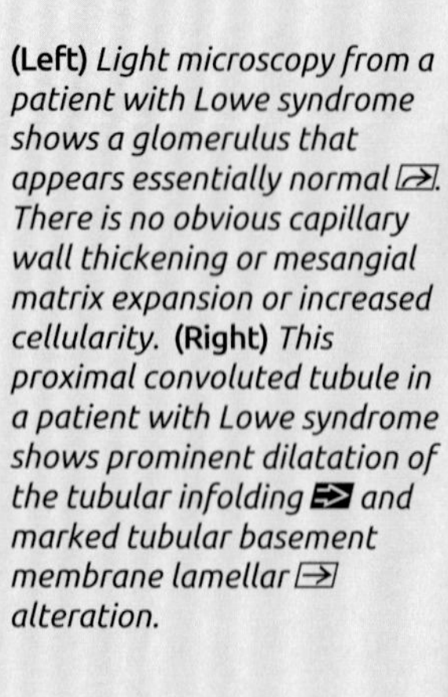

(Left) *Light microscopy from a patient with Lowe syndrome shows a glomerulus that appears essentially normal. There is no obvious capillary wall thickening or mesangial matrix expansion or increased cellularity.* **(Right)** *This proximal convoluted tubule in a patient with Lowe syndrome shows prominent dilatation of the tubular infolding and marked tubular basement membrane lamellar alteration.*

Normal Glomerulus

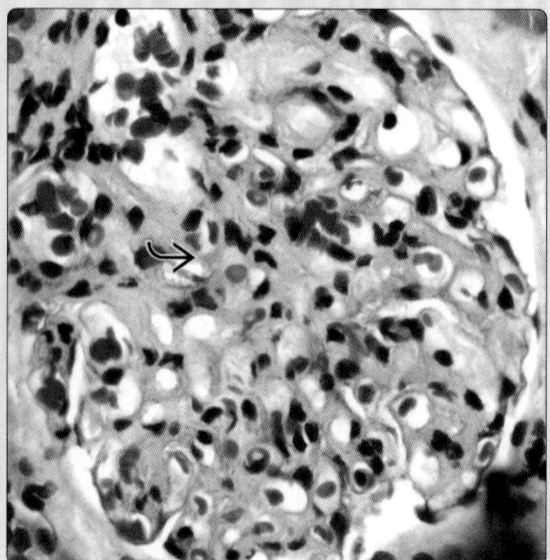

Dilatation of Proximal Tubular Infolding and Basement Membrane Lamellation

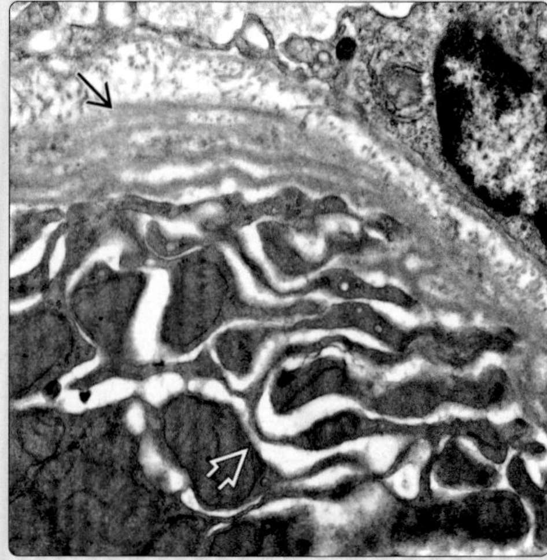

TERMINOLOGY

Abbreviations

- Oculocerebrorenal syndrome of Lowe (OCRL)

Synonyms

- Oculocerebrorenal dystrophy
- Lowe syndrome

Definitions

- Disease triad due to mutations in OCRL
  - Congenital cataracts
  - Cognitive/behavioral impairment
  - Renal proximal tubulopathy

ETIOLOGY/PATHOGENESIS

X-Linked Genetic Disease

- Loss-of-function mutations in *OCRL* gene (Xq26.1)
  - Heterogeneous: Nonsense, insertion/deletion, splice site, and missense mutations
- *OCRL* encodes OCRL1 protein
  - Inositol polyphosphate 5-phosphatase OCRL1
  - Involved in membrane trafficking and actin cytoskeletal organization
  - Affects vesicle-dependent proximal tubule reabsorption and trafficking of transporter proteins
  - Possible role in ciliogenesis and cilia maintenance

CLINICAL ISSUES

Epidemiology

- Incidence
  - 1:200,000-1:500,000 births
  - Pan-ethnic disorder
- Sex
  - Almost all males
  - Females with X-autosomal translocations reported

Presentation

- Hypotonia and cataracts at birth
  - Infantile glaucoma (~ 50%)
- Severe mental retardation (~ 33%)
  - Seizures (~ 50%)
- Renal proximal tubular dysfunction
  - Low molecular weight proteinuria (100%)
  - Aminoaciduria
  - Hypercalciuria
  - Not Fanconi syndrome, no glycosuria, mild phosphaturia
- Cryptorchidism
- Chronic renal failure between 2nd and 4th decade

Laboratory Tests

- Assessment of renal proximal tubule dysfunction
  - Especially low molecular weight proteinuria
- Measurement of OCRL1 activity in cultured skin fibroblasts
- Molecular genetic testing for *OCRL* mutations

Treatment

- Monitor renal function, correct acidosis, and electrolyte replacement
- Oral phosphate and calcitriol for renal rickets

Prognosis

- Chronic renal failure occurs between 2nd and 4th decade
- Dialysis and transplantation plays limited role

IMAGING

Ultrasonographic Findings

- Medullary nephrocalcinosis (~ 50%) and nephrolithiasis

MICROSCOPIC

Histologic Features

- Glomeruli
  - Nonspecific glomerulosclerosis
  - Rarely, diffuse mesangial sclerosis
- Tubules and interstitium
  - Dilated tubules with protein casts
  - Tubular atrophy and interstitial fibrosis
  - Focal calcium phosphate deposition

ANCILLARY TESTS

Immunofluorescence

- Negative for immune reactants and complement

Electron Microscopy

- Proximal tubule
  - Mitochondrial swelling
  - Basement membrane lamellar thickening
  - Dilatation of proximal tubular infolding

DIFFERENTIAL DIAGNOSIS

Dent Disease

- Lacks systemic features (cataracts, mental retardation)
- Nephrolithiasis and nephrocalcinosis prominent
- Mutation in *CLCN5* (Dent-1) or *OCRL* (Dent-2)
  - Genotype does not distinguish Dent-2 from OCRL

Cystinosis

- Multinucleated podocytes
- Thin 1st part of proximal tubule: Swan-neck deformity

Fanconi Syndrome

- Various causes
- Glycosuria present by definition

Hypophosphatemic Rickets

- Inability to establish normal ossification
- Phosphate wasting more severe

SELECTED REFERENCES

1. Recker F et al: Characterization of 28 novel patients expands the mutational and phenotypic spectrum of Lowe syndrome. Pediatr Nephrol. 30(6):931-43, 2015
2. Coon BG et al: The Lowe syndrome protein OCRL1 is involved in primary cilia assembly. Hum Mol Genet. 21(8):1835-47, 2012
3. Cui S et al: OCRL1 function in renal epithelial membrane traffic. Am J Physiol Renal Physiol. 298(2):F335-45, 2010
4. Bockenhauer D et al: Renal phenotype in Lowe Syndrome: a selective proximal tubular dysfunction. Clin J Am Soc Nephrol. 3(5):1430-6, 2008
5. Cho HY et al: Renal manifestations of Dent disease and Lowe syndrome. Pediatr Nephrol. 23(2):243-9, 2008
6. Lewis RA et al: Lowe syndrome, 2001
7. Charnas LR et al: The oculocerebrorenal syndrome of Lowe. Adv Pediatr. 38:75-107, 1991

(Left) *Biopsy from a 37-year-old man with Lowe syndrome and chronic kidney disease shows severe interstitial fibrosis and tubular atrophy with minimal interstitial inflammation. The progressive tubular injury has led to diffuse glomerular injury and scarring* ➡. **(Right)** *There is somewhat milder interstitial fibrosis and tubular atrophy in this biopsy from a 25-year-old man with Lowe syndrome. Patchy tubular atrophy can be seen along with tubular dilatation* ⇨ *and proteinaceous casts* ⇗.

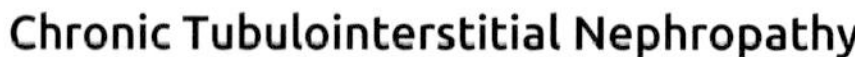

Chronic Tubulointerstitial Nephropathy

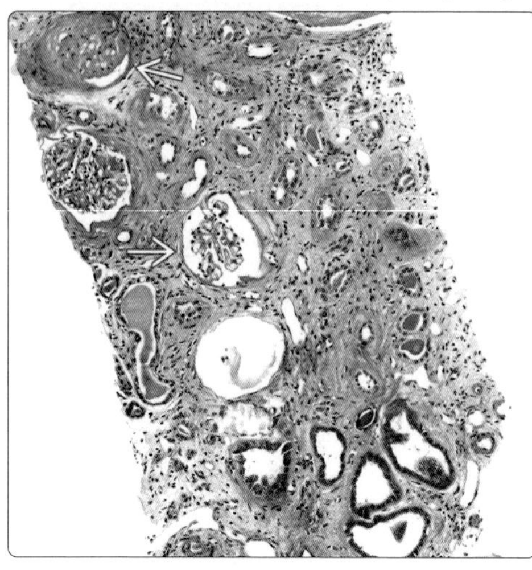

Tubular Atrophy With Dilatation and Proteinaceous Casts

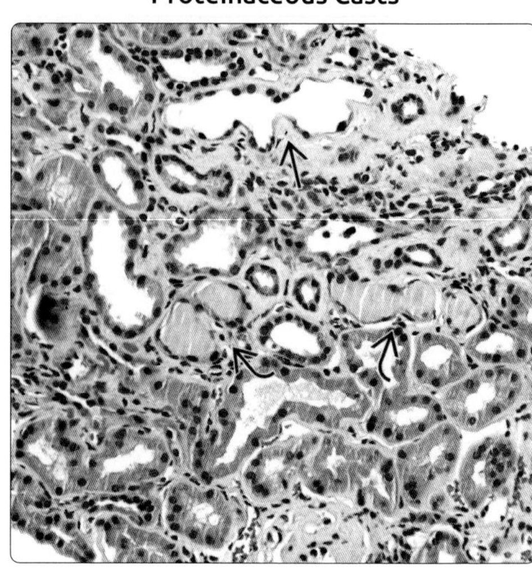

(Left) *Medullary nephrocalcinosis is not uncommon in Lowe syndrome, though it is typically not as prominent as Dent disease. This micrograph shows tubulointerstitial calcium phosphate deposition within the medulla.* **(Right)** *In patients with Lowe syndrome, glomerular lesions by light microscopy are usually not observed until chronic tubulointerstitial disease develops. This biopsy showed largely normal glomeruli with no significant abnormalities of the GBM or mesangial regions.*

Medullary Tubulointerstitial Calcium Phosphate Deposition

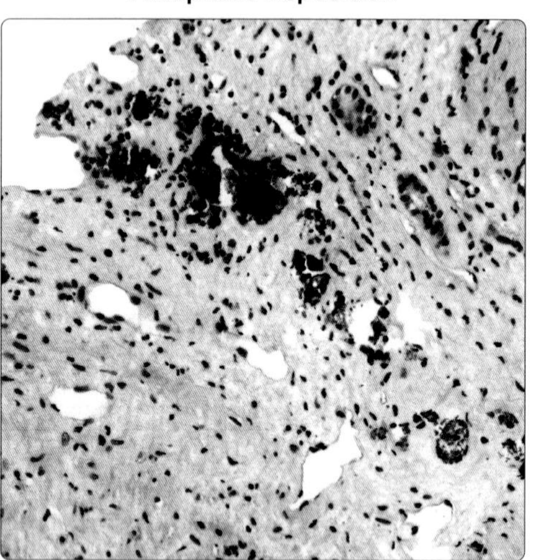

Normal Glomerulus

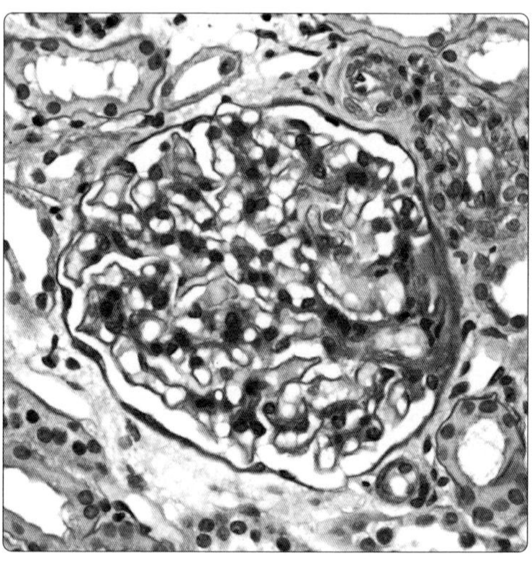

(Left) *This patient with Lowe syndrome has developed progressive renal injury. The glomeruli show prominent periglomerular fibrosis with retraction of the tuft* ⇨*, and there is frequent global glomerulosclerosis.* **(Right)** *Diffuse mesangial sclerosis is rarely encountered in Lowe syndrome. It is characterized by mesangial hypercellularity and increased mesangial matrix* ⇨*. There is distinctive marked epithelial cell hyperplasia and enlargement* ⇨ *with collapse of the capillary loops.*

Progressive Glomerular Injury

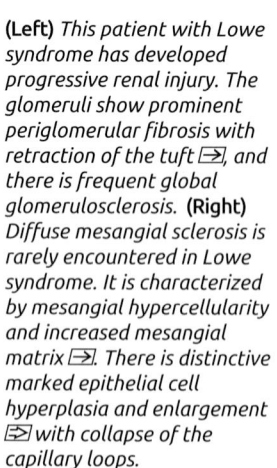

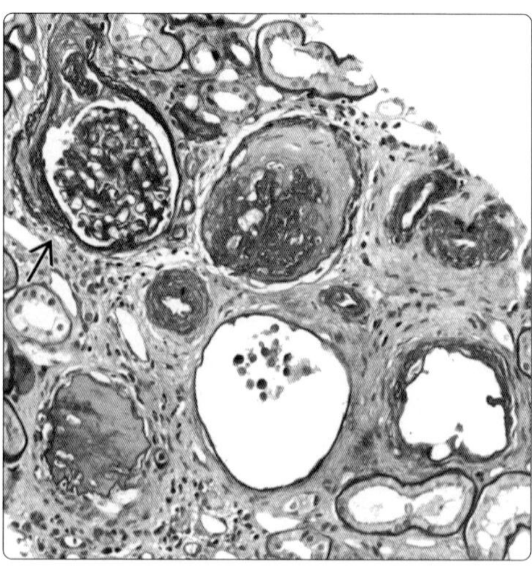

Diffuse Mesangial Sclerosis

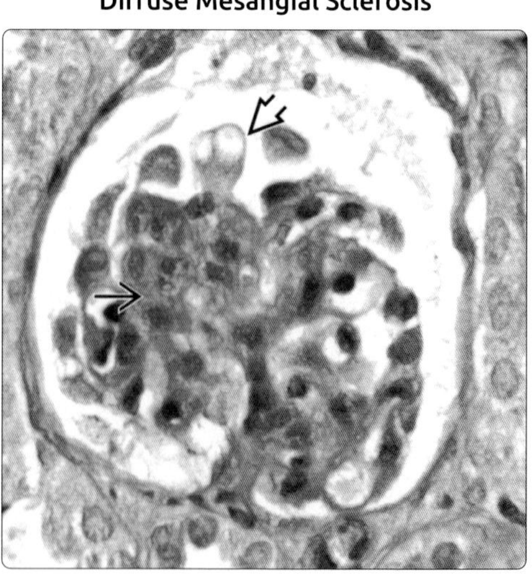

Lamellar Thickening of Tubular Basement Membranes

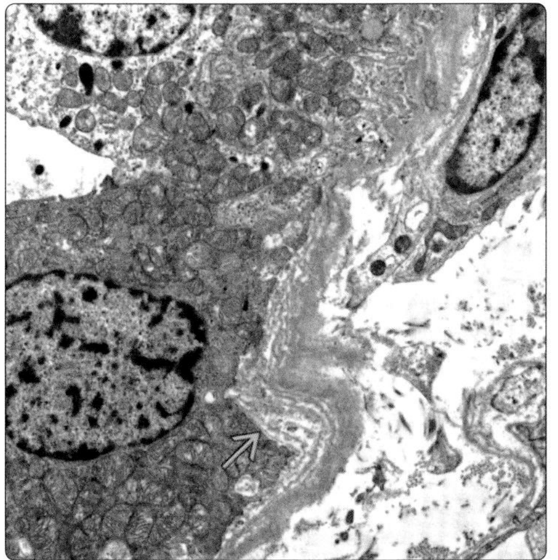

Lamellar Thickening of Tubular Basement Membranes

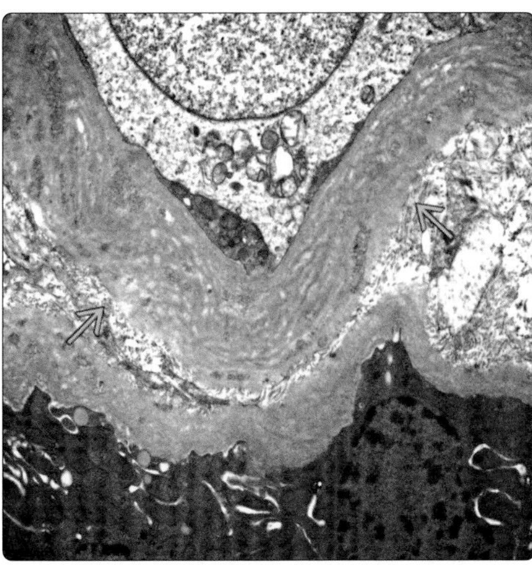

(Left) *In this patient with Lowe syndrome, there is marked thickening and lamellation of the tubular basement membrane →, somewhat similar to glomerular changes in Alport syndrome. The brush border disappears and the cytoplasm may protrude into the tubular lumen.* **(Right)** *This also shows marked thickening and lamellation of the tubular basement membranes →, and while characteristic, this finding is not specific for Lowe syndrome.*

Dilatation of Proximal Tubular Infolding

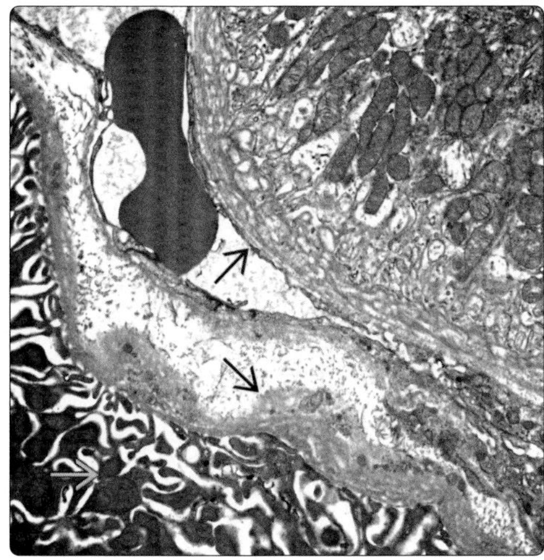

Proximal Tubular Mitochondrial Swelling

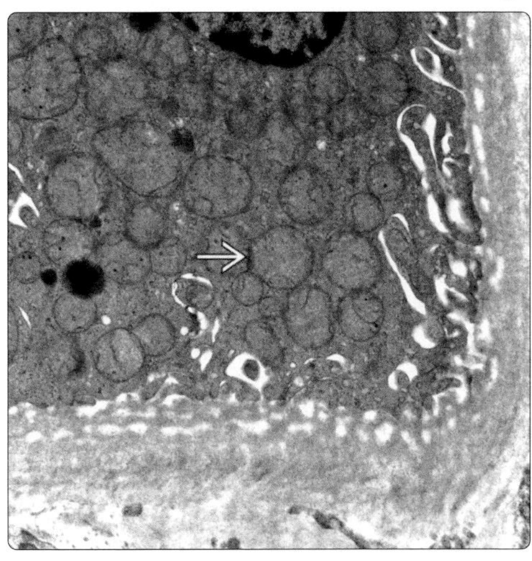

(Left) *The plasma membrane infoldings → of the proximal tubules frequently appear quite dilated in patients with Lowe syndrome. Both tubules in this image also show the characteristic tubular basement membrane thickening and lamellation →.* **(Right)** *Mitochondrial changes in the proximal tubules include swelling and irregularity with a pronounced circular profile ➡. The cristae also appear less numerous, and may be disrupted and shorter or completely absent.*

Mild Glomerular Ultrastructural Alterations

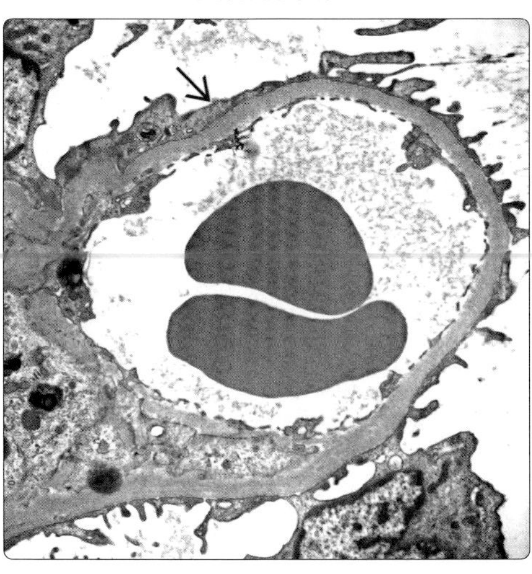

Diffuse Mesangial Sclerosis

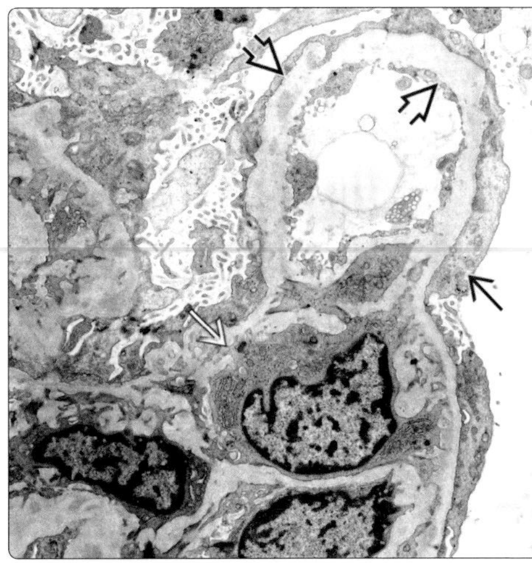

(Left) *The glomerular capillary loops in Lowe syndrome with tubulopathy may be normal or demonstrate mild irregular thickening of the glomerular basement membrane (GBM). Endothelial cell swelling and segmental effacement of podocyte foot processes → are often observed.* **(Right)** *In diffuse mesangial sclerosis there is mesangial hypercellularity ➡, matrix expansion, and marked irregularity of the GBM → with diffuse effacement of the podocyte foot processes →.*

Methylmalonic Acidemia

KEY FACTS

TERMINOLOGY

- Autosomal recessive metabolic defect caused by complete or partial deficiency of adenosylcobalamin-dependent enzyme methylmalonyl-CoA mutase due to mutations in *MUT* or *MMADHC*

ETIOLOGY/PATHOGENESIS

- Impaired metabolism of methylmalonic acid
- Genetic
  - Metabolic defect caused by complete or partial deficiency of adenosylcobalamin-dependent enzyme methylmalonyl-CoA mutase
- Severe vitamin B12 (cobalamin) deficiency
  - Vitamin B12 is cofactor of methylmalonyl-CoA mutase

CLINICAL ISSUES

- Chronic renal failure
- Variable patterns and severity of presentation
- Hydroxy-cobalamin therapy if B12-responsive disease
- Low-protein diet to reduce precursors of methylmalonic acid

MICROSCOPIC

- Interstitial fibrosis and tubular atrophy
- Chronic interstitial nephritis

TOP DIFFERENTIAL DIAGNOSES

- Chronic tubulointerstitial nephropathy
  - Other causes of chronic tubulointerstitial nephropathy/nephritis may have similar histologic appearance
  - Other potential causes include
    - Urinary tract obstruction or infection
    - Vascular diseases
    - Toxins or drugs
    - Renal structural defects and other inherited disorders

Mild Interstitial Fibrosis

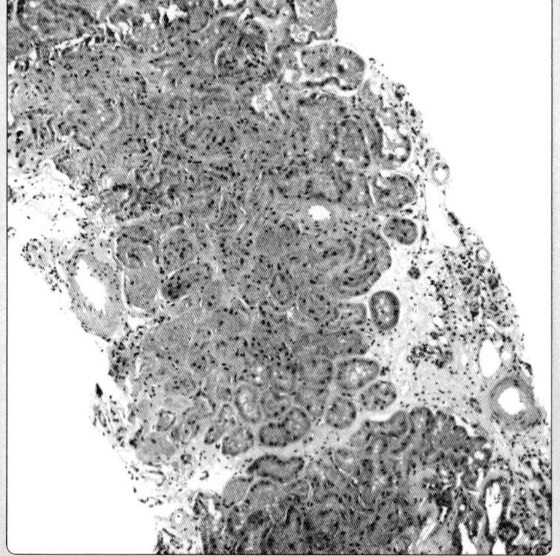

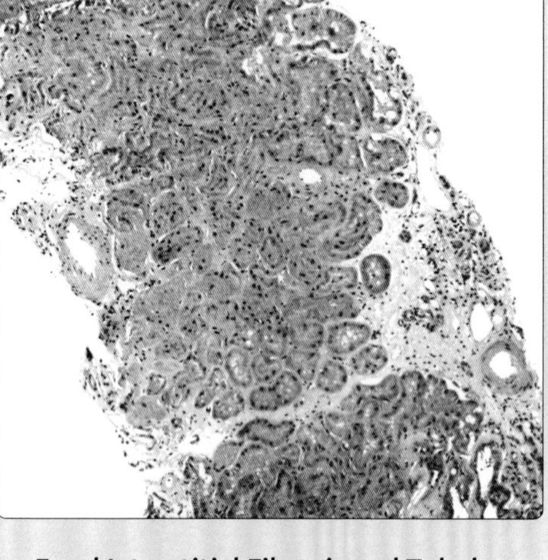

Normal Glomerulus

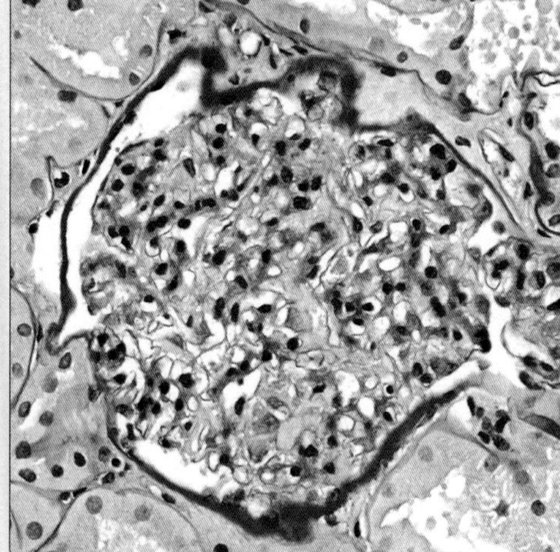

(Left) *H&E shows focal interstitial fibrosis and tubular atrophy in a biopsy from a 26-year-old man with vitamin B12-responsive methylmalonic acidemia. He had chronic renal failure with a serum creatinine of 2.7 mg/dL.* **(Right)** *A nonglobally sclerotic glomerulus appears normal. This case showed focal glomeruli with global sclerosis (not shown).*

Focal Interstitial Fibrosis and Tubular Atrophy

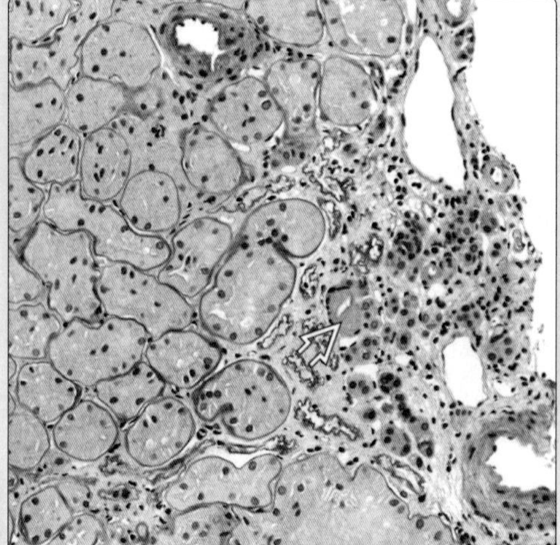

Dropout of Tubules

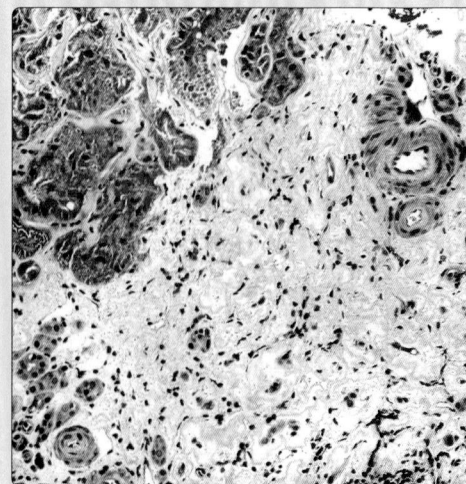

(Left) *Periodic acid-Schiff shows focal interstitial fibrosis and tubular atrophy. Focal arterioles show intimal hyalinosis ➡ in this case.* **(Right)** *The cortex in methylmalonic acidemia (MMA) may show broad areas of interstitial fibrosis and tubular atrophy with little inflammation. The disease may be either genetic or caused by vitamin B12 deficiency.*

TERMINOLOGY

Abbreviations

- Methylmalonic acidemia (MMA)

Synonyms

- Methylmalonic aciduria

Definitions

- Autosomal recessive metabolic defect caused by complete or partial deficiency of adenosylcobalamin-dependent enzyme methylmalonyl-CoA mutase due to mutations in *MUT, MMADHC,* or other genes in cobalamin pathway
- Severe nutritional B12 deficiency

ETIOLOGY/PATHOGENESIS

Impaired Metabolism of Methylmalonic Acid

- Methylmalonic acid generated during metabolism of amino acids isoleucine, methionine, threonine, and valine and odd-chain fatty acids

Genetic

- Metabolic defect caused by complete or partial deficiency of adenosylcobalamin-dependent enzyme methylmalonyl-CoA mutase
  - Several genetic defects identified
    - *MMADHC*
      - Encodes *MMADHC* protein that converts vitamin B12 into adenosylcobalamin or methylcobalamin
    - *MUT*
      - Encodes methylmalonyl-CoA mutase
  - May be detected by newborn screening exams
  - Most methylmalonyl-CoA mutase produced in liver
- Inherited in autosomal recessive fashion

Severe Vitamin B12 (Cobalamin) Deficiency

- Vitamin B12 is cofactor of methylmalonyl-CoA mutase

CLINICAL ISSUES

Epidemiology

- Incidence
  - Approximately 1:48,000
  - Estimated incidence in Europe is 1:115,000 to 1:277,000
- Age
  - Genetic forms have early onset
    - Neonatal period through early childhood

Presentation

- Chronic kidney disease
  - Renal disease develops in patients surviving longer with disease
- Proximal renal tubular acidosis
- Nonrenal manifestations (inherited MMA)
  - Developmental delay, failure to thrive, lethargy, vomiting, seizures, muscular hypotonia
  - Metabolic acidosis, hyperammonemia
- Hypertension
- Variable patterns and severity of presentation

Laboratory Tests

- Plasma and urine concentrations of methylmalonic acid

Treatment

- Surgical approaches
  - Renal transplantation
    - Some methylmalonyl-CoA mutase produced by allograft kidney
      - Treats original metabolic defect, at least in part
  - Liver transplantation
    - Most methylmalonyl-CoA mutase produced in liver
- Drugs
  - Hydroxy-cobalamin therapy if B12-responsive disease
    - Patients with methylmalonyl-CoA mutase mutations do not respond
  - Antibiotics
    - Reduce levels of gut bacteria that produce particular amino acids
  - Angiotensin II inhibition in patients with renal disease
- Low-protein diet to reduce precursors of methylmalonic acid
  - Amino acids
    - Reduced intake of isoleucine, methionine, threonine, valine
  - Reduced intake of odd-chain fatty acids and polyunsaturated fat

MICROSCOPIC

Histologic Features

- Interstitial fibrosis and tubular atrophy
- Chronic interstitial nephritis
  - Sparse inflammation
- Nonspecific histologic findings
  - Biopsy needed to exclude other causes of renal failure

DIFFERENTIAL DIAGNOSIS

Chronic Tubulointerstitial Nephropathy

- Other causes of chronic tubulointerstitial nephropathy/nephritis may have similar histologic appearance
- Other potential causes include urinary tract obstruction or infection, vascular diseases, toxins or drugs, renal structural defects, and other inherited disorders

SELECTED REFERENCES

1. Niemi AK et al: Treatment of Methylmalonic Acidemia by Liver or Combined Liver-Kidney Transplantation. J Pediatr. ePub, 2015
2. Sloan JL et al: Liver or Combined Liver-Kidney Transplantation for Patients with Isolated Methylmalonic Acidemia: Who and When? J Pediatr. ePub, 2015
3. Zsengellér ZK et al: Methylmalonic acidemia: a megamitochondrial disorder affecting the kidney. Pediatr Nephrol. 29(11):2139-46, 2014
4. Manoli I et al: Methylmalonic acidemia. GeneReviews [Internet]. Seattle: University of Washington. Posted August 16, 2006; updated September 28, 2010
5. Ha TS et al: Delay of renal progression in methylmalonic acidemia using angiotensin II inhibition: a case report. J Nephrol. 21(5):793-6, 2008
6. Lubrano R et al: Renal transplant in methylmalonic acidemia: could it be the best option? Report on a case at 10 years and review of the literature. Pediatr Nephrol. 22(8):1209-14, 2007
7. Deodato F et al: Methylmalonic and propionic aciduria. Am J Med Genet C Semin Med Genet. 142C(2):104-12, 2006
8. Lubrano R et al: Kidney transplantation in a girl with methylmalonic acidemia and end stage renal failure. Pediatr Nephrol. 16(11):848-51, 2001
9. Rutledge SL et al: Tubulointerstitial nephritis in methylmalonic acidemia. Pediatr Nephrol. 7(1):81-2, 1993

Systemic Karyomegaly

KEY FACTS

TERMINOLOGY

- Chronic tubulointerstitial nephritis with prominent karyomegaly in tubular epithelium

ETIOLOGY/PATHOGENESIS

- Genetic
  - *FAN1* mutations (9 families)
  - Encodes Fanconi anemia-associated nuclease 1
  - Repairs DNA interstrand crosslink damage
- DNA toxins suspected in some cases (ochratoxin)

CLINICAL ISSUES

- Rare
- Proteinuria, asymptomatic
- Chronic renal failure
- Usually leads to chronic renal failure at 30-40 years of age

MICROSCOPIC

- Karyomegaly in tubules throughout nephron
- Interstitial nephritis, fibrosis, and tubular atrophy
- Karyomegaly in most organs studied
- No associated inflammation or fibrosis except in kidney and rarely lung

ANCILLARY TESTS

- Karyomegalic cells shed in urine
- Cells are aneuploid and nondividing (Ki-67 negative)

TOP DIFFERENTIAL DIAGNOSES

- Viral infection
- Nephronophthisis
- Nuclear atypia from chemotherapy or radiotherapy

DIAGNOSTIC CHECKLIST

- Potential to be misinterpreted as carcinoma in urine cytology
- Probably underdiagnosed

(Left) *Karyomegalic interstitial nephritis has focal, enlarged, abnormal tubular epithelial nuclei ➙ accompanied by tubular atrophy, glomerulosclerosis, interstitial inflammation, and fibrosis. (Courtesy A. Friedl, MD.)* **(Right)** *In karyomegalic interstitial nephritis (KIN), enlarged, hyperchromatic nuclei are most prominent in tubular cells. Similar nuclear changes occur in most other organs, including liver, lung, brain, and endocrine glands. (Courtesy G. Monga, MD.)*

Enlarged Nuclei, Tubular Atrophy, and Fibrosis

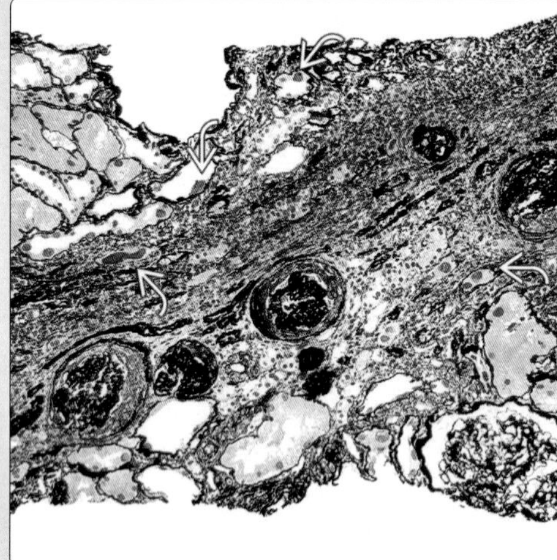

Hyperchromatic Tubular Cell Nuclei

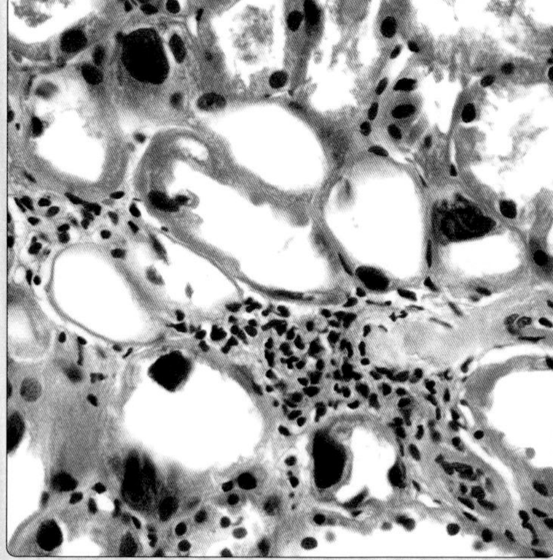

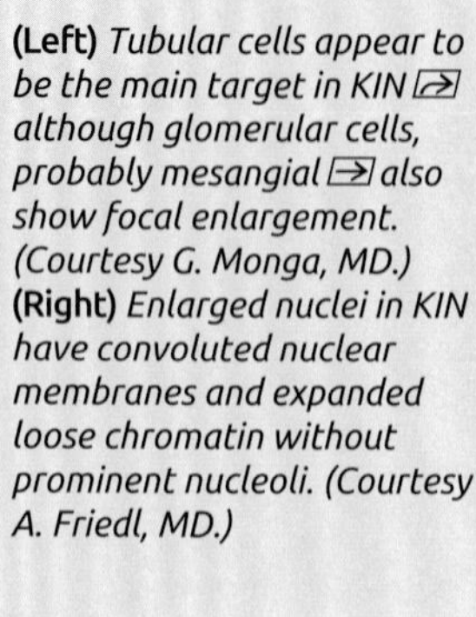

(Left) *Tubular cells appear to be the main target in KIN ➙ although glomerular cells, probably mesangial → also show focal enlargement. (Courtesy G. Monga, MD.)* **(Right)** *Enlarged nuclei in KIN have convoluted nuclear membranes and expanded loose chromatin without prominent nucleoli. (Courtesy A. Friedl, MD.)*

Glomerular Cell Karyomegaly

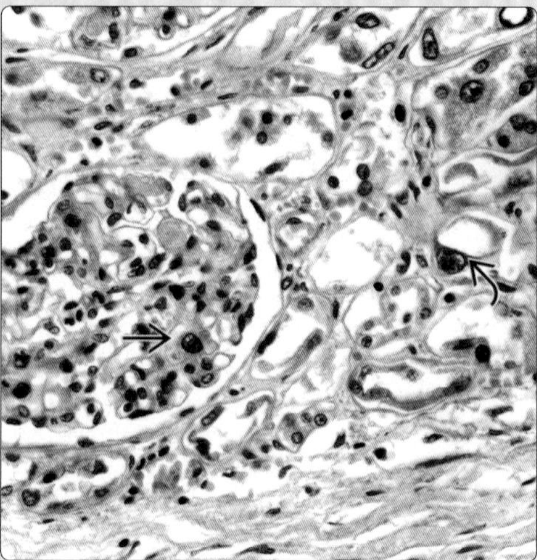

Abnormally Convoluted Nuclear Membrane

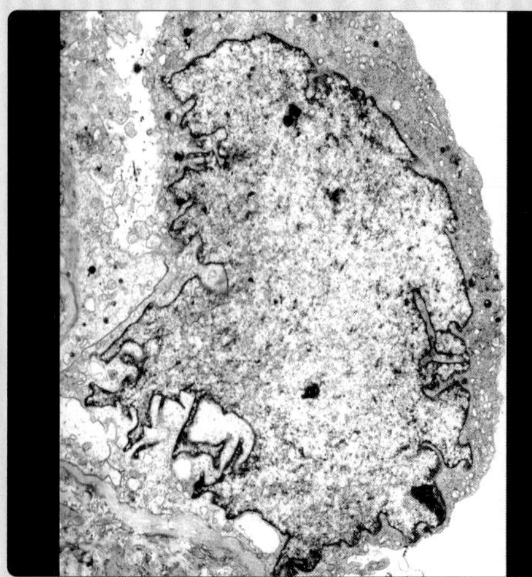

TERMINOLOGY

Synonyms

- Karyomegalic interstitial nephritis (KIN)

Definitions

- Chronic tubulointerstitial nephritis with prominent karyomegaly in tubular epithelium
- Noted by Barry in 1974 and named by Mihatsch in 1979

ETIOLOGY/PATHOGENESIS

Genetic

- *FAN1* mutations (9 families)
  - Autosomal recessive
    - Homozygous or compound heterozygous mutations
    - Truncating, missense and nonsense mutations
  - Encodes Fanconi anemia-associated nuclease 1
    - Complexes with *FANCD2* whose gene is mutated in Fanconi anemia
    - Repairs DNA interstrand crosslink damage
    - Expressed in kidney

Environmental Toxins

- *FAN1* mutations increase susceptibility to DNA toxins
- Ochratoxin implicated in Tunisian cases

CLINICAL ISSUES

Epidemiology

- Incidence
  - Rare; few dozen cases reported
  - Presents at 9-51 years of age (median: 33 years)
  - No gender preference
  - European, Maori

Presentation

- Proteinuria, asymptomatic
  - Low molecular weight (tubular)
- Microhematuria
- Chronic renal failure
- Progressive restrictive lung disease
- Recurrent respiratory infection
- Elevated liver enzymes

Treatment

- None

Prognosis

- Usually leads to chronic renal failure at 30-40 years of age

MICROSCOPIC

Histologic Features

- Glomeruli
  - Global and segmental sclerosis
  - Occasional karyomegaly in glomerular cells
- Tubules
  - Karyomegaly in scattered tubules throughout nephron
    - Nuclei 2-5x larger than normal
    - Hyperchromatic
    - Increased DNA ploidy
    - No mitotic figures
  - Tubular atrophy in affected areas
- Interstitium
  - Fibrosis in areas of tubular atrophy
  - Mononuclear infiltrate
- Vessels
  - Karyomegaly of occasional smooth muscle cells

Other Organs

- Karyomegaly in most organs
  - Smooth muscle cells of vessels and bowel, Schwann cells and astrocytes, pulmonary epithelium, liver
- No associated inflammation or fibrosis except in kidney and rarely lung

ANCILLARY TESTS

Cytology

- Karyomegalic cells shed in urine

Immunohistochemistry

- Ki-67 and PCNA do not stain enlarged nuclei (they are not in cell cycle)

Immunofluorescence

- IgM and C3 in scarred glomeruli

Electron Microscopy

- Abnormal nuclei have expanded loose matrix and convoluted nuclear membranes

DIFFERENTIAL DIAGNOSIS

Viral Infection

- Adenovirus, polyomavirus, cytomegalovirus
- No viral antigens by IHC

Nuclear Atypia From Chemotherapy or Radiotherapy

- Ifosfamide therapy and others
- No viral antigens

Nephronophthisis

- No karyomegaly

DIAGNOSTIC CHECKLIST

Pathologic Interpretation Pearls

- May be misinterpreted as carcinoma in urine cytology
- Probably underdiagnosed

SELECTED REFERENCES

1. Tagliente DJ et al: Systemic karyomegaly with primary pulmonary presentation. Hum Pathol. 45(1):180-4, 2014
2. Zhou W et al: FAN1 mutations cause karyomegalic interstitial nephritis, linking chronic kidney failure to defective DNA damage repair. Nat Genet. 44(8):910-5, 2012
3. McCulloch T et al: Karyomegalic-like nephropathy, Ewing's sarcoma and ifosfamide therapy. Pediatr Nephrol. 26(7):1163-6, 2011
4. Monga G et al: Karyomegalic interstitial nephritis: report of 3 new cases and review of the literature. Clin Nephrol. 65(5):349-55, 2006
5. Hassen W et al: Karyomegaly of tubular kidney cells in human chronic interstitial nephropathy in Tunisia: respective role of Ochratoxin A and possible genetic predisposition. Hum Exp Toxicol. 23(7):339-46, 2004
6. Bhandari S et al: Karyomegalic nephropathy: an uncommon cause of progressive renal failure. Nephrol Dial Transplant. 17(11):1914-20, 2002
7. Mihatsch MJ et al: Systemic karyomegaly associated with chronic interstitial nephritis. A new disease entity? Clin Nephrol. 12(2):54-62, 1979

KEY FACTS

TERMINOLOGY

- Genetic or acquired defect of oxidative phosphorylation due to deficiency of mitochondrial respiratory chain complexes

ETIOLOGY/PATHOGENESIS

- Genetic disorder of mtDNA or nDNA encoding mitochondrial proteins
- Acquired disorder due to drugs (e.g., reverse transcriptase inhibitors)

CLINICAL ISSUES

- Genetic forms clinically and biochemically heterogeneous
  - 50% have renal involvement
    - DeToni-Debré-Fanconi syndrome
    - Chronic renal failure
    - Proteinuria
- Drug induced: Usually responds to drug discontinuation

MICROSCOPIC

- Proximal tubulopathy with dysmorphic mitochondria
  - Eosinophilic/fuchsinophilic coarsely granular cytoplasm indicating large mitochondria
- Tubular atrophy and interstitial fibrosis
- Electron microscopy
  - Abnormal mitochondria in proximal or distal tubules
    - Increased number, large size, irregularly shaped
    - Fragmented, disoriented, or variable loss of cristae
- Histochemistry: Deficiency of respiratory chain enzymes

ANCILLARY TESTS

- Definitive diagnosis based on integration of clinical, electrophysiological, neuroimaging, histopathological, biochemical, and genetic investigations

TOP DIFFERENTIAL DIAGNOSES

- Other forms of tubulointerstitial nephritis

Eosinophilic Giant Mitochondrial Inclusions

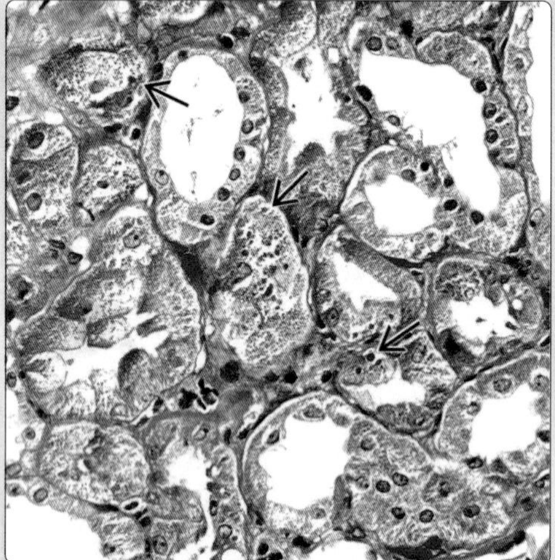

Tubular Cell Giant Irregular Mitochondria

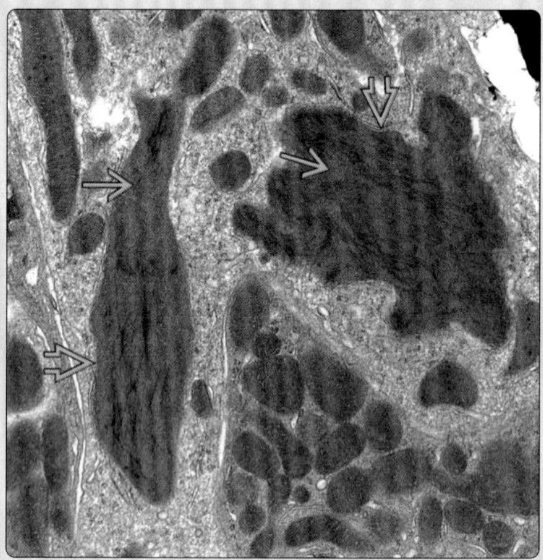

(Left) *Renal tubules show prominent eosinophilic tubular inclusions indicating giant mitochondria ➙ in 9-year-old girl with Fanconi syndrome, opaque cornea, and deafness (traits suggestive of inherited mitochondrial defect).* **(Right)** *Inherited mitochondriopathy in a child showing giant irregular mitochondria with disorganization of the cristae, increased matrix ➙, and thickened membranes ➙.*

Intracellular Fuchsinophilic Giant Mitochondria

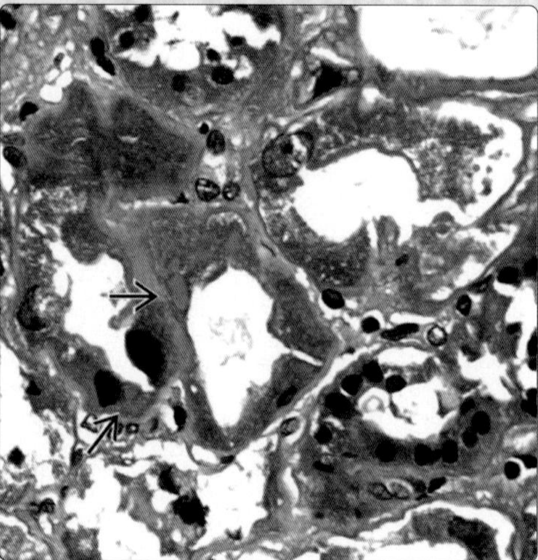

Tubular Cell Abnormal Mitochondria

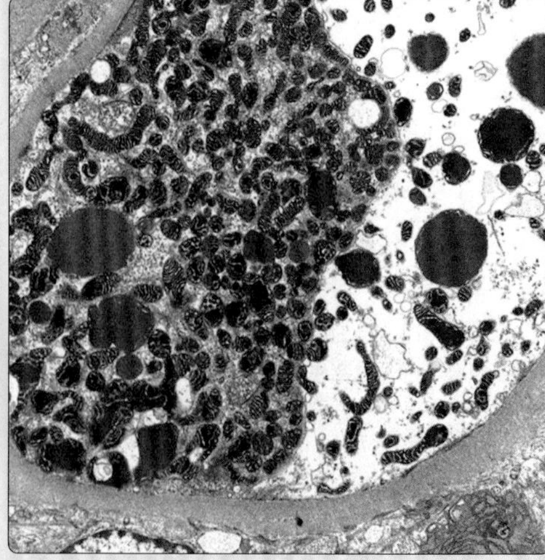

(Left) *A case of Tenofovir toxicity in an HIV(+) patient presenting with acute renal failure shows acute tubular injury, as well as intracytoplasmic round to ovoid eosinophilic inclusions ➙ consistent with enlarged mitochondria. (Courtesy L. Herlitz, MD.)* **(Right)** *In the same case, proximal tubular cells containing a wide range of size and shape of mitochondria, some markedly enlarged, shows disruption of the normal cristae and increased dense matrix. (Courtesy L. Herlitz, MD.)*

TERMINOLOGY

Abbreviations

- Mitochondriopathies (MCP)

Definitions

- Genetic or acquired defect of oxidative phosphorylation due to deficiency of mitochondrial respiratory chain complexes

ETIOLOGY/PATHOGENESIS

Genetic

- Mutated DNA in mitochondria (mtDNA)
  - Each mitochondrion has own circular strand of DNA
  - Encode proteins of electron transport chain, tRNAs, rRNAs, DNA polymerase
  - Biochemical classification based on different types of defects or deficiency in metabolic cell cycle in mitochondria
  - Maternal inheritance pattern
  - Normal at birth
    - Somatic mtDNA mutations accumulate
- Mutations in ≥17 nDNA genes encoding mitochondrial proteins also cause mitochondriopathy with tubulopathy

Drugs

- Reverse transcriptase inhibitors

Mechanism

- Interference with oxidative metabolism

CLINICAL ISSUES

Epidemiology

- Incidence
  - Genetic forms combined: 1/5,000 live births
- Age
  - Children typically have multisystem disease and large-scale deletions of mtDNA or nuclear DNA mutations
  - Adults often present with chronic tubulointerstitial disease without multisystem disease, due to point mutations in mtDNA or nDNA (e.g., *COQ2*)

Presentation

- MCPs clinically, biochemically, and genetically heterogeneous with single or multiorgan involvement
- Pleomorphic signs: Ophthalmoplegia, seizures, lactic acidosis, ataxia, deafness, short stature, cardiomyopathy, hypopituitarism, kyphoscoliosis, anemia, endocrinopathy
- Renal involvement in 50% (particularly)
  - Kearns-Sayre syndrome (KSS); Pearson syndrome; myoclonic epilepsy and ragged red fibers (MERRF); and mitochondrial encephalopathy, lactic acidosis, and stroke-like episodes (MELAS)
- Renal signs
  - DeToni-Debré-Fanconi syndrome
    - Aminoaciduria, glucosuria, phosphaturia, hyperuricemia
  - Chronic renal failure
  - Elevated plasma lactate
  - Nephrotic syndrome (rare)

Treatment

- No specific treatment for inherited form
- Discontinue drugs implicated in acquired MCP
  - Usually reverses renal failure

Prognosis

- High mortality rate for inherited forms
  - Heart and nervous system involvement poor prognostic factors

MICROSCOPIC

Histologic Features

- Glomeruli
  - Usually normal
  - Focal segmental glomerulosclerosis
  - Collapsing glomerulopathy in *COQ2* defect
- Tubules
  - Eosinophilic/fuchsinophilic coarsely granular cytoplasm indicating large mitochondria in proximal tubulopathy
  - Generally PAS and silver stain negative
  - Tubular cystic changes and obstruction by casts
  - Acute proximal tubular injury seen in drug toxicity
- Interstitium
  - Interstitial fibrosis and tubular atrophy
  - Minimal to moderate mononuclear inflammation
- Vessels
  - Premature arterio- and arteriolosclerosis
- Extrarenal
  - Other organs variously affected: Skeletal muscle, heart, liver, central nervous system, and endocrine organs

ANCILLARY TESTS

Histochemistry

- Function of mitochondrial enzymes encoded by mtDNA (e.g., cytochrome C oxidase) or nDNA (succinic dehydrogenase)

Electron Microscopy

- Dysmorphic mitochondria in proximal or distal tubules
  - Increased number, large size, irregularly shaped
  - Fragmented, disoriented, or variable loss of cristae
  - Distended empty core, ring-like
  - Concentric cristae, granular matrix
- Formal criteria for abnormal mitochondria not established

DIFFERENTIAL DIAGNOSIS

Other Forms of Tubulointerstitial Nephritis

- Histologic pattern of MCP may be quite nonspecific
- Mitochondrial EM abnormalities best clue
- Diagnosis requires integration of clinical, biochemical, genetic, histopathological, and electrophysiological results

SELECTED REFERENCES

1. Rahman S et al: Mitochondrial disease–an important cause of end-stage renal failure. Pediatr Nephrol. 28(3):357-61, 2013
2. Herlitz LC et al: Tenofovir nephrotoxicity: acute tubular necrosis with distinctive clinical, pathological, and mitochondrial abnormalities. Kidney Int. 78(11):1171-7, 2010
3. Martín-Hernández E et al: Renal pathology in children with mitochondrial diseases. Pediatr Nephrol. 20(9):1299-305, 2005

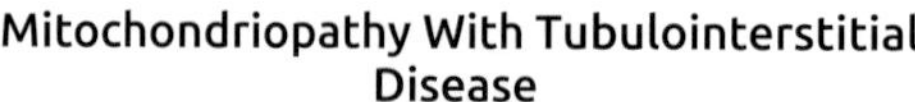

Mitochondriopathy With Tubulointerstitial Disease

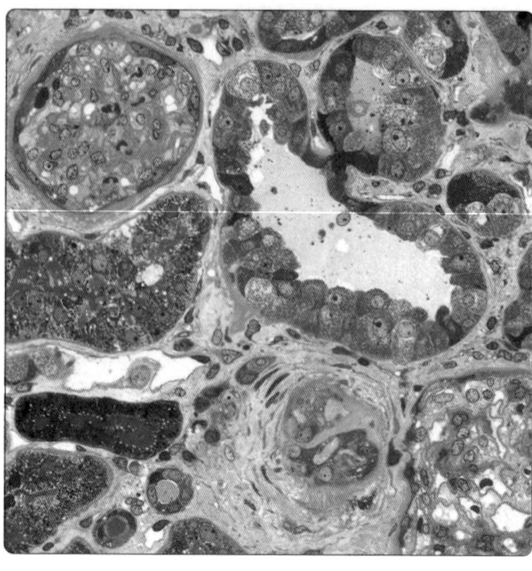

Abnormal Distal Tubular Mitochondria

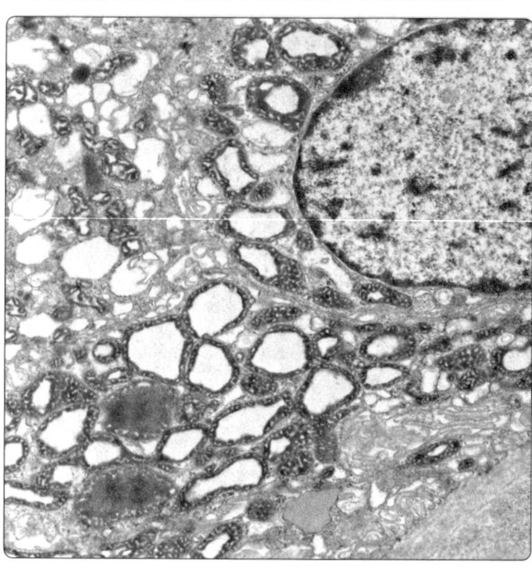

(Left) *A case of familial mitochondrial tubular interstitial nephropathy shows granular tubular epithelial cytoplasm and normal glomeruli. (Courtesy B. Iványi, MD.)* **(Right)** *In the same case, tubular epithelial cells containing mitochondria of varying sizes are shown; some show irregular or concentric cristae forming a peripheral envelope with a clear center and thickened internal membranes. (Courtesy B. Iványi, MD.)*

Distended Mitochondria With Peripheral Cristae

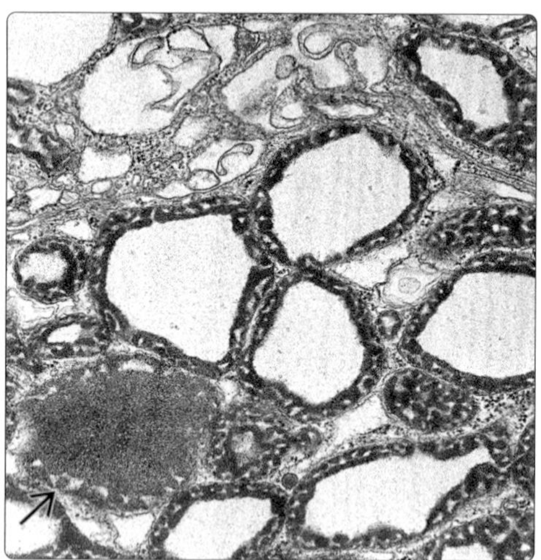

Ragged Red fibers in *COQ2* Myopathy

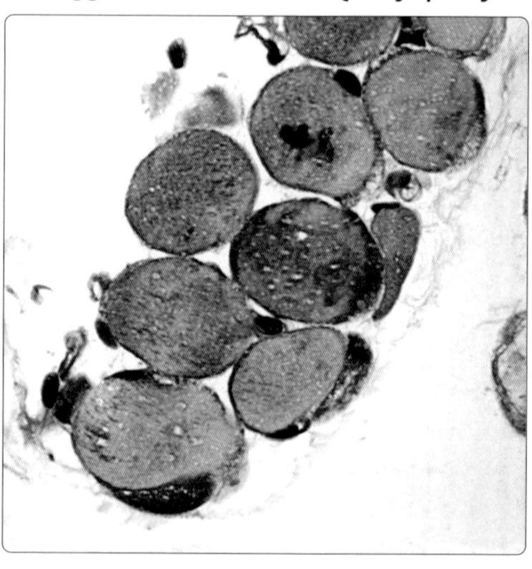

(Left) *In the same case, high magnification of the abnormal mitochondria can be seen, 1 of which shows increased density of the matrix ⇨; the others appear distended with peripherally arranged irregular cristae and a central "empty core." (Courtesy B. Iványi, MD.)* **(Right)** *Myopathy with COQ2 mutation shows ragged red fibers in which PAS(+) granules aggregate and accumulate at the periphery of the myocyte below the sarcolemma. (Courtesy L. Barisoni-Thomas, MD.)*

Collapsing Glomerulopathy in *COQ2* Myopathy

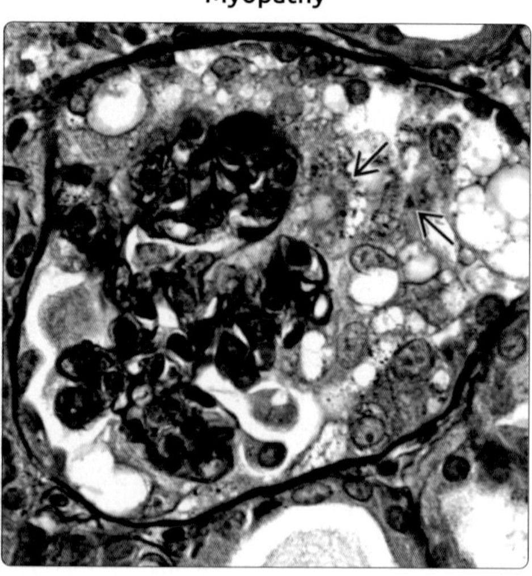

Tubular Vacuolization in *COQ2* Myopathy

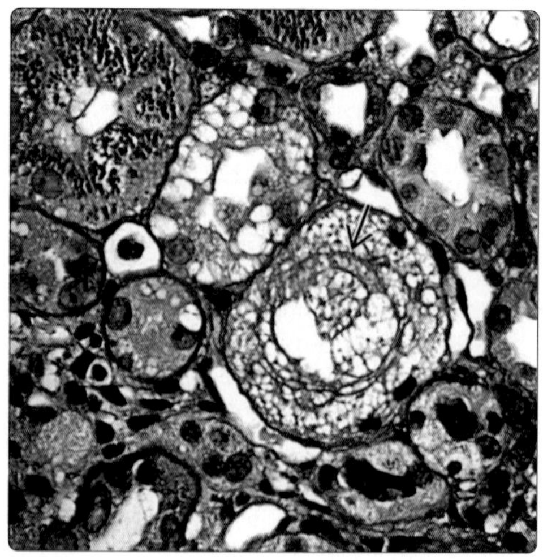

(Left) *Collapsing glomerulopathy with hyperplastic, vacuolated epithelial cells having giant dysmorphic mitochondria seen as coarsely granular inclusion bodies ⇨ in an 18 month old with COQ2 deficiency is seen here. (Courtesy L. Barisoni-Thomas, MD.)* **(Right)** *Proximal tubular cells show vacuolization ⇨ with focal protein resorption droplets in COQ2 defect. (Courtesy L. Barisoni-Thomas, MD.)*

Severe Tubular Injury With Karyomegaly

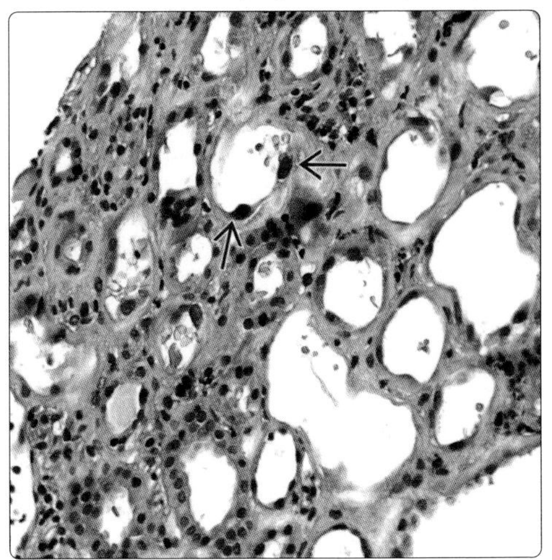

Abnormal Mitochondria in Tenofovir Toxicity

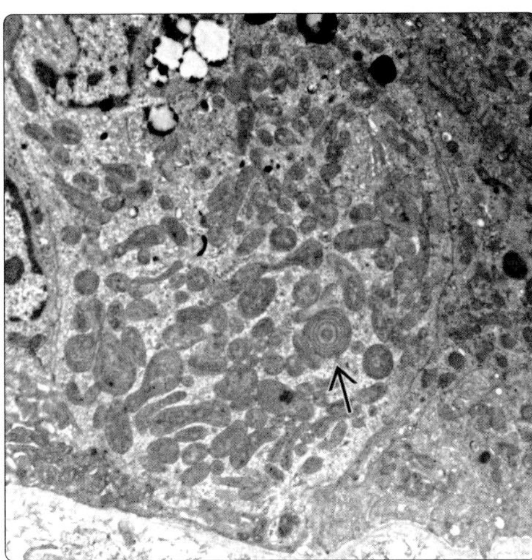

(Left) *An HIV(+) patient on HARRT therapy with Tenofovir, acute renal failure, and metabolic acidosis with glycosuria showing severe tubular epithelial injury, ectasia, loss of brush border, and karyomegaly ⇒ is seen here. (Courtesy B. Fyfe, MD.)* **(Right)** *In the same case, electron micrograph of a renal tubular cell shows varying sizes of mitochondria and shapes with occasional swelling and concentric cristae ⇒.*

Tubular Injury With Granular Cytoplasm

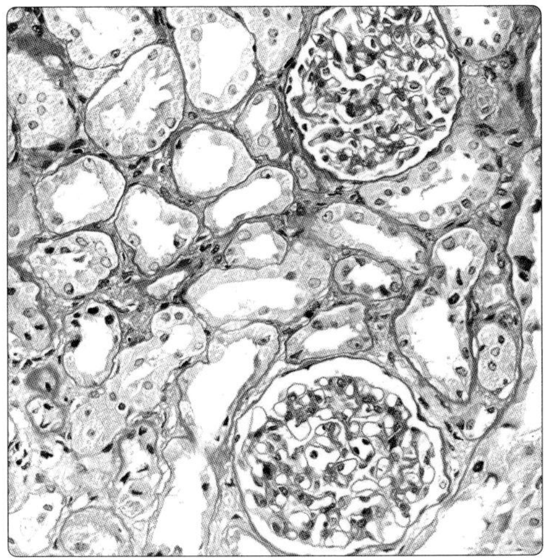

Tubular Cell Abnormally Dense Mitochondria

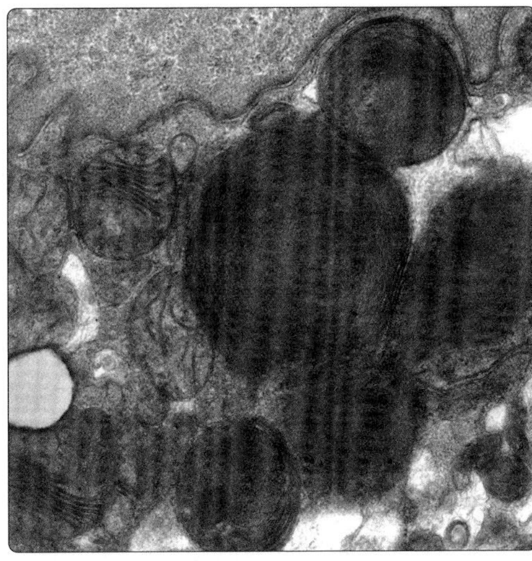

(Left) *A case of MELAS (mitochondrial encephalopathy, lactic acidosis, and stroke-like episodes) presented with a mild Fanconi-like picture and myopathy, showing tubular epithelial injury and fine granularity.* **(Right)** *In the same case, electron micrograph of the tubular cell shows irregularly large mitochondria, dense matrix, and fragmented/concentric cristae. Mitochondria show varied loss of cristae.*

Abnormal Mitochondria in Inherited Cardiomyopathy

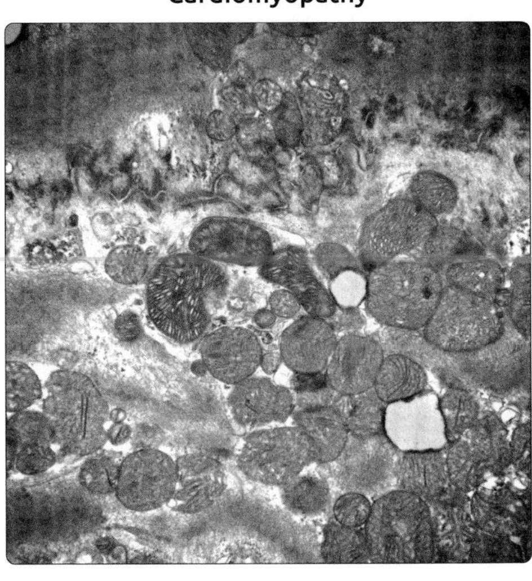

Cardiomyopathy With Abnormal Mitochondria

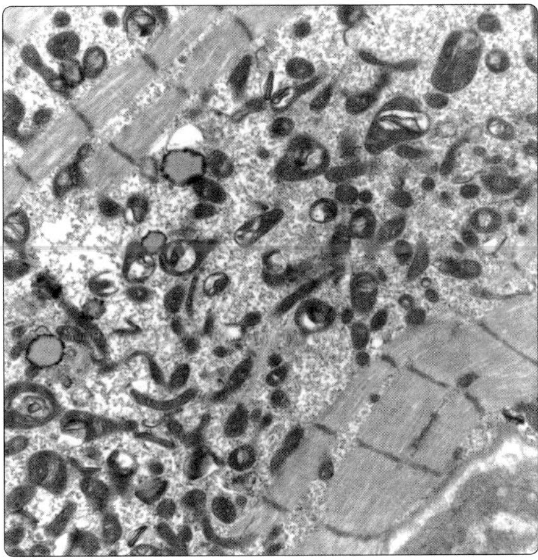

(Left) *A case of MELAS shows ultrastructural features of abnormal mitochondria such as irregular sizes and shapes and a variety of patterns of cristae.* **(Right)** *A 25-year-old male with cardiomyopathy (unknown mutation) shows abnormal mitochondria of varying sizes and irregularly arranged cristae. Several show empty central cores and others show concentric cristae.*

Nephrocalcinosis

KEY FACTS

TERMINOLOGY

- Deposition of abundant calcium phosphate precipitates within renal tubules and interstitium
- "Nephrocalcinosis" usually refers to calcium phosphate deposits in setting of hypercalcemia

ETIOLOGY/PATHOGENESIS

- Hypercalcemia due to various conditions
  - Inherited tubulopathies
  - Nephrocalcinosis usually in chronic hypercalcemia
  - Sarcoidosis
  - Hyperparathyroidism (primary)
  - Hypervitaminosis A or D
  - Hypercalcemia of malignancy
  - Milk-alkali syndrome

CLINICAL ISSUES

- Chronic renal failure
- Hypercalcemia, hypercalciuria

IMAGING

- Diffuse, fine renal parenchymal calcifications

MICROSCOPIC

- Calcium phosphate deposits within tubular lumens, interstitium, and tubular basement membranes
  - Deposits are purple on H&E-stained sections
  - Deposits are positive (black) on von Kossa stain, which stains phosphate
  - Interstitial fibrosis and tubular atrophy and interstitial inflammation

TOP DIFFERENTIAL DIAGNOSES

- Phosphate nephropathy
  - Usually related to ingestion of oral sodium phosphate
- Other tubulopathies causing nephrocalcinosis
- Dent disease
- Medullary sponge kidney
- Nephrogenic systemic fibrosis

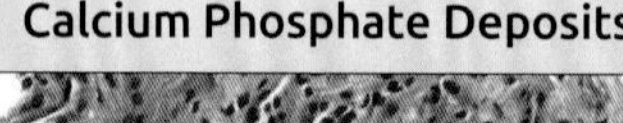

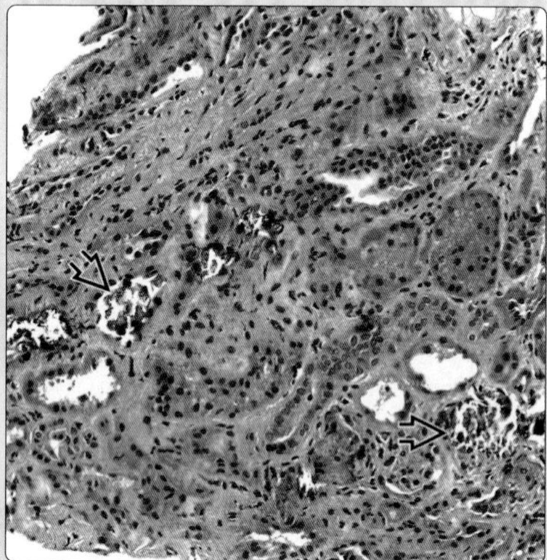

Nephrocalcinosis

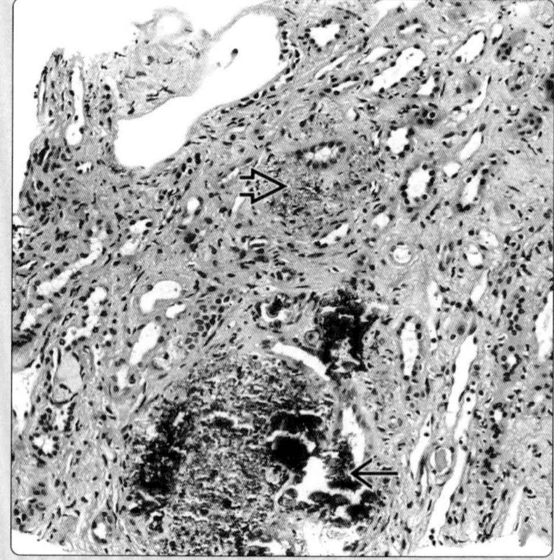

(Left) *H&E shows acute nephrocalcinosis in a patient with acute renal failure, hypercalcemia, and multiple myeloma. Several calcium phosphate ⇨ deposits are within the tubular lumens. There was no evidence of light chain deposition disease or of light chain cast nephropathy.* **(Right)** *Calcium phosphate is deposited in large clumps ⇨ and in finer granules ⇨ in tubular lumina and the interstitium.*

von Kossa

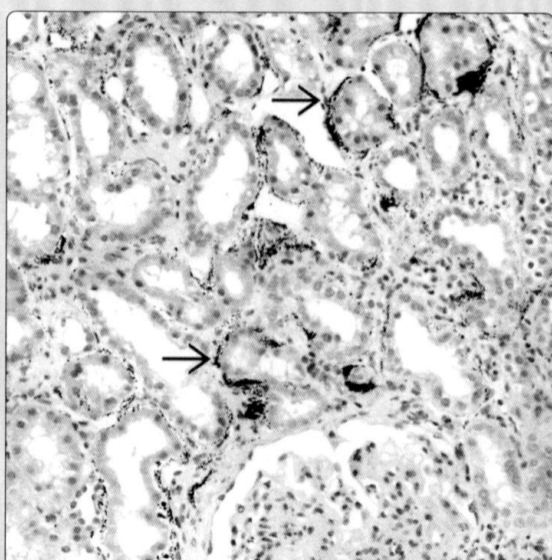

Randall Plaque

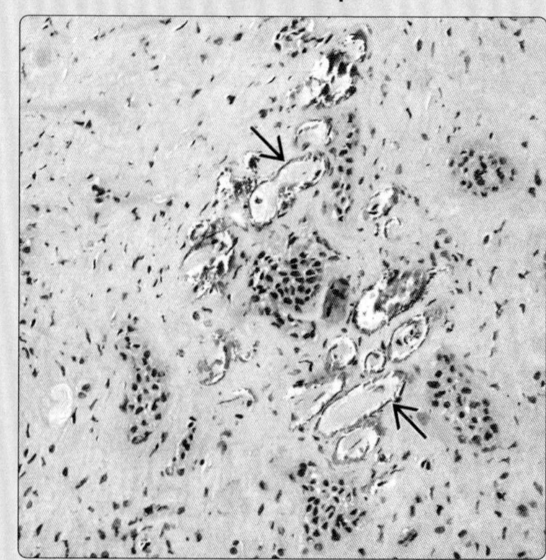

(Left) *A von Kossa stain on a case of diabetic glomerulosclerosis reveals diffuse tubular basement membrane and interstitial calcification ⇨. The patient had a normal serum calcium level at the time of biopsy. The cause of nephrocalcinosis is unknown.* **(Right)** *Randall plaque biopsy shows tubular basement membrane ⇨ calcium phosphate deposits.*

TERMINOLOGY

Definitions

- Deposition of calcium phosphate in renal tubules, tubular basement membrane, and interstitium
- "Nephrocalcinosis" refers to calcium phosphate deposits in setting of hypercalcemia
  - Calcium oxalate deposits in other conditions (e.g., primary hyperoxaluria, termed "oxalosis")

ETIOLOGY/PATHOGENESIS

Calcium Precipitation Within Kidney

- Increased urinary concentration of calcium and phosphate allows precipitation
- Almost all calcium (98%) filtered by glomerulus reabsorbed by tubule
- Randall plaques (calcium deposits at or near papillary tip) may be initial site of calcification
  - Deposits also in interstitium, tubular basement membranes, and tubular lumens

Hypercalcemia Due to Various Conditions

- Nephrocalcinosis can occur in chronic hypercalcemia of any cause
- Sarcoidosis
- Hypercalcemia of malignancy
- Milk-alkali syndrome
- Hypervitaminosis A or D
- Hyperparathyroidism (primary)

Inherited Tubulopathies

- Dent disease, cystinosis, and others

CLINICAL ISSUES

Epidemiology

- Age
  - Childhood through older adulthood
  - Neonates, especially those receiving loop diuretics

Presentation

- Chronic renal failure
- Nephrolithiasis
  - Not always present
- No or little proteinuria
- Benign urine sediment
- Hypercalcemia
- Hypercalciuria
- Nephrocalcinosis may be found in presence of other renal disease

Treatment

- Directed at underlying cause

Prognosis

- Depends on cause

IMAGING

Radiographic Findings

- Diffuse, fine renal parenchymal calcifications

MICROSCOPIC

Histologic Features

- Calcium phosphate deposits within tubular lumens, interstitium, and tubular basement membranes
  - Purple deposits on H&E stained sections
  - Black deposits on von Kossa, which stains phosphate
  - Alizarin red stains calcium specifically
  - Crystals not polarizable
- Interstitial fibrosis and tubular atrophy
- Focal mild interstitial inflammation with mononuclear cells
- No specific glomerular or vascular changes

ANCILLARY TESTS

Metabolic Work-Up

- Hyperparathyroidism
- Hypercalcemia, hyperphosphatemia
- Hypercalciuria, hyperphosphaturia, or hyperoxaluria

DIFFERENTIAL DIAGNOSIS

Acute Phosphate Nephropathy

- Calcium phosphate deposits in tubular lumina
- Usually related to ingestion of oral sodium phosphate

Dent Disease

- X-linked, affects children
- Deposition of calcium phosphate or calcium oxalate crystals in tubulointerstitium
- Renal stone disease, hypercalciuria, proximal tubular dysfunction, low molecular weight proteinuria

Medullary Sponge Kidney

- Medullary nephrocalcinosis
  - Calcium phosphate precipitates within renal cysts

Other Tubulopathies Causing Nephrocalcinosis

- Lowe syndrome, Bartter syndrome, cystic fibrosis, distal renal tubular acidosis, cystic fibrosis, autosomal dominant hypocalcemia, hypomagnesemic hypercalciuric nephrocalcinosis, X-linked hypophosphatemia, Williams syndrome, Wilson disease, Liddle syndrome

Nephrogenic Systemic Fibrosis

- Extensive TBM calcium phosphate deposition
- Calcific deposits in other organs

Calcium Oxalate Deposition in Kidney

- Clear, polarizable crystals on H&E-stained sections

DIAGNOSTIC CHECKLIST

Pathologic Interpretation Pearls

- Nephrocalcinosis may accelerate progression of chronic renal disease

SELECTED REFERENCES

1. Evenepoel P et al: Microscopic nephrocalcinosis in chronic kidney disease patients. Nephrol Dial Transplant. 30(5):843-8, 2015
2. Shavit L et al: What is nephrocalcinosis? Kidney Int. ePub, 2015
3. Koreishi AF et al: Nephrogenic systemic fibrosis: a pathologic study of autopsy cases. Arch Pathol Lab Med. 133(12):1943-8, 2009
4. Troxell ML et al: Glomerular and tubular basement membrane calcinosis: case report and literature review. Am J Kidney Dis. 47(2):e23-6, 2006

KEY FACTS

ETIOLOGY/PATHOGENESIS

- Oxalate accumulation in kidney
  - Enteric malabsorption (gastric bypass)
  - Ingestion of oxalate-containing foods
    - Rhubarb, parsley, spinach, beet greens, starfruit, peanuts, black tea
  - Ingestion of ethylene glycol
  - Excessive vitamin C intake
  - Pyridoxine deficiency

CLINICAL ISSUES

- Acute renal failure
  - Especially with ingestion of ethylene glycol
- Chronic renal failure
  - Slow rise in serum creatinine 1 to several years after gastric bypass
- Nephrolithiasis
  - Calcium oxalate stones
- Progressive nephrocalcinosis

MICROSCOPIC

- Calcium oxalate crystals within tubular lumens, tubular epithelial cytoplasm, and interstitium
  - Crystals translucent and strongly birefringent
- Granulomatous reaction to calcium oxalate crystals

TOP DIFFERENTIAL DIAGNOSES

- Primary oxalosis
- 2,8-dihydroxyadeninuria
- Urate crystals
- Leucine crystals (liver failure)
- Crystals due to monoclonal immunoglobulin
  - Light chain cast nephropathy
  - Light chain Fanconi syndrome
  - Crystal-storing histiocytosis
- Drug crystals
- Acute tubular injury

Calcium Oxalate Under Polarization

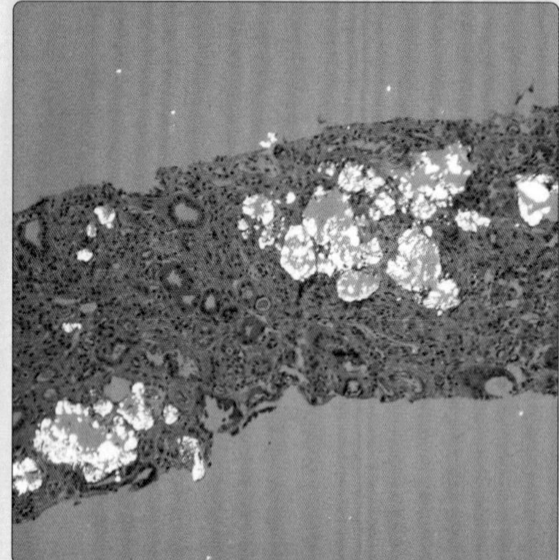

Interstitial Fibrosis With Calcium Oxalate

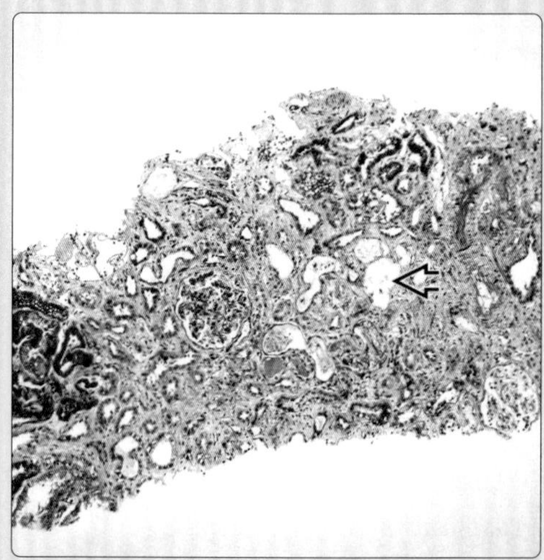

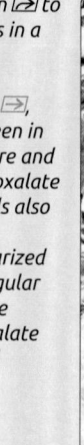

(Left) *Examination under polarized light highlights the abundant calcium oxalate crystals on an H&E stained section. These crystals are best seen on H&E stained sections, as they may dissolve during the staining process for other stains.* **(Right)** *A trichrome stain reveals the extensive interstitial fibrosis in this case. Abundant calcium oxalate crystals ⇨ are seen in areas of fibrosis.*

Granulomatous Reaction

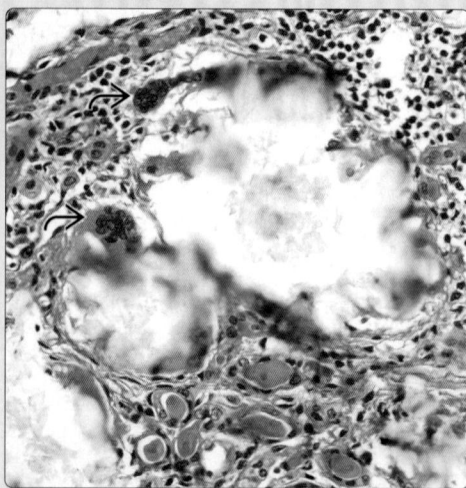

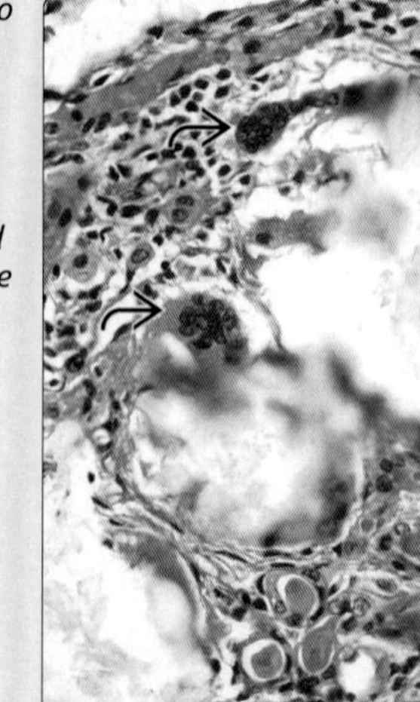

Leucine Crystals

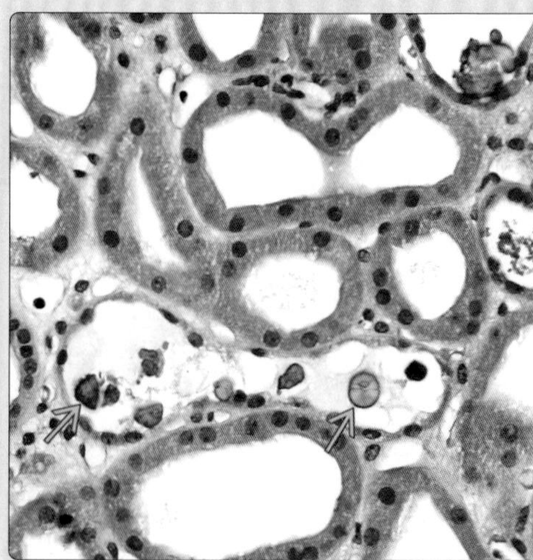

(Left) *Giant cell reaction ⇨ to calcium oxalate crystals in a patient with primary hyperoxaluria is shown.* **(Right)** *Leucine crystals ⇨, pictured here, can be seen in patients with liver failure and may resemble calcium oxalate crystals. Leucine crystals also are birefringent upon examination under polarized light, but have more regular shapes and appear more purple than calcium oxalate crystals on H&E stained sections.*

TERMINOLOGY

Synonyms

- Oxalate nephropathy

Definitions

- Calcium oxalate deposition in kidney parenchyma due to excessive intake or decreased excretion

ETIOLOGY/PATHOGENESIS

Increased Blood Oxalate Levels

- Caused by increased intake, increased absorption, decreased excretion, or vitamin deficiency
- Enteric hyperoxaluria (malabsorptive states)
  - Increased oxalate absorption by gut due to
    - Gastric/intestinal bypass surgery
    - Prolonged use of antibiotics
    - Crohn disease/celiac sprue
    - Pancreatic insufficiency
    - Short bowel syndrome
- Ethylene glycol ingestion
  - Oxalate is metabolite of ethylene glycol
- Increased ingestion of oxalate-containing foods
  - Rhubarb, parsley, spinach, beet greens, starfruit, peanuts, black tea
- Excessive vitamin C intake (rare)
  - Vitamin C is precursor to oxalic acid
- Exposure to methoxyflurane anesthetic
  - Used in 1960s-1970s

CLINICAL ISSUES

Presentation

- Acute renal failure
  - Especially with ingestion of ethylene glycol
- Chronic renal failure
  - Slowly progressive rise in serum Cr
    - 1 to several years after gastric bypass
- Nephrolithiasis
  - Calcium oxalate stones
- Progressive nephrocalcinosis

Treatment

- Remove source of excess oxalates
- Reverse gastric bypass
- Hemodialysis
  - Removes excess oxalate
- Some respond to pyridoxine therapy

Prognosis

- Irreversible renal failure if untreated

MICROSCOPIC

Histologic Features

- Calcium oxalate crystals within tubular lumens, tubular epithelial cytoplasm, and interstitium
  - Crystals translucent on H&E stain and have fan-like or irregular shapes
    - Birefringent under polarized light
  - Massive deposits in advanced cases
  - In oxalosis secondary to gastric bypass, biopsies showed 3.5 calcium oxalate crystals per glomerulus (range: 1.5-7.9) in 1 study
- Tubular injury
- Focal mononuclear cell inflammation in areas of interstitial fibrosis
- Granulomatous reaction to calcium oxalate crystals
- Interstitial fibrosis and tubular atrophy (nonspecific)

DIFFERENTIAL DIAGNOSIS

Primary Oxalosis

- Tends to be younger age of onset (though not necessarily)
- More extensive deposition of oxalate crystals (e.g., arterial media, bone marrow)

2,8-Dihydroxyadeninuria (DHA)

- Polarizable crystals within renal parenchyma, similar to calcium oxalate
- Reddish-brown crystals, vs. clear crystals of calcium oxalate

Tubulointerstitial Nephritis, Granulomatous Interstitial Nephritis

- Usual interstitial nephritis cases do not show calcium oxalate crystals

Urate Crystals

- Large, amorphous deposits; nonpolarizing crystals
- Surrounding granulomatous reaction

Leucine Crystals

- Seen in patients with liver failure
- Polarizable

Drug Crystals

- e.g., triamterene, antibiotics, and antiviral drugs
- Some polarizable

Crystals Due to Monoclonal Immunoglobulin

- Light chain cast nephropathy
- Light chain proximal tubulopathy (light chain Fanconi syndrome)
- Crystal-storing histiocytosis

Acute Tubular Injury

- May have very focal calcium oxalate crystals within tubular lumens

SELECTED REFERENCES

1. Nazzal L et al: Enteric hyperoxaluria: an important cause of end-stage kidney disease. Nephrol Dial Transplant. ePub, 2015
2. Cossey LN et al: Oxalate nephropathy and intravenous vitamin C. Am J Kidney Dis. 61(6):1032-5, 2013
3. Albersmeyer M et al: Acute kidney injury after ingestion of rhubarb: secondary oxalate nephropathy in a patient with type 1 diabetes. BMC Nephrol. 13:141, 2012
4. Bergstralh EJ et al: Transplantation outcomes in primary hyperoxaluria. Am J Transplant. 10(11):2493-501, 2010
5. Hoppe B et al: The primary hyperoxalurias. Kidney Int. 75(12):1264-71, 2009
6. Nasr SH et al: Oxalate nephropathy complicating Roux-en-Y Gastric Bypass: an underrecognized cause of irreversible renal failure. Clin J Am Soc Nephrol. 3(6):1676-83, 2008
7. Nasr SH et al: Secondary oxalosis due to excess vitamin C intake. Kidney Int. 70(10):1672, 2006
8. Alkhunaizi AM et al: Secondary oxalosis: a cause of delayed recovery of renal function in the setting of acute renal failure. J Am Soc Nephrol. 7(11):2320-6, 1996

KEY FACTS

TERMINOLOGY

- Idiopathic chronic kidney disease (CKD) that occurs in Central America particularly among agricultural workers

ETIOLOGY/PATHOGENESIS

- Unknown; many theories
  - Cyclical dehydration
  - Increased fructose/fructokinase metabolism in proximal tubule leads to increased oxidants and chemokines and tubular injury
  - Occupational exposure to toxins (e.g., pesticides)
  - NSAID use

CLINICAL ISSUES

- Most CKD in men in certain geographic areas attributed to Mesoamerican nephropathy
  - Pacific coast in Nicaragua, El Salvador, Costa Rica, Guatemala, Southern Mexico
  - Prevalent in sugar cane workers
- Progressive chronic kidney disease
- Low-grade albuminuria
- No hypertension or edema

MICROSCOPIC

- Glomeruli
  - Global glomerulosclerosis (29-78%)
  - Focal segmental glomerulosclerosis
  - Glomerulomegaly
  - Glomerular ischemic features
- Tubules and Interstitium
  - Interstitial fibrosis and tubular atrophy
  - Mild interstitial chronic inflammation
- Mild or no vascular disease

TOP DIFFERENTIAL DIAGNOSES

- Chronic tubulointerstitial disease from other causes
- Other endemic nephropathies

(Left) *Increased interstitial fibrosis and global glomerulosclerosis ➡ are seen in a case of probable Mesoamerican nephropathy. There is a mild interstitial mononuclear inflammatory infiltrate ➡. Note the normal-appearing artery ➡.* **(Right)** *A focal segmental glomerular scar ➡ is seen in this case of probable Mesoamerican nephropathy in a kidney biopsy from a young man who was an agricultural worker in El Salvador.*

Interstitial Fibrosis and Global Glomerulosclerosis

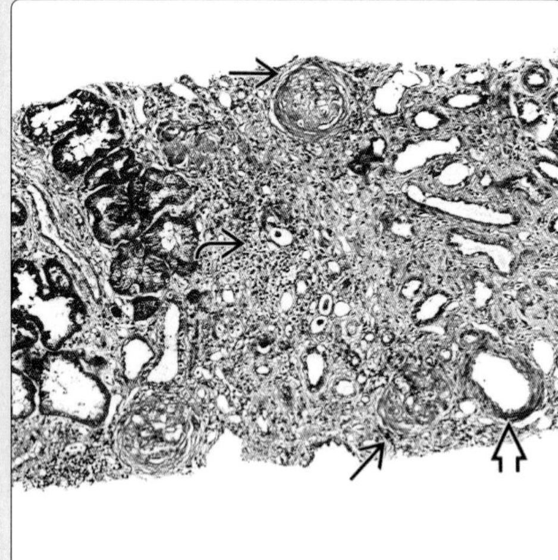

Focal Segmental Glomerular Scarring

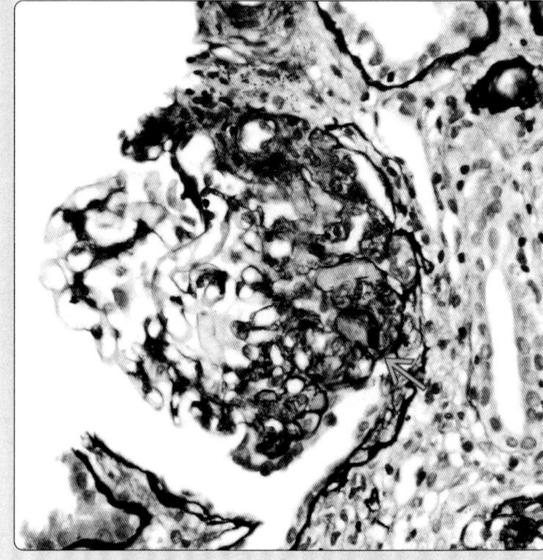

(Left) *Interstitial fibrosis, tubular atrophy, and interstitial inflammation ➡ is seen in a case of Mesoamerican nephropathy.* **(Right)** *Despite global glomerulosclerosis and focal segmental glomerulosclerosis, arteries ➡ appear normal in this biopsy, typical of Mesoamerican nephropathy, which is not associated with hypertension.*

Interstitial Fibrosis and Inflammation

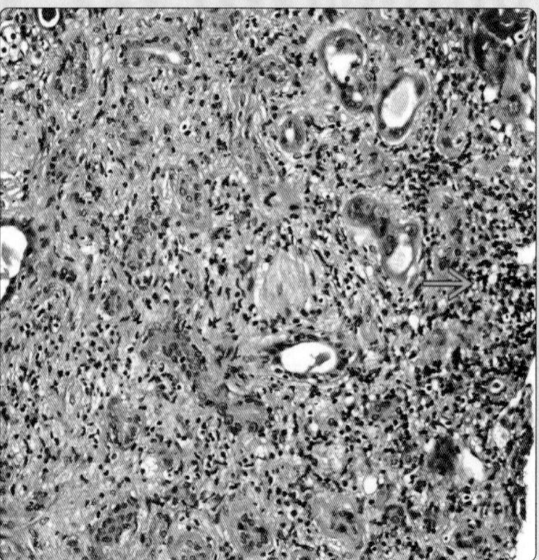

Normal Arteries

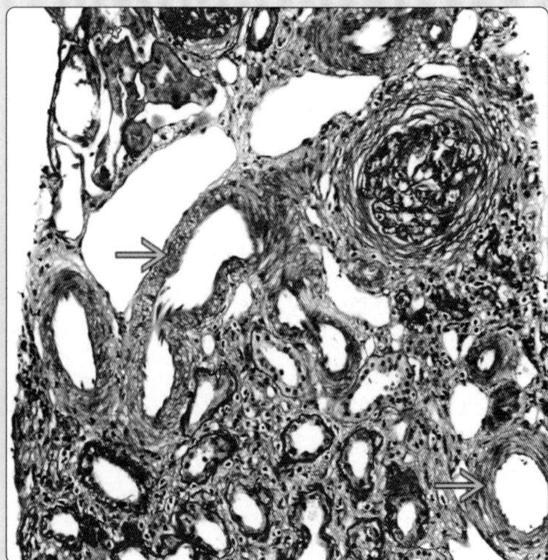

TERMINOLOGY

Abbreviations

- Mesoamerican nephropathy (MeN)

Synonyms

- Agricultural nephropathy
- Chronic agrochemical nephropathy

Definitions

- Idiopathic chronic kidney disease (CKD) that occurs in Central America, particularly among agricultural workers (excludes known causes such as hypertension, diabetes, and polycystic kidney disease)

ETIOLOGY/PATHOGENESIS

Many Potential Causes

- Cyclical dehydration and volume depletion
  - Fructose/fructokinase mechanism
    - Metabolism of fructose to fructokinase in proximal tubule increases oxidants and chemokines
      - Leads to tubular injury and inflammation
      - Fructokinase knockout mice protected from renal injury related to cyclical dehydration
  - Endogenous or exogenous fructose
    - Rehydration with fructose-rich beverages may contribute
- Occupational exposure to toxins (e.g., pesticides)
- NSAID use
- Childhood exposures and low birth weight
- Heavy metal exposure
  - Arsenic and others
- Genetic abnormalities
- Hypokalemia and hyperuricemia (unlikely cause of CKD)
- *Leptospira* infection (unlikely cause of CKD)

Other "Endemic Nephropathies" of Unknown Cause

- Increase in CKD in other agricultural communities in hot climates
- May have similar etiologies as MeN
- CKD in north-central dry zone of Sri Lanka
- "Uddanam nephropathy" in Andhra Pradesh province, India
  - ~ 16% prevalence
- Lack of biopsy or autopsy data for these entities

CLINICAL ISSUES

Epidemiology

- Sex
  - Primarily men
- Occupational disease of agricultural workers in Central America
  - Prevalent in sugar cane workers
  - Not in agricultural workers in higher altitudes
  - Not in sugar cane workers in other geographic locations with hot climates (e.g., Brazil, Cuba, Africa)
- Prevalence
  - CKD prevalence of 13.8% in men in León, Nicaragua
  - CKD up to 50% of men in some El Salvador regions
  - Most CKD in men in certain geographic areas attributed to MeN
- Geographic locations
  - Pacific coast in Nicaragua, El Salvador, Costa Rica, Guatemala, Southern Mexico

Presentation

- Progressive CKD
- Low-grade albuminuria
- Hypokalemia
- No hypertension or edema

MICROSCOPIC

Histologic Features

- Glomeruli
  - Global glomerulosclerosis (29-78%)
  - Ischemic features
    - Periglomerular fibrosis, basement membrane wrinkling
  - Focal segmental glomerulosclerosis
  - Glomerulomegaly
- Tubules
  - Tubular atrophy
- Interstitium
  - Mild interstitial chronic inflammation
  - Increased interstitial fibrosis
- Arteries and arterioles
  - Usually mild or no vascular disease

ANCILLARY TESTS

Electron Microscopy

- Vacuoles in podocytes
- Few glomerular electron-dense deposits in some cases

DIFFERENTIAL DIAGNOSIS

Chronic Tubulointerstitial Disease From Other Causes

- Exclude known toxins and drugs by history
- Exclude infection by culture, special stains

Other Endemic Nephropathies (India, Sri Lanka)

- Geographic area specific but scant pathology data

SELECTED REFERENCES

1. Laux TS et al: Dialysis enrollment patterns in Guatemala: evidence of the chronic kidney disease of non-traditional causes epidemic in Mesoamerica. BMC Nephrol. 16:54, 2015
2. Paula Santos U et al: Burnt sugarcane harvesting is associated with acute renal dysfunction. Kidney Int. 87(4):792-9, 2015
3. Correa-Rotter R et al: CKD of unknown origin in Central America: the case for a Mesoamerican nephropathy. Am J Kidney Dis. 63(3):506-20, 2014
4. Roncal Jimenez CA et al: Fructokinase activity mediates dehydration-induced renal injury. Kidney Int. 86(2):294-302, 2014
5. Wesseling C et al: Resolving the enigma of the mesoamerican nephropathy: a research workshop summary. Am J Kidney Dis. 63(3):396-404, 2014
6. Wijkström J et al: Clinical and pathological characterization of Mesoamerican nephropathy: a new kidney disease in Central America. Am J Kidney Dis. 62(5):908-18, 2013
7. Peraza S et al: Decreased kidney function among agricultural workers in El Salvador. Am J Kidney Dis. 59(4):531-40, 2012
8. Torres C et al: Decreased kidney function of unknown cause in Nicaragua: a community-based survey. Am J Kidney Dis. 55(3):485-96, 2010

Extramedullary Hematopoiesis

KEY FACTS

TERMINOLOGY

- EMH defined as development and growth of hematopoietic tissue outside of bone marrow

ETIOLOGY/PATHOGENESIS

- Underlying hematologic malignancy or other lack of bone marrow hematopoiesis
  - Myelofibrosis (most common)
  - Plasma cell myeloma

CLINICAL ISSUES

- Acute renal insufficiency
- Proteinuria due to concurrent glomerular disease
- EMH at other anatomic locations (especially liver or spleen)
- Renal or perirenal mass lesion (sclerosing extramedullary hematopoietic tumor)

MICROSCOPIC

- Interstitial infiltrate with trilineage hematopoiesis
  - Erythroids, myeloids, and megakaryocytes
- Concurrent glomerulopathy in majority of cases of renal EMH
  - Glomerulopathy associated with myeloproliferative neoplasms
  - Fibrillary-like glomerulopathy
  - Focal segmental glomerulosclerosis (FSGS)

TOP DIFFERENTIAL DIAGNOSES

- Acute tubulointerstitial nephritis (AIN)
  - Presence of eosinophil precursors in renal EMH mimics mature eosinophils in allergic AIN
- Hodgkin lymphoma
  - Megakaryocytes may resemble Reed-Sternberg cells of Hodgkin lymphoma
- Myelolipoma
  - Adipose tissue admixed with hematopoietic elements
- Aggregation of immature hematopoietic cells in vasa recta

EMH in Interstitium

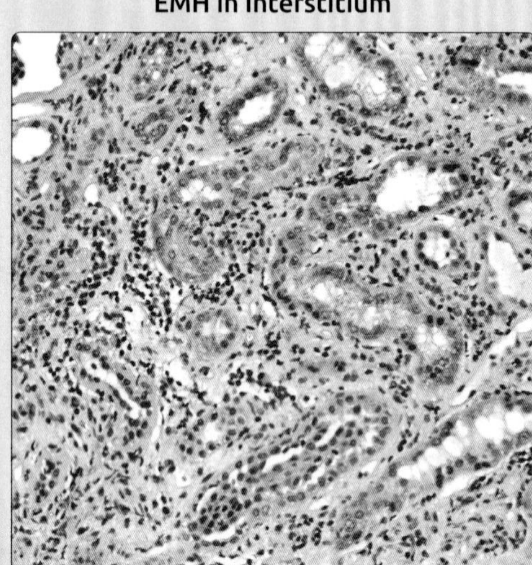

Erythroid Precursors in EMH

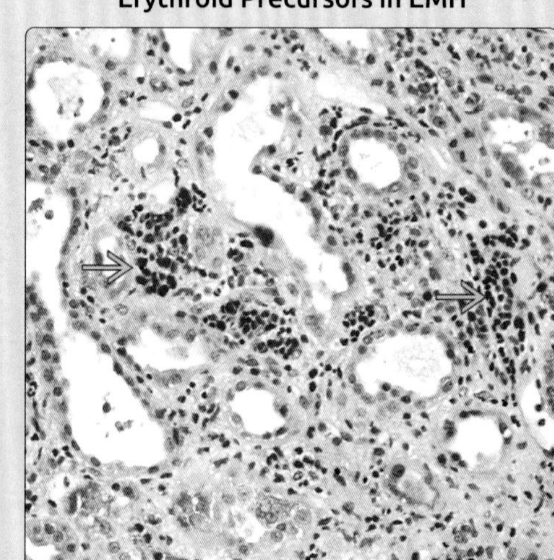

(Left) *EMH in a diffuse infiltrating pattern resembles acute interstitial nephritis.* **(Right)** *Clusters of erythroid precursors ⇒ are seen. These cells have dark nuclei and appear in clusters.*

Megakaryocytes in EMH

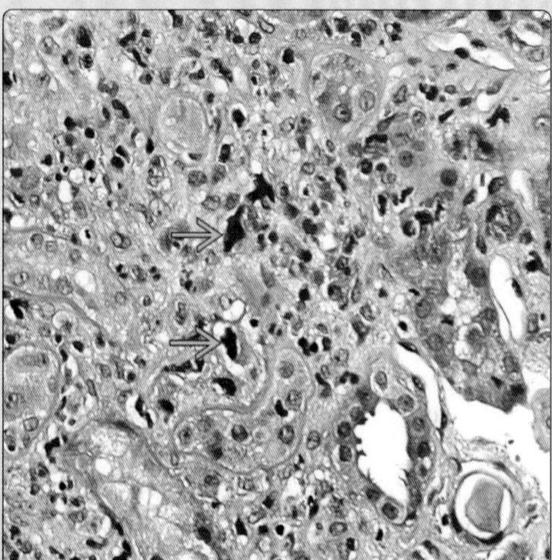

CD61 Stain for Megakaryocytes

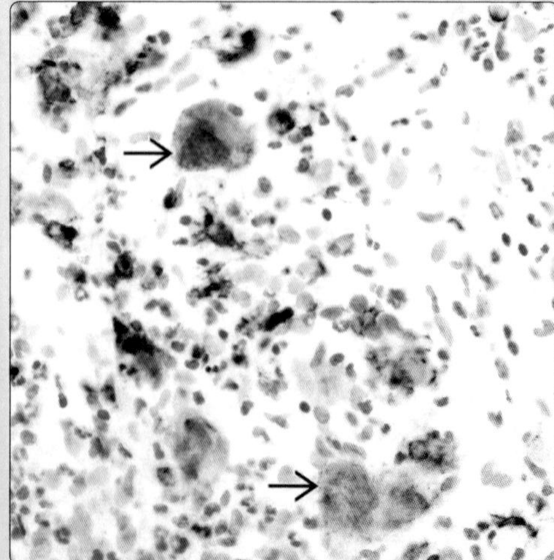

(Left) *Megakaryocytes ⇒ can be seen in the interstitium in renal EMH. Here, the large multilobated nuclei stand out amongst the other infiltrating cells.* **(Right)** *An immunoperoxidase stain for CD61 shows positive staining of megakaryocytes →. The small individual granules are platelets.*

TERMINOLOGY

Abbreviations

- Extramedullary hematopoiesis (EMH)

Definitions

- EMH defined as development and growth of hematopoietic tissue outside of bone marrow

ETIOLOGY/PATHOGENESIS

Underlying Hematologic Malignancy or Impaired Bone Marrow Hematopoiesis

- Myelofibrosis (most common)
- Plasma cell myeloma
- Essential thrombocythemia
- Chronic myeloproliferative neoplasm, not otherwise specified
- Thalassemia

CLINICAL ISSUES

Presentation

- Acute renal insufficiency
- Proteinuria due to concurrent glomerular disease
- Renal or perirenal mass lesion (sclerosing extramedullary hematopoietic tumor)
- EMH at other anatomic locations (especially liver or spleen)
- Renal EMH is more likely to be recognized on post-mortem examination

Treatment

- Treatment directed at underlying hematologic condition

MICROSCOPIC

Histologic Features

- Tubules and interstitium
  - Interstitial infiltrate with trilineage hematopoiesis
    - Erythroid elements
      - Hyperchromatic round nucleus with clear or pink ring of cytoplasm, present in clusters
    - Myeloid elements
      - Includes eosinophils and eosinophil precursors, granulocytes
    - Megakaryocytes
      - Large size, multilobed nuclei, large amount of granular cytoplasm
  - Diffuse infiltrating pattern in interstitium, extrarenal mass lesion, extracapsular extension
  - Lack of significant tubulitis
- Glomeruli
  - Concurrent glomerulopathy in majority of cases of renal EMH
    - Glomerulopathy associated with myeloproliferative neoplasms
      - Chronic thrombotic microangiopathy, mesangial sclerosis
      - Glomerular basement membrane duplication
    - Fibrillary-like glomerulopathy
      - Fibrillary deposits by electron microscopy (EM)
      - Glomerular staining by immunofluorescence for IgM
      - May be weakly congophilic (amyloid type not determined)
    - Focal segmental glomerulosclerosis (FSGS)

ANCILLARY TESTS

Immunohistochemistry

- CD61 for megakaryocytes
- Myeloperoxidase for granulocytes
- Hemoglobin or glycophorin for erythroid elements

Electron Microscopy

- EM reveals features of glomerulopathy
  - Glomerular basement membrane duplication, subendothelial lucency, enlarged endothelial cells in glomeruli
  - Fibrillary deposits in fibrillary-like glomerulopathy
  - Diffuse or segmental podocyte foot process effacement in FSGS

DIFFERENTIAL DIAGNOSIS

Acute Tubulointerstitial Nephritis (AIN)

- Presence of eosinophil precursors in renal EMH mimics mature eosinophils in allergic AIN

Hodgkin Lymphoma

- Megakaryocytes may resemble Reed-Sternberg cells of Hodgkin lymphoma
- Mixed inflammatory infiltrate in background
- Unlike Reed-Sternberg cells, megakaryocytes stain positively for CD61 and are negative for CD15 and CD30

Myelolipoma

- Mass forming; usually present in adrenal gland
- Adipose tissue admixed with hematopoietic elements

Aggregation of Immature Hematopoietic Cells in Vasa Recta

- Intracapillary hematopoietic cells, rather than interstitial cells in "true" renal EMH
- Occurs in sepsis and sometimes in acute tubular necrosis

SELECTED REFERENCES

1. MP Alexander et al: Renal extramedullary hematopoiesis mimics tubulointerstitial nephritis: a study of its clinicopathological spectrum. Submitted, 2015
2. Said SM et al: Myeloproliferative neoplasms cause glomerulopathy. Kidney Int. 80(7):753-9, 2011
3. Sukov WR et al: Sclerosing extramedullary hematopoietic tumor: emphasis on diagnosis by renal biopsy. Ann Diagn Pathol. 13(2):127-31, 2009
4. Nasr SH et al: Myeloma cast nephropathy, direct renal infiltration by myeloma, and renal extramedullary hematopoiesis. Kidney Int. 73(4):517-8, 2008
5. Koch CA et al: Nonhepatosplenic extramedullary hematopoiesis: associated diseases, pathology, clinical course, and treatment. Mayo Clin Proc. 78(10):1223-33, 2003
6. Holt SG et al: Extramedullary haematopoeisis in the renal parenchyma as a cause of acute renal failure in myelofibrosis. Nephrol Dial Transplant. 10(8):1438-40, 1995
7. Nast CC et al: Intrarenal extramedullary erythropoiesis in renal allograft fine-needle aspirates. Am J Kidney Dis. 25(1):46-50, 1995
8. Pitcock JA et al: A clinical and pathological study of seventy cases of myelofibrosis. Ann Intern Med. 57:73-84, 1962

(Left) *In this example of renal EMH, hematopoietic cells are present in the interstitium →, and the EMH extends → beyond the renal capsule.* **(Right)** *Rare tubules show tubulitis → in this example of renal EMH. The presence of focal mild tubulitis does not exclude a diagnosis of EMH.*

Extrarenal EMH

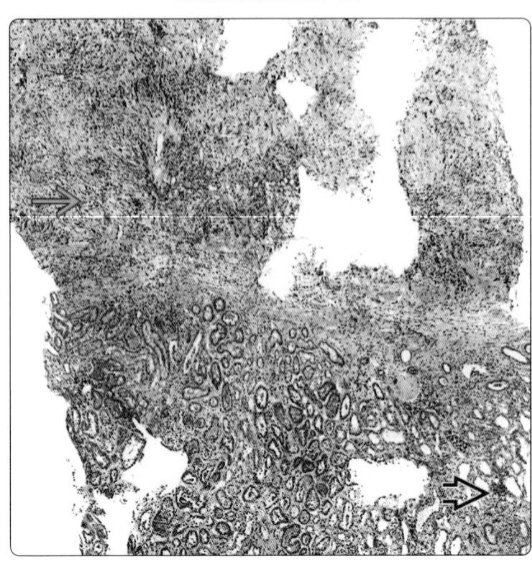

Tubulitis

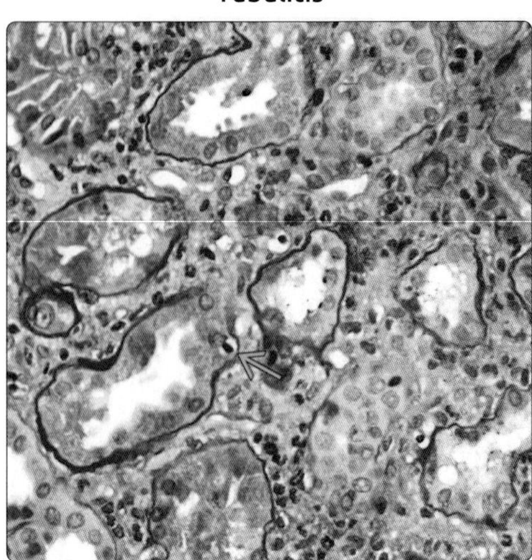

(Left) *An immunoperoxidase stain for glycophorin highlights clusters of erythroid cells →. This stain also detects mature erythrocytes.* **(Right)** *A megakaryocyte → stands out in this field of diffuse infiltrating EMH. Eosinophil precursors → are also present.*

Glycophorin Staining of Erythroid Precursors

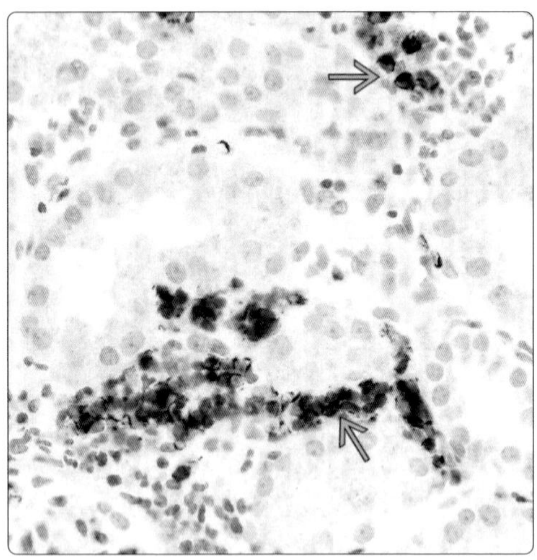

Megakaryocytes in EMH

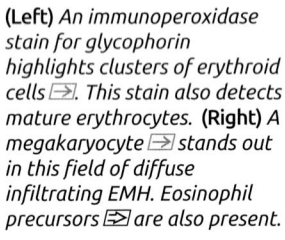

(Left) *EMH may mimic acute allergic interstitial nephritis because of the presence of eosinophils. Upon closer examination, these cells are recognized as immature eosinophils →, many with unilobate nuclei.* **(Right)** *An immunoperoxidase stain for myeloperoxidase (MPO) highlights myeloid cells. There is staining of both neutrophil and eosinophil precursors and mature cells with this stain.*

Eosinophil Precursors

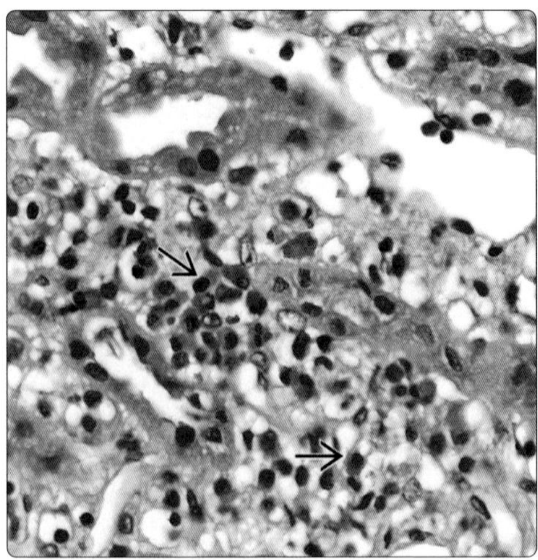

Myeloperoxidase Staining of Myeloid Cells

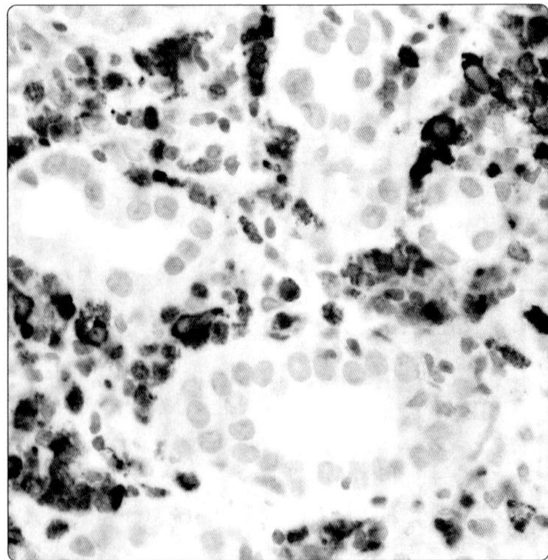

Glomerular Microangiopathy Associated With EMH

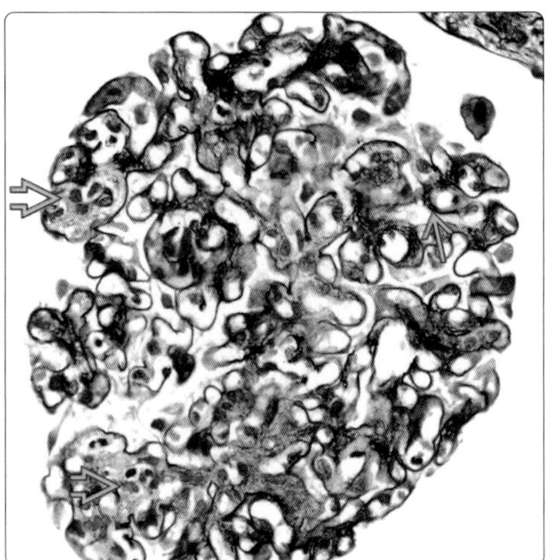

Glomerular Microangiopathy Associated With EMH

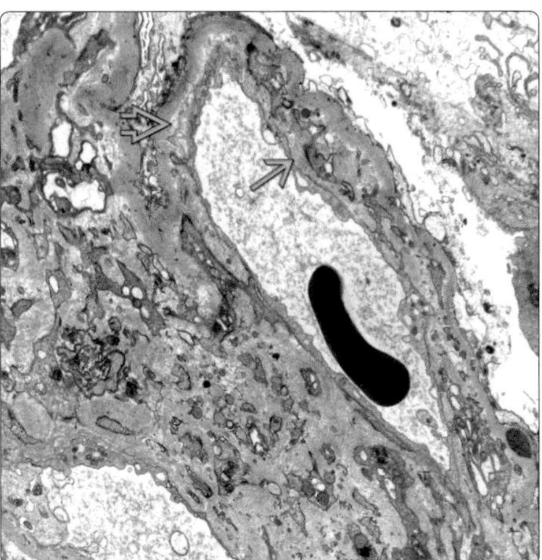

(Left) *Glomeruli show enlarged endothelial cells ➡ and segmental basement membrane duplication ➡.* **(Right)** *Glomerular basement membrane duplication ➡ and subendothelial lucency ➡ are seen in a case of chronic thrombotic microangiopathy associated with EMH.*

Enlarged Endothelial Cells

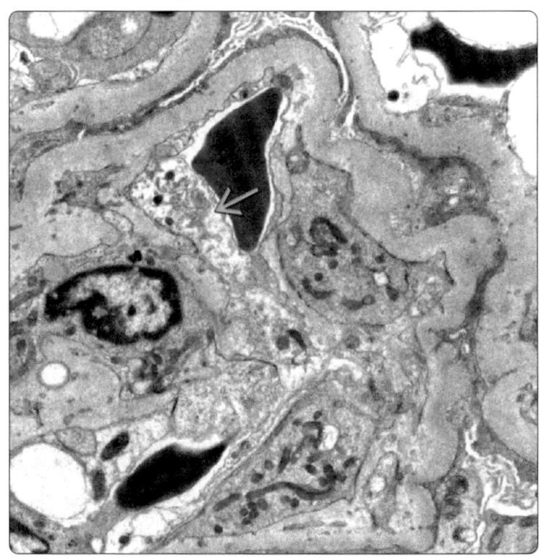

Fibrillary-Like Glomerulonephritis Associated With EMH

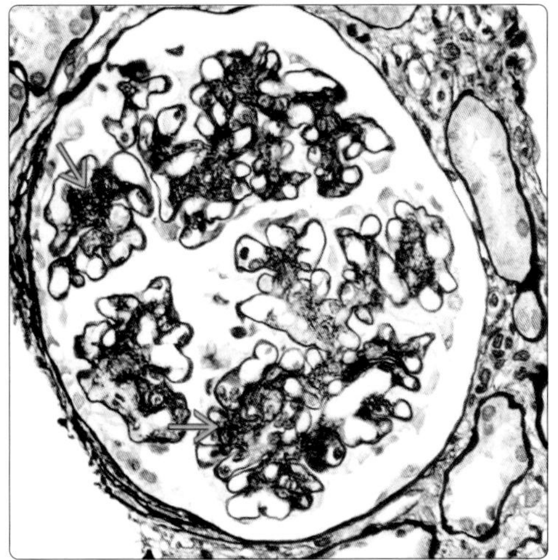

(Left) *Enlarged, reactive-appearing endothelial cells ➡ are seen by electron microscopy in this case of glomerular microangiopathy associated with renal EMH.* **(Right)** *The mesangium is expanded with a fibrillary-like appearance ➡ on this silver stain. By immunofluorescence, glomeruli showed staining for IgM and were negative for IgG; a Congo red stain was negative.*

Fibrillary-Like Glomerulonephritis Associated With EMH

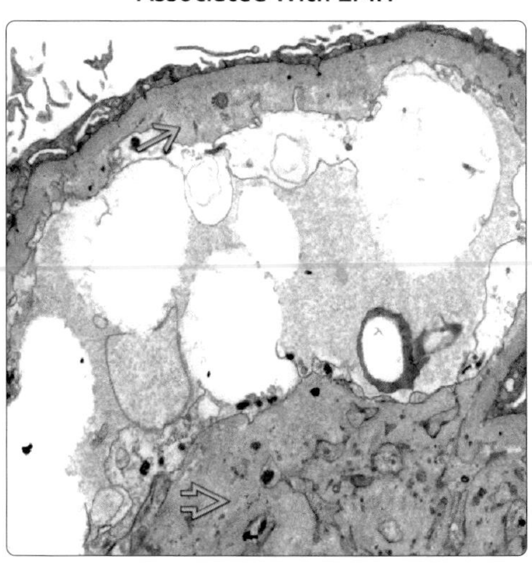

Fibrillary-Like Glomerulonephritis Associated With EMH

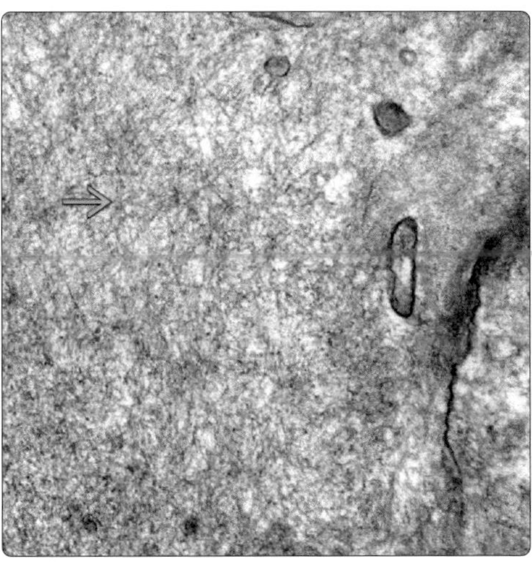

(Left) *The mesangium is expanded ➡ and showed fibrillary deposits on higher magnification. Fibrillary deposits are also present within the glomerular basement membranes ➡.* **(Right)** *By electron microscopy on high magnification, the mesangium shows fibrillary deposits ➡. A Congo red stain was negative.*

SECTION 5
Infections of the Kidney

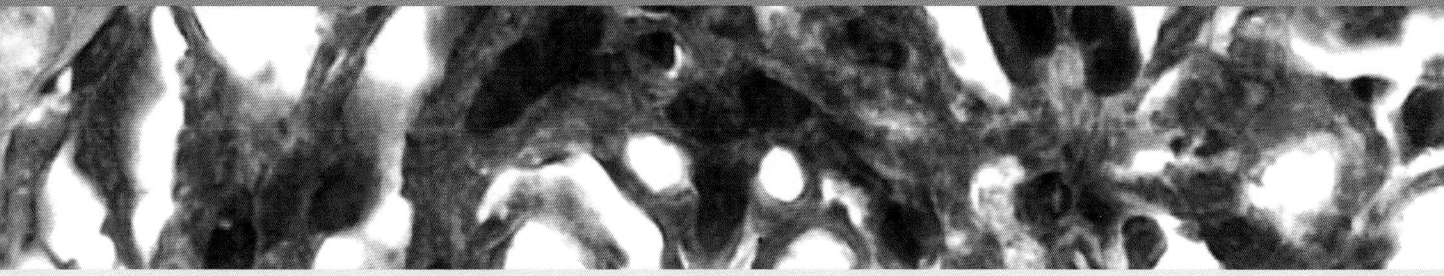

Bacterial Infections of the Kidney

Fungal, Rickettsial, and Parasitic Infections of the Kidney

Viral Infections of the Kidney

Acute Pyelonephritis

KEY FACTS

TERMINOLOGY

- Acute renal parenchymal inflammation due to bacterial or fungal infection

ETIOLOGY/PATHOGENESIS

- Retrograde infection via urethra, bladder, and ureters
  - *Escherichia coli* common organism
- Hematogenous infection in septicemia
  - *Staphylococcus aureus* common organism

CLINICAL ISSUES

- Associated with lower tract problems, obstruction, reflux, pregnancy, diabetes
  - Infants, elderly males and women at risk
- Fever
- Costovertebral angle tenderness
- Leukocyte casts
- Acute uncomplicated pyelonephritis responds to antimicrobial therapy in > 90% of cases

MICROSCOPIC

- Neutrophilic infiltrate and casts in tubules
- Abscesses and papillary necrosis may arise
- Glomeruli and blood vessels relatively spared
- Early infection in medulla and collecting ducts
- Pelvic inflammation in ascending infection
- Special variants
  - Emphysematous pyelonephritis
  - Acute lobar nephronia mimics mass lesion

TOP DIFFERENTIAL DIAGNOSES

- Drug-induced interstitial nephritis
- Glomerulonephritis with severe tubulointerstitial inflammation
- Myeloma cast nephropathy
- Ischemic or toxic tubular injury
- Acute humoral rejection in transplants

Gross Appearance of Acute Pyelonephritis

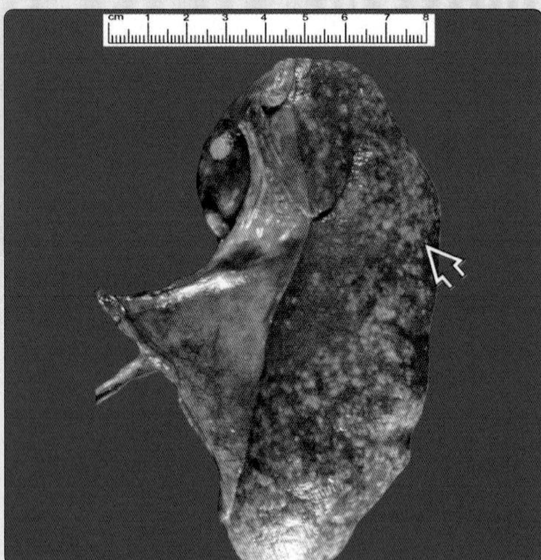

Abscess With Necrosis

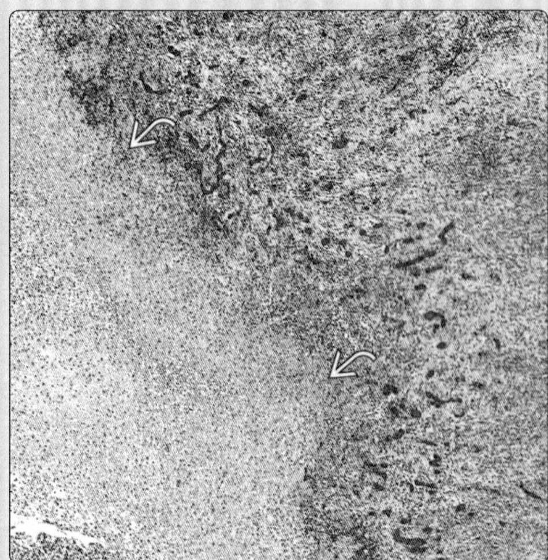

(Left) *Autopsied kidney with acute bacterial pyelonephritis is shown. The renal capsule has been peeled, and the cortical surface shows multiple small abscesses ➡. This is a typical appearance of hematogenous pyelonephritis. (Courtesy L. Fajardo, MD.)* **(Right)** *Autopsied kidney with acute pyelonephritis and a cortical abscess ➡ is shown. The pale area of abscess with neutrophils is surrounded by increased vascularity and chronic inflammation.*

Neutrophil Casts

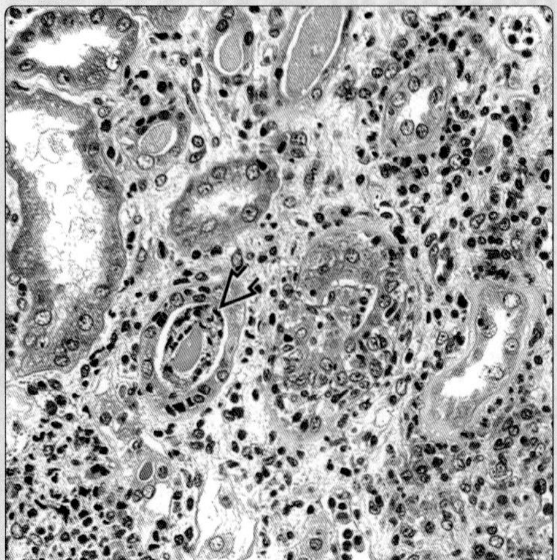

Neutrophil Casts and Chronic Inflammation

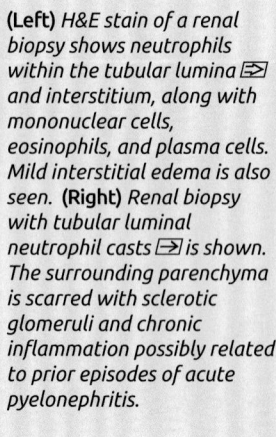

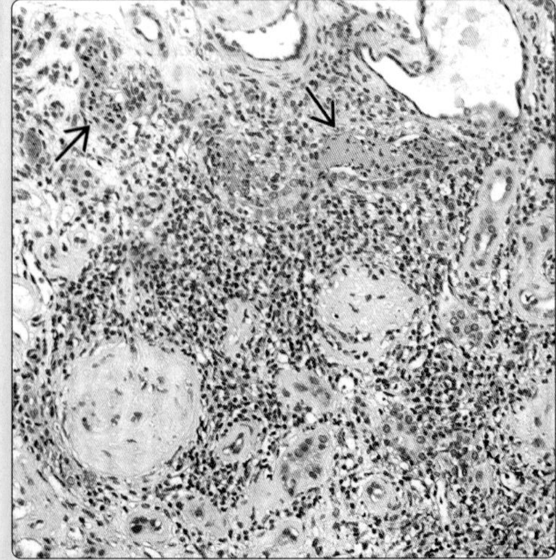

(Left) *H&E stain of a renal biopsy shows neutrophils within the tubular lumina ➡ and interstitium, along with mononuclear cells, eosinophils, and plasma cells. Mild interstitial edema is also seen.* **(Right)** *Renal biopsy with tubular luminal neutrophil casts ➡ is shown. The surrounding parenchyma is scarred with sclerotic glomeruli and chronic inflammation possibly related to prior episodes of acute pyelonephritis.*

TERMINOLOGY

Abbreviations

- Acute pyelonephritis (APN)

Synonyms

- Upper urinary tract infection (UTI)
- Acute bacterial nephritis (used when no pyelitis)

Definitions

- Acute inflammation of kidney parenchyma due to bacterial infection

ETIOLOGY/PATHOGENESIS

Ascending Infection

- Retrograde infection via urethra, bladder, and ureters
- Most common route of infection (95%)
- Usually associated with predisposing factor
  - Obstruction
  - Reflux
  - Instrumentation
  - Urolithiasis
  - Diabetes
  - Pregnancy
  - Renal transplantation immunosuppression
    - APN is the most common bacterial complication
    - Treatment with Cyclosporine A may compromise the host defenses against *Escherichia coli*
- Gram-negative bacteria from gastrointestinal tract (fecal flora) most common
  - *E. coli* most common organism
    - Uropathogenic and virulence factors include fimbriae/pili and serotypes O, K, and H
    - Can colonize urinary bladder efficiently
  - P fimbriae (mannose resistant)
    - Attach to digalactoside residue on urothelial cells and facilitate persistent infection
    - Enhance host innate inflammatory response by interaction with Toll-like receptor 4 (TLR4), resulting in IL-6 and IL-8 production
      - Alpha intercalated cells of the collecting ducts may defend against *E. coli* by acidifying the urine and secreting bacteriostatic protein lipocalin 2 (NGAL)
    - Most important for renal involvement
  - Type 1 fimbriae (mannose sensitive)
    - Binds to Tamm-Horsfall protein
  - *Proteus, Klebsiella, Enterobacter, Pseudomonas, Streptococcus faecalis*
- Fungal organisms can produce similar pathology

Hematogenous Infection

- In septicemia or bacterial endocarditis
  - *Staphylococcus aureus* common pathogen
  - Fungal organisms in immunocompromised hosts
- No obstruction or reflux required for pathogenesis

Asymptomatic Bacteriuria

- Bacterial counts of > 100,000 colony forming units/mL of urine in relatively asymptomatic patient
- Frequently encountered in pregnant women
  - Antimicrobial therapy recommended as it can progress to overt bacteriuria and pyelonephritis

CLINICAL ISSUES

Epidemiology

- Age
  - Infants
    - Often have anatomic abnormalities of urinary tract
  - Elderly males
    - Prostatic hypertrophy is risk factor
- Sex
  - Women more susceptible, especially during pregnancy

Site

- Pelvic urothelium (pyelitis)
- Renal tubules and interstitium (pyelonephritis)
- Renal cortical abscesses (bacterial nephritis)

Presentation

- Fever and chills
- Flank pain
- Nausea and vomiting
- Costovertebral angle tenderness
- May be subclinical
- If lower UTI is present
  - Dysuria, frequency of micturition
  - Suprapubic tenderness may be present
- Acute renal failure
  - Severe and bilateral cases
  - Emphysematous pyelonephritis
  - Single kidney
  - Transplant kidney

Laboratory Tests

- Urine microscopy
  - Pyuria (white blood cells in urine)
  - Leukocyte casts
  - Gram stain may be positive
- Urine cultures
  - Midstream urine needed to minimize contamination
- Blood examination
  - Leukocytosis with shift to left
  - Blood cultures positive in septicemia

Treatment

- Surgical approaches
  - Correction of anatomical defect or source of obstruction
  - Most respond to antibiotics and avoid nephrectomy
  - Nephrectomy may be required in emphysematous pyelonephritis
- Drugs
  - Antimicrobials
  - Empiric antimicrobial therapy with Gram-negative coverage until culture results are obtained

Prognosis

- Severe complications more common in patients with diabetes mellitus and urinary obstruction
  - Papillary necrosis: Coagulative necrosis of papillary tips
  - Pyonephrosis: Pus accumulates in pyelocalyceal system

- Perinephric abscess: Suppurative inflammation extends beyond kidney into perinephric fat
- Emphysematous pyelonephritis: Gas within renal parenchyma, collecting system or perinephritic space
- Septicemia
- Scarring ensues in 30% of children with APN
- Acute uncomplicated pyelonephritis responds to antimicrobial therapy in > 90% of cases
  - Lack of response in
    - Drug-resistant bacterial strains
    - Presence of anatomic abnormality (reflux, etc.)
    - Urinary tract obstruction
- Recurrent episodes of pyelonephritis can lead to chronic pyelonephritis and chronic renal failure

IMAGING

General Features

- Imaging is indicated in select cases
  - Patients with recurrent UTI, especially adult males and children < 5 years of age
  - Patients with diabetes mellitus
- Tests include
  - Cystoscopy
  - Retrograde pyelogram
  - Voiding cystourethrogram
  - Abdominal CT scan and plain radiograph
  - Technetium-99m dimercaptosuccinic acid (DMSA) renal scintigraphy

MACROSCOPIC

General Features

- Enlarged and edematous kidney
- Ascending pyelonephritis
  - Characteristic straight yellow streaks seen in medulla
    - Correspond to collecting ducts filled with pus
    - Typical of ascending APN
  - Pyelitis usual
  - Pyelocalyceal dilatation in obstruction or reflux
  - Scarred areas represent residua of prior episodes
    - Cortical scars in ascending APN overlie pelvic calyces
  - Inflammation may extend into perirenal fat with perinephric abscess
  - Calculi or strictures may be seen in pelvis or ureters
- Hematogenous bacterial nephritis
  - Small subcapsular yellow abscesses measuring a few millimeters in diameter
    - Typical of hematogenous APN
- Emphysematous pyelonephritis
  - Empty (gas-filled) rounded spaces in cortex and perirenal fat; dissection planes under capsule have abscesses

MICROSCOPIC

Histologic Features

- Patchy neutrophilic infiltrate in tubules and interstitium, typically with spared areas
  - Neutrophil casts in tubular lumina, sometimes with associated bacteria
  - Abscesses with tubular destruction in severe cases
- Lymphocytes, plasma cells, eosinophils, and macrophages are seen within a few days
- Acute tubular injury
  - Loss of proximal tubule brush border
  - Simplified tubular epithelium
  - Sloughed epithelial cells in tubular lumens
- Tubular basement membranes disrupted
- Severe cases may have papillary necrosis
  - Usually tip of papilla unlike that in analgesic abuse
- Glomeruli and blood vessels relatively spared
- Bacterial and fungal stains often useful

Variants

- Ascending infection
  - Acute inflammation of pelvis usual
  - Early infection in medulla and collecting ducts
  - Organisms invade via fornix of calyx and intrarenal reflux through collecting ducts
- Hematogenous infection
  - Randomly scattered abscesses in cortex
  - Occasionally, septic emboli in glomeruli containing organisms in endocarditis
  - Little or no inflammation of pelvis
- Emphysematous pyelonephritis
  - Round empty spaces and planes of dissection in tissue due to gas-forming organisms
- Acute lobar nephronia
  - Variant that suggests mass lesions in imaging studies
  - Focal areas of intense inflammation and edema in cortex

ANCILLARY TESTS

Histochemistry

- Tissue Gram stain (Brown-Brenn)
  - Reactivity: Detects gram-positive & -negative organisms
  - Bacteria typically not conspicuous in tubules but can be detected in abscesses
- Grocott methenamine silver
  - Positive in tubules and abscesses if fungal organisms present

Immunofluorescence

- Glomeruli and tubular basement membranes negative for immunoglobulins and complement
- C4d binds to bacterial surfaces in APN via activation of lectin pathway in ring pattern

Electron Microscopy

- Glomerular and tubular basement membranes negative for electron-dense deposits
- Bacteria rarely encountered

DIFFERENTIAL DIAGNOSIS

Drug-Induced Interstitial Nephritis

- Clinical history of drug exposure
  - Neutrophilic infiltrate less prominent
  - Urine and blood cultures are negative

Myeloma Cast Nephropathy

- Neutrophilic infiltrate associated with myeloma casts
- Tubular casts are typically fractured and weakly PAS(+)

Predisposing Factors for Ascending Bacterial Pyelonephritis

Mechanisms	Protective Factors	Predisposing Factors
Bacterial properties	Normal vaginal and urethral flora, such as lactobacilli	P-fimbriated *E. coli*
Entry into bladder	Long urethra (male)	Short urethra (females), trauma (sexual intercourse, catheterization)
Urine properties	Low pH, low glucose, high osmolality, high urea	Diabetes mellitus raises glucose concentration
Flushing mechanism of micturition	Residual volume of urine in bladder only a few mL	Large residual volume (in obstruction, neurogenic bladder, nephrolithiasis)
Ureteral vesicle junction	Competent vesicoureteral valve mechanism	Congenital vesicoureteral reflux, secondary reflux due to obstruction
Intrarenal reflux	Prevented by convex papillae that close with increased pelvic pressures	Compound papillae with flattened tips fail to close, common in the upper and lower poles
Secretion of blood group substances	Secretion of blood group substances (ABO) inhibits bacterial adherence to urothelial cells	Nonsecretor status of host has higher risk of recurrent UTI and scarring
Secreted molecules in urine	Tamm-Horsfall protein binds type 1 fimbriae of *E. coli*	
Bladder epithelium	Anti-adherence mechanisms of bladder mucosa (lining glycosaminoglycans, oligosaccharides)	Denudation and inflammation
Immune system	Cervicovaginal antibody in women; secreted (IgA) or systemic (IgG) antibody to bacterial antigens in urine	Deficiency of antibody, new bacterial strain

- To be excluded in elderly patients with acute renal failure
- Tubular casts are light chain restricted on immunofluorescence microscopy

Glomerulonephritis-Associated Severe Tubulointerstitial Inflammation

- Glomerular hypercellularity seen in primary glomerular process
- Neutrophilic infiltrate less prominent
- No abscesses
- Immunofluorescence and electron microscopy may indicate presence of immune complexes

Ischemic or Toxic Tubular Injury

- Less neutrophilic infiltrate
- No abscesses
- Tubular injury in area without inflammation

Acute Humoral Rejection in Transplants

- Neutrophils in tubules sometimes mimic APN
- C4d in peritubular capillaries
- Abscesses not seen

DIAGNOSTIC CHECKLIST

Clinically Relevant Pathologic Features

- Abscess formation
- Papillary necrosis
- Histological evidence of chronic pyelonephritis
  - Numerous hyaline casts in atrophic tubules reminiscent of thyroidization
  - Can indicate prior episodes of APN or presence of urinary outflow obstruction

Pathologic Interpretation Pearls

- Neutrophils occasionally seen in end-stage kidneys without other evidence of APN, likely due to sterile tubular injury
- Fungal infections can be missed (check PAS and silver stain)
- Persistent infection may have abundant eosinophils

SELECTED REFERENCES

1. Kumar S et al: Acute pyelonephritis in diabetes mellitus: Single center experience. Indian J Nephrol. 24(6):367-71, 2014
2. Paragas N et al: α-Intercalated cells defend the urinary system from bacterial infection. J Clin Invest. 124(12):5521, 2014
3. Tourneur E et al: Cyclosporine A impairs nucleotide binding oligomerization domain (Nod1)-mediated innate antibacterial renal defenses in mice and human transplant recipients. PLoS Pathog. 9(1):e1003152, 2013
4. Pontin AR et al: Current management of emphysematous pyelonephritis. Nat Rev Urol. 6:272-9, 2009
5. Schmidt S et al: Emphysematous pyelonephritis in a kidney allograft. Am J Kidney Dis. 53:895-7, 2009
6. Chung SD et al: Emphysematous pyelonephritis with acute renal failure. Urology. 72:521-2, 2008
7. Hewitt IK et al: Early treatment of acute pyelonephritis in children fails to reduce renal scarring: data from the Italian Renal Infection Study Trials. Pediatrics. 122:486-90, 2008
8. Cheng CH et al: Comparison of urovirulence factors and genotypes for bacteria causing acute lobar nephronia and acute pyelonephritis. Pediatr Infect Dis J. 26:228-32, 2007
9. Lane MC et al: Role of P-fimbrial-mediated adherence in pyelonephritis and persistence of uropathogenic Escherichia coli (UPEC) in the mammalian kidney. Kidney Int. 72(1):19-25, 2007
10. Smaill F: Asymptomatic bacteriuria in pregnancy. Best Pract Res Clin Obstet Gynaecol. 21(3):439-50, 2007
11. Joss N et al: Lobar nephronia in a transplanted kidney. Clin Nephrol. 64:311-4, 2005
12. Webb NJ et al: Cytokines and cell adhesion molecules in the inflammatory response during acute pyelonephritis. Nephron Exp Nephrol. 96(1):e1-6, 2004
13. Hooton TM et al: A prospective study of asymptomatic bacteriuria in sexually active young women. N Engl J Med. 343(14):992-7, 2000
14. Kumar PD et al: Focal bacterial nephritis (lobar nephronia) presenting as renal mass. Am J Med Sci. 320:209-11, 2000
15. Patterson JE et al: Bacterial urinary tract infections in diabetes. Infect Dis Clin North Am. 11(3):735-50, 1997

(Left) *Bivalved kidney with acute bacterial pyelonephritis due to an ascending infection is shown. The pelvic calyceal system is mildly dilated with necrosis of the medullary pyramids. Focal pale abscesses are also seen. (Courtesy L. Fajardo, MD.)* **(Right)** *Cross section of the autopsied kidney shows multiple small, yellow abscesses within the renal cortex. The patient had septicemia due to bacterial endocarditis, which resulted in acute pyelonephritis due to bacterial seeding.*

Gross Appearance of Papillary Necrosis

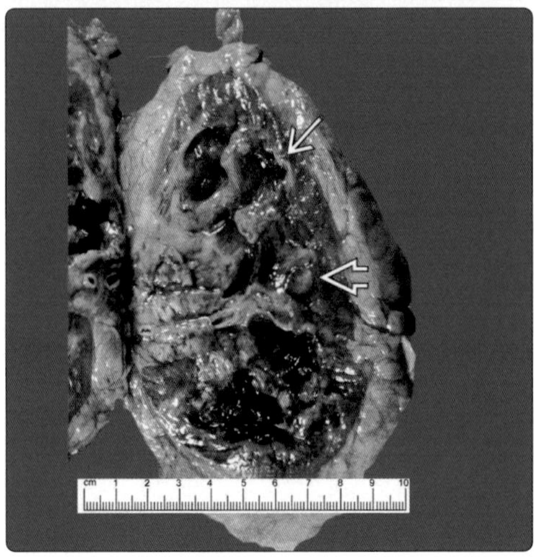

Gross Appearance of Cortical Abscesses

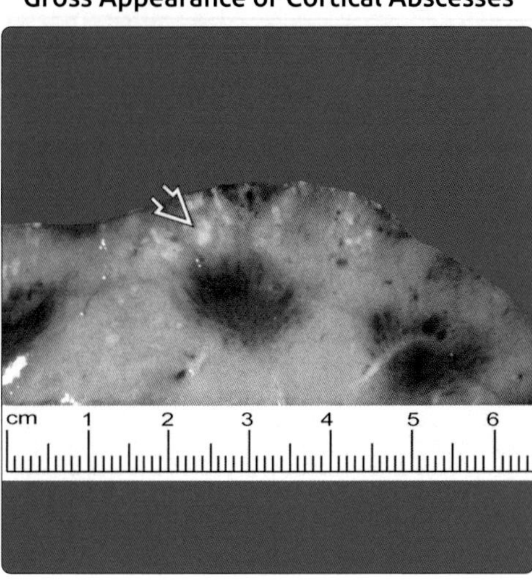

(Left) *Hematoxylin & eosin shows pelvic urothelium infiltrated by neutrophils and lymphocytes, compatible with acute pyelonephritis. Neutrophil exudate is seen in the lumen along with bacteria.* **(Right)** *Periodic acid-Schiff shows neutrophil casts within the collecting ducts of the medulla. Mild interstitial edema is seen. Early acute pyelonephritis due to ascending infection can be localized to the medulla only.*

Acute Pyelitis With Bacteria

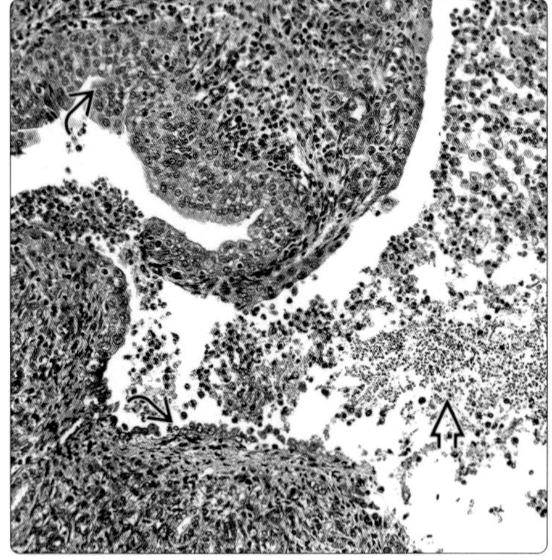

Neutrophil Casts in Medulla

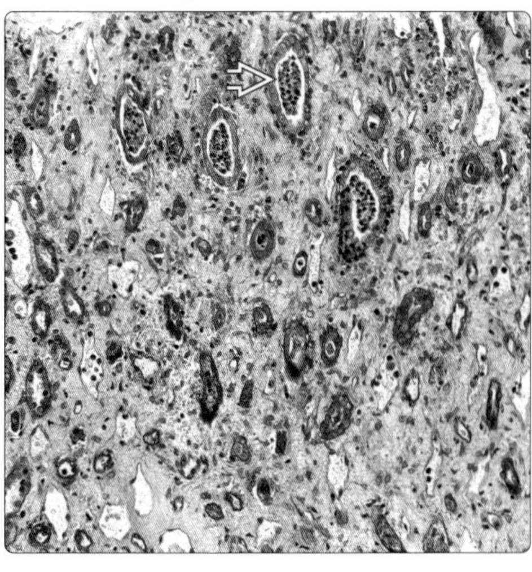

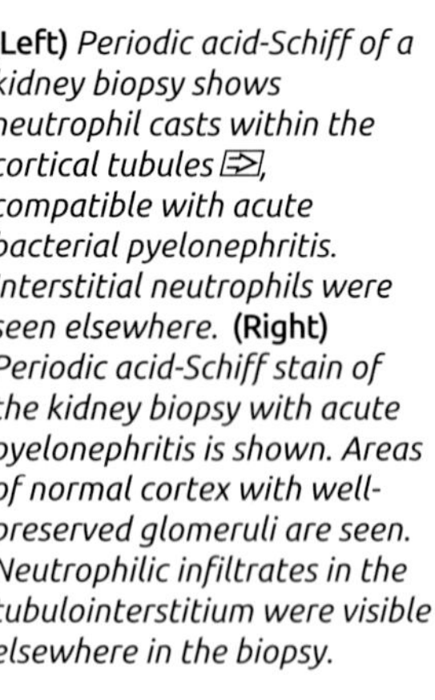

(Left) *Periodic acid-Schiff of a kidney biopsy shows neutrophil casts within the cortical tubules, compatible with acute bacterial pyelonephritis. Interstitial neutrophils were seen elsewhere.* **(Right)** *Periodic acid-Schiff stain of the kidney biopsy with acute pyelonephritis is shown. Areas of normal cortex with well-preserved glomeruli are seen. Neutrophilic infiltrates in the tubulointerstitium were visible elsewhere in the biopsy.*

Neutrophil Casts in Acute Pyelonephritis

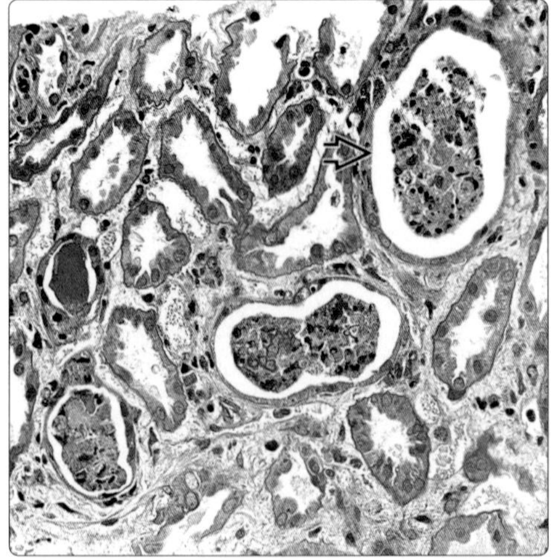

Patchy Cortical Involvement in Acute Pyelonephritis

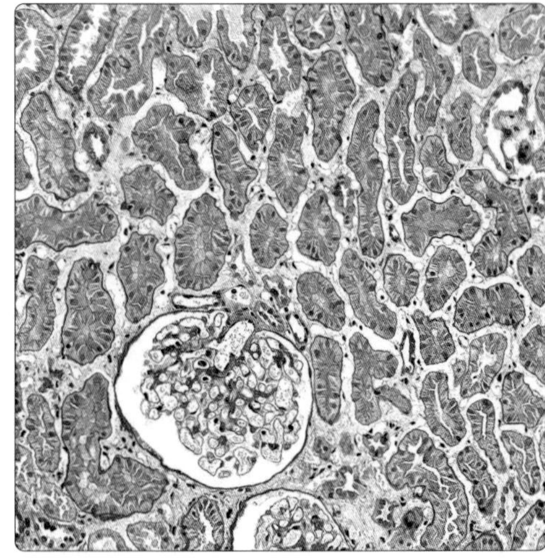

Gross Appearance of Papillary Necrosis

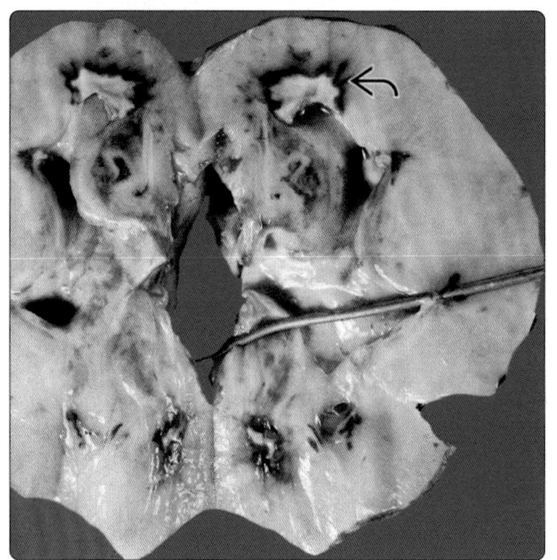

Necrotic Papillae in Acute Pyelonephritis

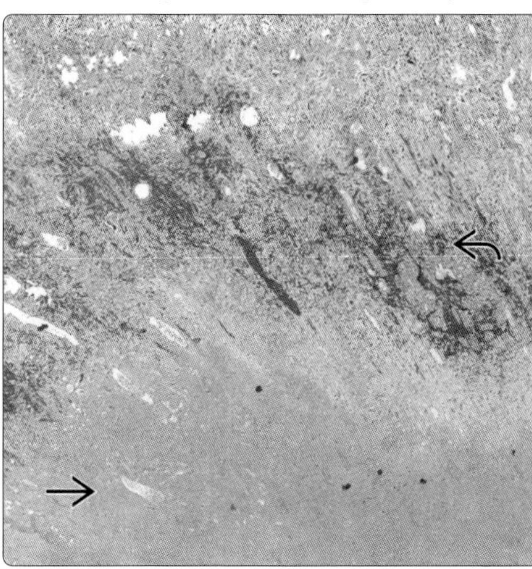

(Left) *Bivalved transplant kidney nephrectomy with severe acute pyelonephritis with papillary necrosis is shown. The necrotic papillae are sharply demarcated by a hemorrhagic zone ➢.* **(Right)** *Transplant kidney nephrectomy with severe acute pyelonephritis with papillary necrosis is shown. The necrotic papillae are sharply demarcated by a hemorrhagic zone ➢. The necrotic area shows no residual viable cells ➡.*

Neutrophil Casts in Transplant Kidney

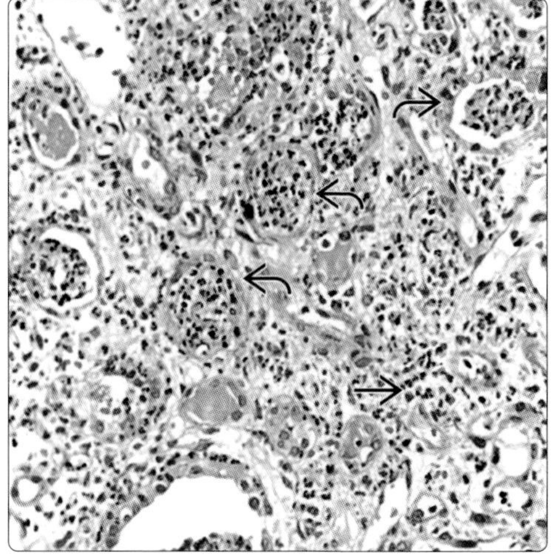

Neutrophil Casts in Transplant Kidney

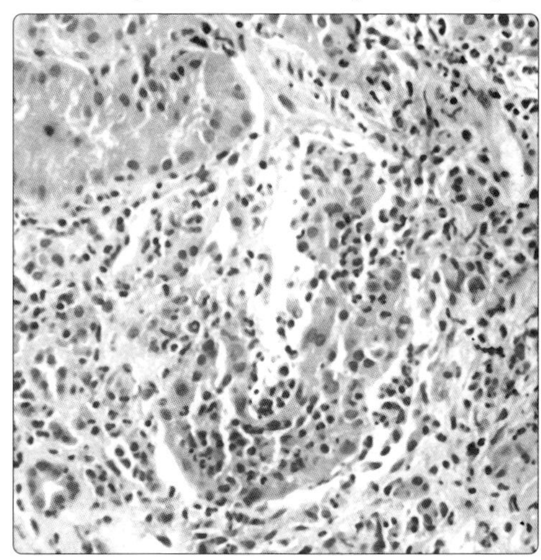

(Left) *Light microscopy shows a case of acute pyelonephritis in a renal transplant. Abundant neutrophils are present in the edematous interstitium ➡, prominently as casts ➢.* **(Right)** *Light microscopy of a renal transplant biopsy shows intense neutrophilic infiltrate forming a cast. The patient had a positive urine culture. This pattern strongly favors APN over rejection, although in acute humoral rejection neutrophils in tubules are not uncommonly observed.*

Bacterial Colonies in Acute Pyelonephritis

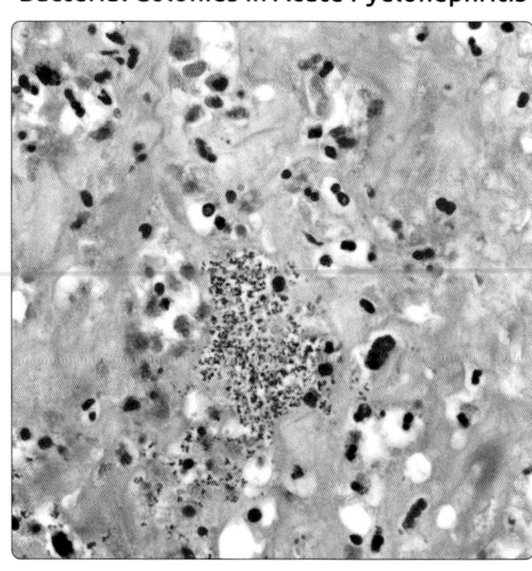

C4d Stain in Acute Pyelonephritis

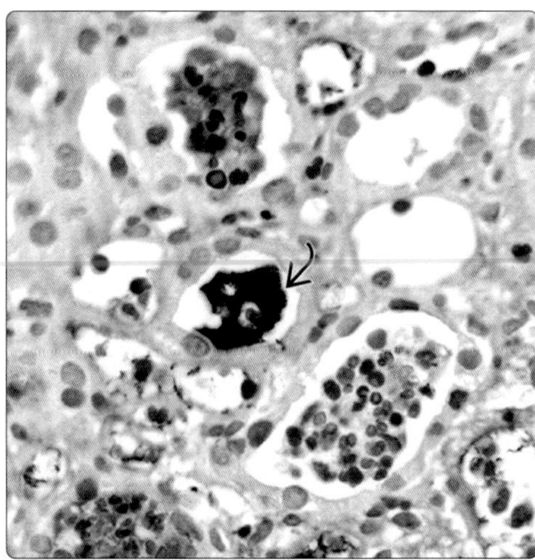

(Left) *Hematoxylin & eosin at high power reveals a cluster of bacteria in the medulla of a transplant kidney with severe pyelonephritis. In contrast to calcium deposits, bacteria are more uniform and are typically smaller.* **(Right)** *C4d stain of a biopsy with acute pyelonephritis shows a cluster of positive-staining cocci in the tubular lumen ➢. C4d is activated by bacterial surface carbohydrates via the lectin pathway (mannose-binding lectin, ficolin).*

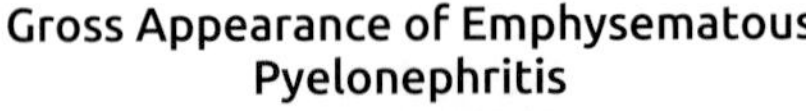

Gross Appearance of Emphysematous Pyelonephritis

Specimen Radiograph of Emphysematous Pyelonephritis

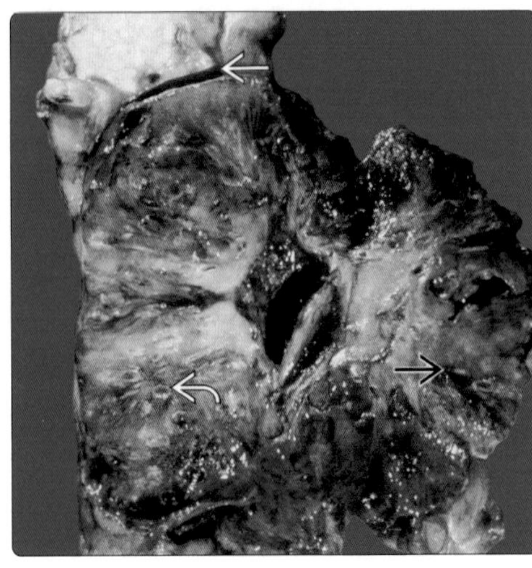

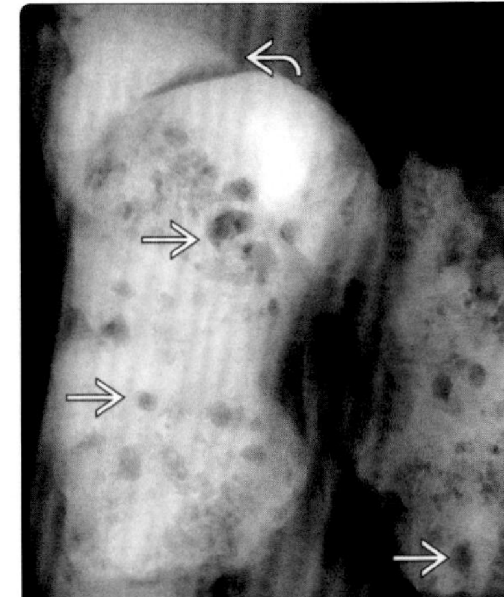

(Left) *Nephrectomy with emphysematous pyelonephritis is shown. Dissection is evident between the kidney and the perinephric fat* ⇒*. Many abscesses are seen with empty centers* ⇒ *that contained gas. A streak of pus in a dilated collecting duct can be seen* ⇒*.* **(Right)** *Specimen radiograph shows bivalved kidney with emphysematous pyelonephritis. Gas has dissected between the kidney and the perinephric fat* ⇒*. The rounded spaces are due to gas-forming E. coli* ⇒*.*

Radiographic Appearance of Emphysematous Pyelonephritis

Cortical Air Spaces in Emphysematous Pyelonephritis

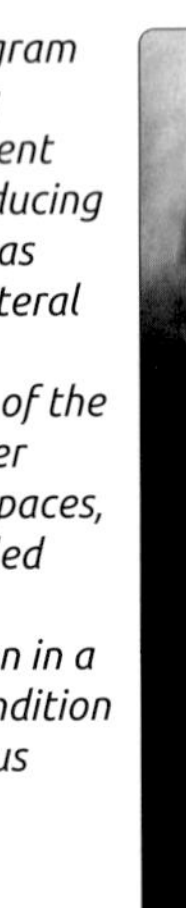

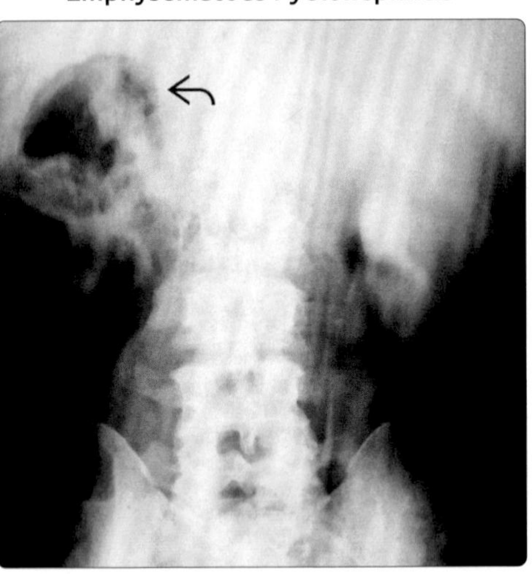

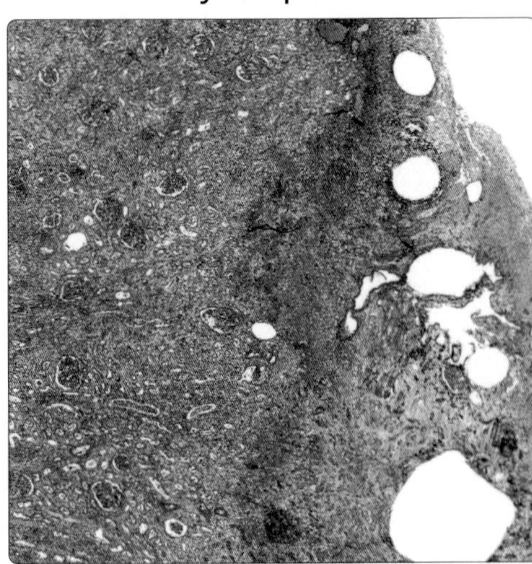

(Left) *Intravenous pyelogram reveals a nonfunctioning kidney* ⇒ *with many lucent areas caused by gas-producing E. coli. A nephrectomy was performed. The contralateral kidney is unremarkable.* **(Right)** *Light microscopy of the outer cortex at low power reveals rounded empty spaces, which were originally filled with gas, due to a gas-producing E. coli infection in a diabetic patient. This condition is termed emphysematous pyelonephritis.*

Abscesses in Emphysematous Pyelonephritis

Medullary Neutrophils in Emphysematous Pyelonephritis

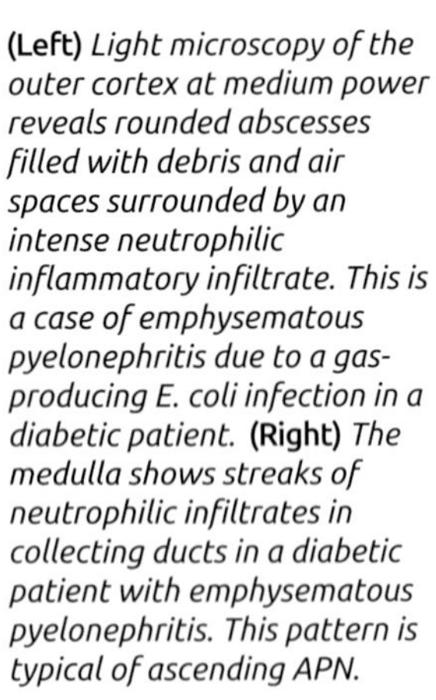

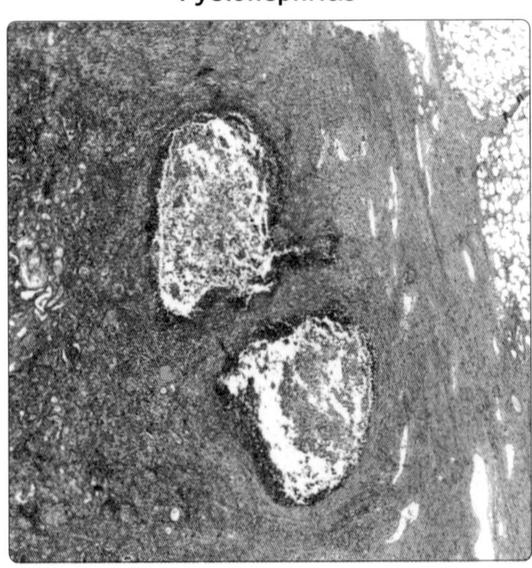

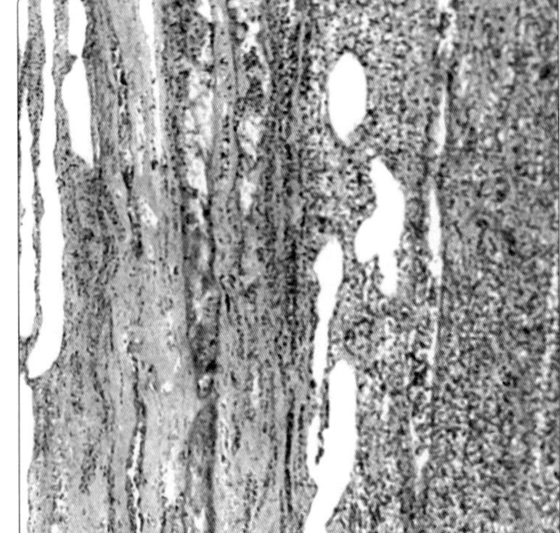

(Left) *Light microscopy of the outer cortex at medium power reveals rounded abscesses filled with debris and air spaces surrounded by an intense neutrophilic inflammatory infiltrate. This is a case of emphysematous pyelonephritis due to a gas-producing E. coli infection in a diabetic patient.* **(Right)** *The medulla shows streaks of neutrophilic infiltrates in collecting ducts in a diabetic patient with emphysematous pyelonephritis. This pattern is typical of ascending APN.*

Radiographic Appearance of Acute Lobar Nephronia

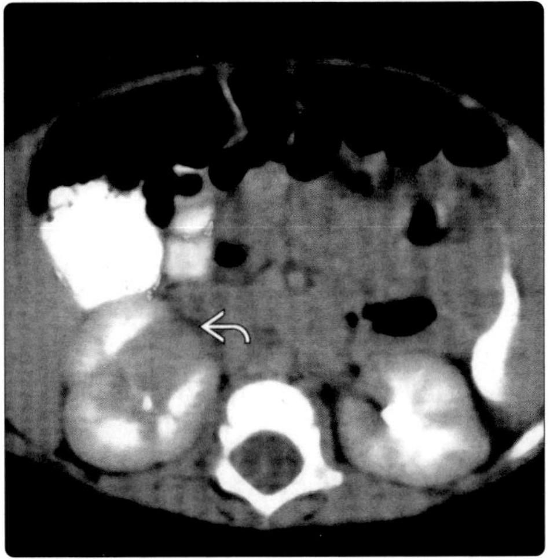

Gross Appearance of Acute Lobar Nephronia

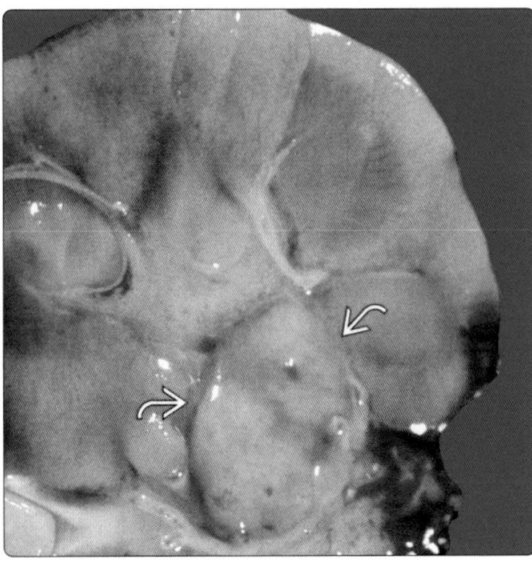

(Left) *Abdomen CT of a 4-year-old girl shows nodular masses in the kidney ➡. These were interpreted as possibly neoplastic, and the kidney was removed. The masses were due to localized bacterial infection (acute lobar nephronia).* **(Right)** *Gross photograph shows a kidney from a 4-year-old girl with acute pyelonephritis presenting as a localized mass on CT. The focus of inflammation is evident as a bulging yellow mass ➡. This form of APN is sometimes termed acute lobar nephronia.*

Inflammation in Acute Lobar Nephronia

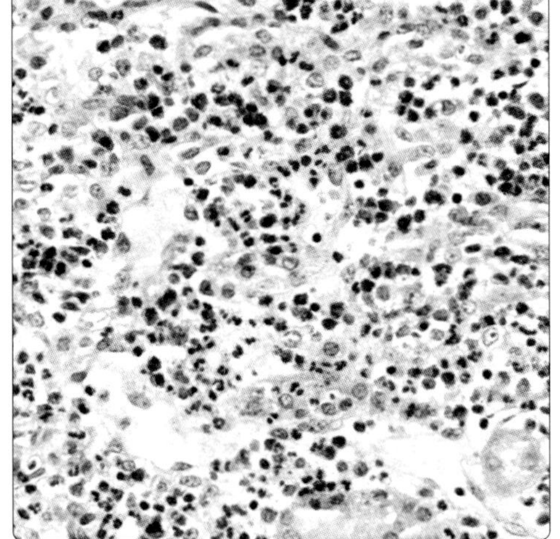

Perinephric Inflammation in Acute Lobar Nephronia

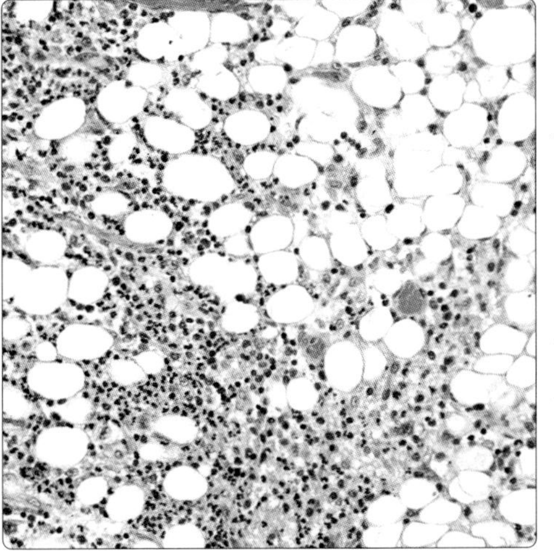

(Left) *Light microscopy of the cortex from a patient with acute lobar nephronia shows intense infiltration by granulocytes, including both eosinophils and neutrophils. Destruction of the tubular architecture is evident.* **(Right)** *Light microscopy shows extension of the inflammation into the perinephric fat in this patient with acute lobar nephronia (focal acute pyelonephritis).*

Interstitial Neutrophils in Acute Lobar Nephronia

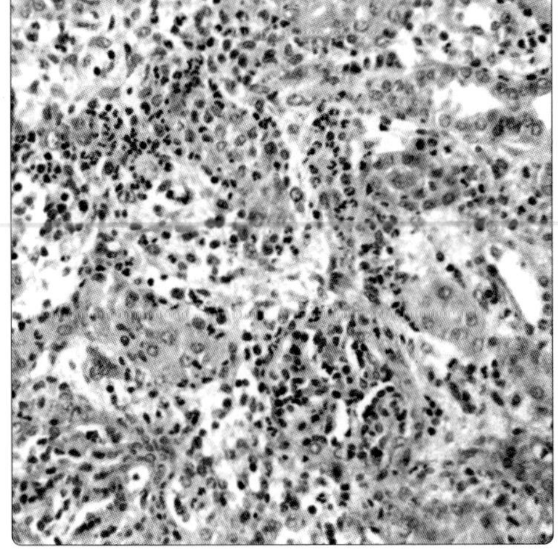

Neutrophil Casts and Tubular Epithelial Reactive Changes

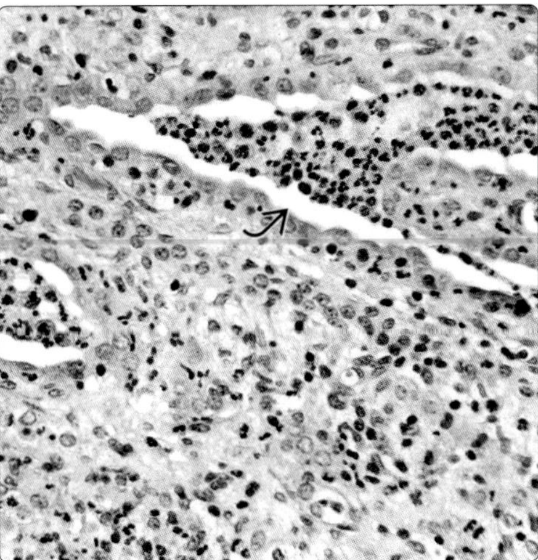

(Left) *Light microscopy shows separation of the tubules by edema and an intense infiltrate of mostly neutrophils in this nephrectomy specimen with acute lobar nephronia.* **(Right)** *Light microscopy of a cortical collecting duct shows a neutrophil cast ➡ filling the lumen. The tubular epithelium is attenuated and basophilic, indicating injury and reactive changes, respectively. The only tubules with branches in the kidney are the collecting ducts.*

Chronic Pyelonephritis

KEY FACTS

TERMINOLOGY

- Renal damage due to repeated bacterial infection and scarring

ETIOLOGY/PATHOGENESIS

- Urinary tract obstruction
- Reflux nephropathy

CLINICAL ISSUES

- Insidious onset of renal insufficiency if bilateral
- Progression to end-stage kidney disease
- Hypertension
- Proteinuria due to secondary FSGS

IMAGING

- Plain radiographs, CT scan of abdomen for obstruction
- Voiding cystourethrogram for reflux nephropathy

MACROSCOPIC

- Large irregular scars on cortical surface
- Dilated pelvis; calyces blunted or deformed
- Cortical scars overlie deformed calyces
- Calculi may be seen in pelvis

MICROSCOPIC

- Patchy chronic tubulointerstitial inflammation
  - Lymphocytes, plasma cells, and monocytes predominate
- Thyroidization of tubules
- Inflammation and scarring involves pelvis and calyces
- Sharp demarcation between inflamed and preserved parenchyma
- Glomeruli relatively spared but often with periglomerular fibrosis
  - Secondary FSGS may be present

TOP DIFFERENTIAL DIAGNOSES

- Chronic tubulointerstitial nephritis
- Primary FSGS
- Hypertensive renal disease

Cortical Scars in Chronic Pyelonephritis

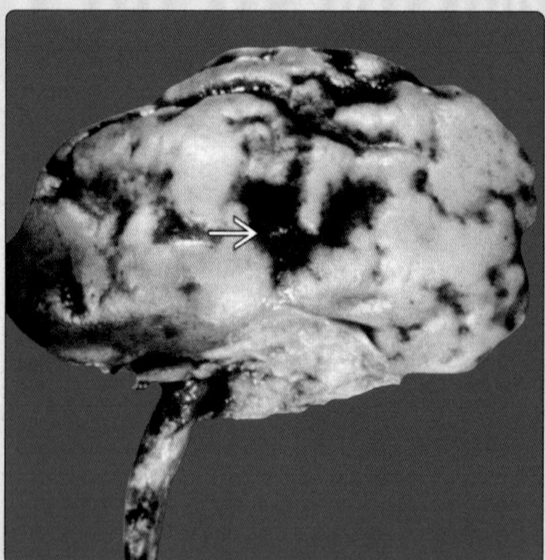

Abrupt Transition to Scarred Parenchyma

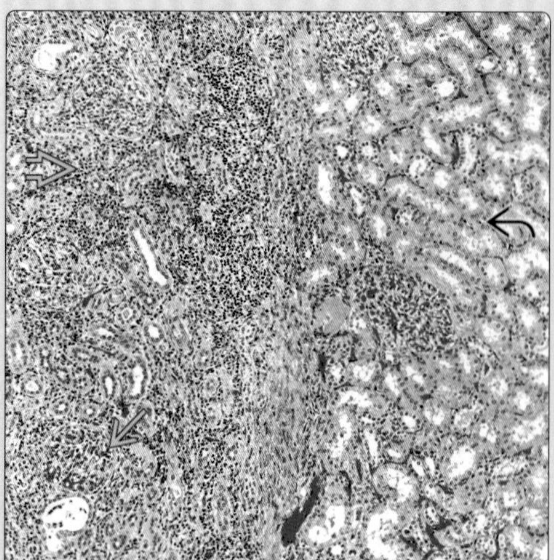

(Left) *Gross photograph of a kidney with chronic pyelonephritis demonstrates large irregular cortical scars ➔ that often overlie the pelvic calyces.* **(Right)** *Hematoxylin and eosin shows an abrupt transition from the normal cortex ➔ to an area of scarring ➔, characterized by tubular atrophy, interstitial fibrosis, and inflammation. Note the sparing of the glomeruli ➔ by sclerosis.*

Thyroidization of Tubules

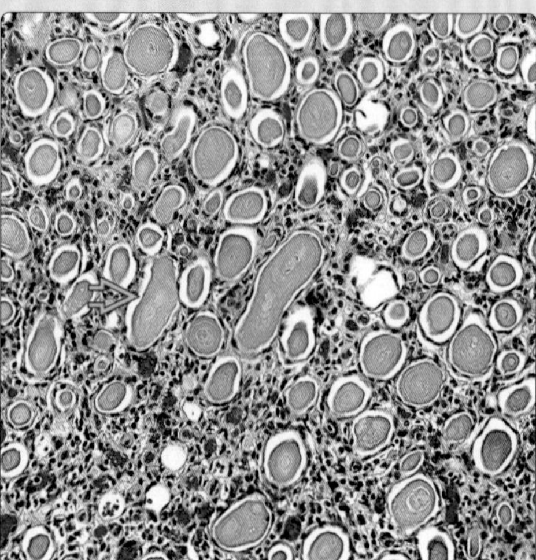

Relative Sparing of Glomeruli

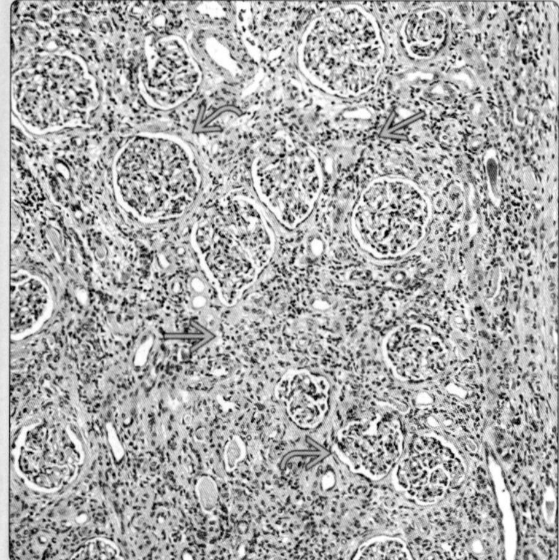

(Left) *Hematoxylin and eosin of nephrectomy performed for chronic pyelonephritis is shown. Although not specific, characteristic hyaline casts ➔ are seen in atrophic tubules (thyroidization).* **(Right)** *Chronic pyelonephritis is characterized by chronic inflammation in scarred tubulointerstitium ➔. The glomeruli are relatively spared in non-end-stage kidney. They demonstrate ischemic retraction and periglomerular fibrosis ➔.*

TERMINOLOGY

Abbreviations

- Chronic pyelonephritis (CPN)

Definitions

- Renal damage due to repeated bacterial infection and scarring

ETIOLOGY/PATHOGENESIS

Urinary Outflow Tract Obstruction or Urinary Reflux

- Prostatic disease
- Nephrolithiasis
- Neurogenic bladder
- Ureteral stenosis or dysfunction
- Vesicoureteral reflux, congenital or acquired
  - Role of infection debated

CLINICAL ISSUES

Epidemiology

- Sex
  - F > M

Presentation

- Chronic renal failure if bilateral
  - Loss of urinary concentration ability
  - Proteinuria, hypertension (HTN)
- Silent clinical course if unilateral; presents as HTN
- Repeated episodes of acute pyelonephritis

Laboratory Tests

- Elevated BUN, serum creatinine
- Urinalysis: Proteinuria, pyuria

Treatment

- Surgical approaches
  - Correct anatomic defect
  - Nephrectomy in unilateral disease to control HTN
- Drugs
  - Antimicrobial therapy if bacterial infection
  - Antihypertensives

Prognosis

- Progression slowed only if detected early

IMAGING

General Features

- Plain radiographs, CT scan of abdomen for obstruction
- Voiding cystourethrogram for reflux nephropathy

MACROSCOPIC

General Features

- Large irregular scars on cortical surface
  - Cortical scars common in upper and lower poles
  - Thickness of cortex can be reduced to 2-3 mm
  - Cortical scars overlie deformed calyces
    - Indicative of ascending infection
- Dilated pelvis and calyces
  - Blunted or deformed calyces
  - Calculi may be in pelvis

MICROSCOPIC

Histologic Features

- Patchy chronic tubulointerstitial inflammation
  - Lymphocytes, plasma cells, and monocytes
  - Sharp demarcation between inflamed and preserved parenchyma
- Tubular atrophy and interstitial fibrosis
  - Atrophic tubules with attenuated epithelium and luminal colloid-like hyaline casts (thyroidization)
    - Not specific for chronic pyelonephritis
- Inflammation and scarring of pelvis and calyces
- Neutrophil casts in setting of acute pyelonephritis
- Extravasated Tamm-Horsfall protein may be abundant
- Glomeruli relatively spared
  - Periglomerular fibrosis common
  - With progression, focal segmental glomerulosclerosis (FSGS) may develop due to loss of renal mass
- Arteriosclerosis, if hypertension

ANCILLARY TESTS

Immunofluorescence

- Segmental glomerular IgM and C3 if FSGS present

Electron Microscopy

- Mild foot process effacement if secondary FSGS

DIFFERENTIAL DIAGNOSIS

Chronic Tubulointerstitial Nephritis

- Pelvicalyceal inflammation and thyroidization more prominent in CPN
- Uniform involvement; no spared lobes

Primary FSGS

- No pelvicalyceal inflammation or medullary destruction

Hypertensive Renal Disease

- No pelvicalyceal inflammation or medullary destruction

DIAGNOSTIC CHECKLIST

Pathologic Interpretation Pearls

- Diagnosis almost impossible on biopsy alone; clinical and radiographic correlations needed
- Sterile reflux produces similar pathology

SELECTED REFERENCES

1. Bhaijee F: Squamous cell carcinoma of the renal pelvis. Ann Diagn Pathol. 16(2):124-7, 2012
2. Watanabe H et al: A case of emphysematous pyelonephritis in a patient with rheumatoid arthritis taking corticosteroid and low-dose methotrexate. Int J Rheum Dis. 13(2):180-3, 2010
3. Craig WD et al: Pyelonephritis: radiologic-pathologic review. Radiographics. 28(1):255-77; quiz 327-8, 2008
4. Roberts JA: Mechanisms of renal damage in chronic pyelonephritis (reflux nephropathy). Curr Top Pathol. 88:265-87, 1995
5. Morita M et al: The glomerular changes in children with reflux nephropathy. J Pathol. 162(3):245-53, 1990
6. Woodard JR et al: Reflux uropathy. Pediatr Clin North Am. 34(5):1349-64, 1987
7. Brenner BM: Nephron adaptation to renal injury or ablation. Am J Physiol. 249(3 Pt 2):F324-37, 1985

(Left) *Hematoxylin and eosin shows dense chronic inflammation involving the pelvis. Lymphocytic infiltrates are seen within the urothelium ➚. Pelvicalyceal involvement is always seen in chronic pyelonephritis.* (Right) *Periodic acid-Schiff of the kidney with CPN shows intense inflammation with a germinal center formation ➜ adjacent to extravasated Tamm-Horsfall protein →. These changes may be due to urinary obstruction.*

Pelvic Inflammation in Pyelonephritis

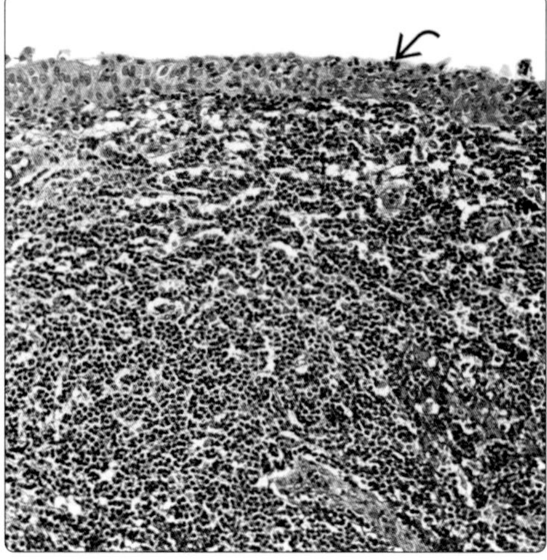

Extravasated Tamm-Horsfall Protein

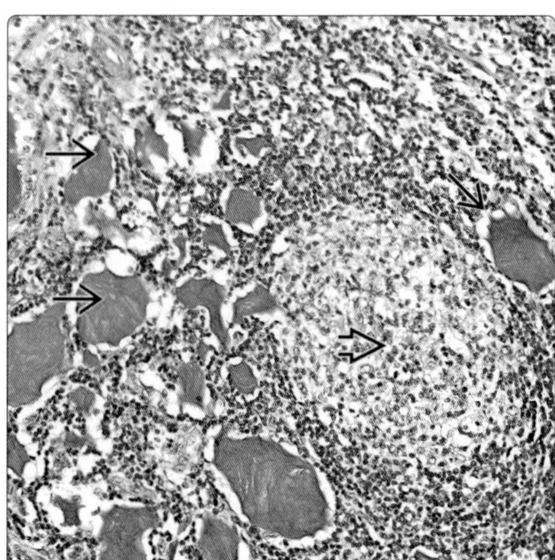

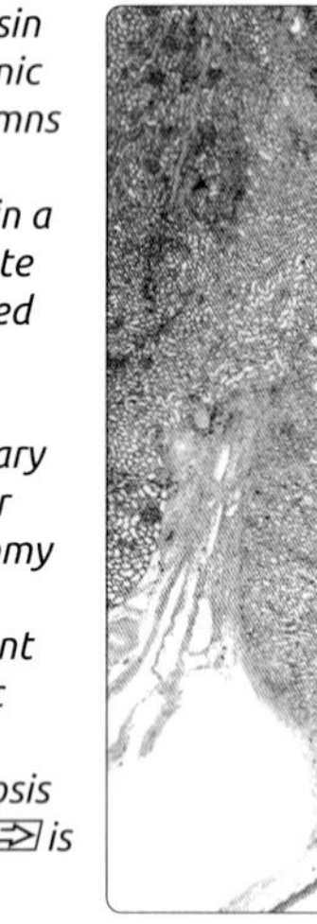

(Left) *Hematoxylin and eosin of nephrectomy with chronic pyelonephritis shows columns of chronic inflammation extending into the cortex in a patchy distribution ⇨. Note the concavity of the blunted papillary tip ➜, which predisposes to intrarenal reflux.* (Right) *The medullary pyramid is replaced by scar tissue → in this nephrectomy performed for chronic pyelonephritis. The adjacent inner cortex shows chronic inflammation, tubular atrophy, & interstitial fibrosis ➚. Flattened urothelium ➜ is seen distal to the scar.*

Inflamed Medulla and Blunted Papillary Tip

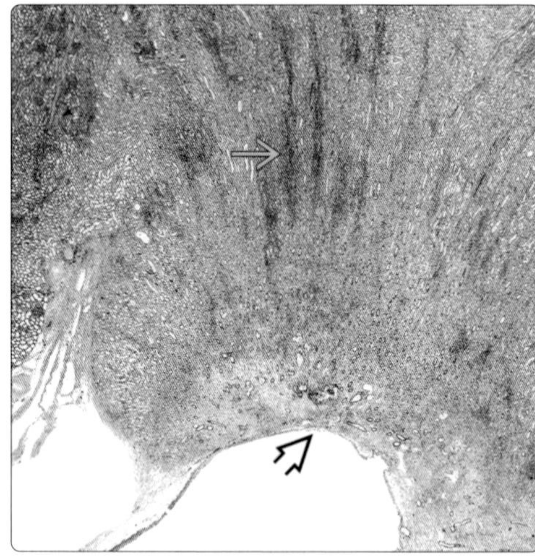

Scarred and Blunted Medullary Pyramid

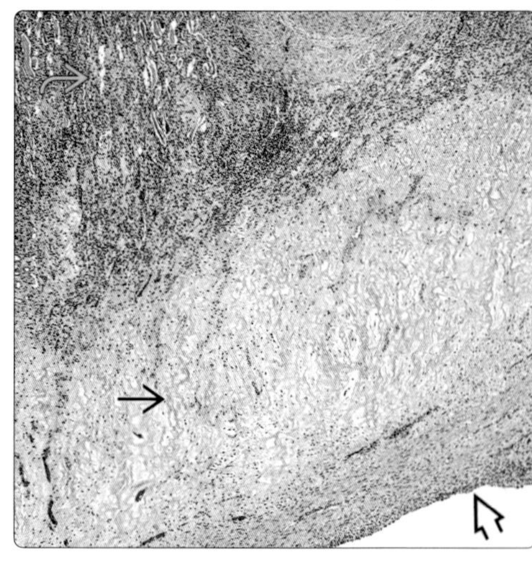

(Left) *Hematoxylin and eosin shows the patchy nature of the tubulointerstitial inflammation in chronic pyelonephritis. Residual proximal tubules show compensatory hypertrophy ➜. A few globally sclerosed glomeruli are seen ➚.* (Right) *Periodic acid-Schiff shows segmental sclerosis ➜ in a glomerulus with Bowman capsular adhesion. Focal segmental glomerulosclerosis is due to the loss of renal mass in chronic pyelonephritis and hyperfiltration in remnant nephrons.*

Patchy Chronic Tubulointerstitial Damage

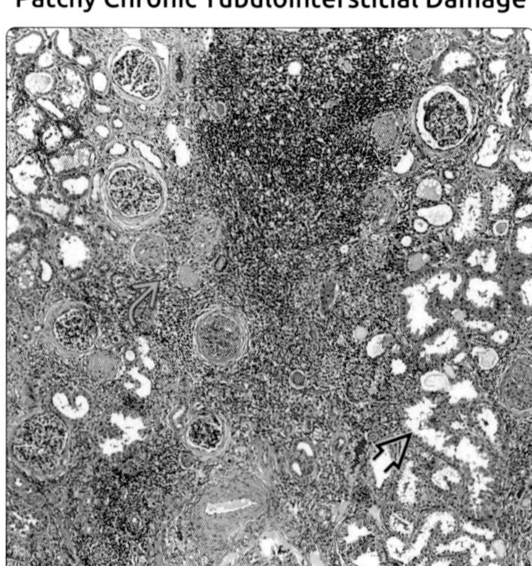

Secondary FSGS in Chronic Pyelonephritis

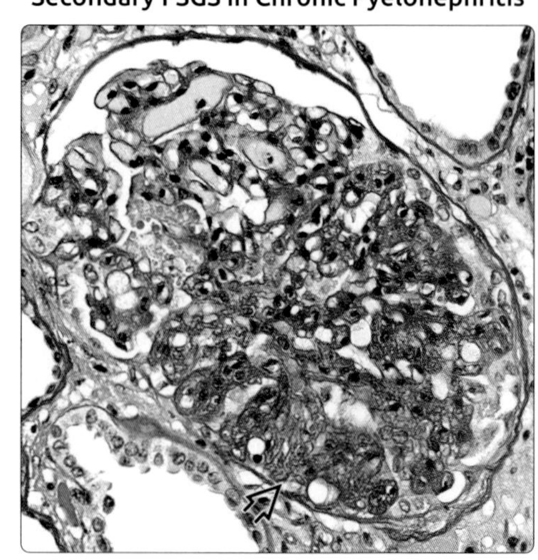

Cortical Surface Distorted by Scars

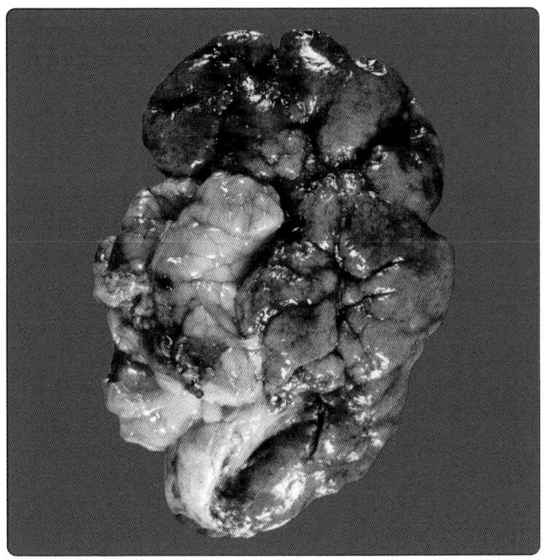

Thinned Cortex Overlying Dilated Calyces

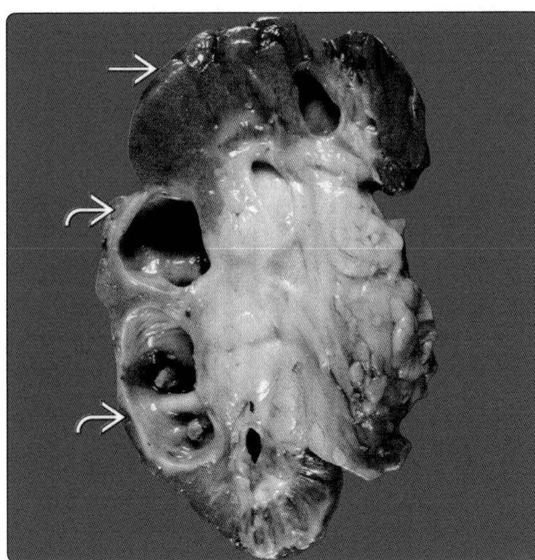

(Left) *External surface of a nephrectomy specimen from a 41-year-old woman with unilateral CPN due to repeated episodes of Enterococcus infections shows a coarsely nodular pattern caused by focal scars with intervening hypertrophy.* **(Right)** *Cross section of a nephrectomy specimen with CPN due to Enterococcus shows a few calyceal stones. The cortex and medulla are markedly thinned in some areas ➡, but other areas are spared ➡.*

Obstructive Chronic Pyelonephritis

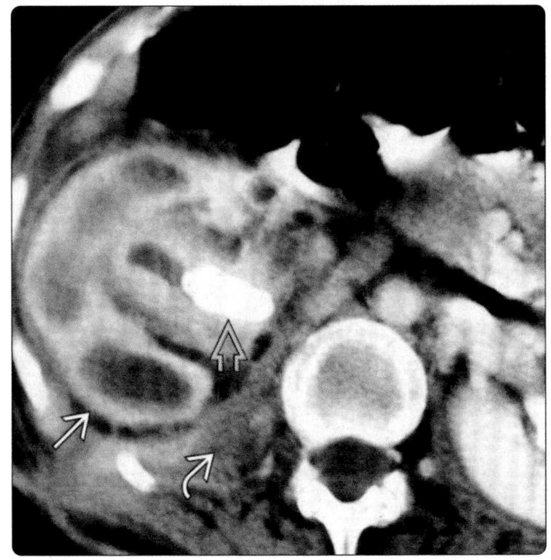

Squamous Metaplasia of Urothelium

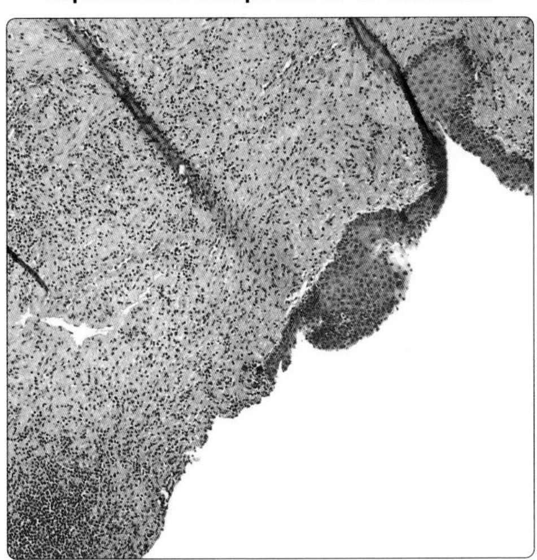

(Left) *Obstructed collecting system due to large central calculus in renal pelvis ⇨ with distorted kidney ➡ is seen on a CT scan. Note also the inflammatory changes in perinephric space ➡.* **(Right)** *Squamous metaplasia of the urothelium is evident in a portion of the pelvis from a nephrectomy specimen with CPN and calyceal stones. Stone disease can lead to squamous metaplasia and increased risk of squamous carcinoma.*

Extensive Global Glomerulosclerosis

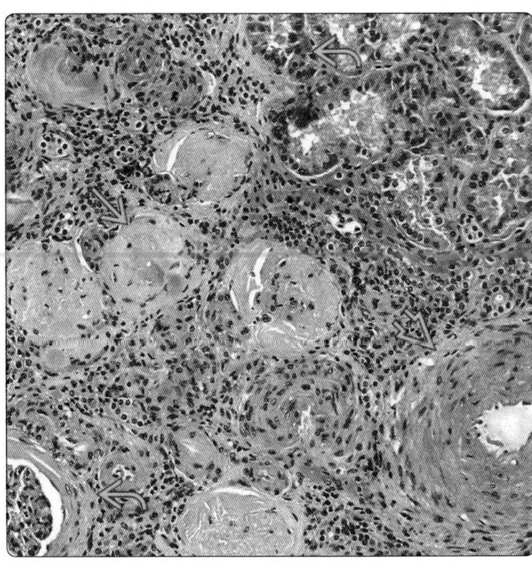

Preferential Involvement of Poles

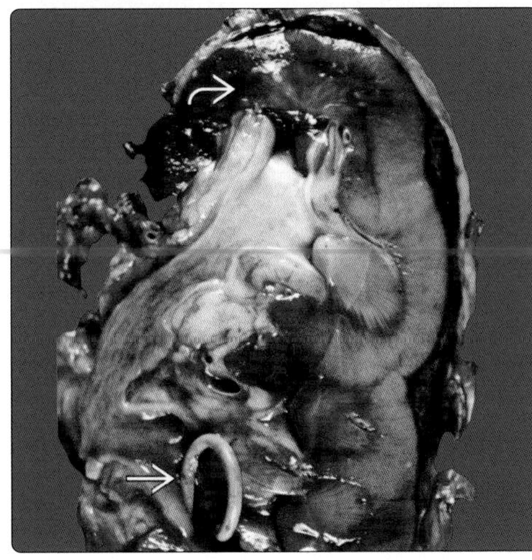

(Left) *Widespread global glomerulosclerosis ⇨ is evident in an area of scarring in CPN. The patient had severe hypertension, and prominent intimal fibrosis is seen in a small artery ⇨. One glomerulus has periglomerular fibrosis ⇨.* **(Right)** *Nephrectomy specimen from a patient with CPN due to inadvertent ureteral injury during ovarian surgery 1 year prior is shown. The poles are most severely affected ➡. A nephrostomy tube is in place in the lower pole ➡.*

Xanthogranulomatous Pyelonephritis

KEY FACTS

TERMINOLOGY

- Variant of chronic pyelonephritis characterized by abundant foamy lipid-laden macrophages

ETIOLOGY/PATHOGENESIS

- *Escherichia coli*, *Proteus* sp, *Pseudomonas* sp, *Klebsiella* sp
- Urinary tract obstruction
- Nephrolithiasis
- Diabetes mellitus

CLINICAL ISSUES

- 5th and 6th decades
- Common in females (M:F = 4:1)
- Predominantly in pelvicalyceal areas
- Often unilateral
- Fever, malaise, flank pain, weight loss, loin tenderness; palpable mass in some patients
- Urine cultures negative in > 30% of patients
- Unilateral nephrectomy is treatment of choice

MACROSCOPIC

- Dilated pelvicalyceal system
- Deformed papillae and yellow necrotic material in calyces
- Large yellow nodules mimic renal cell carcinoma

MICROSCOPIC

- Calyceal areas show sheets of foamy lipid-laden macrophages
- Zonal distribution of inflammation may be seen
  - Neutrophils and necrosis adjacent to collecting system
  - Macrophages and chronic inflammation with fibrosis at periphery

TOP DIFFERENTIAL DIAGNOSES

- Clear cell renal cell carcinoma
- Renal medullary tuberculosis

DIAGNOSTIC CHECKLIST

- Immunostains and bacterial stains helpful in differential

Dilated Pelvicalyceal System

Sheets of Foamy Macrophages

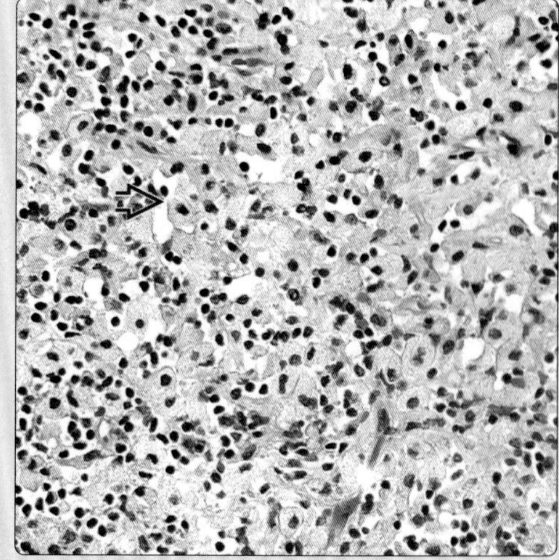

(Left) *Gross photograph shows a kidney with xanthogranulomatous pyelonephritis (XPN). Note the dilated pelvicalyceal system with deformed papillae and also tan-yellow mass lesions.* **(Right)** *Hematoxylin and eosin of a renal "mass" shows foamy histiocytes admixed with lymphocytes. The pelvis is scarred with acute and chronic inflammation in this kidney with xanthogranulomatous pyelonephritis.*

Macrophages Admixed With Lymphocytes

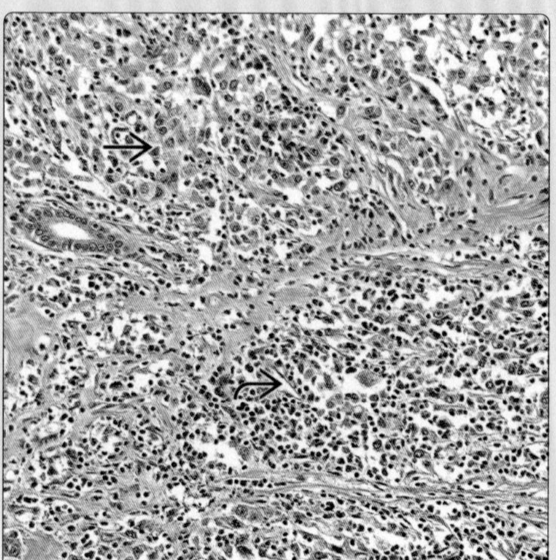

Acute Inflammation in Renal Pelvis

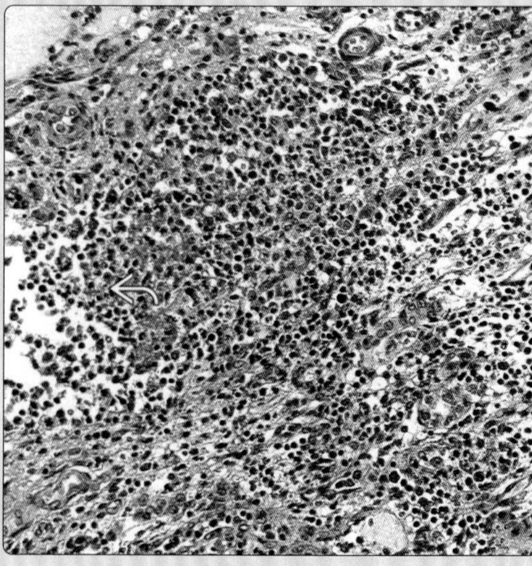

(Left) *Xanthogranulomatous pyelonephritis involving the renal pelvis is shown. Sheets of macrophages and adjacent chronic lymphocytic inflammation can be seen.* **(Right)** *The renal pelvis in XPN shows a neutrophilic infiltrate and necrosis. Xanthogranulomatous inflammation can show a zonal distribution with acute inflammation near the collecting system surrounded by lymphohistiocytic infiltrate at the periphery.*

TERMINOLOGY

Abbreviations

- Xanthogranulomatous pyelonephritis (XPN)

Definitions

- Variant of chronic pyelonephritis characterized by mass lesion with abundant foamy macrophages

ETIOLOGY/PATHOGENESIS

Infectious Agents

- *Proteus mirabilis*, *Escherichia coli*, *Pseudomonas* sp, *Klebsiella* sp
  - *Proteus mirabilis* most common (> 50%)

Predisposing Factors

- Urinary tract obstruction
- Nephrolithiasis
  - Staghorn calculi most common
- Diabetes mellitus

CLINICAL ISSUES

Epidemiology

- Age
  - 5th and 6th decades
  - Can occur in children
- Sex
  - M:F = 1:4

Site

- Predominantly in pelvicalyceal areas
- Often unilateral

Presentation

- Fever, malaise, flank pain, weight loss, loin tenderness
  - Palpable mass in some patients

Laboratory Tests

- Leukocytosis, elevated ESR
- Mild proteinuria, pyuria
- Urine cultures negative in > 30% of patients

Treatment

- Surgical approaches
  - Unilateral nephrectomy is treatment of choice
  - Partial nephrectomy for focal disease
- Drugs
  - Intense antimicrobial therapy may be helpful

IMAGING

General Features

- Ultrasonography, CT scan, and plain radiographs
  - Evidence of urinary tract obstruction, stones
  - Assessment of renal and perirenal involvement

MACROSCOPIC

General Features

- Enlarged kidneys with perirenal adhesions
- Dilated pelvicalyceal system
- Deformed papillae and yellow necrotic material in calyces
- Renal cortical abscesses may be present
- Large yellow nodules mimic renal cell carcinoma
- Large calculi may be present
- Extrarenal extension in ~ 30% (pitfall for malignant gross appearance)

MICROSCOPIC

Histologic Features

- Involved calyces show sheets of foamy, lipid-laden macrophages
- Admixture of mononuclear cells, lymphocytes, and plasma cells
- Neutrophils within necrotic areas
- Zonal distribution of inflammation may be seen
  - Neutrophils and necrosis adjacent to collecting system
  - Macrophages with fibrosis and chronic inflammation at periphery
- Occasional multinucleated giant cells may be present
- Tubular atrophy and interstitial fibrosis in adjacent areas
- Glomeruli relatively spared

DIFFERENTIAL DIAGNOSIS

Renal Cell Carcinoma

- Clinical, gross, and microscopic resemblance to XPN
- Clear cells of renal cell carcinoma may mimic foamy macrophages
- Immunohistochemical stains helpful
  - CD163, CD68 (macrophage markers) negative in neoplastic cells
  - Epithelial markers, such as CKAE1/CAM5.2 and EMA, positive in renal cell carcinoma

Renal Medullary Tuberculosis

- Necrotizing granulomas with epithelioid histiocytes and multinucleated giant cells
- AFB or Fite stain demonstrates acid-fast mycobacteria

DIAGNOSTIC CHECKLIST

Pathologic Interpretation Pearls

- Immunostains and bacterial stains helpful in differential
- Inflammation occurs around calyces
- Macrophages often have indistinct cell borders compared with epithelial cells
- Renal cell carcinoma may coexist with XPN

SELECTED REFERENCES

1. Kim SW et al: Xanthogranulomatous pyelonephritis: clinical experience with 21 cases. J Infect Chemother. 19(6):1221-4, 2013
2. Li L et al: Xanthogranulomatous pyelonephritis. Arch Pathol Lab Med. 135(5):671-4, 2011
3. Afgan F, Mumtaz S, and Ather MH, Preoperative diagnosis of xanthogranulomatous pyelonephritis. Urol J. 4 (3):169-73, 2007
4. Zugor V et al: Xanthogranulomatous pyelonephritis in childhood: a critical analysis of 10 cases and of the literature. Urology. 70(1):157-60, 2007
5. Clapton WK et al: Clinicopathological features of xanthogranulomatous pyelonephritis in infancy. Pathology. 25(2):110-3, 1993
6. Antonakopoulos GN et al: Xanthogranulomatous pyelonephritis. A reappraisal and immunohistochemical study. Arch Pathol Lab Med. 112(3):275-81, 1988
7. Parsons MA et al: Xanthogranulomatous pyelonephritis: a pathological, clinical and aetiological analysis of 87 cases. Diagn Histopathol. 6(3-4):203-19, 1983

(Left) *Gross photograph shows a nephrectomy specimen with XPN associated with a "staghorn" calculus (not shown). Calyces are dilated and lined with yellow nodular plaques ➡.* **(Right)** *Hematoxylin and eosin of a kidney with xanthogranulomatous pyelonephritis shows sheets of lipid-laden foamy histiocytes admixed with lymphocytes. The histiocytes have indistinct cell borders with apparent clearing of cytoplasm.*

Dilated Calyces With Yellow Plaques

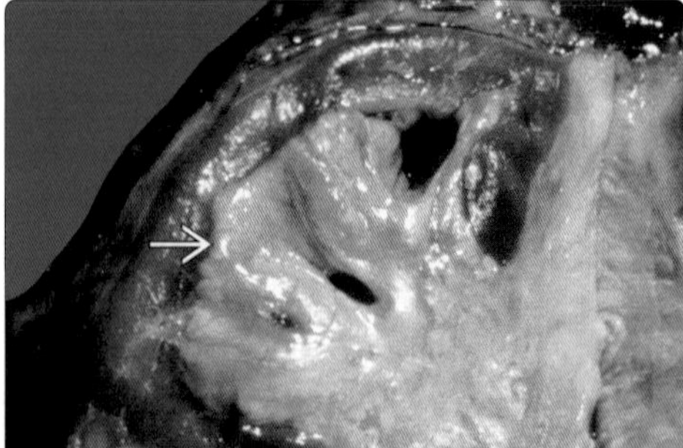

Diffuse Macrophage Infiltrate

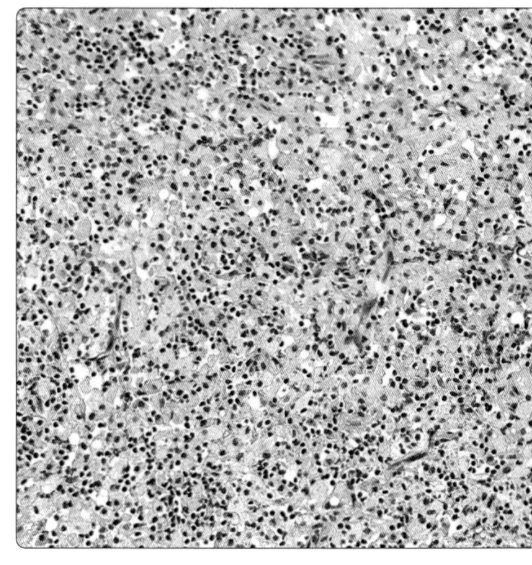

(Left) *XPN appeared as a tan mass lesion composed of spindled cells, mimicking a sarcomatoid renal cell carcinoma. These cells, however, stain positive for CD163, indicative of macrophages.* **(Right)** *CK8/18/CAM5.2 keratin stain shows a renal mass with sheets of spindle cells. Although the histology is suggestive of sarcomatoid renal cell carcinoma, the keratin stain is negative, strongly favoring XPN.*

Macrophages With Spindled Morphology

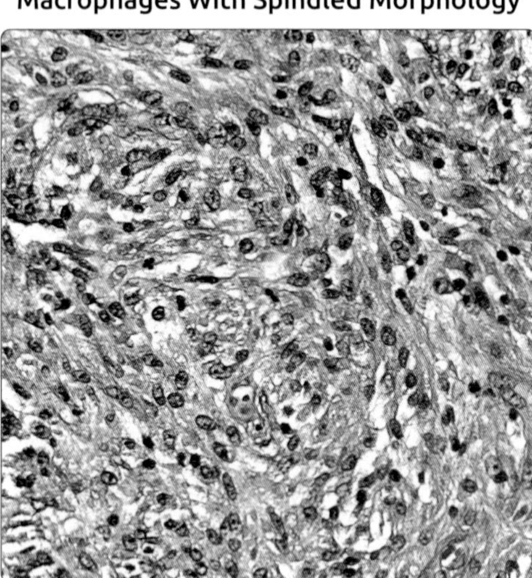

Lack of Epithelial Cells in Renal "Mass"

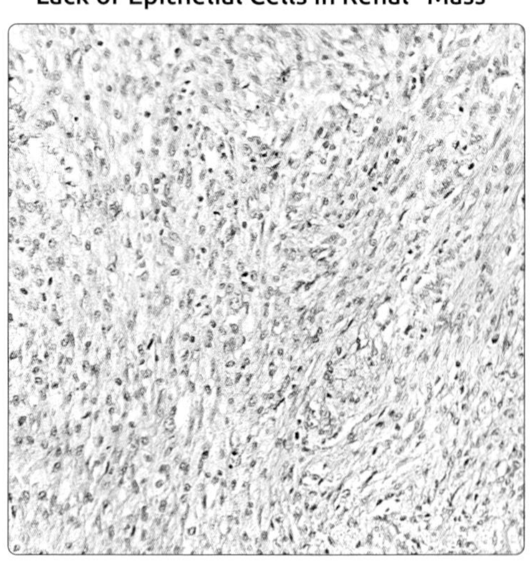

(Left) *A renal mass shows sheets of CD163(+) cells identified as macrophages. The lesional cells were foamy and negative for cytokeratin stain, confirming the diagnosis of XPN.* **(Right)** *The mass lesion of XPN is composed of sheets of macrophages admixed with T lymphocytes, as highlighted by the CD43 immunohistochemical stain.*

Immunohistochemical Confirmation of Macrophages

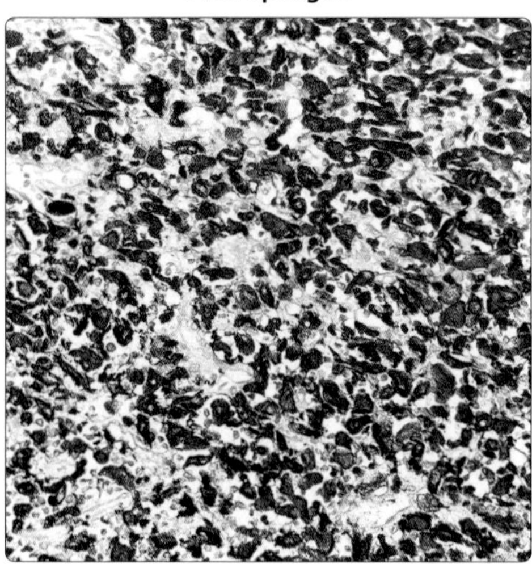

Macrophages Admixed With Lymphocytes

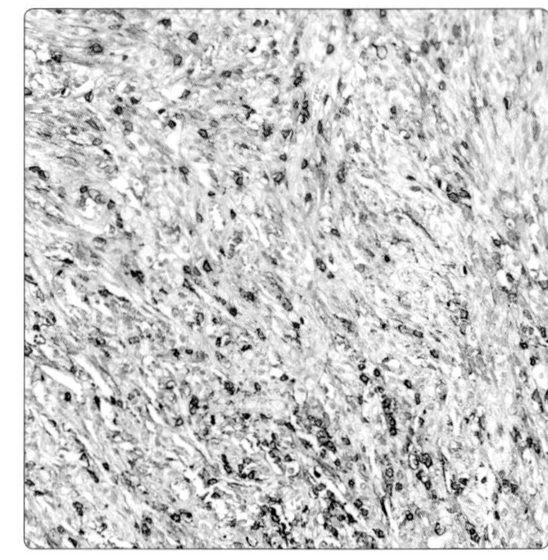

Renal Pelvic Involvement of XPN

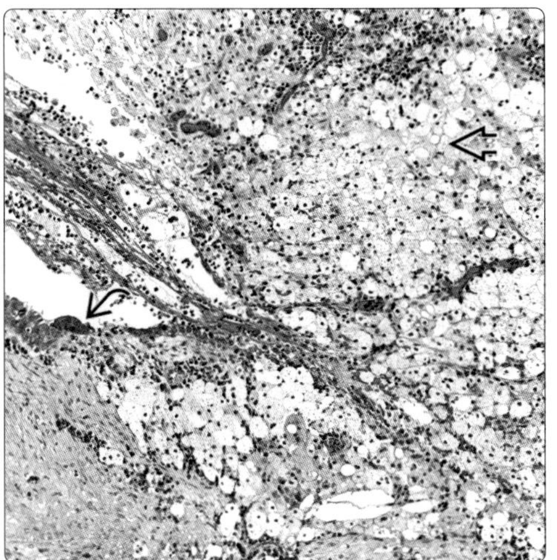

Lipid-Laden Foamy Macrophages

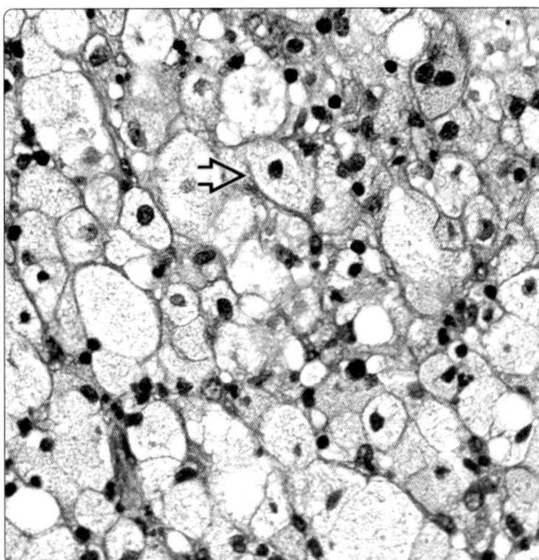

(Left) *Hematoxylin and eosin shows the pelvis ➔ with an adjacent mass lesion composed of clear foamy cells ➔ of XPN. Renal calculi with acute and chronic pyelonephritis were seen elsewhere in the kidney.* **(Right)** *Light microscopy findings of XPN show typical sheets of foamy histiocytes ➔. The clinical, gross, and microscopic findings may resemble a low-grade renal cell carcinoma, clear cell type.*

Renal Cell Carcinoma Mimicking XPN

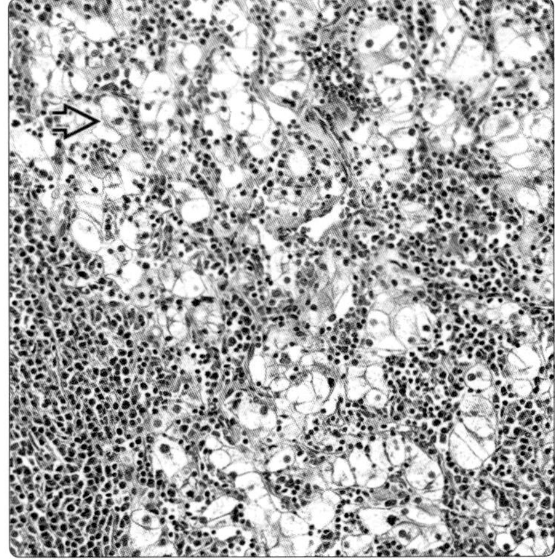

Immunohistochemical Confirmation of Carcinoma

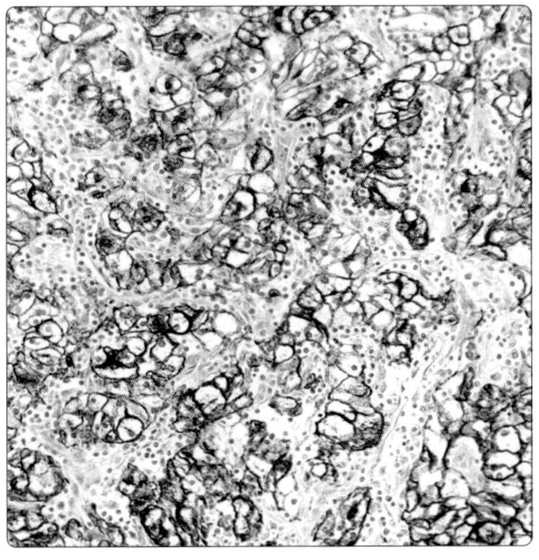

(Left) *Cells in this clear cell renal cell carcinoma have a clear cytoplasm and distinct cell borders ➔. Other areas in the kidney have typical features of XPN, possibly due to obstruction by the renal cell carcinoma.* **(Right)** *Clear cell renal cell carcinoma is positive for CK8/18/CAM5.2 keratins. The neoplastic cells with clear cytoplasm and low-grade nuclei mimic the histiocytes of XPN.*

Collecting Duct Carcinoma Mimicking XPN

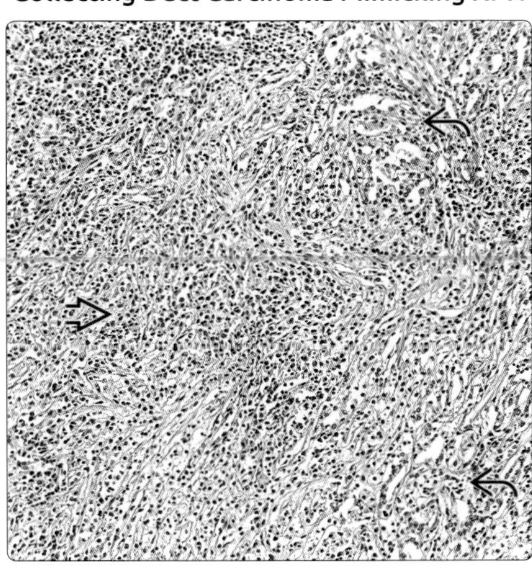

Cytokeratin Stain Highlights Carcinoma

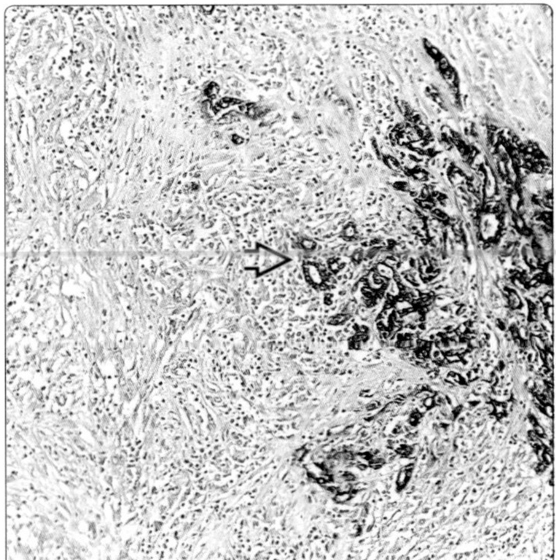

(Left) *This renal cell carcinoma, collecting duct type, has a histiocytic infiltrate ➔ mimicking XPN. Indistinct glands of low-grade collecting duct carcinoma are admixed ➔.* **(Right)** *Glandular structures ➔ of a low-grade collecting duct carcinoma of the kidney are positive for AE1/AE3 keratin. The mass was initially misdiagnosed as XPN due to a prominent histiocytic infiltrate. HMW cytokeratin is also positive.*

Malakoplakia

KEY FACTS

TERMINOLOGY

- Chronic bacterial infection with abundant macrophages containing granular eosinophilic cytoplasm and Michaelis-Gutmann (MG) bodies often forming plaque or mass lesion

ETIOLOGY/PATHOGENESIS

- *E. coli* most common
- Defective intracytoplasmic macrophage bactericidal function
  - Partially digested bacterial products form a nidus for calcium and iron deposition
- Altered immune status is a predisposing factor

CLINICAL ISSUES

- M:F = 1:4
- Involves renal pelvicalyceal system and parenchyma
  - Bilateral involvement common (30-50% of cases)
- Presentation
  - Fever, chills
  - Flank pain, loin tenderness
  - Palpable mass when present; can be mistaken for neoplasm, prompting a nephrectomy
- Surgical therapy now less common with antibiotics and better imaging techniques

MACROSCOPIC

- Yellow-tan nodules in calyces and renal parenchyma

MICROSCOPIC

- Sheets of macrophages with foamy eosinophilic cytoplasm in mass lesion
- Characteristic cytoplasmic inclusions (MG bodies)
  - Calcium positive (von Kossa stain)
  - Iron positive (Prussian blue stain)

TOP DIFFERENTIAL DIAGNOSES

- Renal cell carcinoma
- Xanthogranulomatous pyelonephritis
- Megalocytic interstitial nephritis

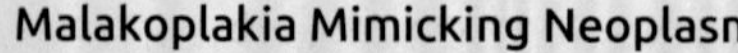

Malakoplakia Mimicking Neoplasm

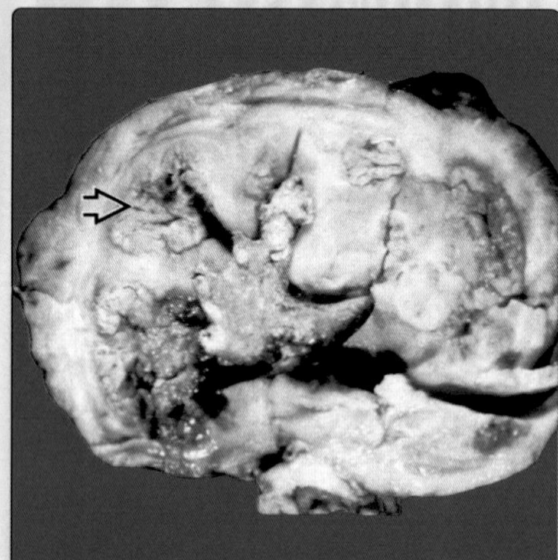

Sheets of Macrophages

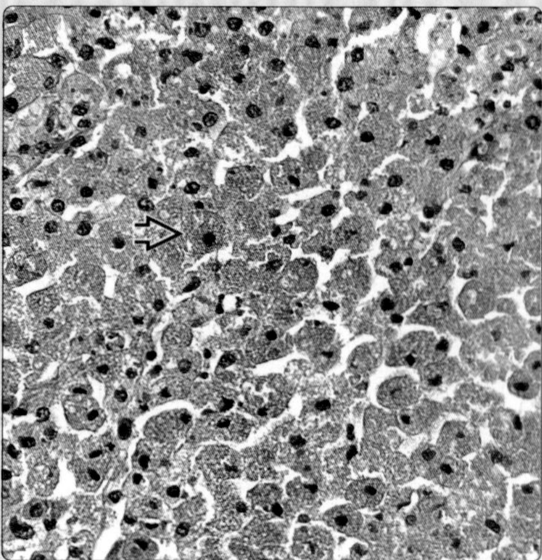

(Left) *Gross photograph of a kidney with malakoplakia shows multiple tan-yellow masses ➡ mimicking a neoplasm. (Courtesy R. Rouse, MD.)* **(Right)** *Hematoxylin and eosin of renal malakoplakia is shown. The mass identified in the nephrectomy specimen is composed of sheets of macrophages with granular eosinophilic cytoplasm ➡.*

Cytoplasmic Granules on PAS Stain

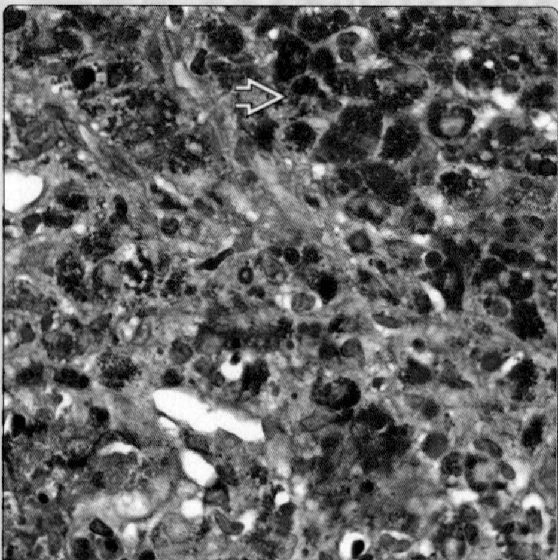

Michaelis-Gutmann Bodies

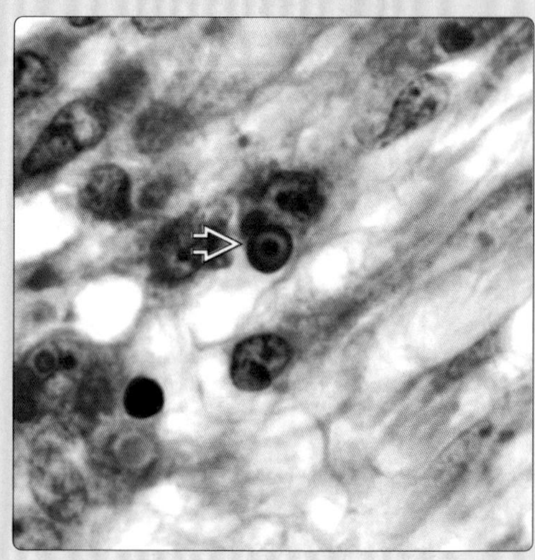

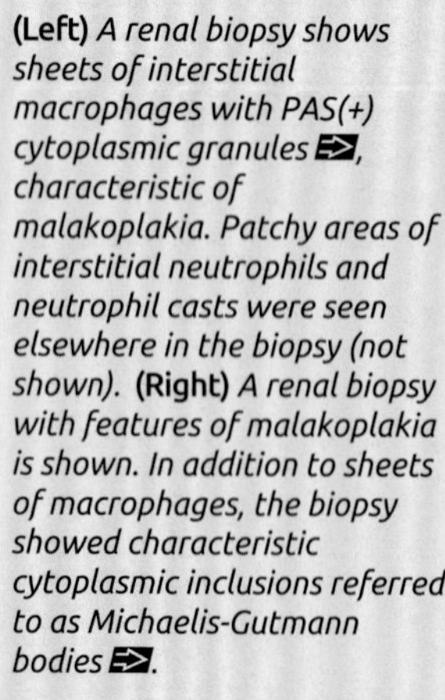

(Left) *A renal biopsy shows sheets of interstitial macrophages with PAS(+) cytoplasmic granules ➡, characteristic of malakoplakia. Patchy areas of interstitial neutrophils and neutrophil casts were seen elsewhere in the biopsy (not shown).* **(Right)** *A renal biopsy with features of malakoplakia is shown. In addition to sheets of macrophages, the biopsy showed characteristic cytoplasmic inclusions referred to as Michaelis-Gutmann bodies ➡.*

TERMINOLOGY

Synonyms

- Malakoplakia

Definitions

- Chronic bacterial infection with abundant macrophages containing granular eosinophilic cytoplasm and Michaelis-Gutmann (MG) bodies often forming plaque or mass lesion

ETIOLOGY/PATHOGENESIS

Infectious Agents

- *E. coli* most common

Defective Intracytoplasmic Macrophage Bactericidal Function

- Decreased lysosomal degradation of bacteria
- Inability of cells to release lysosomal enzymes
- Partially digested bacterial products form a nidus for calcium and iron deposition

Altered Immune Status Is a Predisposing Factor

- AIDS
- Immunosuppressive therapy
- Malignancies

CLINICAL ISSUES

Epidemiology

- Age
  - Infancy to 9th decade
    - 5th decade most common
- Sex
  - M:F = 1:4

Site

- Most common site is urinary bladder
- Renal pelvicalyceal system and parenchyma
  - Bilateral involvement common (30-50% of cases)

Presentation

- Fever, chills
- Flank pain, loin tenderness
- Palpable mass when present, can be mistaken for neoplasm
- Acute renal failure in bilateral disease and renal transplants

Laboratory Tests

- Urinalysis shows pyuria and proteinuria
- Urine cultures may be positive for *E. coli*

Treatment

- Surgical approaches
  - Nephrectomy if suspected malignancy
  - Surgical therapy now less common with antibiotics and better imaging techniques
- Drugs
  - Fluoroquinolone

Prognosis

- High mortality rate (70%) in early reports
- Significant improvement in mortality rate with early diagnosis and antibiotic therapy with fluoroquinolone

MACROSCOPIC

General Features

- Enlarged kidneys
- Yellow-tan nodules in calyces and parenchyma
- Dilated pelvicaliceal system if urinary obstruction
- Renal calculi rare

MICROSCOPIC

Histologic Features

- Sheets of macrophages with foamy eosinophilic cytoplasm in mass lesion
- Characteristic cytoplasmic inclusions, (Michaelis-Gutmann) bodies
  - 4-10 microns in diameter, basophilic
  - Periodic acid-Schiff positive
  - Calcium positive (von Kossa stain positive)
  - Iron positive (Prussian blue stain)
- Admixed lymphocytes and plasma cells

ANCILLARY TESTS

Electron Microscopy

- Michaelis-Gutmann bodies have central crystalline core, intermediate lucent area, and peripheral lamellar rings of deposited mineral

DIFFERENTIAL DIAGNOSIS

Renal Cell Carcinoma

- Immunohistochemistry with CKAE1/CAM5.2 (epithelial cells), CD163, and CD68 (macrophages) is helpful

Xanthogranulomatous Pyelonephritis

- Macrophages foamy and lipid laden
- Absence of Michaelis-Gutmann bodies
- Usually associated with "staghorn" calculus

Megalocytic Interstitial Nephritis

- Macrophages have strongly PAS(+) granular eosinophilic cytoplasm
- Absence of Michaelis-Gutmann bodies

DIAGNOSTIC CHECKLIST

Pathologic Interpretation Pearls

- High level of suspicion needed for biopsy diagnosis
- von Kossa stains and immunostains are useful

SELECTED REFERENCES

1. Kobayashi A et al: Malakoplakia of the kidney. Am J Kidney Dis. 51(2):326-30, 2008
2. Tam VK et al: Renal parenchymal malacoplakia: a rare cause of ARF with a review of recent literature. Am J Kidney Dis. 41(6):E13-7, 2003
3. August C et al: Renal parenchymal malakoplakia: ultrastructural findings in different stages of morphogenesis. Ultrastruct Pathol. 18(5):483-91, 1994
4. al-Sulaiman MH et al: Renal parenchymal malacoplakia and megalocytic interstitial nephritis: clinical and histological features. Report of two cases and review of the literature. Am J Nephrol. 13(6):483-8, 1993
5. Dobyan DC et al: Renal malacoplakia reappraised. Am J Kidney Dis. 22(2):243-52, 1993
6. Esparza AR et al: Renal parenchymal malakoplakia. Histologic spectrum and its relationship to megalocytic interstitial nephritis and xanthogranulomatous pyelonephritis. Am J Surg Pathol. 13(3):225-36, 1989
7. McClure J: Malakoplakia. J Pathol. 140(4):275-330, 1983

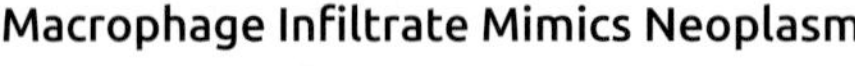

Macrophage Infiltrate Mimics Neoplasm

Basophilic Michaelis-Gutmann Bodies

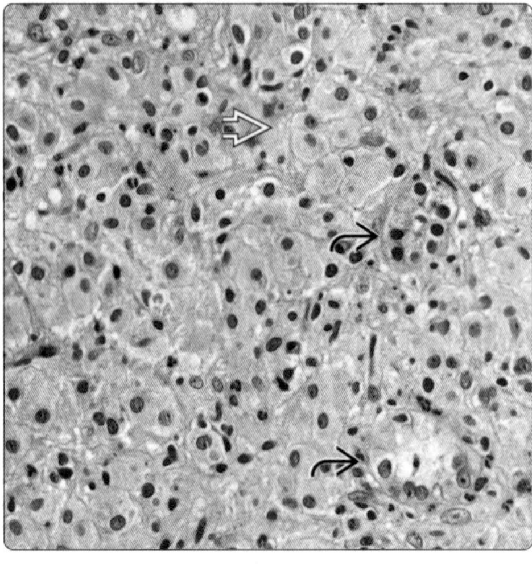

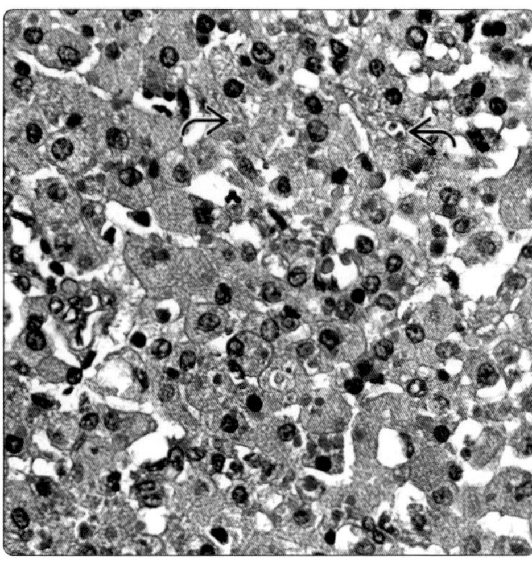

(Left) *Renal malakoplakia as shown here is composed of sheets of plump macrophages with granular cytoplasm mimicking a neoplasm. A few residual preserved renal tubules are also observed.* **(Right)** *Hematoxylin and eosin of renal malakoplakia at high magnification shows the typical basophilic Michaelis-Gutmann bodies within the cytoplasm of the macrophages.*

Necrosis and Acute Inflammation in Malakoplakia

Acute Inflammation in Malakoplakia

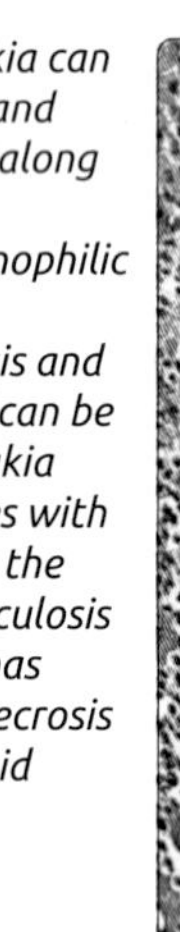

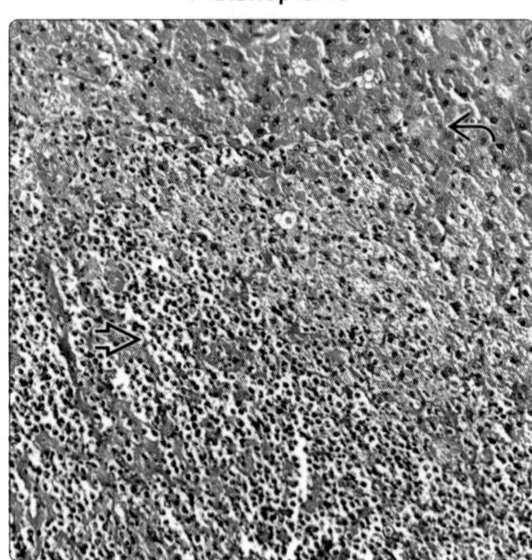

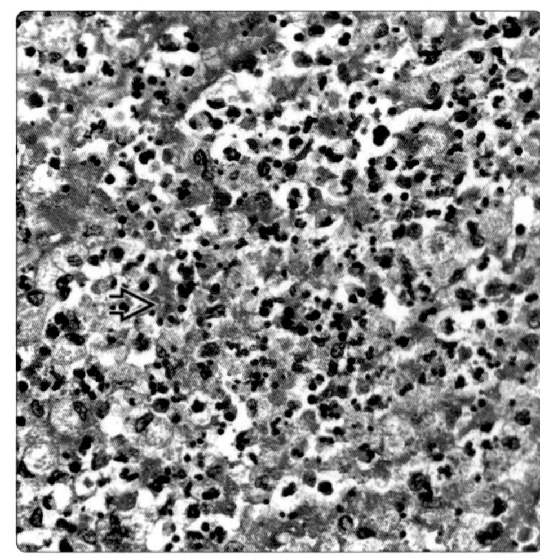

(Left) *Renal malakoplakia can show areas of necrosis and acute inflammation along with the characteristic macrophages with eosinophilic cytoplasm.* **(Right)** *Scattered foci of necrosis and acute inflammation can be seen in renal malakoplakia along with macrophages with granular cytoplasm. On the other hand, renal tuberculosis has caseating granulomas with central acellular necrosis surrounded by epithelioid histiocytes.*

Perinephric Tissue Involvement

Nephrectomy for Suspected Neoplasm

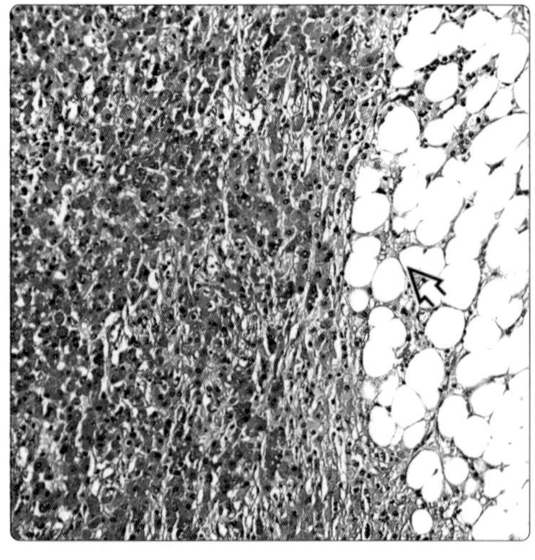

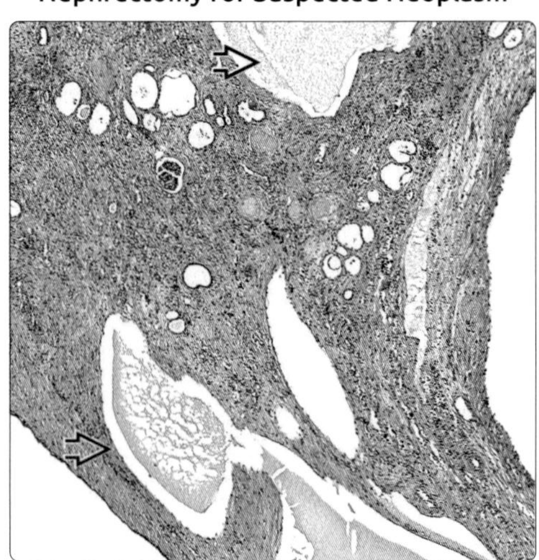

(Left) *Sheets of histiocytes in malakoplakia extending into the pelvic adipose tissue are shown. Similar changes in the capsular surface cause perinephric adhesions. The macroscopic findings of a nephrectomy closely resemble renal cell carcinoma.* **(Right)** *End-stage native kidney with multiple cysts was removed for a suspected renal neoplasm. The microscopic examination of the mass was compatible with renal malakoplakia. The patient had undergone renal transplantation 2 years earlier.*

Immunohistochemical Confirmation of Macrophages

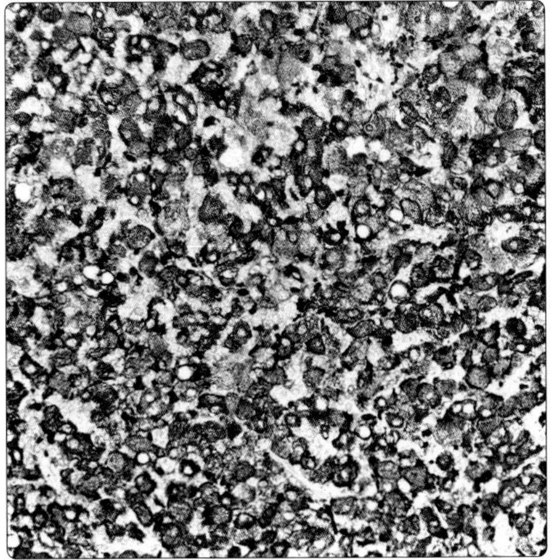

Lack of Epithelial Cell Component

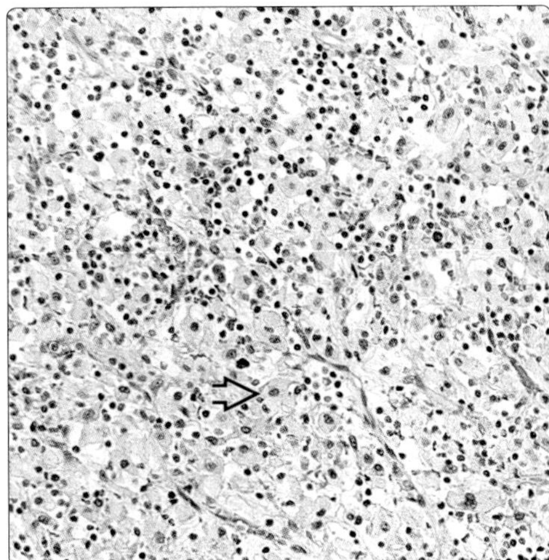

(Left) *CD163 (macrophage marker) of the renal mass lesion diagnosed as malakoplakia is shown. The macrophages are positive for CD163. The cytokeratin stain is negative, ruling out the possibility of renal cell carcinoma.* **(Right)** *CKAE1/AE3 of the native kidney mass diagnosed as renal malakoplakia in a renal transplant recipient is shown. The lesional cells have granular cytoplasm and lack staining for cytokeratin but are positive for CD163 (macrophage marker).*

Macrophages in Renal Cell Carcinoma

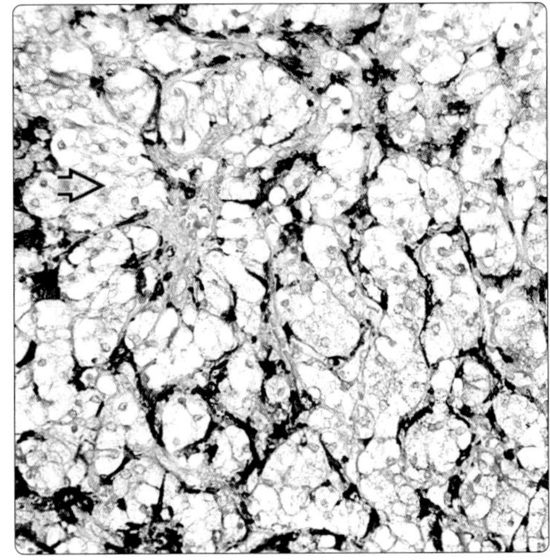

Granular Cytoplasm of Malakoplakia Cells

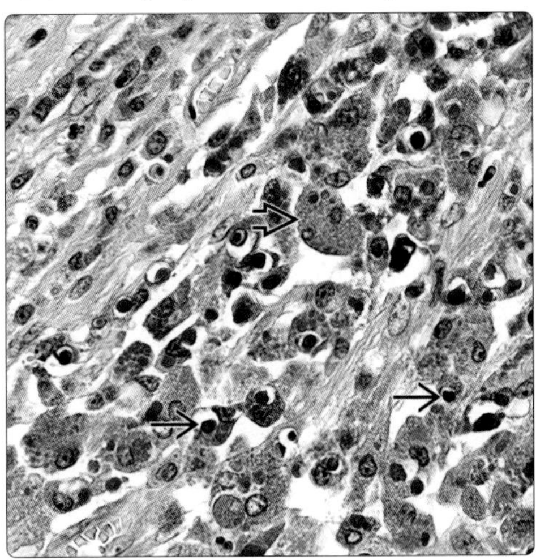

(Left) *CD163 stain of a renal cell carcinoma demonstrates the lack of staining in the lesional neoplastic cells while the admixed histiocytes are positive. Renal malakoplakia is composed of sheets of macrophages, and the histological findings can be mistaken for renal cell carcinoma.* **(Right)** *Periodic acid-Schiff of renal malakoplakia highlights the granular cytoplasm of the macrophages and also stains the characteristic Michaelis-Gutmann bodies.*

Refractile Michaelis-Gutmann Bodies

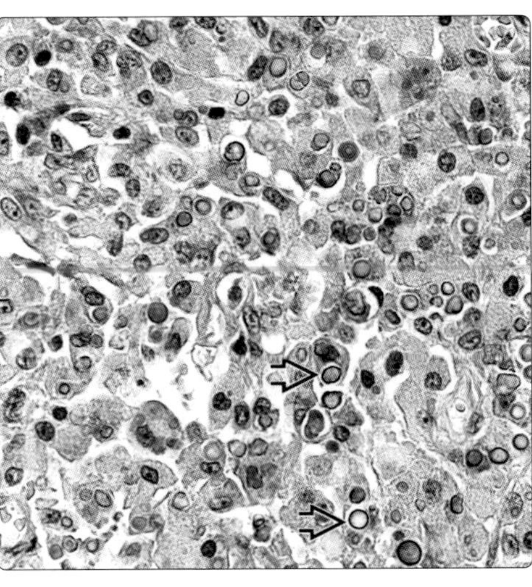

Calcium Deposits in Michaelis-Gutmann Bodies

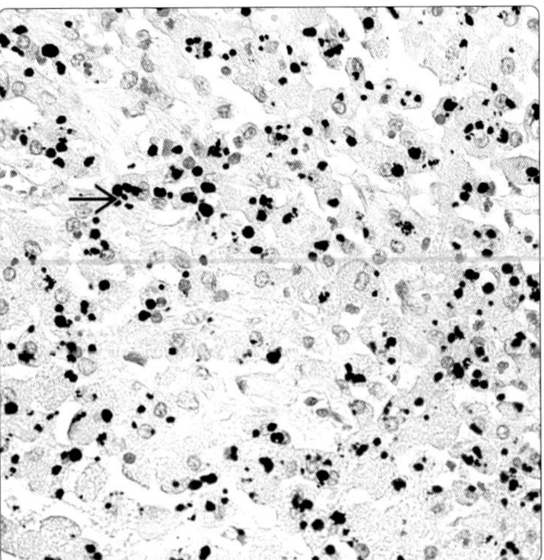

(Left) *Giemsa of renal malakoplakia fails to reveal organisms, but the Michaelis-Gutmann bodies are highlighted by their refractile appearance. Other stains for microorganisms such as AFB, Gram, and Gomori methenamine-silver were also negative.* **(Right)** *von Kossa highlights the Michaelis-Gutmann bodies in malakoplakia. Partially digested bacterial products form the nidus for the calcium (von Kossa[+]) and iron deposition in these bodies.*

Megalocytic Interstitial Nephritis

KEY FACTS

TERMINOLOGY

- MIN is closely related to malakoplakia and characterized by interstitial infiltration of histiocytes

ETIOLOGY/PATHOGENESIS

- *E. coli* and other Gram-negative bacteria
- Leukocyte bactericidal defects, immunodeficiency

CLINICAL ISSUES

- Rare condition affecting middle-aged adults
- Presentation
  - Fever, chills, flank pain
  - Dysuria, urgency
- Urine and blood cultures may be positive for *E. coli*
- Antibiotic therapy directed against Gram-negative bacteria

MACROSCOPIC

- Diffuse involvement of cortex by multiple yellow-gray lesions or discrete nodules

MICROSCOPIC

- Extensive interstitial histiocytic infiltrate with abundant granular eosinophilic cytoplasm

ANCILLARY TESTS

- Periodic acid-Schiff positive cytoplasmic granules

TOP DIFFERENTIAL DIAGNOSES

- Malakoplakia
  - Michaelis-Gutmann bodies identified
- Xanthogranulomatous pyelonephritis
  - Often associated with urinary outflow tract obstruction
- Atypical mycobacterial infection
  - Acid-fast bacilli stain positive for mycobacteria
- Renal cell carcinoma
  - Clear cell carcinoma may have PAS(+) granular cytoplasm
  - Immunohistochemistry for cytokeratin helpful

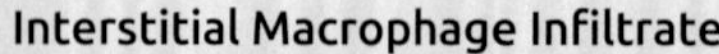

Interstitial Macrophage Infiltrate

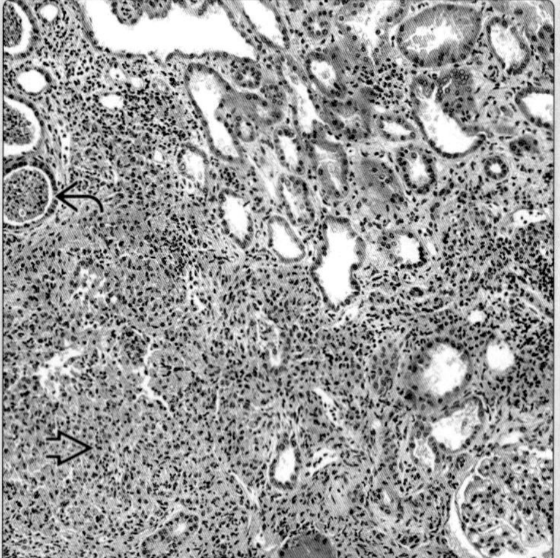

Relative Sparing of Tubules

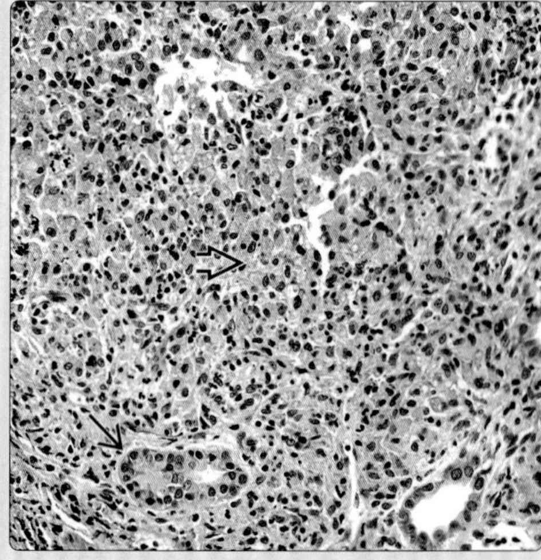

(Left) *Megalocytic interstitial nephritis demonstrates interstitial macrophage infiltrate. A few neutrophil casts are seen within the tubular lumens. (Courtesy C. Nast, MD.)* **(Right)** *Hematoxylin & eosin of a kidney biopsy with megalocytic interstitial nephritis shows diffuse interstitial macrophage infiltrate, but the tubules are spared. (Courtesy C. Nast, MD.)*

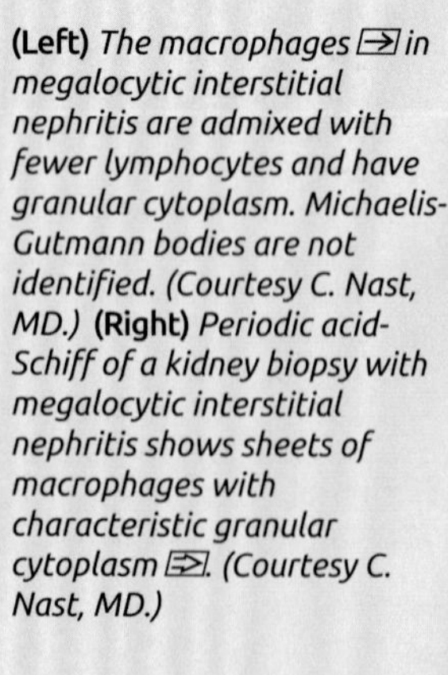

Absence of Michaelis-Gutmann Bodies

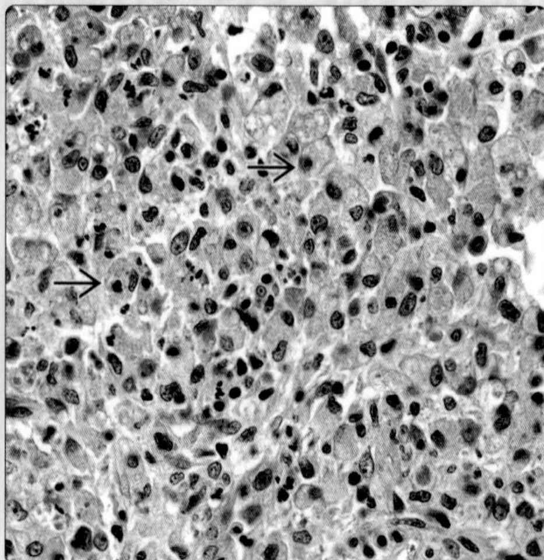

Macrophages With Granular Cytoplasm

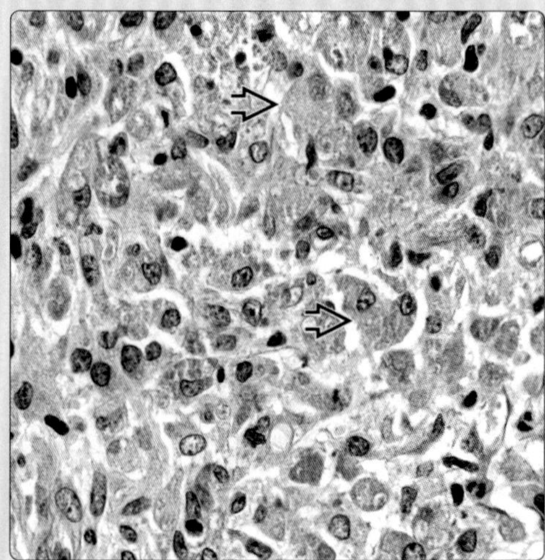

(Left) *The macrophages in megalocytic interstitial nephritis are admixed with fewer lymphocytes and have granular cytoplasm. Michaelis-Gutmann bodies are not identified. (Courtesy C. Nast, MD.)* **(Right)** *Periodic acid-Schiff of a kidney biopsy with megalocytic interstitial nephritis shows sheets of macrophages with characteristic granular cytoplasm. (Courtesy C. Nast, MD.)*

TERMINOLOGY

Abbreviations

- Megalocytic interstitial nephritis (MIN)

Definitions

- MIN is closely related to malakoplakia and characterized by infiltration of histiocytes with eosinophilic granular cytoplasm

ETIOLOGY/PATHOGENESIS

Chronic Bacterial Infection

- *E. coli* and other Gram-negative bacteria

Host Immune Factors

- Leukocyte bactericidal defects
- Immunodeficiency state
  - Transplantation
  - Immunosuppressive therapy
  - Systemic lupus erythematosus
  - Behçet disease

CLINICAL ISSUES

Epidemiology

- Incidence
  - Rare
- Age
  - Middle-aged adults

Presentation

- Fever, chills
- Dysuria, urgency
- Flank pain
- Acute renal failure

Laboratory Tests

- Urinalysis shows white blood cells
- Urine and blood cultures may be positive for *E. coli*

Treatment

- Surgical approaches
  - Nephrectomy if unresponsive to antibiotic therapy
- Drugs
  - Antibiotic therapy against Gram-negative bacteria

Prognosis

- Good with early diagnosis and aggressive antibiotic therapy

IMAGING

Ultrasonographic Findings

- Enlarged kidneys
- Mass lesions may be present

MACROSCOPIC

General Features

- Diffuse involvement of cortex by multiple yellow-gray lesions or discrete nodules
- Can be bilateral

MICROSCOPIC

Histologic Features

- Extensive interstitial histiocytic infiltrate with abundant granular and eosinophilic cytoplasm
- Fewer lymphocytes may be admixed with histiocytes
- Glomeruli uninvolved

ANCILLARY TESTS

Histochemistry

- Periodic acid-Schiff
  - Reactivity: Positive
  - Staining Pattern: Cytoplasmic granules in histiocytes

Immunofluorescence

- Negative for immunoglobulins and complement components

Electron Microscopy

- Macrophages have large intracytoplasmic phagolysosomes filled with granular material and electron-lucent crystalloids

DIFFERENTIAL DIAGNOSIS

Malakoplakia

- Michaelis-Gutmann bodies identified
- Calcium/von Kossa(+)
- PAS(+)

Xanthogranulomatous Pyelonephritis

- Often associated with urinary outflow tract obstruction
- Involvement of pelvicalyceal system
- Often admixed with more lymphocytes & neutrophils

Atypical Mycobacterial Infection

- Acid-fast bacilli stain positive for mycobacteria

Renal Cell Carcinoma

- May have PAS(+) granular cytoplasm
- Immunohistochemistry for cytokeratin helpful

SELECTED REFERENCES

1. Kwon HJ et al: Megalocytic interstitial nephritis following acute pyelonephritis with Escherichia coli bacteremia: a case report. J Korean Med Sci. 30(1):110-4, 2015
2. Jo SK et al: Anuric acute renal failure secondary to megalocytic interstitial nephritis in a patient with Behcet's disease. Clin Nephrol. 54(6):498-500, 2000
3. al-Sulaiman MH et al: Renal parenchymal malacoplakia and megalocytic interstitial nephritis: clinical and histological features. Report of two cases and review of the literature. Am J Nephrol. 13(6):483-8, 1993
4. Esparza AR et al: Renal parenchymal malakoplakia. Histologic spectrum and its relationship to megalocytic interstitial nephritis and xanthogranulomatous pyelonephritis. Am J Surg Pathol. 13(3):225-36, 1989
5. Cledes J et al: Diminished bactericidal activity in megalocytic interstitial nephritis. Clin Nephrol. 23(2):101-4, 1985
6. Garrett IR et al: Renal malakoplakia. Experimental production and evidence of a link with interstitial megalocytic nephritis. J Pathol. 136(2):111-22, 1982
7. Kelly DR et al: Megalocytic interstitial nephritis, xanthogranulomatous pyelonephritis, and malakoplakia. An ultrastructural comparison. Am J Clin Pathol. 75(3):333-44, 1981

Tuberculosis

KEY FACTS

TERMINOLOGY

- Infection by *Mycobacterium tuberculosis*

ETIOLOGY/PATHOGENESIS

- Reactivated latent infection or hematogenous dissemination of active pulmonary infection

CLINICAL ISSUES

- Genitourinary TB accounts for 30% of extrapulmonary TB in developed countries
- Diagnosis
  - Sterile pyuria
  - Mycobacterial cultures positive in 6-8 weeks
  - Mantoux skin test
  - Polymerase chain reaction (PCR) detection of mycobacterial nucleic acid
  - Interferon-γ release assay (ELISA blood test)
    - *M. tuberculosis* antigens in latent and active infection stimulate production of host interferon-γ

MACROSCOPIC

- Destruction of pelvic calyces and papillae with caseous cheesy material
- Large tumor-like nodules of chalky material may replace renal parenchyma

MICROSCOPIC

- Caseating granulomatous inflammation
  - Central necrosis rimmed by histiocytes, plasma cells, lymphocytes, and few multinucleated giant cells
- AA Amyloidosis with longstanding infection
- Cases of glomerulonephritis reported in endemic areas

ANCILLARY TESTS

- Acid-fast bacteria stain (Ziehl-Neelsen)
  - Rare organisms positive at periphery of necrosis

TOP DIFFERENTIAL DIAGNOSES

- *M. avium-intracellulare* infection, sarcoidosis, BCG interstitial nephritis, drug-induced interstitial nephritis

Caseous Necrosis in Renal Pelvis

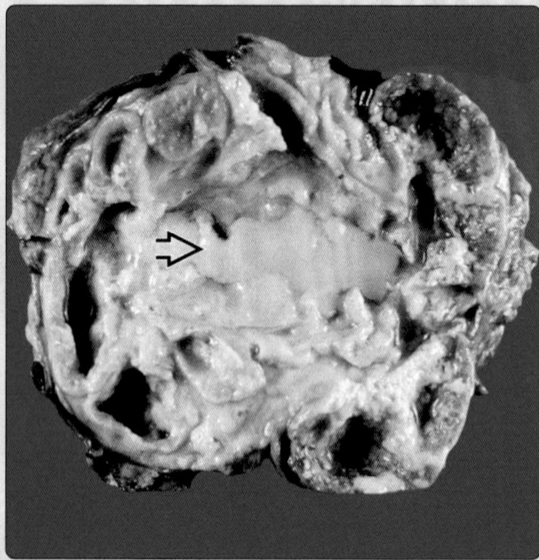

Necrotizing Granulomatous Inflammation

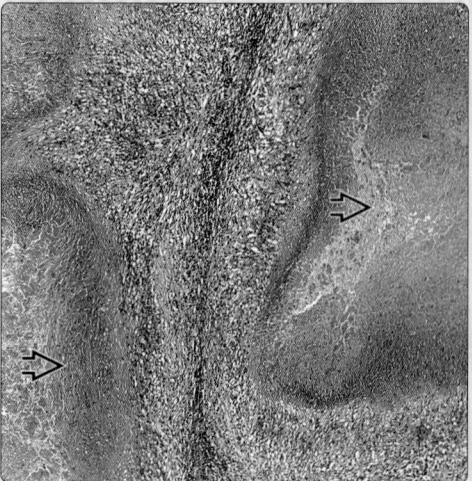

(Left) *Gross photograph of a nephrectomy specimen with renal tuberculosis shows a dilated pelvicalyceal system with ulcerated papillae and caseous necrotic material ➾. (Courtesy L. Fajardo, MD.)* **(Right)** *Caseating granulomatous inflammation is seen in a kidney resected for renal tuberculosis. Extensive necrosis ➾ is present in the granulomas with associated lymphohistiocytic infiltrate.*

Lymphohistiocytic Inflammation and Giant Cells

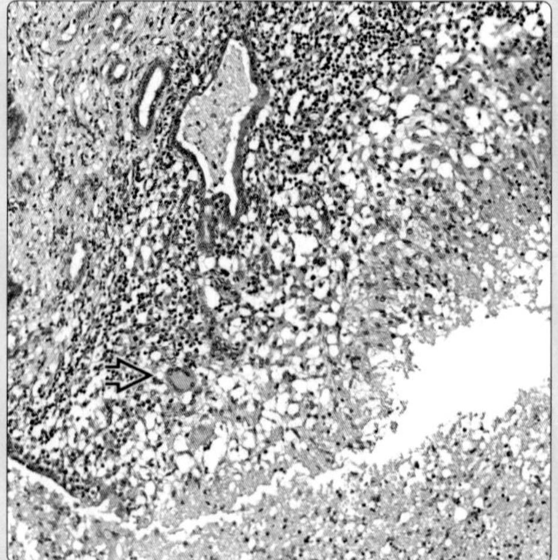

Acid Fast Bacilli in Granulomas

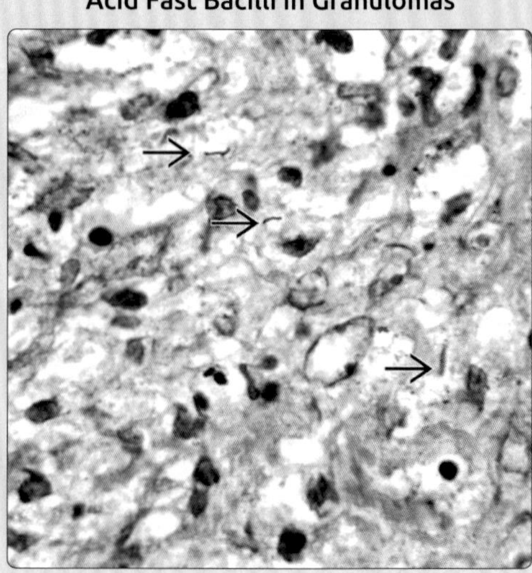

(Left) *Necrotizing granulomas are seen in the pelvic wall, extending into the medulla of a kidney with tuberculous infection. In addition to the histiocytes, occasional multinucleated giant cells ➾ are seen rimming the necrosis.* **(Right)** *Acid-fast bacteria stain of the kidney shows scattered acid-fast bacilli ➙ in the granulomas. (Courtesy G. Berry, MD.)*

TERMINOLOGY

Abbreviations

- Tuberculosis (TB)

Definitions

- Infection of kidney by *Mycobacterium tuberculosis*

ETIOLOGY/PATHOGENESIS

Infectious Agents

- *M. tuberculosis*: Most common organism
- *Mycobacterium bovis*: Bovine bacillus rarely cause disease
- *Mycobacterium avium-intracellulare* in immunosuppressed state

Pathogenesis

- Acute infection
- Hematogenous dissemination of active pulmonary TB
- Reactivated latent infection

CLINICAL ISSUES

Epidemiology

- Incidence
  - Genitourinary TB accounts for 30% of extrapulmonary TB in developed countries
    - Higher frequency in immunosuppressed individuals (HIV, transplantation, dialysis), endemic areas, and drug-resistant TB infection
- Sex
  - More common in men with genital tuberculosis

Site

- Pelvic calyces and renal medulla

Presentation

- Lower urinary tract infection symptoms
- Constitutional symptoms of fever, weight loss unusual

Laboratory Tests

- Urine
  - White blood cells on microscopy
  - Urine bacterial cultures negative (sterile pyuria)
- Mantoux skin test
- PCR detection of mycobacterial nucleic acid
- Interferon-γ release assay (ELISA blood test; QuantiFERON)
  - *M. tuberculosis* antigens in latent and active infection stimulate production of host interferon-γ

Treatment

- Options, risks, complications
  - Hypertension, chronic renal failure
- Surgical approaches
  - Nephrectomy for cavitary lesions
  - Relief of obstruction for ureteral strictures
- Drugs
  - Multidrug therapy with isoniazid, rifampicin, pyrazinamide, and ethambutol (or streptomycin) for several months based on regimen

Prognosis

- Treatment failure due to nonadherence to regimen or drug-resistant organisms

IMAGING

Radiographic Findings

- Calyceal distortion, ureteric strictures on intravenous pyelography (IVP)
- Calcification of necrotic papillae

MACROSCOPIC

General Features

- Ulceration and destruction of pelvic calyces and papillae with caseous cheesy material
- Large tumor-like nodules of chalky material may replace renal parenchyma

MICROSCOPIC

Histologic Features

- Caseating granulomatous inflammation
  - Early infection in medulla but can affect entire kidney
  - Central necrosis rimmed by histiocytes, plasma cells, lymphocytes, and few multinucleated giant cells
- Extensive tubular atrophy, interstitial fibrosis, and variable glomerulosclerosis
- Severe interstitial inflammation may be present
- AA amyloidosis with longstanding infection
- Glomerulonephritis reported with systemic TB in endemic areas
  - Most common is IgA nephropathy

ANCILLARY TESTS

Histochemistry

- Acid-fast bacteria stain (Ziehl-Neelsen)
  - Reactivity: Positive
  - Staining Pattern: Rare organisms at periphery of necrosis

DIFFERENTIAL DIAGNOSIS

M. avium-intracellulare Infection

- Sheets of macrophages, lacks caseation

Sarcoidosis

- Granulomas lack caseating necrosis

BCG Granulomatous Interstitial Nephritis

- Temporal association to BCG therapy

Drug-Induced Interstitial Nephritis

- Granulomas lack caseating necrosis

SELECTED REFERENCES

1. Sun L et al: Be alert to tuberculosis-mediated glomerulonephritis: a retrospective study. Eur J Clin Microbiol Infect Dis. 31(5):775-9, 2012
2. Pai M et al: Systematic review: T-cell-based assays for the diagnosis of latent tuberculosis infection: an update. Ann Intern Med. 149(3):177-84, 2008
3. Wise GJ et al: Genitourinary manifestations of tuberculosis. Urol Clin North Am. 30(1):111-21, 2003
4. Eastwood JB et al: Tuberculosis and the kidney. J Am Soc Nephrol. 12(6):1307-14, 2001

BCG Granulomatous Interstitial Nephritis

KEY FACTS

TERMINOLOGY

- Granulomatous inflammation of kidney due to intracavitary BCG therapy for in situ urothelial carcinoma

ETIOLOGY/PATHOGENESIS

- Hypersensitivity reaction to BCG
- Direct infection of tissues by live attenuated organism in BCG vaccine
- Vesicoureteral and intrarenal reflux is predisposing factor
- Exaggerated immune response combined with host factors may lead to BCG nephritis

CLINICAL ISSUES

- BCG nephritis less frequent than granulomatous cystitis secondary to intravesical BCG therapy
- Presentation
  - Urinary frequency, dysuria
  - Low-grade fever, malaise
  - Flank pain, tenderness
- Temporal association to BCG therapy
- Blood cultures for mycobacteria usually negative
- Treatment
  - Antituberculosis drug regimens
  - Trial of steroid therapy if cultures negative
  - Nephrectomy in therapeutically unresponsive cases

MICROSCOPIC

- Tubulointerstitial inflammation with lymphocytes, histiocytes, plasma cells, and few eosinophils
- Granulomas ± caseating necrosis
- Multinucleated giant cells may be seen

ANCILLARY TESTS

- Ziehl-Neelsen (acid-fast bacteria) stain negative

TOP DIFFERENTIAL DIAGNOSES

- Drug-induced interstitial nephritis
- Sarcoidosis
- Fungal infection

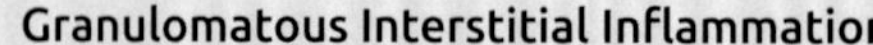

Granulomatous Interstitial Inflammation

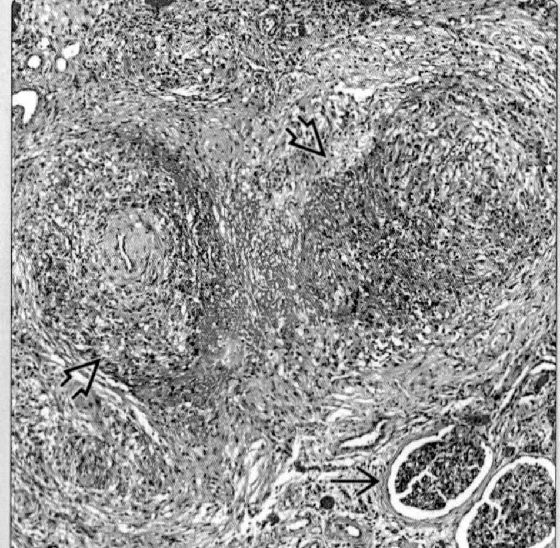

Multinucleated Giant Cells

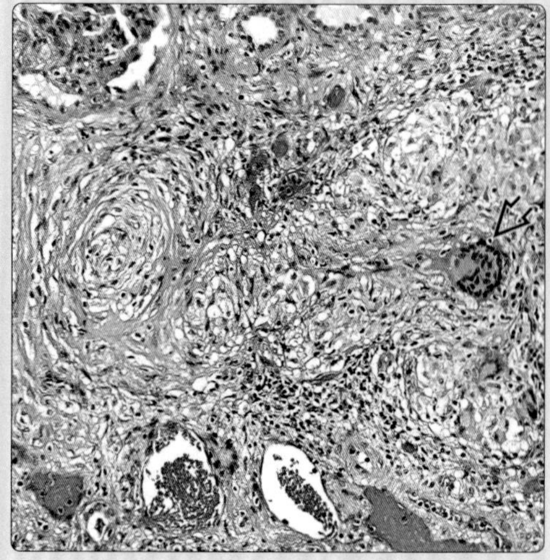

(Left) *Granulomatous inflammation ⇨ of the kidney is seen in a patient treated with intracavitary BCG therapy for in situ urothelial carcinoma of the pelvis. The glomeruli are relatively spared →.* **(Right)** *Hematoxylin & eosin shows granulomatous inflammation due to BCG therapy for in situ urothelial carcinoma of the kidney. The granulomas have scant necrosis but demonstrate lymphohistiocytic infiltrate and multinucleated giant cells ⇨.*

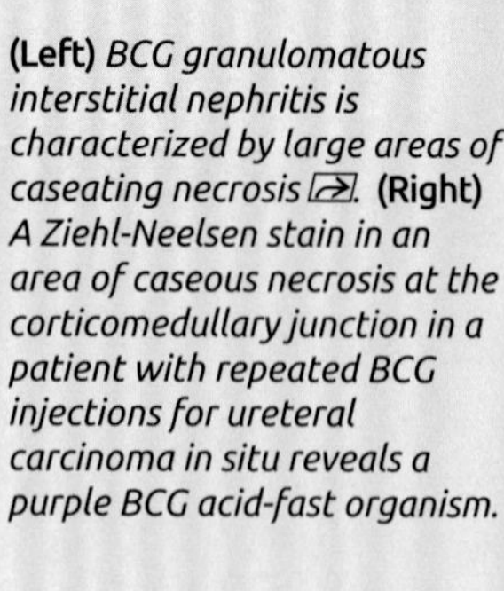

(Left) *BCG granulomatous interstitial nephritis is characterized by large areas of caseating necrosis ⇨.* **(Right)** *A Ziehl-Neelsen stain in an area of caseous necrosis at the corticomedullary junction in a patient with repeated BCG injections for ureteral carcinoma in situ reveals a purple BCG acid-fast organism.*

Caseous Necrosis With BCG

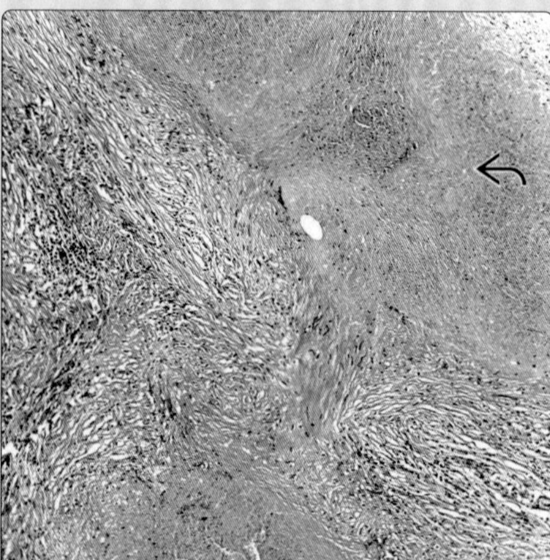

BCG Organism in Caseous Granuloma

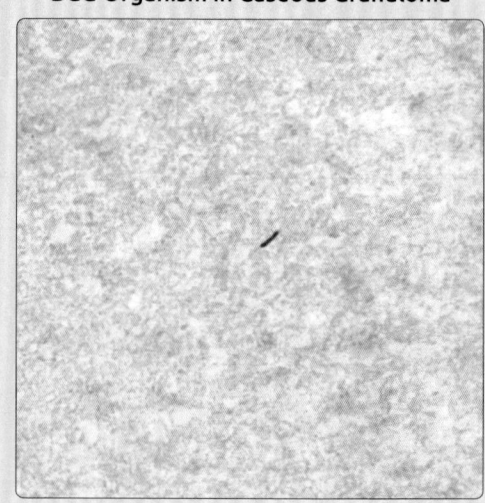

TERMINOLOGY

Abbreviations

- Bacillus Calmette-Guérin (BCG)

Synonyms

- BCG nephritis

Definitions

- Granulomatous inflammation of kidney due to intracavitary BCG for treatment of in situ urothelial carcinoma

ETIOLOGY/PATHOGENESIS

Direct Infection

- Live attenuated organism in BCG vaccine
- Vesicoureteral and intrarenal reflux is predisposing factor

Hypersensitivity Reaction

- Triggered by macrophage phagocytosis of BCG antigen and presentation to helper T cells
- Upregulation of chemokines and cytokines by T cells, macrophages, and neutrophils contribute to antitumor properties of BCG
- Exaggerated immune response combined with host factors may lead to BCG nephritis

CLINICAL ISSUES

Epidemiology

- Incidence
  - Symptomatic BCG nephritis uncommon
    - Asymptomatic granulomatous inflammation of renal pelvis in 25% of patients treated with BCG for noninvasive renal urothelial carcinoma
    - BCG nephritis in 2% of patients who receive intravesical BCG therapy for urothelial carcinoma of bladder

Presentation

- Urinary frequency, dysuria
- Low-grade fever, malaise
- Flank pain, tenderness
- Temporal association to BCG therapy

Laboratory Tests

- Urine
  - White blood cells
  - Cultures often negative
- Blood cultures for mycobacteria usually negative

Treatment

- Surgical approaches
  - Nephrectomy if aggressive medical therapy fails
- Drugs
  - Antituberculosis drug regimens
  - Trial of steroid therapy if cultures negative

Prognosis

- Most respond to combination of antituberculosis therapy and corticosteroids

MACROSCOPIC

Multiple Renal Masses in Cortex and Medulla

- Nephrectomy performed only in therapeutically unresponsive cases

MICROSCOPIC

Histologic Features

- Tubulointerstitial inflammation with lymphocytes, histiocytes, plasma cells, and few eosinophils
- Granulomas ± caseating necrosis
- Multinucleated giant cells may be seen
- Glomeruli relatively spared

ANCILLARY TESTS

Histochemistry

- Ziehl-Neelsen (acid-fast bacteria) stain
  - Reactivity: Negative

Immunofluorescence

- Faint mesangial IgM and C3 staining reported in a few cases (mesangial glomerulonephritis)

Electron Microscopy

- Normal with no electron-dense deposits

DIFFERENTIAL DIAGNOSIS

Drug-Induced Interstitial Nephritis

- Noncaseating granulomas ± eosinophils
- Recent history of drug exposure

Sarcoidosis

- Noncaseating "tight" granulomas with rim of lymphocytes
- Extrarenal manifestations of sarcoidosis may be present

Fungal Infection

- Immunocompromised individuals are susceptible
- GMS (Gomori methenamine-silver) stain positive

SELECTED REFERENCES

1. Airy M et al: Tubulointerstitial nephritis and cancer chemotherapy: update on a neglected clinical entity. Nephrol Dial Transplant. 28(10):2502-9, 2013
2. Kiely B et al: Intravesical bacille Calmette-Guérin-induced multiorgan failure after treatment for transitional cell carcinoma. Scand J Urol Nephrol. 45(4):278-80, 2011
3. Bijol V et al: Granulomatous interstitial nephritis: a clinicopathologic study of 46 cases from a single institution. Int J Surg Pathol. 14(1):57-63, 2006
4. Kennedy SE et al: Acute granulomatous tubulointerstitial nephritis caused by intravesical BCG. Nephrol Dial Transplant. 21(5):1427-9, 2006
5. Tavolini IM et al: Unmanageable fever and granulomatous renal mass after intracavitary upper urinary tract bacillus Calmette-Guerin therapy. J Urol. 167(1):244-5, 2002
6. Prescott S et al: Mechanisms of action of intravesical bacille Calmette-Guérin: local immune mechanisms. Clin Infect Dis. 31 Suppl 3:S91-3, 2000
7. Soda T et al: Granulomatous nephritis as a complication of intrarenal bacille Calmette-Guérin therapy. Urology. 53(6):1228, 1999

Leprosy

KEY FACTS

TERMINOLOGY

- Renal disease caused by *Mycobacterium leprae*: Due to direct infection, host immune response, or treatment effects

ETIOLOGY/PATHOGENESIS

- Obligate intracellular, weakly acid-fast bacillus
- Tuberculoid leprosy has robust cell-mediated immunity with granulomas and paucity of bacilli
- Lepromatous leprosy has poor cell-mediated immunity with abundant bacilli (multibacillary)
  - Robust humoral response has no protective effect but causes immune complex-mediated responses (lepra reaction) such as ENL or glomerulonephritis

CLINICAL ISSUES

- Found worldwide but endemic in tropics
- Presentation
  - Renal insufficiency; rarely, acute renal failure
  - Nephrotic syndrome and edema
  - Hematuria, mild proteinuria
- Treatment: Dapsone, rifampicin, clofazimine
- Steroids and thalidomide in ENL

MICROSCOPIC

- Tubulointerstitial nephritis, may be granulomatous
- Immune-complex mediated and rarely pauci-immune glomerulonephritis
- Amyloidosis (AA type) common in USA

ANCILLARY TESTS

- Fite stain reveals rod-shaped bacilli in infection site
- Granular IgG and C3 deposits in immune-complex GN
- Congo red stain for amyloid

TOP DIFFERENTIAL DIAGNOSES

- Tuberculous granulomatous inflammation
- Drug-induced interstitial nephritis
- Noninfection-related glomerulonephritis

Granulomatous Interstitial Inflammation

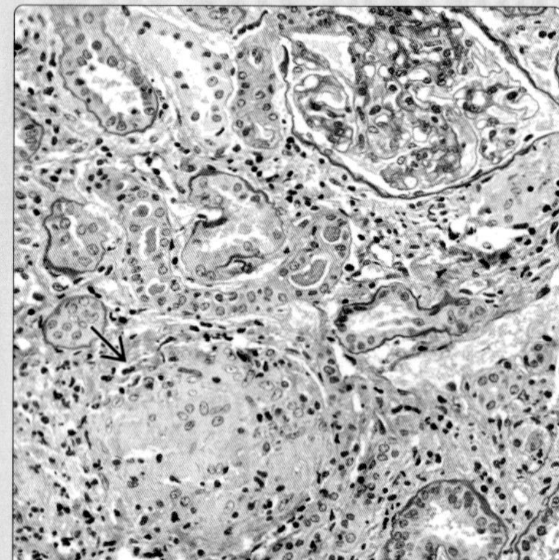

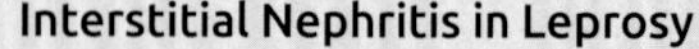

Interstitial Nephritis in Leprosy

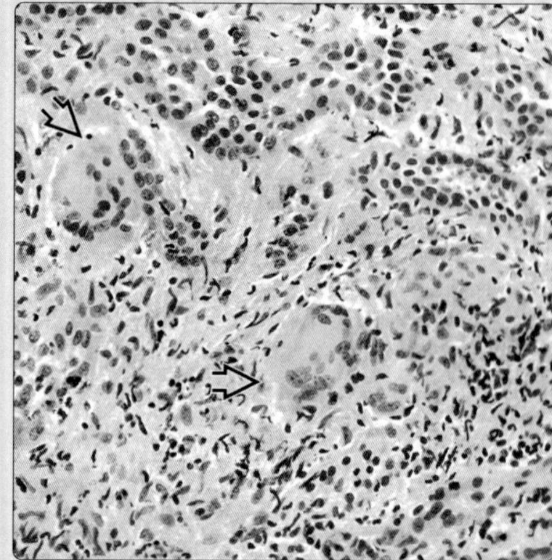

(Left) *PAS stain shows granulomatous interstitial nephritis in a patient with leprosy. A granuloma is present → in a background of diffuse interstitial mononuclear cells and fibrosis.* **(Right)** *H&E shows granulomatous interstitial nephritis → in a patient with chronic renal insufficiency and peripheral nerve involvement by leprosy. Clinical renal involvement is rare in leprosy.*

Leprosy Bacilli in Interstitium

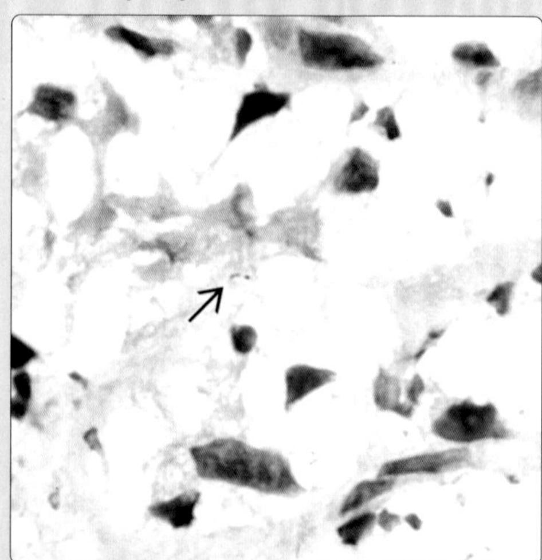

Leprosy Bacillus Ultrastructure

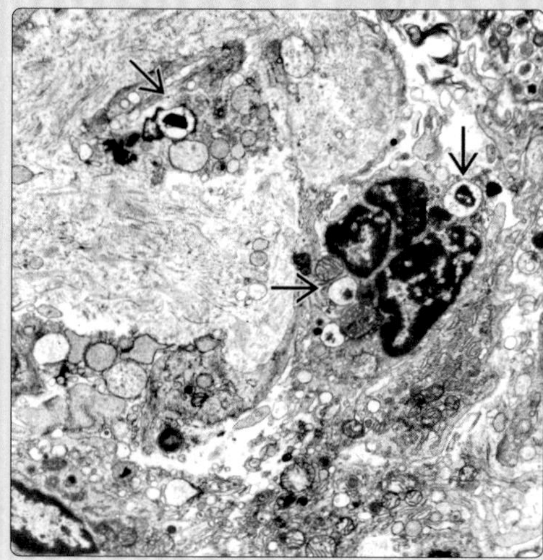

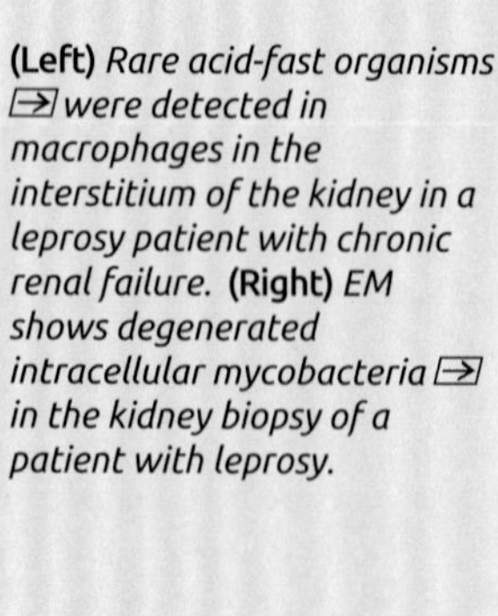

(Left) *Rare acid-fast organisms → were detected in macrophages in the interstitium of the kidney in a leprosy patient with chronic renal failure.* **(Right)** *EM shows degenerated intracellular mycobacteria → in the kidney biopsy of a patient with leprosy.*

TERMINOLOGY

Definitions

- Renal disease caused by *Mycobacterium leprae;* due to direct infection, host immune response, or treatment effects

ETIOLOGY/PATHOGENESIS

Mycobacterium leprae

- Obligate intracellular, weakly acid-fast bacillus
- Disease spectrum from tuberculoid to lepromatous type with intervening borderline categories
  - Tuberculoid leprosy
    - Robust cell-mediated immunity with granulomas and paucity of bacilli
    - Preponderance of T-helper-cell (CD4) response
  - Lepromatous leprosy
    - Poor cell-mediated immunity with abundant bacilli
    - Predominantly cytotoxic T-cell (CD8) response
    - Robust humoral response with high antibody titers
      - No protective effect but causes immune complex-mediated responses such as erythema nodosum leprosum (ENL) or glomerulonephritis

Genetic Factors

- Determine tuberculoid or lepromatous host response

Mechanisms of Glomerular Injury

- Deposition of circulating immune complexes
  - Possible antigens include *M. leprae*, other organisms (coinfection), dapsone
- In situ immune complex deposition
- Cryoglobulinemia

CLINICAL ISSUES

Epidemiology

- Incidence
  - Found worldwide but endemic in tropics

Presentation

- Renal insufficiency and, rarely, acute renal failure
- Hematuria, mild proteinuria
- Nephrotic syndrome and edema
- Functional tubular defects of acidification or urinary concentration ability in few patients

Treatment

- Drugs
  - Antimicrobials: Dapsone, rifampin, clofazimine
  - Steroids and thalidomide helpful in ENL and possibly glomerulonephritis

MICROSCOPIC

Histologic Features

- Tubulointerstitial nephritis
  - Granulomatous nephritis in *M. leprae* infection
    - Associated multinucleated giant cells
- Glomerulonephritis
  - Mesangial, endocapillary proliferative, or membranoproliferative glomerulonephritis
  - Crescents rare but can cause acute renal failure
- Amyloidosis (AA type)
  - Often in lepromatous leprosy with recurrent bouts of ENL or trophic skin ulcers
  - More common in USA than endemic areas
- No histological abnormality with functional tubular defects

ANCILLARY TESTS

Histochemistry

- Modified Ziehl-Neelsen stain (Fite)
  - Reactivity: Positive
  - Staining pattern: Rod-like bacilli in interstitial nephritis
- Congo red
  - Reactivity: Positive in presence of amyloid
  - Staining pattern: Apple-green birefringence under polarized light

Immunofluorescence

- Granular deposits of IgG and C3 in mesangium and capillary walls in glomerulonephritis
- Amyloid subtyping in amyloidosis for amyloid A

Electron Microscopy

- Intracellular degenerated lepra bacilli may be seen within macrophages in interstitial nephritis
- Electron-dense deposits observed in mesangium and subendothelial space in glomerulonephritis
- Randomly oriented amyloid fibrils (8-12 nm) in amyloidosis

DIFFERENTIAL DIAGNOSIS

Tuberculous Granulomatous Inflammation

- Mycobacterial cultures positive
- Lack of response to dapsone therapy

Drug-Induced Interstitial Nephritis

- Clinical history of drug use
- Negative Fite stain

Non-Infection-Related Glomerulonephritis

- Clinicopathologic correlation and positive serology helpful

SELECTED REFERENCES

1. Daher EF et al: Renal dysfunction in leprosy: a historical cohort of 923 patients in Brazil. Trop Doct. 41(3):148-50, 2011
2. Sharma A et al: Renal involvement in leprosy: report of progression from diffuse proliferative to crescentic glomerulonephritis. Clin Exp Nephrol. 14(3):268-71, 2010
3. Guditi S et al: Leprosy in a renal transplant recipient: review of the literature. Transpl Infect Dis. 11(6):557-62, 2009
4. Nakayama EE et al: Renal lesions in leprosy: a retrospective study of 199 autopsies. Am J Kidney Dis. 38(1):26-30, 2001
5. Ahsan N et al: Leprosy-associated renal disease: case report and review of the literature. J Am Soc Nephrol. 5(8):1546-52, 1995
6. Chopra NK et al: Renal involvement in leprosy. J Assoc Physicians India. 39(2):165-7, 1991
7. Weiner ID et al: Leprosy and glomerulonephritis: case report and review of the literature. Am J Kidney Dis. 13(5):424-9, 1989
8. Jain AP et al: Clinico-pathological study of nephrotic syndrome in leprosy. J Assoc Physicians India. 31(7):437-8, 1983
9. Gupta SC et al: A study of percutaneous renal biopsy in lepromatous leprosy. Lepr India. 53(2):179-84, 1981
10. Ng WL et al: Glomerulonephritis in leprosy. Am J Clin Pathol. 76(3):321-9, 1981

KEY FACTS

ETIOLOGY/PATHOGENESIS

- *Nocardia asteroides* most common agent in temperate climates
- Infection due to inhalation of organisms or direct inoculation into skin via trauma
- Opportunistic infection in immunocompromised host
- Can occur in even healthy individuals

CLINICAL ISSUES

- *Nocardia* infection rare
  - Occurs in ≤ 2% of renal transplant recipients
- Kidney involvement rare
  - Secondary to hematogenous spread
- Presentation
  - Fever, chills
  - Pain and tenderness in loin or around renal allograft
  - Skin involvement with draining sinuses may be present
- Laboratory tests
  - Aerobic bacterial cultures of blood, body fluids, or tissue
  - More sensitive molecular detection methods increasingly used
- Sulfonamides are first-line of treatment
  - In sulfonamide resistance, alternative agents, such as amikacin, imipenem, and 3rd generation cephalosporins may be used
  - Treatment for 6-12 months required, especially in immunocompromised patients
- Central nervous system involvement
  - Poor prognostic sign

MICROSCOPIC

- Multiple necrotizing microabscesses with neutrophils
- Rare case of mesangiocapillary glomerulonephritis reported in patient with *Nocardia* pneumonia

ANCILLARY TESTS

- Branched thin filamentous bacteria seen on Grocott-Gomori methenamine-silver stain and Gram stain

Necrotizing Microabscesses in Nocardia Infection

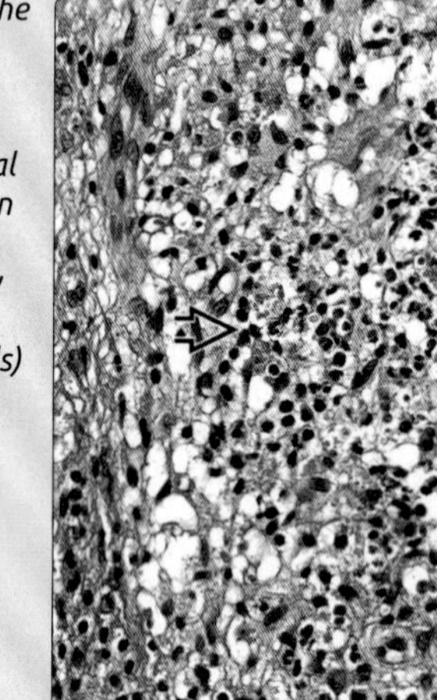

Nocardial Microabscesses With Multinucleated Giant Cells

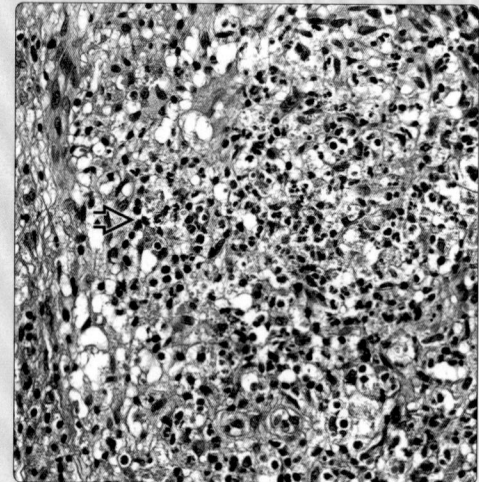

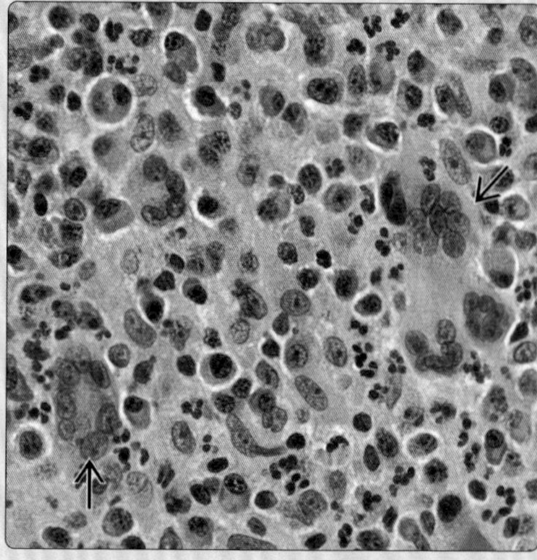

(Left) *Nocardia infection in the kidney is characterized by multiple necrotizing microabscesses ➯ with associated renal parenchymal damage.* **(Right)** *Hematoxylin and eosin characteristically shows a mixed inflammatory infiltrate (neutrophils, lymphocytes and plasma cells) with multinucleated giant cells ➯, which should raise the consideration of nocardiosis. Well-formed granulomas (not shown) are not present. (Courtesy A. Husain, MD).*

Filamentous Nocardial Organisms on GMS Stain

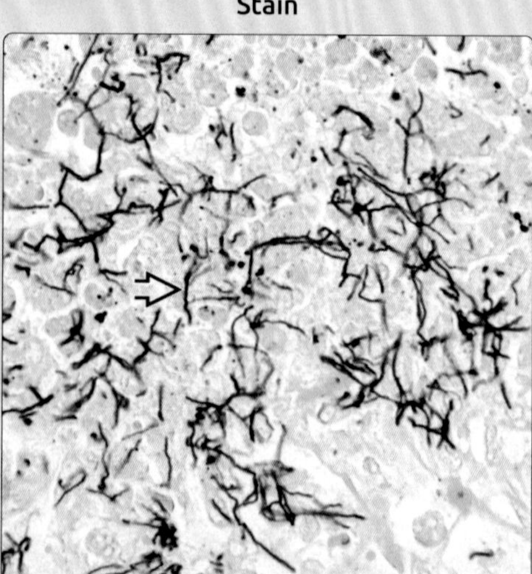

Filamentous Nocardial Organisms on Gram Stain

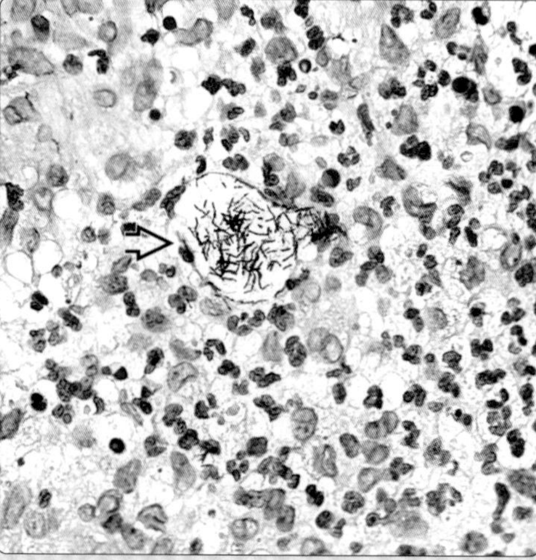

(Left) *A GMS stain shows slender branching filamentous organisms ➯ characteristic of Nocardia infection within the microabscesses. (Courtesy A. Husain, MD.)* **(Right)** *A Gram stain highlights a small collection of tangled filamentous Nocardia organisms ➯ within the microabscesses.*

TERMINOLOGY

Definitions

- Acute inflammation of renal parenchyma by *Nocardia*

ETIOLOGY/PATHOGENESIS

Infectious Agents

- *Nocardia asteroides* most common agent in temperate climates
- *Nippostrongylus brasiliensis* more common in tropical climates
  - Less common species include *Nocardia caviae, Nocardia nova*, and *Nocardia farcinica*
- Ubiquitous organisms in soil
  - Infection route by inhalation or direct inoculation into skin via trauma or animal bite

Predisposing Factors

- Opportunistic infection in immunocompromised host
  - Solid organ transplantation
  - Corticosteroid therapy, HIV infection
- Can occur with chronic lung disease, diabetes, carcinoma, or even in healthy individuals

CLINICAL ISSUES

Epidemiology

- Incidence
  - Nocardia infection rare
    - Occurs in ≤ 2% of renal transplant recipients
    - Lungs most commonly affected organs, followed by skin and disseminated infection
    - Kidney involvement rare
      - Secondary to hematogenous spread

Site

- Kidney parenchyma and perinephric tissues

Presentation

- Fever, chills
- Pulmonary symptoms with septicemia
- Pain and tenderness in loin or around renal allograft
- Skin involvement with draining sinuses may be present

Laboratory Tests

- Aerobic bacterial cultures of blood, body fluids, or tissue
- Urine cultures positive for *Nocardia* if pyelitis present
- More sensitive molecular detection methods increasingly used

Treatment

- Drugs
  - Sulfonamides are first-line of treatment
    - In sulfonamide resistance, alternative agents, such as amikacin, imipenem, and 3rd generation cephalosporins used
  - Prolonged treatment for 6-12 months required, especially in immunocompromised patients

Prognosis

- Central nervous system involvement
  - Poor prognostic sign

IMAGING

General Features

- Renal parenchymal or perinephric abscesses

MICROSCOPIC

Histologic Features

- Multiple necrotizing microabscesses with neutrophils
  - Multinucleated giant cells may be seen
- Acute inflammation may affect glomeruli along with adjacent tubulointerstitium
- Blood vessels usually spared
- Rare case of mesangiocapillary glomerulonephritis reported in patient with *Nocardia* pneumonia

ANCILLARY TESTS

Histochemistry

- Grocott-Gomori methenamine-silver
  - Reactivity: Positive
  - Staining pattern: Branched thin filamentous bacteria
- Gram
  - Reactivity: Positive
  - Staining pattern: Branched thin filamentous bacteria
- Periodic acid-Schiff and acid-fast stains
  - Filamentous bacteria less well seen

DIFFERENTIAL DIAGNOSIS

Non-Nocardial Bacterial Pyelonephritis

- Histochemical stains and cultures useful

Pauci-Immune Glomerulonephritis and Vasculitis

- Glomerular crescents identified and vasculocentric inflammation may be seen
- Neutrophils seen, but well-defined abscesses absent

Acute Tubulointerstitial Nephritis

- Predominantly lymphocytic infiltrate
- Neutrophils seen, but well-defined abscesses absent

Infectious Granulomatous Pyelonephritis

- Epithelioid histiocytes and multinucleated giant cells present at periphery of necrosis
- Mycobacterial and fungal infections should be excluded

SELECTED REFERENCES

1. Santos M et al: Infection by Nocardia in solid organ transplantation: thirty years of experience. Transplant Proc. 43(6):2141-4, 2011
2. Belhocine W et al: Nocardia carnea infection in a kidney transplant recipient. Transplant Proc. 42(10):4359-60, 2010
3. Einollahi B et al: Invasive fungal infections following renal transplantation: a review of 2410 recipients. Ann Transplant. 13(4):55-8, 2008
4. D'Cruz S et al: Isolated nocardial subcapsular and perinephric abscess. Indian J Pathol Microbiol. 47(1):24-6, 2004
5. Frangié C et al: A rare infection in a renal transplant recipient. Nephrol Dial Transplant. 16(6):1285-7, 2001
6. Jose MD et al: Mesangiocapillary glomerulonephritis in a patient with Nocardia pneumonia. Nephrol Dial Transplant. 13(10):2628-9, 1998
7. Raghavan R et al: Fungal and nocardial infections of the kidney. Histopathology. 11(1):9-20, 1987

Leptospirosis

KEY FACTS

TERMINOLOGY

- Zoonotic infectious disease caused by spirochetes of genus *Leptospira*

ETIOLOGY/PATHOGENESIS

- Infection has 2 phases
    - Early: 3-7 days, caused by leptospiremia and direct infection of organs
    - Immunological: 4-20 days, caused by immunologic reaction to *Leptospira* antigens
- Contaminated food/water and direct contact with blood/tissue of infected animals are sources of exposure
- *Leptospira* enter host through abrasions of skin or mucous membranes
- Acute renal failure arises in a number of ways
    - Direct tubular injury: Leptospiral outer membrane protein and endotoxin acting via toll-like receptors
    - Immunologic injury: Tubulointerstitial nephritis
    - Ischemic injury: Peripheral vasodilation, hypovolemia, myocarditis
    - Toxic tubular injury from endogenous toxins
        - Hepatic failure: Bilirubin; rhabdomyolysis, myoglobin

CLINICAL ISSUES

- Anicteric form (80-90% of cases)
- Icteric form (10-20% of cases)
    - Weil disease: Fever, jaundice, acute renal failure
- 40-60% have acute renal failure in course of disease

MICROSCOPIC

- Tubulointerstitial nephritis is characteristic
- Leptospiral organisms or antigen may be detectable in tubules

TOP DIFFERENTIAL DIAGNOSES

- Viral or rickettsial acute interstitial nephritis
- Drug-induced acute interstitial nephritis

Tubulointerstitial Nephritis in Leptospirosis

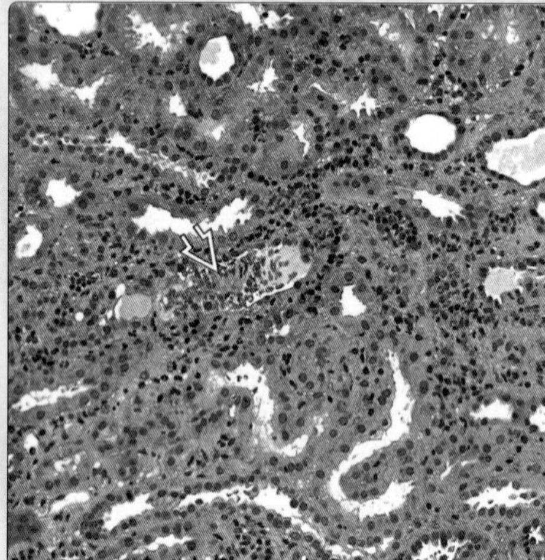

Interstitial Nephritis in Leptospirosis

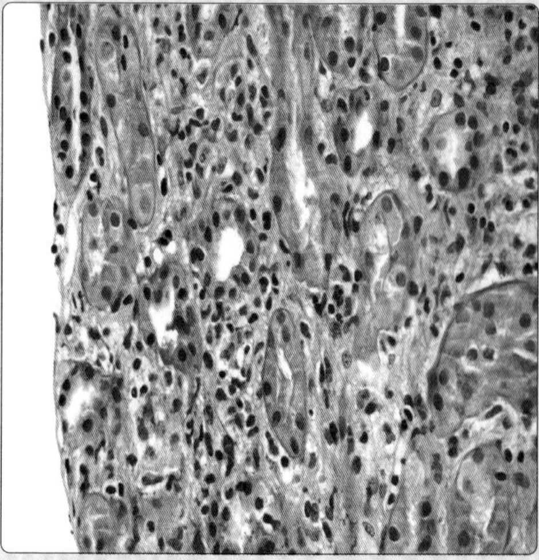

(Left) *Interstitial edema with infiltrates of lymphoid cells and macrophages predominate in interstitial nephritis attributable to leptospirosis. As seen here, a tubule has a bile pigmented cast* ➡ *and the patient, a 17-year-old male, was jaundiced at biopsy. (Courtesy L. Kim, MD.)* **(Right)** *Mononuclear cells, including macrophages and activated lymphoid cells, are seen predominantly in the interstitium. (Courtesy V. Royal, MD.)*

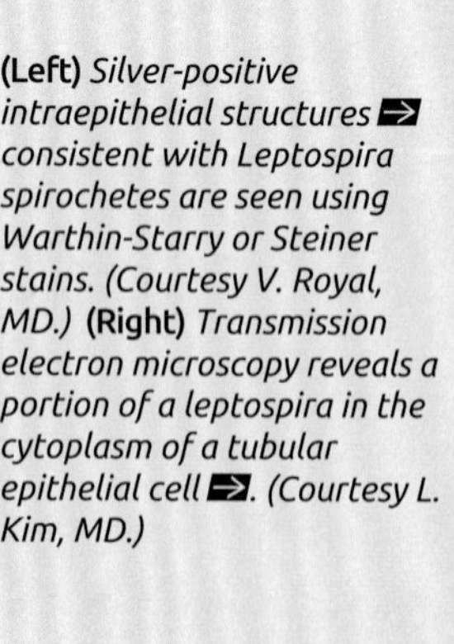

(Left) *Silver-positive intraepithelial structures* ➡ *consistent with Leptospira spirochetes are seen using Warthin-Starry or Steiner stains. (Courtesy V. Royal, MD.)* **(Right)** *Transmission electron microscopy reveals a portion of a leptospira in the cytoplasm of a tubular epithelial cell* ➡*. (Courtesy L. Kim, MD.)*

Spirochetes in Tubular Epithelium

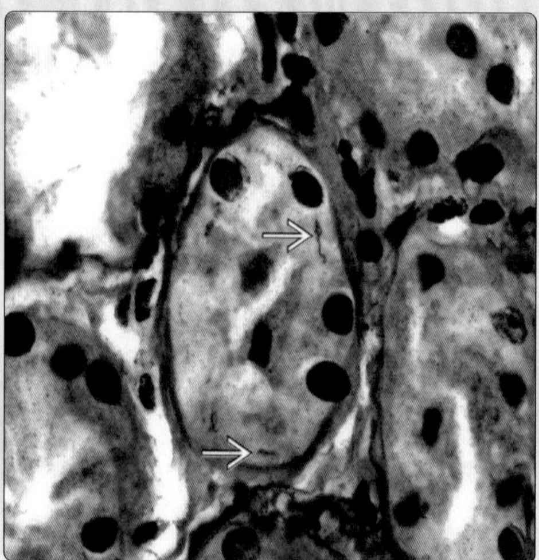

Intraepithelial Leptospira

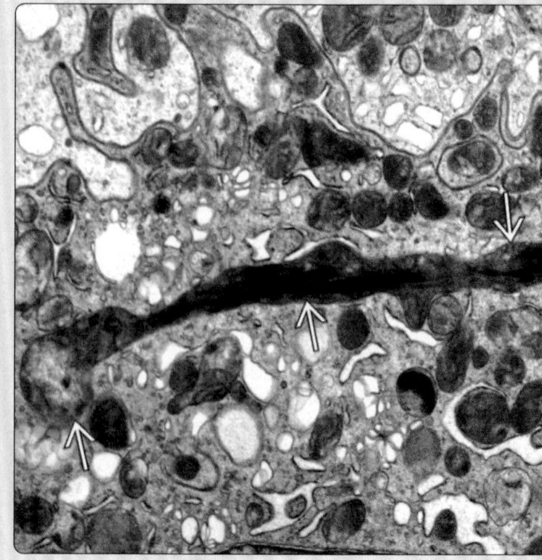

TERMINOLOGY

Definitions

- Zoonotic infectious disease caused by spirochetes of genus *Leptospira*

ETIOLOGY/PATHOGENESIS

Infectious Agents

- Several pathogenic subspecies of *Leptospira interrogans* for humans
  - *L. interrogans* serovars *icterohemorrhagica*, *canicola*, *pomona*, *bataviae*, *grippotyphosa*, and others
- Rats are principal reservoir, also skunks, foxes, ducks, dogs, and frogs
  - *Leptospira* excreted in urine
- Human infection via contaminated food/water or direct contact with blood/tissue of infected animals
  - Outbreaks often coincide with flooding

Pathogenesis

- *Leptospira* enter host through abrasions of skin or mucous membranes
- Wide dissemination of organisms within 48 hours of infection
- 2 phases of disease
  - Early: 3-7 days, caused by leptospiremia and direct infection of organs
  - Immunological: 4-20 days, caused by immunologic reaction to *Leptospira* antigens
- Acute renal failure due to
  - Direct tubular injury: Leptospiral outer membrane protein and endotoxin acting via toll-like receptors
  - Immunologic injury: Tubulointerstitial nephritis
  - Ischemic injury: Peripheral vasodilation, hypovolemia, myocarditis
  - Hepatic failure, rhabdomyolysis from endogenous toxins

CLINICAL ISSUES

Presentation

- Sudden onset after incubation period of 7-12 days
- Anicteric form (80-90% of cases)
  - Self-limited fever, chills, myalgia, headache, conjunctivitis, rash
  - Mild proteinuria, granular casts, hematuria, leukocyturia, bile, and heme casts
- Icteric form (10-20% of cases): Weil disease
  - Fever, jaundice
  - Acute renal failure in 40-60%
  - Thrombocytopenia and pulmonary hemorrhage
- Dark-field microscopy or immunofluorescence with antileptospiral antibodies reveals organisms in weeks 1-4
- *Leptospira* DNA detection by PCR is diagnostic
- Culture on EMcCJH or Fletcher medium takes ≥ 4 weeks

Treatment

- Drugs
  - Penicillin, ceftriaxone, cefotaxime
    - Risk of Jarisch-Herxheimer reaction
  - Steroids used in severe illness

Prognosis

- Mortality in Weil disease (*L. icterohemorrhagica*): 10%
- ~ 25% mortality with acute renal failure
  - 90% of survivors recover renal function

MACROSCOPIC

General Features

- Enlarged kidneys with petechial hemorrhages
  - ± ecchymoses on capsular and cut surfaces, calyceal, and pelvic mucosa
- In Weil disease, brown-yellow discoloration of kidney

MICROSCOPIC

Histologic Features

- Glomeruli: Unremarkable
- Tubules
  - Early acute tubular injury, primarily proximal tubule
  - Tubulitis later with interstitial inflammation
  - Hyaline, necrotic, bile, myoglobin, or hemoglobin casts
- Interstitium
  - Tubulointerstitial inflammation, edema, and hemorrhage
  - Lymphocytes, macrophages, and occasional granulocytes
- Vessels: Unremarkable

ANCILLARY TESTS

Histochemistry

- Warthin-Starry, Steiner, or Levaditi stains reveal 6-20 μm spirochetes

Immunofluorescence

- Leptospiral antigen in interstitium and tubules

Electron Microscopy

- Leptospira seen in tubular lumens, epithelium, and capillaries

DIFFERENTIAL DIAGNOSIS

Viral or Rickettsial Infection

- Rickettsiae, hantavirus, adenovirus, dengue
- Microbial antigens detectable by immunohistochemistry
- Geographic setting, exposure history helpful

Drug-Induced Acute Interstitial Nephritis

- Usually not hemorrhagic, no organisms

DIAGNOSTIC CHECKLIST

Pathologic Interpretation Pearls

- Acute tubular injury and tubulointerstitial nephritis
  - Organisms or leptospiral antigen detectable in situ

SELECTED REFERENCES

1. Goswami RP et al: Predictors of mortality in leptospirosis: an observational study from two hospitals in Kolkata, eastern India. Trans R Soc Trop Med Hyg. 108(12):791-6, 2014
2. Yap DY et al: Cortical necrosis in a kidney transplant recipient due to leptospirosis. Nephrology (Carlton). 19(4):257-8, 2014
3. Yang CW et al: Leptospirosis renal disease. Nephrol Dial Transplant. 16 Suppl 5:73-7, 2001

Mucormycosis

KEY FACTS

TERMINOLOGY

- Fungus infection, typically in immunocompromised patients
- Synonym
  - Invasive zygomycosis

ETIOLOGY/PATHOGENESIS

- *Mucor*
  - Class: Zygomycetes
  - Order: Mucorales
    - Most common species (in descending frequency): *Rhizopus, Rhizomucor, Cunninghamella, Apophysomyces, Saksenaea, Absidia, Mucor*
- Risk factors: Diabetes, immunosuppression, malnutrition, malignancy

CLINICAL ISSUES

- Renal involvement in 20% of disseminated disease patients
- Fever, flank pain
- Rapidly progressive
- Complete debridement of infected tissue
- Amphotericin B
- Reduction of immunosuppression

MACROSCOPIC

- Large infarcts
- Arterial thrombosis
  - Main renal, arcuate, or interlobar artery

MICROSCOPIC

- Nonseptate fungal hyphae with 90° branching
- Cortical necrosis
- Thrombi
- Microabscesses
- Granulomatous interstitial nephritis

TOP DIFFERENTIAL DIAGNOSES

- Aspergillosis
- Candidiasis
- Pseudallescheriasis or fusariosis

(Left) *Jones methenamine silver stain shows numerous hyphae →, typical of mucormycosis in an area of cortical necrosis. (Courtesy E. Bracamonte, MD.)* **(Right)** *Jones methenamine silver stain shows numerous fungal nonseptate branching hyphae → invading the arterial lumen in an area with extensive cortical necrosis. (Courtesy E. Bracamonte, MD.)*

Disseminated Mucormycosis

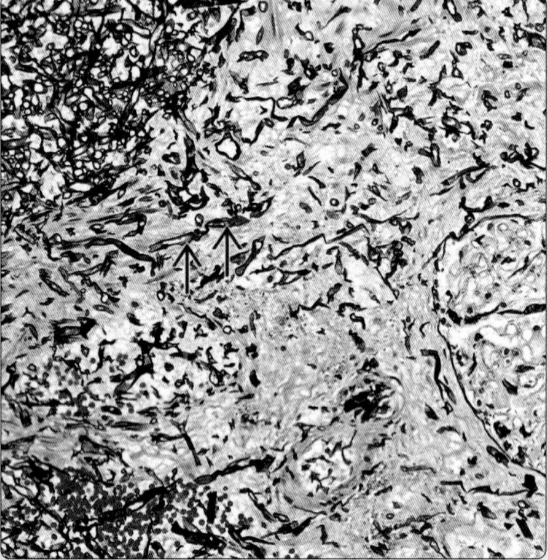

Angioinvasive Mucormycosis

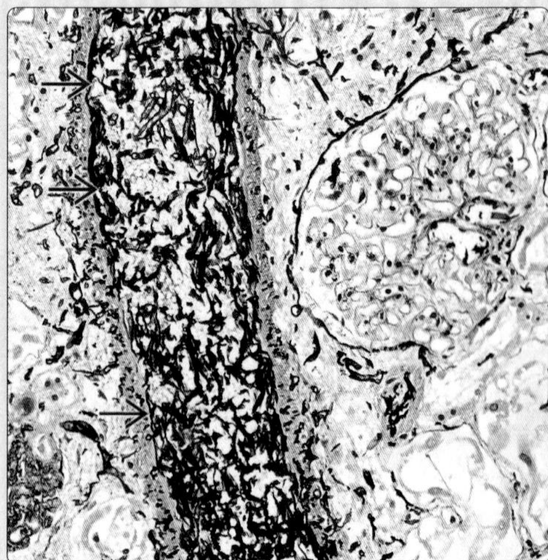

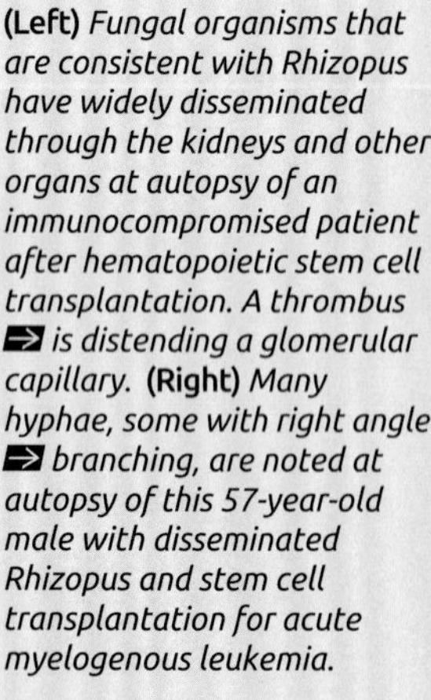

(Left) *Fungal organisms that are consistent with Rhizopus have widely disseminated through the kidneys and other organs at autopsy of an immunocompromised patient after hematopoietic stem cell transplantation. A thrombus → is distending a glomerular capillary.* **(Right)** *Many hyphae, some with right angle → branching, are noted at autopsy of this 57-year-old male with disseminated Rhizopus and stem cell transplantation for acute myelogenous leukemia.*

Glomerular Fungi

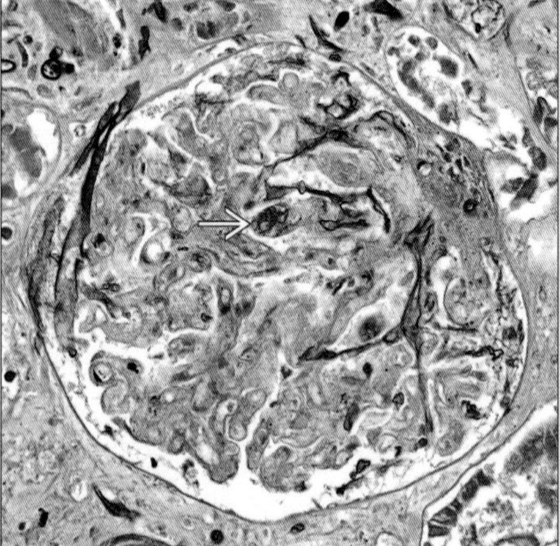

GMS

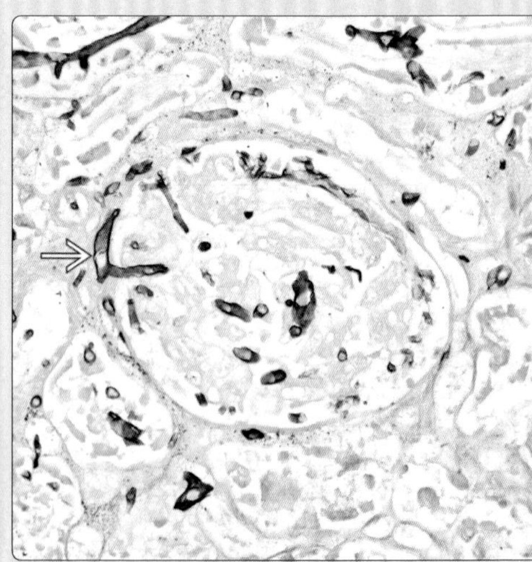

TERMINOLOGY

Synonyms

- Invasive zygomycosis

Definitions

- Fungal infection typically in immunocompromised patients

ETIOLOGY/PATHOGENESIS

Infectious Agents

- *Mucor*
  - Class: Zygomycetes
  - Order: Mucorales
    - Most common species: *Rhizopus*
    - Others (in descending frequency): *Rhizomucor, Cunninghamella, Apophysomyces, Saksenaea, Absidia, Mucor*
  - Ubiquitous organisms found in soil and decaying matter, including moldy bread

CLINICAL ISSUES

Epidemiology

- Incidence
  - Risk factors
    - Diabetes mellitus
    - Leukemia, solid malignancies
    - Immunosuppression
    - Malnourishment

Site

- Sinus and brain (rhinocerebral) ~ 50% of cases
- Lungs, skin
- GI, kidney: Less common

Presentation

- Acute kidney injury
- Fever
- Flank pain
- Rapidly progressive course
- Hematuria

Laboratory Tests

- Fungal cultures
- Biopsy

Treatment

- Surgical approaches
  - Complete debridement of infected tissue
- Drugs
  - Antifungal therapy
    - Amphotericin B
  - Reduction of immunosuppressive agents

Prognosis

- Poor: > 50% mortality in disseminated disease
  - Mucormycosis isolated to kidney may have better prognosis

MACROSCOPIC

General Features

- Arterial thrombosis
  - Main renal artery
  - Arcuate &/or interlobar arteries
- Large infarcts
- Papillary necrosis (rare)

MICROSCOPIC

Histologic Features

- Nonseptate fungal hyphae with 90° branching
  - Found in infarcts, granulomata, thrombi, microabscesses
- Cortical necrosis
- Thrombi
- Arteritis
- Microabscesses
- Granulomatous interstitial nephritis
  - Frequent multinucleated giant cells

DIFFERENTIAL DIAGNOSIS

Aspergillosis

- Septate hyphae with 45° branching

Pseudallescheriasis

- Septate hyphae

Fusariosis

- Septate hyphae

Candidiasis

- Pseudohyphae and budding yeast forms

Tuberculosis

- Caseating necrosis in granulomas with acid-fast bacilli

Bacterial Pyelonephritis

- Prominent neutrophilic infiltrate or abscesses
- No fungal organisms

Sarcoidosis

- Granulomatous inflammation without microorganisms

DIAGNOSTIC CHECKLIST

Pathologic Interpretation Pearls

- Difficult to distinguish fungal species based on morphologic evaluation alone
- Fungal cultures establish diagnosis

SELECTED REFERENCES

1. Park W et al: Allograft mucormycosis due to Rhizopus microsporus in a kidney transplant recipient. Transplant Proc. 46(2):623-5, 2014
2. Gupta KL et al: Mucormycosis of the transplanted kidney with renal papillary necrosis. Exp Clin Transplant. 11(6):554-7, 2013
3. Kuy S et al: Renal mucormycosis: a rare and potentially lethal complication of kidney transplantation. Case Rep Transplant. 2013:915423, 2013
4. Tayyebi N et al: Renal allograft mucormycosis: report of two cases. Surg Infect (Larchmt). 8(5):535-8, 2007
5. Chkhotua A et al: Mucormycosis of the renal allograft: case report and review of the literature. Transpl Int. 14(6):438-41, 2001
6. Gupta KL et al: Renal zygomycosis: an under-diagnosed cause of acute renal failure. Nephrol Dial Transplant. 14(11):2720-5, 1999

KEY FACTS

TERMINOLOGY

- *Candida* infection of kidney
  - Typically in immunocompromised patient

ETIOLOGY/PATHOGENESIS

- *C. albicans*, *glabrata*, *parapsilosis*, and *tropicalis*

CLINICAL ISSUES

- Therapeutic options
  - Fluconazole
  - Amphotericin B
  - Reduction of immunosuppressive agents
  - Transplant nephrectomy

MACROSCOPIC

- Cortical abscesses
- Papillary necrosis
- Pyelitis
- Mycotic pseudoaneurysm

MICROSCOPIC

- Fungal organisms
  - Pseudohyphae
  - Budding yeast forms
- Cortical abscesses
  - May be centered around glomeruli
  - Rare cortical infarcts
- Granulomatous interstitial inflammation

TOP DIFFERENTIAL DIAGNOSES

- Aspergillosis
- Mucormycosis
- Fusariosis
- Pseudallescheriasis

DIAGNOSTIC CHECKLIST

- Budding yeast and pseudohyphae combination characteristic
- Fungal cultures needed for definitive identification

Microabscesses

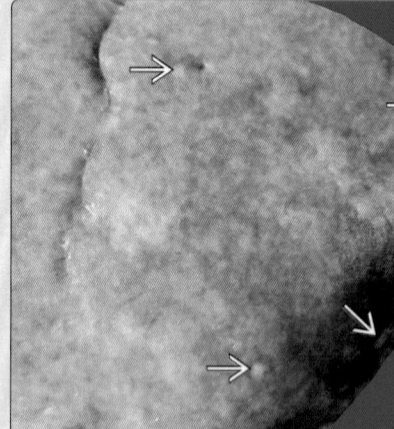

Candida Colonization of Papilla

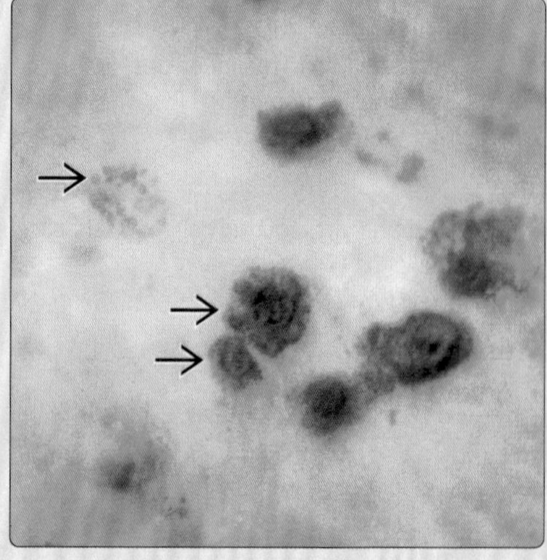

(Left) *Gross photograph of the capsular surface of this kidney at autopsy shows many small abscesses due to disseminated candidiasis from Candida tropicalis.* **(Right)** *Gross photograph shows prominent small and large green lesions on the renal papilla of this autopsy specimen representing colonization by Candida. (Courtesy C. Abrahams, MD.)*

Granulomatous Inflammation

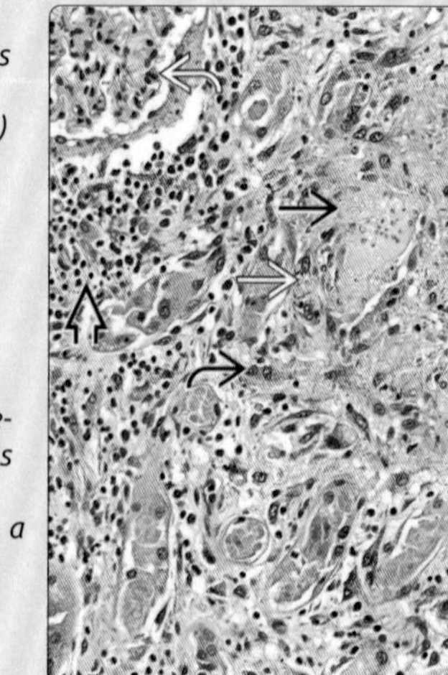

Candida Yeast and Pseudohyphae

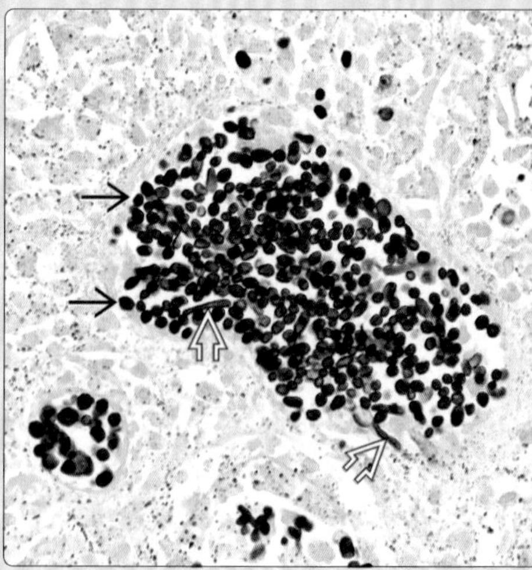

(Left) *Hematoxylin & eosin stain shows fungal organisms intermixed with a Tamm-Horsfall protein (uromodulin) with focal necrosis and rupture of the tubules associated with a granulomatous reaction and scattered interstitial lymphocytes. The glomerulus is normal.* **(Right)** *Gomori methenamine-silver stain shows yeast forms within the renal tubules and a few pseudohyphae, a helpful finding in the identification of Candida.*

TERMINOLOGY

Definitions

- *Candida* infection of kidney
  - Typically in immunocompromised patient

ETIOLOGY/PATHOGENESIS

Infectious Agents

- *C. albicans*
  - Normal flora of skin, gastrointestinal, and genitourinary tracts
- *C. glabrata*
  - Previously named *Torulopsis glabrata* (or torulopsosis)
- *C. parapsilosis*
- *C. tropicalis*
- *C. krusei*

CLINICAL ISSUES

Epidemiology

- Incidence
  - 8 cases per 100,000 persons in United States
  - 4th most common nosocomial bloodstream infection
  - Risk factors include diabetes, chemotherapy, immunosuppression
- Age
  - Neonates
    - Very low birth weight babies susceptible to invasive candidiasis
  - Elderly
    - > 65 years of age
- Ethnicity
  - Higher incidence among African Americans

Presentation

- Renal dysfunction or acute kidney injury
  - May be due to ureteral or bladder obstruction by *Candida*

Laboratory Tests

- Fungal culture
- Direct microscopy

Treatment

- Drugs
  - Fluconazole
  - Echinocandins
  - Voriconazole
  - Amphotericin B
- Reduction of immunosuppression
- Renal allograft nephrectomy

Prognosis

- Up to 50% mortality in disseminated or invasive candidiasis

IMAGING

CT Findings

- Hypodense lesions correspond to renal abscesses
- Fungus balls
- Papillary necrosis

MACROSCOPIC

General Features

- Abscesses
  - Cortical abscesses
    - Miliary distribution
  - Perinephric abscesses
- Pyelitis
  - Fungus balls
- Papillary necrosis
  - 20% of patients with disseminated candidiasis at autopsy
- Mycotic pseudoaneurysm or occlusion of major renal arteries in allograft

MICROSCOPIC

Histologic Features

- Cortical abscesses
  - May be centered around glomeruli
  - Rare cortical infarcts
- Fungal organisms
  - Pseudohyphae
  - Budding yeast forms, 4-6 μm
  - May be in glomerular capillaries &/or arterioles
- Granulomatous interstitial nephritis
  - Multinucleated giant cells (atypical feature)
  - May contain predominantly budding yeast forms

DIFFERENTIAL DIAGNOSIS

Aspergillosis

- Septate hyphae with 45° branching

Mucormycosis

- Nonseptate hyphae with 90° branching

Cryptococcosis

- Capsule-deficient variant mimics *Candida* yeast forms

Fusariosis

- Septate hyphae

Pseudallescheriasis

- Septate hyphae

DIAGNOSTIC CHECKLIST

Pathologic Interpretation Pearls

- Budding yeast and pseudohyphae combination characteristic
- Fungal cultures needed for definitive identification

SELECTED REFERENCES

1. Weerakkody RM et al: Invasive candidiasis complicating renal transplantation. Nephrology (Carlton). 18(2):157, 2013
2. Bagnasco SM et al: Fungal infection presenting as giant cell tubulointerstitial nephritis in kidney allograft. Transpl Infect Dis. 14(3):288-91, 2012
3. Wasi N et al: A rare case of acute renal failure due to massive renal allograft infiltration with Candida glabrata. Nephrol Dial Transplant. 23(1):374-6, 2008
4. Meehan SM et al: Granulomatous tubulointerstitial nephritis in the renal allograft. Am J Kidney Dis. 36(4):E27, 2000

KEY FACTS

TERMINOLOGY

- Synonyms
  - Ohio valley disease
  - Darling disease

ETIOLOGY/PATHOGENESIS

- *Histoplasma capsulatum*
  - Dimorphic fungus
  - Endemic to Mississippi and Ohio river valleys
  - Present in soil
  - Inhalation of airborne conidia (spores)

CLINICAL ISSUES

- M:F = 4:1

MACROSCOPIC

- Discrete nodular masses
- Papillary necrosis
- Diffuse inflammation and necrosis

MICROSCOPIC

- Oval to round fungal organisms, 2-4 μm in diameter
- Granulomatous interstitial nephritis
  - Noncaseating granulomas
  - Focal necrosis, medulla
  - Prominent interstitial inflammation
- Cortical necrosis
- Thrombotic microangiopathy
- Mesangial proliferative glomerulonephritis (rare)

TOP DIFFERENTIAL DIAGNOSES

- Blastomycosis
- Cryptococcosis
- Candidiasis
- Tuberculosis
- Coccidioidomycosis
- Sarcoidosis
- Drug-induced acute interstitial nephritis

(Left) *Hematoxylin and eosin shows extensive cortical necrosis at autopsy in a kidney with numerous round Histoplasma organisms due to disseminated disease in a patient with AIDS. A remnant of a tubule is noted ⮕.* **(Right)** *Gomori methenamine-silver stain highlights numerous fungal organisms from a patient with disseminated histoplasmosis within a necrotic area of the renal cortex.*

Cortical Necrosis

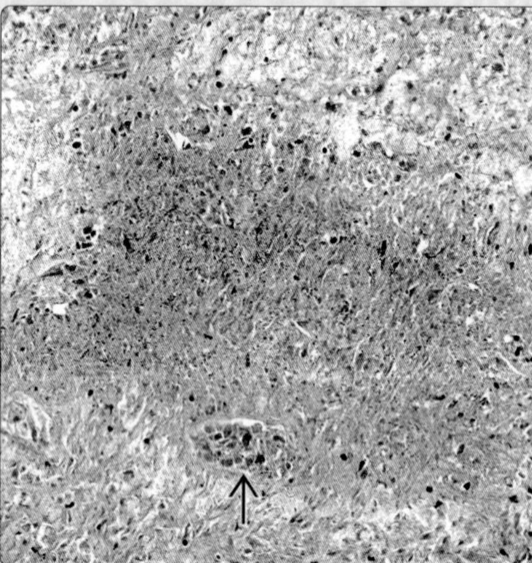

Gomori Methenamine Silver

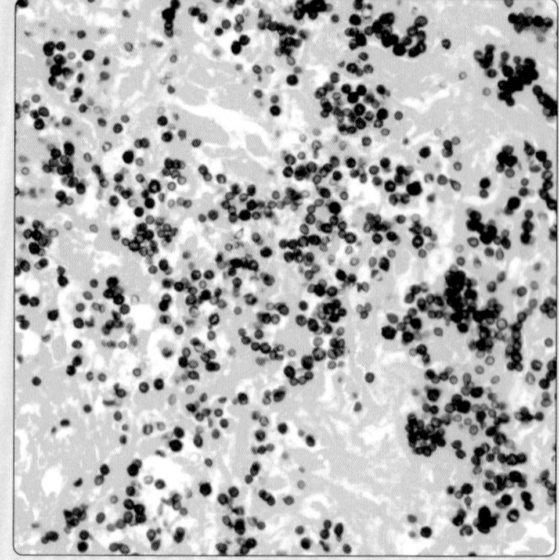

(Left) *Periodic acid-Schiff stain shows numerous clusters of round organisms ⮕ characteristic of Histoplasma capsulatum within the renal tubules.* **(Right)** *Gomori methenamine-silver stain confirms scattered Histoplasma organisms ⮕, which are smaller in diameter than the red blood cells (6-8 μm in diameter) ⇨ within an adjacent peritubular capillary.*

Histoplasma Capsulatum

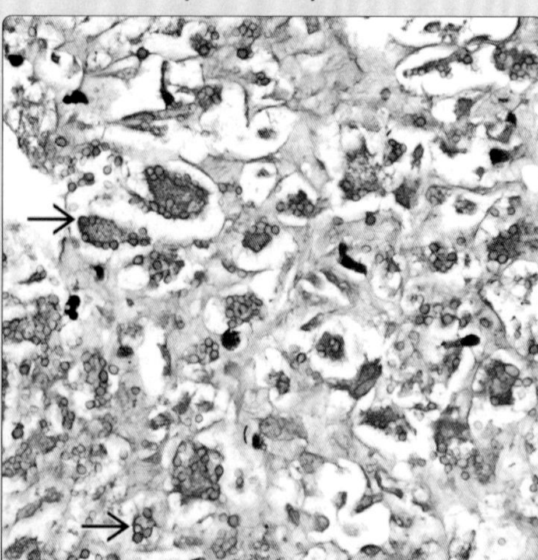

Histoplasma and RBCs

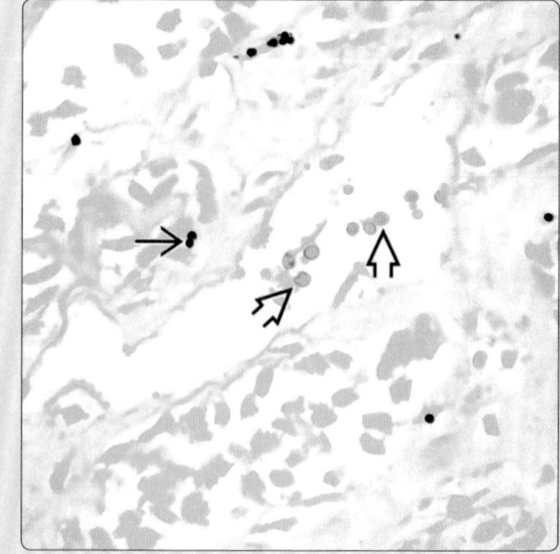

ETIOLOGY/PATHOGENESIS

Environmental Exposure

- Present in soil
  - Bird or bat droppings
- Inhalation of airborne conidia (spores)

Infectious Agents

- *Histoplasma capsulatum*
  - Dimorphic fungus (yeast in body, mycelia in soil)
  - Endemic to Mississippi and Ohio river valleys
  - South and Central America, Africa, Australia, and East Asia

CLINICAL ISSUES

Epidemiology

- Incidence
  - Kidney involved in 40% with disseminated disease
  - AIDS patients in endemic areas at risk (10-25%)
- Sex
  - M:F = 4:1
    - Similar gender exposure based on skin tests

Presentation

- Asymptomatic renal involvement
  - Renal dysfunction unusual
- Flu-like acute respiratory infection
- Hemophagocytic syndrome
- Chronic form mimics tuberculosis

Laboratory Tests

- Radioimmunoassay
  - *Histoplasma capsulatum* polysaccharide antigen
- Complement fixation test
  - More sensitive, less specific than immunodiffusion
  - False-positives from cross-reactivity with antigens from *Blastomyces dermatitidis* and *Coccidioides immitis*
- Immunodiffusion
- Culture
- Biopsy

Treatment

- Drugs
  - Amphotericin B
  - Ketoconazole
  - Itraconazole
  - Fluconazole
  - Decreased immunosuppression

Prognosis

- Disseminated form fatal without treatment
  - May lead to irreversible renal failure
- Localized form in normal individuals (self-limiting)

MACROSCOPIC

General Features

- Discrete nodular masses
- Papillary necrosis
- Diffuse inflammation and necrosis

MICROSCOPIC

Histologic Features

- Fungi are oval to round, 2-4 μm in diameter
- Granulomatous interstitial nephritis
  - Noncaseating granulomas
  - Occasional intratubular granulomas
  - Organisms in macrophages
  - Absence of granulomatous response in severely immunosuppressed patients
  - Focal necrosis, medulla
  - Prominent interstitial inflammation
- Cortical necrosis
- Thrombotic microangiopathy
  - Glomerular capillary thrombi with entrapped fungal organisms may be observed
- Mesangial proliferative glomerulonephritis
  - Rare association with disseminated histoplasmosis
  - *H. capsulatum* antigen detected in mesangial areas

DIFFERENTIAL DIAGNOSIS

Blastomycosis

- 8-15 μm in diameter
- Thick wall and broad-based budding

Cryptococcosis

- 5-10 μm
- Capsule-deficient variant causes granulomatous inflammation
  - Fontana-Masson silver stain positive

Candidiasis

- Budding yeasts may resemble *Histoplasma*

Coccidioidomycosis

- 30-60 μm in diameter
- Endospores (2-5 μm in diameter) resemble *Histoplasma*

Tuberculosis

- Caseating granulomas with acid-fast bacilli

Sarcoidosis

- Noncaseating granulomas without microorganisms

Drug-Induced Acute Interstitial Nephritis

- No microorganisms

DIAGNOSTIC CHECKLIST

Pathologic Interpretation Pearls

- Necrotizing granulomas
- Yeast forms smaller than erythrocytes

SELECTED REFERENCES

1. Nieto-Ríos JF et al: Disseminated histoplasmosis and haemophagocytic syndrome in two kidney transplant patients. Nefrologia. 32(5):683-4, 2012
2. Singh N et al: Donor-derived fungal infections in organ transplant recipients: guidelines of the American Society of Transplantation, infectious diseases community of practice. Am J Transplant. 12(9):2414-28, 2012
3. Sethi S: Acute renal failure in a renal allograft: an unusual infectious cause of thrombotic microangiopathy. Am J Kidney Dis. 46(1):159-62, 2005
4. Burke DG et al: Histoplasmosis and kidney disease in patients with AIDS. Clin Infect Dis. 25(2):281-4, 1997

Coccidioidomycosis

KEY FACTS

ETIOLOGY/PATHOGENESIS

- *Coccidioides immitis*
  - Geographically limited to California San Joaquin valley, southwestern United States, and Mexico
- *C. posadasii*
  - Geographically limited to southwestern United States, Mexico, and South America
- Acquired through inhalation of fungal spores (arthroconidia) in environment
- Dimorphic fungi

CLINICAL ISSUES

- Flu-like symptoms
- Surgical resection for some with pulmonary, bone, or joint involvement
- Fluconazole: First-line agent

MACROSCOPIC

- Perinephric abscess

MICROSCOPIC

- *Coccidioides* spherules
  - Round, thick-walled (PAS & methenamine silver positive)
  - 10-80 μm in diameter
  - Contain numerous endospores (2-5 μm in diameter)
- Necrotic nodules
  - Septate hyphae seen in transitional form
- Granulomatous interstitial inflammation
  - Absent in severely immunocompromised patients

TOP DIFFERENTIAL DIAGNOSES

- Blastomycosis
- Cryptococcoccosis

DIAGNOSTIC CHECKLIST

- Spherules and endospores characteristic for *Coccidioides*
- Rare renal involvement
- Fungal cultures and serologic tests confirm presence of coccidioidomycosis

Immature Coccidioides Spherules

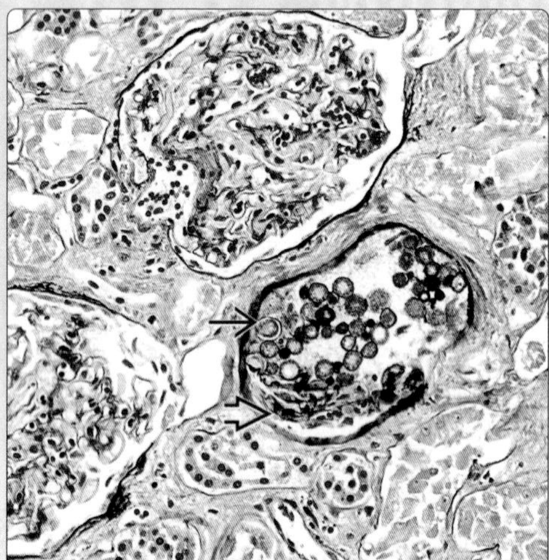

Mature Spherule With Endospores

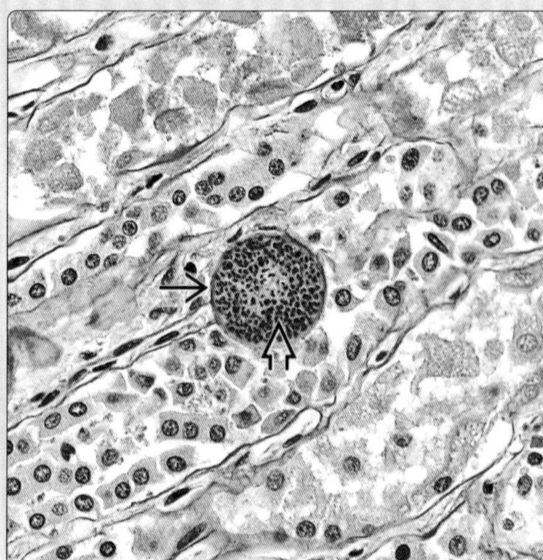

(Left) *Jones methenamine silver shows numerous immature Coccidioides spherules* ⇒ *compressing the glomerulus* ⇒ *within the urinary space in a patient with disseminated disease. (Courtesy E. Bracamonte, MD.)* **(Right)** *Periodic acid-Schiff shows a thick-walled mature spherule* ⇒ *with endospores* ⇒ *characteristic of Coccidioides among the renal tubules (possibly within a peritubular capillary) of this autopsy kidney. (Courtesy E. Bracamonte, MD.)*

Numerous Immature Spherules and Endospores

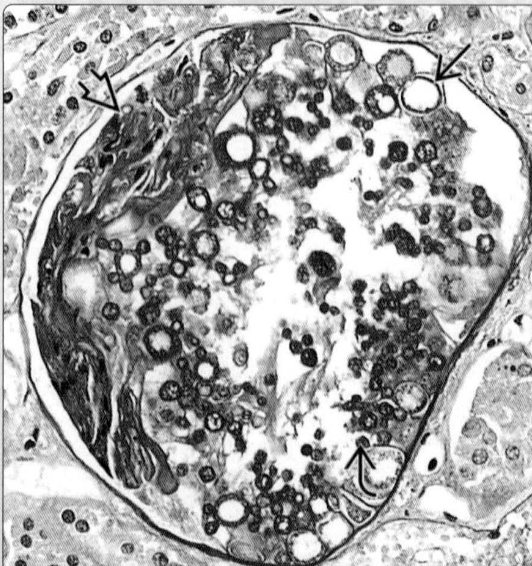

Immature Spherules and Endospores

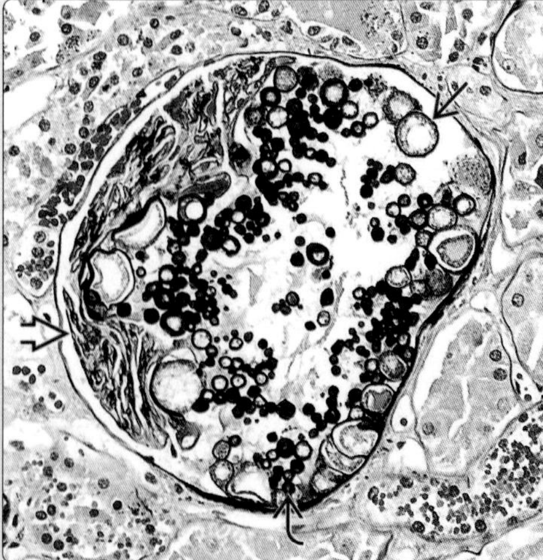

(Left) *Periodic acid-Schiff shows numerous immature spherules* ⇒ *and endospores* ⇒ *that are characteristic of Coccidioides immitis within the Bowman space compressing the adjacent glomerulus* ⇒*. (Courtesy E. Bracamonte, MD.)* **(Right)** *Jones methenamine silver shows immature spherules* ⇒ *and endospores* ⇒ *of Coccidioides within the urinary space and compressing the adjacent glomerulus* ⇒*. (Courtesy E. Bracamonte, MD.)*

TERMINOLOGY

Synonyms

- Valley fever

ETIOLOGY/PATHOGENESIS

Infectious Agents

- *Coccidioides immitis*
  - Geographically limited to California San Joaquin valley, southwestern United States, and Mexico
- *C. posadasii*
  - Geographically limited to southwestern United States, Mexico, and South America
- Acquired through inhalation of fungal spores (arthroconidia)
- Dimorphic fungi

CLINICAL ISSUES

Epidemiology

- Incidence
  - ~ 3% among renal transplant patients in endemic regions
  - Typically occurs within 1st year post transplantation
- Sex
  - Pregnancy is risk factor for disseminated disease
- Ethnicity
  - African, Asian, and Hispanic descent more likely than Caucasians to develop disseminated disease

Presentation

- Flu-like symptoms
  - Fever
  - Cough
  - Myalgia
  - Rash
- Eosinophilia
- Acute renal failure

Laboratory Tests

- Skin test
  - 10-50% of those in endemic areas test positive
  - Coccidioidin
  - Spherulin
- Enzyme immunoassay
  - IgA
  - IgM
    - Antibodies difficult to detect in immunosuppressed patients
- Immunodiffusion assay
- Complement fixation test
- Culture
  - Sputum
  - Other body fluids
- Direct microscopy

Treatment

- Surgical approaches
  - Surgical resection for some with pulmonary, bone, or joint involvement
- Drugs
  - Fluconazole
  - Amphotericin B
    - Second-line agent
    - Used for disseminated disease or azole-resistant strains of *Coccidioides*
  - Reduction of immunosuppressive agents

Prognosis

- Good in limited disease
- Poor in disseminated disease
  - Mortality rate > 50%
  - Up to 75% mortality rate in transplant patients

IMAGING

Radiographic Findings

- Pyelocalyceal alterations similar to tuberculosis in transplant kidneys
- Compression of renal transplant artery may be detected by angiogram

MACROSCOPIC

General Features

- Perinephric abscess

MICROSCOPIC

Histologic Features

- *Coccidioides* spherules
  - Round, thick walled (PAS & methenamine silver positive)
  - 10-80 μm in diameter
  - Contain numerous endospores (2-5 μm in diameter)
- Necrotic nodules
  - Septate hyphae seen in transitional form
- Granulomatous interstitial inflammation
  - Absent in severely immunocompromised patients

DIFFERENTIAL DIAGNOSIS

Blastomycosis

- 8-15 μm in diameter

Cryptococcosis

- Capsule-deficient variant, silver stain positive
- No endospores

DIAGNOSTIC CHECKLIST

Pathologic Interpretation Pearls

- Spherules and endospores characteristic for *Coccidioides*
- Rare renal involvement

SELECTED REFERENCES

1. Singh N et al: Donor-derived fungal infections in organ transplant recipients: guidelines of the American Society of Transplantation, infectious diseases community of practice. Am J Transplant. 12(9):2414-28, 2012
2. Baden LR et al: Case records of the Massachusetts General Hospital. Case 35-2009. A 60-year-old male renal-transplant recipient with renal insufficiency, diabetic ketoacidosis, and mental-status changes. N Engl J Med. 361(20):1980-9, 2009
3. Braddy CM et al: Coccidioidomycosis after renal transplantation in an endemic area. Am J Transplant. 6(2):340-5, 2006

Blastomycosis

KEY FACTS

TERMINOLOGY

- Synonyms
  - North American blastomycosis
  - Gilchrist disease
  - Chicago disease

ETIOLOGY/PATHOGENESIS

- *Blastomyces dermatitidis*
  - Endemic to central/southern United States, Canada
  - Reported in Central/South America, Europe, and Africa
  - Ubiquitous dimorphic fungus in environment
  - Acquired by inhalation

MACROSCOPIC

- Abscesses
  - Cortical > medullary involvement

MICROSCOPIC

- Microorganisms, fungus
  - Thick wall, 8-15 μm in diameter
  - Broad-based budding
  - Some yeast forms are < 8 μm in diameter
  - May be surrounded by or located within multinucleated giant cells
- Granulomatous inflammation
- Neutrophilic inflammation

TOP DIFFERENTIAL DIAGNOSES

- Cryptococcosis
- Coccidioidomycosis
- Paracoccidioidomycosis
- Candidiasis
- Tuberculosis
- Sarcoidosis

DIAGNOSTIC CHECKLIST

- Coinfection with other fungal or viral organisms common

(Left) *Hematoxylin & eosin shows a microabscess with necrosis ⇨, neutrophils ⇨, and numerous round yeast forms ⇨ in the renal cortex of this kidney involved by disseminated blastomycosis.* **(Right)** *Periodic acid-Schiff demonstrates the characteristic thick capsule ⇨ of Blastomyces, which ranges in diameter from 8-15 μm but may be as large as 30 μm.*

Microabscess

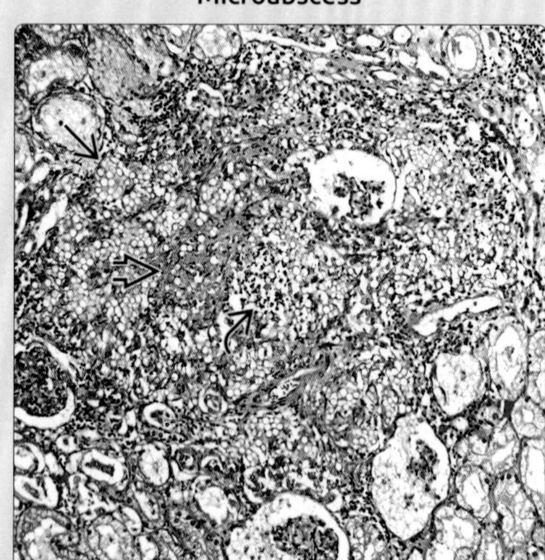

Blastomyces

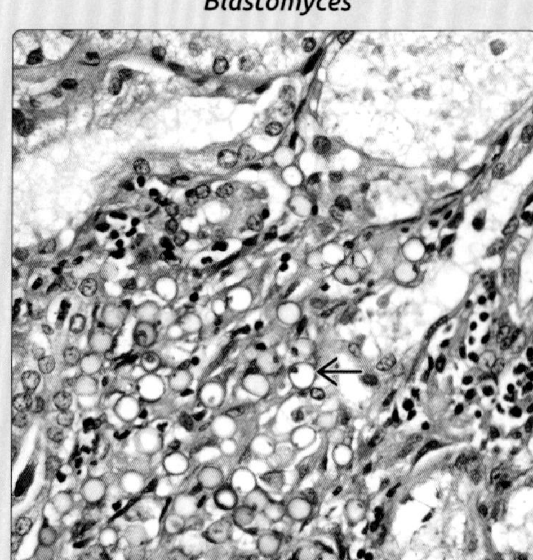

(Left) *GMS (Gomori methenamine-silver) reveals Blastomyces with a broad-based budding yeast form ⇨. The thick capsules ⇨ can resemble those of Cryptococcus and Coccidioides.* **(Right)** *Electron micrograph shows the yeast form of Blastomyces with the outer electron-lucent capsule ⇨ and other internal structures entirely engulfed within a macrophage. (Courtesy J. Taxy, MD.)*

Gomori Methenamine Silver

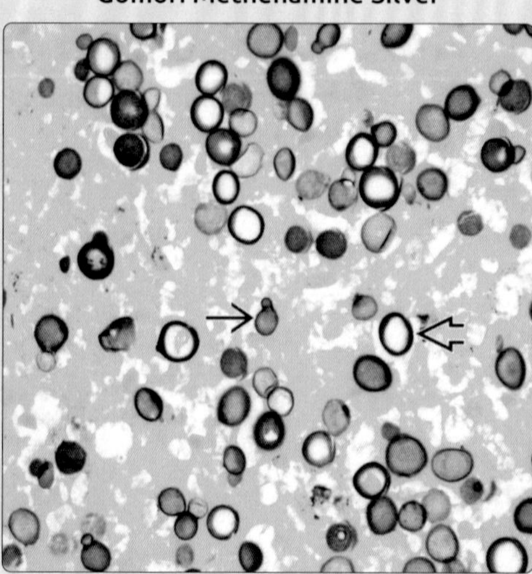

***Blastomyces* Yeast Form**

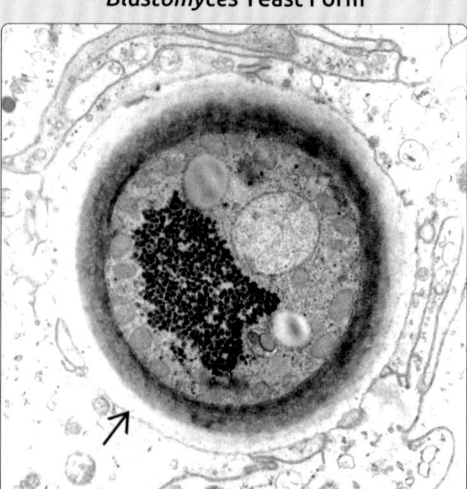

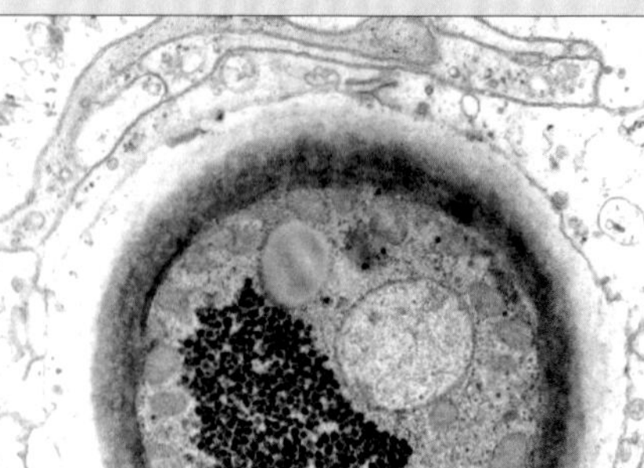

ETIOLOGY/PATHOGENESIS

Environmental Exposure

- Ubiquitous fungus in environment
  - Acquired by inhalation

Infectious Agents

- *Blastomyces dermatitidis*
  - Endemic to central and southern United States and Canada
  - Reported in parts of Central and South America, Europe, and Africa
  - Dimorphic fungus

CLINICAL ISSUES

Epidemiology

- Incidence
  - 1-2 per 100,000 in endemic areas
- Age
  - 30-50 years old
- Sex
  - Male predilection
    - M:F = 2-15:1
- Ethnicity
  - African American predilection

Site

- Lungs
- Skin
- Genitourinary tract
  - Prostate
  - Epididymis
  - Kidney
    - < 10% involvement in disseminated disease

Presentation

- Asymptomatic
  - 50% of cases
- Fever
- Malaise

Laboratory Tests

- Fungal culture
  - Slow growth
- Direct microscopy

Treatment

- Drugs
  - Itraconazole
  - Amphotericin B
  - Ketoconazole
  - Fluconazole
  - Voriconazole

Prognosis

- Overall mortality rate of 4-22%
  - Mortality rate of 90% with kidney involvement
  - Mortality rate of 50% in AIDS patients

MACROSCOPIC

General Features

- Bilateral involvement common
- Abscesses
  - More cortical than medullary involvement
  - Perinephric and sinus

MICROSCOPIC

Histologic Features

- Fungal organisms
  - Thick wall, 8-15 μm in diameter
  - Broad-based budding
  - Some yeast forms are < 8 μm in diameter
  - May be surrounded by or located within multinucleated giant cells
- Granulomatous inflammation
- Neutrophilic inflammation

DIFFERENTIAL DIAGNOSIS

Cryptococcosis

- Capsule or clear halo, mucicarmine positive
- Capsule-deficient variant, silver stain positive

Coccidioidomycosis

- Spherules with characteristic endospores

Paracoccidioidomycosis

- Characteristic clear halos, 12-14 μm in diameter

Candidiasis

- Pseudohyphae and yeasts

Tuberculosis

- Caseating granulomata with acid-fast bacilli

Sarcoidosis

- Granulomatous inflammation without microorganisms

Drug-Induced Acute Interstitial Nephritis

- Granulomatous inflammation without microorganisms

DIAGNOSTIC CHECKLIST

Pathologic Interpretation Pearls

- Coinfection with other fungal or viral organisms common

SELECTED REFERENCES

1. Barocas JA et al: Peritonitis caused by Blastomyces dermatitidis in a kidney transplant recipient: case report and literature review. Transpl Infect Dis. 16(4):634-41, 2014
2. Taxy JB: Blastomycosis: contributions of morphology to diagnosis: a surgical pathology, cytopathology, and autopsy pathology study. Am J Surg Pathol. 31(4):615-23, 2007
3. Dworkin MS et al: The epidemiology of blastomycosis in Illinois and factors associated with death. Clin Infect Dis. 41(12):e107-11, 2005
4. Lemos LB et al: Blastomycosis: organ involvement and etiologic diagnosis. A review of 123 patients from Mississippi. Ann Diagn Pathol. 4(6):391-406, 2000
5. Sekhon AS et al: Blastomycosis: report of three cases from Alberta with a review of Canadian cases. Mycopathologia. 68(1):53-63, 1979

Paracoccidioidomycosis

KEY FACTS

TERMINOLOGY

- Synonyms
  - South American blastomycosis
  - Brazilian blastomycosis

ETIOLOGY/PATHOGENESIS

- *Paracoccidioides brasiliensis*
  - Endemic to South America and Brazil

CLINICAL ISSUES

- Male predilection
- Laboratory testing
  - Enzyme-linked immunoassay
  - Complement fixation test
  - Culture
  - Biopsy
- Drugs
  - Itraconazole: First-line agent

MICROSCOPIC

- Granulomatous interstitial nephritis
- Glomerular granulomas
- Glomerular capillary thrombi
- Glomerular fibrinoid necrosis
- Yeast forms with clear halos

TOP DIFFERENTIAL DIAGNOSES

- Cryptococcosis
- Lobomycosis
- Blastomycosis
- Tuberculosis
- Sarcoidosis
- Drug-induced acute interstitial nephritis

Granulomatous Inflammation

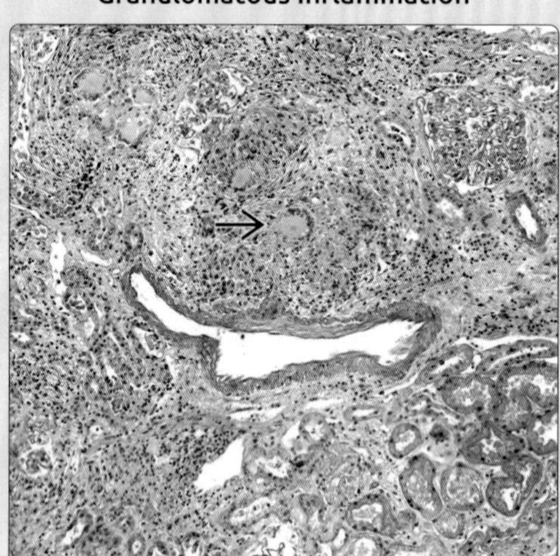

Granulomata

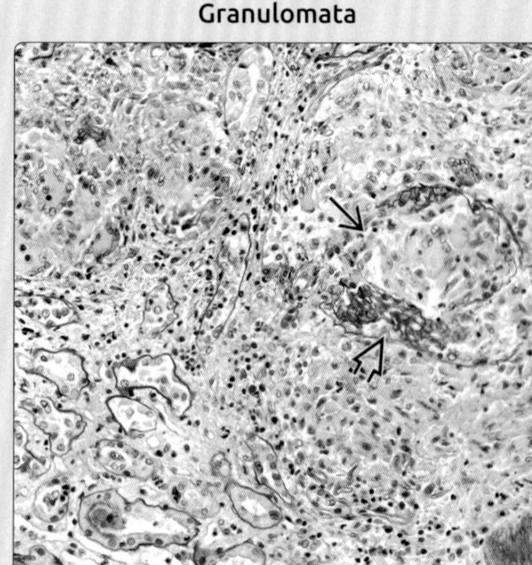

(Left) *Light microscopy shows a granuloma in the cortex with prominent Langhans giant cells ⇨ surrounded by mononuclear cells in a Brazilian male with renal failure. (Courtesy A. Billis, MD.)* **(Right)** *Periodic acid-Schiff shows interstitial and glomerular granulomas ⇨ with glomerular destruction ⇨ in a severe case with a miliary pattern of systemic involvement. Lungs, lymph nodes, and oral mucosa are commonly involved, and less commonly the kidney, spleen, bones, and meninges. (Courtesy A. Billis, MD.)*

Gomori Methenamine Silver

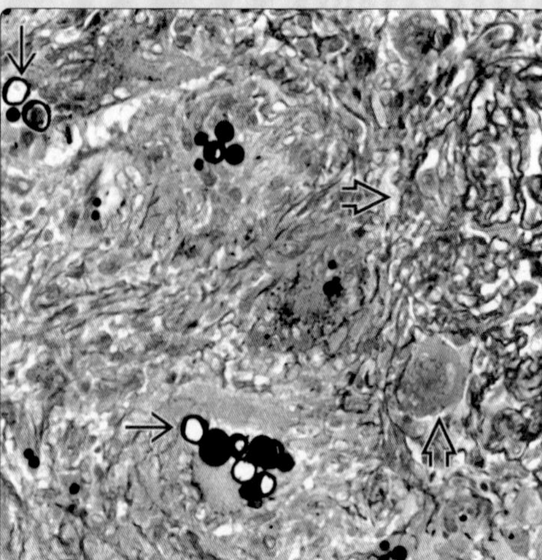

Electron Microscopy

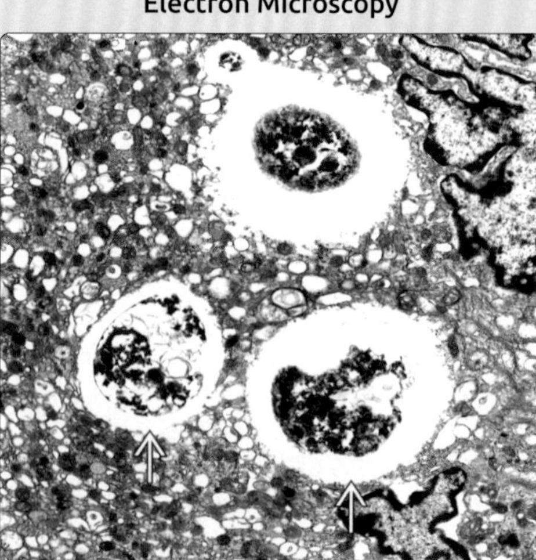

(Left) *Grocott-Gomori methenamine silver stain of granulomas containing fungal bodies shows strong peripheral silver uptake ⇨. An adjacent glomerulus contains a granuloma ⇨. The mechanism of glomerular involvement is believed to be embolic lodging of fungi in the capillaries with subsequent thrombus and inflammation. (Courtesy A. Billis, MD.)* **(Right)** *Electron micrograph of mononuclear giant cells shows 3 Paracoccidioides brasiliensis fungal organisms ➡ with a clear halo. (Courtesy A. Billis, MD.)*

TERMINOLOGY

Abbreviations

- Paracoccidioidomycosis (PCM)

Synonyms

- South American blastomycosis
- Brazilian blastomycosis

ETIOLOGY/PATHOGENESIS

Environmental Exposure

- Agricultural and construction workers

Infectious Agents

- *Paracoccidioides brasiliensis*
  - Endemic in South America
  - Dimorphic fungus
    - Septate hyphae at room temperature
    - Yeast forms at body temperature
  - Acquired through inhalation

CLINICAL ISSUES

Epidemiology

- Incidence
  - Rare
- Age
  - Usually > 30 years of age
  - Rare in children or teenagers
- Sex
  - Strong male predilection
    - M:F = 15-78:1

Presentation

- Asymptomatic
- Acute renal failure

Laboratory Tests

- Skin test
  - Positive result indicates exposure not active disease
- Enzyme-linked immunoassay
  - Detects antibodies to gp43
    - High sensitivity and specificity
- Complement fixation test
  - May cross-react with *Histoplasma capsulatum* antigen
- Immunodiffusion
- Western blot
  - High sensitivity and specificity
- Fungal culture
  - Sabouraud dextrose agar
  - Up to 30 days of growth
    - Growth of yeast form at 37°C confirms diagnosis
- Direct microscopy
  - Wet mount with potassium hydroxide
    - 1 large yeast with budding forms resembles "pilot wheel"
- Biopsy

Natural History

- Generally asymptomatic in immunocompetent hosts

Treatment

- Drugs
  - Itraconazole has low rate of relapse
  - Ketoconazole, sulfonamide, amphotericin B
  - Reduction of immunosuppressive agents in transplant patients

Prognosis

- Poor prognosis in rare juvenile form of disease
- If untreated: Up to 25% mortality rate
- If treated: Good prognosis

MICROSCOPIC

Histologic Features

- Glomeruli
  - Granulomas
    - May resemble cellular crescents
  - Fibrinoid necrosis
  - Capillary thrombi
- Tubules and Interstitium
  - Granulomatous interstitial nephritis
    - Associated with *Paracoccidioides* organisms
    - Caseating necrosis occasionally present
    - Multinucleated giant cells
  - Prominent acute inflammation
    - Pyogenic abscesses
  - Fungal organisms
    - Characteristic clear halos
    - Budding yeast forms, 12-14 μm in diameter
- Vessels: No specific lesions

DIFFERENTIAL DIAGNOSIS

Cryptococcosis

- Capsule positive for mucicarmine stain

Blastomycosis

- 8-15 μm in diameter
- DNA confirmation probe may cross-react with *Paracoccidioides*

Tuberculosis

- Caseating granulomas
- Acid-fast bacilli present
- Coinfection with PCM reported

DIAGNOSTIC CHECKLIST

Pathologic Interpretation Pearls

- Fungal culture or serologic tests confirm infection by *Paracoccidioides brasiliensis*

SELECTED REFERENCES

1. Batista MV et al: Recipient of kidney from donor with asymptomatic infection by Paracoccidioides brasiliensis. Med Mycol. 50(2):187-92, 2012
2. Zavascki AP et al: Paracoccidioidomycosis in organ transplant recipient: case report. Rev Inst Med Trop Sao Paulo. 46(5):279-81, 2004
3. Shikanai-Yasuda MA et al: Paracoccidioidomycosis in a renal transplant recipient. J Med Vet Mycol. 33(6):411-4, 1995

Aspergillosis

KEY FACTS

ETIOLOGY/PATHOGENESIS

- *Aspergillus* species, ubiquitous fungi in environment
  - *A. fumigatus, A. flavus, A. niger*

CLINICAL ISSUES

- Incidence
  - 0.1% in kidney transplant patients after 1 year
  - 30-40% renal involvement in disseminated aspergillosis
    - 50-100% mortality rate for invasive aspergillosis
- Presentation
  - Fever
  - Flank pain
  - Hematuria
- Laboratory tests
  - Cultures
- Treatment
  - Renal allograft nephrectomy
  - Nephrostomy drainage and systemic antifungal therapy
  - Voriconazole

MACROSCOPIC

- Abscesses, cortical or perinephric

MICROSCOPIC

- Microorganisms, fungus
  - Septate hyphae with 45° angle branching
  - Vascular invasion
- Tubulointerstitial inflammation, neutrophil rich

TOP DIFFERENTIAL DIAGNOSES

- Candidiasis
- Mucormycosis
- Pseudallescheriasis
- Fusariosis
- Bacterial pyelonephritis

(Left) *Hematoxylin & eosin shows a necrotic area of renal cortex with prominent neutrophilic inflammation and many acute angle branching hyphae ⇨ that are characteristic of Aspergillus.* **(Right)** *Hematoxylin & eosin shows septate hyphae ⇨ with 45° angle branching, which has entirely replaced a glomerulus in an autopsied kidney of a patient with disseminated aspergillosis.*

Cortical Necrosis

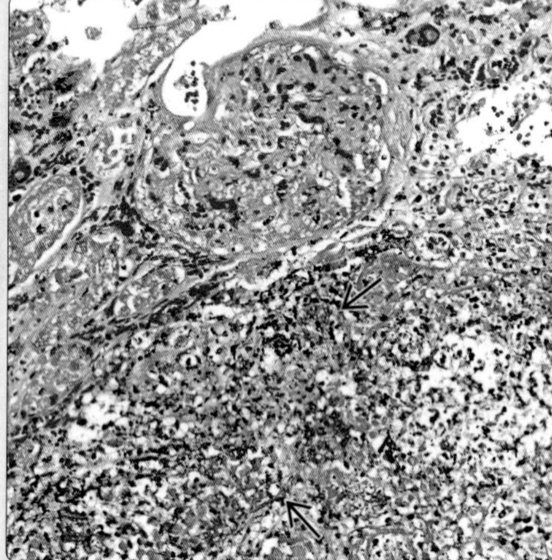

Glomerular Aspergillosis

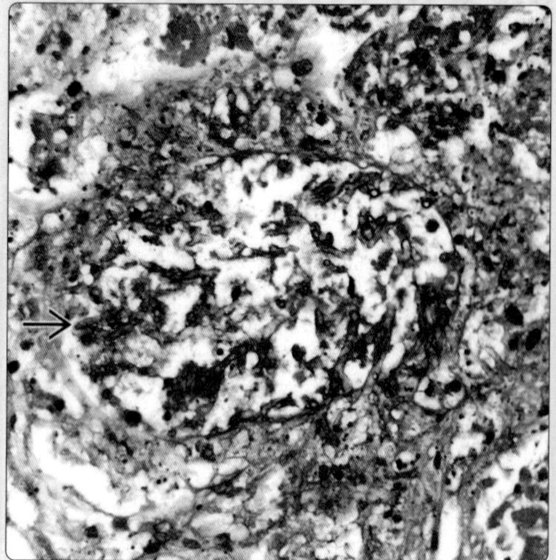

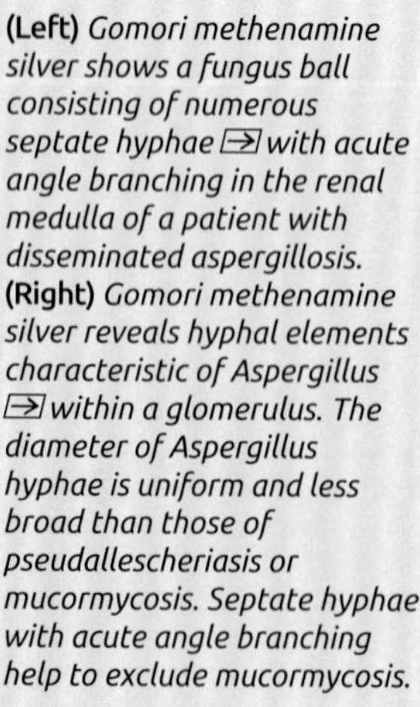

(Left) *Gomori methenamine silver shows a fungus ball consisting of numerous septate hyphae ⇨ with acute angle branching in the renal medulla of a patient with disseminated aspergillosis.* **(Right)** *Gomori methenamine silver reveals hyphal elements characteristic of Aspergillus ⇨ within a glomerulus. The diameter of Aspergillus hyphae is uniform and less broad than those of pseudallescheriasis or mucormycosis. Septate hyphae with acute angle branching help to exclude mucormycosis.*

Gomori Methenamine Silver

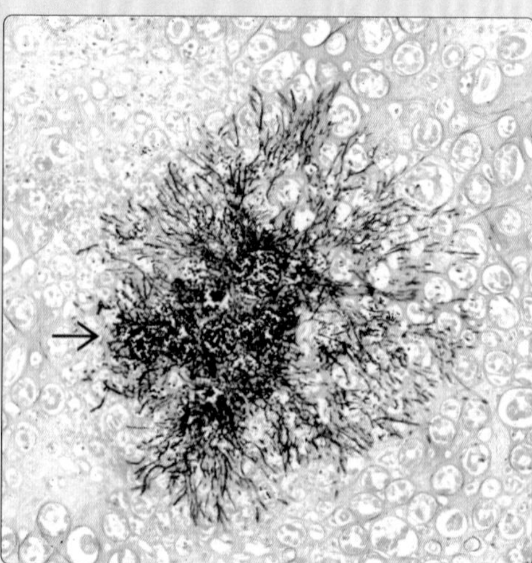

Gomori Methenamine Silver

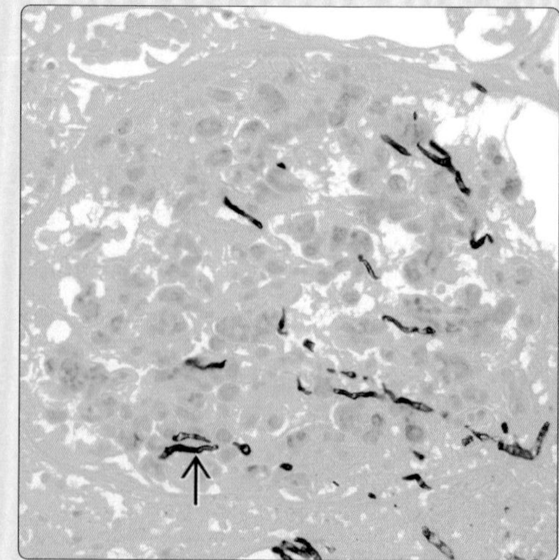

TERMINOLOGY

Definitions

- *Aspergillus* infection of kidney in immunosuppressed or immunocompromised patients

ETIOLOGY/PATHOGENESIS

Environmental Exposure

- Ubiquitous fungus in environment

Infectious Agents

- *Aspergillus*
  - *A. fumigatus*
  - *A. flavus*
  - *A. niger*
  - *A. terreus*
  - *A. nidulans*

CLINICAL ISSUES

Epidemiology

- Incidence
  - 0.1% in kidney transplant patients after 1 year
- Sex
  - M:F = 4:1

Site

- Kidneys
  - 30-40% involvement in disseminated aspergillosis
  - Isolated involvement in some deceased donor allografts
    - Probable transmission from deceased donor or during organ procurement
    - Fungi account for up to 2.5% of isolates cultured from perfusion solutions used for kidney preservation

Presentation

- Fever
- Flank pain
- Hematuria

Laboratory Tests

- Serologic tests
  - Enzyme-linked immunoassay
    - Detection of galactomannan antigen of *Aspergillus*
  - Immunodiffusion
  - Complement fixation
- Cultures
- Direct microscopy

Treatment

- Surgical approaches
  - Renal allograft nephrectomy
  - Nephrostomy drainage and systemic antifungal therapy
- Drugs
  - Voriconazole: First-line agent for invasive aspergillosis
  - Itraconazole, amphotericin B
- Reduction of immunosuppressive agents in transplant patients

Prognosis

- 50-100% mortality rate for invasive aspergillosis
- Risk factors for mortality
  - Disseminated infection, leukopenia, serum galactomannan level

IMAGING

CT Findings

- Hypodense lesions in kidney

MACROSCOPIC

General Features

- Abscesses
  - Cortical
  - Perinephric

MICROSCOPIC

Histologic Features

- Necrosis
- Suppurative inflammation
- Fungal organisms
  - Septate hyphae with 45° angle branching
  - 3-4 μm uniform diameter of hyphae
  - Vascular invasion
- Thrombosis
  - Hemorrhagic infarcts

DIFFERENTIAL DIAGNOSIS

Candidiasis

- Pseudohyphae and budding yeast forms

Mucormycosis

- Nonseptate hyphae with 90° angle branching

Pseudallescheriasis

- Septate hyphae

Fusariosis

- Septate hyphae

Tuberculosis

- Caseating granulomas with acid-fast bacilli

DIAGNOSTIC CHECKLIST

Pathologic Interpretation Pearls

- Fungal cultures useful to confirm diagnosis

SELECTED REFERENCES

1. Heylen L et al: Invasive Aspergillosis after Kidney Transplantation: Case-Control Study. Clin Infect Dis. ePub, 2015
2. Hoyo I et al: Epidemiology, clinical characteristics, and outcome of invasive aspergillosis in renal transplant patients. Transpl Infect Dis. 16(6):951-7, 2014
3. Meng XC et al: Renal aspergillosis after liver transplantation: Clinical and imaging manifestations in two cases. World J Gastroenterol. 20(48):18495-502, 2014
4. Singh N et al: Donor-derived fungal infections in organ transplant recipients: guidelines of the American Society of Transplantation, infectious diseases community of practice. Am J Transplant. 12(9):2414-28, 2012
5. Oosten AW et al: Bilateral renal aspergillosis in a patient with AIDS: a case report and review of reported cases. AIDS Patient Care STDS. 22(1):1-6, 2008
6. Jung SI et al: Surgical treatment of invasive renal aspergillosis after chemotherapy. J Pediatr Urol. 3(3):250-2, 2007

KEY FACTS

ETIOLOGY/PATHOGENESIS

- *Cryptococcus neoformans*
- *Cryptococcus gattii*
  - Found in Pacific Northwest of United States and Canada
- Present in soil
- Inhalation of airborne fungal forms

CLINICAL ISSUES

- 1/100,000 in general population
- 2.8-5% in solid organ transplant patients
  - 0.8-5.8% in renal transplant patients
- Rare in children before puberty
- Male predilection
- Amphotericin B
- Fluconazole

MACROSCOPIC

- Papillary necrosis
  - May be present in cryptococcal pyelonephritis

MICROSCOPIC

- Granulomatous interstitial inflammation
- Fungal organisms
  - Clear halo; mucicarmine, PAS, and silver stain positive
    - Capsule-deficient variant of *Cryptococcus* (all silver stains)
  - 5-10 μm in diameter
  - Narrow-based budding
- Tubulointerstitial inflammation with tubulitis

TOP DIFFERENTIAL DIAGNOSES

- Blastomycosis
- Candidiasis
- Histoplasmosis
- Coccidioidomycosis
- Paracoccidioidomycosis
- Sarcoidosis
- Drug-induced acute interstitial nephritis
- Tuberculosis

Granulomatous Interstitial Nephritis

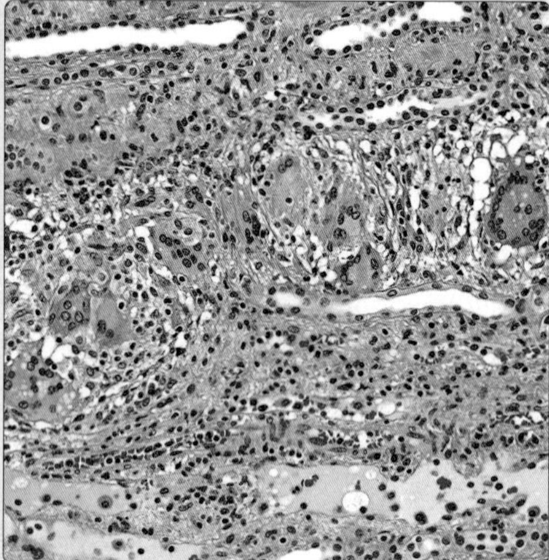

Gomori Methenamine Silver

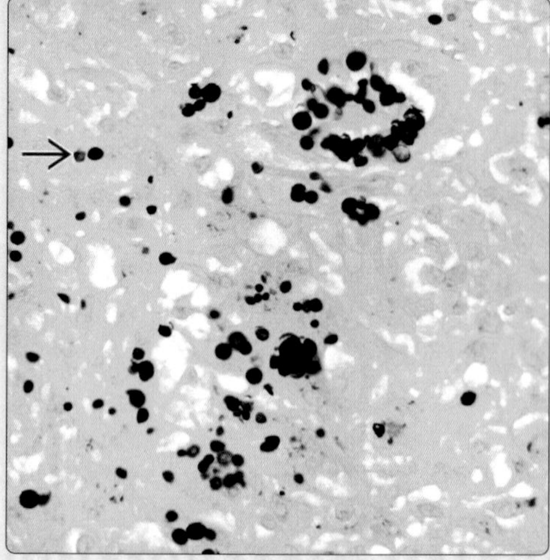

(Left) *Hematoxylin and eosin shows prominent granulomatous interstitial inflammation that involves primarily the renal medulla in a kidney transplant patient.* **(Right)** *Gomori methenamine-silver shows strong staining of numerous round cryptococcal organisms ➡ within the prominent granulomatous inflammation throughout the renal cortex.*

Multinucleated Giant Cells

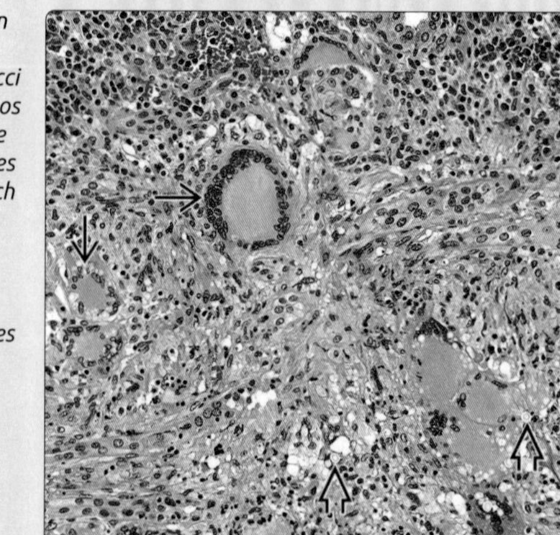

Mucicarmine

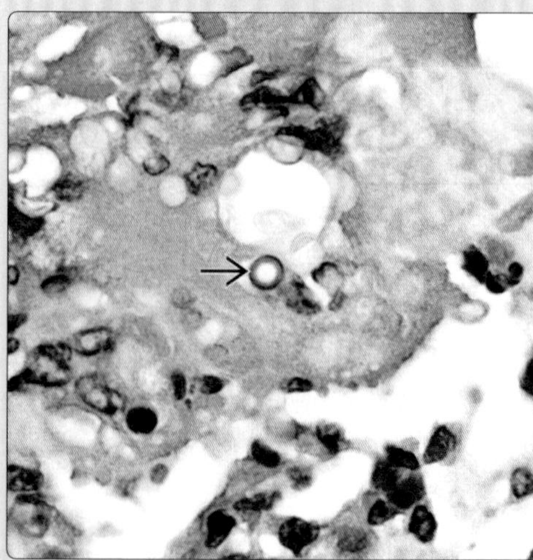

(Left) *Hematoxylin and eosin shows large multinucleated giant cells ➡ and Cryptococci with characteristic clear halos ⇨ that are distinct from the adjacent foamy macrophages in this kidney allograft, which ultimately resulted in a transplant nephrectomy.* **(Right)** *Mucicarmine stain highlights the thick outer capsule ➡ that characterizes Cryptococcus.*

TERMINOLOGY

Definitions

- Cryptococcal infection, typically in immunocompromised patients

ETIOLOGY/PATHOGENESIS

Environmental Exposure

- Present in soil
- Inhalation of airborne fungal forms

Infectious Agents

- *Cryptococcus neoformans*
- *Cryptococcus gattii*
  - Found in Pacific Northwest of United States and Canada
  - Isolated from eucalyptus trees in subtropical and tropical regions
- Rare isolates
  - *Cryptococcus laurentii, Cryptococcus albidus*

Pathogenetic Factors

- Polysaccharide capsule, melanin, urease, laccases, and phospholipase B

CLINICAL ISSUES

Epidemiology

- Incidence
  - 1/100,000 in general population
    - 2-7/1,000 in AIDS patients
  - 2.8-5% in solid organ transplant patients
    - 0.8-5.8% in renal transplant patients
  - Common cause of meningoencephalitis in sub-Saharan Africa
- Age
  - Rare in children before puberty
- Sex
  - Male predilection

Presentation

- Acute renal failure
- Proteinuria

Laboratory Tests

- Cryptococcal antigen test
- Fungal culture

Treatment

- Drugs
  - Amphotericin B, fluconazole
- Reduction of immunosuppressive agents in transplant patients

Prognosis

- Graft loss in 9% of renal transplant patients

MACROSCOPIC

General Features

- Papillary necrosis
  - May be present in cryptococcal pyelonephritis

MICROSCOPIC

Histologic Features

- Granulomatous interstitial inflammation
  - Absence of significant granulomatous or inflammatory response in severely immunocompromised patients
- Fungal organisms
  - Capsule is mucicarmine, PAS, and silver stain positive
  - Capsule-deficient variant of *Cryptococcus* (all silver stains)
  - 5-10 µm in diameter
  - Narrow-based budding
  - May be present in glomerular capillaries within macrophages
- Prominent tubulointerstitial inflammation
- Tubulitis
- Necrotizing and crescentic glomerulonephritis
  - Single report in association with pulmonary cryptococcosis with resolution after antifungal therapy

DIFFERENTIAL DIAGNOSIS

Blastomycosis

- 8-15 µm in diameter
- Broad-based budding

Candidiasis

- Budding yeasts
- Pseudohyphae

Histoplasmosis

- 2-4 µm in diameter
- Endemic to Mississippi and Ohio river valleys

Coccidioidomycosis

- Spherules with characteristic endospores
- Endemic to Southwest USA, Mexico, and South America

Paracoccidioidomycosis

- Endemic to South America and Brazil
- Clear halo, Gomori methenamine silver positive

Tuberculosis

- Caseating necrosis
- Acid-fast bacilli present

SELECTED REFERENCES

1. Pongmekin P et al: Clinical characteristics and mortality risk factors of cryptococcal infection among HIV-negative patients. J Med Assoc Thai. 97(1):36-43, 2014
2. Yang YL et al: Cryptococcosis in kidney transplant recipients in a Chinese university hospital and a review of published cases. Int J Infect Dis. 26:154-61, 2014
3. Kronstad JW et al: Expanding fungal pathogenesis: Cryptococcus breaks out of the opportunistic box. Nat Rev Microbiol. 9(3):193-203, 2011
4. Silveira FP et al: Cryptococcosis in liver and kidney transplant recipients receiving anti-thymocyte globulin or alemtuzumab. Transpl Infect Dis. 9(1):22-7, 2007
5. Iglesias JI et al: AIDS, nephrotic-range proteinuria, and renal failure. Kidney Int. 69(11):2107-10, 2006
6. Nakayama M et al: A case of necrotizing glomerulonephritis presenting with nephrotic syndrome associated with pulmonary cryptococcosis. Clin Exp Nephrol. 9(1):74-8, 2005
7. Singh N et al: Allograft loss in renal transplant recipients with cryptococcus neoformans associated immune reconstitution syndrome. Transplantation. 80(8):1131-3, 2005

Microsporidiosis

KEY FACTS

TERMINOLOGY

- Infection by 1 of many species of *Microsporidia* fungi particularly affecting immunocompromised hosts

ETIOLOGY/PATHOGENESIS

- Kidney involved in minority of cases, typically as part of systemic infection
- 14 species infect humans
- *E. intestinalis* and *E. cuniculi* most common organisms in disseminated cases

CLINICAL ISSUES

- Diarrhea usual presentation
- Acute or chronic renal failure
- Renal allograft dysfunction
- Fever
- Other sites: Lung, brain, heart, liver, eye
- Treatment: Fumagillin, albendazole
- Outcome good if treated with antibiotics and immunocompetence can be improved

MICROSCOPIC

- Acute and chronic interstitial nephritis
- Oval 1 x 2 µm intracellular spores in tubules
    - Purple with Brown-Hopps stain
    - Giemsa-positive central body
- EM identification by unique polar tube
- Acute and chronic interstitial nephritis
- Intraluminal and intracellular 1 x 2 µm ovoid spores in aggregates in tubules

ANCILLARY TESTS

- Electron microscopy reveals pathognomonic coiled polar tube in spores

TOP DIFFERENTIAL DIAGNOSES

- Toxoplasmosis
- Candidiasis and other fungal infections

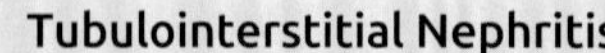

Tubulointerstitial Nephritis

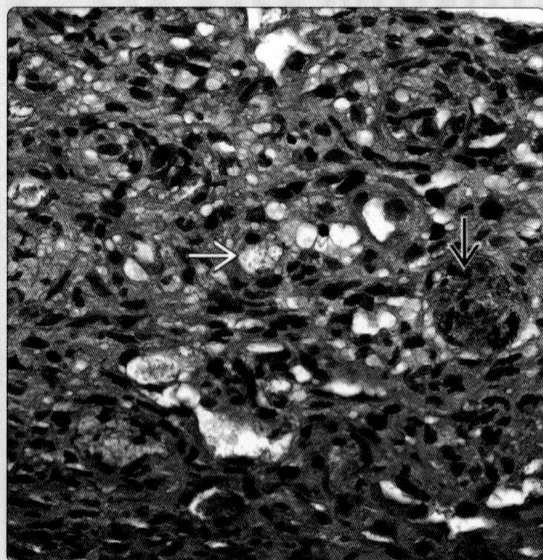

Chronic Tubulointerstitial Nephritis

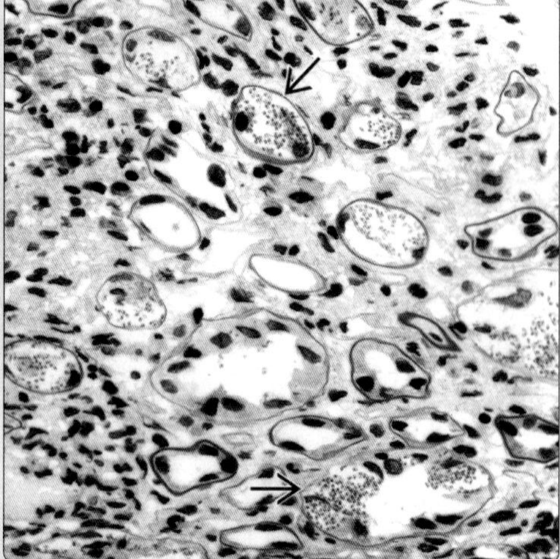

(Left) *Acute and chronic interstitial nephritis due to microsporidiosis is shown. Tubules contain inflammatory cells* ⇨*, debris, and organisms. The tubular epithelium is ballooned and contain aggregates of organisms* ➡*.* **(Right)** *PAS stain of active interstitial nephritis in an HIV(+) patient with microsporidiosis shows that the organisms in tubules* ⇨ *are not strongly stained, which allows differentiation from usual fungi.*

Intracellular Spores

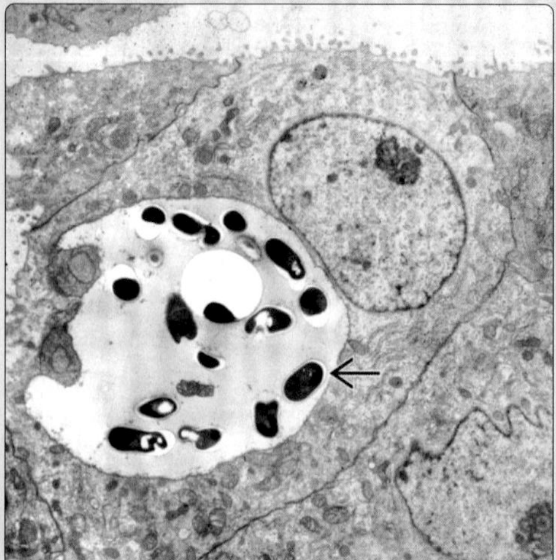

Polar Tube Coil

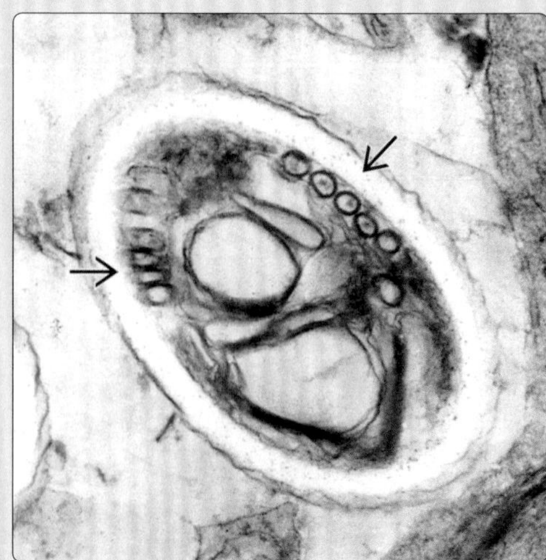

(Left) *Electron micrograph shows intracellular Microsporidia spores* ⇨ *in tubular epithelium.* **(Right)** *High-power electron micrograph shows the pathognomonic polar tube coils* ⇨*, a unique structure of Microsporidia spores. Here, 5 coils are present, typical of E. intestinalis.*

TERMINOLOGY

Definitions

- Infection by 1 of many species of *Microsporidia* fungi particularly affecting immunocompromised hosts

ETIOLOGY/PATHOGENESIS

Infectious Agents

- *Microsporidia*
  - Ubiquitous obligate intracellular eukaryotic pathogens
    - Unique group of fungi with reduced cell organelles (no mitochondria, Golgi)
  - Infects all phyla of organisms
    - Initially identified as silkworm pathogen in 1857 and as human pathogen 50 years ago
  - 14 species infect humans
    - Most common: *Enterocytozoon bieneusi*, *Encephalitozoon intestinalis*, and *Encephalitozoon cuniculi*
  - Unique method of inserting spore contents into cell via a polar tube that behaves like a hypodermic needle
- Kidney involved in minority of cases, typically as part of systemic infection
  - *E. intestinalis* and *E. cuniculi* most common organisms in disseminated cases
  - *E. cuniculi* infects dogs and cats
- *E. bieneusi* limited to GI tract and hepatobiliary system
- Immunodeficiency predisposes to disease
  - HIV patients (CD4 < 100/mm³), transplant recipients (3 weeks to 7 years post transplant)
- Transmission in donor kidneys reported

CLINICAL ISSUES

Presentation

- Acute renal failure
- Chronic renal failure
- Renal allograft dysfunction
  - Kidney involved in ~ 40% of recipients with microsporidiosis
- Fever
- Diarrhea
- Weight loss
- Other sites: Lung, brain, heart, liver, eye

Treatment

- Drugs
  - Fumagillin, albendazole
  - Tapering immunosuppressive drugs

Prognosis

- Good if treated with antibiotics and immunocompetence can be improved

MICROSCOPIC

Histologic Features

- Acute and chronic interstitial nephritis
- Tubules
  - Severe tubular injury, disruption, and destruction
  - Intraluminal and intracellular 1 x 2 μm ovoid spores in aggregates
    - No budding or pseudohyphae
  - Purple with Gram stain (Brown-Hopps, Brown-Brenn)
  - Giemsa stains central body (nucleus)
  - PAS weakly stained in contrast to other fungi
  - Silver positivity in punctate pattern (posterior body)
  - Positive acid-fast stain (red with Ziehl-Neelsen)
  - Calcofluor white fluorochrome stains cell wall polysaccharide (fluoresces blue with DAPI filter)
- Interstitium
  - Acute and chronic inflammation
  - Neutrophils, eosinophils, monocytes, lymphocytes, plasma cells
- Glomeruli
  - No specific feature
  - HIV-associated glomerular disease may be present
- Vessels
  - No specific feature

ANCILLARY TESTS

Immunohistochemistry

- Negative for *Toxoplasma gondii* antigens

PCR

- Identification of species in paraffin-embedded tissues

Electron Microscopy

- Intracellular spores
  - Distinctive and pathognomonic coiled polar tube in spore
    - Allows speciation

DIFFERENTIAL DIAGNOSIS

Toxoplasmosis

- Similar size
- Negative on Brown-Brenn or Brown-Hopps stain
- Positive for anti-*Toxoplasma* antigens by IHC

Candidiasis and Infection by Other Fungi

- PAS(+) cell walls
- Budding spores, pseudohyphae

SELECTED REFERENCES

1. Hocevar SN et al: Microsporidiosis acquired through solid organ transplantation: a public health investigation. Ann Intern Med. 160(4):213-20, 2014
2. Ladapo TA et al: Microsporidiosis in pediatric renal transplant patients in Cape Town, South Africa: two case reports. Pediatr Transplant. 18(7):E220-6, 2014
3. Nagpal A et al: Disseminated microsporidiosis in a renal transplant recipient: case report and review of the literature. Transpl Infect Dis. 15(5):526-32, 2013
4. Lanternier F et al: Microsporidiosis in solid organ transplant recipients: two Enterocytozoon bieneusi cases and review. Transpl Infect Dis. 11(1):83-8, 2009
5. Viriyavejakul P et al: High prevalence of Microsporidium infection in HIV-infected patients. Southeast Asian J Trop Med Public Health. 40(2):223-8, 2009
6. Chan KS et al: Extraction of microsporidial DNA from modified trichrome-stained clinical slides and subsequent species identification using PCR sequencing. Parasitology. 135(6):701-3, 2008
7. Orenstein JM: Diagnostic pathology of microsporidiosis. Ultrastruct Pathol. 27(3):141-9, 2003

Rickettsial Infections

KEY FACTS

TERMINOLOGY

- Systemic infection by rickettsial microorganisms with direct infection of kidney

ETIOLOGY/PATHOGENESIS

- Rocky mountain spotted fever (RMSF): *Rickettsia rickettsii* infection, transmitted by ticks
- Mediterranean spotted fever (MSF): *R. conorii* infection, transmitted by ticks
- Scrub typhus (ST): *Orientia tsutsugamushi* infection, transmitted by mites
- Epidemic typhus (ET): *R. prowazekii* infection, transmitted by body lice
- Organisms directly infect vascular endothelium
- Endothelial injury causes hemorrhage and thrombosis

CLINICAL ISSUES

- Symptoms: Fever, headache, myalgia, rash, acute renal failure
- RMSF: Fever, rash, and history of tick exposure (classic triad)
  - Latency of 2-14 days
  - Rash in 3-5 days; maculopapular or purpuric, involves palms and soles
- Acute renal failure, ± hypovolemic shock, may be associated with any of these infections

MICROSCOPIC

- Nodular perivascular tubulointerstitial inflammation with hemorrhage
- Acute tubular injury
- Vasculitis affecting arteries, capillaries, veins

TOP DIFFERENTIAL DIAGNOSES

- Adenovirus
- Hantavirus and other viral hemorrhagic fevers

(Left) *Peritubular capillary thrombosis ⇒ with interstitial hemorrhage and a predominantly mononuclear inflammatory infiltrate are characteristic of rickettsial tubulointerstitial nephritis (TIN). Focal tubulitis is also evident ⇒. (Courtesy J. Olano, MD.)* **(Right)** *Immunohistochemical staining using a specific antirickettsial antibody reveals rickettsial antigen in the endothelium of a congested interstitial capillary ⇒. The surrounding interstitium is edematous and has numerous mononuclear cells. (Courtesy J. Olano, MD.)*

Capillary Thrombosis and Interstitial Hemorrhage in Rickettsial TIN

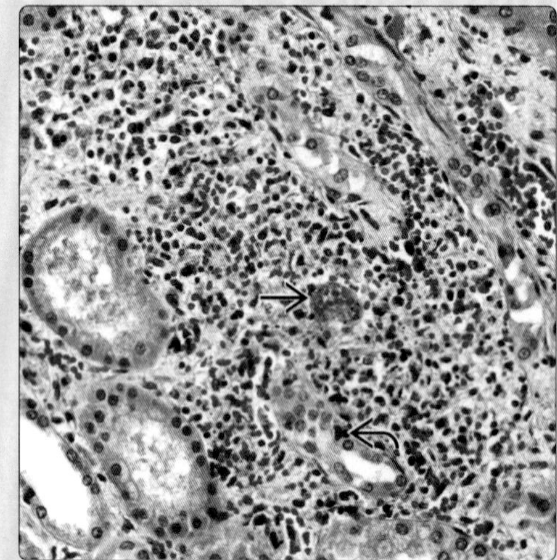

Capillary Endothelial Rickettsial Antigen

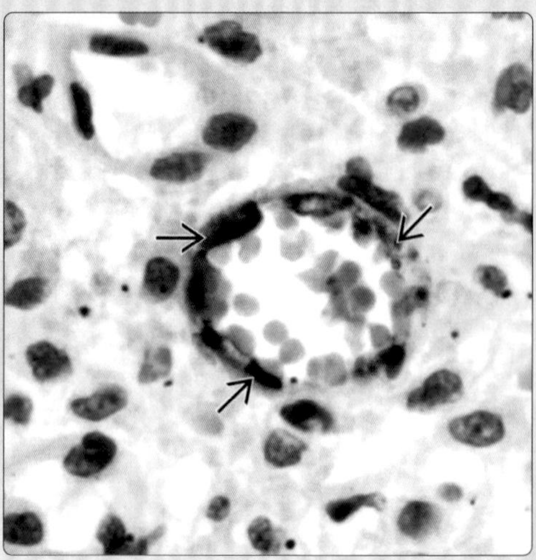

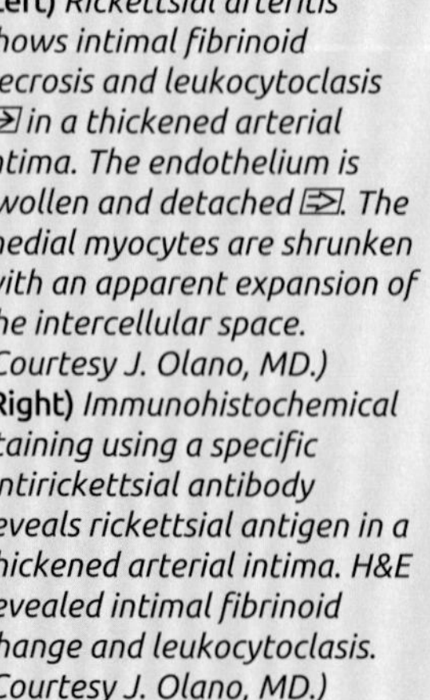

(Left) *Rickettsial arteritis shows intimal fibrinoid necrosis and leukocytoclasis ⇒ in a thickened arterial intima. The endothelium is swollen and detached ⇒. The medial myocytes are shrunken with an apparent expansion of the intercellular space. (Courtesy J. Olano, MD.)* **(Right)** *Immunohistochemical staining using a specific antirickettsial antibody reveals rickettsial antigen in a thickened arterial intima. H&E revealed intimal fibrinoid change and leukocytoclasis. (Courtesy J. Olano, MD.)*

Rickettsial Arteritis

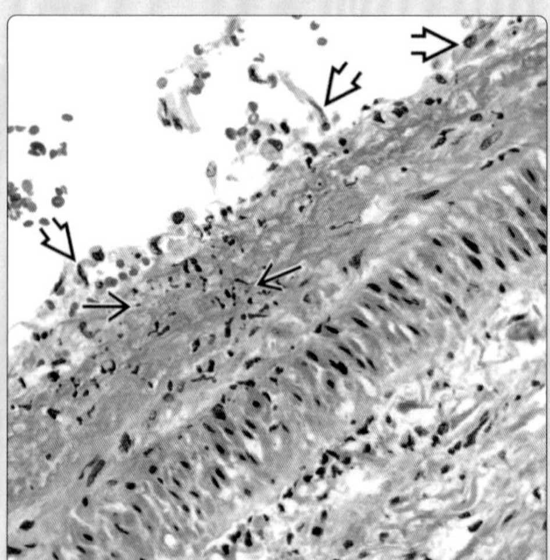

Rickettsial Antigen in Arteritis

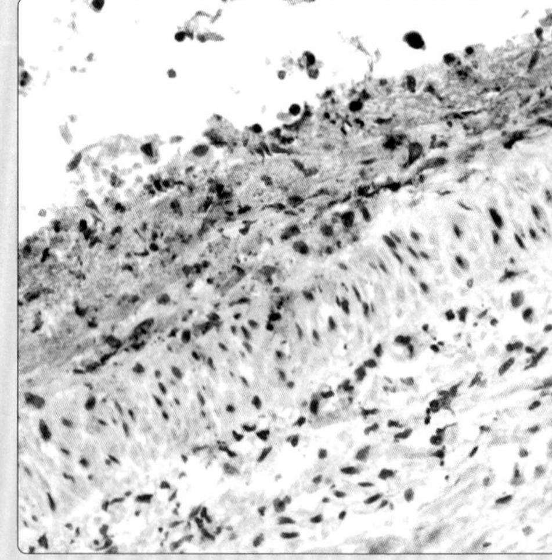

TERMINOLOGY

Abbreviations

- Rocky mountain spotted fever (RMSF)
- Mediterranean spotted fever (MSF) or Boutonneuse fever
- Scrub typhus (ST)
- Epidemic typhus (ET)

Definitions

- Systemic infection by rickettsial microorganisms with direct infection of kidney

ETIOLOGY/PATHOGENESIS

Arthropod-Borne Zoonoses

- Human transmission via arthropod bites
  - RMSF: *Rickettsia rickettsii* transmitted by ticks
  - MSF: *R. conorii* transmitted by ticks
  - ST: *Orientia tsutsugamushi* transmitted by mites
  - ET: *R. prowazekii* transmitted by body lice
- Rickettsial organisms directly infect endothelium, tubular epithelium, smooth muscle
- Uptake into endothelium by cholesterol receptor-mediated endocytosis
  - Endothelial injury causes hemorrhage and thrombosis
- Acute kidney injury
  - Intrarenal vasculitis, acute tubular injury, and tubulointerstitial inflammation

CLINICAL ISSUES

Presentation

- Incidence: ~ 5.6 per 1 million in USA for RMSF
  - Higher in hyperendemic areas (e.g., 18 per 1,000,000 children in Arizona)
- General: Fever, headache, myalgia, and rash
  - RMSF: Fever, rash, and history of tick exposure (classic triad)
    - Peak incidence in spring and early summer
    - Latency of 2-14 days
    - Nausea, vomiting, abdominal pain, and cough
    - Maculopapular &/or purpuric rash involves palms and soles of feet
  - MSF: Eschar, maculopapular rash
  - ST: Eschar, influenza-like illness, lymphadenopathy
  - ET: Influenza-like illness, jaundice, petechiae, hypotension, proteinuria, and hematuria
- Acute renal failure, ± hypovolemic shock, may be associated with any of these infections
- Diagnosis
  - PCR assay to detect *htrA* antigen gene
  - Blood or tissue culture with immunofluorescence (IF) detection of early antigens (results in 48-72 hours)
  - Rising antirickettsial antibody titer: Takes 7-10 days to appear

Treatment

- Tetracycline or chloramphenicol

Prognosis

- Fatality rates 2-25%; typically 9-15 days; 3-5 days in fulminant cases
- Delayed diagnosis, older age, male, glucose-6-phosphate dehydrogenase deficiency, alcoholism → increase risk of severe disease

MACROSCOPIC

Gross Features

- Enlarged kidneys with petechiae, especially outer medulla

MICROSCOPIC

Histologic Features

- Features common to all rickettsial infections
- Glomeruli
  - Capillary thrombi; rarely glomerulonephritis
- Tubules and Interstitium
  - Acute tubular injury
  - Tubulointerstitial nephritis: Corticomedullary junction and outer medulla
    - Lymphoid cells (T cells abundant, few B cells), macrophages, rare eosinophils, edema, tubulitis
    - Nodular perivascular infiltrates
- Vessels
  - Vasculitis: Endothelial necrosis, thrombosis, perivascular hemorrhage
    - Peritubular capillaries, venules; uncommonly in arteries and arterioles
  - *Rickettsia* in endothelium on Giemsa stain (low sensitivity)

ANCILLARY TESTS

Immunohistochemistry

- Rickettsial antigen in endothelium and occasionally in tubules

Electron Microscopy

- Membrane-bound bacilli (1-2 μm) in cytoplasm and nucleus

DIFFERENTIAL DIAGNOSIS

Tubulointerstitial Nephritis With Hemorrhage or Vasculitis

- Hantavirus and other viral hemorrhagic fevers: Viral antigens in vasculature by IHC
- Adenovirus: Tubular nuclear inclusions; viral antigens in tubules by IHC

DIAGNOSTIC CHECKLIST

Pathologic Interpretation Pearls

- Vasculitis, nodular tubulointerstitial inflammation, hemorrhage, acute tubular injury
- Detectable rickettsial antigen by IHC

SELECTED REFERENCES

1. Lee JH et al: A case of Tsutsugamushi disease presenting with nephrotic syndrome. Korean J Intern Med. 28(6):728-31, 2013
2. Kay J et al: Case records of the Massachusetts General Hospital. Case 31-2005. A 60-year-old man with skin lesions and renal insufficiency. N Engl J Med. 353(15):1605-13, 2005
3. Quigg RJ et al: Acute glomerulonephritis in a patient with Rocky Mountain spotted fever. Am J Kidney Dis. 17(3):339-42, 1991
4. Walker DH et al: Acute renal failure in Rocky Mountain spotted fever. Arch Intern Med. 139(4):443-8, 1979

KEY FACTS

TERMINOLOGY

- Renal manifestations due to protozoan *Toxoplasma gondii* infection

ETIOLOGY/PATHOGENESIS

- *Toxoplasma gondii* is an obligate intracellular parasite
  - Ingestion of oocysts shed in cat feces or uncooked meat of infected animals are sources of human infection
- Immunocompetent hosts often have febrile illness with lymphadenopathy and rash
- Immunocompromised hosts are more susceptible
  - Solid organ transplantation of seronegative recipients from seropositive donors is risk factor

CLINICAL ISSUES

- Kidney involvement presents with mild proteinuria
- Laboratory diagnosis
  - Detection of circulating *Toxoplasma* antigens by IgG immunoassay or PCR DNA amplification
  - Increased titers of IgG and IgM anti-*Toxoplasma* antibodies
    - Less sensitive in immunosuppressed patients who fail to develop measurable serological response
  - Parasite isolation from infected tissues or body fluids less sensitive
- Nephrotic syndrome remits after treatment of toxoplasmosis

MICROSCOPIC

- Mesangioproliferative glomerulonephritis
  - Mesangial and segmental capillary wall deposits
- Minimal change disease and FSGS rarely associated with IgM *anti-Toxoplasma* antibodies
- Toxoplasma pseudocysts rare

ANCILLARY TESTS

- Wright-Giemsa stain or *Toxoplasma* immunostain highlights organisms

Necrotic Brain With *Toxoplasma gondii* Tachyzoites

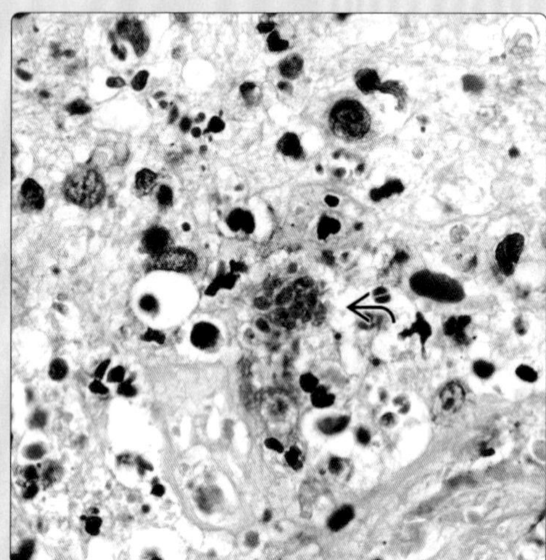

***Toxoplasma* Immunostain**

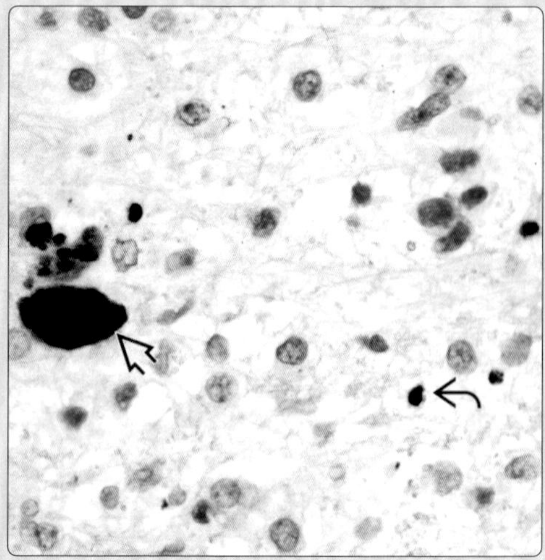

(Left) *Toxoplasma gondii tachyzoites ➔ are seen within foci of extensive necrosis in an immunocompromised patient with encephalitis and disseminated toxoplasma infection. (Courtesy J. Karamchandani, MD.)* **(Right)** *The toxoplasma immunostain highlights a pseudocyst filled with bradyzoites ➔ as well as tachyzoites ➔ in a patient with encephalitis. (Courtesy J. Karamchandani, MD.)*

Cardiac Toxoplasmosis

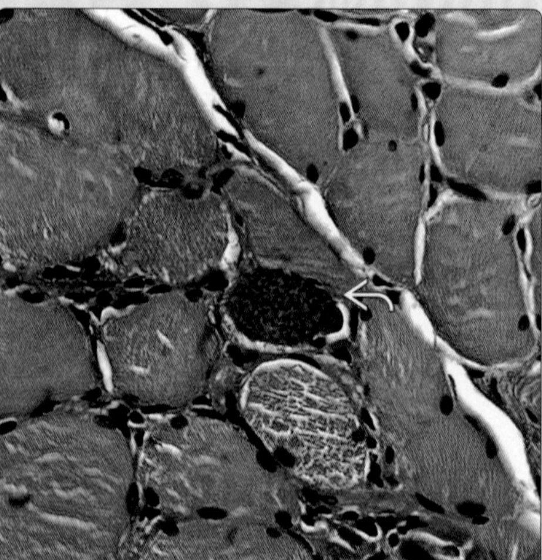

***T. Gondii* Tachyzoites**

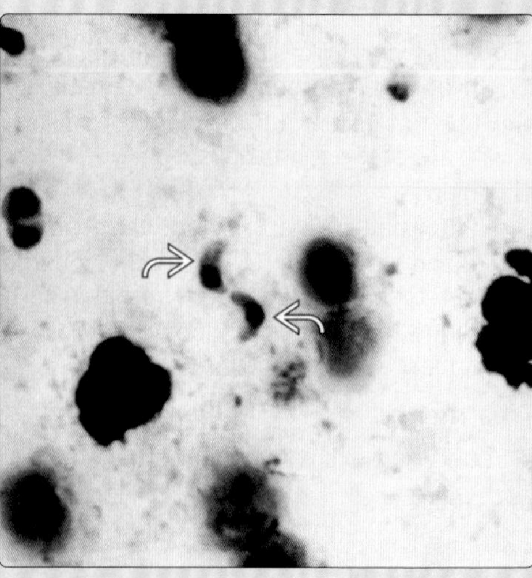

(Left) *H&E-stained section of cardiac muscle from a kidney transplantation recipient shows Toxoplasma gondii pseudocysts ➔. These cysts range 5-50 µm in diameter. (Courtesy J. Montoya, MD.)* **(Right)** *Wright-Giemsa stain highlights T. gondii tachyzoites ➔ in a bronchoalveolar lavage specimen from an AIDS patient with pneumonia. (Courtesy J. Montoya, MD.)*

TERMINOLOGY

Definitions

- Renal manifestations due to protozoan *Toxoplasma gondii*

ETIOLOGY/PATHOGENESIS

Infectious Agents

- *Toxoplasma gondii* is an obligate intracellular parasite
  - Primary host is domestic cat, but can also be transmitted by dogs, rabbits, and guinea pigs
    - Ingestion of oocysts in cat feces or uncooked meat of infected animals are sources of human infection
  - Parasites elicit cellular and humoral host responses

Congenital Infection

- Transplacental transmission occurs
- Often fatal with encephalomyelitis, chorioretinitis, and cerebral calcifications

Acquired Infection

- Primary infection or reactivation of latent infection
  - Immunocompetent hosts asymptomatic or have febrile illness with lymphadenopathy and rash
  - Immunocompromised hosts more susceptible
    - Solid organ transplantation of seronegative recipients from seropositive donors a risk factor
      - Organ involvement may be extensive, including myocarditis, myositis, and encephalitis
    - HIV infection, bone marrow transplantation, and hemodialysis

CLINICAL ISSUES

Epidemiology

- Incidence
  - Worldwide distribution with 20-60% prevalence

Site

- Kidney involvement occasionally
- Transplanted kidney usually not affected

Presentation

- Mild proteinuria with normal renal function
  - Nephrotic syndrome in congenital toxoplasmosis or adults with disseminated disease
- Nephritic syndrome in some patients

Laboratory Tests

- Detection of circulating *Toxoplasma* antigens by IgG immunoassay or PCR DNA amplification
- Increased titers of IgG and IgM anti-*Toxoplasma* antibodies
- Parasite isolation from infected tissues or body fluids

Treatment

- Drugs
  - Pyrimethamine, sulfadiazine, or clindamycin for toxoplasmosis

Prognosis

- If untreated, disseminated toxoplasmosis lethal
- Nephrotic syndrome remits after treatment

MICROSCOPIC

Histologic Features

- Mesangioproliferative glomerulonephritis
  - Glomerular mesangial and endocapillary proliferation
  - Karyorrhectic debris may be seen in glomeruli
  - Interstitial inflammation, fibrosis, and tubular atrophy
- Minimal change disease and focal segmental glomerulosclerosis (FSGS) rarely associated with IgM anti-*Toxoplasma* antibodies
- Toxoplasma pseudocysts rare
  - Packed with round or piriform organisms with distinct cell membranes and homogeneous cytoplasm
- Congenital toxoplasmosis manifests with pseudocysts in glomeruli or tubules, extensive global glomerulosclerosis, and mesangial proliferative glomerulonephritis

ANCILLARY TESTS

Histochemistry

- Wright-Giemsa stain
  - Reactivity: Positive
  - Staining Pattern: Highlights the pseudocysts and tachyzoites of *Toxoplasma*

Immunohistochemistry

- Toxoplasma immunostain can highlight organisms

Immunofluorescence

- Granular mesangial and segmental capillary wall deposits with IgG, IgA, IgM, and C3
  - *Toxoplasma* antigen demonstrated in deposits
- Negative in minimal change disease and FSGS

Electron Microscopy

- Mesangial and subendothelial deposits in proliferative glomerulonephritis
- Podocyte foot process effacement may be observed

DIFFERENTIAL DIAGNOSIS

Non-Toxoplasma-Related Immune Complex-Mediated Glomerulonephritis

- Clinical history may be most helpful
- Laboratory tests to exclude active *Toxoplasma* infection

SELECTED REFERENCES

1. Fernàndez-Sabé N et al: Risk factors, clinical features, and outcomes of toxoplasmosis in solid-organ transplant recipients: a matched case-control study. Clin Infect Dis. 54(3):355-61, 2012
2. Toporovski J et al: Nephrotic syndrome associated with toxoplasmosis: report of seven cases. Rev Inst Med Trop Sao Paulo. 54(2):61-4, 2012
3. Haskell L et al: Disseminated toxoplasmosis presenting as symptomatic orchitis and nephrotic syndrome. Am J Med Sci. 298(3):185-90, 1989
4. Beale MG et al: Congenital glomerulosclerosis and nephrotic syndrome in two infants. Speculations and pathogenesis. Am J Dis Child. 133(8):842-5, 1979
5. Krick JA et al: Toxoplasmosis in the adult–an overview. N Engl J Med. 298(10):550-3, 1978
6. Ginsburg BE et al: Case of glomerulonephritis associated with acute toxoplasmosis. Br Med J. 3(5932):664-5, 1974
7. Shahin B et al: Congenital nephrotic syndrome associated with congenital toxoplasmosis. J Pediatr. 85(3):366-70, 1974

Hydatidosis

KEY FACTS

TERMINOLOGY

- Hydatid cyst or disease
- Echinococcosis
- Cystic parasitic disease caused by larval form of echinococcus granulosus

ETIOLOGY/PATHOGENESIS

- Adult worm lives in small bowel of dog, sheep, cattle (definitive host)
- Excreted eggs ingested by humans (intermediate host)
- Oncospheres hatch from eggs in duodenum, penetrate mucosa, and enter portal vein and disseminate
- Each oncosphere develops into hydatid cyst
- Cysts contain brood capsules and thousands of scolices

CLINICAL ISSUES

- Chronic dull flank pain or mass
- Systemic symptoms of fever and malaise
- Hydatiduria, hematuria, nephrotic syndrome

IMAGING

- Radiograph: Ring-shaped curvilinear calcification
- US/CT: Unicystic to multicystic lesion

MACROSCOPIC

- Thick-walled cyst with numerous cystic brood capsules

MICROSCOPIC

- 3-layered hydatid cyst wall
- Brood capsules contain 5-20 scolices
- Wet prep or Pap stain
  - Scolices with crown or rostellum of hooks
  - Hooks are acid-fast stain positive

ANCILLARY TESTS

- EIA or ELISA assay

TOP DIFFERENTIAL DIAGNOSES

- Cystic nephroma
- Multilocular cystic renal cell carcinoma

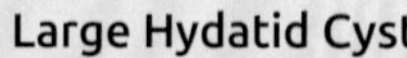

Large Hydatid Cyst

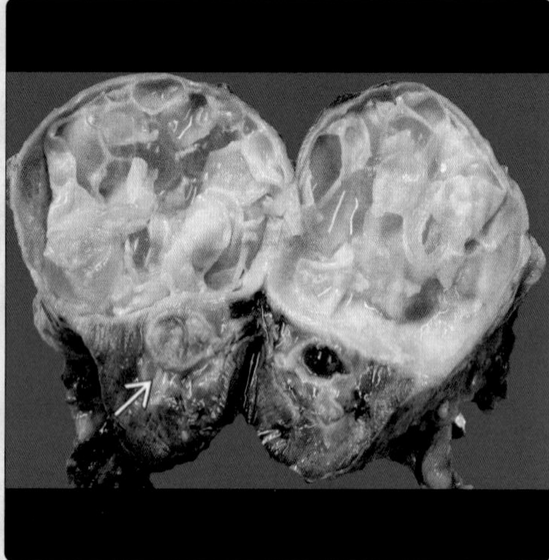

Large Hydatid Cyst

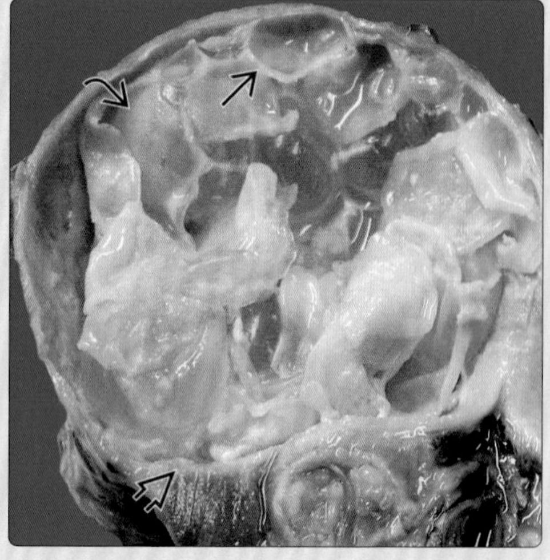

(Left) *This kidney is largely replaced by a large dominant hydatid cyst that necessitated nephrectomy. The cyst has a very thick, fibrous wall with attached cystic brood capsules. There is also a 2nd smaller cyst ➡ adjacent to the large cyst.* **(Right)** *This kidney is largely replaced by a hydatid cyst that has a thick fibrous wall ⇲. Its 3 cyst layers are not discernible grossly. Both opened ➡ and unopened ⇨ brood capsules are present. Within the brood capsules, numerous infective scolices reside.*

Hydatid Cyst With Brood Capsules

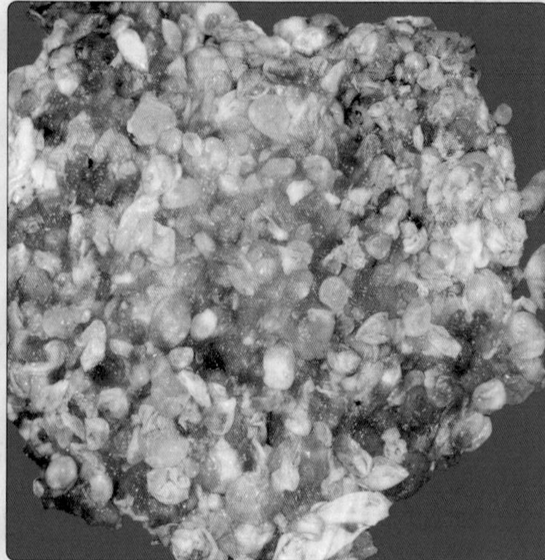

Hydatid Cyst With Brood Capsules

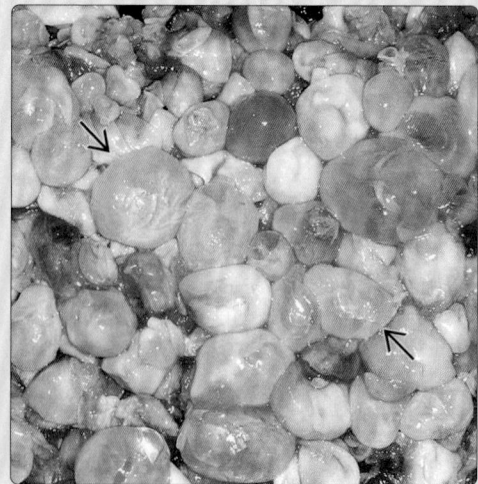

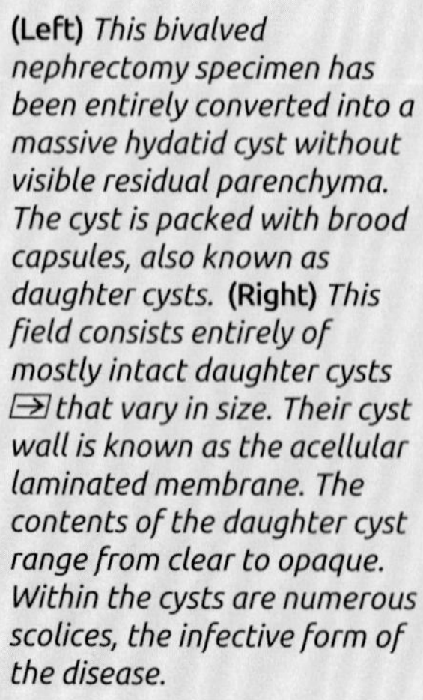

(Left) *This bivalved nephrectomy specimen has been entirely converted into a massive hydatid cyst without visible residual parenchyma. The cyst is packed with brood capsules, also known as daughter cysts.* **(Right)** *This field consists entirely of mostly intact daughter cysts ➡ that vary in size. Their cyst wall is known as the acellular laminated membrane. The contents of the daughter cyst range from clear to opaque. Within the cysts are numerous scolices, the infective form of the disease.*

TERMINOLOGY

Synonyms

- Hydatid cyst or disease
- Echinococcosis

Definitions

- Cystic parasitic disease caused by larval form of cestode *Echinococcus granulosus*

ETIOLOGY/PATHOGENESIS

Infectious Agents

- Adult worm lives in small bowel of dog, sheep, cattle (definitive host)
  - Excreted eggs ingested by humans (intermediate host)
  - Oncospheres hatch from eggs in duodenum
    - Penetrate mucosa and enter portal vein
    - Reach liver (60%), lungs (5-15%), and kidney (2-4%)
- Each oncosphere develops into hydatid cyst
  - Brood capsules develop from inner germinal membrane
    - Contain 5-20 scolices, the infective agent
    - Detach from wall to form daughter cysts
  - Hydatid cysts can contain thousands of scolices
- Kidneys may be involved by direct extension

CLINICAL ISSUES

Epidemiology

- Endemic: Africa, Mediterranean, Eurasia, Canada, South America

Presentation

- Chronic dull flank pain most common: 40% of patients
- Systemic symptoms of fever and malaise
- Hydatiduria: < 10-20%
- Hematuria or nephrotic syndrome: Rare

Laboratory Tests

- ELISA positive in 80%
- Hydatiduria
  - Grape-like daughter cysts enter urine with cyst rupture
- Eosinophilia in 20-50%

Treatment

- Surgical approaches
  - Complete or partial nephrectomy
  - Percutaneous drainage not recommended
  - Antihelmintics
    - Cysts disappear in 33%
    - Cyst size reduced in 30-50%

Prognosis

- Depends upon number of organs affected
- Rare fatal anaphylactic reaction during surgery
- Complications: Cyst rupture, infection, and abscess

IMAGING

Radiographic Findings

- Unilocular or multilocular cystic lesion with ring-shaped, amorphous, or curvilinear calcification

CT Findings

- Unilocular cyst with calcification
- Multivesicular cyst containing daughter cysts

MACROSCOPIC

General Features

- Fluid-filled, thick-walled cyst containing daughter cysts
  - Unilocular cyst typical in children
  - Multivesicular cyst typical in adults

MICROSCOPIC

Histologic Features

- Hydatid cyst wall has 3 layers
  - Pericyst: An adventitial outer fibrous layer of host tissue
  - Hydatid cyst
    - Ectocyst: Acellular laminated membrane
    - Endocyst: Inner germinal membrane
- Closed cyst: All 3 layers intact
- Exposed cyst: Pericyst layer absent
- Open or ruptured cyst: All 3 layers absent
- Brood capsules bud from inner cyst wall
  - Rupture releases scolices into cyst ("hydatid sand")
- Scolex
  - 4 suckers and rostellum of hooks
  - Hooks are acid-fast stain positive
- Glomerulonephritis is a rare complication
  - Membranoproliferative glomerulonephritis
  - Membranous glomerulonephritis

Cytologic Features

- Identifying cyst scolices by wet prep or Pap stain

ANCILLARY TESTS

Serologic Testing

- EIA or ELISA assay

DIFFERENTIAL DIAGNOSIS

Cystic Neoplasms

- Cystic nephroma
- Multilocular cystic renal cell carcinoma

DIAGNOSTIC CHECKLIST

Pathologic Interpretation Pearls

- Cyst containing free-floating cysts is infectious

SELECTED REFERENCES

1. Rexiati M et al: Diagnosis and surgical treatment of renal hydatid disease: a retrospective analysis of 30 cases. PLoS One. 9(5):e96602, 2014
2. da Silva AM: Human echinococcosis: a neglected disease. Gastroenterol Res Pract. pii: 583297, 2010
3. Shukla S et al: Multiple disseminated abdominal hydatidosis presenting with gross hydatiduria: a rare case report. Indian J Pathol Microbiol. 52(2):213-4, 2009
4. Mongha R et al: Primary hydatid cyst of kidney and ureter with gross hydatiduria: A case report and evaluation of radiological features. Indian J Urol. 24(1):116-7, 2008
5. van Velthuysen ML et al: Glomerulopathy associated with parasitic infections. Clin Microbiol Rev. 13(1):55-66, table of contents, 2000

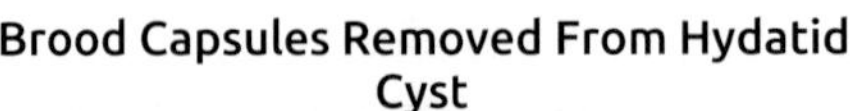

Brood Capsules Removed From Hydatid Cyst

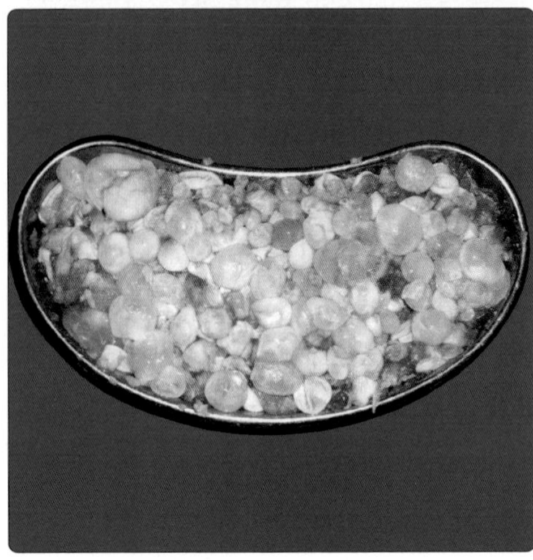

Intact And Ruptured Brood Capsules

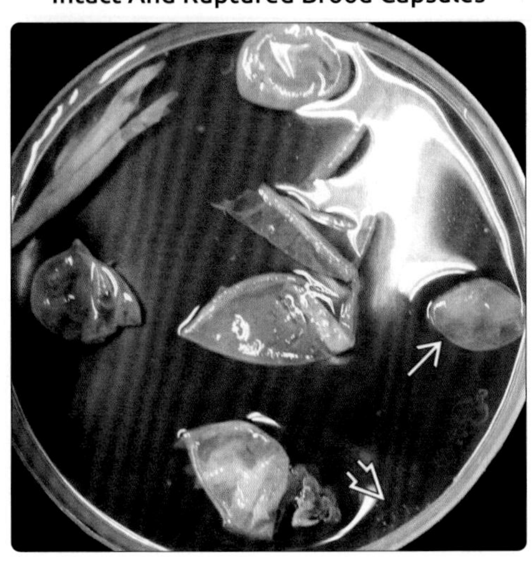

(Left) *The brood capsules or daughter cysts mostly lie free within the large hydatid cyst. This pan contains numerous largely intact daughter cysts. These must be handled with care since each cyst contain highly infective scolices.* **(Right)** *Several daughter cysts have been placed in this dish. Notice the translucent nature of the cyst wall. Notice also the small amount of free scolices often referred to as hydatid sand. These cysts would need careful handling since they each harbor 5-20 infective scolices.*

Brood Capsule Wall

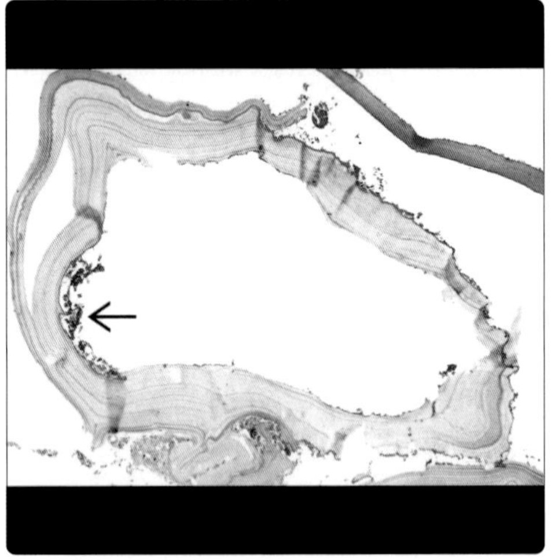

Brood Capsule Wall

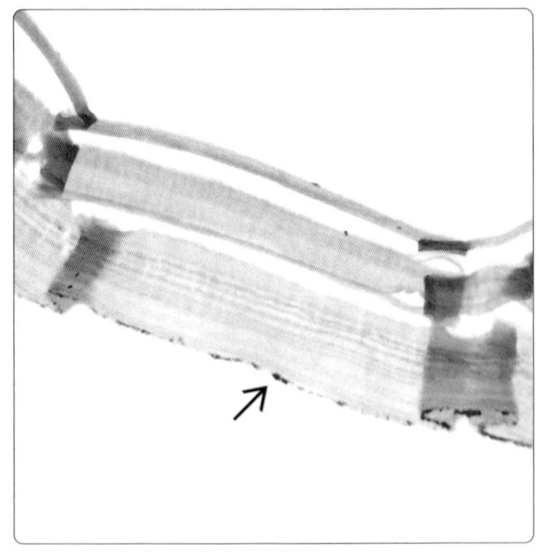

(Left) *This is a daughter cyst or brood capsule. The cyst wall consists of the ectocyst layer, also known as the acellular laminated membrane. Fragments of the internal germinal membrane are visible along the inside of a portion of this daughter cyst.* **(Right)** *This is the ectocyst or acellular laminated membrane. It lacks the pericyst fibrotic membrane formed from atrophic host tissue. A thin remnant of the germinal membrane where brood capsules form is barely visible along its inner surface.*

Germinal Membrane Layer

Daughter Cyst With Scolices

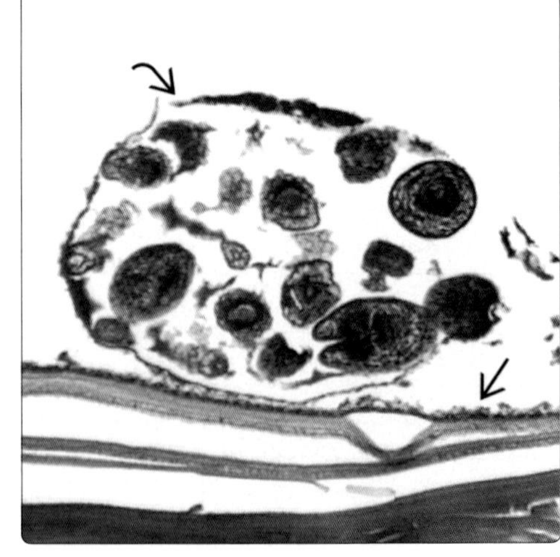

(Left) *Along the inner aspect of the acellular laminated membrane is the germinal membrane layer where daughter cysts or endocysts form. Some of the rounded structures are likely daughter cysts containing the infective agents, the scolices.* **(Right)** *This is a section through a brood capsule. The capsule is partially disrupted. Within the brood capsule are multiple scolices sectioned in various planes. The acellular laminated membrane is at the bottom lined by its germinal matrix.*

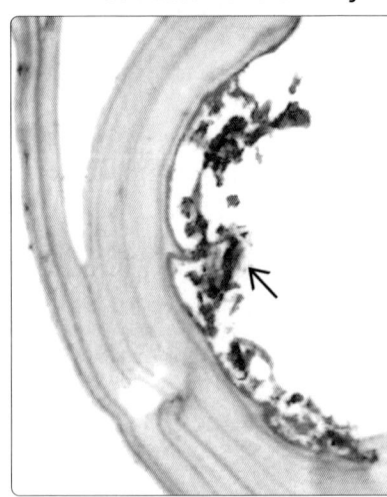

Scolex With Rostellum

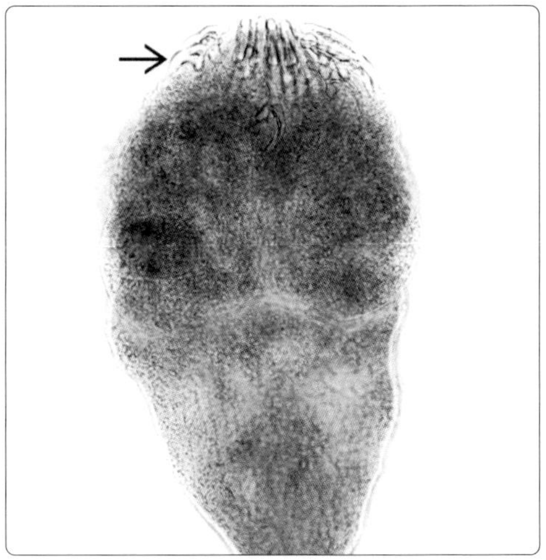

3 Scolices

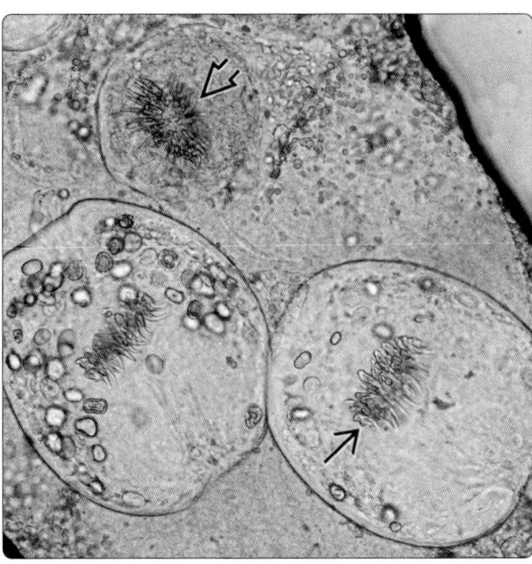

(Left) *This is a Pap-stained pleural effusion that shows a scolex. Each scolex is approximately 100 µm in size. The rostellum, or crown of hooklets, is easily visible at the top of the larva. Each hook ➔ is sickle-shaped and approximately 20-40 µm in size.* **(Right)** *In this wet preparation, 3 scolices are visible. In each scolex the characteristic rostellum or ring of hooks ➔ is visible. The radial arrangement of the hooks is discernible in 1 of the scolices ➔. The other 2 rostellums are viewed laterally.*

Scolex With Rostellum

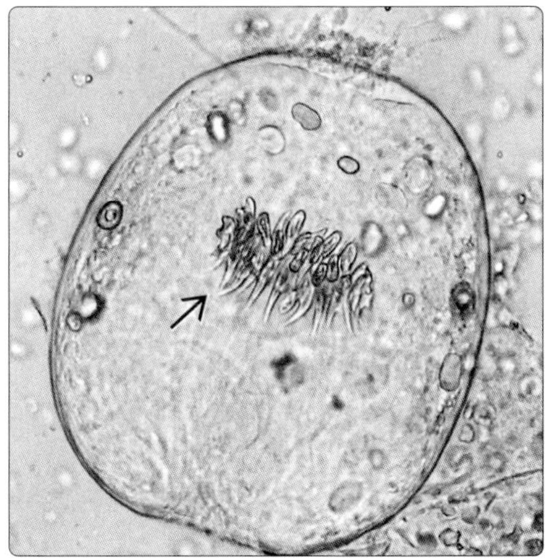

Rostellum

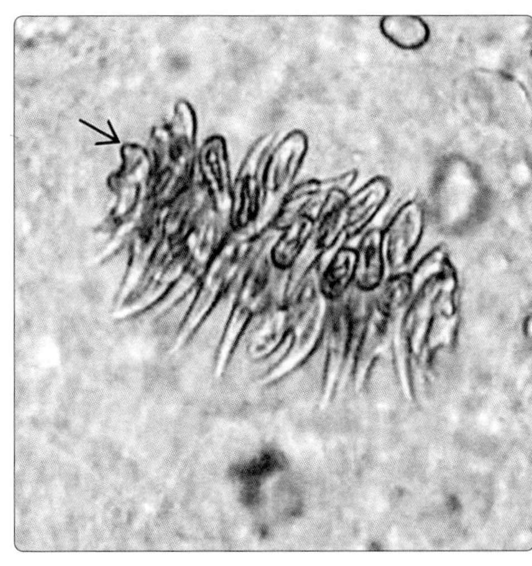

(Left) *This wet preparation of cyst contents shows a scolex, the infective agent of Echinococcus granulosus. Grossly, each scolex appears as a tiny grain of sand. In this scolex, the rostellum or ring of hooks ➔ is visible along with several other organelles. Each hook is sickle-shaped.* **(Right)** *This wet preparation of cyst contents shows the rostellum of a scolex. The hooks of the rostellum are sickle-shaped structures ➔. The rostellum hooks are acid-fast stain positive.*

Multilocular Cystic Renal Cell Carcinoma

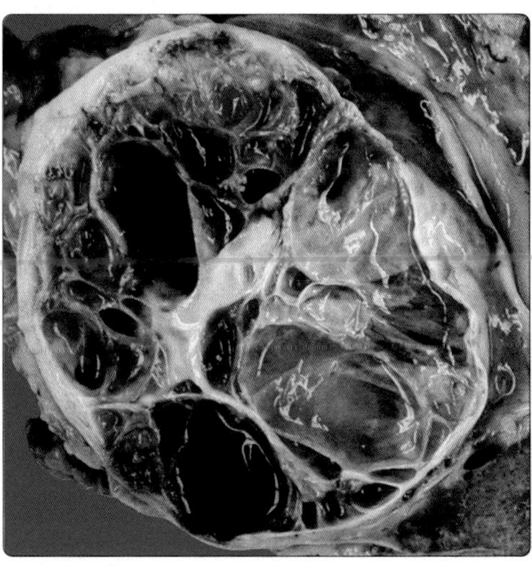

Cystic Nephroma

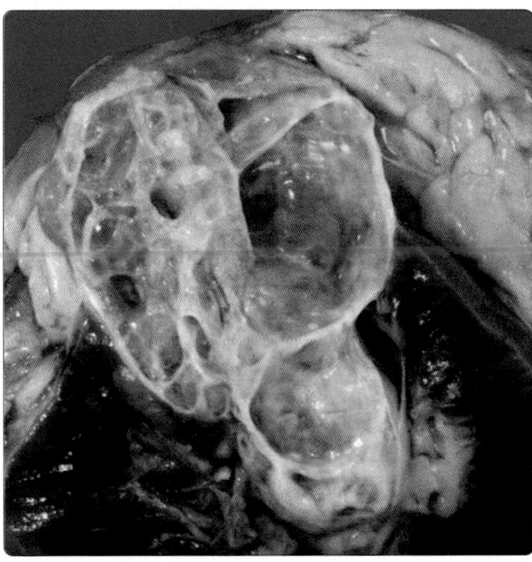

(Left) *This is a multilocular cystic renal cell carcinoma. The WHO defines this lesion as a circumscribed tumor composed entirely of cysts and cyst septae. The septa contain small clusters of clear cells that are indistinguishable from grade 1 clear cell renal cell carcinoma.* **(Right)** *This is a large cystic nephroma, which the WHO defines as a benign cystic neoplasm composed of epithelial and stromal elements. It consists entirely of cystic spaces and cyst septae without solid areas or freely mobile cysts.*

Polyomavirus Nephritis

KEY FACTS

TERMINOLOGY

- Polyomavirus infection in kidney allografts or native kidneys of immunosuppressed or immunocompromised patients

ETIOLOGY/PATHOGENESIS

- BK polyomavirus ~ 85%, JC virus ~ 15%

CLINICAL ISSUES

- Acute renal failure
- ~ 5% prevalence in kidney transplant patients
- Association with ureteral obstruction
- Treated by reduction/change in immunosuppressive drugs
- 7-100% 3-year graft loss, depending on pathologic stage

MICROSCOPIC

- Interstitial inflammation, mononuclear
- Tubulitis
- Nuclear inclusions
- TBM immune complex deposition

ANCILLARY TESTS

- IHC for polyoma large T antigen
- EM for viral particles
- Plasma PCR screen for viral load > 10^4/ml

TOP DIFFERENTIAL DIAGNOSES

- Acute tubulointerstitial (type I) rejection
- Adenovirus nephritis
- Acute tubular necrosis
- Acute interstitial nephritis

DIAGNOSTIC CHECKLIST

- Concurrent PVN and acute rejection occurs, but infrequently
  - Endarteritis or C4d in peritubular capillaries indicates rejection also present
- When borderline inflammatory infiltrate is present, polyoma IHC should be performed even in absence of viral nuclear changes

Zonal Distribution of Inflammation

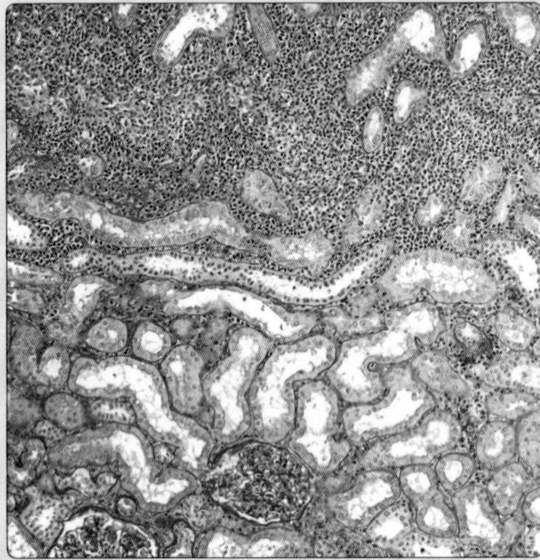

Intranuclear Inclusion

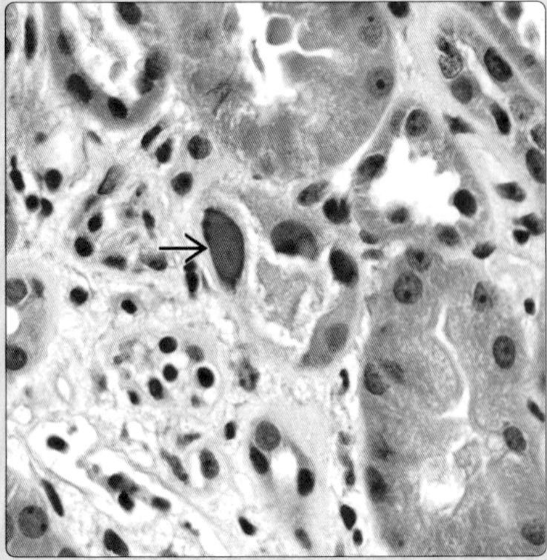

(Left) *Periodic acid-Schiff demonstrates dense zonal or regional interstitial inflammation, which emphasizes the importance of sufficiently sampling an allograft. The diagnosis of PVN would be missed if only the lower 1/2 of this renal cortex were biopsied. The virus is typically found in the areas of inflammation.* **(Right)** *Hematoxylin & eosin shows an intranuclear inclusion ⇨ with a ground-glass appearance in this distal tubule. The adjacent interstitium shows edema and scattered lymphocytes.*

Immunohistochemistry for SV40 Large T Antigen

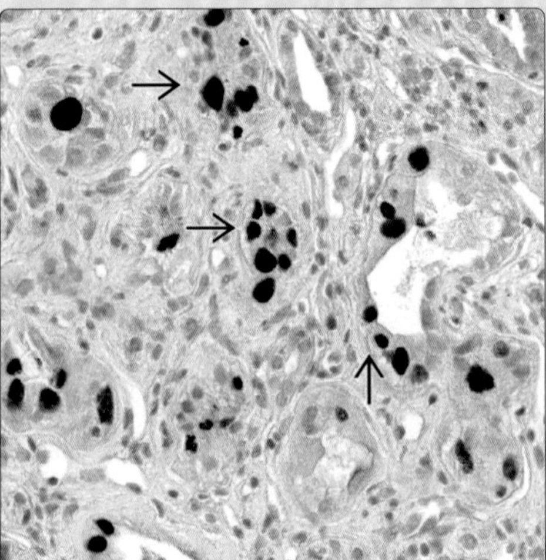

Polyomavirus Virions

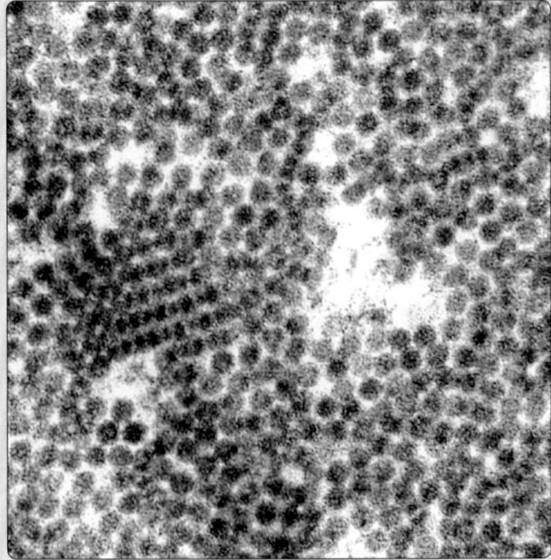

(Left) *Immunohistochemistry for polyoma large T antigen (SV40) stains ⇨ many tubular epithelial cell nuclei accompanied by prominent interstitial inflammation. This diagnostic of polyomavirus infection but does not distinguish the specific agent.* **(Right)** *High-power electron micrograph of a tubular epithelial cell nucleus shows a cluster of polyoma virions that measure about 40 nm. These are significantly smaller than adenovirus or herpes viruses.*

TERMINOLOGY

Abbreviations

- Polyomavirus nephritis (PVN)

Synonyms

- Polyomavirus nephropathy
- BK virus nephropathy

Definitions

- Polyomavirus infection of kidney, usually in immunocompromised host

ETIOLOGY/PATHOGENESIS

Infectious Agents

- Human polyomavirus
  - BK virus
    - Tropism for genitourinary tract epithelium
    - High seroprevalence in adults (80%)
    - Pathogenic only in immunocompromised patients
    - Causes ~ 85% of PVN
  - JC virus
    - Causes ~ 15% of PVN, usually milder than BK
    - Causes progressive multifocal leukoencephalopathy
  - Simian virus 40 (SV40), Merkel cell polyomavirus
    - Rarely, if ever, cause interstitial nephritis in humans

Pathogenesis

- Renal allograft
  - Reactivation of latent virus from donor organ
  - Renal injury promotes viral replication
  - Rejection contributes to pathogenesis
- Native kidney
  - AIDS, genetic immunodeficiency, immunosuppression
  - Rare in recipients of organs other than kidney

CLINICAL ISSUES

Epidemiology

- Incidence
  - ~ 5% in kidney transplant patients on tacrolimus and mycophenolate mofetil (MMF)
- Risk factors
  - Tacrolimus/MMF vs. cyclosporine/MMF (OR 3)
  - Prior rejection episode, older age, male gender

Presentation

- Acute renal failure
- Hemorrhagic cystitis
- Ureteral stenosis
  - Occurs in 5-10% of BK PVN
- Late complication: High-grade urothelial malignancies with expression of viral proteins (large T)

Laboratory Tests

- Plasma PCR
  - > 10^4 virions/ml highly specific for PVN (98%) but not sensitive (64%)
    - About 30% of PVN have plasma levels < 10^4/ml
  - Rare PVN in absence of BK viremia
    - Typical of JC virus PVN
- Urine
  - Decoy cells by cytology
    - Not specific for PVN, but indicate polyoma infection of urinary tract
  - Urine PCR less specific for PVN
  - Viral aggregates ("Haufen") by negative-staining EM
    - High sensitivity and specificity for PVN (> 98%)

Treatment

- Reduce tacrolimus/mycophenolate/switch to low-dose cyclosporine
- Current antivirals not highly effective
  - Cidofovir
  - Leflunomide
- Retransplant generally successful

Prognosis

- Graft loss depends on stage at diagnosis (13-100%)
  - Poorer prognosis with interstitial fibrosis and tubular atrophy
  - Rare graft loss with JC
- Rejection episodes follow in 8-12%
- Residual impairment of renal function common
- BK virus possibly oncogenic
  - Minority of urothelial tumors in renal allografts express large T antigen

MICROSCOPIC

Histologic Features

- Interstitial mononuclear inflammation
  - Lymphocytes and eosinophils
  - Plasma cells usually prominent
  - Associated with viral-infected epithelial cells
- Intranuclear inclusions in tubular epithelium
  - Ground-glass nuclear appearance
  - Nuclear enlargement and hyperchromatism
  - Nuclear inclusions may be present in sloughed cells in tubular lumina
  - Inclusions may not be evident in early PVN
- Tubulitis and tubular injury
  - Plasma cells occasionally in tubules
  - Apoptosis common
- Distal nephron involved more than proximal nephron
  - May involve only renal medulla in early stages, especially collecting ducts
  - Advanced stages involve parietal epithelial cells of glomeruli
- Late changes
  - Interstitial fibrosis and tubular atrophy
  - Extent of tubulointerstitial scarring often correlates with duration of viral infection
  - Correlates with graft survival
  - Dedifferentiated pattern of tubular epithelial cells; appear spindled, possibly reflecting epithelial-mesenchymal transition (EMT)
- High-grade urothelial and renal cell carcinoma reported
  - Expresses large T antigen in all tumor cells (not VP1)

Classifications for PVN

Stage	University of Maryland (2004)	3-Year Graft Loss (Maryland)	Banff Working Group (2009)	3-Year Graft Loss (Banff)
A (early)	Virus infected cells with no or minimal interstitial inflammation or tubular atrophy	13%	Virus-infected cells with no or minimal tubular injury	7%
B (active)	Virus-infected cells with interstitial inflammation/tubular atrophy involving < 25% (B1), 26-50% (B2), or > 50% (B3) of cortex	B1: 40%; B2: 60%; B3: 77%	Tubular epithelial cell necrosis or lysis with denudation of basement membrane spanning > 2 cells	50%
C (inactive/late)	Rare cytopathic effect with extensive interstitial inflammation/tubular atrophy	100%	> 50% interstitial fibrosis with any degree of tubular injury	100%

ANCILLARY TESTS

Immunohistochemistry

- Polyomavirus large T antigen IHC diagnostic
  - Protein of early phase of polyomavirus infection
  - Antibody to SV40 large T antigen detects BK and JC virus
  - Strong nuclear staining of epithelial cells
    - Tubular epithelial cells, often mostly distal tubules and collecting ducts
    - Commonly clustered positive cells
    - Infrequent glomerular parietal epithelial cells
  - Best results reported with PAb416 at concentration > 1/100 and polymer-based detection

Immunofluorescence

- Granular staining of tubular basement membranes (TBM) for IgG, C3, and C4d in ~ 50% of PVN
  - Viral antigens reported in deposits in 1 of 2 studies (not large T or VP1)
  - May persist despite disappearance of polyomavirus by IHC or EM
  - Significance unknown, associated with higher Cr
- C4d in atrophic TBMs may mimic peritubular capillary staining in antibody mediated rejection

Electron Microscopy

- Polyomavirus particles present within epithelial cells
  - ~ 40 nm viral particles in paracrystalline arrays or loose clusters
  - Nuclear and occasionally cytoplasmic location
- Discrete electron-dense deposits within TBMs
  - May be present in atrophic tubules
  - Use IF to confirm that electron-dense deposits represent immune complexes

DIFFERENTIAL DIAGNOSIS

Acute Tubulointerstitial (Type I) Rejection

- Prominent interstitial inflammation with tubulitis unassociated with large T antigen
  - Rare cases of concurrent acute rejection and PVN

Adenovirus Tubulointerstitial Nephritis

- Interstitial hemorrhage, necrosis and granulomas
- Positive adenovirus IHC, negative polyoma IHC

Acute Interstitial Nephritis

- IHC negative for polyoma large T antigen (SV40)

Acute Tubular Necrosis

- Reactive atypia of tubular epithelial cells mimics viral nuclear changes
- IHC negative for polyoma large T antigen (SV40)

DIAGNOSTIC CHECKLIST

Clinically Relevant Pathologic Features

- Stage of disease correlates with outcome
- Viral load scores (Banff) as % IHC positive tubular nuclei
  - pv1 < 1%
  - pv2 1-10%
  - pv3 > 10%

Pathologic Interpretation Pearls

- Predominant medullary inflammation raises PVN suspicion
- When borderline inflammatory infiltrate present, large T antigen IHC is indicated
  - Early PVN may lack viral cytopathic changes
  - Large T antigen in 1 tubular epithelial cell nucleus is diagnostic of infection
- Prominent interstitial inflammation with sparse large T antigen expression suggests concurrent acute rejection
- Concurrent PVN and acute rejection occurs, but infrequently
- TBM immune complexes may persist after viral stains become negative

SELECTED REFERENCES

1. Adam B et al: Banff Initiative for Quality Assurance in Transplantation (BIFQUIT): reproducibility of polyomavirus immunohistochemistry in kidney allografts. Am J Transplant. 14(9):2137-47, 2014
2. Singh HK et al: Polyomavirus Nephropathy: Quantitative Urinary Polyomavirus-Haufen Testing Accurately Predicts the Degree of Intrarenal Viral Disease. Transplantation. ePub, 2014
3. Dadhania D et al: Noninvasive prognostication of polyomavirus BK virus-associated nephropathy. Transplantation. 96(2):131-8, 2013
4. Filler G et al: Native kidney BK virus nephropathy associated with acute lymphocytic leukemia. Pediatr Nephrol. 28(6):979-81, 2013
5. Hirsch HH et al: Polyomavirus BK replication in de novo kidney transplant patients receiving tacrolimus or cyclosporine: a prospective, randomized, multicenter study. Am J Transplant. 13(1):136-45, 2013
6. Jacobi J et al: BK viremia and polyomavirus nephropathy in 352 kidney transplants; risk factors and potential role of mTOR inhibition. BMC Nephrol. 14:207, 2013
7. McDaid J et al: Transitional cell carcinoma arising within a pediatric donor renal transplant in association with BK nephropathy. Transplantation. 95(5):e28-30, 2013
8. Menter T et al: Pathology of resolving polyomavirus-associated nephropathy. Am J Transplant. 13(6):1474-83, 2013
9. Bracamonte E et al: Tubular basement membrane immune deposits in association with BK polyomavirus nephropathy. Am J Transplant. 7(6):1552-60, 2007

Prominent Interstitial Inflammation

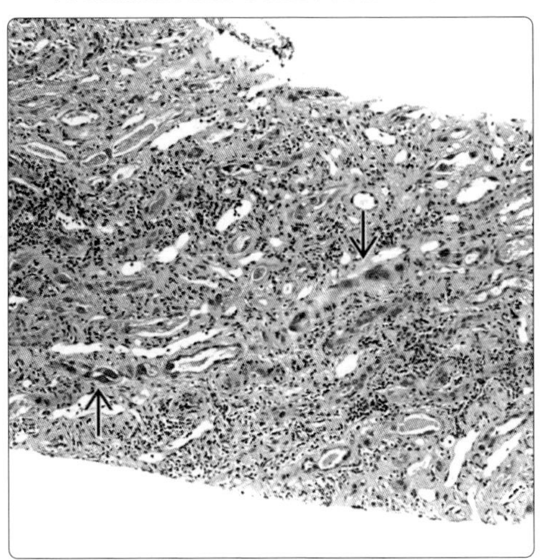

Polyomavirus Large T Antigen

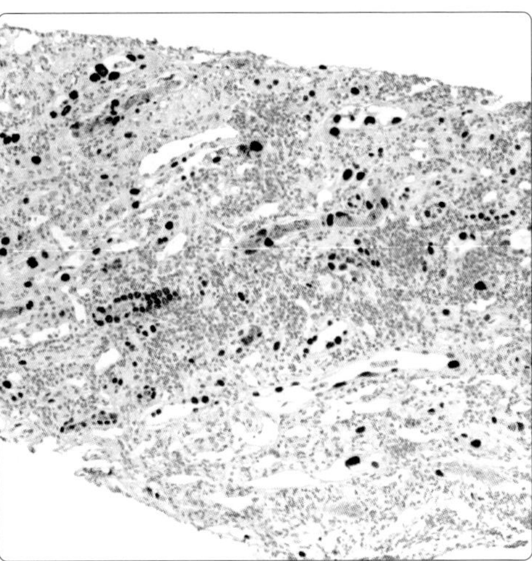

(Left) *Light microscopy of PVN shows widespread tubular changes with large, atypical epithelial cells with spindle shapes and enlarged nuclei* ⇒. *The inflammation is confined to areas with viral cytopathic changes.* **(Right)** *IHC for polyoma large T antigen (SV40) shows widespread infection of tubules, with a characteristic clustering of positive cells within individual tubules. The inflammatory infiltrate is typically in the same area as the virus, arguing that the virus causes the inflammation.*

Intranuclear Inclusion

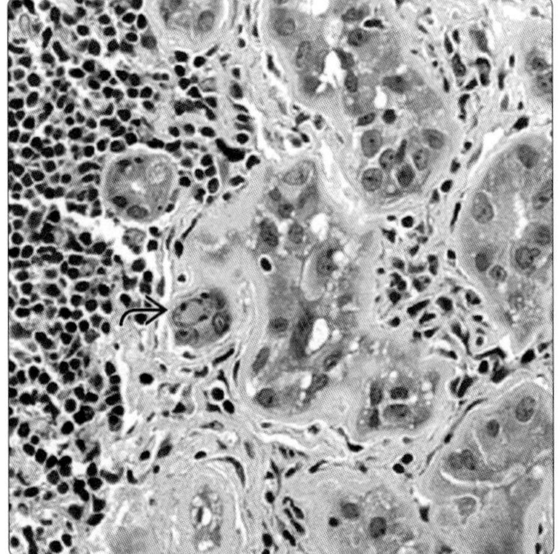

Viral Cytopathic Effect

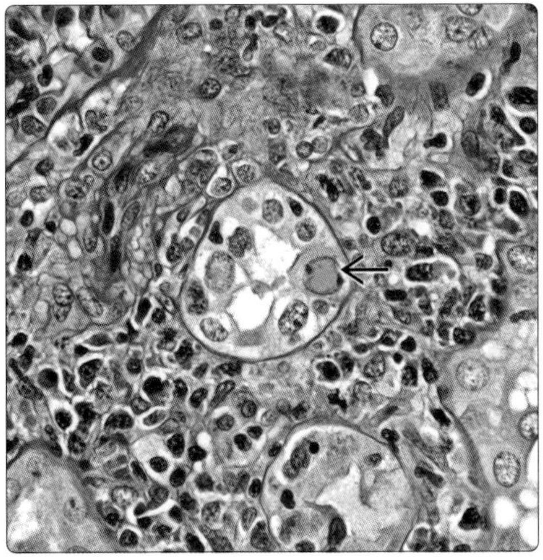

(Left) *In this biopsy from a patient with an advanced stage of PVN, tubular atrophy, interstitial fibrosis, and a focal mononuclear infiltrate are present, which are all nonspecific findings. Only 1 nuclear inclusion was found as a clue to the etiology* ⇒. **(Right)** *Periodic acid-Schiff shows severe interstitial inflammation and a typical, lavender, homogeneous intranuclear inclusion* ⇒ *of polyomavirus. Lymphocytes and plasma cells are in the interstitial infiltrate.*

"Ground-Glass" Intranuclear Inclusions

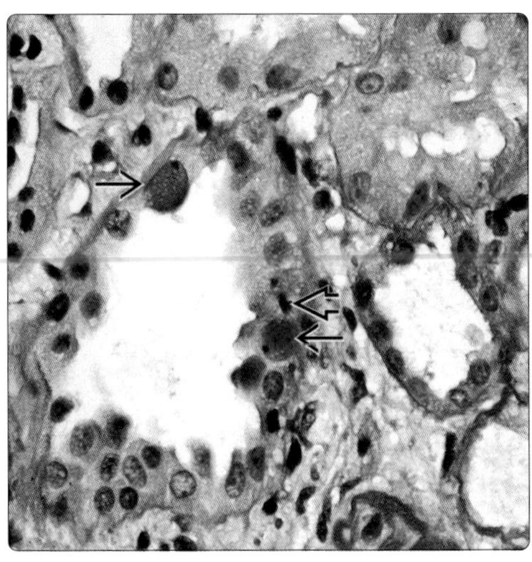

Intranuclear Inclusions

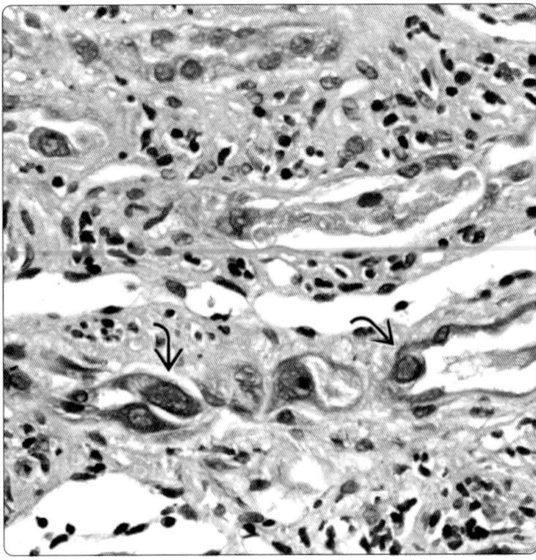

(Left) *Periodic acid-Schiff reveals several tubular epithelial cells with "ground-glass" intranuclear inclusions* ⇒ *and nucleoli displaced against the nuclear membrane. Tubulitis* ⇒ *(or lymphocytes between tubular epithelial cells and tubular basement membrane) is a common finding that mimics acute rejection when viral cytopathic changes are not prominent.* **(Right)** *Spindle-shaped (dedifferentiated) tubular cells show viral inclusions in nuclei* ⇒.

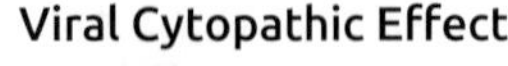

Polyomavirus Nephritis

(Left) *Hematoxylin & eosin shows several nuclei* → *with characteristic cytopathic effect of polyomavirus infection. Nucleoli are often pushed to the nuclear membrane. These features correlate with electron microscopic findings.* **(Right)** *This tubule has largely dedifferentiated or missing epithelium. A plasma cell is present in the tubule* →*, a distinctive finding in PVN. Many plasma cells are in the interstitium, which is also typical of PVN* ↷*.*

Viral Cytopathic Effect

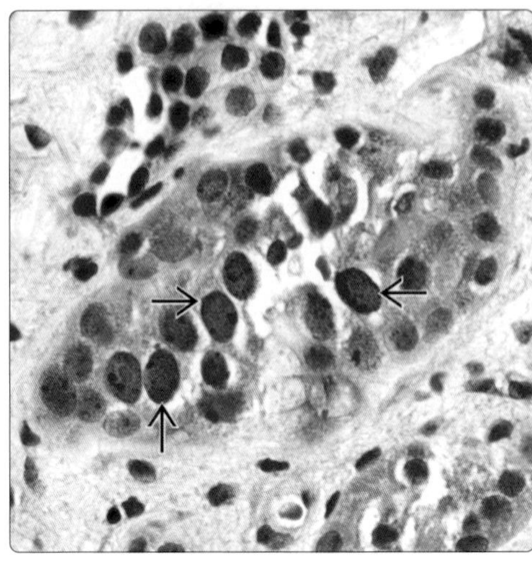

Plasma Cell Tubulitis

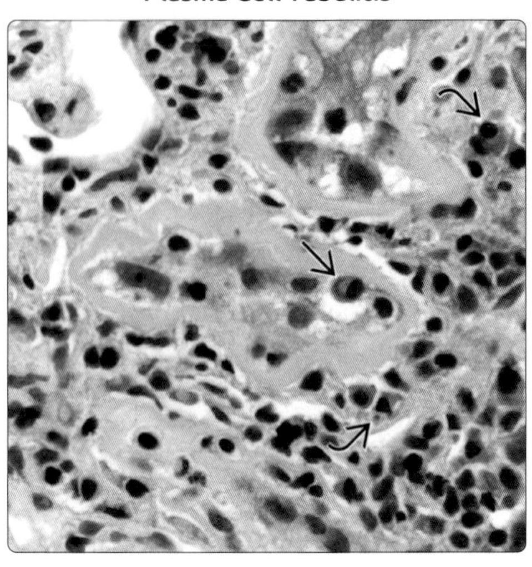

(Left) *Antibody to SV40 large T antigen shows prominent staining of debris in a collecting duct cast. When shed in the urine, these are the origin of the "Haufen" detected by EM. (Courtesy V. Nickeleit, MD.)* **(Right)** *Electron micrograph of a tubular epithelial cell shows shedding of polyomavirus into the lumen* → *and formation of cast-like aggregates* ↷*, which can be detected in the urine as "Haufen" by negative-staining EM.*

Collecting Duct Cast

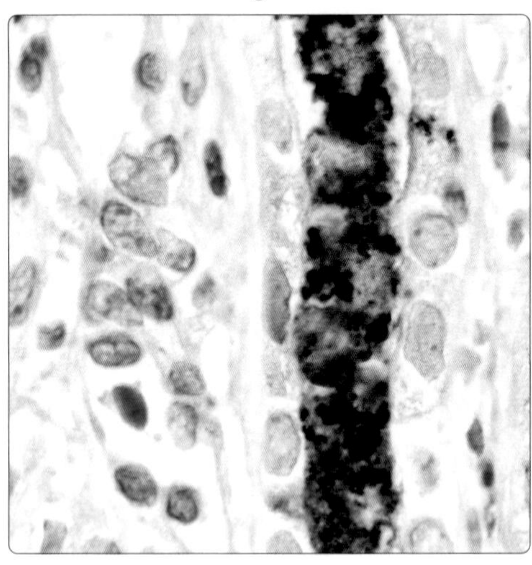

Virion Shedding in Tubule

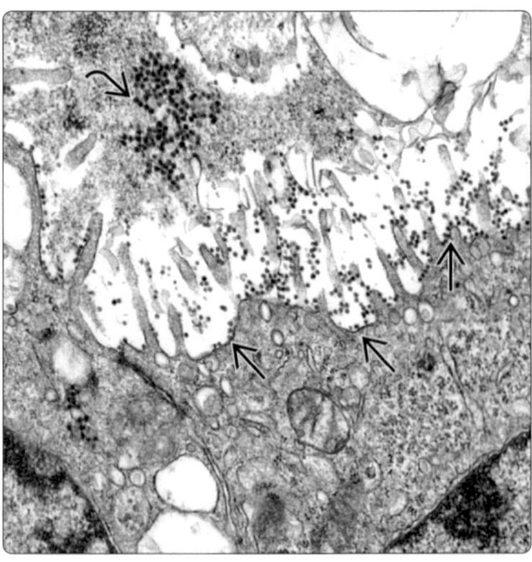

(Left) *Composite image of urine cytology from patients with PVN shows decoy cells with inclusions. These cells, which resemble malignant cells, are not diagnostic of PVN but only of polyoma infection of the urinary tract, which may be asymptomatic.* **(Right)** *Urine sediment examined by negative-staining EM shows an aggregate of virions about 40 nm in diameter, typical of polyomavirus. These aggregates are found almost exclusively in patients with PVN. (Courtesy V. Nickeleit, MD.)*

Decoy Cells

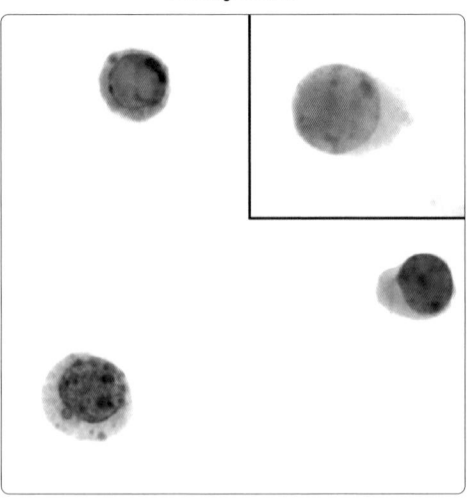

"Haufen" Viral Particles in Urine

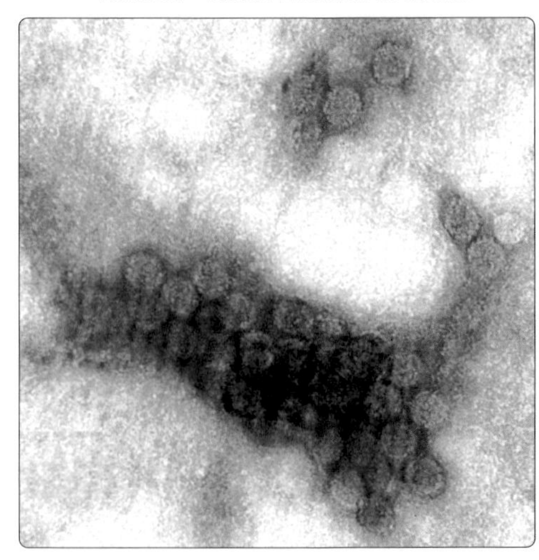

Parietal Epithelial Cells With Inclusions

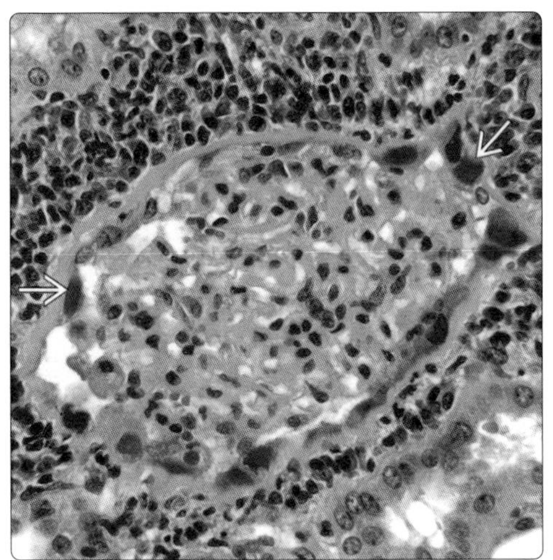

Large T Antigen in Parietal Epithelium

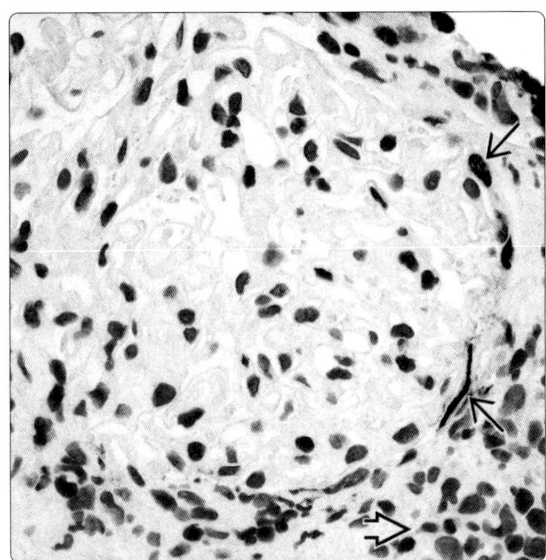

(Left) *Hematoxylin & eosin shows several parietal epithelial cells with enlarged and smudged nuclei* ➡ *and scattered lymphocytes between the Bowman capsule and epithelial cells (or "capsulitis"), which is an uncommon histologic feature of severe PVN.* **(Right)** *SV40 large T immunohistochemistry shows several parietal epithelial cells* ⇨ *infected by polyomavirus without nuclear enlargement. Scattered interstitial inflammation* ⇨ *is present adjacent to this glomerulus.*

Pseudocrescent

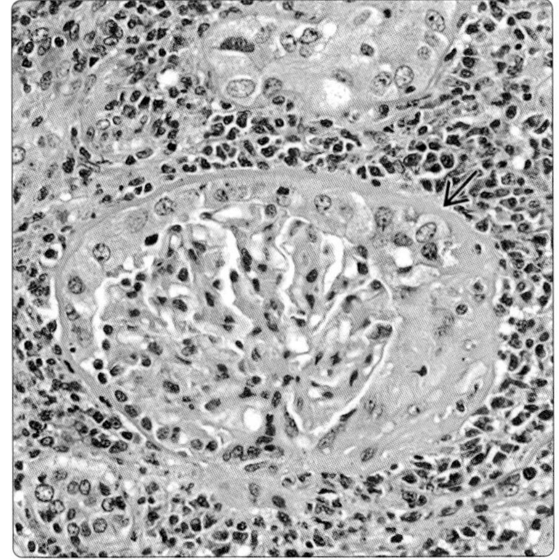

Severe Tubular Atrophy & Loss

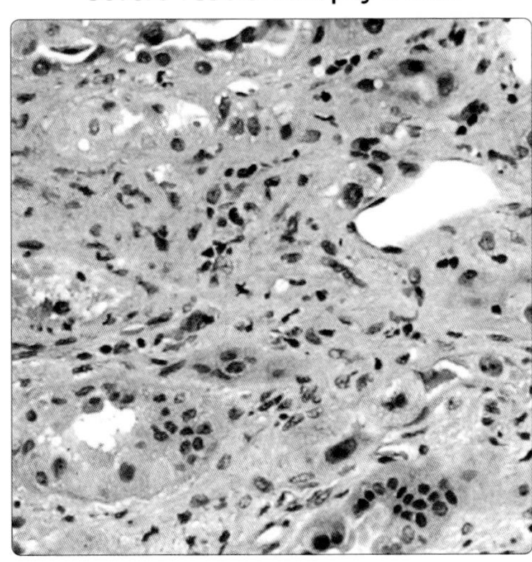

(Left) *Hematoxylin & eosin shows prominence of the parietal epithelial cells* ⇨*, which may be seen in a small subset of PVN and may occasionally mimic cellular crescents. Glomerular fibrinoid necrosis is absent.* **(Right)** *An advanced stage of PVN may show only nonspecific tubular loss, atrophy, and interstitial fibrosis, a.k.a. "chronic allograft nephropathy." Without a prior diagnosis of PVN, the cause would be unknown in this patient.*

Index Case From Patient BK

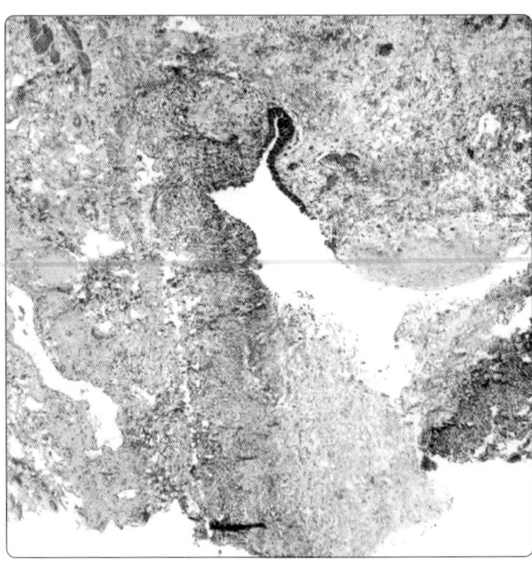

Urothelial Viral Infection

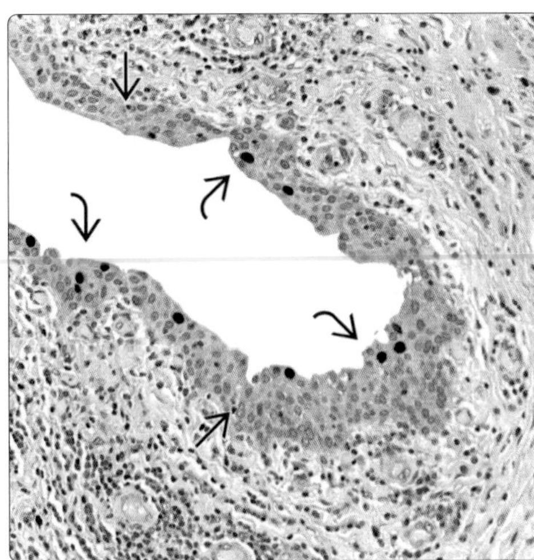

(Left) *This is the original case of polyomavirus infection from an allograft, reported by S.D. Gardner (St. Mary's Hospital, London). The ureter shows intense inflammation and ulceration. The patient's initials were BK, and the then-novel polyomavirus was named. (Courtesy E. Ramos, MD.)* **(Right)** *Ureter from an allograft nephrectomy with PVN shows numerous positive urothelial cells* ⇨ *for SV40 large T antigen. The mucosa shows marked inflammation with scattered lymphocytes invading the epithelium* ⇨*.*

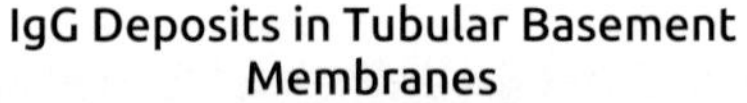

IgG Deposits in Tubular Basement Membranes

Granular C4d Deposits in Tubular Basement Membranes

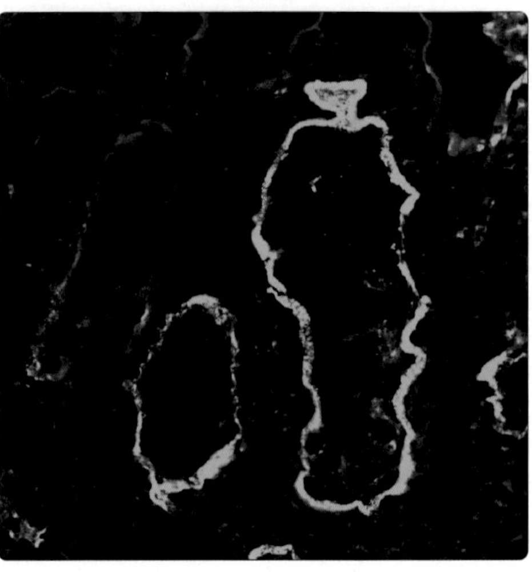

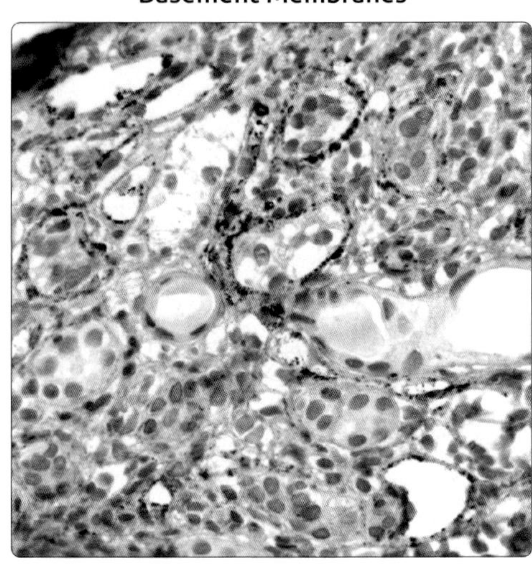

(Left) *Immunofluorescence in a case of PVN shows intense granular deposition of IgG in some but not all tubular basement membranes. Granular IgG in the TBM is indicative of immune complex deposition and is not a nonspecific finding. C3 is similarly deposited, but is not specific, since C3 is commonly detected in the TBM.* **(Right)** *Immunohistochemistry for C4d shows granular deposits along the TBM of a subset of the tubules. The peritubular capillaries are negative.*

JC Polyomavirus Nephropathy

JC Polyomavirus Nephropathy

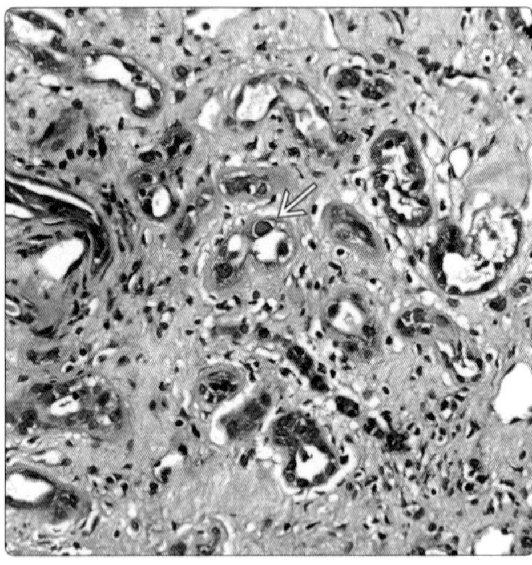

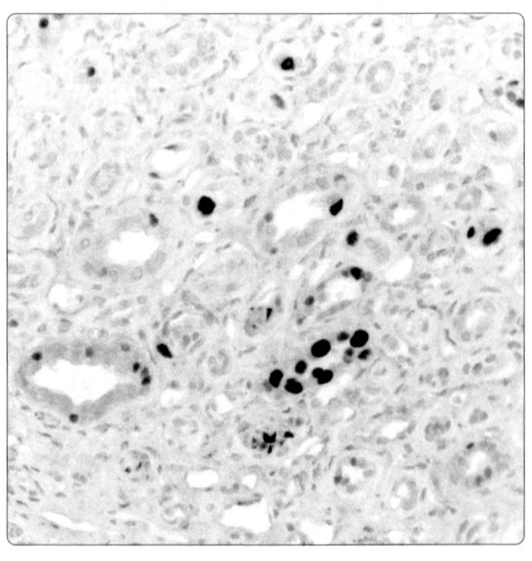

(Left) *JC polyomavirus infections have similar although often milder histologic changes. Viral cytopathic effect is seen in one nucleus ➡. JC virus is suspected when the SV40 large T antigen stain is positive, but the blood PCR for BK virus is negative, since only the latter is specific for BK. (Courtesy R.N. Smith, MD.)* **(Right)** *JC virus large T antigen cross-reacts with the usual antibody to SV40 large T antigen, as shown in the medulla of this case of JC polyomavirus nephropathy. (Courtesy R.N. Smith, MD.)*

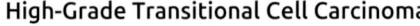

High-Grade Transitional Cell Carcinoma

High-Grade Urothelial Carcinoma Expressing Polyomavirus Large T Antigen

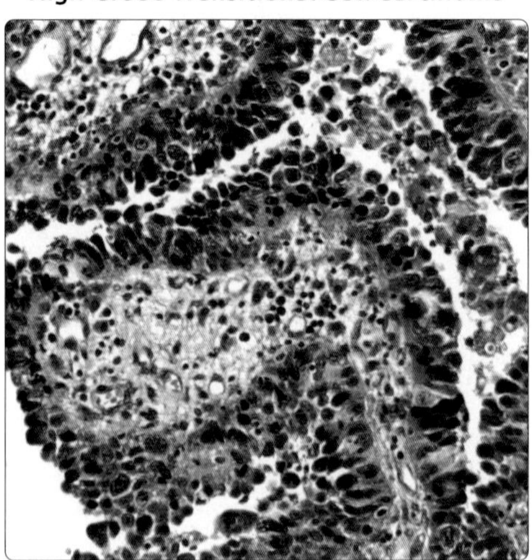

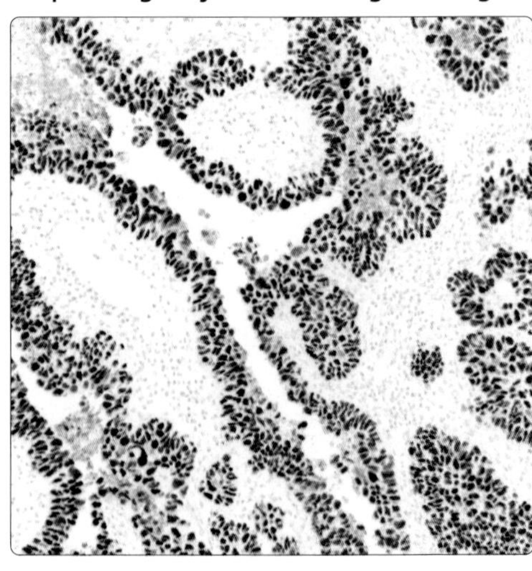

(Left) *High-grade urothelial and renal cell carcinomas have been reported in renal transplants that express the large T antigen in all tumor cells (but not the normal parenchyma). This high-grade papillary pelvic tumor was detected 5 years after an episode of PVN. (Courtesy E. Farkash, MD.)* **(Right)** *About 20% of the urothelial tumors arising in renal transplant recipients express polyomavirus large T antigen. Large T antigens of other polyomaviruses are known to be oncogenic. (Courtesy E. Farkash, MD.)*

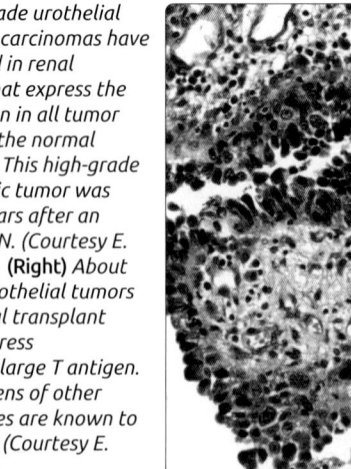

Tubular Basement Membrane Deposits

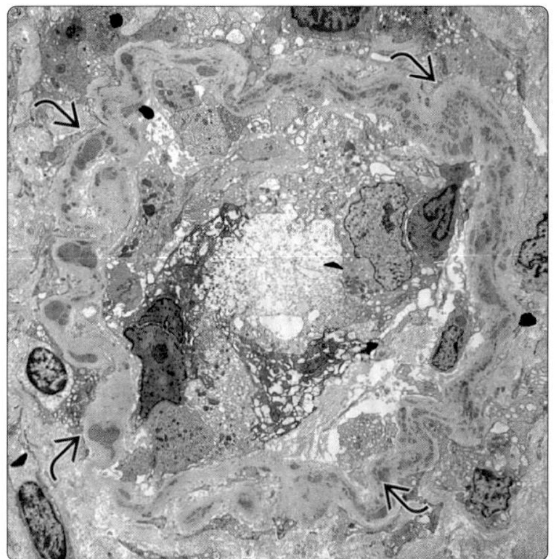

Tubular Basement Membrane Deposits

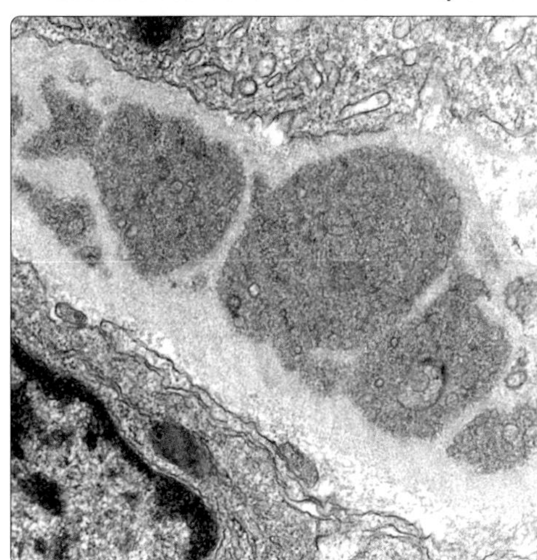

(Left) *Low-power electron micrograph of a cross section of a tubule reveals widespread electron-dense amorphous deposits in the TBM* ➙. **(Right)** *Electron micrograph of the tubular basement membrane deposits at high power shows that the deposits are amorphous and contain scattered membranous debris. No viral particles are evident. SV40 large T antigen has been reported in these deposits using indirect IF microscopy.*

Intranuclear Virions

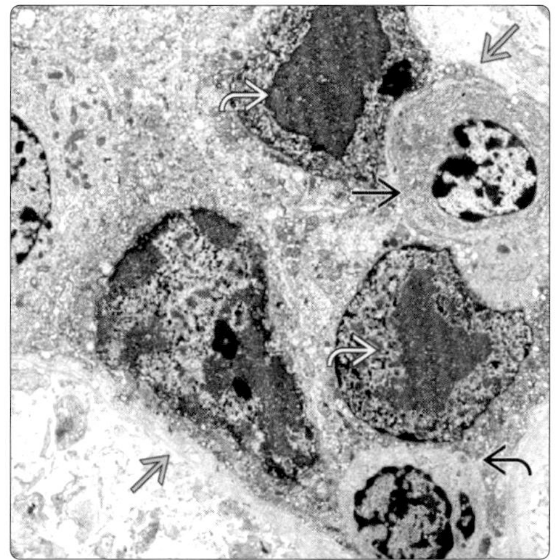

Intranuclear Virions

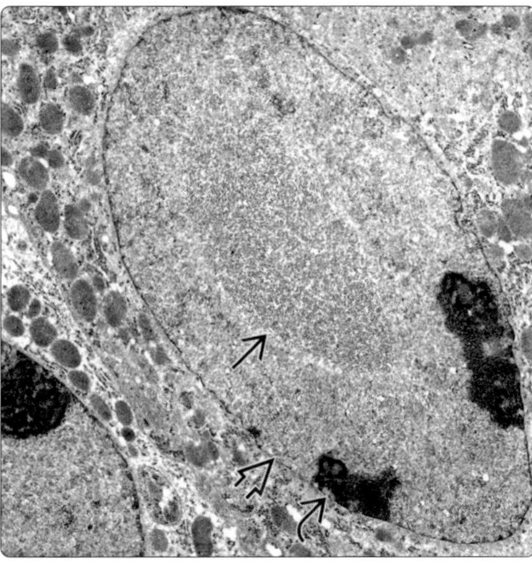

(Left) *Electron micrograph of a severely altered tubule shows large aggregates of polyoma virions in the tubular epithelial nuclei* ➙, *as well as an intratubular plasma cell* ➙ *and lymphocyte* ➙. *The tubular basement membrane is unremarkable* ➙. **(Right)** *Electron micrograph demonstrates numerous individual viral particles* ➙ *within the nucleus* ➙ *of a tubular epithelial cell. Nucleoli* ➙ *are pushed aside against the nuclear membrane. This can also be appreciated on light microscopy.*

Cytoplasmic Virions

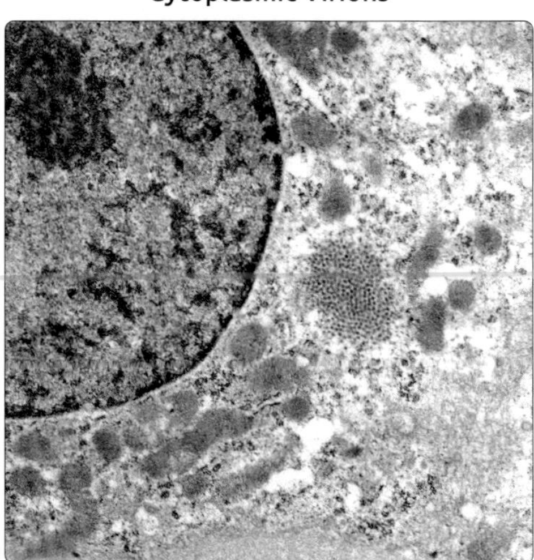

BK Polyoma Virions

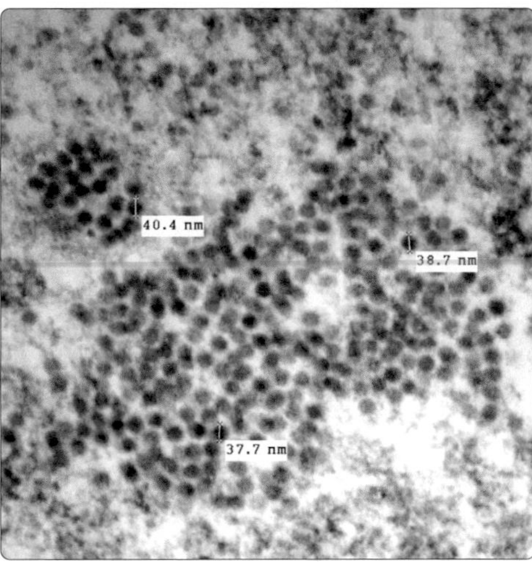

(Left) *EM shows an aggregate of virions within the cytoplasm next to the nucleus of this infected tubular epithelial cell. The viral particles can be closely grouped together or occasionally arranged in a paracrystalline array (not shown).* **(Right)** *Electron microscopy of BK polyomavirus shows viral particles in the nucleus of approximately 40 nm. Polyomavirus is substantially smaller than adenovirus (75-80 nm) or herpes group viruses (150-200 nm).*

Adenovirus Infection

KEY FACTS

TERMINOLOGY

- Synonym
  - Adenovirus nephritis

ETIOLOGY/PATHOGENESIS

- Nonenveloped, double-stranded DNA virus

CLINICAL ISSUES

- Fever
- Graft tenderness
- Hemorrhagic cystitis usual with kidney involvement
  - Gross hematuria
- Acute renal failure
- Blood RT-PCR for diagnosis and surveillance
- Cidofovir, ribavirin, IVIg
- Recovery common if localized
- > 60% fatal if disseminated

MICROSCOPIC

- Granulomatous inflammation
- Necrosis of tubules
- Interstitial hemorrhage
- Smudgy, basophilic, intranuclear inclusions in tubular cells

ANCILLARY TESTS

- Positive for AdV by immunohistochemistry
- EM shows characteristic 60-80 nm virions

TOP DIFFERENTIAL DIAGNOSES

- Acute cellular rejection
- Polyomavirus nephritis
- Drug-induced acute interstitial nephritis

DIAGNOSTIC CHECKLIST

- Coinfection with other organisms common
- Antiviral antibody panel valuable in differential diagnosis (AdV, SV40, CMV)

Necrotizing Granulomata

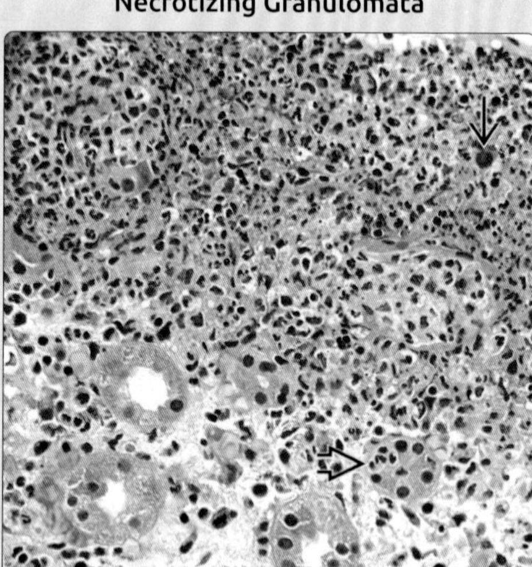

Adenovirus Cytopathic Effect

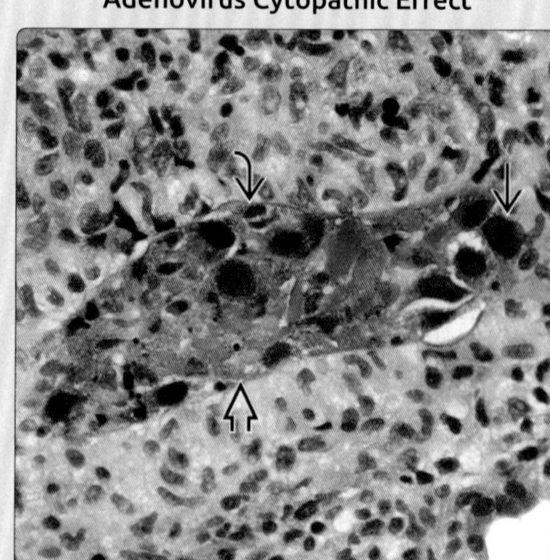

(Left) *Necrotizing granulomata are typical of adenovirus infection, with neutrophils, plasma cells, and lymphocytes in this renal allograft. Viral cytopathic effect ➙ and tubulitis ➙ are noted. (Courtesy L. Novoa-Takara, MD.)* **(Right)** *Hematoxylin & eosin shows viral cytopathic effect ➙ in several tubular epithelial cell nuclei within a tubule with tubulitis ➙ and necrosis ➙, which is surrounded by abundant interstitial inflammation.*

Adenovirus IHC

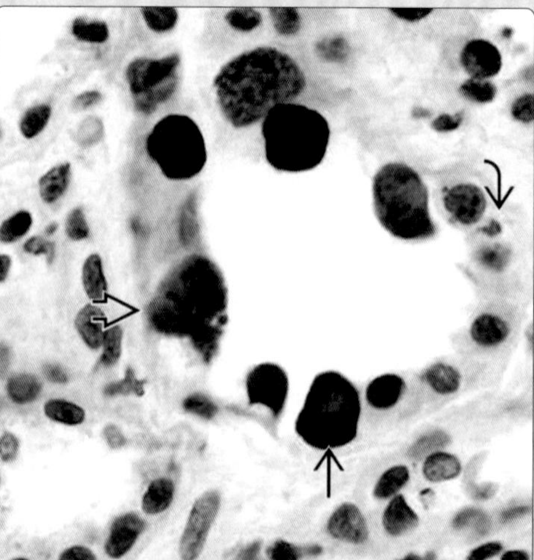

Adenovirus Virions

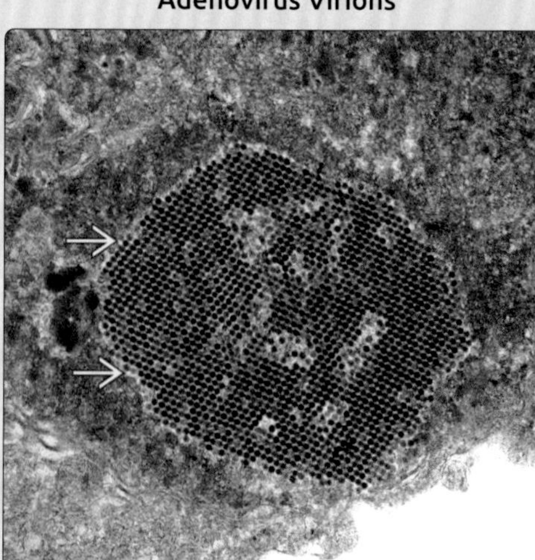

(Left) *Adenovirus immunohistochemistry shows both strong staining ➙ and faint staining ➙ in the nuclei of several tubular epithelial cells in a renal allograft biopsy. Note the scattered interstitial inflammatory cells and focal tubulitis ➙.* **(Right)** *Electron microscopy shows adenovirus virions ➙ in a paracrystalline array within an infected epithelial cell nucleus. The individual virions measure approximately 80 nm in diameter, which is twice the size of human polyomavirus. The scale bar in the bottom left corner measures 500 nm.*

ETIOLOGY/PATHOGENESIS

Infectious Agents

- Adenovirus (Adv)
  - Nonenveloped, double-stranded DNA virus
  - Possible routes of infection
    - Reactivation of endogenous latent infection
    - Transplanted organ or tissue
- Other organs affected: Bladder, lung, liver, GI tract

CLINICAL ISSUES

Epidemiology

- Incidence
  - Rare in kidney transplant recipients (< 1%)
    - Onset typically in 1st 3 months post transplant
  - AdV more common in stem cell recipients (3-7%)
    - Native kidney occasionally involved
- Age
  - Children more susceptible (< 5 years)

Presentation

- Fever
- Hemorrhagic cystitis
  - Gross hematuria
  - AdV rarely causes renal infection in absence of cystitis
- Acute kidney injury
- Graft tenderness
- Bladder and ureter involvement may cause obstructive uropathy

Laboratory Tests

- Real-time polymerase chain reaction (RT-PCR)
  - AdV in blood precedes symptoms by > 3 weeks
- Shell vial assay (culture)
- Enzyme immunoassay for AdV antigen in blood

Treatment

- Drugs
  - Cidofovir, ribavirin; valganciclovir or ganciclovir
  - Intravenous immunoglobulin (IVIg)
- Reduction of immunosuppressive agents

Prognosis

- Disseminated disease often fatal (> 60%)
- Recovery common if localized

MACROSCOPIC

General Features

- White-yellowish streaks with hemorrhagic rim primarily in medulla
- Hemorrhagic mucosal surface in renal pelvis and ureters

MICROSCOPIC

Histologic Features

- Glomeruli
  - Glomerular (visceral and parietal) epithelial cells may be infected
- Tubules and interstitium
  - Acute tubular injury and interstitial nephritis
    - Focal necrosis of tubules
    - Interstitial hemorrhage and edema
  - Granulomas associated with viral-infected tubular epithelial cells and tubular destruction
    - Peritubular location
  - Viral cytopathic effect in tubular epithelial cells
    - Basophilic intranuclear inclusions with smudged appearance
      - Detached infected cells within tubular lumina
      - Distal tubules infected more than proximal tubules
- Vessels: No specific finding

ANCILLARY TESTS

Immunohistochemistry

- Nuclear and cytoplasmic staining for Adv

Immunofluorescence

- No deposits described along TBM

Electron Microscopy

- Viral particles 60-80 nm in diameter in tubular nuclei

DIFFERENTIAL DIAGNOSIS

Acute Cellular Rejection

- Reactive atypia of tubular nuclei may mimic viral inclusions
- Granulomas sometimes seen associated with tubular destruction
- Less severe hemorrhage and tubular necrosis than AdV
- Other evidence of rejection (e.g., endarteritis, C4d deposition)

Polyomavirus Nephritis

- Positive SV40 immunohistochemistry
- Less hemorrhage and tubular necrosis than AdV
- More plasma cells and less granulomatous inflammation

Drug-Induced Acute Interstitial Nephritis

- Hemorrhage and necrosis minimal
- No viral antigen present

DIAGNOSTIC CHECKLIST

Pathologic Interpretation Pearls

- Necrotizing granuloma is distinctive feature
- Panel of antiviral antibodies valuable in differential diagnosis (AdV, SV40, CMV, HSV)
- Coinfection with other fungal or viral organisms may occur

SELECTED REFERENCES

1. Dawood US et al: Disseminated adenovirus infection in kidney transplant recipient. Nephrology (Carlton). 19 Suppl 1:10-3, 2014
2. Lachiewicz AM et al: Adenovirus causing fever, upper respiratory infection, and allograft nephritis complicated by persistent asymptomatic viremia. Transpl Infect Dis. 16(4):648-52, 2014
3. Keddis M et al: Adenovirus-induced interstitial nephritis following umbilical cord blood transplant for chronic lymphocytic leukemia. Am J Kidney Dis. 59(6):886-90, 2012
4. Varma MC et al: Early onset adenovirus infection after simultaneous kidney-pancreas transplant. Am J Transplant. 11(3):623-7, 2011
5. Mazoyer E et al: A case report of adenovirus-related acute interstitial nephritis in a patient with AIDS. Am J Kidney Dis. 51(1):121-6, 2008

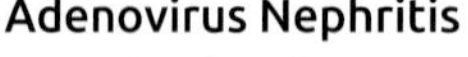

Adenovirus Nephritis

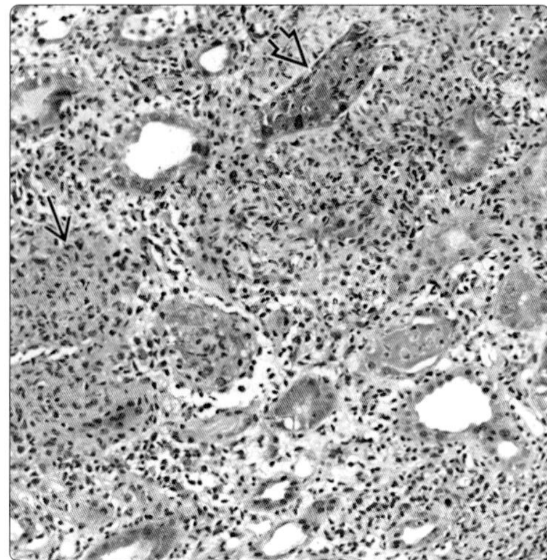

Medullary Interstitial Inflammation

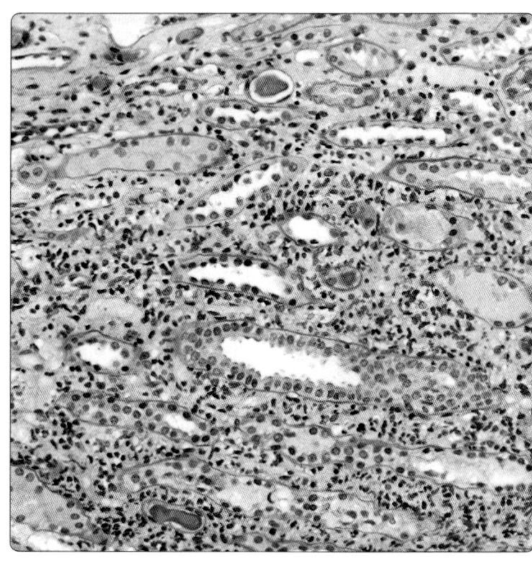

(Left) Hematoxylin & eosin demonstrates severe interstitial inflammation, granulomas →, tubular necrosis ⇨, and interstitial edema in this renal allograft with adenovirus infection. (Right) Periodic acid-Schiff reveals prominent interstitial inflammation and frequent tubulitis in the renal medulla, which is common for adenovirus but atypical for acute rejection. Patchy involvement of the renal cortex (not shown) is also present.

Granulomas

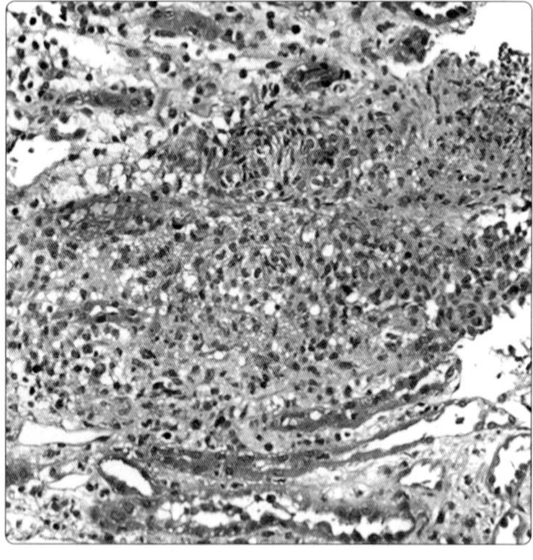

Peritubular Multinucleated Giant Cells

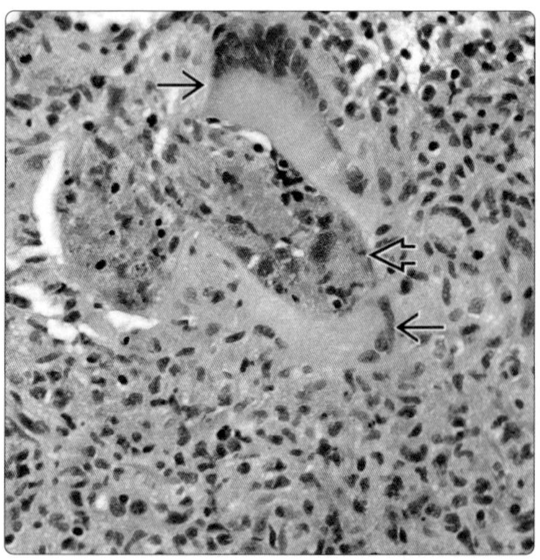

(Left) Granulomas of epithelioid macrophages and tubular destruction are typical of adenovirus infection in the kidney. Granulomas are not common in polyomavirus or cytomegalovirus infections. (Right) Hematoxylin & eosin reveals 2 giant cells → surrounding a severely injured tubule with necrosis ⇨. Interstitial inflammatory cells consist of epithelioid macrophages, lymphocytes, plasma cells, and rare eosinophils.

Adenovirus Smudged Nuclei

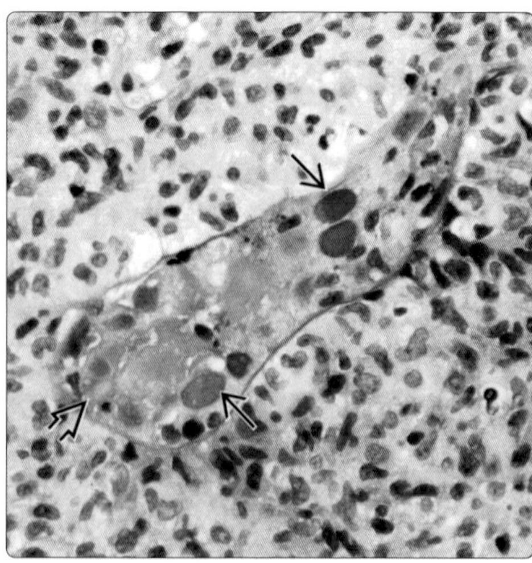

Peritubular Multinucleated Giant Cells

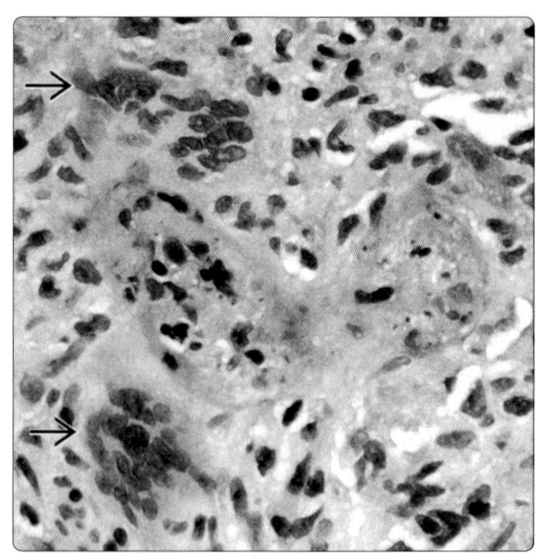

(Left) Periodic acid-Schiff shows enlarged, tubular epithelial cell nuclei with a "smudged" appearance →, which resemble polyomavirus, but the presence of tubular degeneration/necrosis ⇨ and granulomatous inflammation favors adenovirus nephritis. (Right) Periodic acid-Schiff highlights multinucleated giant cells → closely associated with an injured tubule, which contains necrotic and sloughed epithelial cells that are intermixed with lymphocytes in a renal allograft infected with adenovirus.

Adenovirus In Situ Hybridization

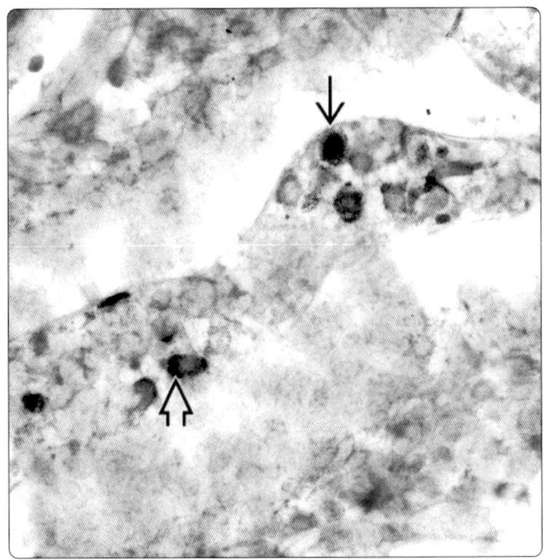

Adenovirus IHC

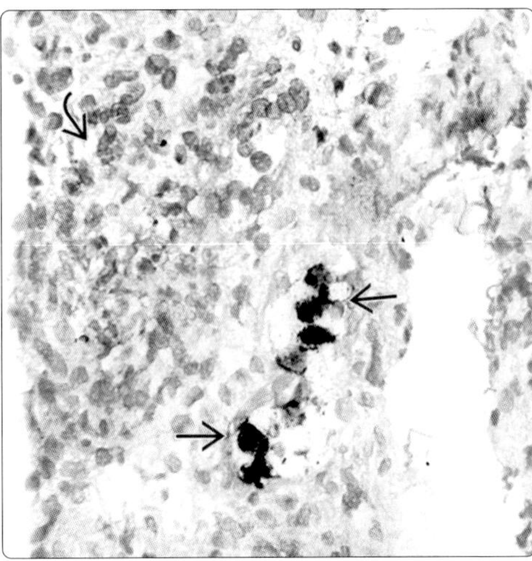

(Left) *In situ hybridization for adenovirus highlights a few tubular epithelial cell nuclei → and cell cytoplasm → within this tubule with extensive injury and necrosis.* **(Right)** *Adenovirus antigens are detected primarily in the nucleus of tubular epithelial cells in the kidney →. Positive cells are typically sparse. A granuloma is seen nearby →.*

Adenovirus Virions

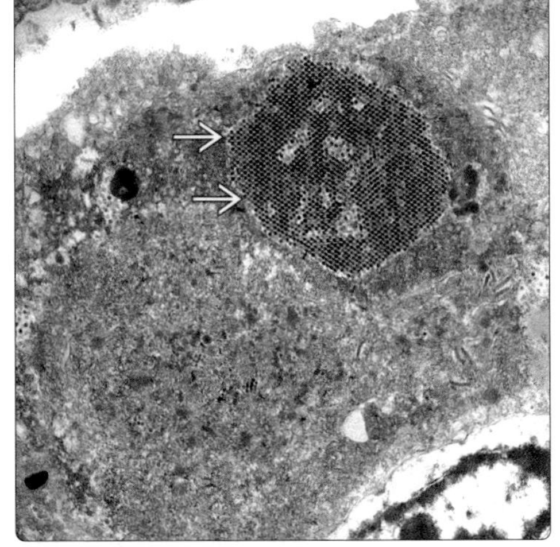

Adenovirus Virions

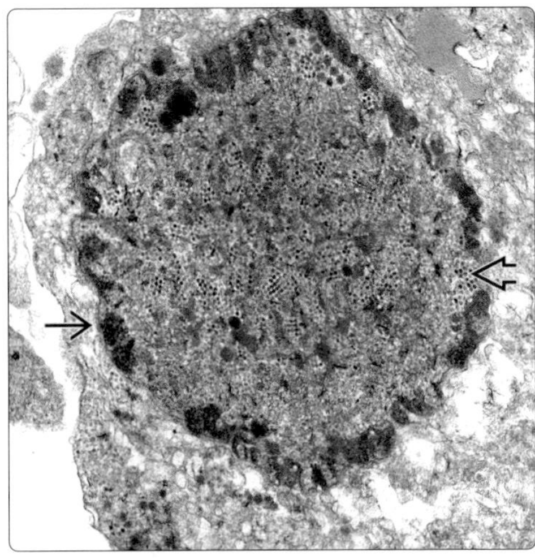

(Left) *Electron microscopy shows numerous adenovirus viral particles forming a paracrystalline array → within the nucleus of this infected epithelial cell.* **(Right)** *Electron microscopy reveals numerous adenovirus virions → that have displaced the nuclear chromatin → against the nuclear membrane within this infected epithelial cell nucleus. The nucleus corresponds with a nuclear inclusion that is observed by light microscopy.*

Adenovirus Virions

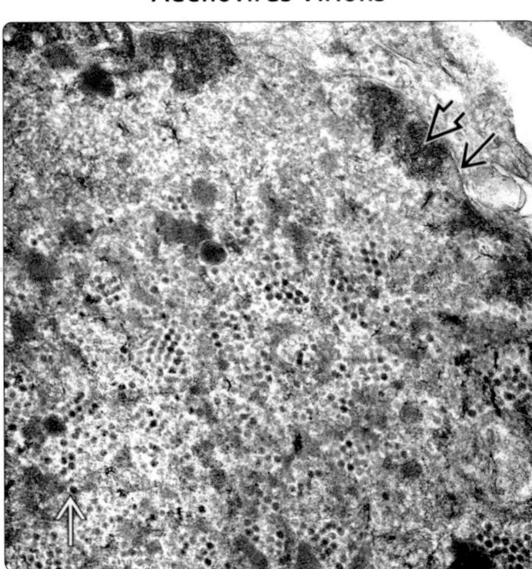

Adenovirus Dimensions

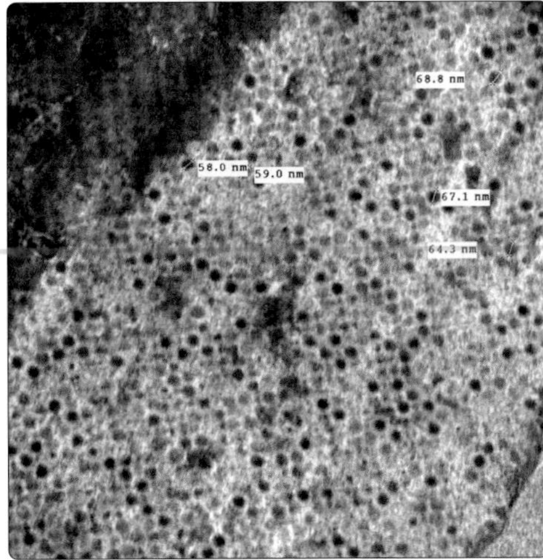

(Left) *Electron microscopy demonstrates numerous individual adenovirus virions → within this nucleus, which has displaced the nuclear chromatin → against the nuclear membrane →.* **(Right)** *Adenovirus virions are 60-80 nm in diameter, as seen here in a nucleus of an infected tubular epithelial cell. The diameter is larger than the ~30-45 nm polyomavirus and smaller than cytomegalovirus (150-200 nm).*

Cytomegalovirus Infection

KEY FACTS

TERMINOLOGY

- Cytomegalovirus (CMV) infection in kidneys, usually associated with systemic CMV in immunocompromised patients

ETIOLOGY/PATHOGENESIS

- Most individuals infected by CMV before adulthood
- Immunocompromised patients at risk
  - Neonatal CMV
  - Transplant CMV

CLINICAL ISSUES

- Presentation
  - Renal dysfunction
  - Flu-like symptoms
- Antiviral agents
  - Ganciclovir or valganciclovir
  - CMV immune globulin
- Reduce or alter immunosuppressive agents

MICROSCOPIC

- "Owl-eye" nuclear inclusions
  - Most prominent in tubular epithelium
  - Glomerular capillary &/or peritubular capillary endothelial cells
- Interstitial inflammation, mononuclear
- Acute glomerulonephritis (rare)

TOP DIFFERENTIAL DIAGNOSES

- Polyomavirus nephropathy
- Adenovirus tubulointerstitial nephritis
- Acute cellular rejection

DIAGNOSTIC CHECKLIST

- CMV intranuclear inclusions present in predominantly endothelial cells or epithelial cells
- Coinfection with other fungal or viral organisms may occur
- Features of foscarnet toxicity may be present in patients treated for CMV infection

(Left) *Hematoxylin and eosin shows characteristic intranuclear ("owl-eye") inclusions → of cytomegalovirus (CMV) infection within the glomerular endothelial cells.* **(Right)** *Hematoxylin and eosin shows CMV intranuclear inclusions → in endothelial cells of a peritubular capillary with basophilic cytoplasmic changes ⇒ that are also present in a tubular epithelial cell ↷.*

Glomerular CMV

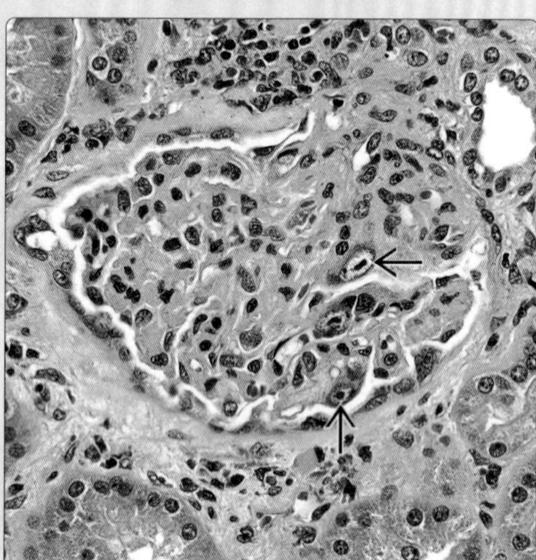

Peritubular Capillary CMV

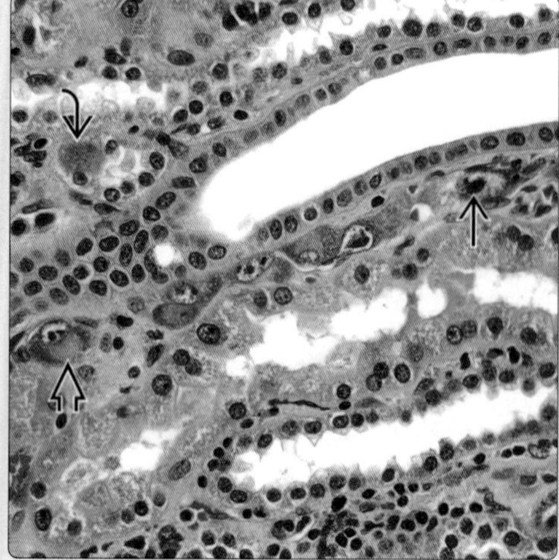

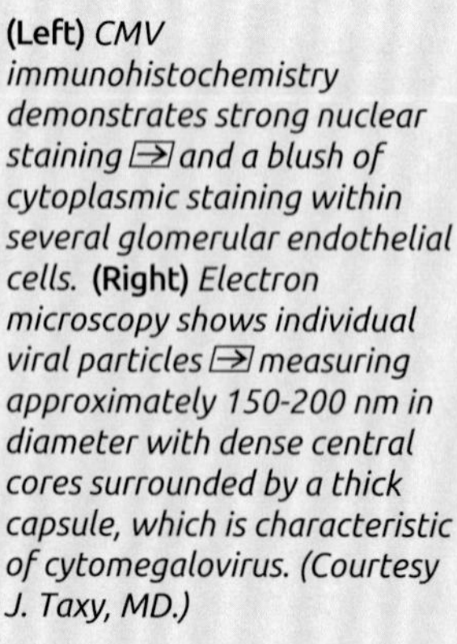

(Left) *CMV immunohistochemistry demonstrates strong nuclear staining → and a blush of cytoplasmic staining within several glomerular endothelial cells.* **(Right)** *Electron microscopy shows individual viral particles → measuring approximately 150-200 nm in diameter with dense central cores surrounded by a thick capsule, which is characteristic of cytomegalovirus. (Courtesy J. Taxy, MD.)*

CMV Immunohistochemistry

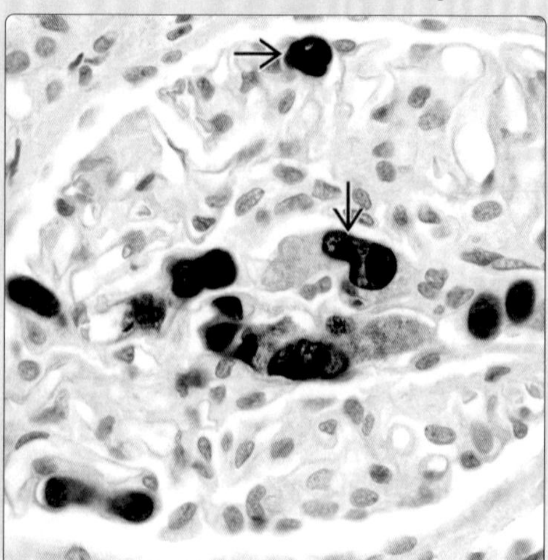

CMV Virions

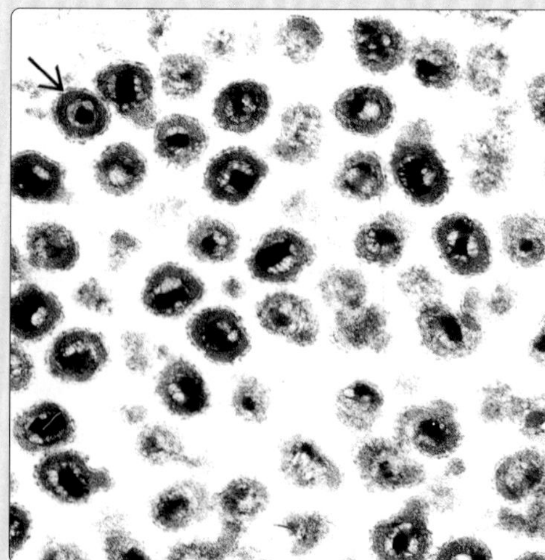

TERMINOLOGY

Abbreviations

- Cytomegalovirus (CMV)

Synonyms

- CMV tubulointerstitial nephritis (TIN)
- CMV glomerulopathy
- CMV nephropathy

Definitions

- Direct CMV infection of kidneys, usually associated with systemic CMV involvement and immunocompromise
  - May promote indirect kidney injury, particularly in renal transplants, including acute allograft glomerulopathy
- Causes benign, self-limited mononucleosis syndrome in normal individuals

ETIOLOGY/PATHOGENESIS

Infectious Agents

- Cytomegalovirus
  - Herpesviridae
    - β-subfamily
    - Double-stranded DNA virus
  - a.k.a. human herpesvirus-5 (HHV-5)

Risk Factors

- Immunocompromised patients at risk for systemic CMV
  - Transplant recipients on immunosuppression
    - Transplant CMV from donor organ or reactivation in recipient
    - Matching CMV serologic status in renal transplant patients has minimized incidence of CMV TIN
  - Infants
    - Neonatal CMV infection from maternal transmission
  - HIV-infected patients

Site of Infection

- Epithelium, endothelium, monocytes
- Renal involvement almost always associated with systemic infection
  - Lungs
  - Liver
  - GI tract
  - Pancreas
  - Adrenals glands
  - Epididymitis
  - Bone marrow
  - Retina

Latent Virus

- Most individuals infected before adulthood
  - Benign self-limited disease in normal individuals
  - Seroprevalence (90%)
  - Virus remains present in latent state lifelong

Effects on Immune System

- Increased IL-6 and IL-10, decreased Th1 cytokines (γ-interferon)
- Decreased expression of HLA antigens

CLINICAL ISSUES

Epidemiology

- Incidence
  - Neonatal CMV
    - Most common neonatal infection
    - 0.2-2% of live births in USA
    - 9.4 per 100,000 infants ages 1-4 years in Australia
  - Transplant CMV
    - ~ 20% incidence of CMV disease with ganciclovir prophylaxis
    - ~ 45% incidence without prophylaxis
    - Frequency of CMV infection in renal transplant biopsies < 1%
- Age
  - Neonatal, intrauterine
  - Immunocompromised adults
- Sex
  - Male predilection
- Ethnicity
  - No ethnic predilection

Presentation

- Fever
- Malaise
- Leukopenia
- Acute kidney injury
- Proteinuria

Laboratory Tests

- CMV IgM antibodies
  - Suggest recent or active infection
  - False-positives due to rheumatoid factor
- CMV IgG antibodies
- CMV antigen test
  - Indirect IF test to detect pp65 protein of CMV in peripheral blood leukocytes
- CMV polymerase chain reaction (PCR)
- Viral culture
  - Shell vial assay

Treatment

- Drugs
  - Ganciclovir or valganciclovir
    - Prophylaxis
    - Intravenous therapy
  - Foscarnet
    - Side effects include crystal formation leading to glomerulopathy
    - Multinucleation of tubular epithelial cell nuclei may persist after foscarnet therapy
  - Cidofovir
  - CMV intravenous immune globulin (IVIG)
- Reduce or alter immunosuppressive agents
- Vaccination to prevent maternal transmission

Prognosis

- Neonatal CMV
  - 30% mortality among symptomatic infants
  - Survivors commonly have neurologic deficits
- CMV disease in transplant recipient

Immunohistochemistry

Antibody	Reactivity	Staining Pattern	Comment
CMV	Positive	Nuclear & cytoplasmic	Epithelial or endothelial cells
SV40	Negative	Not applicable	
Adenovirus	Negative	Not applicable	
EBV-LMP	Negative	Not applicable	
HSV1/2	Negative	Not applicable	

  - Increased graft loss in past (10-20%)
  - Less adverse effect of CMV in patients on current immunosuppressive protocols

MICROSCOPIC

Histologic Features

- Pattern I: Large intranuclear inclusions in tubular epithelial cells with interstitial nephritis
  - Variable interstitial inflammation
  - Occasional granulomatous inflammation
  - Rare or no intranuclear inclusions in endothelial cells
  - Monocyte inclusions in interstitial infiltrate
- Pattern II: Large eosinophilic intranuclear inclusions in endothelial cells
  - Glomerular and peritubular capillary endothelial cells may be infected
  - When endothelial cells are predominant cell infected by CMV, epithelial cells tend to be spared
  - Interstitial inflammation **not** prominent in cases with primarily endothelial cell infection
- Pattern III: Acute glomerulonephritis (rare)
  - Endocapillary hypercellularity
  - Inclusions in glomerular endothelial cells or in circulating monocytes
  - Crescents may be present
  - Scant deposits by EM

ANCILLARY TESTS

In Situ Hybridization

- CMV positive

Electron Microscopy

- Virions in nucleus and cytoplasm
- 150-200 nm in diameter
- Dense core surrounded by thick capsule

DIFFERENTIAL DIAGNOSIS

Polyomavirus Nephritis

- Intranuclear inclusions with "ground-glass" appearance in tubular epithelial cells
- Immunohistochemical for SV40 large T antigen positive
- Prominent interstitial plasmacytic inflammation with tubulitis
- No endothelial inclusions

Adenovirus Tubulointerstitial Nephritis

- Prominent interstitial inflammation and tubular necrosis
- Granulomatous inflammation
- Viral cytopathic effect in tubular epithelial cells
- Immunohistochemical confirmation of adenovirus infection

Acute Cellular Rejection

- Prominent interstitial inflammation with tubulitis
- No viral cytopathic effect
- Endarteritis helpful if present

Acute Allograft Glomerulopathy (Form of Rejection)

- Marked glomerular cell endothelial swelling and activation
- Mesangiolysis: Webs of PAS(+) material
- CD8 T cells in glomeruli
- No inclusions or viral antigens in glomeruli
- May be indirect effect of CMV in some patients
- Endarteritis common
- C4d negative

Acute Glomerulonephritis

- No CMV inclusions or antigens
- Deposits in GBM

Immunotactoid Glomerulopathy

- Microtubular deposits composed of immunoglobulins (often monoclonal)
- Few de novo cases in allografts associated with CMV infection

DIAGNOSTIC CHECKLIST

Pathologic Interpretation Pearls

- Inclusions readily evident at low magnification
- CMV intranuclear inclusions present in predominantly endothelial cells or epithelial cells
- Coinfection with other fungal or viral organisms may occur
- Features of foscarnet toxicity may be present in patients treated for CMV infection

SELECTED REFERENCES

1. Vichot AA et al: Cytomegalovirus glomerulopathy and cytomegalovirus interstitial nephritis on sequential transplant kidney biopsies. Am J Kidney Dis. 63(3):536-9, 2014
2. Rane S et al: Spectrum of cytomegalovirus-induced renal pathology in renal allograft recipients. Transplant Proc. 44(3):713-6, 2012
3. Agrawal V et al: Polyomavirus nephropathy and Cytomegalovirus nephritis in renal allograft recipients. Indian J Pathol Microbiol. 53(4):672-5, 2010
4. Humar A et al: An assessment of herpesvirus co-infections in patients with CMV disease: correlation with clinical and virologic outcomes. Am J Transplant. 9(2):374-81, 2009
5. Pass RF et al: Vaccine prevention of maternal cytomegalovirus infection. N Engl J Med. 360(12):1191-9, 2009
6. Seale H et al: Trends in hospitalizations for diagnosed congenital cytomegalovirus in infants and children in Australia. BMC Pediatr. 9:7, 2009

Proximal Tubules

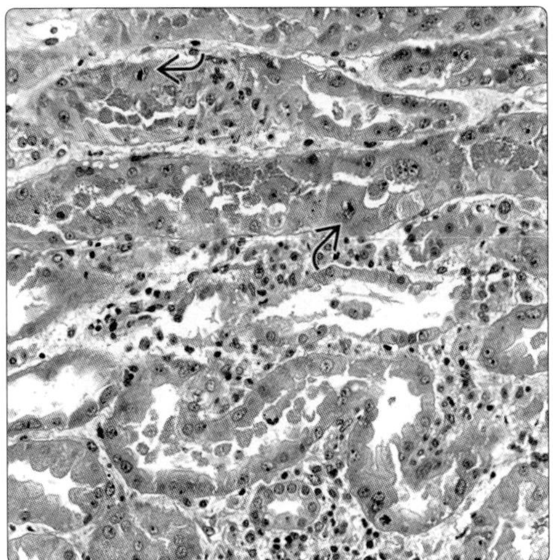

Tubular Epithelial Cells

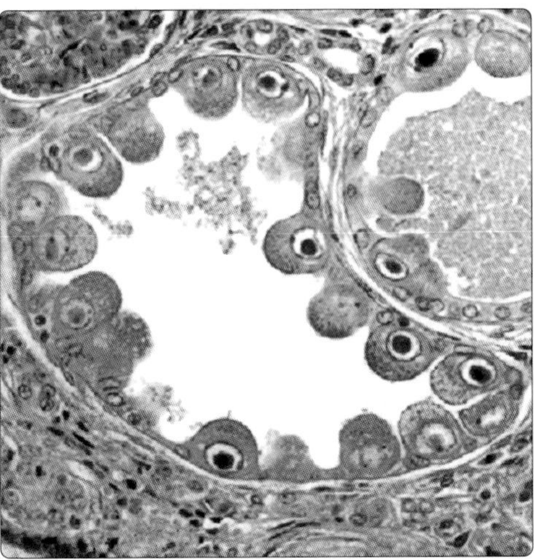

(Left) *Hematoxylin and eosin of a renal transplant biopsy shows a moderately intense mononuclear infiltrate, edema, and tubular injury, resembling acute cellular rejection. Inclusions typical of CMV, however, are seen in the tubules, even at low power* ⮳. **(Right)** *Hematoxylin and eosin of an autopsy from an infant who died from systemic CMV disease shows frequent large eosinophilic inclusions in the tubular epithelial cells, which have a "hobnail" pattern.*

Peritubular Capillary CMV

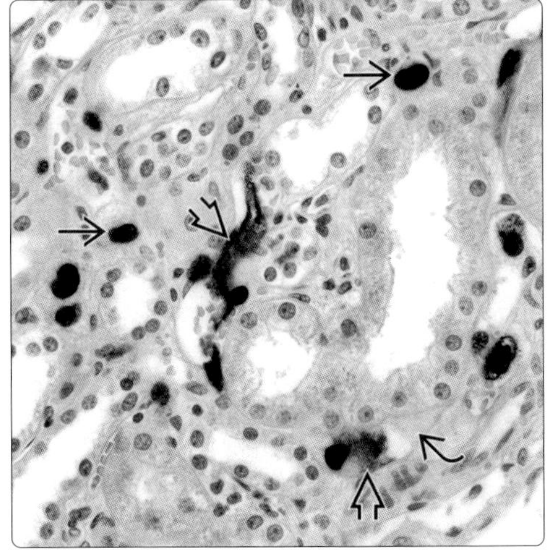

CMV Intranuclear Inclusions

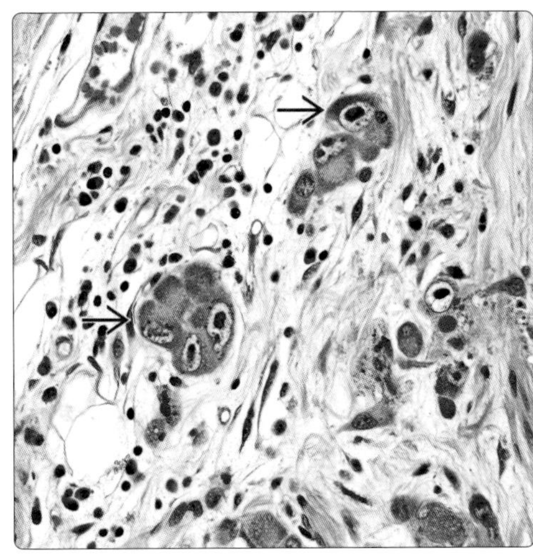

(Left) *CMV immunohistochemistry shows strong nuclear* → *and some cytoplasmic* ⇨ *staining of many peritubular capillary endothelial cells* ⮳ *with marked nuclear enlargement. No CMV staining of the tubular epithelial cells is noted in this photomicrograph.* **(Right)** *Hematoxylin and eosin shows numerous CMV intranuclear inclusions* → *within endothelial cells in small vessels within the renal sinus of this transplant nephrectomy specimen.*

Acute Allograft Glomerulopathy

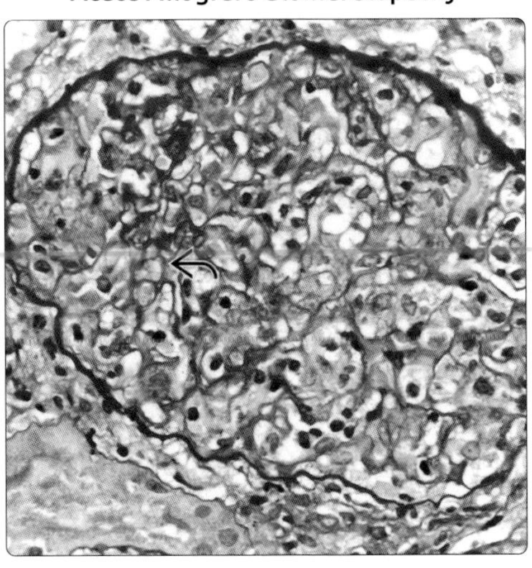

CMV Virions

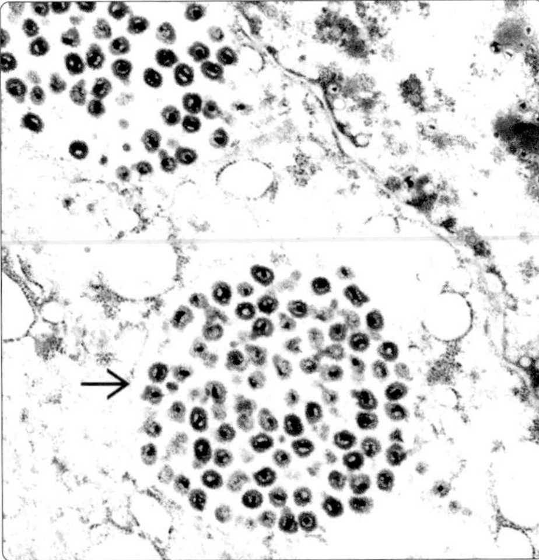

(Left) *Acute allograft glomerulopathy, a form of acute cellular rejection, in a renal transplant recipient with systemic CMV shows endothelial swelling and scattered mononuclear cells in capillary loops. The PAS(+) webs are indicative of mesangiolysis* ⮳. *No CMV inclusions were present. C4d was negative.* **(Right)** *This electron micrograph reveals several clusters of CMV virions that are contained within an electron-lucent membrane* → *in the nucleus of this infected epithelial cell. (Courtesy J. Taxy, MD.)*

Herpes Simplex Acute Nephritis

KEY FACTS

ETIOLOGY/PATHOGENESIS

- Infectious agent
  - HSV1
  - HSV2

CLINICAL ISSUES

- Acute kidney injury
  - Rare kidney involvement
- Treatment
  - Acyclovir
  - Reduction of immunosuppressive agents
- Prognosis
  - Good
    - Worse if herpes simplex virus hepatitis present

MICROSCOPIC

- Prominent interstitial inflammation
- Viral cytopathic effect
  - Tubular epithelial cell nuclei
    - Smudged nuclear appearance
- Tubulitis
- Acute tubular injury &/or necrosis
- Interstitial edema
- Interstitial hemorrhage

ANCILLARY TESTS

- Immunohistochemistry
  - HSV1/2
    - Strong nuclear and cytoplasmic staining
- Electron microscopy
  - HSV virions measure ~ 110 nm in diameter

TOP DIFFERENTIAL DIAGNOSES

- Polyomavirus nephritis
- Adenovirus nephritis
- Acute cellular rejection
- Cytomegalovirus tubulointerstitial nephritis

Interstitial Inflammation

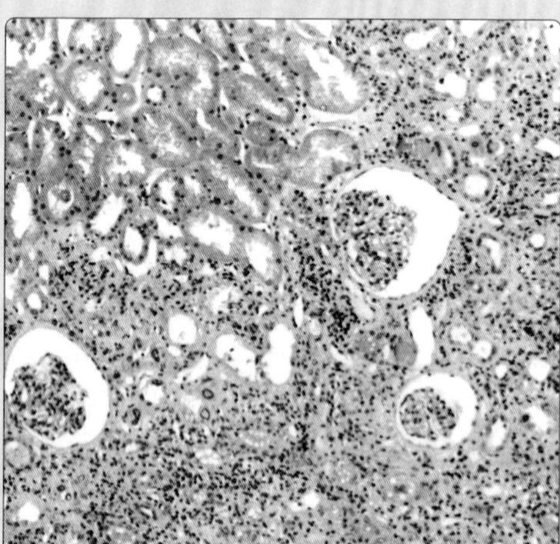

HSV Immunohistochemistry

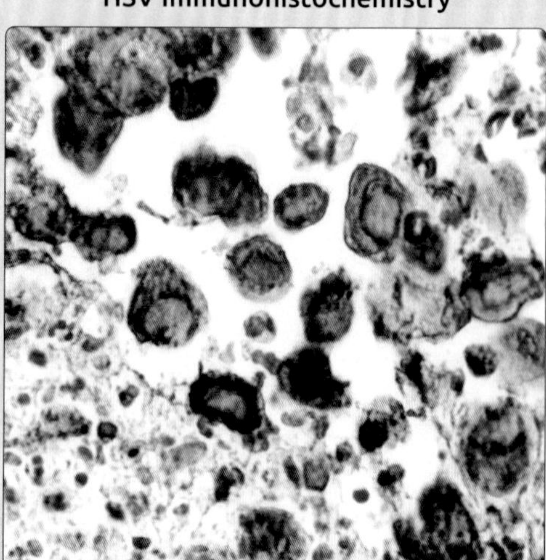

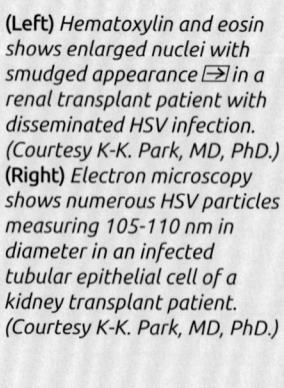

(Left) *Hematoxylin and eosin shows marked interstitial inflammation without apparent viral cytopathic effect in a kidney transplant patient with disseminated herpes simplex virus (HSV). (Courtesy K-K. Park, MD, PhD.)* **(Right)** *HSV1/2 shows strong nuclear and cytoplasmic staining in many sloughed urothelial cells in this renal allograft. (Courtesy K-K. Park, MD, PhD.)*

Viral Cytopathic Effect

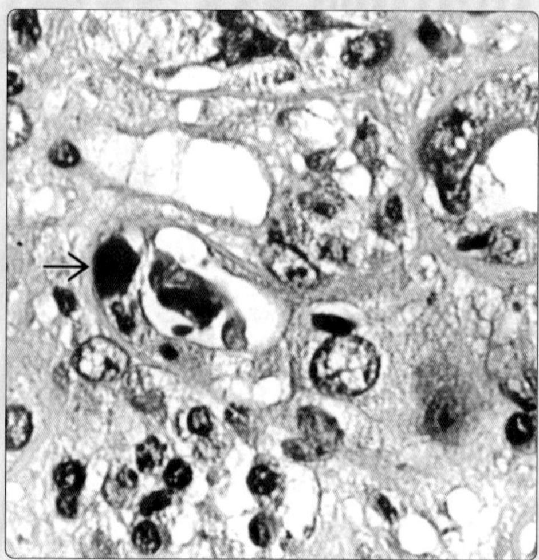

HSV Virions

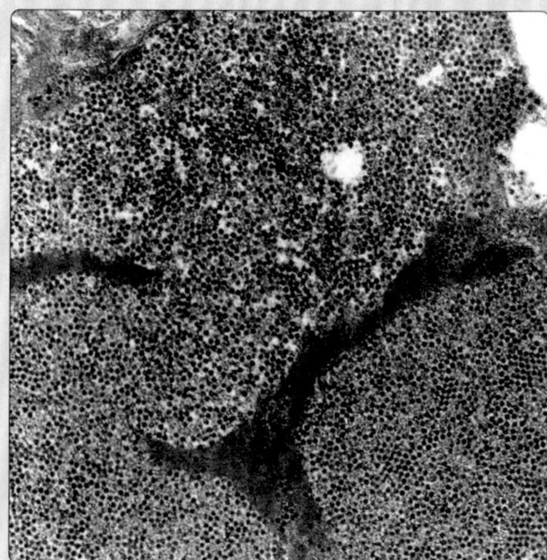

(Left) *Hematoxylin and eosin shows enlarged nuclei with smudged appearance ➔ in a renal transplant patient with disseminated HSV infection. (Courtesy K-K. Park, MD, PhD.)* **(Right)** *Electron microscopy shows numerous HSV particles measuring 105-110 nm in diameter in an infected tubular epithelial cell of a kidney transplant patient. (Courtesy K-K. Park, MD, PhD.)*

TERMINOLOGY

Abbreviations

- Herpes simplex virus (HSV) nephritis

Definitions

- HSV infection in renal allografts

ETIOLOGY/PATHOGENESIS

Infectious Agents

- HSV1
- HSV2
  - 1 possible case without confirmation by kidney biopsy

CLINICAL ISSUES

Epidemiology

- Incidence
  - Rare
- Age
  - No age predilection
- Sex
  - No gender predilection
- Ethnicity
  - No ethnic predilection

Presentation

- Acute kidney injury
- HSV infection in other sites

Laboratory Tests

- Polymerase chain reaction
- Serologic tests
  - Enzyme-linked immunoassay
  - Western blot
    - Anti-gpG1 glycoprotein for HSV1
    - Anti-gpG2 glycoprotein for HSV2
  - Immunofluorescence assays
- Viral culture
  - Shell vial assay

Treatment

- Drugs
  - Acyclovir
- Reduction of immunosuppressive agents

Prognosis

- Good
  - Worse if HSV hepatitis present

MICROSCOPIC

Histologic Features

- Prominent interstitial inflammation
  - Primarily lymphocytes
  - Plasma cells and neutrophils also may be present
- Tubulitis
- Viral cytopathic effect
  - Tubular epithelial cell nuclei
    - Smudged nuclear appearance
- Acute tubular injury
- Interstitial edema
- Interstitial hemorrhage

ANCILLARY TESTS

Immunohistochemistry

- HSV1/2
  - Strong nuclear and cytoplasmic staining

Electron Microscopy

- HSV virions
  - ~ 110 nm in diameter

DIFFERENTIAL DIAGNOSIS

Polyomavirus Nephritis

- Prominent interstitial inflammation with tubulitis
- Viral cytopathic effect
  - Positive SV40 immunohistochemistry
- Virions measure 40 nm in diameter

Adenovirus Nephritis

- Prominent interstitial granulomatous inflammation with tubulitis
- Viral cytopathic effect with smudged nuclei
  - Positive adenovirus immunohistochemistry
  - Individual virions measure ~ 90 nm in diameter
- Tubular necrosis

Cytomegalovirus Tubulointerstitial Nephritis

- Enlarged tubular epithelial cell nuclei
  - Characteristic "owl-eye" nuclear inclusions
  - Basophilic cytoplasmic inclusions
- Prominent interstitial inflammation with tubulitis
- Virions measure 150-200 nm in diameter

Acute Cellular Rejection

- Prominent interstitial inflammation with tubulitis
- Endarteritis may be present
- No viral cytopathic effect

DIAGNOSTIC CHECKLIST

Pathologic Interpretation Pearls

- Coinfection with other viral or fungal microorganisms can occur

SELECTED REFERENCES

1. Capretti MG et al: Herpes Simplex Virus 1 infection: misleading findings in an infant with disseminated disease. New Microbiol. 36(3):307-13, 2013
2. Basse G et al: Disseminated herpes simplex type-2 (HSV-2) infection after solid-organ transplantation. Infection. 36(1):62-4, 2008
3. Kang YN et al: Systemic herpes simplex virus infection following cadaveric renal transplantation: a case report. Transplant Proc. 38(5):1346-7, 2006
4. Sachdeva MU et al: Viral infections of renal allografts--an immunohistochemical and ultrastructural study. Indian J Pathol Microbiol. 47(2):189-94, 2004
5. Sinniah R et al: An in situ hybridization study of herpes simplex and Epstein Barr viruses in IgA nephropathy and non-immune glomerulonephritis. Clin Nephrol. 40(3):137-41, 1993
6. Silbert PL et al: Herpes simplex virus interstitial nephritis in a renal allograft. Clin Nephrol. 33(6):264-8, 1990

Epstein-Barr Virus Nephritis

KEY FACTS

ETIOLOGY/PATHOGENESIS

- Epstein-Barr virus (EBV)
  - a.k.a. human herpes virus 4 (HHV-4)

CLINICAL ISSUES

- EBV infections commonly asymptomatic
- Infectious mononucleosis
  - Usually < 18 years old
  - 60% with subclinical renal involvement
    - Hematuria
    - Proteinuria
- Observed mostly in male pediatric patients
  - M:F = 3:1

MICROSCOPIC

- Interstitial inflammation and edema
  - Lymphocyte predominant (CD8)
- Tubulitis
- Nuclear atypia of tubular epithelial cells (viral cytopathic effect)
- Glomerular alterations
  - Occasional mesangial hypercellularity
  - Glomerular capillary thrombi (rare)
  - Podocyte injury; minimal change disease (rare)
  - Immune complex-mediated glomerulonephritis (rare)

ANCILLARY TESTS

- Immunohistochemistry
  - Positive for EBV-VCA in tubular epithelial cells
  - Negative for EBV-LMP, SV40, or adenovirus
- In situ hybridization
  - EBV-encoded small RNA1 (EBER-1) mRNA

TOP DIFFERENTIAL DIAGNOSES

- Acute interstitial nephritis
- Acute tubular necrosis
- Polyomavirus nephritis

Interstitial Inflammation and Hemorrhage

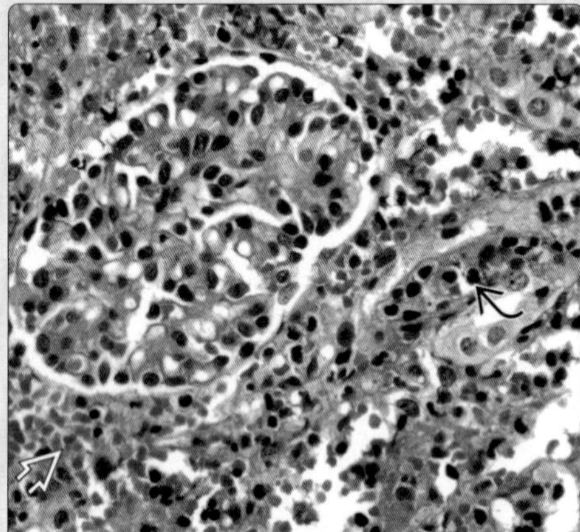

EBER In Situ Hybridization

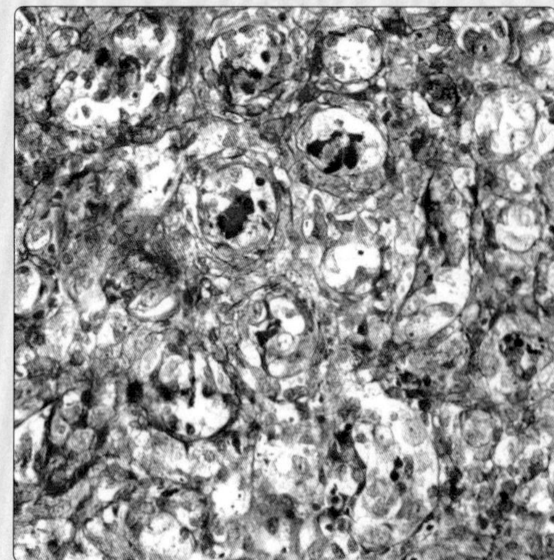

(Left) *Hematoxylin and eosin reveals prominent diffuse interstitial mononuclear cell inflammation and hemorrhage in the kidney of a 16-month-old boy with an acute Epstein-Barr virus (EBV) infection. (Courtesy H. Catthro, MD.)* **(Right)** *In situ hybridization for EBER-1 mRNA is usually negative in tubular epithelial cells. Rare interstitial lymphocytes may stain positive, but none are present. (Courtesy H. Catthro, MD.)*

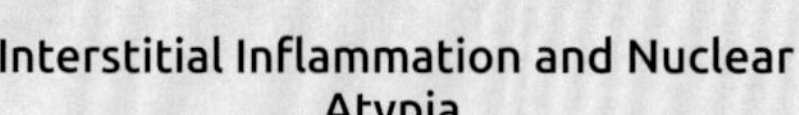

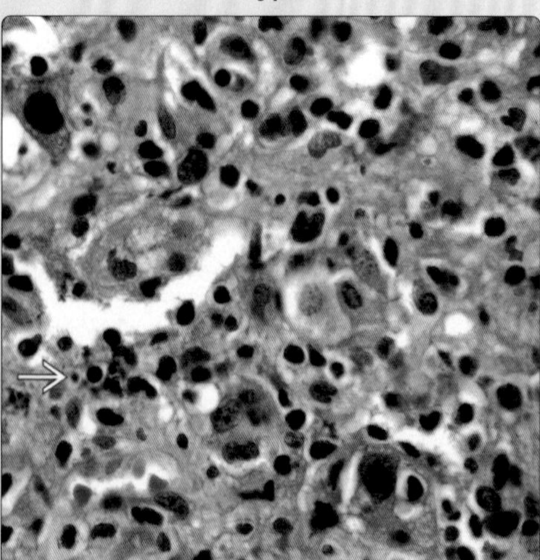

EBV Immunohistochemistry

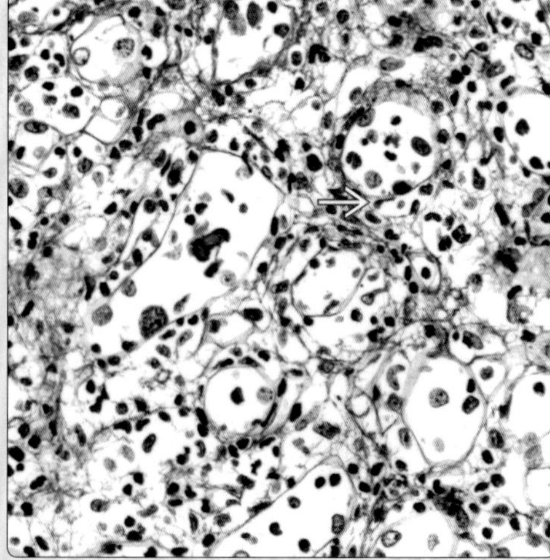

(Left) *Diffuse interstitial inflammation and nuclear atypia in tubular cells are seen in a male toddler with acute EBV infection. (Courtesy H. Catthro, MD.)* **(Right)** *EBV-LMP shows a lymphocyte in a peritubular capillary with faint positive (brown) staining, but most cells are negative. (Courtesy H. Catthro, MD.)*

TERMINOLOGY

Definitions

- Primary Epstein-Barr virus (EBV) infection can result in acute kidney injury

ETIOLOGY/PATHOGENESIS

Infectious Agents

- EBV
  - a.k.a. human herpes virus 4 (HHV-4)
  - 95% of adults infected by age 40
  - Can infect proximal tubular epithelial cells
    - Express CD21 (complement receptor) that binds EBV

CLINICAL ISSUES

Epidemiology

- Incidence
  - EBV infections commonly asymptomatic
    - Infectious mononucleosis
      - Renal involvement in up to 15%
- Age
  - Usually < 18 years old
- Sex
  - M:F = 3:1

Presentation

- Asymptomatic
  - Majority of cases
- Infectious mononucleosis
  - Proteinuria (14%)
  - Hematuria (11%)
- Acute kidney injury
  - Oliguria (rare)
  - May be associated with hepatic failure or rhabdomyolysis

Laboratory Tests

- EBV polymerase chain reaction
- Enzyme-linked immunoassay
  - EBV capsid antigen (VCA)-IgM
  - EBV capsid antigen: IgG
  - EBV nuclear antigen (EBNA)
  - Early antigen (EA)
- Mononucleosis ("monospot") or heterophile antibody test
  - Often negative in children < 10 years old

Treatment

- Drugs
  - Acyclovir
  - Corticosteroids: Variable efficacy

Prognosis

- Good, usually rapid resolution

MICROSCOPIC

Histologic Features

- Interstitial inflammation
  - Lymphocyte predominant (CD8)
- Tubulitis
- Nuclear atypia of tubular epithelial cells (viral cytopathic effect)
- Interstitial edema
- Glomerular alterations
  - Occasional mesangial hypercellularity
  - Glomerular capillary thrombi (rare)
  - Podocyte injury; minimal change disease (rare)
  - Immune complex-mediated glomerulonephritis (rare)

ANCILLARY TESTS

Immunohistochemistry

- Positive
  - EBV-VCA in tubular epithelial cells
    - Positive staining in occasional circulating or interstitial leukocytes
- Negative
  - EBNA
  - EBV latent membrane protein (LMP)

In Situ Hybridization

- EBV-encoded small RNA1 (EBER-1) mRNA
  - Positive staining in rare circulating or interstitial leukocytes

DIFFERENTIAL DIAGNOSIS

Acute Interstitial Nephritis

- Prominent interstitial inflammation
- No viral cytopathic effect
- Absence of acute EBV infection

Acute Tubular Necrosis

- Prominent injury of tubular epithelial cells
- Interstitial inflammation or tubulitis not prominent

Polyomavirus Nephritis

- Prominent plasmacytic interstitial inflammation with tubulitis
- Viral cytopathic effect in tubular epithelial cell nuclei
- Positive SV40 immunohistochemistry in tubular epithelial cell nuclei

Karyomegalic Interstitial Nephritis

- *FAN1* mutation
- Enlarged nuclei

Lead Nephropathy

- Enlarged nuclei and nuclear inclusions

DIAGNOSTIC CHECKLIST

Pathologic Interpretation Pearls

- Clinical and serologic correlation to confirm diagnosis

SELECTED REFERENCES

1. Suzuki J et al: An adult case of fulminant Epstein-Barr virus infection with acute tubulointerstitial nephritis. Intern Med. 51(6):629-34, 2012
2. Tsai JD et al: Epstein-Barr virus-associated acute renal failure: diagnosis, treatment, and follow-up. Pediatr Nephrol. 18(7):667-74, 2003
3. Norwood VF et al: Unexplained acute renal failure in a toddler: a rare complication of Epstein-Barr virus. Pediatr Nephrol. 17(8):628-32, 2002
4. Becker JL et al: Epstein-Barr virus infection of renal proximal tubule cells: possible role in chronic interstitial nephritis. J Clin Invest. 104(12):1673-81, 1999

Hantavirus Nephropathy

KEY FACTS

TERMINOLOGY

- Renal diseases caused by Hantaviruses
- Manifestations vary with strain in geographic area

ETIOLOGY/PATHOGENESIS

- Hantaviruses belong to Bunyaviridae family
- Infection by inhalation of aerosolized rodent excreta
  - Zoonoses from rat, mouse, and vole
- Flu-like syndrome leads to severe multiorgan hemorrhagic microvascular involvement with shock
- Microvascular and immune systems affected
  - Endothelial cells, macrophages, and dendritic cells infected
  - Chemokine/cytokine release and vascular leakage/hemorrhage are 1° pathogenic events

CLINICAL ISSUES

- ~ 150,000/year worldwide; rare in USA
- Acute renal failure
- Disseminated intravascular coagulation with thrombocytopenia and petechiae
- Edema
- Photophobia, abdominal/back pain, and myalgias
- Proteinuria

MICROSCOPIC

- Interstitial inflammation, hemorrhage, or fibrosis
- Acute tubular injury/necrosis
- Membranoproliferative or diffuse proliferative glomerulonephritis (rare)
- Electron microscopy reveals viral nucleocapsid and capillary endothelial injury

TOP DIFFERENTIAL DIAGNOSES

- Other viral hemorrhagic fevers
  - Dengue
  - Ebola
  - Lassa fever

Interstitial Hemorrhage

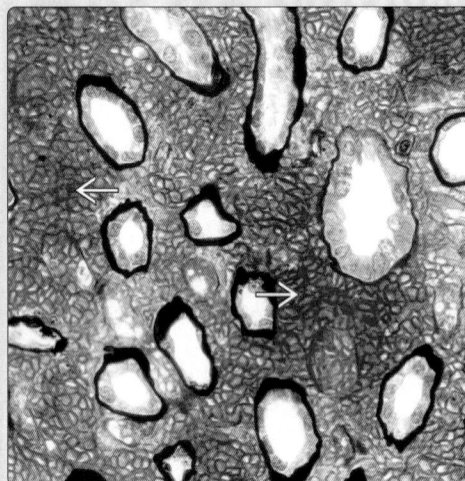

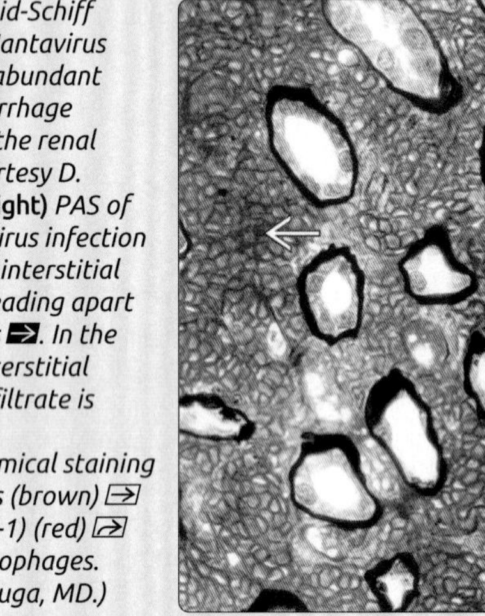

Mixed Interstitial Inflammation Within Hemorrhage

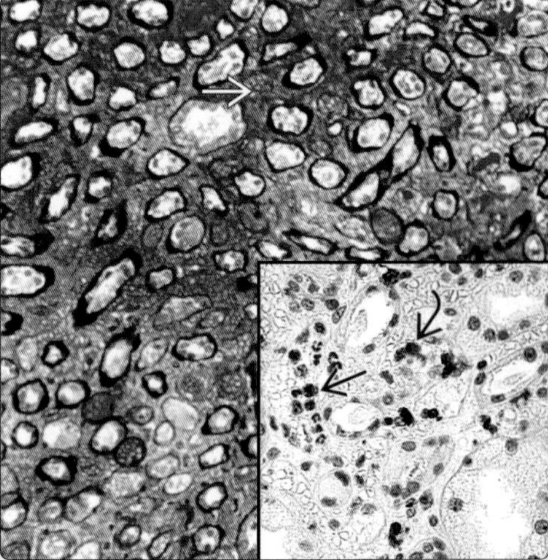

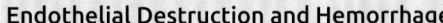

(Left) *Periodic acid-Schiff (PAS) Puumala Hantavirus infection shows abundant interstitial hemorrhage spreading apart the renal tubules ➡. (Courtesy D. Ferluga, MD.)* **(Right)** *PAS of Puumala Hantavirus infection shows abundant interstitial hemorrhage spreading apart the renal tubules ➡. In the inset, a mixed interstitial inflammatory infiltrate is shown with dual immunohistochemical staining for CD8(+) T cells (brown) ➡ and CD68(+) (KP-1) (red) ➡ monocytes/macrophages. (Courtesy D. Ferluga, MD.)*

Peritubular Capillary Congestion and Interstitial Hemorrhage

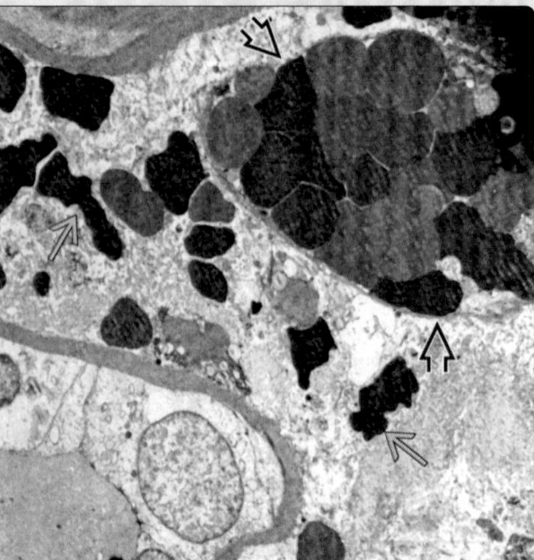

Endothelial Destruction and Hemorrhage

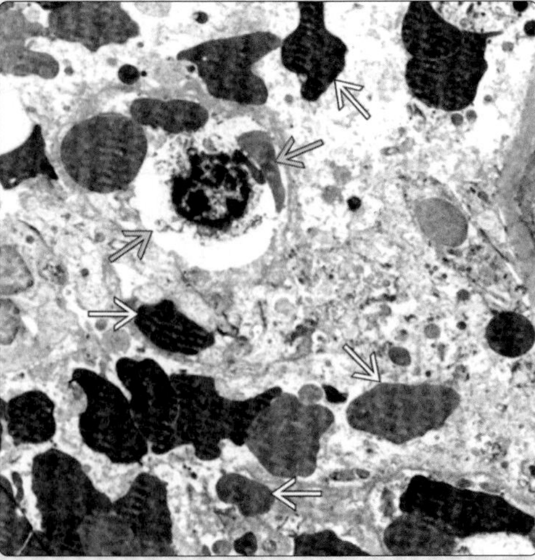

(Left) *EM shows a congested peritubular capillary ➡ with hemorrhage of red blood cells into the interstitium ➡. (Courtesy D. Ferluga, MD.)* **(Right)** *EM shows necrotizing destruction of the endothelium of peritubular capillaries ➡ with hemorrhage of red blood cells into the interstitium ➡. (Courtesy D. Ferluga, MD.)*

TERMINOLOGY

Abbreviations

- Hantavirus nephropathy (HVN)

Synonyms

- Hemorrhagic fever with renal syndrome (HFRS)
- Nephropathia epidemica (NE): Milder form of HFRS

Definitions

- Renal diseases caused by hantaviruses
  - Manifestations vary with strain in geographic area

ETIOLOGY/PATHOGENESIS

Environmental Exposure

- Humans infected by inhaling aerosolized host rodent excreta (urine, saliva, or feces)

Infectious Agents

- Hantaviruses
  - Bunyaviridae, negative-stranded, enveloped RNA viruses
  - > 20 pathogenic strains, worldwide distribution
  - Replicates in endothelium, macrophages, and dendritic cells
- Hantaan virus
  - Severe HFRS in Far East (Russia, China, and Korea)
  - From striped field mouse (*Apodemus agrarius*)
- Seoul virus
  - Moderate HFRS, worldwide including USA
  - From gray rat (*Rattus norvegicus*)
- Dobravirus
  - Severe HFRS in Central and Southeastern Europe (Balkan)
  - From yellow-necked field mouse (*Apodemus flavicollis*)
- Puumala virus
  - 5,000 people annually with NE
    - Milder form of HFRS with lower mortality (< 1%)
  - Throughout Europe (Balkan, Scandinavia, and Russia)
  - From black vole (*Clethrionomys glareolus*)
- Sin Nombre virus
  - Hantavirus pulmonary syndrome (HPS), western USA
  - From deer mouse (*Peromyscus maniculatus*)

Microvascular/Immune System Interaction

- Cytokine release (e.g., TNF-α, VEGF, and γ-interferon)
  - TNF-α and VEGF increase vascular permeability
- Severe microvascular injury and hemorrhage
  - Release of endothelial components into circulation (e.g., VCAM-1, syndecan-1)

CLINICAL ISSUES

Epidemiology

- Incidence
  - ~ 150,000/year worldwide
  - Rare in USA

Presentation

- Fever/chills, hypotensive (hours to 2 days), oliguric renal failure (few days to weeks)
- Nausea/vomiting, abdominal/back pain, and myalgias
- Edema
  - Vascular leak syndrome leads to periorbital edema, retroperitoneal fluid accumulation, hemoconcentration, and postural hypotension
- Thrombocytopenia and petechiae
- Photophobia
- Proteinuria

Prognosis

- Mortality rates
  - > 50% for Sin Nombre
  - 5-15% for Hantaan and Dobravirus
  - 1-5% for Seoul
  - 0.1-1% for Puumala

MICROSCOPIC

Histologic Features

- Glomeruli
  - Diffuse proliferative or membranoproliferative GN (rare)
  - ± mesangial hypercellularity
- Interstitium
  - Interstitial inflammation and hemorrhage; later fibrosis
    - Predominance of lymphocytes and neutrophils
- Tubules
  - Acute tubular injury/necrosis early, atrophy later
- Vessels
  - Congestion of peritubular capillaries
  - Endothelial injury and activation

ANCILLARY TESTS

Electron Microscopy

- Necrotizing endothelial injury, activation and destruction of peritubular capillaries
- Viral particles in endothelium
  - 100 nm in diameter, round or oval viruses
  - Double-layered lipid envelopes with protruding "spikes"
  - Nucleocapsid composed of hollow microfilaments or dense granules
- Golgi apparatus enlarged in infected cells

DIFFERENTIAL DIAGNOSIS

Other Viral Hemorrhagic Fevers

- Flaviviridae (dengue), Arenaviridae (Lassa), and Filoviridae (Ebola)
- Distinctive viral morphology in endothelium
- Detection of specific virus in blood by PCR

Acute Interstitial Nephritis

- More interstitial inflammation, less hemorrhage

SELECTED REFERENCES

1. Latus J et al: Acute kidney injury and tools for risk-stratification in 456 patients with hantavirus-induced nephropathia epidemica. Nephrol Dial Transplant. 30(2):245-51, 2015
2. Krautkrämer E et al: Mobilization of circulating endothelial progenitor cells correlates with the clinical course of hantavirus disease. J Virol. 88(1):483-9, 2014
3. Krautkrämer E et al: Hantavirus infection: an emerging infectious disease causing acute renal failure. Kidney Int. 83(1):23-7, 2013
4. Ferluga D et al: Hantavirus nephropathy. J Am Soc Nephrol. 19(9):1653-8, 2008

SECTION 6
Developmental Diseases

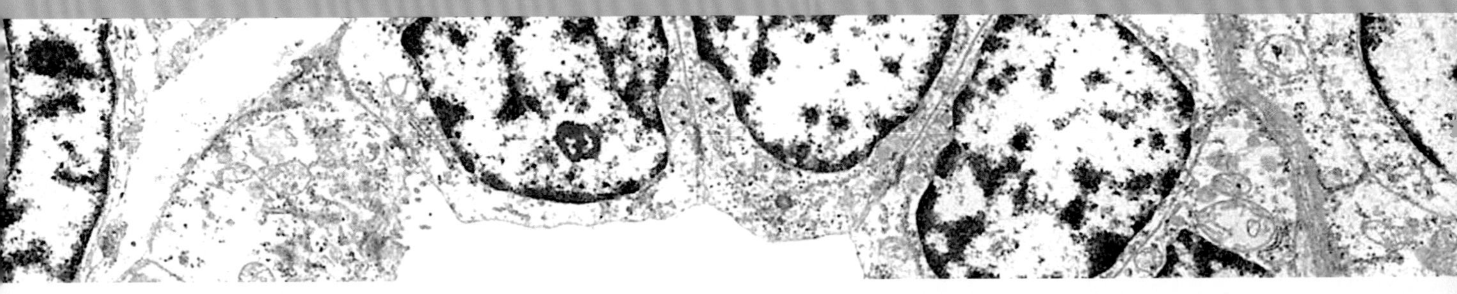

TERMINOLOGY

Definitions

- Defective development of kidney and urinary tract, often referred as congenital anomalies of kidney or urinary tract (CAKUT)

ETIOLOGY/PATHOGENESIS

Developmental Anomaly

- CAKUT occur alone, in combination with another CAKUT, or as a syndrome
  - Categories
    - Renal hypoplasia: Small, architecturally normal kidneys
    - Renal agenesis or aplasia: No kidney formation or involution after early branching
    - Renal dysplasia: Architecturally abnormal kidneys with blastema elements and immature nephrons
    - Duplicated collecting system: Partial or complete duplication of ureter; if complete, then distinct insertions into bladder
    - Ectopic kidneys or malrotation: Abnormal location or orientation of kidney
    - Multicystic dysplasia: Cysts of various sizes across kidney parenchyma and renal dysplasia
    - Duplex or multiple kidneys: Initiation of > 1 kidney
    - Horseshoe or fused kidneys: Joining of kidneys in midline, complete or partial
    - Ureteropelvic junctional (UPJ) abnormalities and hydronephrosis: Proximal narrowing of ureter, dilatation of pelvis
    - Megaureter: Large, tortuous, dilated ureters
    - Hydroureter: Dilated ureter
    - Vesicoureteral reflux (VUR): Backflow of urine from bladder to ureter
    - Ureterovesical junction (UVJ) abnormalities: Narrowing or obstruction of distal ureter-bladder junction
    - Ureterocele: Ureter ending blindly into or outside bladder
    - Posterior urethral valves (PUV): Malpositioned or abnormally developed posterior urethral valves, leads to urinary reflux due to obstruction
- Multisystem involvement
  - May present as syndromes if mutation in gene important for development of many organs
  - May present as complex disease affecting multiple systems if gene defect also results in abnormal function or maintenance of other systems
- Causes
  - Toxins or environmental exposure
    - Dioxins (agent orange): Hydronephrosis
  - Medications
  - Familial or inherited; inheritance may be simple or complex
    - Mendelian: Autosomal recessive or dominant, X-linked genome changes
    - Non-mendelian: Epigenetic, modifier genes with incomplete penetrance and variable expressivity
  - Spontaneous or de novo genomic alterations
  - Maternal nutrition or health
    - Low protein diet, diabetes, excessive high or low salt intake
  - Genetically heterogeneous disorders: Defects in many genes can cause CAKUT
- Etiological classification according to different steps in early kidney development
  - Pronephros and mesonephros defects
    - Nephric duct growth and maturation defects: Renal agenesis, ureter and collecting system defects, male gonadal duct (vas deferens)
    - Failure to repress anterior (mesonephric) buds or timely regression of mesonephros: Supernumerary ureters, gonadal descent defects
  - Metanephros defects
    - Ureteric bud (UB) induction: Renal agenesis, hypoplasia

(Left) *Gross dissection of the urogenital system from a patient with chromosome 4p deletion syndrome shows bilateral hypoplastic kidneys. The ureter on the right was removed before the photograph.* **(Right)** *Histology of hypoplastic kidney from a 4p deletion syndrome patient shows normal kidney architecture but fewer glomerular generations (3-4), as opposed to 13-14 in a normal kidney.*

Bilateral Hypoplastic Kidneys

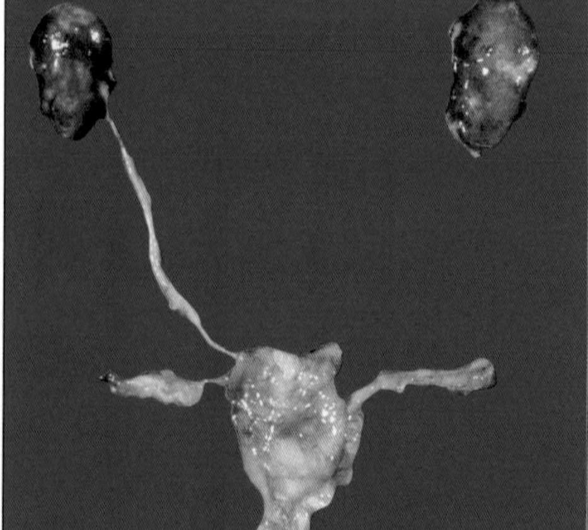

Decreased Nephrons in Hypoplastic Kidneys

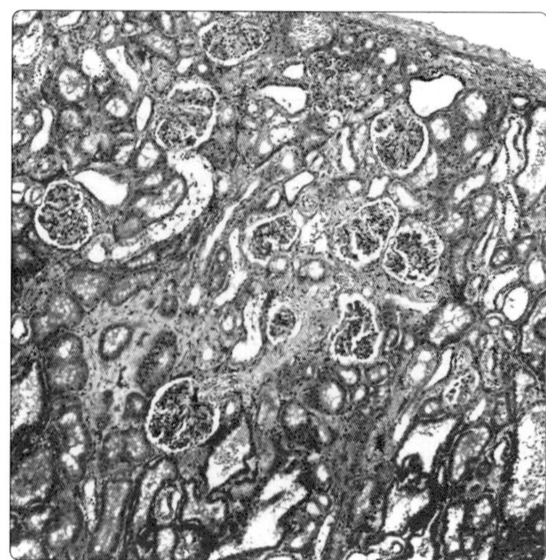

- Branching morphogenesis: Hypoplasia, dysplasia, cysts, tubulogenesis defects, glomerulogenesis defects; encompasses reciprocal interactions among all 3 major components: UB, mesenchyme, and stroma
  - Ureter or UGS maturation defects
    - Proximal or upper ureter: UPJ obstruction, hydronephrosis, bifid ureters
    - Distal or lower urinary tract: UVJ obstruction, VUR, megaureter, hydroureter, ureterocele, PUV
  - Position abnormalities
    - Failure to ascend or rotate: Ectopic kidneys, horseshoe kidneys, crossed renal ectopy
  - Factors extrinsic to kidney primordia
    - Lateral mesoderm and notochord: Ectopic kidneys, fusion, WD maturation, horseshoe kidneys

Genes and Syndromes Associated With CAKUT and Extrarenal Manifestations

- Townes-Brocks syndrome: *SALL1*; limb, sensorineural hearing loss, anal atresia, CAKUT
- CAKUT-Hirschsprung disease or MEN2A: *RET*; intestinal aganglionosis, medullary thyroid carcinoma, pheochromocytoma, CAKUT
- Hypothyroidism, deafness, renal (HDR) syndrome: *GATA3*
- Renal cyst and diabetes syndrome (RCAD): *TCF2*, *HNF1B*; glomerulocystic kidney disease, CAKUT, *MODY5* diabetes, genital defects
- Fraser syndrome: *FRAS1*, *FREM2*; syndactyly, cryptophthalmos, renal agenesis, hypoplasia/dysplasia
- Meckel-Gruber: *MKS1*, *MKS3*; polydactyly, liver malformations, encephalocele, renal dysplasia, cysts
- RHD: *BMP4*, *SIX2*; microphthalmia, cleft lip, renal hypo/dysplasia
- Prune belly syndrome: Gene not known; cryptorchidism, abdominal muscle maldevelopment, CAKUT
- Wolf-Hirschhorn or 4p deletion syndrome: Deletion of end of 4p; dysmorphic facial features, delayed growth, intellectual disability, CAKUT
- Bardet-Biedl syndrome: Many cilia genes; retinopathy, digital anomalies, obesity, male hypogonadism, renal dysplasia
- Fanconi anemia: DNA repair pathway genes *FANCA-M*; anemia, AML, limb malformations, CAKUT
- Smith-Lemli-Opitz syndrome: Cholesterol biosynthesis (*DHCR7*); dysmorphic facial features, microcephaly, syndactyly, mental retardation, dysplastic kidneys
- Branchio-oto-renal syndrome (BOR): *EYA1*, *SIX1*, *SIX5*, *MYOG*; deafness, branchial cysts, CAKUT
- Renal coloboma syndrome: *PAX2*; retinal coloboma, CAKUT

EPIDEMIOLOGY

Incidence

- CAKUT are one of the most common anomalies in antenatal period
- Reported in 0.5-1% of live births (likely underestimation)
- Incidence varies by malformation type; VUR is one of the most common CAKUT
- 25% of ESRD patients have CAKUT

Age Range

- Most diagnosed in utero or perinatally
- Subtle defects may go undetected and present later in life

Gender

- Some malformations have sex preferences
  - PUV only in males
  - VUR more common in females

Ethnicity Relationship

- Affects individuals of any race or ethnicity

CLINICAL IMPLICATIONS

Overview

- CAKUT are most common pediatric cause of renal failure
- Up to 25% cases of ESRD in adults attributed to CAKUT
- Genomic testing often reveal likely pathogenic variants
  - Determining causality challenging

Clinical Presentation

- In utero
  - Oligohydramnios
  - IUGR
  - Routine imaging
- Postnatal
  - Multiple UTI
  - Uremia
  - Renal failure
  - Hypertension
  - Stones
- Clinical issues
  - Spontaneous resolution
  - Surgical/urologic correction
  - Genetic counseling
  - Stricture, scarring, recurrence
  - Medical: Dialysis

MACROSCOPIC

General Features

- Varies depending on phenotype
- Upper urinary tract may be secondarily affected due to lower tract anomaly or may be affected independent of lower tract defects

MICROSCOPIC

General Features

- Varies depending on phenotype

SELECTED REFERENCES

1. Yosypiv IV: Congenital anomalies of the kidney and urinary tract: a genetic disorder? Int J Nephrol. 2012:909083, 2012
2. Song R et al: Genetics of congenital anomalies of the kidney and urinary tract. Pediatr Nephrol. 26(3):353-64, 2011
3. Hildebrandt F: Genetic kidney diseases. Lancet. 375(9722):1287-95, 2010
4. Kerecuk L et al: Renal tract malformations: perspectives for nephrologists. Nat Clin Pract Nephrol. 4(6):312-25, 2008
5. Winyard P et al: Dysplastic kidneys. Semin Fetal Neonatal Med. 13(3):142-51, 2008
6. Vize PD et al: The Kidney: From Normal Development to Congenital Disease. London: Academic Press. 2003

Defects in Mesonephros-WD Development

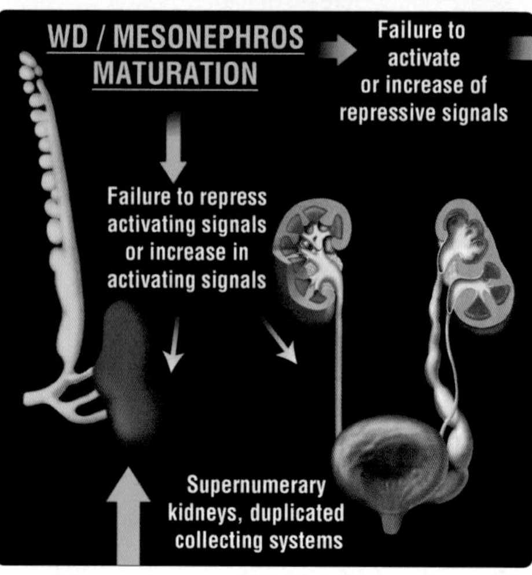

Defects in Induction of Ureteric Bud

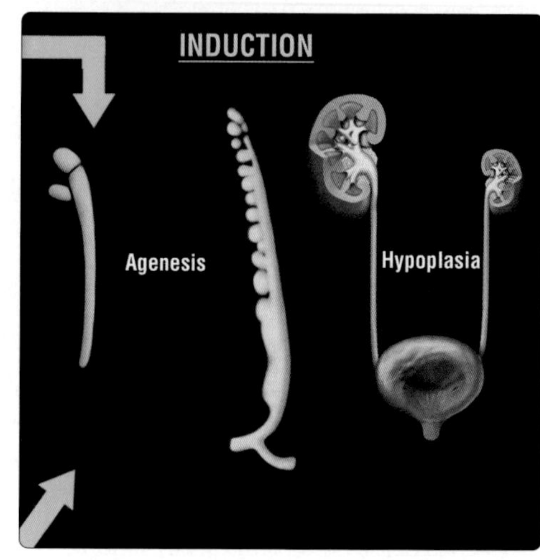

(Left) *Illustration shows renal malformations due to wolffian duct (WD) or mesonephros maturation defects. Increased net signaling from the WD can result in supernumerary ureteric buds (UBs) or duplicated collecting systems.* **(Right)** *Induction defects or net decreased WD maturation or growth can lead to renal agenesis or hypoplasia. Main reasons include failure of distal WD growth, UB induction defects causing failure of UB induction, or malpositioning of UB.*

Early Normal Kidney Development

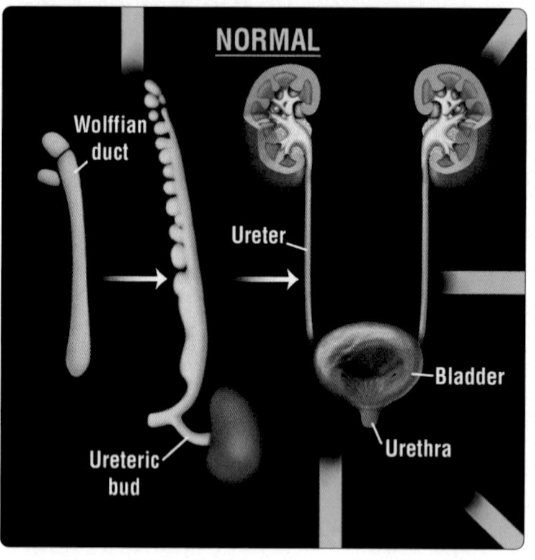

Branching Morphogenesis Defects

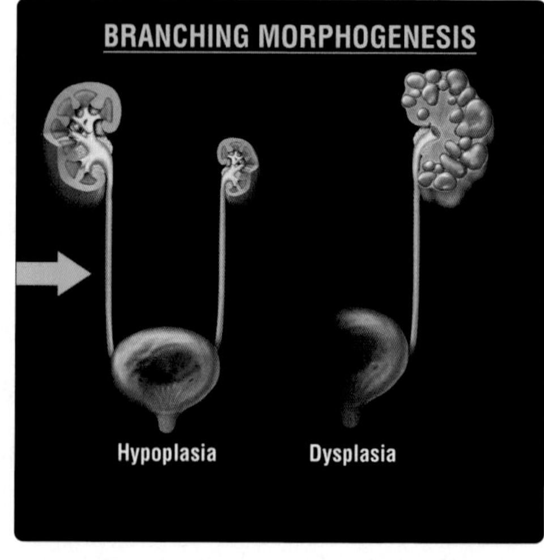

(Left) *Illustration summarizes normal kidney development stages: Pronephros, caudal extension of WD during mesonephros, and induction of ureteric bud (UB) in metanephros followed by branching morphogenesis and ascent. Distal ureter maturation also ensures its normal entry into the bladder.* **(Right)** *Branching morphogenesis defects can cause hypoplasia (reduced nephrons) or dysplasia (abnormally patterned) due to aberrant reciprocal interactions and differentiation defects.*

Upper and Lower Ureter and UGS Defects

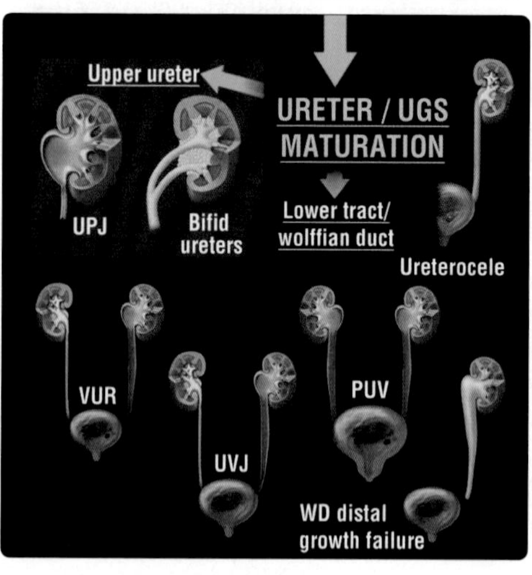

Ascent-Malrotation Defects

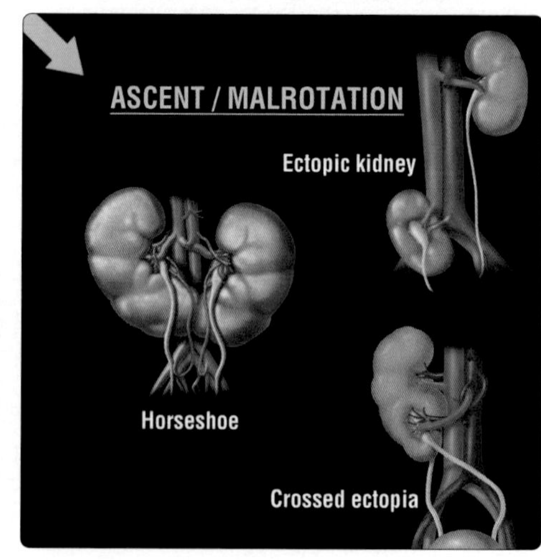

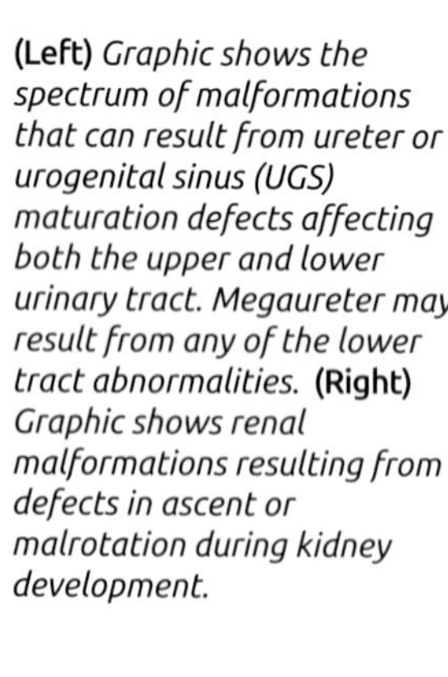

(Left) *Graphic shows the spectrum of malformations that can result from ureter or urogenital sinus (UGS) maturation defects affecting both the upper and lower urinary tract. Megaureter may result from any of the lower tract abnormalities.* **(Right)** *Graphic shows renal malformations resulting from defects in ascent or malrotation during kidney development.*

Meckel-Gruber Syndrome

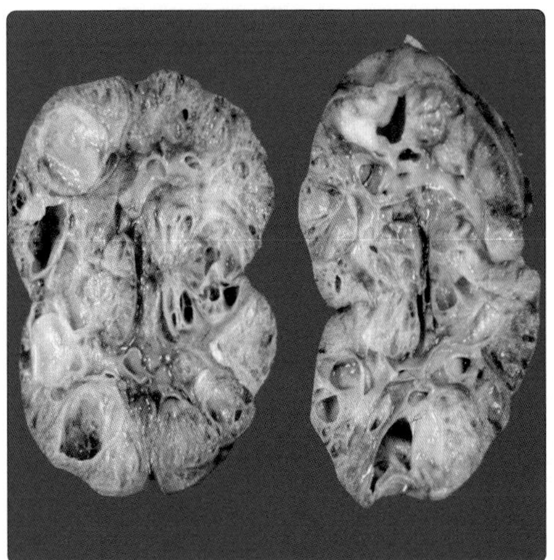

Extra Renal Manifestation in BOR Syndrome

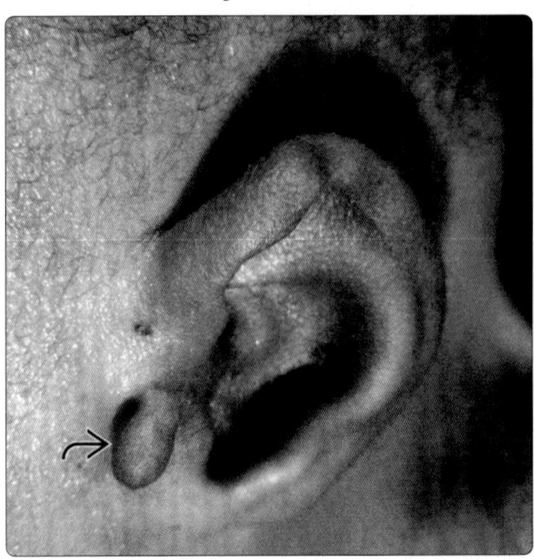

(Left) *Cut surface of kidneys depict macroscopic features of Meckel-Gruber Syndrome. Note enlarged kidney with multiple cysts, histologically confirmed to be multicystic dysplasia.* **(Right)** *Preauricular tag ➲ can be seen frequently in renal malformation syndromes such as branchio-oto-renal and 4p deletion syndrome.*

Megaureter

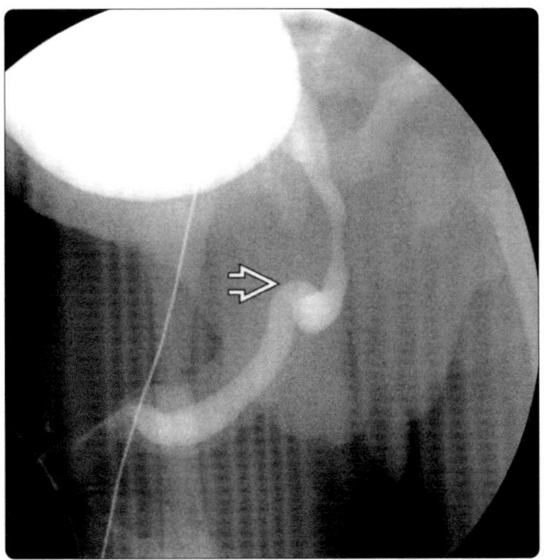

Multiple Renal Cysts in Utero

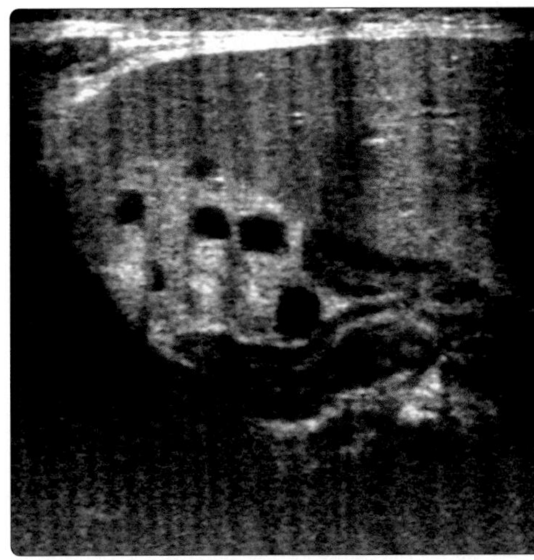

(Left) *Voiding cystoureterogram shows tortuous ureter ➡ and distended bladder in prune belly syndrome.* **(Right)** *Sonogram shows multiple kidney cysts in a patient with prune belly syndrome (cryptorchidism, abdominal muscle maldevelopment, CAKUT).*

Extra Renal Manifestations in CAKUT

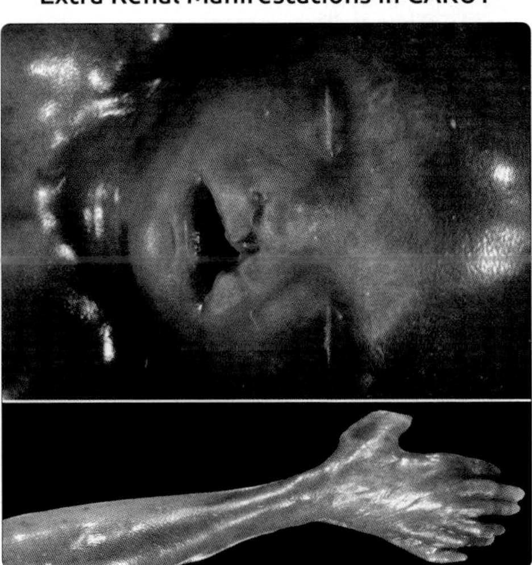

Prune Belly Syndrome

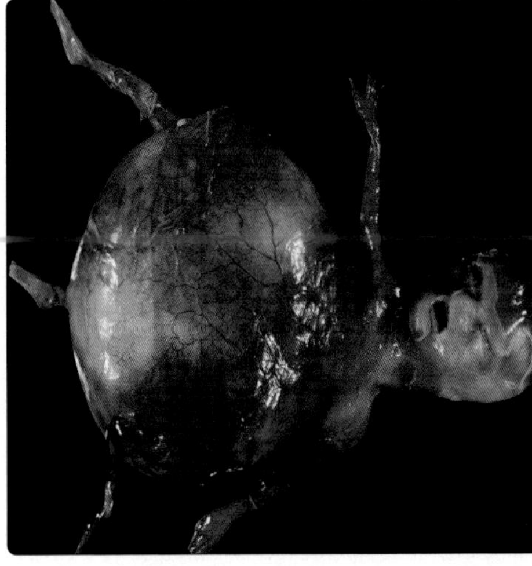

(Left) *Gross images depict extrarenal manifestations of Spitz-Lemli-Opitz syndrome. Note the dysmorphic facial features (cleft palate), syndactyly, and polydactyl.* **(Right)** *Fetopsy shows massively distended abdomen in prune belly syndrome. Normally these patients have a shriveled appearance of abdomen due to muscle maldevelopment; however, this fetus had dilated bladder distending the abdomen, thus masking the typical abdomen appearance.*

Dysplasia/Hypoplasia/Agenesis

KEY FACTS

TERMINOLOGY

- Renal hypoplasia: Small, architecturally normal kidneys, reduced number of nephrons
- Renal agenesis or aplasia: No kidney formation or involution after early branching
- Renal dysplasia: Architecturally abnormal kidneys with varying degree of undifferentiated mesenchyme, stroma, and epithelium

ETIOLOGY/PATHOGENESIS

- Branching morphogenesis defects
- Mechanical, genetic, functional, maternal factors, drugs
- UB induction or position defects
- Nephric duct growth and maturation defects

CLINICAL ISSUES

- Bilateral renal agenesis: Incompatible with life
- Unilateral renal agenesis: Incidentally identified in adults
  - Moderate risk of hypertension, proteinuria
  - 50-70% associated with other genitourinary anomalies
- Bilateral small kidneys may be dysplastic

MICROSCOPIC

- Renal hypoplasia
  - Normal organization into cortex, medulla, and papillae
  - May show compensatory hypertrophy
  - Oligomeganephronia: Glomeruli may be 3x larger than normal
- Renal dysplasia
  - May be segmental, diffuse, or zonal (outer cortex)
  - Little or no proximal nephron components
  - Disorganized architecture
  - Smooth muscle collarettes surrounding primitive collecting ducts
  - Nodules of cartilage in 30%

TOP DIFFERENTIAL DIAGNOSES

- Renal cystic disease

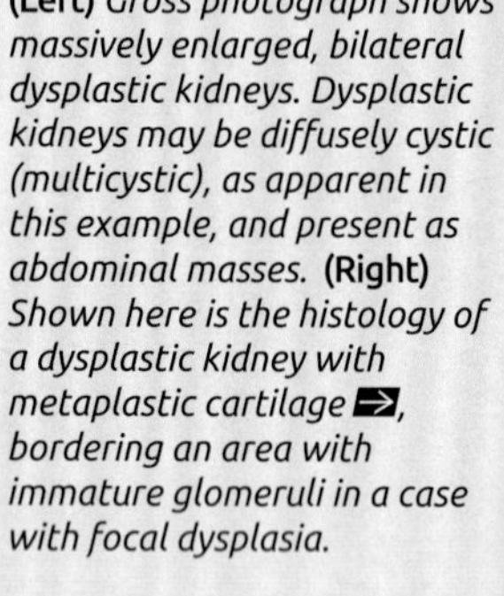

(Left) *Gross photograph shows massively enlarged, bilateral dysplastic kidneys. Dysplastic kidneys may be diffusely cystic (multicystic), as apparent in this example, and present as abdominal masses.* **(Right)** *Shown here is the histology of a dysplastic kidney with metaplastic cartilage* ➡*, bordering an area with immature glomeruli in a case with focal dysplasia.*

Bilateral Dysplastic Kidneys

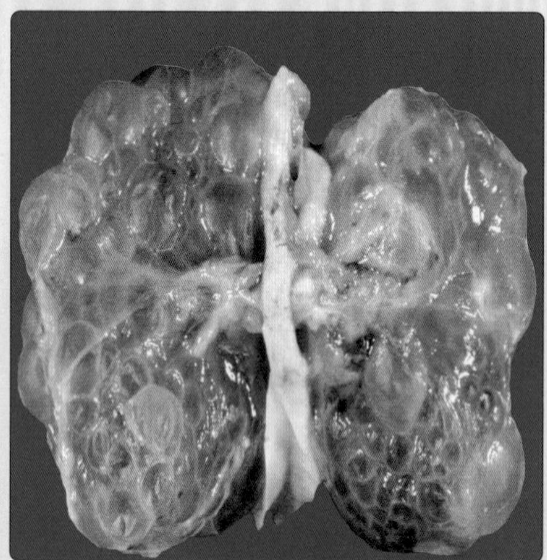

Histology of Kidney Dysplasia

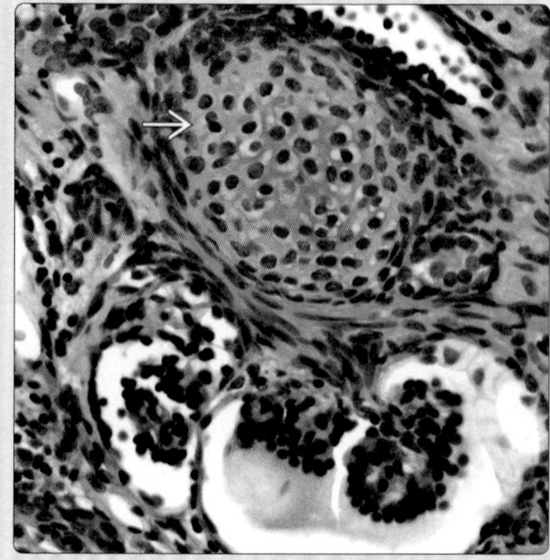

(Left) *Gross image shows right unilateral agenesis. Note the ear-shaped adrenal gland* ➡ *and left hypoplasia* ➡*.* **(Right)** *Ultrasound shows multiple cysts* ➡ *and variable echogenicity in a fetus with prune belly syndrome, consistent with cystic dysplasia.*

Unilateral Agenesis, Hypoplasia

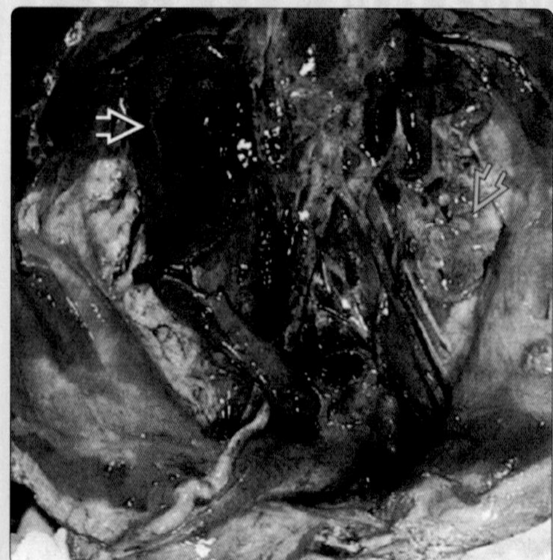

Cystic Dysplasia, Prune Belly Syndrome

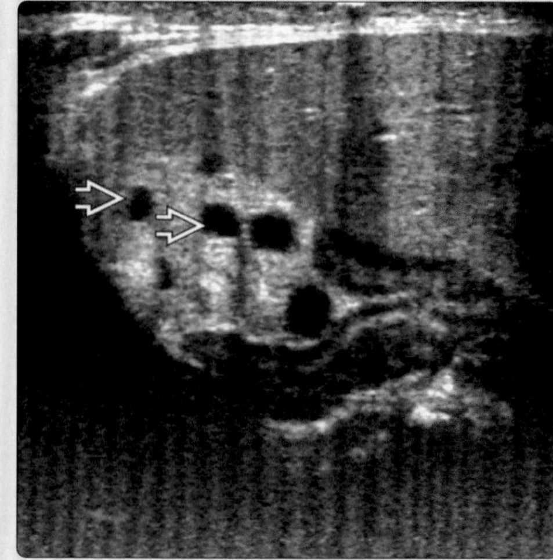

TERMINOLOGY

Abbreviations

- Metanephric mesenchyme (MM)
- Ureteric bud (UB)

Definitions

- Renal hypoplasia: Small, architecturally normal kidneys with decreased number of nephrons 2 standard deviations below age-matched normal kidneys
- Renal agenesis: Absent kidney due to defective kidney induction
- Renal aplasia: Absent or rudimentary kidneys, initially induced but involuted after early branching
- Renal dysplasia
  - Architecturally abnormal kidneys with immature nephrons
  - Abnormal ureteric bud branching or collecting duct remnants
  - Undifferentiated stroma
  - Occasionally with metaplastic cartilage

ETIOLOGY/PATHOGENESIS

Developmental Anomaly

- Defects during different steps in kidney development: Induction, branching, and nephrogenesis

Genetic

- Spontaneous or de novo mutations

In Utero Urinary Obstruction

- Mechanical
  - Ureteropelvic junction (UPJ) obstruction
  - Ureter obstruction
  - Ureterovesical junction (UVJ) obstruction
  - Posterior urethral valves
  - Ectopic ureters
  - Prune belly syndrome (thick bladder wall muscle in absence of physical obstruction)
- Functional (e.g., reflux)

Toxins, Environmental Exposure, Drugs

- Vitamin A deficiency or increase
- ACE-1 inhibitors
- Maternal malnutrition
- Maternal iron deficiency

Renal Agenesis

- Pronephros and mesonephros defects
  - Nephric duct growth and maturation defects
- Metanephros defects
  - UB induction: Failure to form UB or invade MM, early branching
  - UB position: Rostral or caudal to normal budding site, inability to invade MM

Renal Hypoplasia

- UB induction: Slow
- UB position: Rostral or caudal, partly invades MM
- Branching morphogenesis: Slow

Renal Dysplasia and Aplasia

- Branching morphogenesis: Inadequate, disorganized, disrupted reciprocal interactions between MM, stroma, and UB

CLINICAL ISSUES

Presentation

- Bilateral agenesis
  - Oligohydramnios or anhydramnios by ultrasound
- Unilateral agenesis
  - Asymptomatic
  - Later secondary Focal segmental glomerulosclerosis (FSGS) with hypertension, proteinuria
- Dysplasia
  - Identified by routine antenatal ultrasound as increased echogenicity
  - Abdominal mass
  - Entire kidney or only part may be affected
  - Multicystic dysplastic kidneys are nonfunctional
    - Often with underdeveloped ureters or ureteral stenosis
- Bilateral hypoplasia may be idiopathic or associated with oligomeganephronia
  - Term "hypoplasia" often loosely used in radiological exams for small kidneys
    - Grossly or radiographically small kidneys may have glomerular cysts and tubular dysgenesis microscopically
      - May not be truly hypoplastic
- Symptoms and signs in bilateral renal hypoplasia or dysplasia
  - Failure to thrive
  - Growth retardation
  - Hypertension
  - Excessive thirst
  - Increased urine output
  - Kidney failure
  - Salt wasting
- Syndromes associated with renal agenesis or dysplasia or hypoplasia
  - Branchio-oto-renal syndrome (BOR)
  - Renal cysts and diabetes syndrome (RCAD)
  - Fanconi syndrome
  - Kallmann syndrome
  - DiGeorge syndrome
  - Smith-Lemli-Opitz syndrome
  - Hereditary renal adysplasia (unilateral agenesis with contralateral dysplasia)
  - Caudal regression syndrome (imperforate anus, absent bladder, absent urethra)
  - Down syndrome
- Potter sequence
  - Due to oligohydramnios or anhydramnios in some of these conditions, lung hypoplasia ensues, causing neonatal death
  - Musculoskeletal anomalies
    - Wide-set eyes
    - Prominent epicanthal folds
    - Flat nose, ears

- Limb defects

Prognosis

- Bilateral renal agenesis
  - Stillborn or perinatal death
- Unilateral renal agenesis
  - Generally good with no consequences in isolated disease
  - Moderate risk of hypertension and proteinuria due to FSGS
- Hypoplasia
  - Bilateral hypoplasia: Most develop end-stage renal disease (ESRD) in mid to late childhood
  - Increased risk of hypertension and heart disease (oligomeganephronia)
- Dysplasia
  - Unilateral: Good prognosis, treat infections and hypertension
  - Routine surgical removal not recommended
  - Bilateral: Usually nonfunctional kidneys, perinatal death

MACROSCOPIC

Bilateral Agenesis

- Absent kidneys
- Ureters may be absent or truncated
- Hypoplastic lungs

Unilateral Agenesis

- Contralateral kidney may show hypertrophy
- Affected side may have normal, truncated, or absent ureter
- 50-70% associated with other genitourinary anomalies
  - Ureteral ectopia,
  - Renal dysplasia,
  - Absence of vas deferens
  - Reflux nephropathy

Renal Dysplasia

- Small, normal, or slightly enlarged kidneys
  - May be associated with randomly distributed cysts (multicystic)
- Loss of reniform shape
- 50-70% have contralateral kidney defects
- Often associated with other lower urinary tract anomalies
  - Ureterocele
  - Posterior urethral valves
  - Hydronephrosis

Renal Hypoplasia

- Weight usually < 50%
- Normal architecture
- Decreased renal lobes
- May accompany renal artery hypoplasia
- Simple hypoplasia
  - Bilateral greater than unilateral
  - Usually no hypertrophy
  - Reduced kidney volume
- Oligomeganephronia
  - Hypertrophy of nephrons, which are decreased in number

MICROSCOPIC

Histologic Features

- Histology is gold standard to correctly classify these anomalies
  - Biopsies rarely done and diagnosis mainly made from radiological studies, nephrectomies, and autopsies
- Unilateral renal agenesis
  - Normal or compensatory hypertrophy
- Renal hypoplasia
  - Normal organization into cortex, medulla, and papillae
  - Simple hypoplasia: Normal histology
    - May see secondary glomerulosclerosis in severe cases
  - Oligomeganephronia: Glomeruli may be 3x larger than normal
- Renal dysplasia
  - May be segmental (more frequently in adults)
  - Diffuse (almost always in children)
  - Zonal (affecting outer cortex, most recently formed)
    - Thinned cortex
    - Reduced number of nephrons
  - Dysplastic areas have
    - Little or no proximal nephron components (glomeruli, proximal, distal tubules)
    - Only primitive collecting ducts/cysts (ureteric bud)
    - Disorganized architecture with no definitive cortex or medulla
    - Undifferentiated mesenchyme
    - Focal or diffuse cysts
    - Smooth muscle collarettes surrounding primitive collecting ducts
    - Nodules of cartilage in 30%
    - Immature and disorganized tubules may be present, adjacent to dysplastic areas

Cytologic Features

- Reduced epithelial proliferation
- Increased apoptosis
- Cell differentiation defects

ANCILLARY TESTS

Genetic Testing

- Many cases monogenic or familial
  - Depending on family history/phenotype and if syndromic, targeted or whole exome/genome sequencing can be offered
    - Caution should be exercised in interpreting causality
- Genes known to be causative in agenesis, hypoplasia, dysplasia: *RET, PAX2, SIX2, WNT4, SIX1, SALLI, GDNF, FRAS1, GATA3*

DIFFERENTIAL DIAGNOSIS

Renal Agenesis

- Renal aplasia: Solitary kidneys may have contralateral renal aplasia (not true agenesis)
  - Kidneys were induced but regressed or involuted with time
- Renal dysplasia: Dysplastic kidneys may regress over time, making it difficult to differentiate from agenesis

Main Characteristics of Dysplasia, Hypoplasia, and Agenesis

Feature	Dysplasia	Hypoplasia	Agenesis
Incidence	1:7,500 (unilateral), 1:7,500 (bilateral)	1:1,000 (unilateral), 1:4,000 (bilateral)	1:1,000 male = female, left > right (unilateral); 1:10,000 male > female (bilateral)
Mechanism	Defective branching morphogenesis	Slow UB induction, reduced branching, incorrect UB position	WD development defect, UB induction failure
Ultrasonogram findings	Noncommunicating hypoechogenic cysts, small kidney	Small kidney	Absent kidney
Prognosis	Perinatal death or ESRD (if bilateral), normal outcome if unilateral (risk of FSGS)	Most ESRD (bilateral), normal outcome if unilateral (risk of FSGS)	Perinatal death (bilateral), normal outcome if unilateral (risk of FSGS)
Macroscopic	Nonreniform, multicystic; small, normal,or large size	Small, normally shaped kidneys, reduced number of pyramids	No kidneys, earlobe shape, elongated adrenals
Microscopic	Disorganized parenchyma, immature glomeruli and tubules, smooth muscle collarettes around collecting ducts, metaplastic cartilage (30%)	Normal organization, large nephrons in oligomeganephronia	Normal or compensatory hypertrophy in unilateral agenesis

WD = Wolffian duct; UB = ureteric bud; ESRD = end-stage renal disease; FSGS = focal segmental glomerulosclerosis.

  - Need radiology evaluation during embryogenesis and perinatally to rule out dysplasia in child or adult with solitary kidney

Renal Dysplasia

- Renal cystic diseases: May show dysplastic features (glomerulocystic, multicystic dysplasia)
  - Correlate with histological pattern, kidney size, other organ involvement, and genetics
  - Polycystic kidney disease (early onset ADPKD, ARPKD)
  - Primary glomerulocystic kidney disease (autosomal dominant)
- Reflux nephropathy
  - Medulla more affected than cortex
  - Uretero pelvic junction obstruction (UPJO)
  - Uretero vesicle junction obstruction (UVJO)
  - Ureterocele
  - Posterior urethral valves
  - Vesico ureteral reflux (VUR)

Renal Hypoplasia

- Acquired kidney disease
- Aplastic kidney
- Secondary damage: If radiographic exam with contrast shows scarring, calyceal clubbing
- Small kidneys due to dysplasia or atrophy

DIAGNOSTIC CHECKLIST

Clinically Relevant Pathologic Features

- Bilateral dysplasia, agenesis have bad prognosis with perinatal failure

Pathologic Interpretation Pearls

- Dysplastic features in an obstructed kidney suggests congenital anomaly
  - Compared to identifiable normally organized kidney parenchyma in postnatal obstructed kidney (i.e., prostate hyperplasia, stones, tumor)

SELECTED REFERENCES

1. Davis TK et al: To bud or not to bud: the RET perspective in CAKUT. Pediatr Nephrol. 29(4):597-608, 2014
2. Hoshi M et al: Novel mechanisms of early upper and lower urinary tract patterning regulated by RetY1015 docking tyrosine in mice. Development. 139(13):2405-15, 2012
3. Yosypiv IV: Congenital anomalies of the kidney and urinary tract: a genetic disorder? Int J Nephrol. 2012:909083, 2012
4. Song R et al: Genetics of congenital anomalies of the kidney and urinary tract. Pediatr Nephrol. 26(3):353-64, 2011
5. Kerecuk L et al: Renal tract malformations: perspectives for nephrologists. Nat Clin Pract Nephrol. 4(6):312-25, 2008
6. Liapis H et al: Cystic diseases and developmental kidney defects. In Jennette JC et al: Heptinstall's Pathology of the Kidney. 6th ed. Philadelphia: Lippincott Williams & Wilkins. 1257-1306, 2007
7. Vize P et al: The Kidney: From Normal Development to Congenital Disease. London: Academic Press. 2003
8. Hiraoka M et al: Renal aplasia is the predominant cause of congenital solitary kidneys. Kidney Int. 61(5):1840-4, 2002

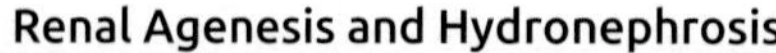

Renal Agenesis and Hydronephrosis

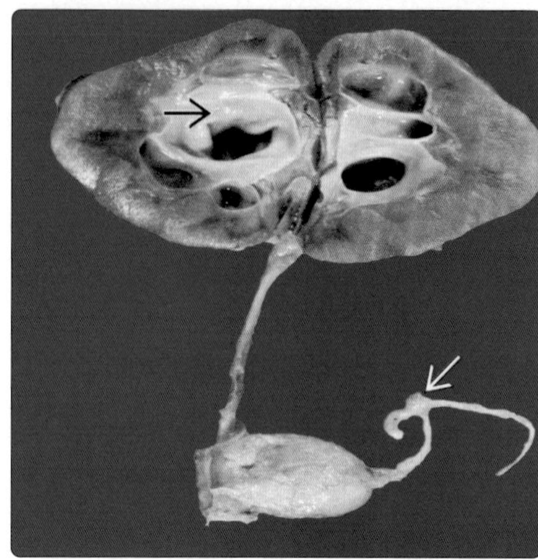

Renal Agenesis and Dysplasia

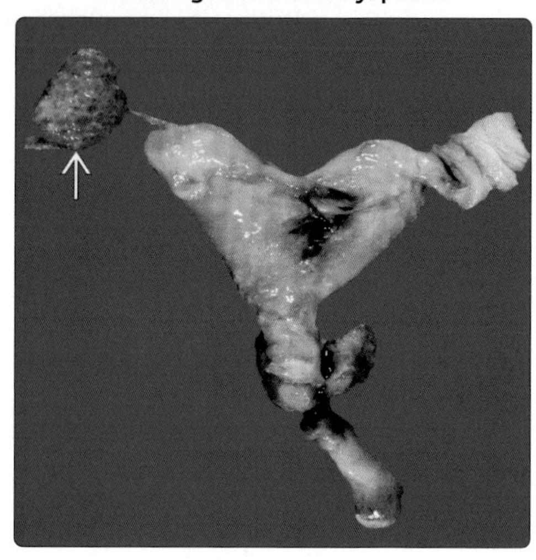

(Left) *This is the gross appearance of the urinary tract from a 4-month-old baby, showing the left unilateral agenesis ➔ and right hydronephrosis ➔.* **(Right)** *Gross appearance of urinary tract depicts left renal agenesis and a small right dysplastic cystic kidney ➔.*

Bilateral Renal Agenesis

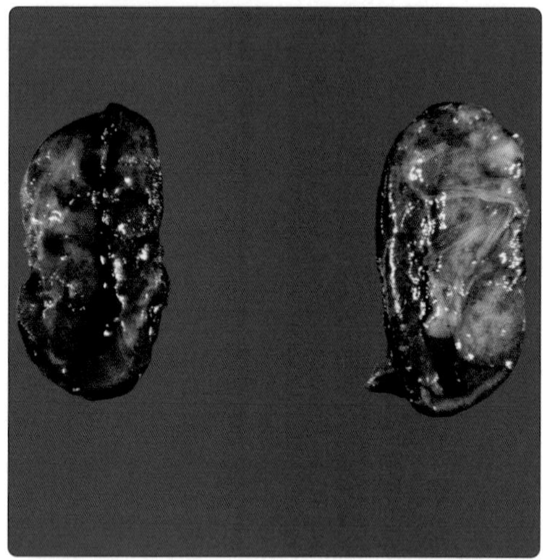

Lung Hypoplasia

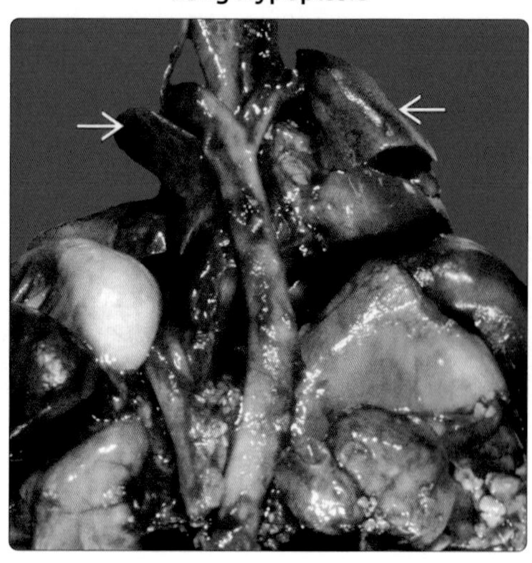

(Left) *Adrenal glands from a baby with bilateral renal agenesis are shown. Note the elongated ear-shaped large adrenal glands due to the absence of caudal resistance by the kidneys.* **(Right)** *Shown here are severely hypoplastic lungs ➔ in a baby due to oligohydramnios resulting from bilateral renal agenesis. This is a component of Potter sequence.*

Mouse Model, Unilateral Agenesis

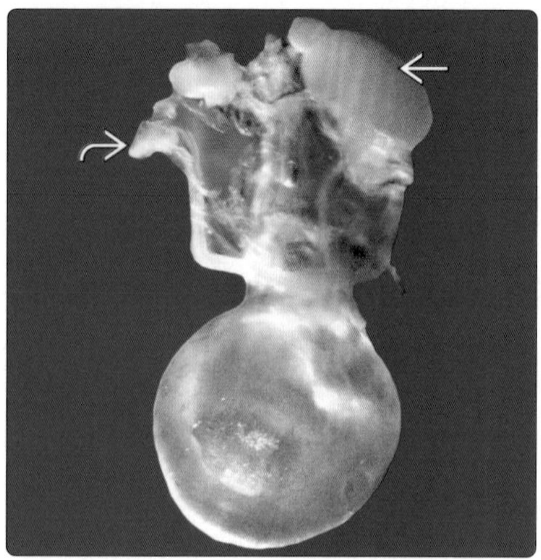

Mouse Model, Unilateral Agenesis

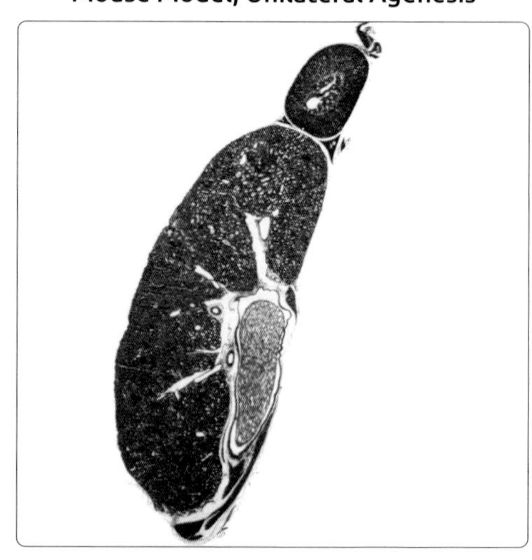

(Left) *Urinary tract of a mutant mouse with reduced receptor tyrosine kinase Ret signaling shows unilateral agenesis ➔ and a hypoplastic kidney ➔. Ret is expressed in the ureteric bud and is involved with ureteric branching. Mutations in Ret are found in 35% of patients with renal agenesis.* **(Right)** *Histological section of hypoplastic kidney from a mouse with decreased Ret signaling shows preserved organization of cortex, medulla, and papilla. An adrenal gland is seen lying on top of the kidney.*

Cystic Dysplasia and Ureter Stenosis

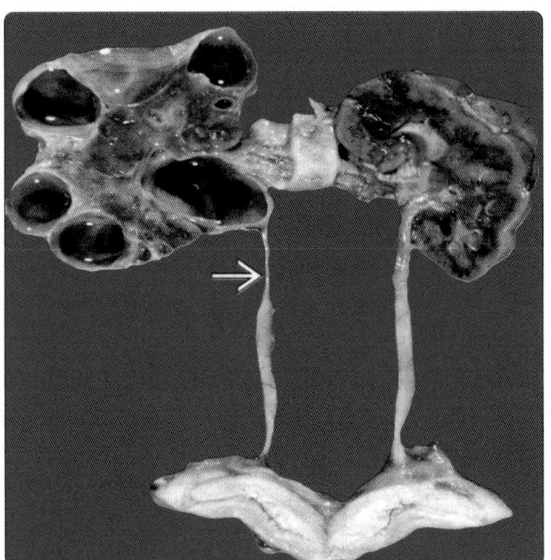

Cartilage in Renal Dysplasia

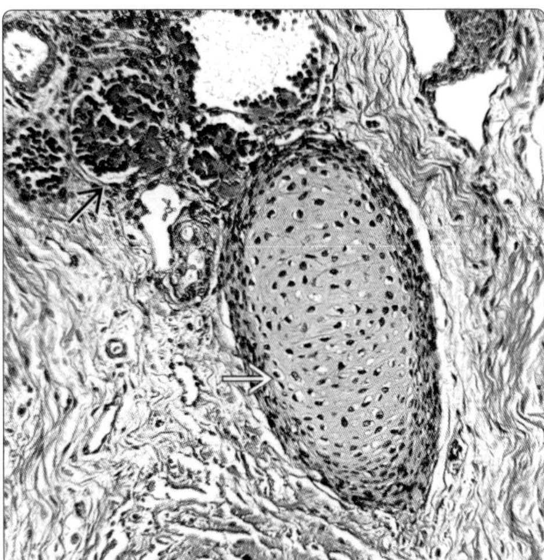

(Left) *Shown here is the coronal section of the urinary tract from a patient with right multicystic dysplasia and proximal ureter stenosis ➡. The left kidney section shows normal architecture with a well-formed cortex and medulla and a normal ureter. Intrauterine obstruction is a common cause of dysplasia.* **(Right)** *Dysplastic kidney with metaplastic cartilage ➡ and an adjacent primitive glomerulus ➡ is shown.*

Small Dysplastic Kidney

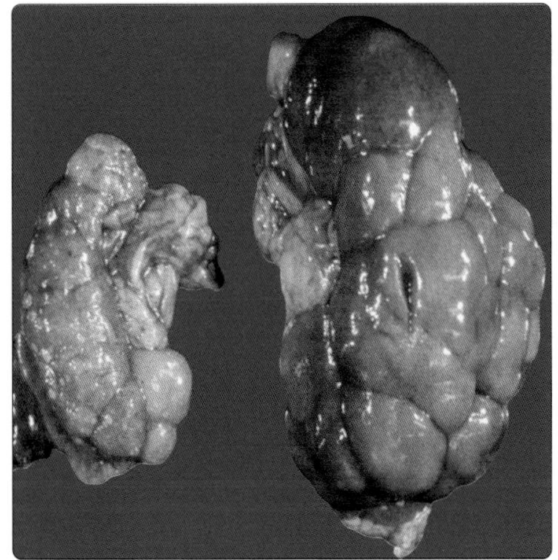

Glomerular Cysts

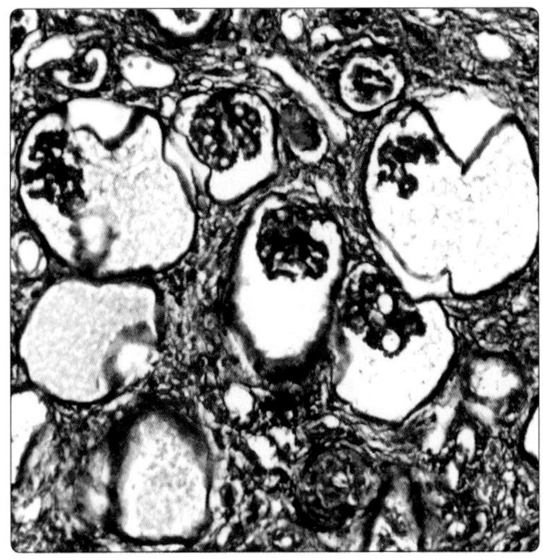

(Left) *Gross photograph shows a small right kidney compared to the normal left kidney. The small kidney showed histological changes of glomerulocystic dysplasia and had UPJ obstruction.* **(Right)** *Histological section of a small kidney shows glomerulocystic dysplasia. Note that cyst size inversely correlates with the cellular component of the glomeruli, eventually leading to complete cystic replacement of the glomerulus.*

Kidney Dysplasia

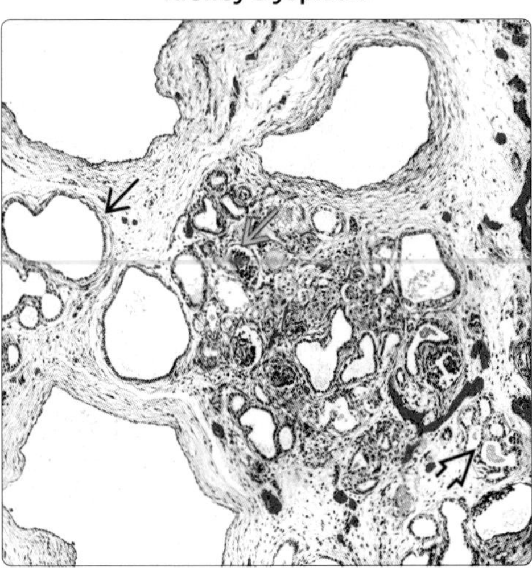

Fibromuscular Collarettes

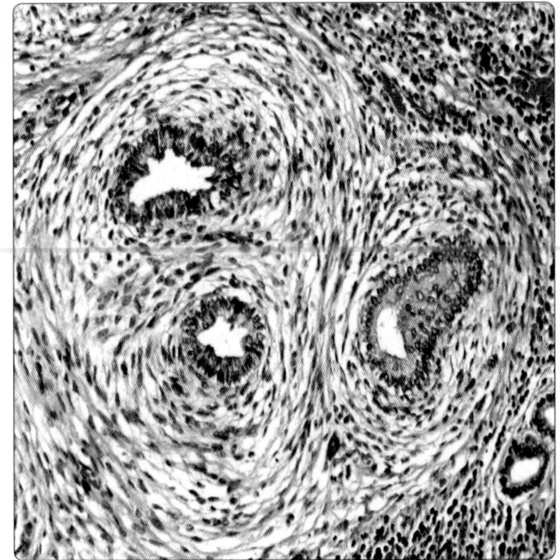

(Left) *Histological section of a dysplastic kidney shows a lack of organization of kidney parenchyma into cortex, medulla, and papilla. Note the random arrangement of immature kidney elements with scattered dilated and atrophic tubules ➡, immature glomeruli ➡, and undifferentiated collecting ducts ➡.* **(Right)** *Dysplastic kidney shows underdeveloped collecting ducts surrounded by smooth muscle-like collarettes.*

Oligomeganephronia

KEY FACTS

TERMINOLOGY

- Bilaterally small kidneys due to renal hypoplasia, which leads to marked compensatory nephron hypertrophy

ETIOLOGY/PATHOGENESIS

- Reduced nephron formation during development leads to nephron hypertrophy, secondary FSGS, and eventually ESRD
- Most cases sporadic
- Genetic causes
  - *PAX2* mutation (Papillorenal syndrome)
  - *EYA1*, *SIX5*, or *SIX1* (Branchio-oto-renal syndrome)
  - *TCF2* mutation
  - Monosomy 4p (Wolf-Hirschhorn syndrome)
  - Acrorenal syndrome

CLINICAL ISSUES

- Usually presents in infancy
  - Growth retardation, polydipsia, polyuria, enuresis
  - Proteinuria
  - Renal function is usually stable for a few years, but later deteriorates to ESRD
- Rarely presents in adulthood with proteinuria, renal insufficiency, and bilateral small kidneys

MACROSCOPIC

- Small, dense kidneys with reduced number of renal lobes
- Weight < 50% of normal

MICROSCOPIC

- Fewer than normal glomeruli
- Hypertrophy of remaining glomeruli and proximal tubules
- Focal interstitial fibrosis and tubular atrophy
- Secondary FSGS

TOP DIFFERENTIAL DIAGNOSES

- Nephronophthisis
- Dysplasia

Reduced Generations of Glomeruli

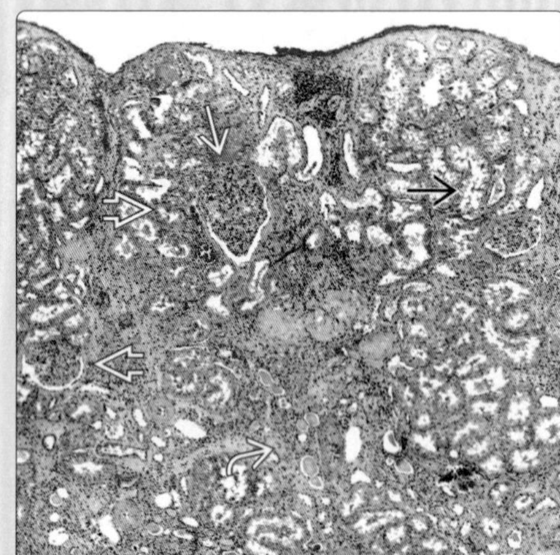

Marked Glomerulomegaly

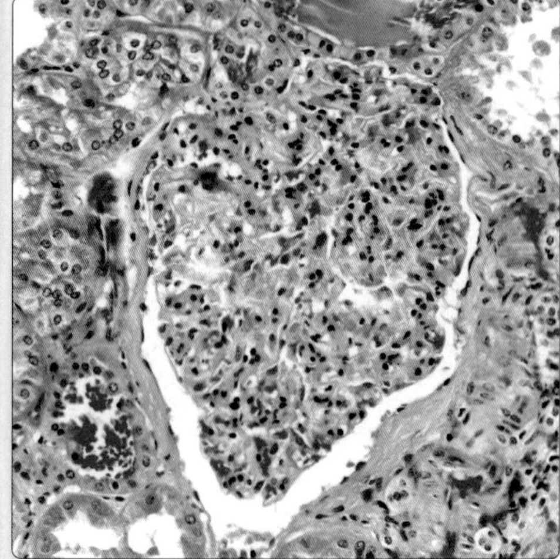

(Left) *OMN shows reduced number of glomeruli, here with only 2 levels of glomeruli in the cortex. The glomeruli and tubules are hypertrophied. Fibrosis and tubular atrophy are present.* **(Right)** *The hallmark of OMN is hypertrophy of the glomeruli due to an adaptive response to a congenital deficiency of nephrons. Glomeruli also have mesangial hypercellularity. A rule of thumb for glomerular hypertrophy is a cross section that is greater than the radius of the usual 400x field (440 µm).*

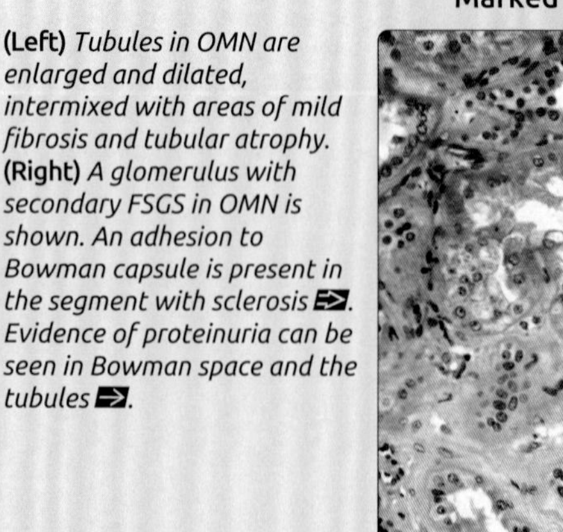

Marked Hypertrophy of Tubules

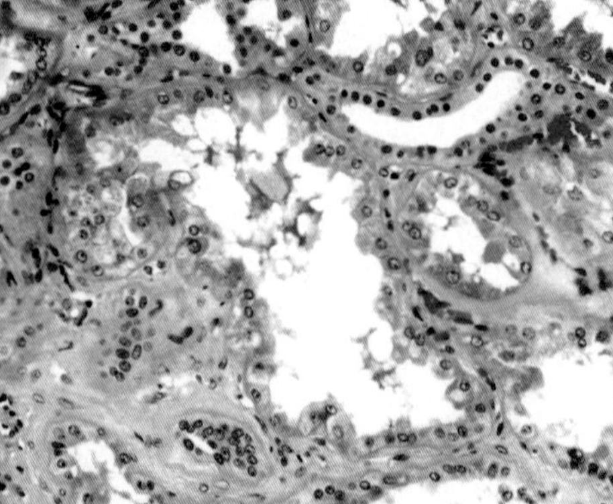

Secondary Focal Segmental Glomerulosclerosis

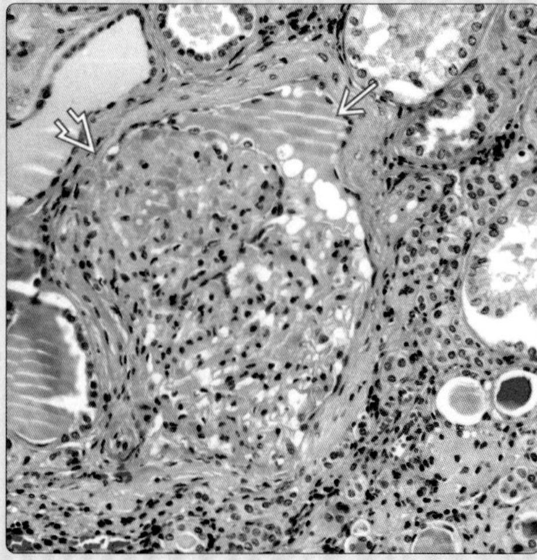

(Left) *Tubules in OMN are enlarged and dilated, intermixed with areas of mild fibrosis and tubular atrophy.* **(Right)** *A glomerulus with secondary FSGS in OMN is shown. An adhesion to Bowman capsule is present in the segment with sclerosis. Evidence of proteinuria can be seen in Bowman space and the tubules.*

TERMINOLOGY

Abbreviations

- Oligomeganephronia (OMN)

Synonyms

- Oligomeganephronic hypoplasia

Definitions

- Histologic pattern of renal hypoplasia with marked compensatory nephron hypertrophy occurring both sporadically and due to known genetic disorders

ETIOLOGY/PATHOGENESIS

Sporadic (Most Common)

- In most cases etiology is unknown

Genetic Disorders (Rare)

- Papillorenal syndrome (OMIM 120330), a.k.a. renal-coloboma syndrome
  - *PAX2* mutation in 50%
    - Associated with optic disc/nerve abnormality
    - Autosomal dominant, chromosome 10q
- Wolf-Hirschhorn syndrome (OMIM 194190)
  - 4p deletion or ring, multiple congenital anomalies
- Branchio-oto-renal syndrome (OMIM 113650, 610896, and 600963), a.k.a. Melnick-Fraser syndrome
  - Brachial fistulae/clefts, ear malformations, and OMN
  - *EYA1* (40%), *SIX5*, and *SIX1* genes combined are involved in about 50% of all cases
  - Autosomal dominant
- *TCF2* mutation (hepatocyte nuclear factor-1β) in POU A domain (DNA binding)
  - Other mutations cause cystic, dysplastic hypoplastic and glomerulocystic kidneys
- Acrorenal syndrome (OMIM 102520)

Pathogenesis

- Abnormal nephron development
  - *PAX2*, *EYA1*, *SIX* transcription factors and *HNF-1B* are necessary for normal kidney development
  - Reduced branching morphogenesis and induction of nephrons
- Secondary FSGS and progression to ESRD

CLINICAL ISSUES

Presentation

- Infancy: Prematurity and low birth weight
  - Growth retardation, polydipsia, polyuria, enuresis
  - May present as ESRD at birth
- Rarely presents in young adulthood (23-33 years) as proteinuria, elevated Cr and bilateral small kidneys

Natural History

- Renal function is usually stable for a few years, but later deteriorates to ESRD
- Proteinuria, a consequence of secondary FSGS

Treatment

- ACE inhibitors may slow progression
- Transplantation

Prognosis

- Renal failure in late childhood to early adulthood
- Presentation in adulthood slower progression

IMAGING

Ultrasonographic Findings

- Small, hyperechoic kidneys bilaterally

CT Findings

- Small kidneys with relatively thick cortex due to hypertrophy

MACROSCOPIC

General Features

- Combined weight 12-45 g (< 50% of normal)
- Surface is smooth to finely granular
- Number of renal lobes is reduced (1-5)
- May have rounded shape

MICROSCOPIC

Histologic Features

- Reduced nephron number with little atrophy or scarring
- Glomerular hypertrophy (increased diameter, cell number)
- Proximal tubule hypertrophy (increased diameter, cell size, cell number)
- Interstitial fibrosis and tubular atrophy are usually only focal
- Secondary FSGS lesions may be evident

DIFFERENTIAL DIAGNOSIS

Nephronophthisis

- Autosomal recessive inheritance
- Prominent cysts and TBM duplication

Dysplasia

- Dysplastic elements (cartilage, smooth muscle, immature tubules)

DIAGNOSTIC CHECKLIST

Clinically Relevant Pathologic Features

- FSGS lesions
- Underlying molecular defects

SELECTED REFERENCES

1. Hopkins K et al: Congenital oligomeganephronia: computed tomography appearance. Clin Pract. 3(2):e31, 2013
2. Fuke Y et al: Oligomeganephronia in an adult without end stage renal failure. Clin Exp Nephrol. 16(2):325-8, 2012
3. Zaffanello M et al: TCF2 gene mutation leads to nephro-urological defects of unequal severity: an open question. Med Sci Monit. 14(6):RA78-86, 2008
4. Bohn S et al: Distinct molecular and morphogenetic properties of mutations in the human HNF1beta gene that lead to defective kidney development. J Am Soc Nephrol. 14(8):2033-41, 2003
5. Sagen JV et al: Enlarged nephrons and severe nondiabetic nephropathy in hepatocyte nuclear factor-1beta (HNF-1beta) mutation carriers. Kidney Int. 64(3):793-800, 2003
6. Salomon R et al: PAX2 mutations in oligomeganephronia. Kidney Int. 59(2):457-62, 2001

KEY FACTS

ETIOLOGY/PATHOGENESIS

- Simple ectopia: Ipsilateral to pelvis
- Crossed ectopia: Contralateral to ureter entering bladder
- Horseshoe kidneys: Usually lower pole fused, fibrous tissue at midline
- Malrotation: Failure of medial rotation during ascent
- Duplication or supernumerary ureters
  - Failure to repress extra ureteric bud (UB) outgrowths from nephric duct (ND)
  - Overactivity of pathways involved in UB and ureter growth

CLINICAL ISSUES

- Duplication
  - 40% complete
  - 80% with upper pole dilation and ureterocele
- Ectopia, malrotation, fusion anomalies, duplication
  - Usually asymptomatic

MACROSCOPIC

- Weigert-Meyer law for duplicated systems
  - Upper ureter enters lower or more distal in outflow tract (inferomedially) in bladder, urethra, or vagina
    - Drains upper pole if kidneys fused
  - Lower ureter (often normal site) enters superolaterally (higher or more proximal in outflow tract) into bladder
    - Drains lower pole if kidneys fused
  - VUR common, usually lower pole/kidney
  - Ureterocele often present in ureter draining upper pole or kidney

TOP DIFFERENTIAL DIAGNOSES

- Duplications
  - Hydronephrosis
  - VUR
  - UPJ obstruction
  - Solitary renal cyst
  - Polycystic kidney disease

Position Abnormalities

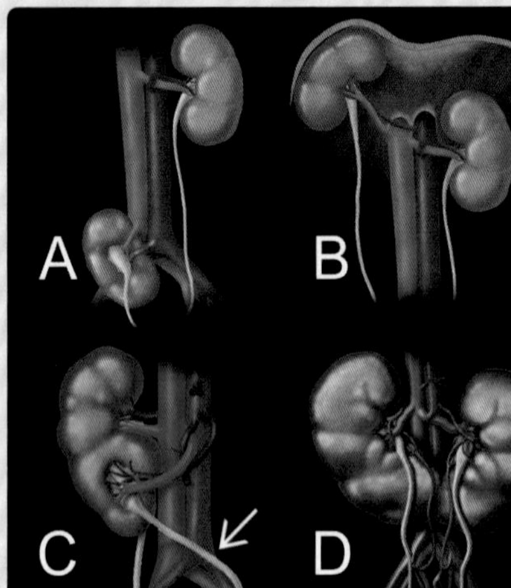

Horseshoe Kidney

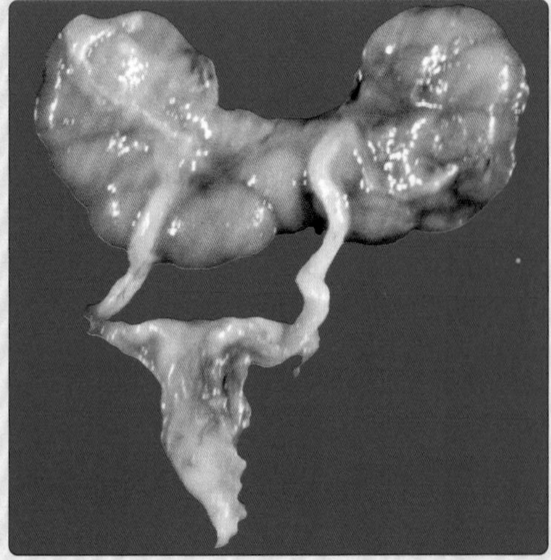

(Left) *Graphic shows ascent and fusion defects: (A) malrotated ectopic right kidney, (B) ectopic right kidney in thoracic cavity, (C) crossed fused ectopy in which left ureter ➔ crosses over and the corresponding kidney is small and fused to the orthotopic kidney, and (D) horseshoe kidney with fused lower poles.* **(Right)** *Gross photograph shows horseshoe kidney. Note the fusion of the 2 kidneys at the lower pole.*

Duplication

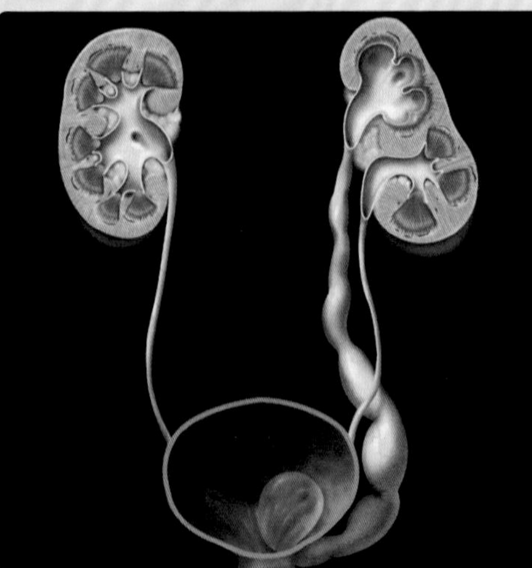

Complete Bilateral Duplication

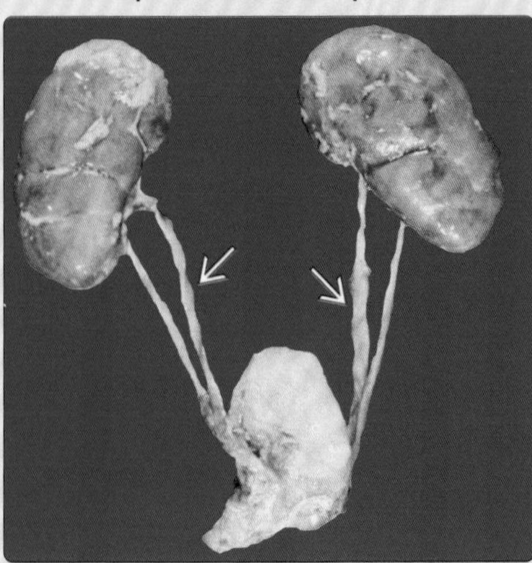

(Left) *Illustration depicts complete duplication of the ureters. Note that the ureter attached to the lower pole of the kidney inserts superomedially into the bladder, as predicted by the Weigert-Meyer rule. The ureter attached to the upper pole of the fused kidney is dilated (megaureter). Hydronephrosis is present in the corresponding upper pole of the kidney.* **(Right)** *Complete bilateral ureteral duplication is shown. The 2 upper pole ureters ➔ are moderately dilated.*

ETIOLOGY/PATHOGENESIS

Developmental Anomaly

- Failure to ascend
  - Ectopia
    - Simple: Ipsilateral to pelvis
    - Crossed: Contralateral to ureter bladder insertion
  - Malrotation
- Fusion anomalies
  - Horseshoe kidneys: Usually lower pole fused, fibrous tissue at midline
  - Crossed fused renal ectopia: Crosses over and fuses with contralateral kidney
  - Fused pelvic kidney: Ectopic kidney and fused; may have horseshoe shape
- Nephric duct (ND) or ureter bud (UB)
  - Duplication
    - Partial ureter duplication: Ureter or UB bifurcate before reaching metanephric mesenchyme or prior to branching of UB ampulla
    - Complete ureter or collecting system duplication: 2 UBs from ND give 2 ureters and 2 kidneys
  - Supernumerary kidneys
    - Multiple kidneys bud separately or growth of multiple UBs into metanephric mesenchyme

Mechanism

- Simple ectopia
  - Ascent failure
- Crossed ectopia
  - Presence of only 1 nephrogenic cord
  - Abnormal ureter migration to contralateral side
  - Abnormal umbilical artery development may prevent ascent, leading to contralateral deviation
- Fusion
  - Abnormal position of mesenchyme or ND (wolffian ducts)
    - In crossed fused ectopia, mesenchyme on only 1 side
- Duplication or supernumerary ureters
  - Failure to repress extra UB outgrowths from ND
  - Overactivity of pathways in UB and ureter growth
- Malrotation
  - Failure of medial rotation during ascent
    - Usually resulting in hilum facing anteriorly

CLINICAL ISSUES

Epidemiology

- Age
  - Antenatally, perinatally, or in adulthood
- Sex
  - Duplication: 65% females; 35% males

Presentation

- Antenatal screening
- Incidentally discovered
- Hydronephrosis
- Vesicoureteral reflux (VUR)
  - 20% could be in ectopic kidney
- Pyelonephritis
- Abdominal pain, cramps
- Mass
- With other syndromes
  - Ectopia
    - Mayer-Rokitansky-Küsher-Hauser syndrome
      - Female reproductive tract, skeletal, cardiac, urinary, and otologic defects
    - Goldenhar syndrome
      - Craniofacial, cardiac, pulmonary, or renal defects
    - Treacher Collins syndrome
      - Craniofacial defects, hearing loss, malformed ears, drooping lower eyelids
- Duplication
  - 20% bilateral
  - 60% bifid ureters
  - 40% complete
  - 80% with upper pole dilation and ureterocele
- Ectopia, malrotation, fusion anomalies, duplication
  - Asymptomatic unless other anomalies develop

Treatment

- Surgical approaches
  - Pyeloplasty if VUR present
  - Reconstruction for fused pelvic kidney
  - Nephrectomy of ectopic nonfunctional kidney
- Drugs
  - Antibiotics to reduce UTIs

Prognosis

- Usually no clinical significance
  - Ectopia
    - Blood pressure usually normal in childhood
    - Ectopic kidney function reduced, overall function may be normal
  - Reflux may resolve if lower grade but monitor if duplication and high grade
  - Duplication
    - Ureteropelvic junction (UPJ)
    - Complete duplication has higher VUR incidence and higher VUR grade
    - Some develop transitional cell carcinoma

MACROSCOPIC

Ectopia

- Simple
  - Kidney usually in pelvis, does not reach adrenal (round inferior end)
  - Ureter may be short
- Crossed
  - Ureter crosses contralaterally from bladder insertion
  - Ectopic kidney may be fused with orthotopic kidney
- Solitary crossed
  - Single crossed ectopic kidney
- May see VUR or hydronephrosis
- May have anomalous blood supply, derived from distal branches of aorta

Fusion Anomalies

- Many variations
- May see VUR or hydronephrosis
- Horseshoe

Summary of Ectopia, Fusion, Malrotation, Duplication, and Supernumerary Kidneys

	Ectopia	Fusion	Malrotation	Duplication	Supernumerary
Definition	Outside renal fossa	Meeting of 2 kidney anlages	Abnormal rotation	> 1 ureter or collecting system	Extra kidneys or ectopic UBs
Types	Simple, crossed, solitary crossed	Horseshoe, crossed fused, fused pelvic	Not applicable	Bifid ureters, complete duplication	Separate or multiplexed
Incidence	1:1,000 (autopsy); 1:10,000 (clinical)	1:400 (horseshoe); 1:2,000 (crossed fused)	1:500	1:25 (autopsy); 1:125 (clinical)	Rare
Mechanism	Failure to ascend, unilateral absence of metanephric mesenchyme, abnormal ureter migration	Abnormal ND or mesenchyme position	Failure of medial rotation during ascent	Failure to repress extra UB from ND, overactivity of ND or UB	Failure to repress extra UB from ND, overactivity of ND or UB
Presentation/treatment	Usually asymptomatic; may have reflux	Follow if associated UPJ, VUR, pyeloplasty, or reconstruction	Asymptomatic, some hydronephrosis and other anomalies	Follow if VUR or ureterocele, most may be asymptomatic	Most asymptomatic, evaluate for reflux or hydroureter
Macroscopic	Pelvic kidney, ureter crossing over to contralateral kidney	Lower poles fused, fusion of pelvic kidneys, crossing over and fusing	Posteriorly facing kidneys	Upper UVJ drains lower kidney/pole (may have VUR), ureter from upper pole enters inferomedially	Extra kidneys, may be fused with normal kidneys

- Frequently lower pole fused
- Ureters enter laterally into bladder
- Fibrous tissue in middle
- Crossed fused renal ectopia
    - Mesenchyme contralateral to ureter bladder insertion and kidney fused
- Fused pelvic kidney

Duplication

- Many variations
    - Bifid ureters may split into 2 before pelvis
        - Single orifice in bladder
    - Complete duplication: 2 ureters/kidneys (may fuse)
    - Ureter may terminate ectopically (e.g., vagina, urethra)
    - May be more than 2 (triplicate)
- Weigert-Meyer law
    - Upper ureter enters lower or more distally in outflow tract (inferomedially) in bladder, urethra, or vagina
        - Drains upper pole if kidneys fused
    - Lower ureter (often normal site) enters superolaterally (higher or more proximal in outflow tract) into bladder
        - Drains lower pole if kidneys fused
- Duplex kidney may be more elongated
- VUR commonly seen, usually lower pole/kidney
- Ureterocele often in ureter, draining upper pole or kidney
- UPJ may be present

Supernumerary Buds

- Extra kidney ectopically located or fused with normally located kidney
- Hydroureter or megaureter or VUR may be present

MICROSCOPIC

Histologic Features

- Duplex or supernumerary kidneys may show hypoplasia or dysplasia
- Horseshoe-fused kidneys may show capsule fusion and fibrous septa
    - Normal parenchyma unless with hydronephrosis or VUR

DIFFERENTIAL DIAGNOSIS

Duplications

- Hydronephrosis
- VUR
- UPJ obstruction
- Solitary renal cyst
- Polycystic kidney disease

DIAGNOSTIC CHECKLIST

Clinically Relevant Pathologic Features

- Complete duplication may pose risk for UTIs due to VUR, or hypertension due to progressive obstructive and reflux nephropathy

Pathologic Interpretation Pearls

- Most cases asymptomatic
- VUR and hydronephrosis may be associated independent anomalies
    - Should be considered as top differential diagnoses

SELECTED REFERENCES

1. Song R et al: Genetics of congenital anomalies of the kidney and urinary tract. Pediatr Nephrol. 26(3):353-64, 2011
2. van den Bosch CM et al: Urological and nephrological findings of renal ectopia. J Urol. 183(4):1574-8, 2010

Ectopic Ureter

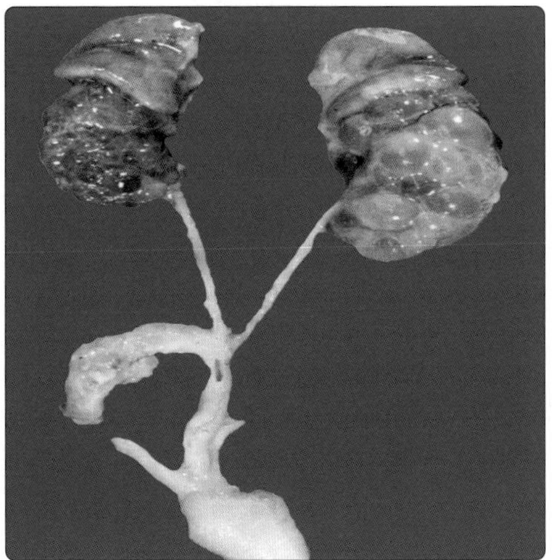

Duplication

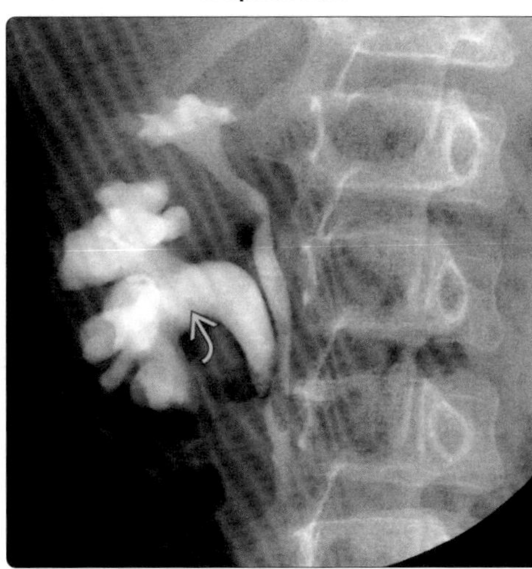

(Left) *Gross photograph shows an example of ureter ectopy where 2 ureters are from the same side. Note that both kidneys are small and multicystic.* **(Right)** *Radiograph shows duplicated collecting system, in this case arising from bifid ureters. The lower ureter shows hydronephrosis ➢.*

Complete Bilateral Duplication

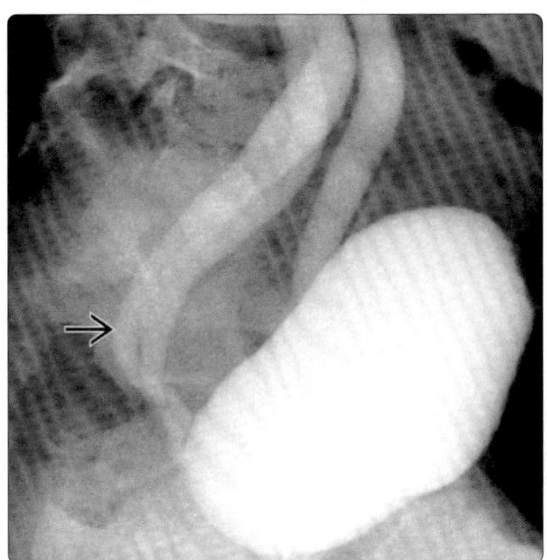

Vesicoureteral Reflux

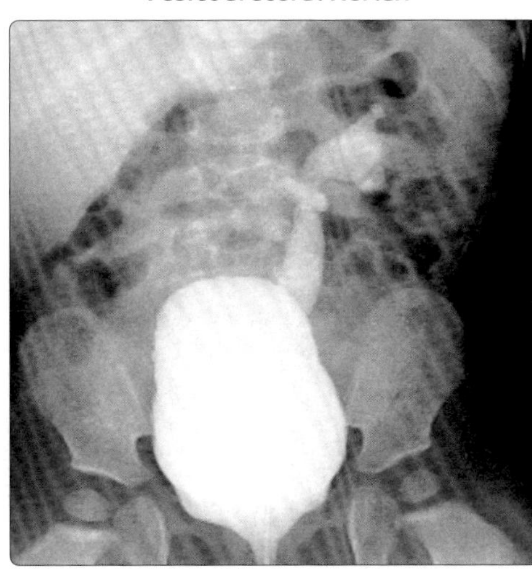

(Left) *Radiograph with contrast material in collecting system shows complete bilateral duplication ➔ in dilated ureters.* **(Right)** *Voiding cystoureterogram shows massively dilated ureter with reflux of dye, indicative of an incompetent ureterovesical valve and vesicoureteral reflux (VUR).*

Ectopic Kidney in Mouse Model

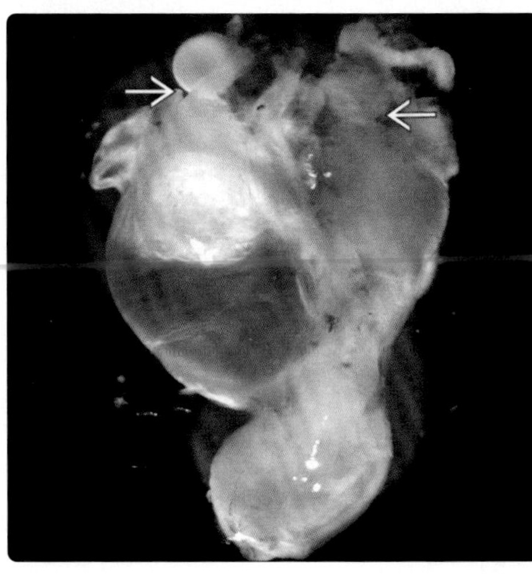

Supernumerary Ectopic Kidneys

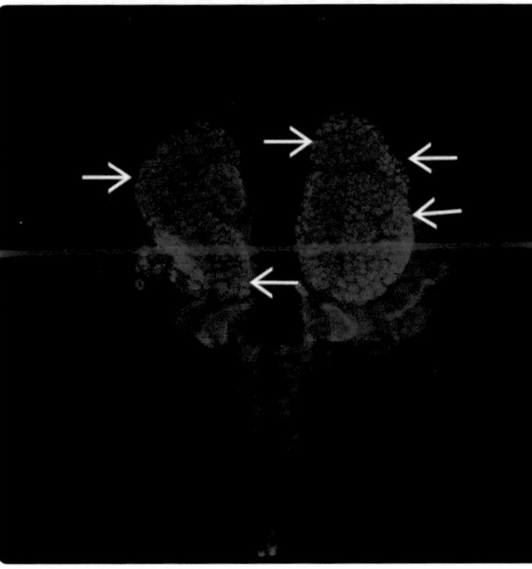

(Left) *Gross image from a Ret signaling mutant mouse shows multilobed pelvic kidneys (do not reach the adrenals normally, round shape ➔) and dilated ureters.* **(Right)** *Whole mount E-cadherin immunofluorescence (labels epithelial cells) from a Ret mutant midgestation mouse genitourinary tract shows multilobed kidneys ➔ due to supernumerary ureters. Round shape of the adrenal gland (faint background) suggests failure of the kidneys to attain normal position.*

Ask-Upmark Kidney

KEY FACTS

TERMINOLOGY

- Congenital or acquired kidney lesion characterized by sharply defined segmental parenchymal hypoplasia of uncertain pathogenesis

ETIOLOGY/PATHOGENESIS

- Ask-Upmark kidney originally regarded as developmental anomaly
  - Chronic reflux or ischemia may represent underlying abnormality
    - If disease due to reflux, process may begin in utero (explains morphology)
    - Segmental renal artery abnormality found in some cases

CLINICAL ISSUES

- Usually discovered in children or young adults
- Hypertension often severe, especially in pediatric cases
  - Usually cured by nephrectomy

MACROSCOPIC

- One or more hypoplastic segments sharply delineated

MICROSCOPIC

- Central groove (hypoplastic area) from cortex to dilated calyx
- Characteristic absence of glomeruli
- Abrupt transition from normal to atrophic cortex with thyroidization of tubules and lack of glomeruli
  - Also seen in cases of focal chronic pyelonephritis
  - Many atrophic tubules in contrast to lack of sclerotic glomeruli

TOP DIFFERENTIAL DIAGNOSES

- Chronic obstruction and reflux nephropathy/pyelonephritis
- Renal dysplasia
- Renal hypoplasia

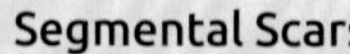

Segmental Scars

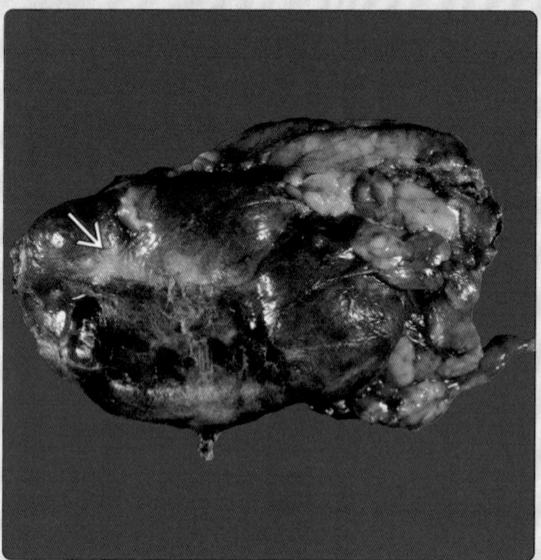

Segmental Hypoplasia

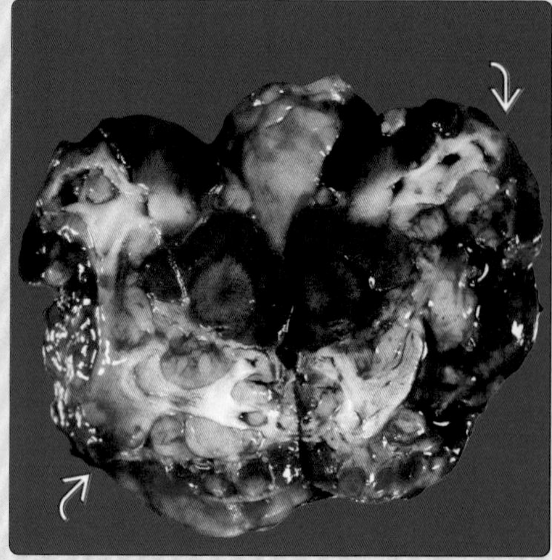

(Left) *Ask-Upmark kidney removed from a 38-year-old woman with recurrent urinary tract infections and nephrolithiasis is shown. Segmental scars can be seen on kidney surface ➡.* **(Right)** *Cross sectioning reveals segmental hypoplasia in several areas ➡ showing absence or marked reduction of normal parenchyma.*

Central Scar

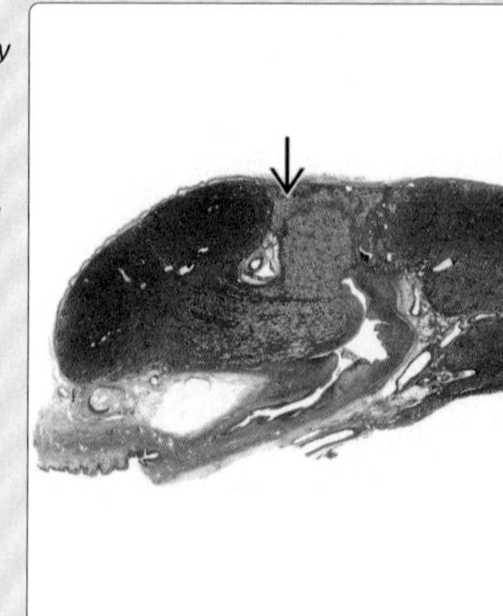

Zonal Scarring

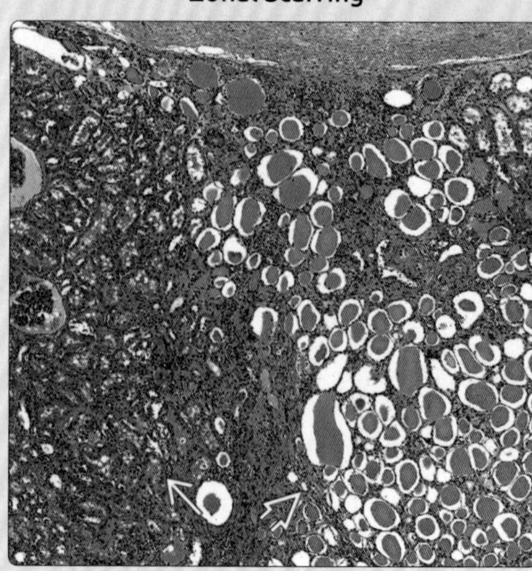

(Left) *Light microscopy of a whole cross section of a kidney shows a central scar ⇨ characteristic of Ask-Upmark kidney.* **(Right)** *Section of an Ask-Upmark kidney shows the abrupt transition from normal cortex ➡ to the atrophic cortex with thyroidization of tubules and lack of glomeruli ➡ in the central scar.*

TERMINOLOGY

Synonyms

- Segmental renal hypoplasia

Definitions

- Congenital or acquired kidney lesion characterized by sharply defined segmental parenchymal hypoplasia of uncertain pathogenesis

ETIOLOGY/PATHOGENESIS

Developmental Anomaly

- Ask-Upmark kidney originally regarded as developmental anomaly
  - Absence of glomeruli (as opposed to glomerular scarring) in affected segments argues for developmental nature of disorder (glomeruli never formed or minimally produced)
  - Challenged by natural history studies suggesting degenerative process

Reflux Hypothesis

- Longitudinal studies show progressive nature of disease
  - Reflux preceded onset of segmental scar by years
- If disease due to reflux, process may begin in utero (would explain morphology)
  - Atrophic cystic tubules and markedly reduced glomeruli also observed in dysplasia secondary to in utero urinary obstruction

Ischemic Hypothesis

- Segmental renal artery abnormality in cases of Ask-Upmark kidney
- Similar to reflux, hypoperfusion might occur early in development to result in absent glomeruli
  - Glomerulogenesis dependent on intact vascular blood flow during nephrogenesis

CLINICAL ISSUES

Epidemiology

- Age
  - Usually children or young adults
- Sex
  - Female predilection

Presentation

- Hypertension
  - Elevated renin levels in some patients
  - Hypertension often severe, especially in pediatric cases
  - Usually cured by nephrectomy
- Usually normal renal function, but can also be decreased
- Recurrent UTI or proteinuria may complicate presentation

IMAGING

Radiographic Findings

- Renal hypoplasia
- Segmental renal artery stenosis or aneurysm may be seen

MACROSCOPIC

General Features

- Small kidney
- One or more hypoplastic segments sharply delineated
  - Thinned parenchyma
  - Dilated, deep calyces underlying parenchymal lesion
- Central groove (hypoplastic area) from cortex to dilated calyx

MICROSCOPIC

Histologic Features

- Glomeruli
  - Characteristic absence of glomeruli
- Tubules and interstitium
  - Abrupt transition from normal to atrophic cortex with thyroidization of tubules and lack of glomeruli
    - Pattern characteristic of Ask-Upmark kidney
      - Also seen in cases of focal chronic pyelonephritis
  - Many atrophic tubules in contrast to lack of sclerotic glomeruli
  - Sparse interstitial inflammation
- Arteries
  - Thickened media and intimal fibrosis
- Electron microscopy and immunofluorescence noncontributory

DIFFERENTIAL DIAGNOSIS

Chronic Obstruction and Reflux Nephropathy/Pyelonephritis

- Ask-Upmark kidney may be form of reflux nephropathy
- Sclerosed rather than absent glomeruli

Renal Dysplasia

- Dysplastic elements including cysts, immature tubules, collecting ducts, and abnormally formed glomeruli
- Presence of cartilage especially helpful in diagnosis
- Renal dysplasia may be focal

Renal Hypoplasia

- Hypoplasia/oligomeganephronia normally not segmental in nature
- Overall reduced nephron number with intact ratio of glomeruli to tubules

SELECTED REFERENCES

1. Babin J et al: The Ask-Upmark kidney: a curable cause of hypertension in young patients. J Hum Hypertens. 19(4):315-6, 2005
2. Marwali MR et al: Ask-Upmark kidney associated with renal and extrarenal arterial aneurysms. Am J Kidney Dis. 33(4):e4, 1999
3. Shindo S et al: Evolution of renal segmental atrophy (Ask-Upmark kidney) in children with vesicoureteric reflux: radiographic and morphologic studies. J Pediatr. 102(6):847-54, 1983
4. Arant BS Jr et al: Segmental "hypoplasia" of the kidney (Ask-Upmark). J Pediatr. 95(6):931-9, 1979
5. Godard C et al: Plasma renin activity in segmental hypoplasia of the kidneys with hypertension. Nephron. 11(5):308-17, 1973
6. Ask-Upmark E: One-sided kidney affections and arterial hypertension. Acta Med Scand. 173:141-6, 1963
7. Ask-Upmark E: Uber juvenile maligne nephrosclerose und ihr verhaltris zu storunger in der nierenentwicklung. Acta Path Microbiol Scand. 6:383–442, 1929

Renal Tubular Dysgenesis

KEY FACTS

TERMINOLOGY

- Congenital absence or incomplete differentiation of proximal tubules

ETIOLOGY/PATHOGENESIS

- Genetic
  - Mutation of renin-angiotensin genes
- Secondary (sporadic) renal tubular dysgenesis
  - Twin-twin transfusion
  - Congenital renal artery stenosis
  - Major cardiac malformations
  - Maternal drug blockage of renal-angiotensin system
  - Congenital hemochromatosis

CLINICAL ISSUES

- Oligohydramnios
- Renal failure at birth
- Respiratory failure at birth

MACROSCOPIC

- Potter oligohydramnios sequence
- Normal, small, or enlarged kidneys
- Skull ossification defects

MICROSCOPIC

- Absence of recognizable proximal tubules

ANCILLARY TESTS

- Negative CD10 stain for proximal tubular differentiation
- Positive EMA stain for distal tubular differentiation

TOP DIFFERENTIAL DIAGNOSES

- Nephronophthisis
- Hypoplasia
- *HNF1B* mutation

DIAGNOSTIC CHECKLIST

- Important to determine cause of RTD

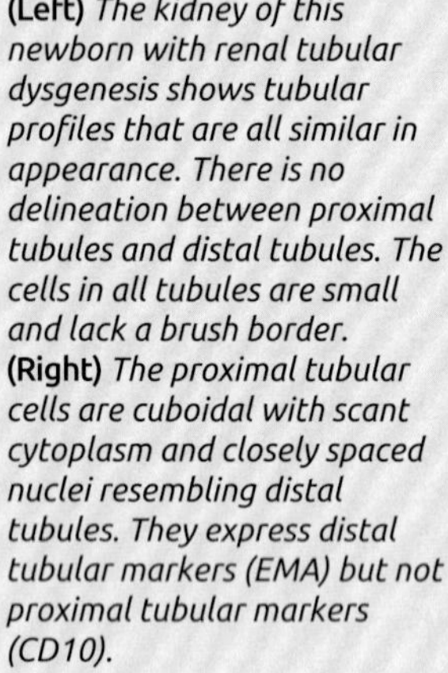
(Left) *The kidney of this newborn with renal tubular dysgenesis shows tubular profiles that are all similar in appearance. There is no delineation between proximal tubules and distal tubules. The cells in all tubules are small and lack a brush border.* **(Right)** *The proximal tubular cells are cuboidal with scant cytoplasm and closely spaced nuclei resembling distal tubules. They express distal tubular markers (EMA) but not proximal tubular markers (CD10).*

Lack of Normal Proximal Tubules and Glomerular Crowding

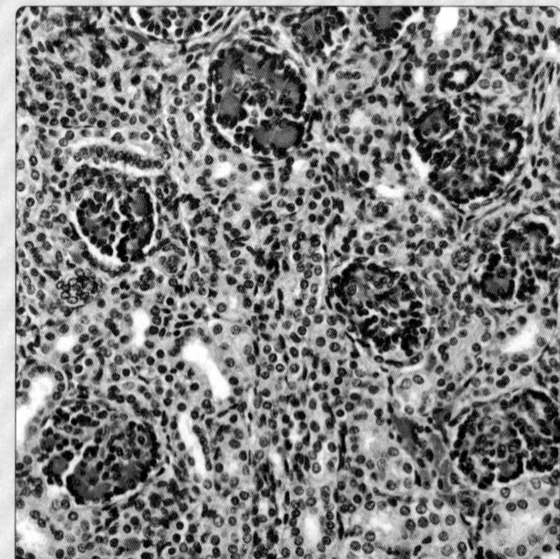

Distal Tubule Phenotype

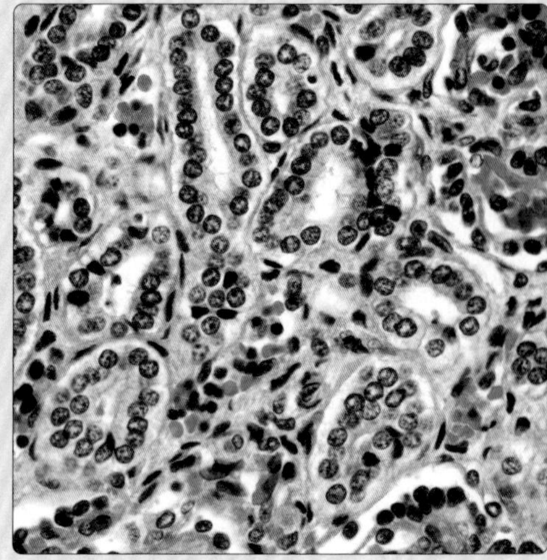

(Left) *In a neonate with renal tubular dysgenesis, proximal tubules exhibit a distal tubule immunophenotype when stained for epithelial membrane antigen →. Normal proximal tubules would not stain.* **(Right)** *The cells lining this proximal tubule in a patient with renal tubular dysgenesis have an ultrastructural appearance identical to a distal tubule cells. They have little cytoplasm, a rounded luminal surface with no microvilli →, and lack complex basal-lateral membrane infoldings.*

Epithelial Membrane Antigen

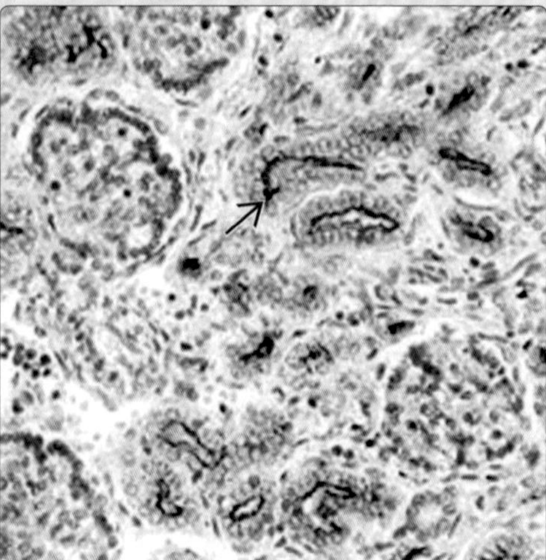

Tubular Ultrastructure With Distal Tubule Phenotype

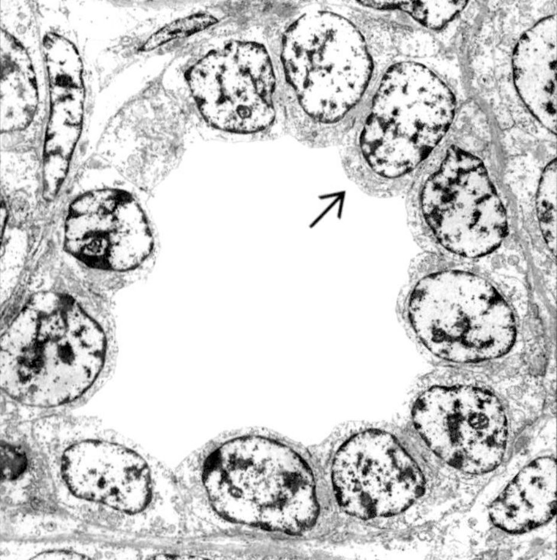

TERMINOLOGY

Abbreviations

- Renal tubular dysgenesis (RTD)

Definitions

- Congenital absence or incomplete differentiation of proximal tubules

ETIOLOGY/PATHOGENESIS

Mutation of Renin-Angiotensin System (*RAS*) Genes

- Autosomal recessive
- Homozygous or compound heterozygous mutations
  - 66% *ACE* (angiotensin-converting enzyme)
  - 20% *REN* (renin)
  - 8% *AGT* (angiotensinogen)
  - 6% *AGTR1* (AT1 receptor gene)
- Truncating or missense
- ~ 40% consanguinity

Secondary (Sporadic) Causes

- RAS blocking drugs during 2nd-3rd trimester of pregnancy
  - ACE inhibitors, ATII receptor antagonists
  - Rare cases attributed to NSAID
- Twin-twin transfusion syndrome
- Congenital renal artery stenosis
- Major cardiac malformation
- Congenital hemochromatosis

Mechanism

- Decreased perfusion of kidneys *in utero*

CLINICAL ISSUES

Epidemiology

- Incidence
  - Rare but probably under recognized

Presentation

- Oligohydramnios after 20-22 weeks gestation
- Respiratory and renal failure at birth
- Intractable hypotension in surviving neonates
- Skull ossification defects with large sutures and fontanelles

Treatment

- Mineralocorticoids and inotropes
- Kidney transplantation curative

Prognosis

- Most neonates die from respiratory failure soon after birth
- Rare childhood survivors
- Variable RTD outcome from RAS inhibitors *in utero*
  - 20% survived but developed chronic renal failure and hypertension age 1-9 years old
  - 5% had normal renal function at 2 years

MACROSCOPIC

Potter Sequence Due to Oligohydramnios

- Facial dysmorphia with low-set ears
- Pulmonary hypoplasia
- Limb positioning defects with arthrogryposis

Normal or Moderately Enlarged Kidneys

- Poor corticomedullary differentiation

MICROSCOPIC

Histologic Features

- Glomeruli
  - Normal but closely spaced
  - May be glomerular cysts with multiple tufts
- Tubules
  - Absence of recognizable proximal tubules
    - Tubules short, straight, and lined by small cuboidal cells, resembling distal tubules
    - No brush border on PAS stains
  - Limited medullary ray-cortical labyrinth differentiation
- Interstitium
  - No inflammation or fibrosis
  - Extramedullary hematopoiesis (17%)
- Arterioles
  - Thickened, disorganized smooth muscle

ANCILLARY TESTS

Immunohistochemistry

- ↑ renin in juxtaglomerular apparatus
  - Except in truncating REN mutations (absence of renin)
- Failure to express proximal tubule markers
  - CD10, winged pea lectin, ACE
  - Normal CD10 in podocytes, Bowman capsule
- Expression of distal tubule/collecting duct markers
  - Epithelial membrane antigen (EMA), cytokeratin 7, *Arachis hypogaea* (peanut) lectin

DIFFERENTIAL DIAGNOSIS

Nephronophthisis

- Normal proximal tubules

Hypoplasia

- Normal proximal tubules

HNF1B Mutation

- Failure to form proximal and distal tubules
- Autosomal dominant

DIAGNOSTIC CHECKLIST

Pathologic Interpretation Pearls

- Important to determine cause of RTD

SELECTED REFERENCES

1. Gubler MC: Renal tubular dysgenesis. Pediatr Nephrol. 29(1):51-9, 2014
2. Plazanet C et al: Fetal renin-angiotensin-system blockade syndrome: renal lesions. Pediatr Nephrol. 29(7):1221-30, 2014
3. Gubler MC et al: Renin-angiotensin system in kidney development: renal tubular dysgenesis. Kidney Int. 77(5):400-6, 2010
4. Delaney D et al: Congenital unilateral renal tubular dysgenesis and severe neonatal hypertension. Pediatr Nephrol. 24(4):863-7, 2009
5. Lacoste M et al: Renal tubular dysgenesis, a not uncommon autosomal recessive disorder leading to oligohydramnios: Role of the Renin-Angiotensin system. J Am Soc Nephrol. 17(8):2253-63, 2006
6. Gribouval O et al: Mutations in genes in the renin-angiotensin system are associated with autosomal recessive renal tubular dysgenesis. Nat Genet. 37(9):964-8, 2005

(**Left**) *Proximal tubules are short, straight, and have a distal tubules phenotype, resulting in glomerular clustering or closer approximation of the glomeruli and a small overall renal size.* (**Right**) *In this newborn with RTD, the glomeruli are closely spaced. The podocytes are prominent and cuboidal-appearing, which is normal at this age. All of the proximal tubules are small and lined by cells with little cytoplasm that are indistinguishable from distal tubular cells.*

Glomerular Clustering

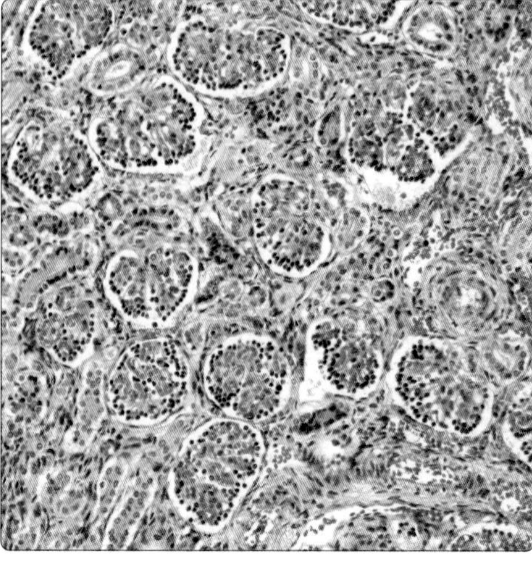

Tubules With Distal Tubule Phenotype

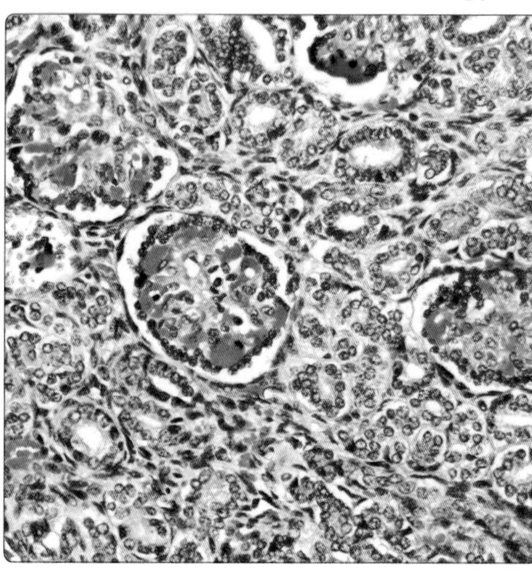

(**Left**) *This fetal kidney shows the nephrogenic zone ➡. There are glomeruli in the S-phase ➡ of formation as well as well-differentiated glomeruli ➡. However, no proximal tubular differentiation is evident. All tubules are small and lined by small cells with little cytoplasm.* (**Right**) *This kidney is from a newborn with renal tubular dysgenesis. All of the tubules ➡ lack the luminal PAS-positive brush border that is characteristic of proximal tubular differentiation. All tubule profiles are small and resemble distal tubules.*

Fetal Kidney With Renal Tubular Dysgenesis

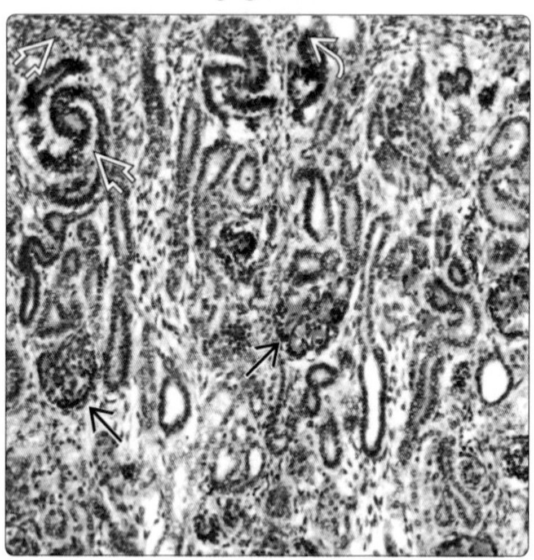

Absent PAS-Positive Brush Border

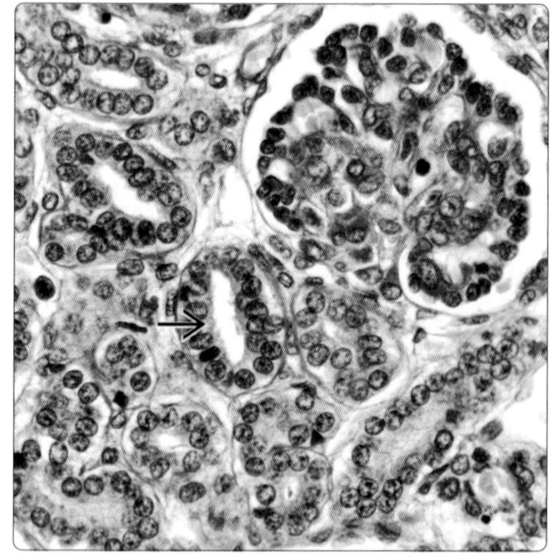

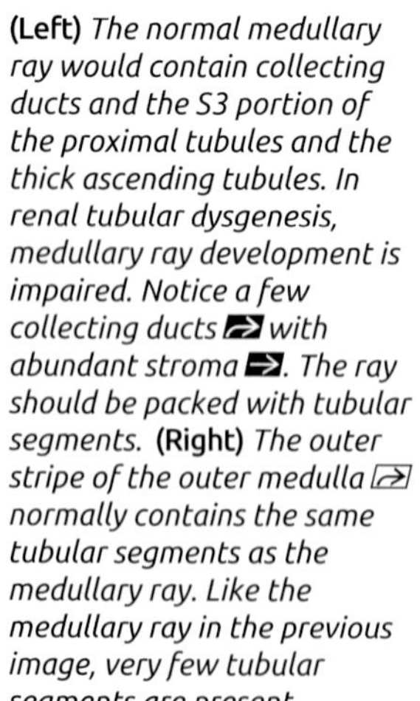

(**Left**) *The normal medullary ray would contain collecting ducts and the S3 portion of the proximal tubules and the thick ascending tubules. In renal tubular dysgenesis, medullary ray development is impaired. Notice a few collecting ducts ➡ with abundant stroma ➡. The ray should be packed with tubular segments.* (**Right**) *The outer stripe of the outer medulla ➡ normally contains the same tubular segments as the medullary ray. Like the medullary ray in the previous image, very few tubular segments are present.*

Medullary Rays Contain Few Tubules

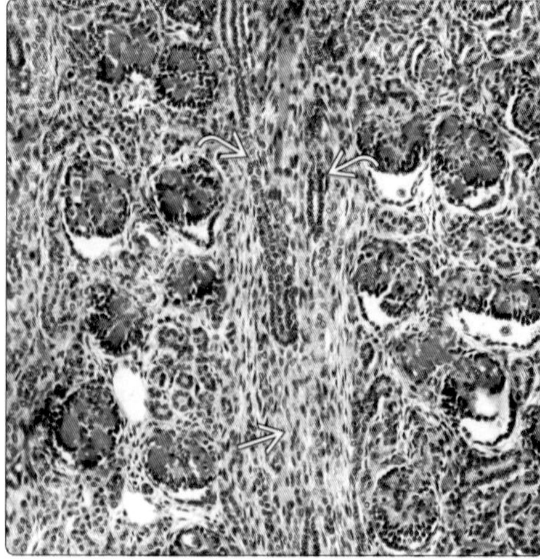

Failure of Formation of Outer Stripe Tubules

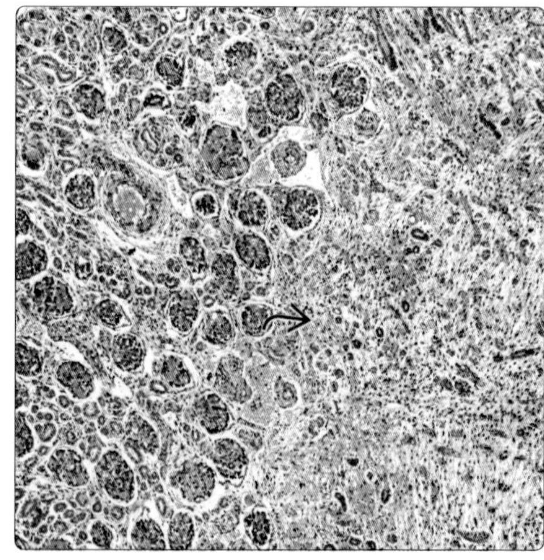

Failure of Formation of Outer Stripe Tubules

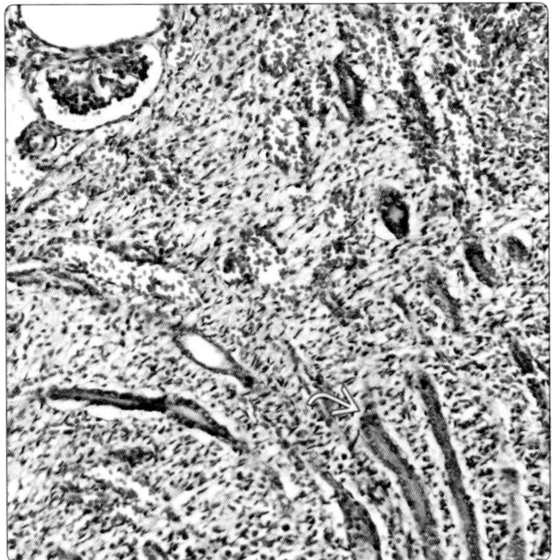

Renal Tubular Dysgenesis May Have Glomerular Cysts

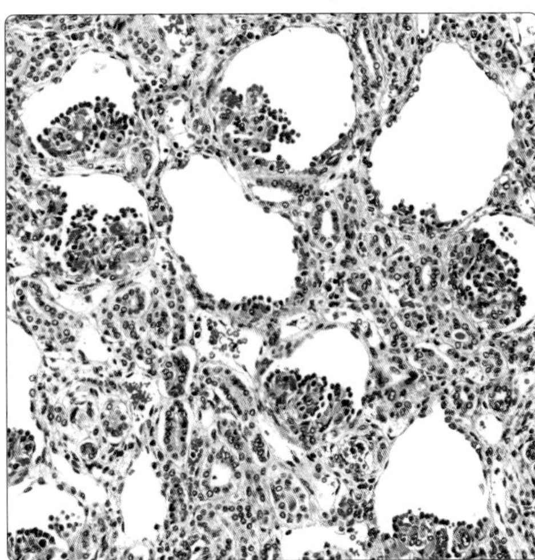

(Left) *Interface between the deep cortex and outer stripe of the outer medulla is shown. The outer stripe contains only a few collecting ducts ➲. There is abundant cellular stroma but only a few ducts without tubules.* **(Right)** *There are many diseases in which glomerular cysts form. When associated with small intervening tubules, chronic renal artery stenosis should be considered. However, diffuse tubular atrophy and interstitial fibrosis would be present and the glomeruli would show ischemic capillary loop wrinkling.*

Glomerular Cysts May Have Abnormal Tufts

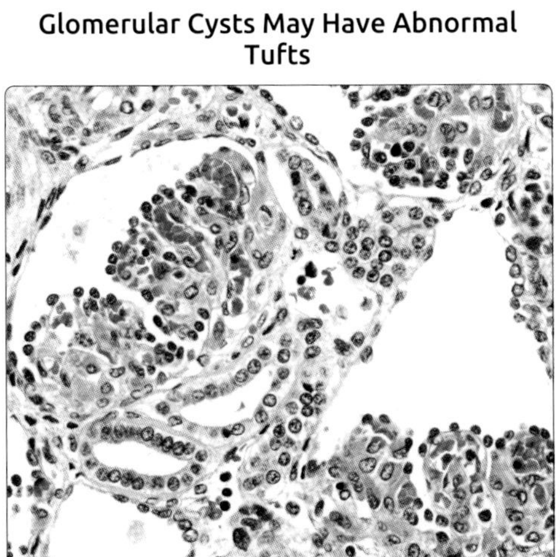

Extramedullary Hematopoiesis

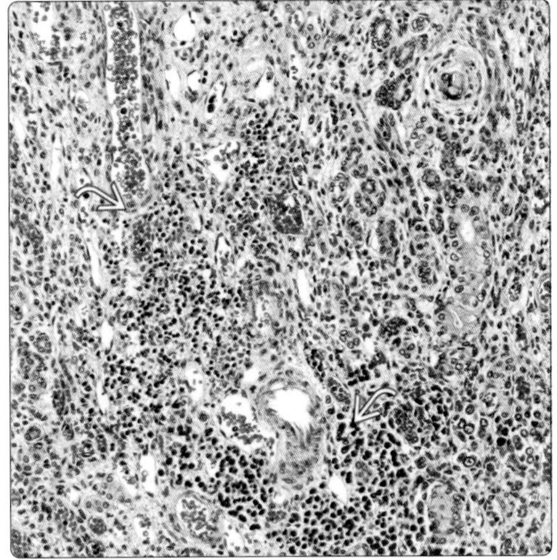

(Left) *Glomerular cysts may be normally developed or maldeveloped. In this case, the glomeruli are abnormal. Notice the odd shape of the glomerular tuft and its surrounding Bowman capsule. The tuft consists of 2-3 lobules that appear to be separately arrayed within Bowman capsule. A similar pattern is seen in HNF1B mutations.* **(Right)** *Extramedullary hematopoiesis ➲ has been observed in approximately 17% of autopsy cases. It may be seen in both cortex and medulla. Both sites were involved in this case.*

Arachis Hypogaea Lectin Binding

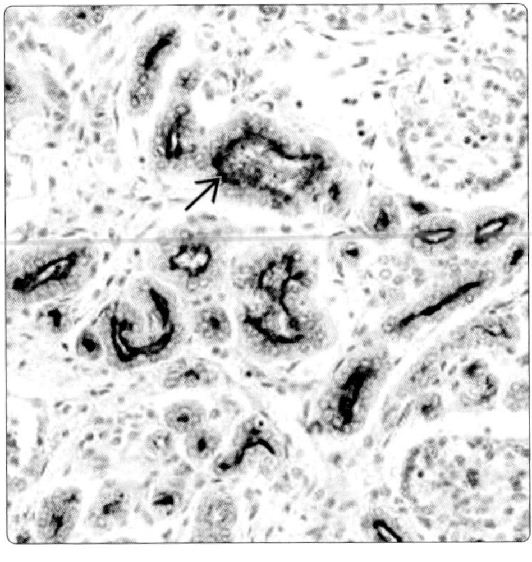

Tubular Ultrastructure With Distal Tubule Phenotype

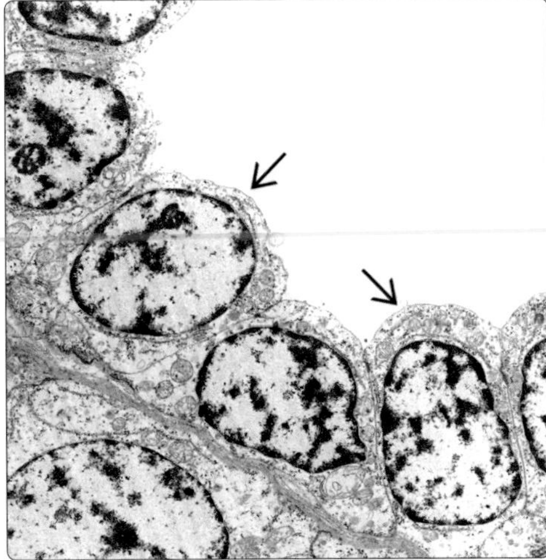

(Left) *The distal tubule/collecting duct marker Arachis hypogaea lectin (peanut agglutinin) stains ➙ the apical cytoplasm of all tubules, indicating distal tubule/collecting duct differentiation.* **(Right)** *This is a typical proximal tubule in renal tubular dysgenesis. It has a distal tubule ultrastructure. It shows little cytoplasm and few intracellular organelles. There are no basal-lateral membrane infoldings or luminal microvilli ➙ present.*

SECTION 7
Cystic Diseases

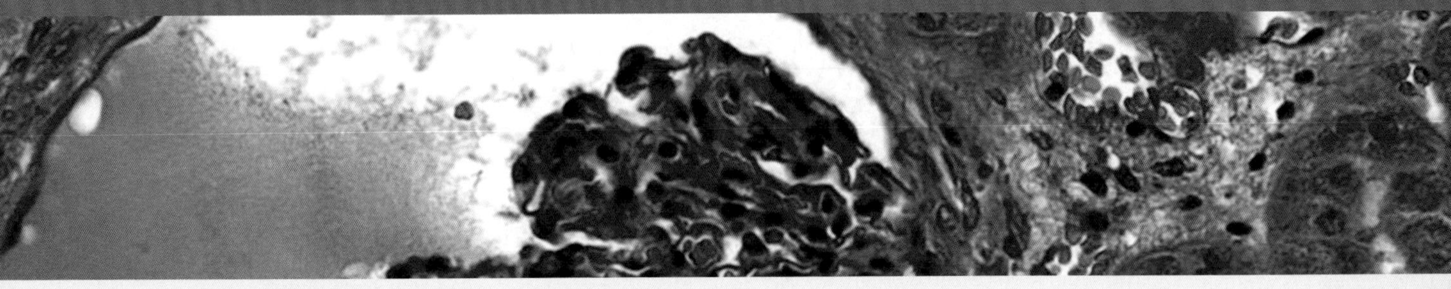

Overview of Cystic Diseases

PATHOGENETIC CLASSIFICATION

Definition

- Renal diseases characterized predominately by cysts
  - Cyst: Closed cavity in previously noncystic structure
    - May arise in any part of nephron but most frequently in tubules
    - May be in cortex, medulla, or both
    - May be diffuse, focal, unilateral, or bilateral
    - Can be randomly or uniformly distributed (e.g., along corticomedullary junction)
    - Bilateral cysts most commonly hereditary
    - Ectasia sometimes present rather than closed cyst
  - Cysts arising in glomeruli called glomerular cysts
  - Term "polycystic" only used for autosomal dominant and autosomal recessive polycystic kidney disease (ADPKD, ARPKD)
  - Location and shape of renal cysts important for classification
  - No universally accepted classification scheme
  - Features considered
    - Genetic basis (genes on cilia)
    - Cystic anatomic structure (tubule, glomerulus, other)
    - Distribution of cysts (cortex, medulla)

Categories

- Hereditary cystic diseases
  - ADPKD
  - ARPKD
  - Autosomal dominant tubulointerstitial disease (ADTKD): UMOD, MUC1, REN, HNF1B
  - Nephronophthisis (NPH)
  - Tuberous sclerosis (TSC)
  - von Hippel-Lindau (VHL) disease
  - Primary glomerulocystic kidney disease (GCKD)
- Acquired cystic diseases
  - Secondary GCKD
  - Acquired cystic kidney disease
  - Medullary sponge kidney
  - Multilocular renal cyst
  - Simple cortical cyst
- Nonnephron renal cystic diseases
  - Pyelocalyceal diverticula
  - Perinephric pseudocyst
  - Lymphangiectasis/lymphangiomatosis

EPIDEMIOLOGY

Incidence

- ADPKD: 1 in 500 live births
- ARPKD: 1 in 20,000 live births
- NPH: 1 in 8 million in USA, 1 in 50,000 in Canada
- TSC: 1 in 10,000-15,000 live births

ETIOLOGY/PATHOGENESIS

Histogenesis

- Cystogenesis: Process involving aberrant formation or maintenance of normally noncystic structure
- Causes of tubular cysts
  - Epithelial cell proliferation
  - Apoptosis and defective clearance of apoptotic cells causing tubular obstruction
  - Scarring of tubule due to inflammation, injury, and fibrosis with consequent obstruction
  - Expansion of luminal contents by vectorial fluid/solute shift
    - Electrolyte contents reveal distal or proximal tubular transport function
  - May begin as ectatic tubule that later becomes cystic space
- Causes of glomerular cysts unclear
  - May involve scarring of outlet
  - Failure of normal proximal tubule formation

MACROSCOPIC

Differential Diagnostic Features

- Spherical cysts in bilaterally enlarged kidneys diagnostic of ADPKD

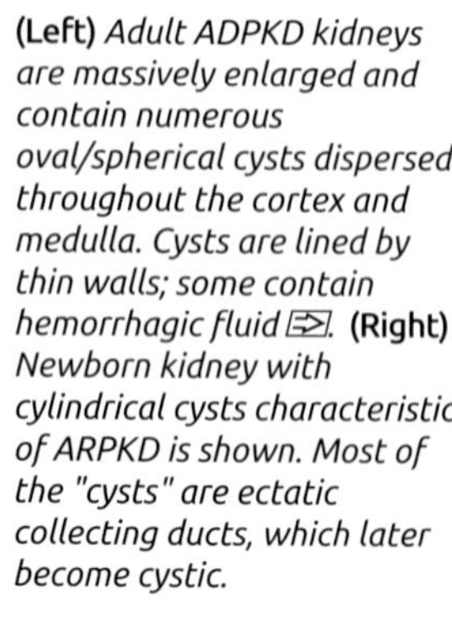

(Left) *Adult ADPKD kidneys are massively enlarged and contain numerous oval/spherical cysts dispersed throughout the cortex and medulla. Cysts are lined by thin walls; some contain hemorrhagic fluid* ➲. **(Right)** *Newborn kidney with cylindrical cysts characteristic of ARPKD is shown. Most of the "cysts" are ectatic collecting ducts, which later become cystic.*

ADPKD Gross Pathology

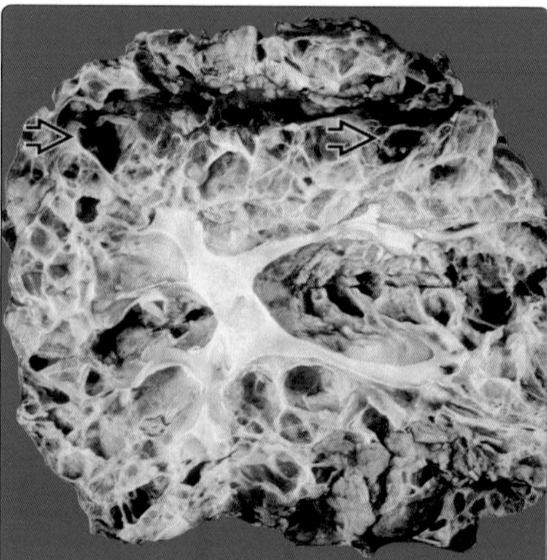

ARPKD Gross Pathology

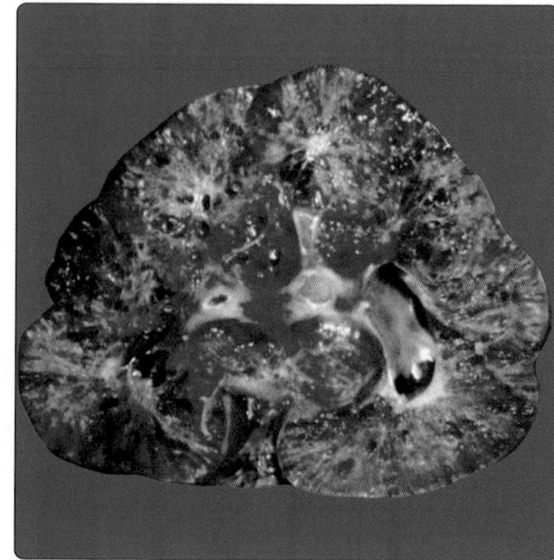

- Cylindrical cysts (really ectatic collecting ducts) in enlarged pediatric kidneys diagnostic of ARPKD
- Few small cysts at corticomedullary junction characteristic of NPH but may be absent in various disorders included in NPH
- Isolated cortical cysts, usually unilateral, are nonhereditary, simple cysts seen in elderly patients without renal disease

MICROSCOPIC

Differential Diagnostic Features

- Cysts contain abundant eosinophilic fluid and micropapillary proliferations characteristic of ADPKD
- Cylindrical cysts characteristic of ARPKD
- Glomerular cysts affecting > 5% of glomeruli define glomerulocystic kidney disease as either primary or secondary
- Secondary GCKD more common than primary and presents in children with ADPKD, ARPKD, or TSC
  - Glomerular cysts defined as Bowman capsule dilation > 3x normal
- Cysts containing renal cell carcinoma characteristic of hereditary neoplasia syndromes (TSC, von Hippel-Lindau disease), ADPKD, or hemodialysis-induced cysts
- Cysts in NPHP/MCDK form are ex vacuo (degenerative)
  - May contain Tamm-Horsfall protein
  - Show tubular basement membrane duplication
- Incidental, simple cysts also degenerative
  - Often lack epithelial lining

HEREDITARY CYSTIC DISEASES

ADPKD

- Classic ADPKD in adults
- Early onset ADPKD in children

ARPKD

- Classic ARPKD in neonates and infants
- Late onset ARPKD in adolescents presenting with medullary ectasia and hepatic fibrosis

GCKD, Primary

- Hereditary GCKD due to *UMOD* or *HNF1B* mutations
- Familial GCKD with unknown gene mutations

Nephronophthisis

- Nephronophthisis (NPH), autosomal recessive
- Genetically heterogeneous with 20 identified genes
- Occurs as isolated kidney disease
  - 15% have extrarenal symptoms affecting central nervous system, eyes, liver, and bones
    - If present, these entities now classified as NPH-related disorders (NPHP-CP)

ADTKD

- Term replaces medullary cystic kidney disease (MCKD) and previous subcategories, such as MCKD 1 and 2
- ADTKD includes uromodulin (ADTKD-UMOD), mucin-1 (ADTKD-MUC-1), renin (ADTKD-Ren), and HNF1B (ADTKD-HNF1B) associated disorders
- Present with polyuria, progressive renal impairment, hyperuricemia, and gout
- Pathologically manifest with tubulointerstitial fibrosis
- Uromodulin, a.k.a. Tamm Horsfall protein, synthesized in thick ascending limb of loop of Henle
  - Also shed in urine and is most abundant protein in human urine
- UMOD protein has high content of cysteine residues frequently affected by *UMOD* gene mutations leading to protein misfolding
  - Misfolded protein accumulates within tubular epithelial cell endoplasmic reticulum
  - Can be detected as fibrillar material by electron microscopy or immunohistochemistry
- Mechanisms leading to renal fibrosis and hyperuricemia remain unclear

von Hippel-Lindau Disease

- Lined by clear cells
- Associated with renal cell carcinoma, clear cell type

Tuberous Sclerosis

- Cysts lined by large plump cells with deeply eosinophilic cytoplasm
  - Nuclear pleomorphism of cyst lining epithelium
- Associated with angiomyolipoma and renal cell carcinoma

NONHEREDITARY CYSTIC DISEASES

Acquired Cystic Disease

- > 50% of dialysis patients develop cysts within 5 years
  - Cysts may appear even before initiation of dialysis
- ≥ 3 cysts in dialysis patient required for diagnosis
- Typically proliferative (Ki-67[+]) and hobnailed cells
- Increased risk for intracystic renal cell carcinoma

Multilocular Renal Cyst

- a.k.a. multilocular cystic nephroma
- Most cases sporadic; some congenital
- Tumor usually encapsulated with noncommunicating cysts filled with gelatinous fluid
- Infrequent lesion; occurs in both children and adults

Localized Cystic Disease

- May be mistaken for ADPKD
- Overall kidney size not increased, unlike ADPKD
- Cysts are naked; intervening renal parenchyma normal
- Uncommon presentation of unilateral, segmental, or bilateral multiple cysts nonhereditary

Simple Cortical Cysts

- Oval or round with smooth outline, located in renal cortex
- Randomly distributed
- 12-15% of adults and common autopsy finding

GCKD, Secondary and Sporadic

- Associated with numerous syndromes
- Can be secondary to other diseases, such as ADPKD, ARPKD, or tuberous sclerosis
- Due to vascular ischemia, such as HUS and renal artery branch stenosis
- Sporadic GCKD

Medullary Sponge Kidney

- Disease of adults
- Genetic basis, if any, unknown

Pathogenetic Classification of Renal Cystic Diseases

Hereditary	Nonhereditary
Polycystic kidney disease	**GCKD**
ADPKD	Secondary
Early onset ADPKD in children	Associated with numerous syndromes
ARPKD	Due to ischemia, e.g., HUS and renal artery branch stenosis
Classic ARPKD in neonates and infants	Sporadic GCKD
Late onset ARPKD in older children with hepatic fibrosis	**Simple cortical cysts**
GCKD	**Localized cystic disease**
Primary	**Acquired cystic disease (end-stage renal disease)**
Familial GCKD with unknown gene mutations	Typically dialysis related
Hereditary GCKD due to *UMOD* or *HNF1B* mutations	**Multilocular renal cyst**
Secondary GCKD	**Medullary sponge kidney**
Associated with ADPKD/ARPKD/TSC	**Nonnephron renal cystic diseases**
Cysts in hereditary cancer syndromes	Pyelocalyceal diverticula
Tuberous sclerosis	Perinephric pseudocyst
von Hippel-Lindau disease	Lymphangiectasis/lymphangiomatosis
Renal medullary cysts	
Nephronophthisis (*NPHP1-4, IQCB1, CEP290, TMEM67* and *OPN5*, others as of 2015	
Autosomal dominant tubulointerstitial kidney disease (ADTKD)	
ADTKD-UMOD	
ADTKD-RENIN	
ADTKD-MUC-1	
ADTKD-HNF1B	

- Characterized by calcium-filled cysts in medullary collecting ducts
- Usually diagnosed radiologically as incidental finding
  - Retention of filtered contrast dye in medullary pyramids

NONNEPHRON CYSTIC DISEASE

Pyelocalyceal Diverticulum

- Associated with nephrolithiasis
- Lined by urothelium
- Echogenic and mobile material within cyst-like lesion

Perinephric Pseudocyst

- No epithelial lining
- May arise from urine leak

Lymphangiectasis/Lymphangiomatosis

- Dilated lymphatics and accumulation of lymph fluid around kidney
  - Hygroma renalis
- May have systemic lymphangiectasis
- Some may be low-grade neoplasms

MIMICS OF CYSTIC DISEASES

Renal Dysplasia

- May be strikingly multicystic
- Cartilage and smooth muscle present
- Absent glomeruli in sites of dysplasia

Pancreatic Pseudocyst

- Sometimes abuts kidney

Perinephric Abscess

- Other signs of abscess evident

SELECTED REFERENCES

1. Antignac C et al: The Future of Polycystic Kidney Disease Research-As Seen By the 12 Kaplan Awardees. J Am Soc Nephrol. ePub, 2015
2. Eckardt KU et al: Autosomal dominant tubulointerstitial kidney disease: diagnosis, classification, and management-A KDIGO consensus report. Kidney Int. ePub, 2015
3. Wolf MT: Nephronophthisis and related syndromes. Curr Opin Pediatr. 27(2):201-11, 2015
4. Gee HY et al: Whole-exome resequencing distinguishes cystic kidney diseases from phenocopies in renal ciliopathies. Kidney Int. 85(4):880-7, 2014
5. Guay-Woodford LM: Autosomal recessive polycystic kidney disease: the prototype of the hepato-renal fibrocystic diseases. J Pediatr Genet. 3(2):89-101, 2014
6. Leung JC: Inherited renal diseases. Curr Pediatr Rev. 10(2):95-100, 2014
7. Liapis H et al: Cystic diseases and developmental kidney defects. In Jennette JC et al: Heptinstall's Pathology of the Kidney. 7th ed. Philadelphia: Lippincott Williams & Wilkins, 2014
8. Northrup H et al: Tuberous sclerosis complex diagnostic criteria update: recommendations of the 2012 Iinternational Tuberous Sclerosis Complex Consensus Conference. Pediatr Neurol. 49(4):243-54, 2013
9. Lennerz JK et al: Glomerulocystic kidney: one hundred-year perspective. Arch Pathol Lab Med. 134(4):583-605, 2010

ADPKD Cysts Are Proliferative

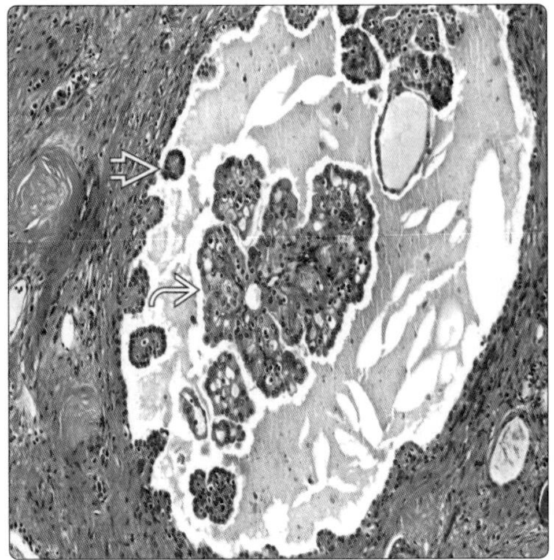

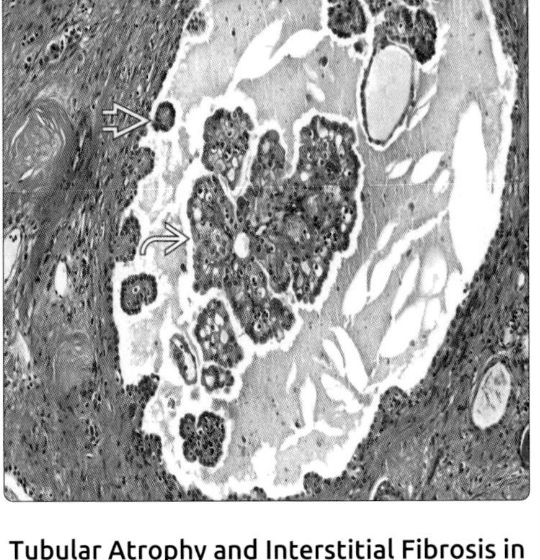

ARPKD Cysts Are Cylindrical

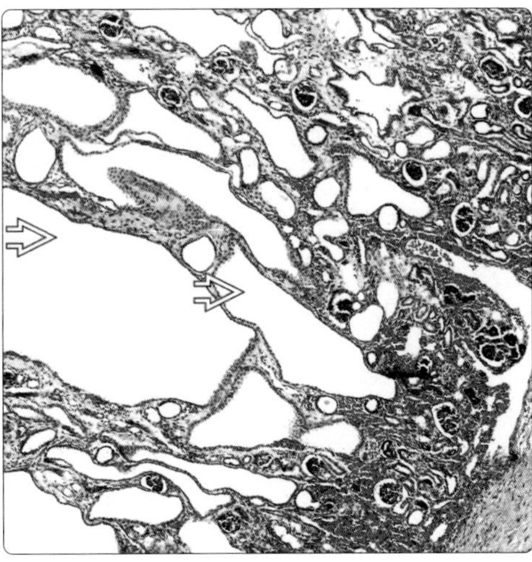

(Left) *In ADPKD, the lining epithelial cells are neoplastic with papillary proliferations and fluid secretion. Micropapillae ➡ and floating papillary fragments ↪ are frequently present.* **(Right)** *Cysts in ARPKD are typically cylindrical ➡ involving the collecting ducts in the medulla and distal cortical tubules.*

Tubular Atrophy and Interstitial Fibrosis in ADTKD

Glomerular Cysts: Bowman Space Dilatation 3x Normal

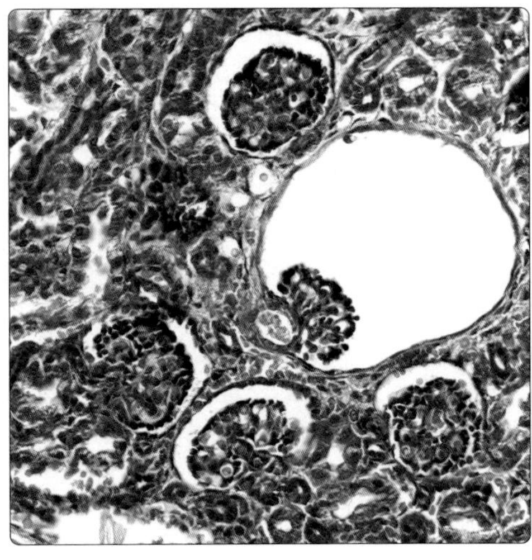

(Left) *Biopsy from a 21-year-old woman with a history of Leber congenital amaurosis who presented with small kidneys, sCr 22 mg/dl, and proteinuria, 3.9 g, is shown. Tubules show basement membrane thickening and duplication ↪.* **(Right)** *Glomerular cysts can be seen in ADPKD, ARPKD, TSC, and renal dysplasia. This case is from an autopsy of a fetus with TSC and fetal cardiomyoma. The kidney shows immature glomeruli and occasional glomerular cysts.*

Cysts in Tuberous Sclerosis

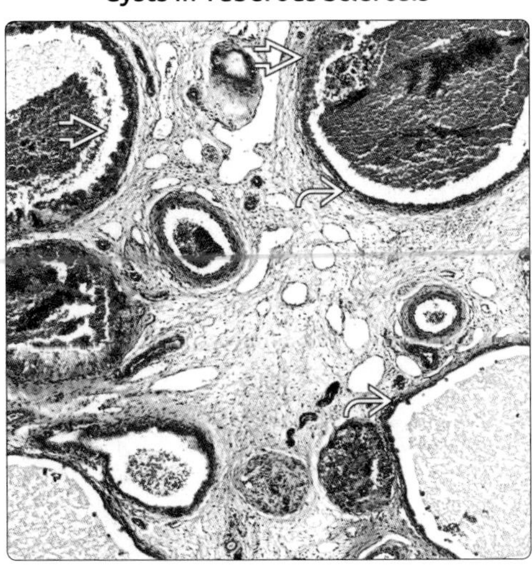

Cysts in Renal Dysplasia

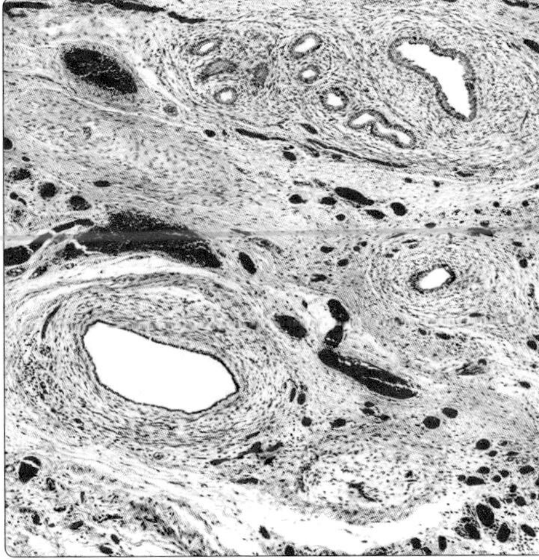

(Left) *This image shows exuberant eosinophilic epithelium, cuboidal ↪, &/or proliferative ➡ in a child with TSC.* **(Right)** *Cysts consist of aborted tubules lined by simplified epithelium surrounded by concentric smooth muscle collarettes.*

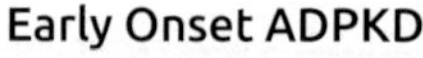

Early Onset ADPKD | **Glomerulocystic Kidney**

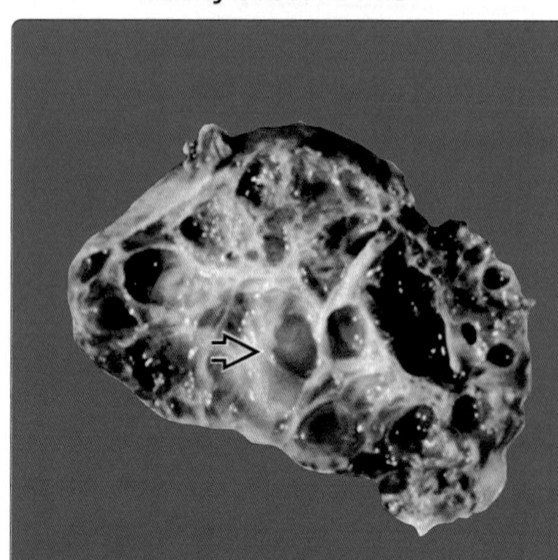

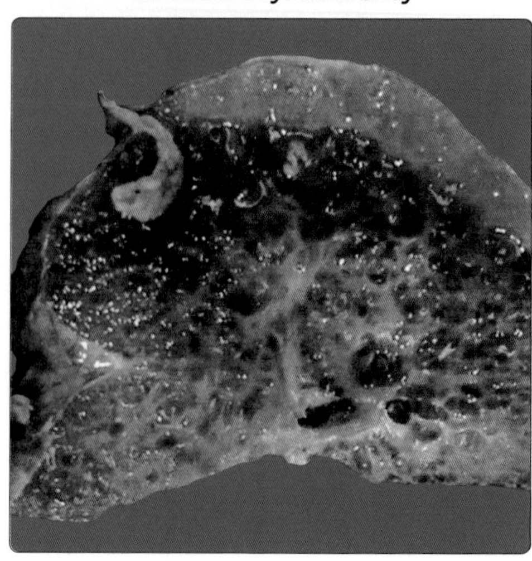

(Left) *Early-onset ADPKD in a young child shows oval cysts varying in size and filled with turbid gelatinous fluid. Overall size of the kidney is moderately large for age.* **(Right)** *Nephrectomy specimen from a newborn with bilateral kidney cysts detected by ultrasound contains numerous small cysts. Microscopically, the majority of the glomerular cysts are of glomerular origin.*

Dialysis-Induced Cysts With RCC | **Multifocal RCCs in VHL**

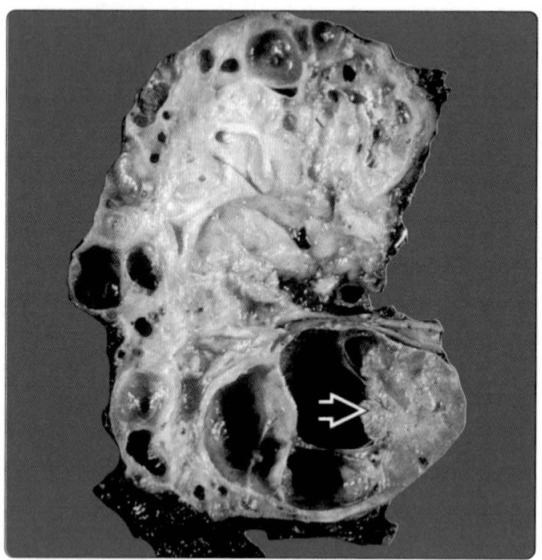

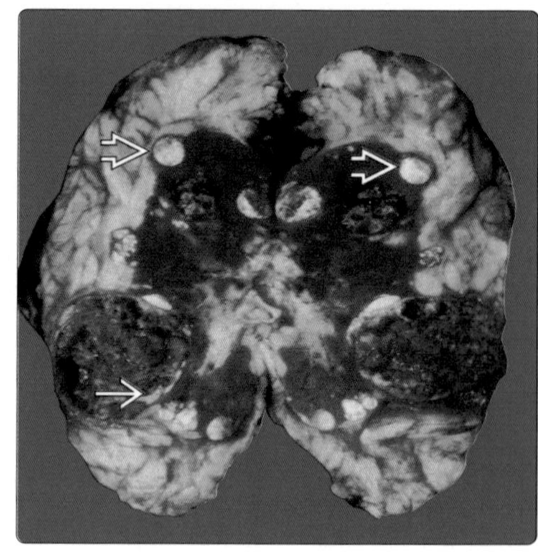

(Left) *This nephrectomy specimen from a patient with dialysis-induced cysts is complicated by renal cell carcinoma. The extensive cysts can mimic ADPKD, but usually the kidneys are not as large.* **(Right)** *Multiple renal cell carcinomas of varying sizes are shown. Yellow color is characteristic of clear cell type. A larger hemorrhagic and necrotic tumor shows a focal yellow rim at the periphery of the cyst.*

Cystic Nephroma | **Cysts and Tumors in TSC**

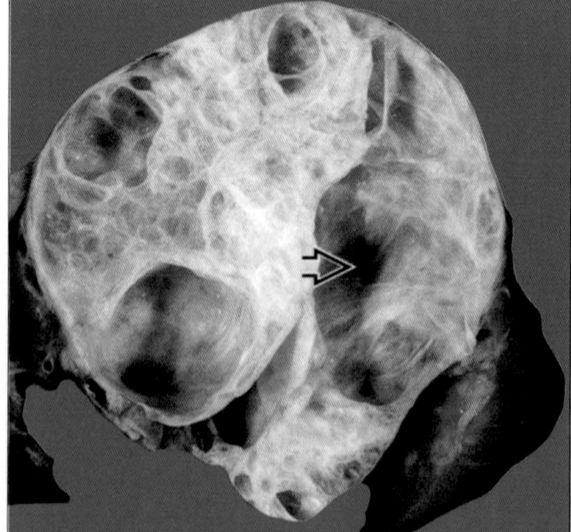

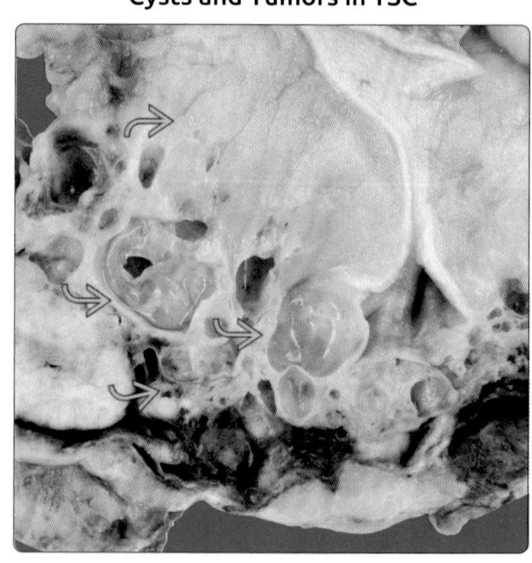

(Left) *Nephrectomy from a young infant shows a well-encapsulated cystic mass with variably sized cysts containing gelatinous fluid. These findings are characteristic of multilocular renal cyst, also called cystic nephroma.* **(Right)** *The yellow mass is angiolipoma. Adjacent to the tumor mass are multiple cysts, small and large, all lined by glistening epithelium.*

Fetal ARPKD

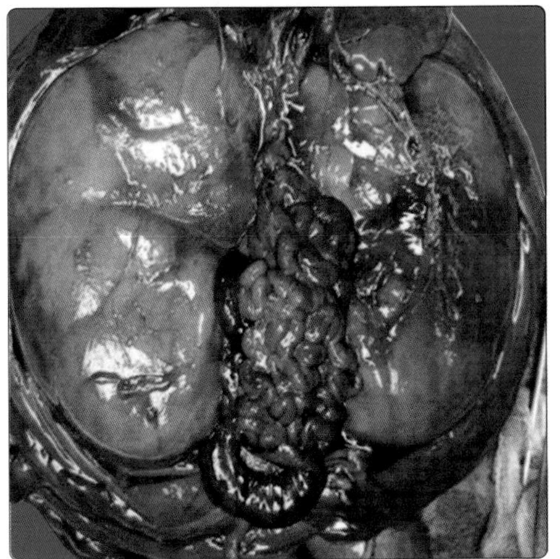

Fetal ARPKD

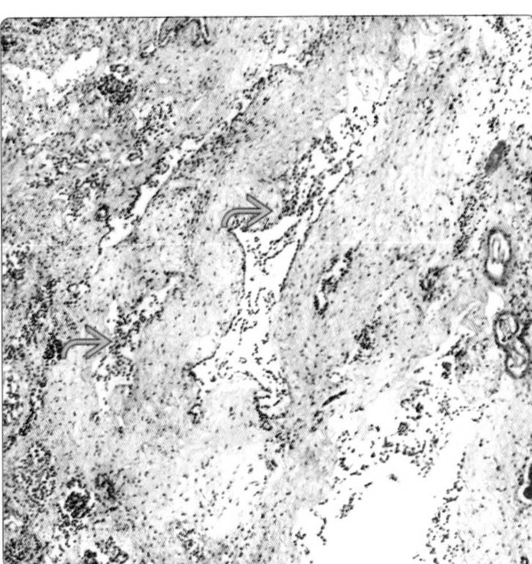

(Left) *31-week stillborn male fetus (mother G6, P2-1-3-4) is shown. Previous spontaneous abortions and pregnancies were complicated by eclampsia. Bilateral kidneys are massively enlarged. Cytogenetics had no results due to tissue.* **(Right)** *Marked interstitial edema and diffuse epithelial degeneration in the same patient is shown; however, a vague cylindrical pattern ⮫ is revealed, consistent with fetal ARPKD.*

Glomerulocystic Ischemic Adult Kidney

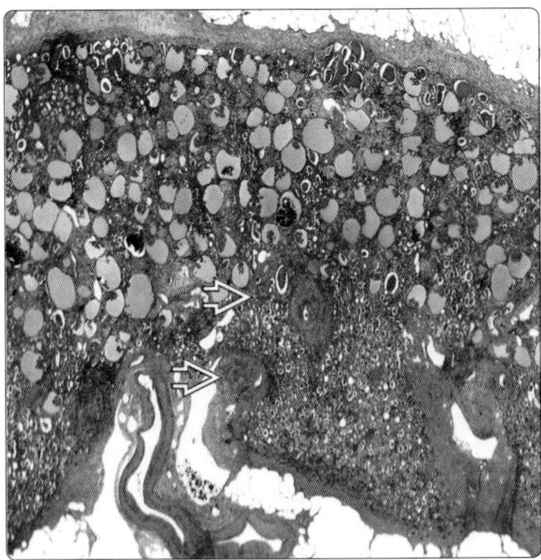

Glomerulocystic Fetal Kidney

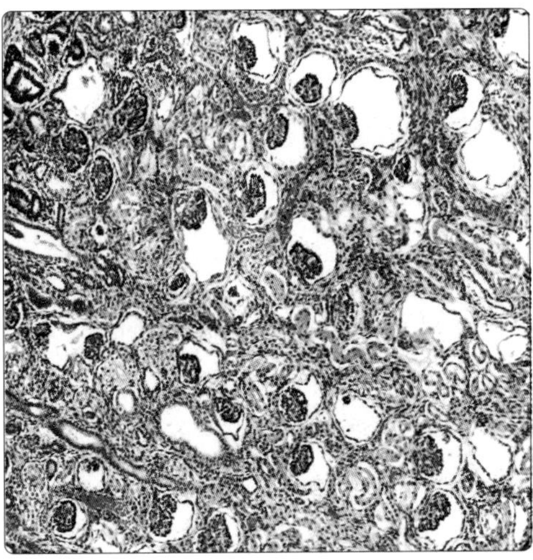

(Left) *All glomeruli are cystic in this kidney with thick parenchymal arteries ➡. The entire cortex and medulla are atrophic.* **(Right)** *Autopsy of 19-week-old girl with Turner syndrome, large kidneys, and multiple anomalies, including pulmonary hypoplasia is shown. The kidneys were enlarged with diffuse glomerular cysts..*

Hydronephrotic, Dysplastic Kidney

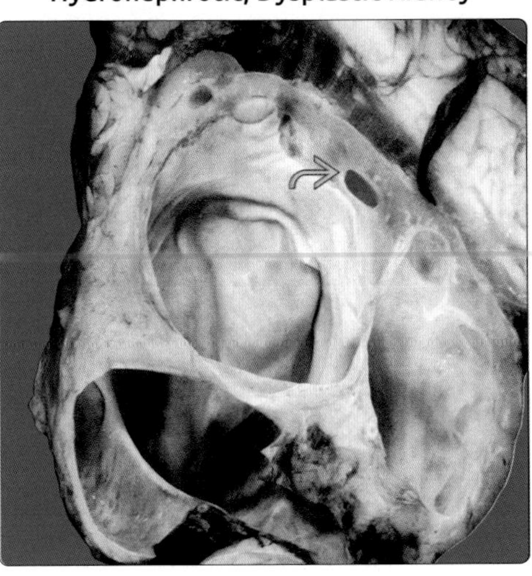

Metaplastic Cartilage in Renal Dysplasia

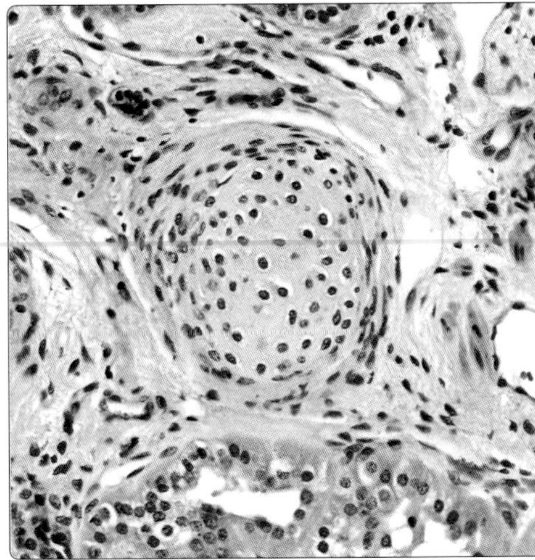

(Left) *The calyces are dilated. The cortex is thin and contains small cysts ⮫.* **(Right)** *Islands of cartilage are pathognomonic of renal dysplasia.*

Autosomal Dominant Polycystic Kidney Disease

KEY FACTS

TERMINOLOGY

- Autosomal dominant polycystic kidney disease (ADPKD)

ETIOLOGY/PATHOGENESIS

- Autosomal dominant inheritance pattern
- Ciliopathy involving proteins of primary cilium
  - *PKD1* (polycystin-1): 85%
  - *PKD2* (polycystin-2): 15%

CLINICAL ISSUES

- 1 in 500 live births
- Symptoms
  - Hypertension
  - Renal failure
  - Abdominal pain/discomfort
  - Hematuria, infections
- No known preventive treatment
- ~ 50% require dialysis or kidney transplant by age 50
- Risk factors for disease progression
  - *PKD1*, particularly truncating mutation
  - Men
  - Early onset of hypertension &/or gross hematuria
  - For women, ≥ 3 pregnancies

MACROSCOPIC

- Numerous cysts throughout both kidneys
  - Kidneys weigh up to 4 kg each
- Cysts in multiple other organs
  - Liver, pancreas, arachnoid, pineal, seminal vesicle

MICROSCOPIC

- Numerous cysts involving all levels of nephron
- Renal cell tumors may be present

TOP DIFFERENTIAL DIAGNOSES

- Autosomal recessive PKD
- Acquired cystic disease

(Left) *Contrast-enhanced CT shows multiple cysts of varying size essentially replacing the renal parenchyma ➡. Cysts are also seen in the liver ➡.* **(Right)** *Numerous cysts are present in this kidney that weighs 2.5 kg and measures 28 cm in length. Only ADPKD leads to such massive enlargement of the kidneys. (Courtesy J. Steinmetz, MD.)*

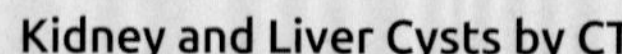

Kidney and Liver Cysts by CT

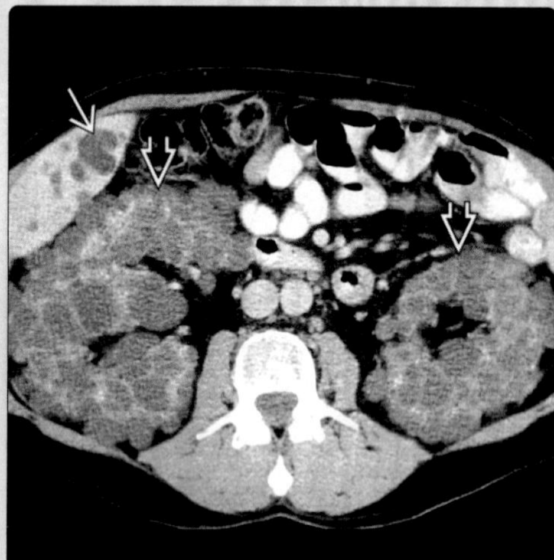

Enlarged Kidney With Numerous Cysts

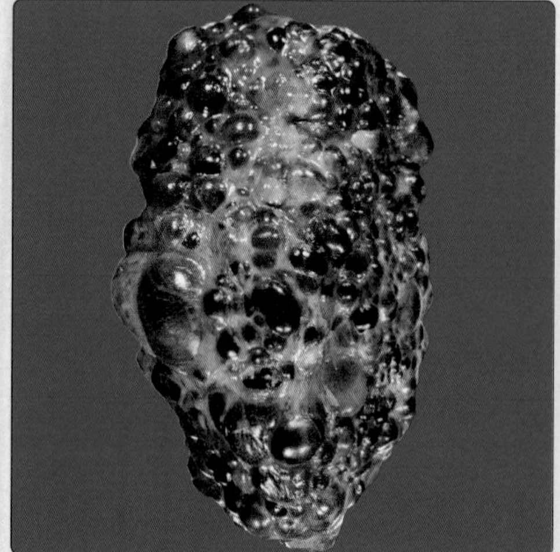

(Left) *Several cysts from a polycystic kidney contain proteinaceous fluid. A globally sclerotic glomerulus ➡ is compressed between several cysts that have mostly replaced the renal parenchyma and resulted in marked and diffuse interstitial fibrosis and tubular atrophy.* **(Right)** *This enlarged cyst is lined by cuboidal to flattened epithelial cells ➡. Diffuse tubular atrophy and interstitial fibrosis with an associated nonspecific inflammatory cell infiltrate are noted.*

Cysts

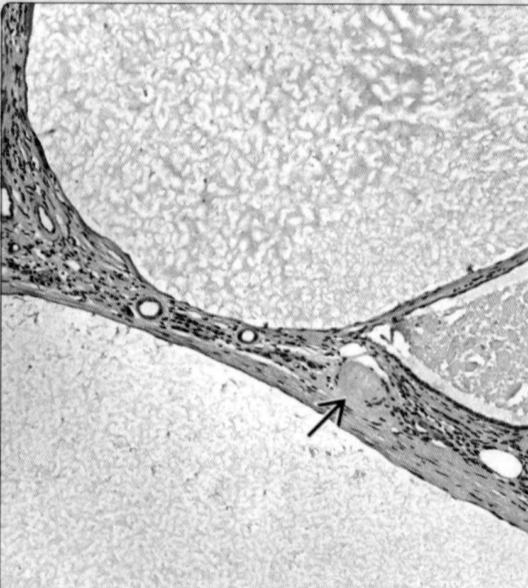

Cysts

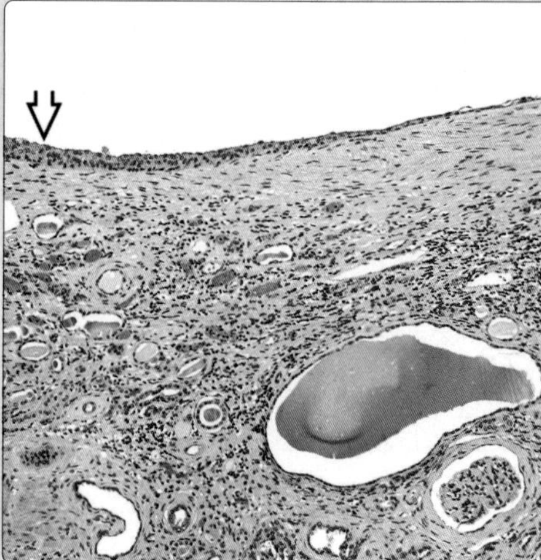

TERMINOLOGY

Abbreviations

- Autosomal dominant polycystic kidney disease (ADPKD)

ETIOLOGY/PATHOGENESIS

Genetic Disease

- Classified as "ciliopathy"
- Autosomal dominant
  - Random somatic mutation of normal allele in individual cells

PKD1 (Polycystin-1) Mutation

- Located on chromosome 16
- Accounts for 85% of ADPKD

PKD2 (Polycystin-2) Mutation

- Located on chromosome 4
- Accounts for 15% of ADPKD
- May act as cation channel for calcium entry into cell

Possible Pathogenic Mechanisms Related to Cilium

- Abnormal cell proliferation
- Deregulated apoptosis
- Defective cellular polarity
- Increased secretion of fluids into tubular lumina

CLINICAL ISSUES

Epidemiology

- Incidence
  - 1 in 500 live births
- Age
  - Usually presents at 30-40 years of age
  - Rarely presents in childhood
  - Cysts develop progressively
- Sex
  - Earlier onset of hypertension and end-stage renal disease in men compared to women at any given age
  - Women have more cysts in liver and develop them at earlier age than men do

Presentation

- Hematuria
- Abdominal pain/discomfort
- Urinary tract infections
- Hypertension
  - Cerebral arterial aneurysms with intracranial hemorrhage in 5-10%

Laboratory Tests

- Genetic tests for *PKD1* or *PKD2* mutations
  - Mutation detection rate: 65-70% for *PKD1*
  - Mutation detection rate: Nearly 90% for *PKD2*

Treatment

- None effective to slow progression
  - Clinical trials of mTOR inhibitors, vasopressin receptor antagonists
- Bilateral nephrectomy if kidneys are too enlarged or if recurrent episodes of pyelonephritis

Prognosis

- ~ 50% of patients will require dialysis or kidney transplant by age 50
- *PKD2* mutations result in milder clinical course compared to *PKD1* mutations
- Risk factors for disease progression
  - *PKD1*, particularly truncating mutation
  - Men
  - Early onset of hypertension &/or gross hematuria
  - For women, ≥ 3 pregnancies

MACROSCOPIC

General Features

- Numerous cysts throughout both kidneys
- Kidneys weigh up to 4 kg each

MICROSCOPIC

Histologic Features

- Cysts in cortex and medulla up to several cm in diameter
  - Arises from any nephron segment or collecting duct
  - Glomerular, tubular cysts
  - Lined by single layer of flattened to cuboidal epithelium
  - Normal intervening parenchyma may be present, depending on stage
- Diffuse interstitial fibrosis and tubular atrophy

Extrarenal Pathology

- Liver cysts (> 90%)
- Cysts in pancreas (10%), seminal vesicles (39%), pineal gland (< 5%), arachnoid, and ovaries
- Mitral valve prolapse or aortic regurgitation in 25%

DIFFERENTIAL DIAGNOSIS

Autosomal Recessive PKD

- Congenital or childhood onset
- Ectatic collecting ducts and bile ducts

Acquired Cystic Disease

- Usually < 1 kg, cysts not as widespread
- Underlying renal disease evident
- May be present in ADPKD

DIAGNOSTIC CHECKLIST

Pathologic Interpretation Pearls

- Bread loaf nephrectomy specimens at 1 cm to exclude neoplasia

SELECTED REFERENCES

1. Cai Y et al: Altered trafficking and stability of polycystins underlie polycystic kidney disease. J Clin Invest. ePub, 2014
2. Schrier RW et al: Predictors of autosomal dominant polycystic kidney disease progression. J Am Soc Nephrol. 25(11):2399-418, 2014
3. Bae KT et al: Imaging for the prognosis of autosomal dominant polycystic kidney disease. Nat Rev Nephrol. 6(2):96-106, 2010
4. Perico N et al: Sirolimus therapy to halt the progression of ADPKD. J Am Soc Nephrol. 21(6):1031-40, 2010
5. Grantham JJ: Clinical practice. Autosomal dominant polycystic kidney disease. N Engl J Med. 359(14):1477-85, 2008

(Left) *Axial CECT shows relatively normal size and function of the kidneys, but with innumerable small cortical and medullary cysts ➡. This is an example of ADPKD due to PKD2 mutation.* **(Right)** *Axial CECT shows innumerable cysts in bilaterally enlarged kidneys in a patient who has been on dialysis for many years. This radiographically mimics autosomal dominant polycystic kidney disease.*

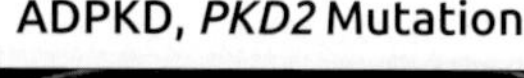

ADPKD, *PKD2* Mutation

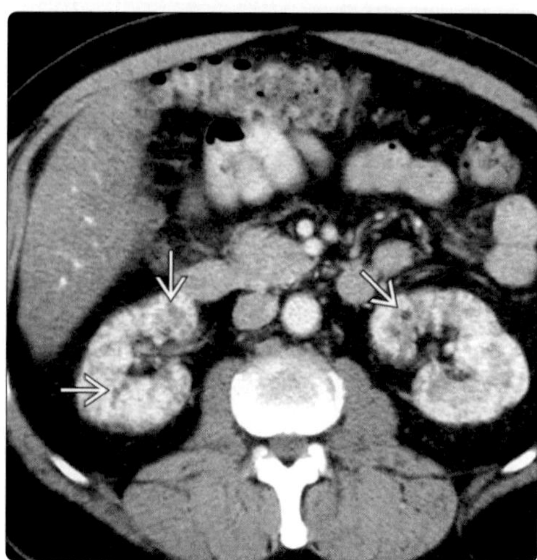

Acquired Cystic Disease

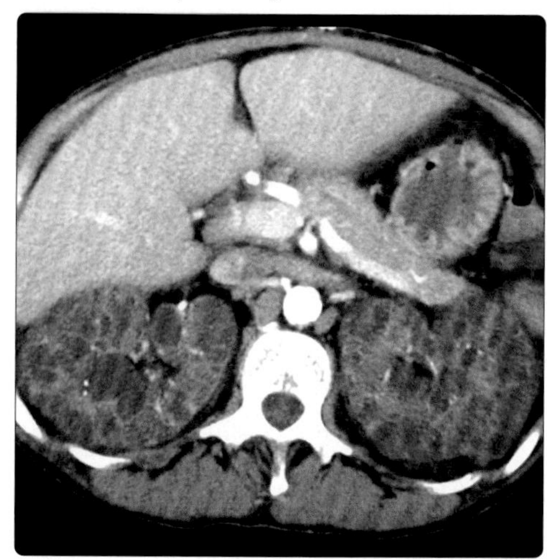

(Left) *Numerous cysts are present throughout this kidney from a patient with ADPKD. Due to the marked enlargement, only half of the kidney is framed within this image. Very little identifiable residual renal parenchyma is seen. Focal hemorrhage is noted within a cyst ➡. (Courtesy J. Moore, MD.)* **(Right)** *This is a kidney from a patient with ADPKD (bivalved). The normal architecture is severely distorted by numerous cysts distributed throughout the renal parenchyma.*

Renal Cysts

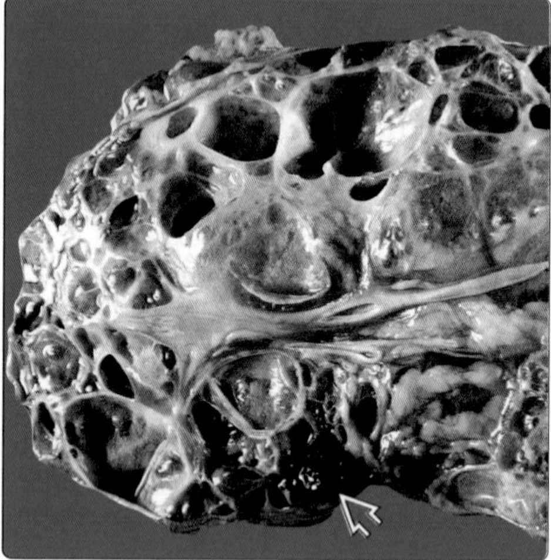

Cysts

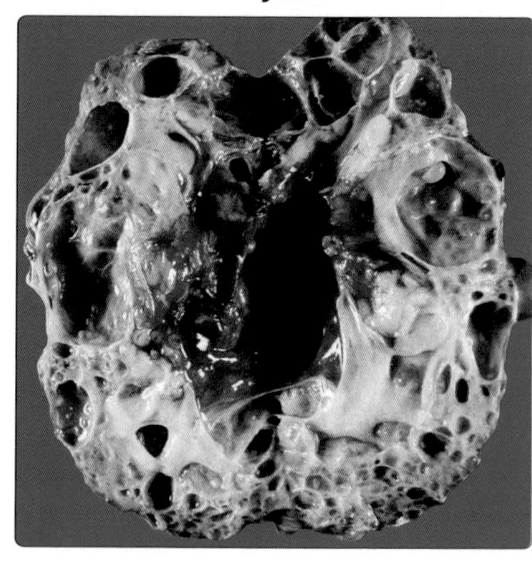

(Left) *These cysts demonstrate the spectrum of findings that may be present within cyst contents. One cyst demonstrates hemorrhage with numerous red blood cells ⇨. The other 2 adjacent cysts → contain proteinaceous material that show varying degrees of eosinophilia.* **(Right)** *Glomerular cysts are a common feature of ADPKD. This should not be confused with glomerulocystic kidney disease.*

Hemorrhagic and Proteinaceous Cysts

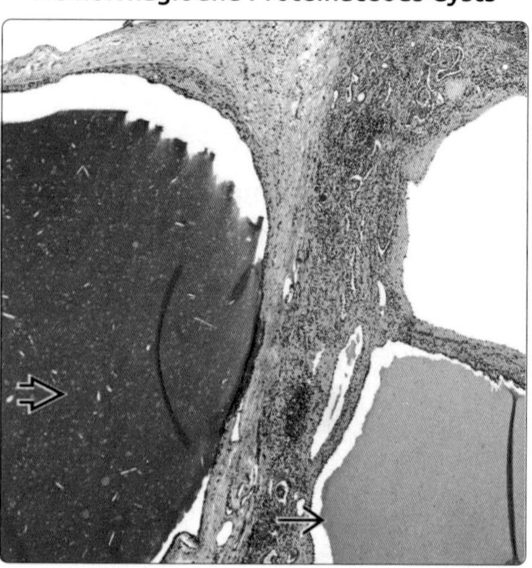

Glomerular Cysts

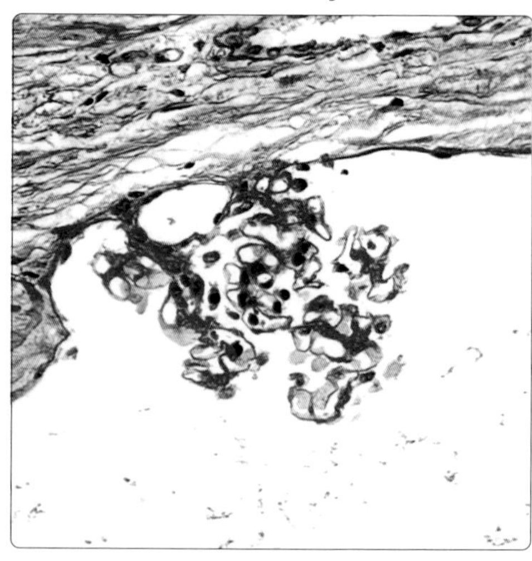

ADPKD, Early Stage

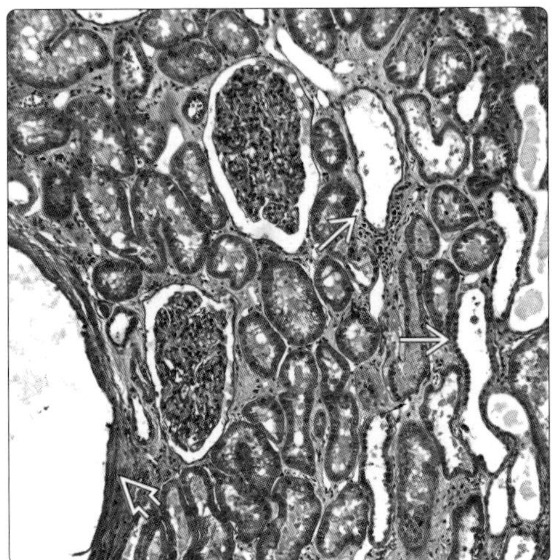

Renal Cysts

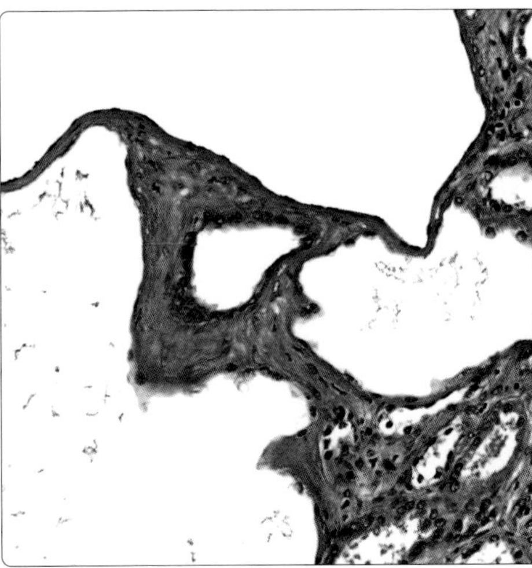

(Left) *In this micrograph of a polycystic kidney, a single cyst lined by flattened epithelium* ➡ *is adjacent to relatively intact renal cortical tissue. Some tubules show flattening of the epithelium, indicating tubular injury* ➡. **(Right)** *Most cysts are lined by flattened epithelia as shown in this micrograph. Cysts affect all levels of the nephron, from the glomerulus to the collecting ducts.*

Columnar Epithelial-Lined Cyst

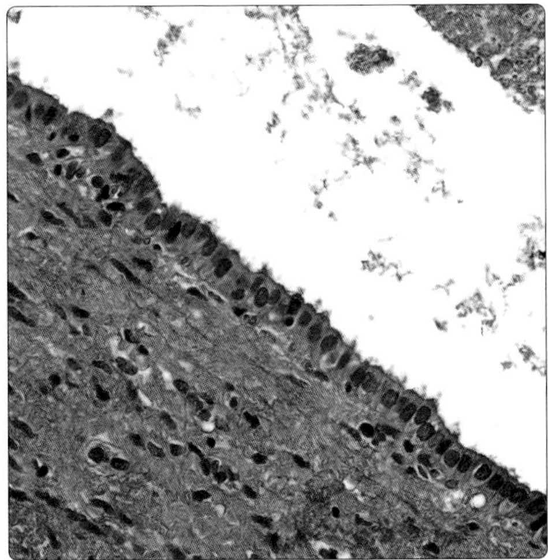

Glomerular Cyst

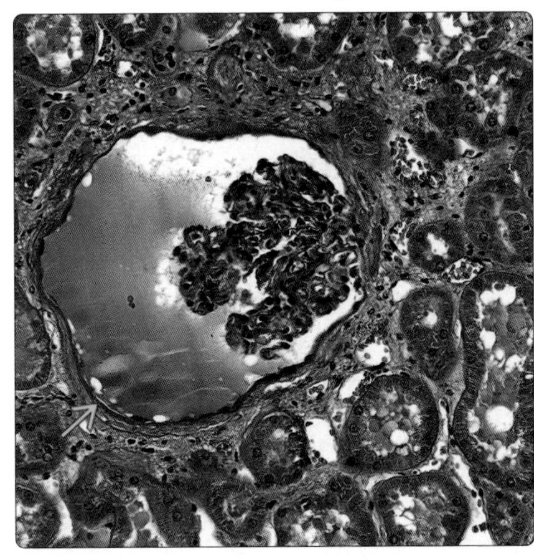

(Left) *Some cysts are lined by epithelia with columnar morphology. This is distinct from the enlarged, hyperplastic hobnailed cells seen in acquired cystic disease.* **(Right)** *This glomerular cyst* ➡ *may have formed as a result of either the distal nephron undergoing cyst formation or secondary distal obstruction by compression of adjacent cysts.*

Tufting of Epithelial Lining Cells

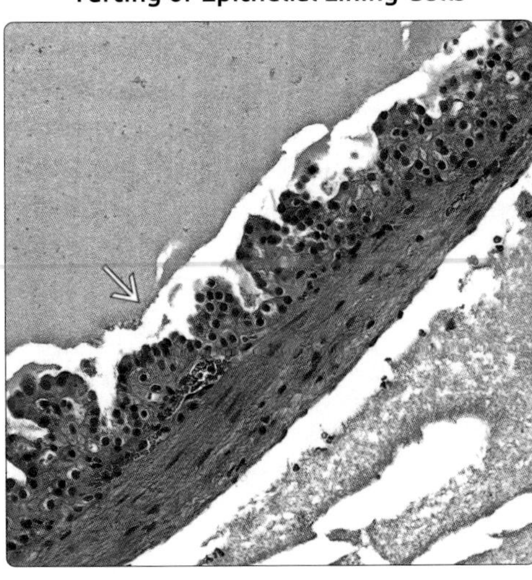

Papillary Neoplasm

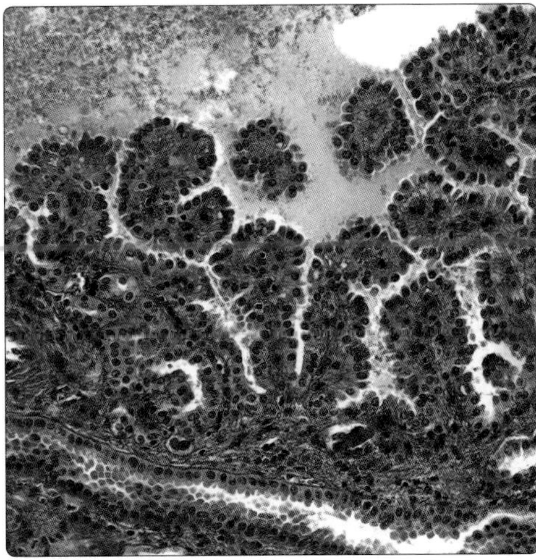

(Left) *A minority of cysts in ADPKD kidneys may be lined by epithelia showing tufting and small papillary projections into the cyst lumen* ➡. **(Right)** *The papillary proliferation of cyst-lining epithelium can be quite exuberant as shown in this micrograph of polycystic kidney. ADPKD kidneys are believed to have an increased probability of developing papillary renal cell carcinoma. Tumors can usually be detected on gross examination after breadloafing at 1 cm, and appear as solid yellow or white nodules.*

Autosomal Recessive Polycystic Kidney Disease

KEY FACTS

TERMINOLOGY

- Autosomal recessive polycystic kidney disease/congenital hepatic fibrosis

ETIOLOGY/PATHOGENESIS

- Mutation of *PKHD1* gene on chromosome 6p12
- *PKHD1* encodes for polyductin/fibrocystin protein

CLINICAL ISSUES

- Neonates present with respiratory failure
- Older children and adults
  - Portal hypertension
  - Renal insufficiency or concentrating defects

IMAGING

- Echogenic large kidneys on ultrasound in neonates
- Normal size ± medullary cysts in older patients

MACROSCOPIC

- Massive, diffusely cystic kidneys in neonates
  - Bilateral hypoplastic lungs
- Medullary cysts ± cortical cysts in older patients
  - Congenital hepatic fibrosis

MICROSCOPIC

- Radially dilated collecting ducts in neonates
  - Bile duct plate malformation in liver
- Medullary collecting duct ectasia in older patients
  - Congenital hepatic fibrosis in children and adults
  - Occasionally Caroli disease: Bile duct dilatation

ANCILLARY TESTS

- Test for *PKHD1* mutation

TOP DIFFERENTIAL DIAGNOSES

- Cystic renal dysplasia
- Medullary sponge kidney
- Autosomal dominant polycystic kidney disease (older patients with ARPKD)

(Left) *A lethal neonatal case of ARPKD has massively enlarged kidneys with persistent fetal lobulation. The dilated ducts are not visible through the renal capsule. The ureters are of normal caliber.* **(Right)** *The radial arrangement of the dilated collecting ducts is apparent. Since most renal pyramids angle toward the collecting system from an anterior or posterior direction, rounded medullary cysts are often seen. The collecting system is completely normal.*

Massively Enlarged Kidneys

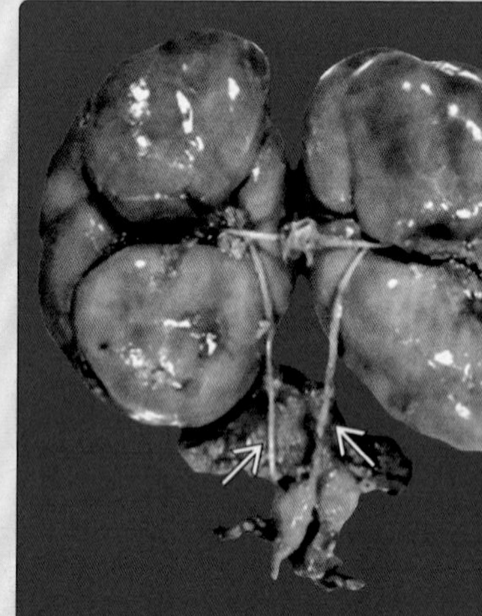

Diffuse Cysts and Dilated Tubules Involving Cortex and Medulla

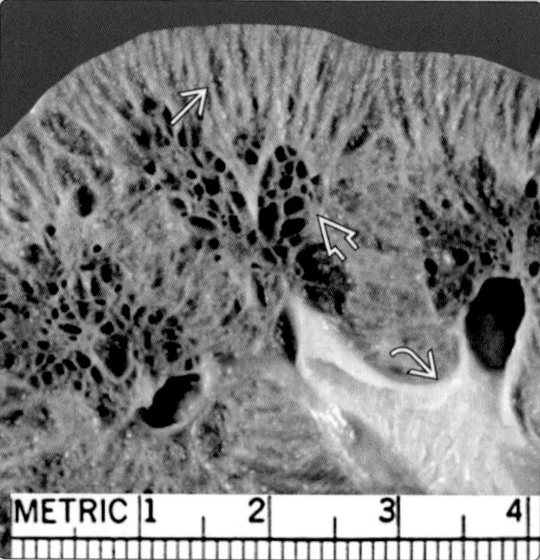

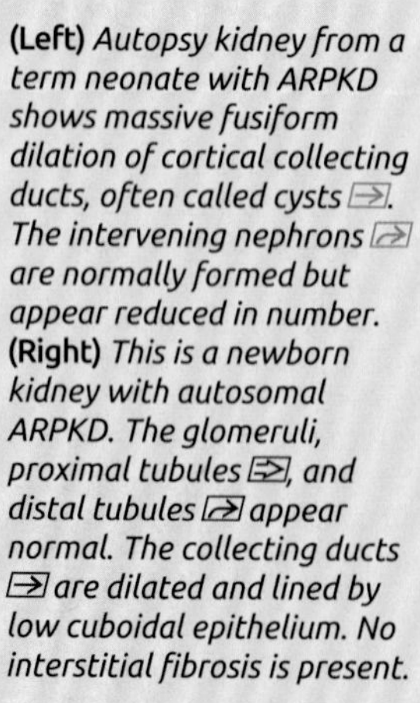

(Left) *Autopsy kidney from a term neonate with ARPKD shows massive fusiform dilation of cortical collecting ducts, often called cysts. The intervening nephrons are normally formed but appear reduced in number.* **(Right)** *This is a newborn kidney with autosomal ARPKD. The glomeruli, proximal tubules, and distal tubules appear normal. The collecting ducts are dilated and lined by low cuboidal epithelium. No interstitial fibrosis is present.*

Radially Oriented Ectatic Collecting Ducts

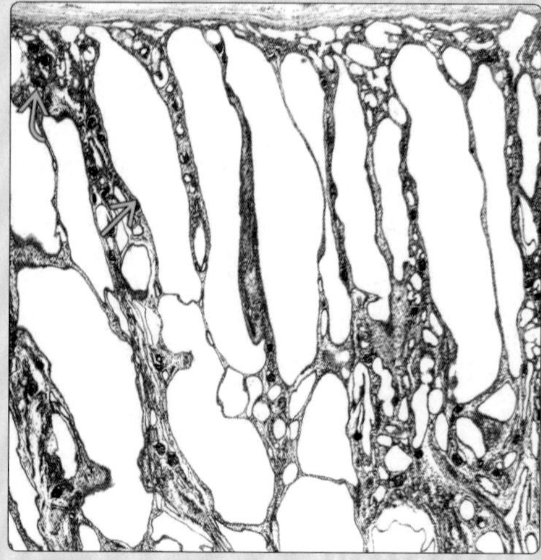

Normal Nephrons Between Collecting Ducts

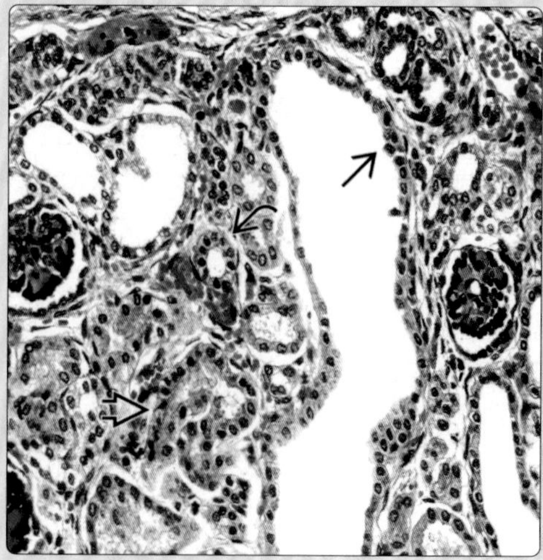

TERMINOLOGY

Abbreviations

- Autosomal recessive polycystic kidney disease (ARPKD)

Synonyms

- Infantile polycystic kidney disease
  - Term not recommended because of adolescent and adult presentations
- Sponge kidney
  - Not to be confused with medullary sponge kidney

Definitions

- Cystic kidney disease/congenital hepatic fibrosis due to *PKHD1* mutation, chromosome 6p12

ETIOLOGY/PATHOGENESIS

Genetic Factors

- *PKHD1* encodes for polyductin/fibrocystin protein
  - Polyductin/fibrocystin protein located in primary cilium
  - > 300 *PKHD1* mutations identified
- Poor genotype-phenotype correlation
  - 2 truncating mutations cause severe neonatal disease

CLINICAL ISSUES

Presentation

- Autosomal recessive, 1:10-40,000 live births
- Newborn
  - Respiratory failure from pulmonary hypoplasia in 30-50%
  - +/- renal failure
  - Abdominal mass
- Childhood to adulthood
  - Systemic hypertension and renal insufficiency in 50%
  - Portal hypertension in 10%
  - Renal concentrating defects ± medullary cysts

Treatment

- Renal &/or liver transplantation in children and adults

Prognosis

- Lethal in 40% of neonates
  - If neonate survives 1st month, 90% 5-year survival

IMAGING

Ultrasonographic Findings

- Neonates: Bilateral enlarged echogenic kidneys with poor corticomedullary differentiation and numerous tiny cysts
- Adolescents to adults: Normal-sized or enlarged kidney with medullary echogenicity ± focal cortical involvement

MACROSCOPIC

General Features

- Lethal neonatal form
  - Potter oligohydramnios phenotype
  - Kidneys massively enlarged
  - Diffuse radially oriented dilated collecting ducts in cortex and medulla
  - Round cysts formed secondarily
  - Small hypoplastic lungs
- Infantile to adult forms
  - Smaller kidneys and larger lungs
  - Medullary cysts and no or few rounded cortical cysts
  - Congenital hepatic fibrosis with hepatosplenomegaly and esophageal varices
  - Occasional patients develop Caroli disease

MICROSCOPIC

Histologic Features

- Nonobstructive fusiform dilatation of cortical and medullary collecting ducts in neonatal cases
  - Nephrons normal without dysgenetic features
- Smaller rounded collecting duct cysts separated by focally atrophic tissue in childhood
- Occasional medullary cysts in older children and adults
- Mild ectasia of proximal tubules (early lesion)

Liver

- Bile duct plate abnormality (retention of embryonic plate configuration)
  - Abnormally shaped and distributed bile ducts
  - Periportal fibrosis and portal-portal bridging without inflammation
  - Abnormal portal vein branching
- Congenital hepatic fibrosis in childhood or adults
- Dilatation of intrahepatic bile ducts (Caroli disease)

ANCILLARY TESTS

Genetic Testing

- *PKHD1* mutations identified in 80-85%

DIFFERENTIAL DIAGNOSIS

Cystic Renal Dysplasia

- Lower urinary tract usually abnormal
- Dysplastic elements: Cartilage, smooth muscle
- Lack of nephrons (glomeruli, proximal and distal tubules)

Medullary Sponge Kidney

- Distal papillary collecting ducts affected
- Papillary tip calcification and nephrolithiasis

Autosomal Dominant Polycystic Kidney Disease

- Older patients: Variably sized and distributed cysts

SELECTED REFERENCES

1. Büscher R et al: Clinical manifestations of autosomal recessive polycystic kidney disease (ARPKD): kidney-related and non-kidney-related phenotypes. Pediatr Nephrol. 29(10):1915-25, 2014
2. Denamur E et al: Genotype-phenotype correlations in fetuses and neonates with autosomal recessive polycystic kidney disease. Kidney Int. 77(4):350-8, 2010
3. Gunay-Aygun M et al: Correlation of kidney function, volume and imaging findings, and PKHD1 mutations in 73 patients with autosomal recessive polycystic kidney disease. Clin J Am Soc Nephrol. 5(6):972-84, 2010
4. Gunay-Aygun M: Liver and kidney disease in ciliopathies. Am J Med Genet C Semin Med Genet. 151C(4):296-306, 2009
5. Guay-Woodford LM: Autosomal recessive PKD in the early years. Nephrol News Issues. 21(12):39, 2007
6. Nakanishi K et al: Proximal tubular cysts in fetal human autosomal recessive polycystic kidney disease. J Am Soc Nephrol. 11(4):760-3, 2000

(Left) *The mother of this newborn with ARPKD presented with oligohydramnios. The newborn had the Potter sequence with Potter facies, which is characterized by low posteriorly rotated ears, recessed chin, broad nose and epicanthic folds, all present in this case.* **(Right)** *This is a lethal neonatal case of ARPKD. The neonate presented with respiratory failure and massive abdominal enlargement due to bilateral cystic kidneys. The kidneys have retained their reniform shape.*

Potter Facies

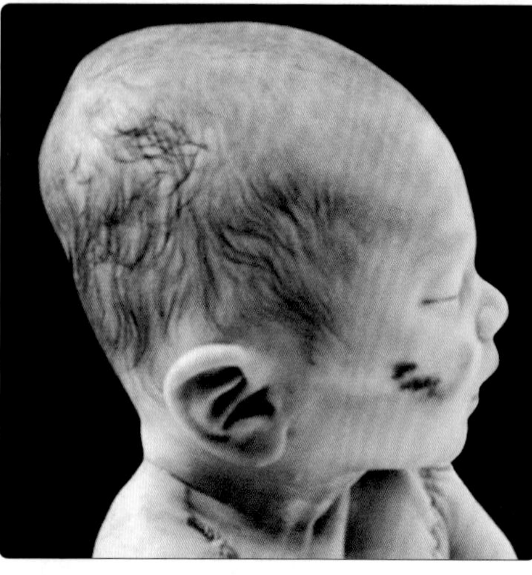

Massively Enlarged Kidneys

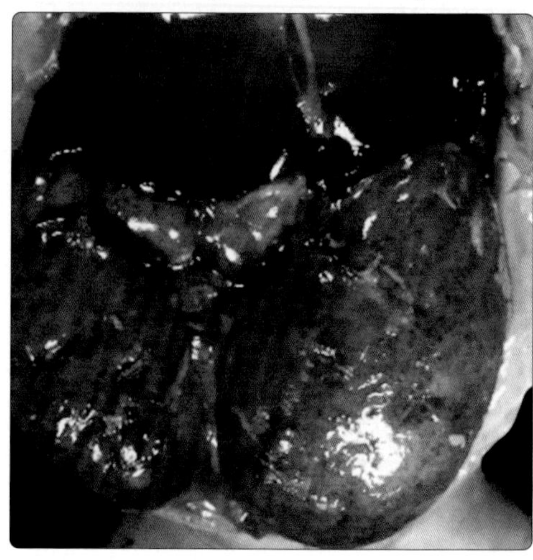

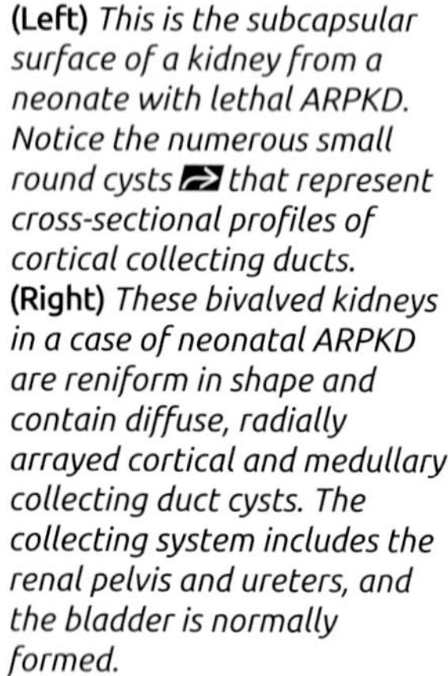

(Left) *This is the subcapsular surface of a kidney from a neonate with lethal ARPKD. Notice the numerous small round cysts ➔ that represent cross-sectional profiles of cortical collecting ducts.* **(Right)** *These bivalved kidneys in a case of neonatal ARPKD are reniform in shape and contain diffuse, radially arrayed cortical and medullary collecting duct cysts. The collecting system includes the renal pelvis and ureters, and the bladder is normally formed.*

Dilated Collecting Ducts Viewed From Capsular Surface

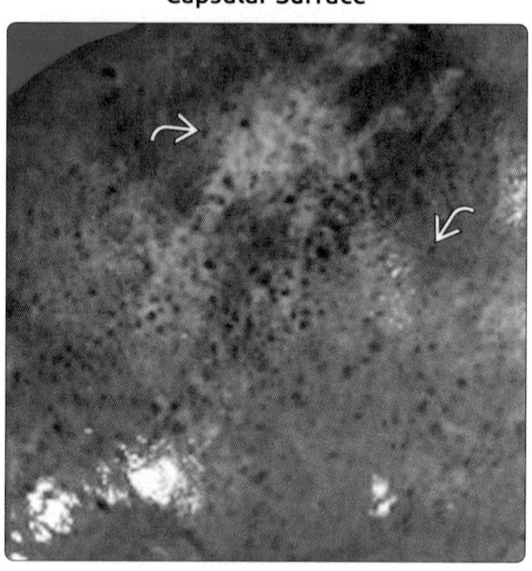

Diffuse Cysts Involving Cortex and Medulla

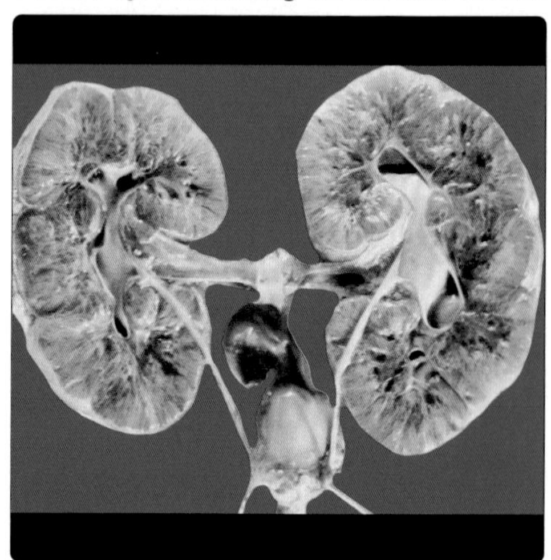

(Left) *The cysts in a lethal neonatal cases of ARPKD are small and very uniform in size. The corticomedullary distinction is lost. The cysts impart a sponge-like quality to the kidneys, not to be confused with medullary sponge kidney.* **(Right)** *This bivalved markedly enlarged kidney in a case of lethal neonatal ARPKD shows radial dilated cortical collecting ducts ➔ and round medullary cysts ➔, which arise secondary to disruption of collecting ducts. Pelvis and calyces were normal but are not in the plane of this section.*

Diffuse Dilated Tubules Involving Cortex and Medulla

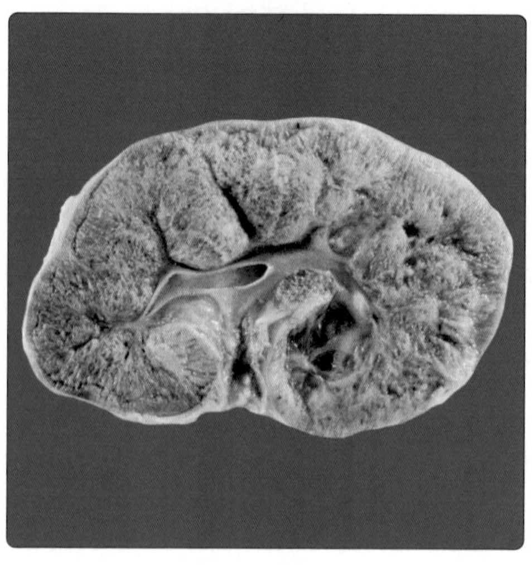

Diffuse Cysts and Dilated Tubules Involving Cortex and Medulla

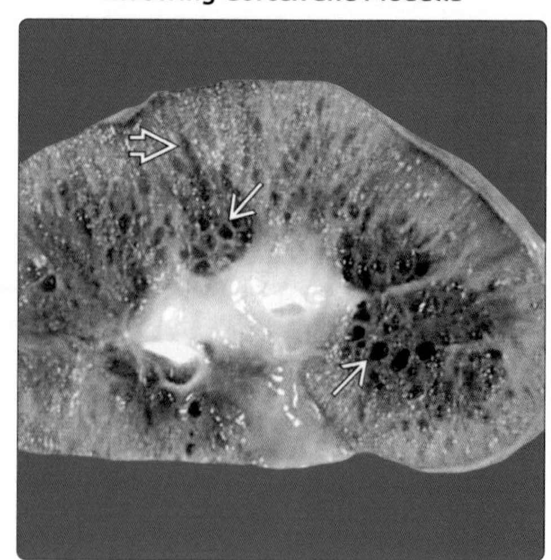

Diffuse Cysts and Dilated Tubules

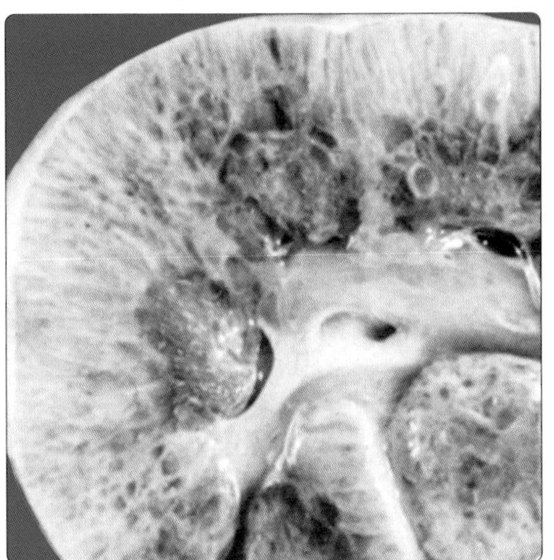

Radially Oriented Dilated Collecting Ducts

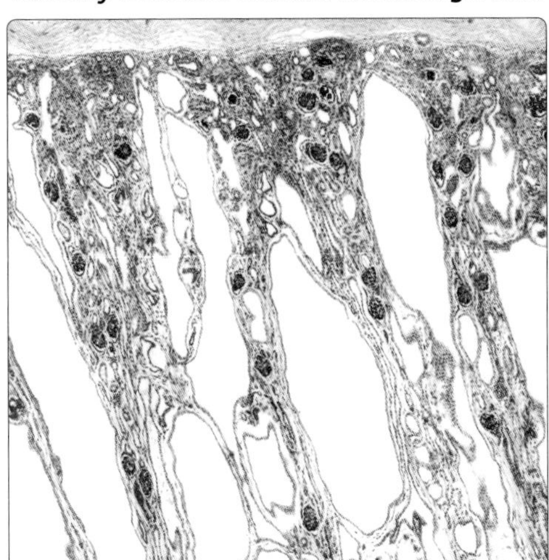

(Left) *Lethal neonatal case of ARPKD shows cortical and medullary cysts. There is very little intervening parenchyma. This creates the sponge-like quality in gross appearance and sponge-like texture of the kidney when handled.* **(Right)** *This lethal neonatal case of ARPKD shows the collecting ducts cysts, which are lined by a low cuboidal epithelium. The intervening parenchyma is not fibrotic or inflamed. It contains morphologically normal nephron components.*

Normal Nephron Between Collecting Ducts

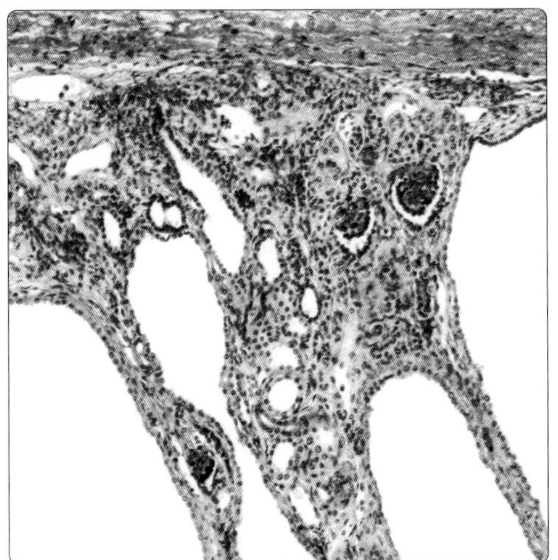

Radially Oriented Collecting Ducts

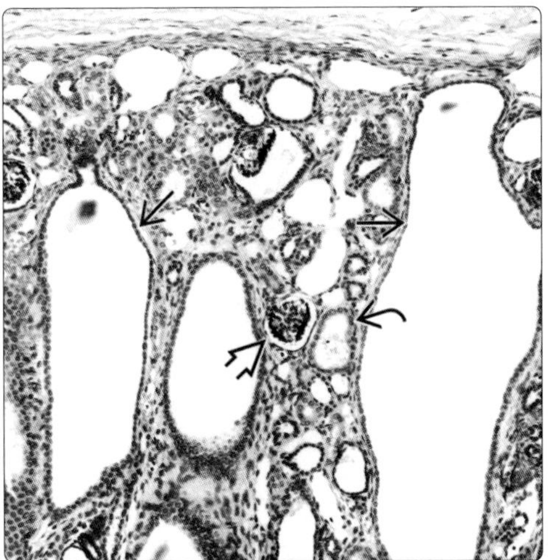

(Left) *In lethal neonatal ARPKD, the nephron elements, glomeruli, and proximal and distal tubules are usually normally formed, appearing most numerous beneath the renal capsule. Abnormalities of metanephric differentiation are not present.* **(Right)** *This term infant with lethal neonatal ARPKD shows the fusiform collecting duct cyst* → *lined by low cuboidal epithelium. Glomeruli* ⇒ *are immature-appearing, as expected in a newborn kidney. There is mild ectasia of the proximal tubules* ↷*, a common finding.*

Radially Oriented Collecting Ducts

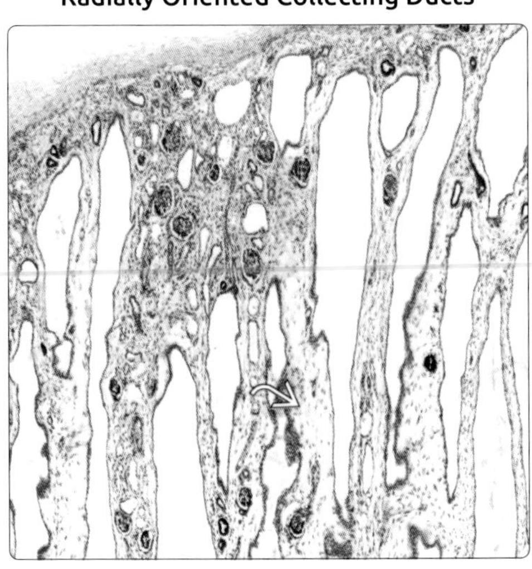

Paucity of Tubules Between Collecting Ducts

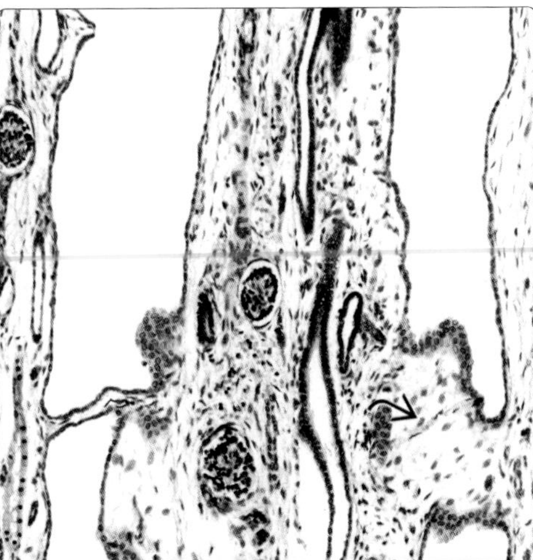

(Left) *This example of lethal neonatal ARPKD shows the radially oriented collecting duct cysts. Notice that the nephron elements vary in the intervening parenchyma. Near the cortex, normally formed glomeruli and tubules are present. However, in the deeper cortex* ↷*, there are glomeruli but few tubules.* **(Right)** *This shows the renal parenchyma between the collecting ducts cysts. There are normally formed glomeruli and abundant loose paucicellular stroma* ↷*. However, the proximal and distal tubules are completely absent.*

Dilated Medullary Collecting Ducts

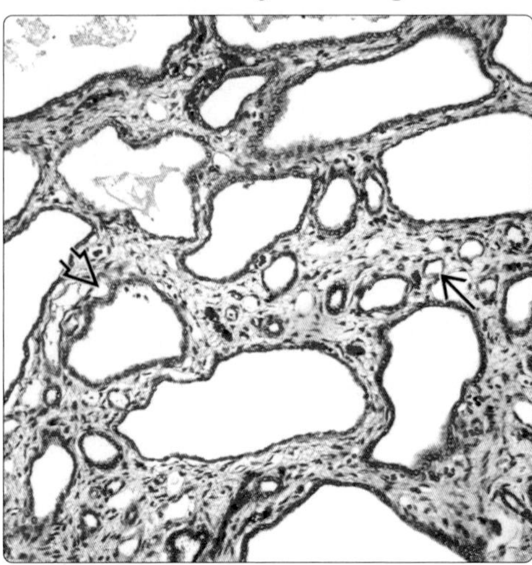

Medullary Collecting Duct Cysts

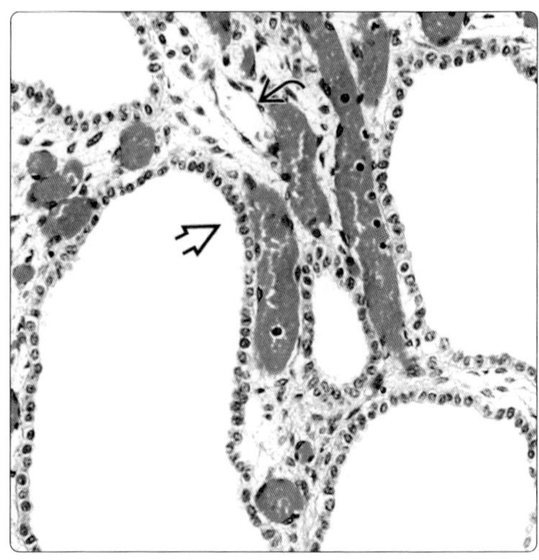

(Left) *Renal medulla from a term neonate with lethal ARPKD shows dilated medullary collecting ducts ⇨ lined by a low cuboidal epithelium. The interstitium is loose and paucicellular with thin loops of Henle ⇨ present.* **(Right)** *Renal medulla from a term neonate with lethal ARPKD shows dilated medullary collecting ducts ⇨ lined by a low cuboidal epithelium. The interstitium is loose and paucicellular. There are peritubular capillaries ⇨ but no thin loops of Henle are present.*

Medullary Collecting Duct Cysts

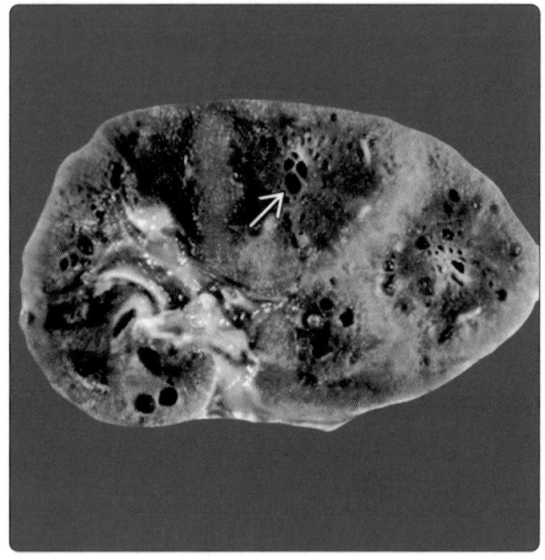

7 Month Old With ARPKD

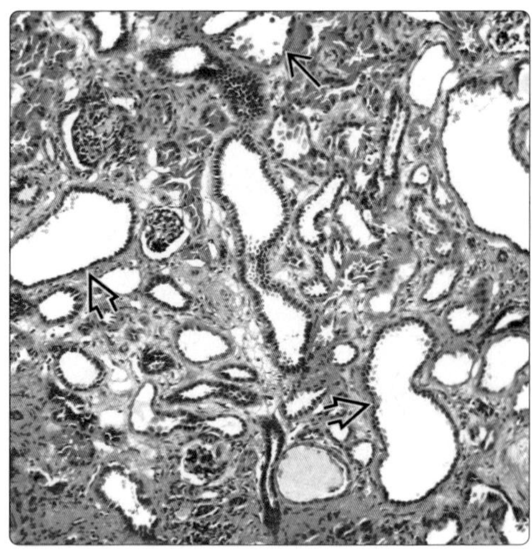

(Left) *This is a childhood case of ARPKD with normal-sized kidneys. The cysts ➡ are predominately located within the renal medulla, and are caused by disruption of the collecting ducts. Cortical cysts are not grossly apparent.* **(Right)** *This is a kidney from a 7 month old with ARPKD. The glomeruli are normal. There is moderate collecting duct ⇨ dilatation and mild proximal tubule dilation ⇨. The cortical interstitium is expanded by fibrosis. Once fibrosis develops it resembles early onset autosomal dominant PKD.*

3 Year Old With ARPKD

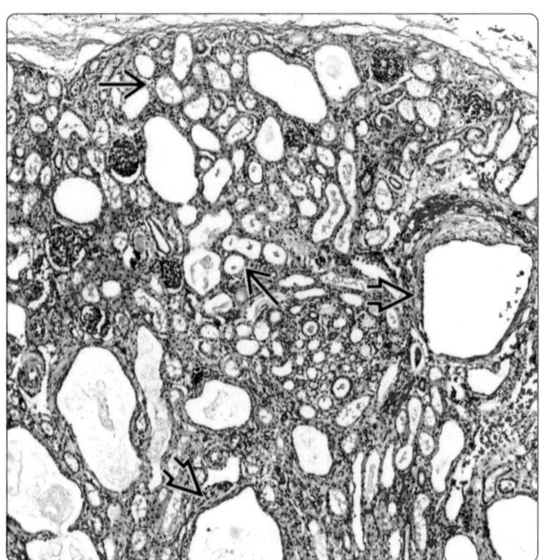

3 Year Old With ARPKD

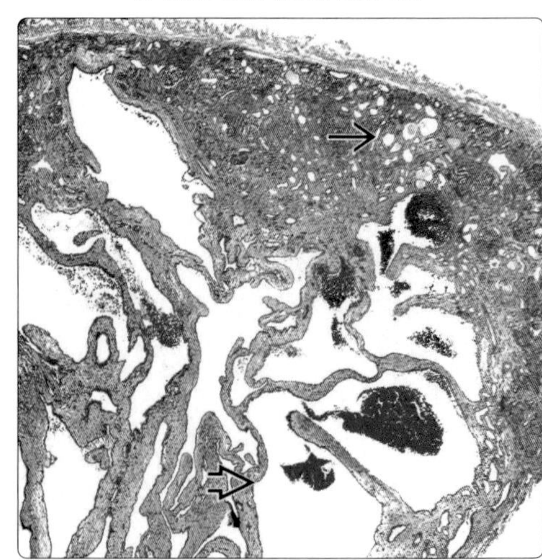

(Left) *This kidney is from a 3 year old with ARPKD. Although the cortex appears well preserved, notice that it is very thin with few nephron generations and there is ectasia of proximal tubules ⇨. There are several rounded ectatic collecting ducts in the cortex and medulla ⇨.* **(Right)** *Kidney from a 3 year old with ARPKD shows mild tubular ectasia ⇨ in an otherwise largely normal superficial cortex. However, there is marked dilation of deep cortical and medullary collecting ducts ⇨.*

Liver With Mild Congenital Hepatic Fibrosis

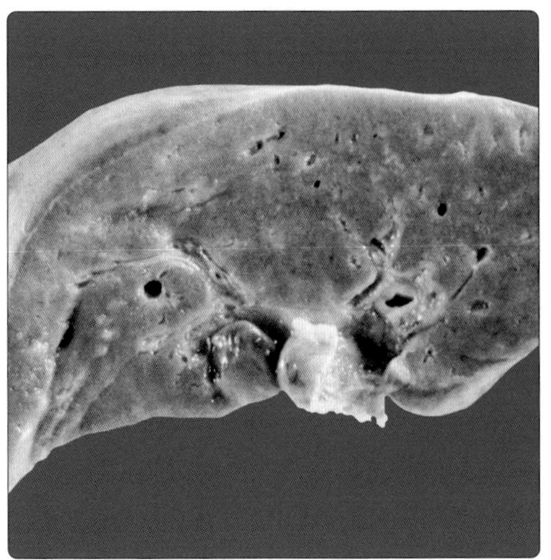

Liver With Congenital Hepatic Fibrosis

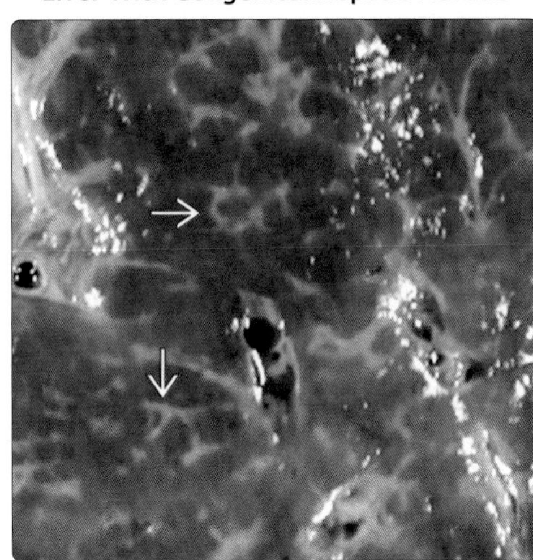

(Left) *This is the liver from a neonate with ARPKD. The cut surface is somewhat pale, rather than red. It has a much firmer texture than normal liver, reflecting the presence of periportal fibrosis. There is subtle portal tract expansion visible.* **(Right)** *This autopsy liver from a 3 year old with ARPKD demonstrates congenital hepatic fibrosis. The liver was grossly very firm. The cut surface shows portal triad to portal triad bridging fibrosis* ➡.

Bile Duct Plate Malformation

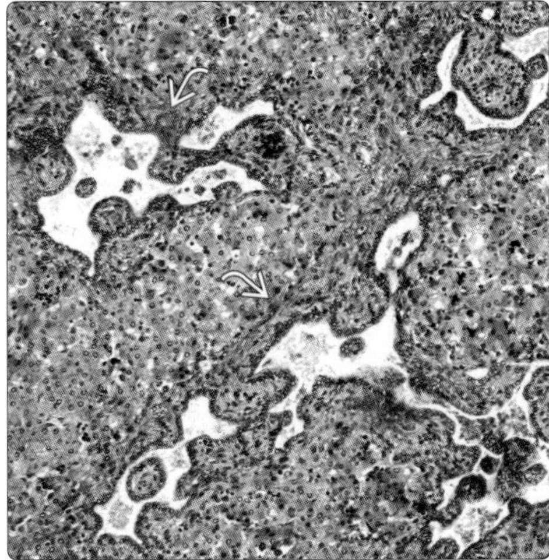

Bile Duct Plate Malformation

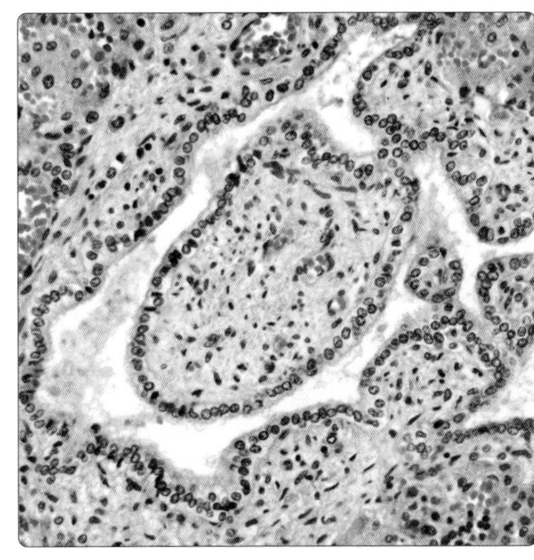

(Left) *Autopsy liver in a case of lethal neonatal ARPKD shows the characteristic bile duct plate malformations. Notice that the bile duct epithelium is cuboidal. The ductules* ➡ *have complex irregular shapes and typically are arrayed at the periphery of the portal triad.* **(Right)** *This portal triad shows a bile duct plate malformation. Rather than the round bile ductules of a normal triad, this duct is markedly irregular with a complex branching conformation. The triad also shows fibrosis.*

Portal Fibrosis

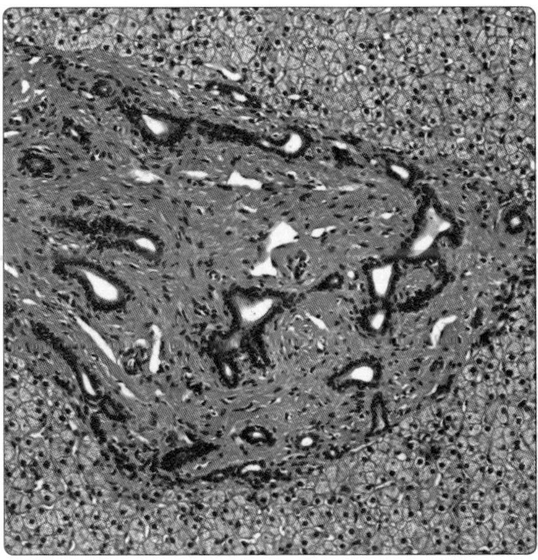

Bridging Portal Fibrosis

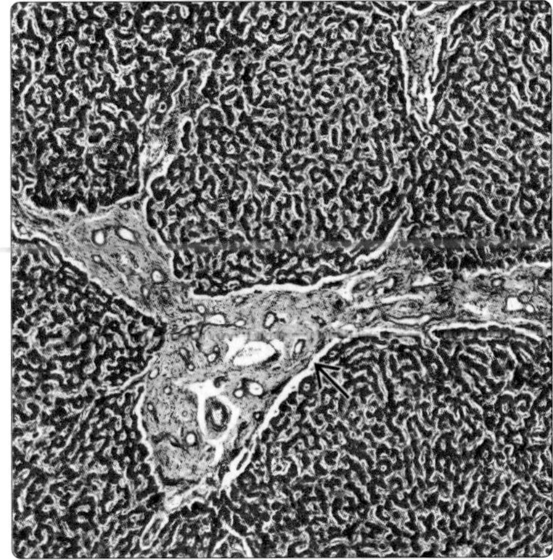

(Left) *ARPKD is found in a three year old presenting with portal hypertension. This portal triad is expanded by dense portal fibrosis. The bile ducts are malformed and more numerous and branched than normal. The hepatocytes are normal.* **(Right)** *Liver of a 3 year old with ARPKD and congenital hepatic fibrosis shows portal triad to portal triad bridging fibrosis* ➡. *There is an increased number of bile ducts throughout the fibrotic portal triad. The hepatocytes are normal.*

Nephronophthisis and Related Ciliopathies

KEY FACTS

TERMINOLOGY

- Autosomal recessive group of inherited renal disorders characterized by tubular atrophy and interstitial fibrosis secondary to mutations in genes encoding proteins of the primary cilium
- Some mutations affect other organs, known as nephronophthisis (NPHP)-related ciliopathies (NPHP-RC) ± affecting kidney

ETIOLOGY/PATHOGENESIS

- Primary cilia are sensory organelles found in almost all cells in vertebrates

CLINICAL ISSUES

- Polyuria, polydipsia, fatigue, anemia, ESRD
- Onset infancy to adolescence
- 15% have extrarenal symptoms (eye, CNS, polydactyly, liver fibrosis)

MICROSCOPIC

- Primarily a tubulointerstitial disease
  - Tubular dilatation, atrophy
  - Tubular atrophy
  - TBM duplication in juvenile and adolescent types
  - Diffuse chronic interstitial inflammation
  - Microcysts in cortex or corticomedullary junction
  - Leakage of uromodulin (Tamm-Horsfall protein)
- Globally sclerosed glomeruli
  - Glomerular cysts in infantile type
- Uromodulin IHC helpful in excluding uromodulin-related kidney disease

TOP DIFFERENTIAL DIAGNOSES

- Autosomal dominant tubuloiinterstitial kidney disease
- Autosomal recessive polycystic kidney disease
- Congenital nephrosis of Finnish type

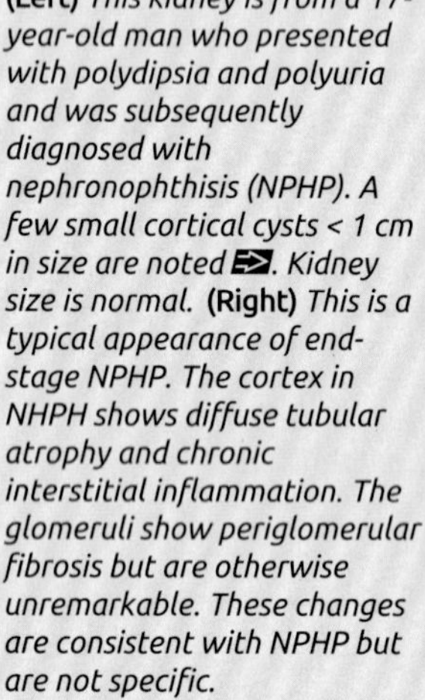

(Left) *This kidney is from a 17-year-old man who presented with polydipsia and polyuria and was subsequently diagnosed with nephronophthisis (NPHP). A few small cortical cysts < 1 cm in size are noted ➡. Kidney size is normal.* **(Right)** *This is a typical appearance of end-stage NPHP. The cortex in NHPH shows diffuse tubular atrophy and chronic interstitial inflammation. The glomeruli show periglomerular fibrosis but are otherwise unremarkable. These changes are consistent with NPHP but are not specific.*

End-Stage NPHP in Adolescent

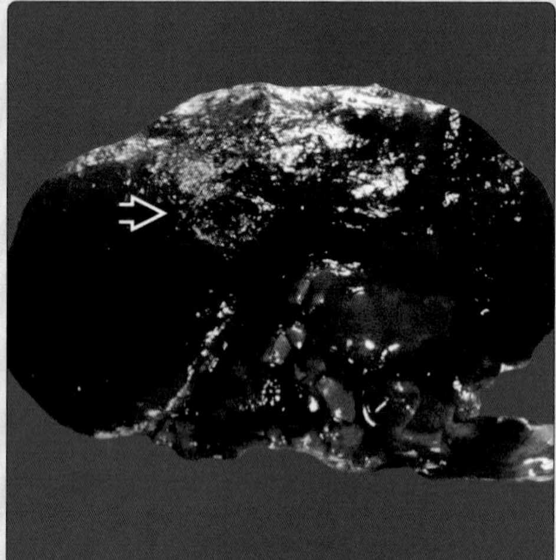

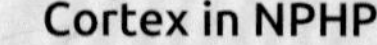

Cortex in NPHP

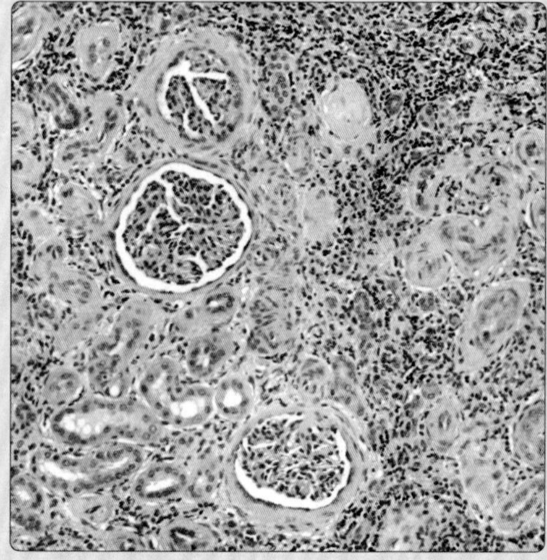

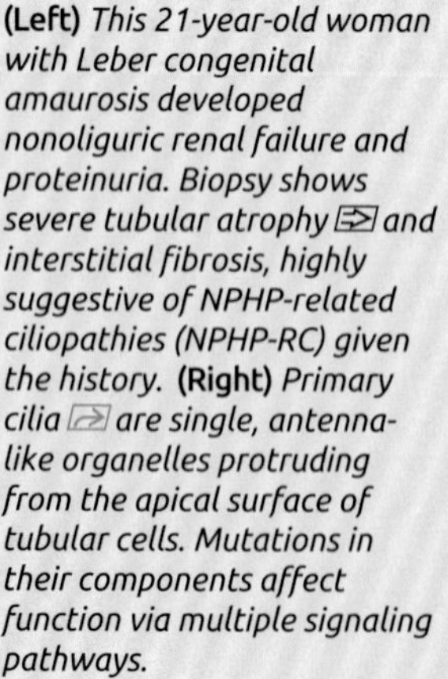

(Left) *This 21-year-old woman with Leber congenital amaurosis developed nonoliguric renal failure and proteinuria. Biopsy shows severe tubular atrophy ➡ and interstitial fibrosis, highly suggestive of NPHP-related ciliopathies (NPHP-RC) given the history.* **(Right)** *Primary cilia ➡ are single, antenna-like organelles protruding from the apical surface of tubular cells. Mutations in their components affect function via multiple signaling pathways.*

TBM Duplication

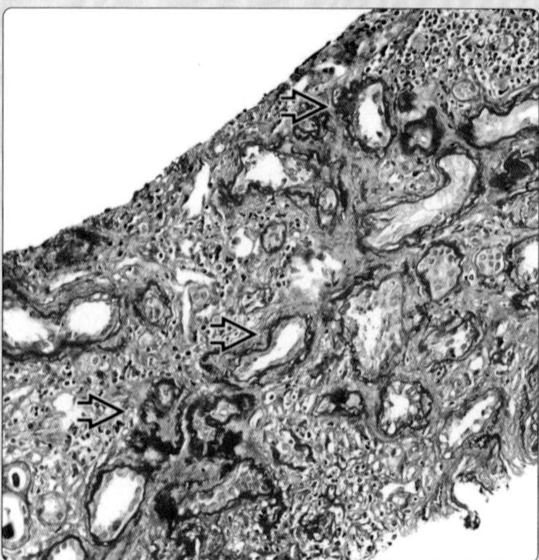

Scanning EM of Primary Cilia

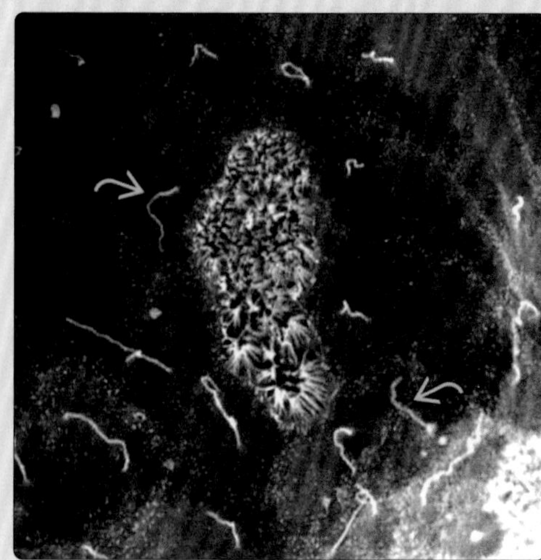

TERMINOLOGY

Abbreviations

- Nephronophthisis (NPHP)

Definitions

- Autosomal recessive group of inherited renal disorders characterized by tubular atrophy and interstitial fibrosis secondary to mutations in genes encoding proteins of primary cilium
- Some mutations affect other organs, known as NPHP-related ciliopathies (NPHP-RC) ± affecting kidney

ETIOLOGY/PATHOGENESIS

Primary Cilia Central in Pathogenesis of NPHP

- All protein products of genes involved in NPHP and NPHP-RC are localized in primary cilia
- Primary cilia are sensory organelles found in almost all cells in vertebrates
  - Primary cilia detect flow, as well as olfactory, chemical, and osmotic stimuli, in contrast to motile cilia drive flow movements
  - Primary cilia consist of basal body and axoneme composed of 9 outer microtubule doublets; motile cilia contain additional inner microtubule doublet
  - In kidney, primary cilia are antenna like, protruding from apical aspect of tubular epithelial cells into tubular lumen
  - Intraciliary transport of proteins takes place within axoneme, also called intraflagellar transport
- Mutations disturb functions of primary cilia in many organs, thus explaining multiorgan involvement
- Genes causing autosomal dominant and recessive polycystic diseases also located in primary cilium

CLINICAL ISSUES

Presentation

- 3 types according to clinical onset
  - Type I: Infantile < 4 years
  - Type II: Juvenile ~ 13 years
  - Type III: Adolescent ~ 19 years
- Polyuria, polydipsia, fatigue, anemia, ESRD
- Majority of patients (~ 85%) have isolated kidney disease
- 15% have extrarenal symptoms
  - Hepatic fibrosis, situs inversus, retinitis pigmentosa, central nervous system (encephalocele, hypopituitarism, vermis aplasia), skeletal anomalies (polydactyly, short ribs, skeletal dysplasia), cardiac defects, ulcerative colitis, bronchiectasis, other neurological abnormalities and attention deficit disorder
- Syndromes with NPHP and other organ involvement
  - Bardet-Biedl (BBS)
    - Retinitis pigmentosa, mental retardation, polydactyly, craniofacial abnormalities
  - Joubert (JS)
    - Developmental delay, muscular hypotonia and ataxia
  - Meckel-Gruber (MGS)
    - Posterior encephalocele, polydactyly, hepatic fibrosis
  - Senior-Loken (SLS)
    - Retinitis pigmentosa

Laboratory Tests

- Genetic testing definitive (next generation, exome sequencing)

Treatment

- Surgical approaches
  - Renal transplantation &/or sequential liver-kidney transplantation is currently treatment of choice

Prognosis

- Prognosis is excellent in patients qualifying for kidney transplantation
- Multiorgan malformations, as in Meckel-Gruber syndrome, are fatal in utero or perinatally
- Loss of function alleles leads to milder disease
- Null mutations likely lead to severe phenotypes
- Emerging evidence suggests that 2nd ciliary gene mutation may affect clinical outcome
- Modifier genes function in conjunction with recessive inheritance patterns

MACROSCOPIC

General Features

- Large kidneys in infantile NPHP
- Small or normal kidneys in juvenile and adolescent NPHP
- Cortical or corticomedullary cysts

MICROSCOPIC

Histologic Features

- Glomeruli
  - Globally sclerosis
  - Glomerular cysts in infantile type
- Tubules
  - Atrophy, dilation
  - Tubular basement membrane duplication in juvenile and adolescent types
  - Microcysts in cortex or corticomedullary junction
- Interstitium
  - Diffuse chronic interstitial inflammation
  - Pools of leaked uromodulin (Tamm-Horsfall protein)

ANCILLARY TESTS

Immunofluorescence

- No specific findings

Electron Microscopy

- Duplication of TBM (nonspecific)

DIFFERENTIAL DIAGNOSIS

Uromodulin, Renin- or MUC1-Related Kidney Disease

- Uromodulin IHC helpful in excluding ADTKD-UROM

Autosomal Recessive Polycystic Kidney Disease

- Prominent cysts and ectatic collecting ducts

Congenital Nephrosis of Finnish Type

- Absent slit diaphragm on EM

Genetic Classification of Ciliopathies Causing Nephronophthisis

Gene (Protein)	Chromosome	ESRD	Clinical Symptoms
NPHP1 (nephrocystin-1)	2q13	~ 13 years	~ 75% isolated kidney disease; retinitis pigmentosa (SLS), oculomotor apraxia (Cogan syndrome)
NPHP3 (nephrocystin-3)	3q22	3-12 years	Situs inversus, liver fibrosis overlap with MGS
NPHP2 (inversion)	9q31	7 months to 5 years	Situs inversus, ventricular septal defect, liver fibrosis
NPHP4 (nephrocystin-4)	1p36	7-33 years	SLS, liver fibrosis, oculomotor apraxia
NPHP5/QCB1 (nephrocystin-5)	3q21	6-47 years	SLS
NPHP6/CEP290 (nephrocystin-6/CEP290)	12q21	2-13 years	Joubert syndrome, MGS
NPHP7/GLIS2 (nephrocystin-7/GLIS2)	16p		NPHP only
NPH8/RPGR1P1L (nephrocystin- 8/RPGRIP1L)	16q	4 months to 17 years	JS, MGS
NPHP9/NEK8 (nephrocystin- 9/NEK8)	17q11	Infants	NPHP only
NPHP10/SDCCAG8 (nephrocystin-10/serologically defined colon cancer antigen 8)	1q44	4-22 years	SLS, obesity (Alstrom syndrome), hypogonadism
NPHP11/TMEM67/MKS3 (nephrocystin-11/Meckelin)	8q22.1	2-22 years	JS, MGS
TTC21B (nephrocystin- *12*/tetratricopeptide repeat-containing hedgehog modulator-1)	2q24.3	Early-onset juvenile	BBS-like, MGS, JS
WDR19/NPHP13 (nephrocystin-13/IFT144)	4p14	Juvenile	BBS-like, Caroli, SLS
ZNF423/NPHP14 (nephrocystin-14/ZNF423)	16q12.1	Infantile	JS, situs inversus
CEP164/NPHP15 (nephrocystin-15/centrosomal protein 164kD)	11q23.3	8-9 years	SLS, JS, hepatic fibrosis
ANKS6/NPHP16 (nephrocystin-16/ ANKS6)	9q22.33	1-4 years	Hepatic fibrosis, situs inversus
IFT172/NPHP17 (nephrocystin-17/IFT172)	2p23.3		JS, Jeune asphyxiating thoracic dysplasia
CEP83/NPHP18 (nephrocystin-18/centrosomal protein 83kD)	12q22	1-4 years	Hydrocephalus, hepatic fibrosis
NPHPL1/XPNPEP3 (nephrocystin-1L/X-prolyl aminopeptidase 3)	22q13	3 to > 29 years	Cardiomyopathy, seizures
NPHP2L/SLC41A1 (nephrocystin-2L/ SLC41A1)	1q32.1		Bronchiectasis
AHI1 (jouberin)	6q23.3	16 to > 20 years	Nephronophthisis, Joubert
CC2D2A (coiled coil and calcium binding protein 2A)	4p15.32		Cerebellar vermis hypoplasia,encephalocele, SLS
MSK1 (mitogen and stress activation protein kinase-1)	17		MGS
ATXN10 (ataxin 10)	19q13.2		Cerebellar aplasia, seizures
B9D2 (B9 containing domain protein 2)	19q13.2		Encephalocele, polydactyly, hepatic fibrosis,

Wolf MT: Nephronophthisis and related syndromes. Curr Opin Pediatr. 27(2):201-11, 2015; Chaki et al: Genotype-phenotype correlation in 440 patients with NPHP-related ciliopathies. Kidney Int 80: 1239, 2011

DIAGNOSTIC CHECKLIST

Clinically Relevant Pathologic Features

- Morphological findings in renal biopsy are nonspecific

Pathologic Interpretation Pearls

- Tubulointerstitial nephritis with TBM thinning or duplication and Tamm-Horsfal pools without lower tract disease in young patients highly suggestive of NHPH
- Should trigger genetic testing in the appropriate clinical scenario

SELECTED REFERENCES

1. Schueler M et al: DCDC2 mutations cause a renal-hepatic ciliopathy by disrupting Wnt signaling. Am J Hum Genet. 96(1):81-92, 2015
2. Wolf MT: Nephronophthisis and related syndromes. Curr Opin Pediatr. 27(2):201-11, 2015
3. Barker AR et al: Meckel-Gruber syndrome and the role of primary cilia in kidney, skeleton, and central nervous system development. Organogenesis. 10(1):96-107, 2014
4. Renkema KY et al: Next-generation sequencing for research and diagnostics in kidney disease. Nat Rev Nephrol. 10(8):433-44, 2014
5. Halbritter J et al: Identification of 99 novel mutations in a worldwide cohort of 1,056 patients with a nephronophthisis-related ciliopathy. Hum Genet. 132(8):865-84, 2013
6. Ronquillo CC et al: Senior-Løken syndrome: a syndromic form of retinal dystrophy associated with nephronophthisis. Vision Res. 75:88-97, 2012
7. Chaki M et al: Genotype-phenotype correlation in 440 patients with NPHP-related ciliopathies. Kidney Int. 80(11):1239-45, 2011
8. Hurd TW et al: Mechanisms of nephronophthisis and related ciliopathies. Nephron Exp Nephrol. 118(1):e9-14, 2011

NPHP Cysts on Ultrasound

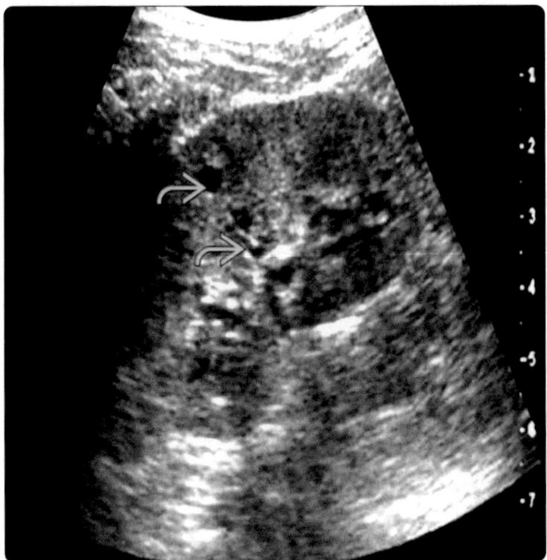

Cysts in NPHP

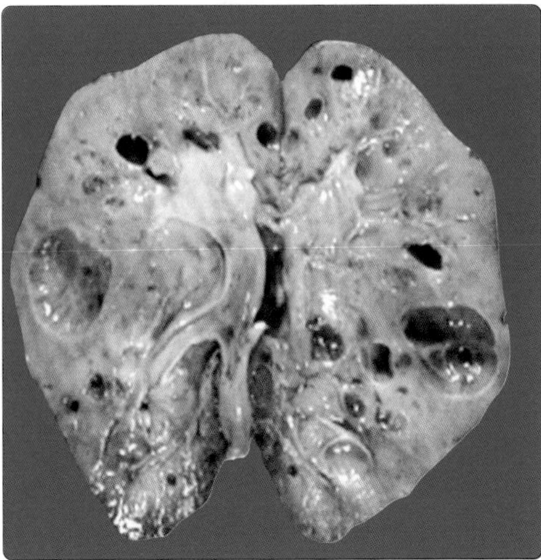

(Left) *Ultrasound in patient with nephronophthisis shows small cortical and corticomedullary cysts ⮫. (Courtesy C. Menias, MD.)* **(Right)** *Kidney from young child with infantile NPHP is shown. The kidney appears edematous and slightly enlarged with prominent corticomedullary cysts. Cysts are not always conspicuous in NPHP.*

NPHP in Child

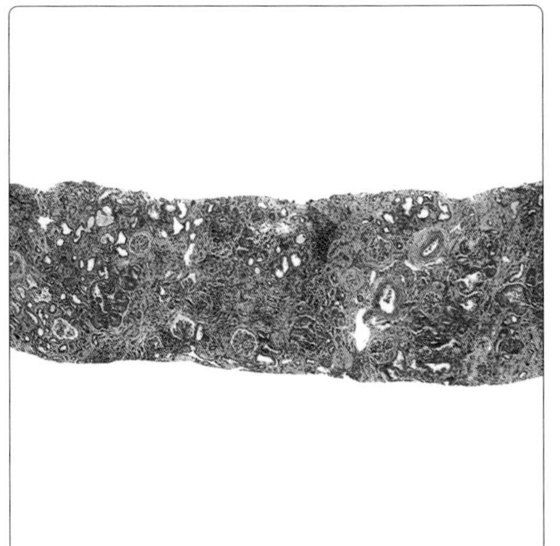

NPHP Due to *NPHP1* Mutation

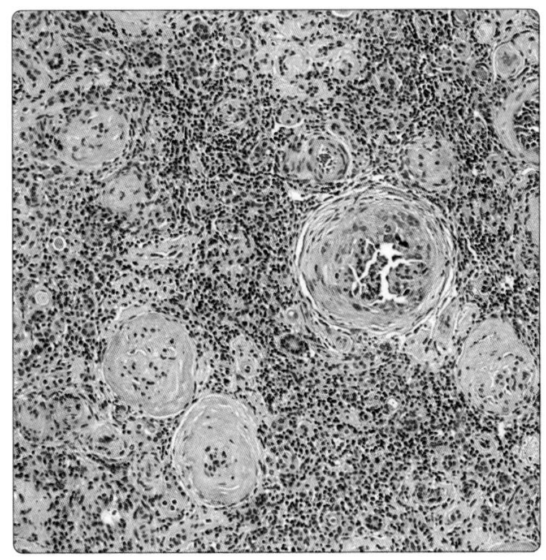

(Left) *H&E from a 4-year-old child with renal biopsy shows marked tubular atrophy, thickening of the TBM, and interstitial inflammation, suggestive of NPHP. The glomeruli are spared. No cysts were evident.* **(Right)** *This nephrectomy from a 7-year-old child shows that most glomeruli are globally sclerosed. The interstitium contains marked chronic inflammation and tubular atrophy consistent with ESRD. The patient was genetically tested and found to have a NPHP1 mutation.*

Cuffing of Tubules

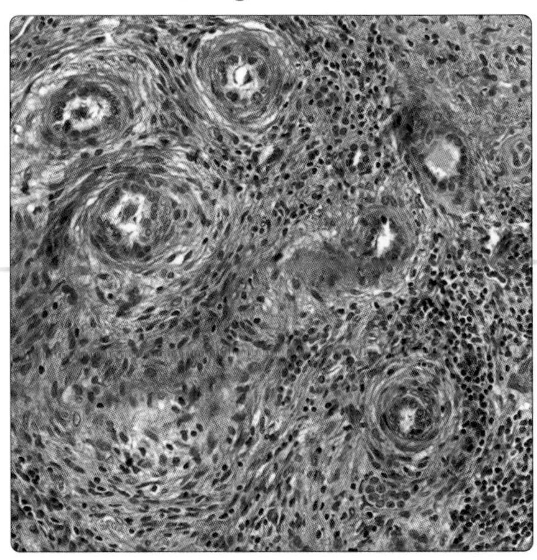

Leakage of Uromodulin Into Interstitium

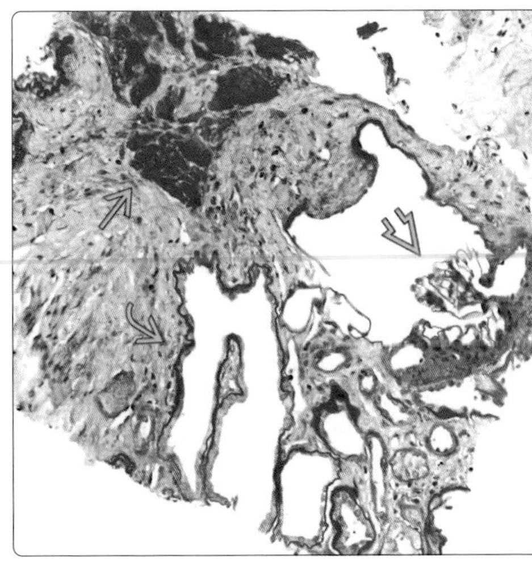

(Left) *Marked peritubular fibroblast proliferation in an adolescent patient with end-stage NPHP is shown.* **(Right)** *In this child with NPHP, leakage of PAS(+) uromodulin (Tamm-Horsfall protein) from tubules into the interstitium can be seen ⮕. This can stimulate an inflammatory reaction. Glomeruli ⮕ and tubules ⮫ are cystic.*

(Left) *An adolescent with NPHP has widespread tubular atrophy and fibrosis with relative sparing of some groups of proximal tubules.* **(Right)** *There is diffuse cortical and medullary inflammation, interstitial fibrosis, tubular atrophy, and scattered hypertrophied tubules. The patient had NPHP1 mutation and attention deficit disorder.*

Sparing of Proximal Tubules in NPHP

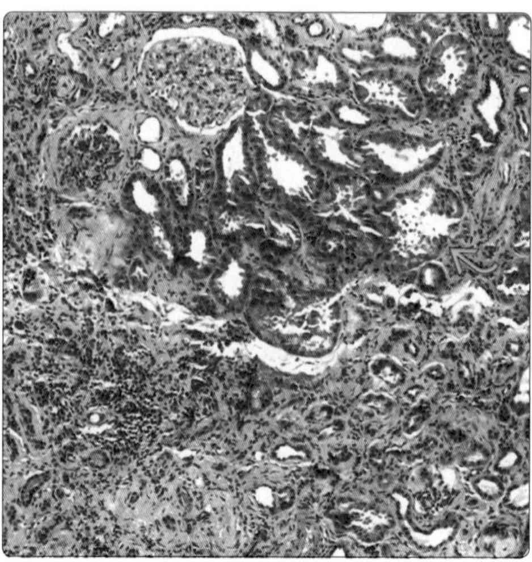

Hypertrophied Proximal Tubules

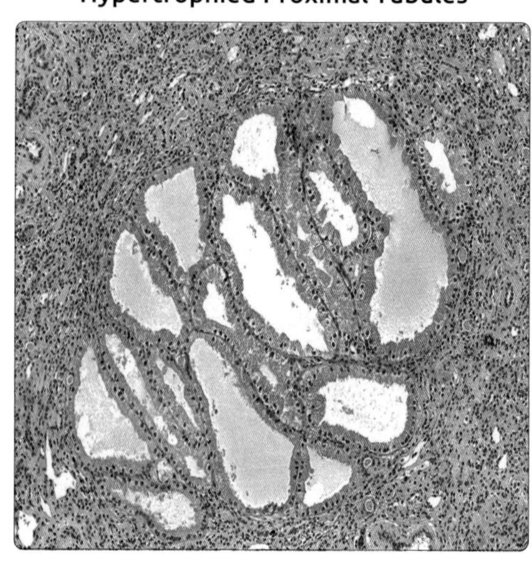

(Left) *Patient with Joubert syndrome has tubular basement membrane duplication highlighted with Jones silver stain. While this is not a specific finding, it is characteristic of this group of diseases.* **(Right)** *Tubular dilation, epithelial cell detachment and thinning, and multilayering of the tubular basement membrane in a child with nephronophthisis is shown.*

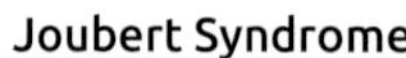

Joubert Syndrome

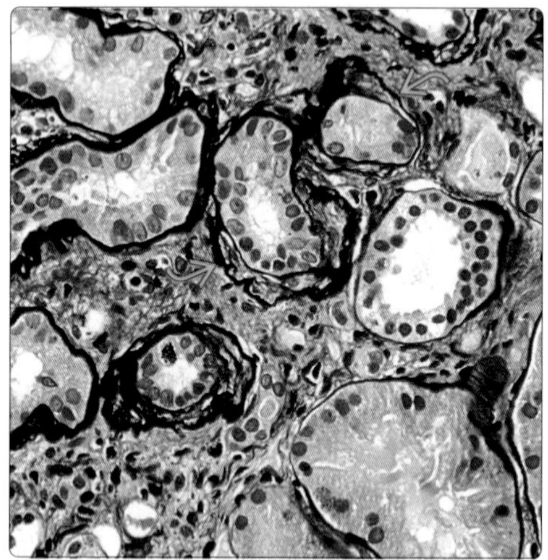

Tubular Cell Detachment and TBM Duplication

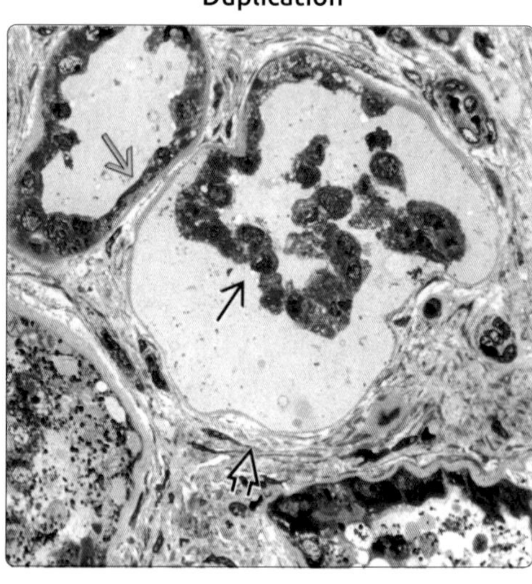

(Left) *A 19-year-old woman with Senior-Løken syndrome (retinitis pigmentosa at age 5) presented with history of hypertension and serum Cr 9.8. Prominent, but nonspecific, thickening and duplication of the TBM is evident.* **(Right)** *The TBM is thick and multilaminated in this case of NPHP with retinitis pigmentosa. The lining epithelium shows degeneration. The adjacent interstitium is fibrotic.*

NPHP in Senior Loken Syndrome

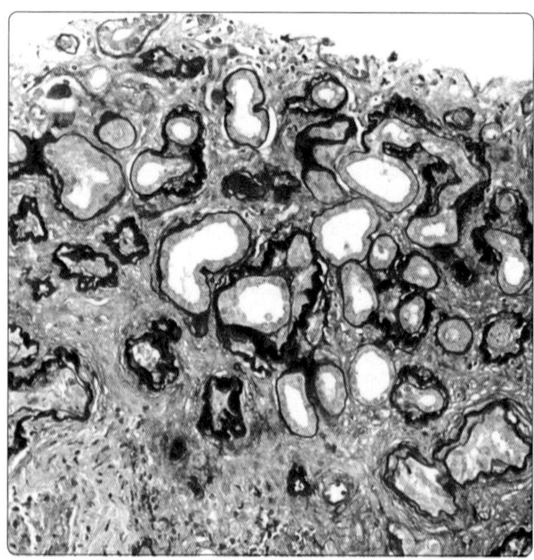

TBM Thickening

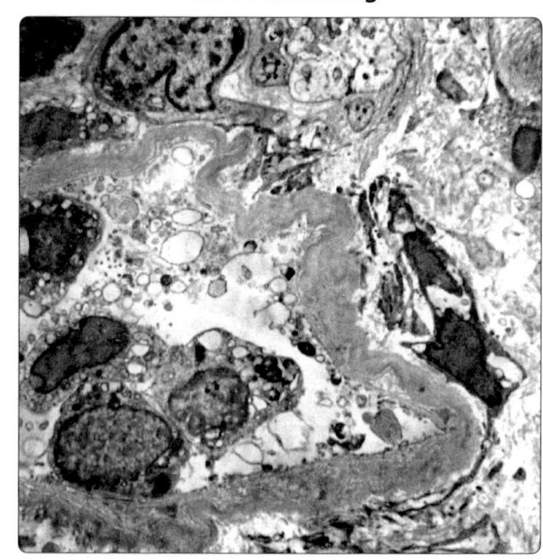

Meckel-Gruber Syndrome

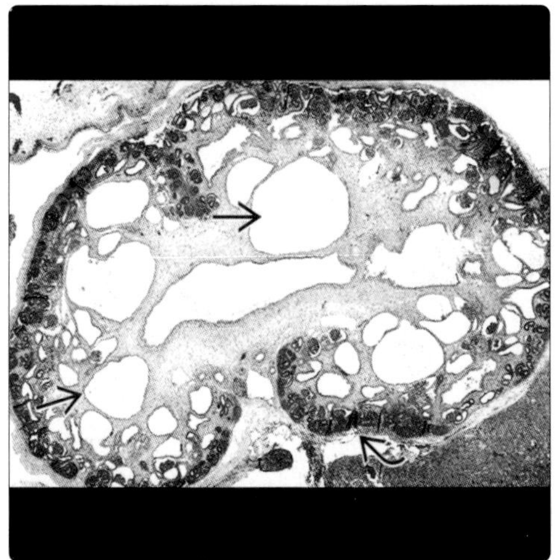

Meckel-Gruber Syndrome

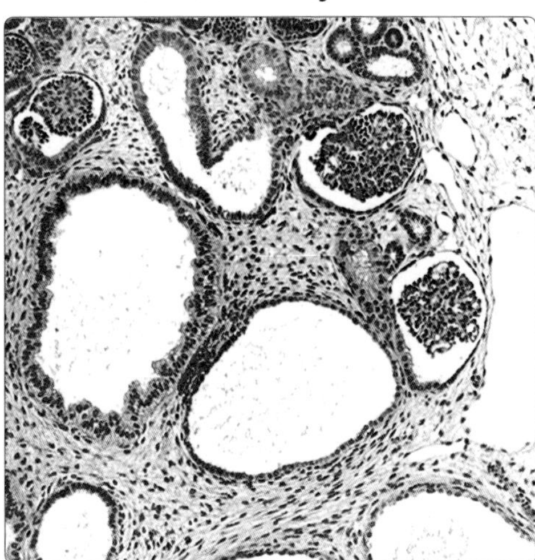

(Left) *A cross section of a kidney from a 12-week-old fetus aborted because of an encephalocele that shows cyst-like dilated collecting ducts ➔ in the medulla and ongoing nephrogenesis ➜ in the outer cortex. Polydactyly was also present.* **(Right)** *High-power view of a kidney from a 12-week-old fetus with an encephalocele and polydactyly shows cyst-like dilated collecting ducts with normal-appearing glomeruli.*

Meckel-Gruber Syndrome

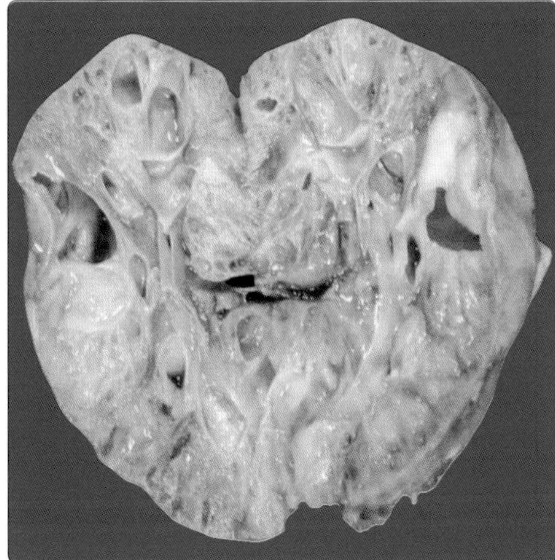

Polydactyly

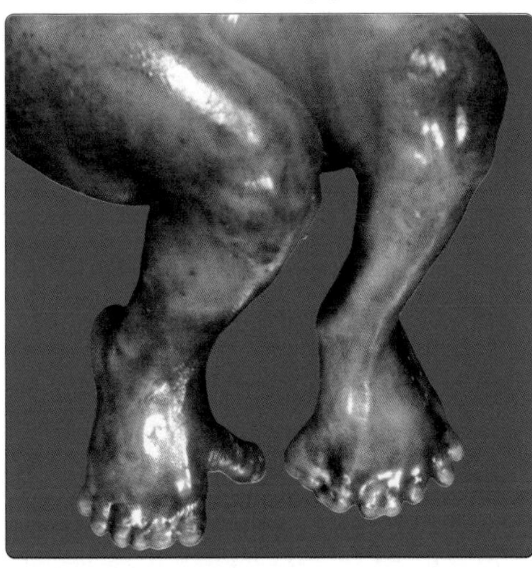

(Left) *A 2-day-old female infant born with multiple anomalies including CNS abnormalities and polydactyly is shown. Both kidneys were enlarged with multiple cortical and medullary cysts. Microscopically, renal dysplasia was found.* **(Right)** *Bilateral polydactyly is one of the complex malformations in Meckel-Gruber syndrome.*

Hepatic Fibrosis

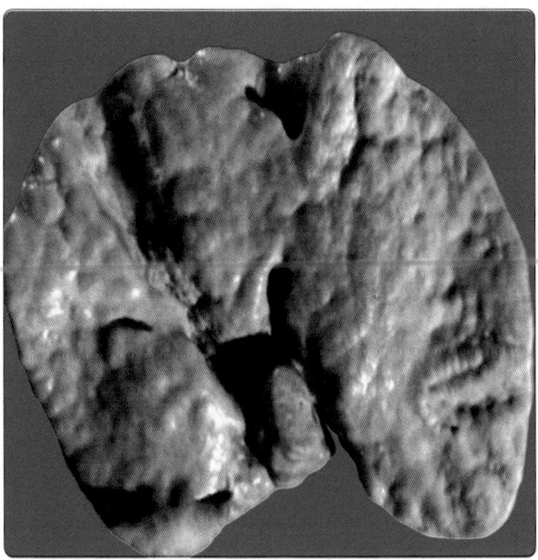

Hepatic Fibrosis

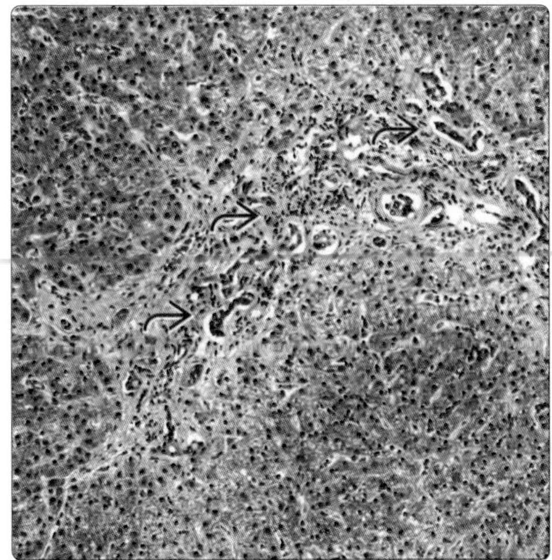

(Left) *The liver is diffusely nodular, diagnostic of cirrhosis. This infant had normal-appearing kidneys and had a family history of NPHP.* **(Right)** *There is bile duct proliferation ➜ without bridging fibrosis, also known as ductal plate malformation.*

KEY FACTS

TERMINOLOGY

- Autosomal dominant familial cancer syndrome due to germline mutation *VHL* gene

ETIOLOGY/PATHOGENESIS

- VHL protein promotes destruction of hypoxia inducible factor 1 alpha via ubiquitin pathway
  - Loss of VHL function leads to increased levels of vascular endothelial growth factor
- 2nd inactivating event predisposes to neoplasms

CLINICAL ISSUES

- Bilateral and multifocal renal cell carcinoma in 40-60%
  - Death from renal cell carcinoma in 50%
- Bilateral and multifocal renal cysts in 70-80%
- Pancreatic cysts in 60-80%
- Hemangioblastoma cerebellum in 60-80%
  - Also retina, spinal cord
- Pheochromocytoma in 10-25%
- Epididymal papillary cystadenoma in 20-50%

MACROSCOPIC

- Multiple cysts with thin yellow lining
- Solid and cystic yellow renal cell carcinomas, sometimes hemorrhagic

MICROSCOPIC

- Cysts lined by clear cells
  - Atypical cysts lined by stratified cells
- Clear cell renal cell carcinoma
  - Cystic or solid

TOP DIFFERENTIAL DIAGNOSES

- Acquired cystic kidney disease
- Tuberous sclerosis/autosomal dominant polycystic kidney disease contiguous gene syndrome
- Dominant polycystic kidney disease

(Left) *This nephrectomy in VHL disease contains numerous variably sized benign renal cysts ⊡. There is also a cystic clear cell renal cell carcinoma ⊡. The benign cyst linings are shiny and translucent. The carcinoma is nodular and yellow with extensive intracystic hemorrhage.* **(Right)** *Renal cyst in VHL is lined by neoplastic clear cells. It also contains a small mural nodule of clear cell renal cell carcinoma. The nuclear grade of the tumor is low, typical of RCCs developing in this disease.*

Multiple Cysts and Renal Cell Carcinoma

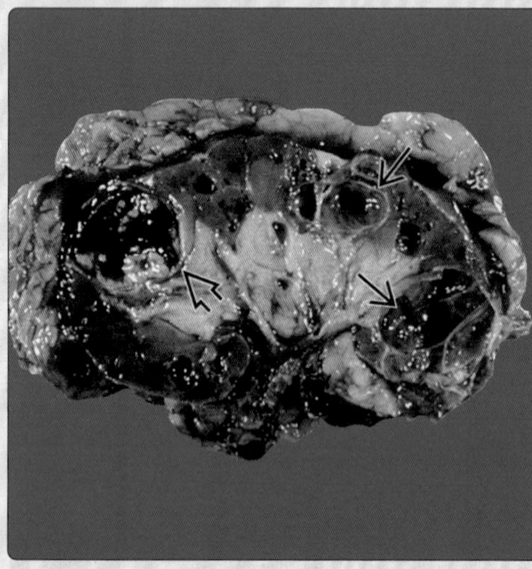

Cyst With Mural Nodule of Renal Cell Carcinoma

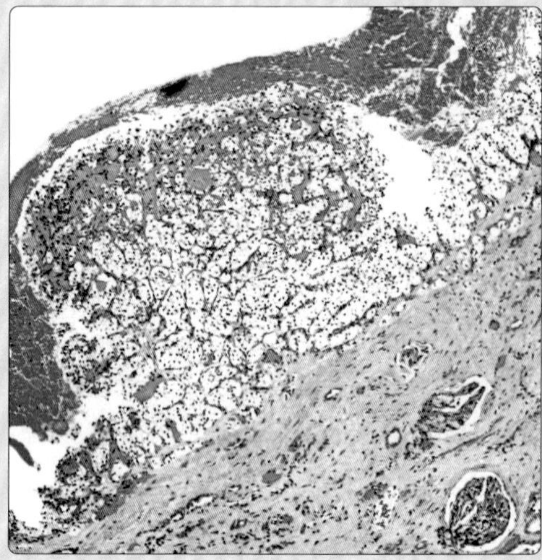

(Left) *This cyst in VHL disease is lined by a single layer of inconspicuous clear cells ⊡. The cells are small and have low-grade nuclei. The cyst is surrounded by a fibrous pseudocapsule ⊡. If a solid nest of clear cells was present then this would be classified as a clear cell renal cell carcinoma.* **(Right)** *This cyst in VHL disease is lined by clear cells that show stratification ⊡. Such cysts have often been referred to as atypical cysts and are believed to be a precursor lesion for clear cell renal cell carcinoma.*

Clear Cell-Lined Cysts

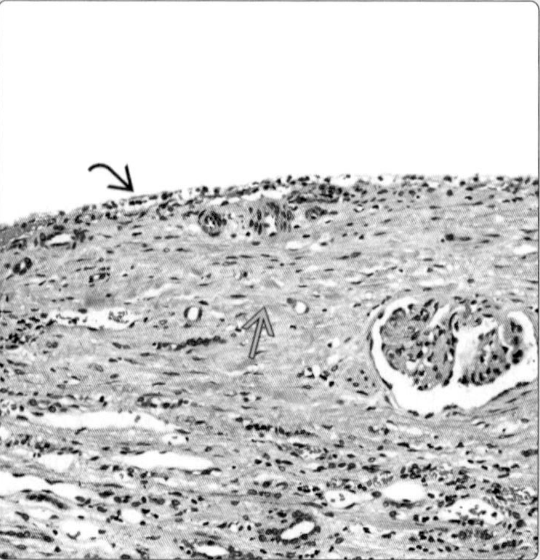

Clear Cell-Lined Cysts

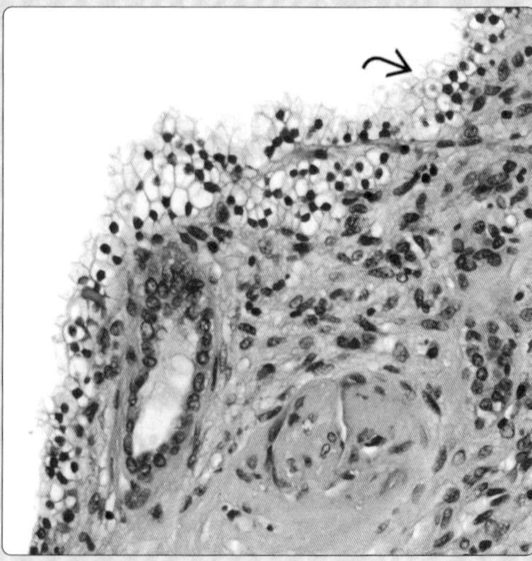

TERMINOLOGY

Abbreviations

- von Hippel-Lindau (VHL) disease

Definitions

- Germline mutation of *VHL* tumor suppressor gene
- Member of phacomatosis familial cancer syndromes
- Diagnosis requires
  - 2 cardinal manifestations, including retinal or CNS disease if no family history, **or**
  - 1 cardinal manifestation, if positive family history

ETIOLOGY/PATHOGENESIS

Molecular Genetics

- Autosomal dominant
- Germline mutation of *VHL* gene, 3p25-26
  - Also present in 50% of sporadic renal cell carcinoma
  - 2nd inactivating event predisposes to neoplasms
- VHL protein
  - Promotes destruction of hypoxia inducible factor 1 alpha (HIF-1-α) via ubiquitin pathway
    - Loss of function leads to increased levels of vascular endothelial growth factor
  - HIF independent regulation of primary cilium and apoptosis via factors NF-kB
    - Loss of function promotes renal cysts
- Genotype-phenotype correlations
  - Type 1 VHL (truncating and exon deletions)
    - Low risk of pheochromocytoma
  - Type 2 VHL (missense mutations)
    - High risk of pheochromocytoma
    - Type 2a: Low risk of RCC
    - Type 2b: High risk of RCC
    - Type 2c: Familial pheochromocytoma without hemangioblastoma or RCC

CLINICAL ISSUES

Epidemiology

- Incidence
  - 1:36,000 live births
  - 90% penetrance by age 65
  - Mean age of renal involvement: 35-40 years

Presentation

- Clear cell renal cell carcinoma (RCC)
  - Bilateral and multifocal in 40-60%
  - Hematuria ± back pain
- Renal cysts
  - Bilateral and multifocal in 70-80%
- Hemangioblastoma is most frequent lesion in VHL
  - Cerebellum in 60-80%
  - Retina in 50-60%
  - Spinal cord in 15-60%
- Pheochromocytoma in 10-25%
- Pancreatic cysts in 60-80%
- Epididymal papillary cystadenoma in 20-50%

Treatment

- Surgical approaches
  - Nephron-sparing surgery
  - Tumor resection when other organs affected

Prognosis

- Death due to metastatic renal cell carcinoma in 50%

MACROSCOPIC

General Features

- Multiple and bilateral cysts
- Multiple and bilateral cystic or solid renal cell carcinomas

MICROSCOPIC

Histologic Features

- Clear cell-lined cysts
  - Benign cyst lined by single cell layer
  - Atypical cysts lined by piled up or stratified cells
- Clear cell renal cell carcinoma
  - Multicystic or solid tumors

DIFFERENTIAL DIAGNOSIS

Cystic Renal Diseases Associated With Renal Neoplasms

- Acquired cystic kidney disease
  - Cyst frequency proportional to duration of ESRD
  - Diverse array of renal cell carcinomas
- Tuberous sclerosis complex/autosomal dominant polycystic kidney disease contiguous gene syndrome
  - Diffusely cystic kidneys identical to ADPKD
  - Multiple and bilateral angiomyolipomas
  - Rarely, renal cell carcinoma
- Autosomal dominant polycystic kidney disease
  - Risk of renal cell carcinoma may be increased
  - Cysts are far more numerous than in VHL

DIAGNOSTIC CHECKLIST

Pathologic Interpretation Pearls

- Bilateral renal cysts and liver cysts: Think ADPKD
- Bilateral renal cysts and pancreatic cysts: Think VHL

SELECTED REFERENCES

1. Hosseini M et al: Pathologic spectrum of cysts in end-stage kidneys: possible precursors to renal neoplasia. Hum Pathol. 45(7):1406-13, 2014
2. Maher ER et al: von Hippel-Lindau disease: a clinical and scientific review. Eur J Hum Genet. 19(6):617-23, 2011
3. Moch H: Cystic renal tumors: new entities and novel concepts. Adv Anat Pathol. 17(3):209-14, 2010
4. Bonsib SM: Renal cystic diseases and renal neoplasms: a mini-review. Clin J Am Soc Nephrol. 4(12):1998-2007, 2009
5. Shehata BM et al: Von Hippel-Lindau (VHL) disease: an update on the clinico-pathologic and genetic aspects. Adv Anat Pathol. 15(3):165-71, 2008
6. Salomé F et al: Renal lesions in Von Hippel-Lindau disease: the benign, the malignant, the unknown. Eur Urol. 34(5):383-92, 1998
7. Neumann HP et al: Renal cysts, renal cancer and von Hippel-Lindau disease. Kidney Int. 51(1):16-26, 1997
8. Chauveau D et al: Renal involvement in von Hippel-Lindau disease. Kidney Int. 50(3):944-51, 1996
9. Solomon D et al: Renal pathology in von Hippel-Lindau disease. Hum Pathol. 19(9):1072-9, 1988

Cyst With Hemorrhage, Likely Renal Cell Carcinoma

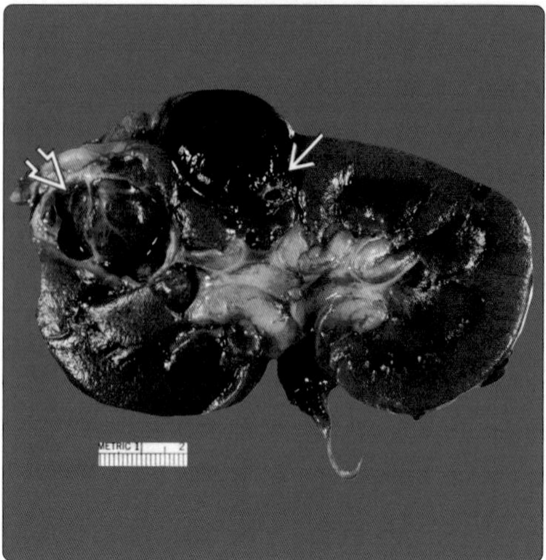

Multiple Renal Cell Carcinomas

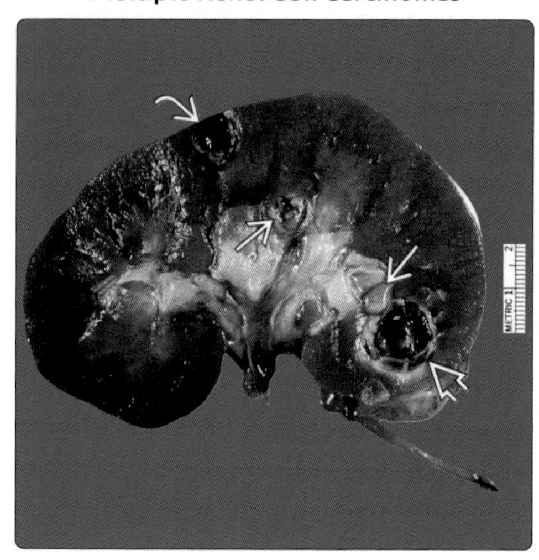

(Left) *Bivalved kidney from a patient with VHL disease contains 2 cystic lesions. One is multicystic with thin, translucent cyst septa indicative of a benign lesion. The other one has a small yellow nodule and is filled with hemorrhage. This lesion is a renal cell carcinoma.* **(Right)** *This kidney shows cysts and 2 small, solid clear cell renal cell carcinomas. The smaller cyst is benign and contains blood. The larger cyst contains blood but also has yellow nodules representing a clear cell renal cell carcinoma.*

Clear Cell-Lined Cyst

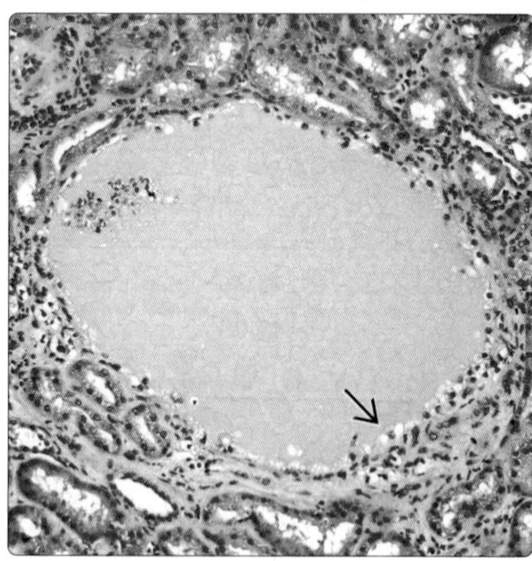

Clear Cell-Lined Cyst

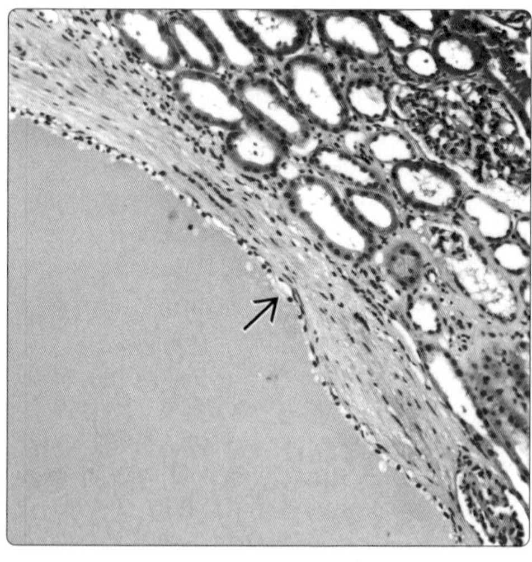

(Left) *This is a small 1 mm benign cyst. In contrast to simple cortical cysts common in adult kidneys, this cyst is lined by cells with complete cytoplasmic clearing and low-grade nuclear features. The lack of stratification qualifies this cyst as benign.* **(Right)** *This is a portion of a benign 2 cm cyst in VHL. The cyst is lined by a single layer of clear cells and has a thin fibrous pseudocapsule. The cells have low-grade nuclear features. Additional cysts and several renal cell carcinomas were present elsewhere.*

Clear Cell-Lined Cyst

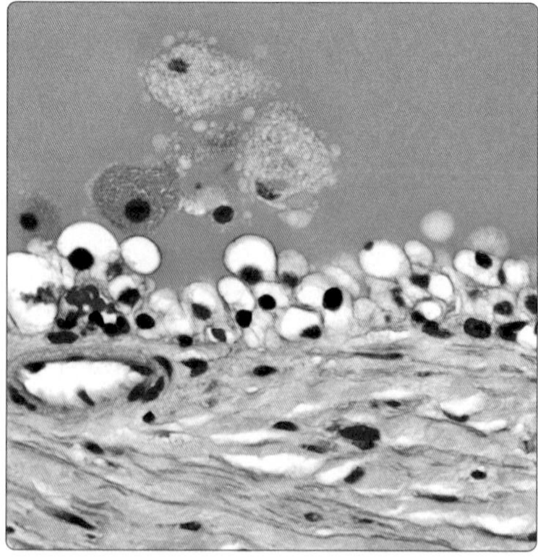

Microscopic Clear Cell Renal Cell Carcinoma

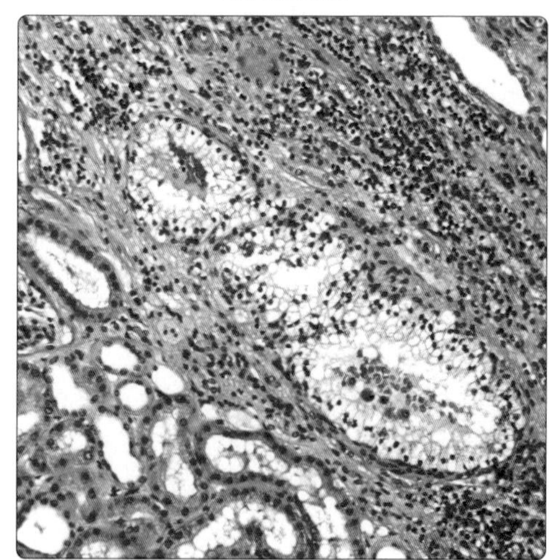

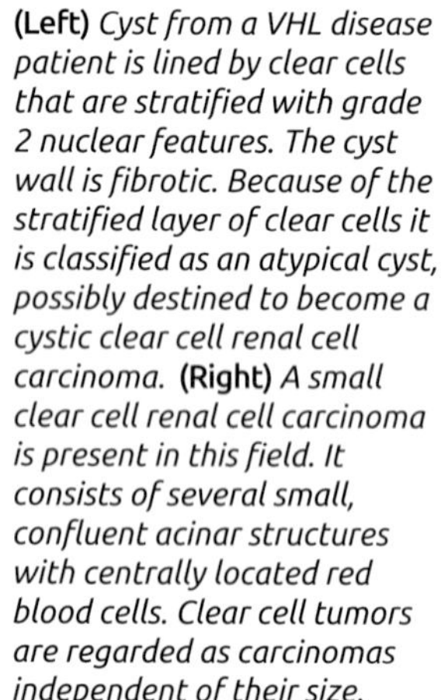

(Left) *Cyst from a VHL disease patient is lined by clear cells that are stratified with grade 2 nuclear features. The cyst wall is fibrotic. Because of the stratified layer of clear cells it is classified as an atypical cyst, possibly destined to become a cystic clear cell renal cell carcinoma.* **(Right)** *A small clear cell renal cell carcinoma is present in this field. It consists of several small, confluent acinar structures with centrally located red blood cells. Clear cell tumors are regarded as carcinomas independent of their size.*

Involuting Renal Cell Carcinoma

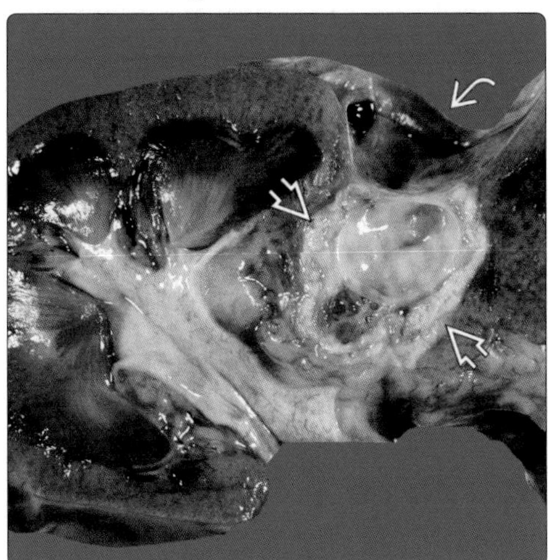

Cystic Hemorrhagic Renal Cell Carcinoma

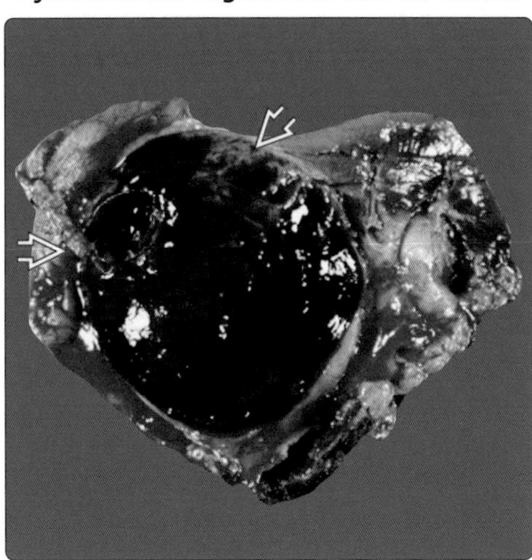

(Left) *This VHL disease patient has 2 cystic lesions. One is a large, superficial, collapsed cyst ➡. The other lesion is associated with prominent sclerosis ➡ and contains a central cyst. The sclerotic areas harbored nests of clear cells, indicating the presence of renal cell carcinoma.* **(Right)** *Nephron-sparing partial nephrectomy in VHL disease contains a renal cell carcinoma. Notice the small yellow nodules of tumor ➡ associated with extensive hemorrhage. Other RCCs were previously resected in this patient.*

Multiple Renal Cell Carcinomas

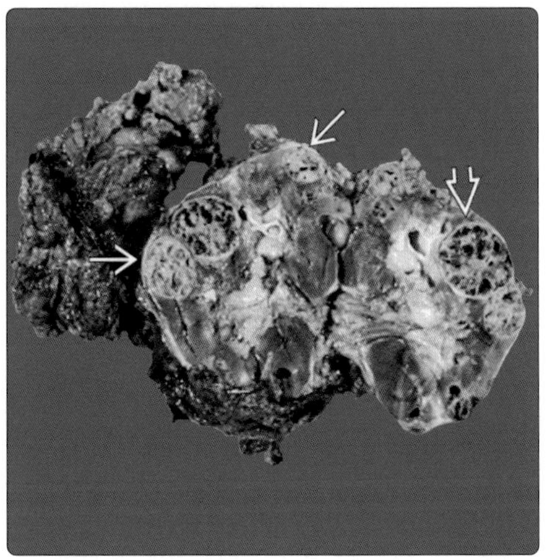

Cystic Clear Cell Renal Cell Carcinoma

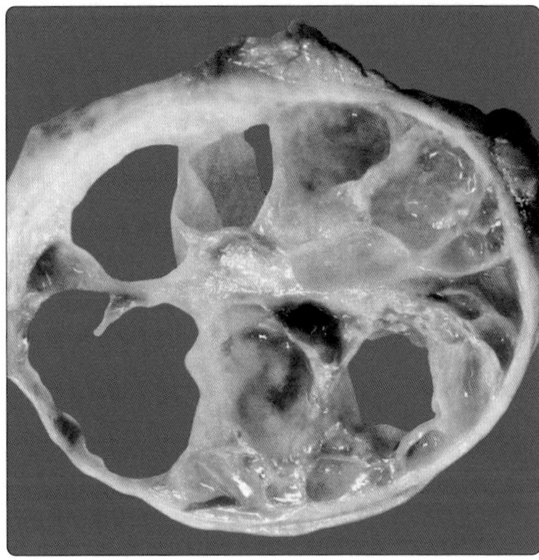

(Left) *This bivalved kidney in VHL disease contains multiple renal cell carcinomas and benign renal cysts. Two of the carcinomas ➡ have both solid and cystic areas and appear yellow. The 3rd carcinoma ➡ is also cystic and yellow but contains hemorrhage.* **(Right)** *This cystic clear cell renal cell carcinoma was 1 of 3 similar tumors in a 28-year-old patient with VHL disease. It appears yellow because the clear cells have a high lipid content. All 3 carcinomas were very cystic and all 3 tumors were renal-limited.*

Cystic Involuting Renal cell Carcinoma

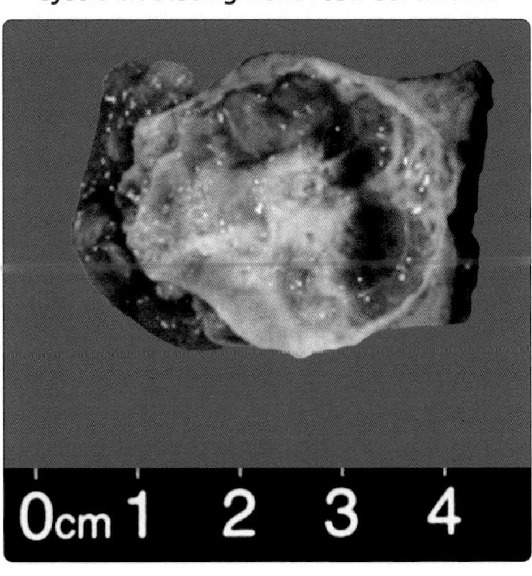

Clear Cell Renal Cell Carcinoma

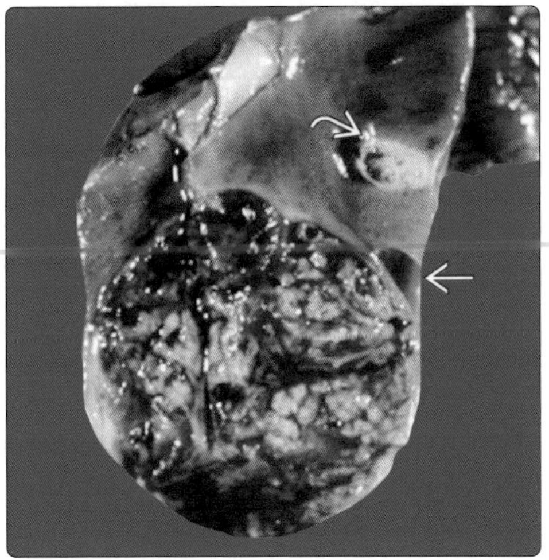

(Left) *This is a partial nephrectomy in a patient with VHL and multiple renal cell carcinomas elsewhere. This particular carcinoma is cystic with sclerotic areas. The sclerosis is a regressive feature and correlates with a low volume of tumor cells.* **(Right)** *This is from a VHL disease patient treated with a partial nephrectomy for multiple renal tumors. Multiple small nodules of clear cell renal cell carcinoma are visible within this hemorrhagic tumor. There is also a small cyst ➡ and a sclerotic lesion that could represent another RCC ➡.*

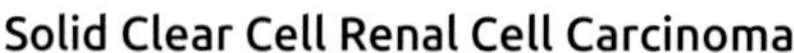

Solid Clear Cell Renal Cell Carcinoma

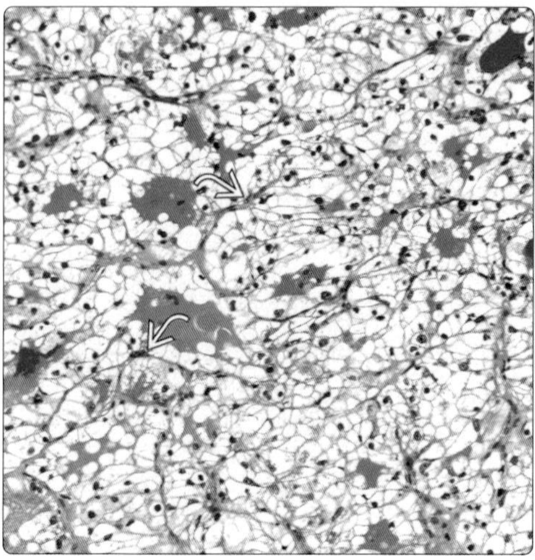

Clear Cell Renal Cell Carcinoma

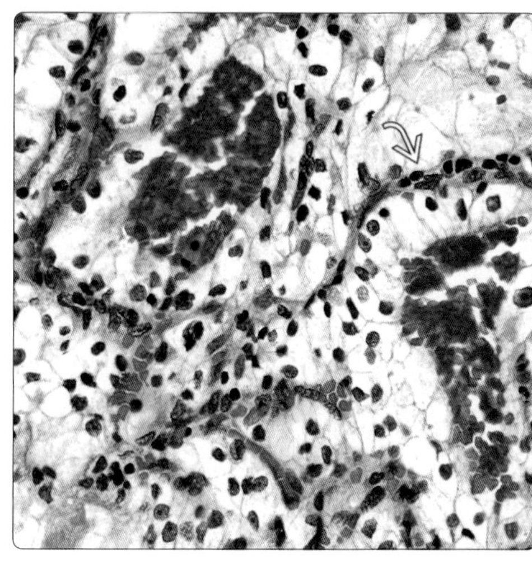

(Left) *This is a solid clear cell renal cell carcinoma in a VHL disease patient. As is typical for a clear cell RCC, this tumor contains a delicate capillary vascular plexus ➔. The tumor cells are arranged in nests and acini and have Fuhrman grade 1 and 2 nuclei.* **(Right)** *Low-grade, nuclear grade 2, clear cell renal cell carcinoma shows the typical delicate vascular capillary plexus ➔ investing the clear cell-lined acini. There is hemorrhage in the acini centers, a common finding in these vascular neoplasms.*

Solid Area in Cystic RCC

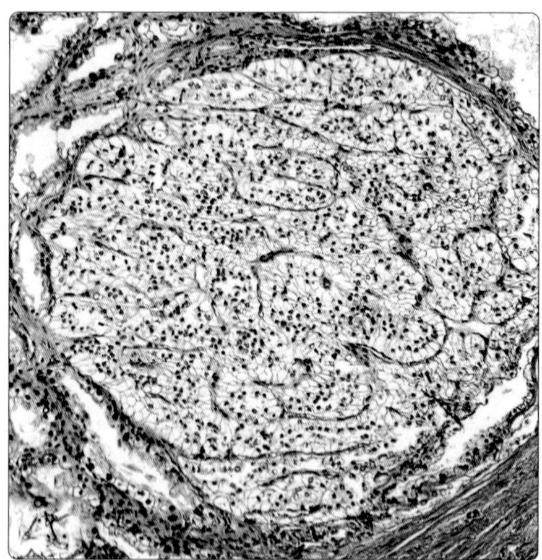

Cystic Clear Cell Renal Cell Carcinoma

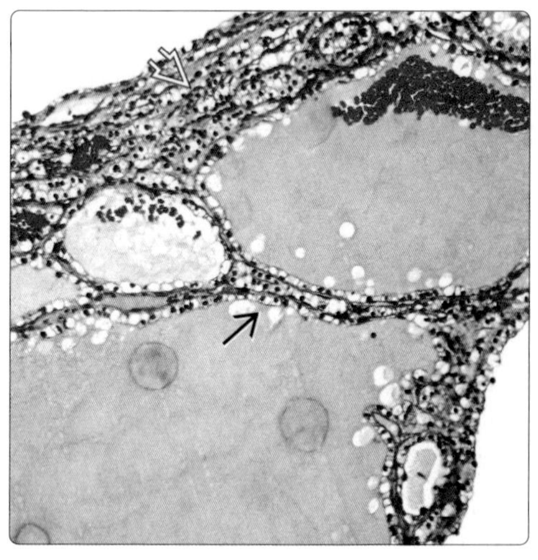

(Left) *This solid nodule of clear cell RCC was present within an extensively cystic cancer. Notice the low nuclear grade with uniform-appearing nuclei. The linear array of nuclei raises the possibility of clear cell papillary RCC, a tumor recently described in VHL disease that lacks the 3p deletions and VHL gene mutations of clear cell RCC.* **(Right)** *This is a cystic clear cell renal cell carcinoma. The cells lining the cystic spaces ➔ and the cells within ➔ the septa appear identical. The solid areas qualify this lesion as a renal cell carcinoma.*

Clear Cell Renal Cell Carcinoma

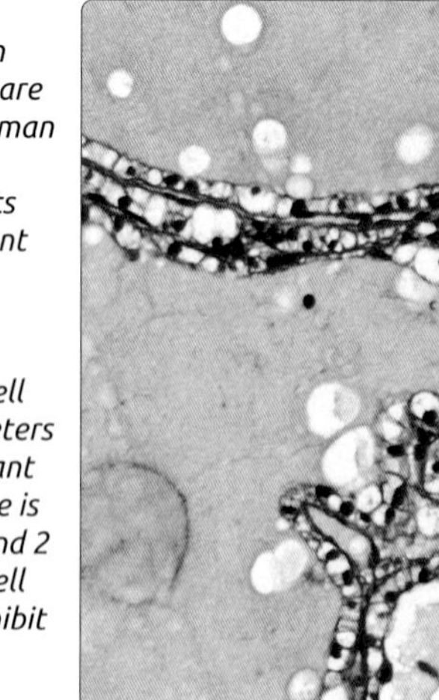

Clear Cell Renal Cell Carcinoma and Cyst

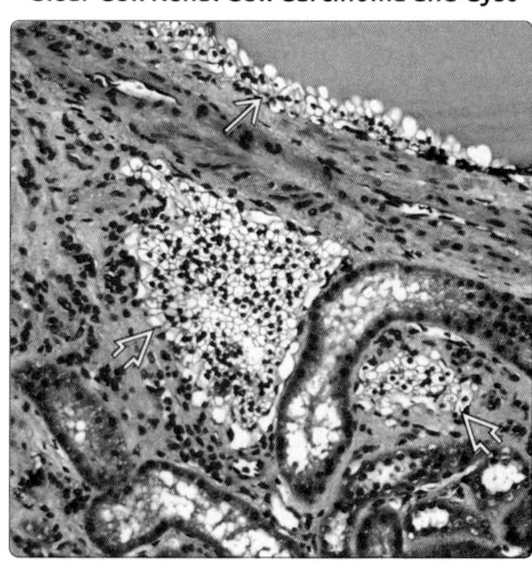

(Left) *Clear cell renal cell carcinomas that develop in patients with VHL disease are often low grade with Fuhrman nuclear grade 1 or 2. The cytoplasmic clearing results from extraction of abundant lipid and glycogen, characteristic of clear cell carcinomas.* **(Right)** *This kidney contained a clear cell carcinoma several centimeters in size. In this section, distant from the main tumor, there is a clear cell-lined cyst ➔ and 2 small solid nests of clear cell carcinoma ➔. All cells exhibit a low nuclear grade.*

Pancreatic Cysts

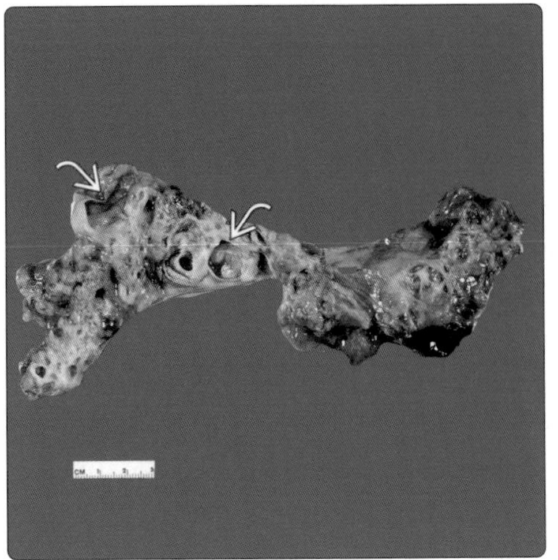

Pancreatic Cysts

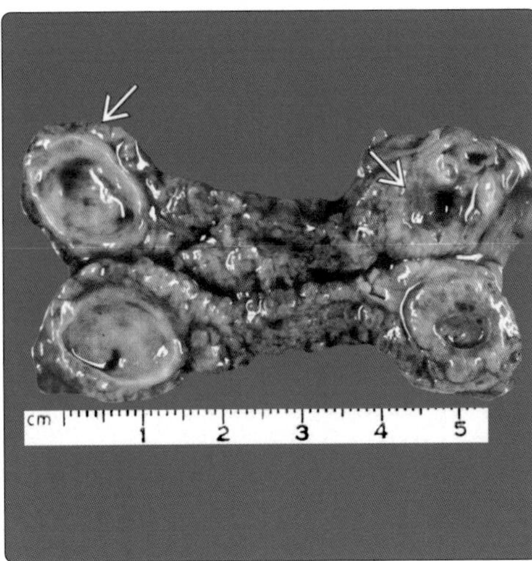

(Left) *This is the pancreas from an autopsy in a patient with VHL disease. The pancreas is diffusely affected by benign cysts ➨. The endocrine function of this gland was unaffected by the cysts. There are no solid tumor nodules present.* **(Right)** *Bivalved pancreas from an autopsied patient with VHL disease contains 2 dominant cysts ➨. There are also several smaller cysts, more difficult to appreciate in this photograph. The central portions of the pancreas appear grossly normal.*

Pancreatic Cysts

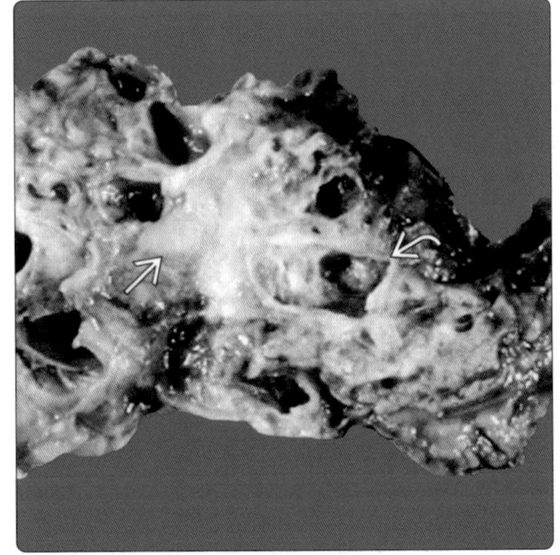

Pancreatic Cysts

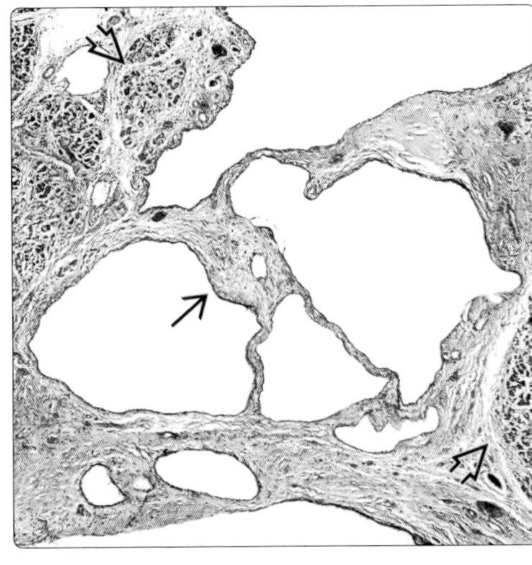

(Left) *Pancreas from an autopsied patient with VHL disease is severely affected. It shows numerous variably sized cysts ➨ and extensive areas of sclerosis ➨; however, no neoplasms were present.* **(Right)** *This is the pancreas from an autopsied patient with VHL disease. The normal pancreatic parenchyma is visible at the edges ➨. The cysts are derived from the pancreatic duct system and lined by a single layer of benign cuboidal duct epithelium ➨ Clear cells do not line the cysts as they do in kidney cysts in VHL disease.*

Pheochromocytoma

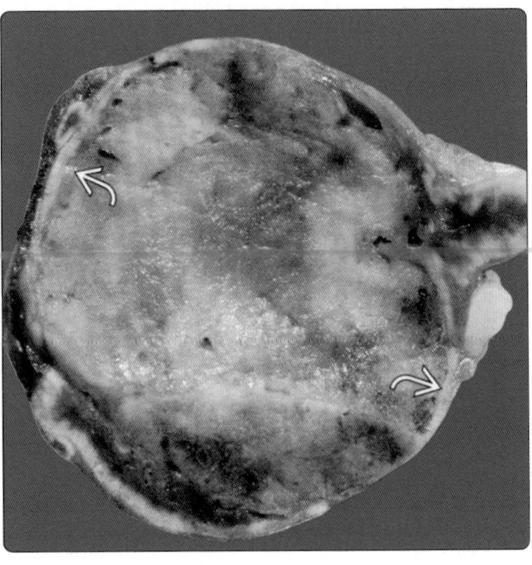

Pheochromocytoma

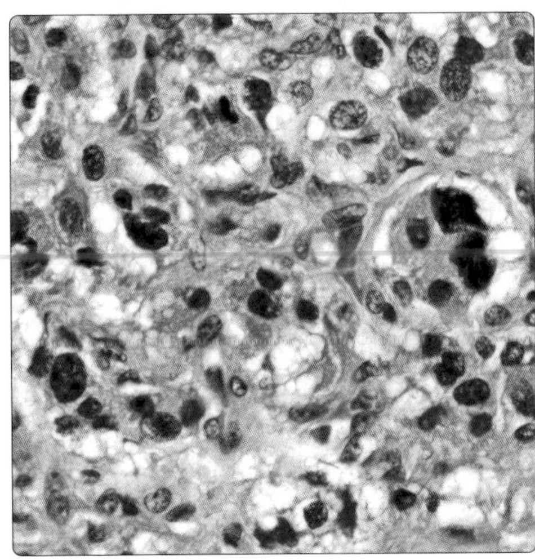

(Left) *This is a pheochromocytoma in a patient with VHL disease. Notice the thin yellow rim ➨ of normal but attenuated adrenal cortex. It was resected along with 3 cystic clear cell RCCs. This combination of findings led to a previously unsuspected diagnosis of VHL disease.* **(Right)** *The cells of a pheochromocytoma can show an extreme degree of nuclear pleomorphism. However, severe nuclear atypia does not indicate malignancy, which is based upon tumor size, presence of necrosis, and invasive behavior.*

Tuberous Sclerosis Complex

KEY FACTS

ETIOLOGY/PATHOGENESIS

- *TSC1* gene, chromosome 9q34: Hamartin
- *TSC2* gene, chromosome 16p13: Tuberin
- Chromosome 16p deletion may result in *TSC2/PKD1* contiguous gene syndrome with early-onset PKD

CLINICAL ISSUES

- Major features
  - Facial angiofibromas, ungual fibroma, shagreen patch, hypomelanotic macules
  - Cortical tuber, subependymal nodule, subependymal giant cell tumor, retinal hamartoma
  - Cardiac rhabdomyoma, renal angiomyolipoma, lymphangioleiomyomatosis
- Minor features
  - Multiple pits in dental enamel, hamartomatous rectal polyps, bone cysts, cerebral white-matter radial migration lines, gingival fibromas, retinal achromic patch, "confetti" skin lesions, multiple renal cysts
- Extreme variability in nature and profile of organ involvement, manifesting over broad age range

MICROSCOPIC

- Multiple and bilateral
  - Angiomyolipomas (45-80%)
  - Cysts (20-30%) and polycystic kidney disease (< 5%)
  - Renal cell carcinoma (2-4%) and oncocytoma (rare)
- Angiomyolipomas and angiomyolipomatous change of renal parenchyma is most common renal finding
- Cysts lined by large plump cells with deeply eosinophilic cytoplasm are characteristic of TSC
- PKD in young pediatric patients sometimes associated with features of metanephric dysgenesis

TOP DIFFERENTIAL DIAGNOSES

- Autosomal dominant polycystic kidney disease
- von Hippel-Lindau disease
- Multicystic dysplasia

(Left) *Cross section of a kidney from a patient with tuberous sclerosis is shown. An angiomyolipoma, many cysts of various sizes, and a renal cell carcinoma are all typical lesions in TSC. Cysts and tumors are often multiple and bilateral.* **(Right)** *Angiomyolipoma in tuberous sclerosis is shown, with all 3 histological components of the tumor, including fat, smooth muscle, and blood vessels. Angiomyolipomas can range from large grossly visible tumors to microscopic tumors.*

Cysts and Tumors

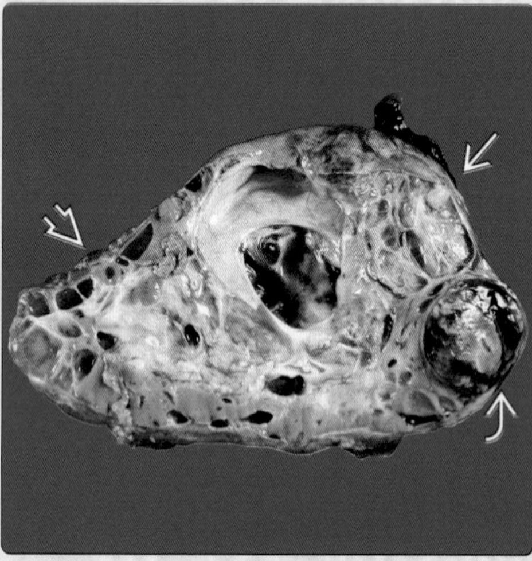

Angiomyolipoma

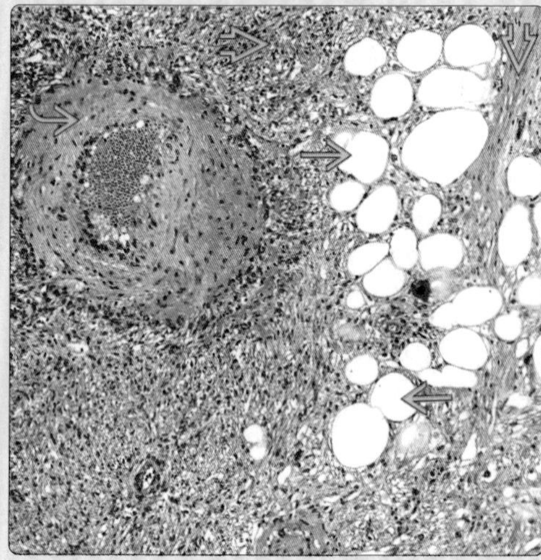

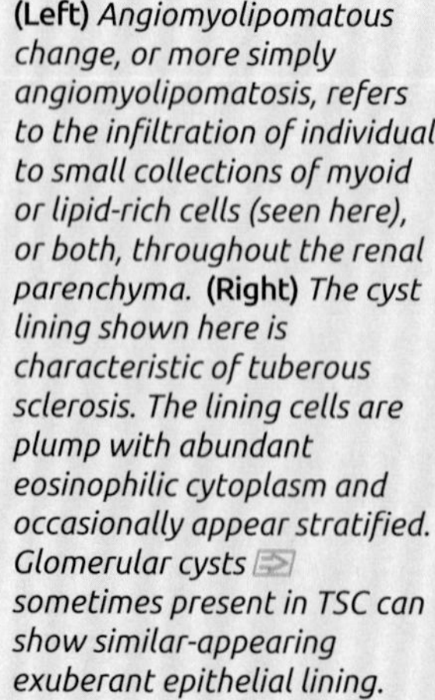

(Left) *Angiomyolipomatous change, or more simply angiomyolipomatosis, refers to the infiltration of individual to small collections of myoid or lipid-rich cells (seen here), or both, throughout the renal parenchyma.* **(Right)** *The cyst lining shown here is characteristic of tuberous sclerosis. The lining cells are plump with abundant eosinophilic cytoplasm and occasionally appear stratified. Glomerular cysts sometimes present in TSC can show similar-appearing exuberant epithelial lining.*

Angiomyolipomatous Change

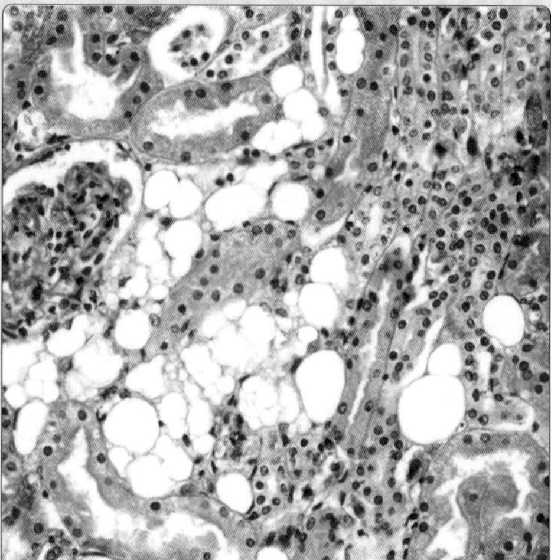

Characteristic Eosinophilic Cyst Lining

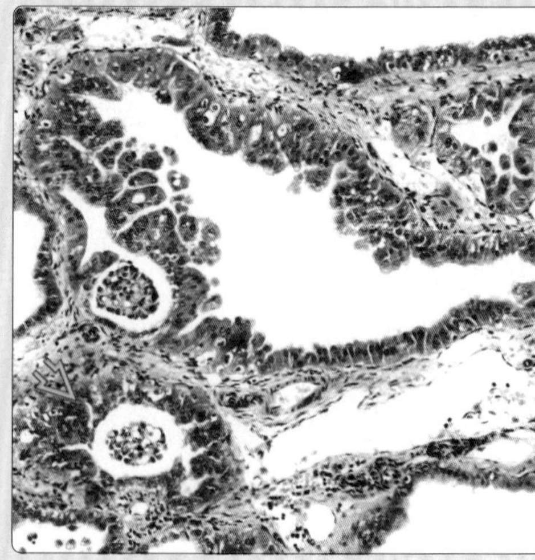

TERMINOLOGY

Abbreviations

- Tuberous sclerosis complex (TSC)

Synonyms

- Tuberous sclerosis

Definitions

- Dominantly inherited syndrome caused by hamartin or tuberin mutations leading to hamartomas, tumors, and cysts of multiple organs (including skin, brain, kidney, heart, lungs)

ETIOLOGY/PATHOGENESIS

Molecular Pathology

- *TSC1* gene, chromosome 9q34: Hamartin
- *TSC2* gene, chromosome 16p13: Tuberin
- 2% of TSC2 patients have large mutations affecting both *TSC2* and *PKD1*, an adjacent gene on chromosome 16, resulting in *TSC2/PKD1* contiguous gene syndrome with early-onset polycystic kidney disease
- Hamartin and tuberin normally interact and inhibit cell growth/proliferation
- In normal cells, TSC complex negatively regulates mammalian target of rapamycin (mTOR), a component of Pi3K/Akt/mTOR pathway, through inhibition of GTP-binding protein Rheb (Ras homolog enriched in brain)

CLINICAL ISSUES

Epidemiology

- Incidence
  - 1 in 6,000
  - Autosomal dominant mode of inheritance
  - 60-80% of cases sporadic
  - *TSC2* mutations account for majority of sporadic cases and are associated with more severe clinical phenotype

Presentation

- Highly variable severity and clinical expression range from minor clinical manifestations to profound cognitive impairment, epilepsy, and infant death
- Extreme variability in nature and profile of organ involvement, manifesting over broad age range
- May develop early (PKD) or late (tumors)
  - Renal cell carcinoma (RCC) diagnosed at younger age in TSC patients compared to general population
- Kidney may be initial organ involved

Treatment

- Annual monitoring with kidney ultrasound
- Control of hypertension
- Nephrectomy if nonremitting pain and hemorrhage or presence of RCC
- Renal transplantation in ESRD: Bilateral nephrectomy should be considered
- mTOR inhibitors (sirolimus [rapamycin], everolimus) for systemic treatment
  - Decrease phosphorylation of downstream effectors of mTOR result in decreased DNA synthesis and cellular proliferation in TSC-derived tumors, including angiomyolipomas (AML) and lymphangioleiomyomatosis
  - Reduce or stabilize other TSC-associated conditions

Prognosis

- Progressive decline of renal function due to progression of AML and cystic disease
- CNS and kidney lesions are main causes of mortality

Diagnosis

- Based on clinical and radiologic features
- Diagnosis requires either 2 major, or 1 major and 2 minor features
  - Major criteria for TSC diagnosis (age at onset)
    - Facial angiofibroma (infancy to adulthood)
    - Ungual fibroma (adolescence to adulthood)
    - Shagreen patch (childhood)
    - Hypomelanotic macules (infancy to childhood)
    - Cortical tuber (fetal life)
    - Subependymal nodule (childhood to adolescence)
    - Subependymal giant cell tumor (childhood to adolescence)
    - Retinal hamartomas (infancy)
    - Cardiac rhabdomyoma (fetal life)
    - Renal AML (childhood to adulthood)
    - Lymphangioleiomyomatosis (adolescence to adulthood)
  - Minor criteria
    - Multiple pits in dental enamel
    - Hamartomatous rectal polyps
    - Bone cysts
    - Cerebral white-matter radial migration lines
    - Gingival fibromas
    - Retinal achromic patch
    - "Confetti" skin lesions
      - Groups of small, lightly pigmented spots
    - Multiple renal cysts
- Genetic testing identifies mutation in 85% of patients

IMAGING

Radiographic Findings

- MR show both bright intensities (cysts) and dark areas (fat in AML)
- Ultrasound used to follow-up progression of lesions

MACROSCOPIC

General Features

- Kidneys often enlarged
- In PKD, external surface often irregular, caused by presence of several variable-sized cysts
  - May be relatively smooth if contains numerous small uniform cysts
  - Cysts randomly distributed throughout cortex and medulla
- If kidneys shrunken and contracted but contain cysts, may represent acquired cystic kidney disease
- Firm to fleshy, tan to yellow AML can be identified
  - Larger lesions usually well demarcated

MICROSCOPIC

Histologic Features

- Renal involvement in TSC
  - Multiple and bilateral
    - AML (45-80%)
    - Cysts (20-30%) and polycystic kidney disease (< 5%)
    - RCC (2-4%) and oncocytoma (rare)
- AML and angiomyolipomatous change of renal parenchyma is most common finding
  - Angiomyolipomatosis is ill-defined uncircumscribed proliferations of tissue consisting of myoid cells, adipocytes, or both
    - Abnormal arteries not usually present
- Grossly visible or microscopic AML, latter referred to as "microhamartoma"
  - Glomerular microhamartomas can be seen
    - Glomerular mass lesions featuring polygonal epithelial cells containing lipid vacuoles
- Smooth muscle proliferations
  - Interstitial, pericystic, collarettes around immature ducts
- Multiple cysts involving both cortex and medulla
  - Cysts and microcysts lined by large plump cells with abundant deeply eosinophilic cytoplasm are characteristic of TSC
    - Variable lining, ranging from flattened to hyperplastic
    - Exuberant, hyperplastic lining with nuclear pleomorphism
    - In some areas appears stratified and forms small papillations
  - Cysts with deeply eosinophilic luminal content
- Ectatic tubules
- Renal cell carcinomas and oncocytomas
  - Most common: Eosinophilic-cystic RCC
  - Chromophobe RCC, renal angiomyoadenomatous tumor, clear cell RCC, and oncocytomas less common
  - Papillary and collecting duct carcinomas rare
- FSGS lesions may develop
- PKD in young pediatric patients associated with features of metanephric dysgenesis
  - Cortical hypoplasia with reduced number of nephron generations
  - Failure of corticomedullary differentiation with medullary islands
    - Medullary islands are rudimentary medullary tissue located within cystic cortex
  - Lack of medullary rays
  - Dimorphic glomerular populations
    - Normal-appearing and immature-appearing glomeruli
  - Glomerular cysts

ANCILLARY TESTS

Immunohistochemistry

- Hamartin and tuberin coexpressed in most human cells and tissues
  - Normal staining patterns in kidney
    - Hamartin
      - Apical staining of proximal tubules
      - Peripheral staining of collecting ducts and distal tubules
      - Hamartin more robust staining than tuberin in distal nephron segments
    - Tuberin
      - Diffuse cytoplasmic staining of proximal and distal tubules
- Hamartin and tuberin IHC staining similar in TSC nonlesional tissue and normal controls despite single functional allele
- Staining of TSC eosinophilic cyst lining similar to proximal tubules, implicating proximal tubule origin of eosinophilic cysts
- Hamartin and tuberin staining pattern of TSC tumors does not permit implication of mutation present

Genetic Testing

- Identifies mutation in 85% of patients

DIFFERENTIAL DIAGNOSIS

Autosomal Dominant Polycystic Kidney Disease

- AML favors tuberous sclerosis
- Clinical history important
- Presence of *TSC2/PKD1* contiguous gene syndrome complicates diagnosis, particularly in juvenile cases

von Hippel-Lindau Disease (VHL)

- Both TSC and VHL may present with kidney cysts and RCC
- VHL does not have AML
- VHL cysts lined by clear cells
- Molecular testing may be required

Multicystic Dysplasia

- Presence of dysplastic elements (immature tubules with loose fibrous collars, cartilage)

DIAGNOSTIC CHECKLIST

Clinically Relevant Pathologic Features

- Extreme variability of phenotypic expression and disease severity makes diagnosis of TSC challenging
  - Confounded by fact that 65% are new mutations

SELECTED REFERENCES

1. Henske EP et al: Tuberous sclerosis complex, mTOR, and the kidney: report of an NIDDK-sponsored workshop. Am J Physiol Renal Physiol. 306(3):F279-83, 2014
2. Yang P et al: Renal cell carcinoma in tuberous sclerosis complex. Am J Surg Pathol. 38(7):895-909, 2014
3. Moavero R et al: Is mTOR inhibition a systemic treatment for tuberous sclerosis? Ital J Pediatr. 39:57, 2013
4. Budde K et al: Tuberous sclerosis complex-associated angiomyolipomas: focus on mTOR inhibition. Am J Kidney Dis. 59(2):276-83, 2012
5. Bonsib SM: Renal cystic diseases and renal neoplasms: a mini-review. Clin J Am Soc Nephrol. 4(12):1998-2007, 2009
6. Rosser T et al: The diverse clinical manifestations of tuberous sclerosis complex: a review. Semin Pediatr Neurol. 13(1):27-36, 2006
7. Henske EP: Tuberous sclerosis and the kidney: from mesenchyme to epithelium, and beyond. Pediatr Nephrol. 20(7):854-7, 2005

Kidney With Multiple Cysts

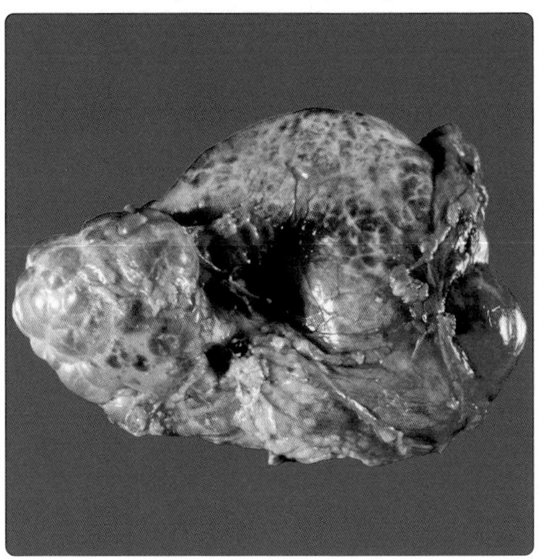

Multiple Cysts and Angiomyolipoma

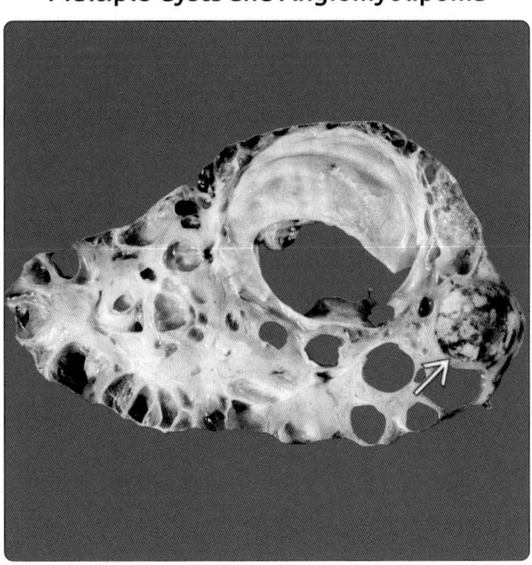

(Left) *External surface of a kidney from a patient with tuberous sclerosis shows multiple cysts of various sizes. This resembles the external appearance of kidneys in autosomal dominant polycystic disease (ADPKD).* **(Right)** *Cross section of a fixed nephrectomy specimen from a patient with tuberous sclerosis shows the extent of the parenchymal involvement by cystic change and an angiomyolipoma* ➡.

Multiple Angiomyolipomas

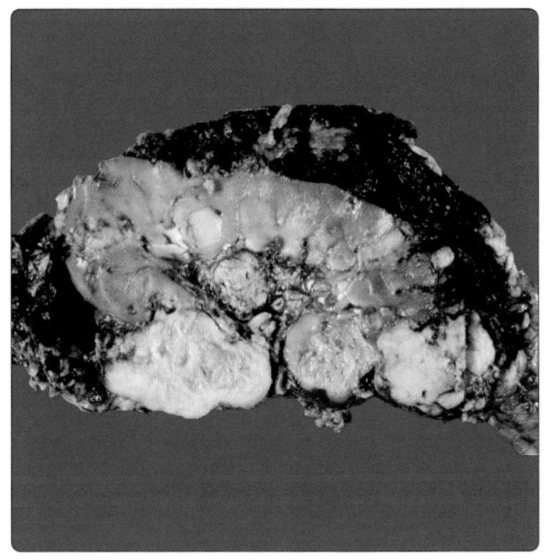

Microscopic Angiomyolipomas

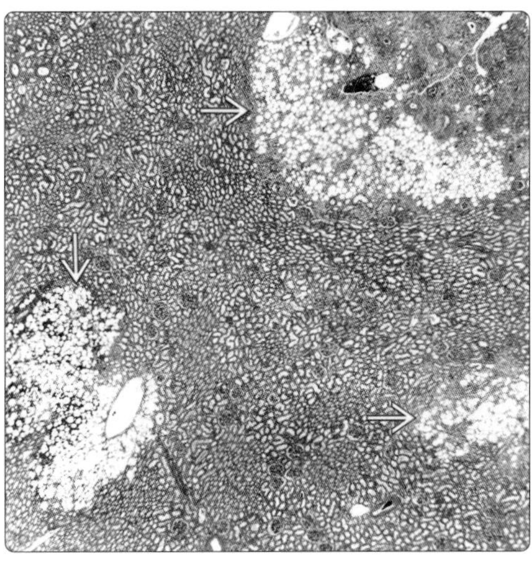

(Left) *Multiple fleshy to fatty-appearing tumors are grossly apparent in this cross section of a kidney from a patient with tuberous sclerosis. The patient presented with flank pain and had retroperitoneal hemorrhage; note the adherent blood surrounding the kidney.* **(Right)** *Three lipid-rich angiomyolipomas* ➡ *are noted here with normal-appearing intervening renal parenchyma; these tumors are small and may not have been visible by gross examination.*

Myoid Cell-Rich Angiomyolipoma

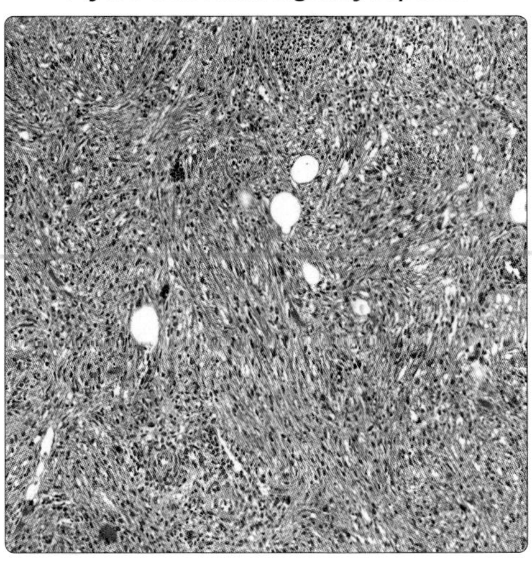

Angiomyolipoma With Epithelial-Lined Cyst

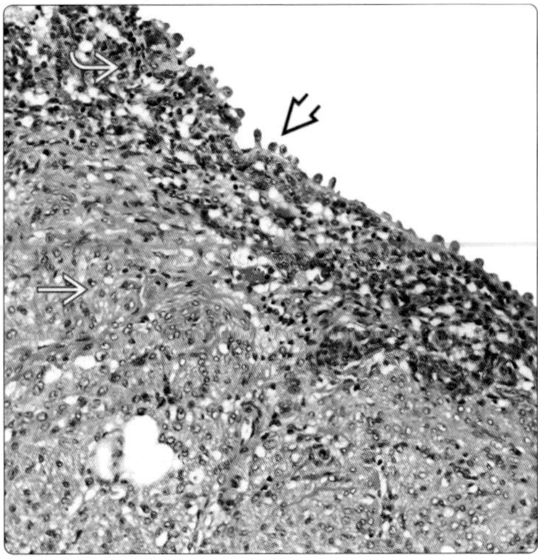

(Left) *Angiomyolipomas can show variable amounts of myoid cells and lipid-rich cells. The section here is myoid predominant.* **(Right)** *An angiomyolipoma with an epithelial-lined cyst (AMLEC) is an angiomyolipoma variant consisting of a myoid predominant AML that contains an epithelial-lined cyst surrounded by a cellular "cambium" layer* ➡ *interposed between the myoid cells* ➡ *and the cyst. The cyst lining* ➡ *is sometimes hobnailed as seen here.*

(Left) *Angiomyolipomatous change can be seen throughout the kidney in tuberous sclerosis. In this micrograph, the abnormal tissue consisting of fat ➡, smooth muscle ➡, and small blood vessels ➡ percolates through the renal cortex.* **(Right)** *Sometimes the angiomyolipomatosis consists mostly of myoid cells ⇨, which are noted here inconspicuously percolating through the cortex.*

Angiomyolipomatous Change

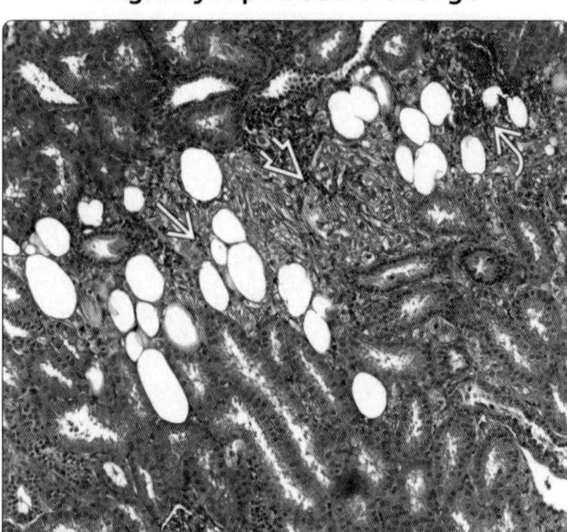

Subtle Angiomyolipomatous Lesions

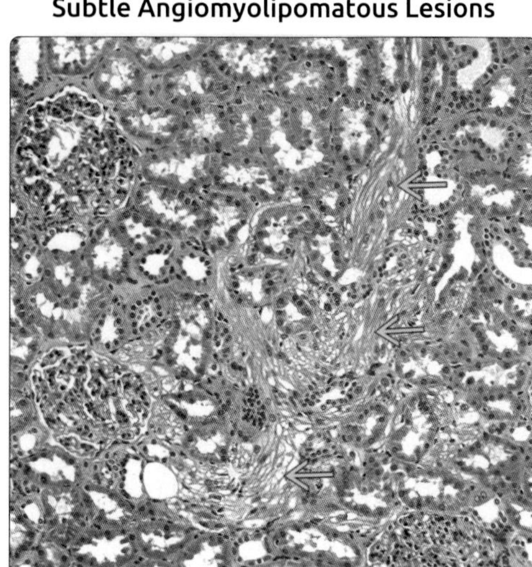

(Left) *This is an example of a relatively intact portion of renal parenchyma. Normal cortex and medullary rays are seen. Note a few small cysts and dilated tubules ➡.* **(Right)** *A characteristic appearance of kidney cysts in TSC is shown. The cells comprising the cystic epithelium have plump eosinophilic cytoplasm with a hobnail pattern and are much larger than cells in noncystic tubules.*

Focal Cysts and Ectatic Tubules

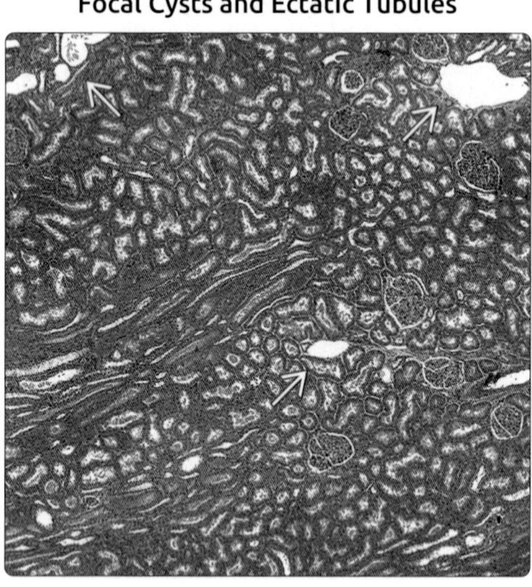

Cyst With Plump Epithelial Lining

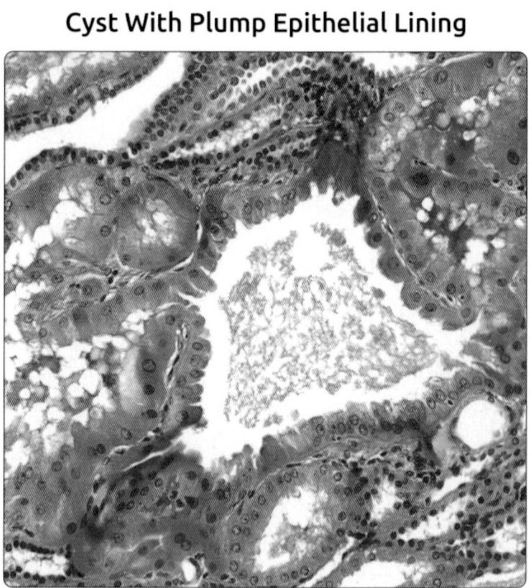

(Left) *The small cyst here is lined by cells with abundant cytoplasm. The hobnailed appearance of the cells is easily noted. The individual cells are much larger than the surrounding proximal and distal tubule cells.* **(Right)** *Many cysts show, in addition to characteristic epithelial cellular changes, an accumulation of deeply eosinophilic material in the cyst lumen.*

Microcyst With Hobnailed Patten

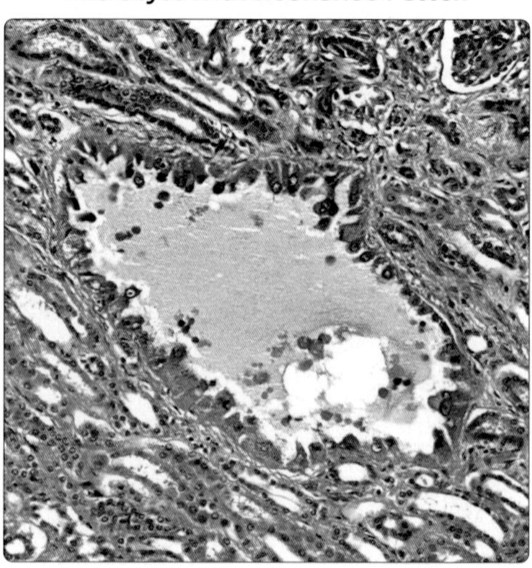

Exuberant Cyst Lining

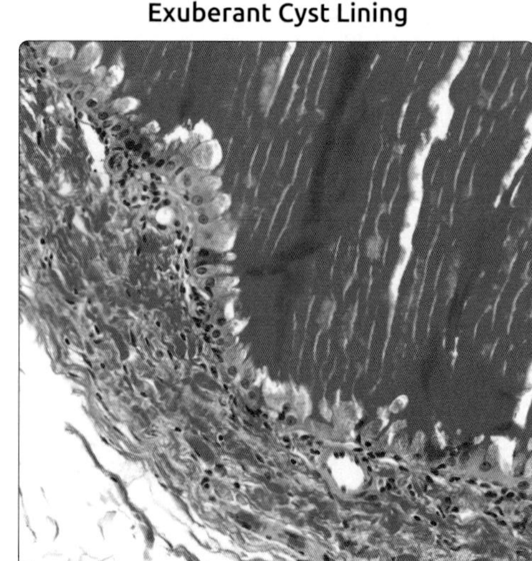

Cystic Kidney Disease

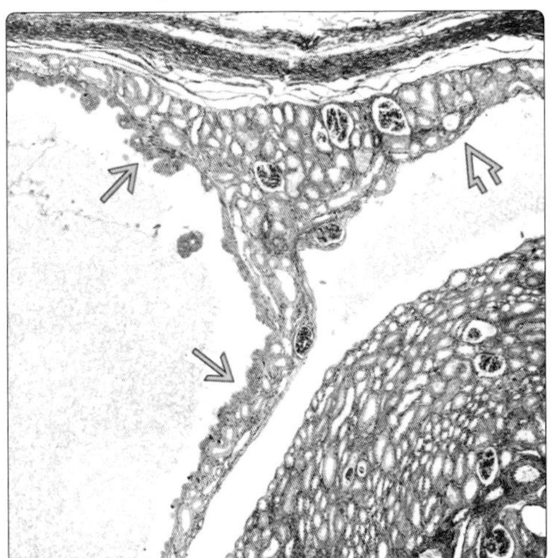

Cystic Kidney Disease in TSC

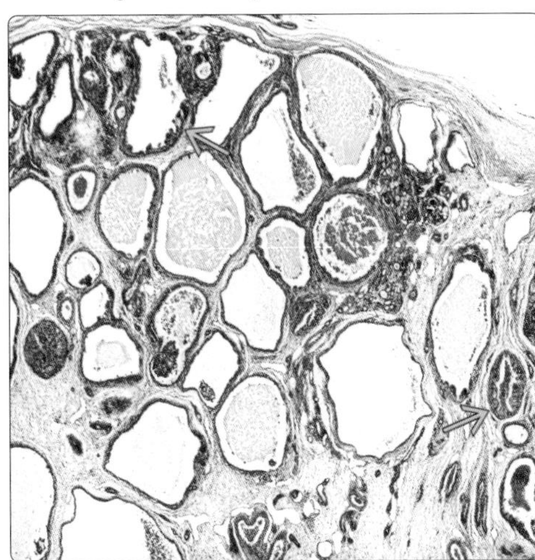

(Left) *This patient with TSC has multiple cysts with variable epithelial lining ranging from attenuated ⇨ to exuberant ⇨. The intervening renal parenchyma is relatively preserved in this patient. In contrast, some patients with cystic disease show marked destruction of the renal parenchyma between and around cysts.* **(Right)** *This patient with TSC shows replacement of the normal parenchyma by multiple cysts, many showing an exuberant epithelial lining ⇨.*

Smooth Muscle Collarettes Around Tubules

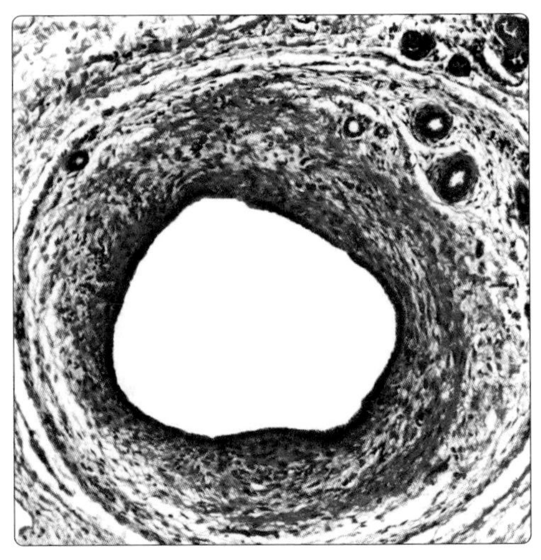

Dimorphic Glomeruli

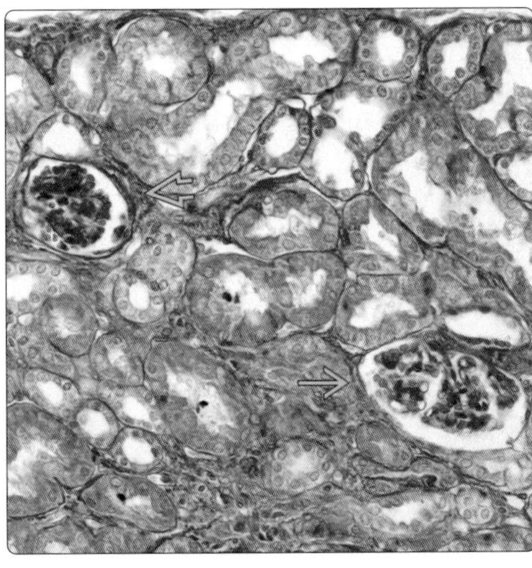

(Left) *Proliferation of smooth muscle in TSC patients includes interstitial and pericystic smooth muscle and collarettes around immature collecting ducts as seen here. Features of metanephric dysgenesis include cortical hypoplasia, lack of medullary rays, dimorphic glomerular populations, and glomerular cysts.* **(Right)** *Some TSC patients with PKD have associated developmental defects including dimorphic glomerular populations of normal ⇨ and immature ⇨ glomeruli.*

Renal Angiomyoadenomatous Tumor

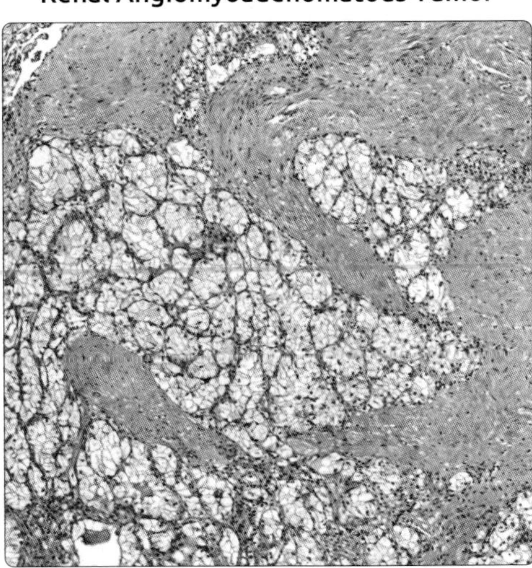

Eosinophilic-Cystic Renal Cell Carcinoma

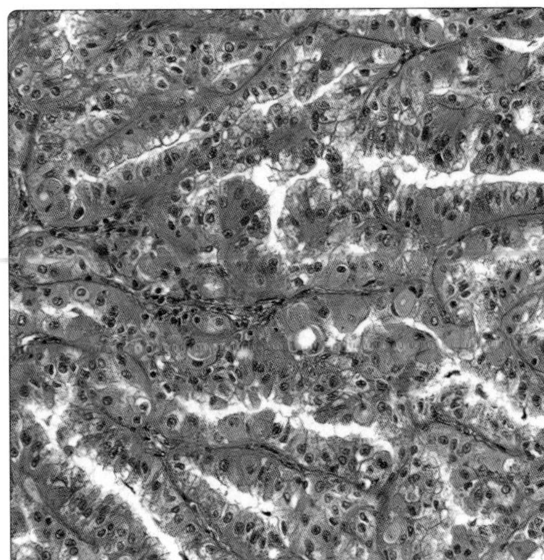

(Left) *This renal angiomyoadenomatous tumor shows clusters of large clear cells with intervening smooth muscle stroma.* **(Right)** *The most common renal cell carcinoma in TSC is the eosinophilic-cystic renal cell carcinoma shown here, followed by the chromophobe type and renal angiomyoadenomatous tumors. Oncocytomas and papillary renal cell carcinomas are rare.*

Zellweger Syndrome

KEY FACTS

TERMINOLOGY

- Autosomal recessive multisystem disease
- 1 of 3 peroxisome biosynthesis disorders

ETIOLOGY/PATHOGENESIS

- *PEX* mutations (13 identified)
- Peroxisome synthesis defect
- Absent or reduced peroxisomes in affected organs

CLINICAL ISSUES

- Craniofacial and limb dysmorphism
- Central nervous system malformations
- Liver dysfunction
- Usually asymptomatic renal cysts, rarely cystic renal dysplasia

IMAGING

- Chondroplasia puncta (stippled epiphyses)
  - Patella and long bones

MACROSCOPIC

- Variable degrees of cystic kidneys
  - Cortical cysts in > 90%
  - Cystic renal dysplasia in rare cases

MICROSCOPIC

- Subcapsular glomerular and tubular cysts to cystic renal dysplasia with severe metanephric dysgenesis
- Hepatic hemosiderosis to micronodular cirrhosis
- Abnormal neuronal migration and myelination

ANCILLARY TESTS

- Elevated plasma very long-chain fatty acids
- Biochemical testing of cultured fetal fibroblasts

TOP DIFFERENTIAL DIAGNOSES

- Enzyme defects of peroxisomal metabolism
  - Acyl-CoA oxidase deficiency
  - Carnitine palmitoyltransferase II deficiency

Zellweger Syndrome With Cortical Cysts

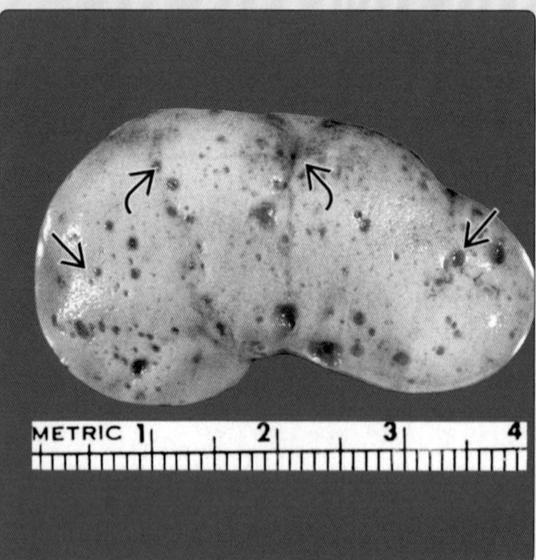

ZS With Small Subcapsular Cysts

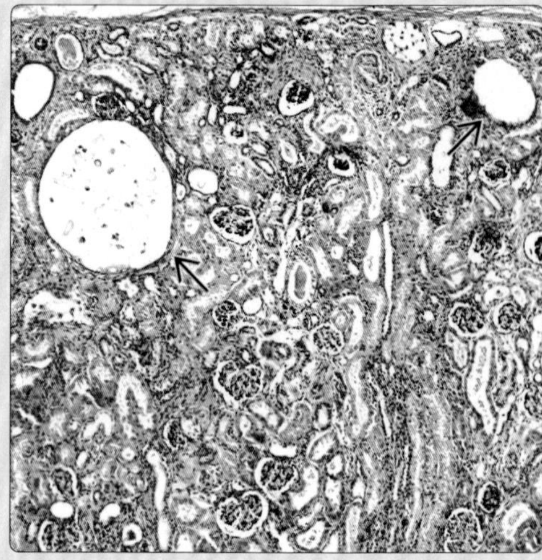

(Left) *This autopsy kidney is from a patient with Zellweger syndrome. The renal capsule has been stripped. It is overall developmentally and functionally normal. There is subtle persistence of fetal lobation ➔. Multiple small, superficial cortical subcapsular cysts are present ➔.* **(Right)** *Autopsy kidney in Zellweger syndrome illustrates that most nephrons are normal. However, there are scattered, small cortical cysts ➔ lined by a thin epithelial cell layer. These resulted in no renal functional impairment.*

ZS With Small Subcapsular Cysts

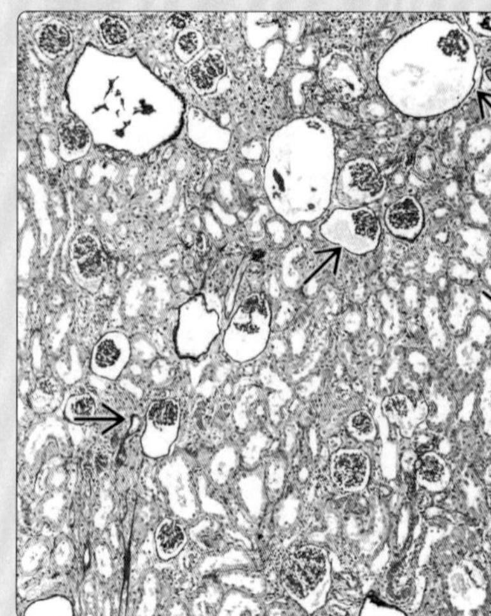

ZS With Glomerular Cyst

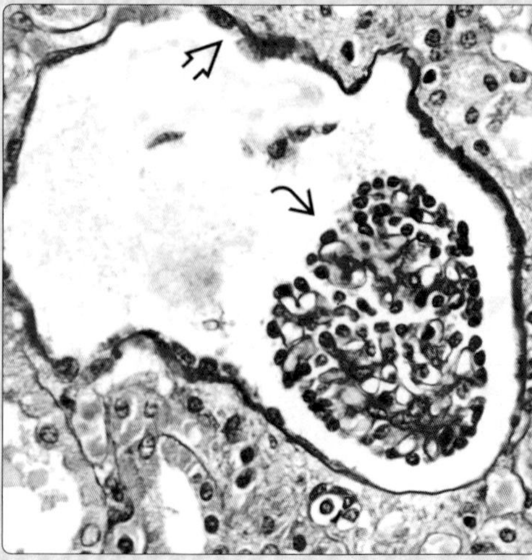

(Left) *Section of kidney from an autopsy in Zellweger syndrome shows that the majority of nephrons are normal. Several microcysts are present. Most of the cysts are glomerular since a glomerular tuft ➔ is visible in the majority of them. Renal function was normal.* **(Right)** *This is a glomerular cyst in Zellweger syndrome. Although Bowman capsule is dilated ➔ and much larger than normal, the glomerular tuft ➔ appears completely normal. The capillary loops are open and the mesangium is inconspicuous.*

TERMINOLOGY

Abbreviations

- Zellweger syndrome (ZS)

Synonyms

- Cerebrohepatorenal syndrome (CHRS)

Definitions

- Autosomal recessive multisystem disease
- 1 of 3 peroxisome biosynthesis disorders
  - Zellweger syndrome is most severe disorder
  - Neonatal adrenoleukodystrophy
  - Infantile Refsum syndrome is least severe disorder

ETIOLOGY/PATHOGENESIS

Mutation of *PEX* Genes

- *PEX* genes encode peroxins
  - Required for peroxisome assembly
    - Cytoplasmic peroxidase enzymes not incorporated into peroxisomes with mutation
- 13 mutations of 16 *PEX* genes identified
  - Most common mutations
    - *PEX1* (70% of cases)
    - *PEX6*
- Absent or reduced peroxisomes in kidney, liver, and other organs

CLINICAL ISSUES

Epidemiology

- Incidence
  - 1 in 50,000 to 1:100,000

Presentation

- In neonates
  - Craniofacial dysmorphism
    - High forehead, large fontanelles, hypotelorism
  - Limb dysmorphism
  - Central nervous system disease
    - Seizures, hypotonia, difficulty feeding
  - Liver dysfunction
    - Jaundice, elevated liver function tests
  - Renal dysfunction
    - Mild azotemia, proteinuria (25%), aminoaciduria (25%)

Laboratory Tests

- Elevated plasma very long-chain fatty acids
- Biochemical testing of cultured fetal fibroblasts

Prognosis

- Most die within 1st year of life

IMAGING

Radiographic Findings

- Chondroplasia puncta (stippled epiphyses)
  - Patellae and long bones

MACROSCOPIC

General Features

- Kidney: Variable degrees of cystic change
  - Cortical cysts in > 90%
    - Subcapsular cysts from < 0.01 to 1 cm
  - Renal cystic dysplasia in some cases
- Central nervous system
  - Macrogyria
  - Cerebellar hypoplasia
- Liver
  - Hepatomegaly at birth
  - Micronodular cirrhosis later

MICROSCOPIC

Histologic Features

- Kidneys
  - Glomerular and tubular microcysts with pericystic fibrosis
  - Rarely, severely altered metanephric differentiation resulting in cystic renal dysplasia
    - Dysgenetic (dysplastic) nephrons
    - Immature collecting ducts with collarettes of spindled cells
    - Poorly formed medulla
- Liver
  - Hemosiderosis, preferentially periportal
  - Micronodular cirrhosis
- Central nervous system
  - Cerebral heterotopias with abnormal neuronal migration and abnormal myelination

ANCILLARY TESTS

Electron Microscopy

- Absent peroxisomes in organs affected

DIFFERENTIAL DIAGNOSIS

Acyl-CoA Oxidase Deficiency (Glutaric Acidemia Type II)

- Dysmorphic features, cystic dysplasia of kidneys, CNS abnormalities, diffuse lipid infiltration of organs

Carnitine Palmitoyltransferase II Deficiency

- Dysmorphic features, cystic dysplasia kidneys and brain, cardiomyopathy, fatty infiltration of organs

SELECTED REFERENCES

1. Salpietro V et al: Zellweger syndrome and secondary mitochondrial myopathy. Eur J Pediatr. 174(4):557-63, 2015
2. Crane DI: Revisiting the neuropathogenesis of Zellweger syndrome. Neurochem Int. 69:1-8, 2014
3. Lee PR et al: Child neurology: Zellweger syndrome. Neurology. 80(20):e207-10, 2013
4. Rafique M et al: Zellweger syndrome - a lethal peroxisome biogenesis disorder. J Pediatr Endocrinol Metab. 26(3-4):377-9, 2013
5. Lindhard A et al: Postmortem findings and prenatal diagnosis of Zellweger syndrome. Case report. APMIS. 101(3):226-8, 1993
6. Powers JM et al: Fetal cerebrohepatorenal (Zellweger) syndrome: dysmorphic, radiologic, biochemical, and pathologic findings in four affected fetuses. Hum Pathol. 16(6):610-20, 1985

ZS With Glomerular Cysts

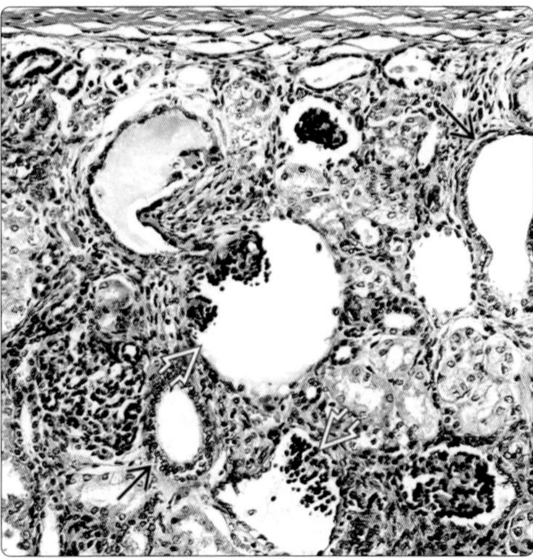

ZS With Large Subcapsular Cysts

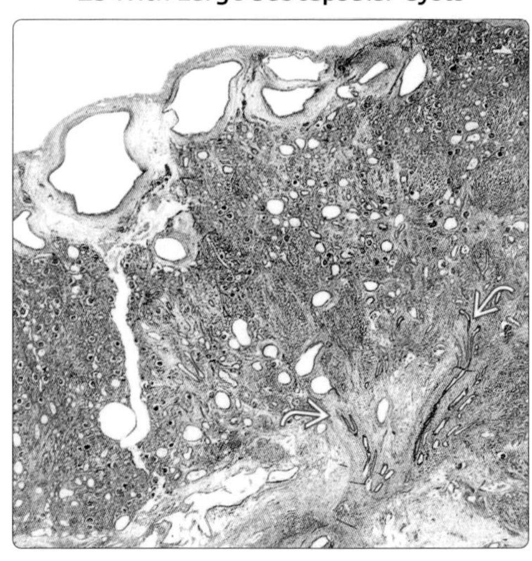

(Left) *Autopsy in Zellweger syndrome shows glomerular cysts and tubular microcysts. The tubular cysts have a shallow, cuboidal cell lining in contrast to the flattened cell lining of the glomerular cysts.* **(Right)** *This section from a patient with Zellweger syndrome shows a row of large subcapsular cysts with pericystic fibrosis. Smaller cysts are scattered throughout the cortex. The medullary tissue is rudimentary containing only a few collecting ducts. Renal failure was present.*

ZS With Severe Cystic Kidney Disease

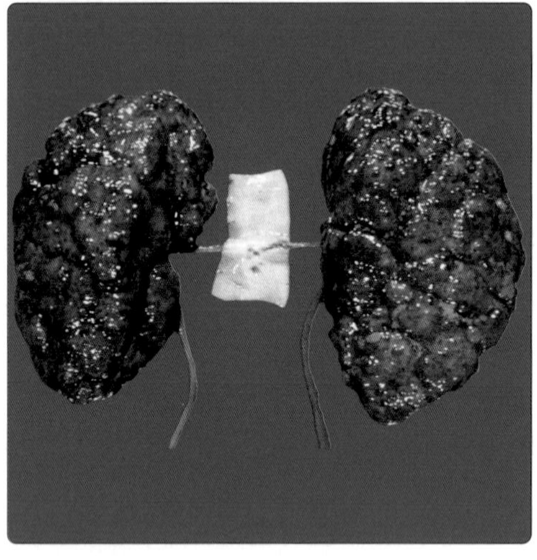

ZS With Severe Cystic Kidney Disease

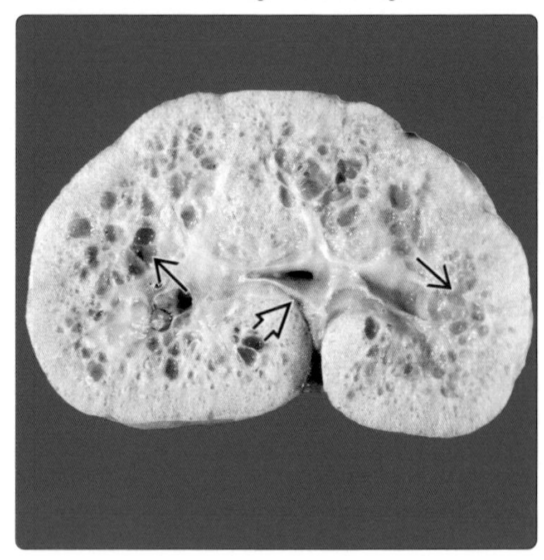

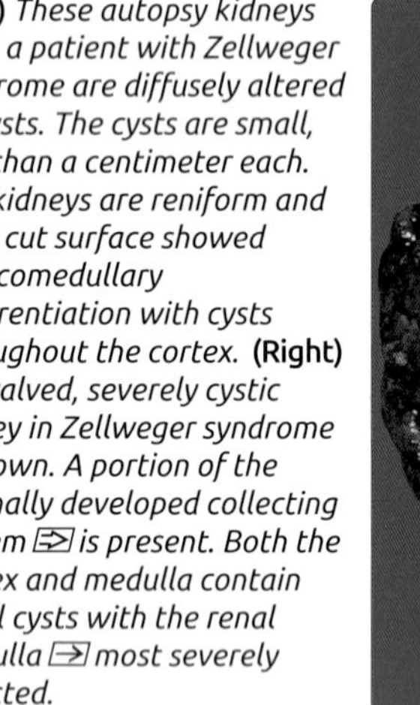

(Left) *These autopsy kidneys from a patient with Zellweger syndrome are diffusely altered by cysts. The cysts are small, less than a centimeter each. The kidneys are reniform and their cut surface showed corticomedullary differentiation with cysts throughout the cortex.* **(Right)** *A bivalved, severely cystic kidney in Zellweger syndrome is shown. A portion of the normally developed collecting system is present. Both the cortex and medulla contain small cysts with the renal medulla most severely affected.*

ZS With Large Subcapsular Cysts

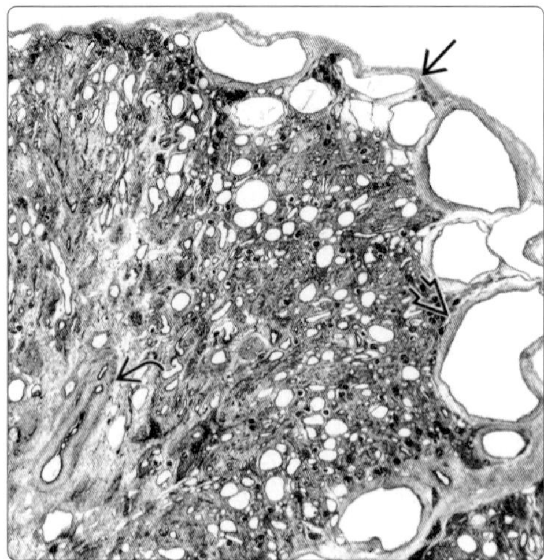

ZS With Large Subcapsular Cysts

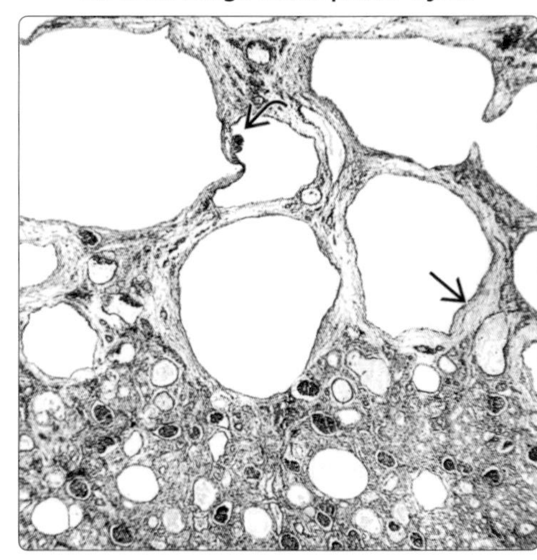

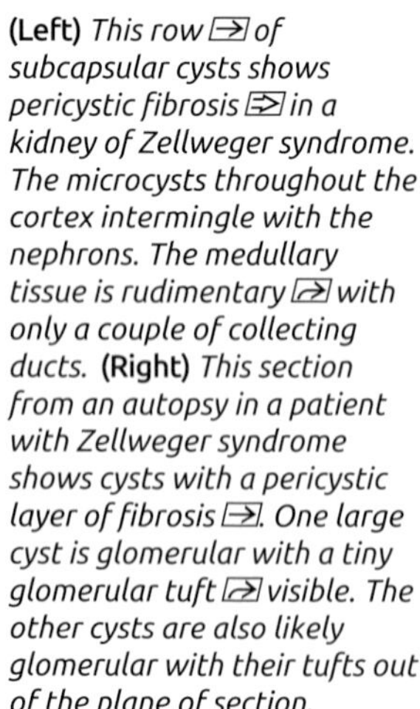

(Left) *This row of subcapsular cysts shows pericystic fibrosis in a kidney of Zellweger syndrome. The microcysts throughout the cortex intermingle with the nephrons. The medullary tissue is rudimentary with only a couple of collecting ducts.* **(Right)** *This section from an autopsy in a patient with Zellweger syndrome shows cysts with a pericystic layer of fibrosis. One large cyst is glomerular with a tiny glomerular tuft visible. The other cysts are also likely glomerular with their tufts out of the plane of section.*

ZS With Large Subcapsular Cysts

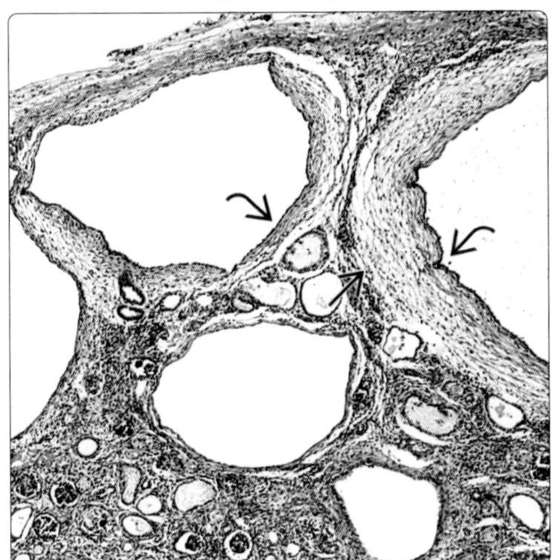

ZS With Severe Metanephric Dysgenesis

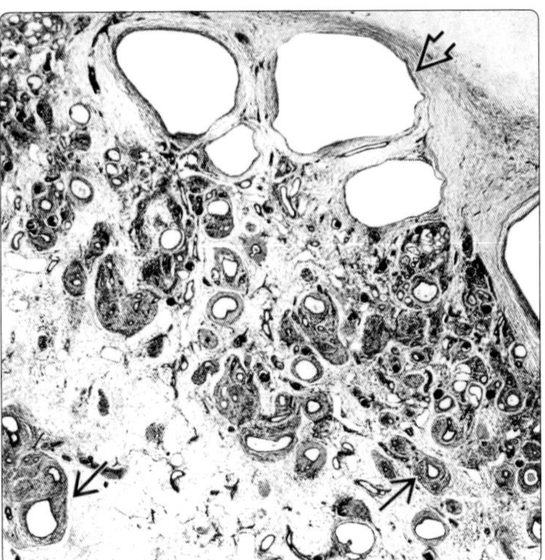

(Left) *There are subcapsular cysts with a pericystic fibrous layer ➡. The cysts are lined by flattened epithelium ➡. The pericystic fibrous tissue is loose and edematous. The nephrons in the deeper cortex appear normal.* **(Right)** *This is a severely affected kidney in a patient Zellweger syndrome. There are subcapsular cysts ➡ and marked failure of metanephric differentiation. Only a few nephron components are present within abundant loose stroma. There are dysplastic collecting ducts with collarettes of spindle cells ➡.*

ZS With Bile Duct Plate Malformation

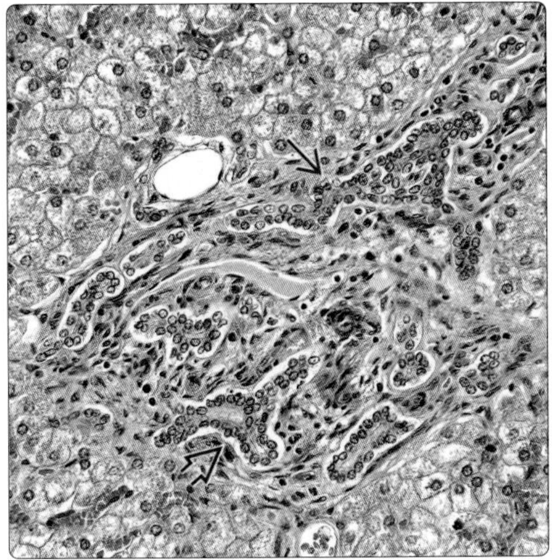

ZS With Hepatic Fibrosis

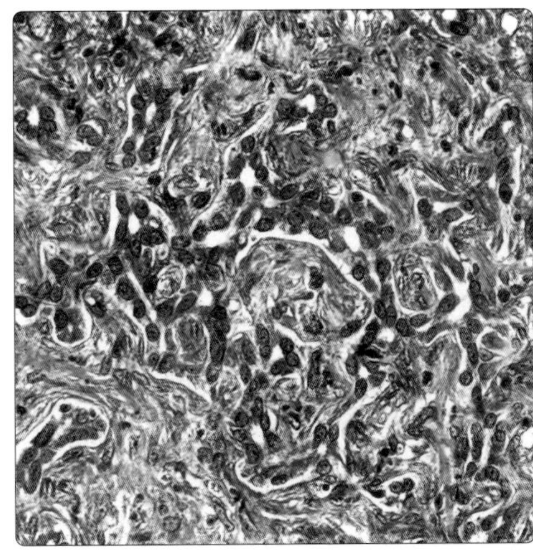

(Left) *This liver is from a neonate with Zellweger syndrome. There is a bile duct plate malformation characterized by a marked increase of portal triad bile ducts ➡ associated with abnormal bile duct branching ➡. There is no fibrous expansion of the portal tract, inflammation, or sinusoidal fibrosis present.* **(Right)** *This liver is from a neonate with Zellweger syndrome. The hepatocytes are small and immature appearing. There is prominent sinusoidal fibrosis through the hepatic parenchyma.*

ZS With Portal Bile Duct Proliferation

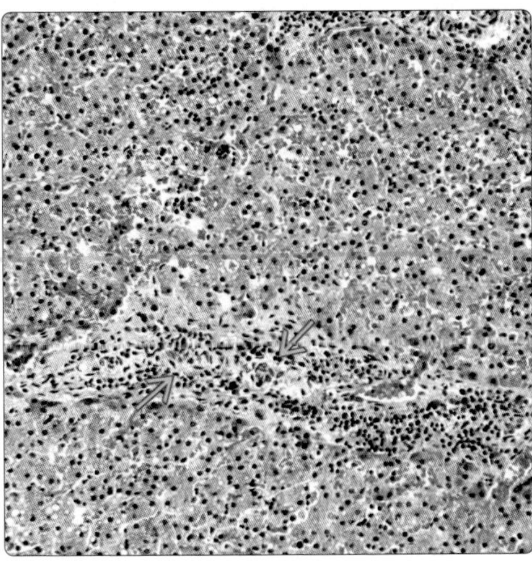

ZS With Hemosiderosis

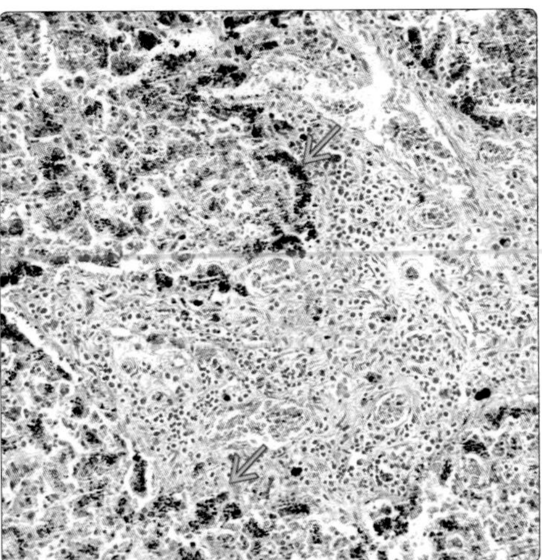

(Left) *Section of liver is from an autopsy in a patient with Zellweger syndrome shows bile duct proliferation ➡. Although the hepatocytes appear normal, there is hemosiderin pigment present most marked in the periportal hepatocytes but visible only at higher magnification.* **(Right)** *This iron stain shows hepatocytes laden with blue-stained hemosiderin granules. The iron in Zellweger syndrome affects all hepatocytes but is characteristically most heavily deposited in periportal hepatocytes ➡.*

Medullary Sponge Kidney

KEY FACTS

TERMINOLOGY

- Medullary sponge kidney (MSK)
- Cystic disease of medulla characterized by ectasia of terminal collecting ducts

ETIOLOGY/PATHOGENESIS

- Developmental defect of collecting system
- Associated with Wilms tumor, urinary tract developmental abnormalities, hemihypertrophy and Beckwith-Wiedemann syndrome, Rabson-Mendenhall syndrome, congenital hepatic fibrosis, Ehlers-Danlos syndrome, pyloric stenosis, multiple endocrine neoplasia type 2 (MEN2), Marfan syndrome

CLINICAL ISSUES

- Recurrent calcium oxalate &/or calcium phosphate stones
- Urinary tract infections
- Loin pain
- If infections and stone formation controlled, course is indolent

IMAGING

- "Paintbrush" ureteral ectasia also sometimes referred to as "bouquet of flowers"

MACROSCOPIC

- Cysts of various sizes (most < 10 mm) observed in medullary pyramids
- Renal papillae most affected

TOP DIFFERENTIAL DIAGNOSES

- Autosomal dominant tubulointerstitial kidney disease
- Autosomal dominant polycystic kidney disease
- Loin pain hematuria syndrome
    - Subset of MSK patients present with loin pain

(Left) *Excretory urogram shows the classic "paintbrush" appearance of tubular ectasia bilaterally in a patient with medullary sponge kidney (MSK).* **(Right)** *Gross photograph of an autopsy kidney specimen shows lesions of medullary sponge kidney. Cysts of various sizes can be seen in the medulla →.*

Radiographic Features of MSK

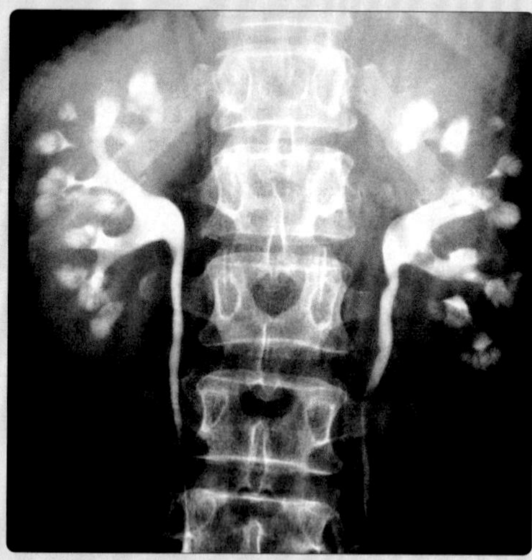

Medullary Sponge Kidney

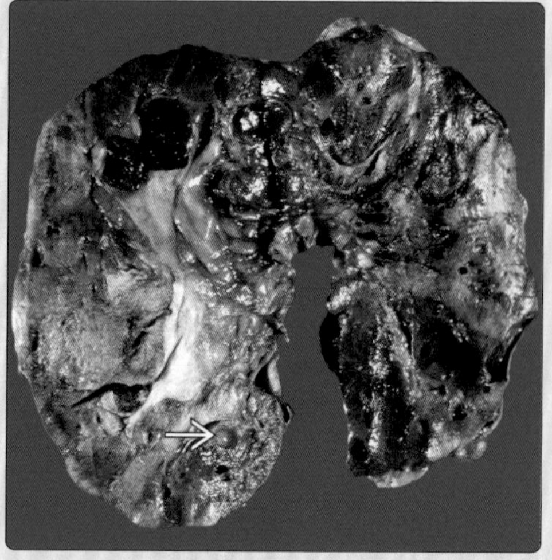

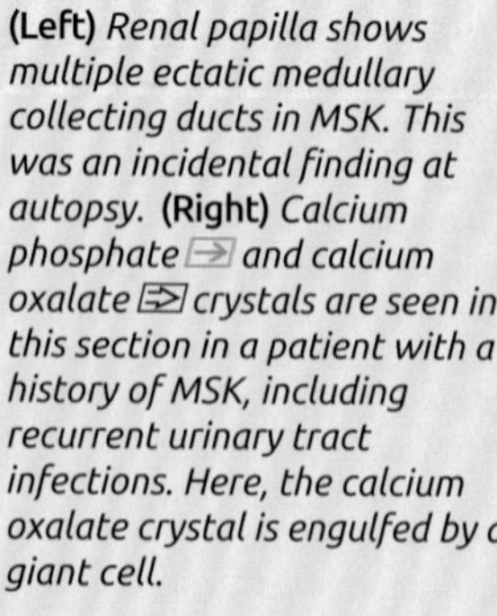

(Left) *Renal papilla shows multiple ectatic medullary collecting ducts in MSK. This was an incidental finding at autopsy.* **(Right)** *Calcium phosphate → and calcium oxalate → crystals are seen in this section in a patient with a history of MSK, including recurrent urinary tract infections. Here, the calcium oxalate crystal is engulfed by a giant cell.*

Dilated Collecting Ducts

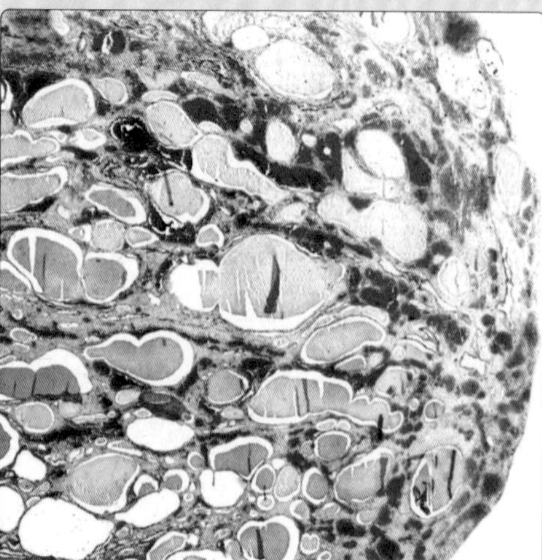

Calcium Crystals

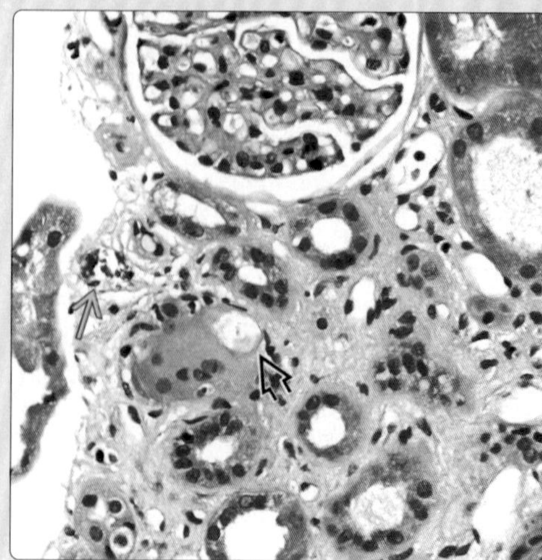

TERMINOLOGY

Abbreviations

- Medullary sponge kidney (MSK)

Synonyms

- Cystic disease of renal pyramids
- Precalyceal canalicular ectasia
- Lenarduzzi's kidney or Cacchi and Ricci's disease

Definitions

- Cystic disease of renal medulla characterized by ectasia of terminal collecting ducts

ETIOLOGY/PATHOGENESIS

Developmental Anomaly

- Developmental defect of collecting system
  - Despite manifesting in 2nd-3rd decades of life, MSK thought to originate as developmental abnormality of collecting system
- Most cases sporadic

Genetics

- ~ 5% hereditary
  - Autosomal dominant mode of inheritance
- Possible implication of mutations or polymorphisms of glial cell line-derived neurotrophic factor (*GDNF*) and receptor tyrosine kinase (*RET*) genes
  - *GDNF* and *RET* receptor interaction important in development of kidney and urinary tract
- Associated with Wilms tumor, urinary tract developmental abnormalities, hemihypertrophy and Beckwith-Wiedemann syndrome, Rabson-Mendenhall syndrome, congenital hepatis fibrosis, Ehlers-Danlos syndrome, pyloric stenosis, multiple endocrine neoplasia type 2 (MEN2), Marfan syndrome

CLINICAL ISSUES

Epidemiology

- Incidence
  - < 0.5-1% of general population
    - Accounts for 12-20% of recurrent calcium stone formers
- Age
  - Usually diagnosed in young adults

Presentation

- Recurrent calcium stones
  - Calcium phosphate &/or calcium oxalate stones
  - Hypercalciuria and hypocitraturia in patients with stone disease
- Urinary tract infection
  - MSK greatly increases risk of developing pyelonephritis
- Distal renal tubular acidosis present in ~ 1/3
- Hematuria
- Loin pain, which may or may not be associated with stones

Treatment

- Prevention and control of infection and stone formation
  - Hydration, thiazide diuretics, antibiotics

Prognosis

- If infections and stone formation controlled, course is indolent

IMAGING

Radiographic Findings

- Excretory urogram
  - "Paintbrush" ureteral ectasia also sometimes referred to as "bouquet of flowers"
- Urinary stones frequently detected, usually bilateral

MACROSCOPIC

Size

- Normal kidneys for most
- Slight enlargement in ~ 1/3 of cases

Gross Cysts

- Cysts of various sizes (most < a few millimeters) observed in medullary pyramids
- Renal papillae most affected
- Degree of involvement of kidneys varies, but disease usually bilateral

MICROSCOPIC

Histologic Features

- Cysts in medullary pyramids lined by cuboidal to columnar epithelium
- Stratification of epithelium may be observed in proximity to urothelial surface (transitional or metaplastic squamous)
- Cyst lumens may contain calculi, RBCs, or inflammatory cells
- Stroma may be expanded with increased cellularity
- Stone formation of infection may lead to stromal inflammation
- Cysts outside of medullary pyramids normally not observed

DIFFERENTIAL DIAGNOSIS

Autosomal Dominant Tubulointerstitial Kidney Disease (ADTKD)

- ADTKD rarely involves deep medulla (commonly involves medullary rays)
  - In MSK, papillary tips most involved
- Calcifications associated with MSK but not ADTKD

Autosomal Dominant Polycystic Kidney Disease (ADPKD)

- May exhibit pericaliceal canalicular ectasia
- Presence of cortical cysts and family history separates ADPKD since most cases of MSK sporadic

Loin Pain Hematuria Syndrome

- Subset of MSK patients present with loin pain

SELECTED REFERENCES

1. Gambaro G et al: Medullary sponge kidney. Curr Opin Nephrol Hypertens. 22(4):421-6, 2013
2. Pritchard MJ: Medullary sponge kidney: causes and treatments. Br J Nurs. 19(15):972-6, 2010
3. Bisceglia M et al: Renal cystic diseases: a review. Adv Anat Pathol. 13(1):26-56, 2006

Cystic Nephroma

KEY FACTS

TERMINOLOGY

- Encapsulated neoplasm composed entirely of epithelial lined cysts and thin cyst septa
- a.k.a. multilocular cyst or multilocular cystic nephroma

ETIOLOGY/PATHOGENESIS

- Adult and childhood cystic nephroma are distinct entities
  - Adult cystic nephroma: Female predominance 8:1
    - No mutations reported
  - Childhood cystic nephroma: Male predominance 2:1
    - *DICER1* mutations in 90%

CLINICAL ISSUES

- Asymptomatic or presents with flank or abdominal pain, hematuria
- Conservative, complete surgical excision is curative

MICROSCOPIC

- Fibrous pseudocapsule
- Fibrous septa range from paucicellular, hyalinized to cellular ovarian stroma-like
- Stromal calcifications, corpora albicans-like structures may be present
- Cyst epithelial lining varies: Flat, cuboidal, or hobnail

ANCILLARY TESTS

- Estrogen &/or progesterone receptor stain commonly positive in ovarian-like stroma

TOP DIFFERENTIAL DIAGNOSES

- Mixed epithelial and stromal tumor
- Cystic partially differentiated nephroblastoma
- Multilocular cystic renal cell carcinoma
- Tubulocystic carcinoma
- Cystic kidney disease
  - Isolated polycystic kidney disease
  - Early-onset autosomal dominant polycystic kidney disease

Cystic Nephroma is Entirely Cystic

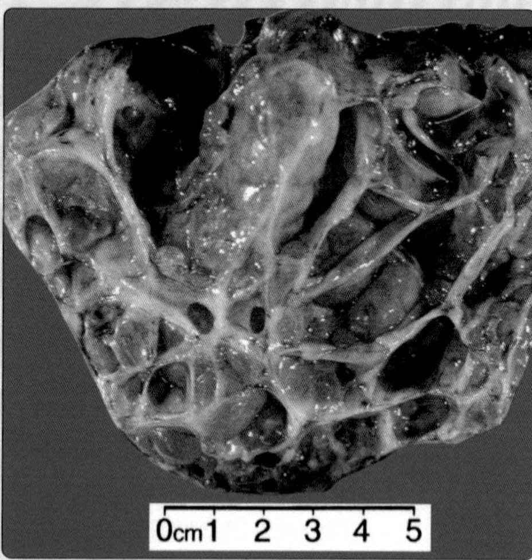

Cystic Nephroma With Variable Cellularity and Cyst Lining

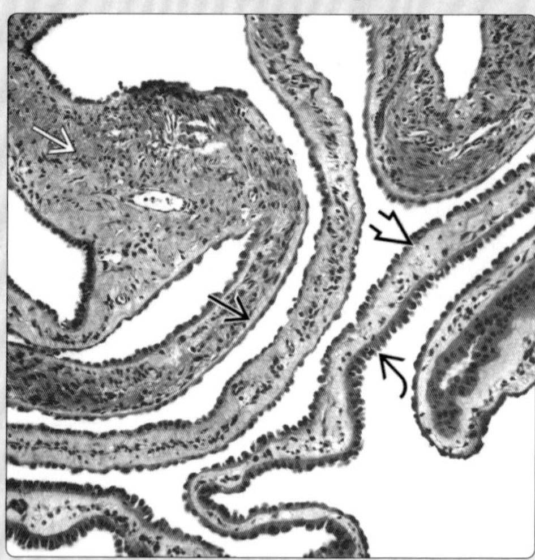

(Left) *This enucleated specimen illustrates the typical gross appearance of a cystic nephroma (CN). It is well demarcated & diffusely cystic. The cyst septa are thin and uniform without solid areas or septal nodularity.* **(Right)** *The cyst epithelium and septa cellularity in CNs are variable. In this example, the epithelial lining varies from flat → and hobnailed to cuboidal →. The septal stroma varies from thin with a loose matrix and relatively paucicellular → to thicker with collagenous matrix and increased cellularity →.*

Cystic Nephroma With Hobnail Cells

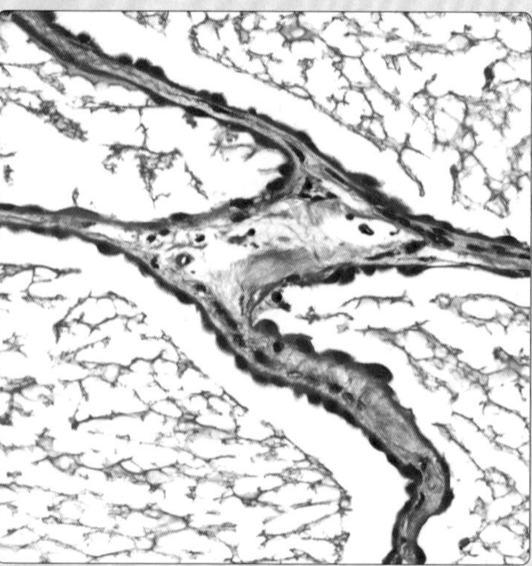

Estrogen Receptor Stain

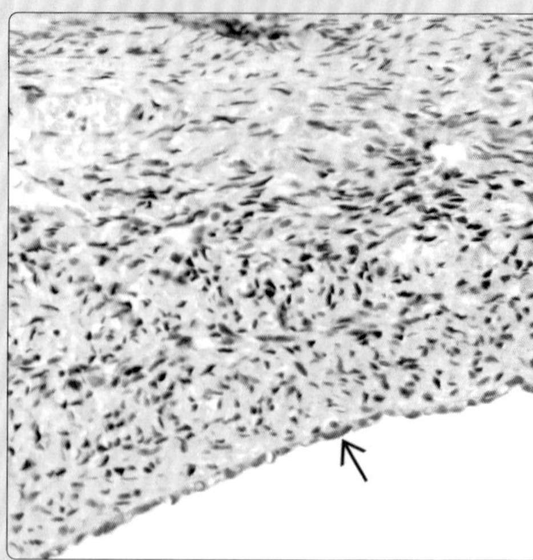

(Left) *Cysts in CN are separated by thin-walled septa with minimal stroma. In this example, the septa are extremely thin with very few stromal cells. The lining epithelium is hobnailed. The cyst contents are mucoid in appearance.* **(Right)** *Most CNs contain foci of septal cellularity in which the stromal cells have a slightly wavy appearance similar to ovarian stroma. The cells are typically estrogen receptor &/or progesterone receptor positive. Notice that the cyst lining cells are negative →.*

TERMINOLOGY

Synonyms

- Multilocular cyst
- Multilocular cystic nephroma

Definitions

- Encapsulated neoplasm composed entirely of epithelial lined cysts and thin cyst septa

ETIOLOGY/PATHOGENESIS

Childhood Cystic Nephroma

- *DICER1* mutations in 90%
- Associated with pleuropulmonary blastoma, which also has *DICER1* mutations

Adult Cystic Nephroma

- No mutations identified
- Distinct neoplasm from childhood type

CLINICAL ISSUES

Epidemiology

- Age
  - Childhood cystic nephroma
    - Rare > 2 years of age
  - Adult cystic nephroma
    - Rare < 30 years of age
- Sex
  - Childhood cystic nephroma: Male predominance 2:1
  - Adult cystic nephroma: Female predominance 8:1

Presentation

- Commonly an incidental finding
- Flank or abdominal pain, hematuria

Treatment

- Surgical approaches
  - Conservative excision is curative

Prognosis

- Excellent after complete excision
  - Recurs with incomplete excision
- Rare cases harbor malignant component

IMAGING

Ultrasound, CT, or MR Studies

- Cystic nephroma resembles other multicystic tumors

MACROSCOPIC

General Features

- Well circumscribed, encapsulated, diffusely cystic
- Cysts contain clear serous fluid

MICROSCOPIC

Histologic Features

- Fibrous pseudocapsule surrounds lesion
- Fibrous septa range from paucicellular or hyalinized to cellular, reminiscent of ovarian stroma
- Stromal calcifications and corpora albicans-like structures may be present
- Epithelial cyst lining ranges from flat to cuboidal to hobnail

ANCILLARY TESTS

Immunohistochemistry

- Ovarian-like stromal cells positive for estrogen &/or progesterone receptor in most cases
- Epithelial cells positive for CK19, AE1/3, EMA, often positive for CD10, CK7, HMWCK

DIFFERENTIAL DIAGNOSIS

Mixed Epithelial and Stromal Tumor (MEST)

- MEST and CN regarded as closely related or same entity
  - Similar mRNA expression, treatment, and prognosis
- MEST architecture and epithelium more complex than CN
  - Solid component often contains smooth muscle
  - Epithelium has complex architecture with papillae and branching glands
  - Epithelium often columnar or eosinophilic to clear and may be stratified
- MEST shows malignant transformation more often than CN

Cystic Partially Differentiated Nephroblastoma (CPDN)

- Previously regarded as closed related to childhood CN
- CPDN lacks *DICER1* mutations found in CN

Multilocular Cystic Clear Cell Renal Cell Carcinoma

- Diffusely cystic, grossly identical to CN
- Clear cells of low nuclear grade line cysts and form solid aggregates in septa

Tubulocystic Carcinoma

- Densely eosinophilic cells with large round nucleolus

Cystic Kidney Disease

- Isolated cystic kidney disease
  - Nonhereditary, unilateral, histologically resembles autosomal dominant polycystic kidney disease
- Autosomal dominant polycystic kidney disease
  - Occasionally presents as unilateral, multicystic mass, especially in children

SELECTED REFERENCES

1. Doros LA et al: DICER1 mutations in childhood cystic nephroma and its relationship to DICER1-renal sarcoma. Mod Pathol. 27(9):1267-80, 2014
2. Wilkinson C et al: Adult multilocular cystic nephroma: Report of six cases with clinical, radio-pathologic correlation and review of literature. Urol Ann. 5(1):13-7, 2013
3. Michal M et al: What is a cystic nephroma? Am J Surg Pathol. 34(1):126-7; author reply 127, 2010
4. Zhou M et al: Adult cystic nephroma and mixed epithelial and stromal tumor of the kidney are the same disease entity: molecular and histologic evidence. Am J Surg Pathol. 33(1):72-80, 2009
5. Mukhopadhyay S et al: Cystic nephroma: a histologic and immunohistochemical study of 10 cases. Arch Pathol Lab Med. 128(12):1404-11, 2004
6. Eble JN et al: Extensively cystic renal neoplasms: cystic nephroma, cystic partially differentiated nephroblastoma, multilocular cystic renal cell carcinoma, and cystic hamartoma of renal pelvis. Semin Diagn Pathol. 15(1):2-20, 1998

Cystic Nephroma is Entirely Cystic

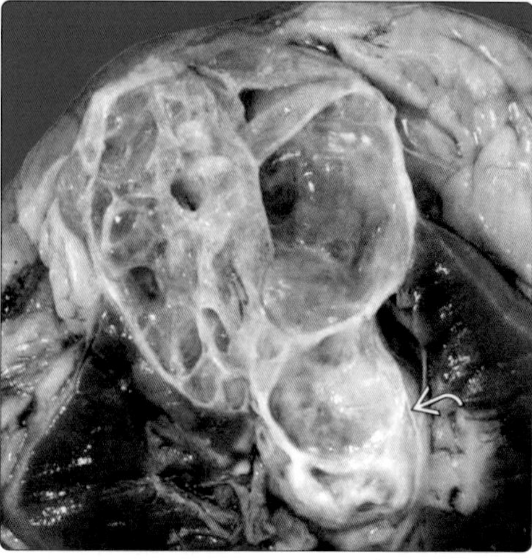

Cystic Nephroma is Entirely Cystic

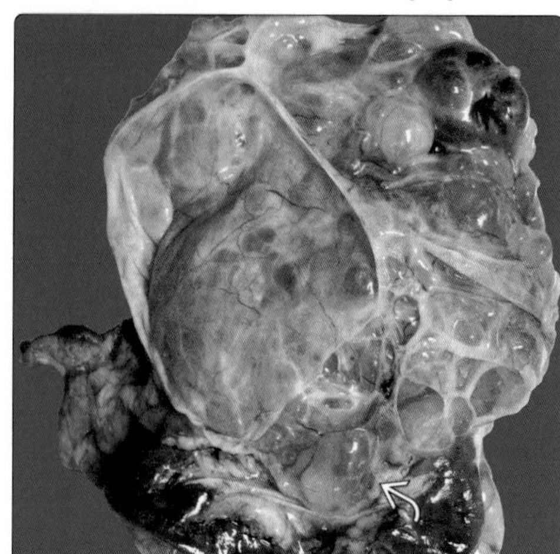

(Left) *This is a typical CN. It is well demarcated and diffusely cystic. It contains thin, delicate and transparent cyst septa. No septal nodularity or solid areas are present. It bulges into the peripheral perinephric fat and also into the renal sinus fat* ➢*.* **(Right)** *This CN is very large with a huge extrarenal component bulging into the peripheral perinephric fat. It also bulges into the sinus fat* ➢*. The cyst size varies. The fibrous septa are uniform, thin, and delicate. No solid areas or septal nodularity are present.*

Cystic Nephroma Consists of Cysts and Thin Septa

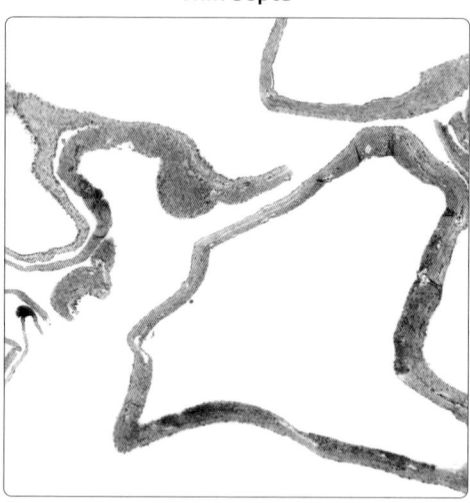

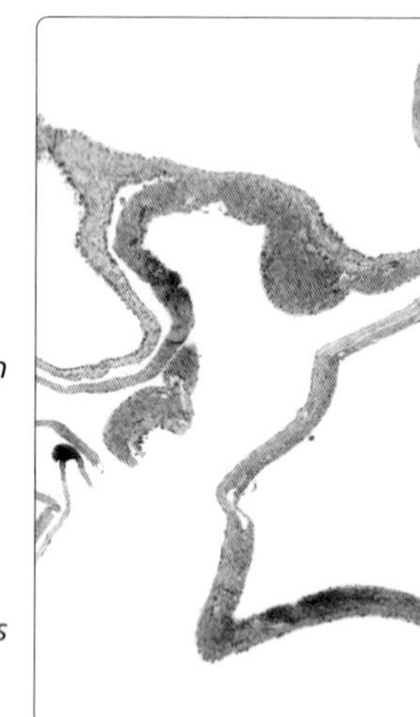

Cytokeratin CAM5.2 Stain

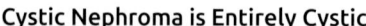

(Left) *A CN consists solely of cysts and thin cyst septa. The cysts usually contain thin, translucent serous fluid. The septa in this case are collagenous with small numbers of bland spindled cells. Ovarian-like stroma is not present.* **(Right)** *The epithelial cyst lining cells stain with a variety of epithelial markers, such as the pancytokeratins AE1/3 and CAM5.2, CK19 and epithelial membrane antigen. In addition, CD10, CK7, and high molecular weight cytokeratins may be positive.*

Cystic Nephroma With Hobnail Cells

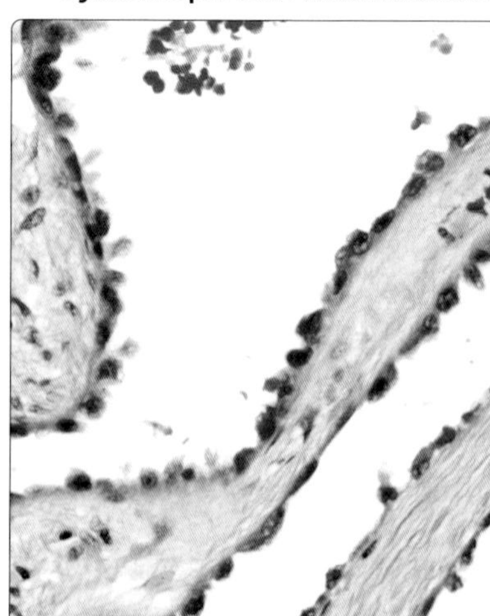

Cystic Nephroma With Septal Calcification

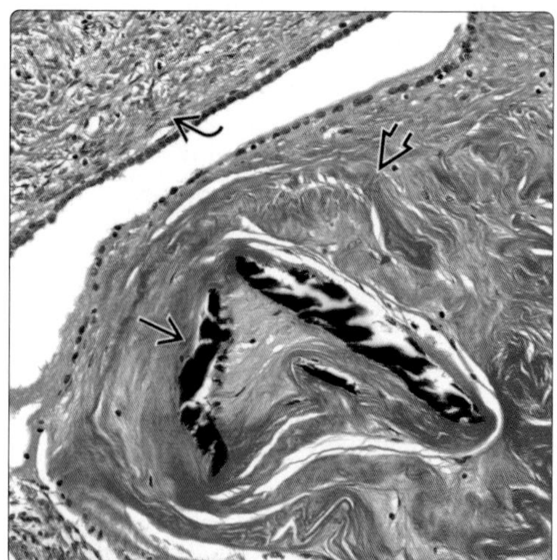

(Left) *Cysts in CN are separated by thin-walled septa. The stromal cellularity is variable. In this example, the septa are extremely thin with few to no stromal cells. The lining epithelium is hobnailed with attenuated cytoplasm resulting in nuclear prominence.* **(Right)** *The septal stroma in this CN varies from cellular* ➢ *to densely hyalinized* ➢*. Basophilic calcifications* ➢ *are commonly observed as in this case. The hyalinized stroma can resemble ovarian corpora albicans.*

Cystic Nephroma With Ovarian-Like Stroma

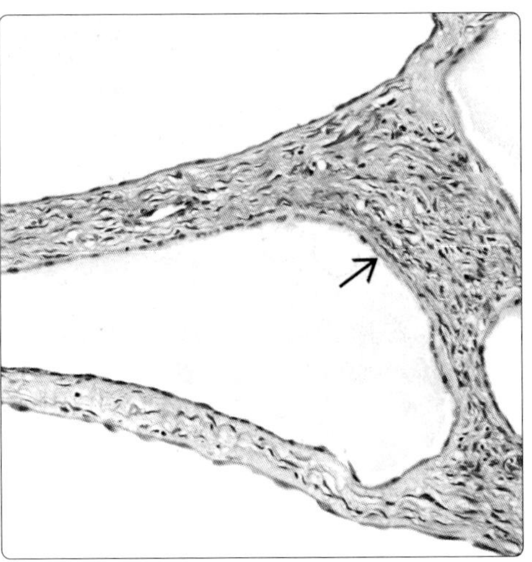

Cystic Nephroma: Progesterone Receptor Stain

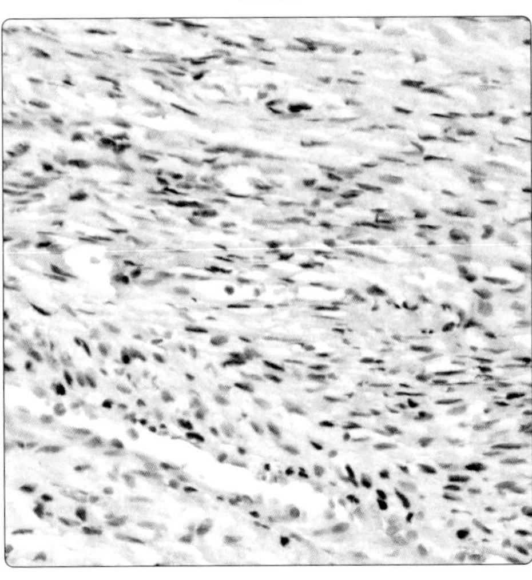

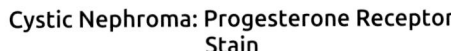

(Left) *Cysts in CN are separated by thin-walled septa with variable stroma. In this example, the septa are thin with spindled stromal cells that have elongated nuclei resembling ovarian stroma ➔. The lining epithelium is flattened to hobnailed.* **(Right)** *Most CNs contain foci of septal cellularity in which the stromal cells have a slightly wavy appearance similar to ovarian stroma. The cells are typically estrogen receptor &/or progesterone receptor positive. This shows a progesterone receptor stain.*

Cystic Partially Differentiated Nephroblastoma

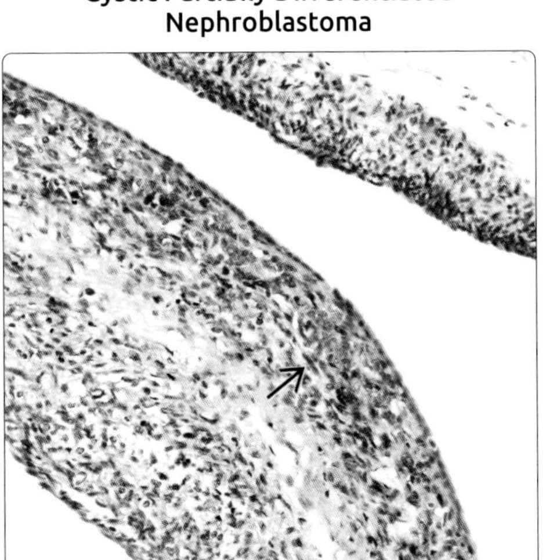

Cystic Partially Differentiated Nephroblastoma

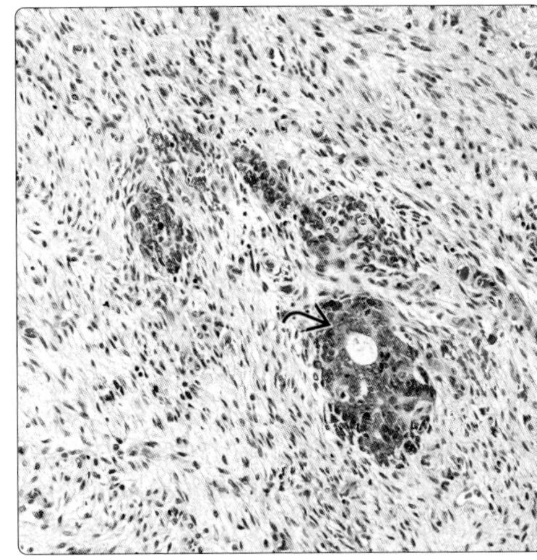

(Left) *This partially differentiated nephroblastoma is diffusely cystic and had a gross appearance similar to a CN. The septal stroma is very cellular with cambian layer of immature cells ➔ having an embryonal appearance similar to the stroma in a Wilms tumor.* **(Right)** *This cystic partially differentiated nephroblastoma shows cellular septal stroma with immature-appearing cellular blastemal cell condensations that demonstrate focal epithelial differentiation ➔.*

Mixed Epithelial and Stromal Tumor

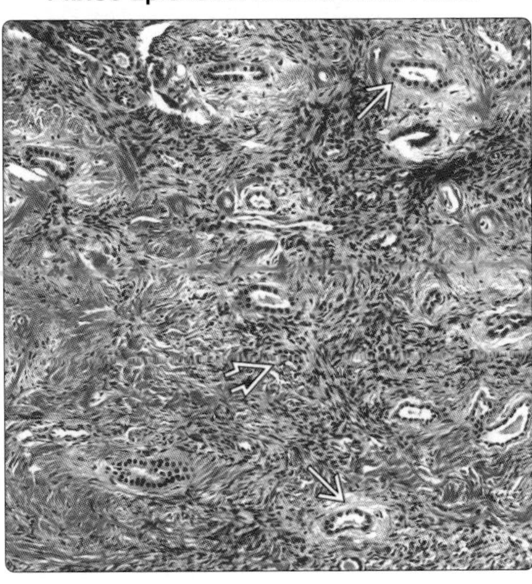

Mixed Epithelial and Stromal Tumor

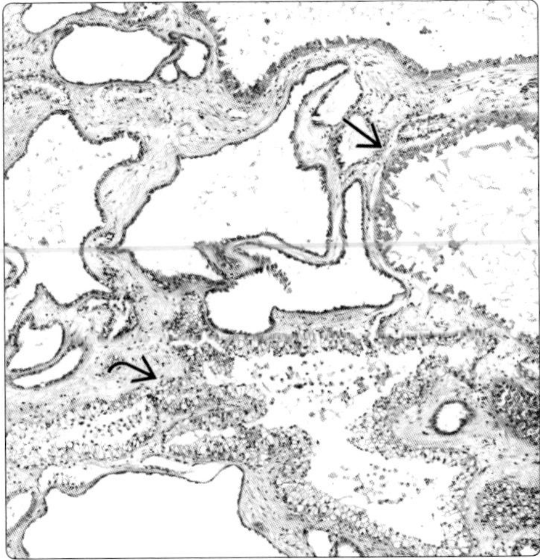

(Left) *Mixed epithelial and stromal tumors contain solid areas and septa of variable thickness. The solid areas may contain small tubules ➔, dense hyaline stroma and cellular stroma, resembling ovarian stroma ➔. In addition, smooth muscle fascicles may be present.* **(Right)** *The epithelium of mixed epithelial and stromal tumors is variable. Note the stratified eosinophilic ➔ and clear cell ➔ epithelium. The cysts may be small and irregularly shaped, as shown here, or exhibit branching or papillary structures.*

Acquired Cystic Disease

KEY FACTS

TERMINOLOGY

- ≥ 3 or more cysts in native kidneys of end-stage renal disease (ESRD) patients whose original cause for renal failure was not cystic kidney disease

ETIOLOGY/PATHOGENESIS

- Possibly physiologic response to chronic renal failure
- Increased proliferation of cyst-lining epithelium

CLINICAL ISSUES

- 8% of patients starting dialysis have acquired cystic kidney disease (ACKD)
- 90% of patient on dialysis for 10 years have ACKD
- Risk of developing renal cell carcinoma (RCC) increases with time
  - 2-7% of patients with ACKD will develop RCC
  - ESRD patients without cysts are at risk for RCC
- Renal transplantation may decrease cyst size
  - Effect of transplantation on RCC risk unknown

MACROSCOPIC

- ACKD kidney weighs < 1,000 g (average: 130 g)
- Cysts involve cortex and medulla, size from mm to cm
- RCCs may be solid or cystic

MICROSCOPIC

- Advanced glomerulosclerosis, tubulointerstitial scarring and arterial sclerosis
- Cysts are lined by flattened to cuboidal cells ± stratification or papillary growth
  - Lining cells may be clear, foamy, or eosinophilic
- Calcium oxalate crystal deposition common
- RCC, adenomas, hemangiomas may be present
  - ACKD-associated RCC is most common
  - Clear cell papillary RCC is 2nd most common
  - Any type of RCC can be present

TOP DIFFERENTIAL DIAGNOSES

- Autosomal dominant polycystic kidney disease

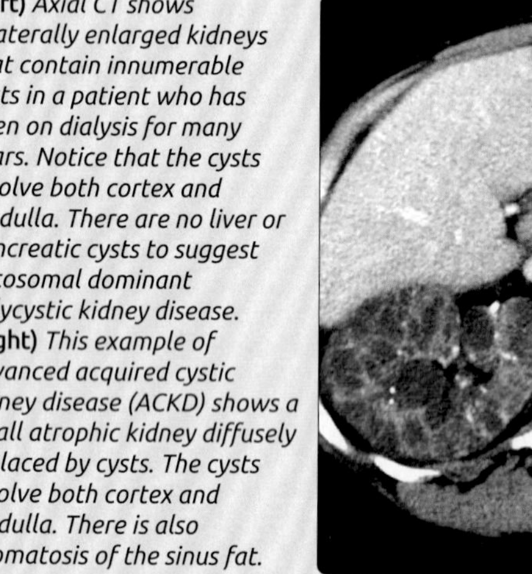

(Left) *Axial CT shows bilaterally enlarged kidneys that contain innumerable cysts in a patient who has been on dialysis for many years. Notice that the cysts involve both cortex and medulla. There are no liver or pancreatic cysts to suggest autosomal dominant polycystic kidney disease.* **(Right)** *This example of advanced acquired cystic kidney disease (ACKD) shows a small atrophic kidney diffusely replaced by cysts. The cysts involve both cortex and medulla. There is also lipomatosis of the sinus fat.*

Acquired Cystic Kidney Disease

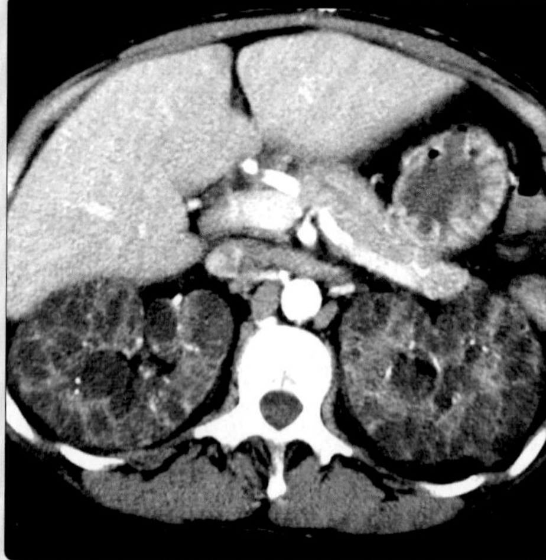

Small Atrophic, Diffusely Cystic Kidney

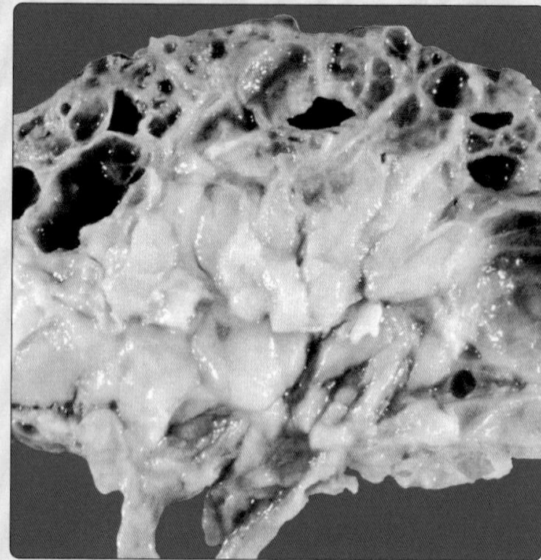

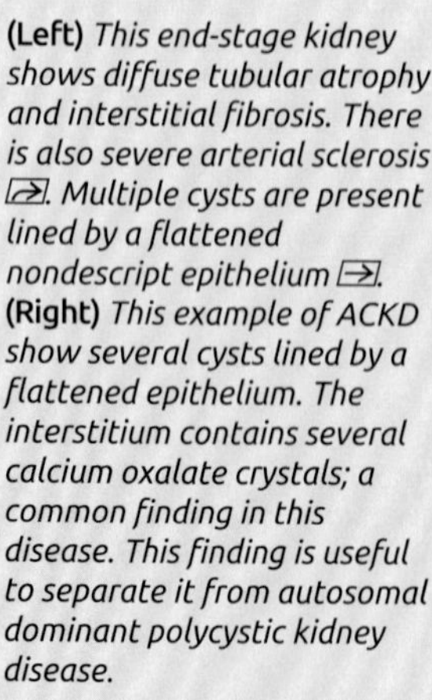

(Left) *This end-stage kidney shows diffuse tubular atrophy and interstitial fibrosis. There is also severe arterial sclerosis ➩. Multiple cysts are present lined by a flattened nondescript epithelium ➔.* **(Right)** *This example of ACKD show several cysts lined by a flattened epithelium. The interstitium contains several calcium oxalate crystals; a common finding in this disease. This finding is useful to separate it from autosomal dominant polycystic kidney disease.*

End-Stage Kidney With Cysts

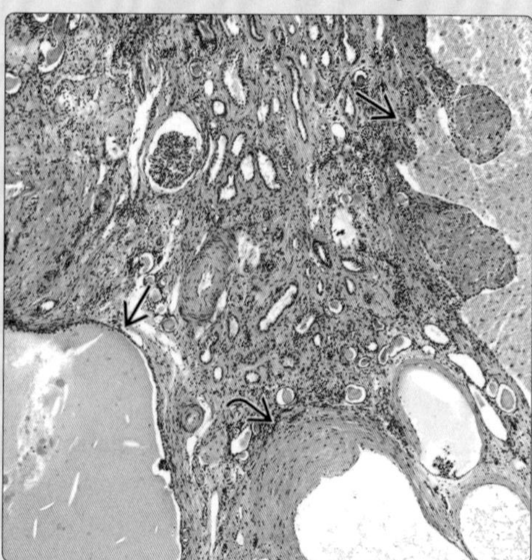

Calcium Oxalate

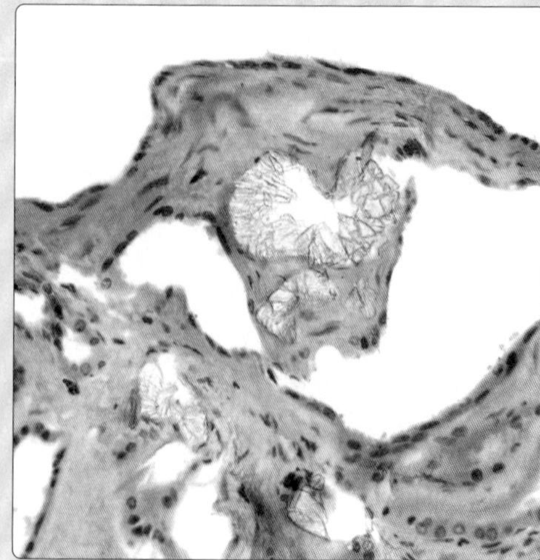

TERMINOLOGY

Abbreviations

- Acquired cystic kidney disease (ACKD)

Definitions

- ≥ 3 cysts in native kidneys of end-stage renal disease (ESRD) patients whose original cause for renal failure was not cystic kidney disease

ETIOLOGY/PATHOGENESIS

Pathogenesis is Unknown

- Possibly physiologic response to chronic renal failure
  - Increased proliferation of cyst-lining epithelium
- Not secondary to dialysis
  - Cyst formation occurs in some patients before dialysis

CLINICAL ISSUES

Epidemiology

- Incidence
  - 8% of patients starting dialysis
  - 90% after 10 years on dialysis
- Age
  - All ages
- Sex
  - More common in males
- Ethnicity
  - More common in African Americans than Caucasians

Presentation

- Usually asymptomatic
- Back pain with hemorrhage or infection of cysts
- Back pain or hematuria with renal cell carcinoma (RCC)

Natural History

- Kidney size, cyst size, and cyst number increase over time
- Risk of RCC increases over time
  - ACKD-associated RCC is most common cancer
  - Clear cell papillary RCC is 2nd most common cancer
  - Any RCC type may develop, such as clear cell RCC, papillary RCC, chromophobe cell RCC
  - Medullary hemangiomas, often multiple, may develop
- ESRD patients without cysts also at risk for RCC

Treatment

- Options, risks, complications
  - Infected cysts require antibiotics
  - Large ± painful cysts may require drainage
  - Periodic surveillance for RCC
- Surgical approaches
  - Nephrectomy for neoplasm or symptomatic cysts
  - Renal transplantation reverses cystic kidney disease
    - Effect of transplantation on risk of RCC unknown

Prognosis

- 2-7% of ACKD patients will develop RCC
  - 40-100x increased risk for RCC compared to population
- Kidneys > 150 g have increased prevalence of RCC (~ 50%)

MACROSCOPIC

General Features

- Kidneys may be enlarged or small with multiple variably sized cysts
  - Weighs < 1,000 g with average of 130 g
  - Cysts involve cortex and medulla
    - Size ranges from mm to several cm
- Neoplasms may be cystic or solid
  - Often multiple and bilateral
  - Multifocal neoplasms may be of more than 1 type

MICROSCOPIC

Histologic Features

- Advanced glomerulosclerosis, tubulointerstitial scarring and arterial sclerosis
- Cysts lined by flattened to cuboidal cells ± stratification or papillary growth
  - Lining cells may be clear, foamy, or eosinophilic
- Calcium oxalate crystal deposition common
- RCC, adenomas, hemangiomas may be present

ANCILLARY TESTS

Immunohistochemistry

- Useful to establish RCC type
  - ACKD-associated RCC: CD10(+), RCC ag, AMACR/CK7(-)
  - Clear cell papillary RCC: CK7(+), AMACR(-), CD10, RCC ag
  - Clear cell RCC: CD10(+), RCC ag, CK7(-), AMACR
  - Papillary RCC: CD10(+), CK7, RCC ag, AMACR

DIFFERENTIAL DIAGNOSIS

Autosomal Dominant Polycystic Kidney Disease

- Kidney typically much larger than ACKD (> 800 g)
- Family history often present
- Liver or pancreatic cysts, colonic diverticula, cerebral aneurysms, cardiac valve defects may be present

DIAGNOSTIC CHECKLIST

Pathologic Interpretation Pearls

- Careful macroscopic evaluation is essential to identify RCC
  - Section kidney at 1 cm intervals recommended

SELECTED REFERENCES

1. Hosseini M et al: Pathologic spectrum of cysts in end-stage kidneys: possible precursors to renal neoplasia. Hum Pathol. 45(7):1406-13, 2014
2. Kryvenko ON et al: Haemangiomas in kidneys with end-stage renal disease: a novel clinicopathological association. Histopathology. 65(3):309-18, 2014
3. Chen YB et al: Spectrum of preneoplastic and neoplastic cystic lesions of the kidney. Arch Pathol Lab Med. 136(4):400-9, 2012
4. Costa MZ et al: Histogenesis of the acquired cystic kidney disease: an immunohistochemical study. Appl Immunohistochem Mol Morphol. 14(3):348-52, 2006
5. Tickoo SK et al: Spectrum of epithelial neoplasms in end-stage renal disease: an experience from 66 tumor-bearing kidneys with emphasis on histologic patterns distinct from those in sporadic adult renal neoplasia. Am J Surg Pathol. 30(2):141-53, 2006
6. Nadasdy T et al: Proliferative activity of cyst epithelium in human renal cystic diseases. J Am Soc Nephrol. 5(7):1462-8, 1995
7. MacDougall ML et al: Prediction of carcinoma in acquired cystic disease as a function of kidney weight. J Am Soc Nephrol. 1(5):828-31, 1990

(Left) *This is an example of an early stage of ACKD. There is no distinct corticomedullary differentiation because of the severe interstitial fibrosis. The cysts are infrequent and small. Although the cystic disease is early, there are several small, solid renal neoplasms →.* **(Right)** *This is an example of more advanced ACKD. The cysts are numerous and vary in size. There are several large cysts. The cysts have a smooth glistening lining. No solid nodules are present to suggest a renal neoplasm.*

Early Stage of Acquired Cystic Kidney Disease

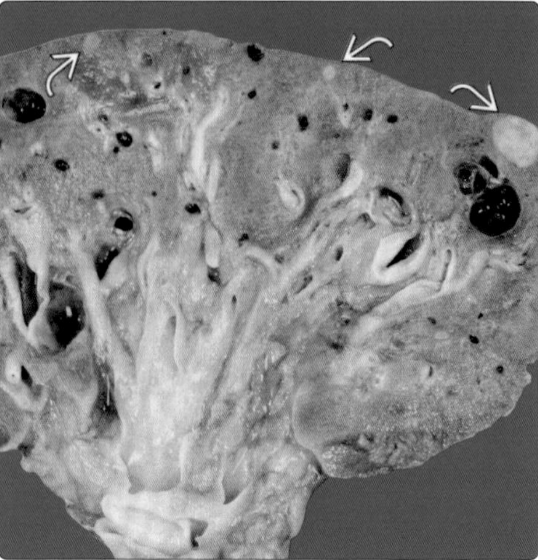

More Advanced Stage of Acquired Cystic Kidney Disease

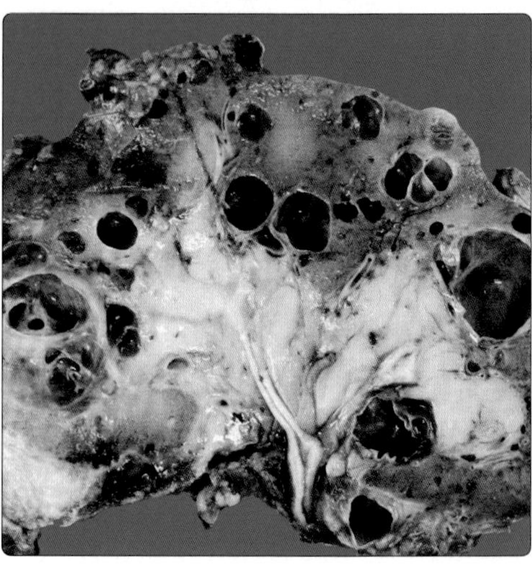

(Left) *This example of advanced ACKD shows small atrophic tubules → and diffuse interstitial fibrosis. The cysts are large. The cyst lining cells are flattened → and inconspicuous.* **(Right)** *There is diffuse interstitial fibrosis and tubular atrophy between the large cysts, consistent with an end-stage kidney. Some cysts are lined by flattened epithelial cells whereas others are lined by cells with clear cytoplasm →. The cysts contain eosinophilic proteinaceous material.*

Diffusely Cystic Kidney

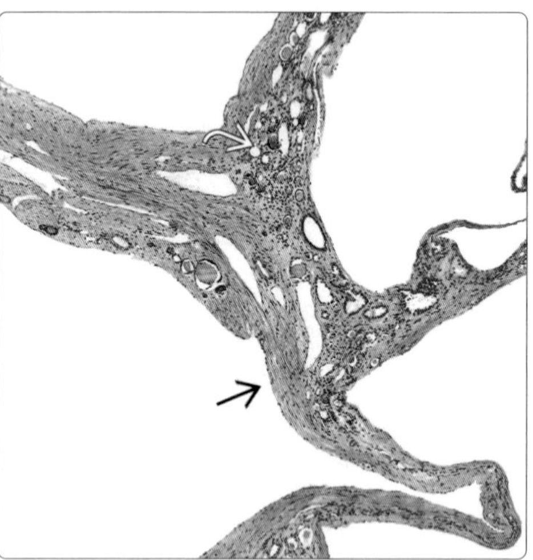

Cysts Containing Proteinaceous Fluid

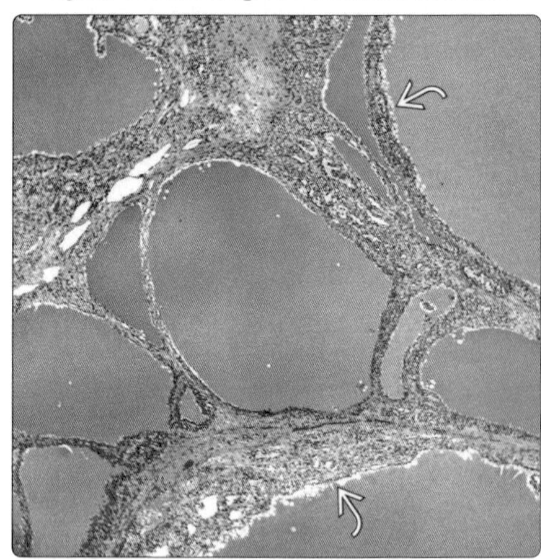

(Left) *One cyst is lined by a single layer of cuboidal eosinophilic cells →. A 2nd cyst is lined by a flattened, nondescript epithelium →. Most cysts appear derived from proximal tubules based upon immunohistochemical and lectin stains.* **(Right)** *This cyst is lined by a single layer of epithelial cells with optically clear cytoplasm. Notice how the nuclei are lined up in a row →. This cell lining is identical to the cells found in clear cell papillary RCC suggesting that this type of cyst may represent a precursor lesion.*

Cyst Lined by Eosinophilic Epithelium

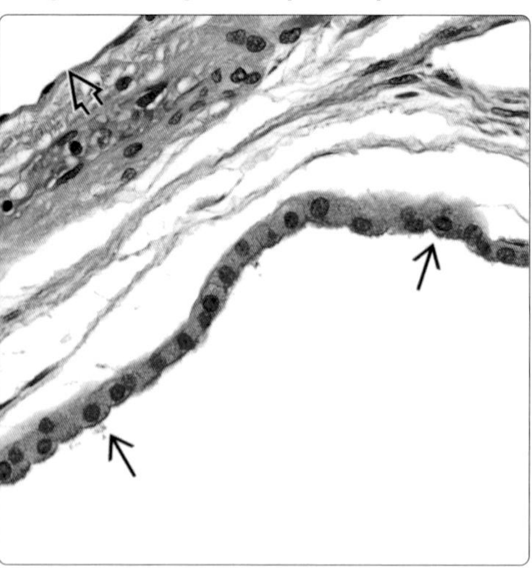

Clear Cell-Lined Cyst

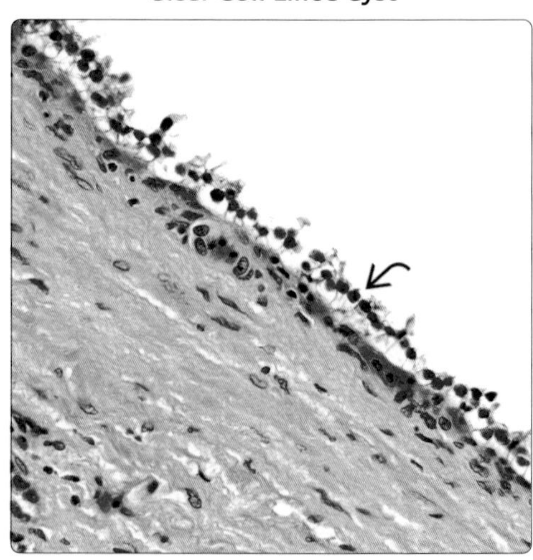

Cysts and Solid Neoplasms

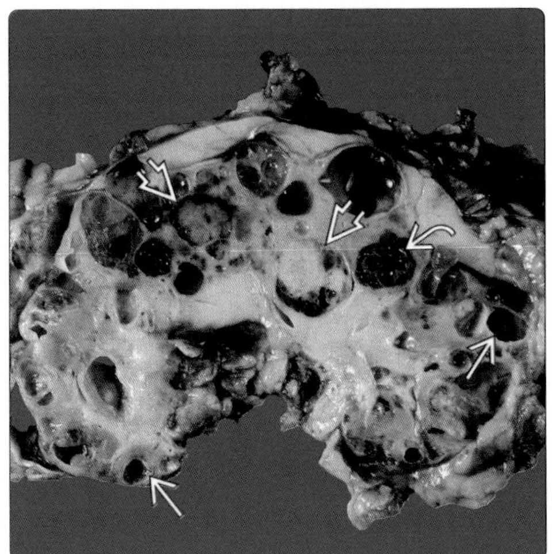

Cysts and Solid Neoplasms

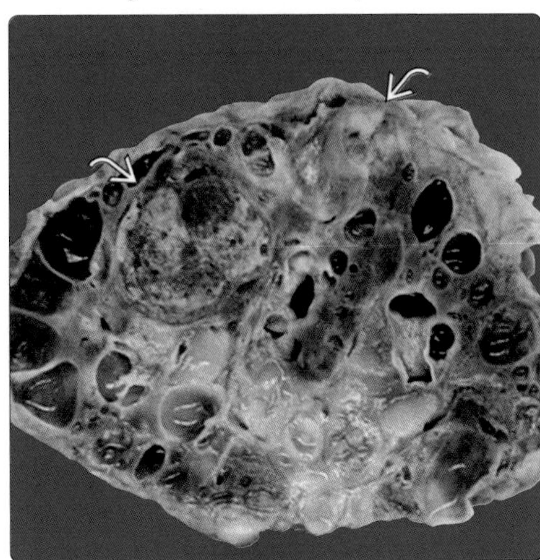

(Left) *Numerous cysts ➡ are present in this kidney with ACKD. Removal of the native kidney is usually performed when imaging studies identify potential renal neoplasms. Notice the presence of 2 mostly solid, but focally cystic, RCCs ➡. There is also a partially solid and cystic RCC ➡.* **(Right)** *This example of advanced ACKD shows both cortical and medullary cysts. There are 2 solid, yellow-appearing RCCs present, which led to the nephrectomy ➡.*

Cyst Lined by Papillary Proliferation

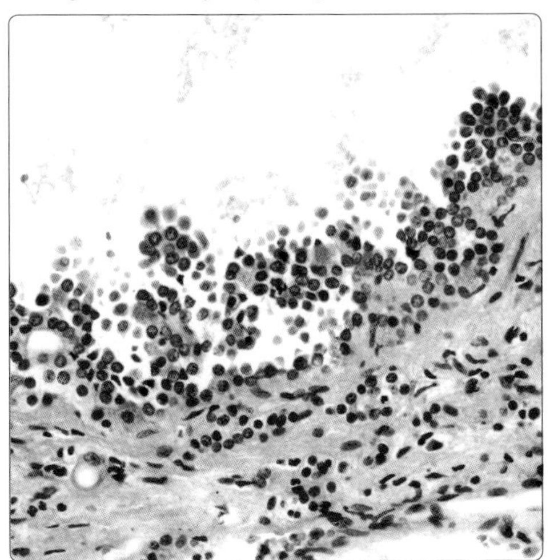

Papillary Adenoma

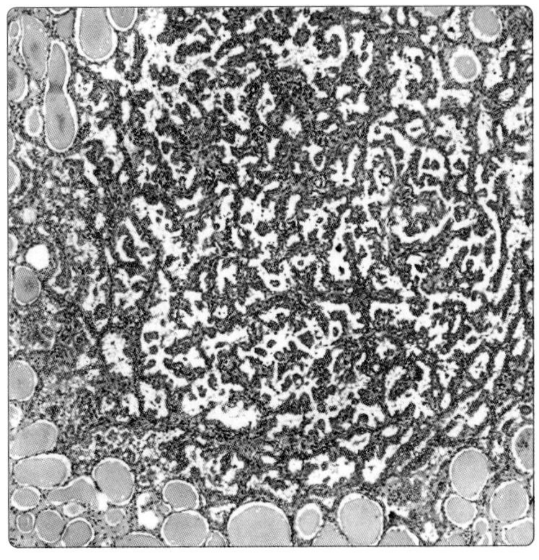

(Left) *The cells that line this cyst are stratified and form small papillary structures. They may present a precursor lesion of papillary adenomas and papillary RCC. The cells contain brown hemosiderin pigment, a common finding in papillary adenomas and papillary RCC.* **(Right)** *This is a papillary adenoma. It is by definition low grade and circumscribed. Its size is well below the 5 mm threshold arbitrarily established for papillary RCC. The surrounding tubules are atrophic and demonstrate so-called thyroidization.*

Acquired Cystic Kidney Disease-Associated Renal Cell Carcinoma

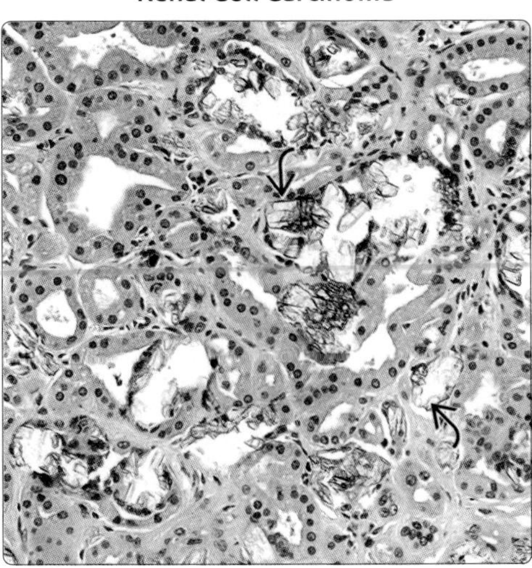

Clear Cell Papillary Renal Cell Carcinoma

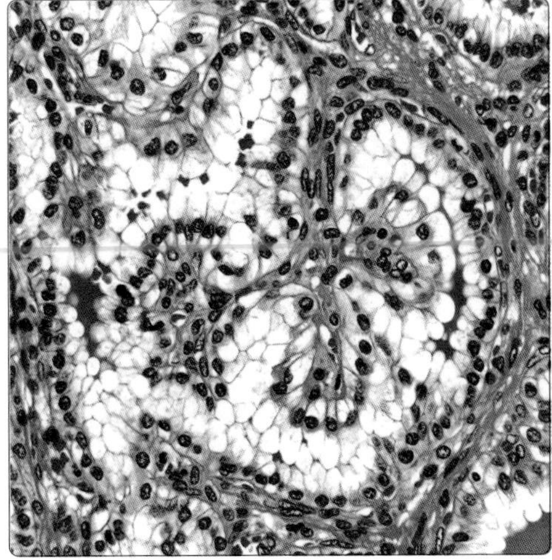

(Left) *This is an ACKD-associated RCC. The tumor is composed of large cells with eosinophilic cytoplasm. The cell are often vacuolated, a feature not present in this field. This RCC typically contains numerous calcium oxalate crystals ➡.* **(Right)** *This is a clear cell papillary RCC. It was originally regarded as limited to ACKD. It is now known to more frequently occur sporadically. In addition to clear cytoplasm and papillary architecture, its nuclei line up in neat rows.*

Simple and Miscellaneous Cysts

KEY FACTS

CLINICAL ISSUES

- Asymptomatic usually
  - Common incidental finding on radiography or autopsy
- Rarely associated with
  - Pain
  - Hematuria
  - Rupture
  - Infection
- Occur in ~ 12% of adult population (5% overall)
- Incidence increases with age (~ 33% > 80 years old)
  - Cyst size and number also increase
- M:F = 2:1

MACROSCOPIC

- Normal kidney size
- Cysts
  - Single or multiple
  - Predominantly unilocular
  - Smooth-walled cyst filled with clear fluid
  - Size: < 0.1 to > 10 cm

MICROSCOPIC

- Cyst epithelial lining attenuated and commonly absent
  - Lined by single layer of epithelial cells
    - May be cuboidal or flattened
- Dense fibrous tissue surrounds cyst

TOP DIFFERENTIAL DIAGNOSES

- Cystic nephroma
  - Simple cysts with incomplete septa
    - Rarely septated
- Cystic renal cell carcinoma
  - Cysts lined by cells with clear cytoplasm
- Acquired cystic kidney disease
  - Arise in prolonged uremia
- Autosomal dominant polycystic kidney disease
- Localized/unilateral renal cystic disease

(Left) *Most simple cysts are incidental findings. This kidney was removed due to hydronephrosis and recurrent infections. A solitary simple deep cortical cyst can be seen in the specimen ⇨.* **(Right)** *Typical histology of a simple cortical cyst is shown. The cyst lining epithelium is attenuated ⇨ and is often absent. A dense fibrous tissue surrounds the cyst ⇨.*

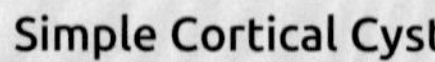

Simple Cortical Cyst

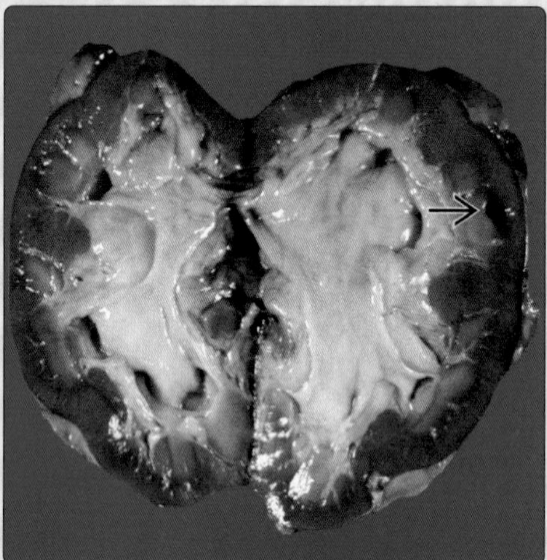

Simple Cyst

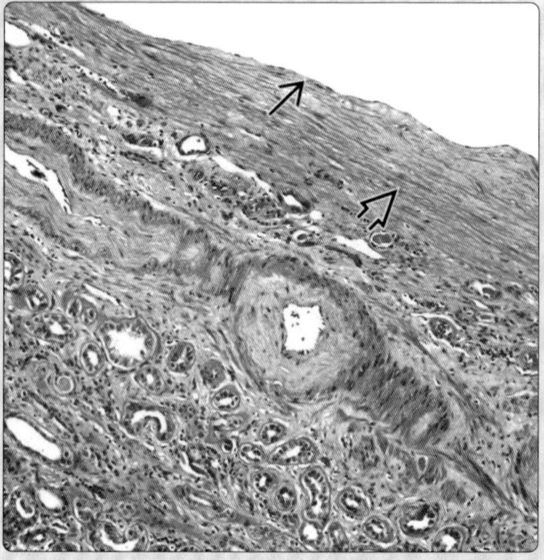

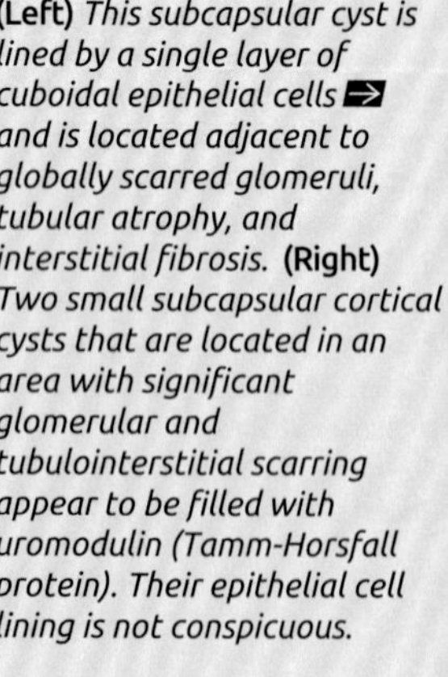

(Left) *This subcapsular cyst is lined by a single layer of cuboidal epithelial cells ➡ and is located adjacent to globally scarred glomeruli, tubular atrophy, and interstitial fibrosis.* **(Right)** *Two small subcapsular cortical cysts that are located in an area with significant glomerular and tubulointerstitial scarring appear to be filled with uromodulin (Tamm-Horsfall protein). Their epithelial cell lining is not conspicuous.*

Simple Cyst

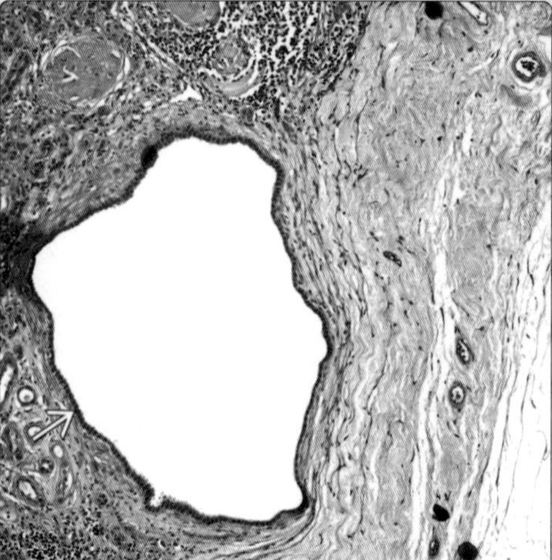

Subcapsular Cysts

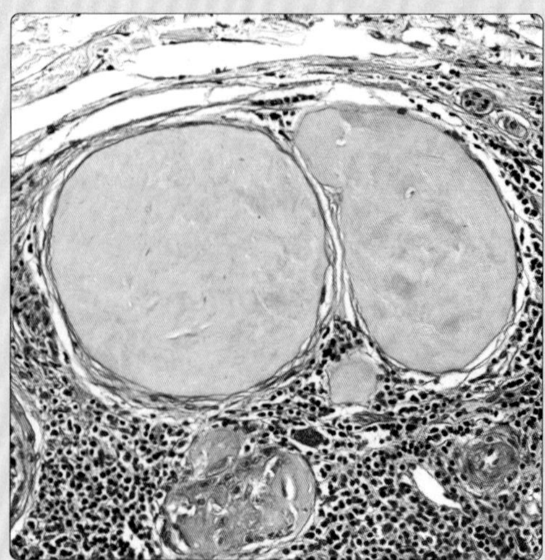

ETIOLOGY/PATHOGENESIS

Acquired Defect

- Cysts originate from diverticula of cortical tubules secondary to weakened basement membrane
  - Primarily proximal tubules
    - May also develop from distal nephron segments
  - Connection to tubular segments often maintained

CLINICAL ISSUES

Epidemiology

- Incidence
  - ~ 12% of adult population (5% overall)
- Age
  - Incidence increases with age
    - Cyst size and number also increase
    - 33% > 80 years old
- Sex
  - M:F = 2:1

Presentation

- Asymptomatic
  - Common incidental finding on radiography or autopsy
- Rarely associated with
  - Pain
  - Hematuria
  - Rupture
  - Infection
- Hypertension
  - Rarely due to compression on renal parenchyma

Treatment

- None in most patients
- Cyst drainage and marsupialization if symptomatic

Prognosis

- No significant health consequences

MACROSCOPIC

General Features

- Cysts
  - Single or multiple
  - Predominantly unilocular
  - Smooth-walled cyst filled with clear fluid
  - Randomly distributed

Size

- Normal kidneys
- Cysts: < 0.1 to > 10 cm

MICROSCOPIC

Histologic Features

- Cyst
  - Lined by single layer of epithelial cells
    - May be cuboidal or flattened
    - May be absent altogether
- Dense fibrous tissue surrounds cyst

DIFFERENTIAL DIAGNOSIS

Cystic Nephroma

- Simple cysts with incomplete septa
- Variability of stroma and presence of cellular stroma in septa strongly favors cystic nephroma

Cystic Renal Cell Carcinoma

- Radiographic discrimination not possible
- Cysts lined by cells with clear cytoplasm

Acquired Cystic Kidney Disease

- Arise with prolonged uremia
- Many simple to possibly complex cysts
  - May have epithelial "hobnailing" and papillary projections

Autosomal Dominant Polycystic Kidney Disease

- Enlarged kidneys with numerous cysts
- Family history and other manifestations, such as liver cysts

Localized/Unilateral Renal Cystic Disease

- Rare benign condition
  - Perhaps an extreme form of multiple simple cysts
- Innumerable cysts usually replace normal kidney

SELECTED REFERENCES

1. Hosseini M et al: Pathologic spectrum of cysts in end-stage kidneys: possible precursors to renal neoplasia. Hum Pathol. 45(7):1406-13, 2014
2. Simms RJ et al: How simple are 'simple renal cysts'? Nephrol Dial Transplant. 29 Suppl 4:iv106-12, 2014
3. Bisceglia M et al: Renal cystic diseases: a review. Adv Anat Pathol. 13(1):26-56, 2006
4. Terada N et al: The natural history of simple renal cysts. J Urol. 167(1):21-3, 2002
5. Caglioti A et al: Prevalence of symptoms in patients with simple renal cysts. BMJ. 306(6875):430-1, 1993
6. Baert L et al: Is the diverticulum of the distal and collecting tubules a preliminary stage of the simple cyst in the adult? J Urol. 118(5):707-10, 1977

Other Localized Cystic Kidney Diseases

Name	Etiology	Clinical Considerations	Pathology
Perinephric pseudocyst	Trauma	Localized, often painful, may cause mass effect; history of trauma or abdominal surgery	No lining epithelium; fat and fibrous tissue with variable amounts of inflammation
Renal calyceal diverticulum	May originate from developmental defect in collecting system	May be an incidental radiographic finding; may produce pain, hematuria due to urinary stone formation, UTI	Cyst wall lined by flat urothelium and smooth muscle; inflammation and calcifications may be present in complicated cases
Localized/unilateral cystic kidney disease	Unknown	Rare, perhaps variant of multiple simple cysts; usually nonprogressive	1 kidney diffusely replaced by innumerable cysts; other kidney may show simple cysts

Renal Lymphangioma/Lymphangiectasia

KEY FACTS

TERMINOLOGY

- Collection of developmental, acquired, and neoplastic lesions of lymphatics
- Sometimes manifested as TEMPI syndrome: Telangiectasias, erythrocytosis, monoclonal gammopathy, perinephric-fluid collections, and intrapulmonary shunting

ETIOLOGY/PATHOGENESIS

- Failure of lymphatics to connect with lymphatic outflow
- Lymphatic obstruction due to trauma or inflammation
- Neoplastic: Karyotypic abnormalities reported

CLINICAL ISSUES

- May present in children or adults
- May present with ascites, flank pain, hematuria, proteinuria, hypertension, polycythemia, renal vein thrombosis

IMAGING

- Kidney may be normal or enlarged
- May be unilateral or bilateral

MACROSCOPIC

- May involve part or all of kidney, renal sinus, renal capsule or be perinephric

MICROSCOPIC

- Thin-walled cysts lined by flattened endothelium
  - Endothelium expresses lymphatic markers
  - May contain smooth muscle and entrapped tubules
- Localized collection (tumor) of cysts and cyst septa
- May produce massive interstitial lymphedema with dilated proximal lymphatics

TOP DIFFERENTIAL DIAGNOSES

- Cystic kidney diseases, especially autosomal dominant polycystic kidney disease
- Cystic renal dysplasia
- Cystic nephroma and mixed epithelial stromal tumor
- Multilocular cystic renal cell carcinoma

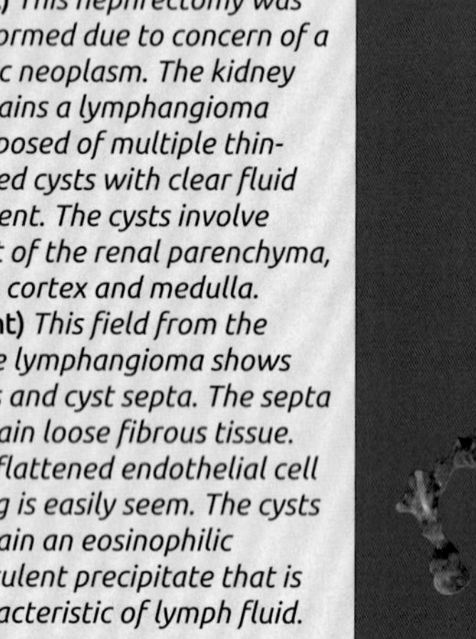

(Left) *This nephrectomy was performed due to concern of a cystic neoplasm. The kidney contains a lymphangioma composed of multiple thin-walled cysts with clear fluid content. The cysts involve most of the renal parenchyma, both cortex and medulla.* **(Right)** *This field from the same lymphangioma shows cysts and cyst septa. The septa contain loose fibrous tissue. The flattened endothelial cell lining is easily seem. The cysts contain an eosinophilic flocculent precipitate that is characteristic of lymph fluid.*

Lymphangioma

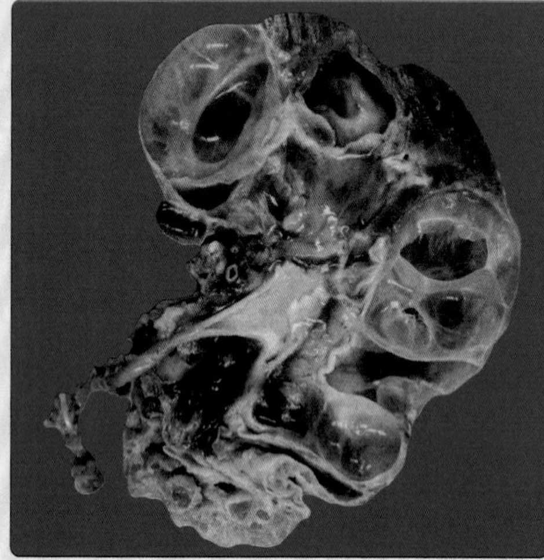

Lymphangioma Containing Lymph Fluid

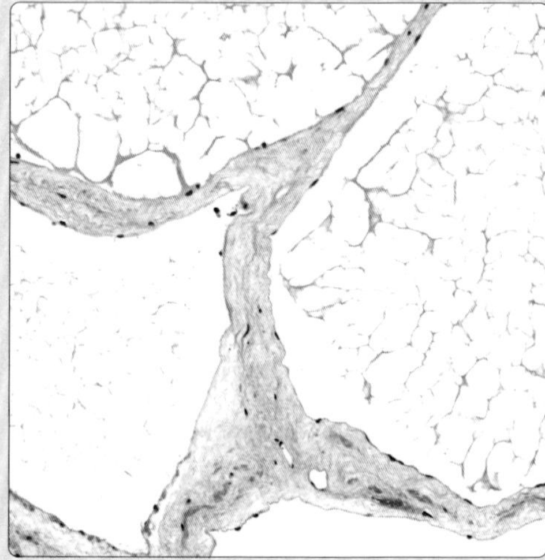

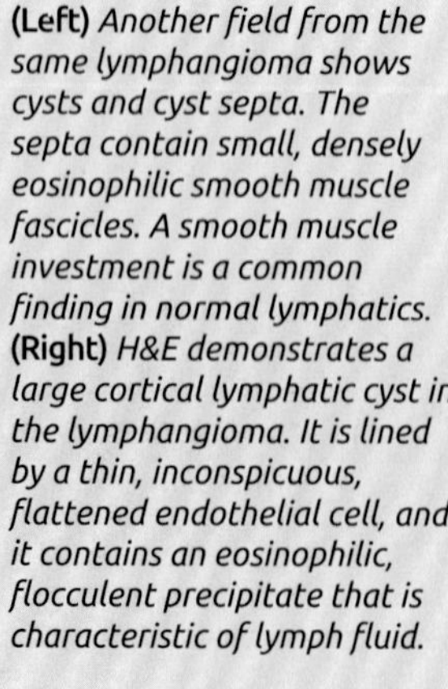

(Left) *Another field from the same lymphangioma shows cysts and cyst septa. The septa contain small, densely eosinophilic smooth muscle fascicles. A smooth muscle investment is a common finding in normal lymphatics.* **(Right)** *H&E demonstrates a large cortical lymphatic cyst in the lymphangioma. It is lined by a thin, inconspicuous, flattened endothelial cell, and it contains an eosinophilic, flocculent precipitate that is characteristic of lymph fluid.*

Smooth Muscle in Septa

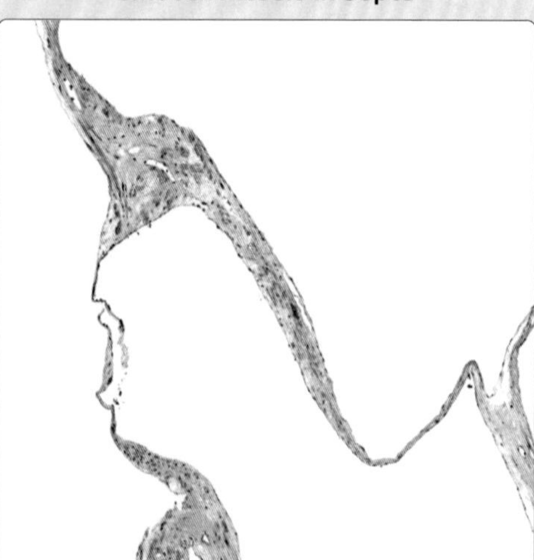

Lymphangioma Involving the Cortex

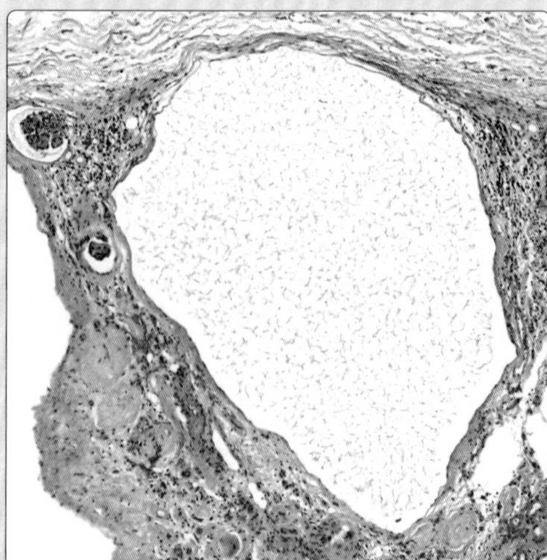

TERMINOLOGY

Definitions

- Collection of developmental, acquired, and neoplastic lesions of renal lymphatics not always distinguishable
  - Lymphangiectasia: Cystic dilatation of lymphatics
  - Lymphangiomatosis: Bilateral disease
  - Lymphangioma: Lymphatic-derived tumor or neoplasm
- Sometimes manifested as TEMPI syndrome: Telangiectasias, erythrocytosis, monoclonal gammopathy, perinephric-fluid collections, and intrapulmonary shunting

ETIOLOGY/PATHOGENESIS

Developmental Anomaly

- Renal lymphatics fail to connect normally with lymphatic outflow
- Rare occurrence in siblings suggests genetic component
- Associated with systemic lymphangiomatosis

Lymphatic Obstruction

- Lymphatic obstruction due to trauma or inflammation

Lymphatic Neoplasm

- Karyotypic abnormalities: Monosomy X, trisomy 7q, and von Hippel-Lindau gene defects

CLINICAL ISSUES

Epidemiology

- Incidence
  - Rare disorders: ~ 60 cases reported in literature
  - More common in adults (2/3) than children (1/3)

Presentation

- Collectively, abnormalities of renal lymphatics have diverse presentations
  - May be asymptomatic
  - If large, flank pain or abdominal mass
  - Ascites
  - Hematuria, proteinuria, chyluria, renal vein thrombosis
  - Hypertension: Renin-dependent due to mass effect and decreased kidney perfusion
  - TEMPI syndrome: Telangiectasias, elevated erythropoietin level and erythrocytosis, monoclonal gammopathy, perinephric-fluid collections, and intrapulmonary shunting

Laboratory Tests

- TEMPI syndrome: Monoclonal gammopathy and elevated erythropoietin

Treatment

- Observation sufficient in many cases
- Cyst aspiration and marsupialization if symptomatic
- Nephrectomy in refractory symptomatic cases or concern for cystic neoplasm
- Bortezomib for TEMPI syndrome

Prognosis

- Stable, slowly progressive or partial regression reported

MACROSCOPIC

General Features

- Kidney normal size or enlarged
- Multiple cysts or cystic mass may be present
- Located in a portion of kidney or entire kidney, renal sinus (peripelvic), renal capsule, or perirenal
- Bilateral or unilateral

MICROSCOPIC

Histologic Features

- Thin-walled cysts lined by flat lymphatic endothelium
  - Cyst lining negative for epithelial markers and positive for vascular ± lymphatic markers: CD31, CD34, podoplanin (D2-40)
  - Fascicles of smooth muscle may be present in septa
  - Entrapped nephron elements may be in septa
- May form localized collection (tumor or mass) involving renal capsule, cortex, or sinus fat
- Cortical edema/lymphedema may be pronounced, with large spaces not lined by endothelial cells

DIFFERENTIAL DIAGNOSIS

Cystic Kidney Diseases, Especially Autosomal Dominant Polycystic Kidney Disease

- Unilateral, bilateral, segmental presentations possible without lower urinary tract abnormalities
- Liver cysts common
- Cyst lining cells are epithelial markers positive, lymphovascular markers negative

Cystic Renal Dysplasia

- Metanephric dysgenesis (dysplasia), immature ducts with cellular collars, ± cartilage, +/- LUT disease

Multilocular Cystic Renal Cell Carcinoma

- Composed entirely of clear cell-lined cysts and cyst septa with no solid areas

Cystic Nephroma

- Composed entirely of epithelial-lined cysts and cyst septa with no solid areas

Mixed Epithelial and Stromal Tumor

- Composed of cysts lined by complex epithelium and solid areas that may contain smooth muscle or fat

Miscellaneous Renal Neoplasms

- Many renal neoplasms may occasionally be diffusely cystic

SELECTED REFERENCES

1. Rosado FG et al: Bone marrow findings of the newly described TEMPI syndrome: when erythrocytosis and plasma cell dyscrasia coexist. Mod Pathol. 28(3):367-72, 2015
2. Ahmad K et al: Mediastino-hepato-renal cystic lymphangiomas-diagnostic and surgical considerations. J Thorac Dis. 6(9):E173-5, 2014
3. Sykes DB et al: The TEMPI syndrome–a novel multisystem disease. N Engl J Med. 365(5):475-7, 2011
4. Bazari H et al: Case records of the Massachusetts General Hospital. Case 23-2010. A 49-year-old man with erythrocytosis, perinephric fluid collections, and renal failure. N Engl J Med. 363(5):463-75, 2010
5. Upreti L et al: Imaging in renal lymphangiectasia: report of two cases and review of literature. Clin Radiol. 63(9):1057-62, 2008

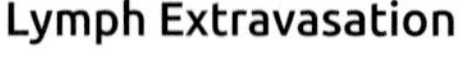

Lymph Extravasation

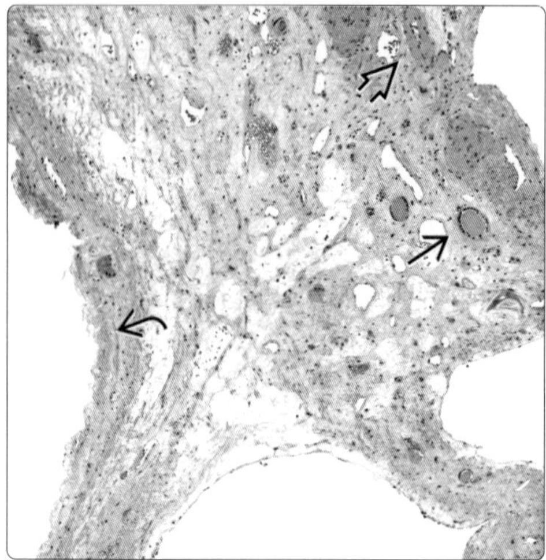

Smooth Muscle and Tubules in Septa

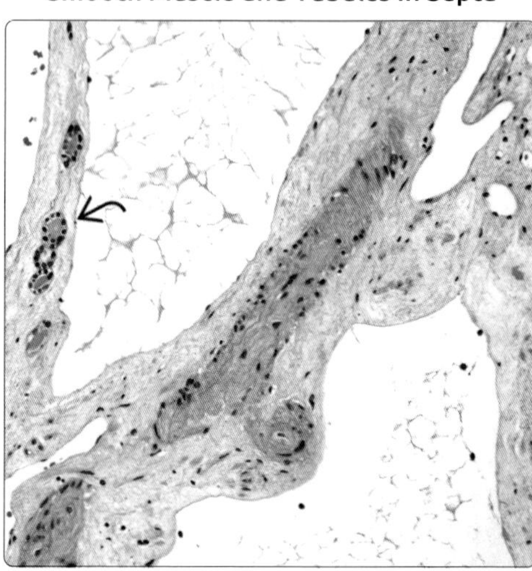

(Left) *In this field, the septa contain bundles of eosinophilic smooth muscle cells and individual smooth muscle cells. Some muscle is pericystic →, some septal stroma and some arterial-related →. There are also small tubules → and lucent foci representing extravasation of lymph fluid.* **(Right)** *The septa in this lymphangioma contain bundles of eosinophilic smooth muscle, possibly arterial-related, and single individual smooth muscle cells. There is also a collection of small, entrapped renal tubules →.*

Podoplanin

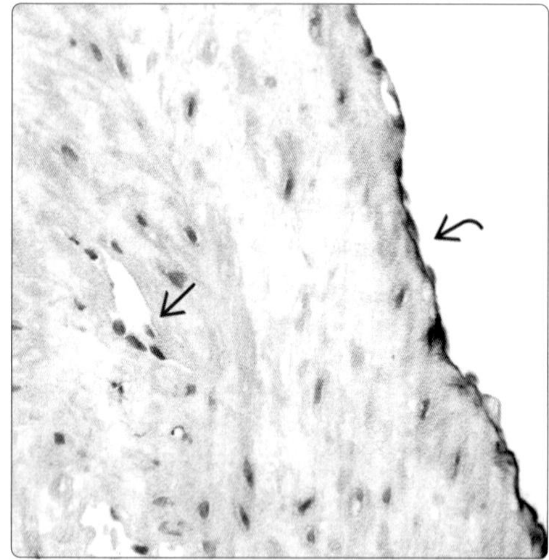

CD31

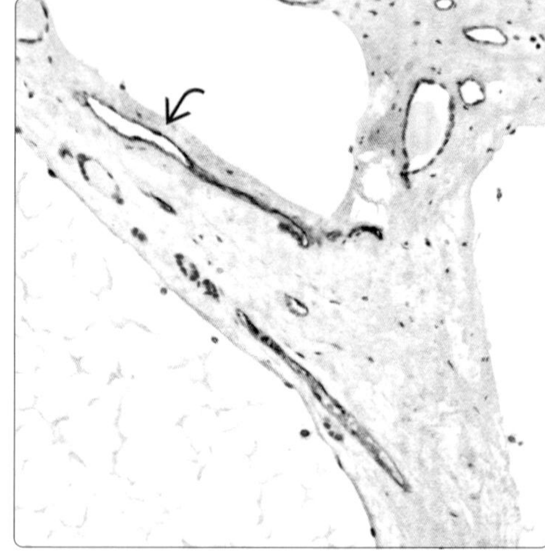

(Left) *This lymphangioma is stained for podoplanin. Hematogenous and lymphatic epithelium cannot be distinguished by routine histochemical stains; however, lymphatic epithelium is podoplanin positive →. Notice that the vascular endothelium is podoplanin negative →.* **(Right)** *Lymphangioma is stained with CD31, a general endothelial cell marker. Normal lymphatic epithelium will be positive. The hematogenous endothelium in the septae are positive → while the lymphatic endothelium failed to stain.*

Normal Lymphatic Stained for Podoplanin

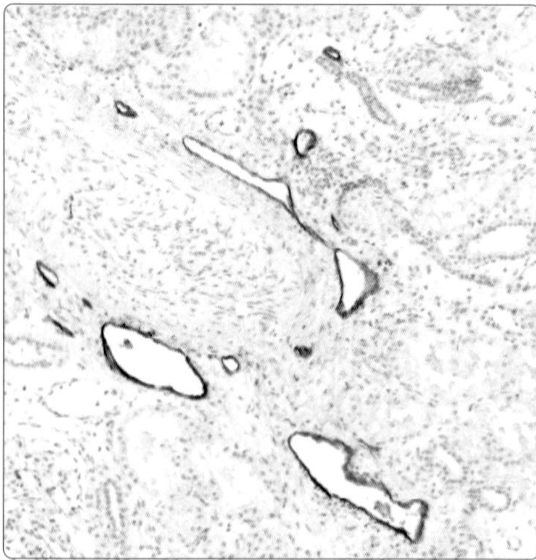

Lymphangiectasia Within Renal Sinus

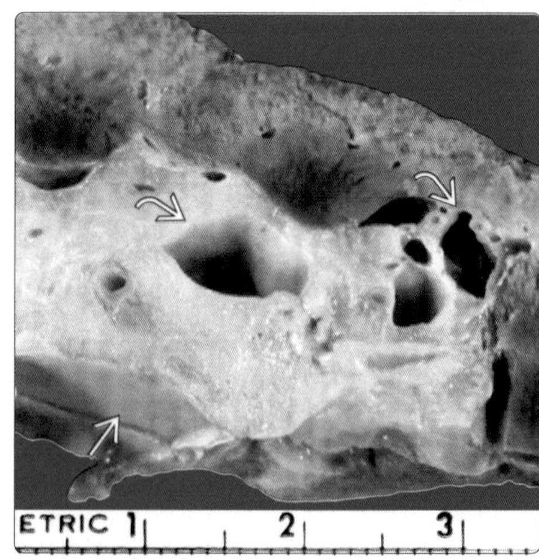

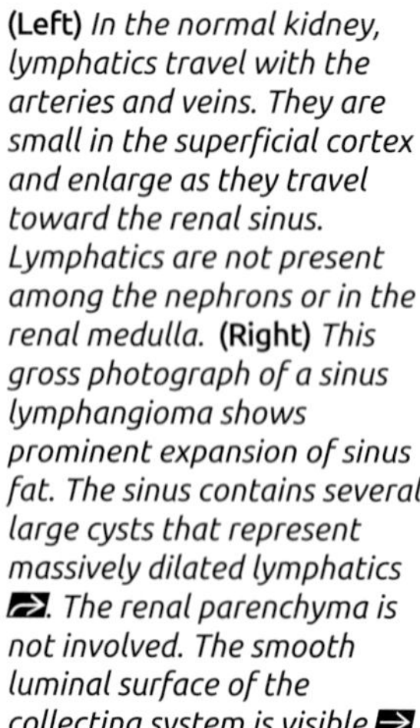

(Left) *In the normal kidney, lymphatics travel with the arteries and veins. They are small in the superficial cortex and enlarge as they travel toward the renal sinus. Lymphatics are not present among the nephrons or in the renal medulla.* **(Right)** *This gross photograph of a sinus lymphangioma shows prominent expansion of sinus fat. The sinus contains several large cysts that represent massively dilated lymphatics →. The renal parenchyma is not involved. The smooth luminal surface of the collecting system is visible →.*

Sinus Lymphangiectasia

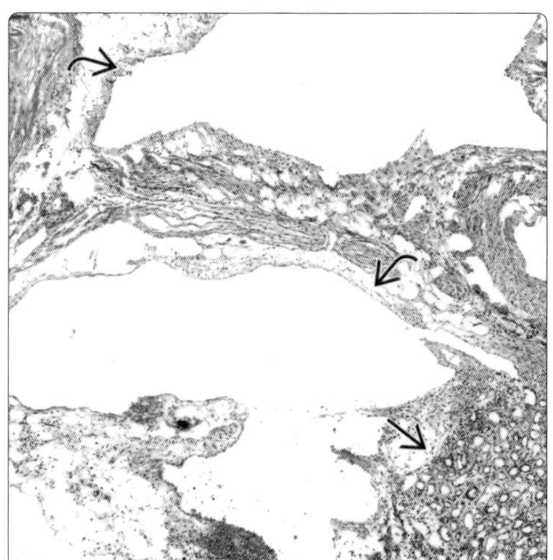

Perinephric Lymph Accumulation

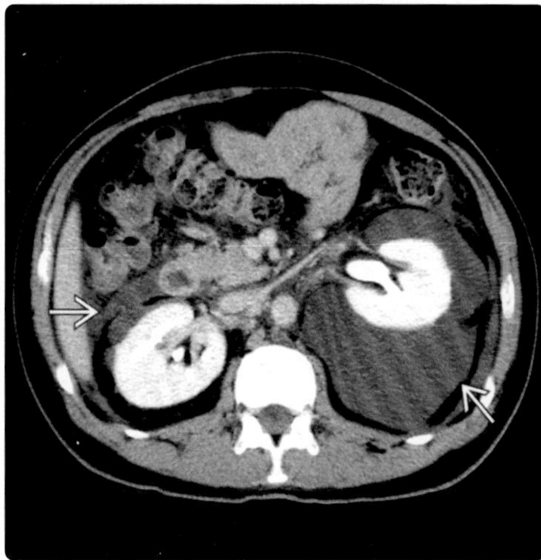

(Left) *Renal sinus lymphangiectasia in a child shows two massively dilated lymphatics within the sinus fat ➔. The lymphatics appear identical to dilated veins. A small portion of the renal parenchyma is present ➔.* **(Right)** *CT scan in a patient with bilateral renal lymphangiectasis shows perinephric accumulations of fluid bilaterally ➔. The kidneys themselves appear unaffected by the fluid accumulation. There is significant asymmetry in the degree of fluid accumulation.*

Interstitial Fluid Believed to Represent Lymph Fluid

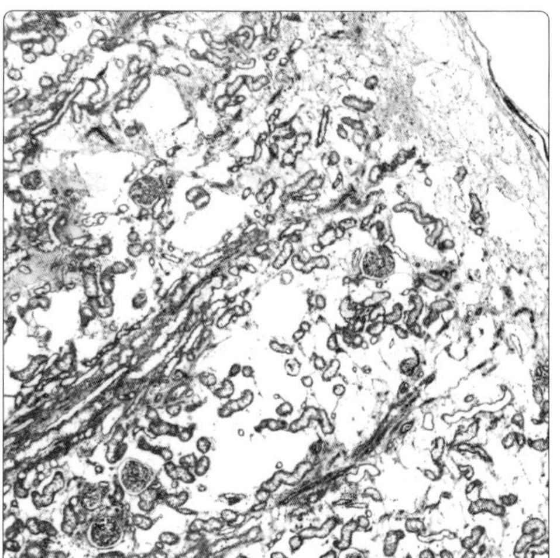

Interstitial Fluid Believed to Represent Lymph Fluid

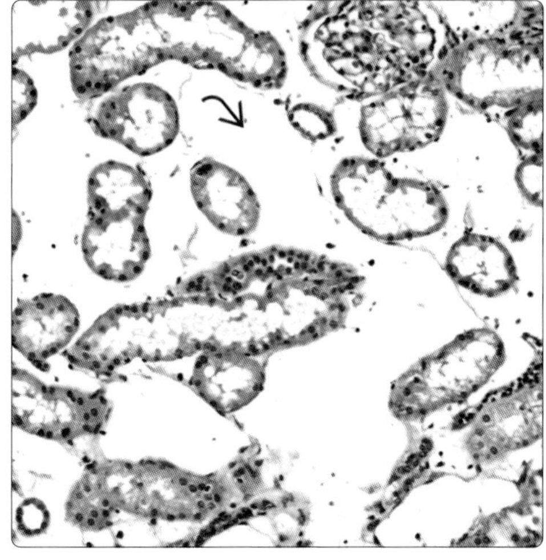

(Left) *H&E shows massive interstitial fluid, believed to represent lymph, that was associated with massive ascites in a renal transplant patient. The fluid was visibly "weeping" from the kidney and flowing into the peritoneal space.* **(Right)** *Massive interstitial lymph fluid accumulation is shown. The interstitial fluid is acellular and is in not within an endothelial lined space ➔. Its origin is presumed to result from lymph extravasation secondary to impaired lymph outflow, possibly a surgical complication.*

Interstitial Fluid Believed to Represent Lymph Fluid

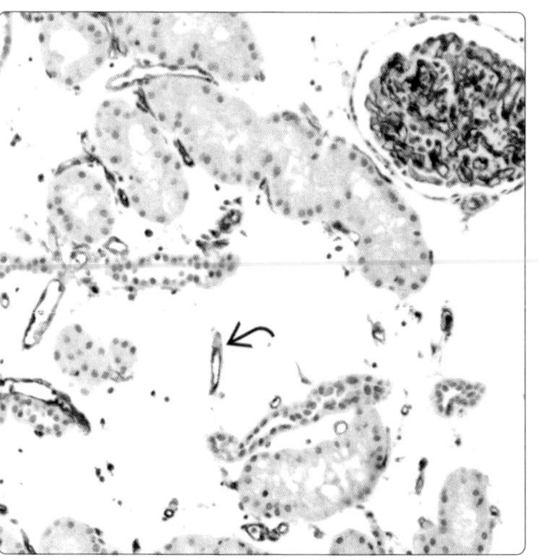

Dilated Lymphatic

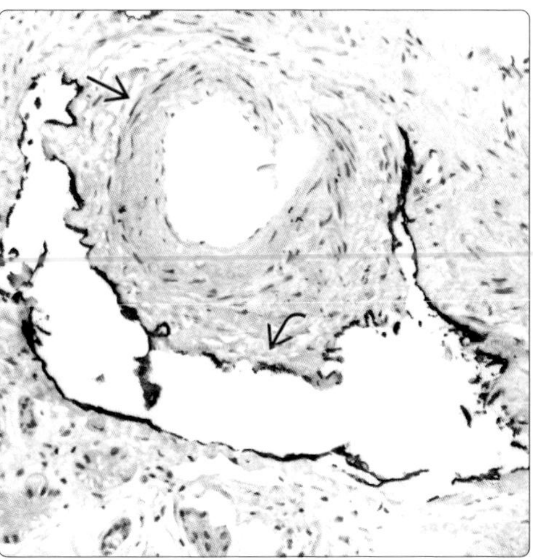

(Left) *The peritubular interstitial fluid is not confined within endothelial-lined spaces. This CD31 stain shows numerous small, intact, nondilated peritubular capillaries floating within the massive interstitial lymph fluid ➔. Normally, there are no lymphatics within the cortical labyrinth.* **(Right)** *Podoplanin stain in a patient with lymphangiectasia and massive cortical interstitial lymph fluid accumulation shows a dilated lymphatic channel in the inner cortex ➔. A normal interlobular artery is also present ➔.*

SECTION 8

Diseases of the Collecting System

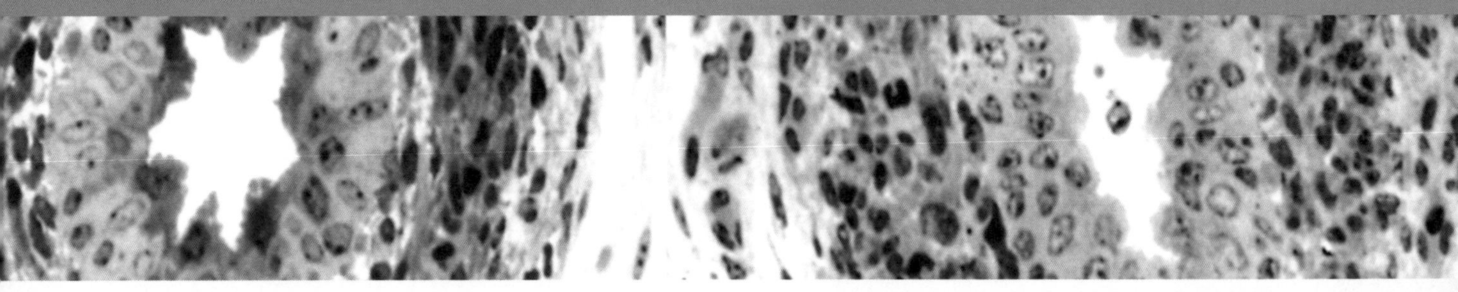

TERMINOLOGY

Definitions

- Impediment to urine flow: Retrograde or hindered urine flow due to obstructive or nonobstructive causes
- Reflux: Retrograde urine flow from bladder into ureters or kidneys due to functional or physical defects of lower urinary tract
- Hydronephrosis: Dilatation of renal pelvis or calyces due to functional or physical impediment to urine flow
- Obstructive nephropathy: Damage to kidney due to obstruction of urine flow
- Reflux nephropathy: Damage to kidney due to urine reflux

CLASSIFICATION

Type of Impediment

- Obstructive
    - Physical
        - Internal urinary system obstruction: Stones, tumors of urinary tract, infections
        - External compression of urinary system: Tumors, pregnancy, retroperitoneal fibrosis, endometriosis, crossing vessels, BPH
    - Functional
        - Ureter or collecting duct dysfunction
    - Congenital
        - Ureteropelvic junction obstruction (UPJO)
        - Primary obstructive megaureter or ureterovesical junction obstruction (UVJO)
        - Ureterocele
        - Posterior urethral valves (PUV)
    - Acquired
- Nonobstructive: Vesicoureteral reflux (VUR)
    - Primary VUR
    - Secondary VUR

Major Impediments to Urine Flow

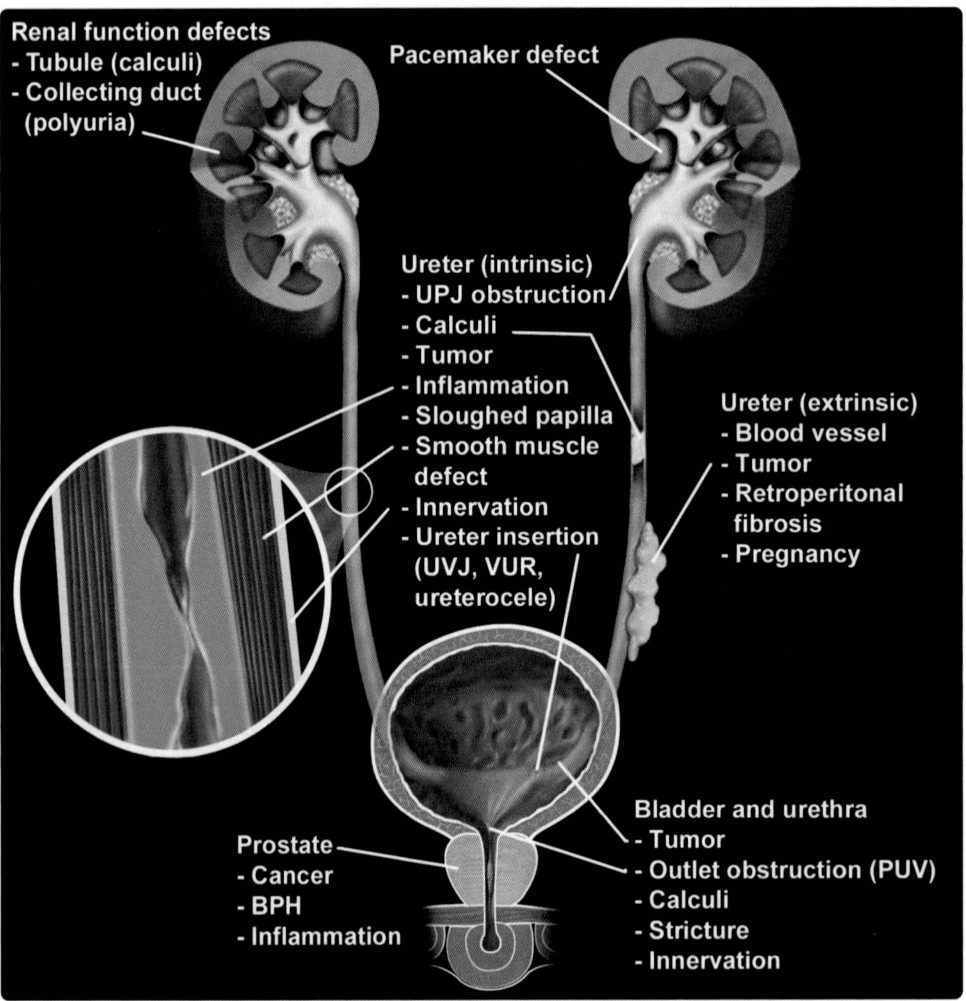

Illustration depicts the different causes (urinary tract intrinsic or extrinsic) of impediment to urine flow. The lesions can arise anywhere along the path of urine flow, beginning in the kidney and extending through the ureters to the bladder and urethra. The major consequences on the kidney are obstructive or reflux nephropathy, which is manifested by dilation of the pelvis and calyces (hydronephrosis), loss of the medullary pyramids, and secondary atrophy of the cortex. These conditions increase the risk of urinary tract infection, which leads to further injury in the form of acute and chronic pyelonephritis.

Region of Impediment and Associated Major Abnormalities

- Upper urinary tract
  - Kidney (tubules, collecting duct)
    - UPJO
- Lower urinary tract
  - Ureter
    - UPJO
    - UVJO or megaureter
    - Ureterocele
  - Bladder and ureter
    - VUR
  - Bladder and urethra
    - PUV

ETIOLOGY/PATHOGENESIS

Developmental Mechanisms

- UPJO
  - Most common cause of obstructive nephropathy
  - Kidney
    - Abnormal water absorption or collecting duct cell function (functional obstruction)
    - Abnormal pacemaker function regulating peristalsis (functional obstruction)
  - Ureter
    - Abnormal ureter or pelvic wall development (increased extracellular matrix, disorganized smooth muscle) leading to defective peristalsis (functional obstruction)
  - Extrinsic
    - Crossing by lower pole renal vessels (physical obstruction)
    - Nervous system (pyeloureteral innervation) mediated defects in peristalsis (functional obstruction)
- Megaureter
  - UVJO, abnormal muscular development or stricture, ureter insertion into bladder may occur normally
  - Supernumerary ureters ectopically inserted into bladder
  - Refluxing megaureter due to primary or secondary reflux
- Ureterocele
  - Distal blind-ending ureter often in duplicated collecting system but can occur in single ureters
- Primary VUR
  - Distal wolffian duct (WD) &/or ureter maturation
    - Abnormal ureteric bud (UB) budding site
    - Failure of ureter insertion into bladder, abnormality of vesicoureteral junction
    - Failure of ureter to separate from WD
    - Abnormal common nephric duct (CND) degeneration
  - Most common congenital anomalies of kidney and urinary tract (CAKUT)
    - 50% of children with UTIs may have VUR
    - 15-34% of children with asymptomatic bacteriuria may have VUR
- PUV
  - Failure of urogenital membrane disintegration

Genetic Mechanisms

- UPJO
  - Autosomal dominant inheritance reported
    - Other modes of inheritance not excluded
  - Genes associated or mutated
    - *Shh*, *Bmp4*, *Tshz3*, *Adamts1*, *Dlgh1*, *Calcineurin*, renin-angiotensin system (*RAS*), *Tbx18*, *Id2*, *Limp2*
- Primary VUR
  - Genetically heterogeneous
    - Inheritance patterns include autosomal dominant, autosomal recessive, polygenic, sporadic, recessive X-linked with incomplete penetrance and variable expressivity
    - May skip generations
  - Individuals in same family may have VUR or other CAKUT
  - Modifier genes or epigenetics can affect phenotype
  - 80% chance in monozygotic twin
  - 32% in siblings
  - Known genetic mutations account for small number of cases
    - Genome-wide association studies (GWAS) identified several common variants of primary VUR
      - In most cases, unknown if associated genes are causal
    - Long-range effects of common variants
    - Rare deleterious variant burden in coding, splice junctions, or insertions/deletions may underlie genetic causes
    - About 10% cases associated with rare genomic imbalances, copy number variations
  - Genes associated and mutated
    - *UPK3A*, *ROBO2*, *RET*, HLA complex, *ACE*, *AGTR2*, *UPK1A*, ABO blood group, *TNFα*, *TGFβ*, *PTGS2*, *IGF1*, *IGF1R*, *EGF*, *CCL2*
- PUV
  - Autosomal dominant, incomplete penetrance, variable expressivity, compound recessive with modifier genes, de novo

Nongenetic Mechanisms

- Environmental: Toxins, drugs, nutrition
- Epigenetic: Methylation, acetylation

CLINICAL IMPLICATIONS

Clinical Presentation

- Lung hypoplasia, oligohydramnios
- Acute pyelonephritis
- Chronic pyelonephritis
- Cystitis
- Hypertension
- Nausea and vomiting
- Failure to thrive
- Flank pain
- Abdominal distension
- Weak stream
- Proteinuria

MACROSCOPIC

General Features

- UPJO
  - Dilatation of pelvis, blunting of calyces
  - Compression of cortex

Characteristics of Major Congenital Impediments to Urine Flow

	UPJ	Megaureter	VUR	PUV
Definition	Severe narrowing of ureter at junction of ureter and pelvis	Large, dilated, and often tortuous ureter	Retrograde urine flow from bladder to kidneys	Abnormal persistence of urogenital membrane causing severe narrowing of proximal urethra
Incidence	1:500 (left > right)	1:10,000 (left > right)	At least 1:100	1:5,000 males
Mechanism	Kidney collecting duct defect, pacemaker abnormality, ureter smooth muscle defect	Abnormal lower ureter wall (UVJ), abnormal insertion of ectopic ureters, secondary to reflux	Distal WD/ureter maturation or developmental defects leading to failure of valve mechanism	Abnormal mesenchymal development resulting in failure of urogenital membrane disintegration
Radiological findings	Hydronephrosis	Dilated, tortuous ureter	Different grades of VUR	Narrow to obliterated distal urethral lumen, dilated proximal urethra, huge irregular bladder shape, reflux
Pathological outcome	Obstructive nephropathy	Obstructive or reflux nephropathy depending on etiology	Reflux nephropathy	Obstructive or reflux nephropathy
Macroscopic	Dilatation of pelvis, calyceal blunting, compression of cortex	Large ureteral lumen; dilated, tortuous, long ureter	Different degrees of ureter dilatation with renal parenchymal compression in grade 5; abnormal entry of ureter into bladder or intravesicular tunnel	Large trabeculated bladder in addition to dilated urethra and reflux
Microscopic	Ureter smooth muscle disorganization (if ureter etiology); obstructive nephropathy changes including tubular atrophy, tubulointerstitial inflammation, fibrosis, atubular glomeruli, glomerulosclerosis, compressed cortex, dysplasia (if congenital)	Similar changes as UPJ; if megaureter due to primary reflux, then reflux nephropathy changes such as segmental renal scarring	Reflux nephropathy changes in primary or secondary VUR including renal scarring, tubulointerstitial inflammation, chronic or acute pyelonephritis, cortical thinning; may see dysplasia if congenital	Thick bladder muscle wall, histopathological changes of obstructive or reflux nephropathy

- Compensatory hypertrophy in contralateral kidney
- Megaureter
  - Segmental or complete ureteral dilatation
  - Tortuous ureter
- VUR
  - Different grades of reflux causing ureter and pelvicalyceal dilatation
- Other CAKUT may be present
- Defects in other organ systems in syndromic cases
- Enlarged trabeculated bladder in PUV
- Segmental or diffuse scarring if progresses to nephropathy and cortical thinning

MICROSCOPIC

General Features

- Primary UPJO or UVJO ureter histology
  - Disorganized smooth muscle layer
  - Increased extracellular matrix
  - Reduced innervation
  - Increased fibrosis
  - Lumen narrow and irregular
  - Intravesical tunnel typically normal in UVJ unless coexisting reflux
- VUR
  - Intravesicular tunnel typically not evaluated for histology
- PUV
  - Thick-walled bladder
- If severe, histopathological changes of reflux or obstructive nephropathy in kidney

SELECTED REFERENCES

1. Klein J et al: Congenital ureteropelvic junction obstruction: human disease and animal models. Int J Exp Pathol. Epub ahead of print, 2010
2. Chen F: Genetic and developmental basis for urinary tract obstruction. Pediatr Nephrol. 24(9):1621-32, 2009
3. Uetani N et al: Plumbing in the embryo: developmental defects of the urinary tracts. Clin Genet. 75(4):307-17, 2009
4. Murawski IJ et al: Gene discovery and vesicoureteric reflux. Pediatr Nephrol. 23(7):1021-7, 2008
5. Rosen S et al: The kidney in congenital ureteropelvic junction obstruction: a spectrum from normal to nephrectomy. J Urol. 179(4):1257-63, 2008
6. Williams G et al: Vesicoureteral reflux. J Am Soc Nephrol. 19(5):847-62, 2008

Ureteropelvic Junction Obstruction (UPJO)

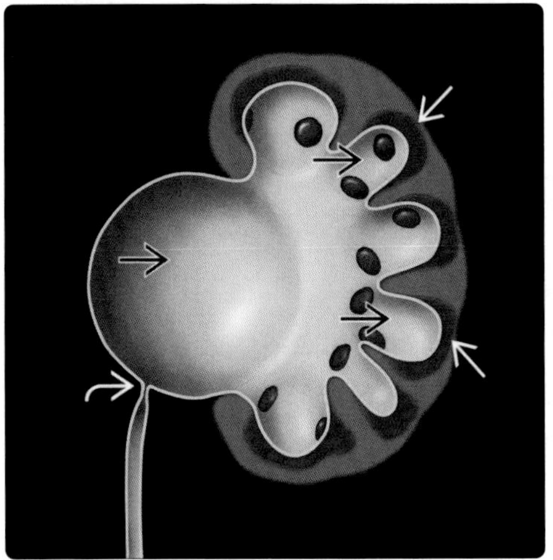

Ureter From Child With UPJO

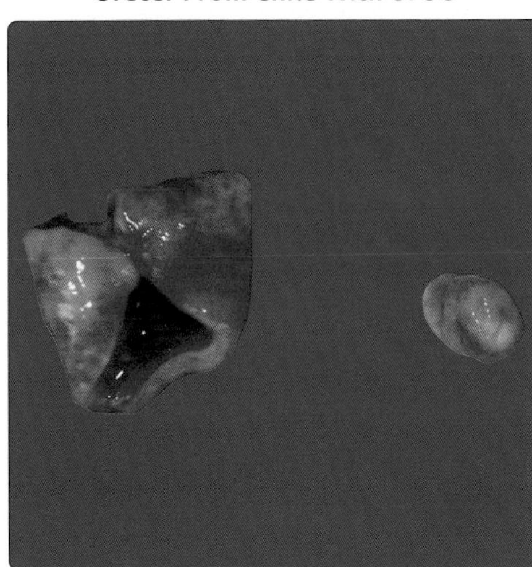

(Left) *Illustration shows typical features of UPJO ➩, including hydronephrosis with dilatation of the pelvis and calyces ➙ due to increased back pressure. This leads to secondary thinning of the cortex ➨.* **(Right)** *This case depicts cross sections of the ureter in a child with UPJO. Note the massively dilated ureter (left) proximal to obstruction and ureter with narrow lumen distal to the obstruction (right).*

Vesicoureteral Reflux (VUR)

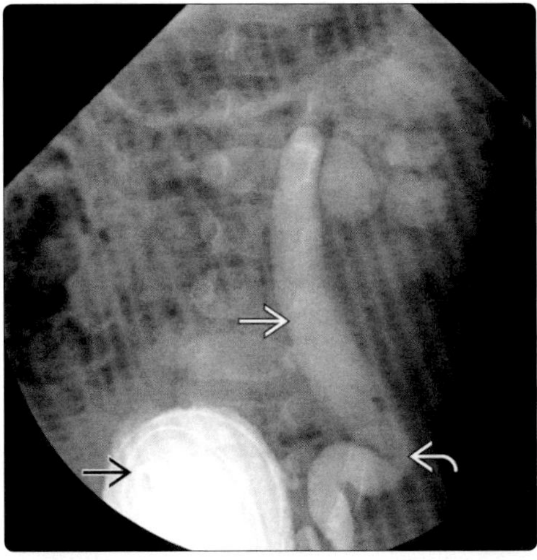

Ureterocele

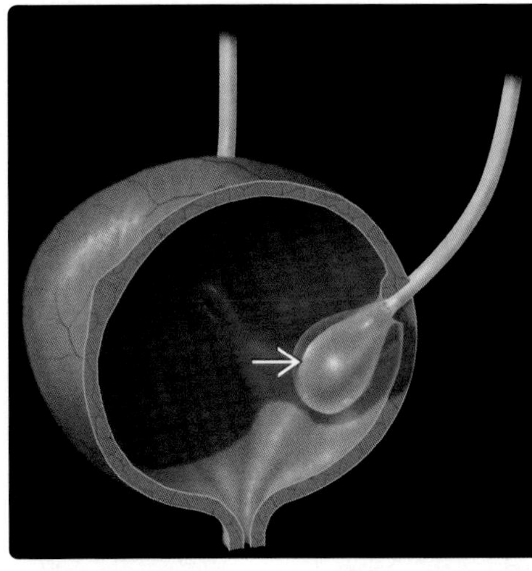

(Left) *Voiding cystourethrogram shows primary reflux of urine from the bladder ➙ into the ureter ➨, resulting in a massively dilated and tortuous ureter ➩. Vesicoureteral reflux (VUR) is one of the most common kidney anomalies; however, it is a rare cause of end-stage renal disease.* **(Right)** *Illustration shows a ureterocele ➨ (blind-ending ureter) that can cause obstruction to urine flow. Ureteroceles are rare and are typically seen in ectopic ureters.*

Posterior Urethral Valve (PUV)

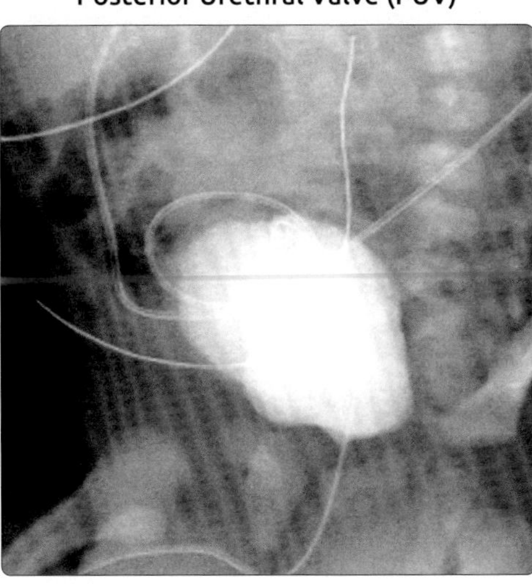

Posterior Urethral Valve Anatomy

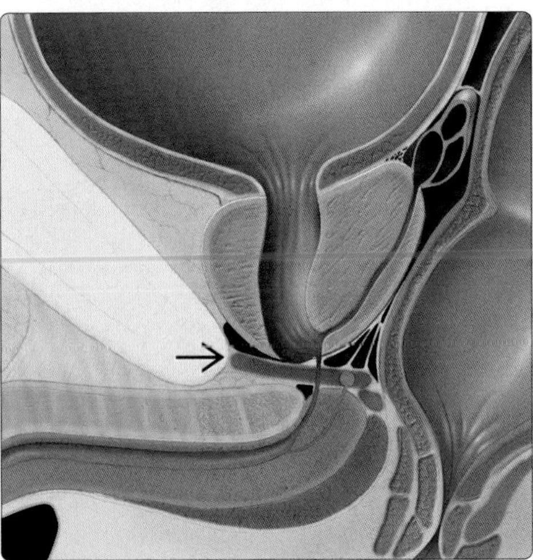

(Left) *Voiding cystourethrogram shows an enlarged bladder with trabeculations in a patient with posterior urethral valves (PUV). PUVs are a major cause of renal insufficiency in male children.* **(Right)** *Illustration shows an anatomical defect in PUV. There is narrowing of the prostatic urethra ➙ (keyhole sign) due to abnormal development of the mesenchymal component of the urogenital sinus causing obstruction. The result is bladder hypertrophy and reflux.*

Reflux Nephropathy

KEY FACTS

TERMINOLOGY

- Reflux nephropathy: Renal parenchymal scarring due to urine reflux

ETIOLOGY/PATHOGENESIS

- Vesicoureteral reflux (VUR), urinary tract infections (UTIs) may accelerate scarring but not necessarily required
- Exposure of kidneys to high-pressure urine reflux or bacteria causes tubulointerstitial damage and scarring
- Intrarenal reflux in utero affects kidney development
- Gene or structural variations in the genome

CLINICAL ISSUES

- Most common cause of severe hypertension in children
- Children with febrile UTIs have high incidence of VUR
- Manage UTIs, acute pyelonephritis, chronic pyelonephritis, and VUR
- Diagnosis: DMSA scan, need adequate blood flow and cellular uptake, utility is debatable
- Prophylactic antibiotics should not be universally mandated as long-term outcome is debatable in progression to nephropathy

MICROSCOPIC

- Tubulointerstitial inflammation, fibrosis, atrophy, and global glomerulosclerosis
- Dysplasia indicates congenital component leading to reflux
- Histological features in primary and secondary urine reflux may be similar and overlap with features of obstructive nephropathy
- Clinical and radiological correlation necessary

TOP DIFFERENTIAL DIAGNOSES

- Obstructive nephropathy
- Ask-Upmark kidney
- Chronic pyelonephritis

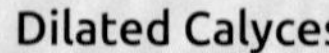

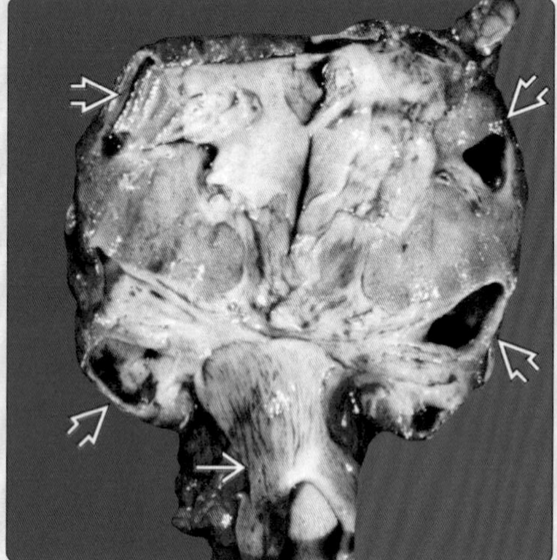

VUR Grades

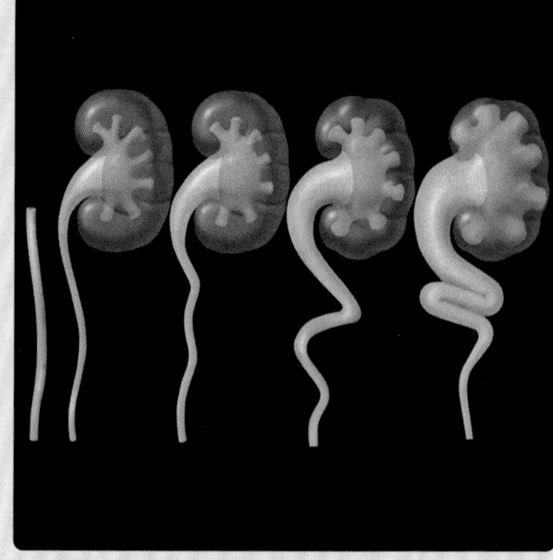

(Left) *Reflux nephropathy with megaureter ➡ shows marked thinning of the cortex and loss of the medulla, especially at the poles ➡.* **(Right)** *Schematic depicts different grades of vesicoureteral reflux (VUR) (1-5). The leftmost image depicts grade 1, and the rightmost image depicts grade 5.*

Severely Thinned Cortex and Medulla

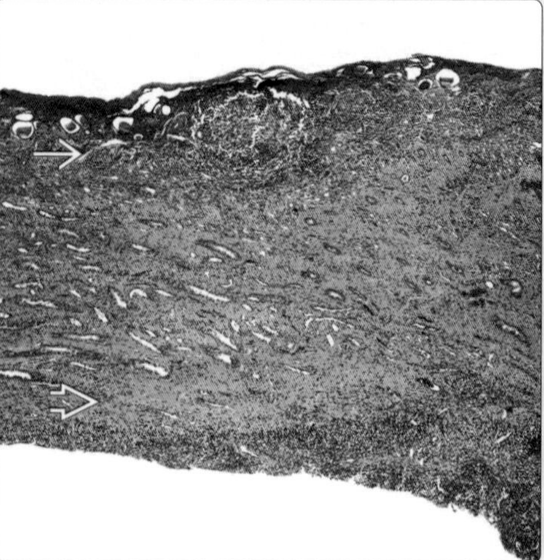

Adaptive FSGS and Glomerular Hypertrophy

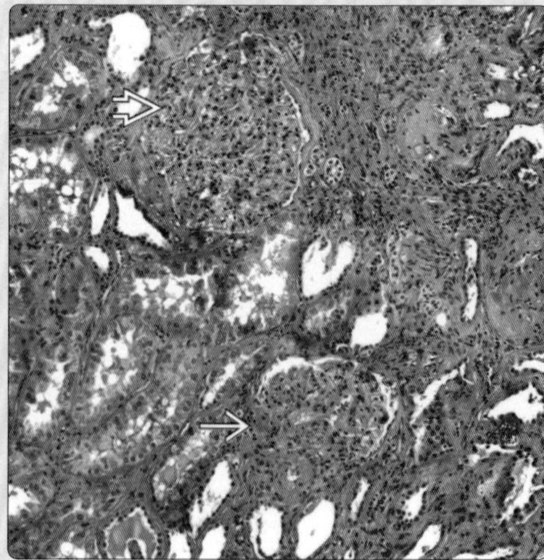

(Left) *Cross section through full thickness of cortex ➡ and medulla ➡ in a 7-year-old boy with reflux nephropathy shows the markedly thin parenchyma corresponding to the gross appearance.* **(Right)** *Glomerular hypertrophy ➡ and secondary FSGS are commonly present in the late stages of bilateral reflux nephropathy. The adhesion and hyaline are typically in a perihilar location ➡.*

TERMINOLOGY

Definitions

- Reflux: Retrograde urine flow from bladder into ureters or kidney due to functional or physical lower tract defects
- Reflux nephropathy: Renal parenchymal scarring due to urine reflux

ETIOLOGY/PATHOGENESIS

Causes

- Vesicoureteral reflux (VUR)
  - Primary VUR
    - Congenital anomaly, unilateral, or bilateral
    - Abnormal insertion of ureter into bladder, abnormal intravesicular tunnel length of ureter
    - Incompetent valve
    - If familial, usually autosomal dominant transmission with variable expressivity and penetrance
  - Secondary VUR
    - Distal obstruction, neurogenic bladder: Posterior urethral valves (PUV), multiple sclerosis, spinal cord injury, stroke, diabetic neuropathy, pelvic surgery, B12 deficiency
    - Dysfunctional elimination syndrome: Abnormal holding of urine and voiding pattern
- Acquired: Urinary tract infections (UTI)

Genetics

- Genes associated with VUR phenotype in humans
  - *TNF, TGFB1, ACE, PTGS2, IGF1, IGF1R, EGF, CCL2, ROBO2, UPK1A, UPK3A, GNB3, AGTR2, RET*
  - Many genes causing reflux are important in kidney development

Pathophysiology

- Reflux urine enters renal parenchyma via compound papillae (2-3 fused papillae at poles with concave orifices)
- Reflux gives bacteria access to kidney
- Continued exposure of kidneys to high-pressure urine reflux or bacteria causes acute or chronic immune response
- Tubulointerstitial damage ensues with these events leading to edema, ischemia, necrosis, inflammation, tubular atrophy, fibrosis, and scar formation
  - Focal scars in compound papillae
  - Ongoing damage can alter anatomy of simple papillae (dome shaped with slit-like orifice and drain single lobe) to compound type and cause more diffuse scars
- Glomerulosclerosis secondary to loss of nephrons
- Activated renin-angiotensin system causes hypertension
- Etiology of scar formation not fully understood
  - Reflux may not be prerequisite for scar formation
    - Scar can develop in kidneys without reflux
  - Bacterial colonization of kidneys may not be necessary to induce kidney damage
    - Scars observed in patients without UTI history
  - New renal scars can develop in presence of reflux and pyelonephritis
- Intrarenal reflux during development can lead to partial or complete developmental arrest of kidney resulting in dysplasia

CLINICAL ISSUES

Epidemiology

- Incidence
  - Reflux nephropathy is cause of renal failure in 3-5% of renal dialysis or transplant patients
  - Most common cause of severe hypertension in children

Presentation

- Hypertension
- Proteinuria
- UTI, acute pyelonephritis, chronic pyelonephritis
  - 50-80% of children with febrile UTI have renal scarring
- Primary or secondary VUR

Laboratory Tests

- Renal parenchyma scintigraphy: Tc-99m dimercaptosuccinic acid (DMSA) scan
  - Depends on adequate renal blood flow and cellular uptake
- Voiding cystourethrogram (VCUG) for lower urinary tract disorder

Treatment

- Surgical repair of VUR vs. prophylactic antibiotics
- Dialysis, transplantation

Prognosis

- High-grade reflux more likely to cause nephropathy than low grade
  - 5% of pediatric renal failure due to reflux nephropathy
- Proteinuria, reduced creatinine clearance and GFR, hypertension, high-grade reflux, and bilateral VUR increase likelihood of chronic kidney disease progression
- Management criteria debatable
  - Monitor for nephropathy in grades 4 and 5 of reflux
- Functional development of kidney may be affected if reflux in early embryogenesis
- 20% of renal failure in boys with reflux due to PUV

IMAGING

Radiographic Findings

- Voiding cystourethrogram shows dye in ureters that may extend into pelvis and kidneys, depending on severity

MACROSCOPIC

General Features

- Irregular kidney surface due to segmental or diffuse cortical scarring
- Dilation of ureters and calyces
- Other congenital anomalies of kidney and urinary tract may be present

MICROSCOPIC

Histologic Features

- Glomeruli
  - Focal segmental or global glomerulosclerosis
  - Compensatory hypertrophy of viable glomeruli
- Tubules
  - Tubular atrophy

Etiology of Reflux Nephropathy

Primary VUR (Congenital)	Secondary VUR (Congenital)	Secondary VUR (Acquired)
Abnormal ureter intravesicular tunnel	Posterior urethral valves	Neurogenic bladder, spinal cord injury, multiple sclerosis
Ectopic ureter	Ureterocele	Benign prostate hyperplasia
Primary ureter	Diverticula	Diabetic neuropathy
	Urethral stricture	Vitamin B12 deficiency
	Primary megaureter	Pelvic surgery
		Dysfunctional elimination syndrome

Key Differences in Reflux and Obstructive Nephropathy

Type	Reflux Nephropathy	Obstructive Nephropathy
Impediment	Patent ureterovesical junction	Physical obstruction, functional, anywhere in urinary tract
Mechanism	Mild to medium hydrostatic pressure, affect compound papillae in lobes 1st	Severe hydrostatic pressure affects all collecting system units
Early pathology	Segmental cortical thinning, scarring	Diffuse dilatation and compression, scarring
Late pathology	Diffuse scarring, end-stage kidney	Diffuse scarring, end-stage kidney

VUR Grading

Grade	Extent of Reflux	Nephropathy Risk
1	Confined to ureter	None
2	Ureter and into pelvis	None
3	Grade 2 and mild increase in tortuosity of ureter	Minimal
4	Grade 3, moderate tortuosity, and blunting of calyces	Moderate
5	Grade 4 with marked collecting system tortuosity and compression of renal parenchyma	High

  - Thyroidization of tubules
  - Dilated collecting ducts
- Interstitium
  - Interstitial fibrosis
  - Interstitial inflammation, particularly in areas of tubular rupture
  - Segmental or diffuse scarring
- Vessels
  - No specific features
- Other features that may be present
  - Dysplasia indicates congenital component leading to reflux
  - Acute pyelonephritis: Neutrophils in tubular lumen or interstitium
  - Peripelvic inflammation
- Histologic features overlap with features of obstructive nephropathy

ANCILLARY TESTS

Genetic Testing

- Consider targeted or whole exome/genome sequencing
  - Unaffected individuals may be carriers with incomplete penetrance

DIFFERENTIAL DIAGNOSIS

Obstructive Nephropathy

- Clinical and radiological correlation necessary

Chronic Pyelonephritis

- Often coexists with reflux, difficult to exclude or include
- Suggested by more severe inflammation around calyces

Ask-Upmark Kidney

- Segmental well-demarcated scar without glomeruli

DIAGNOSTIC CHECKLIST

Pathologic Interpretation Pearls

- Dysplasia suggests congenital VUR as cause of nephropathy

SELECTED REFERENCES

1. Tullus K: Vesicoureteric reflux in children. Lancet. 385(9965):371-9, 2015
2. Peters C et al: Vesicoureteral reflux associated renal damage: congenital reflux nephropathy and acquired renal scarring. J Urol. 184(1):265-73, 2010
3. Uetani N et al: Plumbing in the embryo: developmental defects of the urinary tracts. Clin Genet. 75(4):307-17, 2009
4. Brakeman P: Vesicoureteral reflux, reflux nephropathy, and end-stage renal disease. Adv Urol. PubMed Central PMCID:PMC2478704, 2008
5. Murawski IJ et al: Gene discovery and vesicoureteric reflux. Pediatr Nephrol. 23(7):1021-7, 2008
6. Smith EA: Pyelonephritis, renal scarring, and reflux nephropathy: a pediatric urologist's perspective. Pediatr Radiol. 38 Suppl 1:S76-82, 2008
7. Williams G et al: Vesicoureteral reflux. J Am Soc Nephrol. 19(5):847-62, 2008

Congenital Vesicoureteral Reflux

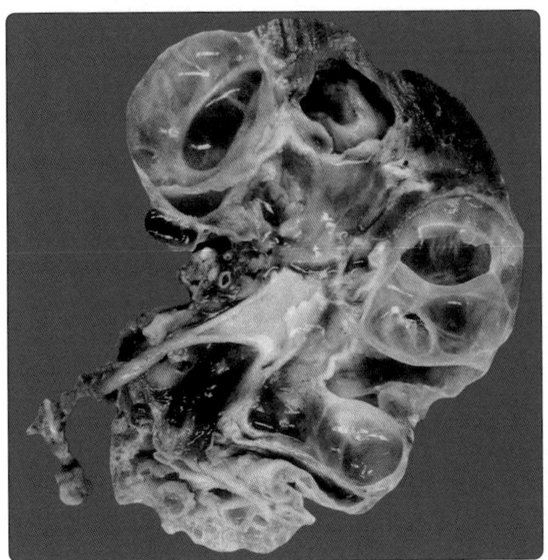

Segmental Scar Reflux Nephropathy

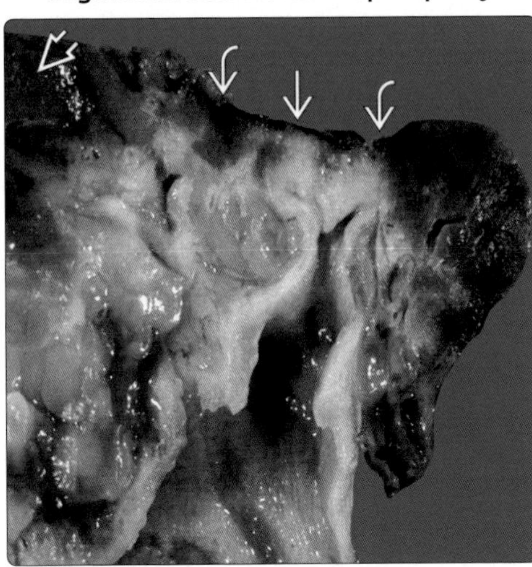

(Left) *Gross image depicts multiple cysts and malformed kidney consistent with cystic dysplasia and vesicoureteral reflux in utero. Dysplasia in this setting indicates congenital etiology of reflux nephropathy.* **(Right)** *Gross image depicts a segmental scar ➔ overlying the dilated calyx in reflux nephropathy. Note the thinning of cortex ➔ and adjoining normal parenchyma ➔.*

Infant Kidney Dilated Calyces and Ureter

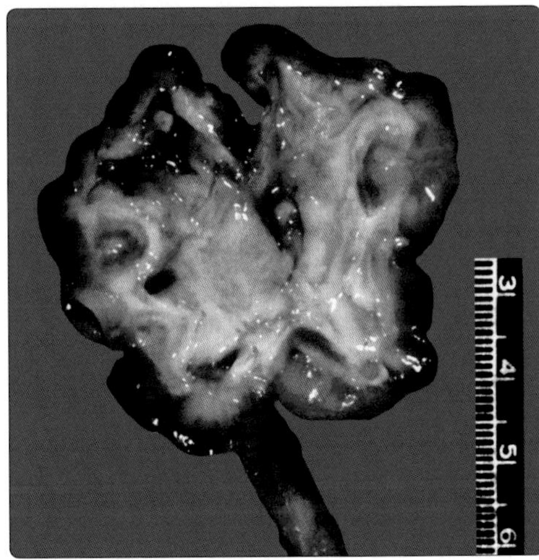

Cortical Thinning at Poles in Early Reflux Nephropathy

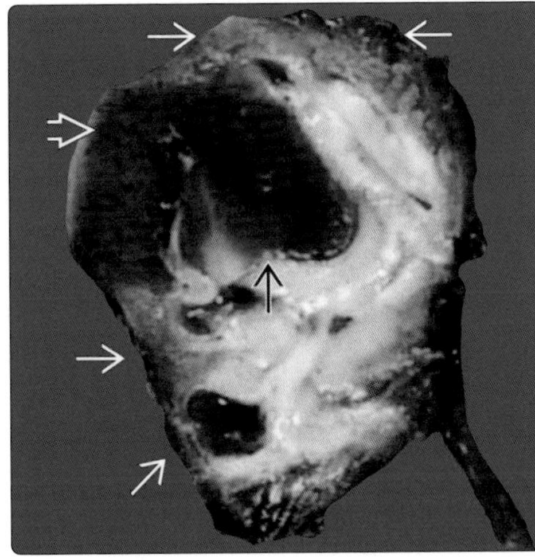

(Left) *Gross image from a 23-month-old boy with reflux nephropathy shows moderate thinning of the cortex and a dilated ureter and pelvis.* **(Right)** *Image depicts both upper and lower lobe cortical thinning ➔ and obliteration of the medulla in a reflux nephropathy patient. The middle lobe cortex ➔ is relatively normal. The middle lobe simple papillae are on the verge of being deformed by encroachment from the scarred upper and lower lobes ➔.*

Grade 5 VUR

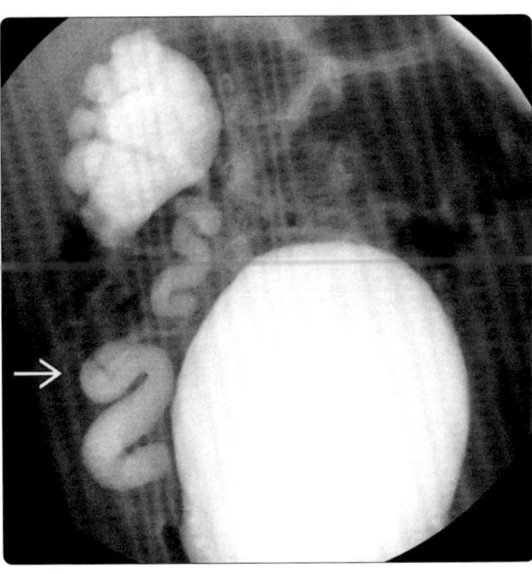

Ureterocele

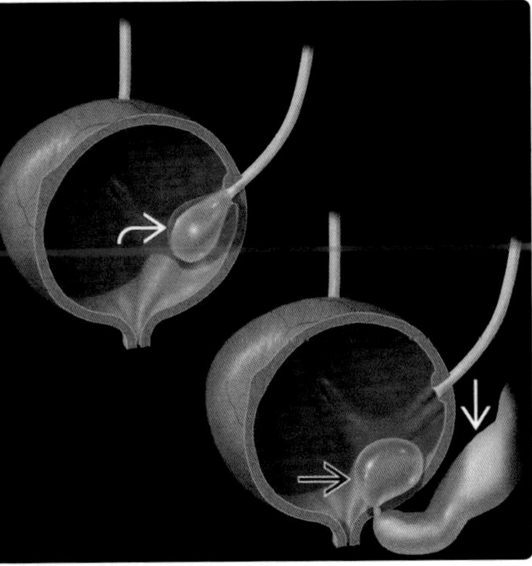

(Left) *Voiding cystourethrogram of a 4-month-old infant with grade 5 VUR secondary to posterior urethral valves shows the severely tortuous ureter ➔ and dye extending into the kidney with severe dilatation of the collecting system.* **(Right)** *Illustration shows a ureterocele as an example of a lower tract obstruction causing reflux. The graphic on top shows a ureterocele ➔ in a single ureter, and the bottom depicts a ureterocele ➔ in an ectopic ureter ➔ causing reflux.*

(Left) *In reflux, the damage to the kidney can be quite segmental, as illustrated here at low power, with a band of almost completely destroyed tubules ➡ adjacent to a relatively normal cortex ➡. The outer cortex is preferentially involved ➡.* **(Right)** *Glomeruli are relatively spared in reflux nephropathy but secondary FSGS commonly arises in the late stages and characteristically is perihilar in distribution ➡. Global glomerulosclerosis is also present ➡. Tubules are completely destroyed in most of this field.*

Segmental Scarring in Reflux Nephropathy

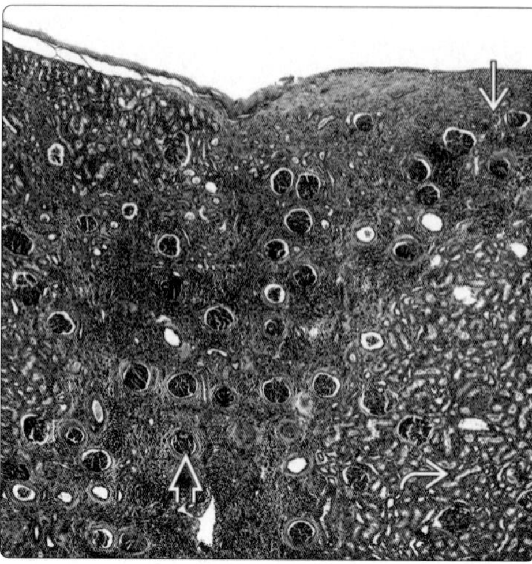

Periglomerular Fibrosis

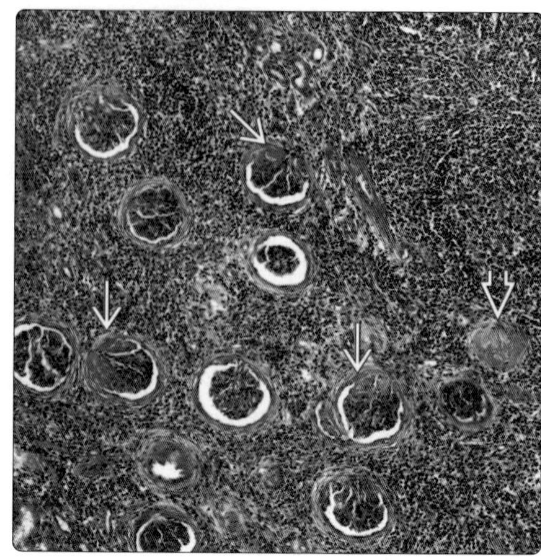

(Left) *With the loss of nephrons due to reflux nephropathy, the remaining glomeruli hypertrophy, as shown here in a 25-year-old woman with end-stage disease after onset of reflux in childhood.* **(Right)** *Kidney section shows segmental scar with dysplastic tubules (left of the dashed line) as a result of high-grade VUR. Relatively unaffected parenchyma is shown on the right.*

Glomerular Hypertrophy Reflux Nephropathy

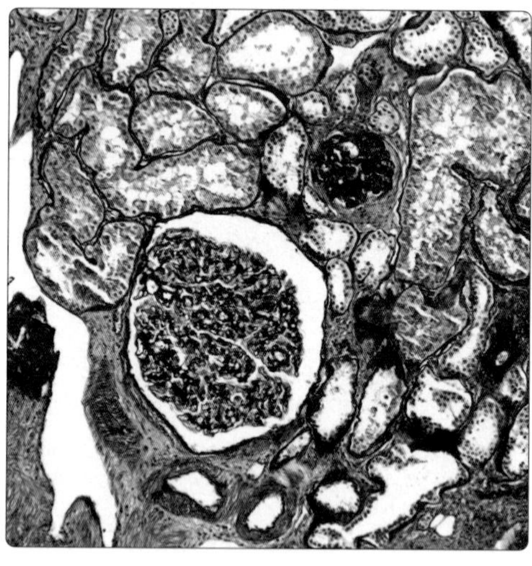

Segmental Scar Reflux Nephropathy

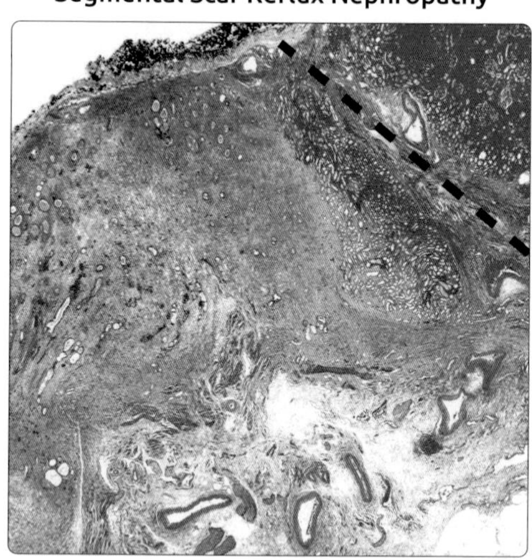

(Left) *Reflux nephropathy characteristically has atrophic tubules with a microcystic appearance (thyroidization) and loss of epithelium ➡. There are several globally sclerosed glomeruli ➡.* **(Right)** *Rupture and leakage of tubular contents, including PAS(+) Tamm-Horsfall protein ➡, is characteristic of reflux nephropathy and commonly elicits local inflammation, sometimes granulomatous.*

Severe Reflux Nephropathy Tubular Atrophy

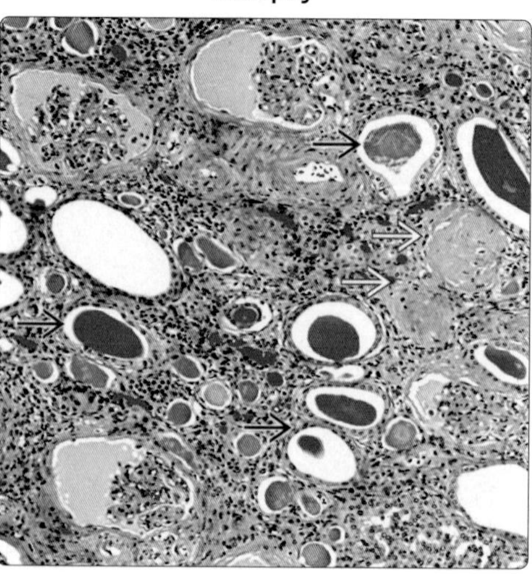

Interstitial Inflammation Tubular Leakage Reflux Nephropathy

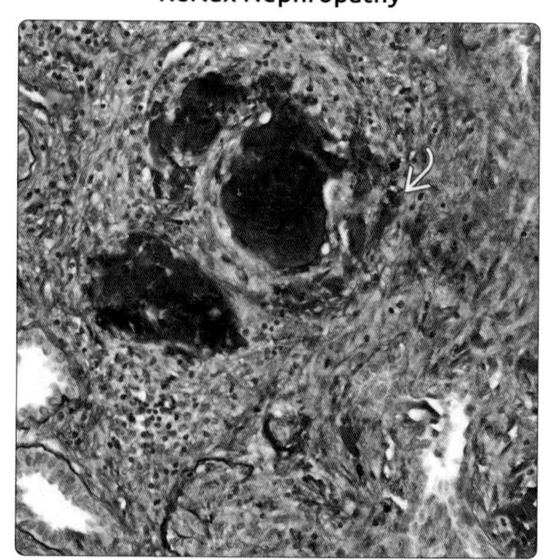

Grade 3 VUR

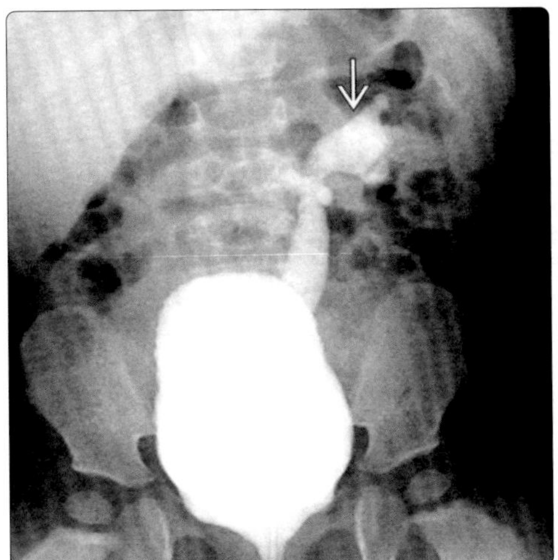

Vesicoureteral Reflux

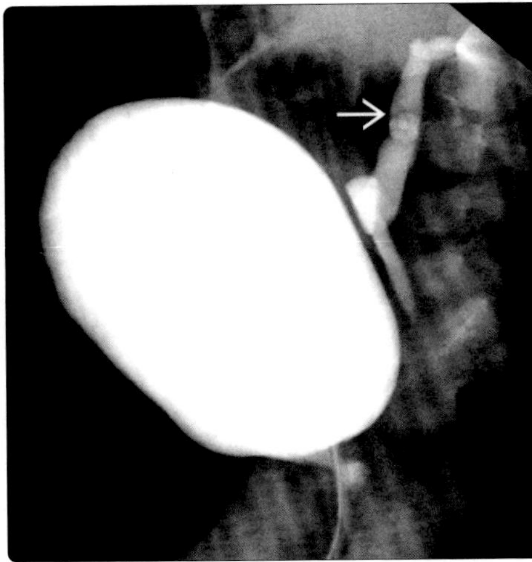

(Left) *Voiding cystoureterogram shows urine in the ureter due to vesicoureteral reflux. The presence of dye in the pelvis* ➡ *denotes grade 3 reflux.* **(Right)** *Voiding cystourethrogram shows vesicoureteral reflux. Note the reflux from the bladder into the ureter* ➡.

VUR Duplication

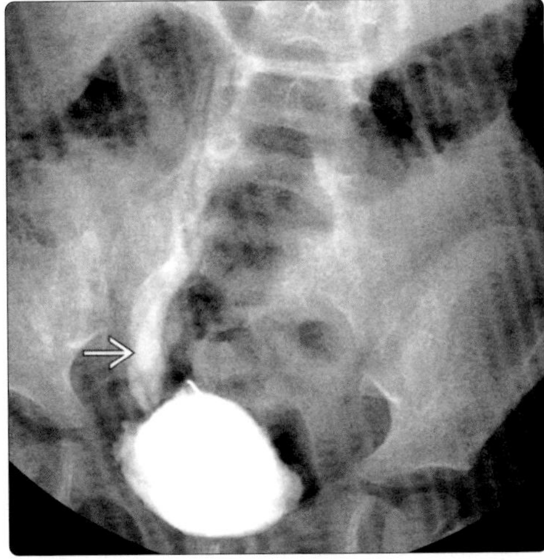

Vesicoureteral Reflux

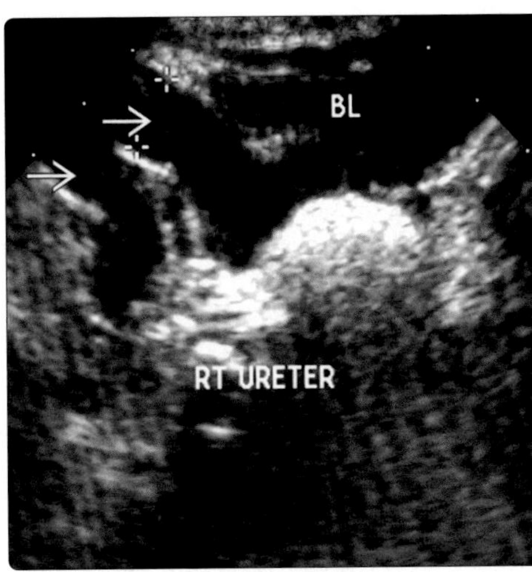

(Left) *Radiologic image shows vesicoureteral reflux in a patient with a duplicated collecting system* ➡. **(Right)** *Ultrasound shows a tortuous megaureter* ➡ *in a patient with primary high-grade VUR. Bladder is abbreviated as BL.*

Grade 5 VUR

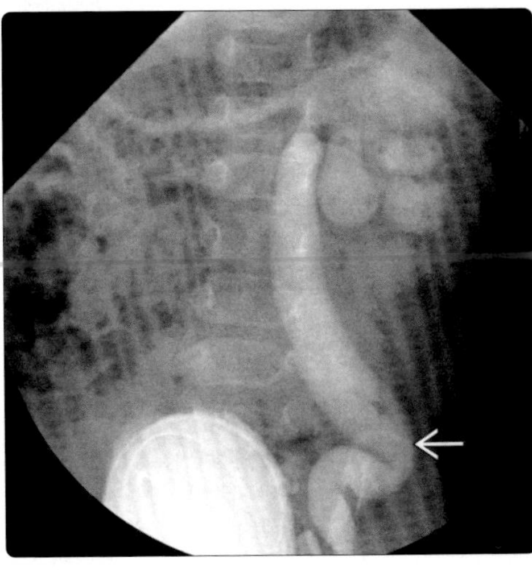

Kidney Scarring

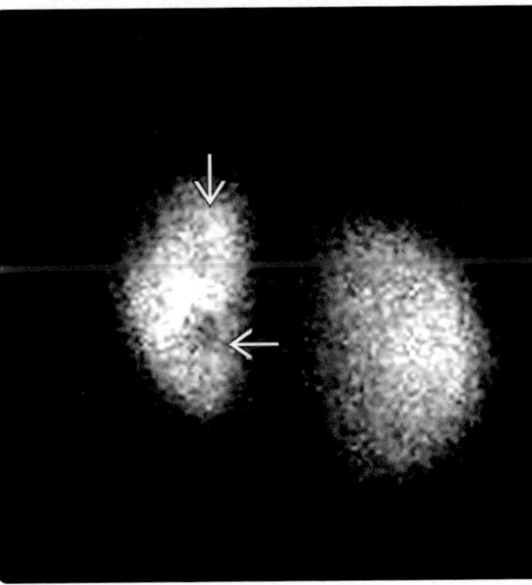

(Left) *Radiologic image shows grade 5 reflux in a 4-year-old child. Note the extreme tortuosity of the ureter* ➡. **(Right)** *DMSA scan from a 2-year-old child with a urinary tract infection shows 2 areas of low uptake* ➡ *suggestive of scarring in the lower and upper poles of the left kidney.*

Obstructive Nephropathy

KEY FACTS

TERMINOLOGY

- Acute or chronic damage to kidney due to obstruction of urine flow

ETIOLOGY/PATHOGENESIS

- Congenital and acquired causes
  - Developmental defect
  - Neoplasia
  - Stones
- Ureteropelvic junction obstruction (UPJO) most common cause

CLINICAL ISSUES

- Chronic or repeated pyelonephritis
- Flank pain
- Hypertension
- Renal failure (bilateral)
- Surgical repair, decompression
  - Deterioration may continue despite surgical correction

MACROSCOPIC

- Dilatation of pelvis (hydronephrosis)
- Blunting of calyces
- Marked loss of medulla, cortical thinning

MICROSCOPIC

- Marked loss of tubules
- Global and segmental glomerulosclerosis
- Interstitial fibrosis, chronic inflammation
- Dilation of collecting ducts
- Cartilage or smooth muscle indicates dysplasia
  - Dysplasia indicates congenital origin

TOP DIFFERENTIAL DIAGNOSES

- Reflux nephropathy
- Ask-Upmark kidney
- Tubulointerstitial diseases

Chronic Obstruction

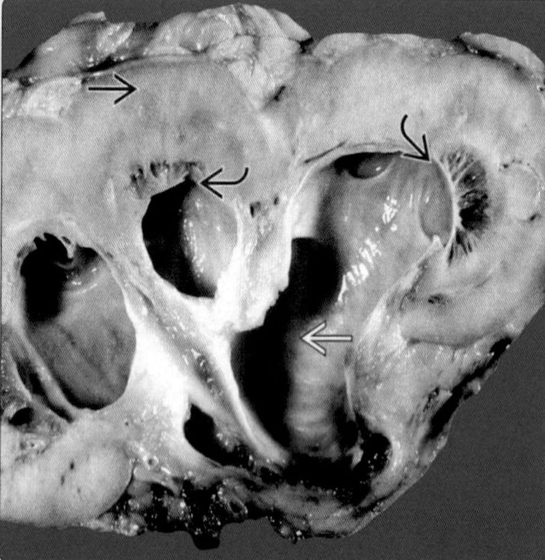

Collecting Duct Dilation UPJO

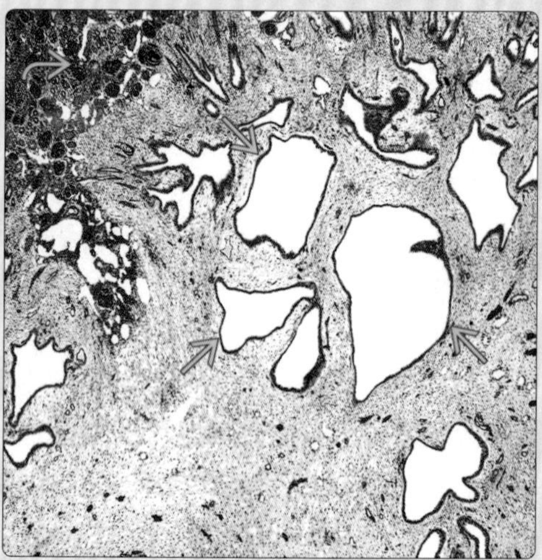

(Left) *The typical features of chronic obstruction include dilation of the pelvis and calyces (hydronephrosis) ➡, loss of the medullary pyramids ➡, and secondary thinning of the cortex ➡.* **(Right)** *A section of the medulla from a child with ureteropelvic junction obstruction (UPJO) shows dilation of the larger medullary collecting ducts ➡ due to increased urine back pressure. The cortex is relatively spared ➡.*

Right UPJ Obstruction

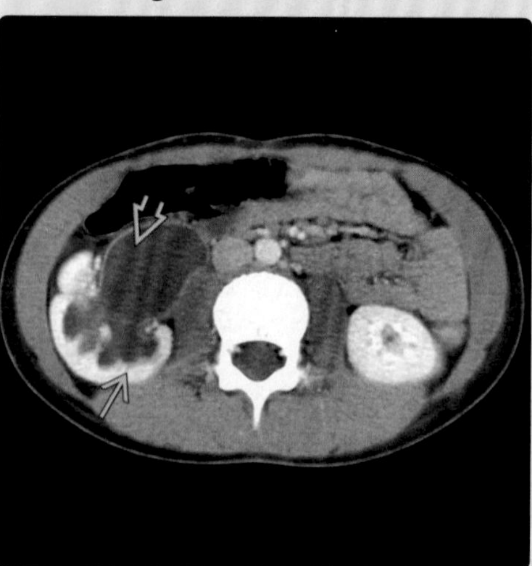

Periglomerular Fibrosis Obstruction

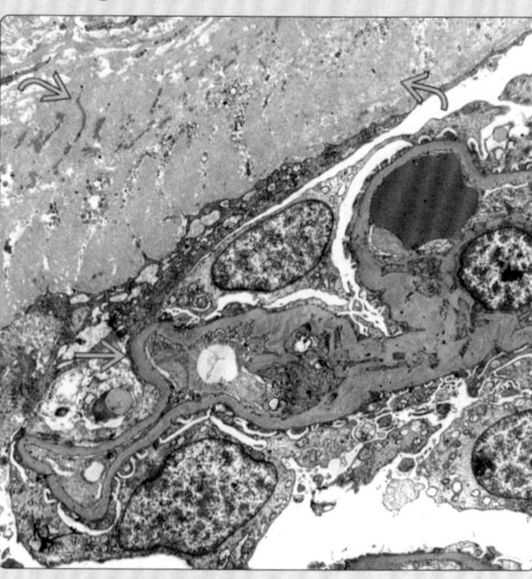

(Left) *CT scan of a 9 year old with right side UPJO shows marked pelvic dilatation ➡. Note the compression of the cortex due to increased distention ➡ of the collecting system.* **(Right)** *EM of the glomerulus in a patient with obstructive nephropathy and proteinuria is shown. Glomerular pathology in obstruction includes podocyte foot process effacement ➡ and periglomerular fibrosis ➡.*

TERMINOLOGY

Definitions

- Obstructive nephropathy: Damage to kidney due to urine flow obstruction
- Hydronephrosis: Dilatation of renal pelvis due to functional or physical impediment to urine flow

ETIOLOGY/PATHOGENESIS

Causes

- Physical obstruction
  - Stone
  - Tumors of urinary tract
    - Prostate, bladder, ureter
  - Benign prostate hyperplasia
  - External compression (tumors, pregnancy, retroperitoneal fibrosis, endometriosis, crossing vessels)
- Functional obstruction
  - Developmental anomalies: Posterior urethral valves (PUV), ureterocele, ureteropelvic junction obstruction (UPJO), primary megaureter
    - UPJO most common cause of obstructive nephropathy

Pathophysiology

- Impediment to urine flow causes dilatation and increase in back pressure into collecting system and tubules
- Compression of renal parenchyma accompanies vascular compromise and inflammatory response
- Cellular changes in interstitium and nephrons lead to varying degrees of scarring
- Intrauterine obstruction during nephrogenesis can cause renal dysplasia

Animal Models

- Unilateral ureteral obstruction (UUO)
  - Commonly used in rodents, marsupials

CLINICAL ISSUES

Presentation

- Acute obstruction (flank pain, nausea, vomiting)
- Chronic obstruction (recurrent pyelonephritis, hypertension, renal failure if bilateral)

Treatment

- Surgical repair, decompression

Prognosis

- Prognostic criteria for congenital impediments to urine flow not well defined
  - Management criteria debatable
- Kidney failure ensues if dysplasia present
  - Deterioration may continue despite surgical correction

IMAGING

Ultrasonographic Findings

- Dilated pelvis

MACROSCOPIC

General Features

- Dilatation of pelvis (hydronephrosis), blunting of calyces
- Compression of cortex
- Irregular kidney surface due to scarring
- Other concurrent anomalies or syndromes: Hydronephrosis, small kidneys, duplicated collecting system, megaureter, hydroureter, dysplastic kidneys
- Compensatory hypertrophy in contralateral kidney

MICROSCOPIC

Histologic Features

- Glomeruli
  - Relatively spared but eventually become globally sclerotic
    - Periglomerular fibrosis prominent
    - Atubular glomeruli (cystic dilation of Bowman space)
  - Crescents rare
  - Increased glomerular size in contralateral kidney
- Tubules
  - Tubular atrophy, apoptosis
  - Microcystic dilatation of distal nephron segments
  - Dilation may be more prominent in subcapsular collecting ducts
- Interstitium
  - Fibrosis, diffuse
  - Mononuclear inflammation, plasma cells
  - Cartilage or smooth muscle indicates dysplasia
- Vessels
  - Arterial medial hypertrophy and intimal fibroelastosis indicate hypertension
- Pelvis and ureter
  - Pelvic dilatation, papillae effacement
  - Hypertrophy and dilation of ureter
  - Chronic inflammation mucosa of pelvis and ureter

DIFFERENTIAL DIAGNOSIS

Reflux Nephropathy

- Generally less hydronephrosis

Ask-Upmark Kidney

- Segmental scar with atrophic tubules and no glomeruli

Chronic Tubulointerstitial Diseases

- No calyceal dilation or hydronephrosis
- Medulla shows less severe destruction

SELECTED REFERENCES

1. Chevalier RL et al: Mechanisms of renal injury and progression of renal disease in congenital obstructive nephropathy. Pediatr Nephrol. 25(4):687-97, 2010
2. Klein J et al: Congenital ureteropelvic junction obstruction: human disease and animal models. Int J Exp Pathol. Epub ahead of print, 2010
3. Rosen S et al: The kidney in congenital ureteropelvic junction obstruction: a spectrum from normal to nephrectomy. J Urol. 179(4):1257-63, 2008
4. Zhang PL et al: Ureteropelvic junction obstruction: morphological and clinical studies. Pediatr Nephrol. 14(8-9):820-6, 2000

Hydronephrosis

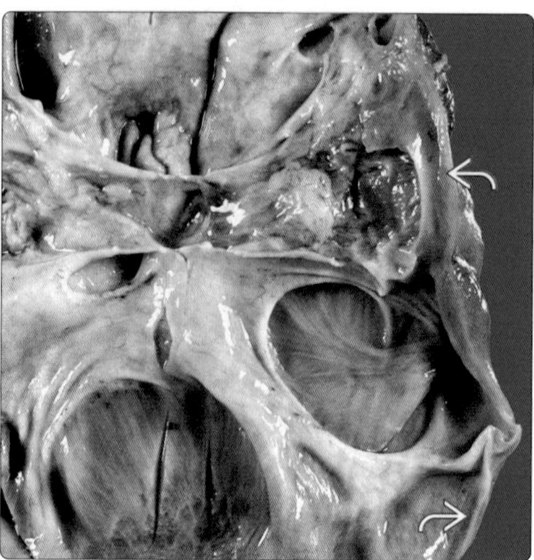

Cortical Thinning Due to Obstruction

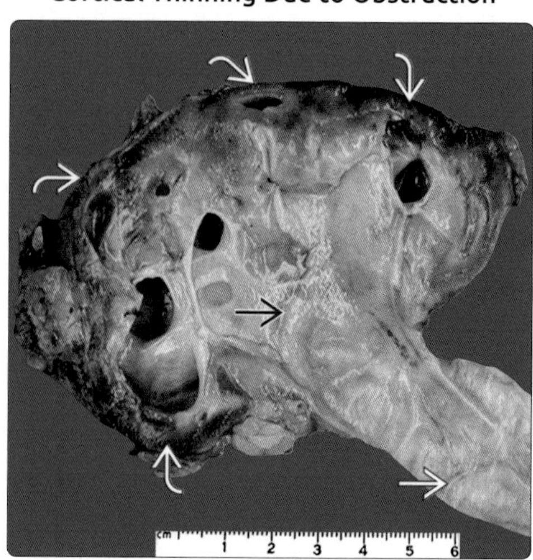

(Left) *Extreme hydronephrosis results in a kidney with a bag-like appearance and almost complete loss of parenchyma. In this case, the cortex and medulla in the lobes are just a few millimeters thick* ➢. **(Right)** *This case of chronic obstructive nephropathy depicts severe dilatation of the ureter* ➡ *indicative of distal obstruction. Note the several areas of cortical thinning and absent pyramids* ➢ *with marked dilation of the pelvis* ⇨.

Primary Megaureter

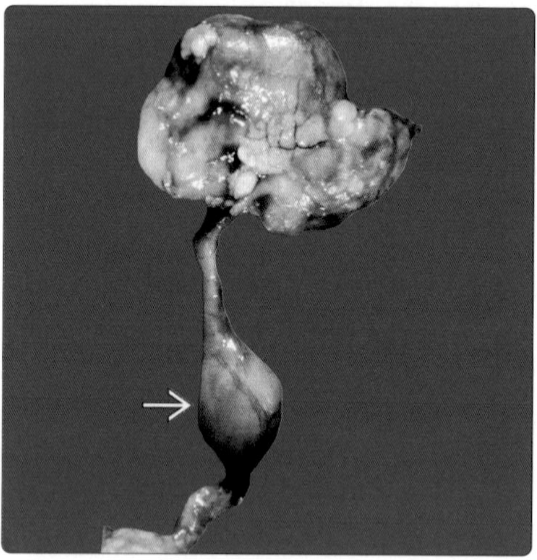

Papillae Blunting and Scarring

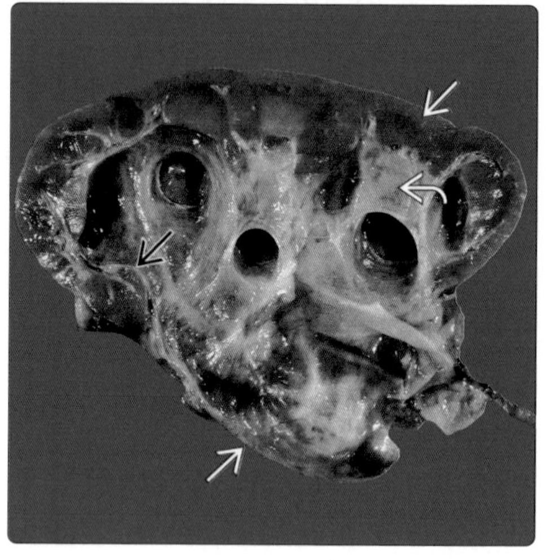

(Left) *Primary megaureter in a child is highlighted by overall ureter dilation with a segment with marked dilation* ➡. *The kidney does not have a normal reniform shape due to abnormal development. Intrauterine obstruction is a known cause of renal dysplasia.* **(Right)** *Gross image of a kidney shows features of obstructive nephropathy. There are varying degrees of corticomedullary thinning* ➡. *There are regions of papillae flattening* ⇨ *and scarring* ➢.

Obstructive Nephropathy Stones

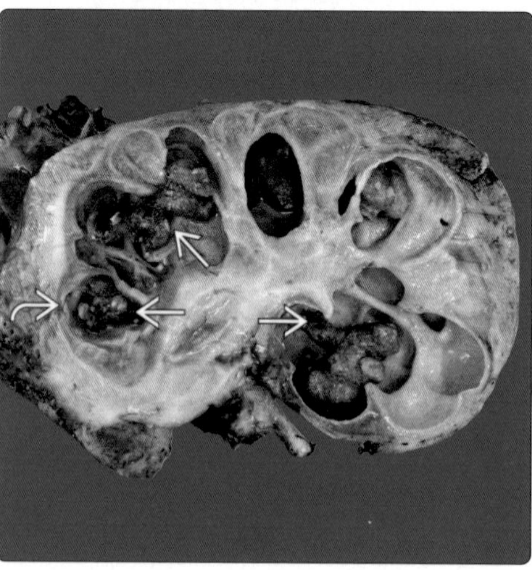

Hydronephrosis

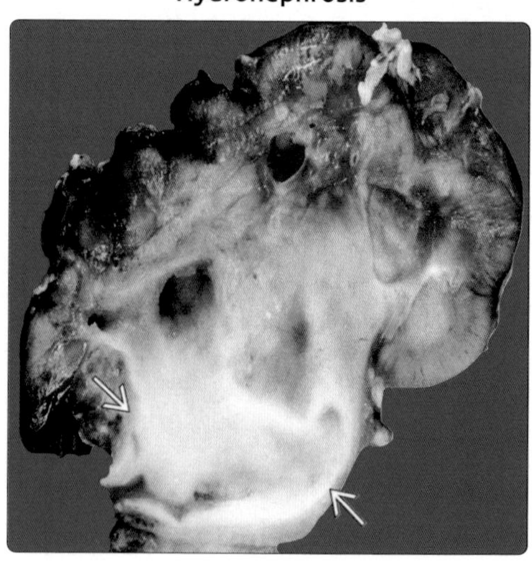

(Left) *Xanthogranulomatous pyelonephritis and staghorn calculi can complicate obstructive nephropathy. This pelvicalyceal system is dilated and filled with staghorn calculi* ➡. *The yellow chronic infection can be seen in the medullary areas* ➢. **(Right)** *Section of a kidney with UPJO causing hydronephrosis demonstrates marked dilatation of the pelvis* ➡.

Hydronephrosis

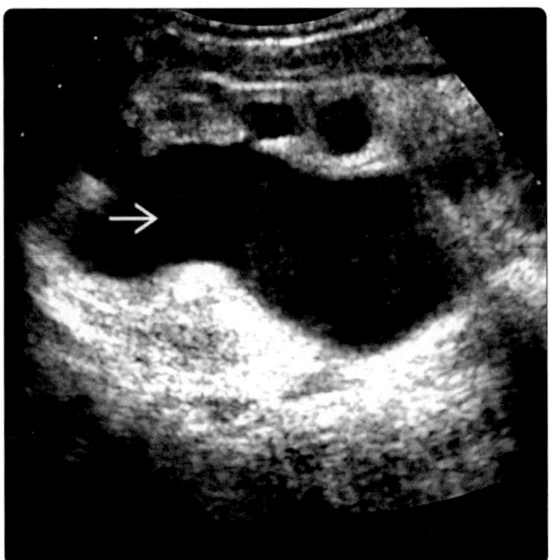

Duplicated Ureters in UPJO

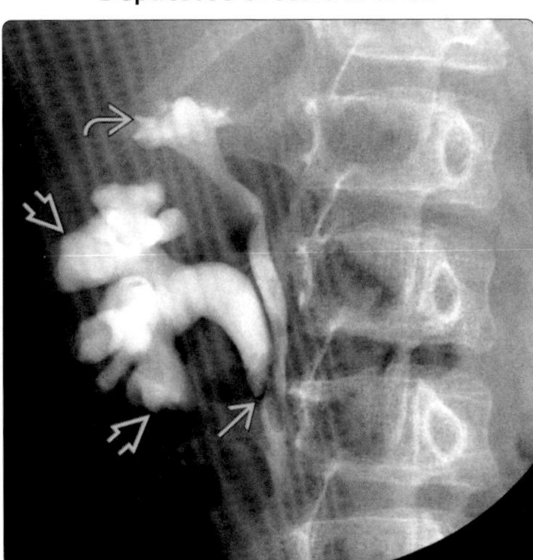

(Left) *Ultrasound can demonstrate hydronephrosis in revealing a dilated pelvis* ➡*, here shown in a child with UPJO.* **(Right)** *In this image of duplicated ureters, the lower ureter has UPJO* ➡ *causing urine backflow and hydronephrosis, as revealed by contrast material in the clubbed calyces* ➡*. The calyces drained by the other ureter are relatively normal and have sharp fornices* ➡*.*

Dilated Ureter Due to Obstruction

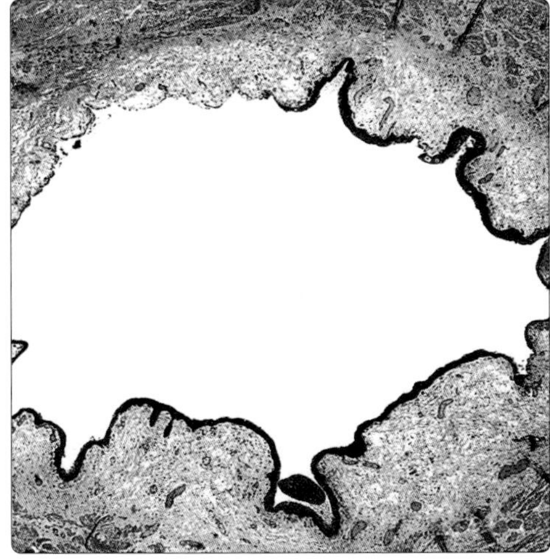

Obstructive Nephropathy

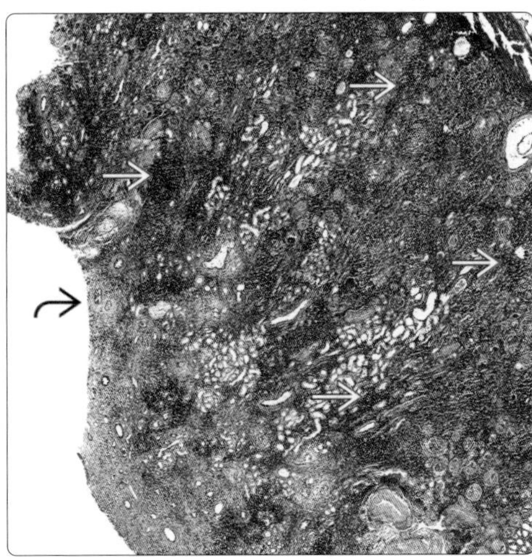

(Left) *This ureter cross section is dilated, moderately inflamed, and hypertrophied, an appearance typical of chronic obstruction.* **(Right)** *Histopathological changes of obstructive nephropathy due to UPJO are highlighted in this low-power image. Note that pelvicalyceal expansion causes effacement of the papillae* ➡ *and diffuse inflammation involving the entire cortex* ➡*. No dysplasia is present, consistent with postnatal onset of obstruction.*

Collecting Duct Dilatation

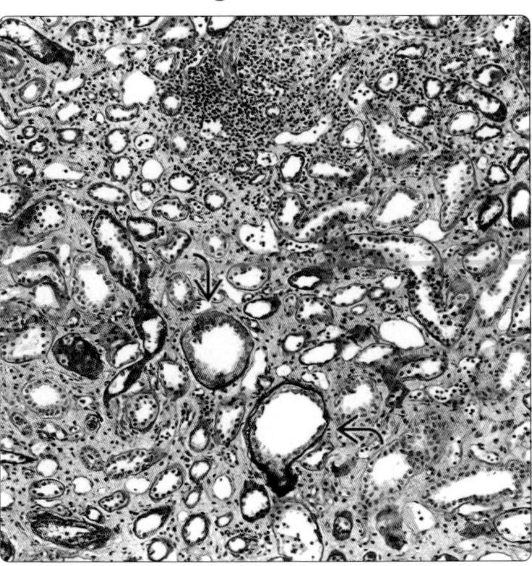

Tubular Atrophy and Interstitial Fibrosis

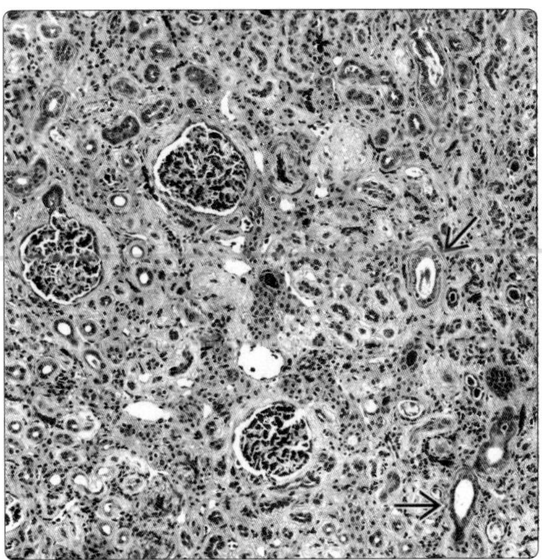

(Left) *Histologic evidence of obstruction on biopsy can be subtle. Here, there is diffuse edema, mild mononuclear inflammation, and dilation of the medullary collecting ducts* ➡*.* **(Right)** *Trichrome stain in a chronically obstructed kidney shows marked loss and atrophy of tubules, with diffuse fine interstitial fibrosis. The glomeruli are relatively spared, although they are probably "atubular" glomeruli. A few residual collecting ducts are seen* ➡*.*

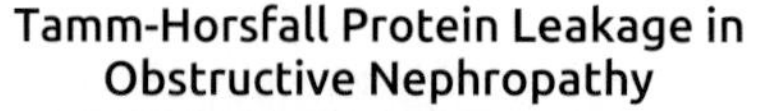

Tamm-Horsfall Protein Leakage in Obstructive Nephropathy

Glomerulosclerosis in Obstructive Nephropathy

(Left) *Leakage of Tamm-Horsfall protein (THP), which is produced in the distal tubule, occurs as a consequence of obstruction and elicits an inflammatory response. Here, THP can be seen in the interstitium around a collecting duct and in the lymphatics.* **(Right)** *This kidney section shows globally sclerosed glomeruli and extensive cortical interstitial inflammation in the cortex in a patient with urinary tract obstruction.*

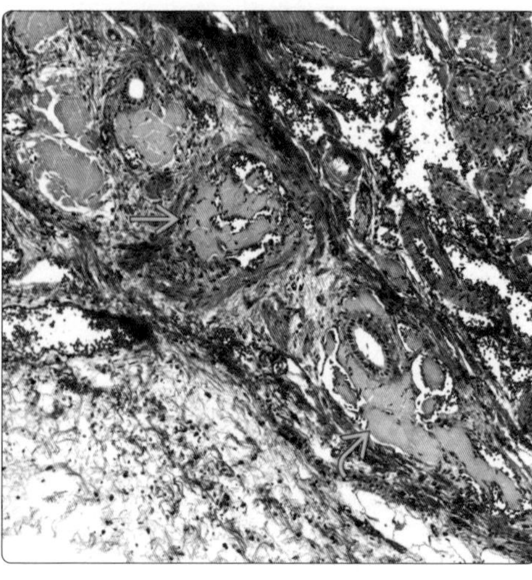

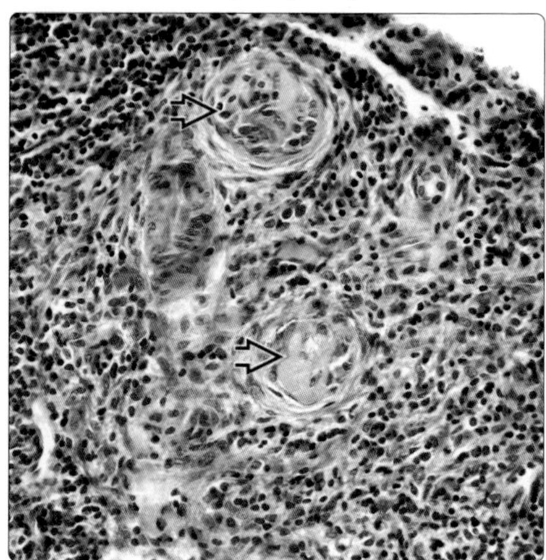

Fibrocellular Crescent Obstructive Nephropathy UPJO

Dysplasia Congenital Obstruction

(Left) *Occasionally in chronic obstruction, especially in children, cellular crescents are found (here with a squamous appearance). This was initially described in UPJO by Seymour Rosen et al and should not be mistaken for a coincidental glomerulonephritis.* **(Right)** *Obstruction in utero not uncommonly leads to dysplasia in the developing kidney. One form it takes is zonal dysplasia, where the outer cortex (subcapsular and in the columns of Bertin) shows cartilage or smooth muscle.*

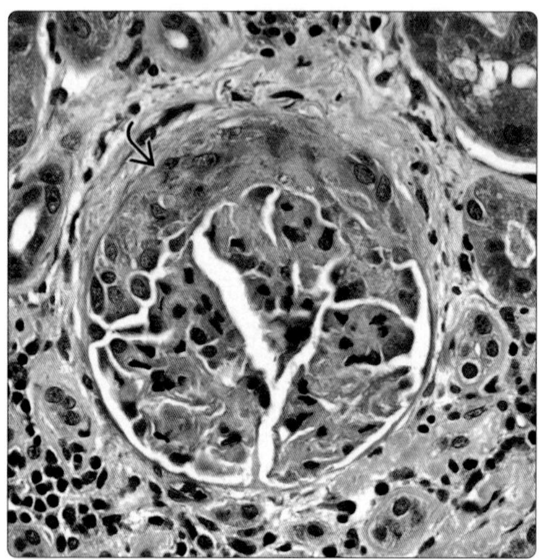

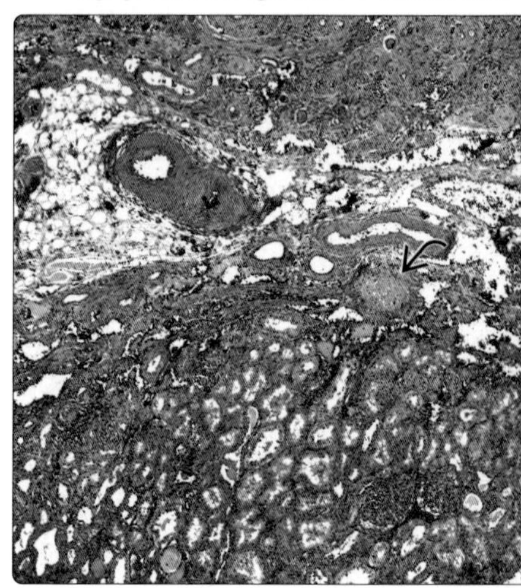

Glomerular Hypertrophy

Glomerular Changes in Obstructive Nephropathy

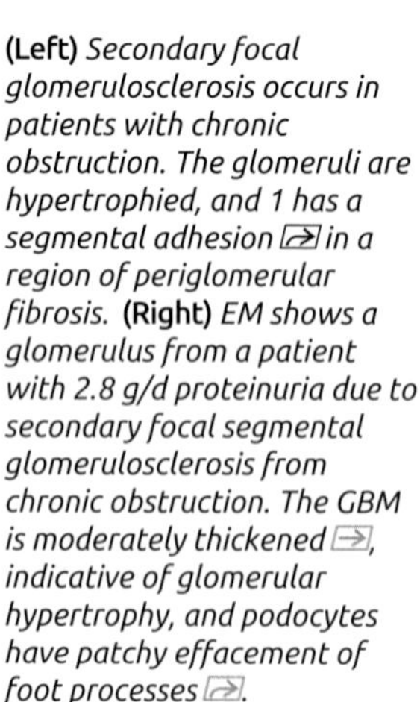

(Left) *Secondary focal glomerulosclerosis occurs in patients with chronic obstruction. The glomeruli are hypertrophied, and 1 has a segmental adhesion in a region of periglomerular fibrosis.* **(Right)** *EM shows a glomerulus from a patient with 2.8 g/d proteinuria due to secondary focal segmental glomerulosclerosis from chronic obstruction. The GBM is moderately thickened, indicative of glomerular hypertrophy, and podocytes have patchy effacement of foot processes.*

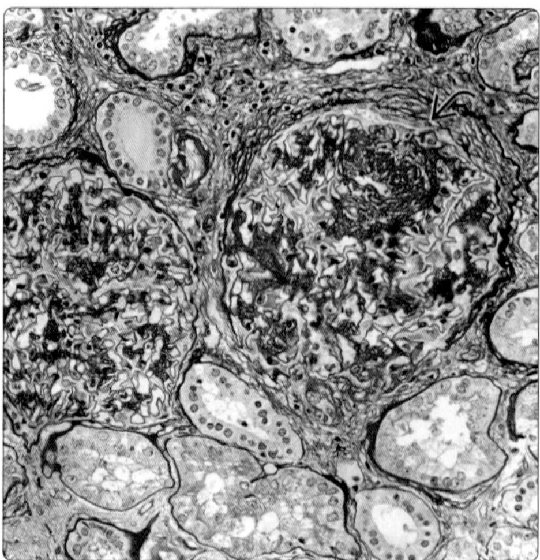

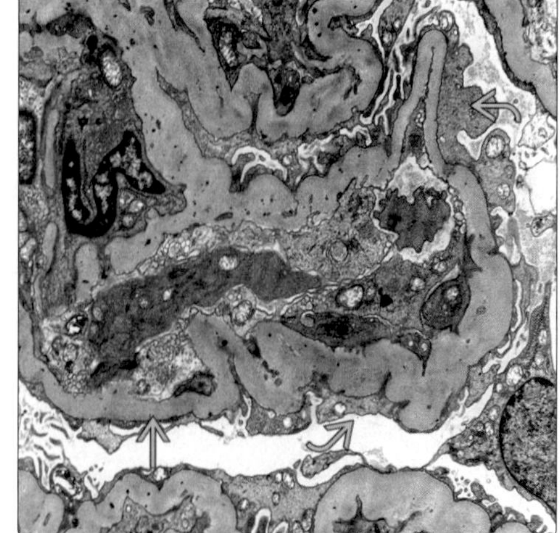

Animal Model of Ureteral Obstruction

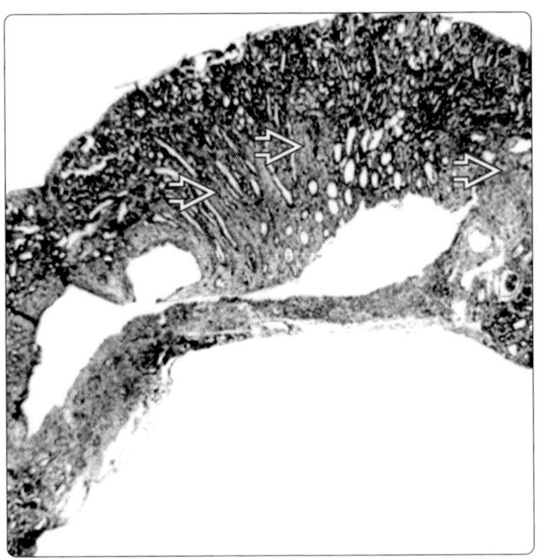

Ureter Smooth Muscle Defect in Mouse Model of Hydronephrosis

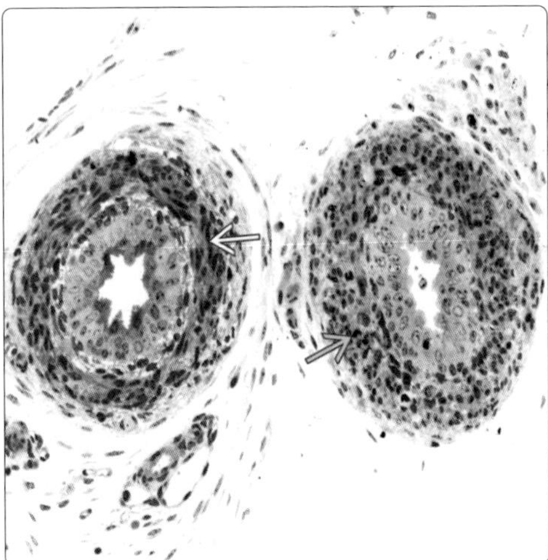

(Left) *Increased fibrosis ➡ is highlighted by trichrome stain in a opossum model of ureteral obstruction. Note the hydronephrosis.* **(Right)** *Section shows ureter wall abnormalities in UPJO in a Dlg1 knockout mouse. Left image from a normal mouse shows normal ureter with a well-formed lumen and well-organized inner longitudinal and outer circular smooth muscles ➡. Right image from Dlg1 knockout mouse shows a narrow lumen and disorganized smooth muscle ⇨. (Courtesy J. Miner, PhD.)*

Apoptosis in Obstruction

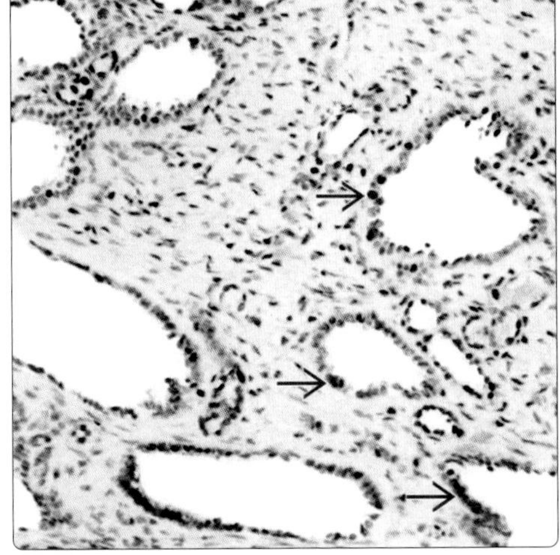

SMA(+) Interstitial Cells

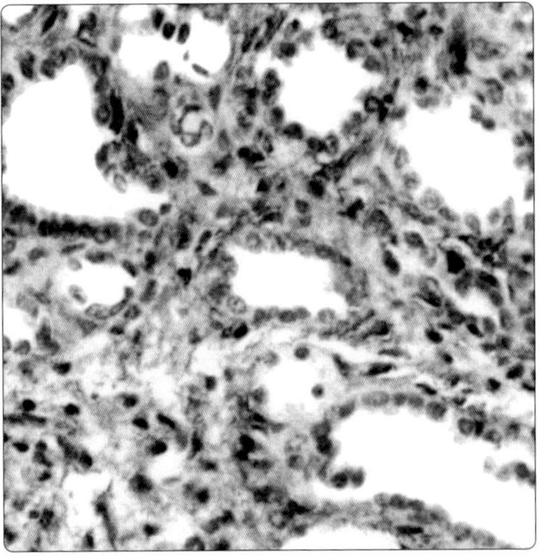

(Left) *Apoptosis (TUNEL) stain of a kidney section shows increased apoptosis ⇨ in obstructive nephropathy in an opossum. Tubular epithelial apoptosis is an early response to acute obstruction.* **(Right)** *Immunoperoxidase staining of kidney sections with antismooth muscle actin (SMA) antibody shows increased labeling in interstitial cells in ureteral obstruction in the opossum.*

Megaureter in Ret Mutant Mice

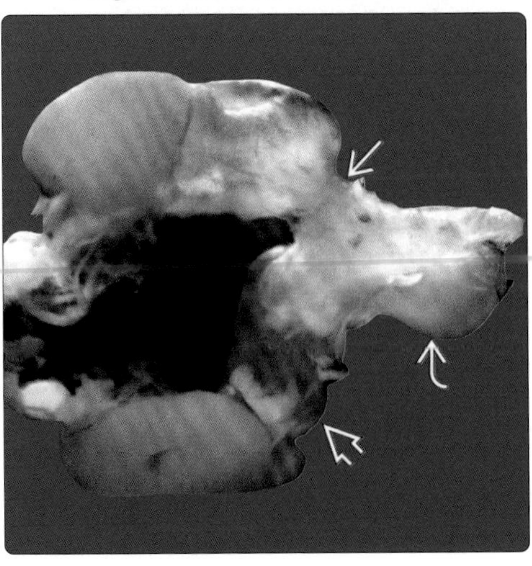

Cystic Dysplasia in Congenital Obstruction Ret Mutant Mouse

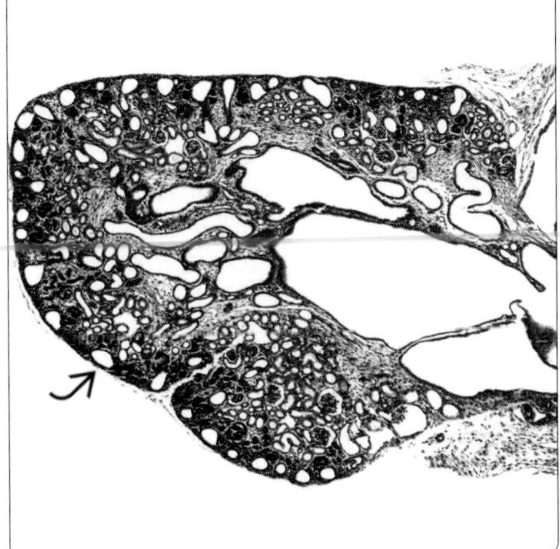

(Left) *The urinary tract from a mouse lacking Ret-activated Plc-γ signaling shows lower ureter obstruction ➡ near the bladder ➡, which caused megaureter ➡.* **(Right)** *Kidney from a mouse with ureteral obstruction due to lack of Ret-activated Plc-γ signaling during development shows pelvicalyceal dilation and cystic dysplasia, a consequence of obstruction in utero. Subcapsular dilation of collecting ducts ⇨ is also a characteristic of obstruction in humans.*

Nephrolithiasis

KEY FACTS

TERMINOLOGY

- Concretion of urinary mineral or organic crystals in kidney

ETIOLOGY/PATHOGENESIS

- Causes
  - 25% known cause
  - 50% idiopathic hypercalciuria
  - 25% unknown cause

CLINICAL ISSUES

- Frequency: 5% of females and 12% of males in USA
- Symptoms include renal colic and hematuria
- Stones recur in ~ 50% of instances
- Treatment includes hydration, thiazide diuretics, shock wave lithotripsy, and nephrolithotomy
- Stone mineral content (stone type) is determined by infrared spectroscopy or x-ray diffraction

MICROSCOPIC

- Calcium oxalate forms pale yellow, refractile, sheaves: Birefringent by polarization microscopy
- Randall plaque is papillary suburothelial confluent apatite deposits
- Bellini and medullary collecting ducts plugged with mineral in most calcium and cystine stone formers
- Interstitial urate deposits have giant cell reaction (gouty tophus)
- Struvite stones (staghorn) associated with acute, chronic, or xanthogranulomatous pyelonephritis
- Small medullary apatite deposits in basement membranes of loops of Henle may be seen in nonstone formers

ANCILLARY TESTS

- von Kossa stain (phosphate)
- Yasue stain (calcium)
- Accurate identification of tissue mineral deposits requires infrared spectroscopy

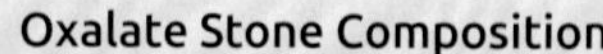

Oxalate Stone Composition

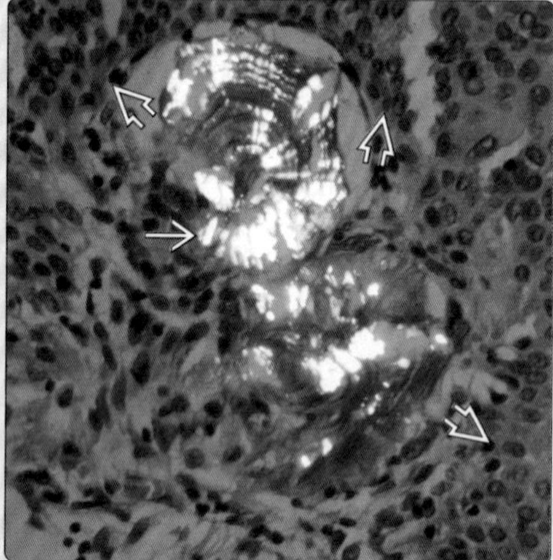

Oxalate Stone Organic Matrix

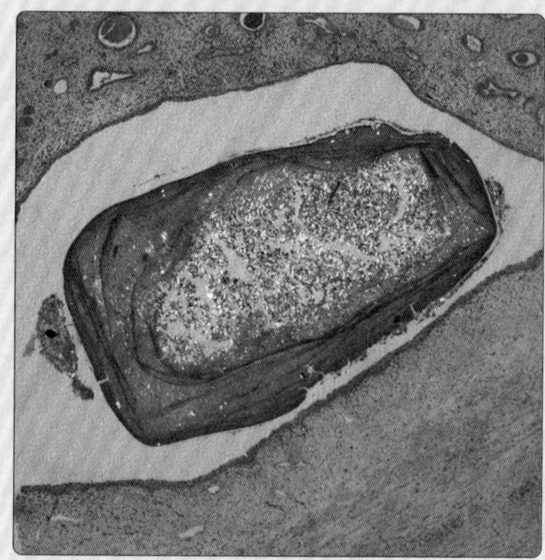

(Left) *Polarized light reveals spiderweb-like organic matrix with calcium oxalate crystals in radial arrays ➡, located in the suburothelium of the renal pelvis ➡.* **(Right)** *Renal calculi may form in a supersaturated solution in the renal calyx. Using partially polarized light, the calculus contains refractile crystalline material embedded in organic matrix material with an irregular laminated structure.*

Peritubular Apatite Deposits

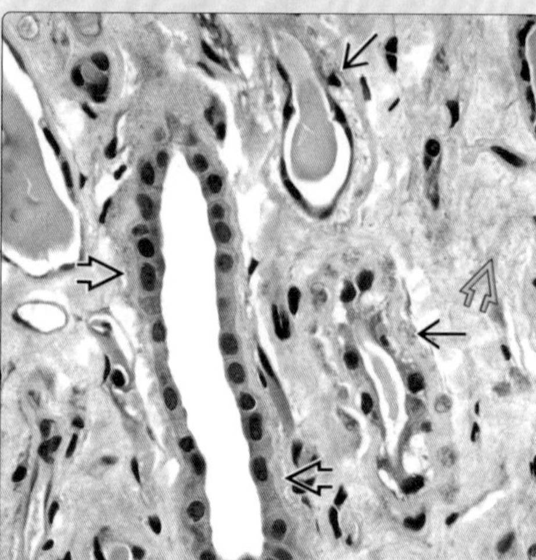

Peritubular Apatite, von Kossa

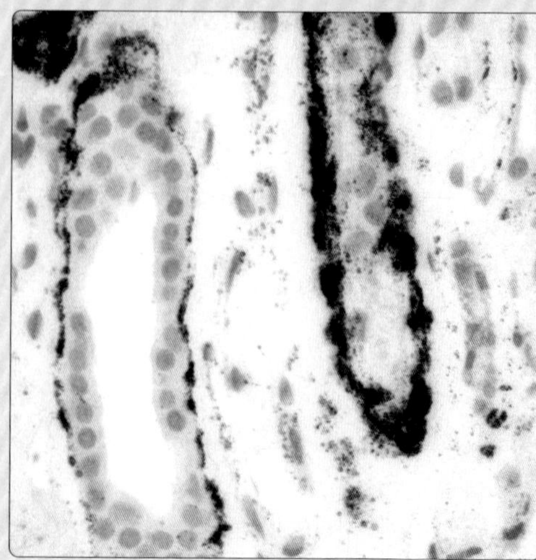

(Left) *The earliest recognizable lesions of Randall plaque have subtle apatite deposits seen as basophilic dust-like particles along the basement membranes of the loops of Henle ➡ and the collecting duct ➡ and in the interstitium ➡.* **(Right)** *The von Kossa histochemical stain for phosphate highlights peritubular and interstitial calcium phosphate (apatite) deposits with a brown-black appearance in this image of an early Randall plaque.*

TERMINOLOGY

Synonyms

- Kidney stone disease, renal stone disease, renal calculi, urolithiasis, lithiasis

Definitions

- Concretion of urinary mineral or organic crystals in collecting system of kidney

ETIOLOGY/PATHOGENESIS

Stone Types by Mineral Content

- Calcium-containing stones (~ 80% of all stones) are composed of the following compounds
  - Calcium oxalate (30%)
  - Calcium oxalate and calcium phosphate (35-45%)
  - Calcium phosphate: Hydroxyapatite (3.75-6%)
  - Calcium monohydrogen phosphate: Brushite (1.25-2%)
- Struvite (magnesium-ammonium phosphate and calcium carbonate-apatite) (5-10%)
- Uric acid (5-10%)
- Cystine (1-2%)
- Miscellaneous: Xanthine, 2,8-dihydroxyadenine, drugs (e.g., indinavir, sulphadiazine, silica-containing antacids), melamine

Predisposing Factors

- Calcium stones
  - Hypercalciuria (defined as > 4 mg Ca/kg/day in urine) without hypercalcemia
    - Idiopathic
    - Renal tubular acidosis
    - Medullary sponge kidney
    - Cadmium and beryllium nephrotoxicity
  - Hypercalcemia and hypercalciuria: Primary and secondary hyperparathyroidism
  - Hyperoxaluria
    - Primary: Autosomal recessive types 1 and 2
    - Secondary: Enteric, due to small intestinal malabsorption or excess intake; dietary, due to poisoning (ethylene glycol)
- Struvite stones
  - Infection by urea-splitting organisms: *Proteus*, *Pseudomonas*, *Providencia* species and others
  - Alkaline urine increases risk
- Uric acid stones
  - Hyperuricosuria
    - Associated with uric acid lithiasis and with ~ 40% of calcium oxalate lithiasis
  - Acidic urine with pH < 5.5
- Cystine stones
  - Hereditary disorders of tubular transport with mutations of solute-linked carriers *3A1* and *7A9* genes
- General
  - Low urine volume

Pathophysiology of Stone Formation

- Urine is supersaturated with stone constituents
- Nucleation is condensation of dissolved salts to solid phase crystals
  - Homogeneous nucleation: When solubility limits are exceeded
  - Heterogeneous nucleation: Cell membranes, cell debris, or other types of crystal form a nidus; occurs at lower supersaturation
- Stones form in at least 3 different ways
  - Concretion of constituents in a supersaturated solution
  - Heterogenous nucleation at Randall plaques
  - Stone growth from crystalline plugs in ectatic Bellini ducts
- Stone composition: About 95% aggregated crystals and 5% organic mucoprotein matrix

Causes of Nephrolithiasis

- 25% known causes, most commonly
  - Primary hyperparathyroidism and other causes of hypercalcemia
  - Renal tubular acidosis
  - Hyperoxaluria
  - Cystinuria
  - Medullary sponge kidney
  - Drugs: Antivirals (acyclovir, ganciclovir, indinavir), sulfonamide derivatives, triamterene, glafenine, pyridoxylate
- 50% idiopathic hypercalciuria
- 25% unknown cause

CLINICAL ISSUES

Presentation

- Frequency: 5% of females and 12% of males in USA
- Nonobstructive stones have only hematuria without other symptoms or signs
- Renal colic is associated with stone passage, which is dependent on stone size
  - < 5 mm: High chance of passage
  - 5-7 mm: ~ 50% chance of passage
  - > 7 mm: Requires intervention for removal

Treatment

- Extracorporeal shock wave lithotripsy utilizes ultrasonic waves to break up stones
- Endoscopic laser-guided stone disruption
- Percutaneous nephrostomy permits removal of larger stones
- Medical treatment includes hydration to increase urinary volume and thiazide diuretics to reduce calcium excretion

Prognosis

- Stones recur in ~ 50% of instances
- Stone formers have higher blood pressure than nonstone formers
- Stone formers with high body mass index (> 27) have lower GFR than matched nonstone formers
- Almost any stone type can be complicated by urinary obstruction or infection

MACROSCOPIC

Morphology of Common Stone Types

- Calcium oxalate and apatite
  - Solitary or multiple; hard, radiopaque; yellow-brown

- Struvite
  - Large and branched ("staghorn"); hard, gray-white, radiopacity dependent on calcium content
- Uric acid
  - Multiple; seldom > 2 cm; hard, smooth surface, yellow-brown; mainly radiolucent
- Cystine
  - Multiple; small, smooth, rounded (rarely "staghorn"); yellow, waxy, radiopaque
- 80% of stones are unilateral
- Stones protrude from ectatic Bellini ducts in calcium, uric acid, cystine, and some cases of enteric oxaluria associated lithiasis
- Stones are attached to papillae at grossly visible Randall plaques in most calcium lithiasis

MICROSCOPIC

Histologic Features

- Mineral deposits
  - Calcium oxalate forms pale yellow, refractile, sheaves: Birefringent by polarization microscopy
  - Apatite is basophilic, laminated, and angulate: Confirmed by von Kossa or Yasue staining
  - Accurate identification of tissue mineral deposits requires infrared spectroscopy
- Medullary histology
  - Randall plaque is papillary suburothelial confluent apatite deposits
    - Possibly evolve from punctate apatite deposits in basement membranes of loops of Henle
    - Nidus for calcium oxalate, phosphate, and mixed stones
    - Found in most calcium stone formers
  - Bellini and medullary collecting ducts plugged with mineral in most calcium and cystine stone formers
    - Stones may grow from plugged terminal ducts
    - Plugged ducts have epithelial injury, ectasia, periductal inflammation, and fibrosis
  - Uric acid lithiasis is associated with intratubular sodium and ammonium urate crystal plugs
    - Interstitial urate deposits have giant cell reaction (gouty tophus)
  - Struvite stones are associated with changes of acute, chronic, or xanthogranulomatous pyelonephritis
  - Small medullary apatite deposits in basement membranes of loops of Henle may be seen in nonstone formers
- Cortical histology
  - Cortical calcium phosphate deposits are evident in hypercalcemia and in cystine lithiasis
  - Cortical interstitial fibrosis, tubular atrophy, and glomerular sclerosis are prominent in brushite and cystine lithiasis
- Most stone disease can be complicated by obstruction and infection (acute, chronic, and xanthogranulomatous pyelonephritis)
- Cortical scarring may occur as a result of crystal deposits, obstruction, infection, shock wave lithotripsy, or surgical intervention

ANCILLARY TESTS

Histochemistry

- von Kossa
  - Reactivity: Positive reaction with phosphate deposit
  - Staining pattern: Black precipitate in areas of calcium phosphate deposits
- Yasue
  - Reactivity: Positive reaction with calcium deposit
  - Staining pattern: Black precipitate in areas of calcium deposits

DIFFERENTIAL DIAGNOSIS

Stone Identification

- Stone mineral content and, therefore, stone type are determined by infrared spectroscopy or x-ray diffraction

Cause of Lithiasis

- Stone type determines investigation of secondary causes

DIAGNOSTIC CHECKLIST

Clinically Relevant Pathologic Features

- Stones grow at papillary tip from Randall plaques, from crystal plugs in ectatic Bellini ducts and in free supersaturated solution
- Randall plaque is observed in calcium and cystine lithiasis
- Bellini duct dilation and stone protrusion seen in calcium phosphate, uric acid, cystine, and some oxalate (enteric) lithiasis

Pathologic Interpretation Pearls

- Randall plaque is medullary subepithelial apatite deposit
- Cortical scarring may occur as a result of crystal deposits, obstruction, infection, lithotripsy, or surgical intervention

SELECTED REFERENCES

1. Linnes MP et al: Phenotypic characterization of kidney stone formers by endoscopic and histological quantification of intrarenal calcification. Kidney Int. 84(4):818-25, 2013
2. Monico CG et al: Genetic determinants of urolithiasis. Nat Rev Nephrol. 8(3):151-62, 2011
3. Coe FL et al: Plaque and deposits in nine human stone diseases. Urol Res. 38(4):239-47, 2010
4. Coe FL et al: Three pathways for human kidney stone formation. Urol Res. 38(3):147-60, 2010
5. Krambeck AE et al: Profile of the brushite stone former. J Urol. 184(4):1367-71, 2010
6. Miller NL et al: A formal test of the hypothesis that idiopathic calcium oxalate stones grow on Randall's plaque. BJU Int. 103(7):966-71, 2009
7. Evan AP et al: Role of interstitial apatite plaque in the pathogenesis of the common calcium oxalate stone. Semin Nephrol. 28(2):111-9, 2008
8. Miller NL et al: Pathogenesis of renal calculi. Urol Clin North Am. 34(3):295-313, 2007
9. Coe FL et al: Kidney stone disease. J Clin Invest. 115(10):2598-608, 2005
10. Evan AP et al: Insights on the pathology of kidney stone formation. Urol Res. 33(5):383-9, 2005

Kidney Stones: Composition, Frequency, Causes, and Associated Disorders

Composition	Frequency	Causes	Associated Disorders
Calcium oxalate and phosphate	80%	Idiopathic hypercalciuria	Excess calcium excretion ± uricosuria
		Hypercalcemia and hypercalciuria	Primary hyperparathyroidism: Parathyroid adenoma, hyperplasia
			Secondary hyperparathyroidism: Chronic renal failure, malabsorption
			Sarcoidosis, malignancy, milk-alkali syndrome
		Distal renal tubular acidosis with hypercalciuria	Autosomal dominant, autosomal recessive, secondary forms (dysproteinemia, Sjögren, SLE, Wilson, primary biliary cirrhosis, drugs/toxins [cadmium, lithium, amphotericin B])
		Medullary sponge kidney with hypercalciuria, stasis, renal tubular acidosis	Some autosomal dominant inheritance; many unknown
		Monogenic mutations	Ion channel and calcium sensor gene mutations (e.g., Dent disease)
		Enteric hyperoxaluria	Malabsorption (Crohn, celiac, ileal resection); dietary excess
		Peroxisomal enzyme gene mutations	Primary oxalosis (types 1-3)
Struvite	5-10%	Urea-splitting bacterial infection (e.g., proteus)	Pyelonephritis (may be xanthogranulomatous) "staghorn" calculus
Uric acid	5-10%	Hyperuricosuria	Uric acid nephropathy (primary or secondary)
Cystine	1-2%	Cystinuria	Amino acid transporter gene mutations
Xanthine	< 1%	Xanthinuria	Xanthine dehydrogenase gene mutations
Dihydroxyadenine	< 1%	2,8-dihydroxyadeninuria	Adenine phosphoribosyl transferase gene mutations
Drugs	< 1%	Drug crystallization	Sulfadiazine, indinavir, acyclovir, triamterene, others

Main Causes, Supersaturations, Medullary Histology, and Stone Composition in Calcium Lithiasis

Stone-Forming Disease	Urinary Supersaturation	Interstitium	Tubules	LH TBM	Stone Composition
Idiopathic CaOx lithiasis	CaOx, CaP, uric acid	Apatite plaque	Apatite, CaOx	Apatite	CaOx, CaP
Brushite lithiasis	CaOx, CaP	Apatite plaque	Apatite	Apatite	Calcium monohydrogen phosphate (brushite)
Hyperparathyroidism	CaOx, CaP	Apatite plaque	Apatite	Apatite	CaOx, CaP
Sarcoidosis	CaOx, CaP	Unknown	Unknown	Unknown	CaOx, CaP
Small intestinal resection	CaOx, uric acid	Apatite plaque	Apatite, CaOx	Apatite	CaOx
Ileostomy	CaOx, uric acid	Apatite plaque	Apatite, urates	Apatite	CaOx, uric acid
Obesity bypass	CaOx	No plaque	Apatite, CaOx	Normal	CaOx
Distal renal tubular acidosis	CaP	No plaque	Apatite, CaOx	Normal	CaP
Nonstone former	None	± apatite	None	Apatite±	None

LH TBM = loop of Henle tubular basement membrane; CaOx = calcium oxalate; CaP = calcium phosphate; ± = present in small amounts.

(**Left**) *Electron micrograph reveals spherical electron-dense apatite particles ⇨ in the thickened and lamellated (injured) basement membrane of a loop of Henle ⇨. The epithelium appears intact. These are thought to be the earliest lesions of Randall plaque. (Courtesy A. Evan, MD.)* (**Right**) *This electron micrograph shows a mixture of matrix material and spherical apatite deposit ⇨ in the medullary interstitium in early Randall plaque formation. (Courtesy A. Evan, MD.)*

Loop Of Henle Basement Membrane Apatite

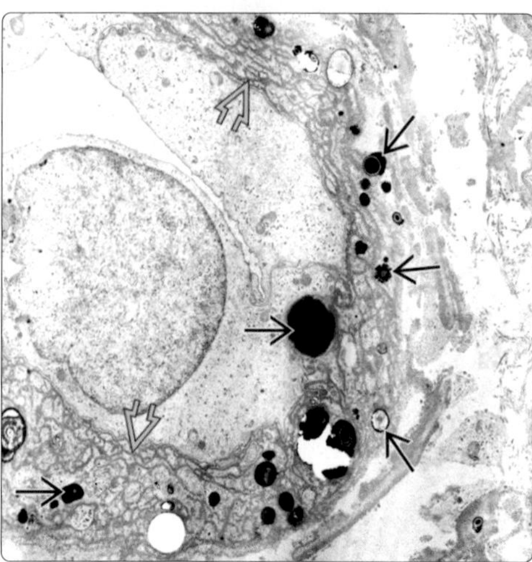

Minute Interstitial Apatite Deposits

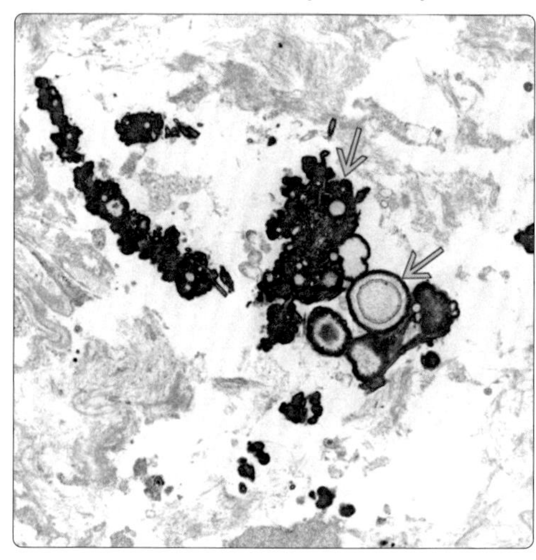

(**Left**) *Electron micrograph reveals the multilayered structure of the spherical apatite deposit. The crystalline material is apatite. The matrix is electron dense. (Courtesy A. Evan, MD.)* (**Right**) *Apatite deposits are shown around loops of Henle ⇨ and vasa recta ⇨ at the papillary tip in a nonstone former. The suburothelium is devoid of apatite.*

Apatite and Matrix

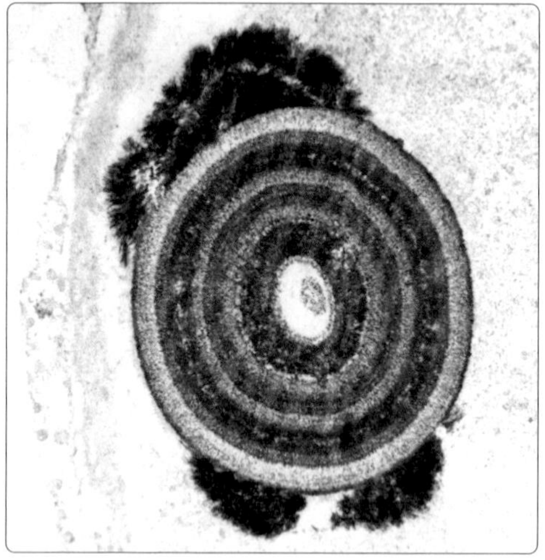

Apatite Deposits In Nonstone Former

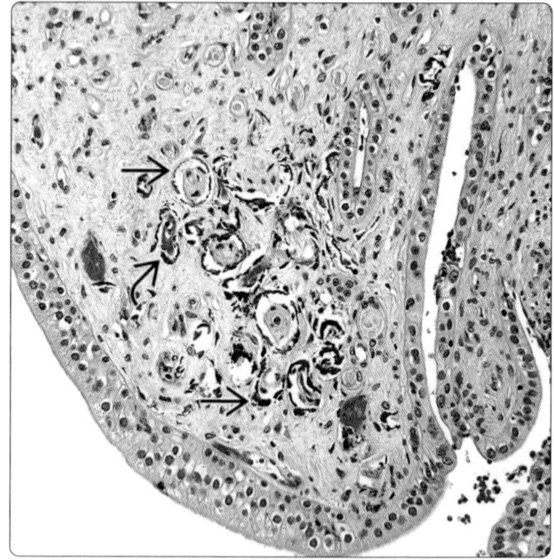

(**Left**) *Suburothelial ⇨ and medullary interstitial ⇨ fine granular apatite deposits are seen in the process of early Randall plaque formation.* (**Right**) *Subepithelial apatite plaque ⇨ with peritubular apatite deposits ⇨ are characteristic of Randall plaques. These are typically seen in calcium oxalate and brushite stone formers.*

Early Subepithelial Apatite

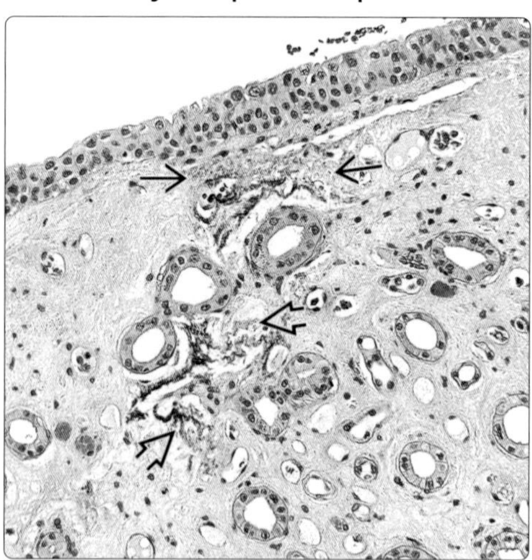

Randall Plaque

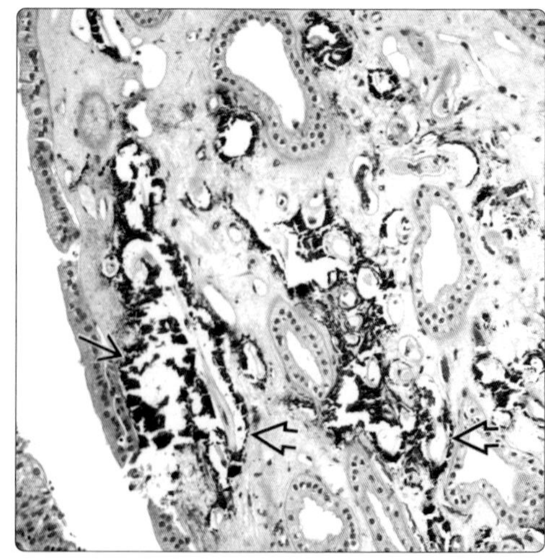

Calcium Oxalate Stone In Situ

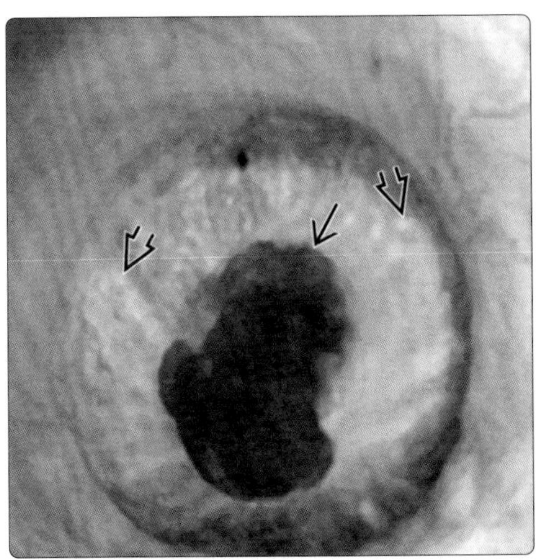

Interstitial Apatite Plaque

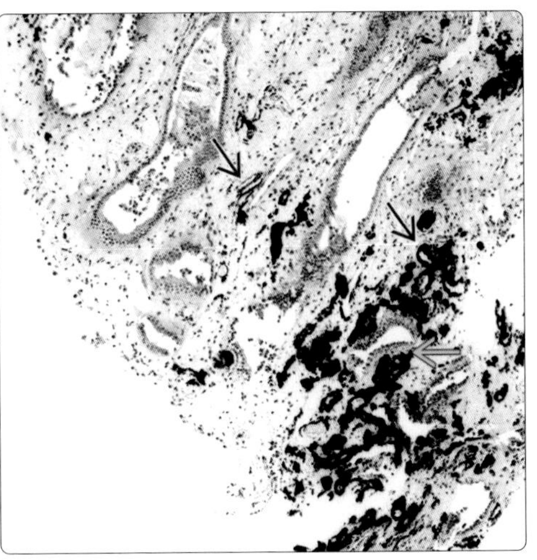

(Left) *This endoscopic gross photograph shows a calcium oxalate stone attached at the papillary tip ⇨. The sides of the papilla have white suburothelial (Randall) plaque ⇨. (Courtesy A. Evan, MD.)* **(Right)** *A papillary biopsy stained for calcium (Yasue) reveals abundant apatite around the loops of Henle ⇨ and the collecting ducts ⇨ and in the interstitium, forming part of a Randall plaque. The papillary urothelium is not sampled in this biopsy. (Courtesy A. Evan, MD.)*

Apatite Stone in Hyperparathyroidism

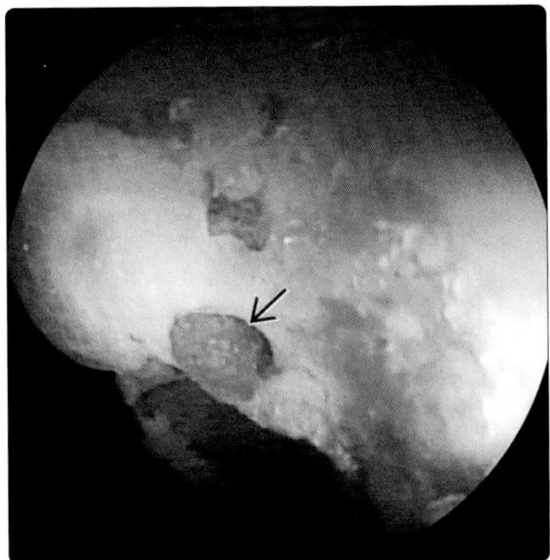

Papillary Apatite in Hyperparathyroidism

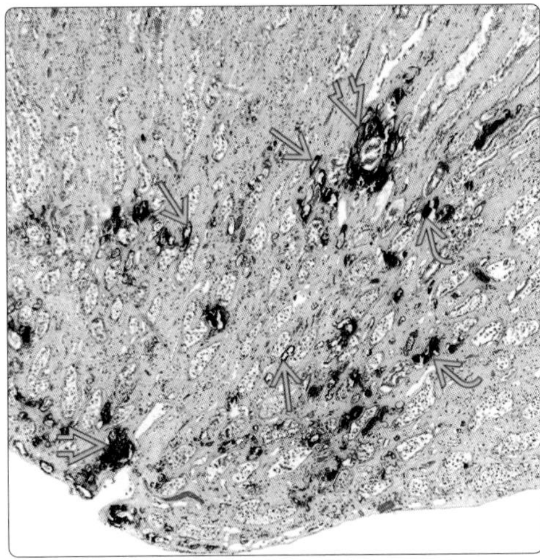

(Left) *Endoscopic gross photograph from a patient with primary hyperparathyroidism demonstrates a protruding brown calcium stone ⇨ in a flattened medullary papilla. (Courtesy A. Evan, MD.)* **(Right)** *The medullary papilla has peritubular ⇨, interstitial ⇨, and intratubular ⇨ apatite deposits in a patient with hypercalcemia and hypercalciuria due to hyperparathyroidism.*

Primary Hyperparathyroidism

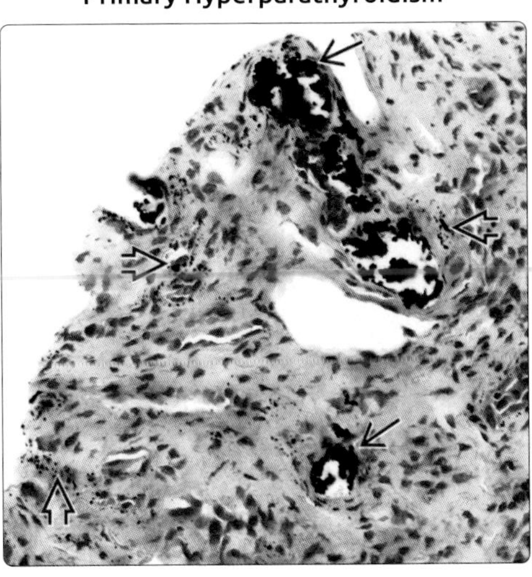

Outer Medullary Apatite in Hyperparathyroidism

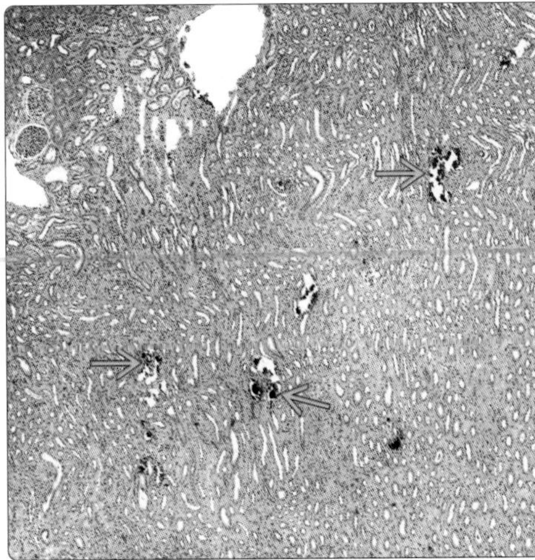

(Left) *Yasue stain for calcium reveals intratubular apatite plugs ⇨ and fine interstitial deposits ⇨ in a papillary biopsy from a patient with primary hyperparathyroidism. (Courtesy A. Evan, MD.)* **(Right)** *Calcium phosphate (apatite) deposits are seen as hematoxyphilic crystalline deposits in the outer medullary tubules ⇨ in hyperparathyroidism. Similar deposits may be seen in the cortex.*

(Left) *Peritubular and interstitial basophilic apatite deposits in Randall plaque from an idiopathic calcium oxalate stone former are shown. In this specimen, the papillary urothelium is absent (lower right), and the tubular epithelium is autolyzed.* **(Right)** *An effaced medullary papilla with dilated Bellini ducts → is shown. Tubules are plugged with apatite → and oxalate →. The interstitium has inflammation and fibrosis in a mixed oxalate and apatite stone former, viewed using partially polarized light.*

Interstitial Apatite Plaque

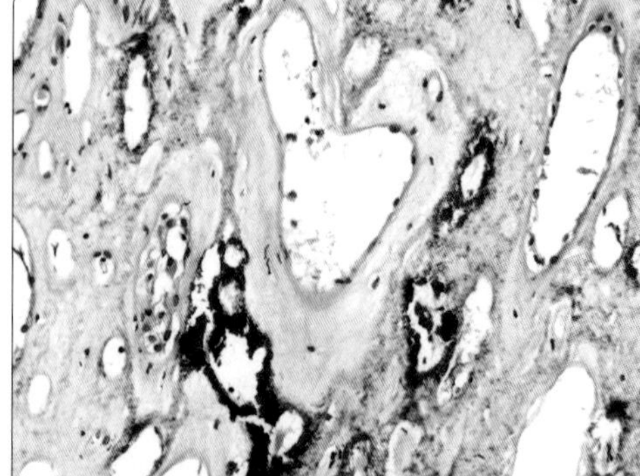

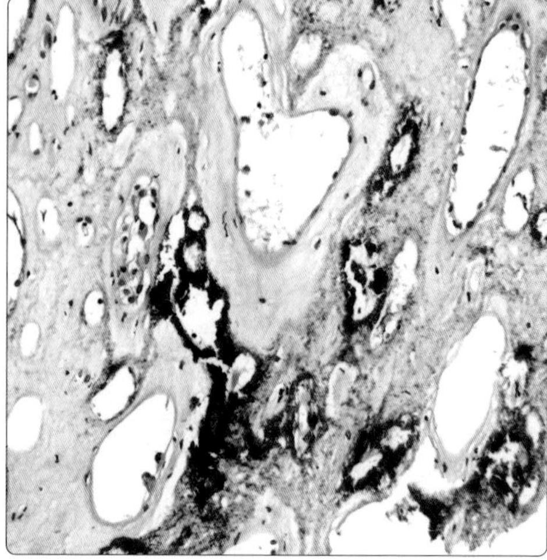

Medullary Inflammation and Fibrosis

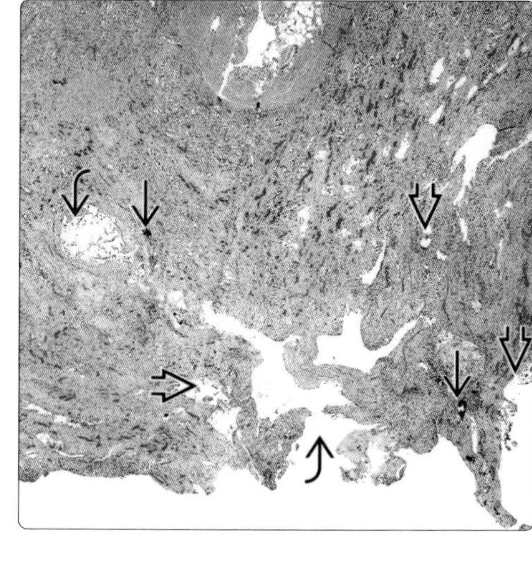

(Left) *Endoscopic gross photograph from a patient with intestinal bypass surgery for obesity reveals a dilated duct of Bellini at the papillary tip →. Small yellow deposits of apatite are also evident →. (Courtesy A. Evan, MD.)* **(Right)** *Yasue stain for calcium reveals tubular plugging with apatite → and medullary fibrosis in a papillary biopsy specimen from a patient with intestinal bypass surgery for obesity and calcium oxalate kidney stones. (Courtesy A. Evan, MD.)*

Obesity Bypass Calcium Oxalate Stone Former

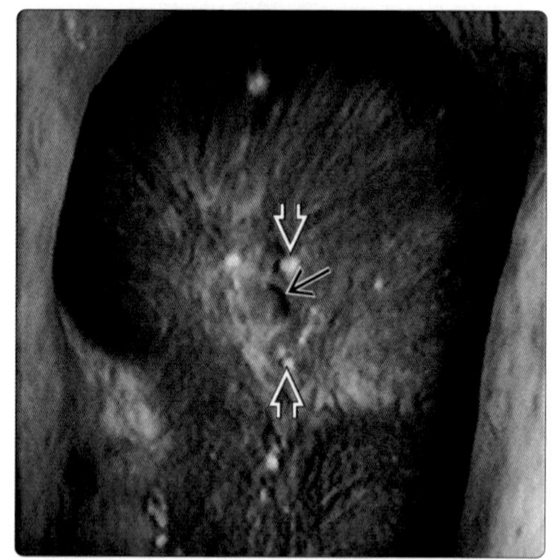

Calcium Oxalate Lithiasis, Intestinal Bypass

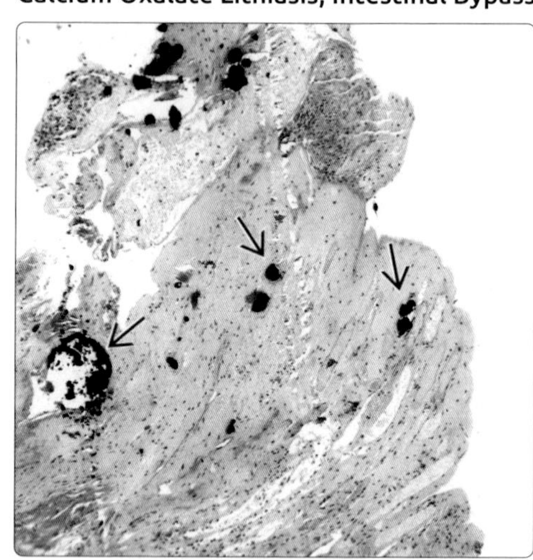

(Left) *Endoscopic gross photograph shows a cystine stone protruding from the opening of a Bellini duct →. Dilated openings of the ducts of Bellini are also evident →. (Courtesy A. Evan, MD.)* **(Right)** *Yasue stain for calcium reveals a tubule plugged with apatite → in a fibrotic medullary papilla in a papillary biopsy from a cystine stone former. Cystine deposits typically fill the ducts of Bellini (not shown). (Courtesy A. Evan, MD.)*

Cystine Stone in Situ

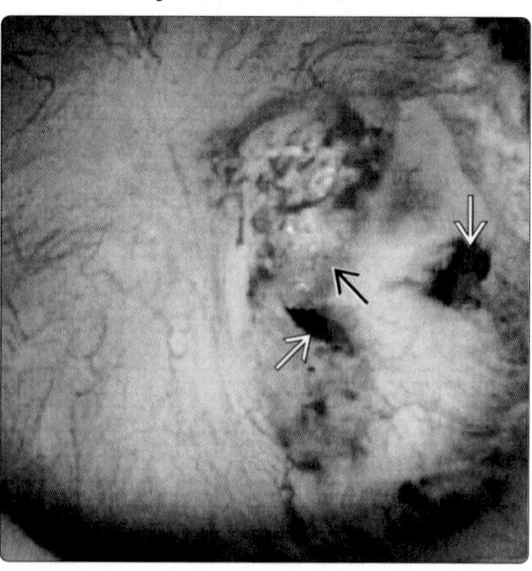

Apatite Plug In Cystine Stone Former

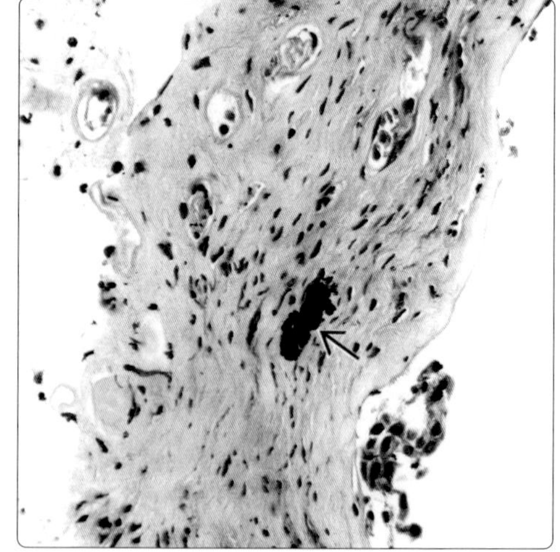

Calcium Oxalate Lithiasis, Crohn Disease

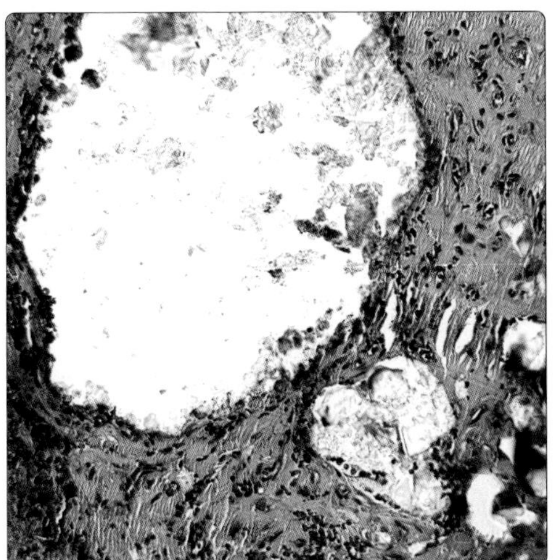

Primary Hyperoxaluria

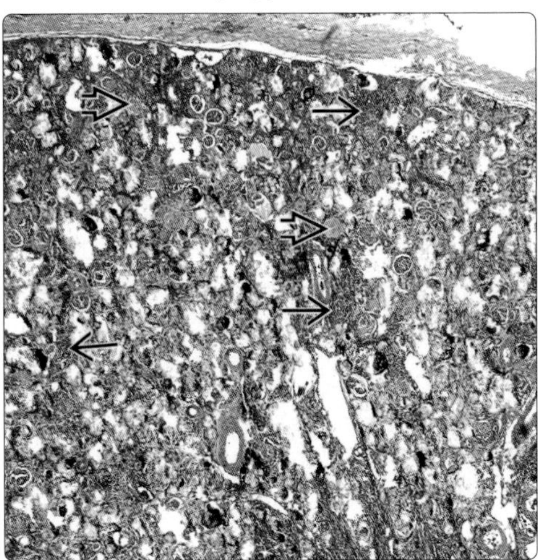

(Left) *Fractured, refractile, clear yellow crystals in a scarred papilla are shown in this patient with Crohn disease, a history of small intestinal resection, and calcium oxalate lithiasis.* **(Right)** *The cortex is filled with refractile pale yellow crystalline material in this kidney from 1 year old with primary hyperoxaluria. Many glomeruli are sclerotic ⇨, and the interstitium is inflamed →. These young patients have oxalate stones in the lower urinary tract.*

Renal Oxalosis in Primary Hyperoxaluria

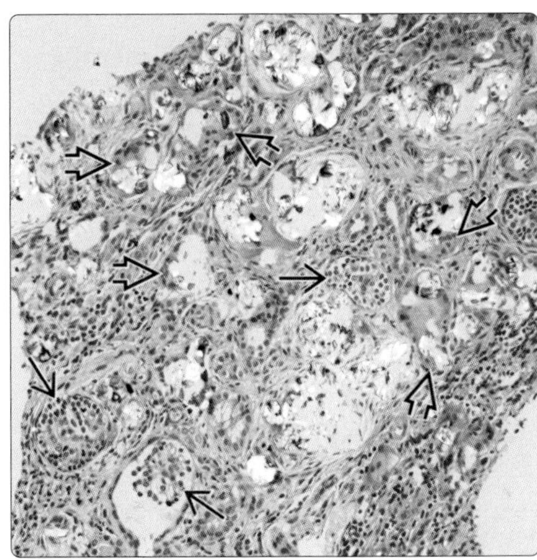

Gouty Tophus in Uric Acid Nephropathy

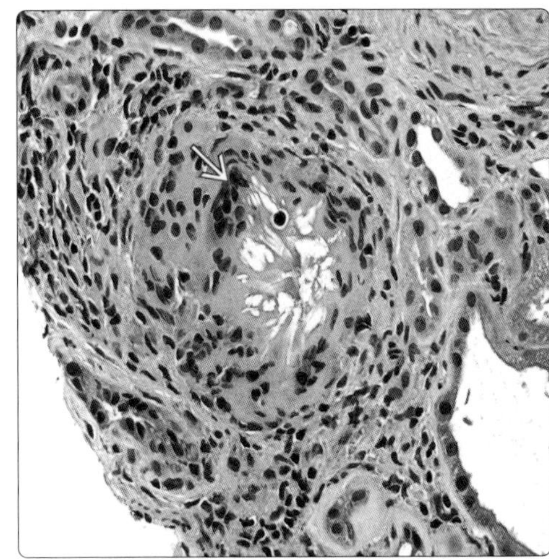

(Left) *Partially polarized light reveals abundant birefringent crystalline material in the interstitium associated with giant cells ⇨. There is extensive tubular atrophy and interstitial inflammation. Glomeruli → are immature but uninvolved.* **(Right)** *The section shows a granuloma with giant cells ➡ and clear central clefts. The interstitium is expanded and has mononuclear and eosinophilic infiltrates.*

Uric Acid Deposit

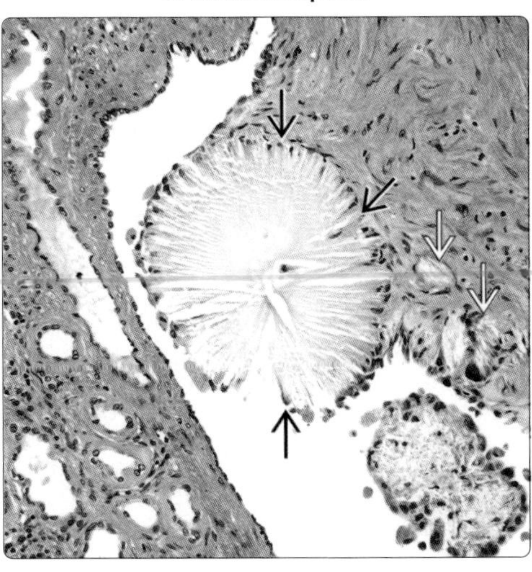

Dihydroxyadenine Deposit

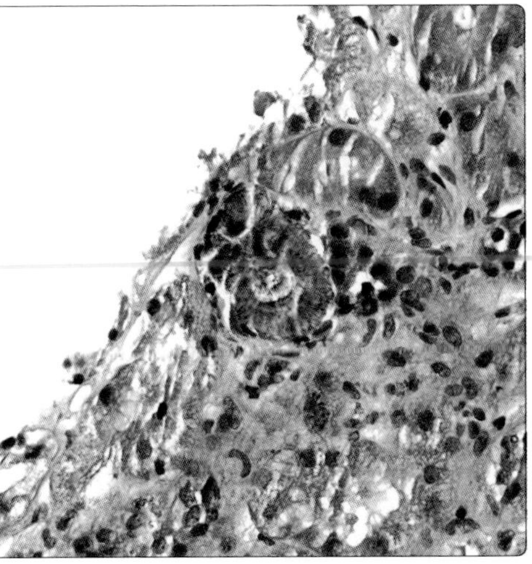

(Left) *A calyceal uric acid deposit at the fornix is shown. An epithelial-lined, radially clefted, organic matrix is highlighted →. The uric acid crystals are dissolved by aqueous fixative. Other smaller deposits are also evident ➡.* **(Right)** *Adenine phosphoribosyltransferase deficiency is associated with 2,8-dihydroxyadenine stone formation. Deposits of 2,8-DHA may be seen in the cortical tubules as golden brown radial arrays. These are difficult to distinguish from triamterene crystals.*

Loin Pain Hematuria Syndrome

KEY FACTS

TERMINOLOGY

- Severe flank (loin) pain associated with hematuria

ETIOLOGY/PATHOGENESIS

- Idiopathic: No identifiable cause
- Secondary: Occurring with many primary renal diseases

CLINICAL ISSUES

- Severe flank pain associated with hematuria
  - Idiopathic: Unexplained glomerular capillary leakage
  - Secondary: Many renal diseases can present with flank pain and hematuria
    - IgA nephropathy and other glomerulonephritides
    - Thin glomerular basement membrane disease and Alport syndrome
    - Occult nephrolithiasis
    - Vascular malformation
    - Vasculitis
    - Urinary tract infection

IMAGING

- Normal or nonspecific minor vascular alterations

MICROSCOPIC

- Idiopathic: Normal or nonspecific findings
- Secondary: Diverse findings dependent upon renal disease

TOP DIFFERENTIAL DIAGNOSES

- Urologic causes
  - Neoplasms
  - Occult renal lithiasis
  - Kidney or bladder infection
- Diverse nephritic glomerular diseases
- Renal vascular diseases
  - Isolated polyarteritis nodosa
  - Vascular malformations

DIAGNOSTIC CHECKLIST

- Biopsy important to identify secondary causes

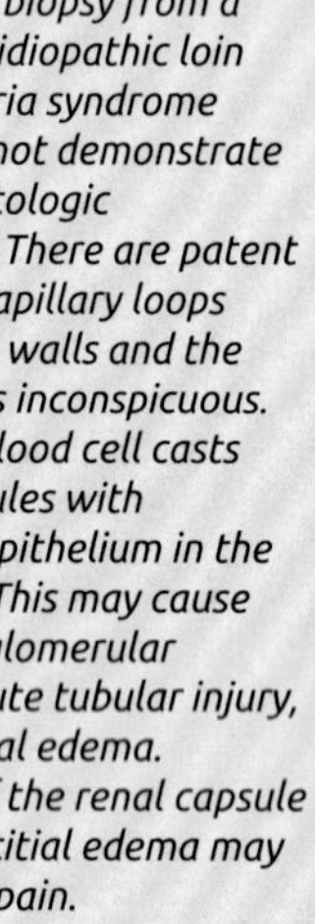

(Left) *Kidney biopsy from a patient with idiopathic loin pain hematuria syndrome (LPHS) does not demonstrate a specific histologic abnormality. There are patent glomerular capillary loops with delicate walls and the mesangium is inconspicuous.* **(Right)** *Red blood cell casts obstruct tubules with attenuated epithelium in the medulla →. This may cause backleak of glomerular filtration, acute tubular injury, and interstitial edema. Distension of the renal capsule due to interstitial edema may result in loin pain.*

Normal Glomerulus

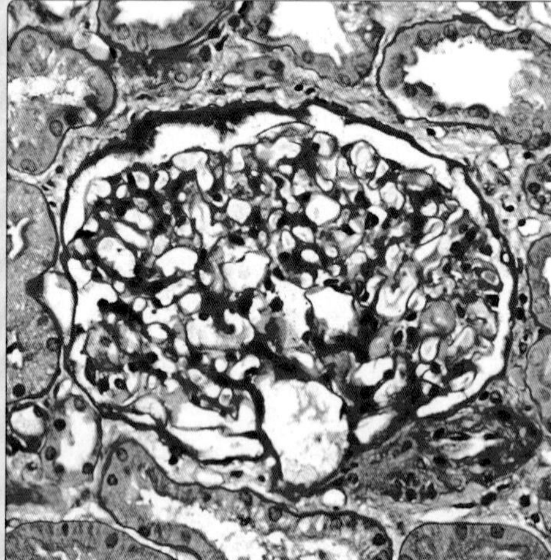

Red Cell Casts

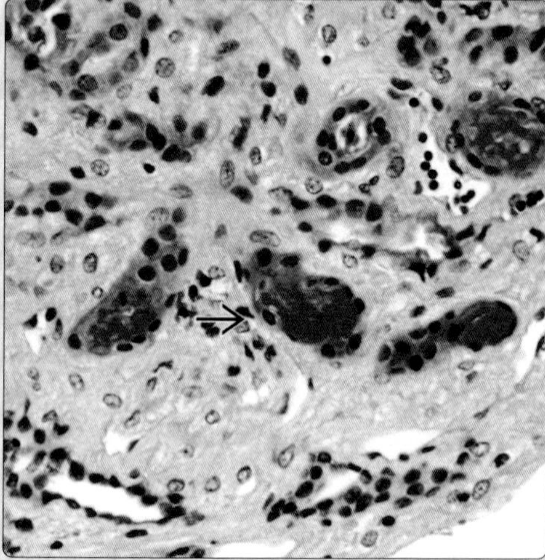

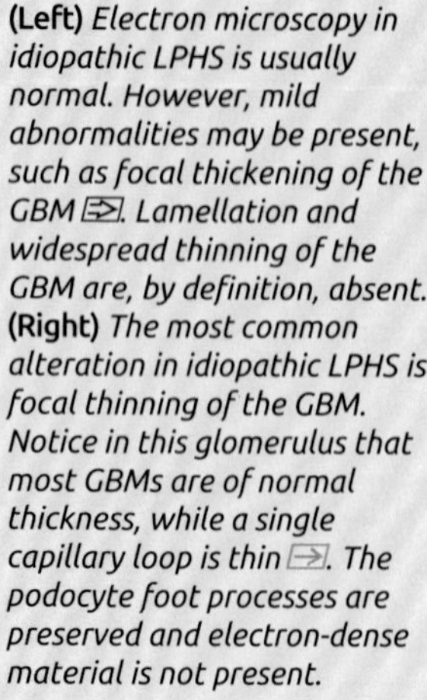

(Left) *Electron microscopy in idiopathic LPHS is usually normal. However, mild abnormalities may be present, such as focal thickening of the GBM →. Lamellation and widespread thinning of the GBM are, by definition, absent.* **(Right)** *The most common alteration in idiopathic LPHS is focal thinning of the GBM. Notice in this glomerulus that most GBMs are of normal thickness, while a single capillary loop is thin →. The podocyte foot processes are preserved and electron-dense material is not present.*

Nonspecific Ultrastructural Abnormalities

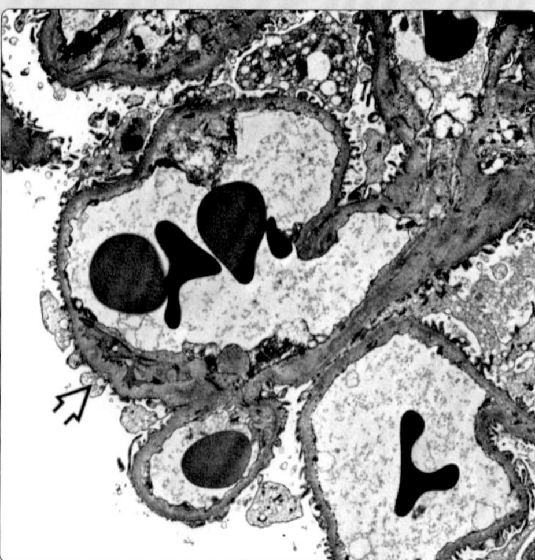

Nonspecific Ultrastructural Abnormalities

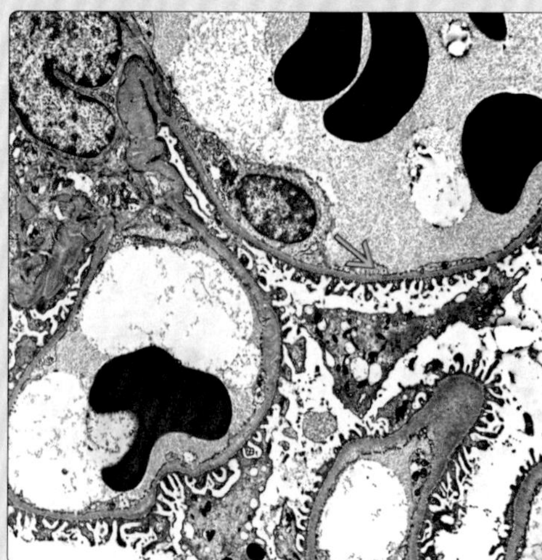

TERMINOLOGY

Abbreviations

- Loin pain hematuria syndrome (LPHS)

Definitions

- Severe flank (loin) pain associated with hematuria

ETIOLOGY/PATHOGENESIS

Idiopathic or Secondary in Context of Primary Renal Diseases

- Idiopathic loin pain hematuria syndrome
  - Possibly idiopathic glomerular capillary hemorrhage
    - RBCs and RBC casts obstruct and injure tubules
    - Interstitial edema with capsular distension and pain
- Renal diseases that may present with flank pain and hematuria
  - IgA nephropathy and other glomerulonephritides
  - Collagen type IV abnormalities: Thin basement membrane nephropathy and Alport syndrome
  - Occult nephrolithiasis
  - Vascular malformation
  - Vasculitis
  - Urinary tract infection

CLINICAL ISSUES

Epidemiology

- Incidence
  - Rarely reported, so true incidence unknown
- Age
  - Children and adults from 1st to 6th decades
  - Median age: Mid 30s
- Sex
  - Females (70%) > males (30%)

Presentation

- Severe recurrent flank pain with hematuria
  - Pain, unilateral or bilateral, radiates to groin or thigh
    - Not always associated with hematuria
  - Hematuria may be gross or microscopic
- Physical exam unremarkable and nonspecific
  - Costovertebral angle tenderness
  - Low-grade fever, dysuria, vomiting may be present
  - Pain persists for hours or may be constant

Laboratory Tests

- Urine analysis shows RBCs and RBC casts

Treatment

- Options, risks, complications
  - Multidisciplinary pain management
    - Analgesia: NSAIDs and opioids
    - Intraureteric and renal pelvic capsaicin
    - Nerve blockade or denervation
    - ACE inhibitors
    - Nephrectomy with autotransplantation

Prognosis

- Long-term renal function well preserved
- Spontaneous resolution in 30%

IMAGING

Radiographic Findings

- Normal or nonspecific minor vascular alterations

MICROSCOPIC

Histologic Features

- Idiopathic causes: Normal or nonspecific
  - Glomerulosclerosis with tubulointerstitial scarring
  - Arterial and arteriolar sclerosis
  - Tubular red cells and RBC casts with interstitial edema
- Secondary causes: Diverse dependent upon renal disease

ANCILLARY TESTS

Immunofluorescence

- Idiopathic: Negative or nonspecific reactions
- Secondary: Dependent upon underlying primary disease

Electron Microscopy

- Idiopathic causes: Normal or minor GBM alterations
- Secondary: Dependent upon underlying primary disease

DIFFERENTIAL DIAGNOSIS

Urologic Causes of Hematuria

- Neoplasms
- Occult nephrolithiasis
- Infection of kidney or bladder

Renal Glomerular Diseases

- IgA nephropathy and other glomerulonephritides
  - 20% of LPHS show IgA nephropathy
- Thin basement membrane nephropathy and Alport syndrome
- Diverse glomerulonephritides with nephritic presentation

Renal Vascular Diseases

- Isolated polyarteritis nodosa
- Vascular malformations

DIAGNOSTIC CHECKLIST

Clinically Relevant Pathologic Features

- Idiopathic: No diagnostic histological abnormalities
- Secondary: Evidence of specific medical renal disease

Pathologic Interpretation Pearls

- Negative biopsy: Idiopathic loin pain hematuria syndrome
- Positive biopsy: Secondary loin pain hematuria syndrome

SELECTED REFERENCES

1. Taba Taba Vakili S et al: Loin pain hematuria syndrome. Am J Kidney Dis. 64(3):460-72, 2014
2. Gambaro G et al: Percutaneous renal sympathetic nerve ablation for loin pain haematuria syndrome. Nephrol Dial Transplant. 28(9):2393-5, 2013
3. Coffman KL: Loin pain hematuria syndrome: a psychiatric and surgical conundrum. Curr Opin Organ Transplant. 14(2):186-90, 2009
4. Dube GK et al: Loin pain hematuria syndrome. Kidney Int. 70(12):2152-5, 2006
5. Ghanem AN: Intra-ureteric capsaicin in loin pain haematuria syndrome: efficacy and complications. BJU Int. 91(4):429-30, 2003
6. Bultitude M et al: Loin pain haematuria syndrome: distress resolved by pain relief. Pain. 76(1-2):209-13, 1998

(Left) *A wide spectrum of nonspecific changes may be encountered in kidney biopsies from patients with LPHS representing age-related changes of hypertension. Isolated glomerulosclerosis* ⇒ *in the subcapsular cortex may be seen in young patients.* **(Right)** *Focal arteriolosclerosis* ⇒*, ischemia-induced glomerular capillary changes, and tubulointerstitial scarring may be present even in patients with no history of hypertension. A localized vascular lesion may be the cause for this phenomenon.*

Nonspecific Histologic Abnormalities

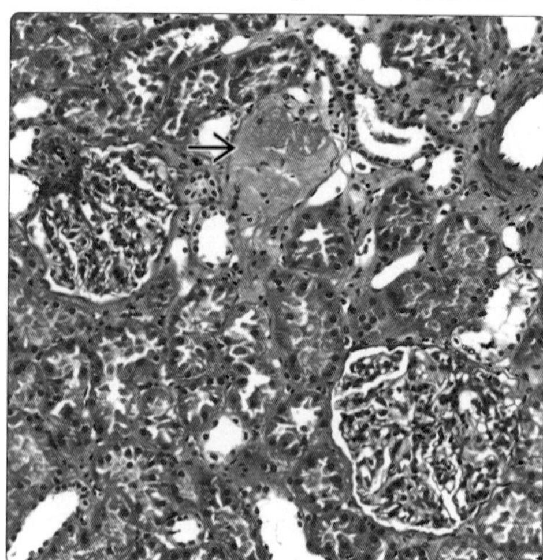

Nonspecific Histologic Abnormalities

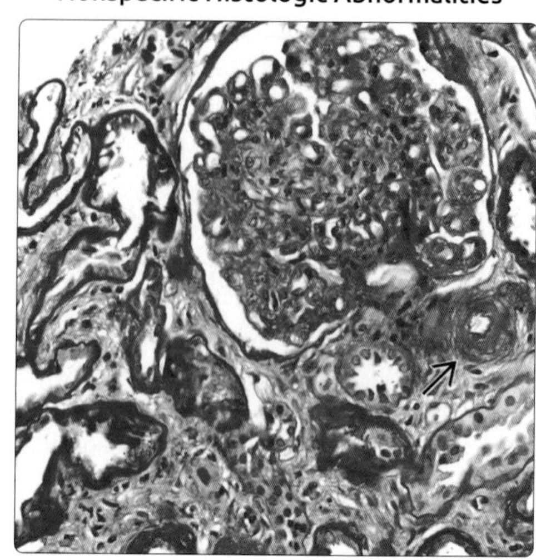

(Left) *In this case, light microscopy revealed red blood cells within tubules leading to obstruction of tubular lumens* ➡*. The tubules otherwise appear unaffected.* **(Right)** *This biopsy from an idiopathic LPHS patient shows a histologically normal cortical tubulointerstitium. The proximal tubules show preserved brush borders. The tubules are back-to-back, and the interstitium is inconspicuous.*

Nonspecific Histologic Abnormalities

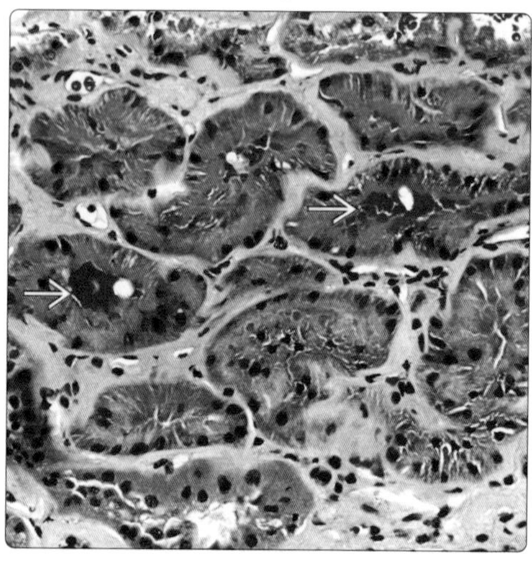

Normal Tubulointerstitium

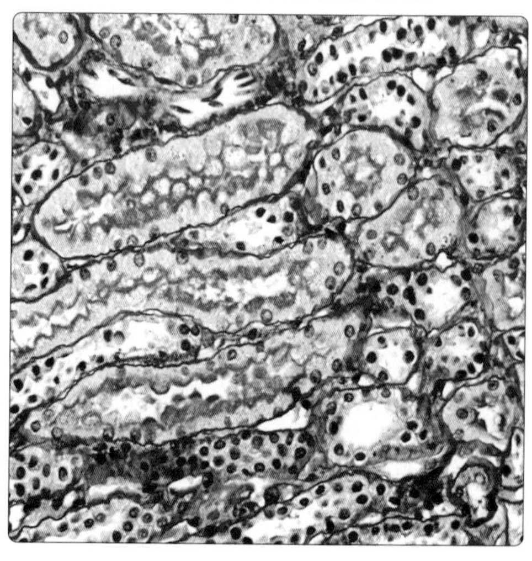

(Left) *In idiopathic LPHS, the biopsy should be normal or only show nonspecific (nondiagnostic) abnormalities. This is an immunofluorescent stain for IgG. There are no IgG deposits. Similarly, the stains for IgA, IgM, C3, C1q, kappa, lambda, and fibrinogen were negative.* **(Right)** *The immunofluorescence in this case demonstrates arteriolar C3 deposition* ➡ *without glomerular immune deposits. Arteriolar C3 deposition is not a marker of any specific disease and is commonly in adults and correlates with arteriolar hyalinosis.*

Negative Glomerular Immunofluorescence

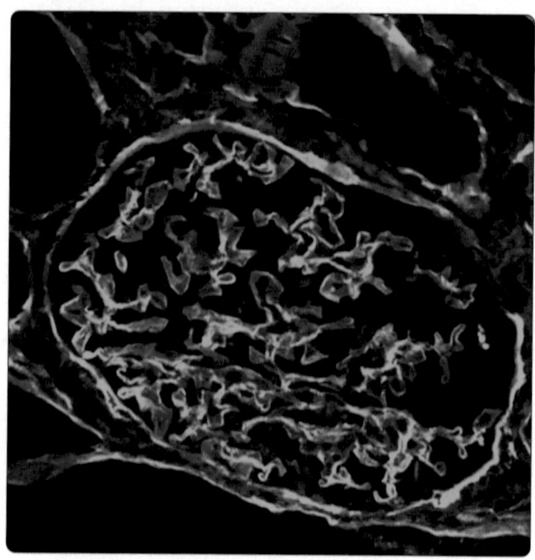

Nonspecific Immunofluorescent Findings

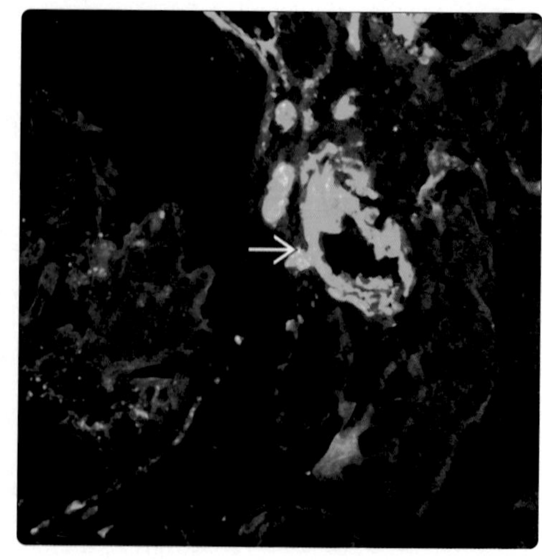

Mesangial IgA Nephropathy

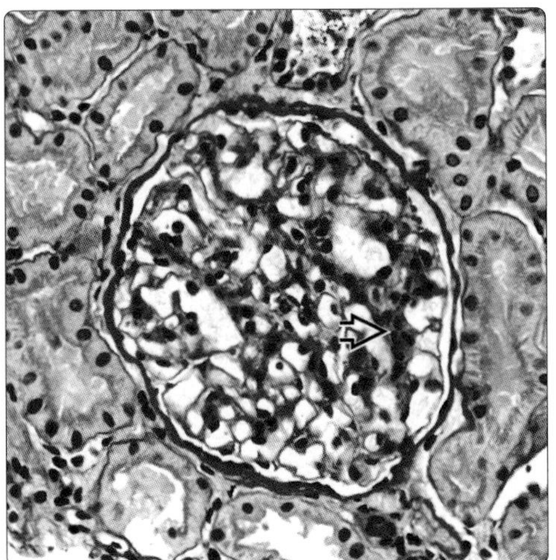

Mesangial IgA Nephropathy

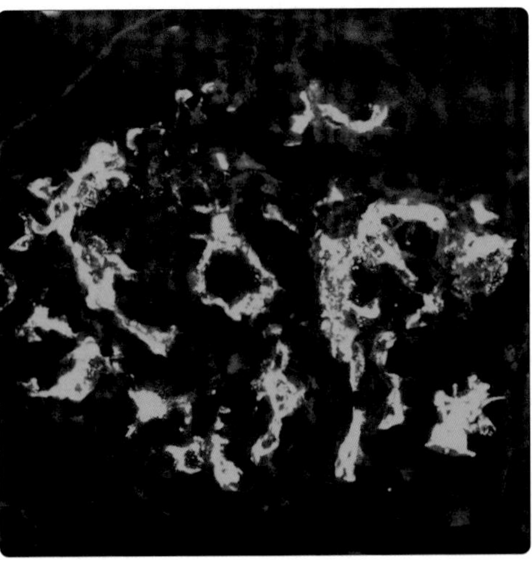

(Left) *LPHS needs to be differentiated from IgAN, seen in 20% of kidney biopsies from clinically diagnosed LPHS. Although IgAN demonstrates mesangial hypercellularity ➩, a wide spectrum of histologic phenotypes may be seen, from no lesion, as in this case, to endocapillary proliferation to crescentic glomerulonephritis.* **(Right)** *There is abundant granular mesangial deposition of IgA, which is the diagnostic immunofluorescence finding in IgA nephropathy. Capillary loops are characteristically negative.*

Mesangial IgA Nephropathy

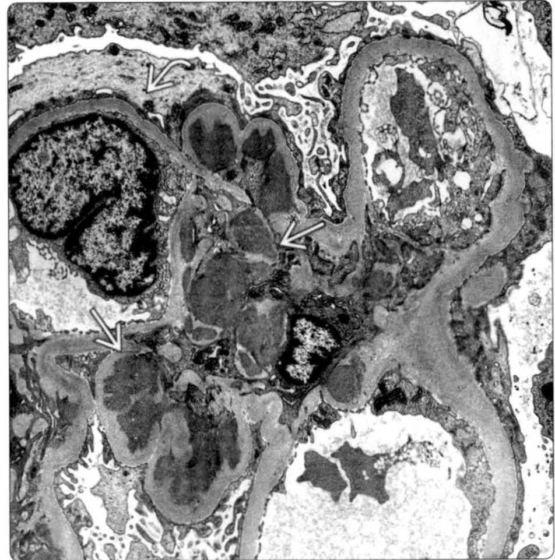

Thin Glomerular Basement Membrane Nephropathy

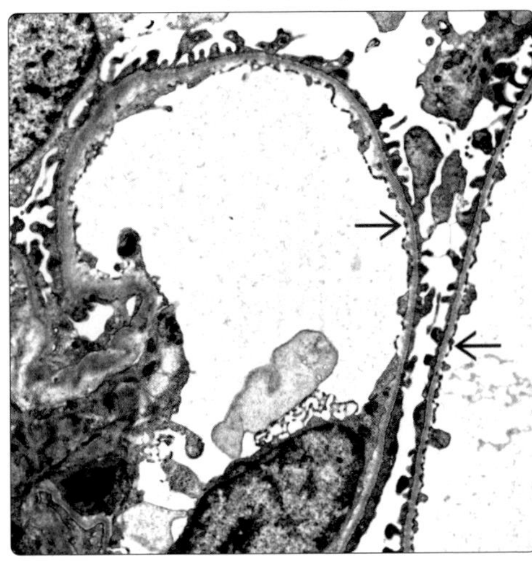

(Left) *This electron micrograph demonstrates findings typically encountered in IgA nephropathy. There is diffuse podocyte foot process effacement ➩. There are also numerous mesangial electron-dense deposits ➩ representing IgA deposition.* **(Right)** *LPHS needs to be differentiated from thin basement membrane nephropathy and from Alport syndrome. This example of TBMN shows widespread thinning of the GBM ➩. No lamellations characteristic of Alport syndrome are present.*

Alport Hereditary Nephritis

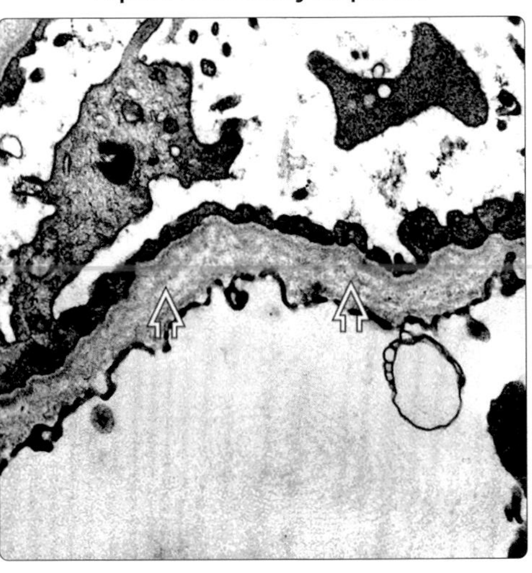

Necrotizing Arteritis

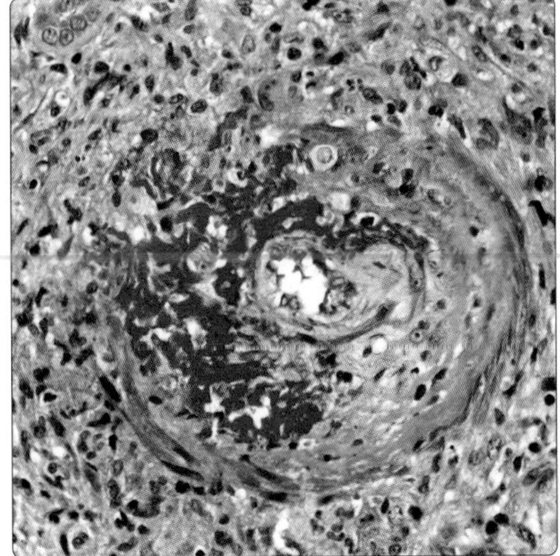

(Left) *In Alport syndrome, there are diffuse alterations of the GBM with irregular thickening and thinning with lamellations ➩. In early stages, only GBM thinning may be present. Immunofluorescence stains for collagen IV a-chains may support a diagnosis of Alport syndrome in some cases.* **(Right)** *Necrotizing arteritis can cause secondary LPHS. The likely cause is tubulointerstitial injury with interstitial edema leading to capsular distension and pain. This shows an interlobular artery with fibrinoid necrosis.*

SECTION 9
Diseases of the Renal Allograft

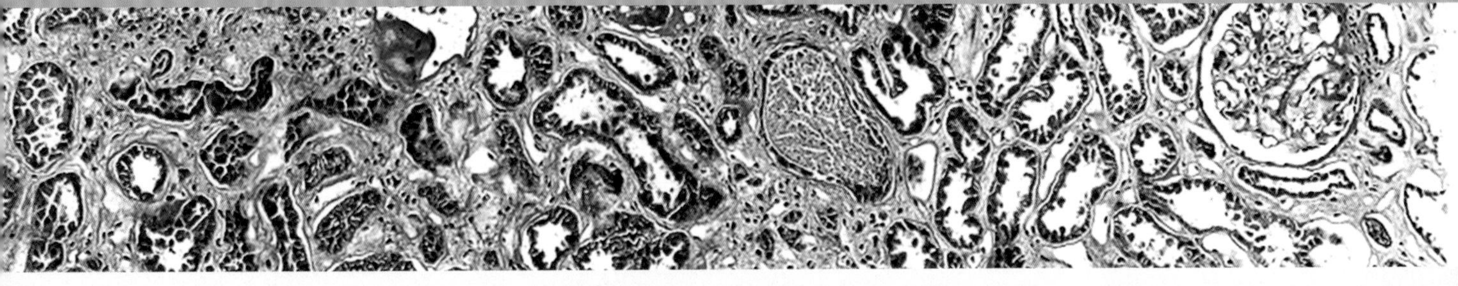

TERMINOLOGY

Pathogenetic Classification

- Based on pathogenesis, divided into broad categories of alloimmune, drug-related, nonalloimmune, and donor-derived diseases

Abbreviations

- T-cell-mediated rejection (TCMR)
- Antibody-mediated rejection (AMR)
- Peritubular capillaries (PTC)
- Focal segmental glomerulosclerosis (FSGS)
- Membranous glomerulonephritis (MGN)
- Membranoproliferative glomerulonephritis (MPGN)
- Interstitial fibrosis and tubular atrophy (IFTA), not otherwise specified (NOS)
- Epstein-Barr virus (EBV)
- Thrombotic microangiopathy (TMA)
- Mammalian target of rapamycin (mTOR)

DEFINITIONS

T-Cell-Mediated Rejection

- Target antigens expressed on cell surfaces of endothelial and parenchymal cells
- Accessory cells, such as macrophages participate
- Alloimmune reaction of T cells to donor alloantigens, predominantly those of major histocompatibility complex (MHC), in humans termed HLA
- Non-HLA antigens are also target (e.g., in HLA-identical siblings)

Antibody-Mediated Rejection

- Alloantibody-mediated injury to cells expressing donor alloantigens, predominantly HLA class I and II antigens
- Accessory mechanisms include complement activation and cells with Fc receptors including macrophages, NK cells, and neutrophils

HLA Molecules

- Polymorphic antigens encoded in MHC locus on chromosome 6
  - Class I molecules (A, B, C) widely expressed on all nucleated cells
  - Class II molecules (DR, DQ, DP), limited expression, B cells, dendritic cells, endothelial cells, macrophages, and activated T cells
- Increased expression by interferon-γ

Minor Histocompatibility Antigens

- Non-MHC antigens that are polymorphic
- Able to trigger allograft rejection in MHC identical recipients

C4d

- Fragment of C4 produced by complement activation that binds covalently to nearby molecules
- No known physiologic function

Multilamination

- Multilayered basement membranes, typically > 4 layers

Transplant Glomerulopathy

- Glomerular disease seen in transplants defined by duplication of GBM
- Has several causes, including chronic AMR, TMA, and recurrent MPGN

Transplant Glomerulitis

- Mononuclear or polymorphonuclear cells in glomerular capillary loops
- Glomerular endothelial swelling and mesangiolysis in more severe cases

Endarteritis/Endothelialitis

- Mononuclear cell infiltration under arterial endothelium

Tubulitis

- Mononuclear infiltration in tubules

CATEGORY 1: ALLOIMMUNE RESPONSES

T-Cell-Mediated Rejection

- Acute T-cell-mediated rejection (acute cellular rejection)
  - Tubulointerstitial (Banff type I)
  - Endarteritis/endothelialitis (Banff type II)
  - Arterial transmural inflammation or fibrinoid necrosis (Banff type III)
  - Transplant glomerulitis (no Banff type)
- Chronic T-cell-mediated rejection
  - Tubulointerstitial (Banff I + fibrosis and tubular atrophy)
  - Transplant arteriopathy (Banff II + intimal fibrosis/foam cells)

Antibody-Mediated Rejection

- Hyperacute rejection
  - Usually C4d(+) PTC (early samples may be negative)
  - Pathology similar to AHR, but occurring < 24 hours post transplant
- Acute antibody-mediated rejection (acute humoral rejection)
  - Tubular injury (Banff type I)
  - Capillaritis with neutrophils (Banff type II)
  - Arterial fibrinoid necrosis (Banff type III)
  - C4d(+) PTC
  - May also be manifested by endarteritis or thrombotic microangiopathy
- Chronic antibody-mediated rejection (chronic humoral rejection)
  - Transplant glomerulopathy and glomerulitis
  - PTC multilamination and capillaritis
  - Transplant arteriopathy
  - Usually C4d(+) PTC, may be C4d(-)
- Variants
  - Smoldering/indolent (mononuclear capillaritis)
  - C4d negative (mostly chronic or smoldering)
  - C4d positive without evidence of active rejection (accommodation)

CATEGORY 2: DRUG TOXICITY AND HYPERSENSITIVITY

Calcineurin Inhibitor Toxicity

- Cyclosporine and tacrolimus

- Chronic (hyaline arteriolopathy, fibrosis, tubular atrophy, FSGS, TMA)
- Functional (vacuolar vasospasm)
- Acute (tubulopathy, TMA)

mTOR Inhibitor Toxicity

- Rapamycin (sirolimus) and related drugs
- Acute tubular injury
- FSGS
- TMA

Antiviral Tubular Toxicity

- Crystal formation (foscarnet)
- Mitochondrial toxicity (adefovir, tenofovir)

Drug-Associated Acute Interstitial Nephritis

- Antibiotics and others

CATEGORY 3: INFECTION

Viral Infection

- Polyomavirus
- Cytomegalovirus
- Adenovirus
- Herpes simplex

Bacterial and Fungal Infection (Partial List)

- Acute pyelonephritis
- Chronic pyelonephritis
- Tuberculosis
- Malacoplakia
- Microsporidiosis

CATEGORY 4: ANATOMIC COMPLICATIONS

Major Vessel Disease

- Arterial thrombosis
- Venous thrombosis
- Arterial dissection
- Arterial stenosis

Pelvis/Ureter

- Urine leak
- Obstruction

CATEGORY 5: RECURRENT AND DE NOVO DISEASES

Recurrent Primary Disease (Partial List)

- FSGS
- Atypical hemolytic-uremic syndrome
- C3 glomerulopathy
- IgA nephropathy
- Primary oxalosis
- Membranous glomerulonephritis
- Diabetic nephropathy

De Novo Disease (Partial List)

- Membranous glomerulonephritis (probably alloimmune)
- FSGS, adaptive
- Diabetic nephropathy
- Anti-angiotensin II type 1 receptor autoantibody syndrome

Recipient-Specific De Novo Diseases

- Anti-GBM disease in Alport syndrome
- Nephrotic syndrome in congenital nephrosis, Finnish type
- Anti-TBM disease in TBM antigen-deficient recipients

CATEGORY 6: DONOR DISEASE

Present at Time of Transplant (Partial List)

- Acute tubular injury (ischemia)
- Arteriosclerosis
- Thrombotic microangiopathy
- Rhabdomyolysis (trauma)
- Pyelonephritis
- Glomerular disease
  - Global glomerulosclerosis due to hypertension/aging
  - IgA nephropathy, MGN, and others
- Neoplasia
  - Primary (renal cell carcinoma)
  - Metastatic tumor

CATEGORY 7: OTHER DISEASES

Neoplasia (Often Viral Related)

- Post-transplant lymphoproliferative disease

Idiopathic

- Interstitial fibrosis and tubular atrophy, not otherwise specified (IFTA, NOS)

NOTES

Comments

- Rejection may be manifested by clinical signs or be subclinical (normal renal function)
- Biopsy specimens often show combinations of diseases
- Knowledge of original native kidney disease, drug regimen, and time post transplant are essential for diagnostic interpretation

SELECTED REFERENCES

1. Nickeleit V et al: Renal transplant pathology. In Jennette JC et al: Heptinstall's Pathology of the Kidney. 7th ed. Philadelphia: Lippincott Williams & Wilkins. 1321-1459, 2015
2. Haas M et al: Banff 2013 meeting report: inclusion of C4d-negative antibody-mediated rejection and antibody-associated arterial lesions. Am J Transplant. 14(2):272-83, 2014
3. Mengel M et al: Banff 2011 Meeting report: new concepts in antibody-mediated rejection. Am J Transplant. 12(3):563-70, 2012

TERMINOLOGY

Definitions

- Major histocompatibility complex (MHC)
  - Locus on chromosome 6
    - Contains genes encoding class I and class II human leukocyte antigens (HLA)
      - MHC antigens are primary target of graft rejection
- Minor histocompatibility antigens
  - Molecules other than MHC antigens that are polymorphic
  - Can elicit immune response in same species
- Class I MHC antigens
  - Heterodimeric protein universally expressed by nucleated cells
    - Consist of polymorphic α chain and monomorphic β2-microglobulin
    - Recognized by CD8(+) T cells and NK cells
    - Encoded by 3 loci (A, B, C)
- Class II MHC antigens
  - Heterodimeric protein expressed constitutively by dendritic cells, B cells, monocytes, and endothelial cells,
    - Consist of polymorphic α chain and a β chain
    - Recognized by CD4(+) T cells
    - Encoded by 3 loci (DR, DP, DQ)
    - Increased by interferon gamma on many cell types

ETIOLOGY/PATHOGENESIS

Afferent Phase

- Donor MHC antigens elicit immune response by recipient T cells and B cells
  - On donor cells (direct pathway)
  - Processed and presented by recipient dendritic cells (indirect pathway)

Efferent Phase

- Donor-reactive T cells infiltrate graft
  - Direct injury to donor cells (cytotoxicity)
  - Indirect injury (via secreted cytokines and other mediators)
  - Other cells recruited and participate
    - Macrophages, granulocytes, NK cells
  - Target cells include arterial and capillary endothelium, tubular epithelium, and others
- Antibodies to donor HLA antigens bind to graft endothelium
  - Complement fixation
    - Release of chemotactic and vasoconstrictive mediators
    - Lysis and loss of endothelial cells
    - Activation of endothelial cells
  - Non-complement-dependent mechanisms possible
    - Activation of endothelial cells
    - Induction of proliferation
  - Cellular participation via Fc receptors
    - Monocytes, NK cells, granulocytes

Effects Determined by Many Variables

- Cellular target (endothelium of arteries, tubular epithelium, glomeruli)
- Type of immune response (antibodies vs. T cells)
- Intensity of immune response
- Resistance of graft to injury
- Immunosuppressive drug therapy

Consequences

- Ischemia
- Loss of nephron integrity
- Promotion of fibrosis
- Repair and recovery

CLINICAL IMPLICATIONS

Clinical Risk Factors

- HLA mismatch
  - HLA identical sibling graft half-life = 29 years
  - HLA haplo-identical living donor graft half-life = 19 years
- Deceased vs. living donor kidneys
  - Deceased

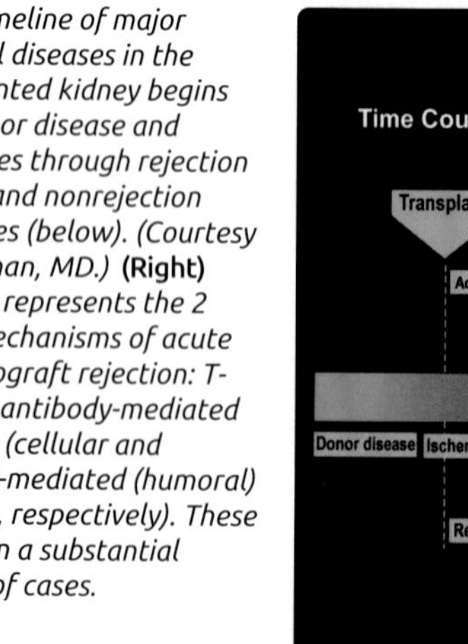

(Left) *Timeline of major potential diseases in the transplanted kidney begins with donor disease and progresses through rejection (above) and nonrejection categories (below). (Courtesy J. Chapman, MD.)* **(Right)** *Diagram represents the 2 major mechanisms of acute renal allograft rejection: T-cell- and antibody-mediated rejection (cellular and antibody-mediated (humoral) rejection, respectively). These overlap in a substantial number of cases.*

Timeline of Diseases in Renal Transplant

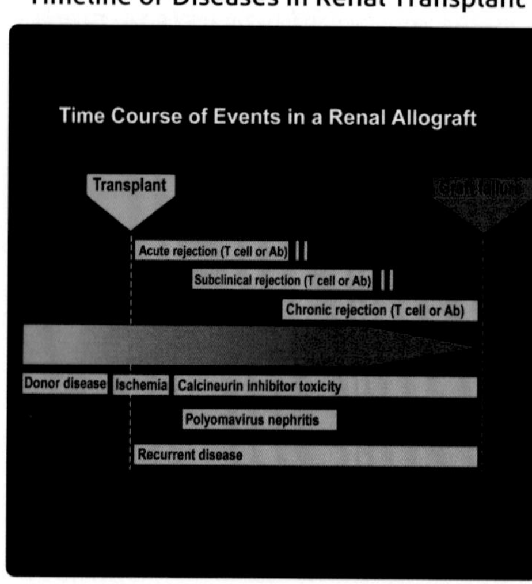

Mechanisms of Acute Rejection

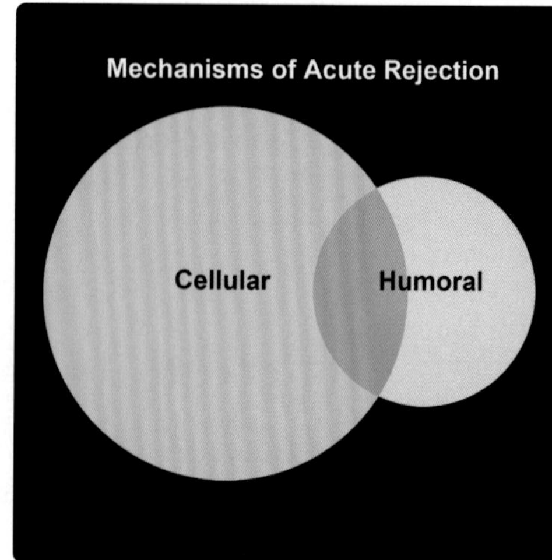

- Graft half-life = 10 years
- 1-year graft survival = 89%
- Living unrelated
  - Graft half-life = 18 years
  - 1-year graft survival = 95%
- Older vs. younger donor
- Presensitization
- Delayed graft function
- Certain recipient diseases that recur
- Inadequate or over-immunosuppression

Current Drug Therapy

- Induction
  - Anti-T-cell antibody (Thymoglobulin, alemtuzumab)
  - Anti-CD25 antibody (basiliximab, daclizumab)
- Maintenance
  - Calcineurin inhibitors (cyclosporine, tacrolimus)
  - Corticosteroids (prednisone)
  - Antiproliferative agent (azathioprine, mycophenolate mofetil)
  - Alternatives
    - Inhibitors of mTOR (rapamycin, everolimus)
    - Steroid-free regimens
    - CTLA4-Ig based therapy (belatacept)
- Acute rejection treatment
  - Pulse steroids
  - Anti-T-cell antibody
  - Plasmapheresis
  - Intravenous immunoglobulin (IVIg)

BIOPSY PROCESSING

Sample

- 16-gauge needle better than 18-gauge for sample adequacy; no great complication rate
  - 47% of 18-gauge single cores are inadequate (< 7 glomeruli and 1 artery) vs. 24% for 16-gauge
- 2 cores needed for adequacy
  - Single core has ~ 90% sensitivity for acute rejection; 2 cores approach 99% sensitivity

Adequacy

- Minimal sample of 7 glomeruli, 1 artery (Banff)
- Adequate sample of 10 glomeruli, 2 arteries (Banff)
- Depends on disease to be identified
  - Some diagnoses can be made in medulla (antibody-mediated rejection, polyomavirus infection)

Routine Pathology Techniques

- Light microscopy (LM): Multiple levels (2-3 microns); stained with H&E, PAS, trichrome, and other stains
  - IHC for viruses, cell phenotype as needed
  - IHC for C4d on paraffin if no frozen tissue
- Immunofluorescence (IF) microscopy on frozen tissue: C4d, full panel if glomerular disease suspected
- Electron microscopy (EM), especially if glomerular disease or chronic antibody-mediated rejection suspected

EVALUATION OF BIOPSY

Careful Examination of All 4 Components

- Glomeruli, tubules, interstitium, and vessels
- Multiple levels important, since most processes are focal (e.g., endarteritis)

Assess and Report Extent of Changes

- Give number of glomeruli, arteries, cores
- Quantitate pathologic features (% affected)
  - Cortex (fibrosis, infiltrate)
  - Glomeruli (sclerosis, glomerulitis, glomerular basement membrane [GBM] duplication)
  - Tubules (atrophy, tubulitis)
  - Arteries (endarteritis, fibrinoid necrosis, intimal fibrosis)
- Compare with previous biopsy if any
- Report diagnostic findings according to current consensus definitions
  - Banff recommended and widely used
- Interpretation of findings needs to be made in conjunction with clinical information

SPECIAL CONSIDERATIONS IN TRANSPLANT BIOPSIES

Important Clinical Information

- Donor source
- Time post transplant
- Whether kidney had good initial function
- Drug therapy
- Original disease
- Renal function
- Anti-donor HLA antibodies

Multiple Diseases May Be Present

- Rejection, drug toxicity, viral infection, donor disease

Important to Compare With Previous Biopsies

- Progression or resolution of process
- Late samples may be nondiagnostic of cause

NEW APPROACHES

Insights Emerging from Research Studies May Have Future Application

- Gene expression in tissue, blood, and urine
- Proteomics urine, blood, tissue
- Systems analysis of pathologic data ("pathomics")
  - Morphometry
  - Active pathways (e.g., phosphorylation of signaling molecules)

Expected Added Value

- Assessment of drug effects
- Measurement of activity
- Assessment of pathways involved in tissue injury

PROTOCOL BIOPSIES (SURVEILLANCE BIOPSIES)

Definition

- Biopsies taken according to predetermined schedule
  - Not for abnormal renal function

Purpose

- Used to monitor status of graft in high-risk patients
  - Some use surveillance biopsies in routine care

- Common in clinical trials to assess efficacy and toxicity
- Provides insights into mechanisms and prevalence of graft pathology

Value

- Identification of subclinical graft pathology
- Trace evolution of chronic progressive diseases
- Validation of tolerance

BANFF CLASSIFICATION

Background

- Classification currently based on LM, IF, or immunohistochemistry, and in some instances, EM
  - Diagnostic categories defined by semiquantitative scores
  - Opportunity to add other modalities, e.g., gene expression
- Refinement occurs through biannual open meetings to reach consensus on additions/changes based on published, confirmed evidence
- Widely used in drug trials
- Adequacy is 10 glomeruli and 2 arteries and should be noted

Banff Categories (2014)

- **1: Normal**
- **2: Antibody-mediated rejection**
  - Hyperacute rejection
  - Acute/active antibody-mediated rejection (all 3 features must be present for diagnosis)
    - Histologic evidence of acute tissue injury, including one or more of the following:
      - Microvascular inflammation (g > 0 or ptc > 0)
      - Intimal or transmural arteritis (v > 0)
      - Acute TMA, in absence of any other cause
      - Acute tubular injury in absence of any other apparent cause
    - Evidence of current/recent antibody interaction with vascular endothelium, including at least 1 of the following
      - Linear C4d staining in peritubular capillaries (C4d2 or C4d3 by IF on frozen sections, or C4d>0 by IHC on paraffin sections)
      - At least moderate microvascular inflammation (g + ptc ≥ 2), unless T-cell-mediated rejection present then g > 1 required
      - Increased expression of gene transcripts in biopsy tissue indicative of endothelial injury, if thoroughly validated
    - Serologic evidence of donor-specific antibodies (DSAs) (HLA or other antigens)
  - Chronic, active antibody-mediated rejection (all 3 features must be present for diagnosis)
    - Morphologic evidence of chronic tissue injury, including 1 or more of the following
      - Transplant glomerulopathy (TG) (cg > 0), if no evidence of chronic thrombotic microangiopathy
      - Severe peritubular capillary basement membrane multilayering (requires EM)
      - Arterial intimal fibrosis of new onset, excluding other causes
    - Often manifested by mononuclear cells in PTC (capillaritis) &/or glomeruli (transplant glomerulitis)
    - Evidence of current/recent antibody interaction with vascular endothelium, including at least 1 of the following
      - Linear C4d staining in peritubular capillaries (C4d2 or C4d3 by IF on frozen sections or C4d > 0 by IHC on paraffin sections)
      - At least moderate microvascular inflammation (g + ptc ≥ 2); unless T-cell-mediated rejection present, then g > 1 required
      - Increased expression of gene transcripts in biopsy tissue indicative of endothelial injury, if thoroughly validated
    - Serologic evidence of donor-specific antibodies (DSAs) (HLA or other antigens)
  - C4d deposition without evidence of rejection (all 3 features must be present for diagnosis)
    - Linear C4d staining in peritubular capillaries (C4d2 or C4d3 by IF on frozen sections or C4d > 0 by IHC on paraffin sections)
    - g = 0, ptc = 0, cg = 0 (by LM and by EM if available), v = 0; no TMA, no PTC basement membrane multilayering, no acute tubular injury
    - No acute cell-mediated rejection (Banff 97 type 1A or greater) or borderline changes
- **3: Borderline or suspicious for acute cellular rejection**
  - Defined by t > 0 and i1 or t1 and i > 0
- **4: T-cell-mediated rejection**
  - Requires > i1 and ≥ t2 or > v0; C4d negative for pure T-cell-mediated rejection
  - Acute T-cell-mediated rejection
    - IA: Interstitial inflammation (> 25% of unscarred cortex) and foci of moderate tubulitis (5-10 mononuclear cells per tubular cross section)
    - IB: Interstitial inflammation (> 25% of unscarred cortex) and foci of severe tubulitis (> 10 mononuclear cells per tubular cross section)
    - IIA: Mild to moderate intimal arteritis (< 25% of luminal area) (v1)
    - IIB: Severe intimal arteritis (> 25% of luminal area) (v2)
    - III: Transmural arteritis &/or fibrinoid necrosis of medial smooth muscle (v3)
  - Chronic active T-cell-mediated rejection
    - Chronic allograft arteriopathy (arterial intimal fibrosis with mononuclear cell infiltration in fibrosis, formation of neo-intima)
- **5: Interstitial fibrosis and tubular atrophy, no evidence of any specific etiology**
  - Use only when unknown etiology of IF/TA
  - Formerly known as chronic allograft nephropathy (CAN)
- **6: Other**
  - Changes considered not due to rejection
    - Calcineurin inhibitor toxicity, polyomavirus infection, and others

Caveats

- Biopsies may meet criteria for 2 or more diagnoses
- Detailed criteria established only for rejection categories
- Reproducibility of certain categories and features is limited

BANFF SCORING CATEGORIES

Interstitial Inflammation (i)

- Mononuclear inflammation in nonfibrotic areas; excludes subcapsular cortex and perivascular infiltrates
  - i0: < 10% of nonfibrotic cortex
  - i1: 10-25%
  - i2: 26-50%
  - i3: > 50%
- Do not include fibrotic areas in denominator

Tubulitis (t)

- Mononuclear cells in tubules; for longitudinal sections count per 10 tubular epithelial nuclei
  - t0: No mononuclear cells in tubules
  - t1: Foci with 1-4 cells/tubular cross section
  - t2: Foci with 5-10 cells/tubular cross section
  - t3: Foci with > 10 cells/tubular cross section
- Need at least 2 foci of tubulitis to be present

Vascular Inflammation (v)

- Mononuclear cells in intima or media of arteries or medial necrosis
  - v0: No arteritis
  - v1: Intimal arteritis in < 25% of lumen (minimum = 1 cell, 1 artery)
  - v2: Intimal arteritis in ≥ 25% of lumen in ≥ 1 artery
  - v3: Transmural arteritis &/or medial smooth muscle necrosis (fibrinoid necrosis)

Glomerulitis (g)

- % of glomeruli with increased mononuclear cells in capillaries
  - g0: No glomerulitis
  - g1: < 25% of glomeruli (mostly segmental)
  - g2: 25-75% of glomeruli (segmental to global)
  - g3: > 75% of glomeruli (mostly global)

Interstitial Fibrosis (ci)

- % of cortex with fibrosis
  - ci0: ≤ 5%
  - ci1: 6-25%
  - ci2: 26-50%
  - ci3: > 50%

Tubular Atrophy (ct)

- % of cortex with atrophic tubules
  - ct0: 0%
  - ct1: ≤ 25%
  - ct2: 26-50%
  - ct3: > 50%

Arterial Fibrointimal Thickening (cv)

- % of narrowing of lumen of most severely affected artery
  - cv0: 0%
  - cv1: ≤ 25%
  - cv2: 26-50%
  - cv3: > 50%
- Note if lesions characteristic of chronic cellular rejection are present (inflammatory cells in intima, foam cells, lack of fibroelastosis in intima)

Transplant Glomerulopathy (cg)

- % of glomerular capillary loops with duplication of GBM in most affected nonsclerotic glomerulus by LM
  - cg0: No GBM double contours by LM or EM
  - cg1: ≤ 25% GBM double contours by LM or EM
    - cg1a: Duplication seen by EM only, in at least 3 glomerular capillaries
    - cg1b: 1 or more glomerular capillaries with GBM double contours by LM
  - cg2: 26-50%
  - cg3: > 50%

Mesangial Matrix Increase (mm)

- % of glomeruli with mesangial increase, at least moderate increase in at least 2 glomerular lobules
  - mm0: 0%
  - mm1: ≤ 25%
  - mm2: 26-50%
  - mm3: > 50%

Arteriolar Hyalinosis (ah)

- Circumferential or noncircumferential (focal) hyaline
  - ah0: No arterioles with hyaline
  - ah1: 1 arteriole with noncircumferential hyaline
  - ah2: ≥ 1 arteriole with noncircumferential hyaline
  - ah3: ≥ 1 arteriole with circumferential hyaline
- Note if peripheral nodules are present

Peritubular Capillary Inflammation (ptc)

- % of cortical PTC with neutrophils or mononuclear cells
  - ptc0: < 10% PTC with > 2 cells/PTC
  - ptc1: > 10% with 3-4 cells/PTC
  - ptc2: > 10% with 5-10 cells/PTC
  - ptc3: > 10% with > 10 cells/PTC
- Note whether only mononuclear cells, < 50% neutrophils, or > 50% neutrophils

C4d Score in PTC (C4d)

- % of PTC with C4d deposition scored in at least 5 HPF
  - C4d0: 0%
  - C4d1: 1-9%
  - C4d2: 10-50%
  - C4d3: > 50%
- Note technique used (frozen vs. paraffin)

Total Inflammation (ti)

- Includes all cortical inflammation, even subcapsular, perivascular, nodular, and fibrotic areas
  - ti0: < 10% of cortex
  - ti1: 10-25%
  - ti2: 26-50%
  - ti3: > 50%

SELECTED REFERENCES

1. Haas M et al: Banff 2013 meeting report: inclusion of C4d-negative antibody-mediated rejection and antibody-associated arterial lesions. Am J Transplant. 14(2):272-83, 2014
2. Mengel M et al: Banff 2011 Meeting report: new concepts in antibody-mediated rejection. Am J Transplant. 12(3):563-70, 2012
3. Williams WW et al: Clinical role of the renal transplant biopsy. Nat Rev Nephrol. 8(2):110-21, 2012
4. Racusen LC et al: The Banff 97 working classification of renal allograft pathology. Kidney Int. 55(2):713-23, 1999

Evaluation of the Donor Kidney

KEY FACTS

CLINICAL ISSUES

- Suitability of ECD kidney
  - Judgment of clinician based on pathological report and patient
  - No absolute cutoff established for any pathologic criteria
- Baseline for clinical trials

MICROSCOPIC

- Sample adequacy
  - ≥ 25 glomeruli including deep cortex
  - ≥ 2 arteries should be present
- > 20% globally sclerotic glomeruli often cited
  - Higher incidence of DGF
  - Higher Cr at 3-24 months
  - Variable effect on graft survival
  - No effect if donor Cr clearance is > 80 mL/min
- Moderate arteriosclerosis (> 25% luminal narrowing)
  - Predictor of worse graft outcome (graft loss, DGF, higher Cr)
- Composite histologic can predict graft function at 1-3 years
  - Maryland Aggregate Pathology Index
  - French Clinicopathologic Composite Score
- Many donor diseases have full recovery
  - IgA nephropathy, membranous glomerulonephritis, acute poststreptococcal glomerulonephritis, lupus nephritis, thrombotic microangiopathy, preeclampsia, hepatorenal syndrome

DIAGNOSTIC CHECKLIST

- Difficulties in interpretation of frozen sections
  - Interstitium looks edematous, resembles fibrosis
  - Glomeruli appear hypercellular
  - Difficult to appreciate acute tubular injury
- Globally sclerotic glomeruli overestimated with wedge biopsies
- Risk of overestimating renal pathology and discarding potentially beneficial donor kidneys

(Left) *This deceased donor kidney biopsy appears edematous and the glomeruli appear hypercellular, common artifacts of frozen sections. The percentage of globally sclerotic glomeruli ➔ is routinely reported.* **(Right)** *After routine permanent processing, the kidney shows only focal fine interstitial edema and normal glomeruli.*

Global Glomerulosclerosis (Donor Biopsy)

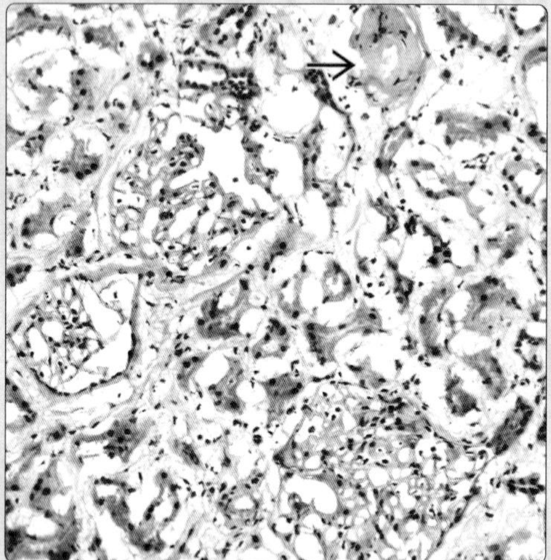

Permanent Section of Donor Kidney

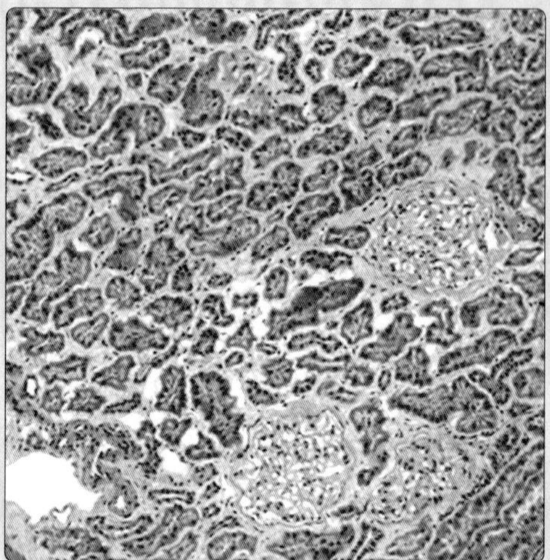

(Left) *Light microscopy shows glomerular thrombi ➔ in a donor biopsy specimen from a 52-year-old woman who died from a subarachnoid hemorrhage. Thrombi are common in donors who died from stroke or head injury. Scattered thrombi do not contraindicate use of the kidney.* **(Right)** *Time zero (implantation) biopsy from a living donor shows moderate arteriosclerosis ➔.*

Glomerular Thrombi

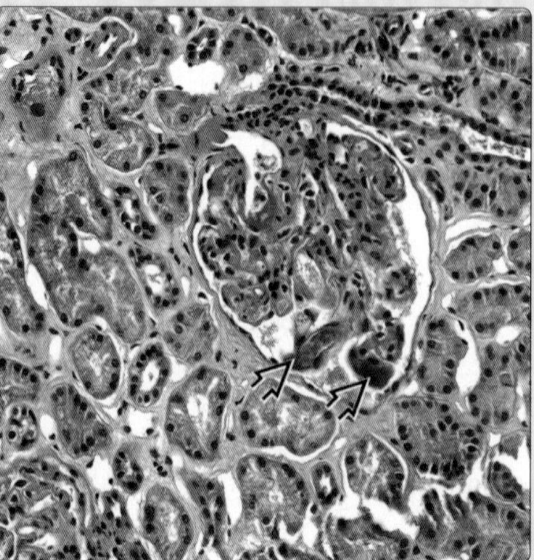

Donor Arteriosclerosis

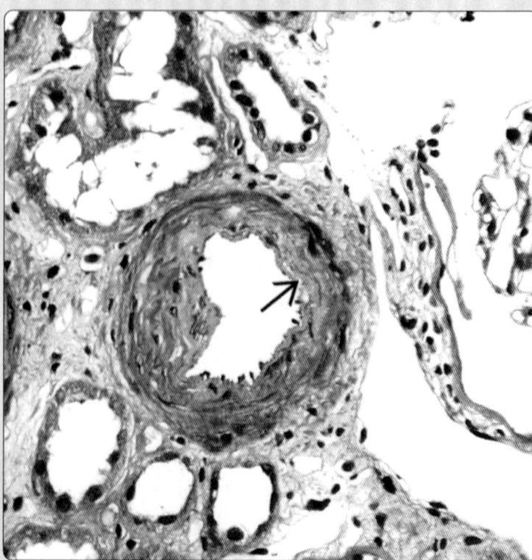

TERMINOLOGY

Definitions

- Donor biopsy
  - Biopsy performed prior to implantation
    - Evaluated by frozen section
  - Used to determine suitability of kidney for transplantation
  - Performed on deceased donor kidneys
- Implantation biopsy, zero-hour biopsy
  - Biopsy performed immediately before or after implantation
    - Evaluated on permanent sections
  - Used in clinical trials to determine baseline histologic features of donor kidney or subclinical renal disease
  - May be performed on either deceased or living donor kidneys
- Expanded criteria donor (ECD)
  - Donor age ≥ 60 years
  - Donor age 50-59 years and at least 2 of the following
    - Death from cerebrovascular accident
    - Hypertension
    - Serum creatinine (Cr) > 1.5 mg/dL
  - Increased risk of graft failure (relative hazard ratio 1.70) and delayed graft function compared to standard-criteria donor
    - Survival benefit for recipients of ECD kidneys compared to continued dialysis
- Donation after cardiac death (DCD)
  - Donors do not meet criteria for brain death
  - Absence of cardiac function prior to organ procurement

CLINICAL ISSUES

Purpose of Donor Biopsy

- Suitability of ECD kidney
  - ~ 40% of ECD kidneys discarded
- Suspected donor renal disease
- Evaluation of neoplasm

Kidney Acceptance Criteria

- Judgment of clinician based on pathological report and status of donor and recipient
  - Older or highly sensitized recipient may benefit from marginal kidney
  - No absolute cut-off established for any pathologic criteria
    - Risk of overestimating damage and discarding useful kidneys
  - Can do double transplant in setting of pediatric to adult or ECD kidney

Purpose of Implantation Biopsy

- Evaluation of donor disease for comparison to later post-transplant pathologic features
- Baseline for clinical trials
- Evidence of antibody-mediated injury in presensitized recipient

Interobserver Variability

- Significant interobserver variability in scoring ECD biopsies
  - In one study, histologic scoring by experienced renal pathologist correlated with graft outcome at 1 year, while on-call pathologist scoring did not

MICROSCOPIC

Evaluation of Donor Biopsy on Frozen Section

- Sample adequacy
  - On donor biopsy, ≥ 25 glomeruli should be present, including from deep cortex
  - ≥ 2 arteries should be present
- Some degree of mild chronic changes present in many time-zero or donor kidney biopsies
- Chronic changes usually mild in living donors and increase with donor age
  - Histologic features of nephrosclerosis present in older healthy living donors despite normal donor function
- Percentage of globally sclerotic glomeruli
  - If > 20% globally sclerotic glomeruli, higher incidence of delayed graft function (DGF) requiring transient dialysis, higher Cr at 3-24 months, variable effect on graft survival
  - > 20% global sclerosis has minimal effect on 1-year graft survival and only if donor Cr clearance is ≤ 80 mL/min (83% vs. 79%)
  - No universally accepted cutoff
  - Sclerotic glomeruli predominate in subcapsular cortex in arteriosclerosis
    - Overestimated in wedge biopsies
  - Strong correlation with donor age
- Arteriosclerosis
  - Moderate arteriosclerosis (> 25% luminal narrowing)
    - Predictor of worse graft outcome (graft loss, DGF, higher Cr)
- Interstitial fibrosis and tubular atrophy
  - Not consistently predictive
- Thrombi in glomeruli, arteries
  - Head trauma in donor can precipitate thrombotic microangiopathy
  - Even with glomerular thrombi, good outcome possible
    - Thrombi usually dissolve by intact fibrinolytic system
  - Glomerular thrombi may be associated with DGF
    - Especially if > 50% of glomeruli have thrombi
  - Cholesterol emboli may be contraindication

Maryland Aggregate Pathology Index (MAPI)

- Aggregate score predictive of graft survival (each given points if present)
  - Periglomerular fibrosis (4 points)
  - Arteriolar hyalinosis (4 points)
  - Scar (focus of scar or atrophy in > 10 tubules) (3 points)
  - Global glomerulosclerosis ≥ 15% (4 points)
  - Wall-to-lumen ratio of interlobular arteries ≥ 0.5 (2 points)
- MAPI = sum of points
- Graft survival at 3 years (validation study)
  - Low MAPI (0-7): 83-84%
  - Intermediate MAPI (8-11): 33-56%
  - High MAPI (12-15): 33-50%
  - Greater predictive value than DGF, cold ischemia, ECD, or donor Cr > 1.5

Classification of Donors

Donor Type	Definition
Expanded criteria donor (ECD)	Donor is either (1) ≥ age 60 at time of death; or (2) age 50-59 years and has 2 of the 3 following criteria: (1) Cerebrovascular accident as cause of death, (2) history of hypertension, or (3) serum creatinine > 1.5 mg/dL
Standard criteria donor (SCD)	Donor who does not fulfill criteria of ECD
Donation after brain death (DBD)	Donor who has primarily brain death with maintained cardiac and respiratory circulation by medical measures; DBD may be SCD or ECD
Donation after cardiac death (DCD)	Patients who do not meet criteria for brain death but had cessation of cardiac function before organ procurement

French Clinicopathologic Composite Score

- Clinical and histopathologic scores combined predicts graft GFR at 1 year
  - Glomerulosclerosis > 10% (absent/present)
  - Donor hypertension &/or donor serum creatinine ≥ 150 mmol/L (~ 1.7 mg/dL) (absent/present)
  - Either present increases odds of eGFR at 1 year < 25mL/min/1.73m^2 by 5x; both present by 27x

Donor Diseases With Documented Full Recovery

- IgA nephropathy
  - IgA present in ~ 10% of donor biopsies
- Membranous glomerulonephritis
- Lupus nephritis
- Acute poststreptococcal infection glomerulonephritis
- Membranoproliferative glomerulonephritis
- Thrombotic microangiopathy
- Preeclampsia
- Hepatorenal syndrome

Implantation Biopsy

- Process and score same as indication transplant biopsies on paraffin process material
- C4d in presensitized recipient
- Immunofluorescence and EM if considering donor glomerular disease
  - Routine EM processing required to evaluate for thin glomerular basement membrane nephropathy (in living donor with hematuria)

ANCILLARY TESTS

Molecular Evaluation of Donor Biopsies

- Molecular studies have been proposed to evaluate suitability of donor kidney
- Detect changes associated with tissue injury and repair, such as
  - Inflammation-associated transcripts
  - Complement gene expression
- Differences detected between living donor and deceased donor kidneys
- Gene expression changes may be more sensitive than current clinical and histologic markers with respect to acute tissue injury

DIAGNOSTIC CHECKLIST

Pathologic Interpretation Pearls

- Sclerotic glomeruli overestimated in wedge biopsies
- Difficulties in interpretation of frozen sections
  - Interstitium looks edematous, resembles fibrosis
  - Glomeruli appear hypercellular
  - Difficult to appreciate acute tubular injury
  - Red cell casts lyse on freezing

REPORTING

Donor Biopsy (Frozen or Permanent)

- Site/type of biopsy
  - Wedge or needle biopsy
  - Presence of capsule, cortex, medulla
- Number of glomeruli and arteries
- Number of globally sclerotic glomeruli
- Intimal fibrosis and arteriolar hyalinosis
- Percentage interstitial fibrosis/tubular atrophy
- Thrombi in glomeruli or vessels
- Any other notable features

Implantation Biopsy

- Standard scoring of transplant biopsies (Banff)

SELECTED REFERENCES

1. Azancot MA et al: The reproducibility and predictive value on outcome of renal biopsies from expanded criteria donors. Kidney Int. 85(5):1161-8, 2014
2. Haas M: Donor kidney biopsies: pathology matters, and so does the pathologist. Kidney Int. 85(5):1016-9, 2014
3. Philosophe B et al: Validation of the Maryland Aggregate Pathology Index (MAPI), a pre-implantation scoring system that predicts graft outcome. Clin Transplant. 28(8):897-905, 2014
4. Rule AD et al: The association between age and nephrosclerosis on renal biopsy among healthy adults. Ann Intern Med. 152(9):561-7, 2010
5. Naesens M et al: Expression of complement components differs between kidney allografts from living and deceased donors. J Am Soc Nephrol. 20(8):1839-51, 2009
6. Nickeleit V: Pathology: donor biopsy evaluation at time of renal grafting. Nat Rev Nephrol. 5(5):249-51, 2009
7. Rao PS et al: The alphabet soup of kidney transplantation: SCD, DCD, ECD--fundamentals for the practicing nephrologist. Clin J Am Soc Nephrol. 4(11):1827-31, 2009
8. Anglicheau D et al: A simple clinico-histopathological composite scoring system is highly predictive of graft outcomes in marginal donors. Am J Transplant. 8(11):2325-34, 2008
9. Kayler LK et al: Correlation of histologic findings on preimplant biopsy with kidney graft survival. Transpl Int. 21(9):892-8, 2008
10. Mueller TF et al: The transcriptome of the implant biopsy identifies donor kidneys at increased risk of delayed graft function. Am J Transplant. 8(1):78-85, 2008
11. Munivenkatappa RB et al: The Maryland aggregate pathology index: a deceased donor kidney biopsy scoring system for predicting graft failure. Am J Transplant. 8(11):2316-24, 2008
12. El-Husseini A et al: Can donor implantation renal biopsy predict long-term renal allograft outcome?. Am J Nephrol. 27(2):144-51, 2007
13. Mohamed N and Cornell LD: Donor Kidney Evaluation. Surgical Pathology Clinics: Pathology of the Medical Kidney, Volume 7, Issue 3, September 2014, Pages 357–365

Arteriolar Hyalinosis on Donor Biopsy

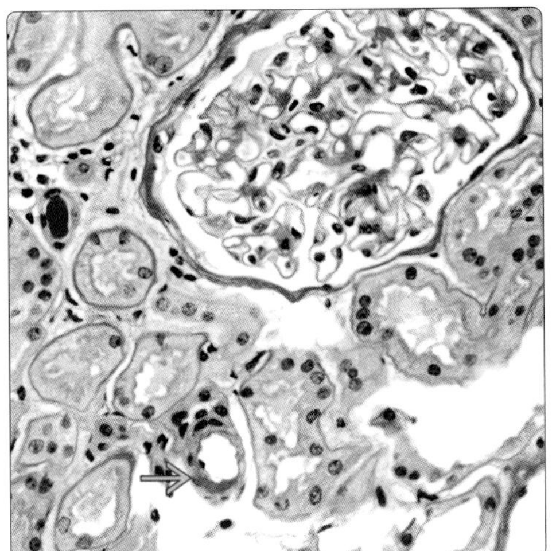

Donor Arteriolar Hyalinosis

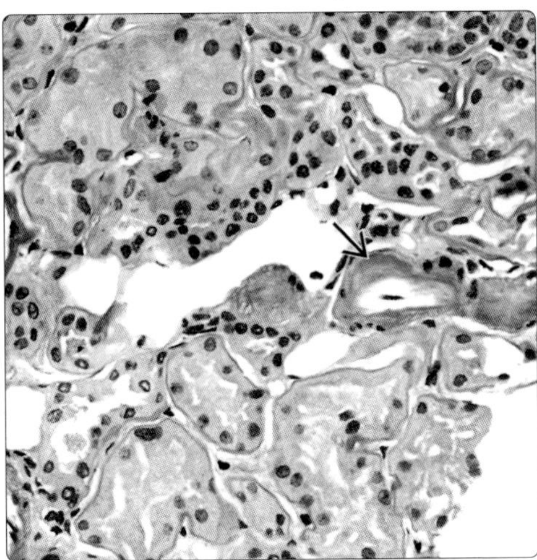

(Left) *Periodic acid-Schiff on a permanent section shows mild intimal arteriolar hyalinosis ⇨, a feature difficult to identify on frozen section. A glomerulus appears normal on the permanent section.* **(Right)** *Periodic acid-Schiff on the corresponding permanent section shows intimal arteriolar hyalinosis ➡, a feature difficult to identify on a frozen section. This feature was seen in several arterioles on the permanent section.*

Myoglobin Cast

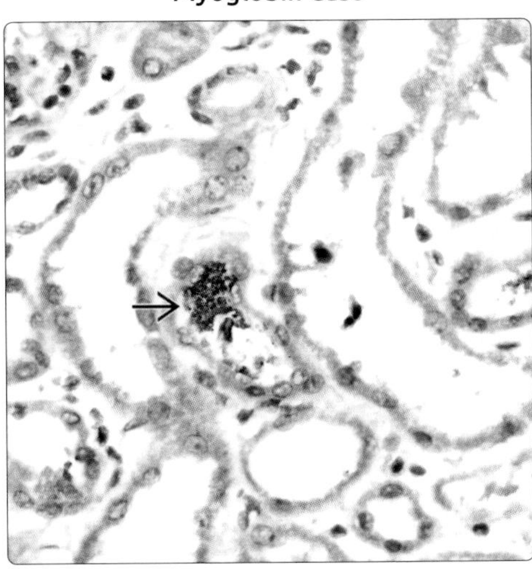

Diabetic Glomerulosclerosis (Permanent Section)

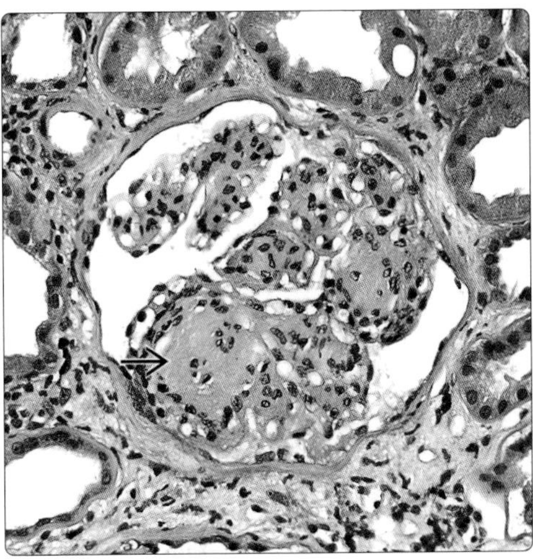

(Left) *The donor of this kidney died from trauma and the kidney had severe tubular injury, with granular eosinophilic casts that stained for myoglobin ➡.* **(Right)** *Biopsy taken 17 days after transplant shows prominent nodular diabetic glomerulopathy ➡. The donor and the recipient were diabetic. The nodules were not apparent in a donor frozen section, even in retrospect. The graft was eventually lost. Donation to a nondiabetic recipient might have been more salutary.*

Normal Glomeruli on Frozen Section

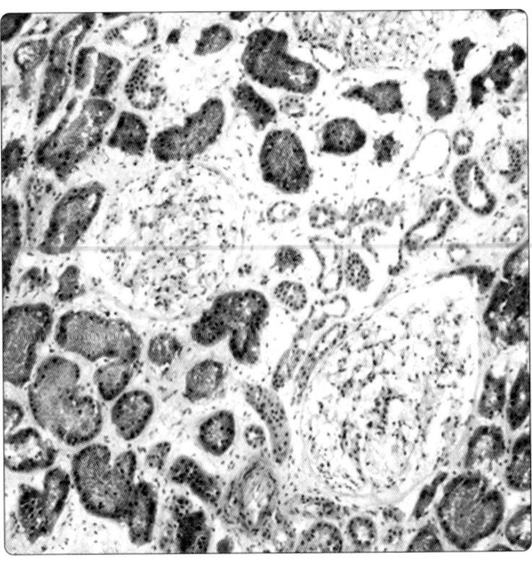

Arteriolar Hyalinosis in Donor Biopsy

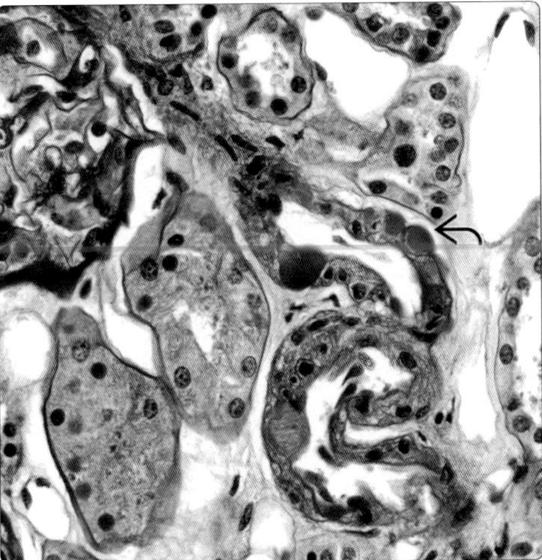

(Left) *Glomeruli often normally appear hypercellular on frozen sections, as illustrated in this donor kidney biopsy; glomeruli were not hypercellular on permanent sections. The interstitium appears edematous.* **(Right)** *Nodular peripheral arteriolar hyalinosis ↩ in a donor biopsy looks exactly like the hyalinosis commonly found in chronic calcineurin inhibitor (CNI) toxicity and once thought to be specific for CNI. This feature, however, is uncommonly seen in the absence of CNI administration.*

Acute T-Cell-Mediated Rejection

KEY FACTS

TERMINOLOGY

- Acute immunologic reaction to renal alloantigens mediated by T cells directed at MHC or non-MHC donor alloantigens

ETIOLOGY/PATHOGENESIS

- Alloreactive T cells against donor antigens expressed on donor cells or on recipient antigen presenting cells
- Secondary participants, macrophages, granulocytes, chemokines, cytokines

CLINICAL ISSUES

- Acute renal failure
- 5-10% in 1st year post transplant in conventional transplants
- Oliguria or decreased urine output or subclinical
- ACR type I and borderline/suspicious for ACR cases are usually responsive to pulse steroid therapy
- ACR type II usually resistant to pulse steroid therapy; additional treatment may consist of anti-T-cell agent

MICROSCOPIC

- Mixed mononuclear interstitial inflammation and tubulitis (type I TCMR)
- Mononuclear cell accumulation under endothelium of arteries (type II TCMR)
- Fibrinoid necrosis of arteries (type III TCMR)
- Interstitial edema and sometimes hemorrhage
- Glomerular involvement is usually mild
- C4d is negative in pure TCMR, but positive if combined with antibody-mediated rejection

TOP DIFFERENTIAL DIAGNOSES

- Acute antibody-mediated rejection
- BK polyomavirus interstitial nephritis
- Pyelonephritis
- Acute allergic tubulointerstitial nephritis
- Post-transplant lymphoproliferative disorder

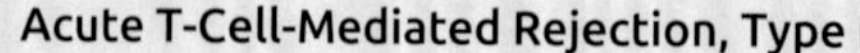

Acute T-Cell-Mediated Rejection, Type I

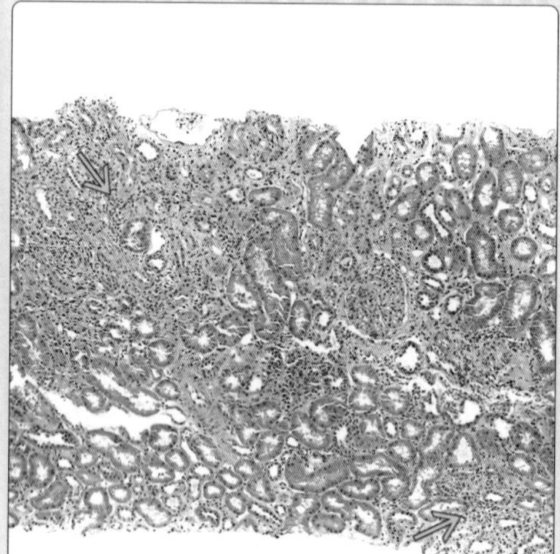

Tubulitis in TCMR

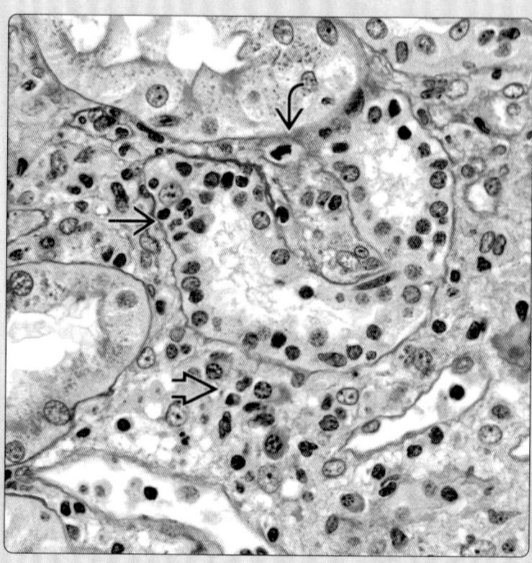

(Left) *This biopsy, taken 3 weeks post transplant for a rising Cr (2.3), shows a patchy interstitial mononuclear infiltrate* ⇨ *and edema typical of acute TCMR. Tubulitis was also present. The patchy nature of the infiltrate makes it important to take 2 cores for diagnostic sensitivity.* **(Right)** *Tubulitis* → *and interstitial mononuclear inflammation* ⇨ *are the defining features of type I acute cellular rejection. The infiltrating cells appear activated, and mitotic figures are present* ↷.

Endothelialitis

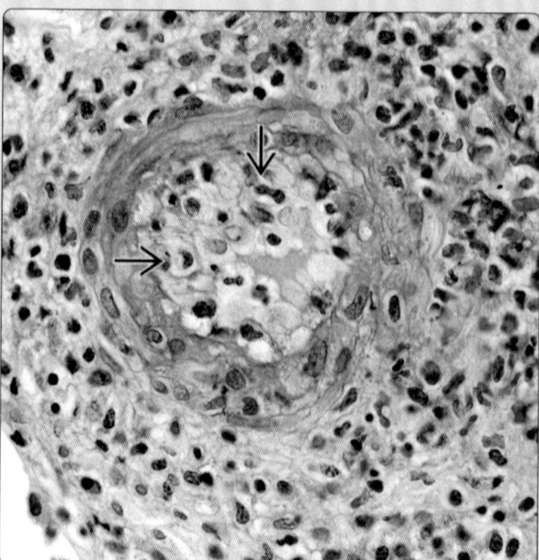

T Cells in ACR

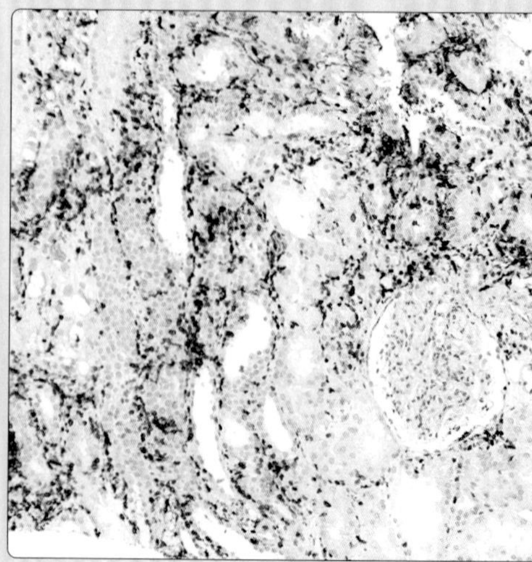

(Left) *Endothelialitis (endarteritis) in a renal transplant biopsy, the defining feature of type II TCMR, is shown. Many mononuclear cells* → *are in the intima. The cells are primarily T cells and monocytes.* **(Right)** *An immunohistochemical stain for CD3 shows numerous infiltrating T cells, typical of TCMR. A C4d stain was also positive, indicative of an additional component of acute AMR.*

TERMINOLOGY

Abbreviations

- Acute T-cell-mediated rejection (TCMR)

Synonyms

- Acute cellular rejection (ACR)

Definitions

- Acute immunologic reaction to renal alloantigens mediated by T cells
  - Type I: Tubulointerstitial
  - Type II: Endarteritis
  - Type III: Fibrinoid arterial necrosis or transmural inflammation of arteries

ETIOLOGY/PATHOGENESIS

T-Cell-Mediated Rejection

- Alloreactive T cells against donor antigens
  - MHC (HLA) or non-MHC
- Target varies and includes capillary and arterial endothelium, tubules, and glomeruli
- Ongoing tubulointerstitial inflammation commonly present in follow-up biopsies 1-2 months after TCMR episode
  - Argues that while TCMR may be of acute onset, inflammation may persist and give chronic cellular rejection phenotype

CLINICAL ISSUES

Epidemiology

- Incidence
  - 5-10% in 1st year post transplant in conventional transplants
    - Type I: ~ 65% of TCMR cases
    - Type II: ~ 30%
    - Type III: < 5%

Presentation

- Acute renal failure
- Oliguria or decreased urine output
- Graft tenderness (severe cases)
- May also be seen on protocol (surveillance) biopsies with normal renal function

Treatment

- Drugs
  - Type I and cases borderline/suspicious for TCMR are usually responsive to pulse steroid therapy
  - Type II usually resistant to pulse steroid therapy; additional treatment may consist of anti-T-cell agent
  - Type III resistant to current therapies

Prognosis

- 1-year graft survival
  - Type I: ~ 95%
  - Type II: ~ 75%
  - Type III: ~ 15%

MICROSCOPIC

Histologic Features

- Glomeruli
  - Usually spared
  - Occasional cases show glomerulitis with mononuclear cells in glomerular capillaries
    - Glomerulitis more commonly found in antibody-mediated rejection (AMR), where macrophages predominate
    - Not currently included as criterion for TCMR
  - Acute allograft glomerulopathy in < 5%
    - Markedly swollen endothelial cells occluding capillary lumen
    - Mesangiolysis with PAS-positive webs
    - When present, usually associated with type II TCMR
- Interstitium
  - Mononuclear cell inflammation in interstitium
    - Diagnosis of rejection by Banff criteria requires > 25% of nonscarred cortex to have mononuclear infiltrate
    - Lesser degrees of inflammation considered "suspicious" or "borderline" for rejection
    - Cells mostly CD4(+) and CD8(+) T cells and CD68(+) macrophages
  - Eosinophils, plasma cells, and a few neutrophils may also be present in infiltrate
    - Plasma cell-rich rejection has worse prognosis
    - Some studies show that eosinophils portend worse outcome
  - Interstitial edema
  - Hemorrhage in more severe cases
- Tubules
  - T cells and macrophages within tubule ("tubulitis")
    - Only nonatrophic tubules are evaluated by Banff criteria
  - Tubular cell injury (loss of brush border, apoptosis)
  - Tubular basement membranes sometimes rupture with severe tubulitis
    - May form granulomas
- Arteries
  - Mononuclear inflammatory cells beneath endothelium in arteries ("endarteritis" or "endothelialitis")
    - CD3(+) T cells and CD68(+) monocytes/macrophages
    - Focal process, affecting ~ 25% of cross sections of arteries and ~ 12% of arterioles
    - Larger vessels affected more than arterioles
    - Endothelialitis in arterioles sometimes seen in conjunction with endothelialitis in arteries; has same significance
  - Marginated mononuclear cells along endothelial surface
    - Does not count for endarteritis, but associated with it
  - Venulitis found in some cases of TCMR, but not prognostically significant
  - Endothelium may develop signs of "activation," with basophilic cytoplasm, enlarged active nuclei
  - Transmural inflammation in more severe cases
    - Fibrinoid necrosis also occasionally seen in severe cases, but more commonly associated with antibody-mediated rejection

ANCILLARY TESTS

Immunofluorescence

- Generally little or no immunoglobulin or C3 deposition in glomeruli or interstitium
  - Fibrin diffusely present in edematous interstitium
- C4d negative in pure T-cell-mediated rejection
- TCMR cases with C4d deposition have superimposed acute &/or chronic AMR

Electron Microscopy

- Not generally needed for diagnosis
- Glomeruli in acute allograft glomerulopathy show marked endothelial reaction (swollen cytoplasm, loss of fenestrations)

DIFFERENTIAL DIAGNOSIS

BK Polyomavirus Interstitial Nephritis

- Plasma cells in infiltrate
- Intranuclear inclusions in tubular epithelial cells
- Inflammation primarily in sites with viral infection (IHC)

Pyelonephritis

- Neutrophilic casts and abscesses
- Positive urine culture for bacterial infection

"Isolated Endothelialitis"

- Variant of TCMR
- Recent study shows that endothelialitis with mild or no interstitial inflammation/tubulitis behaves as TCMR

Thrombotic Microangiopathy (TMA)

- Endothelialitis and luminal fibrin may be present
- Fragmented erythrocytes in intima favor TMA
- Thrombi with minimal endothelial inflammation and mucoid intimal thickening favor TMA

Acute Allergic Tubulointerstitial Nephritis

- May represent an allergic drug reaction
- Difficult or impossible to distinguish from tubulointerstitial acute cellular rejection (type I)

Obstruction

- Edema and collecting duct dilation may be present
- Usually not more than "borderline" infiltrates (< 25% of cortex)
- Dilated lymphatics, sometimes containing Tamm-Horsfall protein
- Can never rule out by morphology

Resolving/Partially Treated TCMR

- Disproportionately more severe tubulitis compared to interstitial inflammation
- Inflammation in areas of interstitial fibrosis

Acute Antibody-Mediated Rejection (Acute AMR)

- C4d deposition in peritubular capillaries, circulating anti-donor antibodies
- May be superimposed on acute TCMR

Peritubular Capillaritis

- Marginated mononuclear cells and a few neutrophils in peritubular capillaries
- Common finding on protocol biopsy in patients with donor-specific anti-HLA antibody
  - C4d stain usually negative (~ 90% of cases)
- Associated with later development of transplant glomerulopathy

Post-Transplant Lymphoproliferative Disorder (PTLD)

- Little edema and predominance of atypical B cells rather than T cells
  - Monoclonal B cell infiltrate most common
- Most cases are EBER positive

Atheromatous Embolism

- Endothelialitis and luminal fibrin may be present
- Unusual finding; thorough examination of tissue levels should reveal cholesterol clefts in arteries with inflammation

DIAGNOSTIC CHECKLIST

Pathologic Interpretation Pearls

- Multiple levels need to be examined to detect focal lesions, such as endarteritis, which are more specific for TCMR
- 1 biopsy core has false-negative rate of about 10%
- Biopsies may meet criteria for ACR and antibody-mediated rejection (C4d[+]), in which case outcome is dominated by latter

GRADING

Banff Grading of ACR

- Borderline/suspicious for acute TCMR
  - Interstitial inflammation in 10-25% of unscarred cortex and foci of mild tubulitis **or** < 10% interstitial inflammation and foci of moderate to severe tubulitis (t2 or t3)
- Tubulointerstitial TCMR (type I)
  - Banff type IA: Interstitial inflammation in > 25% of unscarred cortex and foci of moderate tubulitis (4-10 mononuclear cells per tubular cross section)
  - Banff type IB: Interstitial inflammation in > 25% of unscarred cortex and foci of severe tubulitis (> 10 mononuclear cells per tubular cross section)
- TCMR with endothelialitis (type II)
  - Banff type IIA: Mild to moderate endothelialitis
  - Banff type IIB: Severe endothelialitis
- TCMR with transmural arterial inflammation (type III)
  - Banff type III: Transmural arteritis, &/or arterial fibrinoid change and necrosis of medial smooth muscle

SELECTED REFERENCES

1. Sis B et al: Isolated endarteritis and kidney transplant survival: a multicenter collaborative study. J Am Soc Nephrol. ePub, 2014
2. El Ters M et al: Kidney allograft survival after acute rejection, the value of follow-up biopsies. Am J Transplant. 13(9):2334-41, 2013
3. Gago M et al: Kidney allograft inflammation and fibrosis, causes and consequences. Am J Transplant. 12(5):1199-207, 2012
4. Mannon RB et al: Inflammation in areas of tubular atrophy in kidney allograft biopsies: a potent predictor of allograft failure. Am J Transplant. 10(9):2066-73, 2010
5. Nickeleit V et al: Polyomavirus allograft nephropathy and concurrent acute rejection: a diagnostic and therapeutic challenge. Am J Transplant. 4(5):838-9, 2004

ACR With Increased Eosinophils

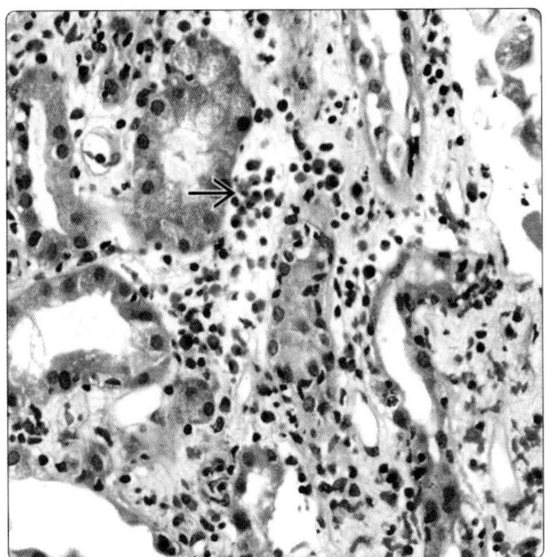

Tubulitis

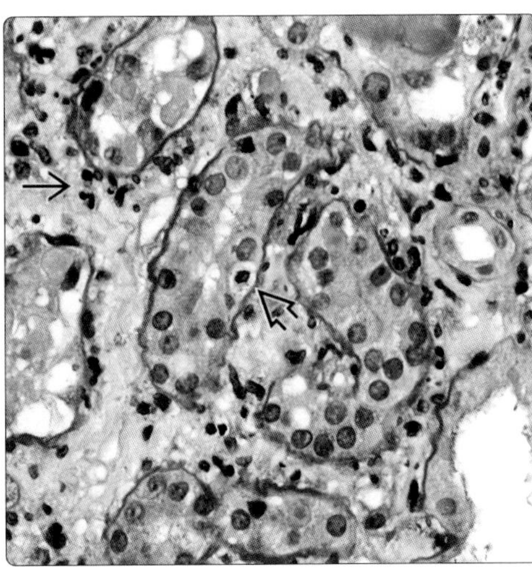

(Left) *Numerous eosinophils ➡ are seen in this case of TCMR. This finding can be part of TCMR and does not necessarily indicate an allergic drug reaction in the transplant.* **(Right)** *Mild tubulitis (t1 lesion) in TCMR type IA is shown. A mononuclear inflammatory cell ⇨ can be recognized by its dark nucleus and surrounding halo. Interstitial inflammation is also present ➡.*

Severe Tubulitis

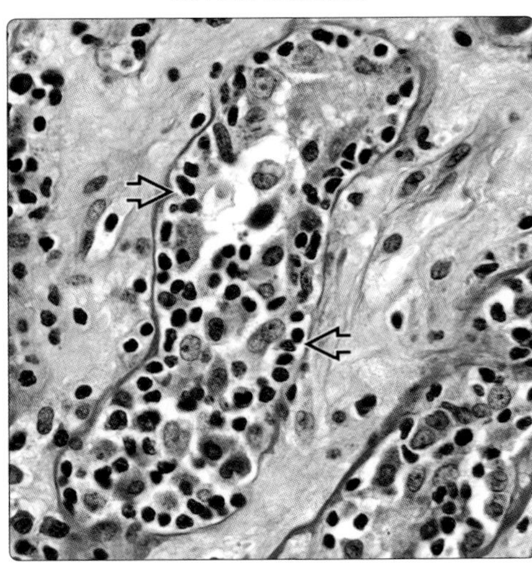

Tubulitis With Basement Membrane Rupture

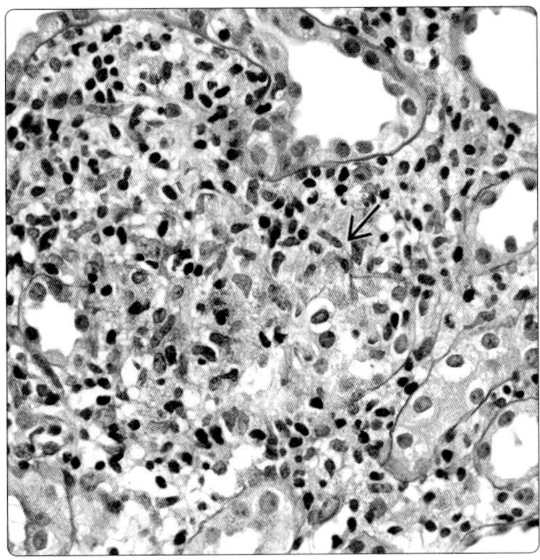

(Left) *Severe tubulitis (t3 lesion) in a case of TCMR type IB shows numerous mononuclear cells ⇨ within the tubule. The tubular epithelium is displaced from the tubular basement membrane. This is not uncommonly seen in grafts after withdrawal of immunosuppressive drugs.* **(Right)** *In tubulitis, tubular basement membrane rupture ➡ is associated with a poorer outcome. A granulomatous response to rupture may develop and should not be confused with an infection.*

Borderline/Suspicious Pattern

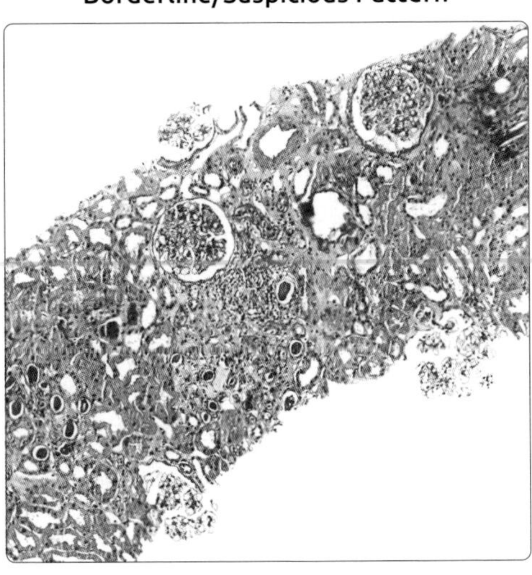

Destructive Tubulitis

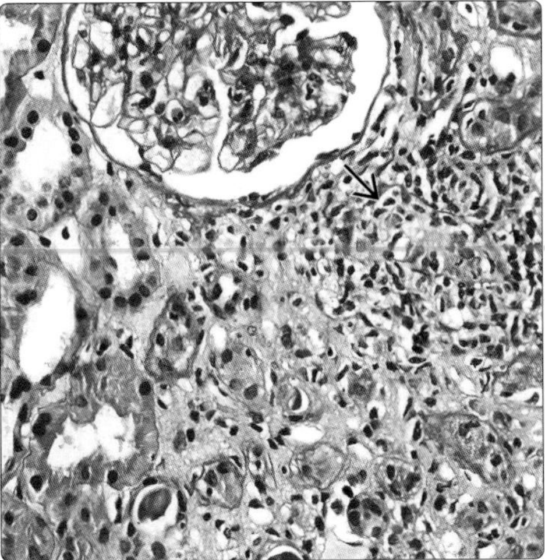

(Left) *Findings are borderline/suspicious for TCMR. Note patchy interstitial inflammation in ≤ 25% of the cortex, with associated tubulitis. This is a 4-month transplant protocol biopsy in a patient on a steroid-free immunosuppressive protocol with normal renal function.* **(Right)** *Focally severe tubulitis ➡ in tubules that are nonatrophic or no more than mildly atrophic are borderline/suspicious for TCMR.*

(Left) *Endothelialitis ➡ is present on this 4 month post-transplant biopsy. The patient's creatinine was elevated to 1.7 mg/dL (baseline of 1.3-1.7 mg/dL). No significant interstitial inflammation or tubulitis was present.* **(Right)** *Transmural inflammation ➡ is shown in a small artery in an allograft 10 years post transplant. Immunosuppression was reduced 4 months previously due to T-cell PTLD. C4d staining was negative.*

Isolated Endothelialitis

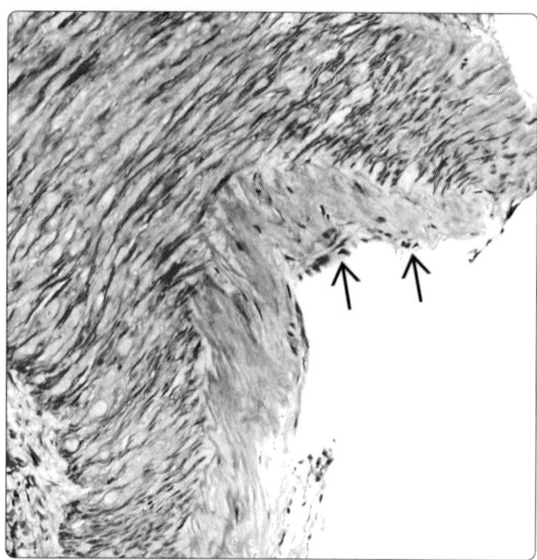

Transmural Arterial Inflammation (Type III TCMR)

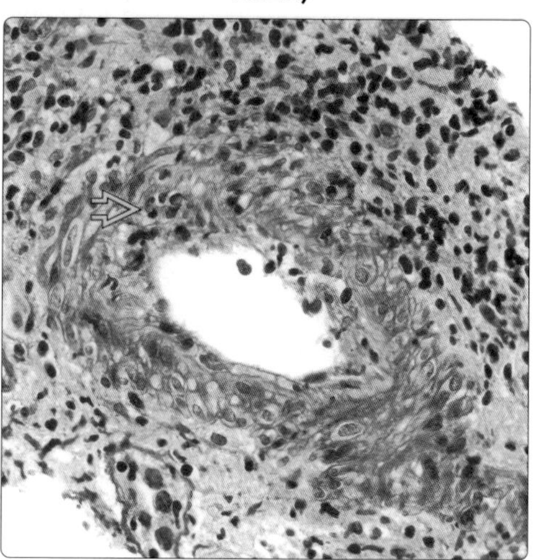

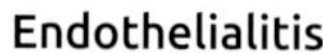

(Left) *An apoptotic cell ➡ is seen in an artery with endothelialitis.* **(Right)** *Fibrinoid necrosis ➡ is seen in a small artery in an allograft 10 years post transplant. Immunosuppression was reduced 4 months previously due to T-cell PTLD. While fibrinoid necrosis is more commonly associated with humoral rejection, this biopsy was C4d(-).*

Endothelialitis

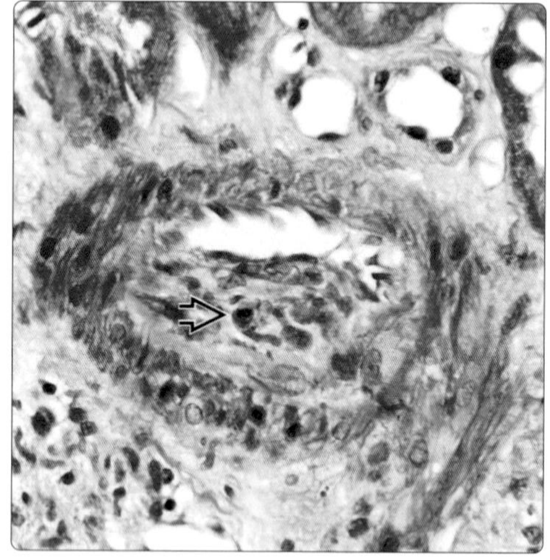

Fibrinoid Necrosis

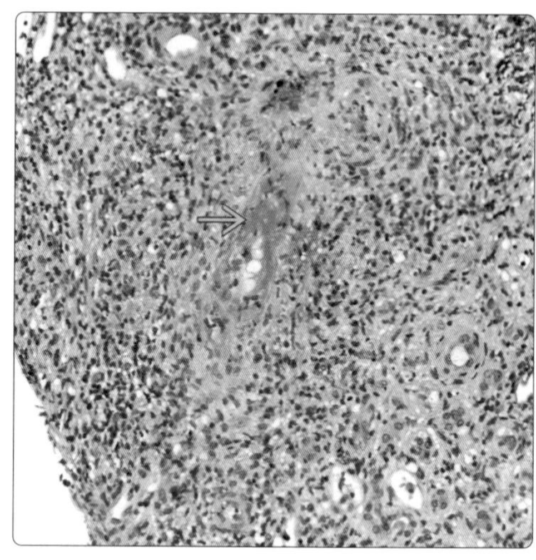

(Left) *This arterial lesion, which occurs in the very early (< 2 weeks) post-transplant period, may resemble endothelialitis. Endothelial cells are enlarged and show areas of vacuolization ➡* **(Right)** *Periodic acid-Schiff shows thrombotic microangiopathy in a native kidney due to factor H deficiency. The intimal inflammation ➡ resembles endarteritis due to rejection. Endothelial cells are markedly reactive.*

Acute Transient Arteriopathy

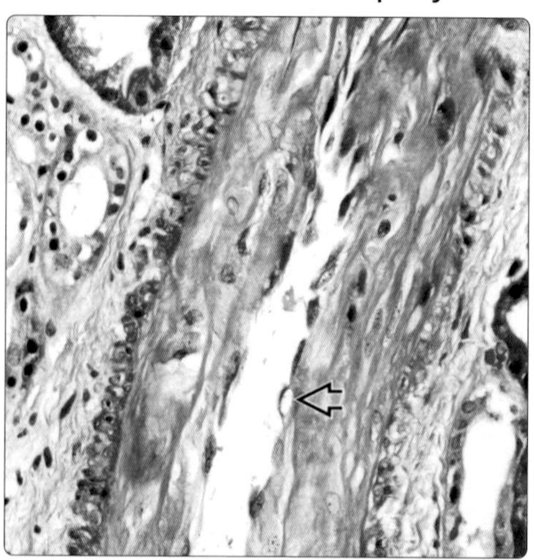

Thrombotic Microangiopathy

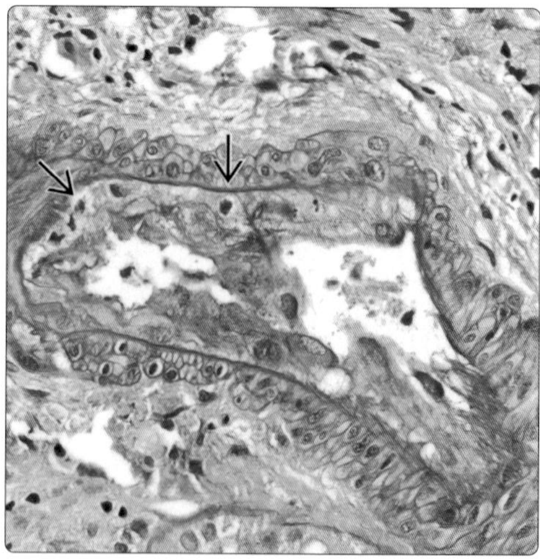

Interstitial Inflammation

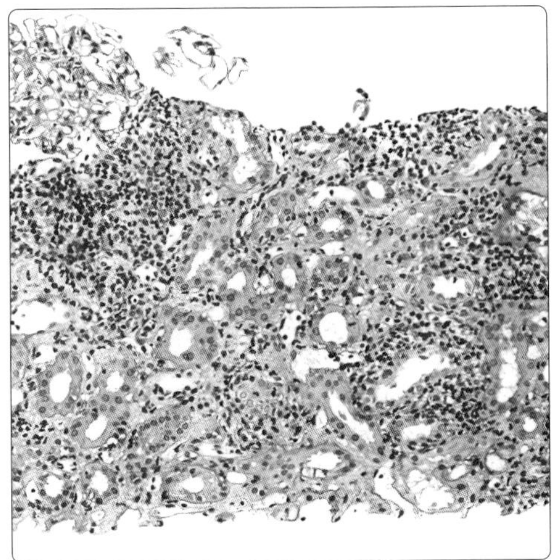

Combined TCMR and Polyomavirus Nephropathy

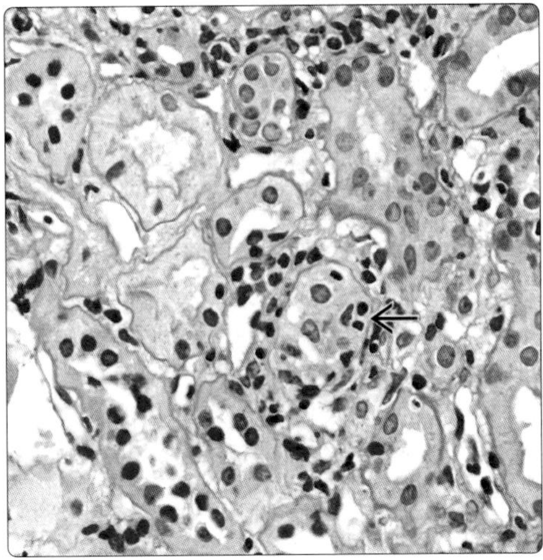

(Left) *Both TCMR and BK polyomavirus infection are manifested by interstitial inflammatory cell infiltrate within the cortex.* **(Right)** *On higher magnification of TCMR and BK polyomavirus infection, mononuclear cell tubulitis is apparent ➡. No viral inclusions are identified in this area. Of note, this patient had low-level BK viremia.*

TCMR IB With Focal BK Infection

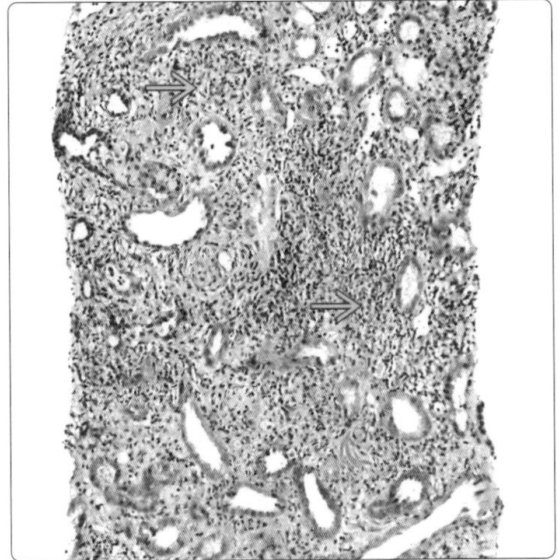

TCMR-IB With Focal BK Infection

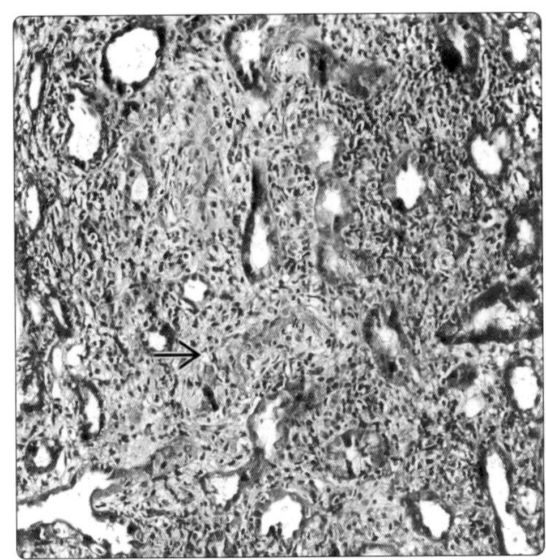

(Left) *Kidney biopsy from a patient 4 months post transplant with slightly elevated serum creatinine and BK viremia shows diffuse interstitial inflammation ➡ and tubulitis.* **(Right)** *Kidney biopsy from a patient 4 months post transplant with slightly elevated serum creatinine and BK viremia shows severe tubulitis ➡.*

TCMR-IB With Focal BK Infection

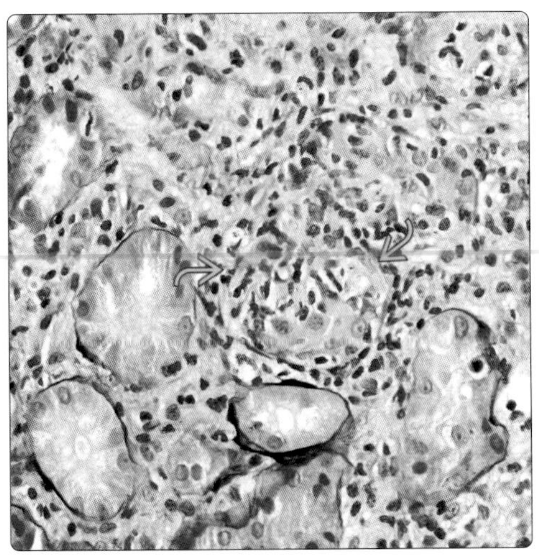

TCMR-IB With Focal BK Infection

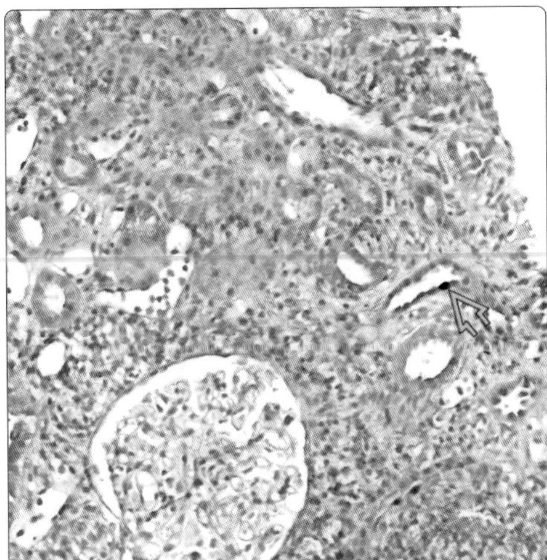

(Left) *Kidney biopsy from a patient 4 months post transplant with slightly elevated serum creatinine and BK viremia shows severe tubulitis with basement membrane disruption ➡ (Banff t3 lesion).* **(Right)** *BK in situ hybridization shows rare BK(+) epithelial cell nuclei ➡. The presence of diffuse interstitial inflammation, physically separated from the BK(+) cells, allows one to make the diagnosis of both TCMR and focal BK infection.*

Ongoing TCMR

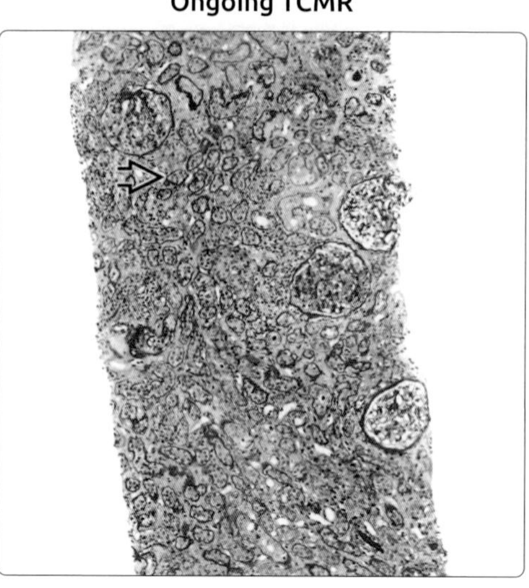

Ongoing TCMR

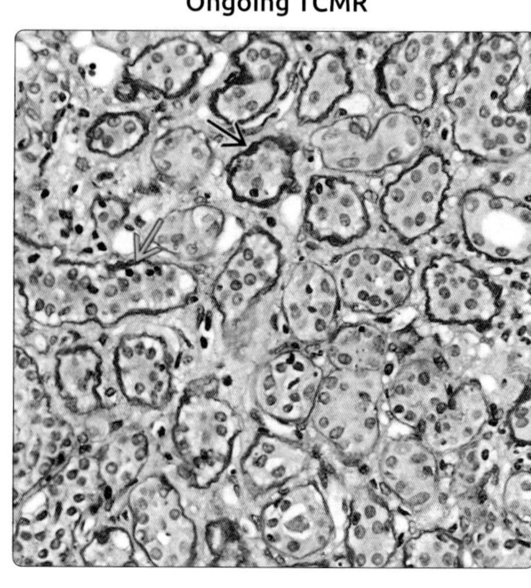

(Left) *This was a follow-up biopsy 6 weeks following TCMR. On low magnification, there is early diffuse interstitial fibrosis and tubular atrophy ⇨, as well as interstitial inflammation.* **(Right)** *This follow-up biopsy 6 weeks following TCMR shows fine interstitial fibrosis, partial tubular atrophy with thickened tubular basement membranes →, and tubulitis ⇨ in partially atrophic tubules. The patient's creatinine had been persistently elevated at ~ 2.3 mg/dL since the previous biopsy.*

Ongoing TCMR

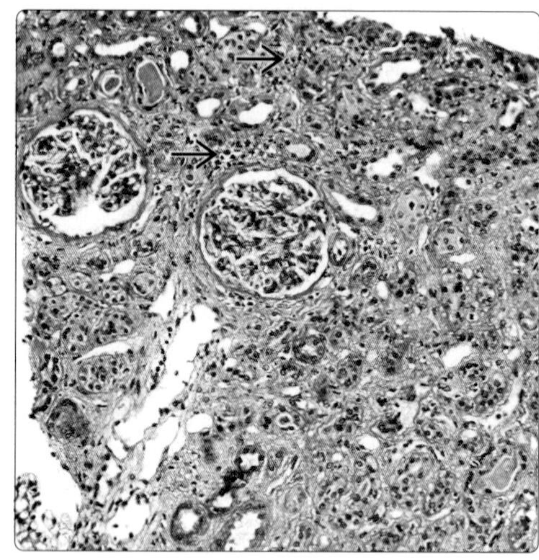

Persistent TCMR

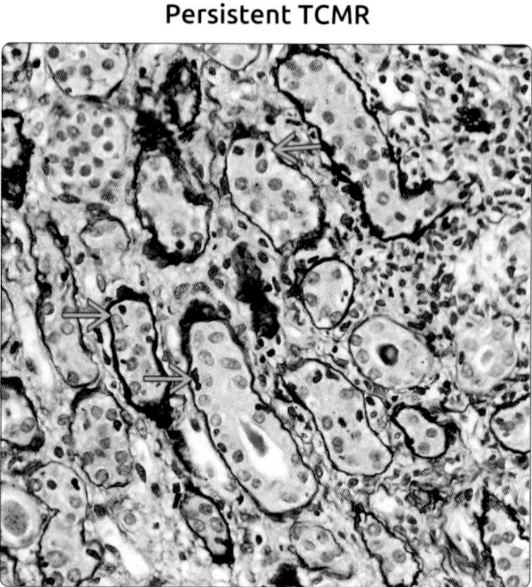

(Left) *Ongoing TCMR 6 weeks following a biopsy that showed TCMR is seen. A trichrome stain highlights the increased interstitial fibrosis. Increased interstitial inflammation → is present as well.* **(Right)** *A silver stain highlights thickened tubular basement membranes; mononuclear cell tubulitis ⇨ is apparent.*

Treated TCMR

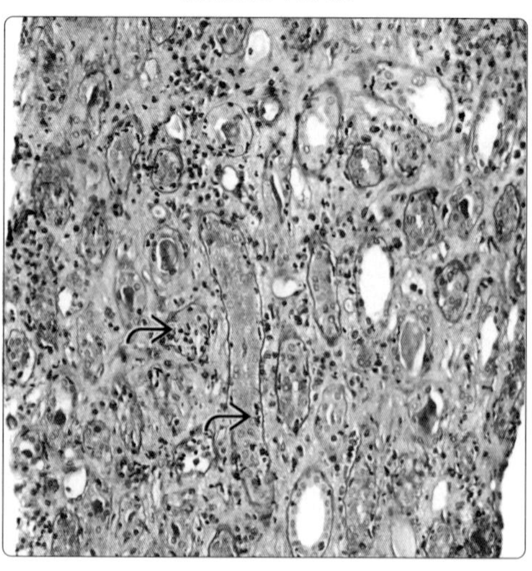

Residual Tubulitis and Edema after Treatment

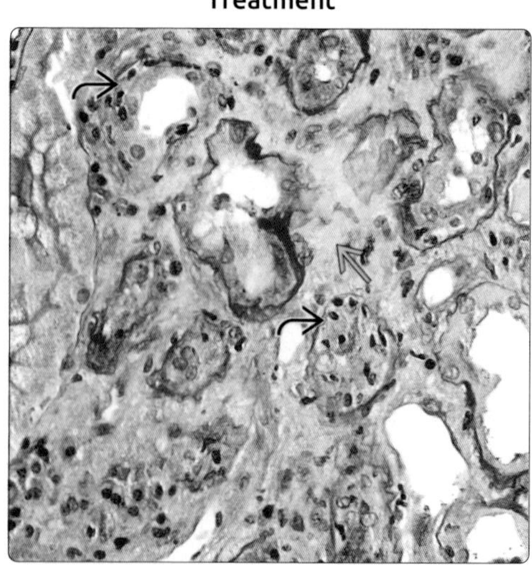

(Left) *This biopsy is from a patient 8 days after being treated with antithymocyte globulin and steroids for TCMR, Banff type IB. This biopsy shows persistent tubulitis ↪ with somewhat lesser interstitial inflammation, typical of a treated rejection.* **(Right)** *This biopsy is from a patient 8 days after being treated with antithymocyte globulin and steroids for TCMR, Banff type IB. Repeat biopsy shows severe tubulitis ↪ with somewhat lesser interstitial inflammation. Note interstitial edema ⇨.*

Borderline TCMR

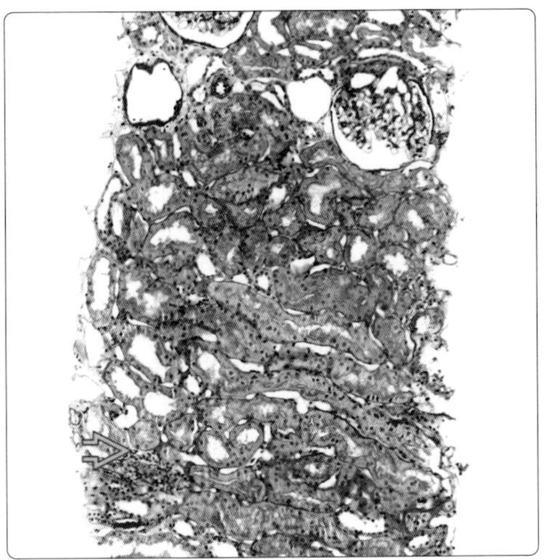

Borderline/Suspicious TCMR

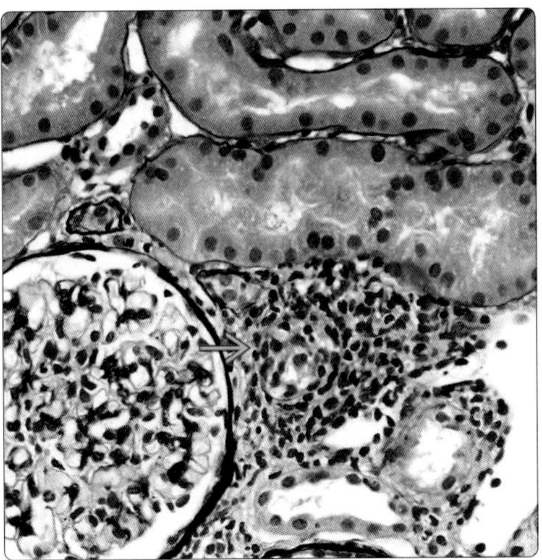

(Left) *This 1-year post-transplant protocol biopsy shows focal mild interstitial inflammation ⇨. There was focal severe tubulitis, indicative of a borderline TCMR. No endothelialitis was present.* **(Right)** *This 1-year post-transplant protocol biopsy shows focal severe tubulitis ⇨ (Banff t3 lesion) with tubular basement membrane disruption. There was only mild interstitial inflammation (~ 5%) in the biopsy. The presence of severe tubulitis qualifies the biopsy for the borderline/suspicious category of TCMR.*

Plasma Cell-Rich Acute TCMR and AMR

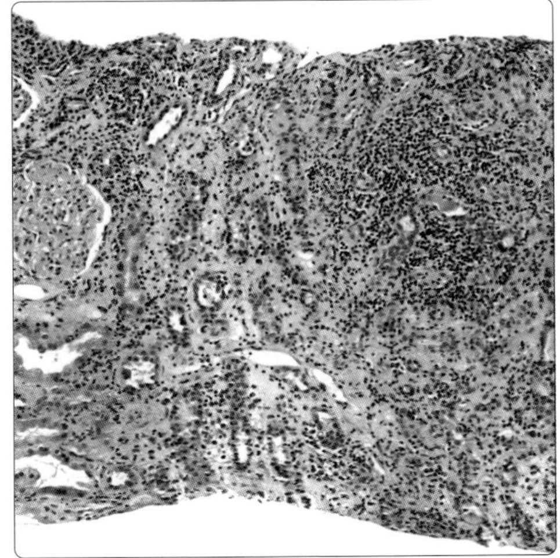

ACR With Plasma Cells

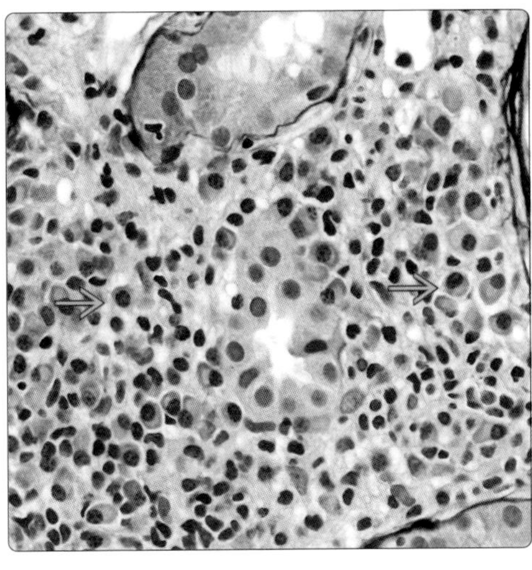

(Left) *This biopsy shows a combination of TCMR and acute antibody-mediated rejection (AMR). Numerous plasma cells within the interstitial infiltrate are present in this variant of acute rejection. Most cases of plasma cell-rich acute rejection are C4d positive.* **(Right)** *In this example of TCMR type I, there were increased numbers of plasma cells ⇨ in the interstitial infiltrate. A stain for BK polyoma virus was negative.*

Plasma Cell Tubulitis

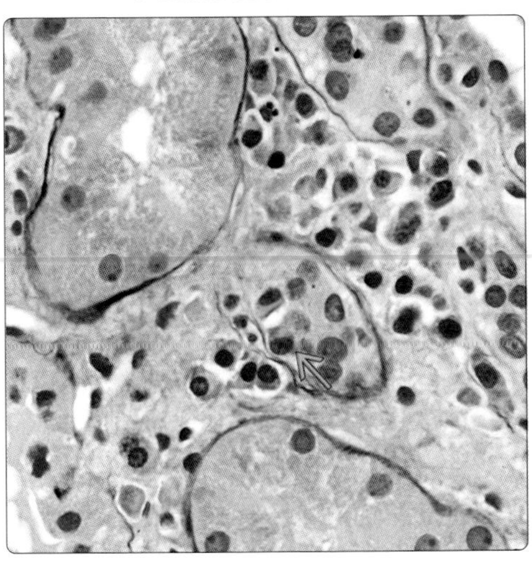

TCMR With Florid Tubulitis

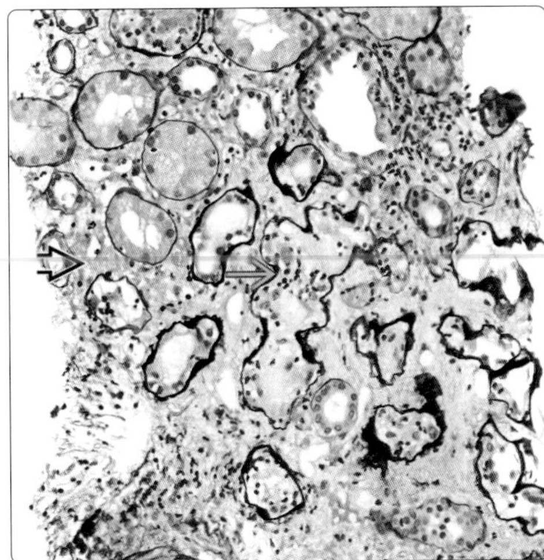

(Left) *A lesion of plasma cell tubulitis ⇨ is seen in this example of TCMR type I with increased interstitial plasma cells. While plasma cell tubulitis is most commonly seen in BK polyoma virus infection, it may occasionally be seen in other entities.* **(Right)** *This case of TCMR type IIA shows severe tubulitis ⇨ and interstitial hemorrhage ⇨. Transplant glomerulopathy was present, a feature of chronic antibody-mediated rejection, but the C4d stain was negative.*

TCMR Type III

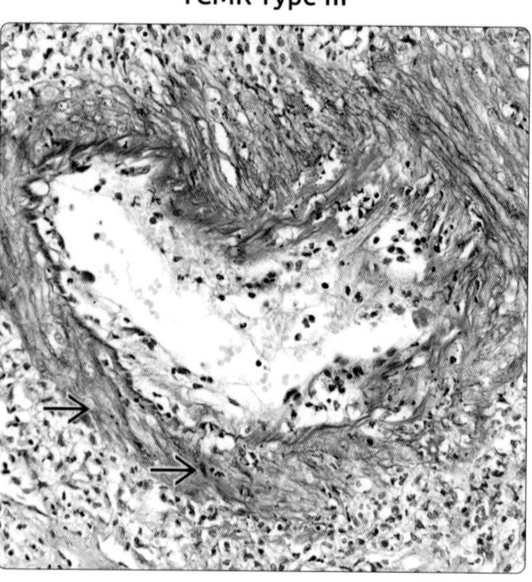

Endothelialitis and Arteriosclerosis

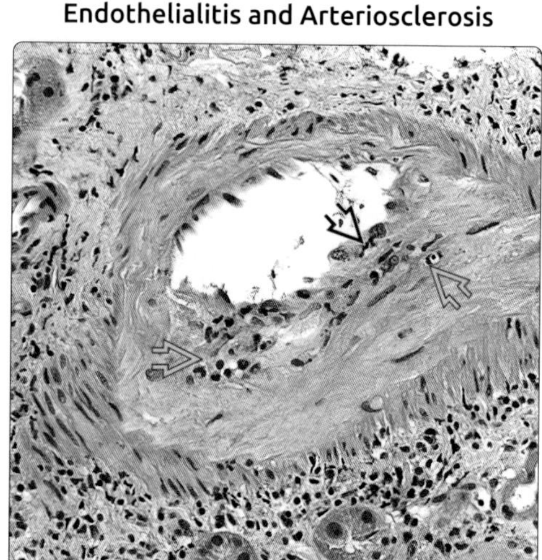

(Left) *Type III acute cellular rejection with transmural inflammation of an arcuate-sized artery is shown. Inflammatory cells can be seen in the media as round dark nuclei ➡.* **(Right)** *Endothelialitis ➡ along with inflammation in a thickened arterial intima ➡ due to donor arteriosclerosis is shown. This may be confused with chronic transplant arteriopathy.*

Resolving TCMR Type II

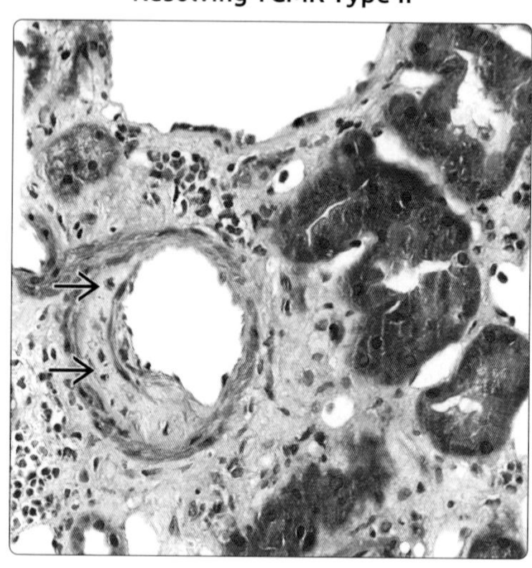

Endothelialitis

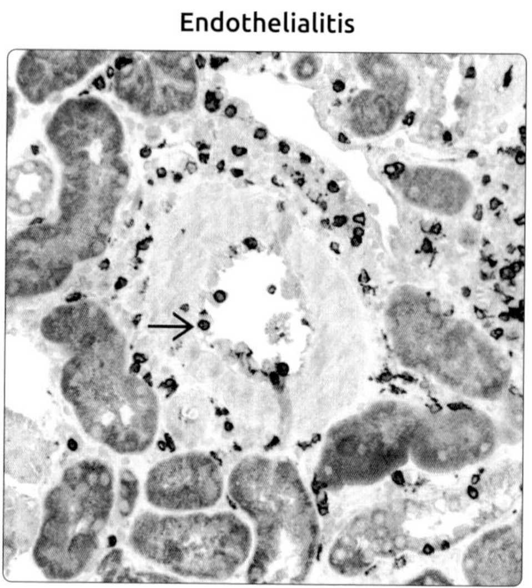

(Left) *Resolving ACR type II shows a few inflammatory cells within a "loose" intima ➡, likely representing early transplant arteriopathy. A biopsy from this patient 2 months earlier showed endothelialitis.* **(Right)** *A stain for CD3 reveals CD3(+) T cells in endothelialitis ➡. The majority of the T cells in these lesions are CD8(+).*

Acute AMR

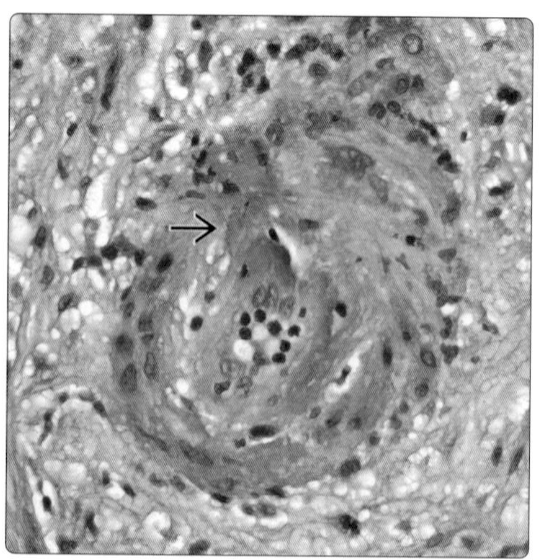

Inflammation in Renal Vein Thrombosis

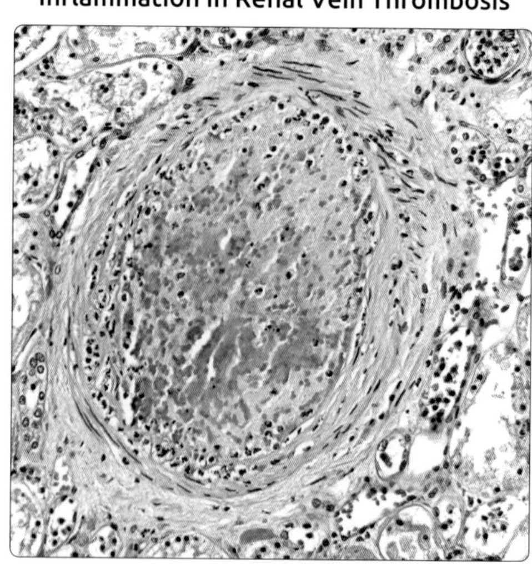

(Left) *Fibrinoid necrosis in a small artery ➡ is shown. Loss of smooth muscle nuclei is present focally. This patient had acute AMR, which accounts for the majority of cases with type III arterial lesions. When the C4d is positive, this is considered acute humoral rejection.* **(Right)** *Arterial inflammation resembles endarteritis in a renal transplant with acute renal vein thrombosis and cortical necrosis; this is not a lesion of rejection.*

Malakoplakia

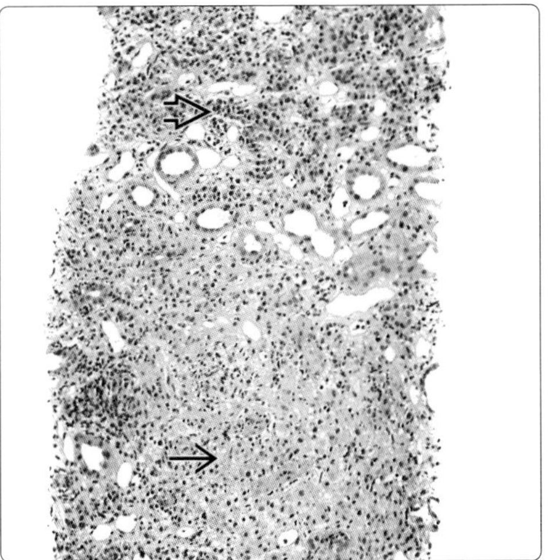

Plasma Cells

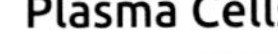

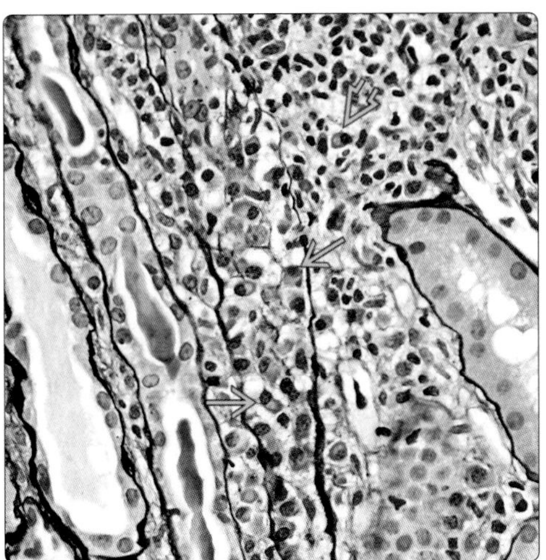

(Left) *Malakoplakia is seen in a transplant biopsy, where there is a diffuse infiltrate of large macrophages →, along with lymphocytes and plasma cells →.* **(Right)** *A transplant biopsy shows numerous plasma cells in the interstitium → and plasma cell tubulitis →, features that raise the possibility of BK polyoma virus infection. The patient had BK viremia, but in situ hybridization was negative for BK polyoma virus. A focal BK infection cannot be excluded.*

Post-Transplant Lymphoproliferative Disorder (PTLD)

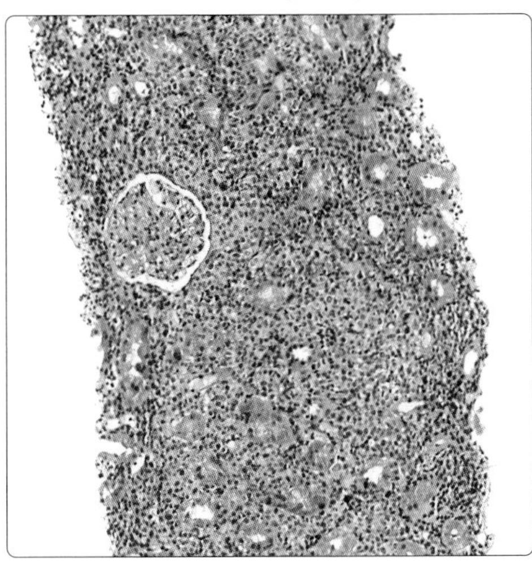

PTLD

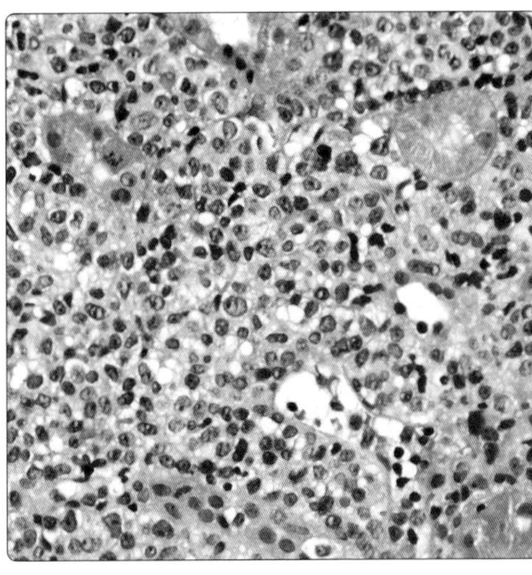

(Left) *PTLD is in the differential diagnosis of TCMR. This biopsy shows a dense lymphoid infiltrate.* **(Right)** *The infiltrating cells of PTLD are atypical, including some large cells. Immunostaining revealed atypical CD20(+) B cells; the patient had a post-transplant marginal zone lymphoma. This case also showed tubulitis with CD3(+) T cells, and so a component of TCMR may have been present. PTLD treatment usually includes decreased immunosuppression.*

Acute Allograft Glomerulopathy (AAG)

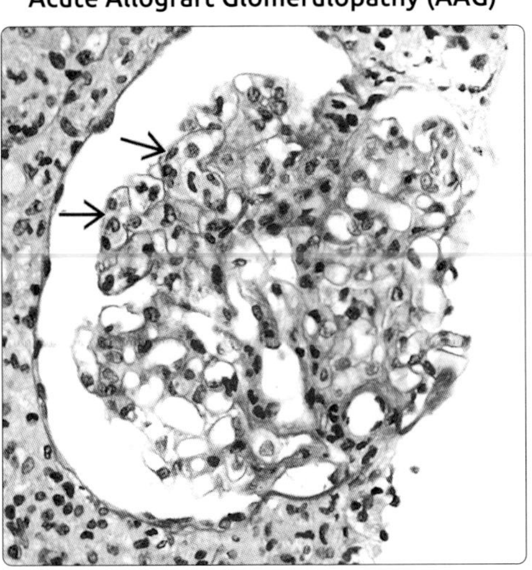

Reactive Endothelial Cells in Arteriole

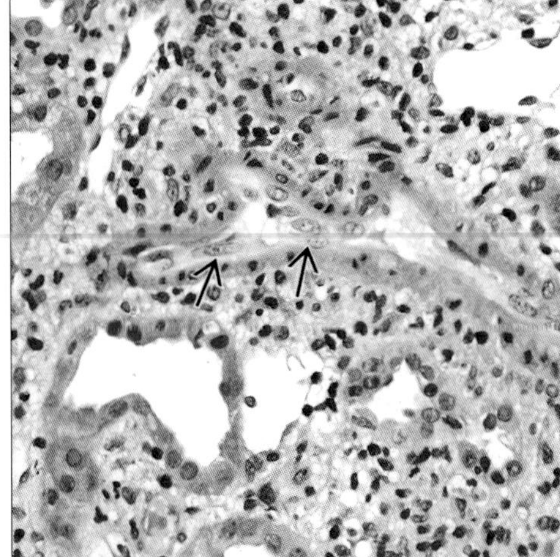

(Left) *An example of AAG shows glomerulitis and marked swelling of endothelial cells →, resembling endocapillary hypercellularity of proliferative lupus nephritis. This glomerular finding can be a lesion of cellular rejection and is nearly always associated with endothelialitis. The C4d stain was negative.* **(Right)** *This arteriole shows markedly enlarged endothelial cells →. Elsewhere this biopsy showed acute allograft glomerulopathy and endothelialitis in arteries.*

Chronic T-Cell-Mediated Rejection

KEY FACTS

TERMINOLOGY

- Persistent or recurrent T-cell-mediated rejection leading to chronic changes in allograft, including transplant arteriopathy, interstitial fibrosis, and tubular atrophy

ETIOLOGY/PATHOGENESIS

- T-cell-mediated injury due to recognition of alloantigens on parenchyma or vessels

CLINICAL ISSUES

- Presents as chronic renal failure, often with proteinuria and hypertension
- May be asymptomatic or seen on protocol biopsy
- Interstitial fibrosis with inflammation shortens graft survival more than either alone
- Presence of chronic transplant arteriopathy also shortens graft survival

MICROSCOPIC

- Tubules and interstitium
  - Mononuclear infiltrate and tubulitis
  - Inflammation in areas of fibrosis
- Arteries
  - Intimal fibrosis
    - Little or no fibroelastosis
  - Mononuclear cells in intima

ANCILLARY TESTS

- Negative stain for C4d in PTCs

TOP DIFFERENTIAL DIAGNOSES

- Chronic antibody-mediated rejection
- Chronic calcineurin inhibitor toxicity
- Late stage of BK polyoma virus nephropathy
- Hypertensive arteriosclerosis
- Chronic pyelonephritis

DIAGNOSTIC CHECKLIST

- Inflammation in areas of fibrosis correlates with progressive graft injury

Inflammation in Fibrotic Areas

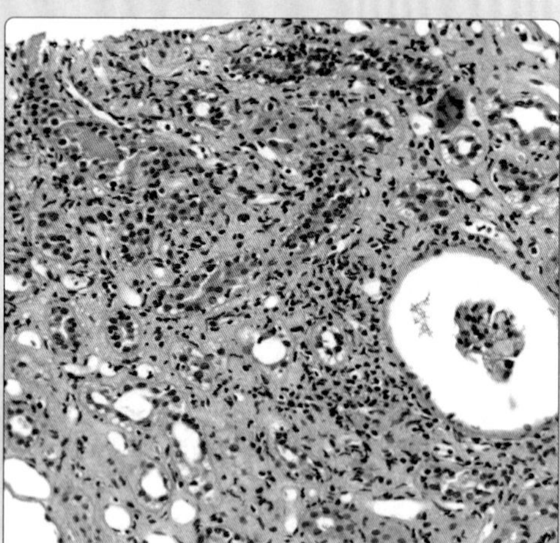

Tubulitis

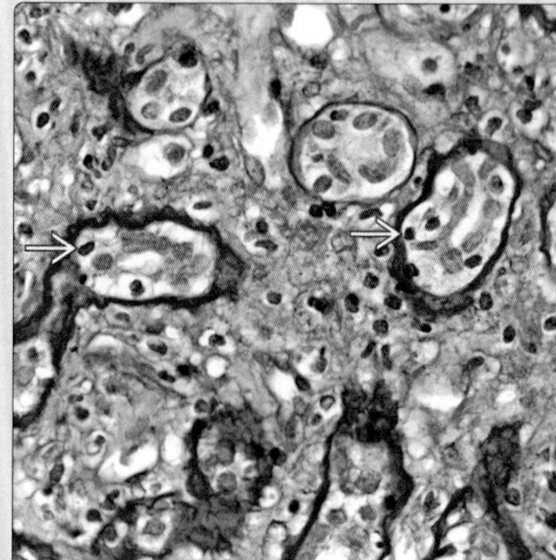

(Left) *A late graft biopsy with chronic cellular rejection shows a diffuse infiltrate of mononuclear cells in areas with interstitial fibrosis, a combination that has a poor prognosis.* **(Right)** *Tubulitis ➡ in atrophic tubules in allografts with late dysfunction is often associated with tubulitis in nonatrophic tubules.*

Transplant Arteriopathy and Endothelialitis

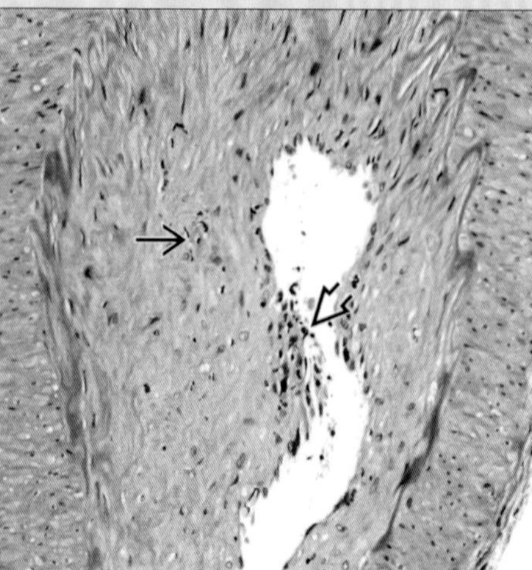

Transplant Arteriopathy

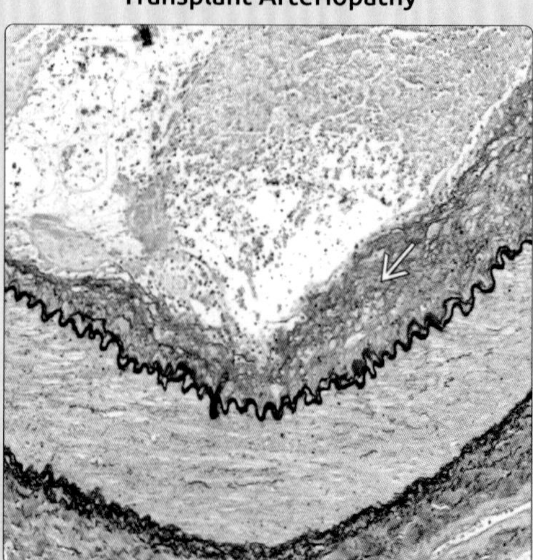

(Left) *This biopsy shows transplant arteriopathy with superimposed endothelialitis ➡. Inflammatory cells are seen within the thickened intima ➡. The biopsy did not show significant tubulointerstitial inflammation. This was a 2-year post-transplant protocol biopsy.* **(Right)** *Arteries with chronic T-cell-mediated rejection have a thickened intima with fibrosis and a sparse infiltrate ➡. In contrast to intimal fibrosis due to hypertension, duplication of the elastica is not prominent.*

TERMINOLOGY

Synonyms

- Chronic cellular rejection
- Chronic active T-cell-mediated rejection

Definitions

- Persistent or recurrent T-cell-mediated rejection leading to chronic changes in allograft
  - e.g., transplant arteriopathy, interstitial fibrosis, and tubular atrophy

ETIOLOGY/PATHOGENESIS

T-Cell-Mediated Injury to Arteries, Tubules, and Vasculature

- Alloresponse to HLA antigens
- Other antigens, including autoantigens, may be relevant
- Macrophages, mast cells also participate
- Fibrosis postulated to be from mediators of tubular cells and inflammatory cells
  - Transforming growth factor (TGF)-beta, bone morphogenic protein (BMP), platelet-derived growth factor (PDGF), and hepatocyte growth factor (HGF)

CLINICAL ISSUES

Presentation

- Chronic renal failure
- May be asymptomatic (subclinical)

Prognosis

- Interstitial fibrosis with inflammation shortens graft survival more than either alone
- Presence of chronic transplant arteriopathy also shortens graft survival

MICROSCOPIC

Histologic Features

- Glomeruli
  - Global glomerulosclerosis
  - Focal segmental glomerulosclerosis
- Interstitium
  - Mononuclear infiltrate meeting criteria of acute cellular rejection
  - Interstitial fibrosis
  - Inflammation in areas of fibrosis
    - Not counted in standard Banff i score
  - Plasma cells may be prominent
- Tubules
  - Tubulitis in nonatrophic tubules
  - Tubulitis also in atrophic tubules
    - Not counted in Banff t score
- Arteries
  - Intimal fibrosis
    - Lacks duplication of elastica in intima, typical of hypertension
  - Mononuclear cells in intima
    - Typically most concentrated under intima
    - Also present in media and adventitia
  - Foam cells in intima
    - Typically lined up against internal elastica

ANCILLARY TESTS

Immunofluorescence

- Negative stain for C4d in peritubular capillaries (PTCs) if no concurrent antibody-mediated rejection

DIFFERENTIAL DIAGNOSIS

Chronic Antibody-Mediated Rejection

- Transplant arteriopathy is a pattern seen in chronic AMR or chronic cellular rejection
  - Histologic patterns indistinguishable
- C4d positive in PTCs in subset of cases
  - Many cases are C4d negative; correlate with presence of circulating donor-specific antibody
- Transplant glomerulopathy often present; not seen in chronic cellular rejection
- Multilamination of basement membrane of PTCs

Chronic Calcineurin Inhibitor Toxicity

- Severe arteriolar hyalinosis
  - Peripheral nodular hyalinosis
- "Striped" fibrosis pattern generally not discriminatory

Hypertensive Arteriosclerosis

- Abundant duplication of elastica in intima
- Minimal or no mononuclear infiltrate

Late Stage of BK Polyoma Virus Nephropathy

- Prior biopsies showing polyoma virus infection give best clue

Chronic Pyelonephritis

- Plasma cells, mononuclear cells, and fewer neutrophils in interstitial infiltrate

DIAGNOSTIC CHECKLIST

Pathologic Interpretation Pearls

- Chronic cellular and antibody-mediated rejection may coexist
- Tubulitis in atrophic tubules is not specific but may be responsible for tubular damage
- Inflammation in areas of fibrosis is not counted in standard Banff i score, but it correlates with progressive graft injury and is therefore likely to be relevant
  - Proposed Banff "total inflammation (ti)" score to account for inflammation in areas of fibrosis
- Late stages of diseases often lose their specific diagnostic features

SELECTED REFERENCES

1. El Ters M et al: Kidney allograft survival after acute rejection, the value of follow-up biopsies. Am J Transplant. 13(9):2334-41, 2013
2. Farris AB et al: Renal interstitial fibrosis: mechanisms and evaluation. Curr Opin Nephrol Hypertens. 21(3):289-300, 2012
3. Gago M et al: Kidney allograft inflammation and fibrosis, causes and consequences. Am J Transplant. 12(5):1199-207, 2012
4. Park WD et al: Fibrosis with inflammation at one year predicts transplant functional decline. J Am Soc Nephrol. 21(11):1987-97, 2010
5. Moreso F et al: Subclinical rejection associated with chronic allograft nephropathy in protocol biopsies as a risk factor for late graft loss. Am J Transplant. 6(4):747-52, 2006

Hyperacute Rejection

KEY FACTS

TERMINOLOGY

- Rejection immediately upon implantation and perfusion of graft

ETIOLOGY/PATHOGENESIS

- Preexisting donor-reactive HLA or blood group antibodies at time of implantation

CLINICAL ISSUES

- Graft primary nonfunction
- Rare
  - < 0.5% of transplants
- Decreased incidence due to improved pre-transplant testing for antibody
- Becomes apparent hours to few days after graft implantation
- No effective treatment currently

MACROSCOPIC

- Cyanosis of graft minutes to hours after perfusion
  - Becomes swollen, hemorrhagic, and necrotic

MICROSCOPIC

- Resemble severe acute humoral rejection
- Platelet and neutrophil margination in capillaries
- Thrombi in glomeruli and arterioles
- Interstitial edema and hemorrhage
- Cortical necrosis in 12-24 hours
- Usually C4d positive peritubular capillaries
  - May be negative

TOP DIFFERENTIAL DIAGNOSES

- Major vascular thrombosis (renal artery &/or vein)
- Perfusion nephropathy
- Donor thrombotic microangiopathy
- Sickle cell trait

Hemorrhagic and Necrotic Kidney

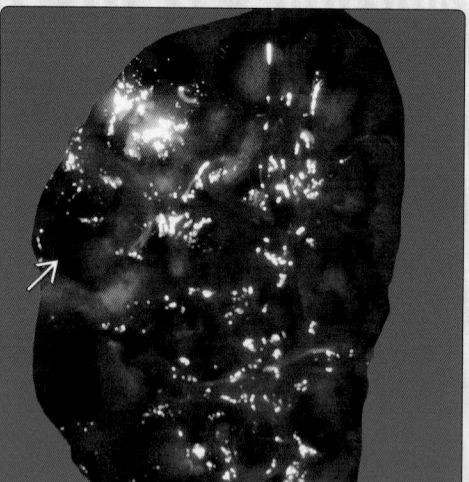

Glomerular Capillaritis

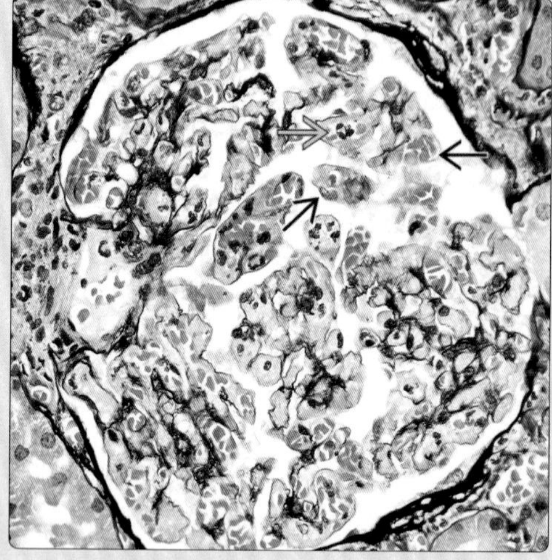

(Left) *Nephrectomy specimen with hyperacute rejection shows edema, as indicated by the glistening cut surface, and hemorrhage. The dark zones at the corticomedullary junction are due to marked congestion. The medullary areas are pale due to ischemia.* **(Right)** *Shown here are neutrophils within glomerular capillaries within a few hours post implantation in hyperacute rejection. Capillaries are congested and some have lost endothelial nuclei. These are the first histological signs of hyperacute rejection.*

Glomerular Thrombi

C4d

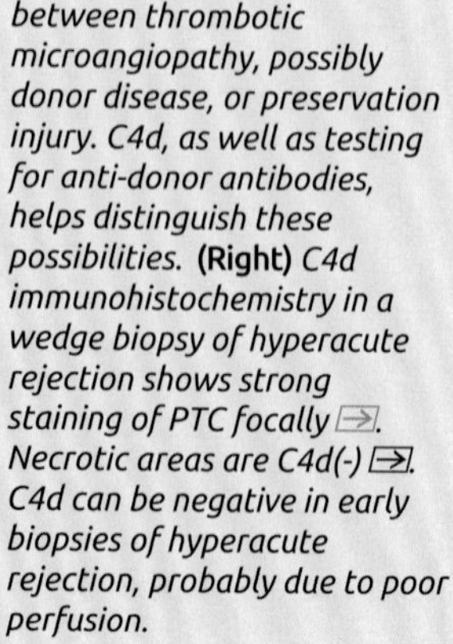

(Left) *H&E shows glomerular thrombi in hyperacute rejection. The differential is between thrombotic microangiopathy, possibly donor disease, or preservation injury. C4d, as well as testing for anti-donor antibodies, helps distinguish these possibilities.* **(Right)** *C4d immunohistochemistry in a wedge biopsy of hyperacute rejection shows strong staining of PTC focally. Necrotic areas are C4d(-). C4d can be negative in early biopsies of hyperacute rejection, probably due to poor perfusion.*

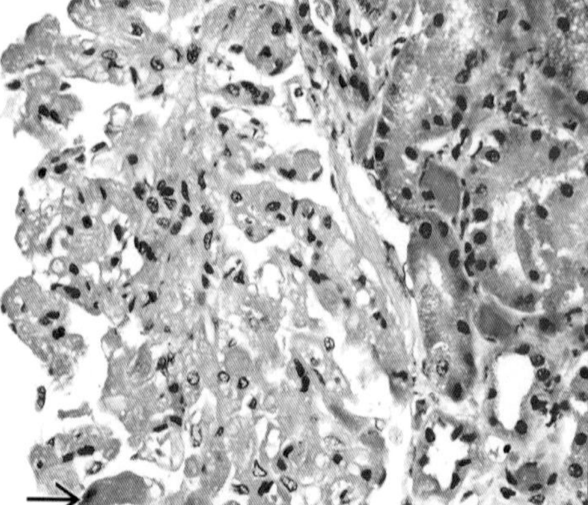

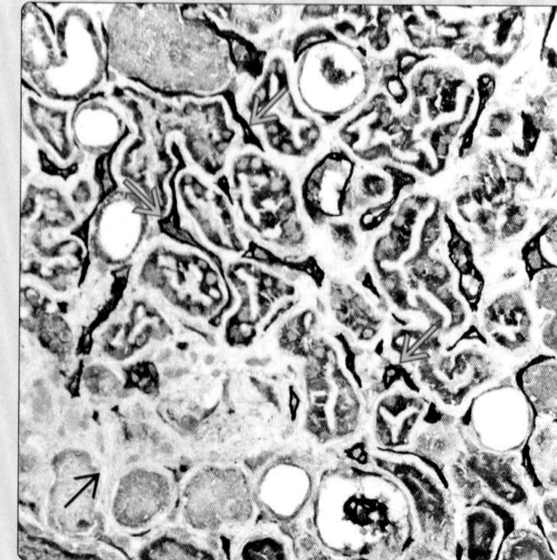

TERMINOLOGY

Definitions

- Rapid rejection (minutes to hours) upon graft implantation

ETIOLOGY/PATHOGENESIS

Antibody Mediated (Usual)

- Preexisting antibodies to donor endothelium
  - Anti-donor ABO blood group or HLA antibody (class I or class II)
    - Rare cases due to other or unidentified endothelial antigens
  - Anti-donor antibody titers high enough to cause immediate rejection
    - Lower levels may delay onset as acute humoral rejection (days)
- Complement activation by antibody, endothelial activation, platelet activation
- Rare cases without complement fixation

T-Cell Mediated (Rare)

- Primed cytotoxic T cells

Exogenous Antibody (Rare)

- Rare cases associated with anti-thymocyte globulin or 3rd party plasma

CLINICAL ISSUES

Epidemiology

- Incidence
  - < 0.5% of transplants
  - Decreased incidence due to improved pretransplant testing for antibody against donor

Presentation

- Graft primary nonfunction
  - Or within hours after graft implantation
- Fever

Treatment

- No effective treatment
- Preventive therapy in ABO-incompatible or positive crossmatch transplants
  - Plasmapheresis to remove donor-specific antibody
  - Intravenous immunoglobulin (IVIG)
  - Rituximab (anti-CD20)
  - Anti-complement drug (experimental)

Prognosis

- Rapid graft loss

MACROSCOPIC

Gross Pathology

- Cyanosis of graft minutes to hours after perfusion
  - Swollen, hemorrhagic with necrosis over 12-24 hours

MICROSCOPIC

Histologic Features

- Early (1-12 hours)
  - Platelet and neutrophil margination in glomerular or peritubular capillaries (PTC)
  - Scattered thrombi in glomeruli and arterioles
- Later (12-24 hours)
  - Widespread thrombi in glomeruli and arteries
  - Fibrinoid necrosis of arteries
    - Larger arteries may be spared (e.g., HLA-DR antibodies)
  - Cortical and medullary necrosis
- Features resemble severe acute humoral rejection

ANCILLARY TESTS

Immunohistochemistry

- PTC and glomeruli
  - C4d and CD61 (platelets)

Immunofluorescence

- Most show C4d-positive PTC
  - Negative or granular luminal PTC C4d staining does not exclude diagnosis of hyperacute rejection
    - Technical difficulties due to poor perfusion early and lack of viable tissue late
    - Possible C4d-negative antibody-mediated rejection
    - Possible T-cell-mediated rejection
- IgG, IgM, &/or C3 may be present in capillaries
  - IgM most common in ABO-incompatible grafts

DIFFERENTIAL DIAGNOSIS

Major Vascular Thrombosis (Renal Artery or Vein)

- May be technical issues of anastomosis or due to hypercoagulable state
  - Thrombi due to technical problems often limited to larger vessels
- Infarction may be present
- C4d negative in viable tissue

Donor Thrombotic Microangiopathy

- C4d negative

Perfusion Nephropathy

- Thrombi and congestion within capillaries
- C4d negative

Sickle Cell Trait

- Rare cases of severe thrombosis at implantation

SELECTED REFERENCES

1. Jackson AM et al: Multiple hyperacute rejections in the absence of detectable complement activation in a patient with endothelial cell reactive antibody. Am J Transplant. 12(6):1643-9, 2012
2. Kim L et al: Intragraft vascular occlusive sickle crisis with early renal allograft loss in occult sickle cell trait. Hum Pathol. 42(7):1027-33, 2011
3. Racusen LC et al: Antibody-mediated rejection in renal allografts: lessons from pathology. Clin J Am Soc Nephrol. 1(3):415-20, 2006
4. Colovai AI et al: Acute and hyperacute humoral rejection in kidney allograft recipients treated with anti-human thymocyte antibodies. Hum Immunol. 66(5):501-12, 2005
5. Ahern AT et al: Hyperacute rejection of HLA-AB-identical renal allografts associated with B lymphocyte and endothelial reactive antibodies. Transplantation. 33(1):103-6, 1982
6. Kissmeyer-Nielsen F et al: Hyperacute rejection of kidney allografts, associated with pre-existing humoral antibodies against donor cells. Lancet. 2(7465):662-5, 1966

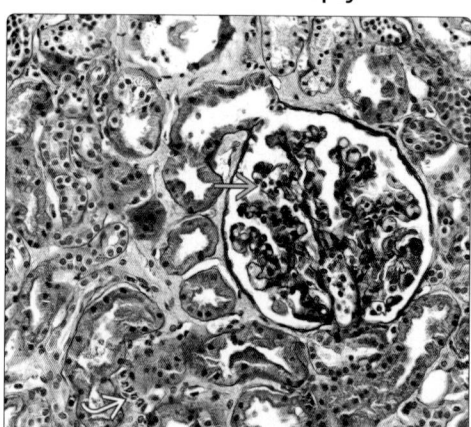

(Left) *This presensitized patient developed hyperacute rejection. Post-perfusion biopsy shows neutrophils in peritubular* ➔ *and glomerular* → *capillaries. The C4d stain was focally positive.* **(Right)** *C4d can be positive* ↪ *on post-perfusion biopsies, as shown in this biopsy from a patient with pre-transplant donor-specific HLA antibodies. The neutrophils in the capillaries also show some staining.*

Post-Perfusion Biopsy

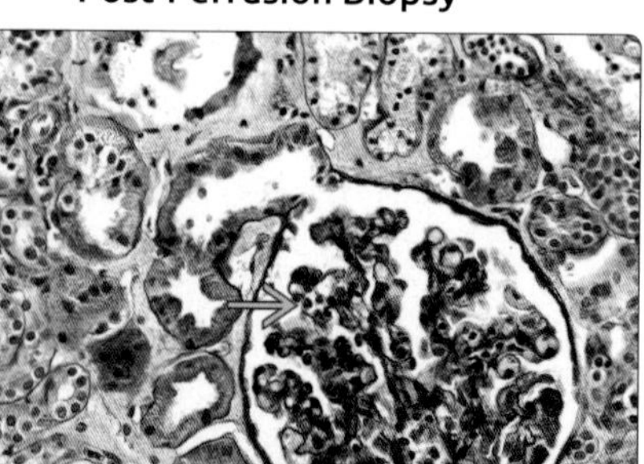

Focal C4d Deposition Post Perfusion

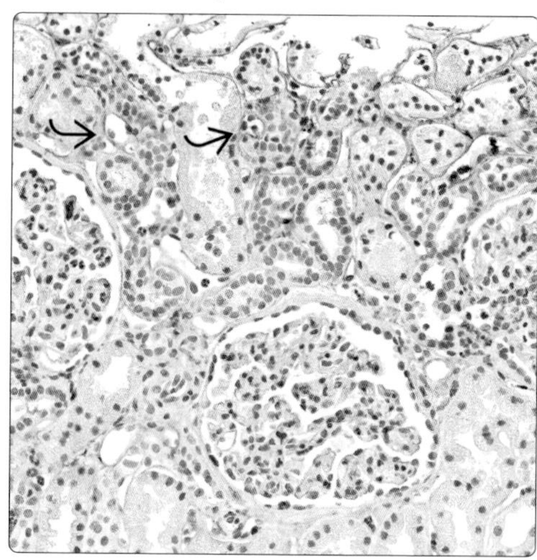

(Left) *Hyperacute rejection, post-perfusion biopsy, shows a 3rd kidney in a patient who received a 6-antigen deceased donor match and was crossmatch negative. Neutrophils are prominent in glomeruli* →. **(Right)** *H&E shows neutrophils within peritubular capillaries (PTC) in hyperacute rejection* →. *This biopsy was taken a few hours after implantation. The PTC are markedly congested. Similar but milder congestion may be due to ischemia reperfusion injury and may be present at the time of implantation.*

Glomerular Capillaritis

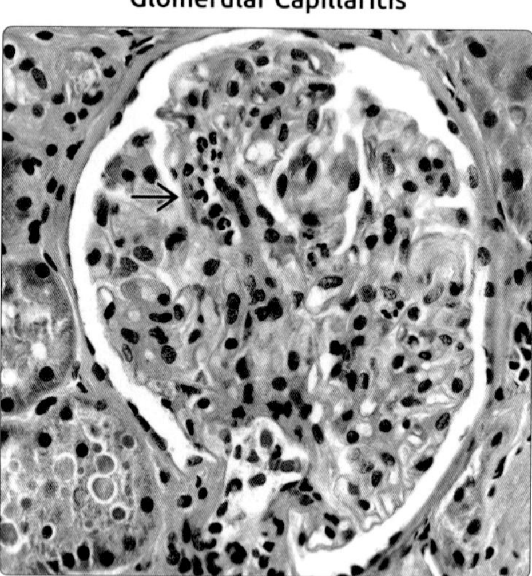

Peritubular Capillaritis

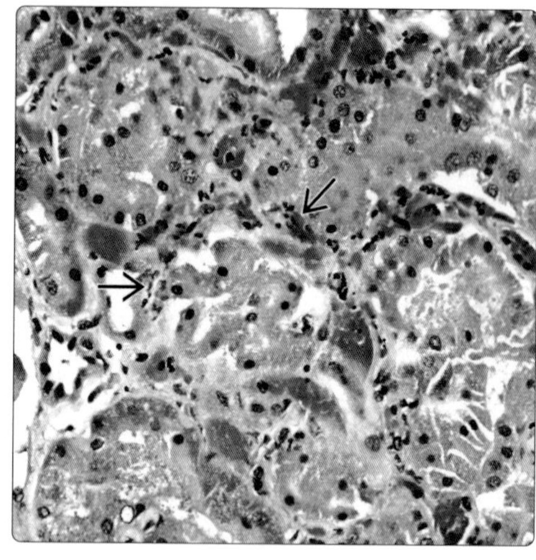

(Left) *Post-perfusion biopsy (hours) in a patient shows patchy C4d staining in peritubular capillaries* →. *Several capillaries are negative* ➔. *Immunofluorescence on frozen tissue was nondiagnostic.* **(Right)** *Post-perfusion biopsy shows prominent CD61 staining in peritubular capillaries, indicating the presence of platelets* →. *CD61 detects the platelet receptor for fibrinogen (IIb/IIIa) and may be a useful test to detect hyperacute rejection.*

C4d

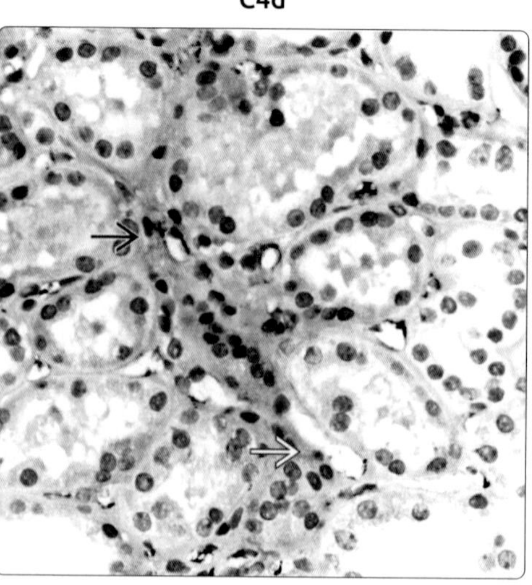

CD61

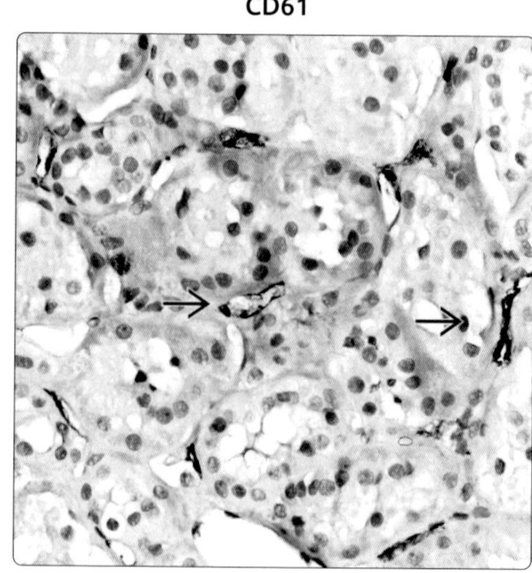

Early Cortical Necrosis in Day 1 Biopsy

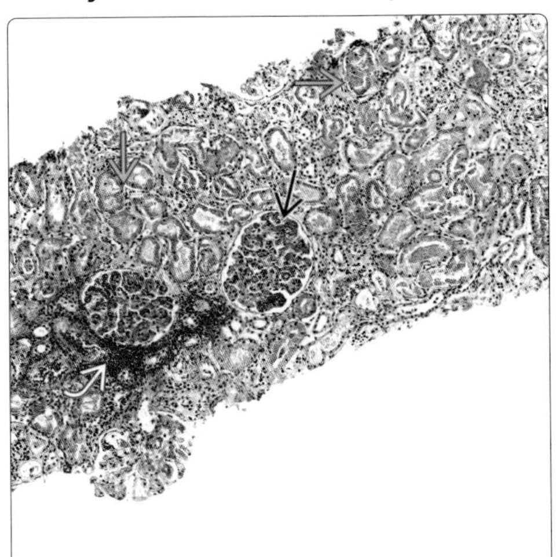

Hyperacute Rejection in Day 1 Biopsy

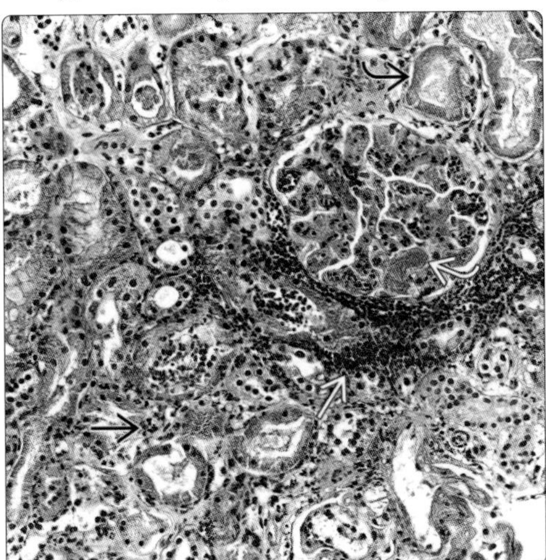

(Left) *Loss of nuclei in proximal tubules ⇨ indicates early cortical necrosis. Interstitial hemorrhage due to peritubular capillary destruction is also evident ➡ as well as glomerular thrombi ⇨. This graft was removed 3 days later.* **(Right)** *This biopsy one day after transplantation shows the classic features of hyperacute rejection: interstitial hemorrhage ➡, glomerular thrombi ➡ and neutrophils in peritubular ⇨ and glomerular capillaries and focal tubular necrosis ⇨.*

Hyperacute Rejection in Day 1 Biopsy

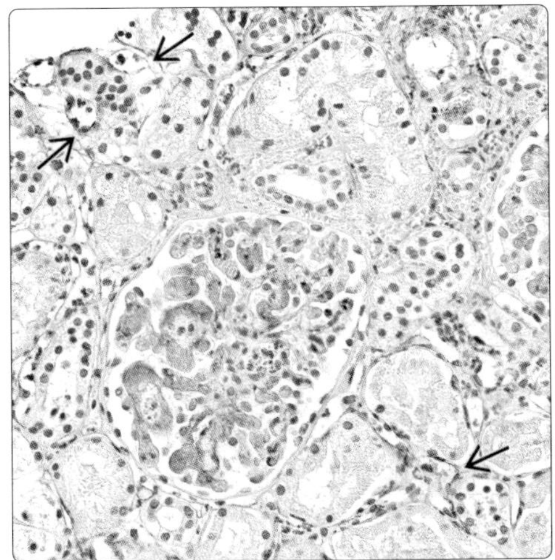

Nephrectomy Specimen With Hyperacute Rejection

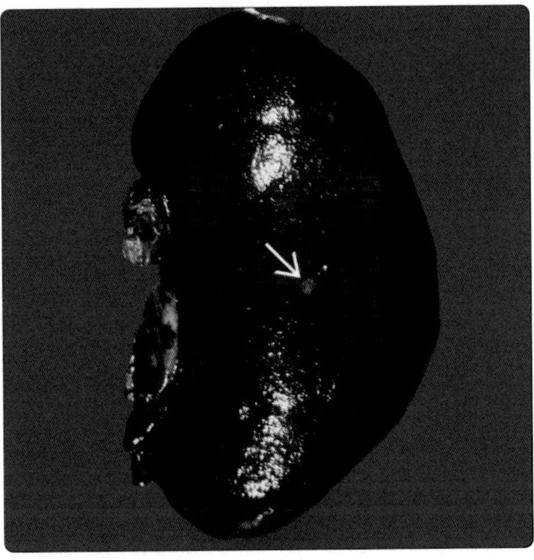

(Left) *C4d is focally positive in peritubular capillaries ⇨ in this biopsy taken one day after transplantation in a presensitized patient. Glomerular capillaries are filled with diffusely staining material corresponding to fibrin and cell debris. Some neutrophils also stain, which may be an artifact.* **(Right)** *This kidney is swollen, hemorrhagic, dusky, and has pale focal areas of necrosis ➡.*

Cortical Necrosis

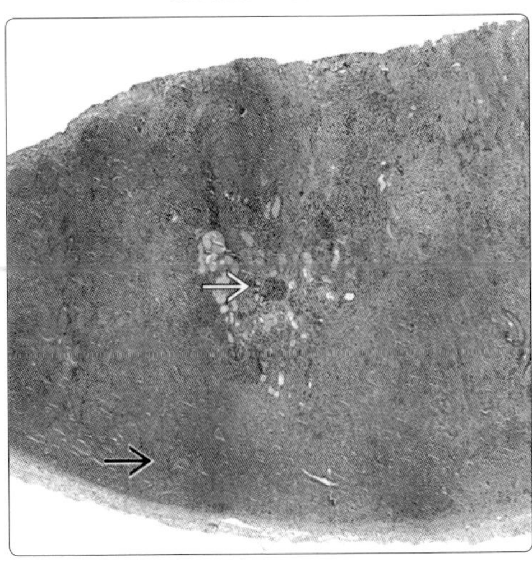

Diffuse Hemorrhage and Necrosis

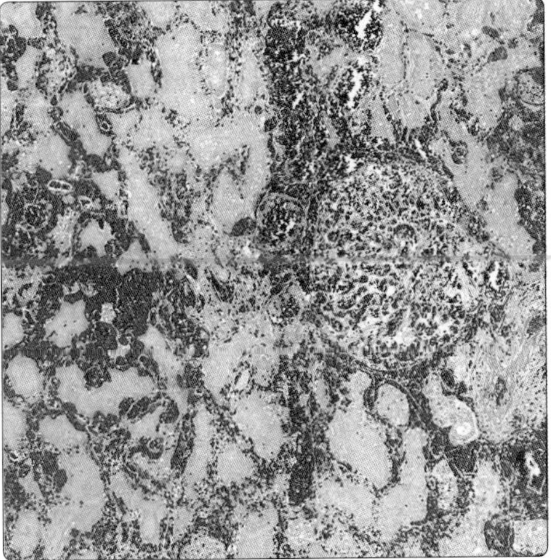

(Left) *H&E shows low-magnification view of a renal allograft with hyperacute rejection. Cortical necrosis and hemorrhage are widespread ⇨. C4d stain was negative in the necrotic areas, comprising 95% of the sample. Nonnecrotic areas were selected from the paraffin-embedded material for C4d staining ➡.* **(Right)** *This nephrectomy specimen from a patient with hyperacute rejection 3 days post transplant shows congestion and necrosis involving all elements of the kidney.*

Acute Humoral Rejection

KEY FACTS

TERMINOLOGY

- Acute allograft rejection caused by anti-donor specific antibodies (DSA) reactive to graft endothelium

ETIOLOGY/PATHOGENESIS

- DSA usually directed against HLA class I or II on endothelium
  - Activates complement via classical pathway
    - Early acute AMR in recipients with preformed DSA is complement mediated
- Mechanism of AMR likely varies with time post transplant and type of DSA

CLINICAL ISSUES

- Acute renal failure
- Serum donor-specific antibody (DSA)
  - Usually donor specific anti-HLA antibody
  - Acute AMR may occur in ABO blood group-incompatible allografts or with antiendothelial cell or other DSA
- Worse allograft survival in acute AMR compared to C4d negative ACR

MICROSCOPIC

- Glomerulitis, neutrophils, monocytes, fibrin
- Glomerular thrombi or mesangiolysis
- Peritubular capillary neutrophils
- Dilated peritubular capillaries (PTCs)
- Acute tubular injury
- Diffuse, bright positive staining of peritubular capillaries for C4d by IF or focal or diffuse for C4d staining by IHC

TOP DIFFERENTIAL DIAGNOSES

- Acute cellular rejection
- Acute tubular necrosis
- Chronic active AMR
- Accommodation
- Pyelonephritis

(Left) *Acute AMR is seen 1 week post transplant. Neutrophils are present within peritubular capillaries ➔, and tubules show acute injury ⇨.* **(Right)** *Diffuse, bright circumferential staining ➔ of PTCs for C4d by immunofluorescence is shown. A positive C4d stain is defined as linear and diffuse PTC staining, usually taken as > 50%.*

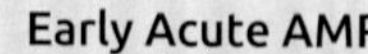

Early Acute AMR

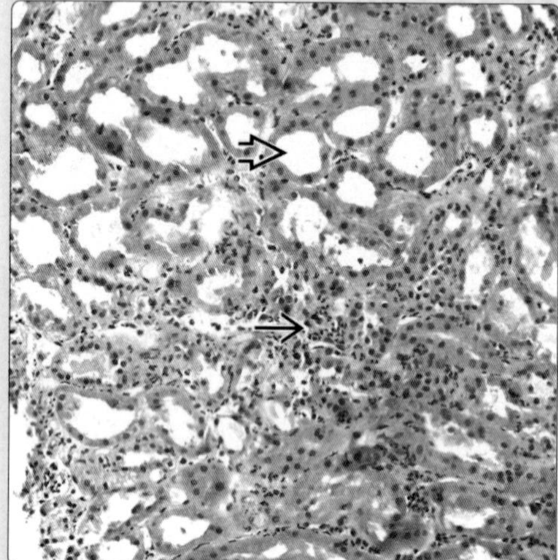

C4d(+) Peritubular Capillaries (PTC)

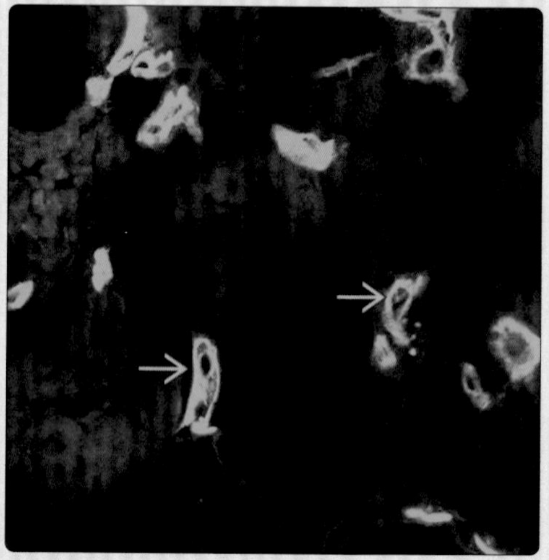

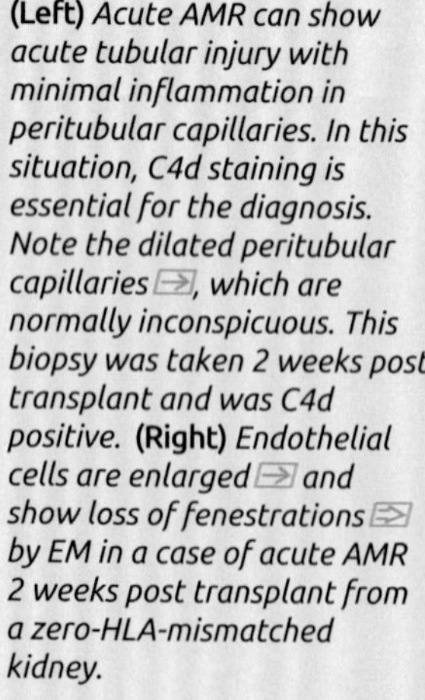

(Left) *Acute AMR can show acute tubular injury with minimal inflammation in peritubular capillaries. In this situation, C4d staining is essential for the diagnosis. Note the dilated peritubular capillaries ➔, which are normally inconspicuous. This biopsy was taken 2 weeks post transplant and was C4d positive.* **(Right)** *Endothelial cells are enlarged ➔ and show loss of fenestrations ⇨ by EM in a case of acute AMR 2 weeks post transplant from a zero-HLA-mismatched kidney.*

Acute AMR With Minimal Inflammation

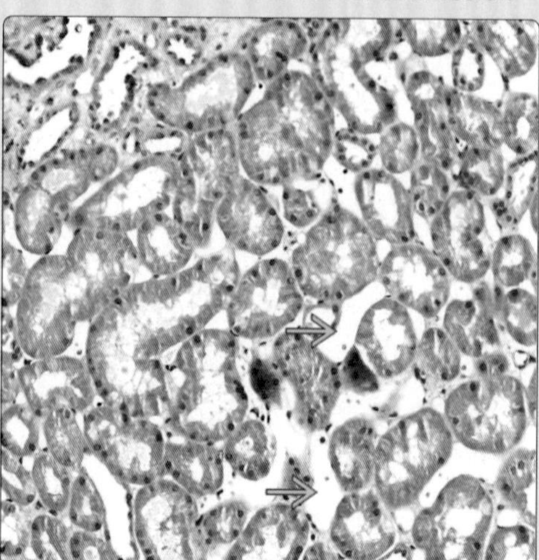

Reactive Endothelial Cells in Acute AMR

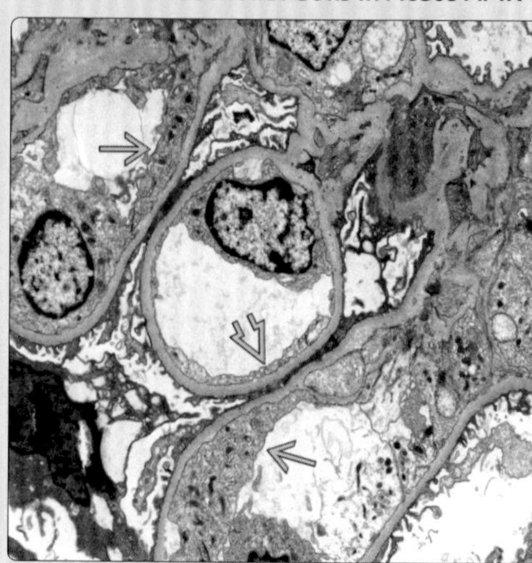

TERMINOLOGY

Abbreviations

- Acute antibody-mediated rejection (acute AMR)

Synonyms

- Acute humoral rejection (AHR)

Definitions

- Acute allograft rejection caused by anti-donor specific antibodies (DSA) reactive to graft endothelium

ETIOLOGY/PATHOGENESIS

Donor-Specific Antibody (DSA) and Complement

- DSA usually directed against HLA class I or II on endothelium
  - ABO blood group antigen in ABO-incompatible grafts
  - Endothelial cell-specific antigens and antiendothelial cell antibodies (AECA)
    - Identified AECAs include endoglin, Fms-like tyrosine kinase-3 ligand, EGF-like repeats and discoidin I-like domains 3, and intercellular adhesion molecule 4
    - Most patients with AECAs also have anti-HLA alloantibody
  - Angiotensin II type 1 receptor
  - Other and unknown non-MHC antigens on endothelium
- DSA activates complement via classical pathway
  - C4d is inactive fragment of C4b of classical complement pathway
    - Covalently bound at site of complement activation on endothelium
  - Complement-fixing DSA and IgG3 subclass of DSA associated with greater acute graft injury
- Mechanism of AMR likely varies with time post transplant and type of DSA
  - Early acute AMR in positive-crossmatch (+XM) kidney transplant recipients with preformed DSA
    - Complement-mediated rejection
    - C4d deposition in capillaries
    - High serum DSA levels
    - Prevention of acute AMR by terminal complement inhibition
    - "Pure" acute AMR phenotype, not combined with T-cell-mediated rejection
  - Later progressive chronic active AMR in +XM recipients
    - More likely C4d negative (~ 10% C4d[+] on protocol biopsy, may be focal)
    - Histologically manifest as glomerular and peritubular capillaritis on protocol biopsy
    - May be mediated by direct endothelial damage by alloantibody
    - May be due to proximal complement pathway components or lower levels of complement activation
    - Also "pure" AMR phenotype, without concurrent T-cell-mediated rejection
    - Chronic active AMR and TG may occur ± preceding acute AMR
  - Late post-transplant acute AMR present in patients with de novo DSA
    - Often combined with T-cell-mediated rejection (tubulitis, interstitial inflammation)

CLINICAL ISSUES

Epidemiology

- Incidence
  - ~ 25% of acute rejection episodes due to antibody
    - Overall acute AMR rate is ~ 6%
      - Early (< 1 month post transplant) rate is ~ 30-40% among +XM patients with preformed anti-HLA DSA

Presentation

- Acute renal failure
- Oliguria

Laboratory Tests

- High levels of circulating serum anti-HLA class I or class II DSA
  - Serum DSA level at time of biopsy correlates with severity of biopsy changes
    - Early acute AMR associated with
      - B-cell flow crossmatch channel shift > 359
      - Bead assay with molecules of equivalent soluble fluorochrome units (MESF) of > 34,000
  - Increased risk of early acute AMR with higher level of pretransplant (baseline) serum DSA
- Minority (5-10%) have undetectable DSA
  - May be due to non-HLA antibody, such as antiendothelial cell antibody
  - Possible antibody absorption by graft

Treatment

- Plasmapheresis
- Intravenous immunoglobulin (IVIG)
- Complement inhibition
  - Eculizumab (C5 inhibitor)
- Rituximab (anti-CD20, B cell)
- Anti-plasma cell therapy (experimental)
  - Bortezomib (proteosome inhibitor)
- Splenectomy in severe cases that are resistant to other treatment

Prognosis

- Worse allograft survival in acute AMR compared to C4d(-) acute cellular rejection (ACR)
  - ~ 30% graft loss within 1 year, vs. 4% graft loss for ACR
- Risk of developing chronic AMR (transplant glomerulopathy [TG]) with anti-HLA DSA, regardless of preceding acute AMR episode
  - Acute AMR episode is indicator of presence of DSA
- Plasma cell-rich variant resistant to treatment
  - Poor clinical outcome

MICROSCOPIC

Histologic Features

- Glomeruli
  - Glomerulitis, neutrophils, monocytes, fibrin
  - Glomerular thrombi or mesangiolysis
    - Particularly in ABO blood group-incompatible grafts
- Peritubular capillaries (PTC)
  - Dilated
  - Neutrophils and mononuclear cells
    - Termed "peritubular capillaritis"

- Arteries
  - Fibrinoid necrosis in minority of cases
  - Endothelialitis (also feature of T-cell-mediated rejection)
- Interstitium
  - Edema, sparse infiltrate
  - Hemorrhage occasionally
  - Plasma cell rich variant
    - Associated with edema and high interferon-γ
- Tubules
  - Acute tubular injury
  - Little or no tubulitis
  - Sometimes neutrophils in lumen

Banff Classification of Acute/Active AMR

- Histologic patterns
  - Type I: Acute tubular injury, minimal inflammation
  - Type II: PTC &/or glomerular capillary inflammation, &/or thromboses
  - Type III: Arterial fibrinoid necrosis or transmural inflammation (v3 lesion)
- In addition to these histologic patterns, biopsies should show evidence of recent antibody interaction with endothelium including
  - PTC C4d deposition
    - Score of C4d2 or C4d3 by immunofluorescence (IF) on frozen sections
    - Or C4d > 0 by immunohistochemistry (IHC) on paraffin sections
  - At least moderate microvascular inflammation ([g + ptc] ≥ 2)
  - Increased expression of gene transcripts in biopsy tissue indicative of endothelial injury
- Serologic evidence of DSA (anti-HLA or other antigens)
- All 3 preceding features **required** for diagnosis of acute/active AMR
  - If 2 present, then "suspicious" for acute/active AMR
- Banff 2013 classification thus allows for C4d-negative acute/active AMR
  - Clinically apparent acute AMR nearly always C4d(+)
  - C4d(-) AMR may be immunologically "active" but with more slowly progressive course

ANCILLARY TESTS

Immunohistochemistry

- Diffuse PTC staining for C4d
  - Less sensitive than IF

Immunofluorescence

- Diffuse, bright positive C4d staining of PTC
  - Small minority of probable acute AMR are C4d(-)
  - Focal C4d (10-50%) less commonly has detectable DSA
  - C4d staining remains positive ~ 5-7 days after antibody removal from circulation

Electron Microscopy

- PTC and glomerular capillary endothelial changes
  - Cell enlargement, loss of fenestrations, microvillus changes, detachment from basement membrane, lysis, apoptosis

DIFFERENTIAL DIAGNOSIS

Chronic Active AMR

- Chronic rejection features: Transplant glomerulopathy, peritubular capillaropathy, transplant arteriopathy
- Mononuclear cells in capillaries with fewer neutrophils, more severe peritubular capillaritis with time post transplant in chronic AMR
  - Increased Banff PTC score not indicator of acute (vs. chronic) AMR
- Usually stable or slowly declining clinical course initially

Acute Cellular Rejection

- Interstitial inflammation and tubulitis
- 20-30% of ACR cases are C4d(+), indicative of concurrent antibody-mediated rejection
  - Late combined acute and chronic cellular and antibody-mediated rejection is associated with medication nonadherence

Accommodation

- C4d deposition without histologic evidence of graft injury and without graft dysfunction
- Commonly seen in ABO blood group-incompatible grafts

Acute Pyelonephritis

- Neutrophils and neutrophilic tubulitis may be seen in acute AMR or in pyelonephritis
- Neutrophilic casts on biopsy and positive urine culture for bacterial infection favor pyelonephritis
- C4d negative

Acute Tubular Necrosis/Injury

- C4d negative

SELECTED REFERENCES

1. Jackson AM et al: Endothelial cell antibodies associated with novel targets and increased rejection. J Am Soc Nephrol. 26(5):1161-71, 2015
2. Haas M et al: Banff 2013 meeting report: inclusion of C4d-negative antibody-mediated rejection and antibody-associated arterial lesions. Am J Transplant. 14(2):272-83, 2014
3. Sellarés J et al: Understanding the causes of kidney transplant failure: the dominant role of antibody-mediated rejection and nonadherence. Am J Transplant. 12(2):388-99, 2012
4. Stegall MD et al: Terminal complement inhibition decreases antibody-mediated rejection in sensitized renal transplant recipients. Am J Transplant. 11(11):2405-13, 2011
5. Hidalgo LG et al: NK cell transcripts and NK cells in kidney biopsies from patients with donor-specific antibodies: evidence for NK cell involvement in antibody-mediated rejection. Am J Transplant. 10(8):1812-22, 2010
6. Burns JM et al: Alloantibody levels and acute humoral rejection early after positive crossmatch kidney transplantation. Am J Transplant. 8(12):2684-94, 2008
7. Lipták P et al: Peritubular capillary damage in acute humoral rejection: an ultrastructural study on human renal allografts. Am J Transplant. 5(12):2870-6, 2005
8. Mauiyyedi S et al: Acute humoral rejection in kidney transplantation: II. Morphology, immunopathology, and pathologic classification. J Am Soc Nephrol. 13(3):779-87, 2002

Acute Tubular Injury in Acute AMR

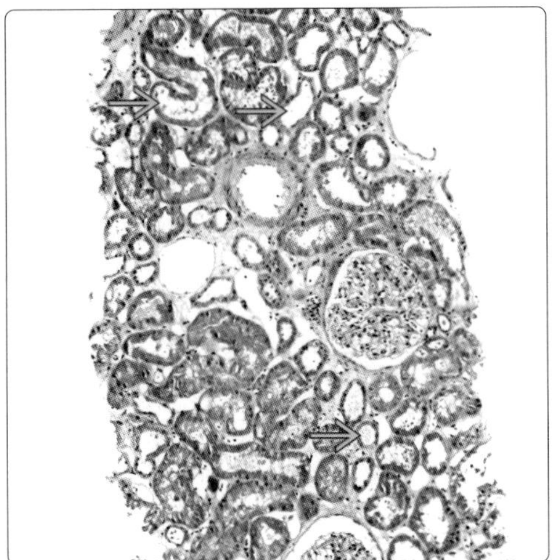

Dilated PTC

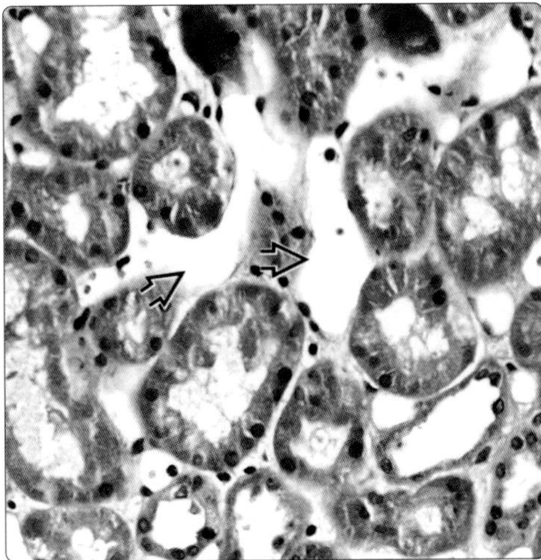

(Left) *In this example of acute AMR 2 weeks post transplant, the tubules are dilated and show flattening of the epithelium* → . **(Right)** *Peritubular capillaries are dilated* → *in this example of early acute AMR. There is scant inflammation in the capillaries. The C4d stain was positive.*

Mesangiolysis and Glomerulitis

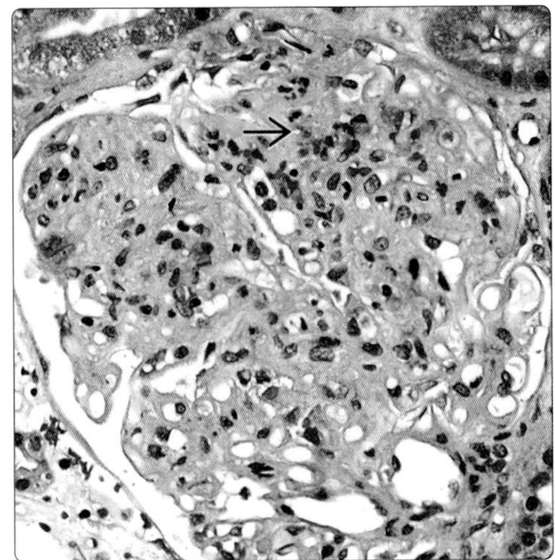

Glomerular Thrombus

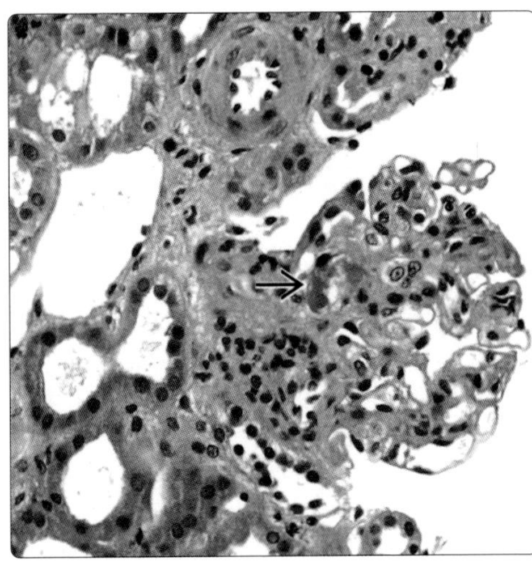

(Left) *Mesangiolysis is seen in this example of acute and chronic AMR. Fragmented red blood cells* → *are present in the expanded mesangium.* **(Right)** *A glomerular thrombus* → *is seen in a case of acute AMR 1 week post transplant in a patient with preformed DSA. This pattern of early acute AMR is typically accompanied by high serum DSA levels and C4d deposition in peritubular capillaries.*

Plasma Cell-Rich Acute AMR

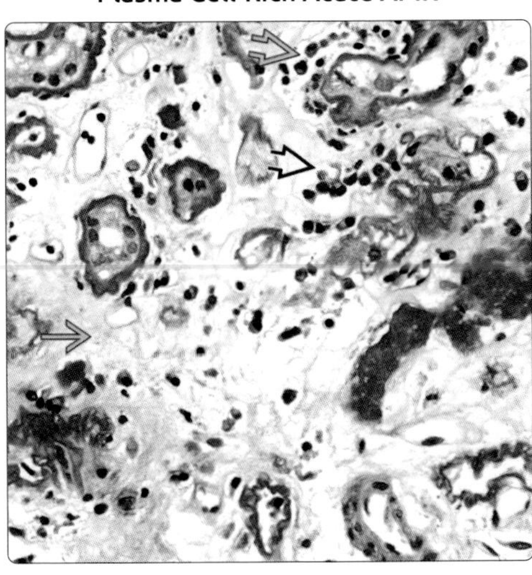

Plasma Cell-Rich Acute AMR

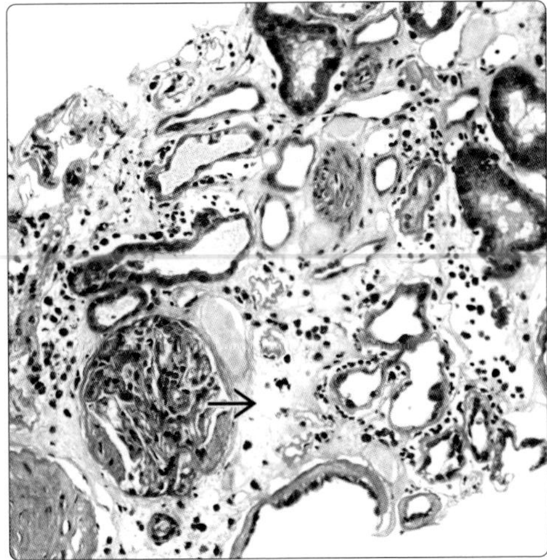

(Left) *This variant of acute AMR shows marked interstitial edema* → *and numerous interstitial* → *and peritubular capillary* → *plasma cells. C4d staining was positive in peritubular capillaries.* **(Right)** *Interstitial edema* → *is seen as pale blue on the trichrome stain in this case of plasma cell-rich acute AMR.*

(Left) *Pure acute AMR commonly shows accumulation of neutrophils in PTC ➔. The histological changes of acute AMR can be subtle.* (Right) *By IHC, peritubular capillaries ➔ show circumferential positive staining for C4d in this example of acute AMR 1 week post transplant. Glomerular capillaries ➔ are also positive.*

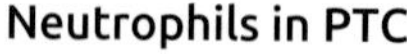

Neutrophils in PTC

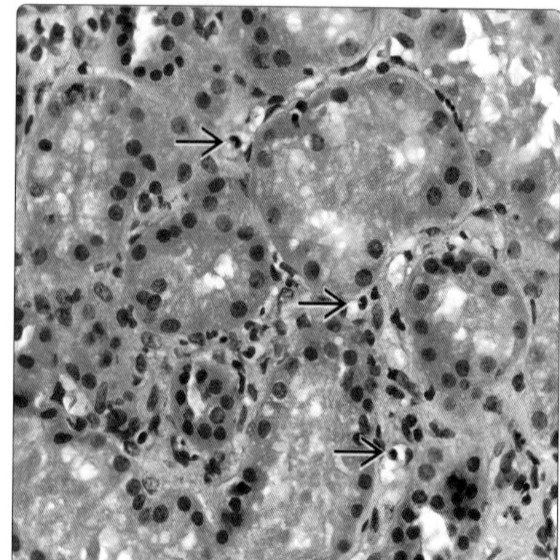

C4d by Immunohistochemistry

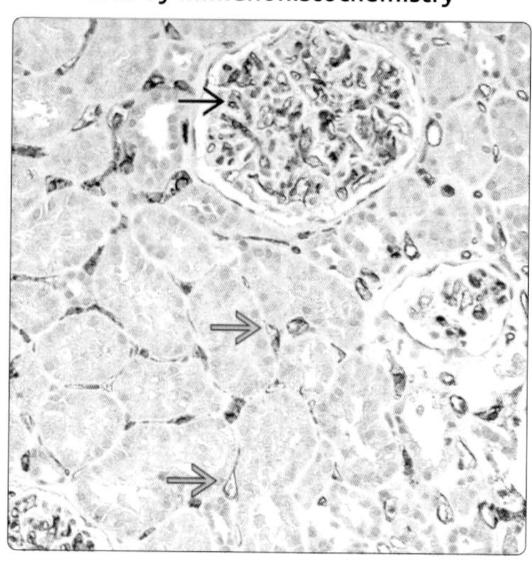

(Left) *In acute AMR, PTCs show enlarged endothelial cells by EM. Microvillus projections are seen ➔, a reactive change.* (Right) *The glomerular endothelial cells have lost their fenestrations and have a shaggy appearance, a sign of injury and activation ➔. Segmental dehiscence from the GBM is also seen ➔. This patient received a liver and kidney transplant 2 weeks previously and had pretransplant DSA to donor class II HLA.*

PTC Reactive Endothelial Cells

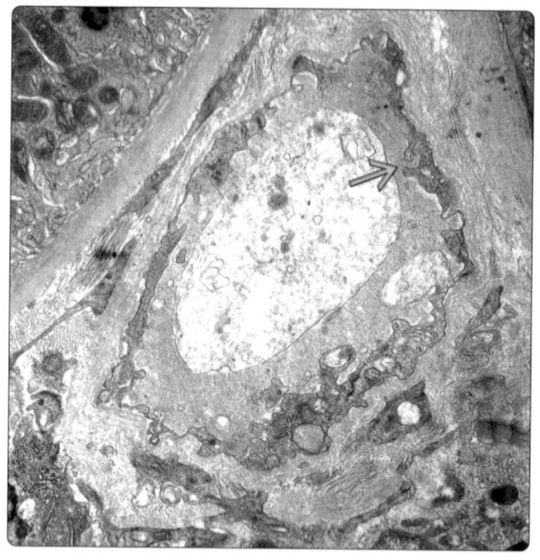

Glomerular Endothelial Injury

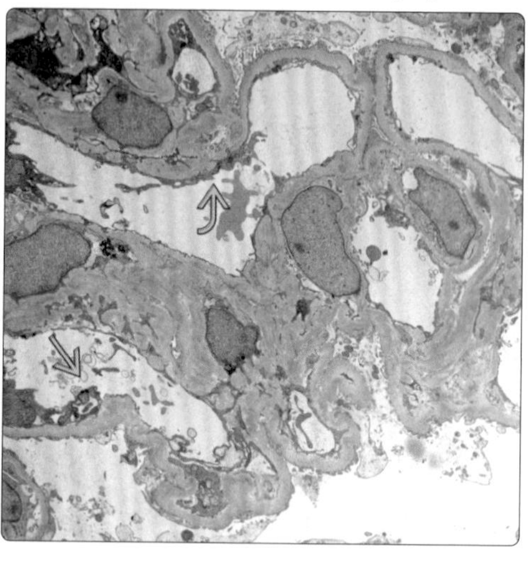

(Left) *This case of severe acute AMR shows fibrin ➔ in an artery along with intimal edema and inflammation. The C4d stain was positive.* (Right) *Endarteritis in patients with DSA may be due to antibody-mediated vascular injury, as shown in animal studies. Here the infiltrate in the intima includes neutrophils ➔ and eosinophils ➔, not usual features of TCMR.*

Arterial Fibrin in Acute AMR

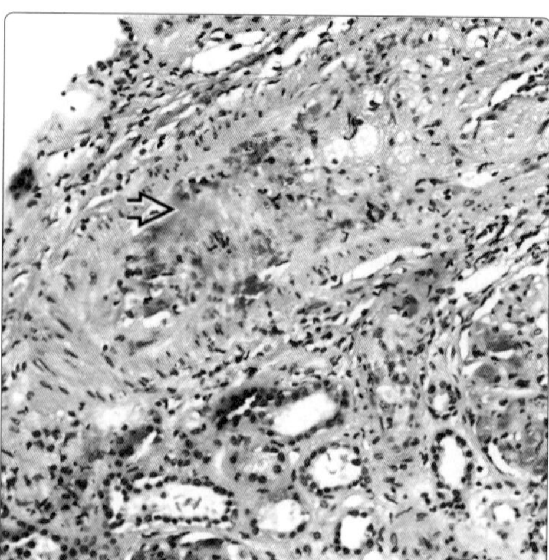

Endarteritis in Acute AMR

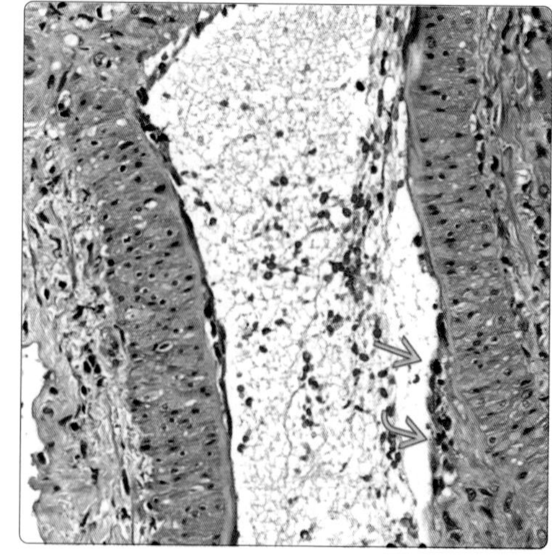

Cortical Necrosis

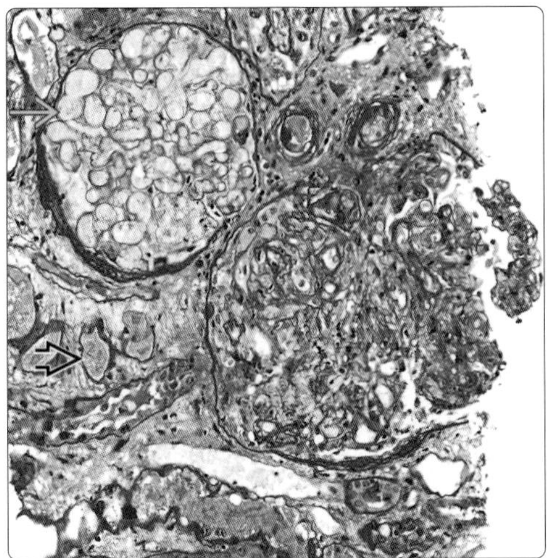

Combined Acute AMR and Acute TCMR

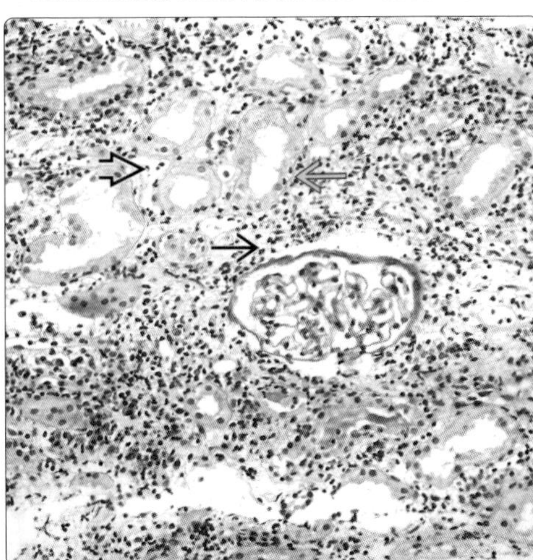

(Left) *Cortical necrosis is manifested by karyolysis in tubules ⮕ and in glomeruli ➡. This case had both acute and chronic AMR. There was focal C4d staining in PTCs; C4d cannot be assessed in necrotic areas.* **(Right)** *Acute AMR and TCMR is often seen in patients with de novo DSA and medication nonadherence. "Pure" AMR is more common in presensitized patients. Interstitial inflammation ➡, tubulitis ➡, and peritubular capillaritis ⮕ are present. C4d was positive.*

Resolution of Acute AMR

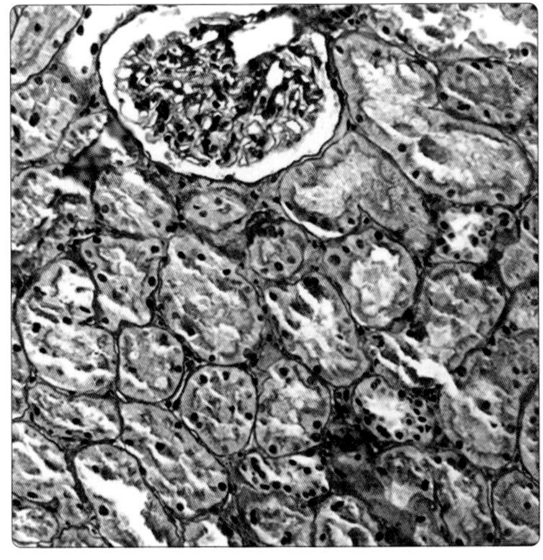

Normal Glomerulus After Acute AMR

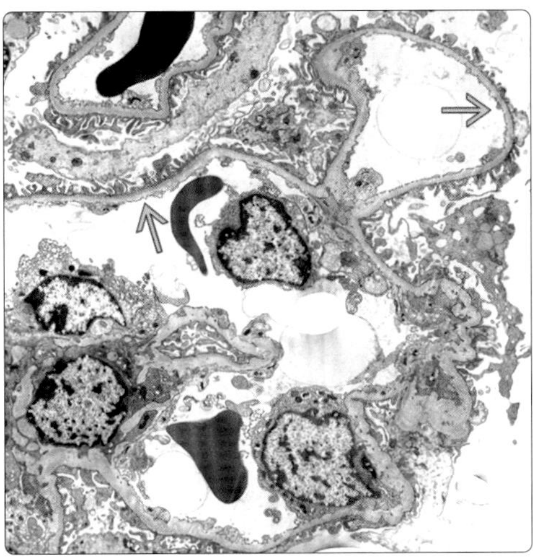

(Left) *Follow-up biopsy was performed 90 days post transplant, after an episode of acute AMR at 2 weeks. The congestion and neutrophils in peritubular capillaries have disappeared since the 14-day biopsy. Glomeruli appear normal. Full recovery can be observed in acute AMR, but patients with persistent DSA often show continued capillaritis.* **(Right)** *Follow-up biopsy occurred 90 days post transplant, after an episode of acute AMR at 2 weeks. Here, endothelium has recovered ➡ from the previous biopsy with acute AMR.*

Peritubular Capillaritis in Smoldering AMR

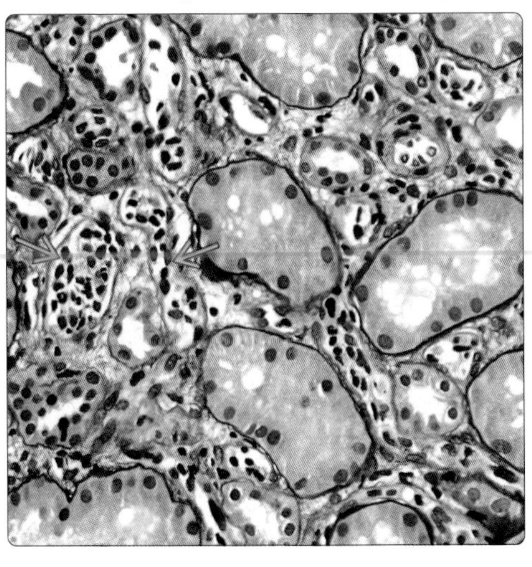

Chronic AMR Sequela of Acute AMR

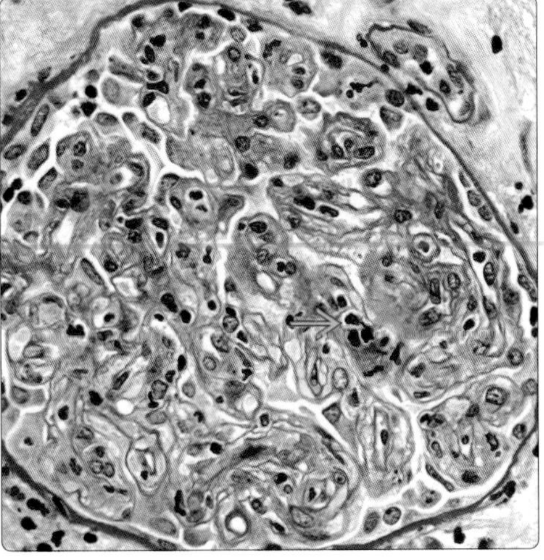

(Left) *Severe peritubular capillaritis ➡ is seen in a 1-year protocol biopsy in a positive-crossmatch transplant with stable creatinine of 1.2 mg/dL. C4d was negative. Counterintuitively, severe capillaritis does not indicate acute AMR, but instead is seen in chronic or smoldering AMR.* **(Right)** *TG developed 6 years after an acute AMR episode. Glomeruli show many mononuclear leukocytes ➡ and duplicated GBM. Anti-class II DSA was present. Chronic AMR may develop with or without preceding acute AMR.*

Chronic Antibody-Mediated Rejection

KEY FACTS

TERMINOLOGY

- Chronic allograft injury mediated by donor-specific antibodies reactive to endothelium, particularly glomerular and peritubular capillaries

ETIOLOGY/PATHOGENESIS

- DSA against HLA class II most common

CLINICAL ISSUES

- Insidious onset > 1 year post transplant; later post transplant with de novo DSA
  - Proteinuria, chronic renal failure
- Cause of ~ 60% of late graft dysfunction

MICROSCOPIC

- Glomeruli
  - Duplication of GBM (transplant glomerulopathy)
  - Mononuclear glomerulitis
  - Mesangial hypercellularity (variable)
- Peritubular capillaritis, mononuclear
- Arteries: Neointimal proliferation (transplant arteriopathy)

ANCILLARY TESTS

- Immunofluorescence or IHC
  - PTC C4d may be diffuse, focal, or negative
- Electron microscopy
  - Duplication of GBM
  - Hypertrophied endothelium and loss of fenestrae
  - Multilamination of PTC basement membranes

TOP DIFFERENTIAL DIAGNOSES

- Thrombotic microangiopathy
- Recurrent or de novo glomerulonephritis

DIAGNOSTIC CHECKLIST

- Diagnostic criteria (Banff)
  - Histologic evidence of chronic tissue injury
  - Evidence for antibody-mediated injury in tissue
  - Serologic evidence of DSA

Transplant Glomerulopathy Due to Chronic AMR

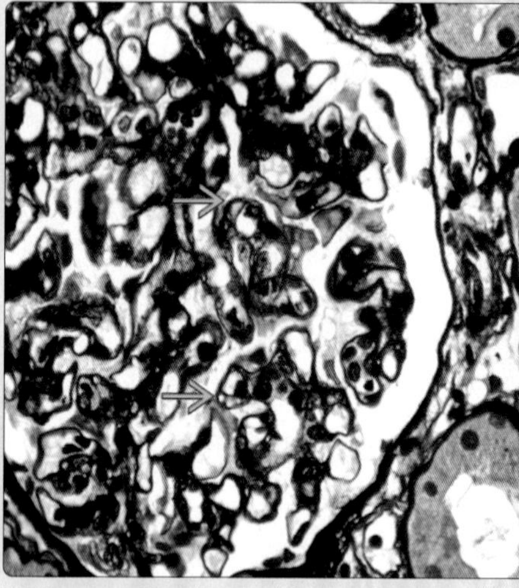

Transplant Glomerulopathy

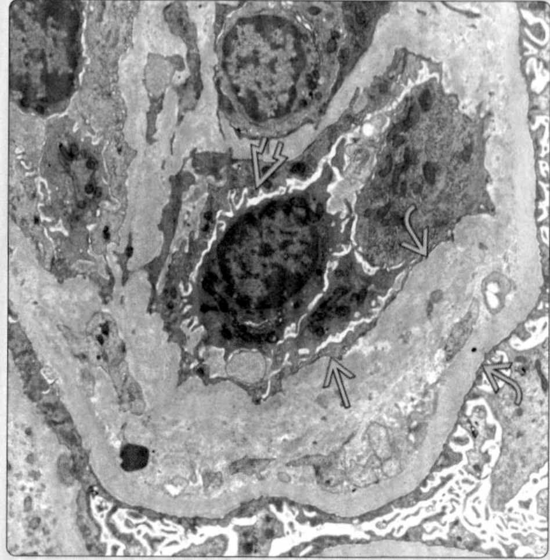

(Left) *Transplant glomerulopathy with glomerular basement membrane duplication ➡ is seen in a case that also showed transplant arteriopathy. Both TG and TA lesions can be seen in chronic AMR but do not necessarily occur together.* **(Right)** *Duplication of the GBM ➡ is striking in this case of chronic AMR, 10 years post transplant. The endothelium is reactive, with loss of fenestrations ➡. Electron-dense deposits are not conspicuous. A lymphocyte in the lumen is in contact with the endothelium ➡.*

PTC Capillaritis With C4d

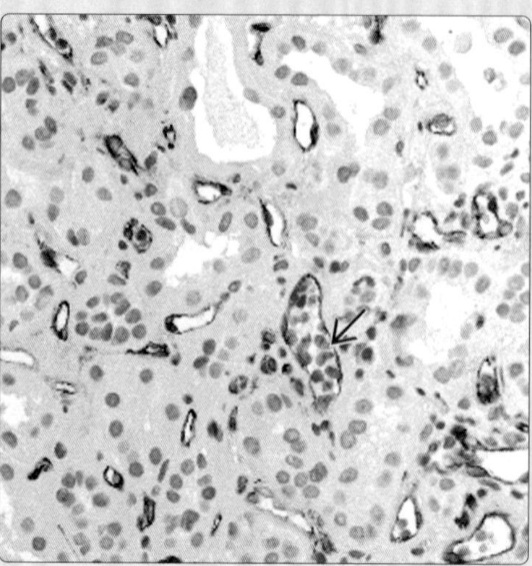

Multilamination of Peritubular Capillary Basement Membrane

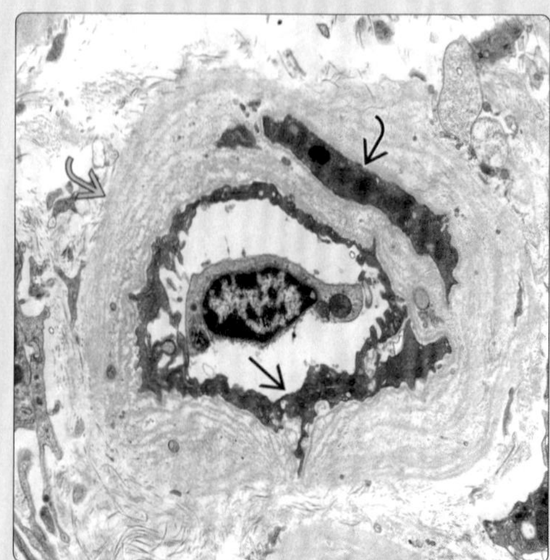

(Left) *Immunoperoxidase stain of case with CHR shows extensive staining of PTCs for C4d; > 90% were positive. Cells in PTC were also evident ➡.* **(Right)** *Chronic AMR characteristically has multilamination of PTC basement membranes as shown here in a severe example with 9-10 layers ➡. A pericyte is embedded between the layers ➡. The endothelium is markedly reactive with increased cytoplasm and organelles ➡. The lumen contains a lymphocyte.*

TERMINOLOGY

Abbreviations

- Chronic antibody-mediated rejection (chronic AMR)
- Transplant glomerulopathy (TG)

Synonyms

- Chronic humoral rejection (CHR)

Definitions

- Chronic allograft injury mediated by donor-specific antibodies reactive to endothelium, particularly glomerular and peritubular capillaries

ETIOLOGY/PATHOGENESIS

Donor-Specific Antibody (DSA) and Complement

- Donor-specific antibody (DSA) against HLA antigens
  - Chronic AMR more strongly associated with anti-HLA class II DSA but may occur with class I DSA alone
- Episodic antibody-mediated endothelial injury/activation/repair
- DSA activates complement by classical pathway in "active" AMR
  - C4d deposition in graft is marker of complement activation
- DSA may also mediate injury via Fc receptors on NK or monocytes or via early complement components (C3)
  - Progressive capillaritis and transplant glomerulopathy occurs even when patients receive terminal complement inhibitor (C5)
  - Evidence for complement-independent, NK-cell-dependent mechanism in chronic AMR in murine heart transplants (transplant arteriopathy)

Capillaritis

- Microvascular inflammation (MVI)
- T cells and monocytes/macrophages
- NK cells
  - Increased NK-cell transcripts and NK cells in capillaries of chronic AMR biopsies

CLINICAL ISSUES

Epidemiology

- ~ 60% of late graft dysfunction is due to chronic AMR
- Risk factors
  - Nonadherence
  - Presensitization
  - Younger age, higher HLA mismatches

Presentation

- Insidious onset > 1 year post transplant; later post transplant (5-8 years) with de novo DSA
- Indolent dysfunction (38%)
- Stable function (32%) (protocol biopsy)
- Proteinuria (86% ≥ 0.5 g/d)
- Hypertension

Laboratory Tests

- Serum donor-specific HLA antibody
  - May be undetectable at time of biopsy
  - Single antigen bead (Luminex) most sensitive

Natural History

- Sequential stages observed in protocol biopsies of nonhuman primates with de novo DSA
  - Stage I: Circulating DSA, no tissue abnormality
  - Stage II: C4d deposition &/or capillaritis without obvious injury
  - Stage III: Transplant glomerulopathy, PTC lamination, and arteriopathy but normal renal function
  - Stage IV: Proteinuria, loss of function
- Prospective studies of de novo DSA (Wiebe, Everly)
  - ~ 15-25% develop de novo DSA
    - Mean: 4.6 years post transplant (6-130 months) in one study
    - Median: 1.6 years post transplant in another study
  - IgM DSA precedes development of IgG DSA
  - Proteinuria follows onset of DSA by ~ 9 months
  - Elevated Cr follows DSA by ~ 12 months
- Chronic AMR with preformed DSA in positive-crossmatch (+XM) kidney transplant recipients
  - Glomerulitis and peritubular capillaritis prevalent on protocol biopsies, precede development of TG
    - Glomerulitis in ~ 30%, peritubular capillaritis in ~ 60% at 1 year post transplant
    - C4d deposition present in only ~ 10% of protocol biopsies with capillaritis
    - Capillaritis present more frequently post transplant in patients with anti-HLA class II DSA
    - Capillaritis and TG tend to increase in severity with time post transplant

Treatment

- Drugs
  - No known effective treatments
  - Rituximab (anti-CD20)
  - Intravenous immunoglobulin (IVIG)
  - Bortezomib (proteosome inhibitor) to deplete plasma cells that produce alloantibody

Prognosis

- 50% graft loss rate at 5 years after diagnosis of transplant glomerulopathy (TG)
  - C4d-positive cases have poorer graft survival
  - Subset with molecular markers of endothelial activation show poorer survival, even if C4d(-)
- Greater graft loss with acute (57%) or indolent dysfunction (40%) compared with stable function (0%) over mean of 19 months follow-up

MICROSCOPIC

Histologic Features

- Glomeruli
  - Duplication of glomerular basement membrane (GBM)
    - Transplant glomerulopathy (TG) (chronic allograft glomerulopathy)
  - Mononuclear cell glomerulitis often present
  - May have segmental glomerulosclerosis, mesangial expansion, or glomerular hypertrophy
- Tubules and interstitium
  - No specific changes, tubular atrophy, and interstitial fibrosis common

- Correlates with loss of PTCs
  - Advanced TG may occur with minimal interstitial fibrosis/tubular atrophy
- Peritubular capillaries
  - Peritubular capillaropathy
    - Duplicated/thickened PTC BM sometimes appreciable by light microscopy when severe
    - Disappearance of PTCs over time
      - Loss of PTCs may be appreciated with stain for endothelial cells (e.g., CD34)
      - PTC loss correlates with increasing serum creatinine
  - Peritubular capillaritis
    - Mononuclear cells in PTCs, particularly moderate to severe (Banff ptc > 1), often seen in chronic AMR
    - May precede development of TG or other chronic AMR features in presensitized patients with normal graft function
      - Often seen on protocol biopsy of presensitized patients (sometimes termed "smoldering" or "indolent" AMR)
- Arteries
  - Transplant arteriopathy (chronic allograft arteriopathy)
    - Fibrous intimal thickening of arteries
    - Inflammatory cells present within thickened intima
      - CD3(+) T cells &/or CD68(+) monocytes/macrophages

ANCILLARY TESTS

Immunohistochemistry

- C4d deposition in PTCs
  - Can be quite focal or absent
  - Not required for diagnosis of chronic AMR if other evidence of antibody interacting with endothelium (e.g., capillaritis)
- Glomerular capillary C4d
  - Glomerular staining for C4d in paraffin sections suggestive of chronic AMR
    - Also seen in immune complex glomerulonephritis
- Cells in peritubular and glomerular capillaries are CD16(+) (many), CD68(+) (many), CD56(+) (few), CD3(+) (few)

Immunofluorescence

- PTC C4d may be diffuse, focal, or negative
  - Not required for diagnosis of chronic AMR if other evidence of antibody interacting with endothelium (e.g., capillaritis)
  - ~ 60% of TG cases are C4d(-) on biopsy
    - Antibody levels and C4d deposition can fluctuate with time
    - May be less active process at time of biopsy
    - C4d(-) cases may represent non-complement-fixing DSA
- IF more sensitive and easier to interpret than IHC on formalin-fixed, paraffin-embedded tissue except for glomeruli
  - Mesangium normally positive for C4d in frozen tissue, not fixed tissue
- Immunoglobulins usually negative, except for segmental IgM and C3
  - Chronic AMR can be associated with de novo membranous glomerulonephritis

Electron Microscopy

- Duplication of GBM, often with multilamination extending circumferentially
  - Hypertrophied endothelium, loss of fenestrae and vacuolization
  - Mesangial cell interposition
  - Early changes detected by EM before development of TG by light microscopy (Banff cg 1a)
    - Subendothelial lucency
    - Subendothelial serration of GBM with early GBM duplication
    - Present as early as 3 months post transplant
- Circumferential PTC basement membrane multilamination (PTCBMML)
  - Grading
    - Mild: 2-4 layers
    - Moderate: 5-6 layers
    - Severe: 7 or more layers
  - Greater specificity for chronic AMR with higher grade
  - Proposed criteria for severe PTCBMML
    - 1 PTC with ≥ 7 layers and at least 2 with ≥ 5 layers
    - Based on 3 most affected of 15-20 PTC examined
    - Present in 83% with C4d(+) chronic AMR
    - 1% of native kidneys

Gene Expression

- Endothelial gene expression (mRNA microarrays)
  - von Willebrand factor, *CD31*, *CD34*, *CD62e*, *CAV-1*, and others
- NK gene expression (*CXCR1*, *NKp80*, *MYBL1*, and others)
- Can detect evidence of chronic AMR in absence of C4d

DIFFERENTIAL DIAGNOSIS

Transplant Glomerulopathy

- Chronic thrombotic microangiopathy
  - Lacks capillaritis and C4d in PTC
- Recurrent or de novo immune complex glomerulonephritis (MPGN, HCV, and others)
  - GBM immune deposits seen by immunofluorescence and electron microscopy

Transplant Arteriopathy

- Arteriosclerosis
  - Fibroelastosis more prominent than transplant arteriopathy
  - Paucity of inflammatory cells
  - Transplant arteriopathy may be indistinguishable from arteriosclerosis due to hypertension
- May be due to AMR, T-cell-mediated rejection, or both
  - C4d and presence of DSA argue for component of chronic AMR
- Thrombotic microangiopathy
  - Arteries may show endothelialitis and intimal thickening

Peritubular Capillaropathy

- Mild or segmental PTCBMML seen in various nonspecific causes (e.g., acute tubular injury)

Peritubular Capillary Margination

- Acute T-cell-mediated rejection type 1 (TCMR)
  - 50% of TCMR has capillaritis

Scoring of Chronic AMR Lesions

Score	Description
Transplant Glomerulopathy	
cg0	No GBM double contours by light microscopy or EM
cg1a	No GBM double contours by light microscopy but GBM double contours in ≥ 3 glomerular capillaries by EM with associated endothelial swelling &/or subendothelial electron lucent widening
cg1b	≥ 1 glomerular capillary with GBM double contours in 1 glomerulus by light microscopy; EM confirmation recommended, if available
cg2	GBM double contours in 26-50% of peripheral capillary loops in most affected nonsclerotic glomerulus
cg3	GBM double contours in > 50% of peripheral capillary loops in most affected nonsclerotic glomerulus
Peritubular Capillaritis	
ptc0	Peritubular capillary (PTC) inflammation in < 10% of cortex
ptc1	PTC inflammation in ≥ 10% of cortex, with 3-4 marginated luminal inflammatory cells in most affected capillary
ptc2	PTC inflammation in ≥ 10% of cortex, with 5-10 marginated luminal inflammatory cells in most affected capillary
ptc3	PTC inflammation in ≥ 10% of cortex, with > 10 marginated luminal inflammatory cells in most affected capillary
Peritubular Capillaropathy (by EM)	
Mild	≤ 3 circumferential layers in 3 PTCs
Moderate	4-6 circumferential layers in 1 or 2 PTCs
Severe	1 PTC with ≥ 7 layers and at least 2 with ≥ 5 layers by EM

- Also has interstitial inflammation and tubulitis
- May be superimposed on chronic AMR
- Acute AMR
    - Usually more neutrophils and less capillaritis
    - Clinical presentation of acute renal failure
    - May superimposed on chronic AMR

Accommodation

- C4d deposition without histologic evidence of rejection
    - 2-6% of HLA incompatible grafts in protocol biopsies
        - Probably not "stable" accommodation
        - Considered stage II of chronic AMR
    - Present in > 90% of ABO incompatible grafts
        - Apparently stable if no concurrent anti-HLA DSA

DIAGNOSTIC CHECKLIST

Pathologic Interpretation Pearls

- Less extensive (or negative) C4d deposition in chronic AMR compared with acute AMR

REPORTING

Diagnostic Criteria for Chronic AMR (Banff 2013)

- 1. Histologic evidence of tissue injury
    - Transplant glomerulopathy
    - Severe PTC membrane multilamination
    - Transplant arteriopathy
- 2. Evidence of current or recent antibody interaction with vascular endothelium
    - At least 1 of the following must be present
        - C4d deposition in PTCs (≥ C4d2 by IF or > C4d0 by IHC)
        - Microvascular inflammation (g+ptc ≥ 2)
        - Molecular markers of endothelial activation (if validated)
- 3. Serologic evidence of DSA
- All 3 criteria required for diagnosis; if only 2 present, considered "suspicious" for chronic AMR

SELECTED REFERENCES

1. Cornell LD et al: Positive crossmatch kidney transplant recipients treated with eculizumab: outcomes beyond 1 year. Am J Transplant. 15(5):1293-302, 2015
2. Haas M et al: Banff 2013 meeting report: inclusion of c4d-negative antibody-mediated rejection and antibody-associated arterial lesions. Am J Transplant. 14(2):272-83, 2014
3. Bentall A et al: Five-year outcomes in living donor kidney transplants with a positive crossmatch. Am J Transplant. 13(1):76-85, 2013
4. Everly MJ et al: Incidence and impact of de novo donor-specific alloantibody in primary renal allografts. Transplantation. 95(3):410-7, 2013
5. Hirohashi T et al: A novel pathway of chronic allograft rejection mediated by NK cells and alloantibody. Am J Transplant. 12(2):313-21, 2012
6. Liapis G et al: Diagnostic significance of peritubular capillary basement membrane multilaminations in kidney allografts: old concepts revisited. Transplantation. 94(6):620-9, 2012
7. Wiebe C et al: Evolution and clinical pathologic correlations of de novo donor-specific HLA antibody post kidney transplant. Am J Transplant. 12(5):1157-67, 2012
8. Baid-Agrawal S et al: Overlapping pathways to transplant glomerulopathy: chronic humoral rejection, hepatitis C infection, and thrombotic microangiopathy. Kidney Int. 80(8):879-85, 2011
9. Hill GS et al: Donor-specific antibodies accelerate arteriosclerosis after kidney transplantation. J Am Soc Nephrol. 22(5):975-83, 2011
10. Gaston RS et al: Evidence for antibody-mediated injury as a major determinant of late kidney allograft failure. Transplantation. 90(1):68-74, 2010
11. Loupy A et al: Outcome of subclinical antibody-mediated rejection in kidney transplant recipients with preformed donor-specific antibodies. Am J Transplant. 9(11):2561-70, 2009
12. Sis B et al: Endothelial gene expression in kidney transplants with alloantibody indicates antibody-mediated damage despite lack of C4d staining. Am J Transplant. 9(10):2312-23, 2009
13. Issa N et al: Transplant glomerulopathy: risk and prognosis related to anti-human leukocyte antigen class II antibody levels. Transplantation. 86(5):681-5, 2008
14. Smith RN et al: Four stages and lack of stable accommodation in chronic alloantibody-mediated renal allograft rejection in Cynomolgus monkeys. Am J Transplant. 8(8):1662-72, 2008
15. Regele H et al: Capillary deposition of complement split product C4d in renal allografts is associated with basement membrane injury in peritubular and glomerular capillaries: a contribution of humoral immunity to chronic allograft rejection. J Am Soc Nephrol. 13(9):2371-80, 2002

(Left) *From low magnification, peritubular capillaritis may be inconspicuous; here, focal PTCs are dilated → and contain marginated inflammatory cells ⇨. There is minimal interstitial fibrosis.* **(Right)** *Intracapillary mononuclear cells → are typically prominent in chronic AMR, with fewer neutrophils. PTCs are dilated in both as shown here. This patient was 4 years post kidney/liver transplantation and had TG and positive C4d. The liver does not completely protect the kidney from AMR.*

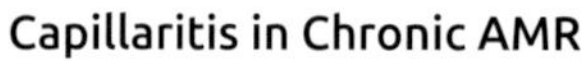

Capillaritis in Chronic AMR

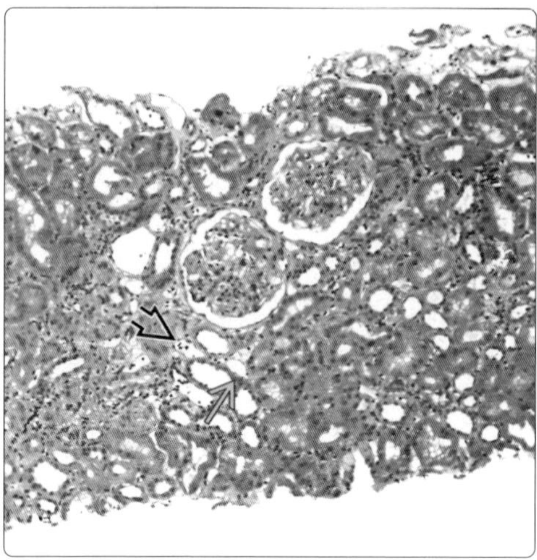

Peritubular Capillaritis

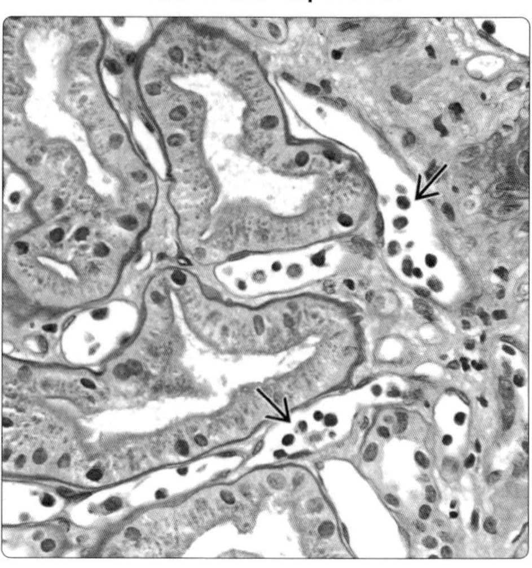

(Left) *Immunoperoxidase stain in paraffin-embedded tissue from a patient with TG and DSA shows rare PTCs positive for C4d →. In contrast, the frozen tissue, which is usually more sensitive, was more extensively positive.* **(Right)** *C4d may be extensive (as in this case) or even negative in chronic AMR. Diffuse C4d in this setting is associated with noncompliance, a more acute onset of graft dysfunction and later graft loss. This patient also had de novo membranous GN.*

Focal C4d Positivity in Chronic AMR

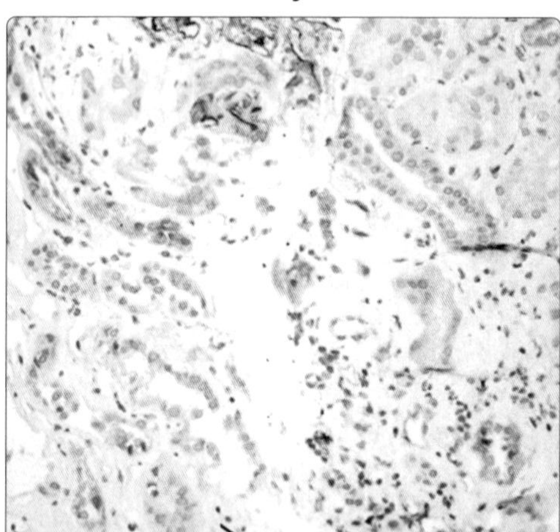

Prominent C4d in Chronic AMR

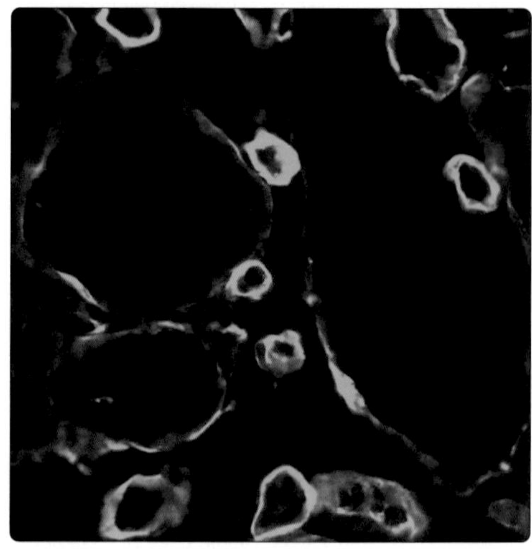

(Left) *The cells in PTC are mostly mononuclear cells, which stain for CD68, typical of monocytes/macrophages. The other cells detected by IHC include NK cells and T cells.* **(Right)** *Occasional mononuclear CD56(+) cells ↷, presumably NK cells, can be seen in PTC in chronic AMR. CD56 is on immature NK cells and is lost as the NK cell becomes activated and increases CD16. NK cells are difficult to identify by IHC or IF, since they have no unique surface marker.*

Macrophages in PTC

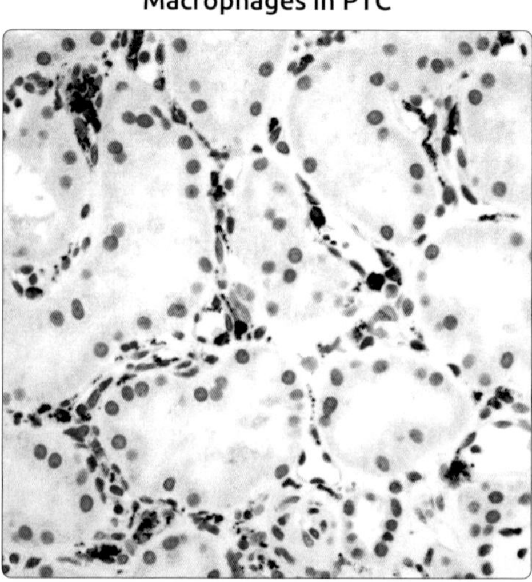

NK Cells in PTC

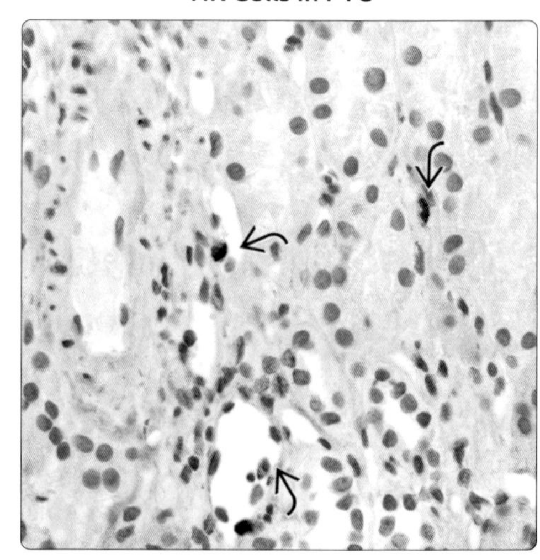

Transplant Glomerulopathy and Glomerulitis

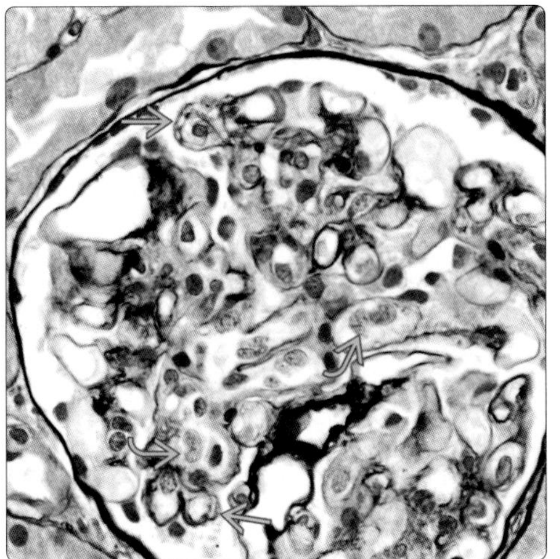

Glomerulitis and TG

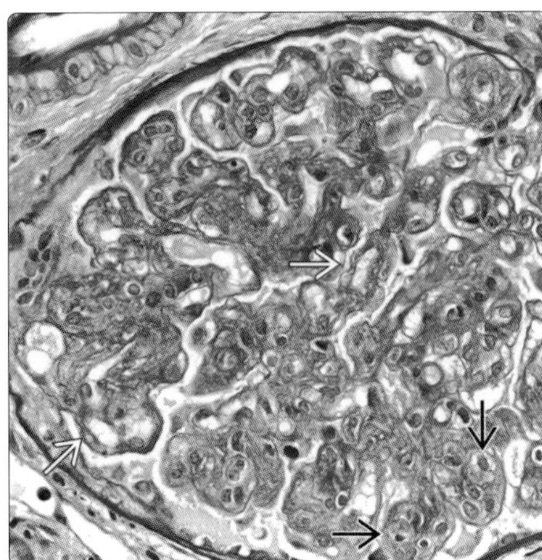

(Left) *Glomerular basement membrane duplication ⇨ is seen in this example of TG due to chronic AMR 11 years after positive-crossmatch kidney transplantation. Endothelial cells are enlarged. Endocapillary hypercellularity is also present ⇨. By IF, there was focal C4d positivity in PTC.* **(Right)** *PAS shows TG with prominent intracapillary mononuclear inflammatory cells (glomerulitis) ⇨, a common feature. Duplication of the GBM is also evident ➡. Patient had class II DSA, and PTCs were positive for C4d.*

CD16(+) (FcγRIII) Cells in Chronic AMR

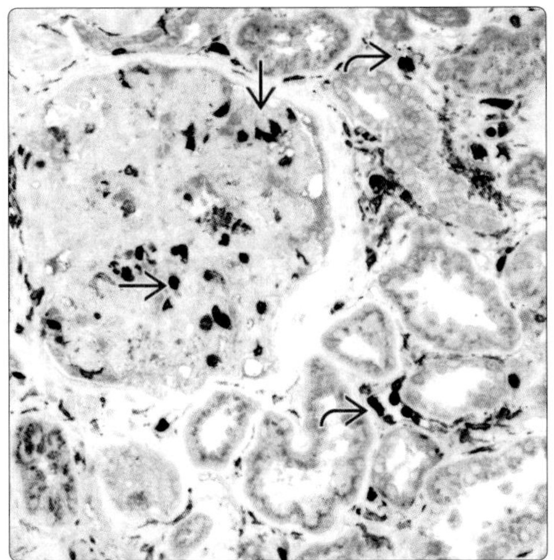

Duplication of GBM

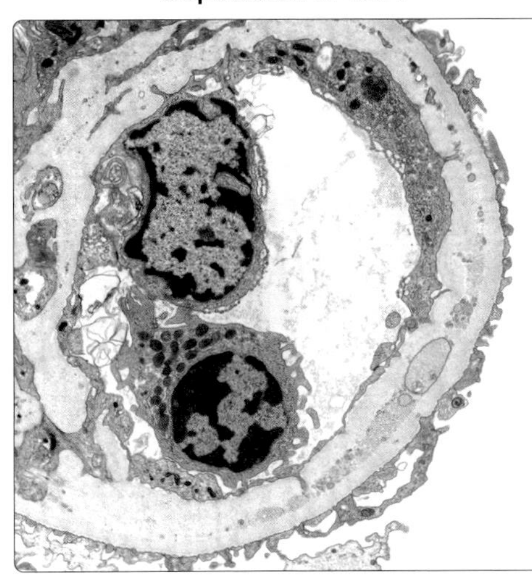

(Left) *Numerous leukocytes stain for the FcγRIII receptor (CD16) in glomerular ⇨ and peritubular capillaries ⇨ in a case of chronic AMR 23 years post transplant. Monocytes and NK cells express CD16.* **(Right)** *Transplant glomerulopathy is defined as duplication of the GBM as shown here in a biopsy 5 years post transplant. The endothelium is reactive with increased organelles and loss of fenestrations. A lymphocyte is in the lumen in contact with the endothelium. C4d was focally positive.*

Advances Transplant Glomerulopathy

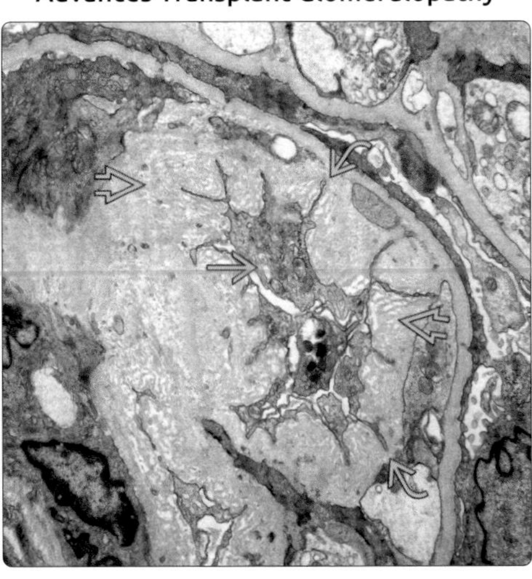

Starburst Activated Endothelium

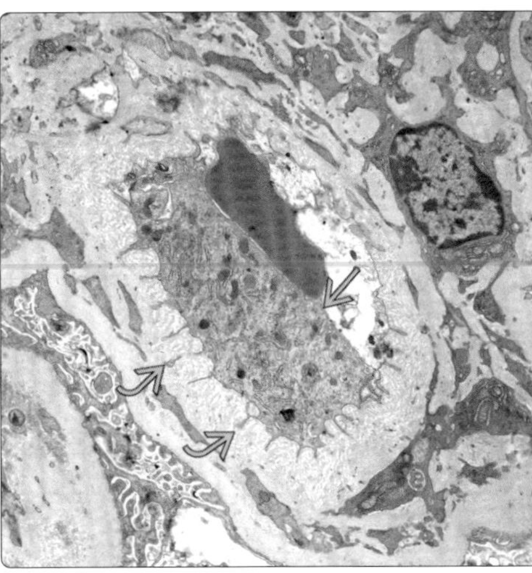

(Left) *Some capillary loops show GBM duplication and multilamination ⇨. Note the enlarged endothelial cell ⇨ with processes extending into crevasses in the GBM layers ⇨.* **(Right)** *Activation of the glomerular endothelium shown here is manifested by loss of fenestrations and increase in the volume and organelles of the cytoplasm ⇨. Cell processes extend ⇨ into the neo-GBM in a distinctive starburst pattern.*

(Left) *Chronic AMR evolves through stages, beginning with production of de novo DSA and progressing to clinically evident chronic AMR. C4d and DSA may be intermittently present during this time. The time between stages is unknown.* **(Right)** *A 4-month protocol biopsy from a positive-crossmatch transplant patient with stable renal function is shown. Mononuclear cells are marginated within peritubular capillaries ⇒. Glomeruli show no evidence of TG. A C4d stain was negative.*

Stages of Chronic AMR

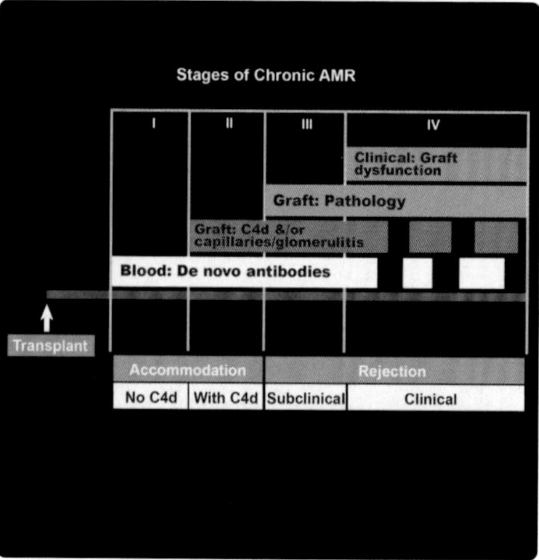

Stage II: Peritubular Capillaritis and Glomerulitis

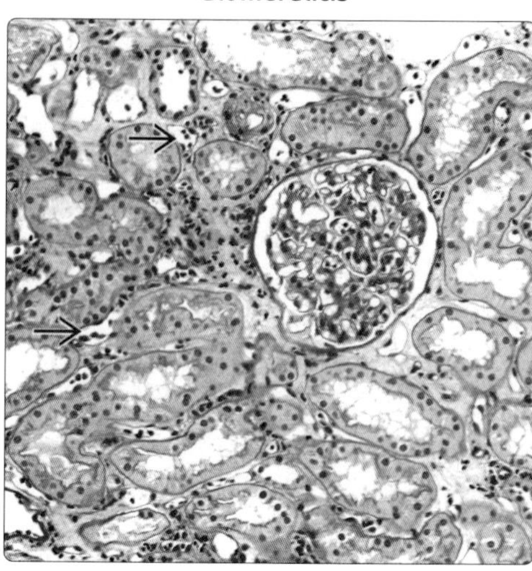

(Left) *This protocol biopsy is from a patient with normal renal function and a positive DSA (class II). The only abnormality is the presence of prominent C4d in PTC ⇒ and glomeruli. No capillaritis was evident. Four years later, the patient developed chronic AMR.* **(Right)** *Electron microscopy can reveal early features predictive of later development of TG: Subendothelial lucency ⇒, enlarged endothelial cells ⇒, and corrugation of the GBM ⇒ are seen here before duplication is evident on light microscopy.*

Stage II With C4d and No Injury

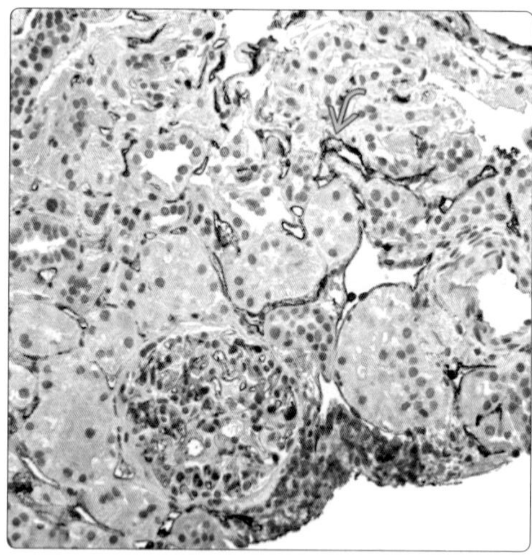

Early Ultrastructural Lesions (cg1a)

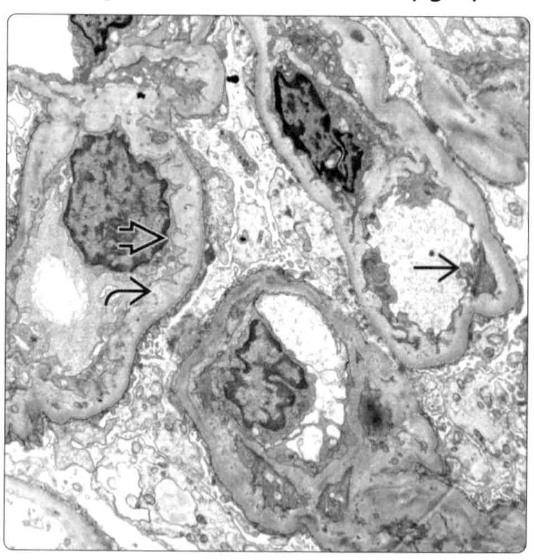

(Left) *A normal glomerulus is seen on biopsy 6 months post transplant from a patient with graft dysfunction due to acute AMR. There was class II DSA and C4d deposition.* **(Right)** *Evolution of glomerular changes is seen 6 years after an acute AMR episode. The patient presented with elevated Cr, proteinuria, persistent class II DSA, and positive C4d. Glomerulitis ⇒ and GBM duplication ⇒ are prominent in this hypertrophied glomerulus. The graft was lost 18 months later.*

Acute AMR With Normal Glomerulus

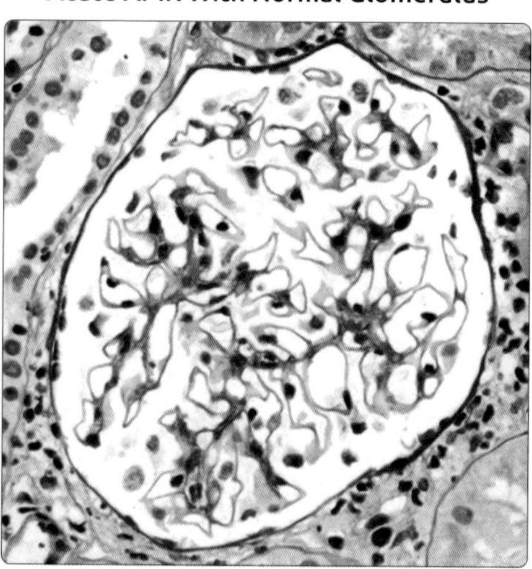

Acute AMR Sequelae of Chronic AMR

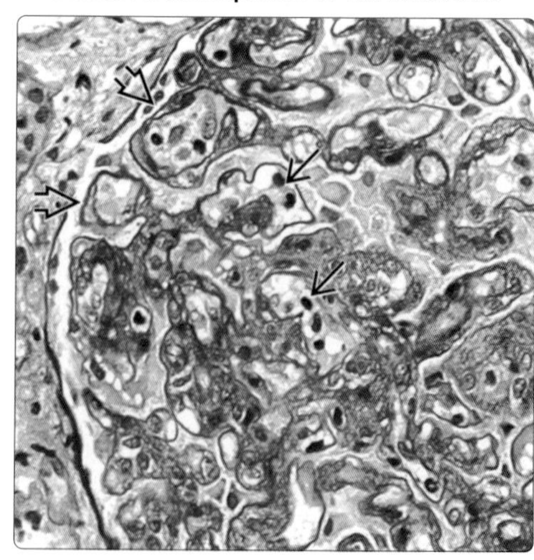

Peritubular Capillaropathy

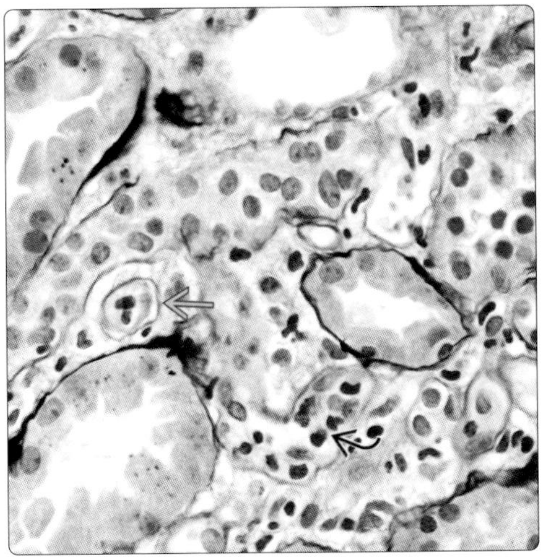

Peritubular Capillaropathy

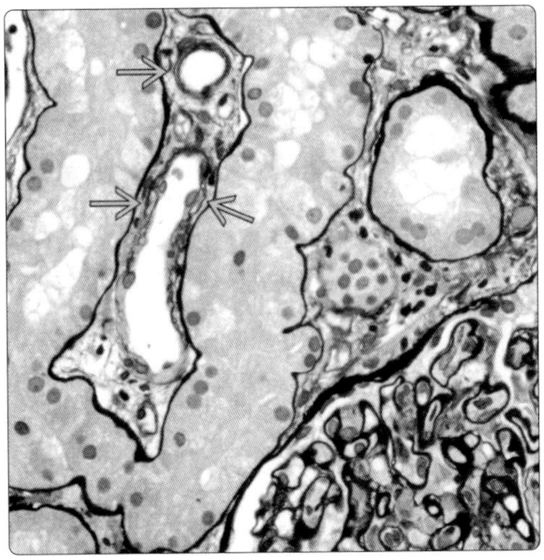

(Left) *Sometimes peritubular capillaropathy can be seen on a silver stains, with basement membrane duplication ➔ or multilayering, although this finding is best seen by EM. Peritubular capillaritis ➔ is also seen here.* **(Right)** *Peritubular capillary basement membrane duplication and multilayering ➔ is seen on a silver stain. These capillaries do not show marginated mononuclear cells, although they are typically present.*

Reactive Endothelium in PTCs

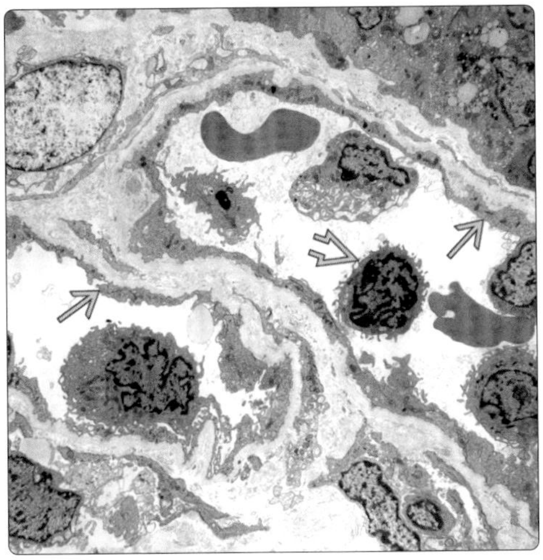

Severe Peritubular Capillaropathy

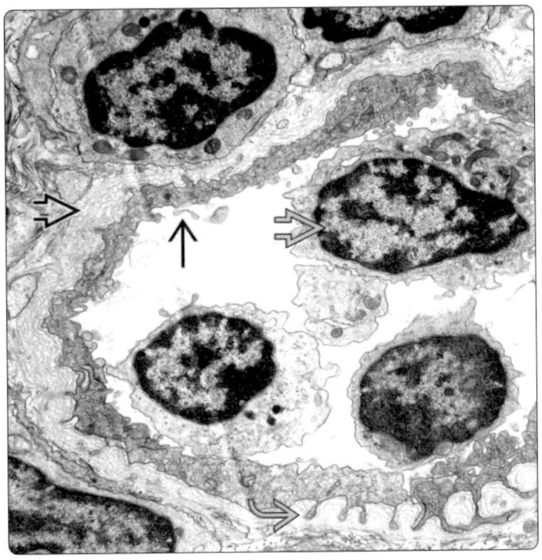

(Left) *Mononuclear cells ➔ in PTC are associated with reactive endothelium ➔. This patient presented with proteinuria (2.8 g/day) and elevated Cr (2 mg/dL) 6 years post transplant. C4d was positive.* **(Right)** *This case shows circumferential PTCBMML ➔ along with activated endothelial cells and marginated mononuclear leukocytes ➔ within the capillary. Endothelial cells are enlarged and show loss of fenestrations, microvillus changes ➔, and a starburst pattern ➔ of extension into the neo-BM.*

Mixed TCMR and AMR

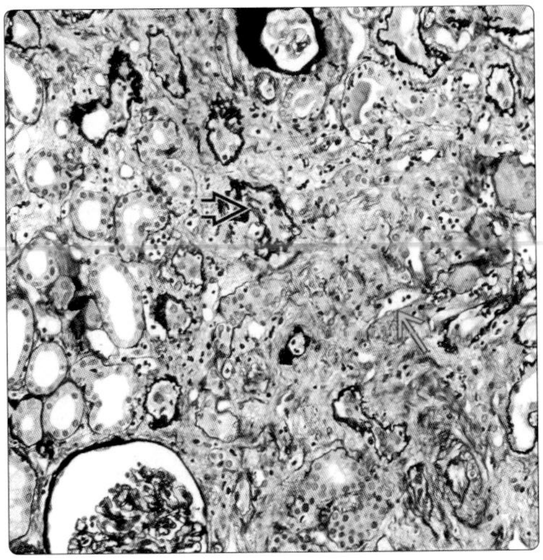

Mixed TCMR and AMR

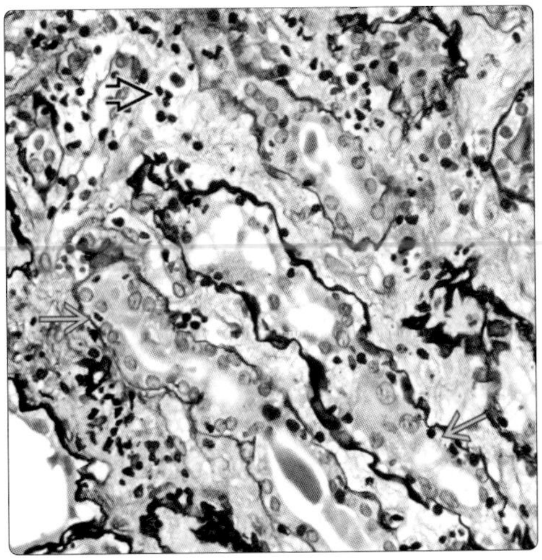

(Left) *Mixed chronic TCMR and AMR is shown, with interstitial inflammation and early fibrosis, tubulitis ➔ in partially atrophic tubules, and peritubular capillaritis ➔. The C4d stain was positive in focal PTCs by IF.* **(Right)** *Tubulitis ➔ is present in partially atrophic tubules, a feature often seen in mixed cellular and humoral rejection that is ongoing. Peritubular capillaritis ➔ is present as well.*

(Left) *Venn diagram shows differential diagnosis of TG. Most cases are due to CHR (57% C4d[+], DSA), but other causes include chronic TMA (13%), hepatitis C virus (4%), MPGN (2%), and idiopathic (24%).* **(Right)** *Renal transplant biopsy with TG is due to TMA, associated with calcineurin inhibitor toxicity and severe arteriolar hyalinosis collapsing FSGS. Duplication of GBM and intracapillary leukocytes are conspicuous, but the C4d stain was negative.*

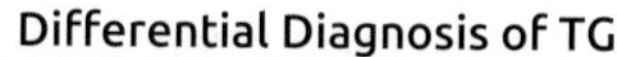

Differential Diagnosis of TG

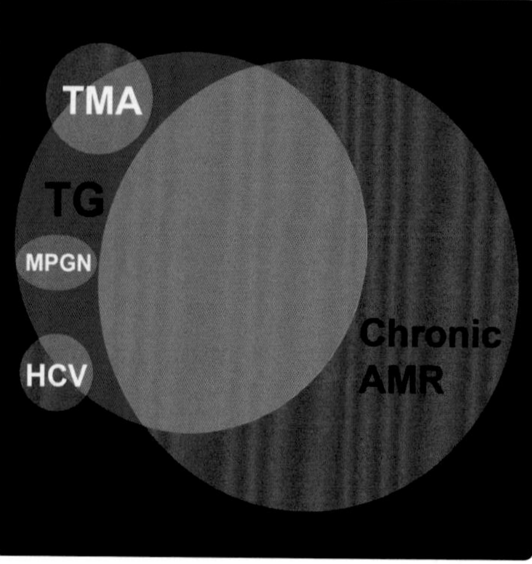

Chronic Thrombotic Microangiopathy

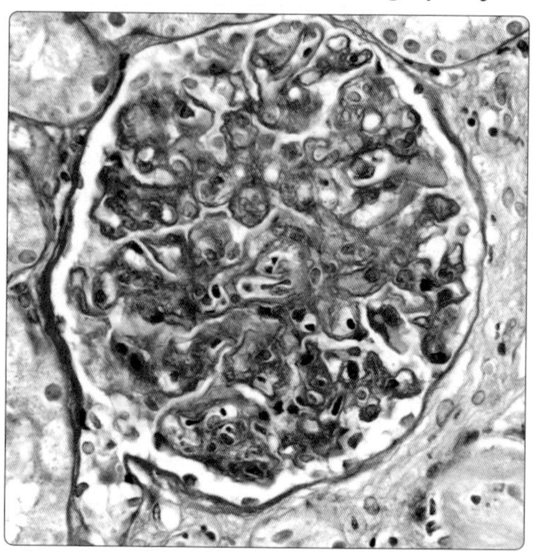

(Left) *Collapsing glomerulopathy and thrombotic microangiopathy in an allograft with chronic calcineurin inhibitor toxicity. GBM duplication ⇒ due to TMA can resemble chronic AMR and is one of the causes of transplant glomerulopathy.* **(Right)** *MPGN, which may mimic transplant glomerulopathy, is distinguished by prominent mesangial and subendothelial deposits by EM ⇒ and C3 ± immunoglobulin by IF.*

Collapsing Glomerulopathy

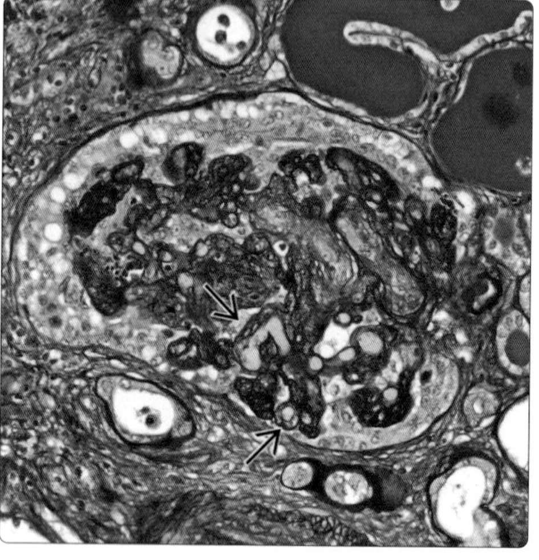

Membranoproliferative Glomerulonephritis (MPGN)

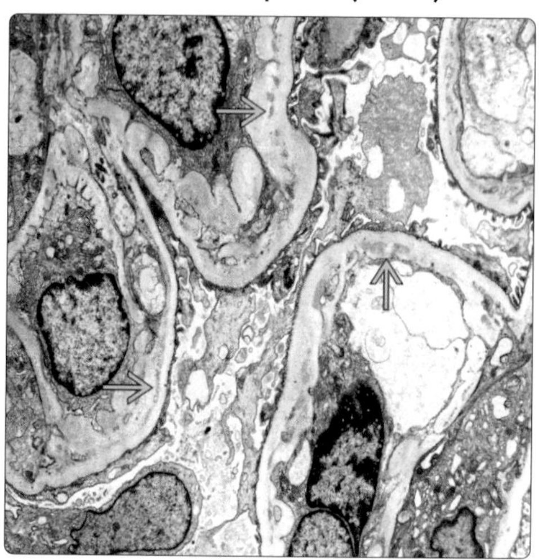

(Left) *This biopsy 6 years post transplant from a nonadherent recipient shows duplication of the GBM ⇗, endothelial swelling and loss of fenestrations ⇒, and foot process effacement ⇒. The serrated subepithelial GBM ⇨ is due to de novo membranous GN* **(Right)** *This patient developed proteinuria 6 years post transplant (original disease obstructive uropathy). The prominent IgG along the GBM is not typical of chronic AMR alone. PTCs were C4d(+). EM showed subepithelial serrations and occasional deposits.*

Transplant Glomerulopathy With De Novo Membranous GN

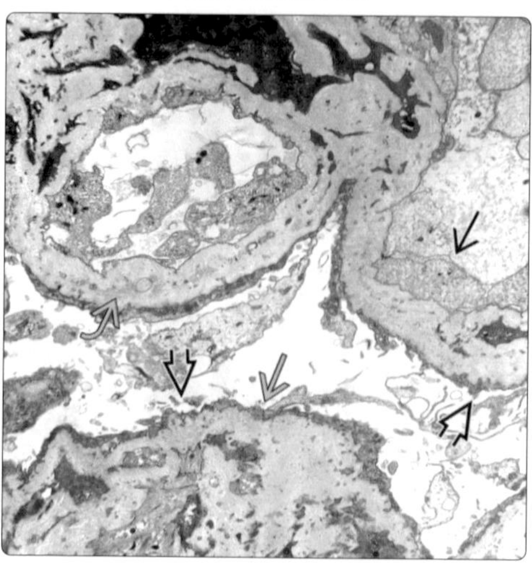

De Novo Membranous GN and Chronic AMR

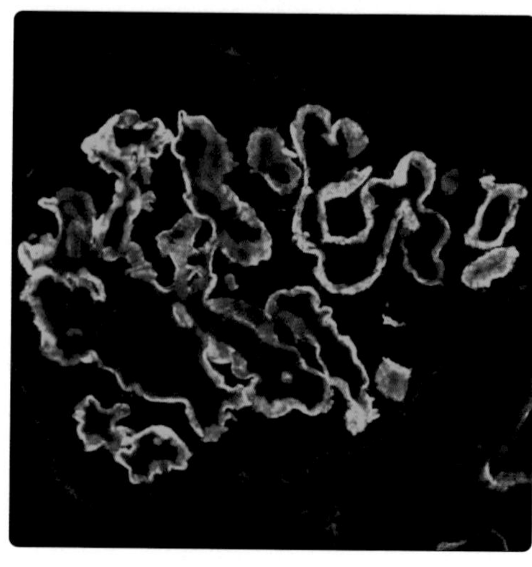

Acute and Chronic TCMR and AMR

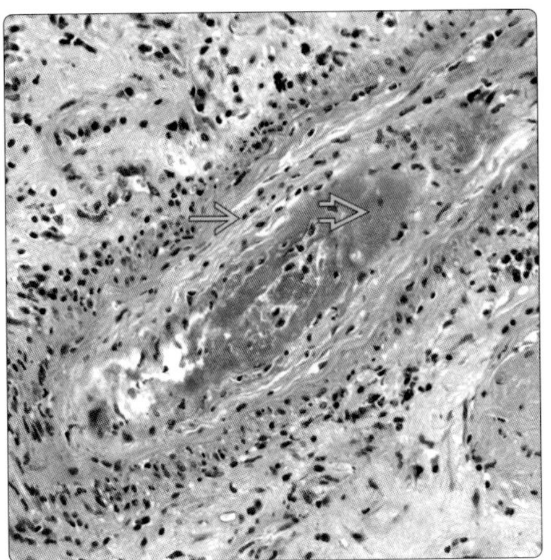

Transplant Arteriopathy

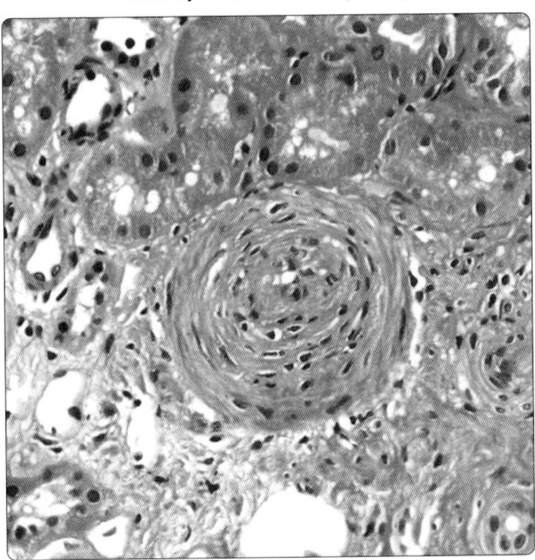

(Left) *This case shows features of acute and chronic rejection, with T-cell-mediated and antibody-mediated rejection. Intimal thickening with inflammatory cells ⇒ is a lesion of chronic rejection, while fibrin ⇒ is a feature seen in acute AMR. A C4d stain was positive.* **(Right)** *Transplant arteriopathy has severe narrowing of the arterial lumen. This biopsy also showed transplant glomerulopathy. The C4d was negative; the patient had a donor-specific HLA class II antibody.*

Arteriosclerosis

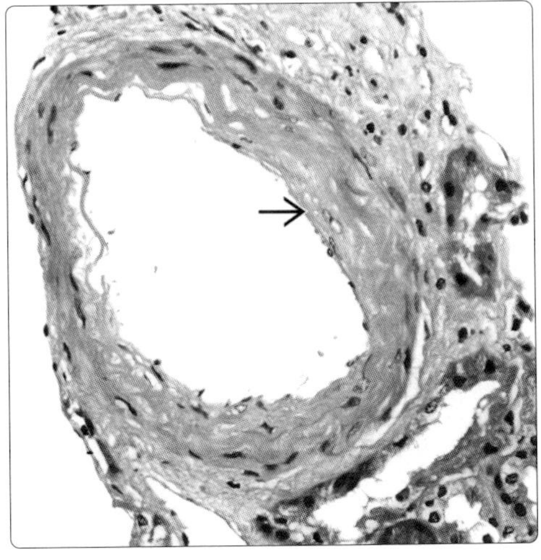

Accelerated Arteriosclerosis

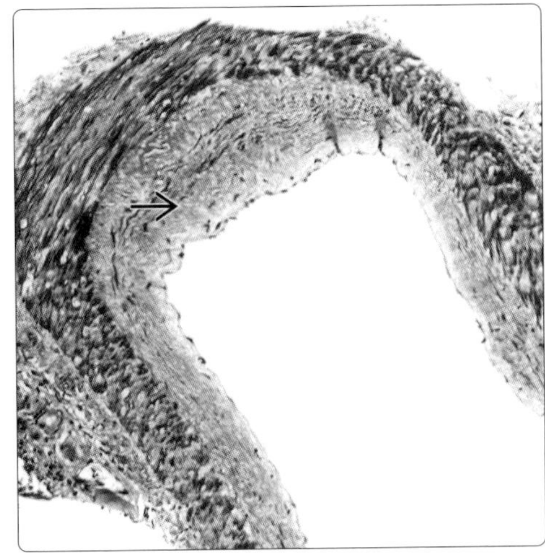

(Left) *A typical lesion of arteriosclerosis due to hypertension shows intimal thickening ⇒, but without inflammation.* **(Right)** *A biopsy from a positive-crossmatch transplant patient shows accelerated arteriosclerosis with a thickened intima ⇒ of an artery. This appearance can be identical to arteriosclerosis due to hypertension but still may represent transplant arteriopathy.*

Transplant Arteriopathy

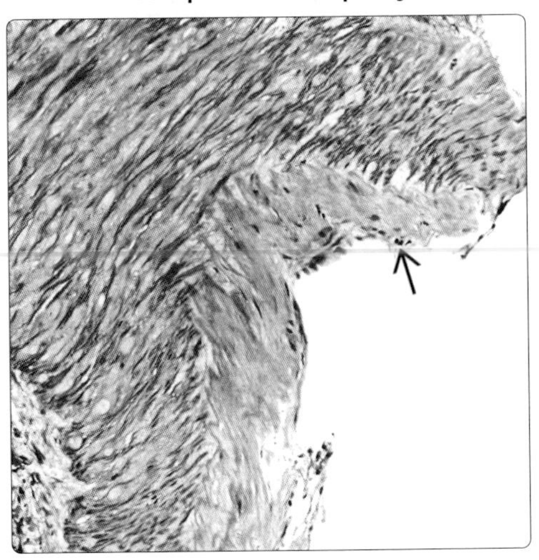

Thrombotic Microangiopathy

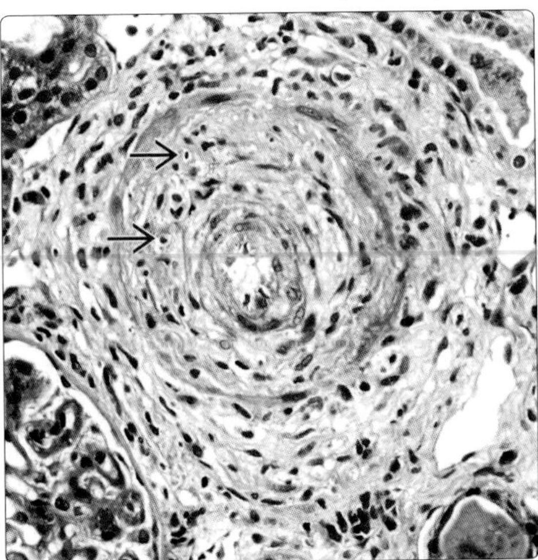

(Left) *This artery shows fibrous intimal thickening and segmental endothelialitis ⇒; the minimal endothelialitis represents a lesion of rejection (either AMR or TCMR).* **(Right)** *This example of arterial intimal thickening resembles transplant arteriopathy, even with inflammatory cells in the thickened intima ⇒ but was seen in a native kidney. This lesion is suggestive of antiphospholipid antibody syndrome in the native kidney.*

Diseases That Recur in Allografts

KEY FACTS

CLINICAL ISSUES

- Recurrent glomerular disease is 3rd leading cause of graft failure
  - Recurrence rates vary by specific disease
  - FSGS, atypical HUS and MPGN have greatest impact on graft survival
  - Timing of recurrence varies from minutes (FSGS) to years (diabetic glomerulopathy)
- Diseases may recur subclinically
- Documentation of primary cause of ESRD essential to diagnose recurrence

MICROSCOPIC

- Pathology resembles primary disease but not identical
  - Diagnosis of recurrent glomerular disease usually requires IF and EM
- Superimposed features of chronic rejection or drug toxicity may be present
- Early stages of recurrent disease appreciated on early protocol biopsies or biopsies performed for other indication (e.g., with acute rejection)

TOP DIFFERENTIAL DIAGNOSES

- De novo disease
  - Early onset (< 1-2 years) favors recurrence of immune complex glomerulonephritis
- Acute transplant glomerulitis
- Transplant glomerulopathy (chronic humoral rejection, hepatitis C infection, &/or chronic thrombotic microangiopathy)

DIAGNOSTIC CHECKLIST

- Must ascertain primary kidney disease
- Prepare to perform IF and EM, particularly if signs of glomerular disease on biopsy > 1 year post transplant

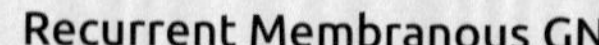

Recurrent Membranous GN

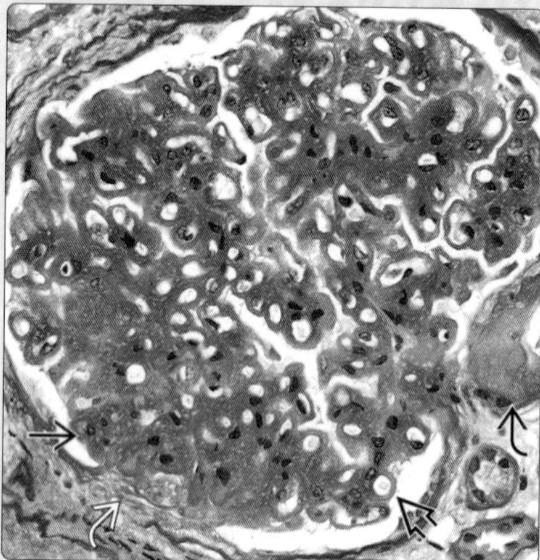

Recurrent Membranous GN, IgG

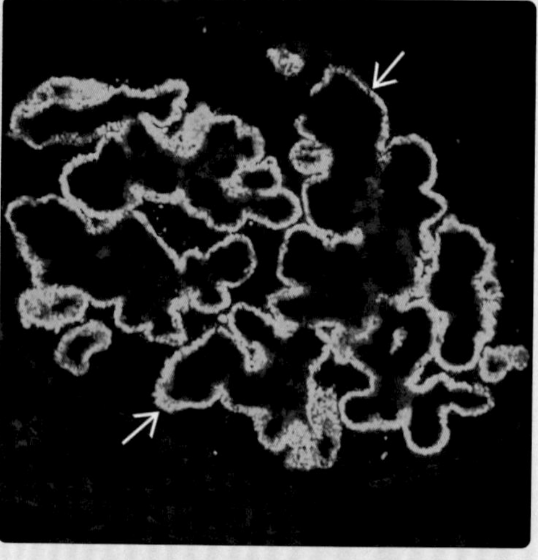

(Left) *Periodic acid-Schiff shows marked thickening of the GBMs → with a vacuolated appearance, characteristic of membranous GN. Other injuries include segmental glomerular scarring → with a fibrous attachment → to the Bowman capsule and marked arteriolar hyalinosis → in this 7-year-old allograft.* **(Right)** *Immunofluorescence for IgG shows strong granular staining of the glomerular capillary walls → in an allograft with recurrent membranous GN.*

Recurrent FSGS

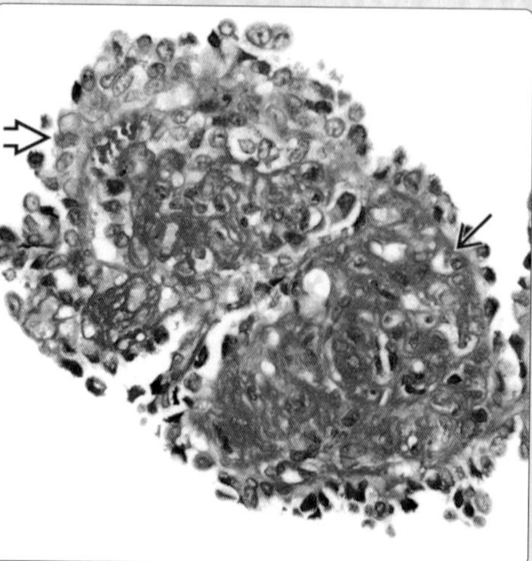

Diffuse Foot Process Effacement

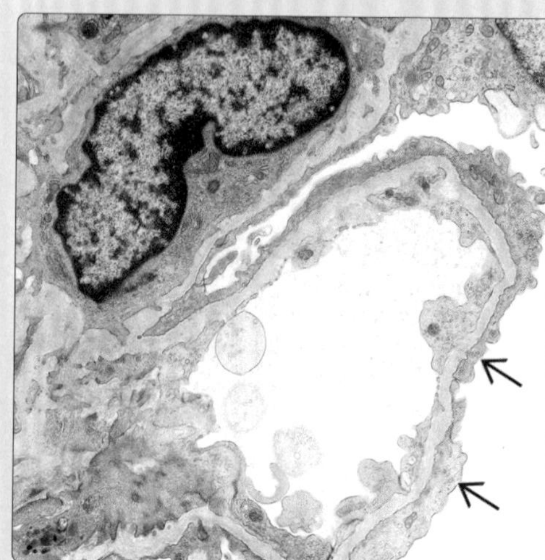

(Left) *Periodic acid-Schiff highlights collapsed glomerular tufts → with prominence of podocytes →. Recurrence of collapsing FSGS may manifest with either collapsing or noncollapsing segmental sclerosis.* **(Right)** *Electron microscopy shows extensive effacement of the podocyte foot processes → in this biopsy with recurrence of FSGS within 2 weeks after renal transplantation.*

TERMINOLOGY

Abbreviations

- Membranous glomerulonephritis (MGN)
- Focal segmental glomerulosclerosis (FSGS)
- Membranoproliferative glomerulonephritis (MPGN)
- Hemolytic uremic syndrome (HUS)

Definitions

- Recurrence of original cause of end-stage renal disease after kidney transplantation

ETIOLOGY/PATHOGENESIS

Proposed Mechanisms

- Pathogenesis of recurrence presumably same as original disease
  - Recurrence often as evidence for circulating factor
    - Give insights into mechanism and early stages
  - Immunosuppressive medications and allogeneic kidney may alter pathogenesis and disease course in allograft
- Primary FSGS (nonfamilial)
  - Humoral or permeability factor postulated due to rapid recurrence after kidney transplantation in nonhereditary etiologies
    - Soluble urokinase-type plasminogen activator receptor (suPAR) as possible candidate
      - Recent significant doubts on specificity of suPAR for primary FSGS
    - Cardiotrophin-like cytokine-1 also possible candidate
  - Hereditary causes generally do not recur
    - *NPHS1* (nephrin) mutation: Antinephrin alloantibodies lead to podocyte injury and proteinuria (not true "recurrence")
    - *NPHS2* (podocin) mutation: Recurrence may be steroid responsive, even if original disease was steroid resistant
- MGN
  - Circulating antibodies against antiphospholipase A2 receptor (PLA2R) in most adults
    - Anti-PLA2R at transplant associated with disease recurrence in allograft
- MPGN
  - Varying causes; some due to defect in complement regulation
  - Immunoglobulin and complement deposits in glomeruli
- C3 glomerulopathy
  - Includes dense deposit disease and C3 GN
  - Due to inherited or acquired defect in regulation of alternative complement pathway
  - Immunofluorescence (IF) staining for C3 only or C3 with sparse immunoglobulin deposits
    - Native kidney disease often misdiagnosed as postinfectious GN or MPGN before description of C3 GN
- Atypical HUS
  - *CFH* (complement factor H) and *FI* (factor I) mutations
    - Recurrence rate is 80% for *CFH* and 90% for *FI* mutations
    - CFH and FI synthesized by liver
    - Simultaneous liver and kidney transplantation is treatment option
  - *CD46* (membrane cofactor protein) mutation
    - 20% recurrence rate
    - Normal CD46 in kidney allograft corrects defect
  - Some immunosuppressive medications cause thrombotic microangiopathy
    - May potentiate underlying propensity to form thrombi
- Proliferative GN with monoclonal IgG deposits (PGMID)
  - Deposition of monoclonal immunoglobulin in glomeruli of allograft
  - Monoclonal protein may not be detectable in serum or in urine pre- or post transplant
    - Detectable in allograft
    - IgG3-kappa (most common)
  - Recurrent PGMID with more aggressive clinical course
    - May recur in absence of detectable monoclonal protein
- Primary hyperoxaluria (PH) type 1
  - Gene defect for liver peroxisomal enzyme alanine:glyoxylate aminotransferase (AGT)
  - Impaired metabolism of glyoxylate to glycine
  - End-stage renal disease due to oxalate nephropathy
  - Liver transplantation cures enzyme defect
    - Performed in combination with kidney transplantation for patients not responsive to pyridoxine therapy
    - Kidney transplantation alone considered for patients with pyridoxine responsiveness

CLINICAL ISSUES

Epidemiology

- Incidence
  - Recurrent disease causes > 15% of allograft loss
    - Most common recurrent diseases that cause graft loss are FSGS, IgA nephropathy, MGN, and MPGN

Presentation

- Acute renal failure
- Chronic renal failure
- Proteinuria
  - MGN
    - High recurrence rate (~ 42%)
    - Recurrence detected by biopsy as early as 2 weeks even in absence of proteinuria
      - Histologic or immunophenotypic recurrence precedes proteinuria
  - FSGS
    - Proteinuria, may be nephrotic range
    - Recurrence 5x more likely in childhood onset FSGS vs. adult-onset FSGS
      - Independent of age at transplantation
    - Increased recurrence rate with living-related organ donation
    - Severe proteinuria may occur immediately post transplant
      - Lesser proteinuria may develop and become progressive over first 1-2 years post transplant
  - Amyloidosis
  - Diabetic glomerulosclerosis

- Common cause of end-stage renal disease
- Recurs later post transplant (5-10 years)
  - Common in 5- and 10-year allograft protocol biopsies
  - Recurrence more prevalent with increased graft survival
- Other glomerular diseases
- Hematuria
  - IgA nephropathy
  - MPGN
  - Lupus nephritis
  - Pauci-immune (antineutrophil cytoplasmic antibody [ANCA]-associated) crescentic GN
  - Antiglomerular basement membrane (GBM) nephritis

Laboratory Tests

- Serologic tests
  - ANCA titer
  - Anti-GBM antibody titer
- Serum or urine protein electrophoresis, serum-free light chains

Treatment

- Surgical approaches
  - Orthotopic liver transplantation
    - Familial HUS patients with *CFH* or *FI* mutations
    - Primary hyperoxaluria
- Drugs
  - Treatment depends on specific glomerular disease
    - Increased steroids
    - Cyclophosphamide
    - Rituximab
    - Eculizumab (experimental for atypical HUS and some complement-mediated glomerulopathies)
- Plasmapheresis
  - FSGS
  - Anti-GBM disease
  - Pauci-immune (ANCA-associated) crescentic GN
  - Hemolytic uremic syndrome

Prognosis

- Variable
  - Depends on original renal disease
  - Lupus nephritis tends not to recur or recurs with minor clinical significance
- 3 diseases with worst prognosis
  - Primary FSGS
  - MPGN
  - Atypical HUS

MICROSCOPIC

Histologic Features

- Morphologic features similar to primary disease
  - May be seen at earlier stages due to concurrent immunosuppression
- MGN
  - Early recurrent MGN
    - Normal glomeruli by light microscopy
    - IF: Granular capillary wall staining for C4d, IgG, kappa, lambda
      - C3 often negative or faint
    - EM: No or very few tiny subepithelial deposits
  - Late recurrent MGN
    - Thickened appearance of GBM
    - GBM "spike" formation seen with silver stains
    - IF: Granular capillary wall IgG, kappa, lambda, C4d
      - Unlike native kidneys, C3 often negative or faint on IF
    - EM: Well-formed subepithelial deposits, like MGN in native kidney
- FSGS
  - Podocyte injury or foot process effacement precedes histologic finding of segmental sclerosis
    - Appears as minimal change disease prior to development of FSGS lesions
  - Segmental glomerular sclerosis with either similar or different features to FSGS prior to transplantation
- Lupus nephritis
  - Mesangial hypercellularity or sclerosis
  - Crescent formation or fibrinoid necrosis
  - Segmental sclerosis or prominent podocyte injury may represent unusual manifestation of recurrent disease
- IgA nephropathy
  - Glomerular alterations range from normal to marked mesangial hypercellularity with cellular crescent formation similar to disease in native kidneys
  - IF: Glomerular IgA-dominant deposits
- Complement-mediated glomerular disease

DIFFERENTIAL DIAGNOSIS

De Novo Glomerular Disease

- Biopsy documentation helps distinguish de novo from recurrent disease
- De novo MGN
  - Often occurs late (~ 5 years) post transplant
  - Associated with features of chronic humoral rejection
  - Negative for PLA2R
- De novo C1q nephropathy
  - C1q-dominant deposits in glomeruli
  - Usually clinically insignificant
- De novo diabetic glomerulosclerosis
  - Often occurs late post transplant
  - In patients who develop post-transplant diabetes (may be due to steroid use)

Acute Transplant Glomerulitis

- Prominent glomerular capillary leukocytic infiltration
  - Resembles endocapillary hypercellularity
- No glomerular immune complex deposition
- Usually associated with endothelialitis

Transplant Glomerulopathy (TG)

- Due to chronic humoral rejection or chronic thrombotic microangiopathy or associated with hepatitis C infection
- Duplication of GBM without immune complexes
- Rare immune complex deposits may be present in TG

Donor-Transmitted Glomerular Diseases

- Implantation (time zero) biopsy helps diagnose donor disease
- IgA nephropathy

- Glomerular IgA deposits in ~ 10% of normal donor biopsies
- Donor IgA nephropathy with mesangial proliferation may occur
  - IgA deposits disappear with time post transplant
- MGN
- Diabetic glomerulosclerosis

DIAGNOSTIC CHECKLIST

Pathologic Interpretation Pearls

- Knowledge of original cause of end-stage renal disease usually necessary for accurate evaluation
- Granular C4d glomerular deposition on IF raises consideration of de novo or recurrent GN
  - Mesangial C4d glomerular IF staining is normal
- Significant glomerular alterations (endocapillary proliferation, basement membrane alterations, increased circulating leukocytes) should trigger additional IF and EM studies
  - Characteristic features may not be present in early stages of recurrent GN

SELECTED REFERENCES

1. Barbour S et al: Advances in the understanding of complement mediated glomerular disease: implications for recurrence in the transplant setting. Am J Transplant. 15(2):312-9, 2015
2. Kattah A et al: Anti-phospholipase A2 receptor antibodies in recurrent membranous nephropathy. Am J Transplant. ePub, 2015
3. Green H et al: Recurrent membranoproliferative glomerulonephritis type I after kidney transplantation: a 17-year single-center experience. Transplantation. ePub, 2014
4. Von Visger JR et al: The risk of recurrent IgA nephropathy in a steroid-free protocol and other modifying immunosuppression. Clin Transplant. 28(8):845-54, 2014
5. Wühl E et al: Renal replacement therapy for rare diseases affecting the kidney: an analysis of the ERA-EDTA Registry. Nephrol Dial Transplant. 29 Suppl 4:iv1-8, 2014
6. Zand L et al: Clinical findings, pathology, and outcomes of C3GN after kidney transplantation. J Am Soc Nephrol. 25(5):1110-7, 2014
7. Kowalewska J: Pathology of recurrent diseases in kidney allografts: membranous nephropathy and focal segmental glomerulosclerosis. Curr Opin Organ Transplant. 18(3):313-8, 2013
8. Servais A et al: C3 glomerulopathy. Contrib Nephrol. 181:185-93, 2013
9. Blosser CD et al: Very early recurrence of anti-Phospholipase A2 receptor-positive membranous nephropathy after transplantation. Am J Transplant. 12(6):1637-42, 2012
10. Canaud G et al: Recurrence from primary and secondary glomerulopathy after renal transplant. Transpl Int. 25(8):812-24, 2012
11. Rodriguez EF et al: The pathology and clinical features of early recurrent membranous glomerulonephritis. Am J Transplant. 12(4):1029-38, 2012
12. Nasr SH et al: Proliferative glomerulonephritis with monoclonal IgG deposits recurs in the allograft. Clin J Am Soc Nephrol. 6(1):122-32, 2011
13. Lorenz EC et al: Recurrent membranoproliferative glomerulonephritis after kidney transplantation. Kidney Int. 77(8):721-8, 2010
14. Ponticelli C et al: Posttransplant recurrence of primary glomerulonephritis. Clin J Am Soc Nephrol. 5(12):2363-72, 2010
15. Said SM et al: C1q deposition in the renal allograft: a report of 24 cases. Mod Pathol. 23(8):1080-8, 2010
16. Czarnecki PG et al: Long-term outcome of kidney transplantation in patients with fibrillary glomerulonephritis or monoclonal gammopathy with fibrillary deposits. Kidney Int. 75(4):420-7, 2009
17. El-Zoghby ZM et al: Identifying specific causes of kidney allograft loss. Am J Transplant. 9(3):527-35, 2009
18. Boyer O et al: Complement factor H deficiency and posttransplantation glomerulonephritis with isolated C3 deposits. Am J Kidney Dis. 51(4):671-7, 2008
19. Ivanyi B: A primer on recurrent and de novo glomerulonephritis in renal allografts. Nat Clin Pract Nephrol. 4(8):446-57, 2008
20. Jeong HJ et al: Progression of renal allograft histology after renal transplantation in recurrent and nonrecurrent immunoglobulin A nephropathy. Hum Pathol. 39(10):1511-8, 2008
21. Meehan SM et al: Pauci-immune and immune glomerular lesions in kidney transplants for systemic lupus erythematosus. Clin J Am Soc Nephrol. 3(5):1469-78, 2008
22. Joshi K et al: Recurrent glomerulopathy in the renal allograft. Transplant Proc. 39(3):734-6, 2007
23. Casquero A et al: Recurrent acute postinfectious glomerulonephritis. Clin Nephrol. 66(1):51-3, 2006
24. Choy BY et al: Recurrent glomerulonephritis after kidney transplantation. Am J Transplant. 6(11):2535-42, 2006
25. Little MA et al: Severity of primary MPGN, rather than MPGN type, determines renal survival and post-transplantation recurrence risk. Kidney Int. 69(3):504-11, 2006
26. Braun MC et al: Recurrence of membranoproliferative glomerulonephritis type II in renal allografts: The North American Pediatric Renal Transplant Cooperative Study experience. J Am Soc Nephrol. 16(7):2225-33, 2005
27. Couser W: Recurrent glomerulonephritis in the renal allograft: an update of selected areas. Exp Clin Transplant. 3(1):283-8, 2005
28. Kowalewska J et al: IgA nephropathy with crescents in kidney transplant recipients. Am J Kidney Dis. 45(1):167-75, 2005
29. Soler MJ et al: Recurrence of IgA nephropathy and Henoch-Schönlein purpura after kidney transplantation: risk factors and graft survival. Transplant Proc. 37(9):3705-9, 2005
30. Floege J: Recurrent glomerulonephritis following renal transplantation: an update. Nephrol Dial Transplant. 18(7):1260-5, 2003
31. Briganti EM et al: Risk of renal allograft loss from recurrent glomerulonephritis. N Engl J Med. 347(2):103-9, 2002

Recurrent Disease After Kidney Transplantation

Renal Disease	Recurrence Rate	5-10-Year Graft Loss	Additional Features
Immune Complex Mediated			
MGN	40-50%	10-15% (10 year)	PLA2R+ in most primary MGN; GBM shows granular C4d staining with little or no C3 in recurrent MGN
IgA nephropathy/Henoch-Schönlein purpura	13-50%	10% (10 year)	IgA deposits may be seen in protocol biopsies in patients with normal function; higher rate of disease recurrence in patients on steroid-free immunosuppressive regimens
MPGN type I	19-24%	10-40%	Recurrence rate increases with successive allografts
Lupus nephritis	Up to 30%	< 5%	Glomerular immune complex deposits may be seen in protocol biopsies in patients with normal function; podocytopathy or FSGS may represent manifestation of recurrent lupus nephritis
Nonimmune Complex Mediated			
FSGS	20-40%	15-20% (10 year)	May recur with features of collapsing glomerulopathy
Diabetic nephropathy	> 50%	5%	Recurs late post transplant (5-10 years)
Complement Mediated			
Dense deposit disease (formerly MPGN type II)	> 80%	10-20%	10-20% Living-related grafts do better than deceased-donor grafts
C3 glomerulonephritis	67%	50% (~ 3 years)	
Atypical or non-Shiga toxin HUS	33-82%	40-50%	High recurrence rate for *CFH* and *FI* mutations; 20% recurrence for *CD46* mutation
Deposits With Substructure or Monoclonality			
Amyloidosis, AL type	10-30%	35%	Recurrence depends on treatment responsiveness of underlying disease
Amyloidosis, AA type	< 10%	Rare	
Proliferative glomerulonephritis with monoclonal IgG deposits	66%	50% graft loss within 2-3 years	May recur even in absence of detectable circulating monoclonal protein
Fibrillary GN	50%	20%	Monoclonal gammopathy-associated fibrillary GN likely to recur; other fibrillary GN less likely to recur; fibrillary GN may recur very late post transplant (> 15 years)
Immunotactoid glomerulopathy	Rare	Not available	
Monoclonal immunoglobulin deposition disease	70-85%	> 50%	
Crescentic GN			
Anti-GBM disease	< 5%	Rare	
Pauci-immune (ANCA-associated) crescentic GN	0-20%	10% (10 year)	Recurrent disease may spare kidney allograft
Genetic/Metabolic Disorders			
Primary hyperoxaluria type 1	90-100% if kidney transplant alone in pyridoxine-resistant patients	80-100%	Liver transplantation is curative and may obviate need for kidney transplantation; excretion of oxalate may simulate disease recurrence
Fabry disease	Low	Rare	Decreasing recurrence with advent of enzyme replacement therapy
Cystinosis	Rare	0%	Macrophages with cystine crystals may deposit in interstitium or mesangium; cystine accumulates in other organs
Sickle cell nephropathy	Rare	Not available	Sickle cell crisis common within 1st year of transplantation

Percentages are approximate, some based on combined reported series.

Recurrent IgA Nephropathy

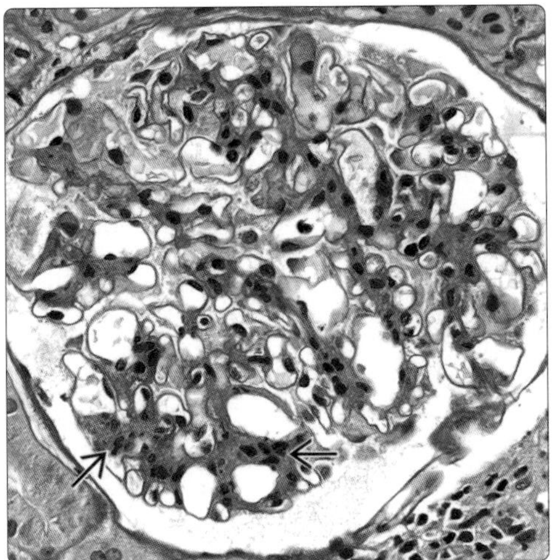

IgA

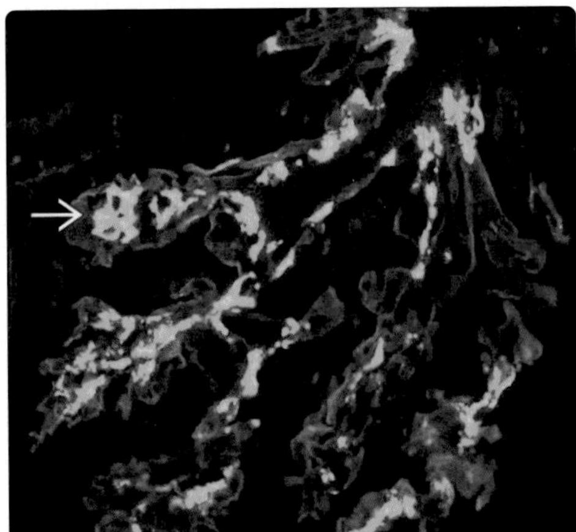

(Left) *Mild mesangial hypercellularity* ⇨ *is the predominant finding in this glomerulus from an allograft with recurrent IgA nephropathy (PAS).* **(Right)** *Immunofluorescence for IgA shows strong granular mesangial* ➡ *staining in a kidney allograft with recurrent IgA nephropathy. This is identical to the pattern of involvement in the native kidneys.*

Recurrent Lupus Nephritis

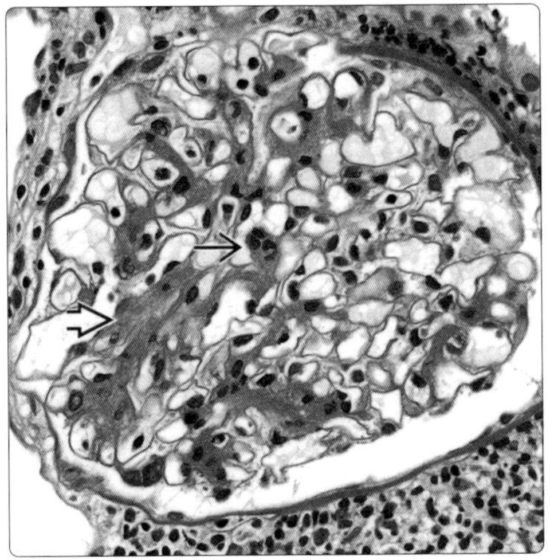

Recurrent Lupus Nephritis

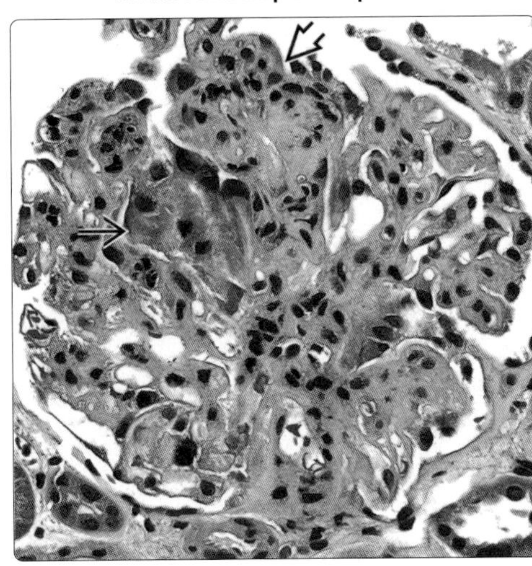

(Left) *Periodic acid-Schiff shows focal mesangial hypercellularity* ⇨ *and mesangial sclerosis* ⇨*, which are common alterations in the early phase of recurrent lupus nephritis. When glomeruli are normal on light microscopy, immunofluorescence microscopy may detect the presence of immune complexes in patients with lupus.* **(Right)** *Segmental fibrinoid necrosis* ⇨ *and endocapillary hypercellularity* ⇨ *are present in this case of recurrent lupus nephritis.*

IgG

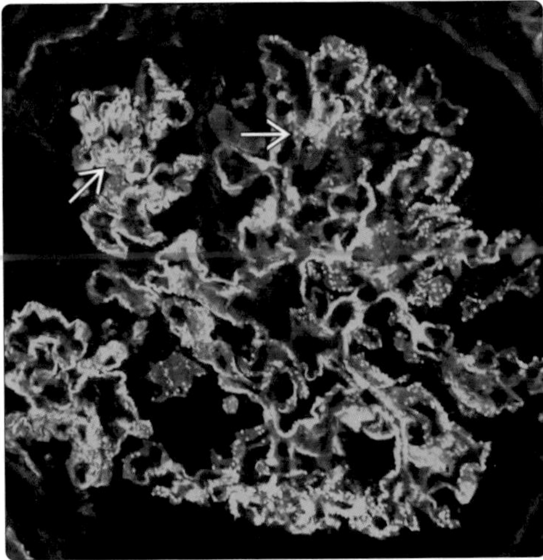

C4d

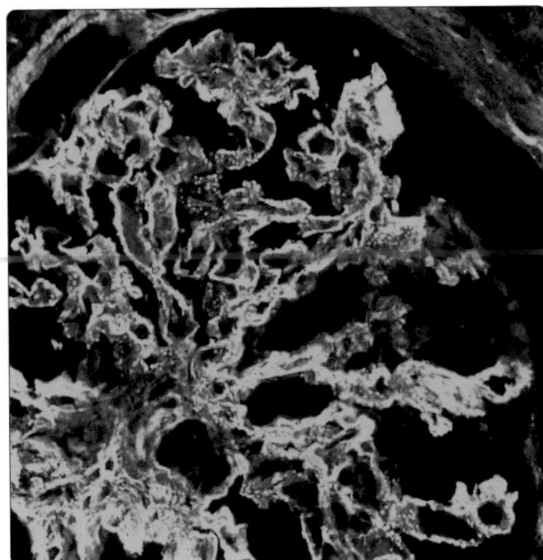

(Left) *IF for IgG reveals discrete granular and confluent staining along the capillary walls and some mesangial regions* ➡ *in this kidney allograft with lupus nephritis with proliferative and membranous features.* **(Right)** *IF shows granular C4d staining along the GBM, which is suggestive of lupus MGN. This staining pattern is distinct from the mesangial C4d staining that may be present in normal glomeruli.*

(Left) *At 2 months post transplant, this glomerulus appears normal by light microscopy. By IF, there was bright granular glomerular basement membrane staining for C4d and less staining for IgG, kappa, and lambda (with negative C3), indicative of recurrent MGN. No deposits were identified by EM.* **(Right)** *Periodic acid-Schiff reveals thick GBMs, characteristic of MGN, in an allograft with recurrent disease. Duplicated GBMs ➡ indicate chronic transplant glomerulopathy.*

Early Recurrent MGN

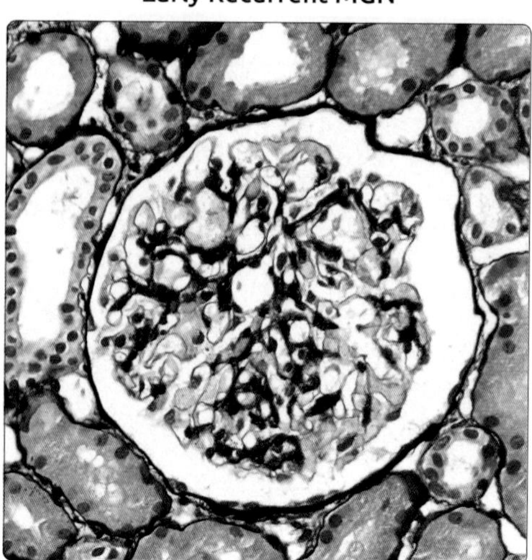

Recurrent MGN

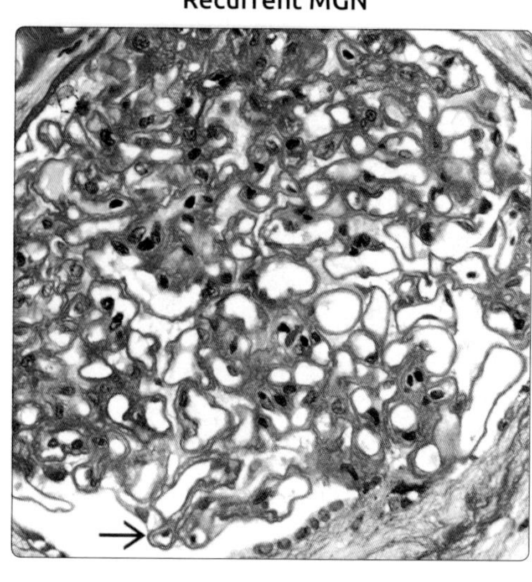

(Left) *There is severe infiltration by inflammatory cells ➡ within this glomerulus and duplication of the glomerular basement membranes ➡ in an allograft with recurrence of MPGN.* **(Right)** *Periodic acid-Schiff reveals a cellular crescent ➡ that accompanies marked endocapillary hypercellularity with numerous inflammatory cells ➡ and duplication of the GBM ➡ in an allograft with recurrent MPGN type I.*

Recurrent MPGN

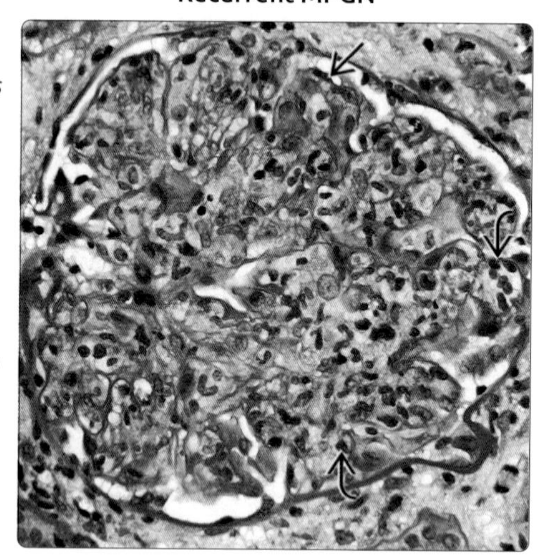

Recurrent MPGN

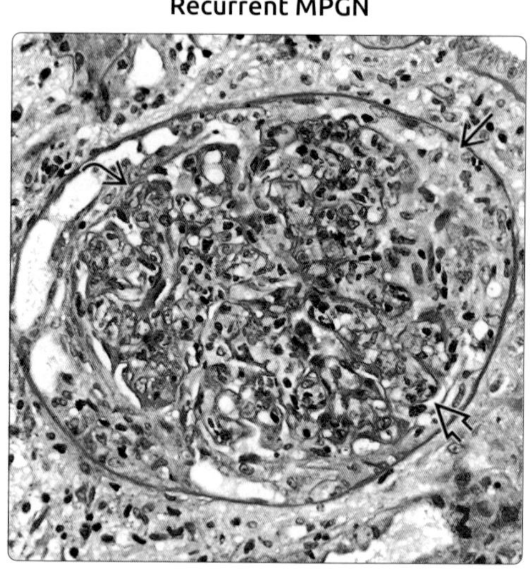

(Left) *Periodic acid-Schiff shows segmental occlusion of glomerular capillaries by hyaline and matrix ➡ in this allograft with recurrent FSGS 6 years after transplantation. Focal duplication of GBM ➡ suggests chronic transplant glomerulopathy.* **(Right)** *In this biopsy from an adult man with recurrent FSGS in a transplant, a podocyte ➡ appears to have "fallen off" the glomerular basement membrane. Urinary podocyte excretion has been found to be increased in patients with FSGS.*

Recurrent FSGS

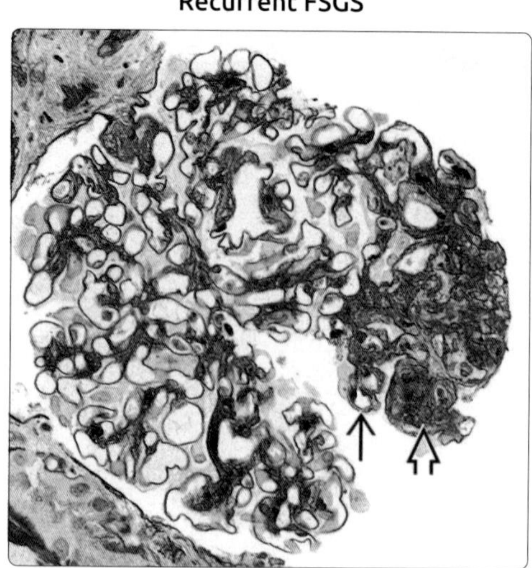

Electron Microscopy in Recurrent FSGS

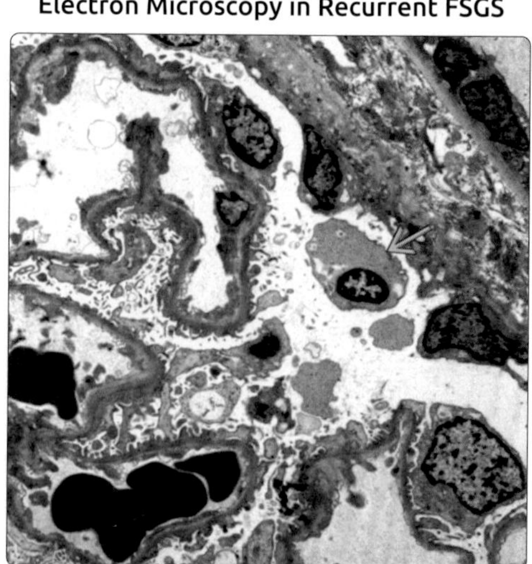

Recurrent Pauci-Immune GN

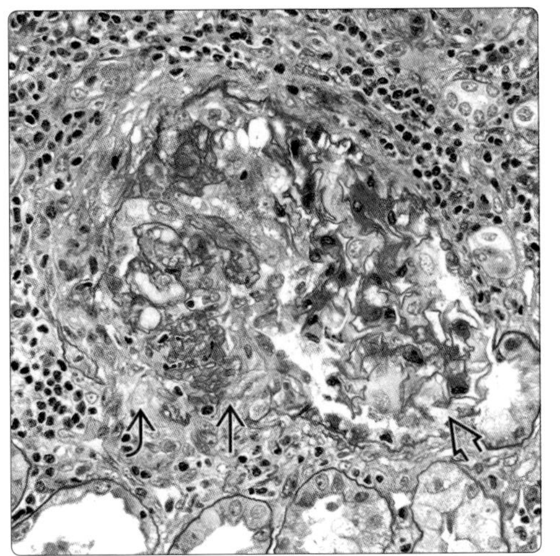

Recurrent Pauci-Immune GN

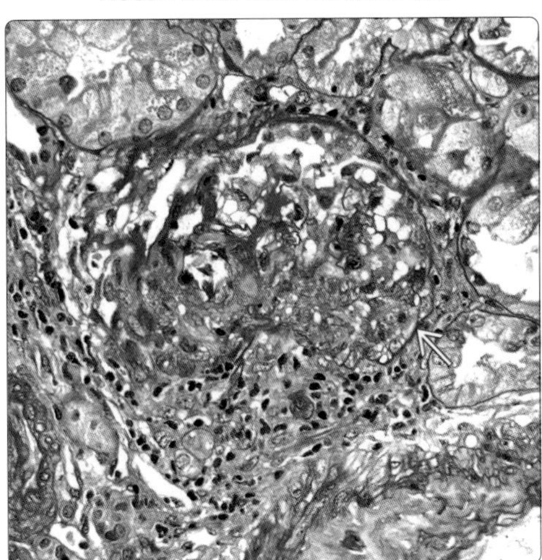

(Left) *Recurrent ANCA-associated disease has a fibrocellular crescent ⇨ and a spared segment of the glomerulus ⇨. The Bowman capsule is disrupted ⇨, a useful sign of crescents. The patient had post-transplant pulmonary hemorrhage, positive myeloperoxidase antibody, and recurrent pauci-immune crescentic GN.* **(Right)** *Periodic acid-Schiff reveals a cellular crescent ➡ in this allograft from a 57-year-old woman with recurrent ANCA-associated pauci-immune crescentic GN.*

Recurrent Diabetic Nephropathy

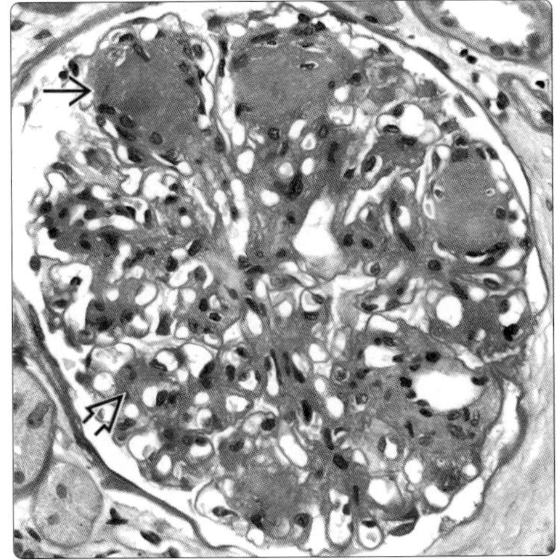

Arteriolar Hyalinosis

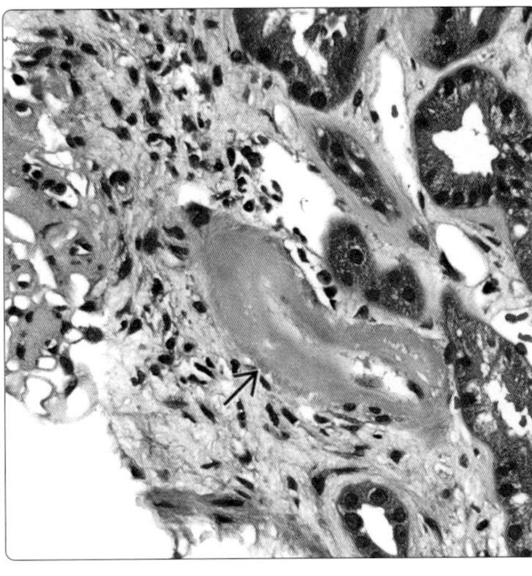

(Left) *Periodic acid-Schiff shows diffuse mesangial ⇨ and nodular sclerosis ⇨, which characterizes recurrence of diabetic nephropathy in an allograft.* **(Right)** *Severe arteriolar hyalinosis is present ⇨ in this allograft with recurrent diabetic nephropathy 6 years after transplantation. Calcineurin inhibitor toxicity and hypertension may also contribute, as their histologic features can be indistinguishable from diabetic vascular injury.*

Recurrent Amyloidosis

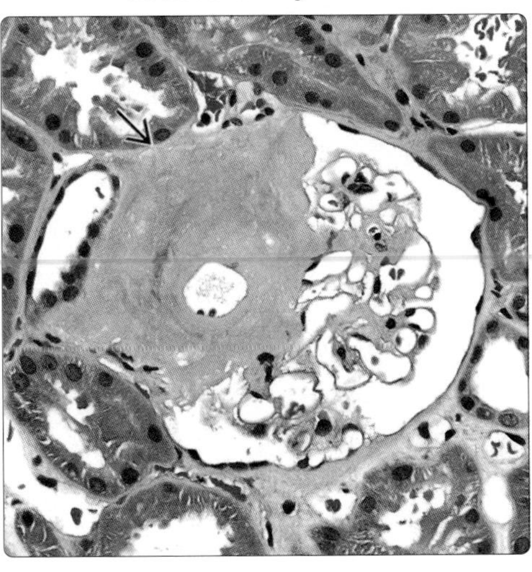

Amyloid A Immunohistochemistry

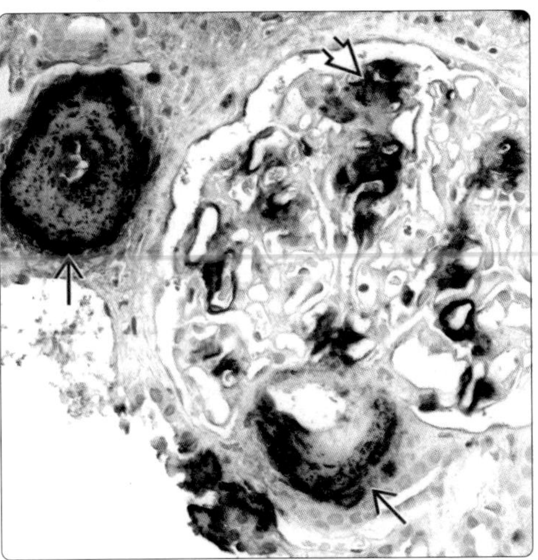

(Left) *Hematoxylin & eosin shows prominent deposition of amorphous eosinophilic material ⇨ in a hilar arteriole, suggestive of recurrent amyloidosis in this 9-year-old allograft from a 47-year-old man with ankylosing spondylitis.* **(Right)** *IHC confirms the presence of AA amyloid deposits in a 47-year-old man with ankylosing spondylitis. Note the prominent amyloid deposition within the arterioles ⇨ and much less involvement of mesangial areas ⇨ in the glomeruli.*

De Novo Focal Segmental Glomerulosclerosis

KEY FACTS

TERMINOLOGY

- Definition
  - Focal segmental glomerulosclerosis (FSGS) or its variants in kidney transplant patients with original disease **not** due to FSGS

ETIOLOGY/PATHOGENESIS

- Hyperfiltration
  - Observed in longstanding allografts with severe nephron loss
  - Pediatric kidneys transplanted into adult recipients
- Severe vascular disease
  - De novo collapsing glomerulopathy (CG) associated with deceased donor kidneys
  - Zonal distribution of CG
- Drug-induced
  - Higher frequency with calcineurin inhibitors (CNI)
    - CNI may contribute via microvascular disease
  - Mammalian target of rapamycin (mTOR) inhibitors

CLINICAL ISSUES

- Proteinuria, nephrotic range
- Chronic renal failure
- De novo FSGS: 60% graft survival within 5 years of diagnosis
- De novo CG: 50% loss of graft within 1 year of diagnosis

MICROSCOPIC

- Focal, segmental glomerulosclerosis or collapsing glomerulopathy
- Arterial or arteriolar sclerosis

TOP DIFFERENTIAL DIAGNOSES

- Recurrent FSGS
- Chronic transplant glomerulopathy
- Calcineurin inhibitor toxicity
- Immune complex-mediated glomerulonephritis, de novo or recurrent

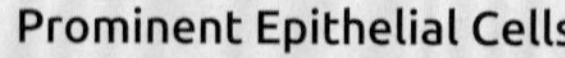

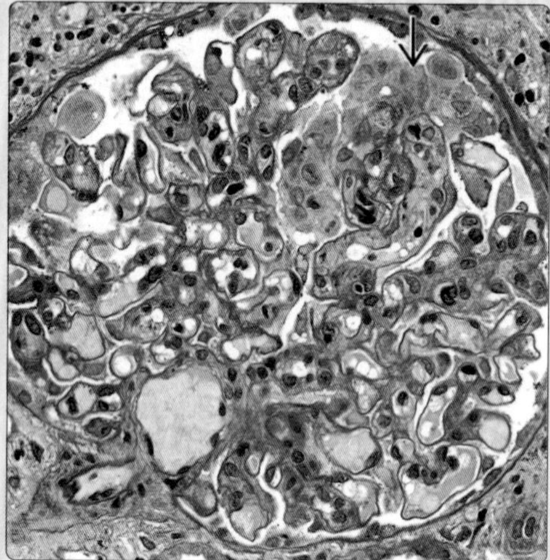

Segmental Sclerosis

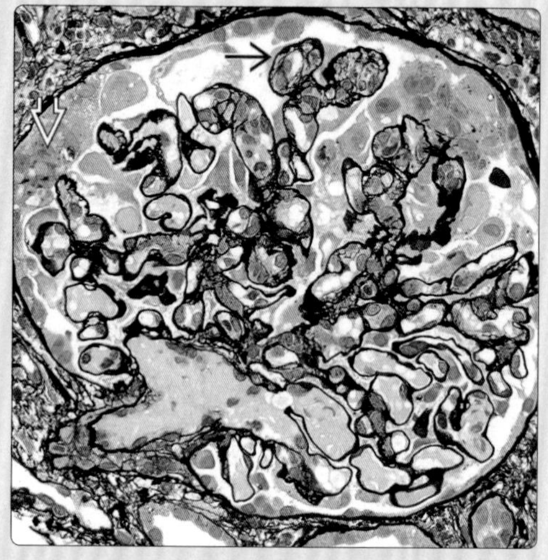

(Left) *Collapsing type de novo focal segmental glomerulosclerosis (FSGS) in a renal transplant patient with nephrotic-range proteinuria shows prominent adjacent visceral epithelial cells (podocytes) →.* **(Right)** *Protein reabsorption droplets ➡ accentuate a few prominent podocytes, which correlate with proteinuria. Duplication of the glomerular basement membranes is present →, which raises the consideration of chronic transplant glomerulopathy (Jones methenamine silver).*

Collapsing FSGS

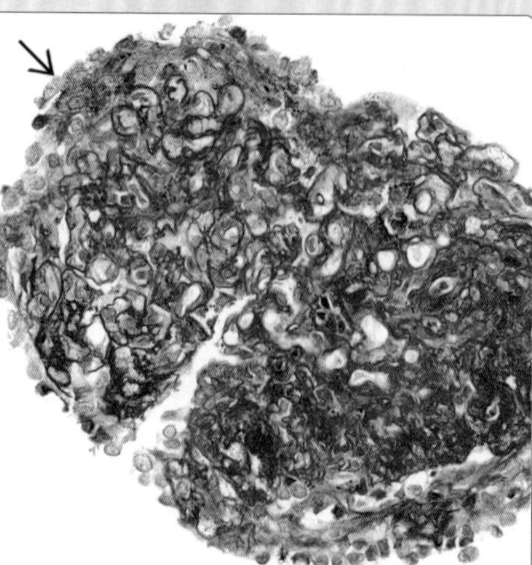

Severe Arteriolar Hyalinosis

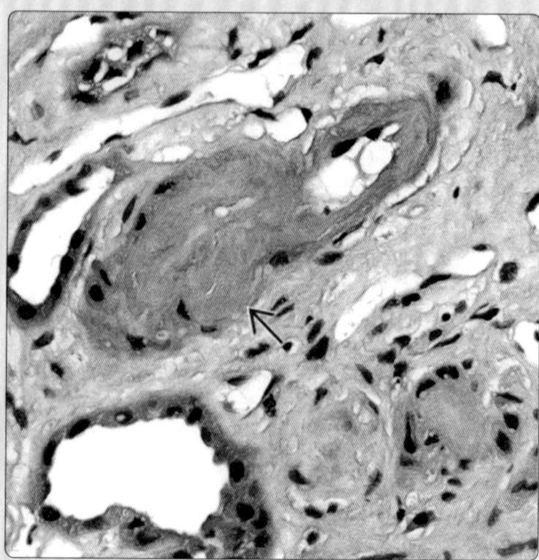

(Left) *Prominent podocytes → overlie a collapsed tuft in this case of de novo collapsing glomerulopathy in a transplant patient with severe proteinuria whose original disease was diabetic nephropathy.* **(Right)** *Prominent subendothelial hyalinosis → of an arteriole is present in an allograft biopsy with collapsing glomerulopathy, implying that it may be related to calcineurin inhibitor toxicity.*

TERMINOLOGY

Abbreviations

- Focal segmental glomerulosclerosis (FSGS)

Synonyms

- Collapsing glomerulopathy (CG)
  - Variant of FSGS

Definitions

- FSGS or its variants in kidney transplant patients with original disease **not** due to FSGS

ETIOLOGY/PATHOGENESIS

Hyperfiltration

- Pediatric kidneys transplanted into adult recipients
- Longstanding allografts with severe nephron loss
- Severe vascular disease

Severe Vascular Disease

- De novo CG associated with deceased donor kidneys
- Zonal distribution of CG

Drug Induced

- Higher frequency with calcineurin inhibitors (CNI)
  - CNI may contribute via microvascular disease
- Mammalian target of rapamycin (mTOR) inhibitors

CLINICAL ISSUES

Presentation

- Proteinuria
  - Variable, unlike recurrent FSGS
- Chronic renal failure

Laboratory Tests

- Urinalysis
- 24 hour urine protein collection

Treatment

- Not well defined
- If CNI implicated, alter drug regimen

Prognosis

- De novo FSGS
  - 60% graft survival within 5 years of diagnosis
- De novo CG
  - 50% loss of graft within 1 year of diagnosis

MICROSCOPIC

Histologic Features

- Segmental glomerulosclerosis with any of following findings
  - Synechial or fibrous attachments to Bowman capsules
  - Obliteration of glomerular capillary lumina by foam cells &/or hyaline
  - Segmental accumulation of mesangial matrix
  - Prominence of visceral epithelial cells (podocytes)
  - Protein reabsorption droplets in podocytes
  - Foot process effacement
- Collapsing glomerulopathy (variant of FSGS)
  - Collapse of glomerulus with podocyte hypercellularity
  - Associated with severe vascular disease and CNI toxicity
  - Zonal distribution
- Global glomerulosclerosis
- Interstitial fibrosis and tubular atrophy
  - Often severe
- Interstitial foam cells can be correlate of severe proteinuria
- Arteriolar hyalinosis
  - Subendothelial hyalinosis
  - Adventitial hyaline nodules may be present

ANCILLARY TESTS

Immunofluorescence

- IgM and C3 in segmental scars

Electron Microscopy

- Podocyte foot process effacement
- Separation of podocytes from GBM if CG

DIFFERENTIAL DIAGNOSIS

Recurrent FSGS

- Usually presents earlier (< 1 year)

Chronic Transplant Glomerulopathy

- Duplication of GBM without immune complex deposition
- Variable C4d peritubular capillary deposition
- May occur concurrently with de novo FSGS

Calcineurin Inhibitor Toxicity

- Isometric vacuolization of tubular epithelial cells
- Adventitial hyaline nodules

Immune Complex-Mediated Glomerulonephritis, De Novo or Recurrent

- Positive immunofluorescence staining for immunoglobulins (immune complex deposition)

DIAGNOSTIC CHECKLIST

Pathologic Interpretation Pearls

- FSGS should trigger IF and EM work-up
- CG may mimic crescentic glomerulonephritis

SELECTED REFERENCES

1. Ponticelli C et al: De novo glomerular diseases after renal transplantation. Clin J Am Soc Nephrol. 9(8):1479-87, 2014
2. Ikeda Y et al: A case of de novo focal segmental glomerulosclerosis occurred one and half years after kidney transplantation supposed to be caused by calcineurin inhibitor. Clin Transplant. 26 Suppl 24:76-80, 2012
3. Nadasdy T et al: Zonal distribution of glomerular collapse in renal allografts: possible role of vascular changes. Hum Pathol. 33(4):437-41, 2002
4. Cosio FG et al: Focal segmental glomerulosclerosis in renal allografts with chronic nephropathy: implications for graft survival. Am J Kidney Dis. 34(4):731-8, 1999
5. Trimarchi HM et al: Focal segmental glomerulosclerosis in a 32-year-old kidney allograft after 7 years without immunosuppression. Nephron. 82(3):270-3, 1999
6. Meehan SM et al: De novo collapsing glomerulopathy in renal allografts. Transplantation. 65(9):1192-7, 1998
7. Barama A et al: Focal segmental glomerulosclerosis in one of two "en bloc" pediatric transplanted kidneys. Am J Kidney Dis. 30(2):271-4, 1997
8. Woolley AC et al: De novo focal glomerulosclerosis after kidney transplantation. Am J Med. 84(2):310-4, 1988

De Novo Membranous Glomerulonephritis

KEY FACTS

ETIOLOGY/PATHOGENESIS

- May represent unusual manifestation of chronic humoral rejection
  - Associated with C4d peritubular capillary deposition and anti-HLA-DQ
  - 1 autopsy showed de novo MGN involving **only** kidney allograft and not native kidneys
  - May recur in subsequent renal allografts

CLINICAL ISSUES

- 0.5-9% of kidney transplant patients
  - Manifests late (> 3 years)
  - Proteinuria
  - Renal dysfunction
  - Unfavorable prognosis
    - 67% require renal replacement therapy

MICROSCOPIC

- Glomerular basement membrane thickening
  - Diffuse or segmental
  - GBM "spike" formation
    - ± "Swiss cheese" appearance depending on stage of MGN
- Mesangial hypercellularity in 1/3 of cases
- Granular IgG staining in glomerular capillary walls
  - C4d and C3 may also stain glomerular capillaries in similar pattern
  - Careful evaluation of C4d glomerular staining pattern if only antibody tested in transplant kidney biopsies
  - C4d in peritubular capillaries found in ~ 70% of cases
- Subepithelial electron-dense deposits seen by electron microscopy ± basement membrane "spike" formation

TOP DIFFERENTIAL DIAGNOSES

- Recurrent MGN
- Donor-derived MGN
- Chronic transplant glomerulopathy

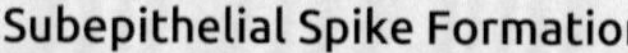

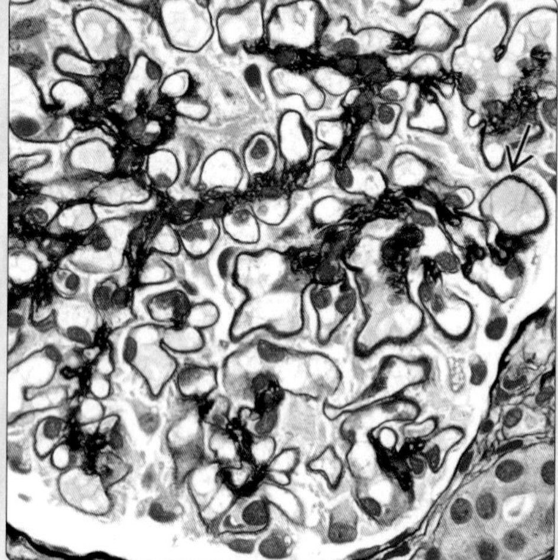

Duplication of GBM

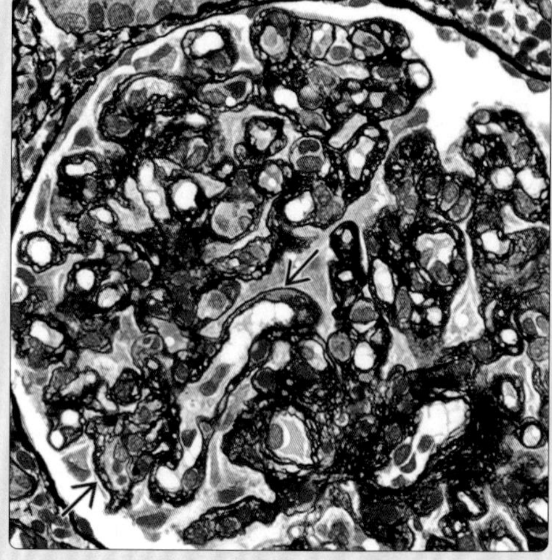

(Left) *Jones methenamine silver shows a hint of subepithelial "spike" formation → along some of the glomerular basement membranes.* **(Right)** *Chronic transplant glomerulopathy or duplication of the GBMs → can affect 50% of de novo MGN, as demonstrated in this glomerulus from a pediatric patient with renal transplant due to renal dysplasia (Jones methenamine silver).*

IgG

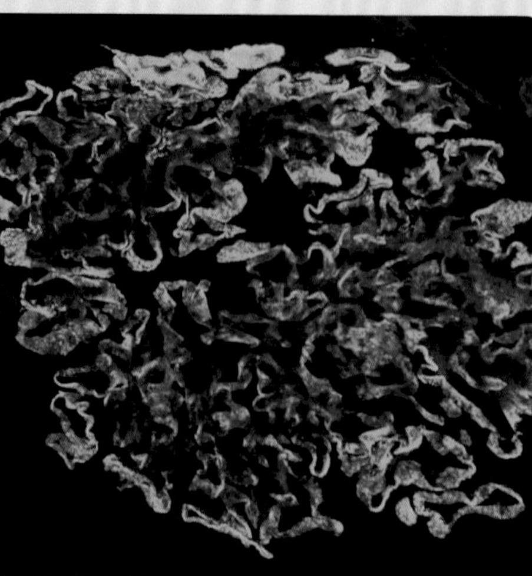

Subepithelial Deposits

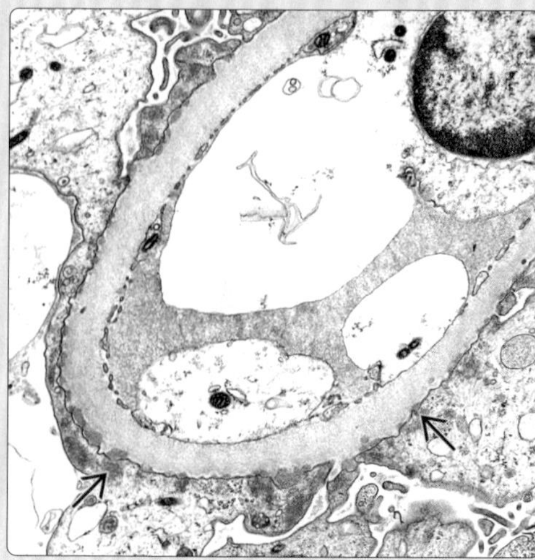

(Left) *Immunofluorescence microscopy for IgG demonstrates granular staining of all glomerular capillaries. Clinical correlation is necessary to confirm whether this represents recurrent or de novo MGN.* **(Right)** *EM of a glomerulus with de novo MGN shows very small deposits in contact with the podocyte → with only minimal spike formation, typical of early and mild MGN. The patient was transplanted 4 years previously for diabetic nephropathy.*

TERMINOLOGY

Abbreviations

- Membranous glomerulonephritis (MGN), de novo

Definitions

- MGN in kidney allograft when primary cause of end-stage renal disease is **not** MGN

ETIOLOGY/PATHOGENESIS

Allo-/Autoantibody

- May represent unusual manifestation of chronic humoral rejection
  - Associated with C4d peritubular capillary deposition and anti-HLA-DQ
  - 1 autopsy showed de novo MGN involving only kidney allograft **without** MGN in native kidneys
    - May recur in subsequent renal allografts
  - 1 de novo MGN case with donor specific antibodies against HLA-DQ7
- Can occur in HLA identical grafts, presumably due to non-HLA antigen
  - Rat model of de novo MGN occurs only in transplant not native kidney
- No autoantibodies to PLA2R1

CLINICAL ISSUES

Epidemiology

- Incidence
  - 0.5-9% of kidney transplant patients

Presentation

- Manifests late (> 3 years)
- Proteinuria
  - 2nd most common cause in renal allograft patients
  - Often nephrotic range (> 3 g/24 hours), may be intermittent or persistent

Prognosis

- 5-year graft loss > 50%
- 67% progress to renal failure

MACROSCOPIC

General Features

- Renal vein thrombosis occasional present
  - Less common than idiopathic MGN in native kidneys

MICROSCOPIC

Histologic Features

- GBM thickening
  - Focal &/or segmental thickening common
- Glomerular capillaritis in ~ 50%
- Mesangial hypercellularity in ~ 33%
- Double contours or duplication of GBM in 50%
  - Possibly due to concurrent chronic transplant glomerulopathy (chronic humoral rejection)
- Prominent interstitial inflammation
  - Often sufficient for diagnosis of acute (cell-mediated) rejection
- Intimal arteritis
  - Acute (type 2) rejection found in subset

ANCILLARY TESTS

Immunofluorescence

- Positive granular capillary wall staining for IgG, kappa and lambda light chains
  - IgG1 predominant subclass
    - IgG4 predominant subclass in primary MGN
  - Variable capillary wall staining for C4d, C3, C1q, and IgM
- C4d(+) PTC in ~ 70%

Electron Microscopy

- Subepithelial amorphous electron-dense deposits
  - Often small and relatively sparse
  - Stage I (Ehrenreich-Churg) deposits common
- Duplication of GBMs
  - Subendothelial space widening when injured endothelial cells detach from GBM

DIFFERENTIAL DIAGNOSIS

Recurrent MGN

- Clinical history of MGN
- Earlier onset (< 3 months)
- IgG4 predominant

Donor-Derived MGN

- Present in donor biopsy, disappears in months

Chronic Transplant Glomerulopathy

- Duplication of GBM without immune complexes
- Occurs concurrently in 50% of de novo MGN cases
- C4d(+) in peritubular capillaries
- Multilamination of peritubular capillaries on EM

DIAGNOSTIC CHECKLIST

Pathologic Interpretation Pearls

- Significant proteinuria should trigger additional evaluation by IF &/or EM
- Thickening or duplication of GBMs or segmental glomerular sclerosis should trigger additional IF &/or EM
- C4d immunofluorescence microscopy may reveal granular glomerular capillary wall staining

SELECTED REFERENCES

1. Ponticelli C et al: De novo glomerular diseases after renal transplantation. Clin J Am Soc Nephrol. 9(8):1479-87, 2014
2. Patel K et al: De novo membranous nephropathy in renal allograft associated with antibody-mediated rejection and review of the literature. Transplant Proc. 45(9):3424 8, 2013
3. Honda K et al: De novo membranous nephropathy and antibody-mediated rejection in transplanted kidney. Clin Transplant. 25(2):191-200, 2011
4. Lal SM: De novo membranous nephropathy in renal allografts with unusual histology. Arch Pathol Lab Med. 131(1):17, 2007
5. Monga G et al: Membranous glomerulonephritis (MGN) in transplanted kidneys: morphologic investigation on 256 renal allografts. Mod Pathol. 6(3):249-58, 1993
6. Truong L et al: De novo membranous glomerulonephropathy in renal allografts: a report of ten cases and review of the literature. Am J Kidney Dis. 14(2):131-44, 1989

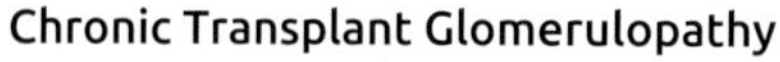

Chronic Transplant Glomerulopathy

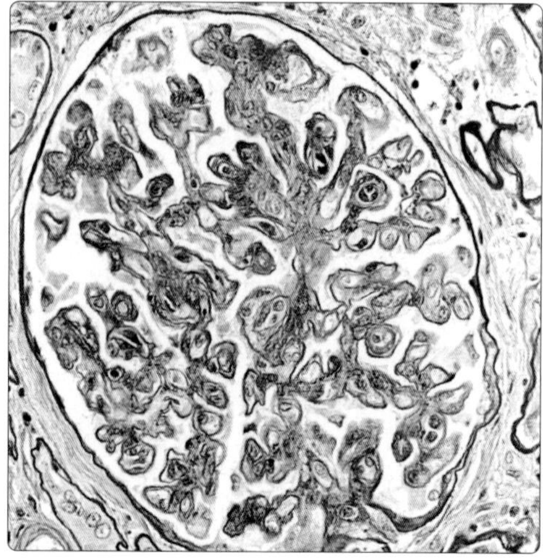

Segmental Sclerosis

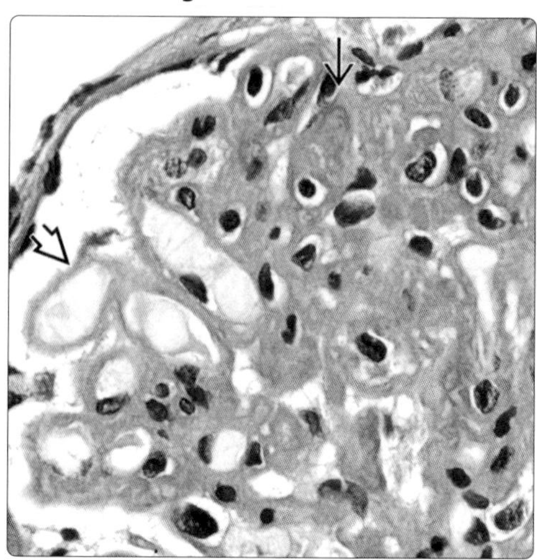

(Left) *Glomerulus with de novo MGN and chronic humoral rejection shows prominent and widespread duplication of the GBM.* **(Right)** *Periodic acid-Schiff of a biopsy with de novo MGN reveals thick GBMs with a vacuolated appearance ⇨ in a glomerulus with segmental accumulation of matrix and hyaline →, which obscures the capillary lumina.*

Segmental IgG

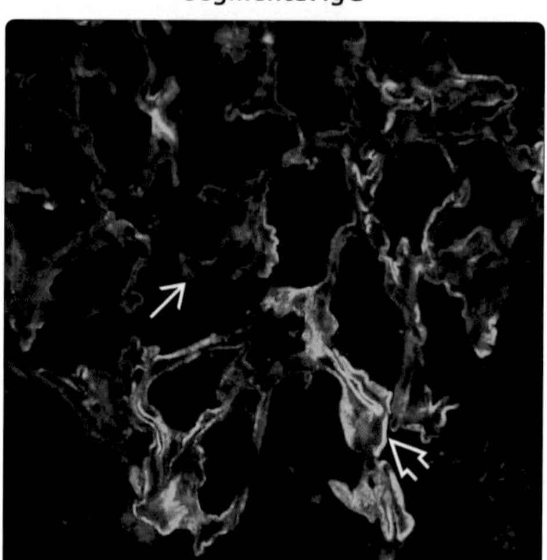

C4d

(Left) *Immunofluorescence for IgG highlights the segmental distribution of immune complex deposition along the glomerular capillaries ⇨. Several glomerular capillaries or segments of GBM show no significant staining →. A similar pattern but less intense staining was also seen with kappa and lambda light chains.* **(Right)** *Immunofluorescence shows granular C4d staining along the glomerular basement membranes, which may be the only hint of MGN, which should trigger additional IF and EM studies.*

C4d

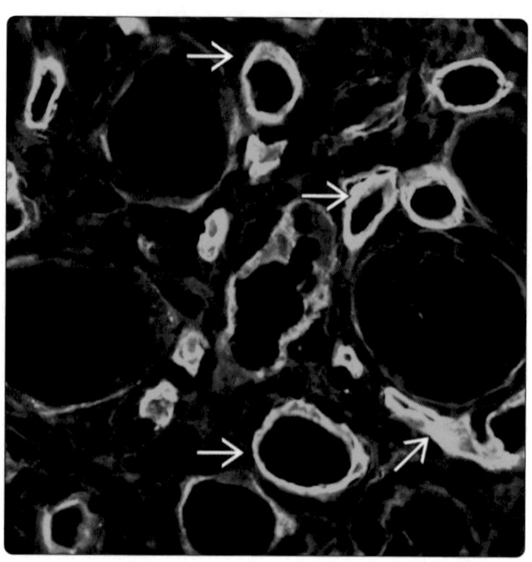

C4d Immunohistochemistry

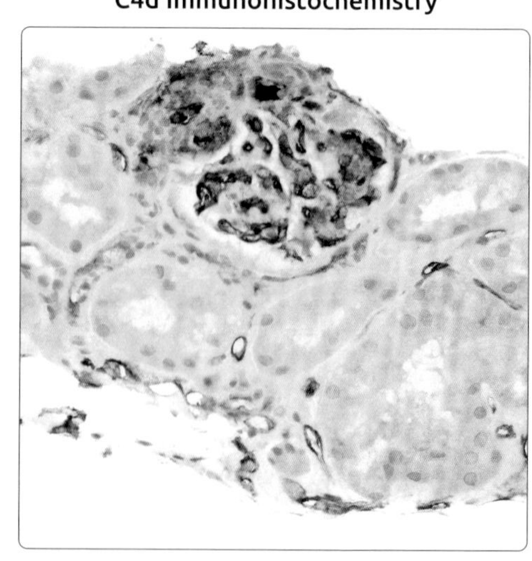

(Left) *C4d deposition is present in the peritubular capillaries in a patient with donor-reactive HLA antibodies and de novo MGN. The peritubular capillaries have widespread linear deposits of C4d, typical of antibody-mediated rejection →.* **(Right)** *C4d deposits are detected in the GBM and in peritubular capillaries in this patient with de novo MGN in a 2nd transplant. The 1st graft was lost to de novo MGN and chronic humoral rejection. Prior de novo MGN is a risk factor for a 2nd episode.*

Subepithelial Immune Complexes

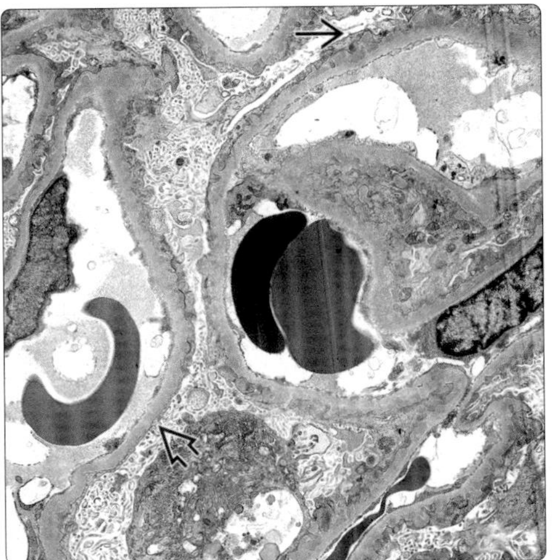

Subepithelial "Spikes"

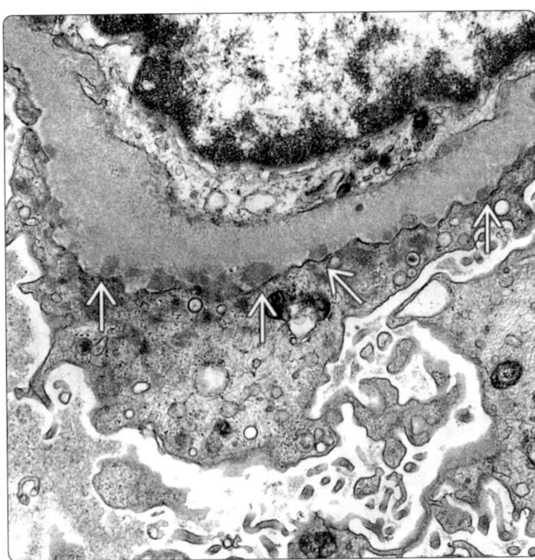

(Left) *Electron microscopy reveals segmental distribution of many small subepithelial electron-dense deposits →. The podocyte foot processes demonstrate diffuse effacement →.* **(Right)** *Electron micrograph of a glomerulus with de novo MGN shows very small deposits in contact with the podocyte → with only minimal spike formation, typical of early and mild MGN. This pattern is not uncommon in de novo MGN.*

Segmental Distribution of "Spikes"

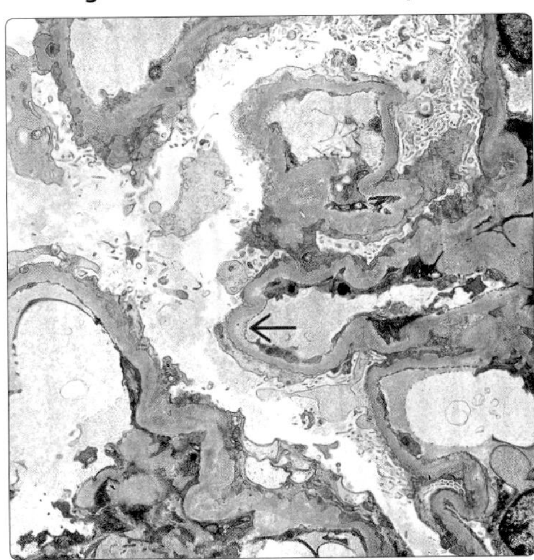

Subepithelial Deposits

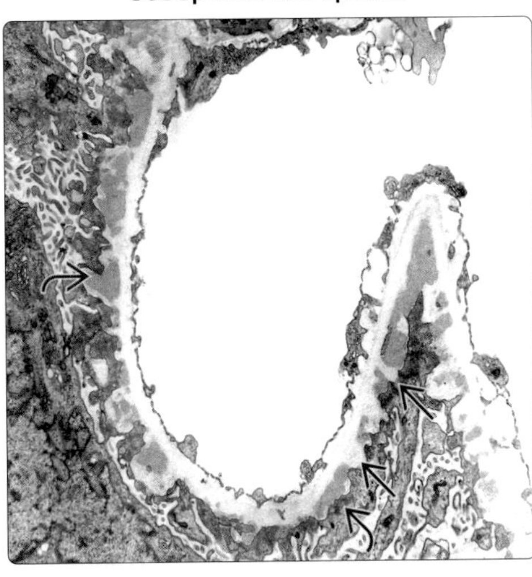

(Left) *Electron microscopy reveals many discrete electron dense deposits in subepithelial locations. Focal separation of the endothelial cell from the GBM → is noted, but duplication of the GBM is not apparent in this or other glomerular capillaries.* **(Right)** *EM of a glomerulus with de novo MGN from a patient transplanted 6 years ago for FSGS shows subepithelial deposits → surrounded by GBM spikes →, typical of stage II MGN.*

Subepithelial and Intramembranous Deposits

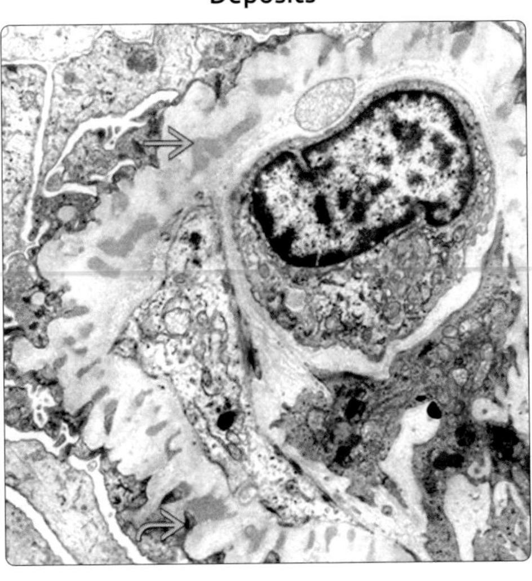

Peritubular Capillary BM Multilayering

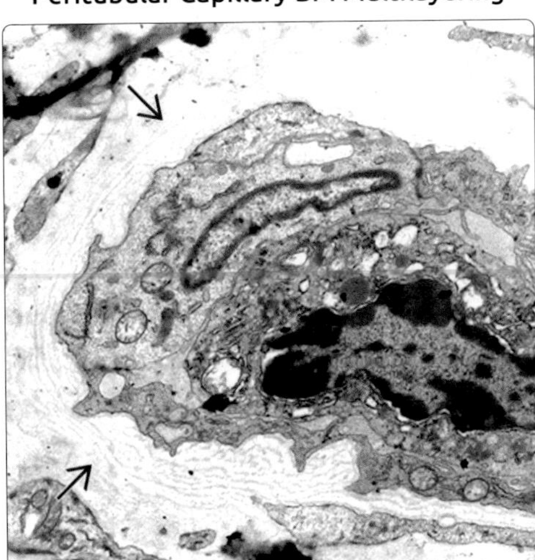

(Left) *Electron micrograph of a glomerulus from a patient with both chronic humoral rejection and de novo MGN shows duplication of the GBM and amorphous electron-dense deposits within the GBM → and in subepithelial locations →.* **(Right)** *Electron micrograph shows multilamination of the peritubular capillary basement membrane → in a patient with donor-reactive HLA antibodies and de novo MGN.*

Anti-GBM Disease in Alport Syndrome

KEY FACTS

TERMINOLOGY

- Alport post-transplant nephritis

ETIOLOGY/PATHOGENESIS

- Antibodies develop against α-3, α-4, or α-5 chains of collagen IV of transplant kidney
  - Larger *COL4A5* deletions may be more susceptible to anti-GBM disease
- X-linked AS patients target NC1 domain of *COL4A5*
- Autosomal recessive AS patients target NC1 domain of *COL4A3* or *COL4A4*

CLINICAL ISSUES

- 3-5% of Alport recipients reported to develop de novo anti-GBM after kidney transplantation
- 0.4% of AS patients develop de novo anti-GBM disease in recent series (2014)
- Acute renal failure
  - 75% of cases occur in 1st post-transplant year
- Hematuria
- Male predominance
- 90% of grafts fail within months after onset
  - Anti-GBM disease often recurs in subsequent allografts with an accelerated course
- Plasmapheresis

MICROSCOPIC

- Cellular crescents &/or fibrinoid necrosis, typically > 80% of glomeruli
- Strong linear IgG immunofluorescence staining of GBM
- Intratubular red blood cell casts
- Acute tubular injury

TOP DIFFERENTIAL DIAGNOSES

- Pauci-immune (ANCA-associated) crescentic glomerulonephritis
- Diabetic nephropathy

Transplant Nephrectomy

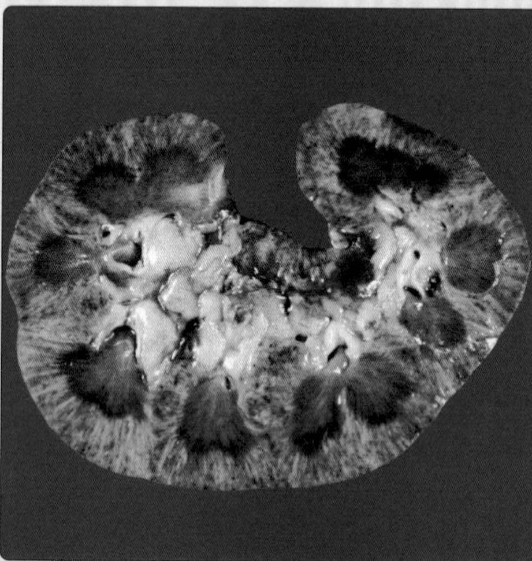

Red Blood Cell Casts

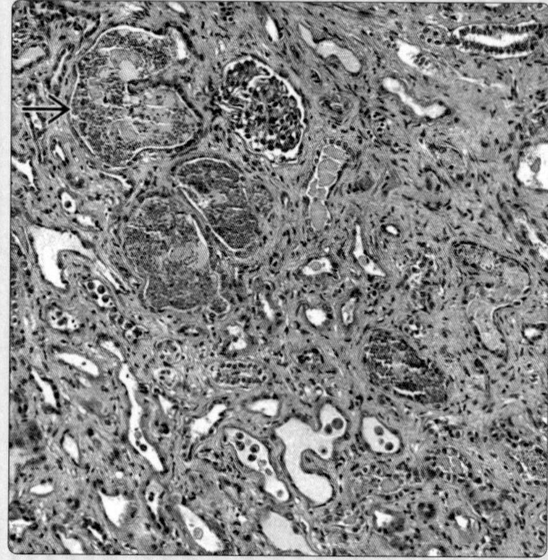

(Left) *Gross photograph shows an allograft nephrectomy from a 37-year-old woman with ESRD due to X-linked Alport syndrome. Eighteen months post-transplant, the patient presented with allograft tenderness and renal failure. Anti-GBM titers were equivocal by ELISA and western blot.* **(Right)** *Hematoxylin & eosin shows several red blood cell and pigmented casts ➔ in the cortex, widespread interstitial fibrosis, and tubular injury in this Alport patient with anti-GBM nephritis after kidney transplantation.*

Cellular Crescent

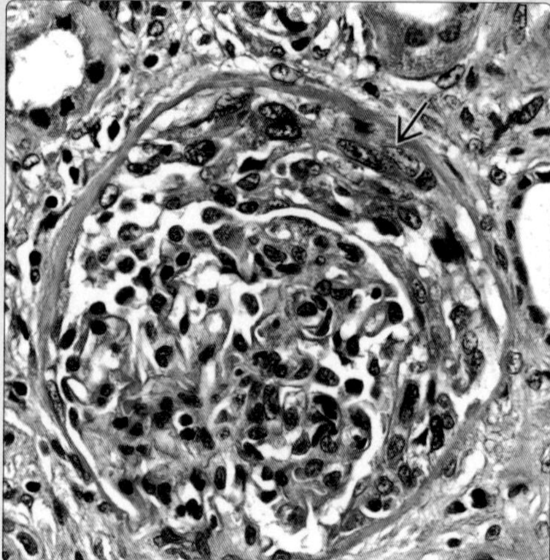

Linear IgG Deposition

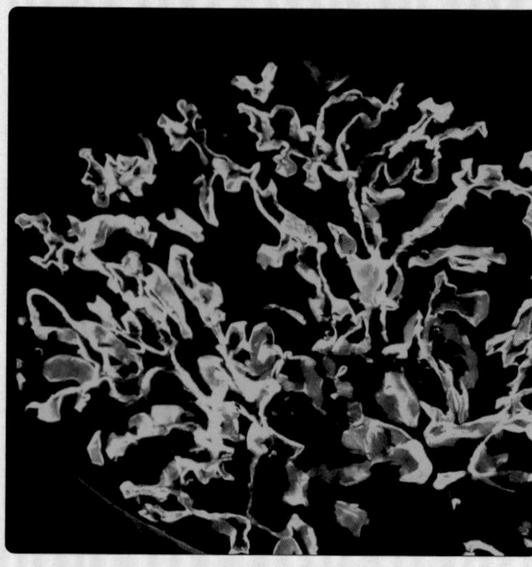

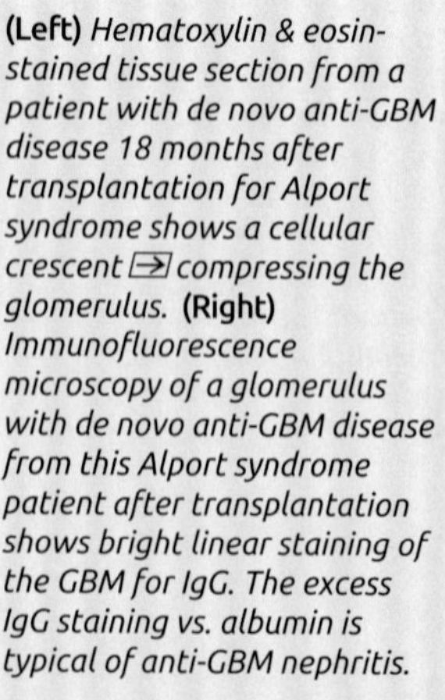

(Left) *Hematoxylin & eosin-stained tissue section from a patient with de novo anti-GBM disease 18 months after transplantation for Alport syndrome shows a cellular crescent ➔ compressing the glomerulus.* **(Right)** *Immunofluorescence microscopy of a glomerulus with de novo anti-GBM disease from this Alport syndrome patient after transplantation shows bright linear staining of the GBM for IgG. The excess IgG staining vs. albumin is typical of anti-GBM nephritis.*

TERMINOLOGY

Abbreviations

- Anti-glomerular basement membrane (anti-GBM) disease in Alport syndrome (AS)

Synonyms

- Alport post-transplant nephritis
- De novo anti-GBM nephritis

Definitions

- Glomerulonephritis (GN) mediated by anti-GBM antibodies in AS renal transplant recipients

ETIOLOGY/PATHOGENESIS

Exposure to Nonendogenous GBM Antigens After Kidney Transplantation

- Antibodies develop against NC1 domains of intact α345NC1 (hexamer of α-3, α-4, or α-5 chains of collagen IV) of allograft in AS patients due to mutated endogenous antigen
  - Larger deletions of *COL4A5* at higher risk for GN
  - Target quaternary epitopes of intact α345NC1
    - Target alloantigen of all alloantibodies that mediate de novo anti-GBM nephritis
    - Distinct antigenic target from Goodpasture syndrome
    - X-linked AS target NC1 domain of COL4A5
    - Autosomal recessive AS patients target NC1 domain of COL4A3 or COL4A4

CLINICAL ISSUES

Epidemiology

- Incidence
  - De novo anti-GBM disease reported after kidney transplantation in 3-5% of Alport recipients in older series
  - 0.4% of AS patients developed clinical de novo anti-GBM disease in 2014 series of 58 patients
- Sex
  - Male predominance
  - Females with X-linked AS have 1 normal allele of α chains of collagen IV and rarely develop anti-GBM disease
    - Only 2 reports involving females with autosomal recessive AS

Presentation

- Acute renal failure
  - 75% within 1st year after kidney transplantation
- Hematuria

Laboratory Tests

- Serum anti-GBM assay by western blot or ELISA

Treatment

- Drugs
  - Cyclophosphamide
  - High-dose corticosteroids
  - Bortezomib (experimental)
  - Rituximab (experimental)
- Plasmapheresis

Prognosis

- 90% of kidney allografts fail within weeks to months after onset of anti-GBM disease
  - Anti-GBM disease often recurs in subsequent allografts with accelerated course
- Overall graft and patient survival after transplant similar to non-Alport recipients

MICROSCOPIC

Histologic Features

- Cellular crescents &/or fibrinoid necrosis (typically > 80% of glomeruli)
  - Glomerular tufts not involved by crescent formation or fibrinoid necrosis appear normal
- Acute tubular injury
- Red blood cell casts
- Cellular or humoral rejection may also be present

ANCILLARY TESTS

Immunofluorescence

- Strong, linear IgG immunofluorescence staining of GBMs
  - Observed in up to 15% of AS patients after kidney transplantation
  - Kappa and lambda light chains and often C3 stain GBMs in similar pattern with lower intensity
  - Intensity of linear IgG staining >>> albumin
  - Bowman capsules and distal tubular basement membranes may also show linear staining

DIFFERENTIAL DIAGNOSIS

Pauci-Immune (ANCA-Associated) Crescentic GN

- Lacks strong linear immunoglobulin deposition in GBM

Diabetic Nephropathy

- Strong linear IgG and albumin IF staining of GBM

DIAGNOSTIC CHECKLIST

Pathologic Interpretation Pearls

- Linear IgG GBM staining may be present without nephritis

SELECTED REFERENCES

1. Mallett A et al: End-stage kidney disease due to Alport syndrome: outcomes in 296 consecutive Australia and New Zealand Dialysis and Transplant Registry cases. Nephrol Dial Transplant. 29(12):2277-86, 2014
2. Olaru F et al: Quaternary epitopes of α345(IV) collagen initiate Alport post-transplant anti-GBM nephritis. J Am Soc Nephrol. 24(6):889-95, 2013
3. Pedchenko V et al: Molecular architecture of the Goodpasture autoantigen in anti-GBM nephritis. N Engl J Med. 363(4):343-54, 2010
4. Kashtan CE: Renal transplantation in patients with Alport syndrome. Pediatr Transplant. 10(6):651-7, 2006
5. Wang XP et al: Distinct epitopes for anti-glomerular basement membrane alport alloantibodies and goodpasture autoantibodies within the noncollagenous domain of alpha3(IV) collagen: a janus-faced antigen. J Am Soc Nephrol. 16(12):3563-71, 2005
6. Browne G et al: Retransplantation in Alport post-transplant anti-GBM disease. Kidney Int. 65(2):675-81, 2004
7. Byrne MC et al: Renal transplant in patients with Alport's syndrome. Am J Kidney Dis. 39(4):769-75, 2002
8. Kalluri R et al: Identification of alpha3, alpha4, and alpha5 chains of type IV collagen as alloantigens for Alport posttransplant anti-glomerular basement membrane antibodies. Transplantation. 69(4):679-83, 2000

Hyperperfusion Injury

KEY FACTS

ETIOLOGY/PATHOGENESIS

- 10% of pediatric kidneys (< 10 years of age) develop this injury
  - Infant kidneys (< 1 year of age) more susceptible
  - En bloc (2 kidneys) transplantation may be less susceptible
- Possible contributing factors
  - Higher blood volume and systemic blood pressure in adults compared with children
  - Smaller glomeruli and thinner glomerular basement membrane thickness in children compared to adults
  - Altered composition of α chains of collagen IV in pediatric glomeruli

CLINICAL ISSUES

- Renal dysfunction
- Proteinuria

MICROSCOPIC

- Global &/or segmental glomerulosclerosis
- Variable mesangial sclerosis &/or hypercellularity
- Interstitial fibrosis and tubular atrophy

ANCILLARY TESTS

- Immunofluorescence microscopy
  - Indirect IF for α-3 and α-5 chains of collagen IV demonstrates strong linear staining of GBM (normal)
- Electron microscopy
  - Prominent glomerular basement membrane alterations
    - Diffuse lamellation and splitting
    - Marked thinning
  - Foot process effacement and microvillous transformation of podocytes

TOP DIFFERENTIAL DIAGNOSES

- Alport syndrome
- Recurrent focal segmental glomerulosclerosis

Glomerular & Tubulointerstitial Scarring

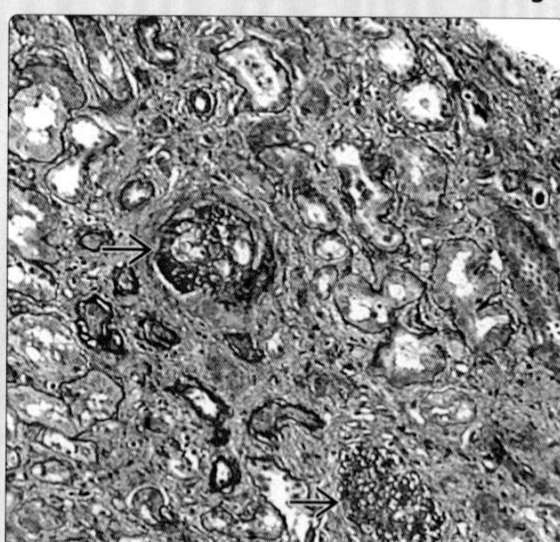

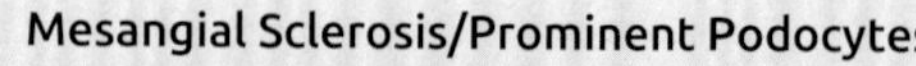

Mesangial Sclerosis/Prominent Podocytes

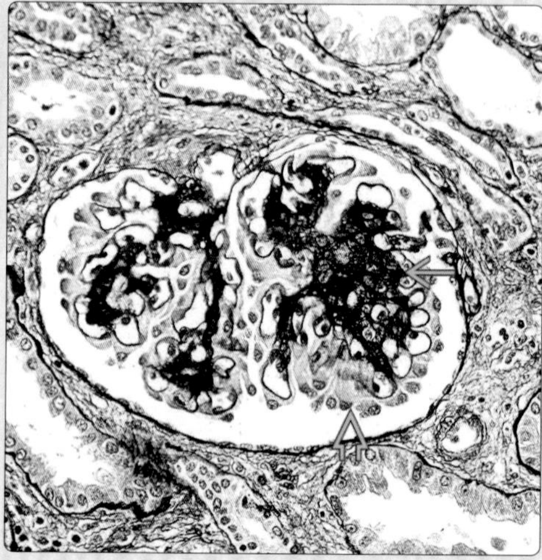

(Left) *Periodic acid-Schiff shows 2 globally sclerotic glomeruli surrounded by severe and diffuse interstitial fibrosis and tubular atrophy in this pediatric kidney allograft. (Courtesy T. Nadasdy, MD.)* **(Right)** *Jones methenamine silver stain shows mesangial sclerosis with prominence of the adjacent visceral epithelial cells. There is also segmental mesangial hypercellularity. (Courtesy T. Nadasdy, MD.)*

Segmental Sclerosis

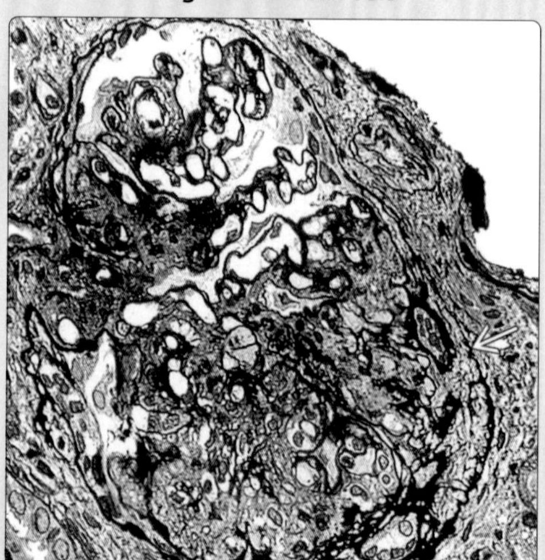

Prominent GBM Alterations

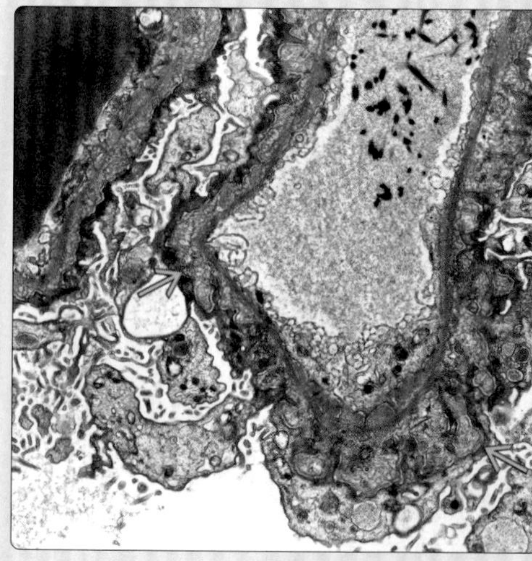

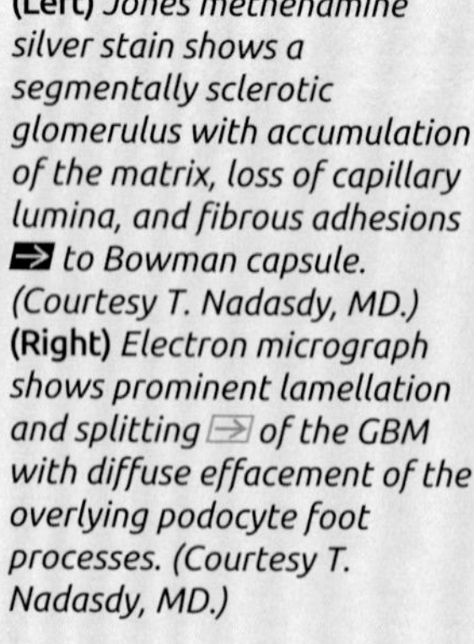

(Left) *Jones methenamine silver stain shows a segmentally sclerotic glomerulus with accumulation of the matrix, loss of capillary lumina, and fibrous adhesions to Bowman capsule. (Courtesy T. Nadasdy, MD.)* **(Right)** *Electron micrograph shows prominent lamellation and splitting of the GBM with diffuse effacement of the overlying podocyte foot processes. (Courtesy T. Nadasdy, MD.)*

TERMINOLOGY

Synonyms

- Hyperfiltration injury

Definitions

- Acute and chronic glomerular injury caused by transplantation of very young pediatric kidneys into adult recipients

ETIOLOGY/PATHOGENESIS

Hyperperfusion Injury

- 10% of pediatric kidneys (< 10 years of age) develop hyperperfusion injury when transplanted into adult recipients
  - Infant kidneys (< 1 year of age) more susceptible
  - En bloc (2 kidneys) transplantation may be less susceptible
- Possible contributing factors
  - Greater blood volume in adults compared with children
  - Higher systemic blood pressure in adults compared with children
  - Smaller glomeruli in children compared to adults
  - Thinner glomerular basement membrane (GBM) in children compared to adults
    - GBM thickness reaches maximum thickness at age 12-13
  - Altered composition of α chains of collagen IV in pediatric glomeruli
    - Embryonic GBM consists of α-1 and α-2 chains of collagen IV, gradually replaced by α-3, α-4, and α-5 chains as glomerulus matures

CLINICAL ISSUES

Epidemiology

- Incidence
  - Rare

Presentation

- Renal dysfunction
- Proteinuria
  - Often nephrotic range
- May develop as early as 10 weeks after transplantation

Laboratory Tests

- None
  - Kidney biopsy with electron microscopy only method to establish diagnosis

Prognosis

- Higher vascular complication rate
- Poor
  - Infant donor kidneys often fail within 1 year of transplantation

MICROSCOPIC

Histologic Features

- Glomerulus
  - Global &/or segmental glomerulosclerosis
    - Variable mesangial sclerosis &/or hypercellularity
  - Variable prominence of podocytes
- Tubulointerstitium
  - Interstitial fibrosis and tubular atrophy

ANCILLARY TESTS

Immunofluorescence

- Indirect IF for α-3 and α-5 chains of collagen IV demonstrates strong linear staining of GBM (normal)

Electron Microscopy

- Prominent glomerular basement membrane alterations
  - Diffuse lamellation and splitting
  - Marked thinning
- Podocyte injury
  - Diffuse foot process effacement
  - Microvillous transformation

DIFFERENTIAL DIAGNOSIS

Alport Syndrome

- Full thickness diffuse lamellation and splitting of GBM without normal segments by EM
- Indirect IF shows absence of GBM α-3 &/or α-5 chains of collagen IV
- Extensive donor work-up minimizes this clinical scenario

Recurrent Focal Segmental Glomerulosclerosis

- History of primary focal segmental glomerulosclerosis as original native renal disease
- Diffuse effacement of podocyte foot processes
- Normal GBM by EM

DIAGNOSTIC CHECKLIST

Pathologic Interpretation Pearls

- Clinical information of kidney donor needed to raise consideration of hyperperfusion injury
- EM essential for diagnosis
- Without EM finding of GBM alterations, light microscopic features of glomerular and tubulointerstitial scarring are nonspecific

SELECTED REFERENCES

1. Feltran Lde S et al: Does graft mass impact on pediatric kidney transplant outcomes? Pediatr Nephrol. 29(2):297-304, 2014
2. Friedersdorff F et al: Outcome of single pediatric deceased donor renal transplantation to adult kidney transplant recipients. Urol Int. 92(3):323-7, 2014
3. Borboroglu PG et al: Solitary renal allografts from pediatric cadaver donors less than 2 years of age transplanted into adult recipients. Transplantation. 77(5):698-702, 2004
4. Nadasdy T et al: Diffuse glomerular basement membrane lamellation in renal allografts from pediatric donors to adult recipients. Am J Surg Pathol. 23(4):437-42, 1999
5. Ratner LE et al: Transplantation of single and paired pediatric kidneys into adult recipients. J Am Coll Surg. 185(5):437-45, 1997
6. Satterthwaite R et al: Outcome of en bloc and single kidney transplantation from very young cadaveric donors. Transplantation. 63(10):1405-10, 1997
7. Hayes JM et al: The development of proteinuria and focal-segmental glomerulosclerosis in recipients of pediatric donor kidneys. Transplantation. 52(5):813-7, 1991
8. Truong LD et al: Electron microscopic study of an unusual posttransplant glomerular lesion. Arch Pathol Lab Med. 115(4):382-5, 1991

Engraftment Syndrome

KEY FACTS

TERMINOLOGY

- Systemic syndrome described in association with hematopoietic cell transplantation
  - Primarily observed in combined nonmyeloablative bone marrow transplant (BMT)/kidney transplant recipients
  - Can probably be seen in a variety of autologous or allogeneic transplants
- Synonyms: Capillary leak syndrome (CLS), marrow activation, or recovery syndrome (MAS)

CLINICAL ISSUES

- Renal dysfunction, fever, pulmonary edema, rash
- Recent regimens have seen less pronounced ES

MICROSCOPIC

- Acute tubular injury (ATI)
- Interstitial hemorrhage
- Congestion of peritubular capillaries (PTCs)

ANCILLARY TESTS

- Ki-67 positive in many cells in PTCs
- Cells include T cells (CD3[+], CD8[+]), macrophages (CD68[+]), & granulocytes (MPO[+])
- Cells in capillaries are of recipient origin by XY FISH
- EM shows severe damage to PTC endothelium & fibrin tactoids
- C4d usually negative

TOP DIFFERENTIAL DIAGNOSES

- Acute tubular injury due to ischemia
- Acute antibody-mediated (humoral) rejection
- Acute cellular rejection
- Thrombotic microangiopathy

DIAGNOSTIC CHECKLIST

- Ki-67(+) cells in glomeruli & PTCs distinguish ES from rejection & ATI

(Left) *PAS stain of a simultaneous bone marrow/kidney transplant patient shows loss of brush borders, flattened epithelial cells, cells in peritubular capillaries ⇨, and tubular mitoses ⇨.* **(Right)** *Light microscopy of a simultaneous bone marrow transplant/kidney transplant tolerance protocol patient shows a slightly hypercellular glomerulus with occasional cells in glomerular capillary loops ➡.*

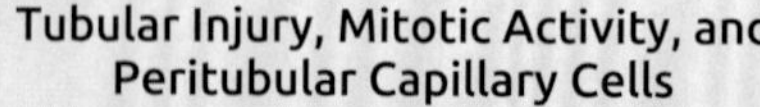

Tubular Injury, Mitotic Activity, and Peritubular Capillary Cells

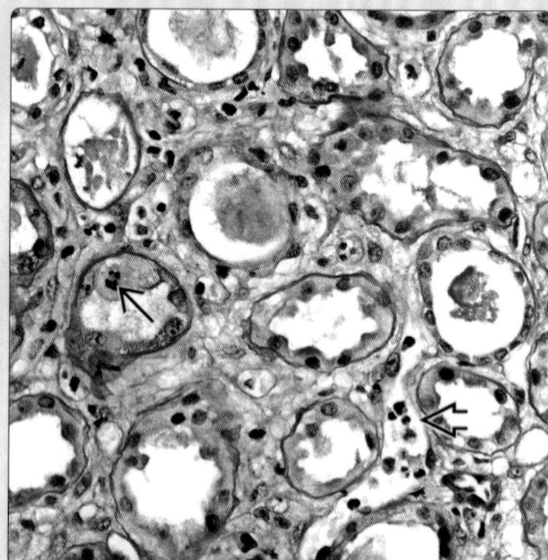

Glomerular Capillary Loop Inflammatory Cells

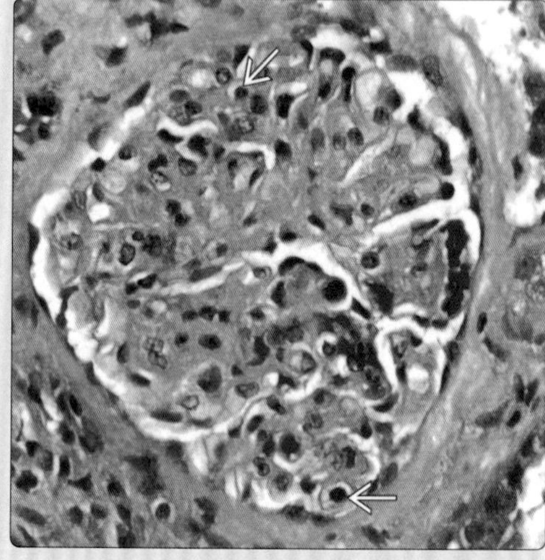

(Left) *Electron micrograph of a simultaneous bone marrow/kidney recipient in a protocol devised to induce tolerance shows "sludging/stasis" of erythrocytes in the peritubular capillaries and an attenuated peritubular capillary endothelium ➡.* **(Right)** *Ki-67 stain of a bone marrow/kidney transplant recipient in a protocol devised to induce tolerance shows numerous positive cells in peritubular capillaries and glomeruli ⇨.*

Erythrocyte Stasis in Peritubular Capillaries

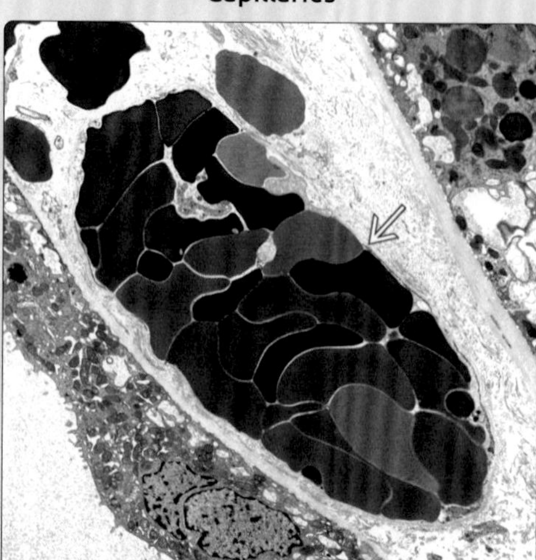

Ki-67(+) Cells in Glomeruli and Peritubular Capillaries

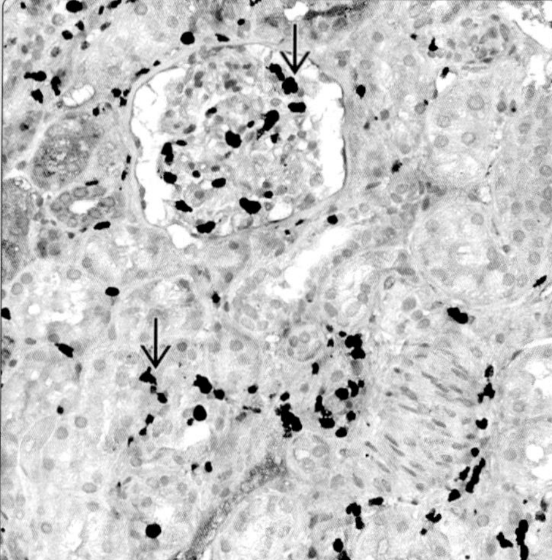

TERMINOLOGY

Abbreviations

- Engraftment syndrome (ES)

Definitions

- Systemic inflammatory syndrome described after bone marrow transplant (BMT)

ETIOLOGY/PATHOGENESIS

Postulated Mechanisms of BMT-Associated ES

- Cytokine release during recipient bone marrow recovery
- Auto-/alloreactivity to endothelium
- Homeostatic proliferation of lymphocytes
- Distinct from graft-vs.-host reaction

CLINICAL ISSUES

Epidemiology

- Incidence
  - Renal dysfunction in ~ 20% of cases in which BMT, either autologous or allogenic, is the only procedure
    - Occurs during recovery of donor marrow
    - Biopsies not typically performed to explain renal dysfunction in isolated BMT
  - ES is common in nonmyeloablative BMT combined with renal transplant
    - Occurs during recovery of recipient marrow, as chimerism declines
    - Although ES has primarily been observed in combined BMT/kidney transplants, the procedure of combined BMT/kidney is uncommon
    - Renal biopsies are more often available in combined BMT/kidney transplant, & findings can be extrapolated to dysfunction in other BMT

Presentation

- Acute renal failure
  - Creatinine rises 10-12 days after combined BMT/kidney transplant
- Fever, pulmonary edema (noncardiogenic), rash

Treatment

- Supportive, sometimes ↑ or ↓ in immunosuppression

Prognosis

- Typically transient

MICROSCOPIC

Histologic Features

- Glomeruli
  - Glomerular capillary mononuclear cells & neutrophils
  - No thrombi or hypercellularity
- Tubules
  - Acute tubular injury (ATI)
- Peritubular capillaries (PTCs)
  - Congestion & occasional inflammatory cells, including neutrophils & mononuclear cells
- Interstitium
  - Interstitial hemorrhage, focal
  - Little or no interstitial infiltrate
- Arteries
  - Usually normal
  - Endarteritis in minority of cases
  - Thrombi not conspicuous

ANCILLARY TESTS

Immunohistochemistry

- PTCs
  - Ki-67 shows numerous positive cells in PTCs & glomeruli
  - Intracapillary cells positive for CD3, CD68, & MPO
  - T cells are frequently CD8(+) with rare CD4(+) T cells; rare cells also FOXP3(+)
- Glomeruli
  - Similar to PTC, with Ki-67(+), CD3(+), CD8(+), & CD68(+) cells

Immunofluorescence

- C4d usually negative by both immunofluorescence (IF) & immunohistochemistry (IHC)
  - C4d(+) in association with donor-reactive antibodies

In Situ Hybridization

- XY FISH shows intracapillary cells are of recipient origin
- Over time, endothelial cells still remain of donor origin

Electron Microscopy

- Severe PTC endothelial damage & loss
- Fibrin tactoids can be seen in many PTCs

DIFFERENTIAL DIAGNOSIS

ATI From Other Causes

- ATI from other causes, such as ischemia, typically will have fewer Ki-67(+) cells in PTC

Acute Antibody-Mediated Rejection (AMR)

- C4d in PTCs by IF or IHC in AMR
- Neutrophils in PTCs & more prominent C4d positivity have been found in some cases of ES in combined BMT-kidney transplant
- No fibrinoid necrosis of arteries in ES

Acute Cellular Rejection (ACR)

- Endarteritis & tubulointerstitial infiltrates

Thrombotic Microangiopathy

- Thrombi in small blood vessels, sometimes accompanied by endothelial swelling, edema, &/or fibrinoid necrosis
- Schistocytes (fragmented red blood cells), particularly in walls of blood vessels
- Electron microscopy (EM) shows subendothelial widening &/or lucencies

SELECTED REFERENCES

1. Kawai T et al: Long-term results in recipients of combined HLA-mismatched kidney and bone marrow transplantation without maintenance immunosuppression. Am J Transplant. 14(7):1599-611, 2014
2. Farris AB et al: Acute renal endothelial injury during marrow recovery in a cohort of combined kidney and bone marrow allografts. Am J Transplant. 11(7):1464-77, 2011
3. Troxell ML et al: Renal pathology in hematopoietic cell transplantation recipients. Mod Pathol. 21(4):396-406, 2008

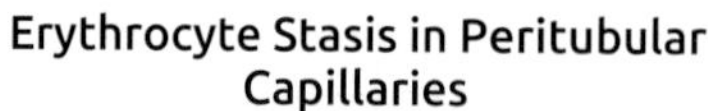

Erythrocyte Stasis in Peritubular Capillaries

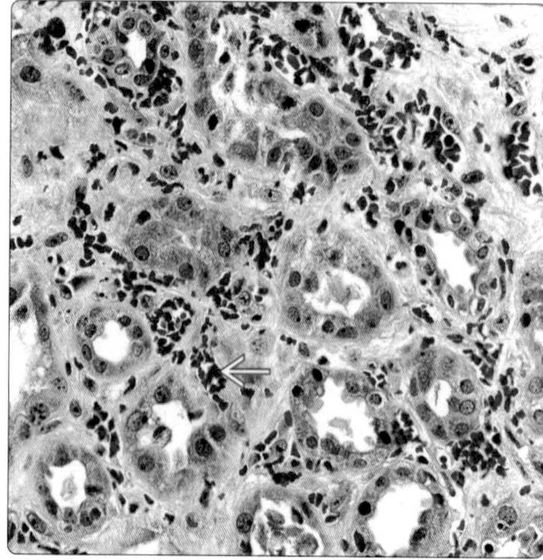

Erythrocyte Stasis in Peritubular Capillaries

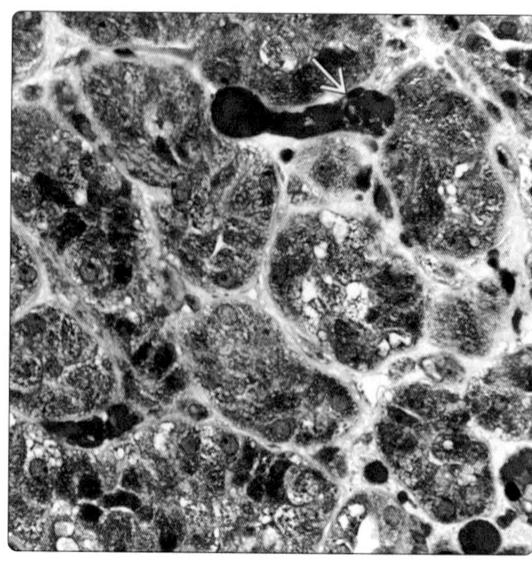

(Left) *Trichrome stain of a patient undergoing simultaneous bone marrow/kidney transplant in a protocol devised to induce tolerance shows widespread erythrocyte stasis* ➡. **(Right)** *Trichrome stain of a bone marrow-kidney allograft recipient in a tolerance protocol shows erythrocyte stasis with occasional cells that can be appreciated in peritubular capillaries on light microscopy* ➡.

Focal Endarteritis During ES Episode

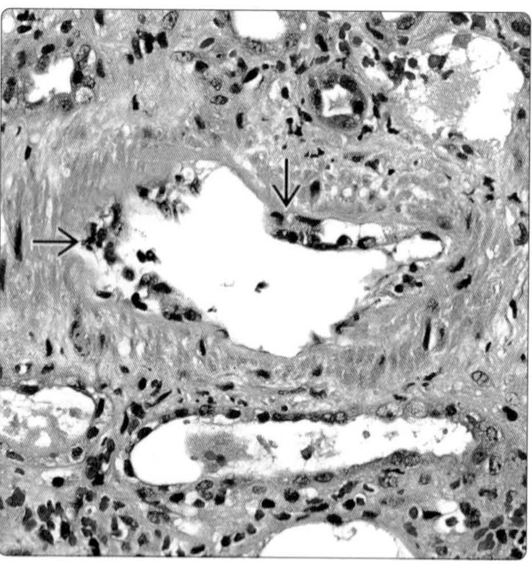

CD3(+) Cells in Glomeruli and Peritubular Capillaries

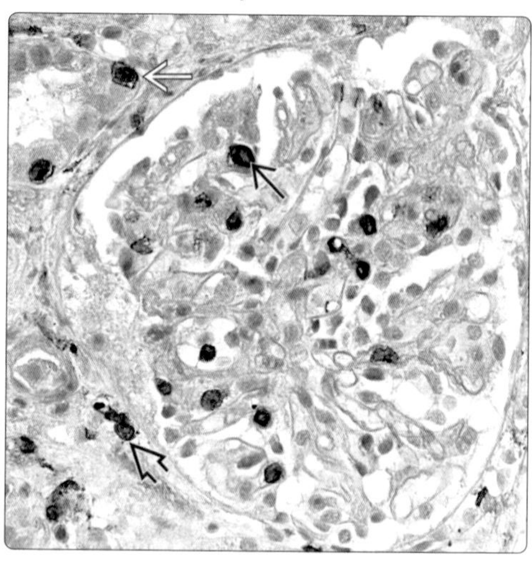

(Left) *Focal endarteritis* → *is seen in a small artery from a bone marrow/kidney recipient in a tolerance protocol biopsied 10 days post transplant during an episode of engraftment syndrome (ES). It is not clear whether this represents cellular rejection or a manifestation of the endothelial injury from ES.* **(Right)** *CD3(+) cells in glomeruli* →*, peritubular capillaries* ⇨*, and a focus of tubulitis* ➡ *can be seen by immunohistochemistry in a bone marrow/kidney transplant recipient in a tolerance protocol.*

CD68(+) Cells in Peritubular Capillaries

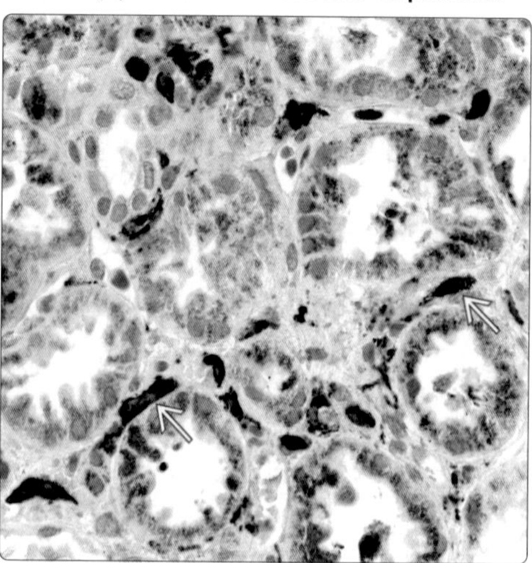

CD34 Stains Peritubular Capillary Endothelium and Cells

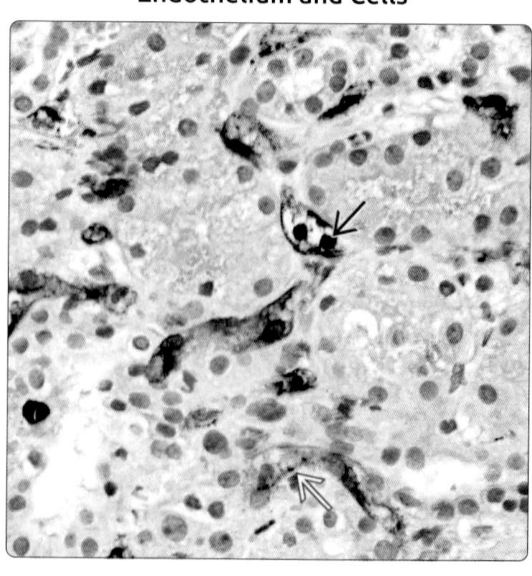

(Left) *CD68 stain shows numerous positive cells in peritubular capillaries* ➡ *in a bone marrow/kidney transplant recipient in a protocol devised to induce tolerance.* **(Right)** *CD34 stain of a bone marrow/kidney transplant recipient in a protocol devised to induce tolerance shows CD34(+) cells in peritubular capillaries* →*, possibly immature bone marrow cells, and patchy loss of CD34 staining of PTC endothelium* ➡*, suggesting endothelial damage.*

Peritubular Capillary Fibrin

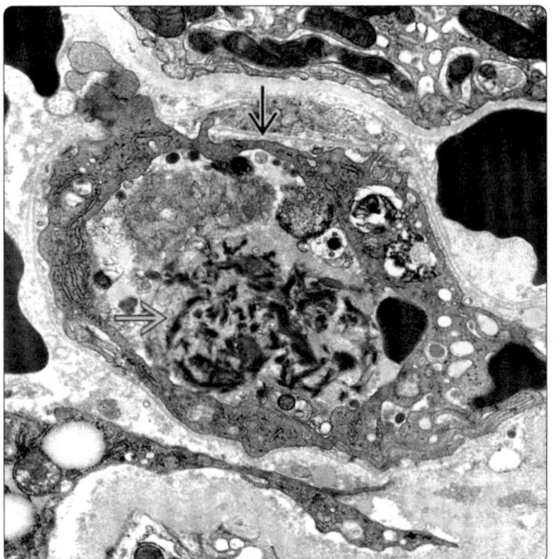

Red Blood Cell Stasis in Peritubular Capillaries

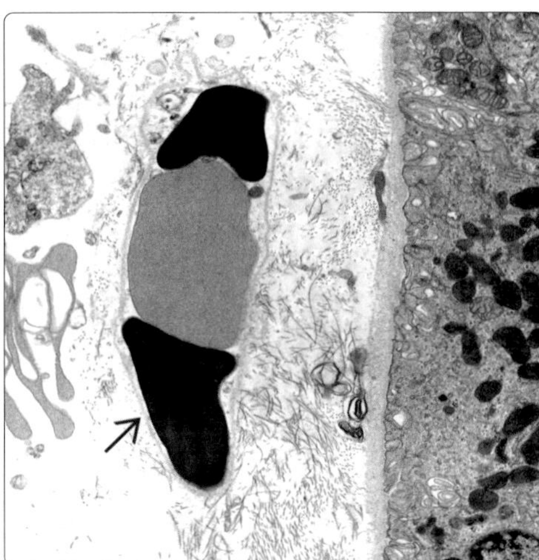

(Left) *Electron micrograph of a peritubular capillary in a bone marrow/kidney transplant recipient in a protocol devised to induce tolerance shows fibrin tactoids ⇒ and a reactive endothelium →.* **(Right)** *Electron micrograph of a simultaneous bone marrow/kidney transplant recipient in a protocol devised to induce tolerance shows a peritubular capillary engorged with erythrocytes with a denuded endothelium →.*

Erythrocytes in Glomerular Capillaries

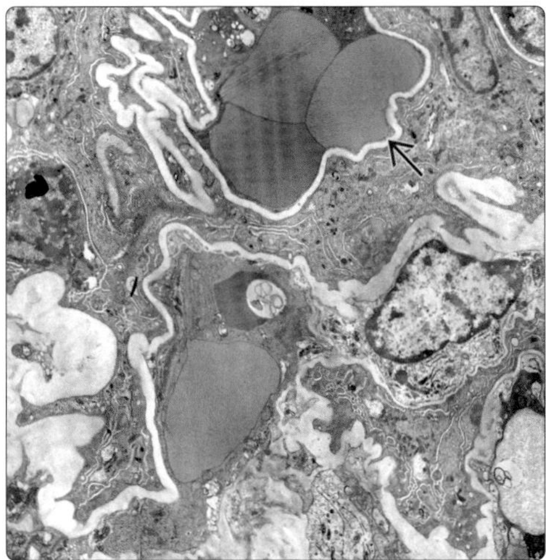

XY FISH Recipient Cells

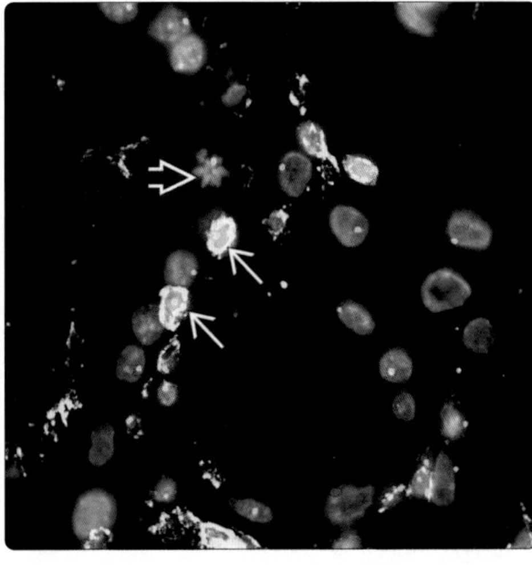

(Left) *Electron micrograph in a tolerance protocol patient status post simultaneous bone marrow/kidney transplant shows that glomerular capillaries are engorged by erythrocytes and that there is focal thinning of the glomerular basement membrane →.* **(Right)** *FISH in a female tolerance protocol recipient of a male renal and bone marrow allograft shows that CD45(+) cells in PTC are from the recipient → (green X chromosome, red Y chromosome, yellow CD45, blue DAPI). A mitotic figure can be seen ⇒.*

XY FISH Recipient Cells

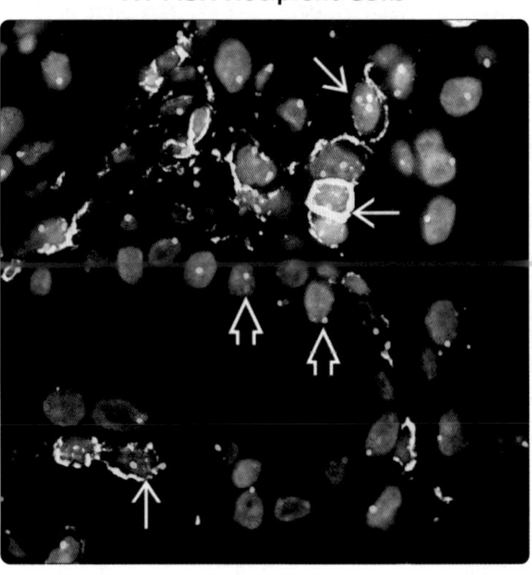

XY FISH Shows Recipient Cells

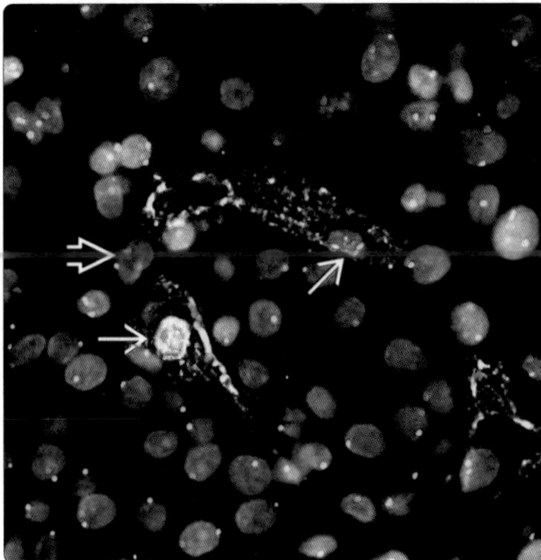

(Left) *FISH in a female tolerance protocol recipient of a male renal and bone marrow allograft shows recipient CD45(+) cells → in PTCs. Donor tubular epithelial cells can be appreciated ⇒ (green X, red Y, yellow CD45, blue DAPI).* **(Right)** *FISH in a female bone marrow/kidney transplant protocol recipient from a male donor shows several recipient cells in peritubular capillaries →. Donor cells can also be seen ⇒ (green X, red Y, yellow CD34, blue DAPI).*

Acute Tubular Injury in Allografts

KEY FACTS

TERMINOLOGY

- Ischemic graft injury in early post-transplant period
- Delayed graft function (DGF) defined by need for dialysis in 1st week
- Primary nonfunction (PNF) grafts never function

ETIOLOGY/PATHOGENESIS

- ↑ risk from deceased cardiac death (DCD) donors as opposed to heart-beating donation after brain death (DBD)
- Glomerular and other microvascular injury through various mediators and complement activation
- Anastomotic site complications and other causes of ischemia (such as poor preservation)

CLINICAL ISSUES

- 95-98% of grafts with DGF recover
- Rejection risk increased
- ↑ with drug toxicity (e.g., calcineurin inhibitors)

MICROSCOPIC

- Tubular epithelial cell flattening, vacuolization, & mitoses
- Interstitial edema & minimal inflammation
- Glomerular injury with variable intracapillary endothelial swelling, neutrophils, and fibrin thrombi
- Medullary vessels dilated and filled with mononuclear cells, erythrocytes, and neutrophils

ANCILLARY TESTS

- C4d negative in peritubular capillaries

TOP DIFFERENTIAL DIAGNOSES

- Calcineurin inhibitor toxicity
- Acute antibody-mediated rejection
- Acute obstruction
- Renal artery or vein thrombosis

DIAGNOSTIC CHECKLIST

- Biopsy to determine cause of DGF after 10 days

Renal Tubular Injury

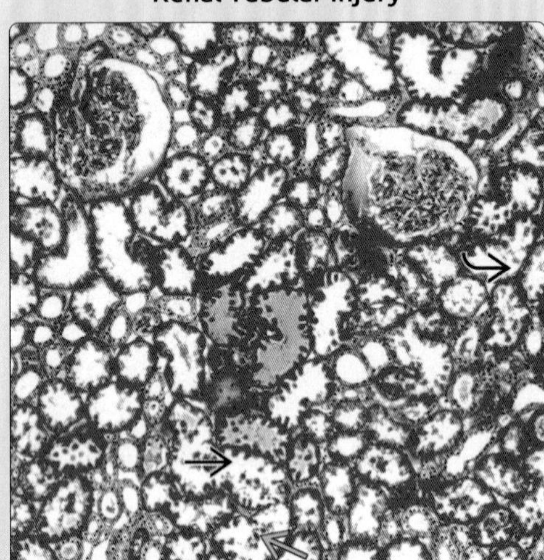

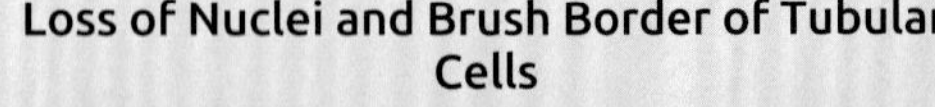

Loss of Nuclei and Brush Border of Tubular Cells

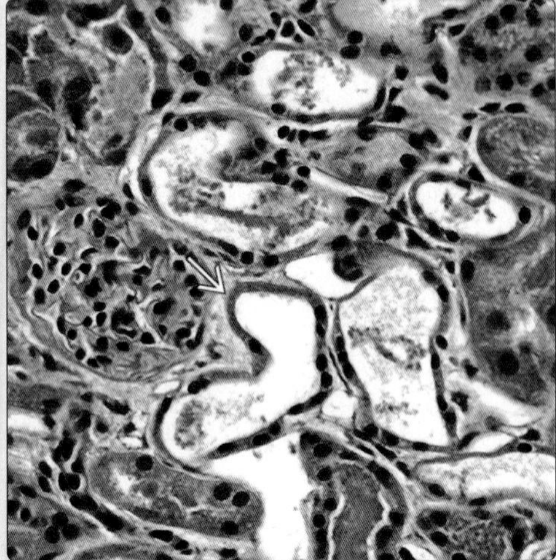

(Left) *Low-power view shows a kidney with ischemic injury, possessing dilated tubules and epithelial injury in a hobnail pattern ⮕. Some glomerular basement membranes are bare ⮕, lacking tubular epithelial cells. Sloughed cells ⮕ can be seen within the renal tubules.* **(Right)** *In a deceased donor renal allograft with oliguria on day 2, there is acute tubular injury with marked tubular cytoplasmic thinning, cellular loss, and debris, showing loss of tubular nuclei ⮕.*

Focal Interstitial Inflammation

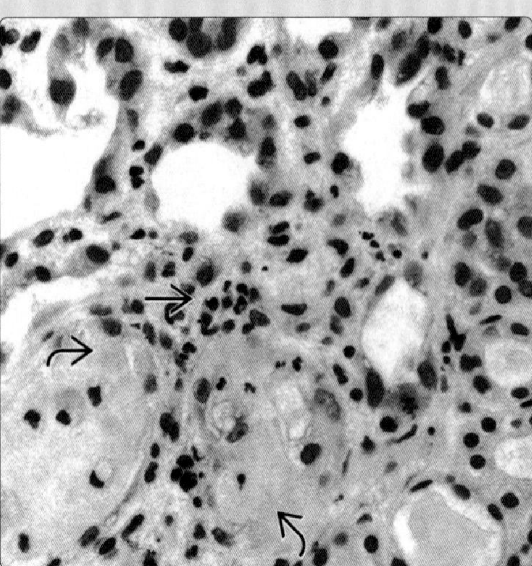

Ki-67 Stains Tubular Nuclei

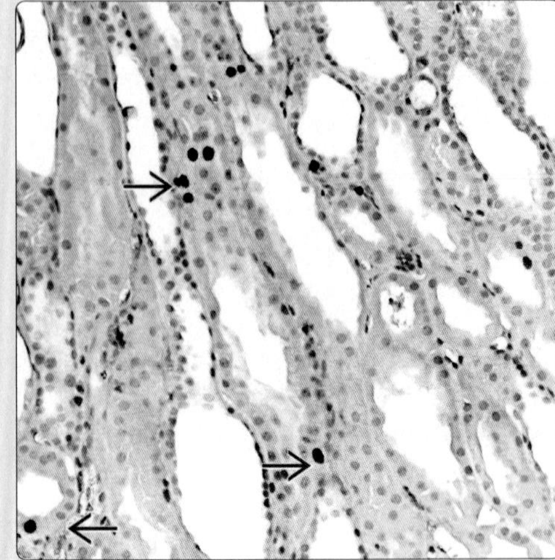

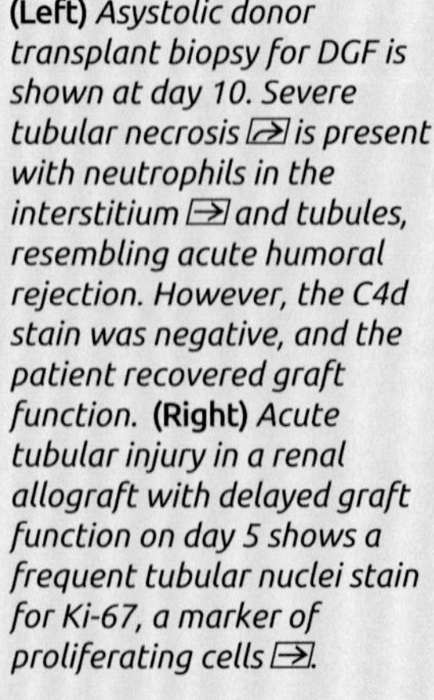

(Left) *Asystolic donor transplant biopsy for DGF is shown at day 10. Severe tubular necrosis ⮕ is present with neutrophils in the interstitium ⮕ and tubules, resembling acute humoral rejection. However, the C4d stain was negative, and the patient recovered graft function.* **(Right)** *Acute tubular injury in a renal allograft with delayed graft function on day 5 shows a frequent tubular nuclei stain for Ki-67, a marker of proliferating cells ⮕.*

TERMINOLOGY

Synonyms

- Acute tubular injury (ATI)

Definitions

- Ischemic graft injury in early post-transplant period
- Delayed graft function (DGF) usually defined by need for transient dialysis in 1st week post transplantation
- Primary nonfunction (PNF) grafts never function

ETIOLOGY/PATHOGENESIS

Acute Ischemic Injury

- ↓ oxygen delivery/perfusion
  - ↑ risk with ↑ warm (> 40 min) & cold (> 24 hr) ischemia times
  - Apoptosis & necroptosis, a regulated necrosis pathway, may participate in cell death
- NK & T cells produce mediators, such as IFN-γ → adhesion molecules upregulation
  - Dying cells release danger signals, alarming toll-like receptors (TLRs), leading to cell recruitment
- Complement activation
  - Colocalization of mannose binding lectins (MBL) with complement in ischemia-reperfusion injury (IRI)
- Calcineurin inhibitor toxicity may augment ATI
- Compromised vascular anastomosis
- Renal artery dissection

CLINICAL ISSUES

Epidemiology

- Incidence
  - DGF in 2-25% of deceased donor grafts & PNF in 1-2%; varies with center
    - Asystolic donors have ↑ DGF (19-84%) & PNF (4-18%)
  - ↑ risk from DCD donors as opposed to DBD

Treatment

- Transient dialysis
- Reduce calcineurin inhibitors
- Complement inhibitors and other inhibitors under investigation

Prognosis

- 95-98% of grafts with DGF recover
  - DGF typically lasts 10-15 days; < 2% last > 4 weeks
- DGF ↑ incidence of acute rejection and later fibrosis
  - 50% increased risk of T-cell-mediated rejection (16% vs. 11%) or antibody-mediated rejection (10% vs. 7%)

MACROSCOPIC

General Features

- Blotchy, mottled appearance with darker areas that are poorly perfused

MICROSCOPIC

Histologic Features

- Glomeruli variably affected
  - Endothelial swelling and vacuolization, capillary collapse
  - Neutrophils correlate with cold ischemia time and subsequent graft loss
  - Fibrin thrombi do not affect overall outcome
- Tubules
  - Brush border and nuclear loss, thinning, and dilation, particularly in proximal tubules
    - Nonisometric tubular cell vacuolization
    - Intratubular cellular debris and neutrophils
    - In severe cases, bare tubular basement membrane (TBM) from desquamation of tubular epithelial cells ("nonreplacement phenomenon")
  - Regeneration features (later): Basophilic cytoplasm, prominent nucleoli, mitosis
- Interstitium
  - Edema & minimal inflammation with a few neutrophils & mononuclear cells
- Vessels
  - Dilated medullary vessels filled with mononuclear cells & erythroid precursors
  - C4d negative in peritubular capillaries

ANCILLARY TESTS

Immunofluorescence

- C4d negative in peritubular capillaries

DIFFERENTIAL DIAGNOSIS

Calcineurin Inhibitor (CNI) Toxicity

- Difficult to distinguish on histologic grounds alone
- Classically, isometric vacuolization plus ATI
- Associated with high levels of CNI

Acute Antibody-Mediated Rejection

- Can present as ATI but peritubular capillaries usually C4d positive
- Donor-specific antibody assays positive in > 90%

Acute T-Cell-Mediated Rejection

- Interstitial mononuclear cells, tubulitis, &/or endarteritis

Acute Obstruction

- Collection ducts dilated with little tubular necrosis
- Tamm-Horsfall protein in lymphatics

Arterial or Venous Thrombosis

- Ultrasound imaging and Doppler to determine blood flow

DIAGNOSTIC CHECKLIST

Pathologic Interpretation Pearls

- Biopsy recommended to determine cause after 10 days

SELECTED REFERENCES

1. Wu WK et al: Delayed graft function and the risk of acute rejection in the modern era of kidney transplantation. Kidney Int. ePub, 2015
2. Zhang ZX et al: Natural killer cells mediate long-term kidney allograft injury. Transplantation. ePub, 2015
3. Ponticelli C: Ischaemia-reperfusion injury: a major protagonist in kidney transplantation. Nephrol Dial Transplant. 29(6):1134-40, 2014
4. Lau A et al: RIPK3-mediated necroptosis promotes donor kidney inflammatory injury and reduces allograft survival. Am J Transplant. 13(11):2805-18, 2013
5. Linkermann A et al: Necroptosis in immunity and ischemia-reperfusion injury. Am J Transplant. 13(11):2797-804, 2013

KEY FACTS

ETIOLOGY/PATHOGENESIS

- Dysfunctional ureterovesical anastomosis, ischemic injury, or rejection episodes
- Laparoscopic techniques previously associated with higher complication rate, but has declined as technique matured

CLINICAL ISSUES

- Urine leak complicates 3-5% of renal transplants
- Presentation in postoperative period, usually within 4 months (84%), within 24 hours if due to a technical error, within 2-3 weeks if ischemia
  - Hematuria, oliguria/renal dysfunction, and fistulas
- Treatment: Percutaneous nephrostomy, dilatation/stent placement, surgical exploration/reanastomosis, endoscopic methods, special catheter placement
- Prognosis: If corrected, does not typically impact 10-year patient or graft survival

IMAGING

- Radiology may demonstrate fluid leak (urinoma)
- Renal scintigraphy tracer urinary extravasation
- Antegrade pyelograph may allow leak localization

MICROSCOPIC

- Interstitial inflammation and tubular injury may be present
  - Inflammation in surrounding soft tissue
- Edema in renal parenchyma and in soft tissue surrounding urine leak
- Vascular thrombosis of periureteral vessels (80%)
  - Productive CMV (15%) or BK virus (8%) infection

TOP DIFFERENTIAL DIAGNOSES

- Lymphocele: Cr and potassium concentrations lower and sodium concentration higher

Ultrasound of Urine Leak

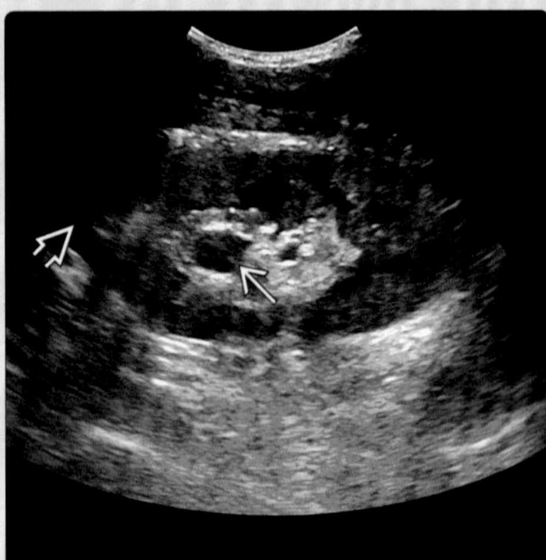

Tubular Injury

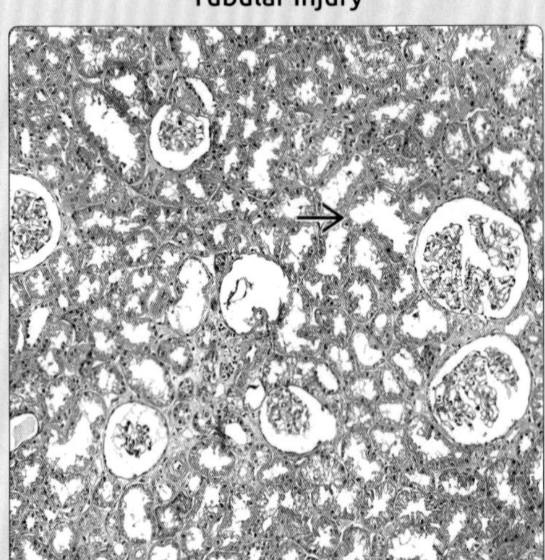

(Left) *Ultrasound of a graft that developed a urine leak, taken 7 days post transplant, shows a collection of perinephric fluid ➡ along one pole. The dilated pelvis ➡ is a sign of obstruction.* **(Right)** *Low-power hematoxylin & eosin of a biopsy specimen from a patient with urine leak shows irregular, dilated renal tubules ➡ with mild tubular injury.*

Tubular Injury

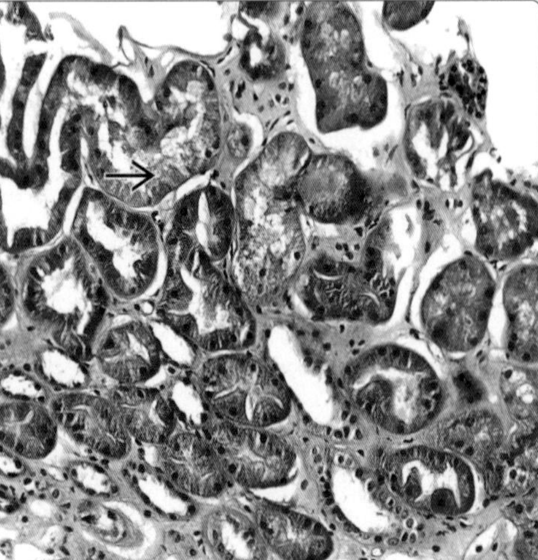

Focal Inflammation

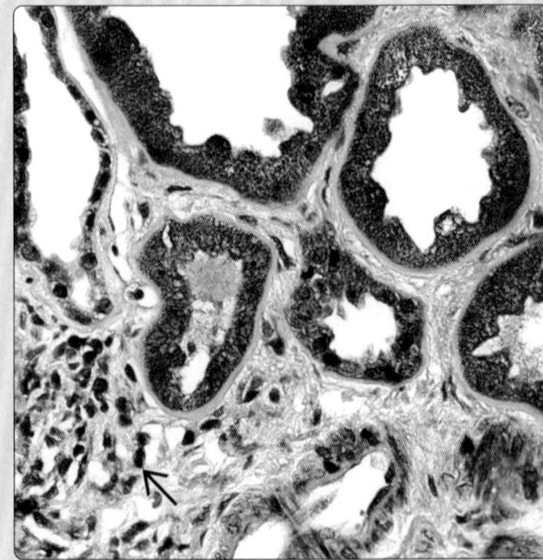

(Left) *Medium power of a biopsy specimen from a patient with urine leak shows focal nuclear loss ➡ and tubular irregularities, both of which are findings of mild tubular injury.* **(Right)** *Medium-power trichome shows a focal lymphoid infiltrate ➡ amidst an edematous stroma and irregular tubules in a urine leak.*

TERMINOLOGY

Definitions

- Urine collection due to numerous causes, often as anastomotic "leak" in setting of transplantation

ETIOLOGY/PATHOGENESIS

Dysfunctional Anastomosis

- May cause reflux/leakage
- Surgical technical error may be cause
  - Misplacement of ureteral sutures (often at ureterovesical location)
  - Insufficient ureteral length
  - Ureter or renal pelvis laceration
  - Often evident within 24 hours

Ureteral Ischemic Injury

- Risk of proximal ureter devascularization since renal pelvic vessels provide its blood supply
- Ureter ischemic more distally from kidney
- Renal allograft pelvic placement allows minimal length of transplant ureter
  - Special techniques: Psoas hitch, Boari flap, ureteroureterostomy, pyelovesicostomy, and ileal ureter
- Lowest risk when "golden triangle" of perirenal fat bordered by ureter and lower renal pole preserved
- Ischemic necrosis leaks usually occur 2-3 weeks after transplantation

Rejection Episodes

- With transplant endarteritis, may involve ureteral graft vessels

Laparoscopic Technique

- Living donor procurement initially associated with high incidence
- Complication rate now almost as low as open donors

CLINICAL ISSUES

Epidemiology

- Incidence
  - 1-15% of renal transplant recipients have urologic complications
    - Urine leak complicates 3-5% of renal transplants
  - 1-3% of renal transplant recipients have ureteral leak

Site

- Renal calyx, bladder, or ureter

Presentation

- Oliguria
  - Sudden decrease in urinary output
- Hematuria
- Urinary fistula
  - May result from necrosis of distal ureter
- Creatinine (Cr) and plasma urea increase
  - Due to solute resorption across peritoneum
- Scrotal swelling
- Wound drain
  - Difficult to determine if fluid production from preexisting seroma or lymph draining

Laboratory Tests

- Provided good renal excretory function, Cr concentration in leak fluid several times higher than serum Cr

Natural History

- Postoperative period: Majority in 1st 4 months (84%)

Treatment

- Percutaneous nephrostomy
- Dilatation/stent placement
- Urgent surgical exploration/reanastomosis
- Endoscopic methods
- 3-way Foley catheter with irrigation that intermittently fills and empties bladder

Prognosis

- Does not typically impact 10-year patient or graft survival

IMAGING

General Features

- Ultrasound shows fluid collection (urinoma) but not its source
- Renal scintigraphy tracer urinary extravasation
- Antegrade pyelograph may allow leak localization

MICROSCOPIC

Histologic Features

- Limited data on renal histopathologic changes
  - Interstitial inflammation and tubular injury may be present
    - Inflammation in surrounding soft tissue
  - Edema in renal parenchyma and soft tissue surrounding urine leak
- In study of 25 surgically removed, necrotic, ureteral segments
  - Vascular thrombosis of periureteral vessels (80%), productive CMV (15%), or BK virus (8%)

DIFFERENTIAL DIAGNOSIS

Lymphocele

- Cr and potassium concentrations lower and sodium concentration higher

SELECTED REFERENCES

1. Hedegard W et al: Management of vascular and nonvascular complications after renal transplantation. Tech Vasc Interv Radiol. 12(4):240-62, 2009
2. Kobayashi K et al: Interventional radiologic management of renal transplant dysfunction: indications, limitations, and technical considerations. Radiographics. 27(4):1109-30, 2007
3. Karam G et al: Ureteral necrosis after kidney transplantation: risk factors and impact on graft and patient survival. Transplantation. 78(5):725-9, 2004
4. Streeter EH et al: The urological complications of renal transplantation: a series of 1535 patients. BJU Int. 90(7):627-34, 2002
5. Fontaine AB et al: Update on the use of percutaneous nephrostomy/balloon dilation for the treatment of renal transplant leak/obstruction. J Vasc Interv Radiol. 8(4):649-53, 1997

Lymphocele

KEY FACTS

TERMINOLOGY

- Collections of lymphatic fluid in perinephric space

ETIOLOGY/PATHOGENESIS

- Incomplete lymphatic anastomosis
  - Donor renal lymphatics at hilum fail to anastomose with recipient lymphatics
  - Normally lymphatics spontaneously reconnect
- Rejection episodes
  - Lead to increased vascular permeability, edema, lymph fluid, and promote lymphocele formation

CLINICAL ISSUES

- Around 34% of transplant patients have clinically significant lymphocele
- Infection can lead to obstruction and infectious complications if large

MICROSCOPIC

- Typically fibrous tissue with internal cystic formation with inflammatory cells in wall
  - Predominantly composed of mononuclear lymphoid cells
- Renal biopsy may show changes of obstruction
- Collecting duct dilation
- Interstitial edema
- Dilation of lymphatics, present normally along larger vessels

DIAGNOSTIC CHECKLIST

- Consider lymphocele when no obvious change in biopsy accounts for renal transplant dysfunction
  - Particularly when obstructive features are seen
  - Microscopic features include chronic inflammation, edema, and dilated lymphatics

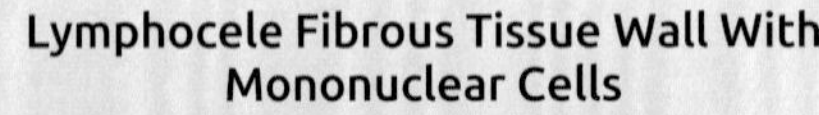

Lymphocele Fibrous Tissue Wall With Mononuclear Cells

Tubular Injury and Focal Interstitial Inflammation

(Left) *Light microscopy of a lymphocele wall shows that it is composed of fibrous tissue with a focus of mononuclear chronic inflammatory cells.* **(Right)** *Kidney biopsy at low power shows a minimal focal interstitial inflammation ⇒ and tubular injury in a case of lymphocele.*

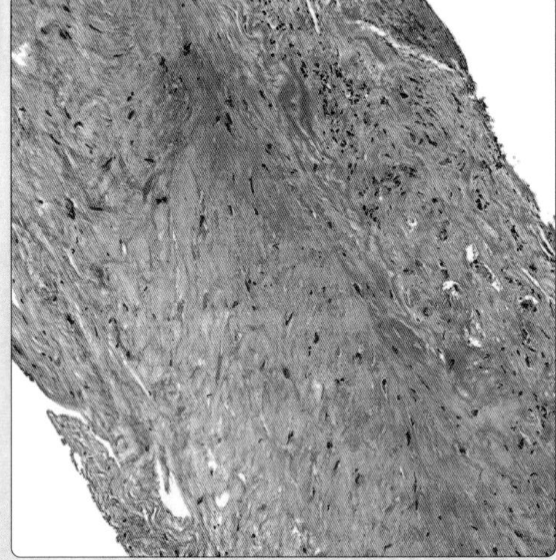

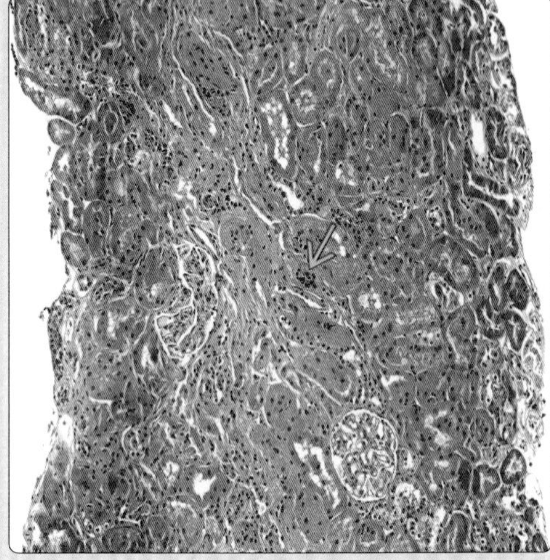

Tubular Injury

Lymphocele Fibrous Tissue Wall With Focal Chronic Inflammation

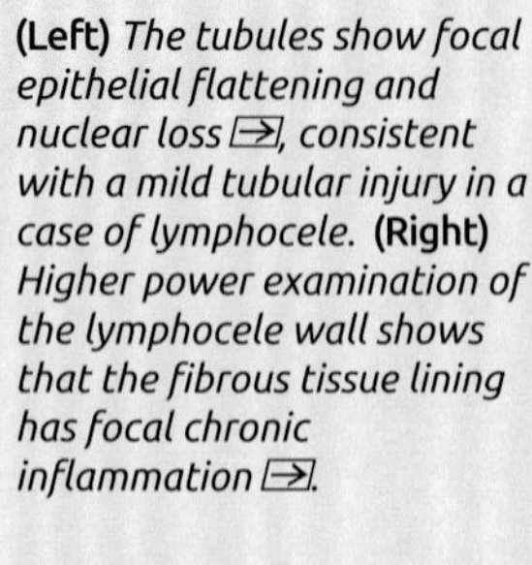

(Left) *The tubules show focal epithelial flattening and nuclear loss ⇒, consistent with a mild tubular injury in a case of lymphocele.* **(Right)** *Higher power examination of the lymphocele wall shows that the fibrous tissue lining has focal chronic inflammation ⇒.*

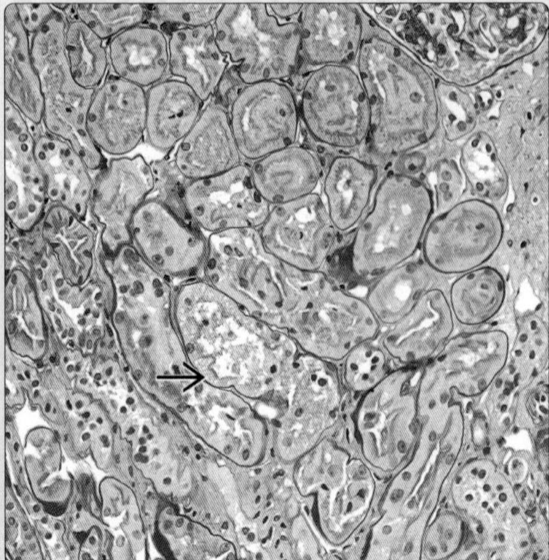

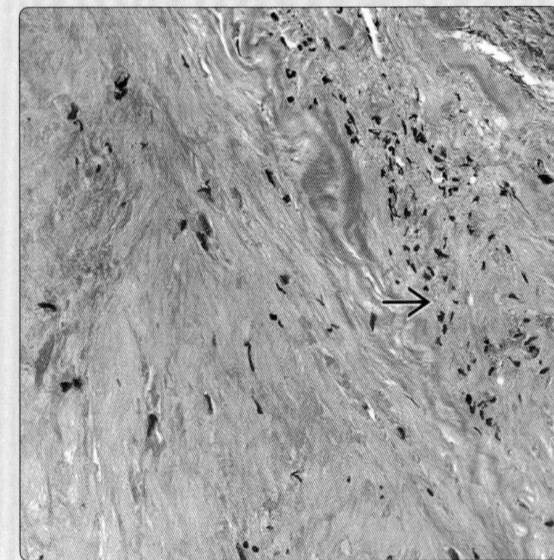

TERMINOLOGY

Definitions

- Collection of lymphatic fluid in nonepithelialized cavity in perinephric space, typically in postoperative field

ETIOLOGY/PATHOGENESIS

Incomplete Lymphatic Anastomoses

- Donor renal lymphatics at hilum fail to anastomose with recipient lymphatics
- Normally lymphatics spontaneously reconnect
- Careful surgical ligation of lymphatic vessels is necessary to prevent lymphocele formation

Rejection Episodes

- Lead to increased vascular permeability, edema, lymph fluid, and promote lymphocele formation

CLINICAL ISSUES

Epidemiology

- Incidence
  - Most occur within 6 weeks after transplantation
  - Occur in 1-26% of transplant recipients
  - Large series indicated incidence is usually around 2%
    - Can occur 2-11 years post transplantation
    - 1/3 had rejection episodes
    - Another series revealed that some lymphoceles are subclinical
  - Obesity a risk factor

Presentation

- May be painful
- Urinary frequency may occur if there is bladder compression
- Lower extremity edema and deep venous thrombosis can be seen
- Infection can lead to obstruction and infectious complications if large

Laboratory Tests

- Creatinine level is similar to serum

Treatment

- Surgical approaches
  - Laparoscopic or open drainage, sometimes with marsupialization
- Ultrasound-guided or CT-guided percutaneous drainage, sometimes combined with sclerotherapy

Prognosis

- 5-10% recur but does not affect graft survival

IMAGING

Ultrasonographic Findings

- Most are small and detected only on ultrasound
- Some are large and may be multilocular or multiple in number
- Hydronephrosis with dilated calyces and hydroureter due to obstruction of ureter may be present

MACROSCOPIC

General Features

- Perinephric nonsanguinous and nonpurulent fluid collection
- Most occur adjacent to lower pole of kidney posterolateral to transplant ureter

MICROSCOPIC

Histologic Features

- Typically fibrous tissue with internal cystic formation with inflammatory cells in wall
  - Inflammation predominantly composed of mononuclear lymphoid cells
  - No epithelial lining
- Renal biopsy may show changes of obstruction
  - Collecting duct dilation
  - Interstitial edema
  - Dilation of lymphatics, present normally along larger vessels
    - Lymphatics are in kidney proper or in operative field
  - Mild interstitial mononuclear inflammation ("borderline" rejection pattern)
- Microscopic pathologic descriptions are limited

DIFFERENTIAL DIAGNOSIS

Abscess

- High numbers of neutrophils are appreciated on aspirate samples
- Cultures of aspirates useful

Hematoma

- Occur earlier, often in immediate postsurgical period

Urine Leak

- Has higher creatinine and potassium concentration and lower sodium concentration

DIAGNOSTIC CHECKLIST

Pathologic Interpretation Pearls

- Lymphocele should be considered when no obvious change in biopsy accounts for renal transplant dysfunction
  - Particularly when obstructive features are seen
- May be mimicked by other perigraft fluid collections

SELECTED REFERENCES

1. Kostro JZ et al: The use of tenckhoff catheters for draining of symptomatic lymphoceles: a review of literature and our experience. Transplant Proc. 47(2):384-7, 2015
2. Giuliani S et al: Lymphocele after pediatric kidney transplantation: incidence and risk factors. Pediatr Transplant. 18(7):720-5, 2014
3. Khater N et al: Pseudorejection and true rejection after kidney transplantation: classification and clinical significance. Urol Int. 90(4):373-80, 2013
4. Lucewicz A et al: Management of primary symptomatic lymphocele after kidney transplantation: a systematic review. Transplantation. 92(6):663-73, 2011
5. Minetti EE: Lymphocele after renal transplantation, a medical complication. J Nephrol. 24(6):707-16, 2011

Renal Artery or Vein Thrombosis

KEY FACTS

TERMINOLOGY

- Thrombosis of renal artery (RAT) or vein (RVT)

ETIOLOGY/PATHOGENESIS

- Anastomotic problems
- Multiple arteries or arterial stenosis
- Hypercoagulability
- External compression by hematoma, lymphocele, or other lesions

CLINICAL ISSUES

- Macrohematuria
- Acute renal failure
- Prevalence highly variable by center
- Early treatment essential
  - Surgical correction or drugs
- Arterial thrombosis usually occurs within 30 days of transplant
- RVT early or late

MICROSCOPIC

- Thrombosis in vessel lumina
- Loss of endothelium
- Infarction of cortex, particularly in RAT
- Sparse neutrophils in capillaries
- Recanalization if chronic

TOP DIFFERENTIAL DIAGNOSES

- Hyperacute and acute humoral rejection
  - C4d(+) in peritubular capillaries
  - Usually no large vessel thrombosis
- Acute cellular rejection
  - Endothelial mononuclear inflammation

DIAGNOSTIC CHECKLIST

- C4d(-) in peritubular capillaries

(Left) *Thrombosis of the renal vein ➡ 2 days post living donor transplant is shown. The cortex is congested. Arterial thrombosis developed hours post transplant. Despite an arterial thrombectomy, RVT ensued.* **(Right)** *An acute thrombus ⇨ is attached to the internal elastic lamina ➡ of the renal artery with loss of endothelium. No inflammation is evident, in contrast to acute humoral or cellular rejection.*

Renal Vein Thrombosis (RVT)

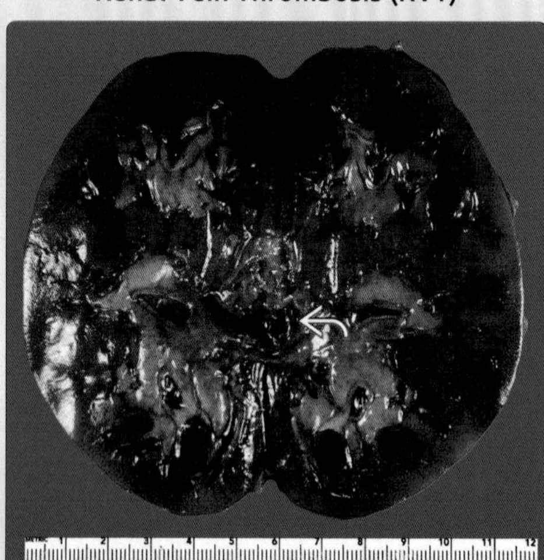

Renal Artery Stenosis

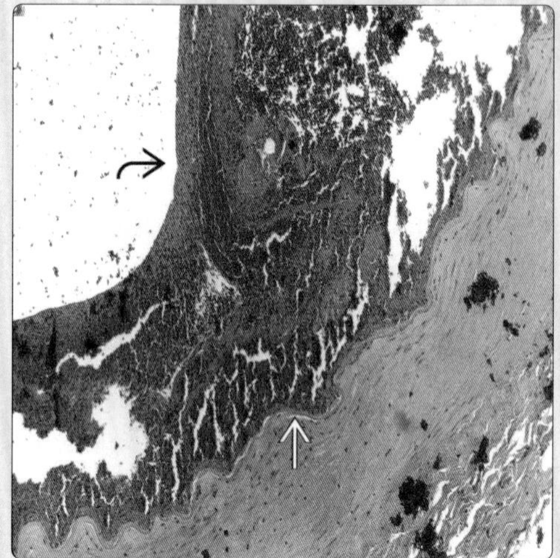

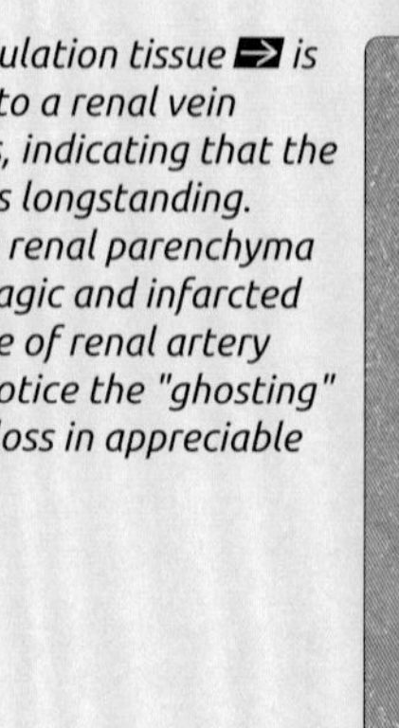

(Left) *Granulation tissue ➡ is growing into a renal vein thrombosis, indicating that the thrombus is longstanding.* **(Right)** *The renal parenchyma is hemorrhagic and infarcted ➡ in a case of renal artery stenosis. Notice the "ghosting" &/or total loss in appreciable tubules.*

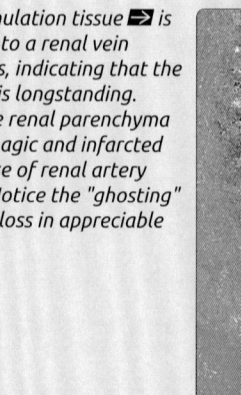

Chronic Renal Vein Thrombosis

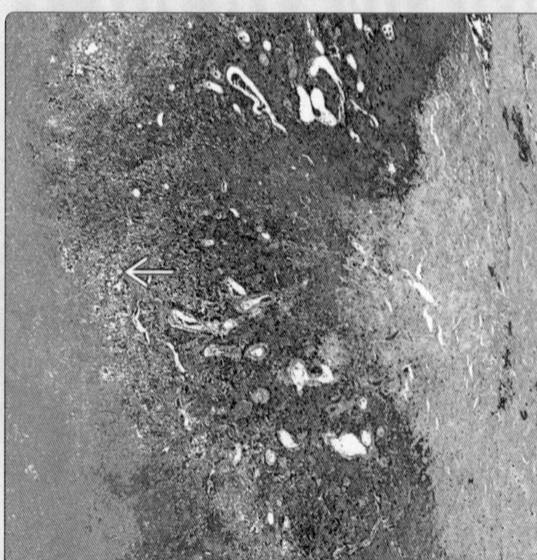

Infarction in Renal Artery Stenosis

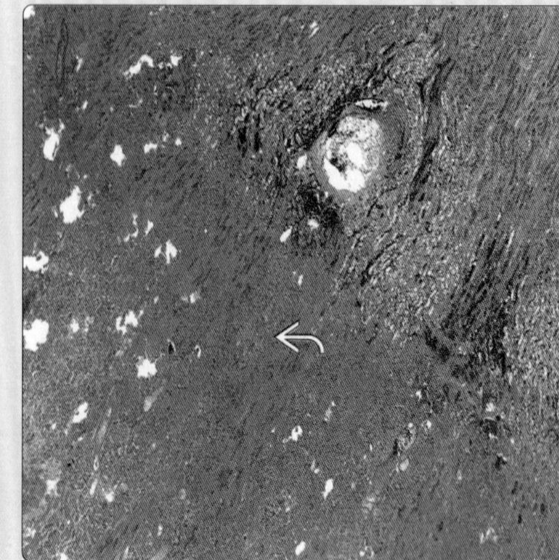

TERMINOLOGY

Abbreviations

- Renal vein thrombosis (RVT)
- Renal artery thrombosis (RAT)

ETIOLOGY/PATHOGENESIS

Surgical Technical Problems

- Intimal injury during procurement
- Difficult anastomosis or stenosis of anastomosis
- Trauma to vessels with dissection
- Narrow, twisted, or compressed renal vein

Hypercoagulable State

- Antiphospholipid antibody syndrome
- Nephrotic syndrome
- Factor V Leiden mutation

Risk Factors

- Multiple arteries
  - Especially if accessory artery supplies lower pole or ureter
- Placement of graft on left side
- Renal artery stenosis can be risk factor for RAT
- Compression of renal vein ↑ risk for RVT (e.g., by lymphocele, hematoma, or other lesion)

CLINICAL ISSUES

Epidemiology

- Incidence
  - Prevalence highly variable by center
    - Primary arterial thrombosis: 0.2-1.9%
    - Primary venous thrombosis: 0.1-3.4%
  - Arterial thrombosis usually occurs within 30 days of transplant
  - RVT early or late

Site

- Hilar vessels
  - Intraparenchymal arteries and glomeruli are spared
- May extend into inferior vena cava

Presentation

- Macrohematuria
- Proteinuria
- Acute renal failure/anuria
  - Sudden decrease in urine output may result from both RVT and RAT
- Pain in transplant
- Graft swelling

Treatment

- Surgical approaches
  - Thrombectomy or revision of anastomosis
- Drugs
  - Thrombolytics, anticoagulation, &/or aspirin

Prognosis

- Usually causes graft loss
- Early treatment essential

IMAGING

Radiographic Findings

- Angiography demonstrates thrombosis and loss of cortical perfusion, usually wedge-shaped

Ultrasonographic Findings

- Doppler ultrasound may demonstrate thrombus and absent flow
- Renal vein thrombosis
  - Diastolic reversal of flow in renal artery
  - Kidney may be enlarged with surrounding blood

MACROSCOPIC

General Features

- RVT: Engorged and purple
- RAT: Pale, infarcted

MICROSCOPIC

Histologic Features

- Both arterial thrombosis and venous thrombosis display
  - Loss of endothelium
  - Adherence of platelets
  - Recanalization if chronic
- Arterial thrombosis in particular displays
  - Dissection of media
  - Infarction of cortex
- Cortex
  - Neutrophils peritubular and glomerular capillaries
  - Edema
  - Congestion

DIFFERENTIAL DIAGNOSIS

Hyperacute and Acute Humoral Rejection

- Usually more neutrophils
- C4d(+) in peritubular capillaries
- Usually no large vessel thrombosis

Acute Cellular Rejection

- Endothelial mononuclear inflammation

DIAGNOSTIC CHECKLIST

Pathologic Interpretation Pearls

- C4d(-) in peritubular capillaries

SELECTED REFERENCES

1. Fallahzadeh MK et al: Acute transplant renal artery thrombosis due to distal renal artery stenosis: A case report and review of the literature. J Nephropathol. 3(3):105-8, 2014
2. Aktas S et al: Analysis of vascular complications after renal transplantation. Transplant Proc. 43(2):557-61, 2011
3. Ripert T et al: Preventing graft thrombosis after renal transplantation: a multicenter survey of clinical practice. Transplant Proc. 41(10):4193-6, 2009
4. Aschwanden M et al: Renal vein thrombosis after renal transplantation–early diagnosis by duplex sonography prevented fatal outcome. Nephrol Dial Transplant. 21(3):825-6, 2006
5. Osman Y et al: Vascular complications after live donor renal transplantation: study of risk factors and effects on graft and patient survival. J Urol. 169(3):859-62, 2003
6. Bakir N et al: Primary renal graft thrombosis. Nephrol Dial Transplant. 11(1):140-7, 1996

Transplant Renal Artery Stenosis

KEY FACTS

TERMINOLOGY

- Post-transplant stenosis of major renal arteries, typically causing refractory hypertension due to increased renin production
- Caused by atherosclerosis, intimal flap, kinking, and chronic rejection

ETIOLOGY/PATHOGENESIS

- Surgical complication
- Donor artery atherosclerosis
- Chronic transplant arteriopathy

CLINICAL ISSUES

- Renal dysfunction/delayed graft function, bruit, hypertension
- Clinically significant in 1-5% of recipients
- Treatment
  - Percutaneous transluminal angioplasty (PTA) ± stent
  - Surgical approaches, including anastomosis revision

MACROSCOPIC

- Stenosis usually occurs at or near anastomosis, such as renal-iliac artery anastomosis

MICROSCOPIC

- Cholesterol emboli may be present if stenosis due to atheroma
- Tubular atrophy with little fibrosis is typical pattern
- Acute tubular injury if acute or intermittent stenosis
- May have prominent juxtaglomerular apparati

TOP DIFFERENTIAL DIAGNOSES

- Calcineurin inhibitor toxicity
- Obstruction

DIAGNOSTIC CHECKLIST

- Histologic findings bland, subtle, and nonspecific
- Diagnosis easily missed
- Atherosclerosis: Cholesterol emboli provide clue

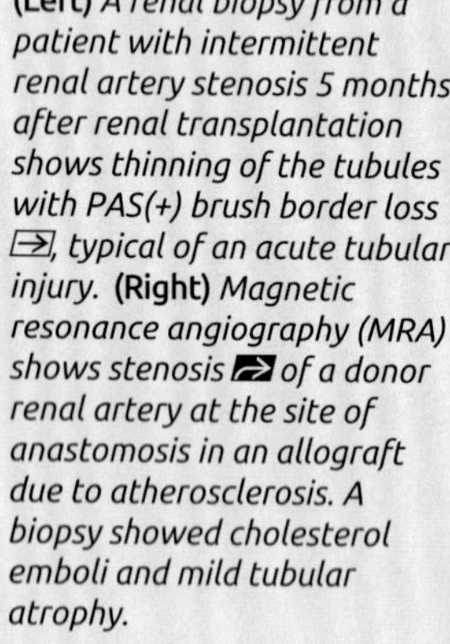
(Left) *A renal biopsy from a patient with intermittent renal artery stenosis 5 months after renal transplantation shows thinning of the tubules with PAS(+) brush border loss ➔, typical of an acute tubular injury.* **(Right)** *Magnetic resonance angiography (MRA) shows stenosis ➔ of a donor renal artery at the site of anastomosis in an allograft due to atherosclerosis. A biopsy showed cholesterol emboli and mild tubular atrophy.*

Brush Border Loss in Tubular Injury

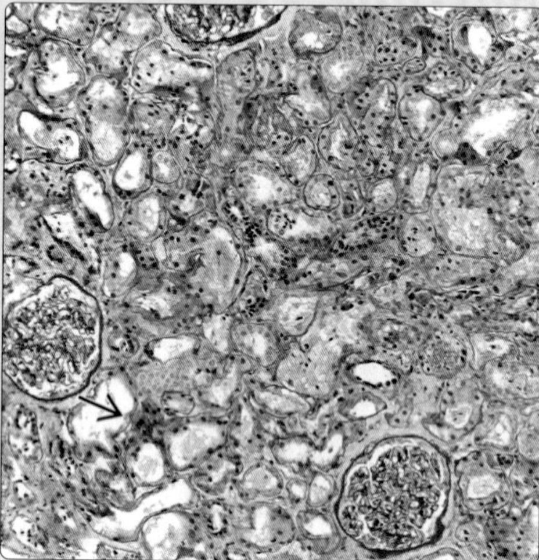

Renal Artery Stenosis on MRA

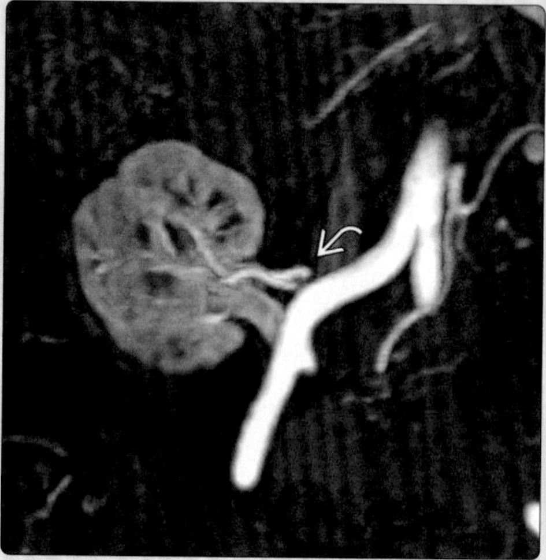

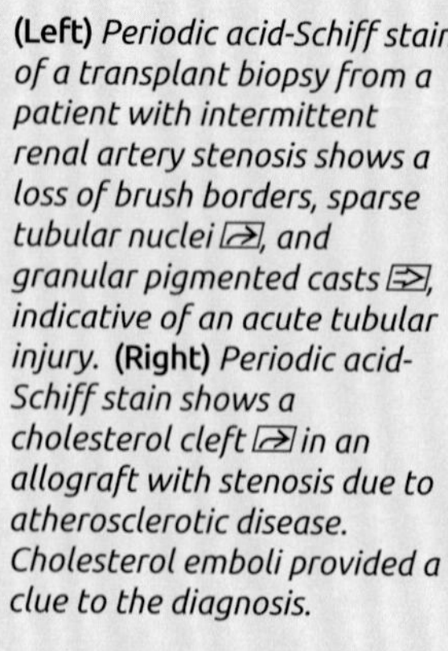
(Left) *Periodic acid-Schiff stain of a transplant biopsy from a patient with intermittent renal artery stenosis shows a loss of brush borders, sparse tubular nuclei ➔, and granular pigmented casts ➔, indicative of an acute tubular injury.* **(Right)** *Periodic acid-Schiff stain shows a cholesterol cleft ➔ in an allograft with stenosis due to atherosclerotic disease. Cholesterol emboli provided a clue to the diagnosis.*

Tubular Casts and Injury

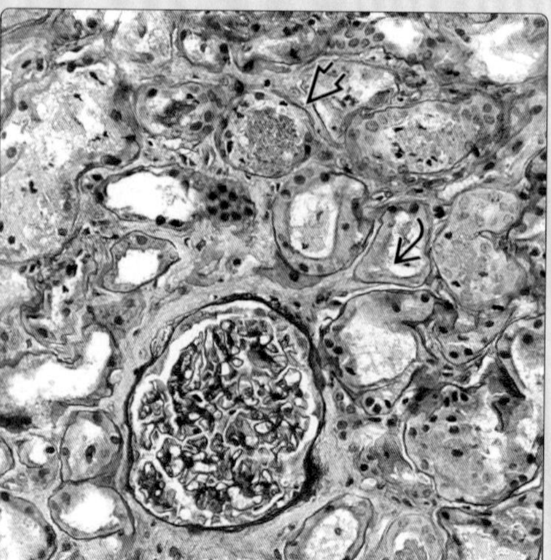

Cholesterol Embolus

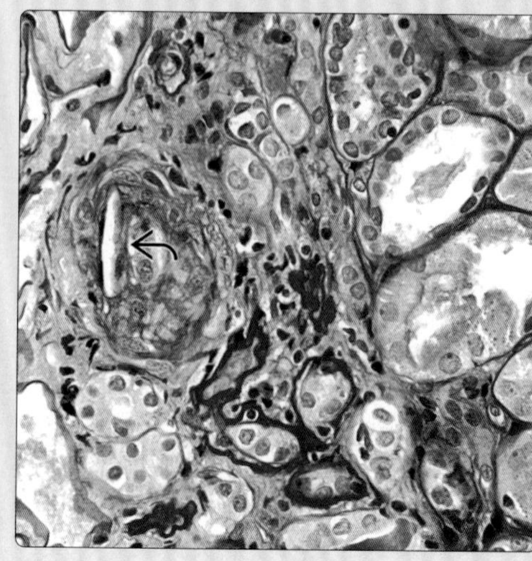

TERMINOLOGY

Abbreviations

- Transplant renal artery stenosis (TRAS)

Definitions

- Post-transplant stenosis of major renal arteries, typically causing refractory hypertension due to increased renin production

ETIOLOGY/PATHOGENESIS

Surgical Complication

- Subintimal dissection or flap created at harvest or reanastomosis
- Kinking or twisting of renal artery at transplantation
- End-to-side anastomoses are higher risk than end-to-end anastomoses
- Trauma may induce arterial intimal fibrosis

Donor Artery Atherosclerosis

- Can be complicated by atherosclerosis in recipient
- Must be distinguished from de novo atherosclerosis and chronic transplant arteriopathy

Chronic Transplant Arteriopathy

- Typically diffuse stenosis
- Episodes of acute rejection more common in recipients with TRAS

CLINICAL ISSUES

Epidemiology

- Incidence
  - Clinically significant in 1-5% of recipients
    - Up to 23% if milder cases included
  - Most common vascular complication after kidney transplantation

Presentation

- Delayed graft function
- Hypertension typically refractory to drugs
- Bruit over transplanted kidney
- Renal dysfunction
  - Progressive deterioration may be intermittent
  - Renin-angiotensin inhibitors worsen function

Natural History

- Usually presents 3-24 months after transplantation

Treatment

- Percutaneous transluminal angioplasty (PTA) ± stent
- Saphenous vein or recipient iliac artery grafts
- Revision of anastomosis

Prognosis

- Percutaneous transluminal angioplasty restenosis rate 10-60%
- Surgical correction difficult; graft loss ~ 20%

IMAGING

Ultrasonographic Findings

- Color flow duplex ultrasound reveals flow abnormalities
  - Stenosis may be incidental finding without hypertension or graft dysfunction
  - "Parvus-tardus" waveform and decreased resistive index, pulsatility index, and acceleration index
- CT, MR, and conventional angiography may also be useful

MACROSCOPIC

General Features

- Stenosis usually occurs at or near anastomosis, such as renal-iliac artery anastomosis
- Uniform atrophy

MICROSCOPIC

Histologic Features

- Transplant kidney
  - Tubular atrophy with little fibrosis if stenosis chronic
  - Acute tubular injury may occur if stenosis intermittent
  - May have prominent juxtaglomerular apparati
  - Cholesterol emboli present if stenosis due to atheroma
  - Normal glomeruli, arteries, and arterioles
- Renal-iliac artery anastomosis
  - Rarely sampled for histology
  - Atherosclerosis
  - Medial dissection
  - Intimal flap
  - Intimal hyperplasia with inflammation (allograft arteriopathy)

DIFFERENTIAL DIAGNOSIS

Calcineurin Inhibitor Toxicity

- Arteriolar hyalinosis and isometric tubular vacuolization

Obstruction

- Collecting duct dilation and Tamm-Horsfall protein leakage into interstitium
- Dilated lymphatics

DIAGNOSTIC CHECKLIST

Pathologic Interpretation Pearls

- Histologic findings bland, subtle, and nonspecific
- Diagnosis easily missed
- Atherosclerosis: Cholesterol emboli provides clue

SELECTED REFERENCES

1. Tso PL et al. Kidney transplantation procedure and surgical technique. In Kirk AD et al. Textbook of Organ Transplantation. Hoboken, NJ: John Wiley and Sons, Ltd. 2014
2. Hurst FP et al: Incidence, predictors and outcomes of transplant renal artery stenosis after kidney transplantation: analysis of USRDS. Am J Nephrol. 30(5):459-67, 2009
3. Geddes CC et al: Long-term outcome of transplant renal artery stenosis managed conservatively or by radiological intervention. Clin Transplant. 22(5):572-8, 2008
4. Audard V et al: Risk factors and long-term outcome of transplant renal artery stenosis in adult recipients after treatment by percutaneous transluminal angioplasty. Am J Transplant. 6(1):95-9, 2006

Post-Transplant Lymphoproliferative Disease

KEY FACTS

TERMINOLOGY

- Post-transplant lymphoproliferative disorder (PTLD)
- Frank lymphoma sometimes manifests in immunocompromised hosts in solid organ or bone marrow allograft recipients

CLINICAL ISSUES

- Occurs in ~ 1% of renal allograft recipients
- Treatment
  - Reduction in immunosuppression, antiviral drugs (acyclovir, ganciclovir, α-interferon), chemotherapy, anti-CD20 (rituximab)
- Reported mortality of 40-60%

MACROSCOPIC

- Swollen kidneys
- Blurring of corticomedullary junction & diffuse petechiae with vaguely nodular involvement

MICROSCOPIC

- Mononuclear cells ("activated" lymphocytes) with enlarged nuclei, prominent nucleoli, & mitoses
- Cells of PTLD may be monomorphic or polymorphic
- Necrosis, often described as being in serpiginous pattern, is often present

ANCILLARY TESTS

- Most express CD20 (~ 85-90%)
- Immunohistochemical stains for EBV-associated antigens (such as LMP-1 & EBNA-2)
- In situ hybridization for EBV-encoded RNA (EBER) usually shows prominent staining in atypical lymphoid cells

TOP DIFFERENTIAL DIAGNOSES

- Allograft rejection
  - CD3(+) T cells, granulocytes, & macrophages are more commonly seen in rejection

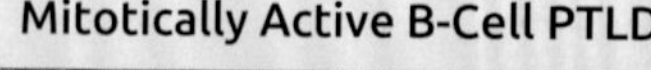

Mitotically Active B-Cell PTLD

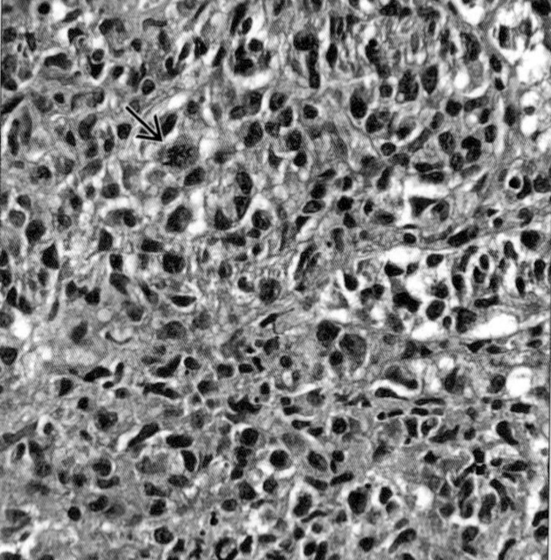

EBV ISH in EBV-Driven B-Cell PTLD

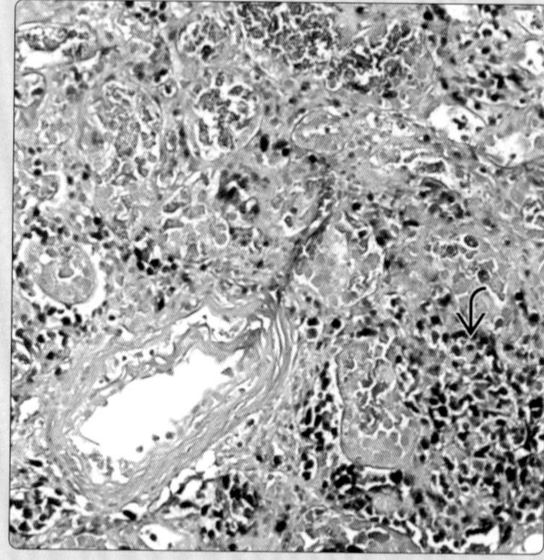

(Left) *High-power view of a monomorphic EBV-driven B-cell PTLD shows pleomorphic cells, many of which are enlarged & have irregular nuclear contours, prominent nucleoli, & mitoses →.* **(Right)** *In situ hybridization (ISH) of Epstein-Barr virus-encoded RNA (EBER) shows that many cells in the lymphoid infiltrate are positive →, indicating that this is a monomorphic EBV-driven B-cell PTLD, diffuse large B-cell lymphoma type.*

PTLD, Diffuse Large B-Cell Lymphoma Type

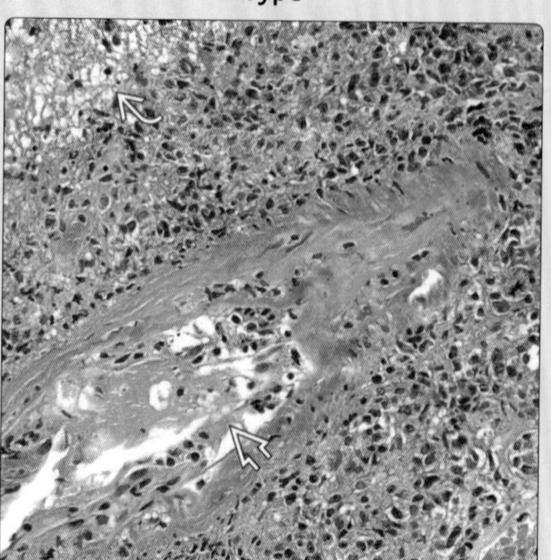

PTLD, Hodgkin Lymphoma Type

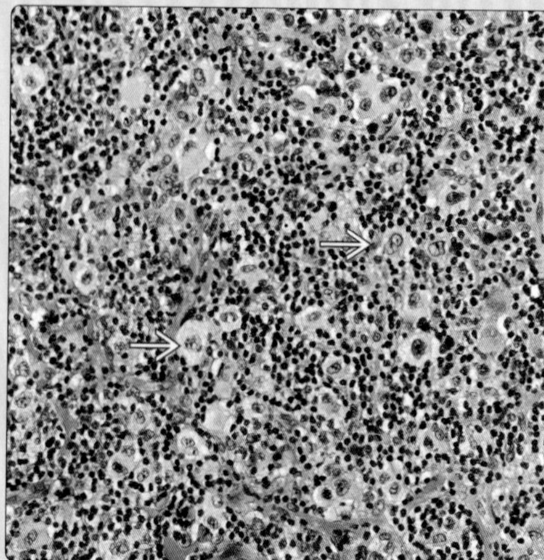

(Left) *At medium power, one can appreciate an arterial wall involved by monomorphic EBV-driven B-cell PTLD, diffuse large B-cell lymphoma type, with adjacent necrosis →, with malignant lymphoid cells & admixed fibrin →.* **(Right)** *This Hodgkin lymphoma-type PTLD contains many Reed-Sternberg variant cells →. (Courtesy N.L. Harris, MD.)*

TERMINOLOGY

Abbreviations

- Post-transplant lymphoproliferative disease (PTLD)

Synonyms

- Post-transplant lymphoproliferative disorder

Definitions

- Lymphoproliferative proliferation that in many cases manifests as a frank lymphoma arising in immunocompromised hosts who are recipients of solid organ or bone marrow allografts

ETIOLOGY/PATHOGENESIS

Immunosuppression

- Risk for PTLD increases with increasing immunosuppression
  - < 1% peripheral blood, stem cell, & bone marrow allograft recipients
  - 1% renal allograft recipients
  - 1-2% cardiac allograft recipients
  - ≥ 5% heart-lung or intestinal allograft recipients

Epstein-Barr Virus (EBV)

- Most important risk factor is EBV seronegativity at time of transplantation
  - Primary EBV infection increases the risk for PTLD by 10-76x
- Epstein-Barr virus (EBV)
  - 70% of PTLD are EBV(+)

B-Cell PTLD

- Most PTLD are B-cell type
- Usually driven by EBV
- Monomorphic B-cell PTLD are monoclonal transformed B lymphocytic or plasmacytic proliferations fulfilling diffuse large B-cell lymphoma criteria (& less commonly Burkitt lymphoma or plasma cell neoplasms)
- Can also be polyclonal

T-Cell & NK-Cell PTLD

- T/NK-cell PTLD account for 7-15% of PTLDs (larger reported range in 1 Japanese series of 2-45%)
- Occur longer after transplant (median of 66 months) & are usually extranodal
- ~ 1/3 are EBV(+)
- Median survival is 6 months
- EBV(+) cases survive longer
- Types
  - Peripheral T-cell lymphoma, unspecified
  - Hepatosplenic T-cell lymphoma
  - T-cell large granular lymphocytic leukemia (EBV[-])

CLINICAL ISSUES

Epidemiology

- Incidence
  - Estimated to occur in ~ 1% of renal allograft recipients (1.4% of 25,127 recipients from 1996-2000)
  - In renal allograft patients with PTLD, allograft kidney is affected in > 30% of patients
  - Kidney more often involved in kidney transplant patients (14%) than in heart transplant patients (0.7%)
    - Conversely, heart is involved more in heart (18%) than kidney (7%) transplant patients
    - Suggests immunologic reaction in allograft is pathogenic factor
  - 67% of PTLDs involving kidney allograft are donor origin
    - Donor origin PTLD appears more common in liver & lung allograft recipients & frequently involves allograft
  - PTLD account for 15% of tumors among adult transplant recipients (~ 51% in children)

Presentation

- Malaise
- Weight loss
- Lethargy
- Fever
  - Fever of unknown origin/unexplained fever
- Mononucleosis-type syndrome
  - Fever & malaise
  - Pharyngitis or tonsillitis
    - Sometimes recognized incidentally on tonsillectomy specimens ± lymphadenopathy
- Abdominal mass
- Hepatocellular or pancreatic dysfunction
- Central nervous system disease

Laboratory Tests

- Quantitative EBV viral load testing with polymerase chain reaction (PCR)
  - Serial assays are more useful in individual patient than specific viral load measurements
  - Assays are not standardized & cannot typically be compared between centers
- Serological testing is not typically thought to be useful

Natural History

- PTLD restricted to kidney transplant (~ 12% of cases) tend to occur early (~ 5 months) after surgery
- EBV(-) PTLD & T/NK-cell PTLD tend to present later (median time to occurrence 4-5 years & 6.5 years, respectively)

Treatment

- Drugs
  - Reduction in immunosuppression
  - Antiviral drugs (acyclovir, ganciclovir, α-interferon)
  - Chemotherapy
    - Often: CHOP (cyclophosphamide, hydroxydaunomycin, vincristine [Oncovin], prednisone)
  - Anti-CD20 (rituximab)
    - Has helped contribute to complete remission
- Radiation
  - Localized radiation may be combined with chemotherapy
- Graft nephrectomy
  - Permits discontinuation of immunosuppression
- Cell immunotherapy (investigative)
  - EBV-specific cytotoxic T cells

Prognosis

- Overall reported 5-year survival: 40-70%
  - 87% 5-year survival in children
  - Recent series show improvement in outcome
- "Early" lesions tend to regress when ↓ immunosuppression
- Polymorphic & less often monomorphic PTLD may also regress with reduction in immune suppression
- Acute & chronic rejection may occur when immunosuppression is reduced, leading to graft loss & mortality
- Associated with adverse outcome
  - Multiple disease sites (not in pediatric patients)
  - Advanced stage
  - Older age at diagnosis
  - Late-onset disease
  - Higher international prognostic index
  - Elevated lactate dehydrogenase
  - Bone marrow vs. solid organ allograft recipients

IMAGING

General Features

- May show up as mass on radiology studies

MACROSCOPIC

General Features

- Swollen kidneys
- Blurring of corticomedullary junction & diffuse petechiae
- Vaguely nodular involvement
- Localized mass

MICROSCOPIC

Histologic Features

- WHO classification (2008)
  - 4 major categories
    - Early lesions
    - Polymorphic PTLD
    - Monomorphic PTLD (T, B, NK)
    - Classical Hodgkin lymphoma
  - First 2 are specific for transplant recipients
- **Early lesions**
  - Plasmacytic hyperplasia & infectious mononucleosis-like PTLD
  - Involved tissue has architectural preservation
  - Nodal sinuses or tonsillar crypts are still present
  - Follicles are often floridly reactive or hyperplastic
  - In plasmacytic hyperplasia, plasma cells are prominently admixed with small lymphocytes
  - In infectious mononucleosis-like lesion, there is paracortical expansion with numerous immunoblasts admixed with T cells & plasma cells
  - Lesions may form masses
  - Occur at a younger age than other PTLD types (children or adult solid organ recipients who have not had prior EBV infections)
  - Lymph nodes or tonsils are common sites
  - Often EBV(+)
- **Polymorphic PTLD**
  - Immunoblasts, plasma cells, & small to intermediate-sized lymphoid cells effacing architecture of lymph nodes
  - Full range of B-cell maturation is present
  - Large, bizarre cells may resemble Reed-Sternberg cells (atypical immunoblasts [may be Hodgkin-like])
  - Areas of geographic necrosis may be present
  - Distinction of polymorphic from monomorphic PTLD is not always clear-cut
  - Frequency: 20-80%, depending on institution
  - Polymorphic variant is most common type in children & frequently follows a primary EBV infection
  - Polymorphic variant is more common in PTLD involving kidney
  - Often EBV(+)
- **Monomorphic PTLD**
  - Fulfills criteria for 1 of the B-cell or T/NK-cell neoplasms recognized in immunocompetent hosts
  - Small B-cell lymphoid neoplasms, such as follicular lymphomas or MALT lymphomas, are not designated as PTLD
    - Despite fact that some have recognized that these occur in post-transplant setting (e.g., MALT lymphoma)
- **Monomorphic B-cell PTLD**
  - Necrosis, often described as being in serpiginous pattern, is often present
  - Monomorphic B-cell PTLD often fulfill criteria for diffuse large B-cell lymphoma
  - Burkitt lymphoma or plasma cell neoplasms occur less commonly
  - Cells are often collected in vaguely nodular pattern in sheets
  - Mononuclear cells ("activated" lymphocytes) with enlarged nuclei, prominent nucleoli, & frequent mitoses
  - Cells may have blast-like features
  - Term "monomorphic" does not imply cellular monotony since cells may be bizarre, multinucleated, & Reed-Sternberg-like
  - May also be plasmacytic or plasmacytoid features
  - Burkitt lymphomas have monomorphic medium-sized transformed cells, often with multiple small nucleoli & dispersed chromatin, & may possess *MYC* gene translocations
    - e.g., characteristically t(8;14) but also t(8;22) or t(2;8)
- **Monomorphic T/NK-cell PTLD**
  - Fulfill criteria for T/NK-cell lymphomas
  - Most present at extranodal sites
  - Largest group consists of peripheral T-cell lymphoma, not otherwise specified (NOS) category
  - Peripheral T-cell lymphoma, NOS has wide range in morphology
  - Peripheral T-cell lymphoma, NOS is often accompanied by eosinophilia, pruritus, or hemophagocytic syndrome
  - Up to 20% of hepatosplenic T-cell lymphomas arise in setting of chronic immunosuppression
    - Mostly long-term immunosuppression for solid organ transplantation in which it is regarded as late-onset PTLD of host origin
  - Hepatosplenic T-cell lymphoma is thought to arise from cytotoxic T cells (usually of γ/δ variety)

- Hepatosplenic T-cell lymphoma demonstrates medium-sized lymphoid cells infiltrating bone marrow, spleen, & liver
- **Classical Hodgkin lymphoma (CHL) type PTLD**
  - Least common form of PTLD
  - Occurs more commonly in renal transplant patients than in other transplant recipients
  - Reed-Sternberg-like cells may be seen in early, polymorphic, & some monomorphic PTLDs & cause diagnostic confusion
  - Cases should fulfill criteria for CHL
  - Usually both CD15 & CD30 are positive
  - CD15(-) cases can occur but must be distinguished from Hodgkin-like lesions

ANCILLARY TESTS

Immunohistochemistry

- Most are B cell derived & express B-cell markers
  - CD20 (~ 85-90%)
  - CD30 is positive in many B-cell PTLD cases (± anaplastic morphology)
  - CD138(+) in a minority
  - EBV(+) cases usually have late germinal center/post germinal center phenotype (CD10[-], Bcl-6[+/-], IRF/MUM1[+])
  - EBV(-) cases often have germinal center phenotype (CD10[+/-], Bcl-6[+], IRF/MUM1[-], CD138[-])
  - EBV(-) monomorphic PTLD frequently lacks expression of cyclin-dependent kinase inhibitor (CDKN2A [p16INK4A])
  - Monotypic immunoglobulin often with expression of γ or α heavy chain in ~ 50% of monomorphic B-cell PTLD
  - EBV replication in tumor (BZLF1[+] or BMRF1[+]) & plasma cell differentiation (XBP1[+]) predictive of poor prognosis (18% vs. 48% 1-year survival)
- Classical Hodgkin lymphoma type PTLD
  - Typically CD15(+) & CD30(+) & EBV(+)
  - CD15(-) classical Hodgkin lymphoma case occur & should be distinguished from other Hodgkin-like lesions
  - CD15, when present, often gives Golgi-type pattern of expression
- T/NK-cell PTLD have pan-T-cell & NK-cell antigens
  - CD4 or 8, CD30, ALK, & α/β or γ/δ T cell
    - Hepatosplenic T-cell lymphoma is usually of γ/δ variety
  - ~ 1/3 are EBV(+)
- Immunohistochemical stains for EBV-associated antigens (such as LMP-1 & EBNA-2)

In Situ Hybridization

- Most EBV(+) (~ 85%)
  - In situ hybridization for EBV-encoded RNA (EBER) usually shows prominent staining in atypical lymphoid cells
- In situ hybridization for kappa & lambda light chains may demonstrate light chain restriction
  - Occurs in ~ 50% of monomorphic PTLD & usually only focal in polymorphic PTLD

PCR

- Gene rearrangement studies can demonstrate clonally rearranged immunoglobulin genes
  - More prominent in monomorphic B-cell PTLD
  - Can occur in polymorphic B-cell PTLD
    - Some have reported immunoglobulin gene variable regions without ongoing mutations in 75% of polymorphic PTLDs
- Monomorphic B-cell PTLDs have oncogene abnormalities, such as *PAS*, *TP53*, & *MYC* rearrangements, *BCL6* somatic hypermutation, & aberrant promoter methylation
- Cases of T-cell origin have clonal T-cell receptor gene rearrangements

Genetic Testing

- Clonal cytogenetic abnormalities are common, particularly in monomorphic PTLD

Array CGH

- Demonstrate additions, gains, & losses

DIFFERENTIAL DIAGNOSIS

Allograft Rejection

- PTLD may be confused with allograft rejection because features mimicking rejection, such as tubulitis & endarteritis, may be present
- Mixed infiltrate typical of rejection, including granulocytes & macrophages, rather than monotonous sheets of mononuclear cells of PTLD
- Rejection predominantly of CD3(+) T-lymphocytes & CD68(+) macrophages, vs. CD20 (+) B cells in PTLD
- Concurrent rejection & PTLD may occur
- Necrosis of infiltrate rare in rejection
- Edema not typical of PTLD

Smooth Muscle Tumors

- Spindle cell neoplasms may be seen in post-transplant setting & may be EBV(+)
- Histologic examination usually confirms prominent spindling, which is not typical of PTLD
- Immunohistochemical studies usually demonstrate smooth muscle differentiation (actin & desmin)

DIAGNOSTIC CHECKLIST

Pathologic Interpretation Pearls

- Detection of rare EBV(+) cells without lymphoid/plasmacytic proliferation is not diagnostic of PTLD

REPORTING

Key Elements to Report

- Categories of PTLD according to 2008 WHO classification
  - Early lesions
    - Plasmacytic hyperplasia
    - Infectious mononucleosis-like lesion
  - Polymorphic PTLD
  - Monomorphic PTLD
    - B-cell neoplasms: Diffuse large B-cell lymphoma (DLBCL), Burkitt lymphoma, plasma cell myeloma, plasmacytoma-like lesion, other (e.g., indolent small B-cell lymphomas arising in transplant recipients)
    - T-cell neoplasms: Peripheral T-cell lymphoma, NOS; hepatosplenic T-cell lymphoma; other
  - Classical Hodgkin lymphoma-type PTLD

Classification & Features of Post-Transplant Lymphoproliferative Disease (PTLD)

Category	Morphology	EBV	Immunophenotype and Genetics
Early Lesions			
Plasmacytic hyperplasia	Plasma cells & lymphocytes	Often +	Usually polyclonal
Infectious mononucleosis-like lesion	Mixture: Lymphocytes ± plasma cells, ± immunoblasts	Often +	Usually polyclonal
Polymorphic PTLD	Mixture: Lymphocytes ± plasma cells ± immunoblasts (full spectrum of maturation)	Often +	May have monoclonal B cells
Monomorphic PTLD			
B-cell neoplasms			Express B-cell markers
Diffuse large B-cell lymphoma	Large B cells	Variable	Clonal
Burkitt lymphoma	Medium-sized B cells with multiple nucleoli & finely dispersed chromatin	Variable	Clonal, may have translocations, e.g., t(8;14) but also t(8;22) or t(2;8)
Plasma cell myeloma	Diffuse plasma cell infiltrate with criteria sufficient to diagnose myeloma	Variable	Clonal
Plasmacytoma-like lesion	Localized site with a diffuse plasma cell infiltrate	Usually -	Monotypic immunoglobulin
T-cell neoplasms			Express T-cell (& less commonly NK-cell) markers
Peripheral T-cell lymphoma, NOS	May be polymorphous or polymorphous with medium to large-sized cells & Reed-Sternberg (RS)-type cells	Minority +	Typically clonal with rearranged T-cell receptor genes
Hepatosplenic T-cell lymphoma	Liver, spleen, & bone marrow are diffusely involved with monotonous medium-sized cells with inconspicuous nucleoli	Minority +	Typically clonal with rearranged T-cell receptor genes (usually of the γ/δ type), may have +8 chromosomal modification
Classical Hodgkin lymphoma-type PTLD	Fulfills criteria for diagnosis of CHL & classically may have RS cells	Often +	Clonality usually cannot be shown, e.g., with IgH rearrangement studies

Swerdlow SH et al: Post-transplant lymphoproliferative disorders. In Swerdlow SH et al: *WHO Classification of Tumours of Haematopoietic and Lymphoid Tissues.* Lyon: IARC. 343-48, 2008

SELECTED REFERENCES

1. Morton M et al: Post-Transplant Lymphoproliferative Disorder in Adult Renal Transplant Recipients: Survival and Prognosis. Leuk Lymphoma. 1-23, 2015
2. Singavi AK et al: Post-transplant lymphoproliferative disorders. Cancer Treat Res. 165:305-27, 2015
3. Gonzalez-Farre B et al: In vivo intratumoral Epstein-Barr virus replication is associated with XBP1 activation and early-onset post-transplant lymphoproliferative disorders with prognostic implications. Mod Pathol. 27(12):1599-611, 2014
4. Serre JE et al: Maintaining calcineurin inhibition after the diagnosis of post-transplant lymphoproliferative disorder improves renal graft survival. Kidney Int. 85(1):182-90, 2014
5. Al-Mansour Z et al: Post-transplant lymphoproliferative disease (PTLD): risk factors, diagnosis, and current treatment strategies. Curr Hematol Malig Rep. 8(3):173-83, 2013
6. Bagg A et al: Immunosuppressive and immunomodulatory therapy-associated lymphoproliferative disorders. Semin Diagn Pathol. 30(2):102-12, 2013
7. Wistinghausen B et al: Post-transplant lymphoproliferative disease in pediatric solid organ transplant recipients. Pediatr Hematol Oncol. 30(6):520-31, 2013
8. Bollard CM et al: T-cell therapy in the treatment of post-transplant lymphoproliferative disease. Nat Rev Clin Oncol. 9(9):510-9, 2012
9. Trappe R et al: Sequential treatment with rituximab followed by CHOP chemotherapy in adult B-cell post-transplant lymphoproliferative disorder (PTLD): the prospective international multicentre phase 2 PTLD-1 trial. Lancet Oncol. 13(2):196-206, 2012
10. Dharnidharka VR et al: Improved survival with recent Post-Transplant Lymphoproliferative Disorder (PTLD) in children with kidney transplants. Am J Transplant. 11(4):751-8, 2011
11. Ibrahim HA et al: Presence of monoclonal T-cell populations in B-cell post-transplant lymphoproliferative disorders. Mod Pathol. 24(2):232-40, 2011
12. Olagne J et al: Post-transplant lymphoproliferative disorders: determination of donor/recipient origin in a large cohort of kidney recipients. Am J Transplant. 11(6):1260-9, 2011
13. Picarsic J et al: Post-transplant Burkitt lymphoma is a more aggressive and distinct form of post-transplant lymphoproliferative disorder. Cancer. 117(19):4540-50, 2011
14. Khedmat H et al: Characteristics and prognosis of post-transplant lymphoproliferative disorders within renal allograft: Report from the PTLD.Int. Survey. Ann Transplant. 15(3):80-6, 2010
15. Parker A et al: Diagnosis of post-transplant lymphoproliferative disorder in solid organ transplant recipients - BCSH and BTS Guidelines. Br J Haematol. 149(5):675-92, 2010
16. Swerdlow SH et al: Post-transplant lymphoproliferative disorders. In Swerdlow SH et al: WHO Classification of Tumours of Haematopoietic and Lymphoid Tissues. Lyon: IARC. 343-48, 2008
17. Swerdlow SH: T-cell and NK-cell posttransplantation lymphoproliferative disorders. Am J Clin Pathol. 127(6):887-95, 2007

Plasmacytic Hyperplasia (Early Post-Transplant Lymphoproliferative Disorder)

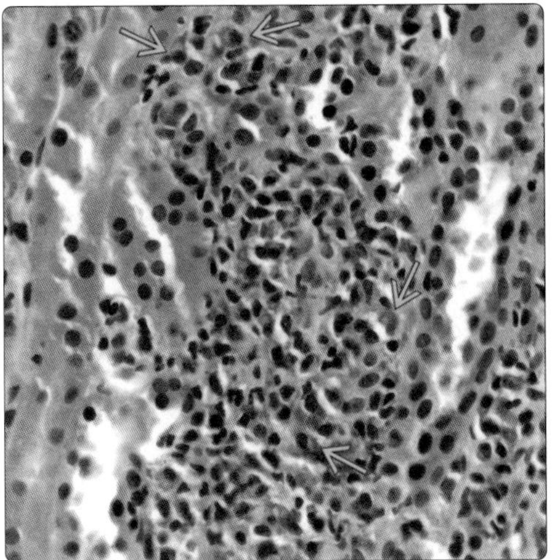

PTLD, Immunoblastic Plasmacytoid Type

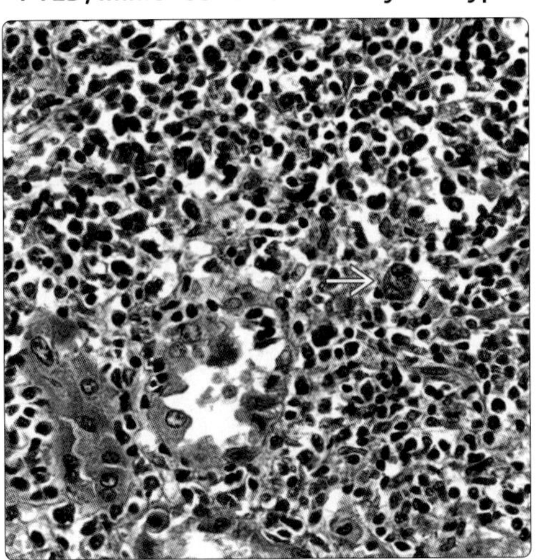

(Left) *Renal allograft protocol biopsy in a 3-year-old girl shows numerous plasma cells ⇒ amidst a hematolymphoid infiltrate, much of which was CD20(+), CD79a(+), & EBV ISH(+), compatible with the diagnosis of plasmacytic hyperplasia.* **(Right)** *High-power view of the allograft from the autopsy of the recipient of a renal allograft shows involvement by PTLD with large atypical cells ➡ among renal tubules. This PTLD was classified as an immunoblastic plasmacytoid PTLD. (Courtesy J.A. Ferry, MD.)*

PTLD, Immunoblastic Plasmacytoid Type

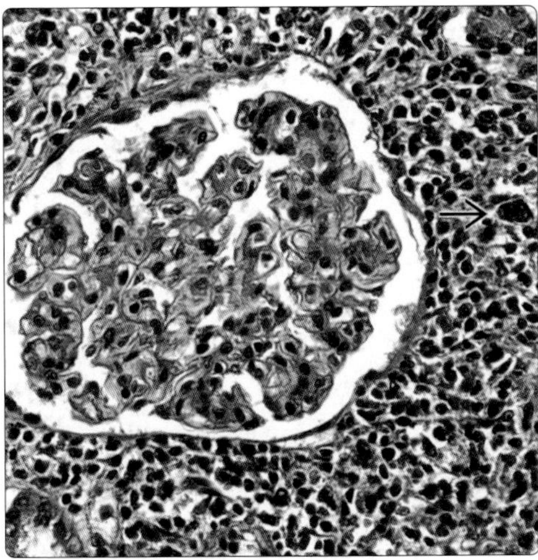

PTLD, Infectious Mononucleosis-Like, Involving Tonsil

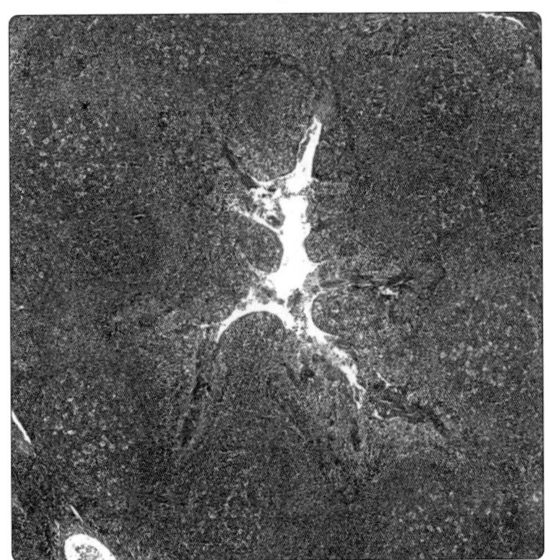

(Left) *High-power view of a renal allograft from the recipient's autopsy shows involvement by immunoblastic plasmacytoid PTLD with large atypical cells ⇒. (Courtesy J.A. Ferry, MD.)* **(Right)** *Low-power view of a tonsil in a pediatric renal allograft recipient shows involvement by an infectious mononucleosis-like PTLD. The architecture is overall preserved, but it can be appreciated that lymphoid follicles show attenuated mantles. (Courtesy J.A. Ferry, MD.)*

Tingible Body Macrophages, Immunoblasts, & Apoptotic Cells in Mononucleosis-Like PTLD

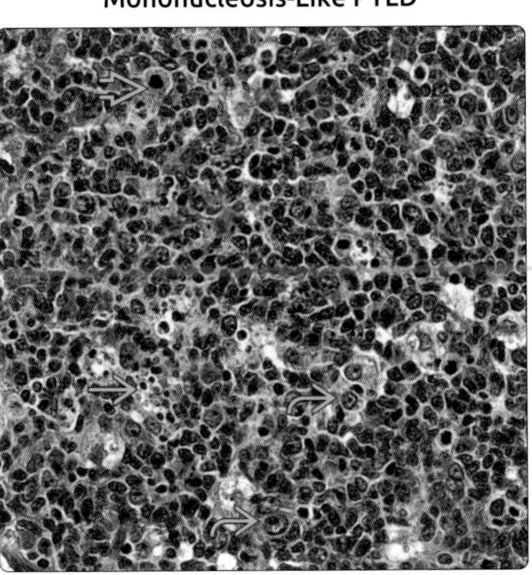

Immunoblasts in PTLD, Mononucleosis-Like

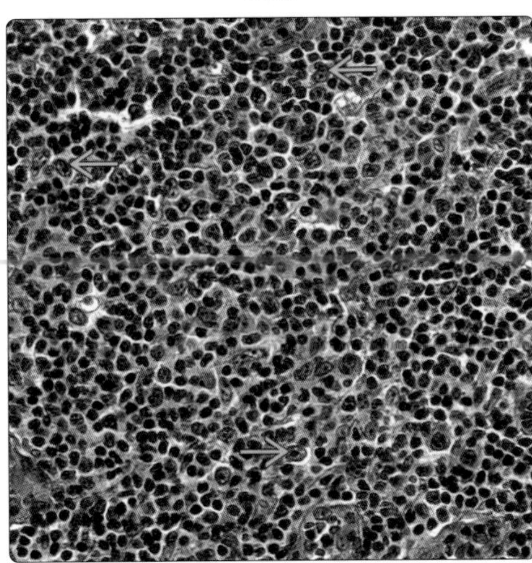

(Left) *High-power view of the tonsil involved by mononucleosis-like PTLD shows that lymphoid follicles are floridly reactive with mostly small lymphocytes & scattered tingible body macrophages ⇒, immunoblasts ⇒, & apoptotic cells ⇒. (Courtesy J.A. Ferry, MD.)* **(Right)** *Higher power view of the interfollicular area of the tonsil with mononucleosis-like PTLD shows mostly small lymphocytes & scattered immunoblasts ⇒. (Courtesy J.A. Ferry, MD.)*

(Left) *A gross photograph shows nodular involvement of an allograft kidney by PTLD. (Courtesy P. Randhawa, MD.)* **(Right)** *A low-power view of the allograft from the autopsy of the recipient of a renal allograft shows involvement by PTLD with an area of necrosis ➡. (Courtesy J.A. Ferry, MD.)*

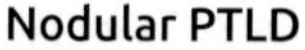

Nodular PTLD

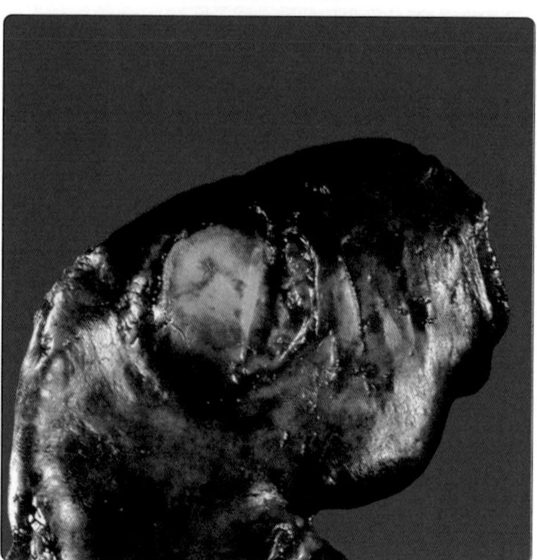

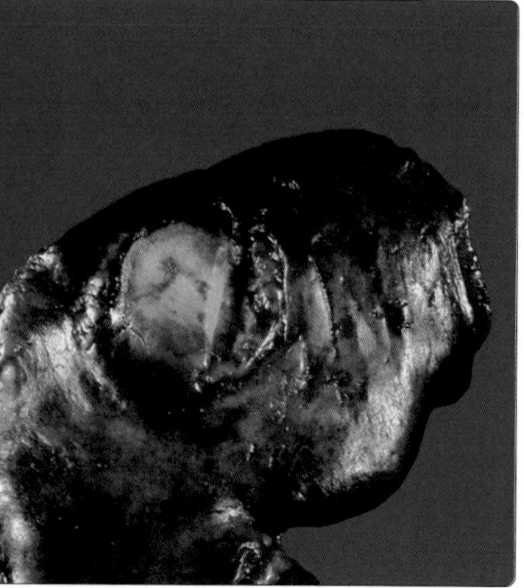

PTLD With Necrosis

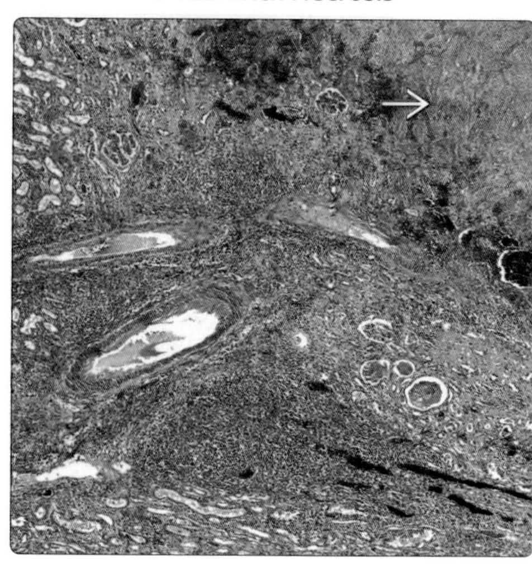

(Left) *PAS stain of a monomorphic EBV-driven B-cell PTLD, diffuse large B-cell lymphoma type, shows a relatively normal glomerulus ⇨ amidst a necrotic parenchyma ⇨ with a dense lymphoid infiltrate ⇨.* **(Right)** *This PTLD shows fatty infiltration in the surrounding soft tissues. (Courtesy P. Randhawa, MD.)*

PTLD, Diffuse Large B-Cell Lymphoma Type, With Necrosis

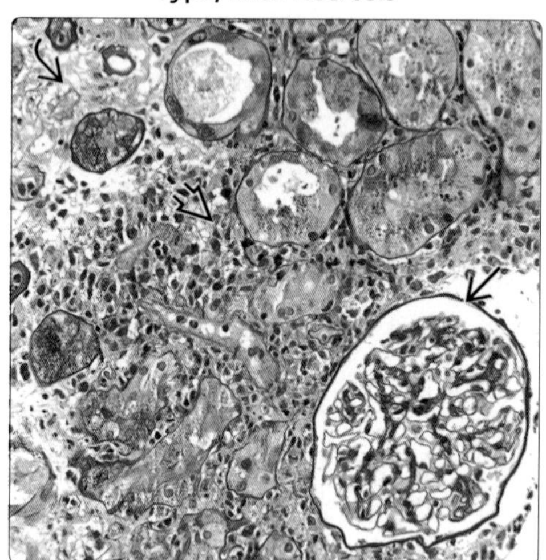

Infiltration of Fat by PTLD

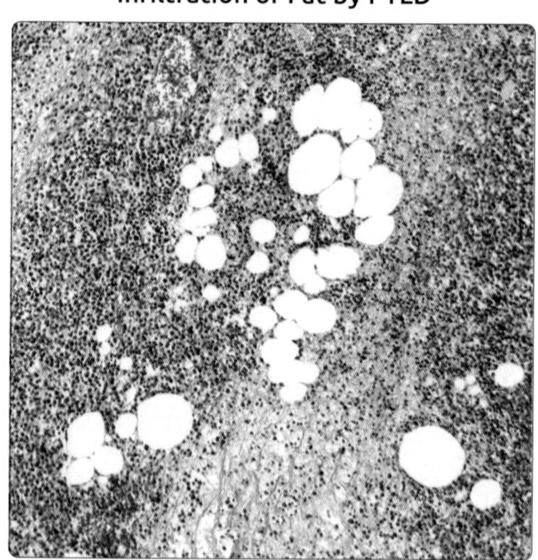

(Left) *This B-cell PTLD has foci of tubulitis, illustrating that this pattern can be seen in PTLD as well as cellular rejection. (Courtesy P. Randhawa, MD.)* **(Right)** *EBER RNA stain shows tubulitis with EBV-infected cells, demonstrating that this PTLD is an EBV-driven process. (Courtesy P. Randhawa, MD.)*

Tubulitis in PTLD

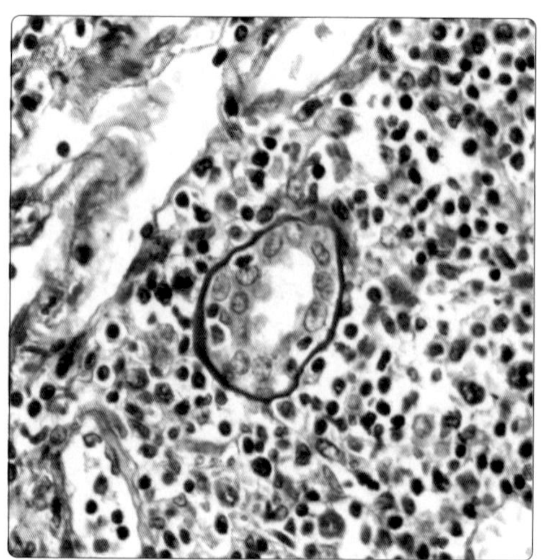

EBV-Driven PTLD

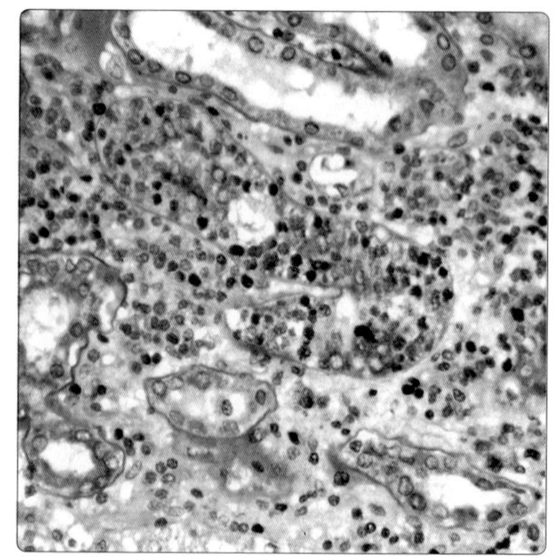

PTLD, Diffuse Large B-Cell Lymphoma Type

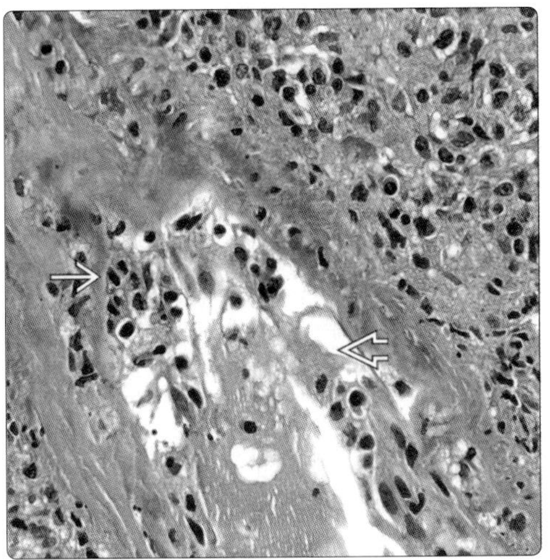

Vascular Involvement by PTLD Simulating Endarteritis

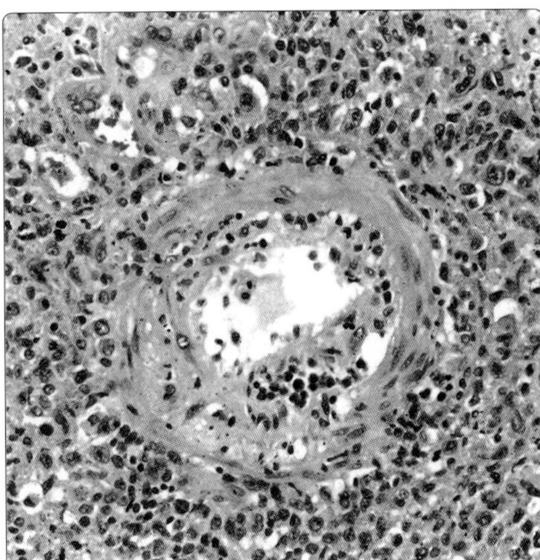

(Left) *High-power examination shows an arterial wall involved by monomorphic EBV-driven B-cell PTLD, diffuse large B-cell lymphoma type, with malignant lymphoid cells ➡ & admixed fibrin ➡.* **(Right)** *Hematoxylin & eosin stain shows vascular involvement by a B-cell PTLD, illustrating the fact that this can occur in PTLD, simulating endarteritis that can be seen in cellular rejection. (Courtesy P. R*

CD20(+) B-Cell PTLD

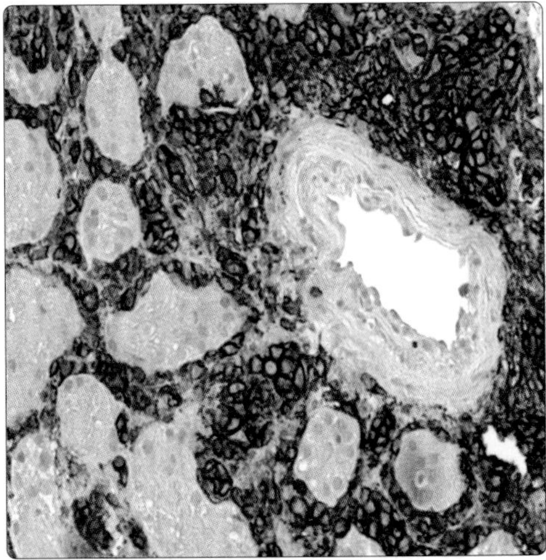

Ki-67 Shows High Proliferation in PTLD

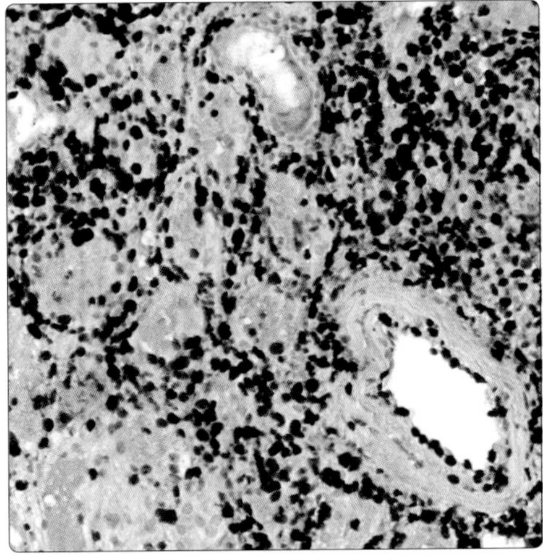

(Left) *CD20 immunohistochemistry of a monomorphic EBV-driven B-cell PTLD, diffuse large B-cell lymphoma type, shows that almost all of the atypical lymphoid infiltrate consists of CD20(+) B cells.* **(Right)** *A Ki-67 immunohistochemical stain is positive in most of the atypical lymphoid infiltrate in this monomorphic EBV-driven B-cell PTLD, diffuse large B-cell lymphoma type, indicating that it is highly proliferative.*

PTLD, Burkitt Lymphoma-Type, Monomorphic, Involving Submandibular Gland

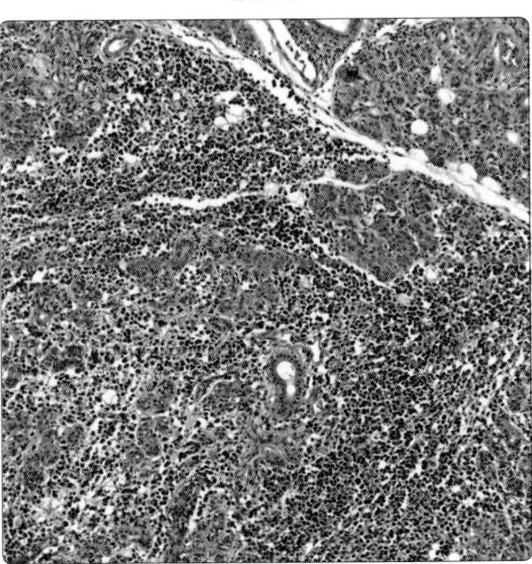

PTLD, Burkitt Lymphoma Type

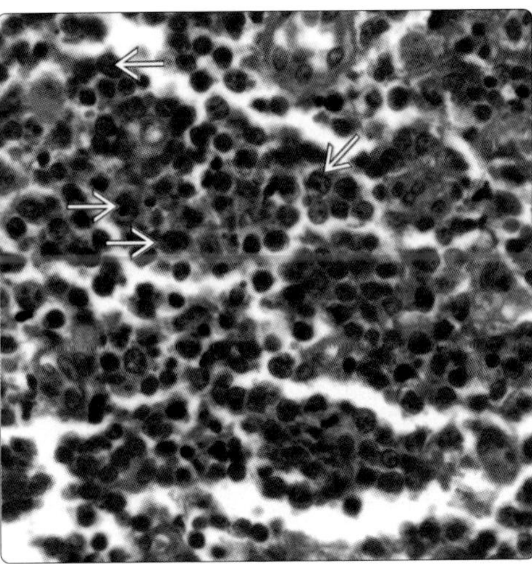

(Left) *Low-power view of a submandibular gland in a patient with history of a renal allograft shows diffuse involvement by a lymphoid infiltrate in a Burkitt lymphoma-type monomorphic PTLD. (Courtesy J.A. Ferry, MD.)* **(Right)** *Giemsa stain of a Burkitt lymphoma-type PTLD shows that many of the cells have prominent nucleoli ➡. (Courtesy J.A. Ferry, MD.)*

(Left) *High-power view shows an atypical lymphoid infiltrate in a case of T-cell PTLD with a mixed pleomorphic cell population containing a mixture of small & large cells with a variety of shapes.* **(Right)** *High-power view of a T-cell PTLD shows large atypical cells ↗, mitotic figures →, & admixed eosinophils ➡.*

Pleomorphism in T-Cell PTLD

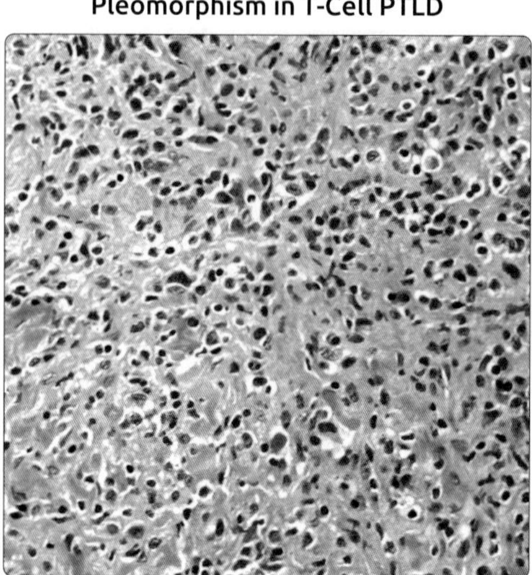

T-Cell PTLD

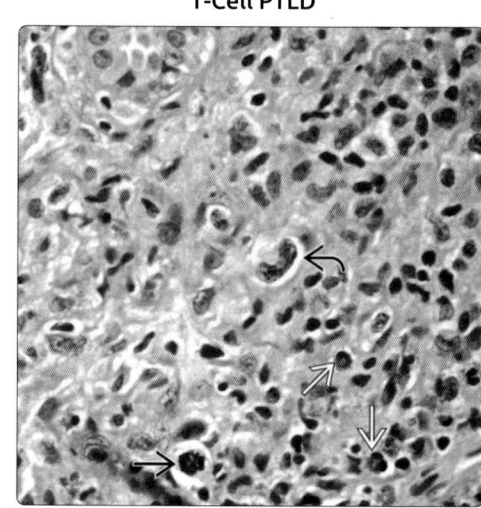

(Left) *Immunohistochemical stain of T-cell PTLD shows that most of the atypical infiltrate is composed of CD3(+) T cells with a variety of shapes & sizes.* **(Right)** *A liver biopsy in a renal allograft recipient with hepatosplenic T-cell lymphoma has diffuse portal & lobular involvement by a lymphoid infiltrate of small to medium lymphoid cells mimicking hepatitis. (Courtesy J.A. Ferry, MD.)*

T-Cell PTLD

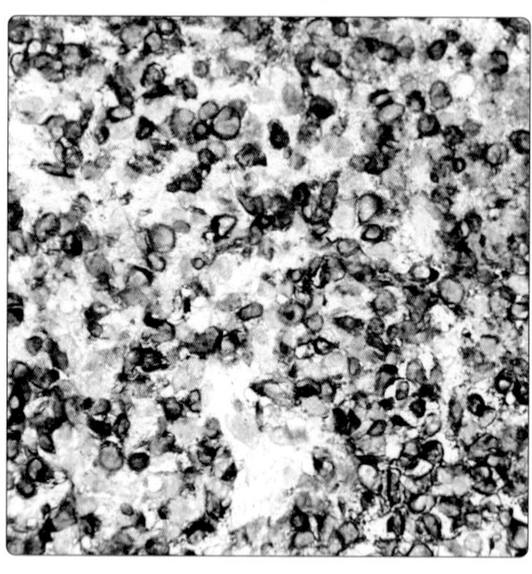

Hepatosplenic T-Cell Lymphoma

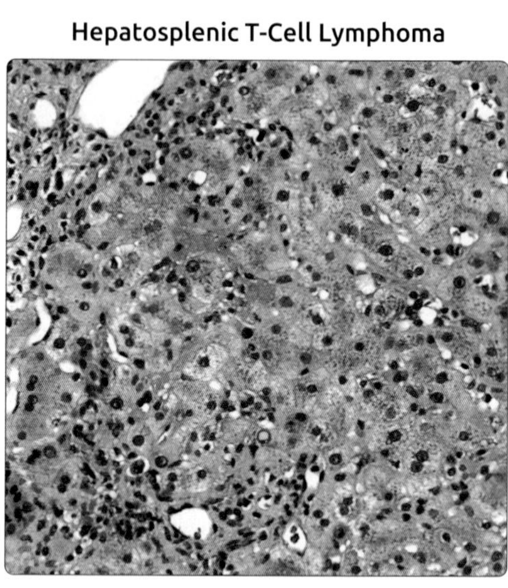

(Left) *A portal tract has a number of small to medium-sized lymphoid cells with only mild cytologic atypia that infiltrate into the lobules in a hepatosplenic T-cell lymphoma in a renal allograft recipient. (Courtesy J.A. Ferry, MD.)* **(Right)** *It can be appreciated in this image that the lymphoid cells primarily travel along the hepatic sinusoids ↓ in the hepatic lobules in a hepatosplenic T-cell lymphoma in a renal allograft recipient. (Courtesy J.A. Ferry, MD.)*

Hepatosplenic T-Cell Lymphoma

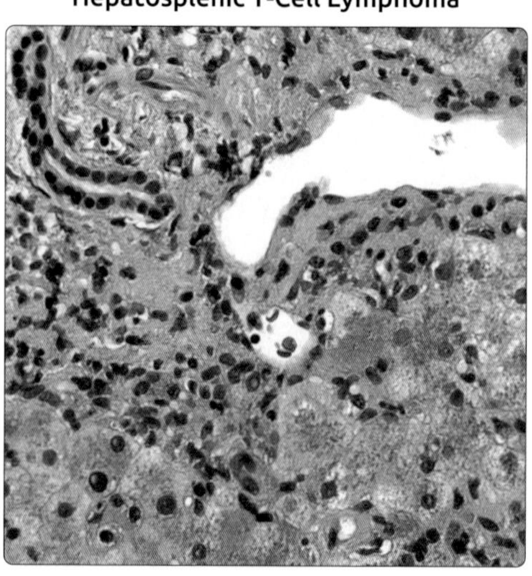

Hepatosplenic T-Cell Lymphoma

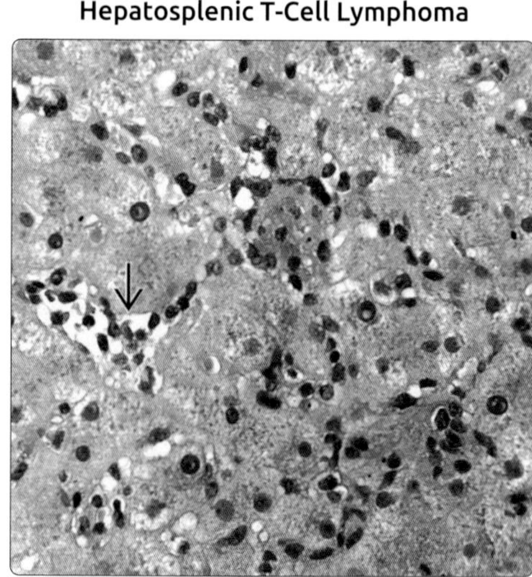

PTLD, Hodgkin Lymphoma Type

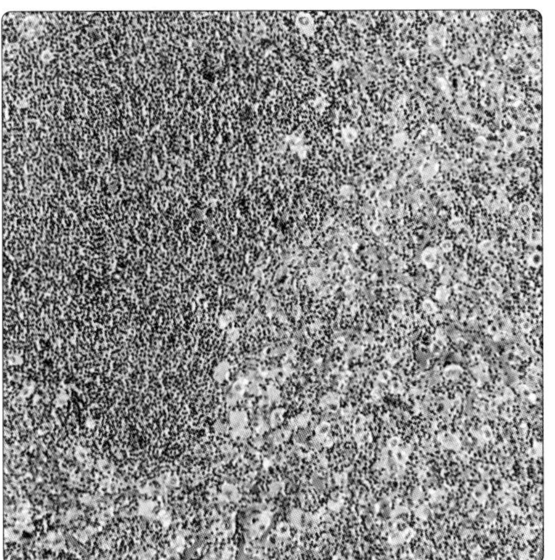

Reed-Sternberg Variant Cells in PTLD, Hodgkin Lymphoma Type

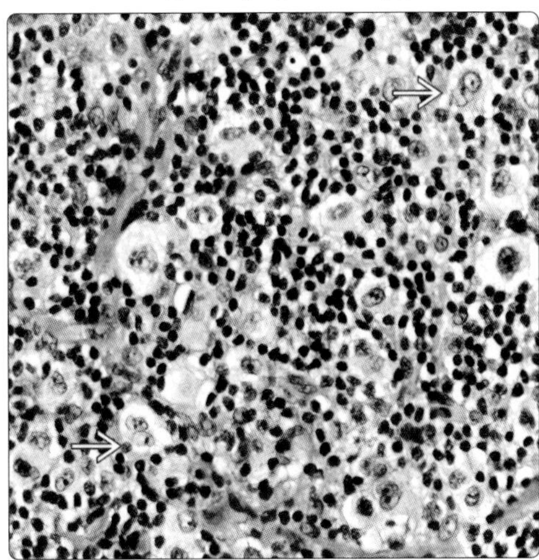

(Left) *At low power, a Hodgkin lymphoma-type PTLD involving the tongue base can be appreciated with a heterogeneous cell population. (Courtesy N.L. Harris, MD.)* **(Right)** *Throughout this Hodgkin lymphoma-type PTLD, there are many Reed-Sternberg variant cells ➡. (Courtesy N.L. Harris, MD.)*

Reed-Sternberg Variant Cells in PTLD, Hodgkin Lymphoma Type

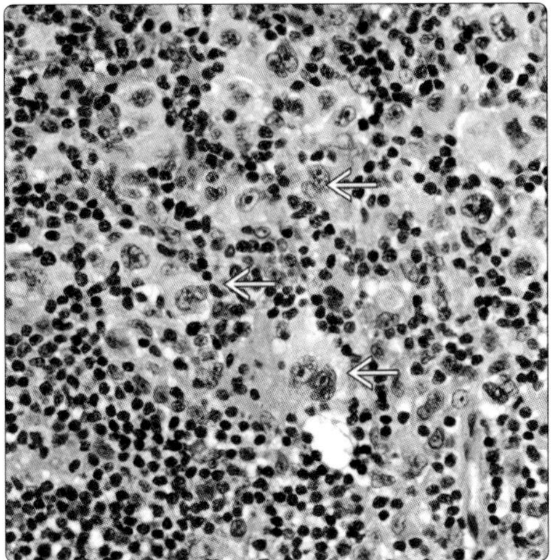

Neural Involvement by PTLD

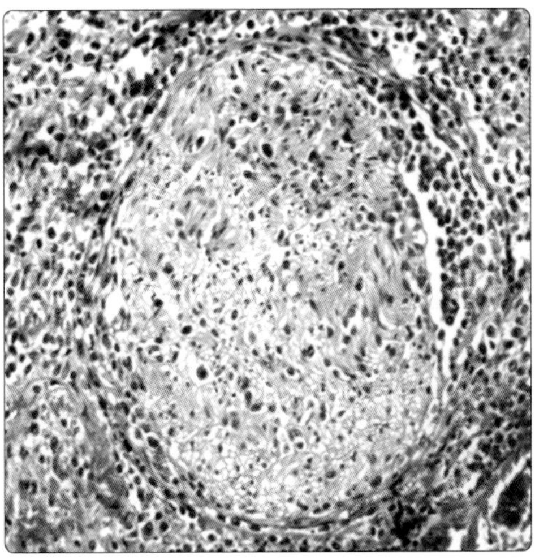

(Left) *This Hodgkin lymphoma-type PTLD contains many Reed-Sternberg variant cells ➡. (Courtesy N.L. Harris, MD.)* **(Right)** *At medium-power examination, one can observe a nerve with involvement by B-cell PTLD. (Courtesy P. Randhawa, MD.)*

Post-Transplant Spindle Cell Tumor

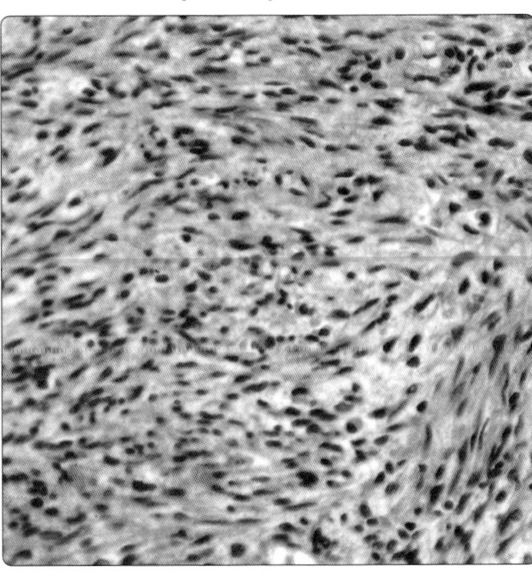

EBER ISH in EBV-Associated Post-Transplant Spindle Cell Tumor

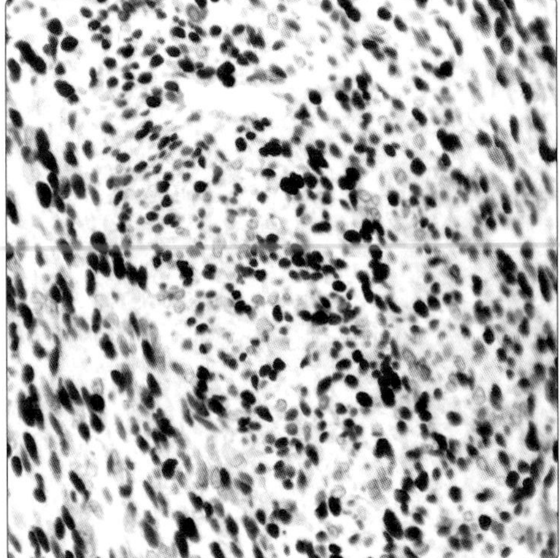

(Left) *Light microscopy shows post-transplant spindle cell tumor. In this case, immunohistochemistry showed smooth muscle differentiation. (Courtesy P. Randhawa, MD.)* **(Right)** *In situ hybridization for EBER shows EBV-infected cells in a spindle cell tumor. Lymphoid markers would demonstrate that this is not a PTLD but rather a post transplant spindle cell tumor caused by EBV. (Courtesy P. Randhawa, MD.)*

TERMINOLOGY

Synonyms

- Surveillance biopsies

Definitions

- Renal allograft biopsies performed at predetermined intervals, unrelated to graft dysfunction

CLINICAL IMPLICATIONS

Value of Protocol Biopsies

- Useful in monitoring highly sensitized patients
- Ability to detect and potentially treat subclinical disease when it may be reversible
  - Includes subclinical rejection, infection, and recurrent disease
- Findings on earlier protocol biopsies may identify cause of later graft loss
  - Specific cause of graft loss can be identified in ~ 95% of cases, largely based on earlier biopsies
- Frequency of subclinical rejection low in modern era
  - Other diseases may be detected: Drug toxicity, polyomavirus infection, recurrent disease
- Clinical trials
  - Document outcome
  - Detect toxicity
- Used more commonly in high-risk (presensitized) patients

Risk of Biopsy Procedure

- 0.4% risk of major complications
  - Hemorrhage
  - Peritonitis from bowel perforation
  - Graft loss (< 0.05%)

Timing

- Implantation ("time zero")
- Early biopsies in highly sensitized patients
- 3-4, 6, 12, 24 months
- Later post-transplant (5 and 10 years) biopsies may give insights into late graft loss

MICROSCOPIC

General Features

- Variable findings depending on diagnosis

Glomeruli

- Normal
- Duplication of glomerular basement membrane
- Mesangial hypercellularity
- Focal segmental glomerulosclerosis
- Immune complex deposition if recurrent or de novo disease
- Late (~ 10 years) post-transplant biopsies show high rate of glomerular disease
  - Mesangial sclerosis, glomerulomegaly, focal segmental glomerulosclerosis, diabetic glomerulosclerosis, increased global glomerulosclerosis

Tubules

- Normal
- Tubular atrophy
- Tubulitis
- Viral inclusions

Interstitium

- Normal
- Fibrosis
- Inflammation
  - Inflammation in areas of fibrosis associated with increased risk of graft loss
  - Inflammation outside areas of fibrosis may indicate subclinical cellular rejection

Arteries and Arterioles

- Normal
- Arteriosclerosis
- Endarteritis
  - More likely to find endothelialitis without significant tubulointerstitial inflammation ("isolated V lesion") on protocol biopsy than on biopsy for cause
- Hyalinosis in arterioles

Peritubular Capillaritis on Protocol Biopsy

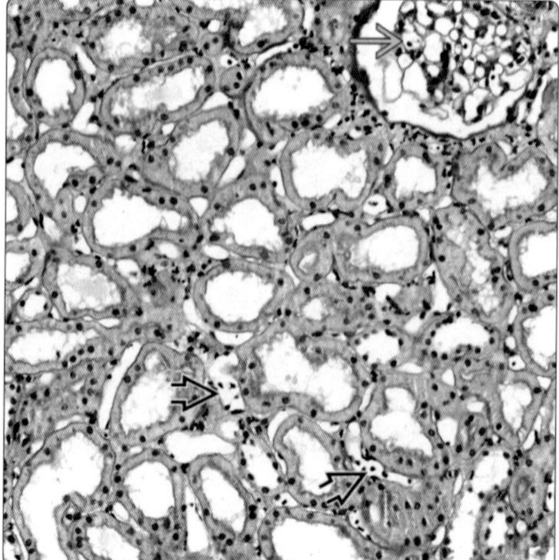

ACR on Protocol Biopsy

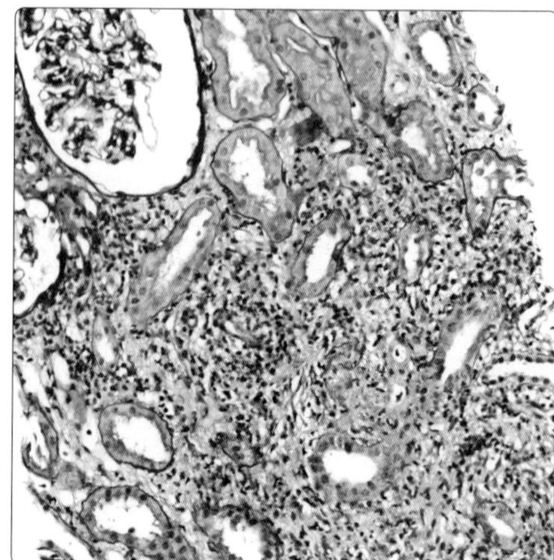

(Left) *Peritubular capillaritis (PTCitis) ➡ and glomerulitis ➡, features of subclinical AMR, are seen in this protocol biopsy, 4 months post transplant, from a patient with preformed donor-specific antibody and normal renal function. PTCitis should not be confused with acute cellular rejection.* **(Right)** *Acute cellular rejection, Banff type IB, is seen on this 4-month post-transplant protocol biopsy. The serum creatinine was stable at 1.6 mg/dL. The patient was on a steroid-free maintenance immunosuppressive protocol.*

Peritubular Capillaries (PTC)

- Normal
- C4d(+) PTC
  - Particularly in ABO blood group-incompatible transplants
- Peritubular capillaritis (mononuclear cells and neutrophils)

DIAGNOSES

Normal Histology

- Comprises majority of protocol biopsies

Subclinical Acute Cellular Rejection (ACR)

- 12-17% of protocol biopsies within first 6 months post transplant; incidence lower after 1st year and on tacrolimus (5%)
- 5-13% prevalence on 1-year protocol biopsies
  - Includes borderline/suspicious ACR, type I ACR (tubulointerstitial), and type II ACR (with endothelialitis)

Subclinical BK Polyomavirus Nephropathy

- 5% prevalence on 1-year protocol biopsies

Chronic Calcineurin Inhibitor Toxicity

- Arteriolar hyalinosis in 61.3%, 90.5%, and 100% of biopsies at 1, 5, and 10 years, respectively, in patients on cyclosporine in 1 study
  - Not necessarily specific for CNI toxicity
- Arteriolar hyalinosis may be less prevalent and less severe in patients on tacrolimus or sirolimus vs. cyclosporine
  - In another study, 19% prevalence of moderate to severe hyalinosis on 5-year protocol biopsies in a series of patients on tacrolimus-based immunosuppression
    - 5% of sirolimus-based, CNI-free immunosuppression showed moderate to severe hyalinosis

Arteriosclerosis

- May be donor disease or de novo
  - Comparison to time-zero (implantation) biopsy is helpful

Interstitial Fibrosis and Tubular Atrophy (IFTA), NOS

- 81% of cases of graft loss with IFTA have identifiable cause, in part detected on earlier biopsies
- ~ 60% of functioning grafts at 5 years have some IFTA (ct or ci > 0)
  - Moderate to severe IFTA (Banff ci > 1, ct > 1) in 17% of biopsies at 5 years
    - Associated with previous acute cellular rejection and BK polyomavirus infection episodes
- IFTA does not necessarily progress with time
  - In study of conventional transplants, allografts with mild fibrosis (ci1) on 1-year protocol biopsy often had different findings on 5-year biopsy
    - 39% showed no fibrosis (ci0) on 5-year biopsy
    - Only 23% showed more severe fibrosis on 5-year biopsy
  - Of patients with moderate fibrosis (ci2) on 1-year protocol biopsy, > 50% show mild or no fibrosis at 5 years
  - Findings may in part represent sampling error
- Combination of interstitial fibrosis and mononuclear inflammation increases risk of later graft loss
  - Shown in several independent studies
  - All types of inflammation are considered in Banff ti score

Chronic Humoral Rejection (Chronic Antibody-Mediated Rejection)

- ~ 2-5% prevalence of transplant glomerulopathy in 1-year protocol biopsies of conventional transplant patients
  - Increased risk in patients with anti-donor HLA antibodies
- Reduced graft survival with TG finding on protocol biopsy
- 14% prevalence of subclinical antibody-mediated rejection (SAMR) on 1-year protocol biopsies in one series
  - SAMR mostly seen in patients with donor-specific antibody (DSA) present prior to transplant (preformed DSA), only 22% with de novo DSA
  - SAMR histologically characterized by glomerular &/or peritubular capillaritis
    - Minority (32%) are C4d positive
  - Worse graft survival (56% at 8 years post transplant) compared to subclinical T-cell-mediated rejection
    - C4d positivity also confers worse graft survival

Accommodation

- No active rejection
- C4d(+) PTC
- Common in ABO-blood-group-incompatible transplants

Recurrent Glomerular Disease

- Early recurrent membranous glomerulonephritis and IgA nephropathy are commonly subclinical

De Novo Glomerular Disease

- Focal glomerulosclerosis and membranous glomerulonephritis are most common
- De novo C1q nephropathy common, usually of little clinical significance

SELECTED REFERENCES

1. de Sandes-Freitas TV et al: Subclinical lesions and donor-specific antibodies in kidney transplant recipients receiving tacrolimus-based immunosuppressive regimen followed by early conversion to sirolimus. Transplantation. ePub, 2015
2. Loupy A et al: Subclinical rejection phenotypes at 1 year post-transplant and outcome of kidney allografts. J Am Soc Nephrol. ePub, 2015
3. Sis B et al: Isolated Endarteritis and Kidney Transplant Survival: A Multicenter Collaborative Study. J Am Soc Nephrol. ePub, 2014
4. Caplin B et al: Early changes in scores of chronic damage on transplant kidney protocol biopsies reflect donor characteristics, but not future graft function. Clin Transplant. 27(6):E669-78, 2013
5. Mengel M et al: The molecular phenotype of 6-week protocol biopsies from human renal allografts: reflections of prior injury but not future course. Am J Transplant. 11(4):708-18, 2011
6. Stegall MD et al: The Histology of Solitary Renal Allografts at 1 and 5 Years After Transplantation. Am J Transplant. 2010 Nov 9. doi: 10.1111/j.1600-6143. 2010. Epub ahead of print, 0331
7. Park WD et al: Fibrosis with inflammation at one year predicts transplant functional decline. J Am Soc Nephrol. 21(11):1987-97, 2010
8. Said SM et al: C1q deposition in the renal allograft: a report of 24 cases. Mod Pathol. 23(8):1080-8, 2010
9. El-Zoghby ZM et al: Identifying specific causes of kidney allograft loss. Am J Transplant. 9(3):527-35, 2009
10. Mengel M et al: Infiltrates in protocol biopsies from renal allografts. Am J Transplant. 7(2):356-65, 2007
11. Moreso F et al: Subclinical rejection associated with chronic allograft nephropathy in protocol biopsies as a risk factor for late graft loss. Am J Transplant. 6(4):747-52, 2006
12. Furness PN et al: Protocol biopsy of the stable renal transplant: a multicenter study of methods and complication rates. Transplantation. 76(6):969-73, 2003
13. Cornell L et al: Banff Criteria Are Inadequate to Assess Chronic Renal Allograft Injury 10 Years Post-Transplantation [abstract]. Am J Transplant. 2015; 15 (suppl 3). Accessed May 3, 2015.

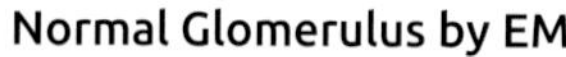

(Left) *A normal glomerulus is seen in a protocol biopsy. Podocyte foot processes are preserved ⇒. No glomerular basement membrane (GBM) duplication or subendothelial lucency is present. No immune deposits are noted. Endothelial cells appear normal, with preserved fenestrations ⇒.* (Right) *Here, a normal peritubular capillary is seen in a protocol biopsy specimen. The capillary shows a single basement membrane layer ⇒ and normal-appearing endothelial cells.*

Normal Glomerulus by EM

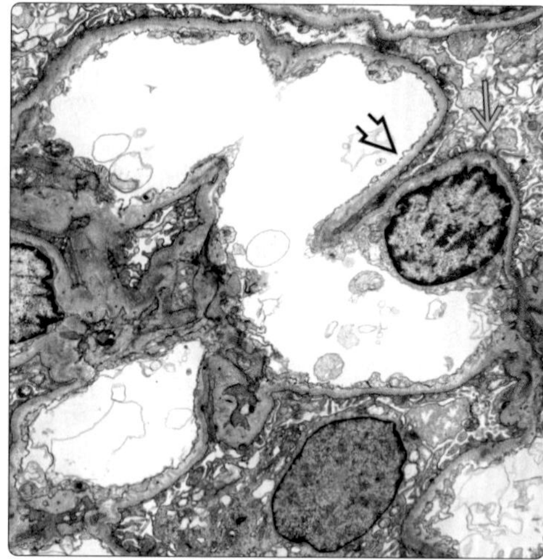

Normal Peritubular Capillary by EM

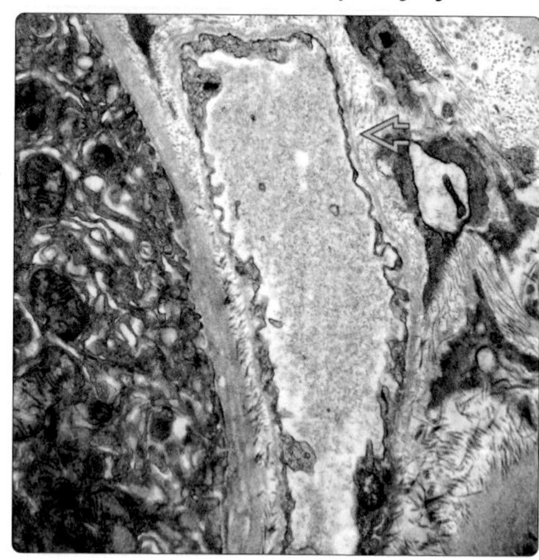

(Left) *Enlarged endothelial cells ⇒ with loss of fenestrations are seen by EM on a protocol biopsy 1 month post transplant in a patient with preformed donor-specific antibodies. This finding may precede development of transplant glomerulopathy. The biopsy appeared normal by light microscopy.* (Right) *A 1-year protocol biopsy specimen in a patient with normal renal function is shown. The biopsy appears normal.*

Reactive Endothelium by EM

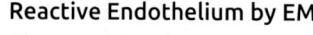

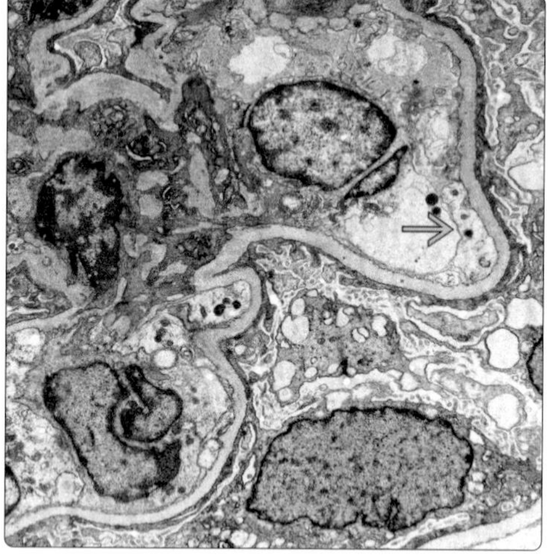

Normal Protocol Biopsy

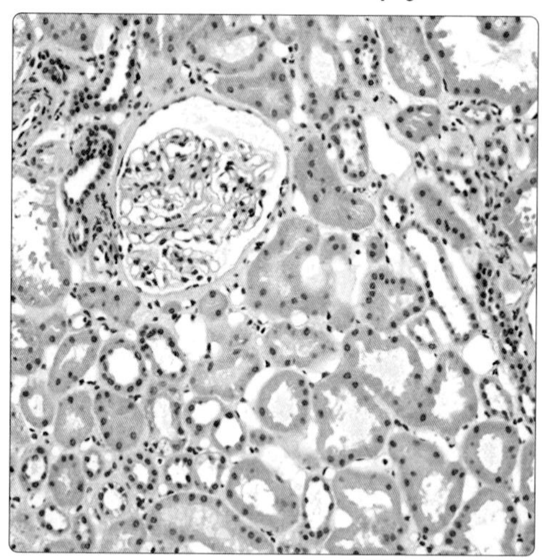

(Left) *This 10-year post-transplant protocol biopsy shows moderate mesangial sclerosis ⇒, which can be nodular and is a feature often present on late post-transplant biopsies even in patients without diabetes.* (Right) *Rare arterioles show intimal ⇒ and peripheral nodular ⇒ hyalinosis, likely due to subclinical calcineurin inhibitor toxicity. Arteriolar hyalinosis becomes more common with time post transplant.*

Mesangial Sclerosis on Late Protocol Biopsy

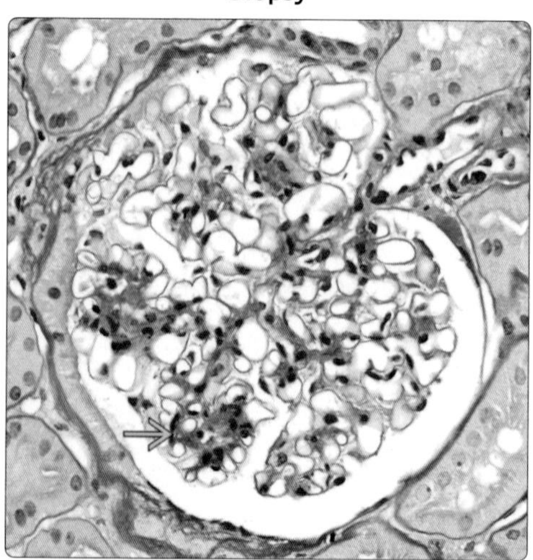

Arteriolar Hyalinosis

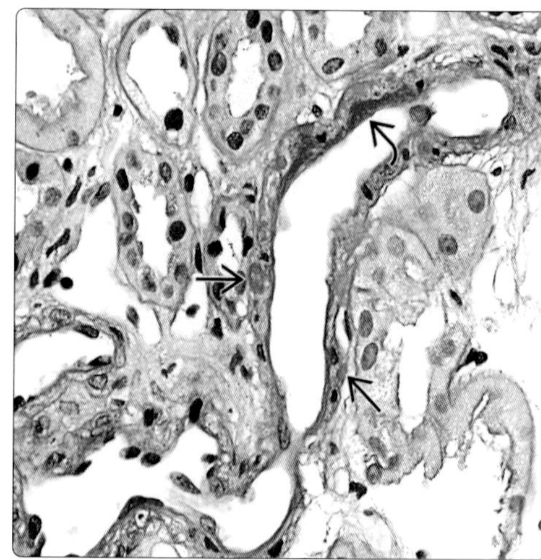

IgA Deposits on Protocol Biopsy

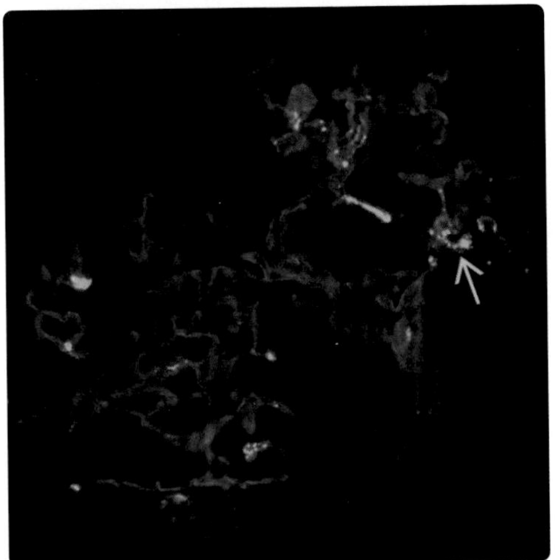

De Novo C1q Nephropathy

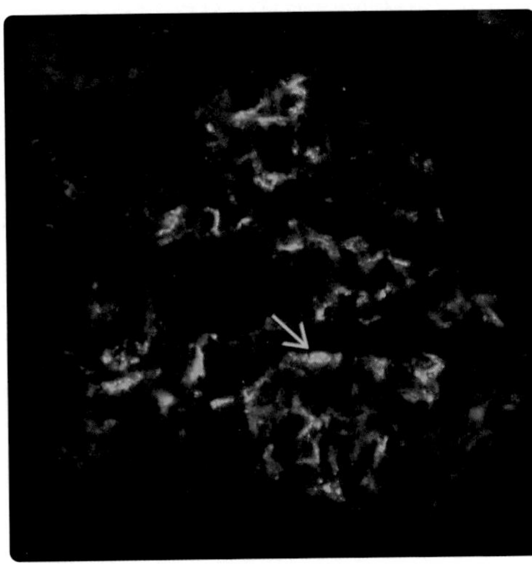

(Left) *Segmental granular mesangial ⇨ staining for IgA is seen on this protocol biopsy 5 years post transplant in a patient with a history of IgA nephropathy in the native kidney. The glomeruli showed mild mesangial hypercellularity by LM.* **(Right)** *IF staining for C1q shows 2+ granular mesangial staining ⇨ on a protocol biopsy 10 years post transplant. By LM, glomeruli showed mesangial hypercellularity. This finding is usually of no clinical significance.*

Early Transplant Glomerulopathy (TG)

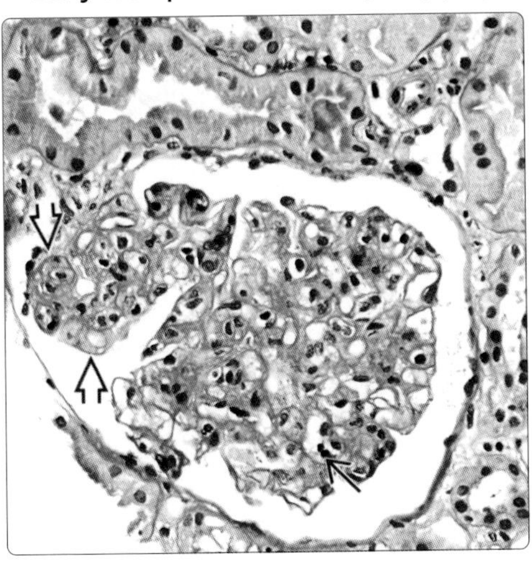

Early Recurrent Membranous Nephropathy (MGN)

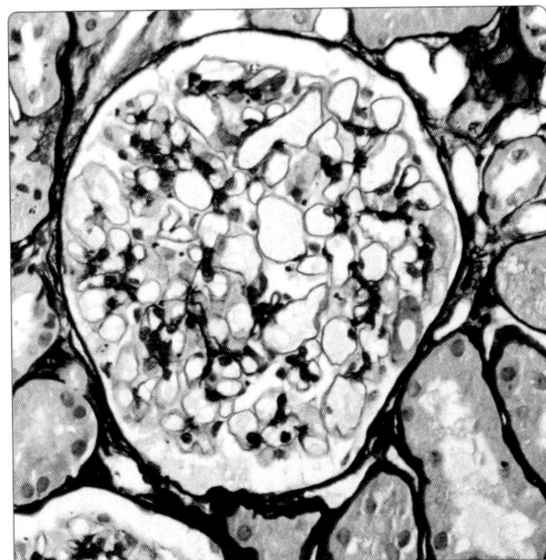

(Left) *Early TG is seen in a 1-year protocol biopsy. Glomerulitis ⇨ and segmental GBM duplication ⇨ are seen. This patient also had preformed donor-specific HLA antibody but normal renal function.* **(Right)** *This glomerulus from early recurrent MGN does not show evidence of GBM abnormalities ("spikes" or "pinholes") on high magnification. No deposits were noted on a trichrome stain.*

Early Recurrent MGN by IF

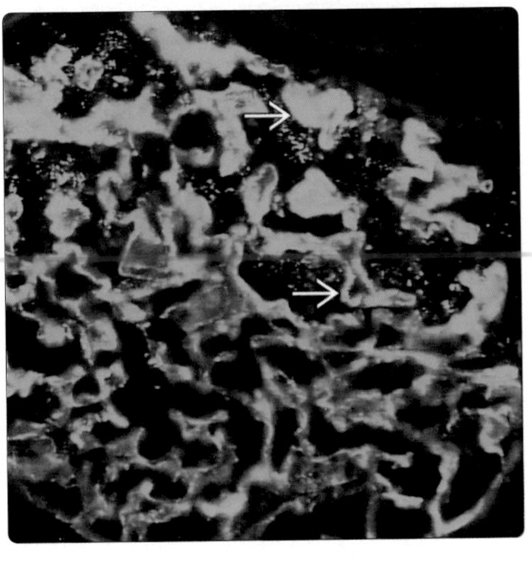

Early Recurrent MGN on EM

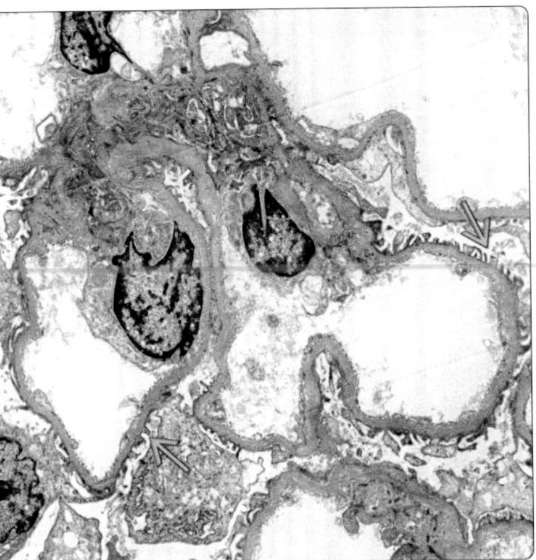

(Left) *In early recurrent MGN, IF staining for C4d reveals granular GBM staining in a membranous pattern ➡, in contrast to usual and normal glomerular C4d staining restricted to the mesangium. Similar staining was seen for IgG.* **(Right)** *A 4-month protocol biopsy specimen in a patient with early recurrent MGN and minimal proteinuria shows no electron-dense deposits by EM, despite IgG and complement deposits by IF. Podocyte foot processes are intact ⇨.*

KEY FACTS

TERMINOLOGY

- Accommodation refers to lack of graft injury in presence of donor-reactive immune response, usually detected by circulating anti-donor antibodies
  - Commonly but not always occurring in ABO-incompatible (ABOi) grafts (> 80%)
- Corresponding Banff definition: Peritubular capillary C4d deposition without evidence of rejection

CLINICAL ISSUES

- Normal graft function
- No treatment indicated for ABOi transplants
- No established treatment in patients with preformed anti-HLA DSA and normal graft function

MICROSCOPIC

- Normal graft biopsy
- C4d deposition in PTC
- No capillaritis
- Normal endothelial cells, GBM, and PTC by electron microscopy

TOP DIFFERENTIAL DIAGNOSES

- Chronic antibody-mediated rejection
  - Glomerulitis and peritubular capillaritis
  - Multilamination of PTC basement membrane and GBM

DIAGNOSTIC CHECKLIST

- Accommodation generally stable in ABO-incompatible (ABOi) grafts, while not stable in kidney transplant recipients with anti-HLA DSA
- Allograft recipients that have circulating anti-HLA DSA, especially if associated with C4d(+) on biopsy, generally progress to transplant glomerulopathy with time

Normal Cortex

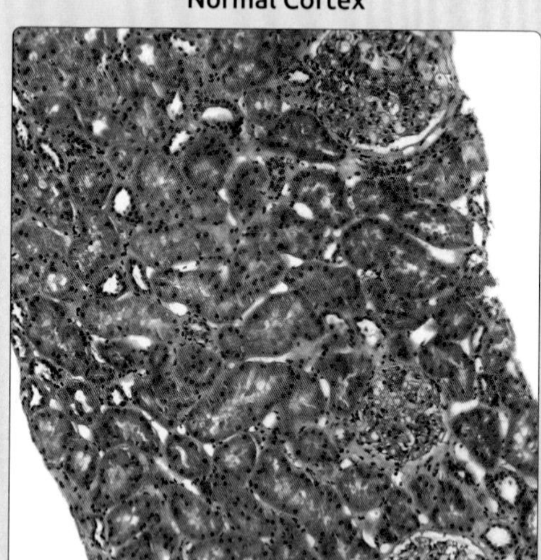

Normal Parenchyma

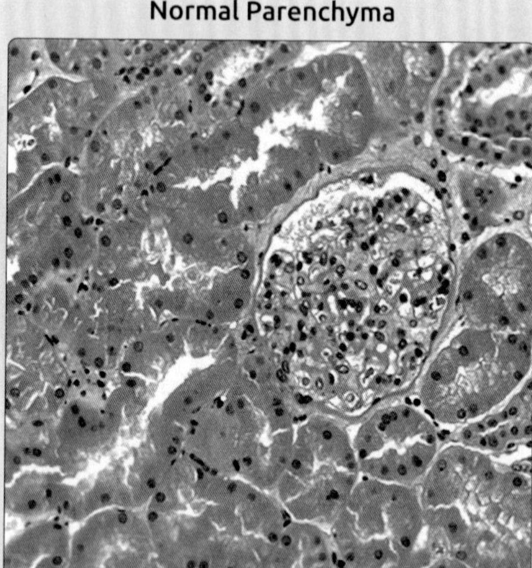

(Left) *Protocol biopsy of an ABO-incompatible graft 3 months after transplantation appears entirely normal by light microscopy.* **(Right)** *Protocol biopsy is shown from a patient with stable renal function with an HLA-incompatible, ABO-compatible graft. The appearance by light microscopy is entirely normal, although C4d was present in PTC.*

C4d

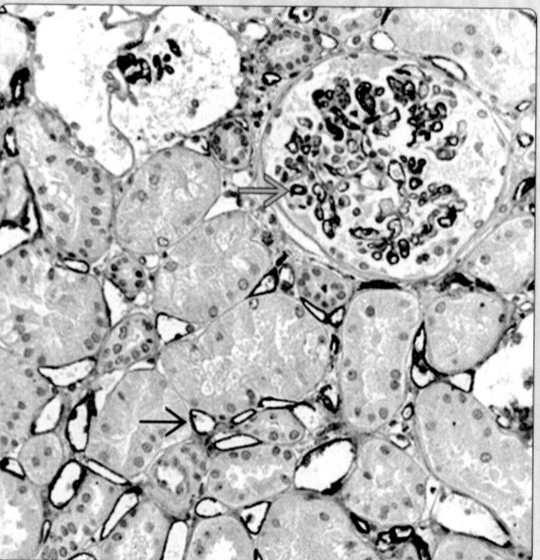

Peritubular Capillary

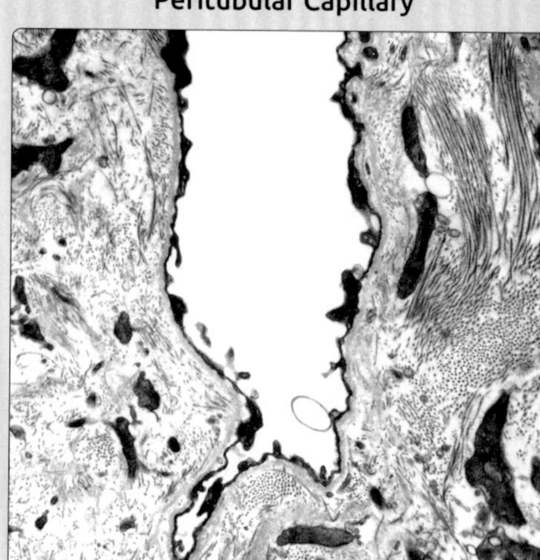

(Left) *Protocol biopsy is shown from a patient with stable renal function with an HLA-incompatible, ABO-compatible graft. C4d is in the PTC ➔ and glomerular ⇨ basement membranes in the absence of inflammation.* **(Right)** *Protocol biopsy of a C4d(+), normal-appearing ABO-incompatible graft 3 months after transplantation shows entirely normal PTC endothelium, indicative of accommodation.*

TERMINOLOGY

Definitions

- Refers to lack of graft injury in presence of donor-reactive immune response, usually by circulating anti-donor antibody detection
  - Commonly but not always occurring in ABO-incompatible (ABOi) grafts
- Corresponding Banff definition: Peritubular capillary C4d without evidence of rejection

ETIOLOGY/PATHOGENESIS

Endothelial Response to Antibodies Reactive to Surface Components

- Increased antiapoptotic molecules (Bcl-xL)
- Increased complement regulatory proteins (CD55, decay accelerating factor)
- Increased MUC1

Animal Models

- In nonhuman primates, 4 stages of chronic antibody-mediated rejection defined with de novo donor-specific antibody (DSA)
  - Stage I: Circulating DSA (accommodation 1)
  - Stage II: DSA + C4d in peritubular capillaries (PTC) (accommodation 2)
  - Stage III: DSA + C4d + pathologic changes (subclinical chronic humoral rejection [CHR])
  - Stage IV: DSA + C4d + pathology + functional impairment
- Time course between stages variable and unpredictable

CLINICAL ISSUES

Epidemiology

- Incidence
  - Commonly occurs in ABOi grafts (> 80% C4d[+] on protocol biopsies)
  - Incidence in HLA incompatible grafts uncertain (2-4% in early protocol biopsies), unstable long term

Presentation

- Normal graft function
- Positive circulating DSA either HLA or ABO blood group antibodies

Treatment

- No treatment indicated for ABOi transplants
- No established treatment in patients with preformed anti-HLA DSA and normal graft function
  - IVIG, rituximab, bortezomib used without clear long-term benefit

Prognosis

- In ABOi grafts, similar long-term graft survival as conventional transplants
- Positive-crossmatch (+XM) patients with preformed anti-HLA DSA
  - Early protocol biopsies (< 3 months) may show minor changes by light microscopy
  - Majority of +XM recipients develop chronic antibody-mediated rejection, increasing incidence with time post transplant

MICROSCOPIC

Histologic Features

- Normal graft biopsy, no evidence of rejection
- Glomeruli
  - No glomerulitis, no GBM duplication
- Interstitium
  - No interstitial infiltrate (< 10%)
- Tubules
  - No tubulitis (< 5 cells/tubule)
- Arteries
  - No arteritis (endothelialitis)
- Peritubular capillaries
  - No capillaritis

ANCILLARY TESTS

Immunohistochemistry

- Positive C4d staining in peritubular and glomerular capillaries

Immunofluorescence

- Positive C4d staining in PTC
- C3d staining by IF in ABOi grafts correlates with capillaritis
  - Presence of C3 in TBM confounds interpretation
  - C3d staining not helpful in grafts with anti-HLA DSA

Electron Microscopy

- Lack of reactive endothelial cells in glomeruli and PTC
- Lack of multilamination of PTC basement membranes
- Lack of glomerular basement membrane duplication

DIFFERENTIAL DIAGNOSIS

Chronic Antibody-Mediated Rejection

- Glomerulitis and peritubular capillaritis
- Multilamination of PTC basement membrane and GBM

DIAGNOSTIC CHECKLIST

Pathologic Interpretation Pearls

- Stability of accommodation
  - Accommodation generally stable in ABO-incompatible (ABOi) grafts, while unstable in kidney transplant recipients with anti-HLA DSA
    - Allografts with circulating anti-HLA DSA, especially if C4d(+) on biopsy, generally progress to transplant glomerulopathy over time
- Clinicians should not overtreat but should not dismiss as benign

SELECTED REFERENCES

1. Bentall A et al: Differences in chronic intragraft inflammation between positive crossmatch and ABO-incompatible kidney transplantation. Transplantation. 98(10):1089-96, 2014
2. Haas M: An updated Banff schema for diagnosis of antibody-mediated rejection in renal allografts. Curr Opin Organ Transplant. 19(3):315-22, 2014
3. Rose ML et al: Accommodation: does it apply to human leukocyte antigens? Transplantation. 93(3):244-6, 2012
4. Smith RN et al: Four stages and lack of stable accommodation in chronic alloantibody-mediated renal allograft rejection in Cynomolgus monkeys. Am J Transplant. 8(8):1662-72, 2008
5. Mengel M et al: Incidence of C4d stain in protocol biopsies from renal allografts: results from a multicenter trial. Am J Transplant. 5(5):1050-6, 2005

KEY FACTS

TERMINOLOGY

- Tolerance: State of immunologically specific acceptance of tissue or organs without destructive immune response, without immunosuppressive drugs, & with full immunologic reactivity to other antigens (e.g., microbes or 3rd-party allografts)

ETIOLOGY/PATHOGENESIS

- Mixed chimerism
  - Bone marrow & kidney allografts from same living donor given to recipient conditioned with thymic irradiation, cyclophosphamide (or whole body irradiation), calcineurin inhibitors, rituximab, & T-cell depleting antibodies
- Ad hoc withdrawal of immunosuppression
  - In some (unpredictable) cases, allografts have continued to function normally
  - Increased number of circulating transitional B cells
- Mechanisms
  - Deletional tolerance (central tolerance)
    - Normal mechanism for preventing autoimmunity
  - Regulatory tolerance (peripheral tolerance)
    - Mediated by regulatory cells (Treg), FOXP3(+)

MICROSCOPIC

- Protocol biopsies of stable kidney allografts off immunosuppression limited in number but revealed spectrum of patterns
- Normal kidney
- FOXP3(+) cells in interstitial and perivascular aggregates
  - Treg-rich organized lymphoid structures (TOLS)
- Accommodation (C4d[+])
- Slowly progressive subclinical chronic antibody-mediated rejection
- Recurrent glomerular disease

DIAGNOSTIC CHECKLIST

- Renal biopsy essential in proving state of tolerance

Normal Kidney Protocol Biopsy

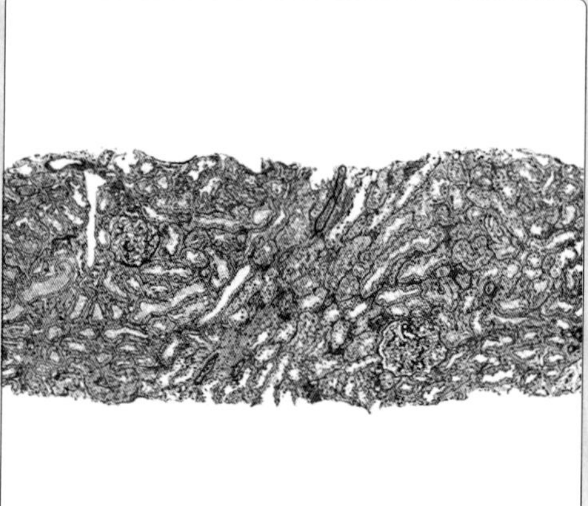

Lymphoid Aggregates in Accepted Allograft

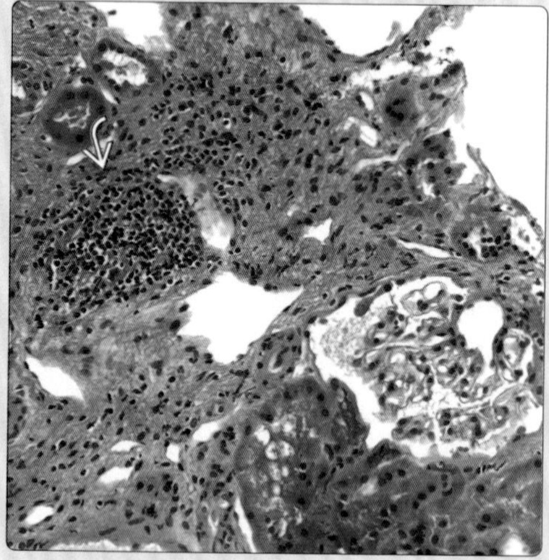

(Left) *This is a 2-year protocol biopsy on patient with normal renal function who has been off immunosuppression for 18 months. Tolerance was induced with donor bone marrow and the mixed chimerism conditioning protocol. The kidney is normal.* **(Right)** *This protocol biopsy in an accepted renal allograft from a patient with normal renal function off immunosuppression 7 years after transplantation shows aggregates of lymphoid cells ➔, which typically contain (Treg) FOXP3(+) cells.*

Aggregates of FOXP3(+) Cells in Accepted Allograft

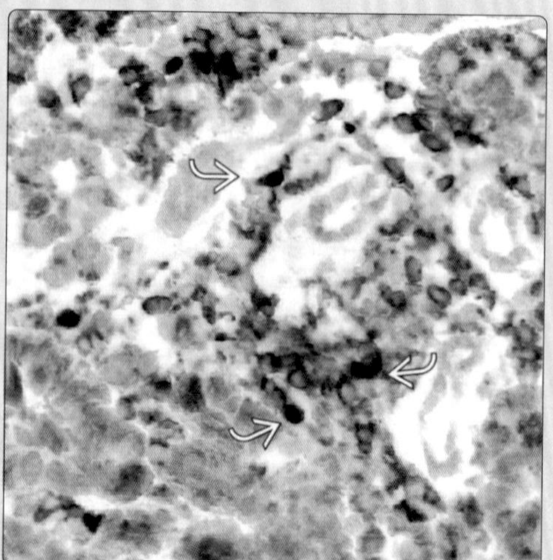

Treg-Rich Organized Lymphoid Structure (TOLS)

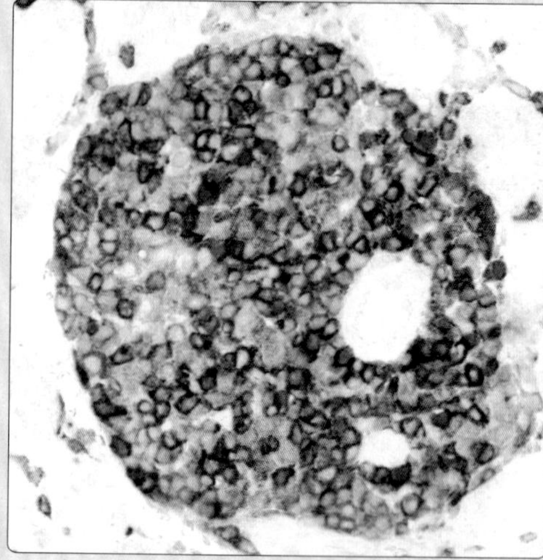

(Left) *Protocol biopsies from accepted renal allografts off immunosuppression often show aggregates of lymphoid cells rich in FOXP3(+) cells ➔. Double stain for FOXP3 (blue) and CD4 (brown).* **(Right)** *TOLS are common in recipients who are tolerant of their renal allografts. These are seen in human, nonhuman primate, pig, and mouse renal allografts (shown) after tolerance induction by a variety of protocols. Double stain for FOXP3 (blue) and CD3 (brown).*

TERMINOLOGY

Definitions

- Tolerance: State of immunologically specific acceptance of tissue or organs without destructive immune response, without immunosuppressive drugs, and with full immunologic reactivity to other antigens, such as microbes or 3rd-party allografts
- While achieved in inbred mice with variety of protocols, only recently tolerance intentionally induced in human kidney allografts

ETIOLOGY/PATHOGENESIS

Protocols to Induce Tolerance in Mice

- Many strategies, such as neonatal injection of donor cells (Medawar et al) costimulation blockade and donor transfusion work in inbred mice
  - Only successful protocol in humans administered donor bone marrow cells
- Administration of donor bone marrow with nonmyeloablative regimen in mice leads to stable leukocyte mixed chimerism and tolerance of organ or skin grafts (Sachs and Sykes)

Protocols to Induce Tolerance in Humans

- Mixed chimerism
  - Applied in clinical trials in kidney transplantation by Kawai, Sachs, Cosimi and colleagues
  - Bone marrow and kidney allografts from same living donor given to recipient conditioned with thymic irradiation, cyclophosphamide (or whole body irradiation), calcineurin inhibitors, rituximab, and T-cell depleting antibodies
  - Transient mixed chimerism in humans
    - Long-term graft survival achieved in substantial fraction of HLA identical and haplo-identical recipients after immunosuppressive drugs withdrawn
- Spontaneous tolerance
  - Occasional kidney allograft recipients have discontinued immunosuppressive drugs after several years for various reasons, and, in some cases, their allografts have continued to function normally
- Cell therapy
  - Administration of bone marrow-derived facilitator cells or induced donor-specific Treg currently under investigation

Mechanisms

- 2 principal physiological mechanisms to avoid autoimmunity or hypersensitivity
- Deletional tolerance (central tolerance)
  - Newly formed self-reactive T cells deleted in thymus
  - Irreversible
- Regulatory tolerance (peripheral tolerance)
  - Effector T cells inhibited by antigen-specific T cells (Treg)
    - Best defined subpopulation expresses Foxp3
  - This form of tolerance may be lost if Treg depleted or if their function impaired
  - Experimental evidence that Treg in allografts can mediate tolerance

CLINICAL ISSUES

Laboratory Tests

- Patients who are spontaneously tolerant have increased number of transitional B cells compared to those on immunosuppression
- No current test predicts which patients can successfully withdraw immunosuppression

MICROSCOPIC

Histologic Features

- Protocol biopsies of stable kidney allografts off immunosuppression are limited in number but revealed spectrum of patterns
  - Normal kidney
    - Reported in HLA-identical grafts in myeloma patients on mixed chimerism protocol
    - No appreciable lymphoid infiltrate, no evidence of antibody-mediated rejection (C4d)
    - Compatible with deletional tolerance
  - Treg-rich organized lymphoid structures (TOLS)
    - Foxp3(+) cells in interstitial and perivascular aggregates
    - Observed in HLA-haplo-identical kidney allografts in humans and nonhuman primates on mixed chimerism protocol
    - Probable signature pattern of regulatory tolerance
  - Accommodation
    - Several recipients developed donor-specific HLA antibodies and had deposition of C4d in peritubular capillaries without simultaneous evidence of rejection either pathologically or clinically
  - Subclinical chronic antibody-mediated rejection (AMR)
    - Progression to chronic AMR manifested by transplant glomerulopathy has occurred in patients with donor-specific HLA antibodies, over 5 or more years
  - Recurrent glomerular disease
    - Tolerance inducing protocols have little or no effect on recurrent disease, such as C3 nephropathy

DIAGNOSTIC CHECKLIST

Clinically Relevant Pathologic Features

- Renal biopsy essential in proving state of tolerance

SELECTED REFERENCES

1. Leventhal JR et al: Immune reconstitution/immunocompetence in recipients of kidney plus hematopoietic stem/facilitating cell transplants. Transplantation. 99(2):288-98, 2015
2. Kawai T et al: Long-term results in recipients of combined HLA-mismatched kidney and bone marrow transplantation without maintenance immunosuppression. Am J Transplant. 14(7):1599-611, 2014
3. Sachs DH et al: Induction of tolerance through mixed chimerism. Cold Spring Harb Perspect Med. 4(1):a015529, 2014
4. Miyajima M et al: Early acceptance of renal allografts in mice is dependent on foxp3(+) cells. Am J Pathol. 178(4):1635-45, 2011
5. Newell KA et al: Identification of a B cell signature associated with renal transplant tolerance in humans. J Clin Invest. 120(6):1836-47, 2010
6. Fudaba Y et al: Myeloma responses and tolerance following combined kidney and nonmyeloablative marrow transplantation: in vivo and in vitro analyses. Am J Transplant. 6(9):2121-33, 2006
7. Billingham RE et al: Actively acquired tolerance of foreign cells. Nature. 172(4379):603-6, 1953

Kidney Diseases in Non-Renal Transplant Recipients

KEY FACTS

TERMINOLOGY

- Renal disease developing in native kidneys after transplantation of other organs or hematopoietic cells

ETIOLOGY/PATHOGENESIS

- Calcineurin inhibitors (cyclosporine, tacrolimus)
- Antiviral drugs
- Polyomavirus
- Diabetic nephropathy
- Hypertensive nephrosclerosis
- Associated with GVHD in hematopoietic transplants

CLINICAL ISSUES

- 16% of recipients of nonkidney organ transplants develop chronic renal failure in 10 years
- Progressive renal failure
- Proteinuria, nephrotic syndrome
- Schistocytes, thrombocytopenia, elevated LDH

MICROSCOPIC

- Varies with cause, small percentage biopsied (1-4%)
  - CNIT, chronic vascular and tubulointerstitial
    - Nodular arteriolar hyalinosis, interstitial fibrosis, tubular atrophy, glomerulosclerosis
  - CNIT, thrombotic microangiopathy
    - GBM duplication, thrombi endothelial injury
  - Membranous GN
    - GBM deposits and "spikes" along GBM
  - Minimal change disease
    - Foot process effacement
  - Drug toxicity
    - Crystals, oxalates, interstitial nephritis
  - Viral infection
    - Nuclear inclusions, positive viral antigens by IHC

DIAGNOSTIC CHECKLIST

- Cause for most cases assumed to be CNIT but without biopsy evidence

(Left) *Peripheral nodular hyaline in arterioles is characteristic, although not pathognomic of calcineurin inhibitor toxicity (CNIT). This is a native kidney biopsy from a heart-lung transplant recipient.* **(Right)** *Fibrosis appears "striped" because it is along the medullary rays in the cortex, a watershed area prone to ischemia from many causes. This is a native kidney from a lung transplant recipient. (Courtesy S. Rosen, MD.)*

Peripheral Nodular Hyaline of CNIT

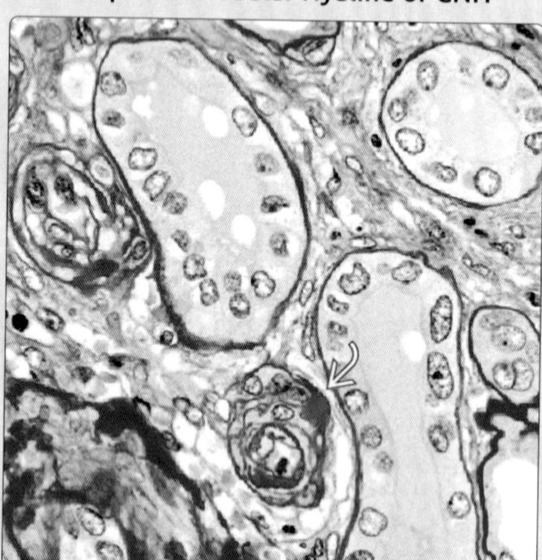

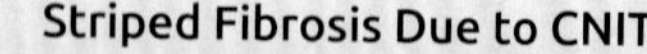

Striped Fibrosis Due to CNIT

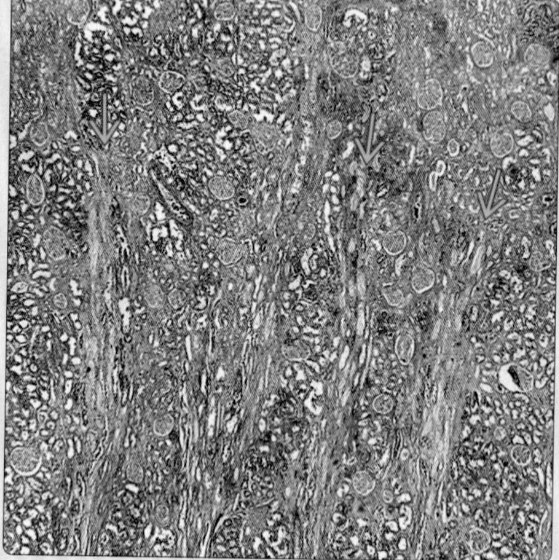

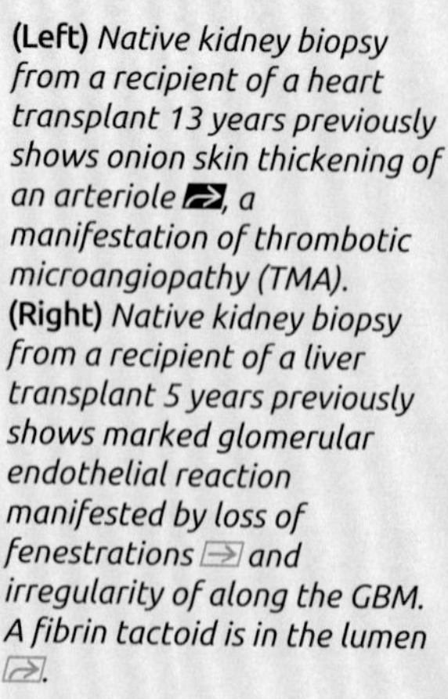

(Left) *Native kidney biopsy from a recipient of a heart transplant 13 years previously shows onion skin thickening of an arteriole , a manifestation of thrombotic microangiopathy (TMA).* **(Right)** *Native kidney biopsy from a recipient of a liver transplant 5 years previously shows marked glomerular endothelial reaction manifested by loss of fenestrations and irregularity of along the GBM. A fibrin tactoid is in the lumen .*

Onion Skin Intimal Thickening of TMA

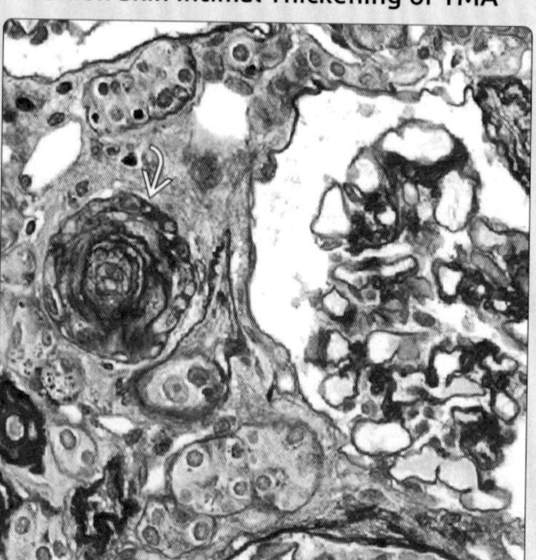

Subclinical Thrombotic Microangiopathy

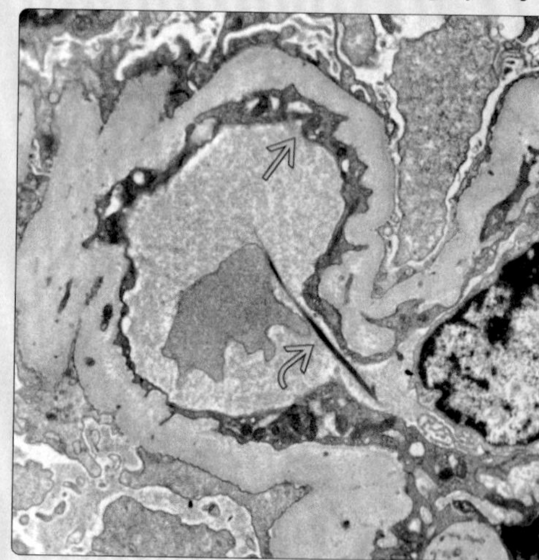

TERMINOLOGY

Abbreviations

- Calcineurin inhibitor (CNI)

Definitions

- Renal disease developing in native kidneys after transplantation of other organs or hematopoietic cells

ETIOLOGY/PATHOGENESIS

Drug Toxicity

- Calcineurin inhibitors (CNI, cyclosporine, tacrolimus)
  - Thrombotic microangiopathy
  - Interstitial fibrosis/tubular atrophy
  - Arteriolar hyalinosis
  - Focal segmental glomerulosclerosis
  - Acute tubular injury
  - Therapeutic levels usually much higher than kidney transplantation
- Antiviral drugs
- Hydroxyethyl starch nephrotoxicity

Infection

- Polyomavirus
  - BK virus
  - JC virus
- Epstein-Barr virus (post-transplant lymphoproliferative disease)
- Adenovirus
- Cytomegalovirus

Progression of Recipient Disease

- Diabetic nephropathy
- Hypertensive nephrosclerosis
- HCV related glomerular disease
- Myeloma cast nephropathy
- Amyloidosis

Immunologic Reaction

- Membranous glomerulonephritis
  - Associated with graft-vs.-host-disease (GVHD)
    - Rare report with autologous stem cell transplantation
- Minimal change disease
  - Associated with GVHD

CLINICAL ISSUES

Epidemiology

- 16.5% of recipients of nonkidney organ transplants develop chronic renal failure in 10 years (GFR < 30 mL/m1.73m^2)
  - At 5 years: 18% of liver recipients, 16% of lung recipients, 11% of heart recipients

Presentation

- Progressive renal failure
  - Calcineurin inhibitor toxicity
  - Hypertensive nephrosclerosis
  - Polyomavirus nephropathy
- Proteinuria, nephrotic syndrome
  - Diabetic nephropathy
  - Focal segmental glomerulosclerosis
  - Membranous glomerulonephritis
  - Minimal change disease
  - HCV-related glomerular disease
- Schistocytes, thrombocytopenia, elevated LDH
  - Calcineurin inhibitor toxicity
  - May also be subclinical thrombotic microangiopathy

Treatment

- Varies with cause
- Reduction or alternation of immunosuppressive therapy

Prognosis

- Varies with cause
- 4.5% develop ESRD overall

MICROSCOPIC

Histologic Features

- Calcineurin inhibitor toxicity
  - Interstitial fibrosis, tubular atrophy, global or segmental glomerulosclerosis, nodular arteriolar hyalinosis
  - Acute tubular injury
  - Thrombotic microangiopathy
    - Acute
      - Thrombi glomerular capillaries, arterioles
      - Acute endothelial injury
    - Chronic
      - Duplication of GBM
      - Nodular arteriolar hyalinosis
- Diabetic nephropathy
  - Arteriolar hyalinosis, nodular glomerulosclerosis
- Hypertensive nephrosclerosis
  - Arterial intimal fibroelastosis, global or segmental glomerulosclerosis, interstitial fibrosis, tubular atrophy
- Membranous glomerulonephritis
  - Thickened glomerular capillaries with deposits and "spikes" along GBM
- HCV related glomerular disease
  - Duplication of GBM, mesangial hypercellularity, pseudothrombi
- Minimal change disease
  - Normal glomeruli, reabsorption droplets in tubules
- Viral drug toxicity
  - Crystals in tubules and sometimes in glomerular capillaries
  - Oxalate deposition and pigmented casts
- Drug reaction
  - Interstitial nephritis
    - Interstitial manifestation of GVHD in kidney not defined
- Viral infection
  - Nuclear inclusions, hyperchromaticity, interstitial inflammation, granuloma (adenovirus)

ANCILLARY TESTS

Immunohistochemistry

- Viral infection
  - Viral antigens (polyoma, adenovirus, cytomegalovirus)

Immunofluorescence

- Membranous GN

Kidney Disease in Recipients of Non-Renal Transplants

	Liver	Heart	Lung	Hematopoietic
Number	210	28	49	49
Vascular Disease				
Arteriosclerosis/hypertensive vascular disease	34%	71%	47%	8%
CNIT/arteriolar hyalinosis	22%	25%	69%	6%
TMA	9%	7%	24%	16%
Glomerular Disease				
FSGS	19%	36%	24%	2%
MPGN	6%	4%		
DM	19%		6%	
IgAN	4%	7%		
Minimal change disease	1%			16% (25% with tip lesion)
Membranous glomerulonephritis	4%			22%
Crescentic GN, NOS	0.5%			
Amyloidosis	0.5%			4%
Tubulointerstitial Disease				
Polyomavirus infection			2%	6%
Oxalate deposition			10%	
Pigmented casts			16%	
Nephrocalcinosis		21%		4%
ATN	10%	50%	43%	27%
Hydroxyethyl starch nephrotoxicity		8%		
Myeloma cast nephropathy				2%

More than 1 diagnosis in some biopsies; categories not uniformly identified or defined; criteria for biopsy not consistent.

Combined data from Pillebout, O'Riordan, Schwarz, Lafaucheur, Kambham, Gutierrez, Chang, Kim, and Taheri and Colvin (unpublished).

  - IgG, C3, granular deposits along GBM
  - PLA2R negative
- HCV-related glomerular disease
  - IgM, IgG, C3, C1q granular deposits along GBM and in mesangium
- Recurrent AL amyloid and cast nephropathy
  - Light chain restriction

Electron Microscopy

- Minimal change disease
  - Effacement of podocyte foot processes
- Diabetic nephropathy
  - Diffuse thickening of GBM
- Membranous GN
  - Subepithelial deposits and GBM "spikes"
- Calcineurin inhibitor toxicity (thrombotic microangiopathy)
  - Loss of fenestrations of glomerular endothelial cells
  - Duplication of GBM

DIAGNOSTIC CHECKLIST

Pathologic Interpretation Pearls

- More than 1 disease may be present
- Renal biopsies are rare in setting of nonrenal transplants, yet renal dysfunction common
  - Cause for most cases assumed to be CNIT but without direct evidence

SELECTED REFERENCES

1. Terzi A et al: Clinicopathologic study of kidney biopsies in patients before or after liver transplant. Exp Clin Transplant. 12 Suppl 1:129-35, 2014
2. White M et al: Sirolimus immunoprophylaxis and renal histological changes in long-term cardiac transplant recipients: A pilot study. Ann Pharmacother. 48(7):837-846, 2014
3. Kim JY et al: The variable pathology of kidney disease after liver transplantation. Transplantation. 89(2):215-21, 2010
4. Schwarz A et al: Biopsy-diagnosed renal disease in patients after transplantation of other organs and tissues. Am J Transplant. 10(9):2017-25, 2010
5. Araya CE et al: Native kidney post-transplant lymphoproliferative disorder in a non-renal transplant patient. Pediatr Transplant. 13(4):495-8, 2009
6. O'Riordan A et al: Renal biopsy in liver transplant recipients. Nephrol Dial Transplant. 24(7):2276-82, 2009
7. Lefaucheur C et al: Renal histopathological lesions after lung transplantation in patients with cystic fibrosis. Am J Transplant. 8(9):1901-10, 2008
8. Troxell ML et al: Renal pathology in hematopoietic cell transplantation recipients. Mod Pathol. 21(4):396-406, 2008
9. Chang A et al: Spectrum of renal pathology in hematopoietic cell transplantation: a series of 20 patients and review of the literature. Clin J Am Soc Nephrol. 2(5):1014-23, 2007
10. Pillebout E et al: Renal histopathological lesions after orthotopic liver transplantation (OLT). Am J Transplant. 5(5):1120-9, 2005

Chronic CNIT

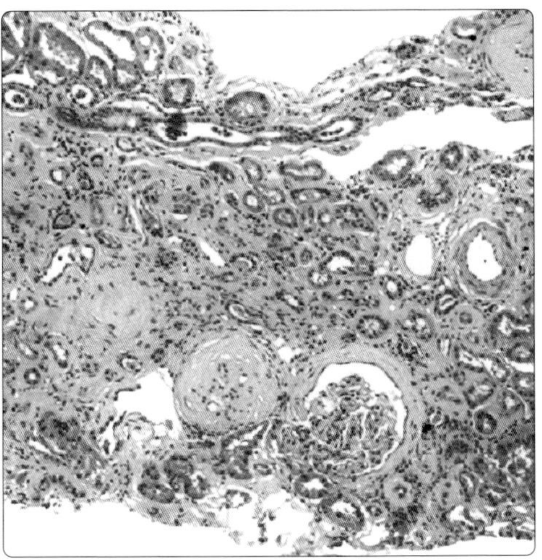

Collapsing FSGS Due to CNIT

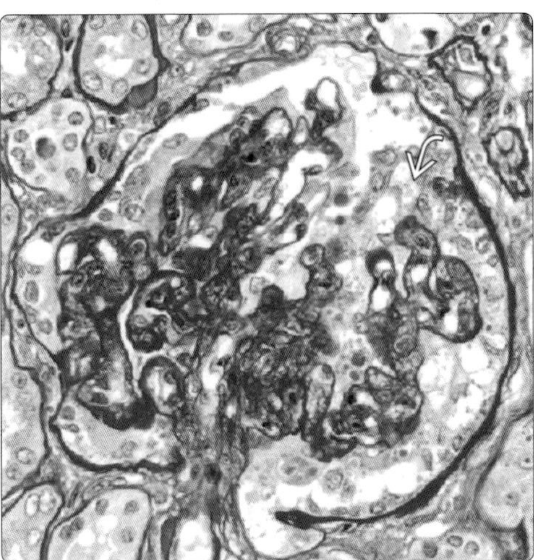

(Left) *This native kidney biopsy from a recipient of a liver transplant 4 years previously, maintained on cyclosporine, shows patchy interstitial fibrosis, tubular atrophy, and global glomerulosclerosis. A small artery is normal. These findings are typical, but not diagnostic, of chronic CNIT.* **(Right)** *This native kidney from a heart-lung transplant recipient shows collapsing FSGS with reactive epithelial cells bridging between the GBM and Bowman capsule* ➡. *Marked arteriolar hyalinosis was evident.*

Diabetic Glomerulopathy

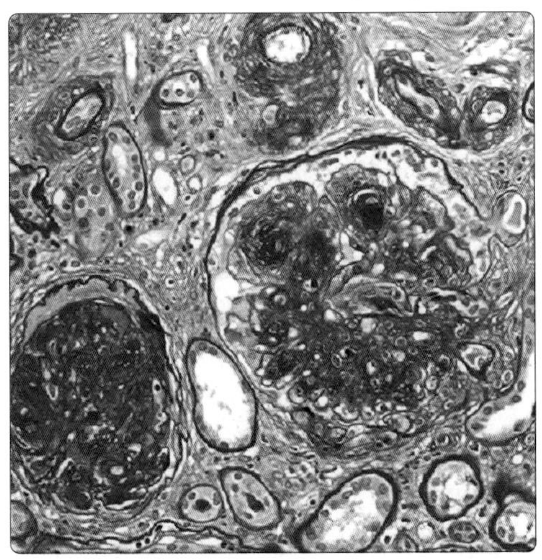

Immune Complex Glomerular Disease

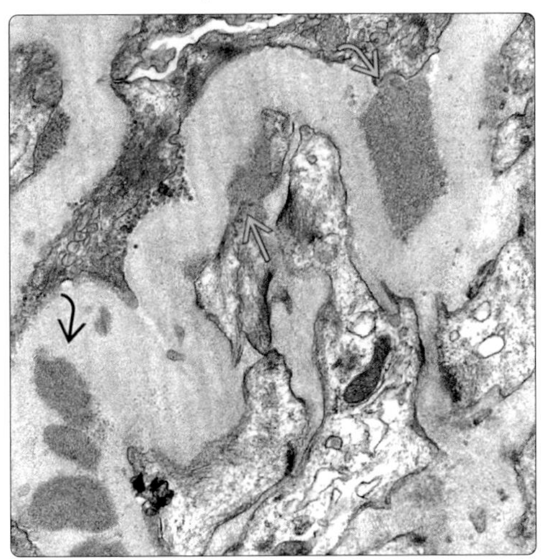

(Left) *This is a native kidney biopsy from a recipient of a liver transplant 10 years previously for HCV. The biopsy also had immune complexes presumably related to the HCV, which are reported to exacerbate diabetic glomerulopathy.* **(Right)** *A native kidney from a recipient of liver transplant shows subepithelial* ➡, *mesangial* ➡, *and intramembranous* ➡ *amorphous deposits, indicative of an immune complex glomerulopathy, probably related to HCV. Diabetic glomerulopathy was also present.*

Acute Thrombotic Microangiopathy (TMA) Due to CNIT

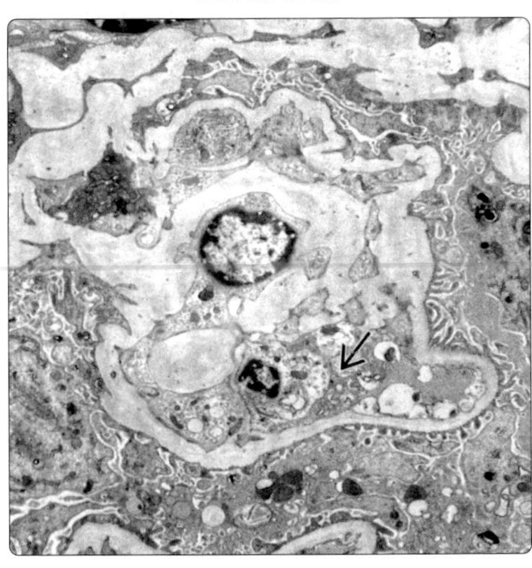

Subclinical TMA Due to CNIT

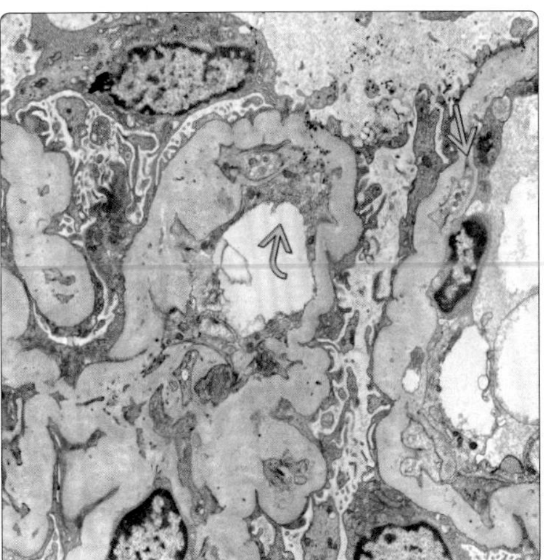

(Left) *This native kidney biopsy is from a heart transplant 6 days previously, maintained on tacrolimus. Cr rose to 4.2 mg/dL. Marked glomerular endothelial cell injury is present* ➡, *manifested by swelling and loss of fenestrations.* **(Right)** *TMA may present without the usual signs, such as schistocytes and thrombocytopenia. This biopsy is from a recipient of a heart transplant 13 years ago with a Cr of 6 mg/dL. Marked glomerular endothelial injury is present, with loss of fenestrations* ➡ *and duplication of the GBM* ➡.

Graft-vs.-Host Glomerulopathies

KEY FACTS

TERMINOLOGY

- Graft-vs.-host disease (GVHD) glomerulopathy
- Glomerular injury in setting of hematopoietic cell transplantation and GVHD
  - Rare after autologous HCT

ETIOLOGY/PATHOGENESIS

- Hematopoietic cell transplantation
  - Mostly allogeneic (80-100%)
- Radiation &/or chemotherapy may be contributing factors

CLINICAL ISSUES

- Proteinuria, nephrotic-range
  - Onset associated with decreased immunosuppression
- Drugs
  - Corticosteroids
  - Mycophenolate mofetil
  - Rituximab
- MCD: ~ 90% complete remission
- MGN: ~ 27% complete remission

MICROSCOPIC

- 3 major patterns
  - Membranous glomerulonephritis
    - PLA2R negative
      - Rare positive case
  - Minimal change lesions
  - Focal segmental glomerulosclerosis
- Concurrent interstitial nephritis, acute tubular injury, polyomavirus nephropathy, or thrombotic microangiopathy may be present

TOP DIFFERENTIAL DIAGNOSES

- MGN, primary
- Recurrent lymphoma
- Thrombotic microangiopathy

(Left) *Jones methenamine silver demonstrates thick glomerular basement membrane with sparse silver staining due to the prominent extent of subepithelial immune complex deposition.* **(Right)** *IgG demonstrates strong granular to confluent staining of the capillary walls in this hematopoietic cell transplant patient with MGN and GVHD.*

Membranous GN

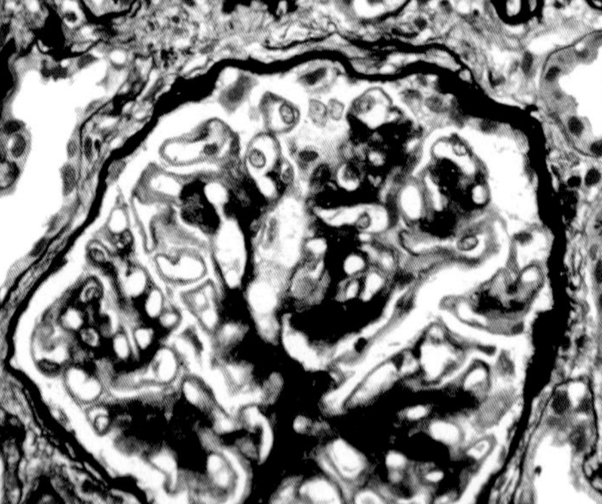

IgG

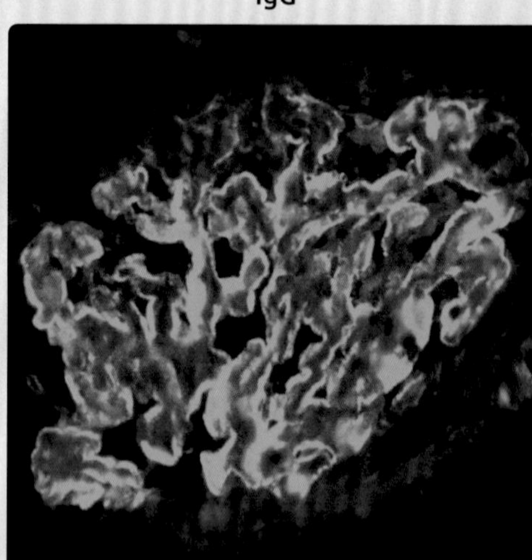

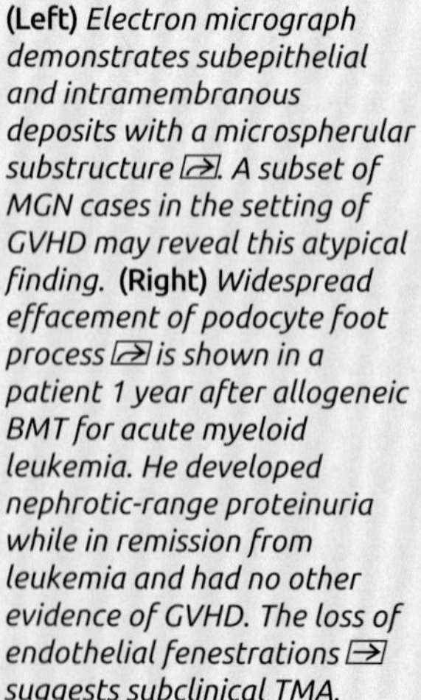

(Left) *Electron micrograph demonstrates subepithelial and intramembranous deposits with a microspherular substructure ➘. A subset of MGN cases in the setting of GVHD may reveal this atypical finding.* **(Right)** *Widespread effacement of podocyte foot process ➘ is shown in a patient 1 year after allogeneic BMT for acute myeloid leukemia. He developed nephrotic-range proteinuria while in remission from leukemia and had no other evidence of GVHD. The loss of endothelial fenestrations ➔ suggests subclinical TMA.*

Microspherular Electron-Dense Deposits

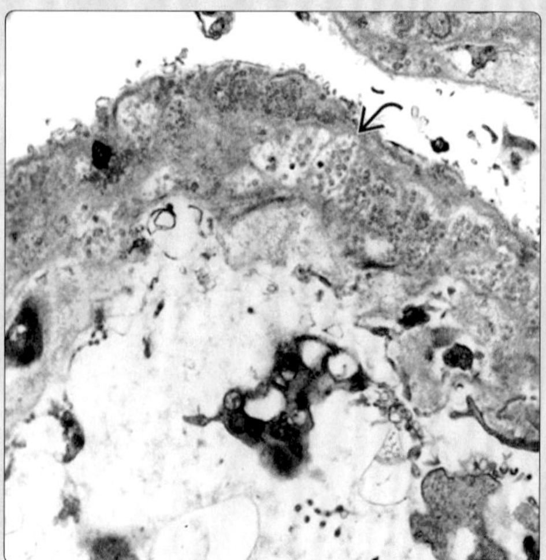

Minimal Change Disease

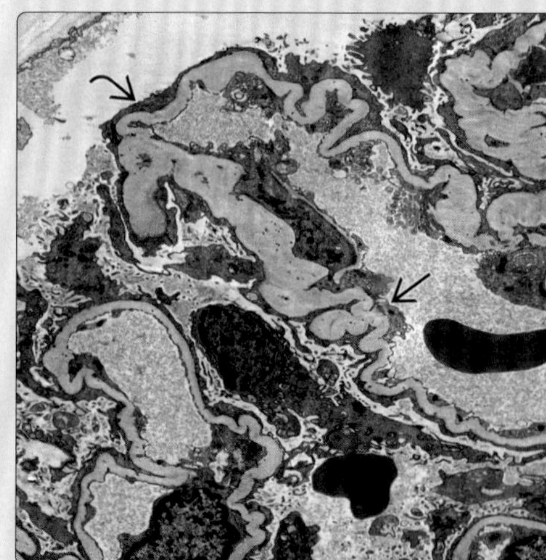

TERMINOLOGY

Abbreviations

- Graft-vs.-host disease (GVHD) glomerulopathy

Definitions

- Glomerular injury in setting of hematopoietic cell transplantation (HCT)

ETIOLOGY/PATHOGENESIS

Hematopoietic Cell Transplantation

- Mostly allogeneic (80-100%)
- 3 patterns
  - Membranous glomerulonephritis (MGN)
    - Rare report in autologous HCT
  - Minimal change disease (MCD)
  - Focal segmental glomerulosclerosis
- Radiation &/or chemotherapy may be contributing factors

Experimental Model

- Chronic GVHD (parent to F1 bone marrow transplant) in mice leads to MGN due to antibodies to minor MHC antigens

CLINICAL ISSUES

Presentation

- Proteinuria, nephrotic-range
  - Usual onset
    - MCD: ~ 8 months post transplant
    - MGN: ~ 14 months post transplant
  - Onset associated with decreased immunosuppression
- Associated with GVHD
  - Skin, mucous membranes, GI tract, lungs
  - Acute GVHD
    - MCD: ~ 40%
    - MGN: ~ 80%
  - Chronic GVHD
    - MCD: ~ 50%
    - MGN: ~ 90%

Treatment

- Drugs
  - Corticosteroids
  - Mycophenolate mofetil
  - Rituximab

Prognosis

- MCD: ~ 90% complete remission
- MGN: ~ 27% complete remission

MICROSCOPIC

Histologic Features

- 3 major patterns
  - Membranous GN (~ 60%)
    - Subepithelial "spike" formation by Jones silver stain
  - Minimal change lesion (~ 25%)
    - Podocyte hypertrophy
    - Tubular reabsorption droplets
  - Focal segmental glomerulosclerosis (~ 15%)
    - Segmental adhesions and sclerosis
    - Tip lesions described
    - Patchy tubular atrophy and fibrosis
- Other diseases may be present
  - Interstitial nephritis, acute tubular injury, polyomavirus nephropathy, thrombotic microangiopathy, recurrent amyloidosis, myeloma cast nephropathy

ANCILLARY TESTS

Immunofluorescence

- Membranous GN
  - Fine granular deposits diffusely along GBM for IgG and variably for other immunoglobulins and C3
  - Kappa and lambda stain equally
  - No staining of deposits for phospholipase A2 receptor 1
- Minimal change lesion
  - No deposits
- Focal segmental glomerulosclerosis
  - Segmental IgM, C3 in scarred glomeruli

Electron Microscopy

- Membranous GN
  - Subepithelial electron-dense deposits
    - Microspherule substructure may be present
    - Stage I or II (Ehrenreich-Churg)
  - Mesangial electron-dense deposits
    - Variably present
- Minimal change lesion
  - Diffuse podocyte foot process effacement
  - No deposits
- Focal segmental glomerulosclerosis
  - Same as MCD plus segmental adhesions
- Endothelial tubuloreticular inclusions (rare)

DIFFERENTIAL DIAGNOSIS

MGN, Primary

- Absence of mesangial immune complexes

Recurrent Lymphoma

- Manifested as MCD or MGN
- Lack of GVHD history

Thrombotic Microangiopathy

- Chronic phase shows double contours
- Fibrin and nonspecific trapping of IgM/C3

SELECTED REFERENCES

1. Byrne-Dugan CJ et al: Membranous nephropathy as a manifestation of graft-versus-host disease: association with HLA antigen typing, phospholipase A2 receptor, and C4d. Am J Kidney Dis. 64(6):987-93, 2014
2. Fraile P et al: Chronic graft-versus-host disease of the kidney in patients with allogenic hematopoietic stem cell transplant. Eur J Haematol. 91(2):129-34, 2013
3. Mii A et al: Renal thrombotic microangiopathy associated with chronic graft-versus-host disease after allogeneic hematopoietic stem cell transplantation. Pathol Int. 61(9):518-27, 2011
4. Chang A et al: Spectrum of renal pathology in hematopoietic cell transplantation: a series of 20 patients and review of the literature. Clin J Am Soc Nephrol. 2(5):1014-23, 2007
5. Brukamp K et al: Nephrotic syndrome after hematopoietic cell transplantation: do glomerular lesions represent renal graft-versus-host disease?. Clin J Am Soc Nephrol. 1(4):685-94, 2006

SECTION 10

Protocols

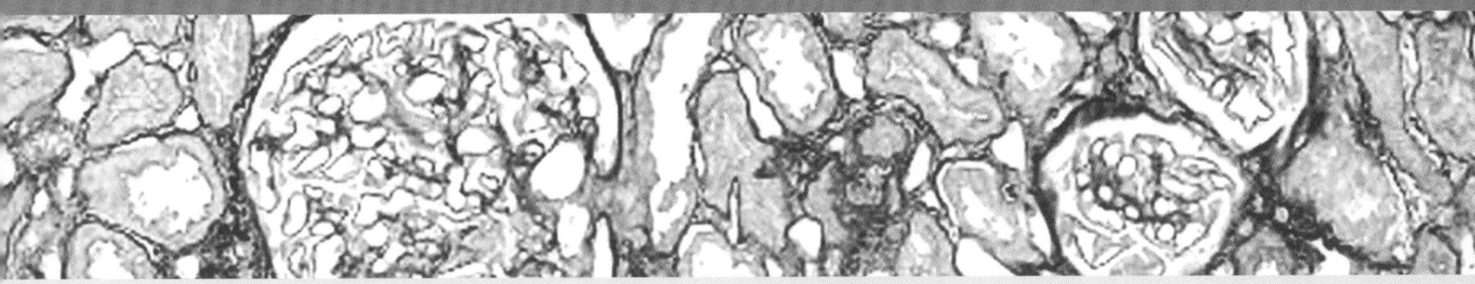

TERMINOLOGY

Definitions

- Renal biopsy report contains clinical, laboratory, and histopathologic data and its integration and interpretation
- Standardization of biopsy report provides
  - Systematic approach
  - Etiologic and pathophysiologic diagnosis
  - Clinicopathologic correlations
  - Good and poor prognostic features
  - Facilitate communication with clinician
  - Improved diagnostic accuracy
  - Guide for appropriate therapy
  - Uniformity of reports for multi-center studies

COMPONENTS OF BIOPSY REPORT

Demographic Data

- Patient information
  - Name, age, gender, date of birth
- Specimen identifiers
  - Institution, pathology number, specimen type
- Ordering physician information
  - Name, address, phone number, fax number

Clinical Data

- Obtain data from clinician or medical record
- Clinical history
  - Hypertension, diabetes, heart disease
  - Family
  - Social/occupational
  - Medications
- Physical examination
  - Body habitus
  - Edema
  - Skin rash
- Vital signs
  - Blood pressure
  - Body temperature
- Imaging studies
- Laboratory data
  - Hematuria, proteinuria, urine sediment exam
  - Serum chemistry: Creatinine, BUN, glucose
  - Serologic testing: Infections, autoimmune diseases and monoclonal proteins
  - Complete blood counts
- Specific data for allograft biopsies
  - Transplant date
  - Type of donor
  - Donor specific antibodies
  - Renal function
  - Proteinuria
  - Native kidney disease
  - Current treatment protocol
  - Relevant serologic testing
  - History of prior transplants for allograft biopsies
  - Calcineurin inhibitor level
  - Indication for biopsy: Baseline, for cause, protocol, follow-up after therapy

Gross Description

- Type of solution for each received sample
- Number of cores, length, and appearance
- Document proper labeling
- Document triaging, if applicable
  - Light microscopy
  - Immunofluorescence microscopy
  - Electron microscopy, when necessary

Microscopic Description

- Document tissue and cellular findings
  - Record both qualitative and quantitative data
    - Whenever possible, give specific numbers or % rather than vague terms like "mild" or "severe"
    - Can be free text or synoptic form
- Light microscopy (LM)
  - Histochemical stains
    - H&E, periodic acid-Schiff, Masson trichrome, Jones methenamine silver, Congo red
    - State when additional levels obtained to exclude focal lesions, such as focal segmental glomerulosclerosis (FSGS)
    - Any additional stains for infectious agents
  - Record presence of cortex, medulla, capsule, calyceal mucosa
    - Number of cores or length of tissue on glass slide should match gross description
  - Record number of total glomeruli
    - Number (%) globally sclerosed
    - Number (%) segmentally sclerosed
  - Number (%) and type of glomerular crescents, necrosis
  - Other glomerular findings
    - Type of proliferative lesions, segmental, global
  - Tubulointerstitial findings
    - Interstitial edema, inflammation and fibrosis
    - Tubular epithelial injury, atrophy
    - Tubular content: Cells, all types of casts, e.g., protein, hemoglobin, myoglobin, bile, monoclonal protein
  - Arteries/arterioles: Medial hypertrophy, intimal fibrosis, hyalinosis
    - Extent of vascular narrowing
    - Thrombi
    - Vasculitis, fibrinoid necrosis
  - Note extrarenal tissue when present
    - Treat as urgent value and notify treating physician
    - Liver
    - Spleen
    - Small/large intestine
    - Pancreas

Immunofluorescence (IF) Microscopy

- Type of tissue
  - Brief histologic description
- Number of glomeruli
  - Number globally or segmentally sclerosed
- Specify semiquantitative scale used (0-3+ or 0-4+)
- Antibody and tissue/glomerular location
  - Staining pattern: Linear, granular, smudgy, lumpy, scattered
  - Distribution: Focal diffuse, segmental, global

- State positive internal controls, when present
  - Tubular casts (IgA)
  - Tubular reabsorption droplets (IgG, kappa, lambda, albumin)
  - Arterioles (C3)
  - Mesangial regions (C4d)
- IF results on paraffin sections
  - If performed as salvage technique or unmask antigens

Immunohistochemistry on Paraffin Sections

- C4d in transplant biopsies
- Immunophenotype inflammatory cells
- Type specific amyloid proteins
- Test for hemoglobin, myoglobin
- Test for specific viral antigens
  - CMV, BKV, adenovirus, EBV
- Test for podocyte antigens
  - WT-1, podocin, synaptopodin

Electron Microscopy (EM)

- Type of tissue
  - Brief histologic description
  - State when tissue processed from paraffin block
- Number of glomeruli, segmental and globally sclerosed in Toluidine blue 1 μm thick sections
  - State whether some or all of submitted tissue examined
    - Reminds pathologist to examine all submitted tissue for focal lesions (e.g., FSGS)
  - Other glomerular findings documented in 1 μm section
- State number of glomeruli examined by EM
- Status of glomerular basement membranes
  - Organization and thickness
    - Duplication, cellular interposition if present
- Absence or extent of foot process effacement
  - Expressed as % of capillary surface
- Any endothelial and mesangial cell abnormalities
- Visceral epithelial cell abnormalities
  - Swelling, vacuolization, protein droplets, other inclusions
- Absence or presence and frequency of electron-dense deposits
- Location of electron-dense deposits
  - Substructure of deposits, if present
    - Granular
    - Extremely dense
    - Fibrils with measurement
    - Crystalline material
- Indicate tubulointerstitium evaluated
  - Tubular basement membranes
    - Thickening, layering, deposits
  - Tubular epithelial cells
    - Evidence of injury, inclusions
  - Indicate peritubular capillary basement membrane evaluation (for transplant biopsies)
    - Specify if multilayering present, severity and extent (focal or diffuse)

Final Diagnosis

- Concise and disease-specific diagnosis recommended
  - Diagnosis based on clinical data, LM, IF, and EM and discussions with nephrologist
- Etio-pathogenesis based diagnosis of glomerulonephritis rather than based entirely on glomerular pattern, where possible
  - e.g., PLA2R(+) membranous GN, IgA nephropathy, HIV-associated nephropathy, HCV-associated glomerulonephritis, ANCA-associated crescentic GN, etc.
- Concomitant co-primary or secondary disease, if present
  - Glomerular, tubulointerstitial or vascular lesions
- State specific classification or scoring systems used for specific diseases
- Morphologic descriptions suggested in the absence of specific diseases
- State activity and chronicity of the disease entity

Comment/Clinicopathological Correlations

- Discuss limitations of evaluation
  - Absence of renal parenchyma or paucity of glomeruli
  - Absence of glomeruli for IF/EM
  - Performing IF/EM on paraffin tissue
- Comparison with previous biopsies
  - Degree of recovery of specific histological parameters
  - Degree and extent of progression
  - Any new findings
- Correlate pathology with major clinical findings
- Discuss possible etiology or differential diagnosis, if pertinent
- Recommend relevant tests to confirm diagnosis
- Cite relevant references, such as the following classifications
  - 2003: ISN/RPS lupus nephritis
  - 2004: Columbia FSGS
  - 2009: Oxford IgA nephropathy
  - 2013: Banff allograft
  - 2011: Leiden diabetic nephropathy

SELECTED REFERENCES

1. Haas M et al: Banff 2013 meeting report: inclusion of C4d-negative antibody-mediated rejection and antibody-associated arterial lesions. Am J Transplant. 14(2):272-83, 2014
2. Sethi S: Etiology-based diagnostic approach to proliferative glomerulonephritis. Am J Kidney Dis. 63(4):561-6, 2014
3. Chang A et al: A position paper on standardizing the nonneoplastic kidney biopsy report. Clin J Am Soc Nephrol. 7(8):1365-8, 2012
4. Berden AE et al: Histopathologic classification of ANCA-associated glomerulonephritis. J Am Soc Nephrol. 21(10):1628-36, 2010
5. Tervaert TW et al: Pathologic classification of diabetic nephropathy. J Am Soc Nephrol. 21(4):556-63, 2010
6. Working Group of the International IgA Nephropathy Network and the Renal Pathology Society et al: The Oxford classification of IgA nephropathy: rationale, clinicopathological correlations, and classification. Kidney Int. 76(5):534-45, 2009
7. D'Agati VD et al: Pathologic classification of focal segmental glomerulosclerosis: a working proposal. Am J Kidney Dis. 43(2):368-82, 2004
8. Walker PD et al: Practice guidelines for the renal biopsy. Mod Pathol. 17(12):1555-63, 2004
9. Weening JJ et al: The classification of glomerulonephritis in systemic lupus erythematosus revisited. J Am Soc Nephrol. 2004 Feb;15(2):241-50. Erratum in: J Am Soc Nephrol. 15(3):835-6, 2004

Examination of the End-Stage Kidney

TERMINOLOGY

Synonyms

- End-stage renal disease (ESRD)
- End-stage kidney disease (ESKD)

Definitions

- ESRD defined as renal failure lasting ≥ 3 months, with a glomerular filtration rate (GFR) of ≤ 15 mL/min/1.73m², requiring renal replacement therapy
- Pathologic correlates include diffuse glomerular sclerosis, interstitial fibrosis, tubular atrophy, and vascular sclerosis ± cyst formation

EPIDEMIOLOGY

Prevalence

- Approximately 0.2% of United States population has ESKD

Age Range

- Median age: 64.2 years
- May occur in either children or adults

Ethnicity Relationship

- Cumulative lifetime risk of ESKD
  - 7.3% for black men; 2.5% for white men
  - 7.8% for black women; 1.5% for white women

ETIOLOGY/PATHOGENESIS

Causes of ESKD in Adults (In Decreasing Order of Frequency)

- Diabetic nephropathy
- Hypertensive nephrosclerosis
- Glomerular diseases
  - Focal segmental glomerulosclerosis (FSGS)
  - Glomerulonephritis (GN)
    - IgA nephropathy
    - Membranoproliferative GN
    - Crescentic GN
      - Pauci-immune (antineutrophil cytoplasmic autoantigen [ANCA]-associated) GN
      - Antiglomerular basement membrane GN
  - Membranous nephropathy
- Hereditary renal diseases
  - Autosomal dominant polycystic kidney disease (ADPKD)
  - Alport nephropathy and others
- Tubulointerstitial diseases
  - Chronic pyelonephritis ± reflux
  - Obstructive nephropathy
  - Acute tubular necrosis/injury
  - Chronic interstitial nephritis
- Secondary glomerulonephritis, vasculitis, and thrombotic microangiopathies
  - Lupus nephritis
  - Systemic ANCA vasculitides including microscopic polyangiitis and granulomatosis with polyangiitis
  - Hemolytic uremic syndrome/thrombotic thrombocytopenic purpura
- Neoplasia
  - Light chain (myeloma) cast nephropathy
  - Primary renal cell carcinoma or urothelial carcinoma
- Other disorders

Causes of ESKD in Children Aged < 20 Years (In Decreasing Order of Frequency)

- Glomerular diseases
  - GN
    - Membranoproliferative GN
    - Crescentic GN, mainly ANCA associated
    - IgA nephropathy
  - FSGS
- Congenital or hereditary diseases
  - Renal hypoplasia or dysplasia
  - Congenital obstructive uropathy
  - Cystic diseases
    - Autosomal recessive polycystic kidney disease (infantile)
    - Medullary cystic disease
    - Nephronophthisis
  - Other hereditary disorders including podocytopathies and cystinosis

Diffuse Granular Cortical Surface

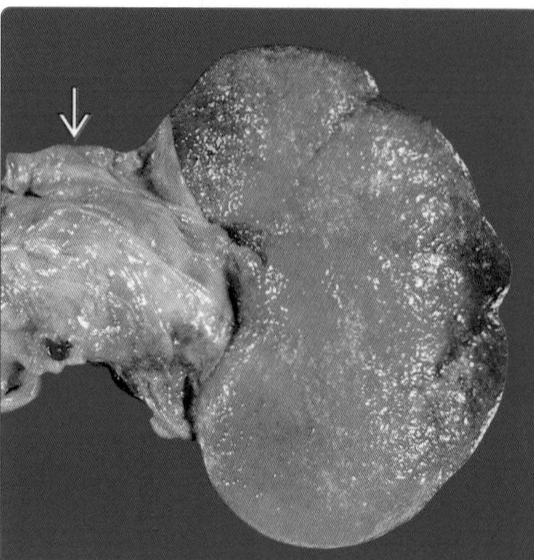

Ischemic Glomerular Obsolescence

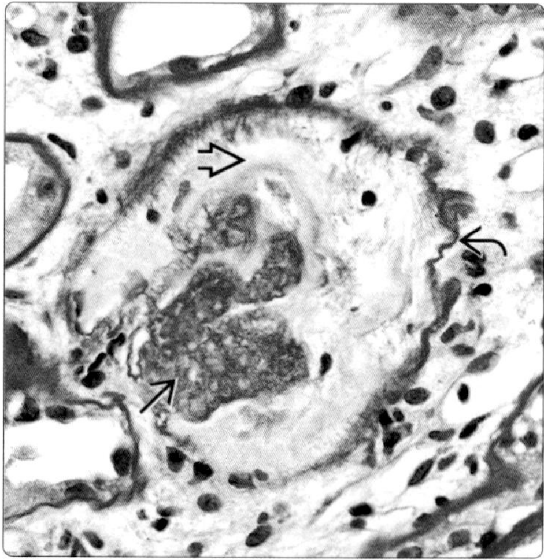

(Left) *The outer surface of an end-stage kidney due to chronic GN or hypertensive nephrosclerosis has a diffusely fine granular appearance after removal of the capsule ➡. The depressed areas are due to fibrosis and tubular atrophy.* **(Right)** *Ischemic glomerular obsolescence has a shriveled hypocellular capillary tuft ➡ and collagen deposition in Bowman space ➡. Bowman capsule is wrinkled ➡ and sometimes frayed.*

- Tubulointerstitial diseases
  - Chronic pyelonephritis ± reflux
  - Obstructive nephropathy
- Secondary GN or vasculitis
  - Lupus nephritis
  - Henoch-Schönlein GN
  - Hemolytic uremic syndrome
- Hypertensive nephrosclerosis
- Diabetic nephropathy
- Neoplasms
  - Primary renal sarcomas, Wilms tumor, and others
- Both adult and pediatric groups have many other miscellaneous causes
  - e.g., sickle cell nephropathy and HIV-associated nephropathy

Pathogenesis of ESKD

- Initial disease causes progressive damage of nephrons and chronic kidney dysfunction
- When GFR decreases to ~ 30% of normal, subsequent renal function declines along a final common pathway
  - Independent of original injury
  - Loss of functioning nephrons results in hyperperfusion of remnant glomeruli
    - Increased individual glomerular filtration (hyperfiltration)
  - Hyperfiltration accelerates podocyte senescence and loss
    - Leads to segmental glomerular sclerosis and proteinuria
    - Progressive glomerular sclerosis, tubular atrophy, and interstitial fibrosis
- Long-term nonselective proteinuria has toxic effects on tubules
  - Plasma proteins injure the epithelium, leading to local inflammation, tubular atrophy, and interstitial fibrosis
- Hypertension, hyperfiltration, and proteinuria-induced tubular injury lead to recruitment of pericytes
- Pericytes are thought to transform to myofibroblasts
  - Myofibroblasts are the source of collagen in interstitial fibrosis

MACROSCOPIC

Kidney Size

- Very small (< 50 g) kidneys
  - Congenital hypoplasia, renal artery stenosis, and advanced hypertensive nephrosclerosis
  - Few pyramids (≤ 5) in congenital hypoplasia
  - Renal artery stenosis has normal numbers of pyramids
- Small (< 125 g) kidneys
  - Surface findings after stripping the capsule may be helpful
    - Discrete and wedge-shaped cortical depressions
      - Prior infarction
      - Thromboembolism or medium-sized vessel vasculitis (e.g., polyarteritis nodosa)
    - Irregular broad depressions at poles typical of chronic pyelonephritis
    - Diffuse and finely granular subcapsular surface
      - Chronic glomerular or tubulointerstitial diseases or hypertensive nephrosclerosis
  - Unilateral small kidney typical of renal artery stenosis
- Small or large kidneys with dilated pelvicalyceal system characteristic of hydronephrosis
  - Common causes of obstruction
    - Ureteral stenosis: Pelviureteric junction or bladder wall
    - Urolithiasis
    - Prostatic enlargement: Hyperplasia or carcinoma
    - Retroperitoneal tumors or fibrosis
    - Urothelial carcinoma
- Large kidneys may or may not have parenchymal cyst formation
  - Large kidneys without cysts suggest diabetic nephropathy or amyloidosis
  - Very large kidneys (500-2,000 g)
    - Multiple cysts (0.5-3 cm) replacing parenchyma are characteristic of ADPKD
- Large or small kidneys with irregularly distributed, predominantly cortical cysts are seen in acquired cystic disease

Pathologic Features of Renal Medulla

- Medullary papillae
  - Effaced in hydronephrosis
  - Necrotic, ragged or calcified in papillary necrosis
    - Due to diabetic nephropathy ± acute obstructive pyelonephritis
      - Also fungal infections, sickle cell nephropathy, nonsteroidal anti-inflammatory agents

Secondary Changes in ESKD

- Secondary changes of acquired cystic disease and hypertensive renal disease are common to ESKD from any cause
  - Increased frequency of renal cell carcinoma (RCC)
- Calcium oxalate or phosphate deposition may be nonspecific feature of ESKD
  - Exclude hyperoxaluria and hyperparathyroidism
- Gross findings must be correlated with clinical history

MICROSCOPIC

General Features

- Glomerular sclerosis may have glomerulopathic or ischemic patterns
- Tubular atrophy has 4 main morphologic types
  - Classic: Luminal shrinkage with thickening and lamination of tubular basement membrane
  - Thyroidization: Microcystic changes with attenuation of epithelium and inspissation of luminal casts
  - Endocrine: Small solid tubules with thin basement membranes
  - Super tubules: Enlarged tubules with increased angularity of tubular profiles and epithelial apical snouts

Diabetic Nephropathy

- Nodular mesangial sclerosis (Kimmelstiel-Wilson nodules)
  - Thickened capillary basement membranes on PAS or silver stains
- Hyaline deposits in glomerular tufts ("fibrin caps")

- Along Bowman capsule ("capsular drops")
- Hyalinosis of afferent and efferent arterioles

Hypertensive Nephrosclerosis

- Arterial and arteriolar sclerosis are relatively nonspecific
  - Can be primary or secondary
- Ischemic glomerular obsolescence, interstitial fibrosis, and tubular atrophy
  - Most prominent in outer cortex
- Prominent juxtaglomerular apparatuses in hyperreninemic states

Glomerular Diseases

- Global glomerular sclerosis
  - End-stage FSGS: Primary or secondary
  - End-stage GN
- Nonsclerosed glomeruli may have diagnostic features of the original glomerular disease
- Immune complex GN may be detectable by immunofluorescence (IF) and electron microscopy
  - Useful for lupus nephritis, IgA nephropathy, or other forms of GN
  - Nonspecific coarse granular IgM and C3 ± C1q
    - In globally sclerotic glomeruli (so-called scar pattern)
- Fibrous crescents with synechiae and destruction of Bowman capsules
  - May indicate crescentic GN

Tubulointerstitial Diseases

- Extensive interstitial fibrosis and tubular atrophy
  - Relative sparing of glomeruli
- Medullary effacement and transparenchymal scars with thinning/atrophy of cortex in obstructive nephropathy
- Thyroidization of cortical tubules, lymphoid aggregates, and lymphocytic pyelitis in chronic pyelonephritis
- Multiple thin-walled cysts lined by flat or cuboidal epithelium in ADPKD

Vascular Diseases

- Vessels of all calibers may be affected in thromboembolism
  - Fibrin-platelet thrombi or cholesterol atheroemboli
- Wedge-shaped remote cortical infarcts
  - Condensed globally sclerotic glomeruli with interstitial fibrosis and tubular loss

Secondary Changes of ESKD

- Hypertensive vascular disease
  - Advanced renal scarring is complicated by secondary hypertension
  - Arterial and arteriolar sclerosis may be severe and progressive
  - Progressive vascular narrowing enhances renal ischemia
- Secondary FSGS
  - Characterized by enlarged glomeruli with perihilar segmental sclerosis
  - Tubules are hypertrophic (super tubules)
- Calcium salt deposits
  - Calcium phosphate or oxalate in tubules and interstitium
- Acquired cystic kidney disease
  - Occurs in patients on hemodialysis or peritoneal dialysis or in nondialyzed patients with chronic uremia
  - Frequency is ~ 20% at 3 years increasing to ~ 90% at 10 years of dialysis
  - 3-5 cysts per kidney or replacement of 10% of parenchyma are acceptable minimal criteria
  - Cysts may be cortical, medullary, or both
    - Lined by flattened to low cuboidal epithelium
  - Areas of epithelial crowding or proliferation, taller epithelium, and nuclear atypia may be associated with development of RCC
  - Intervening parenchyma typically has ESKD changes
- Renal cell carcinoma
  - Risk of RCC in ESKD markedly increases with duration of dialysis and persists after transplantation
  - RCC is seen in ~ 17% of end-stage kidneys and multifocal in ~ 10%
    - 41% clear cell, chromophobe, or papillary RCC in largest series
    - 36% acquired cystic disease-associated RCC
      - Acini or solid tubules with high-grade nuclear features; abundant calcium oxalate crystals
    - 23% clear cell papillary RCC
  - 85% CD57(+); suggests thin ascending limb of Henle origin
  - Rarely present with metastasis (< 5%)

SELECTED REFERENCES

1. Bhatnagar R et al: Renal-cell carcinomas in end-stage kidneys: a clinicopathological study with emphasis on clear-cell papillary renal-cell carcinoma and acquired cystic kidney disease-associated carcinoma. Int J Surg Pathol. 20(1):19-28, 2012
2. Enoki Y et al: Clinicopathological features and CD57 expression in renal cell carcinoma in acquired cystic disease of the kidneys: with special emphasis on a relation to the duration of haemodialysis, the degree of calcium oxalate deposition, histological type, and possible tumorigenesis. Histopathology. 56(3):384-94, 2010
3. Tickoo SK et al: Spectrum of epithelial neoplasms in end-stage renal disease: an experience from 66 tumor-bearing kidneys with emphasis on histologic patterns distinct from those in sporadic adult renal neoplasia. Am J Surg Pathol. 30(2):141-53, 2006
4. Dunnill MS et al: Acquired cystic disease of the kidneys: a hazard of long-term intermittent maintenance haemodialysis. J Clin Pathol. 30(9):868-77, 1977
5. Schwartz MM et al: Primary renal disease in transplant recipients. Hum Pathol. 7(4):455-9, 1976
6. Heptinstall RH: Pathology of end-stage kidney disease. Am J Med. 44(5):656-63, 1968

Diabetic Global Glomerular Sclerosis

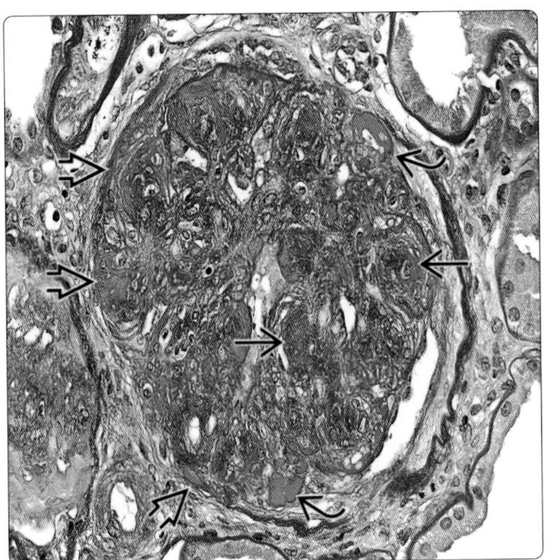

End-Stage Membranoproliferative Glomerulonephritis

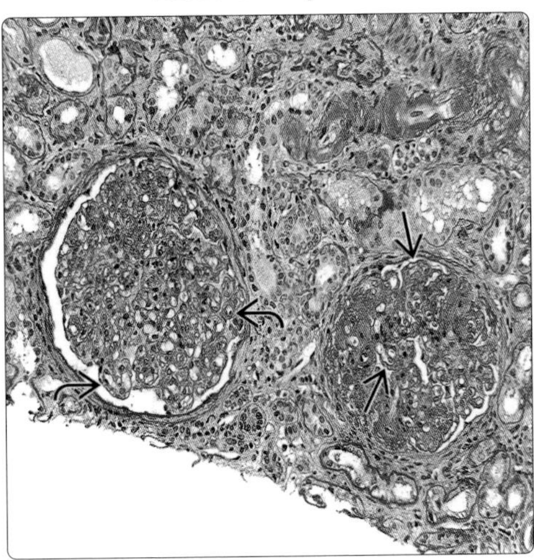

(Left) *End-stage diabetic glomerulosclerosis has solidified glomeruli and broad adhesions to Bowman capsule ⇨. Kimmelstiel-Wilson nodules → and fibrin caps ↷ are also apparent.* **(Right)** *Chronic membranoproliferative GN shows segmental sclerosis and some capillary double contours →. The glomerulus on the left has active GN with endocapillary hypercellularity and double contours ↷.*

End-Stage Crescentic GN

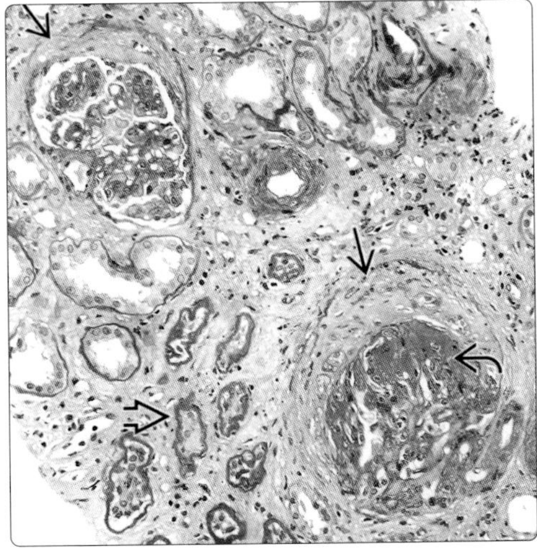

Thyroidization, Calcification, Glomerulosclerosis, Arteriosclerosis

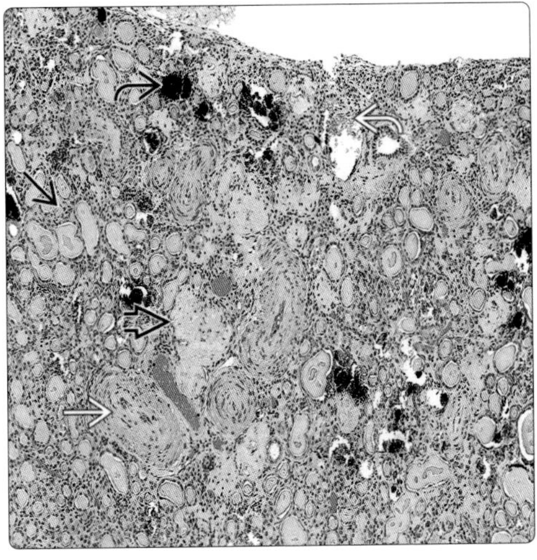

(Left) *Fibrous crescents → and fragmentation of Bowman capsule are evident in this example of pauci-immune crescentic GN. One glomerulus has extensive sclerosis ↷. Classical tubular atrophy and interstitial fibrosis is also evident ⇨.* **(Right)** *Thyroidization → with tubular casts, calcium phosphate ↷ and oxalate ↷ deposition, global glomerular ⇨ sclerosis, and severe arteriosclerosis ➡ are evident in this example of ESKD, which is difficult to classify further.*

Tubular Atrophy

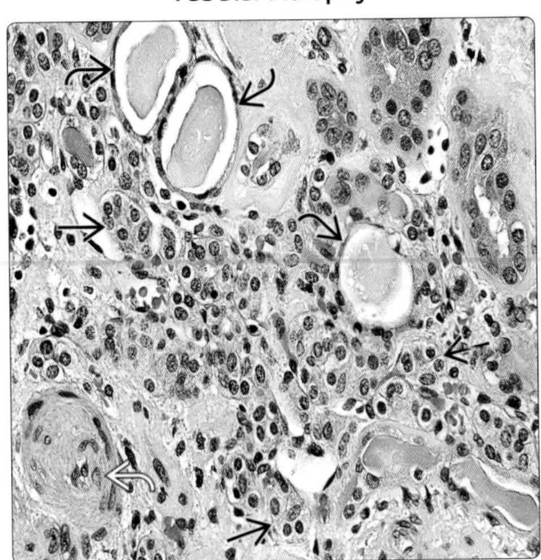

"Super" Tubules

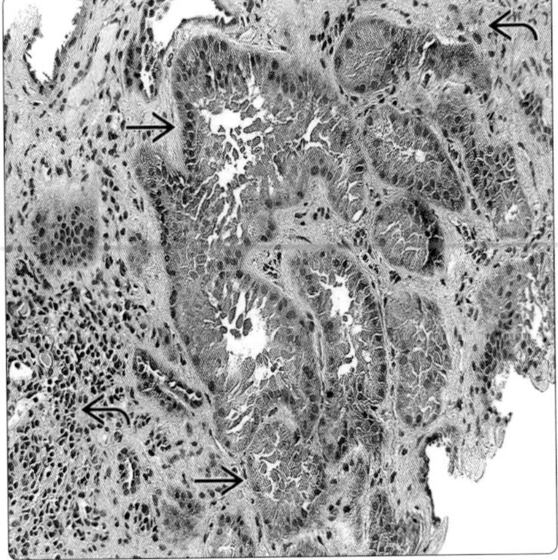

(Left) *Endocrine-type tubular atrophy → has small solid tubules with uniform rounded nuclei and thin basement membranes. "Thyroidization" ↷ is evident beside these atrophic tubules, and there is severe arteriolosclerosis ↷.* **(Right)** *Super tubules have complex profiles, hypercellularity, voluminous cytoplasm, and apical snouts →. These are the features of compensatory hypertrophy. There is extensive interstitial fibrosis and focal mononuclear inflammatory infiltrates ↷.*

(Left) *Severe arteriosclerosis is characterized by marked intimal thickening, myofibroblastic proliferation →, focal fragmentation of the internal elastic lamina →, and medial thickening.* **(Right)** *Severe hyaline arteriolosclerosis with intimal hyaline and luminal occlusion → is evident in this example of ESKD. Hypertension or diabetes may be responsible for these changes.*

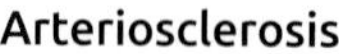

Arteriosclerosis

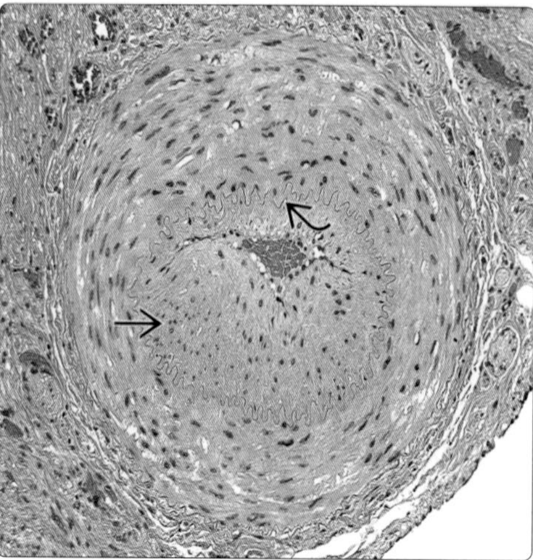

Arteriolar Hyalinosis

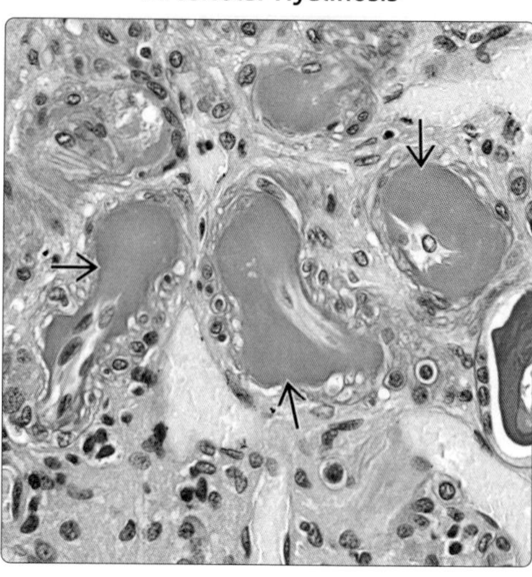

(Left) *A nonfunctioning kidney removed from a 44-year-old woman shows lower ureteral stenosis, obstruction, and marked hydronephrosis. There is marked dilation of the collecting system and parenchymal atrophy.* **(Right)** *A kidney with obstructive hydronephrosis shows diffuse interstitial fibrosis and tubular atrophy affecting pars convoluta → and medullary rays →. Dense outer cortical mononuclear inflammation is also present. Glomeruli are generally spared.*

End-Stage Hydronephrosis

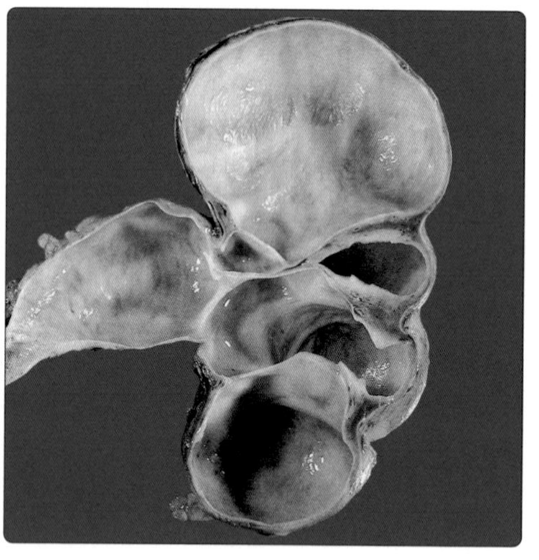

Renal Cortical Fibrosis in Hydronephrosis

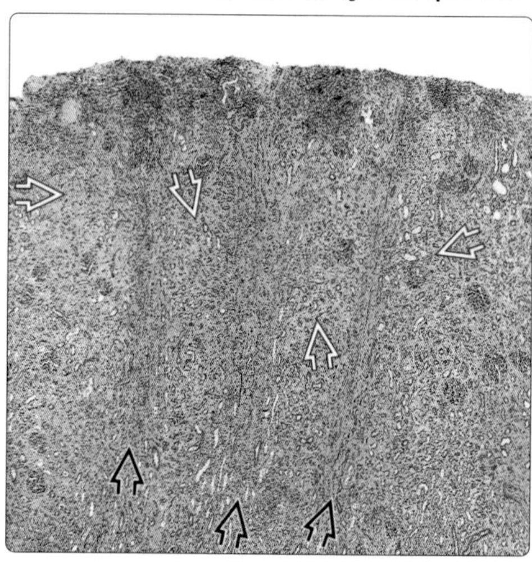

(Left) *Autosomal dominant polycystic kidney disease typically has diffuse enlargement (2,310 g in this example), and both the cortex and medulla are entirely replaced by thin-walled unilocular cysts.* **(Right)** *Characteristic thin-walled cysts are lined by flat → or cuboidal → epithelium in ADPKD. Small papillary proliferations → may also be evident. The intervening renal parenchyma → has shrunken or atubular glomeruli, with interstitial fibrosis, tubular atrophy, and mononuclear infiltrates →.*

Autosomal Dominant Polycystic Kidney Disease

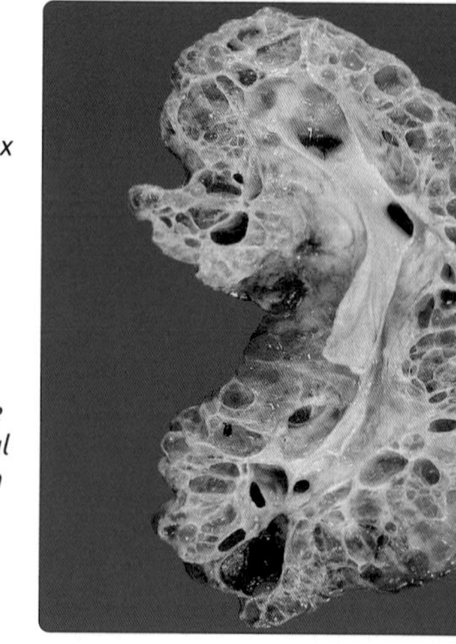

Polycystic Kidney Disease

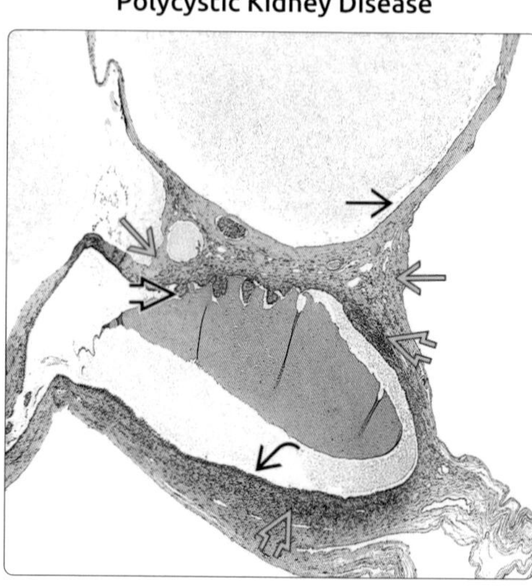

Secondary (Adaptive) FSGS

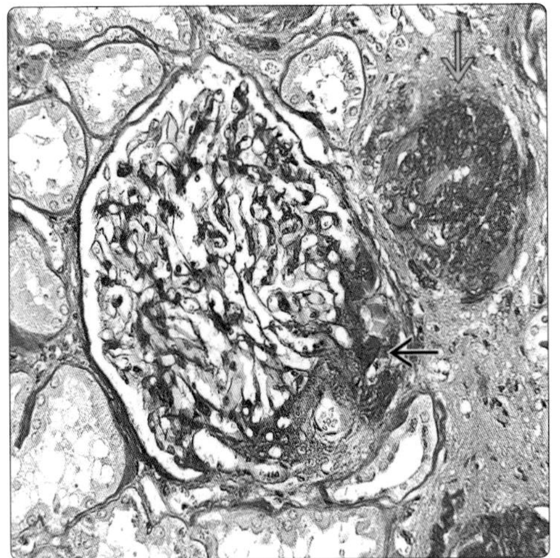

Acquired Cystic Kidney Disease

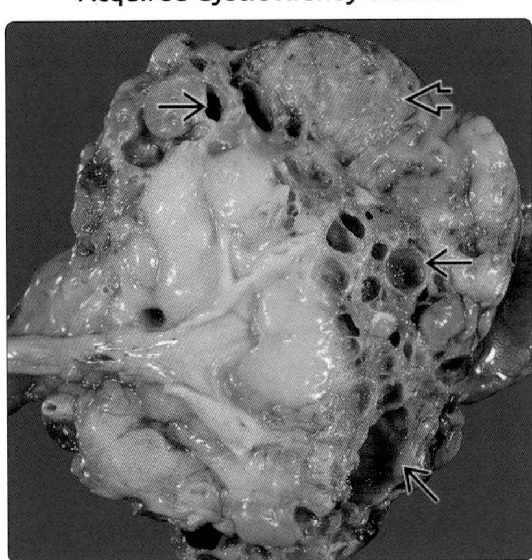

(Left) *Secondary focal segmental glomerular sclerosis may be evident when there is advanced nephron loss from any primary renal disease. Typically the glomeruli are enlarged and have perihilar hyalinization ➡. Adjacent is a globally sclerotic glomerulus ➡.* **(Right)** *A bisected kidney with acquired cystic disease has multiple cysts of varying size ➡ and a circumscribed mass in the upper pole ➡. Adipose tissue is prominent in the renal sinus, a common finding in ESKD.*

Acquired Cystic Kidney Disease

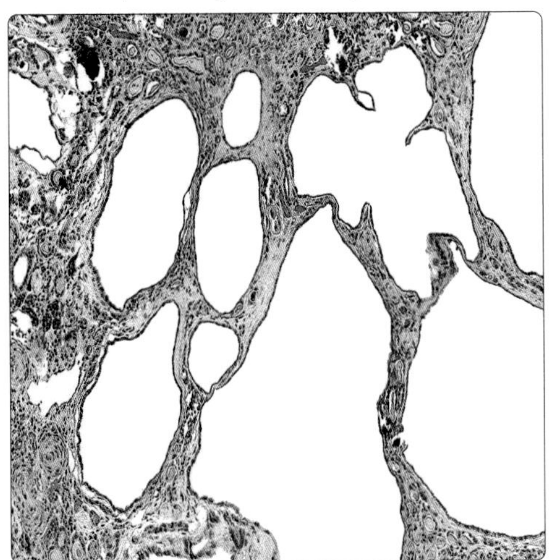

Acquired Cystic Disease in Medulla

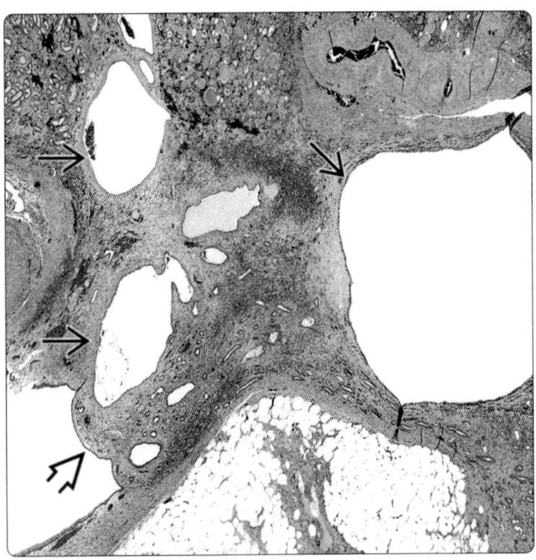

(Left) *Multiple irregularly shaped cysts of variable size and with flattened epithelial lining are present in the cortex of this example of acquired cystic kidney disease. The surrounding tissue has tubular atrophy, interstitial fibrosis, and calcium deposits.* **(Right)** *Multiple medullary cysts of variable size with a flat epithelial lining ➡ are also a feature of acquired cystic kidney disease. The medullary papilla is effaced ➡.*

Acquired Cystic Disease-Associated RCC

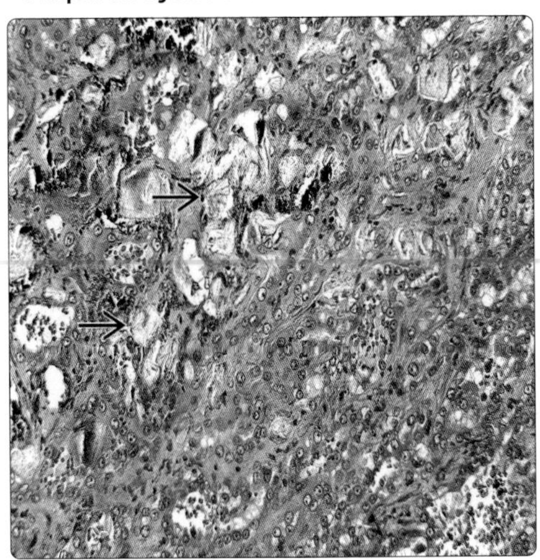

Clear Cell Papillary RCC in ESKD

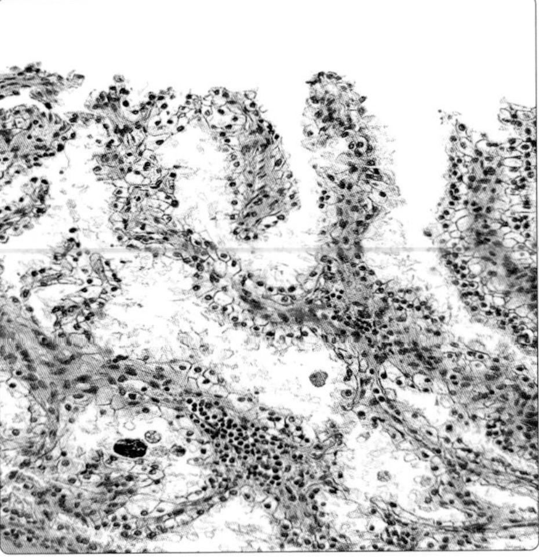

(Left) *Acquired cystic kidney disease-associated renal cell carcinoma is composed of acini with high-grade nuclei and abundant calcium oxalate crystal deposition ➡ within the tumor. Basophilic calcium phosphate is also evident.* **(Right)** *Clear cell papillary renal cell carcinoma is also observed with high frequency in ESKD. The tumors tend to be multicystic. Papillary fronds lined by clear cells with low-grade nuclei are characteristic.*

TERMINOLOGY

Definitions

- Nephron-sparing surgery (partial nephrectomy, radiofrequency or cryoablation) for small (≤ 4 cm) or surgically accessible renal cell carcinoma (RCCs) to maximize preservation of renal function
  - Oncologic control comparable to radical nephrectomy
  - Preserves renal function better than radical nephrectomy
- Chronic kidney disease (CKD): Presence of kidney damage
  - Abnormal imaging, elevated creatinine, albuminuria, or glomerular filtration rate (GFR) < 60 mL/min/1.73^2 for 3 months

EPIDEMIOLOGY

Age Range

- Wilms tumor (nephroblastoma)
  - Represents 85% of renal malignancy of childhood
- Renal cell carcinomas
  - Account for 85% of renal malignancies (12% are urothelial cancers)
  - Includes many phenotypically and genotypically distinct cancers

ETIOLOGY/PATHOGENESIS

Syndromes With *WT1* Mutations and Risk of Wilms Tumor

- WAGR syndrome: Wilms tumor, aniridia, genitourinary tract malformations, and mental retardation
- Denys-Drash syndrome: Wilms tumor, pseudohermaphroditism, nephropathy (most often diffuse mesangial sclerosis)
- Beckwith-Wiedemann syndrome: Wilms tumor, hemihypertrophy, macroglossia, omphalocele, and visceromegaly
- Isolated hemihypertrophy

Renal Cell Carcinomas

- Most common types
  - Clear cell renal cell carcinoma: 3p deletions and von Hippel-Lindau mutation
  - Papillary renal cell carcinoma: Trisomy 7 and 17, loss of Y chromosome in males
  - Chromophobe cell renal cell carcinoma: Multiple monosomies

CLINICAL IMPLICATIONS

Clinical Presentation

- 26% of adults with RCC have chronic kidney disease
  - Major consequences are end-stage kidney disease (ESKD) and cardiovascular disease
- RCC patients more likely to have diabetes, hypertension, obesity, and smoking risk factors for both RCC and ESKD

Clinical Risk Factors

- Impact of unilateral nephrectomy for renal transplantation
  - 15.5-year follow-up of 1,195 donors showed 0.33% incidence of ESKD
  - GFR reduced by only 20-25% because of compensatory hypertrophy of contralateral kidney
- Impact of partial or complete nephrectomy on renal function in children with Wilms tumor
  - In absence of bilateral disease, nephrogenic rests or syndromic disease with renal disease, unilateral nephrectomy is benign procedure
  - 20-year follow-up indicates 2% ESKD and 0.6% ESKD if no syndromic disease or genitourinary anomalies present, respectively
- Impact of partial or complete nephrectomy on renal function in adults with benign or malignant neoplasm
  - Contralateral kidney in adults with RCC is not normal
  - CKD at 10 years develops in 22% with radical nephrectomy and 11.2% with partial nephrectomy

Partial Nephrectomy for Renal Cell Carcinoma

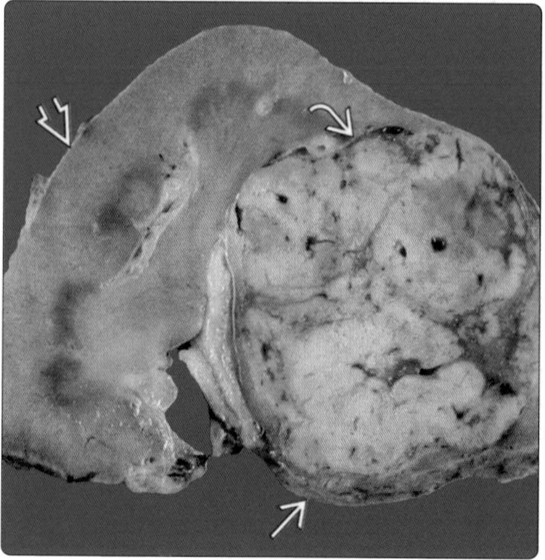

Peritumoral Pseudocapsule

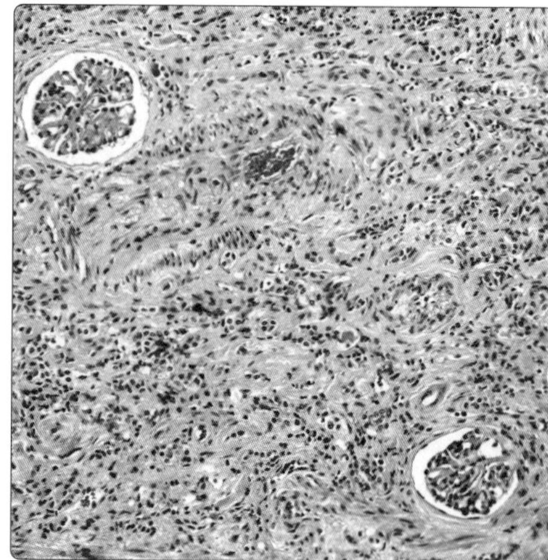

(Left) *This partial nephrectomy contains a clear cell RCC ➡. The deep surgical resection margin is typically thin ➡. However, the lateral margin contains ample tissue to provide accurate assessment of native kidney disease ➡. A section 1 cm from tumor is recommended.* **(Right)** *Fibrous pseudocapsule from a large RCC is shown. There is diffuse tubulointerstitial scarring with inflammation. This is a peritumoral effect and not representative of the nonneoplastic renal parenchyma distant to tumor.*

MACROSCOPIC

Specimen Handling

- International Society of Urologic Pathology 2012 recommendations
  - 1 block of tumor-uninvolved kidney interface
  - 1 block of uninvolved cortex distant to tumor
    - Can be challenging in partial nephrectomy when only thin rim of uninvolved kidney included
  - Assess background glomerular, tubulointerstitial, and vascular disease
    - PAS-stained section recommended by Renal Pathology Society

MICROSCOPIC

Peritumoral Pseudocapsule

- Pseudocapsule of 5 mm or less of atrophic parenchyma invests most RCCs
  - Glomerulosclerosis, tubular atrophy, and interstitial fibrosis are most severe at tumor interface
    - Due to tumor-related centripetal growth and vascular and tubular obstruction
  - Peripheral to pseudocapsule, zone of acute tubular injury is common
- Some tumors, especially benign tumors, do not form pseudocapsule

Retrograde Cortical Venous Invasion

- Especially common with clear cell RCC
  - Can occur with any venous invasive cancer
- Occurs when sinus and main renal veins occluded by tumor
  - RCC grows into venous tributaries of occluded veins and extends proximally into nonneoplastic cortex
  - Cortical veins in retrograde venous invasion may resemble 2nd primary tumor
    - Nodules of involved veins located in venous outflow tract, between pyramids and at cortico-medullary junction, and can involve interlobular veins

Host-Related Changes in Children With Wilms Tumor

- Nephrogenic rests: Abnormal persistence of embryonic cells capable of developing into Wilms tumor
- Nephrogenic rests: Identify patients at risk of contralateral Wilms tumor
  - Perilobar rests: Circumscribed rests located at periphery of a renal lobe
  - Intralobar rests: Located in center of a renal lobe
- Syndromic glomerulopathies
  - Denys-Drash syndrome-related diffuse mesangial sclerosis (common) and focal segmental glomerulosclerosis (rare)

Host-Related Changes in Adults

- Arterial and arteriolar nephrosclerosis
  - Kidneys of hypertensive patients have coarsely granular subcapsular surface
  - Arteriolar hyalinosis and arterial fibrointimal thickening with glomerulosclerosis and tubulointerstitial scarring
    - Subcapsular accentuation of nephrosclerosis results in granular surface
    - Glomerulosclerosis is "normal" aging process; severity proportional to age
      - □ Age/2-10 = % "normal" glomerulosclerosis
- Diabetic glomerulopathy
  - 2nd most common glomerular abnormality
  - Mild diabetic glomerulopathy easily overlooked on H&E stain
    - PAS stain will show mild mesangial expansion and small mesangial nodules

Cystic Diseases Associated With Malignancy

- Acquired cystic kidney disease (ACKD)
  - 10% of ACKD will develop RCC
    - Patients with ESKD but no cysts still at risk for RCC
- von Hippel-Lindau disease (VHL)
  - 40-60% of patients have multifocal and bilateral RCC
    - Clear cell RCC is most common carcinoma
  - 70-80% of patients have renal cysts
    - Cysts lined by clear cell identical to clear cell RCC
- Tuberous sclerosis complex (TSC)
  - 50-80% of patient with TSC have multiple and bilateral angiomyolipomas
    - Microscopic AMLs (so-called microhamartomas) are common in nonneoplastic cortex
  - Renal cysts are 2nd most common lesion in TSC
    - Cysts lined by large, densely eosinophilic cells
  - 1-2% of TSC have mutation of *TSC2* and *PKD1* genes resulting in *TSC2/PKD1* contiguous gene syndrome
    - Patients develop PKD at early age and progress to renal failure at early age
  - 1-2% of TSC patients may also have RCC

SELECTED REFERENCES

1. González J et al: Nephron-sparing surgery in renal cell carcinoma: current perspectives on technical issues. Curr Urol Rep. 16(2):6, 2015
2. Salvatore SP et al: Nonneoplastic renal cortical scarring at tumor nephrectomy predicts decline in kidney function. Arch Pathol Lab Med. 137(4):531-40, 2013
3. Sarsık B et al: Spectrum of nontumoral renal pathologies in tumor nephrectomies: nontumoral renal parenchyma changes. Ann Diagn Pathol. 17(2):176-82, 2013
4. Trpkov K et al: Handling and staging of renal cell carcinoma: the International Society of Urological Pathology Consensus (ISUP) conference recommendations. Am J Surg Pathol. 37(10):1505-17, 2013
5. Chen YB et al: Spectrum of preneoplastic and neoplastic cystic lesions of the kidney. Arch Pathol Lab Med. 136(4):400-9, 2012
6. Bonsib SM et al: Retrograde venous invasion in renal cell carcinoma: a complication of sinus vein and main renal vein invasion. Mod Pathol. 24(12):1578-85, 2011
7. Bonsib SM et al: The non-neoplastic kidney in tumor nephrectomy specimens: what can it show and what is important? Adv Anat Pathol. 17(4):235-50, 2010
8. Henriksen KJ et al: Nonneoplastic kidney diseases in adult tumor nephrectomy and nephroureterectomy specimens: common, harmful, yet underappreciated. Arch Pathol Lab Med. 133(7):1012-25, 2009
9. Henriksen KJ et al: Non-neoplastic renal diseases are often unrecognized in adult tumor nephrectomy specimens: a review of 246 cases. Am J Surg Pathol. 31(11):1703-8, 2007
10. Bijol V et al: Evaluation of the nonneoplastic pathology in tumor nephrectomy specimens: predicting the risk of progressive renal failure. Am J Surg Pathol. 30(5):575-84, 2006

(Left) *Acute tubular injury with tubular epithelial attenuation and interstitial expansion by edema is shown, a common finding outside the pseudocapsule. It may extend for several millimeters but is not representative of the nonneoplastic renal parenchyma.* **(Right)** *This is a large clear cell renal cell carcinoma with thin fibrous pseudocapsule. The main renal vein is occluded by tumor. There is secondary retrograde venous invasion just extending into the nonneoplastic cortical column of Bertin.*

Peritumoral Zone of Acute Tubular Injury

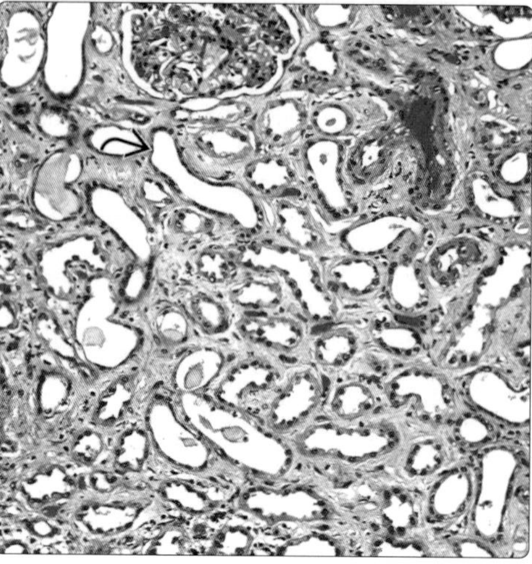

Renal Cell Carcinoma With Retrograde Venous Invasion

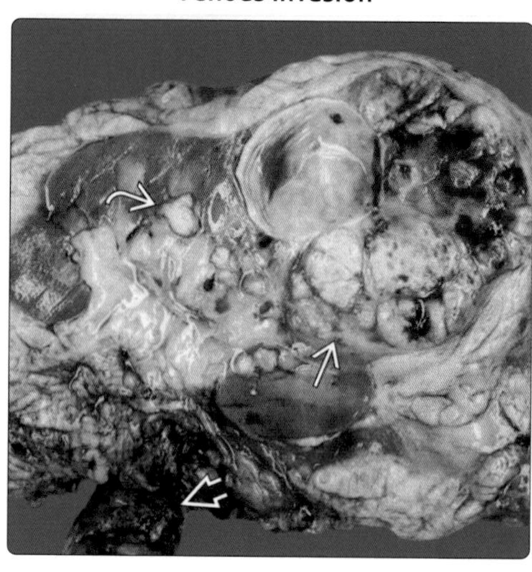

(Left) *Normal cortical veins lack a smooth muscle media. This actin (red) and CD31 (black) immunoperoxidase stain demonstrates a cortical vein with endothelium but no smooth muscle media. This can make it difficult to recognize a cortical vein involved by retrograde venous invasion.* **(Right)** *H&E shows a vein occluded by renal cell carcinoma found separate from the primary tumor. Its rounded contour and location at the cortico-medullary junction in a venous location provide clues to its nature.*

Normal Cortical Interlobular Vein

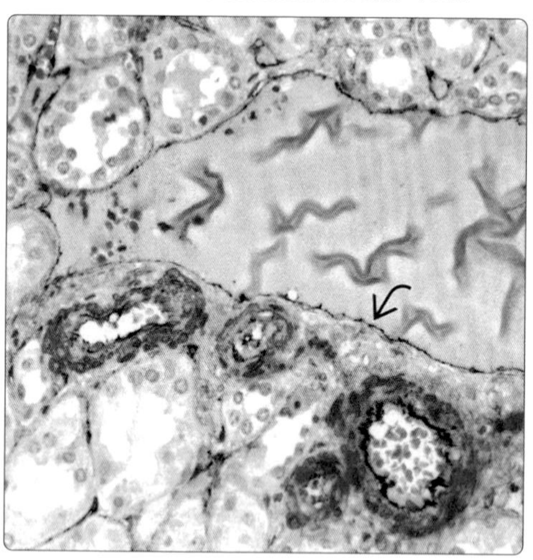

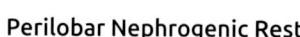

Cortical Vein Showing Retrograde Venous Invasion

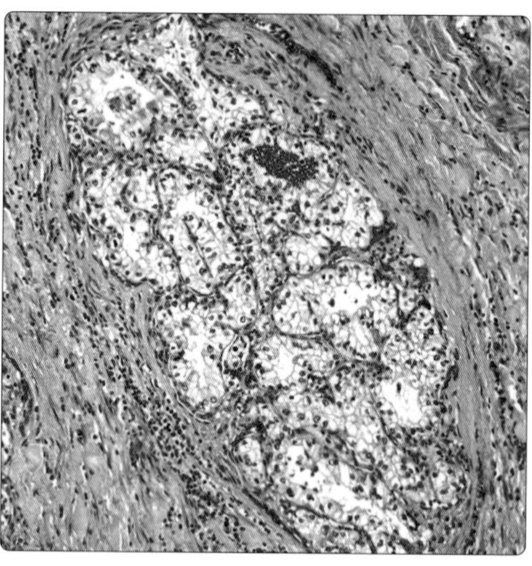

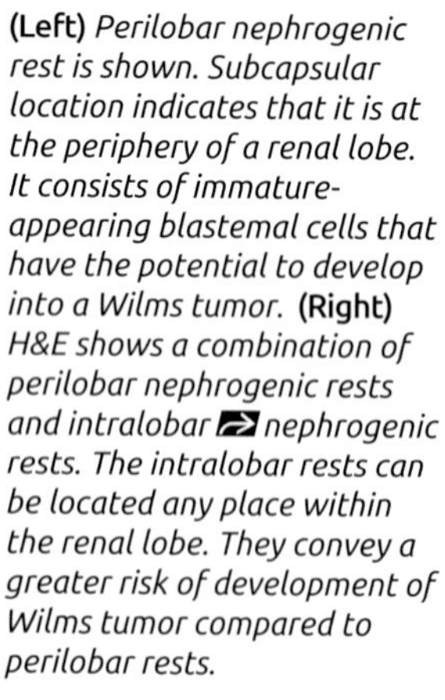

(Left) *Perilobar nephrogenic rest is shown. Subcapsular location indicates that it is at the periphery of a renal lobe. It consists of immature-appearing blastemal cells that have the potential to develop into a Wilms tumor.* **(Right)** *H&E shows a combination of perilobar nephrogenic rests and intralobar nephrogenic rests. The intralobar rests can be located any place within the renal lobe. They convey a greater risk of development of Wilms tumor compared to perilobar rests.*

Perilobar Nephrogenic Rest

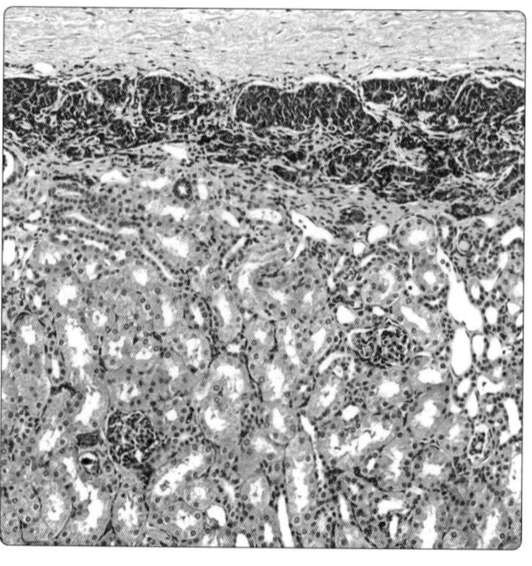

Perilobar and Intralobar Nephrogenic Rests

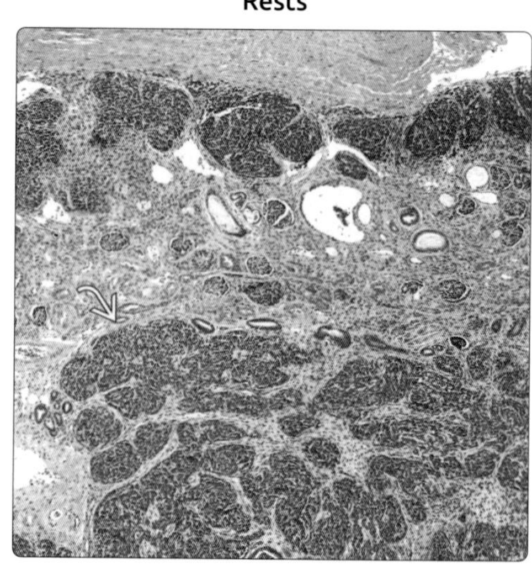

Diffuse Mesangial Sclerosis

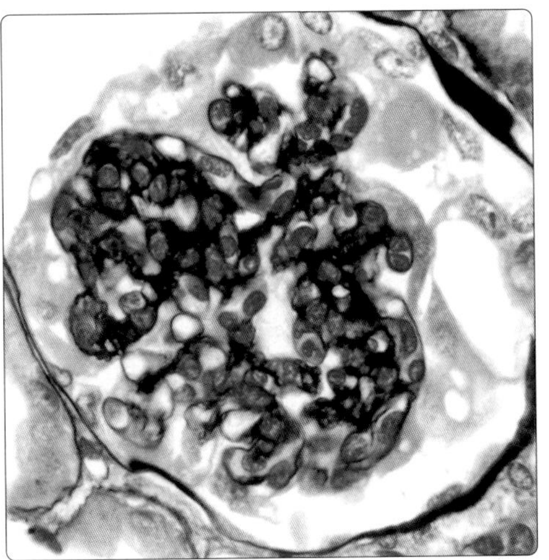

Autopsy Kidney With Hypertension-Related Subcapsular Granularity

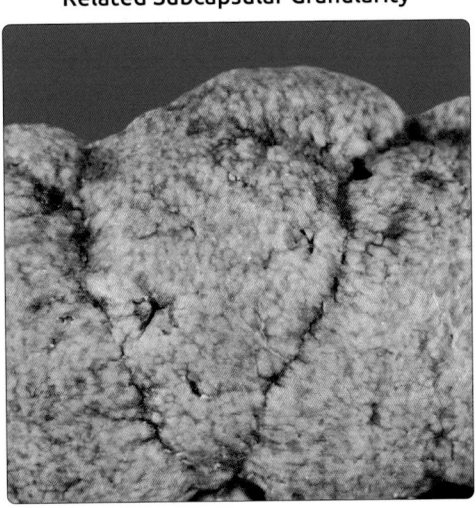

(Left) *Glomerulus with diffuse mesangial sclerosis is shown in a patient with Denys-Drash syndrome. There is mesangial expansion, capillary loop collapse, and vacuolated hyperplastic epithelial cells. Since these patients can have an incomplete form of DDS limited to Wilms tumor and glomerulopathy, any patient with a presumed sporadic Wilms tumor may have Denys-Drash syndrome.* **(Right)** *Autopsy kidney is shown with a coarsely granular subcapsular surface, typical of prolonged hypertensive injury.*

Hypertensive Subcapsular Scar

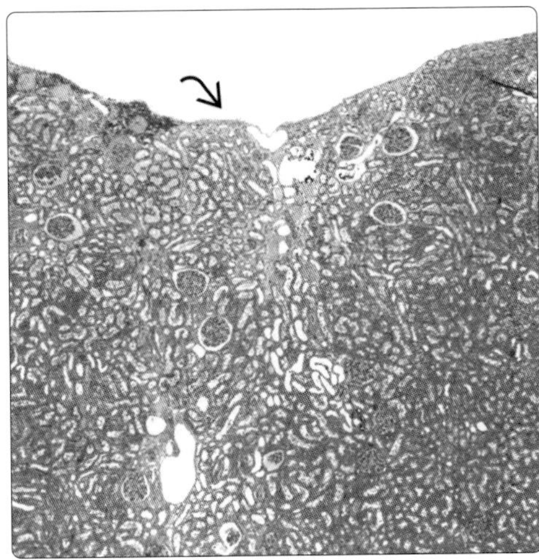

Hypertensive Subcapsular Scar

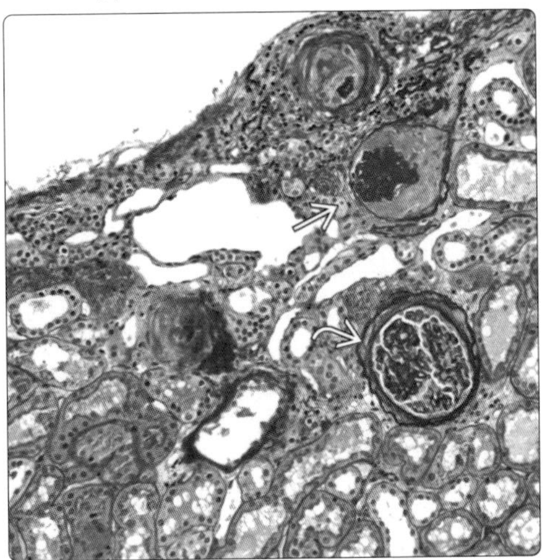

(Left) *Autopsy kidney from a hypertensive patient shows a shallow subcapsular scar ➔ that results in the coarsely granular surface noted grossly, representing the normal non-scarred cortex.* **(Right)** *The subcapsular scar contains an ischemic glomerulus ➔ with wrinkled capillary loops and a sclerotic glomerulus ➔. In addition, there is tubular atrophy responsible for the tissue contraction, interstitial fibrosis, and a bland lymphoid infiltrate*

Hypertensive Arterial Sclerosis

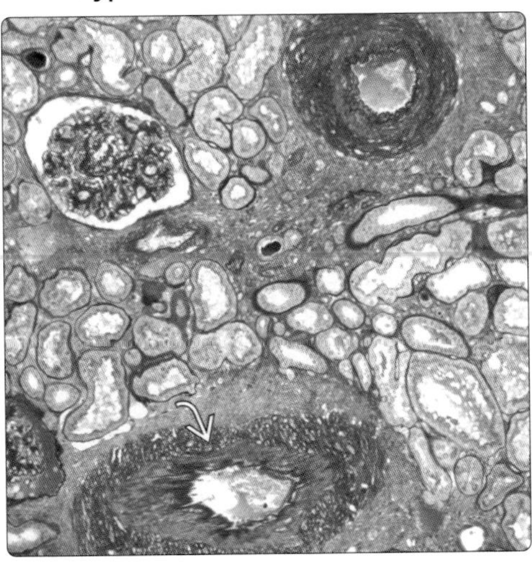

Cholesterol Microembolus

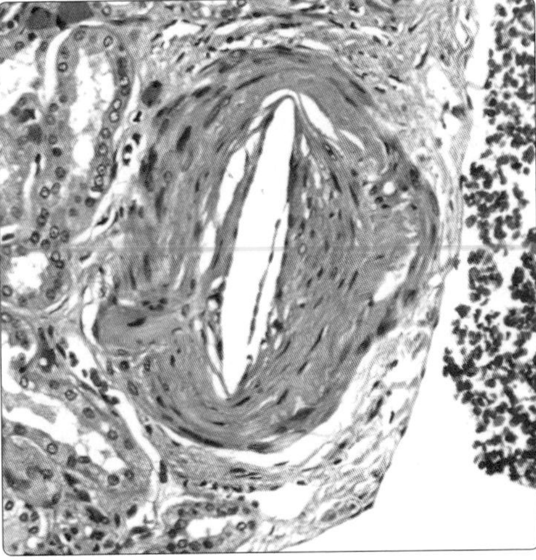

(Left) *The deep cortex of hypertensive kidneys will typically show pronounced arteriosclerotic vascular disease as larger arteries are more severely affected. There is severe arterial fibrointimal thickening ➔, a finding in a tumor nephrectomy that indicates risk of a cardiovascular event.* **(Right)** *H&E shows an interlobular artery occluded by a cholesterol microembolus. This is not an uncommon finding in older hypertensive patients with severe aortic atherosclerotic vascular disease.*

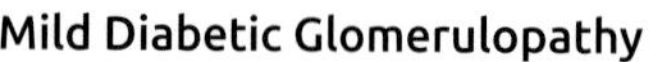

Mild Diabetic Glomerulopathy

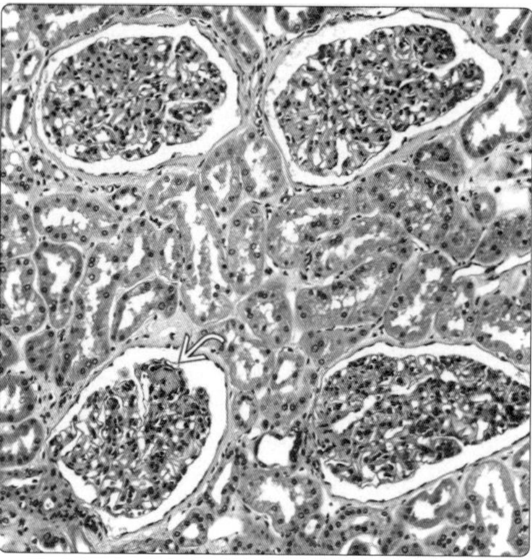

Mild Diabetic Glomerulopathy

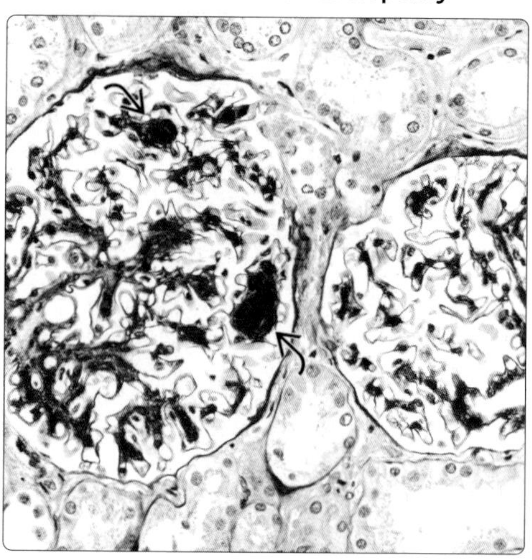

(Left) *Mild diabetic glomerulopathy is shown. The findings can be subtle on conventional H&E-stained sections. Notice that there is a single small Kimmelstiel-Wilson mesangial nodule ➡ typical of mild diabetic glomerulopathy.* **(Right)** *Same glomerulus on PAS-stained section not only makes the diabetic nodules easy to identify ➡, it also shows that there is more generalized mesangial matrix increase indicative of early diabetic glomerulopathy.*

Severe Diabetic Glomerulopathy

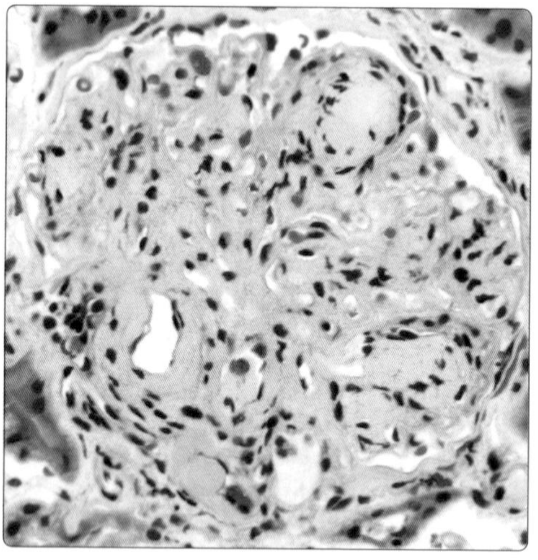

Severe Diabetic Glomerulopathy

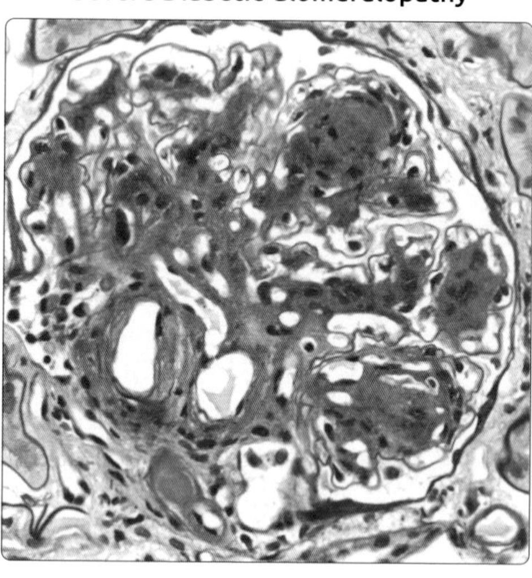

(Left) *Advanced diabetic glomerulopathy is shown. When diabetes severely affects the glomeruli, its recognition is straightforward on H&E-stained sections; however, one has to look for this finding to see it. It must be reported because of its severe prognostic importance for risk of subsequent renal failure.* **(Right)** *This PAS-stained section again enhances the recognition of diabetic glomerulopathy. This severe example shows diffuse mesangial matrix increase and several prominent diabetic mesangial nodules.*

Acquired Cystic Kidney Disease With Renal Cell Carcinomas

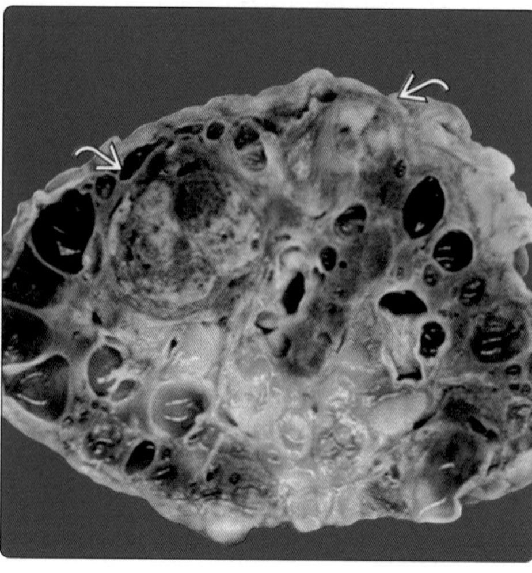

Acquired Cystic Kidney Disease

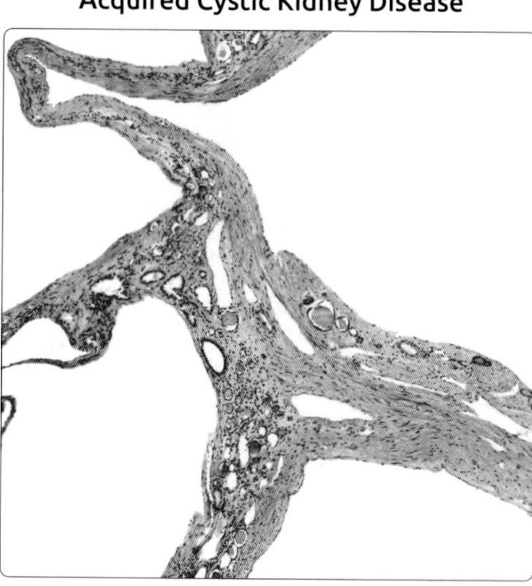

(Left) *This nephrectomy shows acquired cystic kidney disease with two RCCs ➡. The cysts affect the cortex and medulla while the kidney itself is not significantly enlarged. Approximately 10% of patients with acquired cystic kidney disease will develop a renal cell carcinoma.* **(Right)** *Acquired cystic kidney disease shows cysts with thin septa of atrophic cortex. This field is indistinguishable from autosomal dominant polycystic kidney disease; however, the kidneys were not enlarged.*

End-Stage Kidney With Papillary Adenoma

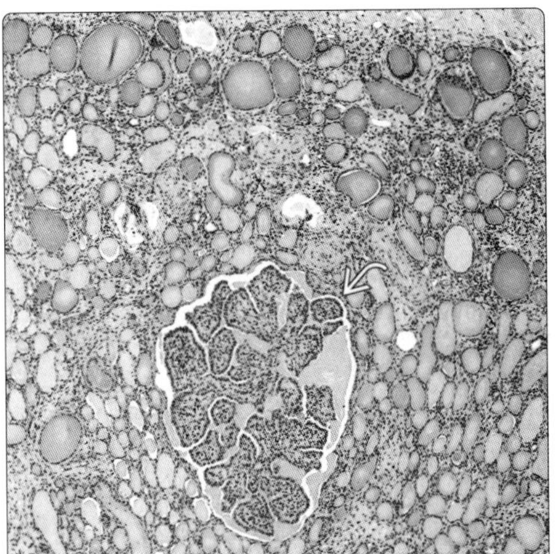

TSC With Microscopic Angiomyolipoma and Eosinophilic Cyst

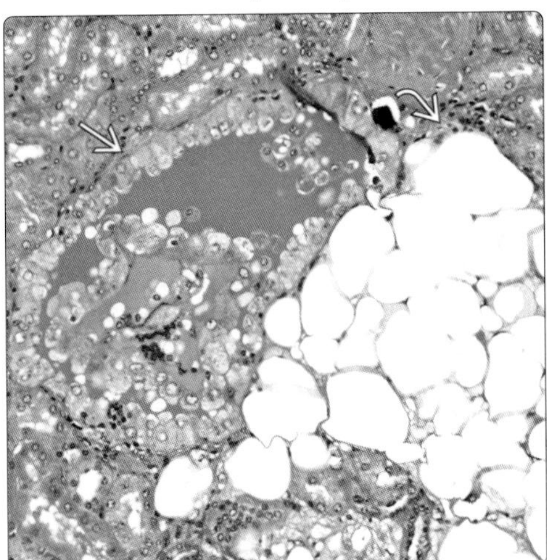

(Left) *ESKD is a risk factor for renal neoplasms. Approximately 1/3 of patients with RCC and ESKD do not have cysts. In this ESK resected for a RCC, the nonneoplastic cortex contained a small papillary adenoma.* **(Right)** *Most patients with tuberous sclerosis have multiple and bilateral angiomyolipomas. In resections, the uninvolved cortex will commonly have microscopic angiomyolipomas that may be lipid cell or myoid cell predominant and may contain cysts lined by large cells with eosinophilic cytoplasm.*

TSC With Eosinophilic Cysts

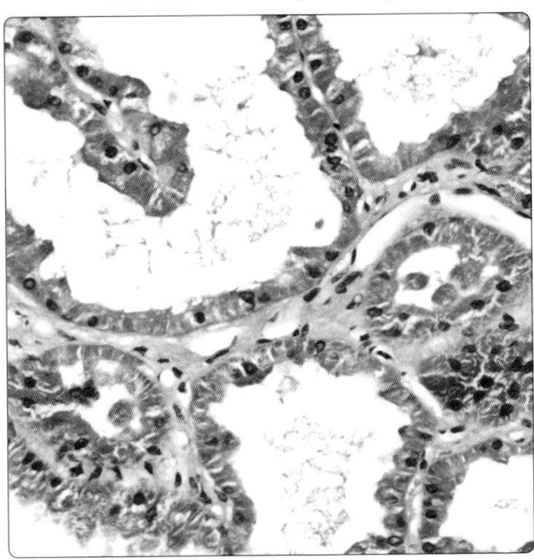

TSC2/PKD1 Contiguous Gene Syndrome

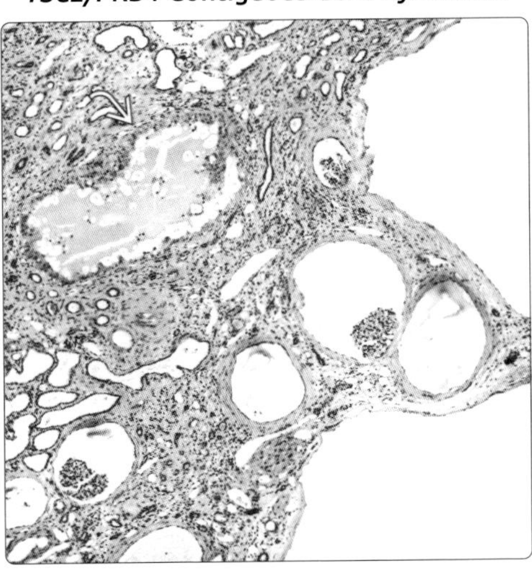

(Left) *Patients with tuberous sclerosis frequently have cysts, and 1-2% develop polycystic kidney disease because of contiguous mutations of TSC2 and PKD1. The cysts in TSC are often lined by large, distinctive cells with densely eosinophilic cytoplasm.* **(Right)** *TSC2/PKD1 contiguous gene syndrome is shown. Microscopically, it looks identical to autosomal dominant polycystic kidney disease. It may also contain cysts lined by the distinctive eosinophilic TSC epithelium and contain angiomyolipomas.*

von Hippel-Lindau Disease

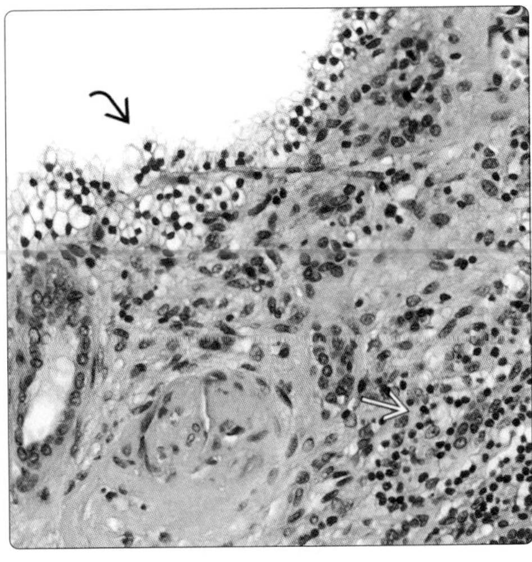

von Hippel-Lindau Disease

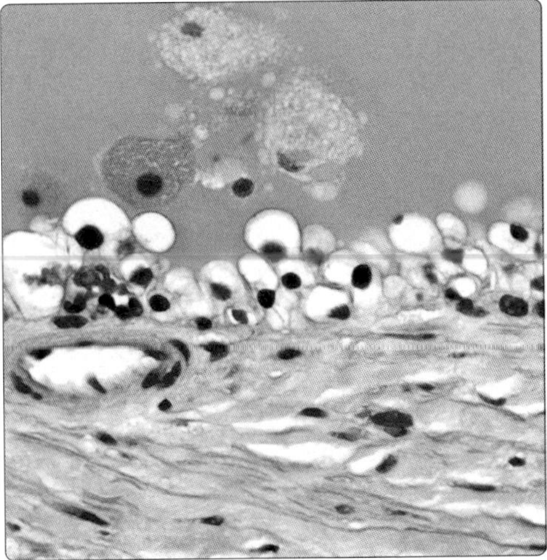

(Left) *Most patients with von Hippel-Lindau disease will develop clear cell renal cell carcinoma. Their nonneoplastic kidney will usually also harbor presumed precursor lesions with clear cell-lined cysts and solid interstitial nests of clear cells.* **(Right)** *In von Hippel-Lindau disease, the cysts are lined by cells with optically clear cytoplasm. They may form a single layer of cells or may be stratified as in this case. These cells are identical in appearance to the cells that comprise clear cell renal cell carcinoma.*

TERMINOLOGY

Synonyms

- Kidney explant

Definitions

- Irreversible renal allograft failure necessitating nephrectomy

ETIOLOGY/PATHOGENESIS

Causes of Early Allograft Loss (< 6 Months Post Transplantation)

- Allograft thrombosis
  - Venous thrombosis ~ 2x more frequent than arterial thrombosis
  - Hypercoagulable/thrombophilic states are important underlying causes of thrombosis
    - Inherited disorders
      - Factor V Leiden (G1691A mutation)
      - Prothrombin (factor II) mutation
      - Protein S, protein C, or antithrombin III deficiency
    - Acquired disorders
      - Tissue factor release from surgery or trauma, antiphospholipid antibodies, hyperhomocysteinemia
    - Sickle cell disease or trait may give rise to intragraft sickle crisis and graft thrombosis
  - Poor blood flow and vessel wall injury also important factors
    - Surgical difficulties arising from anatomical discrepancies between donor and recipient vessels
    - Large vessel injury from torsion, kinks, and compression
    - Small vessel or endothelial injury related to prolonged ischemia or reperfusion injury
- Thrombotic microangiopathy
  - Causes include antibody-mediated rejection and recurrent hemolytic uremic syndrome
- Acute allograft rejection (AR)
  - Cell-mediated rejection &/or antibody-mediated rejection
- Recurrent disease, such as primary oxalosis and hemolytic uremic syndrome
- Primary nonfunction
  - Clinical term for graft that never functioned
  - Causes include
    - Acute tubular necrosis/injury
    - Perfusion nephropathy
    - Atheroembolism arising from plaque rupture at graft harvest
    - Prolonged cold graft ischemia and marginal donor kidneys are predisposing factors

Causes of Late Allograft Loss (> 6 Months Post Transplantation)

- Recurrent disease
  - Focal segmental glomerulosclerosis
  - Glomerulonephritis: IgA nephropathy, membranous nephropathy, membranoproliferative glomerulonephritis (GN)
- De novo glomerulopathies
  - Focal segmental glomerulosclerosis (FSGS)
  - Transplant glomerulopathy
- Allograft rejection
  - Antibody-mediated rejection may account for 2/3 of late allograft losses
  - Antibody ± T-cell-mediated rejection
- Vascular disease
  - Hypertensive nephrosclerosis
- Drug toxicity
  - Calcineurin inhibitor toxicity
- Infection
  - Polyomavirus, cytomegalovirus, or adenovirus
  - Recurrent episodes of pyelonephritis
- Urinary obstruction
- Neoplasms
  - Post-transplantation lymphoproliferative disease
  - Renal cell carcinoma
  - Sarcoma

Transplant Nephrectomy

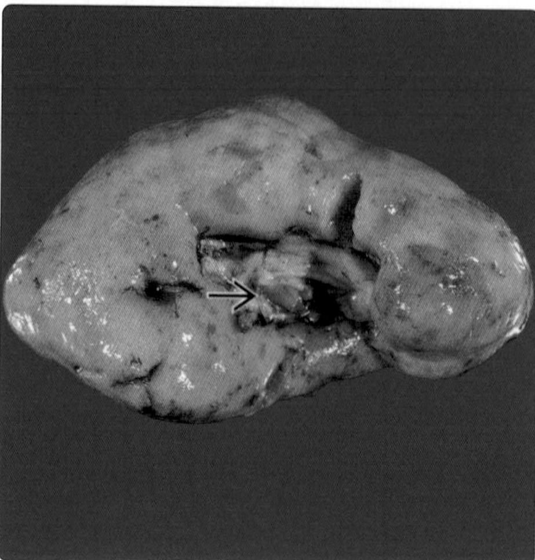

Early Allograft Loss

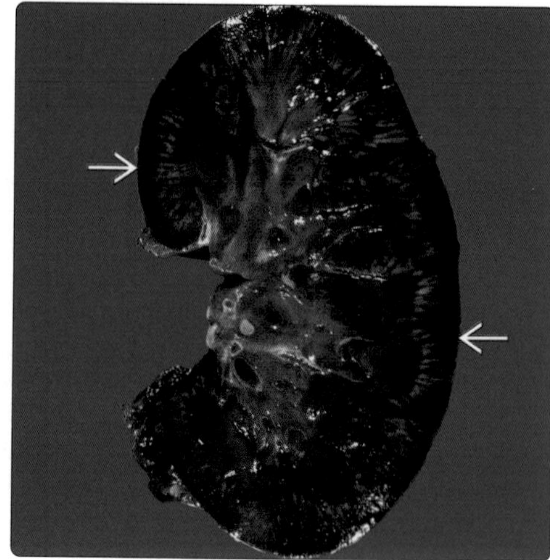

(Left) *Hilar arteries, veins, and the renal pelvis and ureter are often absent ⇒ from kidney transplant nephrectomy specimens.* **(Right)** *Allograft loss on day 2 after transplantation demonstrates enlargement (298 g) with diffuse cortical and medullary hemorrhage. Note also the radial pattern of pallor (necrosis) in the cortex ➡.*

CLINICAL IMPLICATIONS

Clinical Presentation

- Oliguria or anuria
- Flank pain
- Hematuria
- Asymptomatic

Clinicopathologic Correlation

- Detailed clinical and operative history necessary for final diagnosis
- Elective allograft removal often preceded by cessation of immunosuppressive therapy for weeks

MACROSCOPIC

General Features

- Size
  - Enlargement may be associated with
    - Acute tubular necrosis (ATN)
    - AR
    - Renal vein thrombosis (RVT)
  - Thrombosis, torsion, and anatomical discrepancies of donor and recipient vasculature are important features
  - Allograft rupture may be seen in first 2-3 weeks after transplantation due to
    - AR
    - ATN
    - Ureteral obstruction
    - Biopsy procedure
    - Trauma
  - Small renal allograft is feature of chronic disease (e.g., chronic rejection, infection, and chronic ischemia)

Anatomic Features

- Hilar vessels and pelvis frequently not resected at transplant removal
- Thrombi may be seen in hilar vascular remnants or in intraparenchymal vessels
- Location and extent of necrosis and hemorrhage should be described

Specimen Handling

- Save a portion of viable cortex for immunofluorescence and electron microscopy

MICROSCOPIC

General Features

- Necrosis
  - Hemorrhagic or anemic
  - Cortical, or both cortical and medullary
- Large vessel thrombosis may affect arteries or veins or both
- Microvascular thromboses in glomeruli and arterioles are diagnostic of thrombotic microangiopathy
- Acute rejection
  - T-cell mediated: Interstitial edema, mononuclear infiltrates, and tubulitis
    - Intimal or transmural arteritis
  - Antibody mediated: Glomerulitis, peritubular capillaritis, and transmural arteritis with necrosis
  - Features of AR may be superimposed on other disease processes because of discontinuation of immunosuppression
  - AR may obscure underlying cause of end-stage graft failure, especially if necrosis
- Chronic rejection
  - Transplant glomerulopathy and peritubular capillaritis with multilayering of capillary basement membrane
  - Chronic allograft arteriopathy (chronic intimal arteritis)
- Allograft fibrosis
  - Infarct scars are wedge-shaped in outer cortex
  - Biopsy sites are linear or band-like coarse scars and may have hemosiderin deposition
  - Large or medium vessel arteriosclerosis &/or stenosis result in chronic allograft ischemia
    - Subcapsular fibrosis, glomerular obsolescence, and ischemic glomerulopathy
  - Chronic calcineurin inhibitor toxicity results in striped cortical fibrosis
    - Accompanied by nodular arteriolar hyalinization
  - Chronic rejection or polyomavirus nephropathy: Patchy or diffuse interstitial fibrosis and tubular atrophy

Ancillary Studies

- Direct immunofluorescence
  - Detection of immunoglobulins and complement for recurrent and de novo immune complex glomerulonephritis
- Indirect immunofluorescence
  - Detection of C4d important in antibody-mediated rejection
- Immunohistochemistry
  - Detection of C4d, polyomavirus large T antigen, adenovirus, and Cytomegalovirus in paraffin sections
- Electron microscopy
  - Podocyte injury detected in recurrent or de novo FSGS
  - Immune complex deposits in recurrent or de novo glomerulonephritis
- Serology
  - Donor-specific antibodies to histocompatibility antigens essential diagnostic feature of antibody-mediated rejection

SELECTED REFERENCES

1. Morales JM et al: Association of early kidney allograft failure with preformed IgA antibodies to β2-glycoprotein I. J Am Soc Nephrol. 26(3):735-45, 2015
2. Loupy A et al: The impact of donor-specific anti-HLA antibodies on late kidney allograft failure. Nat Rev Nephrol. 8(6):348-57, 2012
3. Phelan PJ et al: Renal allograft loss in the first post-operative month: causes and consequences. Clin Transplant. 26(4):544-9, 2012
4. Sellarés J et al: Understanding the causes of kidney transplant failure: the dominant role of antibody-mediated rejection and nonadherence. Am J Transplant. 12(2):388-99, 2012
5. El-Zoghby ZM et al: Identifying specific causes of kidney allograft loss. Am J Transplant. 9(3):527-35, 2009

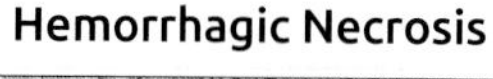

Hemorrhagic Necrosis

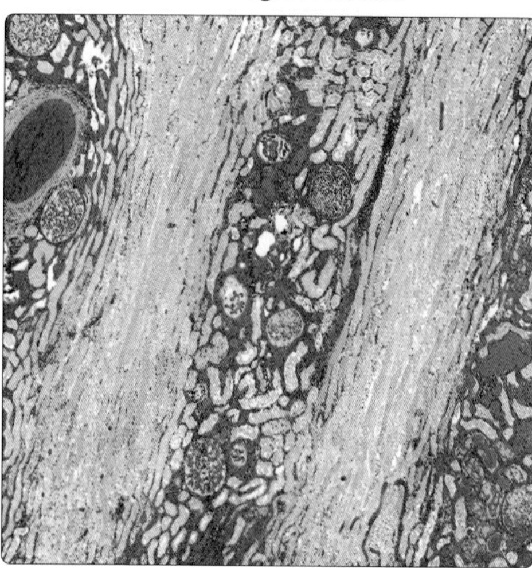

Reperfusion Injury Mimicking Arteritis

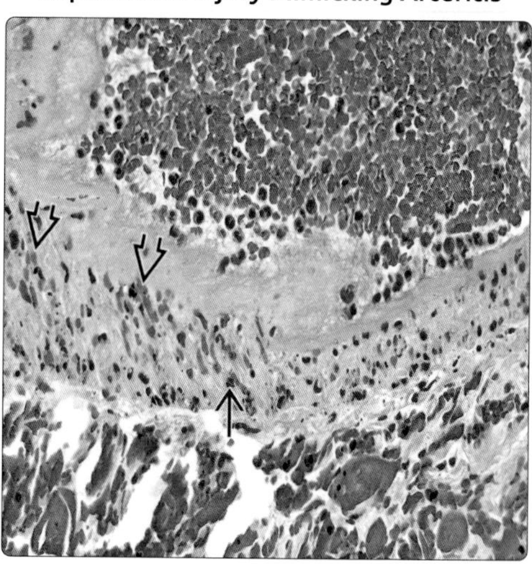

(Left) *H&E shows diffuse cortical necrosis with hemorrhage in the pars convoluta from a renal allograft removed on post-transplant day 2. Medullary rays have necrosis without hemorrhage. Large arteries have occlusive thrombi. Protein S deficiency and oral contraceptive use contributed to graft thrombosis.* **(Right)** *Necrotic arteries often have neutrophils ➡ and erythrocytes ➡ in the media and intima and a lot of karyorrhexis. This is a form of reperfusion injury and should not be mistaken for vasculitis.*

Renal Allograft Venous Thrombosis

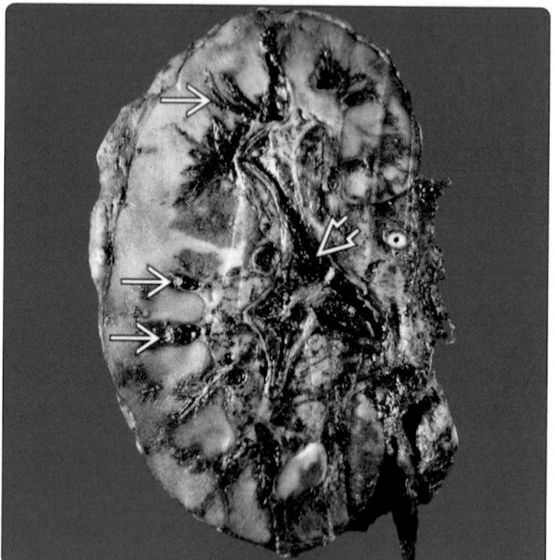

Allograft Hilar Venous Thrombus

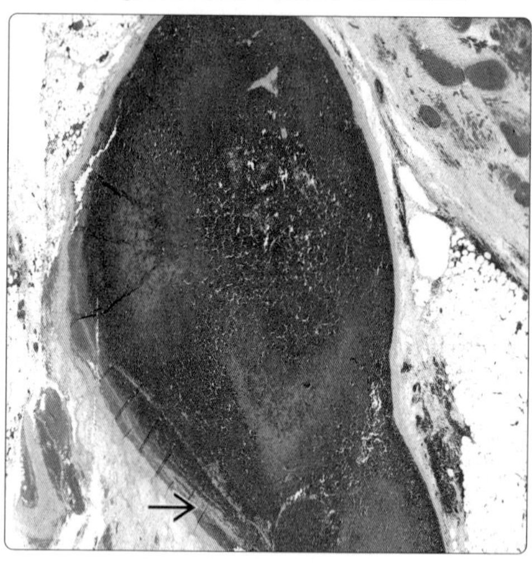

(Left) *A formalin-fixed renal allograft was removed on day 4 post transplant for renal vein thrombosis related to vein injury at implantation. Occlusive thrombi ➡ and diffuse pallor of the cortex are consistent with necrosis. The pelvis is filled with blood clot ➡.* **(Right)** *H&E shows erythrocyte-rich occlusive venous thrombosis in a renal hilar vein from an allograft removed on day 4 post transplant. Layers of fibrin can be seen ➡.*

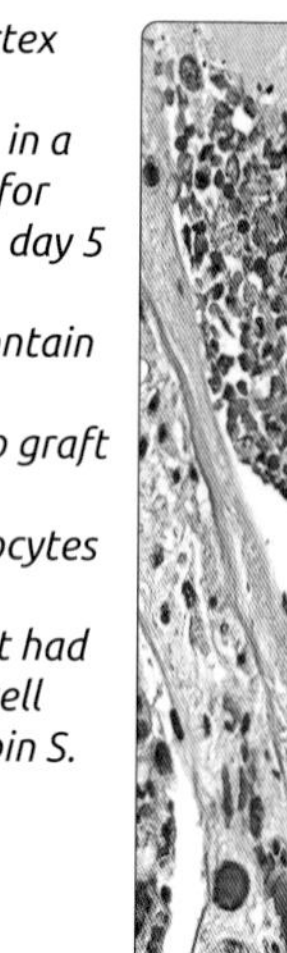

Hemorrhagic Necrosis From Venous Thrombosis

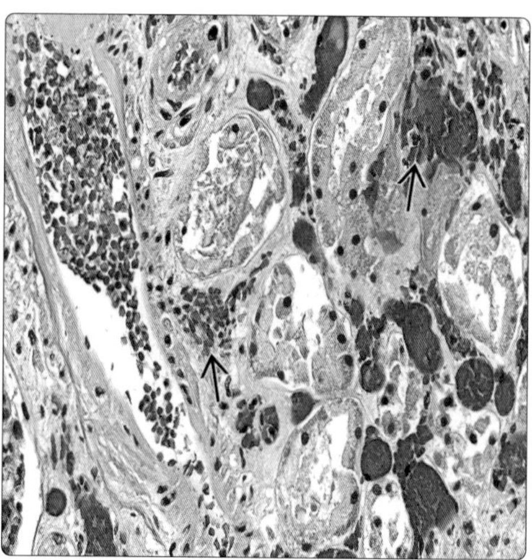

Sickle Cell Thrombosis

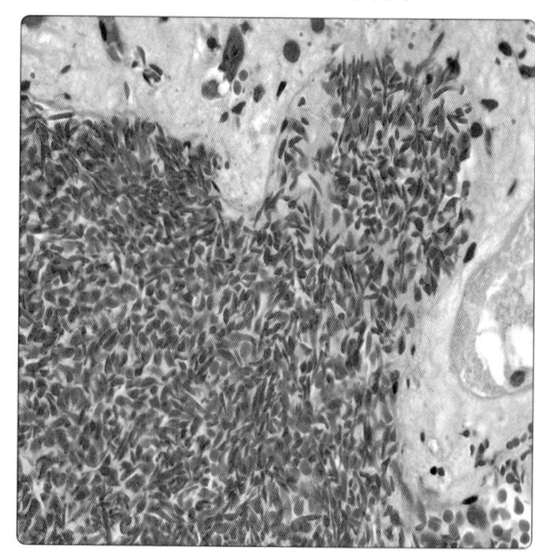

(Left) *Necrosis of the cortex with congestion and hemorrhage ➡ are seen in a renal allograft removed for renal vein thrombosis on day 5 post transplant.* **(Right)** *Vascular thrombi may contain clues to the underlying condition predisposing to graft thrombosis. Multiple refractile, sickled erythrocytes are seen on high-power examination. This patient had a clinically occult sickle cell trait with 26% hemoglobin S.*

Late-Onset Allograft Hemorrhagic Necrosis

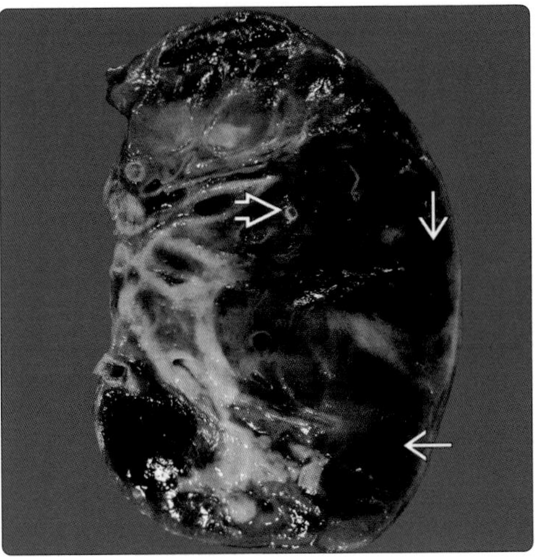

Late Allograft Loss With Segmental Scar

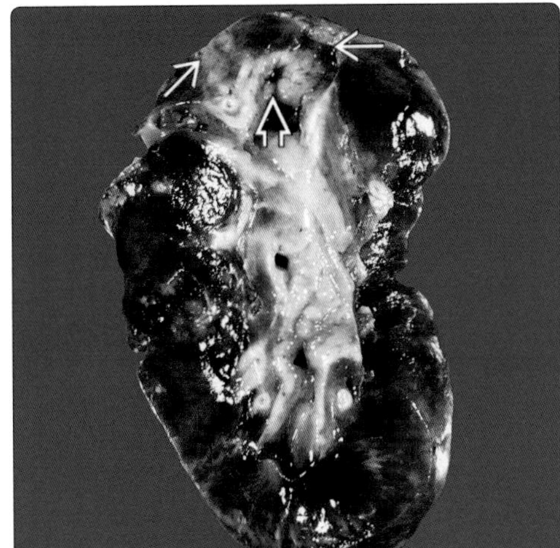

(Left) *Extensive cortical hemorrhage ➡ and necrosis is shown in a 160 g renal allograft removed 4 years after transplantation. There was severe arterial ➡ and arteriolar nephrosclerosis with superimposed severe rejection resulting in hemorrhagic necrosis.* **(Right)** *A 186 g renal allograft removed after 8.5 years shows a segmental scar ➡ and effacement of the pyramid ➡. The parenchyma is hemorrhagic. Histologically, there was severe rejection and recurrent lupus nephritis.*

Late Rejection Without Immunosuppression

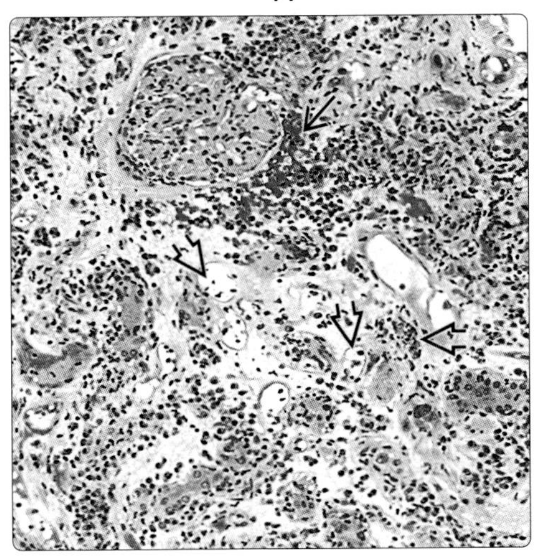

Plasma Cell-Rich Late Rejection

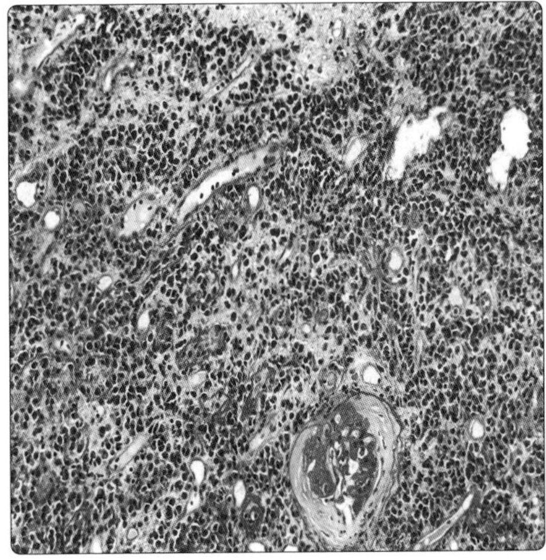

(Left) *Late rejection often has interstitial edema, hemorrhage ➡, plasma cells, eosinophils, and peritubular capillaritis ➡. C4d was present in capillary walls. Tubules are atrophic. The findings are indicative of cell- and antibody-mediated rejection.* **(Right)** *Abundant plasma cells are a feature of late-onset allograft rejection. The tubules are severely atrophic, and the glomerulus is obsolescent. These dense infiltrates must be distinguished from post-transplantation lymphoproliferative disorders.*

Kappa Light Chain RNA ISH

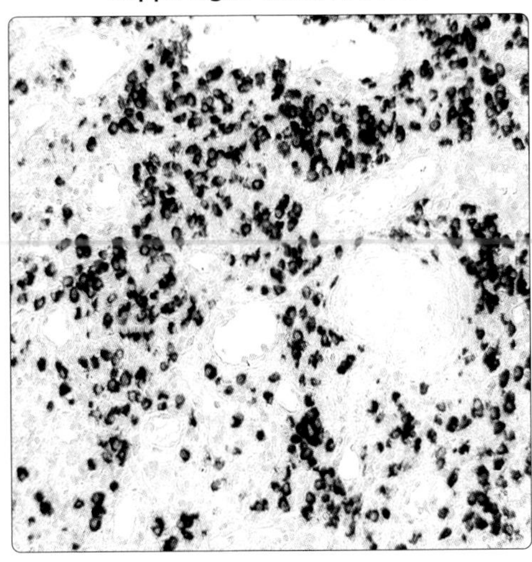

Lambda Light Chain RNA ISH

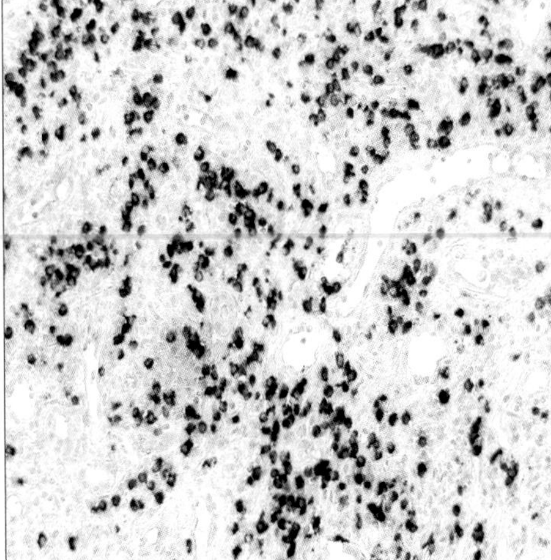

(Left) *Sheets of infiltrating plasma cells raise the possibility of post-transplantation lymphoproliferative disease. In situ hybridization can differentiate reactive from neoplastic plasma cells. κ light chain RNA is evident in this section.* **(Right)** *λ light chain RNA can be detected in conjunction with kappa light chain RNA to help differentiate reactive from neoplastic plasma cell infiltrates in renal allografts. Reactive infiltrates have kappa:lambda ratios of ~ 5-8:1.*

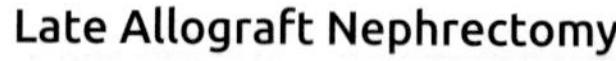

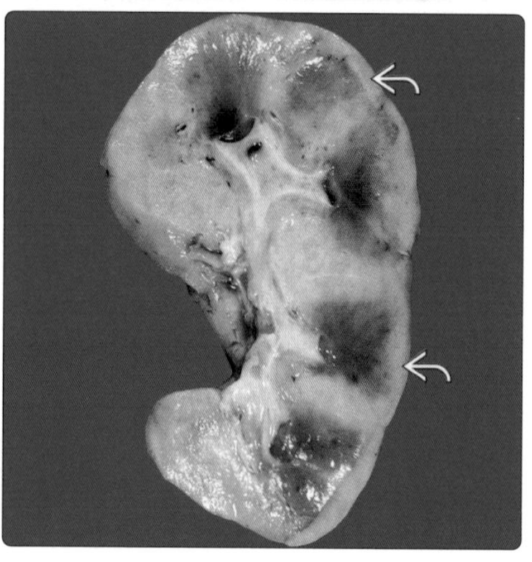

Active Chronic Allograft Arteriopathy

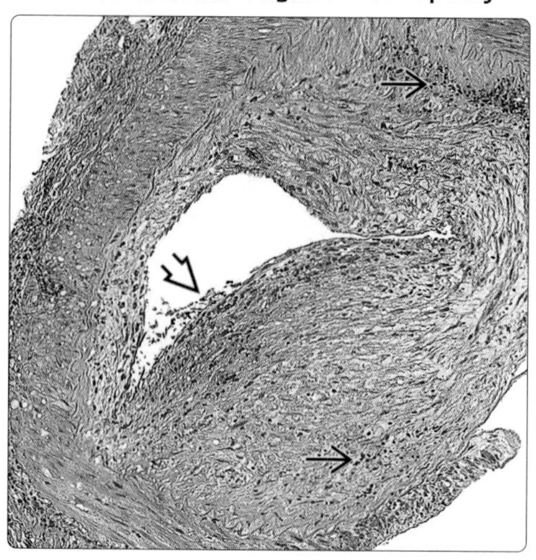

(Left) *Renal allograft removed 5.75 years post transplant demonstrates variable thinning and global pallor ➔ of the cortex. Acute and chronic rejection was evident histologically.* **(Right)** *Acute and chronic intimal arteritis from an allograft removed after 5 months post transplant shows mononuclear infiltrates deep within the fibrotic intima →. The endothelium is undermined by similar infiltrates ⇨.*

Chronic Allograft Arteriopathy

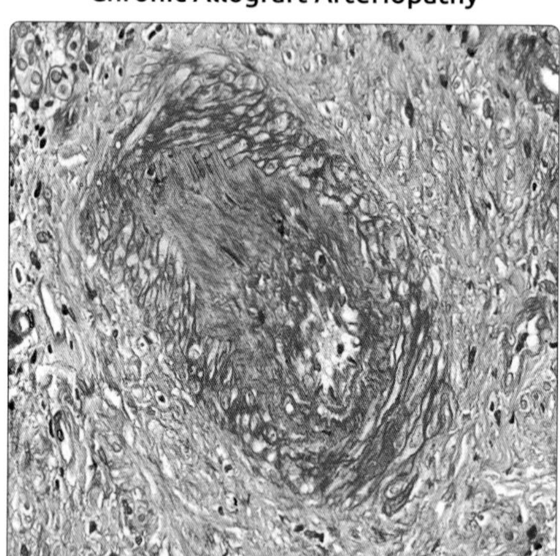

T Cells in Chronic Arteriopathy

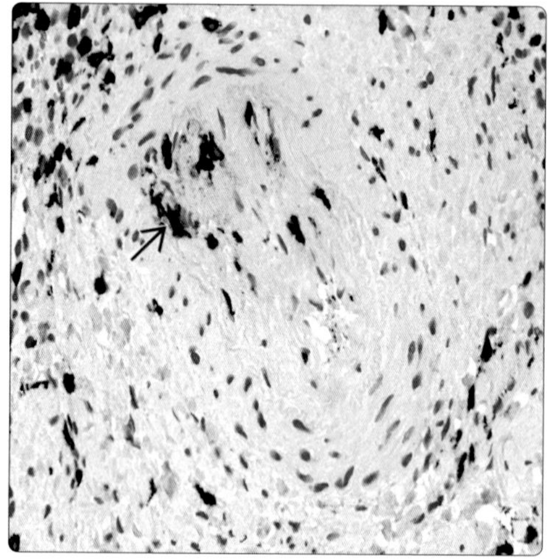

(Left) *Chronic allograft arteriopathy can have a subtle appearance with intimal fibrosis and scattered nuclei within the fibrotic intima. Immunohistochemistry for CD3 may be necessary to identify T-cell infiltrates.* **(Right)** *This artery has CD3(+) T cells deep within the fibrotic intima →, indicative of chronic allograft arteriopathy (chronic intimal arteritis).*

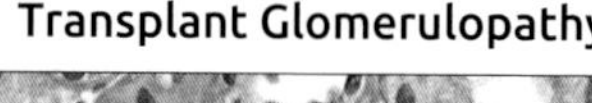

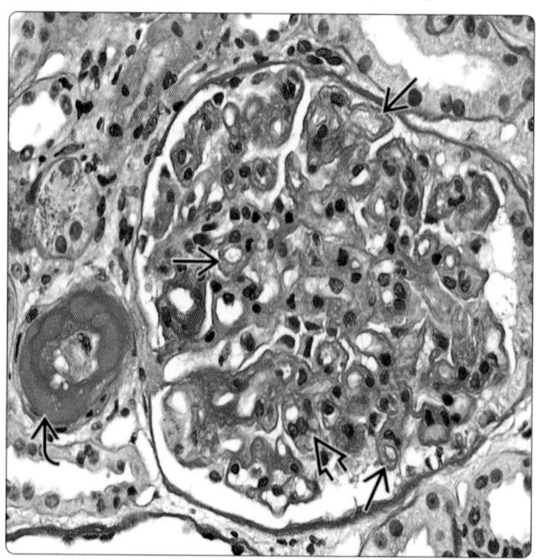

Chronic Transplant Glomerulopathy

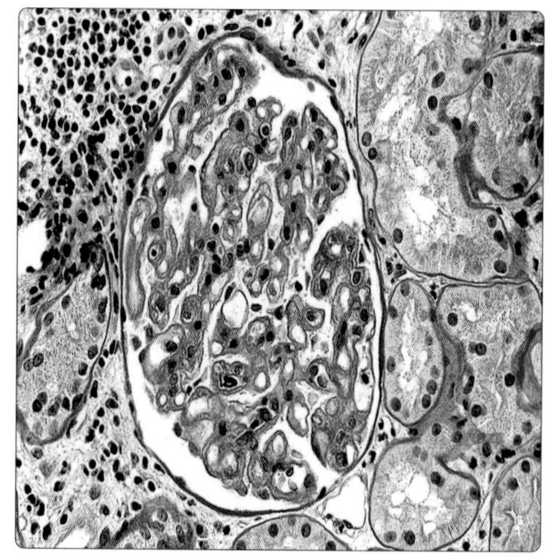

(Left) *Transplant glomerulopathy has global capillary double contours → and segmental hypercellularity ⇨. Hyaline arteriolosclerosis is often a prominent feature ↶. Antibody-mediated rejection accounts for about 80% of cases.* **(Right)** *Morphologic identification of transplant glomerulopathy raises a differential diagnosis of membranoproliferative glomerulonephritis, chronic thrombotic microangiopathy, and antibody-mediated rejection. Hepatitis C infection often has a contributory role.*

Chronic Allograft Ischemia

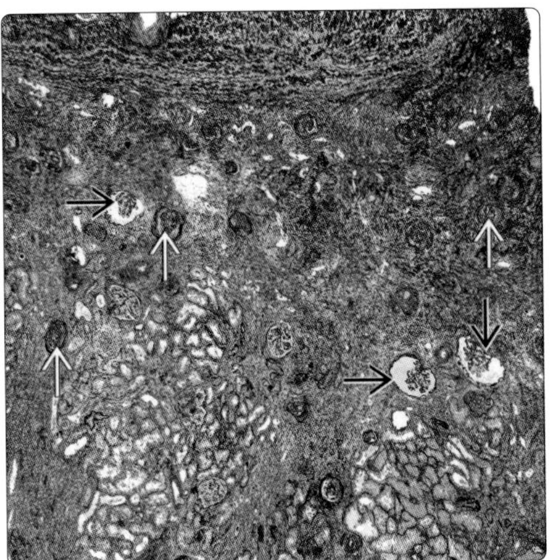

Striped Fibrosis

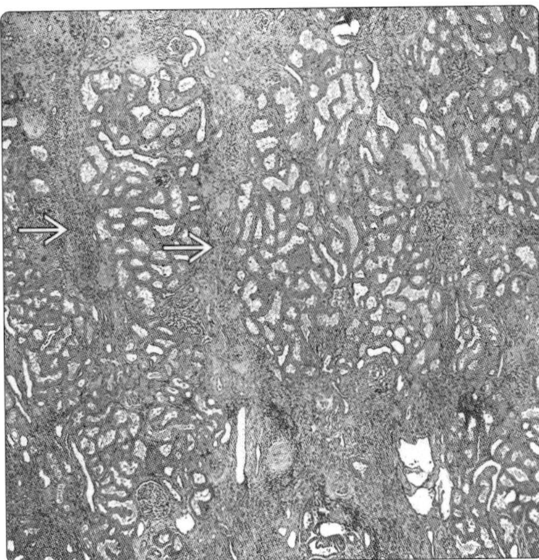

(Left) *Chronic allograft ischemia associated with arteriosclerosis may be associated with outer cortical interstitial fibrosis, tubular atrophy, ischemic glomerulopathy ⇨, & global glomerular obsolescence ➡.* **(Right)** *A striped pattern of interstitial fibrosis and tubular atrophy ➡ is characteristic of chronic calcineurin inhibitor toxicity. Hyaline arteriolosclerosis is found in these cases. Other causes of arteriolosclerosis, such as hypertension and diabetes mellitus, may also give rise to this pattern of fibrosis.*

Borderline Infiltrates

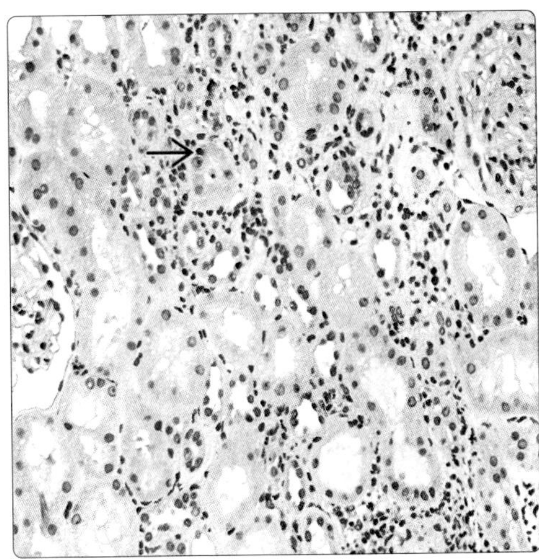

Subtle Polyomavirus Infection

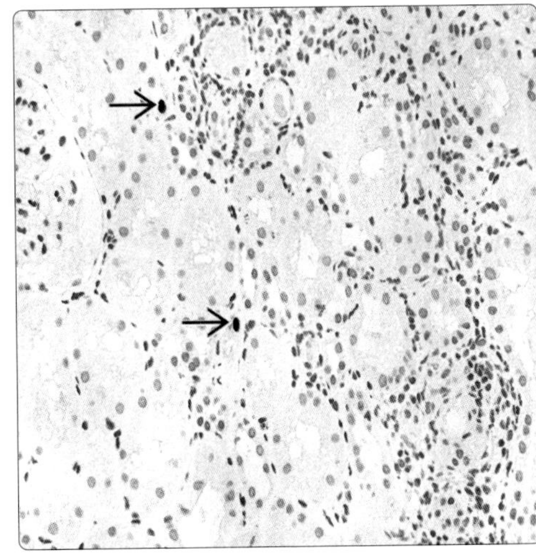

(Left) *Tubulointerstitial mononuclear inflammation affected ~ 20% of the cortex in this 4-year-old allograft. There is also mild tubulitis ⇨. The findings are consistent with a borderline infiltrate by the Banff criteria, but raise the differential diagnosis of viral infection.* **(Right)** *A kidney allograft with a borderline infiltrate has focal tubular nuclear staining for polyomavirus large T antigen ⇨ indicative of active viral replication without viral cytopathic changes. This is a subtle example of polyomavirus nephropathy.*

Acute Pyelonephritis

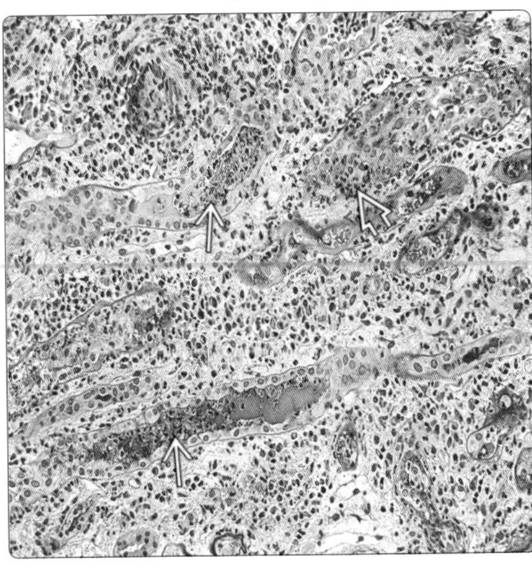

Recurrent Lupus Glomerulonephritis

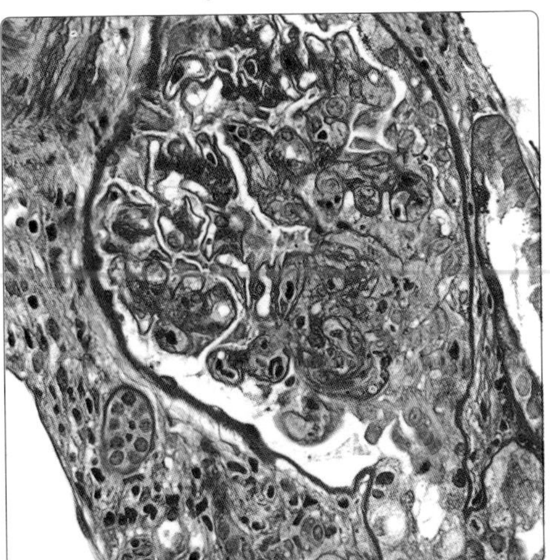

(Left) *This allograft was removed from a 63-year-old man 5 years post transplant. Urine cultures were positive for E. coli. Prominent neutrophilic infiltrates ➡ and casts ➡ are typical of acute pyelonephritis.* **(Right)** *Segmental crescentic glomerulonephritis is evident in this allograft removed 7.75 years post transplant. Immunofluorescence showed granular IgG and C3 deposits. The patient had history of systemic lupus erythematosus (SLE). Findings indicate recurrent lupus nephritis.*

SURGICAL/CLINICAL CONSIDERATION

Goal of Consultation

- Determine if adequate needle biopsy for final diagnosis
- Allocate tissue for special studies
  - Light microscopy (LM)
  - Immunofluorescence (IF)
  - Electron microscopy (EM)
  - Other studies depending on clinical situation
    - Culture for organisms
    - Tissue for molecular studies (e.g., tissue saved in fixatives such as RNAlater for RNA isolation)

Change in Patient Management

- If specimen deemed inadequate, additional needle biopsies will be taken

Clinical Setting

- Medical renal biopsy
  - Generally performed for abnormal renal function or urinary abnormalities (hematuria, proteinuria)
  - Should include renal cortex with glomeruli
  - Also performed to evaluate renal allografts
    - Allograft biopsies often benefit from IF and EM studies
    - Some centers perform surveillance (protocol) allograft biopsies at predetermined time points after transplant
    - Surveillance biopsies evaluate for subclinical rejection, viral infection, recurrent disease, etc.
- Biopsies usually performed under ultrasound guidance or CT guidance
  - Percutaneous (needle) biopsy
    - Ultrasound-guided, automated gun 16- to 18-gauge needle
    - 3 biopsy passes provide adequate sample (by Banff adequacy criteria) in 84% of native and transplant biopsies
    - Compared to 18-gauge needle biopsies, 16-gauge needle biopsies provide more glomeruli & higher percentage of adequate biopsies with fewer passes
  - Transjugular renal biopsy may be performed in high-risk patients for bleeding (coagulopathy or thrombocytopenia)
    - Typically yields smaller sample than percutaneous biopsy, but sufficient for diagnosis in > 90% of cases
- Generally regarded as safe outpatient procedure
  - Hematuria may occur
    - Post-biopsy microscopic hematuria common
    - Gross hematuria in ~ 3.5%
  - Other complications in 1-3% (varies with technique)
    - Higher bleeding risk with 14-gauge needle biopsy
      - 16- and 18-gauge needle biopsies have lower bleeding risk
    - Perirenal hematoma: ~ 2.5%
    - Bleeding requiring transfusion: 0.9%
    - Hemorrhage requiring nephrectomy: 0.01%
    - Death in 0.02% (2 of 8,971 patients in meta-analysis)
  - Intrarenal arteriovenous fistulas in ~ 7% of allograft biopsies
    - Usually resolve
    - No apparent effect on renal function
  - Page kidney (described by Dr. Irwin Page)
    - Most commonly due to trauma, but rare cases occur due to bleeding after kidney biopsy
    - Compression of kidney by accumulation of blood in perinephric or subcapsular space
    - Usually manifests with renin-dependent reactive hypertension due to renal ischemia; occasionally presents with renal insufficiency

SPECIMEN EVALUATION

Gross

- Biopsies must only be touched by clean forceps
  - Minute amounts of formalin can alter antigenicity of tissue used for immunofluorescence
  - Glutaraldehyde contamination can complicate interpretation by light microscopy and on immunoperoxidase stains

Gross Photograph of Kidney Needle Biopsy

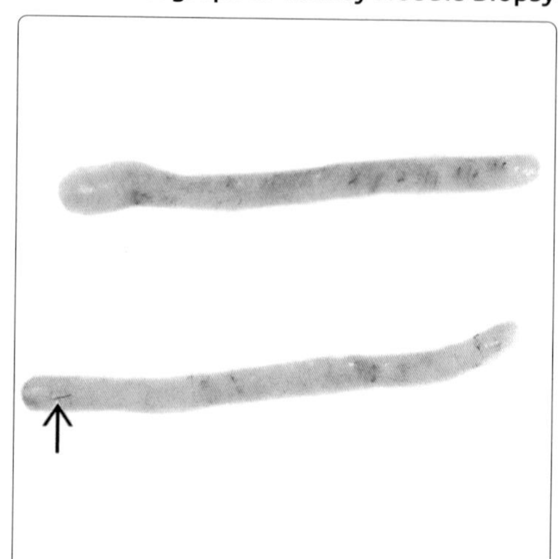

Low Magnification of Needle Biopsy

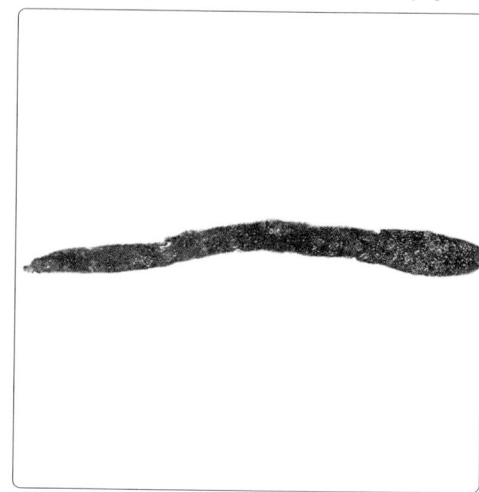

(Left) *Renal 16-g cores are typically 1 mm in diameter x 10-20 mm in length (these are ~ 13 mm). Glomeruli are pale or congested bulges; red cell casts are brown streaks ⇨ or dots. Representative tissue is then allocated for LM, IF, and EM. (Courtesy C. Swetts, MD.)* **(Right)** *The renal biopsy is first examined under low-power magnification to determine the quality of the sample and search for focal lesions.*

- Needle biopsies best examined under stereomicroscopy (dissecting microscope)
  - If not available, renal biopsies can be examined using magnifying glass
- For evaluation of allografts, ≥ 10 glomeruli and 2 arteries considered adequate sample for light microscopy (Banff criteria)
  - Marginal adequacy: 7 glomeruli and 1 artery
  - Glomeruli are pink to red nodules ("raspberries") in pale tan background

Allocation of Tissue

- In majority of cases, tissue saved for light microscopy, IF, and EM
  - Appropriate allocation of tissue depends on several factors
    - Clinical differential diagnosis
    - Focality of expected disease
    - Amount of tissue available
  - Evaluation of tissue by on-site pathologist, compared to no evaluation, yields higher percentage of adequate samples
- Light microscopy
  - Tissue fixed in formalin
  - Standard histochemical stains are H&E, PAS, Jones-methenamine silver, and trichrome
  - Additional stains ordered depending on clinical setting and light microscopy appearance
- Immunofluorescence
  - Cortex and medulla placed in Zeus transport solution (Michel solution)
  - Standard immunohistochemical studies are IgA, IgG, IgM, kappa, lambda, C3, C1q, albumin, and fibrin
    - C4d added for allograft biopsies to evaluate for antibody-mediated rejection
  - If no glomeruli present in tissue submitted in Zeus medium, IF staining may still be contributory
    - Detection of monoclonal immunoglobulin deposition disease, light chain cast nephropathy, AL or AH amyloidosis, etc.
    - C4d staining of peritubular capillaries for transplant biopsies (C4d may also be performed by immunoperoxidase staining)
  - If no glomeruli present in frozen IF tissue, IF can be performed on pronase-digested paraffin sections
    - Pronase-digested paraffin IF less sensitive than routine IF on frozen tissue
- Electron microscopy
  - Tissue with few glomeruli are saved in Karnovsky glutaraldehyde/paraformaldehyde fixative
  - If limited tissue, tissue processed for light microscopy can be deparaffinized for electron microscopy
    - Technique shows artifacts that can inhibit interpretation
      - Artifactual glomerular basement membrane thinning does not allow for diagnosis of thin glomerular basement membrane nephropathy on deparaffinized samples
      - Loss of cellular detail
      - Podocyte foot processes and endothelial cells may not be evaluable

Frozen Section

- In general, tissue should be allocated for special studies and not frozen for histologic examination

REPORTING

Gross

- Reports should include
  - Fixative or transport media in which specimens were received
  - Specimen measurements
  - Adequacy of sample
  - Allocation of tissue

PITFALLS

Evaluation of Number of Glomeruli

- In limited samples, arteries may look like glomeruli grossly
  - Helpful to look for at least 2 glomeruli near each other
- Very small ischemic glomeruli may not be apparent grossly, even under dissection microscope

SELECTED REFERENCES

1. Chung S et al: Safety and tissue yield for percutaneous native kidney biopsy according to practitioner and ultrasound technique. BMC Nephrol. 15:96, 2014
2. Gilani SM et al: Role of on-site microscopic evaluation of kidney biopsy for adequacy and allocation of glomeruli: comparison of renal biopsies with and without on-site microscopic evaluation. Pathologica. 105(6):342-5, 2013
3. Goldstein MA et al: Nonfocal renal biopsies: adequacy and factors affecting a successful outcome. J Comput Assist Tomogr. 37(2):176-82, 2013
4. Mai J et al: Is bigger better? A retrospective analysis of native renal biopsies with 16 Gauge versus 18 Gauge automatic needles. Nephrology (Carlton). 18(7):525-30, 2013
5. Corapi KM et al: Bleeding complications of native kidney biopsy: a systematic review and meta-analysis. Am J Kidney Dis. 60(1):62-73, 2012
6. Kurban G et al: Needle core biopsies provide ample material for genomic and proteomic studies of kidney cancer: observations on DNA, RNA, protein extractions and VHL mutation detection. Pathol Res Pract. 208(1):22-31, 2012
7. Sis B et al: Banff '09 meeting report: antibody mediated graft deterioration and implementation of Banff working groups. Am J Transplant. 10(3):464-71, 2010
8. Kamar N et al: Acute Page kidney after a kidney allograft biopsy: successful outcome from observation and medical treatment. Transplantation. 87(3):453-4, 2009
9. Misra S et al: Safety and diagnostic yield of transjugular renal biopsy. J Vasc Interv Radiol. 19(4):546-51, 2008
10. Solez K et al: Banff 07 classification of renal allograft pathology: updates and future directions. Am J Transplant. 8(4):753-60, 2008
11. Nasr SH et al: Thin basement membrane nephropathy cannot be diagnosed reliably in deparaffinized, formalin-fixed tissue. Nephrol Dial Transplant. 22(4):1228-32, 2007
12. Durkan AM et al: Renal transplant biopsy specimen adequacy in a paediatric population. Pediatr Nephrol. 21(2):265-9, 2006
13. Nasr SH et al: Immunofluorescence on pronase-digested paraffin sections: a valuable salvage technique for renal biopsies. Kidney Int. 70(12):2148-51, 2006
14. Schwarz A et al: Safety and adequacy of renal transplant protocol biopsies. Am J Transplant. 5(8):1992-6, 2005
15. Cluzel P et al: Transjugular versus percutaneous renal biopsy for the diagnosis of parenchymal disease: comparison of sampling effectiveness and complications. Radiology. 215(3):689-93, 2000
16. Racusen LC et al: The Banff 97 working classification of renal allograft pathology. Kidney Int. 55(2):713-23, 1999
17. McCune TR et al: Page kidney: case report and review of the literature. Am J Kidney Dis. 18(5):593-9, 1991

(Left) *The kidney is often biopsied percutaneously under ultrasound or CT guidance using a posterior approach.* **(Right)** *Sagittal image of the left kidney obtained during an ultrasound-guided biopsy shows a core biopsy needle that has been introduced into the cortex of the lower renal pole using real-time guidance. The needle trajectory is directed away from the renal hilum to reduce the risk of injury to hilar vessels and the urinary collecting system.*

Renal Biopsy Procedure

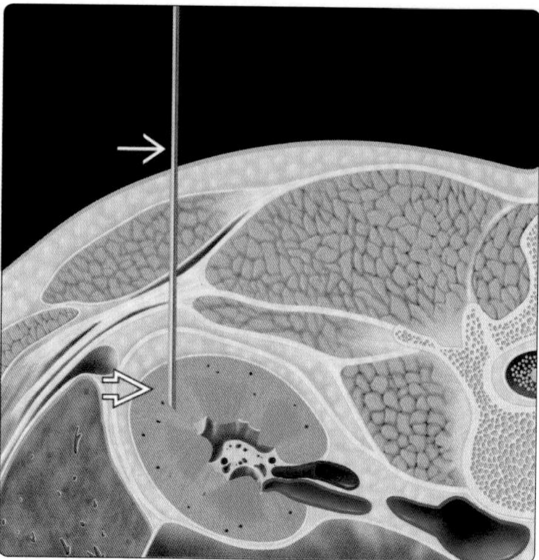

Renal Biopsy Under Ultrasound Guidance

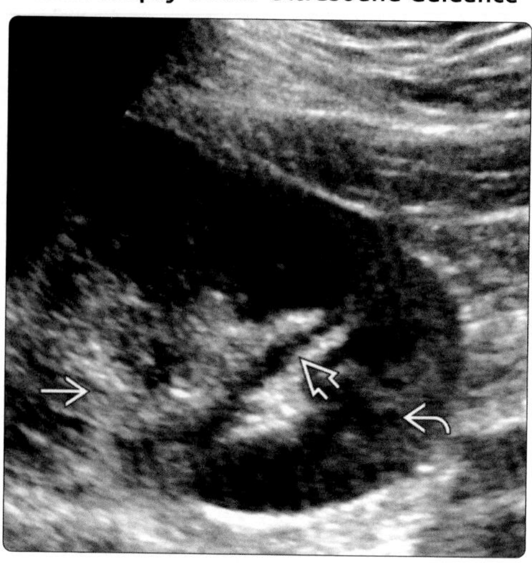

(Left) *A 39-year-old man underwent percutaneous kidney biopsy for chronic renal failure. He subsequently developed hypertension (180s/100s) and renal failure. A CT scan showed a subcapsular hematoma, which resulted in decreased renal perfusion (acute Page kidney).* **(Right)** *An ultrasound image shows an AV fistula at a recent biopsy site in the lower pole of a renal transplant. Doppler waveform at the fistula shows typical high-velocity, low-resistance blood flow. (Courtesy T. Atwell, MD.)*

Acute Page Kidney Following Biopsy

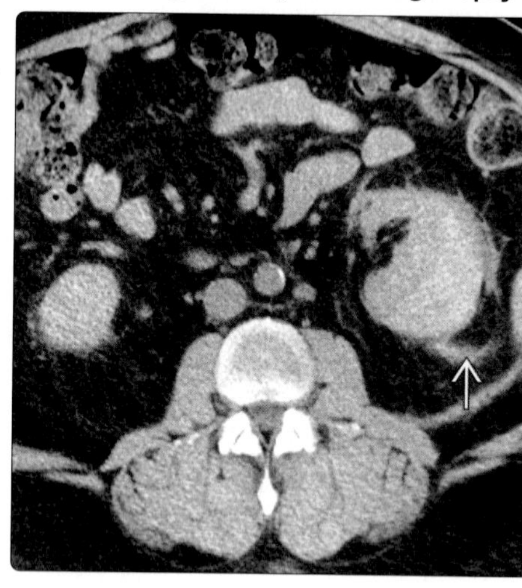

Arteriovenous Fistula Following Kidney Biopsy

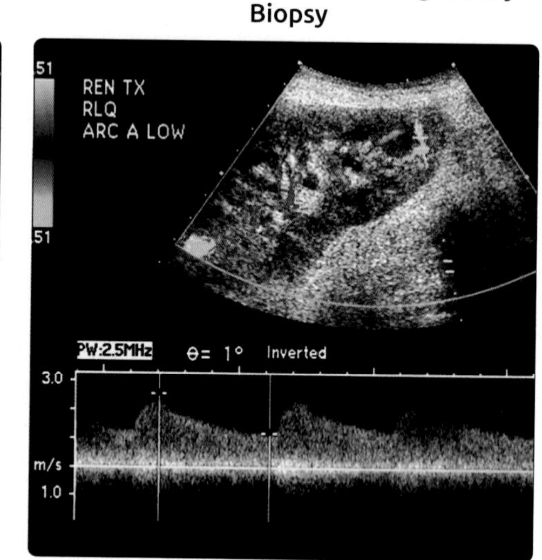

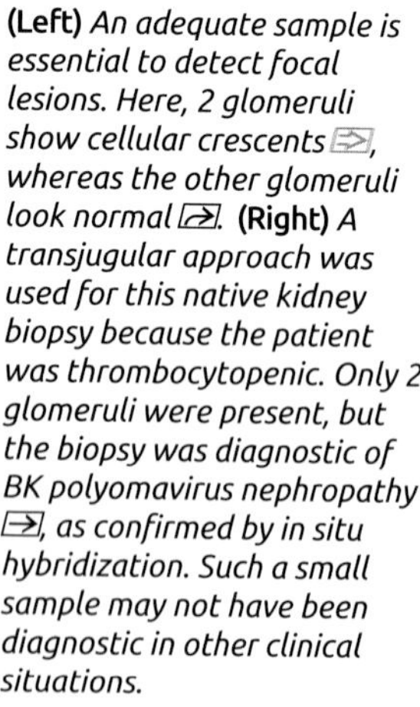

(Left) *An adequate sample is essential to detect focal lesions. Here, 2 glomeruli show cellular crescents, whereas the other glomeruli look normal.* **(Right)** *A transjugular approach was used for this native kidney biopsy because the patient was thrombocytopenic. Only 2 glomeruli were present, but the biopsy was diagnostic of BK polyomavirus nephropathy, as confirmed by in situ hybridization. Such a small sample may not have been diagnostic in other clinical situations.*

Focal Necrotizing and Crescentic Glomerulonephritis, Pauci-Immune

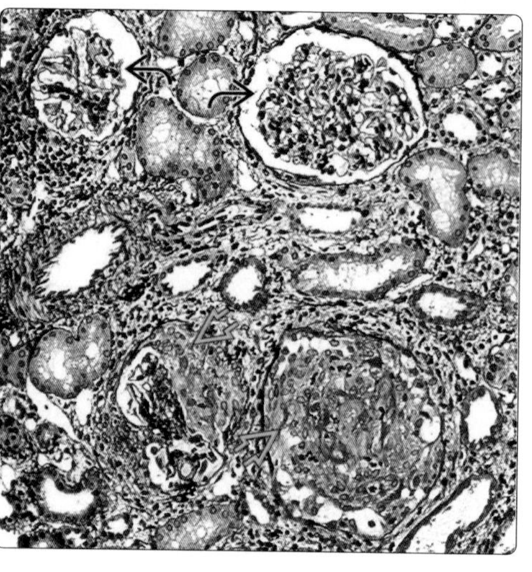

Transjugular Biopsy

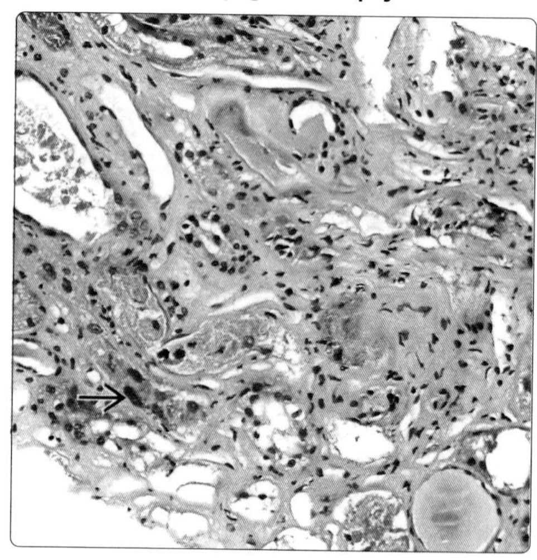

IgA Nephropathy

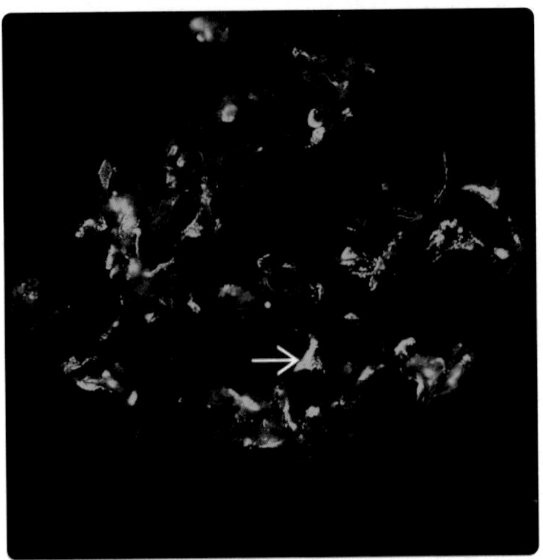

Cryoglobulinemic Glomerulonephritis

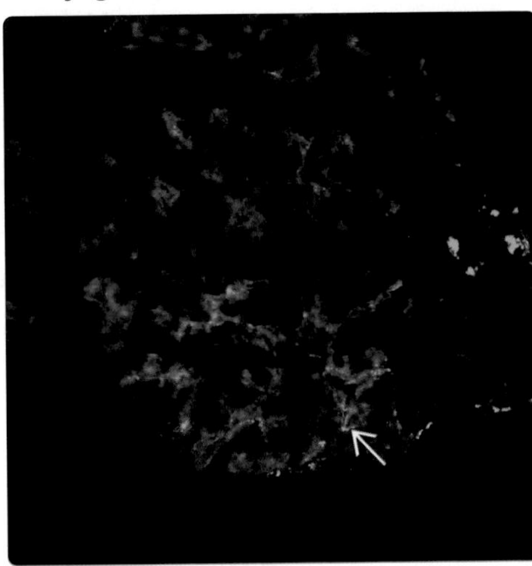

(Left) *Immunofluorescence staining for IgA is diffuse in IgA nephropathy, so even 1 glomerulus present in IF tissue should be sufficient to make a diagnosis of IgA nephropathy with correlating features by light microscopy and EM. This image shows granular mesangial staining for IgA ➡.* **(Right)** *IF staining in cryoglobulinemic glomerulonephritis can be variable between glomeruli. In this glomerulus, there is only trace segmental staining for C3 ➡. A larger IF sample would be helpful to support this diagnosis.*

IF on Limited Tissue Sample

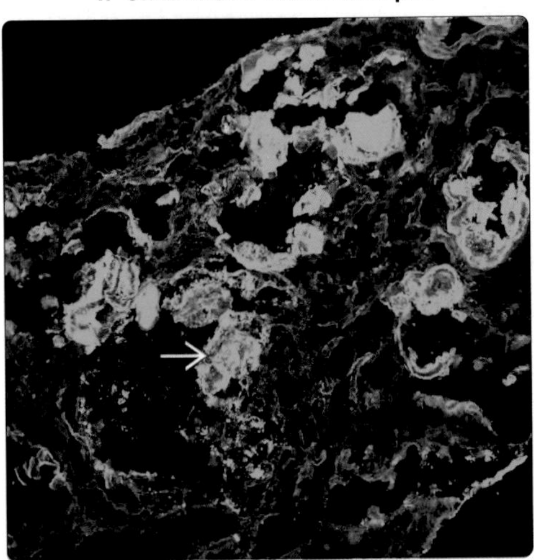

Thin Glomerular Basement Membrane (GBM) Nephropathy

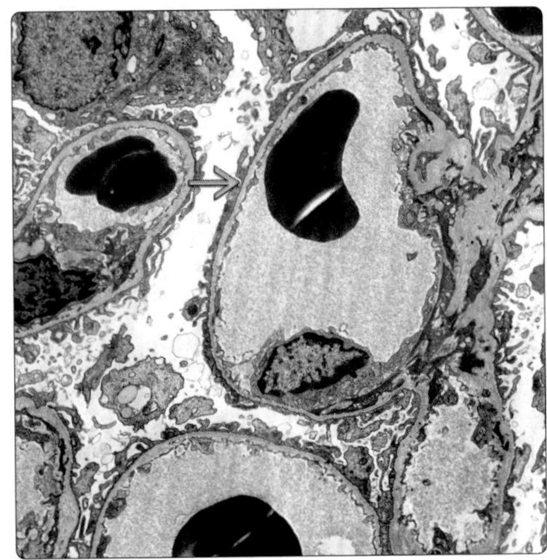

(Left) *IF can be contributory for some diseases, even in biopsies without glomeruli. This patient with acute renal failure had cast nephropathy with casts that stain for lambda ➡ but not kappa light chain.* **(Right)** *A woman underwent biopsy for a history of longstanding microscopic hematuria. By light microscopy and IF, the glomeruli were normal. Electron microscopy shows thin GBMs ➡ (mean: 240 nm). This diagnosis of thin GBM nephropathy cannot be made by EM on deparaffinized tissue due to thinning artifact.*

C4d Stain on Medulla

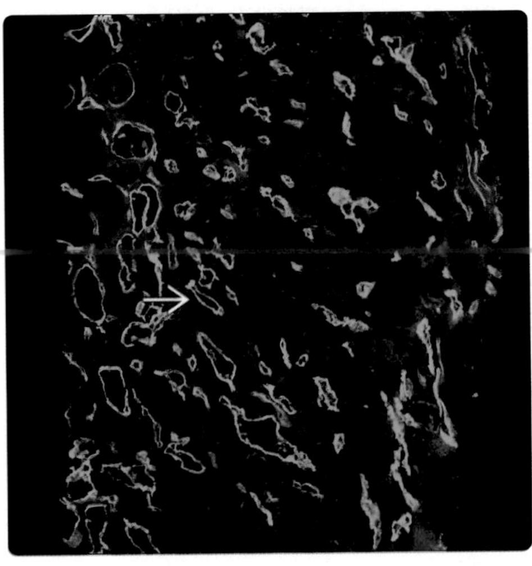

Alport Syndrome

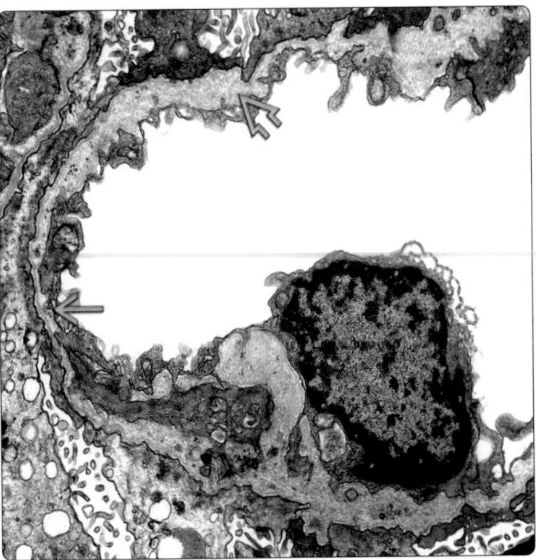

(Left) *C4d staining to evaluate humoral rejection can be interpreted on specimens with medulla and without glomeruli. In this case, there is diffuse bright peritubular capillary staining for C4d ➡.* **(Right)** *This biopsy is from a 13-year-old boy with a history of hematuria, mild proteinuria, and hearing loss. By EM, there is marked basement membrane thinning ➡ with lamellations or "basketweaving" ➡. This diagnosis is best made on tissue fixed in glutaraldehyde rather than on deparaffinized tissue.*

TERMINOLOGY

Definitions

- Interstitial fibrosis: Accumulation of collagen and related molecules in interstitium

VALUE

Prognosis

- Outcome of a wide variety of renal diseases correlates with extent of interstitial fibrosis, often even after a multivariate analysis
  - Studies show reciprocal correlation between kidney function and fibrosis extent
- In renal allografts, extent of fibrosis predicts outcome and may be considered a surrogate marker
  - Many applications have been reported
  - Fibrosis and tubular atrophy (IF/TA) have been associated with
    - Cold ischemia time
    - Clinical & subclinical acute rejection
    - Preexisting donor damage
    - Degree of sensitization
    - Cyclosporine exposure
    - Renal calcifications
  - IF/TA associated with transplant vasculopathy, ↑ serum creatinine, or transplant glomerulopathy implies poorer prognosis than IF/TA without additional lesions
- Fibrosis shows prognostic value in renal donor biopsies
  - ↑ risk of adverse outcome at 6 months
    - 1.9x greater prediction from age alone with Banff index for IF (ci score > 0)
  - Morphometric interstitial volume: Correlates with graft function at 1 year
- Protocol biopsies to assess fibrosis progression can demonstrate baseline state of allograft as well as stepwise changes that occur
  - Useful in clinical trials to assess outcome

MECHANISMS

Molecular Mediators

- Transforming growth factor (TGF)-β
- Bone morphogenetic protein (BMP)
- Platelet-derived growth factor (PDGF)
- Hepatocyte growth factor (HGF)
- Recent genomic approaches show altered molecular factors in IF

Cellular Mediators

- Epithelial cells
- Fibroblasts/myofibroblasts & fibrocytes
- Inflammatory cells: Lymphocytes, monocyte/macrophages, dendritic cells, mast cells
- Endothelial cells

Epithelial-to-Mesenchymal Phenotype (EMP)

- Chronically injured epithelial cells may undergo transition to mesenchymal cells
  - Process termed "epithelial-to-mesenchymal transition (EMT)" in past
  - So-called "EMT" may simply reflect change in protein expression rather than true transition
- Injured epithelium may change morphology and express mesenchymal-like markers, but actual EMT process not observed in vivo
- Mesenchymal markers are not entirely specific, making research questionable (per recent Banff conference and other publications)
  - "EMP" may be more appropriate since changes may simply be observation of altered phenotype

METHODS FOR ASSESSMENT

Qualitative Visual Assessment

- Not all fibrosis is "equal" or "same" in quality & quantity
  - "Early," "young," or "active" fibrosis may have greater potential for remodeling
  - Broad scars: Pyelonephritis & infarcts can produce severe focal injury & parenchymal destruction

Collagen III Immunohistochemistry

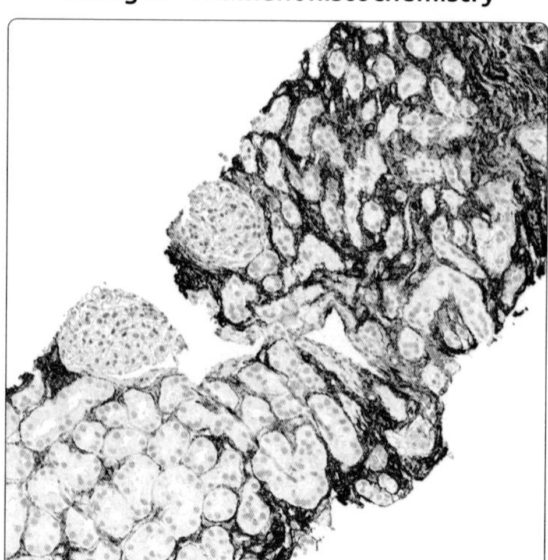

Collagen III Immunohistochemistry Quantitation "Markup"

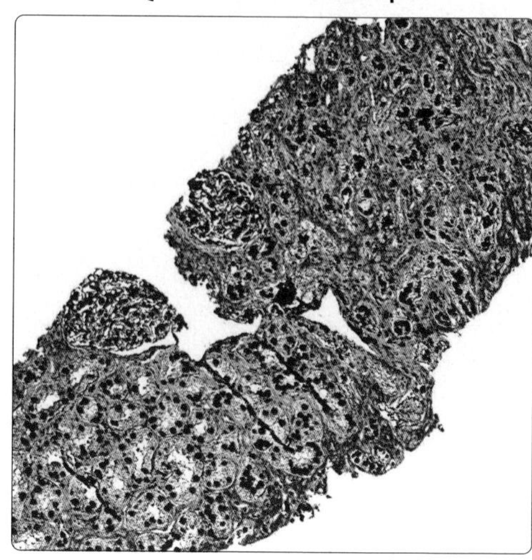

(Left) *Collagen III immunohistochemistry stains fibrous tissue brown.* **(Right)** *A positive pixel count algorithm is applied to the immunohistochemistry, and a "markup" image shows areas that are strongly positive (red), medium positive (orange), and negative (blue).*

- Diffuse, fine fibrosis: Diffuse disease of glomeruli, tubules, & vessels
- Fibrosis patterns may have different implications
  - "Striped," patchy fibrosis described with calcineurin inhibitor use, possibly due to preferential medullary ray involvement
  - Chronic obstructive pattern: Atubular glomeruli, dilated tubules, & intratubular Tamm-Horsfall protein casts with interstitial extravasation
- Inflammation in areas of IF noted to be adverse risk factor for renal disease progression
- Fibrosis and tubular atrophy (TA) typically correlate
  - TA may be profound in renal artery stenosis, with little or no accompanying fibrosis
  - IF/TA (graded I-III based on same cutoffs as ci) has replaced term "chronic allograft nephropathy (CAN)"
- Subcapsular, perivascular, & periglomerular fibrosis typically not included, but objective exclusionary criteria lacking
- Fibrosis assessment typically focuses on cortex, but many emphasize that medullary fibrosis also important

Quantitative Visual Assessment

- Most fibrosis scoring systems (notably Banff) based on quantitation of % of cortical parenchyma involved
  - Banff fibrosis [termed "**ci score**"] uses following cutoffs
    - ci0: ≤ 5%, ci1: 6-25%, ci2: 26-50%, ci3: > 50%
- Special stains
  - Trichrome
    - Visual assessment of trichrome-stained slides often standard practice
    - Stains glomerular and tubular basement membranes in addition to areas of fibrosis
  - Periodic acid-Schiff (PAS)
    - PAS stains glomerular & tubular basement membranes "hot pink" with less staining in interstitium
    - Trichrome also stains glomerular & tubular basement membranes; thus, assessment of stains such as PAS can take these basement membranes into account and allow pathologist to appreciate only interstitium
    - Morphometric methods used to "subtract" basement membranes from trichrome using PAS (so-called "trichrome-PAS" or "T-P" method)
  - Sirius red
    - Pink staining of most tissues under white light
    - Dye molecule intercalates into tertiary groove of collagen I & III
    - Collagen I & III strongly birefringent when observed under polarized light
      - Considered specific for these collagens
  - Collagen immunohistochemistry (IHC)
    - Collagen type III IHC particularly useful for assessing fibrosis in kidney
- Repeat biopsies may show different measured level of fibrosis, presumably due to sampling
  - 1 study estimated that repeat biopsies show decreased IF in 12% of cases
- Visual fibrosis assessment is susceptible to inter- & intraobserver variability
  - Some pathologists consistently overgrade & some undergrade
  - Kappa values (statistical measure of interobserver agreement) on order of 0.3-0.6 reported

Morphometric Quantitative Assessment

- Analysis in morphometric studies correlated with function (e.g., eGFR)
- Point counting techniques on static images traditionally utilized
- Computer-assisted morphometry has shown utility in analysis of variety of stains (e.g., trichrome, Sirius red, & collagen immunohistochemistry)
  - Many methods use pixel-counting algorithms (also called "positive pixel count algorithm")
    - Available algorithms supplied by commercial vendors & "open sources" (e.g., ImageJ provided by National Institutes of Health [NIH])
  - Customized algorithms written by individual researchers also employed
    - Kappa value of 0.68 compared to expert Banff quantification obtained with analysis method described by Meas-Yedid, Servais, et al
  - Methods currently utilize whole slide images as opposed to static images
- May provide more objective, reproducible measurement method

SELECTED REFERENCES

1. Farris AB et al: Banff fibrosis study: multicenter visual assessment and computerized analysis of interstitial fibrosis in kidney biopsies. Am J Transplant. 14(4):897-907, 2014
2. Haas M: Chronic allograft nephropathy or interstitial fibrosis and tubular atrophy: what is in a name? Curr Opin Nephrol Hypertens. 23(3):245-50, 2014
3. Farris AB et al: Renal interstitial fibrosis: mechanisms and evaluation. Curr Opin Nephrol Hypertens. 21(3):289-300, 2012
4. Farris AB et al: Morphometric and visual evaluation of fibrosis in renal biopsies. J Am Soc Nephrol. 22(1):176-86, 2011
5. Kriz W et al: Epithelial-mesenchymal transition (EMT) in kidney fibrosis: fact or fantasy? J Clin Invest. 121(2):468-74, 2011
6. Liu Y: Cellular and molecular mechanisms of renal fibrosis. Nat Rev Nephrol. 7(12):684-96, 2011
7. Meas-Yedid V et al: New computerized color image analysis for the quantification of interstitial fibrosis in renal transplantation. Transplantation. 92(8):890-9, 2011
8. Scian MJ et al: Gene expression changes are associated with loss of kidney graft function and interstitial fibrosis and tubular atrophy: diagnosis versus prediction. Transplantation. 91(6):657-65, 2011
9. Boor P et al: Renal fibrosis: novel insights into mechanisms and therapeutic targets. Nat Rev Nephrol. 6(11):643-56, 2010
10. Mannon RB et al: Inflammation in areas of tubular atrophy in kidney allograft biopsies: a potent predictor of allograft failure. Am J Transplant. 10(9):2066-73, 2010
11. Park WD et al: Fibrosis with inflammation at one year predicts transplant functional decline. J Am Soc Nephrol. 21(11):1987-97, 2010
12. Zeisberg M et al: Mechanisms of tubulointerstitial fibrosis. J Am Soc Nephrol. 21(11):1819-34, 2010
13. Serón D et al: Protocol biopsies in renal transplantation: prognostic value of structural monitoring. Kidney Int. 72(6):690-7, 2007
14. Furness PN et al: International variation in the interpretation of renal transplant biopsies: report of the CERTPAP Project. Kidney Int. 60(5):1998-2012, 2001
15. Marcussen N et al: Reproducibility of the Banff classification of renal allograft pathology. Inter- and intraobserver variation. Transplantation. 60(10):1083-9, 1995

(Left) *Medium-power view of trichrome of a wedge donor biopsy shows subcapsular fibrosis ➡ with chronic inflammation, a finding that is not uncommon.* **(Right)** *Higher power trichrome image shows the subcapsular fibrosis with chronic inflammation ➡ as well as segmental ➡ and global ➡ glomerulosclerosis.*

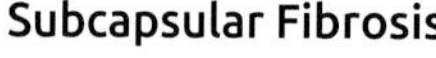

Subcapsular Fibrosis

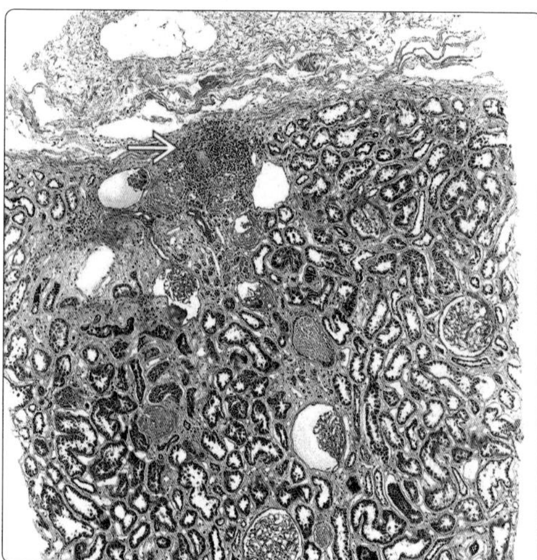

Subcapsular Fibrosis

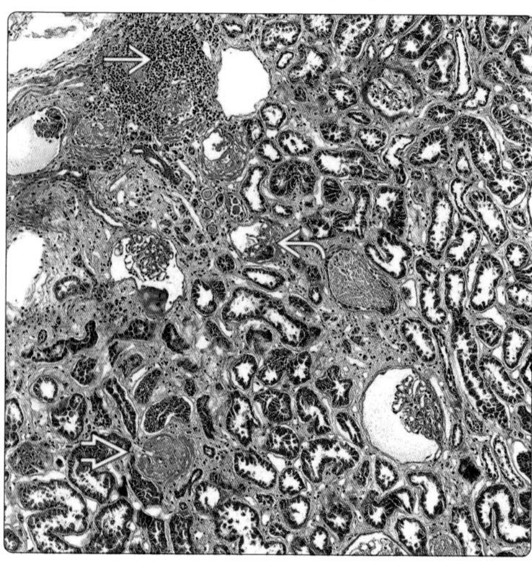

(Left) *Trichrome-stained kidney section from an autopsy of a patient with a history of lung transplantation and longstanding cyclosporine use shows prominent medullary ray fibrosis ➡, so-called "striped" fibrosis. (Courtesy S. Rosen, MD.)* **(Right)** *Two approaches for assessing fibrosis used by pathologists include (A) the percentage of tissue occupied by fibrous tissue and (B) the percentage of morphologically abnormal tissue.*

"Striped" Fibrosis

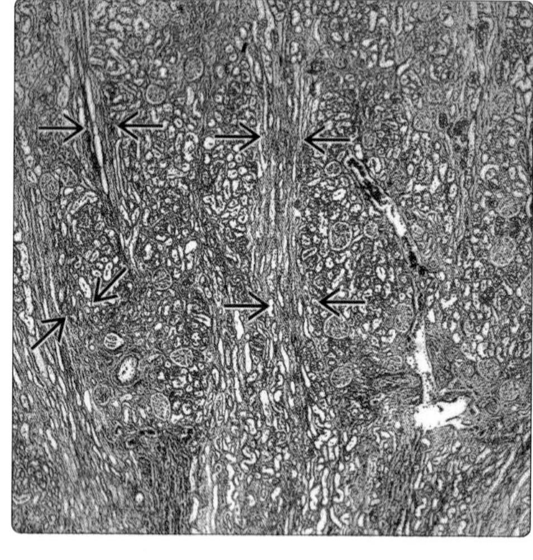

Fibrosis Quantitation Approaches Used by Pathologists

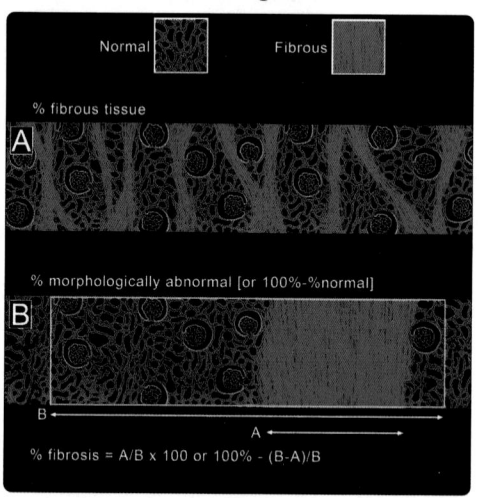

Normal

Fibrous

% fibrous tissue

A

% morphologically abnormal [or 100%-%normal]

B

B

A

% fibrosis = A/B x 100 or 100% - (B-A)/B

(Left) *A case with an essentially baseline level of fibrosis shows diffuse, fine fibrous tissue ➡ between the renal tubules on trichrome stain.* **(Right)** *Quantitation of the blue-staining areas of the trichrome stain is accomplished by using a positive pixel count algorithm tuned to the blue fibrous tissue. Markup image shows areas that are considered positive by the algorithm in orange, resulting in a measurement of the percentage of tissue involved by fibrosis.*

Fibrosis Level at Baseline

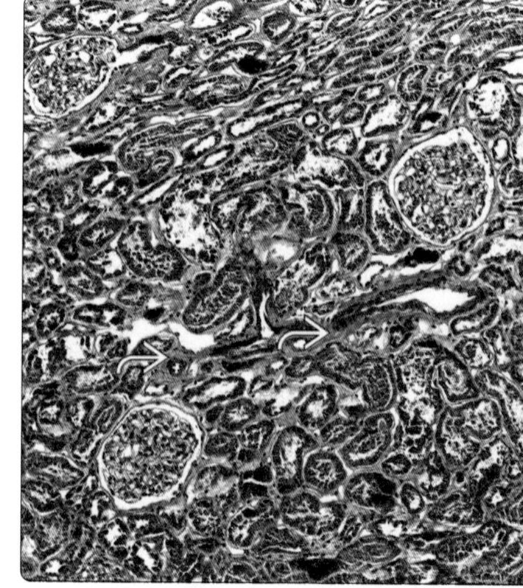

Quantitation "Markup" of Fibrosis at Baseline Level

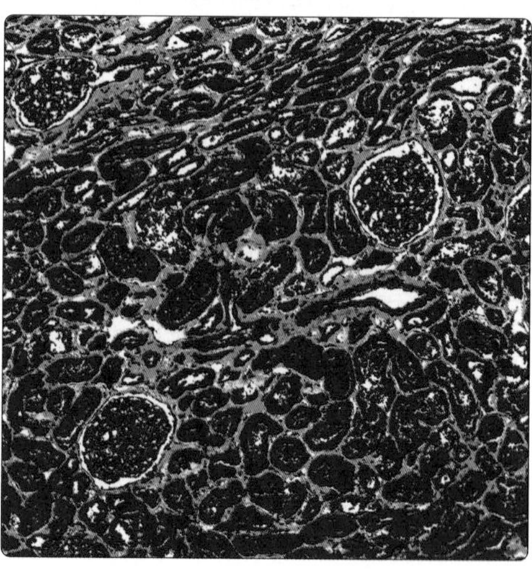

Trichrome and PAS in Fibrosis Assessment

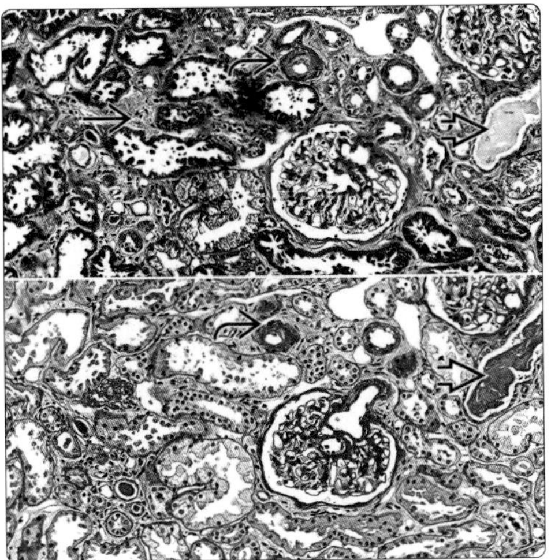

Quantitation "Markup" of Trichrome and PAS (T-P) in Fibrosis Assessment

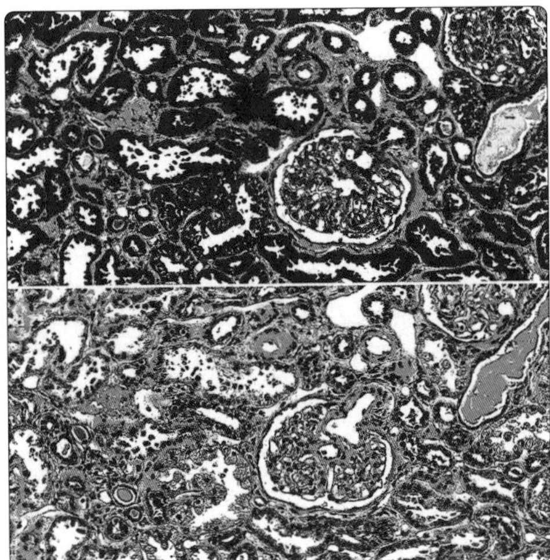

(Left) *Trichrome (upper half) stains focal areas of fibrous tissue* ➔*, basement membranes, vessels* ➔*, and proteinaceous casts* ➔*. The latter 3 can be subtracted through their detection on a PAS stain (lower half) to determine degree of fibrosis.* **(Right)** *Markup images detect areas (yellow, orange) on a positive pixel count algorithm tuned for blue on trichrome (upper half) & pink on PAS (lower half). Subtracting PAS from trichrome using so-called "Trichrome-PAS (T-P)" method gives a measurement of interstitium.*

Sirius Red Fibrosis Staining

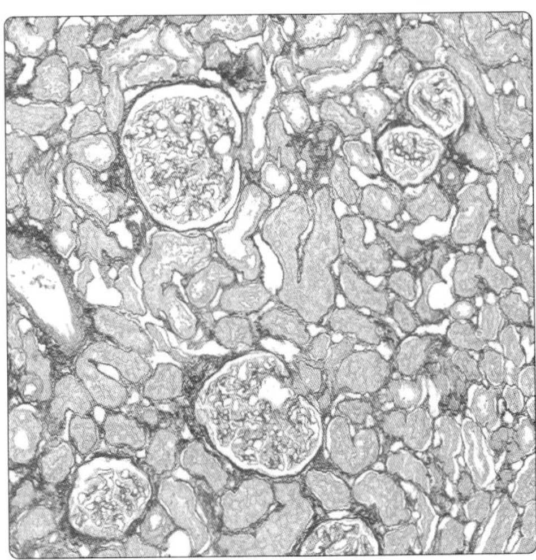

Sirius Red Fibrosis Areas Detected

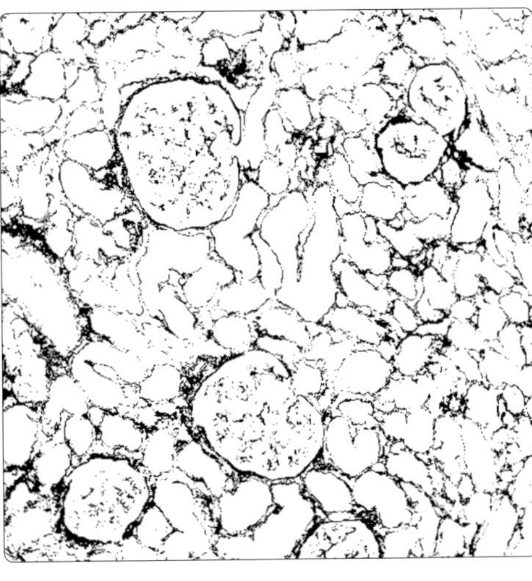

(Left) *Sirius red stains areas of fibrosis red.* **(Right)** *Detection of the red-staining areas on a Sirius red stain provides a measurement of the areas of fibrosis. The quantitation in this case is performed without polarization, and this markup image shows the areas considered positive in black, illustrating the fibrous tissue "skeleton" of the kidney. (Courtesy P. Grimm, MD.)*

Sirius Red Polarization Detects Fibrosis

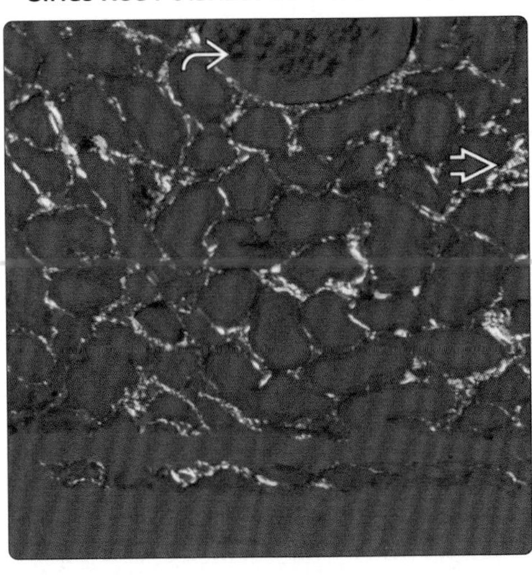

Sirius Red Polarized Fibrotic Areas Detected

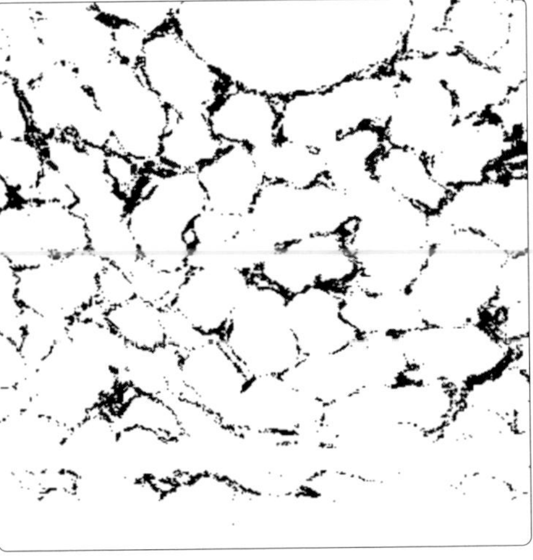

(Left) *Polarization of a Sirius red-stained kidney shows areas of fibrous tissue deposition. Note the absence of staining in the glomerular basement membrane* ➔*, demonstrating how the glomerular basement membrane is composed of collagen type IV as opposed to collagens type I and III in the interstitium. Interstitial fibrous tissue has a characteristic birefringence* ➔*.* **(Right)** *Markup image is used in the quantitation of the fibrous tissue birefringent on the Sirius red stain.*

TERMINOLOGY

Definitions

- Direct immunofluorescence (IF) performed on formalin-fixed, paraffin-embedded tissue
  - Different protocols may use EDTA-trypsin, pronase, or proteinase during digestion phase

DIAGNOSTIC VALUE

Limited Frozen Tissue

- Paraffin IF may be used as salvage method when insufficient frozen material is available
- Identify immune complex-mediated disorders or paraprotein-associated diseases

"Unmask" Occult Deposits

- Used when immunoglobulin components expected, but not detected in frozen tissue, typically in settings with monoclonal immunoglobulin
- Indications
  - Suspected C3 glomerulopathy in frozen section immunofluorescence
    - MPGN with monoclonal Ig deposits
    - Membranous-like glomerulopathy with masked IgG kappa deposits
  - Light chain proximal tubulopathy with crystals
  - Suspected light or heavy chain deposits by EM but negative IF
  - Cryoglobulinemia (type I or II)
  - Atypical pauci-immune crescentic glomerulonephritis

Application and Interpretation

- ~ 6% of native renal biopsies submitted to paraffin IF in largest series describing use of this technique
  - 68% for salvage, 32% for unmasking
- Most successful when applied against immunoglobulins heavy and light chains
  - C3 staining through paraffin IF is not reliable
- Paraffin IF should not be used for diagnosis of anti-GBM disease, as it tends to have heavy background
  - May lead to false-positive results
- Interpretation of paraffin IF requires experience
  - Plasma in capillary loops can stain positively
    - Should not be interpreted as positive result

PROTOCOLS

Proteinase K Method

- Cut 3 mm serial sections on organosilane-coated slides
- Oven dry at 37°C overnight (or at 60°C for 15 min)
- Deparaffinize: Xylene for 10 min (2), ethanol 100% for 5 min (2), 95% for 5 min
- Wash in distilled water (20 dips)
- Rinse in EnVision Flex Wash Buffer (Dako)
- Incubate with Proteinase K (Dako) 20 min
- Incubate in wet chamber at 40°C 30 min with FITC-labeled antibodies (Dako)
- Rinse with PBS 40° C for 10 min
- Mount in aqueous mounting media and examine under fluorescence microscope

EDTA-Trypsin Method

- Cut paraffin tissue section at 2 μm
- Air dry slides for 20 min at 60-80° C
- Deparaffinize as above
- Digest with 0.25% trypsin-EDTA for 90 min at 37°C
- Wash 5x with distilled water and place in PBS 5 min
- Stain with FITC-conjugated antibodies (IgG, IgA, IgM, kappa, lambda, or albumin; 1:10 dilution) 1 hr in moist chamber
- Wash in PBS for 1 min
- Coverslip and examine above

SELECTED REFERENCES

1. Messias NC et al: Paraffin immunofluorescence in the renal pathology laboratory: more than a salvage technique. Mod Pathol. ePub, 2015
2. Larsen CP et al: Membranous-like glomerulopathy with masked IgG kappa deposits. Kidney Int. 86(1):154-61, 2014
3. Nasr SH et al: Immunofluorescence on pronase-digested paraffin sections: a valuable salvage technique for renal biopsies. Kidney Int. 70(12):2148-51, 2006

Membranous Nephropathy With No Glomeruli on Frozen Sections

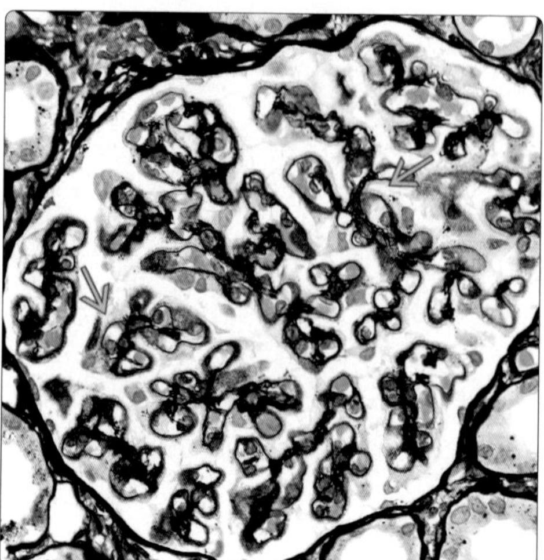

Paraffin IF Used as Salvage Technique

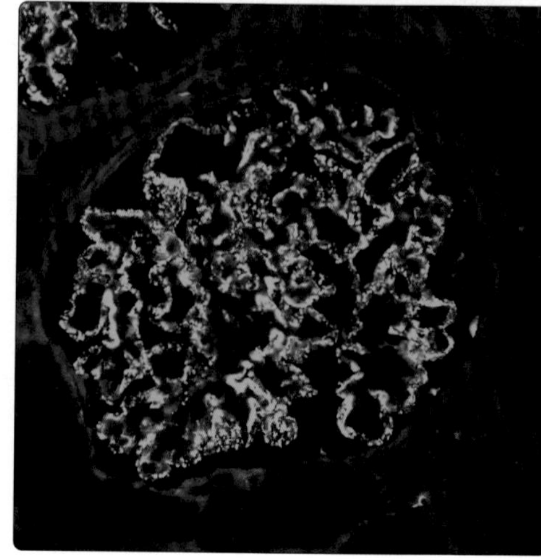

(Left) *Glomerulus in a case of membranous nephropathy shows "spikes" ⇒ on silver stain. The case did not have glomeruli on frozen sections submitted for IF.* **(Right)** *Paraffin IF was used as a salvage technique and made a significant contribution to the diagnosis. Granular capillary loop deposits are shown on paraffin immunofluorescence for IgG, following protease digestion.*

Proliferative Glomerulonephritis With Masked Immune Deposits

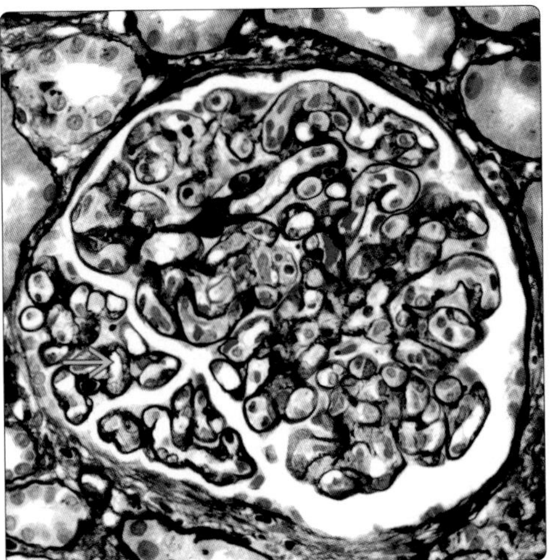

Subendothelial Deposits on EM

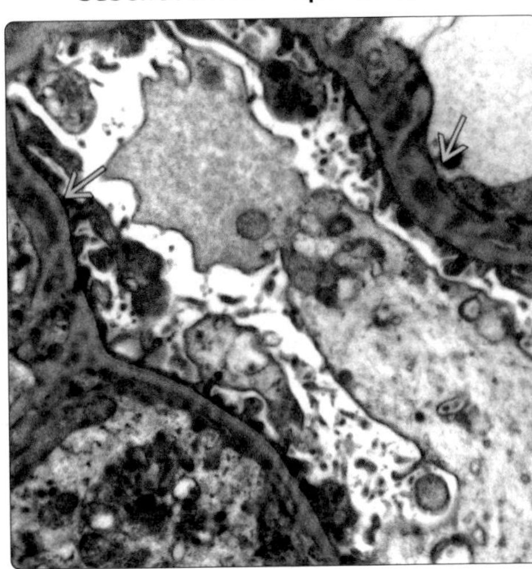

(Left) *Proliferative glomerulonephritis with membranoproliferative features is shown in a case of cryoglobulinemic GN. Note duplication of the GBM ⇒. There is also global endocapillary hypercellularity. Paraffin IF in this case revealed masked immune complex deposits.* **(Right)** *Electron microscopy evaluation demonstrates subendothelial electron-dense deposits and duplication of the basement membranes ⇒ in the same patient.*

Negative IgG on Frozen Sections

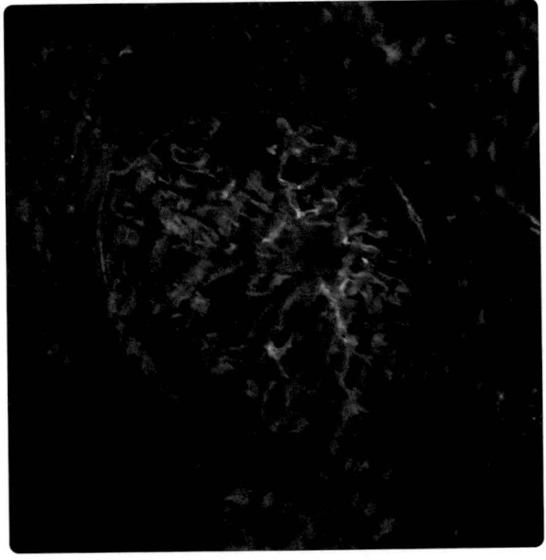

Paraffin IF Positive for IgG

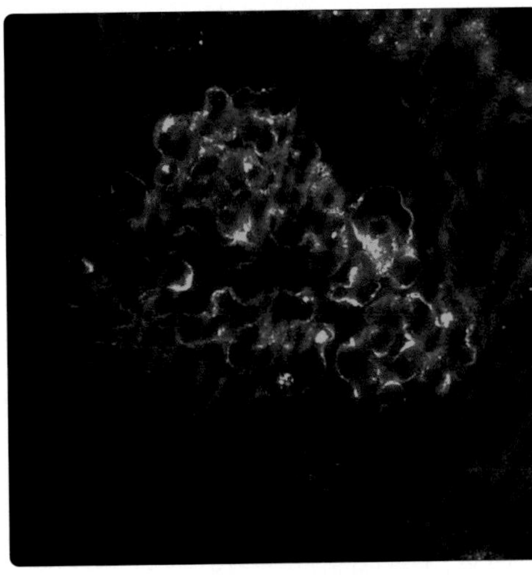

(Left) *IgG performed on frozen section in the same patient shows no significant immunofluorescence detected. As the case had proliferative features and deposits on EM, paraffin IF was performed.* **(Right)** *Paraffin immunofluorescence for IgG following protease digestion is shown in the same patient. Mesangial and capillary loop deposits may be observed, confirming electron microscopy findings.*

False-Positive IgA Stain

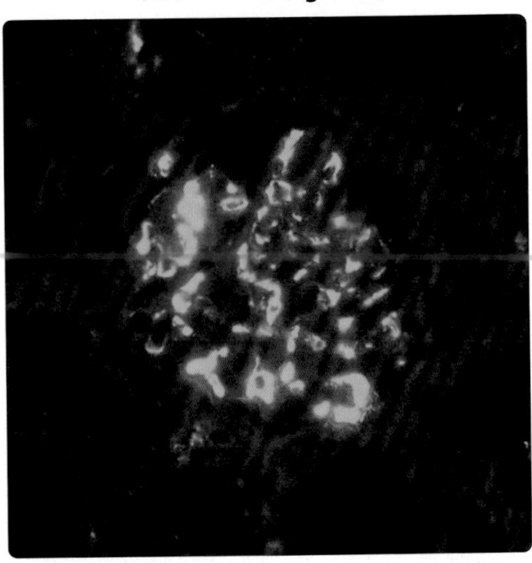

False-Positive IgG Stain

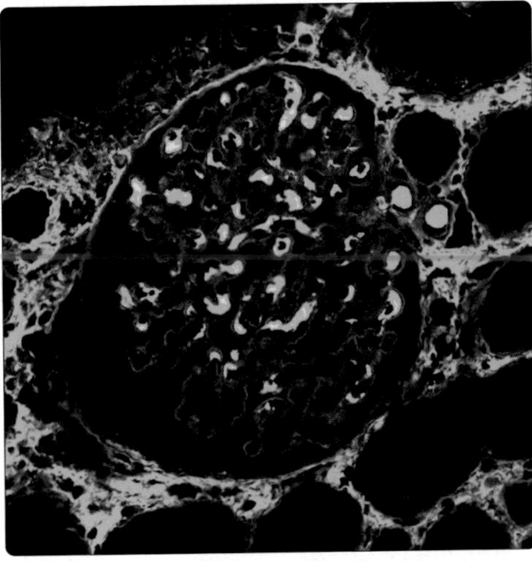

(Left) *Serum within capillary loops may be mistaken for immune-type deposits and lead to erroneous interpretation and false-positive diagnosis. This example illustrates IgA, in which this phenomenon is often observed.* **(Right)** *Serum within capillary loops may be seem with all immunoglobulins, including IgG as in this case.*

TERMINOLOGY

Definitions

- Formalin-fixed paraffin-embedded (FFPE) tissue reprocessed for electron microscopy (EM)

Synonyms

- "Rescued" material, salvage technique

CLINICAL IMPLICATIONS

Utility

- When it is realized too late that EM is needed for diagnosis
- If higher magnification desired for cells seen on light microscopy
  - To look for immune-type deposits
  - To investigate whether inclusions are viral
  - To identify other microbial organisms (e.g., bacteria, parasites, fungus, etc.)
- If specific item of interest (e.g., inclusions, cells, etc.) is rare
  - May be difficult to obtain in small amount of material submitted for EM when specimen divided in random manner

MACROSCOPIC

Specimen Handling

- Based on anecdotal experience, order of preference for obtaining tissue for EM is
  - Tissue immediately into glutaraldehyde or Karnovsky fixative
  - Well-fixed tissue saved in formalin
  - Paraffin-embedded tissue
  - Frozen-embedded tissue
- Obtaining material
  - FFPE block examined in conjunction with light microscopy (hematoxylin & eosin [H&E]) slide
    - Preferably compared to last section cut from block
  - Area of interest is cut from paraffin block and put in vial

PROTOCOLS

"Pop-Off" Technique

- Used for EM of precise areas from stained sections of paraffin-embedded tissue
- Decoverslipped paraffin section "popped-off" after heating on 100° C hot plate for 15 seconds
  - Another technique involves immersion removal of cover glass overnight by immersion in xylene
    - Likely gentler and preferable
- "Popping-off" takes place into inverted Been capsule containing polymerized epoxy resin

Processing FFPE Material for EM

- Includes following, which integrates several methods in literature
- Paraffin removed by xylene immersion (dewaxing)
  - Instead of xylene, chloroform sometimes used
  - Some advocate heating to melt paraffin
    - In 60° C oven for 30 min
- Rehydrated in decreasing alcohol concentrations to buffer
  - Xylene
  - 100% ethanol
  - 95% ethanol
  - 80% ethanol
    - Afterwards, some wash and soak in cacodylate buffer (0.1 M pH 7.4) for couple of hours or phosphate buffer (0.1 M) for 10 minutes
- Material cut into 1 mm cubes
- Postfixed in osmium tetroxide (1% buffered aqueous)
- Dehydrated through graded alcohols
  - 50%, 70%, 80%, 90%, 95%, 100%
  - After this, some specify propylene oxide step
- Embed for electron microscopy
  - In Epon Araldite or Epox 812
- Sectioning and staining
  - Semithin sections cut in usual way
    - 1 μm "thick" survey sections cut with ultramicrotome using glass knife

Immune-Type Deposits on Material Originally in Paraffin

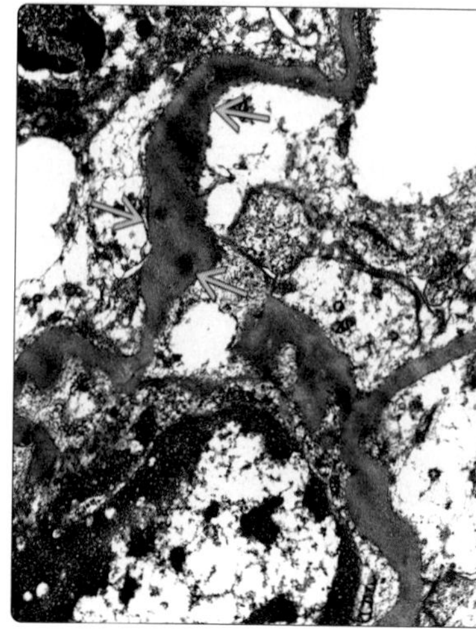

Tubuloreticular Inclusions on Material Originally Frozen

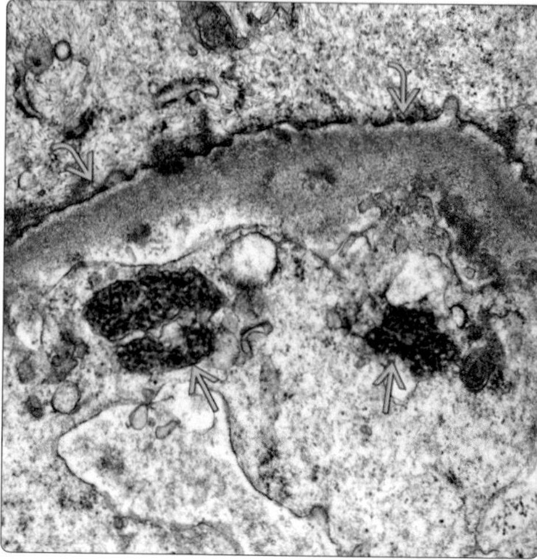

(Left) *Immune-type deposits* ➡ *could be identified after EM was performed on material originally embedded in paraffin. This was a case of ANCA-associated necrotizing, crescentic GN; however, the deposits prompted consideration of an infection.* **(Right)** *After EM on material frozen for immunofluorescence, tubuloreticular inclusions* ➡ *could be identified in addition to extensive podocyte foot process effacement* ➡ *in this case of diffuse proliferative lupus nephritis (ISN/RPS class IV-S [A]).*

- Toluidine blue staining performed (e.g., with 1% toluidine blue) and compared to H&E to relocate area of interest
- Ultrathin sections cut with diamond knife, mounted on copper grids, stained (e.g., with uranyl acetate in 70% alcohol and lead citrate), and examined with EM

Processing Frozen Tissue for EM

- Thaw in standard glutaraldehyde/paraformaldehyde fixative ~ 4 hr
- Dice into 1-2 mm fragments
- Wash in cacodylate buffer
- Proceed from osmication step above

Low-Vacuum Scanning Electron Microscopy (LV-SEM)

- Provides another alternative for performing EM on paraffin-embedded sections
- Also useful for glutaraldehyde-osmium tetroxide-fixed epoxy resin sections
- LV-SEM is used in backscattered electron (BSE) mode
- Can evaluate 3-dimensional ultrastructural changes of glomerulus and extracellular matrix
- Sections stained with periodic acid silver-methenamine (PAM) or platinum blue (Pt-blue) have typically been used
- Can achieve magnifications on the order of 10,000x
- Can visualize deposits in immune complex glomerulonephritis (e.g., membranous glomerulonephritis and IgA nephropathy)
- Can identify basement membrane irregularities (e.g., in Alport syndrome)
- Available in only limited number of centers

Immunoelectron Microscopy

- Has been used on paraffin-embedded biopsies
- Inferior to conventional methods (immediate fixation in paraformaldehyde with low concentration of glutaraldehyde and embedding in LR Gold)
- Gold particles can still be examined with reasonable confidence in localization

MICROSCOPIC

Retrieved Material

- Initial techniques involved slow processing by soaking in changes of xylene for up to 1 week
  - Resulted in loss of most structures
    - Except for hardy intermediate filaments, desmosomes, and viral particles
  - Structures such as sarcomeres and melanosomes reasonably well preserved
- More rapid techniques eventually developed
  - Found better results if tissue properly fixed in formaldehyde, dehydrated, and cleared
  - Fine structures sometimes altered only minimally
  - As well as viral particles, additional structures retain detail (e.g., secretory granules, zymogen granules, desmosomes, tonofilaments, and neuroendocrine granules)
  - Immune deposits can still be identified
  - Foot process effacement degree can still sometimes be assessed

Glomerular Basement Membrane (GBM) Width

- Thin basement membrane nephropathy (TBMN) diagnosis compromised on deparaffinized, formalin-fixed tissue
  - GBM thickness reduced in deparaffinized FFPE tissue compared to glutaraldehyde-fixed, plastic resin-embedded tissue
    - e.g., 23% reduction of TBMN cases vs. 40% normal/minimal change disease cases vs. 34% for diabetic nephropathy cases
      - Some normal/minimal change disease cases would erroneously fall into TBMN category

Virus-Like Particles

- Particles that look like virus can be difficult to distinguish from true viruses

Cytoplasmic Organelles

- Can still visualize a variety of organelles such as mitochondria and vesicles as well as nucleus
  - Mitochondrial cristae can sometimes be difficult to assess
  - Example: Utility demonstrated in distinguishing renal tumors in which oncocytomas have numerous mitochondria and chromophobe renal cell carcinomas have numerous intracytoplasmic vesicles
- Aggregates of a few dense bodies can be difficult to distinguish from lysosomes or secretory granules

SELECTED REFERENCES

1. Masuda Y et al: Glomerular basement membrane injuries in IgA nephropathy evaluated by double immunostaining for α5(IV) and α2(IV) chains of type IV collagen and low-vacuum scanning electron microscopy. Clin Exp Nephrol. ePub, 2014
2. Okada S et al: A novel approach to the histological diagnosis of pediatric nephrotic syndrome by low vacuum scanning electron microscopy. Biomed Res. 35(4):227-36, 2014
3. Miyazaki H et al: Application of low-vacuum scanning electron microscopy for renal biopsy specimens. Pathol Res Pract. 208(9):503-9, 2012
4. Inaga S et al: Rapid three-dimensional analysis of renal biopsy sections by low vacuum scanning electron microscopy. Arch Histol Cytol. 73(3):113-25, 2010
5. Johnson NB et al: Use of electron microscopy in core biopsy diagnosis of oncocytic renal tumors. Ultrastruct Pathol. 34(4):189-94, 2010
6. Lighezan R et al: The value of the reprocessing method of paraffin-embedded biopsies for transmission electron microscopy. Rom J Morphol Embryol. 50(4):613-7, 2009
7. Nasr SH et al: Thin basement membrane nephropathy cannot be diagnosed reliably in deparaffinized, formalin-fixed tissue. Nephrol Dial Transplant. 22(4):1228-32, 2007
8. Dingemans KP et al: Immunoelectron microscopy on material retrieved from paraffin: accurate sampling on the basis of stained paraffin sections. Ultrastruct Pathol. 25(3):201-6, 2001
9. Collar J et al: Paraffin-processed material is unsuitable for diagnosis of thin-membrane disease. Nephron. 69(2):187-8, 1995
10. Ogiyama Y et al: Electron microscopic examination of cutaneous lesions by the quick re-embedding method from paraffin-embedded blocks. J Cutan Pathol. 21(3):239-46, 1994
11. Widéhn S et al: A rapid and simple method for electron microscopy of paraffin-embedded tissue. Ultrastruct Pathol. 12(1):131-6, 1988
12. Wang NS et al: The formaldehyde-fixed and paraffin-embedded tissues for diagnostic transmission electron microscopy: a retrospective and prospective study. Hum Pathol. 18(7):715-27, 1987
13. van den Bergh Weerman MA et al: Rapid deparaffinization for electron microscopy. Ultrastruct Pathol. 7(1):55-7, 1984
14. Bretschneider A et al: "Pop-off" technic. The ultrastructure of paraffin-embedded sections. Am J Clin Pathol. 76(4):450-3, 1981
15. Johannessen JV: Use of paraffin material for electron microscopy. Pathol Annu. 12 Pt 2:189-224, 1977

TERMINOLOGY

Abbreviations

- Phospholipase A2 receptor (PLA2R)

Definitions

- Autoantibodies against PLA2R: Most common etiology of primary membranous glomerulonephritis (MGN)

CLINICAL VALUE

Tissue Stain to Identify PLA2R-Associated MGN

- Positive stain in ~ 75% of adults with primary MGN
- Positive in ~ 45% of pediatric MGN
- Positive in 83% of recurrent vs. 8% of de novo MGN
- Good agreement between tissue stain and circulating antibodies
  - Glomerular PLA2R deposits can be present in seronegative patients, probably due to absorption of circulating anti-PLA2R

Monitoring Disease Activity by Serum Testing for PLA2R Autoantibodies in MGN

- PLA2R autoantibody levels decreased in patients with spontaneous remission but not in those without remission
- Antibody status after treatment predictive of long-term outcome
  - Independent risk factor for not achieving remission
- Positive serology can first become detectable after onset of MGN

PROTOCOLS

Formalin-Fixed Paraffin-Embedded Tissue

- Cut 3 μm thick section; deparaffinize
- Enzyme pretreatment with proteinase K, 30min
- Rabbit polyclonal anti-PLA2R1 antibody (Sigma-Aldrich), 1:50 (diluted in PBS), 30min
- Alexa Fluor 488 goat anti-rabbit IgG (Life Technologies), 1:100 (diluted in PBS), 30min
- Cover slip with aqueous mounting media
- PBS rinse between above steps, all at room temperature
- Interpretation
  - Positive PLA2R staining is a granular GBM pattern identical to IgG
  - Positive interpreted as PLA2R-associated MGN
  - Negative control (anti-rabbit IgG only) compared to ensure that staining not due to secondary antibody
  - FFPE has less background PLA2R staining than fresh tissue and is easier to interpret with a single stain

Double Stain on Frozen Tissue

- Cut 3 frozen sections 2-4 μm in thickness
  - For IgG4 + PLA2R, IgG + PLA2R, and PBS control
  - Air dry slides for 30 min
- 150 μL Avidin D 100 μg/mL in PBS) pre-block for 20 min (Vector Labs)
- 150 μL d-biotin 10 μg/mL in PBS) pre-block for 20 min (Sigma-Aldrich)
- 150 μL rabbit anti-PLA2R1 antibody diluted 1:50 for 1 hour (Sigma-Aldrich)
  - Omit from PBS control
- 150 μL biotinylated anti-rabbit IgG (H&L) diluted 1:100 for 45 min
- 150 μL Cy3 Streptavidin (GE Healthcare) diluted 1:6,000 for 45 min
- 150 μL anti-human IgG4-FITC antibody diluted 1:50 to IgG4 + PLA2R slide and anti-human IgG-FITC 1:30 to IgG + PLA2R slide and incubate for 1 hour
- Cover slip with Aqua-Mount
- Wash in PBS (3x over 2-3 min) between above steps
- Interpretation
  - Positive colocalization of PLA2R and IgG or IgG4 manifested by yellow fluorescence of deposits
  - Can be morphometrically analyzed in digital images for % co-localization of IgG with PLA2R
    - Serologically positive cases have 79±17% colocalization (52-100%; n=18) (A.B. Collins, unpublished)
  - Compare with PBS negative control and a concurrent positive control

Serological Tests for PLA2R Antibodies

- PLA2R transfected cell line
  - Substrate for test is human embryonic kidney cell line (HEK293) transfected with human PLA2R cDNA grown in biochips with multiple chambers (Euroimmun)
    - Non-transfected HEK293 cells serve as controls
  - 30 μL of patient's serum diluted 1:10 in PBS-tween added to test and control well; incubate 30 min
  - Add 25 μL FITC-goat anti-human IgG, incubate 30 min
  - PBS-Tween 20 wash for 5 min between steps
  - Add mounting medium and cover slip
  - All steps at room temperature
  - Examine with fluorescence microscope at 400x
  - Interpretation
    - Positive result is strong fluorescence staining of transfected cells compared with control cells
- ELISA (Euroimmun)
  - Plates coated with PLA2R
  - Standard ELISA assay as per manufacturer
  - Interpretation
    - Results given as relative units (RU)
    - Threshold as per manufacturer
      - Positive ≥ 20 RU/mL, Borderline ≥ 14 to < 20 RU/mL
      - Sensitivity 96%, specificity 99.9%
    - Quantitative, useful for following therapy response

SELECTED REFERENCES

1. VanBeek C et al: Anti-PLA2R-associated membranous nephropathy: a review with emphasis on diagnostic testing methods. Clin Nephrol. ePub, 2015
2. Hoxha E et al: Phospholipase A2 receptor autoantibodies and clinical outcome in patients with primary membranous nephropathy. J Am Soc Nephrol. 25(6):1357-66, 2014
3. Behnert A et al: An anti-phospholipase A2 receptor quantitative immunoassay and epitope analysis in membranous nephropathy reveals different antigenic domains of the receptor. PLoS One. 8(4):e61669, 2013
4. Larsen CP et al: Determination of primary versus secondary membranous glomerulopathy utilizing phospholipase A2 receptor staining in renal biopsies. Mod Pathol. 26(5):709-15, 2013
5. Hoxha E et al: Enhanced expression of the M-type phospholipase A2 receptor in glomeruli correlates with serum receptor antibodies in primary membranous nephropathy. Kidney Int. 82(7):797-804, 2012
6. Beck LH Jr et al: M-type phospholipase A2 receptor as target antigen in idiopathic membranous nephropathy. N Engl J Med. 361(1):11-21, 2009

PLA2R Deposits in MGN

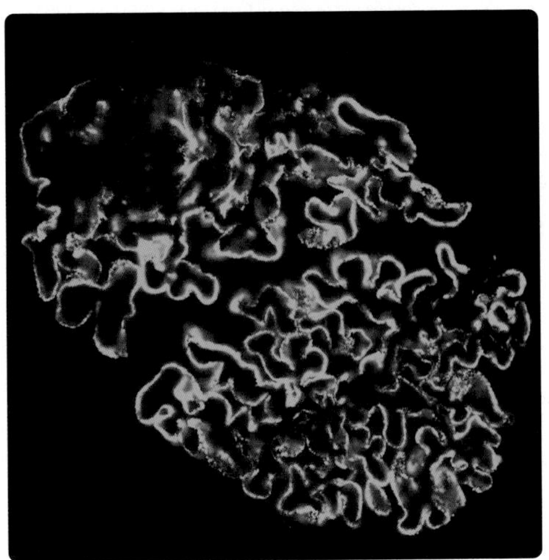

Negative PLA2R Deposits in MGN

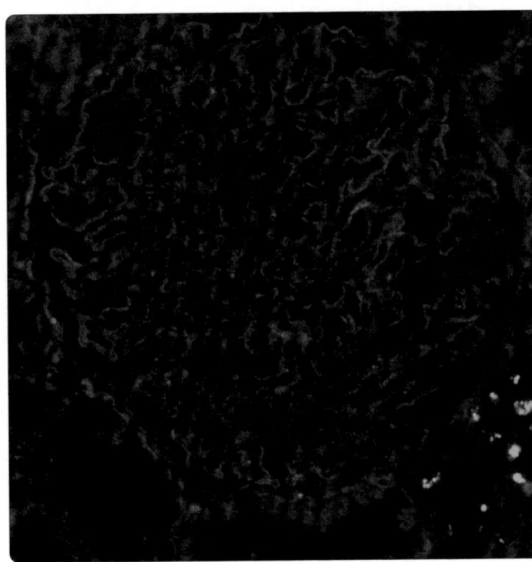

(Left) *Glomerulus from formalin-fixed paraffin-embedded tissue shows strong granular capillary loop staining by PLA2R.* **(Right)** *Negative PLA2R staining in a glomerulus from formalin-fixed paraffin-embedded tissue is shown. The patient had idiopathic membranous glomerulopathy. Approximately 25% of idiopathic membranous cases will stain negative for PLA2R.*

Colocalization of PLA2R and IgG4

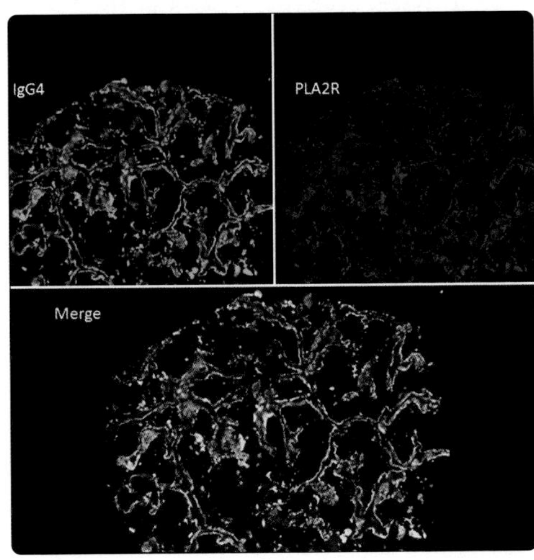

No Colocalization of PLA2R and IgG4

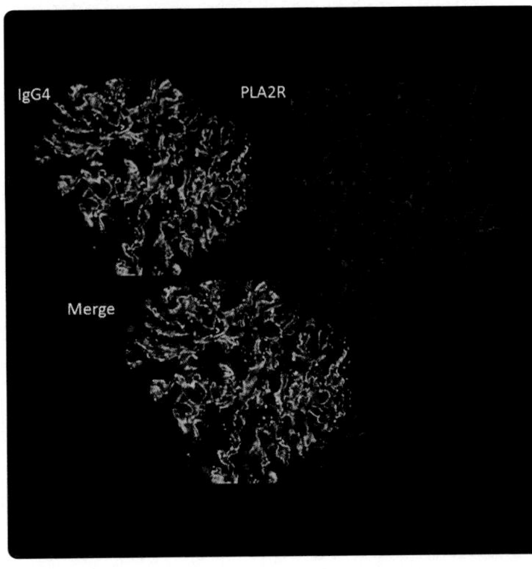

(Left) *Double stain with anti-IgG4-FITC (green) and anti-PLA2R-Cy3 (red) shows the granular deposits of PLA2R co-localize with IgG4 in the merged image, giving a yellow color. This is diagnostic of anti-PLA2R related MGN* **(Right)** *Double stain with anti-IgG4-FITC (green) and anti-PLA2R-Cy3 (red) shows the granular deposits of PLA2R do not co-localize with IgG4 in the merged image. This patient was suspected of having SLE, although the serologies for ANA and dsDNA were negative.*

Positive MGN Serum Staining HEK293 Cells

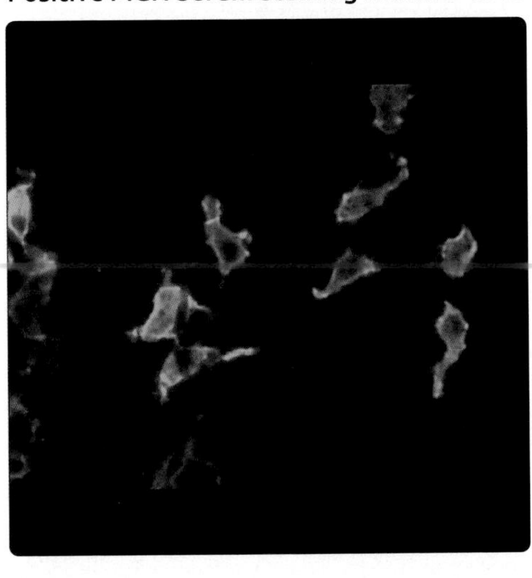

Negative Patient Serum on HEK293 Cells

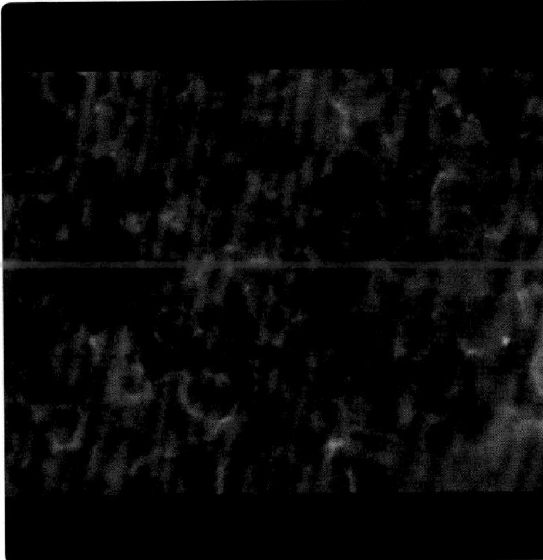

(Left) *Primary MGN serum shows positive staining by indirect immunofluorescence on HEK293 cells on BIOCHIPS (Euroimmun) transfected with a recombinant construct of PLA2R.* **(Right)** *Serum tested by indirect immunofluorescence on HEK293 cells on BIOCHIPS (Euroimmun) transfected with a recombinant construct of PLA2R shows a negative result.*

TERMINOLOGY

Basement Membrane Type IV Collagen

- 3 α chains form triple helix which dimerize via C terminal noncollagenous domain 1 (NC1)
  - 4 dimers cross-link via disulfide bonds at N terminus
  - 6 α chains assembled in 3 matrices
    - α1(IV), α2(IV)
      - In most basement membranes (BM) of endothelium and epithelium, also mesangium as α1.α1.α2(IV)-α1.α1.α2(IV)
      - *COL4A1* and *COL4A2* on chromosome 13q34
    - α3(IV), α4(IV), α5(IV)
      - Principal type in glomerular BM, distal tubule BM, alveolar BM, cochlea, and lens as α3.α4.α5(IV)-α3.α4.α5(IV)
      - *COL4A3* and *COL4A4* on chromosome 2q35-37; *COL4A5* on chromosome X
    - α5(IV), α6(IV)
      - In Bowman capsule, collecting duct, smooth muscle, and epidermal BM as α1.α1.α2(IV)-α5.α5.α6(IV)
      - *COL4A5* and *COL4A6* on chromosome X

IMMUNOFLUORESCENCE TECHNIQUE

Kidney

- Frozen sections 2-4 μm; fix in acetone 10 min
- Denature α5(IV) section in 0.1M glycine/6.0M urea, pH 3.5 solution at 2-8° C for 10 min
- Incubate with 1° antibodies for 1 hr, room temp (RT)
  - MAB1 mouse monoclonal antibody to NC1 α1(IV); 1:25 dilution
  - MAB3 mouse monoclonal antibody to NC1 α3(IV); 1:25 dilution
  - MAB5 rat monoclonal antibody to NC1 α1(IV); 1:50 dilution
  - Source: Wieslab (Thermo-Fisher)
- 2nd antibody
  - Anti-mouse FITC (1:50) (MAB1, 3), 1 hr, RT
  - Anti-rat biotinylated (1:50) (MAB5), 30 min, RT
- Third incubation (MAB5)
  - FITC-streptavidin (1:50), 30 min, RT
- Wash between steps with PBS (2 min x 3)

Skin

- Frozen sections stained in same manner and epidermal BM scored for expression of α5(IV)

IHC Alternative

- Paraffin sections after antigen retrieval using rat monoclonal antibodies that recognize α2 and α5 chains (H22 and H52) (Hashimura 2014)

INTERPRETATION

Staining Pattern Compared With Normal Control

- Diffuse ↓ α3(IV) and α5(IV) in GBM: Homozygotic *COL4A3/4* or male *COL4A5* mutation
- Loss of α5(IV) in Bowman capsule or skin BM: Male *COL4A5* or female homozygotic *COL4A5* mutation
- Segmental ↓ α3(IV) and α5(IV) in GBM: *COL4A5* heterozygote

Correlations

- Segmental or absent α3(IV) in GBM have earlier onset of proteinuria and ESRD compared with diffuse α3 (IV)

Pitfalls

- False negative
  - Nontruncating or somatic mutations in *COL4A5* may have normal staining
  - Overall 20-30% of males with *COL4A5* mutations
- False positive
  - Poor antigenic preservation
    - Detected by loss of normal α1(IV) staining

SELECTED REFERENCES

1. Hashimura Y et al: Milder clinical aspects of X-linked Alport syndrome in men positive for the collagen IV α5 chain. Kidney Int. 85(5):1208-13, 2014
2. Massella L et al: Prognostic value of glomerular collagen IV immunofluorescence studies in male patients with X-linked Alport syndrome. Clin J Am Soc Nephrol. 8(5):749-55, 2013

Normal Glomerular α(IV)

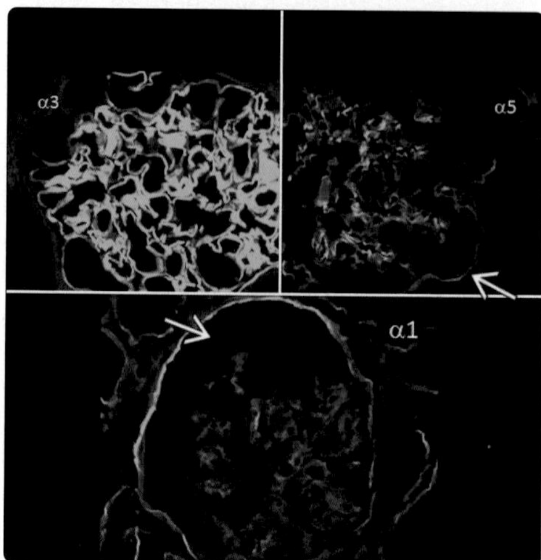

X-Linked Alport Syndrome α(IV)

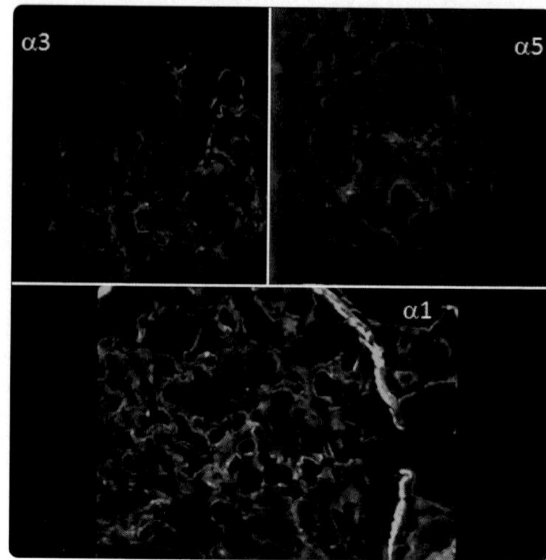

(Left) *The normal glomerular basement membrane (GBM) stains in a linear pattern for α3(IV) and α5(IV). Bowman capsule stains only for α5(IV)* ➡*. α1(IV) is present in Bowman capsule, tubular basement membrane, and the mesangium.* **(Right)** *In men with X-linked Alport syndrome (COL4A5), ~ 70% have complete loss of staining for α3(IV) and α5(IV) in the GBM and loss of α5(IV) from Bowman capsule. This is typical of truncating or nonsense mutations. α1(IV) can be increased in the GBM compared with normals.*

X-Linked Alport Syndrome in Male

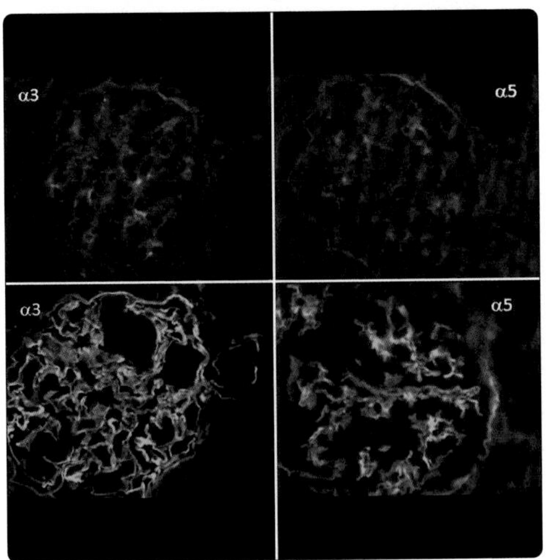

Autosomal Recessive Alport Syndrome

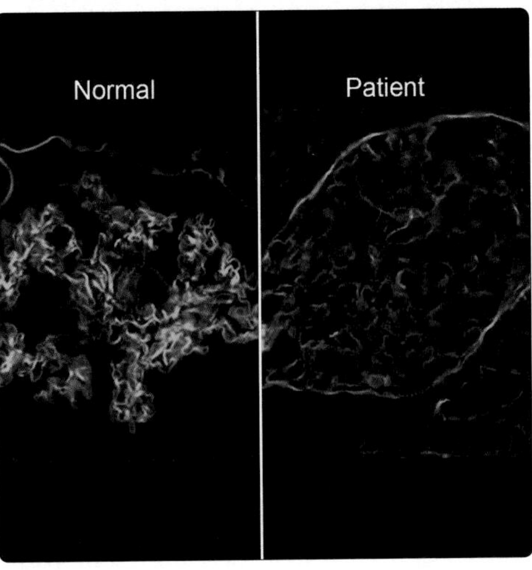

(Left) *This is a biopsy from a 3-year-old boy with hematuria. Markedly reduced staining for a3(IV) is seen in the GBM and TBM and reduced a5(IV) in the GBM and Bowman capsule compared to the concurrent control in the lower row.* **(Right)** *The characteristic findings in autosomal recessive Alport syndrome (due to mutations in COL4A3 or COL4A4 genes) are the loss of a5(IV) from the GBM and preservation in Bowman capsule and collecting ducts.*

X-Linked Alport Syndrome in Female

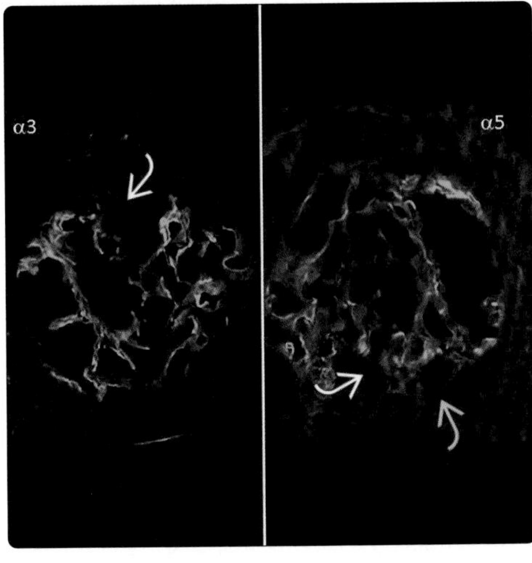

Segmental Loss of a5(IV) in Distal TBM

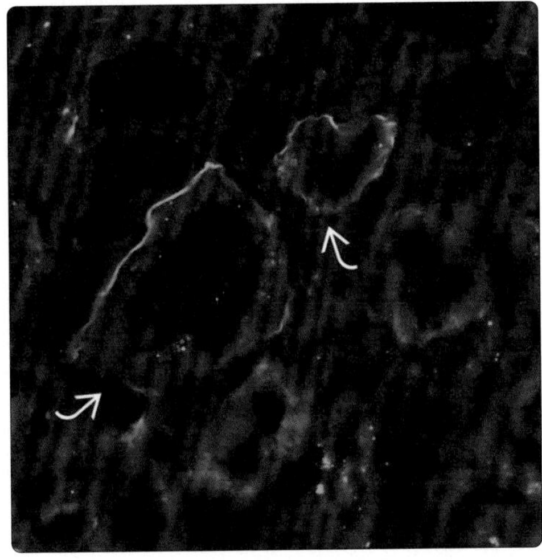

(Left) *Segmental loss of a3(IV) and a5(IV) along the GBM ➡ and a5(IV) in Bowman capsule ➡ are typical of women with 1 mutated COL4A5 gene, due to random inactivation of the X chromosome. Biopsy from a 7-year-old girl with family history of kidney disease in maternal male relatives is shown.* **(Right)** *Segmental loss of a5(IV) in distal tubular basement membranes can be appreciated in women with X-linked Alport syndrome. In this case, the only glomerular changes were thin basement membranes ➡.*

a5(IV) in Normal Skin

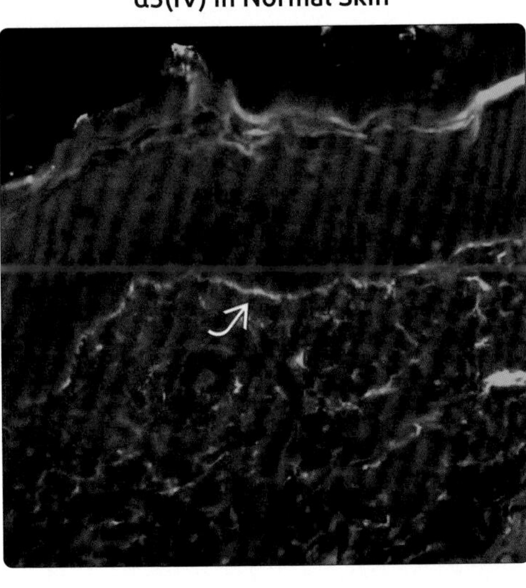

Skin in Woman With X-Linked Alport Syndrome

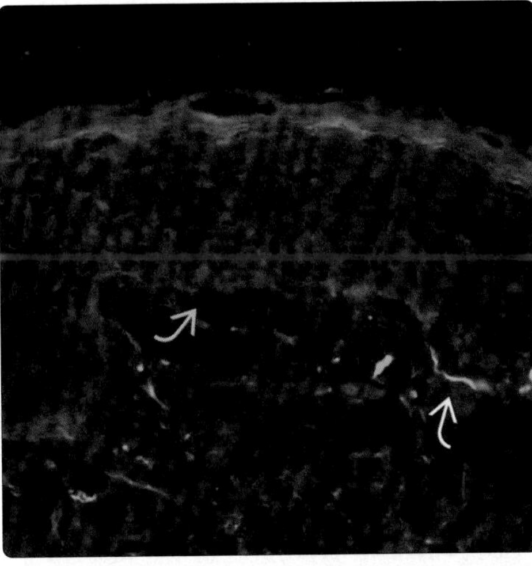

(Left) *The normal epidermal basement membrane stains in a continuous linear pattern for a(IV) ➡, due to the presence of a5(IV).a6(IV) chains.* **(Right)** *a5(IV) chains are segmentally present ➡ and lost ➡ in the epidermal basement membrane in women with a heterozygous mutation in COL4A5, due to the random inactivation of the X chromosome. Patients with mutations in COL4A3 or COL4A4 have normal staining for a5(IV) in the skin. This can distinguish X-linked from autosomal Alport syndrome.*

TERMINOLOGY

Abbreviations

- Peritubular capillaries (PTC)
- Antibody-mediated rejection (AMR)

COMPLEMENT COMPONENTS

C4d

- Cleavage fragment of C4b that contains thiol group, which forms covalent bond with proteins and carbohydrates near site of complement activation
- Cleaved by activated C1qsr esterase to C4b, the active enzyme that in turn combines with C2 and cleaves C3
- C4d itself has no known function

DIAGNOSTIC VALUE

Renal Transplant Biopsies

- Presence of C4d in peritubular cortical or medullary capillaries correlates almost perfectly with presence of antibody in circulation reactive to donor endothelium (HLA or ABO antibodies)
- C4d persists at site of complement activation by classic (or lectin) pathways, while immunoglobulin that initiated complement fixation generally does not
- C4d eventually is cleared from capillaries 1-2 weeks after activation
  - C4d in tissues indicates local complement fixation in the last 1-2 weeks, even in chronic setting

IMMUNOFLUORESCENCE TECHNIQUE (IF)

2-Step Method

- Tissue
  - Frozen sections, 2-4 μm thick, air dry
- Primary antibody
  - Monoclonal anti-C4d (10 μg/mL; Quidel Corp, clone 033II-317.1.3.X), 30 min
- Secondary antibody
  - FITC-horse or goat anti-mouse IgG

3-Step Method

- Tissue
  - Frozen sections, 2-4 μm thick, air dry
- Block endogenous biotin
  - Avidin D in buffered saline, 1% bovine serum albumin, 20 min
  - d-biotin, 20 min
- Primary antibody
  - Monoclonal anti-C4d (10 μg/mL; Quidel Corp, clone 033II-317.1.3.X), 30 min
- Secondary antibody
  - Biotinylated horse anti-mouse IgG 1:100, 30 min (Vector)
- Fluorochrome conjugate
  - FITC-streptavidin 1:50, 30 min (Vector)
- Wash with phosphate buffered saline between steps
- All steps at room temperature
- Higher sensitivity and lower background with 3-step vs. 2-step method

Advantages

- Low background, more easily interpreted than IHC
- Rapid technique

Disadvantages

- Requires frozen tissue
- More difficult to appreciate tissue structure

Pitfalls

- Glomeruli stain in normal kidneys in frozen sections, mostly in mesangium
- Arteriosclerotic intima stains variably for C4d, even in native kidneys
- Segmental TBM staining is sometimes seen and can be misinterpreted as capillary staining, especially in atrophic tubules
- Polyomavirus infections sometimes have granular C4d deposits along TBM
- Areas of necrosis are not interpretable (negative)
- Immune complex deposition in glomerulus is often strongly positive for C4d

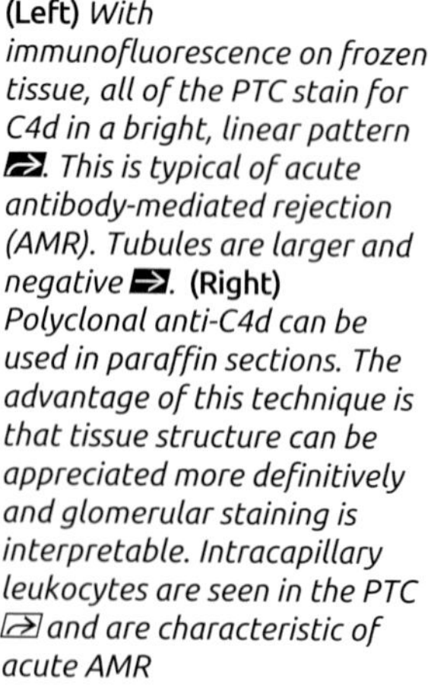

(Left) *With immunofluorescence on frozen tissue, all of the PTC stain for C4d in a bright, linear pattern. This is typical of acute antibody-mediated rejection (AMR). Tubules are larger and negative.* **(Right)** *Polyclonal anti-C4d can be used in paraffin sections. The advantage of this technique is that tissue structure can be appreciated more definitively and glomerular staining is interpretable. Intracapillary leukocytes are seen in the PTC and are characteristic of acute AMR*

Peritubular Capillary C4d in Acute AMR

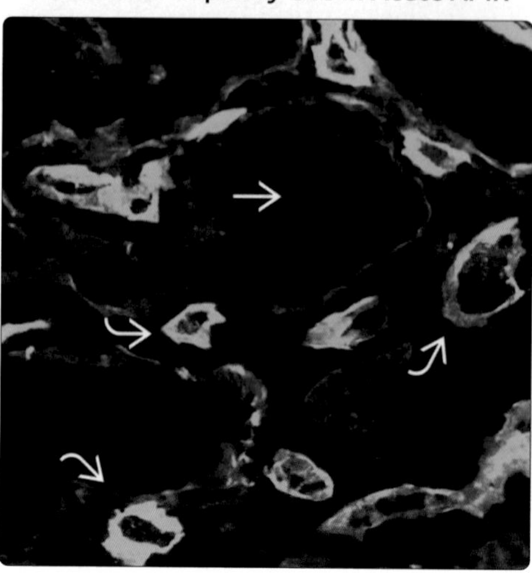

Acute Antibody-Mediated Rejection (AMR)

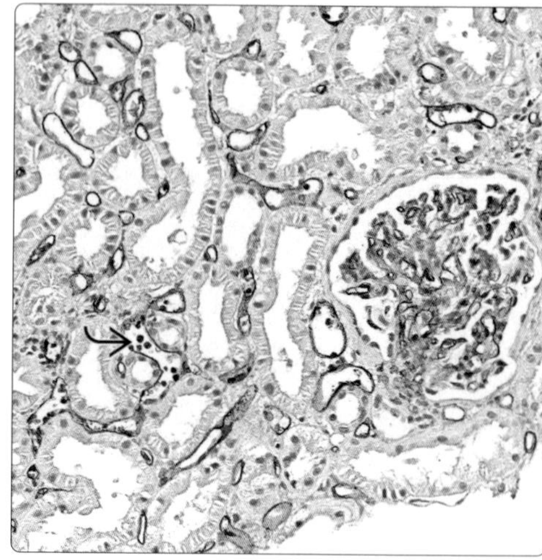

IMMUNOHISTOCHEMICAL TECHNIQUE (IHC)

Method

- Tissue
  - Formalin-fixed, paraffin-embedded tissue
  - 4 μm thick sections on Superfrost Plus slides
  - Deparaffinize, rehydrate sections
- Antigen retrieval
  - 15 min, pressure cooker, 110° C, Citrate, pH 6.0 (e.g., Decloaker Solution, BioCare Medical)
- Block endogenous peroxidase
  - Dual Endogenous Enzyme Block (Dako), 5 min
- Primary anti-C4d antibody (e.g., rabbit polyclonal anti-human C4d 12-500, American Research Products)
  - 30 min, diluted 1:100
- Secondary antibody and enzyme
  - Peroxidase-polymer linked to anti-rabbit IgG (e.g., Envision + Dual Link System, DAKO), 30 min
- Substrate
  - 3,3'-diaminobenzidine solution (DAKO), 10 min
- All rinses between steps in tris-buffered saline/Tween 20
- All staining and washing steps at room temperature
- Alternatives
  - Biotinylated anti-rabbit IgG, then avidin-biotin peroxidase complex (Elite ABC, Vector)
  - 3-amino-9-ethylcarbazole chromogen (BioCare Medical)
  - Overnight incubation with primary antibody

Advantages

- Can be done on routine formalin-fixed tissue
- Better identification of tissue localization
- Normal glomeruli are negative for C4d in fixed tissue, and therefore glomerular staining can be evaluated

Disadvantages

- Less sensitive and less reproducible than IF

Pitfalls

- Plasma C4 in capillaries is fixed by formalin and can give high background that obscures or mimics positive endothelial staining
- Some fixatives destroy immunoreactivity (e.g., alcohol, Bouin)
- Optimal antigen retrieval is important; acid citrate and heat seem best in comparative studies
- Over dilution of primary antibody affects results
- *Granular* PTC C4d deposits correlate with decreased graft survival and delayed graft function, but not with other evidence of AMR

DIAGNOSTIC SPECIFICITY

Definition of Positive

- Immunofluorescence on frozen tissue sections
  - Strong (bright) linear, circumferential stain of ≥ 10% PTC (C4d2-3)
- Immunohistochemistry on formalin-fixed, paraffin embedded tissue sections
  - Linear circumferential stain of > 0% of PTC (C4d1-3), of any intensity

Reported as Banff C4d Scores

- C4d0 (0%, negative), C4d1 (1-9%, minimal), C4d2 (10-50%, focal), C4d3 (> 50%, diffuse)
- Among 1,531 unselected indication transplant biopsies, 73% were C4d0, 3% were C4d1, 7% were C4d2, and 17% were C4d3 (Colvin and Collins, unpublished data)

False-Positives

- Lupus erythematosus, PTC immune complex deposits (IF)
  - Granular vs. more linear pattern in antibody-mediated rejection
- TBM staining in atrophic tubules (IF)
- Vasa recta arterioles (IF)
- Plasma in lumen of capillaries (IHC)
- Plasma fixation of C4 along endothelium (IHC)
- Granular staining of PTC (IHC)

False-Negatives

- Minority of antibody-mediated rejection has negative or minimal C4d deposition
  - 20-50% of chronic AMR, depending on technique
  - Need to look for other signs of AMR, notably capillaritis or glomerulitis
- Poor tissue processing or harsh fixation
- Areas of necrosis

CONTROLS

Positive Controls (IF or IHC)

- Prior case of antibody-mediated rejection (PTC)
- Membranous glomerulonephritis (glomerular deposits)

Negative Controls

- PTC staining, any native kidney (except lupus nephritis)

SELECTED REFERENCES

1. Kikić Z et al: Clinicopathological relevance of granular C4d deposition in peritubular capillaries of kidney allografts. Transpl Int. 27(3):312-21, 2014
2. Mengel M et al: Banff initiative for quality assurance in transplantation (BIFQUIT): reproducibility of C4d immunohistochemistry in kidney allografts. Am J Transplant. 13(5):1235-45, 2013
3. Cohen D et al: Pros and cons for C4d as a biomarker. Kidney Int. 81(7):628-39, 2012
4. Jen KY et al: C4d/CD34 double-immunofluorescence staining of renal allograft biopsies for assessing peritubular capillary C4d positivity. Mod Pathol. 25(3):434-8, 2012
5. Crary GS et al: Optimal cutoff point for immunoperoxidase detection of C4d in the renal allograft: results from a multicenter study. Transplantation. 90(10):1099-105, 2010
6. Seemayer CA et al: C4d staining of renal allograft biopsies: a comparative analysis of different staining techniques. Nephrol Dial Transplant. 22(2):568-76, 2007
7. Troxell ML et al: Comparison of C4d immunostaining methods in renal allograft biopsies. Clin J Am Soc Nephrol. 1(3):583-91, 2006
8. Nadasdy GM et al: Comparative study for the detection of peritubular capillary C4d deposition in human renal allografts using different methodologies. Hum Pathol. 36(11):1178-85, 2005
9. Collins AB et al: Complement activation in acute humoral renal allograft rejection: diagnostic significance of C4d deposits in peritubular capillaries. J Am Soc Nephrol. 10(10):2208-14, 1999

(Left) *No PTC show C4d staining in this donor biopsy. Focal segmental staining is along the TBM* ➡. **(Right)** *This biopsy shows minimal PTC staining (1-9%)* ➡*, Banff C4d1. The patient had no donor-specific antibody by Luminex. The biopsy showed polyomavirus nephropathy. This is not diagnostic of AMR.*

Negative C4d (C4d0)

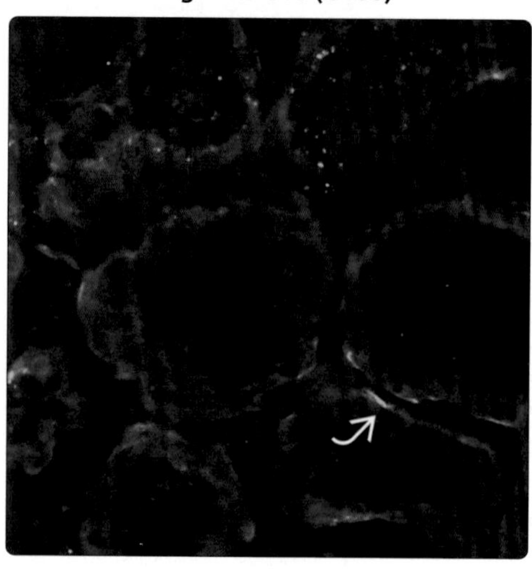

C4d1

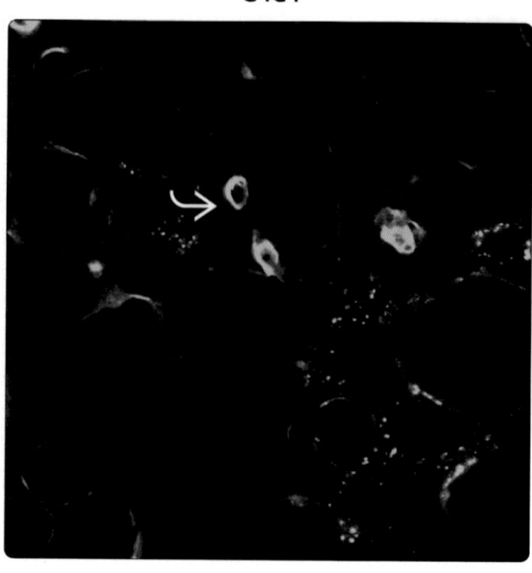

(Left) *About 30% of the PTC in this sample stained for C4d* ➡*, and the rest are negative* ➡*. C4d2 is defined as 10-50% positivity. The staining in this case is very weak, which sometimes happens with the IHC technique and is not considered in the assessment of positive or negative.* **(Right)** *This image shows that ~ 100% of the peritubular capillaries (PTC) are positive for C4d, meeting the threshold for C4d3 (> 50% of PTC). Capillaritis is focally present* ➡*. Linear C4d staining of the GBM is also prominent* ➡*.*

C4d2

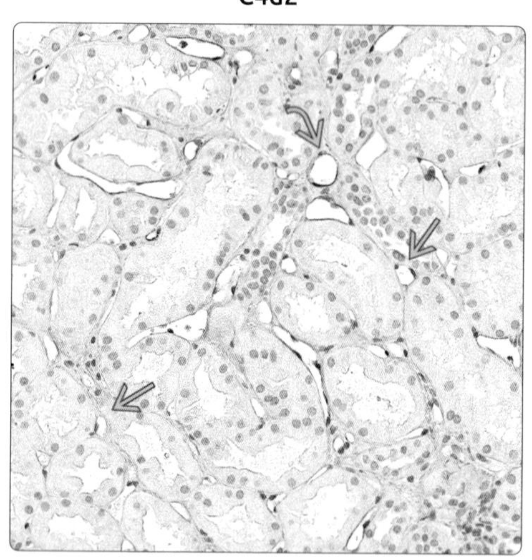

C4d3

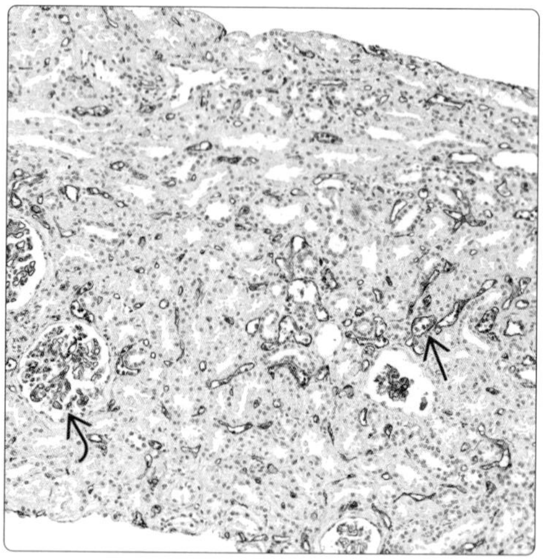

(Left) *In formalin-fixed tissue, the circulating C4 is sometimes fixed in the lumen* ➡ *or along the capillary endothelial surface, which makes interpretation problematic. These cases should be reported as "indeterminant." Frozen tissue does not have this artifact.* **(Right)** *In this sample, the medulla on the right had more easily appreciated capillary C4d deposition* ➡ *than the cortex on the left.*

Plasma Artifact

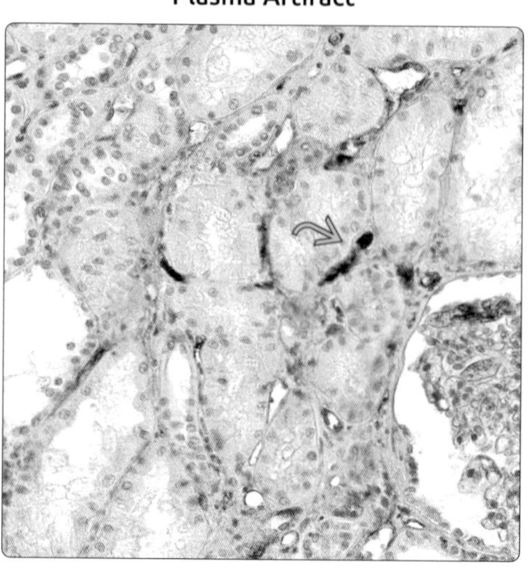

Medulla Stronger C4d Staining Than Cortex

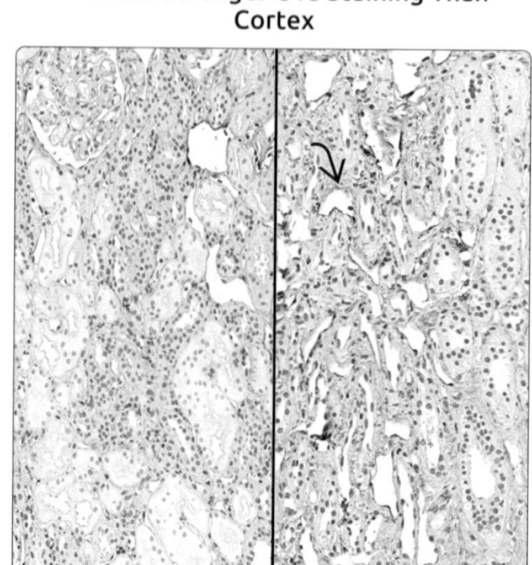

Normal C4d in Mesangium

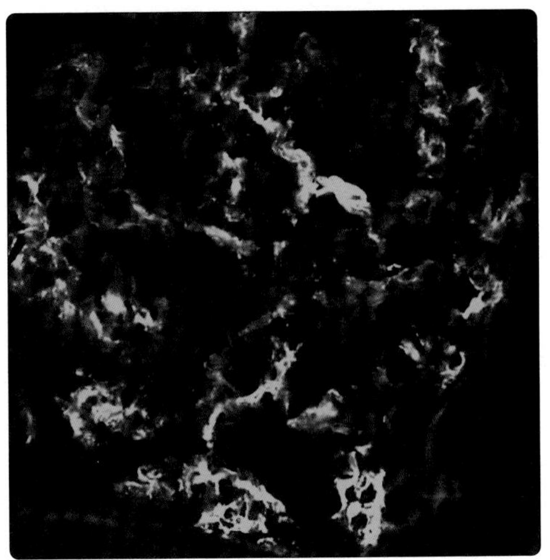

Normal Kidney C4d

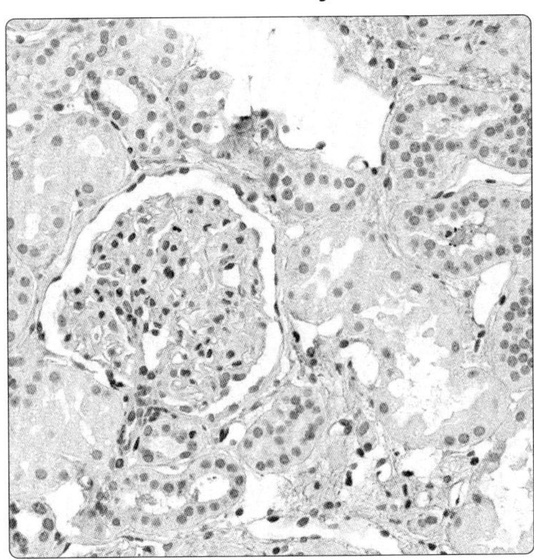

(Left) *Normal glomeruli in frozen sections show C4d in the mesangium, as illustrated in this donor biopsy. This makes interpretation of glomerular C4d difficult. In contrast, glomeruli from formalin-fixed paraffin-embedded samples are negative.* **(Right)** *Glomerular staining for C4d is negative in normal formalin-fixed paraffin-embedded tissue, in contrast to the mesangial C4d seen in frozen sections, which allows interpretation of C4d deposits in pathological samples. This is a donor biopsy with normal histology.*

Recurrent Membranous Glomerulonephritis

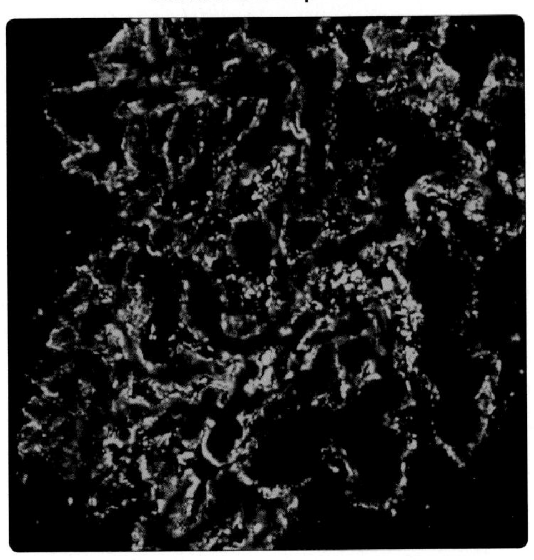

SLE With PTC and TBM C4d Deposits

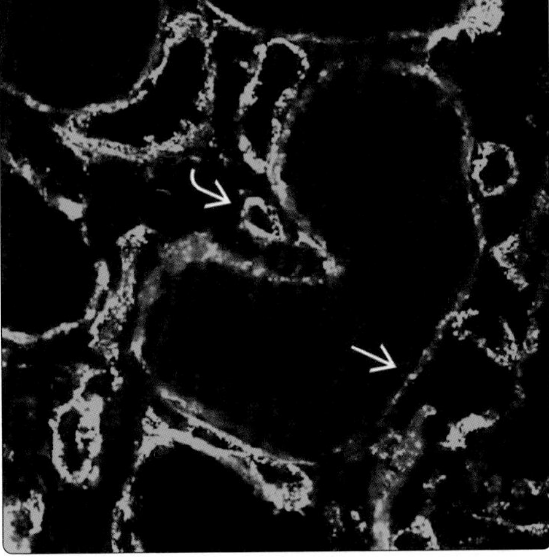

(Left) *This biopsy 4 years after renal transplantation shows granular C4d along the GBM, due to recurrent membranous glomerulonephritis. The pattern is more granular than that in AMR.* **(Right)** *This is a native kidney biopsy from a patient with lupus nephritis. Immune complexes in the tubular basement membrane (TBM) ➡ and peritubular capillaries ➡ stain for C4d. The pattern is more granular than in AMR.*

C4d TBM Deposits in Polyomavirus Nephropathy

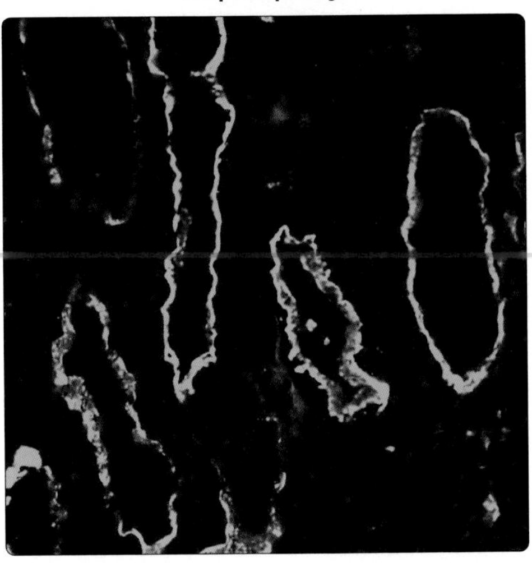

Double Stain for C4d and CD34

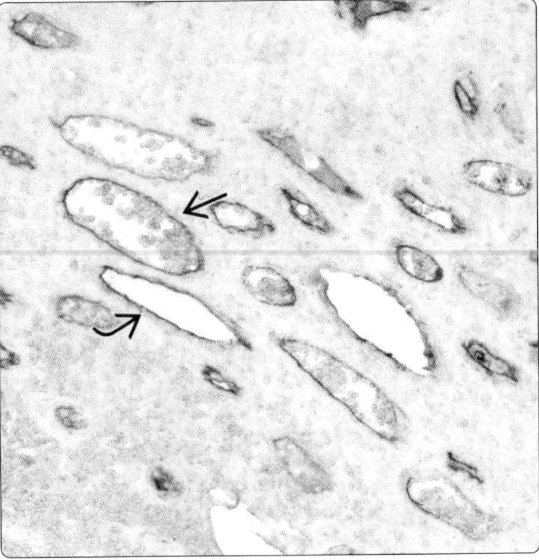

(Left) *About 50% of biopsies with polyomavirus nephropathy have granular deposits of IgG, C3, &/or C4d along the TBM, corresponding to amorphous electron-dense deposits by EM. The nature of the antigen is unknown.* **(Right)** *A CD34 stain is useful to identify capillaries. In this sample, anti-C4d was applied first and developed with diaminobenzidine (DAB, brown), followed by anti-CD34 (blue). The DAB precipitate in C4d(+) capillaries ➡ blocks anti-CD34; those that are blue were C4d(-) ➡. With double IF, no blocking is evident.*

TERMINOLOGY

Polyomavirus Immunohistochemistry

- SV40 large T antigen
  - Most common target
  - Present in lytic and latent infections
  - Mouse IgG2a monoclonal antibodies Pab416 or Pab419
    - Pab416 used by 68% of laboratories in Banff survey
    - Cross reacts with BK and JC polyomavirus
  - Suppliers: Santa Cruz, CalBiochem, Abcam, and others
- VP1
  - Capsid protein expressed in lytic, not latent infections
  - Can give false-negative stain
- Whole virion
  - Lee Biomolecular, Access Biomedical

PROTOCOLS

Polymer Technique (Automated, DAKO)

- Borg decloaker (Biocare Medical Products), 15 min 110° C, pressure cooker
- Cool to room temp, rinse in distilled water and tris-buffered saline/Tween
- Dual endogenous enzyme block (DAKO), 5 min
- Pab419 antibody 1:50, 30 min
- L Polymer (DAKO), 30 min
- Diaminobenzidine, 5-10 min
- Counterstain in Harris hematoxylin, 10 sec
- Rinse, lithium carbonate dip
- Wash in tris-buffered saline between incubation steps
- Alcohol, xylene, Permount

Rapid Polymer Technique (Automated, Leica)

- Antigen retrieval: EDTA 100° C, 40 min
- Antibody Pab419, diluted 1:100, 15 min
- Rabbit polyclonal anti-mouse IgG, 8 min
- Bond polymer refine detection (Kit DS9800), 8 min
- Block with hydrogen peroxide, 5 min
- Develop in diaminobenzidine, 10 min
- Counterstain with hematoxylin, 5 min
- All steps at room temperature unless noted otherwise
- Wash 2x between each step with phosphate-buffered saline (PBS)

Avidin-Biotin Complex Method (Manual)

- Borg Decloaker, 15 min, 110° C, cool in distilled water, PBS
- Block with normal horse serum/avidin 20 min
- Mouse anti-SV40 Pab419, diluted 1:50, overnight at 4° C or 2 hr at room temp, wash PBS
- Biotin/H2O2 block 20 min, wash PBS
- Biotinylated horse anti-mouse IgG (1:200), 35 min, wash PBS
- Elite ABC, 1 hr, wash PBS
- Permanent AEC, 5 min
- Stain with hematoxylin as above

Best Practices

- Banff quality assurance survey using tissue arrays processed, stained, and interpreted at 78 pathology laboratories worldwide concluded
  - Pressure cooker more reproducible than microwave
  - Monoclonal more reproducible than polyclonal antibodies
  - Dilutions of Pab416 ≤ 1:100 more reproducible
  - Polymer-based detection had better results than avidin-biotin
  - Good reproducibility for (+) vs. (-) (kappa 0.78)
  - Reproducibility for intensity and percentage only moderate (kappa 0.49 and 0.42, respectively)

Interpretation

- Positive = nuclear stain of tubular epithelium (≥ 1 nucleus)
- Can be due to either BK or JC polyomavirus (or both)
- Casts sometimes stain due to shed epithelial cells and virus
- Staining possible on decoverslipped slides stained with H&E

SELECTED REFERENCES

1. Adam B et al: Banff Initiative for Quality Assurance in Transplantation (BIFQUIT): reproducibility of polyomavirus immunohistochemistry in kidney allografts. Am J Transplant. 14(9):2137-47, 2014

Typical Nuclear Pattern for Large T Antigen

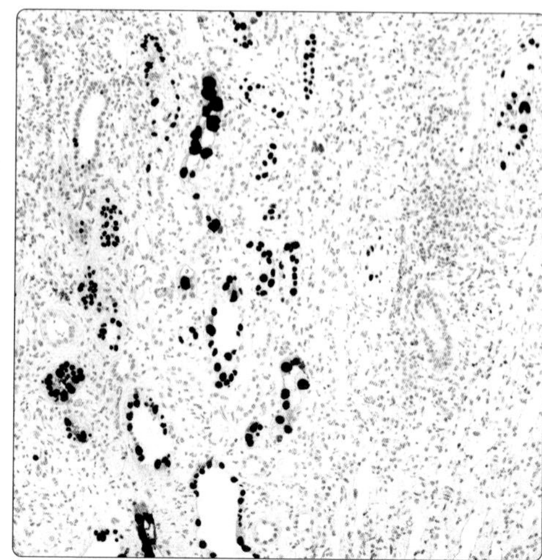

Sparse Nuclear Positivity

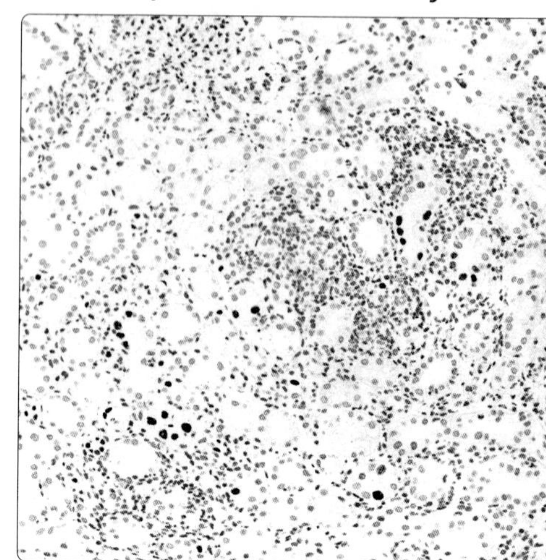

(Left) *The nuclear stain for polyomavirus large T antigen in polyomavirus nephropathy is typically strongly positive, concentrated in individual tubules (particularly collecting ducts) and is associated with inflammation.* **(Right)** *The positive nuclei are sparse, but associated with an interstitial infiltrate, an argument that the polyomavirus is inciting the inflammation rather than rejection.*

Severe Polyomavirus Nephropathy

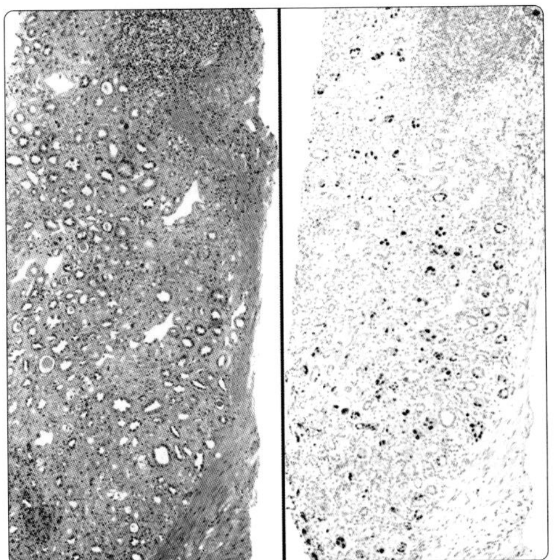

Enlarged Tubular Epithelial Cells With Large T Antigen

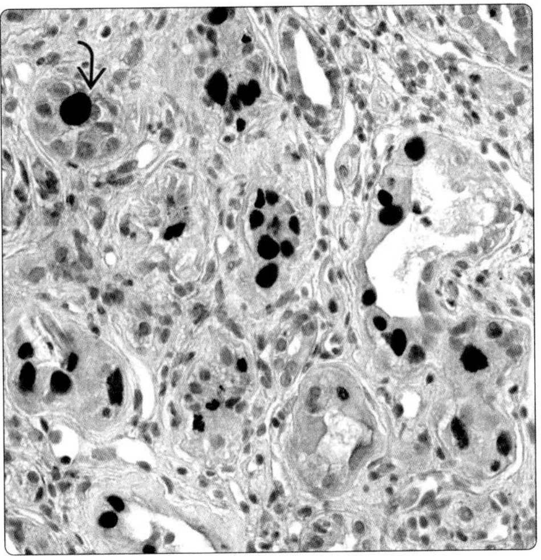

(Left) *The medulla has numerous positive tubules and a diffuse mononuclear infiltrate in this patient 4 months post transplant on a steroid-free regimen (tacrolimus and mycophenolate). Plasma BK-DNA was 5,640,000 copies/mL, Cr 2.7 mg/dL.* **(Right)** *The infected cells typically have larger nuclei than uninfected cells. Occasionally these cells are shed in the lumen ⇨ and can appear in the urine.*

TCMR With Minimal Polyomavirus

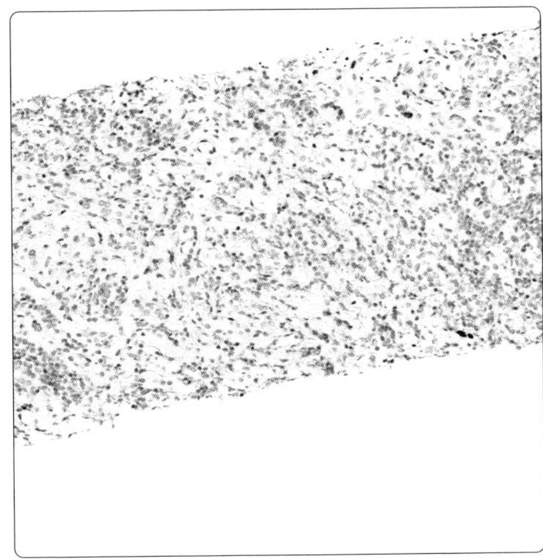

Mixed Acute TCMR and Polyomavirus Nephropathy

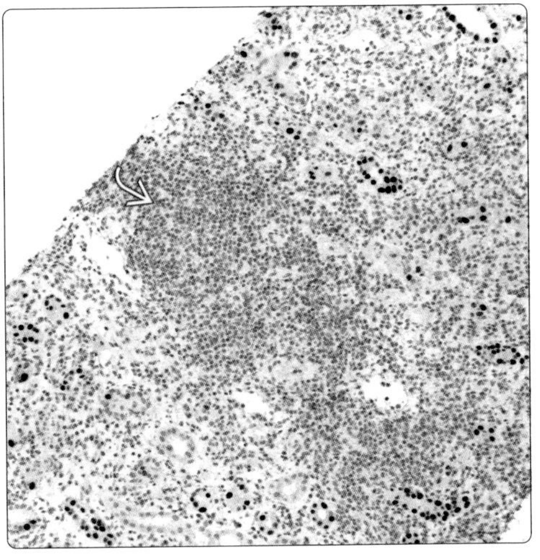

(Left) *Rare positive nuclei is shown with inflammation separated from the areas of polyomavirus, suggesting that the inflammation is related to rejection rather than the virus.* **(Right)** *This patient presented with a rising Cr and a rising BK viremia. Biopsy shows an intense mononuclear infiltrate in an area without virus ⇨. This is a clue that rejection may also be present. This was confirmed by documentation of endothelialitis in a renal artery.*

JC Virus

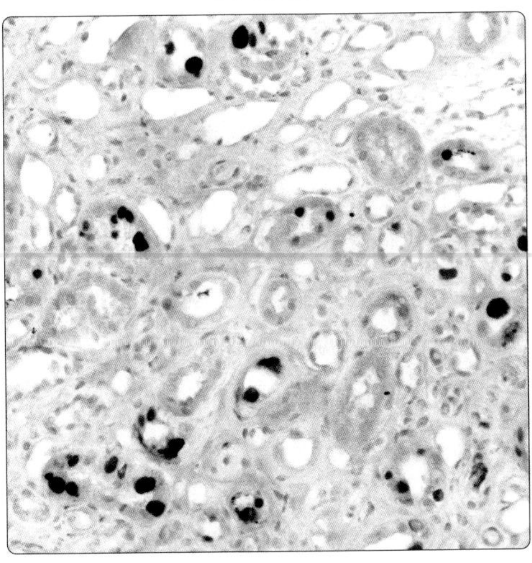

Minimal BK Polyomavirus Nephropathy

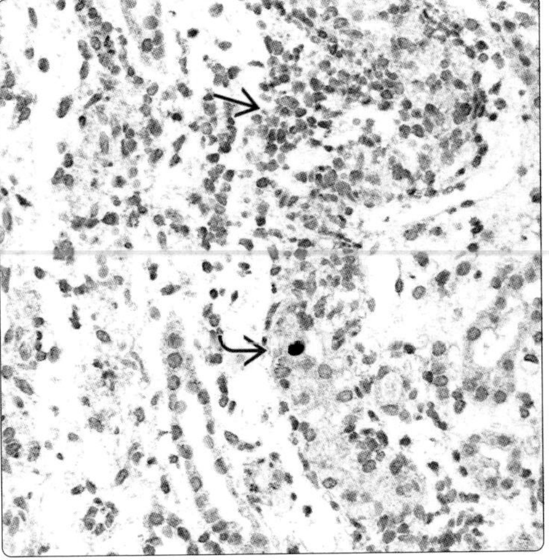

(Left) *This patient had a renal transplant 4 years ago and presented with a rising Cr (2.9 mg/dL). The medulla has numerous tubules positive for SV40 large T antigen when stained with Pab419. The plasma PCR was negative for BK polyomavirus and positive for JC virus (170,00 copies/mL).* **(Right)** *This native kidney biopsy from a patient 9 months after double lung transplant, who presented with rising Cr and rising BK-DNA, 326,000 copies/mL plasma, had one positive cell ⇨ in the medulla associated with focal inflammation ⇨.*

TERMINOLOGY

Abbreviations

- Next generation sequencing (NGS)
- Whole exome sequencing (WES)
- Whole genome sequencing (WGS)
- Single nucleotide polymorphism (SNP)
- Comparative genomic hybridization (CGH)
- Multiplex ligation-dependent probe amplification (MLPA)
- Copy number variations (CNV)

Definitions

- NGS: Various high throughput sequencing approaches in use post mapping of human genome instead of 1 DNA strand at a time
- Exome: Region of genome that codes for proteins (exons); about 1% of whole genome
- CNV: Structural change in genome referring to number of copies in specific regions of genome, usually > 500 bp
- Indels: Insertions and deletions of nucleotides

KIDNEY DISEASES AMENABLE TO DIAGNOSTIC CLINICAL SEQUENCING

Single Gene or Pathway in Kidney Diseases

- Typically large effect, almost fully penetrant; rare
  - Syndromes
    - Steroid-resistant nephrotic syndrome: One of many podocyte genes (e.g., *NPHS1, NPHS2, PLCE1,* WT1*)*
    - Alport syndrome: Collagen 4A3, 4, 5 mutations
    - CAKUT as part of syndrome: *WT1* (WAGR), *PAX2* (renal coloboma syndrome), *SALL1* (Townes-Brocks syndrome), *RET* (agenesis/dysplasia and MEN2 or Hirschsprung disease)
  - Glomerular
    - FSGS pattern: ~ 30% can be explained by variations in ~ 30 podocyte genes
    - IgA nephropathy
  - Metabolic disorders
    - Proximal tubules (PT): Renal tubular acidosis (*CA2*), glucosuria (*SLC5A1/2, SGLT1/2*), aminoaciduria
    - Thin ascending loop of Henle (TAL): Bartter syndrome (*SLC12A1, KCNJ1, ROMK, CLCNKB, NKCC2*)
    - Distal convoluted tubules (DCT): Gitelman syndrome (*SLC12A3*), hypomagnesemia (*CLDN16,* ATP1G1, *FXYD2*)
    - Collecting duct (CD): Liddle syndrome, pseudohypoaldosteronism type 1 (*SCNN1B, G, MLR1*), Gordon syndrome (*WNK4, WNK1*), distal RTA (*SLC4A1*), nephrogenic diabetes insipidus (*AQP2, AVPR2, AVP2R*)
  - Ciliopathies or cystic diseases: ARPKD, ADPKD, nephronophthisis
  - Tubulointerstitial kidney diseases: *UMOD, MUC1, HNF1B, REN*
  - Immune/vascular: Atypical hemolytic uremic syndrome (e.g., *CFH, ADAMTS13, CFHR1, DGKE*)
  - CAKUT: One of several hundred genes important in kidney development (*RET, PAX2, GDNF, WT1, ROBO2, SLIT2, UPKIII, SALL1, DLG1, DYSTK, ATGR2*), rare CNVs
  - Nephrolithiasis: Cystinuria (*SLX3A1, CSNU1, SLC7A9*), Dent disease (*CLCN5*), primary hyperoxaluria (*AGXT, GRHPR*)

Polygenic or Complex Diseases

- Common variations or SNPs may modify kidney disease, low penetrance of individual variants, difficult to assign causality and mechanisms
  - FSGS in African Americans
    - APOL1 G1 and G2 variants
  - Type 2 diabetic nephropathy
    - *ELMO1* variants
    - *ACE, AKRB1, PPARG2* (decreased risk), *SLC2A1, CNDP1* (decreased risk) SNPs

ETIOLOGY/PATHOGENESIS

Monogenic Diseases

- Large effect or causality
- High penetrance
- May or may not be influenced by environmental factors

Flowchart of WES Pipeline

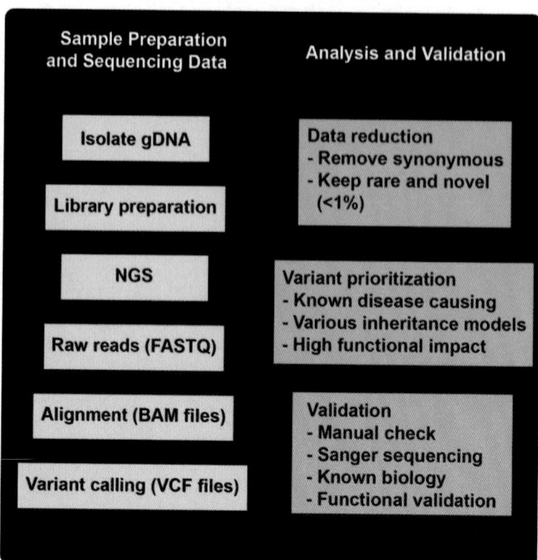

Exome Sequencing Identifies Cause of CAKUT

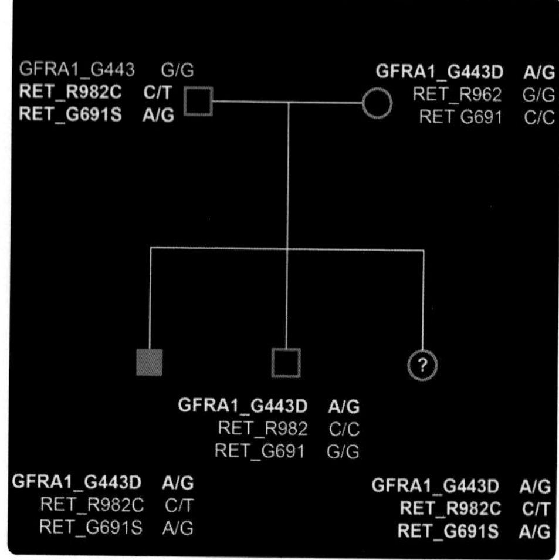

(Left) *Chart shows steps in sample preparation and NGS and sequencing data analysis and validation for discovery of rare or novel causative variants.* **(Right)** *The affected male (black box) was diagnosed with bilateral renal dysplasia, megaureters, and cryptorchidism. WES analysis revealed nonsynonymous RET variants from the father and a GFRA1 variant from the mother (bold font), not present in unaffected brother. The sister's disease status is unknown. Functional studies showed reduced MAPK activity.*

Polygenic or Common Diseases

- Small effect of each genetic change
- Manifest later in life
- Environmental factors may have strong influence

DIAGNOSTIC METHODS AND APPLICATIONS

Sanger Sequencing

- Point mutations, confirmations, ideal for single gene or small genetic regions

Array CGH

- CNVs

Targeted PCR

- Common and rare mutations or indels (use with taqman, RFLP), repeat expansions
- Rapid, preferable in clinical diagnostics for suspected or known regions

MLPA

- CNVs, deletions

SNP Arrays

- Common variants, GWAS, CNVs to examine association between these changes and susceptibility or progression of disease

Linkage Analysis

- Identifying genomic regions of susceptibility with use of markers segregating by trait, requires large families, mendelian disorders with high penetrance

NGS

- Targeted sequencing of several genes, exomes or defined genomic regions by hybridizing targets to customized baits
  - Based on phenotype or linkage analysis, one can focus on where causative variants or mutations are likely to reside
  - Common and rare variants, indels
- Amplicon-based NGS
  - Several PCR amplicons multiplexed and subjected to NGS for small number of genes or genomic regions
  - Cheaper than hybridization methods but limited by target size (up to few hundred amplicons)
  - Common and rare variants, indels
- Whole exome sequencing
  - New or atypical case, no leads from simpler or candidate tests
  - Common and rare or novel variants, indels, de novo mutations, family members/parents may facilitate analysis
  - Analysis challenging, causality uncertain, limited by sensitivity and specificity, expensive
- Whole genome sequencing
  - New or atypical case
  - Common and rare or novel variants, indels, de novo mutations, family members/parents may facilitate analysis
  - Analysis more challenging than WES, causality uncertain, limited by sensitivity and specificity, expensive
    - Expected to supersede WES as analysis and sequencing costs decrease
  - Interpretation of result is more challenging than WES due to added difficulty in interpreting noncoding variants

TYPICAL STEPS IN WES ANALYSIS

Library Preparation

- Fragment DNA and hybridize with baits, followed by series of ligation, PCR and purification steps
- Can prepool several samples by tagging each with unique adaptors or indexed barcodes and then pooling for molecular preparation to increase efficiency and reduce costs

NGS on One of NGS Platforms

- Sequencing technology and machines constantly changing with newer platforms with more sequencing power with overall less costs per base

Demultiplexing Reads

- Parses out reads of each patient aided by the barcodes of unique nucleotides introduced in library preparation
- One of output file is in FASTQ format (retains basic information about sequencing and informs on quality of reads)
  - Retain raw files for future use since downstream softwares of analyses are constantly improved

Aligning With Reference Genome

- Commonly used aligners include NovoAlign, BWA, Bowtie
- Results vary depending on parameters and platform used for NGS
  - Output commonly in "bam" format

Generate SNP or Variant Calls

- Many commercial and public softwares available including GATK
  - Output usually in "vcf" format

Data Reduction Steps

- Depends on purpose, filter to retain rare (< 1%) variants, those known to be disease associated (eliminate those frequent in public databases (1000 genome, institution own database, dbSNP; although latest versions of dbSNP may result in overfiltering, recommend db132 or earlier)
- If multiple affected individuals in same family, can filter to retain common variants in all
- If recessive model, filter for retaining homozygous or compound recessive
- If dominant model, filter away those found in unaffected individuals assuming fully penetrant disorder
- If parents available, can analyze for de novo variations as mechanism for disease

Variant Prioritization

- Can use one or many of several pathogenicity prediction tools (CADD, PolyPhen2, SIFT, MutationTaster, species conservation)
  - Stopgain, stoploss, splicesite, frameshift, nonsynonymous
  - Prediction tools are not perfect, may overcall or undercall

- Recommend burden test to examine statistical significance of excess variants in gene in patients over "controls" to strengthen confidence in association with disease
- Manual examination of reads on integrated genomics viewer (IGV) to filter out false-positives or ambiguous reads

Validation

- Confirmation by Sanger sequencing or other means
- Known biology of gene with mutation, expression pattern supports phenotype
- In vitro or model system to gain confidence and assign causality

CLINICAL IMPLICATIONS

Utility in Patient Care

- Newborn or prenatal screening
- Carrier status
- Diagnosis
- Prognosis
- Pharmacogenomics: To tailor therapy based on variant (mutations in SRNS genes or Alport can prevent unnecessary treatment)
- Mechanisms

Interpretation Challenges and Reporting

- Causation criteria for variants identified
    - Known disease causing: Previously shown to cause disease
    - Likely disease causing: Novel variant in gene known to cause disease and informatics or experimental validation favors pathogenicity
    - Possibly disease causing: No prior information but prioritization analysis based on pathogenicity suggests it could be pathogenic
    - Likely not disease causing: Not previously reported and informatics analysis does not support pathogenicity
    - Not disease causing: Reported and confirmed as neutral or nonpathogenic
    - Variant of unknown clinical significance: Unknown or not expected to be pathogenic but found to be associated with disease
- Beneficial aspects of identified variants in management
    - Protective effect
    - Prediction of drug response
- Interpretation for determining causation remains significant problem
    - Continue to improve with biological testing, clinicopathologic correlations, multidisciplinary teams

Considerations for Order Clinical Sequencing

- Level of urgency for diagnosis
    - For rapid diagnosis, some NGS approaches may not be feasible
        - For example, prenatal testing where short turnaround expected
- Age of patient
- Phenotypic characteristics, atypical or clinical conundrum
- Family history of disease, need carrier status
- Feasibility to obtain specimen
- Bigger genome being interrogated raises larger challenges in interpretation
    - Better to be hypothesis driven based on clinicopathological information and family history
- WES/WGS better if suspect high degree of genetic heterogeneity

Ethical Concerns

- Privacy and discriminations
    - Denial of long-term disability insurance or life insurance
- Secondary findings
    - May find variants associated with adult or other diseases that patient may not want to know
    - Standards to report should be high to avoid burdening health care system with false-positive results
- Ethical dilemmas of implications or reporting to other family members, affected or unaffected and to children with potential risk for adult disease

Data Storage

- Large data files; identify storage space of raw archived material and curated alignment and variant files; how to report to patients and genomic education for interpretation

Costs

- Prohibitively high for NGS and validation limits scope
    - Insurance companies may not cover

SELECTED REFERENCES

1. Scholl UI et al: Recurrent gain of function mutation in calcium channel CACNA1H causes early-onset hypertension with primary aldosteronism. Elife. 4, 2015
2. Schueler M et al: DCDC2 mutations cause a renal-hepatic ciliopathy by disrupting Wnt signaling. Am J Hum Genet. 96(1):81-92, 2015
3. Kiryluk K et al: Discovery of new risk loci for IgA nephropathy implicates genes involved in immunity against intestinal pathogens. Nat Genet. 46(11):1187-96, 2014
4. Sadowski CE et al: A single-gene cause in 29.5% of cases of steroid-resistant nephrotic syndrome. J Am Soc Nephrol. ePub, 2014
5. Ashraf S et al: ADCK4 mutations promote steroid-resistant nephrotic syndrome through CoQ10 biosynthesis disruption. J Clin Invest. 123(12):5179-89, 2013
6. Chatterjee R et al: Targeted exome sequencing integrated with clinicopathological information reveals novel and rare mutations in atypical, suspected and unknown cases of Alport syndrome or proteinuria. PLoS One. 8(10):e76360, 2013
7. Katsanis SH et al: Molecular genetic testing and the future of clinical genomics. Nat Rev Genet. 14(6):415-26, 2013
8. Lemaire M et al: Recessive mutations in DGKE cause atypical hemolytic-uremic syndrome. Nat Genet. 45(5):531-6, 2013
9. Sanna-Cherchi S et al: Mutations in DSTYK and dominant urinary tract malformations. N Engl J Med. 369(7):621-9, 2013
10. Scholl UI et al: Somatic and germline CACNA1D calcium channel mutations in aldosterone-producing adenomas and primary aldosteronism. Nat Genet. 45(9):1050-4, 2013
11. Boyden LM et al: Mutations in kelch-like 3 and cullin 3 cause hypertension and electrolyte abnormalities. Nature. 482(7383):98-102, 2012
12. Chatterjee R et al: Traditional and targeted exome sequencing reveals common, rare and novel functional deleterious variants in RET-signaling complex in a cohort of living US patients with urinary tract malformations. Hum Genet. 131(11):1725-38, 2012
13. Sanna-Cherchi S et al: Copy-number disorders are a common cause of congenital kidney malformations. Am J Hum Genet. 91(6):987-97, 2012
14. Choi M et al: K+ channel mutations in adrenal aldosterone-producing adenomas and hereditary hypertension. Science. 331(6018):768-72, 2011
15. Hildebrandt F: Genetic kidney diseases. Lancet. 375: 1287-1295, 2010
16. Granier C et al: Gene and protein markers of diabetic nephropathy. Nephrol Dial Transplant. 23(3):792-9, 2008
17. Ji W et al: Rare independent mutations in renal salt handling genes contribute to blood pressure variation. Nat Genet. 40(5):592-9, 2008

Types of Genomic Tests, Advantages and Limitations

Test	Common Variants, SNPs	Rare or Novel Variants	CNVs	Exon Deletion or Insertions	Chromosomal Changes	Cost	Time Taken	Scenario	Limitations
Sanger sequencing	X	X				Medium to high	Short to long	NPHS1	Few genes
MLPA	X	X	X	X	X	Low	Low	Missing exons Alport	Size, known mutations
Targeted PCR, Taqman	X	X				Low	Short	G1-G2 variants in APOL1	Multiplexing, size
Array CGH			X		Unbalanced	Medium	Average	CAKUT	No nt data
SNP arrays	X		X			Low	Average	GWAS	Miss rare
FISH			X		X	Low	Short	CAKUT	No nt data
NGS Methods									
Amplicon-based NGS	X	X				medium	average	Known genes	size, sensitivity, specific
Targeted capture ES, amplicon	X	X				Medium	Average	SRNS	Size
WES	X	X	X	X		Medium to high	Average to long	Novel and known disease, monogenic	Sensitivity, specificity, analysis
WGS	X	X	X	X	X	High	Long	Novel and known diseases, others fail	Sensitivity, specificity, analysis

Cost: Low (< $250), medium (< $500), high (> $500) per specimen. Time: Short (< 7 days), average (7 days to 1 month), long (> 1 month).

Modified from Katsanis et al. Nature Reviews, 426, 2013:415.

INDEX

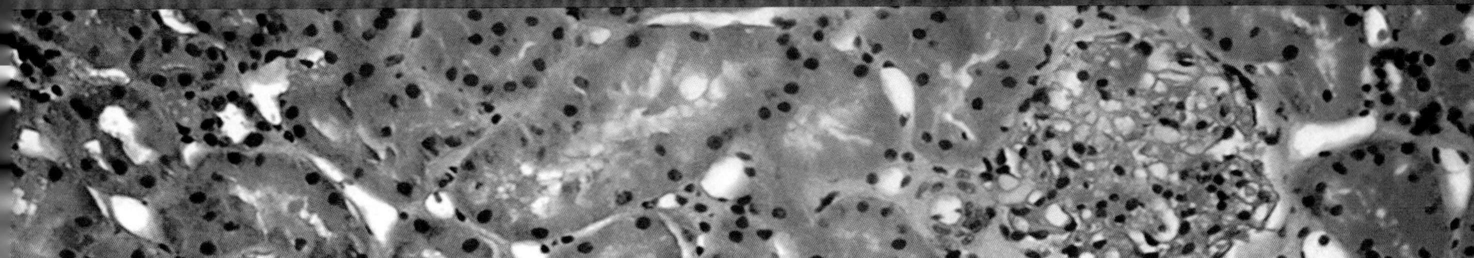

A

INDEX

INDEX

INDEX

B

C

INDEX

INDEX

D

E

F

INDEX

G

H

I

INDEX

M

INDEX

N

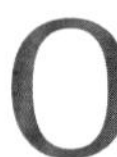

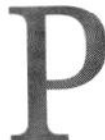

INDEX

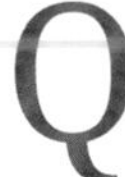

R

S

INDEX

W

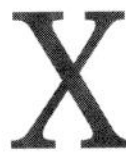

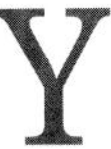

Z